Abrams' Angiography
Interventional Radiology

SECOND EDITION

Abrams' Angiography Interventional Radiology

SECOND EDITION

EDITORS

■ **STANLEY BAUM, MD**

Professor of Radiology
Department of Radiology
University of Pennsylvania
Hospital of the University of Pennsylvania
Philadelphia, Pennsylvania

■ **MICHAEL J. PENTECOST, MD**

Professor of Radiology
Georgetown University School of Medicine
Washington, D.C.
Mid-Atlantic Permanente Medical Group, PC
Kaiser Permanente
Rockville, MD

◆ LIPPINCOTT WILLIAMS & WILKINS
A **Wolters Kluwer** Company

Philadelphia • Baltimore • New York • London
Buenos Aires • Hong Kong • Sydney • Tokyo

Acquisitions Editor: Lisa McAllister
Developmental Editor: Rebecca Barroso
Managing Editor: Jenny Kim
Project Manager: Dave Murphy
Design Coordinator: Doug Smock
Marketing Manager: Angela Panetta
Manufacturing Manager: Ben Rivera
Production Services: Schawk, Inc.
Printer: Edwards Brothers, Inc.

© 2006 by LIPPINCOTT WILLIAMS & WILKINS
530 Walnut Street
Philadelphia, Pennsylvania 19106 USA
351 West Camden Street
Baltimore, Maryland 21201-2436 USA
LWW.com

Printed in the USA

Library of Congress Cataloging-in-Publication Data
Abrams' angiography : interventional radiology / editors, Stanley Baum, Michael J.
Pentecost.— 2nd ed.
    p. ; cm.
    Rev. ed. of: Interventional radiology, which was issued as v. 3 of Abrams' angiography.
4th ed. c1997.
    Includes bibliographical references and index.
    ISBN 0-7817-4089-4 (alk. paper)
    1. Angiography. 2. Interventional radiology. I. Abrams, Herbert L. II. Baum,
Stanley, 1929- III. Pentecost, Michael J. IV. Title: Angiography. V. Title:
Interventional radiology,
    [DNLM: 1. Angiography. 2. Radiology, Interventional. WG 500 A157a 2006]
RC691.6.A53A27 2006
616.1'307572—dc22

                                                                    2005017546

The publishers have made every effort to trace copyright holders for borrowed
material. If they have inadvertently overlooked any, they will be pleased to make the
necessary arrangements at the first opportunity. To purchase additional copies of this
book, call our customer service department at (800) 638-3030 or fax orders to (301)
824-7390. International customers should call (301) 714-2324. Visit Lippincott
Williams & Wilkins on the Internet: at LWW.com. Lippincott Williams & Wilkins
customer service representatives are available from 8:30 am to 6pm, EST.

Care has been taken to confirm the accuracy of the information presented and to
describe generally accepted practices. However, the authors, editors, and publisher
are not responsible for errors or omissions or for any consequences from application
of the information in this book and make no warranty, expressed or implied, with
respect to the currency, completeness, or accuracy of the contents of the publication.
Application of the information in a particular situation remains the professional
responsibility of the practitioner.

The authors, editors, and publisher have exerted every effort to ensure that drug
selection and dosage set forth in this text are in accordance with current recommendations and practice at the time of publication. However, in view of ongoing research,
changes in government regulations, and the constant flow of information relating to
drug therapy and drug reaction, the reader is urged to check the package insert for
each drug for any change in indications and dosage and for added warnings and precautions. This is particularly important when the recommended agent is a new or
infrequently employed drug.

Some drugs and medical devices presented in this publication have Food and
Drug Administration (FDA) clearance for limited use in restricted research settings.
It is the responsibility of the health care provider to ascertain the FDA status of each
drug or device planned for use in their clinical practice.

10 9 8 7 6 5 4 3 2

To Jeanne
and Judy

Contributing Authors

MICHAEL J. ALEXANDER, MD, FACS Director, Duke Neurovascular Center, Division of Neurosurgery, Duke University Medical Center, Durham, North Carolina

JASON ALLEN, MD, PhD Fellow, Departments of Radiology and Neurology, New York University School of Medicine; Fellow, Departments of Radiology and Neurology, New York University Medical Center, New York, New York

J. FRITZ ANGLE, MD Assistant Professor, Division of Angiography, Interventional Radiology and Special Procedures, University of Virginia Health Sciences Center, Charlottesville, Virginia

FILIP BANOVAC, MD Assistant Professor, Department of Radiology, Georgetown University Medical Center, Washington, D.C.; Staff Radiologist, Department of Radiology, Georgetown University Hospital, Washington, D.C.

REBECCA A. BARNETT MBChB Assistant Professor, Department of Anesthesia, University of Pennsylvania; University of Pennsylvania Health System, Philadelphia, Pennsylvania

KLEMENS H. BARTH, MD, FACR Professor of Radiology and Medicine, Georgetown University, Washington, D.C.; Georgetown University Hospital; Associate Professor of Radiology, Department of Radiology, Johns Hopkins Medical Institution, Baltimore, Maryland

RICHARD A. BAUM, MD Associate Professor, Department of Radiology, Harvard Medical School, Boston, Massachusetts; The Herbert L. Abrams Director of Angiography and Interventional Radiology, Department of Radiology, Brigham and Women's Hospital, Boston, Massachusetts

STANLEY BAUM, MD Professor of Radiology, Department of Radiology, University of Pennsylvania; Former Chairman, Department of Radiology, Hospital of the University of Pennsylvania, Philadelphia, Pennsylvania

GARY J. BECKER, MD Branch Chief, Image-Guided Intervention, Cancer Imaging Program, National Cancer Institute, National Institutes of Health, Bethesda, Maryland

TIBOR BECSKE, MD Assistant Professor, Department of Neurology, Neurointerventional Service, New York University School of Medicine, New York, New York; Assistant Attending, Department of Neurology, NYU Medical Center and Bellevue Hospital, New York, New York

CHRISTOPH A. BINKERT, MD Assistant Professor, Department of Radiology, Harvard Medical School, Boston, Massachusetts; Interventional Radiologist, Department of Radiology, Brigham and Women's Hospital, Boston, Massachusetts

FRANCINE BLEI, MD Associate Professor of Pediatrics and Plastic Surgery, New York University School of Medicine, New York; Medical Director, Vascular Anomalies Program, Stephen D. Hassenfeld Center of New York University Medical Center, New York, New York

GILES W. BOLAND, MD Associate Professor, Department of Radiology, Harvard Medical School, Boston, Massachusetts; Vice Chairman of Radiology Business Development, Department of Radiology, Massachusetts General Hospital, Boston, Massachusetts

DANIEL B. BROWN, MD Assistant Professor, Department of Radiology and Surgery, Washington University School of Medicine, St. Louis, Missouri; Assistant Professor, Department of Radiology and Surgery, Mallinckrodt Institute of Radiology, St. Louis, Missouri

CHARLES T. BURKE, MD Assistant Professor, Department of Radiology, University of North Carolina School of Medicine, Chapel Hill, North Carolina

ALLEN W. BURTON, MD Associate Professor and Section Chief, Section of Cancer Pain Management, Department of Anesthesiology and Pain Medicine, University of Texas MD Anderson Cancer Center, Houston, Texas

JEFFREY P. CARPENTER, MD Professor, Department of Surgery, University of Pennsylvania Medical Center; Director, Vascular Laboratory, Hospital of the University of Pennsylvania, Philadelphia, Pennsylvania

SEAN M. CARR, MD Fellow, Vascular and Interventional Radiology, Dotter Interventional Institute, Oregon Health & Science University, Portland, Oregon; Director of Interventional Radiology, Department of Diagnostic Radiology, St. Luke's Regional Medical Center, Boise, Idaho

WILFRIDO R. CASTAÑEDA-ZUÑIGA, MD Professor and Chairman of Radiology Department, Louisiana State University, New Orleans, Louisiana

FLAVIO CASTAÑEDA, MD Clinical Professor of Radiology and Surgery, Department of Radiology, University of Illinois College of Medicine at Peoria, Peoria, Illinois

CONSTANTIN COPE, MD, FSIR Professor Emeritus in Radiology, Department of Radiology, University of Pennsylvania, Philadelphia, Pennsylvania; Staff, Section of Interventional Radiology, Hospital of the University of Pennsylvania, Philadelphia, Pennsylvania

J. A. GORDON CULHAM, MD, FRCPC Professor, Department of Radiology, University of British Columbia, Vancouver, British Columbia, Canada; Director, Department of Radiology, British Columbia's Children's Hospital, Vancouver, British Columbia, Canada

MICHAEL D. DAKE, MD Professor, Department of Radiology, Medicine, and Surgery, University of Virginia–Charlottesville, Virginia; Chairman, Department of Radiology, University of Virginia Health System, Charlottesville, Virginia

MICHAEL DARCY, MD Professor of Radiology, Mallinckrodt Institute of Radiology, Washington University in St. Louis; Chief of Interventional Radiology, Mallinckrodt Institute of Radiology, Barnes-Jewish Hospital, St. Louis, Missouri

STEVEN L. DAWSON, MD Associate Professor, Department of Radiology, Harvard Medical School, Boston, Massachusetts; Program Lead, SimGroup, CIMIT, Department of Radiology, Massachusetts General Hospital, Boston, Massachusetts

JOSÉE DUBOIS, MD Professor, Department of Radiology, University of Montreal, Montreal, Quebec, Canada; Radiologist, Department of Medical Imaging, St. Justine Hospital, Montreal, Quebec, Canada

AVERY J. EVANS, MD Associate Professor, Departments of Radiology and Neurosurgery, University of Virginia Health System; Faculty, Interventional Neuroradiology, Department of Radiology, University of Virginia Health System, Charlottesville, Virginia

GEOFFREY A. GARDINER, JR., MD Assistant Chairman for Interventional Procedures, Department of Radiology, Lahey Clinic Medical Center, Burlington, Massachusetts

LAURENT GAREL, MD Professor of Radiology, Department of Radiology, University of Montreal, Montreal, Quebec, Canada; Head of Department of Radiology, St. Justine Hospital, Montreal, Quebec, Canada

DEBRA A. GERVAIS, MD Assistant Professor, Department of Radiology, Harvard Medical School, Boston, Massachusetts; Director, Abdominal Intervention, Department of Radiology, Massachusetts General Hospital, Boston, Massachusetts

ROY L. GORDON, MD Professor of Radiology, Chief of Interventional Radiology, Department of Radiology, University of California–San Francisco, San Francisco, California

EDWARD G. GRANT MD, FACR Professor and Chairman, Department of Radiology, University of Southern California, Keck School of Medicine, Los Angeles, California

ROY K. GREENBERG, MD Director of Endovascular Research, Department of Vascular Surgery, Cleveland Clinic Foundation, Cleveland, Ohio

MIGUEL A. DE GREGORIO, MD, PhD Professor of Radiology, Department of Radiology, University of Zaragoza, Zaragoza, Spain; Chief of Minimally Invasive Imaging Guided Surgery, Hospital Clinico Universitario Lozano Blesa, Zaragoza, Spain

THOMAS M. GRIST, MD Professor of Radiology, Department of Radiology, University of Wisconsin–Madison, Madison, Wisconsin

KLAUS D. HAGSPIEL, MD Associate Professor of Radiology, Department of Radiology, University of Virginia Health System, Charlottesville, Virginia

SUE E. HANKS, MD Associate Professor of Clinical Radiology, Department of Radiology, Keck School of Medicine, University of Southern California, Los Angeles, California; Chief of Radiology, Department of Radiology, LAC and USC Medical Center, Los Angeles, California

ZIV J. HASKAL, MD, FAHA, FSIR Professor of Radiology and Surgery, Division of Vascular and Interventional Radiology, Columbia University College of Physicians and Surgeons, New York; Director, Division of Vascular and Interventional Radiology, New York Presbyterian Hospital/Columbia, New York, New York

JEFFREY C. HELLINGER, MD Department of Radiology, Stanford University, Stanford, California

JOSÉ M. HERNANDEZ-GRAULAU, MD, FACS Clinical Associate Professor of Surgery, Department of Surgery (Urology), University of Illinois School of Medicine; Staff, Department of Surgery (Urology), St. Francis Medical Center, University of Illinois School of Medicine, Peoria, Illinois

HOWARD C. HERRMANN, MD Professor of Medicine, Cardiovascular Division, University of Pennsylvania School of Medicine, Philadelphia, Pennsylvania; Director, Interventional Cardiology and Cardiac Catheterization Laboratories, Hospital of the University of Pennsylvania, Philadelphia, Pennsylvania

JOHN W. HIRSHFELD, JR., MD Professor of Medicine, Department of Medicine, University of Pennsylvania; Cardiac Catheterization Laboratory, Department of Medicine, University of Pennsylvania Medical Center, Philadelphia, Pennsylvania

ROBERT W. HURST, MD Professor, Department of Radiology, Neurosurgery, and Neurology, University of Pennsylvania, Philadelphia, Pennsylvania

ELIZABETH A. IGNACIO, MD Associate Professor of Radiology, Department of Radiology, The George Washington University, Washington, D.C.; Associate Professor of Radiology, Department of Radiology, The George Washington University Medical Center, Washington, D.C.

MARCY B. JAGUST, MD Assistant Professor of Radiology, Cornell University Medical College; Assistant Attending, Department of Interventional Radiology, The New York Hospital, New York, New York

PAUL F. JAQUES, MD, MRCP, FRCR Professor, Department of Radiology and Surgery, University of North Carolina School of Medicine, Chapel Hill, North Carolina

MARY E. JENSEN, MD Professor, Departments of Radiology and Neurosurgery, University of Virginia Health System; Director, Interventional Neuroradiology, Department of

Radiology, University of Virginia Health System, Charlottesville, Virginia

SUNG-GWON KANG, MD, PhD Assistant Professor, Department of Interventional Radiology, Seoul National University, Bundang Hospital, Seongnam-si, Gyeonggi-do, South Korea

MICHAEL D. KATZ, MD Associate Professor, Department of Radiology, University of Southern California, Los Angeles, California; Chief, Interventional Radiology, LAC & USC Medical Center, Los Angeles, California

JOHN A. KAUFMAN, MD Professor of Interventional Radiology, Dotter Interventional Institute, Oregon Health and Science University, Portland, Oregon; Chief of Vascular and Interventional Radiology, Oregon Health and Science University Hospital, Portland, Oregon

FREDERICK S. KELLER, MD Cook Professor and Director, Dotter Interventional Institute, Oregon Health and Science University, Portland, Oregon; Cook Professor and Director, Dotter Interventional Institute, Oregon Health and Science University Hospital, Portland, Oregon

ROBERT K. KERLAN, JR., MD Professor of Clinical Radiology, Department of Radiology, University of California–San Francisco, San Francisco, California; Interventional Radiologist, Department of Radiology, UCSF Medical Center, San Francisco, California

GI-YOUNG KO, MD, PhD Assistant Professor, Department of Radiology, University of Ulsan College of Medicine, Asan Medical Center, Seoul, Republic of Korea

JEANNE M. LABERGE, MD Professor of Radiology, Department of Radiology, University of California–San Francisco; Interventional Radiology, Department of Radiology, University of California–San Francisco Medical Center, San Francisco, California

PAUL C. LAKIN, MD Professor of Interventional and Diagnostic Radiology and Surgery, Dotter Interventional Institute, Oregon Health and Science University; Attending Physician, Interventional and Diagnostic Radiology, Oregon Health and Science University Hospital, Portland, Oregon

DEOK HEE LEE, MD Professor, Department of Radiology, University of Ulsan College of Medicine, Seoul, Republic of Korea; Asan Medical Center, Seoul, Republic of Korea

CHRISTOPHER J. LEONI, MD Staff Interventionalist, Department of Radiology, St. Anthony Hospital, Denver, Colorado

DANIEL A. LEUNG, MD Assistant Professor, Department of Radiology, University of Virginia, Charlottesville, Virginia

ELLIOT B. LEVY, MD Assistant Professor, Department of Radiology, Medstar-Georgetown University Hospital, Washington, D. C.

HERB LUSTBERG, MD Clinical Assistant Professor, Radiology, Section of Vascular and Interventional Radiology, Yale University School of Medicine, New Haven, Connecticut; Section Chief, Radiology, Section of Vascular and Interventional Radiology, The William W. Backus Hospital, Norwich, Connecticut

ANTONIO MAINAR, MD Faculty, Minimally Invasive Imaging Guided Surgery, Hospital Clinico Universitario Lozano Blesa, Zaragoza, Spain

ERIC C. MARTIN, DM (OXON.), FRCP Emeritus Professor of Radiology, The College of Physicians and Surgeons of Columbia University, New York, New York; Senior Attending, Department of Radiology, Roosevelt Hospital, New York, New York

ALAN H. MATSUMOTO, MD Professor and Vice Chair, Department of Radiology, University of Virginia Health System, Charlottesville, Virginia

MATTHEW A. MAURO, MD, FACR, FSIR, FAHA Professor, Department of Radiology and Surgery, University of North Carolina School of Medicine; Vice-Chairman, Department of Radiology, University of North Carolina Hospitals, Chapel Hill, North Carolina

MANUEL MAYNAR, MD Professor, Diagnostic and Therapeutic Endoluminal Unit, University of Las Palmaz, Canary Islands, Spain; Director, Diagnostic and Therapeutic Endoluminal Unit, Hospitten, Tenerife, Canary Islands

ROBERT J. MIN, MD Associate Professor, Department of Radiology, Weill Medical College of Cornell University, New York, New York; Chief, Department of Radiology, New York Presbyterien Hospital, New York, New York

JEFFREY S. MOULTON, MD Clinical Assistant Professor, Department of Radiology, University of Colorado School of Medicine; Director of Vascular and Interventional Radiology, Department of Radiology, St. Anthony Hospital, Denver, Colorado

TIMOTHY P. MURPHY, MD Professor, Diagnostic Imaging, Brown University, Providence, Rhode Island; Staff Radiologist, Interventional Radiology, Rhode Island Hospital, Providence, Rhode Island

PETER KIM NELSON, MD Associate Professor, Departments of Radiology and Neurosurgery, New York University School of Medicine; Associate Attending, Departments of Radiology and Neurosurgery, NYU Medical Center, New York, New York

JANICE M. NEWSOME, MD Staff Physician, Cardiovascular Interventional Radiology, Inova Alexandria Hospital, Alexandria, Virginia

AALPEN A. PATEL, MD Assistant Professor of Radiology and Surgery, Department of Radiology/Interventional Radiology, University of Pennsylvania, Hospital of the University of Pennsylvania, Philadelphia, Pennsylvania

MICHAEL J. PENTECOST, MD Professor of Radiology, Georgetown University School of Medicine, Washington,

D.C.; Mid-Atlantic Permanente Medical Group, PC, Kaiser Permanente, Rockville, Maryland

PHILLIP C. PHAN, MD Director of Interventional Pain Management, Department of Anesthesiology and Pain Medicine, University of Texas MD Anderson Cancer Center, Houston, Texas

DANIEL PICUS, MD Professor of Radiology and Surgery, Chief of Diagnostic Radiology, Mallinckrodt Institute of Radiology, Washington University School of Medicine, St. Louis, Missouri; Diagnostic Radiologist-in-Chief, Department of Radiology, Barnes-Jewish Hospital, St. Louis, Missouri

JEFFREY S. POLLAK, MD Associate Professor of Radiology, Section of Vascular and Interventional Radiology, Yale University School of Medicine, New Haven, Connecticut; Co-Section Chief, Vascular and Interventional Radiology, Department of Radiology, Yale-New Haven Hospital, New Haven, Connecticut

STEVEN D. QUARFORDT, MD Staff Interventionalist, Department of Radiology, St. Anthony Hospital, Denver, Colorado

DHEERAJ K. RAJAN, MD, FRCPC, FSIR Assistant Professor, Department of Medical Imaging, University of Toronto; Assistant Professor, Department of Vascular and Interventional Radiology, University Health Network and Mount Sinai Hospital, Toronto, Ontario, Canada

PARVATI RAMCHANDANI, MD Professor of Radiology and Surgery, Department of Radiology, University of Pennsylvania Medical Center, Philadelphia, Pennsylvania; Department of Radiology, Section of Genitourinary Radiology, Hospital of the University of Pennsylvania, Philadelphia, Pennsylvania

KENNETH S. RHOLL, MD Associate Clinical Professor, Department of Radiology, George Washington University, Washington D.C.; Staff Physician, Department of Interventional Radiology, Inova Alexandria Hospital, Alexandria, Virginia

ANNE C. ROBERTS, MD Professor, Department of Radiology, University of California, SanDiego, La Jolla, California; Chief of Vascular and Interventional Radiology, Department of Radiology, Thornton Hospital/UCSD Medical Center, La Jolla, California

SAMEER ROHATGI, MD Fellow in Interventional Cardiology, Hospital of the University of Pennsylvania, Philadelphia, Pennsylvania

JOSEF RÖSCH, MD Director and Professor, Research Laboratory, Dotter Interventional Institute, Oregon Health and Science University, Portland, Oregon

ROBERT J. ROSEN, MD Associate Professor, Department of Radiology, New York University School of Medicine; Co-Director, Peripheral and Endovascular Institute, Lenox Hill Cardiac and Vascular Institute, New York, New York

GEOFFREY D. RUBIN, MD Department of Radiology, Stanford University Medical Center, Stanford, California

JEFFREY A. SAAL, MD SOAR, Physiatry Medical Group, Redwood City, California

JI HOON SHIN, MD, PhD Assistant Professor, Department of Radiology, University of Ulsan College of Medicine, Asan Medical Center, Seoul, Republic of Korea

RICHARD SHLANSKY-GOLDBERG, MD Associate Professor, Department of Radiology, University of Pennsylvania; Staff Interventional Radiologist, Division of Interventional Radiology, Hospital of the University of Pennsylvania, Philadelphia, Pennsylvania

TONY P. SMITH, MD Professor and Chief of Division of Interventional Radiology, Department of Radiology, Duke University Medical Center, Durham, North Carolina

GREGORY M. SOARES, MD Assistant Professor of Diagnostic Imaging, Brown Medical School, Providence, Rhode Island; Chief of Vascular and Interventional Radiology Division, Rhode Island Hospital, Providence, Rhode Island

JEFFERY ADAM SOLOMON, MD, MBA Assistant Professor, Department of Radiology, University of Pennsylvania School of Medicine, Philadelphia, Pennsylvania; Assistant Professor, Department of Radiology, Hospital of the University of Pennsylvania, Philadelphia, Pennsylvania

AMY P. SOLTES, RN, MSN, ACNP-BC Nurse Practitioner, Interventional Radiology, Department of Radiology, The George Washington University Medical Center, Washington, D.C.

HO-YOUNG SONG, MD, PhD Professor, Department of Radiology, University of Ulsan College of Medicine, Asan Medical Center, Seoul, Republic of Korea

THOMAS A. SOS, MD Professor of Radiology, Cornell University Medical College; Director, Interventional Radiology, The New York Hospital, New York, New York

MICHAEL C. SOULEN, MD Professor of Radiology and Surgery, Department of Radiology, University of Pennsylvania; Interventional Radiology, Hospital of the University of Pennsylvania, Philadelphia, Pennsylvania

JAMES B. SPIES, MD Professor of Radiology, Department of Radiology, Georgetown University School of Medicine; Chairman and Chief of Service, Department of Radiology, Georgetown University Hospital, Washington, D.C.

DAVID J. SPINOSA, MD Keck School of Medicine, University of Southern California, Los Angeles, California

BRIAN F. STAINKEN, MD Adjunct Professor, Department of Radiology, Boston University School of Medicine, Boston, Massachusetts; Chairman, Department of Diagnostic Imaging, Roger Williams Medical Center, Providence, Rhode Island

S. WILLIAM STAVROPOULOS, MD Assistant Professor of Radiology, Department of Radiology/Interventional Radiology, University of Pennsylvania School of Medicine, Philadelphia, Pennsylvania

KYU-BO SUNG, MD, PhD Professor, Department of Radiology, University of Ulsan College of Medicine, Asan Medical Center, Seoul, Republic of Korea

ELOY TEJERO, MD Associate Professor, Department of Surgery, University of Zaragoza; Medical Assistant, Department of Surgery, Hospital Clinico Universitario Lozano Blesa, Zaragoza, Spain

FRANK J. THORNTON MD, FFRRCSI Assistant Professor, Departments of Radiology and Medical Physics, University of Wisconsin–Madison, Madison, Wisconsin

RENAN UFLACKER, MD, MSc Professor, Department of Interventional Radiology, Medical University of South Carolina, Charleston, South Carolina; Director, Department of Radiology, Medical University of South Carolina Universtiy Hospital, Charleston, South Carolina

ANTHONY C. VENBRUX, MD Professor of Radiology and Surgery, Department of Radiology, The George Washington University, Washington, D.C.; Director of Cardiovascular and Interventional Radiology, Department of Radiology, The George Washington University Medical Center, Washington, D.C.

STEVEN C. WAGNER, MD Interventional Radiologist, Doylestown Hospital, Doylestown, Pennsylvania

ARTHUR C. WALTMAN, MD Associate Professor, Department of Radiology, Harvard Medical School, Boston, Massachusetts; Radiologist, Department of Radiology, Massachusetts General Hospital, Boston, Massachusetts

DAVID S. WANG, MD Howard Hughes Medical Institute Fellow, Section of Cardiovascular and Interventional Radiology, Stanford University School of Medicine, Stanford, California; Resident Physician, Department of Radiology, Stanford University Medical Center, Stanford, California

STANLEY B. WASHINGTON, MD Physician, Department of Radiology, The George Washington University Medical Center, Washington, D.C.

SUSAN M. WEEKS, MD Associate Professor, Department of Radiology, University of North Carolina–Chapel Hill School of Medicine, Chapel Hill, North Carolina

ROBERT I. WHITE, JR., MD Professor of Radiology, Department of Diagnostic Radiology, Yale University School of Medicine; Director of Yale AVM Center, Department of Diagnostic Imaging, Yale New Haven Hospital, New Haven, Connecticut

EDWARD Y. WOO, MD Assistant Professor of Surgery, Divison of Vascular Surgery, University of Pennsylvania Medical Center, Philadelphia, Pennsylvania

STEVEN WORTH, MD Staff Pathologist, Department of Pathology, St. Anthony Hospital, Denver, Colorado

HYUN KI YOON, MD, PhD Associate Professor, Department of Radiology, University of Ulsan College of Medicine, Asan Medical Center, Seoul, Republic of Korea

Foreword

The 20th century was a period of great turbulence, much of it already recorded in history books that will constantly be revised. World Wars I and II, the Great Depression, the rise and fall of fascism and communism, the nuclear planet, hundreds of regional conflicts, the United Nations, the Cold War, and the unmet challenges of hunger and disease were enough to dominate the experience and thinking of thoughtful citizens in all countries.

Along with the violence and disasters, there was an explosion of the creative capacities of individuals and groups—in art, literature, philosophy, physics, engineering, architecture—and not least in the biomedical sciences. For the first time, infectious disease, the course and outcome of which had depended largely on the virulence of organisms and the resistance of hosts, became the subject of rational therapy, with new and different antibiotics introduced almost in a continuum. Molecular biology, genetics, open heart surgery, and an augmented understanding of the science that underlies systemic and organ disorders opened the doors to transplantation and increasing control of heart disease, cancer, diabetes, and even AIDS.

Side by side with these advances, there has evolved an extraordinary capacity to decrease the morbidity of an unusual range of illnesses, accelerated in the past few decades. These forward steps, part of the development of the field of *interventional radiology*, have affected the cardiovascular system from top to bottom and a host of disorders of the gastrointestinal, genitourinary, central nervous, and other systems. Thoracotomies and laparotomies—with all of the insult to the organism that they represent—have been avoided for millions of patients through the skills, ingenuity, and masterful technical achievements of the leaders in this field.

To my great pleasure and the readers' great profit, Dr. Stanley Baum, a former fellow of mine in cardiovascular radiology many years ago and today one of the great figures in the field of radiology, has served as the editor of the last two editions of this text. Together with his co-editor, Dr. Michael J. Pentecost, he has organized and edited this edition with a keen eye for noteworthy progress and for the finest contributors in the world. The timing could not be more spectacular, with new technologies and new methods introduced since the last edition crying for the kind of explication that the authors of each of these 72 chapters have provided.

The reader will find this volume a treasure chest of timely and valuable information, fully encompassing the present state of the art and encouraging another generation to go forward, learning and leading the way in interventional radiology.

Herbert L. Abrams, MD

Preface

Volume III of *Abrams' Angiography*, published in 1997, was a stand-alone text devoted entirely to interventional radiology.

This new 2nd Edition of Volume III highlights the significant changes in the practice of interventional radiology that have occurred during these past 8 years. We include 15 new chapters describing procedures and techniques that were not routinely performed in 1997. For example, there are chapters on helical CT angiography, transluminal placement of endovascular stent grafts for the treatment of abdominal aortic aneurysms, and arterial embolization of uterine fibroids. Our authors also describe new procedures used for pain management, the management of chylothorax, and the treatment of venous insufficiency. Fifty-seven of the 72 chapters in the current edition have been completely updated and revised and illustrate the current state of the art of our specialty.

The accuracy of noninvasive techniques such as vascular ultrasound, CT angiography, and MR angiography has continued to improve. Many diagnoses that could only be made by conventional contrast arteriography now require only these less invasive procedures. This has resulted in a decrease in the number of diagnostic angiograms performed at a time when there has been a significant increase in the number and complexity of interventional procedures overall. The interventionalist, parenthetically, has assumed new clinical responsibilities. This new brand of medical specialist has office hours, admits and cares for inpatients, and assumes the responsibility of these patients after discharge.

This transition to more clinical involvement has presented challenges to the traditional radiology department. Radiology residents choosing interventional radiology as a subspecialty must now be trained, not only in diagnostic imaging, but also in the clinical skills required to care for patients. Since it is unlikely that these clinical skills will be learned in a radiology department, the training of interventional radiologists will almost certainly become much more interdisciplinary. This will require revamping traditional fellowship programs to allow rotation through vascular surgery, intensive care units, and so on. For this to occur, the interventional radiologist, in a reciprocal manner, will have to participate in the training of other specialists.

The first edition of *Abrams' Angiography*, published in 1961, has become a classic work. The subsequent editions presented over the last 44 years have provided an authoritative voice in the emergence of this new subspecialty. The current editors approached the task of updating and re-editing this text with a great deal of caution and humility. We hope that the results capture the excitement that has been the hallmark of the earlier editions. We are appreciative of Herb Abrams' encouragement.

Multi-authored texts can lack cohesion and risk being redundant. In an effort to avoid this, the editors have made changes in the format, organization, and language of some of the contributions. Hopefully this new edition will not squander its inheritance and will be as enthusiastically accepted as its predecessors.

Our wives, Jeanne and Judy, deserve special credit for their willingness to put up with the hours of preparation, often on working weekends and during vacations, which were required to bring this project to completion. Without their encouragement and support, this work would not have happened.

An authoritative text of this magnitude requires the willingness of authors of 72 chapters to meet deadlines, conform to the required editorial changes, and tolerate the editor's frequent evening and weekend calls. We have asked favors of many of our longtime friends and colleagues. We are appreciative and grateful to all of them.

We are thankful to our assistant, Flora Cauley, who managed to keep track of the chapters, authors, and deadlines. We are also grateful for the advice of Lisa McAllister, Acquisitions Editor, and the Managing Editors Jenny Kim, Kerry Barret, and Rebecca Barroso. In addition, we thank David Murphy and Pat Dewey, the Editorial Project Managers, and the excellent editorial staff of Lippincott, Williams & Wilkins.

Stanley Baum
Michael J. Pentecost

Preface to *Abrams' Angiography,* 4th Edition, Volume III

The third volume of the fourth edition of *Abrams' Angiography* is new—a stand-alone text devoted to interventional radiology rather than scattered chapters as in the previous editions. This separate volume was chosen after considerable deliberation and, in many ways, it symbolizes another stage in the growth and evolution of interventional radiology practice.

Increasingly, alternative imaging methods permit accurate and less invasive diagnosis of many conditions. With advances in ultrasound, magnetic resonance imaging, and helical CT, the number of diagnostic angiograms is declining in most practices; to some extent, this decrease has been offset by the growth in interventional procedures. In fact, in most practices interventional procedures are more common than diagnostic examinations.

Whatever the numbers, the rise of interventional radiology has certainly changed the tenor of practice. While some of the tools may be the same, interventional radiology is different than angiography. When attempting to change the course of disease rather than simply study its appearance, a radiologist assumes a whole different level of responsibility—from outpatient clinics to rounds to admitting services. And all of these changes have been good for radiology.

Creating a new field of medicine such as interventional radiology took intelligence, self-confidence, and vision—all traits that characterized our pioneers, many of whom contributed to the first, second, and third editions of *Abrams' Angiography.* The ensuing wave of radiologists are similar to those who fall in the ranks behind forerunners in other disciplines—perhaps less individualistic than their forebears, greater in number, a little narrower in scope, more engineers than pioneers. Their work—filling in the clinical and scientific gaps, quantifying the risks and benefits, developing and codifying training programs, haranguing insurers—is no less important. Whatever their contributions, these two groups gave birth to a new branch of medicine. This volume, to which many of them contributed, is a tribute to them all.

A physician can hope for two great professional pleasures. First, and always foremost, is the satisfaction of caring for an individual patient. The other is a contribution to society—the expansion of scientific knowledge, a public policy initiative, an organizational change that optimizes and improves health care. Those involved in the inception of this field over the past two decades have been fortunate to sample both pleasures.

Of course, interventional radiology is only one facet of the much larger field of minimally invasive therapy. These powerful trends—to less violative surgery, to a smaller incision, a shorter hospitalization, a quicker return to the normal function—are fueled by ever more knowledgeable patients. Fittingly, patients are the prime beneficiaries of interventional techniques as well as advances in allied fields of cardiology, gastroenterology, urology, and laparoscopic and arthroscopic surgery.

A labor of this size requires many hands. A great debt is owed to our administrative assistants, Flora Cauley and Jennifer Waechter, who handled the organization of this project in Philadelphia. The editorial assistance of Mary Frawley and Julie Sullivan was enlightening, understanding and, frankly, indispensable. A task of this magnitude would have been impossible without the steadfast encouragement of Nancy Chorpenning and Deeth Ellis at Little, Brown in Boston. In concert with Little, Brown and Dr. Abrams, we selected a satin enamel finish over more "traditional" enamel gloss papers, as we determined that it provides superior definition and gray-scale reproduction. We hope you find it easier on your eyes!

The counsel and aid of the interventional radiology attendings at the University of Pennsylvania, Drs. Constantin Cope, Ken Fellows, Parvi Ramchandani, Robert Hurst, Richard Shlansky-Goldberg, Michael Soulen, Ziv Haskal, Richard Baum, and Doug Redd, were critical to this effort. Finally, we appreciate the faith and confidence of Dr. Herb Abrams in entrusting us with this important duty.

Stanley Baum
Michael J. Pentecost

Contents

Patient Management

Preintervention Assessment, Intraprocedure Management, Postintervention Care

Klemens H. Barth

PREINTERVENTION ASSESSMENT

Interventional radiology (IR) procedures are minimally invasive surgical procedures that inflict less pain and procedure-related morbidity and mortality than conventional open surgery. Most IR procedures require less than 24 hours of hospitalization and are primarily considered to be outpatient procedures. They do not pose significant cardiovascular risks and do not produce the circulatory and metabolic changes caused by open surgical procedures, particularly those of the major arteries. Because IR procedures are infrequently performed under general anesthesia, they avoid the anesthetic impact on respiratory, cardiac, and hepatorenal function.

The Scope of Clinical Responsibilities

Interventional radiology is in constant evolution. IR techniques are less standardized than surgical techniques, many of which have been passed on through several generations of physicians. IR is largely represented by the first and second generation of practitioners who dedicated most of their professional efforts to developing IR procedures. A third generation has emerged from training programs with a variety of practice styles. This lack of tradition and a limited database on outcomes of IR procedures have certainly had an impact on risk and benefit assessments, which influence their acceptance by referring physicians and patients. Transjugular intrahepatic portosystemic shunting (TIPS) and embolization therapy for uterine leiomyomata (UAE) are particularly prominent examples of procedures receiving intense scrutiny for their indications, complications, and longevity by competing medical specialists and by public health organizations (1,2).

For many interventional radiologists, the idea that an IR procedure poses a much lower risk than surgery and does not preclude its subsequent successful performance provides a powerful rationale for applying it, even though failure or limited success may be encountered, for example, in renal and femoropopliteal artery transluminal angioplasty and in chemoembolization (3–5). It is also clear that interventional radiologists strive to perform these procedures as true alternatives to more invasive therapy and not merely as temporizing or preoperative measures.

In view of the potential benefits gained for the patient through state-of-the-art IR therapy, the radiologist's clinical responsibility becomes obvious (6). Unlike the diagnostic radiologist, whose recognition of pathology constitutes the essence of consultation to the referring physician, who in turn has full responsibility to convert the radiologic findings into clinical care, the interventional radiologist is a clinical consultant, like a surgeon, who converts diagnostic findings directly into clinical care and remains involved from the time a consultation is requested until such time when the consequences of the IR procedure are no longer relevant to the patient's care. This clinical involvement includes preprocedure workup, patient preparation, performance of the procedure, and postprocedure follow-up, which may extend over days or years (7). Most IR procedures do not require the assistance of an anesthesiologist, so the radiologist also prescribes and supervises sedation, pain control, and, if necessary, emergency measures to treat complications during the procedure.

In the hospital setting, the interventional radiologist may function as a member of a clinical team, working primarily as a procedure-oriented specialist who delegates pre- and postprocedure care to medical and surgical team members. While this practice style is still prevalent as it has been when IR evolved from diagnostic radiology, it will not be sustainable in an environment of intense competition for the most attractive IR procedures, such as transluminal angioplasty (PTA) and related interventions. Furthermore, only within the framework of an established team and with the patient's understanding is delegation of clinical responsibility appropriate. In any other situation, the radiologist needs to personally prepare and follow the patient. This statement is made expressly with respect to therapeutic procedures. For diagnostic procedures, the interventional radiologist's role as consultant is generally limited to the immediate procedure-related preparation, the procedure, and follow-up, typically less than 12 hours.

In the environment of managed care, the interventional radiologist may need to play the role of a gatekeeper who prevents overuse of IR procedures. Perceived overuse of inferior vena cava filter placement and PTA have already become prominent examples (8,9). Presentations to hospital staff, weekly specialty conferences, and grand rounds are important forums in which the interventional radiologist can inform clinical colleagues about the proper indications for IR procedures (7).

Diagnostic radiologists will infrequently question the appropriateness of an ordered examination. This posture may be understandable because transmission of information about the patient is usually limited, and research on the complete clinical background may be impossible within the context of a busy practice. However, this does not apply to therapeutic IR procedures. Interventional radiologists, therefore, must understand the different role they play in that part of their practice (7).

These postulates appear straightforward, yet the priorities of radiologic practice do not necessarily favor them. If IR procedures are performed within the daily routine of diagnostic radiology, most of which are diagnostic image interpretations, it may be difficult or impossible to personally review every requested procedure, pay an inpatient visit or conduct an office visit, discuss the procedure, and finally perform the procedure in an appropriate time frame. This situation goes to the heart of the way radiologists practice outside subspecialized practices, typically university hospitals, and has no easy solution. It is often a question of personnel, sharing of responsibility among the members of a group, distribution of specialty skills, maintenance of those skills, sharing of on-call responsibilities, and so forth.

Training of interventional radiologists in accredited programs, subspecialty boards, and practice standards set by professional organizations are all serving to assert quality of professional care. A new education pathway, which includes a broader clinical experience for radiology residents who wish to subspecialize in IR, stems from the rather belated recognition that clinical responsibilities are to be taken more seriously or IR practice may be lost to other clinical specialties (10). Interventional radiologists will have to practice their craft full time or devote enough time to procedures and clinical obligations to receive full recognition as clinical specialists (11). In turn, opposition will lessen to interventional radiologists seeking clinical privileges or maintaining privileges, particularly for those procedures that have gained competing interests among physicians of other specialties (12,13).

A growing number of cardiologists, vascular surgeons, and (to a lesser degree) other specialists, such as nephrologists and gastroenterologists, are already performing IR-endovascular procedures in a competitive environment where clinical care provision and patient access determine who controls which procedure. Not to be underestimated is the role of the device industry, whose sales interests support procedure volume regardless of which specialist provides that care.

A number of practice models have emerged in an attempt to bring the skills of interventional radiologists and other specialists together, most notably those between interventional radiologists and vascular surgeons (14,15). Some are thriving; others failed. It became clear that no universally acceptable model has emerged, and the future of such ventures rests on the preservation of each specialty with perpetuation of sufficient training opportunities by the partners. Under the current condition of reduced recruitment of radiology residents into IR training programs and the increasing efforts by other specialties to incorporate percutaneous catheter skills into their own training, the future of IR as a subspecialty of radiology in its current form is uncertain. The blame for this evolution may be laid on a number of factors or may simply be attributed to evolution in medical care whereby new procedures spawned by one kind of physician become accepted by others who have a vested interest in applying those procedures to "their own" patients. For those radiologists who want to continue practicing IR, being a clinical specialist, like a vascular surgeon or a cardiologist, is a matter of professional survival.

The Interventional Radiology Clinic and Outpatient Consultation

A successful IR practice is served best by an office- or clinic-style operation where patients referred by primary- or secondary-care physicians or self-referrals are seen regularly as outpatients prior to performing any IR procedure. The clinic also serves as a place for follow-up visits and needs to be staffed and equipped according to the needs of the practice (7,16). How to set up such a practice is beyond the scope of this chapter. The interested reader is referred to resources provided by professional organizations such as the Society of Interventional Radiology and the American College of Radiology.

During the office visit, all the necessary preparatory workup can be arranged or performed. Pertinent medical and imaging studies have been sent to the interventional radiologist before that visit or are brought along by the patient. The interventional radiologist may request further workup. For example, if a patient is referred for renal angioplasty, computerized tomographic angiography (CTA) or magnetic resonance angiography (MRA) may serve as definitive diagnostic test on which the decision to intervene is directly based. Similarly, magnetic resonance imaging (MRI) of the pelvis serves as guidance to subsequent UAE, and a patient scheduled for hepatic chemoembolization may need immediate preprocedure

contrast-enhanced CTA as baseline for matching postprocedure Lipiodol retention to individual tumor nodules and for planning follow-up procedures.

The interventional radiologist needs to obtain clinical admission privileges. Patients, after chemoembolizations or UAE (2), are generally admitted. While these admissions may be short, less than 24 hours, several days may be necessary, and in such cases the interventional radiologist serves as the attending physician who, in turn, may seek consultation from an oncologist, gynecologist, or others, depending on circumstances.

Inpatient Consultation

The clinical consultation is initiated for each patient by direct contact with the referring physician unless practice routine has been established between a referring physician or group of such physicians with the interventional radiologist so that typical diagnostic findings prompt a prearranged therapeutic intervention. For instance, after angiographic identification of a significant iliac artery stenosis by invasive arteriography, angioplasty follows immediately because a decision was made with the referring physician to proceed in such fashion. This is communicated with the patient in advance, and consent is obtained. With noninvasive vascular workup by MRA or CTA becoming more prevalent, this type of on-the-spot decision to move from diagnostic to therapeutic intervention may become obsolete.

The initial physician contact gives the radiologist opportunity to review the reason for referral, the essential history, physical findings, and pertinent diagnostic workup. Here the radiologist can clarify the approach and treatment planning. For example, if placement of an inferior vena cava filter is requested, questions to be answered are documented pulmonary emboli, relative or absolute contraindication to anticoagulation, the patient's age and expected longevity, or permanent versus temporary filter placement. During the conversation with the referring physician, the radiologist can also make an initial decision about the appropriateness of the procedure, suggest a modification, request further workup, or determine whether the intervention should be performed emergently to realize its full benefit. The outcome of such conversation, particularly if disagreement as to the proper indication exists, will be heavily influenced by the radiologist's professional stature, clinical competence, and reasoning skills. It is important to ascertain that the referring physician has told the patient about the referral to an interventional radiologist; otherwise, the patient may refuse treatment for not having been able to discuss the matter with his or her physician.

When a problem-focused history is taken, specific questions are asked about such issues as onset of claudication on either side, bilateral symptoms, and which side may be preferable for angioplasty. Other specific questions will pertain to allergy against contrast agents, sedation and analgesia, antibiotics, latex, and so on. A procedure-oriented physical examination includes the entire pulse status for all vascular interventions and auscultation for possible bruits over the groin and in the neck. Finding a loud bruit over the carotid artery, for example, would prompt further workup for carotid stenosis before renal angioplasty to assess the risk of stroke following sudden decrease in blood pressure. All patients undergoing peripheral angioplasty have ankle and brachial indices obtained and documented in the chart.

Additional patient information is obtained from the patient's chart, the nurses, and the house staff. If a change of plans results, the referring physician is immediately notified. For example, a patient scheduled to have a chronic catheter placed for hepatic artery chemotherapy infusion via the left transbrachial access may refuse to have any catheter placed through that arm because she was told by the surgeon "not to have any needles in the arm" after axillary node dissection.

Procedure Consent

After the radiologist has established the "game plan," he or she obtains the patient's written consent. This consent needs to be secured in some temporary relationship to the procedure, most often within 24 hours. Individual state or hospital regulations may prevail. Many patients are more comfortable having the consent interview conducted in the presence of a next of kin or caretaker, and the interventional radiologist should encourage this practice. It is important to conduct explanation of the procedure and the conversation leading to informed consent in a noncoercive fashion and not rushed so that the patient is given adequate time for decision making unless the situation is an emergency.

The main elements in the consent conversation are the nature of the procedure, the most frequent risks, and the alternatives (17,18). In some jurisdictions it is a requirement to put these three elements in writing and to hand a copy to the patient. What constitutes a significant complication is determined by its expected frequency and severity, which may vary depending on the clinical circumstances. For example, small peripheral emboli during peripheral angioplasty are usually of minimal significance if the trifurcation artery runoff is intact. However, if a patient has only a single trifurcation artery, even a small peripheral embolus could have serious consequences. Conversely, a patient with a history of asthma, a condition suggesting an allergic diathesis, may not have a significant risk of contrast-related allergy if the procedure involves nonvascular contrast injection or if carbon dioxide is used in place of iodinated contrast. Informed written consent documents the existence of a contract between physician and patient.

Immediate Preprocedure Preparation

After the consent conversation, the radiologist completes the consultation report with a treatment recommendation and enters specific preparation orders into the patient's chart, which include the type of food to be withheld, the type of hydration, the antibiotic prophylaxis, and additional laboratory tests if needed. Most IR procedures do not require an extended fast. Solid food should be avoided for at least eight hours before the procedure, whereas clear liquids can be maintained up to two hours before the procedure. If anesthesia is requested, anesthesiologists generally require a more extended fasting period.

The intramuscular administration of sedatives or narcotic analgesics on the patient's floor before transfer to the interventional laboratory should be discouraged because the patient is not likely to be monitored adequately (exceptions are given below under "Allergy Preparation"). Instead, it is better practice to have the patient connected to monitoring devices in the angiographic laboratory before sedation is administered and after baseline vital signs have been recorded. Comforting behavior by the physician, technical staff, and nursing staff during such preparation will go a long way to alleviate patient anxiety (19).

The night before or the day of the IR procedure, certain medication adjustments, fasting periods, assessment of vital signs, and a review of the patient's laboratory tests, such as a renal function test, clotting status test, white blood cell count, hematocrit, and so on, are instituted. Also reviewed are changes in pulse status or venous patency for potential access. Outpatients may have the necessary laboratory tests performed immediately before the procedure, such as a creatinine level test for renal tolerance of vascular contrast or a full clotting status test for fluid drainages and large-caliber needle biopsies. If not yet done, the definitive written consent is then finalized, with the patient having already been informed verbally about the procedure. This is not the time for the initial patient-to-physician contact. The patient should be prepared to undergo the procedure after having had reasonable time for decision making (see above).

Prophylaxis Against Contrast-Induced Nephropathy (CIN)

Although nonionic, and particularly nonionic isosmolar iodinated, contrast agents have reduced CIN (20,21), patients undergoing procedures with vascular contrast should not be dehydrated, and oral intake of clear fluids is generally allowed to within 2–3 hours of the IR procedure. Diuretics are withheld, which in most instances are prescribed for control of hypertension. Diabetic patients and those with borderline renal function who have creatinine levels greater than 1.5 mg/dL are prepared with intravenous hydration of normal saline solution (NSS) for 12 hours before and after the procedure (22). The addition of fenoldopam has no proven benefit; instead, N-acetylcysteine (Mucomyst) may be beneficial (23). The most recently recommended regimen following a randomized study consists of sodium bicarbonate solution infused at a rate of 3 mL/kg per hour for 1 hour before and for 6 hours after contrast administration (24). Induced postprocedure diuresis is no longer recommended (25). The only caveat regarding hydration is for patients with limited cardiac function. In these instances, cardiology consultation is advised.

Insulin Adjustment

The insulin dose in diabetic patients is reduced during procedure-related fasting. For morning procedures, the author reduces the morning dose by one half. Blood sugar levels can be monitored during the procedure, and a 50% glucose injection should be available in case of hypoglycemia.

Testing and Adjustment of Spontaneous or Induced Coagulation Deficits

Screening for hemostatic function usually includes tests for coagulation function (Table 1–1). The partial thromboplastin time (PTT) test represents the *intrinsic pathway,* and the prothrombin time (PT), the *extrinsic pathway.* The platelet count completes the assessment. If a platelet deficiency is assumed (platelet aggregation inhibitors, renal failure), the bleeding time (BT) can be checked to assess the *primary hemostatic function.*

For nonvascular percutaneous procedures such as needle chest or abdominal needle biopsies, deep-seated drainages, creation of port pockets or catheter tracts (tunnels), translumbar aortic or inferior vena cava, and transhepatic venous, and for the poorly compressible axillary or brachial artery access, normal coagulation is required.

For transfemoral arterial procedures with catheter or sheath calibers <9 French, a PT <16 seconds (International Normalized Ratio [INR] <1.5), a PTT <40 seconds, and normally functioning platelets >40,000 are acceptable.

TABLE 1–1
TESTING AND MANAGEMENT OF COMMON COAGULATION DEFICIENCIES

Test	Normal Value	Cause of Abnormal Tests	Treatment
Prothrombin time (PT)—"extrinsic coagulation system"	Within 3 sec of control value	1. Warfarin treatment 2. Parenchymal liver disease 3. Vitamin K absorption deficiency: parenteral nutrition, biliary obstruction, malabsorption, antibiotics 4. Consumption of factors: disseminated intravascular coagulation, thrombolytic therapy 5. Congenital: hemophilia	1. Vitamin K 10–15 mg IM or SQ q8h for 3 doses or FFP[a] 2. FFP[a] 3–4 units or 10–20 mL/kg 3. Vitamin K 10–15 mg IM or SQ q8h for 3 doses or FFP[a] 3–4 units 4. Treat initiating cause 5. Consult hematologist
Partial thromboplastin time (PTT)—"intrinsic coagulation system"	Within 6 sec of control value	1. Warfarin treatment 2. Heparin treatment 3. Lupus anticoagulant	1. As above 2. Wait 3–4 hr after stopping heparin, check PTT, or give protamine (1 mg/100 U heparin) IV very slowly (cave anaphylaxis) 3. No treatment necessary
Bleeding time (BT; indicates platelet function if PT and PTT are normal)	Less than 8 min	Platelet deficiency 1. Quantitative platelet count less than 50,000/μL 2. Qualitative: a. uremia; b. ASA, dipyridamole, NSAID[b] 3. Spontaneous	1. Platelet transfusion (10 U), hemodialysis, cryoprecipitate (0.1–0.2 bags/kg), and/or DDAVP[c] (0.4 mcg/kg over 30 min) 2. Stop medication (requires days to weeks to reverse effect) 3. Consult hematologist

[a]FFP = fresh-frozen plasma.
[b]ASA (aspirin), dipyridamole, and NSAID (nonsteroidal anti-inflammatory drugs) generally do not influence the indication for percutaneous vascular procedures, but may do so for deep-seated drainages, percutaneous stone extractions, and so forth.
[c]DDAVP = 1-deamino-(18-D-arginine)-vasopressin.

However, other bleeding risk factors, such as severe hypertension, renal failure, or inadequate hemodialysis, need to be taken into account. Closure devices are a convenient adjunct for postprocedure hemostasis at femoral artery entries; however, their added benefit over mechanical compression—hemostasis with the use of diagnostic-caliber catheters—is questionable (26). Procedures through compressible veins with small-caliber diagnostic catheters, placement of nontunneled transjugular catheters, or placement of peripherally inserted central venous catheters can be performed under abnormal coagulation, including therapeutic anticoagulation.

Depending on the above approaches, patients receiving heparin anticoagulation may need the dose halted or reduced to achieve a PTT <40 seconds for procedures requiring arterial entry. Heparin can be restarted about 2 hours following hemostasis after catheter pullout. The effect of subcutaneous low-molecular-weight heparin (e.g., Lovenox) cannot be reliably tested by PTT; therefore, if critical, testing of the bleeding time is necessary. Allowing a 12-hour interval following the latest administration is a safe way to avoid the anticoagulation effect.

Patients receiving Coumadin generally require several days of treatment-free interval before the coagulation returns to normal or nearly normal levels. If continuation of anticoagulation is critical, as for patients with atrial fibrillation and artificial heart valves, switching to intravenous heparin is the preferred procedure. The above policy is then followed; otherwise, treatment with vitamin K is necessary. For urgent Coumadin reversal, fresh frozen plasma (FFP) is given usually in increments of 2 units followed by check of the PT. FFP administration is also frequently necessary to correct coagulation defects of patients with severe liver disease, for example, in preparation for TIPS or percutaneous biliary drainage.

Patients who have severe coagulation deficits require adjustment for vascular and nonvascular procedures. Patients likely to present these deficiencies have received chemotherapy, bone marrow transplantation, or high-volume blood transfusions (27), or they have severe liver disease, hypersplenism, renal failure, or disseminated intravascular coagulation after severe trauma or sepsis (28). Much rarer in the general hospital environment are patients encountered with congenital hemophilias, spontaneous thrombocytopenias, and von Willebrand disease. Although the referring physician or the clinical service is generally aware of the patient's problem, the interventional radiologist needs to be equally aware and at least familiar with basic steps to correct the coagulation status. Specific tests are available for most deficiencies. For platelet function, other than the overall count, determination of the bleeding time is usually the best test. In many instances, the underlying process cannot readily be corrected; therefore, specific factors, FFP, or single-donor platelets are transfused in close temporal relationship to the IR procedure.

Patients may receive platelet aggregation inhibitors such as aspirin and clopidogrel for prophylaxis of stroke or myocardial infarction or after percutaneous transluminal angioplasty or vascular surgery. Correction of this platelet deficiency is not required for percutaneous vascular procedures performed through compressible arterial access. However, deep-seated drainages with larger-caliber catheters or access sheath placement for renal stone extraction may well encounter unusual bleeding in those patients. Correction of the platelet defect requires medication suspension for 7–10 days before the IR procedure.

Adjustment of Cardiac Rhythm Abnormalities in High-Risk Cardiac Patients

Patients with cardiac arrhythmias, particularly those scheduled to undergo pulmonary arteriography or intrapulmonary thrombolysis by catheter, thrombus aspiration, embolization, and so on, should be adequately prepared by cardiology. If a left bundle branch block is present, a temporary transvenous pacemaker is inserted to treat a potential complete heart block.

Patients with severe ischemic (29) heart disease (unstable angina, ejection fraction less than 30%) belong to the high-risk group for any intervention and should be so identified in the preparatory process.

Allergy Preparation

For patients allergic to contrast agents, appropriate regimens have been designed over the years and consist of steroids or steroids with H_1- or H_2-receptor antagonists (30,31).

It is generally recognized that the incidence of serious allergic reactions to nonionic contrast is rare and roughly equal to that in patients receiving high-osmolality contrast agents after preparatory medication (32). It is also recognized that arterial contrast injections are less likely to evoke allergic reactions than intravenous contrast injections. However, even with routine use of nonionic low osmolar and isosmolar contrast agents, prophylaxis for patients with a documented contrast allergy is necessary.

Patients with a history of asthma have a higher tendency for allergic reactions in general, and prophylaxis before first-time use of parenteral contrast appears prudent.

Preprocedure preparation with benzodiazepines is recommended for patients who have had recent seizures (33).

Prophylactic Antibiotics

Prophylactic antibiotics (Table 1–2) are not routinely required for sterile vascular procedures (34). However, practices vary among practitioners (34,35). Procedures for which administration of prophylactic antibiotics is generally accepted include TIPS, port placements, embolizations to infarct tissue, such as chemoembolization and thermal ablation (33). Those patients are covered with antibiotics to avoid or reduce the bacterial seeding of necrosing tissue through the bloodstream or, more importantly, through bile ducts or the renal collecting system if included in the infracted volume (35). Several such procedural protocols have been established (35). Prophylaxis starts within the hour of the procedure and is usually carried on over 24 to 48 hours. For vascular procedures with percutaneous entry through synthetic grafts, prophylactic antibiotics effective against skin pathogens reduce the possibility of graft infection.

It is best to set up a protocol for the use of prophylactic antibiotics with the infectious disease service of a particular hospital environment. By doing so, specific experience with bacterial resistances is accommodated, and the best routine is established.

The expected benefit of antibacterial prophylaxis needs to be weighed against the risk of contributing to the growing problem of bacterial resistance. More important is strict adherence to sterile technique, including proper skin preparation with 2% chlorhexidine solution and sufficient sterile draping; operator and assistants performing surgical scrubbing (5 minutes for hands and forearms before the first case and 3 minutes for each subsequent case that day), and wearing full operative gear. Many interventional procedure rooms do not provide an operating room environment but require an operating room-type cleaning routine after each procedure, avoidance of alternating sterile with nonsterile procedures, allowing no one to enter the room without wearing scrubs, and removing all soiled clothing and linen from patients outside the procedure room. Technologists need to be trained in sterile procedure preparation, wearing mask and cap when setting up tables and properly draping the equipment. Nurses monitoring the patient and administering sedation and other medications during the procedure need to wear scrubs and mask and/or cap.

Infected Fluid Drainages

Obstructed biliary or urinary tracts may be infected or colonized by bacteria with or without clinical evidence of such infection. This concept also applies to internal fluid collections in proximity to the respiratory, gastrointestinal, and urogenital tracts. Percutaneous drainage of such obstructed fluids by IR procedures is most frequently the preferred technique. Prophylactic antibiotics should be administered (Table 1–2). The procedures are considered "contaminated" or at least "clean-contaminated" (34). Even with antimicrobial protection, patients are still at risk for procedure-induced bacteremia and septic shock. The shock syndrome may be triggered by endotoxin release and not necessarily by overwhelming infection and is therefore unrelated to the immediate effect of bacteriocidal antibiotics (36). If patients develop rigor, 25–50 mg of meperidine intravenously provides an effective countermeasure and can be dosed repeatedly. The interventional radiologist can minimize the risk of seeding endotoxin or bacteria-laden fluid into the bloodstream by inducing the minimal trauma necessary for effective external drainage, by avoiding pressure during contrast opacification, and by postponing a more definitive entry, crossing of the obstruction, introduction of a larger-caliber drain, internal drainage, or other procedure to a later time.

TABLE 1–2
ANTIBIOTIC PROPHYLAXIS FOR INTERVENTIONAL RADIOLOGY PROCEDURES

Vascular Procedures and Biopsies
Patients undergoing sterile vascular procedures do not require prophylactic antibiotics, including those with a history of bacterial endocarditis and prosthetic implants. Strictly adhere to sterile procedure rules.
Exception: Chronic venous catheter implants, catheter introduction through area within 48 hours prior to surgery. Prophylaxis: cefotetan, 2 g IV; start 1 hour before the procedure. (For organ ablation by embolization and chemoembolization, specific procedure protocols apply.)

Biliary and Urinary Drainage Procedures
Antibiotics are administered within the hour before percutaneous biliary, urinary, and other fluid drainages not previously identified as infected (otherwise therapeutic antibiotics should already have been administered). Routine catheter checks during unimpaired drainage and routine catheter exchanges through established tracts do not require such prophylaxis unless the patient is immunocompromised.
Prophylaxis for biliary procedures: Inpatients receive cefoperazone sodium, 2 g IV, or ampicillin, 2 g IV, and gentamicin, 1.5 mg/kg IV. Outpatients receive a single dose of ceftriaxone sodium, 2 g IV. A bile specimen for culture and sensitivity is obtained as soon as the bile ducts are entered.
Prophylaxis for urinary tract procedures: Ampicillin, 2 g IV, and gentamicin, 1.5 mg/kg IV. Patients with limited renal function may receive cefoperazone, 2 g IV. Preferably, urinalysis and urine culture have been performed before the procedure; if not, a urine culture is performed from the first aspirated urine specimen.

Alternative Antibiotic Prophylaxis
Patients allergic to penicillins and cephalosporins receive vancomycin, 1 g IV, and gentamicin, 1.5 mg/kg IV.

INTRAPROCEDURE MANAGEMENT

This section contains general management guidelines that are common to most interventional radiology procedures, both diagnostic and therapeutic. Procedure-specific management is dealt with in individual sections describing those procedures.

In most interventional radiology (IR) procedure rooms, as in operating rooms, endoscopy rooms, and invasive cardiology rooms, a team of physicians, nurses, and technologists works together. Such team efforts, to which every team member contributes specific skills, require coordination by the team leader. In this instance, the interventional radiologist retains the overall responsibility for the care of each patient. Although coordination may be based on mutual understanding and work experience, most hospitals through their accreditation procedures require some written policy on standards of care, credentialing, continued education, conscious sedation, emergency procedures, and quality assurance (37,38). Beyond that it is prudent to compile a laboratory manual that contains current procedure protocols, basic equipment needs, a step-by-step description of infrequently performed procedures, listings of specific precautions, management of complications, and standard dilutions for frequently infused medications such as thrombolytics, vasopressin, and nitroglycerin. Periodic in-service meetings are held to address problems, update protocols, and discuss new ideas and developments in the field, such as those gathered from national meetings. All team members should be certified in basic life support (BLS) and advanced cardiovascular life support (ACLS) with biannual recertification. Occasional emergency preparedness drills are an excellent way to keep the team up to the task. Computer-based simulation of critical events during IR procedures has been developed (39).

Combined efforts among nurses, technologists, and physicians to collect data on quality assurance issues including radiation exposure, duration of procedures, room turnover time, in–out catheter time, total volume of contrast used, as well as complications such as blood loss, hematoma formation, and allergic reactions are most efficient if a computerized format is used, such as the one developed by the Society of Interventional Radiology (40). A computer-based inventory system is also valuable for keeping track of supplies and for facilitating timely restocking (40).

Immediate Preprocedure Assessment

Preparation of patients for procedures performed under conscious sedation requires a problem-focused history and physical exam (H and P). The patients is then classified according to the American Society of Anesthesiologists classification for surgical procedures (41).

Before entering the procedure room, the patient is positively identified and reassessed with regard to change in clinical status and medications taken before arriving in the laboratory, particularly antihypertensive medications, antibiotics, oral hypoglycemic agents, or insulin (see the previous section). An allergy history is confirmed, and compliance with the prescribed allergy preparation is verified. Results of pertinent blood tests are reviewed. The procedure-specific informed consent signed by the patient and witnessed is verified. The site-specific indications for the procedure are also verified independently by at least two members of the team. Examples of this verification include laterality, as in right versus left nephrostomy, iliac carotid versus femoral angioplasty, or upper- versus lower-GI bleeding investigation.

Once the patient enters the IR procedure room, the nurse is usually the first member of the team to assist. His or her posture should be initially geared to lessen the patient's anxiety by providing comfort and compassion. The nurse obtains and records the patient's vital signs. (Periodic monitoring data are added to the written record as well as to the final nursing assessment at the conclusion of the procedure.) The nurse then connects the patient to the monitoring equipment, which includes a pulse oximeter, electrocardiogram (ECG), and blood pressure recorder (Table 1–3). Monitoring devices should be capable of producing a continuously updated digital and analog display as well as hard-copy printout, with the device's display unit clearly visible to the nurse and the physician operator during the procedure. The same unit or an additional console should allow dual-channel pressure recording with hard-copy printout for invasive pressure measurements and should have variable scales for systemic arterial, pulmonary arterial, systemic venous, portal venous, biliary, and urinary tract pressures. Color-coded simultaneous display of at least two pressure tracings is most desirable. The printout copies should display graphics of such scale that pressure differences of <5 mm Hg are readily identifiable and pressure peaks are sharply defined. Monitor readouts are not reliable for defining pressure gradients.

After the patient's baseline vital signs are recorded, an intravenous catheter of preferably 20-gauge caliber is placed into a forearm or antecubital vein to allow rapid intravenous fluid infusion if necessary. This line is kept open by continuous infusion of normal saline, 5% glucose, 5% glucose with one half normal saline solution, or lactated Ringer's

---

TABLE 1–3

AUTOMATED PATIENT MONITORING DURING INTERVENTIONAL RADIOLOGY PROCEDURES

1. Pulse oximetry (with adjustable alarm, e.g., < 92%).
2. ECG (with alarm for bradycardia, tachycardia, arrhythmias).
3. Blood pressure (by cuff, with automatic inflation/deflation cycle and alarm).
4. Have oxygen supply and suction available.

solution as appropriate. An existing peripheral venous access should be used only if it is of sufficient caliber. For elderly male patients, placing a male external catheter is recommended. This catheter allows the patient to void during and immediately after the procedure without invasive catheterization and without the patient being afraid of soiling himself or the surroundings.

Once intravenous access is established, it is appropriate to start intravenous sedation before further patient preparation is performed. With the radiologist's consent, the nurse may give a standard dose of a sedative (see the following section). The initial dose should take into account the patient's height and weight, age (advanced age reduces medication tolerance), respiratory status, cardiac status (arrhythmias including medication-induced bradycardia and limited cardiac output), blood pressure, level of consciousness, narcotic tolerance (patients on chronic narcotic medications or those with current or previous drug dependency may require unusually high doses), and hepatic function (reduced benzodiazepine and narcotics metabolism in patients with decreased liver function). After the initial sedation, the patient is prepared and draped for the procedure, and the radiologist administers local anesthesia by skin infiltration.

Sedation and Pain Control

Although minimally invasive compared with open surgery, IR procedures require percutaneous tracts and cause pain. The extent of manipulation rarely requires general anesthesia in adults; however, some procedures, such as biliary drainage with sizable transhepatic tracts, percutaneous kidney stone extraction, and dilation of biliary and urinary tract strictures, are known to elicit more pain than most patients are able to tolerate under the combination of local anesthesia and neuroleptic sedation and analgesia. Nerve blocks can be employed by those experienced in the technique; otherwise, epidural or general endotracheal anesthesia, administered by anesthesiology, is advisable (41,42). Intraductal lidocaine (1% solution) has been found to reduce pain during biliary duct dilatation (43).

In addition to employing local anesthesia that is always used at the cutaneous entry site and as deep as possible to the intended target (see also the discussion in the "Local Anesthesia" section), IR procedures are typically performed under *conscious sedation*, with exceptions noted above (42). Note that IR procedures in the United States are more likely performed under sedation than those in Europe, according to a European practice survey (44).

Conscious sedation places the patient in a state of diminished apprehension (anxiolysis), of drowsiness with slurred speech but appropriate reaction to verbal stimuli, with eyes open or closed but readily arousable. This state may be categorized as moderate sedation in contrast to light and deep sedation. However, sedation is a continuum, and the individual patient's reaction to medication given to achieve a particular sedation level is highly variable. Therefore, the most important aspect of sedation is continuous monitoring of the patient by a qualified person, usually a nurse who administers medication incrementally as needed (42).

Sedation in most instances is performed with *benzodiazepines* intravenously (Table 1–4). This group of drugs has a dose-related anxiolytic, hypnotic, and amnestic but no analgesic effect. The preferred drug has rapid onset of action and a relatively short biological half-life with minimal or modest cardiorespiratory side effects in effective doses. For this reason, *midazolam* has become the drug of choice by most IR-practices (see also discussion below).

Intravenous analgesia in addition to sedation is desirable in most circumstances. Short-acting *morphine derivatives* are added (Table 1–4). The selection follows the same criteria indicated above. Both medications together have a potentiating effect resulting in deepened sedation with increased risk of respiratory depression. Benzodiazepines are given first, typically before the start of the procedure, and then morphine derivatives are added in increments until a reasonable level of sedation and pain control is achieved. If little pain is expected during the procedure, a benzodiazepine alone may be sufficient.

As a group, benzodiazepines have an excellent sedative effect but differ in potency, duration of action, amnestic effects, and cardiovascular effects. A potent, short-acting, amnestic sedative with relatively mild cardiovascular suppressive effect is midazolam. Agitated patients may benefit from initial intravenous administration of 25–50 mg of diphenhydramine, which has both antihistaminic and mild sedative effects and is generally well tolerated, even by severely debilitated patients. Its administration may reduce the dose of subsequent benzodiazepines and narcotic analgesics. As a matter of general policy, the choice of drugs used should be limited so that the team becomes familiar with the wide variation of response among patients. Although the emphasis in this section is on adult conscious sedation, a suggested approach to the sedation of children is given in Table 1–5.

Blood oxygenation is the key parameter to monitor during conscious sedation (45). A decrease in oxygen saturation because of respiratory depression may trigger carbon dioxide retention, deeper anesthesia, myocardial ischemia, cardiac arrhythmias, and cardiorespiratory arrest. Supplemental oxygen should be immediately available if oxygen saturation drops to the low 90% levels (Table 1–6). Encouraging the patient to take deeper breaths may be all that is needed in many situations. Oxygen saturation levels in patients with chronic lung disease may read below 90% at baseline. Nasal oxygen should be withheld unless the saturation drops further.

With adequate monitoring and incremental dosing of medications, unexpected respiratory depression and cardiovascular effects should be minimal. Once an adequate level of sedation and pain control is achieved, supplemental

TABLE 1–4

SEDATIVES AND ANALGESICS FOR INTERVENTIONAL RADIOLOGY PROCEDURES IN ADULTS

Agents	Initial Intravenous Dose	Total Dose*	Onset	Duration	Comments
Benzodiazepines					
Midazolam	0.5–2.0 mg	0.035–0.150 mg/kg	2 min	1–2 hr	Good amnestic agent, potent, short-acting.
Diazepam	1–5 mg	10–25 mg	2–3 min	6–24 hr	Delayed sedation from metabolites; do not give intramuscularly.
Lorazepam	0.5–2.0 mg	2–4 mg	10–20 min	6–16 hr	Best amnestic agent.
Flumazenil (antagonist)	0.2 mg over 15 sec	3 mg	15–60 sec	20–60 min	Resedation may occur due to short half-life. Repeat dose; monitor closely. If patient is a chronic benzodiazepine user, seizures may occur. Titrate dose.
Narcotic analgesics					
Fentanyl	25–100 μg	1–3 μg/kg	2 min	30–60 min	Minimal cardiovascular effects; chest wall rigidity, if given rapidly.
Morphine	1–5 mg	0.05–0.20 mg/kg	5–10 min	3–4 hr	May cause histamine release and/or a rise in common bile duct pressure.
Meperidine	12.5–50.0	0.5–1.0 mg/kg	3–5 min	2–4 hr	Less effect on common bile duct pressure.
Naloxone (antagonist)	0.1–0.4 mg	Repeat dose in 1–2 min if no response	1–2 min	20–30 min	May need to repeat effective dose every 20 minutes; can precipitate pulmonary edema in higher doses.

*Dose may need to be reduced in elderly or frail patients and in patients with renal or hepatic insufficiency.

doses may be given every 15 minutes after the patient's level of consciousness has been assessed. Timing of drug dosing becomes critical toward the end of the procedure because the lack of pain stimulus may lead to deeper than anticipated sedation. Postprocedure monitoring is therefore important until the patient's level of consciousness has returned to baseline condition. In addition to monitoring the patient's vital signs, the nurse establishes verbal contact with the patient at least every 10 minutes. The nurse also routinely communicates with the physician during the procedure about the patient's clinical status. The interventional radiologist needs to keep the nurse informed about the need for additional analgesics if a period of increased pain is anticipated, such as access tract dilatation, subcutaneous tunneling, catheter manipulation inside the peritoneal cavity, embolization-induced ischemia, and so on.

Patients who descend into deep sedation or respiratory depression and fail to respond to verbal stimuli may need *reversal agents* (Table 1–4). These agents rapidly reverse the effects of benzodiazepines or narcotic analgesics, respectively, but may lead to acute anxiety and pain attacks as well as to withdrawal symptoms in patients with a history of substance abuse. Therefore, overdosing is to be reduced

TABLE 1–5

SEDATION OF EUVOLEMIC CHILDREN WITHOUT CARDIOPULMONARY DISEASE

Sedative	Route	Initial Dose
Chloral hydrate with diphen- hydramine	PO	50–75 mg/kg with 1 mg/kg
Benzodiazepines Midazolam Diazepam	IV (IM) IV only	0.01–0.03 mg/kg 0.1–0.2 mg/kg
Narcotic analgesics Fentanyl Morphine	IV IV (IM)	2–5 μg/kg 0.05–0.10 mg/kg

Barbiturates, ketamine, and propofol reserved for application and monitoring by anesthesiology (21).

TABLE 1–6

OXYGEN THERAPY (APPROXIMATE PERCENTAGE OF OXYGEN IN INSPIRATORY AIR)

By Nasal Cannula		By Mask	
1 liter	24%	5–6 liters	40%
2 liters	28%	6–7 liters	50%
3 liters	32%	7–8 liters	60%
4 liters	36%		
5 liters	40%		
6 liters	44%		

by following the recommended levels (Table 1–4). Reversal agents (antagonists) are also shorter acting than their respective agonists and may need to be repeated. Therefore, very close monitoring is required (42). For ease of communication between the IR nurse and the receiving counterpart on the floor, the Ramsey scale that categorizes the degree of sedation is helpful (42).

It is important to account for postpullout vascular compression or application of closure devices. Femoral artery compression can be a particularly painful experience for an exhausted patient. It is also important to realize that a full bladder can make femoral compression even more painful and is also a potent hypertensive stimulus that should always be considered if the patient's blood pressure keeps rising. If the patient is unable to void spontaneously in the recumbent position, catheter drainage should be provided. This can be done expeditiously with a straight in-and-out catheter. The advantage of fitting particularly elderly male patients with a male external catheter prior to the procedure has been explained earlier.

Nausea may complicate sedation and analgesia, particularly if the patient had food intake within the 6-hour minimum fasting period for solid food or 2-hour period for clear liquids. Nausea may also be triggered by contrast injection, chemoembolization, or pain. Suction equipment should be readily available (46). Potent antiemetics can be administered intravenously, but all of them enhance sedation (Table 1–7). Also see Table 1–7 for other side effects.

Children require sedation for virtually all IR procedures. Those who rarely perform IR procedures in children are advised to seek assistance from pediatric intensivists or anesthesiologists. For a busy pediatric service, the Boston Children's Hospital regimen is readily applicable (47).

Local Anesthesia

In addition to intravenous sedation and analgesia, local anesthesia is provided at the intended needle and catheter entry site. For vascular procedures, it is desirable to place anesthesia on both sides of the entry vessel to reduce vasospasm. If the catheter is to traverse the parietal peritoneum or the pleura, local anesthesia of that surface should be attempted with a small-caliber needle.

Frequently, patients experience an initial burning sensation when the local anesthetic is infiltrated into the skin. This burning can be reduced by neutralizing the acidic anesthesia compound by mixing 10 mL of 1% lidocaine with 1 mL of 8.4% sodium bicarbonate immediately before use (48). The amount of the diluted agent has to be increased proportionally. Occasionally a patient is allergic to a local anesthetic. If the allergenic agent belongs to the chemical group of esters, it can be substituted with an agent from the amide group or vice versa (Table 1–8). In addition, the rare allergy to solution preservatives (e.g., methylparaben) may occur, in which instance preservative-free preparations should be substituted.

It is critical to note that local anesthetics have different potencies and thresholds for central nervous system toxicity (Table 1–8). Similarly, agents with lower toxicity thresholds increase the risk of hypoxia during sedation (42).

Supplemental injections of a local anesthetic should be considered if the catheterization time exceeds 60 minutes, particularly if catheter exchanges are undertaken without protection by an introducer sheath. The effect of lidocaine can be extended for approximately 1 hour to 2–3 hours with the addition of epinephrine (42). This addition is not advised in patients who have significant ischemic heart disease and is typically applied to skin incisions for port pockets. At times, biliary or nephrostomy tube tracts remain

TABLE 1–7

ANTIEMETICS FOR INTERVENTIONAL RADIOLOGY PROCEDURES

Agent*	Single Intravenous Dose	Total Dose	Onset (min)	Duration (hr)	Comments
Metoclopramide	10 mg	0.5–1.0 mg/kg	1–3	1–2	Stimulates upper GI tract motility.
Prochlorperazine	2.5–10.0 mg	10 mg	10–20	4–6	Use a lower dose for elderly patients.
Promethazine	12.5–25.0 mg	25 mg	10–20	4–6	Enhances central nervous system depressant effect of narcotics and benzodiazepines; extravasation can cause tissue necrosis.
Droperidol	0.625–1.250 mg	Higher doses for sedative effect	10–15	4–6	Higher doses may cause dysphoria; potent antiemetic at low doses.
Ondansetron	10 mg over 15 min	0.15 mg/kg	<30	4–6	Very effective; use for chemoembolization; may be combined with dexamethasone (20 mg IV) once.

*All can cause extrapyramidal side effects.

TABLE 1–8
LOCAL ANESTHETICS

Drug	Chemical Group	Relative Potency	CNS Toxicity Threshold (mg/kg)
Procaine	Ester	1	19.2
Chloroprocaine	Ester	1	12.8
Lidocaine	Amide	2	6.4
Mepivacaine	Amide	2	9.8
Etidocaine	Amide	6	3.4
Bupivacaine	Amide	8	1.6
Tetracaine	Ester	8	2.5

Note: When substituting amides for esters or vice versa in allergic patients, also consider preservative-free preparations, since an allergy may exist to the preservative of the individual preparation.

very painful after the procedure. Relief can be provided by local infiltration with a long-acting local anesthetic such as bupivacaine (Table 1–8).

In the special circumstance of chemoembolization, the use of intra-arterial lidocaine (30 mg) immediately before the embolization can significantly reduce the pain associated with the postinfarction syndrome (49).

Fluid Balance

While the patient is under sedation, fluid requirements are assessed. Patients undergoing procedures early in the morning often have a low fluid balance from overnight fasting. Crystalloid infusion of 200–300 mL in the first hour may be required to maintain adequate renal tubular function during contrast injection. A hypotensive reaction with tachycardia early after routine sedation can be corrected by rapid saline infusion in many instances. For patients with reduced renal tubular function, hydration becomes even more critical. Patients undergoing visceral arteriography; visceral artery, bronchial artery, and neuroembolization procedures; and pulmonary arteriography

are likely to receive large amounts of intravascular contrast that challenge renal tolerance.

Adjustment of Blood Pressure, Heart Rate, Renal Function, and Blood Sugar Levels

Hypertensive Reactions

Many patients undergoing IR procedures have hypertension. They should be advised to take their usual dose of antihypertensive medication before most IR procedures. Preprocedure anxiety often increases the blood pressure further (50), and sedation helps suppress that stimulus (51). Therefore, the administration of additional antihypertensive medication should be delayed until the effect of sedation is established. Antihypertensive medication taken by the patient before the procedure may not have reached its peak effect; this, compounded by anxiety, may make the patient's blood pressure appear to be out of control. Before resorting to antihypertensive mediation, adequate pain control is provided, and bladder distention is ruled out (Table 1–9). As initial medication for hypertension, or if the patient has a history of or develops angina, a 1- to 2-inch nitroglycerin patch (Nitropaste) is applied to the chest or shoulder. The second choice or an alternative to the patch is labetalol given intravenously (Table 1–9). Hydralazine is less preferable because of the greater number of side effects. Nitroprusside needs to be carefully titrated with continuous blood pressure monitoring. Toxic effects are a risk, and nitroprusside is not a frontline medication in the IR lab. Intravenous antihypertensive medication should be administered by the radiologist only if he or she has experience in its use because blood pressure changes may be precipitous unless the doses are carefully titrated (41,51). Otherwise, emergency consultation with cardiology or critical care medicine should be undertaken. It is always best to become familiar with the use of a few effective drugs given the variation in patient response.

A hypertensive crisis triggered by selective arteriography for the localization of a pheochromocytoma is probably

TABLE 1–9
TREATMENT OF HYPERTENSIVE CRISIS (NOT SECONDARY TO PHEOCHROMOCYTOMA)

1. Reduce pain, anxiety.
2. Empty bladder.
3. Nifedipine 10 mg PO q30 min; adjust to effect (pierce capsule, have patient swallow it) in older patients; give 5 mg PO and repeat q15 min, if necessary.
4. Nitropaste 1–2 inches on shoulder or chest.
5. Labetalol 0.2 mg/kg IV over 2 min, 40–80 mg repeat injection every 10 min up to desired effect, maximum dose 300 mg. Maximum effect 5 min after injection (can worsen congestive heart failure, possible hepatotoxicity).
6. Hydralazine 10–20 mg IV (can cause hypotension and reflex tachycardia).
7. Nitroprusside IV, 5–10 mg/min initially, titrate (monitor blood pressure via arterial line).

no longer encountered because of the availability of other diagnostic tests. Those arteriograms were always performed with phentolamine available as an adrenergic blocker (41).

Hypotensive Reactions

Hypotensive reactions during IR procedures are most likely the result of oversedation, vasovagal reaction, or blood loss. Hypotension on the basis of septic shock is rarely encountered during or immediately after an IR procedure; however, the prodromes of chills and fever are. These prodromes should be regarded as an indication for treatment with intravenous antibiotics (Table 1–2) and fluids. Meperidine (25–50 mg intravenously) can be administered to temporarily suppress chills and rigor.

Hypotension on the basis of oversedation is usually the result of cardiorespiratory depression. Nasal oxygen, intravenous fluids, and a narcotic or sedative antagonist (Table 1–4) should be given.

Bradycardic hypotension in connection with a vasovagal reaction should be readily recognizable; nausea may be a precursor. Atropine and fluids are the established countermeasures. The atropine dose should be at least 0.6 mg because lower doses may aggravate bradycardia. If hypotension remains unresponsive to atropine and a fluid challenge, dopamine (2–5 micrograms per kilogram per minute via large peripheral veins or preferably a central venous catheter) is started. The dopamine dose is titrated to the desired pressor effect. Above 10 micrograms per kilogram per minute, significant renal, peripheral, and mesenteric vasoconstriction occurs. Peripheral venous infusion of dopamine entails the risk of skin necrosis upon extravasation.

Hypotension secondary to volume loss is usually secondary to bleeding from the vascular entry site or from deep-seated organs such as the kidneys during nephrostomies or the liver during biliary drainage procedures. Frequently, these bleeding sources can be tamponaded by the insertion of a larger-caliber sheath or catheter after pullout of the arterial catheter or by appropriate manual compression. Rapid crystalloid infusion is indicated, and the patient should be typed and cross-matched for blood transfusion (51).

Heparin Reversal

If the patient is anticoagulated with heparin, the effect can be reversed promptly with protamine sulfate (1 mg for each 90 units of heparin). Protamine should be given slowly at a rate of 2 mg per minute intravenously to avoid a hypotensive reaction. Because excess protamine acts as an anticoagulant, the dose should be carefully titrated. The half-life of heparin depends on the dose administered and should average 30–60 minutes for doses customarily administered (3,000–5,000 units as bolus) during IR procedures (52). Protamine can also cause anaphylactoid reactions, particularly in insulin-dependent diabetics (53). Patients undergoing

IR procedures with a high potential for bleeding (e.g., transluminal angioplasty with large introducer sheaths, large-bore nephrostomy, and stone retrieval procedures) should be typed and cross-matched for two units of packed red blood cells before the procedure.

Arrhythmias

Sustained ventricular ectopy, new-onset supraventricular tachycardia, symptomatic sinus bradycardia, heart block, and ventricular tachycardia require immediate management (Table 1–10). A detailed description of treating cardiac emergencies is beyond the scope of this chapter. If a situation arises that is not generally dealt with in the IR laboratory, help should be called as soon as possible. Cardiac lifesaving measures are well established (54). Each hospital has a resuscitation team ("code team"). This team should be called as soon as tachyarrhythmias are observed that are unrelieved by initial therapy (Table 1–10). While the interventional team is waiting for the code team, and if the patient becomes pulseless and stops breathing, the IR team should be ready to start assisted ventilation, apply chest compressions, and maintain an airway. The interventional radiologist and nurse are certified in ACLS (see above). Early initiation of treatment to correct a dysrhythmia is crucial (55). The radiologist may apply defibrillation as soon as ventricular fibrillation is seen on the monitor (Table 1–10).

An adequate supply of emergency medication in the IR laboratory is essential and should be kept up to date by the IR nurse (Table 1–11). The IR lab should have a crash cart that is checked daily, and the defibrillator batteries must be kept charged. Because virtually all emergency drugs are administered intravenously, the importance of a large-caliber venous access becomes obvious. The arterial catheter should not be forgotten for emergency fluid administration or for continuous blood pressure monitoring.

Hypoglycemic Reactions

Oral hypoglycemic agents and insulin may induce hypoglycemia in diabetic patients. Oral agents of the sulfonylurea group (e.g., tolbutamide) are subject to potentiating effects by aspirin, certain other nonsteroidal anti-inflammatory drugs, Coumadin, and sulfonamide, which deepen and prolong hypoglycemia. This potential problem should be apparent from the patient's medication record. Dose reduction for insulin in preparation for an IR procedure is discussed earlier in the chapter. A prudent measure is to determine any diabetic patient's blood glucose levels before and at regular intervals during the procedure. If the blood sugar level falls below normal (≤80–100 mg/100 mL) while the patient remains alert, oral glucose or sugar-containing liquids (orange juice) should be given, with continued close monitoring

TABLE 1–10

DRUG TREATMENT OF CARDIAC ARRYTHMIAS

Symptoms	Medication	Dose	Dose Frequency	Maximum Dosage	Comments
Symptomatic sinus brady-cardia	Atropine	0.6–1.0 mg IV	5-min intervals	2 mg IV	Doses smaller than 0.5 mg may cause a paradoxical bradycardia and lead to ventricular fibrillation; demand pacemaker for refractory bradycardia.
Supraventricular tachycardia[a]	Adenosine	6-mg rapid IV bolus; if no response, repeat	1–2 min	12-mg IV bolus	
	Verapamil	0.1 mg/kg IV slowly (maximum of 10 mg)	0.15 mg/kg IV slowly 30 min after first dose	20 mg IV	Use is contraindicated in patients on β blockers; can be used with patients receiving digitalis.
Ventricular tachyarrythmia[a]	Lidocaine	1-mg/kg bolus IV	Repeat 0.5 mg/kg IV every 8–10 min	3-mg/kg total bolus dose	Once arrhythmia is controlled, continuous infusion of lidocaine at 2–4 mg/min; if circulatory arrest occurs, call code team and defibrillate.
Ventricular fibrillation	Defibrillate: start with 200 joules, then follow ACLS[b] protocol (this treatment should only be administered by ACLS-certified interventional radiologists).				

[a]Consider cardioversion.
[b]ACLS = advanced cardiac life support.

of glucose levels. If the patient's mental function is impaired (confusion, stupor or tremors, seizures), 50 mL of 50% dextrose is injected intravenously, followed by infusion of 5–10% dextrose; blood glucose levels are adjusted to more than 150 mg/100 mL. The administration of high-osmolarity glucose can easily damage a small-caliber vein, a problem that, again, can be reduced by a larger-caliber venous access. Because mental impairment in the early stages of hypoglycemia is masked by intravenous sedation, infusion of 10% dextrose may be instituted even at normal to low-normal blood glucose levels.

Protection of Renal Function

See also the previous section for pre- and postprocedure hydration. Euvolemic patients with normal renal function should be able to tolerate intravascular contrast volumes as needed for virtually all IR procedures. The author limits the contrast dose for a single procedure to 5 mg/kg with a maximum of 300 mL of a 60% contrast solution and uses only isosmolar contrast for all imaging studies as well as dilute, minimally hyperosmolar nonionic contrast for test injections. Patients with impaired renal function (creatinine ≥ 1.5 mg/dL) are at increased risk for contrast-induced nephrotoxicity. Older age is an additional independent risk factor, but Diabetes Mellitus with proven normal renal function is not. However, with the high incidence of diabetic nephropathy at a stage where it has not given rise to serum creatinine, it is wise to regard all patients with known diabetes as potential contrast risks.

Although carbon dioxide can be substituted for ionic contrast for certain diagnostic arteriograms, particularly in the extremities, this contrast agent does not appear practical for many IR procedures. Gadolinium (Gd) compounds are also considered safer than iodinated contrast; however, they provide poor fluoroscopic and radiographic opacification, and the quantities required in most IR procedures exceed the limits currently allowed for MRI studies. There is no safety profile established for higher doses of Gd compounds.

Patients on dialysis should receive contrast soon after or immediately before hemodialysis. In the first instance, patients are best able to tolerate the contrast-induced increased intravascular volume; in the latter instance, the volume overload is immediately corrected. There is no need, however, to provide dialysis specifically to remove contrast.

Management of Anaphylactoid Reactions

Allergic or anaphylactoid reactions are encountered most frequently after intravascular contrast administration and are not unique to IR procedures. Such reactions are more likely to occur in patients who have an allergic diathesis (bronchial asthma) and are typically unpredictable in their severity. What starts out as hives may progress to laryngeal

TABLE 1–11
SUGGESTED EMERGENCY DRUGS AND EQUIPMENT FOR ADULTS (INDIVIDUAL NEEDS MAY VARY)

Drugs	Equipment
Adenosine	Intravenous access and infusion sets,
Albuterol (by	including 22-, 20-, 18-, and 16-gauge
inhalation)	IV catheters
Aminophylline	Intravenous fluids: lactated Ringer's
Ammonia spirits	solution, normal saline
Atropine	Defribrillator
Diazepam	Face masks (small, medium, large),
Digitalis	breathing bag and valve set
Diphenhydramine	Nasal airways (small, medium, large)
Dopamine	Laryngoscope handles
Epinephrine	Laryngoscope blades (straight, curved)
(1:1000, 1:10,000)	Endotracheal tubes and stylets (cuffed
Flumazenil	and uncuffed)
Glucose (50% bolus,	Suction catheters
10% infusion)	Nasogastric tubes
Hydrocortisone	Nebulizer with medication kits
Labetalol	Wall suction
Lidocaine (cardiac)	Nasal cannulas
Naloxone	
Nifedipine	
Nitroglycerin	
(sublingual spray)	
Oxygen	
Phentolamine	
Sodium bicarbonate	
Verapamil	

edema and cardiopulmonary arrest. However, most allergic reactions are limited to urticaria and are typically treated with 50 mg of diphenhydramine intravenously as soon as itching or the first urticaria is noted, typically in the face

and neck area. Various guidelines have been issued for treating allergic reactions, and any of these can be posted in the laboratory or contained in the laboratory manual. Table 1–12 gives a sample regimen.

POSTINTERVENTION CARE

This brief review of postprocedure care is intended to lay down the essentials. Procedure-specific requirements are dealt with in the individual chapters. The idea of the interventional radiologist functioning as a clinical consultant cannot be overemphasized as basis for all of his or her involvement in the care of patients.

Postprocedure Routine for Inpatients and Outpatients

After the interventional radiology (IR) procedure is completed, the patient's monitoring records and the timed and dated medication orders are signed by the interventional radiologist. An entry into the patient's record briefly describes the type and results of the procedure, the amount of contrast used, the medications administered, the body fluids removed, blood loss, complications, and any recommendations for observation and treatment. Verbal instructions may be given to the patient, depending on his or her level of alertness. Verbal instructions are always in addition to, not in lieu of, written postprocedure instructions. For outpatients, the written instructions include a plan for postprocedure care, emergency phone numbers, and a follow-up appointment, if applicable (Figure 1–1). Follow-up by the interventional radiologist is particularly important for angioplasties, transjugular intrahepatic portosystemic shunting (TIPS),

TABLE 1–12
TREATMENT OF ANAPHYLACTIC REACTIONS

Symptom	Drug	Initial Dose	Dose Frequency	Comments
Urticaria	Diphenhydramine	25–50 mg IV	May repeat once	Treat if symptomatic or progressive.
Angioneurotic edema	Diphenhydramine or hydroxyzine	25–50 mg IM	May repeat once	For symptomatic subcutaneous angioedema.
	Epinephrine	0.3 mg SC or IM	Repeat every 10 min as needed	For mucocutaneous swelling or airway compromise.
Bronchospasm	Albuterol	2.5 mg inhaled over 5–15 min		
	Aminophylline	6 mg/kg IV over 20 min	Maintenance, 0.6 mg/kg/hr IV	For suboptimal response or recurrent symptoms after epinephrine. Reduce maintenance dose by ½ in cardiac-risk and debilitated patients.
	Epinephrine	0.3 mg SC or IM	As above	May induce angina in patients with coronary artery disease.
Laryngospasm	Epinephrine	0.3 mg SC or IM	As above	For severe reaction, give 0.5 mL of 1:1000 diluted in 10 mL of normal saline IV slowly; call code team.

To perform your . . . . procedure, it was necessary to puncture a major artery/vein. To prevent complications, the following precautions are recommended:

- Do not drive for at least 12 hours. If walking is necessary, walk slowly.

- Return home and relax on the bed or couch for the rest of the day.

- If possible, arrange for someone to stay with you.

- Avoid any strenuous activity such as bending over, long walks, stair climbing, housework, or lifting heavy objects.

- You may return to work the day after your procedure, if your job is sedentary. Do not perform rigorous or heavy physical activity for 3 days.

- The bandage covering the vessel entry site may be removed in one day. To keep the puncture site dry, wait until the bandage is removed to shower or bathe. If the bandage becomes wet or soiled, it should be changed.

- You may eat and take your medications as usual. Fluid intake is encouraged unless you have been advised otherwise.

- The puncture site may be sore, but if pain develops at the puncture site, observe the site for bleeding or swelling. Should bleeding develop, lie flat and apply *firm pressure* to the area for 10 to 15 minutes without interruption. Have someone contact us at the number below if bleeding occurs.

- If pain develops in the extremity of the vessel entered, inspect the extremity for change in color, coolness, or decreased sensation. Should these symptoms be present, contact us immediately at the number below.

- Contact us or your doctor if you develop fever, chills, or vomiting within 48 hours, or if you have any questions.

If you have problems or questions call: _____
Person or Institution

at _____ between _____
Tel   hours Mon-Friday, Sat/Sun or after _____ call _____
                                                          hour

_____   _____
PATIENT SIGNATURE   RADIOLOGY STAFF SIGNATURE

_____
DATE

Figure 1–1 Discharge instructions for outpatient vascular procedures.

control venous access catheters, and long-term drainage catheter placements. Besides being good medical practice, follow-up provides essential information for any outcome assessment (56).

The IR nurse communicates with his or her counterpart on the inpatient service or the nurse taking care of the outpatient in recovery unless the IR laboratory is equipped and staffed with its own postprocedure outpatient recovery unit (57). In that area, monitoring continues until the patient is able to ambulate and is ready to be discharged. It is wise to leave the intravenous access line in place until the patient ambulates because postural hypotension is not unusual after intravenous sedation and hours of recumbency. Rapid fluid infusion will help to correct this condition. Evaluation of the vascular entry site for hematoma formation is always included in the postangiogram follow-up, as are frequent peripheral pulse checks. The patient is given a written sheet of postprocedure instructions (Figure 1–1). The nurse should review that information with the patient before discharge and have the patient sign the paper, with a copy to be kept in the medical record.

Intermediate and Long-Term Follow-up

Depending on the type of IR procedure, the follow-up may involve days to years. IR procedures with a short follow-up period of 1 day–1 week are typically needle biopsies, needle aspiration of fluid, collections, inferior vena cava filter placements, foreign-body removals, embolization for acute bleeding, vasopressin infusion, and all procedures in which another clinical service typically provides most of the procedure-related follow-up as an integral part of its routine (e.g., urinary tract stone removal, central venous access catheters and ports). Some referring physicians insist on providing routine follow-up themselves and refer to the interventional radiologist only if problems arise.

Procedures requiring extended follow-up are transluminal angioplasties, TIPS, internal and external biliary drainages, nephrostomies, abscess drainages, and tumor embolizations. Biliary, urinary, and abscess drainage must be monitored, and the drainage catheters should be flushed periodically. Unless a team approach exists between interventional radiologist and clinical staff, the radiologist should perform his or her own follow-up on these patients

Clean the tube (catheter) insertion site with soap and water every 24 to 48 hours or whenever the dressing becomes wet or soiled. (Wash hands before and after handling the tube.) Dry the insertion site carefully. You may leave the insertion site open to air or apply a light dressing. Do not use a tight, occlusive dressing because moisture will accumulate and increase the risk of infection.

Avoid baths, but you may shower.

If you experience discomfort at the insertion site, you may take Tylenol, 1 to 2 tablets every 4 to 6 hours.

If you develop any of the following symptoms, notify your physician or present to an emergency department immediately.
  1. Drainage emerging around the tube.
  2. Pain and/or swelling at the insertion site, bleeding from the tube or at the insertion site, dizziness, fainting, weakness, or a rapid pulse (greater than 100 beats per minute).
  3. Fever or chills.
  4. Lack of drainage from the tube.
Drainage catheters require periodic exchange by the interventional radiologist who placed the tube. Your next catheter exchange needs to be done before _____. Please call our number below about 10 days before that date for an appointment. After the drainage tube exchange, you should resume caring for the tube as previously instructed, unless redirected by the radiologist.

If you require sedation for the tube change, you may not drive or operate heavy machinery for at least 12 hours after the procedure. You will need to arrange for transportation home.

If you have problems or questions call: _____
Person or Institution

at _____ between _____
Tel   hours Mon-Friday, Sat/Sun or after _____ call _____
hour

_____   _____
PATIENT SIGNATURE   RADIOLOGY STAFF SIGNATURE

_____
DATE

Figure 1–2 Ambulatory care and precautions for patients with percutaneous drainage catheters.

and communicate directly with the referring physician on the results, both verbally and in writing (58).

Some controversies exist about the need to provide antibiotic prophylaxis each time manipulation and exchanges of chronic catheters such as a biliary or urinary tract drainage catheter are performed. Once a tract is mature, the manipulation per se is not an indication for antibiotic prophylaxis. However, each time drainage is impaired, the fluid is considered infected, and the pressure exerted by contrast injection alone can lead to bacteremia. Therefore, appropriate antibiotics are administered intravenously before the procedure (Table 1–2).

The main aim of routine follow-up for patients with chronic drainage catheters is to avoid obstructive complications and sepsis. Because the interval for which a patient may maintain adequate patency of a drainage catheter varies considerably, initial follow-ups are made at relatively short intervals (3–4 weeks) until a patient's individual tolerance is established. Although some patients with nephrostomy tubes may go unobstructed for 6 months, most nephrostomy and biliary drainage catheters require exchange at least every 3 months. The patient should receive written instructions about catheter care, precautions, warning signs of complications (Figure 1–2), and a phone number to call if a problem arises.

After transluminal angioplasty and TIPS procedures, patients are followed at 3-month intervals up to a year, and thereafter semiannually or annually. The frequent initial follow-up is maintained to cover the critical time of the reaction of the vascular or stent wall to the transluminal procedure and potential restenosis or shunt stenosis. Ankle-to-brachial blood pressure comparison and duplex ultrasound are often valuable for qualitative and quantitative assessment of functional impairment before symptoms reappear.

REFERENCES

1. National Digestive Diseases Advisory Board. Role of transjugular intrahepatic portal systemic shunt (TIPS) in therapy of portal hypertension. Workshop, Feb. 28–March 1, 1994, Bethesda, MD.
2. Andrews ET, Spies JB, Sacks D, et al. Patient care and uterine artery embolization for leiomyomata. J Vasc Interv Radiol 2004;15:115–120.
3. Krijnen P, vanJaarsveld BC, Deinum J, et al. Which patients with hypertension and atherosclerotic renal artery stenosis benefit from immediate intervention? J Hum Hypertens 2004;18:91–96.
4. Grenacher L, Saam T, Geier A, et al. PTA versus Palmaz stent placement in femoropopliteal artery stenoses: results of a multicenter prospective randomized study (REFSA). Rofo 2004;176:1302–1310.
5. Ramsey DE, Kernagis LY, Soulen MC, et al. Chemoembolization of hepatocellular carcinoma. J Vasc Interv Radiol 2002;13:S211–S221.

6. Becker GJ. 2000 RSNA annual oration in diagnostic radiology: the future of interventional radiology. Radiology 2001;220:281–292.

7. Katzen BT, Kaplan JO, Dake MD. Developing an interventional radiology practice in a community hospital: the interventional radiologist as an equal partner in patient care. Radiology 1989; 170:955–958.

8. Arnold TE, Karabinis VD, Mehta V, et al. Potential of overuse of the inferior vena cava filter. Gynecol Obstet 1993;177:463–467.

9. Tunis SR, Bass EB, Steinberg EP. The use of angioplasty, bypass surgery, and amputation in the management of peripheral vascular disease. N Engl J Med 1991;325:556–562.

10. Pentecost MJ. Graduate medical education in radiology: a proposal for subspecialty training during residency. Acad Radiol 1995;2:816–819.

11. White RI, Denny DF, Osterman FA, et al. Logistics of a university interventional radiology practice. Radiology 1989;170:951–954.

12. Williams GM. Who should blow up balloons in arteries? Radiology 1988;169:857.

13. White RA. Endovascular credentialing. Endovascular Surgery Credentialing and Training Subcommittee. J Vasc Interv Radiol 1995;6:287–289.

14. Green RM. Collaboration between vascular surgeons and interventional radiologists: reflections after two years. J Vasc Surgery 2000;31: 826–830.

15. Karamlou T, Landry G, Sexton G, et al. Creating a useful vascular center: a statewide survey of what primary care physicians really want. J Vasc Surg 2004;39:763–770.

16. Siskin GP, Bagla S, Sansivero GE, et al. The interventional radiology clinic: key ingredients for success. J Vasc Interv Radiol 2004; 15:681–688.

17. Reuter SR. An overview of informed consent for radiologists. AJR Am J Roentgenol 1987;148:219–227.

18. Morris KJ, Tarico VS, Smith WL, et al. Critical analysis of radiologist–patient interaction. Radiology 1987;163:565–567.

19. Benotch EG, Lutgendorf SK, Watson D, et al. Rapid anxiety assessment in medical patients: evidence for the validity of verbal anxiety ratings. Ann Behav Med 2000;22:199–203.

20. Sterner G, Nyman U, Valdes T. Low risk of contrast-medium-induced nephropathy with modern angiographic technique. J Intern Med 2001;250:429–424.

21. Aspelin P, Aubry P, Fransson SG, et al. Nephrotoxic effects in high-risk patients undergoing angiography. N Engl J Med 2003; 348:491–499.

22. Bader BD, Berger ED, Siberbaur I, et al. What is the best hydration regimen to prevent contrast media induced nephrotoxicity? Clin Nephrol 2004;62:1–7.

23. Walker PD, Brokering KL, Theobald JC. Fenoldopam and N-acetylcysteine for the prevention of radiographic contrast material-induced nephropathy: a review. Pharmacotherapy 2003;23: 1617–1626.

24. Merten GJ, Burgess WP, Gray LV, et al. Prevention of contrast-induced nephropathy with sodium bicarbonate: a randomized controlled trial. JAMA 2004;291:2328–2334.

25. Spies JB, Rosen RJ, Lebowitz AS. Antibiotic prophylaxis in vascular and interventional radiology: a rational approach. Radiology 1988;166:381–387.

26. Stone HH. Basic principles in the use of prophylactic antibiotics. J Antimicrob Chemother 1984;14(Suppl B):33–37.

27. Platt R, Zaleznik DF, Hopkins EP, et al. Perioperative antibiotic prophylaxis for herniorrhaphy and breast surgery. N Engl J Med 1990;322:153–156.

28. Bergquist EJ, Murphey SA. Prophylactic antibiotics for surgery. Med Clin North Am 1987;71:357–368.

29. DiPiro JT, Cheung RPF, Bowden TA, Mansberger JA. Single dose systemic antibiotic prophylaxis of surgical wound infections. Am J Surg 1986;152:552–559.

30. vanSonnenberg E, Varney RR, Casola G. Antibiotic commentary. Radiology 1988;166:901–902.

31. Grossmann W, Baim DS. Cardiac Catheterization, Angiography and Intervention. 4th Ed. Philadelphia: Lea & Febiger, 1991.

32. Greenberg PA, Patterson R. The prevention of immediate generalized reactions to radiocontrast media in high-risk patients. J Allergy Clin Immunol 1991;87:867–872.

33. Kelly JF, Patterson R, Lieberman P, et al. Radiographic contrast media studies in high-risk patients. J Allergy Clin Immunol 1978;62:181–184.

34. King J, Rothenberger KH, Clauss W. Prevention of anaphylactoid reactions after radiographic contrast media infusion by combined histamine H_1 and H_2 receptor antagonists: results in a prospective, controlled trial. Int Arch Allergy Appl Immunol 1985;78:9–14.

35. Bettman MA. Guidelines for use of low osmolality contrast agents. Radiology 1989;17:901–903.

36. Cronan JJ, Horn DL, Marchello A, et al. Antibiotics and nephrostomy tube care: preliminary observations: II. Bacteremia. Radiology 1989;172:1043–1045.

37. Spies JB, Bakal CW, Burke DR, et al. Standards for interventional radiology. Standards of Practice Committee of the Society of Cardiovascular and Interventional Radiology. J Vasc Interv Radiol 1991;2:59–65.

38. Chopra PS, Kandarpa K, Harrington DP. Quality assurance in cardiovascular and interventional radiology. Crit Rev Diagn Imaging 1992;33:183–200.

39. Medina LS, Racaido JM, Schwid HA. Computers in radiology. The sedation, analgesia, and contrast media computerized simulator: a new approach to train and evaluate radiologists' responses to critical incidents. Pediatr Radiol 2000;30: 200–303.

40. Rholl K, Electronic Data Base Committee. HI-IQ 20 Health Information and Inventory for Quality Control. Fairfax: Society of Cardiovascular and Interventional Radiology, 1995.

41. Barth KH, Matsumoto AH. Patient care in interventional radiology: a perspective. Radiology 1991;178:11–17.

42. Martin ML, Lennox PH. Sedation and analgesia in the interventional radiology department. J Vasc Interv Radiol 2003; 14:1119–1128.

43. Cheng YF, Chen TY, Ko SF, et al. Treatment of postoperative residual hepatolithiasis after progressive stenting of associated bile duct strictures through the T-tube tract. Cardiovasc Intervent Radiol 1995;18:77–81.

44. Haslam PJ, Yap B, Mueller PR, et al. Anesthesia practice and clinical trends in interventional radiology: a European survey. Cardiovasc Intervent Radiol 2000;23:256–261.

45. Alexander CM, Teller LE, Gross JB. Principles of pulse oximetry: theoretical and practical considerations. Anesth Analg 1989;68: 368–376.

46. Grunberg SM, Hesketh PJ. Control of chemotherapy induced emesis. N Engl J Med 1993;329:1790–1796.

47. Karian VE, Burrows PE, Zurakowski D, et al. The development of a pediatric sedation program. Pediatr Radiol 2002;32:348–353.

48. Matsumoto AH, Reifsnyder AC, Hartwell GD, et al. Reducing the discomfort of lidocaine administration through pH buffering. J Vasc Intervent Radiol 1994;5:171–175.

49. Molgaard CP, Teitelbaum GP, Pentecost MJ, et al. Intraarterial administration of lidocaine for analgesia in hepatic chemoembolization. J Vasc Intervent Radiol 1990;1:81–85.

50. Barth KH. Patient care aspects of vascular and nonvascular interventional radiology procedures. Semin Intervent Radiol 1994; 11:83–88.

51. Kiowski W. Treatment of disturbances in blood-pressure regulation, volume homeostasis, and microcirculation during interventional radiology procedures. In: Steinbrich W, Gross-Fengels W, eds. Interventional Radiology, Adjunctive Medication and Monitoring. Berlin: Springer, 1993:49–58.

52. Olsson P, Lagergren H, Stig EK. The elimination from plasma of intravenous heparin: an experimental study on dogs and humans. Acta Med Scand 1963;173:619–630.

53. Cobb CA, Fung DL. Shock due to protamine hypersensitivity. Surg Neurol 1982;17:245–246.

54. Standards and guidelines for cardiopulmonary resuscitation (CPR) and emergency cardiac care (ECC). JAMA 1986;255: 2905–2989.

55. Tortolani AJ, Risucci DA, Rosati RJ, et al. In-hospital cardiopulmonary resuscitation: patient arrest and resuscitation factors associated with survival. Resuscitation 1990;20:115–128.

56. Geigle R, Jones SB. Outcomes measurement: a report from the front. Inquiry 1990;27:7–13.

57. Barth KH, Matsumoto AH. Patient care in interventional radiology: a perspective. Radiology 1991;178:11–17.

58. Katzen BT, Kaplan JO, Dake MD. Developing an interventional radiology practice in a community hospital: the interventional radiologist as an equal partner in patient care. Radiology 1989; 170:955–958.

The Emergency Treatment of Reactions to Contrast Media

Rebecca A. Barnett

Reactions to contrast materials range from mild inconvenience, such as itching and hives, to severe, life-threatening emergencies. Radiologists should be familiar with the pathophysiology and cause of these reactions, be able to identify patients who are at risk, and be able to modify studies and pretreat if necessary. Radiologists should also be able to recognize a reaction readily and be ready to treat promptly if a reaction is seen. This chapter covers the treatment of reactions to contrast media: the preparation and techniques required and the supplies needed for immediate and adequate resuscitation.

All physicians, by the time they have finished medical school and residency training, have been trained and certified in basic life support (BLS) techniques; indeed, most have completed the Advanced Life Support Techniques course offered by the American Heart Association (1). It is strongly recommended that any physicians involved in direct patient care maintain current certification and therefore have a consistent review of their skills in cardiopulmonary resuscitation.

Perhaps the most important aspect of the treatment of contrast reactions is their prevention. Although severe allergic reaction is uncommon, probably less than 1:1000 (2), all patients should have a detailed history with special attention given to previous exposure to contrast dye, any adverse reaction, and history of asthma, hay fever, or food or medication allergy. In patients with asthma, even well controlled, the incidence of allergic reactions is double that of patients who have no history of asthma (3). In patients with a previous reaction, the incidence rate of another reaction is about 20% (4). It is helpful to have a brief history and a list of current medications that the patient is taking so that in the event of an emergency, this information is readily available to the team treating the patient. If a patient is identified as being at risk for an allergic reaction, pretreatment for prophylaxis should be considered (5,6). Pretreatment may consist of corticosteroids alone (3) or may be combined with an H_1 antihistamine (diphenhydramine). Many physicians advocate the use of an H_2 blocker (cimetidine or ranitidine) in addition to the above regime (7,8).

General measures can be taken to avoid the development of adverse reactions (Table 2–1). All these measures have been advocated to reduce or prevent reactions to contrast media (9,10).

Most reactions occur within minutes of the injection of the contrast material; however, the reaction may occur more than 30 minutes after the injection (3, 9–11). Radiology personnel should be alert to this possibility, and patients should continue to be observed even after their study is complete.

Despite all attempts at the prevention of reactions, at some point radiologists may be faced with an unexpected acute life-threatening anaphylactic reaction to the administration of contrast dye. In this situation, the goal is to treat the patient quickly and effectively so that the patient suffers no permanent injury. The primary goal of cardiopulmonary resuscitation is to prevent irreversible brain damage. Oxygenated blood flow to the brain needs to be restored as soon as possible; damage may begin within 3 minutes of anoxia (12).

TABLE 2–1
GENERAL MEASURES TO PREVENT CONTRAST REACTIONS

Avoidance of unnecessary tests
Careful selection of patients for x-ray studies
Slower infusion of the media
Adequate hydration prior to the procedure
Use of a small test dose
Selection of patients for pretreatment/prophylaxis

The initial response should be to stop the study and go to the patient. Call for help immediately, on the way to the patient, because even an unskilled person can fetch equipment and act as a messenger.

Immediately assess the patient and decide whether the patient is having a major or a minor reaction. Signs of a minor reaction include conjunctivitis, erythema or hives, pruritis, rhinitis, and urticaria. The treatment of minor reactions is discussed in detail in the preceding chapter and includes administration of intramuscular epinephrine and diphenhydramine along with supportive measures.

If the patient is having a major reaction, the initial assessment of the patient will follow the basic and secondary ABCDs of resuscitation (Table 2–2). First determine whether the patient is responsive.

If the patient appears to need any form of cardiopulmonary resuscitation (CPR), then immediately call for more help. In the hospital setting, this probably means an overhead page or call to an emergency response or "code" team who has experience in CPR and should be immediately available to assist. In an outpatient setting, this may mean a 911 emergency response call. In either case, the patient needs immediate care until the team arrives. Basic life support (1) should begin as an attempt to maintain circulation and oxygenation. At the same time, additional personnel can move x-ray and other large pieces of equipment out of the immediate vicinity of the patient and bring emergency supplies to the bedside (Table 2–3).

First examine the patient's airway; is the patient breathing? If not, ensure that the airway is unobstructed. If the patient has received any form of sedation or is unconscious for any other reason, it may be that the patient is now obstructed by soft tissues of the upper airway, palate, or tongue, and all that is required is a jaw thrust or head tilt for the return of spontaneous ventilation (13). To perform this maneuver, the patient's head is tilted back as far as possible with one hand on the forehead and the other behind the patient's neck. Infants and children have pliable necks, and overextension may itself cause upper airway obstruction. If the patient has a large head and neck, it may be necessary to place the fingers of both hands along the patient's mandible and sublux the jaw forward and up. To maintain a patent airway, the placement of an oropharyngeal or nasopharyngeal airway may be necessary (see "Airway Supplies" in Table 2–4). Always be aware that the patient may be obstructed by vomitus or secretions (which should be suctioned immediately) or a foreign body. If a foreign body is suspected, it may be carefully removed under direct vision. Blind suctioning or forceps use may push the foreign body farther into the airway, making removal even more difficult. If the foreign body cannot be visualized, turning the patient and performing a Heimlich maneuver may be necessary. With one of your hands on top of the other, place the heel of your bottom hand on the patient's upper abdomen below the rib cage and above the

TABLE 2–2
INITIAL ASSESSMENT OF THE PATIENT WITH MAJOR REACTION

Basic ABCDs of resuscitation in unresponsive patient:
  A. Airway: Is the airway unobstructed?
  B. Breathing: Is the patient breathing spontaneously? If not, give two breaths.
  C. Circulation: Is a pulse detectable? If not, start compressions.
  D. Attach monitor/defibrillator.

Assess rhythm:
  If VT/VF, perform three defibrillations and proceed to secondary ABCDs.
  If non-VT/VF (asystole or pulseless electrical activity), continue basic CPR.

Secondary ABCDs:
  A. Secure airway with endotracheal tube (if difficult airway—laryngeal or oropharyngeal airway—a skilled operator is needed), or continue ventilation with bag and mask until help arrives.
  B. Confirm airway with end-tidal capnography and secure (CO_2 may be negative with cardiac arrest and no output).
  C. Intravenous access, monitors, and medications.
  D. Differential diagnosis.

TABLE 2–3
EMERGENCY SUPPLIES

Emergency airway box (for detailed contents, see Table 2–4)
Oxygen: Two cylinders with valve for up to 15 liters per minute
Intravenous insertion supplies: Catheters, alcohol wipes, tourniquets, razor, tape, intravenous fluid (lactated Ringer's solution or normal saline) with intravenous administration sets, various stop cocks, and extension tubing
Gloves: Sterile and regular of varying sizes
Stethoscope
Intracardiac needle
Portable defibrillator
Suction with rigid and soft catheters
Emergency drug supply cart (for detailed contents, see Table 2–5)
Orogastric/nasogastric tubes
Needles and syringes for drug administration

TABLE 2-4
AIRWAY SUPPLIES

Required:
  Masks of various sizes
    Bag with valve capable of delivering positive pressure
      ventilation with 100% oxygen
  Oropharyngeal airways
  Nasopharyngeal airways
  Lubrication
  Tongue blades
  Laryngoscope with various size and type blades
  Endotracheal tubes (6.0–8.0 mm) for adults
  Endotracheal tube stylets
  12-gauge intravenous catheter for cricothyrotomy
  Carbon dioxide detection

Optional:
  Tracheotomy set
  Laryngeal mask airway (sizes 3–5)

Note: If children or infants are treated or studied in the department or facility, all the above equipment needs to be available in pediatric sizes as well.

navel. Use your body weight to press into the patient's upper abdomen with a quick upward thrust. Repeat until the object is expelled.

If the airway appears to be open and the patient does not promptly resume spontaneous breathing, then artificial ventilation must begin immediately, preferably with a bag and mask with 100% oxygen (Figure 2–1A, B, C, and D). A bag and mask with an oxygen supply is on the list of essential emergency equipment that should be available in

the radiology suite (Table 2–4). Ventilation is confirmed by seeing the patient's chest rise and fall with each breath but may be difficult to appreciate in large patients. Initially, four quick breaths should be given and then an assessment made as to whether the heart is beating by checking a pulse. The preferred location is the carotid because it is often palpable when peripheral pulses are already absent and is readily accessible when managing the airway. If cardiac arrest is evident by lack of a pulse, closed cardiac compression must begin. Artificial ventilation should continue. At this point, if a code team has arrived, intubation is the preferred method of airway management. Intubation should be attempted only by persons with experience in this technique; otherwise, mask ventilation should continue along with chest compressions. Adequate ventilation is essential because there is little point in providing adequate circulation with good chest compressions if the blood that is circulating is not oxygenated.

Guidelines from the American Heart Association, developed in collaboration with the International Liaison Committee on Resuscitation (ILCOR), should be followed (1). The guidelines recommend compressions at a rate of 100 per minute with a compression to ventilation ratio of 15:2 for adults and 5:1 for infants and small children. These compression rates are more rapid than the ones given in previous guidelines. An increase in the rate of cardiac compressions has been shown to increase mean aortic pressure, coronary perfusion pressure, myocardial blood flow, and 24-hour survival in dogs (15), and in humans the increased rate has been shown to cause a significant increase in end-tidal carbon dioxide level (a surrogate for cardiac output) during CPR (16). Despite optimal conditions, chest compressions probably produce only about

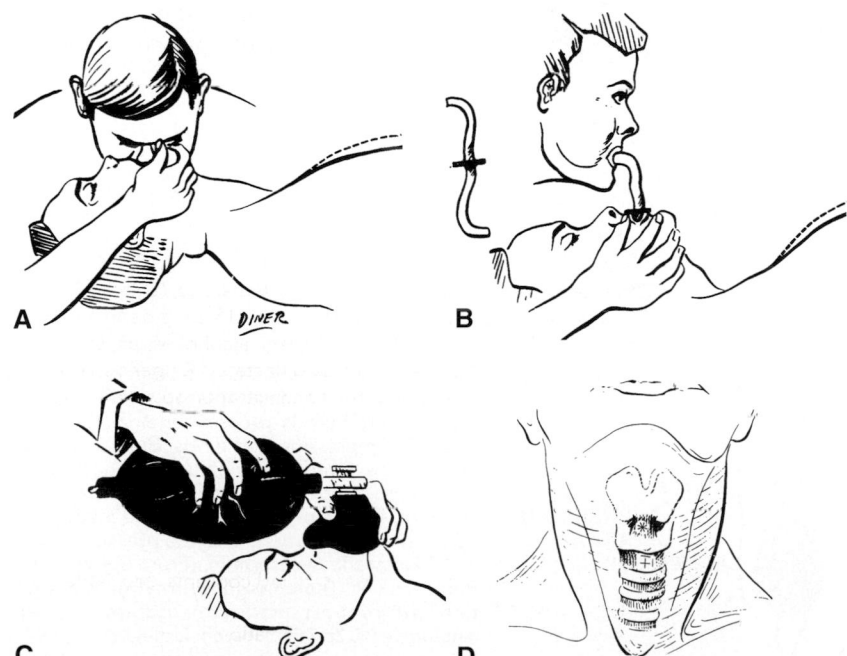

Figure 2–1 Pulmonary resuscitation **A.** If there is no airway, the chin must be pulled forward and the neck extended to free the tongue from obstructing the airway. Note that the rescuer's cheek occludes the victim's nostrils. **B.** Convenient resuscitation with double-ended airway that keeps two sizes available in a single device. The patient's lips should be sealed against the airway. Rise and fall of the chest wall indicates effective air movement. **C.** One type of hand-operated respirator. The mask must be pressed firmly against the face. If an airway is not inserted, the position of the head and neck must be the same as that in mouth-to-mouth resuscitation. **D.** The asterisk (*) marks the location of the cricothyroid membrane, just below the thyroid cartilage, where a quick tracheotomy can be performed. (Modified from Barnhard HJ, Barnahard FM. The emergency treatment of reactions to contrast media. In: Abrams HL, ed. Angiography. 2nd Ed. Boston: Little, Brown, 1971. Used with permission.)

30% of pre-arrest cerebral perfusion and about 10% of pre-arrest myocardial perfusion (17). Thus, the goal is to return the patient to spontaneous circulation as soon as possible.

In most radiology suites, it would be unusual for the radiologist to be the only person present, but you may be the only physician present, and you may be expected at this point to manage the patient's immediate care until help arrives. Immediately begin to delegate tasks to other personnel present. Good intravenous access is essential and should be established as soon as possible and connected to a free-flowing intravenous fluid administration set. A free-flowing set is preferred to a pump because it allows the operator to know that the cannula is in a vein. A pump can force fluid under pressure into the soft tissues for some time before a pressure alarm will sound, depending on the site of insertion, and drug administration will not be effective in the meantime. Central access is preferred for vasoactive drug administration, but a good free-flowing peripheral cannula can save the time required to place a central line in the neck. Other personnel can set up suction, collect the emergency airway drug supplies and defibrillator, and place basic monitoring such as electrocardiogram leads, blood pressure cuff, and pulse oximeter probe.

To be effective, cardiac compressions must be performed correctly (Figure 2–2). First, the patient should always be flat. If the bed or table on which the patient has been placed is even slightly head up, the venous return to the heart may be reduced, and even good compressions may be ineffective. Placing the patient with the head below neutral (Trendelenburg position) has not been found helpful in improving venous return and indeed may hamper resuscitative efforts by forcing the abdominal contents upward against the diaphragm, making adequate ventilation more difficult (14). A firm surface is also preferred. If the surface is soft and cannot be inflated to a firm CPR surface, then a board can be placed under the patient's body to aid correct compressions. Correct compressions are performed by positioning yourself close to the patient's side and placing the heel of one hand on the lower half of the sternum, taking care not to place your hand over the lower tip, or xiphoid process, as this could easily cause fractures with compressions. The other hand should then be placed over the first, with the fingers interlocking. Move your shoulders forward until they are directly over the patient's chest, with your arms straight, and then exert pressure downward to depress the sternum about 1 1/2–2 inches. Release the pressure to allow the sternum to return to the normal resting position, but do not remove your hands from the patient's chest. For children, use only the heel of one hand, and place it over the midsternum. Depression of the chest need be only 3/4–1 1/2 inches. For infants, use only the tips of the first two fingers, and compress only 1/2–3/4 inch. Because the head of a small child or an infant tends to push the back up, slipping one hand behind the back while performing compressions provides more support; alternately, you can encircle the entire chest with your hands and use your thumbs to provide compressions.

Complications of ventilation and chest compressions include gastric insufflation with large quantities of air, aspiration of gastric contents, and fractured ribs or sternum

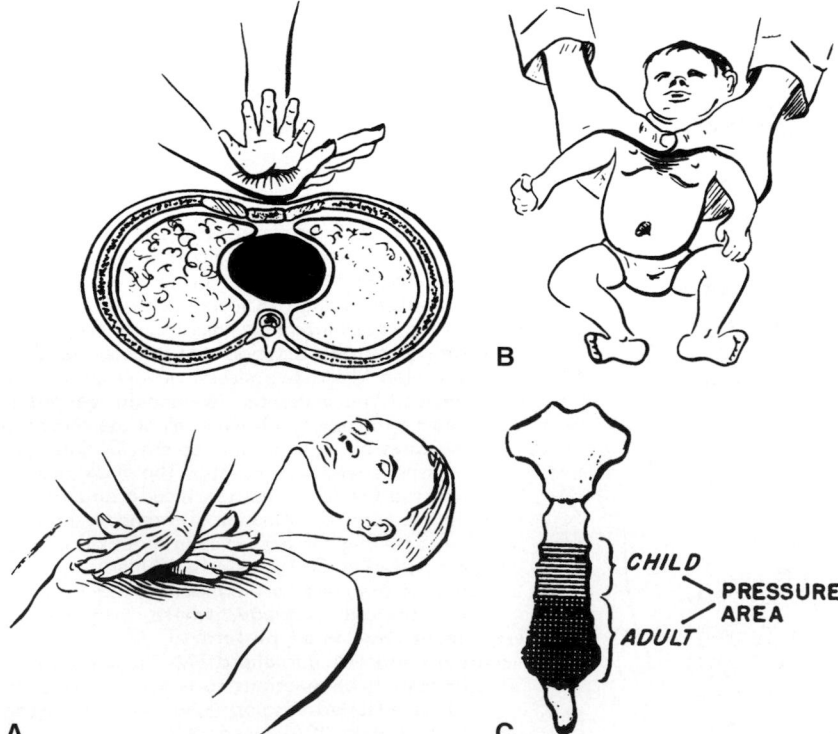

Figure 2–2 External cardiac compression **A.** In an adult, the hands are placed on the chest so that the sternum is pressed against the heart without compression of the ribs. **B.** In a child, the fingers are interlaced behind the back while superimposed thumbs transmit pressure to the sternum. **C.** The pressure area in the adult is just above the xiphisternum, and the pressure area in a child is at the midsternum. (From Barnhard HJ, Barnhard FM. The emergency treatment of reactions to contrast media. In: Abrams HL, ed. Angiography. 2nd Ed. Boston: Little, Brown, 1971. Used with permission.)

(18,19). Rarer complications include rupture of underlying ventricle (20) and rupture of underlying upper abdominal organs, such as the liver or spleen, when too much force is used (21). Complications can even include compression of underlying coronary artery stents (22).

Open cardiac massage has been shown to be superior in providing adequate cardiac output in the porcine model (23) but requires special skills in opening the chest; hence, it is not a widely used technique except in the operating room, in some ICUs, and in trauma centers. More recently, there has been interest in a minimally invasive direct cardiac massage device, which is easy to place through a small substernal incision (24). Again, this requires some specialized training but has been used successfully by paramedics in some cases of cardiac arrest.

Once CPR has been established and help has been called, start thinking about the cause of the arrest and further therapy. The ACLS manual defines a protocol for drug administration and defibrillation in the setting of a cardiac arrest. Although it is not the intent of this chapter to provide complete life support training for radiologists, it is appropriate to give a general outline of the algorithm for resuscitation.

Once pulselessness is established and the airway managed by mask ventilation or intubation, the first drug that should be administered is 1 mg of epinephrine through the intravenous line. If intravenous access is still not available, epinephrine may be given via the endotracheal tube (an easy way to remember drugs that can be given via this route is NAVEL: Narcan, Atropine, Valium, Epinephrine, Lidocaine, the dosage being 2–2½ times the normal dose). Epinephrine is the frontline drug for both ventricular tachycardia/ventricular fibrillation (VT/VF) and non-VT/VF, and so it can be given while waiting for monitor placement to determine rhythm. If VT/VF is seen on placement of monitors, 40 units of vasopressin can be added. Epinephrine can be given in 1 mg doses every 3–5 minutes as needed. After the first dose of epinephrine, if VT/VF is noted, then defibrillation is required. Standard defibrillation is three escalating shocks at 200 joules, 200–300 joules, and 360 joules, or three equivalent biphasic shocks at 150 joules apiece (25). Subsequent shocks, following further drug therapy, should be at 360 joules or monophasic. If there is no response, then bicarbonate, amiodarone, lidocaine, and magnesium may be added. Procainamide and bretylium are acceptable but not recommended in current ACLS guidelines for VT/VF.

Further treatment will now depend on the differential diagnosis and the rhythm assessment seen on the electrocardiogram and should follow current, published ACLS guidelines. Readers are referred to current guidelines established in 2000 by the American Heart Association (1).

One of the hardest decisions a physician may face is deciding when to discontinue resuscitative efforts on a patient with cardiac arrest. On average, only 10–15% of hospitalized patients survive CPR efforts (26), although studies have not been specific to radiology patients receiving contrast dye. The following factors have been associated with survival longer than 24 hours: arrest location other than emergency room or cardiac care unit, CPR duration of less than 15 minutes, noncardiac primary diagnosis, nonasystolic dysrhythmia, less than one intravenous and one drip-administered inotrope, and absence of pacemaker insertion and defibrillation (27).

The AHA ACLS guidelines do not include specific recommendations to trained health providers about when to stop CPR. This decision relies on the clinical judgment of the provider(s) about the individual patient and the underlying cause of the arrest.

In conclusion, health-care providers may be required to provide immediate care to a patient undergoing cardiac arrest. The mainstay of treatment is prevention by careful patient screening and selection. Early recognition is essential. The radiologist should be present during injections and immediately available for at least 30 minutes after an injection. Preparation for a possible arrest is vital; equipment has to be immediately available and well maintained. A policy of routine regular maintenance of all supplies is recommended. In the event of an arrest, the radiologist should know where all emergency equipment is stored and how to quickly get help to come to the area; in most hospitals, there is some form of emergency response team or code team. Know how to call them.

It cannot be stressed enough that keeping up to date with ACLS skills may be lifesaving to a patient in your care.

ACKNOWLEDGMENTS

This chapter appeared in the fourth edition authored by Dr. Stanley Baum and was updated for this edition by Dr. Rebecca Barnett.

REFERENCES

1. American Heart Association International Guidelines for Cardiopulmonary Resuscitation and Emergency Cardiovascular Care. Circulation 2000;102(suppl 8):I1–I370.
2. Katayama H, Yamaguchi K, Kozuka T, et al. Adverse reactions to ionic and nonionic contrast media. A report from the Japanese Committee on the Safety of Contrast Media. Radiology 1990; 175:621–628.
3. Cohen RH, Ellis JH. Iodinated contrast material in uroradiology. Choice of agent and management of complications. Urol Clin North Am 1997;24:471–491.
4. Goldfrank L, Mayer A. Anaphylaxis—the IVP emergency. Hosp Physician 1978;14.28–32.
5. Greenberger PA, Patterson P, Kelly J, et al. Administration of radiographic contrast media in high-risk patients. Invest Radiol 1980;15(Suppl):S40–S43.
6. Lasser EC, Berry CC, Talner LB, et al. Pretreatment with corticosteroids to alleviate reactions to intravenous contrast material. N Engl J Med 1987;317:845–849.
7. Greenberger PA, Patterson R, Tapio CM. Prophylaxis against repeated radiocontrast media reactions in 857 cases. Adverse experiences with cimetidine and safety of beta-adrenergic antagonists. Arch Intern Med 1985;145:2197–2008.

8. Kelly JF, Patterson R, Lieberman P, et al. Radiographic contrast media studies in high-risk patients. J Allergy Clin Immunol 1978;62:181–184.

9. Millburn SM, Bell SD. Prevention of anaphylaxis to contrast medium. Anesthesiology 1979;50:56–57.

10. Patterson R, Schatz M. Administration of radiographic contrast medium after a prior adverse reaction. Ann Intern Med 1975;83:277.

11. Zweiman B, Mishkin MM, Hildreth EA. An approach to the performance of contrast studies in contrast material-reactive persons. Ann Intern Med 1975;83:159–162.

12. Goldberg AH. Cardiopulmonary arrest. N Engl J Med 1974; 290:381–385.

13. Grossman JI, Rubin IL. Cardiopulmonary resuscitation. I. Am Heart J 1969;78:569–572.

14. Johnson S, Henderson SO. Myth: the Trendelenburg position improves circulation in cases of shock. Can J Emerg Med 2004; 6:48–49.

15. Fenely MP, MaierGW, Kem KB, et al. Influence of cardiac compression rate on initial success of resuscitation and 24-hour survival after prolonged manual cardiopulmonary-resuscitation in dogs. Circulation 1988;77:240–250.

16. Kern KB, Sanders AB, Raife J, et al. A study of chest compression rates during cardiopulmonary resuscitation in humans. The importance of rate-directed chest compressions. Arch Intern Med 1992;152:145–149.

17. Niemann JT. Differences in cerebral and myocardial perfusion during closed-chest resuscitation. Ann Emerg Med 1984;13: 849–853.

18. Oschatz E, Wunderbaldinger P, Sterz F, et al. Cardiopulmonary resuscitation performed by bystanders does not increase adverse effects as assessed by chest radiography. Anesth Analg 2001; 93:128–133.

19. Black CJ, Busuttil A, Robertson C. Chest wall injuries following cardiopulmonary resuscitation. Resuscitation 2004;63:339–343.

20. Machii M, Inaba H, Nakae H, et al. Cardiac rupture by penetration of fractured sternum: a rare complication of cardiopulmonary resuscitation. Resuscitation 2000;43:151–153.

21. Patterson RH, Burns WA, Jannotta FS. Complications of external cardiac resuscitation: a retrospective review and survey of the literature. Med Ann DC 1974;42:389–394.

22. Windecker S, Maier W, Eberli FR, et al. Mechanical compression of coronary artery stents: potential hazard for patients undergoing cardiopulmonary resuscitation. Catheter Cardiovasc Interv 2000;51:464–467.

23. Engoren M, Severyn F, Fenn-Buderer N, et al. Cardiac output, coronary blood flow, and blood gases during open-chest standard and compression-active-decompression cardiopulmonary resuscitation. Resuscitation 2002;55:309–316.

24. Rozenberg A, Incagnoli P, Delpech P, et al. Prehospital use of minimally invasive direct cardiac massage (MID-CM): a pilot study. Resuscitation 2001;50:257–262.

25. Schneider T, Martens PR, Paschen H, et al. Multicenter, randomized, controlled trial of 150-J biphasic shocks compared with 200- to 360-J monophasic shocks in the resuscitation of out-of-hospital cardiac arrest victims. Circulation 2000;102: 1780–1787.

26. Rozenbaum EA, Shenkman L. Predicting outcome of in-hospital cardiopulmonary resuscitation. Crit Care Med 1988;16:583–586.

27. Schultz SC, Cullinane DC, Pasquale MD, et al. Predicting in-hospital mortality during cardiopulmonary resuscitation. Resuscitation 1996;33:13–17.

APPENDIX

Dysrhythmia Recognition and Treatment

1. Analyze each ECG rhythm strip in a systematic fashion. Is the rate too fast or slow? Are the atrial and ventricular rates equal (Figure 2–3)?

Are the P-to-P and R-to-R wave intervals regular or irregular? If the rhythm is irregular, is it consistent or is it irregularly irregular?

Is there a P wave before each QRS complex? Are the P waves and the QRS complexes identical and normal in configuration?

Are the P-R and the QRS intervals within normal limits?

What is the significance of the dysrhythmia when it is correlated with clinical observation of the patient?

2. Identify the ECG patterns (Figure 2–3). Rhythms may include the following:

Normal sinus rhythm

Sinus tachycardia

Sinus bradycardia

Premature atrial contractions

Atrial flutter

Atrial fibrillation

Atrioventricular block: first, second, third degree

Premature ventricular contractions

Ventricular tachycardia

Ventricular fibrillation, fine

Ventricular fibrillation, coarse

Cardiac standstill

3. Recognize the significance of the rhythms and begin treatment (31,33).

Normal sinus rhythm

Significance: Normal. No therapy.

Sinus tachycardia

Significance: The rapid rate may increase cardiac output and precipitate congestive heart failure in the damaged heart.

Therapy: Treat underlying cause.

Sinus bradycardia

Significance: A common finding in the early period of acute myocardial infarction (MI), which may predispose to premature beats.

Therapy: Atropine sulfate, to decrease vagal tone, 0.5 mg as a bolus; the dose may be repeated if needed at 5-minute intervals up to a maximum dose of 2 mg. If this fails, try isoproterenol, 1 mg in 500 mL dextrose in water, 1 to 10 mL per minute, titrated. Consider temporary transvenous pacemaker if isoproterenol fails to restore adequate circulation.

Premature atrial contractions (PACs)

Significance: Isolated PACs may occur in normal persons. Frequent PACs may indicate organic heart disease and possibly initiate atrial tachydysrhythmias.

Therapy: Sedation; omission of stimulants (alcohol, caffeine, tobacco); occasionally digitalis, quinidine, propranolol, and procainamide may be employed.

Atrial flutter

Significance: Atrial flutter is most common in the presence of organic heart disease.

Therapy: Directed at slowing ventricular rate. D.C. countershock is effective, especially if clinical status

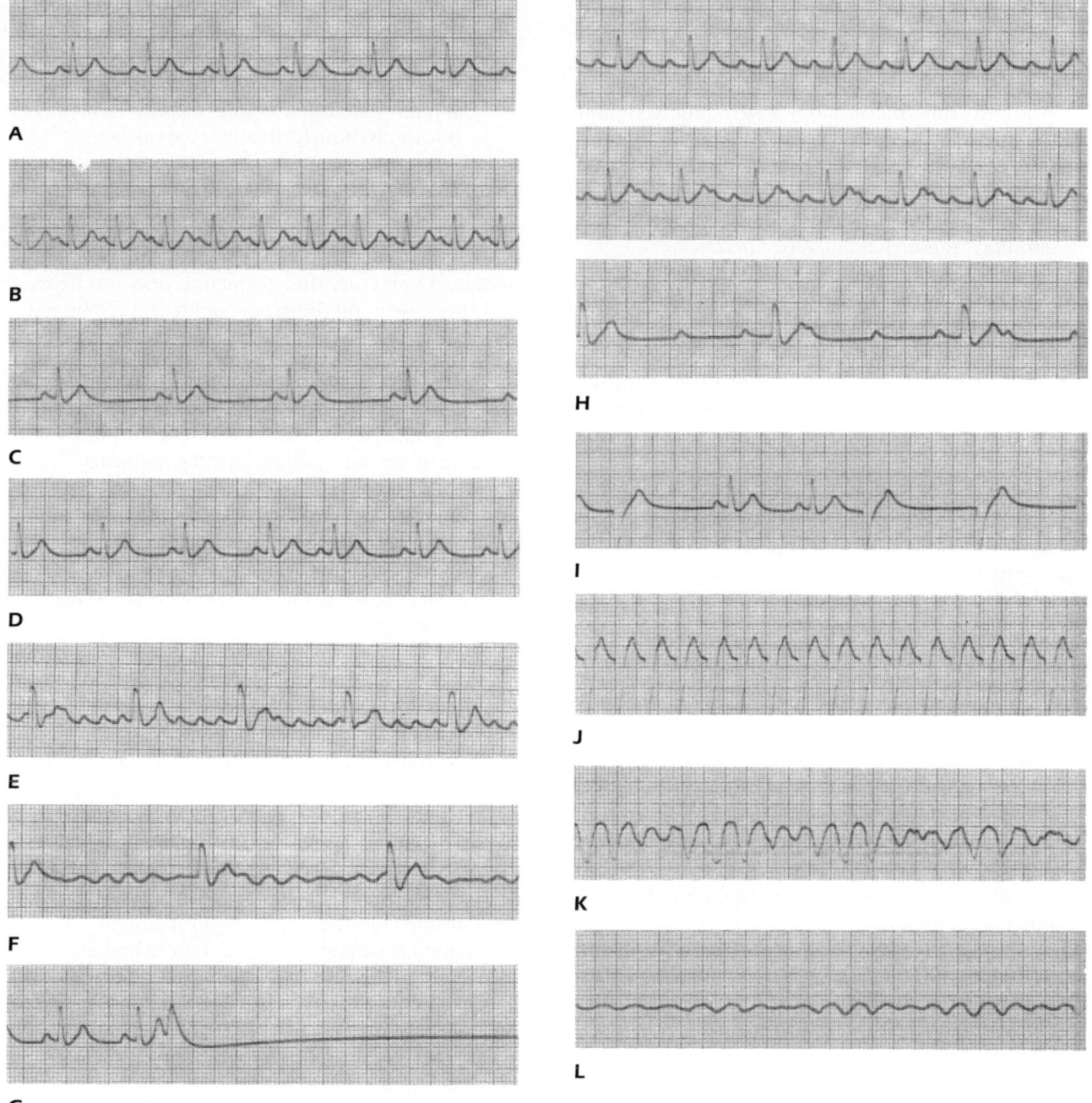

Figure 2–3 ECG rhythms that are commonly seen during cardiopulmonary resuscitation. **A.** Normal sinus rhythm; **B.** sinus tachycardia; **C.** sinus bradycardia; **D.** premature atrial contractions; **E.** atrial flutter; **F.** atrial fibrillation; **G.** cardiac standstill; **H.** atrioventricular block: first, second, third degree; **I.** premature ventricular contractions; **J.** ventricular tachycardia; **K.** ventricular fibrillation, coarse; **L.** ventricular fibrillation, fine.

suggests urgency. Digitalis may slow ventricular rate; propranolol is useful.

Atrial fibrillation

Significance: Atrial fibrillation is usually the result of underlying heart disease.

Therapy: Digitalis, the traditional initial treatment, effectively slows ventricular rate. D.C. shock is usually effective if conversion to normal sinus rhythm (NSR) is essential. Quinidine or propranolol may also be used to convert to NSR.

Atrioventricular block, first degree

Significance: May be the warning of more advanced forms of atrioventricular block in acute MI. It may also be due to digitalis excess.

Therapy: Usually none. Atropine, isoproterenol, occasionally temporary pacemaker for acute MI.

Atrioventricular block, second degree, Mobitz type I

Significance: It is the less serious type of second-degree atrioventricular block, but it is still quite common in patients with acute inferior MI. Generally transient, the type I block does not necessarily require a pacemaker.

Therapy: Observation; if ventricular rate very slow, atropine, isoproterenol; rarely, a pacemaker.

Atrioventricular block, second degree, Mobitz type II

Significance: Type II block occurs in large anterior MIs and is commonly a forerunner of sudden complete atrioventricular block.

Therapy: Standby pacemaker insertion; atropine and so on only until definitive therapy can be employed.

Atrioventricular block, third degree

Significance: The ventricular rate may be so slow that circulation cannot be maintained, and syncope, congestive heart failure, or angina may occur.

Therapy: Pacemaker as soon as possible; atropine and/or isoproterenol to try to maintain ventricular rate of 60.

Premature ventricular contractions (PVCs)

Significance: Dangerous signs are frequent PVCs, runs of PVCs, multifocal PVCs, and the R-on-T phenomenon.

Therapy: Lidocaine, 50–100 mg bolus, may be repeated once if necessary. Lidocaine infusion, 500 mg in 500 ml dextrose in water, titrated to control the PVCs but not more rapidly than 3–4 mg per minute. Other medications—procainamide, phenytoin, propranolol, quinidine, digitalis—may be required.

Ventricular tachycardia

Significance: A most serious and dangerous dysrhythmia. Ventricular tachycardia may be the precursor of ventricular fibrillation.

Therapy: Lidocaine intravenous bolus, 1 mg/kg, followed by infusion of 500 mg in 500-mL dextrose in water. D.C. countershock, beginning with 50 joules.

Ventricular fibrillation

Significance: The patient is clinically dead without effective cardiac output.

Therapy: *Immediate* D.C. defibrillation at maximum setting, 400 joules; otherwise, cardiopulmonary resuscitation until defibrillation is available. Sodium bicarbonate intravenously 50–100 mEq (1 mEq/kg), followed by a second dose 5–10 minutes later if needed and then by one half-dose every 10 minutes if needed. Epinephrine, 5 mL of 1:10,000 solution, repeated every five minutes if needed. Lidocaine, 50–100 mg bolus, followed by second identical dose if needed.

Cardiac standstill

Significance: No cardiac output; the patient is clinically dead.

Therapy: Cardiopulmonary resuscitation, epinephrine, sodium bicarbonate, isoproterenol, calcium chloride intravenously; finally, a pacemaker.

Essential Drugs and Useful Drugs

The national standards for cardiopulmonary resuscitation (13) classify seven drugs as "essential" and nine drugs as "useful." In practice, this distinction does not necessarily apply because useful drugs may suddenly become essential ones. The intent of the distinction is to recognize the drugs most frequently required in emergency cardiac care that are likely to be essential to survival.

1. The objectives of drug treatment during cardiopulmonary resuscitation include the following:
   Correcting hypoxia
   Correcting metabolic acidosis
   Increasing perfusion pressure during cardiac compression
   Stimulating spontaneous or more forceful myocardial contraction
   Accelerating cardiac rate
   Suppressing ventricular ectopic activity

2. The following medications (Table 2–5) must be readily available:

Essential drugs	Useful drugs
Oxygen	Vasoactive drugs
Sodium bicarbonate	Norepinephrine
Epinephrine	Metaraminol
Atropine	Dopamine
Lidocaine	Isoproterenol
Calcium chloride	Propranolol
Morphine sulfate	Procainamide
	Corticosteroids
	Diuretic agents
	Furosemide
	Ethacrynic acid

3. Discussion

   Oxygen heads the list of essential drugs because it protects the brain and other vital organs from irreversible damage. Hypoxia is likely to occur during cardiac arrest because of reduced cardiac output, increased intrapulmonary shunting, and ventilation-perfusion abnormalities. Because oxygen intoxication does not occur for many hours, the concentration of oxygen should be as high as possible until resuscitation is complete or until arterial blood gases and pH indicate that the inspired oxygen concentration can be safely reduced.

   Sodium bicarbonate is used to correct the metabolic acidosis that invariably develops during oxygen deprivation. The usual initial adult dose is 1 mEq/kg intravenously. The dose can be repeated once; thereafter,

TABLE 2–5

RECOMMENDED INTRAVENOUS DOSAGE

Drug	Adults	Infants/Children	Comments
Essential			
Sodium bicarbonate	1 mEq/kg initially (repeat once); 0.5 mEq/kg at 10-min intervals or as indicated by blood gases	1 mL (0.9 mEq)/kg diluted 1:1 with sterile water (repeat after pH obtained and base deficit calculated)	Do not mix with epinephrine, calcium
Epinephrine	0.5–1.0 mL of 1:1,000 solution (repeat at 5-min intervals as needed)	0.1–0.5 mL of 1:1,000 solution (repeat at 5-min intervals as needed)	
Atropine	0.5-mg bolus to be given slowly (repeat at 5-min intervals to total dose of 2 mg)	0.01 mg/kg	Total dose in adults can equal 2 mg when third-degree atrioventricular block present
Lidocaine	1 mg/kg bolus (repeat once); dose then continued as IV drip (1–4 mL/min of 0.1% solution)	Infants: 0.5 mg/kg; children: 5 mg (repeat as needed); dose then continued as IV drip	In adults, infusion rate maximum 4 mg/min; infants and children, rate maximum 100 mg/hr
Calcium chloride 10%	2.5–5.0 mL (3.4–6.8 mEq Ca^{++}); dose may be repeated at 10-min intervals	1 mL/5 kg maximum dose	Calcium salts should never be mixed with sodium bicarbonate
Morphine sulfate	1.0–1.5 mL (3.0–4.5 mg) of 3 mg/mL distilled water solution.		
Useful			
Norepinephrine	Mix 4 mg in 250 mL D5W; start 4 μg/min (¼ mL) and increase to desired effect	Infants: 0.5 mg 1:250 mL D5W; children: 1 mg in 250 mL D5W; titrate to desired effect	First correct blood volume when hypovolemia has led to cardiac arrest
Metaraminol	2–5-mg bolus given slowly; dose may be continued as drip	25 mg/100 mL D5W	Titrate to desired effect
Dopamine	2–20 μg/kg/min in D5W		Titrate to desired effect
Isoproterenol	Mix 1 mg in 500 mL D5W; start 4 μg/min (2 mL) and titrate to desired effect		
Propranolol	0.5–1.0 mg slowly (repeat as needed to maximum of 3 mg)		Lidocaine should be given first; propranolol is given only if lidocaine fails to establish stable cardiac rhythm
Procainamide	25–50 mg/min; total dose range 0.2–1.0 mg		Lidocaine should be given first

Data from Cohen MR, Turco SJ. Parenteral drugs used in cardiopulmonary resuscitation. Bull Parenter Drug Assoc 1975;29:39; and from Hodgkin JE, Foster GL, Nicolay LI. Cardiopulmonary resuscitation: development of an organized protocol. Crit Care Med 1977;5:93. Used with permission.

one half the initial dose can be given at 10-minute intervals until resuscitation is complete or until arterial blood gases and pH are satisfactory. Avoid mixing sodium bicarbonate with either epinephrine or calcium because inotropic agent inactivation will result.

Epinephrine should always be administered early in cardiac arrest to convert fine ventricular fibrillation to coarse ventricular fibrillation, to restore myocardial contractility in the presence of electromechanical dissociation or asystole, and to increase the efficacy of D.C. countershock. The usual adult dose is 0.5–1.0 mg (0.5–1.0 mL of a 1:1,000 solution or 5–10 mL of a 1:10,000 solution) intravenously. Because of its rapid biodegradation, it can be given every 5 minutes. Epinephrine can be injected directly into the ventricles of the heart (a dangerous procedure), and it is also rapidly absorbed by the tracheobronchial tree. The dose when the drug is given by the latter route is 1–2 mg in 10 mL of sterile distilled water.

Atropine sulfate is indicated mainly in hemodynamically significant bradycardia, especially that associated with MI or that complicated by hypotension and PVCs. The initial dose is 0.5 mg given as a bolus, with repeated doses given at 5-minute intervals until the ventricular rate reaches 60 per minute or a maximum dose of 2 mg is reached.

Lidocaine is indispensable in most attempts at cardiac resuscitation although it is of no use to the patient in cardiac standstill. Lidocaine may prevent ventricular fibrillation in the presence of frequent or multifocal PVCs. Control of ventricular tachycardia may be effected with lidocaine, but electrical cardioversion is preferred if the patient also has hypotension. The initial dose of lidocaine is 1 mg/kg IV. Because of the drug's short therapeutic effect, a second bolus may be given, to be followed by a continuous infusion of 1–4 mL/min. Rates faster than 4 mL/min may cause convulsions.

Calcium chloride is effective in reversing electromechanical dissociation because it increases myocardial contractility. It is also useful in asystole and in converting fine fibrillation to coarse fibrillation. The adult dose is 2.5–5.0 mL of a 10 percent calcium chloride solution ($3.4–6.8$ mEq Ca^{++}). As mentioned previously, calcium precipitates with sodium bicarbonate and produces an insoluble salt.

Morphine sulfate is the narcotic of choice for relief of pain in patients with suspected MI. The drug may be prepared by diluting 1 mL (15 mg) morphine sulfate with distilled water to a total volume of 5 mL (3 mg morphine sulfate per mL water). Then 1.0–1.5 mL (3.0–4.5 mg) of the solution should be given as an initial dose and repeated as necessary.

The drugs classified as useful are most often administered in the postresuscitation period, but they may be indicated in impending arrest situations or as part of the immediate therapy of cardiac resuscitation.

Vasoactive drugs, such as norepinephrine and metaraminol, are useful when systemic peripheral resistance is low, as in the hypotension that often accompanies or follows resuscitation.

Norepinephrine in low doses stimulates beta cardiac receptors, which increases the cardiac output and improves the coronary blood flow. In higher doses, the alpha (vasoconstrictive) effect increases peripheral resistance, causing the heart to work harder. Norepinephrine is administered as an intravenous drip by preparing a solution of 4 mg in 250 mL of 5 % dextrose in water (D5W). Administration should begin at a rate of 4 µg/min (¼ mL) and the rate increased until a systolic blood pressure of 90–100 mm Hg is achieved.

Metaraminol will, in a similar fashion, improve inadequate coronary and cerebral blood flow. It may be given as a bolus of 2–5 mg and then continued as a drip.

Dopamine increases β receptor activity, which increases the cardiac output. In low doses (2–10 µg/kg/min), dopamine may increase the heart rate. In high doses (10–20 µg/kg/min), dopamine stimulates α receptors, causing peripheral vasoconstriction and an increase in blood pressure. Splanchnic perfusion is increased by specific dopamine receptors, especially in the kidney. The 5% dextrose drip should be titrated to obtain the desired effect.

Isoproterenol is a very useful drug when atropine fails to increase the heart rate in patients with profound sinus bradycardia. Isoproterenol increases cardiac output through its chronotropic and inotropic effects, but because of its tendency to produce dysrhythmias, especially PVCs, it is a difficult drug to use. It is given intravenously and is prepared as a solution, 1 mg in 500 mL D5W. It should be begun at a rate of 0.4 µg/min and increased to achieve a heart rate of 60 beats per minute.

Propranolol is used to treat specific dysrhythmias, such as ventricular tachycardia and ventricular fibrillation, that after initially responding to standard (lidocaine) therapy repeatedly revert to their original life-threatening character. Propranolol is administered intravenously at a rate not to exceed 1 mg/min. The usual adult dose is 0.5–1.0 mg to a maximum of 3 mg.

Procainamide depresses excitation and conduction in the myocardium. It is useful in treating PVCs and ventricular tachycardia that fail to respond to lidocaine and after countershock when NSR reverts to ventricular fibrillation. Procainamide is infused intravenously at a maximal rate of 25–50 mg/min during ECG monitoring.

Corticosteroids and diuretics may be useful in specific conditions, such as adult respiratory distress syndrome, aspiration, or pulmonary edema, and during the postresuscitation period.

Emergency Cart Equipment and Drugs

The desirability of having emergency equipment and drugs available in your department cannot be overemphasized. Although every hospital certainly possesses such equipment and medications, the nonhospital-based radiologist needs to assemble these materials beforehand, just as the radiologist needs to choose the consulting physicians he or she wishes to call on in the event of cardiac arrest. Emergency carts range in complexity from the most simple, locally designed and stocked carts to the commercially available prefilled cardiopulmonary resuscitation kits (Banyan Emergency Kits). We strongly recommend that the following "essential" equipment be kept close at hand to be used in the event of an emergency; the drugs that are "useful" in providing advanced life support are listed in Table 2–6.

Respiratory Equipment

For airway management and artificial ventilation, the following equipment is essential:

TABLE 2–6
STRENGTHS AND VOLUMES OF DRUGS COMMONLY USED FOR EMERGENCY TREATMENT

Drug	Strength	Volume
Essential		
Atropine	0.1 mg/mL	10 mL ampule
Calcium chloride	100 mg/mL (10%)	10 mL ampule
Epinephrine	1 mg/cc (1:1,000)	1 cc ampule
	OR 0.1 mg/cc (1:10,000)	10 cc injection
Lidocaine HCl	20 mg/mL	5 cc syringe
Sodium bicarbonate	44.6 mEq/50 mL	50 mL syringe
Useful		
Amiodarone	50 mg/mL	3 mL ampule
Aminophylline	500 mg/20 mL	20 mL ampule
Calcium gluconate	10 mg/mL	10 mL ampule
Dexamethasone sodium (Decadron)	4 mg/mL	5 mL vial
Dextrose solution	50%	50 cc syringe
Digoxin	0.25 mg/mL	2 mL ampule
Diphenhydramine HCl (Benadryl)	50 mg/mL	1 mL vial
Dopamine HCl	40 mg/mL	5 mL ampule
Ephedrine sulfate	50 mg/mL	1 mL ampule
Furosemide (Lasix)	10 mg/mL	2 mL or 10 mL ampule
Hydrocortisone succinate (Solu-Cortef)	250 mg	2 mL Mix-O-Vial
Norepinephrine (Levophed)	2 mg/mL	4 mL ampule
Meperidine HCl (Demerol)	50 mg/mL	1 mL ampule
Metaraminol bitartrate (Aramine)	10 mg/mL	1 mL vial
Metoprolol	1 mg/mL	5 mL ampule
Methyl prednisone sodium (Solu-Medrol)	125 mg	2 mL Mix-O-Vial
Morphine sulfate	15 mg/mL	2 mL vial
Naloxone (Narcan)	0.4 mg/mL	1 mL ampule
Pancuronium bromide(Pavulon)	1 mg/mL	10 mL vial
Phenylephrine (Neosynephrine)	10 mg/mL	1 mL ampule
Potassium chloride	2 mEq/cc	20 mL ampule
Procainamide HCl (Pronestyl)	100 mg/mL	10 mL vial
Propranolol HCl (Inderal)	1 mg/mL	1 mL ampule
Succinylcholine chloride (Anectine)	20 mg/mL	10 mL vial

Table compiled by author.

Oxygen cylinders (two E cylinders) with reducing valves capable of delivering 15 liters per minute

Mask for mask-to-mouth ventilation

Oropharyngeal airways

Laryngoscope with blades (curved and straight, for adult, child, and infant) and extra batteries and bulbs

Assorted adult-size (cuffed) and child-size (uncuffed) endotracheal tubes with stylet and 15-mm/22 adapters

Syringe with clamp or plastic valve for endotracheal tube cuff

Bag-valve-mask with provisions for 100 percent oxygen ventilation

Suction device with catheters

Padded tongue depressors

Needle (12-gauge) for cricothyreotomy

The following equipment is optional:

Oxygen reserve equipment (two E cylinders)
Nasogastric tube
Esophageal obturator airway
Tracheotomy tray

Circulatory Equipment

For management of the circulatory system, the following equipment is essential:

Intravenous infusion sets
Indwelling venous catheters
Intravenous solutions (D5W, lactated Ringer)
Cutdown set
Sterile gloves
Assorted syringes and needles, stopcocks, venous extension tubes

Intracardiac needles
Tourniquets, adhesive tape, disposable razor
Sphygmomanometer, stethoscope
Sterile towels, 4 × 4 gauze pads
The following equipment is optional:
  Portable defibrillator—monitor with ECG electrode—
    defibrillator paddles or portable D.C. defibrillator
    and portable ECG monitor

Portable ECG machine, direct writing, with connection to monitor
Central venous pressure catheters
Urinary catheters
Thoracotomy tray

Interventional Pain Procedures for Cancer Pain

3

Phillip Phan, Allen W. Burton

EVALUATION OF CANCER PAIN

Epidemiology

The diagnosis of cancer is distressing to the patient. In the first place, the patient fears that cancer will shorten his or her life. Second, equally as distressing, the patient is apprehensive that the cancer will bring with its progression significant pain and suffering. Indeed, pain has already been experienced by 20–50% of cancer patients at the time of diagnosis. With cancer progression, 75% of patients with advanced cancer will experience pain (1). As many as 80% of cancer patients describe their pain as having moderate to severe intensity.

According to the World Health Organization (WHO), an estimated 6.6 million people worldwide die from cancer every year (2,3). The recent WHO studies pointed out that cancer-related pain continued to be a significant global health concern (2). With advances in therapeutic modalities, about 90% of cancer pain can be controlled easily (4). Unfortunately, even with these advances, cancer pain remains widely undertreated, even in developed countries (5,6). In the United States, the reasons for undertreatment of cancer pain are complex and encompass many barriers, as outlined in Table 3–1.

In recent years, awareness has grown that pain control is an essential part of comprehensive cancer care. Some studies have shown a direct correlation between good pain control and the cancer patient's length of survival as well as responsiveness to timely oncologic treatment (7,8). In addition to

problems stemming from immobility (deep venous thrombosis, pneumonia), uncontrolled pain has also proved to be a major risk factor in cancer-related suicides (9,10).

Etiology

Pain in the cancer patient can have many causes. The large majority of cancer pain is a result of tumor invasion of pain-sensitive structures. This invasion causes a derangement of physiologic processes, including inflammation, edema, and necrosis of pain-sensitive tissues. Further pathologic processes may include invasion of bone or soft tissues, obstruction of lymphatic or vascular vessels, distention of hollow organs, distortion of solid organs, and compression of nervous system structures.

A significant source of pain can also be related to the treatment of cancer itself. Chemotherapy is often associated with sequelae of chronic painful peripheral neuropathy, vascular necrosis of femoral or humoral head, and plexopathy associated with intra-arterial infusion. Radiation treatment may also cause plexopathy, chronic radiation myelopathy, chronic radiation enteritis and proctitis, as well as osteoradionecrosis.

Surgical treatment can cause postoperative pain syndromes. For example, the postradical mastectomy patient often has pain to posterior upper arm, axilla, and anterior chest wall secondary to damage of the intercostobrachial nerve. Similarly, nerve damage during thoracotomy and radical neck dissection can cause pain in the distribution of the affected nerves. Phantom limb pain is especially

TABLE 3-1
BARRIERS TO EFFECTIVE CANCER PAIN CONTROL

I. Barriers by health-care providers
   A. Inadequate assessment by physicians
   B. Lack of knowledge regarding current treatments by providers
   C. Outdated beliefs by practitioners
      1. Cancer pain expected with disease progression
      2. Opioids prescribed only for dying patients
      3. Patient's pain complaints unreliable
   D. Reluctance to prescribe opioids by physicians
      1. Fear of regulatory controls
      2. Fear of increasing liability for overprescribing
      3. Increased work and effort for opioid management
II. Patient- and family-related barriers
   A. Fear of developing addiction to "narcotics"
   B. Reluctance to discuss pain with physician
   C. Fear of acknowledging pain as a disease progression
III. Barriers from health-care system
   A. Lack of coordination for effective treatment of pain
   B. Inadequate resources for dedicated pain treatment

common after an amputation procedure, with burning and cramping sensations in the area of the amputated limb.

Cancer Pain Classification

In assessment of cancer pain, an understanding of pain classification is helpful in delineating both the mechanism of pain and its responsiveness to therapeutic interventions. Pain can be classified broadly into nociceptive and neuropathic pain. Nociceptive pain occurs when non-neurologic tissues suffer insult or injury. The associated neurological structures, however, are not injured and remain functional. Consequently, the injuries of the damaged tissues are detected as noxious stimuli, and these noxious signals are transmitted along the classical pain pathways. The pain perceived by the central nervous system (CNS) is proportional to degree of tissue damage caused by the cancer. This type of pain experienced by the patient is responsive to nonsteroidal anti-inflammatory drugs (NSAIDs) because tissue damage from cancer inevitably initiates activation of cellular phospholipase A2 (PLA2) to release arachidonic acids (AA) from cell lipid membrane. Cyclooxygenase enzymes COX-1 and COX-2 then act on AA to produce potent inflammatory mediators such as thromboxanes, prostaglandins, and leukotrienes. NSAIDs, including COX1 inhibitors and COX2 inhibitors, attenuate this initial inflammatory reaction at the site of the tissue damaged by cancer and thus reduce the initial pain signals.

Opiate therapy is also effective in helping to control nociceptive pain. Opioid analgesics act on pain receptors at the level of the spinal cord and in the brain to modulate pain pathways in the central nervous system. Nociceptive pain responds to opioids in a scaled manner such that pain control is proportional to opioid dosage.

Nociceptive pain can be categorized further into nociceptive somatic pain and nociceptive visceral pain. Nociceptive somatic pain results from activation of nociceptive receptors in somatic tissues (11). These nociceptors are sensitive to mechanical, chemical, and thermal stimuli. They are located in skin, bone, muscle, tendon, joint, and connective tissues. The pain signals from these nociceptors are carried along sensory nerve fibers. The patient's perception of nociceptive somatic pain is characterized typically as aching, dull, sharp, throbbing, and well localized to the injured tissue site.

Nociceptive visceral pain, in contrast, is poorly localized and diffuse (12). It originates typically from solid organs of the chest, abdomen, and pelvis. The nociceptive receptors in these solid organs typically do not respond to cutting or burning stimuli. They are, however, extremely sensitive to any mechanical stress or torsion of organs as well as tension or traction on mesenteric or vascular attachments to organs. The visceral nociceptive pain signals are carried by autonomic sympathetic fibers. The pain is poorly localized by the patient and often described as a vague, dull, aching, or pressurelike pain. The patient often perceives this nociceptive visceral pain as a referred pain that is falsely localizing to a distant site. For example, pancreatic cancer pain often presents as a referred midback pain, and cancer involvement of the diaphragm causes pain in the right shoulder.

The second major class of cancer pain is neuropathic pain. This pain differs from nociceptive pain in that the cancer causes direct injury to the neural tissues (13). Tumor destruction of peripheral nerves will cause abnormal and exaggerated pain signal transmission. Tumor invasion of the peripheral or central nervous system results in abnormal pain signal processing, integration, and perception. The cancer patient often reports extraordinary pain perception, with pain feeling different from the usual pain sensation. Neuropathic pain is often described as diffuse, excessively sensitive (hyperesthesia) pain even with nonnoxious stimuli (dysesthesia). Neuropathic pain is poorly responsive to opioid analgesics and instead requires adjuvant medications and interventional therapy for effective pain control.

Assessment of Cancer Pain

Clinical assessment of pain condition is an essential first step in pain diagnosis. This assessment entails a thorough history and physical exam. Pain history should include details about the pain onset, location, quality, intensity, and duration. The cancer history regarding cancer diagnosis, cancer staging, disease progression, and treatment plan is important. Information about prior treatment of pain, that is, types of medication, is helpful in understanding pain condition. Ancillary laboratory and imaging studies are helpful in assessing the causes of pain and determining an appropriate course of treatment.

The initial physical exam of the patient includes a basic comprehensive exam with special focus on the cancer site as well as the pain location. A complete neurological examination is valuable in finding any cancer involvement of the peripheral or central nervous system. Direct tumor invasion or compression of neurological structures is common with advanced cancer and is often painful. The physical exam helps to reveal the extent of anatomic spread of tumor and the overall physical condition of the patient.

In addition to evaluating the pain symptom, the physician has to focus on a myriad of related symptoms. The cancer patient often experiences fatigue, insomnia, depression, anxiety, somnolence, and even cognitive impairment. The psychosocial symptoms such as anxiety and depression can often have a large impact on the patient's perception and expression of pain. Furthermore, the patient can develop symptoms from side effects of therapeutic intervention such as nausea, vomiting, and headaches. The cancer patient thus commonly presents with a constellation of symptoms that has a profound impact on the patient's psychological well-being, functional status, and quality of life. Any treatment plan for pain must take into consideration these factors. A multimodalities approach treatment of cancer pain is therefore necessary.

PHARMACOLOGIC THERAPY

WHO Guidelines

As discussed earlier, the barriers to effective pain control are multifold. As a result, clinicians have traditionally undertreated cancer pain. There is a growing awareness in the medical community about the problem of undertreating pain. Consequently, the World Health Organization (WHO) and the American Pain Society have established guidelines for treatment of cancer pain (2,14). Although too simple to serve as a treatment algorithm, the principle of treating more resistant cancer-related pain with stronger/higher doses of opioids is generally sound. See Table 3–2.

Nonopioid Analgesics

The nonopioid class of analgesics includes both acetaminophen and nonsteroidal anti-inflammatory drugs (NSAIDs). Nonopioids are commonly used for mild cancer pain, as directed by the WHO analgesic ladder. Even in the patient with advanced cancer, nonopioid analgesics combined with opioid analgesics are effective in treating pain at both central and peripheral sites. Nonopioids help to reduce the dosage requirement of opioids, thus decreasing the opioid-associated side effects of nausea, constipation, somnolence, and cognitive impairment. Nonopioid analgesics must be used with caution, if at all, in the cancer patient who is immunosuppressed. Both acetaminophen and NSAIDs can suppress a fever response indicative of a mounting infection in the immunocompromised patient, that is, while the patient is undergoing immunosuppressive chemotherapy.

Adjuvant Medications

The heterogeneous class of adjuvant medications has a defined role in the WHO three-step analgesic ladder. Adjuvant medications fall into five general categories: antidepressants, anticonvulsants, oral local anesthetics, corticosteroids, and miscellaneous (Table 3–3).

These adjuvant medications act to promote certain desirable effects (or prevent opioid-related side effects) in the cancer patient. Tricyclic antidepressants are useful in certain types of neuropathic pain, especially burning dysesthetic pain. They have a significant side effect of sedation at high dosage. Consequently, they can be helpful in the cancer pain patient who has insomnia and depression. Anticonvulsants and local anesthetics have a membrane-stabilizing effect and are extremely effective in neuropathic pain secondary to nerve injury in both peripheral and central nervous systems. Corticosteroids have a potent anti-inflammatory effect and thus are helpful in cancer patients with spinal cord compression, intracranial tumors, organ capsule distention, and bone infiltration. Steroids also have a CNS effect in improvement of mood and sense of well-being in the cancer patient. Anti-emetics and stool softeners should routinely be prescribed along with opioids. The other miscellaneous adjuvant medications have variable effects and are tailored to the patient's individual pain and associated symptoms.

Opioid Analgesics

Opioid analgesics are a mainstay of treatment for cancer pain. In the WHO three-step analgesic ladder, "weak" opioids are recommended for treatment of moderate cancer pain, and "strong" opioids are prescribed for severe cancer

---

TABLE 3–2

THE WHO THREE-STEP ANALGESIC LADDER FOR CANCER PAIN

Step 1: Mild cancer pain	→	Nonopiod analgesics	±Adjuvant medications
Step 2: Moderate cancer pain	→	"Weak" opioids	±Nonopiod analgesics
			±Adjuvant medications
Step 3: Severe cancer pain	→	"Strong" opioids	±Nonopiod analgesics
			±Adjuvant medications

TABLE 3-3

ADJUVANT DRUGS FOR TREATMENT OF CANCER PAIN

I. Antidepressants:

Amitriptyline	Doxepin
Nortriptyline	Maprotiline
Imipramine	Paroxetine
Desipramine	Venlafaxine

II. Anticonvulsants:

Gabapentin	Valproic Acid
Carbamazepine	Clonazepam
Phenytoin	Topirimate

III. Local Anesthetics:

Mexiletine	Topical lidocaine

IV. Corticosteroids:

Dexamethasone	Prednisolone
Methylprednisolone	Cortisone

V. Miscellaneous:
Psychostimulants—Dextroamphetamine, methylphenidate
GABA-agonist—Baclofen
α-2 antagonist—Clonidine
NMDA-antagonist—Ketamine
Anti-emetics*—metocopramide, ondnsetron
Laxatives/stool softeners*—senna, docusate

*Recommended in all patients receiving opioids

pain. The weak opioids have less potency and also fewer side effects. Table 3–4 lists some common oral weak opioids.

These weak opioids are produced with acetaminophen or aspirin. They are weak because of the limitation of their ceiling dose of acetaminophen or aspirin, above which the patient has a higher risk of renal toxicity and hepatotoxicity.

The strong opioids are more potent because they are made in pure form, without the addition of aspirin or acetaminophen. These opioids thus do not have a maximum ceiling dose. However, at a higher dosage of these strong opioids, the patient tends to experience more significant side effects of nausea and vomiting, constipation, pruritis, somnolence, and cognitive impairment. Table 3–5 lists some common strong opioids.

Failure of Noninterventional Therapies

It has been estimated that as many as 70–90% of patients with cancer pain have satisfactory pain relief

TABLE 3-4

"WEAK" OPIOIDS FOR TREATMENT OF MODERATE CANCER PAIN

Generic Name	Examples
Hydrocodone	Lortab, Vicoden, Lorcet, Norco
Codeine	Tylenol no. 3, no. 4
Propoxyphene	Darvon, Darvocet

TABLE 3-5

"STRONG" OPIOIDS FOR TREATMENT OF SEVERE CANCER PAIN

Generic Name	Examples
Morphine/MS-CR	MSIR, MSContin, Oromorph, Kadian, Avinza
Oxycodone/oxycodone-CR	Roxicodone, Oxycontin
Fentanyl	Duragesic(time-release transdermal), Actiq (PO, immediate release)
Hydromorphone	Dilaudid
Methadone	Dolophine
Oxymorphone	Numorphan

from pharmacologic therapies alone, following the WHO guidelines for cancer pain (15). This, however, means that 10–30% of these patients have pain that cannot be treated with medications alone. The reasons for this failure of pharmacologic treatment are variable (16). They vary from physician-related factors to patient-related factors. The physician-related reasons for pharmacologic failure include inaccurate assessment of pain and deficiency in knowledge of current analgesics and adjuvant medications. Patient-related reasons range from fear of addiction to adverse side effects (17,18). Most commonly, the patient cannot tolerate adverse side effects of the medication regimen, especially with opioid use (18). Failure of pharmacologic control of cancer pain is also commonly seen with progression of cancer. The patients with advanced disease can present with intractable pain from multiple metastases and multiple pain sites.

INTERVENTIONAL THERAPIES

Goal of Intervention

Patients who fail to respond to conservative pharmacologic treatments may be candidates for interventional therapies. A large armamentarium of invasive procedures is available to achieve better control of cancer pain. However, the role of interventional therapies must be placed in the proper context. They cannot be employed as the sole treatment for cancer pain, especially for advanced cancer patients. Rather, they should be used as part of a multimodal approach in the treatment of cancer pain (19,20). As discussed previously, the etiologies of cancer pain are diverse, and the pain symptom is interrelated with the constellation of symptoms experienced by cancer patients. Consequently, a global multimodal approach to the treatment of cancer pain is necessary. Such an approach includes the appropriate antineoplastic therapy, management of analgesics and adjuvant pain medications, behavioral and psychiatric support, and, finally, interventional therapies. Interventional pain procedures will not completely eliminate the need for pain medications. The therapeutic goal of such procedures is to help alleviate cancer pain, reduce the overall analgesic need, and thereby minimize associated opioid-related side effects.

Communication

Prior to proceeding with any invasive pain intervention procedure, communication among the pain physician and the relevant parties is absolutely essential. The patient must first be educated about the risks and benefits of the interventional procedure. He or she must be allowed an opportunity to have any questions about the procedure extensively and satisfactorily answered. The patient, at the same time, must be grounded in realistic expectations in terms of outcomes from the procedure. The patient should be made aware of the efficacy of the procedure, its duration of effectiveness, and the possibility of failure of the procedure to provide complete or even partial pain relief. All the potential complications from the procedure are explained to the patient. The patient must understand that the interventional procedure is part of a multimodal approach for pain control.

With cancer patients, especially those who are critically ill or preterminal, family members and caregivers are often involved in decision-making processes. Family support helps the patient cope emotionally with the cancer disease as well as with undergoing the procedural intervention. Like the patient, the family must also be educated and have realistic expectations about the procedure.

Effective communication with other professional members of the care team is also important. Other members of the team include the patient's oncologists, primary-care providers, and all the relevant consultants. Treatment of cancer is a multidisciplinary effort. The interventional procedure should be planned in coordination with the overall cancer treatment. For example, the cancer patient may undergo chemotherapy with resultant thrombocytopenia. In such a case, the interventional procedure must be carried out prior to chemoinduction or afterward, when the patient's platelet count has normalized. Typically, other members of the patient's care team are informed about the planned interventional procedure and given a chance to voice any input or concern.

Detailed Physical Exam

A thorough physical examination of the patient prior to the procedure is also critical. This entails a complete neurological evaluation. Interventional procedures for pain control are invasive and involve neurologically sensitive tissues such as nerves and central nervous system structures. The objective of intervention is to disrupt or modulate pain pathways involved in nociception. Interventional procedures such as neurolysis of peripheral nerves will not only block pain transmission but also block sensory and motor innervations as well. Consequently, it is important to document before and after the procedure a complete and thorough physical exam with the focus especially on pain and neurological changes. Changes such as sensory and motor blockade are closely monitored after procedures.

Categories of Interventional Techniques

Interventional therapies can be categorized into three groups: neurolytic techniques, neuromodulation techniques, and surgical techniques. Neurolytic or neuroablation techniques are procedures that target destruction of nerves or neural structures that are involved in generation or transmission of pain signals. Neurolytic lesions can be created by a variety of agents. Lysis is achieved with chemicals (glycerol, alcohol, or phenol), heat (radiofrequency coagulation), or cold (cryotherapy).

Neuromodulation techniques have as their basis Wall and Melzack's gate control theory of pain (21). This theory proposes that all nerve fiber endings except those that innervate hair cells are alike and that suprathreshold stimulation of these nonspecific receptors initiates pain signals. According to Melzack and Wall, substantia gelatinosa functions as a primary gatekeeper in the transmission of pain from the periphery to the central nervous system (21). Neuromodulative techniques aim at modulation of pain signals along the transmission pathway. These techniques include local anesthetic blockade; regional infusion of drugs at epidural, intrathecal, intraventricular, or perineural sites; and electrical stimulation of the central nervous system.

Surgical techniques are the third class of interventional pain procedures. These surgical procedures range from the minimally invasive percutaneous vertebroplasty to the extremely invasive neurosurgical destructive techniques. These neurosurgical techniques include percutaneous cordotomy, thalamotomy, cingulotomy, hypophysectomy, and trigeminal tractomy. Most of these procedures are done stereotactically under monitored anesthesia care (MAC) and fluoroscopy or computerized tomographic (CT) guidance.

NEUROLYTIC PROCEDURES

Over the past century, many chemical and physical ablative techniques have been developed with the goal of disrupting the transmission of pain signals along the neural pathways. Chemical neurolysis is achieved with alcohol (100%), phenol (5–15%), and glycerol. These agents produce nerve injury, resulting in degeneration of nerve fiber distal to the lysis lesion (Wallerian degeneration) (22). This disrupts the nerve cell transmission of pain and results in a nociceptive block. However, with Wallerian degeneration, the nerve axon can begin to regenerate within 3 months. Thus, chemical neurolysis provides a temporary block of nociception for about 1–3 months (23).

Alcohol is the chemical that has been classically used in neurolysis in the past (24). Many clinicians today favor use of phenol for peripheral neurolysis because it is less neurotoxic than alcohol (25). Alcohol is used in concentrations up to 100%. It causes nonselective destruction of all nerves as well as surrounding soft tissues. Alcohol is rapidly soluble in blood and is hypobaric relative to cerebrospinal fluid (CSF). If injected into intraspinal space, it will rise rapidly, diffusing away from the initial injection site. Specifically, it damages nerves by extracting fatty substances and precipitating proteins in the nerve axon, resulting in Wallerian degeneration (26). This injury is proportional to both the concentration and volume of alcohol used. There is a higher risk of neuritis associated with alcohol injection (27). Also, patients often experience intense burning pain initially with alcohol injection.

Phenol, now more commonly used, is associated with a lower risk of neuritis (27). Phenol at a 5% concentration is equivalent to alcohol at a 40% concentration in neurolytic potency (28). Phenol is less water soluble than alcohol and thus tends to concentrate more around the injection site. It is diffusible, able to penetrate neural axon and denature proteins, causing Wallerian degeneration (27). Many clinicians prefer phenol because the intensity and duration of neural blockade are less with phenol and thus provide a wider margin of safety.

Less commonly used is glycerol in peripheral neural blockade. It is used primarily for treatment of trigeminal neuralgia. It is injected directly into the trigeminal cistern (Meckel's cave) with good efficacy in blocking trigeminal neuralgia. Other neurolytic chemicals that have been tried in the past include ammonium salt compounds and hypertonic and hypotonic saline solutions, all with variable results (27).

Radiofrequency thermocoagulation is also employed to produce a physical nociceptive block. The lesion created by radiofrequency heating is discreet, and size of lesion is controlled by the temperature of the probe and duration of application (29). Some studies have showed that radiofrequency ablation can produce a longer-lasting block (30).

Cryotherapy can also be used in achieving neurolytic lesioning. Applying extreme cold to the nerve will result in a long-lasting nerve blockade. Cryoneurolysis of intercostal nerves intraoperatively has been reported with good efficacy in controlling postthoracotomy pain (31). Wide application of cryoablation has been hindered by the large size of the probe and relative complexity of the equipment involved.

Patient selection for chemical neurolysis, radiofrequency ablation, and cryoneurolysis is extremely important in achieving the desired outcome. The patient should have an advanced progressive cancer and a limited life expectancy (6–12 months). The pain should be severe, persistent, refractory to conservative treatment, and consistent

---

TABLE 3–6

POTENTIAL RISKS WITH NEUROABLATION TECHNIQUES

Dysesthetic pain—Painful neuralgia as a result of deafferenation, neuritis, or neuroma formation
Tissue damage—Accidental injury to nontargeted neurologic and nonneurologic tissues
Motor paralysis—Especially with intrathecal neurolysis
Sensory deficit—Areas of parasthesia or numbness
Failure to relieve pain—As a result of incomplete ablation or incorrect nerve target
Short-term pain relief—As a result of central nervous system plasticity, axonal regrowth, or tumor progression

---

with a nociceptive somatic or visceral pain. Neuropathic pain usually does not respond well to neuroablation therapy. There are potential risks associated with neuroablation, as outlined in Table 3–6.

Despite the inherent risks of neuroablation, patients with advanced cancer and well-localized nociceptive pain can benefit greatly from neurolytic blockade. Peripheral neurolysis has alleviated suffering of cancer patients with intractable pain (32). Regional blocks are extremely useful in disrupting pain signals transmitted along the sympathetic and parasympathetic nerves.

Neural Blockade in Head and Neck

More than 40,000 patients are diagnosed with head and neck cancer each year in the United States, and more than 500,000 are diagnosed worldwide (33). Cancer of head and neck constitutes about 5% of all malignant diseases in the United States and affects about 6.6 million worldwide (34). Because of dense facial and neck innervations, cancer commonly causes not only disfiguring facial lesions but also disabling pain in the face and neck. Blocking relevant trigeminal nerve or cervical nerve branches can control such pain. Efficacy of interventional nerve block, however, can be affected by tumor distortion of anatomy, radiation-induced fibrosis of local tissues, and possible overlapping sensory innervations of neighboring cranial nerves V, VII, IX, X, and the upper cervical nerves. Careful evaluation of facial pain and proper selection of nerve block will provide patients with relief.

Trigeminal Nerve Block

Indications: Blockade of trigeminal ganglion or specific branches of trigeminal nerves will alleviate somatic and neuropathic pain from cancer.

Anatomy: The trigeminal or gasserian ganglion is formed from two nerve roots that arise from the ventral pons of the brainstem. These roots fuse anteriorly and enter the Meckel's cave, a recess in the middle cranial

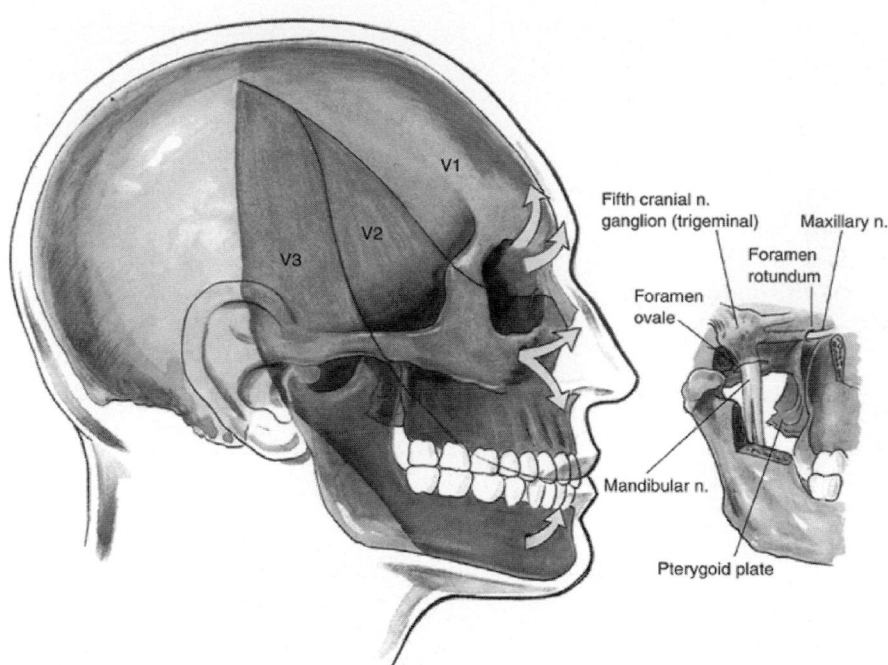

Figure 3–1   Trigeminal nerves and corresponding distribution of V1, V2, and V3. Reproduced with permission from Brown DL. Atlas of Regional Anesthesia. Philadelphia: W.B. Saunders, 1999:149.

fossa. Three sensory divisions then exit anteriorly as the ophthalmic nerve (V1), the maxillary nerve (V2), and the mandibular nerve (V3) (Figure 3–1). Destruction of the gasserian ganglion is useful in intractable pain from invasive tumors of the orbit, maxillary sinus, and mandible (35). Conversely, each individual sensory nerve can be blocked separately if selective blockade is desired.

Techniques: The patient is placed in a supine position, with cervical spine extended on a foam pad or pillow. The cheek skin is prepped with betadine sterilely and then anesthesized with 1% lidocaine at 2.5 cm just lateral to the corner of the mouth. Using C-arm fluoroscopic guidance, a 3.5-inch 20-gauge spinal needle is advanced slowly through the anesthesized skin area, just 2.5 cm from the corner of the lips. The direction of the spinal needle should be cranial, dorsal, and medial with the foramen ovale as the target (Figure 3–2). It may be easier to have the patient gaze straight ahead and then aim the needle in the cephalad direction perpendicular to the midpupillary line. The needle is directed through the pterygopalatine fossa until it reaches the skull base. Then it is walked posteriorly into the foramen ovale. Once the needle enters the foramen ovale, its tip should be located within the Meckel's cave. Careful aspiration of the needle is important to ensure that the needle tip is not in any vascular structure. A sterile solution of 100% alcohol (0.5 mL) is used to achieve neurolysis.

Complications: Inadvertent dural puncture can lead to neurotoxicity, including seizure and death. When the needle is directed through the pterygopalatine fossa, injury to vascular vessels can result in facial hematoma or ocular subscleral hematoma. Postprocedure neuritis can cause significant dysthetic pain in trigeminal sensory areas. Masticator weakness is also possible with trigeminal block.

Occipital Nerve Block

Indications: Occipital nerve block is effective in treating oncologic pain in the posterior scalp and occipital region.

Anatomy: Most of the posterior scalp is innervated by the greater occipital nerve, which arises from the dorsal rami of the C2 nerve root. It emerges subcutaneously in the posterior scalp just slightly inferior to the superior nuchal line and 2–3 cm lateral to the greater occipital protuberance (Figure 3–3). At this point of emergence, it is just medial to the occipital artery (36).

Techniques: The patient is placed in a sitting position, with neck slightly flexed. The greater occipital protuberance and the mastoid process are palpated, and at one-third the distance between these two structures, the greater occipital artery can also be palpated (3–4 cm lateral to the greater occipital protuberance on the superior nuchal line). The greater occipital nerve lies just medial to the greater occipital artery. It can be blocked at this site with local anesthetic or neurolytic injection.

The skin is cleaned with betadine in a sterile manner. A short 1-inch 25-gauge needle is introduced after the skin is infiltrated with local 1% lidocaine.

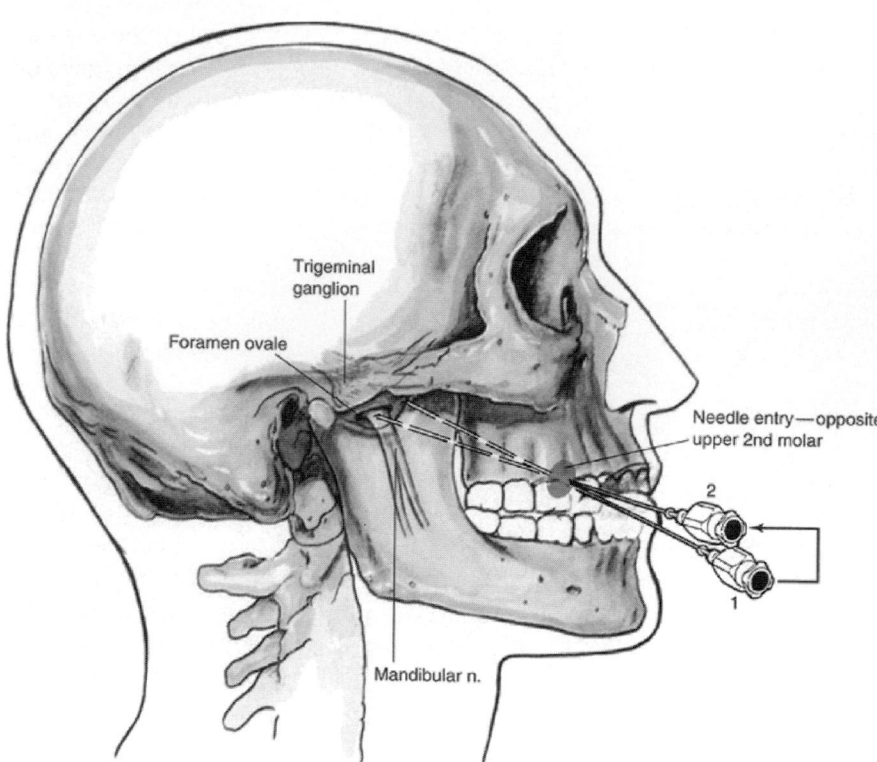

Figure 3–2 Trigeminal nerve block with needle targeting foramen ovale. Reproduced with permission from Brown DL. Atlas of Regional Anesthesia. Philadelphia: W.B. Saunders, 1999:153.

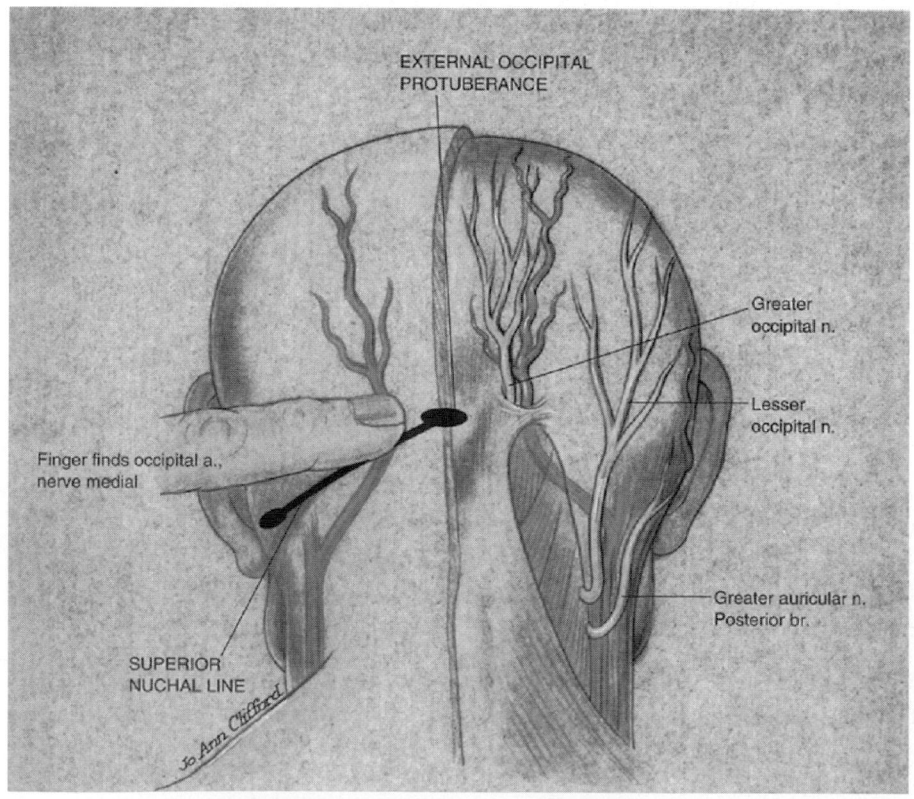

Figure 3–3 Occipital nerve in relationship to occipital artery. Reproduced with permission from Brown DL. Atlas of Regional Anesthesia. Philadelphia: W.B. Saunders, 1999:147.

The bony contact is made at minimal depth of about 2–3 mm. A diagnostic block with 1–2 mL of local anesthetic (1% lidocaine) can be injected. For neurolytic block, a volume of 3–5 mL is used.

Complications: Because of the superficial location of the greater occipital nerve and relative ease of this block, complications are minimal. The close proximity of the greater occipital artery may increase the risk of intravascular injection, which can be avoided by frequent aspiration while slowly injecting the neurolytic solution. Neuritis can also occur with neurolyic agents, especially with alcohol.

Superficial Cervical Plexus Block

Indications: Superficial cervical plexus block is often used to treat cancer pain in the dermatome of the neck innervated by the cervical plexus.

Anatomy: The superficial and deep cervical plexus arises from the first four cervical nerves (Figure 3–4). The cervical plexus lies just lateral to the first cervical vertebrae. It is located anterior to the levator scapulae and middle scalene muscles and posterior to the sternocleidomastoid (SCM) muscle. The plexus gives off both superficial sensory branches and deep motor braches. This anatomic division of sensory and motor nerves allows for selective sensory blockade of the superficial sensory branches of the cervical plexus without compromising the motor function of the neck muscles.

These superficial branches arise from the plexus and pierce the deep fascia of the neck at the posterior border of the SCM muscle. It is at this point, where the bundle of the superficial cervical plexus emerges, that sensory innervation to the plexus can be blocked easily (37). The superficial cervical plexus gives rise to the sensory nerves that supply sensation to the skin and superficial fascia of the head, neck, and shoulder. These nerves include the lesser occipital nerve, the greater auricular nerve, the accessory nerve, the anterior cervical nerve, and the suprascapular nerve (38).

Techniques: The patient is placed in supine position, with head turned away from the site to be blocked. The mastoid process is identified with the attached

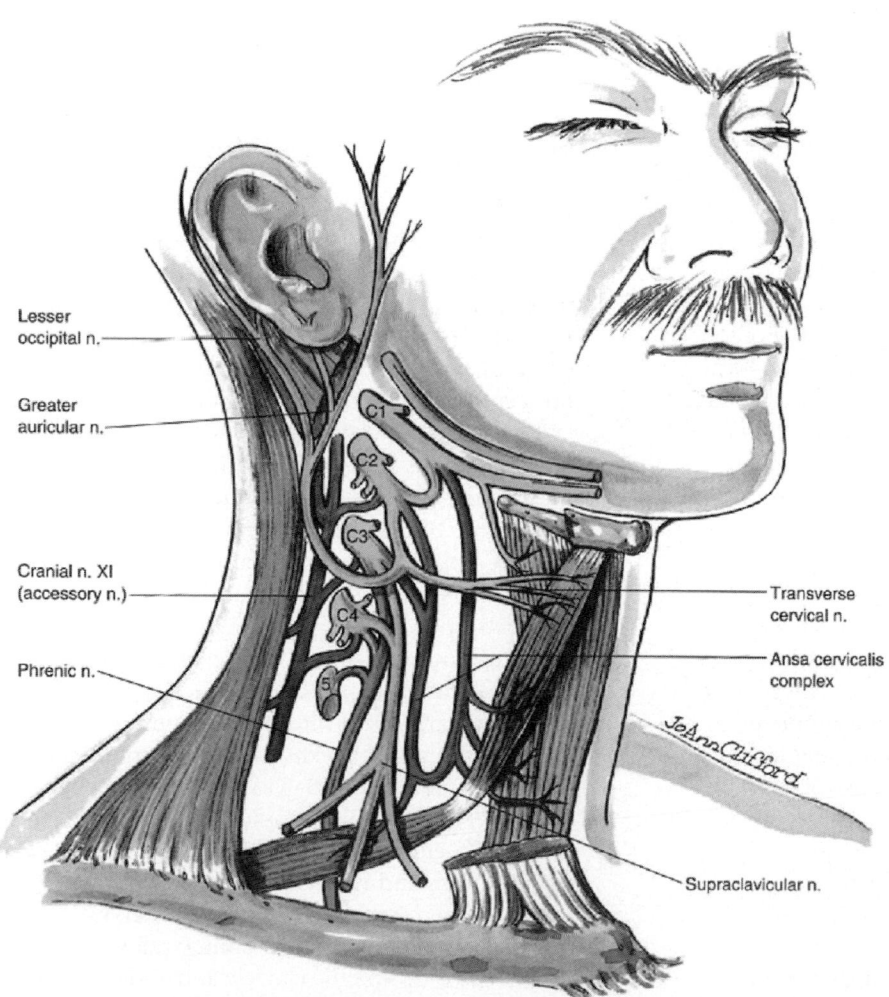

Lesser occipital n.

Greater auricular n.

Cranial n. XI (accessory n.)

Phrenic n.

C1

C2

C3

C4

5

Transverse cervical n.

Ansa cervicalis complex

Supraclavicular n.

Figure 3–4 Superficial and deep cervical plexus arising from the first four cervical nerves. Reproduced with permission from Brown DL. Atlas of Regional Anesthesia. Philadelphia: W.B. Saunders, 1999:182.

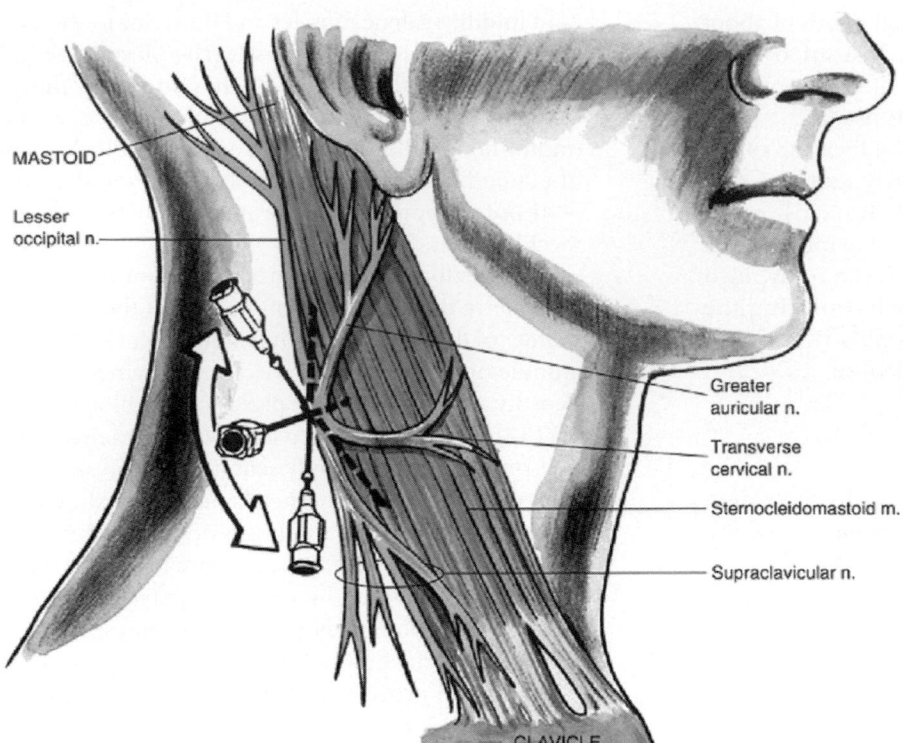

MASTOID

Lesser occipital n.

Greater auricular n.

Transverse cervical n.

Sternocleidomastoid m.

Supraclavicular n.

CLAVICLE

Figure 3–5 Superficial cervical plexus block as it arises at the posterior border of the SCM muscle. Reproduced with permission from Brown DL. Atlas of Regional Anesthesia. Philadelphia: W.B. Saunders, 1999:185.

SCM muscle. The patient may have to raise the head slightly to allow for identification of the SCM muscle. The neck is prepped with betadine in a sterile manner. At the midpoint just lateral to the SCM muscle, a 1-inch, 25-gauge needle is inserted subcutaneously. A volume of 5 mL of local anesthetic (1% lidocaine) is injected subcutaneously at this midpoint (Figure 3–5). The needle is then directed superiorly and inferiorly along the posterior border of the SCM muscle. A total volume of 10–20 mL of local anesthetic can be injected to achieve a diagnostic block. If this is successful, it can be followed with neurolytic agents to achieve a longer blockade. A note of caution is that the external jugular vein crosses the midpoint of the lateral border of the SCM muscle. Careful aspiration prior to infiltration is helpful to avoid intravascular injection (39).

Complications: Few complications occur with this superficial cervical block. The most common complication is intravascular injection into the external or internal jugular vein, with resulting system toxicity. Also, placement of the needle into the jugular vein may result in hematoma or even air embolism.

Neural Blockade of Upper Extremity

Brachial Plexus Block

Indications: Malignancy can involve the upper extremity. Such cancer includes sarcoma of bone as well as soft

tissue sarcoma. In the United States, almost 13,000 new cases of bony sarcoma are diagnosed each year as well as 7,000 new cases of soft tissue sarcomas (40). In most cases, surgical resections of sarcomas with limb-sparing procedures are performed with good result. These patients, however, often have severe pain from direct tumor invasion of a neurovascular bundle or as a consequence of surgical resection of the tumor. Neural blockade of the brachial plexus is effective in controlling somatic nociceptive pain in upper extremity cancer.

For short-term palliation of cancer pain, a brachial plexus block can also be performed with a catheter left in place for continuous infusion of local anesthetic. In cases of severe intractable pain from invasive tumors of the brachial plexus or soft tissues and bone of the shoulder and upper extremity, destruction of the brachial plexus is indicated. The patient should be made aware of the full consequences from neurolysis of the brachial plexus, including paralysis of the upper extremity.

Anatomy: The brachial plexus is formed from fusion of the ventral rami of the C5–T1 nerve roots (Figure 3–6). These nerve roots, with possible contribution from C4 and T2, emerge from the lateral aspect of the vertebral bodies and run laterally and inferiorly in the interscalene compartment. These nerves of the brachial plexus run down the interscalene compartment to pass behind the clavicle and above the top of the first rib and then into the axilla (Figure 3–7).

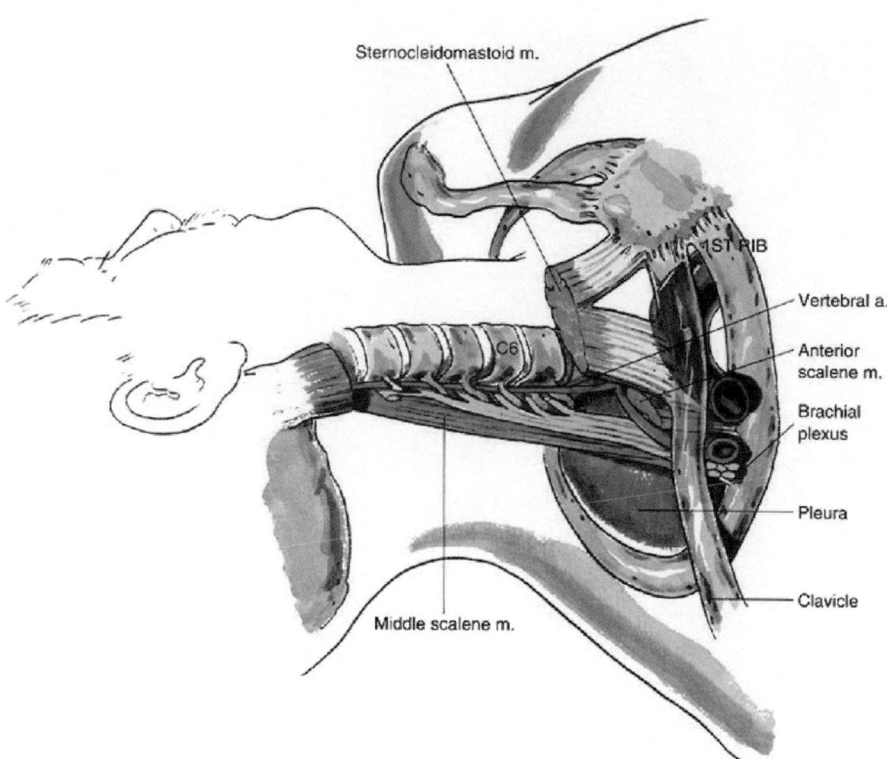

Sternocleidomastoid m.

1ST RIB

Vertebral a.

Anterior
scalene m.

Brachial
plexus

Pleura

Clavicle

C6

Middle scalene m.

Figure 3–6 Brachial plexus formed from fusion of the ventral rami of C5–T1. Reproduced with permission from Brown DL. Atlas of Regional Anesthesia. Philadelphia: W.B. Saunders, 1999:27.

Techniques: The brachial plexus blockade can be approached in a number of ways, including interscalene block, supraclavicular block, and axillary block. In cancer pain from tumor involvement of the shoulder, interscalene block is preferred (41).

The patient is placed in supine position, with head turned away from the site to be blocked. The posterior border of the sternocleidomastoid (SCM) muscle is identified. The patient can cooperate by slightly flexing his or her head. The groove between the posterior border of the SCM muscle and the anterior scalene muscle can be palpated by rolling the fingers posteriorly off the edge of the SCM muscle. The neck is then prepped with betadine in a sterile manner. At the level of the cricoid cartilage (C6) at the interscalene groove, a 1.5-inch, 25-gauge needle is inserted at a slightly caudal and inferior angle (Figure 3–8). The skin is infiltrated with local anesthetic. The needle is then inserted slowly, perpendicular to the skin, until parasthesia of shoulder, arm, or hand is obtained. Such parasthesia is encountered at a needle depth of 3/4–1 inch. Once parasthesia is achieved, the needle is within the brachial plexus. If aspiration is negative for CSF or blood, 30–50 mL of local anesthetic solution can be injected incrementally and with frequent aspiration to rule out intravascular displacement of the needle. Alternatively, a nerve stimulator needle may be used to elicit contraction of arm muscles once the needle is within the brachial plexus compartment. Throughout injection, the patient is monitored for

signs of local anesthetic toxicity or subarachnoid injection.

Once efficacy of local anesthetic blockade in relieving cancer pain has been proved, the patient may wish to proceed with a longer-lasting neurolytic block with phenol. A volume of 20 mL of 6% phenol is slowly injected into the intrascalene compartment of the brachial plexus. Again, motor paralysis of the upper extremity can be expected with this neurolysis of the brachial plexus.

If a shorter prolonged blockade of brachial plexus is desired, a continuous local anesthetic infusion of the brachial plexus can be performed. The infraclavicular approach for this brachial plexus block is preferred because the catheter can remain in the same position for as long as 3 weeks (42). Infraclavicular entry site permits easy catheter threading into the plexus, and the catheter's position is not affected by the patient's movement. For the infraclavicular approach, the patient is placed in supine position with head turned away from the site to be blocked. The clavicle is identified by palpation and by fluoroscopy. The axillary artery is also palpated and marked. The ipsilateral neck, anterior shoulder, and axillary region are prepped with betadine in a sterile manner. At the inferior border of the clavicle at the midpoint, local anesthetic (1% lidocaine) is generously infiltrated subcutaneously. A 16-gauge spinal needle is introduced at this midclavicular point and directed laterally toward the marked axillary artery

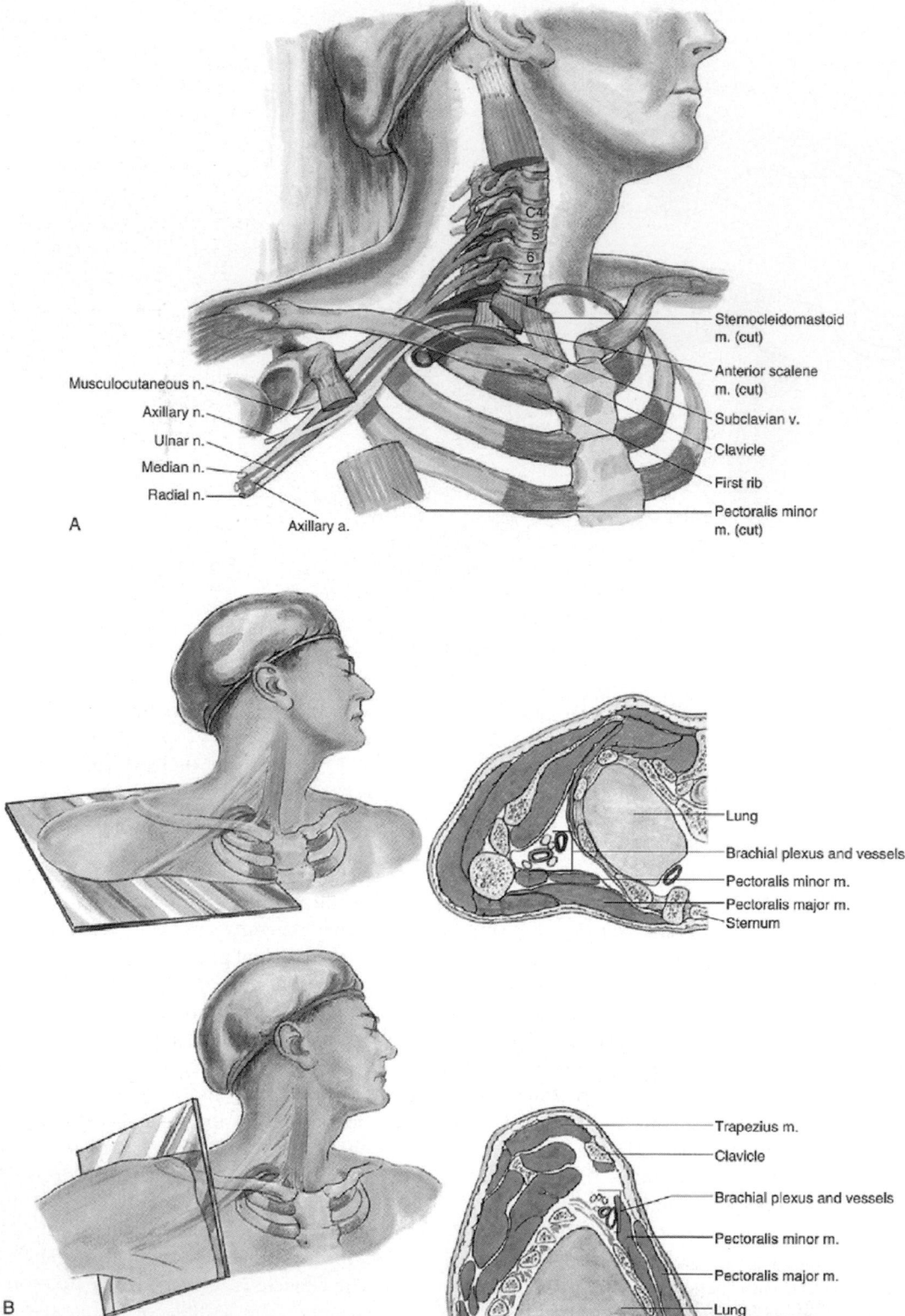

Musculocutaneous n.

Axillary n.

Ulnar n.

Median n.

Radial n.

A

Axillary a.

Sternocleidomastoid m. (cut)

Anterior scalene m. (cut)

Subclavian v.

Clavicle

First rib

Pectoralis minor m. (cut)

Lung

Brachial plexus and vessels

Pectoralis minor m.

Pectoralis major m.

Sternum

Trapezius m.

Clavicle

Brachial plexus and vessels

Pectoralis minor m.

Pectoralis major m.

Lung

B

Figure 3–7   A. Brachial plexus passing behind clavicle, under first rib, and into the axilla. **B.** Cross-sectional views of brachial plexus in the axilla. Reproduced with permission from Brown DL. Atlas of Regional Anesthesia. Philadelphia: W.B. Saunders, 1999:45.

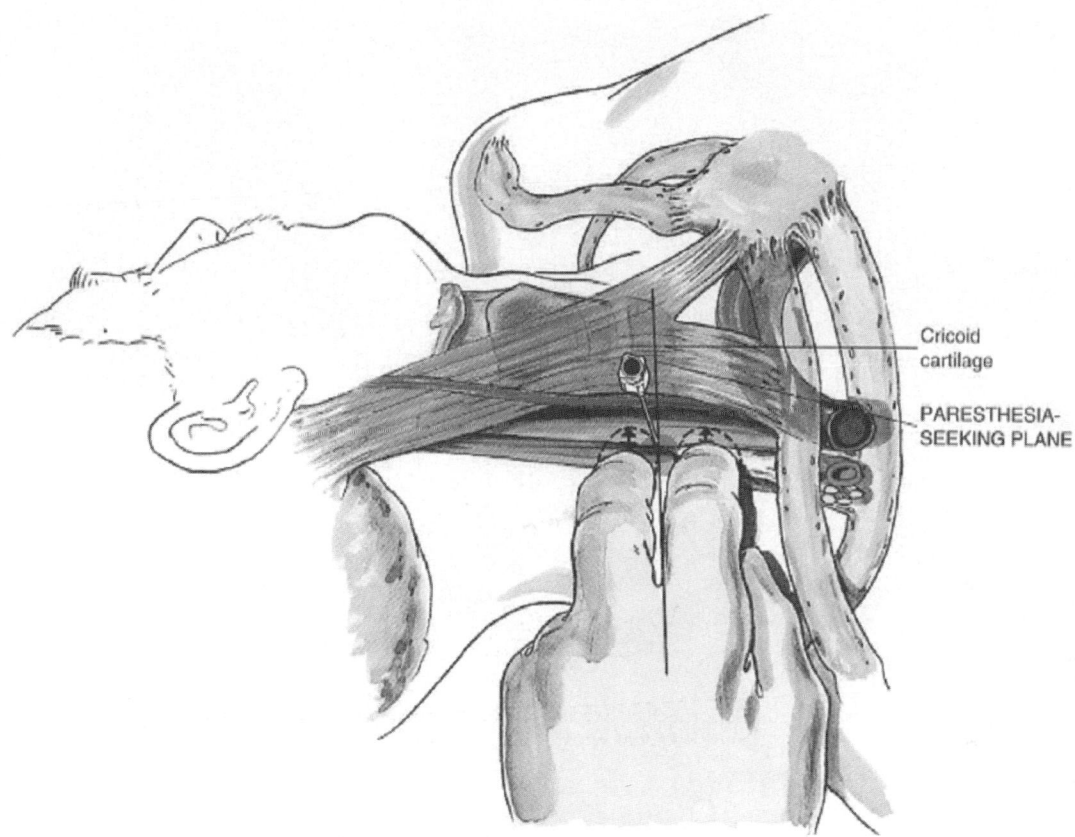

Figure 3–8 Interscalene approach to brachial plexus blockade, with paresthesia achieved once the needle is within the brachial plexus. Reproduced with permission from Brown DL. Atlas of Regional Anesthesia. Philadelphia: W.B. Saunders, 1999:28.

location (Figure 3–9). The needle is directed at a 45-degree angle to the skin and then connected to a nerve stimulator by an alligator clip. As the needle advances, fluoroscopy will allow for visualization of the needle tip. Once the tip enters the brachial plexus, muscles innervated by the plexus will be stimulated, with flexion and extension of elbow, wrist, and fingers visible. At this point, 2–3 mL of contrast dye is injected to confirm under fluoroscopy the spread along the axillary sheath. The catheter is then threaded through the spinal needle and 3–5 cm beyond the tip. The needle is withdrawn, and the catheter is sutured well in place. Infusion of 0.125% or 0.25% bupivacaine is used to provide continuous brachial plexus analgesia. It is effective in controlling somatic pain for several days and sympathetically mediated pain for up to a few weeks.

Complications: Complications from interscalene block are possible because of proximity to many sensitive structures in the neck. Intravascular injection, as mentioned earlier, will lead to systemic toxicity. Subarachnoid injection can cause sensory, motor, and total spinal anesthesia, and even death. Phrenic nerve block is an expected complication of interscalene

block. Ipsilateral phrenic nerve block with hemidiaphragm paralysis is a consideration, especially for patients with respiratory compromise.

Complications from infraclavicular brachial plexus block are similar to those from interscalene block. Proximity to the subclavian artery and vein increases the potential for intravascular injection. The lung apex is also close, so pneumothorax risk is also higher. Probability of phrenic nerve block is lower with an infraclavicular approach, but the risk of recurrent laryngeal nerve blockade and consequent vocal cord paralysis is higher.

Neural Blockade in Thorax

Intercostal Nerve Block

Indications: Lung cancer is the number one cancer killer in both males and females (40). It accounts for 15% of malignant disease in males and 13% in females. Patients diagnosed with lung cancer often require thoracotomy with surgical biopsy or resection of tumor mass. Many such patients experience chest wall pain either from direct tumor involvement of

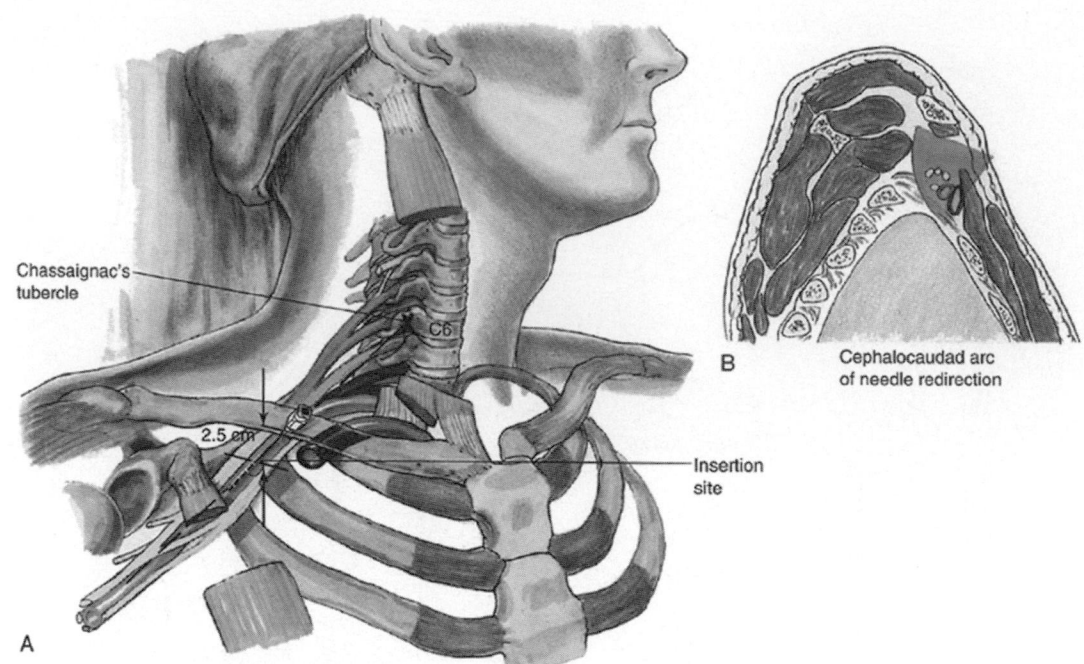

Figure 3–9 Infraclavicular approach to brachial plexus catheter placement. Reproduced with permission from Brown DL. Atlas of Regional Anesthesia. Philadelphia: W.B. Saunders, 1999:47.

the chest wall or from surgical trauma to intercostal nerves. In addition to lung cancer, aggressive breast cancer may also invade ribs and intercostal nerve bundles to cause pain.

Tumor invasion of lung parenchyma and visceral pleura does not cause pain because these are nociceptive-insensitive structures. However, cancer involvement of the parietal pleura will elicit a pain response. Pain is transmitted from the parietal pleura along the somatic nerve, including the intercostal nerves T1–T12. Intercostal nerve blockade is effective in blocking this somatic pain (43).

Anatomy: The intercostal nerves are formed from the ventral rami of the thoracic nerves from T1 through T12 (Figure 3–10). Each nerve, joined by intercostal vein and artery, runs in a neurovascular bundle in the subcostal groove. It gives off four branches as it runs anteriorly in the intercostals space. The first is the gray rami comunicantes, which joins the sympathetic ganglion. The second branch is the posterior cutaneous nerve, which innervates the paravertebral region. The third branch is the lateral cutaneous nerve, which innervates the axillary and lateral chest wall. The fourth is the anterior cutaneous nerve, which innervates the anterior thorax. Considerable sensory overlap occurs among those branches as well as among the intercostal nerves themselves. Thus, pain from one area may require blockade of multiple adjacent intercostal nerves (44).

Techniques: For neurolytic block, the procedure should be performed under fluoroscopic guidance. The patient is placed in a prone position. The relevant ribs are identified by palpation and under fluoroscopy. The inferior border of each rib is marked with a marking pen. The intercostal block is classically performed at the angle of the rib, just lateral to the paraspinal muscle groups. The relevant paraspinal area is prepped with betadine in a sterile manner. The skin is infiltrated subcutaneously with local anesthetic, using a 1-inch, 25-gauge needle (Figure 3–11). By palpation, the clinician should get a gross estimation of the depth from skin to the bone of the rib. The needle is slowly advanced perpendicular to the skin, with fluoroscopic guidance. The C arm should be in anterior-posterior (AP) projection with a caudal tilt. The needle tip should hit the body of the rib and then walk inferiorly off the lower border of the rib into the subcostal groove. Water-soluble contrast dye injected into this groove should show a nice spread along the inferior border of the rib. A neurolytic solution of 10% phenol can be injected, with 3–5 mL for each intercostal block.

Complications: Some common complications with intercostal nerve blockade include pneumothorax and systemic toxicity. Pneumothorax results from needle puncture through parietal and visceral pleura. This will create an air leak from the lung into the pleural space. A simple pneumothorax may progress into a

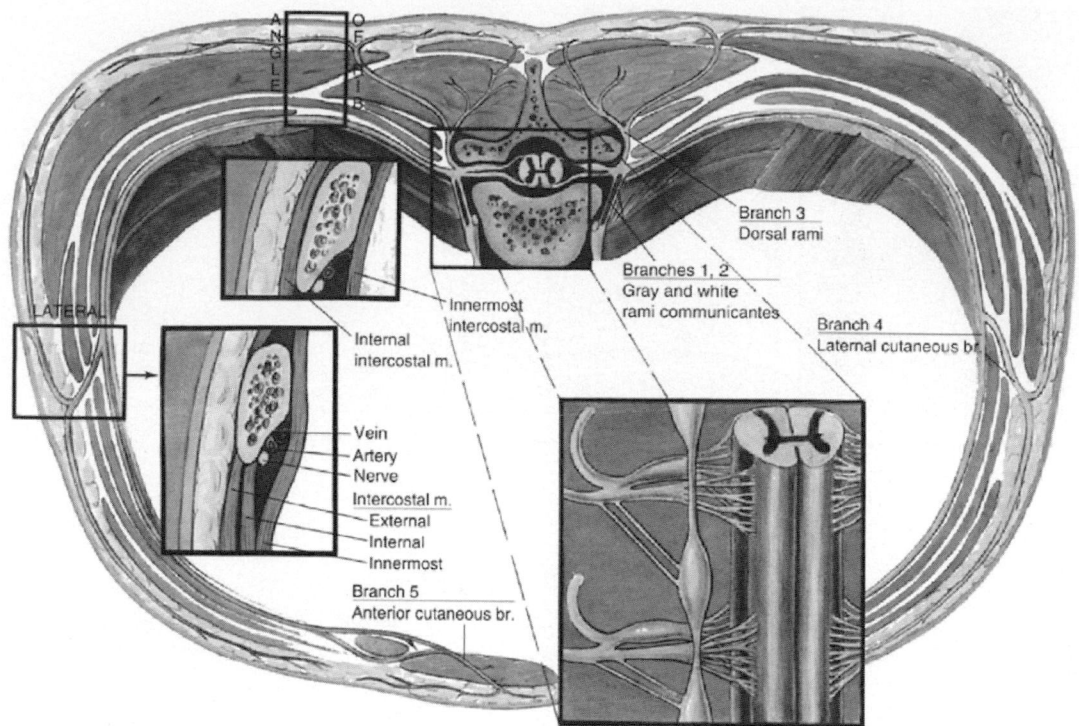

Figure 3–10 Intercostal nerves arising from the spinal cord and giving off peripheral branches. Reproduced with permission from Brown DL. Atlas of Regional Anesthesia. Philadelphia: W.B. Saunders, 1999:242.

tension pneumothorax with its life-threatening implications. The patient should be closely monitored after the procedure, and postprocedure chest radiograph is recommended.

Another complication is systemic toxicity from absorption of anesthetic or neurolytic solution into the intercostal neurovascular bundle. Because of the close proximity of the intercostal artery and vein to the nerve, absorption of injected solution into intercostal space is likely. However, with the small volume used for neurolysis, systemic toxicity is less likely. Another less likely complication is neuroaxis spread of the anesthetic or neurolytic solution.

Instead of chemical neurolysis, cryoanalgesia and radiofrequency ablation have also been used in intercostal nerve blockade. Cryoanalgesia, or freezing of intercostal nerves, has been shown to control pain in postthoracotomy patients if it is done under direct visualization of the intercostal bundle at the termination of surgery (31). After surgery, percutaneous intercostal cryolysis has not been shown to be as effective (45).

Intercostal nerve radiofrequency ablation can also be used for long-lasting blockade. A blunt-tipped 100-mm, 22-gauge radiofrequency electrode with a 5-mm active tip is inserted into the subcostal space. One mL of 2% lidocaine is injected into the elec-trode cannula. Lesioning is then accomplished by coagulation at 80°C for 60 seconds.

Sympathetic Blockade for Cancer Pain

Visceral pain arises from cancer involvement of sympathetically mediated organs. Insults to these organs can be from abnormal distention of organ wall or viscus, tension or torsion on mesenteric vessels, and ischemia. Such visceral pain is commonly seen with gastrointestinal (GI) malignancies such as hepatic metastases, intestinal tract tumor, and pancreatic cancer. Sympathetically mediated pain can involve neuropathic pain, as when there is direct injury to nervous tissue, such as brachial plexopathy and lumbosacral plexopathy. Blockade of sympathetic chain has been shown to be effective in controlling sympathetically mediated pain (46,47).

The sympathetic axis is made up primarily of a pair of ganglionated paravertebral chains that run from the base of the skull to the tip of the coccyx. It also consists of several major vertebral plexuses, including celiac, cardiac, and hyogastric plexuses. Table 3–7 lists major sympathetic structures and the corresponding tissues innervated (48).

These sympathetic structures are attractive targets for blockade of sympathetically mediated pain. Interruption of pain pathways at these discrete sites has been demonstrated to have a useful role in controlling oncologic pain (49,50).

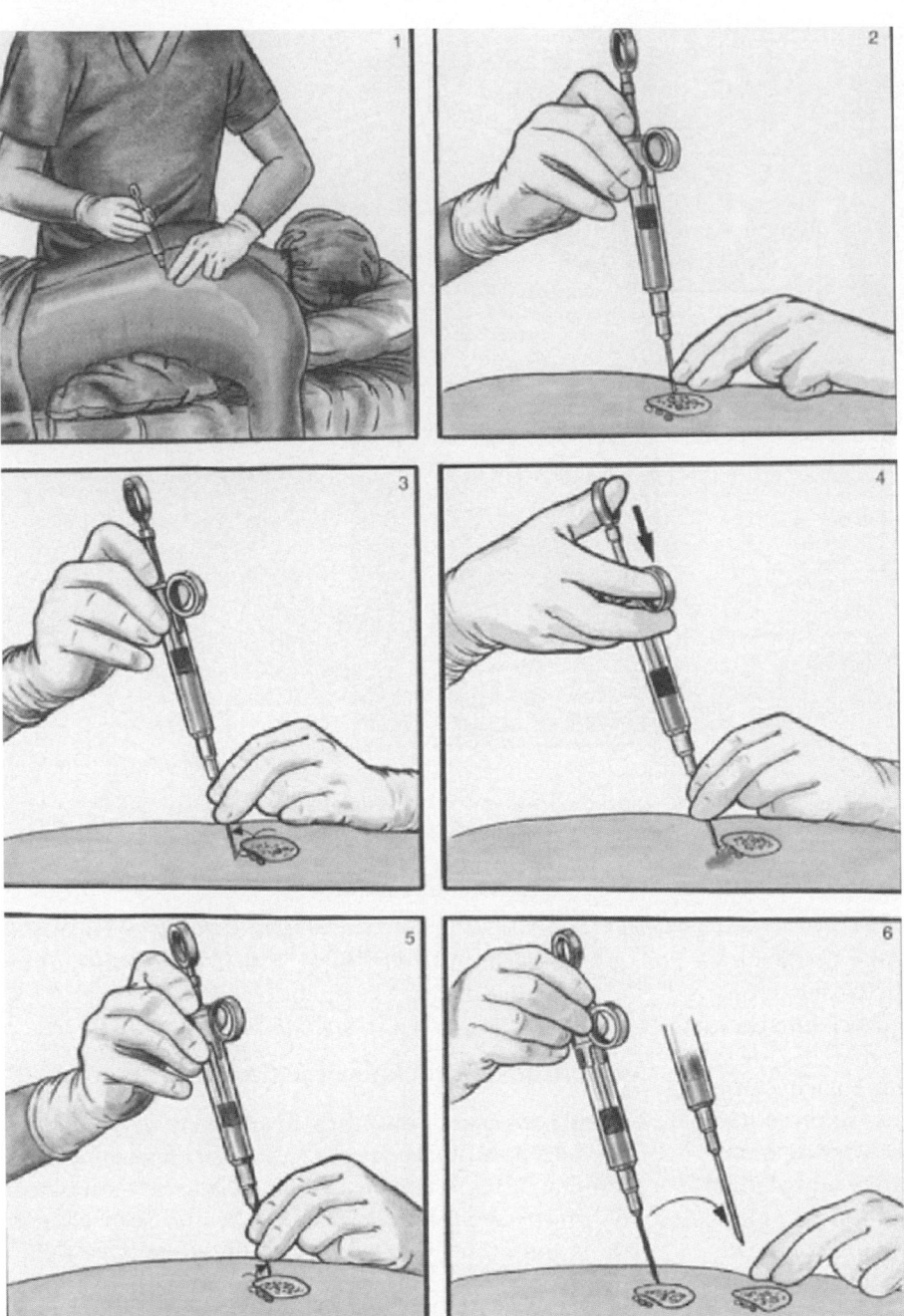

Figure 3–11 Technique of intercostal nerve block, with injection of anesthetic or neurolytic solution into the subcostal groove. Reproduced with permission from Brown DL. Atlas of Regional Anesthesia. Philadelphia: W.B. Saunders, 1999:244.

Stellate Ganglion Block

Indications: Stellate ganglion block helps control sympathetically mediated pain in the head, neck, and upper extremity. Sympathically mediated pain is commonly seen in tumor invasion of brachial plexopathy or in Pancoast syndrome (51).

Anatomy: Stellate or cervicothoracic ganglion is formed from fusion of the inferior cervical and the first sympathetic ganglia. This ganglion controls sympathetic afferent nociceptive signals to the head, neck, and upper extremity. The ganglion is located at the base of the neck and over the neck of the first rib (Figure 3–12).

It is bounded anteriorly by the subclavian artery and the origin of the vertebral artery, posteriorly by the vertebral body and longus colli muscle, laterally by the scalene muscles, and inferiorly by the dome of the pleura.

Techniques: Because of many sensitive structures in the neck adjacent to the stellate ganglion, fluoroscopic imaging is recommended. The patient is placed in a supine position with the neck slightly extended. The classic technique is to identify Chassaignac's tubercle at C6 and enter the needle at this site. However, many clinicians recommend the Racz technique for its improved safety margin (52). The

TABLE 3–7
SYMPATHETIC STRUCTURES

Sympathetic Structures	Innervated Tissues
Stellate ganglia	Brain, ear, tongue, pharynx, larynx; skin of neck, head, and upper extremity
Thoracic ganglia	Mediastinal contents, esophagus, trachea, bronchus, pericardium, heart, lung
Celiac plexus	GI tract (from distal esophagus to midtransverse colon), liver, adrenals, ureters, abdominal vessels
Lumbar ganglia	Skin and vessels of lower extremity, kidneys, ureters, transverse colon, testes
Hypogastric plexus	Descending and sigmoid colon, rectum, vaginal fundus, bladder, prostrate, prostatic urethra, testes, seminal vesicles, uterus, and ovaries
Ganglion impar	Perineum, distal rectum and anus, distalurethra, vulva, and distal third of vagina

patient's neck is prepped in a sterile manner with betadine, and the skin over the C7 vertebral body is anesthetized with local 1% lidocaine. The nondominant hand is used to palpate the carotic artery at the level of C7 and retract it laterally. The dominant hand introduces a 1.5-inch, 22-gauge needle just medial to the palpated carotid artery and directs that needle in a medial direction. The target of the needle tip is the ventrolateral aspect of the C7 vertebral body, not the transverse process as seen in the classic approach. Once the needle tip contacts the C7 vertebral body, it is slightly withdrawn about 1 mm. The needle is then carefully aspirated for CSF or blood. A contrast dye, 1–2 mL, is injected to confirm the caudocephalad spread in front of the prevertebral facia. For gangliolysis, a mixture of 3% phenol, local anesthetic, and steroid is used (i.e., 5 mL of 6% phenol in saline, 5 mL of 0.5% bupivacaine, and 80 mg of methyprednisone).

The volume of this mixture injected is dependent on the blockade desired. Volume of 10 mL of neurolytic mixture is adequate for stellate ganglion blockade of sympathetically mediated pain to head and upper extremity. If blockade of pain from thoracic viscera is desired, a volume of 15–20 mL of neurolytic mixture is necessary. During injection, the clinician must exercise caution to prevent intravascular injection. Even 1 mL of local anesthetic injected into the carotid or vertebral artery can cause loss of consciousness and seizure. An initial test dose, frequent aspiration, and slow injection are good safety measures.

Efficacy: Evidence of sympathetic blockade in the head can include a myriad of symptoms caused by Horner syndrome, such as miosis, ptosis, enopthalmos, facial anhidrosis, and nasal congestion. Sympathetic blockade to upper extremity results in visible engorgement of veins in the hands and forearms. Resolution of prior pain is proof that such pain is sympathetically mediated.

Complications: Because of anatomic proximity to critical structures, serious complications of stellate ganglion block can include pneumothorax, anesthetic-induced seizure from intravascular injection, and total spinal anesthesia from subarachnoid injection. Other less serious problems include localized hematoma, infection, or neck muscle tenderness. Many clinicians fear the complication of permanent Horner syndrome with neurolysis. Racz and colleagues, however, have not observed any long-term Horner syndrome with the modified technique discussed here (52).

Celiac Plexus Blockade

Indications: Celiac plexus blockade continues to be an extremely effective intervention for pain from pancreatic cancer and malignancies involving upper- and midabdomen (49,53). Pancreatic cancer carries such a poor diagnosis and palliation of pain is a priority in these patients, whose survival rate is typically less than 6 months. The patients often present initially with upper abdominal pain with referred pain to the back (54). The pain is described as severe, increasing with disease progression, and poorly relieved by opioids or other medications. Celiac plexus block is the treatment of choice for pain control in these pancreatic cancer patients.

Anatomy: The sympathetic innervations of abdominal organs arise in the anterolateral horn cells in the spinal cord. Preganglionic fibers from T5 to T12 leave the ventral roots of the spinal cord to join with white rami communicans. These fibers do not synapse at the sympathetic chain but instead pass onward to the celiac plexus. Passing from the sympathetic ganglia to the celiac plexus, the preganglionic fibers travel along the discrete splanchnic pathways (Figure 3–13). Preganglionic fibers from T5 to T9 coalesce to form the greater splanchnic nerve. This greater splanchnic nerve will pass through the diaphragm and synapse onto the celiac plexus. Preganglionic nerves from T10 to T11 join together to form the lesser splanchnic nerve before synapsing onto celiac plexus. The least splanchnic nerve arises from the T12 sympathetic ganglion and courses through anteriorly to join the celiac plexus. Blockade of sympathetically mediated pain in this region is accomplished by either neurolysis of the celiac

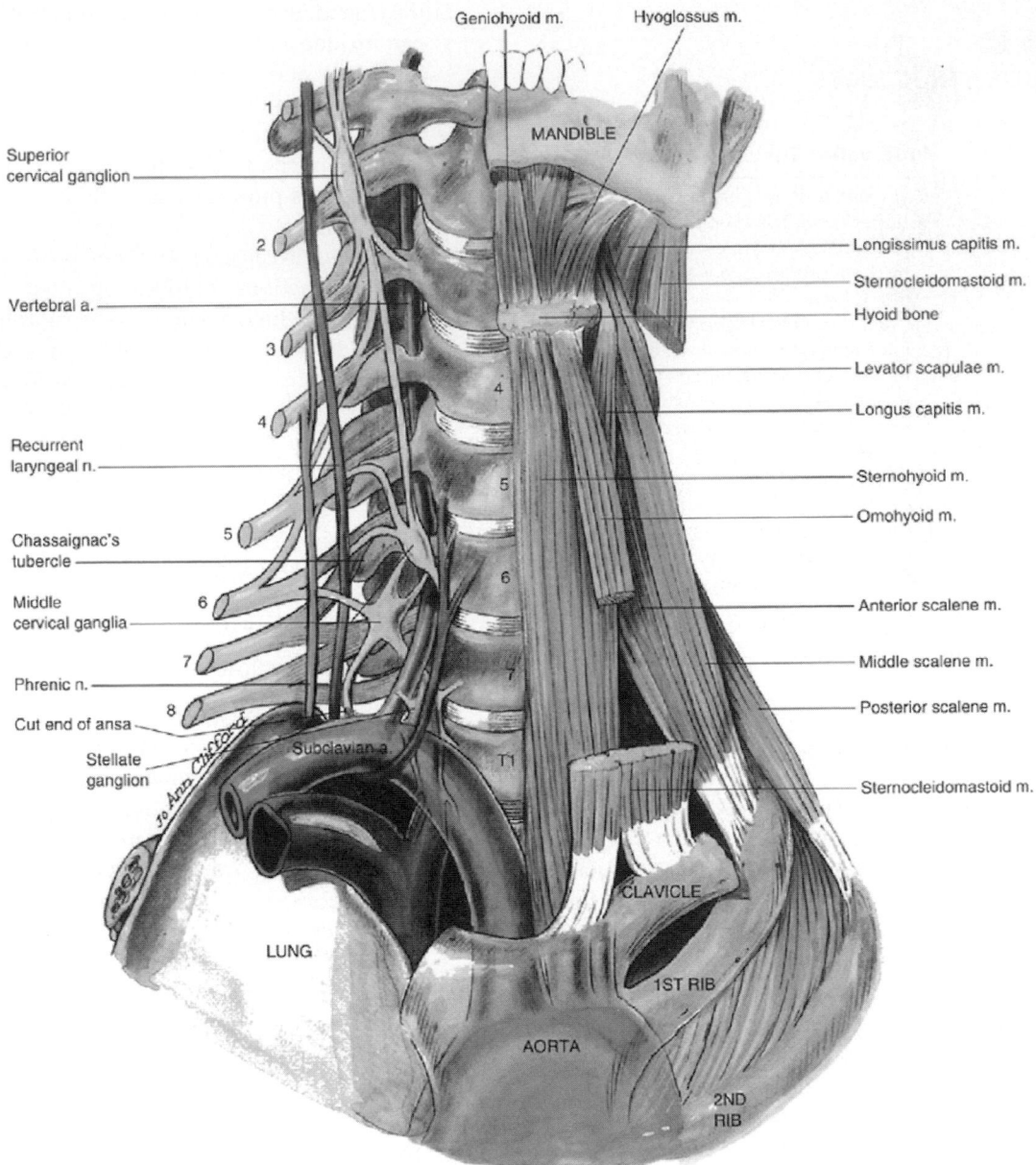

Figure 3–12 Stellate ganglion located at the base of the neck, just posterior to the subclavian artery. Reproduced with permission from Brown DL. Atlas of Regional Anesthesia. Philadelphia: W.B. Saunders, 1999:190.

plexus or the splanchnic nerves that feed into the plexus.

The celiac plexus is located anterior to the aorta at the level of the L1 vertebral body and anterior to the crura of the diaphragm. This plexus contains grossly two large discrete ganglia on either side of the aorta. The left celiac ganglion is slightly lower than the right ganglion.

Techniques: Multiple techniques have been described (as many as 13 approaches) for sympathetic blockade at the level of the celiac plexus (55,56). Posteriorly, the clinician can employ the classic retrocrural, transcural, or transaortic technique. Anteriorly, one can use percutaneous gangliolysis with CT guidance or direct intraoperative celiac gangliolysis.

For the posterior classic retrocrural approach, the patient is placed in a prone position with a pillow under the lower abdomen to minimize lordosis. The midback is prepped with betadine in a sterile manner. Using fluoroscopy, the relevant landmarks are identified and marked. These landmarks are relevant: the spinous processes of T12 and L1 and the inferior border of the twelfth rib. It is extremely

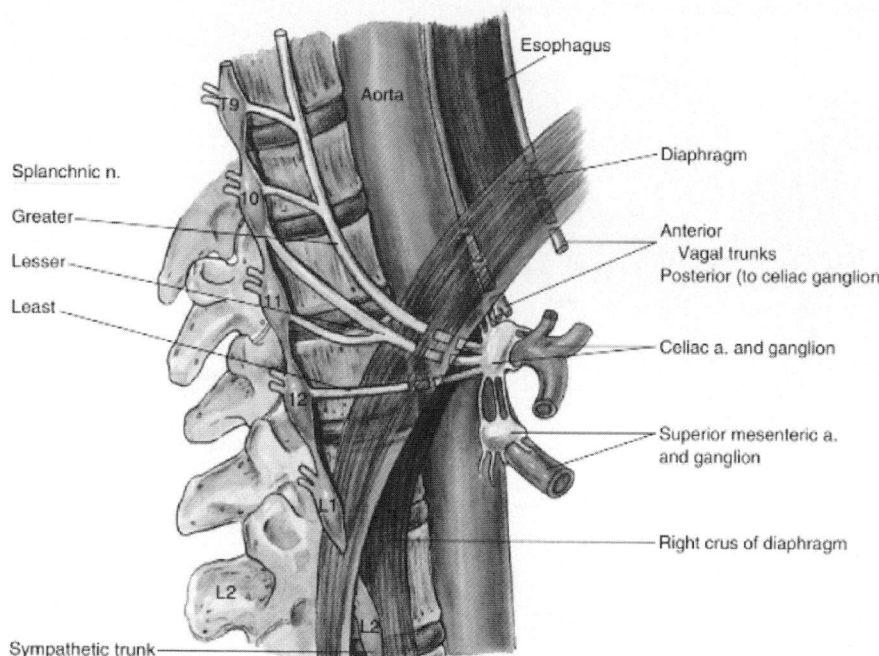

Figure 3–13 Splanchnic nerves passing from sympathetic ganglia to form the celiac plexus. Reproduced with permission from Brown DL. Atlas of Regional Anesthesia. Philadelphia: W.B. Saunders, 1999:285.

important to correctly identify the T12 spinous process by following the twelfth rib medially and also by counting cephalad from the L5 spinous process. Skin is infiltrated with local anesthetic at a distance of 8 cm lateral to the L1 spinous process and inferior to the twelfth rib. The underlying muscle tissue is also infiltrated with local anesthetic. Five-inch, 22-gauge needles are inserted bilaterally. Each needle is advanced slowly, initially oriented at 45 degrees toward midline and about 15 degrees cephalad, using fluoroscopic guidance. The initial target is the L1 vertebral body. Once bony contact is made, the depth of the needle is noted. The needle is then withdrawn and redirected at a steeper angle (60 degrees from midline) so that the needle tip is walked off the L1 vertebral body. The left needle is advanced about 2 cm beyond bony contact, slowly and with frequent aspiration. The right needle is advanced farther, about 4 cm past the vertebral body. The goal is for the left needle tip to be positioned posterior to the aorta and the right needle tip to be positioned anterolateral to the aorta. These positions approximate the location of the celiac ganglia.

A small amount of contrast is injected into both needles to confirm localized dye spread in the proper anatomic location. Local anesthetic solution (12–15 mL of 1% lidocaine) is injected into each side to achieve first a diagnostic block. The patient is awakened from light sedation to confirm pain relief and no adverse motor blockade of the lower extremitites. The patient is again sedated, and neurolysis can be carried out with 10–12 mL of 50% alcohol or 6% phenol to each side.

The splanchnic nerve block is similar to the above classic retrocrural technique. The needles, however, are aimed more cephalad to the anterolateral margin of the T12 vertebral body. The goal is neurolysis of the splanchnic nerves feeding into the celiac plexus.

Efficacy: Celiac plexus blockade has provided significant relief in pancreatic cancer pain. Pain relief has been reported in 70–94% of patients (57). Recent studies show a higher success rate, corresponding to better patient selection and technological advances.

Complications: Although not strictly a complication, sympatholysis with its side effects should be considered in celiac blockade. Significant hypotension, especially orthostatic, may occur and should be anticipated. Unopposed parasympathetic activity will lead to GI hypermotility. The consequent diarrhea is transient and does not last more than 2 days. Serious complications can include visceral injury, renal trauma with hematoma, and intravascular or subarachnoid injection. Pneumothorax is also possible, especially with splanchnic nerve blockade.

Lumbar Sympathetic Block

Indications: Lumbar sympathetic blockade has been used to treat sympathetically mediated cancer pain caused by tumor invasion or metastases to the lumbosacral region, chemotherapy- or radiation therapy-induced lumbar plexopathy, phantom limb pain, and lower extremity neuropathy secondary to malignancy (58).

Anatomy: The lumbar sympathetic chain is highly variable in size and location. The sympathetic ganglia

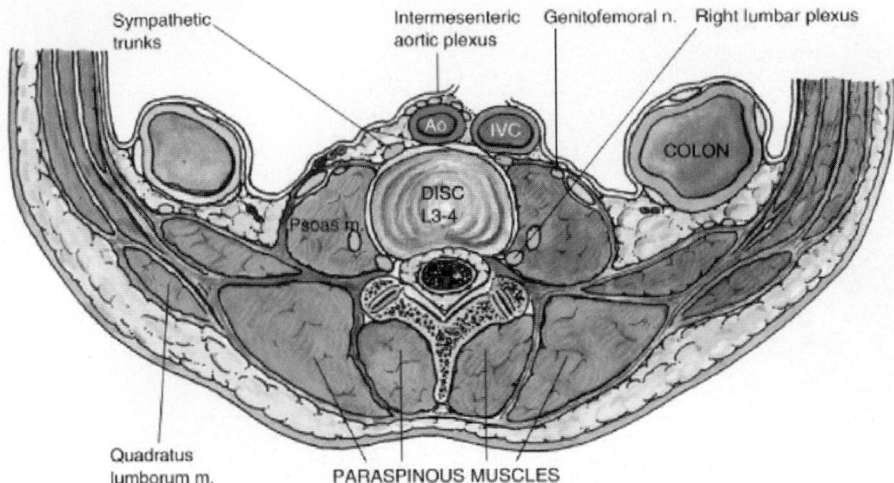

Figure 3–14 Lumbar sympathetic chains lying anterolateral to the vertebral body. Reproduced with permission from Brown DL. Atlas of Regional Anesthesia. Philadelphia: W.B. Saunders, 1999:277.

are usually located between the L2 and L4 vertebral bodies. Classically, the sympathetic chain lies in the fascial plane anterolateral to the lumbar vertebral bodies, just anterior and medial to the psoas muscles (Figure 3–14).

Techniques: The patient is placed in a supine position, with a pillow under the lower abdomen to minimize lordosis. The back is prepped in a sterile manner with betadine. Using fluorosocopy, surface landmarks of L2, L3, and L4 spinous processes are identified and marked. At a distance of 8 cm lateral to each spinous process, the skin and underlying muscle tissue are generously infiltrated with local anesthetic. A 7-inch, 22-gauge needle is introduced at the selected site and directed at a 45-degree angle with midline. The needle is advanced until the vertebral body is confirmed. The depth of the needle is noted, and the needle is withdrawn and redirected at a steeper angle (60 degrees with midline) to walk off the vertebral body. Once it slides past the vertebral body, it is advanced about 1 cm farther into the prevertebral fascial plane. This sequence is repeated bilaterally for the L2, L3, and L4 levels. Contrast dye, 1–3 mL, at each needle site can be used to visualize the spread radiographically. A diagnostic block with 20–30 mL of bupivacaine 0.25% can be done, with the patient awakened to evaluate any neurologic sequelae. Neurolysis can then be performed with 6% phenol at a volume of 5 mL at each needle site.

Complications: Side effects of lumbar sympatholysis include hypotension and diarrhea. Intestinal hypermotility is self-limited to a few days (59). Other complications include psoas muscle necrosis and kidney or visceral damage. The most common complication with lumbar sympatholysis is genitofemoral neuralgia. Most cases are transient and resolve in a few weeks.

Superior Hypogastric Plexus Block

Indications: Pelvic malignancies can affect multiple organs in the pelvis. Such cancers include gynecological cancer and cancer of the prostate. Each year in the United States, 18,400 new cases of gynecological cancer of the uterine cervix, vulva, and vagina occur; and these cancers cause about 6,300 deaths (33). The patient with pelvic malignancy often experiences initial visceral pelvic pain. The pain is often described as vague, poorly localized in the pelvic region, and colicky in character. Surgical destruction of the hypogastric plexus has been shown to relieve pelvic pain (60,61). More recently, Plancarte and colleagues reported a technique for hypogastric blockade with good results for controlling pelvic pain secondary to cancer (50). In this study, all 28 cancer patients with intractable pelvic pain reported good pain relief after the procedure.

Anatomy: The superior hypogastric plexus arises from the coalescence of nerve branches descending from the celiac plexus and lumbar sympathetic chains (Figure 3–15). This hypogastric plexus is a bilateral retroperitoneal structure located usually anterolaterally, extending from the level of the L5 vertebral body to the upper third of the S1 vertebral body. The plexus is just medial to the bifurcation of iliac arteries and veins on each side.

Techniques: The patient is placed in a prone position. A pillow is placed under the lower abdomen to minimize lumbar lordosis. The back is prepped sterilely with betadine. Under fluoroscopy, the spinous processes of L4 and L5 are identified and marked. The entry point is at 5–7 cm off midline at the level of the L4–L5 interspace. The skin and underlying tissue at this point is well anesthetized with local anesthetic (1% lidocaine). A 7-inch, 22-gauge needle is

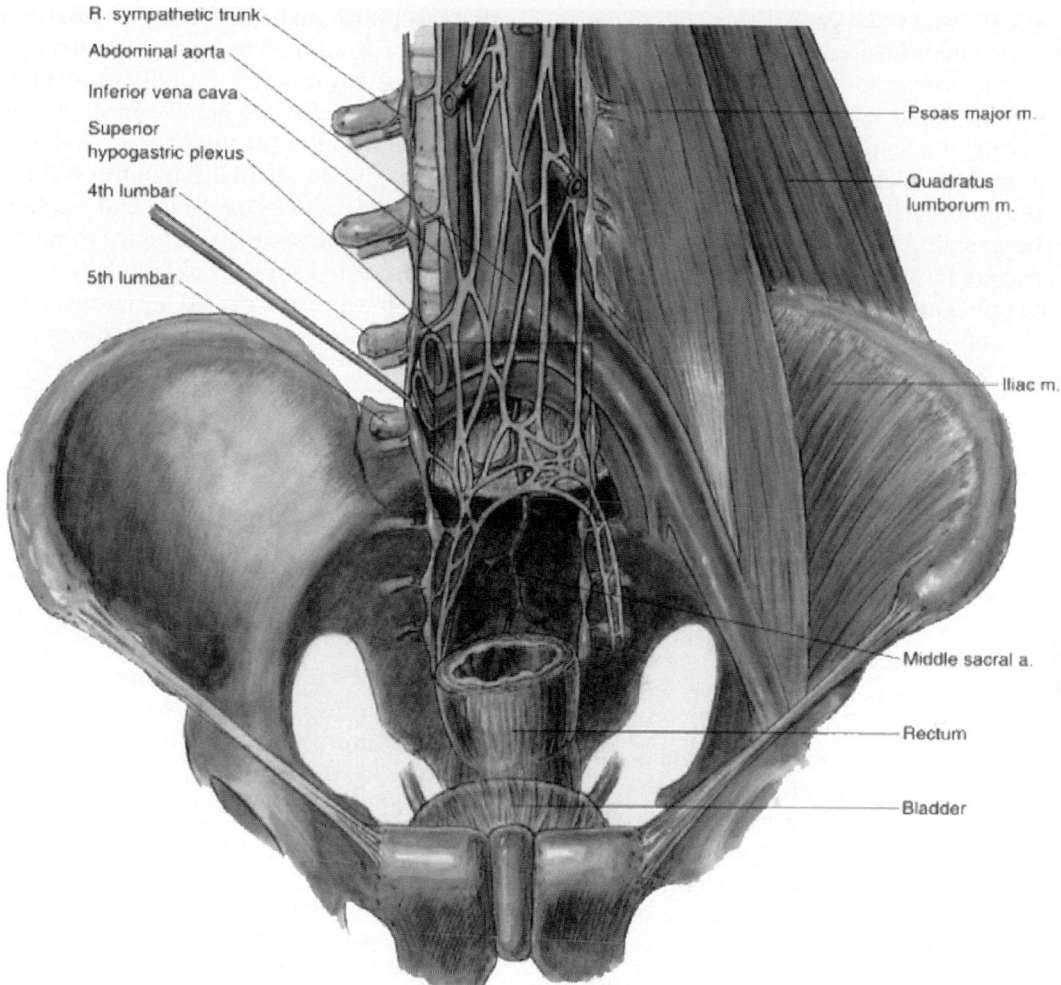

R. sympathetic trunk

Abdominal aorta

Inferior vena cava

Superior
hypogastric plexus

4th lumbar

5th lumbar

Psoas major m.

Quadratus
lumborum m.

Iliac m.

Middle sacral a.

Rectum

Bladder

Figure 3–15 Superior hypogastric plexus in retroperitoneal space, anterolateral to the L5–S1 vertebral bodies. Reproduced with permission from Brown DL. Atlas of Regional Anesthesia. Philadelphia: W.B. Saunders, 1999:296.

introduced at an orientation of 30 degrees caudal and 45 degrees mesiad off midline. Under fluoroscopy in AP and lateral views, the needle is slowly advanced, the target being the anterolateral aspect of the L5 vertebral body. The iliac crest and L5 transverse process can be obstacles along the needle trajectory, and the needle may have to be reoriented slightly to bypass these anatomic structures. Once bony contact is made with the L5 vertebral body, the needle is reoriented to a more mesiad angle to walk the needle tip off the body of the L5 vertebra. The tip of the needle should be advanced about 1 cm past the anterolateral border of the L5 vertebral body. A loss of resistance may be felt as the needle tip passes beyond the psoas muscle fascia and into the retroperitoneal space, where the hypogastrus lies. Because of close proximity to the bifurcation of the iliac vessels, careful aspiration is helpful to ensure that the needle tip is not in intravascular

space. A contrast dye can also be injected to visualize even dye spread to the paramedian space at L5, anterior to the psoas fascia. Each side can be injected with 10 cc of 0.25% bupivacaine for a diagnostic block, and neurolysis can then be achieved with 10 mL of 10% phenol for each site.

Complications: Because of the close proximity of the superior hypogastric plexus to the iliac vessels, the clinician should be cautious about intravascular injection. Vascular puncture may also lead to hemorrhage. Other less likely complications include subarachnoid injection, sacral nerve injury, and bladder or bowel injury.

Ganglion Impar Block

Indications: The perineum contains a diffuse network of mixed sympathetic and somatic innervation. Perineal pain thus usually involves both somatic and sympathetic pathways. Cancer patients with perineal pain can have cancer involvement of the lower colon, rectum, bladder, cervix, and endometrium. Blockage of the ganglion impar with a goal of disrupting the sympathetically mediated pathway has been shown to be effective in managing intractable perineal cancer pain (62).

Anatomy: The ganglion impar is a solitary retroperitoneal structure located at the level of the sacrococcygeal junction. The two parallel sympathetic chains fuse together from the anterior to superior borders of the coccyx to form the ganglion impar, or ganglion of Walther.

Techniques: The patient is placed in a supine position with a pillow placed under the lower abdomen. The buttock area and midsacral area to the anus area are prepped in a sterile manner with betadine. At a site midline and just posterior to the anus, the skin over the anococcygeal ligament is anesthetized using local anesthetic (62). A 3.50-inch, 22-gauge spinal needle is bent at 1 inch from the hub to form a 30-degree angle. This bend of the needle will allow the tip of the needle to maneuver anterior to the concavity of the coccyx and sacrum. Under fluoroscopy, the needle is advanced inferior to the tip of the coccyx and then upward and anterior to the coccyx. The target is the anterior sacrococcygeal junction. A volume of 5 mL of 0.25% bupivacaine is injected for a diagnostic block, and 5 mL of 10% phenol is used for neurolysis.

Complications: This block of the ganglion impar may cause rectal perforation because of the proximity to the rectum. Because most of this region is dually innervated by both somatic and sympathetic fibers, complete pain relief may be difficult to achieve by this block alone.

NEUROMODULATION TECHNIQUES

Intraspinal Drug Delivery

The significant side effects from systemic high-dose opioid administration can be avoided with intraspinal delivery of opioids. Deposition of opioids into close proximity of spinal cord receptors provides for more potent analgesia and fewer side effects. If the opioid dose is delivered into the epidural location, only 20–40% of the systemic dose is required to achieve similar analgesia (63,64). The intrathecal dosage is even lower, requiring only 10% of the systemic dose (63,64).

In cancer patients, an intraspinal opioid dose can be delivered by percutaneously tunneled epidural catherers, tunneled epidural or spinal catheters connected to subcutaneously implanted injection ports, or fully implanted spinal infusion pump systems. The SynchroMed pump system (Medtronic Inc.) is such a fully implantable system

that is sophisticated and yet easy to use. The pump can easily be reprogrammed to meet the patient's changing pain condition. Advantages of a fully implantable intrathecal pump include effective pain control, increased independence and mobility for the patient, and a reduced risk of infection with an internalized pump system. However, the initial cost of system hardware and implantation surgery can be prohibitive and is difficult to justify for patients with a predicted survival of less than 3 months (65,66). With such a short expected survival time, a simple tunneled epidural catheter or subcutaneous infusion is more economically feasible and beneficial for the patient. The epidural space is farther from the spinal cord and thus requires a higher dose or rate of infusion—usually mandating an external pump.

OTHER TECHNIQUES

Vertebroplasty

As mentioned earlier, neurosurgical procedures can be employed to treat intractable pain. Vertebroplasty is one such procedure that provides significant pain relief in patients with vertebral compression fractures secondary to malignant diseases. Such malignant tumors include metastasis, lymphomas, and myeloma. Vertebroplasty involves injection of polymethylmethacrylate (PMMA) cement into the diseased vertebral body (67,68). The full discussion of vertebroplasty, including indications and techniques, is presented in another chapter.

Palliative Care

Palliative care is defined as comprehensive care of the terminally ill patient. In overall oncologic care, much effort and treatment is utilized in the palliative treatment mode. Many patients have meaningful life-extending and life-enhancing palliative (as distinguished from "curative") treatments. These treatments include chemotherapy, radiotherapy, tumor ablative procedures, surgery, and the interventional treatments outlined earlier in this chapter.

Effective palliation in the patient who has advanced cancer always starts with a complete assessment and aggressive pharmacologic management. In some cases where the risk–benefit ratio is favorable and more conservative therapies are failing, interventional pain techniques may be helpful, indeed, extremely helpful. It is wise in treating the advanced cancer patient to keep some tenets of palliative medicine in mind. Among them are these, adopted from Field et al. (69,70): Symptom control is a paramount concern. It is critical to discuss openly and compassionately the patient's goals of care and tailor your treatments in accordance with the patient's wishes. The patient's overall well-being directly impacts the caregiver's quality of life. Be honest with patients and family members while being cautious not to extinguish hope.

SUMMARY

Cancer pain management is a complicated challenge. It requires a thorough understanding of the cancer disease process, the pain diagnosis, and the treatment modalities available to treat the pain condition. In addition to pain, the patient often presents with a constellation of symptoms arising from the cancer and the oncologic treatment. Both pharmacologic and interventional modalities of treatment are necessary to help the patient control pain and reach a satisfactory quality of life. In carefully selected cases, the diverse interventional techniques explained in this chapter help the physician and patient to achieve effective control of cancer pain, thereby optimizing quality of life.

REFERENCES

1. Bonica JJ. Cancer pain: current status and future needs. In: Bonica JJ, ed. The Management of Pain. 2nd Ed. Philadelphia: Lee & Feibiger, 1990:400–455.
2. World Health Organization. Cancer Pain Relief and Palliative Care. 2nd Ed. Geneva: World Health Organization, 1996:12–15.
3. World Health Organization. Fighting disease, fostering development, executive summary. In: The World Health Report 1996. Geneva: The World Health Organization, 1996.
4. Stjernsward J, Teoh N. The scope of the cancer pain problem. In: Foley KM, Bonica JJ, Ventafridda V, eds. Advances in Pain Research and Therapy, vol 16. New York: Raven Press, 1990:7–12.
5. Cleeland CS, Gonin R, Hatfield AK, et al. Pain and its treatment in outpatients with metastatic cancer. N Engl J Med 1994; 330:592–596.
6. Ventafridda V, De Conno F. Status of cancer pain and palliative care worldwide. J Pain Symptom Manage 1996;12:79–81.
7. Leibeskin JC. Pain can kill. Pain 1991;44:3–4.
8. Lillemoe KD, Cameron JL, Kaufman HS, et al. Chemical splanchniectomy in patients with unresectable pancreatic cancer. Ann Surg 1993;217:447–457.
9. Bolund C. Suicide and cancer: II. Medical and care factors in suicides by cancer patients in Sweden, 1973–1976. J Psychosoc Oncol1985;3:31–52.
10. Breitbart W. Suicide in cancer patients. Oncology 1987;1:49–55.
11. Raja SN, Meyer RA, Campbell JN. Peripheral mechanisms of somatic pain. Anesthesiology 1988;68: 571–590.
12. Joshi SK, Gebhart GF. Visceral pain. Curr Rev Pain 2000;4: 499–506.
13. Martin LA, Hagen NA. Neuropathic pain in cancer patients: mechanisms, syndromes, and clinical controversies. J Pain Symptom Manage 1997;14:99–117.
14. Principles of Analgesic Use in the Treatment of Acute Pain and Cancer Pain. Glenview, IL: American Pain Society, 1999.
15. Zech DF, Grond S, Lynch J, et al. Validation of World Health Organization Guidelines for cancer pain relief: a 10-year prospective study. Pain 1995;63:65–76.
16. Portenoy RK. Inadequate outcome of opioid therapy for cancer pain: Influences on practioners and patients. In: Patt RB, ed. Cancer Pain. Philadelphia: Lippincott, 1993:119–128.
17. Colleau SM, Joranson D. Fear of addiction: confronting a barrier to cancer pain relief. Cancer Pain Release 1998;11:1–3.
18. Lyss AP, Portenoy RK. Strategies for limiting the side effects of cancer pain therapy. Semin Oncol 1997;24(Suppl):28–34.
19. Ferrante FM, Bedder M, Caplan RA, et al. Practice guidelines for cancer pain management. Anesthesiology 1996;84:1243–1257.
20. Patt RB, Jain S. Therapeutic decision-making for invasive procedures. In: Patt RB, ed. Cancer Pain. Philadelphia: Lippincott, 1993:275–284.
21. Melzak R, Wall PD. Pain mechanisms: a new theory. Science 1965;150:971–979.
22. Patt RB, Cousins MJ. Neurolytic blockade techniques for chronic and cancer pain. In: Cousins MJ, ed. Neural Blockade in Clinical Anesthesia and Management of Pain. 3rd ed. Philadelphia: Lippincott Williams & Wilkins, 1998: 1007–1061.
23. Ramamurthy S, Walsh NE, Schoenfeld LS, et al. Evaluation of neurolytic blocks using phenol and cryogenic block in management of chronic pain. J Pain Symptom Manage 1989;4:72–75.
24. Swetlow GI, Weingarten B. Alcohol nerve block for pain in malignant disease. Med J Rec 1926; 123:728.
25. Politis MJ, Schaumburg HH, Spencer PS. Neurotoxicity of selected chemicals. In: Spencer PS, Schaumburg HH, eds. Experimental and Chemical Neurotoxicology. Baltimore: William and Wilkins, 1980:613–630.
26. Rumsby MG, Finean JB. The action of organic solvents on the myelin sheath of peripheral nerve tissue. J Neurochem 1966;13:1513–1515.
27. Lipton S. Neurolysis: pharmacology and drug selection. In: Patt RB, ed. Cancer Pain. Philadelphia: Lippincott, 1993:343–358.
28. Moller JE, Helweg-Larsen J, Jacobsen E. Histopathological lesions in the sciatic nerve of the rat following perineural application of phenol and alcohol solutions. Dan Med Bull 1969;16: 116–119.
29. Kline MT. Radiofrequency techniques in clinical practice. In: Waldman SD, Winnie AP, eds. Interventional Pain Management. Philadelphia: WB Saunders, 1996.
30. Cheng TM, Cascino TL, Onofrio BM. Comprehensive study of diagnosis and treatment of trigeminal neuralgia secondary to tumors. Neurology 1993;43:2298–2302.
31. Glynn CJ, Lloyd JW, Barnard JD. Cryoanalgesia in the management of pain after thoracotomy. Thorax 1980;35:325–327.
32. Bonica JJ, Buckley FP, Morrica G, et al. Neurolytic blockade and hypophysectomy. In Bonica JJ, ed. The Management of Pain. 2nd Ed. Philadelphia: Lee & Feibiger, 1990:1980–2039.
33. Landis SH, Murray T, Bolden S, et al. Cancer statistics. CA Cancer J Clin 1999; 49:18–31.
34. Vokes EE, Weichselbaum RR, Lippman SM, et al. Head and neck cancer. N Engl J Med 1993;328: 184–194.
35. Waldman SD. Blockade of the gasserian ganglion. In: Waldman SD, ed. Interventional Pain Management. New York: WB Saunders, 2001; 316–320.
36. Vital JM, Grenier F, Dautheribes M, et al. An anatomic and dynamic study of the greater occipital nerve. Applications to the treatment of Arnold's neuralgia. Surg Radiol Anat 1989;11: 205–210.
37. Pai U, Raj PP. Peripheral nerve blocks: cervical plexus. In: Raj PP, ed. Handbook of Regional Anesthesia. New York: Churchhill Livingstone, 1985;163–167.
38. Wertheim HM, Rovenstine EA. Cervical plexus block. NY State J Med 1939;39:1311–1315.
39. Masters RD, Castresana EJ, Castresana MR. Superficial and deep cervical plexus block: technical considerations. AANA J 1995;63: 235–243.
40. Landis SH, Murray T, Bolden S, et al. Cancer statistics, 1998. CA Cancer J Clin 1998;48:6–29.
41. Bonica JJ. Musculoskeletal disorders of the upper limb. In: Bonica JJ, ed. The Management of Pain. 2nd Ed. Philadelphia: Lee & Feibiger, 1990:891–893.
42. Raj PP. Continuous regional analgesia. In: Raj PP, ed. Practical Management of Pain. 3rd Ed. St.Louis: Mosby, 2000:710–722.
43. Moore DC, Bridenbaugh LD. Intercostal nerve block in 4333 patients: indications, technique, and complications. Anesth Analg 1962;41:1–11.
44. Kopacz DJ, Thompson GE. Intercostal nerve block. In: Waldman SD, ed. Interventional Pain Management. 2nd ed. St. Louis: W.B. Saunders, 2001:401–407.
45. Conacher ID. Percutaneous cryotherapy for post thoracotomy neuralgia. Pain 1986;25:227–228.
46. De Backer LJ, Kienzle WK, Keasling HH. A study of stellate ganglion block for pain relief. Anesthesiology 1959;20:618–623.

47. Bonica JJ. Autonomic innervation of the viscera in relation to nerve block. Anesthesiology 1968;29:793–813.
48. Plancarte R, Velasquez R, Patt RB. Neurolytic blocks of the sympathetic axis. In: Patt RB, ed. Cancer Pain. Philadelphia: Lippincott, 1993:377–425.
49. Brown DL, Bulley CK, Quiel EL. Neurolytic celiac plexus block for pancreatic cancer pain. Anesth Analg 1987;66:869–873.
50. Plancarte R, Amescua C, Patt RB, et al. Superior hypogastric plexus block for pelvic cancer pain. Anesthesiology 1990;73:236–239.
51. Warfield CA, Crews DA. Use of stellate ganglion blocks in the treatment of intractable limb pain in lung cancer. Clin J Pain 1987;3:13–15.
52. Racz GB, Holubec JT. Stellate ganglion neurolysis. In: Racz GB, ed. Techniques of Neurolysis. Boston: Kluwer, 1989:133–144.
53. Thompson GE, Moore DC, Bridenbaugh PO, et al. Abdominal pain and alcohol celiac plexus nerve block. Anesth Analg 1977;56:1–5.
54. Reber HA, Foley KM. Pancreatic cancer pain: presentation, pathogenesis and management. J Pain Symtom Manage 1988;3:163–176.
55. Labat G. Splanchnic analgesia. In: Labat G, ed. Regional Anesthesia: Its Technique and Clinical Application. Philadelphia: W.B. Saunders, 1928:398–402.
56. Moore DC, Bush WH, Burnett LL. Celiac plexus block: a roentgenographic, anatomic study of technique and spread of solution in patients and corpses. Anesth Analg 1981;60:369–79.
57. Eisenberg E, Carr DB, Chalmers TC. Neurolytic celiac plexus block for treatment of cancer pain: a meta-analysis. Anesth Analg 1995;80:290–295.
58. Boas RA. Sympathetic blocks in clinical practice. Int Anesthesiol Clin 1978;16:149–182.
59. Reid W, Watt JK, Gray TG. Phenol injection of the sympathetic chain. Br J Surg 1970;57:45–50.
60. Frier A. Pelvic neurectomy in gynecology. Obstet Gynecol 1965;25:48–59.
61. Lee RB, Stone K, Magelssen D, et al. Presacral neurectomy for chronic pelvic pain. Obstet Gynecol 1986;68:517–521.
62. Plancarte R, Amescua C, Patt RB, et al. Presacral blockade of the ganglion of Walther (ganglion impar). Anesthesiology 1990;73:A751.
63. Lubenow T, Ivankovich A. Intraspinal narcotics for treatment of cancer pain. Semin Surg Oncol 1990;6:173–176.
64. Du Pen SL, Williams AR. The dilemma of conversion from systemic to epidural morphine: a proposed conversion tool for treatment of cancer pain. Pain 1994;56(1):113–118.
65. Bedder MD, Burchiel K, Larson A. Cost analysis of two implantable narcortic delivery systems. J Pain Symptom Manage 1991;6:368–373.
66. Hassenbusch SJ, Paice JA, Patt RB, et al. Clinical realites and economic considerations: economics of intrathecal therapy. J Pain Symptom Manage 1997;14(Suppl): S36—S48.
67. Debusshe-Depriester C, Deramond H, Fardellone P, et al. Percutaneous vertebroplasty with acrylic cement in the treatment of osteoporotic vertebral crush fracture syndrome. Neuroradiology 1991;33(Suppl):149–152.
68. Cotten A, Dewatre F, Cortet B, et al. Percutaneous vertebroplasty for osteolytic metastases and myeloma: effects of the percentage of lesion filling and the leakage of methyl methacrylate at clinical follow-up. Radiology 1996;200:525–530.
69. Field MJ, Behrman RE, eds. When Children Die: Improving Palliative and End-of-Life Care for Children and Their Families. Washington, DC: National Academy Press, 2003.
70. Foley KM, Gelband H, eds. Improving Palliative Care for Cancer. Washington, DC: National Academy Press, 2001.

Intradiskal Electrothermal Therapy (IDET) and Its Role in Spinal Pain Management

4

Jeffrey A. Saal

The treatment of chronic diskogenic low back pain presents the most difficult challenge to the spine specialist. Nonoperative measures frequently are unable to reduce pain and improve function in this patient subgroup (1,2). Interbody fusion for these patients has yielded mixed and often poor results (3,4–6). An alternative therapy to address this problem is therefore desirable. The SpineCATH system to perform intradiskal electrothermal therapy (IDET) was developed to address this difficult clinical dilemma.

PATHOPHYSIOLOGY OF INTERNAL DISK DERANGEMENT

The natural history of the degenerating disk includes loss of nuclear hydrostatic pressure, which leads to buckling of the annular lamellae. This phenomenon leads to increased focal segment mobility and increased shear stress to the annular wall. The process progresses to delamination and fissuring of the annular wall. Annular delamination has been shown to occur as a separate and distinct event from annular fissures (7). Fissures can be radial or concentric. In addition, electron microscopy has demonstrated microfractures of collagen fibrils with disk degeneration. The progressive degeneration of the disk, manifested by any of these morphologic changes, has been shown to alter disk mechanics (8).

Tearing and delamination of the annulus can cause chronic pain. Mechanoreceptors in the disk wall have been shown to discharge with disk mobilization (9). Nociceptive tissue has been shown to be sensitized resulting in a decrease in their firing threshold after treatment with inflammatory enzymes and mediators (10–12).

A scenario for chronic diskogenic pain is created when any combination of annular fissures, delamination, or microfractures of collagen fibrils leads to mechanical distortion of annular lamellae and subsequent sensitization of nociceptors that also may have been sensitized previously by PLA2 (13), nitrous oxide (14,15), interleukin 1 (15), and metalloproteinase enzyme activity (15), or other chemical mediators. Afferent stimuli create substance P release and nociception. Repetitive stimulation of the DRG has been shown to create prolonged neural activity from the dorsal horn receptor fields (10,16–18). As the patient continues to load the disk, the neuronal activity continues. Clinically, the disrupted disk will often cause referral pain into the buttocks and leg because of DRG stimulation, CNS processing, or direct chemical irritation of the nerve roots.

THERMAL IMPACT UPON TISSUE

Innervation of the intervertebral disk has been well documented by researchers since the 1930s. More recently, Bogduk's work illustrated the sources of lumbar disk innervation (19). Coppes et al. found nociceptive properties in nerves of the outer annular wall. In fact, the researchers observed nerve fibers "deeper than the outer third of the annulus fibrosus" (20). Freemont et al. also discovered significant neovascularization with neural expression of substance P and linked that growth to disk degeneration and back pain. They identified nerve fibers as deep as the inner third of the annulus fibrosus and into the nucleus pulposus in several disk samples (21).

Letcher et al. established that irreversible nerve blocks resulting from neural thermocoagulation occur at 45°C in the brain (22), and Cosman et al. used radiofrequency lesioning to produce 45°C isotherms for neural tissue lesioning (23). The intradiskal temperatures generated by the SpineCATH (48°C to 75°C) are in the range necessary to create thermocoagulation of neural tissue in the target zone accessed (24,25).

Collagen contraction, or shrinkage, has been well documented in the use of nonablative laser energy on joint capsular tissue and more recently in RF application in the glenohumeral joint capsule (26,27). Research has shown a direct correlation between the amount of heat and duration of the heating applied to tissue and the resulting collagen contraction (28–32).

The breaking apart of the heat sensitive bonds of the collagen fibrils causes tissue shrinkage. The framework of the intervertebral disk is composed primarily of Types I and II collagen, which have similar molecular structures. The tensile strength of these collagen fibers derives from the extended conformation of the triple helix molecule, which is cross-linked with hydrogen bonds. A portion of these bonds is heat sensitive and breaks apart when exposed to a range of temperatures over time. Disrupting these stabilizing hydrogen bonds releases the molecular strands, which then collapse. This collapse, similar to the release of a taut spring, results in a new contracted state called the denatured or random coil conformation of the collagen fiber.

The optimal temperature for collagen contraction is reported to be 65°C. Sixty degrees (60°C) is the lowest practical temperature at which heat sensitive hydrogen bonds will start to break. As the temperature increases, more bonds break. Whether an additional shrinkage effect occurs above 75°C is unclear.

Kleinstueck et al. attempted to study intradiskal temperature dispersion from the SpineCATH (33). The researchers placed the device in the nucleus rather than in the annulus and were able to measure temperatures greater than 42°C—temperatures sufficient to thermocoagulate unmyelinated nerve fibers—at distances greater than 10 mm from the probe. However, their use of previously frozen cadaverous disks and the placement of the heating element in the

nuclear cavity, rather than in the annulus as is done in clinical practice, may have limited the peak temperatures. Freeman et al. presented temperature maps in vivo on sheep, demonstrating higher peak temperatures (34). The group found temperatures greater than 65°C adjacent to the catheter. In a recent report, Shah et al. found microscopic evidence of acute collagen modulation in cadaverous disks heated with a SpineCATH (25).

Recently, Barendse et al. reported on an RCT evaluating the efficacy of a radiofrequency probe placed into the center of the nucleus and heated (35). The treated group fared no better than the placebo. Houpt et al. has previously demonstrated the inability of temperature dispersion for an RF device to raise intradiskal and annular temperatures (36). For these reasons, the IDET technology, including SpineCATH, does not use RF as a heating element but instead uses a TRC (thermal resistive coil) that produces conductive heat. Additionally, contrary to the RF device studied by Barendse (35), the IDET device is deployed into the annulus and is not deployed in the center of the nucleus (24,37).

CLINICAL RESEARCH REVIEW

The first published series of IDET treated patients reported the six-month outcome results (range 6–9 months, mean 7 months) for 25 patients with chronic low back pain of documented diskogenic origin with a mean duration of preoperative symptoms of 58.5 months. These patients also had failed to adequately improve with a comprehensively applied nonoperative care program, electing IDET rather than chronic pain management or spinal fusion (37). The results demonstrated a statistically significant improvement in functional outcome as measured by VAS SF-36 scores, sitting tolerance times, and narcotic analgesic medication. Sixty-two patients who were treated with IDET and followed for a minimum of one year (mean 16 months, range 12–23 months) postprocedure demonstrated outcome evaluation scores that did not statistically vary from the 6-month group. The mean group change for the SF-36 bodily pain was 17 and physical function was 20. These scores are consistent with significant clinical improvement (37). A two-year follow-up study noted continued improvement in SF-36 scores and in sitting tolerance times (38). Shah et al. noted similar findings in a prospective cohort study (25).

Karasek and Bogduk (39) reported on the one-year outcome of IDET treated patients (24) and compared them to a control group of patients (30) similarly diagnosed but denied insurance authorization for IDET. The researchers used a 50% reduction of VAS scores as an indicator of success. On this basis, 60% were considered successes. Additionally, the researchers noted that 23% of the patients had experienced total relief of symptoms and reported that only one patient in the control group improved, while the remainder continued to have similar pain intensity.

Derby et al. reported that 62.5% of IDET treated patients had a favorable outcome based on the Roland Morris scale, VAS, NASS outcome instrument, and a general activity scale (40). When patients had preserved disk height and had not undergone previous surgery at the index level, the success rate was 76%.

Wetzel et al. presented the two-year results of a multi-center prospective cohort study and found statistically significant improvement in pain reduction and physical function in its study group (41).

Pauza and coworkers completed a sham-controlled, blinded, randomized, clinical trial (RCT) of IDET (42). Their data demonstrated a statistically significant difference in improvement in pain scores within the IDET treated group versus the placebo-sham group. This study proves that IDET is superior to placebo. The study found that 50% of the IDET treated group had at least a 50% reduction in pain. Additionally, 22% of the patients experienced a total cure. Clinically achievable success rates are best judged by the results of the aforementioned case control trials (37–43).

The data regarding IDET is in contrast to studies of spine fusion in the same patient population. A recent RCT demonstrated pain improvement of only 30% in 60% of cases (44). Another arm of the same spine fusion RCT did not demonstrate a statistical difference in outcome between any of the fusion techniques (44). This means that regardless of the screw, plate, cage, or graph used, the results were the same. Brox et al. reported the results of an RCT that compared fusion surgery with physical and cognitive therapy and found no statistical difference between the groups at the 1-year follow-up (3). Despite these findings, the rates of spinal fusion disappointingly have risen by as much as 35% in some states, while associated costs have risen by as much as 300%. Unfortunately, more fusions are performed with more complex and expensive instrumentation despite the lack of evidence to support its use.

Arguably, if IDET can help even 50% of the patients suffering from severe, disabling back pain with a documented diskogenic source avoid spinal fusion, then a tremendous contribution to patient care will have been accomplished. However, attempts to overextend the indications for the procedure to the general population of patients with degenerative disk disease will yield poor outcomes and would be a disservice to patient care.

DIAGNOSTIC WORKUP AND PATIENT SELECTION FOR IDET

The following 10 criteria represent the author's criteria for IDET candidacy (a Pauza RCT tested the key elements):

- Severe, function limiting, chronic low back pain for more than 6 months

- Failure to adequately improve with a comprehensively applied, aggressive, nonoperative treatment program consisting of stabilization exercise training; back education; activity modification; and, when appropriate, fluoroscopically guided, selective, epidural cortisone injections, and in some circumstances, facet injections
- Recommended duration of three months for the nonoperative care program
- Normal neurologic examination
- Negative straight leg raise (SLR) with no reproduction of "true sciatica"
- MRI that does not demonstrate neural compressive disease
- Preservation of disk height at the symptomatic level (<30% disk space collapse)
- No measurable segmental instability
- No lytic or degenerative spondylolisthesis
- Diskogram that demonstrates an annular fissure and reproduces concordant pain at one or more levels at an injection volume of <2.0 cc (low pressure <50 psi) with a documented negative control level
- No irreversible psychosocial barriers to recovery
- Motivated to improve with realistic expectations of outcome

In summary, IDET is intended for psychologically stable and motivated patients with chronic, function limiting, low back pain with a documented diskogenic source of pain and having failed to improve with an aggressive, exercise based, rehabilitation program. Diskography criteria for low volume concordant (or low pressure) pain provocation attempt to separate appropriate patients having focal annular lesions and experiencing pain reproduction at low volumes from questionable candidates (patients with global annular degeneration) who often experience pain reproduction only at larger volumes of injectate (such as >2 cc volumes and higher injection pressures >50 psi). In addition, the effectiveness of IDET on the previously operated segment is an open question.

PROCEDURAL TECHNIQUE

Local anesthesia and conscious, monitored sedation is applied to the patient in an outpatient surgical or radiologic setting. A 17-gauge procedure needle is introduced into the symptomatic disk under multiplane, fluoroscopic guidance. The Smith and Nephew SpineCATH is introduced through the procedure needle and navigated to the offending portion of the annulus. Care must be taken to avoid kinking the catheter, which can lead to catheter breakage. Treatment may be achieved with unilateral catheter deployment, but bilateral deployment is necessary approximately 40% of the time to cover the entire posterior annular wall. The Smith and Nephew autotemperature heat generator controls the catheter heat delivery system. Typically, a maximum catheter temperature of 90°C is attained, which corresponds to tissue temperature of approximately 75°C directly adjacent to the catheter. Occasions do occur in which the temperature profile must be modified to a maximum temperature of 82–89°C to achieve patient comfort. The patient must be alert enough to be observed for the development of radicular pain during the procedure. If this occurs, the catheter must be repositioned or removed. Most patients will experience their typical back pain and referral leg pain during the procedure. However, this pain must be differentiated from radicular pain, especially when the patient experiences it early in the heating cycle, such as a catheter temperature of 65–90°C. If this occurs, it is usually indicative of an extremely attenuated posterolateral annulus or a catheter that is extradiskal. This author prefers to inject 2–5 mg of cefazolin into the disk after treatment and removal of the SpineCATH.

POSTPROCEDURE MANAGEMENT

Experience has taught us to proceed slowly during the postoperative period. The following current postoperative guidelines represent those given to our patients:

- Rest for 7–14 days after your IDET in a comfortable position, such as lying down or reclining, and limit sitting or walking to 10–20 minutes at a time.
- Return to Work Advisory
- Sedentary work—You may return in approximately 2 weeks; however, you may still be sore after your IDET. Be aware of sitting restrictions listed below. For other job types, the decision will be made by your physician.
- Driving—Do not drive for the first 14 days. After that, limit your driving to 20–30 minutes for the first 6 weeks after your IDET. Make sure your seat in the vehicle has good lumbar support. You may need a pillow to help maintain your lumbar lordosis (normal low back curve). If you are a passenger, recline the seat and try to limit driving times to less than 45 minutes for the first 6 weeks. Reclining and being driven home on the day of your procedure or lying down in the back seat is acceptable.
- Sitting—Limit your sitting at any one time to 20–30 minutes for the first 6 weeks. Use a chair that has good support. Avoid sitting on soft couches or chairs. Use a pillow or towel to maintain your lumbar curve when sitting. You may find it helpful to stand and walk around as a break between sitting periods or after short periods of lying down.
- Limit all lifting to no more than 5–10 lb for the first 6 weeks.
- Avoid any bending or twisting of the low back, such as during housework, for the first 6 weeks.

- Avoid chiropractic manipulation, massage (unless otherwise instructed), inversion traction, or traction for the first 12 weeks.

POSTPROCEDURE EXERCISE

- Walk daily for approximately 20 minutes beginning at the end of the first week. Increase to 20 minutes twice per day. If back or leg symptoms increase at any point, reduce the duration of walking.
- Stretch legs gently, including hamstring and pyriformis, with your back flat on the floor (lumbar neutral).
- Do abdominal brace exercises, which may begin at 2–3 weeks in lumbar neutral.
- Swimming may begin at 6 weeks, but avoid excessive kicking (use a pool buoy to support the legs).
- Begin formal physical therapy; a dynamic stablization training program usually begins 6–8 weeks after the procedure.
- Avoid treadmills and stair-climbing machines for the first 6 weeks unless otherwise instructed.
- A lumbar corset with steel stays (or its equivalent) is prescribed for the first 6–8 weeks to be used for all upright activities.

The most important principle appears to be allowing time for a healing reaction and delaying aggressive exercise training for at least 3 months postprocedure. This time frame correlates with the timetable of collagen remodeling and has been observed to be the point at which patients experience a substantial reduction in preprocedure pain.

After the procedure, patients should be able to return to office work within 2–4 weeks and resume light lifting duties at 6 weeks, although returning to heavy work usually requires 5–6 months. The appropriate timing of return to work and postoperative management requires further study (Figure 4–1).

COMPLICATIONS

The potential complications from IDET can be divided into early stage and late stage. The early stage complications may include nerve injury (needle related, thermal, etc.), infection, bleeding, and burns. Complications from five specialty spine centers where IDET is performed regularly were surveyed (45). The researchers sent a questionnaire to each center requesting a report of all patients who had suffered complications from IDET, and they surveyed 1,675 consecutive IDET cases performed at the five locations between July 1997 and February 2001. The results were as follows:

- Six cases of transient nerve injury that resolved (five cases believed to be the result of needle placement and one thermal)

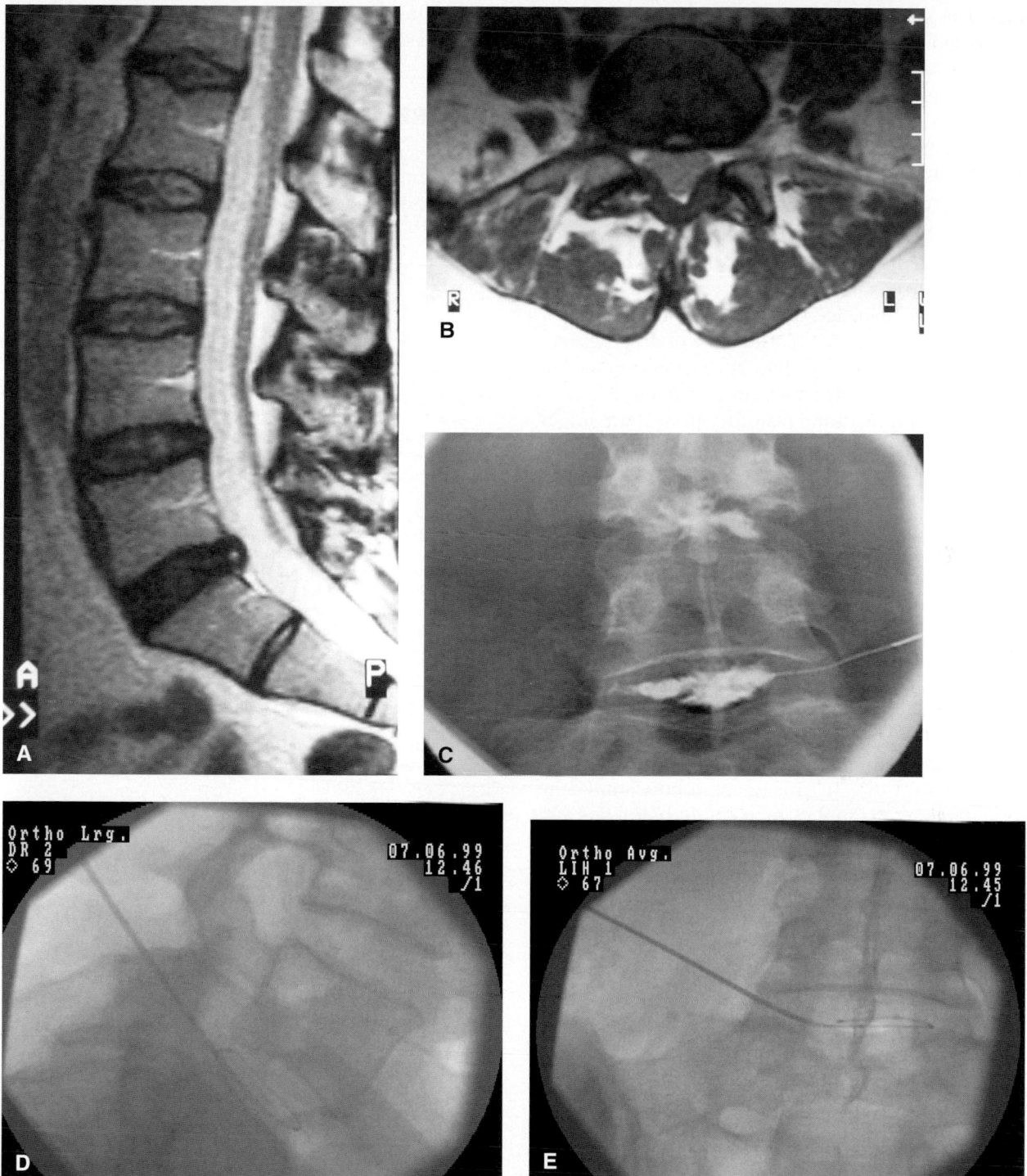

Figure 4–1   A. Clinical history: 45-year-old female with disabling low back pain for 2 years. Sagittal magnetic resonance imaging (MRI) scan, L5-S1 disk protrusion. **B.** L5-S1 axial MRI disk protrusion. **C.** Low volume diskogram with moderately severe concordant pain reproduction. **D.** Lateral radiograph L5-S1, SpineCATH navigated to the posterior annular wall. **E.** Anteroposterior radiograph, L5-S1, SpineCATH navigated to the posterior annular wall.

- One disk space infection in an immunosuppressed gentleman with carcinomatosis on chemotherapy
- No cases of catheter breakage
- No cases of severe pain that required hospitalization
- Five cases of post-IDET disk herniation (three at treated levels at which a new documented injury occurred and two at adjacent levels)

As part of the same report, the researchers reviewed the medical device reports (MDRs) on SpineCATH that had been reported to the FDA. During a period in which more than 35,000 catheters had been used, researchers found 21 cases of catheter breakage. Two were removed percutaneously and one was excised at the time of disk excision. The 18 cases in which a small piece of catheter remained in the disk were not associated with any patient morbidity.

Late-stage complications resulting from IDET might include rapid or accelerated disk space collapse at a treated level or avascular necrosis because of endplate injury. Ho et al. reported at NASS on follow-up MRI scans one and two years post-IDET that no evidence was found of endplate injury or acceleration of the normal degenerative process (46).

One report exists that describes cauda equina injury resulting from IDET (47). This case involved a patient who was overly sedated and whose catheter position prior to heating was not checked in the lateral plane. This resulted in an extradiskal catheter deployment in a nonresponsive patient who suffered a thermal neurologic injury.

A recent report noted that obesity was a negative predictor for IDET (48). In this same cohort study, the authors attempted to tabulate their complication rate and considered any increase in postprocedure discomfort a complication. They reported eight patients with symptoms. Six of eight of these patients resolved their postprocedure symptoms and went on to experience positive outcomes. Two patients had no pain relief with IDET, and whether any persisting new symptoms related to the IDET were present is unclear. If we assume that two patients had new persisting symptoms related to IDET, the complication rate would be 2/79 (2.4%). No cases of persisting neurologic injury, disk space collapse, or infection were reported. Therefore, it is safe to assume that the risk profile of IDET is low, especially when the procedural protocols are observed.

SUMMARY

The cost, morbidity, and observed degree of effectiveness make IDET an attractive alternative to spinal fusion for a specifically diagnosed subset of patients who experience lumbar diskogenic pain. However, the technology was designed to be used only for a specific group of patients by specialists skilled in performing intradiskal techniques who individually or within a team context also possess the ability to accurately diagnose and effectively manage patients with complex spinal disorders.

REFERENCES

1. Carey, TS, Garrett JM, Jackman AM. Beyond good prognosis: examination of an inception cohort of patients with chronic low back pain. Spine 2000;25(1):115.
2. Von Korff M. Studying the natural history of back pain. Spine 1994;19(18S):2041S–2046S.
3. Brox J, Sorenson R, Friis A, et al. Randomized clinical trial of lumbar instrumented fusion and cognitive intervention and exercises in patients with chronic low back pain and disc degeneration. Spine 2003;28(17):1913–1921.
4. Slosar PJ, Reynolds JB, Schofferman J, et al. Patient satisfaction after circumferential lumbar fusion. Spine 2000;25(6):722–726.
5. Wetzel FT, LaRocca SH, Lowery GL, et al. The treatment of lumbar spinal pain syndromes diagnosed by discography: lumbar arthrodesis. Spine 1994;19:792–800.
6. Zdeblick TA. A prospective, randomized study of lumbar fusions: preliminary results. Spine 1993;18:983–991.
7. Moore RJ, Vernon-Roberts B, Fraser RD, et al. The origin and fate of herniated lumbar intervertebral disc tissue. Spine 1996; 21:2149–2155.
8. Schmidt TA, An HS, Lim T, et al. The stiffness of lumbar spinal motion segments with a high intensity zone in the annulus fibrosus. Spine 1998;23(20):2167–2173.
9. Robert S, Eisenstein SM, Menage J, et al. Mechanoreceptors in intervertebral discs. Spine 1995;20:2645–2651.
10. Ozaktay AC, Kallakuri S, Cavanaugh JM. Phospholipase A2 sensitivity of the dorsal root and dorsal root ganglion. Spine 1998; 23(12):1296–1306.
11. Pateromichelakis S, Rood JP. Prostaglandin E increases mechanically evoked potentials in the peripheral nerve. Experientia 1981; 27:282–284.
12. Wall PD, Gutnick M. Ongoing activity in peripheral nerves: the physiology and pharmacology of impulses originating in a neuroma. Exp Neurol 1974;43:580–593.
13. Franson RC, Saal JS, Saal JA. Human disc phospholipase A2 is inflammatory. Spine 1992;17(Suppl):S190–S192.
14. Kang JD, Georgescu HI, McIntyre-Larkin L, et al. Herniated lumbar intervertebral discs spontaneously produce matrix metalloproteinases, nitric oxide, interleukin-6, and prostaglandin E2. Spine 1996;21(3):271–277.
15. Kawakami M, Tamaki T, Weinstein JN, et al. Pathomechanism of pain related behavior produced by allografts of intervertebral disc in the rat. Spine 1996;21:2101–2107.
16. DeLeo JA, Winkelstein BA. Physiology of chronic spinal pain syndromes: from animal models to biomechanics. Spine 2002; 27(22):2526–2537.
17. Devor M. Neuropathic pain and injured nerve: peripheral mechanisms. Br Med Bull 1991;47(3):619–630.
18. Utzschneider D, Kocsis J, Devor M. Mutual excitation among dorsal root ganglion neurons in the rat. Neuroscience Letters 1992;146:53–56.
19. Bogduk N, Tynan W, Wilson AS. The nerve supply to the human lumbar intervertebral discs. J Anat 1981;132:39–56.
20. Coppes, MH, Marani E, Thomeer RT, et al. Innervation of "painful" lumbar discs. Spine 1997;22(20):2342–2350.
21. Freemont AJ, Peacock TE, Goupille P, et al. Nerve ingrowth into diseased intervertebral disc in chronic back pain. Lancet 1997; 350:178–181.
22. Letcher F, Goldring S. The effect of radiofrequency current and heat on peripheral nerve action potential in the cat. J Neurosurg 1968;29:42–47.
23. Cosman ER, Nashold BS, Ovelman-Levitt J. Theoretical aspects of radiofrequency lesions in the dorsal root entry zone. Neurosurgery 1984;15(6):945–950.
24. Saal JA, Saal JS. Thermal characteristics of lumbar disk: evaluation of a novel approach to targeted intradiscal thermal therapy. Presented at the 13th Annual Meeting of the North American Spine Society, 1998. San Francisco, California.

25. Shah R, Lutz GE, Lee J, et al. Intradiscal electrothermal therapy: a preliminary histologic study. Arch Phys Med Rehab 2001;82:1230–1237.

26. Fanton GS, Wall MS, Markel MD. Electrothermally assisted capsule shift (ETAC) procedure for shoulder instability. Am J Sports Med, In Press.

27. Hect P, Hayashi K, Cooley AJ, et al. The thermal effect of radiofrequency on joint capsular properties: an in vivo histological study using a sheep model. Am J Sports Med 1998;26:808–814.

28. Hayashi K, Markel M, Thabit G III, et al. The effect of nonablative laser energy on joint capsular properties: an in vitro mechanical study using a rabbit model. Am J Sports Med 1995;23(4):482–487.

29. Hayashi K, Thabit G III, Bogdanske JJ, et al. The effect of nonablative laser energy on the ultrastructure of joint capsular collagen. Arthroscopy 1996;12(4):474–481.

30. Hayashi K, Thabit G, Vailas AC, et al. The effect of nonablative laser energy on joint capsular properties: an in vitro histologic and biochemical study using a rabbit model. Am J Sports Med 1996;24(5):640–646.

31. Lopez MJ, Hayashi K, Fanton GS, et al. The effect of radiofrequency energy on the ultrastructure of joint capsular collagen. Arthroscopy 1998;14:495–501.

32. Obrzut SL, Hecht P, Hayashi K, et al. The effect of radiofrequency energy on the length and temperature properties of the glenohumeral joint capsule. Arthroscopy 1998;14:395–400.

33. Kleinstueck FS, Diederich CJ, Nau WH, et al. Acute biomechanical and histological effects of intradiscal electrothermal therapy on human lumbar disks. Spine 2001;26:2198–2207.

34. Freeman BJ, Walters R, Moore RJ, et al. In vivo measurement of peak posterior annular and nuclear temperatures obtained during intradiscal electrothermal therapy (IDET) in sheep. Presented at the 28th Annual Meeting of the International Society for the Study of the Lumbar Spine, 2001. Edinburgh, Scotland.

35. Barendse GA, van Den Berg SG, Kessels AH, et al. Randomized controlled trial of percutaneous intradiscal radiofrequency thermocoagulation for chronic discogenic back pain: lack of effect from a 90-second 70 C lesion. Spine 2001;25(3):287–292.

36. Houpt JC, Conner ES, McFarland EW. Experimental study of temperature distributions and thermal transport during radiofrequency current therapy of the intervertebral disc. Spine 1996;21(15):1808–1813.

37. Saal JA, Saal JS. Management of chronic discogenic low back pain with a thermal intradiscal catheter: a preliminary report. Spine 2000;25(3):382–388.

38. Saal JA, Saal JS. Intradiscal electrothermal treatment for chronic discogenic low back pain: a prospective outcome study with minimum two-year follow-up. Spine 2002;27(9):966–974.

39. Karasek M, Bogduk N. Twelve-month follow-up of a controlled trial of intradiscal thermal annuloplasty for back pain due to internal disc disruption. Spine 2000;25(20):2601–2607.

40. Derby R, Eek BC, Chen Y, et al. Intradiscal electrothermal annuloplasty (IDET): a novel approach for treating chronic discogenic back pain. Neuromodulation 2000;3(2):69–75.

41. Wetzel FT, Andersson GBJ, Peloza JH, et al. Intradiscal electrothermal therapy (IDET) to treat discogenic low back pain: two-year results of a multi-center prospective cohort study. Presented at the 16th Annual Meeting of the North American Spine Society, 2001. Seattle, Washington.

42. Pauza K, Howell S, Dreyfuss P, et al. Randomized placebo-controlled trial of intradiscal electrothermal therapy (IDET) for treatment of discogenic low back pain. Spine J 2004;4(1):27–35.

43. Saal JA, Saal JS. Intradiscal electrothermal treatment for chronic discogenic low back pain: a prospective outcome study with minimum one-year follow-up. Spine 2000;25(20):2622–2627.

44. Hagg O, Fritzell P, Eskelius L, et al. Predictors of outcome in fusion surgery for chronic low back pain. A report from the Swedish Lumbar Spine Study. Eur Spine J 2003;12(1):22–33.

45. Maurer P, Wetzel FT, Thompson K, et al. IDET related complications: a multi-center study of 1,675 treated patients and a review of the FDA MDR database. Presented at the 16th Annual Meeting of the North American Spine Society, 2001. Seattle, Washington.

46. Ho C, Kaiser J, Saal JA, et al. Does IDET cause advancement of disc degeneration: a blinded pre- and post-IDET MRI study of 65 patients with a minimum one-year follow-up. Presented at the 16th Annual Meeting of the North American Spine Society 2001. Seattle, Washington.

47. Hsiu AW, Isaac K, Katz JS. Cauda equina syndrome from intradiscal electrothermal therapy. Neurology 2000;55(2):320.

48. Cohen, SP, Larkin T, Abdi S, et al. Risk factors for failure and complications of intradiscal electrothermal therapy: A pilot study. Spine 2003;28(11):1142–1147.

Advances in Diagnostic Angiography

Vascular Ultrasound

5

Edward G. Grant

ULTRASOUND IN VENOUS DISEASE

The Lower Extremities

Lower extremity deep venous thrombosis (DVT) is an important clinical problem. Pulmonary embolism (PE) can occur as an acute complication of DVT, and the postthrombotic syndrome is a potential chronic sequel. The clinical diagnosis of DVT has an imprecise accuracy rate of approximately 50% in symptomatic patients (1). Ultrasound (US) can accurately detect thrombi in the thigh and popliteal fossa, can imply iliac vein patency, and can often differentiate acute from chronic changes. In addition, sonography allows the diagnosis of structural abnormalities that may mimic the clinical manifestations of DVT, such as Baker's cysts, popliteal artery aneurysms, or calf hematomas (2). Because of these advantages and its high accuracy rate, US is now the primary diagnostic modality for DVT.

The deep veins of the lower extremity examined in a routine US study include the caudal aspect of the external iliac vein, the common and superficial femoral veins (SFV), and the popliteal vein. The termination of the greater saphenous vein should be examined because extension of thrombus from this vessel may enter the deep system and serve as a source of PE (3). Debate remains over the benefit of routinely examining the calf veins, because US is frequently technically unsuccessful in these paired, small vessels (4), and there is little evidence in the literature that isolated calf vein thrombosis is a significant source of PE (5).

Grayscale visualization of a clot would seem to be an effective method of diagnosis of acute DVT, but the variability of both clot and blood echogenicity limits the utility of this criterion alone. Acute thrombus may be completely anechoic, and backscatter may mimic solid material in the vessel. Because of this phenomenon, the detection of echogenic material in a vein lumen is only 50% sensitive in the diagnosis of DVT (1). Because normal veins have thin walls, their lumen can be completely collapsed and walls coapted with gentle compression by the US transducer. The inability to completely obliterate the vein lumen with compression is the major sonographic

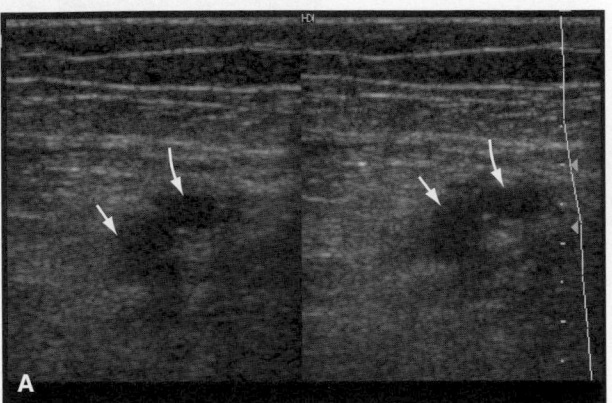

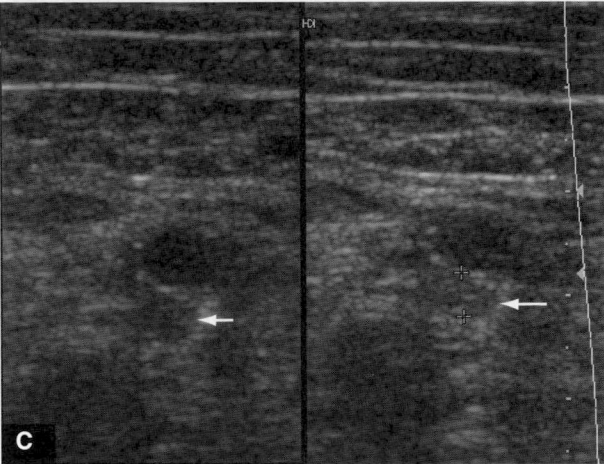

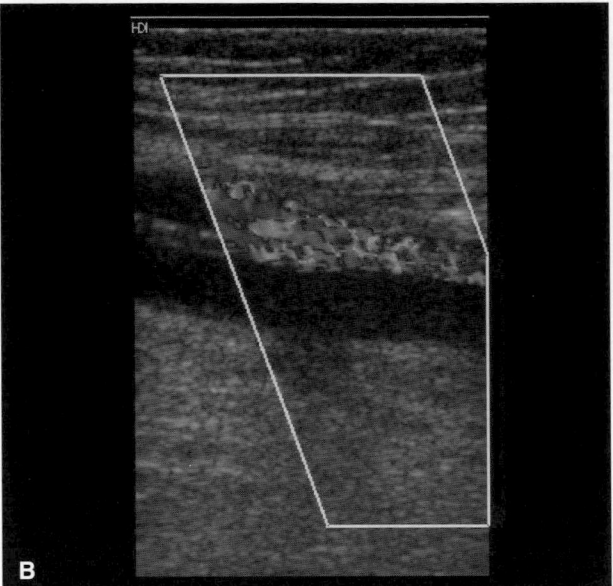

Figure 5–1 A. Transverse images taken at the level of the groin without (*left*) and with (*right*) compression show the left common femoral vein (*arrow*) and artery (*curved arrow*). With compression, there is no change in the appearance of the vein, suggesting thrombosis. **B.** Longitudinal color Doppler image confirms presence of thrombus in the vein; no color is seen. The expansile and anechoic appearance of the vein suggests that the clot is acute. The mixture of colors in the adjacent common femoral artery is because of aliasing, as the scanner is adjusted to identify slow flow. **C.** Transverse images taken at the level of the adductor canal show that the femoral vein is also not compressible. As opposed to the thrombus in the common femoral vein, this clot is likely old. Note the echogenic appearance and small size of the vein compared to the adjacent artery. See Figure 5–1B in color insert.

criterion for diagnosis of venous thrombosis. Color Doppler facilitates vessel identification and confirmation of patency (Figure 5–1). Spectral Doppler allows analysis of flow characteristics—predominately, the identification of depression of cardiac and respiratory phasicity—that indirectly allows assessment of the iliac veins (6).

Distinguishing between acute DVT and chronic residua of venous thrombi is of great clinical importance, because chronic thrombi are epithelialized and adherent to the vein wall and thus unlikely to embolize. Complete clot lysis occurs in only 20% of cases, and unlysed thrombus is organized into fibrous tissue, which may persist indefinitely (7). Differentiating between acute DVT and chronic changes, however, may be difficult with US. Features suggestive of chronic venous disease include thrombus with small caliber (less than or equal to the adjacent artery), echogenic clot, thickened, irregular vein walls, recanalization of vein lumen, and the presence of collateral vessels (8).

THE UPPER EXTREMITIES

US is an excellent technique for evaluating the upper extremity veins and increasingly is recognized as the primary diagnostic technique in their evaluation. The incidence of upper extremity venous thrombosis (UEVT) is growing because of expanded use of chronic central venous catheters. In the series of Kerr et al. (9), 61% of patients with sonograms that were positive for UEVT had some form of venous catheter. Heightened interest in physical fitness has also lead to a greater number of patients developing "spontaneous" or "effort" thrombosis. Effort thrombosis occurs secondary to obstruction of the proximal subclavian vein in patients who have hypertrophied anterior scalene muscles. Diagnosing UEVT is particularly important because it is associated with a high incidence of postthrombotic syndrome (10). Patients with malignancies are also at increased risk for UEVT.

Specifics of the technique of examining the upper extremity veins are described in several publications. Early studies showed good results using color Doppler with the best accuracy in the evaluation of acute effort thrombosis (11–13). The thrombosed vein is visualized as an enlarged, tubular, hypoechoic structure filled with thrombus and, with the exception of the basilic vein, lies adjacent to the artery. Using color Doppler, flow is absent or outlines thrombus. Collaterals often are visualized as prominent venous structures in the soft tissues about the thrombosed main vein and their presence should offer further support for the diagnosis of thrombosis. Care should be taken not to confuse large collaterals with the main vein (14). Spectral analysis is essential in the evaluation of central thromboses where the clot may be impossible to identify. Conversion of the normal triphasic pattern into a dampened or nonphasic signal is strongly suggestive of innominate vein compromise (15).

ULTRASOUND IN THE PERIPHERAL ARTERIES

Noninvasive Evaluation of Peripheral Vascular Disease

Indirect tests can obtain a basic estimation of the extent of peripheral atherosclerotic disease. Color Doppler with spectral analysis may be added to the examination, but whether or not this is performed depends on the laboratory and the needs of the individual patient and the referring physician. Vascular laboratories may differ on the choice of indirect tests, but the most commonly used protocol includes a combination of ankle brachial indices and segmental pressures with a simple, qualitative evaluation of Doppler waveforms. The former provides an estimate of arterial pressure gradients, and the latter gives a rough estimate of flow patterns and the overall status of blood flow throughout the vascular tree. Using the two in combination should yield an adequate physiologic picture of the peripheral vasculature. The information can be extremely useful for differentiating normal patients from those with atherosclerotic disease, for identifying the location of obstructive lesions, and for following up after grafting or angioplasty.

Increasingly, color and spectral Doppler are being used to evaluate peripheral arterial disease. Although this examination requires more time to perform and is more costly, it offers several advantages over the classic physiologic tests, including the ability to localize and characterize stenoses and occlusions, direct therapy, and angiographic approach. Angiography, however, remains the gold standard. It is often performed in patients being considered for intervention and may provide definitive treatment.

The most basic form of indirect testing is the simple comparison of systolic blood pressures in the arms to those taken in the feet; the ankle/brachial (or ankle/arm) index (ABI or AAI). The ABI is an excellent reflection of the amount of perfusion to the feet. Table 5–1 outlines the diagnostic criteria for ankle/brachial indices. Segmental pressures offer an additional refinement of the ABI, because gradients can be localized to specific vascular segments. Table 5–2 outlines normal and abnormal values for segmental pressures. Doppler waveform analysis is an essential adjunct to the segmental pressure/ABI examination and is particularly so in patients with diabetes who may have incompressible arteries and unreliable pressure readings. Waveform analysis is generally a simple visual inspection of the overall waveform shape.

Color sonography and duplex sonography have a number of important advantages over indirect physiologic tests.

TABLE 5–1
ANKLE/BRACHIAL INDEX

Normal	>1.0
Minimal Ischemia (Minimal Symptoms)	= 0.9–1.0
Minimal/Moderate Ischemia (Claudication)	= 0.5–0.9
Moderate/Severe Ischemia (Ischemic Rest Pain)	= 0.3–0.5
Severe Ischemia (Gangrene)	< 0.3

Note: Expected symptoms for degree of vascular compromise shown in parentheses
ABI >1.3 implies noncompressible arteries, unreliable study

These more comprehensive examinations require more time, however, and have several limitations worth considering if they are to be incorporated into the noninvasive testing algorithm. The common and superficial femoral and popliteal arteries can be examined efficiently with color/duplex in the majority of patients (16,17). With a high degree of accuracy, US alone can assess and localize stenoses and occlusions in these vessels. Numerous articles are available in the literature on this subject (18,19). As multisegment disease is common in the legs and peak systolic velocity (PSV) is not constant as one progresses distally, the best diagnostic spectral criteria are ratios calculated from velocities obtained several centimeters proximal to the lesion, to those obtained in or just distal to the stenosis. A good rule of thumb is that an increase in flow velocity of greater than two times baseline is indicative of a hemodynamically significant lesion, and four times baseline is suggestive of a severe stenosis (18,19). Classifying lesion severity exactly is difficult, especially considering the interobserver error inherent in single-plane angiography.

Bypass grafts tend to be easily accessible to US, and duplex sonography is extensively used in their evaluation. Femoropopliteal grafts are the most common type encountered, and they typically lie beneath the skin on the medial side of the thigh. The Doppler diagnosis of patency versus complete thrombosis is straightforward. With synthetic grafts, the echogenic walls are easily located and Doppler used to assess for the presence or absence of flow. Native vein grafts are more challenging because the walls, and therefore the thrombosed graft, are not visible. The diagnosis is based on the inability to depict the graft. Strict Doppler

TABLE 5–2
SEGMENTAL PRESSURES (MM HG)

High thigh (HT)	30–40 >Brachial (Br)
Normal	Ratio HT/Br >1.20
	HT/Br 1.20–0.8 = AI stenosis
	HT/Br <0.8 = Iliac occlusion

Proximal SFA occlusion may also cause drop at high thigh cuff
Other segments	≥20 between segs = stenosis
Toe Pressure—Normal	= 80–90% of brachial

criteria for grading severity of graft stenoses do not exist, but an increase greater than twofold in flow velocity should raise the suspicion of a hemodynamically significant lesion in fem-pop grafts (20). A secondary finding suggestive of graft stenosis/occlusion is the identification of slow flow (<40 cm/sec) proximal to a stenosis. This, however, only applies to larger grafts. Diagnostic criteria for grafts outside the thigh are not well-defined in the literature.

PSEUDOANEURYSMS: DIAGNOSIS AND ABLATION

Peripheral pseudoaneurysms usually occur as a complication of arterial puncture or catheterization, or trauma. They may also occur at anastomotic sites of hemodialysis access grafts or arterial bypass grafts. Pseudoaneurysms present a striking appearance at US, with color Doppler depicting the typical rotating internal flow as the so-called "yin-yang" sign and spectral Doppler defining "to and fro" flow at the neck (21,22). A variable amount of solid thrombus will often be seen in the periphery (Figure 5–2). Just as pseudoaneurysms may occasionally be difficult to differentiate from arteriovenous fistulas, the finding of "to and fro" flow is seen only in the former. Although pseudoaneurysms may spontaneously thrombose (23), they are treated most often with imaging guidance and compression or direct thrombin injection. Both forms of treatment are successful in the majority of postcatheter pseudoaneurysm cases, but thrombin injection is now generally preferred because of its success in a higher percentage of cases, as well as being much faster and less painful. In comparative study, Paulson showed thrombin injection superior to compression with a success rate of 96% for the former versus 74% for the latter (24). Complicating factors with lower chances of success include lesions with multiple loculations, a wide neck, a size greater than 5 cm or an age greater than several weeks. While heparin does lower the chances of success, treatment may be performed in anticoagulated patients when necessary.

ULTRASOUND IN THE ABDOMINAL VESSELS

Renal Artery Stenosis

Renal artery stenosis (RAS) is an uncommon, but potentially correctable, cause of hypertension. Numerous authors have evaluated duplex/color Doppler sonography as a method to screen patients suspected of having RAS. In general, two sonographic methods are used: evaluation of the main renal arteries themselves or identification of slowing of the systolic upstroke of Doppler waveforms obtained from the intrarenal arteries distal to a stenosis (Figure 5–3). With regard to the extrarenal arteries, one seeks an area of velocity elevation that signifies the presence of a stenosis. Diagnostic parameters include peak

systolic velocity (PSV) and renal/aortic ratio (main renal artery PSV compared to aortic velocity). Although some variation exists, most authorities recommend 180 or 200 cm/sec. as the cutoff for normal PSV and a renal/aortic ratio of ≥3.5 as abnormal. House, et al. (25) reported that lowering the renal/aortic ratio to 3.0 considerably improved sensitivity with minimal adverse effect on specificity. In one of the original studies of Doppler and RAS, Kohler et al. found sensitivity of 84%, specificity of 97%, and overall agreement with angiography of 93% (26). A recent study by Olin et al. (27) compared a large amount of patients to angiography and produced excellent results with sensitivity and specificity of 98%. Positive and negative predictive values were 0.99 and 0.97, respectively. Other studies produced very poor results when attempting to evaluate the main renal arteries for stenotic lesions with duplex/color (28,29). Desberg et al. (28) reported 0% sensitivity, largely because of a high quantity of technically inadequate studies. Berland et al. also had similar problems with technically inadequate studies and resultant poor sensitivity (29). For reasons that are not clear, both studies used a very low value (100 cm/sec) as their upper threshold for normal velocity, thereby ensuring a high number of false-positives and a resultant specificity of 37%.

Because the major problem with the extrarenal arterial evaluation lies in the difficulty of depicting the arteries, several authors have evaluated the potential of a US contrast agent to improve their visualization. Melany et al. showed that after administration of contrast, the number of normal patients confidently identified as such increased considerably because of the improved ability to define the main renal arteries (30). The number of patients having RAS identified successfully by US increased by 25%. Scan time decreased, and the number of dual renal arteries identified more than doubled.

The second method of diagnosing RAS relies on identifying the so-called "tardus-parvus" effect, which is essentially the slowing or dampening of the systolic upstroke that occurs distal to an arterial stenosis. Several articles have demonstrated excellent results with this indirect technique (31,32). Diagnostic parameters include the acceleration index (normal >300 cm/sec^2), acceleration time (normal <70 m/sec), and loss of the early systolic peak (ESP). Problems with the tardus-parvus technique include its lack of sensitivity, which has appeared in some studies (33,34), and the intrinsic variability of Doppler waveforms in the normal population (35). Accrediting organizations recommend the use of both intrarenal and extrarenal scanning when one is to perform US for RAS. Among laboratories, great differences seem to exist in the ability to scan the main RA, but those who have produced excellent results agree that the sonographic evaluation of the extrarenal arteries is difficult and time consuming. A growing body of literature suggests that MRA, CTA, or both represent superior methods of evaluating the renal arteries for stenosis (36).

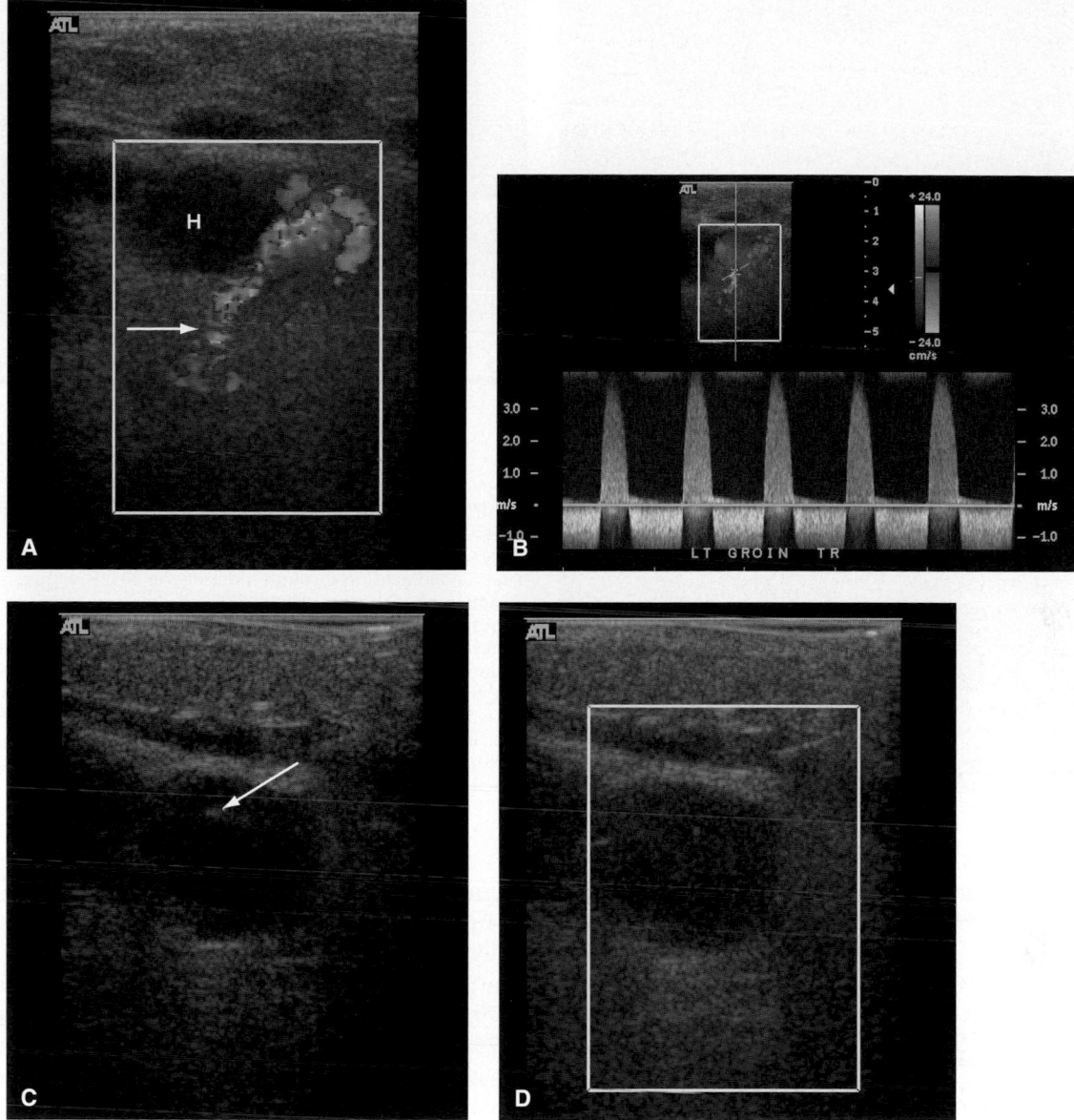

Figure 5–2 Patient 3 days postcardiac catheterization with ecchymotic groin mass. **A.** Color Doppler image shows a typical pseudoaneurysm with a well-defined and narrow neck (*arrow*), swirling flow within (the yin-yang sign) and a hypoechoic area (*H*) representing internal thrombus. **B.** Spectral Doppler image taken at the distal neck of the pseudoaneurysm demonstrates the classic "to and fro" signal. Note sharp upstroke in systole and a holodiastolic flow reversal in diastole. As arterial pressure is higher than that of the pseudoaneurysm during systole, blood flows into the cavity. During diastole blood flows back out as pressure falls in the adjacent artery. **C.** A 23-gauge needle (*arrow*) is advanced into the pseudoaneurysm under ultrasound guidance for injection of thrombin. **D.** Follow-up color Doppler image shows complete absence of flow, confirming successful ablation. See Figure 5–2A, B, and D in color insert.

Prior to ending this discussion, a note should be made about the ability of Doppler to predict the success of interventions, such as surgery or angioplasty/stenting, to lower blood pressure or improve renal function in patients with RAS. A significant number of patients show no clinical improvement despite the opening of the stenotic lesion. The recent Radermacher, et al study determined that when a patient has an RI of greater than 0.80 preoperatively, his

chance of improvement in renal function or of better control of hypertension was poor (37). Doppler may be used, therefore, to differentiate those patients who have irreversible, intrinsic renal disease and will not respond to intervention from those who would and would also avoid the potential complications of a procedure that will yield no benefit. This said, it is likely that all patients being considered for intervention to correct RAS should be evaluated

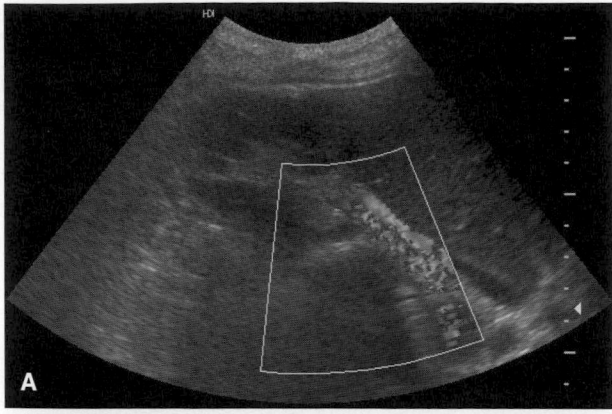

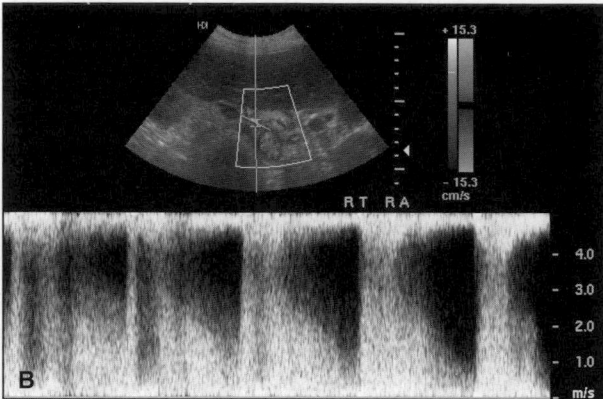

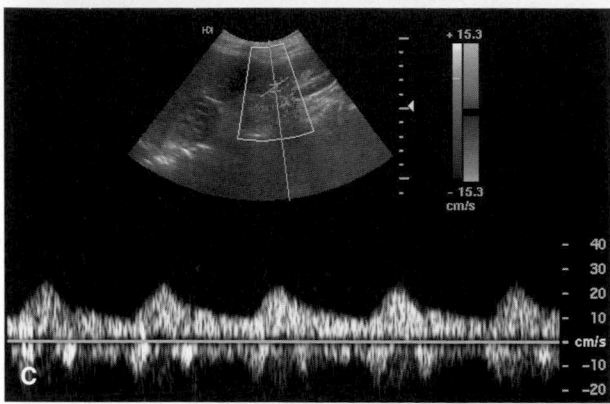

Figure 5–3 Patient with severe, recurrent hypertension, who underwent stenting of left renal artery stenosis 4 years previously. **A.** Color Doppler image of the right renal artery shows pronounced aliasing through most of the vessel suggesting the presence of high speed flow. Curved arrow = aorta, arrows = right renal vein. **B.** Spectral sample from within the proximal right renal artery confirms extremely high velocity of well over 4 meters/second. **C.** Intrarenal spectral examination further suggests renal artery stenosis. Note pyramidal appearance of the waveforms, which show the classic tardus-parvus phenomenon. There is no early systolic peak, and the normal sharp systolic upstroke is delayed. See Figure 5–3A, B, and C in color insert.

with Doppler regardless of whether the radiologist believes that Doppler is the optimum method for diagnosing the lesion itself.

MESENTERIC ISCHEMIA

Chronic intestinal ischemia is an uncommon clinical entity typified by postprandial abdominal pain and weight loss. Most authorities believe that stenosis or occlusion at the origins of the main splanchnic arteries is responsible for the disease and that at least two of the three major vessels supplying the gut—the celiac, superior [SMA] and inferior mesenteric arteries [IMA]—must be compromised. Contrast angiography typically has been the definitive test to diagnose chronic intestinal ischemia, but most clinicians hesitate to subject patients to this test and the disease is likely underdiagnosed. US has been evaluated by a number of authors as a potential noninvasive method of identifying patients with stenoses of the splanchnic arteries. Although the literature is rather sparse on this subject, results of most studies have been positive and many clinicians consider US the initial test of choice.

The US diagnosis of chronic mesenteric ischemia has been approached from two different standpoints: identification of elevated velocities at the site of stenosis or abnormal response to a balanced meal. With regard to the

former, Moneta initially performed a retrospective study of 34 patients and found that significant stenoses could be identified successfully if increased velocity at the celiac and/or SMA origins were found (38). The thresholds for >70% stenoses of these vessels were set at 200 cm/sec and 275 cm/sec, respectively. Moneta et al. further tested this method in a prospective study of 100 patients and found that the overall accuracy of Doppler for the detection of stenosis or occlusion was 96% in the SMA and 82% in the celiac axis (39). A recent study by Lim et al. (40) also tested these thresholds and achieved excellent results with sensitivity, specificity, and accuracy for celiac axis lesions of 100%, 87%, and 89% and for SMA lesions of 100%, 98%, and 99%, respectively.

Others have proposed diagnosing mesenteric ischemia by using Doppler to identify an abnormal response in the SMA to a meal. In the normal state, increased velocity and increased diastolic flow in the postprandial state will be seen. In patients with mesenteric ischemia, little or no change will be seen because of the already maximally dilated state of the vasculature (41). Because no change appears in celiac axis flow with eating, the potential contribution of this vessel and its branches to the disease remains unknown using this technique. Indirect signs of mesenteric ischemia include the identification of an enlarged IMA or reversed flow in the SMA or hepatic artery distal to an occlusion. Both findings occur secondary to the establishment of collateral pathways in response to proximal disease. As experience with direct evaluation of the splanchnic vessels using color and duplex US increases, the postprandial study is increasingly falling out of favor.

VASCULAR IMAGING IN RENAL TRANSPLANTATION

After renal transplantation, US is used extensively for identifying hydronephrosis and peritransplant collections. However, several vascular complications exist in which Doppler plays a significant role. Color Doppler is invaluable in establishing vascular integrity in the immediate postoperative period (42). Acute arterial thrombosis, if not immediately identified, will lead to loss of the graft and ultrasound should be performed on any posttransplant patient who does not immediately produce urine. Absence of color/power Doppler within the kidney should be definitive, and a positive study should prompt immediate intervention.

Renal vein thrombosis is another possible complication of the immediate postoperative period that can lead to loss of the allograft. Several reports have described a characteristic holodiastolic reversal of arterial flow on spectral Doppler in renal vein thrombosis (43). Other causes of diastolic flow reversal include acute rejection and acute tubular necrosis (ATN), but in these entities, the flow reversal does not tend to be holodiastolic. Color Doppler imaging of the renal vein itself also should be used to confirm the diagnosis.

A widely publicized role for Doppler is in the assessment of transplant dysfunction, the major causes of which are acute rejection, ATN, and cyclosporin nephrotoxicity. Unfortunately, despite several initially positive articles, Doppler is unable to differentiate between these entities, and biopsy remains necessary. Renal artery stenosis, on the other hand, can be identified with Doppler, although the diagnostic parameters are not well-defined. An elevated peak systolic velocity (>200 cm/sec) is the most commonly quoted criterion (44), but false-positives are frequent and we do not consider velocities up to 300 cm/sec abnormal at the anastomosis in the immediate postoperative period. Evaluation of the peak systolic velocity in the adjacent iliac artery should occur and be compared to that in the renal artery in order to determine whether focal high-speed flow or systemically increased velocity occurs (45). Several studies suggest that intrarenal arterial spectral patterns (tardusparvus waveforms) may add specificity to the diagnosis of renal artery stenosis in transplants (46).

Arteriovenous fistulas usually are the result of percutaneous biopsy and are identified readily with color Doppler when an area of artifactual color assignment is found in the renal parenchyma (Figure 5–4). This artifactual color assignment has been postulated to be secondary to parenchymal tissue vibration around an area of high-speed flow and has been termed a "color Doppler bruit" (47). Additional evidence of a renal arteriovenous fistula includes finding a decreased resistive index and increased flow velocity in the feeding artery, as well as arterialization of the waveform in the draining vein. Pseudoaneurysm is a rare transplant complication and may be found at the anastomotic site or after biopsy. Color Doppler should be diagnostic and will show similar features to pseudoaneurysms elsewhere.

THE HEPATIC ARTERY

The extrahepatic portions of the artery are best visualized by identifying the celiac axis as it originates from the aorta in the transverse plane and following the branch that runs to the right. In the porta hepatis, the common hepatic artery is usually easily visualized lying anterior to the portal vein when scanning from an oblique intercostal approach. Inside the liver, the hepatic artery branches follow their attendant portal veins in the portal triads and should be visible well into the periphery. The hepatic artery exhibits a typical low resistance pattern with flow throughout diastole.

The hepatic artery plays a subordinate role in parenchymal oxygenation; the portal vein supplies 70–75% of incoming blood. Altered arterial flow to the liver is rarely a primary etiologic factor in hepatic disease in the native liver. Enlargement of the hepatic artery, increased flow, and a tortuous "corkscrew" appearance, however, are commonly observed in patients with cirrhosis and portal hypertension (48). Undoubtedly, the decrease in portal venous flow leads to increased dependence on the arterial system for oxygenation. In such patients, the hepatic artery may be identified more easily with color Doppler than the portal vein. This situation may be particularly troublesome in pre-liver transplant evaluations where identification of a well-defined, patent portal vein is essential.

The hepatic artery is also a potential site for pseudoaneurysm formation. These lesions occur in association with trauma or pancreatitis and have the sonographic appearance of a complex or cystic mass in the liver or along the course of the extrahepatic hepatic artery. When large, they may be mistaken for cysts or abscesses thereby inviting percutaneous drainage. As such, a Doppler examination should be performed in any instance in which pseudoaneurysm could be considered. Small pseudoaneurysms in the liver may be difficult to identify with US. Evidence does exist that CT with contrast may be a superior technique (49).

THE PORTAL VENOUS SYSTEM

Many significant abnormalities of the portal venous system are readily characterized with duplex and color Doppler imaging. Anatomic abnormalities are relatively unusual, but the color features of duplication, several normal variants,

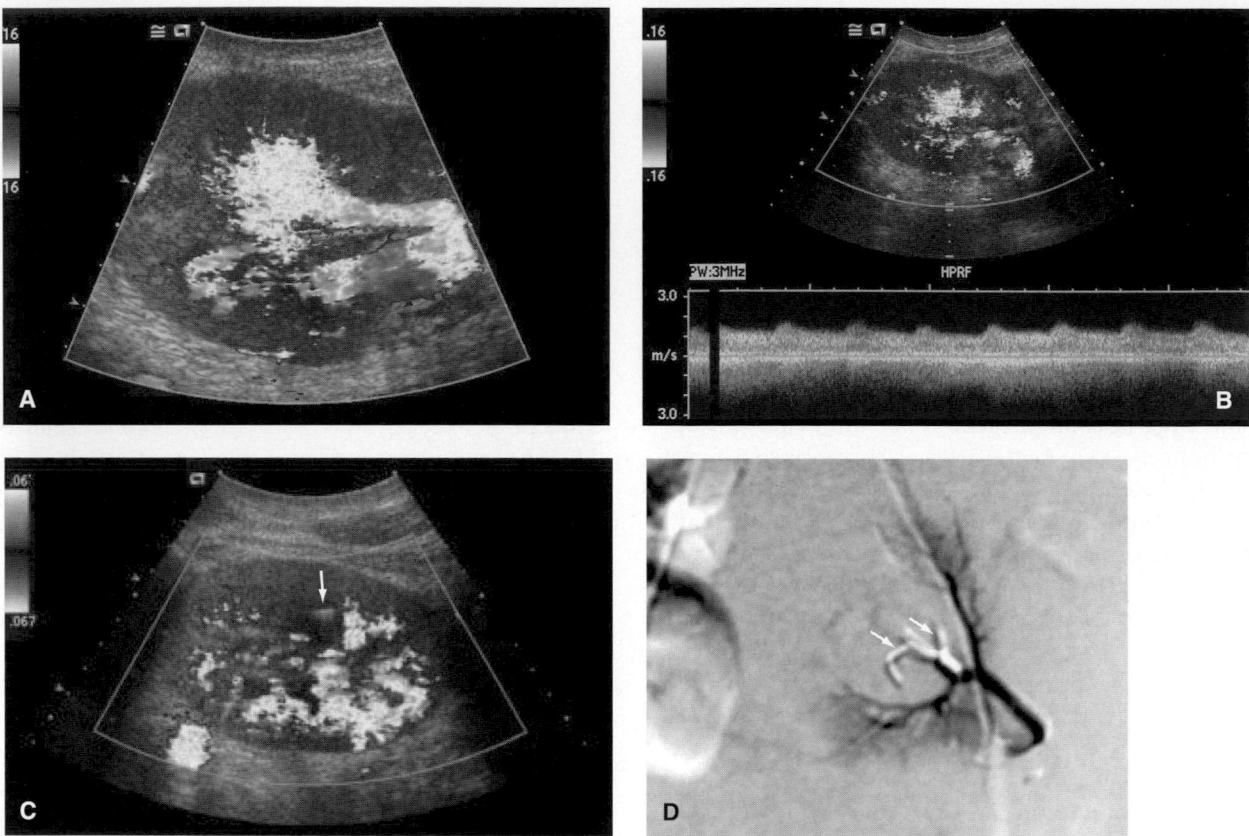

Figure 5–4   Patient with a renal transplant presenting with hematuria following a percutaneous biopsy. **A.** Color Doppler image shows a large color Doppler bruit, typical of an arteriovenous fistula. Note that color is assigned well beyond the expected anatomic location of the renal arteries and veins. **B.** Spectral analysis in the area of the color Doppler bruit shows high speed, extremely low resistance flow, the classic pattern of an AVF. **C.** Postembolization ultrasound reveals a wedge-shaped area of infarction with no color flow, but no evidence of the AVF. Echogenic focus (*arrow*) was believed to represent an embolization coil. **D.** Postembolization angiogram confirms that coils were present (*arrow*) and shows a similar wedge shaped pattern of absent perfusion. There is no longer evidence of an AVF. See Figure 5–4A, B, and C in color insert.

and aneurysms have all been described. In addition, fistulas may affect the portal system, and the communication may be between the portal vein and the hepatic artery or the hepatic veins. Color Doppler imaging should be definitive in both varieties of fistulas. In patients with hepatic artery/portal vein communications, severe portal hypertension with abundant collateral formation is typical (50). Turbulent, high velocity, low resistance arterial flow with a color Doppler "bruit" may be present (48), and portal signals may be arterialized. Portal vein flow is almost invariably reversed. Portal vein/hepatic vein fistulas tend to be asymptomatic as flow proceeds from one low resistance system to another. Cystic spaces may be seen within the liver in the area of the communication. Color Doppler provides the diagnosis by identifying flow in the "cysts" and should be capable of defining the attendant vascular connections (51). The communication between the systemic and portal venous systems often allows the triphasic spectral pattern of the hepatic veins to be reflected back into the portal system.

Thrombosis may affect in the portal vein and is closely associated with hepatocellular carcinoma, hypercoagulable states, and cirrhosis. A significant number of cases have no obvious underlying etiology. The clinical presentation of portal vein thrombosis (PVT) is relatively nonspecific and an effective screening technique would be of considerable value. The study of Tessler, et al showed color Doppler performing well in this role (52). The high negative predictive value (0.98) implies that in patients suspected of having PVT, a normal color Doppler study effectively excludes the diagnosis. On the other hand, severe portal hypertension may reduce flow to the point that Doppler signals are not returned, producing occasional false-positive studies. If the diagnosis of PVT is suggested by color or power Doppler but the lumen appears clear by grayscale evaluation, an alternative imaging modality, such as MRI or CT, should be considered for conformation. Another use of color Doppler sonography in portal vein thrombosis is in differentiating between bland and tumor thrombus. Because such a high association of portal vein thrombosis with HCC exists, identifying tumor thrombus is essentially diagnostic of this lesion. In patients with portal vein thrombus, a meticulous search for arterial flow in the thrombus should be undertaken (53).

Color Doppler is certainly capable of diagnosing portal hypertension, but the global images provided by MR and CT allow a more complete picture of collateral vessels. However, because US is often the initial imaging study in patients with cirrhosis, its characteristics need to be made clear. Certainly, the ability of Doppler to yield directional information allows definitive diagnoses to be made easily when reversed flow is identified in the portal vein. However, patients with reversal of flow represent a relatively small portion of the total patient population with the disease. Several studies have evaluated decrease in velocity as an indicator of portal hypertension (54,55). While successful in selected patients, the normal velocity of the portal vein is extremely variable and the main collateral pathway largely dictates portal vein flow dynamics. Therefore, as with CT and MRI, the most important contribution of color Doppler may be the depiction of portal venous collaterals. Collaterals form in specific locations within the abdomen and in patients suspected of having cirrhosis/portal hypertension, and these areas should be examined carefully. The most common collateral is the coronary vein that arises from the area of the splenic/portal confluence. Other potential pathways of collateralization include the paraumbilical vein (13% of patients) and retroperitoneal/splenorenal vessels (<5% of patients). Again, several recent studies using US contrast agents have shown improved delineation of collaterals in patients with portal hypertension (56).

When complications of portal hypertension cannot be controlled, a portosystemic shunt may be constructed to divert blood from the portal to the systemic veins. Three main types of surgical shunts are used: portocaval, mesocaval, and splenorenal. Portocaval shunts are generally imaged easily using color Doppler but are performed less frequently now because an intact portal vein is highly desirable when a liver transplant is performed. A mesocaval shunt typically is an "H-type" synthetic graft between the midsuperior mesenteric vein and the inferior vena cava (IVC). These shunts may be difficult to identify because they tend to be covered by bowel gas and mesentery. Distal splenorenal, or Warren, shunts are potentially the most difficult to image sonographically. The anastomosis deep in the left upper quadrant but identification of appropriately directed flow in the splenic and renal limbs can be used to imply patency (57).

Percutaneous transjugular placement of a shunt between the hepatic and portal veins (TIPS) has all but replaced surgical shunting in most centers (Figure 5-5). Routine sonographic evaluation of TIPS shunts is important because of a high incidence of stenosis/thrombosis. The evaluation of TIPS thrombosis is relatively uncomplicated, and most centers have reported a high degree of success in this diagnosis. The evaluation of shunt stenosis is more challenging but is of paramount importance if shunt loss is to be prevented. Flow velocities of 100–200 cm/sec within a normally functioning shunt are relatively high (58). Stenosis occasionally manifests as a focal area of increased velocity when the stenosis itself is insonated. More commonly, stenosis is inferred by identifying slow flow (<50 cm/sec) in the intrahepatic portions of the shunt secondary to outflow blockage at the hepatic vein end (59). One can select thresholds in accordance with what is considered an acceptable level of sensitivity or specificity. In the Kanterman, et al article, the lower limit of normal for intrashunt velocity was placed at 90 cm/sec (60). This value maximizes sensitivity. Ancillary findings of shunt dysfunction include return of hepatopedal flow in the intrahepatic portal veins or reversal of flow in the draining hepatic vein(61).

Portal vein flow is normally relatively nonphasic with minor fluctuations in response to cardiac and respiratory motion. Occasionally, however, pulsatile flow may be identified in the portal vein. Any communication between the systemic and portal veins (portosystemic shunts, fistulas) may lead to a pulsatile portal vein. More commonly, however, significant portal vein pulsatility is secondary to right heart failure, tricuspid regurgitation, or both (62,63).

THE HEPATIC VEINS

Compromised hepatic venous outflow may be caused by obstruction located anywhere between the inferior vena cava and the hepatic venules. The resultant symptoms are typically hepatomegaly, ascites, and upper abdominal pain and, when associated with hepatic venous obstruction, are termed Budd-Chiari syndrome. Because symptoms are not specific, an adequate method for screening and characterizing the blockage is desirable, and color Doppler is a reasonable technique in this regard. In its acute form, Budd-Chiari syndrome is diagnosed when flow cannot be identified in all three hepatic veins using color Doppler. Depending on the etiology, actual thrombus may or may not be seen with grayscale (64). After an acute thrombotic episode, collateral pathways open rapidly in and about the liver. Any intrahepatic collateral (a recanalized paraumbilical vein excluded), should suggest Budd-Chiari syndrome as typical portal hypertension diverts blood around not through the liver. The identification of a "bicolored" hepatic vein is pathognomonic and indicates a proximal blockage with one vein draining in the normal direction and the other diverting blood to surface collaterals. In patients with evidence of Budd-Chiari syndrome, the portal vein and IVC should also be carefully evaluated for concurrent thrombosis because of a strong association with hypercoagulable states.

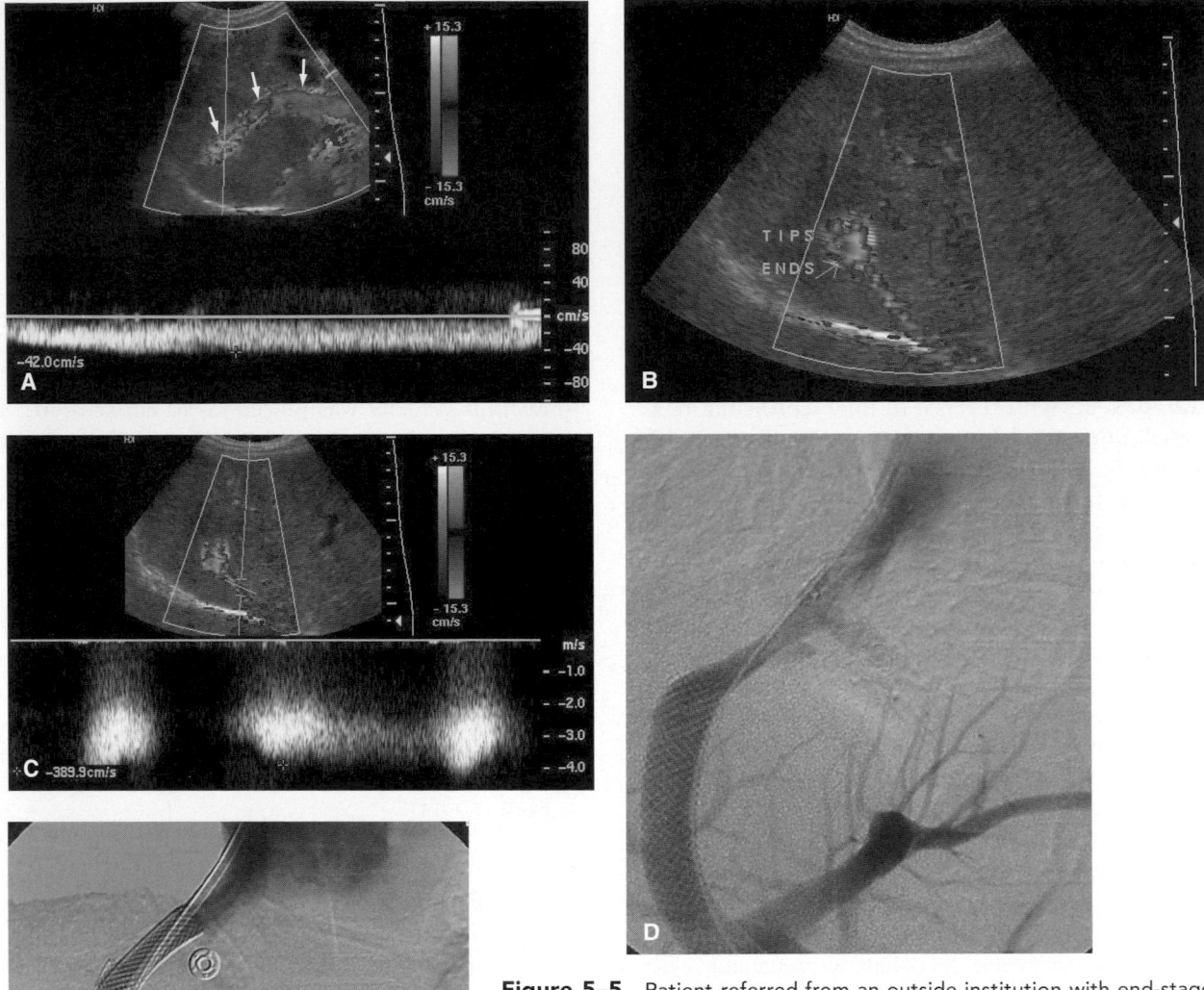

Figure 5–5   Patient referred from an outside institution with end-stage liver disease and multiple episodes of variceal bleeding. **A.** TIPS (*arrows*) is patent but spectral analysis shows flow is abnormally slow at 42 cm/sec. This finding alone will usually prompt intervention as it is highly specific for outlet stenosis. **B.** Color Doppler image demonstrates a diffusely narrowed draining hepatic vein. Aliasing suggests high velocity flow. **C.** Spectral analysis confirms very elevated flow velocity, although signal was intermittent and difficult to obtain. **D.** Angiographic image of TIPS shows narrowing of the hepatic vein, but by visual inspection alone, the degree of stenosis does not appear to be as dramatic as that suggested by the ultrasound. Pressure measurements, however, showed a high gradient, and the TIPS was revised. **E.** Postrevision image shows that the shunt has been extended to almost the level of the IVC. This position is preferred and decreases the propensity for venous stenosis. See Figure 5–5A, B, and C in color insert.

ULTRASOUND IN LIVER TRANSPLANTATION

Hepatic artery thrombosis is the most common vascular complication following liver transplantation. Thrombosis of the hepatic artery, as implied by absent hepatic arterial signal, is a poor prognostic sign and almost invariably dictates retransplantation. Hepatic artery thrombosis occurs most frequently in the first weeks following transplantation. The incidence of hepatic artery thrombosis may occur in 3–12% in adults and 11–42% in children (65), but it

has fallen considerably with improvements in surgical technique and posttransplant care. Duplex/color evaluation of the hepatic artery is usually initially undertaken in the region of the porta hepatis. Color provides images of the artery lying immediately anterior to the main portal vein, and spectral Doppler usually is added to confirm that definitive identification of the artery has happened. Then, most institutions obtain hepatic arterial images with spectral Doppler from both the right and left hepatic arteries. Typically, compromise of the hepatic arterial circulation is associated with parenchymal infarction or ischemic damage to the biliary tree. The former leads to focal hypoechoic lesions, while the latter causes segmental intrahepatic strictures. According to the Worzney et al. study (66), the incidence of hepatic artery thrombosis was 86% in posttransplant patients with focal lesions. The Doppler study should be quite accurate in most cases; the study of Flint et al. (67) demonstrated 92% accuracy in identifying hepatic artery thrombosis.

The ability to form collateral vessels is limited after transplantation but may occur in children and may lead to false-negative studies (65). Arterial collateralization brings flow to the liver, but it is often insufficient and ischemia remains. These children, therefore, are troubled typically by recurrent bouts of sepsis and persistent, focal intrahepatic biliary dilatation and may survive for long periods of time without retransplantation (68,69), despite the ischemic damage. A review of the spectral tracings from these children shows that the resistive index of the hepatic artery is low as an ischemic vascular bed is being sampled (68).

Anastomotic stenoses may also affect the hepatic artery. This complication is another cause of ischemia and can produce clinical findings similar to that in children with chronic thrombosis. Turbulent high velocity flow often accompanied by a color Doppler bruit may be found in the area of the stenosis, if it is visible. As these lesions almost invariably occur in the area of the anastomosis and outside the liver, they may be difficult or impossible to image because of overlying bowel gas. For this reason, indirect signs of ischemia should be sought in the intrahepatic vessels, including low resistance flow (RI ≤0.50) and a tardus-parvus waveform. Combining the intrahepatic and extrahepatic evaluation, Dodd et al. (70) were able to achieve a high degree of success in identifying patients with stenosis or thrombosis with collateralization, both of which will lower RI and require angiography for complete evaluation. Early identification of hepatic artery stenosis is essential if complete thrombosis and extensive parenchymal damage is to be avoided. Once identified, hepatic artery stenosis can be treated successfully by angioplasty, allowing a surgical procedure to be avoided.

Portal vein thrombosis may also occur following transplantation. In our experience, portal vein thrombosis is unusual, even though Dalen et al. (71) report a 7.1% frequency. As with hepatic arterial thrombosis, thrombosis of the portal vein is a devastating vascular complication and usually requires retransplantation (although, when identified rapidly enough, thrombectomy or thrombolysis can be considered). As is true in the native liver, duplex or color Doppler should identify the vast majority of portal vein thromboses (52). The large, normal portal vein is easily visualized in all transplants. A narrow waist with punctate perivascular echogenic foci secondary to surgical clips is frequently noted at the region of the anastomosis and a region of moderate postanastomotic dilatation may be present as well. Although unusual, turbulent spectral patterns are common in patients posttransplantation and are most likely secondary to turbulence originating in the region of the anastomosis. Anastomotic narrowing may occasionally be severe enough the cause high velocity flow, implying the existence of significant stenosis. The clinical implications of such stenoses, however, remain uncertain, but these patients do not appear to progress to frank thrombosis. Hepatic vein thrombosis is quite unusual following transplantation, but patients who have received a large liver for their size may be predisposed to a compromise of the hepatic veins because of compression. Focal narrowing of one hepatic vein at its junction with the IVC is also a recognized complication of patients who have undergone living related or partial liver transplant. This diagnosis typically requires contrast venography, but may be suggested on US examination when dampened hepatic venous pulsatility is identified on spectral Doppler.

REFERENCES

1. Sandler DA, Martin JF, Duncan JS, et al. Diagnosis of deep vein thrombosis: comparison of clinical evaluation, ultrasound, plethysmography, and venoscan with x-ray venogram. Lancet 1984;2:716–720.
2. Fraser JD, Anderson DA. Deep venous thrombosis: recent advances and optimal investigation with US. Radiology 1999; 211:9–24.
3. Sover ER, Brammer HM, Rowedder AM. Thrombosis of the proximal greater saphenous vein: ultrasonographic diagnosis and clinical significance. J Ultrasound Med 1997;16:113–116.
4. Rose SC, Zwiebel WJ, Nelson BD, et al. Symptomatic lower extremity deep venous thrombosis: accuracy, limitations, and role of color duplex flow imaging in diagnosis. Radiology 1990;175: 639–644.
5. Gottlieb RH, Widjaja J, Mehra S, et al. Clinically important pulmonary emboli: does calf vein US alter outcomes? Radiology 1999;211:25–29.
6. Lewis BD, James EM, Welch TJ, et al. Diagnosis of acute deep venous thrombosis of the lower extremities: prospective evaluation of color Doppler flow imaging versus venography. Radiology 1994;192:651–655.
7. Cronan JJ, Leen V. Recurrent deep venous thrombosis: limitations of US. Radiology 1989;170:739–742.
8. Stavros AT, Daigle RJ. Venous duplex imaging of the lower extremities, In: ultrasound categorical course syllabus, American Roentgen Ray Society, 93rd Annu Meet, San Francisco, California, 1993: 333–337.
9. Kerr TM, Lutter KS, Moeller DM, et al. Upper extremity venous thrombosis diagnosed by duplex scanning. Am J Surg 1990;160: 202–206.
10. Donayre CE, White GH, Mehringer SM, et al. Pathogenesis determines late morbidity of axillosubclavian vein thrombosis. Am J Surg 1986;152:179–184.
11. Grassi CJ, Polak JF. Axillary and subclavian venous thrombosis: follow-up evaluation with color Doppler flow US and venography. Radiology 1990;175:651–654.
12. Knudson GJ, Wiedmeyer DA, Erickson SJ, et al. Color Doppler sonographic imaging in the assessment of upper-extremity deep venous thrombosis. AJR 1990;154:399–403.
13. Falk RL, Smith DF. Thrombosis of upper extremity thoracic inlet veins: diagnosis with duplex Doppler sonography. AJR 1987;149: 677–682.
14. Haire WD, Lynch TG, Lieberman RP, et al. Utility of duplex ultrasound in the diagnosis of asymptomatic catheter induced subclavian vein thrombosis. J Ultrasound Med 1991;10:493–496.
15. Patel MC, Berman LH, Moss HA, et al. Subclavian and internal jugular veins at Doppler US: abnormal cardiac pulsatility and

respiratory phasicity as a predictor of complete central occlusion. Radiology 1999;211:579–583.

16. Jager KA, Phillips DJ, Martin RL, et al. Noninvasive mapping of lower limb arterial lesions. Ultrasound Med Biol 1985;11:515.

17. Sacks D, Robinson ML, Marinelli DL, et al. Evaluation of the peripheral arteries with duplex US after angioplasty. Radiology 1990;176:39–44.

18. Cossman DV, Ellison JE, Wagner WH, et al. Comparison of contrast arteriography to arterial mapping with color-flow duplex imaging in the lower extremities. J Vasc Surg 1989;10:522–529.

19. Polak JF, Karmel MI, Mannick JA, et al. Determination of the extent of lower-extremity peripheral arterial disease with color-assisted duplex sonography: comparison with angiography. AJR 1990;155:1085–1089.

20. Polak JF, Donaldson MC, Dobkin GR, et al. Early detection of saphenous vein arterial bypass graft stenosis by color-assisted duplex sonography: a prospective study. AJR 1990;154: 857–861.

21. Mitchell DG. Color Doppler imaging: principles, limitations, and artifacts. Radiology 1990;177;1–10.

22. Abu-Yousef MM, Wiese JA, Shamma AR. The "to and fro" sign: duplex Doppler evidence of femoral artery pseudoaneurysm. AJR 1988;150:632–634.

23. Kotval PS, Khoury A, Shah PM, et al. Doppler sonographic demonstration of the progressive spontaneous thrombosis of pseudoaneurysms. J Ultrasound Med 1990;9:185–190.

24. Paulson EK, Sheafor Dh, Kliewer MA, et al. Treatment of iatrogenic femoral arterial pseudoaneurysms: comparison of US guided thrombin injection with compression repair. Radiology 2000;21:403–408.

25. House MK, Dowling RJ, King P, Gibson RN. Using Doppler sonography to reveal renal artery stenosis: an evaluation of optimal imaging parameters. AJR 1999;173:761–765.

26. Kohler TR, Zierler RE, Martin RL, et al. Noninvasive diagnosis of renal artery stenosis by ultrasonic duplex scanning. J Vasc Surg 1986;4:450–456.

27. Olin JW, Piedmonte MR, Young JR, et al. The utility of duplex ultrasound scanning of the renal arteries for diagnosing significant renal artery stenosis. Ann Intern Med 1995;122: 833–838.

28. Desberg AL, Paushter DM, Lammert GK, et al. Renal artery stenosis: evaluation with color Doppler flow imaging. Radiology 1990;177:749–753.

29. Berland LL, Koslin DB, Routh WD, et al. Renal artery stenosis: prospective evaluation of diagnosis with color duplex US compared with angiography. Radiology 1990;174:421–423.

30. Melany ML, Grant EG, Duerinckx AJ, et al. Initial experience with a phase shift ultrasound contrast agent (dodecafluoropentane) for imaging of the renal arteries. Radiology, 1997;205:147–152.

31. Patriquin HB, Lafortune M, Jequier JC, et al. Stenosis of the renal artery: assessment of slowed systole in the downstream circulation with Doppler sonography. Radiology 1992;184:479–485.

32. Stavros AT, Parker SH, Yakes WF, et al. Segmental stenosis of the renal artery: pattern recognition of tardus and parvus abnormalities with duplex sonography. Radiology 1992;184:487–492.

33. Kliewer MA, Tupler RH, Carroll BA, et al. Renal artery stenosis: analysis of Doppler waveform parameters and tardus parvus pattern. Radiology 1993;189:779–81.

34. Bude RO, Rubin JM, Platt JF, et al. Pulsus tardus: its cause and potential limitations in detection of arterial stenosis. Radiology 1994;190:779–784.

35. Kliewer MA, Hertzberg BS, Keogan MT, et al. Early systole in the healthy kidney: variability of Doppler US in waveform parameters. Radiology 1997;205:109–113.

36. Vasbinder GB, Nelemans PJ, Kessels AG, et al. Diagnostic tests for renal artery stenosis in patients suspected of having renovascular hypertension: a meta-analysis. Ann Intern Med 2001;135:401–411.

37. Radermacher J, Chavan J, Bleck J, et al. Use of Doppler ultrasonography to predict the outcome of therapy for renal artery stenosis. N Engl J Med 2001;344:410–417.

38. Moneta GL, Yeager RA, Dalman R, et al. Duplex ultrasound criteria for diagnosis of splanchnic artery stenosis or occlusion. J Vasc Surg 1991;14:511–520.

39. Moneta GL, Lee RW, Yeager RA, et al. Mesenteric duplex scanning: a blinded prospective study. J Vasc Surg 1993;17:79–86.

40. Lim HK, Lee WJ, Kim SH, et al. Splanchnic arterial stenosis or occlusion: diagnosis at Doppler US. Radiology 1999;211:405–410.

41. Lilly MP, Harward TRS, Flinn WR, et al. Duplex ultrasound measurement of mesenteric flow velocity with pharmacologic and physiologic alteration of intestinal blood flow in man. J Vasc Surg 1989;9:18–25.

42. Taylor KJW, Morse SS, Rigsby CM, et al. Vascular complications in renal allografts: detection with duplex Doppler ultrasound. Radiology 162:31–38, 1987.

43. Kaveggia LP, Perrella RR, Grant EG, et al. Duplex Doppler sonography in renal allografts: the significance of reversed flow in diastole. AJR 1990;155:295–298.

44. Snider JF, Hunter DW, Moradian GP, et al. Transplant renal artery stenosis: evaluation with duplex sonography. Radiology 1989; 172:1027–1030.

45. Gottlieb RH, Lieberman JL, Pabico RC, et al. Diagnosis of renal artery stenosis in transplanted kidneys: value of Doppler waveform analysis of the intrarenal arteries AJR 1995;165:1441–1446.

46. Loubeyre P, Abidi H, Cahen R, et al. Transplanted renal artery: detection of stenosis with color Doppler US. Radiology 1997;203: 661–665.

47. Middleton WD, Kellman GM, Melson GL, et al. Postbiopsy renal transplant arteriovenous fistulas: color Doppler US characteristics. Radiology 1989;171:253–257.

48. Ralls PW. Color Doppler sonography of the hepatic artery and portal venous system. AJR 1990;155:522–526.

49. Soudack M, Epelman M, Gaitini D. Spontaneous thrombosis of hepatic posttraumatic pseudoaneurysms: sonographic and computed tomographic features. J Ultrasound Med 2003;22: 99–103.

50. Endress C, Kling GA, Medrazo BL. Diagnosis of hepatic artery aneurysm with portal vein fistula using image-directed Doppler ultrasound. J Clin Ultrasound 1989;17:206–208.

51. Bezzi M, Mitchell DG, Needleman L, et al. Iatrogenic aneurysmal portal-hepatic venous fistula. Diagnosis by color Doppler imaging. J Ultrasound Med 1988;7:457–459.

52. Tessler FN, Gehring BJ, Gomes AS, et al. Diagnosis of portal vein thrombosis: value of color Doppler imaging. AJR 1991;157: 293–296.

53. Pozniak MA, Baus KM. Hepatofugal arterial signal in the main portal vein: an indicator of intravascular tumor spread. Radiology 1991;180:663–666.

54. Patriquin H, Lafortune M, Burns P, et al. The duplex Doppler examination in portal hypertension: technique and anatomy. AJR 1987;149:71–76.

55. Nelson RC, Lovett KE, Chezmar JL, et al. Comparison of pulsed Doppler sonography and angiography in patients with portal hypertension. AJR 1987;149:77–81.

56. Gebel M, Caselitz M, Bowen-Davies PE, et al. A multicenter, prospective, open label, randomized, controlled phase IIIb study of SHU 508 a (Levovist) for Doppler signal enhancement in the portal vascular system. Ultraschall Med 1998;19:148–156.

57. Grant EG, Tessler FN, Gomes AS, et al. Color Doppler imaging of portosystemic shunts. AJR 1990;154:393–397.

58. Foshager MC, Ferral H, Nazarian GK, et al. Duplex sonography after transjugular intrahepatic portosystemic shunts (TIPS). AJR 1995;165:1–7.

59. Dodd GD, Zajko AB, Orons PD, et al. Detection of transjugular intrahepatic portosystemic shunt dysfunction: value of duplex Doppler sonography. AJR 1995;164:1119–1124.

60. Kanterman RY, Darcy MD, Middleton WD, et al. Doppler sonography findings associated with transjugular portosystemic shunt malfunction. AJR 1997;186:467–472.

61. Feldstein VA, LaBerge JM. Hepatic vein flow reversal at duplex sonography: a sign of transjugular intrahepatic portosystemic shunt dysfunction. AJR 1994;162:839–841.

62. Duerinckx A, Grant E, Perrella R, et al. The pulsatile portal vein: correlation of duplex Doppler with right atrial pressures. Radiology 1990;176:655–658.

63. Abu-Yousef MM, Milam SG, Farner RM. Pulsatile portal vein flow: a sign of tricuspid regurgitation on duplex Doppler sonography. AJR 1990;155:785–788.

64. Millener P, Grant EG, Rose S, Duerinckx A, et al. Color Doppler imaging findings in patients with Budd-Chiari syndrome: correlation with venographic findings. AJR 1993;161:307–312.

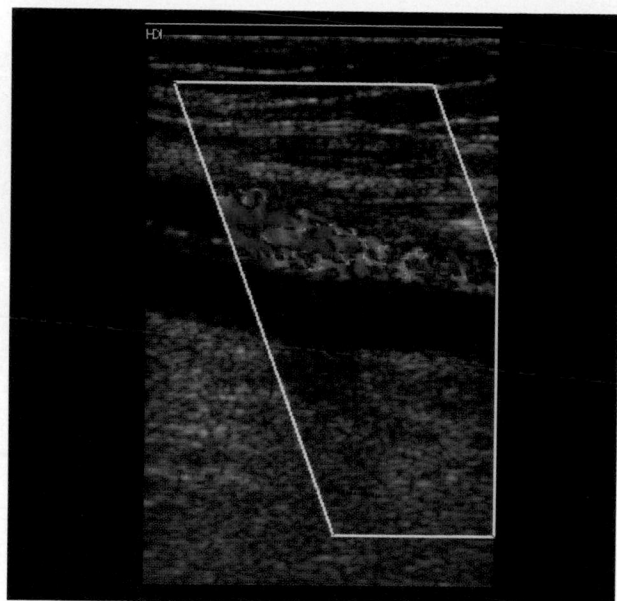

Figure 5–1 B. Longitudinal color Doppler image confirms presence of thrombus in the vein; no color is seen. The expansile and anechoic appearance of the vein suggests that the clot is acute. The mixture of colors in the adjacent common femoral artery is because of aliasing, as the scanner is adjusted to identify slow flow.

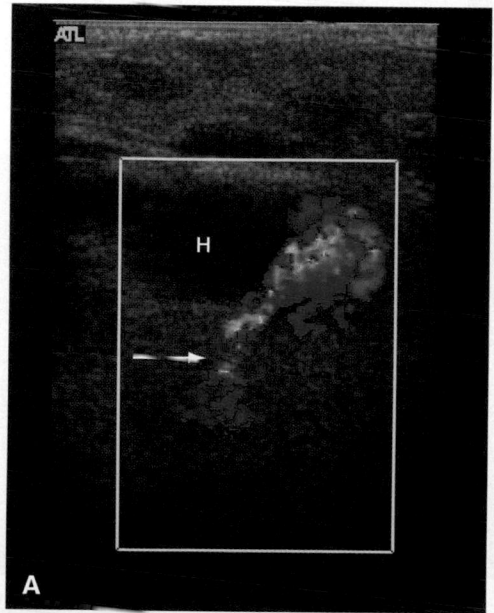

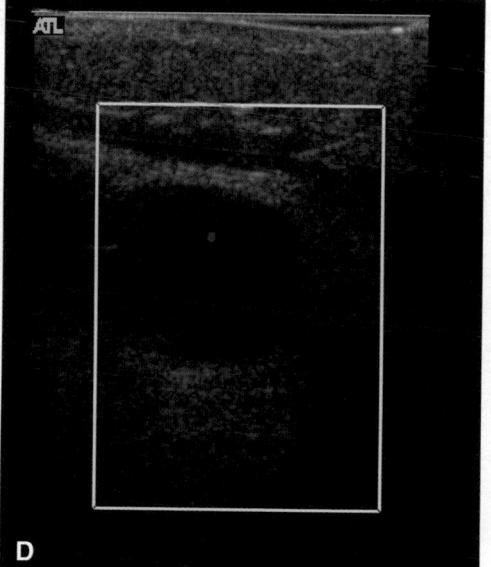

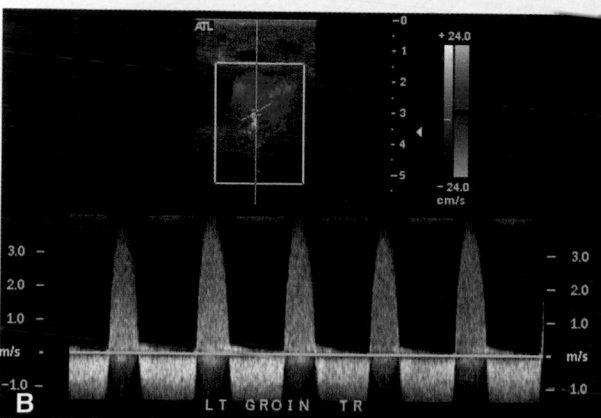

Figure 5–2 Patient 3 days postcardiac catheterization with ecchymotic groin mass. **A.** Color Doppler image shows a typical pseudoaneurysm with a well-defined and narrow neck (*arrow*), swirling flow within (the yin-yang sign) and a hypoechoic area (*H*) representing internal thrombus. **B.** Spectral Doppler image taken at the distal neck of the pseudoaneurysm demonstrates the classic "to and fro" signal. Note sharp upstroke in systole and a holodiastolic flow reversal in diastole. As arterial pressure is higher than that of the pseudoaneurysm during systole, blood flows into the cavity. During diastole blood flows back out as pressure falls in the adjacent artery. **D.** Follow-up color Doppler image shows complete absence of flow, confirming successful ablation.

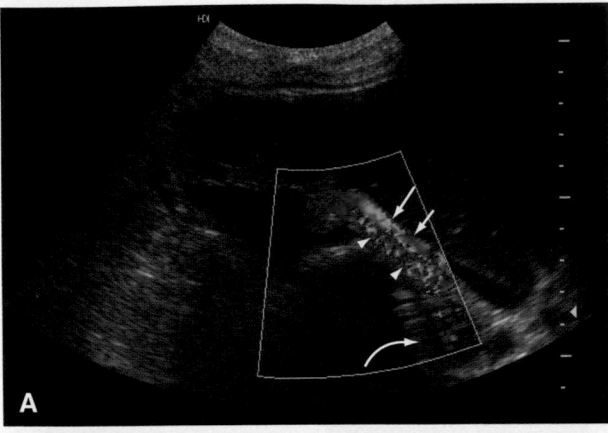

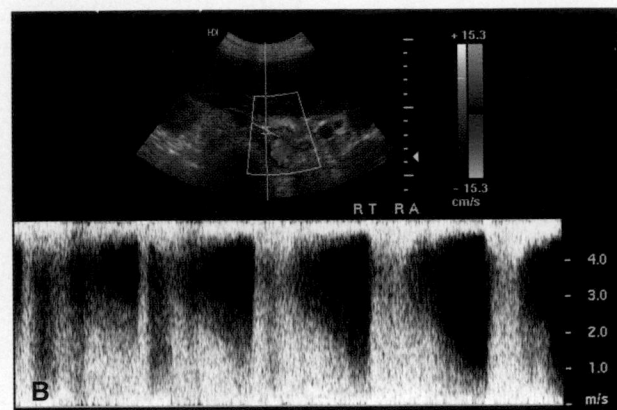

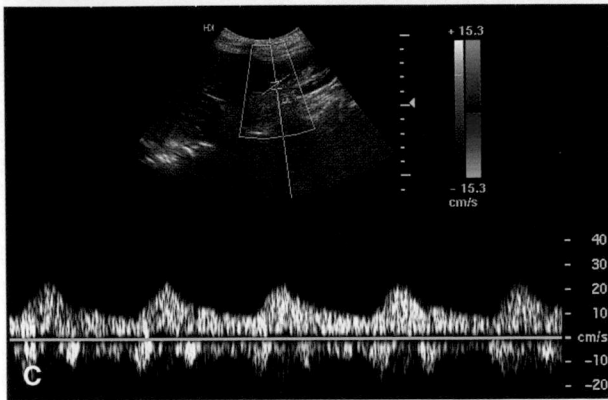

Figure 5–3 Patient with severe, recurrent hypertension, who underwent stenting of left renal artery stenosis 4 years previously. **A.** Color Doppler image of the right renal artery shows pronounced aliasing through most of the vessel suggesting the presence of high speed flow. Curved arrow = aorta, arrows = right renal vein. **B.** Spectral sample from within the proximal right renal artery confirms extremely high velocity of well over 4 meters/second. **C.** Intrarenal spectral examination further suggests renal artery stenosis. Note pyramidal appearance of the waveforms, which show the classic tardus-parvus phenomenon. There is no early systolic peak, and the normal sharp systolic upstroke is delayed.

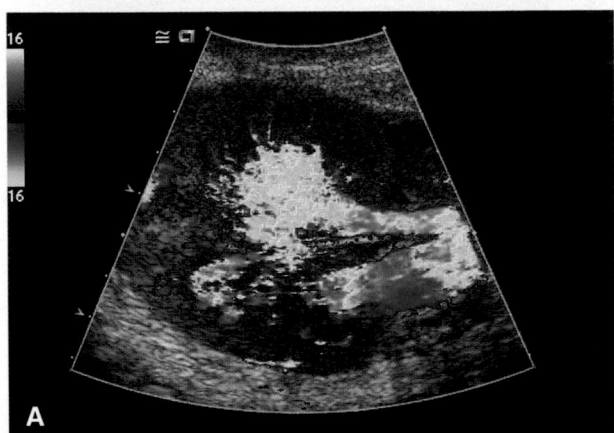

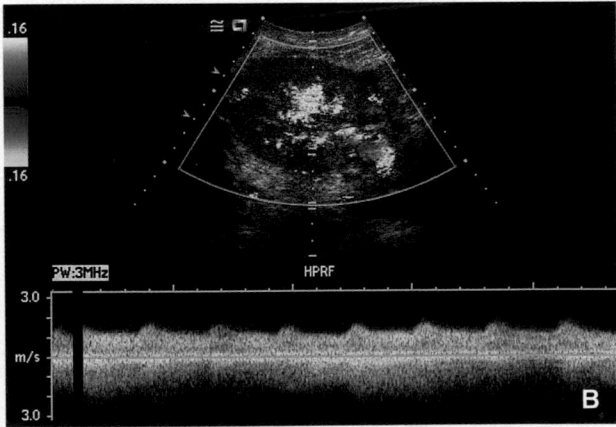

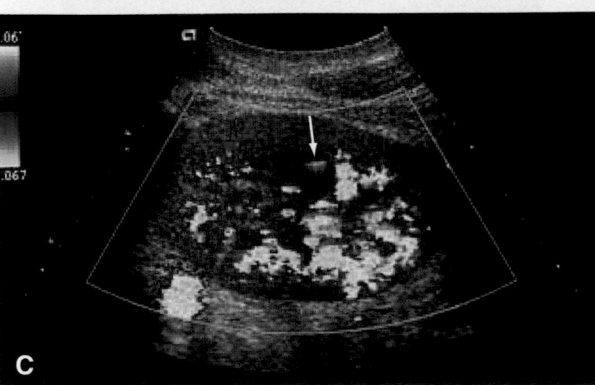

Figure 5–4 Patient with a renal transplant presenting with hematuria following a percutaneous biopsy. **A.** Color Doppler image shows a large color Doppler bruit, typical of an arteriovenous fistula. Note that color is assigned well beyond the expected anatomic location of the renal arteries and veins. **B.** Spectral analysis in the area of the color Doppler bruit shows high speed, extremely low resistance flow, the classic pattern of an AVF. **C.** Postembolization ultrasound reveals a wedge-shaped area of infarction with no color flow, but no evidence of the AVF. Echogenic focus (*arrow*) was believed to represent an embolization coil.

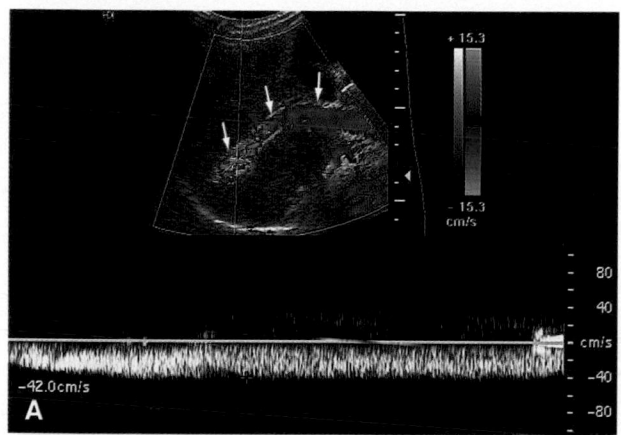

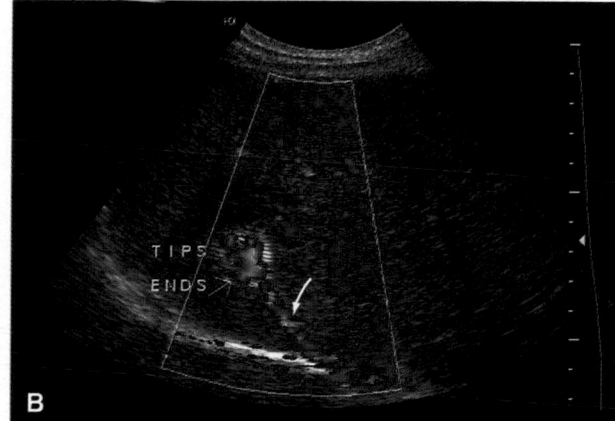

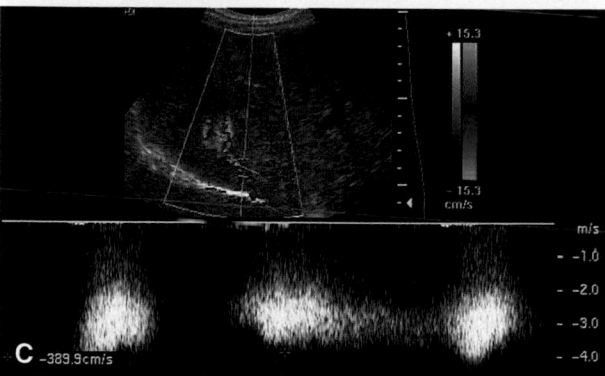

Figure 5–5 Patient referred from an outside institution with end-stage liver disease and multiple episodes of variceal bleeding. **A.** TIPS (*arrows*) is patent but spectral analysis shows flow is abnormally slow at 42 cm/sec. This finding alone will usually prompt intervention as it is highly specific for outlet stenosis. **B.** Color Doppler image demonstrates a diffusely narrowed draining hepatic vein. Aliasing suggests high velocity flow. **C.** Spectral analysis confirms very elevated flow velocity, although signal was intermittent and difficult to obtain.

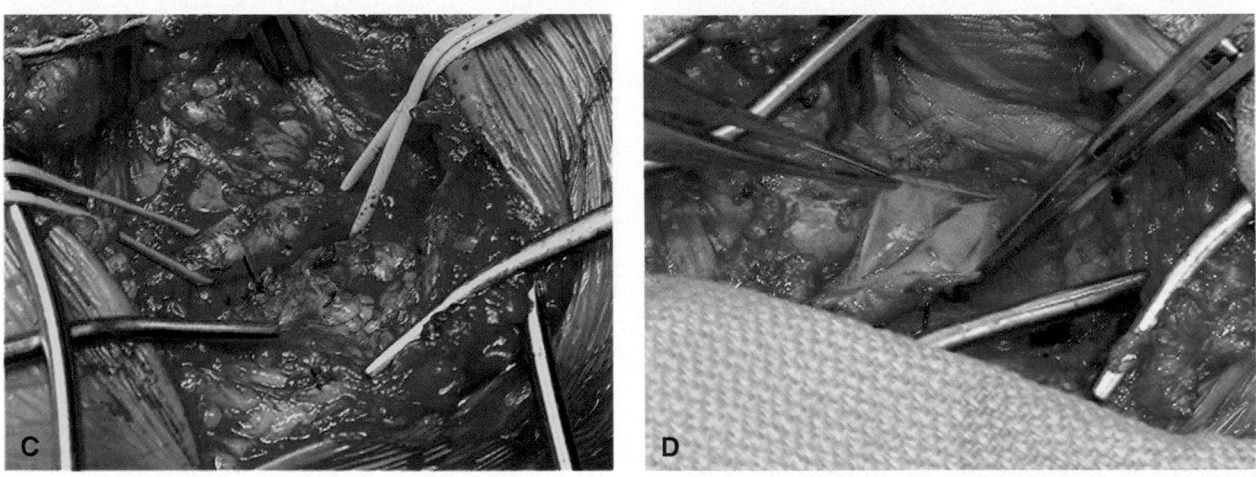

Figure 18–10 C. Localized bulge in the artery with direct visualization at surgery, **D.** with normal underlying artery once decompressed by incision of cyst. (Carin Gosalves, MD—Thomas Jefferson University Hospital)

65. Morton MJ, James EM, Wiesner RH, et al. Applications of duplex ultrasonography in the liver transplant patient. Mayo Clin Proc 1990;65:360–363.

66. Worzney P, Zajko AB, Bron KM, et al. Vascular complications after liver transplantation: a 5-year experience. AJR 1986;147:657–663.

67. Flint EW, Sumkin JH, Zajko AB, et al. Duplex sonography of hepatic artery thrombosis after liver transplantation. AJR 1988;151:481–483.

68. Hall TR, McDiarmid SU, Grant EG, et al. False-negative duplex Doppler studies in children with hepatic artery thrombosis after liver transplantation. AJR 1990;154:573–575.

69. Hoffer FA, Teele RL, Lillehei CW, et al. Infected bilomas and hepatic artery thrombosis in infant recipients of liver transplants. Interventional radiology and medical therapy as an alternative to retransplantation. Radiology 1988;169:435–438.

70. Dodd GD, Memel DS, Zajko AB, et al. Hepatic artery stenosis and thrombosis in transplant recipients: Doppler diagnosis with resistive index and systolic acceleration time. Radiology 1994;192: 657–661.

71. Dalen K, Day DL, Ascher NL, et al. Imaging of vascular complications after hepatic transplantation. AJR 1988;150:1285–1290.

Multidetector Row Computed Tomographic Angiography

6

Technique and Clinical Applications

Jeffrey C. Hellinger, Geoffrey D. Rubin

Endovascular interventions are accepted, minimally invasive alternative therapies to conventional surgical interventions. Parallel with endovascular developments is the application of less invasive diagnostic cardiovascular imaging modalities. Ultrasound, magnetic resonance angiography (MRA), and computed tomographic angiography (CTA) are now integral components of diagnostic algorithms for cardiovascular disease. As a result, catheter angiography is used less for diagnosis and more as an adjunct to endovascular procedures.

Today's cardiovascular imager and interventionalist must have fundamental knowledge of ultrasound, MRA, and CTA, so they can integrate these noninvasive modalities into daily practice for diagnosis and treatment planning. The advantages are many. First, noninvasive imaging benefits patient care as vascular pathology is identified and treatment decisions are made with less risk to the patient and without unwarranted catheter angiography. Second, it affords more widespread vascular screening, allowing diagnoses to be made at an earlier stage. Third, noninvasive imaging can expand clinical volume while optimizing work efficiency in a busy academic or private practice.

Ultrasound and MRA are discussed in Chapters 5 and 7. The purpose of this chapter is to review CTA principles and provide an overview of clinical applications.

HISTORICAL PERSPECTIVE

The introduction of spiral computed tomography (SCT) in 1990 ushered in a new era of diagnostic imaging (1). The ability to acquire large volumes of data more rapidly with improved longitudinal spatial resolution and reduced respiratory motion compared to conventional computed tomography opened the door for new clinical applications of CT. Without question, the most dramatic application has been CT angiography. Initially, clinical use of CTA was restricted to imaging large size vessels, such as central pulmonary arteries, aorta (2,3), and their major branches, including common carotid arteries and renal arteries (4,5). Limited spatial resolution precluded high quality visualization of small caliber vessels (6). In addition, relatively slow acquisition speeds restricted longitudinal coverage. This precluded imaging of entire vascular territories with thin sections in a reasonable duration or single acquisition, such as for the upper and lower extremities (7,8). Technological developments over the course of one and a half decades have addressed these issues. Today, the standard for CTA is defined by submillimeter thickness, subsecond rotation times, and isotropic spatial resolution—capable of imaging larger anatomic regions faster with superior image quality and better optimization of contrast-medium administration. Although improved interpolation algorithms, greater x-ray tube heat capacities, and more rapid gantry rotation have all contributed, the development of multidetector row technology provided the greatest instrumental advancement (9–11). In doing so, CTA has now become a robust, accurate, and reproducible modality for cardiovascular evaluation, affording high clinical confidence among imagers and clinicians.

Currently used multidetector row computed tomography (MDCT) scanners, with 4, 8, 10, 16, 32, 40, and 64 channels, continue to challenge catheter-based angiography as the modality of choice for diagnostic angiography. In fact, at many medical centers, CTA has obviated the need for diagnostic catheter angiography in most clinical algorithms. This includes evaluation of the pulmonary circulation, thoracic and abdominal aorta, extracranial carotid and vertebral arteries, intracranial circulation, mesenteric and renal vessels, and upper and lower extremity vasculature. Although its full clinical potential has yet to be reached, cardiac MDCT, performed with 4- to16-channel scanners, has already had an impact on evaluation and management of adult and pediatric heart disease. Adapting protocols on 32- to 64-channel scanners and beyond will certainly push cardiac MDCT to the front line of diagnostic cardiac evaluation.

PRINCIPLES OF COMPUTED TOMOGRAPHIC ANGIOGRAPHY

Computed tomographic angiography (CTA) occurs by synchronizing a high-flow intravenous contrast-medium injection with a rapid thin section spiral acquisition timed to the arterial or venous phase. From this volumetric dataset, two-dimensional (2D) and three-dimensional (3D) images are generated. As single detector row scanners have advanced to multidetector row scanners with each successive MDCT generation, protocols and techniques have evolved to maximize the capabilities of the scanners, optimize contrast-medium administration, and simplify image display. The three major technical components discussed in the following section—scan acquisition, contrast-medium administration, and image display/postprocessing—will provide a framework for adapting and applying the evolving technology used to acquire CT angiograms.

SCAN ACQUISITION

Scan protocols are designed to provide comprehensive evaluations with high image quality and accurate disease depiction and characterization. To maximize exam efficiency and patient throughput, routine protocols are sufficient in most instances. However, in some cases, scan protocols will require patient-specific modifications to address the clinical questions.

In the context of designing the protocol, several tactical considerations must be addressed. First, in preparation for the exam, patients should not receive any positive oral contrast. The high-density material can limit disease detection and degrade image quality of postprocessed images. Instead, if bowel distention is necessary, water can be administered as a negative contrast agent. To prescribe the exam coverage and field of view, all CT angiograms begin with an anterior-posterior low dose scout view. In some applications, such as upper and lower extremity CTA, prescription is optimized further with a lateral scout view. The next consideration is whether to obtain nonenhanced images (1.25–5.0 mm thickness). The primary role of this possible acquisition is to identify high-density material that may be obscured by or may be confused for injected contrast medium. Images provide valuable information regarding the presence and location of vascular calcifications, aneurysm thrombus calcification, residual intravenous contrast, blood products (such as intramural hematoma), endovascular stents and stent grafts, surgical clips, surgical grafts, mechanical valves, glue material, foreign bodies, and bone fragments (including trauma). By definition, all CT angiograms include the subsequent contrast-enhanced arterial dedicated venous phase acquisition. Among other details, an important technical decision at this step is whether cardiac gating is required. The final consideration to address is the need for delayed contrast-enhanced images, after the initial arterial phase. Clinical applications warranting this phase include those that also necessitate visceral or venous (or both) evaluations and those that require identification of delayed contrast accumulation, including endoleaks and active hemorrhage. In these instances, supplementary contrast-medium administration is not necessary. Scan parameters may vary, depending on the desired spatial resolution, scan duration, and tube heating. When monitoring exams, if the scan gets ahead of the contrast medium, an immediate second phase can be obtained, without infusing more contrast. For other technical limitations, such as excessive noise, poor luminal enhancement, motion artifacts, and streak artifacts, the exam may need to be repeated.

Contrast-Enhanced Phase

CTA parameters can be categorized as those prescribed either for raw data acquisition or those for data reconstruction (Table 6–1). Using the reconstruction parameters, one or more datasets can be generated from the original acquisition. Based on the type of MDCT scanner, parameter selection reflects a balance between desired spatial resolution, temporal resolution, volume coverage, and scan duration. The result is that for some clinical applications, not all MDCT scanners can effectively produce CT angiograms with equal parameters and, as such, protocols must be customized for each scanner. Furthermore, some clinical applications, such as cardiac MDCT, will not be as robust on all scanners. In all instances, the scan durations will influence the breath-hold, opportunity for motion-induced artifacts, and the selection of the contrast-medium protocol.

The parameters fundamental to generating volumetric MDCT datasets with high-quality inplane and longitudinal spatial resolution consist of a thin detector-row configuration, a low pitch, thin reconstruction section thickness, and overlapping reconstruction intervals. This extends from experimental work using phantom models on SDCT scanners that recommended a collimation of 1–2 mm, a pitch of 1–2, and a reconstruction interval of 50% (12–14). For MDCT angiography, the most important of these parameters is the detector-row thickness, because the reconstruction section thickness cannot be less than the detector thickness. The recent introduction of a MDCT scanner that acquires 64 0.4 mm sections using 32 0.6 mm detector rows and an oscillating focal spot within the x-ray tube currently represents the only exception to this rule (Siemens Medical Solutions). Thus, with this one exemption,

it is always possible to reconstruct sections thicker than the detector width, but it is not possible to reconstruct thinner images. Pitch, which is defined as the table increment (mm) per beam width (mm) for each 360-degree rotation, typically ranges between 1.0 and 1.5 for most noncardiac gated MDCTA acquisitions. In general, pitch varies inversely with image quality when multislice linear interpolation algorithms are used, as the effective slice thickness increases. When adaptive axial interpolation algorithms are used, as with Siemens scanners (Siemens Medical Solutions), the effective slice thickness is independent of pitch. Regarding slice thickness and reconstruction increment, for most MDCTA clinical applications, 1–1.5 mm thick images reconstructed every 0.5 mm to 0.8 mm is sufficient. The clinical value for using thin reconstructed sections is illustrated in Figure 6–1. If the exam is performed on a 4-row system, 2.5 mm detectors may be required to cover the entire volume in a reasonable scan duration. In this instance, 2.5–3 mm sections are reconstructed at 1.25–1.5 mm intervals. Depending on the clinical indications, isotropic resolution datasets can be acquired on currently available 16- to 64-channel systems, employing submillimeter collimation/thickness (0.625 mm, for example), and reconstruction intervals (0.5 mm, for example).

Table 6–2 shows hypothetical protocols for 4-, 8-, 16-, and 64-channel MDCT scanners, covering an 800–1,000 mm volume of data. Note how the detector width influences selection of the slice thickness, reconstruction interval, and consequently, image resolution. In addition, note how the number of detector rows influences the table speed (mm/sec) and scan duration (sec). A gain in scan speed can be used to produce high or isotropic resolution datasets. With scanners that have at least 32 detectors, one may consider routine submillimeter acquisitions to produce superior spatial resolution. In this instance, as a result of the scanner speed, volume coverage and scan duration are no longer limiting factors. The downside, however, is the progressive "data overload," whereby the increased number of reconstructed images may potentially limit image reconstruction time, transfer, viewing, and storage. Another shortcoming is that thinner sections will lead to increased image noise.

In addition to detector width, pitch and the gantry speed influence table speed and scan duration. Gantry speed is the time (sec) per each 360-degree rotation of the tube and detectors. Most noncardiac-gated MDCTA acquisitions use a gantry speed of 0.4–0.6. Prescribing a high pitch value and the fastest possible gantry rotation period may be necessary when a shorter scan duration is required to optimize contrast administration or to minimize a patient's breath-hold, as with 4- to 8-row scanners. A faster gantry rotation speed is also required to maximize temporal resolution during cardiac MDCT. The potential limitations with high pitch values are decreased spatial

TABLE 6–1
MDCTA SCAN PARAMETERS

Data Acquisition	Data Reconstruction
Detector row width	Slice thickness
Pitch	Reconstruction interval
Gantry rotation speed	Field of view
Tube current	Reconstruction algorithm
Tube voltage	Half-scan reconstruction
Prospective ECG-gating	Multisector ECG reconstruction
Retrospective ECG-gating	

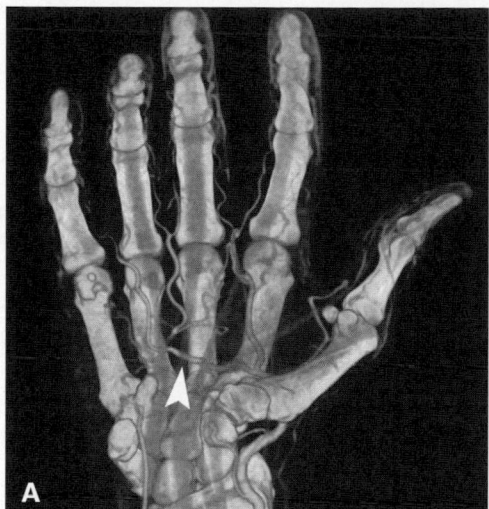
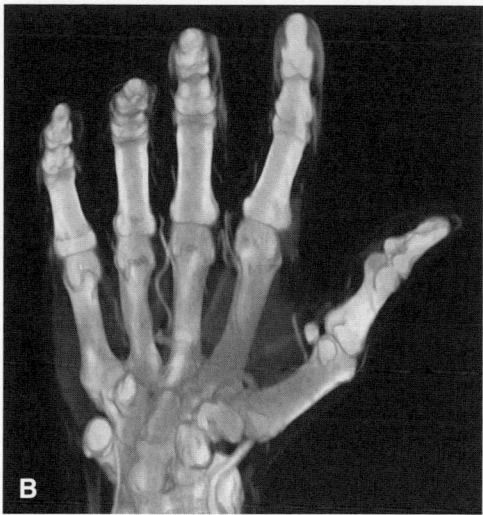
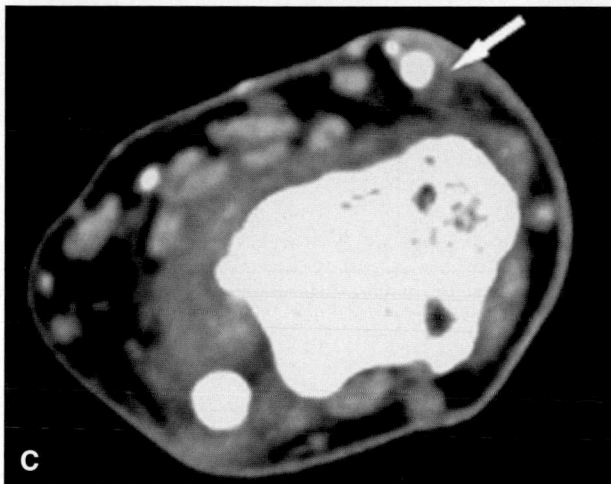

Figure 6–1   Volume-rendered images are from an upper extremity CT angiogram performed in a patient with a focal pulsatile mass at the right wrist. The study was acquired on a 64-channel scanner using a detector width of 0.6 mm, pitch of 0.9, and gantry speed of 0.5 sec/rotation. The original dataset was reconstructed into 1 mm thick sections every 0.7 mm. **A.** A second reconstruction generated 4 mm thick sections at 2 mm intervals. **B.** In comparing the two images, note the loss of distinct bony and vascular detail with the thicker images. The lower spatial resolution in the second reconstruction requires use of lower opacity transfer threshold values to attempt depiction of the 1–2 mm size palmar and digitals vessels. This leads to increased soft tissue visualization, further obscuring vessel depiction. As shown in **C.**, source images reveal a 6 mm x 4.5 mm aneurysm off the proximal radial deep branch with eccentric thrombus (*arrow*). The volume-rendered images from the 1 mm thick dataset are reliable to confirm patency of the deep arch (**A**, *arrowhead*) and common and paired digital arteries, while volume-rendered images from the 4 mm thick sections are nondiagnostic to exclude distal embolization.

resolution and increased image noise. The tradeoff with a faster gantry speed is increased noise. This is because the product of the tube current and the gantry rotation period defines the total number of photons delivered. Lower pitch values are reserved for cardiac imaging and when higher resolution or lower noise datasets are required. Slowing the gantry speed will also reduce noise. The penalties for reducing the pitch or slowing the gantry speed are longer scan durations and increased radiation exposure, for the same tube current.

Minimization of image noise during CT angiogram acquisitions is essential because it improves the contrast-to-background noise ratio and overall quality of the 3D images. In addition to pitch and gantry rotation speed, other factors affecting image noise include tube current, tube voltage, slice thickness and reconstruction algorithm. Of importance is maximizing the tube current, optimizing the voltage, reconstructing thicker sections, or reconstructing images with a soft kernel.

TABLE 6–2
MDCTA PARAMETERS

Number of Rows	Acquisition				Reconstruction			
	Collimation	Pitch	TI	TS	Scan Time	TH	RI	Number of Images
4	4 x 2.5Δ‡ o	1.5	15	30	27–33	2.5	1.25	640–800
	4 x 2.0*	1.375	11	22	36–45	2.0	1.0	800–1,000
	4 x 1.25Δ	1.5	7.5	15	53–67	1.25	0.8	1,000–1,250
	4 x 1.0‡o	1.5	6	12	67–83	1.0	0.8	1,000–1,250
	4 x 1.0 *	1.375	5.5	11	73–91	1.0	0.8	1,000–1,250
8Δ	8 x 2.5	1.35	27	30	14–18.5	2.5	1.25	640–800
	8 x 1.25	1.35	13.5	15	30–37	1.25	0.8	1,000–1,250
16	16 x 1.5o	1.5	36	72	11–14	1.5	0.8	1,000–1,250
	16 x 1.5‡	1.25	30	60	13–17	1.5	0.8	1,000–1,250
	16 x 1.25Δ	1.375	27.5	55	14.5–18	1.25	0.8	1,000–1,250
	16 x 1.0*	1.4375	23	46	17–22	1.0	0.8	1,000–1,250
	16 x 0.75o	1.5	18	36	22–28	0.75	0.5	1,600–2,000
	16 x 0.75‡	1.25	15	30	27–33	0.75	0.5	1,600–2,000
	16 x 0.625Δ	1.375	13.75	27.5	29–36	0.625	0.5	1,600–2,000
	16 x 0.5*	1.4375	11.5	23	35–44	0.5	0.4	2,000–2,500
64	32 x 1.25Δ	0.9375	37.5	75	11–13	1.25	0.8	1,000–1,250
	24 x 1.2o	0.9	26	52	15–19	1.2	0.8	1,000–1,250
	64 x 625Δ	0.9375	37.5	75	11–13	0.625	0.5	1,600–2,000
	2 x 32 x 0.6o	0.9	34.6	69	11.5–14.5	0.6	0.5	1,600–2,000

Note: Parameters shown are for an 800–1,000 mm acquisition with a 0.5 sec gantry rotation. Collimation = Number of channels x detector width (mm); TI = Table Increment/360° gantry rotation; TS = Table speed (mm/sec); Scan time in seconds; TH = Slice thickness (mm).
ΔGE, ‡ Phillips, oSiemens, and *Toshiba scanners.

Cardiac Gating

A vital technical component for cardiac and thoracic aortic CTA is ECG synchronization, which is needed to suppress cardiac and aortic motion, allowing for the evaluation of cardiac structures, the aortic root, coronary vasculature, and bypass grafts (Figure 6–2), as well as for improving the evaluation of dissection flaps (Figure 6–3), subtle intramural hematoma, and aortic injury. Two methods of synchronization are available. The first, prospective ECG triggering, is a nonhelical "step and shoot" technique. Images are acquired at a predetermined phase during the ECG cycle. The number of acquired images per rotation is dependent upon the number of detector rows. This technique is used most often for coronary calcium imaging but is also used when acquiring noncontrast images through the heart to evaluate for pericardial calcification. The second method, retrospective ECG gating, is a low pitch, highly overlapping, volumetric acquisition that generates multiple phases per Z-position. To achieve this, an ECG tracing is recorded simultaneously with the spiral acquisition. The raw data is then reconstructed as a function of both the table position and user-defined phases in the cardiac cycle (15,16). To optimize temporal resolution, the fastest possible gantry rotation speed should be selected. Multisector reconstructions can further improve temporal resolution. These are particularly useful in patients with heart rates of >70 beats per minute. Although the radiation dose increases with retrospective ECG gating (17), advantages include suppression of cardiac and aortic pulsation; time resolved four-dimensional (4D) cine visualization of the heart, thoracic aorta, and great vessels (18); and reliable quantification of ventricular volumes, ejection fractions, and ventricular masses. Thus, with this technique, 3D and 4D cardiac and thoracic aortic renderings can be generated with minimal motion artifacts, providing accurate morphologic and functional assessment.

CONTRAST-MEDIUM ADMINISTRATION

Optimizing contrast-medium administration is an essential element for producing diagnostic images. This is particularly true when using advanced generation scanners, because with rapid volume coverage, there is greater likelihood to miss the bolus. Optimization is achieved by implementing strategies that reflect a balance between physiologic factors, the vascular territory of interest, and

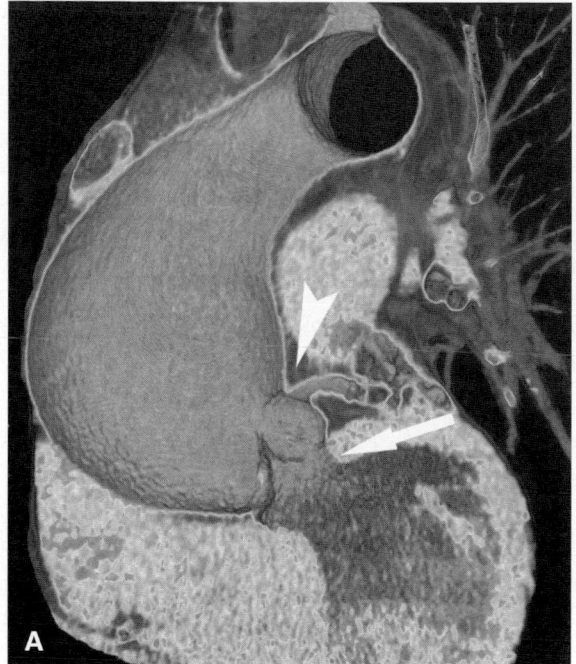

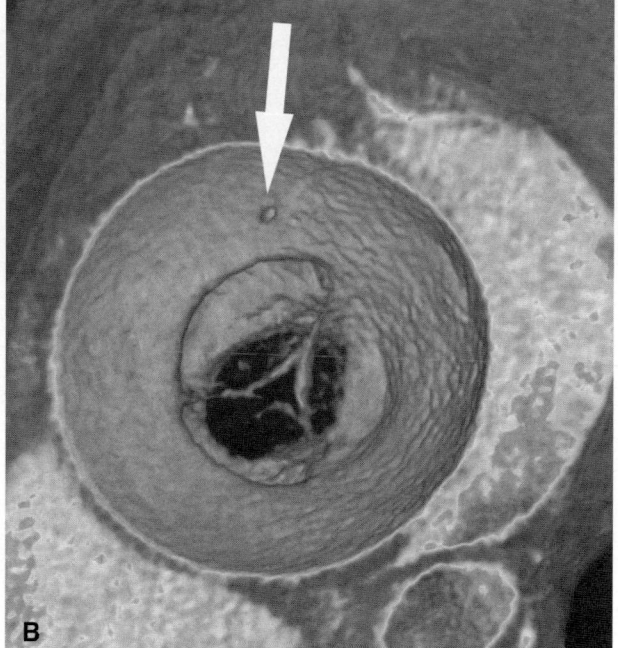

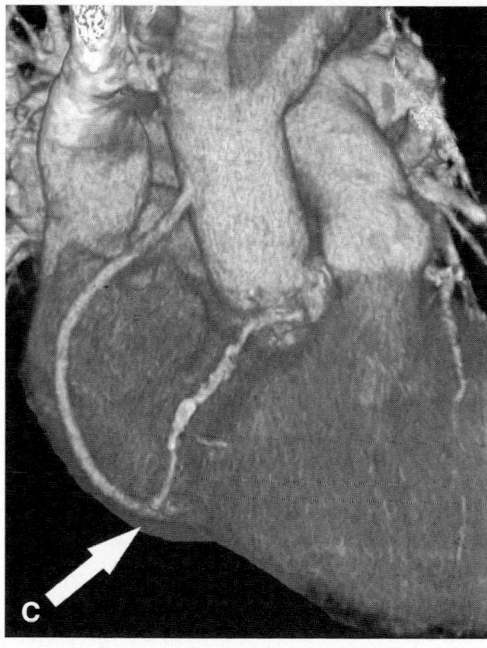

Figure 6–2 CT angiography in a patient with Marfan's disorder demonstrats aneurysmal enlargement of ascending aorta to 8 cm x 8 cm. **A.** Retrospective ECG gating with a 16 mm x 1.25 mm collimation affords precise preoperative evaluation to plan for an aortic composite valve replacement with reimplantation of the left main coronary artery and reversed saphenous bypass grafting to the right coronary artery. In addition to the aneurysm, the volume-rendered image shown here reveals normal size of the aortic annulus (*arrow*) and high origin of the left main coronary artery (*arrowhead*) at the base of the aneurysm. **B.** A short axis projection through the aortic root in diastole. This reveals poor coaptation of the aortic leaflets, consistent with the patient's clinically known aortic insufficiency. This image again reveals left main coronary artery origin from the base of the aneurysm (*arrow*). Postsurgical CT angiography is also performed with retrospective gating. **C.** A selected volume-rendered image from this exam, revealing normal appearance of the ascending aortic graft and patency of the reversed saphenous bypass graft that anastomoses with the second segment of the right coronary artery (*arrow*), distal to a long segment of calcified atherosclerotic plaque.

the scan duration. Before discussing these strategies, a brief overview of relevant contrast-medium pharmacokinetic principles is presented. Fundamental understanding of these principles is important for implementing strategies and quality control purposes.

Contrast-Medium Pharmacokinetics

Intravenously administered contrast medium travels first in the venous circulation to the right heart, through the pulmonary circulation, then the left heart before reaching the systemic arterial circulation (first pass). After circulating through the arterial system, viscera, interstitium, and venous system, contrast reenters the right heart (recirculation). In general, arterial structures are best imaged during first pass kinetics, while venous structures are depicted better during recirculation. However, during a bolus of contrast medium, both first pass and recirculation kinetics affect luminal enhancement quality (Figure 6–4). This affords selection of protocols with either uniphasic or biphasic injections. Uniphasic injections produce a continuous increase in enhancement, followed by an abrupt decrease

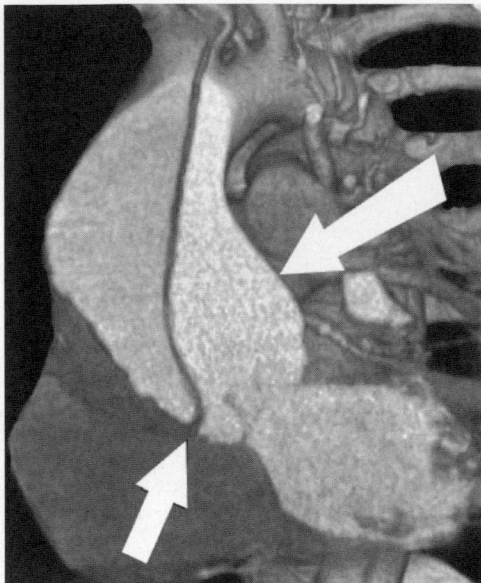

Figure 6–3 A volume-rendered image from 16 mm x 1.25 mm retrospectively ECG-gated CT angiogram depicts a Stanford type A dissection. By suppressing cardiac motion, extension of the dissection flap into the aortic root is demonstrated with high detail (*small arrow*). Note the aneurysmal caliber of the ascending aorta and the differential enhancement of the true lumen (*large arrow*) and false lumen.

in enhancement once the injection is complete, leading to nonuniform enhancement (19). Biphasic injections utilize an initial, higher flow injection (5–8 mL/s) of short duration followed by a second slower flow injection (3–4 mL/s) with a longer duration. This produces more uniform enhancement profiles (20–22).

Once injected, to synchronize the bolus of contrast medium with the scan acquisition, the scan is initiated when contrast reaches the targeted vascular territory. The time for contrast medium to travel from the site of injection to the target site is defined as the contrast-medium transit time (tCMT). After contrast reaches the vascular territory of interest, luminal enhancement, defined by the change in Hounsfield units (HU), depends on the delivery of a sufficient amount of iodine (iodine dose) at an appropriate rate (iodine flux). Each milligram of iodine per milliliter of blood produces a 25 HU attenuation increase (23–24). In general, CTA studies with suitable arterial enhancement should reach at least a minimum of 250–300 HU. However, the minimum threshold for diagnostic studies will vary depending on the noise of the study. For most applications, to reach an acceptable threshold, the recommended minimum iodine dose is 400–600 mgI/kg (1.1–1.7 mL/kg for 350 mgI/mL concentration) (25–29) with a suggested iodine flux of 1.2–1.5 gI/sec, (3.4–4.3 mL/sec for 350 mgI/mL concentration). (29–31). User defined parameters to control both the iodine dose and flux include iodine concentration

(mgI/mL), contrast injection rate (mL/sec), and duration of iodine administration (sec).

Multiple patient-dependent physiologic factors influence luminal enhancement as well. These comprise the site and quality of venous access, vascular pathology, cardiac output, renal function, height, weight, age, and gender. Of these factors, the most important are cardiac output and body weight. Both inversely affect the degree of arterial enhancement, while cardiac output also inversely affects the tCMT. Venous access distance to the targeted vascular territory, stenoses, occlusions, and aneurysms also inversely affect tCMT.

Strategies for Contrast-Medium Administration

Intravenous Access

To achieve more precise, uniform enhancement at the high flow rates, a power injector with a 20-gauge intravenous (IV) catheter is used to administer contrast. An antecubital vein is preferable because this is the least likely peripheral venous site to lead to contrast extravasation. Automated devices are available to detect extravasation and to terminate injection when skin-impedance changes are detected (34–35). When thoracic, cardiac, and carotid CTA are performed, the IV catheter should be placed in the right arm to reduce streak artifacts that may obscure supra-arch vessels. To eliminate streak artifacts when an upper extremity is imaged, IV access is gained in the contralateral upper extremity.

Scanning Delay

To account for the variable tCMT among patients and to ensure continual enhancement during the acquisition window, MDCT angiography requires that the arrival time for contrast medium be determined by a test-bolus injection or automatic bolus triggering. A test bolus is performed by injecting 15–20 cc of contrast at a rate equivalent to that planned for the CTA. Low dose, thick transverse sections are acquired every 2 seconds. A region of interest (ROI) is placed in the reference vessel to generate a time-attenuation curve. The tCMT equals the time to the curve's peak, which then is selected as the minimum delay. Automated triggering is available on all MDCT scanners. During contrast injection, low dose, single level sections are acquired. Reference-vessel attenuation is monitored in near real-time either with an ROI or by visual inspection. The tCMT is defined as the time required to reach a predetermined opacification threshold. The scan then is initiated after a short diagnostic delay. In comparison to a test-bolus injection, the actual scan delay is longer when automated triggering is used. This is because of inherent interscan and image reconstruction delays, in addition to the diagnostic delay. Depending on the scanner, the minimum scan delay may range between 2 and 8 seconds.

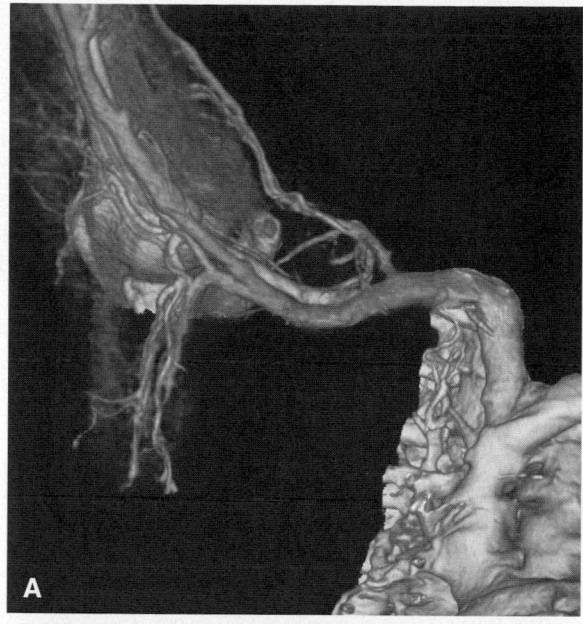

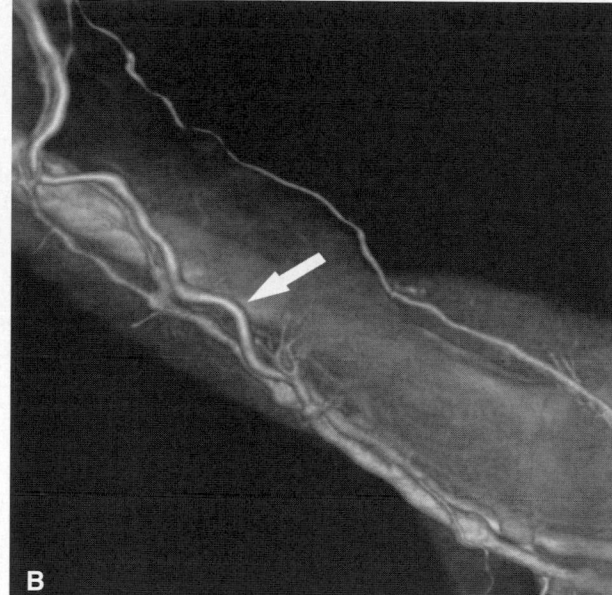

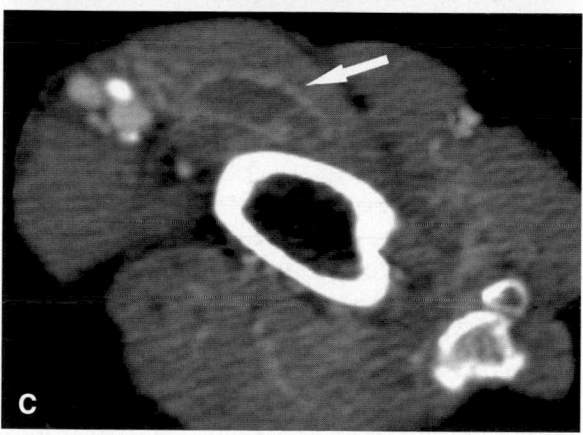

Figure 6–4 A patient with suspected right upper extremity deep venous thrombosis had an equivocal ultrasound examination (*not shown*). Upper extremity CT venography was performed using a biphasic injection protocol with lower injection rates than would be used for imaging the arterial system. A total of 140 cc of contrast medium was administered over 50 seconds. Images were acquired at 60 seconds from the start of contrast administration. Volume-rendered images depict **A.** patent central and **B.** peripheral right upper extremity veins with robust quality. Note also the robust arterial opacification (*arrow*), a product of first pass and recirculation effects. This exam provides an alternative diagnosis to the patient's swelling and erythema—an intramuscular hematoma (*arrow*).

Injection Parameters

Contrast medium with a concentration of at least 300 mg/I should be used. For acquisitions >20 seconds, the injection duration is set to equal the scan duration. As shown in Table 6–3, contrast medium is administered at approximately 3.5–6 mL/sec using a biphasic protocol. Employing these rules will deliver the required iodine dose to most vascular territories for a 60–90 kg patient. It is essential to note that if automated bolus triggering is used to determine the *t*CMT, the injection duration is extended to account for the 2- to 8-second delay intrinsic to the detection and triggering algorithm. For acquisitions that are <20 seconds, if the injection duration is set to equal the scan duration, an insufficient iodine dose may be delivered, leading to decreased peak enhancement. As shown in Table 6–4, strategies to apply for these acquisitions include using high-concentration contrast medium, increasing the injection rate, and increasing the injection duration along with

the scan delay (23–24). Given the short bolus durations, uniphasic injections are sufficient.

The exception to these rules, for both slow and fast acquisitions, occurs when the time for contrast to transit through a vascular territory is longer than the scan duration. In this instance, the injection duration should be set to equal the estimated vascular territory transit time and the diagnostic delay is increased so that the scan and injection durations end simultaneously. Alternatively, by using an effective milliamperage, the pitch can be reduced until the scan duration equals the targeted injection duration. To further optimize contrast-medium administration, high-concentration contrast medium and higher injection rates can be used.

To reduce enhancement variability among patients, particularly those with weights of <60 kg or >90 kg, iodine dose should be selected relative to body weight. In this instance, to administer a patient's ideal dose, the recommendation is to vary the injection rate according to the

TABLE 6–3

MDCTA INJECTION PROTOCOLS FOR ACQUISITIONS >20 SECONDS

Duration			Iodine	300 mg I/mL CM		350 mg I/mL CM		370 mg I/mL CM	
Scan Time (sec)	Scanning Delay (sec)	Total Dose (g)	Iodine Flux (g @ g/s)	Total Volume (mL)	Biphasic Injections (mL @ mL/s)	Total Volume (mL)	Biphasic Injections (mL @ mL/s)	Total Volume (mL)	Biphasic Injections (mL @ mL/s)
45	tCMT+2–8*	55.5	7.5 @ 1.5/48 @ 1.2	185	25 @ 5/160 @ 4	158	21 @ 4.2/137 @ 3.4	150	20 @ 4/130 @ 3.2
40	tCMT+2–8*	49.5	7.5 @ 1.5/42 @ 1.2	165	25 @ 5/140 @ 4	141	21 @ 4.2/120 @ 3.4	134	20 @ 4/114 @ 3.2
35	tCMT+2–8*	43.5	7.5 @ 1.5/36 @ 1.2	145	25 @ 5/120 @ 4	124	21 @ 4.2/103 @ 3.4	117	20 @ 4/97 @ 3.2
30	tCMT+2–8*	37.5	7.5 @ 1.5/30 @ 1.2	125	25 @ 5/100 @ 4	107	21 @ 4.2/86 @ 3.4	101	20 @ 4/81 @ 3.2
25	tCMT+2–8*	35	8.25 @ 1.65/27 @ 1.35	117.5	27.5 @ 5.5/90 @ 4.5	100	23 @ 4.7/77 @ 3.9	95	22 @ 4.5/73 @ 3.6

Note: Parameters reflect iodine dosing for a 70 kg patient in a vascular territory that requires 20 seconds of contrast injection. CM = Contrast medium. tCMT = Contrast medium transit time, established by bolus timing or automated triggering techniques. *When automated triggering is used, the overall scan delay is lengthened by a value equivalent to the inherent diagnostic delay (i.e. 2–8 sec). A longer injection duration is then required (tINJ = tSCAN + tDxDELAY). Biphasic injections are employed. Iodine administration is optimized by controlling the injection rate and/or concentration. Higher concentration CM afford reduced injection rates and volumes.

body weight, rather than the injection duration (28). An individualized injection rate is derived simply by determining the patient's appropriate contrast volume for the selected contrast-medium concentration, such as 1.1–1.7 mL/kg for 350 mgI/mL concentration, and by dividing this amount by the injection duration. If the injection rate exceeds the tolerable limit of the accessed vein, the iodine concentration, the injection duration, or both should be increased. If the injection duration is increased, then the diagnostic delay time should be increased by the same amount.

Saline Flush

Saline flush can be administered with a dual-chamber injector immediately after infusion of contrast medium. This improves contrast utilization as the contrast remaining in the veins is advanced into the central circulation (36–38). Another benefit is reducing perivenous streaks (36–37). This is particularly useful during thoracic, cardiac, upper extremity, and neck CT angiography.

IMAGE DISPLAY AND RENDERING

There are two challenges to CTA display and interpretation. One is the "data explosion." Depending on the coverage, vascular exams may produce 400–2,500 images. Cardiac retrospective ECG-gated studies may generate 2,000–3,500 images. As alluded to earlier, these large datasets influence workload efficiency, not to mention image presentation. The second challenge is that axial display cannot effectively convey every important anatomic relationship. For these reasons, it is necessary to interpret and display the dataset interactively on a workstation using both 2D and 3D displays. While such real-time rendering is the principle means for CTA interpretation, scrolling through the transverse

TABLE 6–4

MDCTA INJECTION PROTOCOLS FOR ACQUISITIONS <20 SECONDS

Duration			Iodine	300 mg I/mL CM		350 mg I/mL CM		370 mg I/mL CM	
Scan Time (sec)	Scanning Delay* (sec)	Total Dose (g)	Iodine Flux (g/s)	Total Volume (mL)	Uniphasic Injection (mL/s)	Total Volume (mL)	Uniphasic Injection (mL@mL/s)	Total Volume (mL)	Uniphasic Injection (mL@mL/s)
20	tCMT	35	1.75	116	5.8	100	5	95	4.7
16	tCMT+4	35	1.75	116	5.8	100	5	95	4.7
12	tCMT+8	35	1.75	116	5.8	100	5	95	4.7
8	tCMT+12	35	1.75	116	5.8	100	5	95	4.7
4	tCMT+16	35	1.75	116	5.8	100	5	95	4.7

Note: Parameters reflect iodine dosing for a 70 kg patient in a vascular territory that requires 20 seconds of contrast injection. CM = Contrast medium. tCMT = Contrast medium transit time, established by bolus timing or automated triggering technique. *A diagnostic delay is added to the beginning of the scan duration so that the CM injection and the scan acquisition conclude together. If automated triggering is used, this delay may vary depending on the inherent diagnostic delay (i.e. 2–8 sec). Iodine administration is further optimized by controlling the concentration. Higher concentration CM affords reduced injection rates and volumes. Saline flush is always used.

source images on a workstation remains essential to confirming vascular pathology identified on the postprocessed images, assessing the vessel wall, and detecting nonvascular abnormalities. As with all radiologic interpretation, viewing the source and the rendered images with correct window and level settings is critical. This includes using a wide window setting to account for vascular calcification, high contrast attenuation, or both.

Four principle visualization techniques exist: multiplanar reformation (MPR), maximum intensity projection (MIP), shaded surface display (SSD), and volume rendering (VR) (39). These techniques and their principle use, advantages, and disadvantages are summarized in Table 6–5. User selection for each technique depends on the cardiovascular territory and clinical issues to be addressed. For most interpretations, MPR, MIP, and VR are the techniques of choice, with the latter two used for generating angiographic-like displays. As emphasized earlier, for display and interpretation, the quality of all postprocessed images depends on the quality of both the CT data acquisition and the contrast-medium administration.

MPRs are 2D displays that can be applied in standard or curved formats. When viewed as image stacks, standard MPRs allow the user to step through the original dataset in coronal, sagittal, or oblique orientations. From an interpretive standpoint, they are useful in assessing stenoses, occlusions, vasculitis, intramural hematoma, dissection, mural thrombus, and stent lumens, in addition to extravascular structures. However, as vessels curve in and out of the planes, standard MPRs are not able to display an entire vascular territory in one image, which can limit precise evaluation, particularly with stenoses. The solution is curved multiplanar reformations (CPR). CPRs are generated by drawing a center line through the vessel on the axial, coronal, or sagittal images. This affords a comprehensive longitudinal cross-sectional display in one 2D image. As curve drawing may be dependent upon an operator, false-positive and false-negative displays are possible. Furthermore, eccentric lesions cannot be depicted accurately by one view alone. Thus, two orthogonal planes, rotating CPR centerline views, or both should always be generated. Automated vessel tracking through the center line of a vascular territory can simplify CPR generation (40).

MIPs project the brightest structures in a 3D volume into a 2D image. Because all selected pixel values in a defined plane are displayed, bone, mural calcium, overlapping vessels, and extravascular structures can obscure visualization. The solution is to either perform prerendering editing or use sliding thin-slab MIP with rotating projectional algorithms. MIP may be limited in the setting of vascular calcifications and in the assessing of stent patency. Depending on the calcium burden, MIP technique may overestimate stenoses. Alternatively, calcifications may lead to the false suggestion of lumen patency. Often with MIP, the stent lumen is obscured.

SSD and VR techniques can appear similar, but they are very different methods for displaying vascular and nonvascular anatomical relationships in a 3D format. SSD relies

TABLE 6–5

VISUALIZATION TECHNIQUES

	Display	Principle Use	Advantages	Disadvantages
MPR	2D	• Structure • Flow lumen • Vessel wall	• "Slice" through dataset in coronal, sagittal, and oblique projections • Simplify image interpretation • Accurate display of stenoses, occlusions, calcification, stents	• Limited spatial display
CPR	2D	• Flow lumen • Vessel wall	• Complete longitudinal vessel display • Accurate display of stenoses, occlusions, calcification, stents	• Operator dependent
MIP	2D	• Angiographic overview	• "Slice" through dataset in axial, coronal, sagittal, and oblique projections • Depict small-caliber vessels • Depict poorly enhancing vessels • Communicate findings	• Vessel/bone/visceral overlap • Limited grading of stent lumen • Limited by heavy calcium burden
SSD	3D	• Angiographic overview	• Depict structural relationships • Communicate findings	• Vessel/bone/visceral overlap • Threshold dependent
VR	3D	• Angiographic overview	• "Slice" through dataset in axial, coronal, sagittal, and oblique projections • Depict structural relationships • Accurate spatial perception • Communicate findings	• Opacity-transfer function dependent

Note: 2D = Two-dimensional, 3D = Three-dimensional

on an absolute voxel threshold to identify surfaces. Grayscale is used to encode surface reflections from an imaging source of illumination, thereby facilitating spatial relationships. Because SSD is threshold dependent, creating or removing lesions is possible. Because of advances in workstation capabilities, SSD is largely of historical significance and VR has replaced it as a more robust 3D technique.

With VR, as distinguished from SSD, the entire dataset is used without thresholding. Voxels are displayed with relative opacity and color as a function of their attenuation values. This opacity transfer function is controlled by user-selected parameters mapped over the histogram of voxel values. The result is that VR produces more reliable and more comprehensive 3D images to interrogate the cardiovascular structures and to show relationships with noncardiovascular anatomy. This is particularly useful for overlapping and tortuous vessels. Compared with other display techniques, phantom model analysis has shown VR to be more accurate in measuring arterial diameters that are <4 mm and, in particular, is superior for severe stenoses, with lumen diameters of 0.5–1.0 mm (41). Similar to MIPs, bone, calcium, endoluminal stents, and adjacent anatomy can obscure visualization. Therefore, to maximize real-time interpretive efficiency, sliding thin-slab VR and rotational projections, with correct opacity and color transfer settings, are important.

Two novel applications for CT vascular display are virtual angioscopy (VA) (39,42) and 4D cine imaging (18). VA is an endoscopic technique that uses SSD or VR techniques first to eliminate (SSD) intraluminal contrast or make it transparent (VR). Perspective renderings then are employed to generate images that depict the structural interface between luminal and extraluminal attenuation. Although its role and usefulness is still being defined, VA

has done much to provide relevant clinical information, including assessment of intracardiac defects, ostia of the pulmonary veins and coronary sinus, aortic root, intimal flaps, complex atherosclerotic lesions, and stent-graft position relative to vessel ostia (Figure 6–5).

Four-dimensional cine imaging provides time-resolved dynamic volumetric MIP or VR depiction for each Z-position. To achieve these acquisitions, retrospective ECG gating is necessary. Four-dimensional cine imaging serves as a useful tool for real-time functional cardiovascular evaluation, in particular for subjective evaluation of myocardial, valvular, and dissection flap motion.

CLINICAL APPLICATION

Compared with catheter angiography, the advantages of CTA include its greater clinical availability, faster acquisition, greater patient convenience, and reduced cost, in addition to being noninvasive. Other important benefits of CTA include the fact that CTA is a volumetric imaging technique, while catheter angiography is a projectional technique. To delineate vascular anatomy and disease with catheter angiography, multiple views routinely are needed, which adds time and contrast volume, as well as radiation exposure and prolonged risk of iatrogenic injury. However, with CTA, image analysis is possible from any projection (including endoluminal), and tortuous, diseased vessels can be interrogated more swiftly. Second, because it is a cross-sectional technique, CTA provides superior tissue characterization of the vessel lumen and wall morphology. This is advantageous when assessing true vessel dimensions, distinguishing soft and calcified atherosclerotic plaque, identifying the burden of

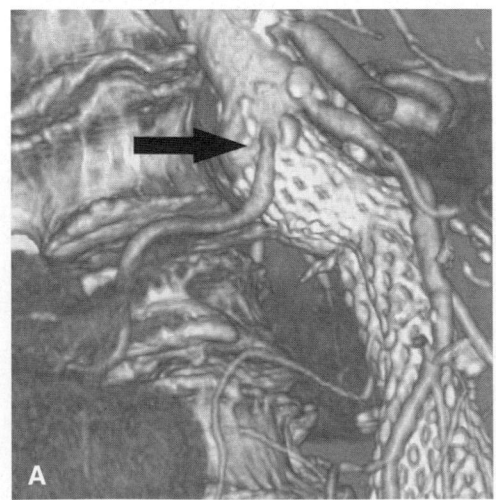 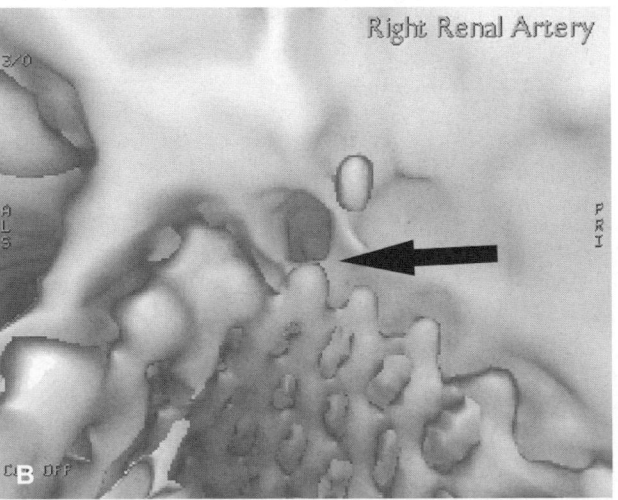

Figure 6–5   An MDCT angiogram is performed in patient who underwent endovascular aneurysm repair with an Aneurx endograft. **A.** The volume-rendered image demonstrates that the superior edge of the body closely approximates the right renal artery ostium (*arrow*). **B.** A virtual angioscopic rendering confirms excellent deployment without compromise of the right renal artery (*arrow*).

mural thrombus, diagnosing acute aortic syndromes, and evaluating for vasculitis. Finally, axial images also offer the distinct advantage of evaluating extravascular disease (Figure 6–4) and vessel relations with adjacent viscera, bone, and soft tissue. This advantage is essential to providing comprehensive vascular evaluations, simplifying the diagnostic workup (such as trauma), planning treatment strategies, and providing alternative diagnoses.

CTA also has several key advantages over ultrasound and MRA. Compared with ultrasound, CTA is less dependent upon an operator and is not limited by an acoustic window. Furthermore, CTA provides complete evaluation of intrathoracic vessels and excellent delineation of extravascular structures. Compared with MRA, from a clinical perspective, CTA is more readily available, is capable of providing information faster, and is tolerated more favorably by patients. From an imaging perspective, CTA has superior spatial resolution and is more reliable at distinguishing vascular calcifications.

As with other CT disciplines, the principle limitations of CTA are radiation and iodinated contrast-medium exposures. Therefore, indications for the study should be clearly defined. Additionally, the diagnostic benefits of CTA should be weighed against subject radiosensitivity, tolerance for iodinated contrast medium, and the strengths of other imaging modalities.

Cardiac MDCT

Cardiac MDCT is a rapidly evolving application. In a single acquisition after administration of contrast medium, coronary vessels, cardiac structure, and myocardial enhancement patterns are evaluated along with function. For adults, the major role is assessing ischemic heart disease (Figure 6–6) and anomalous coronary artery origins (Figure 6–7). Other indications for cardiac MDCT angiography in adults include evaluation of suspected valvular disease, including stenosis and endocarditis, as well as masses, cardiomyopathies, arrythmogenic right ventricular dysplasia (43), and pericardial disease. For pediatric patients, although coronary CTA evaluation for aberrant anatomy and acquired lesions such as Kawasaki's disease is performed frequently, cardiac MDCTA is used primarily for assessing congenital heart disease, including postoperative and postendovascular cardiac surveillance.

Regarding MDCTA evaluation of adult ischemic heart disease, in addition to evaluating stenotic and occlusive lesions, characterization of atherosclerotic plaque (44–47) and assessment of coronary remodeling (48) are possible. This information may be useful for monitoring medical management and predicting lesions at risk for rupture. A promising MDCTA tool is biphasic myocardial perfusion, which can be applied to determine viable myocardium (49–51). Coronary calcium imaging is an essential adjunct to angiographic evaluation. The standard for detection and

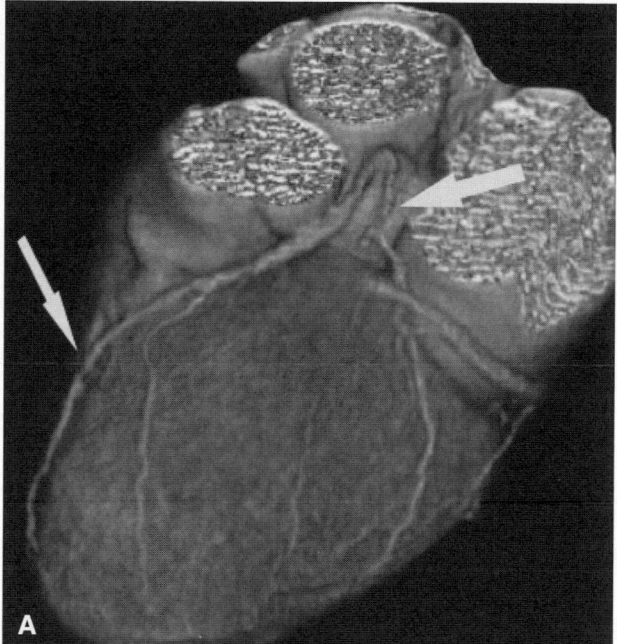

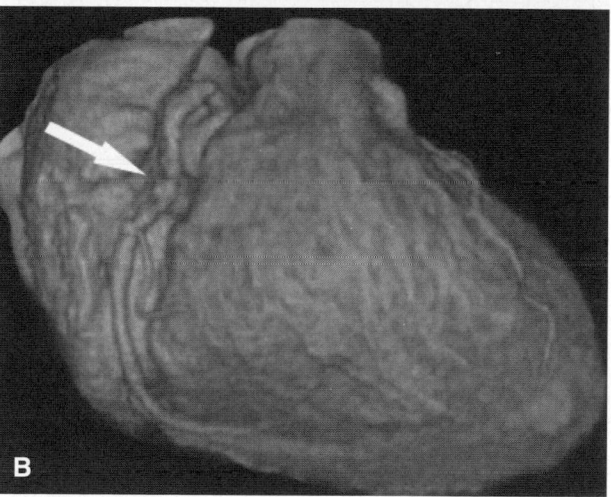

Figure 6–6   Volume-rendered images are from a 16 mm x 1.25 mm retrospectively ECG-gated CT angiogram obtained to evaluate the aorta (*not shown*) and the coronary arteries in a 75-year-old patient with atypical chest pain. **A.** The left main coronary artery bifurcates immediately into the left anterior descending (LAD, *thin arrow*) and circumflex (LCX, *thick arrow*) arteries. The LAD is diffusely diseased with regions of moderate stenoses. Short segment disease involves the proximal LCX, with mild and moderate narrowing. **B.** The right coronary artery has moderate long-segment proximal disease (*arrow*).

quantification of atherosclerotic calcium has been electron beam CT, but MDCT scoring methods achieve comparable results with high inter-reader concordance (52–55). The implications are that MDCT can be used to measure coronary artery calcium noninvasively and, consequently, may be used for cardiac event risk stratification and initiation of preventive management (56–62). MDCT can also serve as a means to

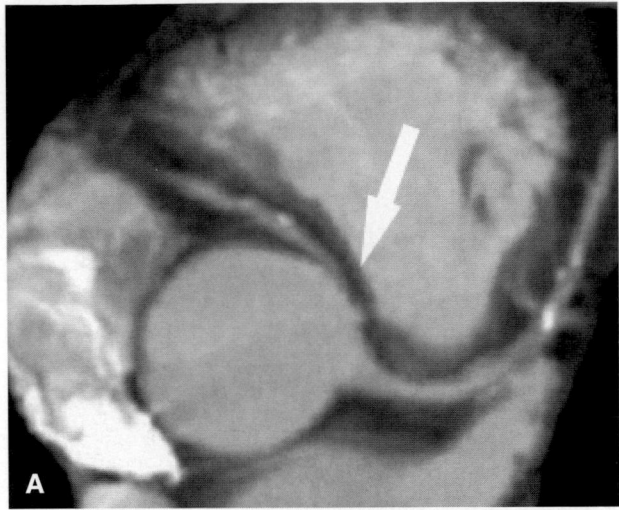

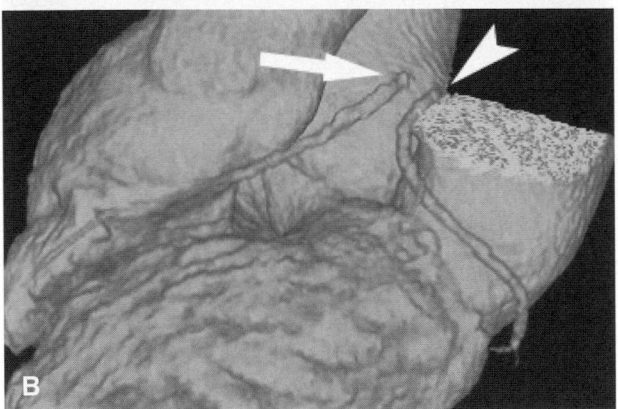

Figure 6–7 Two examples of anomalous coronary arterial anatomy are illustrated. **A.** The right coronary artery (RCA) arises from the left coronary cusp, separate from the left main coronary artery (*arrow*). The RCA courses between the right ventricular out-flow tract and the aortic root. **B.** The LAD (*arrow*) and LCX (*arrowhead*) arise separately from the left coronary cusp.

indicate the burden and location of calcium before MDCT coronary and bypass graft angiography (63).

One emerging application is MDCT coronary venography, which is used to map the coronary venous system before endovascular interventions, such as biventricular pacemaker placement.

Regarding cardiac MDCT protocols, calcium imaging is acquired without contrast, using prospective ECG triggering or retrospective ECG gating at the 70–80% phase of the RR interval (51–54). Standardized images are obtained at a typical slice thickness of 2.5 mm. MDCT coronary angiography, coronary venography, myocardial perfusion, and morphology function studies are all performed using retrospective ECG gating. If coronary bypass grafts require evaluation, in addition to covering the heart, the upper chest is also included. Ideal acquisition parameters for native coronary and bypass graft angiography include submillimeter section thickness and a pitch of 0.3–0.5. If performed on 4- or 8-channel scanners, 1–1.5 mm thickness is prescribed.

When using 16-channel (or greater) scanners, 0.5–0.75 mm thickness is standard. As to contrast-medium administration, iodine dose should reflect the central blood volume. With 4-channel MDCT, an iodine flux of approximately 1.0 g/sec is sufficient to achieve enhancement (64). Higher flux may hinder detection of calcium and consequently, the accuracy of the grading of coronary lesions (64). For faster scanners, the optimum iodine flux will need to be verified. For most applications, tCMT is determined with an ROI placed on the left ventricle or the aortic root. To reduce streak artifacts in the central veins and right heart, images are acquired in an inferior to superior direction, and saline flush is always utilized. One instance in which the imager may decide not to use saline flush is when searching for intracardiac defects or a patent foramen ovale. Dense contrast communicating between cardiac chambers can be used as a diagnostic aid (CT Shunt Sign). A second phase can be obtained during equilibrium to depict the structural anatomy.

Successful cardiac MDCTA application depends on several factors, all of which can impair image quality and interpretation. Pitfalls can be categorized as secondary to cardiac, respiratory, or patient motion artifacts; coronary artery calcification blooming artifact; coronary artery size <1.5 mm; incorrect cardiac reconstruction phase; metallic beam hardening artifacts; low attenuating air streak artifacts; overlapping opacified cardiovascular structures; and suboptimal technical acquisition (65).

Among these factors, it is essential to address cardiac motion, particularly when evaluating coronary arteries and bypass grafts. A principle strategy is controlling the heart rate. Studies using 4-detector row scanners demonstrate that when not controlling for the heart rate, the percentage of diagnostic native coronary arterial segments during retrospectively ECG-gated, 4-channel MDCTA ranges only between 67% and 87% (66–71). An 8-channel MDCT coronary angiogram will show similar results, with only 74% of coronary segments interpretable (72). Superior image quality however, can be achieved at or below a threshold of 65 beats per minute (bpm) (73). If not contraindicated clinically, patients should be premedicated with chronotropic agents to reduce the heart rate below this threshold. Premedicating patients with a β-blocker prior to 4-channel MDCT acquisitions increases the range of interpretable segments to 72–95% (66,74–76). When administering β-blockers prior to 16-channel MDCT acquisitions, 79–100% of coronary arteries are interpretable (77–80). However, it is suggested that with 16-detector row scanners, elevated heart rates may have less negative impact on image quality as a result of improved temporal resolution and use of multiphasic reconstructions. This may allow raising of the heart rate threshold value (for example, 75–80 bpm) and reducing the exam dependence on chronotropic agents (81). Future studies are needed to gauge the impact of 32- to 64-channel scanners on the relationship between heart rate and image quality.

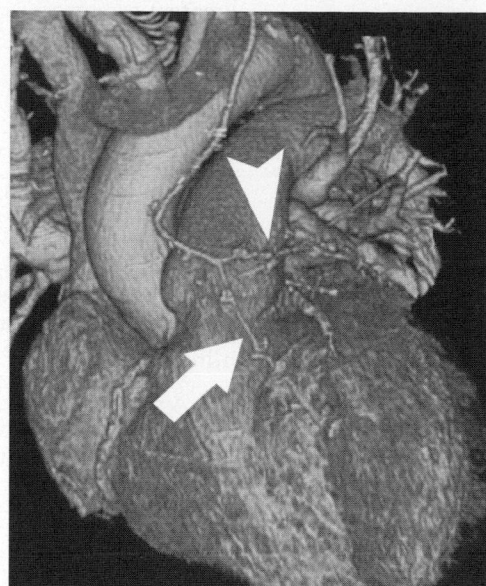

Figure 6–8   A retrospectively ECG-gated chest MDCT angiogram through the chest (16 mm x 1.25 mm collimation) demonstrates a bifurcated left internal mammary artery bypass graft to the LAD (*arrow*) and LCX (*arrowhead*). Although enhancement is seen to the distal vascular segments, the surgical clips limit interpretation using a volume rendered technique. Maximum intensity projection images would also be degraded. In this instance, transverse or longitudinal cross-sectional vessel analysis is required.

The importance of heart rate control has also been demonstrated for bypass graft evaluation. Niemann et al. showed that with 4-channel MDCT, the percentage of interpretable venous grafts and the sensitivity and specificity for detecting graft stenoses diminishes with heart rates >65 bpm (82). The heart rate, however, has less negative effect when assessing for bypass graft occlusions (82–85). Nonetheless, equally important for bypass evaluation is the burden and location of surgical clips (83–85), which potentially can degrade image interpretation regardless whether or not chronotropic agents are required (Figure 6–8).

Once the cardiac MDCT dataset is acquired, the impact of cardiac motion on image interpretation can be minimized further by the reconstruction and viewing of the optimum cardiac phases. Cardiac motion is greatest during end-systole/early diastole (10–30% of the cardiac cycle), when ventricular contraction is synchronized, and also during late diastole (80% of the cardiac cycle), when there is motion at the ventricular base secondary to atrial contraction. Cardiac MDCTA images therefore should be reconstructed during middiastolic phases, because these phases will exhibit less motion. Because the right coronary artery and left circumflex artery lie within the atrioventricular groove, they are subject to greater diastolic motion and image degradation than the left anterior descending coronary artery. Thus, coronary artery interpretation requires specific reconstruction phases. It has been shown that for the right coronary artery, the left circumflex artery, and the left anterior descending artery, the least amount of motion

artifacts occur at 40–50%, 50–60%, and 50–70% of the RR interval, respectively (86–87). Middiastolic phases are best for viewing bypass grafts. Depending on the type of graft and the graft segment, the recommended reconstruction window ranges between 50% and 70% (85).

For MDCT angiography of the coronary arteries, in addition to an elevated heart rate, the severity of coronary calcium and the presence of coronary stents can be major determinants of luminal depiction. This is partly the result of blooming artifacts and volume averaging. However, it also reflects spatial resolution of the scanner. The recommendation is to establish the burden of calcified coronary atherosclerosis disease and the presence of coronary stents before performing the CT angiogram. Using 4-channel scanners, it is advised not to perform an MDCT coronary angiogram whenever the Agatston score equivalent (ASE) exceeds 335 (88). However, Kuettner et al. suggests that because of the improved spatial resolution, this threshold can be set at 1,000 ASE when using 16-channel scanners (80). Advanced generation scanners with superior spatial resolution also improve assessment of stent patency. Accuracy may be improved further with the use of a high-resolution reconstruction kernel (89).

Clinical performance has been reported for several cardiac MDCTA applications. Twelve clinical studies examining the performances of 4-, 8-, and 16- channel MDCT coronary angiography are summarized in Table 6–6. These results support the position that when the majority of segments are of diagnostic quality, isotropic resolution datasets acquired on advanced scanners improve coronary artery depiction and disease detection. With selective β-blocker premedication, 4-channel MDCT achieves a sensitivity of 81–83%, specificity of 90–98%, and accuracy of 89–96% (74–75) in the detection of >50% stenosis. An 8-channel MDCT will achieve a sensitivity of 90%, specificity of 99%, and accuracy of 98% (72), while 16-slice MDCT (12 x 0.75 and 16 x 0.75 collimation) yields a sensitivity of 92–95%, specificity of 86–95%, and accuracy of 90–95% (77–79). Four clinical studies that focused on 4-channel MDCT coronary bypass graft angiography are summarized in Table 6–7. Results indicate that sensitivity, specificity, and accuracy are greater when assessing for occlusions (82–85) than stenoses of greater than 50% (83–100%, 96–98%, 94–98% versus 60–83%, 88–96%, 84–94%) (82–84).

During MDCT coronary angiography, Nikolaou et al. reports that 4-channel scanners are an accurate means to simultaneously depict, localize, and age myocardial infarctions (50). In a retrospective review of 106 patients, this group found a sensitivity of 85%, specificity of 91%, and accuracy of 90%. Volumes of recent infarctions correlated negatively with left ventricular function. The mean Hounsfield units of infarcted myocardium was 54±19 versus 117±28 for noninfarcted regions.

As to MDCTA performance for evaluation of the aortic valve, compared with echocardiography and intraoperative findings, Willmann et al. demonstrated good agreement in

TABLE 6–6

MDCTA DETECTION OF <50% CORONARY ARTERY STENOSIS

Author	Collimation	N	β-Blocker	Diagnostic Segments	Sensitivity	Specificity	Accuracy
Nieman et al. (2001)	4 x 1.0	35	No	73%	81%	97%	95%
Achenbach et al. (2001)	4 x 1.0	64	No	68%	85%	76%	79%
Kopp et al. (2002)*	4 x 1.0	102	No	87%	90–95%	95–96%	94–96%
Vogl et al. (2002)	4 x 1.0	64	No	72%	75%	99%	98%
Nieman et al. (2002	4 x 1.0	78	No	68%	84%	95%	93%
Knez et al. (2001)	4 x 1.0	44	Yes	94%	83%	98%	96%
Becker et al. (2002)	4 x 1.0	28	Yes	95%	81%	90%	89%
Maruyama et al. (2004)	8 x 1.25	25	No	74%	90%	99%	98%
Nieman et al. (2002)	12 x 0.75	59	Yes	100%	95%	86%	90%
Ropers et al. (2002)	12 x 0.75	77	Yes	88%	92%	93%	93%
Mollett et al. (2004)	16 x 0.75	128	Yes	100%	92%	95%	95%
Kuettner et al. (2004)	12 x 0.7.5	60	Yes	79%	72%	97%	NA

Note: Collimation = Number of channels x detector width (mm); N = Number of patients.
*Two-reader analysis without consensus. Reported vessels are either larger than 1.5 mm or 2.0 mm.

determining aortic valve morphology, aortic annulus diameter, and aortic valve calcification in patients with aortic stenosis undergoing evaluation aortic valve replacement (90). Willmann et al. also found MDCTA to have good agreement for evaluating mitral valve thickening, mitral valve calcifications, and mitral annulus calcifications (91). Regarding cardiac function analysis, MDCTA has been shown to correlate well with both conventional left ventriculography (92) and MRI (93–95) in its ability to quantify left ventricular volumes (93–95), right ventricular volumes (94), ejection fractions (92–95), and/or ventricular masses (94) in patients with normal (92–95) and depressed myocardial function (94).

Pulmonary

CT pulmonary arteriography (CTPA) has become a valuable diagnostic modality for assessing acute and chronic pulmonary embolism. With CTPA, one can directly identify thrombi, make alternative diagnoses, and display lung perfusion. This provides a more thorough assessment of symptomatic patients, as compared to ventilation-perfusion scintigraphy or conventional pulmonary angiography alone (96). CTPA also is used to assess vascular causes of pulmonary hypertension and to evaluate pulmonary arterial aneurysms, arteriovenous malformations, and pulmonary slings.

Initial CTPA studies for pulmonary embolism assessment were obtained with single detector row CT (SDCT) scanners, acquiring 3–5 mm thick sections. This yielded variable performance, particularly at the subsegmental level (2,6, 97–102). Thin section, high-resolution MDCT technique, however, is superior and provides improved pulmonary embolism detection. Notably, greater temporal resolution reduces respiratory and cardiac motion artifacts. Combined with the improved spatial resolution, this technique affords better technical adequacy to the subsegmental level, resulting in decreased indeterminate exams and

TABLE 6–7

MDCTA CORONARY BYPASS GRAFT EVALUATION

Author	Collimation	N	β-Blocker	Diagnostic Segments	Sensitivity	Specificity	Accuracy
Ropers et al. (2001)	4 x 1.0	65	Yes				
• Occlusion				100%	97%	98%	98%
• >50% Stenosis				62%	75%	92%	88%
Nieman et al. (2003)*‡	4 x 1.0	20	No				
• Occlusion				95–100%	100%	97.7–97.5%	98%
• >50% Stenosis				90–95%	60–83%	88–90%	84–89%
Marano et al. (2004)	4 x 2.5	57	Yes				
• Occlusion				100%	93%	98%	
• >50% Stenosis				67%	80%	96%	97% 94%
Willmann et al. (2004)*	4 x 2.5	20	No				
• Occlusion				100%	83%	96–98%	94–95%

Note: Collimation = Number of channels x detector width (mm); N = Number of patients.
*Two-reader analysis without consensus; ‡Only venous grafts.

increased interobserver agreement throughout the pulmonary arterial anatomy (103–107). Four–channel MDCT pulmonary angiography has been shown to have a sensitivity of 96–100%, specificity of 89–98%, and a diagnostic accuracy of 91–98% (108–109). Besides using thin sections, additional technical recommendations for CTPA include scanning in an inferior to superior direction, timing to the main pulmonary artery, and injecting contrast medium for at least 15 seconds. Saline flush is useful for

reducing perivenous streaks. Although MIP and VR techniques can be employed, interpretation from the axial source images has been found to be most efficient (Figure 6–9).

Indirect, lower extremity CT venography (LE-CTV) can be combined with CTPA, providing a one-stop, comprehensive exam for evaluating thromboembolism (Figure 6–9). With thick section, single and dual detector row CT, when no pulmonary embolism is detected, deep venous thrombus

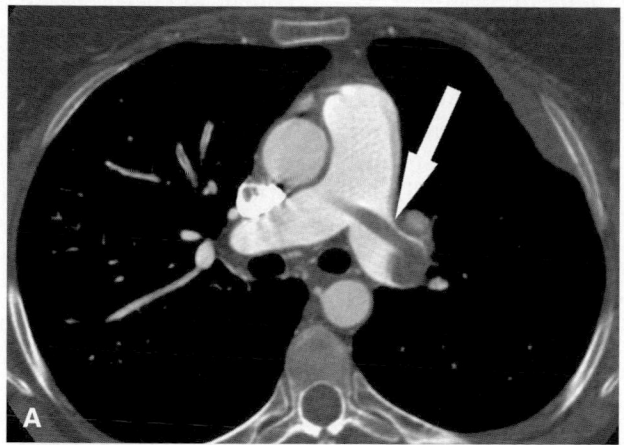
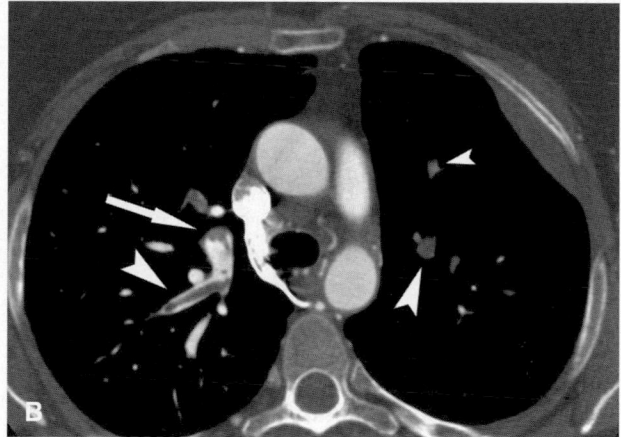

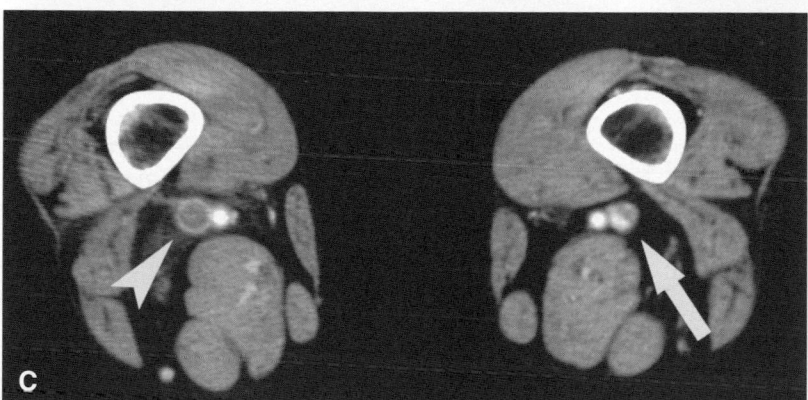

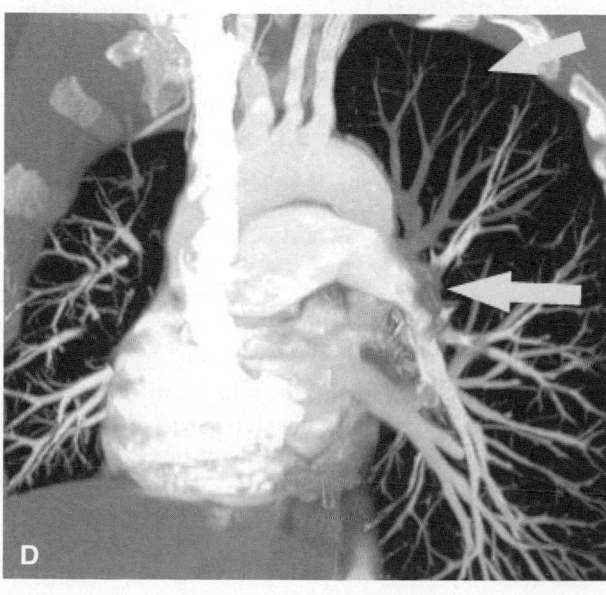

Figure 6–9 **A.** 1.25 mm thick axial sections demonstrate central pulmonary embolism (*arrow*) **B.** with involvement of lobar (*arrow*), segmental (*large arrowhead*), and subsegmental (*small arrowhead*) pulmonary arteries. **C.** Indirect CT venography confirms a residual burden of thrombus in the bilateral superficial femoral veins (*arrow*). **D.** The MIP image demonstrates the occlusive clot burden to the left upper lobe (*arrow*).

(DVT) is reported to be present in 3.5–7% of exams, resulting in a 12–28% increase of thromboembolism detection and management (110–113). However, when acquiring CTPA with thin section MDCT technique, LE-CTV provides less incremental value, suggesting that the addition of CTV should be individualized to each patient. Examining 1,240 consecutive combined CTPA-CTV exams performed on 4-, 8-, and 16-channel MDCT, Hellinger et al. found that when CTPA is acquired with thin section technique (1.25 mm thickness), the prevalence of positive DVT without demonstrable PE, is only 1.1%, resulting in only a 4% increase in thromboembolism detection (114). To perform CTV, at least 120 cc of contrast should be administered. At 3 minutes following administration of the original contrast bolus, 5 mm thick images are acquired from the popliteal fossa through to the mid-IVC.

A modified version of CTPA is used to image the pulmonary veins. One useful application of CT pulmonary venography (CTPV) is evaluation of anomalous pulmonary venous drainage (115). Another indication is mapping the pulmonary venous anatomy prior to radiofrequency catheter ablation for treatment of atrial fibrillation (116–117). In this instance, knowledge of the number, location, diameter, and orientation of the pulmonary veins ostia are important considerations for the electrophysiologist. Important steps are to define the first order branch length for each pulmonary vein; identify anomalous pulmonary venous drainage; and characterize left atrial size, shape, and volume. Finally, preendovascular exclusion of pulmonary venous stenosis and atrial appendage thrombus is essential. Postablation, MDCTA is used to assess for complications, which may include pulmonary venous stenosis, thrombosis, and infarction (118–119). Technically, CTPV is similar to CTPA with exception to using retrospective ECG gating and synchronizing image acquisition to the left atrium. When interpreting pulmonary venous anatomy, VR, VA, and CPR display techniques are used, in addition to review of the source images.

Aorta

Routine indications for thoracic and abdominal aortic MDCTA include evaluation of aneurysms, pseudoaneurysms, dissection, intramural hematoma (IMH), penetrating atherosclerotic ulcers (PAU), traumatic aortic injury (TAI), vasculitis (including Takayasu's arteritis), aortic occlusion, and congenital aortic arch anomalies (120). Without question, for each of these clinical problems, CTA is an integral diagnostic modality for endovascular and surgical planning and postprocedural surveillance.

Evaluation may be limited to the thoracic aorta or the abdominal aorta and iliac vessels, covering approximately 250–350 mm in each dataset. Alternatively, clinical presentation (such as dissection), treatment plans (such as endovascular repair, distal cardiopulmonary bypass), or both may necessitate scanning from the thoracic inlet through to the femoral arteries, resulting in a scan volume of 500–700 mm. In most instances, initial nonenhanced images should be obtained. For the contrast enhanced images, high-resolution technique with a 1.0–1.5 mm detector width is more than adequate to optimize 3D visualization of the aorta and branch vessels. Submillimeter collimation is certainly possible with 16- to 64-channel scanners, but does not provide significant diagnostic benefit. Rather, it may simply increase the image noise and increase the number of images. With 4-channel acquisitions, to cover the chest, abdomen, and pelvis in a reasonable scan duration, selecting a detector width of 2.5 mm may be necessary. Following endovascular stent-graft interventions, it is essential to be able to detect endoleaks, as will be discussed further in this section. With MDCTA, this is best achieved using a triphasic acquisition that consists of noncontrast, immediate arterial, and delayed images. The noncontrast images are key to excluding high attenuation calcium or sequestered contrast medium from previous injections in the surrounding aorta-aneurysm sac, which can cause a pseudoendoleak (121). The delayed images, obtained 70 seconds after contrast administration, may reveal endoleaks that have slow flow (122).

CTA of the aorta has several common pitfalls (123). A few, including timing, luminal opacification, streak artifacts, cardiac pulsation, and aortic pulsation, can be controlled by the user. Timing should be individualized to each patient's tCMT, with the ROI placed at the proximal descending aorta or at the level of the celiac origin, depending on whether the exam is of the thoracic or abdominal aorta, respectively. When imaging the entire aorta, ROI placement defaults to the thoracic level. To achieve optimal opacification, once the iodine dose and flux are defined, contrast medium is administered for at least 15–18 seconds. This rule can be followed for thoracic and abdominal CTA. The injection may need to be extended when aortic occlusion is suspected. As mentioned previously, perivenous streak artifacts in the central veins are minimized when contrast medium is injected from the right arm and a saline flush is used (43). While streak artifacts from indwelling catheters, pacing wires, and surgical clips cannot be controlled, the same cannot be said of artifact from monitoring devices or the upper extremities. Similar to cardiac and pulmonary MDCTA design, external devices and the arms should be excluded from the imaging field. Cardiac pulsations may also cause streak artifacts, while aortic motion may result in curvilinear artifacts simulating dissection. Both cardiac and aortic pulsations are suppressed with retrospective ECG gating (15, 124–125). Roos et al. demonstrated that by using retrospective ECG gating, improvement in image quality is achieved throughout the thoracic aorta, but is greatest at the aortic root (125). When the heart rate is 70 bpm or less, the 75% reconstruction phase provides optimum image quality. When <70 bpm, reconstruction at the 50% phase is recommended (124). An ECG-gated thoracic acquisition can be combined with a nongated abdominal-pelvis CTA to achieve a single contiguous acquisition of the complete aorta using one contrast bolus. In this instance, additional contrast is required to account for the 3–5 second delay between the gated and nongated phases. Given the added radiation exposure, the decision to use ECG gating should always be weighed against the clinical indications, degree of clinical suspicion, and age of the patient.

VR technique provides the most complete 3D display of the aorta, branch vessels, and adjacent vascular and nonvascular structures, particularly with aneurysms and pseudoaneurysms. MIP projections have a limited role in overall aortic display, because extensive editing usually is required to remove extravascular tissues. MIP is also limited in evaluating mural thrombus and dissection flaps. Thin-slab MIP projections are useful for assessing aortic branch vessel stenotic-occlusive disease and for assessing the extent of intimal calcifications as well. Transverse sections, MPRs, and CPRs are most helpful in assessing aortic wall disease (Figure 6-10), mural thrombus, and stenoses. Before surgical or endovascular repair of thoracoabdominal aortic disease, MPR, CPR, MIP, or VR techniques can be applied to map the intercostal artery that supplies the artery of Adamkiewicz (126). Similarly, MIP and VR have been shown to be useful rendering techniques for depicting bronchial arteries in patients undergoing endovascular management of hemoptysis (127).

When evaluating thoracic or abdominal aortic aneurysms with CTA, it is important to measure the maximun diameter, length, area, and volume. All are determinants of aneurysm size, which dictates therapy. For endovascular candidates, evaluation also addresses (1) aortic neck and distal landing zone maximum diameter, length, angulations, thrombus burden, and calcium burden: (2) patency and caliber of relevant aortic branch vessels; (3) iliofemoral arterial diameter, tortuosity, angulation, and calcium burden (Figure 6–11) (128). Similar anatomy is assessed when deciding whether a patient with dissection, IMH, PAU, or TAI is an endovascular candidate (129–134). In all instances, calcification and thrombus can be assessed by visual inspection. Required anatomical measurements are made on a workstation using 3D tools. Double oblique orthogonal tomograms drawn perpendicular to the center of the aortic flow lumen produce the most accurate dimensions and path lengths (135–136). These measurements, along with the burden of calcium and thrombus, serve as means to deciding whether a patient is a suitable endovascular candidate, gauging the degree of endovascular technical difficulty, and predicting immediate and long-term outcomes. In addition, this evaluation is essential in designing the endograft and planning procedural strategies. From a surgical perspective, accurate measurements are also important because this facilitates sizing of a surgical graft.

The aortic syndromes comprise aortic dissection, IMH, PAU, and aortic aneurysm rupture. All of these acute aortic conditions are life threatening and require prompt diagnosis and management. Patients may present with hemodynamic

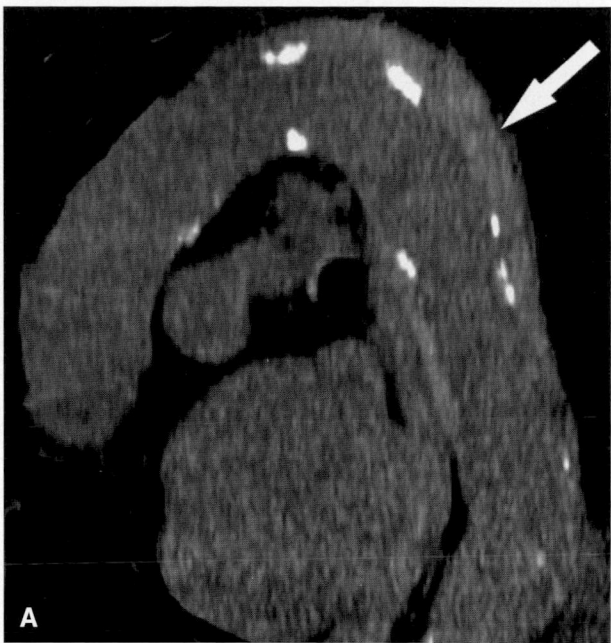

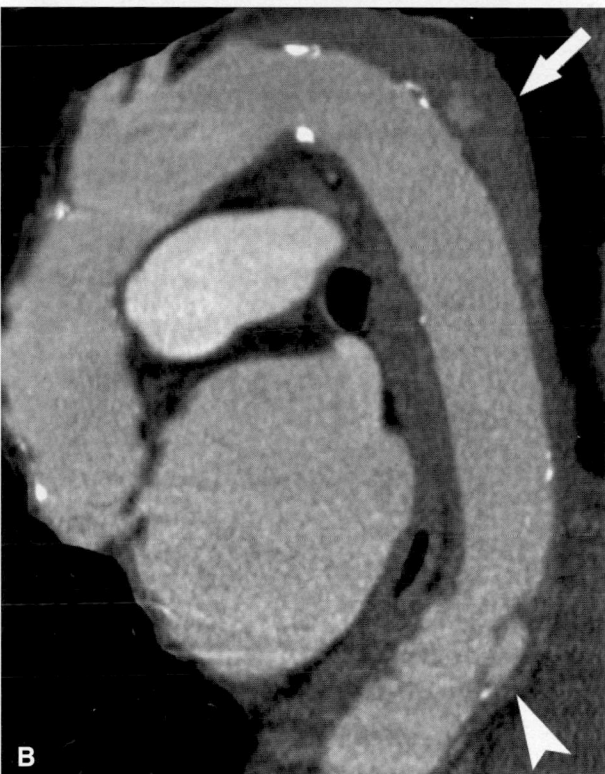

Figure 6–10 MDCT angiography is performed in a patient who presents to the emergency department with acute chest pain. **A.** Noncontrast MPR images reveal high attenuation in the thoracic aortic wall (*arrow*). **B.** Following contrast medium administration, a diagnosis of penetrating ulcers (*arrowhead*) with intramural hematoma (*arrow*) is established. On both acquisitions, note the subintimal location of the intramural hematoma. Calcified and soft atherosclerotic plaque help to define the intimal layer.

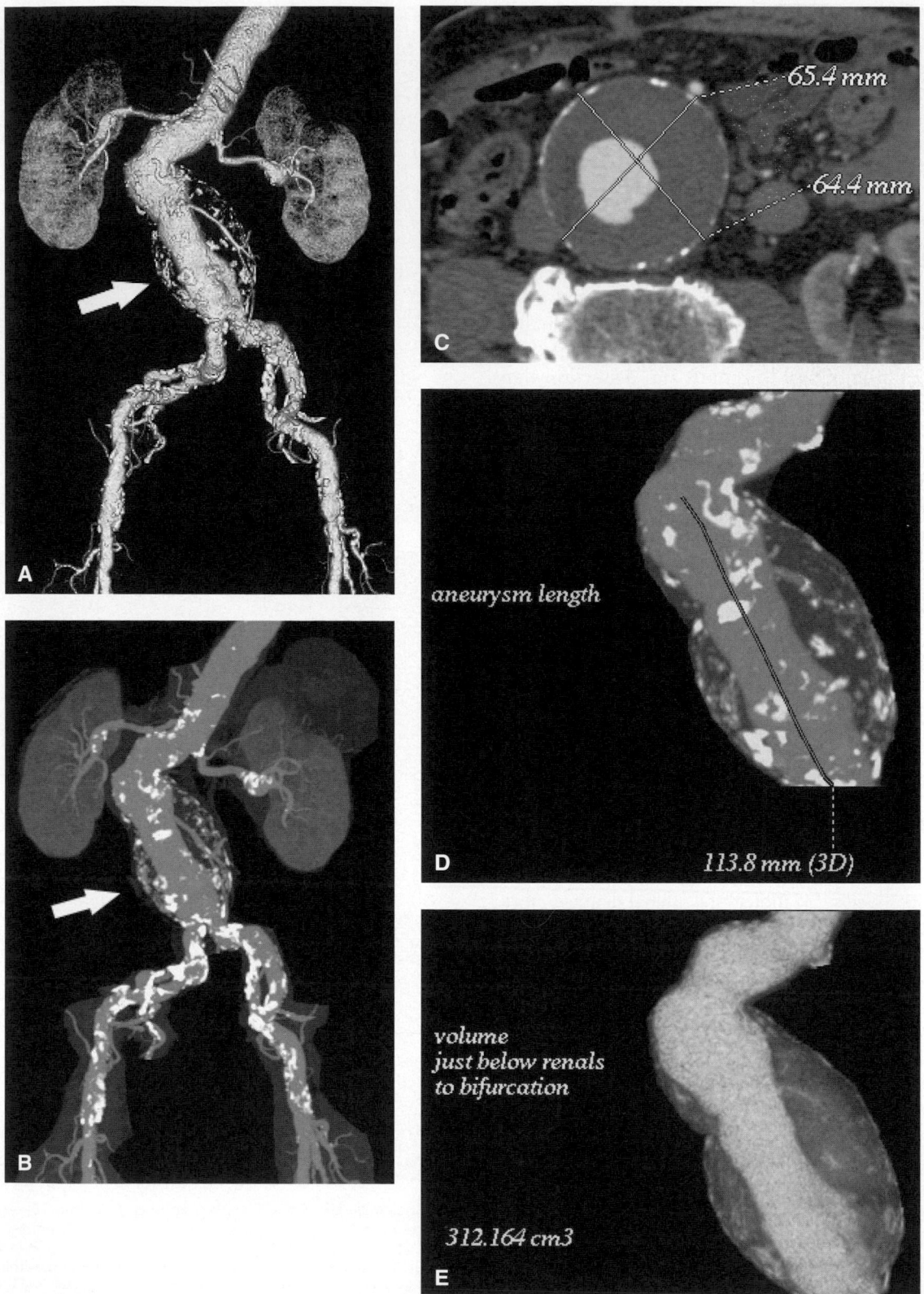

Figure 6–11   A., B. Volume-rendered and MIP images from a 16-channel MDCT angiogram demonstrate an infrarenal abdominal aotic aneurysm (*arrow*), which has maximum transverse dimensions approaching 65 mm x 65 mm, **C.,** a length of nearly 114 mm, **D.,** and a volume of 312 cm³, **E.** Measurements provide a benchmark for subsequent studies. For endovascular aneurysm repair, proximal neck morphology would require suprarenal fixation. The proximal neck has a suitable length (25 mm) and lacks mural thrombus and a significant calcium burden (CPR image, **F.,** *arrowhead*), but has a maximum diameter of 30 mm and exhibits moderate angulation (103 degrees). Overall, the iliofemoral vessels are of adequate morphology for endograft delivery and iliac fixation. The common iliac arteries exhibit moderate tortuosity and mild ectasia. **F.** Despite the diffuse calcified atherosclerosis, as demonstrated by CPR technique, there is neither significant narrowing nor regions of circumferential calcium.

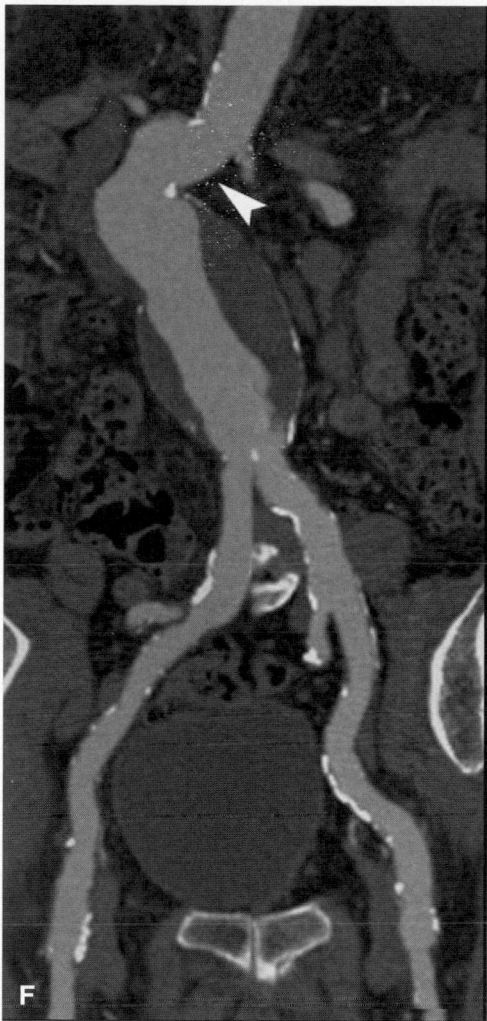

Figure 6–11 *(continued)*

instability, chest pain, abdominal pain, end-organ dysfunction, or all of these. In addition to the aortic aneurysms, dissection, IMH, PAU, and TAI may also lead to rupture. Other complications of the acute diseases, depending on the location and extent of involvement, include aortic insufficiency, pericardial tamponade, and aortic branch vessel compromise. The latter may lead to ischemia or thromboembolism in the coronary, cerebral, mesenteric, renal, upper extremity, or lower extremity vascular territories. The pathogenesis of these acute aortic diseases, in addition to pertinent MDCTA findings, is summarized in Table 6–8. CTA clinical success has been reported for all of these conditions (137–146). Transesophageal echocardiography and MRI are other noninvasive modalities that can be performed. However, because timely diagnosis is paramount, the scanner availability, the scanner proximity to the emergency department, and the exam speed make MDCTA the preferred choice for hemodynamically stable patients (Figure 6–12). In addition, MDCTA provides alternative diagnoses more completely. MDCTA is limited when the aortic root is involved and it cannot evaluate aortic insufficiency dynamically.

MDCTA achieves several clinical goals following endovascular or surgical repair of the thoracic aorta, abdominal aorta, or both. Foremost is establishing a new "baseline" that will serve as a reference for future studies and clinical management. This is particularly important in patients with underlying connective tissue disorders who remain at risk for aortic dilatation, dissection progression, or new dissection.

Interpreting postsurgical exams requires familiarity with procedures and the normal postoperative appearances and pitfalls. For example, after an elephant trunk graft replacement of the aortic arch, a common pitfall is interpreting the transition with native descending thoracic aorta, as a dissection. Infolding of grafts can also simulate a dissection or may appear as a focal pseudoaneurysm. Key surveillance issues to address include anastomotic, graft, and aortic branch vessel patency. Caliber of treated and nontreated vascular segments and reimplanted arteries should be assessed and measured to exclude stenosis, kinking, or enlargement. It is critical to recognize an interposition or inclusion graft anastomotic dehiscence that may have active extravasation, pseudoaneurysm formation, or both. If an inclusion graft has been placed, enhancement in the aneurysm sac would indicate a leak. Retrospective ECG gating is recommended on examinations following a valve sparing aortic root/ascending aorta procedure, because evaluation of leaflet thickening and coaptation are key to assessing surgical success. MDCTA is also an excellent means to evaluate the extravascular structures and their potential complications, as well as the sites for cardiopulmonary bypass cannula placement.

Following endovascular repair, issues to address include endograft position and patency; aortic branch vessel patency; and aorta/aneurysm sac diameter, length, area, and volume (147). In addition, vascular and visceral complications should be excluded (148). Most important, however, is establishing whether the endograft has excluded blood flow and systemic arterial pressure from the treated segment of native aorta, prerequisites for reduction in size of an aneurysm sac (147). Contrast opacification outside the endograft and within the aneurysm sac is defined as an endoleak (149) and is directly seen with MDCTA (Figure 6–13). The concern with endoleaks is the elevated intrasac pressure and the potential risk for aneurysm enlargement and rupture. However, not all endoleaks pose the same risk, which possibly may be related to endoleak flow, aneurysm sac thrombus, and side branch patency.

A classification scheme has evolved to describe the source of endoleaks and elevation of intrasac pressure (150). This scheme is summarized in Table 6–9. Included in it is the phenomenon of endotension (type V endoleak), which is widely discussed but poorly understood. Imaging studies have defined endotension strictly as elevated intrasac pressure without a demonstrable endoleak, and it has been suggested that either the sac thrombus serves as an ineffective barrier to preventing pressure transmission

TABLE 6–8

ACUTE AORTIC PATHOLOGY

	Pathogenesis	MDCTA Features
Aortic Dissection (AD)	• Laceration in aortic intima and inner layer of the aortic media • Predispositions: hypertension, connective tissue disorders • Classification —Acute or chronic —Stanford A or B: Determined by proximal level of dissection flap*; important for management—acute type A. AD requires immediate surgical treatment, type B may be managed medically, unless complications arise for which surgical or endovascular treatment is necessary	• Double channel aorta, separated by an intimomedial flap • Tears may be focal (simple), complex with multiple lacerations, or circumferential • True lumen often distinguished by smaller size, intimal calcification, and acute angled margins • False lumen often larger in size with obtuse angled margins; turbulent density and prolonged enhancement can be seen in the false lumen as a result of slower flow • Important features to characterize: origin of tear and propogation of dissection flap; size and patency of true and false lumens; branch vessel origin and patency; levels of fenestrations and reentry tears; presence of hemorrhagic pleural or pericardial effusions; visceral perfusion
Intramural Hematoma (IMH)	• Primary: Rupture of vasa vasorum into aortic media, as a result of elevated blood pressure • Secondary: PAU, TAI • Weakens aortic wall—risk of dissection and rupture • Classification: Types A or B°; management implications similar to AD	• High attenuation crescent in the aortic wall, best identified on the noncontrast images • Distinguished from luminal mural thrombus by its subintimal location; intima often defined by calcification • Important features to characterize: location and extent of involvement; branch vessel origin and patency; presence of hemorrhagicpleural or pericardial effusions; visceral sequelae
Penetrating Atherosclerotic Ulcers (PAU)	• Atheromatous plaque ulcer disrupts the internal elastic lamina and burrows into the media • Complications: IMH and/or short segment dissection • Progression through adventitia leads to pseudoaneurysm formation/rupture	• Focal contrast-filled excrescence, outside the aortic wall contours • Additional possible findings: IMH; pseudoaneurysm; signs of rupture • Atheromatous ulcers without penetration are distinguished by preservation of the intima: no contrast extends beyond the aortic contours, initima often defined by calcification
Aortic Aneurysm Rupture	• Wall tension and mechanical stress exceeds strength of the aortic wall, as determined by LaPlace's law∆ • Higher risk in setting of hypertension, dissection, ulcers, IMH	• Pseudoaneurysm • Active extravasation • Extravascular hematoma • Hemorrhagic pleural, pericardial effusions
Traumatic Aortic Injury (TAI)	• Rapid deceleration at shear points of aortic attachments (i.e. aortic root, aortic isthmus, diaphragmatic hiatus) • Most common site of injury—aortic root • Most common sites of injury in patients entering the emergency department: aortic isthmus>> distal descending aorta	• Primary findings: IMH; initimal tear; contour and caliber changes; pseudoaneurysm; active extravasation • Secondary findings: periaortic hematoma; mediastinal stranding • Ductus diverticulum distinguished from an aortic isthmus pseudoaneurysm by its anteromedial location, smooth contour transition, and obtuse margins

Note: *Stanford type A—Dissection flap involves ascending aorta; Stanford type B—Dissection flap involvement beyond ascending aorta; °Classification similar to Stanford type A and B; ∆ LaPlace's law: T (wall tension) = P (transmural pressure) x R (vessel radius)

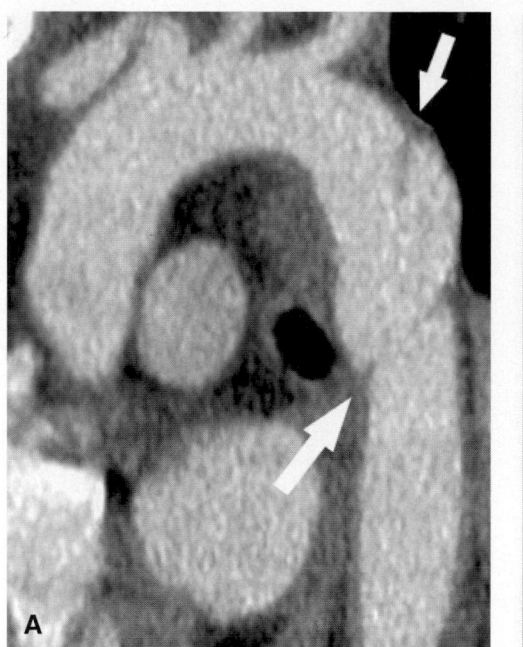 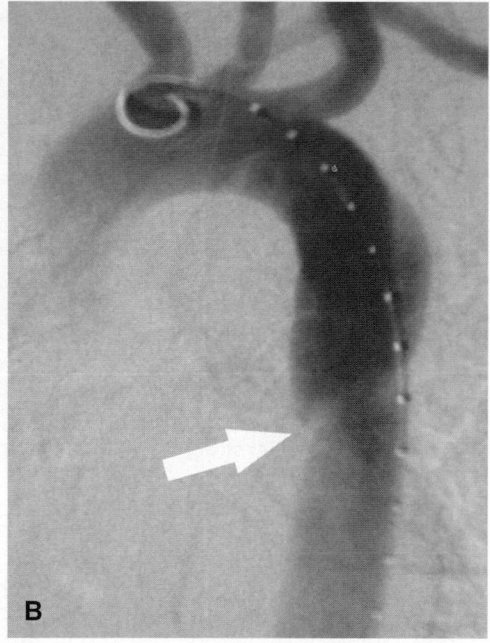

Figure 6–12   Following emergent resuscitation, a patient involved in a motor vehicle collision underwent CT angiography. **A.** This left anterior oblique MPR image of the patient's thoracic aorta reveals a traumatic pseudoaneurysm at the isthmus (*arrow*). The patient subsequently underwent endovascular stent-graft repair. **B.** Predeployment angiography confirms the traumatic aortic injury.

(subtypes A, B), there is intrasac fluid accumulation (subtypes A, B), or the endoleak is occult to imaging, possibly because of slow flow or intermittent endograft malpositioning at the fixation zones (subtypes C, D) (150). The delayed acquisition should be included in all postendograft MDCTA evaluations, because a slow flow endoleak may only be seen as resulting from progressive contrast accumulation. Recognition on serial CT angiograms of a persistently enlarged or an increasing aneurysm sac size without a demonstrable endoleak on the delayed phase would suggest the presence of endotension and may warrant additional investigation, including direct measurement of the arterial sac pressure (151), duplex ultrasound, contrast-enhanced ultrasound (152), and MRA (153) with functional MRI (154).

Cerebrovascular

CT angiography is an established modality for evaluating cerebrovascular disease. SDCT scanners have demonstrated their strength in imaging extracranial and intracranial disease. The most important benefit of MDCT scanners is the ability to image the entire cerebrovascular tree in one caudad-cranial acquisition, with high or isotropic resolution technique (155). The greater speed of 32- to 64-channel scanners should enable arterial-venous biphasic acquisitions, further improving diagnostic quality and providing more functional information. To achieve this, adherence to principles for fast scan durations, including use of high-concentration contrast medium, is necessary. The injection

duration should be at least 10–15 seconds. Although fixed and tailored delays can be used, the recommendation is to determine the *t*CMT with an ROI placed on the transverse aorta.

Carotid atherosclerotic disease is the most common indication for extracranial CTA. Other clinical applications include evaluating carotid stent patency (156), trauma (157–158), and dissection (159–161). With carotid atherosclerosis, the primary imaging goal is to assess the degree and extent of stenotic-occlusive disease, because management decisions for carotid artery stenosis (CAS) depend on accurate measurements (162). Secondary goals are to characterize plaque morphology and predict plaque stability (163–164). CTA is an ideal exam to use for achieving these goals (Figure 6–14). MPR and CPR techniques, as well as the source images, directly show the diseased lumen and wall. MIP and VR techniques display the carotid system in an angiographic-like format. Employing MIP techniques, VR techniques, or both to detect hemodynamically significant 70–99% CAS, single detector CTA has a sensitivity ranging between 81% and 100%, a specificity ranging between 92% and 100%, and an agreement with conventional angiography ranging between 85% and 95% (165–173). Comparing MIP and VR performance in this clinical setting, Leclerc et al. demonstrated that VR has slightly greater sensitivity (169). In the setting of heavy calcification, CPR images should be reviewed in order to more precisely assess the degree of stenosis (Figure 6–15). CTA also has excellent correlation with conventional angiography for occlusive disease. Using MIP and CPR

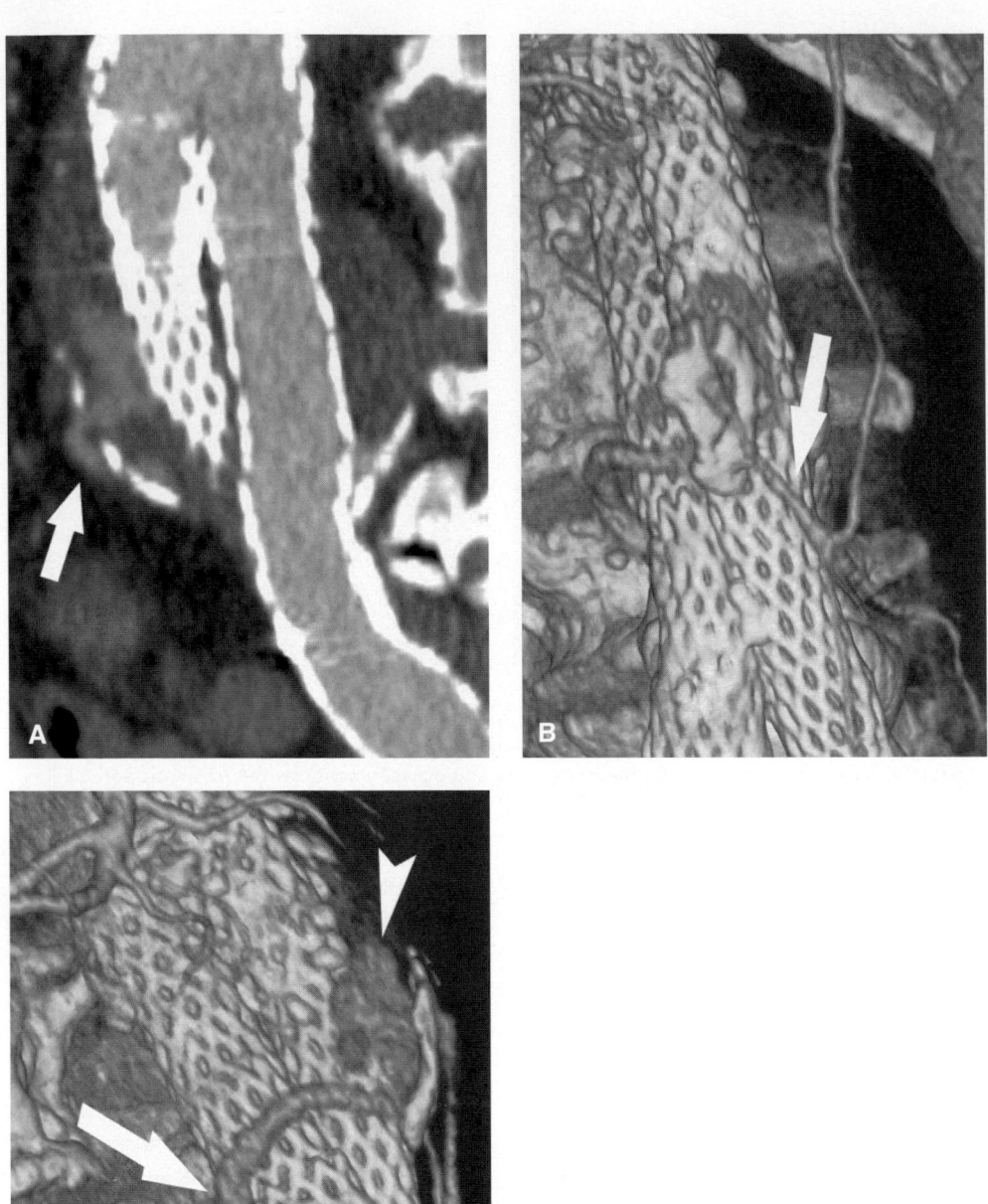

Figure 6–13 A. A sagittal MPR image of an endovascularly repaired infrarenal aneurysm reveals an endoleak accumulating in the anterior portion of the aneurysm sac. The endoleak communicates with the inferior mesenteric artery (*arrow*), consistent with a type II endoleak. **B, C.** This endoleak is further illustrated with volume-rendering technique. As shown, the endoleak also communicates with a lumbar artery, forming a network.

displays to interpret 4-channel MDCTA acquisitions, Chen et al. correctly depicted all 53 extracranial internal carotid arteries with total or near occlusion (173).

Regrading the intracranial vasculature, intracranial CTA is commonly used to evaluate ischemic stroke, to screen for aneurysms, and to search for a cause of subarachnoid hemorrhage. Other applications include evaluation of vasospasm (174–175), vascular malformations, and venous thrombosis

(176), as well as follow-up of surgical (177) and endovascular interventions. As to ischemic stroke, CT protocols provide structural and functional information, which facilitates prompt critical management decisions (178–180). First, noncontrast images are obtained to evaluate for infarction and to exclude nonischemic etiologies of neurologic deficits, such as a hemorrhage or mass. Then, perfusion CT is performed at the level of the basal ganglia to

TABLE 6–9
ENDOLEAK CLASSIFICATION

Types	Mechanism	MDCTA Findings
I	Flow originates from ineffective endograft seal at fixation zones	Periendograft contrast opacification localized to or extending from fixation zone
A	• Proximal	• Important to assess for endograft migration, kinking, and/or buckling
B	• Distal	
C	• Iliac occluder	• Pitfall: Type II–IV endoleak with contrast extending to fixation zone
II	Branch vessel retrograde flow	Periendograft channel or collection of contrast that communicates with patent branch vessel(s):
A	• Single vessel (simple)	
B	• Two or more vessels creating a circuit (complex)	• Thoracic endograft: left subclavian, left common carotid, intercostal arteries
		• Abdominal endograft: lumbar, inferior mesenteric, internal iliac arteries
III	Flow results from structural endograft failure	Periendograft contrast opacification localized to junctional segments (A) or adjacent to the body or limbs (B)
A	• Junctional separation (modular devices)	• MPR and VR display techniques provide direct visual assessment of structural defects
B	• Endograft fracture or holes —Minor (<2 mm) —Major (≥2 mm)	• Important to use wide window settings
IV	Endograft fabric porosity (<30 days after endograft implantation)	Primary periendograft contrast opacification in the immediate postimplantation period, which resolves on follow-up studies
		• Endoleak centered at body or limbs
		• Diagnosis of exclusion
V	Endotension	Elevated intrasac pressure without a demonstrable endoleak seen on MDCTA, including the delayed phase
A	• Without an endoleak	
B	• With a sealed endoleak	• Sac thrombus provides ineffective barrier to pressure transmission (A, B)
C	• With a type I or III endoleak	
D	• With a type II endoleak	• Endoleak occult to imaging (C, D)

Note: Adapted with permission from Veith FJ, Baum RA, Ohki T, et al. Nature and significance of endoleaks and endotension: summary of opinions expressed at an international conference. J Vasc Surg 2002;35:1029–1035.

distinguish infarcted from reversibly impaired ("at risk") brain parenchyma. Finally, the CTA is performed to identify occluded or stenotic vessels as the cause or causes for presenting symptoms. Localization of occlusion is important because it will factor into determining whether a patient is a candidate for intra-arterial or intravenous thrombolysis or anticoagulation therapy (181–182). Agreement between single and dual detector row CTA and conventional angiography for detecting intracranial occlusions ranges between 86% and 100% (181,183–187). CTA interpretation also focuses on identifying collateral pathways. Their extent is a positive predictor of clinical outcome (187).

Regarding CTA diagnosis of intracranial aneurysms, important anatomical features to define are their location, size, shape, neck, and relations with adjacent structures (Figure 6–16). Studies evaluating 4-channel MDCTA detection of intracranial aneurysms demonstrate an overall sensitivity ranging from 81% to 90% and a specificity of 83% to 100% (188–190). While this performance appears similar to SDCT scanners (191), Dammert et al. and Karamessini et al. indicate that 4-channel MDCT scanners have improved sensitivity for detecting small (<3–4 mm) aneurysms, compared to SDCT scanners (68–83% (188, 190) versus 61% (191).

Mesenteric

Common applications for mesenteric CTA are assessment of suspected acute and chronic mesenteric ischemia, vascular mapping, and acute visceral bleeding. CTA can also be used to localize the site and etiology of gastrointestinal bleeding (192). Other indications include assessment of liver transplant vascular patency, evaluation of vascular involvement from pancreatic and mesenteric tumors, and characterization of benign and malignant liver tumors. The latter involves diagnosis prior to and a follow-up after

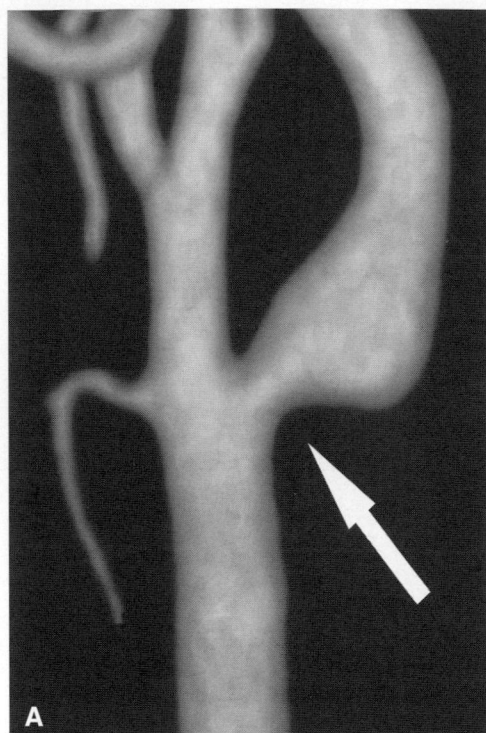

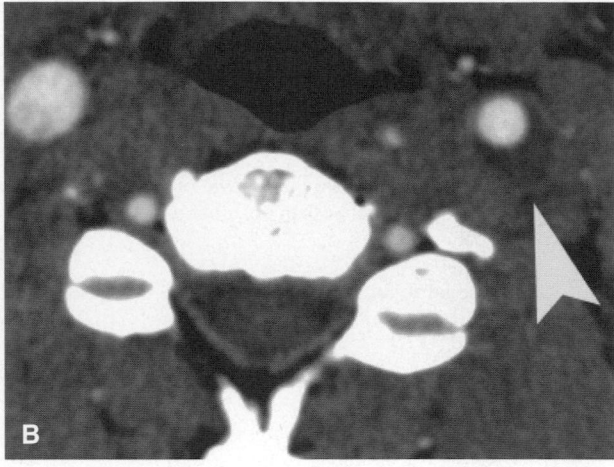

Figure 6–14 **A.** Volume rendering through the left carotid system reveals a 60% stenosis (*arrow*) at the proximal internal carotid artery, associated with poststenotic dilatation. **B.** Review of the axial images identifies a moderate burden of nearly circumferential soft atherosclerotic plaque (*arrowhead*). Ultrasound confirmed the plaque and documented velocity elevations suggestive of at least 50% stenosis (*not shown*).

conventional chemotherapy, surgical resection, or intra-arterial chemoembolization. Frequent, but less common, indications for mesenteric CTA are evaluation of suspected mesenteric aneurysms, dissection, vasculitis, venous thrombosis, aortoenteric fistulae, and angiodysplasia. One novel application is aiding the evaluation of inflammatory bowel disease by identifying vascular sequelae, such as hyperemia and enlarged feeding arteries, as well as by calculating bowel perfusion (193–194).

Mesenteric CTA may be performed as a dedicated exam or in conjunction with abdominal aortoiliac CTA. During the arterial phase, complete vascular territories and collateral pathways are depicted. Subsequently, a visceral phase can be acquired, affording comprehensive vascular and organ evaluation (195). In most instances, high-resolution datasets (1.0–1.5 mm detector width) are sufficient. However, for studies on 16- to 64-channel systems, acquiring isotropic datasets (submillimeter collimation) should always be considered, factoring volume coverage, body habitus, and noise. Biphasic acquisitions, including arterial and visceral phases, are readily achieved through the use of a 40- to 50-second diagnostic delay after the *t*CMT. Recommended collimation detector thickness for the visceral phase is 1.0–1.5 mm with reconstruction into two sets; one with a slice thickness of 2.5–5 mm and the other with thin sections (1.0–1.5 mm). The former is used for axial interpretation, and the latter is used for MPR and VR display. As with every application, complete opacification of the splanchnic vasculature is essential. This requires a 20- to 25-second injection duration. If the scan duration is

less, rules to follow include using a high injection rate, using high concentration contrast medium, and extending the diagnostic scan delay. To optimize parenchymal enhancement, iodine dose is administered in accordance with the patient's body weight. Automated triggering is performed with an ROI at the supraceliac aorta.

Regarding mesenteric ischemia, MDCTA diagnosis relies on the recognition of stenotic-occlusive vessels and end-organ sequelae. Although CTA acquisition is static, identification of the collateral pathways provides a measure of functional status (Figure 6–17). In a retrospective review of 52 patients, each of whom underwent 4-channel MDCTA and conventional angiography, Stueckle et al. concluded that with the correct display technique, MDCTA is an accurate modality for imaging the abdominal aorta and its branch vessels (196). Included in this study group were four superior mesenteric artery (SMA) stenoses and three inferior mesenteric artery (IMA) occlusions, all of which were diagnosed with MDCTA. Kirkpatrick and colleagues validated the clinical performance of biphasic 4-channel MDCT acquisitions in the diagnosis of acute mesenteric ischemia by showing 96% sensitivity and 94% specificity in identification of SMA occlusion, celiac and IMA occlusion with distal SMA disease, arterial embolism, pneumotosis intestinalis, venous gas, bowel wall thickening, lack of bowel wall enhancement, solid organ infarction, and venous thrombosis (197). For patients who undergo endovascular management of mesenteric ischemia, MDCT angiography is an excellent means for surveillance. Instent neointimal hyperplasia (Figure 6–18), stent migration, and untoward

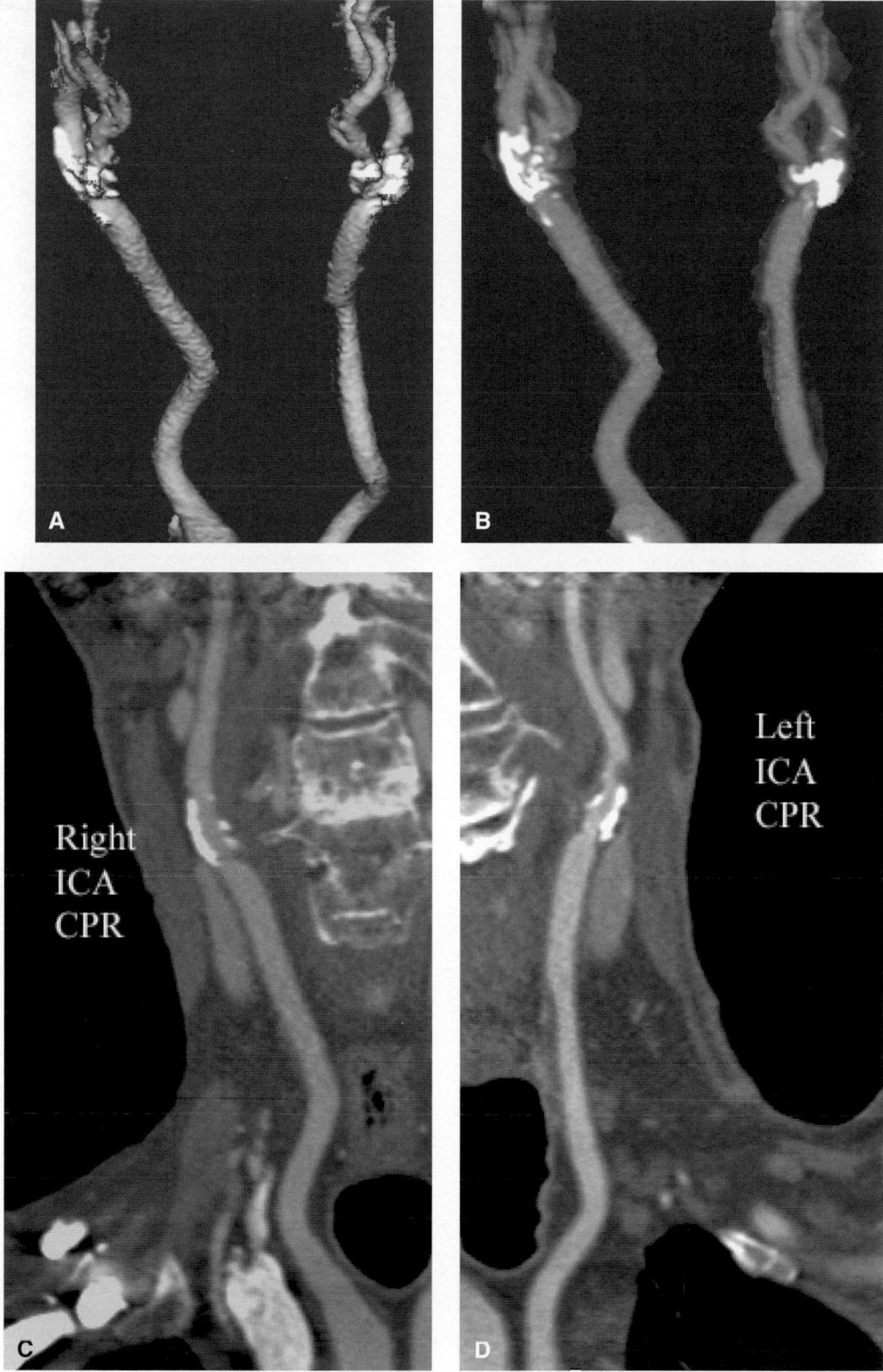

Figure 6–15   An asymptomatic patient was found to have bilateral carotid bruits. Ultrasound suggested severe left and moderate right internal carotid stenosis. However, calcification limited interpretation. A 64-channel MDCT angiogram was performed with 0.6 mm collimation. Interpretation of the **A.** volume-rendered and **B.** MIP images is also degraded by the calcification. CPR images drawn through the center of the lumens provide more precise morphologic evaluation, revealing **C.** approximate 50% right carotid bulb and **D.** a 65% left carotid bulb/proximal internal carotid artery narrowing.

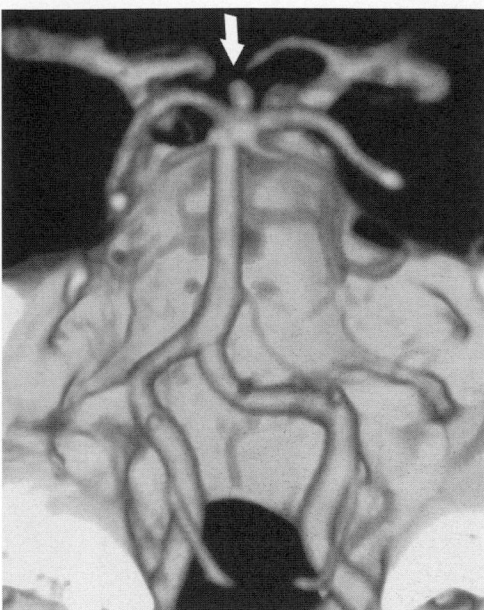

Figure 6–16 A volume-rendered image from an MDCT angiogram (16 mm x 0.625 mm collimation), demonstrates a focal 4 mm basilar tip aneurysm (*arrow*). Based on this study, anatomical features were viewed favorably for possible coil embolization. Transcatheter embolization was subsequently performed without adverse outcome.

complications are evaluated, while the status of visceral anatomy and nontreated vascular segments is gauged.

Regarding mesenteric vascular mapping, identifying normal and variant vascular anatomy is a prerequisite for patients being considered for liver donation, liver transplant, hepatic intra-arterial chemotherapy pump placement, hepatic chemoembolization, laparoscopic gastrectomy, and laparoscopic splenectomy. With a biphasic technique, not only is the roadmap generated, but additional imaging goals for these patients can be met, namely accurate quantification of hepatic and splenic volumes (198–199) and characterization of visceral anatomy and underlying disease (200–203). As to mapping the hepatic vasculature with MDCTA, variant arterial anatomy may be seen in 30–67% of patients (200–207). Variant hepatic and portal venous anatomy is reported to occur in 48–75% and 20–24% of patients, respectively (200,205). Compared with conventional angiography, 4-channel MDCTA is 90–94% sensitive and 93–100% specific for identifying variant hepatic arteries (202,204,206). For displaying the hepatic arteries following a 4-channel high-resolution acquisition, Byun et al. demonstrated that MIP is a more reliable technique compared to VR. This group achieved a sensitivity of 90% and specificity of 93% for MIP, compared to 58% and 88% for VR, respectively (204). MDCTA can achieve excellent results for mapping essential vasculature prior to laparoscopic gastrectomy and splenectomy. In 36 patients undergoing 4-channel MDCTA evaluation prior to laparoscopic gastrectomy, Matsuki et al. reported 100% sensitivity and positive predictive value to correctly

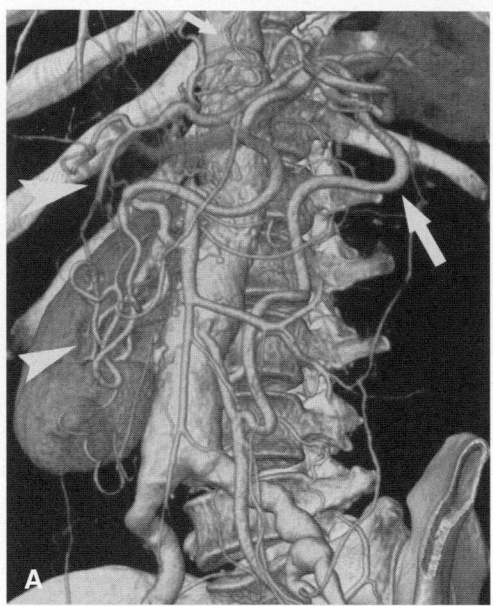

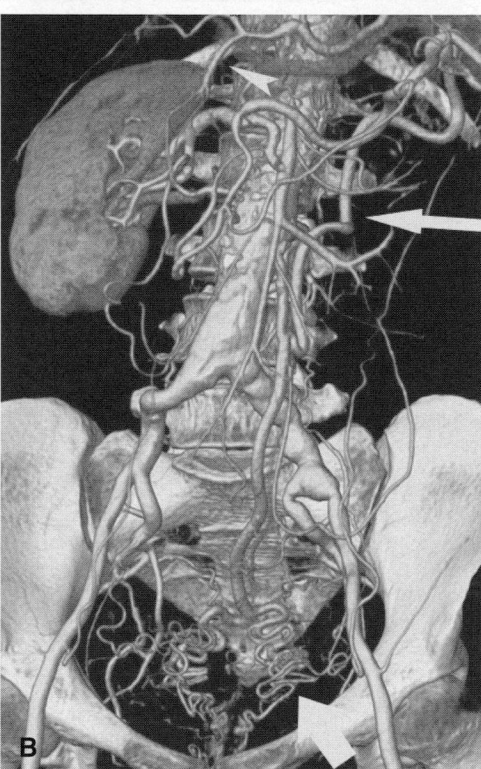

Figure 6–17 This MDCT angiogram (16 mm x 1.25 mm collimation) diagnoses chronic mesenteric ischemia as the cause for a patient's 30-lb weight loss over one year. **A.** Volume-rendered images demonstrate celiac axis and superior mesenteric artery (SMA) occlusion from atherosclerotic plaque. **B.** Prominent rectal collateral vessels have developed to direct flow retrograde from the hypogastric system to inferior mesenteric artery (*broad arrow*). A prominent Arc of Riolan is present (*thin arrow*) for collateral flow between the IMA and SMA territories. Flow into the celiac territory is dependent on the pancreaticoduodenal arcade and an enlarged gastroduodenal artery (*arrowhead*). In addition, there is likely contribution from phrenic arteries (**A.**, *small arrow*).

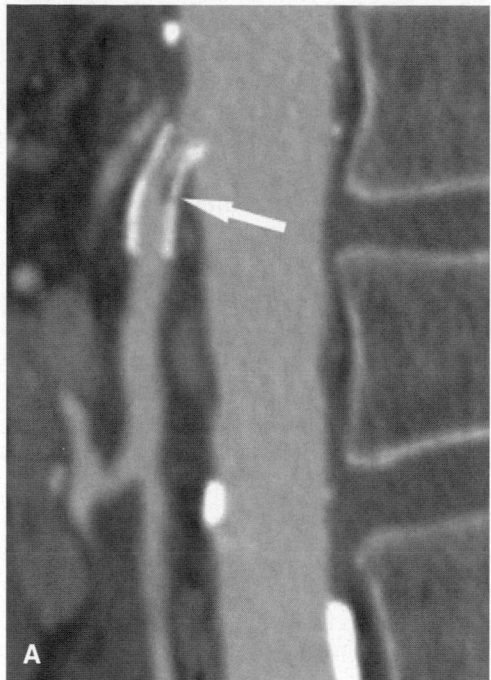

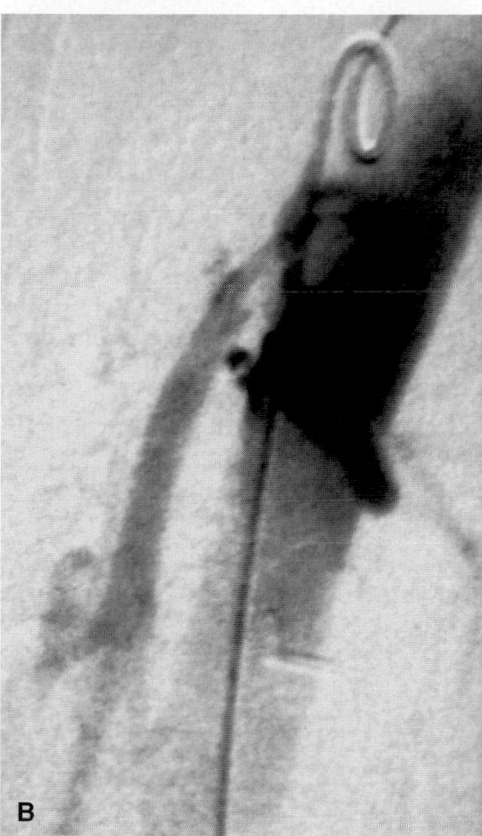

identify the left gastric artery, a replaced left hepatic artery, and the left gastric coronary vein; and 100% sensitivity and 97% positive predictive value to determine the origin of the right gastric artery (208). In 22 patients undergoing 4-channel MDCTA prior to laparoscopic splenectomy, Napoli et al. reported correct identification of splenic artery origins, polar arteries, and an arteria pancreatica magna (199).

Renal

Renal CTA can be applied to address several clinical needs. Two common indications are evaluation of suspected renovascular hypertension (Figure 6–19) and vascular screening for potential living renal donors. In addition to excluding suspected trauma, aneurysms (Figure 6–20), dissection, vasculitis, thromboembolism, and renal masses, other clinical uses involve evaluating renal hemorrhage, assessing endovascular stent patency (209), evaluating renal transplants (210), planning endovascular procedures (211–212), and assessing for a crossed vessel as the cause for ureteropelvic obstruction. Recent work suggests that, by accurately calculating the glomerular filtration rate, MDCTA will become a one-stop shop for the assessment of renal structure and function (213–214).

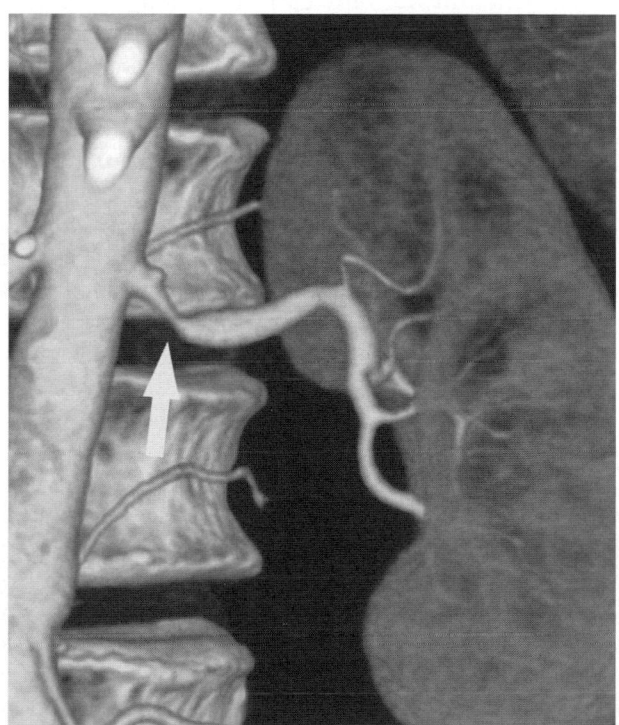

Figure 6–18 **A.** In a patient who had undergone SMA stent placement for mesenteric ischemia 2 years prior, routine CT angiographic surveillance reveals low attenuation soft tissue along the luminal surface of the stent, associated with decreased intrastent luminal caliber (*arrow*). **B.** Findings are consistent with neointimal hyperplasia and moderate restenosis, and were subsequently confirmed with chatheter angiography, obtained at the time of reintervention.

Figure 6–19 A young patient with new onset hypertension underwent a screening MDCT angiogram (16 mm x 0.625 mm collimation). Volume-rendered images reveal a hemodynamically significant stenosis at the left renal artery postostial segment (*arrow*).

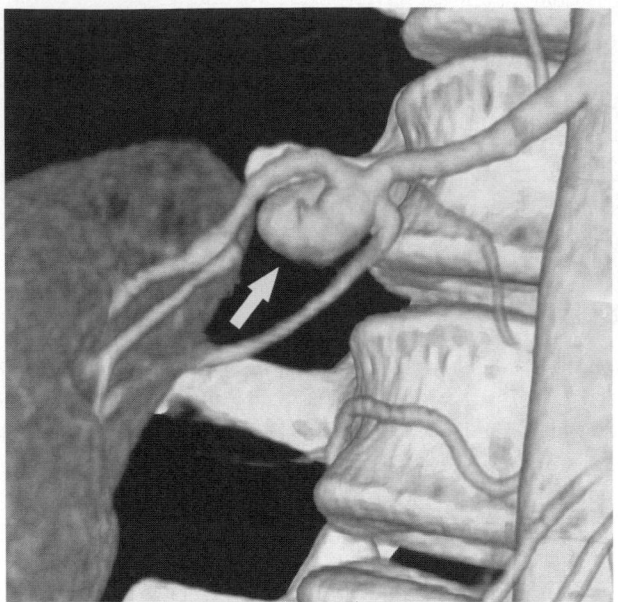

Figure 6–20 Surveillance MDCT angiography for a known right renal aneurysm is acquired with 16 mm x 0.75 mm collimation. Demonstrated with robust detail is a stable, 18 mm aneurysm arising at the renal artery bifurcation (*arrow*). The patient continues to undergo conservative management.

Imaging the complete renovascular system should encompass the abdominal aorta through the common iliac arteries. This will not only cover the kidneys and main renal arteries, but also the accessory arteries that can arise from as high as the inferior phrenic arteries and as low as the common iliac arteries. To accommodate a single breath-hold on an SDCT scanner, this coverage required up to 5-mm thick sections (7). With an MDCT scanner, appropriate coverage can be achieved in a single breath-hold using thin section technique. The increased speed of the MDCT scanners also facilitates designing protocols with arterial, corticomedullary, venous, and urographic phases, a useful benefit in renal donor evaluation.

Similar to mesenteric CTA, MDCT renal angiography is acquired with a detector width of 1.0–1.5 mm or less. Evaluation may take place during routine abdominal aortoiliac CTA or as a dedicated renal CTA. If the exam is performed on 16- to 64-channel systems, it is recommended to acquire isotropic datasets (submillimeter collimation), dependent upon volume coverage, body habitus, and noise. This will provide greater detail of peripheral, small branch vessels. As with mesenteric CTA, enhancement needs to be optimized in both arterial and parenchymal phases. High-concentration contrast medium, weight-based iodine dosing, high injection rate, and an injection duration of at least 15–20 seconds are key. Timing is synchronized to the enhancement of the midabdominal aorta.

Precise diagnosis of renovascular hypertension is important. Renal artery stenosis (RAS) accounts for only 1–5% of hypertension, most commonly from atherosclerosis (90%)

or fibromuscular dysplasia (<10%) (215). When RAS is present and hemodynamically significant, endovascular and surgical intervention can control hypertension and temporize loss in renal parenchyma and function. On the other hand, a negative study will provide the clinical confidence to pursue other secondary causes of hypertension or to appropriately manage essential hypertension. Clinical success for detecting hemodynamically significant, >50% stenoses has been established with SDCT and 4-channel MDCT. For SDCT, studies reveal a sensitivity ranging between 79% and 100%, a specificity of 77% and 100%, and an accuracy of 91–99% (5,7,216–221). Employing two-reader analysis to compare 4-channel MDCTA with conventional angiography in 46 patients, Willman et al. found a sensitivity of 86–93%, specificity of 99–100%, and an accuracy of 98–99% (222). Moderately good results can also be achieved for MDCTA evaluation of renal stent patency. In their early experience, Raza and colleagues demonstrated a sensitivity of 100% and specificity of 80% in detecting renal stent restenosis (209). For native renal arteries and those with stents, VR technique is considered the superior rendering method (223–224). Review of the transverse images will improve CTA performance for assessing the severity of RAS (5,221). When interpreting studies for RAS, it is helpful to search for ancillary findings that indicate the presence of a hemodynamically significant stenosis. These include renal atrophy, cortical thinning, decreased cortical enhancement, and poststenotic dilatation (5,7,225–226).

When screening potential living renal donors, precise assessment of renal arteries, veins, collecting system, and parenchyma is required to plan successful surgical and laparoscopic kidney procurement. The number, location, caliber, branching pattern, and underlying disease of native and variant arteries and veins will determine whether a kidney is suitable (227–229). Nonvascular findings such as hydronephrosis, ureteral duplication, nephrolithiasis, cysts, solid masses, and cortical scarring may also preclude donation (229). Comparing 4-channel MDCT renal angiography with intraoperative findings at the time of donor nephrectomy, Kim et al. has demonstrated a 98% detection rate for all renal arteries and veins (229). A 4-channel MDCTA also attains moderately good to excellent results for detecting accessory renal arteries, prehilar renal artery branching, and renal vein anomalies (228–229).

Lower Extremity

Evaluation of peripheral arterial occlusive disease (PAOD) is the most common indication for lower extremity CTA. Inflow and outflow anatomy (Figures 6–21, 6–22, and 6–23) is assessed in a single injection of contrast medium. As with conventional angiography, key goals include assessing vessel patency, characterizing lesions, and providing strategies for endovascular and surgical intervention. Other clinical applications include preoperative vascular mapping (230);

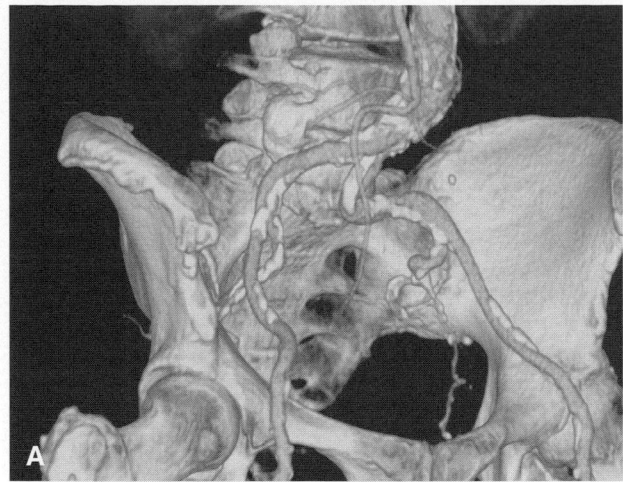

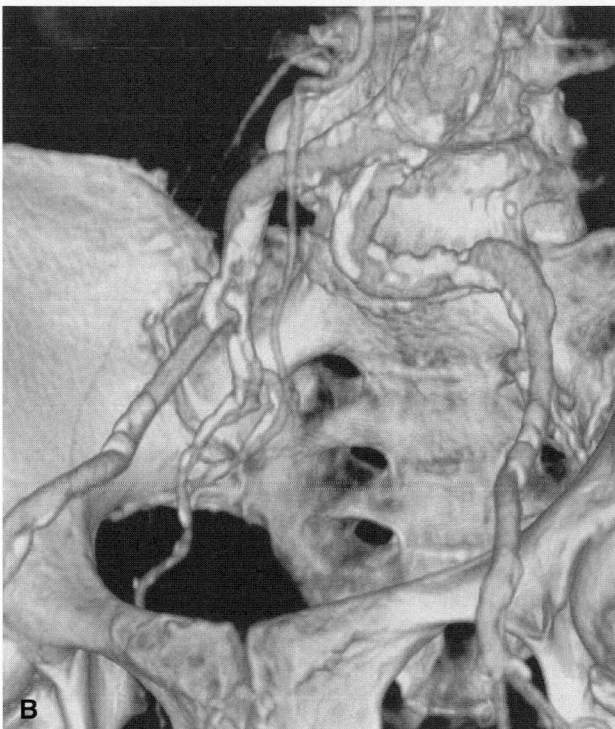

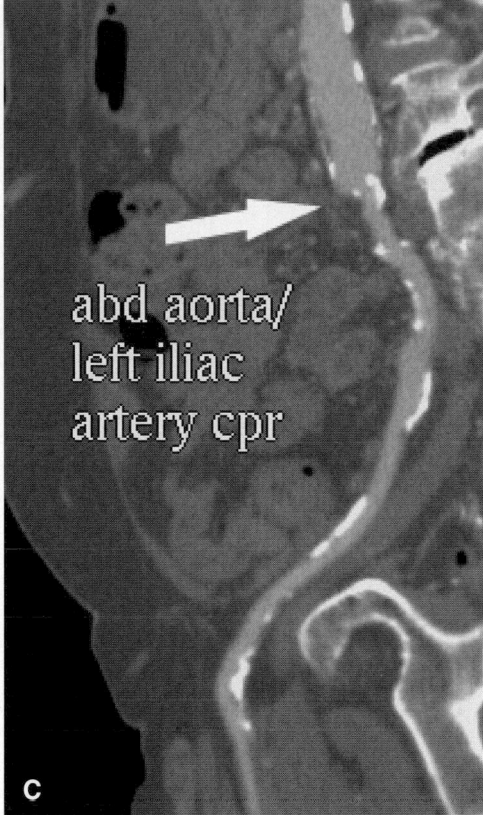

abd aorta/
left iliac
artery cpr

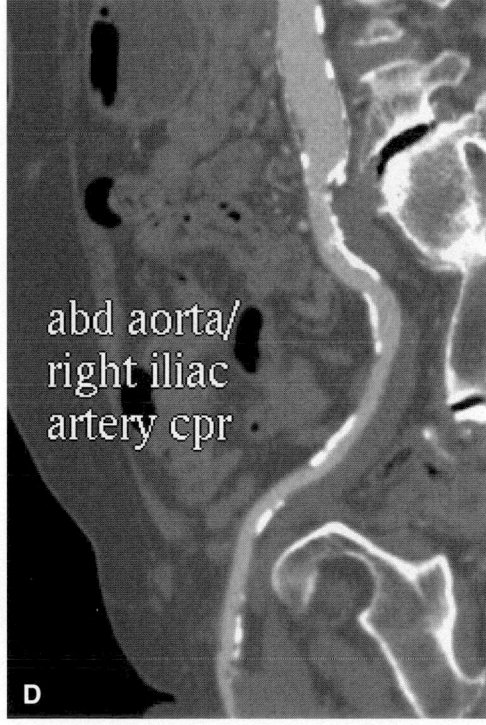

abd aorta/
right iliac
artery cpr

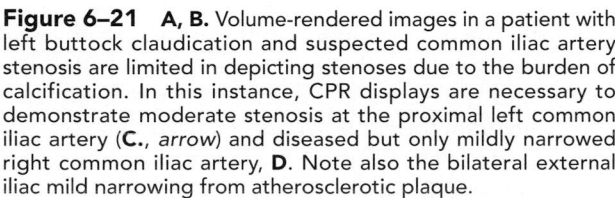

Figure 6–21   A, B. Volume-rendered images in a patient with left buttock claudication and suspected common iliac artery stenosis are limited in depicting stenoses due to the burden of calcification. In this instance, CPR displays are necessary to demonstrate moderate stenosis at the proximal left common iliac artery (**C.**, *arrow*) and diseased but only mildly narrowed right common iliac artery, **D**. Note also the bilateral external iliac mild narrowing from atherosclerotic plaque.

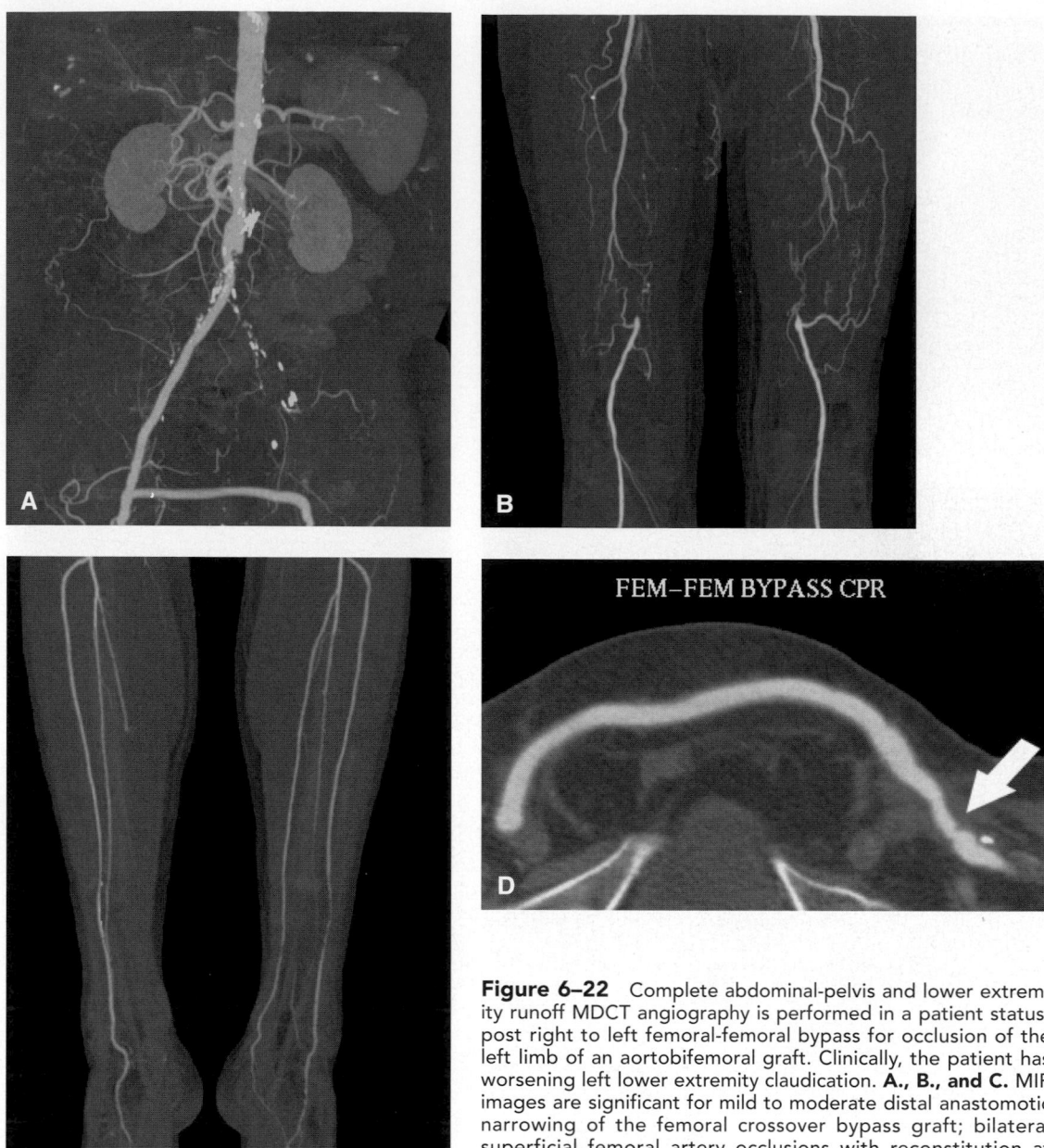

Figure 6–22   Complete abdominal-pelvis and lower extremity runoff MDCT angiography is performed in a patient status-post right to left femoral-femoral bypass for occlusion of the left limb of an aortobifemoral graft. Clinically, the patient has worsening left lower extremity claudication. **A., B., and C.** MIP images are significant for mild to moderate distal anastomotic narrowing of the femoral crossover bypass graft; bilateral superficial femoral artery occlusions with reconstitution at hunter's canal; and a two-vessel right and a three-vessel left mildly diseased runoff. **D.** CPR images confirm the distal graft narrowing (*arrow*).

assessing bypass graft, stent, and angioplasty patency; and evaluating suspected traumatic vascular injury (231–232), vascular masses, arteriovenous malformations, and venous disease, such as May-Thurner syndrome.

Until recently, depending on the exam indications, lower extremity CTA has been one of the most technically challenging vascular applications. PAOD requires complete inflow and outflow coverage, from the supraceliac abdominal aorta through to the feet. For other indications, such as suspected trauma, coverage may begin at the vascular segment of clinical interest and extend through to the feet. The technical issues involving complete coverage result from the large scan volume, which is typically between 1,200 and 1,400 mm. Given the variable flow dynamics over this volume, to achieve robust images in the multiple vascular territories, acquisition and contrast-medium injection parameters need to be precisely selected so that scan duration and contrast administration are synchronized. Furthermore, with the need for high spatial resolution of the small caliber mesenteric, renal, iliac, infrainguinal, infrapopliteal, and collateral branch vessels, the scan volume may yield 1,500–2,000 images for the CTA alone, not to mention the noncontrast images. Such large datasets require advanced computer processors to handle the image reconstruction, networking, viewing, and storage.

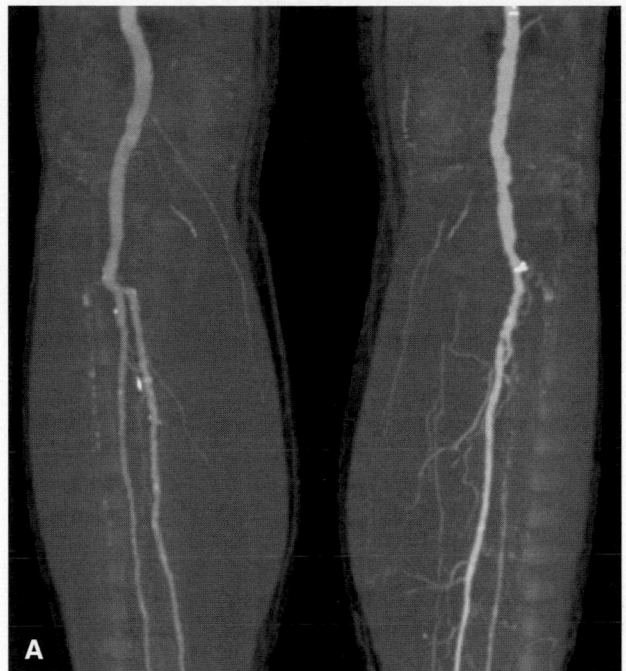

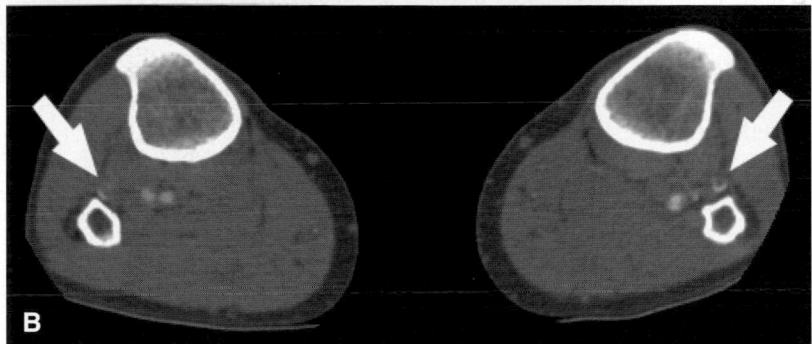

Figure 6–23   Chest, abdominal, pelvis, and bilateral lower extremity MDCT angiography (16 mm x 1.25 mm) is performed in a patient with atrial fibrillation and acute worsening of lower extremity claudication. No source of emboli was seen in the heart or aortoiliac segment (*not shown*). **A.** The runoff is remarkable for acute embolic occlusion of the bilateral anterior tibial arteries. Also shown is proximal left peroneal occlusion. **B.** Anterior tibial artery embolic occlusion is confirmed on the axial source images (*arrow*).

As to the acquisition, patients are placed supine, feet-first into the scanner with the lower extremities positioned at isocenter within the gantry. To maintain this position, cushions and possibly tape may be used. If imaging of only one extremity is required (in the case of trauma, for example), the affected extremity is positioned at isocenter and secured in similar fashion. The contralateral limb is flexed to position it out of the scan field. In general, high-resolution datasets provide sufficient detailed assessment of the inflow and outflow, including the infrapopliteal arteries. However, for complete coverage, this is only feasible on 8- to 64-channel systems. The large volume coverage restricts 4-channel MDCT acquisitions to a detector thickness of 2.5 mm. Isotropic acquisitions are certainly possible on 16- to 64-channel systems, with the disadvantages of increased image noise and number of images. Consequently, submillimeter acquisitions are commonly reserved for targeted coverage of the infrapopliteal segment or for pediatric patients.

Imaging the complete lower extremity vascular tree requires a prolonged contrast injection. For most adult patients, when timing off the supraceliac aorta, the contrast injection duration should be at least 40 seconds (233). When the scan duration is >40, the injection duration equals the scan duration plus additional delay if automated triggering is used. However, for a scan duration ≤40, a diagnostic delay must be added so that once initiated, acquisition coincides with a 40-second injection. For both acquisitions, biphasic injections are used.

With regard to assessment of PAOD, MDCT arteriography is accurate and reproducible with high interobserver agreement for native peripheral arteries (234–236) and bypass grafts (237). As to the native arteries, MDCTA achieves robust arterial enhancement in the lower extremity inflow and outflow, with successive improved contrast efficiency in 4-, 8-, and 16-channel scanners (238–239). Table 6-10 summarizes the reported performance of 4-channel scanners for detection of hemodynamically significant PAOD in native arteries (234–236,240–241). Despite volume coverage precluding thin section, high-resolution imaging, moderately good to excellent results can be achieved. However, the studies suggest that with 4-channel systems, performance is better for detection of occlusions than stenoses of >50%. With 4-channel scanners, studies

TABLE 6–10
PERFORMANCE OF LOWER EXTREMITY MDCTA

Author	Collimation	TH	N	Sensitivity	Specificity	Accuracy
Ofer et al. (2003)	4 x 2.5	3.2	18			
•>50% Stenosis				77%	93%	92%
• Occlusion				91%	98%	97%
Martin et al. (2003)	4 x 2.5	5.0	41			
•>50% Stenosis				76%	93%	91%
• Occlusion				89%	99.8%	98%
Ota et al. (2004)	4 x 2.0	2.0	24			
•>50% Stenosis				99%	99%	99%
• Occlusion				96%	98%	98%
Catalano et al. (2004)	4 x 2.5	3.0	50			
•>50% Stenosis				94%	97%	97%
• Occlusion				97%	99%	99%
‡Romano et al. (2004)	4 x 2.5	3.2	42	93%	95%	94%

Note: Collimation = Number of channels x detector width (mm). TH = Slice thickness. N = Number of patients.
‡ Study only reports overall performance for detecting normal, stenotic, and occlusive arteries.

have indicated that MDCTA performance is greater in the aortoiliac and femoral-popliteal segments, as compared to the infrapopliteal segment (235–236,240,242). This is related to the smaller vessel caliber and to dense calcified plaque, both of which can limit the accurate grading of arterial lesions. Dense calcification can also negatively influence interpretation in the aortoiliac and femoral-popliteal segments. As such, for suspected lesions seen on VR, or MIP images, MPR images, CPR images, or transverse sections (or all), axial images should always be reviewed (241–242). Portugaller et al. stresses the importance of this point by demonstrating that while MIP has slightly greater sensitivity and less specificity compared to VR for detecting hemodynamically significant lesions, MIP combined with axial image interpretation produces the most accurate results (242). Regarding peripheral bypass grafts (Figure 6–24), Willmann et al. analyzed the performance of 4-channel MDCT using two readers. The authors found MDCTA to be reliable in detecting graft stenoses, aneurysmal changes, and arteriovenous fistulas (237). Nintey-nine percent of the graft segments evaluated had good or excellent quality. Compared with conventional angiography, MDCTA detection of hemodynamically significant (>50%) graft stenosis was 98.5% (a range of 97–100%) sensitive and 100% specific (237).

Upper Extremity

CT angiography is an ideal exam for evaluating the complete upper extremity inflow and outflow vascular anatomy (243). The patient's risk of cerebral and digital thromboembolism is rendered obsolete and for some applications, occupational radiation exposure to the interventionalist is needed. Clinical indications include evaluation of arterial

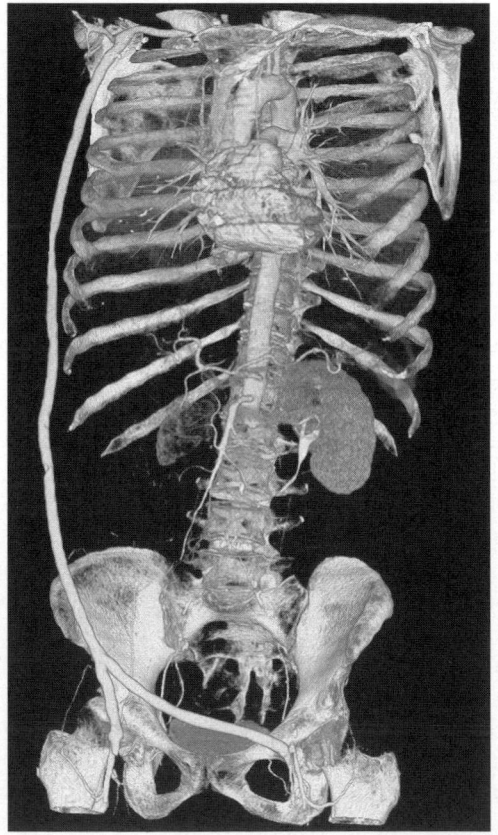

Figure 6–24 A coronal volume-rendered image demonstrates patent axillofemoral and femoral-femoral bypass grafts. MDCT angiography is ideal for this application as blood pool imaging affords complete vascular evaluation in a single bolus.

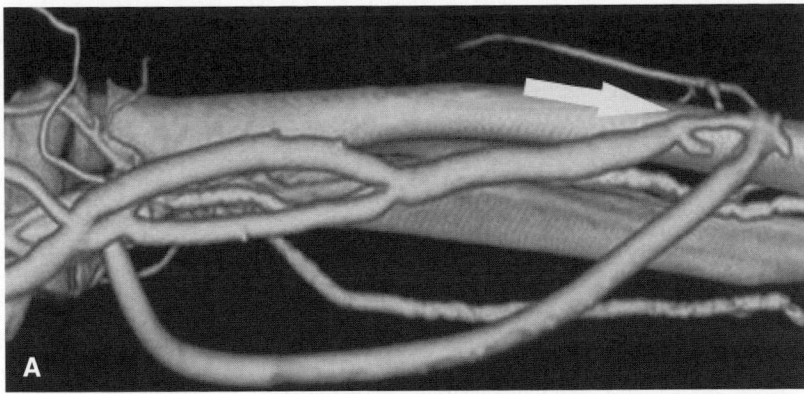

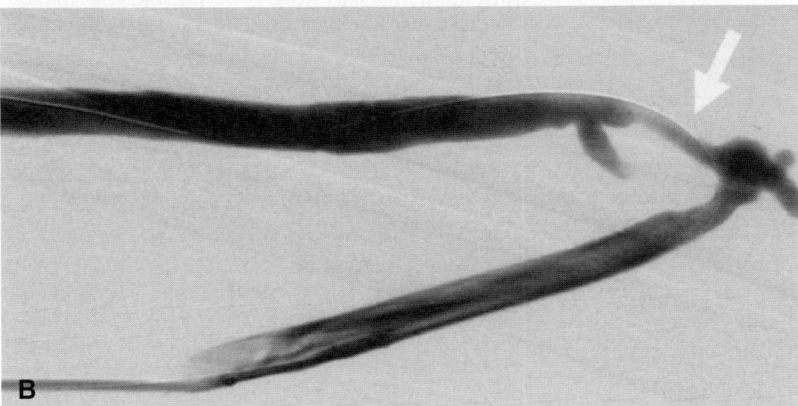

Figure 6–25 An upper extremity CT angiogram (16 mm x 1.25 mm collimation) is performed to evaluate a brachial-cephalic forearm hemodialysis graft. **A.** A volume-rendred image reveals moderate stenosis of the cephalic vein immediately distal to the anastomosis (*arrow*). **B.** Findings are confirmed at the time of angioplasty (*arrow*). Diagnostic catheter venography of the remainder of the peripheral and central veins was not required as these territories were patent on the venous phase of the MDCT angiogram (*not shown*).

occlusive disease; vasculitis; dissection; failing hemodialysis arteriovenous fistulae and grafts (Figure 6–25) (244); trauma (231); vascular masses including aneurysms, pseudoaneurysms, arteriovenous malformations, and hemangiomas; bypass graft patency; and venous occlusive disease. It is also an effective modality for endovascular and surgical treatment planning (230,243). Although complete evaluation of a suspected vasculitis may require intra-arterial vasodilator challenge (245), in our experience, CTA has been beneficial for two important reasons. One is that inflammation within the vessel wall is visualized directly. The other benefit is that when patients with known vasculitis have worsening symptoms, superimposed disease can be excluded noninvasively.

Patients are positioned supine or prone, head-first, with the affected extremity extended above the head. To position the extremity as close to the gantry isocenter as possible, patients may be rotated into a modified swimmer's position. When patients cannot raise the affected extremity, scanning with the extremity next to their side is acceptable, with the risk of increased noise and streak artifacts. Bilateral exams are acquired by scanning both arms together or by scanning each arm individually (16- to 64-channel scanners). Functional CTA can be performed for thoracic outlet syndrome, by imaging first in a neutral position then in a position that duplicates Wright's and Adson's provocative maneuvers.

Routine, complete coverage includes scanning from the aortic arch through to the fingers, yielding a range of approximately 800–1,000 mm. Depending on the clinical indication, scan coverage may be targeted to the region of interest. High-resolution datasets are sufficient for most studies. If acquired on a 4-channel system and required coverage is complete, 2.5 mm detector width collimation may be necessary so that the entire volume is scanned in a reasonable duration. Despite the increased noise and increased number of images, isotropic resolution datasets on 16- to 64-channel systems provide greater detail of small vessels, offering benefit in assessment of vasculitis and pediatric patients.

Extrapolating from lower extremity CTA data (233), to achieve optimal upper extremity arterial enhancement from the aortic arch down to the fingers, the injection duration should be at least 30 seconds, and a biphasic injection protocol should be used, followed by saline flush. *t*CMT is determined with an ROI placed at the transverse aorta. For scan durations >30, the injection duration equals the scan duration plus additional delay if automated triggering is used. For scan durations <30 seconds, a diagnostic delay is added to the beginning of the acquisition, such that the scan duration and injection duration are completed simultaneously. Upper extremity venography is acquired at 60 seconds following initiation of contrast administration. Alternatively, as in studies for treatment planning and assessment of dysfunctioning hemodialysis access, a single acquisition can be obtained and synchronized to the recirculation phase.

Regarding upper extremity MDCTA performance, accurate diagnoses can be made with high interobserver agreement (246). In a retrospective review of 200 vascular segments, of which 39 segments were abnormal based on conventional angiography with either stenoses, occlusions, aneurysms, or dissections, our group found upper extremity MDCT angiography to be 100% sensitive, 98.8% specific, and 99% accurate. For 293 upper extremity vascular segments imaged with MDCTA, excellent interobserver agreement was achieved (Kappa = 0.94) (246).

SUMMARY

The drive for reliable and efficient, less invasive diagnostic imaging has led to rapid technological advancements in spiral computed tomography. At the cornerstone of these developments is multidetector row computed tomography. While each of the body systems has benefited, the most dramatic and exciting application has been CT angiography for the cardiovascular system. Pulmonary, aortic, cerebral, mesenteric, renal, and peripheral vascular territories now are able to be evaluated with robust image quality and high accuracy such that catheter angiography for these vascular territories and their respective diagnostic clinical algorithms are nearly obsolete. Cardiac MDCT has also shown its strength in a very short time. The great promise for widespread use of cardiac MDCT, however, will shine over the next few years during which time there will be growth in clinical volume on the 32- to 64-channel scanners. Continued improvement in image quality, acquisition speed, and cardiac synchronization certainly will aid this transformation. To incorporate MDCTA into daily practice, it is fundamental for the cardiovascular imager and interventionalist to know its strengths and weaknesses, specific to the cardiovascular territories and patients. For the imager, it is equally important to have a sound understanding of MDCTA technical principles. These include principles of scan acquisition, contrast-medium administration, and image display. Combined with the knowledge of cardiovascular anatomy, disease, image findings, and therapy, the cardiovascular imager can play a significant role in strengthening a modern cardiovascular clinical practice.

REFERENCES

1. Kalender WA, Seissler W, Klotz E, et al. Spiral volumetric CT with single-breath-hold technique, continuous transport, and continuous scanner rotation. Radiology 1990;176(1):181–183.
2. Remy-Jardin M, Remy J, Wattinne L, et al. Central pulmonary thromboembolism: diagnosis with spiral volumetric CT with the single-breath-hold technique—comparison with pulmonary angiography. Radiology 1992;185(2):381–387.
3. Rubin GD, Dake MD, Napel SA, et al. Three-dimensional spiral CT angiography of the abdomen: initial clinical experience. Radiology 1993;186(1):147–152.
4. Schwartz RB, Jones KM, Chernoff DM, et al. Common carotid artery bifurcation: evaluation with spiral CT. Work in progress. Radiology 1992;185(2):513–519.
5. Galanski M, Prokop M, Chavan A, et al. Renal arterial stenoses: spiral CT angiography. Radiology 1993;189(1):185–192.
6. Goodman LR, Curtin JJ, Mewissen MW, et al. Detection of pulmonary embolism in patients with unresolved clinical and scintigraphic diagnosis: helical CT versus angiography. AJR Am J Roentgenol 1995;164(6):1369–1374.
7. Rubin GD, Dake MD, Napel S, et al. Spiral CT of renal artery stenosis: comparison of three-dimensional rendering techniques. Radiology 1994;190(1):181–189.
8. Raptopoulos V, Rosen MP, Kent KC, et al. Sequential helical CT angiography of aortoiliac disease. AJR Am J Roentgenol 1996;166(6):1347–1354.
9. Rubin GD, Shiau MC, Schmidt AJ, et al. Computed tomographic angiography: historical perspective and new state-of-the-art using multi detector-row helical computed tomography. J Comput Assist Tomogr 1999;23(Suppl I):S83–S90.
10. Rubin GD, Shiau MC, Leung AN, et al. Aorta and iliac arteries: single versus multiple detector-row helical CT angiography. Radiology 2000;215(3):670–676.
11. Fleischmann D, Rubin GD, Paik DS, et al. Stair-step artifacts with single versus multiple detector-row helical CT. Radiology 2000;216(1):185–196.
12. Brink JA, Lim JT, Wang G, et al. Technical optimization of spiral CT for depiction of renal artery stenosis: in vitro analysis. Radiology 1995;194(1):157–163.
13. Davros WJ, Obuchowski NA, Berman PM, et al. A phantom study: evaluation of renal artery stenosis using helical CT and 3D reconstructions. J Comput Assist Tomogr 1997;21(1):156–161.
14. Kuszyk BS, Heath DG, Johnson PT, et al. CT angiography with volume rendering for quantifying vascular stenoses: in vitro validation of accuracy. AJR Am J Roentgenol 1999;173(2):449–455.
15. Flohr T, Prokop M, Becker C, et al. A retrospectively ECG-gated multislice spiral CT scan and reconstruction technique with suppression of heart pulsation artifacts for cardiothoracic imaging with extended volume coverage. Eur Radiol 2002;12(6):1497–1503.
16. Sato Y, Matsumoto N, Kato M, et al. Noninvasive assessment of coronary artery disease by multislice spiral computed tomography using a new retrospectively ECG-gated image reconstruction technique. Circ J 2003;67(5):401–405.
17. Morin RL Gerber TC, McCollough CH. Radiation dose in computed tomography of the heart. Circulation 2003;107:917–922.
18. Saito K, Saito M, Komatu S, et al. Real-time four-dimensional imaging of the heart with multidetector-row CT. Radiographics 2003;23(1):E8–E8.
19. Bae KT, Heiken JP, Brink JA. Aortic and hepatic peak enhancement at CT: effect of contrast medium injection rate—pharmacokinetic analysis and experimental porcine model. Radiology 1998;206(2):455–464.
20. Bae KT, Tran HQ, Heiken JP. Multiphasic injection method for uniform prolonged vascular enhancement at CT angiography: pharmacokinetic analysis and experimental porcine model. Radiology 2000;216(3):872–880.
21. Fleischmann D, Rubin GD, Bankier AA, et al. Improved uniformity of aortic enhancement with customized contrast medium injection protocols at CT angiography. Radiology 2000;214(2):363–371.
22. Heiken JP, Brink JA, McClennan BL, et al. Dynamic contrast-enhanced CT of the liver: comparison of contrast medium injection rates and uniphasic and biphasic injection protocols. Radiology 1993;187(2):327–331.
23. Fleischmann D. Use of high-concentration contrast media in multiple-detector-row CT: principles and rationale. Eur Radiol 2003;13(Suppl V):M14–M20.
24. Herman S. Computed tomography contrast enhancement principles and the use of high-concentration contrast media. J Comput Assist Tomogr 2004;28(Suppl I):S7–S11.
25. Brink JA, Heiken JP, Forman HP, et al. Hepatic spiral CT: reduction of dose of intravenous contrast material. Radiology 1995;197(1):83–88.
26. Yamashita Y, Komohara Y, Takahashi M, et al. Abdominal helical CT: evaluation of optimal doses of intravenous contrast material—a prospective randomized study. Radiology 2000;216(3):718–723.

27. Heiken JP, Brink JA, McClennan BL, et al. Dynamic incremental CT: effect of volume and concentration of contrast material and patient weight on hepatic enhancement. Radiology 1995; 195(2):353–357.

28. Awai K, Hiraishi K, Hori S. Effect of contrast material injection duration and rate on aortic peak time and peak enhancement at dynamic CT involving injection protocol with dose tailored to patient weight. Radiology 2004;230(1):142–150.

29. Kim T, Murakami T, Takahashi S, et al. Pancreatic CT imaging: effects of different injection rates and doses of contrast material. Radiology 1999;212(1):219–225.

30. Kim T, Murakami T, Takahashi S, et al. Effects of injection rates of contrast material on arterial phase hepatic CT. AJR Am J Roentgenol 1998;171(2):429–432.

31. Mitsuzaki K, Yamashita Y, Ogata I, et al. Multiple-phase helical CT of the liver for detecting small hepatomas in patients with liver cirrhosis: contrast-injection protocol and optimal timing. AJR Am J Roentgenol 1996;167(3):753–757.

32. Bae KT, Heiken JP, Brink JA. Aortic and hepatic contrast medium enhancement at CT. Part II. Effect of reduced cardiac output in a porcine model. Radiology 1998;207(3):657–662.

33. Dawson P, Blomley MJ. Contrast media as extracellular fluid space markers: adaptation of the central volume theorem. Br J Radiol 1996;69(824):717–722.

34. Birnbaum BA, Nelson RC, Chezmar JL, et al. Extravasation detection accessory: clinical evaluation in 500 patients. Radiology 1999;212(2):431–438.

35. Powell CC, Li JM, Rodino L, et al. A new device to limit extravasation during contrast-enhanced CT. AJR Am J Roentgenol 2000;174(2):315–318.

36. Haage P, Schmitz-Rode T, Hubner D, et al. Reduction of contrast material dose and artifacts by a saline flush using a double power injector in helical CT of the thorax. AJR Am J Roentgenol 2000;174(4):1049–1053.

37. Cademartiri F, Mollet N, van der Lugt A, et al. Noninvasive 16-row multislice CT coronary angiography: usefulness of saline chaser. Eur Radiol 2004;14(2):178–183.

38. Schoellnast H, Tillich M, Deutschmann HA, et al. Abdominal multidetector row computed tomography: reduction of cost and contrast material dose using saline flush. J Comput Assist Tomogr 2003;27(6):847–853.

39. Rubin GD. 3D imaging with MDCT. Eur J Radiol 2003;45 (Suppl I):S37–S41.

40. Raman R, Napel S, Beaulieu CF, et al. Automated generation of curved planar reformations from volume data: method and evaluation. Radiology 2002;223(1):275–280.

41. Addis KA, Hopper KD, Iyriboz TA, et al. CT angiography: in vitro comparison of five reconstruction methods. AJR Am J Roentgenol 2001;177(5):1171–1176.

42. Rubin GD, Beaulieu CF, Argiro V, et al. Perspective volume rendering of CT and MR images: applications for endoscopic imaging. Radiology 1996;199(2):321–330.

43. Tandri H, Bomma C, Calkins H, et al. Magnetic resonance and computed tomography imaging of arrhythmogenic right ventricular dysplasia. J Magn Reson Imaging 2004;19(6):848–858.

44. Leber AW, Knez A, Becker A, et al. Accuracy of multidetector spiral computed tomography in identifying and differentiating the composition of coronary atherosclerotic plaques: a comparative study with intracoronary ultrasound. J Am Coll Cardiol 2004; 43(7):1241–1247.

45. Nikolaou K, Sagmeister S, Knez A, et al. Multidetector row computed tomography of the coronary arteries: predictive value and quantitative assessment of noncalcified vessel wall changes. Eur Radiol 2003;13:2502–2512.

46. Schroeder S, Kopp AF, Baumbach A, et al. Noninvasive detection and evaluation of atherosclerotic coronary plaques with multi-slice computed tomography. J Am Coll Cardiol 2001;37(5): 1430–1435.

47. Schroeder S, Kuettner A, Leitritz M, et al. Reliability of differentiating human coronary plaque morphology using contrast-enhanced multislice spiral computed tomography: a comparison with histology. J Comput Assist Tomogr 2004;28(4):449–454.

48. Achenbach S, Ropers D, Hoffmann U, et al. Assessment of coronary remodeling in stenotic and nonstenotic coronary atherosclerotic lesions by multidetector spiral computed tomography. J Am Coll Cardiol 2004;43(5):842–847.

49. Koyama Y, Mochizuki T, Higaki J. Computed tomography assessment of myocardial perfusion, viability, and function. J Magn Reson Imaging 2004;19(6):800–815.

50. Hoffmann U, Millea R, Enzweiler C, et al. Acute myocardial infarction: contrast-enhanced multidetector row CT in a porcine model. Radiology 2004;231(3):697–701.

51. Nikolaou K, Knez A, Sagmeister S, et al. Assessment of myocardial infarctions using multidetector row computed tomography. J Comput Assist Tomogr 2004;28(2):286–292.

52. Horiguchi J, Yamamoto H, Akiyama Y, et al. Coronary artery calcium scoring using 16-MDCT and a retrospective ECG-gating reconstruction algorithm. AJR Am J Roentgenol 2004;183(1): 103–108.

53. Lawler LP, Horton KM, Scatargie JC, et al. Coronary artery calcification scoring by prospectively triggered multidetector row computed tomography: is it reproducible? J Comput Assist Tomogr 2004;28:40–45.

54. Stanford W, Thompson BH, Burns TL, et al. Coronary artery calcium quantification at multidetector-row helical CT versus electron-beam CT. Radiology 2004;230(2):397–402.

55. Kopp AF, Ohnesorge B, Becker C, et al. Reproducibility and accuracy of coronary calcium measurements with multidetector-row versus electron-beam CT. Radiology 2002;225(1):113–119.

56. Stary HC, Chandler AB, Dinsmore RE, et al. A definition of advanced types of atherosclerotic lesions and a histological classification of atherosclerosis. A report from the Committee on Vascular Lesions of the Council on Arteriosclerosis, American Heart Association. Circulation 1995;92(5):1355–1374.

57. Wexler L, Brundage B, Crouse J, et al. Coronary artery calcification: pathophysiology, epidemiology, imaging methods, and clinical implications. A statement for health professionals from the American Heart Association. Writing Group. Circulation 1996;94(5):1175–1192.

58. Arad Y, Spadaro LA, Goodman K, et al. Prediction of coronary events with electron beam computed tomography. J Am Coll Cardiol 2000;36(4):1253–1260.

59. Budoff MJ, Georgiou D, Brody A, et al. Ultra-fast computed tomography as a diagnostic modality in the detection of coronary artery disease: a multicenter study. Circulation 1996;93(5): 898–904.

60. Keelan PC, Bielak LF, Ashai K, et al. Long-term prognostic value of coronary calcification detected by electron-beam computed tomography in patients undergoing coronary angiography. Circulation 2001;104(4):412–417.

61. Shemesh J, Koren-Morag N, Apter S, et al. Accelerated progression of coronary calcification: four-year follow-up in patients with stable coronary artery disease. Radiology 2004;233:201–209.

62. Carr JJ, Nelson JC, Wong ND, et al. Calcified coronary artery plaque measurement with cardiac CT in population-based studies: standardized protocol of multiethnic study of atherosclerosis (MESA) and coronary artery risk development in young adults (CARDIA) study. Radiology 2005;234(1):35–43.

63. Herzog C, Britten M, Balzer JO, et al. Multidetector row cardiac CT: diagnostic value of calcium scoring and CT coronary angiography in patients with symptomatic, but atypical, chest pain. Eur Radiol 2004;14(2):169–177.

64. Becker CR, Hong C, Knez A, et al. Optimal contrast application for cardiac 4-detector row computed tomography. Invest Radiol 2003;38(11):690–694.

65. Choi HS, Choi BW, Choe KO, et al. Pitfalls, artifacts, and remedies in multidetector row CT coronary angiography. Radiographics 2004;24(3):787–800.

66. Giesler T, Baum U, Ropers D, et al. Noninvasive visualization of coronary arteries using contrast-enhanced multidetector CT: influence of heart rate on image quality and stenosis detection. AJR Am J Roentgenol 2002;179(4):911–916.

67. Nieman K RB, van Geuns RJM, Pattynama PMT, et al. Noninvasive coronary angiography with multislice spiral computed tomography: impact of heart rate. Heart 2002;88:470–474.

68. Vogl TJ, Abolmaali ND, Diebold T, et al. Techniques for the detection of coronary atherosclerosis: multidetector row CT coronary angiography. Radiology 2002;223(1):212–220.

69. Achenbach S, Giesler T, Ropers D, et al. Detection of coronary artery stenoses by contrast-enhanced, retrospectively electrocardiographically-gated, multislice spiral computed tomography. Circulation 2001;103(21):2535–2538.

70. Nieman K, Oudkerk M, Rensing BJ, et al. Coronary angiography with multislice computed tomography. Lancet 2001;357(9256): 599–603.

71. Kopp AF, Schroeder S, Kuettner A, et al. Noninvasive coronary angiography with high resolution multidetector row computed tomography. Results in 102 patients. Eur Heart J 2002;23(21): 1714–1725.

72. Maruyama T, Yoshizumi T, Tamura R, et al. Comparison of visibility and diagnostic capability of noninvasive coronary angiography by eight-slice multidetector row computed tomography versus conventional coronary angiography. Am J Cardiol 2004; 93(5):537–542.

73. Schroeder S, Kopp AF, Kuettner A, et al. Influence of heart rate on vessel visibility in noninvasive coronary angiography using new multislice computed tomography: experience in 94 patients. Clin Imaging 2002;26(2):106–111.

74. Becker CR, Knez A, Leber A, et al. Detection of coronary artery stenoses with multislice helical CT angiography. J Comput Assist Tomogr 2002;26(5):750–755.

75. Knez A, Becker CR, Leber A, et al. Usefulness of multislice spiral computed tomography angiography for determination of coronary artery stenoses. Am J Cardiol 2001;88(10):1191–1194.

76. Gerber TC KR, Lane GE, et al. Image quality in a standardized algorithm for minimally invasive coronary angiography with multislice spiral computed tomography. J Comput Assist Tomogr 2003;27(1):62–69.

77. Mollet NR, Cademartiri F, Nieman K, et al. Multislice spiral computed tomography coronary angiography in patients with stable angina pectoris. J Am Coll Cardiol 2004;43(12):2265–2270.

78. Nieman K, Cademartiri F, Lemos PA, et al. Reliable noninvasive coronary angiography with fast submillimeter multislice spiral computed tomography. Circulation 2002;106(16):2051–2054.

79. Ropers D, Baum U, Pohle K, et al. Detection of coronary artery stenoses with thin-slice multidetector row spiral computed tomography and multiplanar reconstruction. Circulation 2003; 107(5):664–666.

80. Kuettner A, Trabold T, Schroeder S, et al. Noninvasive detection of coronary lesions using 16-detector multislice spiral computed tomography technology: initial clinical results. J Am Coll Cardiol 2004;44(6):1230–1237.

81. Hoffmann MHK, Shi H, Manzke R, et al. Noninvasive coronary angiography with 16-detector row CT: effect of heart rate. Radiology 2005;234(1):86–97.

82. Nieman K, Pattynama PM, Rensing BJ, et al. Evaluation of patients after coronary artery bypass surgery: CT angiographic assessment of grafts and coronary arteries. Radiology 2003; 229(3):749–756.

83. Ropers D, Ulzheimer S, Wenkel E, et al. Investigation of aortocoronary artery bypass grafts by multislice spiral computed tomography with electrocardiographic-gated image reconstruction. Am J Cardiol 2001;88(7):792–795.

84. Marano R, Storto ML, Maddestra N, et al. Noninvasive assessment of coronary artery bypass graft with retrospectively ECG-gated four-row multidetector spiral computed tomography. Eur Radiol 2004;14(8):1353–1362.

85. Willmann JK, Weishaupt D, Kobza R, et al. Coronary artery bypass grafts: ECG-gated multidetector row CT angiography—influence of image reconstruction interval on graft visibility. Radiology 2004;232(2):568–577.

86. Hong C, Becker CR, Huber A, et al. ECG-gated reconstructed multidetector row CT coronary angiography: effect of varying trigger delay on image quality. Radiology 2001;220(3):712–717.

87. Kopp AF, Schroeder S, Kuettner A, et al. Coronary arteries: retrospectively ECG-gated multidetector row CT angiography with selective optimization of the image reconstruction window. Radiology 2001;221(3):683–688.

88. Kuettner A, Kopp AF, Schroeder S, et al. Diagnostic accuracy of multidetector computed tomography coronary angiography in patients with angiographically proven coronary artery disease. J Am Coll Cardiol 2004;43(5):831–839.

89. Hong C, Chrysant GS, Woodard PK, et al. Coronary artery stent patency assessed with in-stent contrast enhancement measured at multidetector row CT angiography: initial experience. Radiology 2004;233(1):286–291.

90. Willmann JK, Weishaupt D, Lachat M, et al. Electrocardiographically gated multidetector row CT for assessment of valvular morphology and calcification in aortic stenosis. Radiology 2002;225(1):120–128.

91. Willmann JK, Kobza R, Roos JE, et al. ECG-gated multidetector row CT for assessment of mitral valve disease:initial experience. Eur Radiol 2002;12(11):2662–2669.

92. Juergens KU, Grude M, Fallenberg EM, et al. Using ECG-gated multidetector CT to evaluate global left ventricular myocardial function in patients with coronary artery disease. AJR Am J Roentgenol 2002;179(6):1545–1550.

93. Grude M, Juergens KU, Wichter T, et al. Evaluation of global left ventricular myocardial function with electrocardiogram-gated multidetector computed tomography: comparison with magnetic resonance imaging. Invest Radiol 2003;38(10): 653–661.

94. Hellinger JC, Chan F, Napoli A, et al. Ventricular function and mass quantification with cardiac gated multidetector CT angiography: a valid substitute for MRI. AJR Am J Roentgenol 2004; 182(4):S39.

95. Juergens KU, Grude M, Maintz D, et al. Multidetector row CT of left ventricular function with dedicated analysis software versus MR imaging:initial experience. Radiology 2004;230(2):403–410.

96. Schoepf UJ, Costello P. CT angiography for diagnosis of pulmonary embolism: state of the art. Radiology 2004;230(2): 329–337.

97. Remy-Jardin M, Remy J, Deschildre F, et al. Diagnosis of pulmonary embolism with spiral CT: comparison with pulmonary angiography and scintigraphy. Radiology 1996;200(3):699–706.

98. van Rossum AB, Pattynama PM, Ton ER, et al. Pulmonary embolism: validation of spiral CT angiography in 149 patients. Radiology 1996;201(2):467–470.

99. Mayo JR, Remy-Jardin M, Muller NL, et al. Pulmonary embolism: prospective comparison of spiral CT with ventilation-perfusion scintigraphy. Radiology 1997;205(2):447–452.

100. Garg K, Welsh CH, Feyerabend AJ, et al. Pulmonary embolism: diagnosis with spiral CT and ventilation-perfusion scanning—correlation with pulmonary angiographic results or clinical outcome. Radiology 1998;208(1):201–208.

101. Drucker EA, Rivitz SM, Shepard JA, et al. Acute pulmonary embolism: assessment of helical CT for diagnosis. Radiology 1998;209(1):235–241.

102. Blachere H, Latrabe V, Montaudon M, et al. Pulmonary embolism revealed on helical CT angiography: comparison with ventilation-perfusion radionuclide lung scanning. AJR Am J Roentgenol 2000;174(4):1041–1047.

103. Ghaye B, Szapiro D, Mastora I, et al. Peripheral pulmonary arteries: how far in the lung does multidetector row spiral CT allow analysis? Radiology 2001;219(3):629–636.

104. Patel S, Kazerooni EA, Cascade PN. Pulmonary embolism: optimization of small pulmonary artery visualization at multidetector row CT. Radiology 2003;227(2):455–460.

105. Raptopoulos V, Boiselle PM. Multidetector row spiral CT pulmonary angiography: comparison with single-detector row spiral CT. Radiology 2001;221(3):606–613.

106. Remy-Jardin M, Tillie-Leblond I, Szapiro D, et al. CT angiography of pulmonary embolism in patients with underlying respiratory disease: impact of multislice CT on image quality and negative predictive value. Eur Radiol 2002;12(8):1971–1978.

107. Schoepf UJ, Holzknecht N, Helmberger TK, et al. Subsegmental pulmonary emboli: improved detection with thin-collimation multidetector row spiral CT. Radiology 2002;222(2):483–490.

108. Coche E, Verschuren F, Keyeux A, et al. Diagnosis of acute pulmonary embolism in outpatients: comparison of thin-collimation multidetector row spiral CT and planar ventilation-perfusion scintigraphy. Radiology 2003;229(3):757–765.

109. Winer-Muram HT, Rydberg J, Johnson MS, et al. Suspected acute pulmonary embolism: evaluation with multidetector row CT versus digital subtraction pulmonary arteriography. Radiology 2004;223:806–815.

110. Cham MD, Yankelevitz DF, Shaham D, et al. Deep venous thrombosis: detection by using indirect CT venography. The Pulmonary Angiography-Indirect CT Venography Cooperative Group. Radiology 2000;216(3):744–751.

111. Coche EE, Hamoir XL, Hammer FD, et al. Using dual-detector helical CT angiography to detect deep venous thrombosis in patients with suspicion of pulmonary embolism: diagnostic value and additional findings. AJR Am J Roentgenol 2001;176(4): 1035–1039.

112. Loud PA, Katz DS, Bruce DA, et al. Deep venous thrombosis with suspected pulmonary embolism: detection with combined CT venography and pulmonary angiography. Radiology 2001;219(2): 498–502.

113. Walsh G, Redmond S. Does addition of CT pelvic venography to CT pulmonary angiography protocols contribute to the diagnosis of thromboembolic disease? Clin Radiol 2002;57(6): 462–465.

114. Hellinger JC, Napoli A, Fleischmann D, et al. Multidetector row CT assessment of thromboembolic disease: incremental value of CT venography in 1240 consecutive exams (Abstract). Radiologic Society of North America 2003.

115. Kim TH, Kim YM, Suh CH, et al. Helical CT angiography and three-dimensional reconstruction of total anomalous pulmonary venous connections in neonates and infants. AJR Am J Roentgenol 2000;175(5):1381–1386.

116. Marom EM, Herndon JE, Kim YH, et al. Variations in pulmonary venous drainage to the left atrium: implications for radiofrequency ablation. Radiology 2004;230(3):824–829.

117. Cronin P, Sneider MB, Kazerooni EA, et al. MDCT of the left atrium and pulmonary veins in planning radiofrequency ablation for atrial fibrillation: a how-to guide. AJR Am J Roentgenol 2004;183(3):767–778.

118. Ravenel JG, McAdams HP. Pulmonary venous infarction after radiofrequency ablation for atrial fibrillation. AJR Am J Roentgenol 2002;178(3):664–666.

119. Funabashi N, Yonezawa M, Iesaka Y, et al. Complications of pulmonary vein isolation by catheter ablation evaluated by ECG-gated multislice computed tomography. Heart Vessels 2003; 18(4):220–223.

120. Rubin GD. CT angiography of the thoracic aorta. Semin Roentgenol 2003;38(2):115–134.

121. Lee WA, Rubin GD, Johnson BL, et al. "Pseudoendoleak"—residual intrasaccular contrast after endovascular stent-graft repair. J Endovasc Ther 2002;9(1):119–123.

122. Golzarian J, Dussaussois L, Abada HT, et al. Helical CT of aorta after endoluminal stent-graft therapy: value of biphasic acquisition. AJR Am J Roentgenol 1998;171(2):329–331.

123. Batra P, Bigoni B, Manning J, et al. Pitfalls in the diagnosis of thoracic aortic dissection at CT angiography. Radiographics 2000;20(2):309–320.

124. Morgan-Hughes GJ, Owens PE, Marshall AJ, et al. Thoracic aorta at multidetector row CT: motion artifact with various reconstruction windows. Radiology 2003;228(2):583–588.

125. Roos JE, Willmann JK, Weishaupt D, et al. Thoracic aorta: motion artifact reduction with retrospective and prospective electrocardiography-assisted multidetector row CT. Radiology 2002;222(1):271–277.

126. Yoshioka K, Niinuma H, Ohira A, et al. MR angiography and CT angiography of the artery of Adamkiewicz: noninvasive preoperative assessment of thoracoabdominal aortic aneurysm. Radiographics 2003;23(5):1215–1225.

127. Remy-Jardin M, Bouaziz N, Dumont P, et al. Bronchial and non-bronchial systemic arteries at multidetector row CT angiography: comparison with conventional angiography. Radiology 2004; 233:741–749.

128. Wolf YG, Tillich M, Lee WA, et al. Impact of aortoiliac tortuosity on endovascular repair of abdominal aortic aneurysms: evaluation of 3D computer-based assessment. J Vasc Surg 2001;34(4): 594–599.

129. Dunham MB, Zygun D, Petrasek P, et al. Endovascular stent grafts for acute blunt aortic injury. J Trauma 2004;56(6):1173–1178.

130. Czermak BV, Waldenberger P, Fraedrich G, et al. Treatment of Stanford type B aortic dissection with stent-grafts: preliminary results. Radiology 2000;217(2):544–550.

131. Czermak BV, Waldenberger P, Perkmann R, et al. Placement of endovascular stent grafts for emergency treatment of acute disease of the descending thoracic aorta. AJR Am J Roentgenol 2002;179(2):337–345.

132. Fattori R, Napoli G, Lovato L, et al. Descending thoracic aortic diseases: stent-graft repair. Radiology 2003;229(1):176–183.

133. Schoder M, Grabenwoger M, Holzenbein T, et al. Endovascular stent-graft repair of complicated penetrating atherosclerotic ulcers of the descending thoracic aorta. J Vasc Surg 2002; 36(4):720–726.

134. Demers P, Miller DC, Mitchell RS, et al. Stent-graft repair of penetrating atherosclerotic ulcers in the descending thoracic aorta: midterm results. Ann Thorac Surg 2004;77(1):81–86.

135. Rubin GD, Paik DS, Johnston PC, et al. Measurement of the aorta and its branches with helical CT. Radiology 1998;206(3): 823–829.

136. Tillich M, Hill BB, Paik DS, et al. Prediction of aortoiliac stent-graft length: comparison of measurement methods. Radiology 2001;220(2):475–483.

137. Choi SH, Choi SJ, Kim JH, et al. Useful CT findings for predicting the progression of aortic intramural hematoma to overt aortic dissection. J Comput Assist Tomogr 2001;25(2):295–299.

138. Dyer DS, Moore EE, Mestek MF, et al. Can chest CT be used to exclude aortic injury? Radiology 1999;213(1):195–202.

139. Kazerooni EA, Bree RL, Williams DM. Penetrating atherosclerotic ulcers of the descending thoracic aorta: evaluation with CT and distinction from aortic dissection. Radiology 1992;183(3): 759–765.

140. Parker MS, Matheson TL, Rao AV, et al. Making the transition: the role of helical CT in the evaluation of potentially acute thoracic aortic injuries. AJR Am J Roentgenol 2001;176(5):1267–1272.

141. Quint LE, Francis IR, Williams DM, et al. Evaluation of thoracic aortic disease with the use of helical CT and multiplanar reconstructions: comparison with surgical findings. Radiology 1996; 201(1):37–41.

142. Sebastia C, Pallisa E, Quiroga S, et al. Aortic dissection: diagnosis and follow-up with helical CT. Radiographics 1999;19(1): 45–60;quiz 149–150.

143. Sueyoshi E, Matsuoka Y, Imada T, et al. New development of an ulcerlike projection in aortic intramural hematoma: CT evaluation. Radiology 2002;224(2):536–541.

144. Wong H, Gotway MB, Sasson AD, et al. Periaortic hematoma at diaphragmatic crura at helical CT: sign of blunt aortic injury in patients with mediastinal hematoma. Radiology 2004;231(1): 185–189.

145. Yoshida S, Akiba H, Tamakawa M, et al. Thoracic involvement of type A aortic dissection and intramural hematoma: diagnostic accuracy—comparison of emergency helical CT and surgical findings. Radiology 2003;228(2):430–435.

146. Hayashi H, Matsuoka Y, Sakamoto I, et al. Penetrating atherosclerotic ulcer of the aorta: imaging features and disease concept. Radiographics 2000;20(4):995–1005.

147. Wolf YG, Tillich M, Lee WA, et al. Changes in aneurysm volume after endovascular repair of abdominal aortic aneurysm. J Vasc Surg 2002;36(2):305–309.

148. Harris JR, Fan CM, Geller SC, et al. Renal perfusion defects after endovascular repair of abdominal aortic aneurysms. J Vasc Interv Radiol 2003;14(3):329–333.

149. White GH, May J, Waugh RC, et al. Type III and type IV endoleak: toward a complete definition of blood flow in the sac after endoluminal AAA repair. J Endovasc Surg 1998;5(4):305–309.

150. Veith FJ, Baum RA, Ohki T, et al. Nature and significance of endoleaks and endotension: summary of opinions expressed at an international conference. J Vasc Surg 2002;35:1029–1035.

151. Baum RA, Carpenter JP, Cope C, et al. Aneurysm sac pressure measurements after endovascular repair of abdominal aortic aneurysms. J Vasc Surg 2001;33(1):32–41.

152. Napoli V, Bargellini I, Sardella SG, et al. Abdominal aortic aneurysm: contrast-enhanced US for missed endoleaks after endoluminal repair. Radiology 2004;233(1):217–225.

153. Cejna M, Loewe C, Schoder M, et al. MR angiography versus CT angiography in the follow-up of nitinol stent grafts in the endoluminally treated aortic aneurysms. Eur Radiology 2002;12: 2443–2450.

154. Hellinger JC, Draney M, Markl M, et al. Application of cine phase contrast magnetic resonance imaging and SPAMM-tagging for assessment of endoleaks and aneurysm sac motion (Abstract). Radiologic Society of North America 2003.

155. Klingebiel R, Zimmer C, Rogalla P, et al. Assessment of the arteriovenous cerebrovascular system by multislice CT. A single-bolus, monophasic protocol. Acta Radiol 2001;42(6):560–562.

156. Leclerc X, Gauvrit JY, Pruvo JP. Usefulness of CT angiography with volume rendering after carotid angioplasty and stenting. AJR Am J Roentgenol 2000;174(3):820–822.

157. Munera F, Soto JA, Palacio D, et al. Diagnosis of arterial injuries caused by penetrating trauma to the neck: comparison of helical CT angiography and conventional angiography. Radiology 2000; 216(2):356–362.

158. Munera F, Soto JA, Palacio DM, et al. Penetrating neck injuries: helical CT angiography for initial evaluation. Radiology 2002; 224(2):366–372.

159. Chen CJ, Tseng YC, Lee TH, et al. Multisection CT angiography compared with catheter angiography in diagnosing vertebral artery dissection. AJNR Am J Neuroradiol 2004;25(5):769–774.

160. Leclerc X, Godefroy O, Salhi A, et al. Helical CT for the diagnosis of extracranial internal carotid artery dissection. Stroke 1996; 27(3):461–466.

161. Leclerc X, Lucas C, Godefroy O, et al. Helical CT for the follow-up of cervical internal carotid artery dissections. AJNR Am J Neuroradiol 1998;19(5):831–837.

162. Collaborators NASCET. Beneficial effect of carotid endarterectomy in symptomatic patients with high-grade carotid stenosis. N Engl J Med 1991;325(7):445–453.

163. Berg MH, Manninen HI, Rasanen HT, et al. CT angiography in the assessment of carotid artery atherosclerosis. Acta Radiol 2002;43(2):116–124.

164. Oliver TB, Lammie GA, Wright AR, et al. Atherosclerotic plaque at the carotid bifurcation: CT angiographic appearance with histopathologic correlation. AJNR Am J Neuroradiol 1999; 20(5):897–901.

165. Marks MP, Napel S, Jordan JE, et al. Diagnosis of carotid artery disease: preliminary experience with maximum-intensity-projection spiral CT angiography. AJR Am J Roentgenol 1993;160(6): 1267–1271.

166. Leclerc X, Godefroy O, Pruvo JP, et al. Computed tomographic angiography for the evaluation of carotid artery stenosis. Stroke 1995;26(9):1577–1581.

167. Link J, Brossmann J, Penselin V, et al. Common carotid artery bifurcation: preliminary results of CT angiography and color-coded duplex sonography compared with digital subtraction angiography. AJR Am J Roentgenol 1997;168(2):361–365.

168. Magarelli N, Scarabino T, Simeone AL, et al. Carotid stenosis: a comparison between MR and spiral CT angiography. Neuroradiology 1998;40(6):367–373.

169. Leclerc X, Godefroy O, Lucas C, et al. Internal carotid arterial stenosis: CT angiography with volume rendering. Radiology 1999;210(3):673–682.

170. Marcus CD, Ladam-Marcus VJ, Bigot JL, et al. Carotid arterial stenosis: evaluation at CT angiography with the volume-rendering technique. Radiology 1999;211(3):775–780.

171. Sameshima T, Futami S, Morita Y, et al. Clinical usefulness of and problems with three-dimensional CT angiography for the evaluation of arteriosclerotic stenosis of the carotid artery: comparison with conventional angiography, MRA, and ultrasound sonography. Surg Neurol 1999;51(3):301–308;discussion 308–309.

172. Randoux B, Marro B, Koskas F, et al. Carotid artery stenosis: prospective comparison of CT, three-dimensional gadolinium-enhanced MR, and conventional angiography. Radiology 2001; 220(1):179–185.

173. Chen CJ, Lee TH, Hsu HL, et al. MultiSlice CT angiography in diagnosing total versus near occlusions of the internal carotid artery: comparison with catheter angiography. Stroke 2004;35(1):83–85.

174. Takagi R, Hayashi H, Kobayashi H, et al. Three-dimensional CT angiography of intracranial vasospasm following subarachnoid haemorrhage. Neuroradiology 1998;40(10):631–635.

175. Anderson GB, Ashforth R, Steinke DE, et al. CT angiography for the detection of cerebral vasospasm in patients with acute subarachnoid hemorrhage. AJNR Am J Neuroradiol 2000;21(6):1011–1015.

176. Wetzel SG, Kirsch E, Stock KW, et al. Cerebral veins: comparative study of CT venography with intra-arterial digital subtraction angiography. AJNR Am J Neuroradiol 1999;20(2):249–255.

177. Tsuchiya K, Aoki C, Katase S, et al. Visualization of extracranial-intracranial bypass using multidetector row helical computed tomography angiography. J Comput Assist Tomogr 2003;27(2): 231–234.

178. Schramm P, Schellinger PD, Klotz E, et al. Comparison of perfusion computed tomography and computed tomography angiography source images with perfusion-weighted imaging and diffusion-weighted imaging in patients with acute stroke of less than 6 hours' duration. Stroke 2004;35(7):1652–1658.

179. Tomandl BF, Klotz E, Handschu R, et al. Comprehensive imaging of ischemic stroke with multisection CT. Radiographics 2003; 23(3):565–592.

180. Nabavi DG, Kloska SP, Nam EM, et al. MOSAIC: Multimodal stroke assessment using computed tomography: novel diagnostic approach for the prediction of infarction size and clinical outcome. Stroke 2002;33(12):2819–2826.

181. Verro P, Tanenbaum LN, Borden NM, et al. CT angiography in acute ischemic stroke: preliminary results. Stroke 2002;33(1): 276–278.

182. Tanenbaum LN. CT of acute stroke in the clinical setting. Eur Radiol 2002;12(Suppl II):S25–S31.

183. Brandt T, Knauth M, Wildermuth S, et al. CT angiography and Doppler sonography for emergency assessment in acute basilar artery ischemia. Stroke 1999;30(3):606–612.

184. Knauth M, von Kummer R, Jansen O, et al. Potential of CT angiography in acute ischemic stroke. AJNR Am J Neuroradiol 1997;18(6):1001–1010.

185. Shrier DA, Tanaka H, Numaguchi Y, et al. CT angiography in the evaluation of acute stroke. AJNR Am J Neuroradiol 1997;18(6): 1011–1020.

186. Skutta B, Furst G, Eilers J, et al. Intracranial stenoocclusive disease: double-detector helical CT angiography versus digital subtraction angiography. AJNR Am J Neuroradiol 1999;20(5): 791–799.

187. Wildermuth S, Knauth M, Brandt T, et al. Role of CT angiography in patient selection for thrombolytic therapy in acute hemispheric stroke. Stroke 1998;29(5):935–938.

188. Dammert S, Krings T, Moller-Hartmann W, et al. Detection of intracranial aneurysms with multislice CT: comparison with conventional angiography. Neuroradiology 2004;46(6):427–434.

189. Jayaraman MV, Mayo-Smith WW, Tung GA, et al. Detection of intracranial aneurysms: multidetector row CT angiography compared with DSA. Radiology 2004;230(2):510–518.

190. Karamessini MT, Kagadis GC, Petsas T, et al. CT angiography with three-dimensional techniques for the early diagnosis of intracranial aneurysms. Comparison with intra-arterial DSA and the surgical findings. Eur J Radiol 2004;49(3):212–223.

191. White PM, Wardlaw JM, Easton V. Can noninvasive imaging accurately depict intracranial aneurysms? A systematic review. Radiology 2000;217(2):361–370.

192. Tew K, Davies RP, Jadun CK, et al. MDCT of acute lower gastrointestinal bleeding. AJR Am J Roentgenol 2004;182(2):427–430.

193. Horton KM, Eng J, Fishman EK. Normal enhancement of the small bowel: evaluation with spiral CT. J Comput Assist Tomogr 2000;24(1):67–71.

194. Horton KM, Fishman EK. Volume-rendered 3D CT of the mesenteric vasculature: normal anatomy, anatomic variants, and pathologic conditions. Radiographics 2002;22(1):161–172.

195. Foley WD, Mallisee TA, Hohenwalter MD, et al. Multiphase hepatic CT with a multirow detector CT scanner. AJR Am J Roentgenol 2000;175(3):679–685.

196. Stueckle CA, Haegele KF, Jendreck M, et al. Multislice computed tomography angiography of the abdominal arteries: comparison between computed tomography angiography and digital subtraction angiography findings in 52 cases. Australas Radiol 2004;48(2):142–147.

197. Kirkpatrick ID, Kroeker MA, Greenberg HM. Biphasic CT with mesenteric CT angiography in the evaluation of acute mesenteric ischemia: initial experience. Radiology 2003;229(1):91–98.

198. Kamel IR, Kruskal JB, Warmbrand G, et al. Accuracy of volumetric measurements after virtual right hepatectomy in potential donors undergoing living adult liver transplantation. AJR Am J Roentgenol 2001;176(2):483–487.

199. Napoli A, Catalano C, Silecchia G, et al. Laparoscopic splenectomy: multidetector row CT for preoperative evaluation. Radiology 2004;232(2):361–367.

200. Kamel IR, Kruskal JB, Pomfret EA, et al. Impact of multidetector CT on donor selection and surgical planning before living adult right lobe liver transplantation. AJR Am J Roentgenol 2001; 176(1):193–200.

201. Kapoor V, Brancatelli G, Federle MP, et al. Multidetector CT arteriography with volumetric three-dimensional rendering to evaluate patients with metastatic colorectal disease for placement of a floxuridine infusion pump. AJR Am J Roentgenol 2003; 181(2):455–463.

202. Sahani D, Saini S, Pena C, et al. Using multidetector CT for preoperative vascular evaluation of liver neoplasms: technique and results. AJR Am J Roentgenol 2002;179(1):53–59.

203. Zandrino F, Curone P, Benzi L, et al. Value of an early arteriographic acquisition for evaluating the splanchnic vessels as an adjunct to biphasic CT using a multislice scanner. Eur Radiol 2003;13(5):1072–1079.

204. Byun JH, Kim TK, Lee SS, et al. Evaluation of the hepatic artery in potential donors for living donor liver transplantation by computed tomography angiography using multidetector row computed tomography: comparison of volume rendering and maximum intensity projection techniques. J Comput Assist Tomogr 2003;27(2):125–131.

205. Erbay N, Raptopoulos V, Pomfret EA, et al. Living donor liver transplantation in adults: vascular variants important in surgical planning for donors and recipients. AJR Am J Roentgenol 2003;181(1):109–114.

206. Lee SS, Kim TK, Byun JH, et al. Hepatic arteries in potential donors for living related liver transplantation: evaluation with multidetector row CT angiography. Radiology 2003;227(2): 391–399.

207. Sahani DV, Krishnamurthy SK, Kalva S, et al. Multidetector row computed tomography angiography for planning intra-arterial chemotherapy pump placement in patients with colorectal metastases to the liver. J Comput Assist Tomogr 2004;28(4): 478–484.

208. Matsuki M, Kani H, Tatsugami F, et al. Preoperative assessment of vascular anatomy around the stomach by 3D imaging using MDCT before laparoscopy-assisted gastrectomy. AJR Am J Roentgenol 2004;183(1):145–151.

209. Raza SA, Chughtai AR, Wahba M, et al. Multislice CT angiography in renal artery stent evaluation: prospective comparison with intra-arterial digital subtraction angiography. Cardiovasc Intervent Radiol 2004;27(1):9–15.

210. Hofmann LV, Smith PA, Kuszyk BS, et al. Three-dimensional helical CT angiography in renal transplant recipients: a new problem-solving tool. AJR Am J Roentgenol 1999;173(4):1085–1089.

211. Beregi JP Mauroy B, Willoteaux S, et al. Anatomic variation in the origin of the main renal arteries: spiral CTA evaluation. Eur Radiol 1999;9(7):1330–1334.

212. Hellinger JC, Pezeshkmehr AH, Razavi R, et al. Designing renal artery protection devices: consideration of main renal artery anatomy. J Vasc Interv Radiol 2004;15(2):S159.

213. Hackstein N Cengiz H, Rau WS. Contrast media clearance in a single kidney measured on multiphasic helical CT: results in 50 patients without acute renal disorder. AJR Am J Roentgenol 2002;178(1):111–118.

214. Hackstein N, Wiegand C, Rau WS, et al. Glomerular filtration rate measured by using triphasic helical CT with a two-point Patlak plot technique. Radiology 2004;230(1):221–226.

215. Olin JW. Atherosclerotic renal artery disease. Cardiol Clin 2002; 20(4):547–562, vi.

216. Beregi JP, Elkohen M, Deklunder G, et al. Helical CT angiography compared with arteriography in the detection of renal artery stenosis. AJR Am J Roentgenol 1996;167(2):495–501.

217. Kim TS, Chung JW, Park JH, et al. Renal artery evaluation: comparison of spiral CT angiography to intra-arterial DSA. J Vasc Interv Radiol 1998;9(4):553–559.

218. Olbricht CJ, Paul K, Prokop M, et al. Minimally invasive diagnosis of renal artery stenosis by spiral computed tomography angiography. Kidney Int 1995;48(4):1332–1337.

219. Wittenberg G, Kenn W, Tschammler A, et al. Spiral CT angiography of renal arteries: comparison with angiography. Eur Radiol 1999;9(3):546–551.

220. Kaatee R, Beek FJ, de Lange EE, et al. Renal artery stenosis: detection and quantification with spiral CT angiography versus optimized digital subtraction angiography. Radiology 1997;205(1):121–127.

221. van Hoe L, Vandermeulen D, Gryspeerdt S, et al. Assessment of accuracy of renal artery stenosis grading in helical CT angiography using maximum intensity projections. Eur Radiol 1996; 6(5):658–664.

222. Willmann JK, Wildermuth S, Pfammatter T, et al. Aortoiliac and renal arteries: prospective intraindividual comparison of contrast-enhanced three-dimensional MR angiography and multidetector row CT angiography. Radiology 2003;226(3):798–811.

223. Johnson PT, Halpern EJ, Kuszyk BS, et al. Renal artery stenosis: CT angiography—comparison of real-time volume-rendering and maximum intensity projection algorithms. Radiology 1999; 211(2):337–343.

224. Mallouhi A, Rieger M, Czermak B, et al. Volume-rendered multidetector CT angiography: noninvasive follow-up of patients treated with renal artery stents. AJR Am J Roentgenol 2003; 180(1):233–239.

225. Mounier-Vehier C, Lions C, Devos P, et al. Cortical thickness: an early morphological marker of atherosclerotic renal disease. Kidney Int 2002;61(2):591–598.

226. Mounier-Vehier C, Lions C, Jaboureck O, et al. Parenchymal consequences of fibromuscular dysplasia renal artery stenosis. Am J Kidney Dis 2002;40(6):1138–1145.

227. Rubin GD, Alfrey EJ, Dake MD, et al. Assessment of living renal donors with spiral CT. Radiology 1995;195(2):457–462.

228. Kawamoto S, Montgomery RA, Lawler LP, et al. Multidetector CT angiography for preoperative evaluation of living laparoscopic kidney donors. AJR Am J Roentgenol 2003;180(6): 1633–1638.

229. Kim JK, Park SY, Kim HJ, et al. Living donor kidneys: usefulness of multidetector row CT for comprehensive evaluation. Radiology 2003;229:869–876.

230. Klein MB, Karanas YL, Chow LC, et al. Early experience with computed tomographic angiography in microsurgical reconstruction. Plast Reconstr Surg 2003;112(2):498–503.

231. Hellinger JC WE, Fleischman D, Rubin GD. Assessment for traumatic extremity vascular injury with multidetector row CT angiography: clinical experience in 35 exams. AJR Am J Roentgenol 2004;182(4):S79.

232. Soto JA, Munera F, Morales C, et al. Focal arterial injuries of the proximal extremities: helical CT arteriography as the initial method of diagnosis. Radiology 2001;218:188–194.

233. Fleischmann D, Koechl A, Lomoschitz E, et al. Aortopopliteal bolus transit times in peripheral CTA: can fast acquisitions outrun the bolus. Eur Radiol 2003;13.S268.

234. Catalano C, Fraioli F, Laghi A, et al. Infrarenal aortic and lower-extremity arterial disease: diagnostic performance of multidetector row CT angiography. Radiology 2004;231(2):555–563.

235. Martin ML, Tay KH, Flak B, et al. Multidetector CT angiography of the aortoiliac system and lower extremities: a prospective comparison with digital subtraction angiography. AJR 2003;180: 1085–1091.

236. Romano M, Mainenti PP, Imbriaco M, et al. Multidetector row CT angiography of the abdominal aorta and lower extremities in patients with peripheral arterial occlusive disease: diagnostic accuracy and interobserver agreement. Eur J Radiol 2004;50(3): 303–308.

237. Willmann JK, Mayer D, Banyai M, et al. Evaluation of peripheral arterial bypass grafts with multidetector row CT angiography: comparison with duplex US and digital subtraction angiography. Radiology 2003;229(2):465–474.

238. Napoli A, Rubin GD, Hellinger JC, et al. Multiple detector row CT angiography of peripheral arteries: diagnostic performance of 4-,8-, and 16-row CT scanners. European Radiology 2004;14 (Suppl II):303.

239. Rubin GD, Schmidt AJ, Logan LJ, et al. Multidetector row CT angiography of lower extremity arterial inflow and runoff: initial experience. Radiology 2001;221:146–158.

240. Ofer A, Nitecki SS, Linn S, et al. Multidetector CT angiography of peripheral vascular disease: a prospective comparison with intra-arterial digital subtraction angiography. AJR Am J Roentgenol 2003;180(3):719–724.

241. Ota H, Takase K, Igarashi K, et al. MDCT compared with digital subtraction angiography for assessment of lower extremity arterial occlusive disease: importance of reviewing cross-sectional images. AJR Am J Roentgenol 2004;182(1):201–209.

242. Portugaller HR, Schoellnast H, Hausegger KA, et al. Multislice spiral CT angiography in peripheral arterial occlusive disease: a valuable tool in detecting significant arterial lumen narrowing? Eur Radiol 2004;14(9):1681–1687.

243. Hellinger JC, Napoli A, Willamson E, et al. Upper extremity multidetector row CT angiography: clinical experience in 100 examinations (Abstract). Radiologic Society of North America 2004;SSK04–SSK03:510.

244. Hellinger JC, Frisoli J, Sze DYH, et al. Hemodialysis access evaluation: early experience with upper extremity multidector row CT angiography. J Vasc Interv Radiol 2004;15(2):S252.

245. Stoeckelhuber BM, Suttmann I, Stoeckelhuber M, et al. Comparison of the vasodilating effect of nitroglycerin, verapamil, and tolazoline in hand angiography. J Vasc Interv Radiol 2003;14(6):749–754.

246. Hellinger JC, Napoli A, Schraedley-Desmond P, et al. Multidetector row CT angiography of the upper extremity: comparison with digital subtraction angiography (Abstract). Radiologic Society of North America 2004;SSM04–SSM01: 569.

Magnetic Resonance Angiography

7

Frank J. Thornton, Thomas M. Grist

Clinical magnetic resonance angiography (MRA) has evolved to a point where it now challenges conventional angiography, which previously has been viewed as the gold standard for diagnosis of vascular disease. In many institutions, it is now the primary imaging modality for evaluation of central and peripheral vascular disease. Its rapid ascent in use is credited primarily to the significant advances in MR technology, which stem from the development of gadolinium contrast-enhanced techniques, or CE-MRA (1). The use of intravascular gadolinium chelates in conjunction with three-dimensional (3D) pulse sequences has revolutionized MRA by permitting rapid imaging without saturation effects or flow artifacts that limited previous techniques. Although CE-MRA is currently the core technique in the MRA armamentarium, many protocols still rely in part on noncontrast techniques. Using these strategies and some new emerging techniques, all relevant disease processes of the arteries can be fully depicted. This chapter describes current MRA imaging techniques and focuses on clinical situations in which MRA excels in providing core clinical information. Several new developments will be introduced that promise to improve spatial resolution, acquisition speed, and functional evaluation of vascular disease.

INTRODUCTION

The ubiquitous nature of peripheral vascular disease and the associated morbidity and mortality represent a significant burden on health services worldwide (2,3). The objective of modern clinical practice is to harness modern noninvasive imaging techniques that allow early detection of pathology so that preventative therapies or minimally invasive treatment can be instituted (4). MRA fulfills this role as a noninvasive method for evaluating vascular pathology in many anatomic territories (5). The large body coverage that can now be achieved with absence of ionizing radiation promotes MRA as an ideal imaging modality. Furthermore, gadolinium chelates, which are employed ubiquitously as T_1-shortening contrast agents in CE-MRA, are not nephrotoxic and are well tolerated by patients, making CE-MRA the preferred study for the many vasculopathic patients who suffer from renal insufficiency. The refinement of temporally resolved CE-MRA imaging is another significant realization. These innovations have led to a shift from noncontrast enhanced sequences to CE-MRA, which has less sensitivity to flow artifact and provides superior resolution. Many protocols, however, still employ noncontrast enhanced techniques that, for specific clinical questions, have inherent advantages over CE-MRA. Black-blood imaging provides excellent evaluation of the vessel wall anatomy, particularly when evaluating for intramural hematoma or dissection (6). Two-dimensional (2D) time-of-flight (TOF) imaging can be used as a backup in which CE-MRA images of below knee vessels are degraded by venous contamination (7,8). Steady state free precession (SSFP) provides excellent blood-tissue contrast with rapid evaluation of the major vessel anatomy. Phase contrast imaging is used to interrogate the flow dynamics of vessels, particularly the aorta (9).

All of these techniques are further enhanced by the development of parallel imaging that potentiates more rapid scanning, allowing progress in "bolus chase" image acquisition (10). The increased rate of data collection with multichannel coil design further speeds image acquisition

(11,12). The advent of intravascular contrast agents, which have a prolonged half-life within the circulation, also promises to expand the application of CE-MRA (13).

NONCONTRAST MR ANGIOGRAPHY

Many current MRA protocols include combinations of CE-MRA and noncontrast techniques. The latter group includes bright-blood—TOF, SSFP, black-blood, Double-IR (Inversion Recovery), Triple-IR—and phase-contrast imaging sequences.

Time of Flight Angiography

TOF angiography is well-validated as a vascular imaging technique and continues to be applied clinically, particularly in carotid (14,15) and lower extremity runoff studies (7). The fundamental principal of TOF takes advantage of inflow of the blood into the slice being imaged (16) with the image contrast depending on the blood flow velocity. In this technique, stationary tissue is saturated by the continuous application of selective radiofrequency (RF) pulses that tip the proton spins in a slice or slab into the transverse plane. However, the fully magnetized spins in the moving blood continuously enter the imaging slice. These protons only experience a few RF pulses before exiting; therefore, they generate a high MR signal in contrast to the low signal intensity of the stationary tissue.

The TOF method is very susceptible to blood signal saturation when flow is slow or there is too much within the plane of acquisition (in-plane flow). In cases of slow flow or in-plane flow, the flowing spins experience a greater number of RF pulses before exiting the slab, which will cause relative signal decrease.

A spatial presaturation slab is used to suppress venous signal and is usually placed 5–10 mm away from the slice being imaged for optimal effect. Multiple-thin 2D slices are imaged rapidly, choosing the imaging plane along the direction of blood flow, to generate the highest signal. Postprocessed, rotating, coronal reconstructed images are usually reviewed. Three-dimensional (3D) TOF employs a single-slab or multislab technique and is primarily employed for imaging the carotid bifurcation. Three-dimensional (3D) TOF has several advantages over 2D TOF including shorter TE, thinner slices, and higher signal-to-noise ratio (SNR) as a result of the averaging of noise (17).

TOF scans are usually long, up to 10 minutes, because of the long time recovery (TR) used to optimize image contrast and SNR. This technique provides high SNR and good venous suppression. The disadvantages include in-plane spin saturation seen frequently in the proximal anterior tibial artery, low signal in small vessels resulting from slow flow, and intravoxel dephasing in regions with disturbed flow (18). Dynamic triphasic flow can cause ghosting artifact that can be corrected by the use of cardiac gating. This

further prolongs the acquisition time. When there is inflow compromise, the dampening effect of the stenosis on triphasic flow often results in better image quality. TOF is particularly susceptible to motion and complex flow patterns resulting in pseudolesions. The relatively long TE and large voxels make TOF more susceptible to metallic artifact. More rapid imaging strategies, using shorter echo times, are more reliable when metal hardware is present (Figure 7–1).

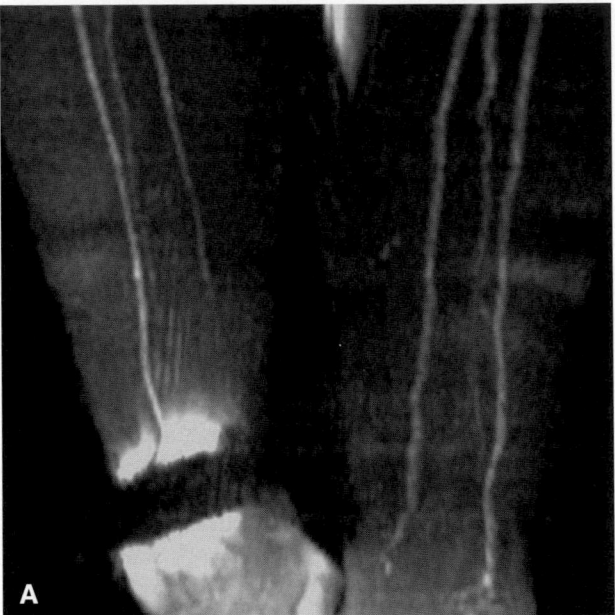

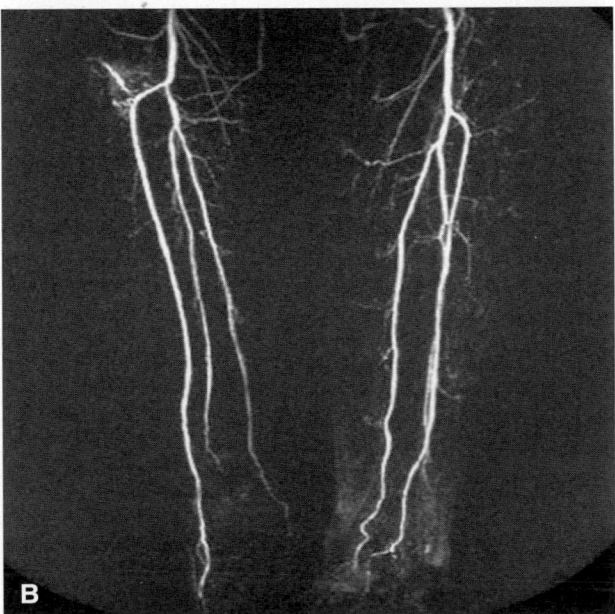

Figure 7–1   A. 2D TOF image from below the knee is degraded by susceptibility artifact from a metallic screw in the right ankle that precludes vessel assessment locally. **B.** The shorter TE and smaller voxel size of PR hyperTRICKS results in images free of artifact with excellent vessel evaluation.

Steady State Free Precession (SSFP, FIESTA, TrueFISP, Balanced FFE)

Steady state free precession (SSFP) has become increasingly important for diagnostic and functional imaging during the past several years. Marketed under several trade names including FIESTA (Fast Imaging Employing Steady State Acquisition—GE Medical Systems), TrueFISP (True Fast Imaging with Steady State Precession—Siemens Medical Systems), or Balanced FFE (Fast Field Echo—Philips Medical Systems), it provides excellent SNR efficiency and a combined T_2 Star/T_1 tissue weighting (excellent blood to tissue contrast) that is flow independent. SSFP is established when a series of closely timed RF pulses are applied to the body (19). All gradients that are subsequently applied are balanced perfectly, causing refocusing rather than spoiling transverse magnetization and leading to a steady state of proton precession. SSFP uses a very short time to recovery (TR), less than 3 ms and TE 1.5, exactly half that of TR, which allows fast imaging and real-time evaluation of the beating heart. When compared with other fast gradient-echo sequences, SSFP imaging has a shorter acquisition time, making breath-holding more feasible.

Currently, this sequence is employed ubiquitously for cardiac imaging where it is mostly used in combination with cardiac gating. Fast, ungated SSFP acquisition is used as a localizer sequence in MRA protocols, which offers excellent contrast resolution. When gated, it offers excellent cine evaluation of aortic dissection anatomy, including intimal flap motion, during the cardiac cycle as well as entry and reentry site mapping (5). The dephasing effect of stenotic flow dynamics at the aortic valve or within a coarctation is also seen well by this technique (Figure 7–2). When applied as an adjunct to the phase contrast technique, it can be used to measure velocity (20). The sequence has been used as a CE-MRA imaging tool, although this is not widely practiced (21). Three-dimensional SSFP is currently being promoted as a reliable method for imaging the coronary arteries (22).

Black-Blood Technique (Double-IR, Triple-IR)

Inversion recovery sequences are spin-echo sequences with magnetization-preparation inversion pulses, which suppress the signal in the vessel lumen (Double-IR) and in both vessel lumen and surrounding fat (Triple-IR), respectively (23). A nonselective 180-degree inversion pulse is first applied followed by a slice-selective 180-degree pulse that immediately restores signal within the slice. A fixed TI of 640 ms, before the imaging sequence, allows time for the signal of blood protons entering the slice to reach their null point. The imaging sequence employed is a fast spin-echo with an echo train length of 8–32. Triple-IR employs a third slice selective 180-degree inversion pulse during the TI for nulling fat signal. The timing allows the null point for fat signal and blood signal to coincide before imaging.

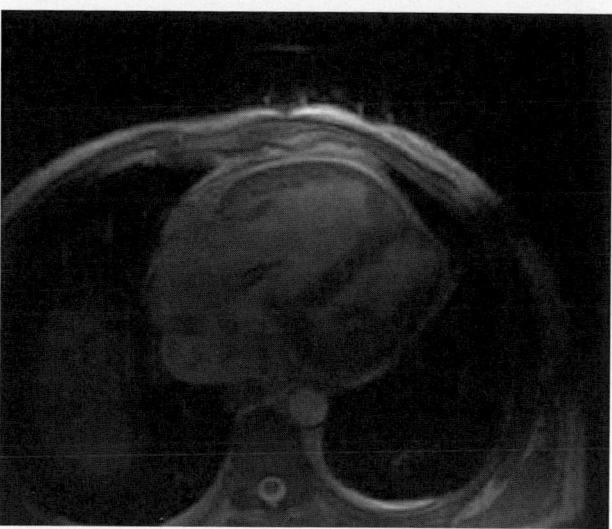

Figure 7–2 Approximate four-chamber view of the heart shows a regurgitant jet at the tricuspid valve. This steady-state free precession (SSFP—"white" blood) sequence is sensitive to the dephasing effect of high velocities as found in a stenotic or regurgitant jet resulting in local loss of signal.

Although black blood techniques may be applied in any plane, blood nulling is optimal when imaging is perpendicular to the flow direction. Cardiac gating and breath holding significantly improve image quality. These imaging strategies are very sensitive to anatomic detail and have been successfully applied to evaluation of the thoracic aorta for intramural hematoma or dissection (24)(Figure 7–3).

Phase Contrast Angiography

Phase contrast imaging uses velocity-encoding gradients prior to data collection to provide a net phase gain to the flowing spins and zero phase gain to the stationary tissue (25,26). For spins with a velocity, the phase-accumulation is nonzero, therefore providing the blood velocity information. For the extraction of unidirectional flow, images are usually acquired with bipolar gradients of equal magnitude and opposite polarity. Phase contrast imaging provides excellent background suppression, therefore high contrast-to-noise ratio (CNR). However, phase contrast imaging often has a long TR and TE because of the bipolar velocity-sensitizing gradients, which results in greater sensitivity to metal artifact and complex flow signal loss.

The velocity encoding dynamic range should be adjusted so that the velocity encoding value (VENC) chosen by the operator is the velocity value that produces a phase difference of 180 degrees when matched to the maximum expected blood flow velocity. The data from a phase contrast sequence is processed into magnitude (anatomic detail) and phase (velocity information) images (Figure 7–4). Postprocessing software allows calculation of the cross-sectional area of the imaged vessel. This information combined with velocity

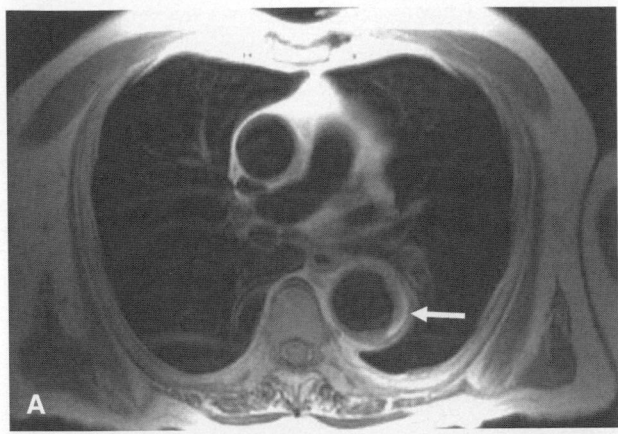

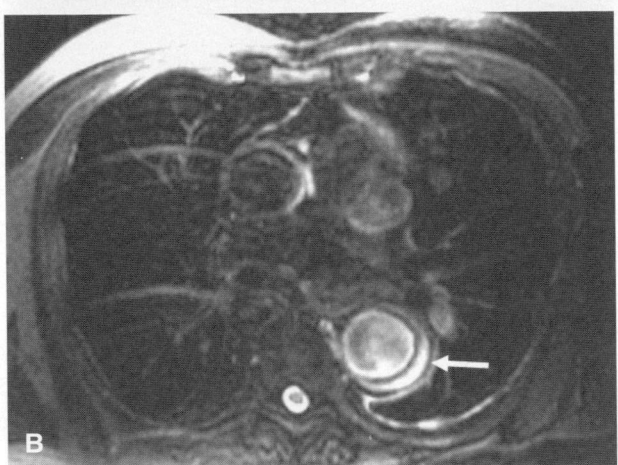

Figure 7–3 Axial Double-IR (black-blood) **A.** and T$_2$-weighted axial image **B.** in a patient who presented with acute aortic syndrome like symptoms of severe interscapular chest pain. The high signal crescent shaped intramural lesion on both sequences represents subacute intramural hematoma.

information intrinsic to each pixel allows calculation of flow volume and profile. If the chosen VENC is too low aliasing occurs, which is similar to that seen in Doppler ultrasound.

Three-dimensional phase contrast has clinical application in evaluating carotid artery flow (27–29) and for characterizing renal artery stenosis (30,31). These methods rely on the velocity-induced signal loss associated with highly turbulent flow near a hemodynamically significant stenosis.

CONTRAST-ENHANCED MRA

First-pass, contrast-enhanced magnetic resonance angiography (CE-MRA) was first introduced by Martin Prince in 1993 (1). Initial studies required prolonged acquisition precluding multistation imaging. The improved performance of current MRI scanners allows shorter repetition times, enabling image acquisition during a single breath-hold and, at multiple stations for a single contrast medium injection.

Paramagnetic contrast agent is administered by intravenous injection, preferably via a right antecubital fossa intravenous catheter. This allows the shortest pathway for contrast passage to the heart, avoiding a compressed brachiocephalic vein and ensuring a tight bolus (5). The contrast material shortens the T$_1$ relaxation time of proton spins in proximity to the paramagnetic molecules. As a result, blood within a vessel in which contrast concentration is high will appear bright on a gradient echo, T$_1$-weighted sequence. Gadolinium is most commonly used because of its high relaxivity and safety profile when bound to a chelator. Although extensive data exist confirming its safety in clinical use (32,33), the use of gadolinium chelate contrast media continues to be an "off label" use in the United States.

A disadvantage of current gadolinium contrast agents is their tendency to leave the intravascular compartment and seek the interstitial space, therefore allowing a narrow window of opportunity to image the vessels before loosing image contrast. Extensive research is underway to design a blood-pool agent that remains in the vessels for a prolonged time. MS-325 (recently completed first phase III trial) is one such gadolinium-based agent that binds reversibly to human serum albumin in plasma thus providing an extended imaging time window (13,34–36). Ultra-small iron particles and polymeric gadolinium chelates have also been evaluated as future blood-pool contrast agents (37,38).

Contrast Material Dose and Injection Timing

Arterial blood gadolinium concentrations in excess of 1 mMolar are required to achieve blood T$_1$ value of <270 ms at 1.5 Tesla (5). This makes blood signal brighter than fat, which is the predominant background tissue having a T$_1$ relaxation time of 270 ms. CE-MRA image quality is influenced by contrast medium dose, rate of injection, and timing of injection. While most MRA researchers advocate doses ranging from 0.1–0.3 mmol/kg, it is important to remember that the dose remains at the discretion of the supervising physician. A total dose of 20–40 mL (approximately 0.3 mmol/kg) is preferred. Arterial gadolinium concentration is proportional to the injection rate and inversely proportional to the cardiac output. To negate the influence of the latter, patients should be relaxed and should avoid exercise and eating immediately before their study. Extreme anxiety should be ameliorated by sedation.

The injection rate should be designed to optimize contrast-to-noise ratio in the acquired images (39–41). The peak contrast concentration within the vessel of interest should coincide with filling of central k-space. The low-spatial frequency data acquired during central k-space filling determines the image contrast. Therefore, for centric or elliptical-centric acquisitions, where central k-space is filled at the beginning of the scan, a more rapid injection

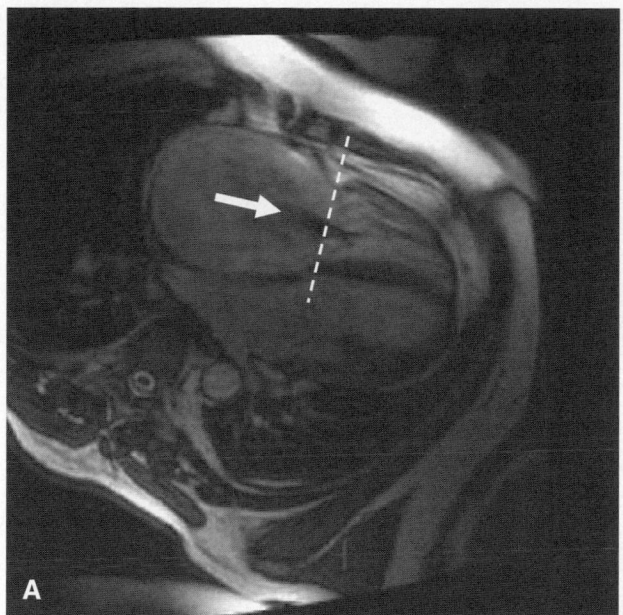

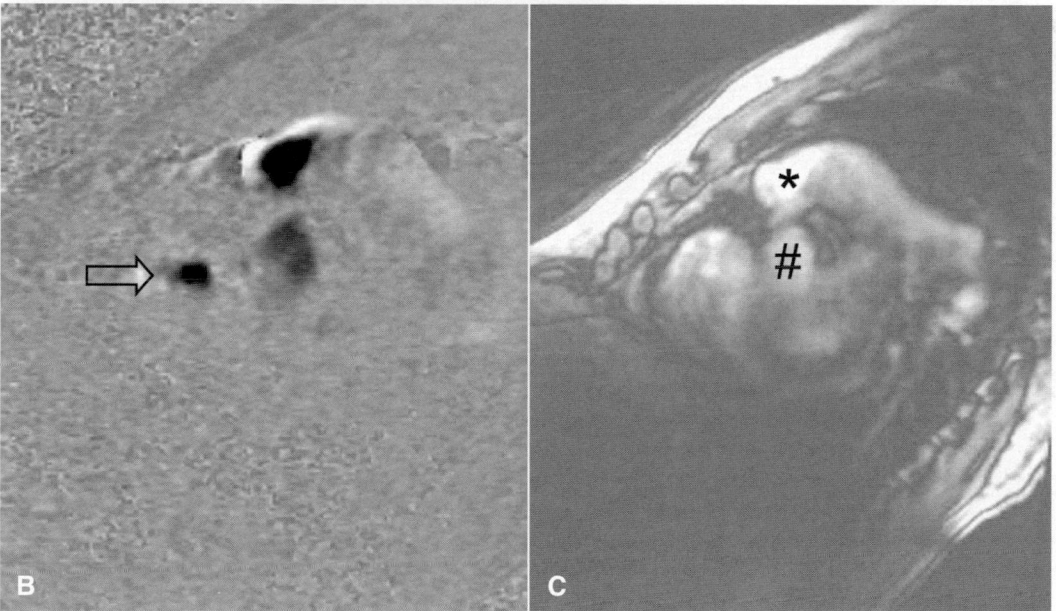

Figure 7–4   **A.** Four-chamber cardiac SSFP image shows a tricuspid valve regurgitant jet (*white arrow*) with associated enlargement of the right atrium. 2D Phase contrast evaluation in the described plane provides a series of phase **B.** and magnitude **C.** images. From the phase images, for which the VENC (velocity encoding value) was set at 400 cm/s, one can calculate the velocity spectrum within the jet (*open arrow*) and, knowing the total right ventricular output, the regurgitant fraction. * = pulmonary artery, # = aorta.

(tight bolus) is desirable because the image contrast is determined in a brief portion of scan time. For the same reason, with shorter acquisition strategies and with more sophisticated pulse sequences, substantially lower contrast doses may be used. With sequential k-space strategies, a slower injection is allowed as central k-space is acquired throughout the scan acquisition, which is a more forgiving technique when accurate timing is not possible or where a power injector is not available. If image acquisition begins too early where T_1 shortening is still in rapid flux, severe

ringing artifact will be present. Most imagers prefer to use a fixed injection rate of 2.0–2.5 mL/second followed by a flush of approximately 30 mL normal saline to ensure that the full contrast dose is delivered.

In our practice, we view MRA as a holistic study that evaluates all structures in the imaged field of view (FOV) and not just vascular pathology. To achieve this, we routinely perform a delayed, postcontrast, gradient-echo axial acquisition with fat suppression. This frequently provides important additional diagnostic information with only a small

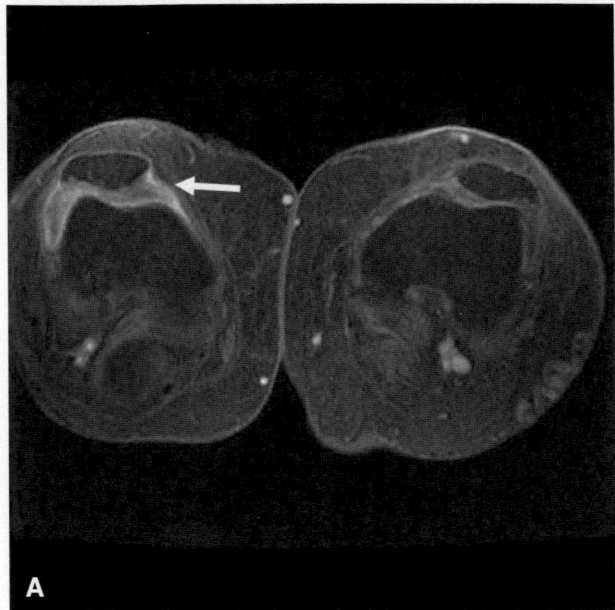

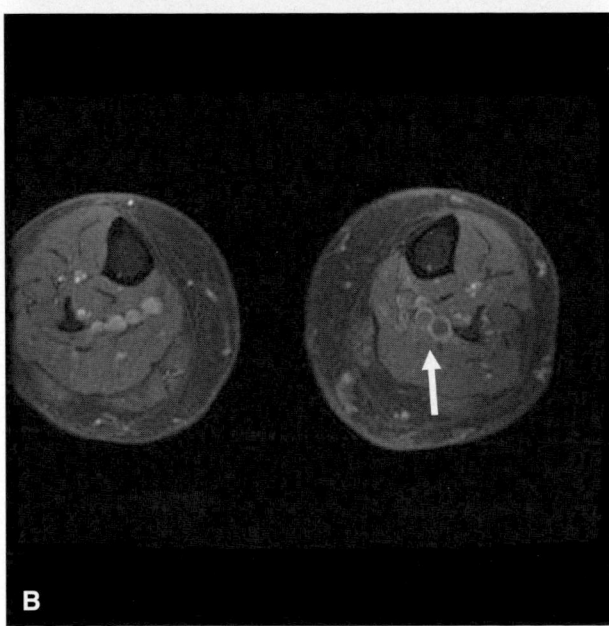

Figure 7–5 Axial fast spoiled gradient echo sequences performed post gadolinium administration in routine peripheral CE-MRA studies show hyper-enhancement of the synovium (*arrow*) in the right patella-femoral joint space **A.** consistent with synovitis and acute expansile and occlusive thrombosis (*arrow*) of the left infrapopliteal deep veins **B.** This rapidly acquired postcontrast sequence frequently shows incidental findings that are clinically relevant.

additional time penalty. Using this additional sequence, inflammatory aneurysms have been evaluated and incidental deep venous thrombosis (Figure 7–5), renal tumors, and liver pathology have been diagnosed. The availability of PACS is advantageous in handling the additional data produced.

Injection Timing Techniques

With the advent of rapid acquisition techniques, timing of the contrast injection is an important prerequisite to

successful imaging (42). Empirical timing, in which the supervising physician "guesstimates" the time from injection to commencement of image acquisition, is fraught with error. In addition, the advent of power injectors and greater sophistication in timing methods ensure that it is used rarely now.

A timing bolus acquisition provides more accuracy, although it does require additional scan time (43). A small contrast material dose (1–2 mL) is administered, followed by a generous normal saline flush. The arrival of contrast is imaged in the vessel of interest using a fast gradient-echo sequence and the time of peak contrast enhancement calculated by graphic analysis. Although a preparatory inversion pulse does require additional scan time, it may be used to null blood signal resulting in greater conspicuity of the contrast signal from the test bolus.

Automatic triggering ("MR SmartPrep" from GE Medical Systems) employs a pulse sequence that can detect change in concentration of contrast medium (44). The operator prescribes a "tracker volume" or region of interest (ROI) that is imaged at 20 ms intervals. After detecting an increase in contrast medium, it commences image acquisition during the arterial phase. A built-in delay of 6–8 seconds usually occurs after contrast detection to allow peak concentration to occur, thus avoiding ringing artifact and maximizing CNR.

Finally, an MRI fluoroscopic technique ("Fluoro-triggering" from GE Medical Systems and "CARE Bolus" from Siemens Medical Systems) allows the operator to choose when image acquisition should begin, by reviewing real-time images of the vessel of interest, during contrast medium injection (45). When optimal contrast is seen on the rapidly acquired 2D images, the operator triggers the 3D MRA acquisition (fluoro-triggering). This technique can be compromised by inter-operator variability, but is, in general, a dependable method for accurate timing. The operator has discretion over starting imaging acquisition and can vary this depending on the k-space filling strategy used.

Compared with x-ray digital subtraction angiography and CT angiography, CE-MRA is free from ionizing radiation. CE-MRA can generate 2D sectional images at any orientation (Maximum Intensity Projection, or MIP, images), 3D volumetric images, or even four-dimensional (4D) images representing spatial-temporal behavior (Time Resolved Imaging of Contrast Kinetics, EC-TRICKS, GE Medical Systems, Milwaukee, WI) or vastly undersampled imaging with projection reconstruction, or VIPR (46). Other advantages of CE-MRA include increased signal-to-noise ratio (SNR), relative resistance to artifact degradation, and the ability to perform in-plane imaging as in conventional angiography.

MRA ADVANCES

CE-MRA has several potential pitfalls including a continuing propensity to err in timing of the contrast bolus, which can result in venous contamination (42,47). In peripheral angiography, this is most evident in below-knee imaging. Many imaging centers continue to use 2D TOF as a backup sequence in lower extremity MRA protocol that has an intrinsic capability to suppress venous signal. Conventional multistation MRA cannot image asymmetric filling of extremity vessels (48), and therefore suffers from limited spatial resolution and SNR because of restricted imaging time per station (8), and may exclude vessels from the FOV because of restrictions in volume prescription (Figure 7–6).

Many new imaging sequences are on the horizon that address the intrinsic deficiencies of "conventional" CE-MRA. Several of these use projection reconstruction techniques to allow radial filling of k-space. The resultant oversampling of central k-space (image contrast) and undersampling of peripheral k-space (image spatial resolution) allows rapid image acquisition. The original TRICKS sequence uses Cartesian strategy to oversample central k-space while acquiring multiple-time frames during passage of contrast material (Figure 7–7). This application is well-used below the knee where venous contamination can be avoided, asymmetric passage of contrast can be appreciated, and overall flow dynamics appreciated (Figure 7–8). It achieves temporal resolution without significant loss of spatial resolution (49). PR-TRICKS and PR-hyperTRICKS, still experimental protocols, have evolved by using projection reconstruction (PR) in two planes and Cartesian strategy in the third imaging plane (46,50). These imaging strategies have better temporal resolution because of the more time efficient PR tactic. All of these techniques benefit from a mask image before arrival of contrast that is subsequently subtracted from the contrasted images similar to digital subtraction angiography (DSA) technique, which further increases image diagnostic quality. PR-hyperTRICKS differs from PR-TRICKS by spending additional time during the equilibrium phase of contrast passage collecting high spatial frequency data (periphery of k-space), which augments the image spatial resolution without loss of contrast or temporal resolution.

VIPR is a further variant of PR strategy that fills k-space radially in all three dimensions. The resultant time series of images provides excellent separation of arterial and venous phases. The variable density k-space sampling intrinsic to this sequence is combined with temporal k-space interpolation to provide time frames as short as 2 seconds. This time resolution reduces the need for exact contrast timing while also providing dynamic information and lending itself to subtraction processing and other more sophisticated postprocessing techniques. Spatial resolution is determined primarily by the projection readout resolution and therefore is isotropic across the FOV, which is also isotropic. This allows for excellent postprocessing as multiprojectional MIP or volume rendered images. Although undersampling the outer regions of k-space introduces aliased

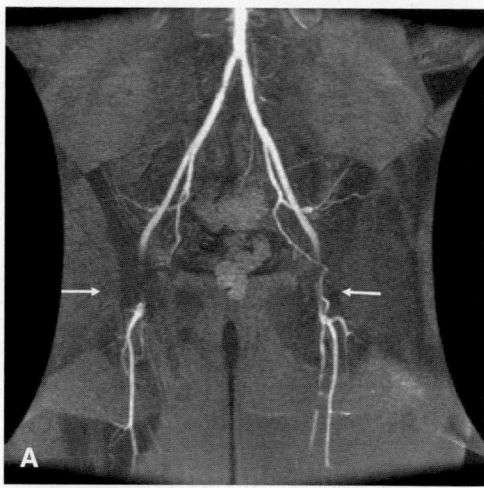

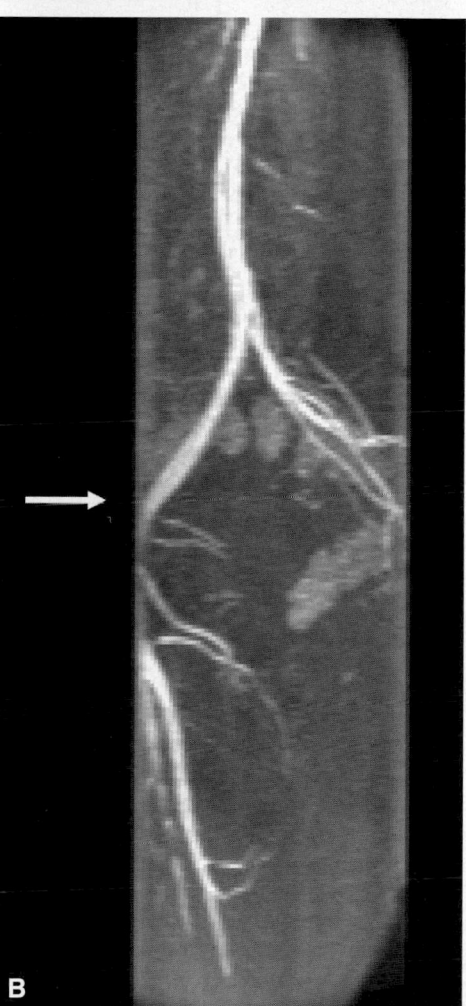

Figure 7–6   A. Apparent occlusion of the common femoral arteries bilaterally (*arrows*) on this coronal MIP image of the pelvic station of a bolus chase peripheral CE-MRA. Note the absence of collateral vessels. **B.** The sagittal MIP reconstruction reveals that the prescribed field of view was inadvertently too small and has excluded the common femoral arteries as they cross anterior to the femoral heads, explaining the findings on the coronal image.

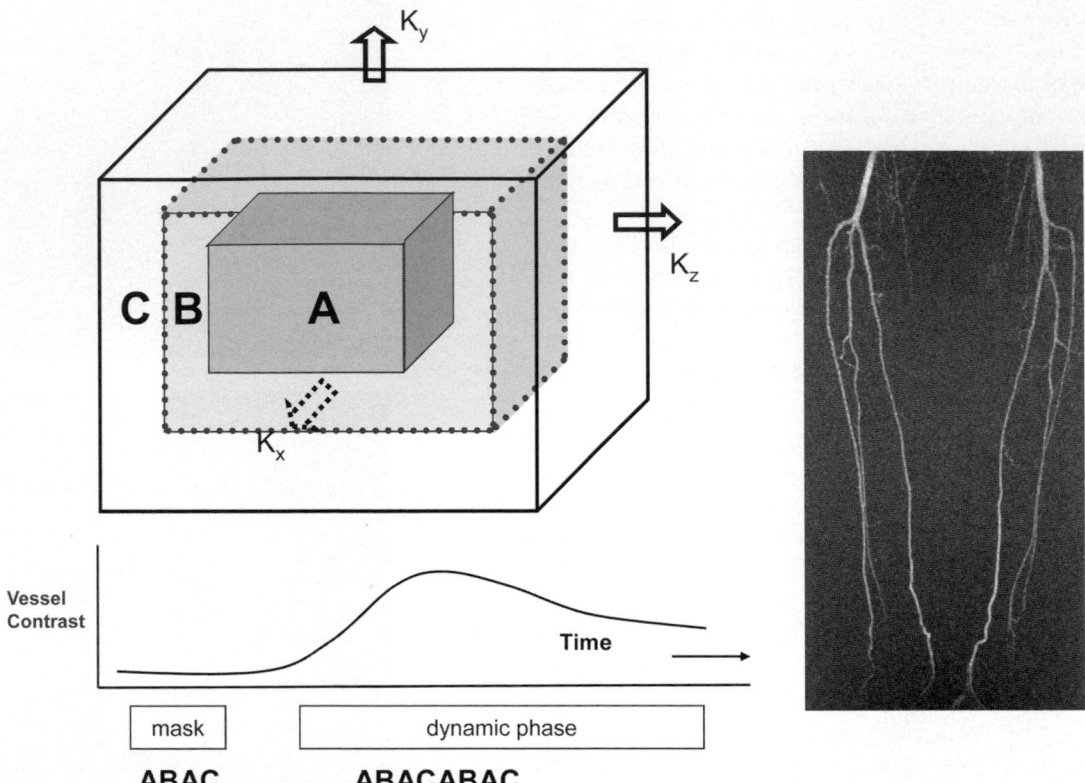

Figure 7–7   Diagrammatic illustration of EC TRICKS that employs cartesian filling of k-space in all planes. The low spatial frequencies (A) centrally in k-space are sampled more frequently than the intermediate and high spatial frequencies (B, C) that are more peripherally located. A similar strategy is used before and after contrast injection to allow for background subtraction. On the right is an example of a normal peak arterial phase image.

energy into the image, which may compromise resolution, this is not a limiting factor in high-contrast applications, such as MRA (51).

These imaging strategies are complemented by almost concurrent development of rapid imaging technology. Foremost among these is parallel imaging, which includes eponyms such as SENSE ("SENSitivity Encoding" from Philips Medical Systems), iPAT ("Integrated Parallel Acquisition Techniques" from Siemens Medical Systems), and ASSET ("Array Spatial Sensitivity Encoding Technique" from GE Medical Systems) (52). These spectacularly quick MR imaging techniques use the unique geometry of phased array coils to spatially encode the image faster (11,53). Simultaneous data are acquired in multiple detectors in the form of arrays of radiofrequency coils. The multifold increase in imaging speed facilitates more rapid injection, and thus higher contrast resolution (54,55). The increased injection rates make timing more critical and prone to error and may lead to greater venous contamination. As SNR increases with the square root of imaging

time, any attempt to increase acquisition speed will adversely influence SNR (56).

Vessel Wall Imaging

Despite the high sensitivity and specificity of imaging modalities to assess the degree of stenosis, evidence suggests that risk of an embolic event is critically dependent on plaque thromboembolic potential. Assessment of atherosclerosis is expanding to include evaluation for "vulnerable" plaques, a concept introduced by Falk in 1992 (57). High-resolution MRI of the vessel wall can now provide important information about the individual makeup of atherosclerotic plaques (58–60). Vulnerable atherosclerotic plaque is rupture prone. Plaques are characterized by assessing the lipid core, fibrous cap, and its thickness and the presence of inflammation within the cap. A vulnerable cap is thought to have a thin fibrous cap, a large lipid rich core that is weakly contained by the fibrous cap, inflammatory cell infiltrate (58), or intraplaque hemorrhage (60).

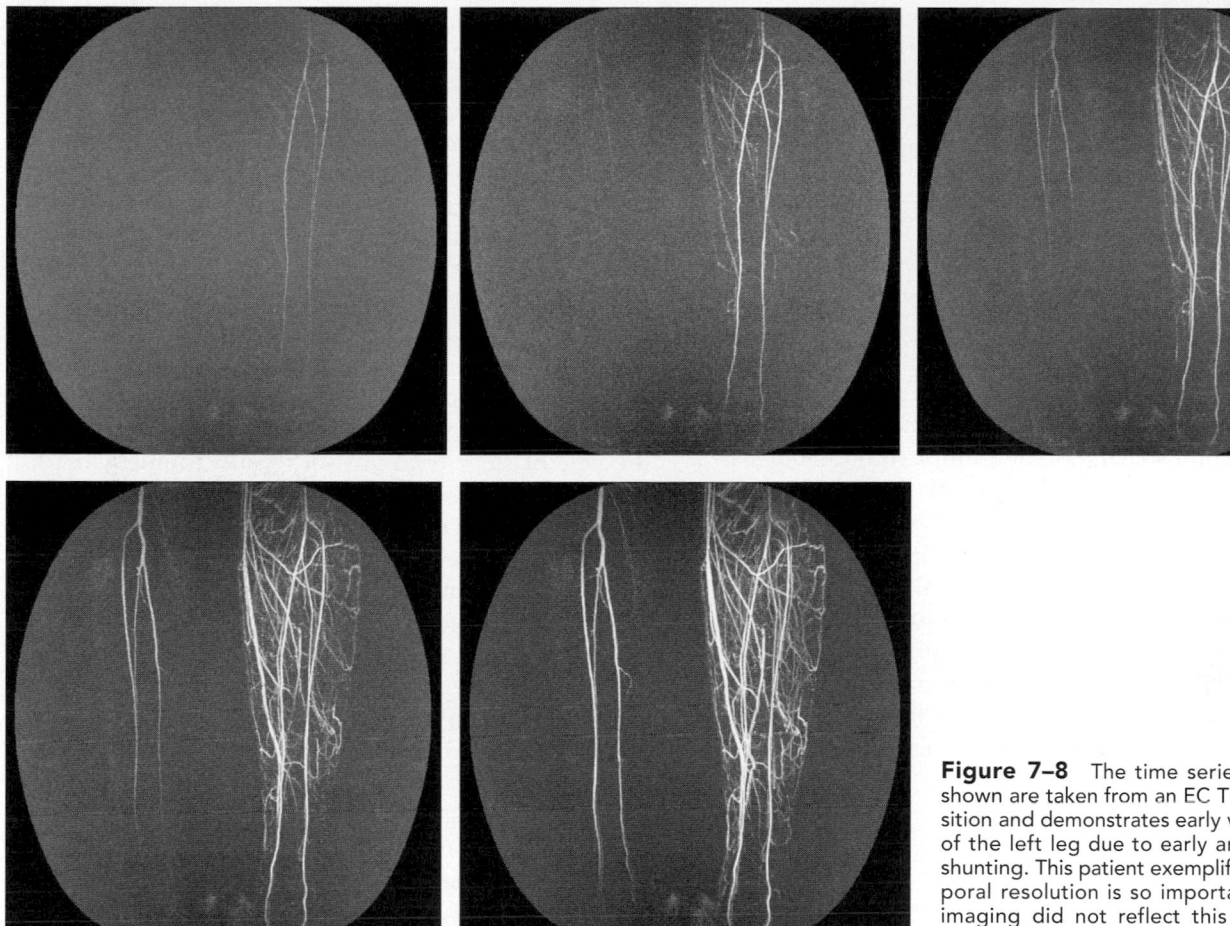

Figure 7–8 The time series of images shown are taken from an EC TRICKS acquisition and demonstrates early venous filling of the left leg due to early arteriovenous shunting. This patient exemplifies why temporal resolution is so important. 2D TOF imaging did not reflect this asymmetric passage of blood.

T_1- and T_2-weighted double inversion SE and PD-weighted FSE imaging are employed to interrogate the vessel wall. A 3D TOF is also used to evaluate differential contrast-weighted images to improve the accuracy of identifying the lipid-rich necrotic core and acute intraplaque hemorrhage. GRE sequences create T_2 Star sensitive tissue signal that improves the depiction of intimal calcifications and fibrous cap.

The superficial anatomic position of the carotid arteries is well-suited for the use of phase array coils. Several dedicated RF coils, both surface and intravascular, have been developed. To detect the early development of plaque, novel contrast agents can be employed as a marker of macrophage activity within the plaque (61).

MRA COILS

Dedicated flexible, surface-phased array coils are now available from most vendors to cover the lower extremities, chest/abdomen, and head/neck. A phased-array coil is an MR receiver radiofrequency coil arrangement containing a combination of local surface coils. Combinations are assembled in a way that electrically isolates each coil with separate and independent signals collected from each element in the array. These signals must be processed independently, each producing a separate image. Finally, these several images are added in a way that optically combines their individual signal patterns. The advantage of a phased-array coil is that it achieves the sensitivity of a small local surface coil, but over a larger FOV. The development of phased-array coils provides for further efficiency in signal-to-noise that can be traded off for faster acquisition times, higher spatial resolution, or lower doses of contrast. Most of these coils are receive-only coils and allow greater uniformity of signal and higher SNR. This results from the closer proximity of the coil segment to the anatomy under study, as well as the averaging of noise between the individual components of the coil. The greater the number of coil elements, the better the SNR; and the more RF channels available, the faster the data transfer. Most phased-array coils still consist of four to eight elements with a maximum of eight RF channels. Significant advances are occurring in coil technology, however, and currently up to 32 data channels have been demonstrated. A dedicated peripheral vascular wrap coil with an array of six elements and four channels is used for lower extremity and pelvis MRA. An eight-channel TORSO coil is used for chest and abdomen imaging and an eight-channel neurovascular phased array coil for head and neck MRA imaging. The body coil has been largely relegated to the role of a transmit tool for MRA purposes.

ARTIFACTS IN CE-MRA

As with other imaging modalities, many variables exist that are detrimental to successful CE-MRA. Those relating to the patient include claustrophobia, inability to remain still during the study, poor cardiac function, and inability to sustain a sufficiently long breath-hold. Technical variables that can degrade image quality include volume of contrast medium administered, rate of administration, and synchronization of image acquisition with the arrival of contrast agent. Human decision is a variable that influences positioning of the patient, choice of scan parameters, and selection of imaging volume. In general, the imaging artifacts present in CE-MRA studies result from a shortcoming in one of the above variables. The ability to accurately report on these studies relies on recognition of the common artifacts encountered and the ability to identify their cause. Knowing the cause of the artifact may permit prevention in future studies.

False Stenoses or Occlusions

Susceptibility Artifact, or Blooming Artifact

This artifact presents as a signal void and occurs at the interface between materials of different magnetic susceptibility (62,63). When materials with a high magnetic susceptibility are juxtaposed with body tissues, local distortion in the magnetic field occurs. In turn, this results in dephasing and frequency shifts in protons from the surrounding tissues. This artifact is commonly seen around implanted metal such as surgical clips, screws, joint prostheses and endovascular stents (64). When occurring in proximity to vessels, susceptibility artifacts can be severely limiting when interpreting 3D MR angiography images.

Magnetic resonance artifacts associated with endovascular stents are related to both stent geometry and the underlying metal composition of the stent (65–69). The effect of the metal composition dominates when imaging the stainless steel Palmer's stent or the cobalt-based alloy Easy Wallstent. Both of these prostheses cause large signal voids on 3D MRA images, making assessment of the stent lumen and patency impossible. The covered Corvita stent is constructed from the same cobalt-based alloy as the Easy Wallstent, although it contains a tantalum core that reduces the associated artifact. Although shortening the TE makes the associated artifact less pronounced, it is still too extensive to exclude the presence of even a significant stenosis. Conversely, stents made from nitinol (Cragg stent, Cragg EndoPro System-1 stent, Passenger stent) cause only

minor artifacts. The stent lumen can be assessed sufficiently to exclude the presence of a hemodynamically significant (>50% lumen narrowing) stenosis. Signal loss because of radiofrequency shielding inside nitinol stents (Faraday cage effect) imaged by CE-MRA can be reduced by applying high flip angles in the order of 70 degrees (67). Vanguard aortic aneurysm stents are also relatively immune to artifact. It would appear that the luminal patency of selected commercially available plain and covered stents indeed can be assessed with 3D contrast MRA. Shortening the TE (minimum) and increasing the flip angle to overcome the RF shielding tendency helps achieve this end. The importance of obtaining full information regarding past endovascular stenting should be stressed, in addition to the type of stent used, for each patient undergoing MR angiographic imaging.

The onus is on the radiologist to acquire a proper surgical history for the patient, particularly a vascular surgical history and any history of endovascular stent placement. Technical parameters may be altered to minimize the effect of susceptibility artifacts. Switching the phase and frequency encoding gradient directions will change the shape of the artifact without eliminating it. Gradient-echo sequences are particularly susceptible to metallic artifact, which is ironic because these sequences are employed ubiquitously for CE-MRA. The Spin Echo sequence employs a refocusing 180-degree pulse that negates the dephasing of stationary protons caused by ferromagnetic objects. When using GRE sequences, minimize artifact by using shorter TE values, which decreases the time for dephasing (refer to Figure 7–1). Reduce the TE by increasing the receiver bandwidth, using asymmetric echo acquisitions, increasing the FOV, reducing matrix size, or increasing the slice thickness. The last three choices, however, also increase voxel size, which may increase intravoxel dephasing.

Pseudostenosis Artifact

Highly concentrated gadolinium contrast medium imparts a paramagnetic affect that results in local magnetic field inhomogeneity, with resultant spin dephasing on gradient-echo images. The normal contrast medium injection route is via a forearm vein. The gadolinium contrast material is adequately dilute on reaching the central vessels or lower extremity so that there is no paramagnetic effect visible. However, when imaging the subclavian or carotid vessels, contrast medium within the subclavian vein ipsilateral to the site of injection produces spin dephasing that extends over several voxels. This effect can cross over from subclavian vein to the adjacent artery causing loss of signal and an apparent stenosis or occlusion of the latter (Figure 7–9) (70). This artifact disappears rapidly as the gadolinium contrast becomes dilute. It is most problematic in centric and elliptical-centric strategies when the data contributing to image contrast is collected at the beginning of the acquisition, or when the gadolinium contrast is not yet adequately

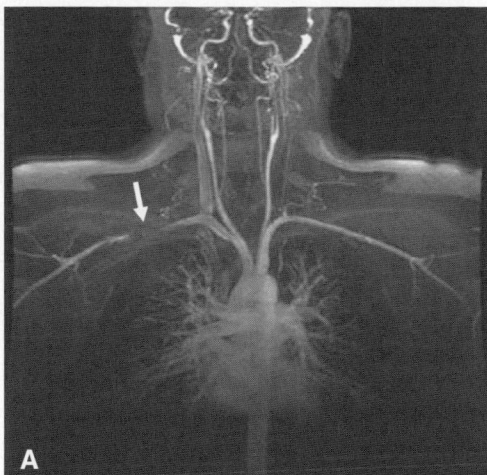

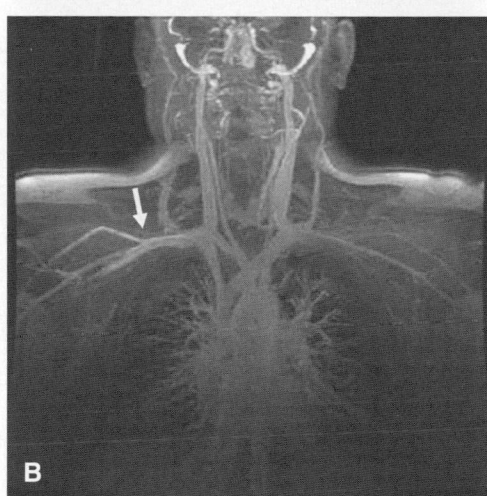

Figure 7–9 3D Coronal MIP during gadolinium injection **A.** shows an apparent stenosis or occlusion of the right subclavian artery. The gadolinium was injected from the right antecubital fossa. The T₂ Star effect from the concentrated gadolinium within the subclavian vein has caused this artifactual appearance in the adjacent artery. The MIP image in the delayed acquisition **B.** shows a patent vessel since the gadolinium within the subclavian vein is now dilute.

dilute. Correlation with delayed imaging will confirm or refute the presence of stenosis.

The best way to avoid this artifact when imaging the subclavian arteries is to inject in the arm contralateral to the vessel of interest. Alternatively, if feasible, inject contrast through a central venous catheter. If injection has to be performed in the same arm as that being evaluated, artifact can be minimized by diluting the contrast agent, using a shorter TE, and using a noncentric, k-space acquisition technique (70).

Postprocessing Artifact

Source images may be combined for interpretation using several techniques. The most commons ones are Maximum Intensity Projection Reconstruction (MIP) and Volume

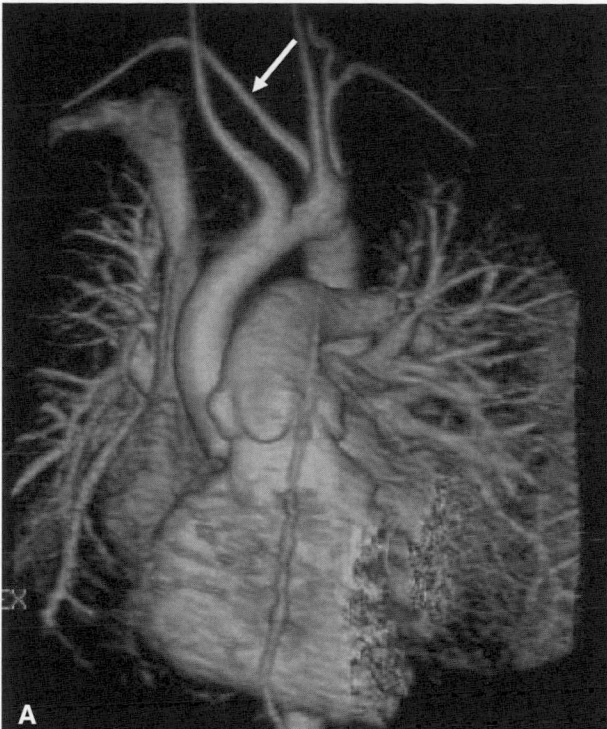

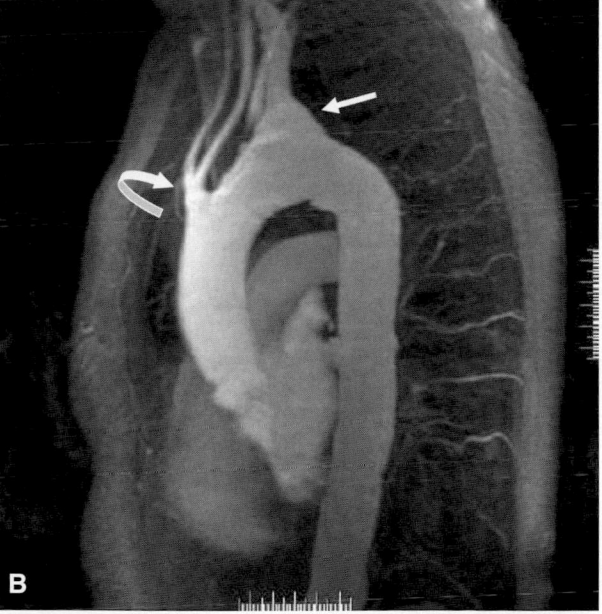

Figure 7–10 **A.** Volume rendered postprocessed image from 3D SPGR CE-MRA demonstrating an aberrant right subclavian artery arising from the distal aortic arch (*arrow*). **B.** Sagittal MIP image from a different patient shows a diverticulum of Kommerell aneurysm at the origin of an aberrant right subclavian artery (*arrow*) with a bovine arch configuration of the common carotid vessels (*curved arrow*).

Rendered Techniques (Figure 7–10). MIP processing reduces a 3D data set to a 2D projection image in any plane, which is achieved by projecting along parallel rays, through the volume data, and recording the maximum pixel intensity encountered along each ray. These can be full-volume or subvolume MIP images. The latter helps avoid artifacts by removing irrelevant data from the 3D volume data set before processing. These images provide an aesthetic overview of the vascular territory being imaged, but should only be interpreted in correlation with source images. A frequent artifact caused by MIP reconstruction is apparent stenosis (pseudostenosis) of a vessel or accentuation of a real stenotic lesion (5). MIP images may also conceal significant intraluminal lesions, such as thrombus or dissection, making it essential to review these images with source images and subvolume MIP images of the region of concern (Figure 7–11). Virtual endoluminal postprocessing can provide additional information in a limited number of clinical situations (Figure 7–12).

Zerofill Interpolation Processing (ZIP) is a widely used postprocessing technique that can improve the apparent resolution by interpolating images between the scanned images. It allows reduction in scan time without loss of resolution. By converting a 256 × 256 matrix to 512 × 512, the "stair-step" artifact can be eliminated from postprocessed images (71).

Anatomy Exclusion Artifact

When prescribing the 3D imaging volume from localizer images, it is important to include the entire vessel of interest within the volume. This can be particularly difficult when the image localizer is noisy, as is often seen in obese

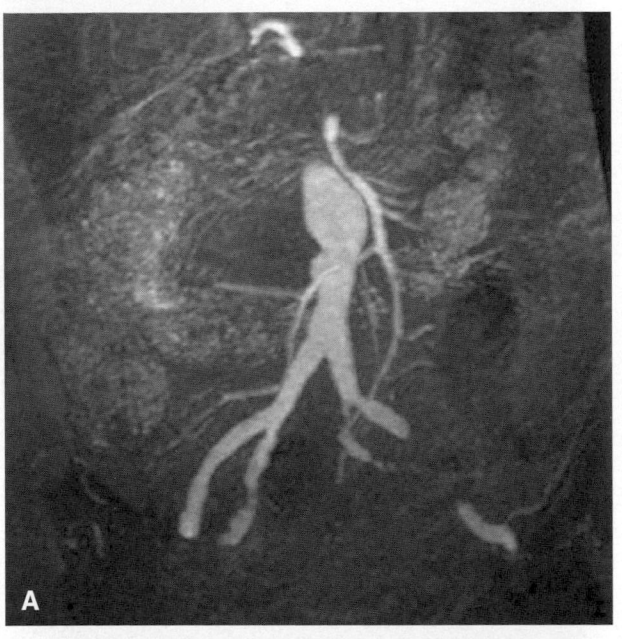

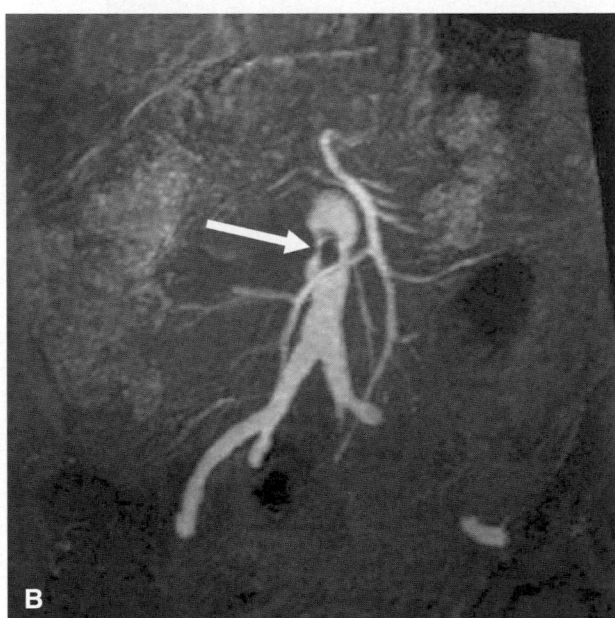

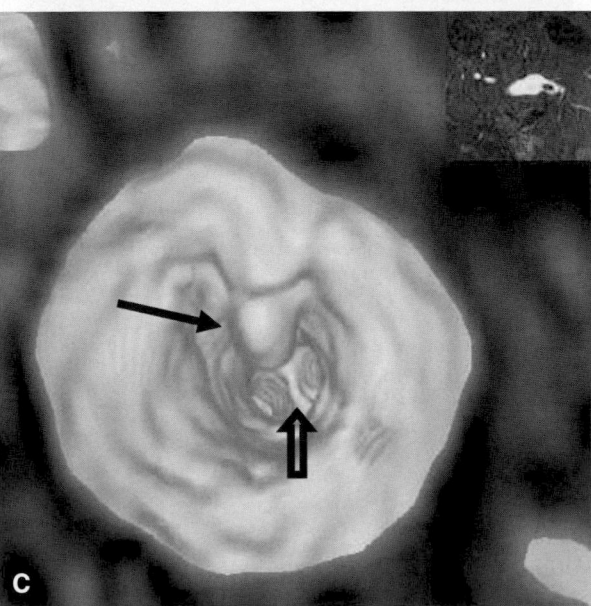

Figure 7–11 This case illustrates the need to review source images or subvolume MIP images. The full MIP image **A.** shows contour irregularity but fails to see the large anterior wall plague (*arrow*) noted in the subvolume MIP **B.** and confirmed on a virtual endoluminal projection image **C.** The iliac artery ostia are seen distally (*open arrow*).

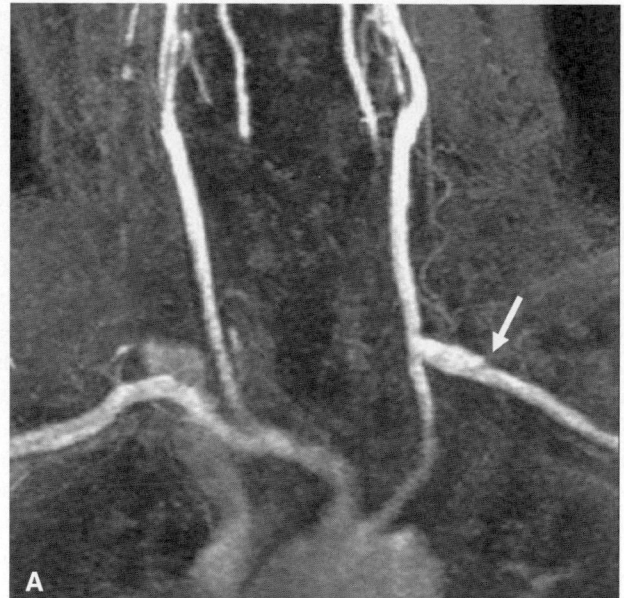

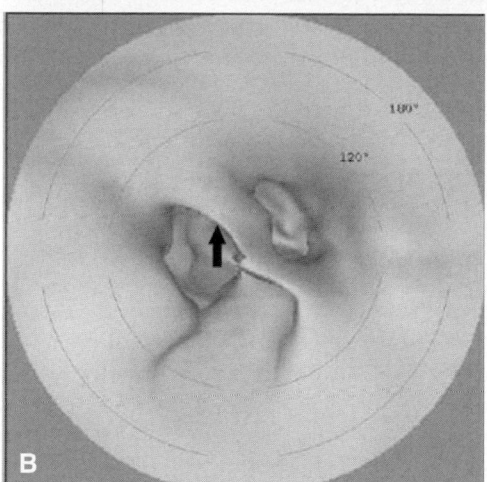

Figure 7–12 **A.** Coronal MIP demonstrates neo-anatomy after left carotid transposition of the subclavian artery and endarterectomy of the left vertebral artery. There is a subtle linear filling defect (*white arrow*) tranversing the lumen distal to the vertebral origin. **B.** Post processing allows virtual endovascular appreciation of a focal, nonobstructing dissection flap (*black arrow*). This postprocessing technique can provide additional diagnostic information in a limited number of cases.

patients. One particular region that is commonly excluded from the volume is the common femoral arteries as they pass anterior to the femoral heads (refer to Figure 7–6) (5). This particular error results in an artifact that can simulate bilateral femoral artery occlusion or possibly bilateral common femoral artery endovascular stents. Correlation with maximum intensity projection or volume rendered images, projected in the sagittal plane, will demonstrate whether the full extent of the vessel has been included in the imaged volume. The absence of collateral vessel formation should always raise suspicion of an anatomic exclusion artifact.

False Intraluminal or Extraluminal Lesions

Image Timing Artifact

Image timing artifacts are the most common artifacts encountered in daily practice (41,72,73). They occur when data acquisition is not synchronized properly with arrival and passage of the contrast material in the vessels of interest. Several different scenarios may present: Contrast material concentration may vary dramatically at the time of imaging, causing rapid alteration in T_1 of blood as k-space is being acquired. The latter presents as one or several dark lines, bright lines, or both along the lumen of the vessel or adjacent to the vessel. This artifact is frequently referred to as "ringing" artifact because of the parallel nature of the lines inside and outside the vessel; also called the Maki artifact (74) (Figure 7–13). Ringing artifact is more frequently encountered when centric or elliptical-centric 3D sequences are employed (74). Too rapid an injection rate can result in similar artifact. The underlying etiology relates to image acquisition while the gadolinium concentration, and thus T_1 relaxation, is still in a state of rapid flux. This artifact may simulate the presence of a dissection when seen in the aorta and its major branches (5). Correlation of the image acquired during passage of contrast agent with an image acquired during recirculation, when the T_1 relaxation of the blood has normalized, should confirm the presence or absence of a dissection. Use of the fluoro-triggering technique helps avoid ringing artifacts, particularly in patients with underlying cardiac failure, in which timing of contrast material is less predictable. It also avoids the problem of renal collecting system opacification seen with the "bolus-timing" technique when imaging the renal arteries.

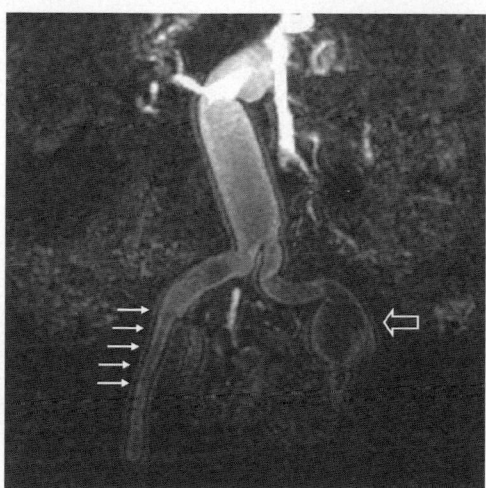

Figure 7–13 Coronal MIP image from an abdominal CE-MRA shows the ringing type artifact that occurs when image acquisition is started too early (*arrows*). The T_1 shortening effect of gadolinium has not stabilized causing this appearance along the vessel wall particularly in the more distal aorta and iliacs. An iliac artery aneurysm is also seen (*open arrow*).

Wraparound Artifact (Aliasing)

When the chosen FOV is smaller than the size of the body part being imaged, wraparound artifact occurs (5). This occurs in the phase encoding direction and is seen as spatial mismapping or wrapping around of the excluded body segment onto the opposite side of the acquired image (Figure 7–14). This artifact can also occur in 3D volume imaging from "front-to-back," if the body volume extends beyond the FOV in the slab-select dimension.

Eliminating wraparound artifact can be accomplished by increasing the FOV to include the entire anatomy. However, this will decrease the spatial resolution unless the number of phase-encoding steps is appropriately increased. Increasing the number of phase encoding steps increases the time of the scan, which in turn increases the risk of movement artifact, particularly in breath-hold situations. The role of the radiologist in these situations is paramount in choosing the parameters that will allow the best study for a particular clinical situation. Alternatively, if the shortest dimension of the body part imaged is not already in the phase-encoding direction, switching the phase and frequency-encoding directions may eliminate wraparound.

Motion Artifact

Movement artifact can be subdivided into those caused by respiratory motion, cardiac motion, or motion of body parts.

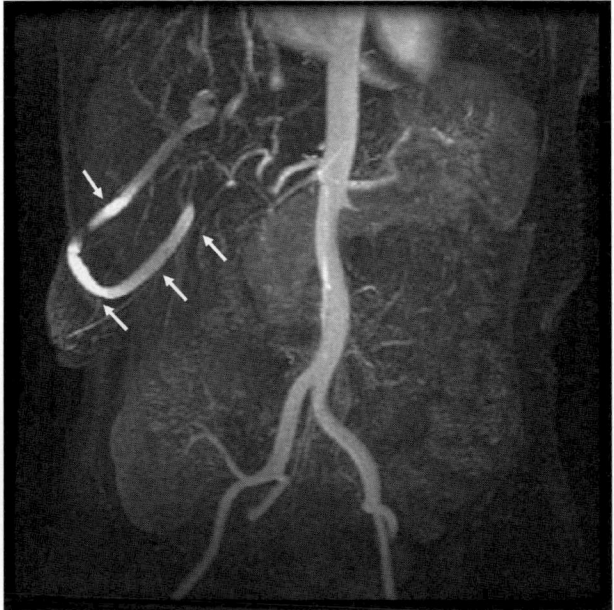

Figure 7–14 This postrenal transplant patient has a tubular, contrast filled structure projected along the right side of the abdomen on this coronal CE-MRA MIP (*arrows*). Post contrast axial survey images showed this to represent a "wraparound" artifact of a left forearm dialysis graft. This resulted from the use of too small a field of view.

Consistent breath-holding technique is essential for achieving diagnostic image quality in 3D MRA of the abdomen and thorax (75). Determining how long a patient can suspend respiration before the examination helps define the maximum possible scan time without incurring respiratory motion artifacts. This can be achieved by evaluating the patient's breathing pattern as recorded by the magnet's respiratory Bellows' system or, alternatively, by performing a trial breath-hold with the patient before entering the scanner. Oxygen administration by nasal canula may improve the patient's breath-holding capacity. An artifact resulting from respiratory motion is most evident in vessels perpendicular to the direction of diaphragmatic motion. Imaging of the renal arteries may be nondiagnostic because of the degree of motion artifact, particularly, in the distal vessel where respiratory motion has maximum influence (76). Tailoring the scan parameters to minimize imaging time can avoid this artifact with parallel imaging techniques playing a pivotal role in achieving this end. Motion experienced in imaging the thoracic vessels may be resolved by cardiac gating although this significantly extends scan time (77,78).

CLINICAL APPLICATIONS

Thoracic Aorta MRA

Thoracic MRA continues to grow in popularity as a noninvasive means to outline the vascular anatomy of the thorax. The many sequences available are well-employed in workup of congenital vascular anomalies. MRA can outline the anomalous vessels, but also may quantitate flow velocities and, in the presence of shunt physiology (Figure 7–15), can determine the $Q_P:Q_S$ ratio. Thoracic MRA is frequently used to evaluate and follow thoracic aortic aneurysms or dissections. Many of these studies arise from a patient presenting with acute onset chest pain in which the differential is wide and includes acute aortic pathology.

Acute Aortic Syndrome

Acute aortic syndromes include all diseases of the aorta that cause overexpansion of the aortic wall and thereby stimulating pain receptors within the adventitia. Thus, aortic aneurysm with and without dissection, aortic rupture, but also inflammation, intramural hematoma, aortic plaque rupture/ulceration, as well as blunt chest trauma with aortic wall laceration, can be involved (79,80). Currently, CT is viewed as the preferred imaging tool when the patient is unstable, particularly, in the context of trauma or acute dissection. For other aortic conditions including acute intramural hematoma (AIH), ulcerating plaque, inflammatory aneurysm, and aortitis, MRA allows

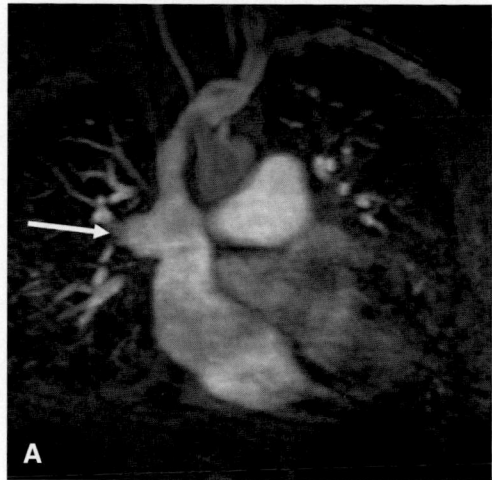

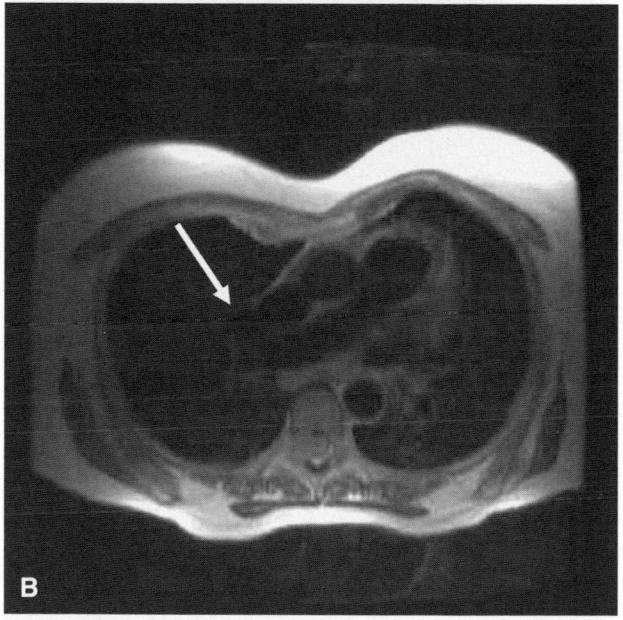

Figure 7–15 **A.** Coronal MIP of 3D SPGR CE-MRA showing partial anomalous pulmonary venous return from the right upper lobe to the superior vena cava (*arrow*). **B.** Double-IR axial image shows the anomalous pulmonary vein entering the superior vena cava (*arrow*).

better characterization because of the diverse enhanced and nonenhanced sequence profile available. In MRI findings of AIH on T_1-weighted MR (Double-IR/black-blood), the intramural hematoma appears as a crescentic to circumferential area of thickened aortic wall that may be isointense (within 3–7 days of onset of symptoms) or hyperintense (after 7 days) relative to skeletal muscle, depending on the age of the lesion (as oxyhemoglobin is converted to methemoglobin). Refer to Figure 7–3. Ability of MRI to define changes in the vessel wall has been utilized to diagnose and follow patients with vasculitis (81).

Routinely, multiplanar SSFP ungated localizers in all thoracic MRA protocols are used. Protocol also includes axial T_2 and Double-IR (black-blood) sequences. Cine SSFP imaging with phase contrast flow assessment can be performed when an aortic valve condition is suspected (refer to Figure 7–2). The latter sequence is also valuable in assessing severity of coarctation by calculating the pressure gradient across the stenosis (82). Standard CE-MRA is a sagittal, 3D, spoiled gradient-echo acquisition. However, if the clinical question implicates the subclavian vessels, a coronal acquisition is performed. Because of the potential for slow flow in an aortic dissection, a standard sequential acquisition order is chosen where dissection is suspected. A centric or elliptical-centric acquisition order can be used in all other cases to avoid venous contamination. Postcontrast, axial, T_1-weighted gradient-echo images are performed routinely. In patients with suspected vasculitis, an inversion-recovery, delayed, postcontrast gradient-echo sequence may be performed in the sagittal plane that demonstrated enhancement and thickening. This may be used to follow response to treatment.

Abdominal MRA

MRA of the abdomen is most frequently performed for evaluation of the aorta (83), renal arteries (30), or mesenteric arteries (84). Multiplanar localizers provide a generalized overview of the anatomy from which an appropriate FOV can be prescribed for the CE-MRA acquisition. In addition, an axial T_2-weighted sequence is performed, which can be invaluable in characterizing many incidental findings such as renal cysts, hemangiomas, and other solid organ pathologic conditions. Most vascular pathology is visible with coronal CE-MRA source, as well as postprocessed MIP images (Figure 7–16). Mesenteric ischemia, however, is best evaluated using sagittal acquisitions during contrast medium injection. A 3D, spoiled gradient recalled echo sequence precontrast, during contrast, and postcontrast passage is routinely performed. Parallel imaging is used to shorten the breath-hold when required. A postcontrast axial survey evaluates the abdominal viscera and can further characterize mycotic aneurysms, noninfected inflammatory aneurysms, and the extent of retroperitoneal fibrosis (Figure 7–17). Abdominal MRA has also been successfully applied to evaluation of native renal (Figure 7–18) (85), transplant renal (Figure 7–19), hepatic and pancreatic vessels, portal venous hypertension (86,87), and follow-up of aneurysm size and vasculitis. CE-MRA is ideal for monitoring the postoperative aorta, particularly for perigraft infection and pseudoaneurysm formation at the anastomosis (Figure 7–20). Current challenges include its application to endovascular stent follow-up for endoleak (Figure 7–21) and reproducible, accurate, aneurysm sac-size measurement.

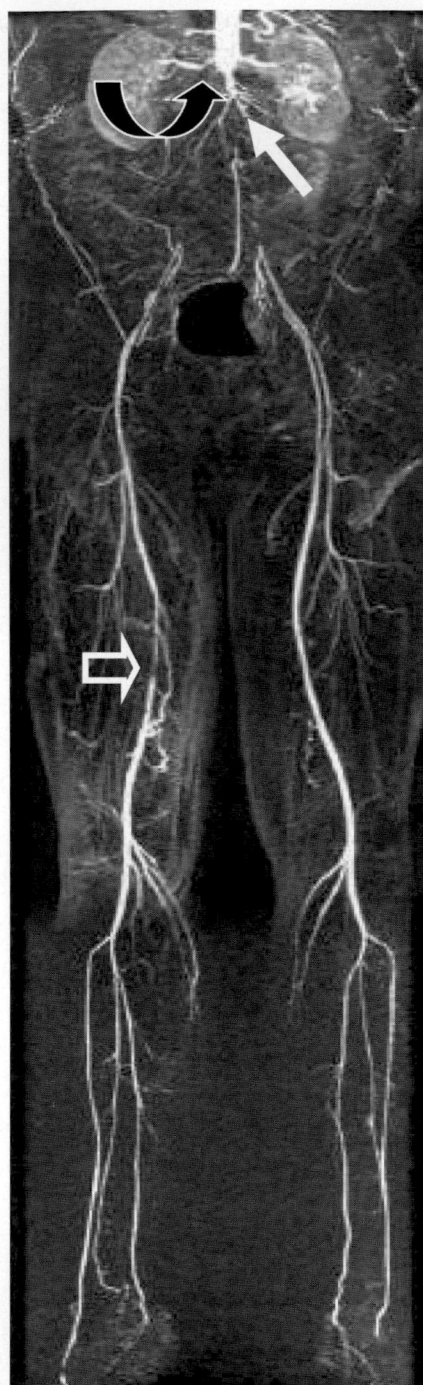

Figure 7–16 Coronal image depicting the entire abdominal and lower extremity circulation. The image is a combination of the MIP images from the pelvis and thigh station and the below-knee EC-TRICKS acquisition. Occlusion of the infrarenal abdominal aorta is shown with collateralization (*white arrow*), right renal artery stenosis (*black arrow*) and right superficial femoral artery occlusion or high-grade stenosis (*open arrow*). Three-vessel run-off is shown bilaterally.

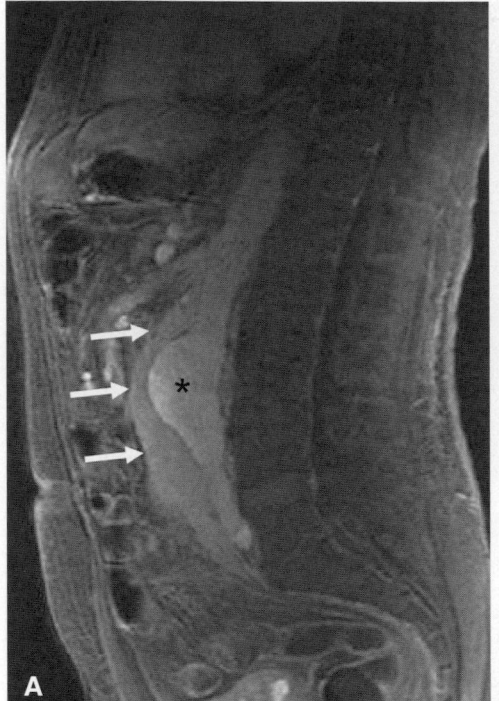

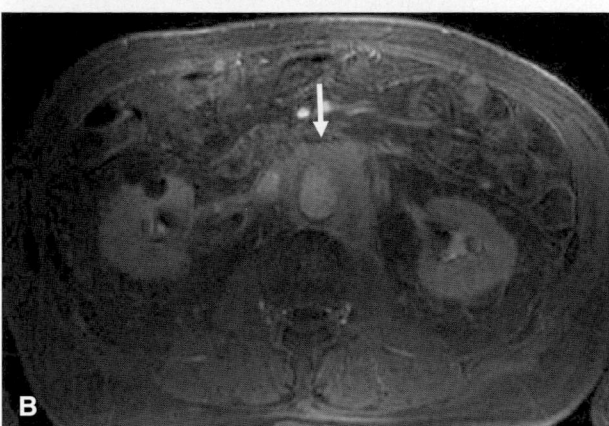

Figure 7–17 Sagittal **A.** and coronal **B.** images demonstrating an enhancing mantle of soft tissue surrounding the aneurysmal (*) abdominal aorta (*arrows*). The appearances represent an inflammatory aneurysm. At surgery, the ureters were encased by the inflammatory process.

Lower Extremity MRA

Assessment of the lower extremity arteries requires coverage from the distal aorta to the pedal arteries. To achieve this, the most routinely employed CE-MRA techniques are variations of the "bolus chase" technique (88–90). These methods, with incorporated table motion algorithms, employ a moving table top ("floating table") to image at more than one station, following a single or dual-phase injection of contrast medium (91). "Bolus chase" technique has now gained widespread acceptance as the foundation

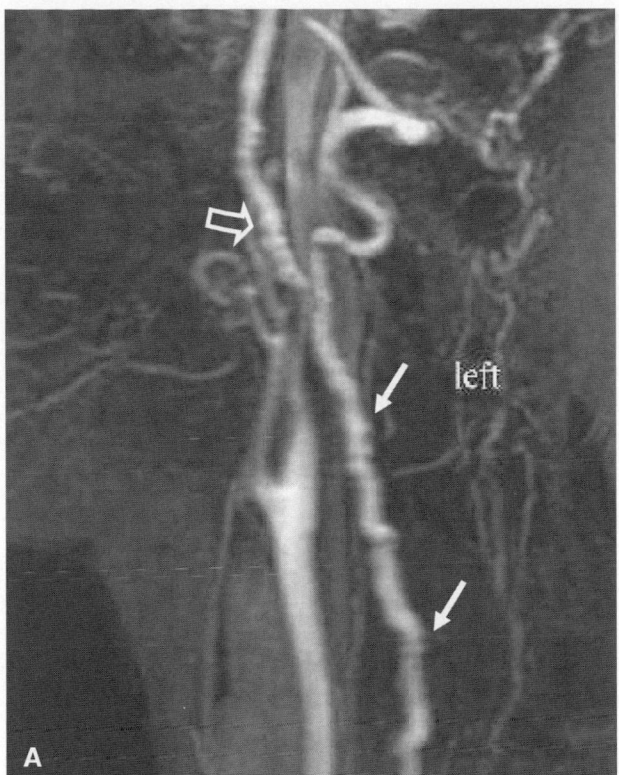

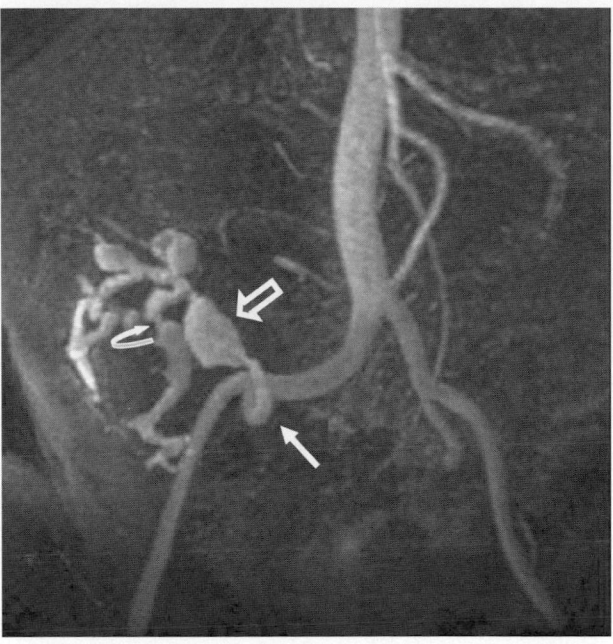

Figure 7–19 Coronal MIP image from 3D SPGR CE-MRA shows arterial phase enhancement of the arterial vessels of a renal transplant. The native right internal iliac artery has a normal appearance (*white arrow*) but there are multiple aneurysms (*open arrow*) and stenoses (*curved arrow*) in the donor transplant vessels consistent with chronic graft rejection.

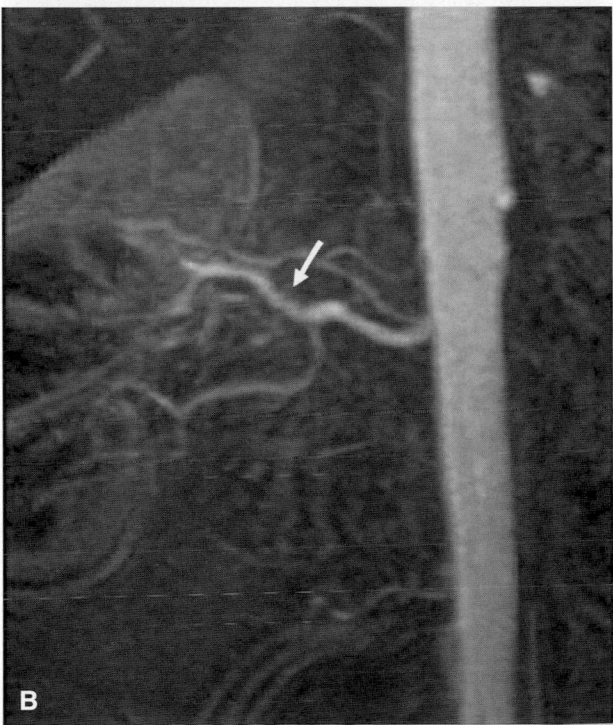

Figure 7–18 This 42-year-old patient presented with hypertension and transient ischemic episode like symptoms. The sagittal CE-MRA MIP image **A.** shows a characteristic "beaded" type appearance in the left vertebral (*white arrows*) and internal carotid vessel (*open arrow*). **B.** A similar appearance is seen on an oblique coronal MIP showing the right renal artery (*white arrow*) consistent with a diagnosis of fibromuscular dysplasia.

of any protocol evaluating peripheral vascular disease (15). This technique can be performed on most current MRI scanners ("Smartstep" from GE Medical Systems; "Mobitrack" from Philips, Best, Netherlands; "AngioSURF" from MR-Innovation and incorporated by Siemens Medical Solutions). Some of these platforms also incorporate automatic switching between coil elements and automatic patient repositioning between stations.

Image subtraction improves vessel to background contrast and for multi-injection studies, eliminates any background soft tissue or vessel enhancement, which may have occurred from the initial injection. Three-dimensional coronal spoiled gradient recalled echo is used as the principal sequence in our extremity MRA protocol and a precontrast (mask), arterial phase (during injection), and venous or delayed phase acquisition is performed. The arterial acquisition is triggered using "fluoro-triggering," and the pelvic and thigh stations are imaged using automated table motion. The addition of parallel imaging techniques, increasing the number of phased-array coil elements and more RF data channels further enhances the diagnostic value of CE-MRA (92).

To evaluate the below-knee vessels, a time-resolved sequence ("EC-TRICKS" from GE Healthcare) is employed. This is performed before imaging the pelvis and thigh stations and requires a separate injection. An average, 70-kg

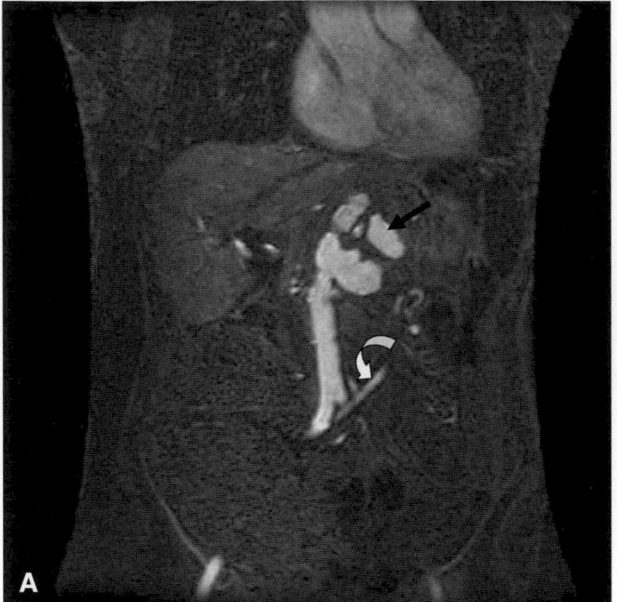

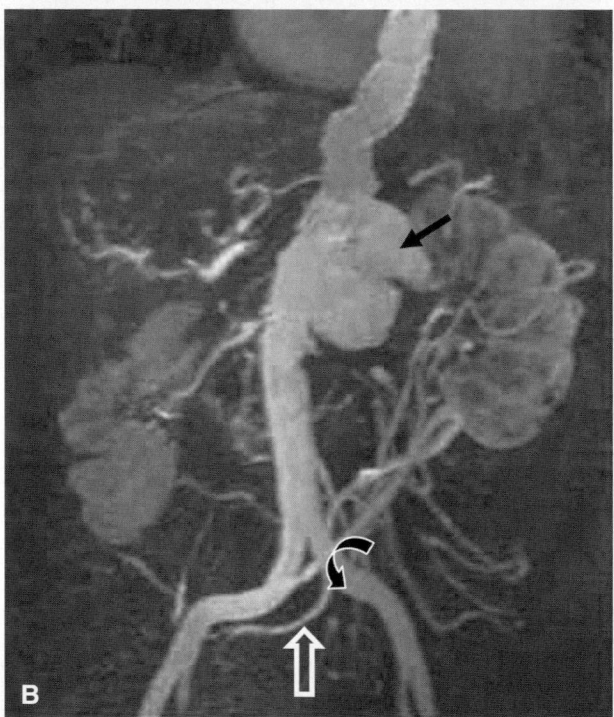

Figure 7–20 CE-MRA abdomen source image **A.** and MIP image **B.** demonstrate a bilobed pseudoaneurysm (*black arrow*) at the proximal anastomosis of an abdominal aneurysm repair. The superior mesenteric artery (*open arrow*) and left renal artery (*curved arrow*) were reimplanted in the common iliac vessels at the original repair.

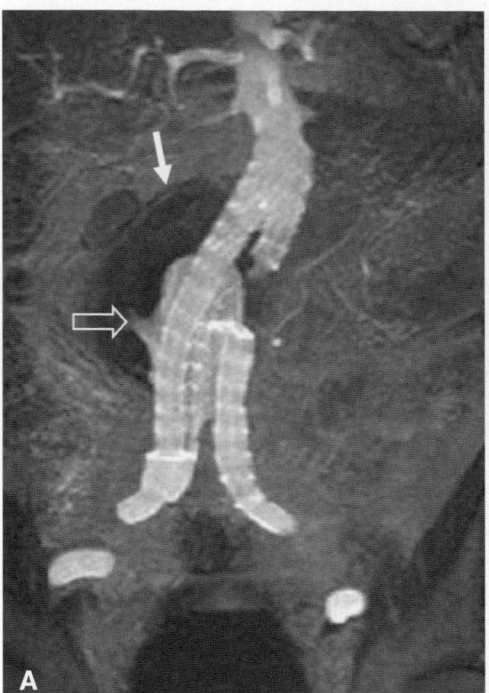

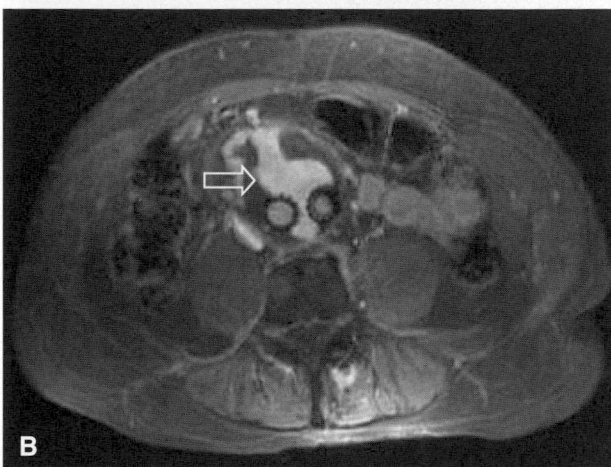

Figure 7–21 Oblique coronal MIP from a CE-MRA **A.** shows endovascular stents in both iliac arteries. There is an aneurysm sac surrounding the right limb of the graft (*white arrow*) and gadolinium contrast surrounds the stent within the sac (*open arrow*). The presence of an endo-leak is easily confirmed on axial postcontrast T_1 images **B.** Review of the source images showed this as a Type 1 endo-leak arising from the distal margin of the right iliac stent.

patient receives 12 mL gadolinium for below-knee imaging and 28 mL for the subsequent pelvis-thigh acquisitions (total 40 mL, approximately 0.3 mmol/kg). The temporal and spatial resolution and contrast-to-noise ratio allows superior evaluation of the distal vessel anatomy and flow dynamics when compared with single injection, multistep techniques or noncontrasted, 2D TOF technique, alone or combined (93). A delayed, postcontrast T_1 survey with fat-suppression, through the abdomen, pelvis, and lower extremities is routinely acquired, which frequently reveals additional clinical diagnostic information. CE-MRA is also useful in the diagnosis of popliteal entrapment syndrome (Figure 7–22).

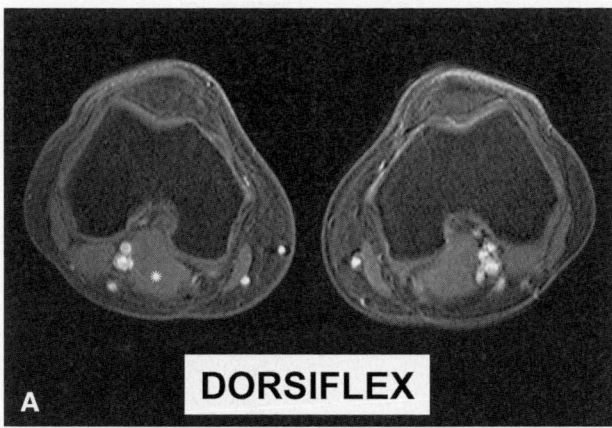

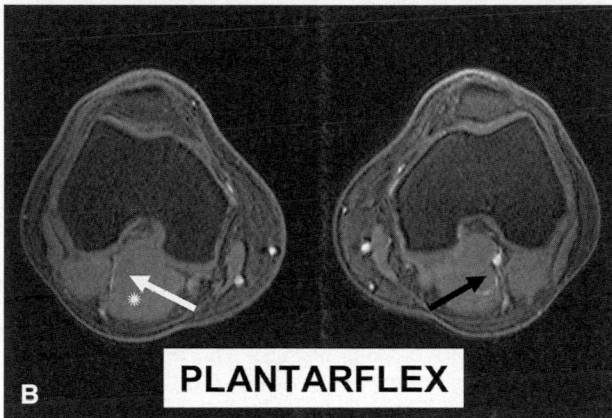

Figure 7–22 Postcontrast axial gradient echo images in a patient with popliteal entrapment syndrome. **A.** In dorsiflexion, the popliteal artery and vein are patent. **B.** Plantarflexion shows effacement of the popliteal artery and vein on the right (*white arrow*) and compression of the vein on the left (*black arrow*). There is hypertrophy of the medial head of gastrocnemius muscle (*) in this 22-year-old soccer player.

INTERVENTIONAL MR (X/MR OR COMBINED FLUOROSCOPY AND MRI INTERVENTION GUIDANCE)

MRI is an attractive means of guiding and monitoring interventional procedures (94–96). Most work on this technique has been experimental until recently, although some clinical applications exist. Fast imaging techniques, including SSFP (94) and projection reconstruction acquisitions (97) allow real-time monitoring with excellent spatial, contrast, and temporal resolution. Initial use of interventional MR has focused on neurosurgery and preliminary findings indicate a substantial benefit from intra-operative MR imaging in this context (98). Many endovascular therapies could potentially benefit from the intrinsic ability of MRI to discriminate between soft tissues and to measure functional parameters including blood flow and oxygenation (99,100). Development of miniature, RF coil-catheter, devices promises the opportunity to achieve high-resolution and high tissue contrast, images of

the vessel wall. This marriage of interventional radiology and MRI has exciting potential as the modality par excellence for imaging the "vulnerable" plaque (101). The vast majority of endovascular procedures, however, are performed with x-ray guidance, and MR currently cannot match the combination of temporal performance and spatial resolution that radiography affords (102). This is currently changing with the advent of parallel imaging and advances in coil technology, as well as introduction of floating table top interventional MRI designs (94,103). Although open, low-field, MRI scanners appear ideal for interventional application because of superior access to the patient, their slower imaging speed and lesser image quality make closed-bore design equipment the current, preferred modality.

SUMMARY

MRA, as currently practiced, represents a momentous advance in vascular imaging. It encompasses a diversity of sequences that can accurately illustrate vessel anatomy and flow dynamics. The rapid advances in MR technology predict the continued improvement in MRA as a diagnostic modality. Parallel advances in MRI compatible vascular interventional equipment predict the combined use of conventional angiography and MRI as a diagnostic and therapeutic tool. Successful implementation of this rapidly evolving technology relies on an understanding of the fundamental MRI sequences and their appropriate application to the clinical question under scrutiny.

REFERENCES

1. Prince MR, Yucel EK, Kaufman JA, et al. Dynamic gadolinium-enhanced three-dimensional abdominal MR arteriography. J Magn Reson Imaging 1993;3(6):877–881.
2. Jones JW, McCullough LB, Richman BW. The ethics of clinical pathways and cost control. J Vasc Surg 2003; 37(6):1341–1342.
3. Turnipseed W, Tefera G, Carr S. Comparison of minimal incision aortic surgery with endovascular aortic repair. Am J Surg 2003; 186(3):287–291.
4. Visser K, de Vries SO, Kitslaar PJ, et al. Cost-effectiveness of diagnostic imaging work-up and treatment for patients with intermittent claudication in The Netherlands. Eur J Vasc Endovasc Surg 2003;25(3):213–223.
5. Prince MR, Grist TM, Debatin JF. 3D Contrast MR Angiography, 3rd Ed. New York: Springer-Verlag, 2003.
6. Tatli S, Lipton MJ, Davison BD, et al. From the RSNA refresher courses: MR imaging of aortic and peripheral vascular disease. Radiographics 2003;23 Spec No: S59–78.
7. Baum RA, Rutter CM, Sunshine JH, et al. Multicenter trial to evaluate vascular magnetic resonance angiography of the lower extremity. American College of Radiology Rapid Technology Assessment Group. JAMA 1995;274(11):875–880.
8. Klein WM, Schlejen PM, Eikelboom BC, et al. MR angiography of the lower extremities with a moving-bed infusion-tracking technique. Cardiovasc Intervent Radiol 2003;26(1):1–8.
9. Fatouraee N, Amini AA. Regularization of flow streamlines in multislice phase-contrast MR imaging. IEEE Trans Med Imaging 2003;22(6):699–709.

10. Weiger M, Pruessmann KP, Kassner A, et al. Contrast-enhanced 3D MRA using SENSE. J Magn Reson Imaging 2000;12(5):671–677.
11. Sodickson DK, McKenzie CA, Ohliger MA, et al. Recent advances in image reconstruction, coil sensitivity calibration, and coil array design for SMASH and generalized parallel MRI. Magma 2002;13(3):158–163.
12. Kyriakos WE, Panych LP, Kacher DF, et al. Sensitivity profiles from an array of coils for encoding and reconstruction in parallel (SPACE RIP). Magn Reson Med 2000;44(2):301–308.
13. Corot C, Violas X, Robert P, et al. Comparison of different types of blood pool agents (P792, MS325, USPIO) in a rabbit MR angiography-like protocol. Invest Radiol 2003;38(6):311–319.
14. Nederkoorn PJ, van der Graaf Y, Eikelboom BC, et al. Time-of-flight MR angiography of carotid artery stenosis: does a flow void represent severe stenosis? AJNR Am J Neuroradiol 2002;23(10):1779–1784.
15. Meaney JF. Magnetic resonance angiography of the peripheral arteries: current status. Eur Radiol 2003;13(4):836–852.
16. Hausmann R. Imaging techniques of magnetic resonance angiography. In Magnetic Resonance Angiography, Arlart IP, Bongartz GM, Marchal G, eds. Berlin, Germany: Springer, 1996.
17. Ross JS, Masaryk TJ, Ruggieri PM. Magnetic resonance angiography of the carotid bifurcation. Top Magn Reson Imaging 1991;3(3):12–22.
18. Korosec FR, Mistretta CA. MR angiography: basic principles and theory. Magn Reson Imaging Clin N Am 1998;6(2):223–256.
19. Scheffler K, Lehnhardt S. Principles and applications of balanced SSFP techniques. Eur Radiol 2003;13(11):2409–2418.
20. Markl M, Alley MT, Pelc NJ. Balanced phase-contrast steady-state free precession (PC-SSFP): a novel technique for velocity encoding by gradient inversion. Magn Reson Med 2003;49(5):945–952.
21. Foo TK, Ho VB, Marcos HB, et al. MR angiography using steady-state free precession. Magn Reson Med. 2002;48(4):699–706.
22. Spuentrup E, Katoh M, Stuber M, et al. Coronary MR Imaging Using Free-Breathing 3D Steady-State Free Precession with Radial k-space Sampling. Rofo 2003;175(10):1330–1334.
23. Ho VB, Corse WR, Hood MN, et al. MRA of the thoracic vessels. Semin Ultrasound CT MR;2003. 24(4):192–216.
24. Stemerman DH, Krinsky GA, Lee VS, et al. Thoracic aorta: rapid black-blood MR imaging with half-Fourier rapid acquisition with relaxation enhancement with or without electrocardiographic triggering. Radiology 1999;213(1):185–191.
25. Reimer P, Boos M. Phase-contrast MR angiography of peripheral arteries: technique and clinical application. Eur Radiol 1999;9(1):22–127.
26. Elster AD. Gradient-echo MR imaging: techniques and acronyms. Radiology 1993;186(1):1–8.
27. Iseda T, Nakano S, Miyahara D, et al. Poststenotic signal attenuation on 3D phase-contrast MR angiography: a useful finding in haemodynamically significant carotid artery stenosis. Neuroradiology 2000;42(12):868–873.
28. Barger AV, Peters DC, Block WF, et al. Phase-contrast with interleaved undersampled projections. Magn Reson Med 2000;43(4):503–509.
29. Papathanasopoulou P, Zhao S, Kohler U, et al. MRI measurement of time-resolved wall shear stress vectors in a carotid bifurcation model, and comparison with CFD predictions. J Magn Reson Imaging 2003;17(2):153–162.
30. Schoenberg SO, Rieger J, Nittka M, et al. Renal MR angiography: current debates and developments in imaging of renal artery stenosis. Semin Ultrasound CT MR 2003;24(4):255–267.
31. Hood MN, Ho VB, Corse WR. Three-dimensional phase-contrast magnetic resonance angiography: a useful clinical adjunct to gadolinium-enhanced three-dimensional renal magnetic resonance angiography? Mil Med 2002;167(4):343–349.
32. Swan SK, Lambrecht LJ, Townsend R, et al. Safety and pharmacokinetic profile of gadobenate dimeglumine in subjects with renal impairment. Invest Radiol 1999;34(7): 443–448.
33. Runge VM, Wells JW. Update: safety, new applications, new MR agents. Top Magn Reson Imaging 1995;7(3):181–195.
34. Mahfouz AE. MS-325 Epix. Curr Opin Investig Drugs 2000;1(4):476–480.
35. Grist TM, Korosec FR, Peters DC, et al. Steady-state and dynamic MR angiography with MS-325: initial experience in humans. Radiology 1998;207(2):539–544.
36. Bluemke DA, Stillman AE, Bis KG, et al. Carotid MR angiography: phase II study of safety and efficacy for MS-325. Radiology 2001;219(1):114–122.
37. Dong Q, Hurst DR, Weinmann HJ, et al. Magnetic resonance angiography with gadomer-17. An animal study original investigation. Invest Radiol 1998;33(9):699–708.
38. Leiner T, Ho KY, Ho VB, et al. Multicenter phase-II trial of safety and efficacy of NC100150 for steady-state contrast-enhanced peripheral magnetic resonance angiography. Eur Radiol 2003;13(7):1620–1627.
39. Svensson J, Petersson JS, Stahlberg F, et al. Image artifacts due to a time-varying contrast medium concentration in 3D contrast-enhanced MRA. J Magn Reson Imaging 1999;10(6):919–928.
40. Maki JH, Prince MR, Chenevert TC. Optimizing three-dimensional gadolinium-enhanced magnetic resonance angiography. Original investigation. Invest Radiol 1998;33(9):528–537.
41. Frayne R, Omary RA, Unal O, et al. Determination of optimal injection parameters for intra-arterial gadolinium-enhanced MR angiography. J Vasc Interv Radiol 2000;11(10):1277–1284.
42. Prince MR, Chabra SG, Watts R, et al. Contrast material travel times in patients undergoing peripheral MR angiography. Radiology 2002;224(1):55–61.
43. Maki JH, Wilson GJ, Eubank WB, et al. Predicting venous enhancement in peripheral MRA using a two station timing bolus. In: Proc Int Soc Magn Reson Med, 11th Annu Meet 2003.
44. Foo TK, Saranathan M, Prince MR, et al. Automated detection of bolus arrival and initiation of data acquisition in fast, three-dimensional, gadolinium-enhanced MR angiography. Radiology 1997;203(1):275–280.
45. Shetty AN, Bis KG, Vrachliotis TG, et al. Contrast-enhanced 3D MRA with centric ordering in k-space: a preliminary clinical experience in imaging the abdominal aorta and renal and peripheral arterial vasculature. J Magn Reson Imaging 1998;8(6):1355.
46. Du J, Carroll TJ, Wagner HJ, et al. Time-resolved, undersampled projection reconstruction imaging for high-resolution CE-MRA of the distal runoff vessels. Magn Reson Med 2002;48(3):516–522.
47. Wang Y, Chen CZ, Chabra SG, et al. Bolus arterial-venous transit in the lower extremity and venous contamination in bolus chase three-dimensional magnetic resonance angiography. Invest Radiol 2002;37(8): 458–463.
48. Yucel EK, SK Reid. Pitfalls of Moving-Table Peripheral MRA. In: XII International Workshop on Magnetic Resonance Angiography, 2002, Lyon, France.
49. Turski PA, Korosec FR, Carroll TJ, et al. Contrast-enhanced magnetic resonance angiography of the carotid bifurcation using the time-resolved imaging of contrast kinetics (TRICKS) technique. Top Magn Reson Imaging 2001;12(3):175–181.
50. Du J, Carroll TJ, Block WF, et al. SNR improvement for multi-injection time-resolved high-resolution CE-MRA of the peripheral vasculature. Magn Reson Med 2003;49(5):909–917.
51. Barger AV, Block WF, Toropov Y, et al. Time-resolved contrast-enhanced imaging with isotropic resolution and broad coverage using an undersampled 3D projection trajectory. Magn Reson Med 2002;48(2):297–305.
52. van den Brink JS, Watanabe Y, Kuhl CK, et al. Implications of SENSE MR in routine clinical practice. Eur J Radiol 2003;46(1):3–27.
53. Madore B. Using UNFOLD to remove artifacts in parallel imaging and in partial-Fourier imaging. Magn Reson Med 2002;48(3):493–501.
54. Goldman JP. Single pass four station peripheral vascular MRA utilizing parallel imaging: imaging from the renal arteries to the foot in 31 seconds. In: International Society for Magnetic Resonance in Medicine, 11th Annu Meet 2003.
55. Maki JH, Wilson GJ, Eubank WB, et al. Utilizing SENSE to achieve lower station sub-millimeter isotropic resolution and minimal venous enhancement in peripheral MR angiography. J Magn Reson Imaging 2002;15(4):484–491.
56. Foo TK, Ho VB, Hood MN, et al. High-spatial-resolution multistation MR imaging of lower-extremity peripheral vasculature

with segmented volume acquisition: feasibility study. Radiology 2001;219(3):835–841.

57. Falk E. Why do plaques rupture? Circulation 1992;86(6 Suppl): III30–42.

58. Choi CJ, Kramer CM. MR imaging of atherosclerotic plaque. Radiol Clin North Am 2002;40(4):887–898.

59. Quick HH, Debatin JF, Ladd ME. MR imaging of the vessel wall. Eur Radiol 2002;12(4):889–900.

60. Yuan C, Miller ZE, Cai J, et al. Carotid atherosclerotic wall imaging by MRI. Neuroimaging Clin N Am 2002;12(3):391–401, vi.

61. Ruehm SG. Magnetic resonance imaging of atherosclerotic plaque. Herz 2003;28(6):513–50.

62. Bartels LW, Bakker CJ, Viergever MA. Improved lumen visualization in metallic vascular implants by reducing RF artifacts. Magn Reson Med 2002;47(1):171–180.

63. Ludeke KM, Roschmann P, Tischler R. Susceptibility artefacts in NMR imaging. Magn Reson Imaging 1985;3(4):329–343.

64. Eustace S, Goldberg R, Williamson D, et al. MR imaging of soft tissues adjacent to orthopaedic hardware: techniques to minimize susceptibility artifact. Clin Radiol 1997;52(8):589–594.

65. Baum F, Vosshenrich R, Fischer U, et al. [Stent artifacts in 3D MR angiography: experimental studies]. Rofo 2000;172(3):278–281.

66. Klemm T, Duda S, Machann J, et al. MR imaging in the presence of vascular stents: a systematic assessment of artifacts for various stent orientations, sequence types, and field strengths. J Magn Reson Imaging 2000;12(4):606–615.

67. Meyer JM, Buecker A, Spuentrup E, et al. Improved in-stent magnetic resonance angiography with high flip angle excitation. Invest Radiol 2001;36(11):677–681.

68. Nitatori T, Hanaoka H, Hachiya J, et al. MRI artifacts of metallic stents derived from imaging sequencing and the ferromagnetic nature of materials. Radiat Med 1999;17(4):329–334.

69. Maintz D, Kugel H, Schellhammer F, et al. In vitro evaluation of intravascular stent artifacts in three-dimensional MR angiography. Invest Radiol 2001;36(4):218–224.

70. Neimatallah MA, Chenevert TL, Carlos RC, et al. Subclavian MR arteriography: reduction of susceptibility artifact with short echo time and dilute gadopentetate dimeglumine. Radiology 2000;217(2):581–586.

71. Elster AD, Burdette JH. Questions and Answers in Magnetic Resonance Imaging. 2nd Ed. St. Louis: Mosby, 2001.

72. Carroll TJ, Korosec FR, Swan JS, et al. The effect of injection rate on time-resolved contrast-enhanced peripheral MRA. J Magn Reson Imaging 2001;14(4):401–410.

73. Lee JJ, Chang Y, Tirman PJ, et al. Optimizing of gadolinium-enhanced MR angiography by manipulation of acquisition and scan delay times. Eur Radiol 2001;11(5):754–766.

74. Maki JH, Prince MR, Londy FJ, et al. The effects of time varying intravascular signal intensity and k-space acquisition order on three-dimensional MR angiography image quality. J Magn Reson Imaging 1996;6(4):642–651.

75. Maki JH, Chenevert TL, Prince MR. The effects of incomplete breath-holding on 3D MR image quality. J Magn Reson Imaging 1997;7(6):1132–1139.

76. Vasbinder GB, Maki JH, Nijenhuis RJ, et al. Motion of the distal renal artery during three-dimensional contrast-enhanced breath-hold MRA. J Magn Reson Imaging 2002;16(6):685–696.

77. Ohno Y, Adachi S, Motoyama A, et al. Multiphase ECG-triggered 3D contrast-enhanced MR angiography: utility for evaluation of hilar and mediastinal invasion of bronchogenic carcinoma. J Magn Reson Imaging 2001;13(2):215–224.

78. Arpasi PJ, Bis KG, Shetty AN, et al. MR angiography of the thoracic aorta with an electrocardiographically triggered breath-hold contrast-enhanced sequence. Radiographics 2000;20(1): 107–120.

79. Svensson LG, Labib SB, Eisenhauer AC, et al. Intimal tear without hematoma: an important variant of aortic dissection that can elude current imaging techniques. Circulation 1999;99(10):1331–1336.

80. van der Loo B, Jenni R. Acute aortic syndrome: proposal for a novel classification. Heart 2003;89(8):928.

81. Angeli E, Vanzulli A, Venturini M, et al. The role of radiology in the diagnosis and management of Takayasu's arteritis. J Nephrol 2001;14(6):514–524.

82. Oshinski JN, Parks WJ, Markou CP, et al. Improved measurement of pressure gradients in aortic coarctation by magnetic resonance imaging. J Am Coll Cardiol 1996;28(7):1818–1826.

83. Ho VB, Corse WR. MR angiography of the abdominal aorta and peripheral vessels. Radiol Clin North Am 2003;41(1):115–144.

84. Chow LC, Chan FP, Li KC. A comprehensive approach to MR imaging of mesenteric ischemia. Abdom Imaging 2002;27(5):507–516.

85. Omary RA, Baden JG, Becker BN, et al. Impact of MR angiography on the diagnosis and management of renal transplant dysfunction. J Vasc Interv Radiol 2000;11(8):991–996.

86. Eubank WB, Wherry KL, Maki JH, et al. Preoperative evaluation of patients awaiting liver transplantation: comparison of multiphasic contrast-enhanced 3D magnetic resonance to helical computed tomography examinations. J Magn Reson Imaging 2002;16(5):565–575.

87. Vosshenrich R, Fischer U, Grabbe E. [MR-angiography in portal hypertension. State of the art]. Radiologe 2001;41(10):868–876.

88. Goldman JP, Andrew S, Teodurescu V. Increased opacification of the pedal vasculature in one run moving table bolus chase MRA by employing a biphasic contrast bolus timed to the aortic bifurcation and the feet. In: International Society for Magnetic Resonance in Medicine, 11th Annu Meet 2003.

89. Ho VB, Choyke PL, Foo TK, et al. Automated bolus chase peripheral MR angiography: initial practical experiences and future directions of this work-in-progress. J Magn Reson Imaging 1999;10(3):376–388.

90. Fain SB, et al. Time-resolved whole body MRA during continuous table motion using floating table isotrophic projection acquisition (FLIPR). In: International Society for Magnetic Resonance in Medicine, 11th Annu Meet 2003.

91. Leiner T, Ho KY, Nelemans PJ, et al. Three-dimensional contrast-enhanced moving-bed infusion-tracking (MoBI-track) peripheral MR angiography with flexible choice of imaging parameters for each field of view. J Magn Reson Imaging 2000;11(4): 368–377.

92. Carroll TJ, Grist TM. Technical developments in MR angiography. Radiol Clin North Am 2002;40(4):921–951.

93. Thornton FJ, Du J, Suleiman SA, et al. High resolution, time-resolved MRA provides superior definition of lower extremity arterial segments. In: International Society for Magnetic Resonance in Medicine, 11th Annu Meet 2003.

94. Quick HH, Kuehl H, Kaiser G, et al. Interventional MRA using actively visualized catheters, TrueFISP, and real-time image fusion. Magn Reson Med 2003;49(1):129–137.

95. Sewell PE, Howard JC, Shingleton WB, et al. Interventional magnetic resonance image-guided percutaneous cryoablation of renal tumors. South Med J 2003;96(7):708–710.

96. Omary RA, Green J, Finn JP, et al. Catheter-directed gadolinium-enhanced MR angiography. Radiol Clin North Am 2002;40(4): 953–963.

97. Fain SB, Du J, Browning FJ, et al. Floating table isotropic projection imaging (FLIPR): a technique for fast extended FOV, contrast enhanced MRA (abstract). In: International Society for Magnetic Resonance in Medicine, Proc 10th Scientific Meeting 2002, Berkley, California.

98. Samset E, Hirschberg E. Image-guided stereotaxy in the interventional MRI. Minim Invasive Neurosurg 2003;46(1):5–10.

99. Rickers C, Jerosch-Herold M, Hu X, et al. Magnetic resonance image-guided transcatheter closure of atrial septal defects. Circulation 2003;107(1):132–138.

100. Wilson MW, Fidelman N, Weber OM, et al. Experimental renal artery embolization in a combined MR imaging/angiographic unit. J Vasc Interv Radiol 2003;14(9 Pt 1):1169–1175.

101. Ladd ME, Quick HH, Debatin JF. Interventional MRA and intravascular imaging. J Magn Reson Imaging 2000;12(4):534–546.

102. Zimmermann-Paul GG, Ladd ME, Pfammatter T, et al. MR versus fluoroscopic guidance of a catheter/guidewire system: in vitro comparison of steerability. J Magn Reson Imaging 1998;8(5): 1177–1181.

103. Quick HH, Kuehl H, Kaiser G, et al. Interventional MR angiography with a floating table. Radiology 2003;229(2):598–602.

Tools of the Trade

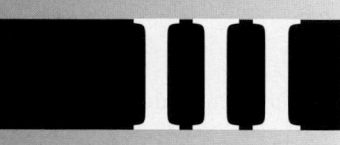

Basic Surgical Techniques for the Interventional Radiologist

8

Edward Y. Woo, Jeffrey P. Carpenter

Traditionally, interventional treatment of vascular disease has been approached through open surgery. With the advent of endovascular techniques, however, minimally invasive therapies have received increasing emphasis. In many cases, iliac angioplasty and stenting, for example, are supplanting open surgery for the treatment of aortoiliac disease. Furthermore, endovascular stent grafting is being used in the treatment of many abdominal aortic aneurysms. Many of these approaches are performed through percutaneous procedures, but they often must combine with open surgical techniques. For example, because of the large sheath size, AAA stent grafting often still requires direct access to the femoral artery. In addition, open techniques continue to be used in endovascular therapy. In repairing common iliac aneurysms that extend to the internal iliac arteries, relocation of the internal iliacs or direct suture to the iliac artery has been performed (1,2). Furthermore, complications can arise during the placement of endovascular devices, which can require urgent or emergent surgical intervention.

Understanding all of the surgical approaches and techniques involved with treating vascular disease requires full training in vascular surgery, which is beyond the scope of this chapter. However, basic surgical techniques, which should be understood fully when endovascular procedures are performed, are addressed in the following sections.

FUNDAMENTALS OF SURGICAL TECHNIQUE

Having a complete grasp of basic surgical technique is critical to performing an operation, and learning about the instruments that are available is an important place to begin. The following is a description of the basic instruments used in vascular procedures.

To start, scalpels are commonly used with #10, #11, and #15 blades. The #10 blade is the standard scalpel blade used for most incisions. The #15 blade is thinner and useful for smaller incisions and curvilinear cuts. The #11 blade comes to a pointed end and is useful for precise incisions, such as for arteriotomy. Sharp dissection is also carried out with scissors, the most common of which are Metzenbaum and Church scissors. These are used most often for tissue dissection. In contrast, Potts scissors are used to incise vessel walls, including during an arteriotomy. In aiding dissection, several different types of forceps are available. Noncrushing or toothed forceps, such as Adson forceps, should be used on the skin to prevent crush injury and subsequent devitalization of the skin. Debakey forceps are useful for dissection and handling of tissues other than skin. Gerald or Potts forceps, which come to a fine tip, aid in precision dissection and suturing.

Sutures are available in absorbable and permanent varieties, including monofilament and braided. They are defined by their diameter and identified by numbers. Smaller numbers indicate a larger suture. For instance, a 2-0 suture is larger than a 4-0. Needles are defined by their shape and size. Varying needles (straight or curved, tapered or cutting) can be attached to varying sutures. Experience will dictate the suture and needle that are most applicable to each situation. Suturing is accomplished with needle

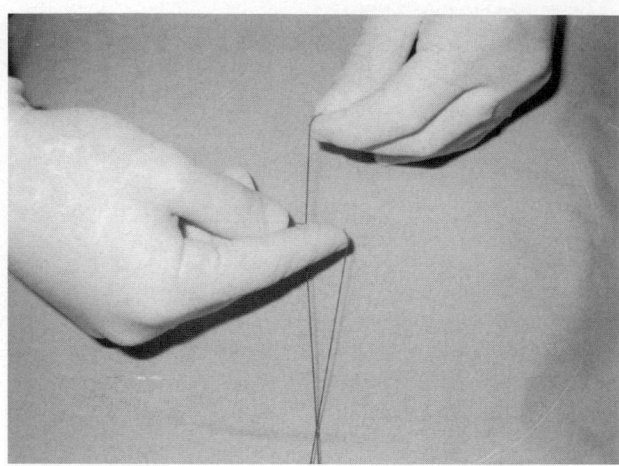

Figure 8–1   Leading with the index finger for a two-handed knot.

holders. These come in many shapes and sizes depending on the suturing to be performed. For example, Castroviejo needle drivers are used for operating with small sutures such as 6-0 or 7-0.

Knot-tying completes the suturing by securing the suture in place. Two-handed and one-handed knots can be performed. The two-handed knot is simpler to perform and begins by leading the suture with the index finger (Figure 8–1). The other hand passes the other end of the suture to the ipsilateral thumb and index finger, which guide the end downward between the two lengths (Figure 8–2). The knot is then pushed down (Figure 8–3). To complete the square knot, the ipsilateral end is led with the thumb (Figure 8–4). The contralateral end is then passed by the other hand to the ipsilateral index finger and thumb, which bring it up and through the two lengths (Figure 8–5). With each throw, it is important to bring the knot all the way down to the point being tied. A one-handed knot is slightly more complex, but it can be per-

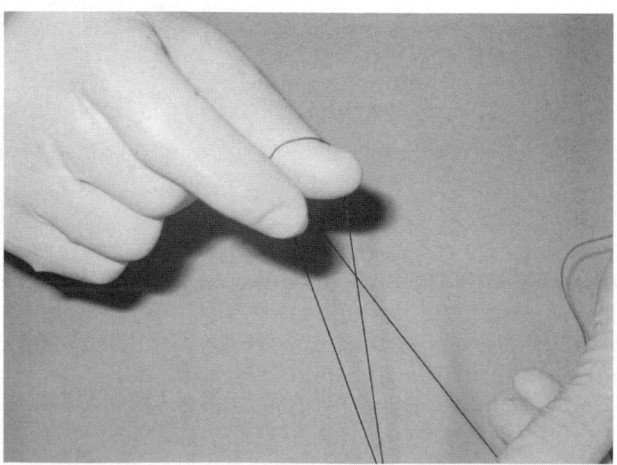

Figure 8–2   Passing the suture through on a two-handed knot.

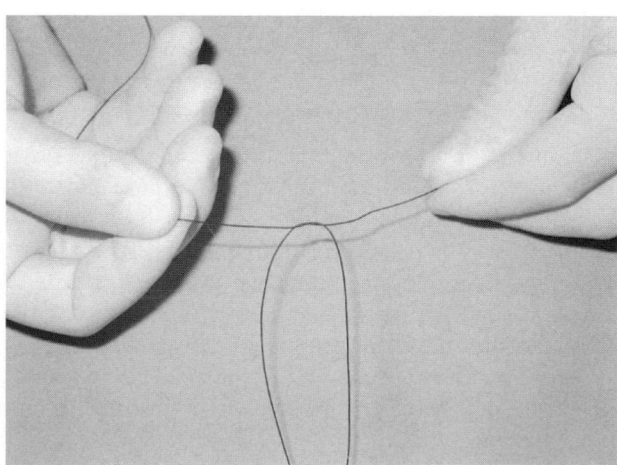

Figure 8–3   Completion of the knot.

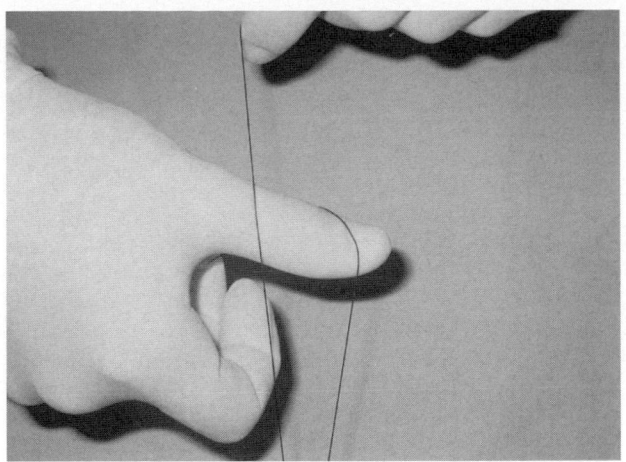

Figure 8–4   Leading with the thumb for a two-handed knot.

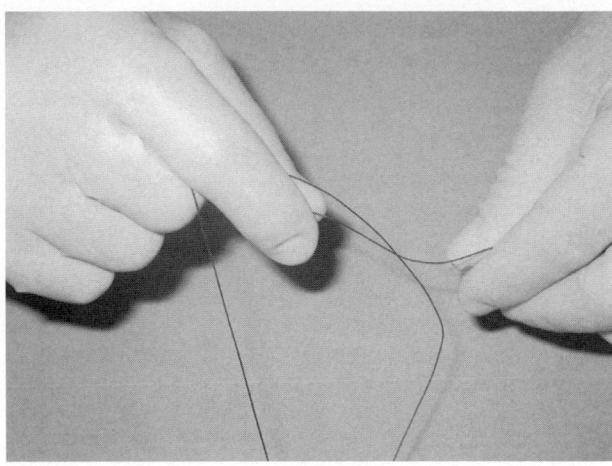

Figure 8–5   Passing the suture through on a two-handed knot.

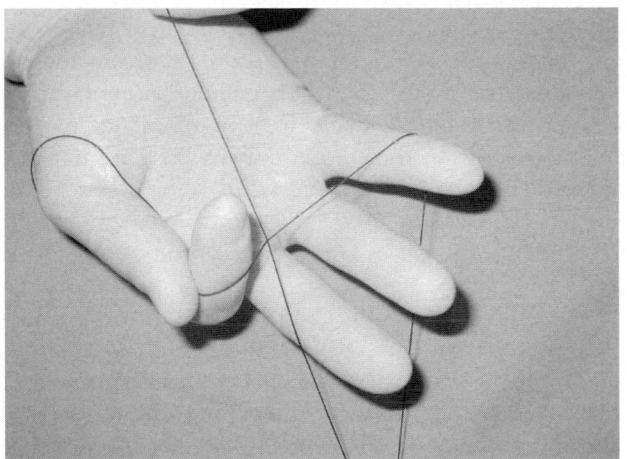

Figure 8–6   First formation of a one-handed knot.

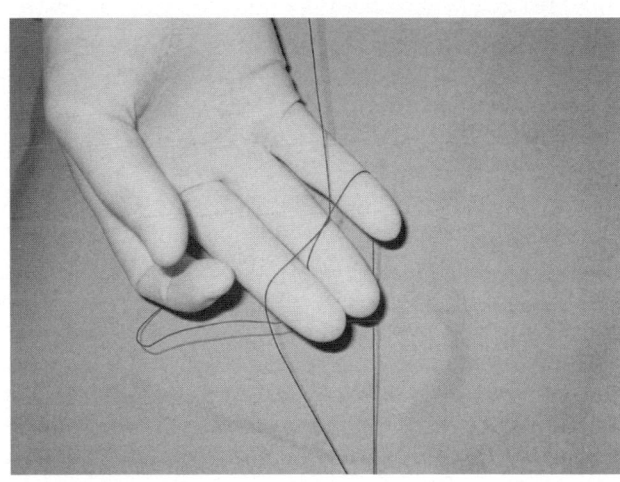

Figure 8–7   Grasping the suture.

formed faster. The ipsilateral end of the suture is bent with the fourth or fifth finger (Figure 8–6). The ipsilateral end is then hooked between the third and fourth finger, and this end is brought down and through the two lengths (Figures 8–7 and 8–8). The knot is then pushed down. The square knot is completed by the ipsilateral index finger being brought down between both lengths (Figure 8–9). The index finger then hooks the ipsilateral end bringing it upward through both lengths (Figure 8–10). Ensuring that the knots are tied down all the way is an important step. The number of knots thrown depends on the suture used. Mastering one-handed and two-handed knots is simple with practice.

Ultimately, all procedures are simplified with appropriate retraction. Except for the extraperitoneal dissection, which requires an abdominal retractor, the vascular exposures described in this chapter can be done with a small self-retaining retractor, such as the Weitlaner (Beckman).

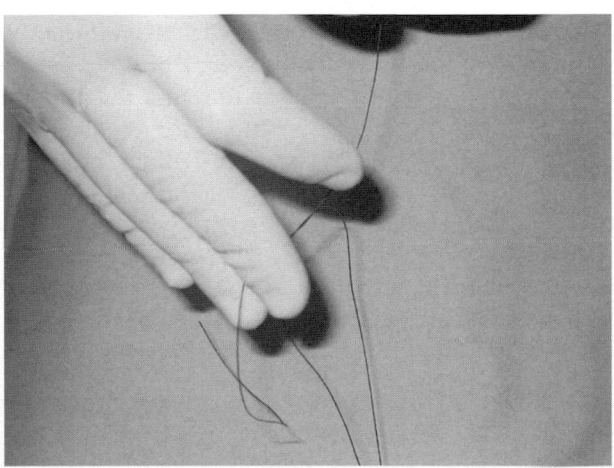

Figure 8–8   Pulling the suture through to complete the knot.

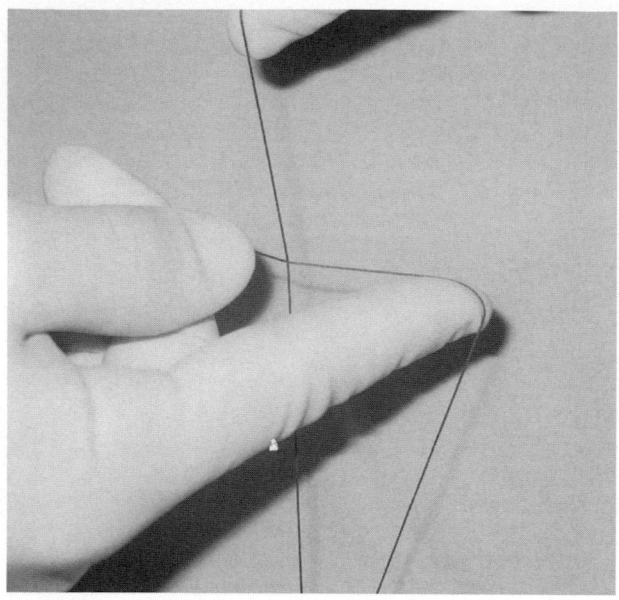

Figure 8–9 Second formation of a one-handed knot.

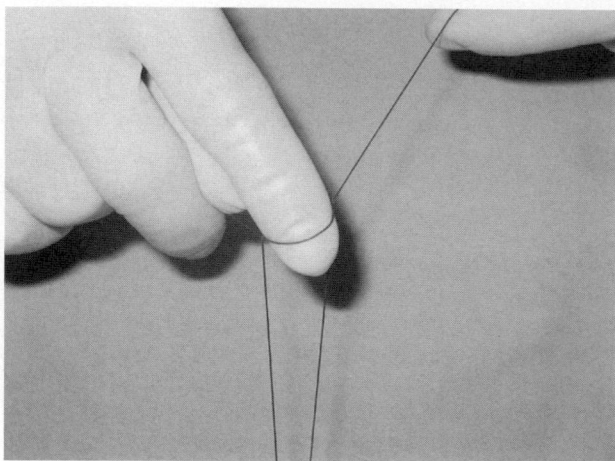

Figure 8–10 Pulling the suture through with the index finger.

ANATOMY

A comprehensive understanding of anatomy is crucial to performing open surgical procedures. Familiarity with the structures of interest, as well as the neighboring structures, is of the utmost importance. It not only allows access to the vessel of interest, but it minimizes injury to the surrounding structures.

Regarding endovascular procedures, the femoral triangle (Figure 8–11) is the most commonly accessed area. It consists of the femoral artery and vein, the femoral nerve, the lateral femoral cutaneous nerve, the femoral branches of the genitofemoral nerve, lymphatic vessels, and superficial inguinal lymph nodes. It is bordered by the inguinal ligament superiorly, the adductor longus medially, and the sartorius laterally. The apex is formed where the latter two muscles meet (3). The iliopsoas and the pectineus muscles form the floor of the triangle. The common femoral artery begins when the external iliac artery traverses beneath the inguinal ligament. It is actually quite short and extends approximately 4 cm before branching into the profunda femoris and superficial femoral artery. The profunda travels posterolaterally off the common femoral artery and supplies most of the blood to the thigh. It also forms collaterals to the pelvis and lower extremity. The superficial femoral artery travels down the leg becoming the popliteal artery and branching to the vessels of the lower leg. The common femoral artery is located lateral to the femoral vein and medial to the femoral nerve posterior to the deep fascia. It overlies the head of the femur.

This concept is important for two reasons. First, it serves as a guide for radiographic location of the artery. Second, compression of the artery against the femoral head allows for hemostasis after percutaneous interventions. The common femoral vein is formed by the confluence of the superficial femoral vein, deep femoral vein, and greater saphenous vein. It lies medial to the common femoral artery and runs posterior to the inguinal ligament where it becomes the external iliac vein. The major nerve in the femoral triangle is the femoral nerve, which lies lateral to the artery. Its main role is innervation of the anterior thigh muscles. The lateral femoral cutaneous nerve and femoral branches of the genitofemoral nerve serve as sensory nerves to the skin.

Although the external iliac vessels are not exposed as often as the femoral vessels, it is important to be familiar with this exposure. The external iliac arteries are the major blood supply to the lower extremities arising from the common iliac arteries. They lie deep in the posterior abdomen in the retroperitoneal space. The psoas muscle is located laterally, over which the genitofemoral nerve travels (3). The external iliac vein is medial to the artery. The ureters cross the iliac arteries approximately at the level of the iliac bifurcation, after which they run medial to the vessels. Lymphatic vessels and the deep inguinal lymph nodes surround the iliac vessels. Unlike the other surrounding structures, the lymphatics can be divided when access to the artery or vein is needed. As the external iliac artery travels distally, it courses upward from the posterior abdomen. At that point, it gives off the inferior epigastric artery just proximal to the inguinal ligament and becomes the femoral artery in the anterior thigh. As it travels anteriorly, accidental injury can occur to it during percutaneous procedures (4). Because tamponading bleeding from the external iliac artery is difficult, these injuries often can be quite morbid and lead to significant blood loss. Thus, during percutaneous procedures, it is vital to ensure that the artery is punctured distal to the inguinal ligament—femoral artery, for example—as this is easily controlled by direct pressure.

The brachial artery is the main blood supply to the upper extremity. It is formed by the continuation of the

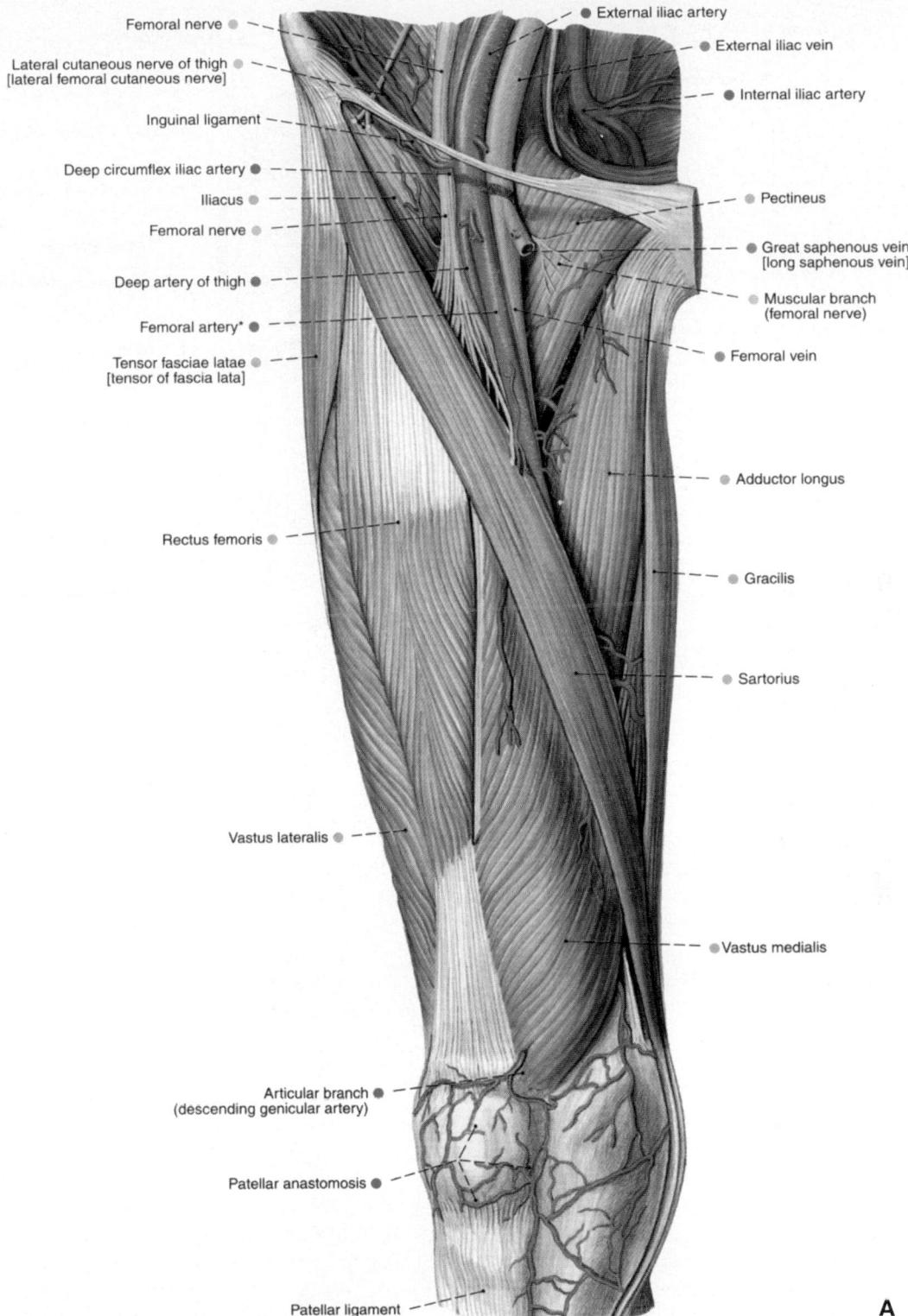

Figure 8–11 A, B. Right femoral triangle (anatomical dissection). (Reprinted with permission from Putz R, Pabst R, eds. Sobotta Atlas of Human Anatomy. 13th Latin Edition [English text with Latin nomenclature]. Baltimore: Lippincott Williams & Wilkins 2001.)

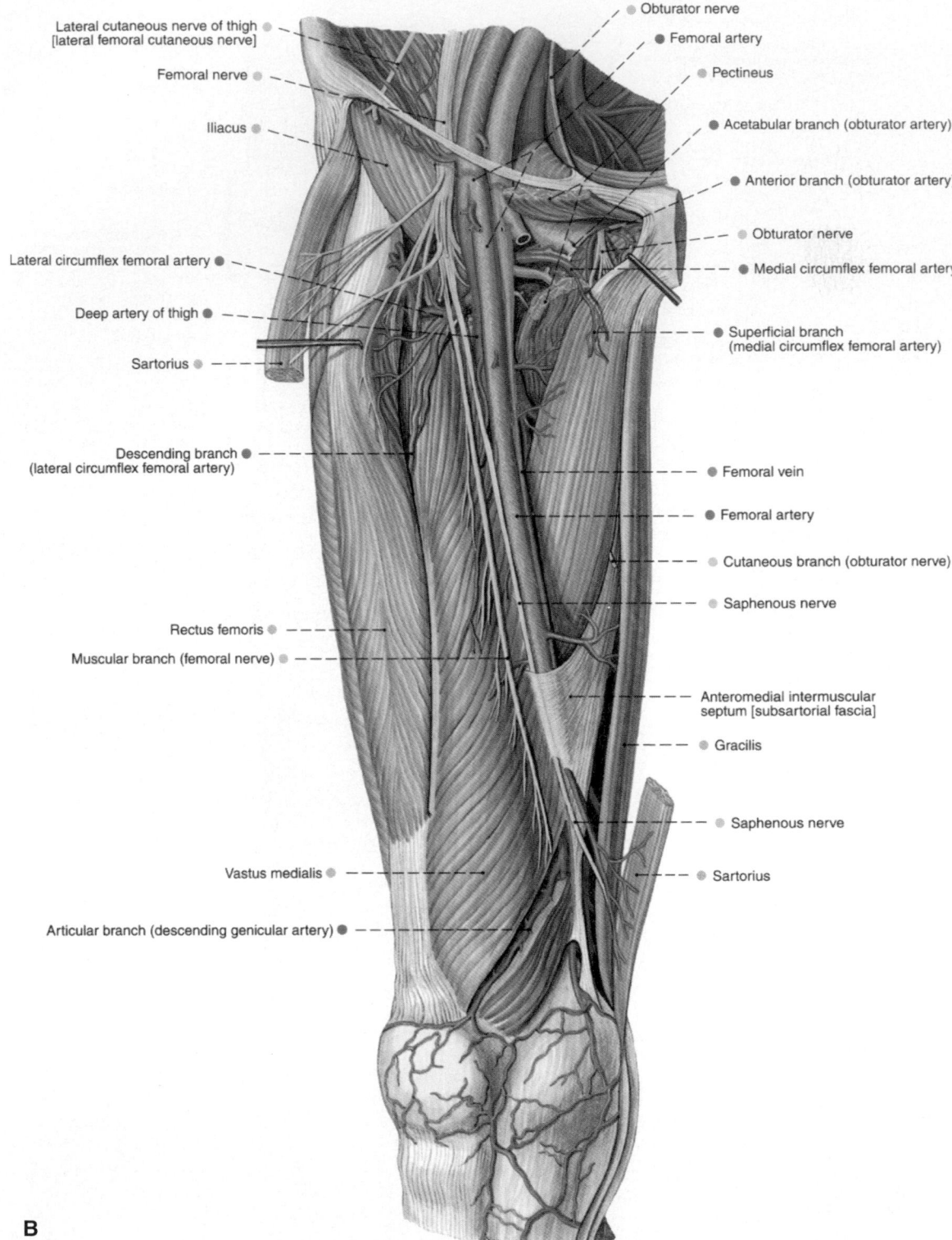

Lateral cutaneous nerve of thigh
[lateral femoral cutaneous nerve]

Femoral nerve

Iliacus

Lateral circumflex femoral artery

Deep artery of thigh

Sartorius

Descending branch
(lateral circumflex femoral artery)

Rectus femoris

Muscular branch (femoral nerve)

Vastus medialis

Articular branch (descending genicular artery)

Obturator nerve

Femoral artery

Pectineus

Acetabular branch (obturator artery)

Anterior branch (obturator artery)

Obturator nerve

Medial circumflex femoral artery

Superficial branch
(medial circumflex femoral artery)

Femoral vein

Femoral artery

Cutaneous branch (obturator nerve)

Saphenous nerve

Anteromedial intermuscular
septum [subsartorial fascia]

Gracilis

Saphenous nerve

Sartorius

B

Figure 8–11 *(continued)*

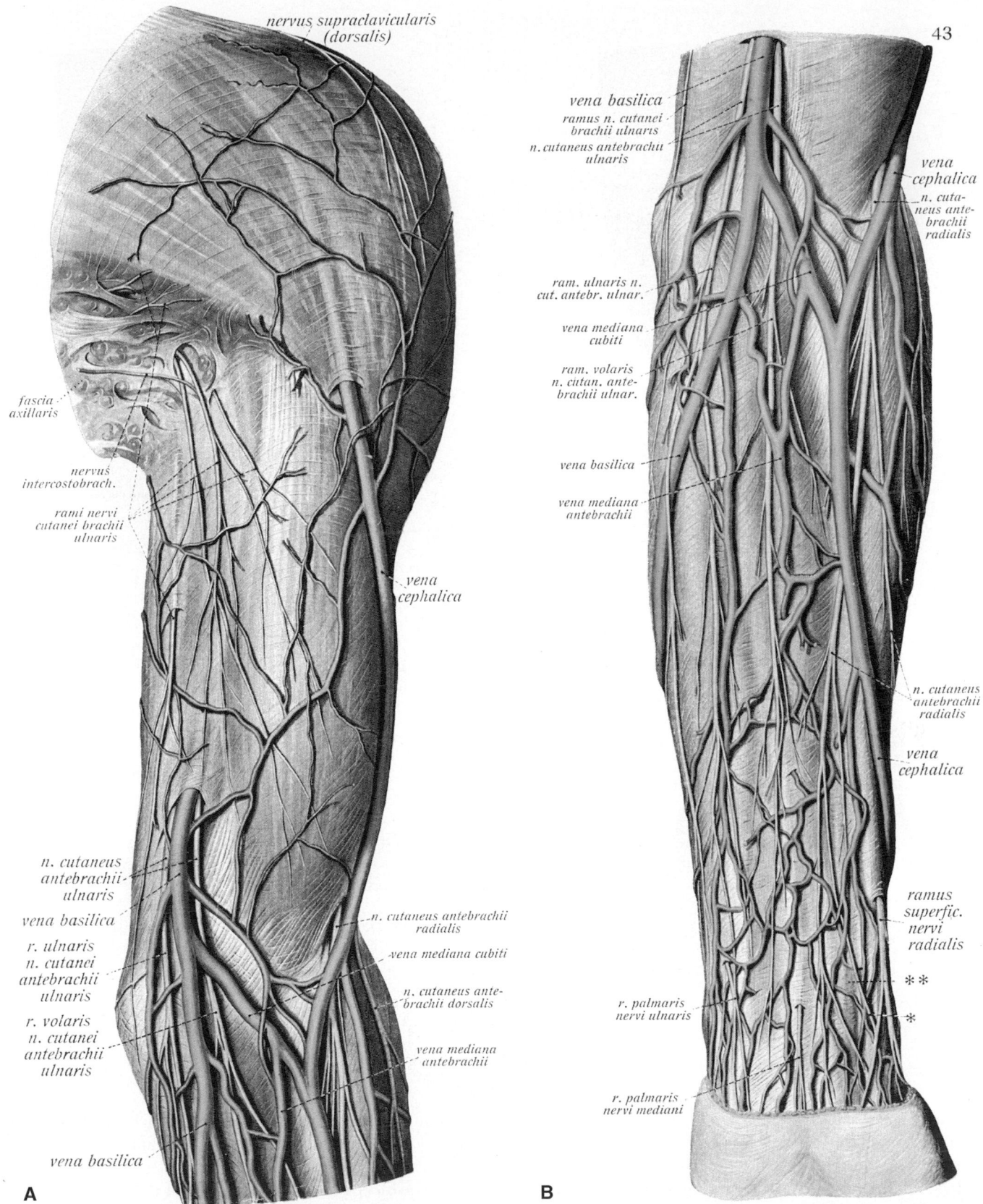

43

nervus supraclavicularis (dorsalis)

vena basilica
ramus n. cutanei brachii ulnaris
n. cutaneus antebrachu ulnaris

vena cephalica
n. cutaneus antebrachii radialis

ram. ulnaris n. cut. antebr. ulnar.

vena mediana cubiti

ram. volaris n. cutan. antebrachii ulnar.

vena basilica

vena mediana antebrachii

fascia axillaris

nervus intercostobrach.

rami nervi cutanei brachii ulnaris

vena cephalica

n. cutaneus antebrachii radialis

vena cephalica

n. cutaneus antebrachii ulnaris

vena basilica

r. ulnaris n. cutanei antebrachii ulnaris

r. volaris n. cutanei antebrachii ulnaris

n. cutaneus antebrachii radialis

vena mediana cubiti

n. cutaneus antebrachii dorsalis

vena mediana antebrachii

ramus superfic. nervi radialis

**

*

r. palmaris nervi ulnaris

r. palmaris nervi mediani

vena basilica

A

B

Figure 8–12 A, B, C, and D. Left antecubital space (anatomical dissection). (Reprinted with permission from Putz R, Pabst R, eds. Sobotta Atlas of Human Anatomy. 13th Latin Edition [English Text with Latin Nomenclature]. Baltimore: Lippincott Williams & Wilkins 2001.)

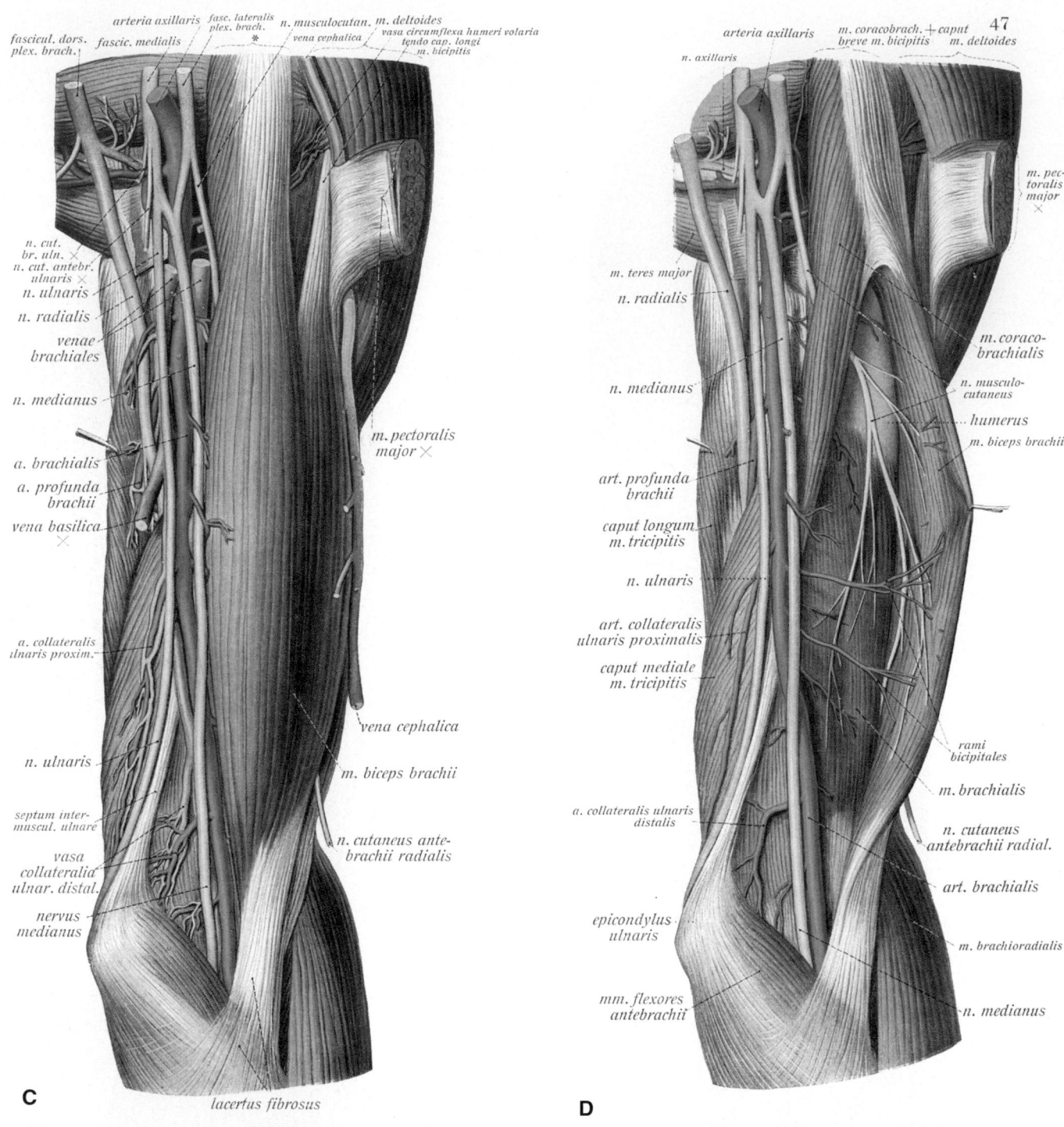

C   *lacertus fibrosus*

D

Figure 8–12   *(continued)*

axillary artery distal to the teres major muscle (Figure 8–12). It extends medial to the biceps brachii muscle until it ends opposite of the radial neck where it bifurcates into the radial and ulnar arteries (3). Exposing the brachial artery is performed most often at its distal aspect in the antecubital fossa. The bicipital aponeurosis provides a superficial covering of this artery. The artery is just deep to this fascial layer and can be palpated easily even through the skin. The

median nerve, although lateral to the brachial artery in the proximal upper arm, is located just medial to the artery in the antecubital fossa. Avoiding injury to this structure is vital. The biceps brachii tendon, which is lateral to the vessel, serves as a good landmark for finding the artery when a pulse cannot be appreciated. The median cubital vein runs superior to the bicipital aponeurosis, and paired brachial veins travel alongside the artery.

ANESTHESIA

Appropriate anesthesia is a fundamental element of any interventional procedure. Ultimately, the choice of anesthetic is made in communication with the anesthesiologist, physician performing the procedure, and the patient. General anesthesia usually is not required for most types of endovascular procedures. Some patients, however, prefer to "be put to sleep." Furthermore, some patients cannot tolerate the procedure or position and need to undergo general anesthesia. As opposed to local anesthesia or local anesthesia with sedation, general anesthesia requires an anesthesiologist. In addition, airway control is mandatory and usually provided via an endotracheal tube. Inhaled agents include nitrous oxide, isoflurane, desflurane, sevoflurane, halothane, and others, although nitrous oxide usually is avoided as it can distend the bowel and interfere with fluoroscopic imaging (5). Careful monitoring of at least the heart rate, blood pressure, respiratory rate, pulse oximetry, and end-tidal CO_2 needs to be performed with more invasive monitoring as needed. Additional intravenous agents can supplement or replace the inhalational anesthetics. These include barbiturates, benzodiazepines, ketamine, propofol, and etomidate (6). Muscle relaxants and opioid analgesics can also be helpful, such as succinylcholine and fentanyl.

The use of local agents usually does not require the presence of an anesthesiologist. The mechanism of action is via blockade of sodium influx of the nerve membrane. This prevents depolarization, and thus, the conductance of a pain stimulus (7). Often, these agents are used locally, and appropriate anesthesia often requires liberal use of these agents. However, toxicity such as seizures and arrhythmias can be associated with overdose. For instance, lidocaine is recommended at a maximum dose of 4 mg/kg (7). Using a 1% solution for a 70 kg person calculates to approximately 28 cc of this agent. Depending on the procedure performed, this may or may not allow adequate pain control. Some maneuvers permit use of greater quantities of anesthetic. Often, diluting the concentration of the agent is done. Also, the addition of epinephrine, which causes local vasoconstriction and decreases absorption, is helpful (8). Ultimately, the maximum dose allowed varies from patient to patient and agent to agent, but one must be aware of these doses.

Monitored anesthesia care (MAC) is simply the addition of conscious sedation. This involves the presence of an anesthesiologist, a physician trained in conscious sedation, or a qualified anesthetist to administer the drugs and monitor the patient. The intravenous agents mentioned previously, including benzodiazepines, are often used. MAC is an adjunct to local anesthesia, is helpful in relaxing the patient, and more importantly, is effective in decreasing the amount of local anesthetic required.

In addition, local agents can be used regionally as a field or nerve block. Knowledge of the anatomic location and distribution of nerves is critical for success in this regard. The choice of anesthetic is determined by the length and type of procedure. Relevant blocks include cervical, brachial, lumbar, and femoral (9). Although an anesthesiologist is not required, the person performing the procedure must be well-trained in performing blocks. Careful follow-up is also important to ensure that the underlying nerves were not injured.

Regional anesthesia also includes spinal and epidural anesthesia. The block is created when the spinal nerves or nerve roots that supply the distribution of the planned procedure are anesthetized. Spinal anesthesia involves direct injection of the subarachnoid space. Entry into this space is confirmed by the return of cerebrospinal fluid (CSF). Dose and baricity of the anesthetic agent affect the degree of anesthesia (10) provided. Altering patient position is also helpful in manipulating the distribution. Spinal anesthesia can be delivered in a single dose or in a continuous manner. Usually, both local agents, such as lidocaine or bupivacaine and opioids are used. Epidural anesthesia takes place in the epidural space by directly acting on the nerve roots as well as indirectly acting on the spinal nerves via diffusion into the subarachnoid space (10). It differs from spinal anesthesia by having a slower onset of action and relatively little dependence upon patient position. In either spinal or epidural anesthesia, adverse events can result from the anesthesia itself, such as hypotension and urinary retention, or from the actual procedure, such as headaches from CSF drainage, infection, or bleeding (11,12).

In summary, various forms of anesthesia can be offered, with each having advantages and disadvantages. General anesthesia offers the best pain control and relaxation; however, it carries the greatest risks and potential complications, including death, pneumonia, and malignant hyperthermia (13,14,15). Local anesthesia with or without MAC is less involved but may not offer appropriate anesthesia. Regional blocks in the form of nerve blocks, spinals, or epidurals have their own advantages and disadvantages. Ideally, the needs of the patient and the requirements of the procedure determine the choice of anesthesia. Preprocedural consultation with an anesthesiologist can be very helpful.

PREPARATION

Preparation of the patient involves all of the preprocedural setup. As discussed, the choice of anesthesia should be made with the patient. The position of the patient is determined by the procedure to be performed. Most endovascular procedures are performed in the supine position, but exceptions exist. For example, the popliteal artery can be approached in the prone position. The placement of the extremities can also be important. When working on the arm, the arm should be abducted on an armboard or table. Finally, any work on the groin must include careful exclusion of the perineal region. Generally, an adhesive drape to cover this region is recommended.

Preparation of the skin is important for antisepsis. Any hair in the region is carefully shaved with an electric razor (16). Sterile providone-iodine 10% solution (Triad Disposables Inc.), or similar preparation, is applied in a circular manner starting at the site of the incision and progressing outward. In the case of an iodine allergy, chlorhexidine gluconate 4% (Steris Corp.) is used. Always prepare a larger field than needed. For example, exposure of the femoral vessels can be facilitated when both groins are prepared above the umbilicus to the knees. This allows for easy extension of the incisions during difficult or emergent procedures as well as access to the other groin when needed. Antibiotics also can be given as a prophylactic agent, especially when prosthetic material is used (17). Creating the surgical field involves surrounding the area of interest with sterile, fluid-resistant drapes. All personnel involved in the procedure should scrub their hands, don sterile gear, and follow universal precautions.

SURGICAL EXPOSURE

Accessing the femoral artery is the most common surgical exposure performed in endovascular surgery. As previously described, the common femoral artery begins at the inguinal ligament, which connects the anterior superior iliac spine to the pubic tubercle. This serves as an important landmark because the skin incision should begin at the inguinal ligament, not the groin crease, in order to gain exposure to the common femoral artery. This allows cannulation in the area with the largest diameter. Traditionally, a longitudinal incision has been used on the skin. Unfortunately, this incision often is trapped within the intertriginous zones of the abdomen and upper thigh, especially in obese patients. This may play a role in predisposing to wound infections. Instead, a transverse or oblique incision can be used, which stays above the lower abdominal fold (Figure 8–13).

This approach keeps the incision out of the intertriginous zones and may help reduce the incidence of wound infections (18). In either case, the skin incision is made with a scalpel. The longitudinal incision is made over the course of the artery determined most easily by palpating the pulse. The transverse incision is made parallel and slightly inferior to the inguinal ligament. Then, electrocautery is used to obtain hemostasis of any subcutaneous bleeding. The subcutaneous tissue, including Scarpa's fascia, is separated with electrocautery. When dissecting through this area, it is important to cauterize or clip any obvious lymphatic vessels because postoperative lymphatic leaks can be quite troublesome (19). Self-retaining retraction is very helpful. After separation of the subcutaneous fat and deep fascia with electrocautery, the artery is located by palpating the pulse. Sharp dissection is performed to

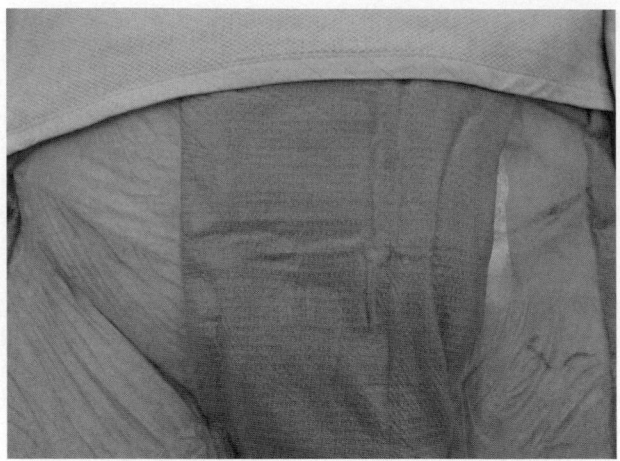

Figure 8–13 Groin prepped and draped with a sterile adhesive covering. Transverse incisions marked just under the inguinal ligaments.

isolate the artery with either Church or Metzenbaum scissors. Care must be taken not to transect the saphenous vein as it travels medially and anteriorly into the femoral vein. When dissecting out the femoral artery, it is easiest to first establish a plane anterior to the artery. This can be carried superiorly up to the inguinal ligament and as far distally as needed. The adventitia of the artery is easily identified by its "bloodshot eye" appearance (Figure 8–14). Attention is then drawn to the lateral and medial aspects of the artery. The connective tissue usually can be separated by a combination of spreading and sharp dissection. Here, it is important to preserve any small branches off the femoral artery because these branches may serve as important vessels for collateral flow. Of note, when handling the artery with forceps, only the adventitia should be grasped to avoid injuring the arterial wall. After the common femoral artery is isolated, attention is drawn to the superficial femoral artery, which extends distally, and profunda artery, which extends posterolaterally. As the common femoral artery is usually only approximately 4 cm in length, it is important to expose the superficial femoral and profunda arteries for control. Only at the points of obtaining control does the artery need to be freed circumferentially. This is done best when the lateral and medial dissections are carried down to the base of the artery and a right-angle dissector is gently passed around the artery. Often, gentle spreading is needed to get around the artery. Passing silastic vessel loops twice around the artery usually is all that is needed to gain control of the vessel and prevent blood flow (Figure 8–14). If this is inadequate, vascular clamps can be used. Because the profunda takes a posterior course, it sometimes is difficult to directly encircle. In these situations, it is easy to exclude the vessel by passing a vessel loop under the common femoral artery superior to the profunda then bringing that end of the loop under the superficial femoral artery inferior to the profunda. Passing this twice allows for hemostatic control of the profunda. Before interrupting

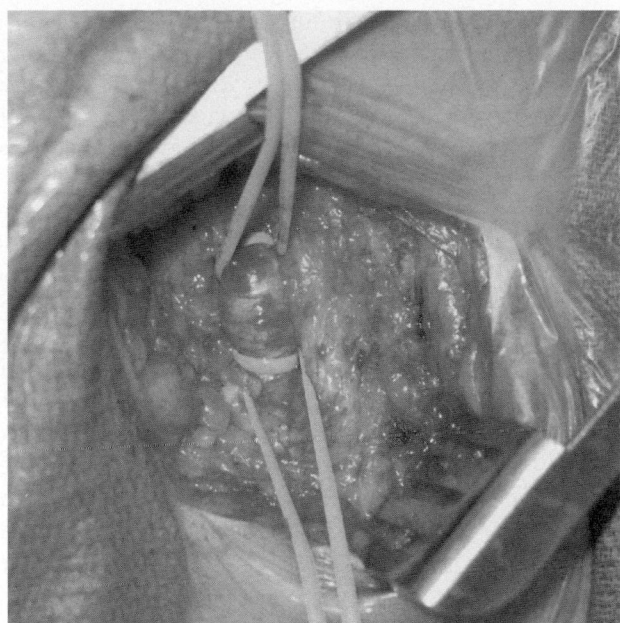

Figure 8–14 Femoral artery exposed.

any blood flow, intravenous heparin is given and allowed to circulate 3–5 minutes.

Different endovascular devices require different access to the vessel. Most simply require direct puncture of the artery (Figure 8–15). In these cases, control of the artery is still needed for proper closure of the vessel. Whenever an arteriotomy is to be made, the vessel loops can be tightened or vascular clamps applied. The procedure to be performed will dictate the type of arteriotomy made. For a strict endovascular procedure, a transverse arteriotomy is preferred. This reduces narrowing of the artery upon closure. However, if a graft is to be sewn into the artery, such as a femorofemoral bypass, a longitudinal arteriotomy is preferred because it allows for a larger anastomosis and proper positioning of the graft. In either case, the arteriotomy

should be made on the common femoral artery. The arteriotomy is started with the insertion of a #11 scalpel into the anterior aspect of the artery. The sharp end of the blade should be pointed up. After insertion, the scalpel is gently pulled up to open a small arteriotomy. It is very important to only insert the scalpel through the anterior wall of the vessel to avoid any injury to the posterior wall of the vessel. Return of blood demonstrates a successful arteriotomy, whereas no blood return usually indicates that the vessel was not entered completely. The arteriotomy is then extended to the appropriate length with Potts scissors. Heparin saline solution at a concentration of 50 units/cc can then be flushed into the vessels to ensure anticoagulation.

Exposure of the femoral vein is similar, as it lies medial to the artery. However, in contrast to the artery, most branches of the vein can be sacrificed without consequence—with the exception of the greater saphenous vein, which should be preserved for possible future use. It is important to recognize that all veins have thinner walls than arteries. Thus, when gaining circumferential exposure of the femoral vein, it is easy to injure this structure, especially along the posterior aspect. Furthermore, when handling the vein with forceps, grasping the vein in total will help avoid tearing the vessel wall.

Closure of an arteriotomy or direct puncture site should be performed with a running nonabsorbable suture after ensuring that the arterial lumen is flushed of any residual debris (Figure 8–16). The suture should be started on one side of the arteriotomy and be finished on the other. All the sutures should be placed with appropriate visualization of each stitch placed to avoid an intimal flap. Sometimes, it is also helpful to place two end-sutures first and use these as holders to prop up the arteriotomy. Particularly fragile or damaged arteries may require repair with individually placed, interrupted sutures, rather than a running closure. For longitudinal arteriotomies, a patch is sometimes necessary to close the defect without narrowing. Either a Dacron patch or a vein patch will suffice. A Dacron patch is simply

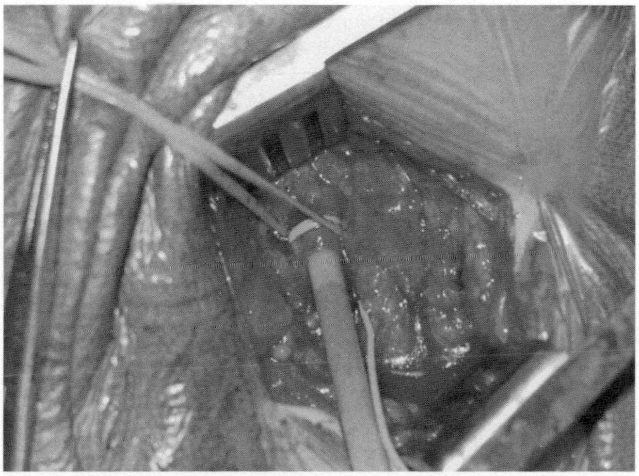

Figure 8–15 Sheath introduced in femoral artery.

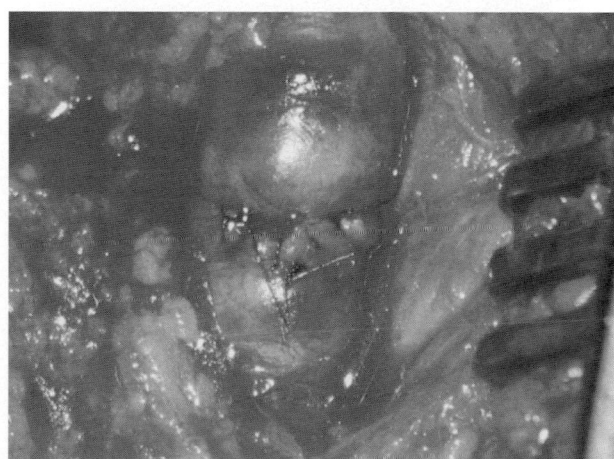

Figure 8–16 Femoral artery closed with nonabsorbable suture.

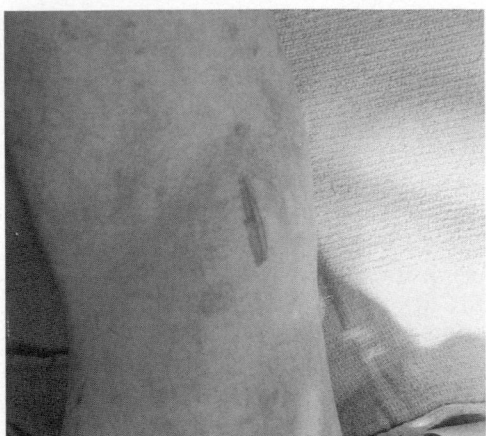

Figure 8–17   Incision marked for brachial artery exposure.

cut to size, whereas a vein is harvested to the appropriate length then opened longitudinally. Both are sewed in with a running-continuous nonabsorbable suture.

After the arteriotomy is repaired, blood flow is restored with the release of clamps or vessel loops. Patch stitches are placed when necessary. Distal flow is checked with palpation of the distal vessels. The entire wound is examined for adequate hemostasis. The deep fascia is closed in a running or interrupted fashion with absorbable sutures. Scarpa's fascia is reapproximated in a similar manner. The skin is best closed with a running absorbable suture, which is performed by taking bites in the subcuticular layer immediately below the skin. A subcuticular closure is preferable to staples because it is more cosmetically appealing and allows for a tight closure of the skin. Finally, many recommend

applying a sealant, collodion (pyroxylin 4%, ether 75%, alcohol 21%) (Amend Drug and Chemical Company, Inc.) or Dermabond Topical Skin Adhesive (2-octyl cyanoacrylate) (Ethicon, Inc.) over the skin closure to create an immediate watertight seal to minimize wound infections, particularly in the groin region (20).

Exposure of the brachial artery is relatively simple. The pulse is palpated and a longitudinal skin incision is made at that site, making sure to stay above the elbow crease (Figure 8–17). Incisions within or across the crease are not well-tolerated and can produce contractures. The subcutaneous tissue is divided with electrocautery. The bicipital aponeurosis is best divided sharply to avoid electrocautery conductance injury to the median nerve. The artery is then isolated, again taking care not to injure the median nerve, which lies medial. Access of this artery is performed in a similar manner to the femoral artery, except that the brachial artery is smaller (Figure 8–18). As a result, it is very important not to narrow the artery upon any closure or repair.

SUMMARY

Although endovascular techniques continue to supplement and supplant open vascular procedures, fundamental surgical skills are still required. Specifically, cutdown procedures are often performed to obtain access to necessary vessels. It is important to learn the manual skills associated with carrying out these procedures. Moreover, understanding the basic anatomy is crucial to achieving success as well as preventing inadvertent injury. This chapter has given a brief summary of the tools and techniques available to accomplish these tasks.

REFERENCES

1. Yano OJ, Faries PL, Morrissey N, et al. Ancillary techniques to facilitate endovascular repair of aortic aneurysms. J Vasc Surg 2001;34(1):69–75.
2. Hinchliffe RJ, Hopkinson BR. A hybrid endovascular procedure to preserve internal iliac artery patency during endovascular repair of aortoiliac aneurysms. J Endovasc Ther 2002;9(4):488–492.
3. Moore K. Clinically Oriented Anatomy. 3rd Ed. Baltimore: Williams and Wilkins, 1992.
4. Franco CD, Goldsmith J, Veith FJ, et al. Management of arterial injuries produced by percutaneous femoral procedures. Surgery 1993;113(4):419–425.
5. O'Keeffe NJ, Healy TE. The role of new anesthetic agents. Pharmacol Ther 1999;84(3):233–248.
6. Kennedy SM. Nonopiod Intravenous Anesthetics. In: Longnecker DE, Murphy FL. Dripps, Eckenhoff, and Vandam's Introduction to Anesthesia. 8th Ed. Philadelphia: W.B. Saunders, 1992:91–101.
7. Covino BJ, Lambert DM. Pharmacology of Local Anesthetics. In: Longnecker DE, Murphy FL. Dripps, Eckenhoff, and Vandam's Introduction to Anesthesia. 8th Ed. Philadelphia: W.B. Saunders, 1992:195–212.
8. Bernards CM, Kopacz DJ. Effect of epinephrine on lidocaine clearance in vivo: a microdialysis study in humans. Anesthesiology 1999;91(4):962–968.
9. Riegler FX. Nerve Blocks. In: Longnecker DE, Murphy FL. Dripps, Eckenhoff, and Vandam's Introduction to Anesthesia. 8th Ed. Philadelphia: W.B. Saunders, 1992:229–246.

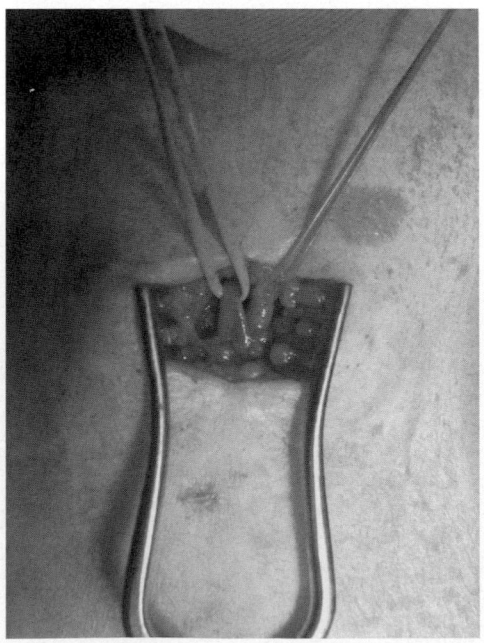

Figure 8–18   Brachial artery (*right*) and brachial vein (*left*).

10. Riegler FX. Spinal and Epidural Anesthesia. In: Longnecker DE, Murphy FL. Dripps, Eckenhoff, and Vandam's Introduction to Anesthesia. 8th Ed. Philadelphia: W.B. Saunders, 1992:213–228.
11. Faccenda KA, Finucane BT. Complications of regional anesthesia: Incidence and prevention. Drug Saf 2001;24(6):413–442.
12. Horlocker TT. Complications of spinal and epidural anesthesia. Anesthesiol Clin North Am 2000;18(2):461–485.
13. Brockwell RC, Andrews JJ. Complications of inhaled anesthesia delivery systems. Anesthesiol Clin North Am 2002;20(3):301–16, vi–vii.
14. Phillips OC, Capizzi LS. Anesthesia mortality. Clin Anesth 1974; 10(3):220–244.
15. Johnson C, Edleman KJ. Malignant hyperthermia: a review. J Perinatol 1992;12(1):61–71.
16. Kjonniksen I, Andersen BM, Sondenaa VG, et al. Preoperative hair removal—a systematic literature review. AORN J 2002;75(5): 928–938, 940.
17. Bandyk DF. Antibiotics—why so many and when should we use them? Semin Vasc Surg. 2002;15(4):268–274.
18. Chuter TA, Reilly LM, Stoney RJ, et al. Femoral artery exposure for endovascular aneurysm repair through oblique incisions. J Endovasc Surg 1998;5(3):259–260.
19. Tyndall SH, Shepard AD, Wilczewski JM, et al. Groin lymphatic complications after arterial reconstruction. J Vasc Surg 1994 May;19(5):858–63; discussion 863–864.
20. Bhende S, Rothenburger S, Spangler DJ, et al. In vitro assessment of microbial barrier properties of Dermabond((R)) Topical Skin Adhesive. Surg Infect (Larchmt) 2002;3(3):251–257.

Catheters, Methods, and Injectors for Superselective Catheterization

9

S. William Stavropoulos, Dheeraj Rajan, Constantin Cope

The principles of percutaneous selective angiography were formulated in the 1950s with the introduction of the Seldinger technique (Figure 9–1) (1) and the development of radiopaque thermoplastic catheters (2). When attempts were made to further advance catheters subselectively, interventional radiologists found that they were better able to opacify and identify small peripheral hypervascular or occult bleeding points that could not be appreciated on standard selective studies (3,4). In addition, this technique provided the interventionalist with the ability to embolize tumors and bleeding sites without sacrificing adjacent clinically sensitive normal tissue. Within the past 15 years, interventional radiologists have learned to probe into the circulation beyond second- and third-order vascular branches with greater depth, precision, and dependability than was ever thought possible as a result of the vast improvement in catheter and guide wire design as well as impressive advances in digital subtraction imaging. Today, skilled interventionists can embolize complex bleeding sites or devascularize and treat peripheral vascular tumors involving the central nervous system, lungs, liver, kidneys, pancreas, bowel, pelvic organs, and extremities with a high success rate and with acceptable risks. This chapter will cover principles, clinical applications, and problems of superselective catheterization beyond first- or second-order vascular branches.

STANDARD CATHETERS AND GUIDE WIRES

Although 4 French to 8 French selective catheters were originally devised for diagnostic arteriography, today they play a central role in interventional procedures either as primary delivery cathethers for use in embolization or drug therapy of third- or even fourth-order branch vessels, or even as guiding conduits for the insertion of coaxial superselective microcatheters and guide wires. The modern selective catheter is composed of a stiff, thin-walled stem to which is welded a more flexible segment set with a pre-shaped curve made of polyethylene, polyurethane, or other soft plastic tubing to obtain better torque control. Steel mesh or a more rigid plastic material such as nylon is incorporated in the shaft during the extrusion process. Because of this composite fabrication, selective catheters are available in a wide range of shapes, flexibility profiles, and dimensions to satisfy most needs. However, because of their construction, catheters may vary in the tolerance of

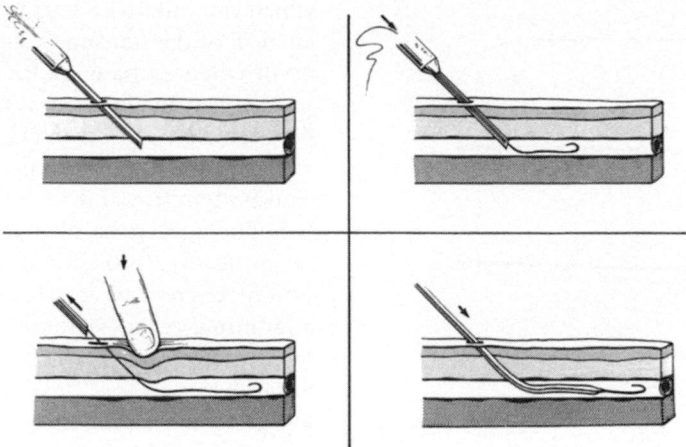

Figure 9–1 The Seldinger technique. After a soft-tipped guide wire is threaded through the arterial introducing needle, the needle is exchanged over the wire for a tapered catheter of the appropriate size.

their internal diameter, not only at the tip but also at the fusion point between the body and the flexible terminal segment. Therefore, catheters and guide wires should always be tested for a smooth fit, especially when purchased from different companies. A high-quality catheter, in addition to having good torque response and radiopacity, should have a flexible atraumatic tip and a low surface frictional resistance for good trackability over a guide wire. Because not all catheters are created equal, interventionists should continue to evaluate new products as they become available to find catheters with the optimal "feel."

Finding a good match between the selective catheter, the guide wire, and the vascular anatomy is the secret to successful superselective catheterization. If the catheter or the guide wire has the wrong flexibility profile, surface characteristics, or torque, the operator may find it impossible to reach the target site, either because the guide wire cannot be properly advanced or because the catheter will not track properly over the guide wire. Standard Teflon-coated helical spring guide wires are available with a fixed or movable core, in a wide range of sizes, tip configurations, floppiness, stem stiffness, and surface coating. The Glidewire (Terumo Medical Corporation) is a wire made of a superelastic nitinol core sheathed in polyurethane and coated with a hydromer compound (Figure 9–2) that has become extremely popular because it can be maneuvered easily and accurately through complex vascular branches (5).

ARTERIAL PUNCTURE AND AORTIC CATHETERIZATION

To perform arterial puncture successfully and safely in a consistent way, the operator should carefully evaluate standard landmarks close to the vessel, palpate the course of the artery for its direction and its point of maximal impulse, and then accurately infiltrate the perivascular sheath with local anesthetic to prevent pain and vascular spasm. The point of the arterial needle used should be as sharp as possible to prevent it from sliding off sclerotic arterial walls. When a compound arterial needle is used, it should be advanced slowly through the soft tissues at an angle of 45 degrees to the vessel toward the point of maximum impulse. When a good transmitted pulse is felt, it is rapidly thrust forward 1–2 cm in order to transfix the vessel. The sharp inner stylet is removed, the cannula is slowly pulled back until a maximum pulsatile jet of blood is obtained (usually a 4- to 6-inch spurt in normotensive individuals), then the cannula is redirected more horizontally and coaxially to enable a guide wire to be advanced smoothly into the vessel without resistance or intimal dissection. When a simple needle is used for a one-wall puncture technique, the same insertion maneuvers are used, except that once the transmitted arterial pulse is felt through the needle, it is advanced forward only 1- to 2-mm steps at a time until there is a good return of blood.

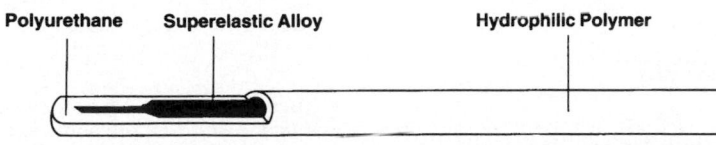

Figure 9–2 Construction of nitinol Glidewire.

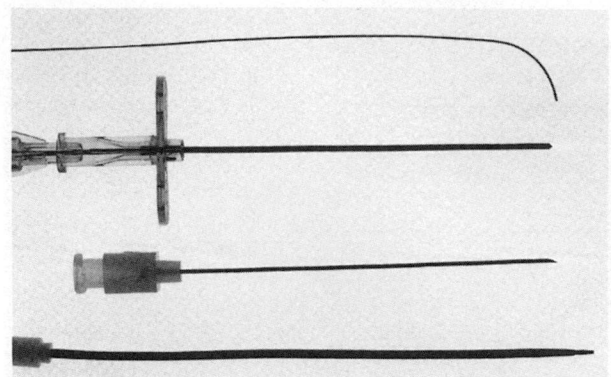

Figure 9–3   The Cook micropuncture introducing set. This set consists of a 0.018-inch guide wire, a 7-cm 21-gauge needle, and a 3 French or 5 French coaxial catheter dilator. Note the significant difference in diameter between a standard 18-gauge arterial needle (*second from top*) and the micropuncture needle.

which can otherwise lead to laceration or irregular overdilatation of the transmural tract. This is especially prone to occur when exchanging for multiple catheters and guide wires, inserting stiff intravascular devices, and removing deflated balloon catheters. These sheaths are also very valuable for introducing nontapered catheters, stents, foreign-body retrieval devices, biopsy forceps, and so forth. Introducing sheaths, also available in longer lengths from 20 cm to over 100 cm, are commonly used to shield the wall of severely atherosclerotic iliac arteries and the lower abdominal aorta (Figure 9–4) from guide wire and selective catheter trauma, which might result in severe atheroembolic disease. More flexible curved catheter introducers less given to kinking have been introduced and are found to be extremely convenient for coaxially passing angioplasty balloon catheters or stents across torutuous vascular anatomy (7,8).

The arterial needle sizes most commonly used are thin-walled 18 gauge or 19 gauge, which allow insertion of standard 0.038- or 0.035-inch stainless steel helical spring guide wires. One should remember not to use plastic-coated nitinol guide wires through an introducing metal needle because the coating may be sheared off by the sharp edge and embolize downstream. Therefore, these wires should be introduced only through a catheter (or through the plastic dilator used to predilate the tract) to prevent the catheter tip from fraying during its movement through the soft tissues.

Although 18-gauge needles are very reliable for puncturing easily palpable large vessels such as the femoral artery, the operator should also be familiar with the use of 21-gauge micropuncture needles (6). These needles are very useful for decreasing the trauma to vessel walls and perivascular vital structures associated with repeated attempts to puncture poorly palpable arteries and grafts; for facilitating puncture of vessels that are slippery or prone to spasm, such as the axillary and brachial arteries; and for decreasing the potential for developing significant hematomas in patients with coagulopathies. The micropuncture needle, by virtue of its smaller diameter and reduced tissue resistance to penetration, is less painful, provides a better feel of the transmitted arterial pulse, and has a sharper bite for the vessel wall. It is available in an introducer set (see Cook micropuncture set in Figure 9–3) that permits the needle to be exchanged for a 4 French or 5 French plastic cannula over a 0.018-inch guide wire, which then allows standard-sized guide wires to be used.

INTRODUCTION SHEATHS

Introduction sheaths are important safeguards used to protect the vascular or graft puncture site from trauma during long and complex diagnostic or interventional procedures,

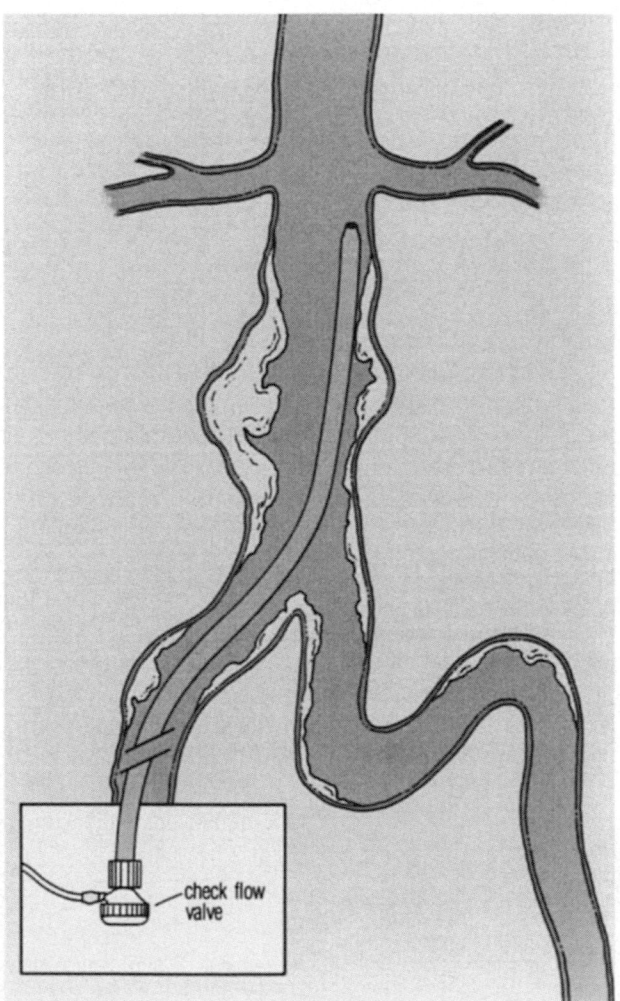

Figure 9–4   A long 7 French catheter-introducing sheath has been advanced past the aortic aneurysm to minimize dislodgment of atheroemboli during selective visceral catheterization. (Reprinted with permission from Cope C, Burke DR, Meranze SG, eds. Atlas of Interventional Radiology. St. Louis: Mosby, 1990.)

ABDOMINAL AORTOGRAPHY

Usually, aortography is performed from the femoral artery. Catheterization of the aorta is normally feasible even in the presence of aneurysms or severe atherosclerotic disease by maneuvering an angled Glidewire (Terumo) to the level of the diaphragm and threading over it a 5 French pigtail catheter with a tightly coiled tip.

Although often bypassed in favor of immediate visceral catheterization, midstream aortography can be a useful step for obtaining a vascular road map before selective studies. Despite the slightly increased load of contrast medium involved, aortography may save catheterization time and lessen later confusion by alerting the angiographer to the presence of anomalous take-off of primary branches and accessory vessels as well as to unsuspected aneurysms and arteriosclerotic stenoses. Aortograms are also very useful in displaying branching vessels in the natural state, an important diagnostic baseline study that allows the operator to distinguish vasospasm secondary to selective catheterization from vascular encasement resulting from tumor.

In the presence of complete obstruction of both iliac arteries or of the lower aorta, aortography can be performed either from the high brachial or axillary route or otherwise by translumbar aortic puncture (Figure 9–5). The left brachial or axillary route is more flexible and generally preferred because it allows the interventionalist to do selective visceral catheterization and interventional procedures. However, if the subclavian artery and the thoracic aorta are very tortuous and atherosclerotic, access to the abdominal aorta from this site can be lengthy, complex, and hazardous because of potential dislodgment of atheroemboli to brachiocephalic vessels, brachial plexus injury, and the development of pseudoaneurysms. With the advent of CTA and MRA as well as modern interventional techniques and equipment, very rarely does translumbar aortography need to be performed. Translumbar aortography is, however, very safe as long as the patient does not have a coagulopathy or severe hypertension (9). Even selective vessel catheterization can be performed from this approach through a 5 French catheter introducer.

SUPERSELECTIVE CATHETERIZATION WITH SIMPLE CATHETERS

Preshaped Catheters

Because most interventional studies begin with the use of a conventional selective catheter, it is always tempting (and less expensive) to see whether this primary catheter can be successfully advanced superselectively, especially in patients with classic vascular anatomy (10). This, in fact, usually can be done with a high degree of success on the arterial side for the control of bleeding or for tumor embolization in the bronchial, gastric, hepatic, renal, pelvic, and extremity circulations (10–15). On the venous side, these catheters are important for venous sampling and embolization procedures (16–17).

The preferred site of entry for most studies of the chest and abdomen is the femoral artery or vein. The brachial or axillary artery route is used for difficult branch vessel angulation. Usually, 5 French or 6 French introduction sheaths are first inserted as a safety precaution to prevent vascular trauma from repetitive guide wire and catheter exchanges. The same standard catheters chosen for catheterization of thoracic and abdominal aortic branches are also used for superselective work; the most commonly used preshaped catheters include those with a C, shepherd's crook, or cobra curve. For catheterizing acutely angled vessels, the author prefers to use a 5 French or 5.5 French Simmons catheter type 1 or 2 or a cobra catheter formed into a "Waltman loop" (Figure 9–6) (18). Simmons catheters can be quickly reformed in the proximal abdominal aorta by simple traction on a 4o plastic suture friction-fitted between the catheter tip and the guide wire (Figure 9–7) (19). If the operator is unable to make the catheter follow the guide wire superselectively because of complex angulation, the catheter should be exchanged for a straight or hockey–stick-curved catheter, preferably with a more flexible and slippery surface.

Balloon Catheters

A quick and easy method for catheterizing high-flow lesions such as arteriovenous fistulas or vascular tumors is

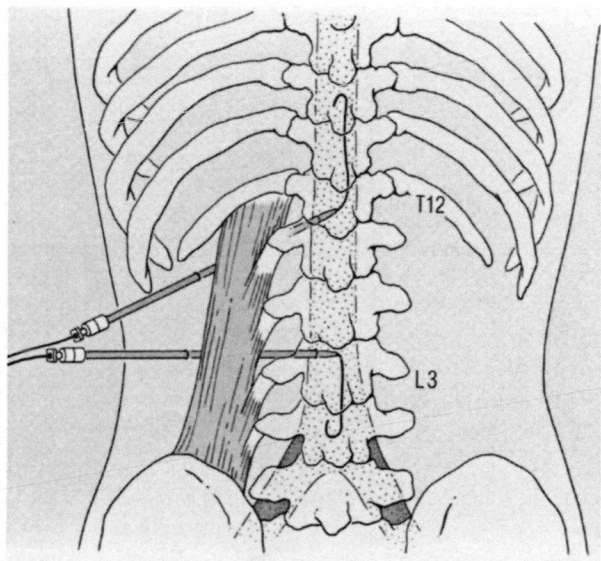

Figure 9–5 Illustration of translumbar aortography performed with 5 French or 6 French over-the-needle catheters introduced at T12 or L3 levels. These can be replaced over a stiff guide wire with an introducing sheath or with longer pigtail or selective catheters. (Reprinted with permission from Cope C, Burke DR., Meranze SG, eds. Atlas of Interventional Radiology. St. Louis: Mosby, 1990.)

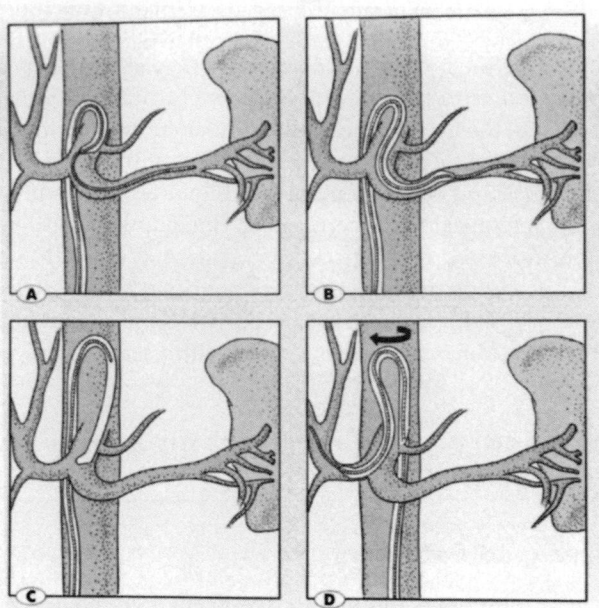

Figure 9–6 The Waltman loop. Following selective catheterization of the splenic artery (or other convenient aortic branches), the Waltman loop is formed by further advancing the guide wire and catheter up the thoracic aorta. The new configuration is convenient for subselective catheterization of the hepatic or left gastric artery. (Reprinted with permission from Cope C, Burke DR, Meranze SG, eds. Atlas of Interventional Radiology. St. Louis: Mosby, 1990.)

to insert a two-lumen occlusion balloon catheter in the major proximal aortic branch feeding the lesion. Once the catheter is sufficiently inflated with carbon dioxide or dilute contrast medium, it will be carried into the lesion by the more rapid blood flow and end well positioned for embolization. Alternatively, a 2 French or 3 French, single-lumen, latex balloon catheter can be threaded through the selective catheter, inflated, and allowed to be carried to the vascular lesion (Figure 9–8) (20). Once in place, the balloon is deflated, and a fine mandrel guide wire is then inserted within its lumen to allow the outer catheter to track over it more easily without kinking. Balloon catheters can also be redirected at bifurcations by infusing a vasoconstricting drug selectively in the unwanted vascular limb to allow the balloon to free-float to the other patent limb (21).

Another functional use of small nondetachable balloons involves diverting blood flow toward the vessel to be embolized. For example, an occasional patient may present with a bleeding duodenal lesion and, because of severe tortuosity or atherosclerotic disease, the operator may find it impossible to selectively catheterize the gastroduodenal artery from the proper hepatic artery. Under these conditions, a 2 French Fogarty balloon catheter can be released from the guiding catheter, and the balloon can be inflated to occlude the common hepatic artery just distal to the gastroduodenal artery. If a contrast test injection shows good

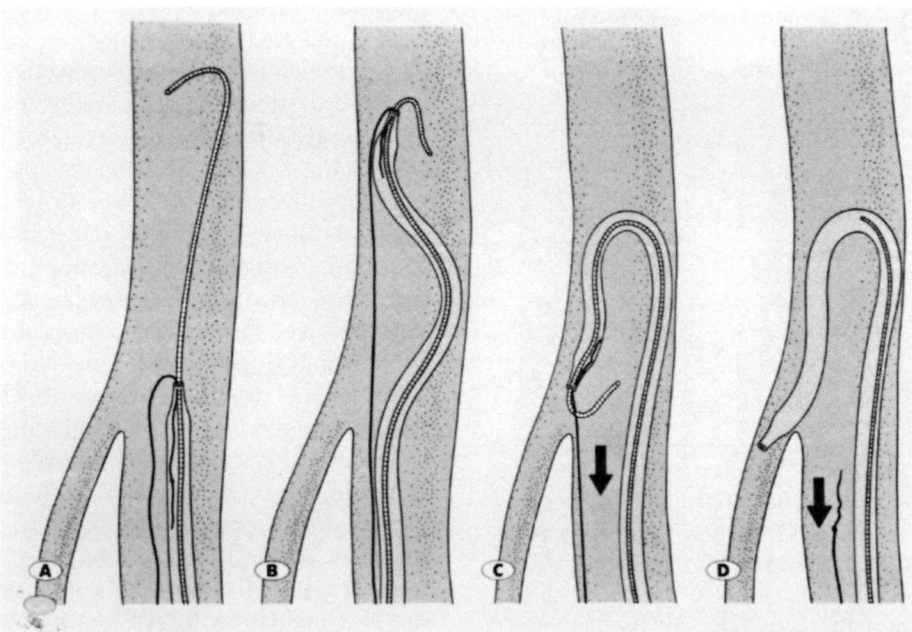

Figure 9–7 Suture technique to reform a Simmons catheter. **A.** A catheter preloaded with a 4ō knotted plastic suture is threaded over a standard guide wire to the lower thoracic aorta. **B.** The guide wire is pulled back to within 1–2 cm of the catheter tip. **C.** The proximal free end of the suture is pulled, while the catheter is slowly advanced until the sidewinder curve is reformed. **D.** Withdrawal of the floppy-tipped guide wire frees the knotted suture and allows selective catheterization. The same technique can be used to form Waltman loops with hockey-stick or cobra-shaped catheters. (Reprinted with permission from Cope C, Burke DR, Meranze SG, eds. Atlas of Interventional Radiology. St. Louis: Mosby, 1990.)

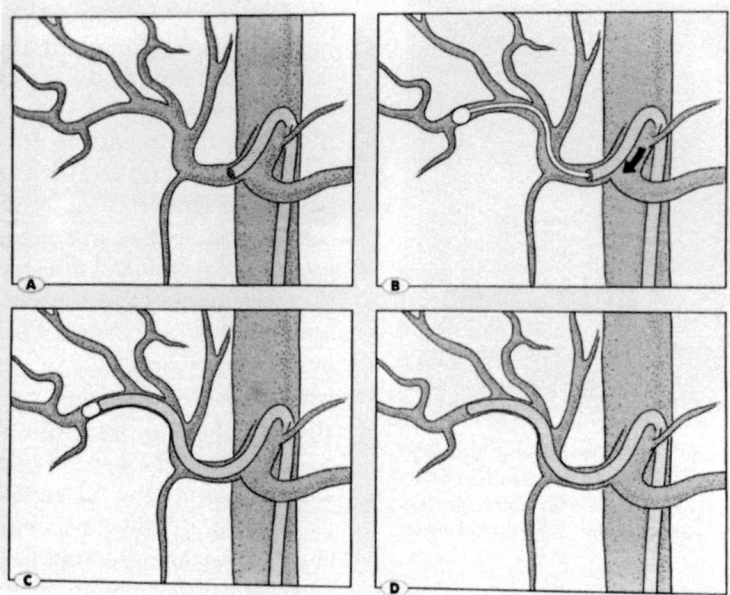

Figure 9–8   Balloon catheter guide wire. A partially inflated 3 French Fogarty balloon catheter has been carried by blood flow through **A.**, a selective celiac catheter to **B.**, a hepatic artery branch. The coaxial catheter can then be advanced over it **C.**, especially if it is stiffened with a fine mandrel wire. **D.** shows final catheter position.

antegrade flow into the gastroduodenal artery, the operator may then safely inject embolic particles through the side arm of the guiding catheter adapter to occlude pancreatico-duodenal branches. Nakamura (22) used a similar princi-ple to redirect blood flow through periportal collaterals for hepatic chemoembolization when the common hepatic artery distal to the gastroduodenal artery was occluded.

SUPERSELECTIVE CATHETERIZATION WITH COAXIAL TECHNIQUE

Because the human body has a great variety of arterial curves and branching patterns further complicated by dis-ease states, the interventionist needs a wide variety of catheter systems to be able to navigate freely through the vascular tree. Four to 6 French preshaped catheters are very practical for superselective catheterization of third- or fourth-order vessels as long as their lumen is of adequate caliber and the branching vascular path is fairly simple. As the tortuosities of the feeding vessels leading to the area of interest increase in number and complexity, these selective catheters become not only less effective because of loss of torque control but also more traumatic to vascular endothelium because of increasing friction between the relatively stiff catheter and the vessel wall, especially at branching points and tight curves. When the diameter of the advancing catheter tip begins to approximate that of the vessel, there is increased friction against the intima and

reduction in blood flow, which can lead to spasm, blood stasis, ischemia of normal adjacent tissue, and occasionally even difficulty in withdrawing the catheter. For these rea-sons, superselective catheterization is performed with as fine and as flexible a catheter as possible that will still retain some operator control, possess adequate radiopac-ity, and have a lumen large enough to allow injection of embolization glues or particles.

GUIDE WIRE-CONTROLLED SUPERSELECTIVE CATHETERIZATION

Early attempts to reach peripheral lesions superselectively with coaxial catheter systems were stymied by the lack of small radiopaque catheters and a suitable torque of guiding wires. In the late 1960s, Eisenberg (23) devised the first com-mercially available, steerable, guide wire-catheter combina-tion for coaxial use (Figure 9–9). The set consisted of a 3.5 French, thin-walled, Teflon catheter with a flexible, shapeable tip connected to a hemostatic irrigation adapter, through which a 0.025-inch torqued guide wire could be fitted. The guide wire consisted of a relatively stiff, 65-cm-long, spring, stainless steel cannula that ended in a very floppy but torqued 15-cm spring segment with a shapeable tip. The sys-tem was used through a 6 French C-shaped thin-walled poly-ethylene guiding catheter that could be introduced selectively into primary or secondary aortic branches with a special torque guide (24). It was successfully used for many years for

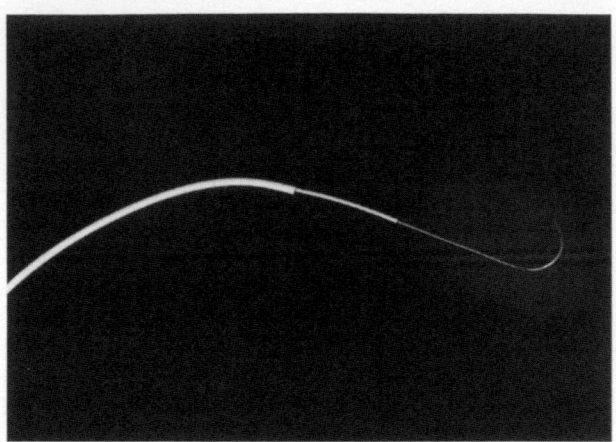

Figure 9–9 Eisenberg coaxial set. The distal floppy segment of the 0.025-inch torqued guide wire is protruding from the 3.5 French Teflon catheter, which has been inserted through a 6 French, nontapered, polyethylene, preshaded, guiding catheter.

superselective catheterization of abdominal visceral arteries (25) and of thyrocervical arteries and for sampling thyroid veins for possible functioning parathyroid tumors (18). A decade later, Cope introduced a simpler, steerable, 0.018-inch guide wire initially designed for transhepatic catheterization but subsequently also used for vascular catheterization (26). It consisted of a core guide wire tapered distally to a very fine flexible tip wrapped with either a stainless steel or a platinum helical spring for improved radiopacity. The tip configuration could be easily reshaped manually.

Today's sophisticated wires, which are based on the same design principles, can vary in diameter from 0.010 to 0.018-inch and in length from 65-cm to exchange lengths. Steerable guide wires are commercially available in a wide array of configurations designed to better fit the needs of various anatomical circulatory patterns. Many variable factors can change the torque characteristics, flexibility, pushability, and tip shape of these fine steerable guide wires. These factors include shaft diameter, length and smoothness of taper, direct connection of core taper to the coil tip versus its attachment through an intermediary safety ribbon, slipperiness of surface coating, thrombogenicity, and degree of tip shape memory (Figure 9-10).

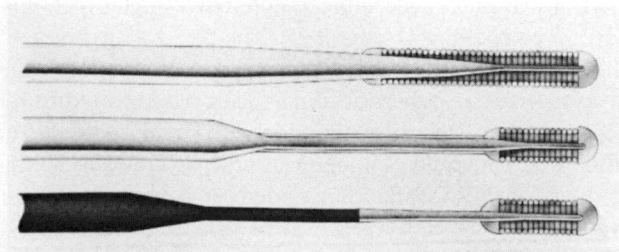

Figure 9–10 Steerable microguide wires (Target). Guide wire characteristics are varied by altering the taper length and thickness of the distal inner core.

Because of the increasing clinical success of percutaneous coronary artery transluminal angioplasty, microwires quickly became a crucial part of the armamentarium of cardiologists for safely guiding balloon catheters through tortuous diseased coronary arteries (27). Steerable wires also began to play a key role in passing microcatheters into the cerebral, hepatic, and peripheral circulation for diagnosis, thrombolysis, or embolization (Figure 9–11). The first 3 French catheters to be tried in conjunction with these specialized wires were made of Teflon for their inherent lubricity, but they were found to be too stiff to negotiate complex curves. More flexible, open-ended, coated, coiled spring guide wires, introduced by Sos, were found to be useful in conjunction with steerable guide wires for superselective thrombolysis and embolization, especially in the abdomen and extremities (28,29). Although these spring-sheathed catheters have excellent radiopacity, high pressure tolerance, good pushability, and the ability to accept relatively large particulate emboli, they are often not flexible enough to follow a fine guide wire through multiple tight vascular curves.

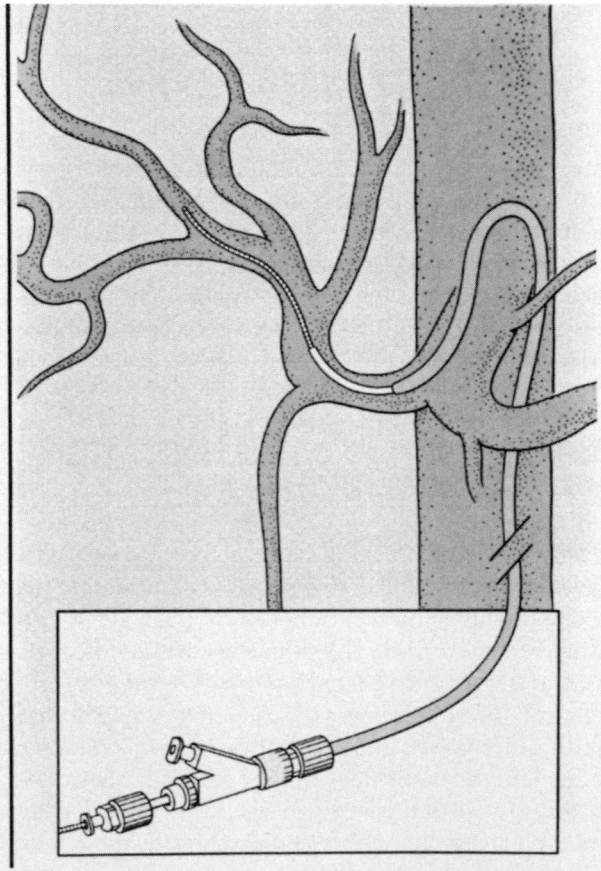

Figure 9–11 Coaxial superselective catheterization requires a 6 French or 7 French introducing catheter through which 3 French or 4 French catheters can be advanced over a fine torqued guide wire. Continuous irrigation between the two catheters is important to prevent clotting. (Reprinted with permission from Cope C, Burke DR, Meranze SG, eds. Atlas of Interventional Radiology. St. Louis: Mosby, 1990.)

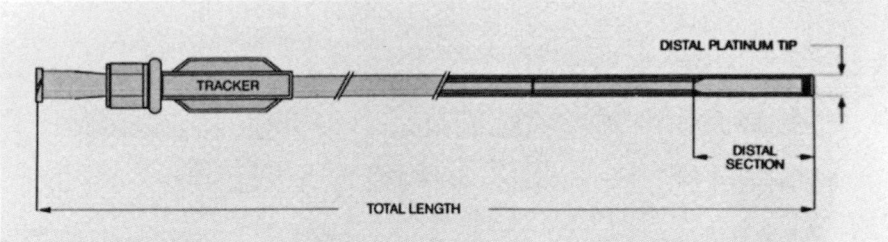

Figure 9–12   Typical microcatheter (Target) made with three increasingly flexible segments.

The modern plastic microcatheter for superselective catheterization is designed with a progressive stiffness profile and consists of a relatively rigid body to provide some torque and pushability, a middle segment of intermediate flexibility, and a floppy distal segment with a radiopaque metal marker at the tip (Figure 9–12). The catheter body wall is made more rigid by using a stiffer plastic, two plastic layers, or incorporating a wire mesh. The distal floppy tail can be made of polyethylene or polyurethane catheter tubing, which have a sufficiently low coefficient of friction to allow the free insertion of a matching steerable guide wire. Microcatheter systems currently in use are available multiple suppliers.

Although these catheters were designed initially for the treatment of neurovascular lesions, interventional radiologists eagerly adopted them for use throughout the body. Representative of a microcatheter system is the Tracker 18 catheter from Target Therapeutics. Extruded from a composite of stiffer polypropylene core and an outer clear polyethylene coat over its proximal and middle sections, the catheter tapers from a 3.2 French body to a floppy, nonradiopaque, polyethylene 2.2 French distal segment through two smooth transition zones with a corresponding diminution in internal diameter from 0.039 to 0.021 inch (30). The platinum radiopaque marker enlarges the catheter tip slightly to 2.7 French (Figure 9–13).

Because its wall surface has a low coefficient of friction, this catheter can be readily threaded through any standard preshaped selective guiding catheter with a 0.038-inch tip opening and will freely track over a 0.018- or 0.016-inch steerable guide wire. Its tip can be manually preshaped to any desirable curve with steam. Despite its limited lumen, it will allow the injection of 60% contrast medium at a rate of 0.4–1.0 mL per second and will accept particulate microemboli up to 600 to 700 m. In addition, it is capable of having various fibered platinum coils (Figure 9–14) threaded through it with a special pusher stylet. As with any coaxial system, it is important to prevent possible backup of blood, microemboli, and binding of the guide wire by using a continuous pressurized flushing system with heparinized saline through both the guide wire and the superselective catheter (Figure 9–15).

Superselective catheterization is usually performed by a series of steps, consisting first of advancing both the microcatheter and the steerable wire through the guiding catheter to the second- or third-order branch, then further manipulating the angled-tip guide wire to the vessel feeding the lesion under study, and finally sliding the catheter over the wire to its tip. The guide wire and the catheter should be advanced in slow, measured steps with frequent back-and-forth maneuvers with the aid of fluoroscopic

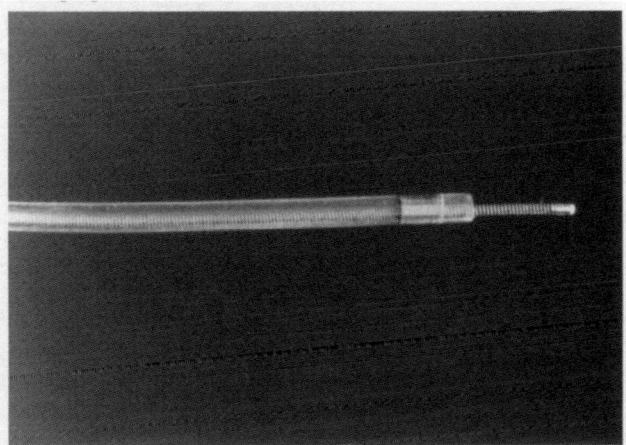

Figure 9–13   Floppy tip of Tracker catheter (Target) with protruding microguide wire (0.016 inch). Note the platinum radiopaque sleeve marker.

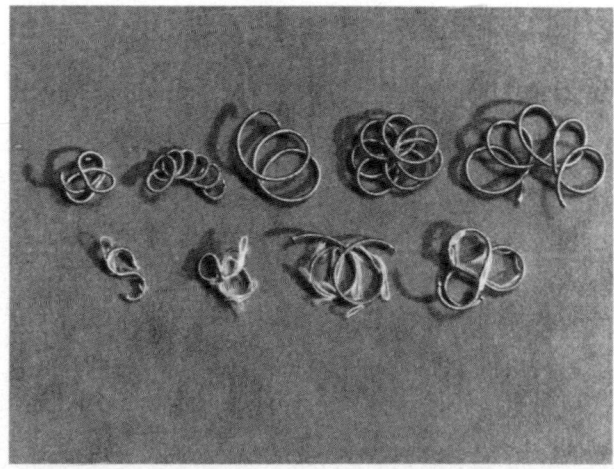

Figure 9–14   Assortment of embolization coils for the Tracker catheter (Target).

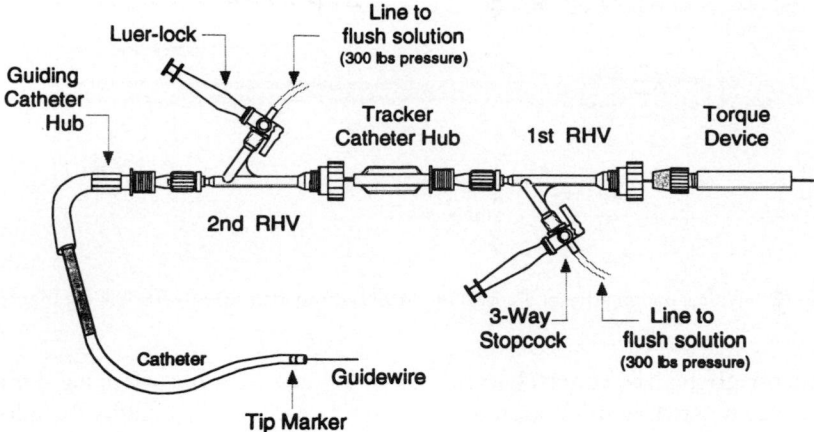

Figure 9–15   Tracker catheter assembly (Target). Note the double irrigation system for the guiding catheter and the inner catheter.

digital road-mapping or with frequent opacifications of the vascular bed to ensure that these devices are following the proper course.

PROBLEMS ASSOCIATED WITH SUPERSELECTIVE CATHETERIZATION

There are definite advantages to using standard-size catheters and guide wires for superselective catheterization whenever possible because of their sturdiness, good radiopacity, torqueability, and large lumen. But a very real risk exists of their inducing vascular spasm, dissection, or occlusion, especially when excessive zeal is used during the procedure (Figure 9–16). Although the use of supple microcatheters and steerable guide wires greatly diminishes the chance of serious vascular trauma, problems inherent in the miniaturization of the system nevertheless can still occur.

CATHETER AND GUIDE WIRE FRAGILITY

Because microcatheters and guide wires are extremely delicate, they must be inspected for defects before use and be handled as carefully as possible to prevent kinking, tearing, or separation. Microcatheters should be inserted with a stylet or a splinting guide wire through the valve of the pressurized directing catheter, and their tips should be followed fluoroscopically until they are in the target artery. All microcatheters should be advanced, or rotated slowly, in measured steps to prevent excessive coiling or kinking. The matching guide wires can have exceedingly fine spring tips that can be easily damaged when they are improperly passed through the irrigating valve or when they are being reshaped by hand. The safety wire or distal weld of these guide wires should be checked repeatedly for integrity

during the course of the procedure. If the tip of the catheter or the guide wire is immobilized by small vessels in spasm, it is possible for the tip of the wire or the catheter to separate whenever the operator tries to withdraw the devices too rapidly (31).

MICROCATHETER PERFORATION, RUPTURE, AND SEPARATION

Although the static burst pressure of a standard microcatheter is in the range of 250 to 350 psi, it can withstand slowly increasing infusion rates at higher pressures. The distal floppy segment of the catheter has the thinnest wall and is the most likely to burst. In the author's experience a flow rate of dilute contrast at 1 mL per second or more can be achieved safely as long as the operator does not use a rapid bolus injection technique. If that thin-walled segment is twisted too quickly or allowed to become redundant by advancing it without a guide wire, it may partially collapse or kink, especially around tight turns. When the operator is unaware that the catheter lumen is thus restricted, the tubing may then rupture at the point of narrowing when he or she subsequently injects contrast medium or embolic particles. If the catheter is kinked unknowingly, reinsertion of the guide wire can easily lead to perforation of the wall. When using coaxial catheters, it is extremely important to ensure that both catheters are irrigated continuously. If for some reason the pressurized system is not functioning, a fibrin coating from refluxing blood can build up very quickly and cause increasing friction either between the two catheters or between the microcatheter and the steerable guide wire (24). If the operator continues to advance the guide wire tip when the wire is bound to the distal catheter, there is a potential risk that the floppy elastic tip may separate from its body.

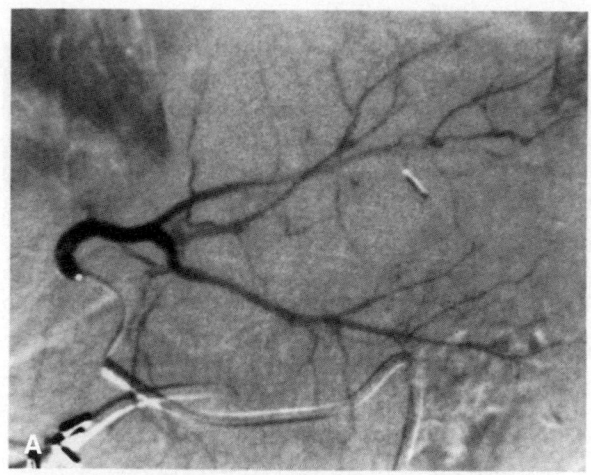

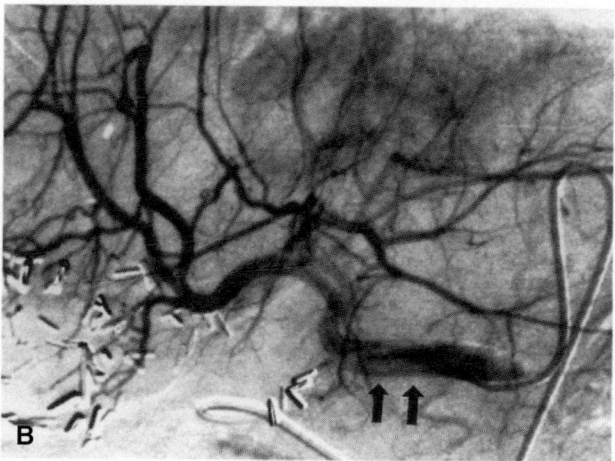

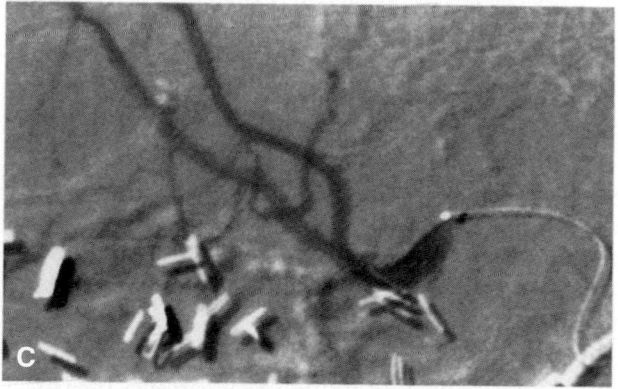

Figure 9–16 Superselective chemoembolization of colonic metastatic disease to the liver. **A.** The Simmons introduction catheter has been successfully advanced to the distal common hepatic artery for introducing a Tracker catheter superselectively in the left hepatic lobe. **B.** On a subsequent visit, the distal common hepatic artery was dissected (*arrows*) by the Simmons introducing catheter and guide wire. **C.** Despite the fresh dissection, it was still possible to pass a Target catheter superselectively through the damaged vessel to the right lobe for continued cheinoembolization.

CATHETER REFLUX AND WHIPPING

Rapid bolus injection through a small very floppy end-hole catheter leads to uncontrolled whipping of the tip. This can cause significant problems such as displacement of the catheter tip from its intended position into a different side branch or else trauma to small peripheral vessels, which can be manifested by spasm or thrombosis or even perforation. If the catheter is being used for fluid sclerosis or particulate embolization, then excessive pressure and flow through it may lead to dislodgment of the tip and accidental infarction of adjacent normal tissue (32). On the other hand, careful, purposeful, and controlled rapid injections of small volumes of contrast medium can be a useful maneuver to redirect angled-tip floppy catheters into target vessels.

CLINICAL USEFULNESS OF SUPERSELECTIVE CATHETERIZATION

Although superselective catheterization dates back to the mid-1960s, it was not widely used clinically for another 10–15 years because of the lack of well-trained interventional radiologists. In addition because the simple catheters and guide wires that were used at that time were relatively stiff and had poor maneuverability and trackability, it often proved difficult even for highly experienced angiographers to catheterize branch vessels superselectively with predictable success. The gradual development of a wide variety of specialized 5 French to 6 French preshaped catheters and more torqued guide wires greatly facilitated the practice of these demanding procedures. As a result, the catheterization of second- to fourth-order aortic branches from the thyrocervical through the bronchial, hepatic, gastroduodenal, pancreatic, renal, pelvic, and large limb arteries eventually became fairly routine in many centers.

The more recent introduction of coaxial microcatheter systems has led to a virtual explosion of superselective procedures for lesions that had previously been technically out of reach or too hazardous to catheterize. The peripheral vessels of virtually any organ of the body down to 1-mm branches can today be catheterized with a great chance of success in a rapid and efficacious manner with a markedly diminished chance of causing vascular spasm and dissection.

The following clinical examples typically seen in a busy angiographic practice will demonstrate the value of coaxial microcatheterization in reaching complex lesions for diagnosis or embolization (Figure 9–17).

Occult Parathyroid Adenoma

The microcatheter system is very useful in sampling for parathormone, not only from the thyroid veins but also from the small cervical and upper mediastinal veins. When an angiographic study demonstrates an adenoma, it can often be defunctionalized with an injection of hypertonic contrast medium (33) if its feeding vessel can be catheterized superselectively.

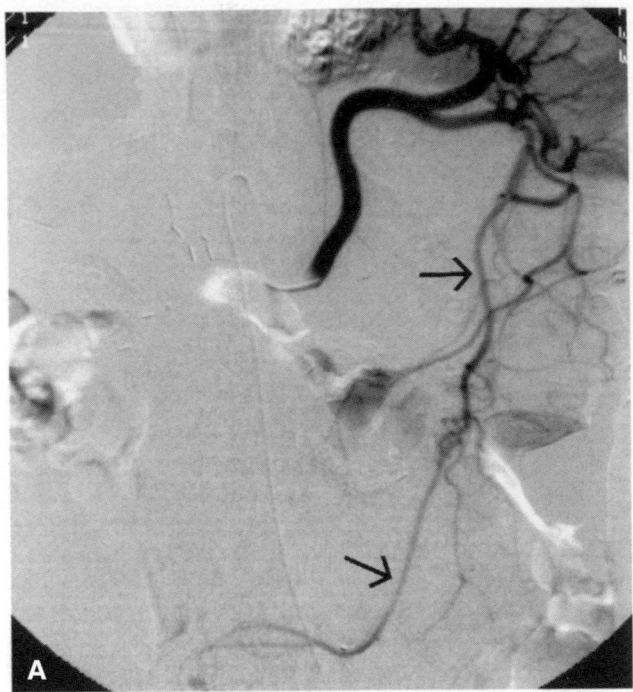

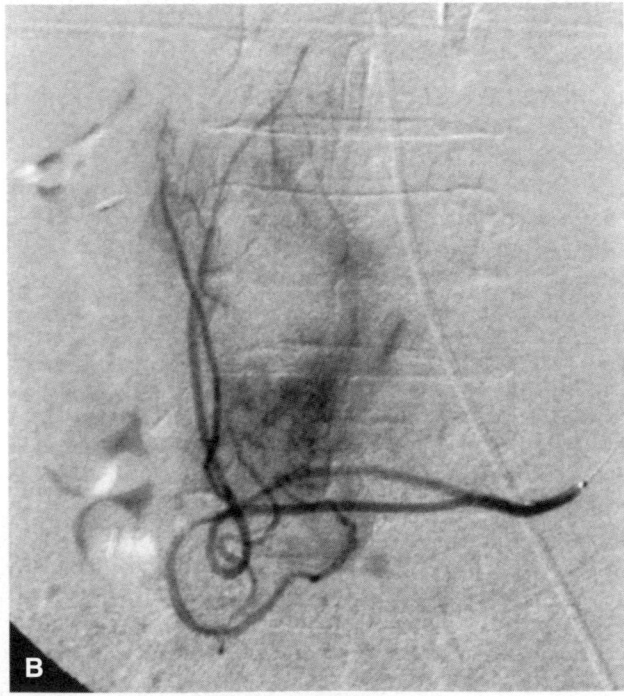

Figure 9–17 Chemoembolization of hepatoma omental metastases. **A.** Selective splenic arteriogram demonstrates the course of the gastroepiploic artery (*arrows*) before superselective catheterization. **B.** Tracker catheter positioned in the distal gastroepiploic artery for chemoembolization.

Hemoptysis

In the evaluation of patients with massive hemoptysis for embolization, the operator needs to be concerned with the exact identification of the bleeding vessel and the prevention of spinal cord ischemia (34).

Because of the small diameter of the microcatheter in relation to the intercostal-bronchial arteries, there is less chance of impairing spinal cord blood supply. In addition, the chances of infarcting the spinal cord diminish greatly when the embolization catheter is advanced past spinal feeders to a safer superselective position. This coaxial system is also very efficacious for catheterizing aberrant bronchial and parasitic vessels arising from subclavian artery branches.

Pancreatic and Gastrointestinal Hemorrhage

The microcatheter system allows very selective embolization of pancreatic and bowel bleeding points or vascular lesions (35). Embolization of the peripheral arcades of the small and large bowel can be performed to arrest bleeding in some cases without requiring subsequent surgery for possible infarction (35).

Patients who are hypotensive from gastrointestinal hemorrhage often have marked vasoconstriction of visceral vessels, a condition that can render subselective catheterization difficult or impossible. Because microcatheters do not usually exacerbate visceral artery spasm, they can often be used very successfully to reach and embolize the vascular bleeding point of these patients.

Liver Trauma and Tumor

Although superselective catheterization of the hepatic artery and its branches can often be performed with preshaped 5 French catheters and Glidewires (Terumo), the coaxial technique is far more dependable for reaching deeply into the liver. By using superselective embolization or chemoembolization, more normal tissue parenchyma is spared, and one minimizes ischemic damage to the duodenum, gallbladder, and central bile ducts from possible reflux embolization (36,37). The coaxial system is especially useful for catheterizing accessory hepatic branches from the superior mesenteric or the left gastric artery. When the celiac axis or proximal hepatic artery is occluded, a microcatheter and guide wire can be used to navigate successfully through dilated pancreatic-duodenal-biliary collateral vessels, phrenic, or internal mammary arteries to reach the reconstituted hepatic branches.

Renal Trauma and Tumor

Because renal arteries branch very early into small-caliber radicals and are very prone to go into spasm, the microcatheter is ideally suited for embolization of third- and fifth-order arterial branches for minimizing loss of functioning parenchyma (Figure 9–18) (38). This is an especially important consideration in the renal allograft, which lacks the potential for collateral flow (Figure 9–19) (39).

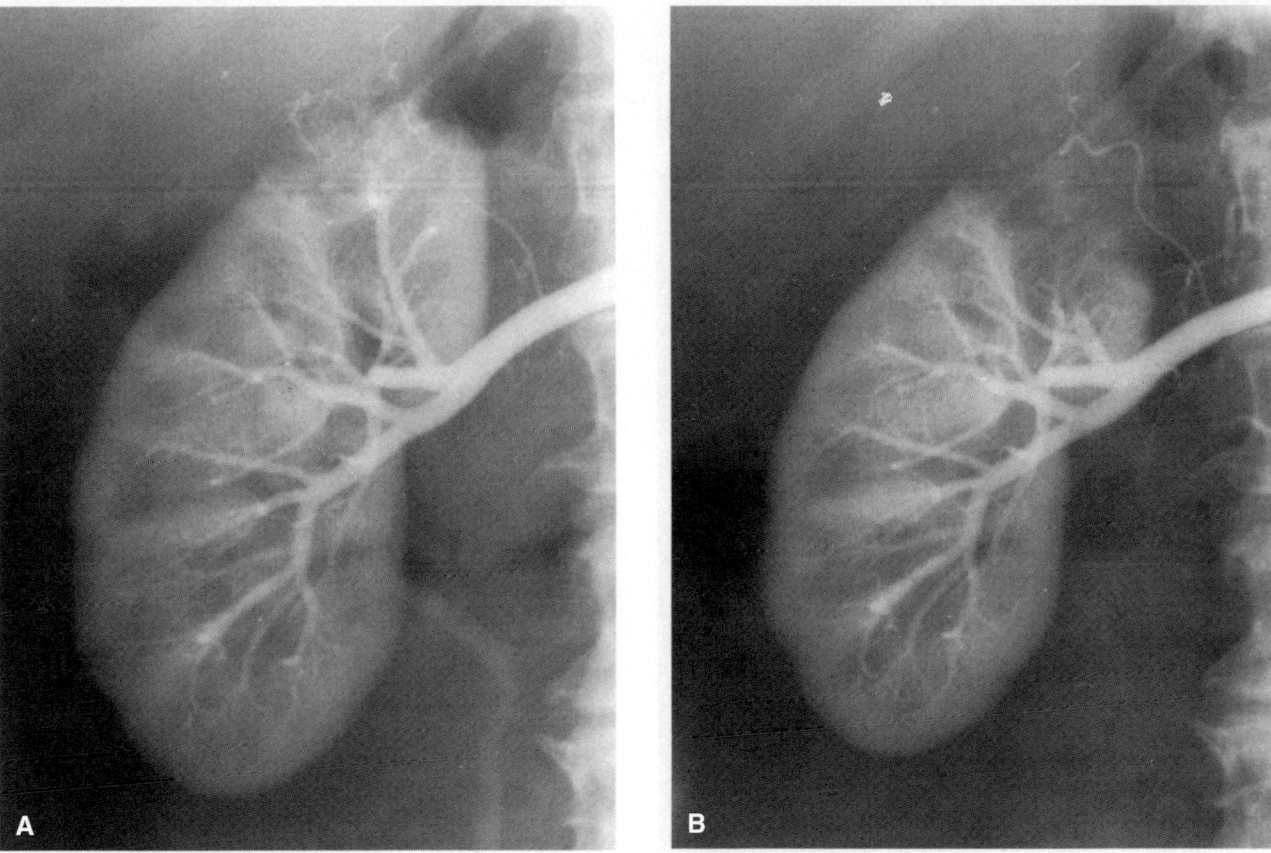

Figure 9–18 Superselective embolization of renal metastatic lesion **A.** with alcohol **B.** in a patient with contralateral nephrectomy.

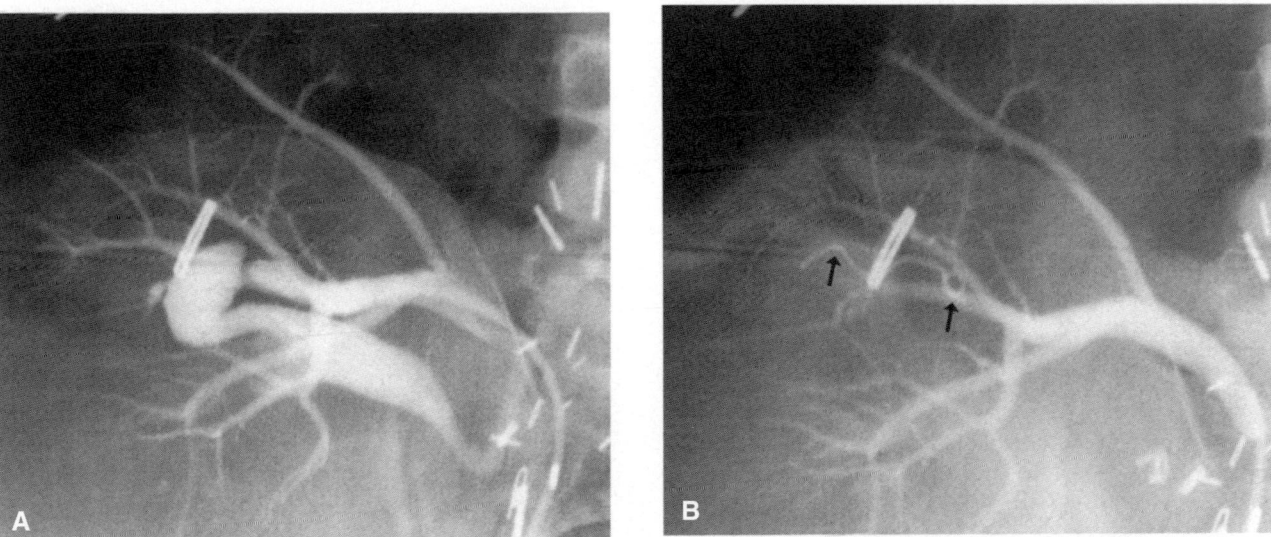

Figure 9–19 Use of microcatheter for renal trauma. **A.** Arteriovenous fistula in renal transplant. **B.** Tissue-sparing superselective occlusion of the fistula with a coil placed across the feeding artery (*arrows*).

Pelvic Trauma, Tumors, and Impotence

Because of the danger of causing spinal cord and major nerve damage, gluteal muscle infarction, and impotence, embolization of pelvic vessels for traumatic arterial bleeding should be as selective as possible to prevent nontarget ischemia (40).

Upper and Lower Extremity Trauma

Microcatheters are ideally suited for reaching wrist and ankle arteries atraumatically without inciting spasm for diagnosis, embolization, or thrombolysis (41).

Because it is possible to seat these microcatheters deeply into 1- to 2-mm branch arteries, one can successfully embolize small traumatic vascular lesions with little danger of refluxing particles to the hand or foot (Figure 9–20).

MECHANICAL INJECTORS

A great deal of dilution occurs when contrast material is injected into the vascular system. The amount of dilution depends on the velocity of blood flow in the vessel or chamber as well as on the rate and amount of contrast material being injected. Selective coronary arteriography can be performed at injection rates of 4 mL per second, and very satisfactory studies can be obtained with hand injections. Thoracic aortography requires injection rates up to 40 mL per second. Obviously, these rates can be accomplished only with a mechanical injector.

The factors controlling flow through nondistensible catheters can be expressed as Poiseuille's law:

$$Q = \frac{pPr4}{8nl}$$

in which

Q = cubic centimeters of contrast material delivered per second

P = hydraulic pressure in dynes per cubic centimeter

r = radius of the catheter lumen in centimeters

n = viscosity coefficient of the contrast material in poises

l = length of catheter in centimeters

This formula assumes that laminar flow is maintained throughout the injection.

One can draw the following conclusions from this information:

1. The speed of injection can be increased by using contrast material with low viscosity. Because the viscosity decreases as the temperature rises, it is important that the contrast be at body temperature at the time of injection.
2. The speed of injection can be increased by using short, thin-walled catheters. As the ratio of lumen to wall thickness increases, there is a corresponding increase in flow rate through the catheter. A short catheter decreases the peripheral resistance and thereby increases the speed of injection. Side holes have a similar effect.

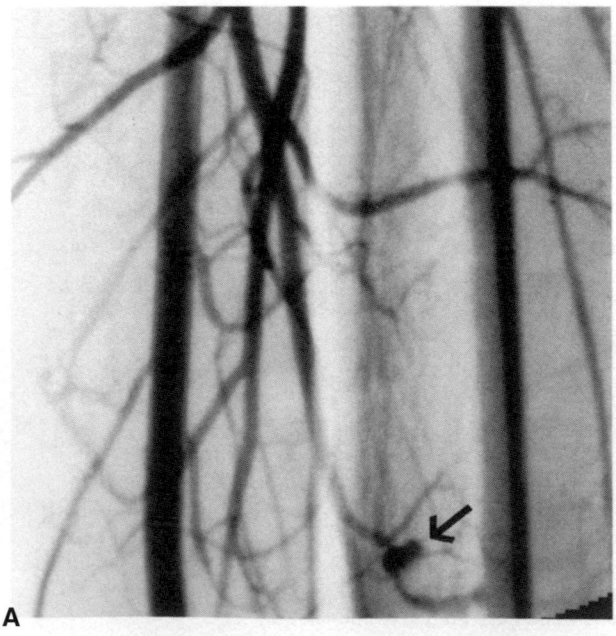

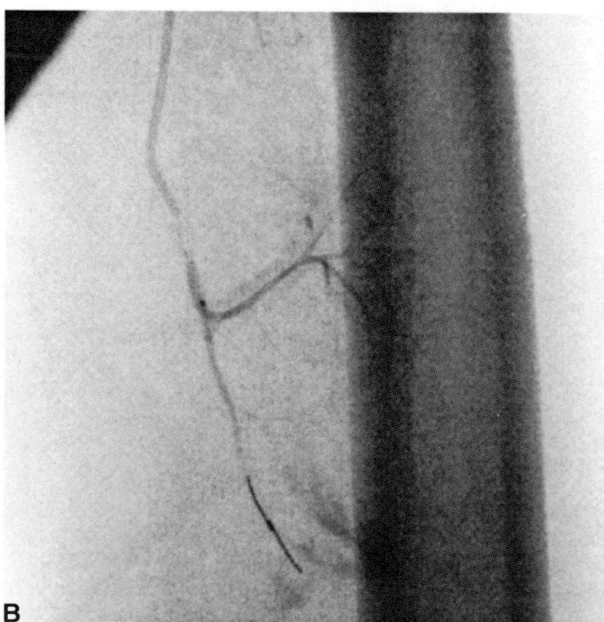

Figure 9–20 Proximity bullet wound in thigh. **A.** Bleeding point (*arrow*) from the superficial femoral artery appears at first glance to arise from the deep femoral artery. **B.** Coaxial superembolization of the pseudoaneurysm arising from a small side branch of the superficial femoral artery.

3. Increasing the pressure of injection will increase the delivery rate. The rupture pressure of the specific catheter is an obvious limiting factor.

BASIC TYPES OF PRESSURE INJECTORS

Hand Injectors

Usually, hand injectors incorporate movable levers that transmit force to a steel or reinforced-glass syringe. These are simple instruments of historical interest only: the force they deliver is inconstant and therefore difficult to reproduce on multiple injections. The maximum pressure is generally inadequate for injections through small catheters.

Pneumatic Power Injectors

These devices use compressed gases to transmit pressure directly to a cylinder, which is connected to the injector syringe. They operate under basic pneumatic and hydraulic principles. In keeping with Pascal's law that pressure applied to a liquid at any point is transmitted equally in all directions, if the area of the pressure cylinder is larger than that of the syringe, a mechanical advantage or power factor is obtained. Thus, a power factor of 5 means that the area of the pressure cylinder is five times the area of the syringe.

Because of the very high pressures that such a system generates, it is necessary to use specially designed stainless steel syringes that tolerate high pressures. Because these syringes are not transparent, special features have to be built in to avoid the inadvertent injection of any air that may enter the syringe while it is being filled with contrast material.

Many injectors have been described that work on the principle of compressed gases. In 1956, Gidlund described a compressed-air injector with a stainless steel syringe that could be placed in a vertical position (42). This position facilitated the addition of a valve for air removal at the top of the syringe. The contrast material was kept at body temperature by a thermostatically controlled water bath that surrounded the injector syringe. Injection pressure could be varied.

In 1960, Amplatz (43) described a cardiovascular injector powered by carbon dioxide cartridges such as those commonly used for the preparation of carbonated beverages (Figure 9–21). The syringe was bathed by a thermostatically controlled water bath so that the contrast material could be kept at 38°C (95°F). The major advantage of this system was that the injector weighed only 5 kg.

Electrically Powered Mechanical-Drive Injectors

Most injectors in use today are mechanical-drive injectors that are electrically powered. They are portable, and the

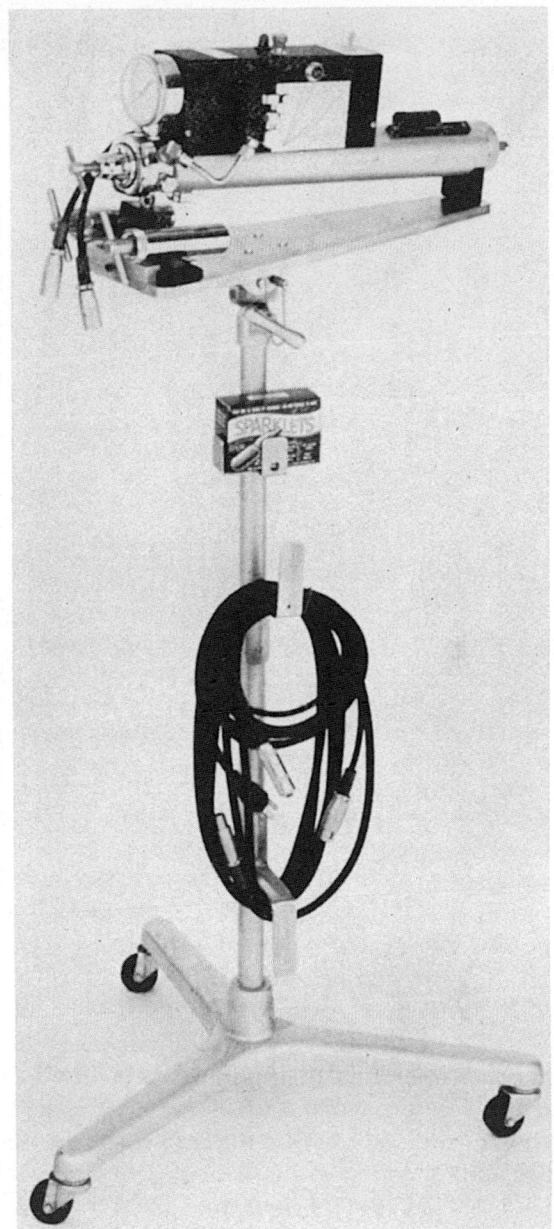

Figure 9–21 Amplatz injector (Nedmac).

only source of power necessary is an electric outlet. They can be programmed with the electrocardiogram so that multiple small injections can be made during very specific phases of the cardiac cycle. The Cordis injector (Johnson and Johnson) was one of the earliest such units available (Figure 9–22).

More recently introduced automatic injectors incorporated built-in safeguards against the hazards of ventricular fibrillation resulting from inadequate grounding of an electric injector at the time the patient's catheter is connected to the syringe (Figures 9–23, 9–24, and 9–25). An

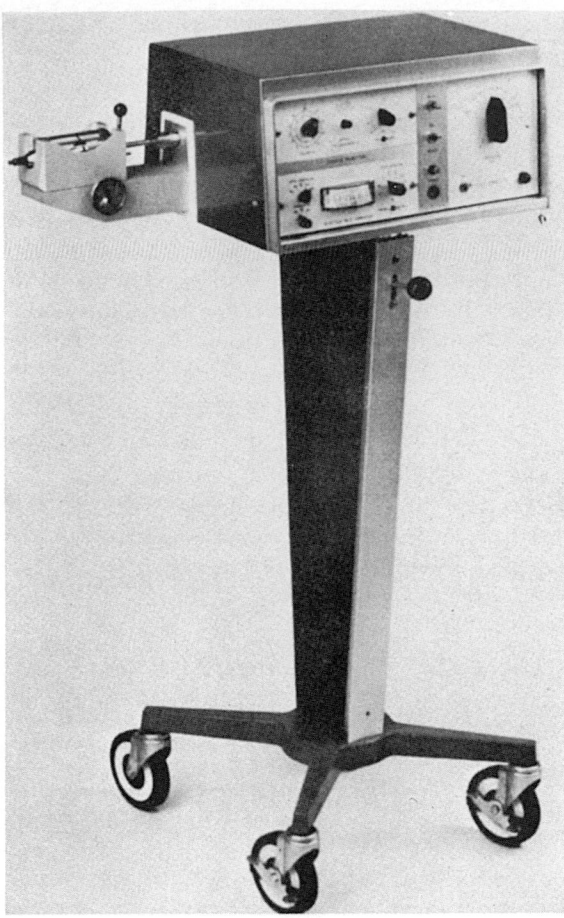

Figure 9–22   Cordis injector (Cordis).

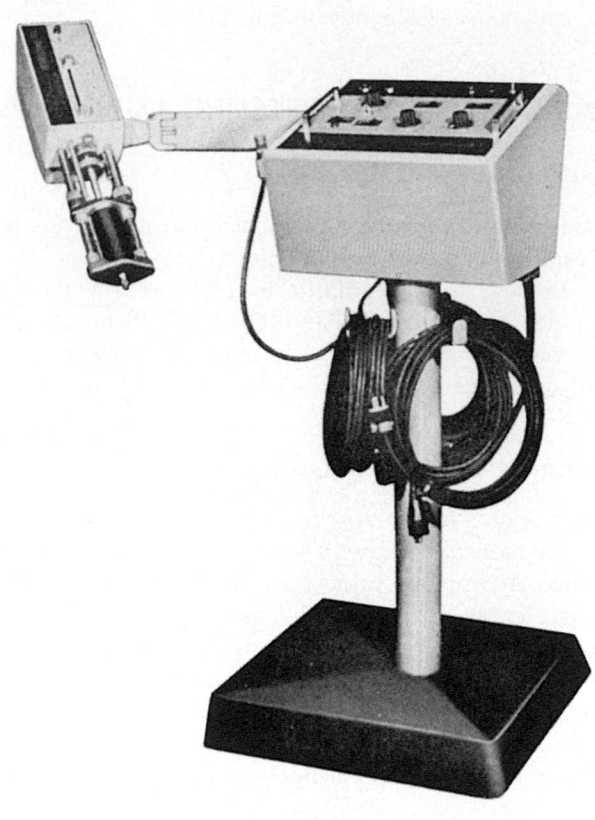

Figure 9–23   Viamonte-Hobbs injector (Barber-Colman Electro-Mechanical Products).

incorporated ground-safe detector detects malfunction of any of the electric circuits in which the preferential voltage ground would be conducted from the patient via the catheter to the injector and to the building ground. The detector has a sensitive sensing circuit that can detect the potential difference of 40 mV or higher; the injector then automatically breaks its ground circuit, the procedure stops, and an audible alarm sounds. Because a catheterization laboratory contains electric equipment that may come in contact with the patient, such as electrocardiograph, electric catheterization tables, pressure transducers, pressure injectors, unsafe grounding is potentially hazardous. Currents as low as 20 mA (60 cycles per second AC) with voltages as low as 60 mVA can induce ventricular fibrillation in dogs. Currents of 1–4 mA (60 cycles per second AC) have fibrillated the human heart during surgery.

These injectors also operate on the principle of metered delivery rate, which not only provides an automatic control of flow rate by compensating for injection variables but also eliminates time-consuming charts. One dial on the control panel selects the duration of the injection

(1–4 seconds), and a second dial selects the delivery rate (2–60 mL per second).

SUMMARY

The skilled interventional radiologist can reach almost any vessel in the body with relative ease and safety as a result of ongoing technological improvements in the material and design of catheter-guide wire systems. Superselective catheterization is vital to the proper evaluation and management of remote lesions amenable to embolization or chemotherapy. By allowing an operator to bypass branch vessels that potentially feed major nerves, the spinal cord, or other susceptible tissues, microcatheters are indispensable for preventing catastrophic complications.

Superselective catheterization is a very powerful method for sampling hormonal blood levels to detect functioning endocrine tumors. In the future, when more sensitive, specific tumor markers are developed, it may play an even more important role for localizing and destroying nascent malignancies of all types.

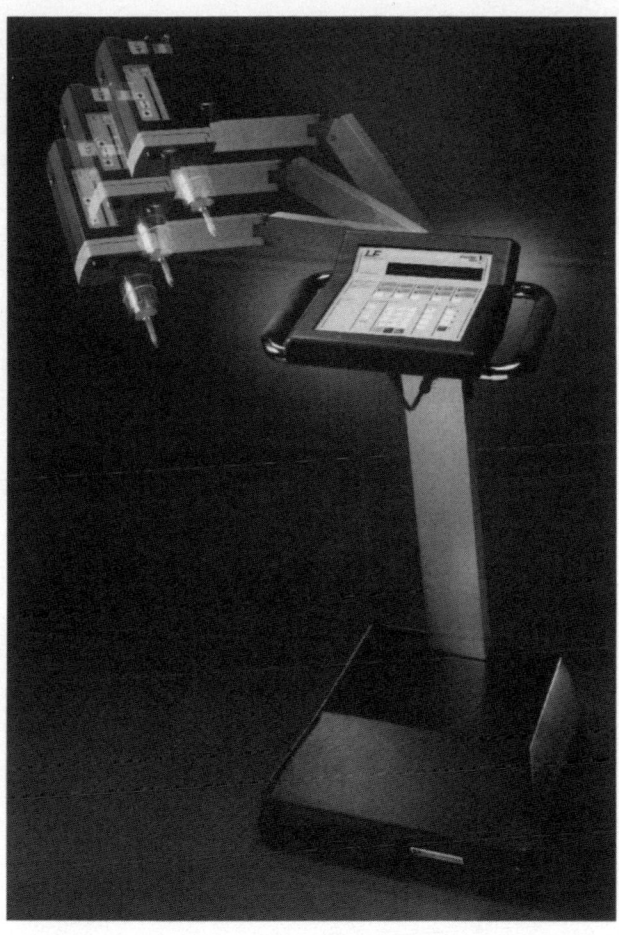

Figure 9–24   Medrad injector (Medrad).

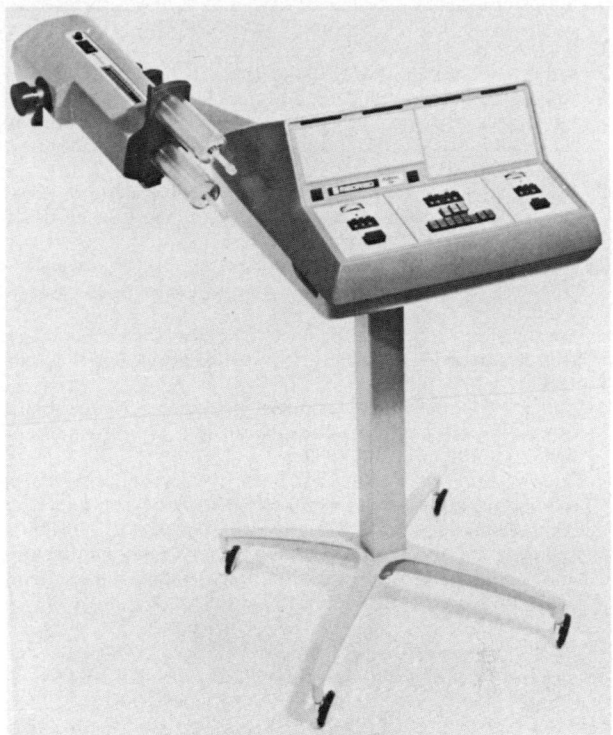

Figure 9–25   Liebel-Florsheim injector.

REFERENCES

1. Seldinger SI. Catheter placement of needles in percutaneous arteriography: a new technique. Acta Radiol 1953;39:368–376.
2. Ödman P. Percutaneous selective angiography of the main branches of the aorta. Acta Radiol 1956;45:1–14.
3. Boijsen E. Selective hepatic angiography in primary and secondary tumors of the liver. Rev Int Hepat 1965;15:385–395.
4. Paul RE, Miller HH, Kahn PC, et al. Pancreatic angiography with application of subselective angiography of the celiac and superior mesenteric artery for the diagnosis of carcinoma of the pancreas. N Engl J Med 1964;272:283–287.
5. Takayasu K, Muramatsu Y, Moriyama N, et al. Plastic-coated guide wire for hepatic arteriography. Radiology 1988;166:545–546.
6. Cope C. Minipuncture angiography. Radiol Clin North Am 1986;24:359–367.
7. Kaufman SL. Angioplasty from the contralateral approach: use of a guiding catheter and coaxial angioplasty balloons. Radiology 1990;177:577.
8. Galli M, Tarantino F, Mameli S, et al. Transradial approach for renal percutaneous transluminal angioplasty and stenting: a feasibility pilot study. J Invasive Cardiol. 2002;14:386–90.
9. Cope C, Burke DR, Meranze SG, eds. Atlas of interventional radiology. St. Louis: Mosby, 1990.
10. Chuang VP, Soo CS, Carrasco CH, et al. Superselective catheterization technique in hepatic angiography. AJR 1983;41:803–811.
11. Richman SD, Green WM, Kroll R, et al. Superselective transcatheter embolization of traumatic renal hemorrhage. AJR 1977;128:843–844.
12. Yu-Tang Goh P, Lin M, Teo N, et al. Embolization for hemoptysis: a six-year review. Cardiovasc Intervent Radiol. 2002;25:17–25.
13. Kramer SC, Gorich J, Rilinger N, et al. Embolization for gastrointestinal hemorrhages. Eur Radiol. 2000;10(5):802–805.
14. Velmahos GC, Toutouzas KG, Vassiliu P, et al. A prospective study on the safety and efficacy of angiographic embolization for pelvic and visceral injuries. J Trauma. 2002;53:303–308.
15. Fisher RG, Ben Menachem Y. Embolization procedures in trauma: the extremities—acute lesions. Semin Intervent Radiol 1985;2:118–124.
16. Rossi GP, Sacchetto A, Chiesura-Corona M, et al. Identification of the etiology of primary aldosteronism with adrenal vein sampling in patients with equivocal computed tomography and magnetic resonance findings: results in 104 consecutive cases. J Clin Endocrinol Metab. 2001;86:1083–1090.
17. Cornud F, Belin X, Amar E, et al. Varicocele: strategies in diagnosis and treatment. Eur Radiol. 1999;9(3):536–545.
18. Waltman AC, Courcy WR, Athanasoulis CA, et al. Technique for left gastric artery catheterization. Radiology 1973;109:732–734.
19. Cope C. Suture technique to reshape the sidewinder catheter curve. J Intervent Radiol 1986;1:63–64.
20. Sawada C. Selective hepatic angiography using a balloon catheter guide. Radiology 1985;156:545–546.
21. Okasaki M, Nakamura T, Higashihara H, et al. Successful transcatheter arterial embolization for the replaced right hepatic artery: a new technique using a balloon catheter and norepinephrine infusion. AJR 1989;152:204.
22. Nakamura H, Hashimoto T, Oi H, et al. Hepatic embolization through periportal collaterals: balloon occlusion technique. AJR 1987;148:626–628.
23. Eisenberg H. Angiography of the pancreas. In: Hilal S, ed. Small vessel angiography. St. Louis: Mosby, 1983:405–409.
24. Cope C. A new one-catheter torque-guide system for percutaneous exploratory abdominal angiography. Radiology 1969;92:174–175.
25. Eisenberg H, Steer HL. The nonoperative treatment of massive pyloroduodenal hemorrhage by retracted autologous clot embolization. Surgery 1976;79:414–420.
26. Cope C. Conversion from small (0.018 in) to large (0.038 in) guide wires in percutaneous drainage procedures. AJR 1982;138:974–976.

27. Simpson JB, Baim DS, Robert EW, et al. A new catheter system for coronary angioplasty. Am J Cardiol 1982;49:1216–1222.

28. Sos TA, Cohn DJ, Srur M, et al. A new open-ended guide wire catheter. Radiology 1985;154:817–818.

29. Bilbao JI, Aqueretta JD, Longo JM, et al. The open-ended guide wire as superselective catheter for intra-arterial chemotherapy: experience in 190 procedures. Cardiovasc Intervent Radiol 1990; 13:375–377.

30. Rüfenacht DA, Latchaus RE. Principles and methodology of intracranial endovascular access. Neuroimag Clin North Am 1992;2:251–268.

31. Wolpert SM, Kwan ESK, Heros D, et al. Selective delivery of chemotherapeutic agents with a new catheter system. Radiology 1980;166:547–549.

32. Encarnacion CE, Kadir S, Malone RB. Subselective embolization with gelatin sponge through an open-ended guide wire. Radiology 1990;174:265–267.

33. Miller DL, Doppman JL, Change R, et al. Angiographic ablation of parathyroid adenomas: lessons from a 10-year experience. Radiology 1987;165:601–657.

34. Yoon W, Kim JK, Kim YH, et al. Bronchial and nonbronchial systemic artery embolization for life-threatening hemoptysis: a comprehensive review. Radiographics. 2002;22:1395–1409.

35. Lefkovitz Z, Cappell MS, Lookstein R, et al. Radiologic diagnosis and treatment of gastrointestinal hemorrhage and ischemia. Med Clin North Am. 2002;86:1357–1399.

36. Savader SJ, Trerotola SO, Merine DS, et al. Hemobilia after percutaneous transhepatic biliary drainage: treatment for transcatheter embolotherapy. J Vasc Interv Radiol 1992;3:345–352.

37. Gee M, Soulen MC. Chemoembolization for hepatic metastases. Tech Vasc Interv Radiol. 2002;5:132–140.

38. Kaufman SL, Martin LG, Zuckerman AM, et al. Peripheral transcatheter embolization with platinum microcoils. Radiology 1992;184:369–372.

39. Maleux G, Messiaen T, Stockx L, et al. Transcatheter embolization of biopsy-related vascular injuries in renal allografts. Long-term technical, clinical and biochemical results. Acta Radiol. 2003;44:13–17.

40. Quinn SF, Frau DM, Saff GN, et al. Neurologic complications of pelvic intra-arterial chemo-embolization performed with collagen material and cisplatin. Radiology 1988;167:55–57.

41. Hanks SE, Pentecost MJ. Angiography and transcatheter treatment of extremity trauma. Semin Interv Radiol 1992;9:19–27.

42. Gidlund A. Development of apparatus and methods for roentgen studies in haemodynamics. Acta Radiol (Stockh) 1956;130 (Suppl):1.

43. Amplatz K. A vascular injector with program selector. Radiology 1960;75:955.

Agents for Small Vessel/Tissue Embolization and Transcatheter Tissue Ablation

Current Status and the Future

Aalpen A. Patel, Michael C. Soulen

Since the first efforts at embolization of vascular territories in the beginning of the 20th century (1), highly sophisticated catheterization tools and numerous embolic materials have been developed that permit interventional radiologists to perform vascular occlusion with suprasurgical precision. The first agents aimed to control hemorrhage and to ablate tumors, organs, and vascular malformations with minimal hazard to nontarget tissues. The mechanism of action was primarily mechanical obstruction of blood vessels. The new generation of embolics currently available or on the horizon capitalizes on the delivery of localized radiation, heat, and chemical or biological therapeutics to

the area or organ of interest. Safe use of these embolics requires the proper use of embolization techniques, which in turn requires an understanding of the vascular anatomy, disease being treated, and the tools used to deliver the embolic agents themselves.

The choice of agent will depend on the organ, the disease process, the size of the vessel to be occluded, and the goal of the therapy. Large vessel occlusion requires mechanical devices such as coils or balloons. Occlusion of higher-order branches on down to the capillary level or tissue ablation can be performed with particulate or liquid agents. This chapter will focus on the embolic or ablative

TABLE 10–1		
EMBOLIC AGENTS		
	Size	Duration
Biodegradable Agents		
Gelatin sponge (Gelfoam or Surgifoam) (powder, slurry, or torpedoes)	40 μ–4 mm	2 days–6 weeks
Microfibrillar collagen (Avitene)	5 μ x 70 μ	1–8 weeks
Starch microspheres (Spherex)	20–70 μ	30–60 min
Permanent Agents		
Polyvinyl alcohol particles (amorphous)	45–1,180 μ	
Spherical embolics		
Spherical PVA (Contour SE Microspheres)	100–1,200 μ	
Bead Block (PVA hydrogel)	100–1,200 μ	
Embospheres	40–1,200 μ	
Pharmaceutical embolics (Pharmembolics) (± encapsulated drugs or radioactivity)	40–500 μ	
Available or in trials:		
SIR-Spheres (Sirtex Medical Limited)		
TheraSphere (MDS Nordion)		
Cells (encapsulated or nonencapsulated)		
Other agents on the horizon or with potential:		
Dox-Spheres		
Thermo-Spheres		
MTC-Dox Spheres (FeRx)		
Liquid Agents		
Commonly used:		
Ethanol (dehydrated)		
Iodized Oil (ethiadol, lipiodol)		
Glue (n-butyl cyanoacrylate [NBCA])		
Rarely Used:		
Sodium tetradecyl sulfate (Sotradecol)		
Boiling contrast		
Hypertonic glucose		

agents for small vasculature. The most commonly used materials are listed in Table 10–1.

The ideal embolic agent is one that is precisely sized, nonaggregating (preventing catheter occlusion), transiently radiopaque (allowing future imaging that is free of artifact), systemically nontoxic (although local, targeted toxicity may be desirable), able to deliver a secondary agent at a prescribed rate, nonallergenic, and inexpensive. It allows easily controlled delivery through conventional or microcatheter systems to a specific vascular territory and provides reliable occlusion for the desired length of time, reliable tissue ablation with attached secondary therapeutics, or both. None of the agents listed in the Table 10–1 meets all these qualifications, but each has its particular niche among the varied clinical indications for embolization. The clinical setting should guide the interventional radiologist to use these agents safely and effectively.

BIODEGRADABLE AGENTS

Gelatin Sponge

Gelfoam (Pharmacia and Upjohn) and Surgifoam (Ethicon) (Figure 10–1A) are inexpensive gelatin sponges packaged as sterile sheets or in powder form. When used as an embolic agent (an off-label use but within the standard of care), gelatin foam causes vascular occlusion by mechanical obstruction, induction of thrombosis, and inflammation of the vessel wall. The gelatin dissolves and permits recanalization of the artery in a matter of days or weeks (2). Because it does not cause permanent occlusion, gelatin foam is useful in the treatment of benign sources of bleeding, such as trauma or peptic ulcer disease, when healing of the underlying lesion is expected. The gelatin may also be useful for temporary devascularization of masses or organs immediately before resection to minimize blood loss.

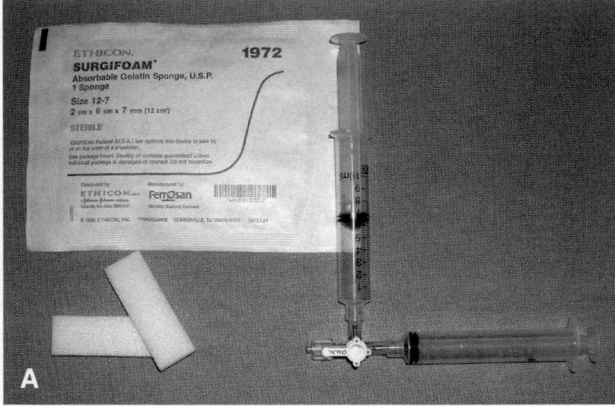

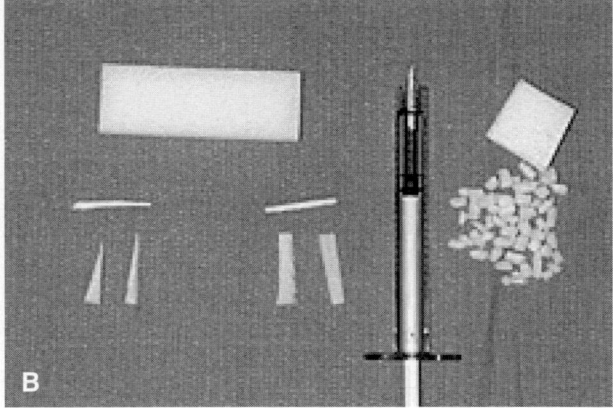

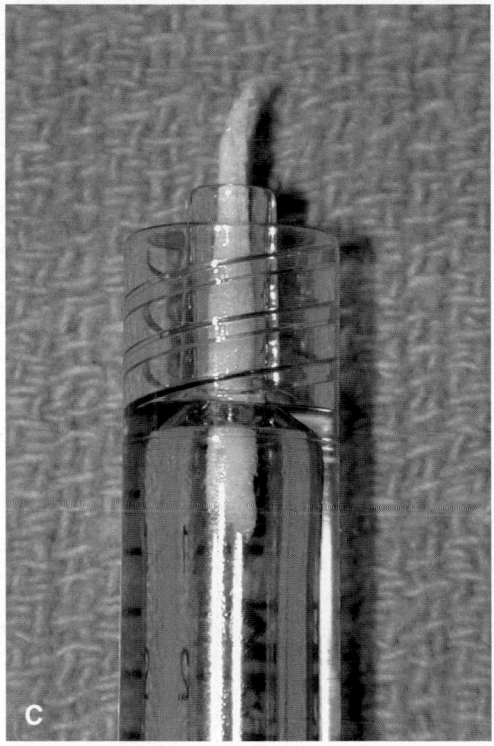

Figure 10–1 **A.** The Surgifoam brand of gelatin foam shown here comes as a sheet of gelatin sponge (*left*). The syringe and three-way stopcock setup (*right*) demonstrates how it should be used for making slurry. **B.** The 1–2 mm cubes illustrated are placed in one syringe and contrast in the other. Vigorous agitation further fragments the pieces and suspends them in a slurry mixture (*not shown*). The strips and triangles may be rolled to form the torpedoes. **C.** This is a magnified view of how a torpedo may be loaded in a 1 mL syringe filled with contrast. For illustration purposes, the tip of the torpedo is partially outside the tip of the syringe. During usage in a procedure, however, the entire torpedo should be fully inside the tip of the syringe. Use caution to keep it from falling into the body of the syringe.

When small branches need to be embolized, such as ramifications of the left gastric artery or pancreaticoduodenal branches of the gastroduodenal artery feeding a peptic ulcer bleed, gelatin foam may be cut into 1–2 mm pieces and loaded into a 10-mL syringe. This is connected to another 10-mL syringe filled with dilute contrast (1:1 ratio) via a three-way stopcock, and the contrast and gelatin foam are agitated rapidly back and forth to create slurry (Figure 10–1B). If more uniform slurry is desired, the stopcock is partially closed to cause more mechanical fragmentation of the gelatin foam pieces. The slurry is injected carefully until the flow in the distal branch vessels is near stasis. Torpedoes may be added to embolize the larger parent artery (Figure 1B and C). Care should be taken not to create complete stasis, because injection at that point will cause reflux of gelatin foam out of the target artery. The slurry is fine enough to pass through a microcatheter. The slurry will have a tendency to float upward in the contrast-filled syringe, so the syringe tip should be pointed up during injection to avoid aggregation of the gelatin foam at the back of the syringe. When using slurry in the gastroduodenal artery to treat duodenal hemorrhage, coil blockade of the proximal right gastroepiploic artery may be performed to protect the greater curve of the stomach and to direct the slurry into the pancreaticoduodenal branches.

Gelfoam powder measures 40–60 μ and, because of particulate aggregation, causes occlusion of vessels 100–200 μ in diameter. This distal level of embolization is beyond most collateral vessels and causes more severe ischemia than slurry or torpedoes. Gelfoam powder is good for preoperative embolization of tumors or organs but should not be used in embolizing the branches that feed the bowel because of the risk of necrosis.

Microfibrillar Collagen

Avitene (Davol, Cranston, RI) is a preparation of collagen fibers derived from cowhide. The fibers are 5 μ in diameter by 70–200 μ in length and cause vascular occlusion at the 25–250 μ level. Avitene causes a granulomatous reaction (more than the gelatin foam) (3–5). Recanalization of the vessels begins at approximately 1 week and continues over 1–2 months. The collagen itself is broken down and reabsorbed after 3 months. As with the Gelfoam powder, the small size of the collagen fibers makes them unsuitable for embolization of the gut because of the risk of infarction. Collagen is useful for tumor embolization, either preoperatively or palliatively, and has been used for chemoembolization in the liver. The small fibers are easily administered when suspended in contrast through microcatheters. However, its use has decreased in favor of new "designer" embolics.

Starch Microspheres

Starch microspheres are biodegradable particles manufactured from potato starch. They are spherical, precisely sized, and deformable to allow easy passage through microcatheters. The starch is metabolized rapidly by amylase and has a half-life of 25 minutes, so the ischemia is short-lived but intense because of the peripheral level of occlusion. The primary application is for chemoembolization, which allows a high level of drug extraction with only transient ischemia. Starch microspheres are not as popular as other microspheres at present (6).

PERMANENT AGENTS

Polyvinyl Alcohol Particles

Polyvinyl alcohol (PVA) is an inert plastic sponge that comes in blocks and sheets or is ground into coarsely shaped particles of graded dimensions from 45–1,180 μ (Figure 10–2). It causes permanent mechanical occlusion of the vessel lumen with subsequent ingrowth of thrombus and fibrin (7). The amorphous particles have a tendency to clump into aggregates so that occlusion occurs at a level of vessels larger than the size of the particles used. Occlusion of the catheter lumen is an occasional problem as well, especially when the suspension of particles is too thick. Suspensions of PVA can be created by pouring a 1 cc vial into 50 mL of dilute contrast in a sterile metal bowl, placing the tip of a 3–5 mL syringe below the surface, and stirring the mixture to suspend the particles. It is important to take care not to cause air bubbles that can trap the particles, which often leads to bigger aggregates.

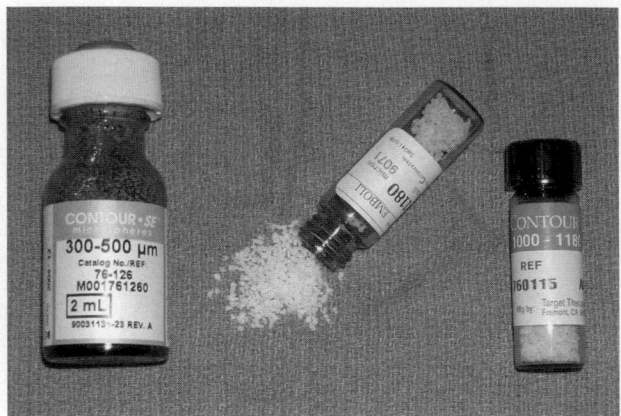

Figure 10–2   Spherical PVA (Contour SE) by Boston Scientific is shown on the left. It is supplied as suspension of particles in saline. On the right, the particles on the towel are the amorphous PVA particles, which are supplied as dry powder. One of the ways a suspension may be formed is by using a similar syringe/stopcock setup as shown in Figure 10–1.

Manufacturers provide a chart of contrast dilution that should be used for the size of particle used. This helps lessen the effect of buoyancy and suspend the particles better. A lower ratio of particles to contrast can be used for smaller or less vascular territories, such as spinal malformations. An alternative method is to pack 0.1–0.2 mL of PVA particles into a 10-mL syringe, then connect via a three-way stopcock to another 10-mL syringe filled with dilute contrast and pump back and forth, in the same way described for making gelatin foam slurry. Only particles less than 250 μ should be injected through microcatheters to avoid clogging the catheter. Like gelatin foam, PVA particles tend to float in contrast, so the syringe must be pointed upward during injection to avoid aggregation or clumping at the back of the barrel. More recently, PVA (nonhydrogel) microspheres have been manufactured and marketed. The permanence and distal level of occlusion caused by PVA makes it well-suited for treatment of hypervascular tumors.

Recently, various spherical embolic agents have become available and have grown increasingly popular. For interventionalists who are accustomed to amorphous PVA particles, the spherical embolics above should be increased in size by 100–200 μ. As these new spherical embolics are compressible, they require the increase in size. Although they may be easier to use, none of the bland variety has proved more efficacious than any other in most applications (8).

Spherical Polyvinyl Alcohol

Contour SE Microspheres (Boston Scientific Natick, MA) combine the biocompatibility of PVA with a spherical conto for better delivery through the catheter. Its structure allows compression to facilitate its delivery. This compressibility also helps achieve a more complete occlusion of the target vessel (9) (Figure 10–2).

Bead Block

Bead Block (Biocompatibles UK Ltd, Farnham, UK) microspheres are manufactured from polyvinyl alcohol (PVA) hydrogel. They are hydrophilic and compressible, facilitating flow through a catheter and microvasculature. For easy visualization in the delivery syringe, Bead Block microspheres are tinted blue (10).

Embospheres

Embospheres (BioSphere Medical Inc., Rockland, MA) are spherical, hydrophilic spheres composed of trisacryl gelatin; the hydrophilic and elastic properties help it prevent aggregation within the catheter lumen, which prevents clogging of the catheter and allows thorough embolization of the vascular territory. The FDA has approved the use of microspheres for embolization of hypervascularized tumors, arteriovenous malformations, and uterine fibroids (8,11–13). Some evidence exists that less operative blood loss occurs when bone tumors are embolized with Embospheres as compared to amorphous PVA (14).

Pharmembolic Particles: Biologically Active Particles

Several different microspheres made from organic compounds, glass, or metal exist or are under development and testing. Features of these particles include smooth, spherical geometry, precise sizing, and coatings or materials that incorporate radioactive or chemotherapeutic agents. Reported applications include treatment of liver tumors (primary or metastatic). On the horizon are drug-eluting beads (embolic microspheres with doxorubicin). Biocompatibles, Inc has developed PVA hydrogel-based microspheres that allow elusion of doxorubicin at a controlled rate. Trials are underway for determining the efficacy of this product in humans. If successful, it may become the chemoembolization technique of the future. Similar technology may be used for other drugs and indications (10). A second product on the horizon is Dox-Spheres (Sirtex Medical Limited). Doxorubicin is incorporated into spheres made from a biodegradable matrix, allowing controlled release of the active drug from the matrix.

Cells

The implantation of cells in diseased organs as a means of treatment holds much promise. Islet cells may be delivered as an embolic through portal vein access to perform islet cell transplant and potentially to cure type I diabetes. Islet cell transplantation has proven to be effective in the treatment of type I Diabetes Mellitus. With new sirolimus-based (steroid free) antirejection protocols and graft cells from two (rarely three donors), more than 80% of patients have been able to discontinue insulin. Although, currently restricted to patients with severe glycemic lability, this process may become the standard of care in the future (15). Alginate hydrogels have been used in the form of microspheres to act as a delivery medium for cells to the tissues via transcatheter injections. Implantable alginate microspheres with genetically engineered cells have been used to deliver insulin, growth hormone, and factor IX in animal models (16–19). Abruzzo et al. showed that microsphere-encapsulated cells may be successfully injected through a properly sized microcatheter without significant changes to microsphere structure, cell viability, or cell function (19). Use of alginate hydrogel microspheres and microcatheter systems may grant some advantage over the nonencapsulated cellular preparations described earlier. Microcatheters permit subselective delivery of cells to precise target vessel branches in the desired locations. The immunoisolation properties of alginate microspheres may allow the microsphere vessels to serve as sanctuaries for the implanted cells (19).

LIQUID AGENTS

Unlike particles that, by virtue of their size, are arrested at a precapillary level, liquid sclerosants can pass to the capillary level and through to the venous circulation. This feature makes them desirable agents when tissue destruction is warranted, such as for ablation of tumors, organs, veins, or vascular malformations. Vascular occlusion occurs from a combination of thrombosis and destruction of the vessel endothelium, which is usually permanent.

The use of liquid sclerosants is more challenging than the use of particulate agents. The lack of radiopacity and their deeper penetration into tissue makes the distribution harder to control and carries an increased risk of nontarget embolization. For example, when using alcohol to ablate a renal tumor, alcohol washing through the tumor is harmless because of rapid dilution in the high-flow renal venous system. However, perfusion of angiographically occult retroperitoneal branches communicating with perineural vasculature can cause paralysis, and undetected reflux into the aorta can lead to visceral infarction. Whenever possible, the use of an occlusion balloon to deliver liquid sclerosants is recommended. The usual technique is to inflate the occlusion balloon in the renal artery and inject enough contrast to determine the volume of contrast needed to fill the tumor to capillary phase. Then, the balloon is deflated, the alcohol drawn up, the balloon reinflated, and the alcohol injected at the same rate as the contrast. The balloon is left up for 3–5 minutes to allow for tissue ablation and thrombosis to occur. The catheter then is aspirated before the balloon is deflated to remove any alcohol or clot debris remaining in the artery and thus prevent reflux into the aorta. If an occlusion balloon cannot be used, then the alcohol can be made partially radiopaque by shaking it with ethiadol in an 8:2 or 7:3 ratio (20). The suspended oil droplets make it possible to observe the flow of the alcohol fluoroscopically. The oil also improves the distribution and embolic effect of the alcohol (21).

Trufill n-BCA Liquid Embolic System (Cordis, Miami Lakes, FL) is an embolization system consisting of N-butylcyanoacrylate, or n-BCA, (two 1-g tubes), ethiadol (10 mL) (Figure 10–3), and tantalum powder (1 g) (22,23). These components are mixed to form a suspension that is injected through a microcatheter to embolize. The approved use is for devascularization of cerebral AVMs before surgical resection. The mixture is liquid during delivery and hardens to form a solid substance on contact with ions. Because of its low viscosity, n-BCA is easy to deliver through microcatheters. However, the lack of radiopacity makes it difficult to use. The embolic can be mixed with ethiadol, tantalum, or tungsten powder to allow visualization of the glue. Tantalum slows the initiation of polymerization, and ethiadol slows the polymerization time. The commonly used mixtures include glue to ethiadol at ratios of 1:1 to 1:4. There is a compromise between visibility and polymerization time. There appears to be a linear relationship between glue dilution and polymerization (1 second at 1:1 and 4 seconds at 1:4 dilution) (22). As the monomer polymerizes when it comes into contact with ions, only D5W would be used for flushes. In addition, polypropylene syringes should be used because polycarbonate can be destroyed by cyanoacrylate. Training is recommended before using n-BCA to achieve effective embolization and to prevent complications. A complete

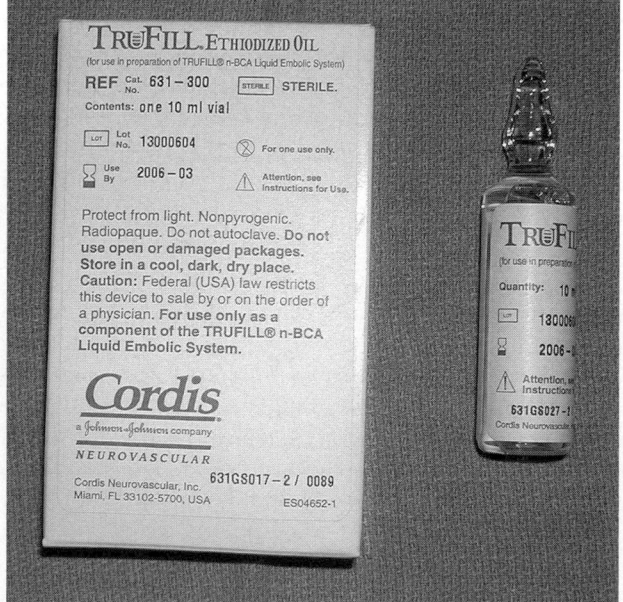

Figure 10–3 A Trufill n-BCA Liquid Embolic System (Cordis) package and supplied ethiadol is shown. The ethiadol may be used with alcohol and some of the chemoembolic protocols.

description of the technique and its nuances is beyond the scope of this chapter. Many off-label uses have been described, including thoracic duct embolization, peripheral AVM embolization, and endoleak embolization after aortic endograft placement (23).

Cyanoacrylate causes acute inflammatory reaction in the wall of the blood vessel and surrounding tissues, progressing to granulomatous reaction with giant cells and fibrosis. If a solid cast of the lesion is not formed, recanalization can occur. Extravascular extrusion of the glue to extravascular space has also been observed (22).

When liquid agents are used to sclerose the gonadal vein in the treatment of a varicocele, the inguinal ring must be compressed to prevent reflux into the scrotum and testicular infarction (24). In the United States, coils and detachable balloons have largely replaced this. In most practices in the United States today, the use of sodium tetradecyl sulfate (Sotradecol), boiling contrast, and hypertonic glucose is rare or nonexistent.

NONEMBOLIC PARTICULATES OR TISSUE ABLATIVE AGENTS

SIR-Spheres (Sirtex Medical Limited, Australia) are biocompatible radioactive microspheres made of resin or ceramic—depending on whether first-generation or second-generation—that contain Yttrium-90 and emit β radiation (25). The microspheres are approximately 35 microns in size (26). On the average the β radiation is only able to penetrate 2.4 mm of tissue. Yttrium-90 has a half-life of approximately 64 hours and, therefore, after 14 days, only 2.5% of the original activity remains (27). The spheres are selectively infused in the blood vessel feeding the area of interest. The SIR-Spheres are trapped in the tumor microvasculature. The primary mode of action for these spheres is radiation, not cessation of blood flow. Irradiating the tumor in this manner is called selective internal radiation therapy (SIRT). SIR-Spheres are indicated for the treatment of unresectable primary and metastic liver tumor (28). When used in conjunction with fluorouracil/leucovorin (FU/LV) therapy, SIRT has been shown to increase response and time to progression (28). In the treatment of unresectable metastatic liver tumors from primary colorectal cancer (US indication) (29), a single dose of SIR-Spheres administered with regional hepatic arterial chemotherapy (floxuridine) is more effective in increasing progression-free survival than the same hepatic arterial chemotherapy alone (30). TheraSphere (MDS Nordion) is a similar product, but it uses 20–30 μm glass microspheres as a delivery agent. The therapeutic agent, however, is the same—Yttrium-90 (31).

Hyperthermia, a well-described technique, destroys cancer cells by raising the temperature of the tumor. Various percutaneous methods include the use of radiofrequency current and focused ultrasound. Thermo-Spheres (Sirtex

Medical Limited) are small magnetic microspheres that can be delivered into the tumor to produce localized heating from within the tumor itself, which works to destroy the tumor. Thermo-Spheres are 0.1–0.2 μm magnetic iron oxide particles encapsulated with a polyester coating to form 32-μm particles (27,32).

MTC-Dox (FeRx), a product under development and testing, uses magnetic targeted carrier (MTC) drug delivery technology. MTCs are 1–3-micron particles made of metallic iron and activated carbon that serve as delivery vehicles for site-specific targeting, retention, and release of pharmaceuticals. The activated carbon component of the particle passively absorbs the drug before the delivery and once delivered, slowly releases it. During the first pass of the particles, an external magnet apparatus is used to extract the particles out of the microvasculature into the tumor. Once trapped, drug elusion destroys the tumor locally. Although FeRx, Inc. is no longer in existence, the concept is still viable and may prove promising in the future (33).

SUMMARY

Interventionalists have many therapeutic agents available to them, and many more are being developed and tested. The intra-arterial therapies are in their infancy, and they hold much promise in fields ranging from oncology to transplantation. As the spectrum of available agents increases, so will the potential applications for catheter-directed therapy. Interventional radiologists must familiarize themselves with the properties of these agents, as well as their mechanisms of action and intended applications, to stay at the forefront of endovascular therapy.

REFERENCES

1. Dawbarn RHM. The starvation operation for malignancy in the external carotid area. JAMA 1904;43:792–795.
2. Barth KH, Strandberg JD, White RI Jr. Long-term follow-up of transcatheter embolization with autologous clot, oxycel, and gelfoam in domestic swine. Invest Radiol 1977;12:273–228.
3. Barbolt TA, Odin M, Leger M, et al. Pre-clinical subdural tissue reaction and absorption study of absorbable hemostatic devices. Neurol Res 2001;Jul;23(5):537–542.
4. Kaufman SL, Strandberg JD, Barth KL, et al. Transcatheter embolization with microfibrillar collagen in swine. Invest Radiol 1978;13:200–204.
5. Daniels JR, Kerlan RK, Dodds L, et al. Peripheral hepatic arterial embolization with crosslinked collagen fibers. Invest Radiol 1987;22:126–131.
6. Civalleri D, Esposito M, Fulco RA, et al. Liver and tumor uptake and plasma pharmacokinetics of arterial cisplatin administered with and without starch microspheres in patients with liver metastases. Cancer 1991;68:988–994.
7. Castañeda-Zuniga WR, Sanchez R, Amplatz K. Experimental observations on short- and long-term effects of arterial occlusion with Ivalon. Radiology 1978;126:783–785.
8. Ryu RK, Omary RA, Sichlau MJ, et al. Comparison of pain after uterine artery embolization using trisacryl gelatin microspheres

9. versus polyvinyl alcohol particles. Cardiovasc Intervent Radiol 2003;26(4):375–378.
9. Available at: http://www.bostonscientific.com/med_specialty/deviceDetail.jsp?task=tskBasicDevice.jsp&sectionId=4&relId=4,178,179,180&deviceId=364&uniqueId=MPDB1519. Accessed June 5,2005.
10. Available at: http://www.biocompatibles.com/us/content.asp?pid=7. Accessed June 5, 2005.
11. Available at: http://www.biospheremed.com/products/index.cfm. Accessed June 5, 2005.
12. Laurent A, Beaujeux R, Wassef M, et al. Trisacryl gelatin microspheres for therapeutic embolization, I: development and in vitro evaluation. AJNR Am J Neuroradiol 1996;17:533–540.
13. Beaujeux R, Laurent A, Wassef M, et al. Trisacryl gelatin microspheres for therapeutic embolization, II: preliminary clinical evaluation in tumors and arteriovenous malformation. AJNR Am J Neuroradiol 1996;17:541–548.
14. Basile A, Rand T, Lomoschitz F, et al. Trisacryl gelatin microspheres versus polyvinyl alcohol particles in the preoperative embolization of bone neoplasms. Cardiovasc Intervent Radiol 2004;27(5):495–502.
15. Shapiro AMJ, Lakey JRT, Ryan EA, et al. Islet Transplantation in Seven Patients with Type 1 Diabetes Mellitus Using a Glucocorticoid-Free Immunosuppresive Regimen. N Engl J Med 2000; 343: 230–238.
16. Chang T. Artificial cells with emphasis on bioencapsulation. Biotechnol Annu Rev 1995;1:267–295. Review.
17. Peirone M, Ross C, Hortelano G, et al. Encapsulation of various recombinant mammalian cell types in different alginate microcapsules. J Biomed Mater Res 1998;42:587–596.
18. Soon-Shiong P, Feldman E, Nelson R, et al. Long-term reversal of diabetes by the injection of immunoprotected islets. Proc Natl Acad Sci USA 1993;90:5843–5847.
19. Abruzzo T, Cloft HJ, Shengelaia GG, et al. In vitro effects of transcatheter injection on structure, cell viability, and cell metabolism in fibroblast-impregnated alginate microspheres. Radiology 2001;220(2):428–435.
20. Soulen MC, Faykus MH, Shlansky-Goldberg RD, et al. Elective embolization for prevention of hemorrhage from renal angiomyolipomas. J Vasc Interv Radiol 1994;5:587–591.
21. Wright KC, Loh G, Wallace S, et al. Experimental evaluation of ethanol-ethiodol for transcatheter renal embolization. Cardiovasc Intervent Radiol 1990;13:309–313.
22. Pollack JA, White RI. The use of cyanoacrylate adhesives in peripheral embolization. J Vasc Interv Radiol 2001;12:907–913.
23. Available at: http://www.jnj.com/news/jnj_news/20020307_1752.htm. Accessed June 5, 2005.
24. Hunter DW, Casteñeda-Zuniga WR, Coleman CC, et al. Spermatic vein embolization with hot contrast medium or detachable balloons. Semin Intervent Radiol 1984;1:163–161.
25. Available at: http://www.sirtex.com/?p=57. Accessed June 5, 2005.
26. Available at: http://www.sirtex.com/?p=72. Accessed June 5, 2005.
27. Available at: http://www.sirtex.com/?p=73. Accessed June 5, 2005.
28. Gray BN, Van Hazel H, et al. Randomised trial of SIR-Spheres + FU/LV versus FU/LV alone in advanced colorectal hepatic metastases. Presented at the 2002 meeting of the American Society of Clinical Oncology (ASCO). Abstract number 599 (100474)
29. Available at: http://www.sirtex.com/?p=75. Accessed June 5, 2005.
30. Gray BN, Van Hazel G et al. Randomised trial of SIR-Spheres plus chemotherapy versus chemotherapy alone for treating patients with liver metastases from primary large bowel cancer. Ann Oncol 2001;12:1711–1720.
31. Available at: http://www.mds.nordion.com/therasphere/documents/package_insert.pdf. Accessed June 5, 2005.
32. Moroz P, Jones SK, Gray BN. Tumor response to arterial embolization hyperthermia and direct injection hyperthermia in a rabbit liver tumor model. J Surg Oncol 2002,80(3). 149–156.
33. Johnson J. Magnetic targeted carriers: an innovative drug delivery technology. Spring 2002;1:1–3. Available at: http://www.magneticsmagazine.com/e-prints/ReRx.pdf. Accessed March 15, 2005.

Mechanical Embolization Agents

11

Herb Lustberg, Jeffrey S. Pollak

Embolization is the act of ceasing flow through endoluminal access. Embolization can be temporary or permanent and can involve particulate or mechanical materials. This chapter will concentrate on the mechanical agents.

TEMPORARY MECHANICAL EMBOLIZATION AGENTS (OCCLUSION BALLOONS)

Temporary mechanical embolization agents are used to prevent flow for a finite period and for a specific purpose. Nondetachable occlusion balloons are the prototypical example (Figures 11–1 and 11–2). Historically, occlusion balloons have been used in several ways, including preoperative occlusion of ruptured abdominal aortic aneurysms (1–5). Other applications have also been explored (6–8).

Surgery on hypervascular organs can lead to great blood loss and risk of life. Occlusion balloons can aid in reducing flow to the target organ and, therefore, reduce intraoperative blood loss. Classic applications include renal and splenic arteries. More recently, temporary internal iliac artery occlusion balloon placement has been used to reduce uterine blood flow during cesarean delivery and possible hysterectomy in the presence of abnormal placentation (9).

An additional application for nondetachable occlusion balloons is used in conjunction with another embolization technique or device for reducing velocity in a high flow state. An arteriovenous malformation may have such a high rate of blood flow within it that imaging may be difficult. An occlusion balloon can slow flow to the point that the inflow of nonopacified blood is reduced, improving imaging quality and making permanent embolization easier, more accurate, or both. High flow states can also make the act of embolization more difficult and dangerous because of the increased risk of migration of embolic material causing nontarget embolization. Once again, a nondetachable balloon can slow or stop flow to the point that precise placement of embolic materials can be achieved with reduced risk of migration.

Occlusion balloons may be used to reduce the reflux and, therefore, nontarget embolization of other embolic agents (10). Finally, nondetachable occlusion balloons have been extremely valuable when used to test occluded carotid arteries before surgery or embolization (11).

The Guardwire Temporary Occlusion and Aspiration System (Medtronic) is worthy of mention in this section because of its ability to prevent flow for a defined amount of time and to achieve a specific purpose (Figure 11–3). The system consists of a 0.014 inch Nitinol wire on which a balloon is mounted. Different balloon sizes are available, including 3–6 mm and 2.5–5 mm, which result in 0.036 inch and 0.028 inch profiles, respectively. Before vascular intervention, the balloon is passed through a lesion and inflated. This causes cessation of flow. An intervention, such as angioplasty or stenting, is then performed. A separate catheter, such as the Export catheter, is needed before balloon deflation and removal to aspirate whatever debris may have collected (12).

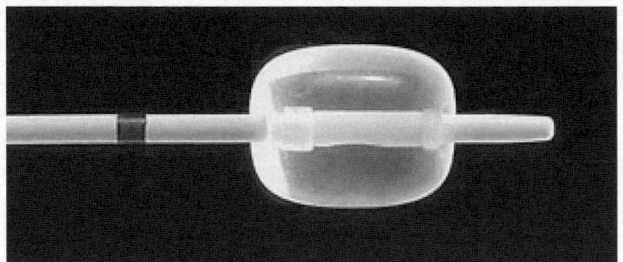

Figure 11–1 Cook's UPJ Occlusion Balloon Catheter can cease flow temporarily.

PERMANENT MECHANICAL EMBOLIZATION AGENTS

Permanent mechanical embolization agents are tools that are routinely used by the interventionalist. Many forms are currently available, including detachable balloons, coils, and stent grafts. Devices used to repair pediatric cardiac defects are also considered embolization agents.

Detachable Balloons

Detachable balloons used to be considered a staple embolization device for the interventionalist, but several factors have contributed to their recent decline in use. Advances in other permanent embolic agents and a lack of developmental attention given to them by the medical device industry have been primary causes. The intended use of detachable balloons for neurointerventional applications meant that the delivery system was never really tailored to peripheral use. The necessity of large guiding catheters for delivery also made the system less desirable. Placement was mostly flow directed with very little steerability. For historical interest and for the sake of completion, the following is a brief overview.

All detachable balloon systems consist of the balloon (Figure 11–4), a delivery inflation catheter, and an introducer

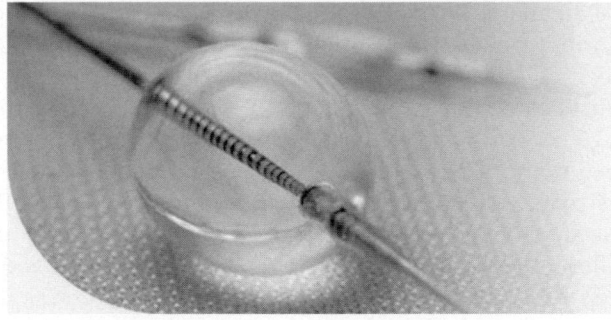

Figure 11–3 Guardwire Temporary Occlusion and Aspiration System by Medtronic Vascular provides temporary occlusion during interventions to prevent embolization of debris. Temporary occlusion is followed by the intervention, then controlled removal of the debris, minimizing distal embolization.

catheter. The balloons may be made of latex or silicone. Silicone is stable and not as subject to degradation as latex (13). Filling the silicone balloons with isosmolar contrast material is important to ensure long-lasting inflation. A hyperosmolar solution can cause the balloon to swell and possibly burst, and a hypo-osmolar solution will likely cause balloon deflation and possible recanalization of the target vessel. Latex balloons do not depend on osmolality; however, deflation has been reported, which may have been related to degraded latex or leaking valve mechanisms (14). Long-term vascular occlusion of systemic vessels appears to occur reliably when the balloon remains inflated for at least 3 weeks (15).

Balloons can be attached to the delivery catheter by several mechanisms that include the elastic grip of the balloon material, elastic ligatures, and self-sealing valves. Clearly, relying on the elastic grip of the balloon material is the least reliable and prone to premature release and immediate deflation of the balloon (16).

Despite the recently declining frequency in the use of detachable balloons, reports of additional applications continue. Some of these include internal iliac artery occlusion before abdominal aortic stent-graft placement (17) and TIPS reduction to reverse worsening hepatic insufficiency (18).

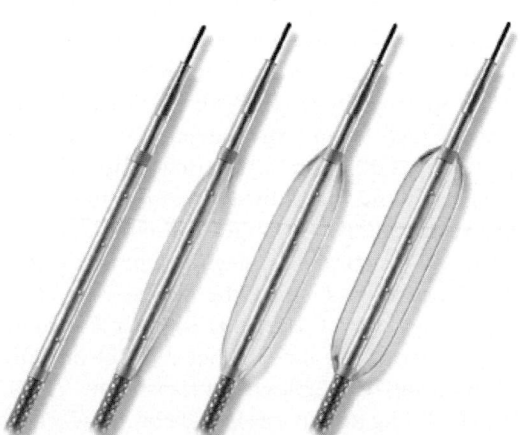

Figure 11–2 Sentry Balloon Catheters by Boston Scientific act as excellent compliant occlusion balloons with low profiles. Image courtesy of Boston Scientific © 2005.

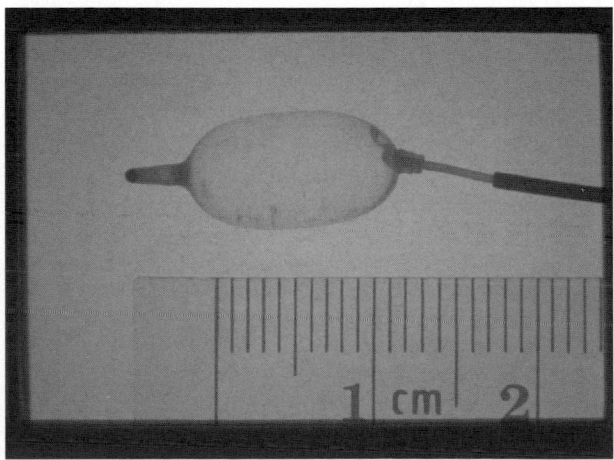

Figure 11–4 Detachable balloons have fallen out of favor because of many factors.

Potential pitfalls of deploying detachable balloons are considerable. Early or unexpected detachment can occur, especially when deploying through a coaxial catheter system. Postdeployment migration is another concern. Migration of a balloon may occur when it is improperly sized to the vessel. Anatomic and physiologic characteristics may also predispose toward balloon instability. A sharply tapered vessel may have a tendency to expel the balloon. Compliant vessels may enlarge in diameter with deep respiratory excursions or in response to the occlusion, particularly as greater hemodynamic forces are transmitted to the wall. Furthermore, drag forces with partial inflation in high flow vessels or arteriovenous fistulae can cause elongation of these deformable detachable balloons. With poor traction against the wall, the balloon may embolize distally, such as across an arteriovenous shunt, or may even reflux into the parent vessel and embolize elsewhere. In the appropriate setting, an alternative to trying to retrieve the balloon is to puncture it percutaneously, permitting its smaller, deflated fragments to travel distally and occlude a smaller territory. Difficulty in detaching a balloon may also occur, usually because of geometric, anatomic, or physical factors. If this difficulty is experienced, controlled deflation and removal may be necessary.

Coil Emboli

Coil emboli (Figure 11–5) have many qualities that make them attractive embolization agents. As a result, coils tend to be the most frequently used mechanical embolization agent. They are readily accessible, relatively easy to use, and reliable.

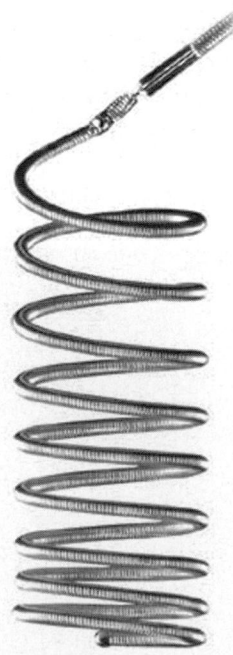

Figure 11–5 GDC coils are delivered and electrolytically detached when satisfactory positioning has been obtained. Image courtesy of Boston Scientific © 2005.

The first of the devices described by Gianturco was a 3-mm-long 19-gauge piece of steel tubing with cotton threads attached to it, while the second was the original steel coil embolus. This consisted of a 5-cm-long coiled piece of 0.038-inch steel guide wire with its central mandril core removed and four 3-cm-long woolen strands attached to its tip. This was introduced into a 7 French nontapered Teflon catheter using a thin mandril extending from 19-gauge steel tubing. The mandril fit inside the core of the wire embolus, straightening it for placement within the catheter. It was then advanced through the catheter using a 0.045- or 0.052-inch guide wire.

Early experience demonstrated the rapid development of complete vascular occlusion of the local segment containing these devices (19–21), although several coils would be needed in larger vessels. While the metal and fabric created physical obstruction of the vessel lumen, more complete occlusion was because of the formation of thrombus. Both animal and clinical studies showed long-term occlusion on follow-up. Late recanalization appeared to be a rare phenomenon (22).

Over the next few years, refinements (23–24) resulted in thinner embolization coils, permitting their use through conventionally tapered 5 French catheters. More recently, coil emboli for use through 3 French or smaller catheter systems have been developed (25–27). Additionally, wool has been replaced by polyester (Dacron), which creates a less severe inflammatory reaction in the vessel wall.

Size

Today, coils can be split into various categories depending on several characteristics. Size is perhaps the simplest to discuss. As stated, coils are made to be delivered through 5 French angiography catheters (0.035- or 0.038-inch coils) and 3 French microcatheters (0.018-inch coils). Obviously, choosing your coil will depend on an adequate size catheter system needed to reach the target vessel.

Small vessels generally are best approached with coaxial microcatheter systems. In addition to permitting superselective, distal catheterization, these systems—when used in conjunction with soft, steerable wires—appear to induce less spasm. The smaller coils (Figure 11–6) can be delivered through them with special coil pushers (Target Therapeutics), 0.025- or 0.018-inch Glidewires (Medi-Tech) that resist kinking or by a forceful saline flush.

Larger vessels allow for larger catheters and 0.035- or 0.038-inch coils. A coaxial catheter system and technique is used when possible, such as the White Lumax Guiding Catheter set (Cook, Inc.). The outer catheter is used for steerability and support. The inner catheter can be advanced and withdrawn during coil deployment to assist in "nesting" the coils, thereby filling any spaces in the coil mass. This system and technique is applicable throughout the body and provides confident deployment with a dense coil mass and little risk of coil extension outside the target vessel. Additionally, if

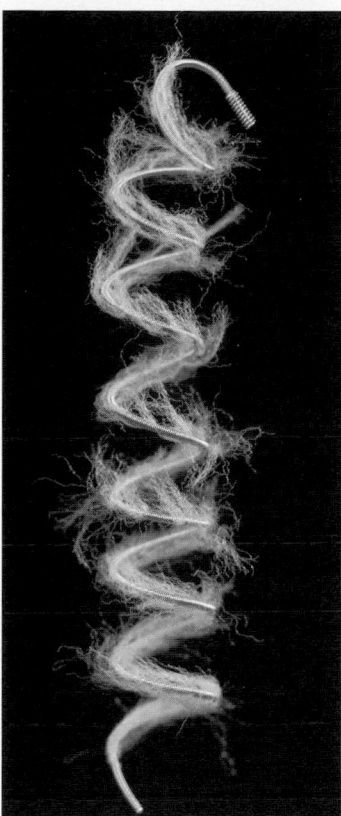

Figure 11–6 Micronester platinum embolization coils utilize 0.018 inch platinum wire with synthetic fibers. Helix diameters are 3–10 mm and wire length is 14 cm.

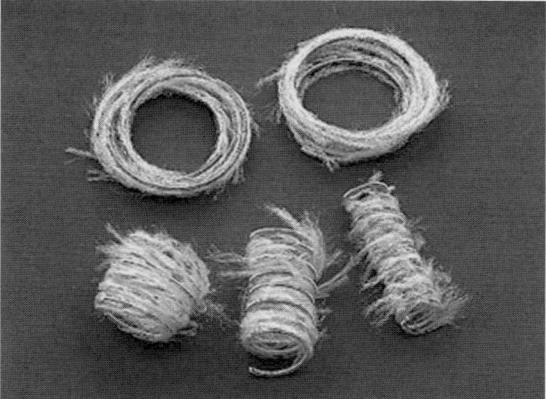

Figure 11–7 Nester embolization coils are 0.035 or 0.038 inch platinum wires with synthetic fibers. Helix diameters are 4–12 mm and wire length is 14 cm.

to be conical or "tornado" shaped. Miconester, Hilal, and Tornado coils are available in 0.018 inch extended embolus diameter. Hilal coils can be coiled or straight; tend to be shorter and smaller in diameter; and are intended for

available, the first portion of the first coil can be "anchored" in a branch vessel to help prevent coil migration.

Material

Coils are made of stainless steel, platinum, and more recently, Nitinol. The conventional steel coil embolus (Cook, Inc.) consists of a short length of guide wire with multiple polyester strands attached transversely along most of its length, between the turns of the wire. These devices are prepackaged and stretched out in metal cartridges to eliminate the need for a special mandril introducer and permit their delivery through conventional 5 French, 0.035- and 0.038-inch, tapered catheters using floppy guide wires. Helical diameters of 3–15 mm and coil lengths of 2–15 cm are available.

Platinum coils are widely used, and they lend to high fluoroscopic visibility. Platinum coils have several other technical advantages over stainless steel, including softer metal allowing tighter packed coil masses and reduced likelihood of vessel wall injury (25,28). Also, they have Dacron fibers that aid thrombogenicity. Macrocoils and microcoils are available. Nester coils (Figure 11–7) are 0.035 and 0.038 inch and are helically shaped. Tornado coils (Figure 11–8) are only 0.035 inch and are intended

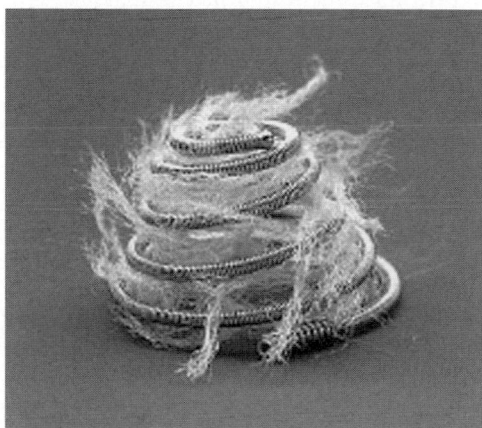

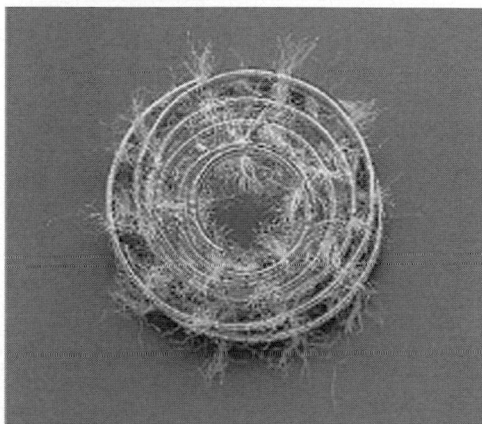

Figure 11–8 Tornado embolization coils are 0.035 inch platinum wires with synthetic fibers and tapered helices. The small diameter ends are 3–5 mm and the large diameter ends are 5–10 mm. Wire lengths are 4–12 cm.

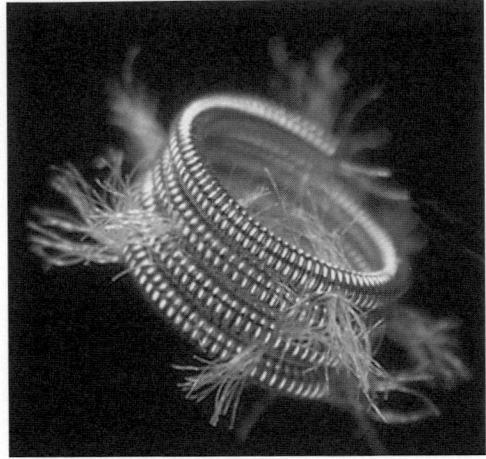

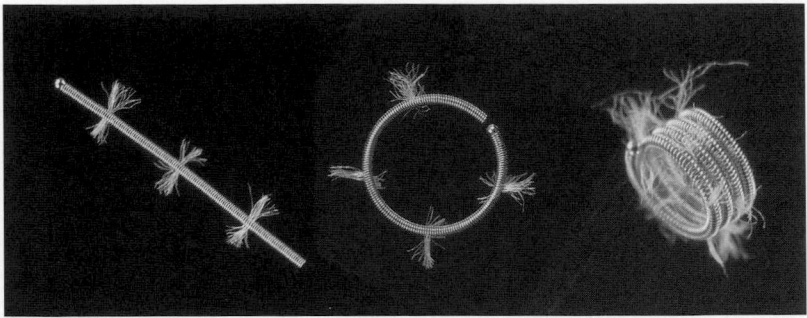

Figure 11-9 Hilal embolization microcoils are 0.018 inch platinum coils with synthetic fibers that come straight, in a single curl, and in multiple curls. Wire lengths are 0.5–3 cm. Coil diameters are 2–5 mm.

small, superselected vessels (Figure 11–9). A wide variety of coil diameters and shapes are available. Choice of coils depends on the vessel morphology and physician preference.

Recently, Nitinol has seen increasing use in interventional radiology in the form of stents, IVC filters, and the like. Newer coil devices have been introduced to take advantage of Nitinol's attributes, including its thermal shape memory. GDC TriSpan detachable coil (Boston Scientific) is an example with three Nitinol pedals that "bridge" a cerebral aneurysm neck to prevent herniation of additional deployed coils into the parent artery (Figure 11–10).

Combination agents are also being studied. The HydroCoil Embolic System (HES; MicroVention) combines a platinum microcoil with a proprietary, highly expandable microporous hydrogel called Intelligel (Figure 11–11). The hydrogel expands after being exposed to blood for a set amount of time. Its intent is to provide improved filling (over traditional platinum coils) of cerebral aneurysms by swelling in the aneurysm after deployment. The significance of this combination mechanical embolization agent is still unclear (29,30).

The platinum-copolymer Matrix detachable coil (Boston Scientific) is another example of a combination embolization agent intended for neurovascular applications. The outer polyglycolic-polylactic acid (PGLA) copolymer is an absorbable material that makes up 70% of the coil volume (Figure 11–12). It is reported to be completely absorbed in 90 days. Other combination material coils

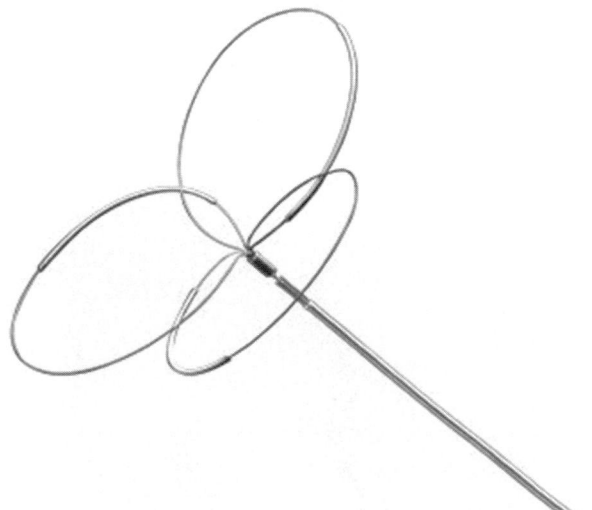

Figure 11-10 TriSpan Nitinol coils are used to confine coils to the aneurysm sack, preventing extension into the parent vessel. The detachment mechanism is similar to that of other GDC coils. Device diameters are 6–16 mm. This device is not yet available in the United States. Image courtesy of Boston Scientific © 2005.

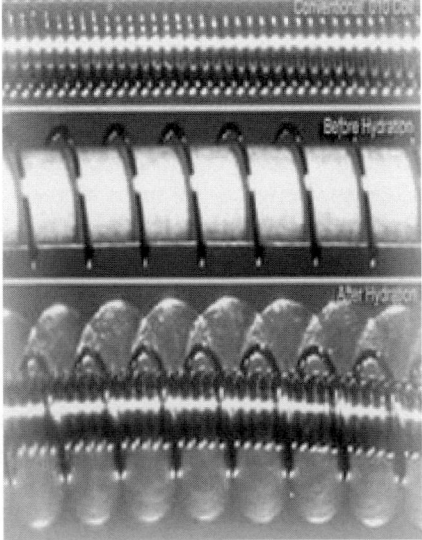

Figure 11-11 The HydroCoil Embolic System is a platinum coil with an outer layer of a hydrophilic, acrylic polymer that expands when exposed to fluid. This image demonstrates the difference in coil volume prior to and after hydration. As a result, coil mass can be more densely packed.

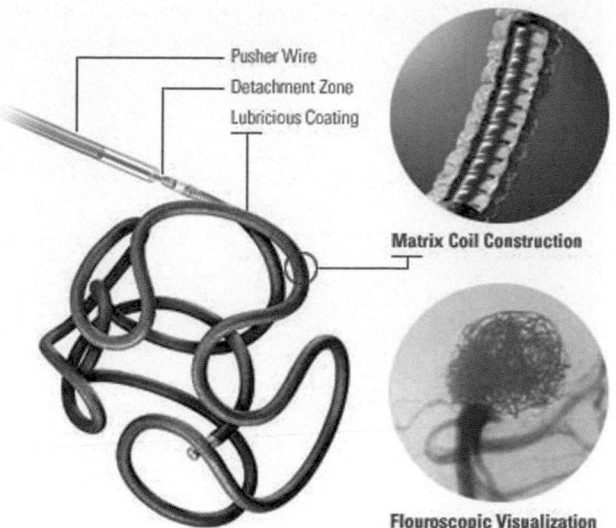

Figure 11-12   Platinum-copolymer Matrix Detachable Coils have a polyglycolic–polylactic acid (PGLA) copolymer outer coating that is resorbable within 90 days of deployment. Image courtesy of Boston Scientific © 2005.

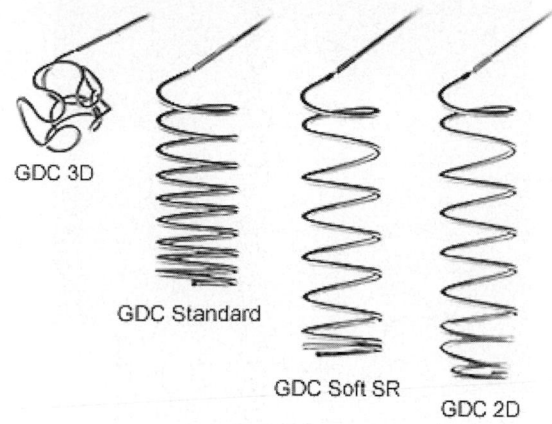

Figure 11-13   Guglielmi Detachable Coils (GDC) come in many shapes, sizes, and softnesses. Available wire lengths are 4–30 cm. Helix diameters are 2–20 mm. Electrolytic detachment is utilized. Image courtesy of Boston Scientific © 2005.

are being investigated, and only scientific evaluation will determine the most efficacious ones.

Deployment

Coil deployment falls into one of two types: pushable and detachable. Pushable coils are used most commonly in peripheral applications and consist of a preloaded, elongated coil inserted into the catheter. Once inserted, a coil pusher or a guide wire can be used to advance the coil into the desired position. Alternatively, a pushable coil can be "injected" by forcefully injecting saline into the catheter once the coil is loaded. A test injection with saline should be performed before loading the coil to assure the interventionalist that the jet effect of the saline exiting the catheter will not force the catheter tip out of position (31).

Detachable coils also can be subdivided into types of detachment mechanisms. The classic Guglielmi detachable coil (Boston Scientific) is electrolytically detached (Figure 11–13). After the coil is in the proper position, a low voltage direct current is applied that results in thrombosis and dissolution of the connecting soft steel segment. Many shapes and sizes are available, including 3D volume-filling shapes (Figure 11–14).

Twist release coils are also available, such as the Flipper (Figure 11–15) and Jackson coils (Cook). The user attaches the coil to the delivery wire and twists the delivery wire to release the coil, once properly positioned. Vascular occlusion applications include treatment of neurovascular disease (32), pediatric cardiac pathology (33), and more atypical examples, such as occluding aorticopulmonary artery fistulae (34).

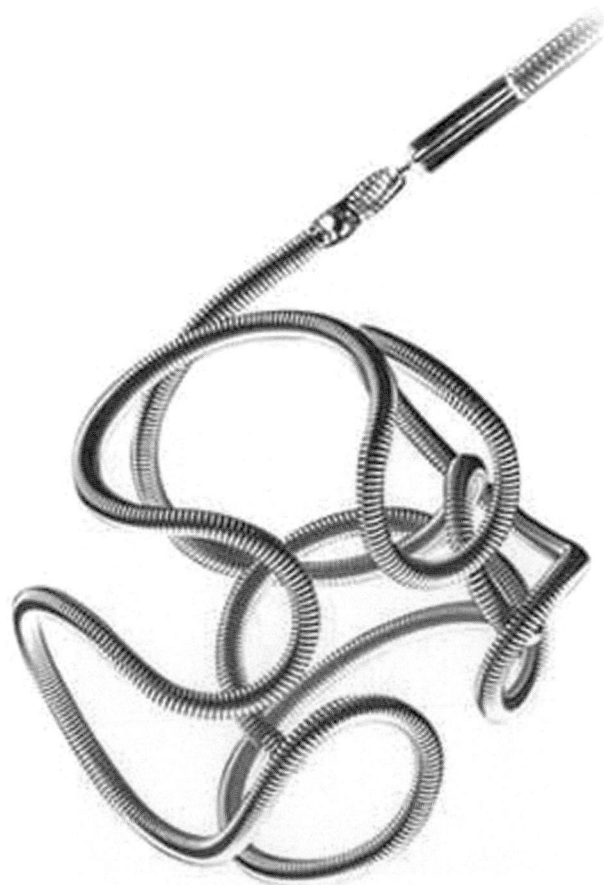

Figure 11-14   GDC 3D Shape Coils can act as scaffolding for additional coil deployment. Outer diameters are available between 3 and 20 mm. Image courtesy of Boston Scientific © 2005.

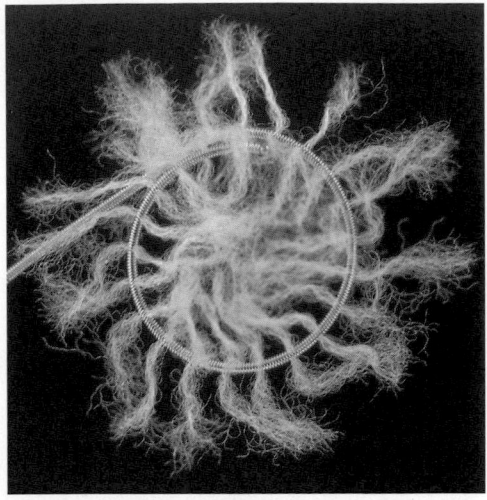

Figure 11–15 Flipper coils from Cook are stainless steel with synthetic fibers to enhance thrombogenicity. Coils are mechanically detached. Coil wire lengths are 3–12 cm, and helices are 3–8 mm.

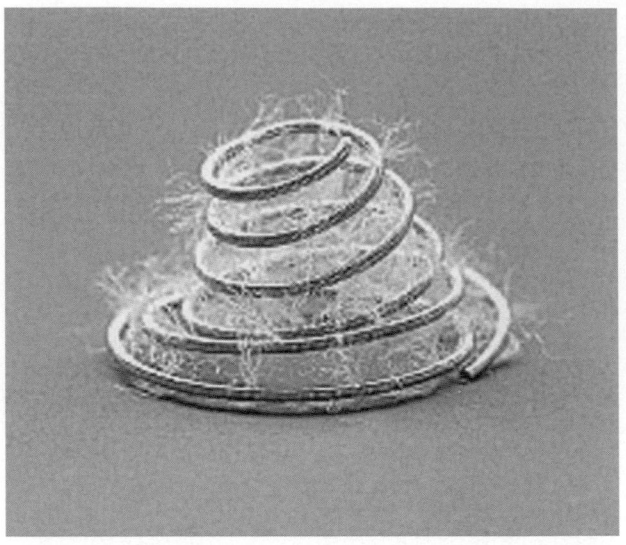

Shape

As one might expect, coil emboli come in all sizes and shapes. The typical shape is helical, but slight variations on this shape are available. Straight coils are common and readily available. Tornado or vortex-shaped coils, mentioned previously, is the descriptive term determined by the manufacturer. The VortXX (Boston Scientific) is shown in Figure 11–16, and the Tornado (Cook) is shown in Figure 11–17. Complex, 3D shapes are also available. TriSpan detachable coils (Boston Scientific) are a unique example, shaped to bridge wide aneurysm necks. Most 3D coils are meant to act as scaffolding through which additional coils are deployed.

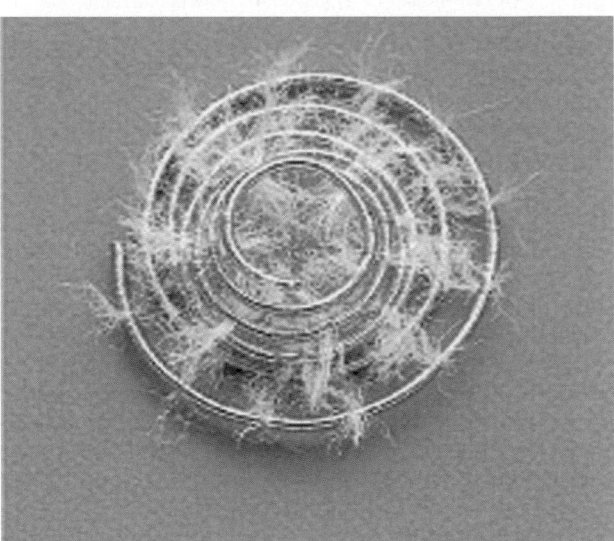

Figure 11–17 Tornado Embolization Microcoils are 0.018 inch platinum wires that are 2–14 cm while extended. Diameters are 2–4 mm on the small end and 3–10 mm on the large end. Synthetic fibers enhance thrombogenicity.

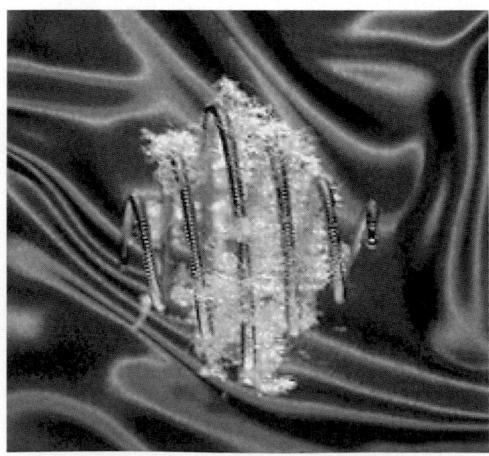

Figure 11–16 VortXX-35 Vascular Occlusion Coils from Boston Scientific are 0.035 inch platinum wires with synthetic fibers. Diameters are 2–3 mm on the small end and 4–7 mm on the large end. Wire lengths range from 30–67 mm while restrained.

Stent Grafts

Covered stents, or stent grafts, are mechanical embolization agents used to exclude a branch vessel while maintaining patency in the parent vessel. Wallgrafts are wallstents covered with PET (polyethylene terephthalate, Boston Scientific). The Fluency product (Figure 11–18) is a Luminexx Nitinol stent covered in ePTFE (expanded polytetrafluoroethylene, Bard). The Viatorr is another example of a covered stent (Gore). Deployment of these products is similar to their uncovered equivalent devices. Applications include trauma, aneurysm exclusion, and TIPS reduction (35–37).

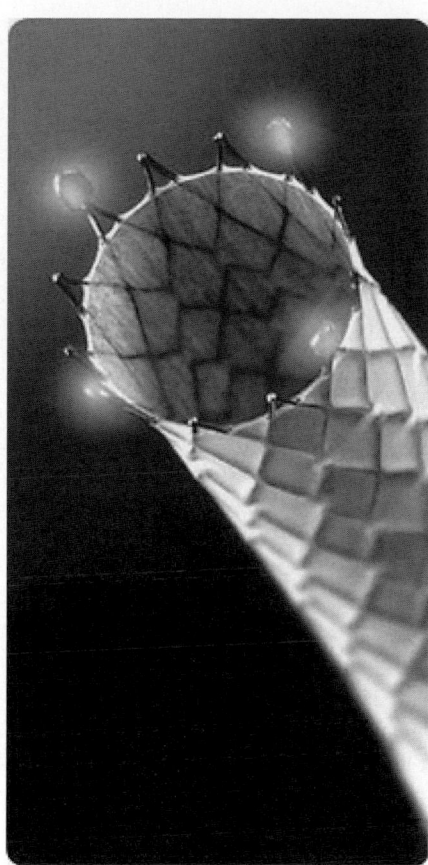

Figure 11–18 The Fluency Stent Graft from Bard is essentially a Luminexx stent covered with ePTFE on both sides. Stent diameters are 6–10 mm and lengths are 4–8 cm.

Pediatric Cardiac Products

Many products have been developed for the purpose of interventional repair of pediatric cardiac anomalies. The devices included here are mechanical embolization devices that can be researched through the reference section at the end of the chapter and through consultation with other chapters in this book.

Since Porstmann's description of transluminal closure of patent ductus arteriosus (PDA) in 1971 (38) using a plug of polyvinyl alcohol foam, a variety of devices and techniques have been described for closing this lesion as well as addressing atrial septal defects (ASD) and small ventricular septal defects (VSD) (39,40).

The FDA has approved the CardioSEAL Septal Occlusion System (Nitinol, Inc.) as a Humanitarian Use Device (HUD) for septal occlusion (Figure 11–19). It consists of a metal framework (MP35N alloy) to which polyester fabric is attached. The device shape is that of a double umbrella, which is intended to straddle a septal defect. It is delivered through a 10 French catheter using an unsheathing technique common in interventional radiology. Although intended for cardiac defect repair, noncardiac uses, such as PAVM occlusion, are reported (41).

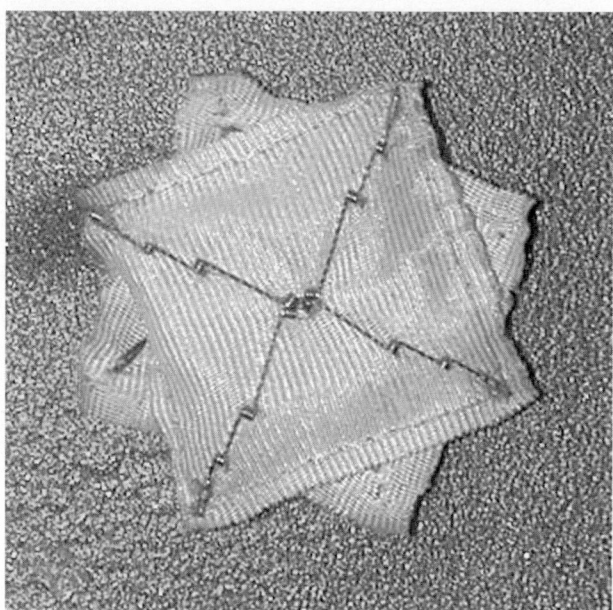

Figure 11–19 The CardioSEAL Septal Occlusion System is made by Nitinol Medical Technologies, Inc., Boston, MA.

An entire family of Amplatzer occlusion devices (AGA Medical Corporation) is intended to tackle the most common congenital cardiac defects. Patent ductus arteriosus (Figure 11–20), atrial septal defect (Figure 11–21), and patent foramen ovale (Figure 11–22) have dedicated specifically designed devices. The Amplatzer vascular plug (Figure 11–23) is more nonspecific and can be used in several places. Again, noncardiac applications, such as portal vein fistula occlusion, have been reported (42).

A uniquely shaped agent of embolization is the Gianturco-Grifka vascular occlusion device (Figure 11–24). This device consists of a nylon sack attached to a coaxial

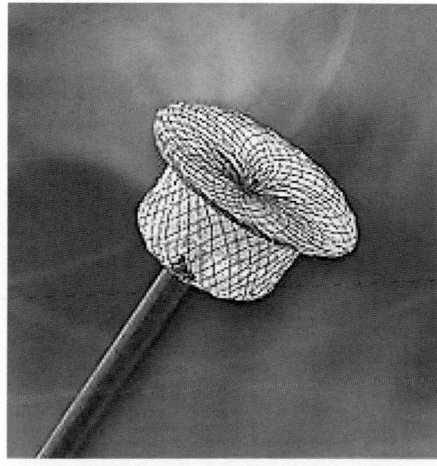

Figure 11–20 Amplatzer PDA occlusion device from AGA Medical Corporation, Golden Valley, MN. The small end (pulmonary artery side) is 4–14 mm. The larger end (aortic side) is 5–16 mm. The retention skirt size is 9–22 mm.

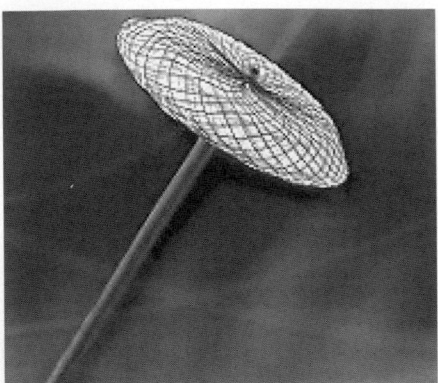

Figure 11–21   Amplatzer ASD occlusion device from AGA Medical Corporation, Golden Valley, MN. Available diameters are 4–38 mm.

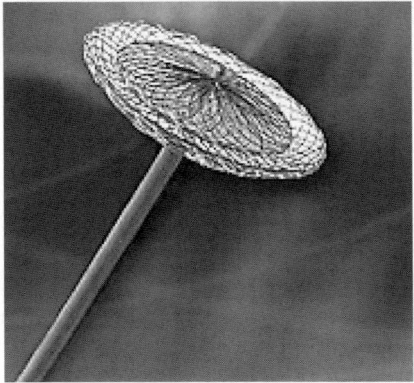

Figure 11–22   Amplatzer PFO occlusion device from AGA Medical Corporation, Golden Valley, MN. Right atrial disks are available in 18, 25, and 35 mm. Left atrial disk sizes are available in 18 or 25 mm.

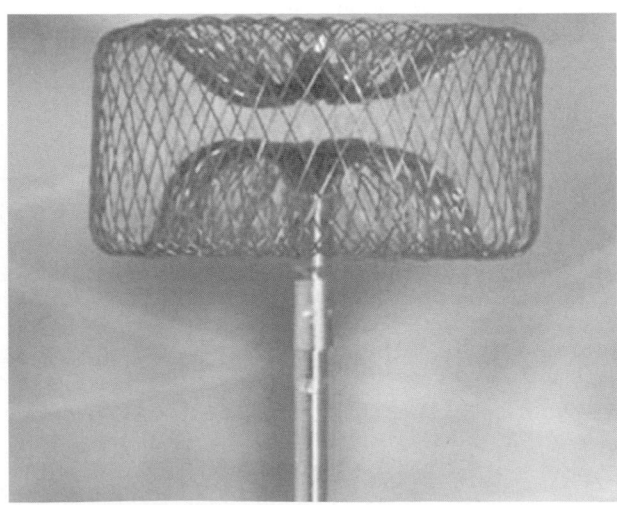

Figure 11–23   Amplatzer vascular plug from AGA Medical Corporation, Golden Valley, MN. Available device diameters are 4–16 mm, with lengths of 7 or 8 mm.

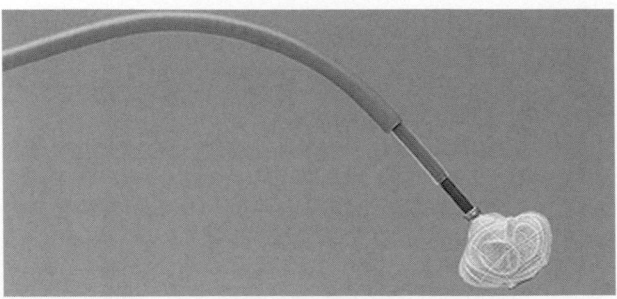

Figure 11–24   The Gianturco-Grifka vascular occlusion device is available in 3, 5, 7, and 9 mm sack diameters.

catheter system. A coil is advanced through the inner catheter to fill the nylon sack. The outer catheter is then used to help release the sack into the targeted vessel for occlusion. This device has been used to occlude cardiac abnormalities, but other applications are inevitable.

Other devices that have been made available include the Lock clamshell device, Rashkind umbrella device, Sideris buttoned device (Figure 11–25), Atrial Septal Defect Occluding System (ASDOS) (Figure 11–26), Angel Wings (Figure 11–27), PFO-Star and Helex devices (Figure 11–28).

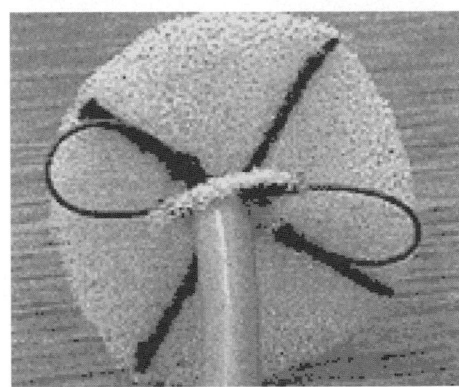

Figure 11–25   Sideris Buttoned Device.

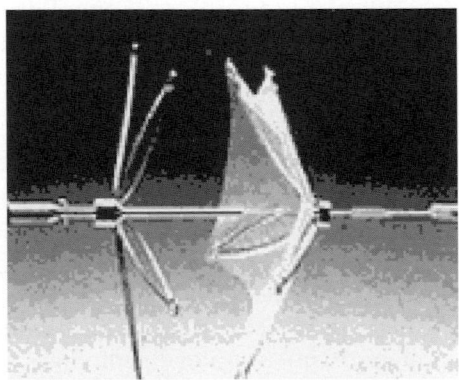

Figure 11–26   Atrial Septal Defect Occluding System (ASDOS).

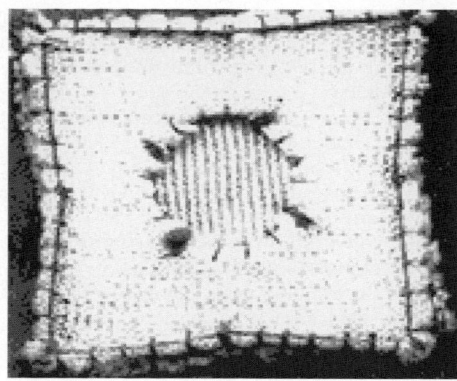

Figure 11–27 Angel Wings from Microvena Corp., White Bear Lake, MN.

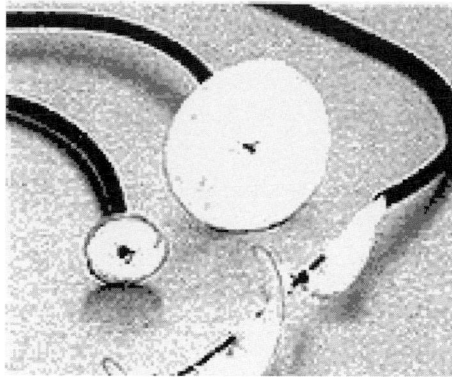

Figure 11–28 Helex device from W.L. Gore and Associates, Flagstaff, AZ.

Radiofrequency or Laser Ablation

Radiofrequency (RF) ablation and laser ablation of varicose veins have become mainstream treatments for lower extremity venous insufficiency disease. Although no occlusion device is left behind at the end of the procedure, as with detachable balloons or coil emboli, these systems still cease flow through endoluminal access. These technologies are covered in greater depth in other chapters of this book.

REFERENCES

1. Dotter CT, Lukas DS. Acute cor pulmonale: an experimental study utilizing a special cardiac catheter. Am J Physiol 1951;164:254–262.
2. Edwards WS, Salter PP, Carnaggio VA. Intraluminal aortic occlusion as a possible mechanism for controlling massive intra-abdominal hemorrhage. Surg Forum 1953;4:496–499.
3. Hesse FG, Kletschka HD. Rupture of abdominal aortic aneurysm: control of hemorrhage by intraluminal balloon tamponade. Ann Surg 1962;155:320–322.
4. Heimbecker RO. An aortic tampon for emergency control of ruptured abdominal aneurysm. Can Med Assoc J 1964;91:1024–1025.
5. Rubenstein RB, Wolvek S. Percutaneous aortic balloon occlusion. Surg Gynecol Obstet 1987;164:561–563.
6. Wholey MH, Stockdale R, Hung TK. A percutaneous balloon catheter for the immediate control of hemorrhage. Radiology 1970;95:65–71.
7. Paster SB, Van Houten FX, Adams DF. Percutaneous balloon catheterization: a technique for the control of arterial hemorrhage caused by pelvic trauma. JAMA 1974;230:573–575.
8. Wholey MH. The technology of balloon catheters in interventional angiography. Radiology 1977;125:671–676.
9. Kidney DD, Nguyen AM, Ahdoot D, et al. Prophylactic perioperative hypogastric artery balloon occlusion in abnormal placentation. AJR Am J Roentgenol 1997;176:1521–1524.
10. Greenfield AJ, Athanasoulis CA, Waltman AC, et al. Transcatheter embolization: prevention of embolic reflux using balloon catheters. AJR Am J Roentgenol 1978;131:651–655.
11. Eckard DA, Purdy PD, Bonte FJ. Temporary balloon occlusion of the carotid artery combined with brain blood flow imaging as a test to predict tolerance prior to permanent carotid sacrifice. AJNR Am J Neuroradiol 1992;13:1565–1569.
12. Baim D, Wahr D, George B, et al. Randomized trial of a distal embolic protection device during percutaneous intervention of saphenous vein aorto-coronary bypass grafts. Circulation 2002;105:1285–1290.
13. Higashida RT, Halbach VV, Dormandy B, et al. Endovascular treatment of intracranial aneurysms with a new silicone microballoon device: technical considerations and indications for therapy. Radiology 1990;174:687–691.
14. Goto K, Halbach VV, Hardin CW, et al. Permanent inflation of detachable balloons with a low viscosity, hydrophilic polymerizing system. Radiology 1988;169:787–790.
15. Kaufman SL, Strandberg JD, Barth KH, et al. Therapeutic embolization with detachable silicone balloons: long-term effects in swine. Invest Radiol 1979;14:156–161.
16. Debrun G, Lacour P, Caron J-P, et al. Detachable balloons and calibrated-leak balloon techniques in the treatment of cerebral vascular lesions. J Neurosurg 1978;49:635–649.
17. Chong A, Soulen MC, Baum RA, et al. Balloon embolization of the internal iliac artery before aneurysm endograft deployment. J Vasc Interv Radiol 2001;12:637–639.
18. Kaufman L, Itkin M, Furth EE, et al. Detachable balloon-modified reducing stent to treat hepatic insufficiency after transjugular intrahepatic portosystemic shunt creation. J Vasc Interv Radiol 2003; 14:635–638.
19. Wallace S, Gianturco C, Anderson JH, et al. Therapeutic vascular occlusion utilizing steel coil technique: clinical applications. AJR Am J Roentgenol 1976;127:381–387.
20. Anderson JH, Wallace S, Gianturco C. Transcatheter intravascular coil occlusion of experimental arteriovenous fistulas. AJR Am J Roentgenol 1977;129:795–798.
21. White RI Jr, Strandberg JV, Gross GS, et al. Therapeutic embolization with long-term occluding agents and their effects on embolized tissues. Radiology 1977;125:677–687.
22. Jhaveri HS, Gerlock AJ Jr, Ekelund L. Failure of steel coil occlusion in a case of hypernephroma. AJR Am J Roentgenol 1978;130:556.
23. Anderson JH, Wallace S, Gianturco C, et al. "Mini" Gianturco stainless steel coils for transcatheter vascular occlusion. Radiology 1979;132:301–303.
24. Chuang VP, Wallace S, Gianturco C. A new improved coil for tapered-tip catheter for arterial occlusion. Radiology 1980;135:507–509.
25. Yang P, Hallbach VV, Higashida RT, et al. Platinum wire: a new transvascular embolic agent. AJNR Am J Neuroradiol 1988;9:547–550.
26. Morse SS, Clark RA, Puffenbarger A. Platinum microcoils for therapeutic embolization: nonneuroradiologic applications. AJR Am J Roentgenol 1990;155:401–403.
27. Teitelbaum GP, Reed RA, Larsen D, et al. Microcatheter embolization of non-neurologic traumatic vascular lesions. J Vasc Interv Radiol 1993;4:149–154.
28. Pugash RA. Pulmonary arteriovenous malformations: overview and transcatheter embolotherapy. Can Assoc Radiol J 2001;52:92–102.

29. Cloft HJ, Kallmes DF. Aneurysm packing with HydroCoil Embolic System versus platinum coils: initial clinical experience. AJNR Am J Neuroradiol 2004;25:60–62.
30. Yoshino Y, Niimi Y, Song JK, et al. Endovascular treatment of intracranial aneurysms: comparative evaluation in a terminal bifurcation aneurysm model in dogs. J Neurosurg 2004;101:996–1003.
31. Makita K, Furui S, Irie T, et al. Embolization with steel coils using a saline flush technique. Br J Radiol 1991;64:708–710.
32. Murphy KJ, Houdart E, Szopinski KT, et al. Mechanical detachable platinum coil: report of the European phase II clinical trial in 60 patients. Radiology 2001;219:541–544.
33. El Sisi A, Tofeig M, Arnold R, et al. Mechanical occlusion of the patent ductus arteriosus with Jackson coils. Pediatr Cardiol 2001;22(1):29–33.
34. Slonim S, Adams MT, Kollmeyer KR. Endovascular repair of an aortopulmonary artery fistula with use of controlled-release coils. J Vasc Interv Radiol 2004;15:861–864.
35. Rundback, JH, Rizvi A, Rozenblit GN, et al. Percutaneous stent-graft management of renal artery aneurysms. J Vasc Interv Radiol 2000;11:1189–1193.
36. Quaretti P, Michieletti E, Rossi S. Successful treatment of TIPS-induced hepatic failure with an hourglass stent graft: a simple new technique for reducing shunt flow. J Vasc Interv Radiol 2001;12:887–890.
37. Saket R, Sze D, Razavi M, et al. TIPS reduction with use of stents or stent grafts. J Vasc Interv Radiol 2004;15:745–751.
38. Porstmann W, Wierny L, Warnke H, et al. Catheter closure of patent ductus arteriosus. 62 cases treated without thoracotomy. Radiol Clin North Am 1971;9:203–218.
39. Hellenbrand WE, Mullins CE. Catheter closure of congenital cardiac defects. Cardiol Clin 1989;7:351–368.
40. Transcatheter occlusion of persistent arterial duct. Report of the European registry. Lancet 1992;340:1062–1066.
41. Apostolopoulou SC, Kelekis NL, Papagiannis J, et al. Transcatheter occlusion of a large pulmonary arteriovenous malformation with use of a CardioSEAL device. J Vasc Interv Radiol 2001;12:767–769.
42. Alonso J, Sierre S, Lipsich J, et al. Endovascular treatment of congenital portal vein fistulas with the Amplatzer occlusion device. J Vasc Interv Radiol 2004;15:989–993.

Balloon Angioplasty Catheters

12

Gary J. Becker

HISTORICAL BACKGROUND

Coaxial Dilating Catheter Method

For nearly a decade after Dotter's and Judkins's introduction of percutaneous transluminal angioplasty, or PTA (1), at a time when little significance was ascribed to therapeutic catheter techniques in the United States and throughout much of the world, Zeitler and colleagues kept the method alive in Europe (2,3). Despite their enthusiasm, Dotter, Judkins, Zeitler, and a few other pioneers in this field recognized that the technique, which employed tapered Teflon coaxial dilating catheters (Figure 12–1), imposed a very real limitation on the size of vessel that could be treated. The larger the vessel to be treated, the larger the catheter shaft required. This meant that the puncture site had to be dilated to very large sizes to treat large arteries, and the result was a greater risk of puncture site complications, particularly hematoma and pseudoaneurysm. Dotter and Judkins recognized this limitation quite early in their experience. They described it and predicted the future development of radially expanding catheters to treat arterial stenoses (1).

In addition to size limitations, the relative inflexibility of the coaxial catheters imposed a limitation on the specific anatomic areas that could be catheterized and treated. Reaching a coronary artery lesion with one of these catheters would have been unthinkable. But in the mid-1960s, the design of coaxial dilating catheters was only one of many limitations, each of which would have made coronary angioplasty unthinkable. Among these limitations were the lack of soft-tipped, steerable, highly radiopaque guide wires; the lack of torque control catheters and guiding catheters; the relatively early point in time of the development of sophisticated cardiac catheterization laboratories; and the relative lack of adjunctive pharmacotherapeutics. Confronted with these very real limitations, Dotter and Judkins still predicted applications of angioplasty in the coronary, renal, and carotid arteries (1).

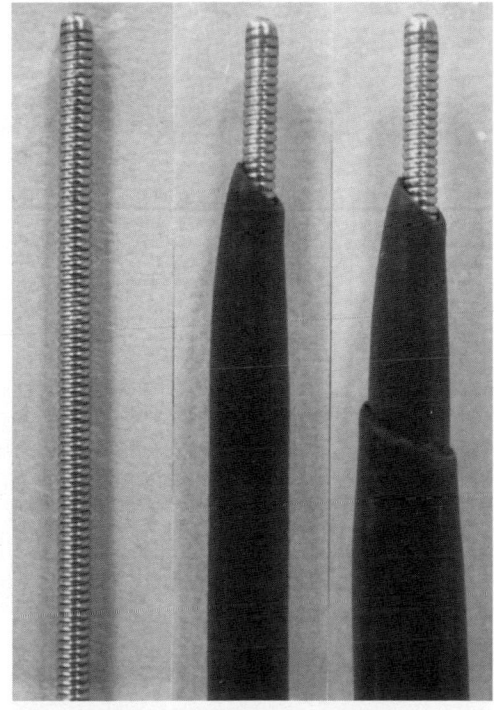

Figure 12–1 Dotter coaxial dilating catheters.

Finally, the coaxial dilator method applied not only a radial force to the diseased vessel wall at the site of the lesion, but an undesirable shearing force as well. Therefore, efforts were undertaken to develop a catheter that would, after delivery to the site of the atherosclerotic lesion, radially expand and thereby deform or mold the plaque and enlarge the vessel lumen.

Early Balloon PTA Catheters

Porstmann's "korsett balloon catheter" (4) and Dotter's reinforced balloon dilating catheter (Figure 12–2) (5,6) and caged balloon catheter (Figure 12–3) (5,7) were early products of these efforts. The last-mentioned device was a Teflon catheter with short parallel slits in its long axis near the leading end that were arranged about the circumference of the catheter shaft. Inside this Teflon catheter, a coaxial latex balloon on a 22-gauge metal cannula positioned at the site of the slits (cage) was expanded at the time of angioplasty. The result of this design was a radial force applied to the stenosis during angioplasty. The cage restricted the size that the balloon could reach and thereby provided a safeguard against bursting. The catheter was dilated up to 9.3 mm from a minimum diameter of 3.0 mm. Dotter and colleagues reported their success with the caged balloon catheter in more than 90% of 48 consecutive cases of atherosclerotic iliac artery obstruction (7). Follow-up in the series was up to 6 years. Despite these results, the use of Dotter's caged balloon catheter was associated with very real limitations, such as inflexibility and occasional thromboembolic complications. These detracted from its clinical utility and encouraged investigators to develop better angioplasty catheters.

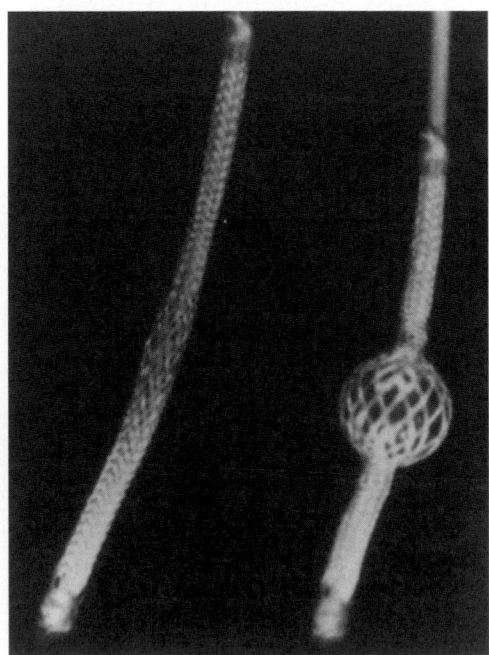

Figure 12–2 Dotter's reinforced balloon dilating catheter.

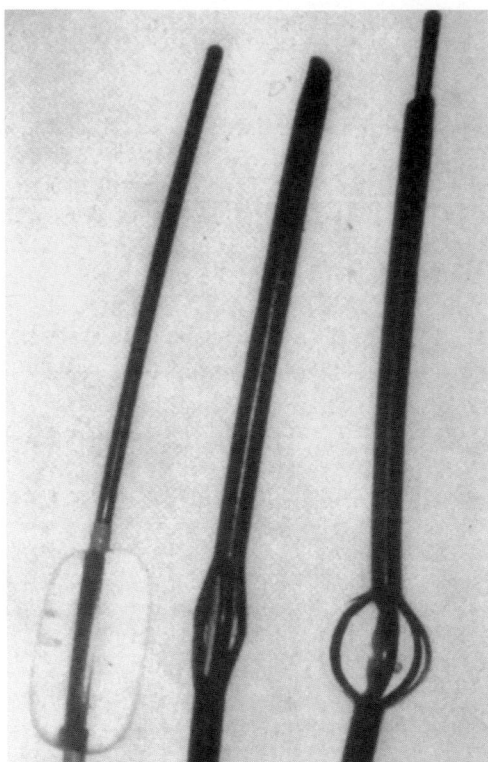

Figure 12–3 The caged balloon catheter.

The Beginnings of Modern Balloon PTA

The first major advance leading to balloon catheters as we know them today was the development of polyvinyl chloride (PVC) balloon PTA catheters by Gruentzig and Hopff. Encouraged by Dotter's work and armed with his own cardiology background, training under Zeitler, and experience with peripheral PTA, Gruentzig had been continuing the search for a more suitable material with which to build a balloon catheter specifically for coronary angioplasty. He teamed up with Hopff, a professor emeritus of organic chemistry from the Eidgenossischen Technischen Hochschule of Zurich and PVC was selected (8). Walter Schlumpf, husband of Maria Schlumpf, Gruentzig's assistant, actually built the first PVC balloon catheters that Gruentzig used on patients for peripheral PTA. The first case series of PTA with use of the new PVC catheters (in 1974) comprised a group of patients with atherosclerotic obstructions in the lower extremities (9). In 1976 and 1977, the new catheters were used intraoperatively to dilate human coronary artery stenoses (10), and on September 16, 1977, Gruentzig performed the first percutaneous transluminal coronary angioplasty (PTCA). He reported his first five patients in a letter to the editor of *Lancet*, which was published in February of 1978 (11). His clinical report of a series of patients followed in 1979 (12). By 1980, angioplasty's flame had been reignited in the United States, preparing the way for all of the ensuing developments we have witnessed.

BASIC PROPERTIES AND FUNCTIONS OF BALLOON PTA CATHETERS

Since the earliest beginnings of balloon PTA, experience has helped to determine the problems with and limitations of existing technologies in various applications. The understanding thus derived has helped manufacturers focus on the most important balloon catheter characteristics and to develop better products.

Balloon compliance and dilating force, hoop strength, profile, trackability, kink resistance, pushability, and balloon inflation and deflation times are the most important attributes of angioplasty balloon catheters. For a modern treatment of balloons, we might add a discussion of stent compatibility. Although stents will be mentioned below, no formal guidelines or standards have been established.

Balloon Compliance and Dilating Force

In the strictest sense, compliance is the change in volume per unit change in pressure. For most PTA balloon catheters, the changes in length that occur in response to increased pressure are negligible. Therefore, volume changes occur primarily because of changes in balloon diameter, and balloon compliance is best represented by the expression

$$C = \frac{dD}{dP}$$

where C is balloon compliance, D is balloon diameter, and P is pressure inside the PTA balloon. Gruentzig's original balloons and all of the early PTA balloons were made of PVC, a relatively compliant balloon material by today's standards. These balloons tended to yield under pressure and increase their diameter significantly before reaching the limits of tensile strength (burst). The result during PTA was often a balloon diameter significantly larger than that stated by the manufacturer. Abele has provided an excellent discussion of how, with increasing force applied to such materials in a severe stenosis, expansion of compliant balloons can result in (1) unpredictable balloon diameters; (2) overstretching of the balloon material not abutting the lesion (for example, the portion contacting the normal vessel wall); (3) overstretching and possible rupture of adjacent normal vessel segments; (4) a poor tactile sense of the lesion; and (5) decreased dilating force at the lesion site (13,14).

Since the introduction of PTA balloons, developments in polymer science and technology have led to thin-walled balloons made of less compliant materials, including polyethylene (PE), polyethylene terephthalate (PET), nylon, and polyurethane. These materials are less compliant than PVC and are, therefore, generally better suited for PTA, although PE is the most compliant among them. Noncompliant balloons increase very little in diameter before reaching the point of burst. Therefore, the selection of the correct balloon size to match the vessel size all but guarantees that a vessel rupture (transmural tear) will not occur during angioplasty. The balloon itself may rupture when the limits of tensile strength are exceeded, but the vessel should remain intact. Figure 12–4, a graph of compliance of various balloon materials, illustrates the differences between some of these materials. Other than the specific balloon material, variables related to compliance and burst include temperature, number of inflations (15), and balloon diameter. PVC balloons tend to stretch before burst, not only in response to increasing pressure, but also in response to repeated inflations (16). Such balloon overstretching has led to vessel rupture in clinical angioplasty (17,18).

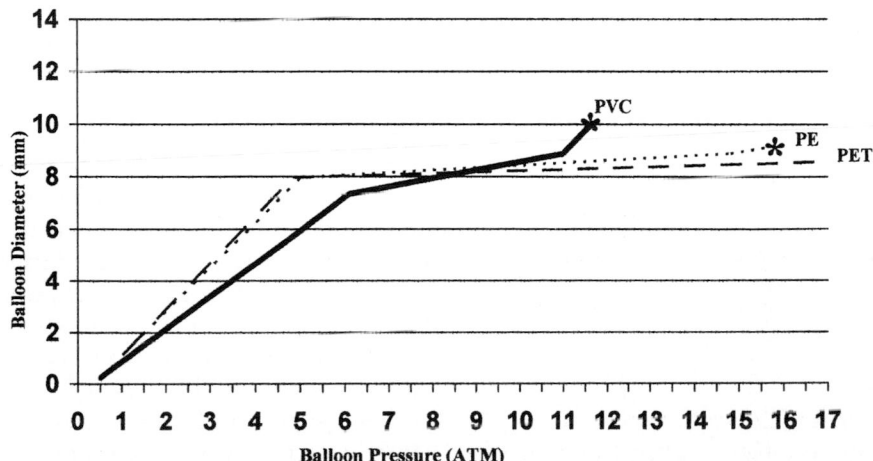

Figure 12–4 Compliance curves for various balloon catheters of 8 mm nominal diameter. Because length is assumed to be constant, compliance is represented by change in balloon diameter as a function of pressure. From most compliant to least compliant: PVC (polyvinyl chloride), PE (polyethylene), PET (polyethylene teraphthalate). The *asterisks* represent burst point.

Hoop Strength

The nonradial force applied to the surface of the balloon circumferentially during balloon expansion is known as *hoop stress*. Because pressure is force per unit area, for a given pressure, a large balloon surface experiences greater hoop stress than does a smaller balloon. The hoop stress, *T*, is the product of pressure, *P*, and balloon diameter, *D*.

$$T = P \times D$$

For a given balloon material and inflation pressure, a balloon of larger diameter has greater hoop stress applied to its surface. Therefore, large balloons burst at lower pressures than small balloons of the same material. Stated another way, in a selection of various balloon sizes of the identical material, each balloon bursts at the same level of hoop stress. However, because of the above relationship, for a given level of hoop stress, the pressure and balloon diameter are inversely related. Therefore, for large balloons, relatively low pressures are required to reach the hoop stress at which burst will occur. Consequently, the largest balloons have the lowest burst pressure ratings. "High-pressure balloons" that withstand up to 20 atm of pressure (but whose advertised maximum inflation pressures are 10–16 atm) are available and in use in clinical PTA.

The most important underlying cause of vessel rupture angioplasty is overdistention of the vessel. The simplest way to ensure that overdistention will not occur and that the maximum dilating force will be applied to the lesion site is to select a noncompliant balloon with the appropriate diameter. Because one uses a noncompliant balloon to perform PTA, dilating force increases linearly with the inflation pressure (14). Finally, one alternative to the ideal noncompliant PTA catheter is a controlled compliance catheter. This concept, which is used by the manufacturers of some of the nylon balloons, entails using a PTA balloon catheter in conjunction with an inflation device. For any inflation pressure chosen, the balloon has a known diameter, because its compliance curves are accurate and reproducible. Using such a system, it is possible, for example, to expand an 8.0-mm balloon to 7.5 or 8.5 mm (or whatever diameter between these two extremes is needed) by choosing the correct pressure to reach the corresponding predicted balloon diameter.

Balloon Profile

Profile may be thought of as the maximum cross-sectional area or diameter of the PTA catheter. It is usually expressed in French size. Thus, a 5 French PTA catheter whose balloon increases the profile slightly may be a true 5.7 French. Most modern PTA is performed through an angiographic sheath with hemostatic valve and side port. A 5.7 French

profile would necessitate use of a 6 French sheath. Balloon catheters with significantly larger profiles at the balloon site than throughout the remainder of the shaft length have a propensity for causing blood leakage at the catheter insertion site when used without an angiographic sheath.

Low profile confers two tangible benefits: a smaller arterial access sheath (and the potential of fewer local entry site complications) and lesion crossability. The latter property refers to the ability of the balloon to cross the target lesion so that PTA can be performed. Aside from profile, another factor related to crossability is the frictional force between the lesion surface and the balloon surface. To decrease this frictional force, some manufacturers have added hydrophilic coatings to the balloon surfaces.

The early PTA catheters had 9 French shafts. Adding the balloon wrap to the catheter shaft often produced a true profile in the 10 French to 11 French range. Such prohibitively large catheters could never have been used to track over a wire through tortuous vessels for visceral or coronary angioplasty. To actually decrease the profile of most PTA catheters, manufacturers have used better catheter materials and modern extrusion technology to reduce the overall catheter shaft size, decreased the diameter of the portion of the catheter shaft beneath the balloon, used very thin but noncompliant balloon materials, and perfected the balloon wrap. The specific balloon catheter design (coaxial, double-lumen, balloon-on-a-wire) is another determinant of profile. All commonly used PTA balloon sizes are available on 5 French catheter shafts. At least two of the manufacturers have balloons up to 12 mm in diameter on a 5 French shaft (Figure 12–5), and two have high-pressure balloons on 5 French shafts. The profile, including the balloon wrap, on these 12 mm balloon catheters is approximately 7 French. Therefore, a 7 French sheath is required to use them.

Some vessels are so small that the most important catheter characteristic is profile. Small-vessel balloon catheters used for tibial PTA, pediatric renal PTA, and renal branch PTA are available on shafts ranging from 3.1–5.0 French (Figure 12–6). These balloon diameters range from 2–6 mm, and the balloons are rated at 6–16 atm, depending on balloon material, diameter, and manufacturer. Problems related to profile exist in interventional cardiology, too. In PTCA, some severe stenoses in mid- to distal-coronary arterial segments are not crossable without extremely low profile balloon catheters. The manufacturers have responded to this challenge, however, and a wide array of low-profile PTCA balloons is now available.

The angiographer also has some control over profile. For almost all balloon catheters, including those that "wing" significantly upon deflation, counterclockwise torque decreases balloon profile to the lowest possible level. Occasionally, when faced with a situation in which the balloon catheter cannot be advanced over a wire through the area of stenosis, minimizing profile with counterclockwise rotation on the catheter enables passage

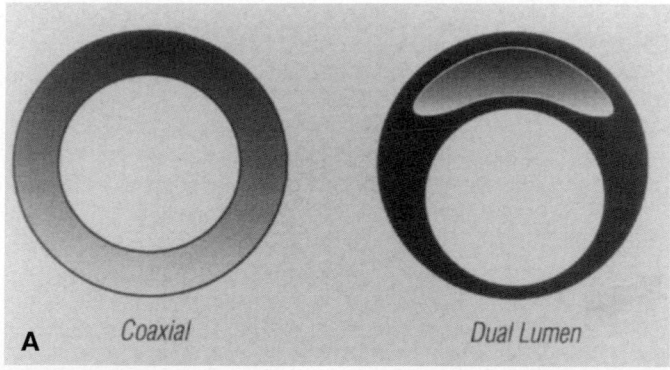

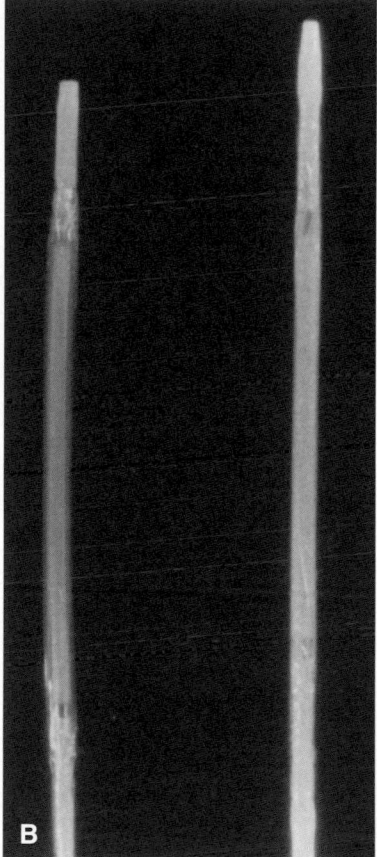

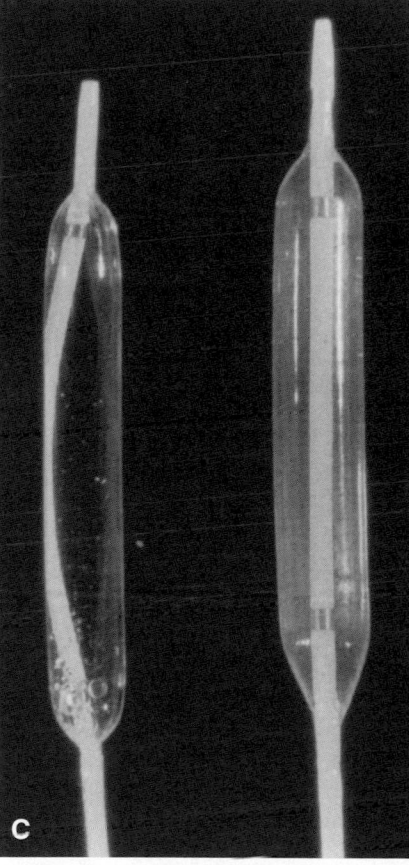

Figure 12–5 Peripheral PTA balloons are available in a variety of designs and sizes on 5 French catheter shafts. **A.** Cross sections of coaxial and double-lumen balloon catheters. **B., C.** Double-lumen (*left*) and coaxial (*right*) 5 French balloon catheters before **(B.)** and after **(C.)** inflation.

of the balloon through the lesion. Profile must be kept in mind even when a balloon has been deflated and is about to be removed from the angiographic sheath. Often, a balloon catheter that resists withdrawal through the sheath may be retrieved successfully once counterclockwise torque is applied. If there is any question about which direction of rotation produces the lowest profile of the balloon catheter, the angiographer should rotate the balloon with one hand and grip it with the index and forefinger of the other hand. Winging should not occur when the proper direction has been selected. In addition, some of the high-pressure balloons wing markedly when negative pressure is applied forcefully to the balloon inflation syringe (Figure 12–7). For the safest, least traumatic

removal of these balloons, it may be necessary to deflate forcefully and patiently and open the balloon port to ambient pressures before withdrawal.

Trackability

Trackability is the tendency of a PTA catheter to follow a guide wire through a tortuous path to the lesion site without loss of wire position. In any given case, the specific anatomy, the skill and experience of the operator, and the guide wire–catheter combination contribute to the likelihood that the catheter will track to the desired location. In the early days of superficial femoral and retrograde iliac angioplasty, trackability was never a necessary feature.

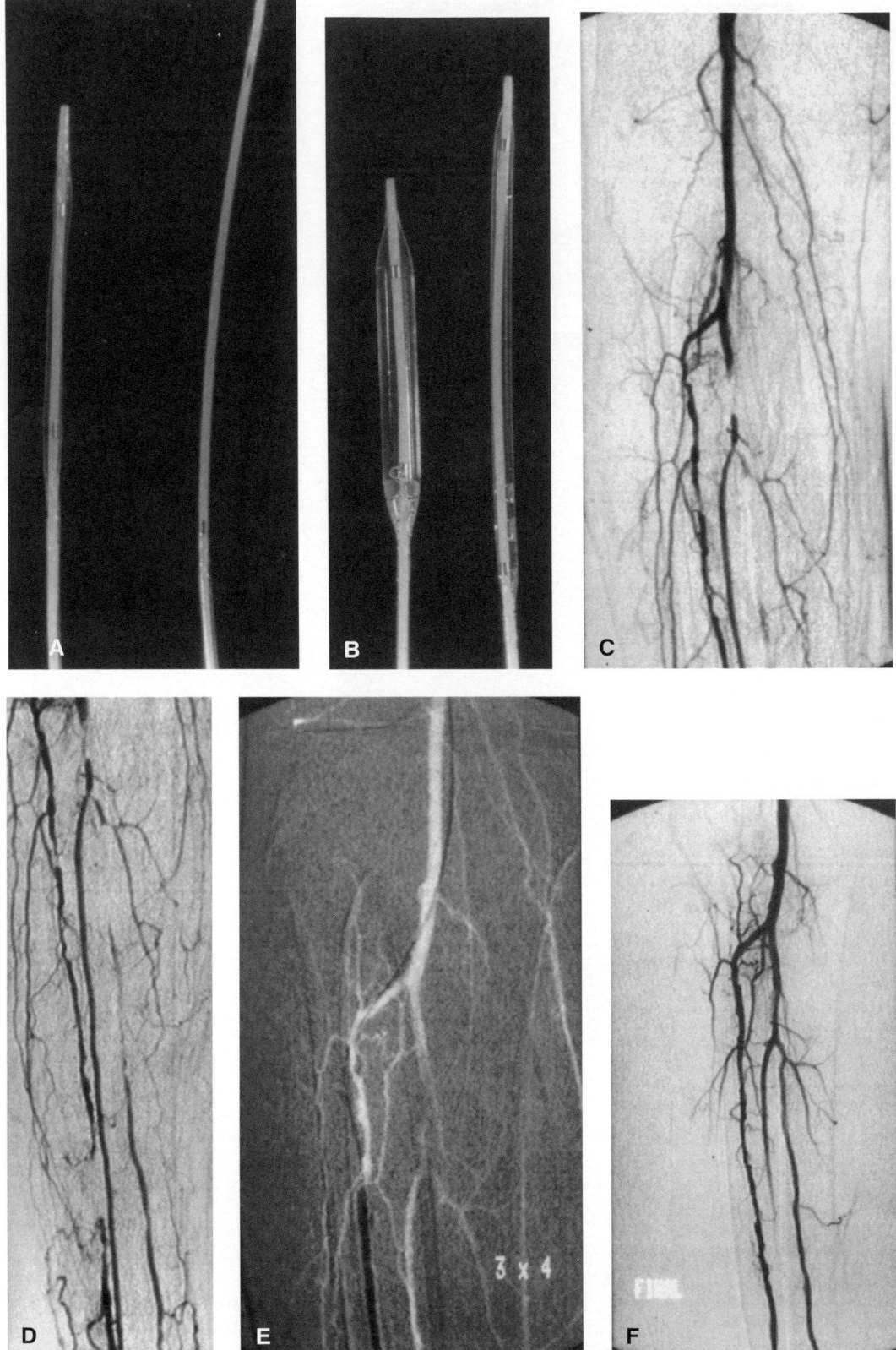

Figure 12–6 **A., B.** Small-vessel angioplasty balloons for tibial and branch renal angioplasty: 4 mm by 2 cm balloon on a 4 French shaft (*left*) and 2 mm by 4 cm balloon on a 3.7 French shaft (*right*) before **(A.)** and after **(B.)** inflation. **C., D.** A patient with a nonhealing ulcer of the right foot. Angiogram before PTA depicts numerous stenoses and segmental occlusions in the anterior tibial and tibioperoneal vessels of the right lower leg. **E.** Roadmap image during PTA of the anterior tibial artery with a 3 mm by 4 cm small-vessel balloon catheter. **F., G., H.** Images from the angiogram after PTA of all trifurcation vessels reveal an excellent morphologic result.

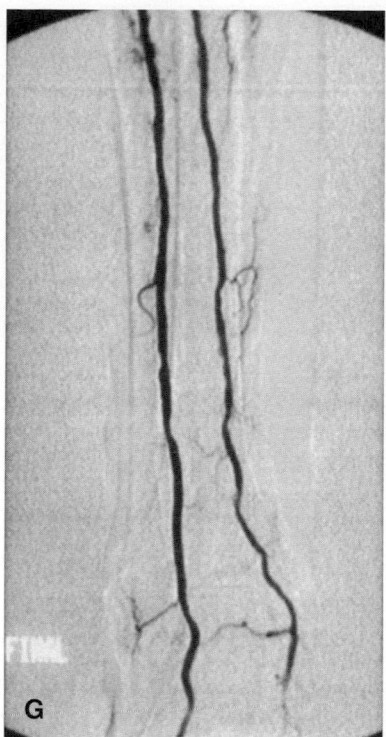
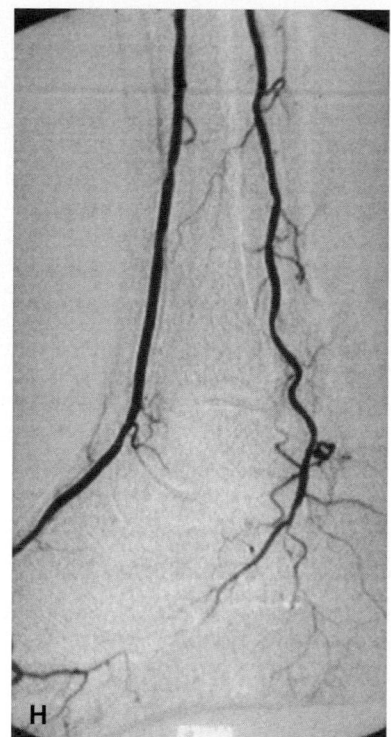

Figure 12–6 *(continued)*

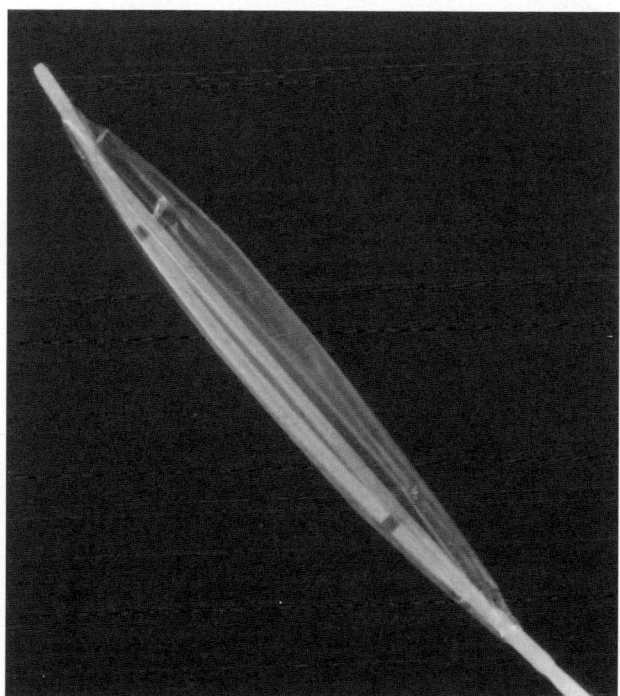

Figure 12–7 "Winging" of a high-pressure balloon during aspiration on the balloon port. This balloon will not rewrap to its original low profile upon deflation and removal. However, the profile can be minimized and the effects of "winging" diminished by aspirating the balloon and opening the balloon port to ambient pressure before removal.

Therefore, the relatively large, stiff PTA catheters seemed quite acceptable. Because their stiffness made them pushable, most lesions could be traversed and dilated. But the need to do over-the-bifurcation iliac and femoral PTA, renal PTA, and visceral PTA placed new demands on the manufacturers (Figure 12–8). Sufficient flexibility had to be incorporated into catheter design to enable angiographers to do these procedures. To a great degree, this flexibility came about with the reduction in profile that the manufacturers achieved. Much of this reduction has been accomplished by the manufacture of thin-walled catheters. However, an increased tendency for the catheter to kink and a decrease in pushability are the prices to be paid. In addition to thinner catheter walls, another factor that has enhanced the trackability of modern PTA catheters is the wide variety of guide wires currently in use. A veritable array of exchange wires and steerable wires in 0.035-inch size are now available. The ideal wire enables the operator to steer across the site and has a flexible, soft, radiopaque tip and a relatively stiff body over which the catheter can track. In practice, however, it is often necessary to use more than one wire to complete a procedure. For instance, in renal PTA (Figure 12–9), crossing a stenosis with a sidewinder catheter led by a Bentson wire may provide the ideal combination of catheter shape and soft wire tip. Once the catheter has crossed the lesion and the correct intraluminal position is confirmed by injection of contrast material, the Bentson wire may be exchanged for a Rosen wire, a TAD (torsional attenuating diameter) wire, or other

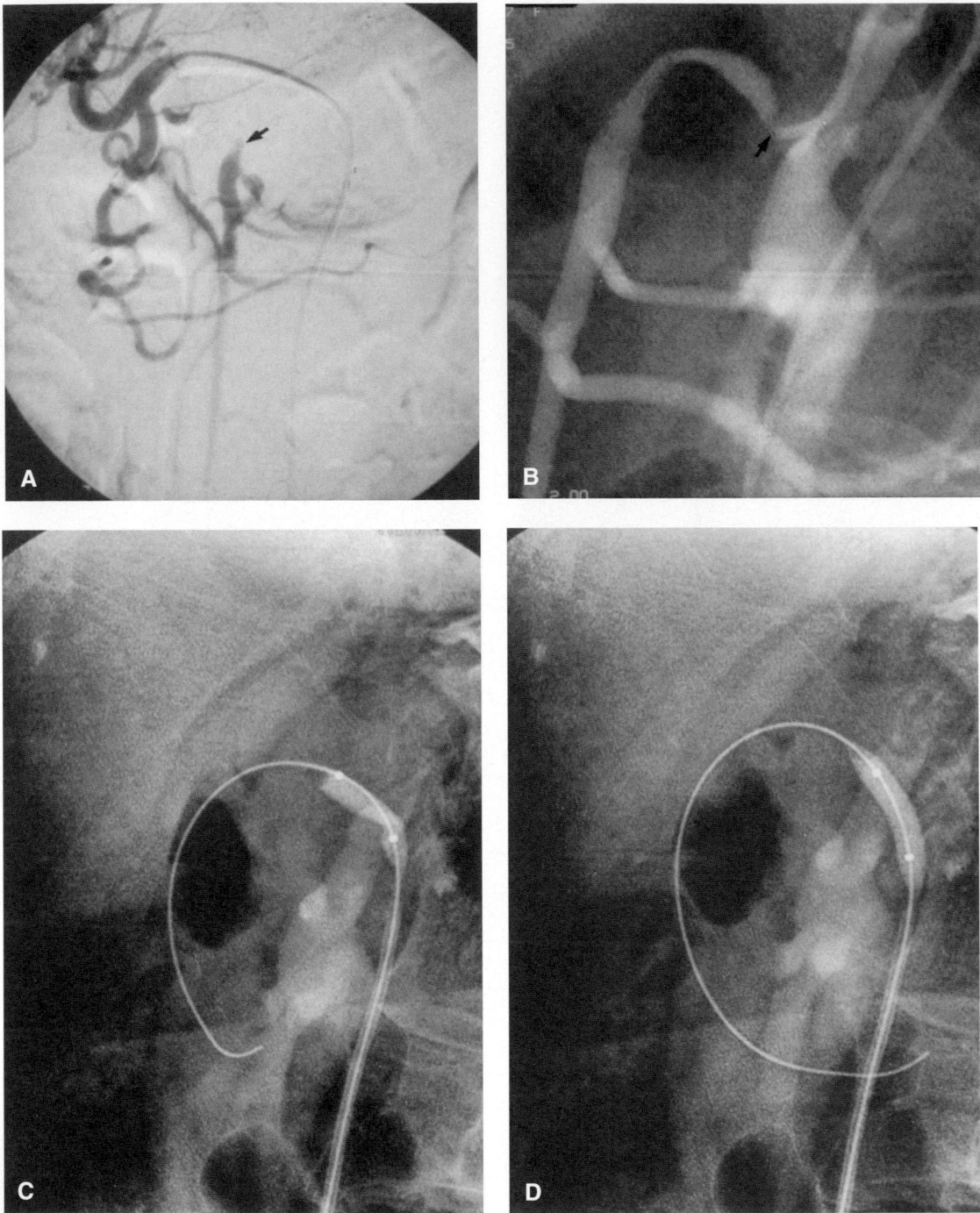

Figure 12–8   Trackability and low profile are two important characteristics that enable peripheral PTA balloon catheters to function in stenoses located along difficult curves, particularly in renal and visceral PTA. **A., B.** Even with these properties, sometimes a guiding catheter is required to success-fully negotiate a difficult stenosis. **A.** Posteroanterior proper hepatic and **B.** lateral selective superior mesenteric artery injections in a patient with abdominal angina attributable to inferior mesenteric artery occlusion (*not shown*), severe superior mesenteric artery (SMA) stenosis (*arrows*), and moder-ate celiac stenosis (*not shown*). **C., D.** PTA with a 6 mm by 2 cm balloon catheter positioned within the SMA stenosis through a guiding catheter. **E., F.** Post-PTA angiograms showing marked angio-graphic improvement. **G.** Artist's rendering of an over-the-bifurcation PTA of a contralateral renal transplant arterial stenosis. The arrows at the bifurcation indicate that the angiographer "shimmies" the catheter shaft over the aortic bifurcation to avoid pulling the wire out of position or pushing it up into the aorta. In so doing, the operator is taking advantage of the fact that the coefficient of dynamic friction is lower than that of static friction. **H.** The over-the-bifurcation iliac guide catheter is a very reasonable alternative that results in a larger arterial puncture site.

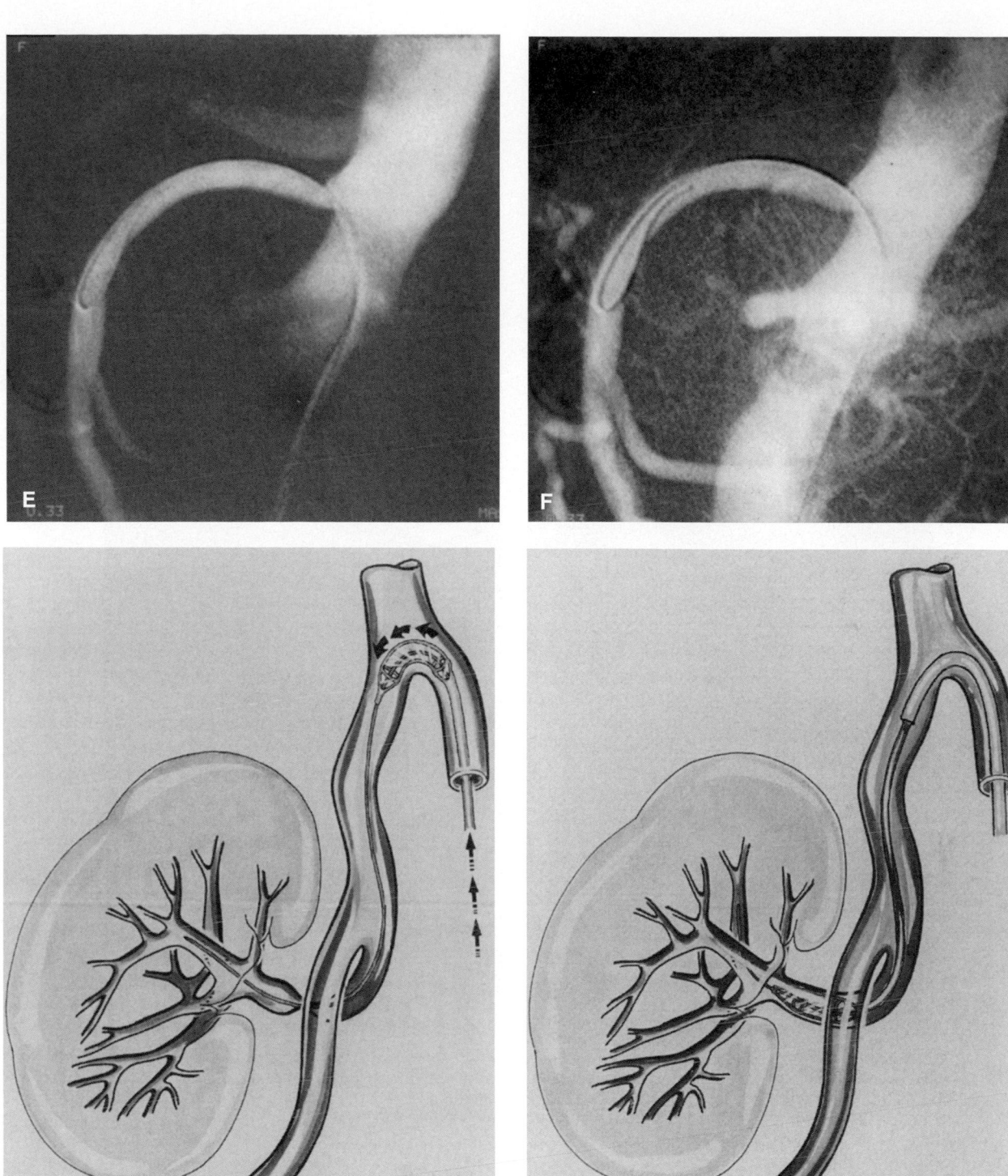

Figure 12–8 *(continued)*

relatively stiff wire with a safe tip, over which the PTA catheter will track through the stenosis. A balloon catheter that tracks poorly will erase the previous selective catheterization efforts by pulling the exchange wire out of the target vessel into the aorta or parent vessel as it is being advanced (Figure 12–10).

Kink Resistance

Ideally, a catheter used to negotiate tortuous paths and severe stenoses should also be able to resist kinking when the shaft is being advanced through a curve with a narrow radius. In PTA, this problem is perhaps most frequently

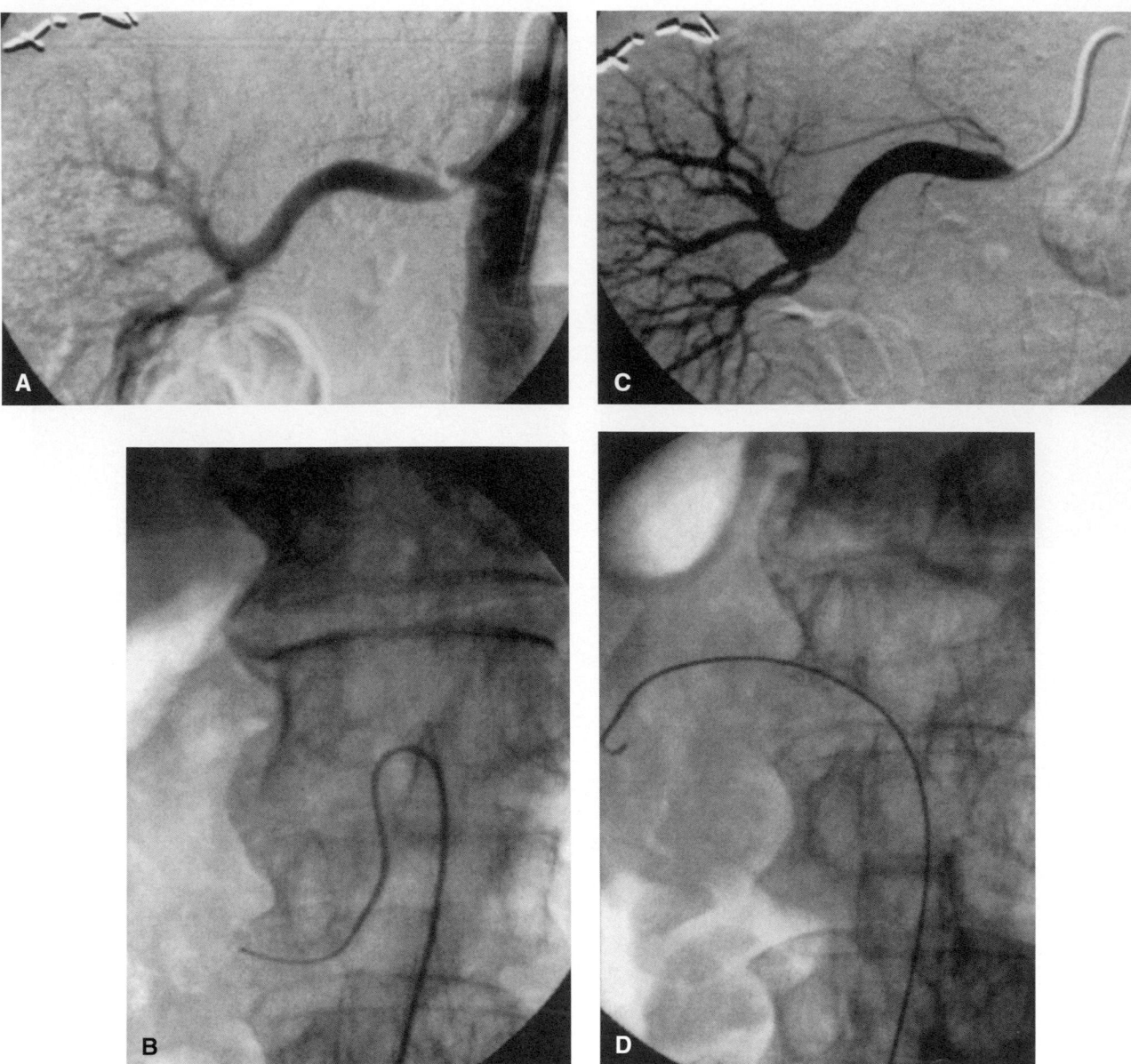

Figure 12–9 **A.** Selective right renal arteriogram in a patient with bilateral renal artery stenosis. The patient was undergoing PTA of both renal arteries on the same day. **B.** A 0.035-inch Bentson wire is used to guide the 5.5 French Simmons-1 catheter tip across the stenosis. **C.** Injection beyond the stenosis confirms the intraluminal catheter position in the renal artery distal to the stenosis. **D.** A 0.035-inch Rosen wire is introduced. **E., F.** Balloon dilatation of the stenosis. **G.** Aortogram immediately after right renal PTA demonstrates marked improvement.

encountered when the operator needs the PTA to also double as a diagnostic angiographic catheter. For instance, in over-the-bifurcation PTA of the superficial femoral artery (SFA), the operator may wish to withdraw the guide wire temporarily so that the guide wire lumen may be used to inject contrast material for the post-PTA arteriogram. When the guide wire is being withdrawn, the catheter shaft (along with its balloon lumen and guide wire lumen) is most susceptible to kinking. In PTCA, kinking is not as much of a problem because of the use of guiding catheters and because the PTCA balloon catheters are never used for injecting contrast material.

Most, if not all, of the 5 French PTA balloon catheters have demonstrated this kinking problem in over-the-bifurcation PTA and other applications. Once kinking occurs, it sometimes can be overcome by withdrawing the catheter in small increments while advancing a tapered-tip guide wire. Usually, however, the catheter must be withdrawn and the vessel must be recatheterized. To avoid this problem, a few maneuvers can be performed. The first is to position a relatively stiff 0.018-inch wire with a soft tip beyond the stenosis and to affix a Y adapter with a hemostatic valve to the injection port of the balloon PTA catheter. A sufficiently trackable balloon PTA catheter may then be brought into

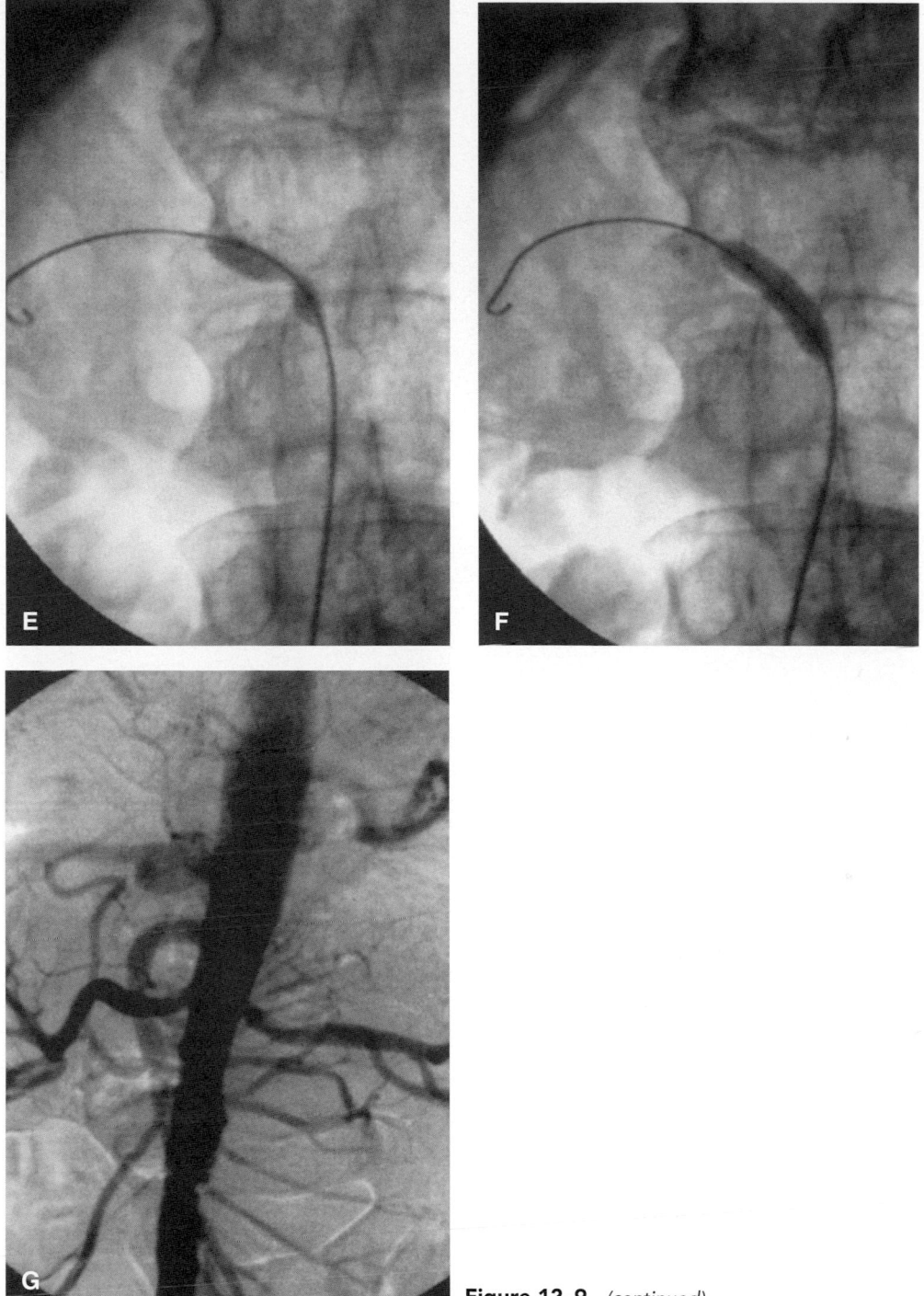

Figure 12–9 *(continued)*

position over the wire, and the side port of the Y adapter may be used to inject contrast material, nitroglycerin, saline flush, or other substances (Figure 12–11). The second is to use an over-the-bifurcation iliac guide or sheath that broadens the curve (increases the radius of curve) required of the 5 French catheter during contralateral work. Kinking thus may be avoided; however, the advantage of low profile at the catheter entry site is lost.

Virtually all materials have a high susceptibility of kinking when the catheter wall is too thin. However, for a given thickness of catheter wall, different materials have different kink resistances. Braided catheters may have the best kink resistance, but limitations exist in profile and trackability. A 5 French braided catheter with a balloon lumen added for PTA would increase profile significantly above 5 French and would be less trackable than a nonbraided catheter.

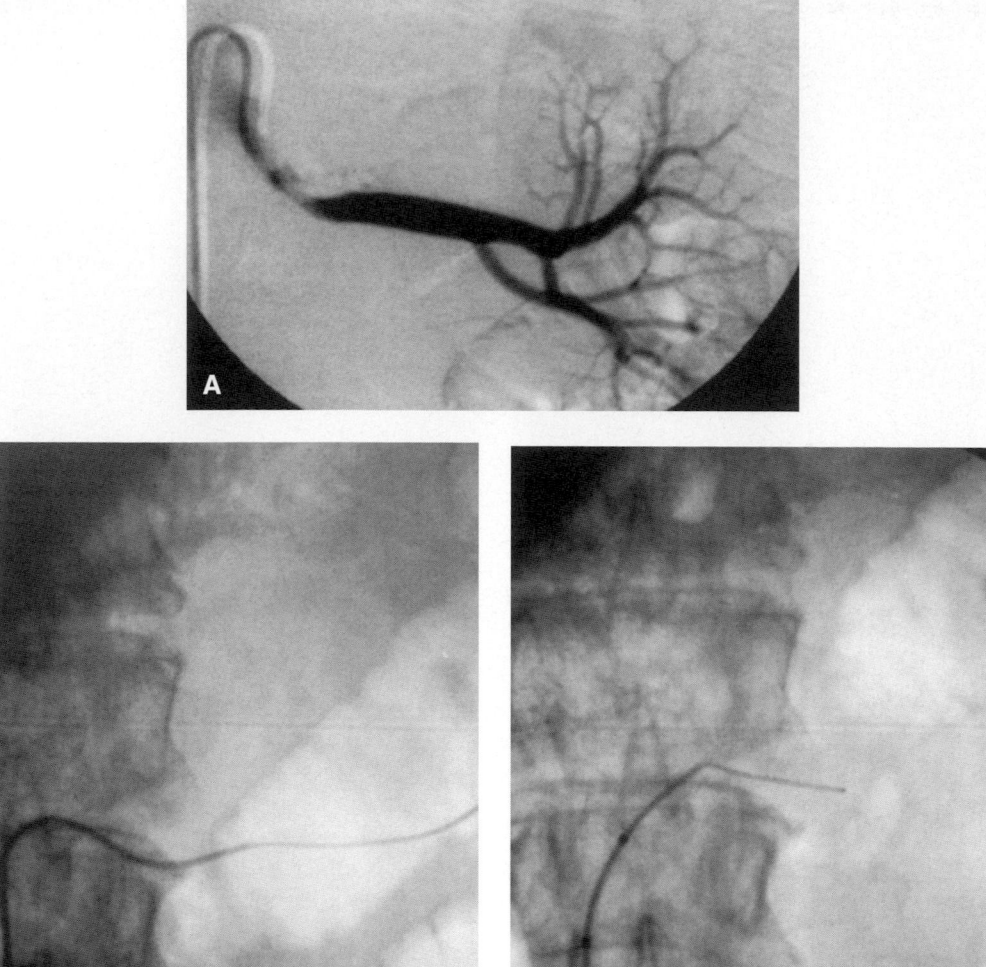

Figure 12–10   Attempted angioplasty of a left renal artery stenosis. **A.** Selective left renal arteriogram demonstrates severe stenosis. **B.** A 5.5 French Simmons-1 catheter is introduced safely through the stenosis over a wire. **C.** The balloon will not track over the straight, fixed-core exchange wire through the stenosis. Rather, it continues up the aorta and, in the process, pulls the wire out of the renal artery.

Therefore, although some sheaths, guide catheters, and many selective catheters are braided, balloon PTA catheter shafts generally are not.

To summarize, low-profile balloon catheters manufactured from very thin materials are susceptible to kinking, particularly when advanced through a curve with a narrow radius and when the guide wire is removed. Currently, no manufacturer has a completely kink-resistant, low-profile PTA catheter. The best way to deal with kinking is to avoid it with one of the maneuvers described earlier.

Pushability

It is perhaps easiest to conceptualize the problem of pushability by considering PTCA rather than PTA, although the principle comes into play in over-the-bifurcation femoropopliteal PTA, in tibial PTA, in renal and visceral PTA, and now in intracranial PTA. The very low-profile PTCA catheters may have no problem reaching a severe stenosis; however, if the catheter lacks pushability, it may not be able to cross the stenosis. To overcome this problem, manufacturers have now come up with very floppy catheters at the balloon end (leading end) that also have a relatively stiffer shaft for pushing at the trailing end. The longer and smoother the transition between stiff portion and floppy portion, the more the catheter is able to resist kinking. The pushability property of PTA catheters takes on a different meaning in over-the-wire applications, including most circumstances encountered in peripheral PTA. Here, the angiographer is able to use the stiffness of the

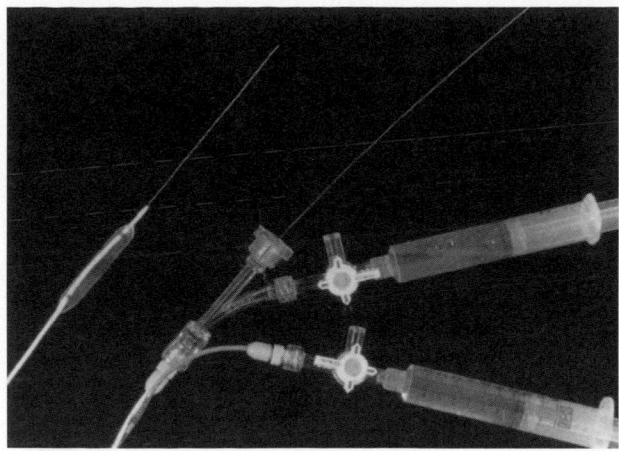

Figure 12–11 Catheter setup for over-the-bifurcation work that enables contrast material injection without losing wire position and without allowing kinking of the balloon port or central lumen at the aortic bifurcation. The procedure for contralateral superficial femoral PTA would be: (1) catheterize the contralateral superficial femoral artery with a cobra or other curved catheter, (2) replace the 0.035-inch guide wire with a 200-cm, 0.018-inch guide wire, (3) place the PTA balloon (5 French) over 0.018-inch wire to the site of lesion, (4) dilate, (5) deflate and withdraw the balloon catheter but leave wire in position across the treated area, and (6) perform angiogram through Y adapter.

guide wire to support the catheter as it is being pushed through the lesion. Even under such circumstances, it is helpful to use an angioplasty balloon catheter with a well-tapered tip and a low profile. Perhaps the epitome of reliance on the guide wire for support as the catheter is pushed through a lesion is the pull-through technique for recanalization PTA and stenting of chronic iliac occlusions (Figure 12–12).

Balloon Catheter Tip

Balloon catheter tips should taper well to fit the guide wire and to aid in crossing stenoses. An excessively bulky or poorly tapered tip design can result in a catheter that will not cross severe stenoses, even over a stiff guide wire. A poorly tapered tip and poor pushability of the shaft make an especially undesirable combination. The only other major property of balloon catheter tips is length. In many applications, such as retrograde balloon PTA of the common iliac artery, tip length may not be an issue. However, wherever branch vessels beyond the catheter tip are susceptible to tip trauma (as in renal artery and tibial applications), a short tip length is required.

Balloon Inflation and Deflation Times

Even though the "flow" of dilute contrast material through the balloon port of a PTA catheter during inflation and deflation is not laminar, it is useful to think of it as such to understand the factors contributing to

observed inflation and deflation times. Modern PTA catheters have a low profile and a proportionately small diameter balloon port or channel. "Flow" of liquid through this channel is proportional to the fourth power of the radius. It is also inversely related to the length of the catheter. Therefore, if we compare two 12-mm-diameter PTA balloon catheters that have the same-diameter balloon ports but different lengths, one 40 cm and the other 80 cm, we find that the 80-cm catheter takes approximately twice as long to deflate as the 40-cm one.

Stent Compatibility

Stent compatibility may be thought of as that property or collection of properties of a balloon catheter that determine its suitability as a delivery device for balloon-expandable stents. Currently, only one balloon-expandable stent, the Palmaz balloon-expandable intraluminal stent (Johnson and Johnson Interventional Systems) is available for use on humans in the United States, although others are in development. Therefore, at present, a stent-compatible balloon catheter is appropriately considered to be one that is suitable for deploying a Palmaz stent. Desirable properties that these balloons should possess for peripheral vascular work include a sufficiently low profile with the stent mounted to pass through a 7 French sheath with hemostatic valve, resistance to slippage of the stent on the balloon surface during passage through the sheath and deployment, and scratch resistance. Most of the 5 French PTA balloon catheters fulfill the profile criterion, and virtually all of these balloons allow manual crimping of the stent sufficient to avoid slippage during passage through the sheath to the target site. However, once balloon inflation begins, two serious problems can still occur. The first, slippage off the balloon surface, can occur with balloons that have coatings to reduce friction and enhance lesion crossability. Therefore, it is unwise to choose these balloons as a first choice for stent deployment. The second problem that can occur is balloon rupture. This tends to happen with scratch-sensitive balloons. These balloons lose their structural integrity when scratched by a stent or even by a sharp, calcified plaque. Balloon rupture during stent deployment and stent slippage off the balloon surface during deployment may lead to loss of the stent in the vessel or in a non-target vessel. Figure 12–13 depicts a situation in which a balloon catheter exchange was required to salvage a stenting procedure after a partial deployment. Although no carefully controlled trials are available to compare the utility and safety of the various balloon types in stent deployment, many experienced interventionalists have concluded that Duralyn (nylon) balloons are the most scratch-resistant (least likely to develop holes and to fail during stent deployment). The next most scratch-resistant balloons are PE. Of the balloon materials in common usage in peripheral PTA, PET is the most scratch-sensitive. The experience in the

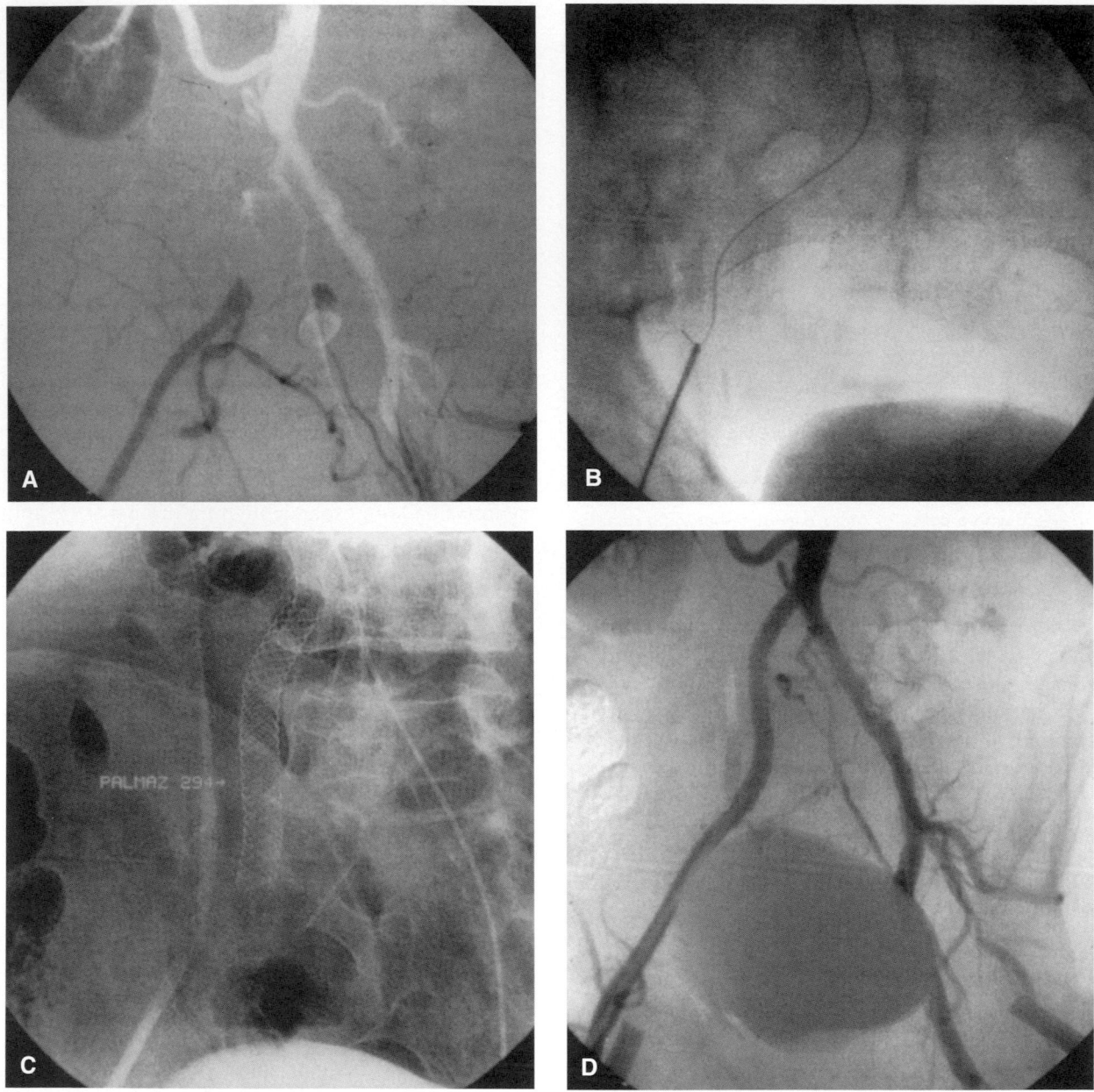

Figure 12–12 Pull-through method for recanalization, PTA, and stenting of chronic iliac artery occlusions. **A.** Arteriogram of right common iliac artery occlusion in a patient with claudication. Early arterial phase film is used for subtraction mask; the result is black and white arteries resulting from late filling of the right external iliac artery by collaterals. **B.** After a sidewinder catheter has been used to successfully pass a wire through the occlusion from a contralateral approach, the wire is snared from the right with a snare through a sheath that has been placed in the right groin. **C.** Stents are placed using a right retrograde approach. **D.** Completion angiogram shows an excellent anatomic result.

author's institution is that approximately 30–40% of attempted stent deployments with PET balloons result in rupture and a need to exchange balloon catheters. With Duralyn, balloon ruptures still occur but much less frequently (5–10% of attempted deployments). Because of these differences, Duralyn is an excellent choice of balloon material for stent deployment. The author has deployed up

to five iliac stents in a procedure using a single 5 French Duralyn balloon.

Other Functions of Balloon PTA Catheters

In recent years, the high frequency of postangioplasty restenosis, the economic impact of restenosis, and the

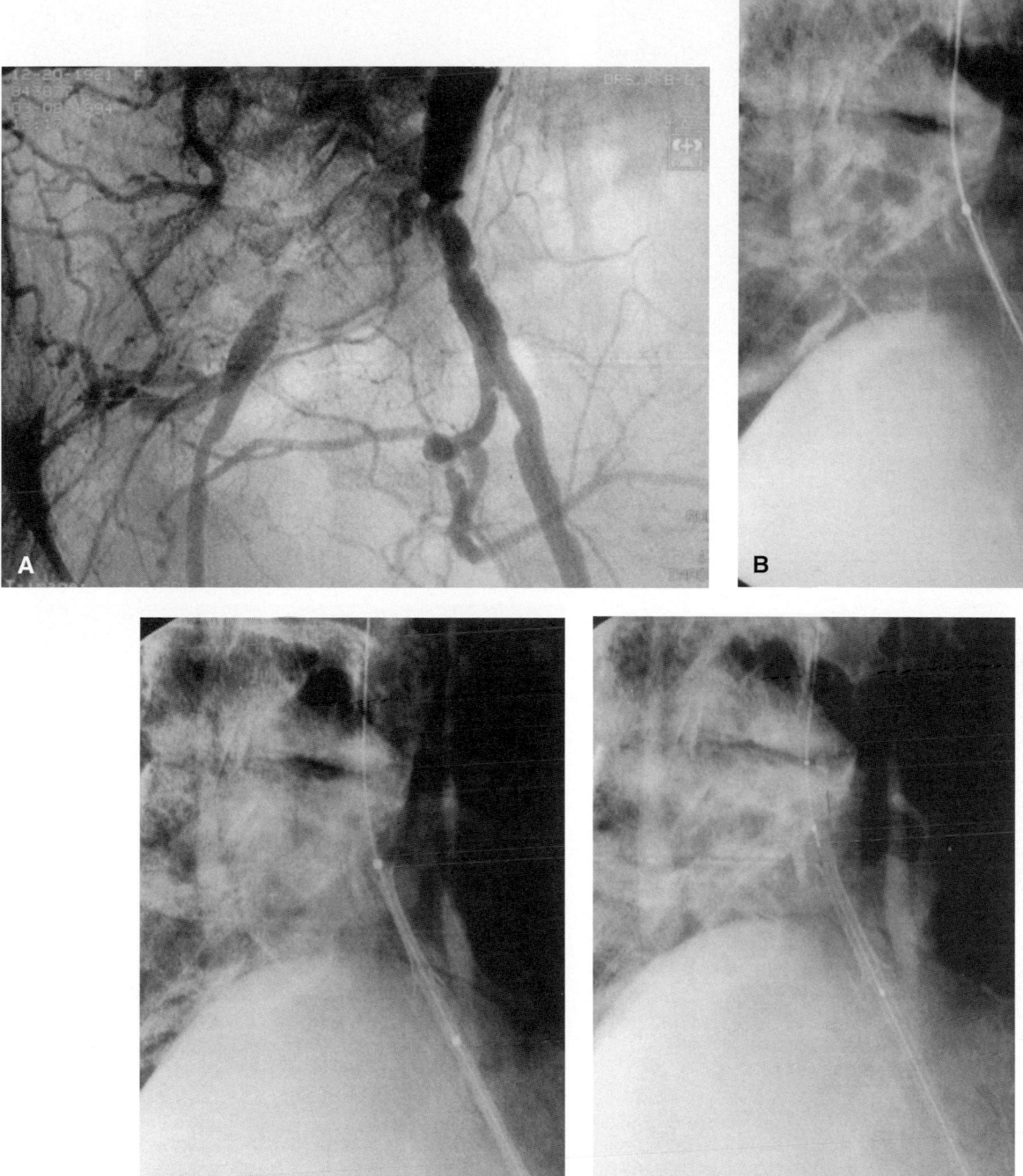

Figure 12–13   Patient with bilateral claudication. **A.** Preliminary angiogram reveals right iliac occlusion and left iliac stenoses. **B.** Attempted stent deployment results in balloon rupture and only partial expansion of the stent (minimal flaring on leading and trailing edges). Attempted rapid expansion of the balloon, first with a 10-mL then with a 5-mL syringe, in an effort to complete stent deployment failed because of a large rent in the balloon. **C.** The sheath was advanced to the trailing edge of the stent to prevent stent migration during subsequent manipulations. A decision was made to exchange balloon catheters; however, a 5 French catheter would have been too large to traverse the stent lumen, so a low-profile balloon was used. In preparation for using a low-profile balloon, the 0.035-inch wire was exchanged for an 0.018-inch guide wire. The balloon was withdrawn as the partially flared stent edge was held against the leading edge of the sheath. **D.** A 5-mm by 4-cm low-profile balloon was brought into position inside the stent. **E., F.** Preliminary deployment was accomplished with the 5-mm balloon. **G.** Deployment was completed with an 8-mm balloon. **H.** Completion angiogram after stenting on left and recanalization and stenting on right.

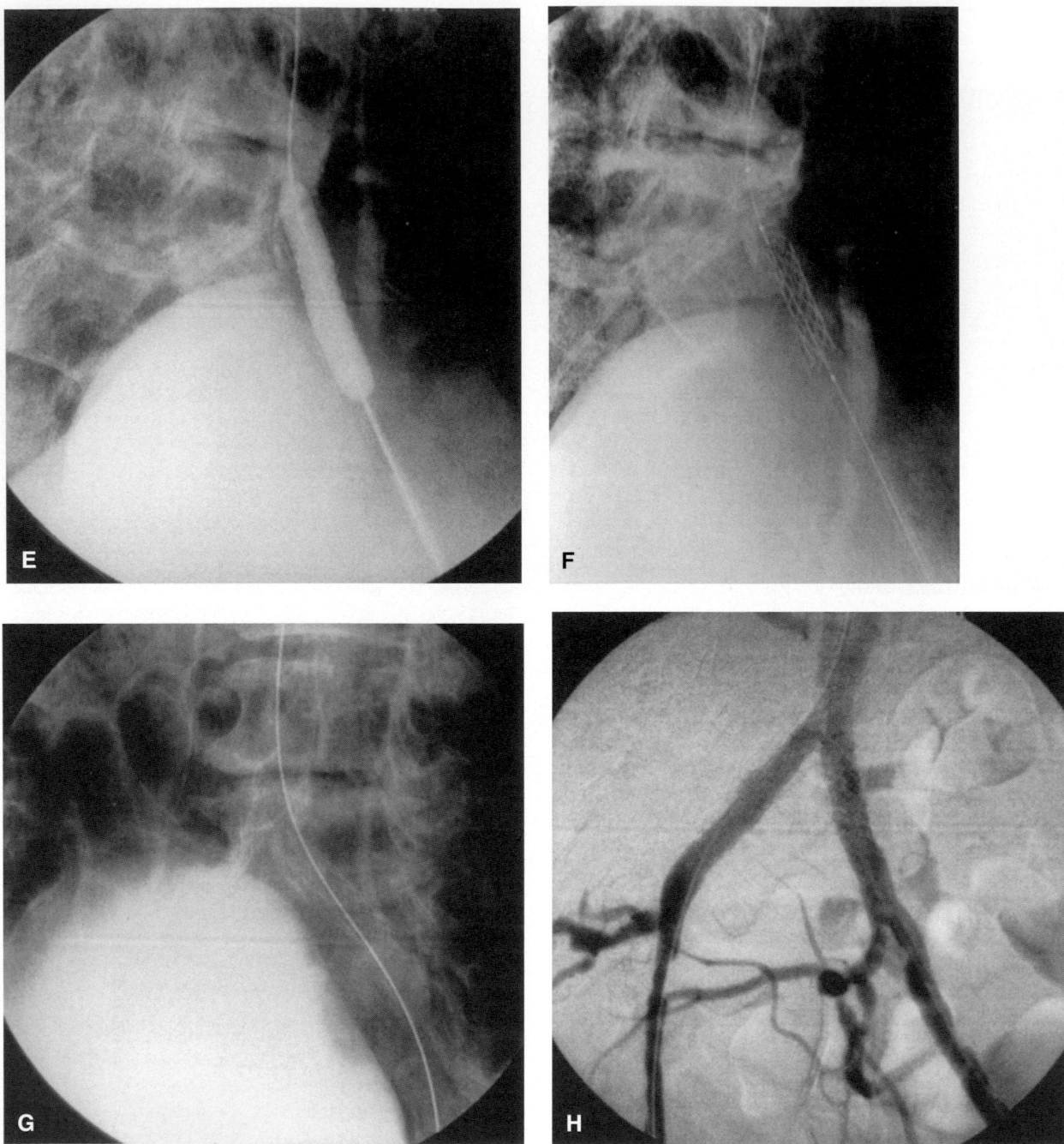

Figure 12–13 *(continued)*

added risk to patients of subsequent revascularization procedures have generated widespread interest in basic and clinical research aimed at reducing or eliminating the problem. Approaches have been mechanical (stents, atherectomy), pharmacologic, and even genetic. Current theory holds that once PTA occurs, growth factors cause a fundamental change in medial smooth muscle cells (SMCs) that result in a synthetic rather than a contractile phenotype. These transformed SMCs migrate into the intima and elaborate an organic matrix that constitutes 90% of the volume of neointimal hyperplastic tissue. The latter is responsible for most cases of restenosis.

Many of the drugs, cytotoxic agents, and other potentially antiproliferative substances that have been investigated for their ability to control restenosis will never be delivered intravenously because their effects in high doses would be too toxic to patients. Others, including oligopeptides, oligonucleotides, and various drugs cannot be given orally because of their susceptibility to digestive enzymes and the various pH conditions of the stomach and intestine. Therefore, an interest has developed in delivering control substances directly into the target site at the time of PTA. Naturally, the PTA balloon has been considered a potential delivery device for such strategies.

Hydrogel-coated angioplasty balloons with the capability of using the hydrogel as a drug delivery vehicle have been used in experiments aimed at this goal (19). Others have used microporous balloon angioplasty catheters of various types in their own experiments to deliver drugs to the vessel wall (20–22).

It is also possible that angioplasty balloons could be used to deliver energy to the vessel wall and thus prevent or inhibit restenosis. Radiofrequency energy delivery via a specially modified angioplasty balloon has been proposed as a means of sealing PTA-induced dissections and of molding the vessel wall with PTA without producing a dissection (23–25). Laser energy has also been delivered via optical fibers in attempts to reduce restenosis (26,27).

Finally, others have proposed using balloons as a delivery device for liquid polymers that would solidify upon endovascular delivery and "pave" the vessel wall injured by PTA, thereby protecting it from growth factors in the circulation and other substances that may induce restenosis (28). At the same time, the paved vessel would be protected against closure because of PTA-induced dissection. Some of the polymers proposed include polylactic acids and other substances degradable by the body. Although the mechanical properties of these substances pose problems for the concept of stenting, they offer the possibility of temporary stenting without having to remove a device.

EMERGING TECHNOLOGIES

New balloon technologies are under development to obviate some of the chronic shortcomings of endovascular therapies: dissection, thrombosis, distal embolization, and restenosis. These technologies include cryoplasty balloons and cutting angioplasty balloons.

Cryoplasty balloons, in addition to the mechanical remodeling of other angioplasty catheters, reduce the temperature of adjacent tissues to –10°C. Experimental evidence suggests that this reduction triggers apoptosis or programmed cell death in the affected tissue and thereby reduces restenosis. This technique has shown preliminary promise in the treatment of refractory recurrent stenosis in hemodialysis grafts (29).

Cutting balloon angioplasty, both in the coronary and peripheral circulation, has been proposed for patients with refractory stenosis after intravascular brachytherapy or recurrent stenoses in hemodialysis fistula (30,31).

NOMENCLATURE

All interventionalists confront the need to describe the various portions of the balloon catheter in clinical dictation, in writing a scientific report, and in verbal communication with a colleague or assistant during a procedure or in oral presentations. Inevitably, the terms *proximal* and *distal*

spring up as the interventionalist attempts to describe the balloon catheter at a critical point of the procedure. Also inevitably, the interventionalist feels uneasy as he or she realizes his or her uncertainty about which end of the balloon is which. For example, in a PTA of the cavoatrial junction for Budd-Chiari syndrome, if the balloon is placed from a transfemoral approach so that it is partially across the cavoatrial junction, partially in the right atrium, and partially in the inferior vena cava, which end of the balloon is proximal? If one said it would be the end in the inferior vena cava, one has probably been consistent with the common practice of referring to the end of the balloon closest to the operator as proximal. However, the truth is that the term *proximal* has no meaning without anatomic reference points. When anatomic references are chosen, proximal always means the central most position; therefore, the right atrial end would be the correct answer. The problem is that because the catheter itself is nonanatomic, it cannot have a proximal or distal end.

In a previous publication, the author made a plea with the interventional community to avoid this confusion by abandoning attempts to use the terms *proximal* and *distal* with respect to devices and to replace them with terms that would be understood consistently in the context of the action that is taking place (32). The terms are *leading* and *trailing*. Whenever a need arises to describe the catheter in use or a portion thereof, it is simple to refer to the leading end and the trailing end. For example, in the case just described, a rather precise description can derive from applying these terms to the radiopaque markers on the balloon catheter: "With the wire tip in the superior vena cava, the trailing marker of the balloon catheter was positioned 2 cm below the stenotic cavoatrial junction, while the leading marker was midatrial." The terminology works for guide wires and diagnostic catheters as well.

Stents and other devices for deployment are unique. The terminology works for stents, as long as they are on the catheter up to and including the time of deployment. As long as a stent is on its delivery catheter, it has a leading and trailing end, to which one can refer until it is delivered. Once deployed, it is free of the operator and of any ongoing action. It therefore assumes the anatomic reference points of the body tube or cavity it inhabits. If a stent were being deployed in the earlier example, during the deployment the end of the stent nearest the leading tip of the catheter would be the leading end of the stent and that end nearest the trailing end of the catheter would be the trailing end of the stent. Once it was deployed, leading and trailing would no longer have meaning. The atrial end of it would be proximal and the inferior vena caval end would be distal. The same principles apply to inferior vena cava filters and other devices that are deployed in the body.

Widespread adoption of these simple rules about nomenclature would improve our spoken and written communications about devices and procedures immeasurably.

SUMMARY

In less than 2 decades since the beginning of balloon angioplasty, balloon catheter and guide wire technology has advanced in response to clinical need and a competitive marketplace. High-pressure, low-compliance, controlled-compliance, low-profile, trackable, pushable, and (for some balloons) scratch-resistant are a few of the terms that can be used to accurately describe the modern peripheral PTA balloon catheters now available. Specialty guide wires that are steerable, radiopaque, stiff, floppy, and variable in stiffness are available. Commonly used wire sizes include 0.014–0.018 inch for small-vessel balloon catheters and 0.035–0.038 inch for low-profile 5 French balloon catheters. Future development should focus on kink resistance, scratch resistance, stent compatibility, and balloons for delivery of pharmacotherapeutic agents, genes, and biodegradable or bioresorbable stents. Research should also focus on miniaturization of all balloon functions for application in intracranial interventions.

Acknowledgments

I wish to thank Carol A. Mascioli and Tony Chirinos for their kind and skillful assistance with the illustrations in this chapter; and Barry Uchida for providing photographs from the Dotter Museum at the Dotter Institute.

REFERENCES

1. Dotter CT, Judkins MP. Transluminal treatment of arteriosclerotic obstructions: description of a new technic and a preliminary report of its application. Circulation 1964;30:654–670.
2. Zeitler E, Schoop W, Zahnow W. The treatment of occlusive arterial disease by transluminal catheter angioplasty. Radiology 1971;99:19.
3. Zeitler E, Schmidtke J, Schoop W. Die perkutane Behandlung von arteriellen Durchblutungsstorungen der Extremitaten mit Katheter. Vasa 1973;2:401.
4. Porstmann W. Ein neuer Korsett-Ballonkatheter zur transluminalen Rekanalisation nach Dotter unter besonderer Berucksichtigung an Obliterationen an der Beckenarterien. Radiol Diagn (Berl) 1973;14:239–244.
5. Geddes LA, Geddes LE, eds. The Catheter Introducers. Chicago: Mobium, 1993:60–61.
6. Dotter CT, Judkins MP, Frische LH, et al. The "nonsurgical" treatment of iliofemoral arteriosclerotic obstruction. Radiology 1966;86:871–875.
7. Dotter CT, Rosch J, Anderson JM, et al. Transluminal iliac artery dilation. JAMA 1974;230:117–124.
8. Geddes LA, Geddes LE, eds. The Catheter Introducers. Chicago: Mobium, 1993:71–77.
9. Gruentzig A, Hopff M. Perkutane Rekanalisation chronischer arterieller Verschlusse mit einem neuen Dilatationskatheter: Modifikation der Dotter-Technik. Dtsch Med Wochenschr 1974;99:2502–2510.
10. Gruentzig AR, Myler RK, Hanna ES, et al. Coronary transluminal angioplasty. Circulation 1977;56(Suppl III):84.
11. Gruentzig A. Transluminal dilation of coronary-artery stenosis. Lancet 1978;1(8058):263.
12. Gruentzig AR, Senning A, Siegenthaler WE. Nonoperative dilatation of coronary-artery stenosis. N Engl J Med 1979;301:61.
13. Abele JE. Balloon catheter technology. In: Castañeda WR, Tadavarthy SM, eds. Interventional Radiology. 2nd Ed. Baltimore: Williams & Wilkins, 1992:345–350.
14. Abele JE. Balloon catheters and transluminal dilatation: technical considerations. AJR Am J Roentgenol 1980;135:901–906.
15. Gerlock AJ, Regen DM, Shaff MI. An examination of the physical characteristics leading to angioplasty balloon rupture. Radiology 1982;144:421–422.
16. Simonetti G, Rossi P, Pasariello R, et al. Iliac artery rupture: a complication of transluminal angioplasty. AJR Am J Roentgenol 1983;140:989–990.
17. Zollikofer CL, Salomonowitz E, Castañeda-Zuniga WR, et al. The relation between arterial and balloon rupture in experimental angioplasty. AJR Am J Roentgenol 1985;144:777–779.
18. Zollikofer CL, Cragg AH, Hunter DW, et al. Mechanism of transluminal angioplasty. In: Castañeda-Zuniga WR, Tadavarthy SM, eds. Interventional Radiology. 2nd Ed. Baltimore: Williams & Wilkins, 1992:249–297.
19. Consigny PM, Barry JJ, Vitali NJ. Local delivery of an antiproliferative drug with use of hydrogel-coated angioplasty balloons. J Vasc Interv Radiol 1994;5(1):9–10.
20. Lambert CR, Leone J, Rowland S. The microporous balloon: a minimal-trauma local drug delivery catheter. Circulation 1992; 86(4):I-381.
21. Hong MK, Farb A, Unger EF, et al. A new PTCA balloon catheter with intramural channels for local delivery of drugs at low pressure. Circulation 1992;86(4):I-380.
22. Wolinsky H, Lin CS. Use of the perforated balloon catheter to infuse marker substances into diseased coronary artery walls after experimental postmortem angioplasty. J Am Coll Cardiol 1991;17(Suppl B):174.
23. Becker GJ, Lee BI, Waller BF, et al. Radiofrequency balloon angioplasty: rationale and proof of principle. Invest Radiol 1988;23:810–817.
24. Becker GJ, Lee BI, Waller BF, et al. Potential of radiofrequency balloon angioplasty: weld strengths, dose response relationships, and correlative histology. Radiology 1990;174: 1003–1008.
25. Lee BI, Becker GJ, Waller BJ, et al. Thermal compression and molding of atherosclerotic vascular tissue with use of radiofrequency energy: implications for radiofrequency balloon angioplasty. J Am Coll Cardiol 1989;13:1167–1175.
26. Spears JR, Reyes VP, James LM, et al. Laser balloon angioplasty: initial clinical experience. Circulation 1988;78(Suppl II):296.
27. Ferguson JJ, Dear WE, Leatherman LL, et al. A multicenter trial of laser balloon angioplasty for abrupt closure following PTCA. J Am Coll Cardiol 1990;15(Suppl A):25.
28. Slepian MJ, Schindler A. Polymeric endoluminal paving/sealing: a biodegradable alternative to intracoronary stenting. Circulation 1988;78(Suppl II):409.
29. Rifkin BS, Brewster UC, Aruny JE, et al. Percutaneous balloon cryoplasty: a new therapy for rapidly recurrent anastomotic venous stenoses of hemodialysis grafts? Am J Kidney Dis 2005; 45:e27–232.
30. Fasseas P, Orford JL, Lennon R, et al. Cutting balloon angioplasty vs. conventional balloon angioplasty in patients receiving brachytherapy for treatment of in-stent restenosis. Catheter Cardiovasc Interv 2004;63:152–157.
31. Singer-Jordon J, Papura S. Cutting balloon angioplasty for primary treatment of hemodialysis venous stenoses: preliminary results. J Vasc Interv Radiol 2005;16:25–29.
32. Becker GJ. Suggested standard terms for interventional procedures. J Vasc Interv Radiol 1993;4:616.

Vascular Stents

13

Elliot Levy

REVIEW OF GENERAL PRINCIPLES OF METALLIC STENTS

The age of metallic stent therapy for cardiovascular disease began officially in the United States with FDA approval of the Gianturco-Roubin stent in 1993 for coronary interventions. The Palmaz-Schatz stent was subsequently approved the following year for treatment of stenoses less than 15 mm in length in the native coronary circulation as defined in the Belgium Netherlands Stent I (BENESTENT I) and Stent Restenosis Study (STRESS) clinical trials. In 1997, the Multi-Link, AVE GFX, and NIR stents were subsequently approved for similar indications. More recent clinical practice has been characterized by the expansion of the variety of stents available as well as indications for stent deployment. The elucidation of the biological response to stent implantation resulting in restenosis has ushered in what many would refer to as the "new age" of stent therapy with drug-eluting and radioactive stents.

BIOLOGICAL RESPONSE TO STENT IMPLANTATION

Metallic stents have generally conformed to five different design configurations: tubular, coil, ring, complex or multicell, and mesh. Metallic stents are further differentiated by their delivery via self-expansion or by balloon-mounted delivery and expansion. Desirable characteristics for the stent delivery system include a low pre-expansion profile, a simple deployment mechanism such as unsheathing of self-expanding stents, reliability and stability of the delivery system, good trackability over guide wires, and a reliable, precise stent deployment procedure. The stent itself must necessarily be rigid enough to resist elastic recoil and provide a durable surface for endothelial growth and stability. Stents should foster blood flow patterns conducive to uniform stent endothelialization. Stent materials should be biocompatible and not provoke a confounding inflammatory reaction.

STENT FLEXIBILITY, HOOP STRENGTH, AND RELATION TO NEOINTIMAL THICKNESS AND MEDIAL ATROPHY

Several investigators have shown a relationship between changes in the vascular intima and media following intra-arterial implantation of different types of metallic stents. Barth et al. (1) observed neointimal hyperplasia occurring in descending order of extent and severity within the Strecker tantalum stent, Wallstent, and Palmaz stent following intra-arterial implantation in a canine model. Medial atrophy was more severe following Palmaz stent implantation compared with the Strecker stent or Wallstent in this study. Schurmann et al. (2) observed the greatest neointimal thickening over and between struts in Wallstents, a lesser extent in the Memotherm stent, and the least in Palmaz stents in a sheep arterial model. Statistical differences, however, were not significant among the stent types. Medial atrophy in the area under the stent struts was most extensive in the Wallstent, less extensive in the Memotherm stent, and least extensive in the Palmaz stent. Statistically significant differences were observed only between Wallstents and Palmaz stents. Schurmann et al. (2) postulated that although a significant increase in medial atrophy appeared to be associated with increased stent flexibility and reduced hoop strength, factors other than mechanical compression likely influence medial atrophy.

Carter et al. (3) compared early thrombosis rates and inflammatory response for nitinol self-expanding and balloon-expandable tubular slotted stainless steel stents in a porcine coronary artery model. Inflammatory response at the 3-day interval was 30% greater for the tubular slotted stainless steel stents than for the nitinol stents. The mean cross-sectional area of the nitinol stents increased 10% during the postimplantation interval, which sufficiently offset the neointimal thickening without inducing greater injury to the vessel than would be expected with a balloon-expandable stent. The authors' suggestion that ". . . the nitinol stent will require adjunctive balloon dilation to optimize deployment when implanted in severely diseased and calcified atherosclerotic human coronary arteries" has subsequently been confirmed in clinical practice.

STENT DESIGN AND ENDOTHELIALIZATION

In-stent restenosis typically occurs as a consequence of excessive acute thrombus deposition or late neointimal hyperplasia. Intimal thickening occurs where endothelial coverage is incomplete or has failed to occur at all. Palmaz (4) showed that endothelial cells migrate from adjacent zones untouched by procedural injury. Sprague (5) observed that stent endothelialization in vitro proceeds in the direction of flow (flow-related wall shear stress) at a rate of 10–15 micrograms per hour under no flow conditions, increasing to 25 micrograms per hour in the direction of flow at high (15 dynes per cm) wall shear stress flow.

Endothelial cells are sensitive to contact guidance by microscopic topographic features of metallic stents (6), and the edge of the implanted stent at the vascular luminal surface theoretically constitutes an important topographic feature or transition zone that would likely influence endothelial cell migration. Hamuro et al. (7) measured endothelial cell migration in vitro on cell culture plates with different edge angles under flow conditions with known shear value. They observed that migration distances on plates with edge angles of 35 degrees were greater at each time interval measured compared with edge angles of 70, 90, and 140 degrees. The rate of migration was greater for an edge angle of 35 degrees compared with all other edge angles. Migration distances were greater at all edges on 35-degree pieces compared with 90-degree pieces at upstream, downstream, right, and left edges. Migration rates differed depending upon edge position relative to flow, with migration rates measuring greater downstream relative to direction of flow.

IN-STENT RESTENOSIS AND PREVENTION STRATEGIES

The elastic recoil of the vascular wall that had previously been observed following balloon angioplasty has been reduced by the placement of metallic stents. As a result of stent deployment, restenosis in relatively large arteries has been reduced to an incidence rate of approximately 10–20%, although restenosis rates in diabetic patients are significantly higher than in normoglycemic patients (8).

The mechanism of restenosis following stent placement is characterized primarily by (a) platelet aggregation on the stent struts, (b) recruitment of inflammatory cells to platelet-rich thrombi, followed by (c) migration and proliferation of smooth muscle cells in response to cytokines, mitogens, and growth factors. The clinical outcomes associated with acute thromboses and recurrent stenoses in the peripheral and coronary circulations are clearly different, as are the reported outcome measures for angioplasty and stent placement in these circulations. One-year patency rates following transluminal angioplasty with or without stent placement range 90–95% in the carotid arteries and 80–95% in the iliac arteries to 22–65% in the superficial femoral arteries (9,10). It is not uncommon for patency rates and patient survival following angioplasty or stent placement in the peripheral circulation to be described using life table analysis. Rates for major adverse cardiac events (MACE) following coronary stent implantation, on the other hand, represent the significant clinical endpoint for coronary stent trials. MACE are most often defined as Q-wave and non–Q-wave infarctions and death. Reported coronary stent patency rates refer to binary in-stent restenosis as greater than 50% luminal reduction within the previously placed stent.

Most of the investigations and trials for treatment of in-stent restenosis have been performed either in animal coronary models or in the human coronary circulation as a consequence of the more significant impact on patient morbidity and mortality resulting from in-stent restenosis. The strategy for overcoming in-stent restenosis had focused initially on prevention of acute thrombosis using orally administered anticoagulants or antiplatelet agents and more recently on prevention of the proliferative response of smooth muscle cells to arterial injury. Initially, metallic stents underwent several modifications to improve the antithrombotic characteristics of the stents. These modifications included structural design changes and employing inorganic elements, such as gold, or coatings, such as polylactic acid or fibrin. Antithrombotic drugs such as heparin and abciximab have been applied to metallic stent struts as well. These modifications resulted in a slight decrease in the rate of acute stent thrombosis, but the incidence of in-stent restenosis was not significantly reduced (11).

Subsequent efforts to prevent in-stent restenosis share a common antiproliferative strategy toward the observed smooth muscle cell proliferation. The two most extensively investigated strategies are deployment of antiproliferative drug-eluting stents and endovascular irradiation. The pharmaceutical-based antiproliferative strategy as well as endovascular radiation are extensions of the antineoplastic cell proliferation paradigm to the problem of neointimal hyperplasia and vascular smooth muscle cell proliferation. The development of drug-eluting and radioactive stents and recent results obtained with these devices are discussed in the remainder of this chapter.

ANTIPROLIFERATIVE AGENTS AND PREVENTION OF RESTENOSIS

Table 13–1 lists the various agents that are currently being tested or are being considered for potential antiproliferative applications to prevent in-stent restenosis.

Rapamycin (Sirolimus)

Rapamycin is characterized as a macrocyclic lactone antibiotic similar in structure to the immunosuppressant

TABLE 13–1

AGENTS BEING TESTED FOR PREVENTING IN-STENT RESTENOSIS

Antineoplastic/Antiproliferative Agents

Paclitaxel
7-hexanoyltaxol
Actinomyin D
ABT 578
Vincristine
Methotrexate
Angiopeptin
Antisense c-myc

Immunosuppressants

Sirolimus
Everolimus
Tacrolimus
Dexamethasone
Mycophenolic acid

Migration Inhibitors

Batimastat
Halofuginone Probucol

Enhanced Healing Agents

17-beta-estradiol
HMG CoA reductase inhibitor
BCP 671
VGEF

tacrolimus, which is naturally produced by *Streptomyces hygroscopicus*. According to the threshold model of cell cycle regulation, progression in the cell cycle is regulated by a balance between cyclin-dependent kinase enzymes and their inhibitors (12,13). E2F is a transcription factor that regulates the expression of genes that encode proteins necessary for the G1-to-S cell cycle transition. Rapamycin specifically binds to an intracellular binding protein called FK-binding protein 12 (FKBP-12). The complex of bound rapamycin and FKBP-12 then binds to and inhibits the activation of mammalian target of rapamycin (mTOR), an important serine-threonine kinase. Inhibition of mTOR function inhibits the translation of a group of mRNAs that code for proteins essential for cell cycle progression. Inhibition of mTOR also results in accumulation of the cyclin-dependent kinase inhibitor p27^{Kip1}. Accumulation of this inhibitor prevents phosphorylation of a complex that activates the transcription factor E2F, resulting in interruption of the cell cycle. In this manner, rapamycin blocks progression of the cell cycle at the G1-to-S transition in smooth muscle cells (14,15).

Rapamycin has been demonstrated to inhibit smooth muscle cell (SMC) proliferation and migration in vitro and to reduce neointima formation in vivo (16).

Paclitaxel

Paclitaxel (Taxol) is a microtubule-stabilizing agent that interferes with cell division and other microtubule-dependent functions. Paclitaxel specifically binds to a portion of the beta-tubulin subunit in microtubules and promotes polymerization of available microtubules. The exact equilibrium between microtubule assembly and degradation is determined by the current phase of the cell cycle, and the presence of a sufficient amount of paclitaxel shifts the equilibrium in favor of microtubule assembly. As a result, cell division is interrupted, and at other phases of the cell cycle, dysfunctional bundles of microtubules are formed that specifically prevent progression through the mitotic phase (17,18).

7-hexanoyltaxol

7-hexanoyltaxol (QP2) is a taxane analog with a metabolism and toxicity similar to those of paclitaxel. This agent is highly lipophilic and insoluble in water. QP2 differs from paclitaxel as its C-7 portion is esterified with caproic acid to slow drug release from a unique polymer sleeve-coated stent delivery system without significantly altering its efficacy as a microtubule inhibitor.

Actinomycin D

Actinomycin D forms a stable complex between the tricyclic ring portion of the molecule (phenoxazone) and DNA at adjacent G-C base pairs and inhibits DNA-dependent RNA synthesis as well as causes single-strand breaks in DNA.

Dexamethasone

Dexamethasone is a synthetic glucocorticoid hormone 9-fluoro-11ß, 17, 21-trihydroxy-16 α-methylpregna-1, 4-diene-3, 20-dione that has considerable anti-inflammatory properties and is capable of inducing apoptosis in neoplastic cells.

Everolimus

Everolimus is an orally active derivative of sirolimus that has been rendered less hydrophobic than sirolimus through alkylation. It has been suggested that a less hydrophobic preparation of rapamycin might result in higher and more durable local concentrations of the antiproliferative agent in vascular endothelial cells (19).

Batimastat

Batimastat is a matrix metalloproteinase inhibitor that blocks the action of matrix metalloproteinase, which is secreted by activated smooth muscle cells to digest the extracellular matrix and facilitate SMC migration.

DRUG-ELUTING STENT DEVELOPMENT

The initial efforts to develop drug-eluting stents began with the selection of available metallic stents that were subsequently modified or treated to serve as drug delivery platforms. The U.S. Food and Drug Administration generally used the original Palmaz-Schatz coronary stent, by virtue of its earlier debut, as the gold standard against which newer coronary stents were evaluated. In the peripheral circulation, the Palmaz and, ultimately, the Wallstent received FDA approval for the treatment of atherosclerotic iliac vascular disease. In the coronary circulation, however, the rigidity of the original Palmaz-Schatz coronary stent occasionally resulted in more difficult passage through tortuous vessels. As a result, alternative stent designs and delivery systems were compared with the Palmaz-Schatz coronary stent. The Bx VELOCITY (Cordis/Johnson & Johnson) and the NIR (Boston Scientific) stents were developed to provide maximum flexibility in the coronary circulation as well as maximum scaffolding following deployment. Consequently, the BX VELOCITY and NIR stents were among the first coronary stents to be modified for endovascular drug delivery.

Selected stainless steel stents must be significantly modified to serve as drug-delivery vehicles. Drug-eluting stents must retain the structural characteristics to resist elastic recoil and remain biocompatible despite the addition of a drug-delivery substrate and an antiproliferative drug as well. Drugs must be bound to the selected stent in a manner that will permit elution of the drug in a predictable and reliable fashion. Any modification of an intra-arterial metallic stent must satisfy several additional conditions. First, if the modification is a coating that is applied to the metallic skeleton, the coating must be durable, both within the delivery system prior to implantation and following expansion of the stent at the intended delivery site. Second, the coating or treatment must be resistant to platelet and fibrin deposition in order to avoid thrombosis. Finally, all elements of the stent must be independently biocompatible.

Diffusion is the principal mechanism by which drugs are released from stents. The selected pharmaceutical is released at a rate according to Fick's law of diffusion (the rate of diffusion of a gas across a membrane is proportional to the difference in partial pressure, proportional to the area of the membrane, and inversely proportional to the thickness of the membrane) where, in this case, the rate of diffusion depends on the difference in drug concentration inside and outside the coating or polymer matrix. In two instances (the V-Flex stent [Cook with Angiotech] and the ACHIEVE system [Cook with Guidant]), proprietary polymer-free methodology is employed to deliver cGMP paclitaxel by local diffusion. Alternatively, drugs can be released by dissolution or diffusion when absorbed into nonbioerodible polymers. A nonerodible polymer is generally preferable for applications such as stents because the polymer coating may fragment and cause embolic occlusions and macrophage-mediated inflammatory reactions. Nonbioerodible (biostable) polymers may also offer a more gradual release of drugs (20).

Stent coatings can be further classified as inorganic agents, biological materials, and synthetic polymers. Inorganic coatings have been recently evaluated as a drug-eluting stent coating. The JoMed Flexmaster stent tested in the Preliminary Safety Evaluation of Nanoporous Tacrolimus-eluting (PRESENT) stents clinical trials consisted of a nanoporous 300-μm ceramic layer (aluminum oxide matrix) containing tacrolimus-loaded nanocavities (21).

Phosphorylcholine, a naturally occurring phospholipid, is an example of a biological polymer stent coating that has been shown not to interfere with stent endothelialization and that does not cause increased neointimal proliferation compared with uncoated metallic stents (22). The BiodivYsio stent (Abbott Vascular) consists of a metallic stent with phosphorylcholine bound to methacrylate. Other biological polymers composed of proteins, carbohydrates, or lipids may be compromised by a relatively low mechanical resistance and more irregular controlled-release parameters.

Synthetic polymers can be either bioerodible or nonbioerodible. In the case of the sirolimus-eluting Cypher stent, two nonerodible polymers, poly n-butyl methacrylate and polytheylene vinyl acetate, are combined as the drug-eluting substrate. Paclitaxel-eluting stents, on the other hand, use poly(lactide-co-caprolactone) polymer.

Stents with Polymer Carriers

QuaDS (Quanam Medical Corp)

The QuaDS drug-eluting stent (Quanam Medical Corp) was the first drug-eluting stent implanted in human coronary arteries. This slotted tube stent has 50% of its surface area covered by multiple nonbiodegradable polyacrylate sleeves that release 7-hexanoyltaxol (called QP2 or taxane). Approximately 800 μg of the drug was loaded per 2.4 mm of sleeve length, such that 13-mm-long stents have a total drug dose of 2,400 μg and 17-mm-long stents contain 3,200 μg of taxane (23). The SCORE trial with the QuaDS-QP2 stent was interrupted after enrolling 266 patients because of a 9.4% incidence of stent thrombosis and a 14.5% incidence of myocardial infarction in the drug-eluting stent group. These unfavorable results were attributed at least partially to very high tissue concentrations of taxane.

NIR Conformer (Medinol and Scimed, Angiotech, Boston Scientific)

The NIR stent has a stainless steel multicell design with strut thickness of 100 micrometers. NIR stents coated with poly(lactide-co-Σ-caprolactone) copolymer containing paclitaxel (200 μg per stent) were initially tested in porcine coronary arteries. Paclitaxel-eluting stents showed a marked reduction in neointimal and medial cell proliferation at all time points (7, 28, 56, and 180 days) (24). However, arteries treated with paclitaxel showed incomplete healing, late persistence of a large number of macrophages, and fibrin deposition. Similar findings were observed with a stent platform coated with cross-linked biodegradable polymer (chondroitin sulfate and gelatin), and 42.0, 20.2, 8.6, or 1.5 μg of paclitaxel in rabbit iliac arteries (25). These studies indicated the need for a more controlled drug release of paclitaxel because of the narrow toxic-therapeutic window and the highly hydrophobic character of this compound (23). This stent design was subsequently specifically tested in the TAXUS I and II trials in humans using reduced total concentrations of paclitaxel as well as slow- and moderate-release formulations.

TAXUS Express (Boston Scientific)

The TAXUS Express stent evaluated in the TAXUS III and IV trials consists of a 316L stainless steel NIR slotted tube stent design, which is coated with the Translute polymer (poly[styrene-b-isobutylene-b-styrene]). This polymer functions similarly to the PEVA/PBMA copolymer used in the CYPHER stent. The pharmacokinetics of the paclitaxel release are slightly different from those of the CYPHER stent; burst release occurs within the first 48 hours, followed by slower release over the next 10 days, and no further drug elution after 30 days.

Cypher (Johnson & Johnson)

The Bx VELOCITY stent (Cordis/Johnson & Johnson) consists of a stainless steel slotted tube design with a strut thickness of 140 μ which features a six-closed ring design and two layers of synthetic nonerodible polymers 51 μm thick. The Cypher drug-eluting stent consists of a 316L

stainless steel Bx VELOCITY framework that is coated with a primer layer of parylene C to which a mixture of two polymers and sirolimus is applied. The two nonerodible polymers (polyethylene-co-vinyl acetate [PEVA] and poly n-butyl methacrylate [PBMA]) are combined in a 67% to 33% ratio, respectively, and then dissolved in tetrahydrofuran (THF—a solvent suitable for dissolving organic molecules). A final drug-free coat of PBMA is dissolved in THF and then applied to the stent to control drug release (26). This outer coating of drug-free PBMA prevents the so-called burst effect that results when the drug on the surface of the polymer is rapidly released following immersion into water or solvent.

The outer layer of PEVA/PBMA slows the rate of sirolimus diffusion, allowing delivery of the drug over a longer period of time. The concentration of the drug subsequently decreases according to first-order elimination kinetics. Approximately 50% of the total drug is eliminated within the first 10 days of implantation. The drug is 90% removed from the stent by approximately 60 days and is completely removed by about 90 days. The peak drug concentration occurs about 4 hours after implantation. Blood levels of sirolimus are 10- to 20-fold lower than those observed after administration of sirolimus by oral solution in healthy volunteers or transplant patients. The terminal half-life of the drug in stent recipients was 213 ± 97 hours, compared with 72.9 ± 19.3 hours in healthy volunteers who received oral solution administration and 58.2 ± 19.2 hours in transplant recipients. The Cypher stent has been evaluated in the RAVEL and SIRIUS stent trials.

Endeavor (Medtronic)

The Endeavor drug-eluting stent system features Medtronic's Driver cobalt chromium alloy coronary stent system with a phosphorylcholine polymer coating containing the drug ABT-578 (10 μg per mm), a rapamycin analog (Abbott Laboratories). The Driver stent features thin struts (0.0036 in, or 0.91mm) that, together with higher strength than stainless steel, maintain good radial strength. The cobalt chromium alloy is more dense than steel and may enjoy better radiopacity than stainless steel.

Multi-Link Tetra (Guidant)

The Multi-Link Tetra stent has functional characteristics that are similar to the Bx Velocity stent and also consists of a stainless steel slotted tube design with a strut thickness of 90–124 micrometers. Compared with the Multi-Link Tetra stent, the Multi-Link Penta stent (Guidant) has a modified link pattern, which improves flexibility and scaffolding and maintains side-branch access with the possibility to expand the stent cell toward the side branch up to 4 mm in diameter. The Tetra stent, modified to elute actinomycin-D, was evaluated in the ACTION study, which was terminated at the 9-month follow-up interval as a result of a higher restenosis rate.

BiodivYsio (Biocompatibles)

The BiodivYsio stent has a stainless steel slotted tube design with strut thickness of 50–90 micrometers, which results in a particularly low metal-to-artery ratio of 9%. This stent was subsequently modified with a phosphorylcholine coating to elute batimastat, a matrix metalloproteinase inhibitor that functions as an antimigration and angiogenesis inhibitor. This drug-eluting stent was subsequently evaluated in the BRILLIANT-EU trial as well as the DISTINCT trial.

Stents Without Polymer Carriers

Supra G and V-Flex Plus (Cook, Inc.)

The Supra G stent has a stainless steel slotted tube design with paclitaxel adhered to the surface of the stent without a polymer that was evaluated in the ASPECTS trial, while the V-Flex Plus stent was specifically tested in the ELUTES trial.

Drug-Eluting Stents: Clinical Trials

Rapamycin

In 2001, Sousa et al. (27) reported the first experience with implantation of the rapamycin-coated Bx Velocity stent in humans. The study group consisted of 30 consecutive patients who received a single 18-mm-long stent between December 1999 and February 2000. Half the patients received a slow-release formulation (SR; $\geq$28-day drug release), and the other half received a fast-release version of the stent (FR; <15-day drug release). Quantitative coronary angiography and intravascular ultrasound (IVUS) imaging were performed at implantation and at 4-month follow-up. No patients were observed to develop $\geq$50% vessel narrowing, and only three patients had >15% intimal hyperplasia by IVUS. No MACE occurred up to the 8-month follow-up interval. In comparing lumen, stent, and neointimal hyperplasia volumes between the two versions of the stent, a slight difference in neointimal hyperplasia volume was noted between the SR and FR groups (p = 0.07), revealing a slightly larger neointimal hyperplasia volume in the SR group. The small number of enrolled patients in each arm of this safety and feasibility study did not provide adequate power to detect significant differences in these outcomes. The authors compared their results with the lower range of intimal hyperplasia observed after implantation of noncoated stents 15 mm or shorter in length of 19.7% (28). At 1 year, in-stent minimal lumen diameter and percent diameter stenosis remained essentially unchanged in the original 30 patients, while neointimal hyperplasia (obstruction volume) was "virtually absent" at 1 year (29). Two-year follow-up data on 15 patients who had received a single, slow-drug-release format sirolimus-eluting Bx Velocity stent (140 μg sirolimus per cm^2 stent surface area) as well as an 8-week course of

antiplatelet therapy revealed a single 60% diameter stenosis in a patient at the 18-month interval. A second patient presented with angina 22 months after the index drug-eluting stent placement and underwent additional stent placement for progression of a preexisting atherosclerotic lesion 12 mm from the distal stent edge. In the remainder of the patients, quantitative coronary angiography revealed that the in-stent luminal diameter and percent diameter stenosis remained unchanged compared with the 6-month follow-up. One patient developed neointimal hyperplasia reaching 10% stent volume (IVUS) that corresponded to an actual lumen loss of 0.29 mm at the 18-month follow-up interval (30). These early trials, while limited by the small number of enrolled patients, did suggest that placement of sirolimus-eluting stents resulted in the remarkable persistent inhibition of restenosis and absence of serious adverse events.

Duda et al. (31) subsequently reported in the same year their early experience with sirolimus-eluting stents for the treatment of long femoral artery stenoses or occlusions. Eighteen patients each received either uncoated Smart stents or Smart stents coated with an elastic copolymer combined with sirolimus in a 30:70 drug:copolymer weight ratio (90 μg sirolimus per cm^2 stent surface area). The patient cohorts differed only in the percentage with Rutherford-Becker classifications of 3 or 4 and the presence of Diabetes Mellitus (both greater for the drug-eluting stent group). This report featured the first deployment of a drug-eluting, *self*-expanding nitinol stent. The stented vessels were studied with quantitative angiography at the 6-month interval. In-stent mean percent diameter stenosis was 22.6% in the sirolimus-eluting stent group and 30.9% in the uncoated stent group (p = 0.294), and the in-stent mean lumen diameter was significantly larger in the drug-eluting stent group (4.95 mm versus 4.31 mm, p = 0.047). The binary in-stent restenosis rate was 0% for the drug-eluting stent population and 23.5% in the bare stent group, and no revascularization procedures were required in either group. Unlike the coronary studies, the long length of the femoral lesions (mean 85 mm in both groups) required deployment of an average of 2.2 stents per lesion in both groups.

The first multicenter trial with stents coated with sirolimus was by Marie-Claude Morice and colleagues (32). In the RAVEL trial of 238 patients at 19 medical centers, revascularization of single, primary lesions in native coronary arteries with sirolimus-coated and bare metal stents were compared. Between August 2000 and January 2001, random assignment yielded a control group of 118 patients and a group of 120 patients to receive the drug-eluting stent. The study was designed to have 90% power to detect a 0.25 mm difference in the mean late luminal loss between the two groups using a two-group t-test and a two-sided significance level of 0.05. The primary study endpoint was in-stent late lumen loss at 6 months, and the secondary endpoints included the rate and percent in-stent restenosis. Restenosis was defined as luminal narrowing of 50% or more. All subjects were treated with antiplatelet agents for 8 weeks. At the 6-month poststent implantation interval, the mean late luminal loss was significantly lower in the sirolimus stent group (-0.01 ± 0.33 mm) than in the bare metal stent group (0.80 ± 0.53 mm)($p <0.001$). Observed restenosis of 50% or more at 6 months was 0% and 27% with sirolimus-coated versus standard stents ($p <0.001$). Neointimal hyperplasia within the stents measured 2 ± 5 mm^3 versus 37 ± 28 mm^3 (control) ($p <0.001$). No aneurysm formation, in-stent thrombosis, persistent dissection, or edge effect was observed. During a follow-up period exceeding 1 year, the overall MACE rate was 5.8% in the sirolimus-coated stent group and 28.8% in the control group ($p <0.001$). The higher MACE rate in the control group was attributed to a higher rate of required revascularization of the target vessels in the bare metal stent group (27 stents). These findings were subsequently corroborated by the data from the "SIRolImUS-coated VELOCITY Stent in treatment of patients with de novo coronary artery lesions (SIRIUS)" trial in the United States in 2003. This randomized, double-blind study compared the outcomes following placement of a sirolimus-coated Bx Velocity stent with a standard Bx Velocity stent to treat a newly diagnosed stenotic lesion in native coronary arteries in 1,058 patients treated at 53 centers (33). The patient population in this trial featured more "complex" lesions resulting from the frequent presence of diabetes (26%) as well as longer lesions (14.4 mm) and small vessels (2.8 mm). The primary endpoint of the study was treatment vessel failure as defined by death from cardiac causes, myocardial infarction, or repeated revascularization of the target vessel within 270 days.

The rate of target vessel failure was reduced to 8.6% in the sirolimus-eluting stent group compared with 21% in the standard stent group ($p <0.001$). Drug-eluting stent (DES) efficacy was further supported by the observed 85% reduction in the rate of "out-of-hospital non-Q-wave myocardial infarction." Revascularization frequency was similarly reduced from 16.6% in the standard stent group to 4.1% in the DES group ($p <0.001$). Binary in-stent restenosis was observed in 3.2% of the DES and 35.4% of the standard stent group ($p <0.001$), but in-segment restenosis was observed in 8.9% of the DES group and in 36.3% of the standard stent group. The higher rate of in-segment restenosis in the DES group compared with the group's observed in-stent restenosis rate was attributed to a smaller reduction in late luminal loss and a higher rate of restenosis at the proximal versus distal margin or in the body of the stent (33). A significant difference ($p <0.001$) was observed in the length of the restenosis occurring after stent placement. Restenotic lesion length averaged 9.1 ± 5.8 mm after placement of a DES, while lesion length measured 14.8 ± 7.4 mm after standard stent placement ($p <0.001$). One subacute stent thrombosis occurred during the 1–30 day postimplantation interval in each group. One

of the four total late stent thromboses (between 31 and 270 days after implantation) occurred in the DES group.

One-year follow-up from the SIRIUS trial has recently been published, although the results focus on clinical restenosis or target lesion revascularization. The absolute difference in rates for target vessel revascularization increased from the 9-month interval, reaching 4.9% for DES and 20% for uncoated stents (34). The MACE rate at 1 year equaled 8.3% in the DES group and 24.8% in the control group.

Paclitaxel

Investigations with paclitaxel-eluting stents consist of comparisons of two forms of drug-eluting stents and bare metal stent controls. The QuaDS-2 taxol-derivative QP2 coronary stent and Quanam stents featured a paclitaxel-eluting nonbiodegradable polymer sleeve, and the TAXUS polymer-coated stents with slow- or moderate-drug-release profiles were assessed in the later TAXUS trials.

Early experience with paclitaxel-eluting stents came in the form of a report in 2001 describing follow-up on a cohort of 13 patients who had received the QuaDS-2 taxol-derivative QP2-eluting coronary stent (35). At a mean follow-up interval of 11.2 months, all 13 QuaDS-QP2 stents were patent by angiography and IVUS.

The QuaDS-QP2 stent was evaluated in 15 consecutive patients with in-stent restenosis. Restenosis occurred in two lesions at the 6-month interval, including one between two drug-eluting stents, and eight lesions (61.5%) at 12 months, suggesting a "late catch-up of restenosis" (36). Five patients who received QuaDS-QP2 stents underwent directional atherectomy for recurrence of in-stent stenosis. The findings of persistent fibrin deposition with varying degrees of inflammation were interpreted by the authors in a subsequent report to represent a delay in healing a neointimal growth associated with the QuaDS-QP2 stent rather than prevention of the neointimal response (37). The larger multicenter randomized SCORE trial initiated in 2000 by the Quanam Medical Corporation enrolled 266 patients at 17 sites in Europe. Patients were randomized to receive a paclitaxel-coated Quanam stent. However, the 30-day MACE rate was reported as 10.2% and attributed to acute stent thrombosis or side branch occlusion. This trial was subsequently terminated after enrollment of 266 patients because of a high incidence of stent thrombosis (9.4%) and MI (14.5%) in the DES group (23). These experiences with the QuaDS-QP2 stent may have been related to the polymer sleeves of the stent combined with extremely high concentrations of taxane (36).

Paclitaxel-eluting stent safety and efficacy was also assessed in the TAXUS I trial using the NIRx stent (85 µg paclitaxel per stent, 1.0 µg per mm^2) and the bare metal NIR stent as a control. Sixty-one patients with single coronary lesions of less than 15 mm were randomized between the two study groups. The primary endpoint of the study,

30-day MACE, ultimately proved to be 0%. The 6-month binary in-stent restenosis rate was 0% for the NIRx stent and 11% for the NIR stent. No instances of stent thrombosis were observed (38). Eighteen-month follow-up data subsequently reported for a subset of the TAXUS I study population revealed that the MACE rate as well as the restenosis rate at 18 months in these 20 patients continued to be 0% (39). At the 2-year follow-up interval, the MACE rate was 3.3% (remote target vessel revascularization), and the stent thrombosis rate remained 0% (40).

The TAXUS II study, a triple-blinded, randomized multicenter study, consisted of two cohorts that compared the efficacy of a slow-release paclitaxel stent preparation and a moderate-release preparation against bare metal control stents in single de novo lesions less than or equal to 12 mm in length (41). The moderate release version of the stent delivered an eightfold greater amount of paclitaxel in the first 10 days. Each cohort consisted of nearly 270 total patients divided nearly equally into DES (slow-release or moderate-release 15-mm NIRx stents) and control groups. Follow-up intervals were 30 and 180 days as well as annually. The primary endpoint of in-stent net volume obstruction (neointimal hyperplasia) at 6 months by IVUS was 7.8% in both the moderate- and the slow-release DES group and 20.5% and 23.2%, respectively, in the associated control groups. At 6 months, the target lesion revascularization rate ($p = 0.002$) and MACE rate ($p = 0.006$) were both significantly reduced in the TAXUS MR group compared with controls. Apparently, both drug elution profiles appeared to effectively reduce in-stent restenosis rates in the study interval. The authors acknowledged, however, that the study was not specifically designed to detect differences in IVUS, angiographic, or clinical outcomes between the two DES formulations. Restenosis at 6 months was observed in the stented segment at a rate of 2.3% for the slow-release formulation and 4.7% for the moderate-release stent (41).

The TAXUS III trial consisted of a single-arm two-center study including 28 patients who were evaluated for treatment of in-stent restenosis with one or more TAXUS NIRx paclitaxel-eluting stents with a total load of 1.0 μg per mm^2 (42). Inclusion criteria included lesion length less than or equal to 30 mm, 50–90% diameter stenosis, and vessel diameter between 3.0 and 3.5 mm. The overall restenosis rate was 16% (4 of 25) (23), but two restenoses occurred at the gap between eluting stents and another within a bare metal stent adjacent to the DES. During the 6-month follow-up period, a total of eight adverse events were noted, for a 6-month MACE rate of 29%.

The TAXUS IV trial studied placement of a slow-release formulation polymer-based paclitaxel-eluting TAXUS stent versus bare metal Express stent placement in a larger study population with single de novo coronary artery lesions measuring 10–28 mm in length, with up to 12-month follow-up (43). One-year follow-up data was available on 639 TAXUS stents and 633 controls. Findings included

significant reductions in target lesion revascularization (15.1% controls to 4.4% TAXUS, p <0.001) and target vessel revascularization (17.1% controls to 7.1% TAXUS, p <0.001). The most significant predictors of target lesion revascularization in both TAXUS and control groups included the total stent length and vessel diameter ($p \leq 0.007$ in both instances). Although a reduction in the rate of repeat revascularization procedures is apparent between 9- and 12-month follow-up intervals in the TAXUS group compared with controls, the *cumulative* rates over 12 months of observation of cardiac death (1.4% versus 1.3%), myocardial infarction (3.5% versus 4.7%), and stent thrombosis (0.6% versus 0.8%) were similar between the two groups (43).

The ELUTES and ASPECT trials evaluated the paclitaxel-eluting version of the V-Flex stent. The ELUTES (European Evaluation of Paclitaxel-Eluting Stent) trial featured a comparison of the V-Flex stent (Cook, Inc.) loaded with four different doses of paclitaxel (0.2, 0.7, 1.4, and 2.7 μg per mm^2) versus bare metal stents for the treatment of de novo coronary lesions. One hundred eighty patients were randomized among the five study groups. Observed late lumen loss varied inversely with the loaded paclitaxel dose, ranging from 0.1 mm (highest dose) to 0.7 mm (in the lowest paclitaxel dose and control groups) (44). Observed binary restenosis decreased from 20.6% to 3.2%. The cumulative MACE rate at 12 months varied directly with the concentration of paclitaxel on the stent, ranging from 5% at 0.2 μg per mm to 14% at 2.7 μg per mm. The ASPECT (Asian Paclitaxel-Eluting Clinical Trial) compared Supra G stents (Cook, Inc.) directly impregnated with two different doses of paclitaxel (1.3 and 3.1 μg per mm^2) and bare metal stents in de novo coronary lesions treated with single stents. The randomized, controlled, triple-blind study was conducted at three centers with a total of 177 patients with coronary lesions less than 15 mm long between January 2000 and March 2001. In-stent late lumen loss, neointimal hyperplasia volume, and restenosis rates varied inversely to the dose of paclitaxel and were maximal in the control group (45).

In contrast to the rapamycin-eluting trials, studies evaluating paclitaxel-eluting stents have used different drug-elution designs as well as doses. Silber (46) analyzed the results of six randomized controlled trials (TAXUS I, II, and IV; ASPECT; ELUTES; DELIVER-I) using paclitaxel-eluting stents to distinguish differences in angiographic and clinical outcomes that could be attributed to paclitaxel dose differences or drug-elution methodology. Silber concluded that stent safety was independent of stent design, including the presence or absence of a polymer drug carrier. Stents using a polymer carrier were highly effective at a paclitaxel dose of 1 μg per mm^2 in terms of binary restenosis rates, whereas stents lacking a polymer coating had a higher minimally effective paclitaxel dose of 3 μg per mm^2. Implantation of non–polymer-based paclitaxel eluting stents in the ASPECT and DELIVER trials apparently was not associated with improved clinical outcomes compared with bare metal stents. In the ASPECT study (Cook Supra G stent), despite the reduction in binary restenosis rates, the clinical outcome (MACE rate) or revascularization rates at 6 months (47) were not improved (using both paclitaxel doses of 1 µg per mm^2 and 3.1 µg per mm^2) compared with a control group that received bare metal stents, although the sample sizes were relatively small. In the Guidant study DELIVER-1 (RX Achieve system; Guidant Multi-Link Penta stent with Cook's paclitaxel coating), although a reduction in the binary restenosis rate from 22% in the controls to 14% in the Achieve group was observed, the reduction in MACE incidence at 9 months was not statistically significantly different (48).

Stent Brachytherapy

Radiation therapy represents another approach to suppress the proliferation of smooth muscle cells and neointimal hyperplasia associated with restenosis. The goal of this intervention is to deliver an antiproliferative radiation dose without exceeding local tissue tolerance. The concept of intravascular brachytherapy to suppress in-stent restenosis was initially evaluated using catheter-based radioactive sources and delivery systems. Catheter-based brachytherapy was initially shown to prevent vascular wall remodeling and neointimal proliferation and inhibit angioplasty-related neointimal hyperplasia in animal studies (49–54). Catheter-based endovascular radiation has been demonstrated to inhibit restenosis in human trials using gamma and β emission sources (55–58).

The results of other studies, however, suggest that tissue tolerance remains somewhat imprecisely defined. Vascular radiation therapy from both high-dose-rate catheter systems (59,60) and low-dose radioactive stents (61,62) inhibits neointima formation but also delays arterial luminal surface re-endothelialization in animal models. Radiation dose-dependency of the delayed re-endothelialization process was also observed in the canine coronary artery studies of Taylor (63), where delayed healing within canine coronary arteries 15 weeks following implantation of 32P stents was observed. Incomplete re-endothelialization in vessels was observed with all 32P stents (3.5–14.4 µCi), manifested as a dose-dependent increase in fibrin area. Delayed endothelialization, fibrin deposition, and platelet recruitment (64) have been implicated as significant contributing factors of late thrombosis. Vodovotz et al. (65) suggest that intra-arterial radiation may affect mural thrombus formation and morphology These authors argue that increased thrombus may adversely affect vessel healing and that postirradiation mural thrombus may lack a cellular component that plays a significant role in the healing process (66–68).

The use of endovascular radiation therapy to prevent restenosis has been associated with several technical limitations, including late occlusion, edge effect, and geographic miss. Late occlusion is represented by thrombosis of the treated vessel more than 1 month after therapy. In Waksman's retrospective review of 473 patients enrolled in brachytherapy protocols, late occlusion occurred in 28 patients compared with two patients in the placebo group (69). In a separate study (70), treatment with the antiplatelet agent clopidogrel for 6 months resulted in a late thrombosis rate of 4.2%, and treatment for 12 months yielded a late thrombosis rate of 3.3%. MACE incidence rate was 21% in the 12-month antiplatelet treatment group and 36% in the 6-month treatment group.

Geographic miss occurs when segments of the coronary artery are injured as a consequence of balloon dilatation and stent placement outside the direct brachytherapy treatment zone, therefore receiving a smaller β radiation dose (71). While the exact clinical consequence of geographic miss cannot be determined, Bonan (72) hypothesizes that if geographic miss occurs in 30% of vascular brachytherapy procedures, geographic miss may contribute up to 10 percentage points to the observed postbrachytherapy restenosis rate.

Multiple authors (73–75) have summarized optimal design requirements for radioactive stents. Tissue exposure and dosimetry provided by radioactive stents should temporally match the pathophysiologic sequence leading to neointimal hyperplasia. As neointimal hyperplasia is known to develop only in the first few weeks after angioplasty (76–78), the ideal isotope half-life should be no more than a few weeks. Stent radioactivity must be high enough everywhere on the stent to achieve the threshold dose rate necessary to prevent restenosis (74,79,80), even at stent margins (81). At the same time, the total dose to the layers of the vessel wall should not exceed doses known to result in late injury to the arterial wall (82). The energy of the emitted particles must be sufficient to penetrate even calcified plaque (83) in order to reach target cells (84).

Stents as Radioactive Sources

The use of an implanted stent as the source for the radiation offers several advantages: stent implantation techniques are relatively simple and standardized, the stent activity and penetrating power of the radioactivity can be low, obviating the need for the presence of a radiation safety officer and/or radiation oncologist as well as reducing the exposure of associated personnel, and the stents provide direct contact between the radiation source and the vessel wall target for a relatively extended period of time (weeks) compared with catheter-based radiation delivery systems. Implantation of radioactive stents may be associated with two significant disadvantages. The delivery of an *inadequate* dose of radiation following angioplasty or stent-related vessel wall injury may result in edge restenosis 2–3 mm proximal and distal to the leading and trailing stent edges (the "candy wrapper" effect) (74,85). The second potential problem is delayed healing and thrombosis at the surface of the stent, which may be caused by *excessive* radiation dose (74,86–89).

Metallic stents can be rendered radioactive by several techniques. First, stents can be placed in a cyclotron and bombarded with charged particles such as deuterons or protons. Second, radioisotopes can be directly implanted on metallic stents or bound to metallic stents as a consequence of electrochemical reactions with or without polymer coatings.

The most widely studied radioisotope for stent applications, Phosphorus-32, which is a pure β particle emitter, is ideally suited for intravascular implantation because of the short penetration distance of the β particles; 95% of the absorbed dose occurs within 4 mm of the stent edge (90). A rapid decline in activity to 1/1,000 of the original level occurs up to 5 months postimplantation. In relative terms, a "low-activity" 32P stent (0.75 μCi) delivers 8 Gy, and a "high-activity" 32P stent (12 μCi) delivers 140 Gy at a distance of up to 5 mm from the stent edge over the initial 28-day exposure period (90). By comparison, the total dose delivered by catheter-based systems ranges 8–50 Gy up to a depth of 1 mm into the vessel wall.

Alternative β-emitting sources include 48V, 198Au, and 90Y, although 48V and 198Au are not pure β emitters. Higher-energy β emissions identified with 90Y result in increased particle range compared with those of 32P. Dose distribution calculations for 90Y suggest a 5–10% increase in radiation dose at distances of 1–2.5 mm from the stent surface. This possible advantage of 90Y over 32P is overshadowed by the findings at 90-day follow-up after 90Y stent implantation, with activities of 16–32 μCi reported by Taylor et al. (88). Alternatively, some have advocated using low-energy photon-emitting species to overcome edge restenosis, including 103Pd and 131Cs (74,91–93). Monte Carlo modeling of tissue dose with 103Pd or 131Cs around the proximal and distal ends of the radioactive stent is enhanced compared with 32P (94). Unfortunately, edge restenosis at lower activities and incomplete vascular healing at higher activities were observed in a rabbit iliac artery model using 103Pd stents (95).

Radioactive Stent Experience

Multiple studies in porcine (96,97) and rabbit models (98) have established the effectiveness of radioactive stents in reducing mean neointimal thickness following stent placement as well as medial smooth muscle proliferation and density.

The Palmaz-Schatz PS 153 stent (Cordis/Johnson & Johnson) was the first stent modified to deliver intracoronary brachytherapy in clinical trials in the United States. The stent contained 32P embedded beneath the surface of the stent (ion implantation) and was subsequently mounted on a delivery balloon and covered with a sheath for protection prior to deployment. The Isostent for Restenosis Intervention Study (IRIS), a nonrandomized

multicenter trial, evaluated the safety and feasibility of 32P radioactive Palmaz-Schatz stent placement in patients with symptomatic de novo coronary stenosis or restenotic lesions. Patients who had single coronary lesions with a maximum length of 28 mm and objective evidence of ischemia were considered eligible. The study was organized as a two-arm dose escalation safety trial featuring low-activity (IRIS IA; 0.5–1.0 μCi, mean 0.7 μCi) and intermediate-activity (IRIS IB; 0.75–1.5 μCi, mean 1.14 μCi) stents. Thirty-two patients were enrolled to receive the low-activity stent, and 25 patients received the intermediate-activity stent. For the IRIS IA arm, the MACE rate at the 30-day postimplantation interval was 0%, and at the 6-month interval, the clinically driven target vessel revascularization rate was 21%. Between 6 and 12 months, no further target vessel revascularization events occurred (99).

The Phase I IRIS IB trial arm was designed to test the effect of higher stent activity, and 30-day follow-up revealed no incidence of MACE in this subgroup (100). Although the initial technical success rate was high, angiographic follow-up in 52 of the original 57 patients revealed binary intralesion and stent edge restenosis in 21 patients (40.4%), approximating the reported results for nonradioactive metallic stents (101). Similar findings were observed in a smaller safety study (102) conducted in Heidelberg with the 15-mm 32P radioactive Palmaz-Schatz stent (1.5–3 μCi) in 11 patients who had restenosis after coronary angioplasty. This study concluded with a 36% "clinically driven" target vessel revascularization rate. At the 6-month follow-up, restenosis was observed in 6 of 11 patients (54%), occurring mainly at the articulation of the stents and, at a lower rate, at the proximal and distal edges.

In their review of the IRIS trial, Fischell et al. suggest several factors that may have influenced the observed restenosis rates (99). First, in 32% (7 of 22) of the patients with de novo coronary stenoses receiving the β-emitting stent, the reference vessel diameter was less than 2.5 mm. Second, optimal stent placement using IVUS was achieved in only 56% of the cases, "due mainly to high plaque burden preventing an optimal ratio of stent to reference vessel cross-sectional area." Third, the design of the Bx stent (Isostent, Inc.) (honeycomb-shaped cells linked by alternating articulation geometries) may favor more uniform distribution of dose compared with the Palmaz-Schatz stent (two 7-mm hemistents connected by a single 1-mm articulating metal filament). Janicki et al. studied dosimetry of the 1.0 μCi Palmaz-Schatz stent and found dose nonuniformity in areas adjacent to stent strut wires and between the wires (103). Their models showed that for a 32P stent of 1.0 μCi that was 15 mm in length, at a distance of 0.1 mm, dose values of 2,500 cGy were delivered at the strut wires (peaks) and 800 cGy between the wires (valleys) over one half-life (14.3 days).

Wardeh et al. (104) subsequently published data from their IRIS trial patient subgroup from Rotterdam, the Netherlands. Twenty-six patients with de novo or restenotic coronary lesions underwent successful implantation of a total of four 32P radioactive Palmaz-Schatz stents and 26 Bx stents with activity ranging from 0.75 to 1.5 μCi. Six-month postimplantation angiographic follow-up was available in 23 patients. Seventeen percent of patients had in-stent restenosis, and 13% required repeat revascularization. No restenosis was observed at the stent edges in this study. Quantitative coronary arteriography, however, revealed no difference in the patterns of cellular proliferation between the Palmaz-Schatz and Bx stents.

Albiero et al. at the EMO Centro Cuore Columbus in Milan performed a single-center nonrandomized dose response study with 32P stents using three categories of activity: 0.75–3.0 μCi, 3.0–6.0 μCi, and 6.0–12.0 μCi. Twenty-seven lesions (93% de novo) in 23 patients were treated by implantation of thirty-one 32P PS 153 stents with initial activity of 0.75–3.0 μCi (Group 1, low activity; mean activity 1.5 μCi) (85). Stent thrombosis and MACE rates were both 0% in this group at the 6-month interval. After 6 months, intralesion binary restenosis (defined as ≥50% luminal reduction) occurred in 10 of 19 lesions (52%) in patients who underwent angiographic follow-up (reported to be 70 of 82 total patients in the three groups). These observations were similar to the group of 11 patients in Heidelberg, with 54% (6 of 11) restenosis that occurred primarily at the articulation of the stents and at a lower rate at the proximal and distal edges (102)

Albiero et al. compared two higher-activity 32P stents by implanting 39 32P Bx stents with initial activity of 3–6 μCi to treat 32 lesions (91% de novo lesions) in 29 patients (Group 2). A second group of 32 lesions (100% de novo lesions) in 30 patients (Group 3) received 31 Bx stents with an initial activity of 6–12 μCi (mean 9.3 μCi) (85). With 80% of patients having angiographic follow-up at up to 6 months, the intralesion restenosis rate was 41% in the lower-stent-activity Group 2 and 50% in the highest-activity Group 3. However pure intrastent stenosis occurred in only one patient in Group 2 and in none in Group 3, even though three patients sustained stent occlusion in the highest-activity Group 3. Restensosis appears to have occurred primarily at stent edges. These authors first suggested the term *candy wrapper* effect to describe a relatively good intrastent patency result combined with stent edge restenosis. In an effort to clarify the mechanism of edge restenosis and to evaluate the relative contributions of decreased radiation dose at the stent margin and balloon injury without subsequent stent coverage, the lesions with and without edge restenosis were compared by univariate analysis. The ratio of the maximum diameter of the longest balloon used to predilate the vessel, deploy, or postdilate the stent to the reference vessel diameter was significantly higher in the lesions with edge restensosis. Additionally, the lesions with edge restenosis had a significantly smaller reference lumen diameter and a smaller final minimum lumen diameter as shown by angiography than the group without edge restenosis. IVUS analysis of the 13 lesions treated with a single stent further confirmed that the late lumen loss in the first 1–3 mm outside the stent was mainly a result of neointimal hyperplasia.

The final arm of the radiation dose escalation was conducted with stents ranging in activity from 12 to 21 μCi. The technique used to deploy radioactive stents in this patient group featured a nonaggressive stent deployment strategy designed to overcome the candy wrapper effect by reducing local balloon-related vessel trauma. Lesion predilitation, stent deployment, and stent dilatation were performed with an undersized, shorter balloon in order to avoid damaging the reference vessel segments. A total of 54 lesions in 40 patients were treated with single 32P Bx stents with activity of 12–21 μCi in this manner (105). Although intrastent neointimal hyperplasia was significantly reduced in this group compared with historical results with nonradioactive stents, edge restenosis as the cause of observed intralesion restenosis occurred at a frequency of 26%. This rate of edge restenosis was comparable to the rate of 33% observed in the cohort of 42 lesions in 40 patients treated with 3–12 μCi 32P stents (106). Serial IVUS analysis (after stenting and at follow-up) determined that late lumen loss in the first 1–3 mm from the stent margins was mainly a result of shrinkage of the vessel (remodeling) as compared with the IVUS observation of neointimal hyperplasia as the cause in the restenotic lesions associated with implantation of 3–12 μCi stents (106). The authors also reported that in-stent intimal hyperplasia was lower in the central 5-mm segment compared with the proximal and distal 5-mm vessel segments. Thus, it would appear that increasing the stent activity and limiting balloon-related vessel injury beyond the margins of the stent reduces the degree of edge restenosis related to intimal hyperplasia but provokes or fails to prevent the negative vessel remodeling component.

To overcome the arteriopathic effects on vascular remodeling observed with higher-activity 32P stents, an alternative approach utilizes a 25-mm Bx stent with a radioactive center segment measuring 15.9 mm, with activity of 6–24 μCi and nonradioactive segments at each end measuring 5.7 mm in length. This "cold ends" stent was evaluated following implantation for 10 de novo lesions (105). Unfortunately, restenosis was observed at 6-month angiographic follow-up in four patients only in the nonradioactive end segments of the stent. One late (3.5 month) symptomatic occlusion occurred after the discontinuation of antiplatelet therapy.

Alternatively, increasing the activity at the stent edges yielded the prototype "hot ends" 32P stent, initially measuring approximately 18 mm in length. The initial segmental maximum stent activity measured 2.6 μCi per mm in the proximal and distal 2 mm of the stent and 0.57 μCi per mm in the central 14 mm of the stent. This design resulted in a maximal total stent activity of approximately 18.5 μCi. Albiero et al. treated 36 patients with 39 de novo native coronary artery lesions with implantation of 39 "hot ends" stents. Six-month angiographic follow-up was available in

24 patients with 26 lesions. Binary restenosis was observed in 31%, occurring at the proximal stent edge in 26% (107).

A summation of the clinical trials with 32P β particle-emitting stents suggests that, although true intrastent neointimal hyperplasia and, consequently, restenosis is limited to 4% at activities between 3 and 21 μCi, a high intralesion restenosis rate resulting from edge or candy wrapper effect occurs in 30–50% of instances. This edge restenosis effect has proved resistant to recent "cold-ends" and "hot ends" stent dosing efforts.

SUMMARY

The initial reports (27,38) of 0% binary restenosis after short-term follow-up following implantation of drug-eluting stents represented a remarkable observation and achievement that generated considerable excitement. Multiple trials have demonstrated that the beneficial effect of local delivery of antiproliferative agents is durable in the intermediate term. As the long-term experience with drug-eluting stents grows, several important considerations will need to be addressed. First, these remarkable innovations do not come without additional significant fixed costs to the coronary and peripheral vascular health-care bill. Kong et al. (108) point out the distinction between the economic impact of relatively expensive drug-eluting stents on hospitals as opposed to "societal cost–benefit analysis." In their model, predicted shifts from medical therapy, conventional stents, and bypass surgery to drug-eluting stents may result in significant and deleterious cash flow problems for major medical centers. Kong et al. argue that the added value derived from drug-eluting stents in reducing the number of revascularization procedures required may be offset by treatment of increased numbers of multilesion and multivessel procedures with DES. Some discussions of potential economic impact have included the concept of rationing of the DES resource for specified indictions (109).

Even though each version of drug-eluting stent has been compared with bare metal stents in terms of safety and efficacy, there have been no direct prospective trials comparing the drug-eluting stents to identify any significant difference in performance or outcome. Kastrati et al. (110) presented their data on their randomized trial in which 100 patients were randomized to one of three treatments for in-stent restenosis: Cypher stent, TAXUS stent, or balloon angioplasty. Outcomes were measured at 1, 9, and 12 months. Maximal late lumen loss was 0.45 mm with the Cypher stent and 0.66 mm with TAXUS stents ($p =$ 0.02). The total vessel revascularization rate was 8% for Cypher stents and 19% for TAXUS stents. Sapra et al. (111) have treated 307 patients in New Dehli, India, with 214 Cypher and 204 TAXUS stents for coronary stenosis and presented 6-month angiographic follow-up data for 79 consecutive patients. Late lumen loss of more than 25% in the stented segment was observed in 24.2% of TAXUS

stents and 18.3% of Cypher stents, although the difference was not statistically significant. In their patients, Sapra et al. observed that the late lumen loss occurred within the stent itself in a majority of the TAXUS stent instances, whereas the majority of the late lumen loss occurring with the Cypher stent was observed at the proximal and, to a lesser extent, the distal 5-mm margin of the stent. As of March 2004, the REALITY trial in progress has enrolled 1,386 patients to receive the Cypher sirolimus-eluting stent or the TAXUS Express[2] paclitaxel-eluting stent. This trial will directly compare the two stents in the treatment of longer lesions in smaller-diameter vessels, including multiple vessel stenting, in a higher percentage of diabetic patients.

Finally, the introduction of drug-eluting stents into mainstream clinical practice has been marred by FDA warnings and voluntary product recalls. An FDA warning on October 29, 2003, advised physicians of 290 reports of acute Cypher stent thrombosis observed 1–30 days following implantation, resulting in 60 reported deaths. In the October 29, 2003, warning, the FDA has also noted more than 50 reports, including some deaths, that the Cordis Corporation considered to be possible hypersensitivity reactions to the Cypher stent. Reported symptoms included pain, rash, respiratory distress, hives, itching, fever, and blood pressure changes. Virmani et al. (112) reported a case of hypersensitivity reaction associated with two Cypher stents identified postmortem manifested by T cell and eosinophilic cellular infiltrates as well as aneurismal dilatation of the stented arterial segment. Polymer fragments surrounded by giant cells and eosinophils were noted as well. Virmani et al. (113) note that hypersensitivity reactions to various polymers as well as uncoated stainless steel stents have been reported as well. Longer-term clinical experience with drug-eluting stents will reveal whether heightened surveillance for the rare hypersensivity-mediated stent thrombosis is required.

The future for stent-based therapy for restenosis may include several interesting concepts that are currently in the early stages of development. Regarding stent brachytherapy, current efforts to eliminate the edge restenosis effect are focused primarily in two areas. Gamma radiation is being employed to provide higher longitudinal depth of penetration, particularly at the stent ends, compared with β irradiation. Second, self-expanding stents are being considered as a replacement for balloon-expandible stents to reduce balloon-related trauma at and beyond the stent edges. Alternatively, a hybrid radioactive stent is being designed with 103Pd at each end and 32P in the central portion of the stent (Implant Sciences Co.). The gamma emitter 103Pd provides more tissue dose in the axial dimension at the stent ends, and the β emitter is ideal for homogeneous dose delivery to the target tissue in the body of the stent.

Prospects exist for gene-based therapy for restenosis in the form of a tissue-engineered stent under development by Medtronic Corporation. In this iteration, the drug delivery occurs via a genetically engineered cellular mechanism. The proposed device uses a Wiktor stent framework coated with fibronectin and seeded with smooth muscle cells that have been transfected with a plasmid, cosmid, YAC vector or retroviral vector. Plasmid-based gene expression can result in locally delivered cellular production of tissue plasminogen activator or activated protein C. The drug-eluting *cells* can be either coated directly on the stent or incorporated into a polymer coating.

REFERENCES

1. Barth KH, Virmani R, Froelich J, et al. Paired comparison of vascular wall reactions to Palmaz stents, Strecker tantalum stents, and Wallstents in canine iliac and femoral arteries. Circulation 1996;93:2161–2169.
2. Schurmann K, Vorserk D, Kulisch A, et al. Neointimal hyperplasia in low-profile Nitinol stents, Palmaz stents, and Wallstents: a comparative experimental study. Cardiovasc Intervent Radiol 1996;19:248–254.
3. Carter AJ, Scott, Laird JR, et al. Progressive vascular remodeling and reduced neointimal formation after placement of a thermoelastic self-expanding nitinol stent in an experimental model. Cathet Cardiovasc Diagn 1998;44:193–201.
4. Palmaz JC. Intravascular stenting: from basic research to clinical application. Cardiovasc Intervent Radiol 1992;15:279–284.
5. Sprague EA, Luo J, Palmaz JC. Human aortic endothelial cell migration onto metal stent surfaces under static and flow conditions. J Vasc Interv Radiol 1997;8:83–92.
6. Palmaz JC, Benson A, Sprague EA. Influence of surface topography on endothelialization of intravascular metallic material. J Vasc Interv Radiol 1999;10:439–444.
7. Hamuro M, Palmaz JC, Sprague EA, et al. Influence of stent edge angle on endothelialization in an in vitro model. J Vasc Interv Radiol 2001;12:607–611.
8. Suselbeck T, Latsch A, Siri H, et al. Role of vessel size as a predictor for the occcurrence of in-stent restenosis in patients with diabetes mellitus. Am J. Cardiol 2001;88:243–247.
9. Gray BH, Olin JW. Limitations of percutaneous transluminal angioplasty with stenting for femoropopliteal arterial occlusive disease. Semin Vasc Surg 1997;10:8–16.
10. Cheng SW, Ting AC, Wong J. Endovascular stenting of superficial femoral artery stenosis and occlusions: results and risk factor analysis. Cardiovasc Surg 2001;9:133–140.
11. Haude M, Konorza T, Kalnins U, et al. Heparin-coated stent placement for the treatment of stenoses in small coronary arteries of symptomatic patients. Circulation 2003;107:1265–1270.
12. Bresnahan WA, Boldogh I, Ma T, et al. Cyclin E/Cdk2 activity is controlled by different mechanisms in the G0 and G1 phases of the cell cycle. Cell Growth Differ 1996;7:1283–1290.
13. Koff A, Polyak K. p27KIP1, an inhibitor of cyclin-dependent kinases. Prog Cell Cycle Res 1995;1:141–147.
14. Jayaraman T, Marks AR. Rapamycin-FKBP12 blocks proliferation, induces differentiation, and inhibits cdc2 kinase activity in a myogenic cell line. J Biol Chem 1993;268: 25385–25388.
15. Marx SO, Jayaraman T, Go LO, et al. Rapamycin FKBP inhibits cell cycle regulators of proliferation in vascular smooth muscle cells. Circ Res 1995;76:412–417.
16. Windecker S, Roffi M, Meier B. Sirolimus eluting stent: a new era in interventional cardiology? Curr Pharm Des 2003;9: 1077–1094.
17. Rowinsky EK, Donehower RC, Jones RJ, et al. Microtubule changes and cytotoxicity in leukemic cell lines treated with taxol. Cancer Res 1988;48:4093–4100.
18. De Brabander M, Geuens G, Nuydens R, et al. Taxol induces the assembly of free microtubules in living cells and blocks the organizing capacity of the centrosomes and kinetochores. Proc Natl Acad Sci USA 1981;78:5608–5612.
19. Grube E, Buellesfeld L. Everolimus for stent-based intracoronary applications. Rev Cardiovasc Med 2004;5(suppl 2):S3–S8.
20. Mathiowitz E, ed. Encyclopedia of Controlled Drug Delivery. Somerset, NJ: John Wiley & Sons, 1999.
21. Grube E. Final tacrolimus outcomes in native coronaries and saphenous vein grafts: PRESENT and EVIDENT. Presented at the Scientific Sessions of the American College of Cardiology, Drug-Eluting Stent Symposium, Chicago, March 29, 2003.
22. Malik N, Gunn J, Shepard L, et al. Phosphorylcholine-coated stents in porcine coronary arteries: in vivo assessment of biocompatibility. J Invasiv Cardiol 2001;13:193–201.
23. Sousa JE, Serruys PW, Costa MA. New frontiers in cardiology: drug-eluting stents: part II. Circulation 2003;107:2383–2389.
24. Drachman DE, Edelman ER, Seifert P, et al. Neointimal thickening after stent delivery of paclitaxel: change in composition and arrest of growth over six months. J Am Coll Cardiol 2000; 36:2325–2332.
25. Farb A, Heller PF, Shroff S, et al. Pathological analysis of local delivery of paclitaxel via a polymer-coated stent. Circulation 2001;104:473–479.
26. Mitchell RD, Skwish S. Method of treating hyperproliferative vascular disease. U.S. Patent No. 5,288,711, April 28, 1992.
27. Sousa JE, Costa MA, Abizaid A, et al. Lack of neointimal proliferation after implantation of sirolimus-coated stents in human coronary arteries. A quantitative coronary angiography and three-dimensional intravascular ultrasound study. Circulation 2001;103:192–195.
28. Dussaillant GR, Mintz GS, Pichard AD, et al. Small stent size and intimal hyperplasia contribute to restenosis: a volumetric intravascular ultrasound analysis. J Am Coll Cardiol 1995: 26:720–724.
29. Sousa JE, Costa MA, Abizaid AC, et al. Sustained suppression of neointimal proliferation by sirolimus-eluting stents: one-year angiographic and intravascular ultrasound follow-up. Circulation 2001;104:2007–2011.
30. Degertekin M, Serruys PW, Foley DP, et al. Persistent inhibition of neointimal hyperplasia after sirolimus-eluting stent implantation: long-term (up to 2 years) clinical, angiographic, and intravascular ultrasound follow-up. Circulation 2002;106: 1610–1613.
31. Duda SH, Pusich B, Richter G, et al. Sirolimus-eluting stents for the treatment of obstructive superficial femoral artery disease: six-month results.Circulation 2002;106:1505–1509.
32. Morice MC, Serruys PW, Sousa JE, et al. A randomized comparison of a sirolimus-eluting stent with a standard stent for coronary revascularizastion. N Engl J Med 2002;346:1773–1780.
33. Moses JW, Leon MB, Popma JJ, et al. Sirolimus-eluting stents versus standard stents in patients with stenosis in a native coronary artery. N Eng J Med 2003;349:1315–1323.
34. Holmes DR, Leon MB, Moses JW, et al. Analysis of 1-year clinical outcomes in the SIRIUS trial: a randomized trial of a sirolimus-eluting stent versus a standard stent in patients at high risk for coronary restensosis. Circulation 2004;109:634–640.
35. de la Fuente LM, Miano J, Mrad J, et al. Initial results of the Quanam drug eluting stent (QuaDS-QP-2) registry (BARDDS) in human subjects. Catheter Cardiovasc Interv 2001;53: 480–488.
36. Liistro F, Stankovic G, Di Mario C, et al. First clinical experience with a paclitaxel derivate-eluting polymer stent system implantation for in-stent restenosis. Immediate and long-term clinical and angiographic outcome. Circulation 2002;105:1883–1886.
37. Virmani R, Liistro F, Stankovic G, et al. Mechanism of late in-stent restenosis after implantation of a paclitaxel derivate-eluting polymer stent system in humans. Circulation 2002;106: 2649–2651.
38. Grube E, Silber S, Hauptmann KE, et al. TAXUS I: six-and twelve-month results from a randomized, double-blind trial on a slow release paclitaxel-eluting stent for de novo coronary lesions. Circulation 2003;107:38–42.
39. Bullesfeld L, Gerckens U, Muller R, et al. Long-term evaluation of paclitaxel-coated stents for treatment of native coronary lesions. First results of both the clinical and angiographic 18 month follow-up of TAXUS I. Z Kardiol 2003;92:825–832.
40. Grube E. TAXUS I two year results—sustained benefit over time. Presentation at the Paris Course of Revascularization (EuroPCR), 2003.

41. Colombo A, Drzewiecki J, Banning A, et al. Randomized study to assess the effectiveness of slow- and moderate-release polymer-based paclitaxel-eluting stent for coronary artery lesions. Circulation 2003;108:788–794.

42. Tanabe K, Serruys PW, Grube E, et al. TAXUS III trial: in-stent restenosis treated with stent-based delivery of paclitaxel incorporated in a slow-release polymer formulation. Circulation 2003; 107:559–564.

43. Stone GW, Ellis SG, Cox DA, et al. One-year clinical results with the slow-release, polymer-based, paclitaxel-eluting TAXUS stent: the TAXUS-IV trial. Circulation 2004;109:1942–1947.

44. Gershlick A, De Scheerder I, Chevalier B, et al. Inhibition of restenosis with a paclitaxel-eluting, polymer-free coronary stent: the European evaluation of paclitaxel eluting stent (ELUTES) trial. Circulation 2004;109:487–493.

45. Park SJ, Shim WH, Ho DS, et al. A paclitaxel-eluting stent for the prevention of coronary restenosis. N Engl J Med 2003;348: 1537–1545.

46. Silber, S. Paclitaxel-eluting stents: are they all equal? An analysis of six randomized controlled trials in de novo lesions of 3,319 patients. J Interv Cardiol 2003;16:485–490.

47. Park SJ, Shim WH, Ho DS, et al. A paclitaxel-eluting stent for the prevention of coronary restenosis. N Engl J Med 2003; 348: 1537–1545.

48. O'Neill WW. The DELIVER trial: a randomized comparison of paclitaxel-coated versus metallic stents for treatment of coronary lesions. Presented at the 52nd Annual Scientific Sessions of the American College of Cardiology (ACC), Chicago, Illinois, March 30, 2003.

49. Wiedermann JG, Marboe C, Amols H, et al. Intracoronary irradiation markedly reduces restenosis after balloon angioplasty in a porcine model. J Am Coll Cardiol 1994;23:1491–1498.

50. Waksman R, Robinson K, Crocker I, et al. Intracoronary radiation before stent implantation inhibits neointima formation after coronary artery balloon injury in the swine restenosis model. Circulation 1995;92:3025–3031.

51. Waksman R, Robinson K, Crocker I, et al. Intracoronary radiation before stent implantation inhibits neointima formation in stented porcine coronary arteries. Circulation 1995;92: 1383–1386.

52. Waksman R, Robinson K, Crocker I, et al.Endovascular low-dose irradition inhibits neointima formation after coronary artery balloon injury in swine: a possible role for radiation therapy in restenosis prevention. Circulation 1995;91:1533–1539.

53. Weinberger J, Amols H, Ennis RD, et al. Intracoronary irradiation: dose response for the prevention of restenosis in swine. Int J Radiat Oncol Biol Phys 1996;36:767–775.

54. Wiedermann JG, Marboe C, Amols H, et al. Intracoronary irradiation markedly reduces neointimal proliferation after balloon angioplasty in swine: persistent benefit at 6-month follow-up. J Am Coll Cardiol 1995;25:1451–1456.

55. Teirstein PS, Massullo V, Jani S, et al. Catheter-based radiotherapy to inhibit restenosis after coronary stenting. N Engl J Med 1997;336:1697–1703.

56. Waksman R, White LR, Chan RC, et al. Intracoronary radiation therapy for patients with in-stent restenosis: 6 month follow-up of a randomized clinical study [abstract]. Circulation 1998;98:I-651.

57. King SB, Williams DO, Chougule P, et al. Endovascular b-radiation to reduce restenosis after coronary balloon angioplasty: results of the Beta Energy Restenosis Trial (BERT). Circulation 1998;97:2025–2030.

58. Teirstein PS, Massullo V, Jani S, et al. Two-year follow-up after catheter-based radiotherapy to inhibit coronary restenosis. Circulation 1999;99:243–247.

59. Waksman R, Robinson KA, Crocker IR, et al. Endovascular low-dose irradiation inhibits neointima formation in stented porcine coronary arteries. Circulation 1995;92:1383–1386.

60. Wiedermann JG, Marboe C, Amols H, et al. Intracoronary irradiation markedly reduces neointimal proliferation after balloon angioplasty in swine: persistent benefit at 6-month follow-up. J Am Coll Cardiol 1995;25:1451–1456.

61. Farb A, Tang A, Virmani R. The neointima is reduced but endothelialization is incomplete 3 months after 32P b-emitting stent placement [abstract]. Circulation 1998;98:I-779.

62. Shroff SS, Farb A, Sweet WL, et al. Sustained neointimal inhibition with delayed healing 6 months after placement of 32P b-emitting stents [abstract]. Circulation 1999;100:I-155.

63. Taylor AJ, Gorman PD, Farb A, et al. Long-term coronary vascular response to (32)P beta-particle-emitting stents in a canine model. Circulation 1999;199:2366–2372.

64. Salame M, Lampkin J, Mulkey SP, et al. Effects of endovascular irradiation on platelet recruitment at sites of balloon angioplasty in pig coronary arteries [abstract]. J Am Coll Cardiol 1999;33 (Suppl):44-A.

65. Vodovotz Y, Waksman R, Kim WH, et al. Effects of intracoronary radiation on thrombosis after balloon overstretch injury in the porcine model. Circulation 1999;100:2527–2533.

66. Dangas G, Fuster V. Management of restenosis after coronary intervention. Am Heart J 1996;132:428–436.

67. Fingerle J, Johnson R, Clowes AW, et al. Role of platelets in smooth muscle cell proliferation and migration after vascular injury in rat carotid artery. Proc Natl Acad Sci USA 1989;86: 8412–8416.

68. Schwartz RS. Pathophysiology of restenosis: interaction of thrombosis, hyperplasia, and/or remodeling. Am J Cardiol 1998;81:14E–17E.

69. Waksman R, Bhargava B, Mintz GS, et al. Late total occlusion after intracoronary brachytherapy for patients with in-stent restenosis. J Am Coll Cardiol 2000;36:65–68.

70. Waksman R, Ajani AE, Pinnow E, et al. Twelve versus six months of clopidogrel to reduce major cardiac events in patients undergoing gamma-radiation therapy for in-stent restenosis: Washington Radiation for In-Stent Restenosis Trial (WRIST) 12 versus WRIST PLUS. Circulation 2002;106: 776–778.

71. Sabate M, Costa MA, Kozuma K, et al. Geographic miss: a cause of treatment failure in radio-oncology applied to intracoronary radiation therapy. Circulation 2000;101:2467–2471.

72. Bonan R. "Geographic miss" in vascular brachytherapy. In Waksman R, ed. Vascular Brachytherapy. Armonk, NY: Futura Publishing, 2002.

73. Carter AJ, Fischell TA. Current status of radioactive stents for the prevention of in-stent restenosis. Int J Radiat Oncol Biol Phys 1998;41:127–133.

74. Serruys PW, Kay IP. I like the candy, I hate the wrapper: the (32P) radioactive stent. Circulation 2000;101:3–7.

75. Amols HI. Designing the ideal radioactive stent [abstract]. Cardiovasc Radiation Therapy IV Symposium. February 16–28, 2000.

76. Clowes AW, Reidy MA, Clowes MM. Mechanisms of stenosis after arterial injury. Lab Invest 1983;49:208–215.

77. Geary RL, Williams JK, Golden D, et al. Time course of cellular proliferation, intimal hyperplasia, and remodeling following angioplasty in monkeys with established atherosclerosis. A non-human primate model of restensosis. Arterioscler Thromb Vasc Biol 1996;16:34–43.

78. Labinaz M, Pels K, Hoffert C, et al. Time course and importance of neoadventitial formation in arterial remodeling following balloon angioplasty of porcine coronary arteries. Cardiovasc Res 1999;41:255–266.

79. Carter AJ, Scott D, Bailey L, et al. Dose-response effects of 32P radioactive stents in an atherosclerotic porcine coronary model. Circulation 1999;100:1548–1554.

80. Carter AJ, Jenkins JS, Bailey LR, et al. Dose rate and cumulative dose effects of P-32 radioactive stents [abstract]. J Am Coll Cardiol 1999;33:20A.

81. Lansky AJ, Popma JJ, Massullo V, et al. Quantitative angiographic analysis of stent restenosis in the Scripps Coronary Radiation to Inhibit Intimal Proliferation Post Stenting (SCRIPPS) Trial. Am J Cardiol 1999;84:410–414.

82. Teirstein PS. Vascular radiation therapy: the devil is in the dose. J Am Coll Cardiol 1999;34:567–569.

83. Sioshansi P, Bricault RJ. Low-energy 103Pd gamma (x-ray) source for vascular brachytherapy. Cardiovasc Radiat Med 1999;1:278–287.

84. Hausleiter J, Li A, Makkar R, et al. Localization of target tissue and the minimum effective dose in intracoronary radiation therapy [abstract]. J Am Coll Cardiol 1999;33:44.

85. Albiero R, Adamian M, Kobayashi N, et al. Short- and intermediate-term results of 32P radioactive beta-emitting stent implantation in patients with coronary artery disease: the Milan Dose-Response Study. Circulation 2000;101.18–26.

86. Carter AJ, Scott D, Bailey LR, et al. Dose-response effects of 32P radioactive stents in an atherosclerotic porcine coronary model. Circulation 1999;100:1548–1554.

87. Waksman R, Mehran R, Bhargava B, et al. Recurrent restenosis after "failed" intracoronary radiation therapy: angiographic patterns and predictors [abstract]. Circulation 1999;100:222.

88. Taylor AJ, Gorman PD, Hudak C, et al. The 90-day Coronary Vascular Response to (90)Y-ß particle-emitting stents in the canine model. Int J Radiat Oncol Biol Phys 2000;46:1019–1024.

89. Schulz C, Niederer MS, Andres C, et al. Endovascular irradiation from beta-particle-emitting gold stents results in increased neointima formation in a porcine restenosis model. Circulation 2000;101:1970–1975.

90. Albiero R, Colombo A. European high-activity (32)P radioactive stent experience. J Invasive Cardiol 2000;12:416–421.

91. Sioshansi P, Bricault RJ. Low-energy 103Pd gamma (X-ray) source for vascular brachytherapy. Cardiovasc Radiat Med 1999;1:278–287.

92. Rahdert DA, Sweet WL, Tio FO, et al. Measurement of density and calcium in human atherosclerotic plaque and implications for arterial brachytherapy. Cardiovasc Radiat Med 1999; 1: 358–367.

93. Amols HI. Methods to improve dose uniformity for radioactive stents in endovascular brachytherapy. Cardiovasc Radiat Med 1999;1:270–277.

94. Coffey CW, Duggan DM. The calculation and measurement of radiation dose surrounding radioactive stents: the effects of radionuclide selection and stent design on dosimetric results. In Waksman R, ed. Vascular Brachytherapy. 2nd Ed. Armonk, NY: Futura Publishing, 1999.

95. Strauss BH, Li C, Whittingham H, et al. Late effects of low-energy gamma-emitting stents in a rabbit iliac artery model. Int J Radiat Oncol Biol Phys 2002;54:551–561.

96. Laird JR, Carter AJ, Kufs WM, et al. Inhibition of neointimal proliferation with low-dose irradiation from a beta-particle-emitting stent. Circulation 1996;93:529–536.

97. Carter AJ, Laird JR, Bailey LR, et al. Effects of endovascular radiation from a beta-particle-emitting stent in a porcine coronary restenosis model. A dose-response study. Circulation 1996; 94:2364–2368.

98. Hehrlein C, Stintz M, Kinscherf R, et al Pure beta-particle-emitting stents inhibit neointima formation in rabbits. Circulation 1996;93:641–645.

99. Fishell Carter A, Foster M. Lessons from the feasibility radioactive (IRIS) stent trials. In Waksman R, ed. Vascular Brachytherapy. 2nd Ed. Armonk, NY: Futura Publishing, 1999:475–481.

100. Moses J, Ellis S, Bailey S, et al. Short-term (1 month) results of the dose response IRIS feasibility study of a beta-particle-emitting radioisotope stent [abstract]. J Am Coll Cardiol 1998;31:350A.

101. Moses J. US IRIS trials low-activity 32P stent [abstract]. In Cardiovascular Radiation Therapy III. Washington, DC: 1999: 387–388.

102. Hehrlein C, Brachmann J, Hardt S, et al. P-32 stents for prevention of restenosis: results of the Heidelberg Safety Trial using the Palmaz-Schatz stent design at moderate activity levels in patients with restenosis after PTCA [abstract]. Circulation 1998;98:I780.

103. Janicki C, Duggan DM, Coffey CW, et al. Radiation dose from a phosphorous-32 impregnated wire mesh vascular stent. Med Phys 1997;24:437–445.

104. Wardeh AJ, Kay IP, Sabate M, et al. Beta-particle-emitting radioactive stent implantation. A safety and feasibility study. Circulation 1999;100:1684–1689.

105. Albiero R, Colombo A. Radioactive stents: the Milan experience. In Waksman R, ed. Vascular Brachytherapy 3rd Ed. Armonk, NY: Futura Publishing, 2002:383.

106. Albiero R, Nishida T, Adamian M, et al. Edge restenosis after implantation of high activity (32)P radioactive beta-emitting stents. Circulation 2000;101:2454–2457.

107. Albiero R,Nishida T, Amato A, et al. Results of "hot ends" 32P radioactive beta-emitting stent implantation in patients with CAD. The Milan experience [abstract]. Circulation 2000;102:II-568.

108. Kong DF, Eisenstein EL, Sketch MH, et al. Economic impact of drug-eluting stents on hospital systems: a disease-state model. Am Heart J 2004;147:449–456.

109. O'Neill WW, Leon MB. Drug-eluting stents: costs versus clincal benefit. Circulation 2003;107:3008–3011.

110. Kastrati A. ISAR-DESIRE: Drug-eluting stents for in-stent restenosis [abstract]. Presented at the European Society of Cardiology Congress, Munich, Germany, 2004.

111. Sapra R, Kaul U, Gupta RK, et al. A comparative analysis of late loss patterns in drug-eluting stents [abstract]. Indian Heart J 2003;55:107.

112. Virmani R, Guagliumi G, Farb A, et al. Localized hypersensitivity and late coronary thrombosis secondary to a sirolimus-eluting stent: should we be cautious? Circulation 2004;109:701–705.

113. Virmani R, Farb A, Guagliumi G, et al. Drug-eluting stents: caution and concerns for long-term outcome. Coron Artery Dis 2004;13:313–318.

Principles of Selective Thrombolysis

14

Anne Roberts

Thrombolysis is an effective therapy for the clinical management of many thromboembolic disorders. Advances in clinical methodology of thrombolysis are derived largely from advances in basic science. This chapter considers some scientific concepts that underlie current thrombolytic therapy.

To exploit current and approaching methodology, the interventionalist should be familiar with (1) thrombosis and the coagulation system; (2) the physiology of endogenous fibrinolytics; (3) the pharmacodynamics of exogenous fibrinolytics; (4) platelet–fibrinolytic relationships; (5) pharmacologic adjuncts of fibrinolysis, including antiplatelet and antithrombic agents; (6) the methodology of fibrinolytic delivery; (7) methods of mechanical thrombolysis; and (8) results of clinical thrombolysis. An overview of these subjects is provided here. In Chapter 15, details of clinical implementation will be emphasized, along with results and complications.

Fibrin constitutes the basic structural component of thrombus; thus, thrombolysis is used synonymously with fibrinolysis, a proteolytic process through which fibrin is cleaved into soluble fibrin degradation products (FDPs). To supplement the endogenous fibrinolytic system, exogenous fibrinolytic agents can be administered for therapeutic purposes. Thrombi can also be treated by mechanical means, a process for which the term mechanical thrombolysis is used.

Systemic administration of fibrinolytics is common, particularly for the treatment of acute myocardial infarction and, more recently, for stroke therapy. However, selective administration generally is used to treat peripheral thromboemboli and venous thrombosis and is more effective in the treatment of stoke than systemic administration. Selective methods provide intrathrombic concentrations of fibrinolytic agents much higher than those achievable by intravenous administration, which allows specific targeting of the thrombus with relative sparing of thrombi elsewhere and with less loss of circulating fibrinogen.

COMPONENTS OF THE FIBRINOLYTIC SYSTEM

The endogenous fibrinolytic system involves several blood and endothelial elements, including fibrin, plasmin, plasminogen, plasminogen activators, plasminogen activator inhibitors, and antiplasmins. To understand the fibrinolytic system (the breakdown of clot), the clotting sequence also must be understood because of the dynamic balance between clot formation and clot breakdown. Understanding the components involved in thrombosis helps to understand the various pharmacological agents that can be used to move the balance point toward clot dissolution.

Thrombosis

Multiple factors are involved in coagulation and the coagulation system may seem overwhelmingly complex (Figure 14–1). The generation of the enzyme thrombin from its precursor prothrombin is the central and pivotal event of the blood coagulation process (1). Thrombin is formed as a result of reactions involving a sequential transformation of coagulation factors, which are present in plasma in an inactive form (2). The *extrinsic pathway* begins when tissue factor and factor VIIa combine to form a VIIa/tissue factor complex. Tissue factor, a cellular receptor for activated factor VII, is a primary trigger (1,3,4). Injury to the arterial or venous wall or the rupturing of an

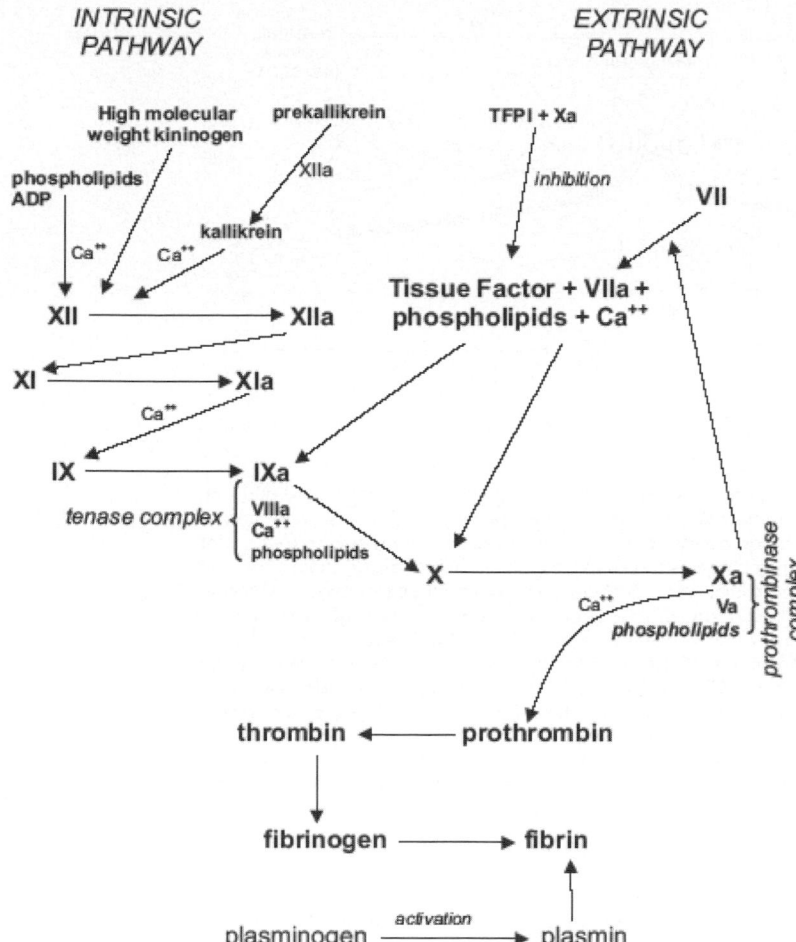

Figure 14-1 The coagulation system consists of the extrinsic and intrinsic pathways. The extrinsic pathway is triggered by the release of tissue factor from the site of injury coming into contact with plasma containing factor VII or factor VIIa. The intrinsic pathway is stimulated by high–molecular-weight kininogen and prekallekrein. Both pathways activate factor IX that then complexes with factor VIIIa, calcium, and phospholipids to activate factor X to Xa that then goes on to convert prothrombin to thrombin.

atherosclerotic plaque exposes nonvascular, tissue factor-expressing cells to blood, and factor VIIa binds to the tissue factor (4). This complex causes the activation of factors IX and X. Factor IXa then binds to factor VIIIa to form a complex that activates factor X. Factor Xa then binds to factor V on the membrane surface, and the factor Va-factor Xa assembles on the membrane surface to form prothrombinase, the prothrombin-activating complex (1). The factor Xa in this complex activates prothrombin to thrombin, which then dissociates from the membrane surface and converts fibrinogen to fibrin monomers (3).

Blood can also coagulate without the activation of tissue factor. This pathway is the *intrinsic pathway*, which begins with the surface activation of factor XII and proceeds, with the accessory components prekallekrein and high–molecular-weight kininogen, to activate factor XI to factor XIa (5). The exposure of negatively charged phospholipids supports the assembly of the "tenase" complex on the surface of activated platelets as part of the intrinsic pathway (5). The "tenase" complex is comprised of IXa, VIIIa, and calcium (4). This tenase complex activates factor X to form factor Xa, the same endpoint as the extrinsic pathway, the complex-forming prothrombinase that generates thrombin. The final common mediator of both the intrinsic and extrinsic

coagulation pathways is thrombin (4). Thrombin triggers platelet activation, as well as the production of factor V, factor VIII, and factor IX, and it mediates the proteolytic cleavage of fibrinogen to fibrin (4).

Fibrinogen and Fibrin

Fibrinogen (Figure 14-2) is a large symmetrical protein with three nonidentical, long polypeptide chains—designated α, β, and γ—in each half of the molecule. Two short central branches, termed *fibrinopeptide A* and *fibrinopeptide B*, are attached to the α or β chains, respectively, connecting the two halves of the molecule with disulfide bridges. Fibrinogen is present in blood plasma in concentrations of 200–400 mg/dL and is released from platelets when platelets are activated.

Molecules of fibrin are formed from fibrinogen after cleavage of fibrinopeptides A and B by thrombin. Fibrinopeptide A can be used as an early marker of fibrinogen-to-fibrin conversion (6). The fibrin molecules aggregate into a three-dimensional mesh via noncovalent interactions. Stabilizing cross-linkages begin to form between γ chains and later between α chains (but not between β chains) under the influence of factor XIII (7).

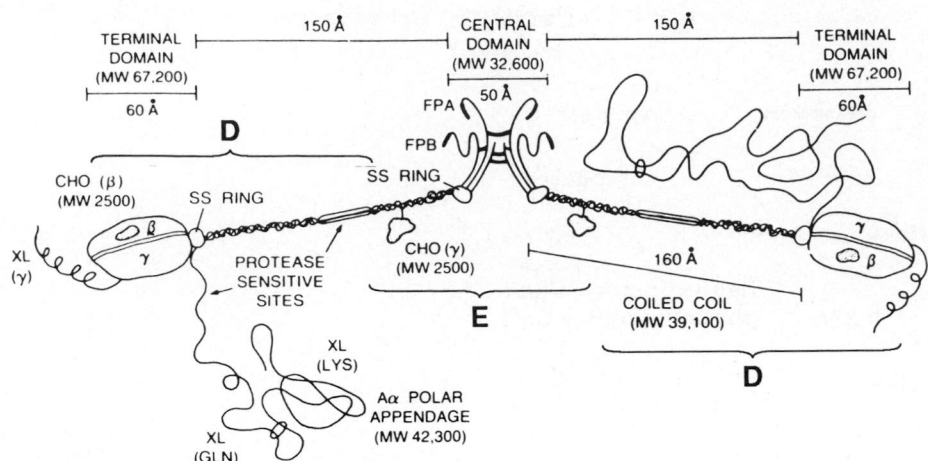

Figure 14–2   Fibrinogen molecule, schematic diagram. Molecular weight is about 340,000 daltons. The symmetrical structure of the molecule is evident, with three separate chains, α, β, and γ, one each side, connected by three disulfide bonds centrally. The molecule is shown with four major protein regions: the *central domain*, which contains the amino-terminal ends of all six chains; the thin connecting α-helical *coiled coils* of three chains each, the two carboxy-*terminal domains*, and the α-chain *polar appendages*. Fibrinopeptides A and B (*FPA* and *FPB*) are noted as slightly thickened parts of the amino-terminal ends of the α and β chains. Factor XIII$_a$—related sites of cross linking (*XLs*) are situated near the carboxy terminus of the γ and α chains. The multiple sites of lysine throughout the molecule are not illustrated. CHO = carbohydrate cluster; SS = disulfide. (Courtesy of R. Doolittle.) During conversion of fibrinogen to fibrin by thrombin, the four A and B fibrinopeptides are cleaved. After proteolysis by plasmin, the molecule is divided into various fibrinogen degradation products, indicated as *D* and *E*. Fragment *D* plus *E* constitute a fragment known as Y. Both *D*s and an *E* constitute a fragment known as X. Fibrin degradation products consist of these same fragments, but cross-linked.

These cross-linkages moderately inhibit, but do not prevent, fibrinolysis. The fibrinogen $\gamma\alpha$ chain plays a critical role in mediating platelet aggregation via the platelet fibrinogen receptor.

In the process of fibrinolysis (the breakdown of clot), fibrin is degraded by plasmin into soluble FDPs.

Plasminogen

Fibrinolysis is initiated by plasminogen activators that convert plasminogen to plasmin, and plasmin then acts to degrade fibrin clots. The major activator of plasminogen in vivo is tissue plasminogen activator (tPA), but there are several pathways of plasminogen activation. Factor XIIa, XIa, and kallikrein are capable of converting plasminogen to plasmin (6). Plasminogen circulates in the blood as an inactive zymogene (6), which is activated to create the active fibrinolytic enzyme plasmin. Plasminogen is a single-chain glycoprotein that is synthesized in the liver and normally circulates in the plasma at concentrations of 20–30 mg/dL. Plasminogen exists in two forms: (1) the lys-plasminogen form with lysine at the amino-terminal end and (2) glu-plasminogen with glutamic acid at the amino-terminal end. The two forms of plasminogen differ somewhat functionally; the lysine form is predominant in fibrin or endothelial-bound plasminogen, and the glutamic acid form is more prevalent in plasma. The estimated biologic half-lives of glu-plasminogen and lys-plasminogen are 2.2 and 0.8 days, respectively. Under the influence of plasmin, glu-plasminogen undergoes partial degradation to the lysine form.

Variable amounts of plasminogen also exist within thrombus, at least partially bound to fibrin. The amount of plasminogen bound to thrombus is sufficient for thrombolysis, regardless of clot age. The plasminogen activators to be effective must interact with clot-bound plasminogen, and the plasminogen activator must be able to get to the clot-bound plasminogen. Because sufficient plasminogen is already bound to fibrin within thrombus means inflow of circulating plasminogen is not necessarily a prerequisite for lysis, this explains the efficacy of intrathrombic administration of fibrinolytic agents.

Plasmin

Under the influence of plasminogen activators, plasminogen is converted into plasmin, its active form, through hydrolysis of the arginine–lysine peptide bond. Simultaneously, the single-chain plasminogen becomes two-chain plasmin. The heavier of the two chains contains five loops (kringles) and retains fibrin-binding capacity, and the light chain contains the protease activity. Under physiologic intravascular conditions, tissue-type plasminogen activator (tPA) is a primary catalyst for the conversion of plasminogen to plasmin. Fibrin-bound plasminogen is converted into fibrin-bound plasmin, which can be neutralized by fibrin-bound α-antiplasmin.

The major substrate of plasmin is fibrin, which is cleaved into various soluble FDPs termed X, Y, D, or E. The X fragment can participate in fibrin polymerization, whereas incorporation of Y, D, or E fragments terminates the polymerization process. Plasmin is a nonspecific proteolytic agent and also digests other coagulation factors, particularly fibrinogen and factors V and VIII. Plasmin, as well as thrombin, is also an extremely potent platelet activator. The half-life of intrathrombic plasmin, when plasmin is partially fibrin-bound and protected from circulating inhibitors, is approximately 10 seconds. On the other hand, plasmin in plasma is neutralized rapidly by a_2-antiplasmin so that the estimated half-life of circulating plasmin is only 100 milliseconds.

The abundance of plasmin inhibitors in plasma and thrombus and the lack of fibrin specificity of plasmin largely explain the difficulty of using plasmin as a direct therapeutic agent.

PLASMINOGEN ACTIVATORS

Streptokinase

Streptokinase (SK) is a single chain glycoprotein derived from β-hemolytic streptococci and has a molecular weight of about 45,000–50,000 daltons. Unlike other plasminogen activators, SK is not an enzyme, but rather an indirect activator of plasminogen that first forms irreversible activator complexes with plasminogen (or plasmin). Once in this complex, streptokinase is transformed into an activated plasminogen possessing a proteolytic active serine site, which then activates any remaining plasminogen (8). The plasminogen SK complex shows slight fibrin selectivity, but much less than that of tPA. Because of the prevalence of prior streptococcal infections, antibodies against SK that inhibit formation of SK-activator complexes are present in many populations. This inhibitory effect can be overcome by a loading dose of SK, typically about 250,000 units in North Americans. For 6 months after SK therapy, antibody titers can be sufficiently elevated to block the fibrinolytic effect of further SK administration. There have been two half-lives identified in the human body. The first is 18 minutes and represents clearance after binding with antibodies or inhibitors, or about 80–85% of a single dose given intravenously (8). The second half-life is approximately 83 minutes, which represents about 10–15% of an administered dose (8).

Other thrombolytics have largely replaced streptokinase in the United States. Disadvantages of SK include its antigenicity, which precludes patients from receiving frequently repeated therapy, and its increased consumption of plasminogen associated with the two-step process of activation. The increased requirement for plasminogen decreases its usefulness when it is administered intrathrombic.

Urokinase

Urokinase (UK) is a two-chain glycoprotein that activates plasminogen in a one-step process. Originally derived from human urine, UK has also been isolated from fetal kidney cells and developed as a recombinant DNA product (though presently not commercially available). There are two major species: a high molecular weight (HMW) is approximately 55,000 daltons and a 33,000 low molecular weight (LMW). Both have similar plasminogen-activator activity (8). The HMW urokinase consists of two polypeptide chains (33,000 and 54,000 daltons) connected by disulfide bonds. The 33,000-dalton chain contains the serine active site (8). The plasma half-life is about 15–20 minutes. The endothelial cells synthesize UK as a relatively inactive single-chain molecule that is activated by plasmin through conversion to a two-chain enzyme. A low–molecular-weight (33,000 dalton) form of UK exists after further plasmin hydrolysis. Urokinase probably plays little physiologic role in fibrinolysis. Few or no natural antibodies exist against UK, and UK seems not to be antigenic.

The single-chain urokinase precursor (scuPA or pro-uPA) may be obtained from endothelial cell tissue culture media, urine, plasma, or transformed bacteria. Molecular weights vary from about 54,000 to 68,000 daltons. The proenzyme is converted into two-chain urokinase by limited hydrolysis by plasmin or kallikrein (8). As a plasminogen activator, scuPA is only about 1% as effective as UK, the two-chain variety. However, scuPA has fibrin selectivity comparable to tPA, and after binding to fibrin, it is activated to produce relatively selective fibrinolysis. Fibrin also enhances the catalytic efficacy of scuPA from 10-fold to 2,000-fold. The half-life of scuPA in blood is about 7 minutes. A human recombinant glycosylated prourokinase (r-pro-UK) is produced by recombinant technology, but is not commercially available.

Despite its limited fibrin specificity, UK was very popular in the United States until the FDA removed it from the market in 1999 because of manufacturing problems. In the 3 years that it was not available in the United States, interventional radiologists began to use other thrombolytic agents and gradually became comfortable with these other agents. When UK returned to the market in 2002, there was resistance to returning to it, primarily because of the increased cost. Gradually, interventionalists had tPA, which decreased complications, and also significantly decreased the cost of the thrombolysis. UK returned to the market at the same price that it left the market, but in the meantime, the cost of using alternative agents was far below that of UK.

UK has a number of desirable features, including lack of antigenicity, high efficacy, and low incidence of serious hemorrhage. Along with tPA, its short biologic half-life allows surgical intervention relatively soon after thrombolysis.

Tissue Plasminogen Activator (tPA)

Under physiologic conditions, tPA, a serine protease produced by endothelial cells and other tissues, is the major activator of plasminogen. Endothelial cells synthesize tPA as a single-chain protein with a molecular weight of 60,000–72,000 daltons. Thrombin, heparin, DDAVP, and other substances augment the release of tPA from endothelial cells. Single-chain tPA binds to fibrin followed by the addition of plasminogen to form a ternary complex (9). In the absence of fibrin, tPA is an inefficient activator of plasminogen, but once bound to fibrin, its efficacy in converting plasminogen to plasmin is markedly accelerated (6,10). Plasmin, in turn, performs a limited hydrolysis on single-chain tPA and converts it into a two-chain molecule of an identical molecular weight. The single- and double-chain forms of tPA have essentially equivalent fibrinolytic and activating-activating properties. The half-life of the single-chain tPA is 5 minutes, and the double-chain tPA has a half-life of 8 minutes.

There are three major derivatives of tissue plasminogen activator that are commercially produced and clinically available: alteplase, reteplase, and tenecteplase.

Alteplase (r-tPA, tPA)

Alteplase (r-tPA) is manufactured commercially by Genentech, using recombinant DNA technology—brand name Activase. The specific activity of alteplase is 550,000–667,000 IU/mg. The biological half-life of alteplase is 3–6 minutes. It has an increased specificity and affinity for fibrin, which led to speculation that r-tPA would have decreased activity in plasma and, therefore, perhaps a better safety profile. However, markedly improved safety has not been evident clinically. In addition, fibrin selectivity is less important when agents are administered by the selective intrathrombic route than when administered systemically. The high molecular weight of tPA (and other plasminogen activators) contributes to slow diffusion within the thrombus, which is one factor limiting the rate of thrombolysis and a reason the intrathrombic administration of thrombolytics may be of critical importance.

Early in the selective use of alteplase, relatively high doses were being used (3–6 mg/hr). Although effective, there was a high bleeding rate associated with this regime (11). Over time and with increasing experience, the dosage gradually has been decreased to 1–1.5 mg/hr, with recommendations of even lower doses of 0.5–1.0 mg/hr. It has been suggested that the total dose not be greater than 40 mg for catheter-directed therapy (12).

The native tPA molecule has been modified in an attempt to achieve improved lytic characteristics with less risk of bleeding (13). These newer agents are described below.

Reteplase (rPA)

Reteplase (brand name Retevase) is manufactured by Centocor and is a third-generation recombinant mutant of tissue-type plasminogen activator in which the finger, epidermal growth factor, and kringle 1 regions have been deleted (14). The kringle 2 region and the protease domains of tPA remain intact (13). Reteplase retains fibrin specificity and preferentially converts clot-bound plasminogen rather than free plasminogen (14). Compared with tPA, reteplase has a lower fibrin binding, which may translate to improved clot penetration. Reteplase has potent in vivo thrombolytic activity and leads to rapid reperfusion; the half-life is similar to that of urokinase 14–18 minutes. In peripheral artery disease, various doses have been tried. One study (15) used three doses: 0.5 units/hr, 0.25 units/hr, and 0.125 units/hr. The 0.125 units/hr group had significantly longer infusion times, while the 0.5 units/hr group had a significantly higher bleeding complication rate. The efficacy was essentially the same in all three groups, and the conclusion of the study was that 0.25 units/hr was the optimal dose. A consensus conference recommended a reteplase dose of 0.25–1.0 U/h, with or without an initial bolus of 2–5 U (14). A total dose of ≤20 U for treatment of a peripheral occlusion was believed to be appropriate (14).

Tenecteplase (TNK)

Tenecteplase (TNK) is manufactured by Genentech and is a third-generation, bioengineered thrombolytic agent. TNK is a triple-point mutation of tPA that has been altered at three different portions of the molecule, in the T, N, and K domains. The substitutions prolong the half-life to approximately 20–24 minutes. It has the highest degree of fibrin specificity of the recombinant tPAs with increased specificity for fibrin. Tenecteplase also has the greater resistance to inhibition by PAI-1 by approximately 80-fold (16). The hope was to decrease the systemic effect and decrease the delayed and remote bleeding seen with alteplase and reteplase. Small numbers of patients with peripheral thromboses have been treated with TNK. Doses of 0.25 mg/hr–0.50 mg/hr appear to be safe and effective (17). Fibrinogen levels dropped by an average of 23% with this type of dose (17).

Plasminogen activators are classified as fibrin-specific or non–fibrin-specific agents. Streptokinase and urokinase are non–fibrin-specific agents and alteplase, reteplase, and tenecteplase are fibrin-specific agents. Although it was anticipated that fibrin specificity would decrease the incidence of hemorrhage relative to non–fibrin-specific fibrinolytics, the clinical incidence of hemorrhagic complications after the use of fibrin-specific fibrinolytics is considerable. Some of these complications may represent a lack of understanding of the proper dosage, particularly for peripheral thrombolysis.

The reasons for the less-than-expected safety of fibrin-specific agents are still being evaluated. Alteplase is 400 times more likely to convert plasminogen to plasmin when plasminogen is fibrin bound than when it is freely circulating (16). Fibrin-bound plasmin then degrades cross-linked fibrin into multiple, soluble, fibrin degradation products (FDPs). The most prolific of the FDPs is D dimer-E complex [(DD)E] (18). A fibrin-specific plasminogen activator (such as alteplase) actively binds to circulating (DD)E with an affinity similar to fibrin. This complex undergoes a conformational change and is 350 times more active in the conversion of free plasminogen to plasmin. The (DD)E itself binds to circulating plasminogen. The bound plasminogen is converted into plasmin by the complex of (DD)E with the fibrin-specific plasminogen activator. This circulating complex degrades fibrinogen and starts a process of fibrinogen depletion (fibrinogenolysis) that is associated with bleeding. The bleeding may be the result of production of a degradation product called fragment X. Fragment X seems to be a by-product of fibrinogen degradation by circulating plasmin. Large amounts of fragment X can persist in the circulation for as long as 24 hours after bolus infusions of alteplase. Fragment X can be incorporated into hemostatic plugs. However, when fragment X is incorporated into hemostatic plugs, the thrombus has lower tensile strength and is more susceptible to lysis. Non–fibrin-specific agents apparently degrade fibrinogen into smaller, nonclottable fragments, so there is no accumulation of fragment X. Without fragment X accumulation, less potential exists for forming distant thrombus of lower tensile strength that may be more prone to bleeding.

Another consideration is that the strong affinity that fibrin-specific agents have for fibrin may result in a prolonged biological half-life, despite its shorter plasma half-life when compared to non–fibrin-specific agents. When the fibrin-specific agents are bound to fibrin and plasmin, plasmin is protected from a_2-antiplasmin, the primary inhibitor of the lytic process. This might explain the delayed and sustained systemic lytic effects seen with alteplase.

Clearly, tPA shows a greater tendency to bind to endothelial cells than streptokinase or urokinase, another possible factor related to hemorrhagic complications of tPA.

REGULATORS OF FIBRINOLYTIC SYSTEM

Plasminogen Activator Inhibitors (PAI)

Inhibitors of plasminogen activator play an important role in regulating fibrinolysis. Four distinct types have been described: PAI-1, PAI-2, PAI-3, and protease nexin (6). PAI-1 is the most important in inhibiting tPA in plasma (3). Synthesis of PAI-1 occurs primarily in endothelial cells (6). PAI is also released from activated platelets. The amount of PAI released from endothelium and platelets is relatively small and probably insufficient to significantly interfere

with the large concentrated doses of plasminogen activator used for selective intrathrombic thrombolysis. Inhibition of PAI-1 results in increased endogenous fibrinolytic activity. One strategy to promote fibrinolysis is the development of small-molecule PAI-1 inhibitors—currently, such agents are being investigated.

Alpha₂-Antiplasmin

Alpha₂-antiplasmin is the primary inhibitor of active plasmin and is found in plasma and thrombus. In plasma, a_2-antiplasmin binds rapidly to plasmin to form an irreversible stable complex: plasmin-antiplasmin complex (6). Free plasmin is much more rapidly bound to a_2-antiplasmin than plasmin attached to fibrin (6). The presence of a_2-antiplasmin enhances resistance to fibrinolysis. However, because fibrin-bound plasmin is protected fairly well from inactivation, fibrinolysis can occur despite physiologic levels of a_2-antiplasmin (10).

Thrombin-Activatable Fibrinolysis Inhibitor

Thrombin-activatable fibrinolysis inhibitor (TAFI) is also known as *plasma carboxypeptidase B* (3,6). Thrombin, when bound to thrombomodulin, can activate TAFI, which can inhibit fibrinolysis by several mechanisms (3). It cleaves the carboxyl terminal end of fibrin, reducing the ability of fibrin to facilitate plasminogen activation via tPA. It can also inhibit plasmin activity directly and be cross-linked to fibrin and incorporated into a fibrin clot, which prevent premature lysis. Inhibitors of procarboxypeptidase B should enhance fibrinolytic activity.

Alpha₂-Macroglobulin

Alpha₂-macroglobulin is a general proteinase inhibitor and slowly inactivates many components of the fibrinolytic system, including plasmin, tcuPA, tPA, and the streptokinase-plasmin(ogen) complex. It plays a limited role as a plasmin inhibitor, becoming important only when the concentration of plasmin exceeds the capacity of a_2-antiplasmin.

The presence of powerful circulating antiplasmins provides some of the rationale for intrathrombic deposition of fibrinolytic agents, in sufficient concentration to overwhelm intrathrombic plasmin inhibitors. The amount of inhibitory agent within thrombus is currently unknown.

COMPOSITION OF THE THROMBUS

Major advances have been made in the understanding of thrombus formation, particularly with regard to the role of platelets and the assembly of fibrin fibrils, as well as their susceptibility of fibrinolysis.

Although much emphasis has been placed on the fibrin network of thrombus, it must be emphasized that thrombus contains other ingredients, including red cells, white cells, and platelets. Platelets play a critical role in hemostatic balance—primarily (but not exclusively) a prothrombotic and antifibrinolytic role. An understanding of thrombolysis requires consideration of the role of platelets. For example, the coagulation cascade activated by the procoagulant activity expressed on the surface of activated platelets is believed to play a crucial role in the formation of occlusive thrombi (19).

Platelets

Platelets contribute to normal hemostasis by adhering to subendothelial surfaces of injured vessels via receptors for von Willebrand factor, collagen, fibrinogen, fibronectin, and perhaps vitronectin, laminin, and thrombospondin (20,21). (Figure 14–3). Activation of platelets also occurs in response to high shear rate within high-flow vascular channels (22). High shear rate causes platelet activation, degranulation, and release of substances that promote activation of surrounding platelets (22). Adhesion activates the platelet, which then undergoes a conformational change exposing the GPIIb/IIIa surface receptor (20). The 40,000–80,000 GPIIb/IIIa receptors on each platelet bind to several proteins, including fibrinogen—the protein primarily responsible for platelet aggregation—and von Willebrand factor. Because fibrinogen and von Willebrand factor have multiple binding sites, they can bind to multiple platelets to cause cross-linking and platelet aggregation (20,23). Platelets release components that activate additional platelets that aggregate and form a growing thrombus (23). Activated platelets release substances including a_2-antiplasmin, plasminogen activator inhibitor-1 (PAI-1), fibrinogen, serotonin, calcium, epinephrine, and ADP, all

of which activate additional platelets (20,24). Platelets also secrete TXA_2, platelet factor 4 (a heparin inhibitor) and factor XIII, which stimulates fibrin cross-linking (24,25). Factor XIII has three antifibrinolytic properties: (1) it strongly promotes fibrin cross-linkages that in turn decrease the rate of fibrinolysis compared to non–cross-linked fibrin, (2) it accelerates cross-linking of a_2-antiplasmin to fibrin, and (3) it promotes cross-linkage of fibronectin to fibrin, in turn facilitating intrathrombic migration of fibroblasts (26). Fibronectin, a structural protein, provides a network along which fibroblasts can migrate into clot to subsequently form collagen (27).

Platelet-rich thrombi have been shown experimentally to be much more resistant to lysis than thrombi rich in red blood cells (RBCs) (28). The platelet-rich thrombi have significantly more fibrin fibers compared with platelet-poor areas, suggesting that the fibrin network is dramatically influenced by the presence of platelets (29). The lysis resistance of platelet-rich clots is related to a reduced r-tPA-binding rate (29). In vitro, GPIIb/IIIa inhibitors have been shown to improve fibrinolysis by uncoupling fibrin from platelet-integrin receptors and promoting fibrinolysis at the platelet-fibrin interface (29).

The platelet concentration and activity in clot vary considerably, and the factors influencing platelet concentration are poorly understood. Arterial thrombi are predominantly composed of platelets, while venous thrombi consist mainly of fibrin and RBCs (3). There tends to be increased platelet concentration at the leading edge of thrombi, as well as regions of concentrated platelets associated with dense fibrin (lines of Zahn) throughout thrombus. Intrathrombic platelets may be incompletely degranulated, suggesting that further activation and secretion may occur during thrombolysis, thus emphasizing the need for concomitant antiplatelet and antithrombic measures during thrombolysis.

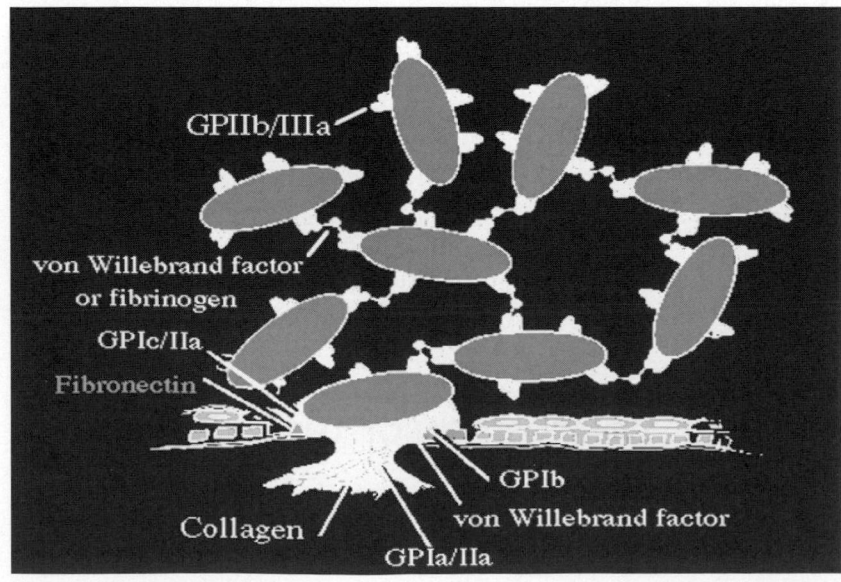

Figure 14–3 Platelet adhesion, activation, and aggregation. Platelets respond to the damage of the arterial wall that exposes collagen, tissue factor, and von Willebrand factor. The platelets adhere to the damaged area. Activation of the platelet occurs with the conformational change of the GPIIb/IIIa receptor. This allows binding to fibrinogen and von Willebrand factor. The binding results in cross-linking of the platelets and aggregation of platelets to form thrombus.

Maturation of Clot

Activation of platelets during fibrin formation results in platelets attaching to fibrin fibers, mediated at least partially by GPIIb/IIIa complex (23). Clot retraction is a dynamic process that leads to reorganization of the cytoskeleton formed by platelets. Clot retraction has been associated with moderately increased lysis resistance, perhaps secondary to shielding of tPA binding sites on fibrin. As the clot retracts, there is decreased binding of the tPA (29).

High platelet foci within the clot contribute significantly to the clinical problem of lysis resistance. Thrombi that form in the arterial system, in an area of rapidly flowing blood, often harbor foci of high platelet concentration, particularly at their leading edges or at sites of rupture of atherosclerosis (30). Upon gross examination, these foci are pale and, hence, are known as white thrombus. Clinically, the lysis-resistant portion of the clot often is situated at the proximal end of an arterial or graft thrombosis. When biopsied, this resistant material has revealed dense collections of fibrin and relatively few red cells, which are features typical of white thrombus (26).

The surface of a thrombus may have greater structural integrity than its depth. Relatively dense fibrin layers at or near the surface of thrombus have been described. There is also experimental evidence that the surface of a clot differs in composition from its deeper structure. It has been observed that the peripheral fibrin fibrils (termed *leptofibrils*) are finer and more tightly woven than the deeper fibrils (termed *pachyfibrils*) (26). It has been postulated that the decreased surface porosity retains intrathrombic thrombin and prevents ingress of plasminogen, plasminogen activators, or both, thus inhibiting thrombolysis..

The relative lysis resistance of the thrombic surface may partially explain the much greater efficacy of intrathrombic over parathrombic infusion of lytic agents. By breaking through a relatively resistant surface with a catheter, the lytic agent is deposited within less resistant thrombus. Dense strands of fibrin can be found throughout thrombus, also in relation to dense columnar accumulation of platelets, and these fibrin strands probably also interfere with the intrathrombic diffusion of fibrinolytic agents. By moving the catheter within thrombus using pulse-spray thrombolysis or combining thrombolytic agents with mechanical devices, diffusion barriers may be disrupted, allowing deposition of material throughout the clot.

It is generally assumed that older clots (>2 weeks) lyse much more slowly than younger ones and that they may become clinically unlysable. Diminished plasminogen concentration has been found in some experimentally aged clots, but other evidence indicates that the plasminogen concentration is adequate for lysis in both fresh and older human thrombi. Lysis resistance has been ascribed to the increase in cross-linkage of fibrin, but experimental evidence demonstrates only about 35–50% slower lysis of cross-linked as compared to non–cross-linked fibrin. As described above, retracted clots are less lysable than nonretracted clots. The markedly increased lysis resistance of platelet-rich clots has been commented on already, and it is possible that sequential layers of platelets bind to thrombus over time. Current postulates explaining relative lysis resistance of older thrombi include progressive binding of albumin to fibrin or early collagen deposition by fibroblasts migrating along fibronectin pathways. Once the clot has become organized with deposition of fibroblasts, the possibility of lysis will be severely reduced or eliminated.

THE DYNAMIC NATURE OF THROMBOLYSIS

There is a dynamic equilibrium between clot formation and clot dissolution and thrombolysis and concurrent rethrombosis. During thrombolysis, thrombin bound to fibrin is released as thrombin-bound FDP. This thrombin retains the capacity to convert fibrinogen to fibrin and is a potent platelet activator (22). Both thrombin and plasmin are powerful platelet activators so that platelet activation and all the sequelae described above are brought into play. Shear activation of platelets almost certainly occurs during pulse-spray methods of thrombolysis, and certainly with mechanical thrombolysis, along with destruction of red cells and the presumed release of platelet-activating ADP and other procoagulants. The use of antiplatelet agents may decrease the rate of recurrent thrombosis.

Preexisting systemic or local conditions also contribute to rethrombosis. Stressful clinical situations, such as myocardial infarction or severe ischemic leg pain, increase epinephrine levels. Epinephrine is an activator of platelets, and epinephrine levels may be related to the shortened bleeding times and aspirin resistance of patients with myocardial infarction. Finally, the underlying vascular conditions that initially predisposed to thrombosis, usually stenosis, exposed mural elements, or both, persist during and immediately following lysis.

To effect a successful thrombolytic procedure, the interventionalist must also be knowledgeable of all parts of the clot forming/clot dissolving equation. Although the coagulation and fibrinolytic cascades generally have been thought of as separate and independent, they are, in fact, linked (31). Thus, it is important to recognize the requirement to pharmacologically address not only the fibrinolytic aspect but also ongoing coagulation and platelet activation.

ANTICOAGULANTS

Fibrinolysis is involved in the breaking down of thrombus, but the process of breaking down thrombus simultaneously activates thrombogenesis. The presence of clot tends to stimulate continued clotting. Anticoagulant strategies are directed toward inhibiting thrombogenesis. These strategies focus primarily on inhibiting thrombin, preventing thrombin generation, or blocking initiation of coagulation (3). Thrombin inhibitors block thrombin activity, whereas agents that target clotting enzymes higher in the coagulation pathways prevent thrombin generation. Anticoagulant drugs suppress the synthesis or function of clotting factors and are used to control thromboembolic disorders.

Thrombin Inhibitors

Thrombin can be inactivated directly—by binding to thrombin and preventing its interaction with substrates. Alternatively, it can be inactivated indirectly—by activating naturally occurring thrombin inhibitors.

Warfarin (Coumadin) is an orally administered agent whose anticoagulant effect is mediated by vitamin K-dependent coagulation factors (32). Vitamin K is an essential cofactor mediating the posttranslational modification of coagulation factors II, VII, IX, and X, the process consisting of the carboxylation of glutamic acid (33). Vitamin K antagonists inhibit this process, thereby producing an anticoagulant effect (33). By exerting its effect on vitamin K-dependent coagulation cofactors, warfarin acts indirectly on the coagulation system and, as a result, has a slow onset of action (4). It also has a slow offset of action because of its long plasma half-life and the half-life of the affected vitamin K-dependent coagulation factors (4).

Heparin is a polymeric glucosaminoglycan. It is available as unfractionated and low–molecular-weight heparins that block thrombin formation and thrombin activity by activating antithrombin, which then complexes and inhibits thrombin and factor Xa (3,34,35). Heparin enhances the activity of antithrombin, and although antithrombin can bind to thrombin in the absence of heparin, the presence of heparin increases the rate more than 1,000-fold (33). Neither type of heparin can inactivate fibrin-bound thrombin or factor Xa bound to activated platelets within the thrombus.

Unfractionated heparin is heterogenous in its molecular size, anticoagulant effect, and pharmacokinetic properties. It also binds nonspecifically to plasma proteins, thereby limiting the amount of heparin available to interact with antithrombin, hepatic macrophages, osteoblasts and osteoclasts, and platelet factor 4—which can produce heparin-induced thrombocytopenia, or HIT (4).

Low–molecular-weight heparins (LMWHs) are derived from unfractionated heparin by chemical or enzymatic degradation (4). They are heterogenous in size, and their principal advantage over unfractionated heparin is that they are less likely to bind to plasma proteins and platelets, which results in a more predictable anticoagulant effect (4). LMWHs can also result in HIT and, with long-term treatment, may cause osteoporosis, but the risk of these

complications appears to be less than with unfractionated heparin.

Full systemic heparinization was commonly used during thrombolysis with UK. Because of concern for bleeding complications, however, heparin levels were kept to a minimum—almost a homeopathic dose when used with other thrombolytics.

Direct thrombin inhibitors have potential advantages over heparin. Thrombin bound to fibrin or fibrin degradation products is relatively protected from inactivation by heparin (3), but direct thrombin inhibitors readily inhibit both fluid- and clot-bound thrombin (3,36). Direct thrombin inhibitors produce a more predictable anticoagulant response than heparin because, unlike heparin, they do not bind to plasma proteins (3). Likewise, direct thrombin inhibitors are not neutralized by platelet factor 4, a highly cationic, heparin-binding protein released from activated platelets (3).

Direct thrombin inhibitors include hirudin and bivalirudin, a semisynthetic hirudin fragment. Both have been approved for clinical use.

Hirudin

Hirudin is a 65-amino acid polypeptide originally isolated from the salivary glands of the medical leech and is now available through recombinant DNA technology. The recombinant form is not sulfated at Tyr 63 and exhibits at least a 10-fold reduced affinity for thrombin (3). Hirudin is a potent and specific inhibitor of thrombin that forms a slowly reversible complex with the enzyme (3). The almost irreversible nature of this complex is a potential weakness of this drug, because no antidote is available should bleeding occur. Hirudin is predominantly cleared by the kidneys and undergoes little hepatic metabolism. It has a plasma half-life of 40 minutes after IV administration and approximately 120 minutes after subcutaneous injection. Hirudin has been used successfully to treat patients with arterial and venous thrombotic complications of heparin-induced thrombocytopenia. The narrow therapeutic window of hirudin limits its utility as an adjunct to thrombolytic therapy.

Bivalirudin

Bivalirudin is a semisynthetic, bivalent thrombin inhibitor. Unlike hirudin, bivalirudin produces only transient inhibition of the active site of thrombin because once bound to thrombin an Arg3-Pro4 bond is cleaved, converting bivalirudin into a lower-affinity inhibitor and reexposing the catalytic center of thrombin (36). The shorter half-life of bivalirudin may make it safer than hirudin. Only a fraction of bivalirudin is renally excreted, suggesting that hepatic metabolism and proteolysis at other sites contribute to its clearance (3). Because renal excretion is not important, bivalirudin is appropriate for patients with compromised renal function. Its stable antithrombotic effect allows it to be administered as a constant infusion.

Other Thrombin Inhibitors

Many other thrombin inhibitors are being investigated. These include natural thrombin inhibitors, such as tick anticoagulant peptide (TAP)—a potent and specific inhibitor of factor Xa (4). A synthetic pentasaccharide with an indirect factor Xa inhibitor, TAP has a rapid onset of action with peak concentrations at 2 hours and a plasma half-life of about 15 hours (4). Noncovalent inhibitors bind noncovalently to the active site of thrombin and act as a competitive inhibitor. Argatroban is a noncovalent inhibitor that has been used as an alternative to heparin in patients with heparin-induced thrombocytopenia and has been approved for this indication. Inhibitors of the factor VIIa/tissue factor complex are undergoing experimentation (4). Other approaches include covalent inhibitors and double-stranded DNA aptamers (3). These various types of inhibitors are undergoing scientific investigations but are not in clinical use at the present time.

ANTIPLATELET AGENTS

Platelets play a major role in causing thrombus formation. They are activated not only by vessel injury but by other factors, including the placement of catheters, balloons, and stents and the process of thrombolysis (36). In thrombolysis, clot-bound thrombin is exposed, resulting in the activation of platelets and initiation of the coagulation cascade, both of which incite new thrombus formation at the same site (37). When thrombogenesis proceeds more quickly than thrombolysis, thrombosis recurs. Inactivating platelets is an important adjuvant therapy to pharmacologic thrombolysis. Antiplatelet agents can augment the rate of thrombus dissolution leading to a reduction in the incidence of recurrent thrombosis (37).

Aspirin

Aspirin irreversibly inhibits the function of cyclooxygenase in platelets by affecting the biosynthesis of thromboxane A2, resulting in the inhibition of platelet aggregation (20,33). Aspirin can reduce the incidence of recurrent thrombosis after interventions. Administered orally, aspirin is absorbed rapidly, with appreciable concentrations in the plasma in less than 30 minutes (38). After a single dose, a peak value is reached in about 2 hours, then gradually declines (38). Although aspirin is cleared from the body within hours, its effects on the platelets are irreversible and, thus, last for the life of the platelet (39).

A number of studies have demonstrated that aspirin enhances fibrinolysis, although other studies have either not shown a benefit or have suggested a negative effect

(24). Some laboratory evidence suggests that the effect of aspirin may be dose dependent and that timing may also be important (24).

Thienopyridines

Oral thienopyridines, including ticlopidine—brand name Ticlid (Roche)—and clopidogrel—brand name Plavix (Sanofi)—are inhibitors of ADP-induced platelet aggregation acting by direct inhibition of ADP binding to its receptor and of the subsequent ADP-mediated activation of the GPIIb/IIIa complex. They act by irreversibly modifying the platelet ADP receptor, so the platelets exposed are affected for the remainder of their lifespan.

Cilostazol

Cilostazol, brand name Pletal (Otsuka America), inhibits the phosphodiesterase pathway, acting as a cyclic AMP (cAMP) phosphodiesterase III inhibitor. This results in an increase of cAMP in platelets, leading to inhibition of platelet aggregation. This inhibition of platelet aggregation is reversible. This agent also causes dilation of vascular beds, which makes it effective in treating patients with claudication. Dipyridamole, or Persantine (Boehringer Ingelheim), also works by this mechanism.

GPIIb/IIIa Receptor Inhibitors

GPIIb/IIIa receptors are the final common pathway for platelet aggregation. When platelets are activated, the 40,000–80,000 GPIIb/IIIa receptors bind fibrinogen and von Willebrand's factor to form the thrombus (40). Inhibition of the GPIIb/IIIa receptor can prevent platelet aggregation and thus inhibit thrombus formation. There are two general classes of GPIIb/IIIa receptor inhibitors: the immunoglobulins (50,000 daltons) and the small molecules (molecular weight 500–800 daltons) (30). Abciximab is the only clinically available antagonist in the immunoglobulin class (30). The second class of antagonists, the small molecules, consists of eptifibatide and tirofiban (30). The immunoglobulins bind tightly to the receptor with a relatively long period of dissociation, and the small molecules move from one receptor to another, accounting for a shorter half-life compared to the immunoglobulins (30). The difference in binding is important in the event of a bleeding complication. The effects of abciximab can be rapidly reversed by platelet transfusions, but the effect of the small molecules cannot be reversed by platelet transfusions (30). The smaller molecules are mostly excreted by the kidneys, and the dose must be adjusted in patients with renal insufficiency (20).

Some early studies using GPIIb/IIIa receptor inhibitors in peripheral vascular disease were performed suggesting that the addition of a systemically administered abciximab may result in increased fibrinolytic efficacy without decreased patient safety (37,40,41).

GPIIb/IIIa receptor inhibitors may also have an antithrombin effect. Abciximab has been shown to dramatically decrease thrombus formation, and adding heparin in the doses usually used for coronary interventions has not had any further reduction in mural thrombus (42).

Abciximab

Abciximab, or ReoPro (Centocor) is a Fab fragment of the chimeric human-mouse monoclonal antibody 7E3. Following IV bolus administration, free plasma concentrations decrease rapidly with a half-life of 10–30 minutes. Platelet function generally recovers within 48 hours, although abciximab remains in the circulation for up to 10 days in a platelet-bound state. Because abciximab circulates for such a long period of time, it may prevent platelet adhesion during the healing process following thrombolysis and angioplasty (14).

Tirofiban

Tirofiban, or Aggrastat (Merck), is a highly selective non-peptide that inhibits ex vivo platelet aggregation in a dose-dependent and concentration-dependent manner. Inhibition persists over the duration of the maintenance infusion and is reversible within 4 hours following infusion. Its half-life is approximately 2 hours.

Eptifibatide

Eptifibatide, or Integrilin (Schering-Plough and COR Therapeutics), is a cyclic heptapeptide with a rapid onset of action (15 minutes). Complete reversal of antiplatelet effects occurs within 4 hours after infusion is stopped. Antithrombotic effects are dose dependent and related to duration of drug administration. It has a plasma half-life of 50–60 minutes in healthy volunteers and 90–120 minutes in elective coronary intervention patients.

Several small studies have evaluated the use of concomitant thrombolysis and the GPIIb/IIIa inhibitors in the peripheral vascular system. These have demonstrated an increased rate of thrombolysis, a decrease in the rate of embolization, and a decreased requirement for surgery without a statistically significant increase in the risk of bleeding (37,40,43,44).

Effective Thrombolysis

Because of clinical observations of concurrent and immediate postthrombolytic rethrombosis, as well as theoretical reasons for a local hypercoagulant state at the site of thrombolysis, antithrombin and antiplatelet measures during thrombolysis have been investigated extensively and now are being incorporated into thrombolytic regimens. Heparin has been shown to accelerate thrombolysis in vitro. Other

thrombin inhibitors, such as hirudin, may be even more effective than heparin. For a long time, aspirin has been used in conjunction with thrombolysis, despite the fact that the benefits may only be moderate; on the other hand, the risk and costs are low. Other antiplatelet agents may significantly augment the rate of thrombolysis by inhibiting the platelet receptors that are involved with thrombosis. Combinations of drugs used in an experimental evaluation of tPA admixed with heparin and PGE_1 (an antiplatelet agent) demonstrated significant advantage over intravenous or nonuse of the adjuvant agents in accelerating thrombolysis.

Experimental, as well as clinical observations, indicate that anticoagulant and antiplatelet therapy should be used during thrombolysis. Heparin can be used liberally with UK thrombolysis but should be used much more cautiously with tPA. Heparin can and should be mixed with UK usually at a dose of 5,000 units admixed with 250,000 units of UK. The mixture of heparin and tPA is not recommended by the manufacturer because of possible precipitation. This may be more of a theoretical concern; one thousand units of heparin have been mixed with 2 mg of tPA on numerous occasions with no evidence of precipitation being witnessed. The rationale for the intrathrombic use of heparin is to activate intrathrombic antithrombin-III. Systemic activated clotting times (ACTs) should be checked during the procedure, particularly when thrombolysis is progressing slowly or rethrombosis becomes evident. The patients should also receive aspirin shortly before the procedure, and depending on the clinical circumstances, the use of GPIIb/IIIa antiplatelet agents should be considered.

Delayed Rethrombosis

In addition to concurrent rethrombosis, delayed rethrombosis may occur within hours or days of technically successful thrombolysis (22). The factors leading to delayed rethrombosis are probably similar to those leading to concurrent rethrombosis. They include: (1) the continued presence of the initiating vascular lesion, (2) incompletely lysed thrombus yielding partial obstruction and enhanced platelet adhesion, (3) residual activation of platelets and clotting factors secondary to thrombolysis, (4) gradual waning of anticoagulant effects of heparin or fibrin(ogen) degradation products, and (5) discontinuance of anticoagulant or antiplatelet therapy (45). Rethrombosis occurs in inverse frequency to the plasma half-life of the fibrinolytic, with the lowest incidence associated with APSAC and urokinase (about 10%), intermediate frequency with SK (about 15%), and the highest incidence with tPA (20%). This emphasizes the importance of regimens directed against rethrombosis, including continuing thrombolysis until as much thrombus as possible has been lysed, early angioplasty/stenting, and use of anticoagulants or antiplatelet agents. Several investigators have reported a significantly reduced incidence of rethrombosis with combined use of tPA and UK.

PERFORMANCE OF SELECTIVE THROMBOLYSIS

In 1974, Dotter et al. suggested selective transcatheter parathrombic infusion of thrombolytic agent. The method enabled lower doses of SK than systemic administration, with augmented safety and efficacy. Selective administration proved much more effective than systemic administration in the management of peripheral vascular occlusion. Early reports after systemic administration of SK demonstrated restoration of patency in only 9–24% of arterial occlusion and required infusions of 1–3 days duration. Dotter's results were much superior to these systemic infusion results, and they made systemic infusion obsolete for peripheral occlusion.

Although parathrombic injection with SK seemed to be an improvement, it still resulted in a significant failure rate of 25%, a high rate of complications approximately 33%, and long lysis times with a mean of 38 hours. In 1985, McNamara described a modified method for selective thrombolysis using intrathrombic infusion of UK and intermittent catheter advancement as the thrombolysis progressed. Lysis times were reduced to 18 ± 20 hours, the failure rate to 17%, and hemorrhagic complications to 4%.

Pulse-spray pharmacomechanical thrombolysis (PSPMT) was then popularized. In vitro experiments demonstrated (1) no relative advantage of SK, UK, tPA or plasmin when used in equimolar concentrations, (2) a significant advantage of high concentrations of UK or tPA but not SK, and (3) a significant advantage of clot maceration. PSPMT involves placement of a multi–side-hole catheter into the clot, followed by high-pressure pulsed injection of concentrated fibrinolytic agent through the catheter. This technique markedly augments the speed, efficacy, and safety of clinical thrombolysis. PSPMT efficacy and speed are increased with the concomitant use of thrombin inhibitors and antiplatelet agents. Admixture of heparin with the thrombolytic, as well as systemic administration of heparin and aspirin, speeds the process.

The principles of PSPMT are as follows:

1. Penetrating intrathrombic injections of fibrinolytic spray to macerate clot and increase the interactive surface area, as well as to penetrate the lysis-resistant surface membranes of the thrombus
2. Circulatory isolation of thrombolytic agents to minimize dilution, inhibition of fibrinolysis by plasmin inhibitors in plasma, and systemic effects
3. Simultaneous treatment of the entire thrombus to increase the rate of lysis
4. Concentrated agent to increase the rate of lysis and to overwhelm intrathrombic inhibitors
5. Intrathrombic heparin and systemic antiplatelet agents to significantly inhibit concurrent rethrombosis
6. Small pulse volumes (0.2–0.4 mL) and briefly delayed treatment of small distal plug of thrombus to minimize embolization
7. Transluminal angioplasty, stenting, or both to eliminate residual luminal compromise and to promote flow after lysis has reached a plateau

Other methods of delivering concentrated thrombolytics intrathrombic have also been popularized, including the lyse-and-wait technique described by Cynamon (46), the lyse-and-go technique described by Semba (16), and other techniques that combine pharmacologic agents with mechanical devices.

The use of mechanical devices for recanalization of clotted structures—arteries, veins, and dialysis grafts—has become popular, and several devices have been approved by the Food and Drug Administration (FDA) for mechanical thrombectomy. By and large, these devices have been tested and approved for treatment of thrombosed hemodialysis grafts, but off-label use of these devices in peripheral arteries and veins is not uncommon. These devices have several mechanisms of action. Some create vortex with suction to circulate fluid within the graft. These devices circulate fluid within the graft and aspirate thrombus by using suction (47). Others create a vortex without suction so that the clot is pulverized but not aspirated (47). Still other devices that use wall contact macerate the clot by using mechanical components to emulsify the thrombus. They may or may not have a suction component. There is a perception, supported by a few small studies, that mechanical devices may increase the removal of a clot. Use of such devices should be accompanied by consideration of the effect of these devices on platelets and the coagulation pathways. These devices will definitely cause major activation of platelets as well as a stimulation of coagulation by all of the mechanisms just outlined. The use of these devices should be accompanied by use of antiplatelet agents and antithrombotics. In some cases, consideration should be given to the use of thrombolytics for a combination approach.

Chapter 15 elaborates further on the clinical aspects of thrombolysis, emphasizing details of the methodology, results, and complications.

REFERENCES

1. Mann KG. Thrombin formation. Chest 2003;124:4S–10S.
2. Verstraete M. Biology and chemistry of thrombosis. In: Haber E, Braunwald E, eds. Thrombolysis: Basic Contributions and Clinical Problems. St. Louis: Mosby Year Book, 1991;3–16.
3. Weitz JI, Hirsh J. New anticoagulant drugs. Chest 2001;119:95S–107S.
4. Hirsh J. Current anticoagulant therapy—unmet clinical needs. Thromb Res 2003;109 (SupplI):S1–8.
5. Spronk HM, Govers-Riemslag JW, ten Cate H. The blood coagulation system as a molecular machine. Bioessays 2003;25:1220–1228.
6. Norris LA. Blood coagulation. Best Pract Res Clin Obstet Gynaecol 2003;17:369–383.
7. Mosesson MW, Siebenlist KR, Meh DA. The structure and biological features of fibrinogen and fibrin. Ann N Y Acad Sci 2001;936:11–30.
8. Bell WR. Present-day thrombolytic therapy: therapeutic agents—pharmacokinetics and pharmacodynamics. Rev Cardiovasc Med 2002;(Suppl II)2:S34–44.

9. Nieuwenhuizen W. Fibrin-mediated plasminogen activation. Ann N Y Acad Sci 2001;936:237–246.

10. Collen D. The plasminogen (fibrinolytic) system. Thromb Haemost 1999;82:259–270.

11. Swischuk JL, Fox PF, Young K, et al. Transcatheter intra-arterial infusion of rt-PA for acute lower limb ischemia: results and complications. J Vasc Interv Radiol 2001;12:423–430.

12. Semba CP, Bakal CW, Calis KA, et al. Alteplase as an alternative to urokinase. Advisory Panel on Catheter-Directed Thrombolytic Therapy. J Vasc Interv Radiol 2000;11:279–287.

13. Smalling RW. Pharmacological and clinical impact of the unique molecular structure of a new plasminogen activator. Eur Heart J 1997;18(Suppl F):F11–16.

14. Benenati JF, Shlansky-Goldberg R, Meglin A, et al. Thrombolytic and antiplatelet therapy in peripheral vascular disease with use of reteplase and/or abciximab. The SCVIR Consultants' Conference; May 22, 2000; Orlando, FL. Society for Cardiovascular and Interventional Radiology. J Vasc Interv Radiol 2001;12:795–805.

15. Castaneda F, Swischuk JL, Li R, et al. Declining-dose study of reteplase treatment for lower extremity arterial occlusions. J Vasc Interv Radiol 2002;13:1093–1098.

16. Semba CP, Sugimoto K, Razavi MK. Alteplase and tenecteplase: applications in the peripheral circulation. Tech Vasc Interv Radiol 2001;4:99–106.

17. Razavi MK, Wong H, Kee ST, et al. Initial clinical results of tenecteplase (TNK) in catheter-directed thrombolytic therapy. J Endovasc Ther 2002;9:593–598.

18. Weitz JI. Limited fibrin specificity of tissue-type plasminogen activator and its potential link to bleeding. J Vasc Interv Radiol 1995;6:19S–23S.

19. Goto S. Understanding the mechanism and prevention of arterial occlusive thrombus formation by anti-platelet agents. Curr Med Chem Cardiovasc Hematol Agents 2004;2:149–156.

20. Shlansky-Goldberg R. Platelet aggregation inhibitors for use in peripheral vascular interventions: what can we learn from the experience in the coronary arteries? J Vasc Interv Radiol 2002;13:229–246.

21. Patel D, Vaananen H, Jirouskova M, et al. Dynamics of GPIIb/IIIa-mediated platelet-platelet interactions in platelet adhesion/thrombus formation on collagen in vitro as revealed by videomicroscopy. Blood 2003;101:929–936.

22. Ouriel K. Use of concomitant glycoprotein IIb/IIIa inhibitors with catheter-directed peripheral arterial thrombolysis. J Vasc Interv Radiol 2004;15:543–546.

23. Mondoro TH, White MM, Jennings LK. Active GPIIb-IIIa conformations that link ligand interaction with cytoskeletal reorganization. Blood 2000;96:2487–2495.

24. Buczko W, Mogielnicki A, Kramkowski K, et al. Aspirin and the fibrinolytic response. Thromb Res 2003;110:331–334.

25. Coller BS. Role of platelets in thrombolytic therapy. In: Haber E, Braunwald E, eds. Thrombolysis: Basic Contributions and Clinical Progress. St. Louis: Mosby Year Book, 1991;155–178.

26. Bookstein JJ, Valji K. Principles of selective thrombolysis. In: Baum S, ed. Abrams' Angiography. 4th Ed. Boston: Little, Brown, and Company 1997;119–131.

27. Mirshahi M, Azzarone B, Soria J, et al. The role of fibroblasts in organization and degradation of a fibrin clot. J Lab Clin Med 1991;117:274–281.

28. Jang IK, Gold HK, Ziskind AA, et al. Differential sensitivity of erythrocyte-rich and platelet-rich arterial thrombi to lysis with recombinant tissue-type plasminogen activator. A possible explanation for resistance to coronary thrombolysis. Circulation 1989;79:920–928.

29. Collet JP, Montalescot G, Lesty C, et al. A structural and dynamic investigation of the facilitating effect of glycoprotein IIb/IIIa inhibitors in dissolving platelet-rich clots. Circ Res 2002;90:428–434.

30. Ouriel K. The use of glycoprotein IIb/IIIa antagonists in peripheral arterial occlusion. Tech Vasc Interv Radiol 2001;4:107–110.

31. Nesheim M. Thrombin and fibrinolysis. Chest 2003;124:33S–39S.

32. Hirsh J. Oral anticoagulant drugs. N Engl J Med 1991;324:1865–1875.

33. Labuzek K, Krysiak R, Okopien B, et al. Progress in pharmacotherapy of thrombosis. Pol J Pharmacol 2003;55:523–533.

34. Weitz JI. Low molecular weight heparins. N Engl J Med 1997;337.

35. Hirsh J. Heparin. N Engl J Med 1991;324:1565–1574.

36. Antman EM. Should bivalirudin replace heparin during percutaneous coronary interventions? JAMA 2003;289:903–905.

37. Ouriel K, Castaneda F, McNamara T, et al. Reteplase monotherapy and reteplase/abciximab combination therapy in peripheral arterial occlusive disease: results from the RELAX trial. J Vasc Interv Radiol 2004;15:229–238.

38. Flower RJ, Moncada S, Vane JR. Analgesic-antipyretics and anti-inflammatory agents: drugs employed in the treatment of gout. In: Gilman AG, Goodman LS, Rall TW, Murad F, eds. The Pharmacological Basis of Therapeutics. 7th Ed. New York: Macmillian, 1985;674–715.

39. O'Reilly RA. Anticoagulant, antithrombotic and thrombolytic drugs. In: Gilman AG, Goodman LS, Rall TW, Murad F, eds. The Pharmacological Basis of Therapeutics. New York: Macmillan, 1985;1338–1359.

40. Drescher P, Crain MR, Rilling WS. Initial experience with the combination of reteplase and abciximab for thrombolytic therapy in peripheral arterial occlusive disease: a pilot study. J Vasc Interv Radiol 2002;13:37–43.

41. Tepe G, Schott U, Erley CM, et al. Platelet glycoprotein IIb/IIIa receptor antagonist used in conjunction with thrombolysis for peripheral arterial thrombosis. AJR Am J Roentgenol 1999;172:1343–1346.

42. Hayes R, Chesebro JH, Fuster V, et al. Antithrombotic effects of abciximab. Am J Cardiol 2000;85:1167–1172.

43. Duda SH, Tepe G, Luz O, et al. Peripheral artery occlusion: treatment with abciximab plus urokinase versus with urokinase alone—a randomized pilot trial (the PROMPT Study). Platelet Receptor Antibodies in Order to Manage Peripheral Artery Thrombosis. Radiology 2001;221:689–696.

44. Hull JE, Hull MK, Urso JA. Reteplase with or without abciximab for peripheral arterial occlusions: efficacy and adverse events. J Vasc Interv Radiol 2004;15:557–564.

45. Cannon CP. Combination therapy for acute myocardial infarction: glycoprotein IIb/IIIa inhibitors plus thrombolysis. Clin Cardiol 1999;22:IV37–43.

46. Cynamon J, Lakritz PS, Wahl SI, et al. Hemodialysis graft declotting: description of the "lyse and wait" technique. J Vasc Interv Radiol 1997;8:825–829.

47. Gibbens DT, Triolo J, Yu T, et al. Contemporary treatment of thrombosed hemodialysis grafts. Tech Vasc Interv Radiol 2001;4:122–126.

Thrombolysis: Clinical Applications

15

Anne Roberts

The pharmacologic dissolution of thrombus is a widely practiced and accepted method for treating vascular occlusions in both the arterial and venous systems. Increased understanding of the fibrinolytic process, the effect of exogenous plasminogen activators, the adjuvant use of anticoagulants and antiplatelet agents, and the development of catheter and mechanical thrombolytic systems have allowed for faster and safer thrombolytic procedures.

The scientific principles and pharmacology of thrombolysis are discussed in Chapter 14. This chapter considers clinical applications of transcatheter thrombolysis.

Arterial and venous thromboses are major causes of morbidity and mortality. In the peripheral vascular system, arterial thrombosis can lead to stroke, claudication, and gangrene. Venous thrombosis can result in dialysis graft failure, pulmonary embolism, and the postthrombotic syndrome. These thrombotic problems can be treated appropriately by thrombolysis.

INDICATIONS

Thrombolytic therapy, often in conjunction with supplementary transcatheter or operative procedures, is appropriate for the following conditions (1):

- Iliac artery occlusions of any length or age in patients with severe claudication, ischemic rest pain, or tissue loss (Rutherford class I-3, II, or III)
- Short (2–20 cm) infrainguinal arterial occlusions of any age in patients with Rutherford class I-3, II, or III symptoms
- Acute peripheral arterial or bypass graft occlusions of any length in the presence of demonstrable runoff vessels

- Upper extremity arterial thromboses of any length or age
- Acute thromboses that occur during diagnostic angiography or transcatheter therapy
- Thrombosed hemodialysis access grafts
- Symptomatic upper extremity venous occlusions
- Symptomatic IVC, iliac, and lower extremity venous thrombosis
- Pulmonary artery embolism in patients with impending cardiorespiratory collapse
- Intracranial arterial thrombosis causing stroke—in selected patients and in the appropriate time frame
- Intracranial venous thrombosis, such as superior sagittal sinus thrombosis
- Treatment of occluded catheters

Thrombolytic therapy is occasionally performed in other vascular beds, such as the aorta, renal arteries and veins, and mesenteric arteries, but the published experience has been limited and the relative benefits and risks in these settings have not been established.

The decision to attempt thrombolysis is based on several factors, including the patient's symptoms, the location and anatomy of the lesion, an assessment of the relative benefit and risk of the procedure compared with alternative therapies and the contraindications to thrombolysis. As a rule, transcatheter therapy has been considered when surgical intervention is indicated. However, because of the lower morbidity and mortality associated with thrombolysis, indications for percutaneous treatment have been liberalized—for example, treatment of peripheral arterial occlusion in patients with mild to moderate claudication, symptomatic upper extremity venous occlusion, symptomatic lower extremity venous occlusion, and stroke therapy. Thrombolysis may be preferable to surgical intervention in patients at high operative risk, in peripheral bypass graft candidates without a suitable autologous vein, and in patients with infection at the proposed operative site without infection in the vicinity of the occluded vessel. Catheter-directed thrombolysis has the theoretical and practical advantages over thromboembolectomy of decreasing endothelial trauma, uncovering the underlying lesions, and visualizing the arterial runoff vessels (2)

CONTRAINDICATIONS

Thrombolysis should be avoided in patients at increased risk for bleeding from the use of anticoagulants or fibrinolytic agents, including:

- Recent intracranial, thoracic, or abdominal surgery
- Recent major trauma
- Recent gastrointestinal hemorrhage
- Recent stroke or presence of intracranial neoplasm
- Pregnancy
- Severe hypertension
- Bleeding diathesis

However, even some of these contraindications must be considered relative and the use of thrombolytics decided in the context of the patient's clinical situation. The major absolute contraindications are an intracranial process, such as hemorrhagic strokes, surgery, trauma, and tumor, within the last 3 months, active bleeding diathesis, and ongoing gastrointestinal bleeding (3).

Patients with suspected infection at the site of thrombosis should not be treated with thrombolytic agents. The sites most likely to harbor infected thrombus include hemodialysis access grafts, the anastomoses of peripheral bypass grafts, and upper extremity and thoracic veins containing vascular access catheters. Infected clot appears to be relatively resistant to exogenous fibrinolytic agents. More importantly, lysis of infected clot may cause systemic sepsis (4).

Patients with profound ischemia from acute arterial or bypass graft occlusion are at high risk for limb loss. Signs of irreversible ischemia include severe pain, gross sensorimotor deficits, lack of arterial or venous Doppler signal, and laboratory evidence of muscle necrosis, including myoglobinuria. Rapid treatment is critical for limiting the amputation level and decreasing mortality; in most instances, thrombolysis is contraindicated because of the time required to open the vessels. Revascularization of patients with profound ischemia may be life threatening because a reperfusion syndrome may occur, manifested by acidosis, hyperkalemia, myoglobinuria leading to renal failure, hemodynamic instability, and death (2). Primary amputation is preferred for patients with irreversible ischemia or when revascularization of the severely ischemic limb could jeopardize the patient's life (3).

In situ thrombosis, in the absence of underlying obstructive disease, is often the result of the presence of a hypercoagulable state. Such occlusions may not benefit from thrombolytic therapy unless the coagulation defect can be temporarily corrected or alleviated.

CHOICE OF FIBRINOLYTIC AGENT

The fibrinolytic agents are discussed thoroughly in Chapter 14. When treating either arterial, venous or dialysis occlusions, the choice of a thrombolytic drug depends on the comfort level of the operator administering the drug. Familiarity with the thrombolytic dosing appropriate for the chosen drug and for the site being treated is very important. Streptokinase (SK) has largely been supplanted by other thrombolytics in the United States. Urokinase (UK) is available, but the manufacturer may discontinue the production of this agent. Tissue plasminogen activator (TPA, alteplase) and the other modifications of tissue plasminogen activators (RPA, reteplase and TNK, tenecteplase) are available, and it is anticipated that more fibrinolytics will be developed in the future.

Although differences exist in the pharmacology and biologic behavior of the plasminogen activators, the complex and tightly regulated endogenous hemostasis/thrombosis system of the human body may minimize the clinical impact of these differences (5). Definitive conclusions regarding the superiority of one agent over another are difficult to establish based on the available literature, and this is magnified by discrepancies in the reporting of methods and results in the literature (5).

METHODS OF THROMBOLYSIS

Different methods of infusing thrombolytics abound, which makes comparing various reports difficult. The Working Party on Thrombolysis in the Management of Limb Ischemia has defined the following methods of delivery (3):

- Systemic intravenous infusion—Intravenous administration of a thrombolytic agent through a peripheral vein
- Regional intra-arterial infusion—Nonselective administration; the catheter is positioned proximal to the occluded vessel. With selective administration, the end of the catheter is within the occluded artery, but its tip is proximal to the thrombus.
- Intrathrombus infusion—The catheter tip is embedded within the thrombus
- Intrathrombus bolusing or lacing—Refers to the initial intrathrombic delivery of a concentrated lytic agent with a view toward saturating the thrombus with the thrombolytic. The catheter (with end hole or with multiple

side holes) is positioned in the distal part of thrombus and retracted proximally as the thrombolytic agent is delivered along the length of the thrombus.

- Stepwise infusion—The catheter tip is placed in the proximal thrombus and lytic agent is infused. As the thrombus dissolves, the catheter is advanced and the process is repeated until the thrombus has dissolved.
- Continuous infusion—Infusion of lytic agent through the catheter using a constant infusion pump; may or may not be preceded by intrathrombus lacing
- Graded infusion—Periodic tapering of the infusion rate with the highest doses given within the first few hours
- Pulse spray infusion—Forceful injection of the lytic agent into the thrombus to increase the working surface area available for the thrombolytic drug
- Pharmacomechanical thrombolysis—Combination of mechanical thrombus disruption with concomitant infiltration of a lytic agent. Pulse spray catheters, balloons designed for local drug delivery, and other mechanical devices can achieve disruption.

Infusion Thrombolysis

The techniques of thrombolysis have steadily evolved over the years. Originally, administration of an intravenous, systemic thrombolytic was the method of clot dissolution. However, systemic intravenous infusion for most peripheral uses has been abandoned because the success rates are lower and the complication rates are higher (2,3).

Dotter et al. (6) suggested selective transcatheter parathrombic infusion of thrombolytics in 1974, allowing lower doses of thrombolytics with improved safety and efficacy. Selective administration has proved to be more effective than intravenous administration in the management of peripheral vascular occlusion (2).

The current techniques for infusion thrombolysis are modified versions of the method originally described by McNamara and Fischer (7). Once the occlusion has been crossed with a guide wire, a therapeutic catheter is placed for infusion. Thrombolysis may be performed with an end-hole catheter embedded in the proximal clot at the top of the obstruction, a multi–side-hole catheter or wire within the clot for intrathrombic infusion, or a coaxial system for split infusion at the proximal and midportions of the occlusion. Intrathrombic infusions optimize the delivery of fibrinolytic agent into the clot. The inability to embed a catheter into the proximal thrombus may be predictive of failure of lysis (8,9). Before infusion, thrombolysis may be initiated by lacing the thrombus with a thrombolytic agent or by performing pulse spray of the thrombolytic agent into the thrombus. Sullivan et al. demonstrated more rapid lysis with a lower overall thrombolytic requirement after initial lacing of thrombi with large doses of thrombolytic before infusing (10–13).

The dose of thrombolytic depends on the thrombolytic agent being used. Table 15-1 gives some commonly used protocols for infusion thrombolysis. The dosages in this table are largely from consensus documents, and as knowledge of thrombolytics improves, these doses undoubtedly will change.

Fibrinogen levels are commonly monitored when TPA is being infused—fibrinogen levels are less likely to become abnormal when UK is the infused agent (14). However, in an individual patient, there is no clear association between the results of any single coagulation or fibrinolytic test and bleeding (3). A low fibrinogen level marks an increased bleeding risk but does not accurately predict hemorrhage, and patients bleed in the presence of a normal fibrinogen level (3,14).

Pulse Spray/Pharmacomechanical Thrombolysis

Acceleration of thrombolysis by forceful pulsed injection of fibrinolytic agents directly into clot has been observed in vitro, in animal experiments, and in clinical applications (15–18). Once the occlusion is traversed with a guide wire, a pulse spray catheter is placed within the thrombus (Figure 15-1). A number of pulse spray systems are commercially available. The essential element of a pulse spray system is a noncompliant catheter with very small side slits or side holes. The active catheter length (length of distal catheter with side slits) is chosen on the basis of the length of the occlusion. The catheter initially is placed with the tip about 1–2 cm above the bottom of the occlusion to leave a small, untreated segment of clot. This plug may prevent embolization of large clot fragments in the early stages of thrombolysis. The catheter is advanced later to treat this distal segment. The end hole is obstructed with a wire that occludes the catheter tip, and the catheter is fitted with a hemostatic valve. The system is purged of air using heparinized saline.

The thrombolytic agent is prepared, usually diluting the agent in a total of approximately 10 cc solution. The solution is injected through the catheter by forceful manual thrusts of a tuberculin syringe in 0.2–0.3 mL increments every 20–30 seconds. Care is taken to keep air bubbles out of the system. Angiograms are used to monitor the progress of lysis. A suitable endpoint for thrombolytic therapy can be defined when serial angiograms show no change in the appearance of residual disease after treatment with additional doses of fibrinolytic agent. The underlying disease may be treated safely at this point with a balloon catheter, provided that large intraluminal filling defects are not present.

Residual disease found after thrombolysis may represent organized clot, lysis-resistant clot, atherosclerotic plaque, intimal hyperplasia, or embolus composed of one or more of these materials. Mural disease can be treated with balloon angioplasty with little risk of distal embolization. Large residual intraluminal material also can be treated by angioplasty but with increased risk of distal embolization. Surgical thrombectomy may be warranted in such cases, particularly when the distal vessels are severely compromised.

TABLE 15-1

DOSAGE SCHEMES FOR CATHETER THROMBOLYSIS

Peripheral Arterial Thrombolysis

Agent	Schemes	Comments	References
Stepwise Infusion			
UK	3,000–4,000 units every 3–5 minutes	Very labor intensive	(3)
Continuous Infusion			
UK (low dose)	Variable up to 100,000 units/hr	Usually 60,000–100,000 units/hr	(3)
UK (high dose)	Mainly graded infusion (see below)		
TPA (alteplase)		Maximum infused dose should not exceed 100 mg	(3)
Weight-based dosing	0.001–0.02 mg/kg per hr	Recommend not to exceed 2 mg/hr	(31)
Non–weight-based dosing	0.12–2.0 mg/hr	Recommend limiting total dose to ≤40 mg	(31)
RPA (reteplase)	0.25–1.0 units/hr	±Initial bolus of 2–5 units Maximum total dose 20 units	(32)
TNK (tenecteplase)	0.25 mg/hr	Initial bolus of 5 mg in 3 mL normal saline Heparin not given	(40) **Pilot study**
Graded Infusion			
UK	4,000 units/min to antegrade flow 1,000 units/min to complete lysis		(3)
	4,000 units/min for 2 hr 2,000 units/min for next 2 hr 1,000 units/min to complete lysis		(3)
Intrathrombus Bolus			
UK	60,000–250,000 bolus followed by 4,000 units/min to antegrade flow 1,000 units/min to complete lysis 250,000 bolus followed by 50,000 units/hr		(3)
TPA	2–5 mg bolus		(3)
RPA	2–5 unit bolus		(32)
TNK	5 mg bolus		(40) **Pilot study**
Pulse Spray			
UK	25,000 units/mL at 0.2 mL every 30 sec for 20 min, every 60 sec thereafter		(3)
	25,000 units/10 cm of thrombus then graded infusion		(3)
TPA	0.5 mg/mL at 0.2 mL every 30 sec for 20 min, every 60 sec thereafter		(3)
Deep Venous Thrombosis			
UK	120,000 units/hr	Large range of infusion 40,000–400,000 units/hr	(177)
TPA	3–5 mg bolus directly into clot followed by continuous infusion 0.5 mg/hr	Infusion concentration 0.01 mg TPA/mL normal saline	(31)
RPA	0.5–1.0 units/hr	Some investigators trying 0.25 units/hr	(32)
TNK	5 mg in 3 mL bolus into clot followed by continuous infusion 0.25 mg/hr	Infusion 5 mg in 400 mL of normal saline (0.0125 mg/mL)	(40) **Pilot study**
Dialysis Graft			
UK	25,000 units/mL at 0.2 mL every 30 sec	250,000 units/10 mL of normal saline	(77)
TPA	1–2 mL diluted in 10 mL of normal saline	Pulse spray or "lyse and wait"	(31)
RPA	1–5 units/10 mL	Pulse spray or "lyse and wait"	(32)
Pulmonary Embolism			
UK	4,400 units/kg bolus, then 4,400 units/min for 12 hours	Systemic intravenous administration	(115)
TPA	100 mg over 2 hours	Systemic intravenous administration	(115)
RPA	10 units over 2 min, wait 28 min then repeat	Systemic intravenous administration (Not FDA approved)	(115)

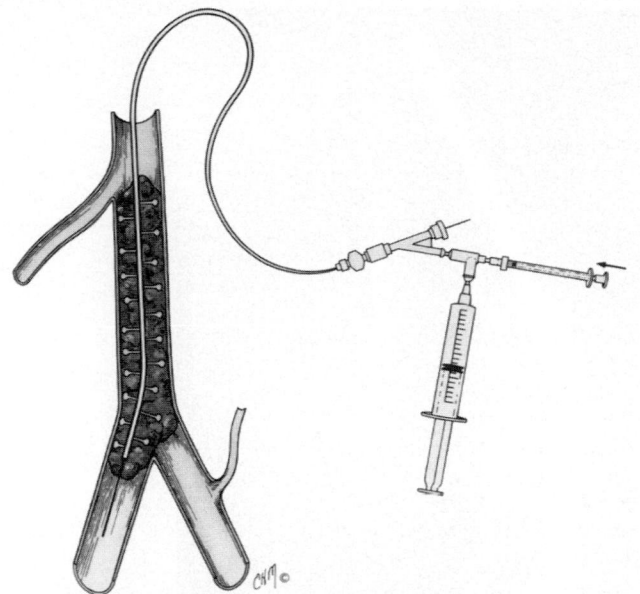

Figure 15–1   Line drawing of pulse spray catheter and tip-occluding wire within arterial occlusion. The catheter is fitted with a hemostatic adapter and three-way stopcock. Injections are made with a tuberculin syringe. The 12-mL syringe serves as a reservoir for the urokinase/heparin mixture. (Reprinted with permission from Valji K, Bookstein JJ. Pulsed spray thrombolysis accelerates clot dissolution. Diagn Imaging (San Franc) 1991;13:58–63.)

Good results with the pulse spray method can be obtained by careful adherence to technique, including the use of appropriate catheters, the inhibition of concurrent rethrombosis with aspirin and intrathrombic heparin, and determination of the appropriate endpoint for thrombolysis (1,19,20).

Although the pulse spray method originally was described as a way to perform the entire thrombolytic procedure in a single session, it is not commonly used in this fashion except for dialysis grafts. Rather, it is used as a method to "jump-start" the thrombolytic procedure by seeding the thrombus with thrombolytic agent and beginning an infusion of thrombolytic.

Arterial Thrombolysis

Thrombolytic therapy is performed only after a diagnostic study is performed. In most cases, this will be a diagnostic angiogram, but in some cases, a magnetic resonance angiogram (MRA) or computed tomography angiogram (CTA) may be the primary diagnostic study (21–23). If a noninvasive vascular study is the diagnostic study, then an appropriate access will be chosen depending on the anatomy seen on the diagnostic study. If the patient is taken to angiography as the initial study, then access is usually obtained through a contralateral femoral artery puncture to perform a diagnostic study. Sometimes, occlusions can be treated from a contralateral side using the access site chosen for the diagnostic arteriogram. This approach avoids

a second arterial puncture, but difficulties crossing the occlusion may arise when a contralateral approach is used. Commonly, the approach to the occluded artery is via an ipsilateral approach. A popliteal artery approach may be advantageous in certain cases, such as with markedly obese patients, graft occlusions without a "nipple" at the proximal anastomosis to allow entry into the graft, or grafts in which the proximal anastomosis is near the top of the common femoral artery (24,25). Occasionally, an occluded synthetic peripheral arterial bypass graft may be accessed directly with a crosscatheter technique identical to the approach for an occluded dialysis graft (26,27) (Figure 15–2). This allows access to both the proximal and distal anastomosis for both thrombolysis and transcatheter angioplasty.

The occlusion initially is crossed with a guide wire. Soft-tipped wires are less likely to produce a subintimal passage and usually are tried first. Hydrophilic guide wires are particularly useful in negotiating difficult occlusions. If other methods fail, the combination of a Rosen wire and straight catheter may be successful. Some controversy exists regarding the value of thrombolytic therapy when the occlusion cannot be traversed with a guide wire. McNamara and others believe that inability to cross an arterial obstruction predicts a poor response to thrombolysis (7,9). However, Smith and coworkers found that the inability to cross an occlusion with a guide wire had no significant bearing on the success of clot lysis (28). Most operators will attempt thrombolytic therapy if at least some portion of the occlusion can be penetrated.

After the catheter has been placed, lacing of the clot or pulse spray may be performed prior to beginning the infusion of the fibrinolytic. The catheter is secured in place, and the patient is transferred to an intermediate or intensive care unit for monitoring. The patient is observed for hemorrhagic complications, with evaluation of the puncture sites and serial hematocrits. The patient should be evaluated frequently for changes in the neurological status of the affected limb, as well as for evidence of bleeding from sites distant from the treatment site. Stools should be tested for evidence of bleeding, and IV sites should also be monitored for bleeding. Intramuscular injections should not be given, and any type of intravenous catheterization should be minimized.

Angiograms should be obtained relatively frequently, usually every 2–6 hours to monitor lysis. This allows for adjustments in dose and catheter position. If thrombolysis is began early in the morning, the patient may return to the angiography suite in the afternoon to assess the extent of clot lysis. Otherwise, infusion is continued overnight, and angiography is repeated the following day. In some cases, such as when a high dose protocol is being used, the infusion rate may be decreased during the evening to permit slow delivery of thrombolytic overnight. If clot lysis is judged complete, with the artery being completely clear of thrombus or no change having occurred since the previous angiographic check, then the underlying stenoses are treated with balloon angioplasty, intravascular stents, or both (Figure 15–3). If the angiogram

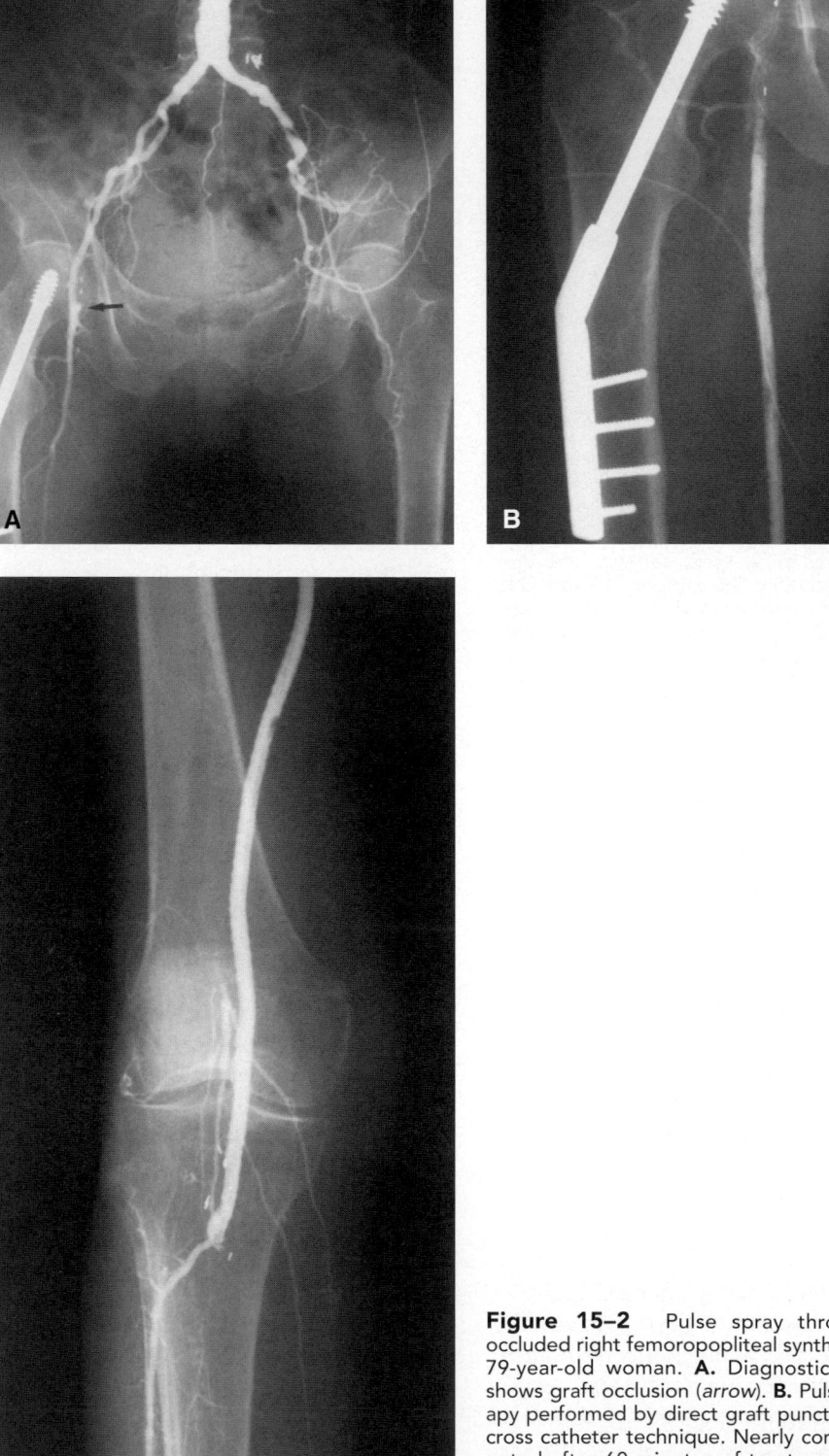

Figure 15–2   Pulse spray thrombolysis of occluded right femoropopliteal synthetic graft in a 79-year-old woman. **A.** Diagnostic arteriogram shows graft occlusion (*arrow*). **B.** Pulse spray therapy performed by direct graft puncture and crisscross catheter technique. Nearly complete lysis is noted after 60 minutes of treatment with urokinase. **C.** Graft and distal anastomosis are widely patent after thrombolysis and balloon angioplasty.

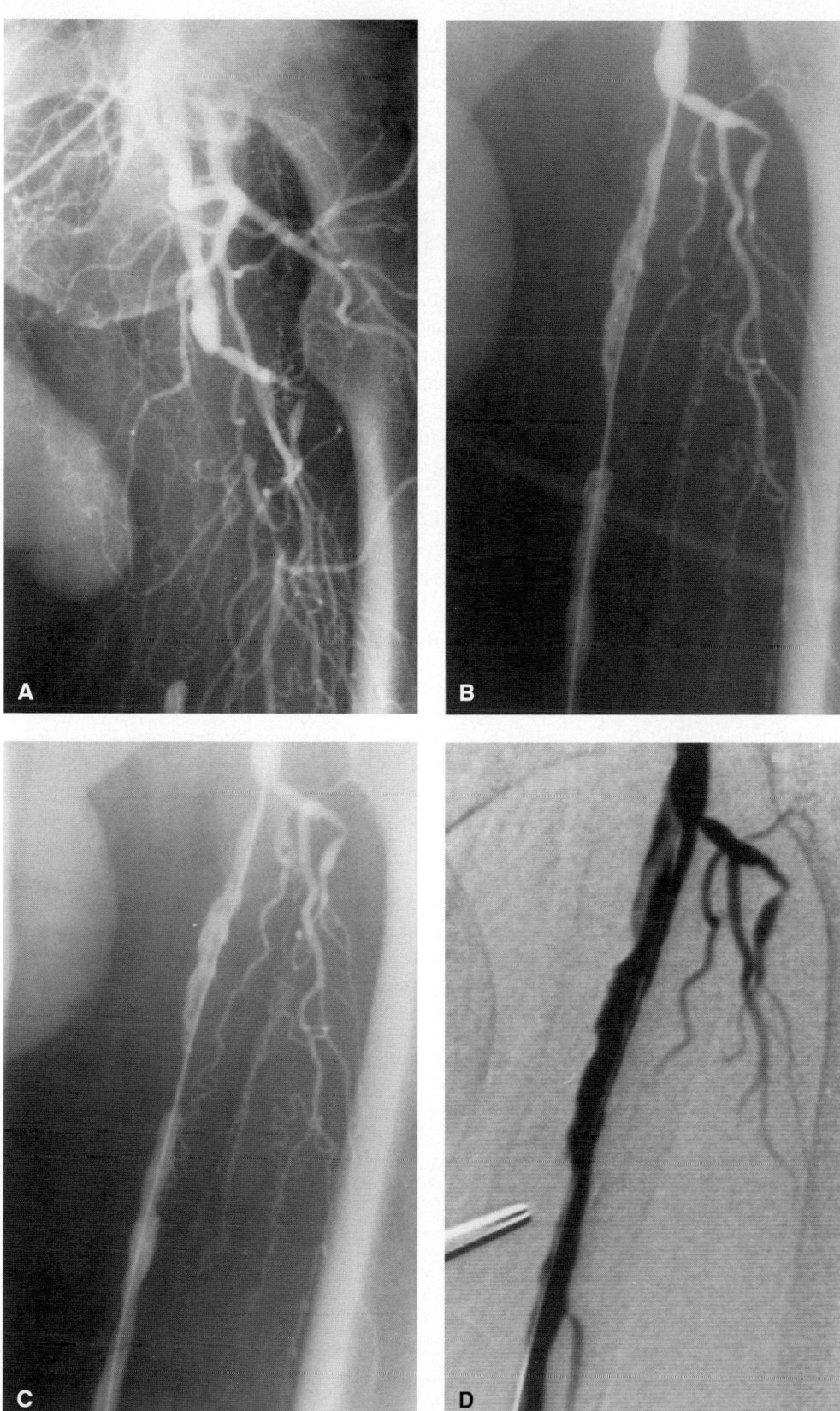

Figure 15–3 A. Arteriogram shows short occlusion of the left superficial femoral artery. **B.** Following treatment with pulse spray thrombolysis with urokinase over 30 minutes, significant lysis has occurred with residual disease present. **C.** Treatment with additional urokinase over 30 minutes produces no change in the appearance of residual disease. **D.** The artery is widely patent following balloon angioplasty.

suggests the presence of residual clot, the infusion may be continued. However, infusions are usually stopped after 36–48 hours of therapy because the risks of the procedure increase with the increasing duration of the procedure (3).

Technical Modifications for Treatment of Hemodialysis Grafts

The anatomy of hemodialysis grafts demands a slightly different approach than arterial or venous thrombolysis. Infusion thrombolysis has proved ineffective in treating thrombosed hemodialysis access grafts. However, pulse spray thrombolysis has been found to be a safe, rapid, and reliable method for recanalizing clotted grafts. Several modifications of the standard pulse spray technique are necessary. Direct punctures are made at two sites in the midportion of the graft, and dilators are placed in a crisscrossed fashion to allow access to the entire clot and to allow graft inflow and outflow for treatment of underlying stenoses (Figure 15–4). The catheter directed toward the venous anastomosis should be inserted first. If the venous anastomosis cannot be crossed, thrombolysis should not be performed. The dilators are replaced with pulse spray catheters. The active catheter length is chosen to allow exposure of the entire clot to fibrinolytic agents while keeping the side slits within the graft.

The thrombolytic mixture is divided between the two catheters and injected over approximately 15 minutes. Additional thrombolytic is only given when large amounts of clot are still present after the first dose has been given. Otherwise, residual clot is macerated with a dilatation balloon.

The composition of clot within a thrombosed dialysis graft is not homogeneous. The body of the graft is filled largely with red, cell-rich thrombus that is quite sensitive to fibrinolytic agents. However, clot at the most proximal end of the graft is relatively insensitive to these agents. Surgeons frequently retrieve a small white plug from the arterial anastomosis of clotted grafts during operative thrombectomy. This residual filling defect is also noted in most cases after thrombolytic therapy (Figure 15–5). In keeping with limited histologic examinations, this plug is thought to consist of dense concentrations of fibrin and few red cells, characteristics of "white" or platelet-rich clot. The plug may be removed by several means. Maceration with a dilatation balloon usually is effective. If the clot is directly opposite the arterial anastomosis, dilation may produce downstream emboli. In such cases, an 8.5 mm occlusion balloon can be inserted beyond the clot into the adjacent artery. When the balloon is gently inflated and pulled back against the plug, the plug will be displaced back into the graft and can be macerated with a dilatation balloon.

Following clot lysis, an underlying cause for graft thrombosis should be sought. Venous anastomotic stenosis is the usual reason for graft failure. Other causes for thrombosis include venous outflow obstruction, arterial anastomotic or inflow stenosis, and intragraft stenosis.

Use of Antithrombin and Antiplatelet Agents

When a thrombus forms in a vessel, a dynamic balance between endogenous fibrinolysis and ongoing thrombosis takes place. When exogenous fibrinolytic agents are infused around or within a clot, concurrent rethrombosis may occur during thrombolysis. Studies in animal models of thrombosis have shown that adjunctive antithrombin and antiplatelet agents used during pulse spray thrombolysis enhance clot lysis (18,29).

The use of anticoagulants during thrombolytic therapy is controversial. Heparin therapy during thrombolysis became routine after thrombus formation around the infusion catheter was reported in a substantial number of

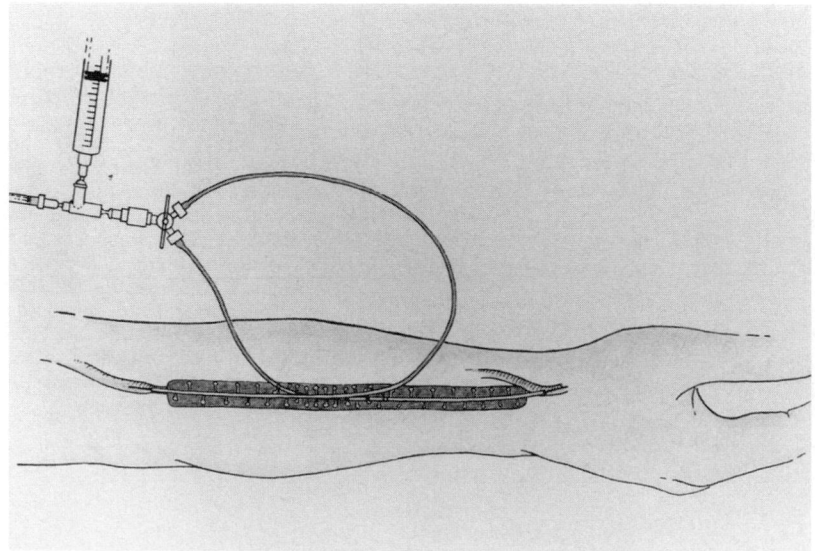

Figure 15–4 Line drawing of crisscross pulse spray catheter technique for treatment of occluded hemodialysis grafts.

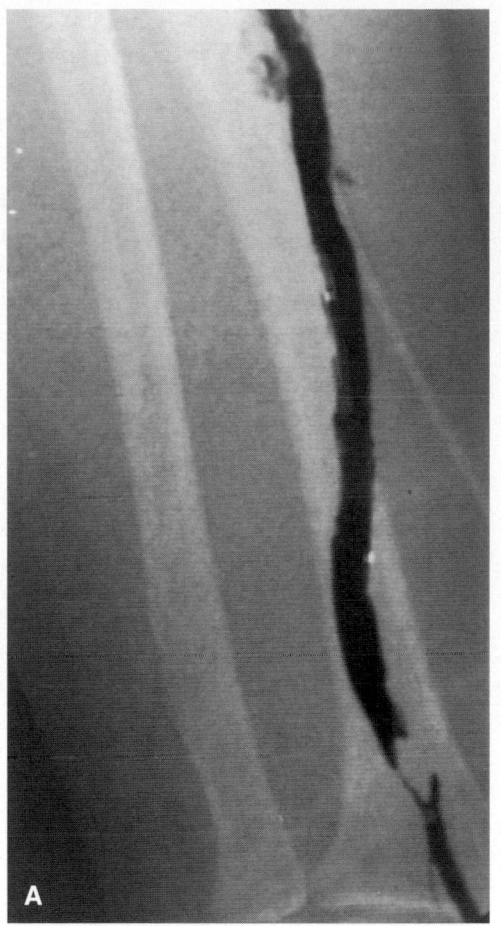
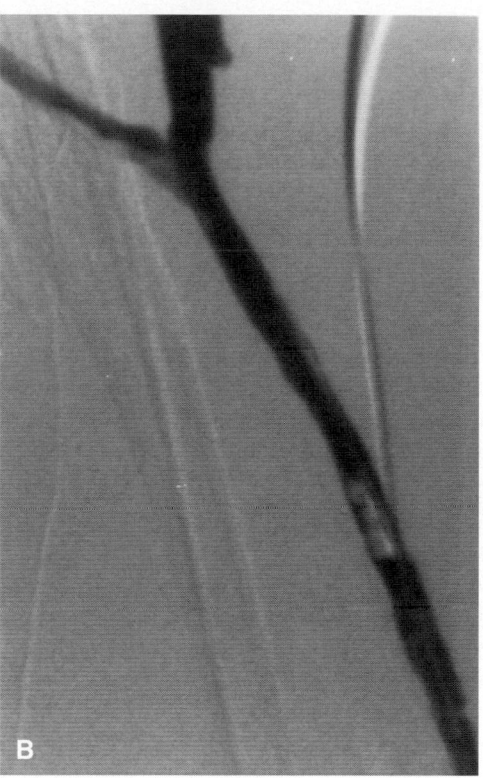

Figure 15–5 Lysis-resistant arterial "plug" presents after thrombolysis of clotted hemodialysis graft. **A.** Oval filling defect in proximal portion of the graft with otherwise complete clot lysis. **B.** Occlusion balloon used to pull plug into midportion of graft; residual material is then macerated with an angioplasty balloon.

patients by early investigators in the field. However, frequent bleeding complications were reported with the use of heparin during thrombolysis with SK, and some operators did not administer anticoagulation because of the bleeding risk. When thrombolysis was being performed with UK, many operators used anticoagulation because of the relative safety of the UK and the lack of bleeding complications. When UK was no longer available and TPA began to be used more extensively, bleeding complications again increased. The standard approach has been to forego anticoagulation or to decrease the amount of heparin to 500 units/hr or less.

Rapid and effective clot lysis during thrombolysis is dependent on inhibition of concurrent rethrombosis using anticoagulation agents and antiplatelet agents. Thrombolytic procedures, by their very nature, activate both coagulation factors and platelets. During thrombolysis, thrombin bound to fibrin is released as thrombin-bound FDP. This thrombin retains the capacity to convert fibrinogen to fibrin and is a potent platelet activator (30). Maintenance doses of heparin (500–1,500 units/hr) are commonly given during

UK thrombolytic procedures. A consensus group has recommended when using TPA to follow a subtherapeutic regimen consisting of a 2,500 unit heparin bolus followed by a continuous drip at 500 units/hr to maintain the PTT time between 1.25 and 1.5 times control values (31). No consensus was reached on the use of heparin when performing thrombolysis with RPA (32). It is important to understand that heparin metabolism varies widely among patients, largely because of its nonspecific binding with plasma proteins. Thus, the anticoagulative response may be unpredictable. Direct thrombin inhibitors produce a more predictable anticoagulation response because unlike heparin, they do not bind to plasma proteins (33).

The activated partial thromboplastin time (aPTT or PTT) can be used to guide heparin therapy. If therapeutic heparinization is being administered, then the heparin dose is adjusted to maintain the PTT at 1.5–2.0 times control. In the angiographic suite, a more rapid method of monitoring anticoagulation may be needed. The activated clotting time (ACT, Medtronic) is an indicator of whole blood clotting and is useful in guiding anticoagulant therapy. An ACT reading in a normal, nonanticoagulated patient is in the range of 120–140 seconds. The ACT reading should be prolonged to 250–300 seconds in a patient who is being therapeutically anticoagulated.

Antiplatelet agents are very important adjuncts in thrombolytic therapy. Platelets are activated by the angiographic procedure, including placement of catheters, balloons, stents, and by the process of thrombolysis. Antiplatelet agents can augment the rate of thrombus dissolution leading to a reduction in the incidence of recurrent thrombosis (34). Various antiplatelet agents are now available, which are described more thoroughly in Chapter 14. Aspirin is the least expensive and a very effective agent (35). It is an appropriate first-line therapy (3). GPIIb/IIIa receptor inhibitors are significantly more expensive, but they may be helpful in selected cases. Studies using GPIIb/IIIa receptor inhibitors suggest that the addition of systemically administered abciximab (ReoPro, Centocor) may result in increased fibrinolytic efficacy without decreased patient safety (34,36,37). Eptifibatide (Integrillin, Schering-Plough and COR Therapeutics) has also been shown in a few small studies to increase the rate of thrombolysis, decrease the rate of embolization, and decrease the requirement for surgery, without a statistically significant increase in the risk of bleeding (38–40).

Use of Vasodilators

Prophylactic use of vasodilators may be a useful adjunct to thrombolysis in arteries that are prone to vasospasm, including renal, mesenteric, upper extremity, tibial, and pedal arteries. Oral or sublingual nifedipine (10 mg) may be given before therapy. In addition, intra-arterial nitroglycerin may be given in 150–200-µg aliquots immediately before or during thrombolysis or angioplasty procedures.

SPECIFIC APPLICATIONS OF THROMBOLYTIC THERAPY

Pelvic and Lower Extremity Arteries

The most frequently treated sites are the iliac and femoropopliteal arteries. Aortic thrombosis has also been managed successfully with thrombolytic techniques. The same general principles apply to occluded tibial and pedal vessels, although experience is less in these arterial beds.

Before any percutaneous therapy is embarked upon, the patient must be evaluated. In most cases, the patient will have acute ischemia of the lower extremity, characterized by a relatively abrupt onset of pain or change in function. It is important to ask whether the patient has a history of claudication or previous interventions and whether the patient has had a previous diagnosis of heart disease (particularly, atrial fibrillation) or aneurysms (another embolic source). The patient should also be asked about other risk factors for atherosclerosis. A physical examination should be performed, focused on the physical findings (pulses, color and temperature, sensory function, motor function) that will define the severity of the ischemia (2,3). The patient needs to be questioned regarding risk factors that would preclude thrombolytic therapy. The degree of ischemia should be categorized, which will help determine the appropriate therapy (Table 15–2).

Thrombolysis is more likely to be successful with short occlusions and with the presence of at least one runoff vessel below the occlusion. Clot age should not be considered a major factor in selecting patients for thrombolysis as long as the thrombus has not organized sufficiently to prevent passage of a guide wire and catheter. However, although clot age may not be an important determinant for success in occlusions less than 6 months old (16), some studies have shown a significant reduction in technical

TABLE 15–2

CLINICAL CATEGORIES OF ACUTE LIMB ISCHEMIA

Category	Description/ Prognosis	Findings			Doppler Signals		
		Capillary Refill	Sensory Loss	Muscle Weakness	Arterial	Venous	Most Appropriate Procedure
I. Viable	Not immediately threatened	Intact	None	None	Audible	Audible	Catheter directed thrombolysis
II. Threatened							
a. Marginal	Salvageable when promptly treated	Intact/slow	Minimal (toes) or none	None	Audible	Inaudible	Catheter directed thrombolysis
b. Immediate	Salvageable with immediate revascularization	Slow/Absent	More than toes, associated with rest pain	Mild, moderate	Audible	Inaudible	Thrombolysis- surgery
III. Irreversible	Major tissue loss or permanent nerve damage inevitable	Absent	Profound, anesthetic	Profound, paralysis (rigor)	Inaudible	Inaudible	Surgery- amputation

success and long-term patency for occlusions older than 6 months (3,8,41).

A poor outcome from transcatheter therapy may be anticipated with (1) an inability to traverse the occlusion with a guide wire, (2) subintimal dissection during therapy, (3) the presence of organized thrombus, (4) rethrombosis occurring during lysis, (5) lack of adequate inflow to or outflow from the treated segment, (6) the presence of a hypercoagulable state (Figure 15–6), or (7) significant residual disease after thrombolysis and angioplasty.

Technical success, defined as recanalization of the artery and clearing of about 90–95% of the occlusion with restoration of antegrade flow, is achieved in about 38–97% of cases using infusion therapy with a variety of thrombolytic agents and methods (3,5,14,42–47). With infusion methods, lysis times usually range from 18–24 hours. High-dose infusion therapy has not been consistently shown to improve technical efficacy over low-dose regimens, although there is some evidence that outcomes can be improved (10,13,48). Technical success can be achieved in 95% of cases using PSPMT (49,50). Pulse spray therapy significantly accelerates clot dissolution and the use of

PSPMT to lace the clot with thrombolytic agent combined with infusion in the proximal portion of the clot seems to improve the speed and efficacy of lysis (10,13,51,52).

Reports of successful thrombolysis using UK has varied widely from 38–95% (5). Alteplase (TPA) and the modifications of TPA, such as reteplase (RPA) and tenecteplase (TNK), have been shown to be effective agents for treating peripheral arterial and bypass graft occlusions. Most of the studies have been performed with alteplase, with a smaller number using reteplase (37,53–55) and very few with tenecteplase (40,56,57). Technical success is achieved in 60–100% of cases, and infusion times range from 3 to 40 hours (5). The difficulty in trying to analyze the reports on thrombolysis is the variability in reporting standards, dosing, technique, and use of concurrent anticoagulation and antiplatelet agents (5,58).

Patients with severe acute limb ischemia pose a difficult challenge. Thrombolysis has been found effective in such patients. At 12 months follow-up, patients treated with thrombolysis had a 68–82% limb salvage rate, essentially equal to the limb salvage rate with surgery and a mortality rate of 13–16% compared to a 15–42% mortality rate with

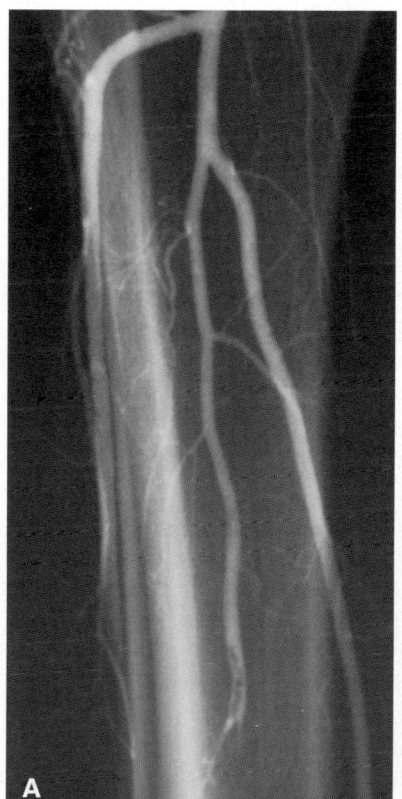
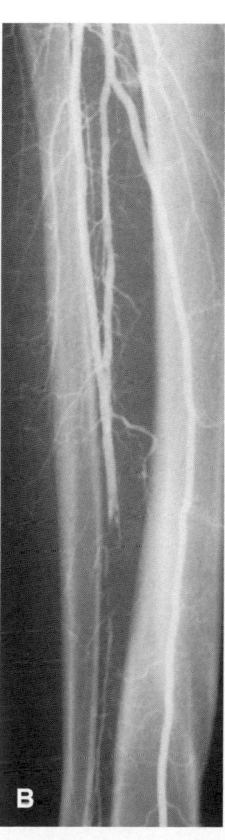
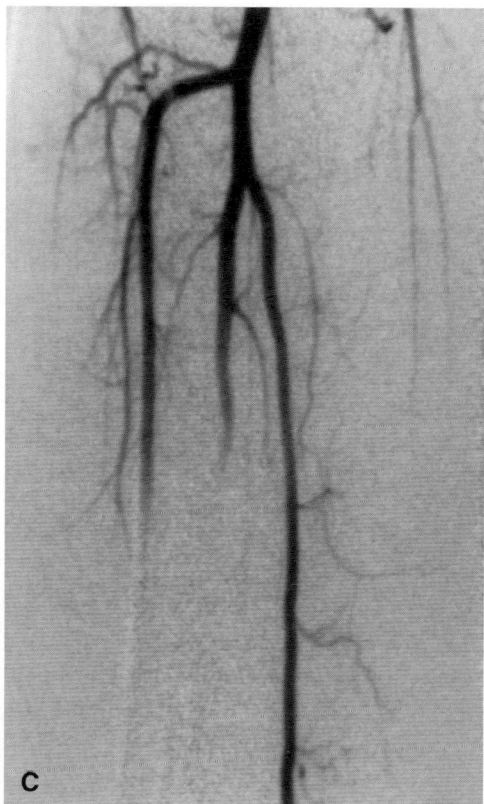

Figure 15–6 Poor response to thrombolysis resulting from hypercoagulable state in a 38-year-old woman with metastatic melanoma and thrombocytosis. **A.** Right lower extremity arteriogram reveals emboli or in situ thrombosis in perineal and anterior tibial arteries. **B.** Almost no response to thrombolysis is noted after pulse spray with thrombolytic. Patient was receiving heparin and aspirin. **C.** After overnight infusion into the popliteal artery, no significant lysis is noted.

surgery (2,59,60). However, the time required for successful infusion thrombolysis may be prohibitive in some of these patients. Many have widespread thrombotic disease with occlusion of several or all of the tibial arteries and extensive disease in pedal vessels. Blood flow must be reestablished without delay to avoid or limit amputation. Accelerated thrombolysis with PSPMT has been found to be useful in this subgroup of patients (61) (Figure 15–7). However, severe acute limb ischemia continues to be associated with substantial limb loss and appreciable mortality (3).

Peripheral embolism represents a special category of peripheral vascular obstruction. Although it may be difficult to distinguish embolic occlusions from thrombotic ones, suggestive features include multiple separate branch occlusions, the absence of large collateral vessels, a convex margin at the proximal extent of occlusion, a history of atrial fibrillation, known left atrial or ventricular thrombus, and acute onset of symptoms. Suprainguinal emboli should be removed preferably surgically (3). If the presenting embolus is fragmented and occludes many vascular branches or where it is complicated by propagated thrombus, thrombolysis may be a useful first choice of treatment (3). Prolonged intra-arterial thrombolytic infusions have the potential to cause further lysis of the original embolic source (usually within the heart), which may lead to repeated embolization. Although this complication has been described in case reports (62), most patients with embolic occlusions treated by thrombolytic infusion have not developed additional emboli during therapy (63).

Several studies have shown significantly higher rates of technical success with embolic occlusions. On the other hand, emboli may consist of material that is not amenable to thrombolysis or balloon angioplasty, such as organized clot or atherosclerotic plaque. Balloon angioplasty poses a significant risk of distal embolization when unlysable intraluminal material is dilated. If large intraluminal residua are present, surgical embolectomy may be required.

Peripheral Bypass Grafts

Thrombolysis should be used as an alternative to an open surgical approach for bypass graft occlusions. It provides a means of restoring arterial perfusion, which provides the opportunity to unmask stenotic lesions responsible for the occlusion. The lesion responsible for the occlusion can then be addressed with either an endovascular procedure or an operative approach (3).

Advances in the practice of vascular surgery have improved the long-term patency of peripheral bypass grafts. Advanced techniques, such as the placement of vein bypass grafts to small vessels in the foot, are relatively routine. The 5-year patency rate of infrainguinal in situ saphenous vein grafts is 70–80% (59). Periodic surveillance of grafts using Doppler sonography can increase their longevity significantly (64). Landry et al. reported a 5-year assisted primary patency rate of 88%, and a 10-year assisted primary patency

rate of 80%, for grafts determined by ultrasound to be failing. This is compared with an occlusion rate of 80% in unrevised grafts with a critical stenosis (65).

However, despite efforts to maintain graft patency, graft thrombosis remains a vexing problem. About 3–5% of in situ saphenous vein grafts fail within 1 month of operation, usually because of inadequate outflow, technical error, or abnormalities of the venous conduit. These grafts usually should be treated with surgical revision (3).

Thrombolysis is an effective means of recanalizing occluded peripheral bypass grafts. Technical success is achieved in about 70–90% of cases (66,67). Thrombolysis is either completed or abandoned in 48 hours (66). PSPMT can be very effective, with graft recanalization in more than 95% of cases with a mean lysis time of just under 2 hours (16).

Thrombolytic therapy has several advantages over surgical thrombectomy and revision. Avoiding Fogarty embolectomy minimizes damage to the endothelium of vein grafts. Fibrinolytic agents may lyse clot in vessels distal to the graft in areas that are inaccessible to embolectomy. In some cases, balloon angioplasty of underlying stenoses will provide definitive therapy. When transcatheter techniques are inadequate, a limited operation may be performed guided by angiographic findings following lysis.

After thrombolysis, an underlying anatomic cause for occlusion can be found in 50–90% of patients (67). The most common reasons for graft failure are intragraft stenoses, distal or proximal anastomotic stenoses, diffuse graft disease, native proximal or distal arterial stenoses, and poor distal runoff (67). Additional causes of graft failure include emboli, technical errors, and persistent fistulas.

Although most grafts can be reopened with thrombolysis, the 1-year primary patency rate after thrombolysis of occluded bypass grafts is about 20–60%. Hye and coworkers noted a 28% primary patency rate at 30 months for 33 occluded grafts treated with PSPMT (68). On the other hand, long-term results after surgical thrombectomy and revision are also poor. Thrombosed vein grafts have a 23%, 3-year secondary patency (64). Even with aggressive surveillance, the 5-year primary patency rate has been reported as 49% (64). These poor results after operative repair are probably because of a combination of factors, including permanent vessel wall injury from ischemia, endothelial injury from Fogarty embolectomy, and incomplete clot extraction. Even with placement of a new bypass graft, patency rates are only modest (67).

Because only modest long-term results can be expected with transcatheter therapy, proper selection of patients is important. Some studies have shown that technical success is more likely with prosthetic graft occlusions, suprainguinal grafts, and recent occlusions (67,69).

Failure of therapy is usually because of rethrombosis, graft infection, organized clot, diffuse graft disease, inability to correct an underlying lesion, or intraprocedural complications that prevent complete therapy (bleeding or graft

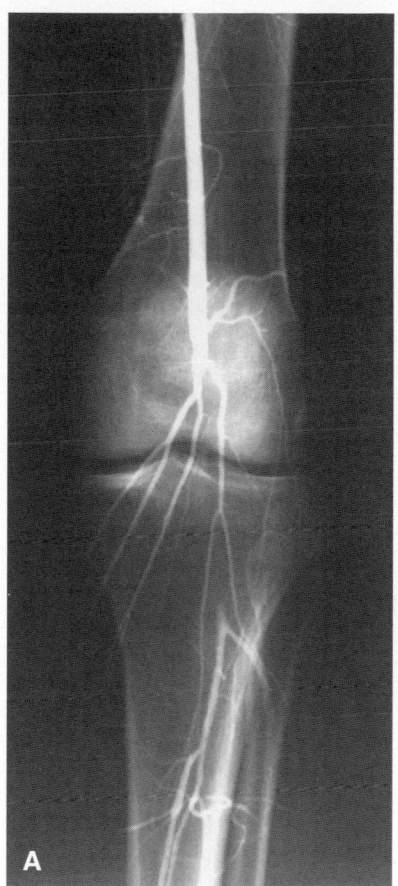

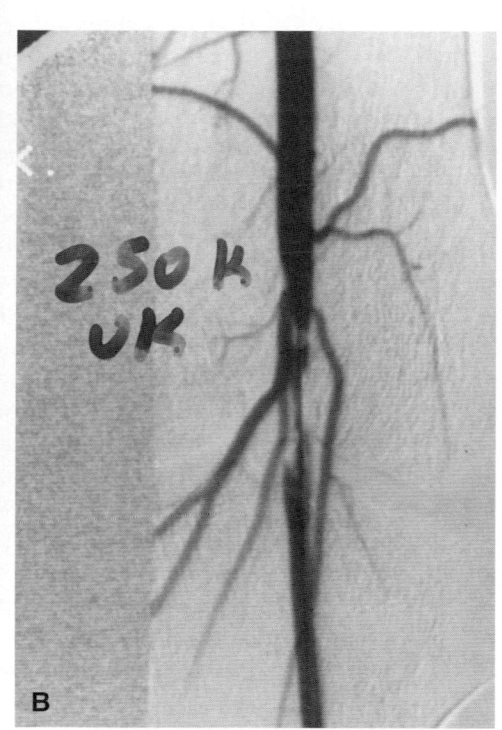

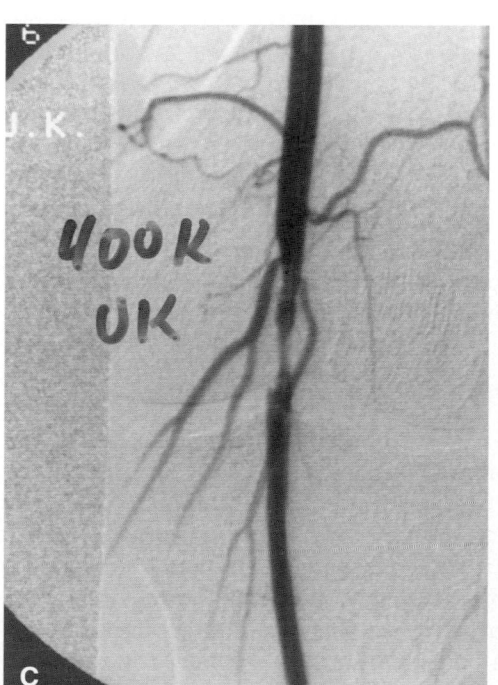

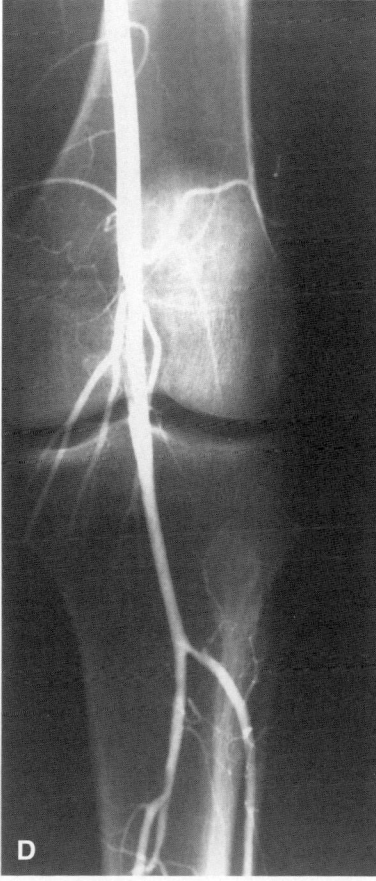

Figure 15–7 Pulse spray thrombolysis of acute popliteal artery occlusion. **A.** Arteriogram shows complete occlusion of left popliteal artery. **B.** Following PSPMT with 250,000 units of urokinase, partial lysis is noted. **C.** Treatment with a total of 400,000 units of urokinase over a total thrombolytic time of 50 minutes demonstrates minimal additional lysis with residual mural disease. **D.** Widely patent popliteal artery following balloon angioplasty. Runoff study did not demonstrate any distal emboli.

dissection). Long-term patency is greater for vein grafts, grafts with underlying correctable lesions, and grafts that have been functional for a long period (67,68). Continued careful graft surveillance using frequent color Doppler sonography is critical to maintaining patency.

Hemodialysis Grafts

Thrombosis of vascular access grafts is a major problem for patients on chronic hemodialysis. Access grafts have a high rate of failure with a 60–70% patency of synthetic grafts at 1 year (70–72). As patients are being maintained on hemodialysis for longer periods of time, the need for preserving access sites has become more critical.

Thrombolysis of clotted hemodialysis access devices was attempted in the 1960s. Early methods of treatment by infusion of SK or UK were often unsuccessful because prolonged infusions were required, bleeding complications were frequent, and the underlying disease was not treated (1). Local infusion therapy followed by balloon angioplasty of stenoses led to better results (73).

Dialysis graft thrombolysis became practical with the development of PSPMT. The features of this method include (1):

- Cross-catheter technique to allow access to the entire clot and graft inflow and outflow
- Rapid intrathrombic injection of a single dose of thrombolytic over 10–15 minutes
- Identification and treatment of underlying stenoses from the arterial inflow to central venous outflow
- Mobilization of lysis-resistant clot at the arterial anastomosis by withdrawal of an inflated occlusion balloon from the artery into the graft
- Maceration of residual clot with a dilatation balloon
- Long-term aspirin therapy to prevent rethrombosis

Thrombosed hemodialysis grafts can be treated with thrombolysis or mechanical thrombolysis. Surgical revision is preferred if operative placement or revision is performed within 2 weeks or, if frequent, repeated percutaneous procedures have been required to maintain graft function.

Other methods of dialysis graft thrombolysis include the "lysis and wait," "lysis and go," and percutaneous mechanical thrombectomy. The "lysis and wait" and "lysis and go" techniques are very similar. The "lysis and wait" technique was described by Cynamon (72,74) as an injection of 250,000 units of UK mixed with 5,000 units of heparin through a standard intravenous catheter inserted within the venous limb of the graft. The graft is manually compressed at the arterial and venous anastomoses while the thrombolytic mixture is infused over 1 minute into the graft. This portion of the procedure could be performed in a holding area outside the interventional radiology suite. After at least 30 minutes, the patient is transferred to the interventional radiology suite, and the

declotting procedure is continued with angioplasty of the venous stenosis and mobilization of the arterial plug. Introducing the thrombolytic mixture into the graft before bringing the patient into the interventional radiology suite resulted in the declotting portion of the procedure requiring little or no room time and avoiding the expense of an infusion catheter. This technique has also been described using TPA as the thrombolytic agent with 2–5 mg of TPA (72,75,76). The "lysis and go" technique is very similar, but the thrombolytic is injected when the patient is in the angiographic room. The patient is then prepped and draped, and the procedure is started without any waiting period.

Thrombolysis of dialysis grafts is very successful, with technical success rates ranging from to 95–100% (72,74,77). Lytic infusion time with PSPMT is usually under 20 minutes, and the mean procedure room time is about 65 minutes (1,72,77,78). The procedure room time for lyse and wait is approximately 45 minutes (72).

Underlying obstructions, presumed to be the cause of the thrombosis, are found most commonly in the venous circulation, at the venous anastomosis (79%), or within the venous outflow (20%) (Figure 15–8). However, the arterial anastomosis or inflow was also involved (13%), and some obstructions were within the graft (6%).

Complications of percutaneous treatment of thrombosed hemodialysis access are relatively uncommon. The most common is bleeding from the catheter site or from recent puncture sites. These are controlled easily with manual compression or with placement of a purse-string suture to stop the bleeding (72). Pulmonary embolism is known to occur when patients are studied with perfusion scans; usually, these emboli are asymptomatic (79,80) and may be less consequential when thrombolytics are used instead of mechanical thrombolysis (81). Arterial embolization can occur with thrombolysis and mechanical thrombolysis and are often associated with attempts to mobilize the arterial plug. Usually, the clot can be pulled back easily into the graft with a Fogerty style balloon catheter (81).

Long-term results with thrombolysis for dialysis grafts have been favorable. The primary and secondary patency rates at 1 year are 23–44% and 57–69%, respectively (82). These results are comparable to the 50–70% patency rate reported for surgical revision at 1 year (83–85).

Upper Extremity Arteries

Although arterial thrombosis is a far less common problem in the arm than in the leg, the management of upper extremity occlusions is often more complex. Operative approaches to occlusive upper extremity disease include embolectomy, proximal bypass surgery, and microvascular reconstruction for distal thromboses. However, attempted surgical therapy has significant mortality and morbidity. Initial surgical technical success is achieved in 99%, but

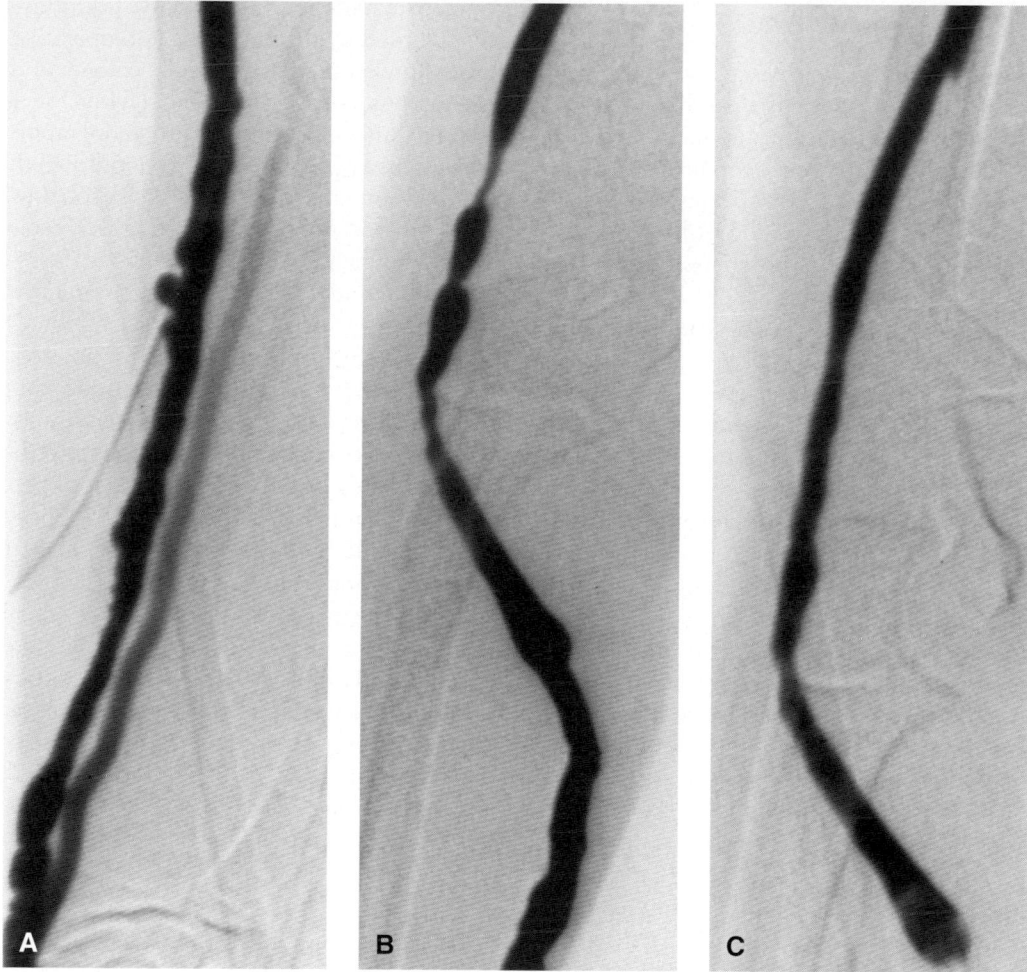

Figure 15–8 Thrombolysis of clotted hemodialysis graft. **A.** Complete clot lysis is noted after treatment with thrombolysis using pulse spray. Small pseudoaneurysms at dialysis puncture sites are seen throughout the graft. **B.** Two significant stenoses are noted at and just beyond the venous anastomosis. **C.** A good result from balloon angioplasty of the stenoses is achieved.

there is a 30-day mortality of 3%, stroke 3%, and total complications of 19% (86).

Early attempts at thrombolytic therapy of upper extremity occlusions using streptokinase (SK) often required 2–4 days of infusion and were often unsuccessful (1). Intraarterial thrombolysis has not been as common a procedure in the upper extremities as in the lower extremities, but it has been used successfully in the treatment of atherosclerotic and embolic occlusions, occluded upper extremity grafts, thoracic outlet syndrome, arteritis, thrombosis of brachial catheterization sites, posttraumatic thrombosis, and thrombosis resulting from self-administration of illicit drugs (87–93). Successful therapy depends significantly on the duration of occlusion, with occlusions less than 2 days old responding most favorably (94,95).

Unlike disease in the leg, thrombosis is often extensive, with involvement of several forearm vessels, the palmar arch, and digital vessels, making operative therapy impractical. Therefore, thrombolytic infusion may be the preferred method of treatment. Acceleration of the thrombolysis with PSPMT may help to jump-start the process. Clinically successful thrombolysis often requires 2–3 days of local infusion. Results of thrombolysis with pulse spray or infusion methods are often incomplete (92). Nonetheless, most patients improve and have long-lasting benefit even when extensive disease is present, probably because the fibrinolytic agent opens collateral vessels (92,94–96). Long-term anticoagulation is often required after successful lytic therapy.

One risk of thrombolysis of upper extremity occlusions not encountered with lower extremity disease is embolic stroke from pericatheter clot. Full anticoagulation with heparin may not prevent this severe complication. Therefore, an antegrade brachial approach should be considered when distal disease is present (95).

Axillary and Subclavian Veins

Upper extremity venous thrombosis is separated into primary and secondary categories. Primary thrombosis occurs in the absence of recognized risk factors and includes effort thrombosis also known as the Paget-Shroetter syndrome. Primary thrombosis accounts for 1–9% of cases (97) and is the result of extrinsic compression on the axillary or subclavian veins by muscles, tendons, or bony structures in the costoclavicular or subcoracoid spaces. In most cases, repeated venous trauma or compression by these structures causes damage to the vein wall with subsequent thrombosis. These patients tend to be young and active. The thrombosis is associated with a repetitive or strenuous exercise or occupation such as painting, chopping wood, baseball, tennis, or surfing.

Secondary thrombosis is much more common and occurs in the setting of recognized thrombotic risk factors. Central venous access devices are now the most frequent cause of subclavian or axillary vein thrombosis responsible for 39–63% of cases (97). Upper extremity thrombosis may also result from systemic disease, hypercoagulable states, trauma, malignancy, or radiation therapy. The patients tend to be older and more often systemically ill (98). A substantial number of these patients will have concomitant lower extremity thrombosis (99,100), and there appears to be an increased risk of symptomatic pulmonary emboli in this group of patients with estimated rates from 9–36% (97,101,102). A substantial number (28–30%) of these patients appear to have an antithrombin III (ATIII) deficiency (100), many of whom will not respond to anticoagulation alone.

The diagnosis of subclavian or axillary vein thrombosis can be established with a high degree of accuracy by color Doppler sonography (103), but this approach may not demonstrate isolated SVC or brachiocephalic vein thrombosis (104). Helical CT phlebography and gadolinium-enhanced magnetic resonance venography may be helpful in establishing the diagnosis (98,104). However, contrast upper arm venography remains the most conclusive test.

Patients with secondary thrombosis often can be treated effectively with long-term anticoagulation and supportive therapy. Patients not responsive to conservative measures, those with underlying disease that predisposes to repeated thrombosis, and those with severe symptoms may benefit from clot dissolution or removal. Persistent symptoms of occlusion, including arm edema, exertional pain, or pulmonary embolism, are present in 47–90% of patients with primary subclavian or axillary vein thrombosis (97,105). Conventional treatment of subclavian or axillary vein thrombosis includes thrombectomy and correction of the underlying anatomic abnormality, such as first rib resection, division of the anterior scalene muscle, and excision of the subclavius muscle (97,106).

Thrombolytic therapy has largely replaced the surgical thrombectomy and has become an important adjunct to surgery in patients with primary thrombosis. Early diagnosis followed by thrombolysis and operative thoracic outlet decompression restores venous patency and relieves extrinsic venous compression, achieving the most favorable results (106). After upper arm venography, local infusion or pulse spray thrombolysis is performed through a sheath placed in an antecubital vein. Occasionally, access from the femoral vein may be necessary. Prolonged infusion over 24–72 hours and cumulatively large doses of thrombolytics are often required to achieve complete clot dissolution. Results of thrombolytic therapy tend to be very good with complete thrombolysis in approximately 80% of cases (97,107,108). Thrombolysis alone rarely provides long-term venous patency, but subsequent thrombolysis surgery can be performed to decompress the vein and minimize the risk of thrombosis (106). Most patients also require long-term anticoagulation to prevent repeated thrombosis.

Transluminal angioplasty is performed after the surgical decompression to treat underlying stenoses. Angioplasty of the venous stenoses before surgery is usually unsuccessful and may have an adverse effect on venous patency (107–109). However, following the surgical decompression angioplasty can be effective at treating persistent subclavian vein stenosis (110). Stents should not be used in the vein before a surgical release because of the stent deformation caused by the musculoskeletal elements (97,111,112). Following decompression, stents may be more appropriate but should be avoided whenever possible (97,110).

Lower Extremity Veins

The standard of care for patients with deep venous thrombosis (DVT) of the lower extremity is anticoagulation with low–molecular-weight heparin (LMWH) followed by a 6-month course of oral warfarin (113). Because anticoagulation does not remove thrombus, the ability of the body to remove the obstructing thrombus depends on the endogenous fibrinolytic system. If this does not occur, the patient is at risk for damage to the venous valves and the subsequent development of a postthrombotic syndrome (PTS). This syndrome is caused by chronically elevated venous pressure in the lower extremities because of venous outflow obstruction, valvular incompetence, or both (114). It may occur in 25–40% of patients with proximal (iliofemoral) DVT (115). Potential advantages of thrombolytic therapy in such patients include prompt symptomatic relief through rapid clot lysis and reduced vein wall and valve damage that predispose to the postthrombotic syndrome. Intravenous thrombolytic therapy with SK has been found to reduce the incidence of postphlebitic symptoms in patients with lower extremity deep venous thrombosis compared with heparin therapy alone (116,117). A recent small study showed 35 patients with iliofemoral venous thrombosis who were randomized to local SK thrombolysis and anticoagulation or to anticoagulation alone. The results indicated that there was complete lysis in 6 months in 72% of the thrombolytic group versus 12% in the anticoagulation group. There was no lysis at 1 week in 100% of the anticoagulation group, but all the thrombolysis patients showed evidence of some lysis with 61% having complete lysis. There was no obstruction or reflux in 72% of the thrombolysis group, but only 12% of the anticoagulation group had no obstruction or reflux, while 59% of the anticoagulation group had severe obstruction, but only 6% of the thrombolysis group had severe obstruction. Reflux was also higher in the anticoagulation group (41%) than in the thrombolytic group (11%). One patient in the anticoagulation group had a symptomatic pulmonary embolus, and three patients in the thrombolysis group had a fever. There was no major bleeding or death (118).

In the National Venous Thrombolysis Registry, UK was found to be efficacious in treating DVT (119). This trial was done without a unified study protocol, dosing regimen, or technical approach, which makes evaluation difficult. It did, however, demonstrate that complete lysis (99–100%) was achieved in 31%, partial lysis (50–99%) in 52%, and no lysis (<50%) in 17% (114,119). In a subsequent study involving a subset of the Registry patients, Comerota et al. demonstrated better functioning and quality of life in patients with iliofemoral DVT treated by catheter-directed thrombolysis than in those treated with anticoagulants alone (120).

Unfortunately, most of the reports on thrombolysis for DVT are systemically delivered thrombolytic that intuitively would seem ineffective. These reports also tend to have higher complication rates. The safety of thrombolytic therapy is the greatest impediment toward adoption of thrombolytic therapy (114). The risk of hemorrhagic complications even with catheter-directed thrombolytic therapy is considerably higher than treatment with LMWH (approximately 1.5%) (114). In the Venous Registry, major bleeding complications were reported in 11%, there was one fatal intracranial hemorrhage and one subdural hematoma, and a fatal pulmonary embolism occurred (114,119).

Although the opportunity to treat uncomplicated iliofemoral thrombus may be somewhat limited, thrombolytic therapy can play an important role in patients with phlegmasia cerulea dolens. This syndrome is marked by complete thrombosis of one or both lower extremity venous systems, leading to pain, edema, cyanosis, and arterial insufficiency. Phlegmasia cerulea dolens is often associated with malignancy or with the presence of an inferior vena cava filter. Amputation is required in a significant number of cases, and the mortality from this disease has been estimated at 25–40%. Thrombolysis is particularly useful in patients presenting with venous gangrene, who virtually never respond to anticoagulation and supportive measures alone.

The technique for treating iliofemoral thrombus is well described by Semba et al. (121). The initial approach usually involves accessing the popliteal vein in the popliteal fossa using ultrasound guidance. An ascending venogram is performed, and a 6 French sheath is inserted. A guide wire is negotiated into the inferior vena cava and a multi–side-hole catheter is embedded into the thrombus. Thrombolytic therapy is initiated, and the patient is monitored in an ICU or intermediate care unit. Low-dose heparin (100–500 units/hr) is given through sheath or peripheral IV. Fibrinogen and PTT values are obtained every 6–8 hours and maintained >100 mg/dL and <60 seconds. Pneumatic compression can be used to massage the limb and improve the edema. The patient is evaluated the next day, and a decision is made about how to proceed:

- Complete thrombolysis and no stenosis, no further intervention
- Complete thrombolysis and a stenosis, then angioplasty followed by stent placement. Avoid stenting over the inflow of the profunda or saphenous vein.
- Complete thrombolysis and femoral vein stenosis, angioplasty only of stenosis
- Partial thrombolysis, infusion continued as long as fibrinogen values are >100 mg/dL and no bleeding complications. Reevaluate patient in late afternoon.
- No thrombolysis of iliac and femoral vein, then considered technical failure and no further intervention

Pulmonary Arteries

Most patients with pulmonary embolism only require treatment to prevent further embolization. Anticoagulation, or an inferior vena cava filter, is the appropriate therapy. However, a small fraction of patients sustain acute massive pulmonary embolism that causes profound cardiovascular compromise and is associated with high mortality. The traditional approach for these patients was a pulmonary embolectomy; however, the overall mortality for surgical embolectomy when performed on patients in cardiac arrest is about 58–74%, although in patients without cardiac arrest the mortality is 3–31% (122). Because of this high mortality rate, noninvasive approaches are critical.

Results from phase I and phase II studies of the multicenter Urokinase Pulmonary Embolism Trial established that intravenous fibrinolytic agents were more effective than anticoagulation alone in the dissolution of pulmonary emboli, especially when clots were massive (123–125). In those studies, significant improvement in angiographic abnormalities was observed in 9% of patients treated with heparin alone and in 53% of patients treated with UK. However, bleeding complications were frequent in both groups (27 and 45%, respectively). In addition, no significant differences in the final degree of resolution by radionuclide scanning, recurrence of pulmonary embolism, or mortality were found between the two treatment regimens.

The introduction of TPA has rekindled interest in thrombolytic therapy for pulmonary embolism. A study comparing TPA to heparin alone demonstrated a rapid improvement of right ventricular function in the TPA group at 24 hours, which was highly significant compared to the heparin group. But there was no effect on survival (126). Another study comparing TPA and heparin in patients with acute submassive and massive PE demonstrated significant reductions of pulmonary artery pressure and total pulmonary resistance together with an increase in cardiac output in the first 12 hours in the TPA but not in the heparin group (127). However, by the end of the first week no difference was present between the groups. The largest prospective randomized thrombolysis trial to date was published recently (128). Enrolled patients had submassive PE with evidence of pulmonary hypertension, right ventricular dysfunction, or both. Patients were randomized to TPA or placebo with concomitant heparin anticoagulation. The primary endpoint of the study was in-hospital death or need for escalation of treatment. Alteplase treatment reduced the incidence of the primary endpoint from 25% to 11%. The in-hospital mortality rate, however, showed no significant difference. No fatal or cerebral bleeding episodes were observed in the alteplase group (129).

The dosing of thrombolytic agents is different than for arterial disease; administration is primarily systemic. UK is used with a 4,400 unit/kg loading dose followed by an infusion of 2,200 units/kg/hr for 12 hours. Alteplase (TPA) is administered as a 100-mg infusion over 2 hours. Reteplase is not approved for use in PE but has been studied at a dose of two intravenous boluses of 10 units, 28 minutes apart (115).

The optimal route for treating massive pulmonary emboli is subject to debate. There has been no clear evidence that catheter-directed thrombolysis is superior to systemic therapy. Directed thrombolysis (130,131), mechanical dissolution by fragmentation (132–134), and direct removal (135) have all been tried but primarily in case reports or small series.

The critical issue is whether the rapid improvement in hemodynamic parameters can affect the prognosis of some patients enough to justify the potential risks of thrombolytic agents. The risk of life-threatening or disabling hemorrhage associated with thrombolysis ranges from the incidence of major bleeding events as high as 36% and that of an intracranial/fatal hemorrhage at 4% (129). Thrombolytic agents are considered potentially dangerous drugs and are reserved for high-risk patients whose condition requires rapid resolution of the emboli. Criteria for percutaneous intervention for an acute PE includes: arterial hypotension (BP <90 mm Hg or a drop of >40 mm Hg), cardiogenic shock with peripheral hypoperfusion and hypoxia, circulatory collapse with the need for cardiopulmonary resuscitation, echocardiographic findings of RV strain or pulmonary hypertension, an A-a gradient of >50 mm Hg (122).

Visceral Arteries and Veins

Thrombolysis has been reported in the arteries and veins of the abdomen. Most of the reports are scattered case reports, making it difficult to draw firm conclusions.

Renal Artery

Renal artery thrombosis usually results from underlying atherosclerotic disease, embolism, blunt abdominal trauma, dissection from catheterization or renal artery angioplasty, or complications of transplantation (136). Thrombolytic therapy has been applied in scattered cases of acute renal artery thrombosis, renal transplant arterial thrombosis, and of occluded renal artery grafts (137–141). Muegge et al. reviewed the published experience with SK infusion in the treatment of renal artery occlusions (142). Although lysis is successful in most cases, full recovery of renal function is unusual, and segmental renal infarctions are common.

Preservation of function largely depends on the extent of preexisting collateral blood flow through periureteric, capsular, lumbar, and inferior adrenal branches. In particular, late reconstitution of the distal renal artery by collateral vessels and the presence of a distinct nephrogram may predict successful return of at least partial renal function after treatment (1). Flow may be insufficient for adequate renal function but sufficient to maintain organ viability. Therefore, thrombolysis is probably warranted even weeks after occlusion in a patient with suspected chronic renal artery disease. However, thrombolysis should not be delayed more than several hours in patients with probable acute occlusion, such as embolism or trauma (143).

Renal Vein

Renal vein thrombosis can be caused by neoplastic disease, trauma, kidney transplant, dehydration, sepsis, and complications of nephritic syndrome (144,145). Most patients are treated with anticoagulation; however, with an acute thrombosis, collateral vein formation may not be adequate, and renal function may be lost (146). There has been limited experience with thrombolytic infusions for native renal vein thrombosis. Direct thrombolytic therapy can be performed into the renal vein (147). Thrombolysis directly into the renal vein but supplemented by renal artery infusion also appears to be effective (146,148).

Thrombosis of the vein in a transplanted kidney is a rare, potentially catastrophic event usually related to kinking of the vein, extension of lower extremity thrombophlebitis into the pelvic veins, or extrinsic compression by hematoma or lymphocele (1). To salvage the transplant and prevent spontaneous rupture, surgical thrombectomy or thrombolysis may be necessary. Thrombolysis for graft salvage by direct venous infusion has been successful, and the native kidney infusion of thrombolytic agents into the artery may also be helpful (149–151).

Mesenteric Arteries

Mesenteric artery thrombolysis has been reported, primarily in case reports and small series (152–157). Thrombolysis in this arterial bed should be undertaken with great care. If the patient has severe ischemia from thrombosis of the mesenteric artery, bowel infarction is going to occur. Prolonged thrombolytic infusion while ischemia is ongoing may lead to bowel necrosis, bowel perforation, and decreased survival.

Acute mesenteric ischemia is primarily caused by an embolus to the superior mesenteric artery (SMA) or thrombosis of the artery (158). In a Swedish autopsy study, the cause of occlusion was embolism in 57.3%, thrombosis in 41.3%, and indeterminate in 1.4% (159). Most of the patients with embolic occlusion (70%) had evidence of a cardiac source. Importantly 68% of the patients with an embolus had one or more emboli within the mesenteric vessels. This study also found that most of the occlusions whether embolic or thrombotic occurred in a proximal location thus leading to more extensive bowel infarction (159,160). Patients with thrombosis from preexisting atherosclerotic disease may be the most appropriate for thrombolytic therapy because they may have formed collaterals, which can support bowel perfusion.

If an attempt at thrombolysis is going to be attempted, there may be certain factors that can contribute to success. An excellent review of thrombolysis of acute superior mesenteric artery thromboembolism is available (160). The patient should have fewer than 72 hours of symptoms and preferably fewer than 12 hours (158,160). The patient should be resuscitated, and if possible, the diagnosis established with dynamic CT (158). The CT must show no evidence of bowel infarction (no intramural air, ileus, pneumoperitoneum, or ascites) (161,162). If there are peritoneal findings, the patient should go immediately to laparotomy (158). On angiography an arterial occlusion is identified, and if there is some filling of SMA, thrombolysis could be performed. If there is no filling, thrombolysis could be tried (and has been successful), but there should be a compelling medical reason for the patient not to go on to surgery and there should be a low threshold for proceeding to surgery if thrombolysis is not proceeding as expected or if the patient's condition changes (158). The thrombolytic agent should be short acting so that surgery is not precluded, pulse spray or another way of rapidly delivering thrombolytic into the thrombus should be used and probably a high dose, because short infusion time is important. Anticoagulation should probably be used, and a vasodilator may be helpful. If at anytime the patient develops peritoneal signs, then the patient should be taken to surgery.

Mesenteric and Portal Vein

Mesenteric venous thrombosis (MVT) accounts for 5–15% of all intestinal ischemic events (158). It is classified according to its etiology, into primary and secondary MVT. When an etiologic factor is found, patients are said to have secondary MVT (163). Primary MCT is probably most commonly because of hereditary or acquired hypercoagulation

disorders, and if one of these disorders is identified, the patient would be considered to have secondary MVT (163,164). Disorders including protein C and S deficiency, antithrombin III deficiency, dysfibrinogenemia, abnormal plasminogen, and factor V Leiden mutation (164). Secondary causes include malignancies, pancreatitis, inflammatory bowel disease, cirrhosis and portal hypertension, splenomegaly, splenectomy or other abdominal surgeries, sclerotherapy for esophageal varices, trauma, and oral contraceptives (158,163,164).

Contrast-enhanced CT is the examination of choice for suspected cases of MVT, and it can demonstrate the thrombus within the mesenteric vein. Well-developed collateral circulation indicates mesenteric venous thrombosis of more than a few weeks duration (163). Other CT findings included thickening of the bowel wall, intestinal pneumatosis, and an ominous finding of mesenteric or portal venous gas (165).

In symptomatic patients with acute MVT, the choice of treatment is determined by the severity of peritoneal signs. Anticoagulation therapy should be started immediately (164). Patients with peritoneal signs will require emergency surgery because bowel infarction has probably occurred. In the other symptomatic patients, thrombolysis can be considered. There have been a number of case reports of thrombolytic treatment for MVT (166–172). The approach for thrombolysis has been variable including via a transjugular approach (170), a transhepatic approach (171), an arterial approach (167,169,172), mechanical thrombolysis (166,171,173) or a combination (171,174). Involvement of the portal vein with thrombosis and the extent of thrombosis may influence the approach. The transjugular approach is particularly appropriate when there is the need for a transjugular intrahepatic portosystemic shunt, such as in a patient with cirrhosis and mesenteric/portal vein thrombosis (173). Thrombolytic therapy should be continued until either the thrombus is resolved, there is no further improvement in the appearance of the thrombus, worsening clinical symptoms, evidence of systemic fibrinolysis, or bleeding complications (172).

COMPLICATIONS

The major complications resulting from thrombolytic therapy are bleeding, distal embolizations, allergic or idiosyncratic drug reactions, reperfusion syndrome, pericatheter thrombosis, and graft extravasation. Comparison of complications among studies is complicated because of the variety of conditions treated, variety of drugs and combination of drugs used, techniques (including time for lysis and method of delivering thrombolytic) involved, and classification of complications.

Most of the data on bleeding complications with thrombolytic therapy are derived from large-scale studies on myocardial infarction with systemic administration of thrombolysis. Although catheter-directed methods of thrombolysis are much less likely to produce a systemic lytic effect, fibrinolysis may occur at a site remote from the occluded vessel. This bleeding may be lysis of a preexisting hemostatic plug, the induced fibrinolytic or anticoagulated state, or loss of vascular integrity via an already established vessel puncture (3). Hemorrhage at remote sites can be minimized by withholding treatment from patients with risk factors for bleeding. The risk of hemorrhage with fibrinolytic therapy is compounded by the use of anticoagulants and antiplatelet agents.

Severe systemic or intracranial bleeding is the most significant clinical risk associated with any thrombolytic therapy. Severe hemorrhage is defined as causing an interruption in therapy, causing hypotension, requiring blood transfusion or surgical evacuation. For directed thrombolysis, such complications have ranged from 0–8% in peripheral arterial thrombolysis (58) to 10% in DVT thrombolysis (175). The incidence of hemorrhagic stroke has been reported at 1–2.3% (3). The frequency of major bleeding complications seems to be connected more closely to the duration of infusion rather than to the total dose of fibrinolytic agent.

Minor bleeding at the puncture site is by far the most common complication of thrombolytic therapy for peripheral vascular occlusions and is reported in ranges of 0–25% of cases (3,58). Bleeding is usually self-limited and requires no further therapy.

It is possible that specific techniques may decrease bleeding complications. Intrathrombic administration of fibrinolytic agents may allow for decreased thrombolytic dose and decreased time of thrombolysis. Using UK for PSPMT in peripheral arteries and bypass grafts, there was a 3% minor and 0.5% major bleeding rate, with no episodes of retroperitoneal or intracranial hemorrhage (16). There have been very few randomized studies comparing various types of thrombolytics and methods of delivering those thrombolytics.

The management of severe bleeding includes discontinuing the thrombolytic agent and anticoagulants, replenishing coagulation factors (for example, fresh frozen plasma and cryoprecipitate) and blood, and intervening surgically only to evacuate hematoma causing pressure phenomena on adjacent tissues or to repair a vascular injury that continues to bleed. Bleeding from the puncture site should be controlled with local compression, an increase in catheter size, and placement of a sheath or surgical stitch on the vessel or graft (3).

Distal embolization is the other major complication from thrombolytic therapy. Embolization is reported in 2–15% of patients treated for peripheral arterial occlusions (1). However, angiographic assessment of distal vessels after the procedure was not performed routinely in all reported series. When large, clearly intraluminal filling defects are present after thrombolysis, avoiding angioplasty can minimize embolization. Thrombolysis should be continued whenever distal embolization occurs. Additional measures to be considered are a more distal repositioning

of the catheter, a new bolus dose, or an increased dose. Thrombus aspiration or surgery may be required if thrombolysis does not improve the clinical condition.

With treatment of thrombosed dialysis grafts embolization of small clot fragments to the lung probably occurs in the majority of cases. However, symptomatic pulmonary embolism is rare observed. Embolization of clot from the proximal portion of the graft into the efferent artery has been reported and can be minimized by careful manipulation of guide wires and catheters within the proximal portion of the graft and by delaying angioplasty of residual clot near the arterial anastomosis until the plug is withdrawn into the body of the graft with an occlusion balloon.

Allergic reactions are a known complication with SK, and some idiosyncratic reactions to UK have been reported. Symptoms develop 30–60 minutes after starting therapy and involve moderate to severe rigors, agitation, tachycardia, and occasionally nausea or vomiting. Reactions to TPA or the other modified analogs appear to be very rare.

Revascularization complications that may occur after thrombolysis include compartment syndrome and the postrevascularization syndrome. Compartment syndrome is a rare complication after infusion thrombolysis and was seen in 4% of patients treated by McNamara et al. for acute lower extremity ischemia (176).

Pericatheter thrombosis was a frequent problem in the early years of thrombolytic therapy. The routine use of systemic heparin with UK had virtually eliminated this problem, but with decreasing doses of heparin with TPA, there may be an increase in this complication. In a small fraction of patients, ongoing rethrombosis may occur, particularly when a hypercoagulable state is present.

REFERENCES

1. Valji K, Bookstein JJ. Thrombolysis: clinical applications. In: Baum S, ed. Abrams' Angiography. 4th Ed. Boston: Little, Brown and Company 1997:132–159.
2. Dormandy JA, Rutherford RB. Management of peripheral arterial disease (PAD). TASC Working Group. TransAtlantic Inter-Society Consensus (TASC). J Vasc Surg 2000;31:S1–S296.
3. Thrombolysis in the management of lower limb peripheral arterial occlusion—a consensus document. J Vasc Interv Radiol 2003;14:S337–S349.
4. Davis GB, Dowd CF, Bookstein JJ, et al. Thrombosed dialysis grafts: efficacy of intrathrombic deposition of concentrated urokinase, clot maceration, and angioplasty. AJR Am J Roentgenol 1987;149:177–181.
5. Razavi MK, Lee DS, Hofmann LV. Catheter-directed thrombolytic therapy for limb ischemia: current status and controversies. J Vasc Interv Radiol 2004;15:13–23.
6. Dotter CT, Rosch J, Seaman AJ. Selective clot lysis with low-dose streptokinase. Radiology 1974;111:31–37.
7. McNamara TO, Fischer JR. Thrombolysis of peripheral arterial and graft occlusions: improved results using high-dose urokinase. AJR Am J Roentgenol 1985;144:769–775.
8. Results of a prospective randomized trial evaluating surgery versus thrombolysis for ischemia of the lower extremity. The STILE trial. Ann Surg 1994;220:251–266 (discussion 266–258).
9. Ouriel K, Shortell CK, Azodo MV, et al. Acute peripheral arterial occlusion: predictors of success in catheter-directed thrombolytic therapy. Radiology 1994;193:561–566.

10. Sullivan KL, Gardiner GA, Jr, Shapiro MJ, et al. Acceleration of thrombolysis with a high-dose transthrombus bolus technique. Radiology 1989;173:805–808.
11. Kandarpa K, Goldhaber SZ, Meyerovitz MF. Pulse spray thrombolysis: the "careful analysis." Radiology 1994;193:320–324.
12. Kandarpa K, Chopra PS, Aruny JE, et al. Intra-arterial thrombolysis of lower extremity occlusions: prospective, randomized comparison of forced periodic infusion and conventional slow continuous infusion. Radiology 1993;188:861–867.
13. Braithwaite BD, Buckenham TM, Galland RB, et al. Prospective randomized trial of high-dose bolus versus low-dose tissue plasminogen activator infusion in the management of acute limb ischaemia. Thrombolysis Study Group. Br J Surg 1997;84:646–650.
14. Valji K. Evolving strategies for thrombolytic therapy of peripheral vascular occlusion. J Vasc Interv Radiol 2000;11:411–420.
15. Bookstein JJ, Saldinger E. Accelerated thrombolysis. In vitro evaluation of agents and methods of administration. Invest Radiol 1985;20:731–735.
16. Bookstein JJ, Valji K. Pulse spray pharmacomechanical thrombolysis: updated clinical and laboratory observations. Semin Intervent Radiol 1992;9:174–182.
17. Valji K, Bookstein JJ. Pulsed spray thrombolysis accelerates clot dissolution. Diagn Imaging (San Franc) 1991;13:58–63.
18. Valji K, Bookstein JJ. Efficacy of adjunctive intrathrombic heparin with pulse spray thrombolysis in rabbit inferior vena cava thrombosis. Invest Radiol 1992;27:912–917.
19. Bookstein JJ, Valji K, Roberts AC. Pulsed versus conventional thrombolytic infusion techniques. Radiology 1994;193:318–320.
20. Bookstein JJ. How does one determine when thrombolysis is sufficient? AJR Am J Roentgenol 1995;164:258.
21. Sharafuddin MJ, Wroblicka JT, Sun S, et al. Percutaneous vascular intervention based on gadolinium-enhanced MR angiography. J Vasc Interv Radiol 2000;11:739–746.
22. Sharafuddin MJ, Stolpen AH, Dixon BS, et al. Value of MR angiography before percutaneous transluminal renal artery angioplasty and stent placement. J Vasc Interv Radiol 2002;13:901–908.
23. Roh BS, Park KH, Kim EA, et al. Prognostic value of CT before thrombolytic therapy in iliofemoral deep venous thrombosis. J Vasc Interv Radiol 2002;13:71–76.
24. Dorros G, Hall P, Iyer SS. Urokinase infusion of chronically occluded femoropopliteal Gortex bypass grafts via the popliteal approach. Cathet Cardiovasc Diagn 1991;24:197–203.
25. Hall P, Iyer SS, Dorros G. Successful thrombolysis of a chronically occluded femoropopliteal synthetic bypass graft via the popliteal approach: case report. Cardiovasc Intervent Radiol 1991;14:352–354.
26. Page JE, Buckenham TM, Taylor RS. Accelerated thrombolysis facilitated by direct puncture of occluded prosthetic femoral grafts. Australas Radiol 1992;36:230–233.
27. Lee DE, Waldman DL, Sumida RK, et al. Direct graft puncture with use of a crossed catheter technique for thrombolysis of peripheral bypass grafts. J Vasc Interv Radiol 2000;11:445–452.
28. Smith DC, McCormick MJ, Jensen DA, et al. Guide wire traversal test: retrospective study of results with fibrinolytic therapy. J Vasc Interv Radiol 1991;2:339–342.
29. Buczko W, Mogielnicki A, Kramkowski K, et al. Aspirin and the fibrinolytic response. Thromb Res 2003;110:331–334.
30. Ouriel K. Use of concomitant glycoprotein IIb/IIIa inhibitors with catheter-directed peripheral arterial thrombolysis. J Vasc Interv Radiol 2004;15:543–546.
31. Semba CP, Bakal CW, Calis KA, et al. Alteplase as an alternative to urokinase. Advisory Panel on Catheter-Directed Thrombolytic Therapy. J Vasc Interv Radiol 2000;11:279–287.
32. Benenati J, Shlansky-Goldberg R, Meglin A, et al. Thrombolytic and antiplatelet therapy in peripheral vascular disease with use of reteplase and/or abciximab. The SCVIR Consultants' Conference; May 22, 2000 (Orlando, FL). Society for Cardiovascular and Interventional Radiology. J Vasc Interv Radiol 2001;12:795–805.
33. Weitz JI, Hirsh J. New anticoagulant drugs. Chest 2001;119:95S–107S.
34. Ouriel K, Castaneda F, McNamara T, et al. Reteplase monotherapy and reteplase/abciximab combination therapy in peripheral arterial occlusive disease: results from the RELAX trial. J Vasc Interv Radiol 2004;15:229–238.
35. Braithwaite BD, Jones L, Yusuf SW, et al. Aspirin improves the outcome of intra-arterial thrombolysis with tissue plasminogen activator. Thrombolysis Study Group. Br J Surg 1995;82:1357–1358.
36. Tepe G, Schott U, Erley CM, et al. Platelet glycoprotein IIb/IIIa receptor antagonist used in conjunction with thrombolysis for peripheral arterial thrombosis. AJR Am J Roentgenol 1999;172:1343–1346.
37. Drescher P, Crain MR, Rilling WS. Initial experience with the combination of reteplase and abciximab for thrombolytic therapy in peripheral arterial occlusive disease: a pilot study. J Vasc Interv Radiol 2002;13:37–43.
38. Yoon HC, Miller FJ Jr. Using a peptide inhibitor of the glycoprotein IIb/IIIa platelet receptor: initial experience in patients with acute peripheral arterial occlusions. AJR Am J Roentgenol 2002;178:617–622.
39. Shlansky-Goldberg R. Platelet aggregation inhibitors for use in peripheral vascular interventions: what can we learn from the experience in the coronary arteries? J Vasc Interv Radiol 2002;13:229–246.
40. Burkart DJ, Borsa JJ, Anthony JP, et al. Thrombolysis of acute peripheral arterial and venous occlusions with tenecteplase and eptifibatide: a pilot study. J Vasc Interv Radiol 2003;14:729–733.
41. Decrinis M, Pilger E, Stark G, et al. A simplified procedure for intra-arterial thrombolysis with tissue-type plasminogen activator in peripheral arterial occlusive disease: primary and long-term results. Eur Heart J 1993;14:297–305.
42. Guest P, Buckenham T. Thrombolysis of the occluded prosthetic graft with tissue-type plasminogen activator—technique, results, and problems in 23 patients. Clin Radiol 1992;46:381–386.
43. Ouriel K, Shortell CK, DeWeese JA, et al. A comparison of thrombolytic therapy with operative revascularization in the initial treatment of acute peripheral arterial ischemia. J Vasc Surg 1994;19:1021–1030.
44. Weaver FA, Comerota AJ, Youngblood M, et al. Surgical revascularization versus thrombolysis for nonembolic lower extremity native artery occlusions: results of a prospective randomized trial. The STILE Investigators. Surgery versus Thrombolysis for Ischemia of the Lower Extremity. J Vasc Surg 1996;24:513–521 (discussion 521–513).
45. Comerota AJ, Weaver FA, Hosking JD, et al. Results of a prospective, randomized trial of surgery versus thrombolysis for occluded lower extremity bypass grafts. Am J Surg 1996;172:105–112.
46. Ouriel K, Veith FJ, Sasahara AA. Thrombolysis or peripheral arterial surgery: phase I results. TOPAS Investigators. J Vasc Surg 1996;23:64–73 (discussion 74–65).
47. Swischuk JL, Fox PF, Young K, et al. Transcatheter intra-arterial infusion of rt-PA for acute lower limb ischemia: results and complications. J Vasc Interv Radiol 2001;12:423–430.
48. Tsetis DK, Kochiadakis GE, Hatzidakis AA, et al. Transcatheter thrombolysis with high-dose bolus tissue plasminogen activator in iatrogenic arterial occlusion after femoral arterial catheterization. Cardiovasc Intervent Radiol 2002;25:36–41.
49. Mewissen MW, Minor PL, Beyer GA, et al. Symptomatic native arterial occlusions: early experience with "over-the-wire" thrombolysis. J Vasc Interv Radiol 1990;1:43–47.
50. Valji K, Roberts AC, Davis GB, et al. Pulsed spray thrombolysis of arterial and bypass graft occlusions. AJR Am J Roentgenol 1991;156:617–621.
51. Yusuf SW, Whitaker SC, Gregson RH, et al. Prospective randomised comparative study of pulse spray and conventional local thrombolysis. Eur J Vasc Endovasc Surg 1995;10:136–141.
52. Yusuf SW, Whitaker SC, Gregson RH, et al. Immediate and early follow-up results of purse spray thrombolysis in patients with peripheral ischaemia. Br J Surg 1995;82:338–340.
53. Hull JE, Hull MK, Urso JA. Reteplase with or without abciximab for peripheral arterial occlusions: efficacy and adverse events. J Vasc Interv Radiol 2004;15:557–564.
54. Nakada MT, Montgomery MO, Nedelman MA, et al. Clot lysis in a primate model of peripheral arterial occlusive disease with use of systemic or intra-arterial reteplase: addition of abciximab results in improved vessel reperfusion. J Vasc Interv Radiol 2004;15:169–176.
55. Davidian MM, Powell A, Benenati JF, et al. Initial results of reteplase in the treatment of acute lower extremity arterial occlusions. J Vasc Interv Radiol 2000;11:289–294.

56. Burkart DJ, Borsa JJ, Anthony JP, et al. Thrombolysis of occluded peripheral arteries and veins with tenecteplase: a pilot study. J Vasc Interv Radiol 2002;13:1099–1102.

57. Razavi MK, Wong H, Kee ST, et al. Initial clinical results of tenecteplase (TNK) in catheter-directed thrombolytic therapy. J Endovasc Ther 2002;9:593–598.

58. Kessel DO, Berridge DC, Robertson I. Infusion techniques for peripheral arterial thrombolysis. Cochrane Database Syst Rev 2004:CD000985.

59. Ouriel K. Comparison of surgical and thrombolytic treatment of peripheral arterial disease. Rev Cardiovasc Med 2002;3(Suppl II):S7–S16.

60. Earnshaw JJ, Whitman B, Foy C. National Audit of Thrombolysis for Acute Leg Ischemia (NATALI): clinical factors associated with early outcome. J Vasc Surg 2004;39:1018–1025.

61. Lang EV, Stevick CA. Transcatheter therapy of severe acute lower extremity ischemia. J Vasc Interv Radiol 1993;4:481–488.

62. Paulson EK, Miller FJ. Embolization of cardiac mural thrombus: complication of intra-arterial fibrinolysis. Radiology 1988;168:95–96.

63. Lonsdale RJ, Berridge DC, Makin GS, et al. Detection of left heart thrombus by echocardiography is not essential before peripheral arterial thrombolysis. J R Coll Surg Edinb 1992;37:19–22.

64. Nguyen LL, Conte MS, Menard MT, et al. Infrainguinal vein bypass graft revision: factors affecting long-term outcome. J Vasc Surg 2004;40:916–923.

65. Landry GJ, Moneta GL, Taylor LM Jr, et al. Long-term outcome of revised lower-extremity bypass grafts. J Vasc Surg 2002;35:56–62 (discussion 62–53).

66. Nehler MR, Mueller RJ, McLafferty RB, et al. Outcome of catheter-directed thrombolysis for lower extremity arterial bypass occlusion. J Vasc Surg 2003;37:72–78.

67. Conrad MF, Shepard AD, Rubinfeld IS, et al. Long-term results of catheter-directed thrombolysis to treat infrainguinal bypass graft occlusion: the urokinase era. J Vasc Surg 2003;37:1009–1016.

68. Hye RJ, Turner C, Valji K, et al. Is thrombolysis of occluded popliteal and tibial bypass grafts worthwhile? J Vasc Surg 1994;20:588–596 (discussion 596–587).

69. Nackman GB, Walsh DB, Fillinger MF, et al. Thrombolysis of occluded infrainguinal vein grafts: predictors of outcome. J Vasc Surg 1997;25:1023–1031 (discussion 1031–1022).

70. Kumpe DA, Cohen MA. Angioplasty/thrombolytic treatment of failing and failed hemodialysis access sites: comparison with surgical treatment. Prog Cardiovasc Dis 1992;34:263–278.

71. Krysl J, Kumpe DA. Failing and failed hemodialysis access sites: management with percutaneous catheter methods. Semin Vasc Surg 1997;10:175–183.

72. Cynamon J, Pierpont CE. Thrombolysis for the treatment of thrombosed hemodialysis access grafts. Rev Cardiovasc Med 2002;3(Suppl II):S84–S91.

73. Zeit R. Clearing of clotted dialysis shunts by streptokinase injection at multiple sites. AJR Am J Roentgenol 1983;141:1053–1054.

74. Cynamon J, Lakritz PS, Wahl SI, et al. Hemodialysis graft declotting: description of the "lyse and wait" technique. J Vasc Interv Radiol 1997;8:825–829.

75. Falk A, Mitty H, Guller J, et al. Thrombolysis of clotted hemodialysis grafts with tissue-type plasminogen activator. J Vasc Interv Radiol 2001;12:305–311.

76. Vogel PM, Bansal V, Marshall MW. Thrombosed hemodialysis grafts: lyse and wait with tissue plasminogen activator or urokinase compared to mechanical thrombolysis with the Arrow-Trerotola percutaneous thrombolytic device. J Vasc Interv Radiol 2001;12:1157–1165.

77. Valji K, Bookstein JJ, Roberts AC, et al. Pulse spray pharmacomechanical thrombolysis of thrombosed hemodialysis access grafts: long-term experience and comparison of original and current techniques. AJR Am J Roentgenol 1995;164:1495–1500 (discussion 1501–1493).

78. Valji K. Transcatheter treatment of thrombosed hemodialysis access grafts. AJR Am J Roentgenol 1995;164:823–829.

79. Kinney TB, Valji K, Rose SC, et al. Pulmonary embolism from pulse spray pharmacomechanical thrombolysis of clotted hemodialysis grafts: urokinase versus heparinized saline. J Vasc Interv Radiol 2000;11:1143–1152.

80. Swan TL, Smyth SH, Ruffenach SJ, et al. Pulmonary embolism following hemodialysis access thrombolysis/thrombectomy. J Vasc Interv Radiol 1995;6:683–686.

81. Weng FL, Berns JS. Complications of percutaneous treatment of thrombosed hemodialysis access grafts. Semin Dial 2003;16:257–262.

82. Aruny JE, Lewis CA, Cardella JF, et al. Quality improvement guidelines for percutaneous management of the thrombosed or dysfunctional dialysis access. J Vasc Interv Radiol 2003;14:S247–S253.

83. Palder S, Kirkman R, Whittemore A, et al. Vascular access for hemodialysis. Ann Surg 1985;202:235–239.

84. Kanterman RY, Vesely TM, Pilgram TK, et al. Dialysis access grafts: anatomic location of venous stenosis and results of angioplasty. Radiology 1995;195:135–139.

85. Patel NH, Revanur VK, Khanna A, et al. Vascular access for hemodialysis: an in-depth review. J Nephrol 2001;14:146–156.

86. Kandarpa K, Becker GJ, Hunink MG, et al. Transcatheter interventions for the treatment of peripheral atherosclerotic lesions: part I. J Vasc Interv Radiol 2001;12:683–695.

87. Kartchner MM, Wilcox WC. Thrombolysis of palmar and digital arterial thrombosis by intra-arterial thrombolysin. J Hand Surg [Am] 1976;1:67–74.

88. Kretz JG, Weiss E, Limuris A, et al. Arterial emboli of the upper extremity: a persisting problem. J Cardiovasc Surg (Torino) 1984;25:233–235.

89. Feldman DR, Vujic I, McKay D, et al. Crutch-induced axillary artery injury. Cardiovasc Intervent Radiol 1995;18:296–299.

90. Martinez R, Rodriguez-Lopez J, Torruella L, et al. Stenting for occlusion of the subclavian arteries. Technical aspects and follow-up results. Tex Heart Inst J 1997;24:23–27.

91. Bucek RA, Schnurer G, Ahmadi A, et al. A severe case of vascular thoracic outlet syndrome. Wien Klin Wochenschr 2000;112:973–977.

92. Cejna M, Salomonowitz E, Wohlschlager H, et al. rt-PA thrombolysis in acute thromboembolic upper-extremity arterial occlusion. Cardiovasc Intervent Radiol 2001;24:218–223.

93. Geschwind JF, Dagli MS, Lambert DL, et al. Thrombolytic therapy in the setting of arterial line-induced ischemia. J Endovasc Ther 2003;10:590–594.

94. Widlus DM, Venbrux AC, Benenati JF, et al. Fibrinolytic therapy for upper-extremity arterial occlusions. Radiology 1990;175:393–399.

95. Lambiase RE, Paolella LP, Haas RA, et al. Extensive thromboembolic disease of the hand and forearm: treatment with thrombolytic therapy. J Vasc Interv Radiol 1991;2:201–208.

96. Lang EV, Bookstein JJ. Accelerated thrombolysis and angioplasty for hand ischemia in Buerger's disease. Cardiovasc Intervent Radiol 1989;12:95–97.

97. Meissner MH. Axillary-subclavian venous thrombosis. Rev Cardiovasc Med 2002;3(Suppl II):S76–S33.

98. Nemcek AA, Jr. Upper extremity deep venous thrombosis: interventional management. Tech Vasc Interv Radiol 2004;7:86–90.

99. Hingorani A, Ascher E, Lorenson E, et al. Upper extremity deep venous thrombosis and its impact on morbidity and mortality rates in a hospital-based population. J Vasc Surg 1997;26:853–860.

100. Hingorani A, Ascher E, Yorkovich W, et al. Upper extremity deep venous thrombosis: an underrecognized manifestation of a hypercoagulable state. Ann Vasc Surg 2000;14:421–426.

101. Bernardi E, Piccioli A, Marchiori A, et al. Upper extremity deep vein thrombosis: risk factors, diagnosis, and management. Semin Vasc Med 2001;1:105–110.

102. Mustafa S, Stein PD, Patel KC, et al. Upper extremity deep venous thrombosis. Chest 2003;123:1953–1956.

103. Kerr TM, Lutter KS, Moeller DM, et al. Upper extremity venous thrombosis diagnosed by duplex scanning. Am J Surg 1990;160:202–206.

104. Otten TR, Stein PD, Patel KC, et al. Thromboembolic disease involving the superior vena cava and brachiocephalic veins. Chest 2003;123:809–812.

105. Druy EM, Trout HH III, Giordano JM, et al. Lytic therapy in the treatment of axillary and subclavian vein thrombosis. J Vasc Surg 1985;2:821–827.

106. Schneider DB, Dimuzio PJ, Martin ND, et al. Combination treatment of venous thoracic outlet syndrome: open surgical

decompression and intraoperative angioplasty. J Vasc Surg 2004;40:599–603.

107. Beygui RE, Olcott Ct, Dalman RL. Subclavian vein thrombosis: outcome analysis based on etiology and modality of treatment. Ann Vasc Surg 1997;11:247–255.

108. Lee MC, Grassi CJ, Belkin M, et al. Early operative intervention after thrombolytic therapy for primary subclavian vein thrombosis: an effective treatment approach. J Vasc Surg 1998;27:1101–1107 (discussion 1107–1108).

109. Azakie A, McElhinney DB, Thompson RW, et al. Surgical management of subclavian-vein effort thrombosis as a result of thoracic outlet compression. J Vasc Surg 1998;28:777–786.

110. Schindler N, Vogelzang RL. Superior vena cava syndrome. Experience with endovascular stents and surgical therapy. Surg Clin North Am 1999;79:683–694, xi.

111. Meier GH, Pollak JS, Rosenblatt M, et al. Initial experience with venous stents in exertional axillary-subclavian vein thrombosis. J Vasc Surg 1996;24:974–981 (discussion 981–973).

112. Maintz D, Landwehr P, Gawenda M, et al. Failure of Wallstents in the subclavian vein due to stent damage. Clin Imaging 2001;25:133–137.

113. Buller HR, Agnelli G, Hull RD, et al. Antithrombotic therapy for venous thromboembolic disease: the Seventh ACCP Conference on Antithrombotic and Thrombolytic Therapy. Chest 2004;126: 401S–428S.

114. Semba CP, Razavi MK, Kee ST, et al. Thrombolysis for lower extremity deep venous thrombosis. Tech Vasc Interv Radiol 2004;7:68–78.

115. Baker WF Jr. Thrombolytic therapy: clinical applications. Hematol Oncol Clin North Am 2003;17:283–311.

116. Elliot MS, Immelman EJ, Jeffery P, et al. A comparative randomized trial of heparin versus streptokinase in the treatment of acute proximal venous thrombosis: an interim report of a prospective trial. Br J Surg 1979;66:838–843.

117. Arnesen H, Hoiseth A, Ly B. Streptokinase of heparin in the treatment of deep vein thrombosis. Follow-up results of a prospective study. Acta Med Scand 1982;211:65–68.

118. Elsharawy M, Elzayat E. Early results of thrombolysis vs. anticoagulation in iliofemoral venous thrombosis. A randomised clinical trial. Eur J Vasc Endovasc Surg 2002;24:209–214.

119. Mewissen MW, Seabrook GR, Meissner MH, et al. Catheter-directed thrombolysis for lower extremity deep venous thrombosis: report of a national multicenter registry. Radiology 1999; 211:39–49.

120. Comerota AJ. Quality-of-life improvement using thrombolytic therapy for iliofemoral deep venous thrombosis. Rev Cardiovasc Med 2002;3(Suppl II):S61–S67.

121. Semba CP, Tam I, Blaney M. Re: catheter-directed thrombolytic therapy for limb ischemia: current status and controversies. J Vasc Interv Radiol 2004;15:517.

122. Rahimtoola A, Bergin JD. Acute pulmonary embolism: an update on diagnosis and management. Curr Probl Cardiol 2005;30: 61–114.

123. Urokinase pulmonary embolism trial. Phase 1 results: a cooperative study. JAMA 1970;214:2163–2172.

124. The urokinase pulmonary embolism trial. A national cooperative study. Circulation 1973;47:II1–108.

125. Urokinase-streptokinase embolism trial. Phase 2 results. A cooperative study. JAMA 1974;229:1606–1613.

126. Goldhaber SZ, Haire WD, Feldstein ML, et al. Alteplase versus heparin in acute pulmonary embolism: randomised trial assessing right-ventricular function and pulmonary perfusion. Lancet 1993;341:507–511.

127. Konstantinides S, Tiede N, Geibel A, et al. Comparison of alteplase versus heparin for resolution of major pulmonary embolism. Am J Cardiol 1998;82:966–970.

128. Konstantinides S, Geibel A, Heusel G, et al. Heparin plus alteplase compared with heparin alone in patients with submassive pulmonary embolism. N Engl J Med 2002;347:1143–1150.

129. Konstantinides S. Thrombolysis in submassive pulmonary embolism? Yes. J Thromb Haemost 2003;1:1127–1129.

130. Sze DY, Carey MB, Razavi MK. Treatment of massive pulmonary embolus with catheter-directed tenecteplase. J Vasc Interv Radiol 2001;12:1456–1457.

131. De Gregorio MA, Gimeno MJ, Mainar A, et al. Mechanical and enzymatic thrombolysis for massive pulmonary embolism. J Vasc Interv Radiol 2002;13:163–169.

132. Schmitz-Rode T, Janssens U, Schild HH, et al. Fragmentation of massive pulmonary embolism using a pigtail rotation catheter. Chest 1998;114:1427–1436.

133. Schmitz-Rode T, Janssens U, Duda SH, et al. Massive pulmonary embolism: percutaneous emergency treatment by pigtail rotation catheter. J Am Coll Cardiol 2000;36:375–380.

134. Muller-Hulsbeck S, Brossmann J, Jahnke T, et al. Mechanical thrombectomy of major and massive pulmonary embolism with use of the Amplatz thrombectomy device. Invest Radiol 2001;36:317–322.

135. Uflacker R. Interventional therapy for pulmonary embolism. J Vasc Interv Radiol 2001;12:147–164.

136. Theiss M, Wirth MP, Dolken W, et al. Spontaneous thrombosis of the renal vessels. Rare entities to be considered in differential diagnosis of patients presenting with lumbar flank pain and hematuria. Urol Int 1992;48:441–445.

137. Cronan JJ, Jr., Dorfman GS. Low dose thrombolysis: a nonoperative approach to renal artery occlusion. J Urol 1983;130:757–759.

138. Pineo GF, Thorndyke WC, Steed BL. Spontaneous renal artery thrombosis: successful lysis with streptokinase. J Urol 1987;138: 1223–1225.

139. Louden JD, Leen GL, Cove-Smith R. Systemic thrombolysis for bilateral atherosclerotic renal artery occlusion resulting in prolonged recovery of renal function. Nephrol Dial Transplant 1998;13:2924–2926.

140. Gluck G, Croitoru M, Deleanu D, et al. Local thrombolytic treatment for renal arterial embolism. Eur Urol 2000;38:339–343.

141. Rathod J, Upadhayay D, Modhe J, et al. Restoration of renal function after prolonged allograft artery occlusion by thrombolysis. Nephrol Dial Transplant 2000;15:287–288.

142. Mugge A, Gulba DC, Frei U, et al. Renal artery embolism: thrombolysis with recombinant tissue-type plasminogen activator. J Intern Med 1990;228:279–286.

143. Blum U, Billmann P, Krause T, et al. Effect of local low-dose thrombolysis on clinical outcome in acute embolic renal artery occlusion. Radiology 1993;189:549–554.

144. Laville M, Aguilera D, Maillet PJ, et al. The prognosis of renal vein thrombosis: a reevaluation of 27 cases. Nephrol Dial Transplant 1988;3:247–256.

145. Witz M, Kantarovsky A, Morag B, et al. Renal vein occlusion: a review. J Urol 1996;155:1173–1179.

146. Huang AB, Glanz S, Hon M, et al. Renal vein thrombolysis with selective simultaneous renal artery and renal vein infusions. J Vasc Interv Radiol 1995;6:581–584.

147. Rowe JM, Rasmussen RL, Mader SL, et al. Successful thrombolytic therapy in two patients with renal vein thrombosis. Am J Med 1984;77:1111–1114.

148. Vogelzang RL, Moel DI, Cohn RA, et al. Acute renal vein thrombosis: successful treatment with intra-arterial urokinase. Radiology 1988;169:681–682.

149. Lee G, Watson CW, Mammen KJ, et al. Successful selective thrombolysis of a spontaneous transplant renal vein thrombosis. BJU Int 1999;83:869–870.

150. Modrall JG, Teitelbaum GP, Diaz-Luna H, et al. Local thrombolysis in a renal allograft threatened by renal vein thrombosis. Transplantation 1993;56:1011–1013.

151. Schwieger J, Reiss R, Cohen JL, et al. Acute renal allograft dysfunction in the setting of deep venous thrombosis: a case of successful urokinase thrombolysis and a review of the literature. Am J Kidney Dis 1993;22:345–350.

152. Hirota S, Matsumoto S, Yoshikawa T, et al. Simultaneous thrombolysis of superior mesenteric artery and bilateral renal artery thromboembolisms with three transfemoral catheters. Cardiovasc Intervent Radiol 1997;20:397–400.

153. Yamaguchi T, Saeki M, Iwasaki Y, et al. Local thrombolytic therapy for superior mesenteric artery embolism: complications and long-term clinical follow-up. Radiat Med 1999;17:27–33.

154. Sternbergh WC III, Ramee SR, DeVun DA, et al. Endovascular treatment of multiple visceral artery paradoxical emboli with mechanical and pharmacological thrombolysis. J Endovasc Ther 2000;7:155–160.

155. Wang G, Lu W, Xia Q, et al. Superior mesenteric arterial embolism: a retrospective study of local thrombolytic treatment with urokinase in West China. Int J Clin Pract 2003;57:588–591.

156. Tsuda M, Nakamura M, Yamada Y, et al. Acute superior mesenteric artery embolism: rapid reperfusion with hydrodynamic thrombectomy and pharmacological thrombolysis. J Endovasc Ther 2003;10:1015–1018.

157. Wakabayashi H, Shiode T, Kurose M, et al. Emergent treatment of acute embolic superior mesenteric ischemia with combination of thrombolysis and angioplasty: report of two cases. Cardiovasc Intervent Radiol 2004;27:389–393.

158. Sreenarasimhaiah J. Diagnosis and management of intestinal ischaemic disorders. Br Med J 2003;326:1372–1376.

159. Acosta S, Ogren M, Sternby NH, et al. Clinical implications for the management of acute thromboembolic occlusion of the superior mesenteric artery: autopsy findings in 213 patients. Ann Surg 2005;241:516–522.

160. Schoots IG, Levi MM, Reekers JA, et al. Thrombolytic therapy for acute superior mesenteric artery occlusion. J Vasc Interv Radiol 2005;16:317–329.

161. Chou YH, Tiu CM, Chen JD. Superior mesenteric thrombophlebitis subsequent to acute appendicitis in an adult. J Clin Ultrasound 2003;31:288–289.

162. Fleischmann D. Multiple detector-row CT angiography of the renal and mesenteric vessels. Eur J Radiol 2003;45(Suppl I):S79–S87.

163. Kumar S, Sarr MG, Kamath PS. Mesenteric venous thrombosis. N Engl J Med 2001;345:1683–1688.

164. Yasuhara H. Acute mesenteric ischemia: the challenge of gastroenterology. Surg Today 2005;35:185–195.

165. Bradbury MS, Kavanagh PV, Bechtold RE, et al. Mesenteric venous thrombosis: diagnosis and noninvasive imaging. Radiographics 2002;22:527–541.

166. Sze DY, O'Sullivan GJ, Johnson DL, et al. Mesenteric and portal venous thrombosis treated by transjugular mechanical thrombolysis. AJR Am J Roentgenol 2000;175:732–734.

167. Antoch G, Taleb N, Hansen O, et al. Transarterial thrombolysis of portal and mesenteric vein thrombosis: a promising alternative to common therapy. Eur J Vasc Endovasc Surg 2001;21:471–472.

168. Ciccarelli O, Goffette P, Laterre PF, et al. Transjugular intrahepatic portosystemic shunt approach and local thrombolysis for treatment of early posttransplant portal vein thrombosis. Transplantation 2001;72:159–161.

169. Tateishi A, Mitsui H, Oki T, et al. Extensive mesenteric vein and portal vein thrombosis successfully treated by thrombolysis and anticoagulation. J Gastroenterol Hepatol 2001;16:1429–1433.

170. Aytekin C, Boyvat F, Kurt A, et al. Catheter-directed thrombolysis with transjugular access in portal vein thrombosis secondary to pancreatitis. Eur J Radiol 2001;39:80–82.

171. Lopera JE, Correa G, Brazzini A, et al. Percutaneous transhepatic treatment of symptomatic mesenteric venous thrombosis. J Vasc Surg 2002;36:1058–1061.

172. Henao EA, Bohannon WT, Silva MB III. Treatment of portal venous thrombosis with selective superior mesenteric artery infusion of recombinant tissue plasminogen activator. J Vasc Surg 2003;38:1411–1415.

173. Uflacker R. Applications of percutaneous mechanical thrombectomy in transjugular intrahepatic portosystemic shunt and portal vein thrombosis. Tech Vasc Interv Radiol 2003;6:59–69.

174. Rosen MP, Sheiman R. Transhepatic mechanical thrombectomy followed by infusion of TPA into the superior mesenteric artery to treat acute mesenteric vein thrombosis. J Vasc Interv Radiol 2000;11:195–198.

175. Watson L, Armon M. Thrombolysis for acute deep vein thrombosis. Cochrane Database Syst Rev 2004:CD002783.

176. McNamara TO, Bomberger RA, Merchant RF. Intra-arterial urokinase as the initial therapy for acutely ischemic lower limbs. Circulation 1991;83:I106–119.

177. Grunwald MR, Hofmann LV. Comparison of urokinase, alteplase, and reteplase for catheter-directed thrombolysis of deep venous thrombosis. J Vasc Interv Radiol 2004;15:347–352.

Percutaneous Image-Guided Biopsy

16

Jeffrey S. Moulton, Christopher J. Leoni
Steven D. Quarfordt, Steven Worth

The first percutaneous needle biopsy procedure was performed in Germany in 1883. At that time, the theoretical foundation for modern techniques was laid, but the pioneers would scarcely recognize the procedure today given its current sophistication. Increasing acceptance by both practitioners and referring physicians has made it the most frequently performed interventional radiological procedure. This continued growth is attributable to three major factors. First, the development and evolution of cytologic techniques have allowed pathologic diagnoses to be made on the basis of the examination of individual cells. Second, recent advances in radiologic guidance techniques permit accurate and minimally invasive access to almost any site in the body. Third, the procedure has proved to be extremely safe when small-caliber aspiration needles are used.

Martin and Ellis from Memorial Hospital in New York are generally acknowledged as the founders of the needle aspiration technique. Martin, a head and neck surgeon, was reluctant to treat cancer patients without a preoperative pathologic diagnosis. He believed that surgery performed only for diagnosis carried an unacceptable risk of tumor dissemination in resectable disease and exposed patients to undue cost and morbidity in unresectable disease. Needle aspiration biopsy emerged as an alternative. The technique, which involved a simple handheld syringe and 18-gauge needle, was refined in the 1920s with initial results published in 1930 (1). The procedure did not initially gain widespread acceptance in the United States, in part because the cytologic specimens from 18-gauge needles were thick and poorly prepared, thus requiring unequivocal evidence of malignancy for diagnosis. At that time, the use of larger cutting needles to obtain histologic cores carried an unacceptably high complication rate.

Ultimately, needle biopsy for the preoperative diagnosis of tumors was replaced by intraoperative frozen section techniques. In the 1950s, percutaneous biopsy techniques were reborn in Europe with the development of small-caliber aspiration needles, which could obtain excellent cytologic specimens with minimal risk. Advancements in specimen preparation, largely refined in Sweden in the 1960s, improved the ability to interpret such specimens. The potential scope of percutaneous biopsy expanded dramatically with the development of cross-sectional guidance modalities, primarily ultrasound and computed tomography (CT). However, it was not until the 1970s that the procedure began to gain more widespread acceptance in the United States.

Throughout the last 20 years, greater evolution of pathologic techniques, biopsy needle technology, and guidance modalities has occurred. Numerous investigators have advanced the technique with continued improvements in accuracy and safety. In the current cost-conscious medical environment, percutaneous biopsy will assume an even greater role as an inexpensive, safe, and effective diagnostic tool. This chapter summarizes the current status of percutaneous biopsy and the theoretical basis of modern techniques.

PATHOLOGIC BASIS FOR BIOPSY TECHNIQUE

The primary indication for percutaneous fine needle aspiration (FNA) biopsy is the nonsurgical diagnosis of cancer. FNA biopsy has earned widespread acceptance due, in part, to the accuracy of cytologic diagnosis. Malignant sensitivity is reported to range from 56 to 95%, with some of the variation dependent upon the biopsy site and the types of tumors included in different series (2–12). Despite this wide range, most series report a diagnostic accuracy rate of greater than 85%.

The accuracy of cytologic diagnosis involves many variables. A pathologist competent in the interpretation of cytologic specimens is an important one. Providing the pathologist with an adequate sample of material from the lesion of interest is important as well. Many lesions, benign or malignant, may not be entirely homogeneous. Areas of fibrosis, necrosis, or cystic change are commonly encountered. Thus, a random sampling of cells from a heterogenous lesion may not be entirely representative of the lesion as a whole. Because FNA sampling error is a major cause of false-negative diagnoses, it is important to understand how sampling error occurs in order to provide adequate specimens and lower false-negative rates

Physical handling of the aspirated material is another important variable in the accuracy of cytologic diagnosis because it has a direct effect upon specimen adequacy. Whenever smears are made at the time of the procedure, care should be taken that they are made well. The smears should be of appropriate thickness, without clots, and either air-dried or fixed according to the wishes of the interpreting pathologist. The development of liquid-based monolayer systems have alleviated many of these concerns by allowing the aspirate to be transferred immediately into a fluid medium for slide preparation sometime later in the pathology laboratory.

Cooperation between the radiologist and pathologist is critical to accurate cytologic diagnosis (13,14). A willingness to communicate cannot be overemphasized. Active dialogue allows the pathologist to make the most of the plethora of ancillary techniques at his or her disposal when analyzing the biopsy material. Communication also helps to avoid some of the limitations of cytologic interpretation by narrowing the focus of the differential diagnosis. This is particularly true when the patient's history or physical/radiographic findings are complicated or difficult to interpret or when the tumor is poorly differentiated. The predictive value of FNA in the classification of poorly differentiated neoplasms can be significantly improved if detailed clinical information accompanies the FNA (15). At some medical facilities, the pathologist is present during the FNA procedure to assess the adequacy of the specimen in real time. The use of a "fast stain technique" allows immediate feedback to the radiologist both in terms of specimen adequacy and in terms of providing a preliminary diagnosis (14,16,17). If the fast stain is interpreted as "nondiagnostic," the radiologist has the opportunity to take steps to obtain diagnostic material. Direct communication becomes especially important in the event an unexpected diagnosis is suggested on the fast stain. For instance, pathologists can request additional specimens at the time of the procedure to aid in the interpretation. Examples include submitting additional aspirates for flow

cytometry for lymphoma immunophenotyping or submitting them as culture material when an infectious etiology is suspected. However, the ability of the radiologist and pathologist to communicate does not require the presence of the pathologist during the biopsy procedure. The requisition that accompanies the specimen to the pathology laboratory can be very helpful if used appropriately. The suspected diagnosis and appropriate clinical/radiographic findings have a tremendous impact on what might be done with the specimen once it leaves the radiology department. In as much as "lung lesion" is generally considered clinical history, expanding the note to read "lung lesion, past history of lymphoma" has much more impact on the cytologic interpretation and increases diagnostic accuracy.

The interpretation of cytologic specimens relies on well-known cytodiagnostic criteria. These include such things as nuclear shape and size, presence or absence of nucleoli, chromatin pattern, and quality of the cytoplasm. Cytologic specimens have a slight edge over histologic specimens (formalin-fixed tissue biopsies) in this regard because they provide better cellular detail. The major disadvantage of cytologic specimens is that the cells are removed from their supporting tissue elements. The architectural context, best appreciated by histologic specimens, is lost. Loss of architectural context can make subclassification of certain neoplasms difficult by cytology. This is especially true of well-differentiated neoplasms. Because cytology depends on morphologic changes in individual cells, the more closely the tumor cells resemble normal cells the more difficult the cytologic diagnosis can be. For this reason, pathologic interpretive error is a more significant problem when dealing with well-differentiated malignant neoplasms. Such tumors may defy cytologic diagnosis because the determination of malignant potential requires histologic architectural changes such as vascular or capsular invasion (18,19). The majority of tumors, however, are less well-differentiated and have such striking cellular morphologic alterations that the diagnosis of malignancy is readily and reliably made by cytologic examination. Using cytologic clues, the pathologist attempts to classify tumors as carcinoma, lymphoma, sarcoma, and melanoma. However, subclassifying can be more difficult. For instance, poorly-differentiated carcinomas may not be defined as easily as squamous cell carcinomas or adenocarcinomas. Similarly, the diagnosis and subtyping of sarcomas and lymphomas often depends on histology and ancillary studies (immunophenotyping and cytogenetics) and, thus, they are more difficult to subclassify by cytology alone (Figure 16–1) (18–22).

In addition to the aforementioned diagnostic limitations of cytology, reasons for false-negative and false-positive diagnoses need to be understood. The reported false-negative rates for percutaneous biopsy range from 7 to 44% (2–11). False-negative diagnoses result from sampling

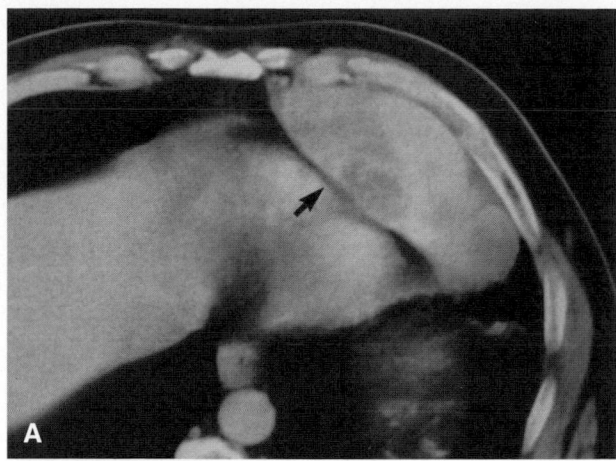

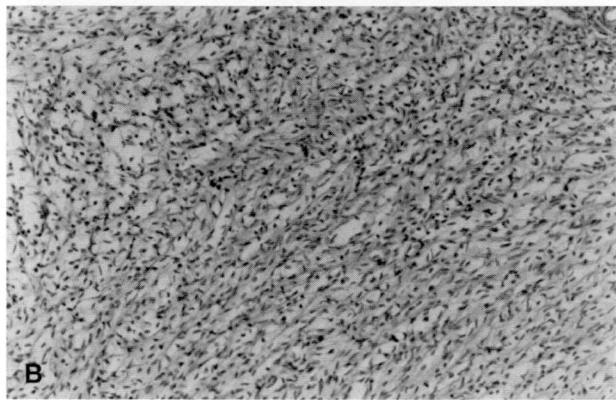

Figure 16–1 A. CT section showing an enhancing mass (*arrow*) arising near the anterolateral pericardium and diaphragm. Coaxial biopsy was performed via an angled subxyphoid approach using an 18-gauge automated gun and a 22-gauge chiba needle. **B.** Histologic section demonstrates a low-grade, malignant, spindle-cell neoplasm representing a primary pericardial fibrosarcoma. The aspiration cytology specimen was nondiagnostic.

error or pathologic interpretive error. Sampling error may occur simply because the target lesion was missed. This is somewhat unusual given modern guidance techniques but can still occur in small deep lesions, poorly visualized lesions, and uncooperative patients. More commonly, sampling error is a result of the retrieval of nonrepresentative tissue from the target lesion. Some large tumors have extensive areas of central necrosis that will not yield recognizable malignant cells when sampled (Figure 16–2). Other tumors elicit a dense, fibrous-tissue reaction or a surrounding reactive inflammatory response. Sampling of these nontumorous areas may yield nonspecific benign reactive tissue without diagnostic malignant cells. Extremely vascular tumors may yield only blood.

False-positive diagnoses are reported to occur in 1–2% of cases and may contribute to the false-negative rate in an indirect way (9,10). Certain benign neoplasms and reactive or inflammatory conditions have enough cellular atypia to mimic a well-differentiated malignancy (18,19).

Because of the clinical and medicolegal implications of a false-positive diagnosis, pathologists are generally more willing to accept a slightly higher false-negative rate rather than risk a false-positive diagnosis when faced with a borderline specimen.

Accuracy in the cytologic diagnosis of benign conditions is low. Literature series report that a specific diagnosis can be made in only 20–65% of benign lesions by cytologic examination alone (4–8,12,23,24). This is not surprising when we remember that many benign lesions are defined histologically with little cytologic differentiation from the parent tissue. A specific diagnosis can be made in conditions with characteristic cellular morphology such as a pulmonary hamartoma or hepatic steatosis, as well as in some infectious lesions and benign simple cysts; but most benign neoplasms, reactive changes, and inflammatory conditions present a greater problem for cytologic diagnosis (Figure 16–3).

A significant limitation of aspiration cytology is a variable negative predictive value that ranges from 17 to 78% (1,5–12,23). The negative predictive value depends on both the false-negative rate and the prevalence of malignancy in a given series. Both a high false-negative rate and a high prevalence of malignancy will lead to a lower negative predictive value. A nonspecific true-negative specimen will appear, by cytologic examination, very similar to a false-negative specimen in which peritumoral inflammation or fibrosis is retrieved. The result is that most nonspecific cancer negative diagnoses must undergo further diagnostic evaluation: either repeat biopsy or surgical excision. If a specific benign diagnosis is made, the negative predictive value improves considerably and no further evaluation is usually necessary (24–26).

Knowledge that the cytologic technique has limitations is central to understanding the areas on which to focus in order to improve the diagnostic accuracy of FNA biopsy. These may be summarized as obtaining more cells and/or tissue for examination, obtaining better quality specimens, and utilizing ancillary studies to aid in pathologic interpretation.

Obtaining more material for cytologic examination will decrease both sampling and interpretive errors. The simplest way to do this is to make a greater number of biopsy passes, often using a tandem or coaxial system for ease of localization. Attempts should be made to sample several different areas within a given lesion to account for heterogeneity. It has also been reported that the use of larger aspiration needles and aspiration needles with modified tip configurations allows one to retrieve more tissue and improve the diagnostic results (27,28). The exception is fibrous lesions where a thinner needle (25-gauge) often performs better (13).

Different methods of pathologic examination of specimens have improved both sensitivity and specificity. Special stains to identify cellular biochemical products have helped in determining tumor subtypes (18,20).

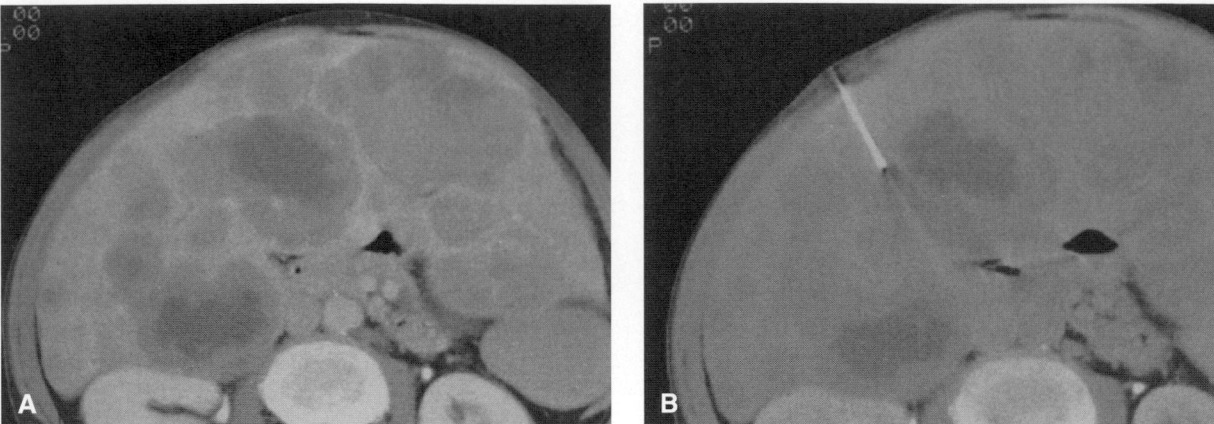

Figure 16–2 Metastatic adenocarcinoma of the colon. **A.** Contrast-enhanced CT section shows multiple hypodense lesions, at least two of which show central necrosis. **B.** A 19-gauge guiding needle is placed through a rim of normal liver parenchyma to the partially enhancing rim of a tumor nodule in order to avoid sampling error resulting from the central necrosis.

Electron microscopy for ultrastructural analysis can also help in this regard but is expensive, cumbersome, and not routinely available (19). Immunoperoxidase stains are becoming increasingly helpful, particularly in the subclassification of lymphomas and poorly differentiated malignancies (19,20). Flow cytometry, performed on "live" cellular aspirates, is especially helpful in subclassifying non-Hodgkin's lymphomas (29). Organism stains and cultures are useful in improving the specificity of diagnosis in benign infectious processes (9).

The most effective method of improving biopsy accuracy is to obtain specimens for histologic as well as cytologic examination. Initial attempts to obtain histologic specimens focused on obtaining microhistologic fragments using modified 20- to 22-gauge aspiration needles (2,9,10,27). These studies showed that, when evaluated separately, the results of cytologic examination were better than the results of microhistologic examination. When the results were combined, however, overall biopsy accuracy improved. Pathologists were subjectively more comfortable in rendering a definitive diagnosis when both types of specimens were available for examination. Most importantly, each series reported cases in which the histology was diagnostic while the cytology was not and vice versa. This difference suggests that improvements in sampling error played a significant role in improved results. The conclusion was that cytologic and histologic examinations were complementary. This conclusion is logical in that

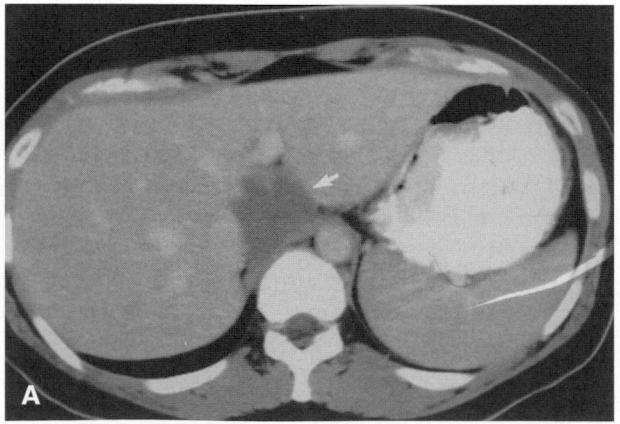
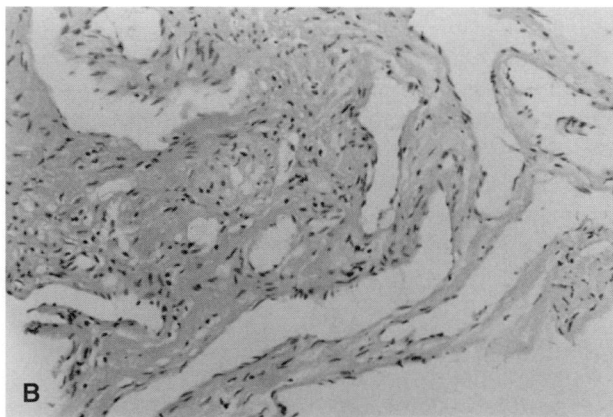

Figure 16–3 **A.** Contrast-enhanced CT section shows an irregular nonenhancing mass (*arrow*) between the liver and the right crus of the diaphragm. **B.** Histologic section reveals irregular dilated lymphatic spaces lined by flattened endothelial cells representing a retroperitoneal lymphangioma. The aspiration cytology specimen revealed only normal lymphocytes.

Spring-loaded automated cutting needles are available that can greatly improve both the histologic recovery rate and the quality of histologic specimens. Obtaining true histologic cores with cutting needles has been shown to improve all aspects of biopsy accuracy (21,22,24–26,30). Malignant sensitivity of greater than 90% can be routinely obtained (6,8,22,24–26,30,31). Accuracy in diagnosing lymphoma and other mesenchymal malignancies can be improved from 20–70% by cytology alone to 80–90% by histology (Figure 16–4) (8,21,22,25,32). There is also a dramatic improvement in the ability to obtain a specific pathologic diagnosis in benign disease (6,8,24–26). The importance of a specific benign diagnosis is probably the single greatest contribution of histology because in such cases the negative predictive value approaches 100% (Figure 16–5). This has the potential

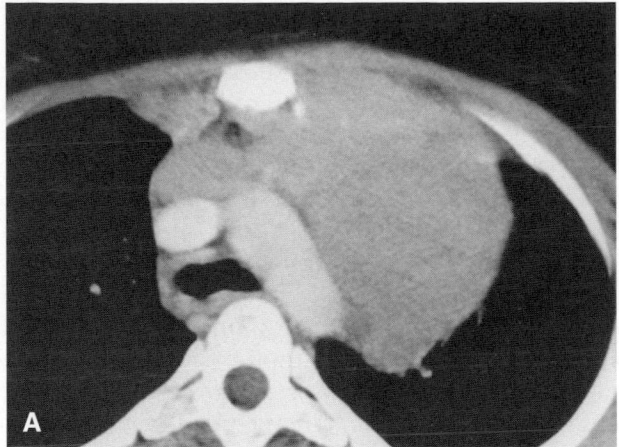

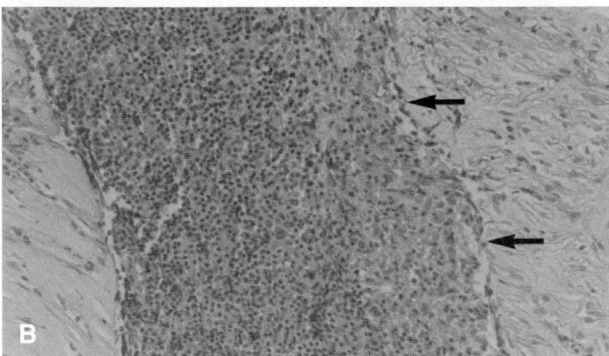

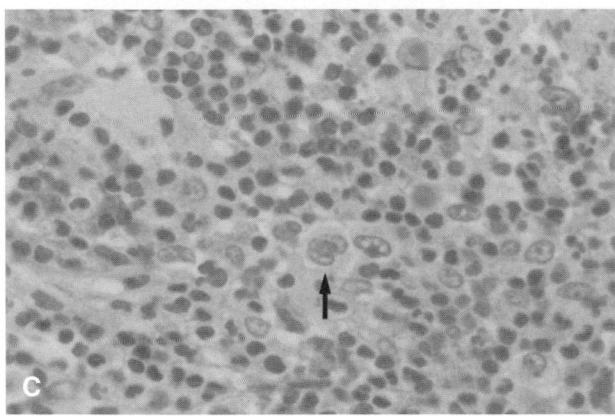

Figure 16–4 Nodular sclerosing Hodgkin's disease. **A.** CT section demonstrates a large anterior mediastinal mass. Biopsy was performed using both an 18-gauge automated biopsy gun and a 22-gauge aspiration needle. The cytology specimen revealed only nonspecific inflammatory cells. **B.** Low-power view of the histologic section shows a lymphoid tumor nodule (*arrows*) surrounded by bands of dense sclerosis. **C.** Higher-power view of the histologic section shows several Reed-Sternberg cells (*arrow*) with a pleomorphic background of inflammatory cells and small lymphocytes.

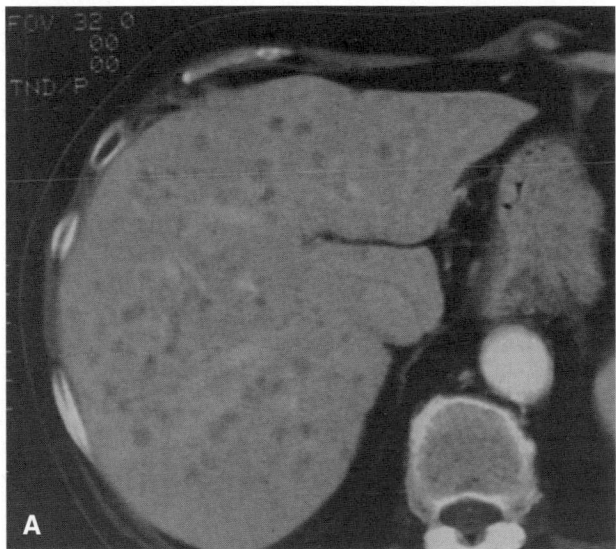

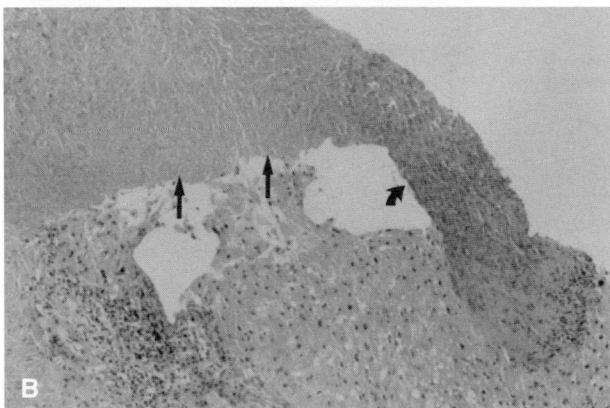

Figure 16–5 **A.** Contrast-enhanced CT section shows multiple low-density liver lesions in a patient with rheumatoid arthritis and elevated liver enzymes. **B.** Histologic section demonstrates pallisading epithelial macrophages (*curved arrow*) and a portion of a necrobiotic rheumatoid nodule (*straight arrows*). The aspiration cytology specimen revealed only nonspecific inflammatory cells. The liver lesions resolved after steroid therapy.

cytologic specimens are best suited to evaluate cellular and nuclear morphologic changes whereas histologic specimens are best suited to evaluate architectural changes. It is unreasonable to expect either technique to optimally evaluate both types of pathologic change.

to eliminate one of the key weaknesses of aspiration biopsy: the need for surgery or repeat biopsy in cancer-negative cases. Accurate subtyping of malignancies, particularly those of mesenchymal origin, is also improved significantly when tumor architecture can be evaluated (6,9,10,21,22,25,26).

The majority of biopsy cases encountered represents metastatic disease from known primary epithelial tumors. It can be argued that the accuracy of cytologic diagnosis is so high in this situation that histologic cores are not necessary. Larger needle core biopsies then may be reserved for more difficult pathologic questions or for repeat biopsies in those cases in which the initial results were inconclusive. In a significant number of cases, however, definite advantages to the addition of histology exist. If histologic specimens can be obtained safely, then there is no advantage to aspiration biopsy alone. We are now at a point at which such specimens can be obtained routinely and safely by percutaneous methods. When high-quality specimens for both cytology and histology are obtained, fewer pathologic interpretive errors and less dependence on an expert cytopathologist will be present. Further improvements in biopsy accuracy will depend on reducing sampling error, which is primarily under the control of the radiologist.

TECHNICAL CONSIDERATIONS

Biopsy devices and techniques have been modified and refined in attempts to increase accuracy, decrease complications, or both, with variable success. Although technique is determined largely by user preference, certain developments have emerged as being more significant in optimizing results.

Biopsy Devices

Biopsy needles may be classified by tip configuration and size. The two primary needle tip configurations are the aspiration needles and the cutting needles. Aspiration needles are thin-walled cannulas with a varying degree of bevel angulation at the tip. The most widely used examples are the spinal and Chiba needles. A gentle to-and-fro motion of the aspiration needle passing through the tissue yields a cellular monolayer for evaluation. Cutting needles are designed to obtain histologic cores rather than cytologic specimens. The two major mechanisms of action of cutting needles are the Menghini and tru-cut mechanisms. The Menghini-type needles are hollow cannulas with a sharpened beveled tip that cuts a cylindrical core of tissue during advancement while suction is maintained in the lumen. The tru–cut-type needles have a

notched central stylet and outer cylindrical cannula. After the stylet is advanced, tissue enters the notch. A semi-cylindrical tissue core then is cut off by advancement of the outer cutting cannula. The majority of automated biopsy devices use a tru–cut-type needle attached to a spring-loaded handle that mechanically performs the steps of tissue retrieval. These devices greatly simplify the biopsy procedure and require less operator experience for optimal use.

There are three general categories of needle size. Small-caliber needles are 21- to 25-gauge, middle-caliber needles are 18- to 20-gauge, and large-caliber needles are 16-gauge or larger. In general, more tissue is retrieved by larger needles. This does not mean, however, that larger needles are always better than smaller needles. If the intention is to obtain a specimen for cytologic evaluation, it will be best to obtain a large number of individual cells separate from the supporting stroma so that a uniform monolayer of cells may be examined. Small-caliber aspiration and modified aspiration needles are best suited for this purpose. A common property of some cancer cells is poor intercellular cohesiveness, a feature that facilitates retrieval of a large number of malignant cells free of the surrounding stromal elements.

Cutting needles are superior to aspiration needles in obtaining tissue cores for histologic examination. Histologic recovery rates of 97–100% are achieved using automated tru–cut-type biopsy devices (25,30,31). Although larger cutting needles obtain larger cores, excellent specimens may be reliably retrieved with middle-caliber automated devices (25,30). The choice depends on the estimated amount of tissue needed for adequate diagnosis and classification of a pathologic lesion and the risk factors attendant in biopsy in any given case.

Biopsy Techniques

Several techniques have been developed to increase the amount of tissue retrieved, the simplest of which is to make multiple biopsy passes. When sequential, separate biopsy passes are made, the needle tip must be localized with every pass. This is a more significant drawback when using CT guidance than when using ultrasound or fluoroscopic guidance. The tandem technique involves initial localization of a small-caliber needle followed by nonguided, parallel placement of one or more biopsy needles to the same depth. The disadvantages of this method are that separate organ punctures are required for each biopsy pass and that tip localization is not precisely controlled. The coaxial technique involves placement of a thin-walled guiding needle, which then is used as a conduit for the biopsy needle. A coaxial system has several advantages. Needle-tip localization is performed only once, and multiple biopsy passes may be made with only one puncture of the target organ. It is relatively simple to use both small-caliber needles to obtain cytologic specimens and middle-caliber needles to obtain histologic cores via the same guiding needle. The most significant advantage is that virtually any needle may be placed through a coaxial guide, including automated devices. The guide and biopsy needle may be angled manually for subsequent biopsy passes to sample different areas of a lesion. The guide also may be used for track embolization when necessary. The only disadvantage of the coaxial method is that the guide must have a larger caliber than the actual biopsy device, but this is not a significant drawback.

The purpose of percutaneous biopsy is to obtain diagnostic tissue samples with minimal risk to the patient. Even given the above advantages and disadvantages, the choice of needles and biopsy technique remains largely one of personal preference and experience. Practitioners should adopt a technique with which they are comfortable and should develop expertise in that technique. Nevertheless, results are the only true measure of success, and physicians should remain open-minded regarding other methods that may improve both the accuracy and safety of biopsies in their particular institution.

Guidance Modalities

The evolution of guidance modalities has been a major factor in the increased acceptance of percutaneous biopsy. Initially percutaneous biopsies were either blind or guided only by palpation. Fluoroscopy was the first imaging tool used to guide biopsy needle placement, followed by ultrasound and CT. Guidance by magnetic resonance imaging (MRI) continues to be explored. Each of these modalities has continued to evolve, becoming both more accurate and easier to use. More than any other aspect of technique, the choice of guidance modality is one of personal preference and experience. The basic tenet of guidance, regardless of the chosen modality, is that it should allow safe and accurate placement of the biopsy needle with absolute documentation that the biopsy specimen was obtained from the target lesion. The best modality usually is the one that best demonstrates the lesion and the adjacent vital structures.

In the past, fluoroscopic guidance was used primarily for lung biopsies, although currently the majority of percutaneous thoracic biopsies are performed using CT or CT-fluoroscopic guidance. The major advantages of fluoroscopic guidance are that needle advancement can be monitored continuously and that the length of time during which the needle is in the patient is relatively short. The main disadvantages of fluoroscopic guidance are radiation

exposure to the operator and difficulty in localizing small lesions or lesions in close proximity to vital soft-tissue density structures.

Ultrasound guidance has advanced tremendously in recent years with the advent of high-resolution scanners and small real-time phased array transducers. Ultrasound probably requires more operator expertise than other modalities but is also extremely flexible. Experienced practitioners favor a "free-hand" approach, controlling the biopsy needle with one hand and the transducer with the other. Mechanical needle guides attached to the transducer are also available if necessary. Ultrasound guidance is used most commonly for biopsies of the kidneys, liver, and thyroid gland. Advantages of ultrasound guidance include real-time visualization of the needle throughout placement, multiplanar approach capabilities, lack of ionizing radiation, speed, and cost (Figure 16–6). The major disadvantage is that even with modern scanners, it is occasionally difficult to precisely localize the needle tip in relation to the lesion. Overlying bone, bowel, or lung will obscure the underlying lesion, and deep or small lesions may be visualized inadequately for effective localization.

CT guidance is the most accurate modality in terms of precise needle tip localization and can be applied to virtually any lesion in the body. It provides the best visualization of intervening and adjacent vital structures so that the safest biopsy path may be chosen. It is quite common to encounter lesions that cannot be approached safely using any other modality. Mediastinal and pleural-based lung lesions can be approached without crossing aerated lung in almost every case (Figure 16–7). Biopsies may be safely performed immediately adjacent to major vascular structures in the mediastinum and retroperitoneum (Figure 16–8). Contrast-enhanced CT images can help in selecting the optimal portion of a given lesion to biopsy, avoiding areas of potential tumor necrosis. CT also provides more sensitive and immediate feedback regarding possible complications such as perilesional bleeding or pneumothorax.

In the past, the most significant drawback of CT guidance has been the longer procedure time and the inability to visualize the needle in real time during placement. The development of CT fluoroscopy has allowed real-time evaluation of needle placement and decreased procedure times (33). However, concerns regarding radiation exposure to patients and personnel may be a factor in the lack of its widespread use. The development of high-speed scanners with much faster image reconstruction times has essentially eliminated the time constraints of CT guidance. The advent of positron emission tomography (CT-PET) will also help to better localize active lesions that may improve pathologic diagnosis.

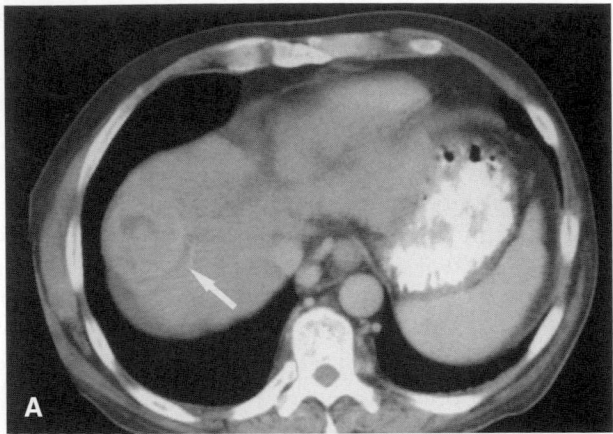

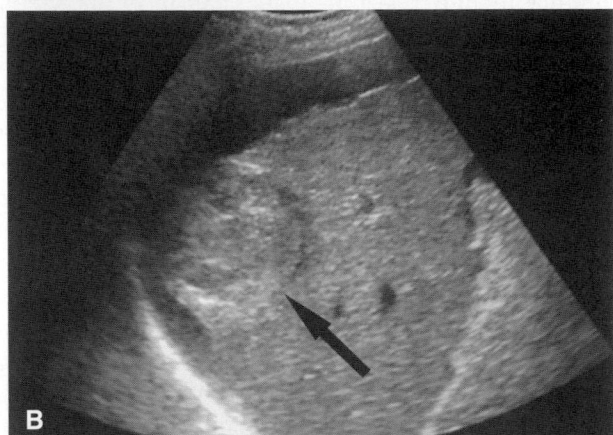

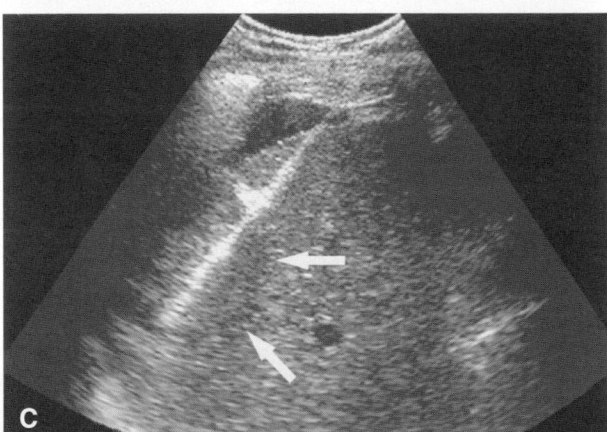

Figure 16–6 Hepatocellular carcinoma complicating cirrhosis. **A.** Contrast-enhanced CT section shows a hypervascular mass (*arrow*) in the dome of the right lobe of the liver. CT-guided biopsy would require that the needle traverse the lower portion of the right lung. **B.** Longitudinal ultrasound image showing an inhomogeneous mass (*arrow*) in the dome of the liver with ascites anterior to the liver. **C.** Longitudinal ultrasound image showing an 18-gauge, automated biopsy needle traversing the hepatic mass (*arrows*). The biopsy needle was placed coaxially through a 17-gauge guiding needle via a subcostal approach. Ultrasound guidance allowed the guiding needle to be placed with cranial angulation in order to avoid traversing the pleura and diaphragm. The biopsy track was subsequently embolized with gelfoam pledgets that were injected through the guiding cannula before guide removal.

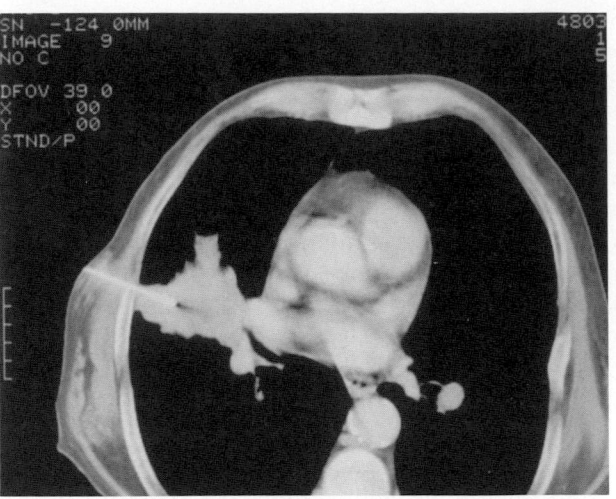

Figure 16–7 Small-cell, anaplastic carcinoma of the right hilum with peripheral postobstructive atelectasis reaching the pleural surface. CT guidance allows precise placement of the guiding needle through the pleural attachment and into the central mass.

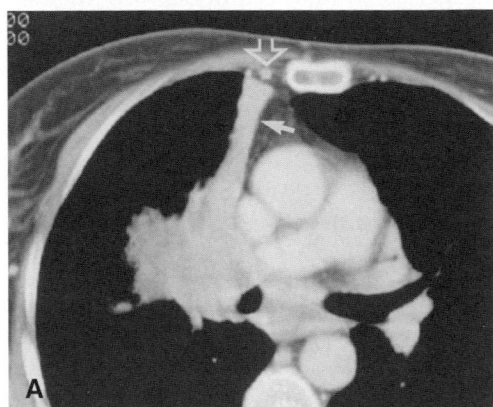

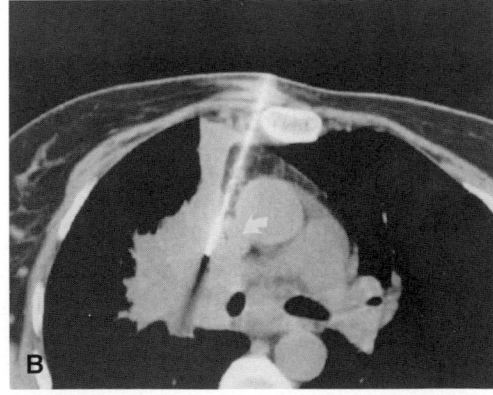

Figure 16–8 Small-cell, anaplastic carcinoma of the right hilum. Bronchoscopic examination was nondiagnostic. **A.** Contrast-enhanced CT section shows a 5-cm right hilar and mediastinal mass with a small linear wedge of collapsed upper lobe (*solid arrow*) extending to the anterior chest wall. Internal mammary vein (*open arrow*). **B.** A 19-gauge guiding needle has been placed medial to the internal mammary vein and through the collapsed upper lobe into the central portion of the mass. The distal aspect of the guiding needle is immediately adjacent to the aorta and superior vena cava (*arrow*).

COMPLICATIONS

The accuracy of percutaneous biopsy techniques has continued to improve because of advances in needle technology, the ability to reliably obtain both cytologic and histologic specimens with small needles, faster and more accurate guidance modalities, and advances in preparation and interpretation of biopsy specimens. It is equally important, however, to accomplish this with an acceptable complication rate. The demonstrated safety of 21- to 22-gauge aspiration needles was a major reason behind the early growth of percutaneous biopsy techniques. Much of the reason that cytologic techniques evolved at all was the concern regarding the high complication rates associated with larger needles. Martin and Ellis (1) stated the problem succinctly in 1930, observing that "larger specimens uniformly fixed and stained offer more satisfactory material upon which to reach a definite opinion, but such a preparation can too often be obtained only at considerable disadvantage to the patient. A postmortem diagnosis never benefits the one most concerned, the donor of the specimen."

All biopsies involve both risk and benefit. The benefits of percutaneous biopsy are clear, providing proper indications for the procedure are met. Contraindications to biopsy, although usually relative, must be considered. To completely justify the use of larger-caliber cutting needles the risk of complications must compare favorably with that of small-caliber aspiration needles. Two complications, pneumothorax and bleeding, are of dominant concern and will be discussed separately. Other less common complications are site-specific and will be discussed with regional biopsy considerations.

Indications and Contraindications

It is difficult to succinctly summarize the various indications that may apply for any given biopsy. The imaging characteristics of a lesion must present a differential diagnosis. If the imaging features are sufficiently characteristic of any given pathologic entity that would be treated by surgical resection, then a preoperative diagnosis is usually not necessary. An example would be a typical renal cell carcinoma in a patient with no contraindications to surgery. Second, entities in the differential diagnosis must be distinguishable by the biopsy method chosen, either cytologic or core histologic examination. An example would be a small nonfunctioning adrenal mass in a patient with no other evidence of malignancy. One should expect considerable difficulty in distinguishing the two main diagnostic considerations, adenoma and nonfunctioning primary adrenal carcinoma, by examination of a needle biopsy specimen.

Third, there must be significantly different treatment regimens for the entities in the differential diagnosis, and the patient should understand these considerations and have agreed to undergo the therapy dictated by the biopsy results. If the results of the biopsy will have no significant bearing on subsequent treatment, then the risk-benefit ratio becomes unacceptable. Finally, percutaneous biopsy should not be performed in lieu of other potential diagnostic modalities that would provide a safer means of securing the diagnosis.

The majority of contraindications to percutaneous biopsy are relative. In an uncooperative patient it will be more difficult to secure a diagnosis and the risks of doing so will be higher. It is also important that a safe access route be available, although with modern guidance techniques this is almost always possible. There are well-defined conditions that would predispose a patient to a higher risk of pneumothorax or bleeding, and these are discussed in the following sections.

Pneumothorax

Pneumothorax is reported to occur in 10 to 60% of transthoracic biopsies (7,9,34–38). Although unusual, it can also complicate biopsy of upper abdominal organs if the pleural space is crossed. Chest tube placement is required after 2–20% of transthoracic biopsies (10–60% of pneumothoraces) (25,36–38).

The decision to place a chest tube is based generally on the size of the pneumothorax and/or the severity of the resultant symptoms. Observation of a small, minimally symptomatic pneumothorax is an option but often requires serial films over several days to ensure that the pneumothorax is not enlarging. A potentially successful alternative is simple aspiration of the pneumothorax without placement of a chest tube. Large pneumothoraces or those associated with significant symptoms should be treated with formal tube thoracostomy, which then may be placed to suction or to a Heimlich valve. Most physicians prefer to observe patients with chest tubes on an inpatient rather than an outpatient basis, although either is acceptable. Management of pneumothoraces is subjective and is based on the experience and personal preferences of the operator, but all radiologists performing transthoracic biopsies must be familiar with the technique of tube thoracostomy should it be needed urgently.

Several risk factors have been identified that may increase either the risk of pneumothorax or the likelihood that chest tube treatment will be needed. The most significant risk factor for the development of a pneumothorax is whether or not aerated lung is crossed by the needle (34,35,39). Theoretically, there should be no risk of pneumothorax if aerated lung is not crossed. In practice, this can occur if a coaxial system is used and the guide needle is placed in the pleural space adjacent to a lesion that abuts but does not invade the pleura (Figure 16–9). One of the most significant advantages of CT over fluoroscopic guidance for thoracic biopsies is the ability to select a needle path that does not cross aerated lung.

The presence of chronic obstructive pulmonary disease (COPD) may impart a slightly greater risk of pneumothorax, but the effect is minimal and COPD should not be considered a contraindication to biopsy (37–41). The biopsy needle path should be chosen carefully in order to avoid puncture of emphysematous bullae. Patients with COPD have diminished pulmonary reserve, and those who develop a pneumothorax are more likely to be symptomatic and to require a chest tube for treatment (39,41). An uncooperative patient is at higher risk, and the inability to suspend respiration during the biopsy should be considered a relative contraindication to biopsy. The use of 16-gauge or larger cutting needles will result in a higher pneumothorax rate, but no significant difference has been

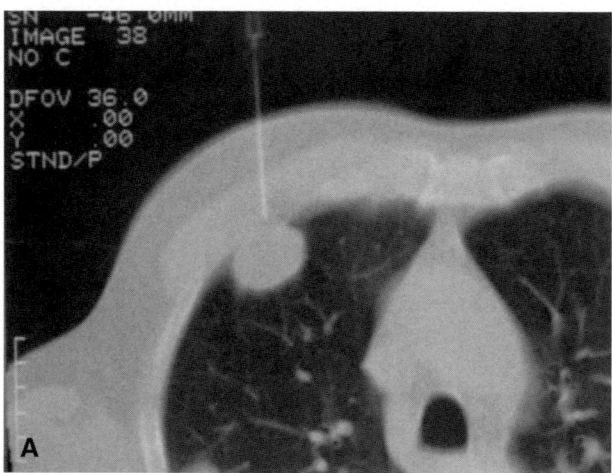

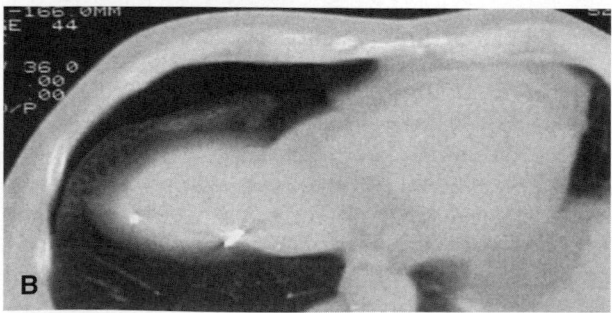

Figure 16–9 Pneumothorax complicating coaxial biopsy of a pleural-based lung mass (metastatic hepatocellular carcinoma). **A.** The tip of the 19-gauge guiding needle is shown at the edge of the lesion where it abuts the pleural surface. **B.** Postbiopsy scan demonstrates a small pneumothorax. This occurred because the lesion abutted but did not invade the pleura, thus allowing air ingress via the guiding needle during the coaxial biopsy.

demonstrated between needles ranging from 18- to 22-gauge (12,25,39,40). A slight increased risk of pneumothorax may appear when multiple pleural punctures are made or when the needle path traverses a pleural fissure (12,38–41). Increasing depth and decreasing size of a lesion have also been implicated in increasing the risk of pneumothorax although data regarding this is conflicting (11,12,37–41). Biopsy of small lung lesions or lesions near the pulmonary hilum is more likely to result in perilesional bleeding and hemoptysis. The coughing response to parenchymal bleeding will increase the chance of developing a pneumothorax.

Several modifications in technique have been proposed to decrease the risk of pneumothorax. The blood patch technique involves injection of autologous clot into the biopsy track during removal of a coaxial guide in an attempt to seal the pleural puncture site. The only controlled studies of this technique have failed to demonstrate any benefit (37,38). Positioning the patient with the biopsy side down immediately after the procedure is theoretically beneficial by creating dependent atelectasis and allowing tamponade of the pleural puncture site against the chest wall. Although the only controlled study has not shown this to be effective in decreasing the incidence of pneumothorax, it does appear to decrease the need for tube thoracostomy (36). A similar effect is seen with the administration of 100% oxygen after the biopsy (40).

The fast-stain method is a technique in which the aspirated cytology specimen is stained and examined during the biopsy procedure. As soon as an adequate cytological specimen is obtained, the procedure is terminated. The rationale behind this technique is to increase the diagnostic yield while decreasing the number of needle passes. Unfortunately, this has not been shown to decrease the pneumothorax rate in controlled studies (17). The coaxial biopsy technique may be used to allow multiple biopsy passes to be made with fewer pleural punctures. This technique also allows the operator to place different biopsy needles through a single coaxial guide in order to obtain specimens for both cytological and histological examination. Regardless of the guidance modality used, some of the higher pneumothorax rates reported in the literature have been in series in which both a coaxial guide and the fast-stain technique were used together (5,11,24,39,41). With this combination the guide needle is left in place across the pleura for an extended period, increasing the likelihood of an air leak or pleural laceration. It may be that one of the most important things that can be done to minimize the pneumothorax rate is to minimize the amount of time that any needle is in the lung.

Some reports have suggested that the use of CT guidance is associated with a higher incidence of pneumothorax (4,5,24). In these studies, both a coaxial system and the fast-stain technique were used together, which resulted in pneumothorax rates of 43–61%. Other potential explanations for the higher pneumothorax rate include the increased sensitivity of CT for small pneumothoraces and the difficult nature of the lesions selected for CT-guided biopsy in these series. In contrast, other studies of CT-guided thoracic biopsy have reported pneumothorax rates of 11–19% (25,34). The fast-stain technique and coaxial system were not used in combination in these series. It would appear that the length of time that a needle is crossing the pleura is a more important factor in the risk of pneumothorax than is the guidance modality. The advent of high-speed scanners with short reconstruction times, in combination with the improved ability to avoid crossing aerated lung, has made CT a more attractive guidance modality without necessarily increasing the risk of pneumothorax.

Bleeding Complications

Bleeding is the second most common complication of percutaneous biopsy. It may occur in up to 12% of cases, although most series report bleeding complication rates of 6% or less (28,30,42–46). Most bleeding complications are minor and require no treatment. Significant bleeding requiring transfusion or surgical or endovascular intervention are reported in 0–3% of cases (30,42,46–48). The mortality rate from bleeding is estimated at 0.01 to 0.10% (49,50). It can be difficult to compare the incidence of bleeding complications in various series because of differences in patient populations, different biopsy sites and technique, varying methods used to detect complications, and inconsistent definitions of what constitutes a minor bleeding complication. Most recent studies have the advantage (or disadvantage) of employing high-resolution imaging modalities that are able to detect much more subtle bleeding. Some amount of perinephric bleeding can be detected after almost all renal biopsies using CT guidance. The great majority is asymptomatic and would probably not be reported in most studies. With this in mind, certain conclusions can be made regarding factors that may place a given patient at a higher risk for significant bleeding.

Coagulation Disorders

The most commonly used measures of coagulation are the prothrombin time, international normalized ratio, partial thromboplastin time, platelet count, and less commonly, the skin bleeding time. Several laboratory and uncontrolled clinical studies have suggested that defects in hemostasis impart an increased risk of bleeding complications (43,51,52). These studies suggested that defects in cellular hemostasis are more significant than defects in thrombin-mediated clot formation. Other studies, however, found no correlation between the commonly used measures of peripheral blood coagulation and the risk of bleeding from surgical or interventional procedures (49,53,54). The fact that skin bleeding time does not correlate well with liver bleeding time raises the possibility that local cellular and

biochemical mediators of hemostasis exist and that these factors cannot be measured peripherally (53,54). Although it seems to defy common sense to assume that a defect in coagulation does not impart an increased risk of bleeding, at the same time, currently available measurements of coagulation status do not allow us to quantify that risk in any given patient. Part of the problem is one of degree, in that the incidence of bleeding complications is so low that it is difficult to demonstrate a statistically significant difference without a very large number of patients, particularly when the coagulation defects are not severe. Controlled clinical studies of this issue would be unacceptable on ethical grounds. Laboratory studies suffer from the uncertainty as to whether controlled in vitro conditions accurately reflect in vivo conditions.

It is clear that our understanding of hemostasis has limitations and that our methods of measuring it are imperfect. Defects in hemostasis do impart an increased risk in general, but the increase is relatively small and certain local tissue factors are more important in individual cases. While currently available measures of hemostasis cannot be used to quantify the risk of bleeding in a given patient, almost all clinical investigators list coagulation defects as a relative contraindication to biopsy, and most continue to perform prebiopsy screening. Significant defects in hemostasis can be detected and steps can be taken to correct or counteract them when necessary.

Local Tissue Factors

Cellular and mechanical tissue factors may be the most important determinant of the risk of bleeding. Normal liver tissue is soft, and the track left by a biopsy needle will collapse and aid in local hemostasis by promoting tamponade. Tumors, on the other hand, often have a very firm fibrous stroma that prevents collapse of the track. Benign processes such as severe cirrhosis also lead to a more fibrous and less pliable liver in which local tamponade may be less effective. This hypothesis is supported by studies demonstrating an increased risk of bleeding in biopsy of malignant nodules or cirrhotic livers independent of coagulation status (43,49). The ability of normal liver to tamponade a biopsy track is also evidenced by an increased risk of bleeding from liver biopsy if the lesion is on the peritoneal surface of the liver (49,50). Biopsy of presumed high-risk lesions of the liver such as a cavernous hemangioma can be performed safely when a rim of normal liver tissue is interposed between the puncture site in the capsule and the edge of the lesion. The lack of local mechanical tamponade is also a factor in the risk of bleeding from nonhepatic lesions that abut either the peritoneal surface or another potential space in which a significant amount of blood could collect.

Both malignant and benign tumors may demonstrate arterial hypervascularity. An increased incidence of bleeding complications has been reported after biopsy of such lesions (50,52). The importance of vascularity is evidenced also by the increased incidence of bleeding following renal biopsy as compared to liver biopsy. Liver tissue is soft and is supplied primarily by low-pressure veins, whereas renal tissue is more firm and has a much more extensive high-pressure arterial blood supply. Another important factor is the inherent pathologic difference between normal arteries and tumor vessels. Normal arteries develop smooth muscle contraction in the vessel wall in response to trauma, thus limiting blood loss. Neoplastic vessels do not have a smooth muscle media and cannot contract. Once severed, the vessel will freely bleed until external tamponade occurs. Increased vascularity of a lesion should not be considered a contraindication to biopsy, although the needle path should be carefully chosen so that local mechanical factors can be exploited to assist in tamponade of the tract.

Biopsy Technique

The diameter of the biopsy needle is generally considered to have some correlation with the risk of bleeding complications. The use of large-caliber cutting needles for biopsy of many different anatomic sites has been reported. However, in these studies, only lesions considered to be at low risk for bleeding complications were selected for biopsy with large-caliber needles. The data that are available indicate that there is a small but real increased risk of bleeding complications with 14- to 16-gauge needles as compared to 18- to 22-gauge needles (6,28,42,44–46). The same studies have demonstrated no significant increase in risk with the use of 18- to 20-gauge needles as compared to 21- to 22-gauge needles. Some data suggest that the use of cutting needles carries a slightly higher risk as compared to aspiration needles of the same gauge, but the difference is small and probably not significant (6,52). The most important conclusion from this literature is that middle-caliber cutting needles can reliably obtain histologic cores with no significant increase in complications.

Protective Measures

The relative potential significance of the above described risk factors in any individual case can be assessed in a subjective, if not quantitative, fashion, and steps may be taken to prevent bleeding complications when a higher risk is foreseen. Deferring biopsy is advisable in patients with a severe coagulopathy when this can be corrected. Cessation of medications affecting either cellular or thrombin-mediated hemostasis is the most obvious example. Transfusion of platelets or cryoprecipitate may be performed before biopsy but is rarely necessary. The single most important preventive step that can be taken is to carefully select a biopsy needle path that will avoid vascular structures and take advantage of the effects of local tamponade. The use of 14- to 16-gauge cutting needles

should probably be avoided except when local mechanical tamponade is ensured.

Transjugular biopsy of the liver has been advocated in cases of severe coagulopathy. The transjugular technique is slightly less reliable than percutaneous cutting-needle biopsy in obtaining adequate histologic specimens but is still acceptable (47,48). The technique is somewhat more cumbersome than percutaneous biopsy. Complication rates are relatively low given the patient population but can be significant. Inadvertent carotid artery puncture, cardiac arrhythmias, or capsular perforation may occur in 2–6% of cases (55,56). One significant advantage of the transjugular biopsy technique in cirrhotic patients is the ability to perform hepatic hemodynamic measurements during the same procedure. Given that many interventional radiologists have experience with transjugular, intrahepatic, portosystemic shunt procedures, it would be expected that the transjugular biopsy technique would be relatively simple for most to perform.

Embolization of percutaneous biopsy tracks is also an alternative when a higher risk of bleeding is anticipated (48,51). This technique requires some form of coaxial system through which the biopsy is performed. After biopsy the guiding needle or cannula is used as a conduit for placing embolic material into the biopsy track (Figure 16–10). The two most common embolic materials used have been gelfoam pledgets and autologous clot. Vascular embolization coils and thrombin tissue sealants have also been used. Biopsy and embolization may be performed with any guidance modality. Real-time control of the embolization is possible under fluoroscopic guidance, whereas embolization is partially "blind" when CT or ultrasound guidance is used (Figure 16–11). The great majority of cases of track embolization reported in the literature have been performed under CT or ultrasound guidance, and with experience, this procedure is simple to perform. Because standard coaxial guiding needles are used, the biopsy can be performed with any automated biopsy gun. The histologic recovery rate and diagnostic accuracy are higher than with transjugular biopsy. This technique can be used following biopsy of any organ or location, not just hepatic biopsies. Although the main indication for embolization is coagulation disorders, it can be used for other indications, such as biopsy of hypervascular lesions or biopsies in which no tissue rim is present to aid in local tamponade. To date there have been no controlled randomized trials demonstrating the efficacy of the track embolization technique, and indeed such trials may not be possible because of ethical concerns. The technique has been used in a large number of patients with coagulation defects in a noncontrolled fashion with very low complication rates (47,48,51). A potential risk exists that small pieces of embolic material could enter a vascular channel and embolize distally, but to date, no adverse effects related specifically to this embolization technique have been reported.

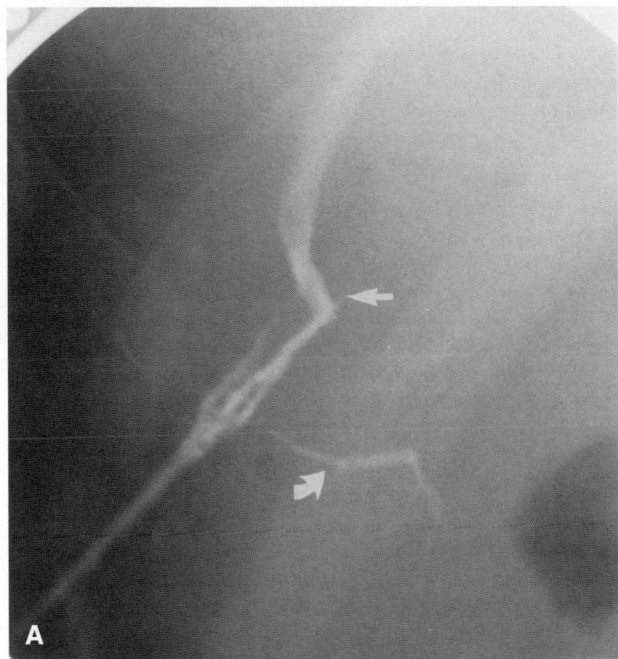

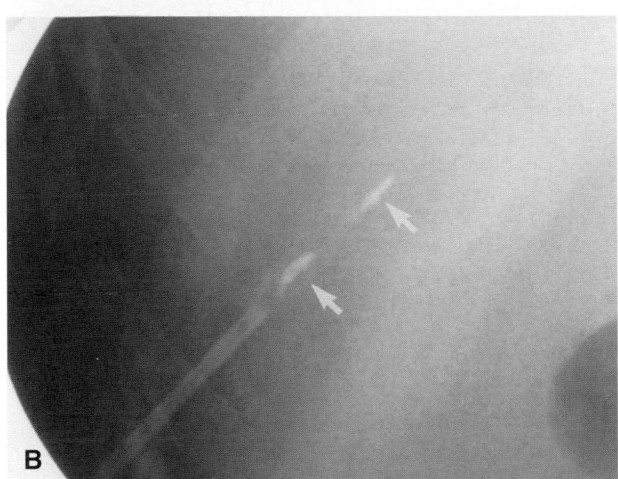

Figure 16–10 Fluoroscopic-guided liver biopsy with track embolization in a patient with suspected hemachromatosis and a moderate coagulopathy. These biopsy passes were performed coaxially with a 15-gauge, automated cutting device through a 6 French hemostatic sheath. **A.** Postbiopsy spot film during contrast injection into the sheath shows the trident shape of the three adjacent biopsy tracks. The inferior track communicates with a small portal vein branch (*curved arrow*), and the middle track communicates with a larger hepatic vein branch (*straight arrow*). **B.** Spot film obtained after track embolization shows two contrast-opacified gelfoam plugs (*arrows*) in the distal and mid portions of the biopsy track. A third gelfoam plug was later placed just below the liver capsule.

REGIONAL BIOPSY CONSIDERATIONS

The previous sections covering pathology, technical considerations, and complications apply to all percutaneous image-guided biopsies regardless of the anatomic site. There are, however, differences in technique, potential complications, and results for each specific anaomic area

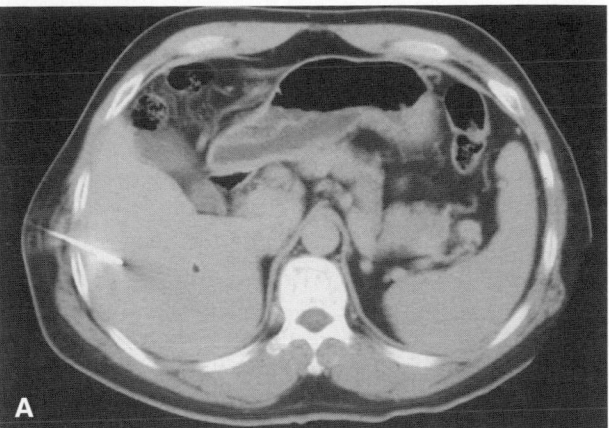

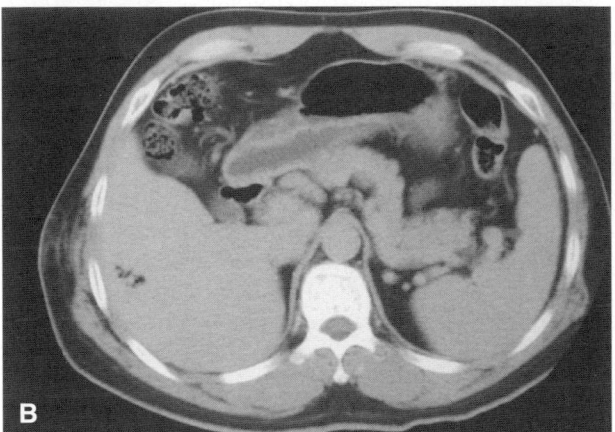

Figure 16–11 Biopsy track embolization with gelfoam under CT guidance. The biopsy was performed for staging of hepatitis C. **A.** CT image showing a 17-gauge, coaxial guiding needle placed into the right lobe of the liver. Three core biopsy specimens were obtained using an 18-gauge, automated biopsy device placed through the coaxial guide. Several small gelfoam pledgets were injected through the guiding cannula before removal of the guide. **B.** Postbiopsy scan showing a small amount of air trapped in the gelfoam in the biopsy tract. There were no complications from the biopsy.

that may be considered for biopsy. The following sections will cover in more detail the specifics of biopsies in the most common anatomic regions.

Thoracic Biopsy

Thoracic lesions may be approached in several ways, including bronchoscopy, thoracoscopy, mediastinoscopy, parasternal mediastinotomy, or thoracotomy. Bronchoscopy is accurate and safe in the diagnosis of central lesions with an endobronchial component but is less accurate for peripheral lung lesions or mediastinal disease (23,57). Thoracoscopy is more invasive but is very accurate in the diagnosis of diffuse parenchymal lung disease, benign lung nodules, and peripheral nodules, particularly those too small for percutaneous needle sampling (11,23). Mediastinoscopy and mediastinotomy have a high diagnostic accuracy but are appropriate only for specific limited nodal chains. The surgical modalities all have superior diagnostic accuracy but also carry significantly higher morbidity and mortality rates than either percutaneous or endoscopic techniques (57). Overall, percutaneous biopsy is the most versatile approach, combining both high diagnostic accuracy and safety. It is important that all diagnostic modalities be considered in each individual case. A close cooperative working relationship between interventional radiologists, pulmonologists, and thoracic surgeons will ensure that the most appropriate diagnostic modality is chosen for any given patient.

Because of the relative predominance of noncarcinomatous masses in the mediastinum, the accuracy of needle biopsy is improved significantly when cutting needles are used to obtain histologic specimens in addition to routine cytologic sampling. The best example of this is in the diagnosis of lymphoma. The reported sensitivity of cytology alone in the diagnosis of non-Hodgkin's lymphoma ranges from 54 to 83% (3,7,8). With the addition of histology, both the diagnosis and subtype can be established in more than 90% of cases (21,22,25,32). Neither cytology nor core biopsy can reliably differentiate follicular from diffuse forms of non-Hodgkin's lymphoma, but this feature has little clinical significance. Results in general are better for non-Hodgkin's lymphoma than for Hodgkin's disease because the latter diagnosis rests in the demonstration of relatively sparse Reed-Sternberg cells. Histologic specimens are also superior in the diagnosis of thymoma, although differentiating benign and malignant forms can be difficult (3,7). Cytology fares well in the diagnosis of carcinomatous mediastinal metastases, but the addition of histology will be of benefit in accurate subtyping, particularly when prior tissue samples are not available for comparison (3,8,9,22,25,26).

For malignant lung lesions, cytology alone fares well and has a reported malignant sensitivity of 80 to 93% (4,5,8,9,11,12,24,26). When adequate histologic specimens are also obtained, the combined malignant sensitivity is increased to 85–97% (9,11,22,24–27). Accurate subtype determination is slightly better with histology, although cytology appears adequate in differentiating small-cell from non–small-cell carcinomas (9,24). The most significant advantage of histology is the ability to obtain a specific diagnosis in benign nodules (5,8,9,24–26). If a specific benign diagnosis is obtained, the negative predictive value approaches 100% (24–26). Cytology alone often provides only a non-specific cancer-negative result in benign disease and in this setting the predictive value negative is much lower. In this situation, further diagnostic evaluation is usually necessary, either a repeat of the biopsy or surgery.

Needle biopsy may also be performed for the diagnosis of diffuse parenchymal lung disease (58,59). Fine-needle aspiration cytology alone can demonstrate an etiologic agent in approximately 75% of diffuse infections but does not fare well in the diagnosis of noninfectious interstitial disease (58–60). The use of larger cutting needles improves accuracy in noninfectious disease but carries an unacceptably high complication rate. Not only are pneumothoraces more frequent, but significant hemoptysis is seen in up to 21% of cases, and mortality rates approaching 1% have been reported (59,60). In selected cases, fine-needle aspiration biopsy seems an acceptable alternative in the diagnosis of infectious disease as long as the patient is not on mechanical positive pressure ventilation. In most cases, however, bronchoscopy and thoracoscopy are both more accurate and safer and should therefore be the primary diagnostic modalities.

Complications specific to thoracic biopsy, in addition to pneumothorax, include hemoptysis and air embolism. Hemoptysis is reported to occur in 2–12% of cases (4,5,9,12,24). Although usually minor and self-limited, hemoptysis can be severe and in very rare cases can be fatal (61). Hemoptysis is more frequent and more severe when larger airways or vessels are traversed, which explains the increased incidence in biopsy of hilar lung lesions (61). Bleeding disorders and pulmonary arterial hypertension are considered relative contraindications to biopsy because of the potential for more severe hemoptysis.

Air embolism may occur when a bronchovascular communication is created in the face of increased intrathoracic pressure, including coughing or positive pressure ventilation, or when a needle is left open to air with the tip in a pulmonary vein in the face of decreased intrathoracic pressure, such as during inspiration. This is an extremely rare complication but can be fatal. To minimize the risk of air embolism, it is important to keep the needle tip within the lesion, particularly when a coaxial guide needle is used. The needle should be in the chest for as short a period as possible and not be left open to air. These precautions assume greater importance in patients who are unable to suspend respiration during the biopsy. Patients on positive pressure mechanical ventilation should not undergo percutaneous thoracic biopsy unless absolutely necessary.

Although fluoroscopy was used for guidance in most early thoracic biopsy studies, CT is now the most commonly used modality. Fluoroscopy is relatively fast and simple but is limited to lesions observed clearly in two planes and is therefore suboptimal in demonstrating small nodules or abnormalities in or adjacent to the mediastinum. It can also be difficult to avoid crossing aerated lung during fluoroscopically guided biopsy of pleural-based lung lesions when the pleural attachment is small. Postobstructive lobar collapse may also obscure a central lesion, predisposing to sampling error.

CT is more accurate in determining the optimal needle path to avoid traversing aerated lung and bronchovascular structures. In the mediastinum, it is almost always possible to traverse an extrapleural path to the lesion (Figure 16–12). Even when an extrapleural access route is

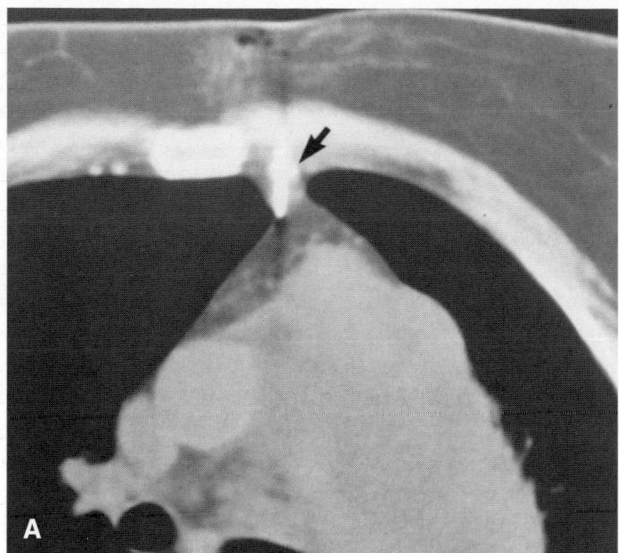

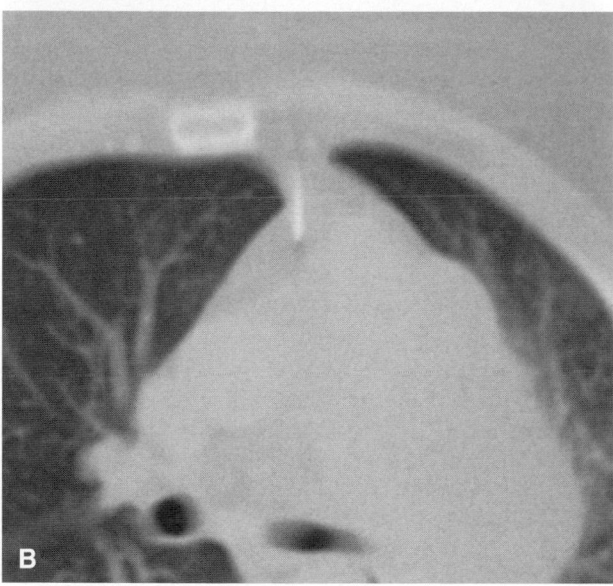

Figure 16–12 Metastatic, small-cell, anaplastic carcinoma in the left superior mediastinum. **A.** A 19-gauge guiding needle has been placed between the internal mammary vein and the internal mammary artery (arrow). **B.** Scan obtained after further advancement of the guiding needle shows the needle path to be within mediastinal fat medial to both the right and left mediastinal pleural reflections, thus avoiding traversal of aerated lung.

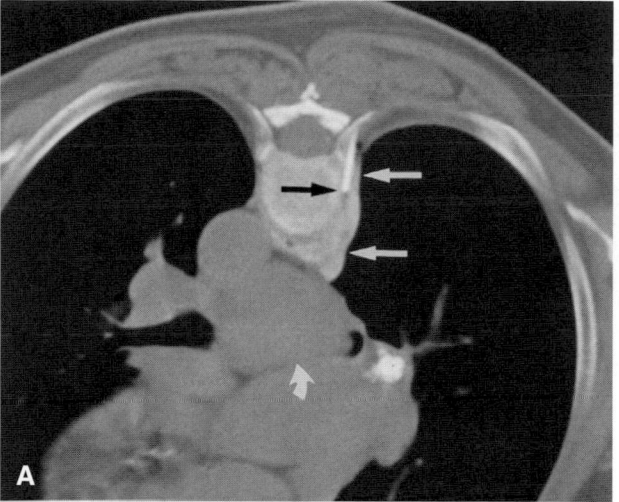

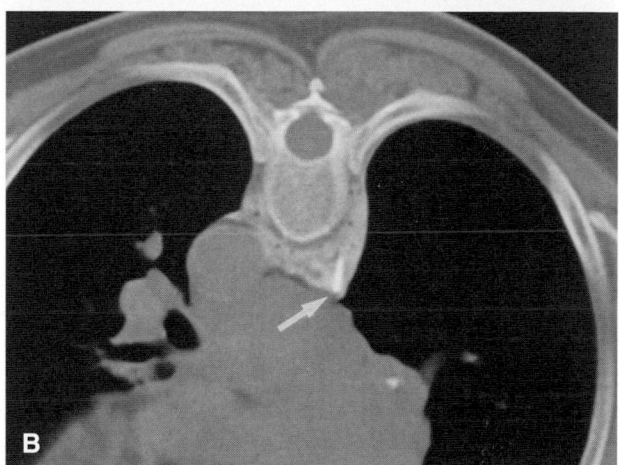

Figure 16–13 Use of an artificial extrapleural window for mediastinal biopsy. **A.** Prone CT section shows a subcarinal mass (*curved white arrow*) and the tip of a 19-gauge guiding needle (*straight black arrow*) in a paraspinous position. Diluted contrast has been injected via the guiding needle to displace the right mediastinal pleura (*straight white arrows*) laterally away from the vertebral body. **B.** Scan obtained after further guide needle advancement shows the needle tip (*arrow*) at the lesion margin. Additional saline was injected before the needle was advanced into the mass so that the needle path was entirely extrapleural. The biopsy revealed metastatic adenocarcinoma.

not obvious, an artificial extrapleural window may be created by injecting saline outside the parietal pleura to displace the adjacent aerated lung away from the intended needle path (Figure 16–13) (62). In pleural masses and peripheral pleural-based lung masses, the pleural attachment can usually be traversed, although this occasionally requires a complex approach (Figure 16–14). Regions of postobstructive collapse may be used also as a nonaerated path to central masses. CT-guided needle tip placement is more precise in both small and large masses and thus allows one to avoid necrotic portions of a tumor. Greater operator experience and the development of high-speed

CT scanners have allowed thoracic biopsies to be performed as quickly with CT as with fluoroscopy and with improved accuracy and safety.

Liver Biopsy

The primary indications for liver biopsy are the diagnosis of suspected primary or secondary malignancy and the investigation of diffuse hepatocellular disease. Fine-needle aspiration cytology has a malignant sensitivity of 70–90% in the diagnosis of metastatic disease from epithelial malignancies (2,6). However, cytology is not as accurate in the diagnosis of well-differentiated hepatocellular carcinoma or of metastases from nonepithelial malignancies such as sarcomas or

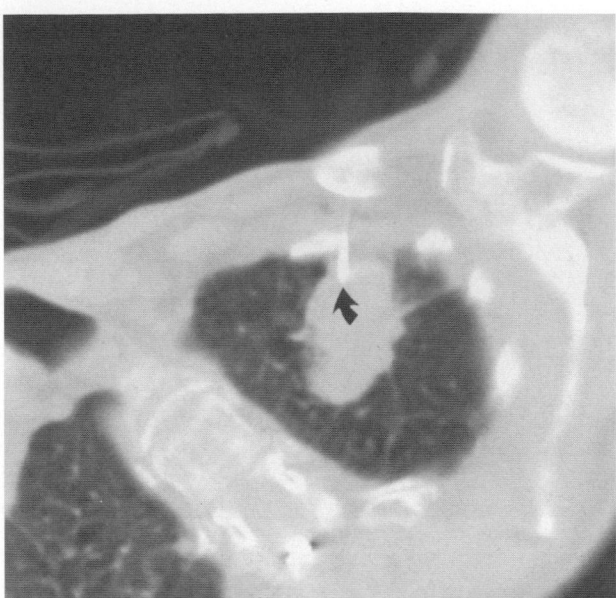

Figure 16–14   Primary left apical adenocarcinoma in a patient with chronic obstructive pulmonary disease. The guiding needle tip (*arrow*) is seen just within the anterior margin of the mass. An oblique supraclavicular approach with caudal needle angulation allowed placement of the guiding needle through the pleural-based portion of the mass.

lymphoma (2,19). Malignant sensitivities of 90–98% have been reported when both cytologic and histologic specimens are obtained (2,6,9,10,18,19,22,25,28,63).

Cytology alone plays no role in the diagnosis of diffuse hepatocellular disease because these entities are defined by histologic architecture in addition to cellular morphologic changes. Cirrhosis presents a very heterogeneous histologic pattern that requires excellent nonfragmented cores for accurate diagnosis (43). Because of this microscopic heterogeneity, it has been common practice to use 14- to 16-gauge cutting needles when investigating suspected diffuse hepatocellular disease such as cirrhosis. Several recent studies, however, have reported excellent results in biopsy of both native hepatocellular disease and liver allografts using 18-gauge automated biopsy devices (31,43). Transjugular hepatic biopsy is a useful alternative to percutaneous biopsy, particularly in patients with impaired coagulation. The diagnostic quality of transjugular biopsy specimens is not quite as good as specimens obtained using percutaneous automatic biopsy devices, but the transjugular approach may be slightly safer and allows for measurement of intrahepatic venous hemodynamics during the same procedure (47,55,56). Regardless of the technique used, it is prudent for physicians performing liver biopsies to review the specimens with the pathology staff to determine the most efficacious technique and needle size in their institution.

Although the advantages of obtaining histologic and cytologic specimens are well-documented, it is equally important that this be accomplished with no increase in complications.

Coaxial systems allow for both cytologic and histologic sampling from a single puncture. Adequate histologic cores can be obtained in almost all cases using 18- to 20-gauge automated biopsy devices, with reported complication rates of 1–3% (25,31,43). This is comparable to the complication rates reported for small-caliber aspiration needles (2,6,28). The use of 14- to 16-gauge cutting needles for diffuse hepatocellular disease is associated with a slight increase in bleeding complications (2,28). When large-caliber percutaneous needles are used, particularly in the face of abnormal coagulation studies, it is helpful to employ precautionary techniques such as biopsy track embolization (48,51).

The best guidance modality is the one that best demonstrates the pathology and adjacent structures. CT and ultrasound are the most commonly used modalities, with the choice between the two being largely based on personal experience and preference. Precise guidance not only increases accuracy but also decreases complications. Bleeding complications can be minimized, even with hypervascular lesions, by ensuring that a rim of normal liver tissue is interposed between the capsular puncture site and the margin of the lesion. Central portal structures, dilated bile ducts, large vessels, lung, and adjacent organs are relatively easy to avoid with either CT or ultrasound. As a result, nonhemorrhagic complications, such as colon or gallbladder perforation, pneumothorax, bile leak, and arteriovenous fistula or pseudoaneurysm formation have dramatically decreased in incidence when compared to blind biopsies (Figure 16–15).

Biopsy of the Pancreas

Most pancreatic biopsies are performed for suspected ductal adenocarcinoma. Occasionally, masses of indeterminate nature are encountered, with the differential diagnosis primarily being adenocarcinoma versus chronic pancreatitis. Cystic neoplasms, rare solid epithelial neoplasms, and neuroendocrine tumors are much less common. Clinical and imaging characteristics are often highly suggestive of a benign or a malignant process, but overlap is sufficient enough to keep a definitive diagnosis from being made without pathology. Because pancreatic carcinoma is usually unresectable at presentation, needle biopsy assumes a prominent role in establishing the diagnosis.

There is significant variability in the reported sensitivity of needle biopsy for the diagnosis of malignant pancreatic lesions, with reported sensitivities ranging from 67% to 93% (2, 63–65). In these series, better results were obtained with 18- to 20-gauge needles than with 22-gauge needles. Cytology fares well in biopsy of the pancreas because the primary diagnostic features of malignancy are primarily cellular morphologic changes rather than histologic architectural changes (18–20). Diagnostic difficulties arise because pancreatic carcinoma often incites an intense desmoplastic fibrotic response as well as a surrounding inflammatory reaction indistinguishable pathologically from chronic pancreatitis (63,64). For this reason, sampling error is the

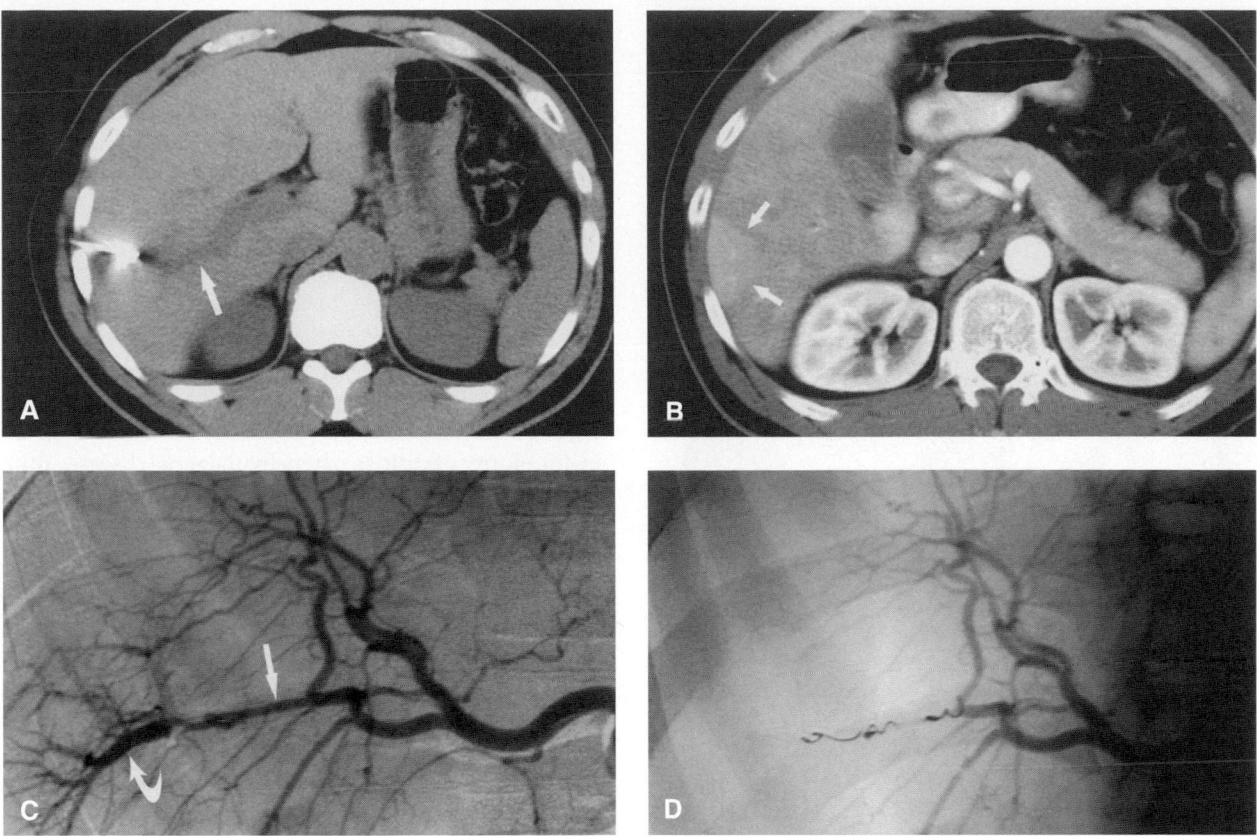

Figure 16–15 Arterial-portal fistula complication liver biopsy. The biopsy was performed for staging of hepatitis C. **A.** CT image showing a 17-gauge, coaxial guiding needle placed into the right lobe of the liver. The tip of the guide needle is near the major branch point of the right portal vein (*arrow*). Three core biopsy specimens were obtained using an 18-gauge, automated biopsy device placed through the coaxial guide. **B.** Arterial-phase, contrast-enhanced CT image obtained two days after the biopsy. The scan was obtained because of intermittent cramping abdominal pain. The clinical suspicion was that the pain resulted from the intermittent biliary obstruction from hemobilia. The CT image shows a blood clot in the gallbladder, presumably from a small vascular-biliary fistula, confirming hemobilia. The scan also shows a wedge-shaped area of early portal vein enhancement (*arrows*) peripheral to the biopsy site. **C.** Hepatic arteriogram confirms a fistula between a branch of the right hepatic artery (*straight arrow*) and a peripheral branch of the right portal vein (*curved arrow*). The vascular-biliary fistula was not demonstrated on the arteriogram. **D.** Angiographic image after coil embolization of the right hepatic artery branch confirms occlusion of the arterial-portal fistula. There were no further adverse clinical sequelae.

most common cause of false negatives and can occur with either cytologic or histologic specimens. A biopsy diagnosis of chronic inflammation and fibrosis cannot therefore be considered diagnostic of chronic pancreatitis (Figure 16–16) (65). Accurate guidance plays an important role in limiting sampling error. When ultrasound guidance is used, the hypoechoic central portion of the mass should be targeted (64). Under CT guidance, it is important to use contrast enhancement so that the lower-density central tumor may be sampled rather than the higher-density surrounding inflammatory mass, although this technique is not infallible.

The primary complications of pancreatic biopsy are bleeding and pancreatitis, which occur in 0–7% of cases (2,28,63–66). In these series, slightly lower complication rates were noted using 20-gauge or smaller needles. Despite

its rarity, pancreatitis following biopsy can be fatal (66). Most reported cases of pancreatitis have occurred after biopsy of small tumors, normal glands, or chronic pancreatitis (64,66). It has been postulated that puncture of ducts or intact pancreatic tissue rather than tumor predisposes to peripancreatic leak of enzymes, leading to pancreatitis. Although this is difficult to prove given the small number of cases, it would still seem wise to avoid puncture of major ducts. The use of needles 16-gauge or larger is neither advisable nor necessary. Bowel loops frequently overlie the pancreas and can be traversed safely, although most practitioners will avoid puncture of the colon with 18-gauge or larger needles. A transcaval approach using small-caliber aspiration needles may be used for biopsy of small lesions in or near the pancreatic head or uncinate process when no other safe access path is available (67).

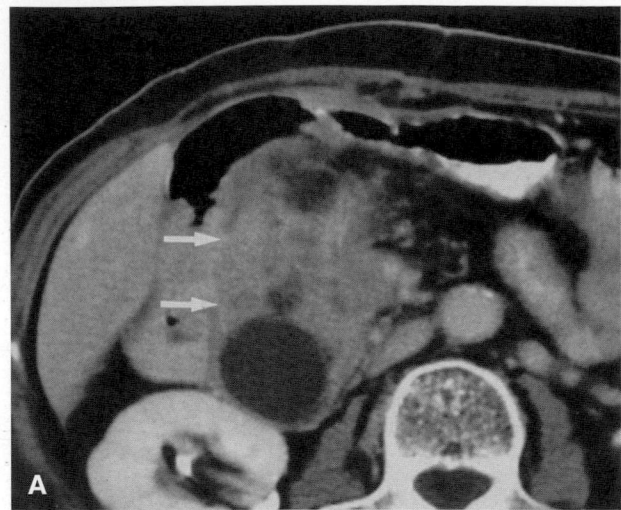

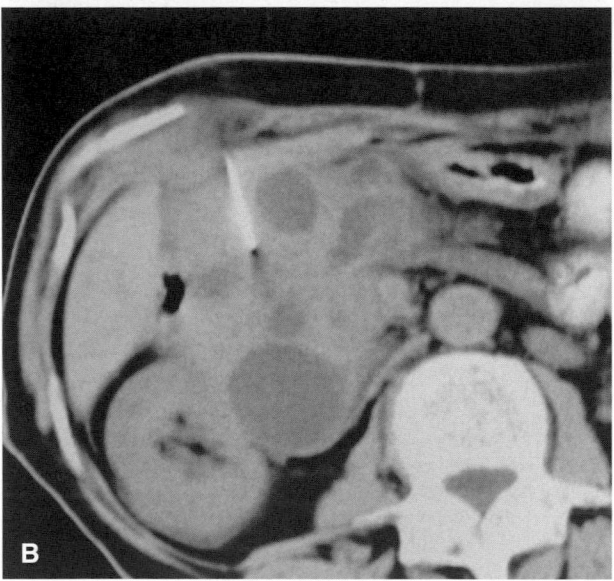

Figure 16–16 Ductal adenocarcinoma of the pancreas. **A.** Contrast-enhanced CT section shows a large mass (*arrows*) in the head of the pancreas with several low-density areas of either necrosis or cystic degeneration. **B.** Scan obtained for guiding needle localization documents specimen retrieval from the noncystic enhancing portion of the mass. Examination of the biopsy specimen revealed chronic pancreatitis and fibrosis. Subsequent open surgical biopsy revealed ductal adenocarcinoma.

Renal Biopsy

The imaging characteristics of large primary renal tumors are usually sufficiently specific to obviate preoperative biopsy. Biopsy is then reserved for small solid masses, for cases in which the imaging features suggest an atypical or noncarcinomatous tumor, for suspected metastatic disease to the kidney, and for the diagnosis of focal infection. Biopsy for the diagnosis of a focal renal mass has results and complications similar to those of other abdominal and retroperitoneal biopsies.

Biopsy for the diagnosis of diffuse parenchymal renal disease is quite different in that histologic cores of renal

cortex with at least 5–10 glomeruli per core are required for adequate diagnosis. Until recently, renal biopsies were performed blind or under fluoroscopic guidance using 14-gauge or larger cutting needles, with diagnostic tissue obtained in 75–95% of cases (46,68). In the majority of inadequate biopsies, no renal tissue was obtained, either because the renal cortex was missed or because the needle did not penetrate the renal capsule. Complications occurred in 6–12% of biopsies, primarily hematuria, perinephric hemorrhage, and arteriovenous fistula formation. More recently, results and complication rates have improved because of advancements in both guidance and needle technology.

Ultrasound is the most commonly used guidance modality for biopsy of diffuse parenchymal renal disease, although occasionally it may be suboptimal in obese patients, for whom CT guidance is preferable (45,68). The use of cross-sectional guidance allows much more accurate targeting of the kidney. Within the kidney, the operator may also selectively biopsy the lower pole cortex and avoid biopsy of the central sinus or medulla.

Automated tru–cut-type biopsy devices are now the preferred needle for renal biopsy. More glomeruli are obtained per core with the larger devices, and for a given size more glomeruli are obtained with automated devices than with manual needles (44,45). Adequate specimens can be obtained in 91–95% of cases with 18-gauge devices, with complication rates of 1–6% (44-46). The use of 14- to 15-gauge devices is recommended by some investigators, who report an accuracy rate approaching 99% and no increase in complications (68). Practitioners should review their own results to determine whether the smaller devices are satisfactory at a given institution.

Biopsy of the Adrenal Glands

Adrenal masses are detected in 2–5% of all abdominal CT scans and thus present a common diagnostic dilemma. Most are nonfunctioning benign adenomas and require neither a pathologic diagnosis nor treatment. Metastases are the second most common entity, and primary adrenal malignancy is quite rare. Although certain tumors, such as myelolipomas, often have diagnostic imaging features, most lesions are nonspecific in appearance. There has been considerable interest in attempting to predict the malignant or benign nature of adrenal masses by contrast-enhanced CT, ultrasound, and magnetic resonance imaging, but results to date show sufficient overlap that a definitive diagnosis is often not possible.

In developing a diagnostic approach to adrenal masses, it is helpful to divide patients into oncologic and nononcologic groups. Oncologic patients are those who have had a prior malignancy or who currently have clinical or radiologic evidence of cancer. Nononcologic patients are those who have no such prior history or current clinical or radiographic suspicions. In the presence of a unilateral adrenal mass, the diagnostic approach differs significantly in the two groups.

In nononcologic patients, the clinically important differential diagnosis includes nonfunctioning adenoma, functioning adenoma, and primary malignancy. Biochemical screening for hormonal activity will detect the functioning adenomas and 85% of the primary adrenocortical carcinomas, which are treated primarily by surgical excision. In nonfunctioning masses, the approach is largely dictated by size. A unilateral adrenal mass smaller than 5 cm will essentially never be a metastatic lesion, and primary carcinoma of this size is exceedingly rare (42,69). Masses of this size often are adenomas and may be followed with serial scans. Masses larger than 5 cm have a slightly greater likelihood of being malignant and require a pathologic diagnosis. Although biopsy may be performed in such cases, it can be difficult to differentiate a well-differentiated adrenocortical carcinoma from an adenoma, particularly by cytology alone (18,19). Histology may be helpful in demonstrating capsular or vascular invasion, but false negatives still occur.

In oncologic patients, the likelihood of an adrenal mass being a metastatic lesion varies with the primary cell type and stage. In patients with carcinoma of the lung, 40–50% of unilateral adrenal masses are metastases and the remainder are benign adenomas (Figure 16–17). The percentage representing metastatic disease will be much lower for other primary malignancies. Percutaneous biopsy is the primary diagnostic procedure in this situation, with a reported sensitivity of more than 90% for epithelial metastases (19,42,69). Retrieval of normal adrenal tissue is highly predictive of benignity (69). Even in this setting, adrenal biopsy is not a common procedure because other more accessible metastatic lesions are often present.

Adrenal biopsy is technically more difficult than other abdominal biopsies because of the deep subphrenic location of the glands. As a result, complication rates are slightly

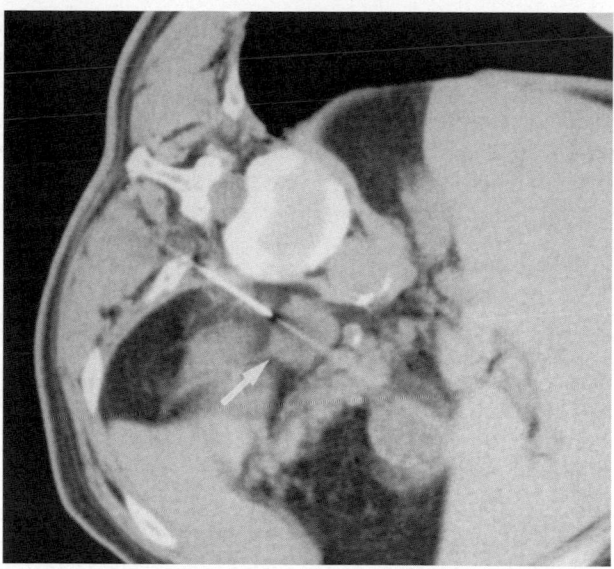

Figure 16–18 Left adrenal metastasis (*arrow*) in a patient with large-cell, undifferentiated carcinoma of the lung. A posterior approach in the left lateral decubitus position was used to collapse the posterior costophrenic sulcus and thus avoid crossing aerated lung with the coaxial guiding needle.

higher, approaching 10% (28,42,69). Minor hemorrhage and pneumothorax are the most common complications. The risk of pneumothorax can be minimized when an angled subcostal approach, right transhepatic approach, or decubitus posterior approach is used (Figure 16–18). A rare but significant complication is hypertensive crisis after biopsy of a pheochromocytomas (70). Although most pheochromocytomas are detected by hormonal screening, up to 14% are occult and may undergo biopsy. Such cases usually proceed without incident, but the need for treatment of a hypertensive crisis should be anticipated.

Biopsy of the Peritoneum and Retroperitoneum

Epithelial metastases, lymphoma, and other rare, primary, mesenchymal tumors constitute the majority of peritoneal and retroperitoneal masses referred for biopsy. In AIDS patients, infection with unusual organisms, such as atypical mycobacterium, is also a consideration. Aspiration cytology has a high sensitivity in the diagnosis of epithelial metastatic disease, whereas histologic specimens are often necessary for accurate diagnosis of mesenchymal tumors, just as in the mediastinum (10,21,32). The major difference between mediastinal and retroperitoneal masses is that the latter are usually much easier to reach. Local mechanical tamponade in the retroperitoneum allows the use of 18-gauge or even larger cutting needles with minimal bleeding complications. Lesions in the peritoneum or mesentery, however, behave more like lesions on the capsular surface of the liver, with minimal effective local

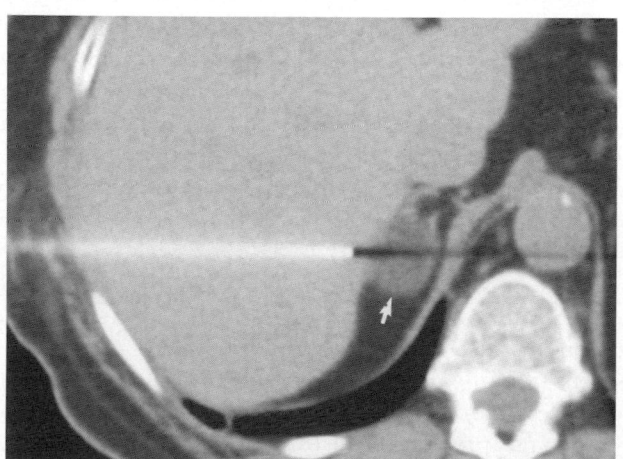

Figure 16–17 Nonfunctioning right adrenal adenoma (*arrow*) in a patient with adenocarcinoma of the lung. A lateral transhepatic approach in the supine position was used to avoid crossing aerated lung with the coaxial guiding needle.

tamponade. Needles of up to 18-gauge in size may be used safely when the access route is chosen carefully to avoid the colon and adjacent solid viscera. The bladder may be traversed safely with such needles when necessary. Track embolization may also be helpful when larger needles are used and when it is expected that local tamponade may be ineffective. Because of overlying bowel and the deep location of most retroperitoneal masses, CT guidance is technically easier than ultrasound.

Biopsy of the Musculoskeletal System

Musculoskeletal lesions in almost any location are amenable to percutaneous biopsy. The technique varies depending on whether the lesion is in bone or soft tissue. If it is in bone, the technique depends on whether the lesion is blastic or lytic. Blastic bone lesions require the use of 10- to 16-gauge trephine biopsy needles (Figure 16–19) (71–73). Soft tissue masses or lytic bone lesions without an intact cortex may be biopsied with standard needles (Figure 16–20). For lytic lesions with an intact cortex, a trephine needle may be placed through the cortex and used as a coaxial guide for standard needles (73).

Lesions of the appendicular skeleton may be biopsied under CT or fluoroscopic guidance, whereas CT is preferred for biopsy of the axial skeleton. CT more accurately depicts the lesion, the planned needle path, associated soft tissue abnormalities, and vital intervening structures. Complex approaches to vertebral body lesions may be necessary, including transforaminal, translaminar, transpedicular, and transcostovertebral paths.

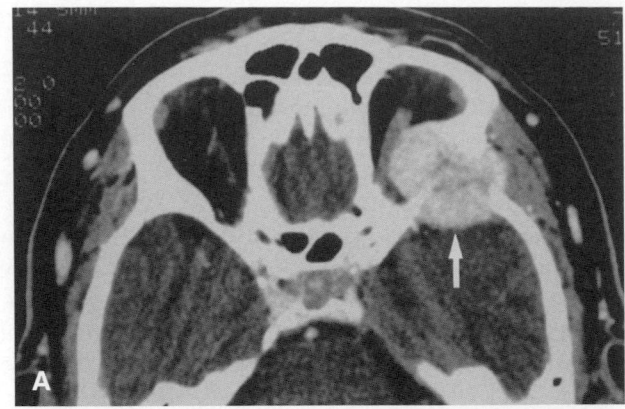

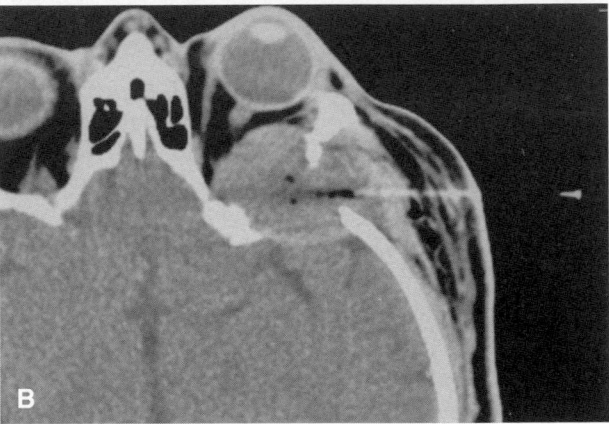

Figure 16-20 Metastatic thyroid carcinoma. **A.** Hypervascular, soft tissue mass (*arrow*) with lytic destruction of the sphenoid bone, intraorbital extension, and displacement of the optic nerve. **B.** Postbiopsy scan with the 19-gauge guiding needle in place. The biopsy was performed coaxially using a 20-gauge automated gun. The two air bubbles in the center of the mass indicate the location from which the cutting needle biopsy specimen was taken.

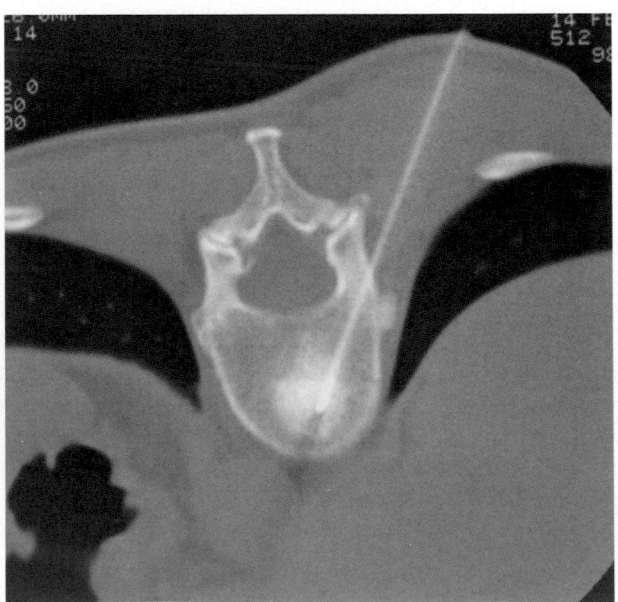

Figure 16–19 Sclerotic metastasis in the T11 vertebral body from carcinoma of the breast. Scan shows a 17-gauge, trephine, bone-coring needle in place via a transpedicular approach.

For optimal results, it is important to obtain specimens for both cytologic and histologic evaluation (72,73). Accuracy depends not only on technique but also on the nature of the lesion. Biopsy for the diagnosis of infection is accurate, but false-negatives may occur if antibiotics have been administered before the biopsy. Cytologic or histologic features may be diagnostic in such cases even when cultures are negative. Accuracy is also high in cases of metastatic disease. Malignant sensitivity of 80–90% may be expected, with lytic lesions being easier to diagnose than blastic lesions (71–73).

Biopsy of suspected primary bone tumors is performed less often for several reasons. Because most primary bone tumors are treated by surgical resection, there may be little benefit from the results of a preoperative biopsy. Whether or not to perform a preoperative biopsy is largely a matter of personal preference on the part of the surgeon, but biopsy can be helpful when preoperative radiation therapy or chemotherapy is anticipated. Diagnosis of bone lesions is more difficult with needle biopsy specimens than with resected specimens, and diagnosis in this area—more than any other area—requires a very skilled pathologist. Certain lesions, such as cartilaginous tumors and soft tissue sarcomas, are extremely difficult to classify by needle biopsy alone (19). There is also tremendous pleomorphism in both malignant and benign bone tumors, and the distinction between the two may not be clear by the study of cellular morphologic changes (18). In centers with a high volume, considerable experience, and expert pathologists, an accuracy of 70–90% may be obtained, but it is doubtful that such results can be obtained at smaller institutions with less experience (71,73). Close cooperation between the radiologist and the orthopedic surgeon is mandatory, not only in selecting patients for biopsy but also in determining the biopsy needle path so that it may be resected along with the tumor at the time of surgery.

Thyroid Biopsy

The likelihood that a thyroid nodule is malignant is approximately 5% (74). However, no single imaging feature is 100% predictive of a thyroid malignancy. Some imaging features are suggestive of thyroid malignancy, and the ultimate decision to biopsy a thyroid nodule should also consider the patients' risk of having a malignancy (75). Biopsy of the thyroid gland to evaluate for diffuse thyroid disease is usually not necessary.

Ultrasound-guided, fine-needle aspiration of the thyroid nodule allows real-time monitoring of the biopsy. Vital structures, such as the carotid artery, can be observed and avoided and small nonpalpable nodules can be found through biopsy. Thyroid nodules are frequently cystic, and the continued visualization of the needle during biopsy allows preferential sampling of solid areas.

To ensure the maximum amount of cellular material and a minimum amount of blood, a small needle is used. A 22- to 25-gauge needle with no or little suction is passed through the nodule with a slow, back-and-forth motion. After approximately eight manipulations, or when material is seen in the hub, the sampling stops and the needle is withdrawn. The specimen smears are reviewed immediately for the presence of cellular material. Each nodule is sampled a minimum of four times, and additional sampling may be required when there is a lack of cellular material.

The complication rate for ultrasound-guided, thyroid-nodule biopsy is very low, and the diagnostic accuracy is between 80 and 95% (76). Some difficulty in cytologic evaluation exists in differentiating a benign microfollicular adenoma from a follicular carcinoma. Also, the presence of Hürthle cells can be seen in benign thyroiditis as well as in some neoplasms (77).

SUMMARY

The accuracy of cytologic diagnosis, the safety of fine-needle aspiration, and advances in guidance are responsible for the development, evolution, and increasing effectiveness of percutaneous biopsy techniques. Cytology is very accurate in the diagnosis of epithelial malignancies, which are the most common lesions encountered in any given biopsy practice. However, the cytologic technique is suboptimal for the diagnosis of noncarcinomatous tumors and benign lesions. These limitations are best addressed by obtaining histologic core specimens, in addition to cytologic aspirates. The improvement in biopsy accuracy realized by the addition of histology depends on the type of lesions encountered and the cytopathologic expertise available in any given practice. It is important to use proper technique to obtain each type of specimen. Small-caliber aspiration needles are best suited to retrieve cytologic specimens, while automated cutting needles allows for the reliable retrieval of high-quality, histologic, core specimens. The roles of histologic and cytologic analysis remain complementary. Obtaining excellent specimens for each makes pathologic interpretation easier and more accurate. With careful technique, it is possible to safely obtain diagnostic tissue in up to 95% of cases referred for biopsy. Sampling error is then the most significant obstacle to even greater biopsy accuracy, thus placing control of accuracy largely in the hands of the radiologist. Future efforts should be directed toward minimizing complications and toward developing methods to sample tissue safely from multiple areas of a lesion to minimize sampling error.

REFERENCES

1. Martin HE, Ellis EB. Biopsy by needle puncture and aspiration. Ann Surg 1930;92:169–181.
2. Schwerk WB, Durr HK, Schmitz-Moormann P. Ultrasound guided fine-needle biopsies in pancreatic and hepatic neoplasms. Gastrointest Radiol 1983;8:219–225.
3. Herman SJ, Holub RV, Weisbrod GL, et al. Anterior mediastinal masses: utility of transthoracic needle biopsy. Radiology 1991; 180:167–170.
4. vanSonnenberg E, Casola G, Ho M, et al. Difficult thoracic lesions: CT-guided biopsy experience in 150 cases. Radiology 1988;167:457–461.
5. Fink I, Gamsu G, Harter LP. CT-guided aspiration biopsy of the thorax. J Comput Assist Tomogr 1982;6:958–962.
6. Martino CR, Haaga JR, Bryan PJ, et al. CT-guided liver biopsies: eight years' experience. Radiology 1984;152:755–757.
7. Weisbrod GL, Lyons DJ, Tao LC, et al. Percutaneous fine-needle aspiration of mediastinal lesions. AJR 1984;143:525–529.
8. Goralnik CH, O'Connell DM, El Yousef SJ, et al. CT-guided cutting needle biopsies of selected chest lesions. AJR 1988;151:903–907.
9. Greene R, Szyfelbein WM, Isler RJ, et al. Supplementary tissue-core histology from fine-needle transthoracic aspiration biopsy. AJR 1985;144:787–792.
10. Lieberman RP, Hafez GR, Crummy AB. Histology from aspiration biopsy: Turner needle experience. AJR 1982;138:561–564.
11. Wallace MJ, Krishnamurthy S, Broemeling LD, et al. CT-guided percutaneous fine-needle aspiration biopsy of small (<1-cm) pulmonary lesions. Radiology 2002;225:823–828.
12. Swischuk JL, Castaneda F, Patel JC, et al. Percutaneous transthoracic needle biopsy of the lung: review of 612 lesions. J Vasc Intervent Radiol 1998;9:347–352.
13. Epstein HD. Fine-needle aspiration of soft tissue lesions. Pathology (Phila) 1996;4:463–492.

14. Jeffrey PB. Fine-needle aspiration of the lung. Pathology (Phila) 1996;4:439–461.
15. Thunnissen FB, Peterse JL, van Pel R, et al. Reliability of fine needle aspiration cytology for distinguishing between carcinoma, lymphoma and sarcoma: the influence of clinical information. Cytopathology 1993;4:107–114.
16. Hughes JH, Cohen MB. Fine-needle aspiration of the pancreas. Pathology (Phila) 1996;4:389–407.
17. Miller DA, Carrasco CH, Katz RL, et al. Fine-needle aspiration biopsy: the role of immediate cytologic assessment. AJR 1986;147:155–158.
18. Hajdu SI, Melamed MR. Limitations of aspiration cytology in the diagnosis of primary neoplasms. Acta Cytol 1984;28:337–345.
19. Katz RL. The scope of fine-needle aspiration biopsy: cytologic diagnosis and techniques. Semin Intervent Radiol 1985;2:207–219.
20. Bocking A. Cytological versus histological evaluation of percutaneous biopsies. Cardiovasc Intervent Radiol 1991;14:5–12.
21. Demharter J, Muller P, Wagner T, et al. Percutaneous core-needle biopsy of enlarged lymph nodes in the diagnosis and subclassification of malignant lymphomas. Eur Radiol 2001;11:276–283.
22. Tikkakoski T, Paivansalo M, Siniluoto T, et al. Percutaneous ultrasound-guided biopsy: fine needle biopsy, cutting needle biopsy, or both? Acta Radiol 1993;34:30–34.
23. Mitruka S, Landreneau RJ, Mack MJ, et al. Diagnosing the indeterminate pulmonary nodule: percutaneous biopsy versus thoracoscopy. Surgery 1995;118:676–684.
24. Klein JS, Salomon G, Stewart EA. Transthoracic needle biopsy with a coaxially placed 20-gauge automated cutting needle: results in 122 patients. Radiology 1996;198:715–720.
25. Moulton JS, Moore PT. Coaxial percutaneous biopsy technique with automated biopsy devices: value in improving accuracy and negative predictive value. Radiology 1993;186:515–522.
26. Hanninen EL, Vogl TJ, Ricke J, et al. CT-guided percutaneous core biopsies of pulmonary lesions. Acta Radiol 2001;42:151–155.
27. Weisbrod GL, Herman SJ, Tao LC. Preliminary experience with a dual cutting edge needle in thoracic percutaneous fine-needle aspiration biopsy. Radiology 1987;163:75–78.
28. Welch TJ, Sheedy PF, Johnson CD, et al. CT-guided biopsy: prospective analysis of 1,000 procedures. Radiology 1989;171:493–496.
29. Cha I, Goates JJ. Fine-needle aspiration of lymph nodes: use of flow cytometry immunophenotyping. Pathology (Phila) 1996;4:337–364.
30. Parker SH, Hopper KD, Yakes WF, et al. Image-directed percutaneous biopsies with a biopsy gun. Radiology 1989;171:663–669.
31. Chezmar JL, Keith LL, Nelson RC, et al. Liver transplant biopsies with a biopsy gun. Radiology 1991;179:447–448.
32. Erwin BC, Brynes RK, Chan WC, et al. Percutaneous needle biopsy in the diagnosis and classification of lymphoma. Cancer 1986;57:1074–1078.
33. Gianfelice D, Lepanto L, Perreault P, et al. Value of CT fluoroscopy for percutaneous biopsy procedures. J Vasc Interv Radiol 2000;11:879–884.
34. Gobien RP, Stanley JH, Vujic I, et al. Thoracic biopsy: CT guidance of thin-needle aspiration. AJR 1984;142:827–830.
35. Haramati LB, Austin JHM. Complications after CT-guided needle biopsy through aerated versus nonaerated lung. Radiology 1991;181:778.
36. Moore EH, LeBlanc J, Montesi SA, et al. Effect of patient positioning after needle aspiration lung biopsy. Radiology 1991;181:385–387.
37. Bourgouin PM, Shepard JA, McLoud TC, et al. Transthoracic needle aspiration biopsy: evaluation of the blood patch technique. Radiology 1988;166:93–95.
38. Herman SJ, Weisbrod GL. Usefulness of the blood patch technique after transthoracic needle aspiration biopsy. Radiology 1990;176:395–397.
39. Cox JE, Chiles C, McManus CM, et al. Transthoracic needle aspiration biopsy: variables that affect risk of pneumothorax. Radiology 1999;212:165–168.
40. Poe RH, Kallay MC, Wicks CM, et al. Predicting risk of pneumothorax in needle biopsy of the lung. Chest 1984;85:232–235.
41. Kazerooni EA, Lim FT, Mikhail A, et al. Risk of pneumothorax in CT-guided transthoracic needle aspiration biopsy of the lung. Radiology 1996;198:371–375.
42. Bernardino ME, Walther MM, Phillips VM, et al. CT-guided adrenal biopsy: accuracy, safety, and indications. AJR 1985;144:67–69.
43. Sheets PW, Brumbaugh CJ, Kopecky KK, et al. Safety and efficacy of a spring-propelled 18-gauge needle for US-guided liver biopsy. J Vasc Intervent Radiol 1991;2:147–149.
44. Bogan ML, Kopecky KK, Kraft JL, et al. Needle biopsy of renal allografts: comparison of two techniques. Radiology 1990;174:273–275.
45. Cozens NJA, Murchison JT, Allan PL, et al. Conventional 15-G needle technique for renal biopsy compared with ultrasound-guided spring-loaded 18-G needle biopsy. Br J Radiol 1992;65:594–597.
46. Mostbeck GH, Wittich GR, Derfler K, et al. Optimal needle size for renal biopsy: in vitro and in vivo evaluation. Radiology 1989;173:819–822.
47. Sawyerr AM, McCormick PA, Tennyson GS, et al. A comparison of transjugular and plugged-percutaneous liver biopsy in patients with impaired coagulation. J Hepatol 1993;17:81–85.
48. Smith TP, McDermott VG, Ayoub DM, et al. Percutaneous transhepatic liver biopsy with tract embolization. Radiology 1996;198:769–774.
49. McDill DB, Rakela J, Zinsmeister AR, et al. A 21-year experience with major hemorrhage after percutaneous liver biopsy. Gastroenterology 1990;99:1396–1400.
50. Smith EH. Complications of percutaneous abdominal fine-needle biopsy. Radiology 1991;178:253–258.
51. Zins M, Vilgrain V, Gayno S, et al. US-guided percutaneous liver biopsy with plugging of the needle track: a prospective study in 72 high-risk patients. Radiology 1992;184:841–843.
52. Gazelle GS, Haaga JR, Rowland DY. Effect of needle gauge, level of anticoagulation, and target organ on bleeding associated with aspiration biopsy: work in progress. Radiology 1992;183:509–513.
53. Ewe K. Bleeding after liver biopsy does not correlate with the indices of peripheral coagulation. Dig Dis Sci 1981;26:388–393.
54. Rodgers RPC, Levin J. A critical reappraisal of the bleeding time. Semin Thromb Hemostasis 1990;16:1–20.
55. Corr P, Beningfield SJ, Davey N. Transjugular liver biopsy: a review of 200 biopsies. Clin Radiol 1992;45:238–239.
56. Gamble P, Colopinto RF, Stronell RD, et al. Transjugular liver biopsy: a review of 461 biopsies. Radiology 1985;157:589–593.
57. Schenk DA, Bower JH, Bryan CL, et al. Transbronchial needle aspiration staging of bronchogenic carcinoma. Am Rev Respir Dis 1986;134:146–148.
58. Zavala DC, Bedell GN. Percutaneous lung biopsy with a cutting needle: an analysis of 40 cases and comparison with other biopsy techniques. Am Rev Respir Dis 1972;106:186–193.
59. Youmans CR, deGroot WJ, Marshall R, et al. Needle biopsy of the lung in diffuse parenchymal disease: an analysis of 151 cases. Am J Surg 1970;120:637–643.
60. Palmer DL, Michael D, Rodney L. Needle aspiration of the lungs in complex pneumonias. Chest 1980;78:16–21.
61. Berquist TH, Bailey PB, Cortese DA, et al. Transthoracic needle biopsy: accuracy and complications in relation to location and type of lesion. Mayo Clin Proc 1980;55:475–481.
62. Moulton JS. Artificial extrapleural window for mediastinal biopsy. J Vasc Intervent Radiol 1993;4:825–829.
63. Hall-Craggs MA, Lees WR. Fine-needle aspiration biopsy: pancreatic and biliary tumors. AJR 1986;147:399–403.
64. Brandt KR, Charboneau JW, Stephens DH, et al. CT- and US-guided biopsy of the pancreas. Radiology 1993;187:99–104.
65. Karlson BM, Forsman CA, Wilander E, et al. Efficiency of percutaneous core biopsy in pancreatic tumor diagnosis. Surgery 1996;120:75–79.
66. Mueller PR, Miketic LM, Simeone JF, et al. Severe acute pancreatitis after percutaneous biopsy of the pancreas. AJR 1988;151:493–494.
67. Gupta S, Ahrar K, Morello FA, et al. Masses in or around the pancreatic head: CT-guided coaxial fine-needle aspiration biopsy with a posterior transcaval approach. Radiology 2002;222.
68. Sateriale M, Cronin JJ, Savadier LD. A 5-year experience with 307 CT-guided renal biopsies: results and complications. J Vasc Intervent Radiol 1991;2:401–407.

69. Silverman SG, Mueller PR, Pinkney LP, et al. Predictive value of image-guided adrenal biopsy: analysis of results of 101 biopsies. Radiology 1993;187:715–718.

70. Casola G, Nicolet V, vanSonnenberg E, et al. Unsuspected pheochromocytoma: risk of blood pressure alterations during percutaneous adrenal biopsy. Radiology 1986;159:733–735.

71. Kattapuram SV, Rosenthal DI. Percutaneous biopsy of skeletal lesions. AJR 1991;157:935–942.

72. Tikkakoski T, Lahde S, Puranen J, et al. Combined CT-guided biopsy and cytology in diagnosis of bony lesions. Acta Radiol 1992;33:225–229.

73. deSantos LA, Lukeman JM, Wallace S, et al. Percutaneous needle biopsy of bone in the cancer patient. AJR 1978;130:641–649.

74. Tollin SR, Mery GM, Jelveh N, et al. The use of fine-needle aspiration biopsy under ultrasound guidance to assess the risk of malignancy in patients with a multinodular goiter. Thyroid 2000;10:235–241.

75. Kim EK, Park CS, Chung WY, et al. New sonographic criteria for recommending fine-needle aspiration biopsy of nonpalpable solid nodules of the thyroid. AJR 2002;178:687–691.

76. Boland GW, Lee MJ, Mueller PR, et al. Efficacy of sonographically guided biopsy of thyroid masses and cervical lymph nodes. AJR 1993;161:1053–1056.

77. Mazzaferri EL. Management of a solitary thyroid nodule. N Engl J Med 1993;328:553–559.

Revascularization of the Aorta and Its Branches

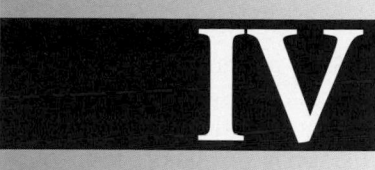

IV

Percutaneous Aortoiliac Intervention in Vascular Disease

17

Janice M. Newsome, Kenneth S. Rholl

Percutaneous transluminal interventional techniques have profoundly changed the management of vascular occlusive disease. Percutaneous transluminal angioplasty (PTA) and stents in the iliac arteries for patients with aortoiliac disease is now one of the most commonly performed and widely accepted interventional procedures (1–3). Its acceptance was gradual and hard fought, and there was significant resistance from the surgical community. Over the last 10 years, interventionalists have demonstrated that catheter-based techniques provide a significant benefit to patients and have a profound impact on the care of the patient with peripheral vascular disease. Today, there is a major shift from surgery (aortofemoral bypass) to stent placement (aortoiliac stents) in patients with aortoiliac insufficiency (4). This is a testament of the contributions made by interventionalists to the treatment of peripheral arterial occlusive disease.

After crossing an occluded iliac segment inadvertently, Dotter first wrote of possible percutaneous treatment of atheromatous occlusive disease in 1964 (5). One year later, Dotter used a series of coaxial polyethylene catheters to restore perfusion in the leg of an elderly woman who had refused amputation (6). Early gangrenous changes were reversed, and the leg was saved. Ten years later, Gruentzig introduced the double-lumen balloon catheter for vessel dilation, which allowed one to dilate lesions to a larger diameter while using a small arteriotomy (7). This paved the way for the technical and medical revolution that has subsequently occurred with rapid advances in balloon technology and the development of balloon systems for any vessel anywhere in the body. Currently, PTA and stenting of iliac lesions have become routine with comparable long-term outcome with bypass surgery (8–13).

Stent technology continues to expand. Self-expandable and balloon-expandable stents have played an important role in treating aortoiliac atherosclerotic disease. Thrombolytic therapy has expanded the role of PTA. Chronic arterial occlusions are being recanalized by subintimal revascularization as well as mechanical thrombectomy devices. Drug-eluting stents are now on the horizon, and although this technology is in its infancy in treating aortoiliac disease, there is no doubt it will play a significant role in the future. Covered stents or "stent grafts" have already revolutionized the treatment of abdominal aortic aneurysm (AAA) and will likely continue to gain significant importance in the treatment of iliac artery disease especially in the setting of arterial rupture. At the time of its initial description, iliac interventions were a portent of the revolutionary potential of nonsurgical treatment of "surgical disease," a promise that is still being fulfilled with the continued evolution of other interventional, minimally invasive therapies. The increased awareness and growing interest in the field of endovascular therapy will continue to benefit patients and create opportunities with new challenges for the future. The current clinical utility and applications of aortoiliac intervention are considered within this chapter.

CLINICAL EVALUATION

Before intervention is considered, a complete evaluation of the patient should be performed, including a directed history and physical examination (H and P). Thereafter, a noninvasive vascular examination may be done to confirm the presence of disease as well as to localize the level of the disease and allow quantification of the disease as it relates to the patient's symptoms. This information is crucial in helping the interventionalist to decide whether invasive therapy is indeed appropriate.

HISTORY AND PHYSICAL EXAMINATION

Patients with aortoiliac disease may present with a variety of symptoms because of the proximal nature of the obstruction. Intermittent claudication is by far the most common presenting symptom. It is usually described as "cramping, aches, tightness, soreness, and even numbness" of a leg that is exacerbated with exercise and relieved by rest. Even though the dominant site is the calf, claudicating may involve the hips, thighs, and buttocks in varying degrees and combinations. The presence of more proximal symptoms should point the clinician toward aortoiliac disease. A directed and detailed H and P can nearly always distinguish between true vascular claudication and nonvascular pseudoclaudication.

It is important to recognize that several causes may exist for leg fatigue and pain with ambulation including musculoskeletal and neurologic disorders (Table 17–1) (14).

TABLE 17–1
CAUSES OF LEG PAIN

Location of Pain	Associated Factor	Clinical Diagnosis
Calf, Buttock, Hip, or Thigh	Aggravated by exercise; relieved by rest	Claudication
Calf, Buttock, Hip, or Thigh	Aggravated by standing + exercise; relieved by back flexion	Lumbar stenosis
Hip, Knee, Ankles	Aggravated by variable factors; relieved by NSAIDs	Arthritis
Calf, Leg Radiation	Aggravated by variable factors; relieved by NSAIDs	Herniated disk

Young women (ages 40–50) with a history of tobacco use have a unique pattern of atherosclerotic vascular disease consisting of diffuse disease of the distal abdominal aorta, or the "small aorta syndrome" (15). The young age and female predilection as well as the nonclassic clinical profile of atherosclerotic disease often lead to a delay in diagnosis. Erectile dysfunction in men may also be a presenting symptom. Impotence may be seen as being in concert with intermittent claudication or as an isolated complaint. Leriche syndrome includes the constellation of symptoms of lower extremity ischemia and impotence secondary to distal aortic occlusion (Figure 17–1). Because presenting symptoms depend on the activity level of the patient, it is important to determine the mobility of the patient at the time of the initial interview. Quantification of distance, time of symptoms, aggravating and relieving factors, degree of activity, and the time course of the evolution of symptoms are all important in assessing the patient's disease.

A sudden onset of ischemic symptoms in one or both lower extremities without preexisting claudication suggests a primary embolic event. A sudden worsening of symptoms in a patient with preexisting symptoms may indicate occlusion of a previously stenotic segment. Microemboli occluding the digital arteries may be caused by aortoiliac disease presenting as focal severe ischemia to the digits, the "blue toe syndrome" (16–18). Bilateral simultaneous "blue toes" suggests an aortic, bilateral iliac, or cardiac source of emboli (Figure 17–2). Alternately, unilateral findings may occur with any lesion distal to the aortic bifurcation.

In addition to a history directed at the current symptomatology, an evaluation of the risk factors for peripheral vascular disease should be undertaken. It is critical to identify cardiovascular risk factors and treat them aggressively (19). Risk factors include smoking, diabetes, hypertension, and obesity, personal or family history of heart disease,

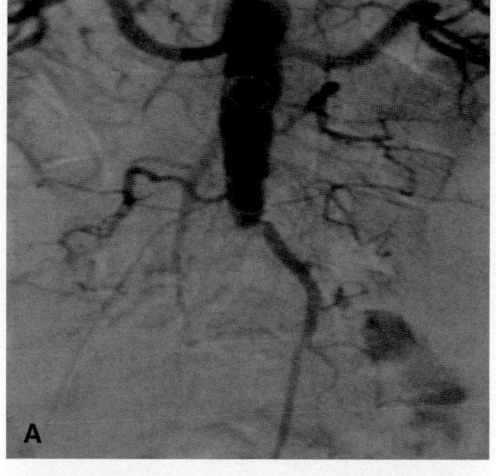
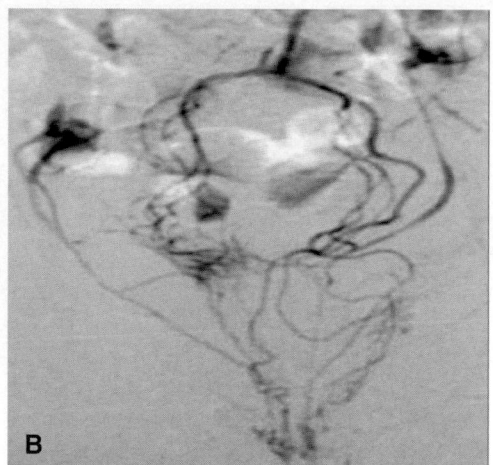
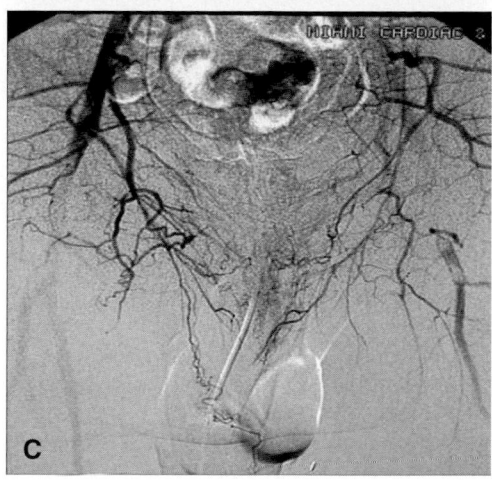

Figure 17–1   Leriche Syndrome. This is a patient with bilateral lower extremity rest pain and impotence secondary to chronic distal aortic occlusion. The patient has perfusion to his legs through collaterals from the inferior mesenteric artery (IMA).

hyperlipidemia, physical inactivity, high levels of homocysteine, and advanced age.

Tobacco consumption is foremost in this evaluation because this is the one truly reversible risk factor. Smoking increases the risk of atherosclerosis by 50%, and it accelerates the rate as well. It damages the endothelium directly, increases vascular tone, and promotes platelet activation (20). Many patients with vasculopathy will improve without intervention when they discontinue smoking and undertake a regular, graded exercise program (21). In the absence of limb-threatening ischemia, patients who continue to smoke should have their intervention postponed until tobacco use is discontinued.

Diabetes Mellitus is an important risk factor for atherosclerosis. It not only increases the risk for atherosclerosis but also increases the rate. The relative risk for cardiovascular disease is twofold to eightfold higher in persons with diabetes compared to those without diabetes when matched for age, sex, and ethnicity (22–26). The pathogenesis is multifactorial, making the exact mechanisms of cause and potential benefit of correcting the offending stress unknown. However, it is widely accepted that early intervention in the form of primary prevention and behavior modification, such as weight management, exercise, and proper nutrition, will reduce the cardiovascular complications in patients with diabetes (22,27).

It has been reported that diabetes increases the rate of amputation by as much as 20% when compared to individuals without diabetes (22,26). Maintaining a blood pressure of 140/90 mm Hg or below imparts significant reduction in cardiovascular mortality (28,29). Hyperlipidemia is one of the most undertreated conditions with well-established risk factors for peripheral vascular disease (30–34). More recently, elevated levels of amino-acid homocysteine have been linked strongly to premature atherosclerosis (35–37). Patients with elevated plasma levels of homocysteine can be modified by oral vitamin supplementation using pyridoxine and folate. This has been shown to decrease plasma levels of homocysteine. If a patient is under the age of 50 with atherosclerotic disease, then the clinician must consider elevated hypoprotein, elevated fibrinogen, and elevated C-reactive protein as possible causes, which are markers for progressive atherosclerosis with familial tendencies, undiagnosed hypercoagulable syndromes, or both (38–40).

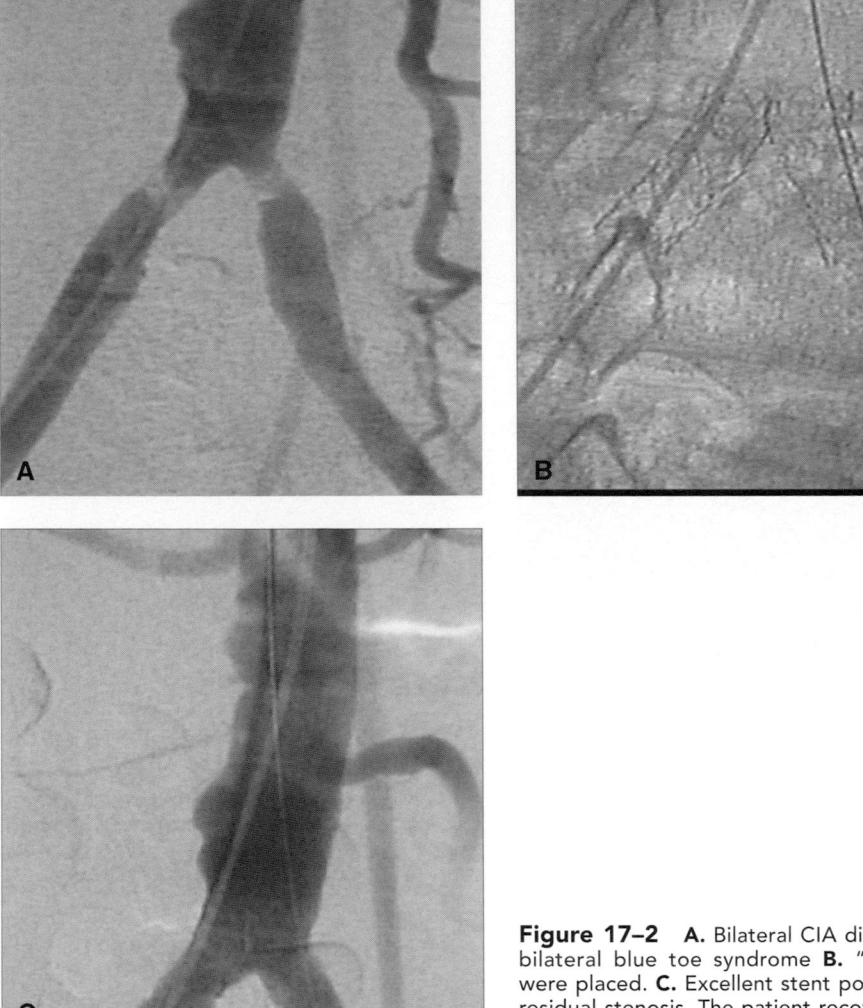

Figure 17–2 **A.** Bilateral CIA disease causing bilateral blue toe syndrome **B.** "Kissing BES" were placed. **C.** Excellent stent position with no residual stenosis. The patient recovered with no further episodes of embolization.

Physical examination of the patient with aortoiliac disease often reveals diffusely decreased or absent femoral, popliteal, and pedal artery pulses. It is true that femoral pulses may be present and "normal" at rest, which can significantly delay the diagnosis. After exercise, the pulse will decrease significantly and disappear frequently, pointing at the value of noninvasive testing with an exercise protocol. A bruit over the aortoiliac segment sometimes can be auscultated. Gentle palpation of the abdomen for the presence of an abdominal aortic aneurysm is also an important part of the routine evaluation of peripheral vascular disease.

The distal extremities should be elevated for both acute and chronic ischemia. Loss of hair over the foot and calf and atrophic changes in the nail bed are signs of chronic ischemia. As the ischemia progresses, dependent rubor with pallor upon elevation may be present in the affected limb. Capillary refill may be noticeably slowed. Finally, the patient may have pain at rest that is often relieved by placing the extremity in the dependent position. With more severe ischemia, tissue breakdown may occur with formation of ischemic ulceration. As this advances, gangrenous changes occur as the tissue breakdown becomes irreversible. When ischemia is more acute, the viability of the extremity should be determined by evaluating capillary refill, sensory and motor function; this assessment is critical in determining the subsequent therapy. The Fontaine and the modified Rutherford-Becker classification system should be used to classify both chronic and acute ischemia (41–43). This system is generally accepted by the surgical and interventional communities and provides a common definition of the clinical status (Tables 17–2 and 17–3).

TABLE 17–2
ACUTE LIMB ISCHEMIA

Category	Description	Capillary Refill	Motor Impairment	Sensory Impairment	Arterial Doppler	Venous Doppler
Viable	Not immediately threatened	Intact	None	None	Audible, ankle greater pressure than 30 mm Hg	Audible
Threatened	Salvageable, if promptly treated	Intact, slow	Mild	Mild	Inaudible	Audible
Irreversible	Major tissue loss, amputation required regardless of treatment	Absent (marbling)	Profound paralysis Rigor	Profound anesthetic	Inaudible	Inaudible

NONINVASIVE VASCULAR TESTING

Although a directed history and physical examination are extremely useful in evaluating patients with suspected peripheral vascular disease, both false-positive and false-negative diagnoses may result from sole reliance on the history and physicals. Noninvasive Vascular Testing (NVT) can be extremely useful, not only in the detection of disease but also in quantifying and localizing the disease (44–59). NVT can correlate the patient's constellation of symptoms to vascular disease if present, because many diseases can present with symptoms very similar to those of vascular disease. Exercise testing can help differentiate vascular from nonvascular symptoms, thus preventing unindicated interventions (60,61). It is important to remember that the mere presence of disease is not an indication for intervention.

Although a complete description of NVT is beyond the scope of this chapter, a brief discussion of the modalities available is presented. NVT modalities generally can be categorized by the information they provide, that is, physiologic or anatomic tests. Common physiologic tests include segmental limb pressures, Doppler waveform analysis, volume plethysmographic tracings (PVRs), and digital photoplethysmographic tracings (PPGs). Anatomic tests include duplex ultrasound, with or without color, Magnetic Resonance Angiography (MRA) and Computed Tomography Angiography (CTA). The choice of testing modality should depend on the information being sought, with some consideration given to the cost and availability of the examination at your institution. Physiologic testing is intended to provide information on the overall perfusion status of the extremity and allows localization and quantification, which are the bases for ischemia classification (Table 17–3). Exercise testing is an important part of physiologic testing in patients with exertional symptoms. It helps to correlate the physiologic change occurring with exercise with the patient's complaints. While anatomic testing confers greater localization and anatomic information,

TABLE 17–3
CHRONIC LIMB ISCHEMIA

Grade	Category	Clinical Description	Objective Criteria
	0	Asymptomatic, no hemodynamically significant lesion	Normal treadmill[a]/stress test
I	1	Mild claudication	Treadmill completed, postexercise AP[b] >50 mm HG but >25 mm HG below normal
	2	Moderate claudication	Symptoms between Categories 1 and 3
	3	Severe claudication	Treadmill test cannot be completed; postexercise AP<50 mm HG
II	4	Ischemic rest pain	Resting AP< or = to 40 mm HG; flat or barely pulsatile metatarsal plethysmography, toe pressure <30 mm HG
III	5	Minor tissue loss, nonhealing ulcer, focal gangrene with diffuse pedal edema	Resting AP< or = to 60 mm HG; ankle or flat or metatarsal plethysmography flat or barely pulsatile, toe pressure <40 mm HG
	6	Major tissue loss, extending above transmetatarsal level, functional foot not salvageable	Same as for Category 5

[a]Treadmill at 2 mph with a 12% grade for 5 minutes
[b]AP = Ankle pressure

it provides little physiologic information. No exercise equivalent is present in anatomic testing. Physiologic testing is particularly suited for determining the presence of vascular disease and relating the disease to the patient's symptomatology. Physiologic testing is also much cheaper than anatomic alternatives. Anatomic testing is more suited to characterizing the disease and, therefore, may play a significant role in differentiating the patients who have lesions amenable to percutaneous therapy (62). In particular, MRA is well-suited for patients with diabetes and renal insufficiency where using noniodinated contrast will often provide the information needed to determine whether a percutaneous or surgical intervention is necessary. Frequently, a modified combination of the two modalities may be useful, such as a limited duplex examination to differentiate arterial occlusion from stenosis after physiologic testing. The authors prefer physiologic testing as the initial evaluation of a patient with suspected peripheral vascular disease. Therefore, anatomic testing is reserved as a complement to physiologic testing in a select group of patients.

PERCUTANEOUS REVASCULARIZATION TECHNIQUES

Patient Preparation and Imaging

After a complete clinical evaluation, those patients who are believed to be candidates for aortoiliac intervention should undergo a thorough diagnostic arteriographic examination. A complete study should include images of the abdominal aorta and iliac arteries. The images are examined carefully not only for stenotic disease but also for aneurysmal disease. Nonvisualization of lumbar arteries, even in the face of an apparently normal-caliber aorta, should raise suspicion about an underlying aneurysm. Oblique views of the aorta are important for imaging the renal ostium when renal artery stenosis is suspected in the face of systemic hypertension or renal insufficiency. Oblique imaging of the pelvis is mandatory for thorough elucidation of iliac and femoral arterial bifurcation lesions. In general, the contralateral oblique projection opens the iliac artery bifurcations, whereas the ipsilateral oblique projection is most useful for the femoral artery bifurcation. Finally, complete imaging of the infrainguinal runoff must be performed before any intervention. If the runoff is imaged only after an intervention is undertaken, then the etiology of a distal occlusion that may represent emboli rather than preexisting occlusive disease may be impossible to know. This is particularly important when, despite a successful aortoiliac intervention, the patient shows little improvement or perhaps worsens in vascular status. Thanks to advances in digital vascular imaging and contrast medium, extensive imaging of the runoff vessels is achievable with lower contrast volumes and, therefore, is less of a risk for renal damage. The use of carbon dioxide

(CO_2) as a contrast agent eliminates or significantly decreases the need for iodinated contrast, in particular with those patients who have compromised renal function or a history of significant contrast allergy (63–65). Gadolinium-based contrast agents may also be used as an alternative to iodine-based agents (66–68). Dose limitations of gadolinium must be considered. The maximum dose is 0.4 mmol/kg (approximately 60 cc) (63,69,70).

The prior noninvasive evaluation will help the interventionalist plan a treatment approach for the patient. Although some prefer to perform the diagnostic angiogram from the side of the suspected disease, thereby possibly obviating a second arteriotomy, this approach has two significant drawbacks. First, if an occlusion is encountered at the onset of the study, the diagnostic examination cannot be completed, and an intervention or a contralateral arteriotomy must first occur. The importance of performing a good angiogram, including the runoff, cannot be overstated. Second, a contralateral approach helps to avoid inadvertent occlusion of an iliac artery with a preexisting stenosis as a consequence of placing the diagnostic catheter through the stenotic region. When this happens unexpectedly and an occlusion is found, the site of stenosis may be difficult to determine, because it could be occurring anywhere from the arteriotomy site to the proximal end of the occlusion. This is especially true of distal external iliac and common femoral artery stenoses (Figure 17–3). In cases of severe bilateral disease, alternative approaches should be considered, including radial, brachial, axillary, and venous digital subtraction angiography. Translumbar approach is rarely done.

Hemodynamic assessment of the aortoiliac segment is crucial in the determination of the significance of morphological disease. Although a lesion is identified angiographically, determining whether that lesion is the source of the patient's symptoms is difficult. Intra-arterial pressure measurements through the aortoiliac segment can quantify the hemodynamic effect of a lesion. Occasionally, intra-arterial pressure monitoring may uncover a lesion at which none was suspected. It is reasonable to judge the significance of an arterial stenosis based on the degree of narrowing it produces. The decision to initiate treatment, however, should be based on the likelihood of that lesion contributing to the patient's clinical symptoms. Contrast angiography is limited in providing any information about the functional significance of a stenosis; therefore, pressure measurements are used as a direct indicator of hemodynamic effect of a stenosis (71,72).

It is commonly accepted that a mean pressure gradient of >5 mm Hg is abnormal; corresponding to a systolic pressure gradient of 10–15 mm Hg. In the absence of a resting gradient, intra-arterial administration of nitroglycerine (100–200 µg), tolazine (25–40 mg) or papaverine (15–30 mg) given distal to the runoff of the extremity in question may reveal the significance of a lesion. The vasodilation produced in the distal vascular beds imitates the arterial demand of exercise (73,74). An augmented gradient of

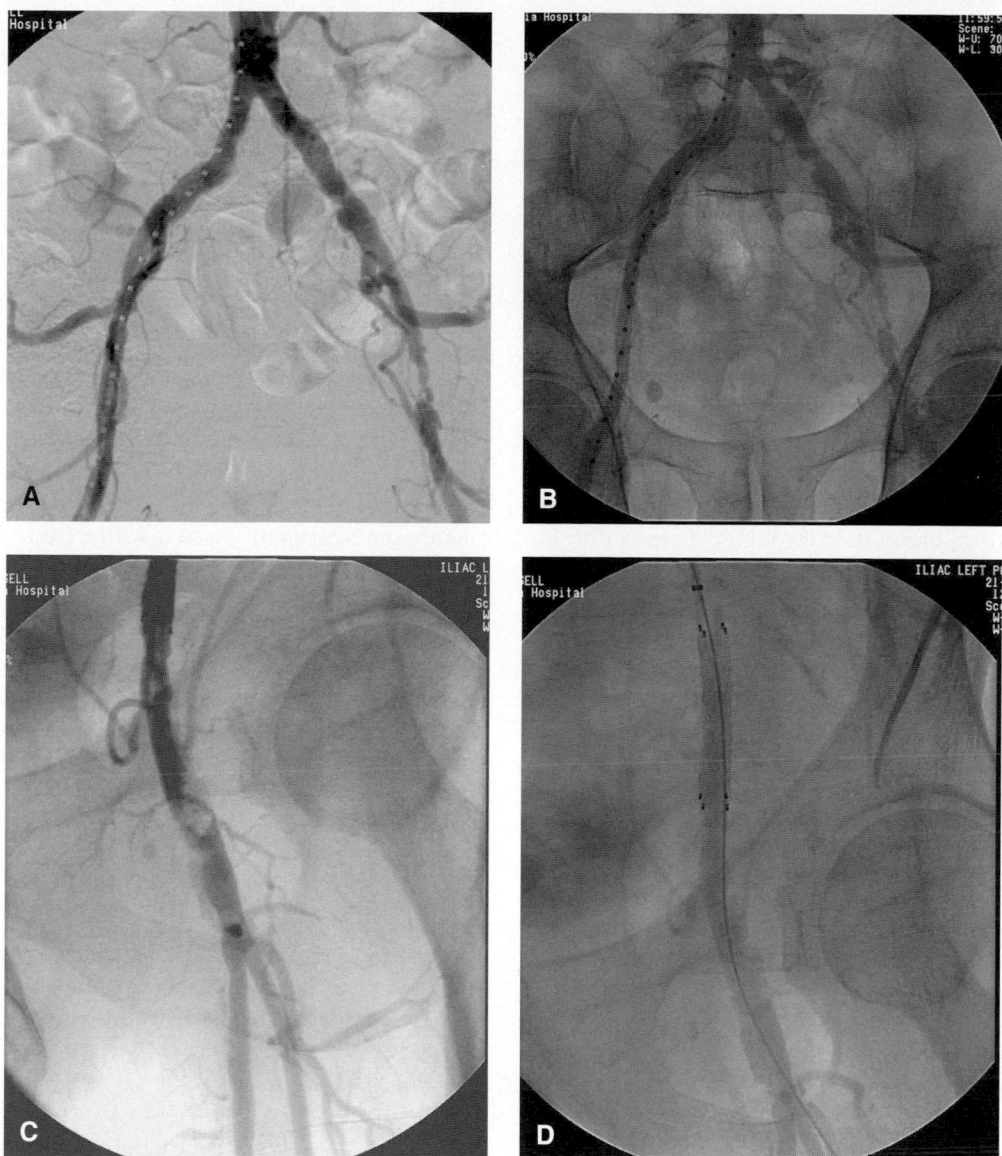

Figure 17–3   This is a 58-year-old male with severe Lt. hip and thigh claudication. On PE, the Lt. pulse is barely palpable. The Rt. CFA was selected for puncture. **A., B.** Arteriography shows critical stenosis and severe ulcerated plaque in the Lt EIA. If the symptomatic side was selected for access, then (i) the angiogram could not be done, (ii) risk of inadvertent occlusion from the catheter, and (iii) treatment could not be performed from this ipsilateral side. **C., D.** The EIA lesion treated with a SES. The CFA stenosis was dilated across the bifurcation to 7 mm with good angiographic and hemodynamic results.

greater than 8–10 mm Hg is generally considered hemodynamically significant. Repeat measurements after interventions, such as PTA, help to decide the technical success of the procedure; or conversely, to pinpoint those areas in which a significant, flow-limiting lesion remains that may necessitate further intervention (75,76).

Despite their usefulness in evaluating stenotic disease, gradients must be evaluated with the entire angiographic and clinical picture in mind. Creation of a gradient requires outflow down from the lesion. When there is no outflow, no gradient can be measured—although there may be severe inflow stenosis (77). This fact becomes extremely important in multilevel disease in which correction of outflow obstruction is being considered. For example, if one relies solely on the hemodynamic data and fails to correct obvious inflow disease before treating the outflow disease, then a distal graft may be compromised because patency of the graft is extremely dependent on adequate inflow.

Many pharmacologic agents are now available to help interventionalists perform revascularization procedures with fewer complications. Recent advances in antiplatelet therapy have permitted more high-risk interventions to be performed successfully. Although aspirin has been the mainstay of antiplatelet therapy for several decades, it is now recognized to be a relatively weak inhibitor of platelets. The discovery of the platelet glycoprotein IIb/IIIa receptor led to development (invention) of new antiplatelet drugs that bond with the glycoprotein receptor, which is critical for platelet aggregation. The three most extensively evaluated drugs are eptifibatide (Integrelin), tirofiban (Aggrastat) and abciximab (ReoPro). Clopidogrel (Plavix), an oral agent, has now become the mainstay therapy for PVD patients (19,78–81). The decision to use anticoagulants during a procedure depends on the complexity of the procedure, including the general blood flow through the vessel during the procedure, the length of time a vessel is expected to be occluded, and the thrombogenicity of the device being used. Heparin is given frequently as a bolus (50–100 u/kg) during aortoiliac stent procedures in order to limit acute thrombosis. This is especially important when the intervention is performed through an ipsilateral femoral sheath because the sheath itself may obstruct outflow through the common femoral artery, potentially promoting stenosis and inciting thrombosis. Angiomax (Bivalirudin) is a direct thrombin inhibitor used instead of heparin for prompt anticoagulation effect and does not require titration to a desired activated clotted time (ACT) (82,83). For most routine aortoiliac interventions, many of the previously mentioned drugs are omitted. Although the routine use of IIb/IIIa inhibitors and new classes of low molecular-weight heparin has resulted in major advances for the coronary circulation, this has not translated to the same benefit in the aortoiliac segment where the cost and potential bleeding complications may not justify their routine use.

Patient Selection

Options available for the treatment of aortoiliac disease include surgical revascularization, percutaneous intervention, and conservative management. When one is contemplating treatment, several factors must be considered. Foremost among them are the severity of the ischemia and its effect on the patient. Mild symptoms of claudication that are not lifestyle limiting do not require aggressive intervention. Alternatively, conservative management with appropriate follow-up is warranted (84–86). Frequently, the last options of conservative management are forgotten even though most patients will improve with a graded exercise program and nicotine abstinence. Accordingly, every patient presenting with symptoms of intermittent claudication deserves a trial of "conservative management" before more invasive therapies are considered. This management must be properly monitored and tailored to the needs of the individual patient and have a mechanism of review of

no less than three months (85). For more severe ischemic presentations, such as rest pain or tissue loss (or in patients with rapidly progressive symptoms), this may not be an option. Patients with lifestyle limiting claudication and who have failed an adequate trial of conservative management may be candidates for percutaneous intervention. Traditionally, these patients have not been candidates for surgical intervention until the limitation has become disabling or a threatened limb is present. In conjunction with the severity of ischemia, the overall health of the patient must be examined. The risks of any intervention must be weighed against potential benefits. Percutaneous procedures, in general, have a lower rate of morbidity and mortality when compared to their corresponding surgical options. As the morbidity and mortality of the procedure increases, so should the severity of the disease that would justify the treatment. Subsequently, it may be appropriate to perform an iliac PTA on a patient who may not be a candidate for a surgical bypass. However, the rare complication of a percutaneous procedure can occur, requiring a surgical procedure that would put the patient at increased risk. No matter how routine, every procedure should be taken seriously with respect to its possible consequences.

When a percutaneous intervention is being considered, the anticipated immediate technical and long-term clinical success should be weighed against the risks and the expected results with surgical revascularization. The morphology of the patient's disease plays a major role in determining these outcomes (87).

A list of factors influencing the outcome of aortoiliac PTA and stenting is included in Table 17–4.

The anatomic distribution of atherosclerosis follows three distinct patterns: (87)

Type 1—Patients with arterial disease limited to the distal abdominal aorta and CIA with good runoff

Type 2—Patients with arterial disease involving the EIA with good runoff

Type 3—Patients with arterial disease extending to the femoral, popliteal, and two or three calf arteries

The common theme is that the more extensive the disease, whether in the treated vessel or the runoff vessels, the worse the outcome (87–90). Also, larger vessels tend to do better than smaller vessels. Many additional factors are also pertinent and interwoven with the extent of the disease (88–95). In general, patients who are sent for intervention with limb salvage as the indication have more diffuse and extensive atherosclerotic disease than those who are intermittent claudicants. Patients with diabetes do worse as a group than those without diabetes (22,96). Even though patients who continue to smoke are generally believed to have a poorer long-term patency rate than those who abstain from tobacco use, little published evidence supports this idea.

The Society of Interventional Radiology (SIR) publishes guidelines for PTA in the aorta (Table 17–5) and iliac arteries (Table 17–6) based on morphologic characteristics of the

TABLE 17–4

FACTORS INFLUENCING INTERVENTIONAL OUTCOMES

Predictive Factors/ Indication	Worse Outcome/Limb Salvage or Tissue Loss	Better Outcome/ Claudication
Site	Distal (external iliac artery)	Proximal (common iliac artery)
Gender	Female	Male
Number of Lesions	Multiple	Single
Lesion Type	Long occlusion, eccentric, calcified	Short stenosis, concentric, noncalcified
Runoff	Diseased	Intact
Diabetes	Present	Absent
Smoking	Yes	No

plaque as well as coexisting disease (97). With each category, suggested treatment is proposed based on the clinical situation and assumed results. The Joint Council of the American Heart Association for iliac interventions (98) and the TASC Working Group (92) have established similar guidelines.

The guidelines propose PTA as the treatment of choice for short focal stenoses. Conversely, in patients with diffuse disease, including long chronic occlusions, PTA has a very limited role. Worth noting is the fact that the recommendations for each category are meant to serve only as a guideline when an intervention is being contemplated. In every case, the patient's entire clinical picture must be assessed and the potential risks versus expected benefits, as well as the alternatives, must be weighed.

Lifestyle limiting claudication is the most common clinical indication for aortoiliac PTA, including categories 1–3 of chronic limb ischemia (Table 17–3). These categories encompass patients with mild claudication to patients with severe disabling pain. Of course, this assessment must be made on an individual basis. For instance, a very active person wishing to play tennis or golf will be limited with much milder disease than will a more sedentary person needing to ambulate only one or two blocks to accomplish his or her routine. Once a regular exercise program is implemented, including reduction of risk factors such as

smoking, and significant limitations remain, both patients may be candidates for percutaneous revascularization.

Patients with categories 4–6 disease (Table 17–3), indicating more severe ischemia of pain at rest and tissue loss, normally will not be able to endure a prolonged trial of conservative management, especially when a suitable alternative intervention is available. Frequently, this category includes patients with extensive disease who are less than optimal candidates for PTA. Unfortunately, anatomic factors and coexisting risk factors frequently make them poor surgical candidates as well. In these cases, the lower morbidity and mortality of a percutaneous revascularization may warrant an attempt, especially because a failed percutaneous procedure does not preclude the surgical alternative; whereas, a failed surgical procedure generally makes any further intervention nearly impossible.

Patients with multilevel disease involving both inflow and outflow obstruction may often benefit from a combined surgical and percutaneous approach. This usually involves PTA and stenting of an iliac stenosis before femoropopliteal bypass (99–101). Stenting of an iliac stenosis in a patient with a contralateral iliac occlusion may also be performed prior to a femorofemoral bypass (102,103) in patients who are not candidates for aortobifemoral or aortoiliac bypass (Figure 17–4).

TABLE 17–5

AORTIC LESION CLASSIFICATION

Category	Description	Guideline for Rx
1	Stenoses <3 cm in length, concentric, noncalcified	PTA is treatment of choice.
2	Stenoses 3–5 cm in length, concentric, noncalcified; stenoses <3 cm, eccentric, calcified	PTA well-suited; includes lesions followed by distal bypass
3	Stenoses 5–10 cm, chronic occlusions <5 cm	Amenable to PTA; moderate chance of success vs. surgery; PTA may be performed in patients with high surgical risk or lack of surgical material
4	Stenoses greater than 10 cm, chronic occlusions >5 cm after thrombolysis; extensive bilateral aortoiliac disease; iliac stenosis associated with aneurysms or other lesions requiring surgery	PTA has a limited role; low technical success; poor long-term benefit; PTA only when no surgical options or in very high risk patients

TABLE 17-6

ILIAC LESION CLASSIFICATION

Category	Description	Guidelines for Rx
1	Stenoses <3 cm in length, concentric, noncalcified	PTA is treatment of choice.
2	Stenoses 3–5 cm in length, concentric, noncalcified; stenoses <3 cm, eccentric, calcified	PTA well-suited; includes lesions followed by distal bypass
3	Stenoses 5–10 cm, chronic occlusions <5 cm	Amenable to PTA; moderate chance of success vs. surgery; PTA may be performed in patients with high surgical risk or lack of surgical material.
4	Stenoses greater than 10 cm chronic occlusions >5 cm after thrombolysis; extensive bilateral aortoiliac disease; iliac stenosis associated with aneurysms or other lesions requiring surgery	PTA has a limited role; low technical success; poor long-term benefit; PTA only when no surgical options or in very high-risk patients

Aortoiliac lesions presenting with distal emboli as seen in blue toe syndrome were first assessed as contraindications to percutaneous intervention. However, these lesions have been treated successfully with PTA and stenting without a significant incidence of intraprocedural embolization (104,105). Angioplasty and stenting generally result in cessation of embolic events from the lesion (probably secondary to some remodeling of the ulcerated lesion), changes in hemodynamic patterns within the stenosis, or both. Occasionally, a high-grade stenosis may be associated with thrombus. If this is suspected during angiography, then thrombolysis should be done before dilation to avoid intraprocedural embolization.

Impotence is quickly becoming an indication for aortoiliac intervention. Many causes of impotence exist, including arterial insufficiency, venous incompetence, and neurogenic etiologies. A noninvasive vascular study of penile blood flow is useful before angiographic evaluation. Because supply to the cavernosal arteries is bilateral, either aortic or bilateral iliac disease must be present to produce impotence. A concurrent history of bilateral claudication, particularly when it involves the thigh, buttocks, or both, is a strong indicator of proximal disease. Disease of the aorta, common iliac arteries, the proximal segments of the hypogastric arteries, or all three may be amenable to percutaneous techniques with good long-term patency rates associated with larger vessels

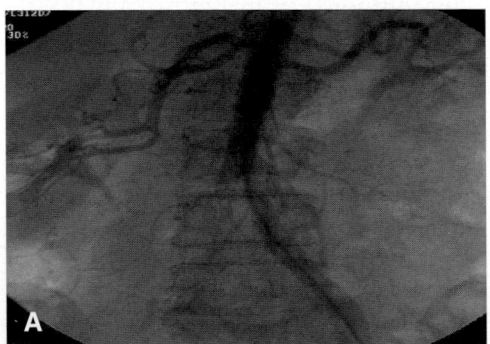
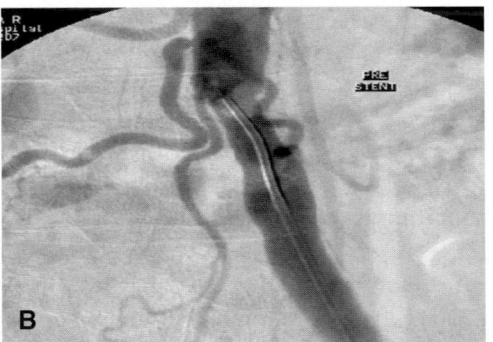
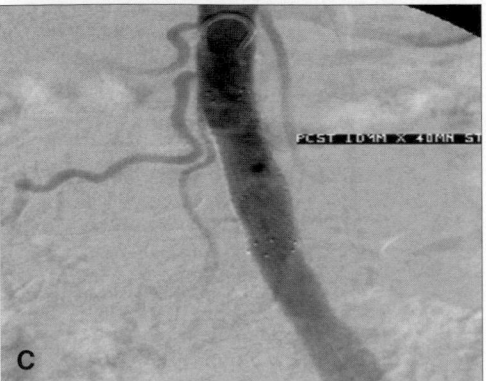

Figure 17-4   A. This is an 88-year-old male with recent MI (EF 20%) and left foot gangrene. Aortogram demostrates occlusion of Rt. CIA and critical stenosis of Lt. CIA. Despite multiple attempts at crossing the Rt. CIA occlusion from an antegrade and retrograde approach, it was not successful. The patient is considered a high surgical risk for aortofemoral bypass. **B.** Magnified view of the aortic bifurcation showing calcified plaque at the ostium of the Lt. CIA and occlusion of Rt. CIA. **C.** An SES was placed to treat the Lt. iliac inflow before bilateral amputations and fem-fem bypass.

(Figure 17–5) (106). A steal phenomenon secondary to an external iliac artery has been reported as a rare cause of impotence (107). In these cases, a history of activity is related to impotence. In most cases, however, arteriosclerotic disease is the culprit, and particularly with concurrent diabetes, the disease is concentrated in a smaller distal branch of the internal iliac artery with little benefit to either surgical or percutaneous revascularization.

Aortoiliac Angioplasty

Increasingly, endovascular techniques are being accepted as the initial treatment of choice for most diseases of the abdominal aorta. Angioplasty of the aorta has been used successfully for several decades to treat stenotic disease of the aorta and its bifurcation. Focal disease of <2 cm (Category 1 in Table 17–6) have been treated successfully with PTA alone (106,108,109). The technical success rate is greater than 90% with low recurrence rates (109). Treatment of lesions greater than 4 cm has been reported in a small number of patients.

Although the technique of balloon angioplasty has been described thoroughly in the literature, aspects of particular importance in aortoiliac disease are addressed in this chapter. The value of adequate patient preparation cannot be overestimated, including informed consent, which is mandatory before any form of intervention may be undertaken.

Historically, an ipsilateral retrograde approach has been preferred for iliac angioplasty (Figure 17–6). Its greatest advantage is that of excellent catheter and guide wire control during the procedure. This approach is also advantageous for recanalization of an obstructed iliac artery and allows for precise stent placement in the iliac segment, especially the common iliac artery ostium. Additionally, the treated region can be imaged through the angioplasty catheter without excessive manipulation or withdrawal of the catheter across the lesion. Ideally, a single access for interventional procedures is preferred because most complications are related to access sites that can be reduced when a single site is used (87). Unfortunately, most significant iliac artery disease is bilateral, and in up to one third of patients, plaque involves the terminal aorta or common iliac artery ostium, therefore making it necessary to perform bilateral femoral punctures in order to stent the contralateral common iliac artery to preserve the ostium. PTA has been performed from a contralateral approach without significant increase in complications (110,111). Patients with less acute angulation of the aortic bifurcation and less tortuosity of the iliac arteries are best-suited for this approach. Approximately two thirds of patients with aortoiliac disease will have occlusive or stenotic disease of the external iliac artery segment. This is best treated from a contralateral approach especially when the lesion is near the inguinal ligament (111). A brachial or axillary approach is rarely necessary, and because of the course of the vessel, there is less

mechanical control over the catheter and guide wires. The choice of angioplasty balloon diameter is important in order to obtain optimal results and yet avoid arterial rupture, which can be catastrophic. Many interventionalists consider slight overdilatation of the vessel necessary. When stent placement is expected, pre-stent angioplasty is not necessary because it is associated with more complications (112). It is somewhat controversial on the treatment of a focal, noncalcified, concentric iliac stenosis. For Category 1 lesions, most interventionalists would perform balloon angioplasty by itself and only stent when an unsatisfactory result is present. It is generally accepted that all other aortoiliac lesions would be treated with stent placement with PTA at the same time or after stent deployment.

Stenting

Intravascular stents have expanded the indicators for percutaneous treatment of aortoiliac disease. Treatment of longer stenoses and occlusions is possible where PTA alone has a low likelihood of long-term success. Both balloon and self-expandable stents have been placed in the iliac artery system. Stents are not only placed in native vessels but also in bypass grafts (Figure 17–7). Regardless of the type of stent selected, the goal is to cover all hemodynamically significant stenoses and preserve nondiseased segments. Precise stent positioning can be achieved when meticulous technique is followed. Using flourofade and digital roadmapping can ensure accurate stent positioning. The most reliable way to guarantee stent positioning is to perform real-time angiography by injecting contrast through the introducer sheath.

Aortic Stenting

The use of stents in the aorta was a natural progression from their initial application in the iliac arteries. The techniques surrounding endovascular placement of stents are well-known to interventionalists. Several technical aspects should be considered to achieve the best results. Intra-aortic stenting can be more challenging than when done in the iliac artery.

Disease of the aortic bifurcation can arise from the distal aorta, common iliac arteries, or both. If the stenosis is predominantly in the terminal aorta and extends into the common iliac ostium, then placement of simultaneous balloon-expandable stents, or "kissing stents," into each common iliac artery and extending into the aorta is preferred (113–120). Aortic stents are usually dilated to 10–15 mm. If the decision is made to place a stent in the terminal aorta, then it is important to consider the location of the origin of the inferior mesenteric artery before deployment. Equally important is the location of the stent distally. This is especially true when a single stent of the distal aorta is being placed. The interventionalist must ensure that the stent does not cover the ostium of the contralateral iliac artery.

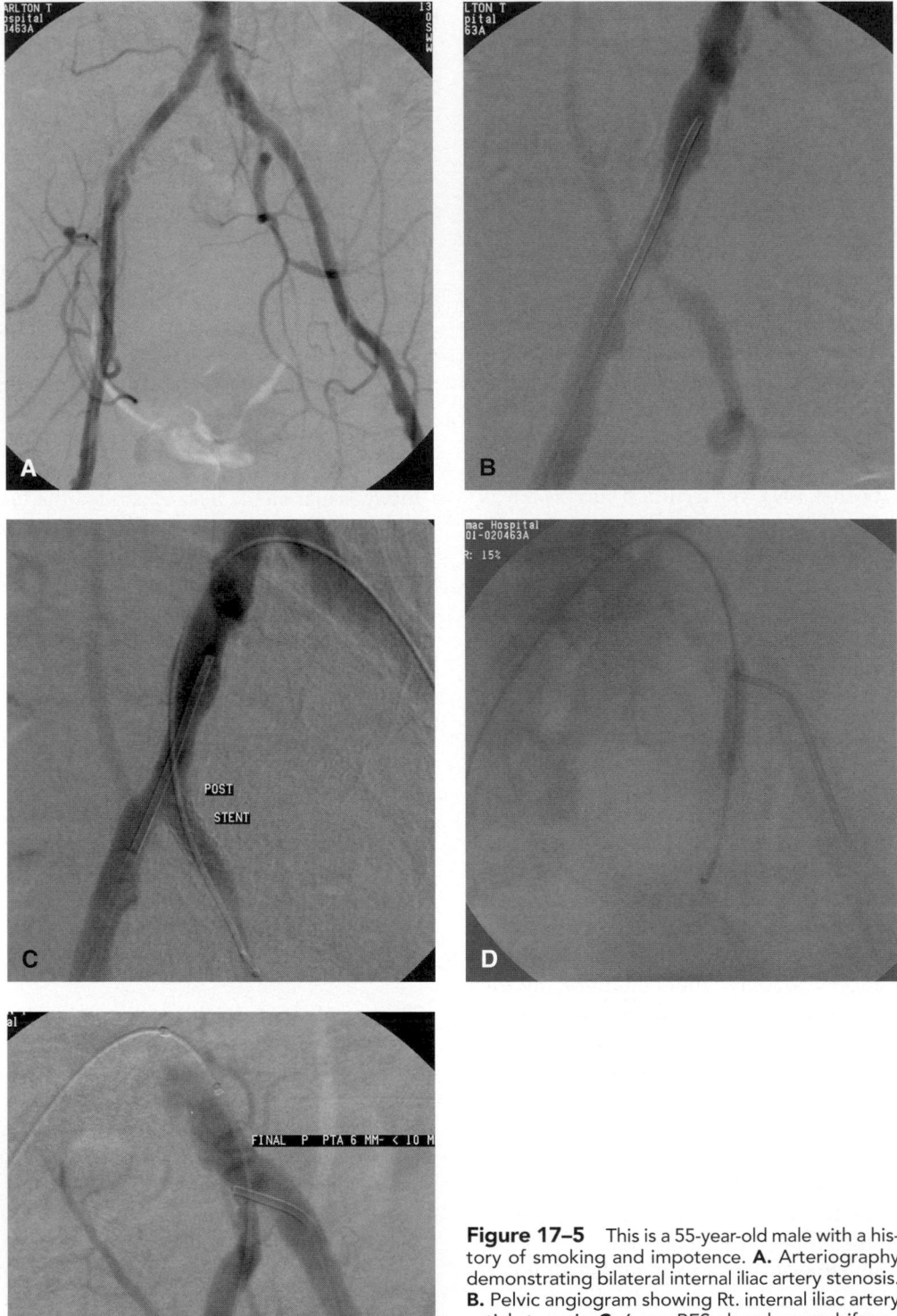

Figure 17–5 This is a 55-year-old male with a history of smoking and impotence. **A.** Arteriography demonstrating bilateral internal iliac artery stenosis. **B.** Pelvic angiogram showing Rt. internal iliac artery ostial stenosis. **C.** 6 mm BES placed across bifurcation into origin with good result. **D., E.** The Lt. internal iliac artery was dilated with a 6 mm balloon with satisfactory angiographic results and <10 mm Hg gradient after NTG. The patient recovered, and his erectile dysfunction resolved. He remains asymptomatic.

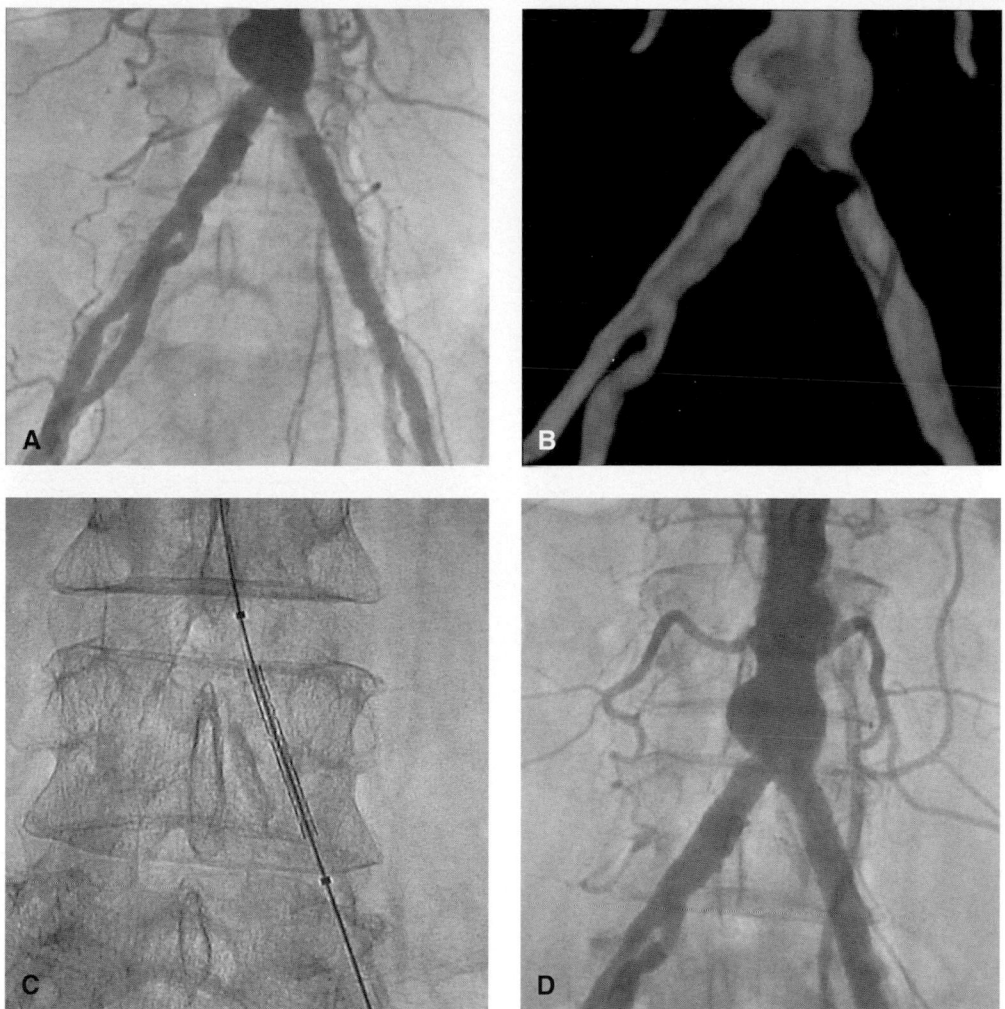

Figure 17–6   This is a 48-year-old runner with limiting Lt. thigh claudication. He is hypertensive and hyperlipidemic and is a former two-pack-a-day smoker. Doppler waveform analysis suggested Lt iliac disease, therefore, the Lt CFA was used for access. **A.** Pelvic angiogram showing eccentric stenosis of CIA. A small AAA is also seen. **B.** 3D rotational angiography better at defining the degree of narrowing. **C., D.** Primary stenting was done using a BES from an ipsilateral approach with excellent angiographic and hemodynamic results. The patient recovered and was back to full activity in 2 weeks.

The length of the stent chosen must completely cover the entire lesion. Good stent-wall opposition is important. It is sometimes necessary to use two simultaneous inflated smaller balloons to gain full expansion of the stent to the vessel wall. This is especially difficult in the heavily calcified distal aorta. Choices of stents include balloon-expandable and self-expandable stents, and each has its own characteristics, advantages, and disadvantages. Takayasu's aortitis is an uncommon cause of aortic stenosis but can be treated successfully with PTA and stenting (121–123). Most physicians agree that interventions should only be done during the quiescent phase of the disease.

Acute Aortic Occlusion

Acute aortic occlusion is seen infrequently. Patients may present with bilateral ischemic limbs, abdominal symptoms, paralysis, and acute hypertension (124–126). Although this clinical scenario can be caused by embolic occlusion (127), more often than not, a preexisting atherosclerotic lesion combined with a low flow state produces acute aortic occlusion (128). Hypercoagulable diseases from various etiologies are associated with abdominal aortic thrombosis (124,125). Urgent revascularization is needed in these cases. Surgical management with thromboembolectomy, aortofemoral

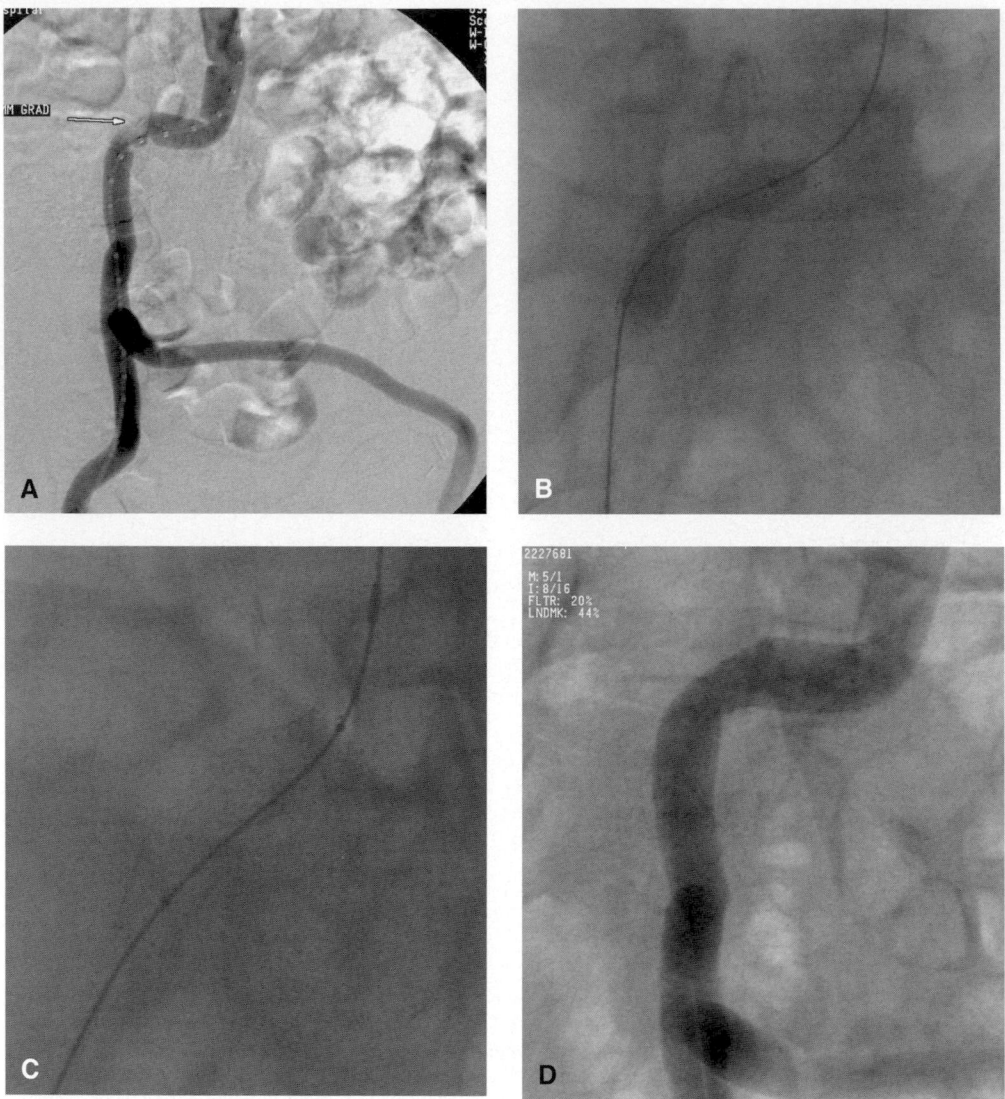

Figure 17–7 This is a 74-year-old male with multiple medical problems and PVD. He underwent Rt. axillo-femorofemoral bypass graft for occlusive aortoiliac disease. One year later, his symptoms of Rt. thigh and leg claudication returned. **A.** Angiogram demonstrating a kink in the graft with a significant pressure gradient. **B.** Avoided surgical revision of the graft by placing an SES. **C., D.** Demonstrate full expansion of the stent. The stenosis resolved with no remaining gradient. The patient was doing well 2 years later.

bypass, or extra-anatomic bypass (axillofemoral) is still the most commonly used method of treatment. Immediate anticoagulation and measures to improve poor cardiac output can change morbidity and mortality outcomes. It is well-recognized that percutaneous management consisting of pharmacological thrombolytic therapy and mechanical thrombectomy followed by stent placement has a lower mortality rate than operative therapy in this high-risk group of patients (Figure 17–8) (129,130). Abdominal aortic aneurysm thrombosis is a rare cause of acute aortic occlusion (131,132). These patients rival aortic rupture as a vascular

emergency, and immediate intervention surgically or percutaneously must be undertaken.

Iliac Stenting

Endovascular stenting of the iliac arteries has become a widely accepted interventional technique with excellent results and limited complications (1–3,8–13,133–135). In 1991, the U.S. Food and Drug Administration (FDA) approved the stents for use in iliac arteries in the United States. The FDA has defined the indication for iliac artery

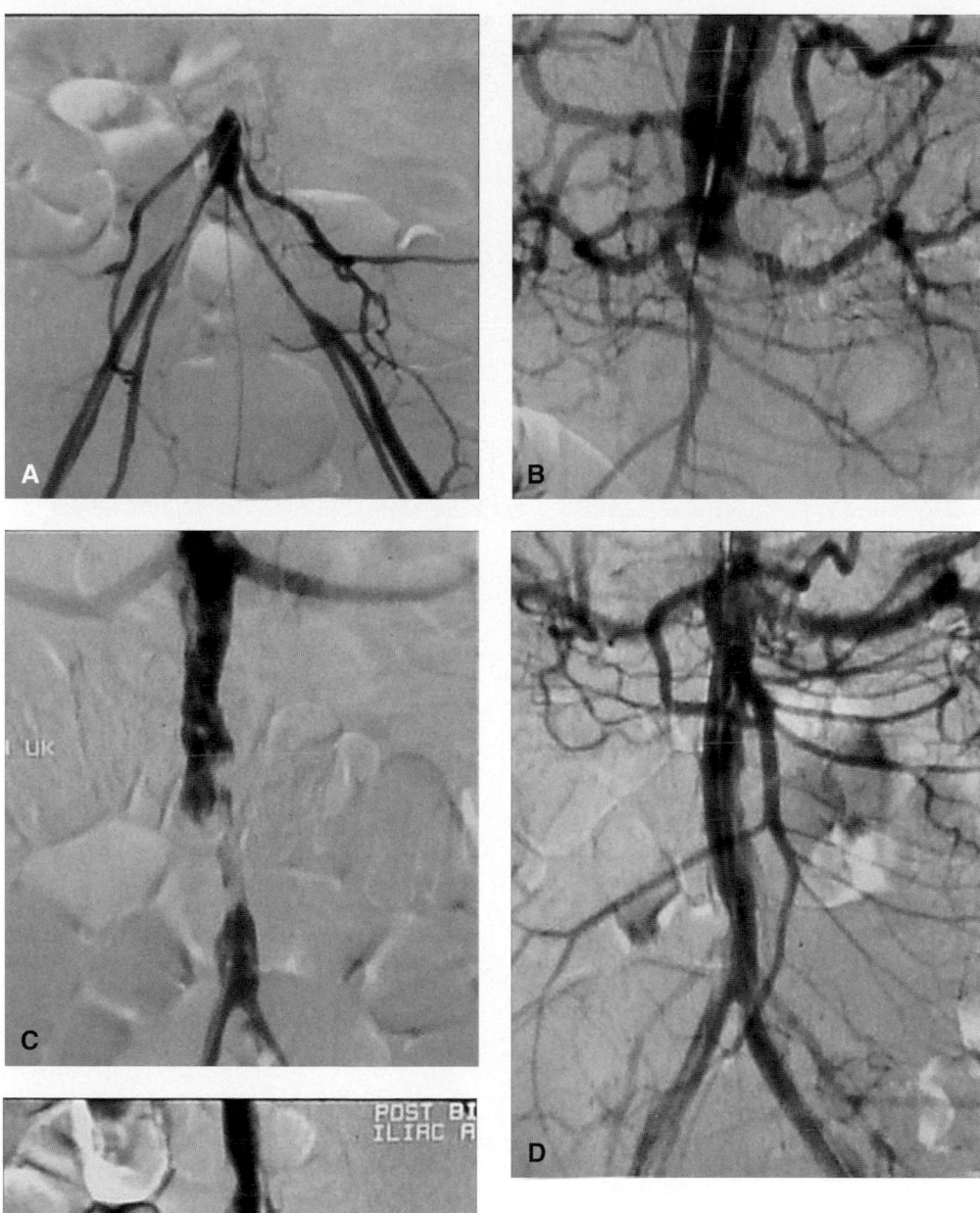

Figure 17–8   While attempting access for a cardiac catheterization, this distal aortic occlusion was encountered. **A.** The patient was transferred from an outside institution with new onset cold and painful legs after a massive MI. He had a long history of bilateral claudication and blue toes. On PE, the femoral pulses were diminished. **B.** Aortography from the Lt. axillary approach confirming distal aortic occlusion. The renals and mesenteric arteries are patent. A guide wire passed easily through the occlusion, and catheter thrombolysis was initiated. **C.** Following 18 hours of lysis, flow was established and an underlying critical stenosis was uncovered. **D.** Following angioplasty and stenting, complete restoration of flow was experienced. **E.** The iliac arteries were treated with PTA. The patient underwent bilateral BKAs for embolic disease to his calf vessels and was discharged from the hospital after 1 month.

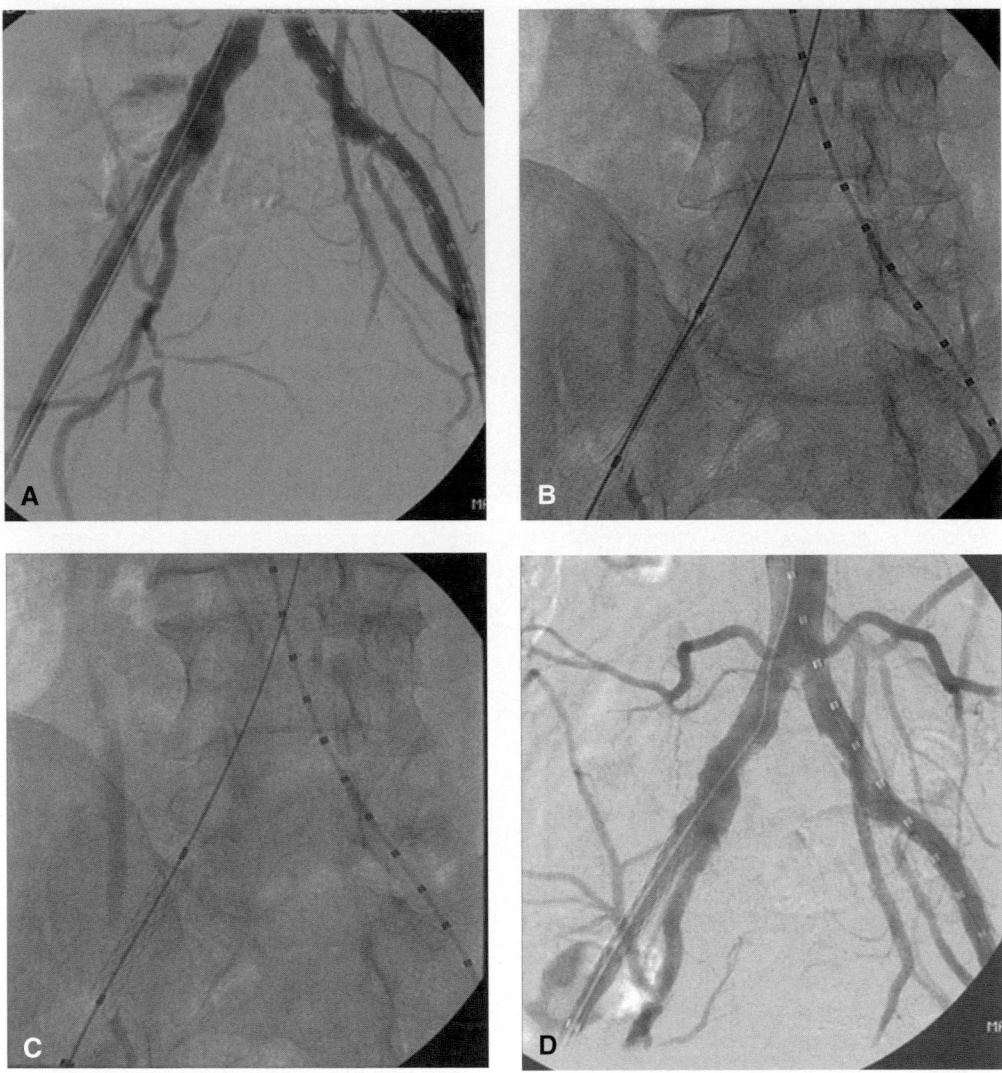

Figure 17–9   This is a 66-year-old with stenotic disease of the Rt. EIA. PTA was done to 8 mm. **A.** Post-PTA angiogram reveals focal hemodynamically significant dissection flap. **B.** Balloon-expandable stent position over the injured area. **C.** Fully expanded BES. **D.** Final angiogram showing coverage of flap and excellent flow through stent.

stenting to be a suboptimal result of PTA caused by dissection (Figure 17–9) or residual pressure gradient, total occlusions, and recurrence of PTA. It is well-known that in clinical practice, primary stenting prior to PTA is often performed with controversial scientific data (8,9,13,136–138).

The Palmaz 308 (Cordis) stent was the first to receive FDA approval for use in the iliac arteries. The Wallstent (Boston Scientific) and the SMART stent (Cordis) are also FDA approved for iliac artery use. Most stents then are used "off label" for treating iliac arterial disease.

Lesions involving the origins of both iliac arteries usually require simultaneous inflation and stenting, referred to as the "kissing balloon" or "kissing stenting" technique (Figure 17–10) (113–118). This provides larger dilatation of the distal aorta, which is frequently diseased, and it avoids the shifting of bifurcation plaque from one side to the other. Unilateral common iliac artery stenosis, when present, can be managed with unilateral stent placement. However, in many of these patients, kissing bilateral stents are placed in order to reduce the chance of plaque being dislodged into the more normal side (118). Additionally, stenting the patient's contralateral common iliac artery prevents the stent placed in the occluded or stenotic iliac artery from covering the ostium of the artery.

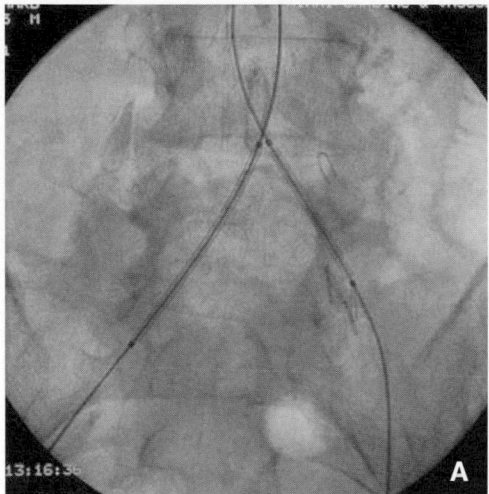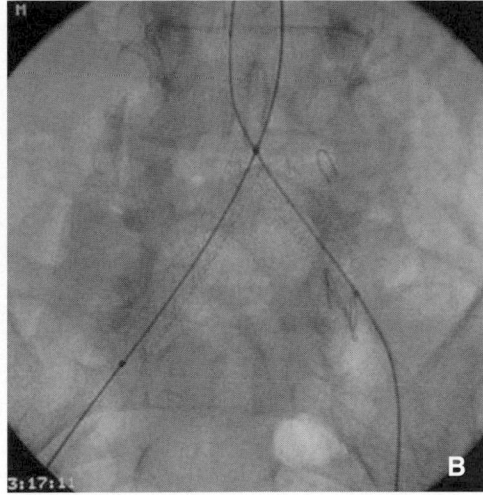

Figure 17–10 **A., B.** Spot radiograph of "kissing stents" in CIAs predeployment and post-deployment.

Significant overdilation of any artery usually results in pronounced discomfort to the patient. Patients should, therefore, be monitored for pain related to the balloon inflation; when excessive, the balloon size should be decreased. Documentation of the results of PTA and stenting should include angiographic and intra-arterial hemodynamic evaluation, discussed earlier in the chapter.

Thrombolysis

Catheter-directed thrombolysis has been widely used for the treatment of occluded arteries and grafts (139–145). In addition to acute occlusive disease, chronic occlusions have been treated successfully with this technique. Deciding whether an occlusion is chronic or acute can be puzzling. The symptoms of chronic severe stenosis progressing to acute occlusion may be indistinguishable for most patients. If the occlusion exceeds three months, then primary recanalization followed by stenting may be acceptable (Figure 17–11). If the guide wire passes relatively smoothly through the occlusion, then this suggests that soft thrombosis is present (8,135). Thrombolysis prior to any other intervention is then indicated in order to avoid distal embolization. If guide wire crossing is difficult, then the occlusion may be chronic and no acute thrombosis is present. Lysis in this group of patients offers little benefit.

Once the occluded segment is traversed with a catheter and guide wire, an infusion system for lysis is positioned in the occluded segment. Placement from the contralateral approach is preferred, however, ipsilateral lysis is acceptable if the occluded segment cannot be crossed except from the ipsilateral side. A single multi–side-hole catheter is usually adequate to infuse the entire length of occlusion. The most proximal side hole is placed at the proximal edge of the thrombus. It is important that the infusion catheter stay within the thrombus enabling the lytic agent to bathe the entire thrombus burden without being occlusive. Although fibrinolysis is not perfect, there are guidelines for therapy. Three agents have been used for peripheral fibrinolysis: activase (t-PA) (Alteplase, Genentech), reteplase (r-PA) (Retavase, Centocor), and urokinase (Abbokinase, Abbott Laboratories), all of which have been used with good success (145). TNKase is a bioengineered variant of t-PA that is also used extensively in the peripheral arterial-venous thromboses. The commonly accepted dose of t-PA is 0.25–0.5 mg/hr or TNKase of 0.25–0.5 mg/hr or UK in doses ranging from 60,000–250,000 IV/hr. The use of concomitant anticoagulation with heparin during fibrinolysis is controversial. Contemporary practices prefer "low dose" (100 u–500 u/hr) heparin infused through the sheath in order to limit pericatheter thrombosis. After removal of the thrombus, the underlying offending atherosclerotic lesion can be evaluated and treated appropriately, usually with PTA and stent. On rare occasions, an occlusion is caused by an embolus, and after thrombolysis, no underlying lesion is identified and a widely patent vessel is restored (Figure 17–12).

Chronic Total Occlusion/Subintimal Revascularization

Although significant advances have been made in mechanical thrombectomy, thrombolysis, lasers, and many elaborate and intricate tools, recanalization of chronic iliac occlusions remains a challenge (146–151). It is often very difficult to find the inner lumen. The liberal use of hydrophilic wires has greatly expedited the success in crossing chronic occlusions

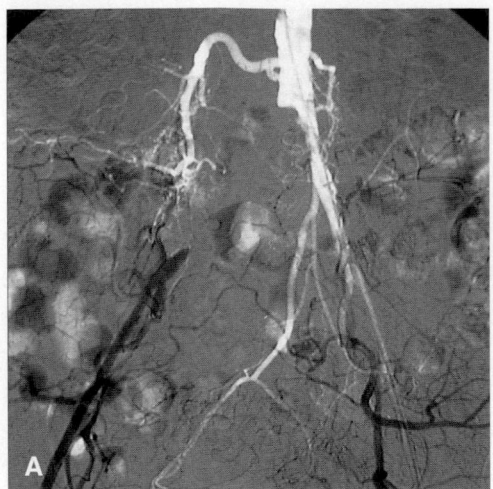

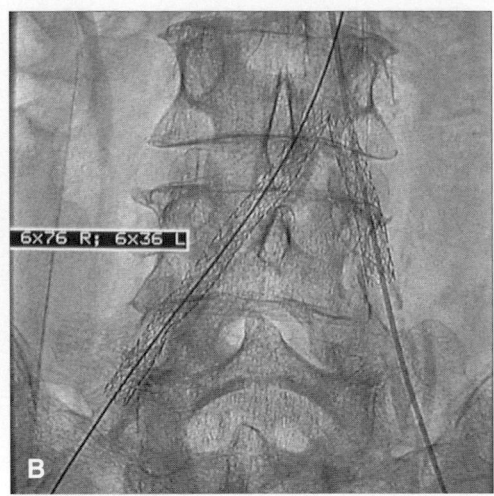

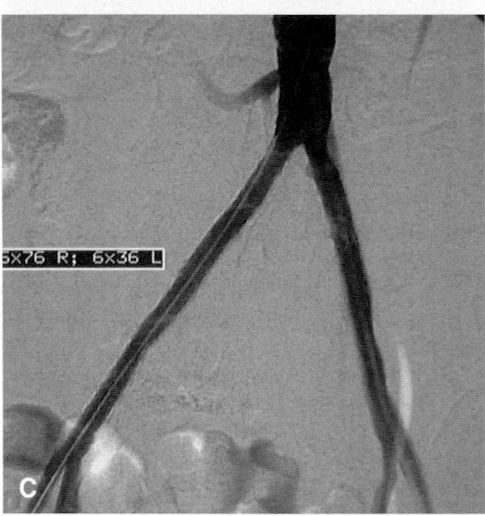

Figure 17–11   A. Diagnostic pelvic angiogram in a patient with chronic occlusion and extensive iliac disease. Without prior diagnostic arteriography from an alternate approach, assessment was difficult as to whether the occlusion at the left iliofemoral junction was preexistent or caused by the catheter placement. **B., C.** Following guide wire recanalization, bilateral "kissing stents" were placed with excellent angiographic results. There was severe spasm of the Lt. iliofemoral junction that was treated successfully with intra-arterial nitroglycerin.

with technical success rates of 81–95% (8). Whenever a subintimal tract is created, establishing reentry into the true lumen can be complicated. The subintimal position of the guide wire is suggested by a large J-configuration of the wire or the spiral course of the wire. The wire is usually navigated with little resistance, and contrast injections demonstrate a crescent-shaped collection in place. Intentional subintimal recanalization is relatively new (152). Worth noting is that the entry point in the subintimal space must be within the occluded segment of the artery and that the true lumen be entered immediately above and below the occlusion. As long as the guide wire finds the true lumen above and below the obstruction, then reconstruction with stents can be done with excellent angiographic, hemodynamic, and clinical results (Figure 17–13). Many published techniques exist to expedite free passage into the true lumen. The combined antegrade-retrograde technique with snaring of the guide wire is the most common (153). A more aggressive

technique using a curved needle to puncture the true lumen blindly has been described (154). The introduction of ultrasound, image-guided, needle puncture (CrossPoint catheter, Medtronic) has provided unprecedented access to treating occluded segments that otherwise would have needed open surgical repair (155,156). Rarely, surgical consultation or surgical vessel repair may become necessary when a flow-limiting dissection plane propagates into the common femoral artery.

Complications related to fatal perforation of the iliac artery have been reported, but they are rare. These injuries can be treated successfully with prolonged balloon inflation (157), additional bare metallic stent placement, or covered stent (1,112).

Distal embolization is a more common problem, and no technique can completely eliminate this difficulty. However, primary stenting will decrease the risk in all patients. Close follow-up is essential with all such patients.

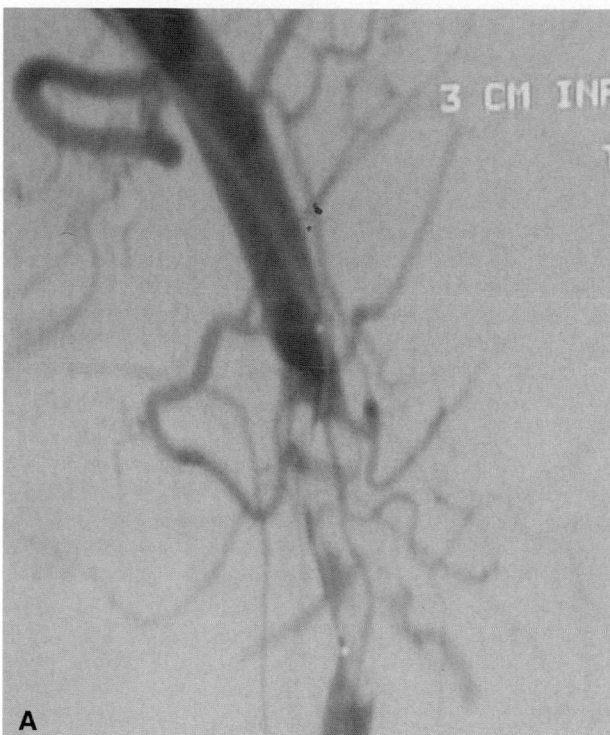 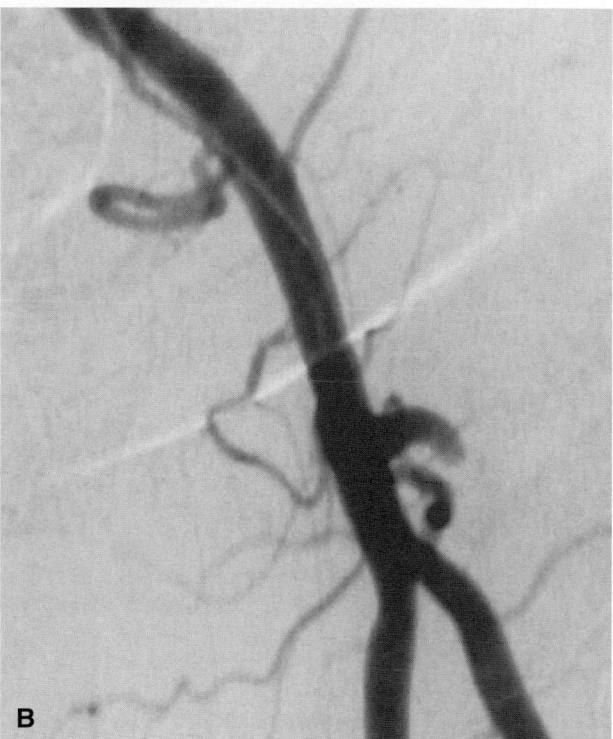

Figure 17–12 This is a 57–year-old male with newly diagnosed a-fib. He presented to ER with a cool, painful, pulseless Lt. foot. **A.** Pelvic angiogram showing embolus at the femoral bifurcation (A). This was treated with overnight thrombolysis. **B.** Eighteen hours after initiation of lysis, the clot was completely dissolved with no distal embolization.

Mechanical Thrombectomy

These devices are designed to disintegrate, pulverize, dislodge, and evacuate thrombus from arteries, veins, and bypass grafts. Mechanical thrombectomy devices can restore patency of the vessel and provide quick reperfusion of ischemic limbs (149,150,158–167). The devices can be used alone or in combination with pharmacologic lytic agents. Many of the devices are not FDA approved for use in the peripheral arterial circulation but have been used "off label" in thrombotic, ischemic limbs. Only the AngioJet Rheolytic Thrombectomy system is currently approved by the FDA for peripheral arterial application. The ones used most commonly in the aortoiliac system include the Oasis (Boston Scientific/Medi-Tech), AngioJet/Xpendior (Possis Medical), Hydrolyser (Cordis Endovascular) and the Amplatz thrombectomy device (Microvena). When dealing with larger thrombus burden as seen in aortic occlusion from embolic disease, hemolysis and fluid overload is more of a problem that is relative to catheter activation time and extended use (168). Distal embolization is also seen (165). Endothelial damage is also an important factor to consider when choosing mechanical thrombectomy devices (MTDs) (169,170). Ultimately, once the blood flow is restored, the underlying lesion can be definitively treated with stents.

Atherectomy

Atherectomy devices remove the atheromatous material (plaque) causing the obstruction without producing elastic recoil. Therefore, in theory, the devices should produce a longer lasting result than PTA (171). Earlier reports were favorable for the Simpson directional atherectomy catheter (172–174), but more recent studies demonstrate improved long-term outcome with balloon angioplasty than atherectomy catheters (133,135,175). A number of different types of atherectomy devices are available and are commonly used in the coronary circulation. The three types of devices now available are directional, rotational, and extractional. With directional devices, the plaque is sliced, stored, and withdrawn from the vessel with the device. Rotational devices use a rapidly turning burr to pulverize the plaque and break it down to sizes comparable to red blood cells. The debris travels distally, which is clinically silent and is disposed of naturally by the body. Extractional atherectomy shaves the plaque and vacuums the debris out of the artery.

These atherectomy devices are valuable cardiology tools but have limited utility in the aortoiliac arteries. The major disadvantages include rigidity and small working diameter. The newest 8F directional atherectomy catheters can only

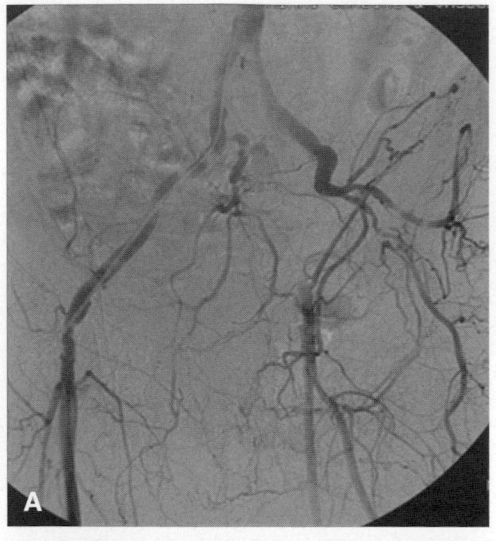
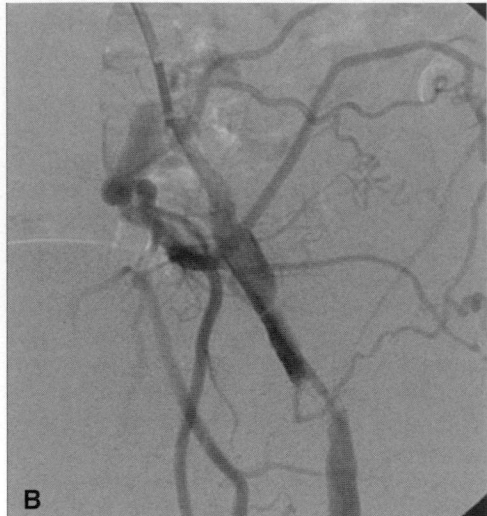
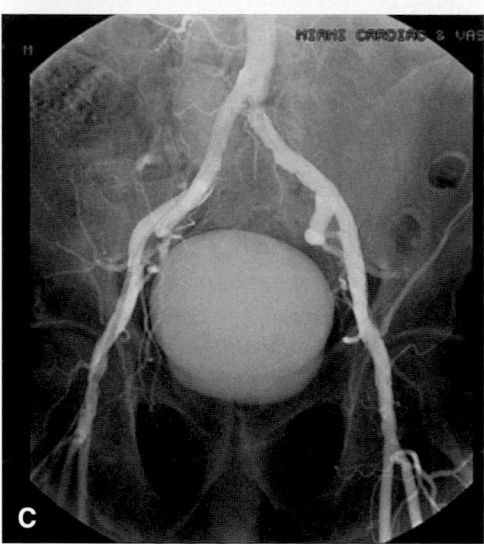

Figure 17–13 This is a 70-year-old with h/o severe PVD. **A.** Pelvic angiogram showing stenotic disease of Rt. CIA and EIA and chronic occlusion of Lt. CIA. **B.** S/P subintimal recanalization with reestablishment of lumen in CFA. **C.** Final angiogram following bilateral iliac stenting. No distal embolization. The patient recovered and was doing well 25 months later.

be used in vessel diameters of 2.75 mm ± 0.5 mm. These devices may play a more important role in the infrageniculate arteries (176,177).

CONTRAINDICATIONS

Contraindications to aortoiliac intervention are relative to the clinical situation at hand. The safety of the patient must be considered first and be balanced against the possible benefits of the procedure. Although these procedures are generally well-tolerated, the extremely debilitated patient may not be able to withstand the strain of even the most benign of procedures. Again, there are no absolute contraindications for most of these procedures. Relative contraindications may include irreversible (or untreated) coagulopathy, severe medical debilitation (such as acute pulmonary edema),

inability to find safe access site (such as an infected groin), and an uncooperative patient. Severely contracted patients can be challenging. Occasionally, lesion morphology itself can be a relative contraindication to percutaneous intervention. Lesions with extensive exophytic plaque that is prone to embolization or disease with involvement of the offending lesion by aneurysmal disease may be better treated by surgical therapy (96,97). Many occlusions once thought to be in the surgical domain are now readily treated by percutaneous methods.

COMPLICATIONS

Although aortoiliac angioplasty and stenting is relatively safe, significant complications may occur. The overall incidence of complications is difficult to assess because of variations in definitions and reporting. Reported rates of complication range from 4% to 20% (1,2,10,112,137,178–182). Complications are divided into minor and major categories. Reports show that disease limited to the common iliac artery has a lower complication rate when compared to disease in the external iliac artery (87). Females experience a higher procedural complication rate than do males (87,178). Some speculate that this is secondary to the smaller size of the female arteries as compared to the size of the percutaneous devices. Most of the complications reported in women were related to the puncture site (178).

Complications directly related to access site represent a significant percentage of all complications of aortoiliac interventions. Up to 40% of all complications are access site related (87). These include hemorrhage, hematoma, or both. It is important to remember that massive blood loss could occur as blood dissects into the retroperitoneal space without immediate visible manifestation. Acute arterial occlusion occurs in approximately 11% of cases (10,183). Possible etiologies include vasospasm, primary thrombosis, or dissection. During stent deployment, dissections can arise from initial difficult wire passage, preliminary PTA, or intima trauma. Prolonged balloon inflation, additional stents, or both have been very successful in the treatment of dissections. Worth noting is that the entire length of the dissection is treated. A pulsatile mass in the groin at or near the puncture site is a hallmark sign of pseudoaneurysm (PSA) or a contained leak. Pseudoaneurysms are now treated universally with ultrasound-guided compression, thrombin injection, or both. Percutaneous thrombin injection is safe, with reported thrombosis rates occurring within seconds and at nearly 100% (184–191). The technique involves placing a skinny needle into the pseudoaneurysm with ultrasound guidance. Once the needle is confirmed to be in the apex of the pseudoaneurysm, thrombin is injected until stenosis of flow is observed. If the PSA cannot be treated with thrombin injection and surgical treatment is not an option, then stent graft repair has been reported (192,193). Arteriovenous fistulae have also been treated with stent graft repair (192,194). Arterial rupture is an infrequent complication but can be quite frightening. The incidence of aortic or iliac rupture during PTA and stenting is extremely low, <0.1% (112,180,195). Severe pain with angiographic evidence of extravasation of contrast signals a tear in the adventitia. Other systemic signs of hypotension, bradycardia, and symptoms of altered or decreased mental status, and diaphoresis will then occur. Once the rupture is recognized, then immediate action must be taken. Resuscitation efforts must occur simultaneously with other therapies. It is critical to maintain wire access across the angioplasty site. The leak can be tamponade with inflation of a balloon across the area of rupture (157). Once the bleeding is controlled and the patient is hemodynamically stable, the definitive therapy can be addressed. The possible therapies include surgical ligation, patching, or bypass. Endovascular stent grafting is now the most commonly used method of treating focal ruptures (Figure 17–14). The risk factors associated with arterial rupture include chronic steroid use, overinflation during angioplasty, calcified plaque that penetrates the arterial wall during PTA, fibromuscular dysplasia, vasculitis/arteritis, or any other changes that influence the strength of the arterial wall. Infection is a dreaded complication of percutaneous therapy but one that is not often encountered. It is nearly always secondary to bacterial contamination at the access site (196–198), although there are reports of stents becoming secondarily infected from injected blood (199). A stent may be infected without local signs of purulence and erythema. Hyperthermia and leukocytosis are common. Septic emboli are an important phenomenon of an infected stent. Although some patients may be managed well with antibiotic therapy usually aimed at staph aureus—the most commonly cultured organism—surgical resection of the infected portion of the artery may become necessary. Fatal outcomes have been reported as well as limb amputations. These are, thankfully, rare. Some interventionalists advocate routine prophylactic use of antibiotics before stent placement.

Distal embolization can occur in up to 3–7% of patients (112,137). According to some speculation, many more cases of embolization are clinically silent. The smaller the size of the embolic particle, the greater the clinical insignificance (137). Embolic particles may be composed of thrombus, atherosclerotic plaque, or cholesterol. Although primary stenting decreases the risk of embolization, it does not eliminate the potential for embolic material to travel downstream from the treated area. Thrombolytic therapy, which is the mainstay of treatment, works poorly on emboli composing of plaque. In those cases, other techniques such as suction embolectomy, either manual or mechanical, can be used (164,169).

STENT SELECTION

Vascular stents are metallic devices designed to maintain patency of the blood vessel. They are divided into two categories of balloon-expandable versus self-expandable types. The metals used include stainless steel, nitinol, platinum, and various metal alloys such as cobalt. Currently, only three stents are FDA approved for placement in the iliac arteries. These are the Palmaz 308 stent, the Wallstent, and the SMART stent. All other stents are used off label in the iliac arteries with biliary and tracheobronchial FDA approval. Several factors influence the type of stent placed in the aortoiliac arterial segment. Whether a lesion is eccentric or concentric, calcified or soft, focal or diffuse, it will influence the type of stent desired. Besides the characteristic of the lesion being stented, several other factors contribute to the type of stent selected for treatment. These include vessel tortuosity, size of the sheath needed for placement, access site, experience of the interventionalist

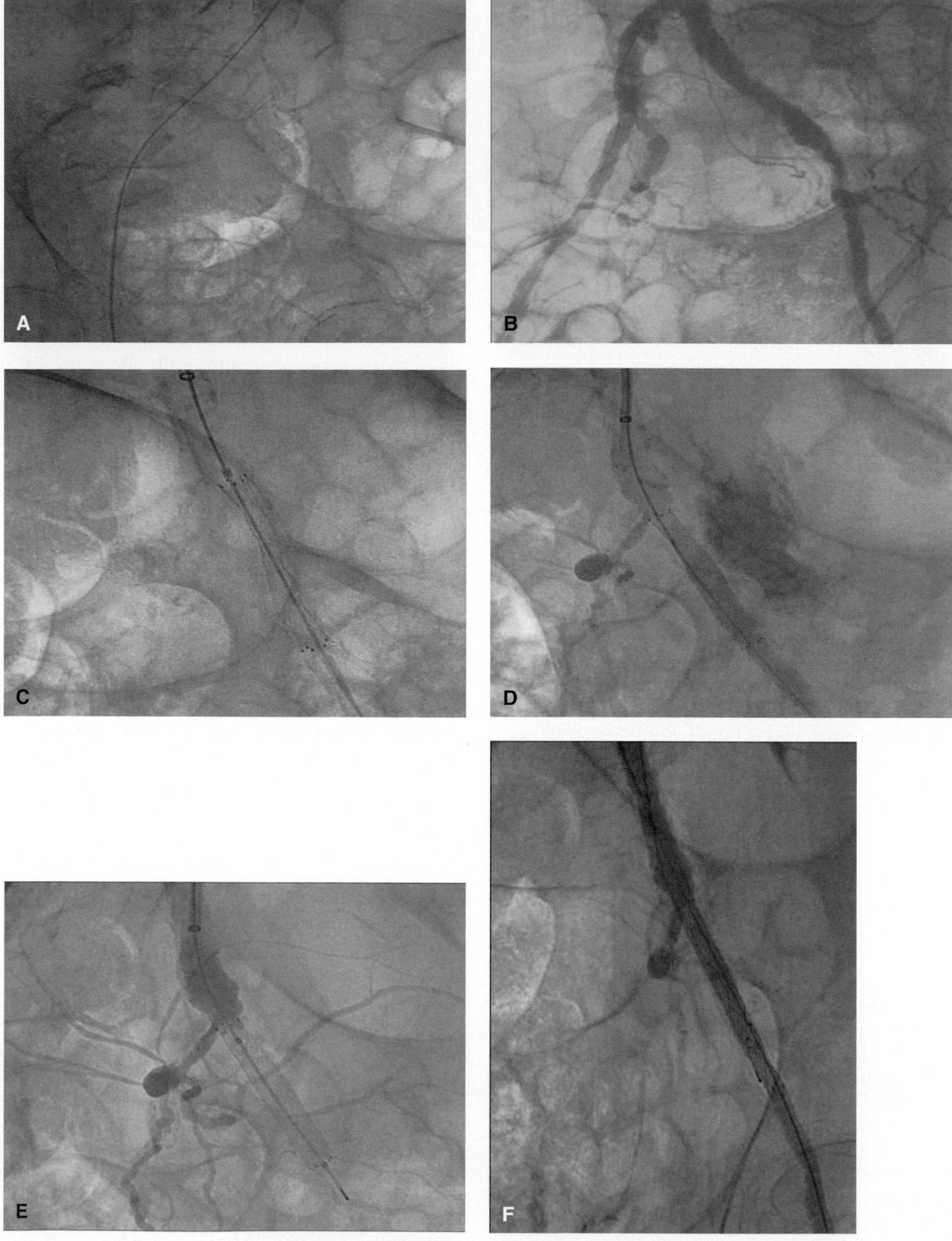

Figure 17–14 This is an 82-year-old female with a nonhealing ulcer of her left foot. **A.** Diagnostic angiogram revealed densely calcified aortoiliac arteries and **B.** high-grade Lt. external iliac artery stenosis. **C.** A nitinol SES was placed and dilated to 7 mm. **D.** Post-deployment angiogram showing ruptured artery with frank extravasation of contrast into soft tissues. The patient complains of pain and becomes hypotensive. **E.** Wire maintained across rupture and balloon inflated in CIA. **F.** Lt. CFA accessed and stent graft placed across rupture. No further bleeding. Patient stabilized.

with that particular product, inventory choices, and the cost of stents. Aortic stenotic disease requiring stent placement is generally treated with balloon expandable stents because of the advantage of hoop strength and precision of placement.

A short focal lesion can be treated with either balloon-expandable or self-expandable stents. In the case of occlusions or long segment disease, self-expandable stents are better suited. If the lesion is heavily calcified or fibrotic, then placing a balloon-expandable stent may be better for the radial strength. When this involves the distal aorta, the common iliac ostium, or both, then the stents are placed using the "kissing" technique (113–120). When the lesion to be stented is located in a tortuous arterial segment, then placement of a balloon-expandable stent will result in straightening of the vessels and may impair good stent-vessel wall apposition, thereby increasing the likelihood of restenosis. This also results in kinking and angulation of the vessel toward the end of the stent. Self-expandable stents are more flexible and better able to conform to the tortuous vessel segment. They are better in tortuous anatomy as well as areas in which there is a quick transition of vessel diameter, such as from the common iliac artery to the external iliac artery. When stenting of the iliac artery is performed from a contralateral approach over the aortic bifurcation, a flexible delivery system is necessary. Historically, a self-expandable stent has been the only option. But because of advances in stent technology, even a balloon-expandable stent can be flexible enough (Figure 17–15) to be placed up and over the bifurcation. Stents in general are not recommended for placement across the joints, however. If no other options for revascularization are present, then a self-expandable stent should be selected because it is more crush-resistant and less likely to have stent fracture (200).

Covered stents are playing an increasing role in treating aortoiliac atherosclerotic disease (201–204). The most common indication is treatment of ruptures (Figure 17–16), aneurysms, and arteriovenous fistulas. Covered stents are usually self-expandable but balloon-expandable covered stents are also available. The major disadvantage to covered stents is the higher profile of the delivery systems. Most stents require sheath sizes of 8 French to 14 French and even larger for aortic stents. If the need arises for placing a covered stent in the aorta, portions of bifurcated endografts designed for repairing aneurysms could be used such as an aortic cuff. If the iliac artery requiring stenting is of large enough diameter, then a prefabricated limb from an endograft could be placed. No covered stents are FDA approved for placement in the iliac arteries. As with metallic base stents, off-label use is prevalent—most of the stents are approved for tracheobronchial use.

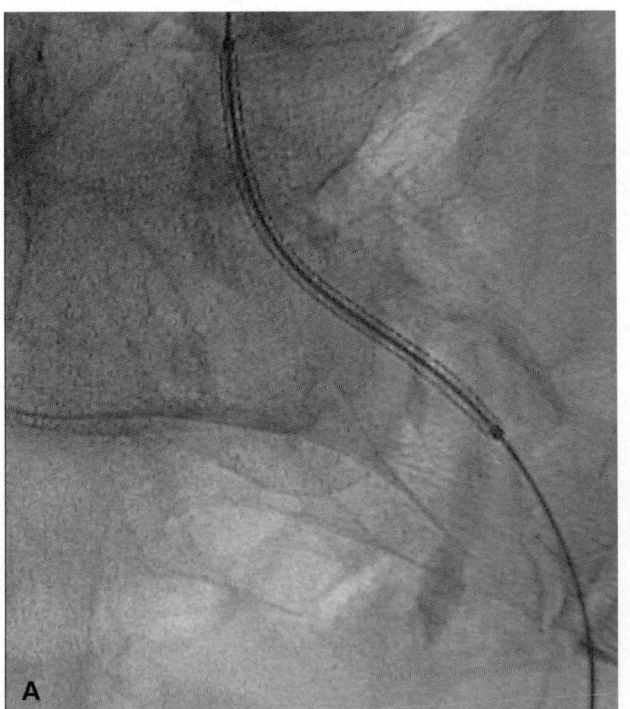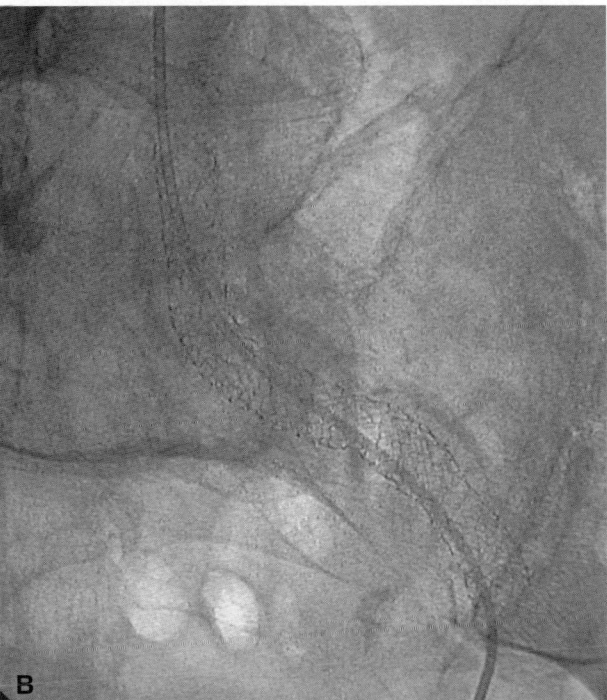

Figure 17–15   **A., B.** showing flexibility and conformabilty of BES in EIA.

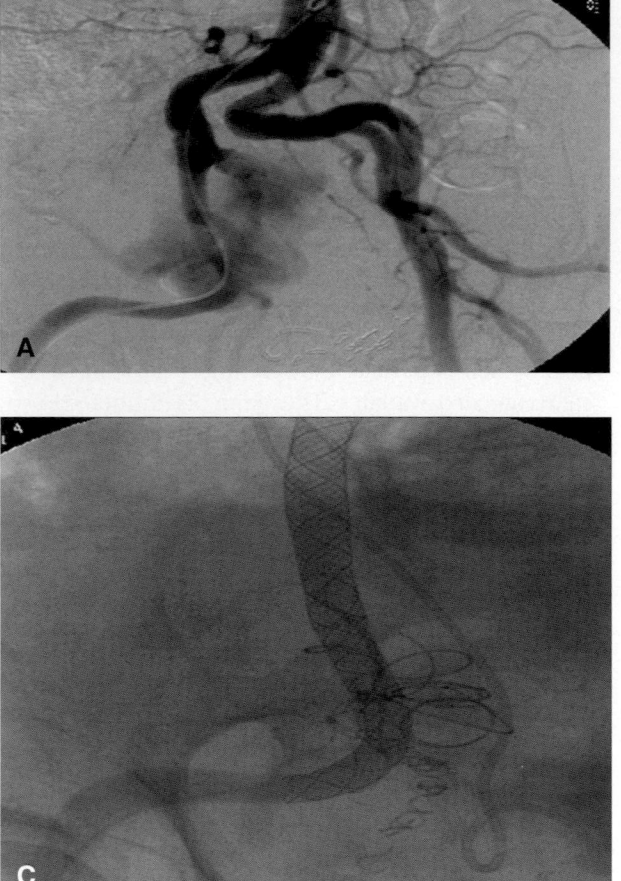

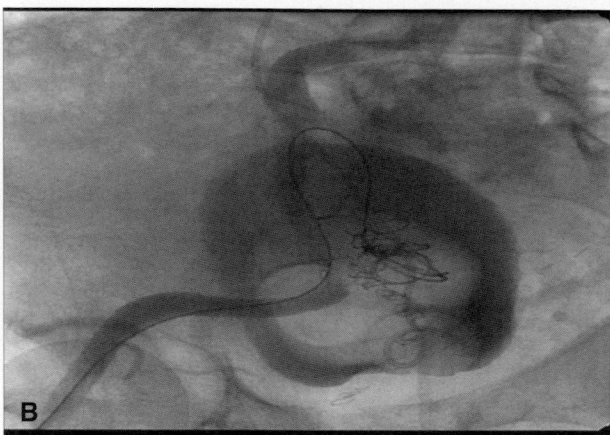

Figure 17–16 An 88-year-old male with bladder cancer and hematuria. **A.** Pelvic angiogram showing large pseudoaneurysm of Rt. internal iliac artery secondary to tumor invasion. After successful coil embolization of the internal iliac artery. **B.** The friable external iliac artery ruptured. **C.** This was successfully treated with a covered stent. The patient's hematuria stopped, but he died of the metastatic cancer 7 months after the procedure.

RESULTS

A thorough discussion of the results of any procedure must include not only the immediate technical success but also long-term success and clinical implication, complications, and cost-effectiveness. Immediate technical success is easily quantified and has been documented well for most procedures. The long-term success rate is tied to patency rates and can be more difficult to quantify. Finally, the direct and indirect cost of any procedure is perhaps the most difficult to quantify, but it plays an important part in evaluating the cost-effectiveness of any procedure.

Technical success rate is defined as the relief of stenosis or occlusion with residual narrowing of <20%. Significant hemodynamic improvement must be present with no major complications. Clinical success is defined as the complete relief of or substantial improvement in symptoms for which treatment is being performed. Patency rate (long-term success) is defined as the percentage of patients who initially had a successful procedure but in a specified period experienced a return of symptoms, restenosis, or both of the treatment site.

The location, morphology, and pathology of a lesion have a significant impact on technical success. Concentric lesions perform better than eccentric lesions. Ostial lesions or lesions at branch points of a vessel may not respond well to PTA. Calcified lesions are more resistant to PTA, thereby requiring higher inflation pressures and have a slightly lower technical success rate and increase chances of complications. Clinical success rate is intimately associated with good technical results and is highest when minimal disease is present elsewhere in the body. Long-term success can be increased when cardiovascular risk factors are well-controlled. In general, larger vessels and short-segment disease have better patency rates than smaller vessels and longer disease segments. It is important to note that the progression of the disease itself affects long-term benefit and patency. Therefore, patency rates of percutaneous procedures must be compared with the parallel surgical therapy.

Although initial reports suggested that the long-term patency rates of iliac artery angioplasty were in the range of 90% at 5 years, subsequent reports have suggested a wide range of patency rates of anywhere from 45% to 95% at 5 years depending on whether stents were placed. The evolution of treatment of the iliac arteries with primary stenting without predilation makes the analysis of PTA alone difficult because of limited up-to-date data. The improvements in techniques and equipment have contributed to marked improvement in technical success rates. However, the absence of uniform reporting standards has been the greatest limitation to a true assessment of efficacy of these procedures.

Patency rates are expressed as primary (those remaining patent without further intervention), primary assisted (those patent with additional intervention to maintain patency), or secondary (those in which patency needs to be reestablished by another intervention). Patency rates quoted in the literature sometimes do not clearly define the rates that are being used. Additionally, rigorous follow-up is not documented in most studies. Noninvasive testing, most commonly the ankle-brachial index (ABI), does not yield the information specific to the PTA stent site. The use of clinical result as an end point, although very important, does not give any information specific to the treatment site. Recurrence of symptoms does not equate to recurrence of disease at the specific treatment site. Conversely, relief of symptoms is not always indicative of a disease-free treatment site because symptomatic improvement can be secondary to collateral development. A "failed" percutaneous procedure can be difficult to define. For example, some interventionists may choose to stent the iliac arteries only when a failed PTA is present. Both procedures are performed at the same angiographic setting, which makes it difficult to define the effectiveness of each individually. A failed percutaneous procedure normally does not carry the same implications as a failed surgical procedure and frequently do not negate the ability to perform a surgical intervention.

The iliac arteries have been the site of most investigations with peripherally placed intravascular stents. The Palmaz stent was the first stent approved in the United States by the FDA for use in the iliac arteries, and therefore, is the stent with the greatest clinical experience. In 1992, Dr. Palmaz et al. published the results of a multicenter trial investigating the Palmaz stent in the iliac arteries (183). The immediate clinical success rate was 99%, with 1- and 2 year clinical success rates of 91% and 84%, respectively. At 3 years, the clinical success rate dropped to 69% even though angiographically, the stent patency rate was 92%. This emphasizes the difficulty in determining the long-term durability of any vascular procedure. Most of the patients with recurrent symptoms were found to have a patent stent but had progression of disease remote to the site of the stented segment.

Dr. Murphy summarized the data of 18 published studies of iliac stent placement. He found that the weighted average technical success rate was 97%. Primary patency rates at 5 years ranged from 58% to 82%, and secondary patency rates at 5 years ranged from 78% to 91% (205).

These patency rates approach those of surgical aortoiliac bypass grafts.

Complex iliac stenotic disease, especially bilateral stenoses or total iliac occlusions, were usually considered "don't touch" lesions for endovascular therapy and are usually treated with aortofemoral or aortobifemoral bypass surgery. The widespread use of the "kissing" balloon-stent technique has allowed for multiple studies documenting their use (13,85,113–20). In 2002, Haulon et al. reported on 106 patients in whom "kissing stents" were used for aortoiliac reconstruction (114). The primary patency rate was 79.4% with a secondary patency rate of 97.7%. Greiner et al. reported 100% technical success rate with primary patency of 92% and secondary patency of 100% (117). Ninety-two percent of patients had continued clinical improvement at 2-year follow-up. Primary stenting of chronic iliac occlusion after guide wire recanalization has a technical success rate of 92% as reported by Reyes et al. (206). The primary patency rate was 73%, and the secondary patency rate was 88%. Scheinert et al. performed primary stenting of the aortoiliac bifurcations with kissing stents after laser recanalization of chronic iliac occlusions (115).

The technical success rate was 90%. The primary patency rates were 84% at 1 year, 81% at 2 years, 78% at 3 years, and 76% at 4 years. Secondary patency rates were 88%, 88%, 86%, and 85% at 1, 2, 3, and 4 years, respectively (115).

Many identified prognostic factors influence the outcome of iliac artery stent patency. Severe multilevel disease was found to be a significant factor of stent patency by Timaran et al. (88). In that study, the primary patency rate for iliac stent at 1, 3, and 5 years was 85%, 72%, and 64% versus 89%, 86%, and 86% after surgical reconstruction, respectively. Poor infrainguinal runoff was found to be the main risk factor for decreased primary patency in both groups; however, it was less so in the surgical bypass group.

The study also reported external iliac artery disease and female gender as independent predictors of poor outcome after iliac stenting. These findings were supported by Powell et al. who found that external iliac artery stenoses adversely affect both the primary and secondary patency rates of iliac interventions (89). Dr. Lee and his colleagues disagree in their published comparison between external iliac and common iliac artery stent patency rates and found no differences in the primary patency rates, even though the EIA stent patients were older and had more ischemic limbs. The primary patency rates were (EIA and CIA) 93% versus 88% at 1 year, 91% versus 85% at 2 years, and 90% versus 78% at 3 years (94).

Anatomic distribution of atherosclerosis was shown to play a significant role in patency rates. Laborde et al. studied 455 patients and stratified them according to the three anatomic distributions of disease. They concluded that type 3 aortoiliac lesions had inferior patency rates at 3 years (60.8%) when compared to type 1 (91.6%) and type 2 (97.9%) disease (87). Bosch et al. evaluated the results of PTA versus stent placement to treat aortoiliac occlusive disease (2). A meta-analysis of the data of six PTA studies and eight stent placement studies was published. Technical success rate was 91% in PTA and 96% for stent placement, but this difference is not statistically significant. Four-year patency rates were higher than 65% for stenoses and 54% for occlusions. The risk of long-term failure was reduced by 39% after stent placement, compared to PTA alone. The authors later published their cost-analysis study comparing PTA and selective stenting to primary stent placement and concluded that selective stent placement is the most cost effective. Tetteroo and his colleagues also found this to be true when they compared the two groups (72). The clinical success rate at 2 years was 78% and 77% for primary stent and selective stenting after PTA, respectively. The primary patency rates were 71% versus 70% at 2 years, respectively.

Aortic stent placement for stenotic or occlusive disease has an excellent technical success rate ranging from 87% to 100%. The primary patency rates on average range from 75% to 91% (207–213). The secondary patency rates range from 89% to 100%. Several factors affect the patency rates as previously mentioned. Therasse et al. found that aortic diameter may be a predictive factor for restenosis (210). Elkouri and his colleagues found the presence of iliac disease and poor runoff to be stronger predictive values of patency failure (211).

Repeat percutaneous transluminal angioplasty and selective stent placement is successful in the treatment of aortic restenosis. Dr. de Vries et al. reported a 17% repeat intervention rate because of hemodynamically significant stenoses in combination with severe clinical symptoms (212). Feugier et al. reported a 9.9% restenosis rate (seven patients) with aortobifemoral bypass as the treatment in 57% of the cases (213).

Restenosis remains a major limitation to percutaneous angioplasty and stenting especially in complex lesions. The extent of restenosis after PTA is a result of negative remodeling and development of neointimal hyperplasia. The implantation of a stent prevents recoil and negates the issue of negative remodeling. However, intimal hyperplasia continues to plague the procedure. Hehrlein and his colleagues correlated the severity of acute vascular injury after PTA and stent with the extent of neointimal hyperplasia and restenosis (214). They concluded that prolonged or chronic vascular expansion, as with implantation of stents, increases smooth muscle cell death that subsequently stimulates neointimal growth. Targeting the smooth muscle cell with antiproliferation drugs delivered in many forms and use of local radiation therapy are promising techniques to prevent or reduce restenosis. Many new endovascular techniques aimed at treating restenosis already are

implemented in clinical cardiology practice, especially drug-elating stents and brachytherapy. Similar studies have been made in the femoropopliteal arterial segment with cryoplasty and photodynamic therapy. Drug-elating stents raise a reasonable optimism, but no studies currently are being done in the aortoiliac arterial segment. The ultimate endovascular technique to reduce or eliminate restenosis may be revealed over the next few years. On the horizon is local gene transfer for inhibition of restenosis. Ongoing basic science and clinical research will clarify and establish new methods for the prevention of restenosis.

SUMMARY

Since the first percutaneous revascularization performed by Dr. Charles Dotter in 1964, aortoiliac interventions have become one of the most frequently performed procedures in the treatment of peripheral vascular disease. Despite early resistance, it has gained widespread acceptance in both the medical and surgical communities as the initial treatment of choice for patients with aortoiliac disease, largely because of its excellent long-term durability and low association with morbidity and mortality.

Currently, aortoiliac intervention is performed by many different specialists; namely, interventional radiologists, interventional cardiologists, and endovascular surgeons. The primary objective, regardless of specialty, is to provide percutaneous revascularization in an efficient and safe manner. The ideal practice involves participation from all three specialties in order to provide optimal benefit to the vascular patient. Setting credentialing criteria for competency is extremely important for ensuring that patients get the best possible care. "Limited competency" is unacceptable, and all cardiovascular specialists should be both well-trained and credentialed to serve as experts in treating peripheral vascular disease.

The excellent safety record of aortoiliac PTA has also led to an expansion of its indication for revascularization beyond the more traditional conservative indications for the corresponding surgical procedures. The guidelines for treating aortoiliac disease, established by the Joint Council of the American Heart Association, the TASC Working Group and the special writing group (authored by Pentecost et al. and published by SIR), are now limited in their clinical application. This is primarily because lesions that had been treated by surgery only (TASC's C and D; Categories 3 and 4) are now successfully treated by percutaneous methods. Advances in the understanding of vascular biology, pharmacologic therapy, and balloon and stent technology have permitted the percutaneous approach to treat increasingly complex lesions. Continued advances in imaging technology, stent grafts, and treatment of restenosis will most certainly continue to expand the indications for and the success of percutaneous treatment of aortoiliac disease.

REFERENCES

1. Murphy TP, Khwaja AA, Webb MS, et al. Aortoiliac stent placement in patients treated for intermittent claudication. J Vasc Interv Radiol 1998;9:421–428.
2. Bosch J, Hunink M. Meta-analysis of the results of percutaneous transluminal angioplasty and stent placement for aortoiliac occlusive disease. Radiology 1997;204:87–96.
3. Martin EC. Percutaneous therapy in the management of aortoiliac disease. Semin Vasc Surg 1994;7:17–27.
4. Ernst CB, Rutkow IM, Cleveland RJ, et al. Vascular surgery in the United States. Report of the Joint Society for Vascular Surgery—International Society for Cardiovascular Surgery Committee on Vascular Surgical Manpower. J Vasc Surg 1987;6:611–621.
5. Dotter CT. Cardiac catheterization and angiographic technics of the future. Cesk Radiol 1965;19:217–236.
6. Dotter CT, Judkins MP. Transluminal treatment of arteriosclerotic obstruction: description of a new technic and a preliminary report of its application. Circulation 1964;30:654–670.
7. Gruentzig A. Die perkatane rekavalisation chrovischer artelieller verschulusse (Dotter-Privzip) mit einem nemen doppellumingen dilatationskather. Rofo 1976;124:80–86.
8. Murphy TP, Webb MS, Lambiase RE, et al. Percutaneous revascularization of complex iliac artery stenoses and occlusions with use of Walstent: 3 years' experience. J Vasc Interv Radiol 1996;7:21–27.
9. Sapoval MR, Chatellier G, Long AL, et al. Self-expandable stents for the treatment of iliac artery obstructive lesions: long-term success and prognostic factors. AJR Am J Roentgenol 1996;166:1173–1179.
10. Martin EC, Katzen BT, Benenati JF, et al. Multicenter trial of the wallstent in the iliac and femoral arteries. J Vasc Interv Radiol 1995;6:843–849.
11. Palmaz JC, Richter GM, Noeldge G, et al. Intraluminal stents in atherosclerotic iliac artery stenosis: Preliminary report of a multicenter study. Radiology 1988;168:727–731.
12. Murphy TP, Ariaratnam NS, Carney WI, et al. Aortoiliac insufficiency: long-term experience with stent placement for treatment. Radiology 2004;231:243–249.
13. Henry M, Amor M, Ethevenot G, et al. Percutuneous endoluminal treatment of iliac occlusions: long-term follow-up in 105 patients. J Endovasc Surg 1998;228–235.
14. Yeager RA. Nonatherosclerotic claudication. Semin Vasc Surg 1993;6:24–35.
15. Cronenwett J, Davis J, Gooch J, et al. Aortoiliac occlusive disease in women. Surg 1980;88:775.
16. Applebaum RM, Kronzon I. Evaluation and management of cholesterol embolization and the blue toe syndrome. Curr Opin Cardiol 1996;11:533–542.
17. Renshaw A, McCowen T, Waltke EA, et al. Angioplasty with stenting is effective in treating blue toe syndrome. Vasc Endovasc Surg 2002;36:155–159.
18. Matchett WJ, McFarland DR, Eidt JF, et al. Blue toe syndrome: treatment with intra-arterial stents and review of therapies. J Vasc Radiol 2000;11:585–592.
19. Hirsch, AT, Criqui MH, Jacobson DT, et al. Peripheral arterial disease detection, awareness, and treatment in primary care. JAMA 2001;286:1317–1324.
20. Hirsch AT, Jacobson DT, Lando HA, et al. The role of tobacco cessation, antiplatelet, and lipid-lowering therapies in the treatment of peripheral arterial disease. Vasc Med 1997;2:243–251.
21. Mukherjee D, Yadav JS. Update on peripheral vascular diseases: from smoking cessation to stenting. Cleve Clin J Med 2001;8:723–733.
22. Aquino R, Johnnides C, Makoun M, et al. Natural history of claudication: long-term serial follow-up study of 1,244 claudicants. J Vasc Surg 2001;34:962–970.
23. Howard BV, Rodriquez BL, Bennett PH, et al. Prevention conference VI: diabetes and cardiovascular disease. AHA conference proceedings. Circulation 2002;105:e132–144.
24. McDaniel MD, Cronenwett JL. Basic data related to the natural history of intermittent claudication. Ann Vasc Surg 1989;3:273–277.
25. Klein R. Hyperglycemia and microvascular and macrovascular disease in diabetes. Diabetes Care. 1995;18:258–268.
26. Kleinman JC, Donahue RP, Harris MI, et al. Mortality among diabetes in a national sample. Am J Epidemiol 1988;128:389–401.
27. Redberg RF, Greenland P, Fuster V, et al. Prevention Conference VI—Diabetes and cardiovascular disease: risk assessment in persons with diabetes. Circulation 2002;105:e144–152.
28. The sixth report of the Joint National Committee on prevention, detection, evaluation, and treatment of high blood pressure (JNC 6). Arch Intern Med 1997;157:2413–2446.
29. Berlowitz DR, Ash AS, Hickey EC, et al. Inadequate management of blood pressure in a hypertensive population. N Engl J Med 1998;339:1957–1963.
30. McNamara DB, Champion HC, Kadowitz PJ. Pharmacologic management of peripheral vascular disease. Surg Clin North Am 1998;447–464.
31. Sacks FM, Pfeffer MA, Mage LA, et al. The effects of pravastatin on coronary events after myocardial infarction in patients with average cholesterol levels. N Engl J Med 1996;335:1001–1009.
32. McDermott M, Guralnik J, Greenland P, et al. Statin use and leg functioning in patients with and without lower-extremity peripheral arterial disease. Circulation 2003;107:757–761.
33. Mohler ER III, Hiatt W, Creager MA. Cholesterol reduction with atorvastatin improves walking distance in patients with peripheral arterial disease. Circulation 2003;108:1481–1486.
34. Mukherjee D, Lingam P, Chetcuti S, et al. Missed opportunity to treat atherosclerosis in patients undergoing peripheral vascular interventions. Circulation 2002;106:1909–1912.
35. Cheng JW, Ting AC, Wong J. Fasting total plasma homocysteine and atherosclerotic peripheral vascular disease. Ann Vasc Surg 1997;217–223.
36. Clarke R, Daly L, Robinson K, et al. Hyperhomocysteinemia: an independent risk factor for vascular disease. N Engl J Med 1999;324:1149–1155.
37. Malinow MR, Kang SS, Taylor LM, et al. Prevalence of homocysteinemia in patients with peripheral arterial occlusive disease. Circulation 1989;79:1180–1188.
38. Fruchart JC, Nierman MC, Stroes ES, et al. New risk factors for atherosclerosis and patient risk assessment. Circulation 2004; 109(Suppl III):1.
39. Ridker PM, Cushman M, Stampfer MJ, et al. Plasma concentration of C-reactive protein and risk of developing peripheral vascular disease. Circulation 1998;97:425–428.
40. Ridker P. Rifai N. Pfeffer M, et al. Long-term effects of provastatin on plasma concentration of C-reactive protein: the cholesterol and recurrent events (CARE) investigators. Circulation 1999;100:230–235.
41. Rutherford RB. Standards for evaluating and reporting the results of interventional therapy for peripheral vascular diseases. Circulation 1991;83(Suppl I):6–11.
42. Rutherford RB, Becker GJ. Standards for evaluating and reporting the results of surgical and percutaneous therapy for peripheral arterial diseases. J Vasc Interv Radiol 1991;2:169–174.
43. Rutherford RB, Flanigan DP, Gupta SK, et al. Suggested standards for reports dealing with lower extremity ischemia. J Vasc Surg 1986;4:80–94.
44. Barretto S, Bullman K, Rooke T, et al. Early-onset peripheral arterial occlusive disease, clinical features and determination of disease severity and location. Vasc Med 2003;2:95–100.
45. Jaff MR. Lower extremity arterial disease: diagnostic aspects. Cardiol Clin 2002;4:491–500.
46. Toursarkissian B, Mejia A, Smilanich RP, et al. Noninvasive localization of infrainguinal arterial occlusive disease in diabetes. Ann Vasc Surg 2001;1:73–78.
47. Steffens J, Schafer F. Oberscheid B, et al. Bolus-chasing contrast-enhanced 3D MRA of the lower extremity. Comparison with intra-arterial DSA. Acta Radiol 2003;44:185–192.
48. Yin D, Baum R, Carpenter J, et al. Cost-effectiveness of MR angiography in cases of limb threatening peripheral vascular disease. Radiology 1995;194:757–764.
49. Goyen M, Ruehm, S, Debatin J. MR angiography for assessment of peripheral vascular disease. Radiol Clin North Am 2002;40:835–846.
50. Vavrik J, Rohrmoser G, Madani B, et al. Comparison of MR angiography versus digital subtraction angiography as a basis for

planning treatment of lower-limb occlusive disease. J Endovasc Ther 2004;11:294–301.

51. Katzen BT. The future of catheter-based angiography: implications for the vascular interventionalist. Radio Clin North Am 2002;40:689–692.

52. Meaney J, Ridgway J, Chakraverty S, et al. Stepping-table gadolinium enhanced digital subtraction MR angiography of the aorta and lower extremities: preliminary experience. Radiology 1999;211:59–67.

53. Sueyoshi E, Sukamoto I, Masuoka Y, et al. Aortoiliac and lower extremity arteries: comparison of three dimensional dynamic contrast-enhanced subtraction MR angiography and conventional angiography. Radiology 1999;210:683–688.

54. Lawler L, Fishman E. Multidetector row computed tomography of the aorta and peripheral arteries. Cardiol Clin 2003;21:607–629.

55. Green D, Parker D. CTA and MRA: visualization without catheterization. Semin Ultrasound CT MR 2003;24:185–191.

56. Rieker O, Duber C, Schmiedt W, et al. Prospective comparison of CT angiography of legs with intra-arterial digital subtraction angiography. AJR Am J Roentgenol 1996;166:269–276.

57. Catalano C, Fraioli F, Laghi A, et al. Infrarenal aortic and lower extremity arterial disease: diagnostic performance of multidetector row CT angiography. Radiology 2004;231:555–563.

58. Rubin G, Schmidt A, Logan L, et al. Multidetector row CT angiography of the lower extremity arterial inflow and runoff: initial experience. Radiology 2001;221:146–158.

59. Koelemay M, Lijmer J, Stoker J, et al. Magnetic resonance angiography for the evaluation of lower extremity arterial disease: a meta-analysis. JAMA 2001;285:1338–1345.

60. Halperin JL. Evaluation of patients with peripheral vascular disease. Thromb Res 2002;106:v303–v311.

61. Gahtan V. The noninvasive vascular laboratory. Surg Clin North Am 1998;4:507–518.

62. Koelemay M, Legemate O, de Vos H, et al. Duplex scanning allows selective use of arteriography in the management of patients with severe lower leg arterial disease. J Vasc Surg 2001;4:661–667.

63. Spinosa D, Angle F, Hagspiel K, et al. Lower extremity angiography with use of iodinated contrast material or gadodiamide to supplement C02 angiography in patients with renal insufficiency. J Vasc Interv Radiol 2000;11:35–45.

64. Rolland Y, Duvauferrier R, Lucas A, et al. Lower limb angiography: a prospective study comparing carbon dioxide with iodinated contrast material in 30 patients. AJR Am J Roentgenol 1998;171:333–337.

65. Weaver FA, Pentecost MJ, Yellin AE, et al. Clinical applications of carbon dioxide/digital subtraction angiography. J Vasc Surg 1991;13:266–272.

66. Spinosa D, Kaufman J, Hartwell G. Gadolinium chelates in angiography and interventional radiology: a useful alternative to iodinated contrast medial for angiography. Radiology 2002;223:319–325.

67. Kaufman J, Geller S, Bazari H, et al. Gadolinium-based contract agents as an alternative at vena cavography in patients with renal insufficiency: early experience. Radiology 1994;212:280–284.

68. Parodi JC, Ferreira LM. Gadolinium-based contrast: an alternative contrast agent for endovascular intervention. Ann Vasc Surg 2000;14:480–483.

69. Prince MR, Arnoldus C, Frisoli J. Nephrotoxicity of high-dose gadolinium compared with iodinated contrast. J Magn Reson Imaging 1996;6:162–166.

70. Tombach B, Bremes C, Reimer P, et al. Renal tolerance of a neutral gadolinium chelate (gadobutrol) in patients with chronic renal failure: results of a randomized study. Radiology 2001;218:651–657.

71. Kinney TB, Rose SC. Intra-arterial pressure measurements during angiographic evaluation of peripheral vascular disease: techniques, interpretation, applications, and limitations. AJR Am J Roentgenol 1996;166:277–284.

72. Tetteroo E, van Engelen AD, Spithoven JH, et al. Stent placement after iliac angioplasty: comparison of hemodynamic and angiographic criteria. Dutch Iliac Stent Trial Study Group. Radiology 1996;201:155–159.

73. Casteneda-Zaniga W, Knight L, Formanek A, et al. Hemodynamic assessment of obstructive aortoiliac disease. AJR Am J Roentgenol 1976;127:559–561.

74. Kamphius AG, van Engelen AD, Tetteroo E, et al. Impact of different hemodynamic criteria for stent placement after suboptimal iliac angioplasty. J Vasc Interv Radiol 1999;10:741–746.

75. Bonn J. Percutaneous vascular intervention: value of hemodynamic measurements. Radiology 1996;201:18–20.

76. Standards of practice committee of the Society of Cardiovascular and Interventional Radiology. Guidelines of percutaneous transluminal angioplasty. J Vasc Interv Radiol 1990;1:5–15.

77. Tetteroo E, Haaring C, van de Graaf Y, et al. Intra-arterial pressure gradients after randomized angioplasty or stenting of iliac artery lesions. Cardiovasc Intervent Radiol 1996;19:411–417.

78. CAPRIE Steering Committee: A randomized, blinded, trial of clopidogrel versus aspirin in patients at risk of ischemic events. (CAPRIE) Lancet 1996;348:1339–1339.

79. Toprol EJ, Moliterno DJ, Herrmann HC, et al. Comparison of two platelet IIb/IIIa inhibitors, tirofiban and abciximab, for the prevention of ischemic events with percutaneous coronary revascularization. N Engl J Med 2001;344:1888–1894.

80. Tepe G, Schottu, Erley CMN, et al. Platelet glycoprotein IIb/IIIa receptor antagonist used in conjunction with thrombolysis for peripheral arterial thrombosis. AJR Am J Roentgenol 1996;176:1343–1346.

81. Stavropoulos SW, Solomon J, Soulen M, et al. Use of abciximab during infrainguinal peripheral vascular interventions: initial experience. Radiology 2003;227:657–661.

82. Lincoff M, Kleiman N, Kereiakes D, et al. Long-term efficacy of bivalirudin and provisional glycoprotein IIb/IIIa blockade vs. heparin and planned glycoprotein IIb/IIIa blockade during percutaneous coronary revascularization. JAMA 2004;292:696–703.

83. Shammas NW, Lemke JH, Dippel DJ, et al. Bivalirudin in peripheral vascular interventions: a single center experience. J Invasive Cardiol 2003;15:401–404.

84. Regensteiner J, Steiner J, Hiatt WR. Exercise training improves functional status in patients with peripheral arterial diseases. J Vasc Surg 1996;23:104–115.

85. Regensteiner J, Hiatt WR. Medical management of peripheral arterial disease. J Vasc Interv Radiol 1994;5:669–677.

86. Weitz J, Byrne J, Clagett P, et al. Diagnosis and treatment of chronic arterial insufficiency of the lower extremities: a critical review. Circulation 1996;94:3026–3049.

87. Laborde JC, Palmaz JC, Rivera FJ, et al. Influence of anatomic distribution on the outcome of revascularization with iliac stent placement. J Vasc Interv Radiol 1995;6:513–521.

88. Timaran CH, Prault TL, Stevens SL, et al. Iliac artery stenting versus surgical reconstruction of TASC (TransAtlantic Inter-Society Consensus) type B and type C iliac lesions. J Vasc Surg 2003;38:272–278.

89. Powell RJ, Fillinger M, Bettman M, et al. The durability of endovascular treatment of multisegment iliac occlusive disease. J Vasc Surg 2000;31:1178–1184.

90. Timaran CH, Ohki T, Gargiulo NJ, et al. Iliac artery stenting in patients with poor distal runoff: influence of concomitant infrainguinal arterial reconstruction. J Vasc Surg 2003;38:479–484.

91. Muluk SC, Muluk VS, Kelley ME, et al. Outcome events in patients with claudication: a 15-year study in 2,777 patients. J Vasc Surg 2001;33:251–258.

92. TASC working group management of peripheral arterial disease (PAD). J Vasc Surg 2000;31:S1–S289.

93. Aquino R, Johnnides C, Makaroun M, et al. Natural history of claudication: long-term serial follow-up study of 1,244 claudicants. J Vasc Surg 2001;34:962–970.

94. Lee E, Steenson CC, Trimble R, et al. Comparing patency rates between external iliac and common iliac artery stents. J Vasc Surg 2000;31:884–894.

95. Brand FN, Abbott RD, Kannel WB. Diabetes, intermittent claudication, and risk of cardiovascular events. The Framingham Study. Diabetes 1989;38:504–509.

96. Spies J, Bakal C, Burke D, et al. Guidelines for percutaneous transluminal angioplasty. J Vasc Interv Radiol 2003;14:S209–S217.

97. Pentecost MJ, Criqui MH, Dorros G, et al. Guideline for peripheral percutaneous transluminal angioplasty of the abdominal

aorta and lower extremity vessels. A statement for health professionals from a special writing group of the councils on Cardiovascular Radiology, Arteriosclerosis, Cardiothoracic and Vascular Surgery, Clinical Cardiology, and Epidemiology and Prevention, the American Heart Association. J Vasc Interv Radiol 2003;14:S49–S515.

98. Faries PL, Brophy D, LoGerfo FW, et al. Combined iliac angioplasty and infrainguinal revascularization surgery are effective in diabetic patients with multilevel disease. Ann Vasc Surg 2001;15:67–72.

99. Demasi RJ, Snyder SO, Wheeler JR, et al. Intraoperative iliac artery stents: combination with infrainguinal revascularization procedures. Am Surg 1994;60:854–859.

100. Nelson PR, Powell RJ, Schermerhorn ML, et al. Early results of external iliac artery stenting combined with common femoral artery endarterectomy. J Vasc Surg 2002;35:1107–1113.

101. Siskin G, Darling C, Stainken B, et al. Combined use of iliac artery angioplasty and infrainguinal revascularization for treatment of multilevel atherosclerotic disease. Ann Vasc Surg 1999;13:45–51.

102. Aburahma A, Robinson P, Cook C, et al. Selecting patients for combined femorofemoral bypass grafting and iliac balloon angioplasty and stenting for bilateral iliac disease. J Vasc Surg 2001;33(Suppl II): S93–S99.

103. Frahm C, Widmer MK, Brossman J, et al. Bilateral leg ischemia due to descending aortic dissection: combined treatment with femoro-femoral cross-over bypass and unilateral aorto-iliac stenting. Cariovasc Intervent Radiol 2002;25:444–446.

104. Matchett WJ, McFarlund DR, Eidt JF, et al. Blue toe syndrome: treatment with intra-arterial stents and review of therapies. J Vasc Interv Radiol 2000;11:585–592.

105. Renshaw A, McCowen T, Waltke EA, et al. Angioplasty with stenting is effective in treating blue toe syndrome. Vasc Endovascular Surg 2002;36:155–159.

106. Ravimandalam K, Rao VR, Kumar S, et al. Obstruction of the infrarenal portion of the abdominal aorta: results of treatment with balloon angioplasty. AJR Am J Roentgenol 1991;6:1257–1260.

107. Goldwasser B, Carson CC, Braum SD, et al. Impotence due to the pelvic steal syndrome: treatment by iliac transluminal angioplasty. J Urol 1985;133:860–861.

108. Audet P, Therasse E, Oliva VL, et al. Infrarenal aortic stenosis: long-term clinical and hemodynamic results of percutaneous transluminal angioplasty. Radiology 1998;209:357–363.

109. Yakes WF, Kumpe DA, Brow SB, et al. Percutaneous transluminal aortic angioplasty: technique and results. Radiology 1989;172:965–970.

110. Kaufman SL. Angioplasty from the contralateral approach: use of guiding catheter and coaxial angioplasty balloons. Radiology 1990;177:577–578.

111. Kashdan BH, Trost DW, Jagust MB, et al. Retrograde approach for contralateral iliac and infrainguinal percutaneous transluminal angioplasty: experience in 100 patients. J Vasc Interv Radiol 1992;3:515–521.

112. Strecker EP, Baos IB, Hagen B. Flexible tantalum stents for the treatment of iliac artery lesions: long-term patency complications, and risk factors. Radiology 1996;199:641–647.

113. Mouanoutoua M, Maddikutana R, Allaquaband S, et al. Endovascular intervention of aortoiliac occlusive disease in high risk patients using the kissing stents technique: long-term results. Catheter Cardiovasc Interv 2003;60:320–326.

114. Haulon S, Mounier-Vehier C, Gaxotte V, et al. Percutaneous reconstruction of the aortoiliac bifurcation with the "kissing stents" technique: long-term follow-up in 106 patients. J Endovasc Ther 2002;9:363–368.

115. Scheinert D, Schroder M, Balzer JO, et al. Stent-supported reconstruction of the aortoiliac bifurcation with the kissing balloon technique. Circulation 1999;100:S295–S300.

116. Mendelsohn FO, Santos RM, Crowley JJ, et al. Kissing stents in the aortic bifurcation. Am Heart J 1998;136:600–605.

117. Greiner A, Dessel A, Klein-Weigel P, et al. Kissing stents for treatment of complex aortoiliac disease. Eur J Vasc Endovasc Surg 2003;26:161–165.

118. Mohamed F, Sarkar B, Timmons G, et al. Outcome of "kissing stents" for aortoiliac atherosclerotic disease, including the effect on the nondiseased contralateral limb. Cardiovasc Intervent Radiol 2002;25:472–475.

119. Rosset E, Malikov S, Magnan PE, et al. Endovascular treatment of occlusive lesions in the distal aorta: mid-term results in a series of 31 consecutive patients. Ann Vasc Surg 2001;15:140–147.

120. Insall RL, Loose HWC, Chamberlain J. Long-term results of double-balloon percutaneous transluminal angioplasty of the aorta and iliac arteries. Eur J Vasc Surg 1993;7:31–36.

121. Sharma S, Bahl VK, Saxena A, et al. Stenosis in the aorta caused by nonspecific aortitis: results of treatment by percutaneous stent placement. Clin Radiol 1999;54:46–50.

122. Sawada S, Tanigawa N, Kobayashi M. Treatment of Takayasu's aortitis with self-expanding metallic stents (Gianturco stents) in two patients. Cardiovasc Intervent Radiol 1994;17:102–105.

123. Tyagi S, Kaul UA, Arora R. Endovascular stenting for unsuccessful angioplasty of the aorta in aortoarteritis. Cardiovasc Intervent Radiol 1999;22:451–456.

124. Johnson M, Gernsheimer T, Johansen K. Essential thrombocytosis: underemphasized cause of large-vessel thrombosis. J Vasc Surg 1995;22:443–449.

125. Bhagia, ST, Livesay J, Ruel G, et al. Hypercoagulable state leading to paraplegia in a middle aged man. Tex Heart Inst J 2002;29:30–32.

126. Meagher AP, Lord RS, Graham AR, et al. Acute aortic occlusion presenting with lower limb paralysis. J Cardiovasc Surg (Torino) 1991;32:643–647.

127. Lee WA. Acute aortic occlusion from a cardiac embolus. J Vasc Surg 2003;38:197.

128. Bell JW. Acute thrombosis of subrenal abdominal aorta. Arch Surg 1967;95:681–684.

129. Mesa A, Villareal R, Krajeer Z. Endoluminal treatment of acute aortoiliac thrombosis. Catheter Cardiovasc Interv 2000;50:78–82.

130. Zeller T, Frank U, Burgelin K, et al. Early experience with a rotational thrombectomy device for treatment of acute and sub-acute infra-aortic arterial occlusion. J Endovasc Ther 2003;10:322–331.

131. Hitoshi H, Masatake T, Naoaka M, et al. Acute occlusion of an abdominal aortic aneurysm. Angiology 200;51:515–523.

132. Criado FJ. Acute thrombosis of abdominal aortic aneurysm. Tex Heart Inst J 1982;9:367–371.

133. Murphy ED, Encarnacion CE, Le VA, et al. Iliac artery stent placement with the Palmaz stent: follow-up study. J Vasc Interv Radiol 1995;6:321–329.

134. Henry M, Amor M, Ethevenot G, et al. Palmaz stent placement in iliac and femoropopliteal arteries: primary and secondary patency in 310 patients with 2–4 year follow-up. Radiology 1995;197:167–174.

135. Vorwerk D, Günther RW, Schürmann K, et al. Aortic and iliac stenoses: follow-up results of stent placement after insufficient balloon angioplasty in 118 cases. Radiology 1996;198:45–48.

136. Bosch JL, Tetteroo E, Mali WP, et al. Iliac arterial occlusive disease: cost-effectiveness analysis of stent placement versus percutaneous transluminal angioplasty. Dutch Iliac Stent Trial Study Group. Radiology 1998;208:641–648.

137. Dyet JF, Gaines PA, Nicholson AN, et al. Treatment of chronic iliac artery occlusions by means of percutaneous endovascular stent placement. J Vasc Interv Radiol 1997;8:349–353.

138. Hoballah J. How adequate are the appropriateness criteria for iliac angioplasty? Currents 2003;4:1–4.

139. Motarjeme A, Gordon GI, Bodenhagen K. Thrombolysis and angioplasty of chronic iliac occlusions. J Vasc Interv Radiol 1995;6:S66–S72.

140. Levy JM, Duszak RL, Akins EW, et al. Thrombolysis for lower extremity arterial and graft occlusions. American College of Radiology. ACR Appropriateness Criteria. Radiology 2000;215:1041–1054.

141. Bucek RA, Schnurer G, Haumer M, et al. Long-term results of sys temic thrombolysis therapy in aortoiliac occlusive disease. Vasa 2001;30:212–218.

142. Suggs WD, Cynamon J, Martin B, et al. When is urokinase treatment an effective sole or adjunctive treatment for acute limb ischemia secondary to native artery occlusion? Am J Serg 1999;178:103–106.

143. DeMaioribus CA, Mills JL, Fujitani RM, et al. A reevaluation of intra-arterial thrombolytic therapy for acute lower extremity ischemia. J Vasc Surg 1993;17:888–895.

144. Barr H, Lancashire MJR, Torrie EPH, et al. Intra-arterial thrombolytic therapy in the management of acute and chronic limb ischemia. Br J Surg 1991;78:284–287.

145. Thrombolysis in the management of lower limb peripheral arterial occlusion—a consensus document. Working Party on Thrombolysis in the Management of Limb Ischemia. Am J Cardiol 1998;81:208–218.

146. Yilmaz S, Sindel T, Luleci E. Subintimal versus intraluminal recanalization of chronic iliac occlusions. J Endovasc Ther 2004;11:107–118.

147. Leu AJ, Schneider E, Canova CR, et al. Long-term results after recanalization of chronic iliac artery occlusions by combined catheter therapy without stent placement. Eur J Vasc Endovasc Surg 1999;18:499–505.

148. Diethrich EB, Timbadia E, Bahadir I. Applications and limitations of laser-assisted angioplasty. Eur J Vasc Surg 1989;3:61–70.

149. Sarac TP, Hilleman D, Arko FR, et al. Clinical and economic evaluation of the trellis thrombectomy device for arterial occlusions: preliminary analysis. J Vasc Surg 2004;39:556–559.

150. Ouriel K. Endovascular techniques in the treatment of acute limb ischemia: thrombolytic agents, trials, and percutaneous mechanical thrombectomy techniques. Semin Vasc Surg 2003;16:270–279.

151. Lipsitz EC, Ohki T, Veith FJ, et al. Does subintimal angioplasty have a role in the treatment of severe lower extremity ischemia? J Vasc Surg 2003;37:389.

152. Murphy TP. Subintimal revascularization of chronic iliac artery occlusions. J Vasc Interv Radiol 1996;7:47–51.

153. Bolia A, Fishwick G. Recanalization of iliac artery occlusion by subintimal dissection using the ipsilateral and the contralateral approach. Clin Radiol 1997;52:684–687.

154. Murphy TP, Marks MJ, Webb MS. Use of a curved needle for true lumen re-entry during subintimal iliac artery revascularization. J Vasc Interv Radiol 1997;8:633–636.

155. Saketkhoo RR, Razavi MK, Padidar A, et al. Percutaneous bypass: subintimal recanalization of peripheral occlusive disease with IVUS guided luminal re-entry. Tech Vasc Interv Radiol 2004;7:23–27.

156. Joye J. Percutaneous lower-extremity bypass. Endovasc Today 2004;26–28.

157. Smith TP, Cragg AH. Nonsurgical treatment of iliac artery rupture following angioplasty. J Vasc Interv Radiol 1989;4:16–18.

158. Olin JW, Graor RA. Thrombolytic therapy in the treatment of peripheral arterial occlusions. Ann Emerg Med 1988;17:1210–1215.

159. Muller-Hulsbeck S, Grimm J, Leidt J, et al. In vitro effectiveness of mechanical thrombectomy devices for large vessel diameter and low pressure fluid dynamic application. J Vasc Inter Radiol 2002;13:831–839.

160. Angle JF, Spinosa DJ, Hagspiel KD, et al. Management of acute lower extremity embolus with use of the oasis thrombectomy device and suction embolectomy. J Vasc Interv Radiol 2000;11:1331–1335.

161. Rilinger N, Gorich J, Scharrer-Pamler R, et al. Short-term results with use of the Amplatz thrombectomy device in the treatment of acute lower limb occlusions. J Vasc Interv Radiol 1997;8:343–348.

162. Henry M, Amor M, Henry I, et al. The Hydrolyser thrombectomy catheter: a single-center experience. J Endovasc Surg 1998;5:24–31.

163. Kasirajan K, Gray B, Beavers FP, et al. Rheolytic thrombectomy in the management of acute and subacute limb threatening ischemia. J Vasc Interv Radiol 2001;12:413–421.

164. Reekers JA, Kromhout JG, Spilhoven HG, et al. Artenal thrombosis below the inguinal ligament: percutaneous treatment with a thrombosuction catheter. Radiology 1996;198:49–53.

165. Muller-Hulsbeck S, Kalinowski M, Heller M, et al. Rheolytic hydrodynamic thrombectomy for percutaneous treatment of acutely occluded infra-aortic native arteries and bypass grafts: midterm follow-up results. Invest Radiol 2000;35:131–140.

166. Stainken BF. Mechanical thrombectomy: basic principles, current devices, and future directions. Tech Vasc Interv Radiol 2003;6:2–5.

167. Muller-Hulsbeck S, Janke T. Peripheral arterial applications of percutaneous mechanical thrombectomy. Tech Vasc Interv Radiol 2003;6:22–34.

168. Nazarian GK, Qian Z, Coleman CC, et al. Hemolytic effect of the Amplatz thrombectomy device. J Vasc Interv Radiol 1994;5:155–160.

169. Haskal ZJ. Mechanical thrombectomy devices for the treatment of peripheral arterial occlusions. Rev Cardiovasc Med 2002;3(Suppl II):S45–S52.

170. Veseley TM, Hovsepian DM, Daray MD, et al. Angioscopic observation after percutaneous thrombectomy of thrombosed hemodialysis grafts. J Vasc Interv Radiol 2000;11:971–977.

171. Maynar M, Reyes R, Cabrera V, et al. Percutaneous atherectomy as an alternative treatment for postangioplasty obstructive intimal flaps. Radiology 1989;170:1029–1031.

172. Simpson JB, Selmon MR, Robertson GC, et al. Transluminal atherectomy for occlusive peripheral vascular disease. Am J Cardiol 1988;61:96–101.

173. Kim D, Gianturco LE, Porter DH, et al. Peripheral directional atherectomy: 4-year experience. Radiology 1992;183:773–778.

174. Wildenhain PM, Wholey MH, Jarmolowski CR, et al. Infrainguinal directional atherectomy: long-term follow-up and comparison with percutaneous transluminal angioplasty. Cardiovasc Interv Radiol 1994;17:305–311.

175. Tielbeek AV, Vroegindeweij D, Buth J, et al. Comparison of balloon angioplasty and Simpson atherectomy for lesions in the femoropopliteal artery: angiographic and clinical results of prospective randomized trial. J Vasc Interv Radiol 1996;7:837–844.

176. Orlic D, Reimers B, Stankovic G, et al. Initial experience with a new 8 French-compatible directional atherectomy catheter: immediate and mid-term results. Catheter Cardiovasc Interv 2003;60:159–166.

177. Zeller T, Frank U, Burgelin K, et al. Initial clinical experience with percutaneous atherectomy in the infrageniculate arteries. J Endovasc Ther 2003;10:987–993.

178. Ballard JL, Spark SR, Taylor FC, et al. Complications of iliac artery stent deployment. J Vasc Surg 1995;24:545–555.

179. Cikrit DF, Gustafson PA, Dalsing MC, et al. Long-term follow-up of the Palmaz stent for iliac occlusive disease. Surg 1995;118:613–614.

180. Gardiner GA, Meyerovitz MF, Stokes KR, et al. Complications of transluminal angioplasty. Radiology 1986;159:201–208.

181. Palmaz JC, Garcia OJ, Schatz RA, et al. Placement of balloon-expandable intraluminal stents in iliac arteries: first 171 procedures. Radiology 1990;174:969–975.

182. Long, AL, Page PE, Raynaud AC, et al. Percutaneous iliac artery stent: angiographic long-term follow-up. Radiology 1991;180:771–778.

183. Palmaz JC, Laborde JC, Rivera FJ, et al. Stenting of the iliac arteries with the Palmaz stent: experience from a multicenter trial. Cardiovasc Intervent Radiol 1992;15:291–297.

184. Padidar AM, Kee ST, Razavi MK. Treatment of femoral artery pseudoaneurysm using ultrasound-guided thrombin injection. Tech Vasc Interv Radiol 2003;6:96–102.

185. Kurz DJ, Jungius KP, Luscher TF. Delayed femoral vein thrombosis after ultrasound-guided thrombin injection of a postcatheterization pseudoaneurysm. J Vasc Interv Radiol 2003;14:1067–1070.

186. Morgan R, Belli AM. Current treatment methods for postcatheterization pseudoaneurysm. J Vasc Interv Radiol 2003;14:697–710.

187. Kruger K, Zahringer M, Sohngen FD, et al. Femoral pseudoaneurysm: management with percutaneous thrombin injections—success rates and effects on systemic coagulation. Radiology 2003;2226:452–458.

188. Kang SS. Thrombin injection for pseudoaneurysm occlusion: technical considerations. J Endovasc Ther 2002;9:36–37.

189. Powell A, Benenati JF, Becker GJ, et al. Percutaneous ultrasound-guided thrombin injection for the treatment of pseudoaneurysms. J Am Coll Surg 2002;194:S53–S57.

190. Reeder SB, Widlus DM, Lazinger M. Low-dose thrombin injection to treat femoral artery pseudoaneurysm. AJR Am J Roentgenol 2001;177:595–598.

191. Sheiman RG, Brophy, DP. Treatment of iatrogenic femoral pseudoaneurysms with percutaneous thrombin injection: experience in 54 patients. Radiology 2002;222–293.

192. Baltacioglu F, Cimjit NC, Cil B, et al. Endovascular stent-graft applications in iatrogenic vascular injuries. Cardiovasc Intervent Radiol 2003;26:434–439.

193. Criado E, Marston WA, Ligush J, et al. Endovascular repair of peripheral aneurysms, pseudoaneurysms, and arteriovenous fistulas. Ann Vasc Surg 1997;11:256–263.

194. Marin WL, Veith FL, Panetta TF, et al. Percutaneous transfemoral insertion of a stented graft to repair a traumatic femoral arteriovenous fistula. J Vasc Surg 1993;18:299–302.

195. Belli AM, Cumberland DC, Knox AM, et al. The complications of percutaneous peripheral balloon angioplasty. Clin Radiol 1990;41:380–383.

196. Deiparine MK, Ballard JL, Taylor FL, et al. Endovascular stent infection. J Vasc Surg 1996;23:529–533.

197. Bukhari RH, Muck PE, Schlueter FH, et al. Bilateral renal stent infection and pseudoaneurysm formation. J Vasc Interv Radiol 2000;11:337–341.

198. Sheeran SR, Gestring MI, Murphy TP, et al. Endovascular graft-related iliac artery infection. J Vasc Interv Radiol 1999;10:877–882.

199. Therasse E, Soulez G, Cartier P, et al. Infection with fatal outcome after endovascular metallic stent placement. Radiology 1994;192:363–365.

200. Leung D, Spinosa D, Klaus D, et al. Selection of stents for treating iliac arterial occlusive disease. J Vasc Interv Radiol 2003;14:137–152.

201. Cynamon J, Marin ML, Veith FJ, et al. Stent-graft repair of aortoiliac occlusive disease coexisting with common femoral artery disease. J Vasc Interv Radiol 1997;8:19–26.

202. Duda SH, Bosiers M, Pusich B, et al. Endovascular treatment of peripheral artery disease with expanded PTFE-covered nitinol stents: interim analysis from a prospective controlled study. Cardiovasc Intervent Radiol 2002;25:413–418.

203. Cragg AH, Dake MD. Treatment of peripheral vascular disease with stent-grafts. Radiology 1996;205:307–314.

204. Lammer J, Dake MD, Bleyn J, et al. Peripheral arterial obstruction: prospective study of treatment with a transluminally placed self-expanding stent-graft. International Trial Study Group. Radio 2000;217:95–104.

205. Murphy TP. The role of stents in aortoiliac occlusive disease. In: Becker GJ, Perler BA, eds. Vascular Disease: Surgical and Interventional Management. New York: Thieme, 1998;111–135.

206. Reyes R, Maynar M, Lopera J, et al. Treatment of chronic iliac artery occlusions with glidewire recanalization and primary stent placement. J Vasc Interv Radiol 1997;8:1049–1055.

207. Schedel H, Wissgott C, Rademaker J, et al. Primary stent placement for infrarenal aortic stenosis: immediate and mid-term results. J Vasc Interv Radiol 2004;15:353–359.

208. Stoeckelhober BM, Meissner O, Stoeckelhober M, et al. Primary endovascular stent placement for focal infrarenal aortic stenosis: initial and mid-term results. J Vasc Interv Radiol 2003;14:1443–1447.

209. Nyman U, Uher P, Lindh M, et al. Primary stenting in infrarenal aortic occlusive disease. Cardiovasc Intervent Radiol 2000;23:97–108.

210. Therasse E, Cote G, Oliva UL, et al. Infrarenal aortic stenosis: value of stent placement after percutaneous transluminal angioplasty failure. Radiology 2001;219:655–662.

211. Elkouri S, Hudon G, Demers P, et al. Early and long-term results of percutaneous transluminal angioplasty of the lower abdominal aorta. J Vasc Surg 1999;30:679–692.

212. de Vries JP, van Den Heuvel DA, Vos JA, et al. Freedom from secondary interventions to treat stenotic disease after percutaneous transluminal angioplasty of infrarenal aorta: long-term results. J Vasc Surg 2004;39:427–431.

213. Feugier P, Toursarkissian B, Chevalier JM, et al. Endovascular treatment of isolated atherosclerotic stenosis of the infrarenal abdominal aortic: long-term results. Ann Vasc Surg 2003;375–385.

214. Hehrlein C, Weinschenk I, Metz J. Long period of balloon inflation and the implantation of stents potentiate smooth muscle cell death. Possible role of chronic vascular injury in restenosis. Int J Cardiovasc Intervent 1999;2:21–26.

Angiography of Lower Extremity Peripheral Vascular Disease

18

Geoffrey A. Gardiner Jr., Steven C. Wagner

The role of catheter angiography in patients with peripheral vascular disease has changed significantly within the last two decades. Although angiography was developed as a diagnostic tool, it is no longer the primary means of diagnosis in patients with symptoms of lower extremity arterial occlusive disease. That role has largely been assumed by noninvasive hemodynamic tests such as the ankle-brachial index (ABI) or segmental pulse-volume recording (PVR) in conjunction with a careful history and physical examination. Although catheter angiography is still occasionally used as a means of diagnosis in cases with confusing physical findings and equivocal results on hemodynamic testing, its primary role is currently related to documentation of the location and extent of vascular disease prior to interventional or surgical therapy.

Once the need for intervention has been established in a patient with peripheral vascular disease, catheter angiography is the gold standard method for demonstrating the precise site and severity of arterial lesions, which is essential for planning the appropriate treatment. Angiographic findings are the principle means of determining whether specific vascular lesions are best suited for surgical or endovascular treatment. In appropriate cases, transluminal interventions can be performed at the time of the diagnostic procedure.

The recent development of magnetic resonance angiography (MRA) and computed tomographic angiography (CTA) has permitted excellent visualization of the peripheral arteries in some patients, although reported sensitivity and specificity vary considerably from study to study when compared to catheter angiography (1,2). However, these techniques have shown rapid improvement in image quality, particularly with the use of multidetector CT and likely will play a major role in imaging patients with peripheral vascular disease in the future.

ANGIOGRAPHIC TECHNIQUES AND IMAGING PITFALLS

Although a clear understanding of arterial anatomy, anomalies, and collateral pathways is essential for adequate imaging and interpretation of lower extremity angiography, it is beyond the scope of this chapter. Also, the technical details of performing angiography, and the associated risks and complications will not be discussed, but should be well understood.

Interpreting angiography correctly depends to a large extent on good image quality. This has been well documented by angiographic studies of the coronary, renal, and carotid arteries, which have shown a direct relationship between reduced image quality and increased errors and variability in interpretations (3–7). Unlike most other methods of vascular imaging, image quality in catheter-based angiography depends greatly on the operator and requires technical skills and effective imaging techniques individualized for each patient. The combination of two factors—good vessel opacification and appropriate projections—is the key to image quality in angiography. This requires adequate contrast injection rates and volumes, multiple views of questionable lesions, and bilateral oblique projections in the pelvis. The use of special techniques to enhance blood vessel opacification in areas with poor blood flow is important.

This often includes selective contrast injections in the distal external iliac or femoral arteries for adequate visualization of the distal arteries below the knee.

Recent technical advances include the use of digital imaging, which has largely replaced film-screen angiography. Digital imaging has greatly simplified the selection of appropriate radiographic techniques and has resulted in much more consistent image quality. Although digital technique sacrifices some degree of spatial resolution, it has several other important advantages. One primary advantage is the reduced procedure time, because images are instantly available for review. Digital imaging also allows techniques such as "roadmapping," which is an invaluable technique to employ when catheterizing a particularly difficult artery or when crossing very narrow or irregular arterial lesions. Digital subtraction techniques also improve contrast resolution compared to film-screen angiography. This provides the ability to adequately visualize vessels that are only faintly opacified and permits the use of dilute contrast agents or CO_2, which may be important in patients with compromised renal function. In addition, nearly every angiographic equipment manufacturer now offers some type of dynamic imaging capability. This feature allows rapid field-of-view changes at the same time that images are being acquired. This permits "rotational angiography" in which the image intensifier rotates rapidly around a fixed axis giving multiple views of the same area from different angles, which could be very important when multiple crossing vessels are present or when arterial lesions are very eccentric or complex. It also permits visualization of the entire arterial system of the lower extremities during a single contrast injection when the field-of-view is moved down the legs as the contrast bolus is carried down the legs by the arterial blood flow.

Improved contrast agents have also had a major impact on the comfort and safety of angiographic procedures. The development of nonionic contrast agents has greatly reduced the frequency and severity of contrast-related reactions and may also contribute to less nephrotoxicity than did the older ionic agents. The most obvious improvement has been the greatly reduced discomfort caused by the injection of contrast agents into arteries supplying muscle or skin. The extreme sensation of heat caused by the older contrast agents was painful enough that patients often refused to have additional angiographic studies after their initial experience. Angiography now is associated with only minor discomfort that results mostly from the injection of the local anesthetic. Contrast injections of isosmolar agents, such as iodixanol, are associated with only a very mild sensation of warmth, with no pain.

Knowing the common imaging pitfalls is an important step in preventing errors in angiographic interpretation. Because atherosclerotic plaques tend to occur along the posterior wall of the aorta and iliac arteries, significant luminal narrowing may occur and yet be difficult to detect on standard AP projections. Also, the anterior-posterior course of the iliac arteries makes oblique views of these vessels essential in avoiding, missing, or underestimating the severity of arterial lesions. The omission of these views may explain, in large part, the lack of correlation between hemodynamic or surgical findings and angiographic imaging (8–13). Oblique views of the pelvic arteries are also necessary to evaluate the femoral and iliac bifurcations adequately (14–20). Overlapping arteries in the pelvis, thighs, and distally in the calves may also require multiple views to visualize each arterial segment clearly. More than one view of eccentric lesions at any location may be necessary in determining true hemodynamic significance (Figures 18–1 and 18–2). In cases in which the significance

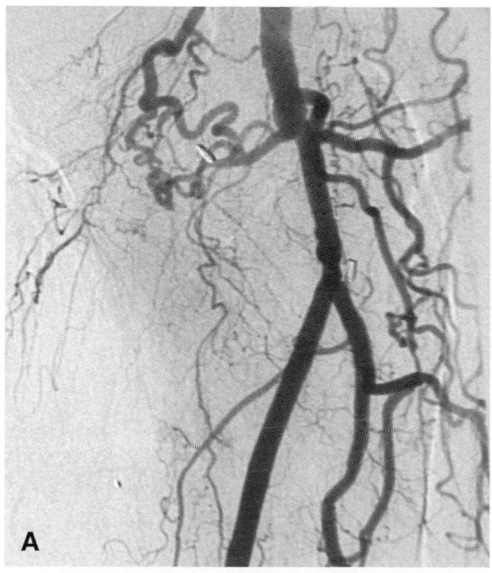 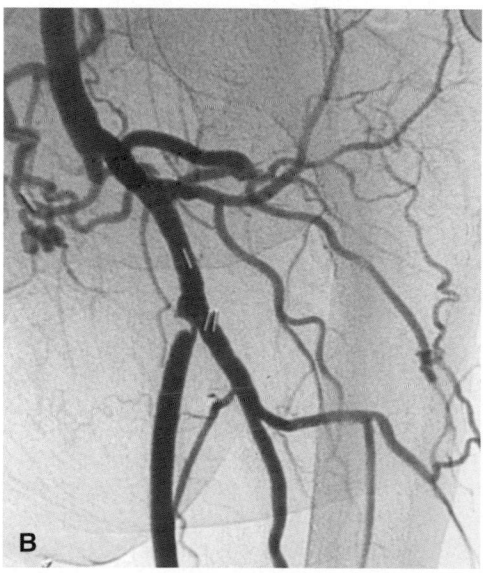

Figure 18–1   Graft origin from the deep femoral artery. **A.** Apparently normal in this view. **B.** Obvious severe stenosis in this oblique view.

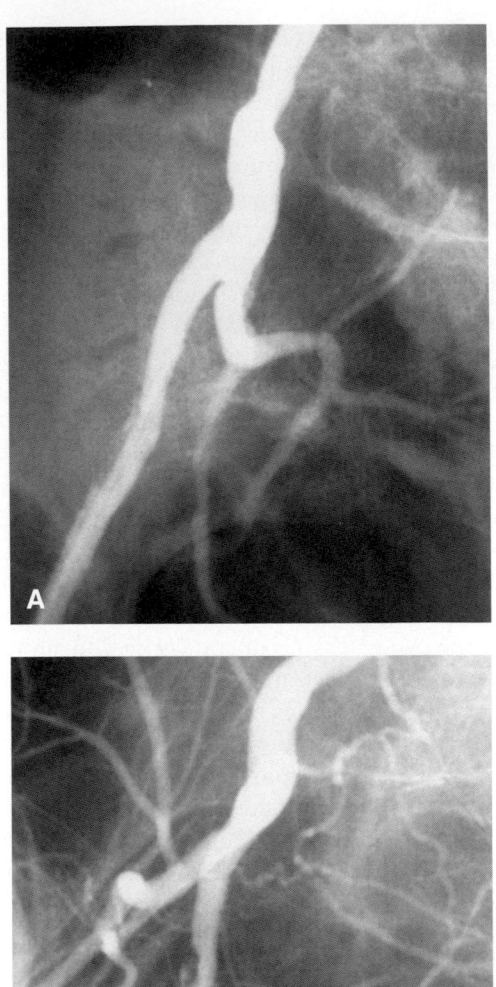

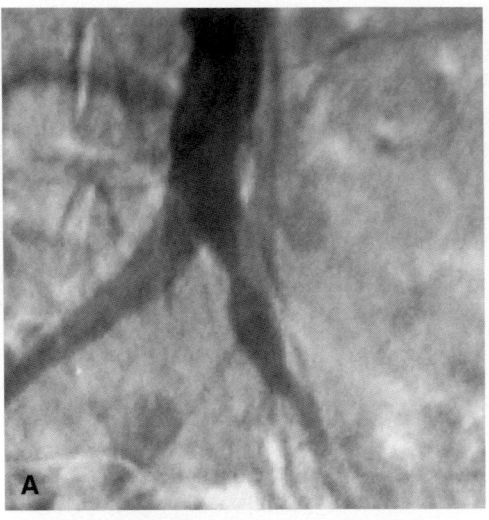

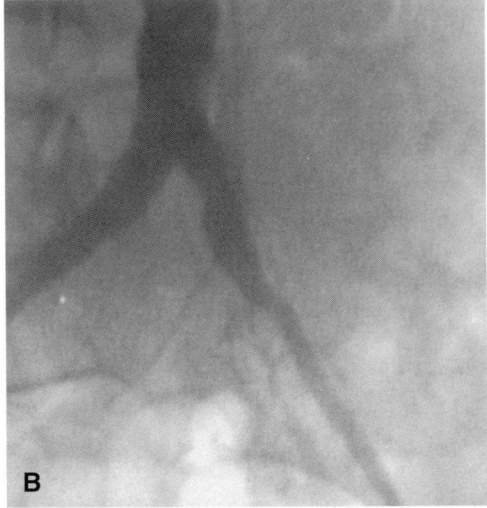

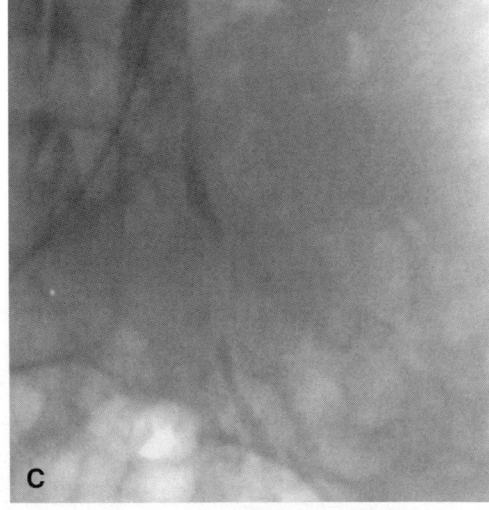

Figure 18–2   Complex plaque in the right external iliac artery. **A.** Only minimal irregularity and no luminal narrowing in this view. **B.** Large, irregular, intraluminal plaque with much greater luminal compromise is evident on this view.

of an arterial lesion is in question, the hemodynamic effect often can be determined by direct catheter measurement of pressure gradients.

Subtraction artifacts may cause the erroneous diagnosis of a vascular lesion produced by overlying densities such as surgical clips, bone cortex, or contrast in the urinary tract (Figure 18–3). The false diagnosis of vascular occlusion (pseudo-occlusion) can occur when severe stenosis prevents or delays adequate opacification or when retrograde filling of a vessel is not appreciated

Figure 18–3   Subtraction artifact. **A.** Digital subtraction arteriogram showing significant left common iliac artery stenosis. **B.** Same image, unsubtracted, showing no narrowing of the left common iliac artery. **C.** Early arterial phase, unsubtracted, showing contrast in left ureter. Superimposed contrast in the ureter caused misdiagnosis of arterial stenosis.

because of the faulty timing of image acquisition. This same factor may also lead to a false interpretation of the length of an occlusion. Also, when opacification of the entire vessel lumen is not accomplished because of inadequate injection rates or dilated (aneurysmal) arteries, flow dynamics and the effects of the specific gravity of contrast may cause layering of contrast posteriorly, which can result in nonopacification of arteries that originate or course anteriorly.

The false impression of an arterial lesion in the distal anterior tibial or dorsalis pedis artery can be caused by extrinsic compression of the artery by underlying bone or external restraints. This is known as the "ballerina defect" (Figure 18–4) and is caused when the foot is forced into excessive plantar flexion (21).

An interesting phenomenon usually seen in the medium-sized arteries of the thigh or calf is known as "standing or stationary waves" (Figure 18–5). This angiographic finding produces an arterial segment of very regular, periodic constrictions and dilatations, which have been described as "corrugated arteries" or "string of pearls"

(22–24). Various theories have been advanced to explain this phenomenon usually based on some form of vascular spasm or response of the vessel wall to the mechanical injection of contrast (25). This appearance is not a fixed deformity and will often resolve with administration of a sympatholytic drug. Because this deformity has not been associated with flow limitation, its only clinical significance seems to be that it not be mistaken for a true vascular lesion.

ATHEROSCLEROTIC VASCULAR DISEASE

Atherosclerosis is the predominant cause of lower extremity ischemia, although in younger patients or in patients with atypical histories or physical findings, nonatherosclerotic diseases should be considered. Atherosclerotic plaques commonly calcify and produce focal, patchy, irregular calcifications in the intima of the arterial wall. These calcifications are easily seen on plain radiographs of the extremities and should be distinguished from the

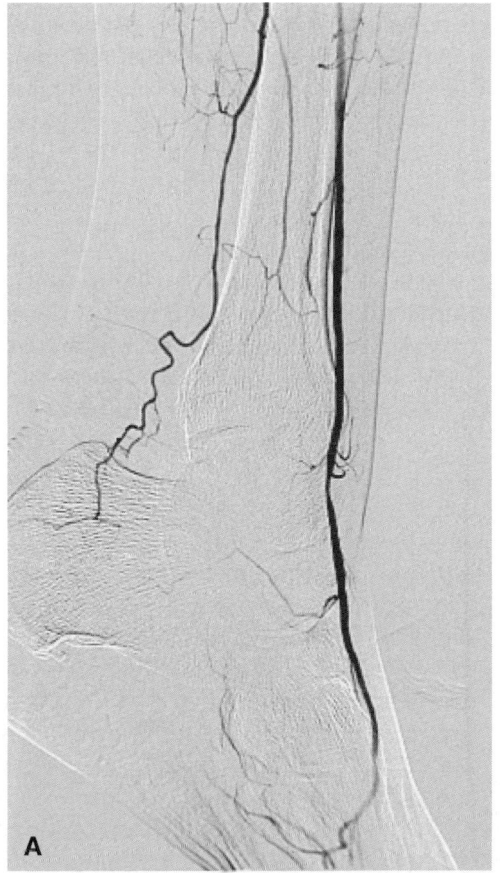
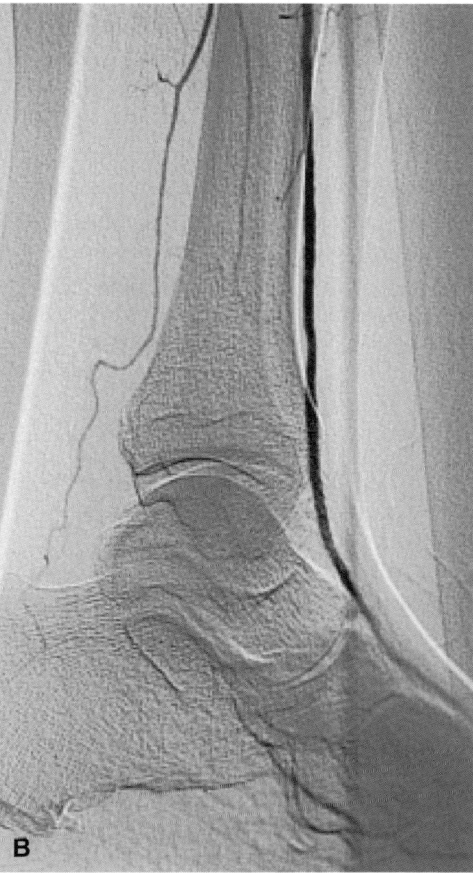

Figure 18–4 Ballerina defect. **A.** With the foot fully planter-flexed, moderate narrowing is evident in the distal anterior tibial artery. **B.** No arterial lesion is present with foot in neutral position.

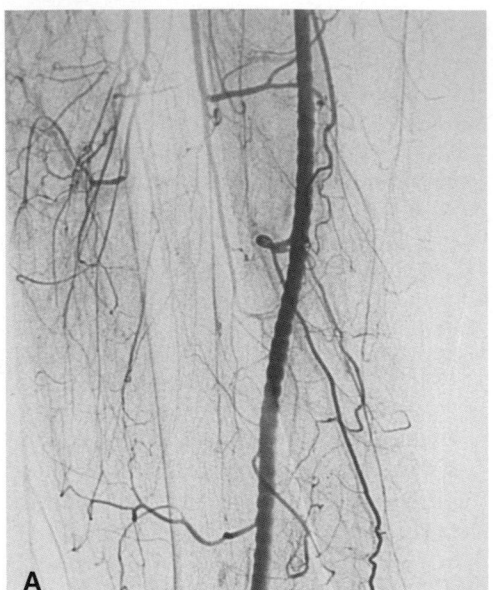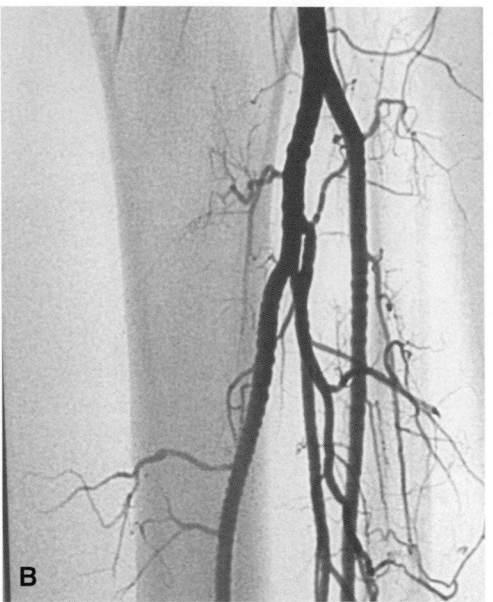

Figure 18-5   Standing waves in the **A.** superficial femoral artery and **B.** proximal tibial arteries.

calcification that occurs in the medial arterial wall, known as Monckeberg's medial sclerosis (Figure 18–6). This type of calcification has a uniform, smooth, or finely granular appearance and is circumferential and diffuse in distribution, often producing an appearance described as a "tramline." It occurs in muscular arteries and is most commonly found in the medium- and small-sized arteries of the extremities, especially in the lower extremity, but has also been reported in the mesenteric and visceral arteries. The precise cause of this phenomenon is unknown, but it is found most frequently in patients with chronic renal failure and type II diabetes, especially when neuropathy is present (26–30). It has also been associated with metabolic bone disease (especially osteoporosis) and chronic corticosteroid therapy (31). Although not associated with luminal narrowing and originally thought to have no clinical significance, it is now believed to be an independent predictor of cardiovascular morbidity and mortality (32–34).

Atherosclerotic plaques are typically classified as eccentric or concentric, simple or complex, and calcified or noncalcified. Plaques may have a wide variety of angiographic appearances, ranging from diffuse, relatively smooth narrowing of long arterial segments to very focal web-like lesions. Occasionally, plaques have a polypoid appearance with a very irregular, rounded mass extending into the lumen from a relatively narrow base. Little is known about the correlation between angiographic lesion morphology and clinical implications, such as long-term plaque stability or progression of disease in lower extremity

arteries. In the coronary arteries, the clinical syndrome of "unstable" or "crescendo" angina has been associated with complex arterial plaques (35). These are plaques that have ruptured or ulcerated and have certain angiographic features, including irregular or poorly defined margins, overhanging edges producing acute angles at the lesion border, and intraluminal filling defects. These plaques are thought to be at high risk of acute thrombotic occlusion. The analogous clinical scenario in the extremities might be blue toe syndrome.

Blue toe syndrome is a condition usually associated with distal microembolization of fibrinoplatelet debris or material containing cholesterol-crystals to the digital arteries from proximal arterial lesions, although other causes of this clinical picture do exist (36,37). In the classic scenario, patients present with rapid onset of discolored and painful toes with intact pedal pulses. Identifying the responsible arterial lesion or lesions is one of the key objectives of successful treatment. Acute occlusion in a proximal artery or an isolated arterial stenosis in the involved extremity is easily identified as the probable source of emboli. Aneurysms may also be the source of emboli. When multiple arterial lesions or diffuse arterial diseases are present, however, localizing the embolic source becomes much more difficult and may sometimes present a formidable clinical challenge. The responsible arterial lesion may or may not be a hemodynamically significant stenosis, but it often displays the characteristics of unstable plaque (complex lesions). Involvement of digits in both feet suggests that the responsible lesion is proximal

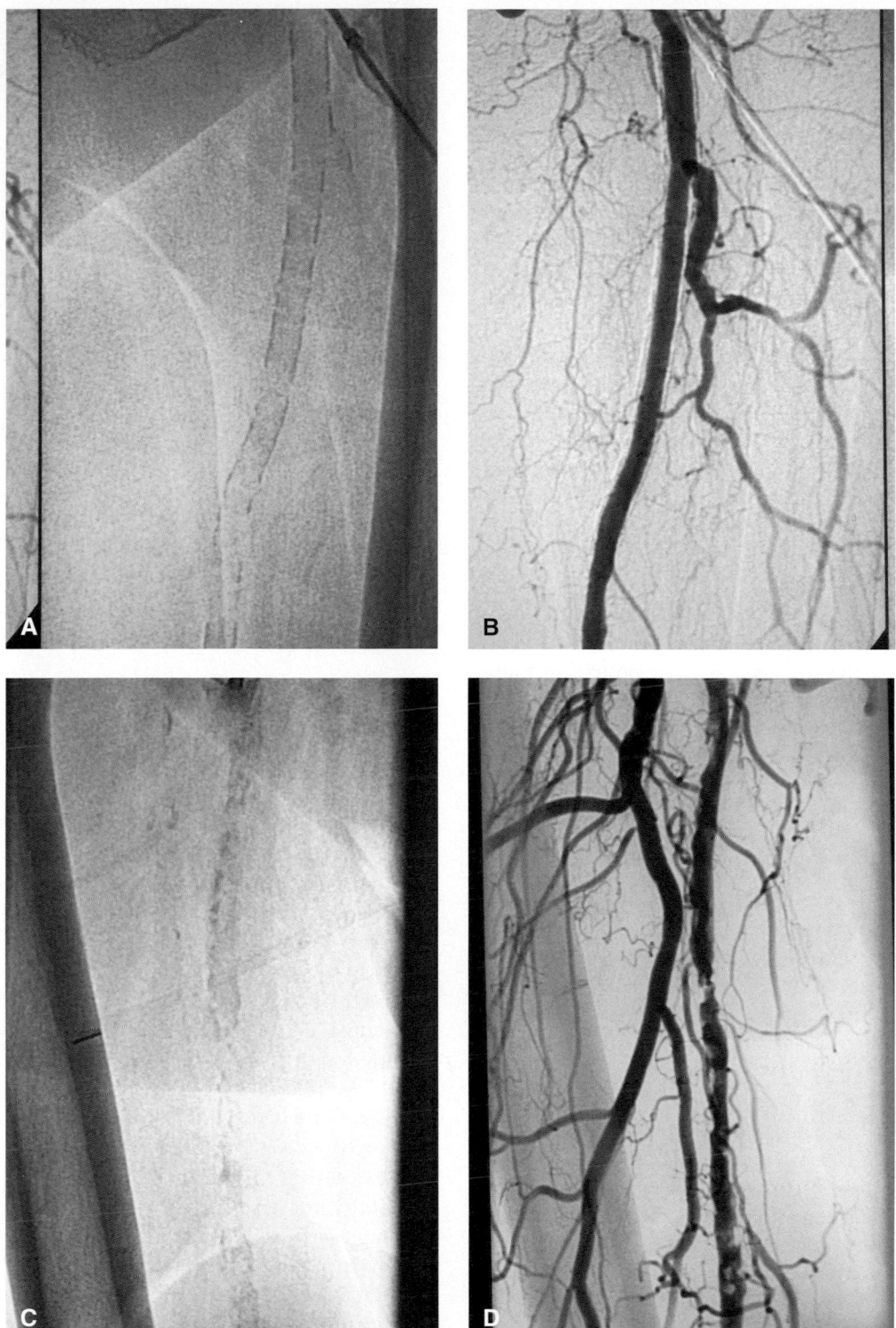

Figure 18–6   Vascular calcification. **A.** Calcification of the superficial femoral artery from Monckeberg's medial sclerosis **B.** with normal arterial lumen. **C.** Calcified superficial femoral artery from atherosclerosis **D.** with narrowing and irregularity of the arterial lumen.

to the aortic bifurcation, although embolic sources from the aorta may produce unilateral symptoms because of flow patterns (38,39). Searches for the embolic source when both feet are involved should always include the descending thoracic aorta. In patients with unilateral symptoms, the source lesions are usually distal to the aortic bifurcation. Medical therapy with antiplatelet agents or anticoagulants remains controversial without surgical or endovascular treatment of the embolic source. Recurrent embolic episodes occur in a high percent of patients (40,41), with the end result being extensive tissue infarction (42,43).

Complex coronary artery plaques have also been associated with more rapid progression of stenosis compared to smooth or simple plaques (44). Similar studies based on lesion morphology have not been performed in the lower extremities, although one study found that in superficial femoral arteries, severity of stenosis was predictive of progression to occlusion and that smooth-asymmetric lesions progressed more slowly than others (45). However, progression of disease is difficult to predict. Severe lesions may remain stable for years, whereas seemingly insignificant lesions may suddenly cause luminal occlusion. Occlusion of the proximal arteries has been noted to protect the more distal arteries, with a result of slower progression of disease (46). The authors have observed several cases in which arteries beyond a proximal occlusion have been entirely free of disease despite severe and widespread atherosclerosis in the other extremity.

The distribution of atherosclerotic lesions in lower extremity arteries is surprisingly symmetrical in most patients. A fairly strong correlation exists between the extent of disease and clinical presentation, although clinical symptoms may not be a good measure of angiographic progression of disease (47). Patients with claudication usually have flow-limiting vascular lesions at one level—pelvis, thighs, or calves—compared to patients with limb-threatening ischemia in which multiple proximal and distal arteries are involved.

In most cases, the earliest angiographic evidence of peripheral vascular disease occurs first in the superficial femoral artery, especially at or near the adductor canal (48). Certain diseases associated with atherosclerosis have atypical and characteristic angiographic patterns of arterial involvement. Patients with diabetes have an increased frequency and severity of symptoms related to peripheral vascular disease. Some have questioned the concept of microvascular disease in diabetes (49,50). Instead, accelerated atherosclerosis largely confined to the infrapopliteal arteries in the calf is commonly demonstrated (51,52). The severity of disease correlates well with the duration of diabetes, independent of patient age (53,54). Interestingly, the proximal lower extremity arteries seem to be relatively spared and, in fact,

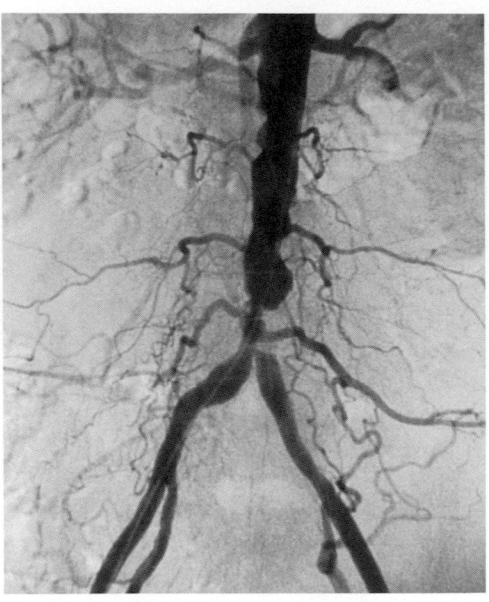

Figure 18–7 Premature atherosclerosis. The distal vessels are entirely normal.

seem to have less involvement than typical nondiabetic patients who have peripheral vascular disease (55), producing the classic angiographic findings of normal proximal vessels with severe disease in the tibial and peroneal arteries. The increased severity of symptoms may be, in part, the result of impaired collateral formation, which has been demonstrated in the heart (56).

Premature atherosclerosis is usually defined as symptomatic arterial obstruction in patients younger than 50 years of age (57). It is often associated with a positive family history (58) and may be associated with hyperlipidemia (59). Some studies have demonstrated a high incidence of hypercoagulable states in these patients (60). As opposed to diabetic vascular disease, premature atherosclerosis usually occurs in the proximal arteries, mainly the distal aorta and iliac arteries (61,62) (Figure 18–7). Within this subgroup of patients, a specific clinical entity known as hypoplastic aortoiliac syndrome has been described. This syndrome occurs almost exclusively in young women who are heavy smokers (63). Characteristically, the infrarenal aorta is tapered with maximum narrowing at the aortic bifurcation. The iliac arteries are diffusely narrowed and straight, forming an acute angle at their origins. Symptoms of lower extremity ischemia are believed to result from the combination of the small-caliber arteries and superimposed atherosclerotic plaque. Traditionally, these patients have been considered difficult to treat because they require multiple procedures and suffer many complications.

DEVELOPMENTAL ANOMALY

Persistent sciatic artery is a rare developmental anomaly that occurs in approximately 0.05% of patients (64). The sciatic artery is the axis artery in the embryo and is replaced almost completely by the femoral artery by the third month of gestation. In cases of a persistent sciatic artery, the femoral arteries are hypoplastic, and the sciatic artery—originating from the internal iliac artery—becomes the dominant blood supply to the lower extremity. The sciatic artery courses posteriorly through the greater sciatic notch, then moves posteriorly down the thigh and joins the popliteal artery at the knee. The anomaly is bilateral in up to one third of patients (65,66). This anomaly may be initially suspected in patients found to have normal distal pulses but a weak or absent femoral pulse. When symptomatic, patients may present with claudication or sciatic neuropathy. The sciatic artery is prone to aneurysmal degeneration and may present as a pulsatile buttock mass or as limb-threatening ischemia, the result of distal embolization (67). Angiography shows an enlarged internal iliac artery with a large anomalous branch extending inferiorly and posteriorly to run lateral to the normal position of the superficial femoral artery in the thigh. The external iliac and femoral arteries are hypoplastic.

ANEURYSMS AND ARTERIOMEGALY

Arteriomegaly is a term used to describe a condition in which diffuse arterial enlargement is associated with slow blood flow. Although the exact criteria for diagnosis remain imprecise, arteriomegaly appears to represent a distinct pathologic entity. For many years, the condition was considered a form of atherosclerosis. However, recent studies have demonstrated loss of elastin in the medial layer of the arterial wall, and a defect in elastin formation is now believed to be related to pathogenesis (68). Arteriomegaly usually involves males (90%) who are at an average age of 70 years. The condition most often involves the lower extremity arteries, but it has been found in other arteries, including the coronary arteries. The incidence of arteriomegaly in one study was approximately 6% of patients who had peripheral vascular disease (69). The process of arterial enlargement is believed to begin centrally (iliac arteries) and progress distally. It mainly affects the major arteries, with relatively normal-sized muscular branch arteries. Patients with arteriomegaly present most often with a history of claudication, but as many as 35% may present with acute ischemia related to the two main complications of arteriomegaly: acute thrombosis with or without distal embolization and arterial aneurysms (70). The slow arterial flow related to the large vessel diameter may be a predisposing factor in the development of

thrombosis and embolization. Up to two thirds of patients with arteriomegaly have multiple aneurysms, which are found most often in the aorta and popliteal arteries (71–73). Aneurysms of the femoral and iliac arteries are also common. Angiographic imaging can be difficult because blood flow is often extraordinarily slow. Findings include large redundant pelvic arteries, diffusely enlarged distal arteries—sometimes extending to the level of the ankle, with minimal luminal irregularity—and multiple aneurysms (Figure 18–8).

Popliteal artery aneurysms are the most common peripheral arterial aneurysm (74). They usually occur in elderly males (95%) and are commonly bilateral (50–70%) (75,76). More than half of all patients with popliteal aneurysms have aneurysms at other locations (21% of unilateral popliteal aneurysm), most commonly in the abdominal aorta (30–50%) (77). Therefore, in the presence of popliteal aneurysms, a careful search for other aneurysms should be performed. Many patients with popliteal aneurysms are asymptomatic. Symptomatic patients may develop claudication, rest pain, or acute limb-threatening ischemia as a result of acute thrombosis and distal embolization. Less often, symptoms are related to venous or nerve compression. Rupture is rare, occurring in only 2–3% (77).

Most popliteal aneurysms are fusiform and involve the proximal popliteal artery. Angiography usually demonstrates an enlarged, tortuous popliteal artery (Figure 18–9A). Rarely, the lumen may be almost normal in diameter because of layered thrombus, and the only sign of an aneurysm may be the absence of the usually popliteal artery side branches. An aneurysm should always be suspected in an occluded popliteal artery when a popliteal aneurysm is found on the opposite side (Figure 18–9B). A key role of angiography in these patients is to document the condition of the distal arteries, because embolization is common and the status of the distal arteries is a major determinant of surgical outcome.

NONATHEROSCLEROTIC VASCULAR OCCLUSIVE DISEASE

There are many interesting nonatherosclerotic causes of vascular disease in the lower extremities. However, they are fairly rare and are usually discovered in younger patients or in patients with other predisposing conditions. Nonatherosclerotic disease should be suspected in the appropriate clinical setting, when angiography shows an isolated lesion and otherwise normal arteries. The etiology can be determined, to a large degree, by knowledge of the clinical history and the arterial segment or segments involved.

Cystic adventitial disease is a rare condition in which a mucin-containing cyst forms in the adventitial layer of the arterial wall, causing luminal narrowing or arterial occlusion.

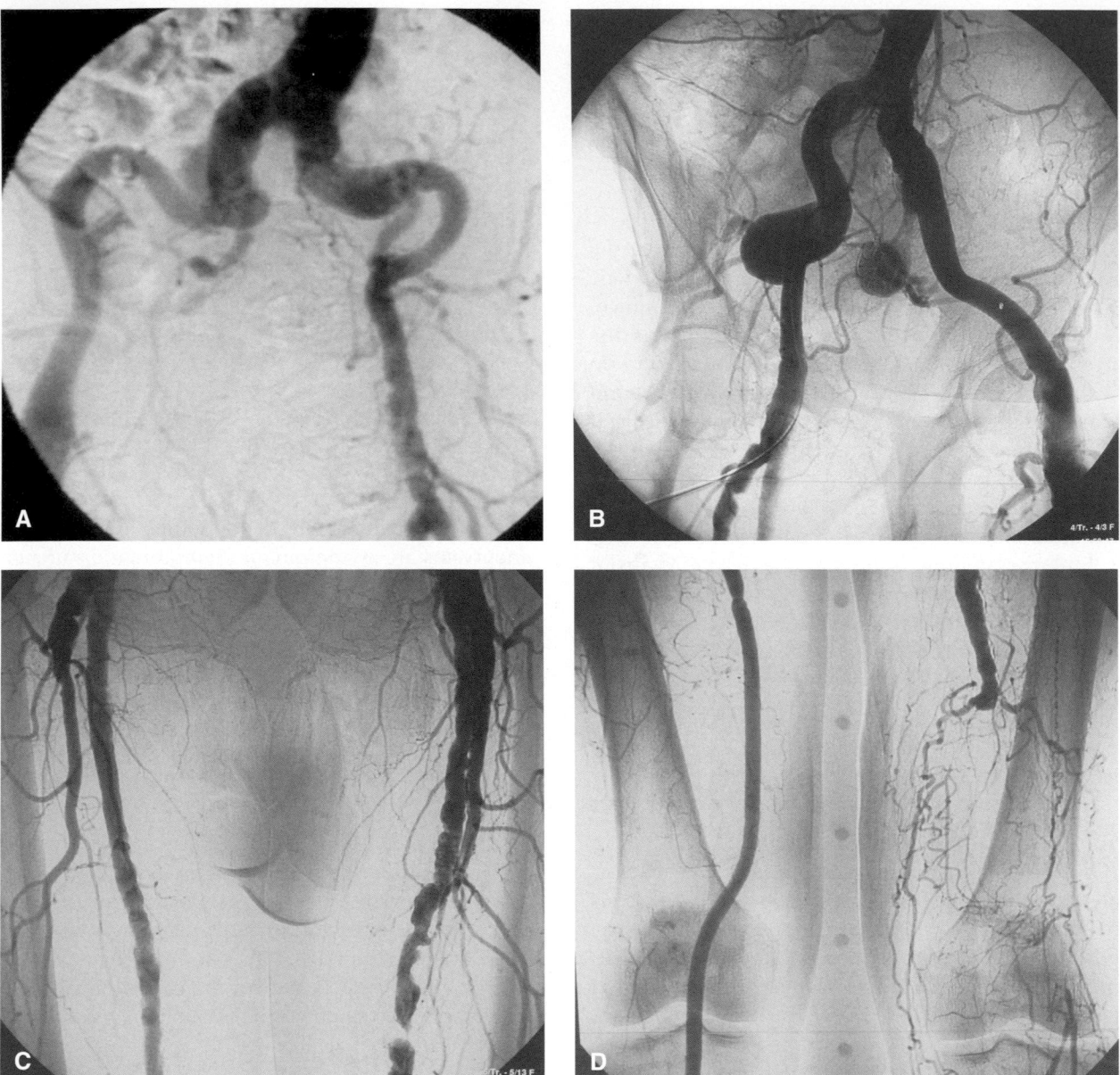

Figure 18–8 Arteriomegaly. **A.** Large iliac arteries may be very tortuous. **B.** Large iliac arteries with aneurysms. **C.** Large superficial femoral arteries with superimposed atherosclerosis. **D.** Occlusion of left popliteal artery from thrombosed aneurysm.

Most cases are found in young males (80–90%) with claudication (78). Typically, patients report a sudden onset of symptoms, and there may be intervals of exacerbation and remission. Although the disease has been reported in various arteries, the majority occurs in the popliteal artery (87%), with the next most frequent site being the external iliac/common femoral arteries (10%) (79). The disease is always a single, unilateral lesion. The cyst itself is rarely palpable, but distal pulses may become diminished or lost with leg flexion (Ishikawa's sign) (80). Several theories have been proposed regarding the cause of the cysts. The two most

popular are the synovial or ganglion theory (81), in which the cysts are believed to represent synovial or ganglion cysts, caused by herniation of synovium from an adjacent joint; and the embryological theory, which suggests that the cysts arise from mesenchymal cell rests incorporated into the vessel wall during development (79). The cysts are always located near joint spaces and, in some cases, have been found to have anatomic communication with the knee joint capsule (82).

Angiography typically shows a smoothly tapered, curvilinear, or spiral stenosis, usually involving the proximal

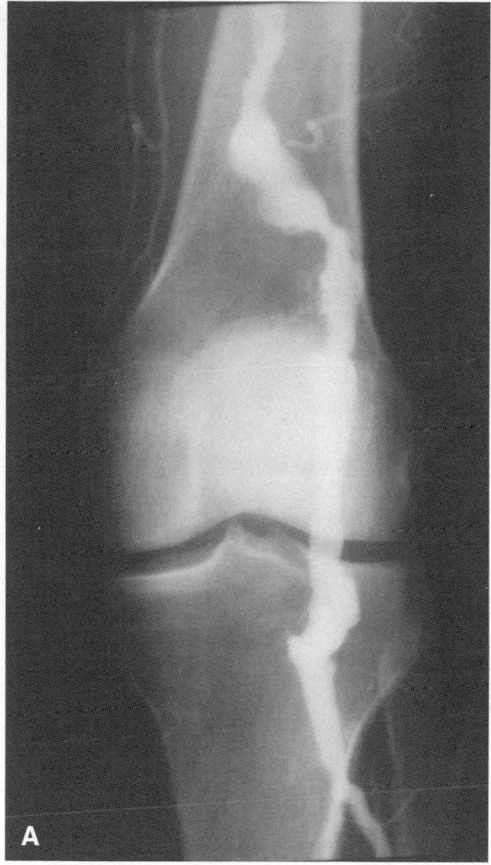

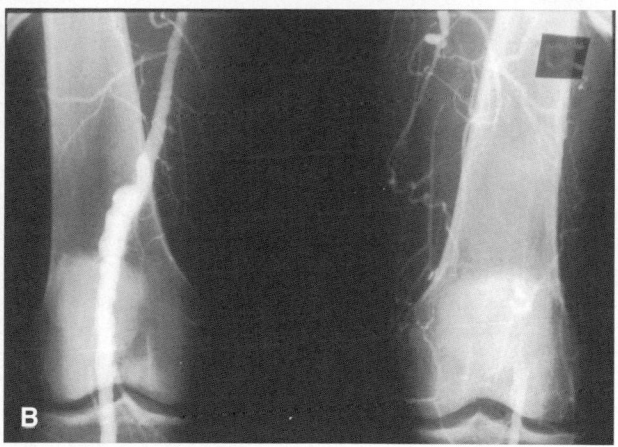

Figure 18–9 Popliteal aneurysm. **A.** Typical appearance of a popliteal aneurysm. In this case, the entire popliteal artery is involved. **B.** Bilateral popliteal aneurysms with thrombosis on one side.

popliteal artery above the level of the knee joint (Figure 18–10). When the cysts are concentric, the stenosis may have an "hourglass" configuration, but more commonly, they are eccentric producing the classic saber- or scimitar-shaped stenosis (83). Characteristically, poststenotic dilatation is absent and collaterals are not well-developed. The cysts may be multiloculated and extend over many centimeters. Because the endothelial layer of the artery wall remains intact, distal embolization is very rare and occlusion often occurs without thrombosis. Therefore, limb-threatening ischemia is rare. Duplex ultrasound examination shows intramural cysts that appear as anechoic or hypoechoic masses (84,85).

Popliteal artery entrapment is a rare disorder caused by an abnormal anatomic relationship between the popliteal artery and the adjacent musculotendinous structures, primarily the medial head of the gastrocnemius. Several classifications of popliteal entrapment have been described. The most commonly used classification defines five major types based on anatomic variations (86,87). However, not all cases fit neatly into any single category. In type 1, the abnormality is based on an anomalous arterial course, with the popliteal artery deviated medially around the normally positioned medial head of the gastrocnemius.

This was originally thought to be the most common type, but better imaging techniques have not confirmed this early claim, which was probably related to the fact that this type is easiest to diagnose. Type 2 occurs when the medial head of the gastrocnemius originates abnormally from the intercondylar notch, lateral to its normal position, and passing between the artery and vein. In type 3, an accessory slip or a portion of the medial gastrocnemius head originates from the intercondylar notch. This is sometimes described as a broad-based attachment of the medical head of the gastrocnemius, which encircles the popliteal artery. Types 2 or 3 are found variously to be the most common types when provocative maneuvers are used for diagnosis. Type 4 occurs when the popliteal artery courses abnormally beneath the popliteus muscle or fibrous band. Type 5 is defined as any abnormality involving both the artery and vein. The popliteal vein is involved in approximately 4–11% of reported cases (88,89). Additionally, "functional" popliteal artery entrapment can occur in patients with normal anatomy; however, these patients are usually asymptomatic (90).

Patients with popliteal entrapment are usually young males who tend to be athletic. They usually present with claudication or complaints of leg weakness. Symptoms are

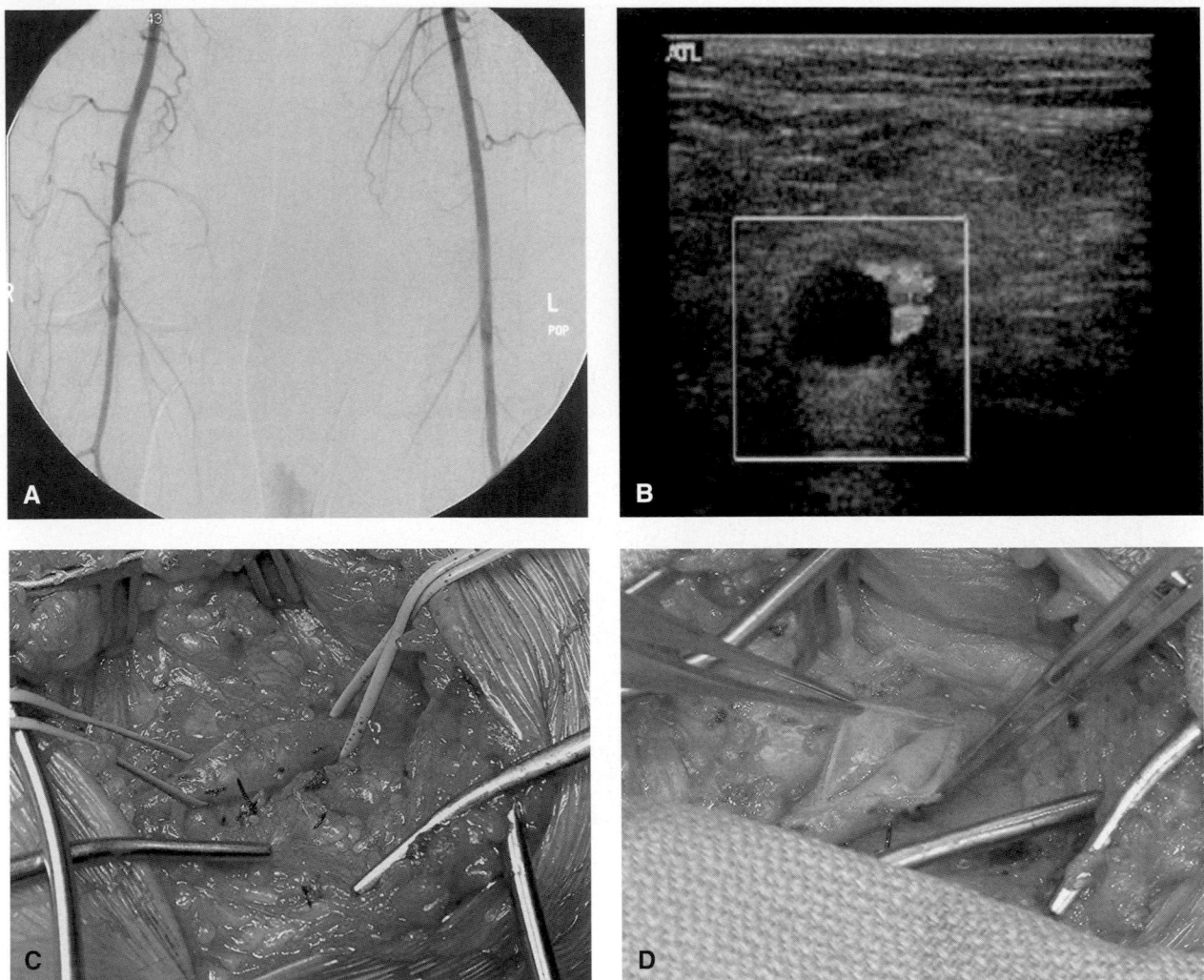

Figure 18–10 **A.** Cystic adventitial disease with eccentric, tapered scimitar-shaped stenosis. **B.** Ultrasound showing compression of lumen by echolucent mass. **C.** Localized bulge in the artery with direct visualization at surgery. **D.** with normal underlying artery once decompressed by incision of cyst. See Figure 18–10C, D in color insert. (Carin Gonsalves, MD—Thomas Jefferson University Hospital)

usually unilateral, despite the presence of the anomaly in both legs in approximately two thirds of patients (89,91). The claudication symptoms, however, may have unusual features. The phrase "paradoxical claudication" has been used to describe symptoms that occur with standing or walking, but not with running or riding a bike; or they may occur in some sports but not others. Claudication may also be associated with paresthesias or numbness of the foot. As opposed to cystic adventitial disease, approximately 5–10% of patients with popliteal entrapment present with acute limb-threatening ischemia (88).

The site of arterial pathology is very similar to cystic adventitial disease, usually located in the proximal popliteal artery and just above the level of the knee joint. Arterial compression and repetitive microtrauma can cause stenosis,

thrombosis with distal embolization, and, rarely, aneurysm formation (Figure 18–11). Angiography may demonstrate poststenotic dilation and extensive collateral formation, rarely seen in cystic adventitial disease. Medial deviation of the popliteal artery may be demonstrated but is present in a minority of cases. Provocative maneuvers with passive dorsiflexion or active plantar flexion are essential for diagnosis (92,93). Multiple views of the popliteal artery may be necessary because the arterial narrowing may be difficult to visualize on the standard AP view. Popliteal artery entrapment is a progressive disorder, and it can result in limb-threatening ischemia if left untreated. Early surgical treatment is indicated and has better results when thrombolysis, thrombectomy, or bypass surgery is not required (94,95).

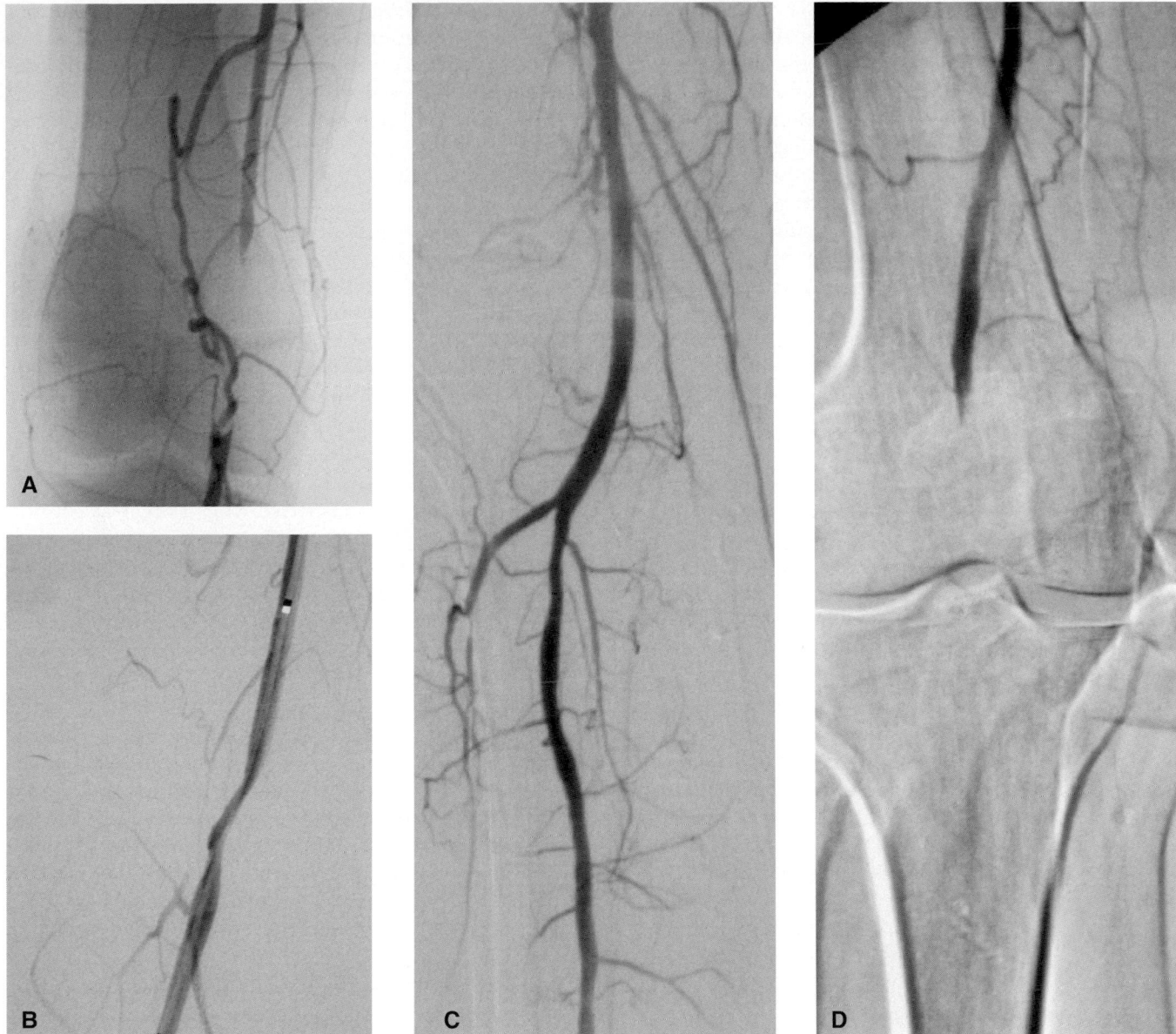

Figure 18–11 Popliteal artery entrapment. **A.** Acute thrombosis of popliteal artery. **B.** Successfully treated by intra-arterial thrombolysis. **C.** Normal-appearing popliteal artery with leg at rest. **D.** Complete occlusion with forceful plantar flexion. (Chris Peeters, MD—University of Pennsylvania)

A similar, but rarely documented, entity has been reported at the adductor canal, known as the adductor canal syndrome (96–99). This syndrome is caused by extrinsic compression of the distal superficial femoral artery by an abnormal musculotendinous band at the outlet of the adductor canal. Clinical presentation and patient population are very similar to popliteal entrapment, with claudication in young, active males. But associated neurologic symptoms, including numbness, tingling, and hypesthesia, seem to be more common. Angiography typically demonstrates a short segment occlusion at the adductor canal, which may occur without thrombosis. Proximally and distally, the arteries are normal.

Lower extremity compartment syndrome may be an acute or chronic condition. Acute compartment syndrome may result from blunt trauma, vascular injury, myositis, or as a complication of arterial revascularization in a severely ischemic extremity. Cases of chronic compartment syndrome are usually related to chronic repetitive overuse injury (100–103). Compartment syndrome may present clinically with parasthesia, pain on passive stretch, and paresis (104). Chronic compartment syndrome often produces atypical claudication associated with isolated muscle cramping and swelling after prolonged activity (100). Patients often are young athletes involved in activities such as soccer and endurance running. Physical examination may reveal diminished pedal pulses, swelling, and firmness of the lower leg. Compartment syndrome is diagnosed by compartment pressure measurements >25 mm Hg (105). ABIs and PVRs may show diminished blood flow to the lower leg. MR imaging of compartment syndrome may show areas of intramuscular edema, hemorrhage, or necrosis (102). Angiography has demonstrated smooth, diffuse, or generalized arterial narrowing with slow blood flow in arteries of the affected compartments (103). Prompt treatment with surgical fasciotomy is required to prevent tissue ischemia.

Radiation arteritis is a rare sequela of radiation therapy and has been reported in various arteries, most frequently in the carotid artery, upper extremity, and lower extremity arteries. In the lower extremities, the external iliac arteries are most commonly affected as a result of patients undergoing external beam radiotherapy for pelvic malignancies, such as cervical or rectal carcinoma. It has been suggested that a dose of 3,950 to 8,000 Gy over a relatively short period is necessary to produce arterial damage (106). Radiation-induced changes in the medium and large arteries are divided into acute and chronic phases. Acute changes involve damage to the endothelial cells with subendothelial accumulation of foam cells and hemorrhage in the arterial wall. Chronic changes include intimal thickening, medial necrosis and fibrosis, and adventitial and periarterial fibrosis associated with obliteration of the vasa vasorum (107). In the acute phase, patients may rarely present with arterial wall disruption and sudden hemorrhage (108). Chronically, symptoms resulting from arterial damage may not develop for years after treatment. Radiation leads to acceleration of atheromatous plaque, producing the typical arteriographic findings associated with atherosclerosis. In the authors' experience, however, angiography more often demonstrates isolated, smooth, segmental, and rather uniform lumenal narrowing probably caused by connective tissue proliferation and compression of the arterial lumen by periarterial fibrosis.

Thromboangiitis obliterans, or Buerger's disease, is a rare, nonatherosclerotic, inflammatory vaso-occlusive disorder of unknown etiology that affects the small- and medium-sized arteries and veins of the arms and legs (109–112), although a variety of vascular beds have been affected. The disease usually begins in the distal arteries of the hands and feet and progresses proximally. The lower extremities are involved earliest, but the upper extremities are eventually involved in nearly 90% of cases, although

fewer than half become symptomatic (111). Typically, patients are male smokers who are younger than 40 years of age (females account for 8–20% of cases). Multiple possible clinical presentations exist; foot claudication in a young male smoker is almost pathognomonic. A characteristic discoloration of the digits is present, and these digits may become cold and painful. Gangrene and ulceration of fingers or toes may precede claudication symptoms. Recurrent migrating, superficial thrombophlebitis is present in approximately 40% of patients (109,111).

The pathologic finding in acute lesions is an occlusive, hypercellular thrombus with giant cells and microabscesses. Inflammatory cells are also present in the arterial wall, but to a lesser extent. The internal elastic membrane remains intact. Chronically, fibrous thickening of the arterial wall and recanalization of the thrombus are present. Angiographic findings typically show long, tapered stenoses ending in occlusion (113). Multiple segmental occlusions may be interspersed with "skip areas" of normal artery. Usually, an extensive collateral network exists with typical "corkscrew," "root-like," or a "spider legs" appearance. The disease is more pronounced distally; proximally, the arteries are normal. Discontinuation of smoking is the only proven means of halting progression of the disease.

Ergotism, or ergotamine-induced vasoconstriction, is a very rare disorder associated with the use of ergot derivatives. The incidence of ergotism is estimated to be 0.001–0.002% of patients using ergotamine preparations (114). These medications are often used in the treatment of migraine headaches. Chronic prolonged therapy is the usual history. Vasoconstriction occurs by stimulation of the alpha-adrenergic and 5–hydroxytryptamine (5–HT) receptors, resulting in ischemic effects. Patients are often young women being treated for migraines who have developed claudication and painful burning of the affected limb. Angiography may show generalized arterial spasm, with areas of long, tapered stenosis, possibly leading to occlusion, filling defects consistent with thrombus, and formation of collateral vessels (114, 115). The use of intra-arterial vasodilators can confirm, but not exclude, the diagnosis of vasospasm. Treatment includes discontinuation of the ergotamine, oral vasodilator therapy, and even the use of anticoagulation and antiplatelet agents as prophylaxis for thrombosis because the vasoconstrictive effects may continue several weeks after discontinuation (114).

Fibromuscular dysplasia is an arteriopathy of unknown etiology in which noninflammatory, fibrotic tissue proliferates within the arterial wall. Fibromuscular dysplasia most commonly occurs in the renal and carotid arteries. In the lower extremities, it usually involves the external iliac arteries, but may occur in the femoral and popliteal arteries as well (116–118). Most patients with external iliac artery

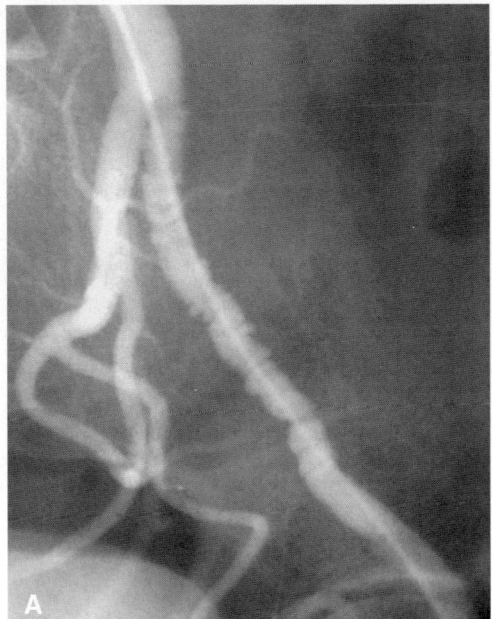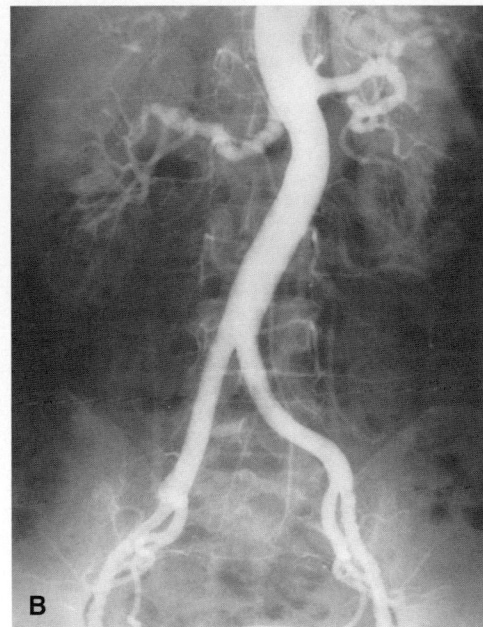

Figure 18–12 **A.** Fibromuscular dysplasia of the external iliac artery. **B.** With involvement of the renal artery.

involvement also have fibromuscular dysplasia in the renal arteries. Patients with fibromuscular dysplasia involving the lower extremity arteries are often asymptomatic, but peripheral embolism, chronic ischemia, or acute dissection can occur (116). Angiography demonstrates the typical "string-of-beads" appearance (Figure 18–12), but may also show the presence of a complication, such as long segment narrowing from arterial dissection, or evidence of distal microembolism.

Endofibrosis is an uncommon arteriopathy that affects the external iliac artery and occurs in high-level athletes, particularly competitive cyclists. The disease is characterized by an isolated, noninflammatory thickening of the endothelium with collagen fibers, fibroblasts, and smooth muscle cells (119). Theories suggest that pathophysiology is related to a combination of hemodynamic injury secondary to shear stresses of increased blood flow, along with repetitive mechanical stresses related to body position and repetitive flexion of the artery. Presentation is typically an athlete with unilateral claudication during prolonged exercise, but often, patients will only complain of easy fatigue, weakness, or deterioration of performance (120). Interestingly, symptoms are nearly always unilateral, with bilateral symptoms in only 15% (121). The fact that lower extremity pulses are usually normal only serves to delay investigation of a vascular explanation for the patient's symptoms. ABIs obtained at rest and after exercise are useful in detecting the arterial lesion (122).

Angiography often shows only diffuse mild to moderate stenosis (<40%); however, the external iliac artery may be elongated or redundant (123), and hemodynamically significant "kinks" have been demonstrated (124). Subtle irregularity of the arterial lumen may require multiple views to visualize (120). Occasionally patients may present with thrombosis and occlusion or dissection of the external iliac artery (120,125,126).

Lower extremity angiography continues to play a critical role as a guide in the treatment of, and sometimes in the diagnosis of, patients with vascular disease involving the lower extremities. However, optimal results require a thorough knowledge of vascular anatomy and radiographic technique, experience in interpreting vascular imaging, an understanding of both atherosclerotic and nonatherosclerotic vascular diseases, and perhaps most importantly, a willingness on the part of the angiographer to spend the necessary time and effort to produce the highest quality angiographic images possible.

REFERENCES

1. Nelemans PJ, Leiner T, de Vet HC, et al. Peripheral arterial disease: meta-analysis of the diagnostic performance of MR angiography. Radiology 2000;217:105–114.
2. Koelemay MJ, Lijmer JG, Stoker J, et al. Magnetic resonance angiography for the evaluation of lower extremity arterial disease: a meta-analysis. JAMA 2001;285(10):1338–1345.

3. Fisher LD, Judkins MP, Lesperance J, et al. Reproducibility of coronary arteriographic reading in the coronary artery surgery study (CASS). Cathet Cardiovasc Diagn 1982;89:565.

4. DeRouen TA, Murray JA, Owen W. Variability in the analysis of coronary arteriograms. Circulation 1977;55(2):324.

5. Paul JF, Cherrak I, Jaulent MC, et al. Interobserver variability in the interpretation of renal digital subtraction angiography. AJR Am J Roentgenol 1999;173:1285.

6. Rothwell PM, Gibson RJ, Villagra R, et al. The effect of angiographic technique and image quality on the reproducibility of measurement of carotid stenosis and assessment of plaque surface morphology. Clin Radiol 1998;53:439.

7. Zir LM, Miller SW, Dinsmore RE, et al. Interobserver variability in coronary angiography. Circulation 1976;53:627.

8. Moore WE, Hall AD. Unrecognized aortoiliac stenosis: a physiologic approach to the diagnosis. Arch Surg 1971;103:633–638.

9. Thompson BW, Read RC, Slayden JE, et al. The role of primary and secondary profundaplasty in the treatment of vascular insufficiency. J Cardiovasc Surg (Torino) 1977;18:55–61.

10. Udoff EJ, Barth KH, Harrington DP, et al. Hemodynamic significance of iliac artery stenosis: pressure measurements during angiography. Radiology 1979;132:289–293.

11. Slot HB, Strijbosch L, Greep JM. Interobserver variability in single-plane aortography. Surgery 1981;90:497–502.

12. Castaneda-Zuniga W, Knight L, Formanek A, et al. Hemodynamic assessment of obstructive aortoiliac disease. AJR Am J Roentgenol 1976;127:559–561.

13. Thiele BL, Strandness DE Jr. Accuracy of angiographic quantification of peripheral atherosclerosis. Prog Cardiovasc Dis 1983;26:223–235.

14. Van Andel GJ, Kan C, Krepel VM. Oblique projections in pelvic and femoral angiography. Medica Mundi 1982;27:2–13.

15. Beales JS, Adcock FA, Frawley JS, et al. The radiological assessment of disease of the profunda femoris artery. Br J Radiol 1971;44:854–859.

16. Thomas ML, Andress RM. Value of oblique projections in translumbar aortography. Am J Roentgenol Radium Ther Nucl Med 1972;116:187–193.

17. Sethi GK, Scott SM, Takaro T. Multiple-plane angiography for more precise evaluation of aortoiliac disease. Surgery 1975;78:154–159.

18. Crummy AB, Rankin RS, Turnipseed WD, et al. Biplane arteriography in ischemia of the lower extremity. Radiology 1978;126:111–115.

19. McDonald EJ Jr, Malone JM, Gooding GW, et al. Stenosis of the deep femoral artery: an evaluation of the accuracy of single-plane, anteroposterior arteriograms. Br J Radiol. 19:932–933.

20. McDonald EJ Jr, Malone JM, Eisenberg RL, et al. Arteriographic evaluation of the femoral bifurcation: Value of the ipsilateral anterior oblique projection. AJR Am J Roentgenol 1976;127:955–956.

21. Thompson MJ, Dorfman GS. Artifactual occlusion of the anterior tibial artery secondary to patient immobilization. J Vasc Interv Radiol 1993;4:287–288.

22. Theander G. Arteriographic demonstration of stationary arterial waves. Acta Radiol 1960;53:417–425.

23. New PF. Arterial stationary waves. Am J Roentgenol Radium Ther Nucl Med 1966;97:488–499.

24. Adams DF, Lebowitz RL. Corrugated arteries: fixed pathology or functional alteration? Arch Surg 1972;104:18–19.

25. Jacobsen JCB, Beierholm U, Mikkelsen R, et al. "Sausage-string" appearance of arteries and arterioles can be caused by an instability of the blood vessel wall. Am J Physiol Regul Integr Comp Physiol 2002;283:R1118–R1130.

26. Moskowitz M, Verani M. Monckeberg's arteriosclerosis revisited: or silver vessels among the old. J Can Assoc Radiol 1976;27:200–202.

27. Meema HE, Oreopoulos DG. Morphology, progression, and regression of arterial and periarterial calcifications in patients with end-stage renal disease. Radiology 1986;158:671–677.

28. Leskinen Y, Salenius JP, Lehtimaki T, et al. The prevalence of peripheral arterial disease and medial arterial calcification in patients with chronic renal failure: requirements for diagnostics. Am J Kidney Dis 2002;40(3):472–479.

29. Edmonds ME, Morrison N, Laws JW, et al. Medial arterial calcification and diabetic neuropathy. Br Med J (Clin Res Ed) 1982;284:928–930.

30. Everhart JE, Pettitt DJ, Knowler WC, et al. Medial arterial calcification and its association with mortality and complications of diabetes. Diabetologia 1988;31:16–23.

31. Amos RS, Wright V. Monckeberg's arteriosclerosis and metabolic bone disease . Lancet 1980 Aug2;2(8188):248–49.

32. Niskanen L, Siitonen O, Suhonen M, et al. Medial artery calcification predicts cardiovascular mortality in patients with NIDDM. Diabetes Care 1994 Nov;17(1):1252–1256.

33. Lehto S, Niskanen L, Suhonen M, et al. Medial artery calcification: a neglected harbinger of cardiovascular complications in non–insulin-dependent diabetes mellitus. Arterioscler Thromb Vasc Biol 1996;16:978–983.

34. Chantelau E, Lee KM, Jungblut R. Association of below-knee atherosclerosis to medial arterial calcification in diabetes mellitus. Diabetes Res Clin Pract 1995;29:169–172.

35. Dangas G, Mehran R, Wallenstein S, et al. Correlation of angiographic morphology and clinical presentation in unstable angina. J Am Coll Cardiol 1997;29:519–525.

36. Blackshear JL, Oldenburg WA, Cohen MD. Making the diagnosis when the patient has "blue toes." Geriatrics 1994;49:37–45.

37. O'Keeffe ST, Woods BO, Breslin DJ, et al. Blue toe syndrome: causes and management. Arch Intern Med 1992;152:2197–2202.

38. Kvilekval KH, Yunis JP, Mason RA, et al. After the blue toe: prognosis of noncardiac arterial embolization in the lower extremities. J Vasc Surg 1993;17:328–335.

39. Kaufman JL, Stah DM, Leather RP. Atheroembolism and microthromboembolic syndromes: blue toe syndrome and disseminated atheroembolism. In: Rutherford RD, ed. Vascular Surgery. Philadelphia: WB Saunders, 1995:669–677.

40. Karmody AM, Powers SR, Monaco VJ, et al. "Blue toe" syndrome: an indication for limb salvage surgery. Arch Surg 1976;111:1263–1268.

41. Morris-Jones W, Preston FE, Greaney M, et al. Gangrene of the toes with palpable peripheral pulses. Ann Surg 1981;193:462.

42. Branowitz JB, Edwards WS. The management of atheromatous emboli to the lower extremities. Surg Gynecol Obstet 1976;143:941.

43. Schecter DC. Atheromatous embolization to lower limbs. NY State J Med 1979;79:1180.

44. Chester MR, Chen L, Tousoulis D, et al. Differential progression of complex and smooth stenosis within the same coronary tree in men with stable coronary artery disease. J Am Coll Cardiol 1995;25:837–842.

45. Walsh DB, Powell RJ, Stukel TA, et al. Superficial femoral artery stenosis: characteristics of progressing lesions. J Vasc Surg 1997;25(3):512–521.

46. Wijendra M, Dodd D, Chalmers N. Proximal arterial occlusion protects the distal lower limb vessels. Eur J Vasc Endovasc Surg 2003;26:354–356.

47. Coran AG, Warren R. Arteriographic changes in femoropopliteal arteriosclerosis obliterans. N Engl J Med 1966;274(12):643–647.

48. Mavor GE. The pattern of occlusion in atheroma of the lower limb arteries: correlation of clinical and arteriographic findings. Brit j surg 1956; 43;352–364.

49. Mozes G, Keresztury G, Kadar A, et al. Atherosclerosis in amputated legs of patients with and without diabetes mellitus. Int Angiol 1998;17(4):282–286.

50. LoGerfo FW, Coffman JD. Current concepts. Vascular and microvascular disease of the foot in diabetes: implications for foot care. N Engl J Med 1984;311(25):1615–1619.

51. Strandness DE, Priest RE, Gibbons GE. Combined clinical and pathological study of diabetic and non-diabetic peripheral arterial disease. Diabetes 1964;13:366–372.

52. Jude EB, Oyibo SO, Chalmers N, et al. Peripheral arterial disease in diabetic and nondiabetic patients. Diabetes Care 2001;24(8):1433–1437.

53. Katsilambros NL, Tsapogas PC, Arvanitis MP, et al. Risk factors for lower extremity arterial disease in non–insulin-dependent diabetic persons. Diabet Med 1996;13(3):243–246.

54. Beach KW, Strandness DE. Arteriosclerosis obliterans and associated risk factors in insulin-dependent and non–insulin-dependent diabetes. Diabetes 1980;29:882–888.

55. Rubba P, Leccia G, Faccenda F, et al. Diabetes mellitus and localizations of obliterating arterial disease of the lower limbs. Angiology 1991;42(4):296–301.

56. Abaci A, Oguzhan A, Kahraman S, et al. Effect of diabetes mellitus on formation of coronary collateral vessels. Circulation 1999;99:2239–2242.

57. Hansen ME, Valentine RJ, McIntire DD, et al. Age-related differences in the distribution of peripheral atherosclerosis: when is atherosclerosis truly premature? Surgery 1995;118(5):834–839.

58. Valentine RJ, Verstraete R, Clagett GP, et al. Premature cardiovascular disease is common in relatives of patients with premature peripheral atherosclerosis. Arch Intern Med 2000;160(9):1343–1348.

59. Valentine RJ, Kaplan HS, Green R, et al. Lipoprotein (a), homocysteine, and hypercoagulable states in young men with premature peripheral atherosclerosis: a prospective, controlled analysis. J Vasc Surg 1996;23(1):53–61.

60. Levy PJ, Gonzalez MF, Hornung CA, et al. A prospective evaluation of atherosclerotic risk factors and hypercoagulability in young adults with premature lower extremity atherosclerosis. J Vasc Surg 1996;23(1):36–43.

61. Barretto S, Ballman KV, Rooke TW, et al. Early-onset peripheral arterial occlusive disease: clinical features and determinants of disease severity and location. Vasc Med 2003;8(2):95–100.

62. Valentine RJ, MacGillivray DC, DeNobile JW, et al. Intermittent claudication caused by atherosclerosis in patients aged forty years and younger. Surgery 1990;107:560–565.

63. Jernigan WR, Fallat ME, Hatfield DR. Hypoplastic aortoiliac syndrome: an entity peculiar to women. Surgery 1983;94(5):752–757.

64. Greebe J. Congenital anomalies of the iliofemoral artery. J Cardiovasc Surg (Torino) 1977; 18:317–323.

65. Noblet E, Gasmi T, Mikati A, et al. Persistent sciatic artery: case report, anatomy, and review of the literature. Ann Vasc Surg 1988;2:390–96.

66. Hassan A. Symptomatic persistent sciatic artery. J Am Coll Surg 2004;199:171–173.

67. Ito H, Okadome K, Odashiro T, et al. Persistent sciatic artery: two case reports and a review of the literature. Cardiovasc Surg 1994;2(2):275–280.

68. Randall PA, Omar RR, Rohner R, et al. Arteria magna revisited. Radiology. 1979;132:295–300.

69. Callum KG, Thomas ML, Browse NL. A definition of arteriomegaly and the size of arteries supplying the lower limbs. Br J Surg 1983;70:524–529.

70. Carlson DH, Gryska P, Seltz J, et al. Arteriomegaly. Am J Roentgenol Radium Ther Nucl Med 1975;125(3):553–558.

71. Kinnunen J, Totterman S, Tervahartiala P. Arteriomegaly. Eur J Radiol 1985;5:156–157.

72. Lawrence PF, Wallis C, Dobrin PB, et al. Peripheral aneurysms and arteriomegaly: is there a familial pattern? J Vasc Surg 1998;28:599–605.

73. Chan O, Thomas ML. The incidence of popliteal aneurysms in patients with arteriomegaly. Clin Radiol 1990;41:185–189.

74. Dent TL, Lindenauer SM, Ernst GB, et al. Multiple arteriosclerotic arterial aneurysms. Arch Surg 1972;105:338.

75. Shortell CK, DeWeese JA, Ouriel K, et al. Popliteal artery aneurysms: a 25-year surgical experience. J Vasc Surg 1991;14:771.

76. Wychulis AR, Spittell JA Jr, Wallace RB, et al. Popliteal aneurysms. Surgery 1970;68:942.

77. Vermillian BD, Dimmis SA, Pace WG, et al. A review of one hundred forty-seven popliteal aneurysms with long-term followup. Surgery 1981;90:1009.

78. Flanigan DP, Burnham SJ, Goodreau JJ, et al. Summary of cases of cystic adventitial disease of the popliteal artery. Ann Surg 1979;189:165–175.

79. Levien LJ, Benn CA. Adventitial cystic disease: a unifying hypothesis. J Vasc Surg 1998;28:193–205.

80. Ishikawa K, Mishima Y, Kobayashi S. Cystic adventitial disease of the popliteal artery. Angiology 1961;12:357.

81. Vanhoenacker FM, Vandevenne JE, De Schepper AM. Regarding "Adventitial cystic disease: a unifying hypothesis." J Vasc Surg 2000;31(3):621–622.

82. Lassonde J, Laurendeau F. Cystic adventitial disease of the popliteal artery: Clinical aspects and etiology. Am Surg 1982;48:341–343.

83. Peterson JJ, Kransdorf MJ, Bancroft LW, et al. Imaging characteristics of cystic adventitial disease of the peripheral arteries: presentation as soft-tissue masses. AJR Am J Roentgenol 2003;621–625.

84. Miller A, Salenius JP, Sacks BA, et al. Noninvasive vascular imaging in the diagnosis and treatment of adventitial cystic disease of the popliteal artery. J Vasc Surg 1997;26:715–720.

85. Brodmann M, Stark G, Pabst E, et al. Cystic adventitial degeneration of the popliteal artery: the diagnostic value of duplex sonography. Eur J Radiol 2001;38:209–212.

86. Rich NM, Collins GJ, McDonald PT, et al. Popliteal vascular entrapment: its increasing interest. Arch Surg 1979;114:1377–1384.

87. Whelan TJ, Haimovici H, eds. Vascular Surgery: Principles and Techniques, 2nd Ed. New York: McGraw-Hill, 1984;557–567.

88. Rosset E, Hartung O, Brunet C, et al. Popliteal artery entrapment syndrome: Anatomic and embryologic bases, diagnostic and therapeutic considerations following a series of 15 cases with a review of the literature. Surg Radiol Anat 1995;17:161–169.

89. Levien LJ, Veller MG. Popliteal artery entrapment syndrome: More common than previously recognized. J Vasc Surg 1999;30:587–598.

90. Chernoff DM, Walker AT, Khorasani R, et al. Asymptomatic functional popliteal artery entrapment: demonstration with MR imaging. Radiology 1995;195:176–180.

91. Collins PS, McDonald PT, Lim RC. Popliteal artery entrapment: an evolving syndrome. J Vasc Surg 1989;10:484–490.

92. Greenwood LH, Yrizarry JM, Hallett JW Jr. Popliteal artery entrapment: Importance of the stress runoff for diagnosis. Cardiovasc Intervent Radiol 1986;9:93–99.

93. Ring DH, Haines GA, Miller DL. Popliteal artery entrapment syndrome: arteriographic findings and thrombolytic therapy. J Vasc Interv Radiol 1999;10:713–721.

94. di Marzo L, Cavallaro A, Sciacca V, et al. Natural history of entrapment of the popliteal artery. J Am Coll Surg 1994;178:553–556.

95. di Marzo L, Cavallaro A, Sciacca V, et al. Popliteal artery entrapment syndrome: the role of early diagnosis and treatment. Surgery 1997;122:26–31.

96. Balaji MR, DeWeese JA. Adductor canal outlet syndrome. JAMA 1981;245(2):167–170.

97. The SH, Wilson RA, Gussenhoven EJ, et al. Extrinsic compression of the superficial femoral artery at the adductor canal: evaluation with intravascular sonography. AJR Am J Roentgenol 1992;159(1):117–120.

98. Verta MJ Jr, Vitello J, Fuller J. Adductor canal compression syndrome. Arch Surg 1984;119(3):345–346.

99. Lee BY, LaPointe DG, Madden JL. The adductor canal syndrome. Am J Surg 1972;123:617.

100. Turnipseed WD. Clinical review of patients treated for atypical claudication: A 28-year-experience. J Vasc Surg 2004;40:79–85.

101. Leppilahti J, Tervonen O, Herva R, et al. Acute bilateral exercise-induced medial compartment syndrome of the thigh: correlation of repeated MRI with clinicopathological findings. Int J Sports Med 2002;23:610–615.

102. Lam R, Lin PH, Alankar S, et al. Acute limb ischemia secondary to myositis-induced compartment syndrome in a patient with human immunodeficiency virus infection. J Vasc Surg 2003;37:1103–1105.

103. Reuss PM, Rosen RJ, Adelman M. Compartment syndrome complicating lower extremity thrombolysis. J Vasc Interv Radiol 1999;10:1075–1082.

104. Ulmer T. The clinical diagnosis of compartment syndrome of the lower leg: are clinical findings predictive of the disorder? J Orthop Trauma 2002;16:572–577.

105. Rorabeck CH, Bourne RB, Fowler PJ, et al. The role of tissue pressure measurement in diagnosing chronic anterior compartment syndrome. Am J Sports Med 1988;2:143–146.

106. Chuang VP. Radiation-induced arteritis. Semin Roentgenol 1994; 29:64–69.

107. Fonkalsrud EW, Sanchez M, Zerubavel R, et al. Serial changes in arterial structure following radiation therapy. Surg Gynecol Obstet 1977;145:395–400.

108. McCready RA, Hyde GL, Bivins BA, et al. Radiation-induced arterial injuries. Surgery 1983;93:306–312.

109. Olin JW, Young JR, Graor RA, et al. The changing clinical spectrum of thromboangiitis obliterans (Buerger's disease). Circulation 1990;82(Suppl IV):3–8.

110. Olin JW. Thromboangiitis obliterans (Buerger's disease). N Engl J Med 2000;343:864–869.

111. Shionoya S. Buerger's disease (thromboangiitis obliterans). In: Rutherford RB, ed. Vascular Surgery. 3rd Ed. Philadelphia: W.B. Saunders, 1989:207–217.

112. Mills JL, Porter JM. Buerger's disease: a review and update. Semin Vasc Surg 1993;6:14–23.

113. Lambeth JT, Yong NK. Arteriographic findings in thromboangiitis obliterans with emphasis on femoropopliteal improvement. AJR Am J Roentgenol 1970;109:553–562.

114. Zavaleta EG, Fernández BB, Grove MK, et al. St. Anthony's fire (ergotamine-induced leg ischemia): a case report and review of the literature. Angiology 2001;52:349–356.

115. Garcia GD, Goff JM Jr, Hadro NC, et al. Chronic ergot toxicity: a rare cause of lower extremity ischemia. J Vasc Surg 2000;31: 1245–1247.

116. Sauer L, Reilly LM, Goldstone J, et al. Clinical spectrum of symptomatic external iliac fibromuscular dysplasia. J Vasc Surg 1990;12: 488–496.

117. van den Dungen JJ, Boontje AH, Oosterhuis JW. Femoropopliteal arterial fibrodysplasia. Br J Surg 1990;77:369–399.

118. Schneider PA, LaBerge JM, Cunningham CG, et al. Isolated thigh claudication as a result of fibromuscular dysplasia of the deep femoral artery. J Vasc Surg 1992;15:657–660.

119. Rousselet MC, Saint-Andre JP, L'Hoste P, et al. Stenotic intimal thickening of the external iliac artery in competition cyclists. Hum Pathol 1990;21(5):524–529.

120. Ford SJ, Rehman A, Bradbury AW. External iliac endofibrosis in endurance athletes: a novel case in an endurance runner and a review of the literature. Eur J Vasc Endovasc Surg 2003;26: 629–634.

121. Abraham P, Saumet JL, Chevalier JM. External iliac artery endofibrosis in athletes. Sports Med 1997;24(4):221–226.

122. Abraham P, Bickert S, Vielle B, et al. Pressure measurements at rest and after heavy exercise to detect moderate arterial lesions in athletes. J Vasc Surg 2001;33:721–727.

123. Chevalier JM, Enon B, Walder J, et al. Endofibrosis of the external iliac artery in bicycle racers: an unrecognized pathological state. Ann Vasc Surg 1986;1(3):297–303.

124. Shep G, Bender MH, van de Tempel G, et al. Detection and treatment of claudication because of functional iliac obstruction in tip endurance athletes: a prospective study. Lancet 2002; 359(9305): 466–473.

125. Cook PS, Erdoes LS, Selzer PM, et al. Dissection of the external iliac artery in highly trained athletes. J Vasc Surg 1995;22(2): 173–717.

126. Kral CA, Han DC, Edwards WD, et al. Obstructive external iliac arteriopathy in avid bicyclists: New and variable histopathologic features in four women. J Vasc Surg 2002;36:565–570.

Femoropopliteal Revascularization

19

Eric C. Martin

In 1964, Dotter and Judkins described the first angioplasty, which was performed in the femoropopliteal system with coaxial systems up to 12 French in diameter (1). These catheters were later modified by Staple (2) and Van Andel, who used serial, tapered dilators (3). But it was not until Grüntzig and Hopff designed the coaxial balloon catheter, which inflated to a fixed diameter, that angioplasty came to be used with any frequency in the United States (4).

There have been significant advances in catheter and balloon technology, particularly in size, trackability, and profile. Advances, too, in guide wires and sheaths, as well as concomitant advances in the pharmacological adjuncts to angioplasty. This progress, when combined with the improvement in image intensification and digital subtraction imaging, has contributed to the increasing efficacy and safety of the procedure and the gradual increase in the number of angioplasties performed (5).

With the acceptance of percutaneous transluminal angioplasty (PTA) came the development of other methods of recanalization, but the seminal technique of angioplasty will be discussed first in this chapter. Although considerable enthusiasm exists for the newer techniques, not least because there has been so little change in angioplasty over the years, the results have certainly not matched the enthusiasm nor have they yet justified the expense. Perhaps more important are the techniques to affect restenosis—a term first used in the coronary circulation and where the results are sometimes dramatic. These techniques have the potential for influencing in a similar way the peripheral circulation and will be discussed under that heading. The real need, however, is for a technique suitable for most patients who suffer with femoropopliteal disease, not mere improvements around the margins in the limited number of patients for whom angioplasty is suitable today.

Fifteen years ago, cardiologists were keen on techniques being tried in the periphery on their way to the heart. This brought lasers and atherectomy. Today, devices, techniques, and even drugs are tried in the heart first, leaving one to wonder about their untried and untested role in the peripheral circulation. Despite the enormous changes in the management of atheroma in the coronary circulation, however, little has been transferable, and few firm advances in the femoropopliteal circulation have been made.

The medical management of peripheral vascular disease, the use of genes expressing endothelial and platelet-derived growth factors, and other gene-based therapies are outside the scope of this chapter.

DISTRIBUTION OF DISEASE

Before considering the techniques and results of percutaneous femoropopliteal revascularization, it is important to know the distribution of peripheral vascular disease. A multicenter study involving 440 consecutive patients demonstrated that femoropopliteal disease was at least three times more frequent than iliac disease (6). Among patients with femoropopliteal disease, occlusions are about three times more frequent than stenoses and, in the iliac system, stenoses predominate by about the same factor. Therefore, the majority of patients with significant peripheral vascular disease have femoropopliteal occlusions. When one plots the relative frequency of lesions against length for femoropopliteal disease, the slope for stenoses is approximately asymptotic, with

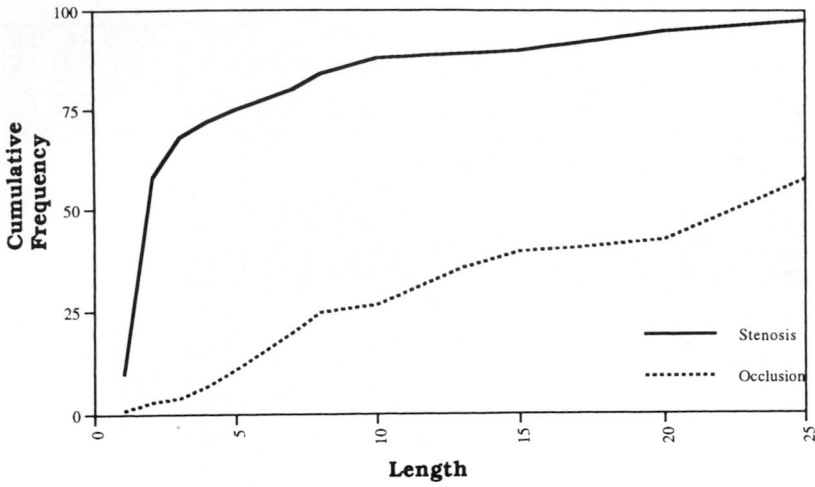

Figure 19–1   Cumulative relative frequency plotted against length for stenoses and occlusions in the femoropopliteal position (Reprinted with permission from Martin EC. Transcatheter therapies in peripheral and noncoronary vascular disease. Introduction. Circulation 1991;83(Suppl II):I1–5.)

about 80% of patients having stenoses 10 cm or less in length (Figure 19–1). But only about 20% of occlusions are 10 cm or less. This would suggest that, because 10 cm is the upper limit of length with good long-term success after angioplasty, only about 25% of patients with femoropopliteal disease and significant symptoms are suitable candidates (5). This should be kept in mind when considering angioplasty, and it makes the comparison of angioplasty with surgery unsatisfactory. It is also important to recall these data when considering the role of the newer endoluminal revascularization devices.

PATIENT CARE DURING ANGIOPLASTY

Standards of care do not differ from those for iliac angioplasty. Guidelines published by the American Heart Association (AHA) should be followed (7).

Standards of care also include suitable equipment, as well as techniques to reduce the radiation dose, large field-of-view intensifiers, and moving-top tables, or gantries. Images should be recorded on a permanent medium. Such standards are defined in the Optimal Resources for the Examination and Endovascular Treatment of the Peripheral and Visceral Vascular Systems guidelines, also promulgated by multiple councils of the AHA (8).

INDICATIONS FOR ANGIOPLASTY

Indications depend first on the clinical status of the patient, specifically the symptoms and the comorbidity factors, which influence the risk of therapy. It is important that the decision to proceed with angioplasty is a clinical one and not based exclusively on the anatomy.

Asymptomatic Patients

Asymptomatic patients should not have angioplasty, because the risks, although small, outweigh the benefits. The exception is to preserve a bypass graft (Figure 19–2).

Symptomatic Patients

Angioplasty may be appropriate for patients with documented peripheral vascular disease, which initially is established by noninvasive flow studies. The objective criteria are outlined in the Society of Vascular Surgery (SVS) clinical categories of chronic ischemia (9) and are seen in Table 19–1. Mild claudication (grade 1, category 1) allows patients to complete a treadmill test but to have an ankle pressure after exercise that is above 50 mm Hg, but 25 mm Hg or more below systemic blood pressure. Category 3 (severe claudication) is defined as patients who cannot complete the treadmill test and whose ankle pressure after exercise is less than 50 mm Hg. Category 2 patients, with moderate claudication, fall between these two parameters.

Most symptomatic patients being considered for femoropopliteal angioplasty have claudication and are in SVS grade 1. Patients are suitable candidates when the claudication is lifestyle limiting and when the patient and physician consider the risk-benefit ratio favorable. This depends on the local interventional experience and the wishes of the patient. Active patients find mild claudication more limiting than patients whose horizons are more limited. Ultimately, the decision depends on the actual risk of angioplasty. In SVS grade 1, the percentage of patients suitable for femoropopliteal angioplasty will be about 30%.

Magnetic Resonance Angiography (MRA) increasingly will define the anatomy and help in the determination of angioplasty as appropriate or inappropriate and even whether

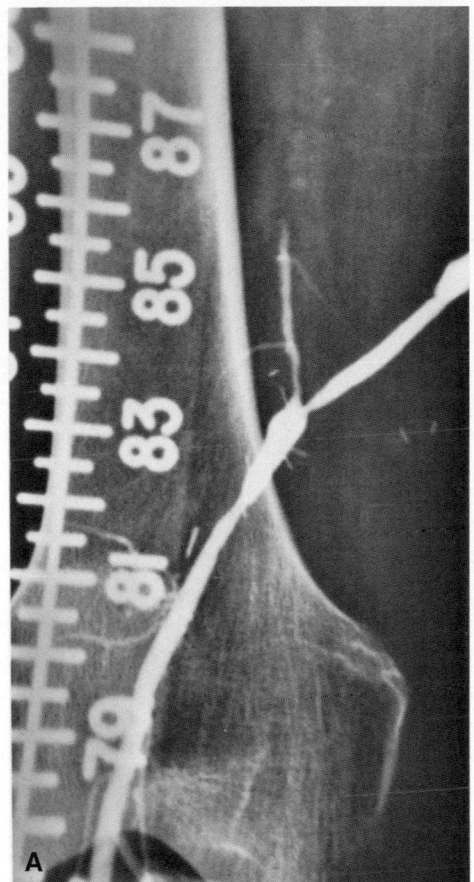 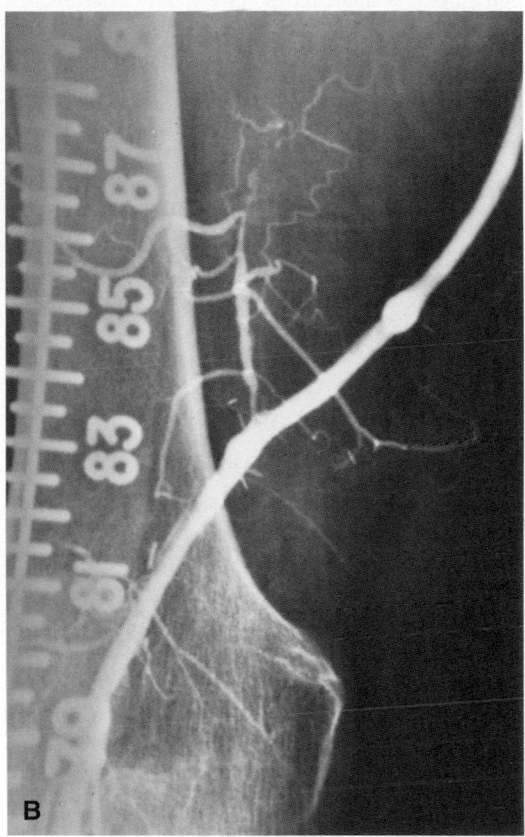

Figure 19–2   **A.** Saphenous vein femoropopliteal artery bypass with a distal anastomotic stenosis. **B.** After treatment with a 6 mm balloon.

intervention should be provided at all. In patients with more severe symptoms, surgery may be performed, based on the MRA, depending on the findings and the quality of the study. Regardless, complete diagnostic arteriography should precede any percutaneous vascular intervention and should be

recorded permanently (7,8). In addition, it will frequently precede surgery.

To be judged suitable for angioplasty in the femoropopliteal system, lesions should be less than 10 cm in length, although for patients who are very high risks for

TABLE 19–1
CLINICAL CATEGORIES OF CHRONIC LIMB ISCHEMIA

Grade	Category	Clinical Description	Objective Criteria
0	0	Asymptomatic: no hemodynamically significant occlusive disease	Normal treadmill/stress test
1	1	Mild claudication	Completes treadmill exercise, AP after exercise <50 mm Hg but >25 mm Hg less than BP
	2	Moderate claudication	Between categories 1 and 3
	3	Severe claudication	Cannot complete treadmill exercise; AP after exercise <50 mm Hg
2	4	Ischemic rest pain	Resting AP <40 mm Hg; flat or barely pulsatile ankle or metatarsal PVR; toe pressure <30 mm Hg
3	5	Minor tissue loss: nonhealing ulcer, focal gangrene with diffuse pedal ischemia	Resting AP <60 mm Hg; ankle metatarsal PVR flat or barely pulsatile; toe pressure <40 mm Hg
	6	Major tissue loss extending above TM level; functional foot no longer salvageable	Same as category 5

Abbreviations: AP = ankle pressure; BP = blood pressure; PVR = pulse volume recording; TM = transmetatarsal.

surgery, this restriction may be extended with the knowledge that the angioplasty is destined to close. The Society of Interventional Radiology (SIR), formerly the Society of Cardiovascular and Interventional Radiology (SCVIR), has developed guidelines for the suitability of angioplasty. The SIR describes four categories (10) promulgated by the American Heart Association in Guidelines for Peripheral Transluminal Angioplasty of the Abdominal Aorta and Lower Extremity Vessels (7), which is endorsed by the Council on Cardiovascular Surgery, the Council on Cardiovascular Radiology, the Council on Clinical Cardiology, and the Council on Epidemiology and Prevention.

In the femoropopliteal system, lesions are classified as follows:

Category 1 (PTA procedure of choice)

A. Single stenosis, up to 5 cm in length, that is not at the superficial femoral origin or distal portion of the popliteal artery
B. Single occlusion, up to 3 cm in length, that does not involve the superficial femoral origin or distal portion of the popliteal artery

Category 2 (well-suited for PTA)

A. Single stenosis, 5–10 cm in length, that does not involve the distal popliteal artery
B. Single occlusion, 3–10 cm in length, that does not involve the distal popliteal artery
C. Heavily calcified stenosis, up to 5 cm
D. Multiple lesions, each less than 3 cm, either stenoses or occlusions
E. Single or multiple lesions where there is no continuous tibial runoff, to improve inflow for distal surgical bypass

Category 3 (PTA under special circumstances only. Surgery superior.)

A. Single occlusion, 3–10 cm in length, involving the distal popliteal artery
B. Multiple focal lesions, each 3–5 cm, that may be heavily calcified
C. Single lesion, either stenosis or occlusion, with a length greater than 10 cm

Category 4 (not suitable for PTA)

A. Complete common femoral occlusions, superficial femoral occlusions, or both
B. Complete popliteal and proximal trifurcation occlusions
C. Severe, diffuse disease with multiple lesions and no intervening normal vascular segments

Common femoral artery disease is excluded from these categories, at least by implication. For the most part, surgery is preferable.

The advantages of angioplasty include low mortality and morbidity compared to surgery (11), decreased hospitalization time, and cost savings (12,13). Angioplasty should also be considered as an adjunct to surgery so that a lesser operation may be performed. All patients in SVS grades 2 or 3 should be considered for angioplasty, although the incidence of patients suitable for angioplasty in this population will be no more than 20%.

Veith et al. reviewed 2,829 patients who had critical lower extremity ischemia, of whom 2,221 were presenting for the first time (14). Thirty-five percent were treated by angioplasty, including iliac PTA, although only 19% had angioplasty by itself. The remainder also had surgery. This illustrates both the complementary nature of angioplasty in multisegment disease and the limitations.

Patients who experience angioplasty and later have a recurrence are seldom worse than before treatment, and it is unusual for angioplasty to alter the scope of the original surgery that it was planned to replace. This is not true for femoropopliteal bypass grafting because, in a significant percentage of patients, close to 25% for patients with polytetrafluorethylene (PTFE) grafts, the popliteal artery will occlude when the femoropopliteal artery bypass closes.

TECHNIQUE OF ANGIOPLASTY

Stenoses

Occasionally, it may be convenient to perform angioplasty of stenoses from the contralateral side, such as when iliac angioplasty is also being performed. But this technique should be used only in short-segment stenoses that appear easy to cross. The most frequent use of a contralateral approach is after thrombolysis has been performed around the bifurcation. Otherwise, all femoropopliteal angioplasties are performed with an antegrade puncture. A sheath should be used, both to reduce trauma to the vessel and to allow an opportunity to inject through the side arm of the sheath for roadmapping, or otherwise delineating, the vessel.

Patients are heparinized once the catheter is in the vessel. For short-segment stenoses, an appropriate catheter is advanced to several centimeters above the stenosis, an image is taken, and the stenosis crossed with a guide wire. The catheter should be parallel to the line of the vessel when approaching the stenosis. When the superficial femoral artery describes a general curve, the catheter must approximate that curve; otherwise the guide wire will not aim at the center of the stenosis. A Van Andel or a Berenstein catheter is appropriate for most eventualities. A soft, angled, hydrophilic guide wire (Terumo) is used to cross the lesion. Great care must be taken not to dissect. The guide wire must be directed through the point of the stenosis no matter how eccentric it is. Once across the obstruction, an exchange is made over a Rosen wire for the balloon catheter, which is inflated for one minute. The catheter may be perfused with saline during this period. When the balloon is deflated, a phasic pressure trace should be observed, but pullback gradients with balloon-mounted catheters in the femoropopliteal system are not reliable. As the balloon is inflated, one should observe the patient for pain, which should be relieved by deflation of the catheter. Persistent pain unrelieved by balloon deflation may indicate vessel rupture, but this is seldom catastrophic—unlike a rupture in the iliac system.

The catheter is then pulled back over a guide wire, and contrast is injected above the lesion to assess the result. If satisfactory, the runoff is filmed to help ensure that no distal embolization (Figure 19–3) has occurred. If the appearances are unsatisfactory, the lesion is recrossed and the balloon reinflated. It may be necessary to change to a larger balloon. Most patients with femoropopliteal disease should be dilated with 6 mm balloons, but occasionally 5 mm, 7 mm, or even 8 mm balloons will be the primary choice. The balloon should be slightly larger than the normal vessel lumen. The same technique may be applied to stenotic bypass grafts (Figure 19–2).

Occlusions

Antegrade punctures are essential for all occlusions, and sheaths are used. Once the lesion is filmed and the point of occlusion and reconstitution (as well as the shape of the proximal portion of the occlusion) is known, a 5 French Van Andel catheter or a hockey stick catheter (Berenstein, Kumpe, Tegtmeyer) is positioned 2–5 cm above the occlusion, and the lesion is gently probed with a Terumo wire. Again, as with stenoses, the catheter should be parallel to the vessel just above the occlusion so that the guide wire is properly centered. The effective radius of the curved guide wire can be changed by an advancement and retraction of the curved catheter to explore different portions of the occlusion. Regardless, exploring the edge of the lesion is likely to lead to a subintimal passage. Once subintimal dissection has occurred, it is frequently difficult to reenter the lumen. If the Terumo wire is unsuccessful, the so-called snowplow technique may be employed. This approach is occasionally necessary because a collateral arises at the site of the obstruction so that the guide wire always passes down the collateral, and the point of obstruction cannot be engaged. With the snowplow technique, a Van Andel catheter is used with a Rosen guide wire just protruding from it so that the tight J of the Rosen wire protects the catheter tip. The catheter and wire then

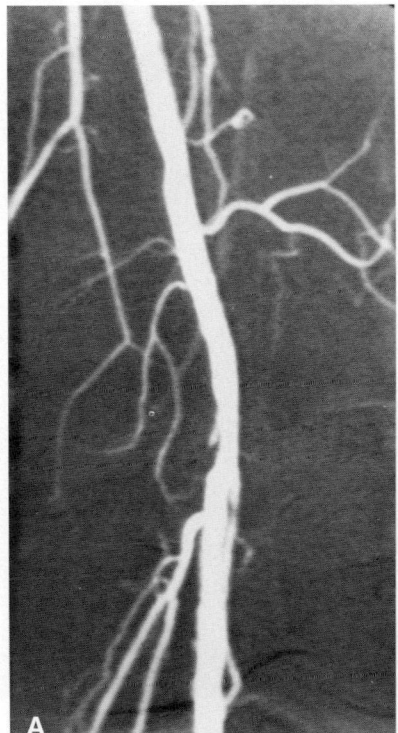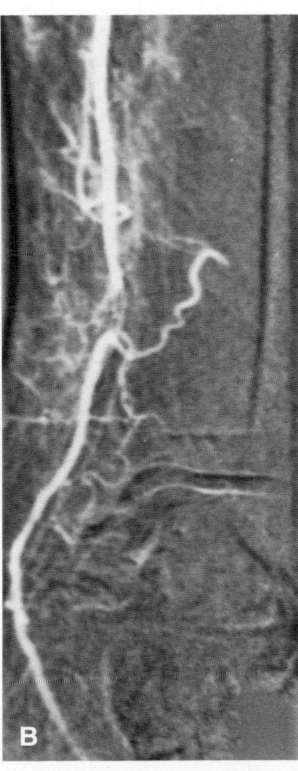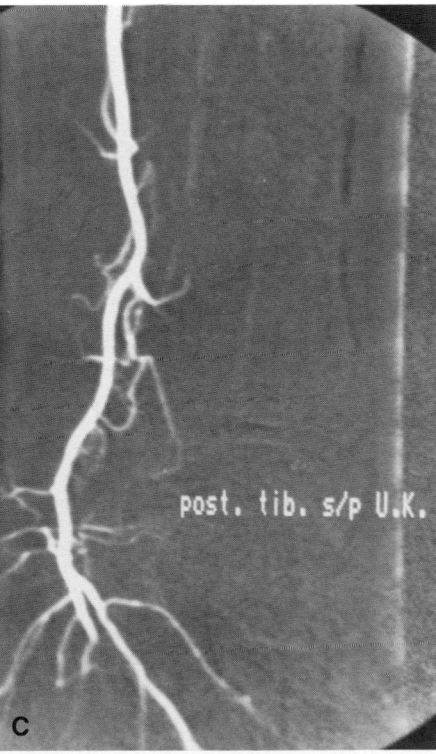

Figure 19–3   **A.** Angiogram after successful angioplasty of a popliteal occlusion. **B.** Angiogram showing distal embolization to the posterior tibial artery. **C.** After 1 hour of urokinase (200,000 units).

are advanced as a unit across the obstruction into the distal vessel. The disadvantage of this technique is that if a subintimal passage occurs, reentry into the true lumen is difficult. If the problem is a collateral, the snowplow technique may be started for the first two centimeters. After that, a switch back to the hydrophilic wire is made to complete the crossing.

Once the distal vessel is entered and confirmation of this is made by a contrast injection, an exchange is made over a Rosen guide wire for the appropriate balloon catheter and inflation is performed from distal to proximal to cover the length of the lesion. Balloons of 4 cm in length are usually satisfactory, but for very long lesions, balloons of 10 cm may be more desirable.

For sequential lesions, it is preferable to cross all lesions and work from distal to proximal. Once dilatation is complete, the operator pulls back over a guide wire and performs a contrast injection. The lesion may then be easily

and safely recrossed for reinflation with either the same or larger balloon when necessary. Again, it is important both to film the angioplasty site and to examine distally for embolization. Emboli will lead to early, or even late, occlusion and usually can be managed with thrombolysis or aspiration (Figure 19–3).

Because a palpable pulse is one of the best predictors of good long-term patency, dilating a single proximal tibial or posterior tibioperoneal trunk stenosis may be done at the same time as the femoral angioplasty. This is a new addition to the technique and springs from the increasing safety of distal angioplasty. Whereas formerly tibial angioplasty was recommended only for limb salvage, a proximal lesion may be dilated with minimal risk and such dilation may improve the long-term patency of the femoropopliteal lesion. However, this approach is recommended only for centers with extensive experience and low complication rates (Figure 19–4).

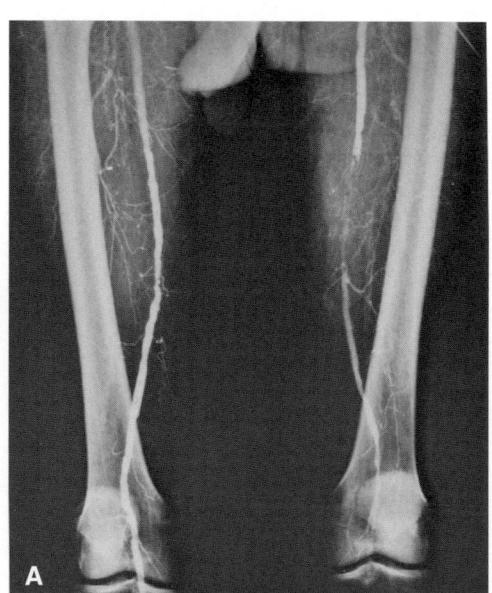
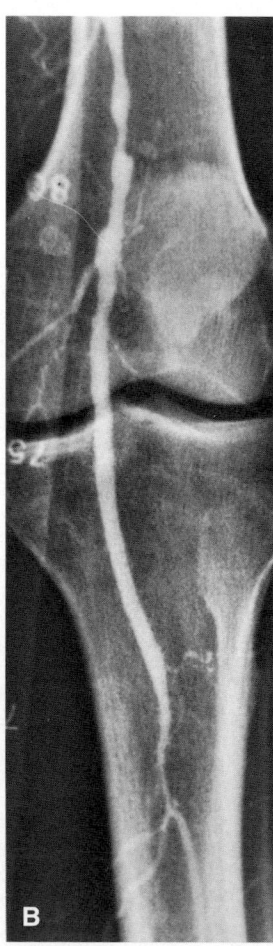
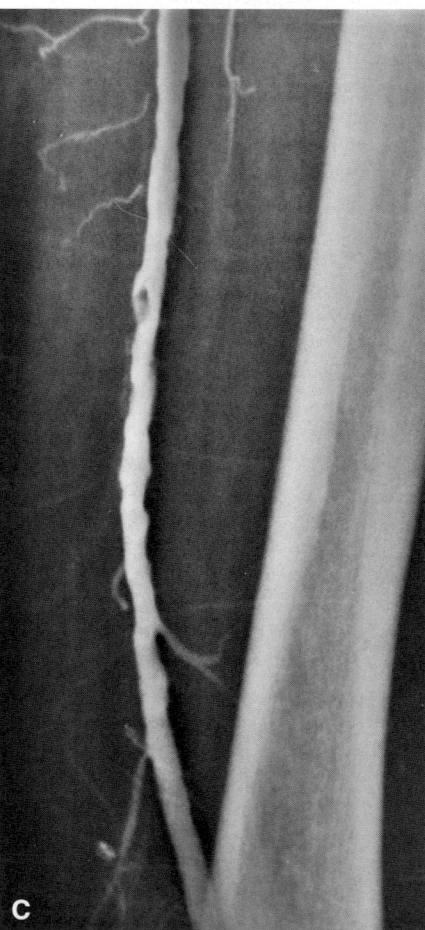

Figure 19–4   **A., B.** Angiograms of a patient with rest pain and an ABI of 0.37.

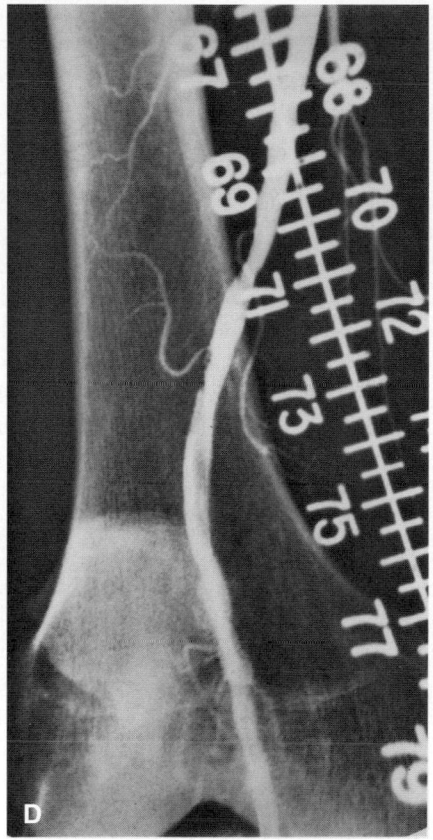
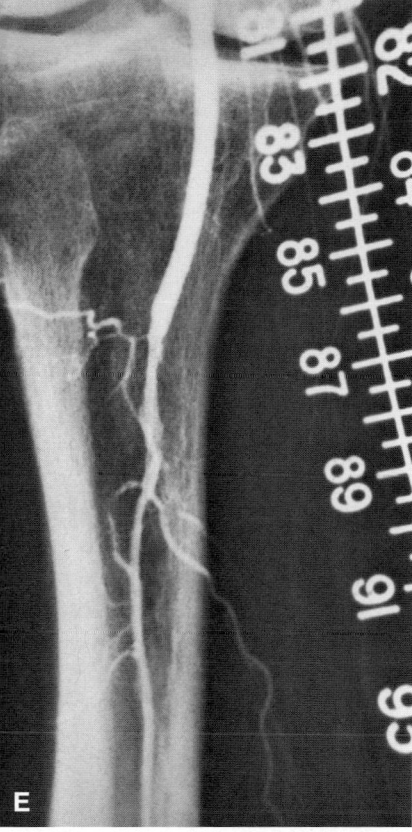
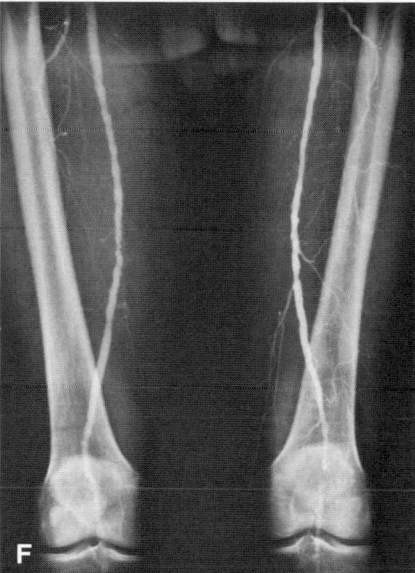

Figure 19–4 *(continued)* **C., D., E.** After treatment. The posterior tibial-peroneal trunk was treated at the same time because of the low ABI. **F.** Two years later. With a return of symptoms, there is a new popliteal stenosis, but the previously treated lesions remain patent.

PHARMACOLOGIC ADJUNCTS TO ANGIOPLASTY

Heparin

All patients are heparinized for femoral popliteal artery revascularization. Three thousand to 5,000 units is the usual dose, and the sheath is removed when the ACT falls below 120 seconds. In patients having long angioplasties, it may be advantageous to restart heparin after 4 hours at a rate of 800 to 1,000 units per hour, later to be modified by the APTT results. The heparin can be continued until the morning.

Nitroglycerin

Intra-arterial nitroglycerin should be used frequently in doses of 100–150 mcg during the angioplasty. It is an excellent vasodilator and very rarely causes significant hypotension. In patients with long angioplasties, or diminished flow, nitropaste may be a useful adjunct overnight.

Calcium Channel Blockers

Oral nifedipine has been used prior to an infrainguinal angioplasty and intra-arterial verapamil, in the case of spasm or slow flow. However, the short-acting dihydropyrodines (DHPs) have been linked to an increased incidence of myocardial infarction (unless beta-blockers are used concomitantly). So, non DHP calcium channel blockers should be used instead (15). Common drugs are diltiazem and verapamil. Because of improvements in antiplatelet drugs, which are used routinely, many use intra-arterial verapamil only in cases of a poor result, slow flow, or spasm, and rely on nitroglycerin as the sole vasodilator during the procedure. Diltiazem is prescribed for 48 hours in patients with long angioplasties, poor runoff, slow flow, or spasm.

Antiplatelet Therapy

Platelets are central to atherothrombosis. Mehta and Yusuf provide an excellent review of short- and long-term therapy, including a nice cartoon depicting platelet activation (16).

Cardiologists have been aggressive in influencing platelet function and have had considerable success, but whether or not such an approach is as valuable in the peripheral circulation is a question yet to be studied. Most likely, its relevance increases as the vessel size diminishes.

Aspirin alone reduces the frequency of ischemic complications after percutaneous cardiac interventions, and it does so largely by reducing thromboxane A2 (17,18) and should be used routinely in the peripheral circulation.

Adenosine Diphosphate Receptor Antagonists

Ticlopidine was used for some years as an inhibitor of platelet function following angioplasty, but because of the rare complication of bone marrow suppression, it has been replaced largely by clopidogrel, or Plavix (19).

In the CAPRIE (Clopidogrel versus Aspirin in Patients at Risk for Ischemic Events) study, clopidogrel was found to significantly reduce death, myocardial infarction (MI), and ischemic stroke by 8.7% compared to aspirin (20). The CREDO trial (Clopidogrel for the Reduction of Events During Observation) involved 2,116 patients having coronary angioplasty (PTCA). Patients were randomized to receive a loading dose of 300 mgm/clopidogrel 3–24 hours before PTCA, or placebo (21). Thereafter, all patients received 75 mgm/daily through day 28. Then, they were randomized to receive placebo or Plavix at 75 mgm/once a day. At 1 year, the long-term clopidogrel group was associated with a 27% relative reduction in the combined risk of death, MI, and stroke, but this translates to only a 3% absolute reduction. Pretreatment did not change these numbers significantly, but subgroup analysis suggested that pretreatment provided 6 hours before PTCA conferred additional benefit.

The CURE trial (Clopidogrel in Unstable angina-Recurrent Events) showed a 20% risk reduction of aspirin and clopidogrel compared to placebo and aspirin over a 12-month period in patients with acute coronary syndromes (22). However, this trial showed that the effects of clopidogrel were apparent very early. At 24 hours, a 34% reduction was seen in cardiovascular death, MI, stroke, and severe ischemia.

How well this information translates to the peripheral circulation is unknown. In some practices, clopidogrel is used for a month after angioplasty and aspirin is continued (or started) indefinitely as the medical condition of the patient permits. The interventional radiologist practicing as an independent physician will also have to consider the long-term treatment of these patients. Equally, he or she will have to consider adding statins, more properly 3-hydroxy-3-methyl-glutaryl coenzyme A reductase inhibitors, to the long-term therapy (23). Yet again, there are no data on the risks and benefits to the peripheral circulation.

Glycoprotein IIb/IIIa Antagonists

Oral agents have been disappointing, with one meta-analysis demonstrating a 37% increase in mortality and a 78% excess of major bleeding (24). This is in contrast to the short-duration therapy during percutaneous coronary interventions. Multiple trials, including CADILLAC (Controlled Abciximab and Device Investigation to Lower Late Angioplasty Complications) (25), ADMIRAL (Abciximab before Direct angioplasty and stenting in Myocardial Infarction Regarding Acute and Long-term follow-up) (26), and EPISTENT (Evaluation of Platelet IIb/IIIa Inhibition in Stenting) (27) showed a benefit to abciximab in *acute* coronary syndromes. But, at the time of writing (September 2003), no data have addressed whether or not the addition of a GPIIb/IIIa receptor antagonist to patients having *elective* percutaneous coronary interventions (who are also pretreated with aspirin and clopidogrel) is beneficial. TOPSTAR (Troponin in planned PTCA/stent implantation with or without administration of GPIIb/IIIa antagonist, tirofiban), designed to rectify this, suggested a benefit (28), but changes in troponin are even less transferable to the peripheral circulation.

Abciximab is used frequently in peripheral vascular laboratories in combination with thrombolysis, but there is no convincing evidence to add it to elective angioplasty. Bleeding at the puncture site is a significant complication and reached 8–15% in the EPIC (Evaluation of c7E3Fab in Preventing Ischemic Complications of High-Risk Angioplasty) trial using a chimeric antibody to platelet GPIIb/IIIa integrin (29). This trial also had a 0.3% incidence of intracranial hemorrhage. This is one of several different IIb/IIIa antagonists now being studied.

CRITERIA FOR ASSESSING THE RESULTS OF ANGIOPLASTY

The angioplasty literature has been inconsistent in its reporting, and comparison between studies is difficult. More difficult still is the comparison between angioplasty and surgery, if, indeed, it is warranted, because of the different patient populations. Rutherford has introduced rigid reporting standards, which are now widely accepted (9). These criteria have been modified by Rutherford and Becker for interventional procedures (30).

The term *long-term patency* is used frequently, yet it is applied with validity only to angiographic patency, patency documented at surgery, and patency documented by color flow Doppler ultrasound, or MRA. Yet, an obvious need exists for clinically derived patency. The Rutherford-Becker criteria supply it (30). However, to confound the issue further, patients with documented patent grafts may be clinically worse, just as patients with occluded grafts may be symptomatically improved. The Rutherford-Becker criteria for reporting improvement are described in Table 19–2.

Criteria for improvement after percutaneous intervention should be divided into early and late success. Early success should be judged by a combination of clinical, hemodynamic, and angiographic factors, with all three necessary to consider the procedure successful. Clinical

TABLE 19–2

CHANGES IN THE CONDITION OF THE EXTREMITY AFTER PERCUTANEOUS INTERVENTION

Grade	Clinical Description
+3	Markedly improved: symptoms gone or markedly improved; ABI increased to more than 0.90
+2	Moderately improved: still symptomatic, but at least a single-category improvement; ABI increased by more than 0.10 but not normalized
+1	Minimally improved: greater than 0.10 increase in ABI but no categorical improvement, or vice versa (i.e., upward categorical shift without an increase in ABI of more than 0.10)
0	No change: no categorical shift and less than 0.10 change in ABI
−1	Mildly worse: no categorical shift but ABI decreased by more than 0.10, or downward categorical shift with ABI decreased less than 0.10
−2	Moderately worse: one category worse or unexpected minor amputation
−3	Markedly worse: more than one category worse or unexpected major amputation

improvement should include symptomatic improvement *and* a change in at least one category on the Rutherford scale. Hemodynamic improvement should be defined as an increase in the ankle-brachial index of 0.1 or greater. In the case of diabetic patients with incompressible vessels, the pulse-volume recording distal to the revascularized site should increase by 5 mm above preprocedural testing. Angiographic success should result in less than a 30% residual stenosis. Changes in the condition of the extremity should be categorized on a scale of +3 to −3.

RESULTS OF ANGIOPLASTY

Although there have been numerous reports of the results of femoropopliteal PTA, most do not meet the reporting standards of Rutherford and Becker.

Adar developed the confidence profile method, a form of meta-analysis, to analyze combined data from 12 selected series. He derived the best estimate of the expected outcome of femoropopliteal angioplasty in patients with intermittent claudication and with more severe limb-threatening ischemia (31). In this report, the early success rate for angioplasty performed for claudication was 89%, compared to 77% for limb salvage. The three-year patency was 62% for patients with claudication and 43% for limb salvage. The largest decline in patency occurred in the first year. The difference in long-term patency between patients with claudication and those with limb-threatening ischemia was assumed to be caused by the difference in runoff.

In 1989, Wilson et al. reported on a randomized trial of angioplasty against surgery from the Veterans Administration that involved 98 patients with femoropopliteal disease (32). Fifty-nine percent of the angioplasties were patent at 3 years, a result that was not statistically different from the surgical results. The criticism of this series is that in order to be randomized, all patients had to be eligible for both angioplasty and surgery (i.e., they had short-segment lesions). It is representative, therefore, of only a small percentage of patients.

The majority of patients in angioplasty series have stenoses instead of occlusions, and multiple or long-segment stenoses fare particularly poorly. In 1987, Murray et al. reported on a group of patients with long-segment stenoses, of which those with greater than 7 cm had a 6-month patency of 23% (33). This is similar to the results of long occlusions (greater than 10 cm), which have similarly disappointing results (34).

Even fewer studies have drawn attention to the capabilities of angioplasty in total femoropopliteal occlusion. The author and colleagues reviewed the initial results of angioplasty in 116 consecutive patients with complete femoropopliteal artery occlusions. Between 1977 and 1980, angioplasty was performed in 46 patients and a technical success rate of 74% was achieved (35). In the subsequent study period between 1981 and 1988, angioplasty was performed in 70 patients and the technical success rate increased to 91% (36). During the study period, equipment quality improved markedly. Balloons now have a lower profile, and 5 French balloons can be used exclusively. Patient selection for angioplasty has also changed as the results have become known. In the first study period, for example, the authors tried to treat occlusions 20 cm in length, whereas in the second series no lesion was longer than 10 cm. During the same period, the skill of the interventionalists also improved. These initial success rates are now standard in recent series, and the procedure is about 20% more successful (primary success) than in series from the early 1980s (33,34,37,38,39–41).

Huninck et al. examined the patency rates of angioplasty and surgery in femoropopliteal disease by a meta-analysis of papers with adequate Kaplan-Meier analyses published between 1985 and 1992 (42). The unadjusted data gave a 5-year patency for angioplasty of 45%. Femoropopliteal bypasses using vein had a 5-year patency of 73%, while PTFE had a five-year patency of 49%. Hazard rate ratios then were created to determine the influence of risk factors in predicting failure. Five-year adjusted patencies were better for stenoses and claudication (68%) than stenoses and critical ischemia (47%). Occlusion and claudication (35%) did better than occlusion and critical ischemia (12%). By way of comparison, the adjusted 5-year patency of PTFE in critical ischemia is 47% above the knee and 33% below.

Huninck et al. (43) also conducted a cost-effectiveness analysis measuring Quality Adjusted Life Expectancy (QUALE), and a lifetime cost analysis was constructed using a Markov process to examine decisions regarding angioplasty and surgery. Sensitivity analysis suggested that angioplasty would be the preferred initial treatment if the five-year patency exceeded 30%. It is, therefore, the preferred treatment in claudication with a stenosis or an occlusion, as well as in critical ischemia with a stenosis.

Two series deserve additional comment. The first is a retrospective review of 217 angioplasties performed on 152 patients between 1978 and 1986 at the Hospital of University of Pennsylvania, with the majority of patients studied in 1979 and 1980 (34). Selection of patients for the series was weighted toward those cases with complete data profiles so that a 10-year follow-up could be obtained. Most patients, therefore, were dilated with polyvinyl balloons and did not have the benefit of pharmacologic assistance. Follow-up in the series was by segmental Doppler arterial leg pressures and pulse-volume recordings initially, and thereafter annually, for an indefinite period. In patients in whom the ankle-brachial pressure index fell by 0.2, compared to the immediate postangioplasty index, a repeat arteriogram was performed, when possible (71 of 152 patients). Most patients were studied for mild to moderate claudication (74%), with only 26% being in SVS grades 2 and 3. Diabetes was present in 33% of patients. Forty percent of the patients had one- or zero-vessel runoff.

Overall, the 10-year primary patency was 38%, and the secondary patency was 40%, with an initial technical success rate of 90% (Figure 19–5). The prognosis for stenoses appears to be considerably better than for occlusions, but these data are confounded by the primary success of crossing lesions in this series (Figure 19–6). Failure to cross a stenosis and perform an angioplasty occurred in 7% of patients, whereas in 18% of occlusions, the lesions could not be crossed. Because the life-table curves for stenoses and occlusions are parallel, with

the occlusions starting 11% lower, it is not unreasonable to assume that with the 91% primary success rate expected today, these two curves would be superimposed. Therefore, if one excludes the technical failures from this series, predominantly from 1979, the 5-year patency rises to 58%. The data also indicate that angioplasty of an occlusion, when technically successful, carries the same prognosis for long-term patency as angioplasty of a stenosis, an observation made previously by others (37,44,45).

This series is valuable for several reasons, not least in demonstrating the durability of angioplasty after the initial drop in patency at one year. It demonstrates that repeat angioplasty carries an identical prognosis to the initial angioplasty. Importantly, it also demonstrates that lesion length correlates with outcome, with shorter lesions doing better than longer ones. Specifically, the series identified lesions greater than 10 cm in length to have only a 20% 1-year patency, but among lesions less than 10 cm, no statistical difference was appreciated in long-term patency when stratified by length (Figure 19–7). Although a superficial glance at the life-table curve would suggest that lesions 0–2 cm in length fared better than those 5–10 cm in length, when one excludes the confounding variable of the higher incidence of failing to cross the longer lesions, no difference is seen (Table 19–3). The series firmly establishes that the upper limit of length with good long-term success for femoral artery occlusions is 10 cm.

These data conform well to an analysis of 984 consecutive angioplasties by Johnston et al., of which 271 were in the femoropopliteal segment (38). Again, most were performed in the early 1980s. The data were reexamined in 1992 (46). The criteria for success were clinical improvement and continued improvement in the ankle-brachial index. The overall 5-year patency in the femoropopliteal position was 40%. Again, a difference was observed between the long-term patency for stenoses and occlusions (Figure 19–8) and between claudication and limb salvage (Figure 19–9), with the curves being parallel.

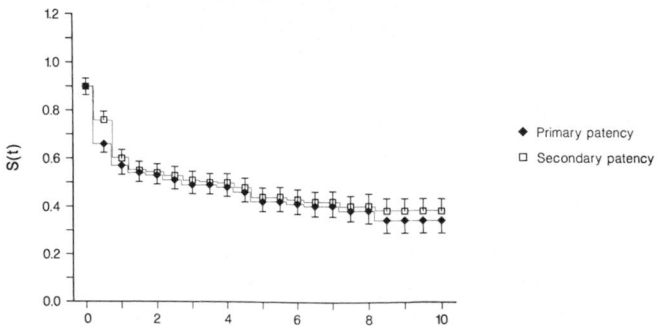

Figure 19–5 Long-term patency of femoropopliteal angioplasty (Reprinted with permission from Capek P, McLean GK, Berkowitz HD. Femoropopliteal angioplasty factors influencing long-term success. Circulation 1991;83 (Suppl II):70–80.)

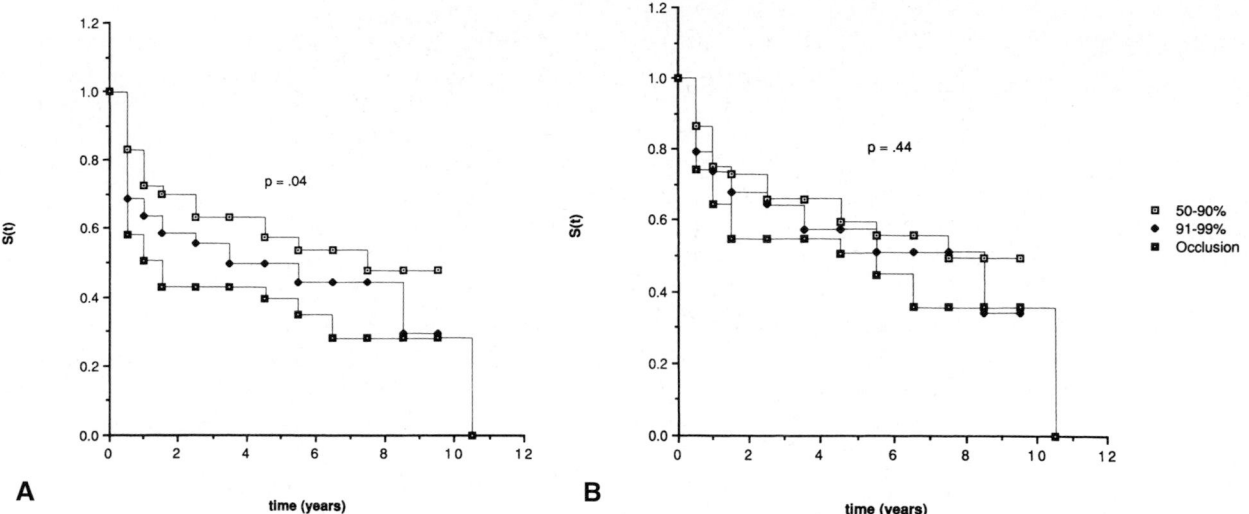

Figure 19–6 Long-term patency. **A.** With technical failures included, stratified by degree of stenosis. Occlusions have a significantly worse prognosis than stenoses (*p* = 0.04). **B.** With technical failures excluded. Occlusions fare as well as stenoses (*p* = 0.44). (Reprinted with permission from Capek P, McLean GK, Berkowitz HD. Femoropopliteal angioplasty: factors influencing long-term success. Circulation 1991;83[Suppl II]:70–80.)

Johnston did not observe that this was because of the difference in primary success rate, but in patients with claudication it was 93% and in limb salvage 74%. Johnston also showed a significant difference between patients with good runoff and poor runoff, which is not related to the primary success (Figure 19–10).

Although extensive comments have been made here about the significance of primary failure, it is important that failures not be excluded from the analysis so that better comparisons may be made from series to series. However, in older series, in which the primary success rate may be 20% worse than today, some recognition should be given to this fact and its influence as a confounding variable.

For a modern series, the STAR (SCVIR Transluminal Angioplasty and Revascularization Registry) was interrogated to consider variables predictive of long-term success with femoropopliteal angioplasty (47). Two hundred fifty-nine limbs were examined. Fifty-seven percent of the patients had claudication, and 79% of the lesions were stenoses. The primary patency was 87% at 1 year and 69% at 3 years. Diabetes and renal failure were independent variables associated with a significantly lower patency. Patency was higher in AHA category 1 lesions, but no difference was seen between categories 2 and 3. Poor tibial runoff is the most predictive factor of lower patency and more dramatically so than in Figure 19–10.

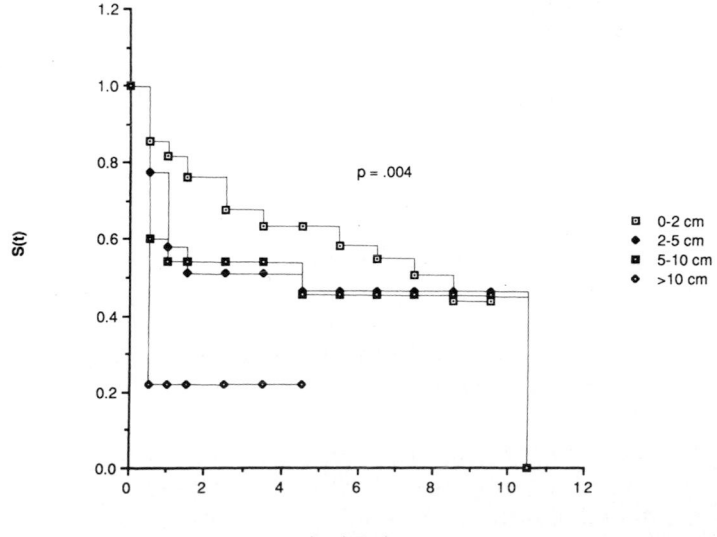

Figure 19–7 Long-term patency stratified for length. (Reprinted with permission from Capek P, McLean GK, Berkowitz HD. Femoropopliteal angioplasty: factors influencing long-term success. Circulation 1991;83[Suppl II]:70–80.)

TABLE 19–3

EFFECT OF LESION LENGTH ON PROGNOSIS

Comparison	P	N
Overall comparison	0.004*	
0–2 cm		56
2–5 cm		31
5–10 cm		21
> 10 cm		9
Comparison between groups		
0–2 vs. 2–5 cm	0.100	
0–2 vs. 5–10 cm	0.060	
2–5 vs. 5–10 cm	0.540	
0–2 vs. > 10 cm	0.007*	
2–5 vs. > 10 cm	0.015*	
5–10 vs. > 10 cm	0.120	

*Statistically significant association.
Reprinted with permission from Capek P, McLean GK, Berkowitz HD. Femoropopliteal angioplasty factors influencing long-term success. Circulation 1991; 83(Suppl II): 70–80.

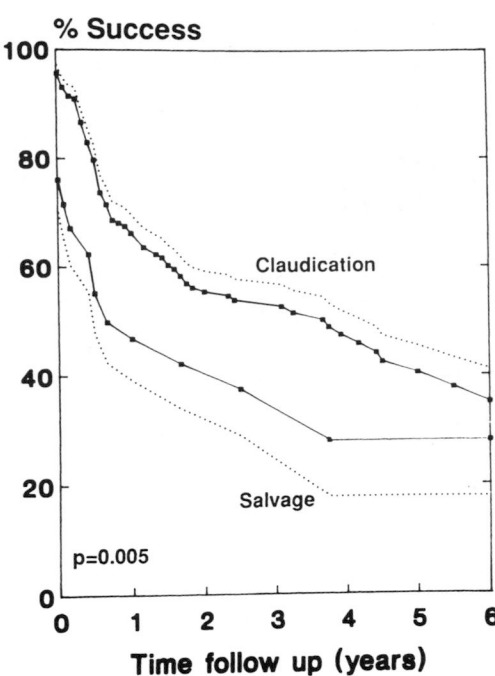

Figure 19–9   Long-term patency of claudication versus limb salvage. (Reprinted with permission from Johnston KW. Femoral and popliteral arteries: reanalysis of results of balloon angioplasty. Radiology 1992;183:767–771.)

COMPLICATIONS

The complications of femoropopliteal angioplasty do not differ significantly from those of iliac angioplasty. However, because occlusions have angioplasty more frequently in the femoropopliteal than in the iliac system, the embolic risk is higher. In one small series, it was 10%, although in five of the six symptomatic patients, urokinase successfully lysed the thrombus (36).

Large series do not separate iliac from femoral angioplasties. For 4,662 patients gathered from series in the literature (including renal angioplasty), Becker et al. reported a mortality of 0.23% with a 2.5% incidence of surgery because of complications of angioplasty (48). The largest single series, with 1,642 patients, reported a mortality of 0.1%. Among patients with ischemia, the incidence of surgery was 2.8% with 0.9% requiring bypass, whereas among those with claudication, the incidence was 0.7% with 0.5% requiring bypass (11).

The guidelines for PTA of the abdominal aorta and lower extremity vessels, approved by multiple councils of the AHA, give thresholds for complications (7) derived from these series (Table 19–4). If the incidence of complications rises above these levels, the site and potentially the physician should be investigated.

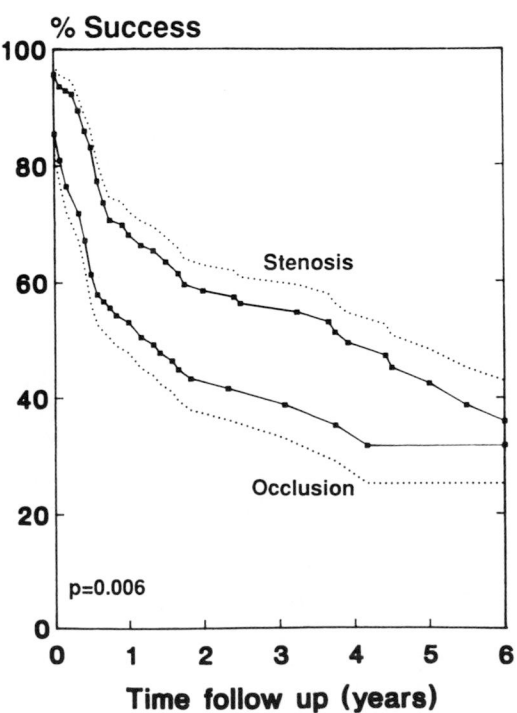

Figure 19–8   Long-term patency of stenoses versus occlusions. The curves are essentially parallel but start at different levels. (Reprinted with permission from Johnston KW. Femoral and popliteral arteries: reanalysis of results of balloon angioplasty. Radiology 1992;183:767–771.)

POTENTIAL IMPROVEMENTS TO ANGIOPLASTY

When the mechanisms of closure of angioplasty are considered, three interrelated factors are paramount: (1) acute thrombosis, (2) elastic recoil with negative vessel remodeling, and (3) intimal hyperplasia.

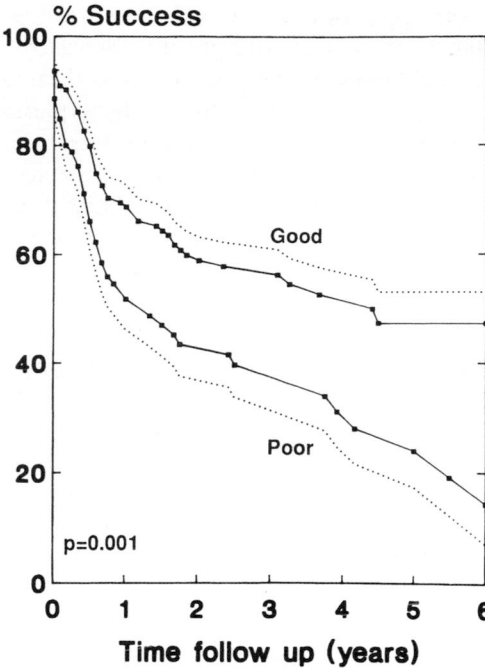

% Success

p=0.001

Good

Poor

Time follow up (years)

Figure 19–10 Long-term patency of good versus poor runoff. (Reprinted with permission from Johnston KW. Femoral and popliteal arteries: reanalysis of results of balloon angioplasty. Radiology 1992;183:767–771.)

TABLE 19–4

THRESHOLDS FOR THE INCIDENCE OF COMPLICATIONS FROM PTA OF THE ABDOMINAL AORTA AND LOWER EXTREMITY VESSELS

Complications	Threshold (%)	
Puncture site		
Bleeding	3.4	
False aneurysm	0.5	
Arteriovenous fistula	0.1	
	4.0	
Angioplasty site		
Thrombus	3.2	
Rupture	0.3	
	3.5	
Distal vessel		
Dissection	0.4	
Embolization	2.3	
	2.7	
Systemic		
Renal failure	0.2	
Myocardial infarction	0.2	(fatal)
Cardiovascular accident	0.05	(fatal)
	0.4	
Consequences		
Surgical repair	2.0	
Limb loss	0.2	
Mortality	0.2	

Reprinted with permission from Pentecost MJ et al. Guidelines for percutaneous transluminal angioplasty of the abdominal aorta and lower extremity vessels. Circulation 1994; 89:511–531.

Acute thrombosis frequently has an underlying mechanical factor, but antiplatelet drugs may influence it. Elastic recoil should be influenced by stents. Finally, after many years of research, progress has been made against intimal hyperplasia using brachytherapy and immunosuppressive drugs.

However, this view is derived from the coronary circulation. In the periphery, an isolated stenosis in an otherwise normal vessel is not what is being referred to. Rather, an inline vessel system, perhaps, a 100 cm in length, much of which is diseased, must be addressed. Closure of a 1 cm angioplasty may lead to an SFA occlusion 25 cm in length. More to the point, even after angiography, it is not always known whether the new symptoms represent failure of the old angioplasty or new disease in the same segment. Certainly, this confounds the results.

Stents

Stents have been moderately successful in the iliac vessels in which elastic recoil and negative vessel remodeling can be influenced significantly. Data from the Wallstent trial in the iliac vessels showed the minimum lumen diameter (MLD) to increase from 1.8 mm before angioplasty to 4.4 mm. After stenting, performed for a poor angioplasty result, the MLD increased to 7.3 mm (53). However, there is an increase in intimal hyperplasia. For this reason, Sapoval et al. showed diminishing patency rates in the iliac system with decreasing diameter (49). He also showed patency

to be related to the stented length, with diminished patency above 75 mm. These caveats are relevant to the femoropopliteal system in which stenting has met with questionable success.

Cejna et al. conducted a multicenter, prospective, randomized trial of angioplasty versus stent placement in femoropopliteal occlusive disease using the Palmaz stent (50). One hundred fifty-four limbs were randomized, 46 of which had ischemia (categories 4 and 5). The mean length of the lesions was 5 cm. The two arms had identical clinical patencies of 65% at 2 years.

A smaller, randomized study by Grimm et al. gave a 3-year primary patency of 68% for angioplasty alone and 62% for angioplasty and stenting, again using the Palmaz stent (51).

Muradin and Huninck's meta-analysis of 19 studies involved 923 angioplasties and 473 stent placements (42,52). For patients with claudication and an SFA stenosis, the 3-year patency for angioplasty was 61% and for stent placement, 63–66%. For occlusions, the 3-year patency was 48% after angioplasty and 64% after stenting.

The Wallstent has fared no better than the Palmaz in the femoropopliteal position. In the Wallstent trial, there were 38 occlusions (mean length 9.4 cm) and 71 stenoses (mean length 3.7 cm) (53). The primary clinical patency at 1 year was 61%, and at 2 years, it was 49%. For stenoses, the primary clinical patency at 1 year was 66%, and for occlusions, it was 53%, which did not reach statistical significance, despite the obvious difference in the complexity of the lesions.

Strecker et al. reported on 80 tantalum stents in the femoropopliteal position (54). Again, no improvement was seen over angioplasty. The 2-year patency was 51%. Shorter stents did better than longer ones, at 59% versus 30%. Stenoses did better than occlusions, at 73% versus 33%.

Stenting does not allow longer lesions to be attempted and does not generally improve the patency. Sapoval has recommended the use of stents only in acute closure during angioplasty (55).

Covered Stents

The notion that covered stents would be successful by blocking the inward migration of smooth muscle cells and, therefore, lead to an improved patency rate, is naïve. Indeed, intimal hyperplasia is more pronounced than after bare stenting (56).

The Endopro was the first covered stent to be used. The polyester (PET) is mounted on a nitinol stent, and the fabric is coated with low molecular-weight heparin. Ahmadi et al. reported on 30 patients (57). Forty percent had the postimplantation syndrome, and 60% had persistent pain. At 1 year, the primary patency was 23%. PET-covered stents have consistently caused pain and fever for several days, but this syndrome is not unknown with PTFE (58).

PTFE stents have fared slightly better. Saxon et al. reported a randomized trial of the Hemobahn stent graft against angioplasty in 28 patients (58). Primary patency at 2 years was 87%, significantly better than angioplasty alone, but most patients had stenoses, good runoff, and a lesion length of 7 cm.

Jahnke et al. reported on 63 Hemobahn stent grafts (59). The mean covered length was 11 cm, and primary patency was 74% at 2 years, but data were available for only 60% of the patients. Bauermeister tackled lesions with a median length of 22 cm (60). Twenty-nine percent were occluded at 6 months.

Certainly, the results do not justify the considerably increased cost nor the increased complication rates because of the larger size. They certainly seem to put paid to the idea of a percutaneously placed femoropopliteal bypass graft—at least one that is endovascular.

TECHNIQUES TO COUNTERACT INTIMAL HYPERPLASIA

Finally, after many years of effort in the coronary system, progress is being made against restenosis, especially when all the causes of angioplasty failure are lumped under this rubric. Elastic recoil and negative vessel remodeling should be mitigated by stenting, despite the increased intimal hyperplasia, although the results, so far, are disappointing in the femoropopliteal position. Intimal hyperplasia, mediated by smooth muscle migration and proliferation, would seem more amenable to a chemical, or even a gene-based influence, but the first success came with brachytherapy.

Brachytherapy

Initial work in the coronary circulation was concerned with finding the ideal technique and dose using the γ emitter ^{192}Iridium (61,62). But, β emitters are easier to use and two commercial platforms have emerged: the ^{90}Strontium-Yttrium BetaCath (Novoste) and the ^{32}Phosphorus Galileo (Guidant) (63). Doses are still not maximized, and trials vary between using 12–18 Gray, 2–3 mm from the center of the source. Nevertheless, radiotherapy has emerged as the preferred treatment for coronary in-stent stenosis. Problems exist with the edge effect, which appear to be soluble by extending the radiation source beyond the stent. Late thrombosis, more than 30 days after radiation therapy, is one of the major complications and requires long-term antiplatelet therapy (64). The technique also has been used in *de novo* lesions, such as in BERT (Beta Energy Restenosis Trial) (65).

In the femoropopliteal position, Minar et al. has conducted several studies using gamma radiation therapy delivered via the MicroSelectron HDR system. One hundred thirteen patients entered one prospective, randomized, placebo-controlled trial in which angioplasty was used for long lesions of the order of 16 cm in length (66). At 6 months, the restenosis rate in the brachytherapy group was 28% and 53% in the angioplasty-alone group ($p < 0.05$). Further refinements have led to the ongoing PARIS (Peripheral Artery Radiation Investigational Study) with the lowest recurrence rate so far—13% at 1 year (67). This is the first inkling that brachytherapy might have broad applicability and might increase the number of angioplasties performed. Long-term data is awaited, but enthusiasm seems well under control. ^{192}IR (intravascular radiation) γ therapy requires that the patient be transported to the radiotherapy department to receive the afterloader. The angioplasty is, therefore, considerably prolonged and at increased risk of infection. Two β-emitter trials currently underway have not yet reported, which is likely to postpone the widespread use of radiotherapy even further.

DRUG-ELUTING STENTS

A polymeric stent coating may be manufactured, and drugs may be eluted from it to influence intimal hyperplasia. Indeed, it may be possible to bind the drug directly to the stent. Two immunosupressant drugs have shown distinct promise—sirolimus and paclitaxil.

Sirolimus

Rapamycin is an antibiotic with a potent immunosuppressive action isolated from streptomycis hygroscopicus. It inhibits cell division early in the cycle and was first approved for the treatment of renal transplant rejection.

The first multicenter, randomized, double-blind trial, RAVEL (Randomized study with the sirolimus-coated Velocity stent), treated *de novo* coronary artery stenoses (68). At 6 months, the restenosis rate in the sirolimus arm was 0%, and there was no loss in minimal lumen diameter. SIRIUS (Sirolimus in the United States), the next randomized trial, involving 1,100 patients, showed in-stent stenosis at 8 months at 2% in the drug-eluting arm and 21% in the noncoated arm ($p < 0.001$) (69). These results are dramatic and have caused considerable excitement in the cardiology community.

Johnson & Johnson (Cordis) has also coated SMART stents, and a prospective randomized trial is underway in the femoropopliteal segment outside the United States. The endpoint of this trial, at least in the preliminary data, is the in-stent mean percent diameter stenosis, as measured by angiography at 6 months—a choice not full of meaning to interventional radiologists. Preliminary findings in 18 patients at 6 months show a lumen of 4.95 mm in the sirolimus group versus 4.31 mm in the bare-stent group—a trial of questionable relevance, with a less than dramatic outcome, so far (70).

Paclitaxil

This is an antitumoral drug extracted from the bark and needles of the Pacific yew tree. It inhibits platelet-derived growth factor and the proliferation of smooth muscle cells further down the pathway than sirolimus. A potential disadvantage is that it delays endothelialization for 3 months. It also has a steep dose response curve, and an optimum dose has yet to be chosen, which is the subject of various trials. Paclitaxil may also be applied directly to the stent without a polymeric coating. TAXUS-2 (Taxol/Taxane-coated stents) uses a NIRx stent (Boston Scientific) coated with paclitaxil (71). In coronary stenoses, in-stent restenosis at 6 months was 36.9% compared with 6.4% in the pacli-taxil arm. The dose of paclitaxil probably has not been worked out adequately nor has another variable, the time of release. There is no study in the peripheral circulation so far (September 2003).

Related drugs, such as evarolimus and tacrolimus, are being investigated, as is a metalloprotease inhibitor, 17-β estradiol and dexamethasone, among others. All may be eluted from stent platforms (72). However, the question arises about whether layer upon layer of expensive additions make peripheral angioplasty a viable alternative to surgery. The answer is only when they significantly increase the number of patients suitable for percutaneous therapy. They do in the coronary circulation, but nothing has yet proved whether they are successful in the femoropopliteal system, not to mention increasing the number of patients suitable for less invasive procedures.

ALTERNATIVE METHODS OF FEMOROPOPLITEAL RECANALIZATION

The major thrust of this chapter has been on angioplasty, because it is the most established technique and certainly is the one with the best long-term follow-up. But other, more sophisticated, endovascular techniques have been developed. In the past, a physician would develop a technique, design a pilot device, test it, then take it to a manufacturer for refinement and distribution. Today, manufacturers thrust finished products on the interventional community. Ring addressed this matter in an editorial in which the lack of adequate studies surrounding many of the new devices was criticized (73). Another voice of criticism, specifically about lasers, came from Strandness who sees their development more in terms of marketing than of medical progress (74).

Perhaps because many of these devices were not developed by the medical community, or perhaps because marketing was perceived as important by the physician end user, their usefulness in peripheral recanalization has not always been seen in perspective. Because femoropopliteal disease is at least three times more prevalent than iliac disease, and because in the femoropopliteal system occlusions predominate over stenoses by a ratio of at least 3:1, it is clear that most patients with significant, symptomatic peripheral vascular disease have femoral occlusions. Furthermore, only about 20% of these lesions are 10 cm or less in length and are suitable for angioplasty (5,7). One would imagine, therefore, that new devices would be developed to expand the role of angioplasty into the previously untreatable patient population. Yet, the modern and sophisticated devices have specifically not done so. To date, no device has significantly expanded the patient population suitable for endovascular therapy and, indeed, many of them are no longer manufactured.

Debulking Devices

Histology studies demonstrate that angioplasty, although widening the lumen, leaves large amounts of atheromatous plaque, indeed, nearly the same volume as before (75). This has been confirmed by intravascular ultrasound (76,77). The concept of excising atheroma and leaving a smooth lumen is, therefore, attractive.

In the past, the Simpson Atherocath, the Auth rotablator, the PAC, the TEC, the low-speed rotational catheter, and the Kensey were described in the literature, but little has been heard of them in more recent years. For those with a historical bent, an excellent review by McLean is recommended (78).

However, in 1995, Henry et al. used the rotablator in 150 patients with stenotic disease with a mean length of 4 cm, although 50% were below the knee (79). He opined that rotational ablation has taken a preeminent position in the treatment in distal leg arteries. Despite that, he has not reported since and much of the enthusiasm for this device has waned. Nevertheless, the development of such devices continues. Yoffe et al. reported preliminary work with a corkscrew cutting device, the Xtrak (80). The device was used on occlusions ranging from 4 to 16 cm (mean–11 cm) followed by balloon angioplasty. Yet again, the preliminary results were similar to balloon angioplasty alone. Distal embolization remains a potential problem with all these devices. Cryotherapy is the latest contender, but results are too preliminary to be reported here.

Enthusiasts believe that it is only a matter of time before one of these devices is successful. People buy lottery tickets on the same principle. Any successful device certainly will not employ adjunctive angioplasty and will have to solve the problem of distal embolization. The manufacturers are usually more sanguine and continue to speak of niche markets, which is a sure sign of the limitations of the devices.

Lasers

Lasers offer another way to debulk, but again have limitations. Fifteen years of laser research has looked at the 308-nanometer Xenon chloride excimer laser, the 488–514 nm Argon laser, the 504 nm dye laser, the 1,064 nm Neodymium-YAG laser, and the 2,090 nm Holmium-YAG laser, among others. Attempts have been made to stain plaque with tetracycline, betacarotine, or hematoporphyrins to improve the absorption of a specific laser wavelength, but none have met with much success. The energy has been continuous-wave and pulsed. Fibers have been bare and bundled. Metal hot tips and laser-lucent sapphires have been tried.

Lammer has carefully reviewed this effort and concluded that "the technique of laser angioplasty was continuously improved until the initial recanalization rates and the long-term patency rates in femoropopliteal artery occlusions were the same as the success rates of percutaneous transluminal angioplasty" (81). Not wishing to denigrate either his own considerable effort over the years or that of others, he concluded that the work should continue. Nevertheless, it has no role as a routine procedure. At most, it has the same deficiency as the Dotter catheter; the lumen achieved is only as big as the catheter. So far, there has been no escape from concomitant balloon angioplasty. Although laser energy is very efficient at vaporizing tissue, with no significant embolic risk, the inhomogeneity of plaque, with its different absorption characteristics, is its ultimate downfall.

Lammer et al. reported a prospective, multicenter trial of the sapphire lens YAG laser (82). He described laser recanalization in 338 patients with femoropopliteal artery occlusions averaging 8.5 cm in length. The initial recanalization rate was 85%, and complications were observed in 14% of patients, with emergency surgery required in 1.5%. The cumulative long-term patency rate was 57% at 3 years; that is, the results were similar to balloon angioplasty, but with a higher complication rate.

Scheinert et al. recently reported on 411 SFA occlusions in 318 consecutive patients treated with the excimer laser with a mean lesion length of 19 cm (83). Although the technical success was 91% after two attempts, the primary patency at 1 year was 33.6%. One hesitates to predict the 5-year primary patency.

Subintimal Angioplasty

The description of the technique of angioplasty earlier in the chapter makes a great point of staying within the vessel lumen and not dissecting it, as well as showing that it is particularly important in short-segment lesions. Nevertheless, it is obvious that when traversing a long-segment occlusion, even though one may have started within the original lumen, it is difficult to know that one has remained within it. It has always been assumed that emerging successfully out of the obstruction and into a patent lumen implies that one has remained intraluminal. This cannot always be the case.

For 15 years, Bolia et al. has championed subintimal angioplasty for long-segment occlusions (84–87). A Van Andel catheter and a floppy-tipped guide wire are used deliberately to exit the lumen above the obstruction and create a subintimal channel, which is dissected away using the snowplough technique. When the bottom of the obstructed lesion is reached, a guide wire is looped into a large U, which, when advanced, reenters the true lumen and balloon dilatation is undertaken in the normal way to reveal a smooth, subintimal lumen. The fact that some practitioners have had difficulty reentering is attested to by the fact that special needles have been designed to facilitate reentry. In the author's experience, reentry is frequently achieved several centimeters below the obstructed segment, thereby extending the length of the reopened segment. Bolia et al. would argue that this is unimportant because the new, smooth lumen contains no atheroma. Bolia also argues that long-segment occlusions are easily recanalized in this fashion, but conventional recanalization of long-segment occlusions has never been the problem. Rather, it has been the long-term patency.

In 1994, London and Bolia reported their experience with 200 consecutive, intentional, subintimal femoropopliteal artery recanalizations with a technical success rate of 80%

(84,85). One hundred fifty-nine lesions were occlusions, 73 of which were 10 cm or less in length, 63 were 11–20 cm and 23 were greater than 20 cm. The primary success rates were essentially the same in the three groups. The overall 3-year patency was 48%. These results are similar to conventional angioplasty, but the complexity of the lesions is surprising. Eighty percent of the lesions were occlusions, and 54% of them were greater than 10 cm in length. Multiple regression analysis showed that each additional 10 cm in length increased the risk by 1.73%, a highly significant factor. The major risk appears to be dissecting off a critical collateral, and this risk increases with length. Nevertheless, there was no limb loss in the series. Each additional runoff vessel decreased the risk by 0.54, again highly significant and no different from conventional angioplasty.

Here is a technique *not* derived from the coronary circulation, which *does* extend the number of patients suitable for treatment *and* gives comparable results. A technique, that allows many patients with ischemia to be treated and legitimately could be randomized against surgery. It deserves considerably more enthusiasm than it has received. Perhaps it needs a different messenger and certainly deserves more trials.

SUMMARY

Millions of dollars have gone toward the development of alternatives to balloon angioplasty. The early driving force was an attempt to capture the lucrative coronary market, not to affect femoropopliteal disease. The second goal was to overcome the very high restenosis rate in the coronary circulation—approximately 50% at 6 months. At last, dramatic results have been achieved in the coronary circulation. Multidrug regimes have improved patency, stents have been highly successful, and intimal hyperplasia has at last been significantly influenced, if not controlled. Few of these techniques are yet particularly influential in the femoropopliteal system, but radiotherapy holds some promise, and different drug regimes may prove beneficial. Subintimal angioplasty certainly should be explored more actively.

It may well be that with bipedalism, we have evolved away from a dominant profunda to a long SFA, which, with any perturbation in the system, atheroma, longevity, and diminished runoff, is destined to close. Perhaps a percutaneously placed, extravascular, unsupported (or only partially supported) femoropopliteal artery bypass graft is needed, although prosthetic bypass grafts themselves are far from ideal. For the present time, however, balloon angioplasty with all its limitations remains the procedure of choice, except in special situations. Unfortunately, there is only a relatively small population of patients with femoropopliteal disease for whom angioplasty is suitable.

REFERENCES

1. Dotter CT, Judkins MP. Transluminal treatment of arteriosclerotic obstruction: description of a new technique and a preliminary report of its application. Circulation 1964;30:654–670.
2. Staple TW. Modified catheter for percutaneous transluminal treatment of arteriosclerotic obstructions. Radiology 1968;91:1041–1043.
3. van Andel GJ. Percutaneous Transluminal Angioplasty (The Dotter Procedure): A Manual for Radiologists. Amsterdam: Elsevier, 1976.
4. Grüntzig A, Hopff H. Perkutane Rekanalisation Chronischer Arterieller Verschlusse Mit Einem Neuen Dilatations-Katheter. Dtsch Med Wochenschr 1974;99:2502–2510.
5. Martin EC. Transcatheter therapies in peripheral and noncoronary vascular disease. Introduction. Circulation 1991;83(Suppl II):I1–5.
6. Martin EC. The impact of angioplasty: a perspective. J Vasc Interv Radiol 1992;3:511–514.
7. Pentecost MJ, Criqui MH, Dorros G, et al. Guidelines for peripheral percutaneous transluminal angioplasty of the abdominal aorta and lower extremity vessels. Circulation 1994;89:511–531.
8. Cardella JF, Casarella WJ, De Weese JA, et al. Optimal resources for the examination and endovascular treatment of the peripheral and visceral vascular systems. AHA Intercouncil report on peripheral and visceral angiographic and interventional laboratories. Circulation 1994;89:481–493.
9. Rutherford RB, Flanigan DP, Gupta SK, et al. Suggested standards for the reports dealing with lower extremity ischemia. J Vasc Surg 1986;4:80–94.
10. Standards of Practice Committee SCVIR. Guidelines for percutaneous transluminal angioplasty. J Vasc Interv Radiol 1990;1:5–15.
11. Belli AM, Cumberland DC, Knoz AM, et al. The complication rate of percutaneous peripheral balloon angioplasty. Clin Radiol 1990;41:380–383.
12. Kinnison ML, White RI Jr, Bowers WP, et al. Cost incentives for peripheral angioplasty. AJR Am J Roentgenol 1985;145:1241–1244.
13. Jeans WD, Danton RM, Baird RN, et al. A comparison of the costs of vascular surgery and balloon dilatation in lower limb ischaemic disease. Br J Radiol 1986;59:453–456.
14. Veith FJ, Gupta SK, Wengerter KR, et al. Changing arteriosclerotic disease patterns and management strategies in lower limb threatening ischemia. Ann Surg 1990;212:402–412.
15. Holland Interuniversity Nifedipine/Metoprolol Trial (HINT) Research Group: British Heart Journal. Br Heart J 1986;56:400–413.
16. Mehta SR, Yusuf S. Short- and long-term oral antiplatelet therapy in acute coronary syndromes and percutaneous coronary intervention. J Am Coll Cardiol 2003;41:79S–88S.
17. Lewis HD, Davis J, Archibald D, et al. Protective effects of aspirin against acute myocardial infarction and death in men with unstable angina. N Engl J Med 1983;309:396–403.
18. Schwartz L, Bourassa MG, Lesperance J, et al. Aspirin and dipyridamole in the prevention of restenosis after percutaneous transluminal coronary angioplasty. N Engl J Med 1988;318:1714–1719.
19. Gill S, Majumdar S, Brown NE, et al. Ticlopidine associated pancytopenia:implications of an acetylsalicylic acid alternative. Can J Cardiol 1997;13:909–13.
20. The CAPRIE steering committee. A randomized, blinded, trial of clopidogrel versus aspirin in patients at risk of ischemic events. Lancet 1996;348:1329–1339.
21. Steinhubl SR, Berger PB, Mann JT III, et al. Early and sustained dual oral antiplatelet therapy following percutaneous coronary intervention: a randomized controlled trial. JAMA 2002;288:2411–2420.
22. Mehta SR, Yusuf S, et al. On behalf of the CURE Investigators. The Clopidogrel in Unstable angina to prevent Recurrent Events (CURE) trial program: rationale, design, and baseline characteristics including a meta-analysis of the effects of thienopyridines in vascular disease. Eur Heart J 2000;21:2033–2041.
23. Messerli AW, Aronow HD, Sprecher DL. The Lescol Intervention Prevention Study (LIPS): starting a statin immediately after PCI. Cleveland Clin J Med 2003;70:561–566.

24. Chew DP, Bhatt DL, Sapp S, et al. Increased mortality with oral platelet glycoprotein IIb/IIIa antagonists: a meta-analysis of Phase III multicenter randomized trials. Circulation 2001;103:201–206.

25. Stone G. The CADILLAC investigators: Controlled Abciximab and Device Investigation to Lower Late Angioplasty Complications (CADILLAC). N Engl J Med 2002;346:957–966.

26. Montalescot G, Barragan P, Wittenberg O, et al. Platelet glycoprotein IIb/IIIa inhibition with coronary stenting for acute myocardial infarction. N Engl J Med 2001;344:1895–1903.

27. The EPISTENT investigators. Randomized placebo-controlled and balloon-angioplasty-controlled trial to assess safety of coronary stenting with use of platelet glycoprotein IIb/IIIa blockade. Lancet 1998;352:87–92.

28. Bonz AW, Lengenfelder B, Strotmann J, et al. Effect of additional temporary glycoprotein IIb/IIIa receptor inhibition on troponin release in elective percutaneous coronary interventions after pretreatment with aspirin and clopidogrel (TOPSTAR trial). J Am Coll Cardiol 2002;40:662–668.

29. Aguirre FV, Topol EJ, Ferguson JJ, et al. Bleeding complications with the chimeric antibody to platelet glycoprotein IIb/IIIa integrin in patients undergoing percutaneous coronary intervention. EPIC Investigators. Circulation 1995;91:2882–2890.

30. Rutherford RB, Becker GJ. Standards for evaluating and reporting the results of surgical and percutaneous therapy for peripheral arterial disease. J Vasc Interv Radiol 1991;2:169–174.

31. Adar R, Critchfield GC, Eddie DM. A confidence profile analysis of the results of femoropopliteal percutaneous transluminal angioplasty in the treatment of lower extremity ischemia. J Vasc Surg 1989;10:57–67.

32. Wilson SE, Wolf GL, Cross AP. Percutaneous transluminal angioplasty versus operation for peripheral arteriosclerosis. J Vasc Surg 1989;9:1–9.

33. Murray RR, Hewes RC, White RJ Jr, et al. Long-segment femoropopliteal stenoses: is angioplasty a boon or a bust? Radiology 1987;162:473–476.

34. Capek P, McLean GK, Berkowitz HD. Femoropopliteal angioplasty factors influencing long-term success. Circulation 1991;83 (Suppl II):70–80.

35. Martin EC, Fankuchen EI, Karlson KB, et al. Angioplasty for femoral artery occlusion: comparison with surgery. AJR Am J Roentgenol 1981;137:915–919.

36. Morgenstern BR, Getrajdman GI, Laffey KJ, et al. Total occlusions of the femoropopliteal artery: high technical success rate of conventional balloon angioplasty. Radiology 1989;172:937–940.

37. Krepel VM, van Andel GJ, van Erp WE, et al. Percutaneous transluminal angioplasty of the femoropopliteal artery: initial long-term results. Radiology 1985;156:325–338.

38. Johnston KW, Rae M, Hogg-Johnston SA, et al. Five-year results of a prospective study of percutaneous transluminal angioplasty. Ann Surg 1987;206:403–413.

39. Zeitler F. Percutaneous dilatation and recanalization of iliac and femoral arteries. Cardiovasc Intervent Radiol 1980;3:207–212.

40. Waltman AC, Greenfield AJ, Noveline RA, et al. Transluminal angioplasty of the iliac and femoropopliteal arteries. Arch Surg 1982;117:1218–1221.

41. Tamura S, Sniderman KW, Beinart C, et al. Percutaneous transluminal angioplasty of the popliteal artery and its branches. Radiology 1982;143:645–648

42. Hunink, MGM, Wong JB, Donaldson MC, et al. Patency results of percutaneous and surgical revascularization for femoropopliteal arterial disease. Med Decis Making 1994;14:71–81.

43. Hunink MGM, Wong JB, Donaldson MC, et al. Revascularization for femoropopliteal disease: a decision and cost-effectiveness analysis. JAMA 1995;274:165–71.

44. Hewes RC, White RI Jr, Murray RR, et al. Long-term results of superficial femoral artery angioplasty. AJR Am J Roentgenol 1986;146:1025–1029.

45. Probst P, Cerny P, Owens A, et al. Patency after femoral angioplasty: correlation of angiographic appearance with clinical findings. AJR Am J Roentgenol 1983;140:1227–1232.

46. Johnston KW. Femoral and popliteal arteries: reanalysis of results of balloon angioplasty. Radiology 1992;183:767–771.

47. Clark TWI, Groffsky JL, Soulen MC. Predictors of long-term patency after femoropopliteal angioplasty: results from the STAR registry. J Vasc Interv Radiol 2001;12:923–933.

48. Becker GJ, Katzen BT, Dake MD. Noncoronary angioplasty. Radiology 1989;170:921–940.

49. Sapoval MR, Chatellier G, Long AL, et al. Self-expandable stents for the treatment of iliac artery obstructive lesions: long-term success and prognostic factors. AJR Am J Roentgenol 1996;166:1173–1179.

50. Cejna M, Thurnher S, Illiasch H, et al. PTA versus Palmaz stent placement in femoropopliteal artery Obstructions: a multicenter prospective randomized study. J Vasc Interv Radiol 2001;12:23–31.

51. Grimm J, Muller-Hulsbeck S, Jahnke T, et al. Randomized study to compare PTA alone versus PTA with Palmaz stent placement for femoropopliteal lesions. J Vasc Interv Radiol 2001;12:935–942.

52. Muradin GS, Bosch JL, Stijnen T, et al. Balloon dilation and stent implantation for treatment of femoropopliteal arterial disease: meta-analysis. Radiology 2001;221:137–145.

53. Martin EC, Katzen BT, Benenati, JF, et al. Multicenter trial of the wallstent in the iliac and femoral arteries. J Vasc Interv Radiol 1995;6:843–849.

54. Strecker EP, Boos IB, Gottman D. Femoropopliteal artery stent placement: evaluation of long-term success. Radiology 1997;205:375–383.

55. Sapoval MR, Long AL, Raynaud AC, et al. Femoropopliteal stent placement: long-term results. Radiology 1992;184:833–839.

56. Cejna M, Virmani R, Jones R, et al. Biocompatibility and performance of the Wallstent and the Wallgraft, Jostent, and Hemobahn stent-grafts in a sheep model. J Vasc Interv Radiol 2002;13:823–30.

57. Ahmadi R, Schillinger M, Maca T, et al. Femoropopliteal arteries: immediate and long-term results with a Dacron-covered stent-graft. Radiology 2002;223:345–350.

58. Saxon RR, Coffman JM, Gooding JM, et al. Long-term results of ePTFE stent-graft versus angioplasty in the femoropopliteal artery: single center experience from a prospective, randomized trial. J Vasc Interv Radiol 2003;14:303–311.

59. Jahnke T, Andresen R, Muller-Hulsbeck S, et al. Hemobahn stent-grafts for treatment of femoropopliteal arterial obstructions: midterm results of a prospective trial. J Vasc Interv Radiol 2003;14:41–51.

60. Bauermeister G. Endovascular stent-grafting in the treatment of superficial femoral artery occlusive disease. J Endovasc Ther 2001;8:315–320.

61. Teirstein PS, Massullo V, Jani S, et al. Catheter-based radiotherapy to inhibit restenosis after coronary stenting. N Engl J Med 1997;336:1697–1703.

62. Waksman R, White RL, Chan RC, et al. Intracoronary gamma radiation therapy after angioplasty inhibits recurrence in patients with in stent restenosis. Circulation 2000;101:2165–2171.

63. Ajani AE, Waksman R. Beta radiation: state of the art. J Interv Cardiol 2001;14:601–609.

64. Waksman R, Bhargava B, Mintz GS, et al. Late total occlusion after intra-coronary brachytherapy for patients with in-stent restenosis. J Am Coll Cardiol 2000;36:65–68.

65. King SB III, Williams DO, Chougule P, et al. Endovascular beta-radiation to reduce restenosis after coronary balloon angioplasty: results of the beta energy restenosis trial (BERT). Circulation 1998;97:2025–2030.

66. Minar E, Pokrajac B, Maca T, et al. Endovascular brachytherapy for prophylaxis of restenosis after femoropopliteal angioplasty: results of a prospective randomized study. Circulation 2000;102:2694–2699.

67. Waksman R, Laird JE, Jurkovitz CT, et al. Intravascular radiation therapy after balloon angioplasty of narrowed femoropopliteal arteries to prevent restenosis: results of the PARIS feasibility trial. J Vasc Interv Radiol 2001;12:915–921.

68. Morice M, Serruys PW, Sousa J et al. The RAVEL study: a randomized study with the sirolimus coated Bx velocity balloon-expandable stent in the treatment of patients with de novo native coronary artery lesions [Abstract]. Eur Heart J 2001;22:484.

69. Moses JW, Leon MB, Popma JJ, et al. Sirolimus-eluting stents versus standard stents in patients with stenosis in a native coronary artery. N Engl J Med 2003;349:1315–1323.

70. Duda SH, Pusich B, Richter G, et al. Sirolimus-eluting stents for the treatment of obstructive superficial femoral artery disease: six-month results. Circulation 2002;106:1505–1509.

71. Colombo A, Drzewiecki J, Banning A, et al. Randomized study to assess the effectiveness of slow- and moderate-release polymer-based paclitaxel-eluting stents for coronary artery lesions. Circulation 2003;108:788–794.

72. Duda SH, Poerner TC, Wiesinger B, et al. Drug-eluting stents: potential applications for peripheral arterial occlusive disease. J Vasc Interv Radiol 2003;14:291–301.

73. Ring EJ. New interventional devices and the need for restraint. Radiology 1989;170:945–946.

74. Strandness DE Jr, Barnes RW, Katzen B, et al. Indiscriminate use of laser angioplasty. Radiology 1989;172:945–946.

75. Castaneda-Zuniga WR, Formanek A, Tadavarthy M, et al. The mechanism of balloon angioplasty. Radiology 1980;135:565–571.

76. Pandian NC, Kreis A, O'Donnell T. Intravascular ultrasound estimation of arterial stenosis. J Am Soc Echocardiogr 1989;2:390–392.

77. Yock PG, Fitzgerald PJ, Linker DT, et al. Intravascular ultrasound guidance for catheter-based coronary interventions. J Am Coll Cardiol 1991;17(VI Suppl B):39–45.

78. McLean GK. Percutaneous peripheral atherectomy. J Vasc Interv Radiol 1993;4:465–480.

79. Henry M, Amor M, Ethevenot G, et al. Percutaneous peripheral atherectomy using the rotablator: a single-center experience. J Endovasc Surg 1995;2:51–66.

80. Yoffe B, Yavnel L, Altshuler A, et al. Preliminary experience with the Xtrak debulking device in the treatment of peripheral occlusions. J Endovasc Ther 2002;9:234–240.

81. Lammer J. Laser angioplasty of peripheral arteries: an epilogue? Cardiovasc Intervent Radiol 1995;18:1–8.

82. Lammer J, Pilger E, Karnel F, et al. Laser angioplasty: results of a prospective multicenter study at 3-year follow-up. Radiology 1991;178:335–337.

83. Scheinert D, Laird JR Jr, Schroder M, et al. Excimer laser-assisted recanalization of long, chronic superficial femoral artery occlusions. J Endovasc Ther 2001;8:156–166.

84. Bolia A, Miles KA, Brennan J, et al. Percutaneous transluminal angioplasty of occlusions of the femoral and popliteal arteries by subintimal dissection. Cardiovasc Intervent Radiol 1990;13:357–363.

85. London NJM, Srinivasan R, Naylor AR, et al. Subintimal angioplasty of femoropopliteal artery occlusion: the long-term results. Eur J Vasc Surg 1994;8:148–155.

86. London NJM, Varty K, Sayers RD, et al. Percutaneous transluminal angioplasty for lower limb critical ischemia. Brit J Surg 1995;82:1232–1235.

87. Varty K, Nydahl S, Butterworth P, et al. Changes in the management of critical limb ischemia. Brit J Surg 1996;83:953–956.

Infrapopliteal Revascularization

20

Marcy B. Jagust, Thomas A. Sos

Since percutaneous transluminal angioplasty (PTA) of peripheral vessels was first described by Dotter and Judkins (1) in 1964, the procedure has been performed with increasing frequency. Initially, dilatation was performed by passage of progressively larger tapered catheters, which evolved into the use of balloon catheters. Although initial results were disappointing, advances in catheter and guide wire technology markedly increased success rates. Today, angioplasty of iliac, superficial femoral, and popliteal arteries is a widely accepted and often performed procedure.

Early results of infrapopliteal angioplasty were not impressive (2,3). The higher risks of procedures in this area kept PTA reserved for limb-threatening ischemia and cases in which surgery was not feasible. Manipulation through tibial vessels became easier with the introduction of small-diameter, low-profile balloon catheters and very radiopaque, soft, steerable guide wires originally developed for use in the coronary vasculature. In addition, advances in radiographic equipment that permitted roadmapping allowed radiologists to consider PTA for small, diseased tibial vessels. Angioplasty of the infrapopliteal vasculature has gained increasing popularity over the past few years as technical advances have made tibial PTA safer and more successful.

PATIENT SELECTION

Patients with tibial occlusive disease may be minimally symptomatic or asymptomatic. The absence of pedal pulses may be an incidental finding in patients with well-developed collateral vessels or limited activity. Ischemic symptoms must be present before any intervention is considered. Disabling claudication, rest pain, toe ulcers, and gangrene are symptoms of severe, limb-threatening ischemia. These symptoms may be grouped according to a classification outlined by Rutherford et al. (4) (Table 20–1). Before treatment, the diagnosis of lower extremity ischemia resulting from tibial vessel disease should be made, and other possible etiologies for pain should be excluded. A thorough history and physical examination should be obtained as well as appropriate noninvasive testing, including pulse volume recordings (PVRs) and ankle-brachial pressure indices (ABIs). Ischemic rest pain is associated with ABIs less than 0.5 mm Hg (5) or resting ankle pressures of less than 40 mm Hg (4). Nonhealing ulcers and gangrene are associated with ankle pressures of less than 60 mm Hg (4). ABIs are not useful in diabetic patients with calcified, noncompressible vessels. PVRs will show marked waveform damping. At some institutions, the decision to perform tibial angioplasty is made in conjunction with the vascular surgeon after careful review of the diagnostic arteriogram. Patients with limb-threatening ischemia often have multilevel disease. Depending on the severity of the inflow lesions, especially occlusions or long-segment severe stenoses, the supratibial disease is often treated first. The limb is then reevaluated 4–6 weeks later, after there has been time for the limb to heal and for collateral vessels to develop.

The type of lesion is also an important determinant in the decision to perform tibial PTA. As in other vessels, long-term patency after dilatation is more favorable for

TABLE 20–1

CLINICAL CATEGORIES OF CHRONIC LIMB ISCHEMIA

Grade	Category	Clinical Description	Objective Criteria
I	0	Asymptomatic, no hemodynamically significant occlusive disease	Normal results of treadmill*/stress test. Completes treadmill exercise*; AP after exercise <50 mm Hg but >25 mm Hg less than BP. Symptoms between those of categories 1 and 3. Cannot complete treadmill exercise and AP after exercise is <50 mm Hg
	1	Mild claudication	
	2	Moderate claudication	
	3	Severe claudication	
II	4	Ischemic rest pain	Resting AP <40 mm Hg, flat or barely pulsatile ankle or metatarsal PVR; TP <30 mm Hg
III	5	Minor tissue loss—nonhealing ulcer, focal gangrene with diffuse pedal ischemia	Resting AP <60 mm Hg, ankle or metatarsal PVR flat or barely pulsatile; TP <40 mm Hg
	6	Major tissue loss—extending above transmetatarsal level, functional foot no longer salvageable	Same as for category 5

AP = Ankle pressure; BP = Brachial pressure; PVR = Pulse volume recording; TP = Toe pressure
* Five minutes at 2 mph on a 12% incline
Reprinted with permission from Rutherford RB, Flanigan DP, Gupta SK, et al. Suggested standards for dealing with lower extremity ischemia. J Vasc Surg 1986;4:80–94.

single focal stenoses (6). Although long-term patency may be limited for diffusely diseased vessels, short-term patency may be sufficient to heal superficial ulcerations or amputation sites. Occlusions can be crossed and dilated; however, the chance of success decreases with increasing length. If chronic occlusions cannot be crossed intraluminally, a subintimal approach may be attempted. Bolia et al. (7) report good technical results with this method, although others have had difficulty in duplicating these results. The use of metal stents in this situation promises to increase the technical success rate.

The time course for the development of symptoms is also an important consideration. Recent onset of symptoms with an occlusion implies associated thrombus, which should be lysed initially. In turn, this may reveal underlying stenoses.

EQUIPMENT

Balloon Catheters

Tibial angioplasty is performed with 2- to 4-mm balloons on catheter shafts of 4 French and smaller. These balloon catheters are available in lengths of 80–135 cm. They accept 0.010–0.018-inch guide wires and differ considerably in stiffness and trackability. The catheter shaft should be stiff enough to allow tracking over a guide wire in a small vessel with extensive atherosclerotic disease and increased friction. Monorail systems are also available and may be useful in patients who have limited focal disease requiring less trackability.

Guide Wires

The ideal guide wire should be easily visible under fluoroscopy, be torqueable to follow curves and maneuver around plaques, have a relatively floppy tip to avoid dissection, and have a stiff body to allow the balloon catheter shaft to follow. The Flex-T (Mallinckrodt), Platinum Plus (Boston Scientific), and the various hydrophilic guide wires are all useful. Some interventionalists prefer the shapeable, soft, radiopaque, hydrophilic tip and a stiff shaft of the V-18 Control Wire (Boston Scientific).

TECHNIQUE

Physical Examination

Before any arteriogram or interventional procedure, it is important to assess the patient's peripheral pulses or Doppler signals as well as extremity color and temperature.

Puncture

The diagnostic arteriogram usually is performed from a retrograde puncture in the groin opposite the affected limb. Vascular access for angioplasty usually is obtained via an antegrade puncture into the common femoral artery on the symptomatic side with placement of a vascular sheath. Puncture of the common femoral artery below the inguinal ligament is essential to reduce the chance of retroperitoneal hemorrhage. It is also important to make the puncture over the bone so that postprocedure compression is against resistance. In obese patients whose body habitus precludes an antegrade puncture, a retrograde puncture of the contralateral groin may be performed for an up-and-over-the-bifurcation procedure. A retrograde approach may also be helpful in those patients who have had extensive surgery in the ipsilateral groin. Drawbacks to this approach include less control of the catheter and guide wire, inability to reach more distal lesions because of limitations in catheter length, and decreased trackability. The use of guiding catheters or sheaths across the aortic bifurcation helps make the retrograde technique easier.

Because the incidence of puncture site complications increases with increasing catheter size, it is important to minimize the size of the vascular sheath. If the procedure is limited to the tibial vessels, a 4 French sheath is inserted. If angioplasty of suprapopliteal lesions is also planned, a 4 French or 5 French sheath is inserted. Several manufacturers have low-profile balloons ranging from 2–6 mm that fit through 4 French sheaths. Therefore, there is often no need to increase the sheath size when an adjunct angioplasty in a supratibial vessel is planned.

Lesion Traversal

Roadmapping may be performed through the balloon catheter or from the side port of the vascular sheath. This capability allows for precise maneuvering through the small, diseased tibial vessels. Some interventionalists advocate placing two guide wires when the lesion is close to a bifurcation (8). The origin of the adjacent vessel may then be dilated if it is narrowed by the first angioplasty. This is rarely a problem and not a routine approach to bifurcation lesions, but it may be reserved for severe stenoses at both origins.

The platinum tip wires are very visible, easily torqueable, very soft, and therefore atraumatic. However, in vessels with extensive and eccentric disease, the wire tip may become lodged under a plaque. In these cases, it may be impossible to withdraw and redirect the wire as it becomes bent and accordioned at the tip. In these instances, an angled hydrophilic wire may be more useful. In the past, the 0.018-inch Terumo hydrophilic wires were difficult to see. But, more recent versions have gold tips to make them more radiopaque. The V-18 Control Wire (Boston Scientific) has a highly radiopaque hydrophilic tip.

An occlusion may be crossed with an 0.018-inch hydrophilic wire. However, on occasion, an 0.018-inch guide wire may not be stiff enough to cross a firm occlusion. In this instance, a 0.035-inch wire is advanced across the lesion followed by a tapered 4 French or 5 French straight catheter. Some interventionalists use the Bentson wire, whose floppy tip becomes rigid when only a small length is passed beyond the catheter tip. If the Bentson wire cannot be passed, a straight or angled hydrophilic

Terumo guide wire (Medi-Tech) may be used. After the catheter is advanced across the lesion, the 0.035-inch guide wire may be exchanged for an 0.018-inch guide wire, and the balloon catheter inserted.

In all these maneuvers, gentleness and finesse are important initially, and more force is applied only when gentler maneuvers have failed. Because "feedback" is less with the hydrophilic wires, there is an increased chance of subintimal passage. On occasion, a firm occlusion cannot be crossed intraluminally. Some operators advocate deliberate subintimal wire passage and the performance of subintimal angioplasty (7). Although there is no data supporting primary stent placement in the infrapopliteal vessels, many interventionalists will use them to rescue a potentially failed procedure.

Balloon Selection

In general, 3- and 4-mm balloons are used in the proximal to midtibial vessels, 2- and 3-mm balloons are used in the mid- to distal tibial vessels, and 2-mm balloons are used in the foot vessels. Balloon size is usually determined by measuring the caliber of the nearest normal segment of vessel. On digital images, the vessel size can be determined through comparison with a known measurement on the image. After many procedures on the same equipment, the authors frequently "eyeball" the balloon size, particularly when the balloon size can be compared with a real-time road map. Some interventionalists inflate a balloon for 30 seconds across an infrapopliteal vessel lesion.

Follow-Up Arteriography

After angioplasty, the balloon catheter is withdrawn into the popliteal artery, and the guide wire is left across the dilated area. The follow-up arteriogram is then performed from the side port of the vascular sheath to avoid having to recross the lesion in the event further intervention is needed. Successful angioplasty is defined as a residual stenosis of 30% or less. If a significant lesion remains, it may be redilated with the same or larger balloon (Figures 20–1, 20–2, 20–3, and 20–4).

Postprocedure Care

After the procedure, patients are brought to the recovery room for observation while the administered heparin is metabolized; use of protamine to reverse anticoagulation is often not recommended. It is very convenient and almost essential to have a Hemochron (International Technidyne Corporation) or similar machine available to measure the activated clotting time (ACT) to ascertain at what point it is safe to pull the sheath or catheter. The

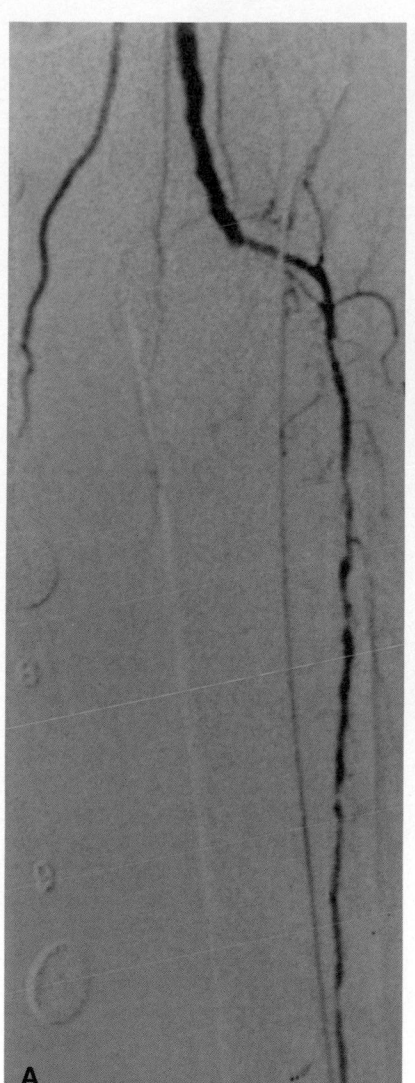
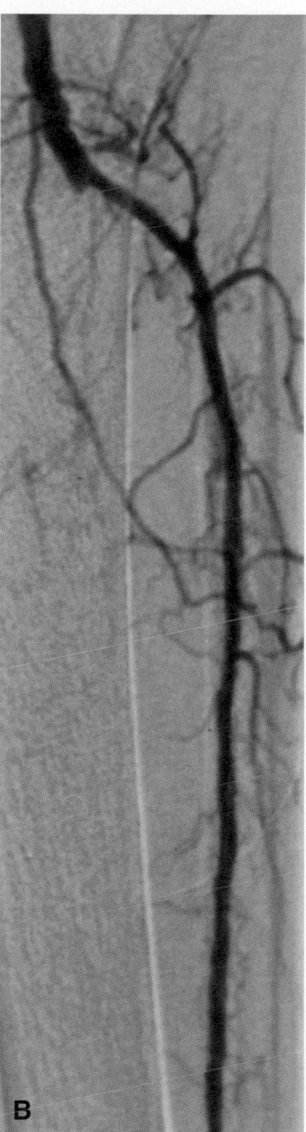

Figure 20-1 A. Angiogram showing multiple stenoses of the anterior tibial artery, which is the sole runoff vessel. **B.** Postangioplasty angiogram. The patient had a palpable dorsalis pedis pulse.

reflects heparin activity and is a means of assessing the anticoagulation status (9). After the heparin has worn off, the vascular sheath is removed and compression is applied until hemostasis is achieved. Closure devices are also available that can be used while the patient is still anticoagulated to limit the patient's time in the interventional area.

Patients are not routinely anticoagulated after the procedure. However, patients with a poor initial angiographic result, extensive distal atherosclerosis with slow flow, or both are often anticoagulated. After successful angioplasty, chronic antiplatelet therapy with aspirin is the recommendation. No consensus exists on the correct dosage (10), but 80–325 mg daily is recommended.

Many physicians also begin patients on clopidogrel (Plavix) after the procedure. This comes from the cardiology data and is standard procedure postcoronary angioplasty

(11). Patients usually are given a loading dose of 300 mg followed by a 75-mg daily dose for the next month.

PHARMACOLOGIC AGENTS

Anticoagulants

After vascular access has been achieved, the patient is systemically anticoagulated. Recommendations for the level of anticoagulation vary. Between 5,000 and 10,000 units of heparin may be given, depending on the extent of tibial disease, the length of the procedure, and the size of the patient. If the procedure is prolonged, additional heparin is given. The activated clotting time (ACT) is kept between 260 and 280 seconds.

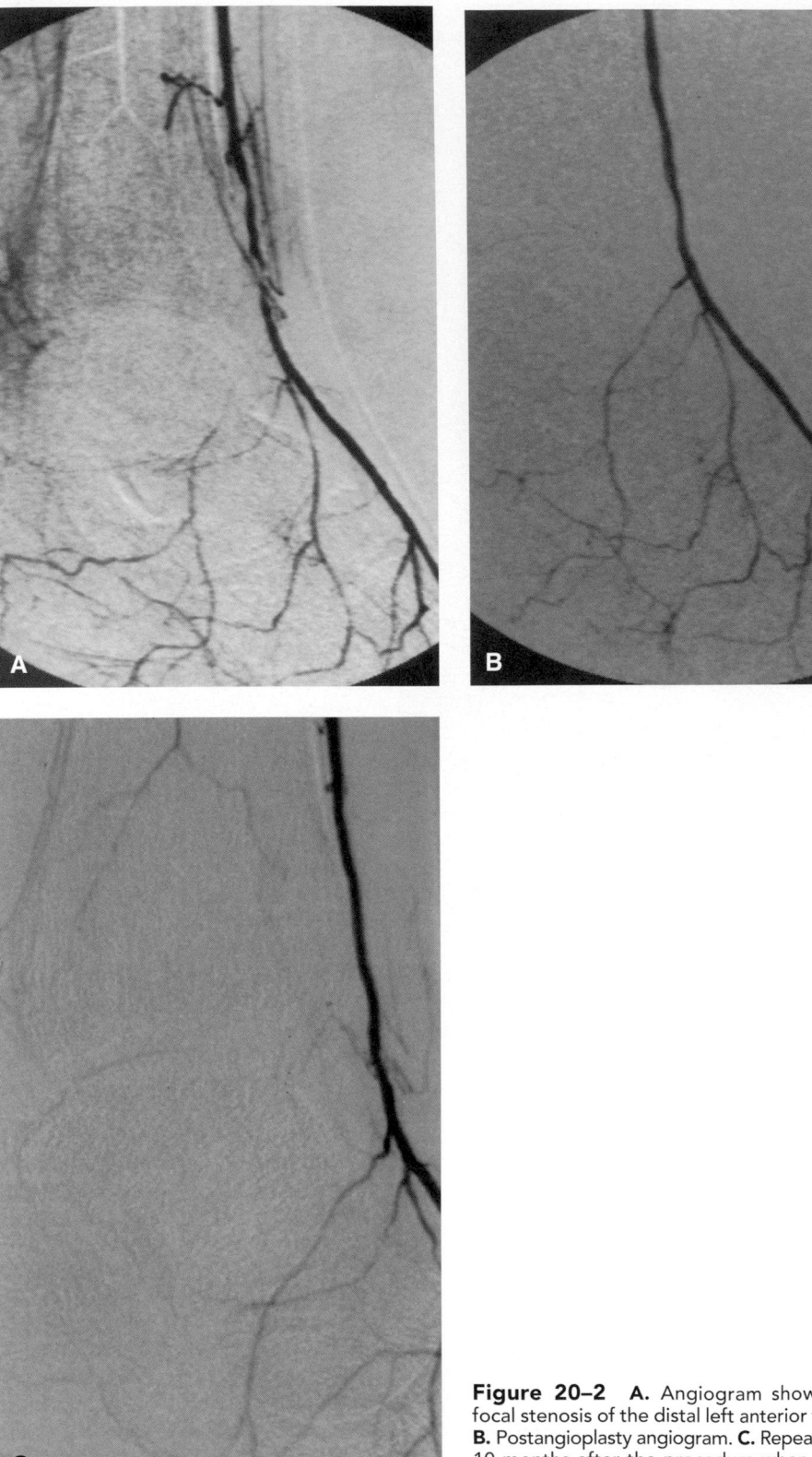

Figure 20–2 A. Angiogram showing severe focal stenosis of the distal left anterior tibial artery. **B.** Postangioplasty angiogram. **C.** Repeat angiogram 10 months after the procedure when the patient presented with symptoms in the other leg.

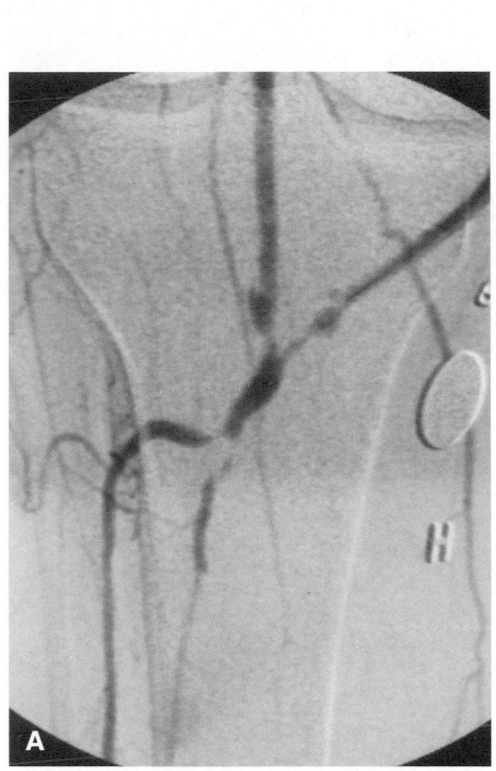

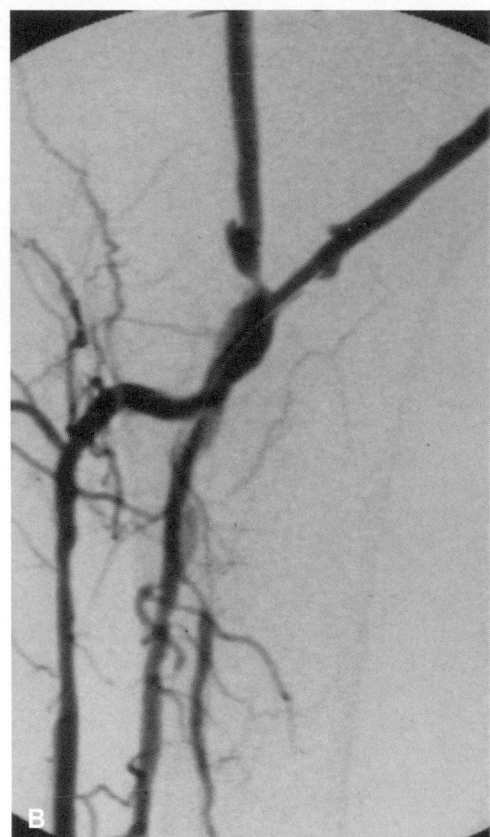

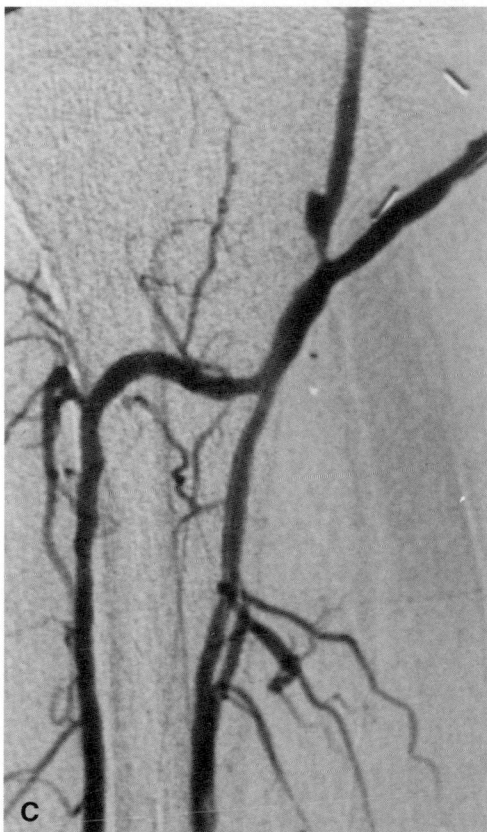

Figure 20–3 **A.** Angiogram showing severe stenoses at the distal anastomosis of a femoropopliteal bypass graft and at the origins of the anterior tibial artery and tibial peroneal trunk. **B.** Postangioplasty angiogram. **C.** Angiogram 2 years later after reangioplasty of the distal graft anastomosis. The native vessels remain patent.

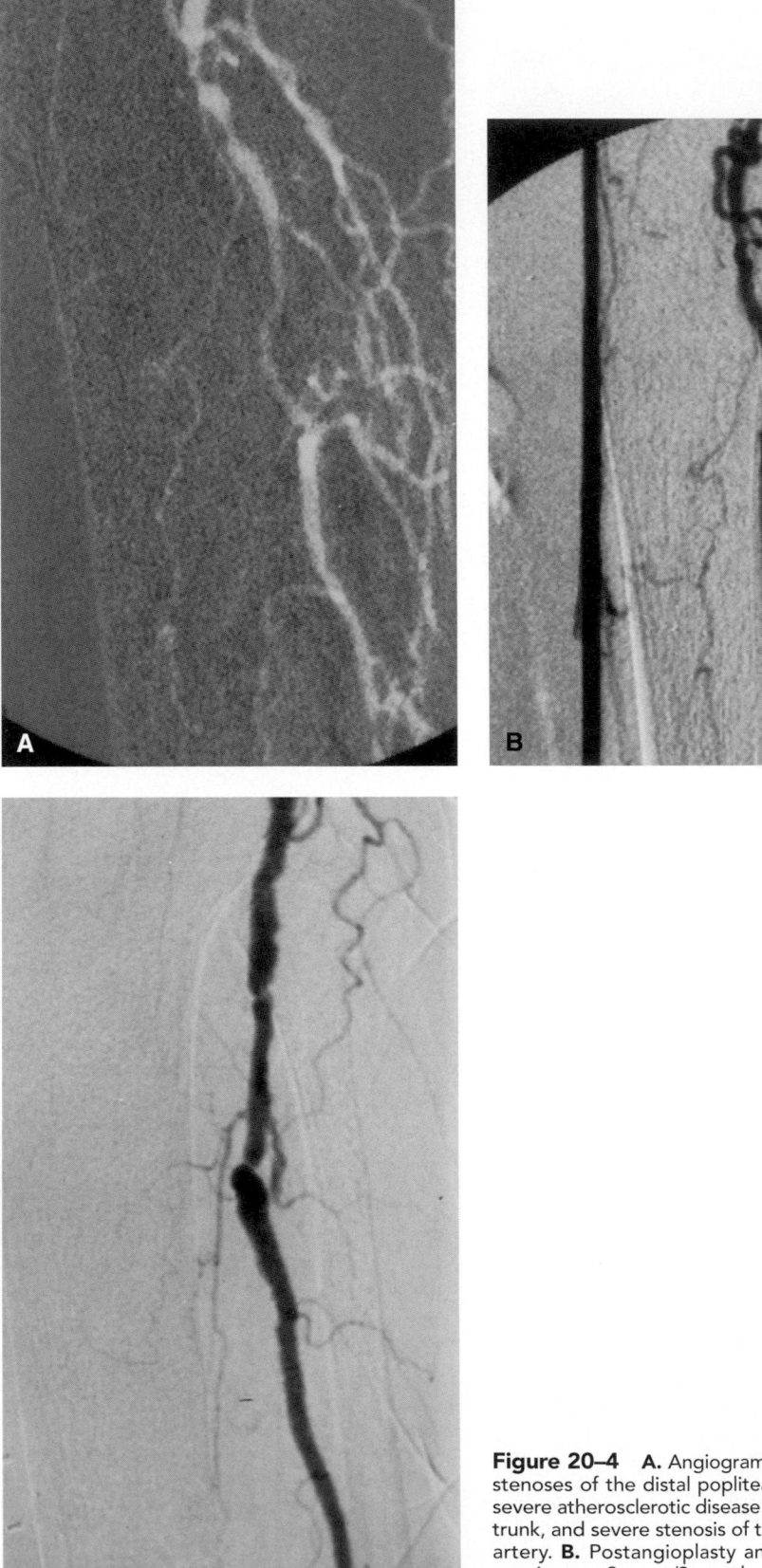

Figure 20–4   **A.** Angiogram showing two severe stenoses of the distal popliteal artery, moderately severe atherosclerotic disease of the tibial peroneal trunk, and severe stenosis of the proximal peroneal artery. **B.** Postangioplasty angiogram. **C.** Repeat arteriogram 3 years/3 months later demonstrates a recurrent moderate stenosis at the origin of the peroneal artery.

Antispasmodics and Vasodilators

The tibial vessels, similar to the coronary arteries, are prone to spasm and occlusion. Patients often are given 10 mg of nifedipine orally before the procedure. Liberal boluses of 100–200 µg of nitroglycerin are also given intra-arterially to prevent spasm. Nitroglycerin is administered before a wire is passed into a tibial vessel, as well as after dilation.

On occasion, significant spasm remains in the tibial vessel after angioplasty despite aliquots of intra-arterial nitroglycerin. In this instance, a 30-mg dose of intra-arterial papaverine is often helpful. This may be given through the balloon catheter or from the side port of the vascular sheath. The papaverine should be diluted in approximately 20 mL of normal saline to diminish pain and burning on administration.

Antiplatelet Agents

Oral aspirin therapy has been shown to benefit patients in the long-term management of stroke or myocardial infarction. In the absence of contraindications, most clinicians treat patients who have coronary artery disease or symptomatic peripheral vascular disease with daily aspirin. Ticlopidine and clopidogrel belong to a class of antiplatelet agents called *thienopyridines*. They interfere with the function of the platelet membrane by inhibiting platelet-fibrinogen binding. Ticlopidine and aspirin have been shown to be superior to warfarin after coronary stent placement (12). Neutropenia occurs in a small percentage of patients who are given ticlopidine, so these individuals need to be monitored. Most cardiologists have therefore switched to clopidogrel, which has a similar antithrombotic effect after coronary stent placement (11). The CAPRIE (clopidogrel versus aspirin in patients at risk of ischemic events) trial (13) demonstrated an 8.7% reduction in risk of a repeat vascular event with clopidogrel compared to aspirin. In patients with peripheral vascular disease, the risk reduction was 23.8% in favor of clopidogrel. There have been recent reports of thrombocytopenic purpura with clopidogrel. Although rare, this risk must be balanced against potential benefits.

The class of agents known as glycoprotein IIb/IIIa inhibitors prevents platelet aggregation and inhibits the formation of platelet thrombus. Abciximab often is used during coronary artery angioplasty and stenting. Although limited data exists on its use after complex peripheral vascular interventions, the initial experience is promising (14).

COMPLICATIONS

The complications of tibial angioplasty are the same as for angioplasty of other vessels, including spasm, thrombosis, subintimal dissection, embolization, perforation, and rupture (Table 20–2).

Thrombosis

Tibial artery thrombosis may occur in situ as the result of slow flow in diseased vessels, as the result of an embolus, or as a complication of angioplasty. In the case of an acute occlusion, a 3 French catheter or an open-lumen guide wire may be passed into the tibial vessel. The vessel is then laced with a bolus of a thrombolytic agent. A drip infusion is started and run from 1–2 hours, either selectively into a single occluded tibial vessel or from the distal popliteal artery if more than one vessel is involved. Also, a 4 French or 5 French multislit catheter (Unifuse Angiodynamics) may be inserted into the vessel and a pulsed lytic infusion performed. Alternatively, mechanical thrombectomy may be performed with a rheolytic device. The most widely used being the Possis AngioJet. Although there is limited data in the peripheral vessels, a glycoprotein IIb/IIIa inhibitor may be tried, either alone or in combination with a lytic agent. If the thrombus has not resolved, an overnight drip of a thrombolytic agent may be started.

Embolization

On occasion, embolization of atherosclerotic plaque or organized thrombus occurs during angioplasty and becomes a persistent filling defect that does not lyse. A nontapered 5 French or 6 French catheter can be used to aspirate this material and then withdrawn from the vessel under continuous suction through a sheath (15).

RESULTS

Early studies of tibial angioplasty were not encouraging. In a series from 1980, Sprayregen et al. (2) performed dilatations with tapered catheters. Technical success was achieved in four of six patients, with good clinical results in just two patients at 19 and 22 months after angioplasty. In a series from 1982, Tamura et al. (3) performed tibial dilatation with either tapered catheters or 3- and 4-mm balloon catheters after popliteal or superficial femoral artery angioplasty. Of the five tibial angioplasties attempted, only three were technically successful. Of the two that were clinically successful in the short term, symptoms recurred at 3 months in one and at 6 months in the other.

Technical success and clinical results have improved with innovations in catheters and guide wires and refinements in radiographic equipment. Since 1990, several series of tibial angioplasty patients have concluded that the results are favorable in selected patients (16–33) (Table 20–3). Recent studies have attempted to define the groups likely to benefit.

Several problems have been encountered when looking at these series. One is the heterogeneity of the populations. In some study groups, patients with lifestyle-limiting claudication are included, while others are limited to rest pain and gangrene. Also, a problem is the inclusion or

TABLE 20–2

COMPLICATIONS OF TIBIAL ANGIOPLASTY IN 1,164 PATIENTS[a]

Complications	Number of Patients
Death Within 30 Days[b,c]	14
Myocardial Infarction	7
Stroke	1
Pulmonary Edema	1
Acute Thrombosis	
Surgical Treatment: Bypass or Thrombectomy	6
Lysis	21
Other Emergency Surgery	6
Major Amputation	8
Other Occlusion/Vessel Dissection	12
Renal Failure	1
Distal Embolization (Clinically Significant)	10
Major Hematoma[d,e]	35
Surgical Repair	13
Transfusion	14
Compartment Syndrome	1
Pseudoaneurysm	8
Access Repair	5
Vessel Perforation	5
Groin Infection	2
Distal Embolization (Clinically Insignificant)[f]	16
Congestive Heart Failure	3
Minor Hematoma	28
Transient Renal Failure	26
Spasm	14

[a]Complications are not divided into major and minor because different authors classify the same complications differently. There is also incomplete reporting of all complications by the individual authors. Varty et al. did not report minor complications.
[b]One death occurred in a patient who had an MI 7 hours after ray amputation under spinal anesthesia 29 days after angioplasty.
[c]One death because of fatal retroperitoneal bleeding promoted by an overdose infusion of heparin in the surgery department after PTA
[d]How the hematoma was managed and was not indicated in the series by Durham et al.
[e]Includes five patients who did not receive transfusions; however, the large hematomas prolonged inpatient stay.
[f]Several authors did not classify whether distal emboli were clinically significant. If the embolus was removed by aspiration, it was grouped with the clinically insignificant. If the embolus required lysis or surgery, it was considered significant.
Adapted from data in the following sources (listed in References section): 16, 17, 19, 21, 22, 23, 24, 25, 26, 27, 28, 29, 31, 32, and 33.

exclusion of patients with preexisting grafts, particularly distal bypass grafts, in which the lesion may be the result of myointimal hyperplasia. Another problem is the inclusion of patients who are too sick for surgery, patients who lack an adequate conduit, or patients who do not have a satisfactory target vessel for bypass. An additional problem is the definition of technical success; some studies define it as <50% residual stenosis, while others define it as <30% residual stenosis.

Clearly, the severity and number of lesions as well as the condition of the distal outflow are influences on the success of the procedure. Bakal et al. (16) used the term *straight-line flow* to indicate continuous flow to the foot through a tibial vessel whose diameter is narrowed by 75% or less. They showed a 97% (28 of 29) clinical response when angioplasty restored straight-line flow to the foot but only a 36% (4 of 11) clinical response when it did not. By life-table analysis, the Bakal series had a 57% PTA-assisted limb salvage rate at 2 years with an 82% PTA-assisted limb salvage rate at 2 years for patients with straight-line flow to the foot (12).

Schwarten and Cutliff (8) reported one of the largest early studies that included below-the-knee popliteal dilatations and excluded patients with acute ischemia. Three years later, Schwarten published a follow-up (19). Of the 96 patients who had angioplasty with balloon catheters, 97% had primary clinical success. By life-table analysis, the cumulative limb salvage at 2 years was 86%, which rivals

TABLE 20-3

TIBIAL ANGIOPLASTY RESULTS

Series	Number of Patients/Limbs/ Vessels	Age (Mean)	Initial Clinical Success (%)	Technical Success (%)	Adjunctive PTA (%)	Cumulative Limb Salvage (% 1 yr/2 yr/3 yr)
Bakal et al. (1990)	53/57/76	36–96 (70)	32 (80)	78	30/57 (53)	60.0/57.0/NA
Horvath et al. (1990)	71/NA/103	44–92 (70.2)	63 (92.5)	96	43/71 (61)	79.8/75.3/64.6
Dorros et al. (1990)	111/151/168	(67)	106 (95)	90	62/111(56)	NA
Schwarten (1991)	96/112/146	35–86 (66)	98 (87)	97	7/96 (7)	88.0/83.0/NA
Bull et al. (1992)	168/168/186	44–89 (67.1)F 27–89(61.6)M	103/168(61)	77	58/168(35)	67/67/NA
Saab et al. (1992)	13/14/17	52–83 (67)	10/14 (71)	100	4/14 (29)	77.0/77.0/NA
Flueckiger et al. (1992)	91/99/125	36–82 (66.2)	81/91 (89)	81	57/99[a]	76.7/71/64.2
Matsi et al. (1993)	103/84/NA[b]	38–90 (72)	NA	83	NA[b]	56/49/49
Brown et al. (1993)	40/55/NA	(67.6) F (68.7) M	46/55 (84)	95	NA[c]	60.0/50.0/NA
Buckenham et al. (1993)	13/13/14	NA	11/13 (85)	100	5/13 (38)	NA
Durham et al. (1994)	14/14/14	39–82 (65)	11/14 (79)	100	8/14 (57)	77[d]
Sivananthan et al. (1994)	38/50/73	40–83 (69.6)	NA	96	44/50 (88)	73/60/54
Varty et al. (1995)	38/40/NA	44–87 (74)	38/40 (98)	98	19/40 (48)	77/68/NA
Lofberg et al. (1996)	82/86/121[e]	37–94 (72)	NA	88	55/94(56)[e]	79/75/72
Dorros et al. (1998)	312/417/657	32–88 (66)	400/417 (96)	92	NA	NA
Boyer et al. (2000)	49/49/NA	42–91 (71.6)	44/49 (90)[f]	92	24/49 (49)	87/87/87
Soder et al. (2000)	60/72/NA	38–92 (72)	45/72 (63)	76	32/60 (53)	80/NA/NA
Dorros et al. (2001)	235/284/NA	40–86 (67)	270/284 (95)	92	169/284 (60)	NA/NA/NA (91)[g]

NA = Not available; F = Female; M = Male
[a]Excluding 22 patients with laser assisted PTA and eight patients with thrombolysis and PTA
[b]The study included patients who had femoropopliteal angioplasty alone and did not specify the ones performed in conjunction with tibial PTA.
[c]Primary thrombolysis was performed in 33% before PTA in four native vessels and in 14 bypass grafts
[d]Limb salvage at 17 months
[e]Ninety-four procedures: Repeat angioplasty was performed on the same leg in six patients (twice in four cases and three times in three cases)
[f]Includes 18 patients who had an additional surgical procedure that had been planned before PTA
[g]Limb salvage rate at 5 years (8% had surgical bypass)

many surgical series. However, only 35 patients were available for follow-up at that interval.

A series by Horvath et al. (17) reported angioplasty procedures on 103 infrapopliteal vessels in 71 patients. The cumulative limb salvage by life-table analysis was 79.8, 75.3, and 64.6% at 1, 2, and 3 years, respectively.

In a large series of 168 patients from Austria, Bull et al. (22) also included below-the-knee popliteal arteries and

femoropopliteal grafts. By life-table analysis, single stenoses had the greatest cumulative clinical success (83%) at 3 years, followed by 76% for multilevel lesions, 44% after lytic therapy, 36% for segmental occlusions, and only 14% for anastomotic stenoses. The patients with rest pain had better clinical success than those with tissue necrosis.

Brown et al. (24) found a 79% long-term success rate (about 25.8 months) in patients who had angioplasty involving native vessels only, but when patients with infrainguinal bypass grafts were included, there was only 36% success. Similar to Bakal et al., Brown et al. found that the success rate was improved when continuous runoff was reestablished. They also found poor results in patients with bypass grafts who required thrombolysis before PTA and had lesions near the distal anastomoses of bypass grafts, despite good cosmetic results on postprocedure arteriograms. Because atherectomy specimens from such locations yielded myointimal hyperplasia, the utility of conventional angioplasty in these areas is doubtful.

Matsi, Lofberg, and Dorros collected the larger of the more recent series. In Matsi et al.'s published series (26), PTA was performed when technically possible and surgery when angioplasty was not possible. They found that the determinants for avoiding major amputation were related to the number of stenoses or occlusions. Patients with 1–5 lesions did significantly better than patients with six or more. They also noted that patients with at least one calf vessel and no stenoses greater than 75% had a better prognosis than patients with no continuous calf vessels. Their limb salvage rate was better after successful recanalization of occluded vessel segments than after dilatation of stenoses.

In a series from Sweden, Lofberg et al. (29) excluded patients with bypasses as well as femoral or popliteal occlusions >10 cm and tibial occlusions >5 cm. The type of lesion or occlusion versus stenosis did not adversely affect their results. In 10 limbs, the patient returned for repeat PTA, which slightly increased limb salvage at 36 months. Thirteen of 82 patients underwent elective bypass after reocclusion at a mean of 7.2 months. Twenty of the 82 patients underwent amputation after reocclusion without an attempt at surgical reconstruction because of severe distal disease.

The largest series over recent years was published by Dorros et al. (33), who reported a clinical 5-year follow-up with 91% of limbs salvaged; however, this series did include 57% severe claudicants. Also, long-term results were computed only for patients who had successful recanalization procedures. Eight percent of angioplasty patients subsequently had bypass surgery, and 9% had major amputations. As other series have noted, this population has a significant morbidity and mortality from comorbid conditions. The 5-year probability of survival was 56%.

Among these series, large differences exist in the number of complications reported. Schwarten (19) reported two intraprocedural thromboses after an initial bolus of 5,000 units of heparin. These were successfully thrombolysed. Bakal (16) reported three major complications: two puncture site hematomas that required surgical repair and one death from cardiopulmonary arrest after the procedure. The Horvath series (17) included three major complications: an anterior tibial artery rupture treated by surgical bypass, an

intimal flap causing vessel occlusion, and a puncture site hematoma that was evacuated. The Bull series (22) showed a much higher incidence of major complications (11.3%) than the others. However, nine cases of spasm were included in this list, as well as 11 cases of thrombosis. This may have been the result of inadequate heparinization because heparin was given at 1,000 units per hour, but no initial bolus was administered. Although complications occurred in 16 of 55 procedures in the Brown series (24), 75% were associated with primary thrombolysis.

DISCUSSION

Because limb loss is a potential consequence of complications from tibial PTA, the patients who were initially chosen for the procedure had to have limb-threatening ischemia with rest pain (grade 2, category 4) or tissue loss (grade 2, category 5). The increasing success resulting from the continued evolution of catheters and guide wires and the increased experience of operators have allowed these indications to be expanded by many to include disabling claudication (grade 1, category 3). Tibial PTA in these patients remains controversial because few patients with claudication will require surgery. Patients with critical limb ischemia, on the other hand, inevitably will need an amputation whenever revascularization with angioplasty or surgery is unsuccessful. In many institutions, angioplasty has become the first approach for patients in these categories. Nonetheless, it is important not to jeopardize a potential surgical option with a technically or clinically unsuccessful procedure.

Restoration of continuous flow to the foot is highly predictive of a beneficial clinical response. Patients with discontinuous flow do significantly less well. This finding has led some to suggest that when an angioplasty procedure will not reestablish straight-line flow, the patient may be better served by receiving surgery for reconstruction when possible (24).

The patient's overall general medical condition is an important consideration when deciding between a surgical or a percutaneous approach with tibial disease. The incidence of cardiac disease in the population with peripheral vascular disease is approximately 60%. Previous studies have demonstrated a significant correlation between early death after arterial reconstruction and the presence of trifurcation disease (34). The numerous comorbidities in this population contribute to the perioperative complications. As with any intervention, the aim is to optimize the risk-benefit ratio. Although surgical revascularization may be more durable, it carries higher risks.

Another consideration is the availability of veins for bypass. Synthetic grafts do poorly when used for infrapopliteal bypass (35,36). If the vein has been used for coronary bypass grafts, it may be possible in some patients to perform a bypass with synthetic material above the knee and to treat the infrapopliteal disease with angioplasty. Also, tibial PTA may allow a vein to be preserved for future use. An additional advantage of angioplasty is that the procedure may be repeated for recurrent disease or disease progression.

Initial tibial angioplasty results approach those of surgical series, although more long-term follow-up is needed. The associated mortality and morbidity of surgery make PTA an important option in selected patients.

OTHER MODALITIES

Although angioplasty remains the primary percutaneous modality for recanalization of the infrapopliteal arteries, many new devices have been developed in recent years for this purpose.

Atherectomy

Atherectomy was developed to remove plaque from the vessel and, theoretically, was superior to PTA because it avoided subintimal dissection and would decrease the restenosis rate by reducing the plaque burden. Although some interventionalists advocated atherectomy for eccentric or calcified lesions or occlusions, there was limited experience in the tibial vessels. Older directional atherectomy catheters such as the AtheroCath (Simpson) and AtheroTrack (Peripheral Systems Group) were best suited for short, eccentric, or calcified lesions (37). The cutting assembly was brought against the vessel wall by inflation of a balloon. These devices were limited to vessel diameters of at least 4 mm, and their results did not exceed conventional angioplasty.

The Silverhawk catheter (Fox Hollow) is a newer directional atherectomy device designed for treatment of stenoses in native peripheral arteries. When the Silverhawk catheter is connected to the drive unit, pulling back the lever turns on the motor and causes the distal portion of the cutter assembly to deflect. Longer lesions can be treated in less time. The Silverhawk device has become available in 6 French and may be used in vessels of at least 2 mm. Although there is limited experience, preliminary midterm results with this device in the infrapopliteal vessels involving 33 patients have been published (38). Additional balloon angioplasty was performed in 15 lesions, and in two cases, stents had to be placed because of dissection. The technical success rate was 97%. One technical failure was because of calcification in a diabetic patient in which the lesion could not be reached despite predilation. Follow-up at 6 months was evaluated by duplex resulting in a restenosis rate of 22%. Of the 32 patients available after 6 months, 24 were clinically improved. Two of the six patients with stage 5 lesions had recurrent ulcers after initial healing because of recurrent ischemia. The 6-month cumulative

patency rate was 94% ± 3.3%. This device should not be used when subintimal passage is suspected, because of the risk of perforation.

A circumferential atherectomy catheter, the Arrow-Fischell pullback atherectomy catheter (Arrow International), has undergone clinical trials, primarily in the cardiac vessels. It obtained less tissue than directional atherectomy and was found to be more difficult to use (39).

A multicenter trial looking at the safety and efficacy of the pullback atherectomy catheter (PAC) was performed for lower extremity arterial disease (40), and no major complications were found. The advantage of this catheter was its utility in diffuse disease as well as in eccentric and concentric lesions. Despite a high rate of technical success, the catheter cannot create a lumen greater than its own diameter without extrinsic compression. Without compression, it is limited to vessels <4 mm. It may be used in vessels up to 6 mm that can be compressed with a blood pressure cuff. There is currently no data referring to its use in the infrapopliteal vessels.

Laser Angioplasty

Laser angioplasty was developed for photothermal plaque ablation. Early studies on laser angioplasty had significant complications including dissection, perforation, and thermal vessel injury. Several studies with hot tip laser probes did not demonstrate improved long-term success over balloon angioplasty (41). The results in the tibial vessels were poor. Over the past 25 years, the technique was improved. The excimer laser uses pulsed wave ultraviolet energy, which is believed to reduce arterial injury. The CLiRpath cool laser revascularization catheter (Spectranetics) for peripheral artery therapy uses an excimer laser. The LACI II—laser angioplasty for critical limb ischemia—trial (42) contained 145 patients who were poor surgical candidates and not candidates for PTA because the lesions could not be crossed with a guide wire. In the 155 critically ischemic limbs, 41% of the lesions were in the infrapopliteal arteries. Laser treatment was delivered in 99%, and adjunctive PTA was performed in 96% of cases. There was limb salvage in 95% of patients at 6 months. At this point, clinical trials are ongoing. Although laser use may be a last resort when other modalities fail, no studies have yet demonstrated that it surpasses the clinical success of angioplasty in a similar cohort of patients. Also, it is an expensive procedure.

Cutting Balloon Angioplasty

Cutting balloons contain 3 or 4 microsurgical atherotomes mounted on the surface of a noncompliant balloon. They score the plaque and dilate at lower pressures. Cutting balloon angioplasty (CBA) aims to control balloon-induced injury to the vessel wall. These balloons were introduced in coronary angioplasty to treat heavily calcified lesions.

Proponents now advocate CBA as being superior to conventional PTA for in-stent restenosis in coronary arteries. This is because of its decreased tendency to move during inflation from the slipperiness of the surface of the hyperplastic tissue.

Ansel et al. (43) looked at CBA for peripheral angioplasty. Most patients were in categories 3 and 4. Seventy-one percent presented with limb-threatening ischemia. Eighty-two percent were de novo lesions. Eighteen percent were in-stent restenoses. At 1 year, there was limb salvage in 89.5% of patients. Ansel and colleagues concluded that CBA was safe and immediately technically successful. Further evaluation is still needed to determine whether CBA provides any benefits beyond those associated with standard angioplasty. Cutting balloon angioplasty may have a role in treating stenoses at graft anastomoses (44).

Drug-Eluting Stents

Drug-eluting stents have been used with excellent results in the coronary arteries; however, there is only limited data on their use in peripheral vessels. In the SCIROCCO trial (45), the study group contained 36 patients with critical limb ischemia and SFA disease. Eighteen patients received sirolimus-eluting nitinol SMART stents (Cordis), and 18 patients received uncoated SMART stents. The endpoint was in-stent mean diameter stenosis as measured by angiography. At 6 months, mean percent diameter stenosis was 22.6 in the sirolimus-eluting stent group and 30.9 in the uncoated stent group. Three patients refused angiography.

Despite similar sizes, the infrapopliteal arteries differ significantly from the cardiac vessels. The tibial arteries have lower flow rates and generally longer lesions. The inhibition of in-stent neointimal hyperplasia in this location remains to be seen before primary stent placement can become an alternative to PTA.

Brachytherapy

Intravascular radiation is another method of reducing stenosis, which has been shown to be effective in coronary arteries. Although studies have been performed in the femoropopliteal segment, no data on infrapopliteal brachytherapy currently exists.

A series of studies on the superficial femoral artery were conducted at the University of Vienna (46). The Vienna II trial included 113 patients with de novo or recurrent femoropopliteal lesions, 57 of whom were randomized to PTA and brachytherapy, while 56 were randomized to PTA alone. The cumulative patency rates were 63.6% in the PTA and vascular brachytherapy group versus 35.3% in the PTA alone at 12 months follow-up.

Krueger et al. (47) performed a randomized controlled trial on centered gamma irradiation following angioplasty of de novo femoropopliteal stenoses in 15 patients. The control group also contained 15 patients. At 24 months, five patients in the control group and two in the irradiation group had <50% restenosis. The degree of stenosis was 9.6 ± 43.5 in the irradiation group versus 34.9 ± 28.1 in the control group. At 24 months, four repeat angioplasty procedures were performed in the target vessel of the irradiation group versus two in the control group, mainly because of edge stenoses.

REFERENCES

1. Dotter CT, Judkins MP. Transluminal treatment of arteriosclerotic obstruction: description of a new technique and a preliminary report of its application. Circulation 1964;30:654–670.
2. Sprayregen S, Sniderman KW, Sos TA, et al. Popliteal artery branches: percutaneous transluminal angioplasty. AJR Am J Roentgenol 1980;135:945–950.
3. Tamura S, Sniderman KW, Beinart C, et al. Percutaneous transluminal angioplasty of the popliteal artery and its branches. Radiology 1982;143:645–648.
4. Rutherford RB, Flanigan DP, Gupta SK, et al. Suggested standards for dealing with lower extremity ischemia. J Vasc Surg 1986;4:80–94.
5. Barnes RW. Noninvasive diagnostic assessment of peripheral vascular disease. Circulation 1991;83(Suppl I):20–27.
6. Johnston KW, Rae M, Hogg-Johnston SA, et al. 5-year results of a prospective study of percutaneous transluminal angioplasty. Ann Surg 1987;206:403–413.
7. Bolia A, Sayers R, Thompson M, et al. Subintimal and intraluminal recanalization of occluded crural arteries by percutaneous balloon angioplasty. Eur J Vasc Surg 1994;8:214–219.
8. Schwarten DE, Cutliff WB. Arterial occlusive disease below the knee: treatment with percutaneous transluminal angioplasty performed with low profile catheters and steerable guide wires. Radiology 1988;169:71–74.
9. Rath B, Bennett DH. Monitoring the effect of heparin by measurement of activated clotting time during and after percutaneous transluminal angioplasty. Br Heart J 1990;63:18–21.
10. Bochner F, Lloyd J. Is there an optimal dose and formulation of aspirin to prevent arterial thrombo-embolism in man? Clin Sci 1986;71:625–631.
11. Bertrand ME, Rupprecht HJ, Urban P, et al. Double-blind study of the safety of clopidogrel with and without a loading dose in combination with aspirin compared with ticlopidine in combination with aspirin after coronary stenting: the clopidogrel aspirin stent international cooperative study (CLASSICS). Circulation 2000;102: 624–629.
12. Leon MB, Baim DS, Donald S, et al. A clinical trial comparing three antithrombotic drug regimens after coronary artery stenting. N Engl J Med 1998;339:1665–1671.
13. CAPRIE Steering Committee. A randomized, blinded trial of clopidogrel versus aspirin in patients at risk of ischemic events (CAPRIE). Lancet 1996;348:1329–1339.
14. Stavropoulos SW, Solomon JA, Soulen MC, et al. Use of abciximab during infrainguinal peripheral vascular interventions: initial experience. Radiology 2003;227:657–661.
15. Sniderman KW, Bodner L, Saddekni S, et al. Percutaneous embolectomy by transcatheter aspiration. Work in progress. Radiology 1984;150:357–361.
16. Bakal CW, Sprayregen S, Scheinbaum K, et al. Percutaneous transluminal angioplasty of the infrapopliteal arteries: results in 53 patients. AJR Am J Roentgenol 1990;154:171–174.
17. Horvath W, Oertl M, Haidinger D. Percutaneous transluminal angioplasty of crural arteries. Radiology 1990;177:565–569.
18. Dorros G, Lewin R, Jamnadas P, et al. Below-the-knee angioplasty: tibioperoneal vessels, the acute outcome. Cathet Cardiovasc Diagn 1990;19:170–178.
19. Schwarten DE. Clinical and anatomical considerations for nonoperative therapy in tibial disease and the results of angioplasty. Circulation 1991;83(Suppl I):86–90.

20. Bakal CW, Cynamon J, Sprayregen S, et al. Infrapopliteal artery angioplasty: follow-up and factors influencing clinical response. Presented at SCVIR 17th Annual Meeting, April 4–9, 1992.

21. Saab MH, Smith DC, Aka PK, et al. Percutaneous transluminal angioplasty of tibial arteries for limb salvage. Cardiovasc Intervent Radiol 1992;15:211–216.

22. Bull PG, Mendel H, Hold M, et al. Distal popliteal and tibioperoneal transluminal angioplasty: long-term follow-up. J Vasc Interv Radiol 1992;3:45–53.

23. Flueckiger F, Lammer J, Klein G, et al. Percutaneous transluminal angioplasty of crural arteries. Acta Radiol 1992;33:152–155.

24. Brown KT, Moore ED, Getrajdman GI, et al. Infrapopliteal angioplasty: long-term follow-up. J Vasc Interv Radiol 1993;4:139–144.

25. Buckenham TM, Loh A, Dormandy JA. Infrapopliteal angioplasty for limb salvage. Eur J Vasc Surg 1993;7:21–25.

26. Matsi P, Manninen H, Suhonen M, et al. Chronic critical lower limb ischemia: prospective trial of angioplasty with 1–36 months follow-up. Radiology 1993;188:381–387.

27. Durham J, Horowitz J, Wright J, et al. Percutaneous transluminal angioplasty of tibial arteries for limb salvage in the high risk diabetic patient. Ann Vasc Surg 1994;8:48–53.

28. Sivananthan U, Browne T, Thorley P, et al. Percutaneous transluminal angioplasty of the tibial arteries. Br J Surg 1994;81:1282–1285.

29. Lofberg A, Lorelius L, Karacagil S, et al. The use of below-knee percutaneous transluminal angioplasty in arterial occlusive disease. causing chronic critical limb ischemia. Cardiovasc Intervent Radiol 1996;19:317–322.

30. Dorros G, Jaff M, Murphy K, et al. The acute outcome of tibioperoneal vessel angioplasty in 417 cases with claudication and critical limb ischemia. Cathet Cardiovasc Diagn 1998;45:251–256.

31. Boyer L, Therre T, Garcier J, et al. Infrapopliteal percutaneous transluminal angioplasty for limb. Acta Radiol 2000;41:73–77.

32. Soder H, Manninen H, Jaakkola P, et al. Prospective trial of infrapopliteal artery balloon angioplasty for critical limb ischemia: angiographic and clinical results. J Vasc Interv Radiol 2000;11:1021–1031.

33. Dorros G, Jaff M, Dorros A, et al. Tibioperoneal (outflow lesion) angioplasty can be used as primary treatment in 235 patients with critical limb ischemia. Circulation 2001;104:2057–2062.

34. Kallero KS, Bergqvist D, Cederholm C, et al. Late mortality and morbidity after arterial reconstruction: the influence of arteriosclerosis in popliteal artery trifurcation. J Vasc Surg 1985;2:541–546.

35. Veith FJ, Gupta SK, Ascer E, et al. Six-year prospective multicenter randomized comparison of autologous saphenous vein and expanded polytetrafluoroethylene grafts in infrainguinal arterial reconstructions. J Vasc Surg 1986;3:104–114.

36. Veterans Administration Cooperative Study Group 141. Comparative evaluation of prosthetic, reversed, and in situ vein bypass grafts in distal popliteal and tibial-peroneal revascularization. Arch Surg 1988;123:434–438.

37. Ahn SS. Status of peripheral atherectomy. Surg Clin North Am 1992;72:869–878.

38. Zeller T, Rastan A, Schwarzwalder U, et al. Midterm results after atherectomy-assisted angioplasty of below-knee arteries with use of the Silverhawk device. J Vasc Interv Radiol 2004;15:1391–1397.

39. Webb J, Carere R, Lau E, et al. Pullback atherectomy with the Arrow-Fischell atherectomy device. Cathet Cardiovasc Diagn 1997;42:70–83.

40. White CJ. Peripheral atherectomy with the Pullback atherectomy catheter: procedural safety and efficacy in a multicenter trial. PAC Investigators. J Endovasc Surg 1998;5:9–17.

41. Self SB, Seeger JM. Laser angioplasty. Surg Clin North Am 1992;72:851–869.

42. Laird JR, Reiser C, Biamino G, et al. Excimer laser-assisted angioplasty for the treatment of critical limb ischemia. J Cardiovasc Surg (Torino) 2004;45:239–248.

43. Ansel GM, Sample NS, Botti III CF Jr, et al. Cutting balloon angioplasty of the popliteal and infrapopliteal vessels for symptomatic limb ischemia. Catheter Cardiovasc Interv 2004;61:1–4.

44. Engelke C, Morgan RA, Belli AM. Cutting balloon percutaneous transluminal angioplasty for salvage of lower limb arterial bypass grafts: feasibility. Radiology 2002;223(1):106–14.

45. Duda SH, Pusich B, Richter G, et al. Sirolimus-eluting stents for the treatment of obstructive superficial femoral artery disease superficial femoral artery disease: six month results. Circulation 2002;106:1505–1509.

46. Minar E, Pokrajac B, Maca T, et al. Endovascular brachytherapy for prophylaxis of restenosis after femoropopliteal angioplasty: results of a prospective randomized study. Circulation 2000;102:2694–2699.

47. Krueger K, Zaehringer M, Bendel M, et al. De novo femoropopliteal stenoses: endovascular gamma irradiation following angioplasty—angiographic and clinical follow-up in a prospective randomized controlled trial. Radiology 2004;231:546–554.

Evaluation and Endovascular Therapy for Renal Artery Stenosis

21

Alan H. Matsumoto, David J. Spinosa, J. Fritz Angle,
Klaus D. Hagspiel, Daniel A. Leung

During the past 25 years, the percentage of Americans who are aware that they have hypertension has increased from 51% to 73%, and those chosing to be treated have increased from 32% to 55% (1,2). With the aging of our patient population, the prevalence of renovascular disease as a cause of hypertension has also increased (3,4). However, patients with physiologically significant renal artery stenosis (RAS) often go undetected because hypertension can be well-controlled by medical therapy, and renal function will usually remain stable (5). Yet, delaying the diagnosis and treatment of significant RAS may be detrimental to patient outcomes. It has also become evident that patients with atherosclerotic RAS (ARAS) have higher rates of cardiovascular events and a decrease in survival when compared to patients with essential hypertension (6–9). In one study, 68 hypertensive patients with greater than 70% ARAS documented by angiography were treated without revascularization (10). Although 85% (58/68) of the patients had stable creatinine levels at 39 months of follow-up, patients with stenoses affecting their entire renal mass (global ischemia) experienced a 43% mortality rate versus a 21% mortality rate for patients with unilateral RAS. Most deaths were secondary to cardiovascular events. The survival data in this study mirror patient survival rates following renal artery stent therapy (RAST) (11). In contrast, a cohort of patients without ARAS on abdominal aortography had a 4-year mortality rate of 14% (12). Therefore, the presence of ARAS (and not the

treatment) appears to be the most powerful independent predictor of survival. In addition, "flash" pulmonary edema and renal insufficiency may occur as a physiological consequence of RAS (2,4,13–15). Chronic renal ischemia caused by ARAS is also recognized as an independent predictor of cardiovascular morbidity and mortality, independent from its association with hypertension or atherosclerosis in other vascular territories (6).

The mechanisms that lead to an increase risk in cardiovascular morbidity in patients with ARAS are complex. The following contribute to the cardiovascular morbidity in this patient population (16–22):

- Vasomotor tone regulation by angiotensin II and nitrous oxide
- Cytokine- and mitogen-mediated migration of vascular smooth muscle cells in the heart and peripheral arteries
- Angiotensin II mediated interstitial fibrosis in the heart and kidneys
- Endothelin
- Growth factors
- Inflammation
- Leukotrienes
- Oxidative stress
- Endothelial cell dysfunction
- Prothrombogenic state mediated by endothelial cell dysfunction
- Other yet-to-be-determined factors

In addition, ARAS has been implicated as an important cause of end-stage renal disease (ESRD), which in and of itself, is associated with a poor prognosis (23,24). Therefore, the ability to detect and manage patients appropriately with RAS is becoming more and more important.

ETIOLOGIES FOR RENAL ARTERY STENOSIS

Disease entities that can lead to clinically significant RAS can be divided into three broad categories: (1) atherosclerosis, (2) fibromuscular dysplasia (FMD), and (3) miscellaneous. Atherosclerosis and FMD account for more than 95% of the cases of significant RAS in the United States, with ARAS accounting for more than 85% of the cases. A miscellaneous group of patients can also present with clinically significant RAS: postoperative (renal allografts, post-bypass surgery), neurofibromatosis, Takayasu's arteritis (vasculitis), radiation-induced, and aortic dissection. This chapter presents a review of RAS secondary to atherosclerosis, FMD, neurofibromatosis, Takayasu's arteritis, and renal allografts.

NATURAL HISTORY OF ATHEROSCLEROTIC RENAL ARTERY STENOSIS

The true prevalence of ARAS in an unselected patient population is unknown, but it does increase with advancing age. Autopsy studies have demonstrated a 5% incidence of significant RAS in individuals younger than 64 years old, increasing to greater than 40% in individuals 75 years or older (25,26). Autopsy series from a hypertensive patient population reveal an incidence of RAS of 56%, compared to 17% in a nonhypertensive patient population (25). In patients with suspected cardiovascular disease who are undergoing cardiac catheterization or peripheral angiography, the incidence of RAS ranges from 14 to 45% (27–33).

Although ARAS is considered a progressive disorder, not all lesions will progress. Therefore, the challenge is to determine which lesions will progress in which patients and whether or not aggressive lipid therapy, blood pressure control, smoking cessation, or endovascular intervention will alter the progressive nature of these stenotic lesions and affect patient survival rates (34). In a study of 170 patients (295 kidneys), serial renal duplex scans were performed for a mean of 33 months (35). In renal arteries initially classified as normal, less than 60% stenosis and greater than or equal to 60% stenosis, the three-year progression rates—defined as any detectable increase in the degree of diameter reduction affecting at least one renal artery—were 18%, 28%, and 49%, respectively. Renal artery occlusions occurred in nine (3.1%) arteries in which a greater than 60% stenosis on the initial evaluation was noted. In another study, eight of 50

patients (16%) with ARAS greater than or equal to 50% and who managed with medical therapy progressed to total occlusion at 12 months (36). Renal atrophy, defined as a reduction of greater than 1 cm in renal length at follow-up duplex scan at 2 years, occurred in 5.5% of kidneys with renal arteries initially classified as normal, 17% of kidneys with RAS less than 60%, and 21% of kidneys with ARAS greater than or equal to 60% (37). The occurrence of atrophy correlated with changes in serum creatinine levels, suggesting a relationship between the progression of RAS and worsening renal parenchymal disease. However, in a review of 821 abdominal angiograms, 38% of normotensive patients had significant RAS (38). Therefore, the presence of ARAS does *not* imply a cause-and-effect relationship between the RAS and the presence of hypertension, renal insufficiency, or both. Rather, the presence of ARAS in asymptomatic patients should be considered a marker for more diffuse cardiovascular disease, and aggressive treatment to reduce cardiovascular morbidity and risk factors should be instituted.

PATHOPHYSIOLOGY OF RENOVASCULAR DISEASE

Renal hypoperfusion induces the release of renin and a subsequent increase in plasma angiotensin II levels. Angiotensin II, a potent vasoconstrictor, also stimulates the release of aldosterone. Aldosterone causes sodium and water resorption and an increase in extracellular fluid volume. Therefore, renovascular hypertension, in its simplest form, appears to be related to vasoconstriction that occurs because of an increase in angiotensin II levels and an increase in extracellular fluid volume resulting from aldosterone-mediated sodium and water retention. However, the acute changes that are mediated by the renin-angiotensin II-aldosterone mechanisms are overcome by changes in the intrarenal hemodynamics and local endothelial pressor mechanisms that lead to a transition into a chronic phase of renovascular hypertension (39–41). The reasons why the acute phase of renovascular hypertension evolves into a chronic phase are poorly understood, and the time frame is poorly defined. However, once the chronic phase of renovascular hypertension develops and multiple local pressor mechanisms have been recruited, renin release may become suppressed, the hypertension may not respond to an ACE inhibitor, and any test utilized for detecting RAS that relies on the renin-angiotensin axis is relatively insensitive (39).

In addition, in the presence of RAS, renal perfusion may be adequate to maintain tissue viability but is insufficient to sustain effective glomerular function. Intratubular urine flow may cease, and autoregulatory mechanisms may become nonfunctional (41). Further reductions in systemic pressure with medical therapy may lead to a greater reduction of renal perfusion and an incremental decrease in the glomerular filtration rate (GFR). Therefore, despite adequate blood pressure control, ongoing renal ischemia may cause progressive renal insufficiency (41–44). It has also been suggested that renal insufficiency could arise from significant unilateral RAS. In this setting, the ipsilateral kidney has a decrease in GFR while the contralateral, unaffected kidney begins to hyperfiltrate. The need to chronically hyperfiltrate leads to interstitial fibrosis in the contralateral kidney and a subsequent decrease in its function (45).

INDICATIONS FOR EVALUATION AND TREATMENT

As a general rule, patients should undergo evaluation only when the detection of RAS will alter the therapy. Three broad clinical situations exist in which patients should undergo evaluation and treatment for RAS:

1. Hypertension—Patients with the onset of hypertension before the age of 40, especially those without a family history (think FMD); recent onset of hypertension after age 55, especially in association with an abdominal bruit (and particularly when the bruit continues into diastole and lateralizes); and accelerated or resistant hypertension
2. Renal insufficiency—Patients with worsening renal function precipitated by an angiotensin-converting enzyme (ACE) inhibitor or angiotensin receptor blocker (ARB); patients beyond the age of 60 years who coexist with coexistent diffuse atherosclerotic vascular disease, especially in the setting of a normal urine sediment; and asymmetric kidney size or a decrease in the size of a solitary kidney, especially in the presence of a flank bruit (Note: The absence of hypertension does not exclude ischemic nephropathy.) (24,46–50)
3. Cardiac disturbance syndromes—Patients with recurrent "flash" pulmonary edema not secondary to cardiac ischemia, especially in patients with relatively normal left ventricular function who have coexistent renal insufficiency, poorly controlled hypertension, or both (2,13,14)
4. Prophylactic therapy—Although ARAS is considered a progressive disorder, determining the lesion that will progress is difficult. Because any revascularization procedure is associated with some morbidity and costs, routine treatment of all asymptomatic RAS is not recommended. However, if the stenosis is severe enough to be considered "preocclusive," revascularization may be undertaken when there is a solitary kidney, severe RAS is present bilaterally, progression of RAS is documented, kidney size decreases, renal function deteriorates, or blood pressure control becomes more difficult. As noted earlier, patients with "asymptomatic" RAS should be managed aggressively to reduce cardiovascular risk factors and be followed very closely.

NONINVASIVE DIAGNOSTIC EVALUATION

The gold standard for the diagnosis of RAS is catheter-based angiography. However, it is invasive and costly and, therefore, cannot be used as a screening test in the majority of patients. Of the noninvasive diagnostic tests that have been used over the years, only four are routinely used in clinical practice: (1) ACE inhibitor scintigraphy, (2) Doppler sonography, (3) computed tomographic angiography (CTA), and (4) magnetic resonance angiography (MRA) (39,51–55).

It is important to understand that renovascular hypertension (RVH) and chronic renal failure due to RAS and ischemic nephropathy, respectively, are not synonymous. As noted earlier, stenoses of the renal arteries are common in patients without hypertension or renal insufficiency and can be associated, but not necessarily etiologic. Thus, an ideal screening test would allow for the detection of RAS, while establishing its role as the cause for RVH, ischemic nephropathy, or both. Furthermore, the test should allow for the prediction of treatment response. Unfortunately, such a test does not currently exist.

Angiotensin Converting Enzyme Inhibitor Renography/Scintigraphy

Renal scintigraphy quantitatively assesses the renal clearance of radiotracers. The combination of scintigraphy with the administration of an ACE inhibitor, such as captopril (PO) or enalapril (IV), gives optimum diagnostic results (56–64). ACE inhibitors reduce the angiotensin-mediated constriction of the efferent arterioles. The glomerular pressure is lowered, resulting in a reduction in the GFR in the kidney ipsilateral to the RAS with or without a delay in renal excretion. The disruption of the renin-angiotensin system can improve function of the contralateral kidney and thus, will enhance the asymmetry between the normal and affected kidney, making the detection of abnormalities easier (61,62).

ACE inhibitor scintigraphy has several pitfalls. Patients with urinary obstruction, large ampullary collecting systems, bilateral RAS, renal insufficiency, segmental or accessory RAS, or on certain medications (ARBs, ACEIs, diuretics, or sympatholytics), can give misleading test results (64–66). Hypotension during the examination can also render the test nondiagnostic. Nevertheless, ACE inhibitor scintigraphy is used in many centers as one of the primary noninvasive screening methods. Reports on ACE inhibitor scintigraphy show sensitivity and specificity values of 64–91% and 44–98%, respectively (56–66). ACE inhibitor scintigraphy has also been shown to establish RAS as the etiological factor responsible for hypertension (57). However, the absence of a nonlateralizing ACE inhibitor scintigraphy test does not exclude the presence of significant RAS. Therefore, many institutions do not utilize ACE inhibitor scintigraphy in the evaluation of patients with RAS (59).

Doppler Sonography

Doppler sonography is the least expensive diagnostic test, but it is also the most dependent on an operator. Two approaches to diagnose RAS with Doppler techniques exist. The first approach relies on the detection of Doppler abnormalities at the site of the stenosis and utilizes the well-established concept that arterial stenoses produce high flow velocities at and immediately distal to the area of stenosis (67,68). However, for an adequate examination, it is important to evaluate the main renal arteries in their entire course, which is not feasible because of body habitus, bowel gas, or both in a significant number of patients. Peak systolic velocities in the renal arteries exceeding 150–200 cm/sec or a renal artery to aortic peak systolic velocity ratio exceeding 3.5 are considered indicative of significant RAS (Figure 21–1) (68,69).

Changes in the Doppler signal within the intrarenal vasculature distal to the stenosis can also be measured. Unlike the main renal arteries, the intrarenal vasculature can be visualized in the vast majority of patients. The distance of the vessel being interrogated with Doppler is usually too far from the stenosis to allow detection of high-velocity signals. However, sampling of Doppler signals distal to the stenosis takes advantage of the changes in the configuration of the renal waveform into an abnormal tardus-parvus pattern. Doppler signals distal to a stenosis typically show both a dampened waveform with slow systolic acceleration and a diminished amplitude of the systolic peak (69–72).

It appears that a combination of the two approaches of Doppler evaluation offers the highest sensitivity for detecting RAS. The complexity and duration (60–90 minutes) of the examination only allow performance of reliable studies in very dedicated vascular labs. However, even in dedicated labs, Doppler studies do not detect the majority of accessory renal arteries (73,74). Reported sensitivities for the detection of significant RAS range from 17% to 100%, with specificities ranging from 47 to 100% (56,67–76). It should

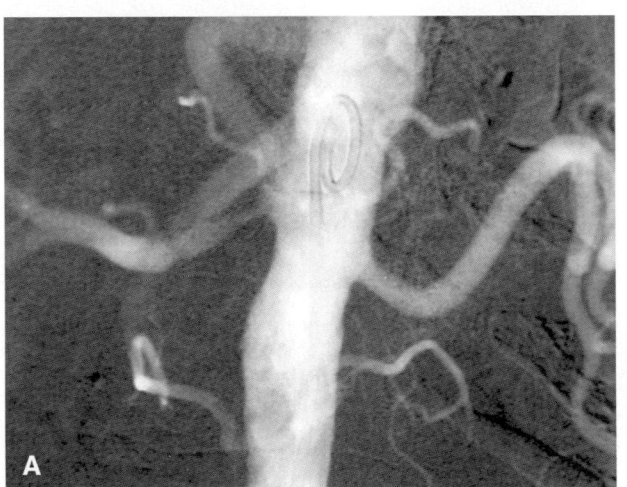

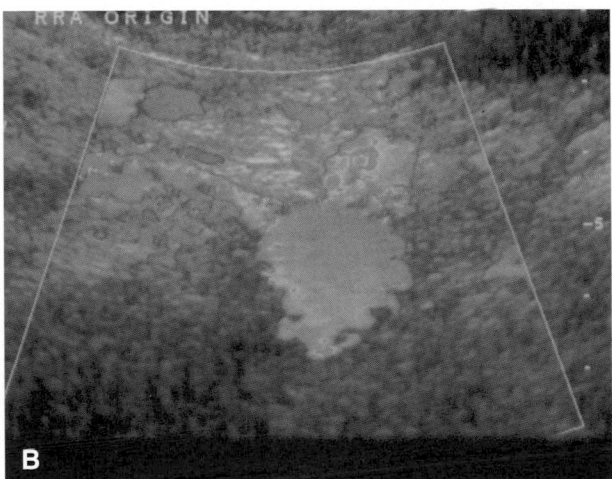

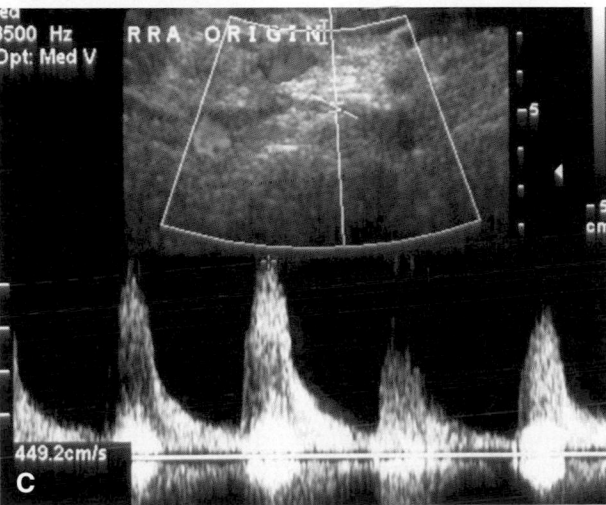

Figure 21–1 A. In-stent restenosis resulting from intimal hyperplasia in a right renal artery Palmaz stent. **B.** Ultrasound shows narrowing of the lumen of the proximal stent because of hyperechogenic hyperplastic intima (*arrow*). **C.** Doppler sonography shows velocity in stenotic segment of 450 cm/sec. The velocity in the aorta was 90 cm/sec resulting in a renal artery to aortic peak systolic velocity ratio of 5.0.

be kept in mind that these data almost never include patients whose examinations are nondiagnostic.

The measurement of intrarenal resistive indices with Doppler sonography may allow for the prediction of treatment outcomes in both RVH and ischemic nephropathy, but this suggestion remains controversial (77,78). Duplex ultrasound is also suitable to follow patients after renal PTA (PTRA) and RAST (see Figure 21–1) (79). Contrast-enhanced renal sonography and renal blood flow reserve measurements using Doppler flow wires are new developments that have shown some promising results, but their true role remains to be determined (80,81).

Computed Tomographic Angiography (CTA)

Volume acquisition of CT data using spiral scanning is the basic technological prerequisite for the performance of CTA (82–84). The data are sampled during the peak arterial enhancement phase of an intravenous contrast bolus and during a breath-hold. Rapid scanning covering the aorta, the renal arteries, and the kidneys with isotrophic resolution is possible in 10 seconds (85–88). Multiple reconstruction algorithms exist to display the raw data in a more "angiographic" fashion (87–90). The examination requires a well-timed contrast bolus given at a rapid injection rate (between 2.5 cc/sec and 7 cc/sec) using a total volume of contrast of approximately 80–150 cc. The contrast requirement limits the application of this technique in patients with impaired renal function. However, research has shown that CTA performed for the detection of RAS may not be associated with an increased risk of contrast-induced nephropathy (CIN) when compared with intra-arterial digital subtraction arteriography (DSA) (91). The use of a thin collimation (0.5–3 mm) technique is essential. Reported sensitivities range from 67 to 100%, with specificities of 83–98% (84,85,87,92–103). One prospective study comparing CTA with Doppler sonography also found CTA to be superior for the detection of RAS (92).

The correct choice of reconstruction parameters is of utmost importance. Research has shown that maximal intensity projections (MIPs) performed better than the three-dimensional shaded surface display method (3D SSD), and one study reported a sensitivity of 92% for MIPs and 59% for 3D SSD displays (92). Volume rendering (VR) techniques are superior to MIP algorithms, mainly because of increased test specificity. The combination of MIP and VR techniques and quantitative measurements generally gives optimum results (87,89,90,104). The latest generation of multidetector scanners (currently, 64 channels) has dramatically improved the diagnostic capabilities of CTA. However, the advancement in CT technology is not reflected in the current, published literature. At the UVA Health System, for example, the authors routinely demonstrate subtle FMD changes with CTA (Figure 21–2).

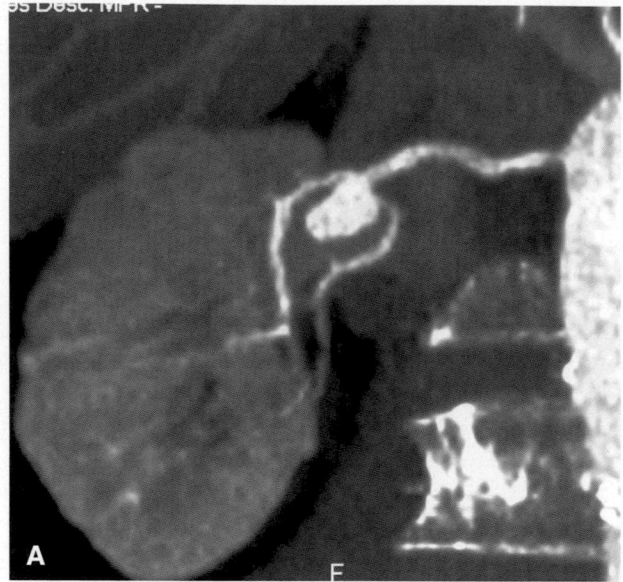

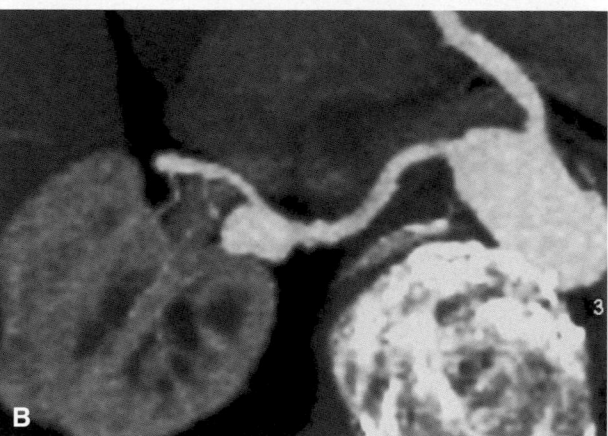

Figure 21–2 A. Renal artery aneurysm resulting from fibromuscular dysplasia. CTA shows aneurysm off the right renal artery bifurcation. **B.** Note subtle pleats in the main renal artery.

Magnetic Resonance Angiography (MRA)

Because of its sensitivity in detecting flow, MRA is used extensively for the depiction of renal arteries. However, lengthy imaging times, inconsistent visualization of the distal portions of the renal arteries, and difficulty in grading a stenosis because of flow phenomena initially resulted in limited acceptance of MRA as a screening test (105–112). However, advances in scanner technology, as well as the development of ultra-fast, three-dimensional sequences, has allowed 3D contrast-enhanced MRA of the renal arteries to replace all other previously published MRA techniques. The technique is robust and not operator dependent (113). Similar to CTA, the technique is based on an intravenous injection of a contrast bolus with rapid acquisition of a 3D data set during a breath-hold in the arterial enhancement phase. Typically, each patient receives

30–40 cc of a gadolinium chelate-based contrast (Gd). In addition, Gd has been shown to be safe in patients with impaired renal function (114,115). Determining the degree of RAS can be problematic with 3D MRA techniques, but strategies have been developed to ascertain the hemodynamic significance of a renal artery lesion (116–120). A number of variations in the basic sequence have been evaluated (121–126). Reported sensitivities and specificities for detecting RAS range (Figure 21–3A, B) between 88 to 100% and 75 to 100%, respectively (56,72, 127–141). In addition, unlike Doppler ultrasound, most accessory renal arteries are detected with MRA. However, its relative unreliability in the detection of FMD remains a weakness of the technique.

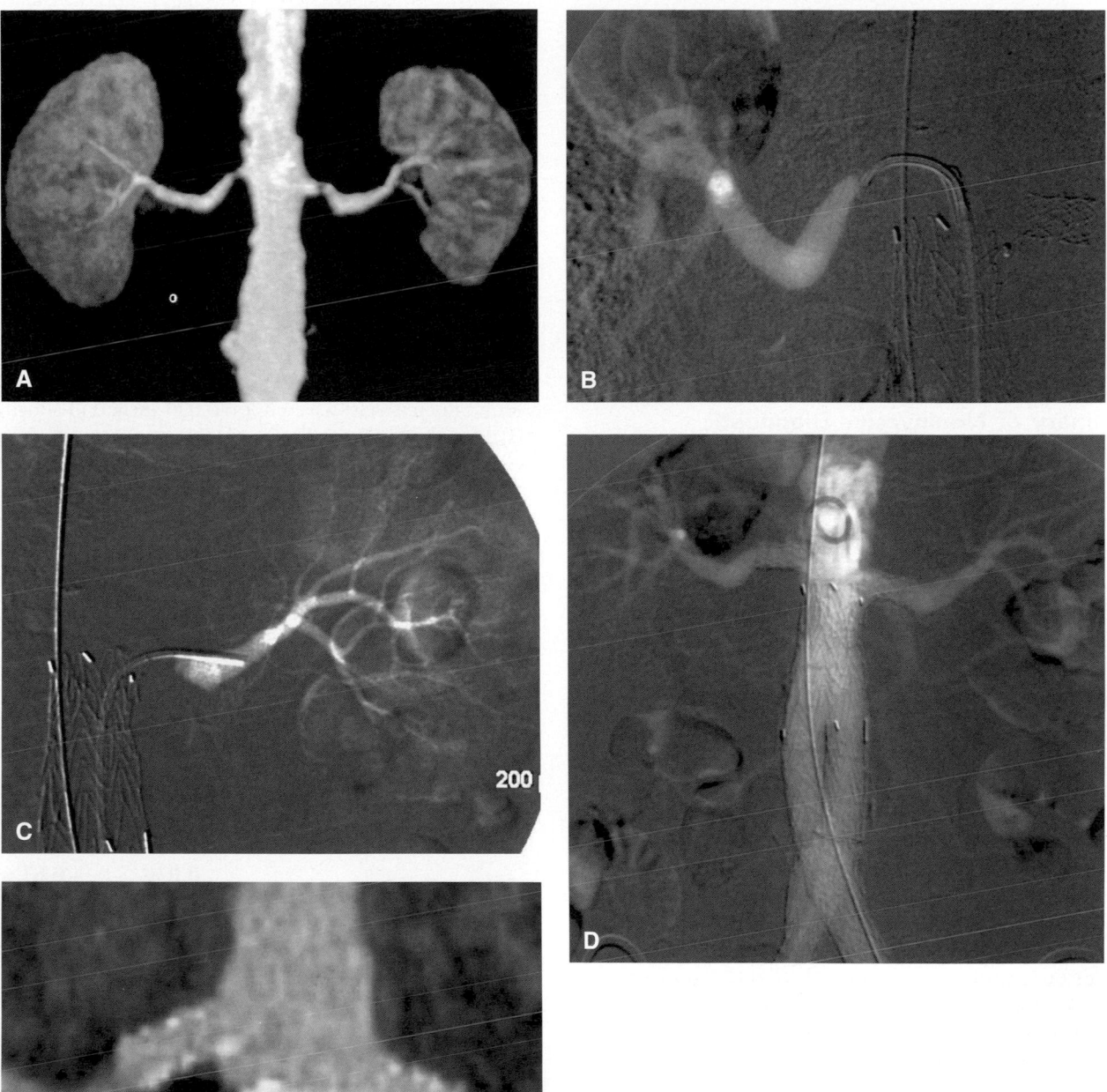

Figure 21–3 Patient with bilateral ARAS. **A.** 3D CE MRA shows severe bilateral ostial ARAS. Note the small saccular aneurysm of the abdominal aorta. Selective **B.** right, **C.** left renal arteriograms confirm high-grade stenoses. **D.** Angiogram after bilateral stent placement (and aortic endograft placement) shows 100% patency of both renal arteries. **E.** CTA performed after renal stenting and placement of a stent graft for the saccular aortic aneurysm also demonstrates patency of the stents.

Limitations also exist in patients with claustrophobia, which precludes the performance of MRA in approximately 2–5% of patients. Pacemakers, defibrillator devices, certain implants, and metallic fragments in the eyes are also general contraindications for MRA. In addition, the majority of patients who have undergone stent placement in the renal arteries cannot be followed because of artifacts caused by the stent (142). In these patients, ultrasound and CTA (Figure 21–3C) are preferable for evaluating the renal arteries (143).

A major advantage of MRA is that it allows for the visualization of the aorta and the iliac and femoral arteries at the time of renal artery imaging. Thus, MRA helps to visualize potential access sites for the procedure and to estimate the risk of cholesterol embolization based upon the amount of plaque burden in the aorta. Studies have shown that pre-procedural planning using the Gd-enhanced MRA significantly reduces the volume of iodinated contrast required during percutaneous renal artery interventions and significantly shortens the procedure time (144). In order to achieve optimum diagnostic performance with MRA, the use of a high-performance 1.5 T system and review of all source images are necessary.

Summary of Noninvasive Diagnostic Evaluation

A large meta-analysis found that CTA and Gd-enhanced MRA are preferred for the evaluation of RVH (56). However, a prospective multicenter trial comparing CTA and MRA with DSA in 356 patients produced somewhat disappointing results (145). The prevalence of significant RAS (>50%) in this study population was 20%. Two panels of three observers each judged CTA and MRA studies, blinded to the results of all other modalities. The sensitivity for CTA ranged from 61 to 69%, with a specificity of 89–97%. MRA fared even worse, with sensitivities from 57–67%, and specificities of 77–90%. Also, reproducibility of the two techniques was disappointing, with a kappa value of 0.59–0.64 for CTA and 0.40–0.51 for MRA. The patients in this study had their examinations done using single-detector CT scanners (rather than MDCT scanners) and MR systems that were not high-performance cardiovascular systems. As such, the data are not representative of the results that can be achieved with current state-of-the-art systems. However, the results do emphasize that the evaluation of renal arteries should be performed on the latest generation CT and MR scanners. The authors currently perform breath-hold, contrast-enhanced, 3D MRA using a dedicated 1.5 T cardiovascular high-performance gradient system (Sonata, Siemens Med). Contrast-enhanced MRA is fast, is not dependent on an operator, allows for reliable detection of accessory renal arteries, and avoids the use of iodinated contrast. Contrast MRA provides morphological assessment of a stenotic lesion, but different techniques assess for the hemodynamic significance of a detected lesion (perfusion MRI and 3D-phase contrast techniques). Doppler sonography provides information about the hemodynamic significance of a lesion and is well-suited to follow patients after stent placement, but is heavily dependent on an operator. The authors also perform multi-detector CTA using a 16-channel system in patients who have normal renal function, which has been as accurate as MRA in detecting RAS. CTA also allows for assessment of stent patency. The best test for evaluating patients suspected of having FMD has not yet been determined. Whenever a high index of suspicion exists for FMD, the diagnostic test of choice continues to be angiography.

TECHNICAL CONSIDERATIONS FOR PTRA AND STENTING

In the appropriate clinical setting, revascularization should be pursued once RAS has been detected. Before performing PTRA, RAST, or both, becoming familiar with the various devices and techniques is mandatory. Over the past 10 years, balloon catheter, guide wire, sheath, guiding catheter, stent technology, and contrast agents for application in the renovascular system have changed significantly. A variety of balloon catheters exist based upon 0.035-inch, 0.018-inch, and 0.014-inch platforms. As would be expected, smaller systems are more flexible, have a lower profile, can track better, and are available in both coaxial and monorail (rapid exchange) systems. However, with smaller systems, the stents are often less visible and have less hoop strength. In addition, most of the published data on RAST are based upon 0.035-inch systems (Figures 21–4 and 21–5).

With premounted stent technology, the stents are "nested" on the balloon material. This nesting improves the security of the stent on the balloon, lowers the profile of the balloon/stent system, and optimizes the relationship between the stent and balloon length. Many of the premounted stent systems are secure enough to allow for the advancement of

	0.035	0.014/18
• HOOP STRENGTH	+	--
• NON-COMPLIANCE	+	--
• COSTS	+	--
• VISIBILITY	+	--
• DATA	+	--
• PROFILE	--	+
• TRACK/FLEXIBILITY	--	+
• MONORAIL/RAP X	--	+

Figure 21–4 Comparison of relative device characteristics between 0.035-inch and 0.014/18-inch renal artery stent systems. (+) means relatively better versus (–) meaning relatively worse.

	OTW	RAP X
• **0.035 INCH**	+	−
• **GW EXCHANGE**	+	−
• **COST**	+	−
• **0.014/18 INCH**	+	+
• **WIRE LENGTH**	±	+
• **ARM ACCESS**	−	+
• **EASE OF USE**	−	+

Figure 21–5 Comparison of over-the-wire and rapid exchange/monorail renal artery stent systems. (+) means relatively better versus (−) meaning relatively worse.

the balloon and stent directly through a lesion, with minimal concern for displacement of the stent off the balloon. With use of a monorail/rapid exchange system, shorter guide wires can be used, making the procedure easier to perform (Figure 21–6). In addition, many of the smaller systems are now quite visible fluoroscopically (Figure 21–7).

In general, 0.035-inch balloon catheter systems employ less compliant balloons, whereas the smaller profile and rapid exchange systems are based usually on more compliant balloon technology. Many of the 0.014/0.018-inch systems involve the use of a stent that has less hoop strength when compared to a 0.035-inch system. However, the industry is trying to address this issue by developing more robust stents (chromium and cobalt-based stents) for use with the smaller systems, so that recoil of the stent within a very resistant ostial RAS is minimized.

Many of the systems utilized for PTRA and RAST involve the use of 6 French to 8 French outer diameter (OD) guiding sheaths or catheters that are preshaped; have soft, radiopaque tips; come with tapered dilators; and have side ports to allow for contrast injection around guide wires

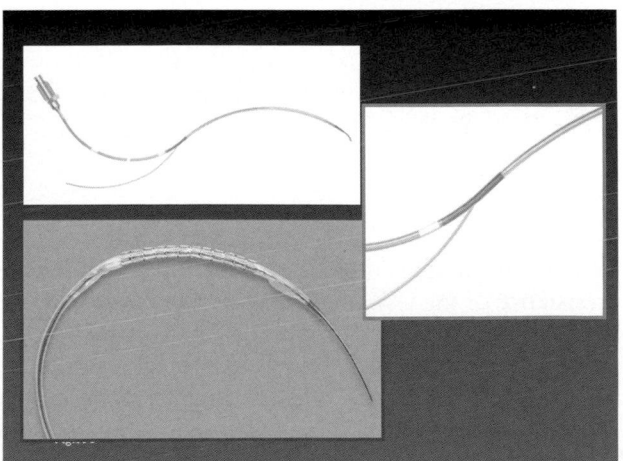

Figure 21–6 Rapid exchange 0.018-inch renal artery system showing the premounted stent on a monorail system.

(Figures 21–8 and 21–9). Therefore, during the PTRA/RAST procedure, repeat contrast injections can be performed to optimize stent placement (Figure 21–10).

Many different guide wires are now available. Some are preshaped, straight-tipped, or J-tipped, and very radiopaque. Each guide wire has its own advantages and disadvantages. Familiarity with the transition and other characteristics specific to the guide wire is necessary (Figure 21–11).

Because of advancements in device technology, most renal artery interventions can be performed from a femoral artery approach. However, in the rare circumstance of infrarenal abdominal aorta occlusion or an acutely angulated renal artery, performing the procedure from a brachial or radial artery approach may become necessary. If a brachial artery approach is used, guiding sheaths in 6 French, 70–80 cm lengths are available to facilitate performance of the procedure (Cook, Inc.). Use of the left radial artery as an access site for PTRA/RAST has also been reported (146).

Before performance of an endovascular intervention, nonselective abdominal aortography is mandatory. On occasion, the availability of a high-quality MRA or CTA study that defines the aortic and proximal renal artery anatomy obviates the need for abdominal aortography. However, at our institution, aortography typically is performed before selective renal artery catheterization. In patients with renal insufficiency, aortography can be performed with carbon dioxide (CO_2) and selective angiography with either Gd or dilute iodixanol (Visipaque, Amersham Health). Defining the underlying lesion is critical, whether or not an ostial ARAS or a branch RAS exists because of FMD.

The orientation of the renal artery origins from the aorta can be determined from a prior MRA or CTA. Most often, the right renal artery originates in a slight anterior orientation off the abdominal aorta, whereas the left renal artery most often originates from a relatively posterior location. In the absence of a prior noninvasive study, an abdominal aortogram performed in a 15°–20° left anterior oblique projection will often profile the origins of the renal arteries. Defining the origin of each renal artery to optimize therapy and to ensure accurate placement of a stent is extremely important. If the renal artery ostium is not profiled, the stent may not cover the entire lesion (Figure 21–12). Another critical step is to delineate the number of renal arteries and the more distal main renal artery and its branches, especially in young patients in whom FMD is a concern.

Once the lesion has been adequately defined, the intervention can be undertaken. In most instances, a reverse-curve catheter (SOS 2 Omni, AngioDynamics) can be used to select the renal artery. At some institutions, the lesion is traversed with either a soft-tip guide wire (Bentson, Cook, Inc.) or a steerable guide wire (Terumo, Boston Scientific or Wholey, Mallinckrodt), and an effort is made to keep the distal tip of the guide wire within the main renal artery as the catheter is advanced across the lesion. Once the tip of the catheter traverses the lesion and an intraluminal

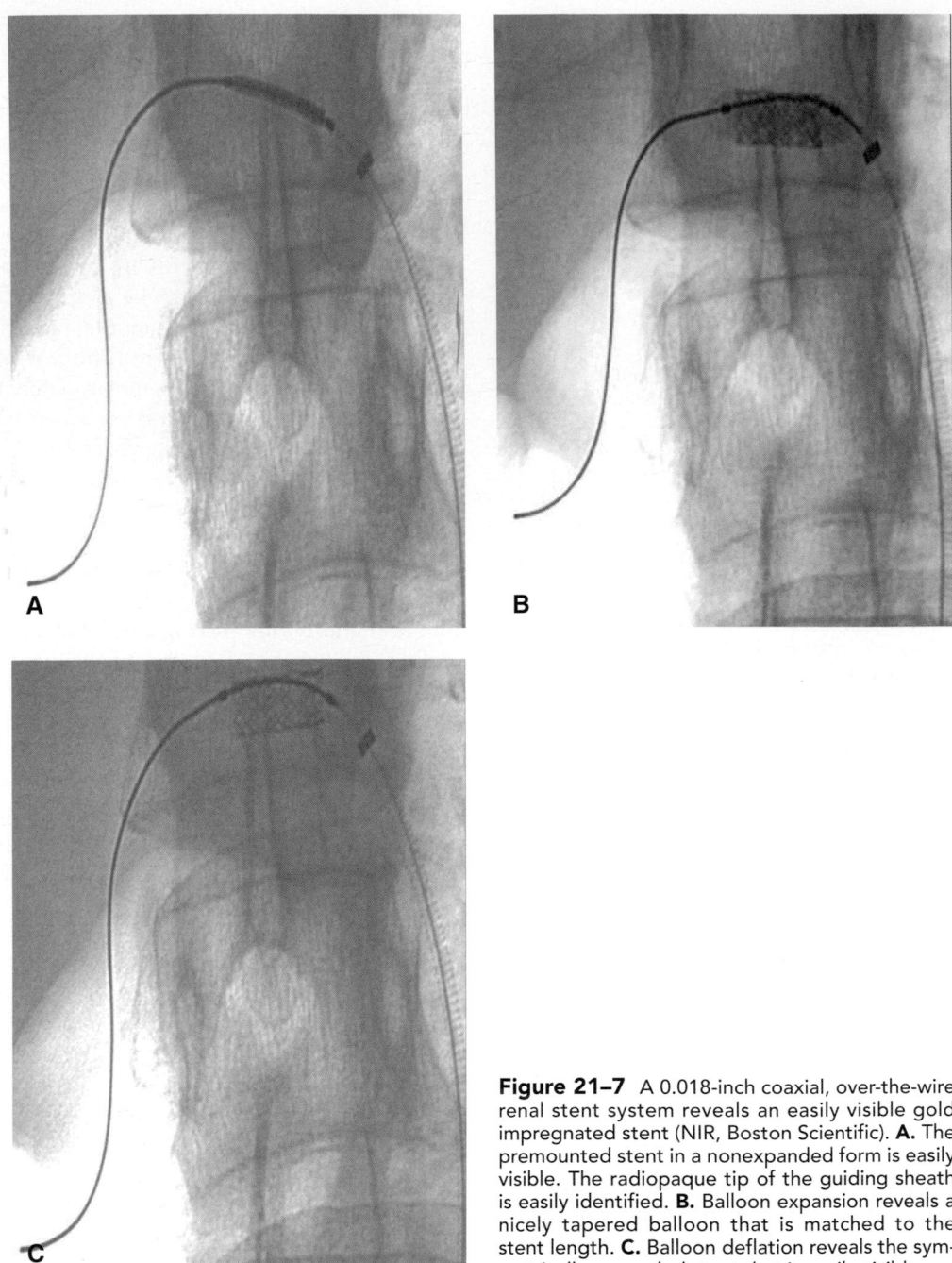

Figure 21–7 A 0.018-inch coaxial, over-the-wire renal stent system reveals an easily visible gold impregnated stent (NIR, Boston Scientific). **A.** The premounted stent in a nonexpanded form is easily visible. The radiopaque tip of the guiding sheath is easily identified. **B.** Balloon expansion reveals a nicely tapered balloon that is matched to the stent length. **C.** Balloon deflation reveals the symmetrically expanded stent that is easily visible.

location is documented, a decision is made to use either a 0.035-inch or 0.014/0.018-inch system. In most instances, a 0.035-inch Rosen guide wire (Cook or AngioDynamics) is inserted. A 6 French preshaped guidesheath (0.035-inch system) is advanced over the guide wire, followed by balloon dilatation of the lesion. For ostial lesions, stent placement is performed. The presence of the 6 French guide sheath facilitates contrast injections, balloon advancement, and stent placement (Figure 21–10).

Predilatation of ostial lesions allows the determination of resistance of the lesion, the appropriate size of the balloon, the stability of the balloon in the lesion (i.e., whether the balloon jumps forward or backward during its inflation), and the amount of discomfort the patient has with balloon inflation. The advantage of predilatation should be weighed against the risk of creating a problematic dissection, the need for additional manipulations within the renal artery, and the risk of embolization.

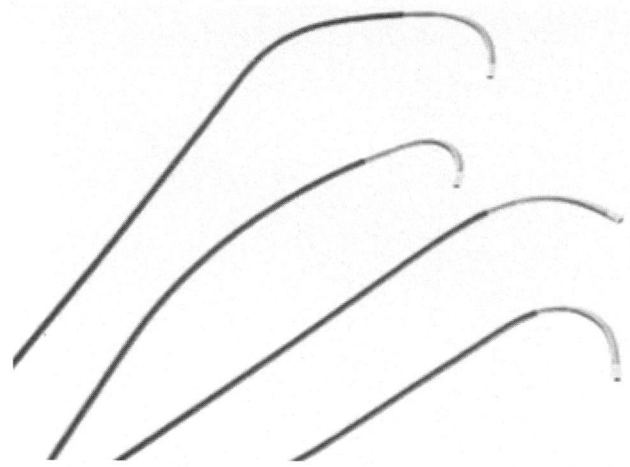

Figure 21–8 Several shapes and configurations of guiding sheaths for renal artery stent therapy are shown.

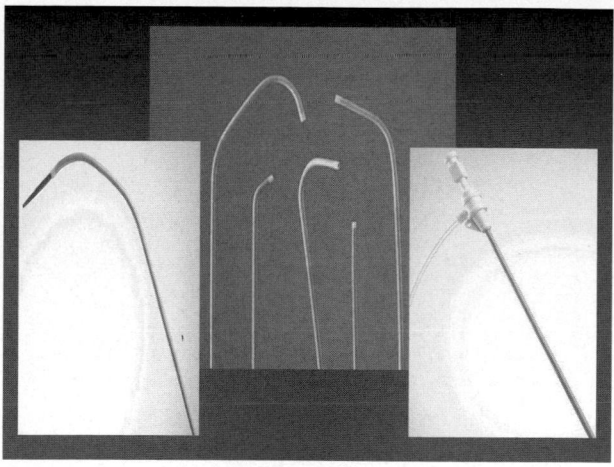

Figure 21–9 Several 6 French to 8 French guiding catheters for renal artery stent placement are displayed.

Primary RAST is performed when there is a high risk of cholesterol embolization, manipulations need to be minimized, or an atherosclerotic lesion recurs shortly after a previous PTRA.

If a 0.014/0.018-inch system is chosen, an appropriate platinum-tip guide wire is inserted through the reverse-curve catheter. Current guide catheters and guide sheath systems come with dilators tapered to 0.018 inch and can be advanced over the platinum guide wires to the renal ostium. The procedure then is performed in a fashion similar to that described above for the 0.035-inch system, often with the use of a rapid exchange system.

If the diseased artery has an early bifurcation or more complex anatomy is uncovered, use of double guide wire access and a "kissing balloon" technique may become necessary. In order to facilitate use of double guide wire access, access via both femoral arteries may become necessary to have. However, it has been found that two 0.014-inch monorail systems can be advanced through a 6 French guiding sheath or 7 French guiding catheter. An early bifurcation of the main renal artery often obviates the ability to utilize a renal stent. However, PTRA in this situation may still prove to be very useful (Figure 21–13). In addition, not all atherosclerotic lesions are the same. Some of the lesions are the result of an aortic plaque, whereas other lesions may be truncal and may primarily involve the main renal artery (Figure 21–14). Therefore, some atherosclerotic lesions may respond to PTRA alone (Figure 21–15) and may not require placement of a stent (147).

When treating more peripheral main renal artery lesions, such as FMD, the lesion is traversed with a Wholey wire, with subsequent placement of a 5 French or 6 French guiding sheath or a 6 French or 7 French guide catheter into the proximal renal artery, followed by balloon dilatation with an appropriate size balloon catheter. If the lesion involves a small renal artery, a tortuous vessel, difficult access, or a branch vessel, a 0.014/0.018-inch wire is advanced across the lesion. An appropriately shaped 6 French guide catheter is chosen and advanced over the guide wire (with the tapered dilator in place) into the proximal renal artery. The balloon diameter chosen depends upon the lesion being treated. For very resistant, intimal, fibroplasia lesions (very young patients with FMD, radiation-induced lesions, or neurofibromatosis), a smaller balloon diameter size is initially chosen and gradually increased, as necessary, to minimize the risk of rupture. For more traditional medial fibroplastic FMD or atherosclerotic lesions, a balloon size is chosen that corresponds to the size of the adjacent normal vessel. In these situations, the balloon may be oversized by as much as 20–25%, as long as it is done gradually and carefully, while monitoring the patient's discomfort during balloon inflation. For atherosclerotic lesions, ostial lesions are often dilated with a balloon slightly smaller than the anticipated vessel size to minimize the risk of creating a dissection. However, once the ostial lesion is opened, an appropriate diameter balloon—premounted with a stent—is used to treat the lesion. Whenever possible, the lesion is overdilated by approximately 20% to facilitate optimum approximation of the stent to the vessel wall and to optimize the poststent minimal lumen diameter (MLD). Quantitative vascular angiography has confirmed the correlation between the MLD following RAST and stent patency (50). In addition, restenosis rates can be stratified by reference vessel diameter. Vessels that measure 4.5 mm or less have a restenosis rate of 36%, compared to 15.8% for vessels 4.5–6 mm ($p = 0.068$), versus 6.5% for vessels greater than 6 mm in diameter ($p < 0.01$) (50). Indeed, some operators routinely use intravascular ultrasound (IVUS) to optimize MLD and stent to vessel wall apposition (148).

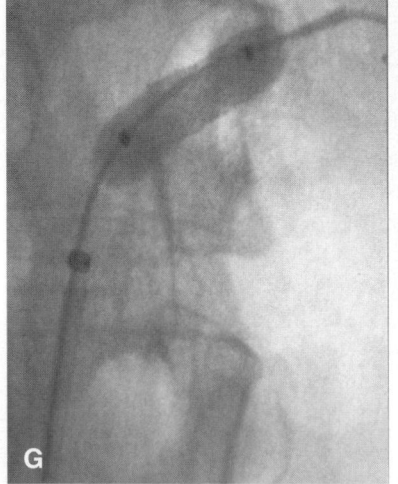

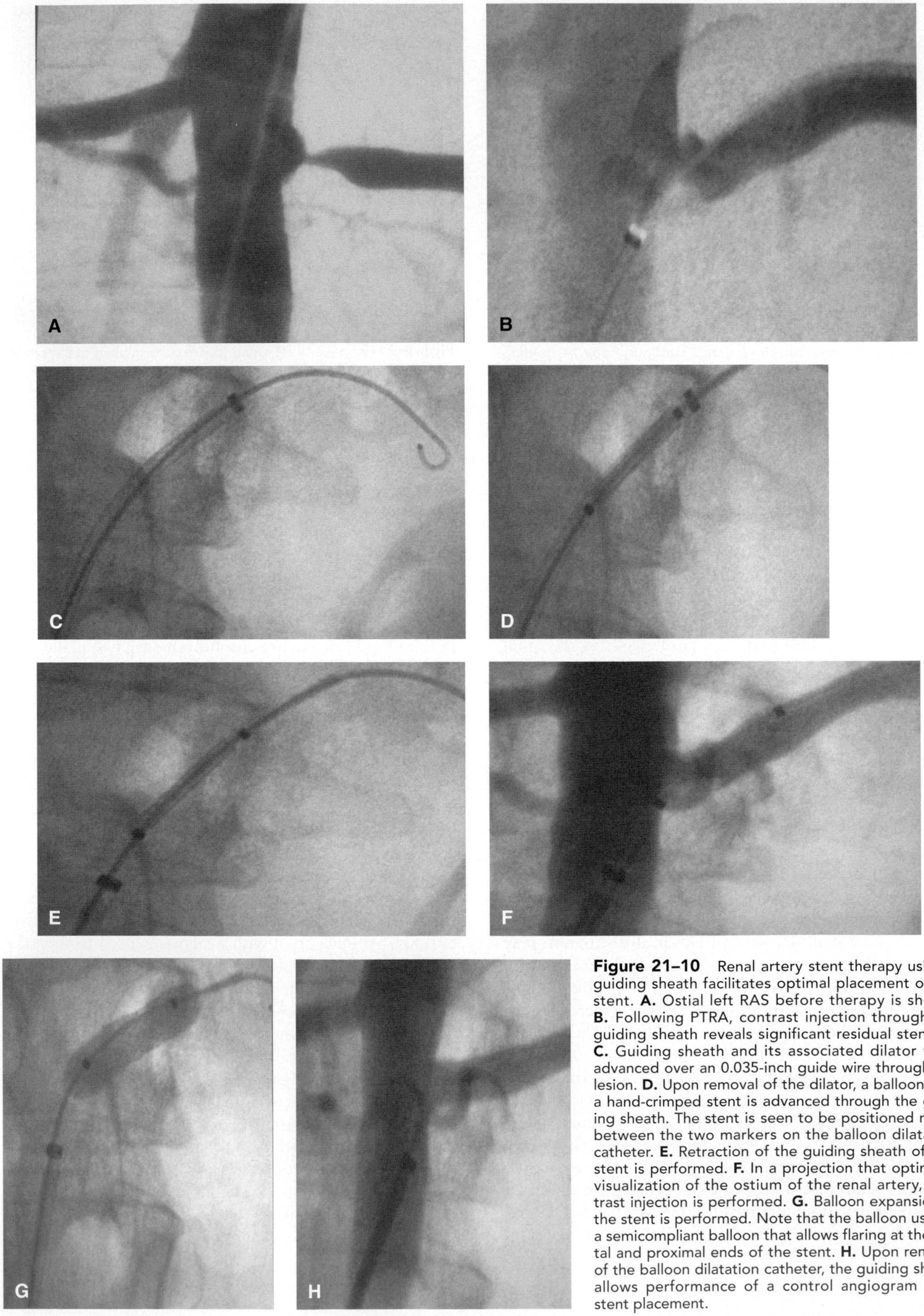

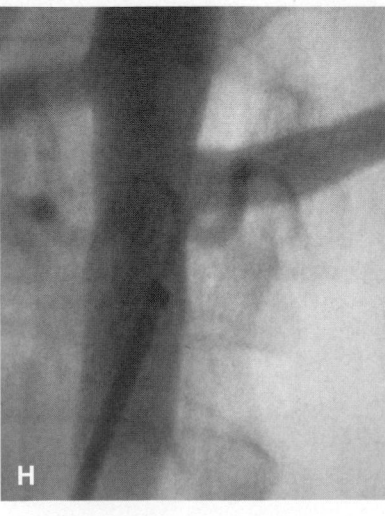

Figure 21–10 Renal artery stent therapy using a guiding sheath facilitates optimal placement of the stent. **A.** Ostial left RAS before therapy is shown. **B.** Following PTRA, contrast injection through the guiding sheath reveals significant residual stenosis. **C.** Guiding sheath and its associated dilator were advanced over an 0.035-inch guide wire through the lesion. **D.** Upon removal of the dilator, a balloon with a hand-crimped stent is advanced through the guiding sheath. The stent is seen to be positioned nicely between the two markers on the balloon dilatation catheter. **E.** Retraction of the guiding sheath off the stent is performed. **F.** In a projection that optimizes visualization of the ostium of the renal artery, contrast injection is performed. **G.** Balloon expansion of the stent is performed. Note that the balloon used is a semicompliant balloon that allows flaring at the distal and proximal ends of the stent. **H.** Upon removal of the balloon dilatation catheter, the guiding sheath allows performance of a control angiogram after stent placement.

	J	**STRAIGHT**
• PERFORATIONS ↓	+	--
• PURCHASE NEEDED	+	--
• STABILITY	+	+
• SPASM	--	+
• SMALL VESSELS	--	+
• STEERABILITY	--	+

Figure 21–11 Knowledge of the characteristics of the various guide wires used for PTRA and RAST is important. Comparison of the benefits versus drawbacks between a J-tipped guide wire and a straight-tipped guide wire are noted. A (+) indicates relatively better versus (–) indicating relatively worse.

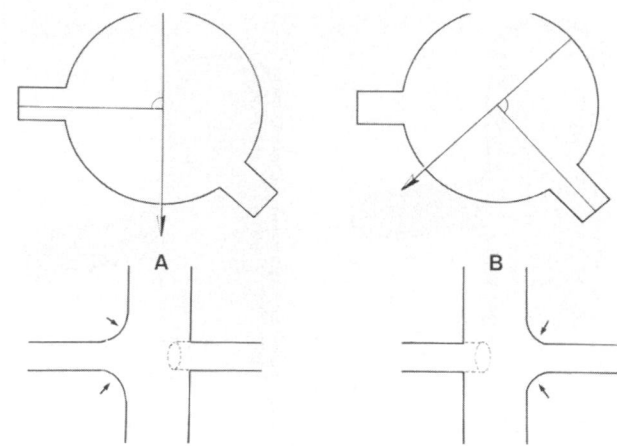

Figure 21–12 When the x-ray beam is oriented at a 90° angle to the renal artery origin, the renal artery origin can be well-profiled. **A.** An anterior-posterior projection profiles the right renal artery origin. Note: When the renal artery origin is profiled, it "funnels open" toward the aorta (*arrow*). The left renal artery is foreshortened in this projection, and its origin is not well delineated. **B.** A left anterior oblique projection profiles the left renal artery (*arrow*), whereas the right origin is not well-defined.

During renal artery interventions, routine use of pharmacotherapy is recommended. Whenever possible, patients are initiated on 325 mg of aspirin at least one day prior to the procedure. If there is a high index of suspicion that the patient has ARAS, the patient is also initiated on clopidogrel (Plavix, Sanofi-Synthelabo Inc.) 300 mg the day before the procedure and 75 mg the day of the procedure. Before the procedure, the patient is hydrated with at least 300 cc of normal saline. During the intervention, the patient receives heparin to maintain an activated clotting time (ACT) level greater than 220 or bivalirudin (Angiomax, The Medicines Co.) using a weight-adjusted dose. Intra-arterial vasodilators (nitroglycerin 100–200 micrograms and/or verapamil 2.5 mg increments) are given directly into the renal artery to minimize vasospasm. Glycoprotein IIb-IIIa inhibitors are not routinely used unless in situ thrombosis develops.

After a successful PTRA procedure, patients are maintained on 325 mg of aspirin for life. If stent implantation is performed, the patient is also given a 1- to 3-month course of clopidogrel (75 mg/day). There is no evidence that aspirin or clopidogrel reduces restenosis or acute thrombosis rates, but evidence does show that these medications improve cardiovascular outcomes (149).

Depending upon the characteristics of the stenotic lesion, such as length, irregularity, multiplicity, and the resistance of the distal vascular bed, lesions that narrow the vessel cross-sectional area by at least 75% or the diameter by at least 50% are considered hemodynamically significant. The physiological significance of a borderline lesion probably depends upon the resistance of the peripheral renovascular bed and the underlying intrarenal autoregulatory mechanisms (150,151). In cases of borderline RAS, intra-arterial pressure measurements are obtained. Simultaneous pressures are measured from the abdominal aorta and from the renovascular bed peripheral to the stenotic lesion. The two pressure curves from both transducers (aortic and renal) should be superimposed so that the variability in measurements is minimized. A peak systolic pressure gradient of greater than 10% of the systemic systolic blood pressure or

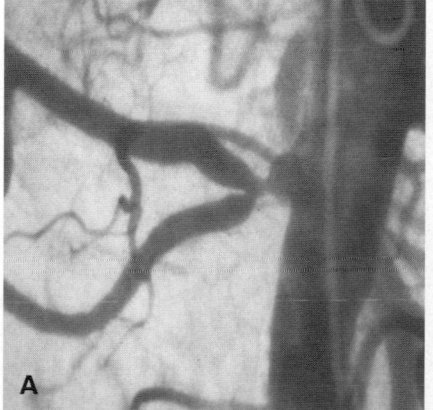
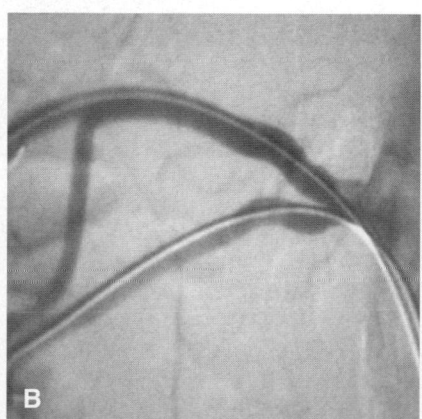
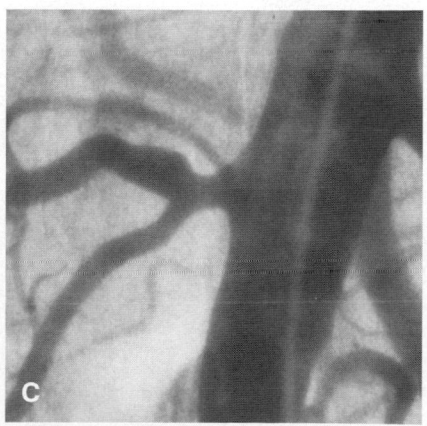

Figure 21–13 Complicated renal artery lesions may require use of a kissing balloon technique. **A.** Arteriogram reveals an ostial right RAS with a very early bifurcation. **B.** Double guide wire access was obtained, and a "kissing balloon" technique was performed. **C.** Follow-up angiogram 17 months later reveals a satisfactory appearance to the previously dilated right renal artery lesion.

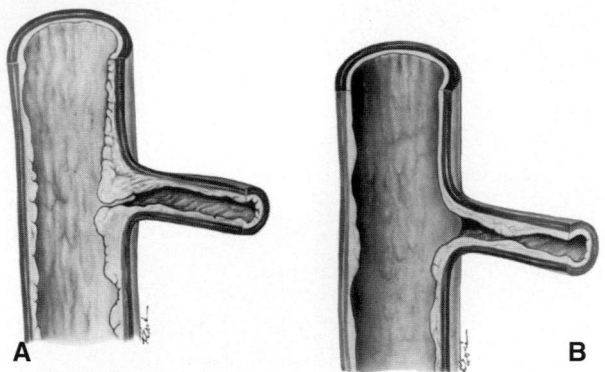

Figure 21–14 Not all atherosclerotic renal artery lesions are equivalent. **A.** A true ostial lesion is often related to an aortic plaque that prolapses over the ostium of the renal artery. These lesions require use of a stent for optimum results. **B.** A nonostial, truncal ARAS represents a lesion within the renal artery, rather than an aortic plaque. Truncal lesions may respond to PTRA alone.

20 mm Hg is generally accepted as indicating a hemodynamically significant stenosis (152,153). However, these recommended values are arbitrary and no objective outcomes data exist to support these recommendations—but it has been reported that a 50% diameter stenosis is associated with a systolic pressure gradient of 22 mm Hg (153). The effect of pharmacological vasodilatation on the peripheral renal vascular bed for determining the physiological significance of a stenosis is also unknown. Other tests that can lend support to the clinical significance of a borderline RAS include lateralizing renal vein renins, a lateralizing ACE inhibitor renal nuclear medicine study, or an abnormal

renal Doppler study (57,77,78,154,155). As noted earlier, use of the renal resistive index from a meticulously performed Doppler ultrasound has provided mixed results. One study suggests that a resistive index greater than 80 predicts a poor outcome following revascularization (77). Whereas, in another report, patients undergoing RAST for significant RAS demonstrated a statistically significant improvement in blood pressure at 1 year of follow-up despite a resistive index greater than 80 (78). Therefore, each interventionist must evaluate the clinical, anatomic, and hemodynamic data available and make an appropriate decision. Following intervention, a residual pressure gradient less than 5 mm Hg systolic is considered satisfactory. In general, a de novo lesion that creates less than a 10 mm Hg systolic gradient preintervention in a patient with hypertension or renal insufficiency is not treated.

Although the use of embolic protection devices in carotid stent therapy has become popular, the application of distal protection devices for PTRA and RAST is still evolving. The incidence of clinically significant atheroemboli following PTRA, RAST, or both is not clearly defined. However, any embolization to kidneys in patients with renal insufficiency may have significant implications. To date, there are two small reports on the use of distal protection devices during RAST (156,157). In the largest study, 46 renal arteries in 37 patients with ischemic nephropathy underwent PTRA and RAST with distal main renal artery protection (157). All lesions were considered greater than 80% (diameter) narrowed, and no lesion required predilatation. The distal protection device used was the AngioGuard Filter Wire (Cordis Corp.). The device consists of a 0.014-inch guide wire with a polyurethane

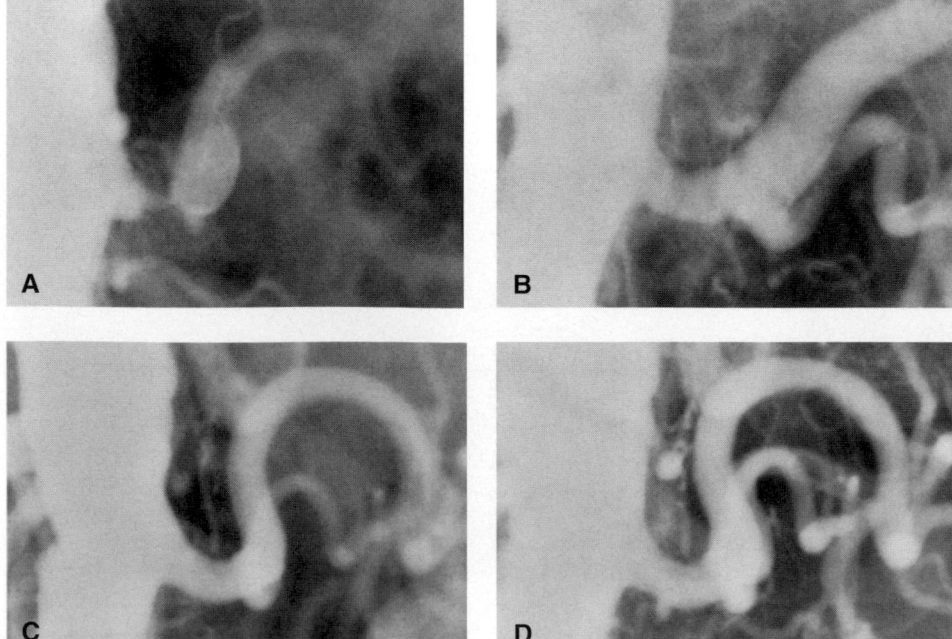

Figure 21–15 Some atherosclerotic renal artery lesions will respond to PTRA alone. **A.** Atherosclerotic, proximal left RAS. **B.** Following PTRA, there is a satisfactory appearance. **C.** Eighteen-month follow-up angiogram reveals a satisfactory appearance to the previously dilated left renal artery. **D.** A 53-month follow-up angiogram reveals that the left main renal artery remains widely patent after PTRA.

basket at the distal end that contains 100 micron pores and is supported by 8 nitinol wire struts. The device was deployed in the distal main renal artery. All stents were dilated to 6–7 mm in diameter. In 65% of the cases, the distal protection filter contained macroscopic or microscopic contents, which included fresh thrombus, chronic thrombus, atheromatous fragments, and cholesterol clefts. The remainder of the filter baskets (16 of 46, or 35%) were either empty or contained insufficient material. Overall, 95% of the patients treated with distal protection had improvement or stabilization of renal function during a mean follow-up of 12.5 months. The results of this study were compared to a retrospective analysis of 22 arteries treated in 20 patients without distal protection. Only 75% of the patients treated without a distal protective device experienced improvement or stabilization in renal function. Although this data is encouraging, the study involved two different patient cohorts. In the group that did not receive distal protection, no efforts to minimize contrast-induced nephropathy—hydration, use of N-acetyl cysteine, use of Gd as the contrast—were made, and the degree of stenosis and the vessel diameters treated were not defined (157).

RESTENOSIS AFTER RAST

The incidence of significant restenosis following RAST varies depending upon the diameter of the renal artery treated—the larger the diameter, the less percentage restenosis observed. Other factors include the gender of the patient (females have higher restenosis rates), whether the patient continues to smoke (smoking is associated with higher restenosis rates), how well the stent is apposed to the vessel wall, and whether the lesion is completely covered. Many biomolecular and mechanical rheologic factors that affect restenosis rates are yet to be determined. Once in-stent restenosis occurs, PTRA alone is often successful at further expanding the stent and obliterating the hemodynamically significant pressure gradient. With in-stent restenosis, the hyperplastic tissue is often very resistant and "slippery." Therefore, use of a noncompliant, high-pressure balloon is necessary to achieve a satisfactory result. In addition, the balloon should be centered within the lesion in order to keep the balloon from "squirting" in or out of the stent.

Brachytherapy for coronary stent applications is associated with a 50% reduction in in-stent restenosis (158). Use of endovascular brachytherapy has been used for treatment of in-stent restenosis in the renal artery (159). However, brachytherapy for the renal arteries remains challenging and of unproved benefit.

In situations in which PTRA with a traditional balloon is unsuccessful for treating in-stent restenosis, cutting balloons have been used. The so-called cutting balloon (Boston Scientific) is currently FDA-approved for use in coronary artery saphenous vein grafts and is available in diameters up to 8.0 mm. The cutting balloons may also have a role in treating very resistant lesions, as seen with the intimal fibroplasia-type of FMD, radiation-induced stenoses, and neurofibromatosis. Cutting balloons should be routinely undersized. If oversized, the razor-sharp blades on the cutting balloon could easily create a longitudinal, transmural "cut" through the vessel wall. The risks of cutting balloon use should be weighed against other therapeutic alternatives, such as surgical revascularization. Cryoplasty balloons (Boston Scientific) represent another a possible avenue of therapy, but no published data exist regarding its use for restenosis.

COMPLICATIONS

Complication rates related to endovascular therapy for RAS depend upon the criteria used for patient selection and the experience of the operator. When reviewing data from two large series and two meta-analyses, the weighted mean complication rate was 14% (160–164). The most frequently reported complications included groin hematomas and puncture site trauma. The 30-day mortality rate was 1%, which usually related to either renal artery rupture, cholesterol embolization, acute renal failure, or bleeding resulting from a puncture site above the inguinal ligament. The need for subsequent secondary nephrectomy occurred in less than 1% of cases. The need for a surgical salvage procedure appears to be less than 1% (162,163). The incidence of symptomatic embolization varies from 1 to 8% (160,162). However, the incidence of cholesterol embolization during renal interventions may be underestimated (165). Inadvertent occlusion of the main renal artery varies between 0.8% and 2.5%. Occlusion of a renal artery branch causing a segmental infarction occurs in 1.1–1.7% of patients (162,163). Experience and refinements in technology also affect complication rates. Martin et al. found that the total complication rate fell from 20% in the first hundred to 13% in the second hundred cases of PTRA (166).

Technical complications occurring during a procedure that ultimately have no clinical consequences but lead to an increase in procedural time, cost, or the use of an additional stent or device can occur in as many as 25% of patients (166,167). In addition, an infrequent but documented complication of renal artery stent placement is stent infection (168,169). Therefore, prior to placement of an intravascular stent, patients may be given an IV dose of an appropriate antibiotic.

The incidence of deterioration in renal function following endovascular therapy depends upon the population of patients treated. With the advent of alternative contrast agents, preprocedure hydration, and preprocedure medications (discussed later in the chapter), the authors have been able to reduce the incidence of acute deterioration in renal function to less than 5% in patients with underlying renal insufficiency (170).

In summary, the mean incidence of complications associated with endovascular therapy for the treatment of RAS is about 14%. Most of these complications are not life threatening nor do they result in a significant loss in renal function, but rather, they are most often the result of complications related to the access site. The combined incidence of 30-day mortality, loss of a kidney, rupture of a renal artery, occlusion of the main renal artery, and the need for surgical intervention should be less than 4% (160–163).

CONTRAST-INDUCED NEPHROPATHY

Background

Contrast-induced nephropathy (CIN) is a form of acute renal failure that begins shortly after the administration of iodinated contrast media and usually resolves after 1–2 weeks. However, some patients with CIN develop permanent deterioration in renal function (171–173). The incidence of CIN after the administration of iodinated contrast media varies from 10 to 30%, depending on the studied patient population, risk factors, and the definition of CIN used (174–177). The definition of CIN varies because of the variability in reporting—20% versus 50%, 0.5 mg/dL versus 1.0 mg/dL, or 44.2 µmol/L versus 88.4 µmol/L change in serum creatinine—and the time period during which renal function is observed—24, 48, 72 hours, or longer. Risk factors for developing CIN include underlying renal insufficiency, diabetes, dehydration, multiple myeloma, higher volumes of contrast used, and multiple iodinated contrast exams within 48 hours. The pathophysiology of CIN is complex and not well understood. However, evidence suggests that CIN is the result of multiple factors, including osmotic, direct toxic, and hemodynamic effects on the kidney (174,175,178). A detailed discussion of the pathophysiology of CIN is beyond the scope of this chapter, but the significance of CIN should not be overlooked. Patients who develop CIN have higher in-hospital mortality rates when compared to patients with similar comorbidities who do not develop CIN (173,179).

Several approaches to reducing the risk of CIN during renal angiography can be employed. Preprocedure patient preparation, contrast media selection, catheter techniques, and total contrast media volume used are important considerations when trying to prevent CIN.

HYDRATION AND ADJUNCT MEDICATIONS

Adequate hydration repeatedly has been shown to reduce the risk of CIN (180–182). Most hydration protocols recommend administering 1–1.5 cc/kg per hour of normal or half-normal saline for 12 hours before and after the procedure. Adjunct medications, such as diuretics and mannitol, may not reduce the risk of CIN (180). Other agents, such as theophylline, nifedipine, and adenosine also do not appear to be effective in preventing CIN (183–187). However, treatment with sodium bicarbonate may reduce the risk for CIN (188).

Recently, N-acetylcysteine (Mucomyst, Roxane Lab) and fenoldopam mesylate (Corlapam, Abbott Labs) were used with the intent of reducing the risk of CIN. N-acetylcysteine, a potent antioxidant, has been shown to be a free-radical scavenger that may prevent oxidative tissue damage (189–191). N-acetylcysteine usually is administered in two separate 600 mg doses on the day before and the day of the procedure. Birck et al. performed a meta-analysis of studies evaluating the role of N-acetylcysteine administration in reducing CIN. It showed that N-acetylcysteine administration resulted in a significant reduction in the risk of CIN (191).

Fenoldopam mesylate is a specific dopamine A-1 receptor agonist that produces systemic, peripheral, and renal vasodilatation and increases plasma renal blood flow in patients with or without renal insufficiency (192–194). Protocols for fenoldopam mesylate administration typically start at a dose of 0.05 µg/kg per minute. Doses are increased every 20 minutes by 0.05–0.1 µg/kg per minute up to a maximum of 0.5 µg/kg per minute as long as the patient's blood pressure does not drop more than 40% from baseline. Fenoldopam is administered preprocedure, intraprocedure, and (for 4–6 hours) postprocedure. Patients with a documented allergy to sulfites should not receive fenoldopam. Single and multicenter registry studies, as well as several smaller studies, have shown a benefit following fenoldopam mesylate administration (195–199).

However, a review of the literature shows that results are mixed regarding the risk reduction of CIN with the use of N-acetylcysteine and fenoldopam. The few prospective, randomized trials available at the present time have failed to show a benefit of either N-acetylcysteine or fenoldopam in reducing the risk of CIN, compared with adequate hydration alone (200,201). Clearly, additional studies are needed to determine whether either of these agents will prove useful in reducing CIN, especially in patients with ischemic nephropathy undergoing an endovascular procedure.

TYPE OF IODINATED CONTRAST MEDIA

Several prospective studies comparing the use of low-osmolarity contrast media (LOCM) with high-osmolarity contrast media (HOCM) have failed to demonstrate a clinically significant reduction in the incidence of CIN (202–206). However, relatively few patients at risk for CIN were included in these studies. When patients at high risk for CIN were studied, the incidence of CIN was significantly reduced when LOCM was used instead of HOCM (207). Therefore, in patients with normal renal function, the incidence of CIN is equally low with either LOCM or HOCM, but in patients with increased risk of developing CIN, LOCM is less likely to cause CIN. Isosmolar contrast media (IOCM) (Iodixanol, Amersham Health) may also provide additional benefit in reducing CIN when compared with LOCM (208).

IODINATED CONTRAST MEDIA VOLUME

Iodinated contrast media volume should be limited in patients at risk for developing CIN (209–212). Unfortunately, determining a threshold dose that is likely to cause CIN in an individual patient is difficult. However, reports have shown CIN to occur in high-risk patients receiving as little as 20 mL of iodinated contrast media (213). Therefore, in patients with renal insufficiency undergoing angiography with iodinated contrast media, total contrast dose should be minimized. A successful strategy to help minimize the use of iodinated contrast media includes diluting the contrast media to 1/3–1/2 of its normal concentration before injection.

ALTERNATIVE CONTRAST AGENTS

Carbon dioxide (CO_2) and Gd are noniodinated alternative contrast agents that can be used in place of iodinated contrast media. The intra-arterial use of CO_2 was pioneered by Hawkins and has been demonstrated to be an effective agent with DSA and renal interventions (214–219). CO_2 is a nontoxic, noncombustible, odorless, and colorless gas that is buoyant, invisible, compressible, nonviscous, and heavier than room air. Understanding these properties allows for the successful use of CO_2 as an intravascular contrast agent. CO_2 does not mix with blood; rather it must replace/displace the blood in a vessel to accurately image the vessel. Because CO_2 floats, patient positioning is important to maximize the visualization of the vessel under investigation. Insufficient displacement of blood will result in incomplete vessel delineation. Delivering the CO_2 in a controlled, uncontaminated manner is important. Prepping the catheter with 3–5 cc of CO_2 can facilitate a more controlled, less explosive delivery of the CO_2 during image acquisition. Use of a bag delivery system (AngioDynamics) minimizes the risk of contamination of the CO_2 with room air (220). Because of its low viscosity, CO_2 can be injected around guide wires in catheters much more easily than liquid contrast agents.

Pitfalls with CO_2 DSA include over-estimation of the degree of vessel stenosis, bowel and motion artifacts that deteriorate the radiographic image, and "trapping" of CO_2 in nondependent vessels (221,222). Transient mesenteric ischemia and cardiac arrest resulting from trapping of CO_2 in the mesenteric and main pulmonary arteries, respectively, have been reported (222,223).

Gadolinium-based (Gd) contrast provides another intravascular agent as an alternative to iodinated contrast media. Off-label, intra-arterial use of Gd, whether alone or in conjunction with CO_2, can be helpful in reducing the need for iodinated contrast media during diagnostic studies and percutaneous interventions (224–227). Gadolinium is a rare earth metal that has a higher atomic number ($Z = 64$) and k-edge (50 keV) than iodine (53 and 33 keV, respectively). A higher kilovolt peak (96 kVp versus 73 kVp) can be used when acquiring DSA images with Gd in order to reduce radiation exposure to the patient, without reducing the quality of the radiographic image (228). Nevertheless, images with Gd-based contrast agents are inferior to those obtained with iodinated contrast media because of reduced signal to noise. When performing renal angiography using CO_2 and Gd as the contrast agents, Gd is best used as a problem solver (229,230). CO_2 angiograms can identify the number of renal arteries and the projection that best profiles their origins. If necessary, findings from the CO_2 angiogram can be confirmed with a 10 cc bolus of Gd injected by a power injector over 0.5 seconds. Selective renal artery angiograms can be performed with 3–5 cc of Gd to confirm the presence of a stenosis and to guide and monitor the progress of a PTRA and RAST procedure. Using Gd in this manner allows the total dose of these agents to stay within the intravenous dose guidelines (0.03 mmol/kg), because no intra-arterial guidelines currently exist (231–234).

RENOVASCULAR HYPERTENSION

Results of Therapy

Since the early 1980s, new classes of antihypertensive medications have become available and widely used. The impact of these agents is enormous. Medical regimens employing these agents for the treatment of RVH have increased the likelihood of achieving good blood pressure control from 46% to higher than 90% (235,236). Therefore, many patients with RAS and hypertension likely will remain undetected because blood pressure is well-controlled and renal function remains stable on these medical regimens (236,237). Therefore, the decision to refer a specific patient for renal artery revascularization depends on the expected outcome of an intervention versus medical therapy alone. Unfortunately, very few prospective, randomized data comparing the results of medical therapy versus revascularization exist (36,238,239). The investigators of these randomized trials should be complimented for their attempts to acquire meaningful information, but several problems occur with all three trials:

- Small sample sizes—the three trials recruited a total of 210 patients
- Short follow up—the follow-up period for these three studies varied from 6 to 12 months

- No use of stents and variability in what was defined as an "intervention"—less than 5% of the patients received renal artery stents, yet the lesions treated were atherosclerotic in most of the patients, and an intervention was often defined as a nephrectomy, surgical bypass, or no treatment in patients with total renal artery occlusions that were randomized to PTRA
- Crossover of patients from the medical therapy group to the intervention group—this approached 50% in the largest study

Despite the heterogeneity between the trials, a meta-analysis of these three randomized trials revealed a statistically significant reduction in systolic and diastolic blood pressure in the angioplasty population versus the medical therapy patients (240).

Percutaneous Transluminal Renal Angioplasty (PTRA)

A more detailed analysis of the largest randomized trial involving 106 patients randomly assigned to either PTRA or medical therapy revealed some interesting findings (36). In this study, 56 patients were randomized to PTRA and 50 patients were randomized to medical therapy alone. Of the 106 patients, 10 (9.4%) had less than 50% stenosis but were still entered into the trial. Of the 56 patients undergoing PTRA, seven (12.5%) were not fully treated (three patients with renal artery occlusions were not treated and four PTRA failures were not treated with stents). At the 3-month assessment point, patients who underwent PTRA were on fewer blood pressure medications (2.1 versus 3.2, $p < 0.001$), had a better creatinine clearance (70 cc/min, $p = 0.03$), and had fewer abnormal renal nuclear medicine studies (36% versus 70%, $p = 0.002$). At the end of 12 months, 44% of the medical therapy group (22 of 50) crossed over to PTRA but were analyzed on the basis of intention-to-treat. Yet, patients who underwent PTRA primarily were on fewer blood pressure medications (1.9 versus 2.4, $p = 0.002$), had fewer lesions progress to total renal artery occlusions (0 versus 16%), and had a decrease incidence of worsening renal function (3.6% versus 12%). In addition, more PTRA patients had improved blood pressure control (68% versus 38%) at 12 months and fewer had worsening blood pressure control (9% versus 33%).

In a meta-analysis of 10 nonrandomized PTRA series that included a total of 644 patients with ARAS, hypertension was either improved or cured in 53% and 10% of patients, respectively, at a mean follow-up of 19 months (163). In another study, only one of six patients whose diastolic blood pressure was controlled with two antihypertensive medications versus 24 of 25 for patients with more severe hypertension ($p = 0.004$) had improvement in blood pressure control following PTRA. In addition, patients over age 65 had a response rate of only 40% (2 of 5) versus more than 90% (22 of 24) in younger patients ($p = 0.024$). Therefore, this study suggests that middle-aged patients

with easily controlled hypertension and elderly patients with hypertension and no renal insufficiency are less likely to benefit from an intervention (241).

In summary, PTRA appears to be beneficial in the treatment of renovascular hypertension in a defined subset of patients. Patients with easily controlled hypertension, older patients with hypertension without renal insufficiency, and patients with RAS less than 50% diameter are least likely to benefit from an intervention. In addition, a question not clearly defined so far is whether PTRA for RAS actually alters cardiovascular morbidity and survival. At the time of this writing, a multicenter, NIH-funded trial involving 1,080 patients is specifically addressing the cardiovascular outcomes of renal artery interventions (CORAL Trial) for ARAS.

Renal Artery Stent Therapy (RAST)

In a meta-analysis of 14 renal stent trials published between 1991 and 1998 involving 678 stent patients, high blood pressure was cured in 20% of patients and improved in 49%, for an overall benefit of 69%. Noteworthy is the fact that patients undergoing RAST had a technically successful procedure in more than 95% of procedures versus a technical success rate of 73% for PTRA (163). In a randomized trial comparing PTRA versus stenting, 85 patients were randomized between PTRA and RAST for ostial ARAS (242). In this trial, the technical success rates, restenosis rates, and primary patencies were better for patients undergoing RAST versus PTRA (90% versus 63%, 14% versus 48%, and 79% versus 28%, respectively).

In summary, use of RAST for ostial ARAS in whom there is high clinical suspicion for renovascular disease proves beneficial in blood pressure control in about 70% of patients. Restenosis rates within renal stents are higher in patients with renal arteries less than 6 mm in diameter, in female patients, and in patients who continue to smoke (50,243).

Surgery Versus Endovascular Therapy

Few series exist in which a direct comparison is made between the results of PTRA, RAST, and surgery. In one retrospective analysis of patients who underwent either PTRA or surgical bypass for treatment of RVH, 10 of 12 (83%) patients with nonostial ARAS and 10 of 22 (45%) patients with ostial ARAS experienced a clinical benefit after PTRA alone. In the patients undergoing surgery, 5 of 10 (50%) patients with ARAS benefited from the surgical procedure. All patients had a minimum of 6 months of follow-up. Major complications occurred in 20% of the surgical patients and in 3% of the PTRA patients (244).

In a prospective, randomized trial involving 58 patients, PTRA or surgery was performed for the treatment of "severe" hypertension. Only nondiabetic patients with unilateral RAS were included in this study (245). In this study, 90% of patients undergoing PTRA had improvement or cure of their hypertension versus 86% of the surgical patients. PTRA was technically successful in 83% of patients versus 97% of the surgical patients. Primary and secondary patency rates at 24 months for PTRA versus surgical patients were 75% versus 96%, and 90% versus 97%, respectively. Major complications occurred in 17% of the PTRA patients and in 31% of the surgical patients.

Results of Therapy for Ischemic Nephropathy

The progressive course of renovascular disease with worsening RAS, renal atrophy, and reduction in GFR was first described in 1973 by Deane (246). In 1988, Jacobson introduced the term "ischemic nephropathy" to define the reduction in GFR or loss of renal parenchyma resulting from significant RAS (247). Ischemic nephropathy can cause either rapid or gradual loss of renal function (248–250). Atherosclerosis accounts for about 80% of renal artery lesions and is the most common cause of ischemic nephropathy (251,252). Once ischemic nephropathy progresses to chronic renal failure, the survival rate in this patient population is very low (24,253).

Clinical Features

The clinical presentation of patients with ischemic nephropathy typically includes both hypertension and renal dysfunction, but renal dysfunction can be seen in the absence of hypertension. Renal dysfunction usually has a progressive pattern in patients with ischemic nephropathy (254). However, some patients with ischemic nephropathy can present with acute renal failure, especially when the administration of an ACE inhibitor or ARB or renal artery thrombosis of an underlying stenotic lesion occurs (255–258). Acute renal failure resulting from an ACE inhibitor or ARB typically resolves after withdrawal of the offending medication. However, these agents can cause acute renal failure in about 6 to 38% of patients with severe renovascular disease (259,260).

Treatment

The goal of treating ischemic nephropathy is to stabilize or improve renal function. Treatment options include surgical revascularization, PTRA with or without RAST, and medical therapy alone. Because no consensus exists regarding which patients with RAS are best treated or who will benefit from renal artery revascularization, the following considerations should be recognized:

- Clinical and anatomic evidence suggesting that renal function is deteriorating on the basis of RAS should be present.
- A diameter stenosis of at least 70% is needed to cause hemodynamic and physiologic changes sufficient to cause ischemic nephropathy (251,261,262).
- A pattern of progressive deterioration in renal function should exist—a patient with stable renal insufficiency is unlikely to benefit from revascularization.

- The extent of renal parenchymal disease should be determined before revascularization. Traditionally, kidney size and degree of echogenicity by ultrasound examination have been used. Resistive index (RI) measurements have been proposed as another method to evaluate the extent of preexisting renal parenchymal disease (77). However, the predictive role of the RI has come into question, because patients with renal insufficiency, significant RAS, and elevated RI values have benefited from renal revascularization (78).
- Finally, timing of revascularization is important. Revascularization is best performed before progression to irreversible parenchymal injury occurs. Patients with a serum creatinine of less than 3 mg/dL before renal revascularization appear to have the best chance for improvement after revascularization (263,264). However, patients with serum creatinine levels greater than 3 mg/dL have responded favorably to revascularization.

The risks of renal artery intervention are significant. Complications have been discussed previously in this chapter, but a few complications are worth being reemphasized. Cholesterol embolization is probably under-recognized and under-reported (265). Renal reserve in patients with ischemic nephropathy is severely limited. This limited reserve results in a much lower margin of safety in patients with renal insufficiency. An additional 10% loss of functioning renal parenchyma in some patients with renal insufficiency can result in the need for dialysis (Figure 21–16).

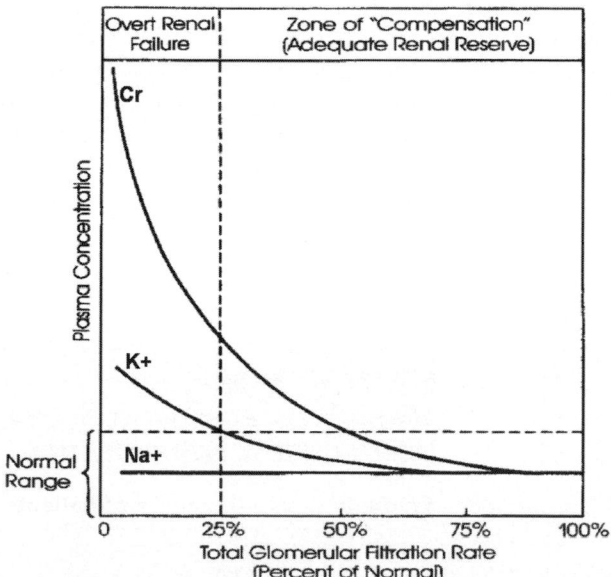

Figure 21–16 The relationship between serum creatinine and functional renal reserve is demonstrated in this chart. Although the total glomerular filtration rate may be reduced by as much as 50%, the serum creatinine level may actually be within the normal range. However, once the glomerular filtration rate falls below 50%, the serum creatinine level will change exponentially despite small losses in renal function.

TABLE 21–1

RESULTS OF SURGICAL REVASCULARIZATION FOR ISCHEMIC NEPHROPATHY

Study	# of Patients	Improved (%)	Stable (%)	Worse (%)
Alcazar et al. (261)	32	62	23	15
Bredenberg et al. (266)	40	55	25	20
Chaikoff et al. (267)	30	47	47	6
Crinniou (268)	21	43	43	14
Fergany et al. (269)	158	35	47	18
Hallet et al. (270)	91	22	53	25
Hansen et al. (271)	70	49	36	15
Hansen et al. (272)	232	58	35	7
Libertino et al. (273)	91	49	35	16
Novick et al. (274)	16	58	31	11
van Damme et al. (275)	23	56	26	18

Contrast-induced nephropathy (CIN) is of particular significance in patients with renal insufficiency and may occur in up to 30% of cases, especially in patients with diabetes. Efforts to minimize the risk of CIN have been discussed in this chapter. The risk of CIN can be reduced to less than 5% when alternative contrast agents are employed (227,229,231).

Surgical Revascularization

Reported benefit of surgical revascularization in patients with presumed ischemic nephropathy is 70 to 90% (Table 21–1). Criteria for surgical revascularization include: (1) kidney size greater than 8 cm, (2) patency of the distal main renal artery and its intrarenal branches, (3) viability of the involved kidney shown by isotope renography, and (4) a biopsy demonstrating well-preserved renal tubules and minimally sclerosed glomeruli (266–275). Although most investigators consider stabilization or a slowing of the rate of decline in renal function a success, Hansen et al. reported that in patients with ischemic nephropathy undergoing surgical revascularization, patients with improved renal function after surgery

had a significant and independent increase in dialysis-free survival compared to patients whose renal function stabilized (271).

The morbidity and mortality rates associated with renovascular surgery are reported to be about 30% and 3 to 13%, respectively, although surgical series often include patients undergoing concomitant abdominal aortic reconstruction (261,271,275,276). However, patients selected for surgery tend to be healthier than those who undergo percutaneous renal revascularization (271,276,277).

Percutaneous Angioplasty and Stenting

Several authors have reported on the benefits of PTRA for ischemic nephropathy (261,278–283). See Table 21–2. Because most atherosclerotic lesions involve the renal ostium, technical success rates following PTRA alone have been reported to be as low as 50%, with recurrence rates as high as 40% (279–289). Results from these studies demonstrate that improvement or stabilization in renal function is in the range of 65–75% of patients, with deterioration of renal function in the range of 5–35% (279–290).

TABLE 21–2

RESULTS OF ANGIOPLASTY (PTRA) ALONE FOR ISCHEMIC NEPHROPATHY

Study	# of Patients	Improved (%)	Stable (%)	Worse (%)
Alcazar et al. (261)	23	31	38	31
Karagiannis et al. (278)	27	22	50	28
Lossino et al. (279)	60	27	67	6
O'Donovan et al. (280)	17	53	12	35
Paulsen et al. (281)	135	38	42	20
Pickering et al. (282)	55	47	30	23
Weibull et al. (245)	24	20	74	5

TABLE 21–3

RESULTS OF RENAL STENTS FOR ISCHEMIC NEPHROPATHY

Study	# of Patients	Improved (%)	Stable (%)	Worse (%)
Boisclair et al. (291)	17	41	35	24
Harden et al. (292)	32	36	36	28
Rees et al. (293)	14	36	36	28
Runback et al. (294)	45	25	43	32
Spinosa et al. (295)	96	26	37	37
Tuttle et al. (296)	74	15	81	4
van de Ven et al. (242)	29	17	55	28

The failure of PTRA to produce satisfactory and durable results in ostial atherosclerotic RAS has led to the introduction of RAST as an adjunct to PTRA. Recent literature demonstrates technical success rates with RAST to be greater than 95%, with in-stent restenosis rates of about 20% (11,50,163,243). In nonrandomized and uncontrolled series, the reported incidence of improvement or stabilization in renal function following RAST is 63–96% (Table 21–3) (163,242,291–296).

Critics of renal artery revascularization, whether it is surgical or percutaneous, point to the randomized, controlled trials comparing medical therapy alone to renal revascularization that demonstrate no significant difference in outcomes between the two (Table 21–4) (36,238,239,242). In addition, others argue that despite initial clinical benefit, within five years, no initial benefit obtained with revascularization is maintained (242).

The authors recently reviewed their experience in 96 consecutive patients with renal insufficiency (creatinine = 1.5–7.6 mg/dL, mean = 2.7 mg/dL) who underwent PTRA, RAST, or both (295). All procedures were performed using CO_2 and Gd as the contrast agents. Clinical, survival, and creatinine data were obtained in 96 of 99 (97%) patients at a minimum follow-up of 30 months. The cohort of 99 patients had a significant improvement in renal function ($p = 0.015$). However, three distinct groups of patients were identified: In Group 1, 26% had a ≥20% improvement in renal function; in Group 2, 37% had a stabilization in serum creatinine, and in Group 3, 37% had a continued decline in renal function (Figure 21–17). Patients in Groups 1 and 2 had a dialysis-free survival (DFS) rate at 30 months of about 80%; whereas, patients in Group 3 experienced a DFS of 44% at 30 months (Figure 21–18). Predictors of a favorable outcome included lesions involving renal arteries ≥6 mm diameter, lesions ≥80% diameter stenosis, and mean kidney length of 9 cm. Therefore, a definite subgroup of these patients with renal insufficiency appeared to benefit from revascularization (Figure 21–19).

TABLE 21–4

RESULTS FROM RANDOMIZED CONTROL STUDIES: MEDICAL THERAPY VERSUS PTRA FOR ISCHEMIC NEPHROPATHY

Study	Total # of Patients	# of Patients Randomized to PTRA	Effect on Renal Function
van Jaarsveld et al. (36)	106	56	Increase in creatinine level @ 12 months in 12% of medical patients and 3.6% of PTRA patients
van de Ven et al. (242)	84	42	Increase in creatinine level in 15% of patients in both groups
Plouin et al. (239)	49	29	No difference in renal function
Webster et al. (238)	55	30	No difference in creatinine level in medicine or PTRA group

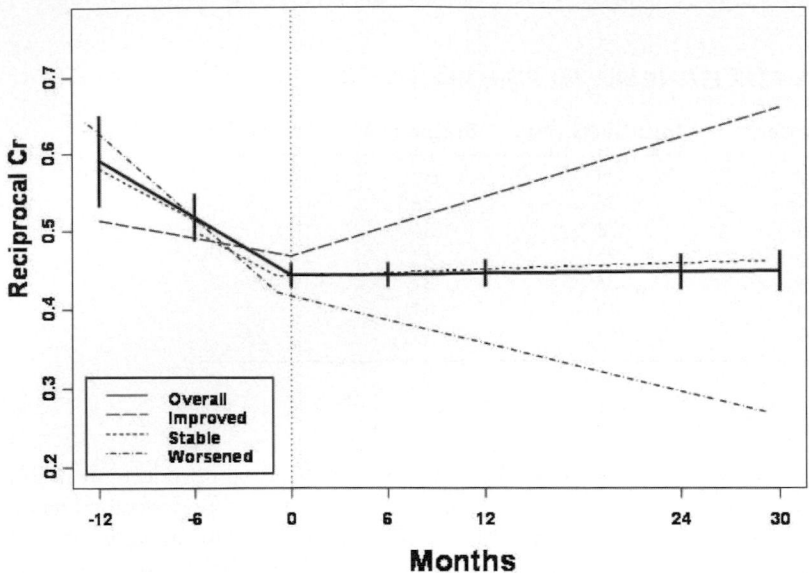

Figure 21–17 A graph of the reciprocal of serum creatinine versus time reveals a linear downward slope for the patient cohort (*solid line*) at the time of intervention (0 months). Following intervention, the renal function of the cohort appears to stabilize as reflected by flattening of the slope of the curve. Three distinct patient populations within the patient cohort are identified. One group clearly demonstrates an improvement in renal function after intervention (*dashed line-upward slope following intervention*). One group reveals stabilization of renal function (*dotted line*). The third group demonstrates persistent deterioration in renal function (*downward slope of curve*) despite the intervention (*dash intermittent with dot line*).

Medical Therapy

Once renovascular disease progresses to chronic renal failure, survival is poor. Older, atherosclerotic, and hypertensive patients undergoing dialysis have 3- and 5-year survival rates of less than 50% and 20%, respectively (24, 253). Therefore, preserving renal function and altering cardiovascular risk factors in patients with renovascular disease is critical. Blood pressure control or lack thereof, has been shown to be a strong predictor for the development of renal failure in diabetic and nondiabetic patients (297). A linear relationship has been demonstrated between blood pressure control and the rate of decline in renal function (298). The addition of ACE inhibitors or ARBs has also been shown to have a renal protective effect that appears to extend beyond their antihy-

pertensive effect (299–303). Therefore, aggressive and attentive medical management of patients with ischemic nephropathy helps to stabilize renal function.

Controlling proteinuria also plays a role in renal protection. The amount of proteinuria has been shown to consistently determine the rate of loss of renal function (304,305). A low-protein diet lowers proteinuria and reduces the rate of renal function loss (306). In addition, medications such as ACE inhibitors, ARBs, nonsteroidal anti-inflammatory drugs, and COX-2 inhibitors may also play a role in proteinuria reduction (300–305). However, caution is necessary with use of medications, because all of these medications can exacerbate renal insufficiency. Finally, increasing evidence points out that controlling hyperlipidemia decreases coronary morbidity and mortality (307–309). Controlling

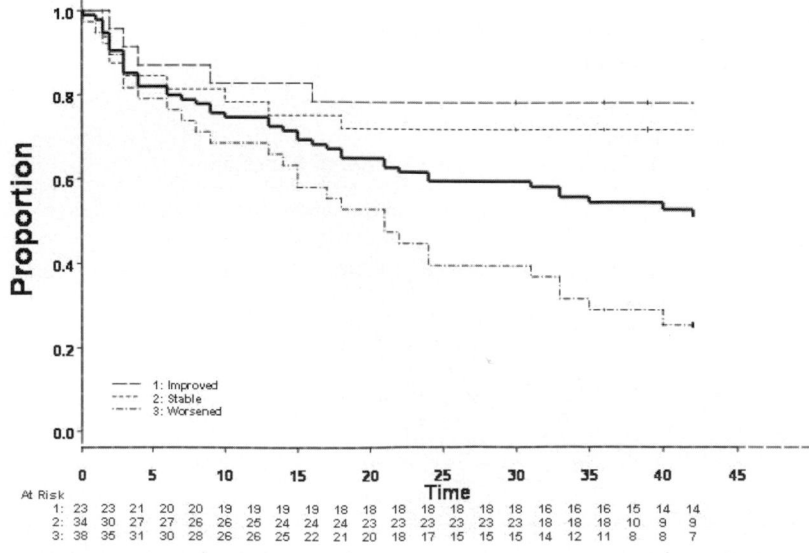

Figure 21–18 Life-table analysis for dialysis-free survival reveals that post-PTRA/RAST, the patients with improved (*dashed line*) and stabilized (*dotted line*) renal function have significantly improved dialysis-free survival when compared to patients who had continuing deterioration in renal function (*dashed/dotted line*).

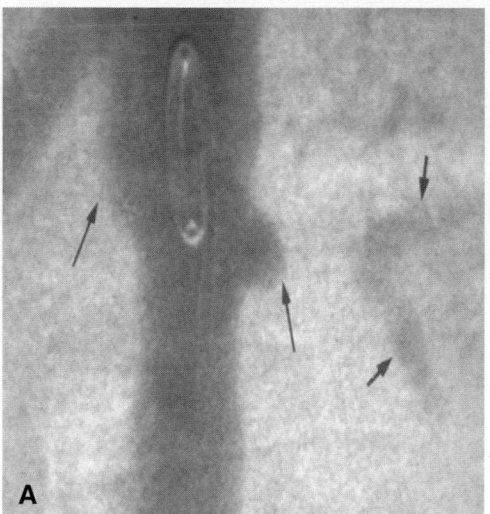 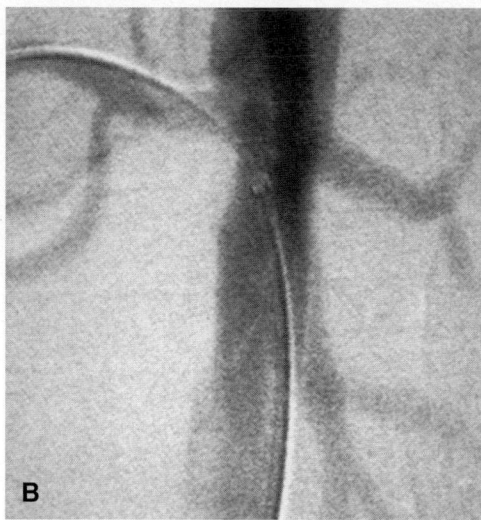

Figure 21–19 A 66-year-old female with a sudden increase in serum creatinine to 3.2 mg/dL presents with congestive heart failure. **A.** Carbon dioxide angiography reveals bilateral renal artery occlusions (*large arrow*) with reconstitution of the intrarenal branches in the left kidney (*small arrows*). **B.** Following recanalization and RAST of the right and left renal artery occlusions, the patient was seen in follow-up 8 weeks later. The serum creatinine had decreased to 1.2 mg/dL, and the patient had no further episodes of congestive heart failure.

hyperlipidemia could decrease the progression of atherosclerotic renovascular disease and potentially delay the appearance of ischemic nephropathy. However, no evidence exists to prove this hypothesis at the present time.

In summary, ischemic nephropathy is being recognized increasingly as a cause for renal failure. Some patients demonstrate progressive RAS leading to deterioration in renal function. Renal revascularization, whether performed surgically or percutaneously, improves or stabilizes renal function in most patients when judicious selection criteria are employed. However, not all patients will benefit from revascularization. The time has come for a well-designed clinical trial to evaluate "best" medical therapy, with or without renal revascularization, to determine which patients are most likely to benefit from an intervention, thereby limiting unnecessary procedures, complications, and expenses. As noted earlier, the role of distal protection devices during PTRA and stenting is yet to be defined (158).

Fibromuscular Dysplasia (FMD)

Fibromuscular dysplasia (FMD) of the renal arteries is a less common cause of renovascular hypertension than atherosclerosis. Patients who present with hypertension and FMD have a median age of 33 years and are more often women (>75%) (310,311). About two thirds of these patients have bilateral stenosis. FMD lesions can be classified based upon the angiographic appearance (312–314). About 80% of patients will have the medial fibroplasia type of FMD, with the characteristic angiographic findings of a "string of beads" appearance, and on occasion, frank aneurysms (Figure 21–20). Focal narrowing of the mid or distal artery

in conjunction with saccular outpouchings smaller than the native vessel diameter can be seen with the perimedial hyperplasia type of FMD and accounts for about 15% of cases. The underlying histopathology in these lesions reveals disorganization and disruption of the normal medial smooth muscle architecture. Excessive accumulation of fibrous tissue leads to the formation of "webs." The webs alternate with areas of medial thinning and aneurysmal dilatation, accounting for the classic "string of beads" appearance. The natural history of medial fibroplastic and perimedial hyperplastic FMD lesions of the renal artery is not well-defined, but some evidence does show that medial fibroplastic lesions are slowly progressive in 12 to 16% of patients, but rarely do they lead to renal artery occlusion or renal atrophy (315–317). However, in one series, 21% of patients (14 of 66) with FMD had renal insufficiency and 83% (12 of 14) of these patients experienced improvement in renal function after PTRA (318). Medial hyperplasia and intimal fibroplasia types of FMD are seen in <5% of cases. Intimal fibroplastic lesions are seen most often in very young patients, and the lesions tend to be very fibrotic. These lesions have a characteristic long, high-grade, symmetric stenoses of the mid to proximal renal artery. The underlying histopathology with these lesions reveals hyperplastic intima. If left untreated, this lesion often leads to progressive renal atrophy.

Results of PTRA

A summary of 25 published series on PTRA in the treatment of FMD of the renal arteries reveals an overall technical success rate of 82–100%, (mean of 94%) for PTRA

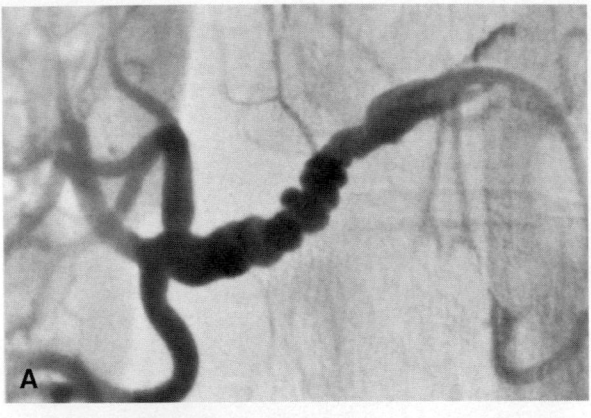
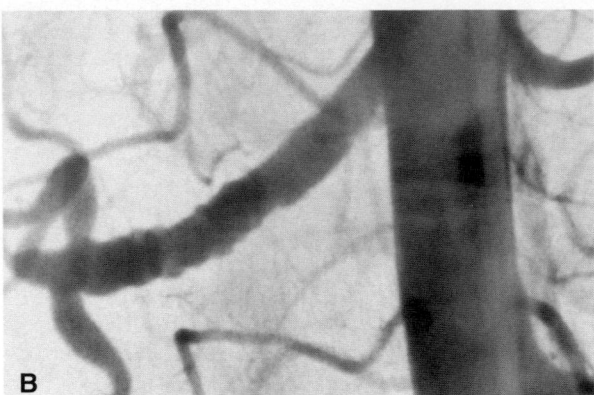
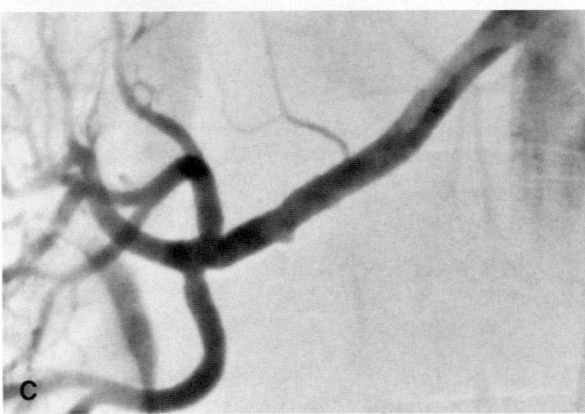

Figure 21–20 A 51-year-old woman presents with hypertension. **A.** Renal arteriogram reveals extensive FMD of the right renal artery. **B.** Immediately after dilatation with a 5 mm balloon, the vessel appears irregular, but rapid flow is present. This appearance is typical immediately after PTRA for FMD. **C.** Arteriogram obtained 12.5 months later shows smooth healing of the vessel. This response to successful PTRA is the usual long-term appearance after dilatation of FMD lesions. (Reprinted with permission from Tegtmeyer CJ, Kellum CD, Ayers C. Percutaneous transluminal angioplasty of the renal artery: results and long-term follow-up. Radiology 1984;153:77–84.)

(Table 21–5) (318–343). The clinical response to a technically successful PTRA in patients with hypertension is very good—about 42% are cured and an additional 45% have improved blood pressure control. The durability of PTRA in FMD reveals a long-term primary patency rate of about 84% and a secondary patency rate of 93%. Restenosis following PTRA of FMD lesions occurs in about 10 to 15% of patients. Therefore, repeat angiography and PTRA should be undertaken in patients in whom a poor initial response after PTRA or recurrence of symptoms occurs.

The benefits of PTRA are particularly evident in the treatment of medial fibroplastic lesions (318,340). Balloon sizing can be difficult in patients who have medial fibroplasia and in whom multiple aneurysms may be present or the entire length of the vessel is involved with dysplastic changes. Choosing a balloon size based on an aneurysmal segment can lead to vessel rupture, so it is best to start with a conservative balloon size and redilate with a larger diameter balloon as needed.

Patients with multiple lesions, branch vessel stenoses or intimal fibroplasia lesions require careful planning before an intervention (322,343,344). Branch vessel stenoses occur in 25–39% of cases, so a detailed diagnostic evaluation must be performed preintervention. Technical success can be expected in 84% of branch vessel lesions; however, meticulous technique, judicious use of anticoagulation and vasodilators, as well as experience, are needed to avoid the complications of branch vessel spasm, dissection, or occlusion (345,346) (Figure 21–21). In some cases, the use of "kissing" balloons to treat bifurcation lesions optimally, while protecting the affected branches, is required. PTRA is the treatment of choice for most patients with FMD and hypertension. With appropriate patient selection and technical expertise, the clinical outcomes should be excellent.

Renal Allografts

Stenoses in transplant renal arteries (TRAS) can cause hypertension or deterioration in allograft function and have been reported in as many as 23% of transplant recipients (347–349). The apparent high prevalence of TRAS may result from two factors: (1) an increased rate of detection because of the use of MRA to screen patients and (2) new immunosuppressive agents that may be associated with vascular injury, which increases the incidence of TRAS (349). The causes of TRAS differ according to the location of the stenosis: preanastomotic (atherosclerosis, vessel clamp injury), anastomotic (technical, perfusion injury, reaction to suture material, intimal hyperplasia), postanastomotic (intimal hyperplasia, immunologic, turbulent flow, kinking, twisting, or compression), or more distal (rejection).

Eighty percent of renal transplant recipients have hypertension 6 months after transplantation (351). The etiology of hypertension in this population is multifactorial and includes essential hypertension, renin secretion by the

TABLE 21-5
RESULTS OF PTRA ON HYPERTENSION IN FIBROMUSCULAR DYSPLASIA

Series	# of Patients	Technical Success*	Long-Term Patency**		Clinical Results**			Follow-up (mo)***	
			1°	2°	Cure	Improvement	Benefit	Mean	Range
Surowiec (319)	14	13/14 93%	87%	5/14 36%	6/14 43%	11/14 79%		96	8–84
Kumar (320)	20	19/20 95%	18/20 90%		10/20 50%	7/20 35%	17/20 85%	50	1–204
de Fraissinette (321)	70	66/70 95%	58/66 88%		9/66 14%	49/66 74%	58/66 88%	39	
Birrer (322)	27	27/27a 100%	25/31 81%	26/27 96%	21/47b 23%		20/27 74%	10	6–14
Lovaria (323)	69	72/88c 82%	58/69 84%		7/28b 25%	11/47 23%	32/47 68%	6	
Klow (324)	49	48/49 98%	32/48 67%	45/48 93%	4/13 31%	12/28 43%	19/28 68%	11	0–108
Baumgartner (325)	13		11/15c 73%	13/15c 87%	5/11b 45%	7/13 54%	11/13 85%	11	
Von Knorring (326)	12	12/12 103%				6/11 55%	11/11 100%	48	
Jensen (327)	30	29/30 97%	28/29 97%		11/29 38%	13/29 45%	24/29 83%	12	
Bonelli (328)	105	93/105 89%			22%	63%	85%	43	
Rodriguez-Perez (329)	27	25/27 92%	19/25 76%	19/25 75%	6/12b 50%	3/12 25%	9/12 75%		3–96
Tegtmeyer (318)	66	66/66 100%	60/66 91%	65/66 98%	26/66 39%	39/66 59%	65/66 98%	39	1–121
Baert (330)	22	19/22 86%	15/19 79%		11/19 58%	4/19 21%	15/19 79%	26	6–72
Greminger (331)	34	30/34 88%	23/30 77%	30/30 100%	14/30 47%	16/30 53%	30/30 100%	20	6–48
Klinge (332)	52	47/52 90%		42/47 89%	18/47 38%	26/47 55%	44/47 94%	6	
Beebe (333)	9	9/9 100%	4/9 44%	8/9 89%	3/9 33%	5/9 55%	8/9 88%	23	6–60
Simmonetti (334)	25				15/25 60%	6/25 24%	21/25 84%	48	
Bell (335)	8	7/8 88%	7/7 100%		5/7 71%	2/7 29%	7/7 100%	19	12–48
Kremer Hovingaa (336)	10	10/10 100%	7/9 77%	6/6 100%				19	4–45
Grim (337)	26	26/26 100%	24/26 92%		15/26 58%	9/26 35%	24/26 92%	26	1–60
L.G. Martin (338)	20	20/20 100%	17/20 85%		5/20 25%	12/20 60%	17/20 85%	16	3–39
Miller (339)	15	15/15 100%	13/13b 100%		11/13b 85%	2/13 15%	13/13 100%		6–36
Sos (340)	31	27/31 87%	25/27 93%		16/27 59%	9/27 33%	25/27 93%	16	4–40
Mahler (341)	6	6/6 100%	4/6 66%		5/6 83%	1/6 17%	6/6 100%	29	12–47
Colapinto (342)	11	9/11 82%	9/9 100%		4/9b 44%	5/9 55%	9/9 100%	11	1–36
Martin (343)	8	8/8 100%	6/8 75%		5/8 63%	1/8 13%	6/8 75%	13	4–25
Totals	779	654/697 94%	463/552 84%	241/258 93%	231/552 42%	248/552 45%	482/579 83%	27	1–204

* Results converted to patients rather than vessels treated where possible
** Initial technical failures excluded
*** Clinical and/or vascular imaging follow-up
a Includes a PTRA rescued with stent placement
b Some patients not having follow-up
c Lesions rather than patients

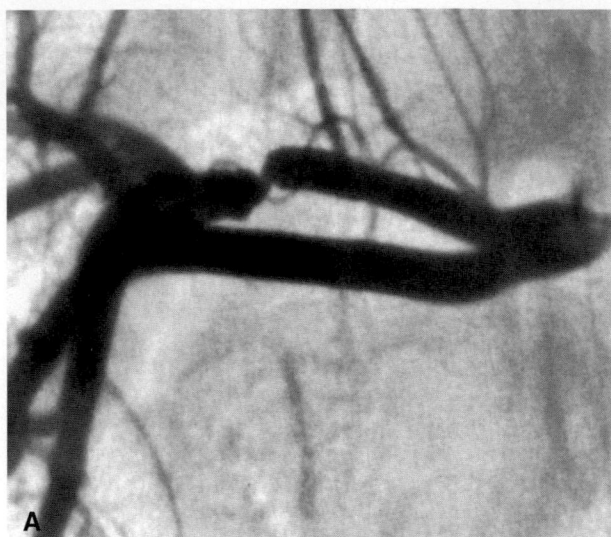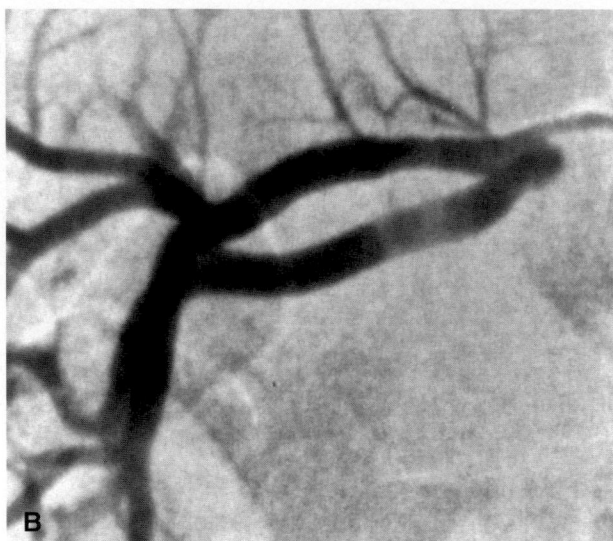

Figure 21–21   A 27-year-old female presents with a 4-year history of worsening hypertension. **A.** Selective right renal angiogram reveals a segmental branch stenosis of the right renal artery (the lesion is characteristic of FMD, although not the classic medial fibroplasias). **B.** Follow-up angiogram 27 months after PTRA reveals a widely patent right renal artery at the angioplasty site. Mild spasm of the proximal segmental renal arteries resulting from catheter manipulation was identified. The patient remains normotensive off all medications.

native kidneys, transplant rejection, cyclosporine-induced hypercalcemia, steroids, progression of the underlying disease, and TRAS (352). Therefore, once TRAS is detected, determining the physiologic significance of the lesion may be difficult. Similarly, renal insufficiency is most often the result of rejection, obstruction, infection, or progression of the underlying disease, rather than ischemia resulting from TRAS. However, it is clear that TRAS can be responsible for physiologic effects.

Three types of therapy are available for management of TRAS: medical, surgical, and PTRA/RAST. Hypertension usually can be controlled medically, but drug intolerance and progressive renal failure may occur. Surgical correction of TRAS is successful in approximately 92% of cases (353). However, the extensive fibrosis that ensues after renal allograft surgery makes reoperation on these vessels difficult. In addition, surgical repair requires a transabdominal approach, and there is a high risk of significant injury to the allograft. The third treatment option is endovascular therapy. A review of the literature reveals that in patients with TRAS treated with PTRA, RAST, or both, 63–100% of the procedures were technically successful (Table 21–6) (323,324,347,353–372). Blood pressure control improved in 58 to 100% (mean of 80%), and transplant renal function stabilized or improved in 38 to 100% (mean of 87%). PTRA/RAST has become the first choice of therapy for TRAS, except for cases in which lesions are caused by kinking, twisting, or poor surgical anastamoses.

Renal transplant angiography can be performed using CO_2 and small amounts of Gd or iodinated contrast (373,374). For transplants placed with an end-to-side anastomosis, an ipsilateral retrograde femoral access is usually the best approach (Figure 21–22). For an end-to-end anastomosis to the internal iliac artery, an "up-and-over" approach from the contralateral femoral artery is preferred. A screening MRA before intervention provides information on the course of the transplant renal artery, the patency of the iliac arteries, and the views that will best demonstrate the lesion during angiography. Intra-arterial pressure measurements can be obtained in cases of equivocal lesions, although the translesion pressure gradient that is considered significant is not standardized. As in native renal artery angioplasty, anticoagulation and the administration of intra-arterial vasodilators should be routine. PTRA and stenting are appropriate for treating iliac artery lesions proximal to the transplant anastomosis. Stents are indicated in TRAS lesions that do not respond to PTRA alone or in recurrent TRAS after a previous PTRA (374,375).

Takayasu's Arteritis

Takayasu's arteritis is an uncommon chronic inflammatory disease that most often affects the thoracic aorta and brachiocephalic arteries but can also affect the pulmonary arteries, abdominal aorta, and the renal arteries. When the renal arteries are affected, the disease is often bilateral, and 70% of the patients will have angiographic findings of aortic involvement.

TABLE 21–6
RESULTS OF PTRA AND/OR STENTING IN RENAL ALLOGRAFTS

Series	# of Patients	Technical Success		Blood Pressure Improved		Allograft Function Stable or Improved		Follow-up (mo) Mean	Range
Patel (347)	17	16/17	94%	13/14	93%			27	
Tang (354)	22	21/22	95%					73	13–110
Lovaria (323)	15	14/15	93%	7/8	87%			6	
Rundback (355)	23	18/23	78%	18/18	100%	15/18	83%	6	
Klow (324)	74	62/74	84%		70%		38%		
Sankan (356)	16	12/16	75%	7/12	58%	11/12	92%	45	
Lo (357)	14	13/14	93%	8/12	67%			24	3–42
Rodriguez-Perez (329)	28	21/28	75%	14/16	88%			12	
Thomas (358)	15	14/15	93%	10/11	91%	10/11	91%	34	12–74
Fauchal (359)	25	22/25	88%	10/16	63%	14/21	67%	24	6–78
Bover (360)	27	25/27	93%	19/25	76%			6	
Matalon (361)	18	16/18*	89%	11/18	61%	16/18	89%	12	2–32
Benoit (353)	49	34/49	69%	26/34	76%			32	1–110
Kirst (362)	32	25/32	78%	25/32	78%				
De Meyer (363)	17	14/17	82%	8/11	73%	13/14	93%	12	
Aliabadi (364)	7	7/7	100%	5/7	72%	6/7	86%	30	12–96
Greenstein (365)	39	33/39	85%	25/30	83%			30	1–72
Raynaud (366)	43	35/43	81%	23/35	66%	33/35	94%	12	
Lohr (367)	4	4/4	100%	4/4	100%	4/4	100%	15	6–23
Curry (368)	8	5/8	63%	3/5	60%	3/5	60%		
Tegtmeyer (369)	7	6/7	86%	5/6	83%			24	5–51
Gerlock (370)	7	7/7	100%	7/7	100%	7/7	100%	7	3–12
Sniderman (371)	12	10/12	83%	10/11	91%			9	1–15
Totals	519	434/519	84%	269/332	84%	132/152	87%	21	—

* Includes two patients requiring two attempts at PTRA resulting in initial success

Clinically, there is an early disease phase characterized by arthralgias, fevers, night sweats, chest or abdominal pain, and rashes. In the late phase, or pulseless phase, symptoms resulting from vascular occlusions develop. The early phase usually is managed medically with steroids and other immunosuppressive medications. The later phase often is managed with revascularization when symptoms are present. Hypertension and renal failure can develop in patients with Takayasu's arteritis secondary to renal artery occlusive disease. If the erythrocyte sedimentation rate (ESR) is elevated, use of steroids may be helpful to suppress the active inflammatory process. However, the ESR is not a sensitive indicator of disease activity. In most cases, when percutaneous therapy is undertaken and the lesion can be crossed with a guide wire, technical success can be achieved. Technical success rates with PTA and stenting approach 95% (376–384). Even in cases of complete occlusion (Figure 21–23), angioplasty can be successful and provide dramatic relief of symptoms (381). Technical failures because of lesion recoil or early restenosis can be treated with stents, particularly in large vessels (376). Long-term follow-up reveals a restenosis rate of 16% (384). Surgical bypass can also be performed with a high technical success rate. Late complications after surgery are rare, but they may include anastomotic stenoses or aneurysms (385).

Neurofibromatosis

Hypertension in patients with neurofibromatosis (NF) may result from coarctation of the aorta, pheochromocytoma, or RAS. In older patients, the hypertension associated with NF is often secondary to a pheochromocytoma. In younger patients, it is usually a result of RAS.

The abdominal aorta and renal arteries are the most common sites of arterial compromise in NF (386). The vascular involvement in NF can be divided into two groups: large vessel involvement, which is most often due to ganglioneuromatous tissue surrounding the aorta and renal arteries, and small vessel involvement, with mesodermal dysplasia of the vessel wall.

Success with PTRA in the treatment of RAS in patients with NF was first reported in 1981 (387). Subsequently, mixed results have been reported in very small series (344,387–390). In general, RAS seen in patients with NF appear to be very fibrous and often require the use of high-pressure, noncompliant balloons (Figure 21–24). Use of a cutting balloon (Boston Scientific) may also be considered. Overall, experience with PTRA in patients with NF is limited. However, small case series and anecdotal reports have demonstrated that endovascular therapy can sometimes provide an alternative to surgery (391).

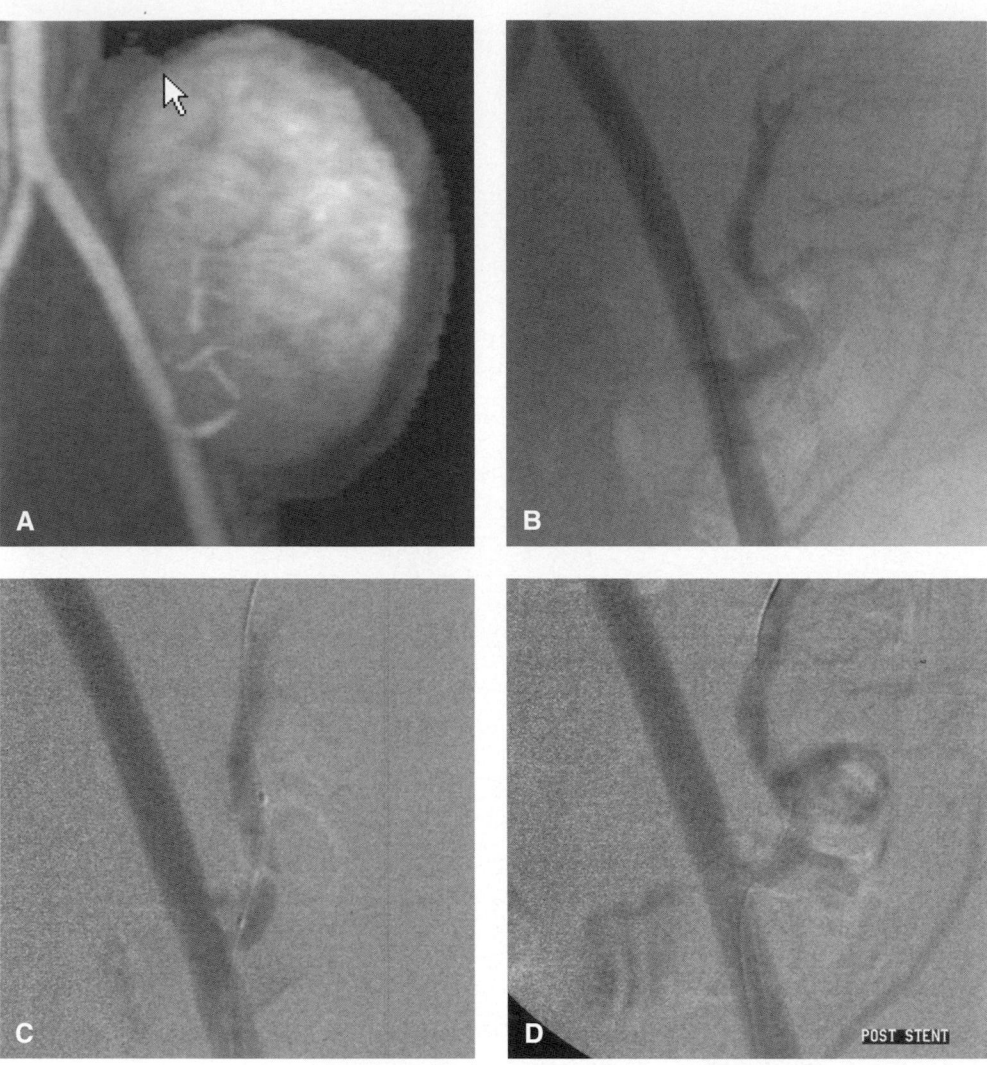

Figure 21–22 **A.** End-to-side anastomosis of a renal allograft artery to the external iliac artery as seen on Gd-enhanced MRA demonstrates a midrenal artery stenosis. **B.** Angiogram performed with Gd confirms the RAS. **C.** Stent is placed from an ipsilateral approach. **D.** Poststent angiogram demonstrates a good angiographic result. Kidney function is stabilized and blood pressure control improved.

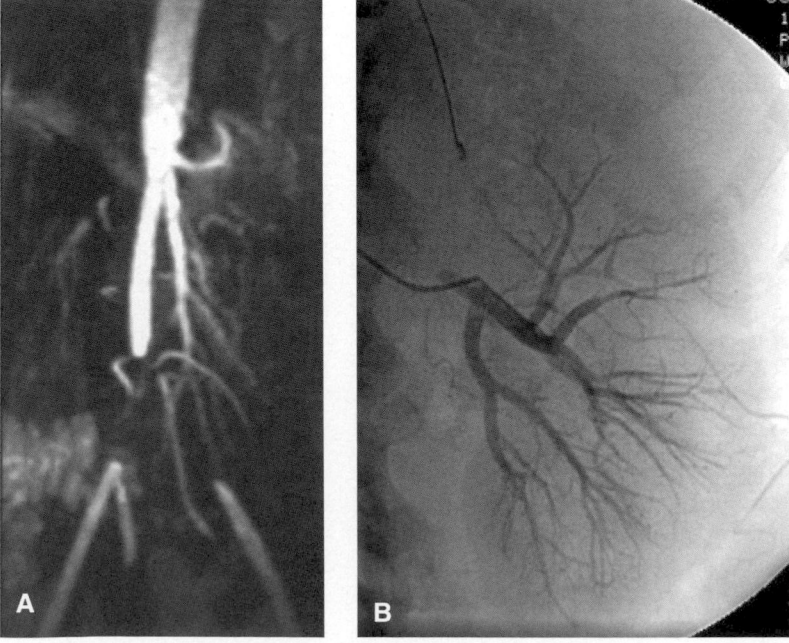

Figure 21–23 A 22-year-old female presents with the recent onset of acute renal failure. **A.** MRA demonstrates occlusions of renal and common iliac arteries. **B.** The left renal artery occlusion was crossed.

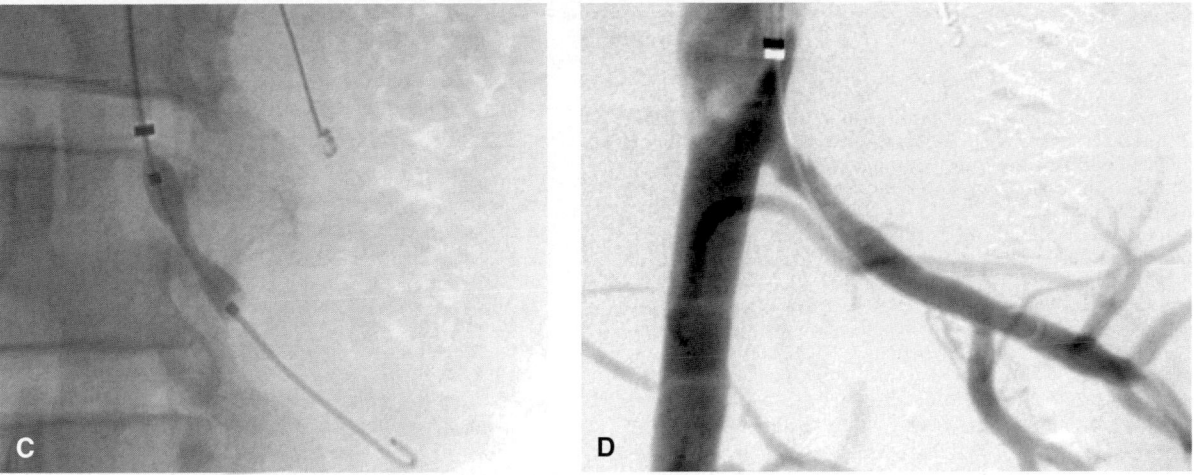

Figure 21–23 *(Continued)* **C.** The lesion balloon is dilated. **D.** Post-PTRA, no residual stenosis is seen. The right lesion could not be crossed. The patient's renal function returned and remained normal at 10 months follow-up. (Reprinted with permission from Savage BJ, Gupta RK, Angle JF. Okusa MD. Takayasu arteritis presenting as a pulmonary-renal syndrome. Am J Med Sci 2003;5:275–281.)

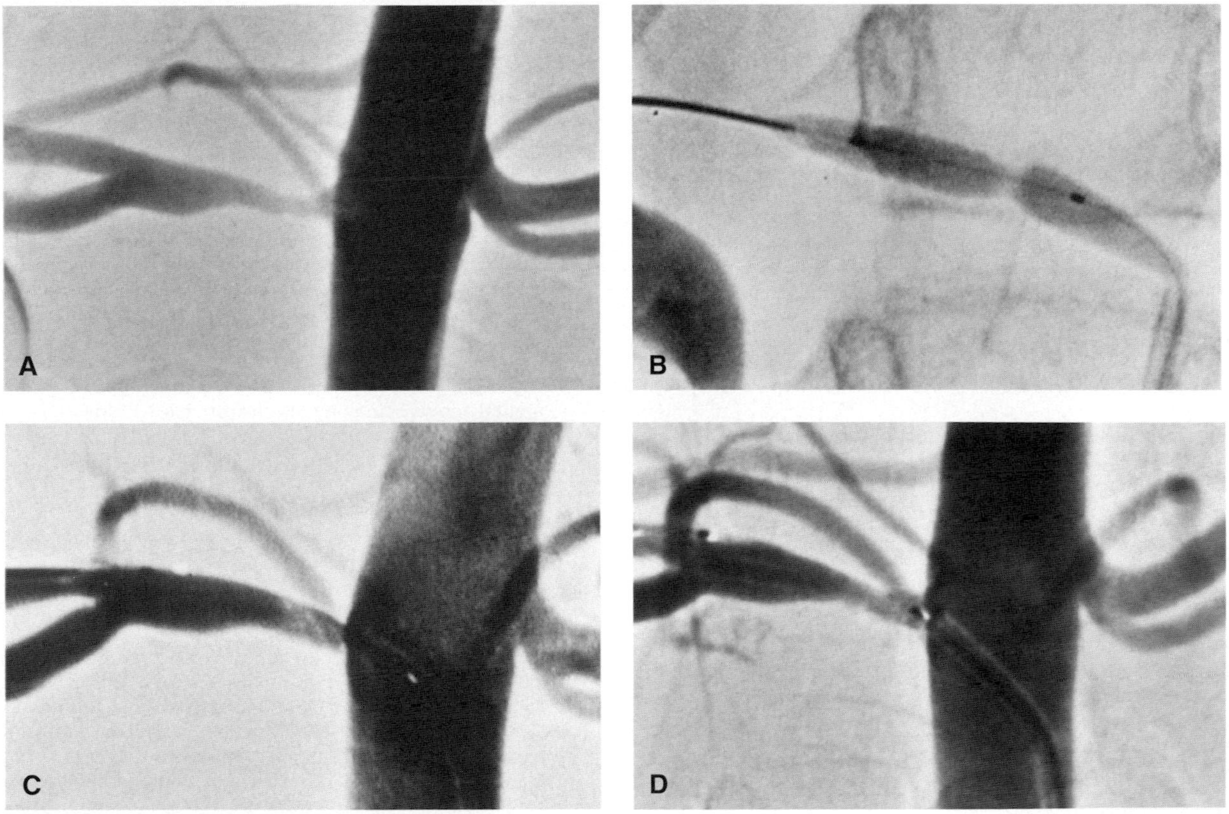

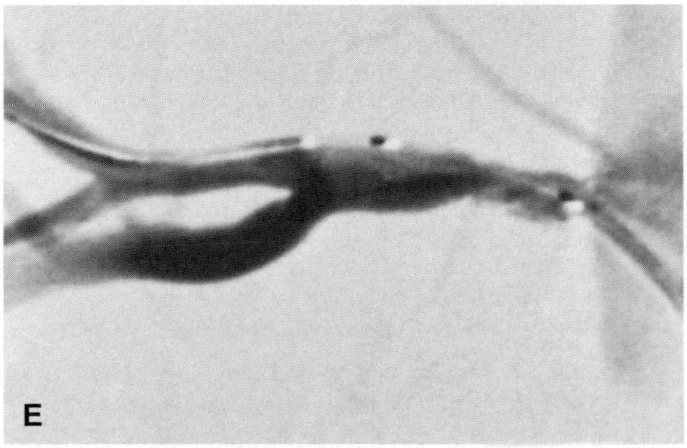

Figure 21–24 Results of PTRA in a 9-year-old child with NF. **A.** The entire proximal segment of the right renal artery is narrowed. **B.** The inflated balloon has a persistent waist, despite the use of high-pressure inflation. **C.** Post-PTRA image demonstrates modest improvement. **D.** 15-month follow-up angiogram reveals improvement in the proximal portion of the lesion and some narrowing distally. **E.** Following redilatation, the vessel caliber is improved, but a residual stenosis remains. The patient was normotensive 50 months after the original procedure.

REFERENCES

1. Burt VL, Cutler JA, Higgins M, et al. Trends in the prevalence, awareness, treatment, and control of hypertension in the adult US population. Data from the health examination surveys, 1960 to 1991. Hypertension 1995;26:60–69.
2. The Sixth Report of the Joint National Committee on prevention, detection, evaluation, and treatment of high blood pressure. Arch Intern Med 1997;2413–2446.
3. Gifford RW Jr. Evaluation of the hypertensive patient with emphasis on detecting curable causes. Milbank Mem Fund Q 1969;47:170–186.
4. Anderson GH Jr, Blakeman N, Streeten DH. The effect of age on prevalence of secondary forms of hypertension in 4,429 consecutively referred patients. Am J Hypertens 1994;12:609–615.
5. Rihal CS, Textor SC, Breen JF, et al. Incidental renal artery stenosis among a prospective cohort of hypertensive patients undergoing coronary angiography. Mayo Clin Proc 2002;77:309–316.
6. Valentine RJ, Clagett P, Miller GL, et al. The coronary risk of unsuspected renal artery stenosis. J Vasc Surg 1993;18:433–440.
7. Isles C, Main J, O'Connell J, et al. Survival associated with renal vascular disease in Glasgow and New Castle: a collaborative study. Scott Med J 1990;35:70–73.
8. Losito A, Faguguli RM, Zampi I, et al. Comparison of target organ damage and renal vascular essential hypertension. Am J Hypertens 1996;9:1062–1067.
9. Meissner MD, Wilson AR, Jessup M. Renal artery stenosis and heart failure. Am J Cardiol 1988;62:1307–1308.
10. Chabova V, Schirger A, Stanson AW, et al. Outcomes of atherosclerotic renal artery stenosis managed without revascularization. Mayo Clin Proc 2000;75:437–444.
11. Dorros G, Jaff M, Mathiak L, et al. Four-year follow-up of Palmaz-Schatz stent revascularization as treatment for atherosclerotic renal artery stenosis. Circulation 1998;98:642–647.
12. Conlon PJ, Athirakul K, Kovalik E, et al. Survival in renal vascular disease. J Am Soc Nephrol 1998;9:252–256.
13. Khosla S, White CJ, Collins DJ, et al. The effects of renal artery stent implantation in patients with renovascular hypertension presenting with unstable angina or congestive heart failure. Am J Cardiol 1997;80:363–366.
14. Bloch MJ, Trost DW, Pickering TG, et al. Prevention of recurrent pulmonary edema in patients with bilateral renal vascular disease through renal artery stent placement. Am J Hypertens 1999;12:1–7.
15. Winker MA. The emerging epidemic of atherosclerosis. JAMA 1999;281:84–85.
16. Dzau VJ. Tissue angiotensin and pathology of vascular disease: a unifying hypothesis. Hypertension 2001;37:1047–1052.
17. Higashi Y, Sasaki S, Nakagawa K, et al. Endothelial function and oxidative stress in renal vascular hypertension. N Engl J Med 2002;36:1954–62.
18. Meyier A. [Vascular mechanisms of renal fibrosis. Vasculonephropathies and arterial hypertension.] Bull Acad Natl Med 1999;183:33–45.
19. Yusuf S, Sleight P, Pogue J, et al. Effects of an angiotensin-converting-enzyme inhibitor, ramipril, on cardiovascular events in high-risk patients. The Heart Outcomes Prevention Evaluation Study Investigators. N Engl J Med 2000;342:145–153.
20. Lerman LO, Nath KA, Rodriguez-Porcel MG, et al. Increased oxidative stress in experimental renal vascular hypertension. Hypertension 2001;37:541–546.
21. Johansson M, Herlitz H, Jensen G, et al. Increased cardiovascular mortality in hypertensive patients with renal artery stenosis. Relation to sympathetic activation, renal function and treatment regimens. Am J Hypertens 1999;17:1743–1750.
22. Romero JC, Feldstein AE, Rodriguez-Porcel MG, et al. New insights into the pathophysiology of renal vascular hypertension. Mayo Clin Proc 1997;72:251–260.
23. Conlon J, O'Riordan E, Kalra PA. New insights into the epidemiologic in clinical management stations of atherosclerotic renal vascular disease. Am J Kidney Dis 2000;35:573–587.
24. Mailloux LU. Atherosclerotic ischemic renal vascular disease: do published outcomes justify the over-zealous diagnostic approaches? Semin Nephrol 2003;23:278–282.
25. Holley KE, Hunt JC, Brown AI. Renal artery stenosis: a clinical-pathological study in normotensive and hypertensive patients. Am J Med 1964;37:14–22.
26. Schwartz CJ, White TA. Stenosis of the renal artery: an unselected necropsy study. Br Med J 1964;2:1415–1421.
27. Missouris CG, Buckenham T, Cappuccio FP, et al. Renal artery stenosis: a common important problem in patients with peripheral vascular disease. Am J Med 1994;96:10–14.
28. Valentine RJ, Clagett GP, Miller GL, et al. The coronary risk of unsuspected renal artery stenosis. J Vasc Surg 1993;18:433–439.
29. Swartbol P, Thorvinger BO, Parsson H, et al. Renal artery stenosis in patients with peripheral vascular disease and its correlation to hypertension: a retrospective study. Int Angiol 1992;11:195–199.
30. Olin JW, Melia M, Young JR, et al. Prevalence of atherosclerotic renal artery stenosis in patients with atherosclerosis elsewhere. Am J Med 1990;88:46N–51N.
31. Choudhri AH, Cleland JG, Rowlands PC, et al. Unsuspected renal artery stenosis in peripheral vascular disease. Br Med J 1990;301:1197–1198.
32. Wachtell K, Ibsen H, Olsen H, et al. Prevalence of renal artery stenosis in patients with peripheral vascular disease and hypertension. J Hum Hypertens 1996;10:83–85.
33. Rihal CS, Textor SC, Breen JF, et al. Incidental renal artery stenosis among a prospective cohort of hypertensive patients undergoing coronary angiography. Mayo Clin Proc 2002;77:309–316.
34. Williamson WK, Abou-Zamzam AM, Monet GL, et al. Prophylactic repair of renal artery stenosis is not just a fight in patients who require infrarenal aortic reconstructions. J Vasc Surg 1998;28:14–22.
35. Caps MT, Perissinotto C, Zierler RE, et al. Prospective study of atherosclerotic disease progression in the renal artery. Circulation 1998;98:2866–2872.
36. van Jaarsveld BC, Krijnen P, Pieteran H, et al. The effect of balloon angioplasty on hypertension and atherosclerotic renal artery stenosis. Dutch Renal Artery Stenosis Intervention Cooperative Study Group. N Engl J Med 2000;342:1007–1014.
37. Zierler RE, Bergelin RO, Davidson RC, et al. A prospective study of disease progressive in patients with atherosclerotic renal artery stenosis. Am J Hypertens 1996;9:1055–61.
38. Vanvelzer DA. Atherosclerotic narrowing of renal arteries associated with hypertension. AJR Am J Roentgenol 1961;86:806–818.
39. Detection, evaluation, and treatment of renovascular hypertension: final report. Working Group on Renovascular Hypertension. Arch Intern Med 1987;147:820–829.
40. Nabel EG, Gibbons GH, Dzau VJ. Pathophysiology of an experimental renovascular hypertension. Am J Kidney Dis 1985;5:A111–A119.
41. Schreiber MJ Jr, Pohl MA, Novick AC. Preserving renal function by revascularization. Ann Rev Med 1990;41:423–429.
42. Dean RH, Kieffer RW, Smith BM, et al. Renovascular hypertension: anatomic and renal function changes during drug therapy. Arch Surg 1981;116:1408–1415.
43. de Leeuw PW. Renal function in the elderly: results from the European Working Party on high blood pressure in the elderly trial. Am J Med 1991;90(3a):45S–49S.
44. Rimmer JM, Gennari FJ. Atherosclerotic renovascular disease and progressive renal failure. Ann Int Med 1993;118:712–719.
45. La Batide-Alanore A, Azizi M, Froissart M, et al. Split renal function outcome after renal angioplasty in patients with unilateral renal artery stenosis. J Am Soc Nephrol 2001;12:1235–1241.
46. Mann SJ, Pickering TG. Detection of renovascular hypertension. State-of-the-art. Ann Intern Med 1992;117:845–853.
47. Albers FJ. Clinical characteristics of atherosclerotic renovascular disease. Am J Kidney Dis 1994;24:636–641.
48. Fergany A. Ischemic nephropathy: epidemiology and clinical implications. Urol Clin North Am 2001;28:805–813.
49. O'Neill EA, Hansen KJ, Canzanello VJ, et al. Prevalence of ischemic nephropathy in patients with renal insufficiency. Am Surg 1992;58:485–490.
50. Lederman RJ, Mendelsohn FO, Santos R, et al. Primary renal artery stenting: characteristics and outcomes after 363 procedures. Am Heart J 2001;142:314–323.
51. Textor SC. Renovascular hypertension. Endocrinol Metab Clin North Am 1994;33:227–234.
52. Wilcox CS. Ischemic nephropathy: noninvasive testing. Semin Nephrol 1996;16:43–52.
53. Khauli RB. Defining the role of renal angiography in the diagnosis of renal artery disease. Am J Kidney Dis 1994;24:679–684.

54. Mann SJ, Pickering TG. Detection of renovascular hypenension. Ann Intern Med 1992;117:845–853.
55. Canzanello VJ, Textor SC. Noninvasive diagnosis of renovascular disease. Mayo Clin Proc 1994;69:1172–1181.
56. Vasbinder GBC, Nelemans PJ, Kessels AG, et al. Diagnostic tests for renal artery stenosis in patients suspected of having renovascular hypertension: a meta-analysis. Ann Intern Med 2001;135(6): 401–11.
57. Geyskes GG, de Bruyn AJ. Captopril renography and the effect of percutaneous transluminal angioplasty on blood pressure in 94 patients with renal artery stenosis. Am J Hypertens 1991;4(12 Pt 2):685S–689S.
58. Dondi M, Monetti N, Fanti S, et al. Use of technetium-99m-MAG3 for renal scintigraphy after angiotensin-converting enzyme inhibition. J Nucl Med 1999;32(3):424–428.
59. van Jaarsveld BC, Krijnen P, Derkx FH, et al. The place of renal scintigraphy in the diagnosis of renal artery stenosis. Fifteen years of clinical experience. Arch Intern Med 1997;157(11):1226–1234.
60. Fernandez P, Morel D, Jeandot R, et al. Value of captopril renal scintigraphy in hypertensive patients with renal failure. J Nucl Med 1999;40(3):412–417.
61. Taylor A, Nally J, Aurell M, et al. Consensus report on ACE inhibitor renography for detecting renovascular hypertension. Radionuclides in Nephrourology Group. Consensus Group on ACEI Renography. J Nucl Med 1996;37(11):1876–1882.
62. Taylor AT, Fletcher JW, Nally JV, et al. Procedure guidelines for diagnosis of renovascular hypertension. J Nucl Med 1998;39: 1297–1302.
63. Bourgoignie JJ, Rubbert K, Sfakianakis GN. Angiotensin-converting enzyme-inhibited renography for the diagnosis of ischemic kidneys. Am J Kidney Dis 1994;24:665–673.
64. Mann SJ, Pickering TG, Sos TA, et al. Captopril renography in the diagnosis of renal artery stenosis: accuracy and limitations. Am J Med 1991;90:30–40.
65. Working Group on Renovascular Hypertension. Final report of the Working Group on Renovascular Hypertension. Arch Intern Med 1987;147:820.
66. Claveau-Tremblay R, Turpin S, De Braekeleer M, et al. False–positive captopril renography in patients taking calcium antagonists. J Nucl Med 1998;39(9):1621–1626.
67. Strandness ED Jr. Duplex imaging for the detection of renal artery stenosis. Am J Kidney Dis 1994;24:674–678.
68. Hoffmann U, Edwards JM, Carter S, et al. Role of duplex scanning for the detection of atherosclerotic renal artery disease. Kidney Int 1991;39:1232–1239.
69. House MK, Dowling RJ, King P, et al. Using Doppler sonography to reveal renal artery stenosis: an evaluation of optimal imaging parameters. AJR Am J Roentgenol 1999;173:761–765.
70. Olin JW, Piedmonte MR, Young JR, et al. The utility of duplex ultrasound of the renal arteries for diagnosing significant renal artery stenosis. Ann Intern Med 1995;122:833–838.
71. Schwerk WB, Restrepo IK, Stellwaag M, et al. Renal artery stenosis: grading with image-directed Doppler US evaluation of renal resistive index. Radiology 1994;190:785–790.
72. Leung DA, Hoffmann U, Pfammatter T, et al. Magnetic resonance angiography versus duplex sonography for diagnosing renovascular disease. Hypertension 1999;33:726–731.
73. Berland LL, Koslin DB, Routh WD, et al. Renal artery stenosis: prospective evaluation of diagnosis with color duplex US compared with angiography. Work in progress. Radiology 1990;174: 421–423.
74. Desberg AL, Paushter DM, Lammert GK, et al. Renal artery stenosis: evaluation with color Doppler flow imaging. Radiology 1990;177:749–753.
75. Riehl J, Schmitt H, Bongartz D, et al. Renal artery stenosis: evaluation with colour duplex ultrasonography. Nephrol Dial Transplant 1997;12:1608–1614.
76. Taylor DC, Kettler MD, Monet GL. Duplex ultrasound scanning in the diagnosis of renal artery stenosis: a prospective evaluation. J Vasc Surg 1986;7:363–369.
77. Radermacher J, Chavan A, Bleck J, et al. Use of Doppler ultrasonography to predict the outcome of therapy for renal-artery stenosis. N Engl J Med 2001;344:410–417.
78. Zeller T, Müller C, Frank U, et al. Stent angioplasty of severe atherosclerotic ostial renal artery stenosis in patients with diabetes mellitus and nephrosclerosis. Catheter Cardiovasc Interv 2003;58:510–515.
79. Sharafuddin MJ, Raboi CA, Abu-Yousef M, et al. Renal artery stenosis: duplex US after angioplasty and stent placement. Radiology 2001;220:168–173.
80. Beregi JP, Mounier-Vehier C, Devos P, et al. Doppler flow wire evaluation of renal blood flow reserve in hypertensive patients with normal renal arteries. Cardiovasc Intervent Radiol 2000; 23:340–346.
81. Lencioni R, Pinto S, Cioni D, et al. Contrast-enhanced Doppler ultrasound of renal artery stenosis: prologue to a promising future. Echocardiography 1999;16:767–773.
82. Zeman RK, Silverman PM, Vieco PT, et al. CT angiography. AJR Am J Roentgenol 1995;165:1079–1088.
83. Rubin GD, Walker PJ, Dake MD, et al. Three-dimensional spiral computed tomographic angiography: an alternative imaging modality for the abdominal aorta and its branches. J Vasc Surg 1993;18:656–665.
84. Galanski M, Prokop M, Chavan A, et al. Renal arterial stenoses: spiral CT angiography. Radiology 1993;189:185–192.
85. Olbricht CJ, Galanski M, Chavan A, et al. Spiral CT angiography—can we forget about arteriography to diagnose renal artery stenosis? Nephrol Dial Transplant 1996;11(7):1227–1231.
86. Beregi JP, Louvegny S, Ceugnart L, et al. [Helical x-ray computed tomography of renal arteries. Apropos of 300 patients.] J Radiol 1997;78(8):549–556.
87. Berg MH, Manninen HI, Vanninen RL, et al. Assessment of renal artery stenosis with CT angiography: usefulness of multiplanar reformation, quantitative stenosis measurements, and densitometric analysis of renal parenchymal enhancement as adjuncts to MIP film reading. J Comput Assist Tomogr 1998;22(4):533–540.
88. Brink JA, Lim JT, Wang G, et al. Technical optimization of spiral CT for depiction of renal artery stenosis: in vitro analysis. Radiology 1995;194(1):157–163.
89. Van Hoe L, Vandermeulen D, Gryspeerdt S, et al. Assessment of accuracy of renal artery stenosis grading in helical CT angiography using maximum intensity projections. Eur Radiol 1996;6(5): 658–664.
90. Johnson PT, Halpern EJ, Kuszyk BS, et al. Renal artery stenosis: CT angiography—comparison of real-time volume-rendering and maximum intensity projection algorithms. Radiology 1999;211(2): 337–343.
91. Lufft V, Hoogestraat-Lufft L, Fels LM, et al. Contrast media nephropathy: intravenous CT angiography versus intra-arterial digital subtraction angiography in renal artery stenosis: a prospective randomized trial. Am J Kidney Dis 2000;40(2):236–242.
92. Halpern EJ, Rutter CM, Gardiner GA Jr, et al. Comparison of Doppler US and CT angiography for evaluation of renal artery stenosis. Acad Radiol 1998;5(8):524–532.
93. Elkohen M, Beregi JP, Deklunder G, et al. A prospective study of helical computed tomography angiography versus angiography for the detection of renal artery stenoses in hypertensive patients. J Hypertens 1996;14(4):525–528.
94. Farres MT, Lammer J, Schima W, et al. Spiral computed tomographic angiography of the renal arteries: a prospective comparison with intravenous and intra-arterial digital subtraction angiography. Cardiovasc Intervent Radiol 1996;19(2):101–106.
95. Beregi JP, Elkohen M, Deklunder G, et al. Helical CT angiography compared with arteriography in the detection of renal artery stenosis. AJR Am J Roentgenol 1996;167(2):495–501.
96. Cikrit DF, Harris VJ, Hemmer CG, et al. Comparison of spiral CT scan and arteriography for evaluation of renal and visceral arteries. Ann Vasc Surg 1996;10(2):109–116.
97. Olbricht CJ, Paul K, Prokop M, et al. Minimally invasive diagnosis of renal artery stenosis by spiral computed tomography angiography. Kidney Int 1995;48(4):1332–1337.
98. Elkohen M, Beregi JP, Deklunder G, et al. Evaluation of spiral computed tomography of the renal arteries alone or combined with Doppler ultrasonography in the detection of renal artery stenosis. Prospective study of 114 renal arteries. Arch Mal Coeur Vaiss 1995;88(8):1159–1164.
99. Kaatee R, Beek FJ, de Lange EE, et al. Renal artery stenosis: detection and quantification with spiral CT angiography versus optimized digital subtraction angiography. Radiology 1997; 205(1):121–127.
100. Rubin GD, Napel S. Helical CT angiography of renal artery stenosis. AJR Am J Roentgenol 1997;168(4):1109 1111.

101. Kim TS, Chung JW, Park JH, et al. Renal artery evaluation: comparison of spiral CT angiography to intra-arterial DSA. J Vasc Interv Radiol 1998;9(4):553–559.

102. Wittenberg G, Kenn W, Tschammler A, et al. Spiral CT angiography of renal arteries: comparison with angiography. Eur Radiol 1999;9(3):546–551.

103. Van Hoe L, Gryspeerdt S. Helical CT angiography of renal artery stenosis. AJR Am J Roentgenol 1997;168(5):1380–1381.

104. Rubin GD, Dake MD, Napel S, et al. Spiral CT of renal artery stenosis: comparison of three-dimensional rendering techniques. Radiology 1994;190:181–189.

105. Arlart IP, Guhl L, Hausmann R. [The evaluation of 2D- and 3D-"time of flight" magnetic resonance angiography (MRA) in the diagnosis of renal artery stenoses.] Rofo 1992;157(1):59–64.

106. Lewin JS. Time-of-flight magnetic resonance angiography of the aorta and renal arteries. Invest Radiol 1992;27(Suppl II):S84–S89.

107. Yucel EK, Kaufman JA, Prince M, et al. Time of flight renal MR angiography: utility in patients with renal insufficiency. J Magn Reson Imaging 1993;11(7):925–930.

108. Duda SH, Schick F, Teufl F, et al. Phase-contrast MR angiography for detection of arteriosclerotic renal artery stenosis. Acta Radiol 1997;38(2):287–291.

109. Miller S, Hahn U, Schick F, et al. [Diagnosis of renal artery stenosis in 1.0 T using 3D phase contrast magnetic resonance angiography and dynamic contrast medium perfusion]. Rofo 1999;170(2):163–167.

110. Kim D, Edelman RR, Rent KC, et al. Abdominal aorta and renal artery stenosis: evaluation with MR angiography. Radiology 1990;174:727–731.

111. Debatin JF, Spritzer CE, Grist TM, et al. Imaging of the renal arteries: value of MR angiography. AJR Am J Roentgenol 1991;157:981–990.

112. De Cobelli F, Mellone R, Salvioni M, et al. Renal artery stenosis: value of screening with three-dimensional phase-contrast MR angiography with a phased-array multicoil. Radiology 1996;201:697–703.

113. Leung DA, Hagspiel KD, Angle JF, et al. Value of image subtraction in 3D gadolinium-enhanced MR angiography of the renal arteries. J Magn Reson Imaging 2002;8(3):598–602.

114. Niendorf HP, Haustein J, Cornelius I, et al. Safety of gadolinium-DTPA: extended clinical experience. Magn Reson Med 1991;22:222–228.

115. Prince MR, Arnoldus C. Frisoli JK. Nephrotoxicity of high-dose gadolinium compared with iodinated contrast. J Magn Reson Imaging 1996;6:162–166.

116. Debatin IF, Ting RH, Wegmuller H, et al. Renal artery blood flow: quantitation with phase-contrast MR imaging with and without breath holding. Radiology 1994;190:371–378.

117. Schoenberg SO, Knopp MV, Bock M, et al. Renal artery stenosis: grading of hemodynamic changes with cine phase-contrast MR blood flow measurements. Radiology 1997;203:45–53.

118. Wasser MN, Westenberg J, van der Hulst VP, et al. Hemodynamic significance of renal artery stenosis: digital subtraction angiography versus systolically gated three-dimensional phase-contrast MR angiography. Radiology 1997;202:333–338.

119. Prince MR, Schoenberg SO, Ward JS, et al. Hemodynamically significant atherosclerotic renal artery stenosis: MR angiographic features. Radiology 1997;205:128–136.

120. Hagspiel KD, Spinosa DJ, Angle JF, et al. Comprehensive evaluation of renal artery stenosis: combination of gadolinium-enhanced MR angiography and MR perfusion imaging of the kidney using extraslice spin tagging. J Vasc Interv Radiol 1999;10(2):211.

121. Wilman AH, Riederer SJ, King BF, et al. Fluoroscopically triggered contrast-enhanced three-dimensional MR angiography with elliptical centric view order: application to the renal arteries. Radiology 1997;205:137–146.

122. Volk M, Strotzer M, Lenhart M, et al. Renal time-resolved MR angiography: quantitative comparison of gadobenate dimeglumine and gadopentetate meglumine with different doses. Radiology 2001;220:484–488.

123. Korst MB, Joosten FB, Postma CT, et al. Accuracy of normal-dose contrast-enhanced MR angiography in assessing renal artery stenosis and accessory renal arteries. AJR Am J Roentgenol 2000;174(3):629–634.

124. Leung DA, Pelkonen P, Hany TF, et al. Value of image subtraction in 3D gadolinium-enhanced MR angiography of the renal arteries. J Magn Reson Imaging 1998;8(3):598–602.

125. Prince MR. Gadolinium-enhanced MR aortography. Radiology 1994;91:155–164.

126. Hany TF, McKinnon GC. Leung DA, et al. Optimization of contrast timing for breath-hold three-dimensional MR angiography. J Magn Reson Imaging 1997;7:551–556.

127. Prince MR, Narasimhan DL, Stanley IC, et al. Breath-hold gadolinium-enhanced MR angiography of the abdominal aorta and its major branches. Radiology 1995;197:785–792.

128. Leung DA, McKinnon GC, Davis CP, et al. Breath-hold contrast-enhanced three-dimensional MR angiography. Radiology 1996;201:569–571.

129. Mittal TK, Evans C, Perkins T, et al. Renal arteriography using gadolinium-enhanced 3D MR angiography—clinical experience with the technique, its limitations and pitfalls. Br J Radiol 2001;74:495–502.

130. Bakker J, Beek FJ, Beuder JJ, et al. Renal artery stenosis and accessory renal arteries: accuracy of detection and visualization with gadolinium-enhanced breath-hold MR angiography. Radiology 1998;207:497–504.

131. Bongers V, Bakker J, Beutler JJ, et al. Assessment of renal artery stenosis: comparison of captopril renography and gadolinium-enhanced breath-hold MR angiography. Clin Radiol 2000;55(5):346–353.

132. De Cobelli F, Venturini M, Vanzulli A, et al. Renal arterial stenosis: prospective comparison of color Doppler US and breath-hold, three-dimensional, dynamic, gadolinium-enhanced MR angiography. Radiology 2000;214(2):373–380.

133. Gilfeather M, Yoon HC, Siegelman ES, et al. Renal artery stenosis: evaluation with conventional angiography versus gadolinium-enhanced MR angiography. Radiology 1999;210(2):367–372.

134. Masunaga H, Takehara Y, Isoda H, et al. Assessment of gadolinium-enhanced time-resolved three-dimensional MR angiography for evaluating renal artery stenosis. AJR Am J Roentgenol 2001;176(5):1213–1219.

135. Qanadli SD, Soulez G, Therasse E, et al. Detection of renal artery stenosis: prospective comparison of captopril-enhanced Doppler sonography, captopril-enhanced scintigraphy, and MR angiography. AJR Am J Roentgenol 2001;177(5):1123–1129.

136. Schoenberg SO, Bock M, Knopp MV, et al. Renal arteries: optimization of three-dimensional gadolinium-enhanced MR angiography with bolus-timing-independent fast multiphase acquisition in a single breath hold. Radiology 1999;211(3):667–679.

137. Schoenberg SO, Knopp MV, Londy F, et al. Morphologic and functional magnetic resonance imaging of renal artery stenosis: a multireader tricenter study. J Am Soc Nephrol 2002;13(1):158–169.

138. Tan KT, van Beek EJ, Brown, PW, et al. Magnetic resonance angiography for the diagnosis of renal artery stenosis: a meta-analysis. Clin Radiol 2002;57(7):617–624.

139. Willmann JK, Wildermuth S, Pfammatter T, et al. Aortoiliac and renal arteries: prospective intra-individual comparison of contrast-enhanced three-dimensional MR angiography and multidetector row CT angiography. Radiology 2003;226(3):798–811.

140. Volk M, Strotzer M, Lenhart M, et al. Time-resolved contrast-enhanced MR angiography of renal artery stenosis: diagnostic accuracy and interobserver variability. AJR Am J Roentgenol 2000;174(6):1583–1588.

141. Baskaran V, Pereles FS, Nemcek AA Jr, et al. Gadolinium-enhanced 3D MR angiography of renal artery stenosis: a pilot comparison of maximum intensity projection, multiplanar reformatting, and 3D volume-rendering postprocessing algorithms. Acad Radiol 2002;9(1):50–59.

142. Hagspiel KD, Dulai S, Leung D, et al. MR Angiography in patients after implantation of platinum stents: comparison with conventional stent designs. In: Book of Abstracts, 10th Annual Scientific Meeting of the International Society of Magnetic Resonance in Medicine 2002, Hawaii.

143. Behar JV, Nelson RC, Zidar JP, et al. Thin-section multidetector CT angiography of renal artery stents. AJR Am J Roentgenol 2002;178:1155–1159.

144. Sharafuddin MJ, Stolpen AH, Dixon BS, et al. Value of MR angiography before percutaneous transluminal renal artery angioplasty and stent placement. J Vasc Interv Radiol 2002;13(9 Pt 1):901–908.

145. Vasbinder GBC, Nelemans PJ, Kessels AGH, et al. Computed tomographic angiography and magnetic resonance angiography

for the diagnosis of renal artery stenosis: a comparative study with digital subtraction angiography. In: Vasbinder GDC. Evaluation of CT and MR Angiography for the Diagnosis of Renal Artery Stenosis, pp. 36–52. PhD Thesis, Universiteit Maastricht, Netherlands, Oct 30 2003.

146. Kessel DO, Robertson I, Taylor EJ, et al. Renal stenting from the radial artery: a novel approach. Cardiovasc Intervent Radiol 2003;26:146–149.

147. Baumgartner I, von Aesch K, Do DD, et al. Stent placement in ostial and nonostial atherosclerotic renal artery stenosis: a prospective follow-up study. Radiology 2000;216:498–505.

148. Leertouwer TC, van Overhagen HV, van Jaarsveld BC, et al. Intravascular ultrasound (IVUS) to guide percutaneous renal artery stent placement. J Vasc Interv Radiol 1998;9(Suppl I):213.

149. A randomised, blinded, trial of clopidogrel versus aspirin in patients at risk of ischaemic events (CAPRIE). CAPRIE Steering Committee. Lancet 1996;348:1329–1339.

150. May AG, van de Berg L, De Weese JA, et al. Critical arterial stenosis. Surgery 1963;54:250–259.

151. Haimovici H, Zinicola N. Experimental renal artery stenosis: diagnostic significance of arterial hemodynamics. J Cardiovasc Surg (Torino) 1962;3:259–262.

152. Archie JP Jr. Analysis and comparison of pressure gradients and ratios for predicting iliac stenosis. Ann Vasc Surg 1994;8:271–280.

153. Gross CM, Kramer J, Weingartner O, et al. Determination of renal arterial stenosis severity: comparison of pressure gradient and vessel diameter. Radiology 2001;220:751–756.

154. Simon G. What is critical renal artery stenosis? Implications for treatment. Am J Hypertens 2000;13:1189–1193.

155. Harward TR, Poindexter B, Huber TS, et al. Selection of patients for renal artery repair using captopril testing. Am J Surg 1995;170: 183–187.

156. Henry M, Clonaris C, Henry I, et al. Protected renal stenting with the PercuSurge Guardwire device: a pilot study. J Endovasc Ther 2001;8:227–237.

157. Holden A, Hill A. Renal angioplasty and stenting with distal protection of the main renal artery in ischemic nephropathy: early experience. J Vasc Surg 2003;38:762–768.

158. Williams DO. Intracoronary brachytherapy: past, present, and future. Circulation 2002;105:2699–2700.

159. Chrysant Gs, Goldstein JA, Caserly IP, et al. Endovascular brachytherapy for treatment of bilateral renal artery in-stent restenosis. Catheter Cardiovasc Interv 2003;59:251–254.

160. Martin LG, Rundback JH, Sacks D, et al. Quality improvement guidelines for angiography, angioplasty, and stent placement in the diagnosis and treatment of renal artery stenosis in adults. J Vasc Interv Radiol 2002;13:1069–1083.

161. Beek FJ, Kaatee R, Beutler JJ, et al. Complications during renal artery stent placement for atherosclerotic ostial stenosis. Cardiovasc Intervent Radiol 1997;20:184–190.

162. Bakker J, Goffette PP, Henry M, et al. The ERASME study: a multicenter study on the safety and technical results of the Palmaz stent use for the treatment of atherosclerotic ostial renal artery stenosis. Cardiovasc Intervent Radiol 1999;22:468–474.

163. Leertouwer TC, Gussenhovien EJ, Bosch JL, et al. Stent placement for renal arterial stenosis: where do we stand? a meta-analysis. Radiology 2000;216:78–85.

164. Martin LG. Renal revascularization using percutaneous balloon angioplasty for fibromuscular dysplasia and atherosclerotic disease. In: Calligaro KD, Dougherty MJ, eds. Modern management of renovascular hypertension and renal salvage. Philadelphia PA: Williams and Wilkins, 1996, pp. 125–144.

165. Scolari F, Tardanico R, Zani R, et al. Cholesterol crystal embolization: a recognizable cause of renal disease. Am J Kidney Dis 2000; 36:1089–1109.

166. Martin LG, Casarella WJ, Alspaugh JP, et al. Renal artery angioplasty: increase technical success and decreased complications in the second 100 patients. Radiology 1986;159:631–634.

167. Kuhn FP, Kutkuhn B, Torsello G, et al. Renal artery stenosis: preliminary results of treatment with the Strecker stent. Radiology 1991;180:367–372.

168. DeMaioribus CA, Anderson CA, Popham SS. Mycotic renal artery degeneration and systemic sepsis caused by infected renal artery stent. J Vasc Surg 1998;28:547–550.

169. Deparine MK, Ballard JL, Taylor FC, et al. Endovascular stent infection. J Vasc Surg 1996;23:529–533.

170. Spinosa DJ, Matsumoto AH, Angle JF, et al. Safety of CO(2)- and gadodiamide-enhanced angiography for the evaluation and percutaneous treatment of renal artery stenosis in patients with chronic renal insufficiency. AJR Am J Roentgenol 2001; 176:1305–1311.

171. Barrett BJ. Contrast nephropathy. J Am Soc Nephrol 1994;5: 125–137.

172. Solomon R. Contrast-medium-induced acute renal failure. Kidney Int 1998;53:230–242.

173. Parfrey PS, Griffiths SM, Barrett BJ, et al. Contrast-material induced renal failure in patients with diabetes mellitus, renal insufficiency or both. A prospective controlled study. N Engl J Med 1989;320:143–149.

174. Brezis M. Epstein FH. A closer look at radiocontrast-induced nephropathy. N Engl J Med 1989;320:179–181.

175. Porter GA. Contrast-associated nephropathy. Am J Cardiol 1989;64:22E–26E.

176. Fenves AZ, Allgren RI. Radiocontrast dye-induced acute tubular necrosis (ATN). Natriuretic peptide ANP vs placebo [Abstract]. Am J Nephrol 1995;6:463.

177. Rihal CS, Textor SC, Gril DE, et al. Incidence and prognostic importance of acute renal failure after percutaneous coronary intervention. Circulation 2002;105:2259–2264.

178. Briguori C, Tavano D, Colombo A. Contrast agent-associated nephrotoxicity. Prog Cardiovasc Dis 2003;45:493–503.

179. Levy EM, Viscoli CM, Horwitz RI. The effect of acute renal failure on mortality: a cohort analysis. JAMA 1996;275:1489–1494.

180. Solomon R, Werner C, Mann D, et al. Effects of saline, mannitol, and furosemide to prevent acute decreases in renal function induced by radiocontrast agents. N Engl J Med 1994;331: 1416–1420.

181. Mueller C, Buerkle G, Buettner HJ, et al. Prevention of contrast media-associated nephropathy: randomized comparison of 2 hydration regimens in 1,620 patients undergoing coronary angioplasty. Arch Intern Med 2002;162:329–336.

182. Taylor AJ, Hotchkiss D, Moric RW, et al. PREPARED: Preparation for Angiography in Renal Dysfunction: a randomized trial of inpatient vs outpatient hydration protocols for cardiac catheterization in mild-to-moderate renal dysfunction. Chest 1998;114: 1570–1574.

183. Brooks DP, DePalma PD. Blockade of radiocontrast-induced nephrotoxicity by the endothelin receptor antagonist, SB 209670. Nephron 1996;72:629–636.

184. Erley CM, Duda SH, Rehfuss D, et al. Prevention of radiocontrast-media-induced nephropathy in patients with preexisting renal insufficiency by hydration or in combination with the adenosine antagonist theophylline. Radiology 1999;14:1146–1149.

185. Katholi RE, Taylor GJ, McCann WP, et al. Nephrotoxicity from contrast media: attenuation with theophylline. Radiology 1995; 195:17–22.

186. Bakris GO, Burnett JC. The role of calcium in radiocontrast-induced reduction in renal hemodynamics. Kidney Int 1995; 27:465–468.

187. Pflueger A, Larson TS, Nath KA, et al. Role of adenosine in contrast media-induced acute renal failure in diabetes mellitus. Mayo Clin Proc 2000;75:1275–1283.

188. Morton GJ, Burgess, WP, Gray LV, et al. Prevention of contrast-induced nephropathy with sodium bicarbonate: a randomized controlled trial. JAMA 2004;291:2328–2334.

189. Dimari J, Megyesi J, Udvarhelyi N, et al. N-acetyl cysteine ameliorates ischemic renal failure. Am J Physiol 1997;272:F929–F298.

190. Tariq M, Morais C, Sobki A, et al. N-acetylcysteine attenuates cyclosporine-induced nephrotoxicity in rats. Nephrol Dial Transplant 1999;14:923–929.

191. Birck R, Krzossok S, Markowetz F, et al. Acetylcysteine for prevention of contrast nephropathy: meta-analysis. Lancet 2003; 362:598–603.

192. Singer I, Epstein M. Potential of dopamine A-1 agonists in the management of acute renal failure. Am J Kidney Dis 1998; 31:743–755.

193. Mathur BS, Swan SK, Lambrecht LJ, et al. The effects of fenoldopam, an elective dopamine receptor agonist, on systemic and renal hemodynamics in normotensive subjects. Crit Care Med 1999;27:1832–1837.

194. Murphy MB, McCoy CE, Weber RR, et al. Augmentation of renal blood flow and sodium excretion in hypertensive patients during blood pressure reduction by intravenous administration of dopamine A-1 agonist fenoldopam. Circulation 1987;76: 1312–1318.

195. Madyoon H. Clinical experience with the use of fenoldopam for prevention of radiocontrast nephropathy in high-risk patients. Rev Cardiovasc Med 2001;2(Suppl I):S26–S30.

196. Kini AS, Mitre CA, Kamran M, et al. Changing trends in incidence and predictors of radiographic contrast nephropathy after percutaneous coronary intervention with use of fenoldopam. Am J Cardiol 2002;89:999–1002.

197. Carey RM, Siragy HM, Ragsdale NV, et al. Dopamine-1 and dopamine-2 mechanisms in the control of renal function. Am J Hypertens 1990;3:59S-63S.

198. Allison NL, Dubb JW, Ziemniak JA, et al. The effect of fenoldopam, a dopaminergic agonist on renal hemodynamics. Clin Pharmacol Ther 1987;11:282–288.

199. Bakris GL, Lass NA, Glock D. Renal hemodynamics in radiocontrast medium-induced renal dysfunction: a role for dopamine-1 receptors. Kidney Int 1999;56:206–210.

200. Allaqaband S, Tumuluri R, Malik AM, et al. Prospective randomized study of N-acetyl cysteine, fenoldopam, and saline for prevention of radiocontrast-induced nephropathy. Catheter Cardiovasc Interv 2002;57:279–283.

201. Stone GW, McCullough PA, Tumlin JA, et al. Fenoldopam mesylate for the prevention of contrast-induced nephropathy. JAMA 2003;290:2284–2291.

202. Harris KG, Smith TP, Cragg AH. Nephrotoxicity from contrast material in renal insufficiency: ionic versus nonionic agents. Radiology 179:849–852, 1991.

203. Taliercio CP, Vlietstra RE, Ilstrup DM, et al. A randomized comparison of the nephrotoxicity of iopamidol and diatrizoate in high-risk patients undergoing cardiac angiography. J Am Coll Cardiol 1991;17:384–390.

204. Barrett BJ, Parfrey PS, Vavasour HM, et al. Contrast nephropathy in patients with impaired renal function: high versus low osmolar media. Kidney Int 1992;41:1274–1279.

205. Moore RD, Steinberg P, Powe NR, et al. Nephrotoxicity of high-osmolality versus low-osmolality contrast media: randomized clinical trial. Radiology 1992;182:649.

206. Schwab SJ, Hlatky MA, Pieper KS, et al. Contrast nephrotoxocity: a randomized clinical trial of a nonionic and ionic radiographic contrast agent. N Engl J Med 1989;320:149–153.

207. Rudnick MR, Goldfarb S, Wexler L, et al. Nephrotoxicity of ionic and nonionic contrast media in 1196 patients: a randomized trial. The Iohexol Cooperative Study. Kidney Int 1995;47:254–261.

208. Aspelin P, Aubry P, Fransson SG, et al. Nephrotoxicity in high-risk patients. A double-blind randomized multicenter study of isosmolar and low-osmolar nonionic contrast media: the nephrotoxicity, high risk, isosmolar contrast media (NEPHRIC) study. N Engl J Med 2003;348:491–499.

209. Cigarroa RG, Lange RA, Williams RH, et al. Dosing of contrast material to prevent contrast nephropathy in patients with renal disease. Am J Med 1989;86:649–552.

210. McCullough PA, Wolyn R, Rocher LO, et al. Acute renal failure after coronary intervention: incidence, risk factors, and relationship to mortality. Am J Med 1997;103:368–375.

211. Freeman RV, O'Donnell M, Share D, et al. Nephropathy requiring dialysis after percutaneous coronary intervention and the critical role of an adjusted contrast dose. Am J Cardiol 2002; 90:1068–1073.

212. Vliestre RE, Nunn CM, Naverte J, et al. Contrast nephropathy after coronary angioplasty and chronic renal insufficiency. Am Heart J 1996;32:1049–1050.

213. Manske CL, Sprafka JM, Strong JH, et al. Contrast nephropathy in azotemic diabetic patients undergoing coronary angiography. Am J Med 1990;89:260–615.

214. Hawkins IF. Carbon dioxide digital subtraction angiography. AJR Am J Roentgenol 1982;139:19–24.

215. Caridi JG, Stavropoulos SW, Hawkins IF Jr. Carbon dioxide digital subtraction angiography for renal artery stent placement. J Vasc Interv Radiol 1999;10:635–640.

216. Caridi JG, Stavropoulos W, Hawkins IF Jr. CO2 digital subtraction angiography for renal artery angioplasty in high-risk patients. AJR Am J Roentgenol 1999;173:1555–1556.

217. Hawkins IF Jr, Wilcox CS, Kerns SR, et al. CO2 digital angiography: a safer contrast agent for renovascular imaging? Am J Kidney Dis 1994;24:685–694.

218. Frankhouse JG, Ryan MG, Papanicolaou G, et al. Carbon dioxide/digital subtraction arteriography-assisted transluminal angioplasty. Ann Vasc Surg 1995;9:448–452.

219. Weaver FA, Pentecost MJ, Yellin AE, et al. Clinical applications of carbon dioxide-digital substraction arteriography. J Vasc Surg 1991;13:266–272.

220. Hawkins IF Jr, Caridi JK, Kerns SR. Plastic bag delivery system for hand injection of carbon dioxide. AJR Am J Roentgenol 1995;165: 1487–1489.

221. Ehrman KL, Tabor TE, Gaylord GNM, et al. Comparison of diagnostic accuracy with carbon dioxide vs iodinated contrast material in imaging of hemodialysis access fistulas. J Vasc Interv Radiol 1994;5:771–775.

222. Spinosa DJ, Matsumoto AH, Angle JF, et al. Transient mesenteric ischemic: a complication of carbon dioxide angiography. J Vasc Interv Radiol 1998;9:561–564.

223. Caridi JG, Hawkins IF Jr. CO2 digital subtraction angiography: potential complications and their prevention. J Vasc Interv Radiol 1997;8:383–391.

224. Kinno Y, Odagiri K, Andoh K, et al. Gadopentetate dimeglumine as an alternative contrast agent for the use in angiography. AJR Am J Roentgenol 1993;160:1293–1294.

225. Kaufman JA, Geller SC, Waltman AC. Renal insufficiency: gadopentetate dimeglumine as a radiographic contrast during peripheral vascular interventional procedures. Radiology 1996; 198:579–581.

226. Matchett WJ, McFarland DR, Russell DK, et al. Azotemia: gadopentetate dimeglumine as contrast agent at digital subtraction angiography. Radiology 1996;201:569–571.

227. Spinosa DJ, Matsumoto AH, Angle JF, et al. Renal insufficiency: usefulness of gadodiamide-enhanced renal angiography to supplement CO2–enhanced renal angiography for diagnosis and percutaneous treatment. Radiology 1999;210:663–672.

228. Spinosa DJ, Hartwell GD, Angle JF, et al. Optimizing imaging technique for gadolinium contrast angiography [Abstract]. J Vasc Interv Radiol 1998;9(Suppl I):S192.

229. Spinosa DJ, Matsumoto AH, Hagspiel KD, et al. Gadolinium-based contrast agents in angiography and interventional radiology. AJR Am J Roentgenol 1999;173:1403–1409.

230. Spinosa DJ, Kaufman JA, Hartwell GD. Gadolinium chelates in angiography and interventional radiology: a useful alternative to iodinated contrast media for angiography. Radiology 2002;223: 319–325.

231. Prince MR, Arnoldus C, Frisoli JK. Nephrotoxocity of high-dose gadolinium compared with iodinated contrast. J Magn Reson Imaging 1996;6:162–166.

232. Arsenault TM, Kang BF, Marsh JW, et al. Systemic gadolinium toxicity in patients with renal insufficiency and renal failure. Retrospective analysis of an initial experience. Mayo Clin Proc 1996;71:1150–1154.

233. Berg KJ, Lundby B, Reinton V, et al. Gadodiamide in renal transplant patients: effects on renal function and usefulness of a glomerular filtration rate marker. Nephron 1996;72:212–217.

234. Tombach B, Bermer C, Reiner P, et al. Renal tolerance of a neutral gadolinium chelate (gadobutrol) in patients with chronic renal failure: results of a randomized study. Radiology 2001;218: 651–657.

235. Hollenberg NK. Medical therapy for renovascular hypertension: a review. Am J Hypertens 1988;1:338S–343S.

236. Textor SC. ACE inhibitors in renovascular hypertension. Cardiovasc Drugs Ther 1990;4:229–235.

237. Rihal CS, Textor SC, Breen JF, et al. Incidental renal artery stenosis among a perspective cohort of hypertensive patients undergoing coronary angiography. Mayo Clin Proc 2002;77:309–316.

238. Webster J, Marshall F, Abdalla M, et al. Randomized comparison of percutaneous angioplasty versus continued medical therapy for hypertensive patients with atheromatous renal artery stenosis. J Hum Hypertens 1998;12:329–335.

239. Plouin PF, Chatellier G, Darne B, et al. Blood pressure outcome of angioplasty in atherosclerotic renal artery stenosis: a randomized trial. Essai Multicentrique Medicaments vs Angioplastie (EMMA) Study Group. Hypertension 1998;31:823–829.

240. Ives NJ, Wheatley K, Stowe RL, et al. Continuing uncertainty about the value of percutaneous revascularization in atherosclerotic renovascular disease: a meta-analysis of randomized trials. Nephrol Dial Transplant 2003;18:298–304.

241. Helin KH, Lepantalo M, Edgren J, et al. Predicting the outcome of invasive treatment of renal artery disease. J Intern Med 2000; 247:105–110.

242. van de Ven PJ, Kaatee R, Beutler JJ, et al. Arterial stenting and balloon angioplasty in ostial atherosclerotic renovascular disease: a randomized trial. Lancet 1999;363:282–286.

243. Rees CR. Stents for atherosclerotic renovascular disease: state-of-the-art. J Vasc Interv Radiol 1999;10:689–705.

244. Miller GA, Ford KK, Braun SD, et al. Percutaneous transluminal angioplasty versus surgery for renovascular hypertension. AJR Am J Roentgenol 1985;144:447–450.

245. Weibull H, Bergqvist D, Bergentz SE, et al. Percutanous transluminal renal angioplasty versus surgical reconstruction of atherosclerotic renal artery stenosis: a perspective randomized study. J Vasc Surg 1993;18:841–851.

246. Deane RH, Foster JH. Criteria for the diagnosis of renovascular hypervascular hypertension. Surgery 1973;74:926–929.

247. Jacobson AR. Ischemic renal disease: an overlooked clinical entity? Kidney Int 1988;34:729–743.

248. Scoble ZE, Maher ER, Hamilton R, et al. Atherosclerotic renovascular disease causing renal impairment: a cause for treatment. Clin Nephrol 1989;31:119–122.

249. Appel RG, Bleyer AJ, Reavis S, et al. Renovascular disease in older patients beginning renal replacement therapy. Kidney Int 1995;48:171–176.

250. Fergany A. Ischemic nephropathy. Epidemiology and clinical implications. Urol Clin North Am 2001;28:805–813.

251. Greco BA, Breyer JA. Atherosclerotic ischemic renal disease. Am J Kidney Dis 1997;29:167–187.

252. Wollenweber J, Sheps SG, Davis GD. Clinical course of atherosclerotic renovascular disease. Am J Cardiol 1968;91:60–71.

253. Mailloux LU, Napolitano B, Bellucci AG, et al. Renal vascular disease causing end-stage renal disease, incidence, clinical correlates, and outcomes: a 20-year clinical experience. Am J Kidney Dis 1994;24:622–629.

254. Rimmer J, Jennari F. Atherosclerosis renovascular disease in progressive renal failure. Ann Intern Med 1993;118:712–719.

255. Murray S, Martin M, Amoedo L, et al. Rapid decline in renal function reflects reversibility and predicts the outcome after angioplasty in renal artery stenosis. Am J Kidney Dis 2002;39:60–66.

256. Hricik DE, Browning PJ, Kopelman R, et al. Captopril-induced functional renal insufficiency in patients with bilateral renal-artery stenoses or renal-artery stenosis in a solitary kidney. N Engl J Med 1983;30:373–376.

257. Alcazar JM, Mazuecos A, Garcia E, et al. Renal insufficiency and renovascular hypertension. G Ital Nefrol 1992;12:99–106.

258. Le Goff C, Ryckelynck JP, Levaltier B, et al. Reversible acute renal failure following aortic thrombosis inducing bilateral renal-artery occlusive disease. Nephrol Dial Transplant 1995;10:879–881.

259. Jackson B, McGrath BP, Matthews PG, et al. Differential renal function during angiotensin converting enzyme inhibition in renovascular hypertension. Hypertension 1986;8:650–654.

260. Toto RD, Mitchell HC, Lee HC, et al. Reversible renal insufficiency due to angiotensin converting enzyme inhibitors in hypertensive nephrosclerosis. Ann Intern Med 1991;115:513–119.

261. Alcazar JM, Rodicio JL. Ischemic nephropathy: clinical characteristics and treatment. Am J Kidney Dis 2000;36:883–893.

262. Tuttle KR. Toward more rational management of ischemic nephropathy: the need for clinical evidence. Am J Kidney Dis 2000;36:863–865.

263. Steinbach F, Novick AC, Campbell S, et al. Long-term survival after surgical revascularization for atherosclerotic renal artery disease. J Urol 1997;158:38–41.

264. Campo A, Boero B, Stratta P. et al. Selective stenting and the course of atherosclerotic renovascular nephropathy. J Nephrol 2002;15:525–529.

265. Thadhani RI, Camargo C, Xavier RJ, et al. Atheroembolic renal failure after invasive procedures:natural history based on 52 pathologically proven cases. Medicine 1995;74:350–358.

266. Bredenberg CE, Sampson LN, Ray FS, et al. Changing patterns in surgery for chronic renal artery occlusive disease. J Vasc Surg 1992;15:1018–1024.

267. Chaikof EL, Smith RV, Salam AA, et al. Ischemic nephropathy in concomitant aortic disease: a 10-year experience. J Vasc Surg 1994;19:135–148.

268. Crinniou JN, Gough MJ. Bilateral renal artery atherosclerosis. The results of surgical treatment. Eur J Vasc Endovasc Surg 1996;11:353–358.

269. Fergany A, Kolettis P, Novick AC. The contemporary role of extra-anatomical surgical revascularization in patients with atherosclerotic renal artery disease. J Urol 1995;153:1798–1801.

270. Hallett JW, Textor SC, Kos PB, et al. Advanced renovascular hypertension and renal insufficiency: trends in medical comorbidity and surgical approach from 1970 to 1993. J Vasc Surg 1995;21:750–760.

271. Hansen KJ, Starr SM, Sands RE, et al. Contemporary surgical management of renovascular disease. J Vasc Surg 1992;16:319–331.

272. Hansen KJ, Cherr GS, Craven TE, et al. Management of ischemic nephropathy: dialysis-free survival after surgical repair. J Vasc Surg 2000;32:472–478.

273. Libertino JA, Bosco PJ, Ying CY, et al. Renal revascularization to preserve and restore renal function. J Urol 1992;147:1485–1487.

274. Novick AZ, Ziegelbaum M. Vidt DG, et al. Trends in surgical revascularization for renal artery disease: 10-years experience. JAMA 1987;257:498–501.

275. van Dammee H, Jeusette F, Pans A, et al. The impact of renal revascularization on renal dysfunction. Eur J Vasc Endovasc Surg 1995;10:330–337.

276. Hansen KJ, Thomason RB, Craven TE, et al. Surgical management of dialysis dependent ischemic neuropathy. J Vasc Surg 1995;21:197–211.

277. Hallett JW Jr, Fowl R, O'Brien PC, et al. Renovascular operations in patients with chronic renal insufficiency: do the benefits justify the risks? J Vasc Surg 1987;5:622–627.

278. Karagiannis A, Douma S, Voyiatzis K, et al. Percutaneous transluminal renal angioplasty in patients with renal vascular hypertension: long-term results. Hypertens Res 1995;18:27–31.

279. Lossino F, Zuccalá A, Busato F, et al. Renal artery angioplasty for renal vascular hypertension and preservation of renal function: long-term angiographic and clinical follow up. AJR Am J Roentgenol 1994;162:853–857.

280. O'Donovan RM, Guierrezoh SOS, Izzo JOL Jr. Preservation of renal function by percutaneous renal angioplasty and high-risk LOA patients: short-term outcome. Nephron 1992;60:187–192.

281. Paulsen D, Klow NE, Rogstad B, et al. Preservation of renal function by percutaneous transluminal angioplasty in ischemic renal disease. Nephrol Dial Transplant 1999;14:1454–1461.

282. Pickering TG, Sos TA, Suddekni S, et al. Renal angioplasty in patients with azotemia and renovascular hypertension. Am J Hypertens 1986;(Suppl VI)4:S667–S679.

283. Beutler JJ, Van Ampting JMA, van de ven PJG, et al. Long-term effects of arterial stenting on kidney function for patients with ostial atherosclerotic renal artery stenosis and renal insufficiency. J Am Soc Nephrol 2001;12:1475–1481.

284. Martin LG, Casarella WG, Gaylord GMM. Azotemia caused by renal artery stenosis. Treatment by percutaneous angioplasty. AJR Am J Roentgenol 1988;150:839–844.

285. Canzanello UJ, Millan VG, Spiegel JE, et al. Percutaneous transluminal renal angioplasty and management of atherosclerotic renovascular hypertension: results in 100 patients. Hypertension 1989;13:163–172.

286. Pattison JM, Reidy JF, Rafferty MJ, et al. Percutaneous transluminal renal angioplasty in patients with renal failure. Q J Med 1992;308:883–888.

287. Martin LG, Cork RD, Kaufmann SL. Long-term results of angioplasty in 110 patients with renal artery stenosis. J Vasc Interv Radiol 1992;3:619–626.

288. Plouin PF, Darne B, Chatellier G, et al. Restenosis after a first percutaneous transluminal angioplasty. Hypertension 1993;21:89–96.

289. Patty NA, Wa PM, Becker GJ, et al. Percutaneous angioplasty for atherosclerotic renal artery disease effect on renal function in azotemic patients. Cardiovasc Intervent Radiol 1994;17:143–146.

290. Byrd R, Warwick R, Hilson A, et al. Renal artery angioplasty in severe atherosclerotic renovascular disease. Brit J Surg 1995;82:561–566.

291. Boisclair C, Therasse E, Oliva LV, et al. Treatment of renal angioplasty failure by percutaneous renal artery stenting with Palmaz stents: midterm technical and clinical results. AJR Am J Roentgenol 1997;168:245–251.

292. Harden PN, MacLeod MJ, Rodger RS, et al. Effect of renal artery stenting on progression of renovascular renal failure. Lancet 1997;349:1133–1136.

293. Rees CR, Palmaz JC, Becker GJ, et al. Palmaz stent in atherosclerotic stenoses involving the ostia of the renal arteries: primarily report of multicenter study. Radiology 1991;181:507–514.

294. Rundback JH, Manoni T, Rozenblit GN, et al. Balloon angioplasty or stent placement in patients with azotemic renovascular disease: a retrospective comparison of clinical outcomes. Heart Dis 1999;1:121–125.

295. Spinosa DJ, Matsumoto AH, Bissonette E, et al. PTA/stenting for renal insufficiency: 30 month results. Presented at 15th Annual International Symposium on Endovascular Therapy 2003. Miami, FL, pp.165–166.

296. Tuttle KR, Chouinard RF, Webber JT, et al. Treatment of atherosclerotic ostial renal artery stenosis with the intravascular stent. Am J Kidney Dis 1998;32:611–622.

297. Bakris GL, Williams M, Dworkin L, et al. Preserving renal function in adults with hypertension and diabetes: a consensus approach. Am J Kidney Dis 2000;36:646–661.

298. Vogt L, Navis G, De Zeeuw D. Renoprotection: a matter of blood pressure reduction or agent-characteristics? J Am Soc Nephrol 2002;13:S202–S207.

299. Parving HH, Hommel E, Damkjaer Nielsen M, et al. Effect of captopril on blood pressure and kidney function in normotensive insulin dependent diabetes with nephropathy. Br Med J 1989; 299:533–536.

300. Ravid M, Lang R, Rachmani R, et al. Long-term renoprotective effect of angiotensin converting enzyme inhibition on noninsulin dependent diabetes mellitus. A seven-year follow-up study. Arch Intern Med 1996;156:286–289.

301. Brenner BM, Cooper Me, de Zeeuw D, et al. Effects of Losartan on renal and cardiovascular outcomes in patients with type 2 diabetes and nephropathy. N Engl J Med 2001;345:861–869.

302. Maschio G, Alberti D, Janin G, et al. Effect of the angiotensin-converting-enzyme inhibitor benazepril on the progression chronic renal insufficiency. N Engl J Med 1996;334:939–945.

303. Gisen Group: Randomized placebo control trial of effect of Ramipril on decline of glomerular infiltration rate and risk of terminal renal failure in proteinuric, nondiabetic nephrography. Lancet 1997;349:1857–1863.

304. Williams PS, Fass G, Bone JM. Renal pathology and proteinuria to determine progression in untreated mild-moderate chronic renal failure. Q J Med 1988;67:343–354.

305. Remuzzi G, Bertani T. Is glomerulosclerosis a consequence of altered glomerular permeability to macromolecules? Kidney Int 1990;38:384–394.

306. El Nahas AM, Masters-Thomas A, Brady SA, et al. Selective effect of low protein diets in chronic renal diseases. Br Med J 1984; 289:1337–1341.

307. Russouw JE, Lewis B, Rifkind BM. The value of lowering cholesterol after myocardial infarction. N Engl J Med 1990;323: 1112–1119.

308. Brown BG, Zhao XQ, Sacco DE, et al. New insights into prevention of plaque disruption and clinical events in coronary disease. Circulation 1993;87:1781–1791.

309. Downs JR, Clearfield M, Weis S, et al. Primary prevention of acute coronary events with lovastatin in men and women with average cholesterol levels: results of AFCAPS/TexCAPS. Air Force/Texas Coronary Atherosclerosis Prevention Study. JAMA. 1998;279: 1615–1622.

310. Bergentz SE. Natural history of renal artery stenosis. Ann Chir Gynaecol 1992;81:98–101.

311. Simon N, Franklin SS, Bleifer KH, et al. Clinical characteristics of renovascular hypertension. JAMA 1972;220:1209–1218.

312. McCormack LJ, Poutasee EF, Meaney TF, et al. A pathologic arteriographic correlation of renal artery disease. Am Heart J 1966; 72:188–198.

313. McCormick LJ, Dustan HP, Meaney TF. Selected pathology of the renal artery. Semin Roentgenol 1967;2:126–138.

314. Meaney TF, Dustan HP, McCormick LJ. Natural history of renal artery disease. Radiology 1968;91:881–887.

315. Pohl MA, Novick AC. Natural history of atherosclerotic and fibrous renal artery disease: clinical implications. Am J Kidney Dis 1985;5:A120–A130.

316. Stanley JC. Renal artery fibroplasia. In: Novick A, Scoble J, Hamilton G, eds. Renal Vascular Disease. Philadelphia: W.B.Saunders, 1996.

317. Cragg AH, Smith TP, Thompson BH, et al. Incidental fibromuscular dysplasia in potential renal donors: long-term follow-up. Radiology 1989;172:145–147.

318. Tegtmeyer CJ, Selby JB, Hartwell GD, et al. Results and complications of angioplasty in fibromuscular disease. Circulation 1991;83(Suppl I):155–161.

319. Surowiec SM, Sivamurthy N, Rhodes JM, et al. Percutaneous therapy for renal artery fibromuscular dysplasia. Ann Vasc Surg 2003;17:650–655.

320. Kumar A, Dubey D, Bansal P, et al. Surgical and radiological management of renovascular hypertension in a developing country. J Urol 2003;170:727–730.

321. de Fraissinette B, Garcier JM, Diew V, et al. Percutaneous transluminal angioplasty of dysplastic stenosis of the renal artery: results on 70 adults. Cardiovasc Intervent Radiol 2003;26:46–51.

322. Birrer M, Do DD, Mahler F, et al. Treatment of renal artery fibromuscular dysplasia with balloon angioplasty: a prospective follow-up study. Eur J Vasc Endovasc Surg 2002;23:146–152.

323. Lovaria A, Nicolini A, Meregaglia D, et al. Interventional radiology in the treatment of renal artery stenosis. Ann Urol (Paris) 1999;33:146–155.

324. Klow NE, Paulsen D, Vatne K, et al. Percutaneous transluminal renal artery angioplasty using the coaxial technique. Acta Radiol 1998;39:594–603.

325. Baumgartner I, Triller J, Mahler F. Patency of percutaneous transluminal renal angioplasty: a prospective sonographic study. Kidney Int 1997;51:798–803.

326. von Knorring J, Edgren J, Lepantalo M. Long-term results of percutaneous transluminal angioplasty in renovascular hypertension. Acta Radiol 1996;37:36–40.

327. Jensen G, Zachrisson BF, Delin K, et al. Treatment of renovascular hypertension: one-year results with renal angioplasty. Kidney Int 1995;48:1936–1945.

328. Bonelli FS, McKusick MA, Textor SC, et al. Renal artery angioplasty: technical results and clinical outcome in 320 patients. Mayo Clin Proc 1995;70:1041–1052.

329. Rodriquez-Perez, JC, Plaza C, Reyes R, et al. Treatment of renovascular hypertension with percutaneous transluminal angioplasty: experience in Spain. J Vasc Interv Radiol 1994;5:1010–109.

330. Baert AL, Wilms G, Amery A, et al. Percutaneous transluminal renal angioplasty: initial results and long-term follow-up in 202 patients. Cardiovasc Intervent Radiol 1990;13:22–28.

331. Greminger P, Steiner A, Schneider E, et al. Cure and improvement of renovascular hypertension after percutaneous transluminal angioplasty of renal artery stenosis. Nephron 1989;51:362–366.

332. Klinge J, Mali WPTM, Puijlawet CBAJ, et al. Percutaneous transluminal renal angioplasty: initial and long-term results. Radiology 1989;171:501–506.

333. Beebe HG, Chsesbro K. Merchant F, et al. Results of renal artery balloon angioplasty limit its indications J Vasc Surg 1988;8: 300–306.

334. Simonetti G, Urigo F, Sergiacomi GL, etal. Percutaneous transluminal renal angioplasty: follow-up at 48 months. In: Glorioso N, et al. eds. Renovascular Hypertension. New York: Raven, 1987; 499–509.

335. Bell GM, Reid J, Buist TAS. Percutaneous transluminal angioplasty improves blood pressure and renal function in renovascular hypertension. Q J Med 1987;241:393–403.

336. Kremer Hovinga TK, de Jong PE, de Zeeuw D, et al. Restenosis: prevalence and long-term effects on renal function after percutaneous transluminal renal angioplasty. Nephron 1986;44(Suppl I): 64–67.

337. Grim CE, Yune HY, Donohue JP, et al. Renal vascular hypertension: surgery vs. dilation. Nephron 1986;44(Suppl I):96–100.

338. Martin LG, Price RB, Cassarella WJ, et al. Percutaneous angioplasty in clinical management of renovascular hypertension: initial and long-term results. Radiology 1985;155:629-633.

339. Miller GA, Ford KK, Braun SD, et al. Percutaneous transluminal angioplasty vs. surgery for renovascular hypertension. AJR Am J Roentgenol 1985;144:447–450.

340. Sos, TA, Pickering TG, Sniderman K, et al. Percutaneous transluminal renal angioplasty in renovascular hypertension due to atheroma or fibromuscular dysplasia. N Engl J Med 1983;309: 274–279.

341. Mahler F, Probst P, Haertel M. et al. Lasting improvement of renovascular hypertension by transluminal dilatation of atherosclerotic and nonatherosclerotic renal artery stenoses: a follow-up study. Circulation 1982;65:611–617.

342. Colapinto RF, Stronell RD, Harries-Jones EP, et al. Percutaneous transluminal dilatation of the renal artery: follow-up studies of renovascular hypertension. AJR Am J Roentgenol 1982;139: 727–732.

343. Martin EC, Mattern RF, Baer L, et al. Renal angioplasty for hypertension: predictive factors for long-term success. AJR 1981; 137:921–924.

344. Courtel JV, Soto B, Niaudet P, et al. Percutaneous transluminal angioplasty of renal artery stenosis in children. Pediatr Radiol 1998;28:59–63.

345. Cluzel P, Raynaud A, Beyssen B, et al. Stenoses of renal branch arteries in fibromuscular dysplasia: results of percutaneous transluminal angioplasty. Radiology 1994;193:227–232.

346. Mounier-Vehier C, Haulon S, Devos P, et al. Renal atrophy outcome after revascularization in fibromuscular dysplasia disease. J Endovasc Ther 2002;9:605–613.

347. Patel NH, Jindal RM, Wilkin T, et al. Renal arterial stenosis in renal allografts: retrospective study of predisposing factors and outcome after percutaneous transluminal angioplasty. Radiology 2001;219:663–667.

348. Fervenza FC, Layfayett RA, Alfrey EJ, et al. Renal artery stenosis in kidney transplantation. Am J Kidney Dis 1998;31:142–148.

349. Roberts JP, Ascher NL, Fryd DS, et al. Transplant renal artery stenosis. Transplantation 1989;48:580–583.

350. Wong W, Fynn SP, Higgins RM, et al. Transplant renal artery stenosis in 77 patients: does it have an immunological cause? Transplantation 1996;61:215–219.

351. Linas SL, Miller PD, McDonald KM, et al. Role of the renin angiotensin system in posttransplant hypertension in patients with multiple kidneys. N Engl J Med 1978;298:1440.

352. Halimi JM, Al-Najjar A, Buchler M, et al. Transplant renal artery stenosis: potential role of ischemia/reperfusion injury and long-term outcome following angioplasty. J Urol 1999;161:28–32.

353. Benoit G, Moukarzel M, Hiesse C, et al. Transplant renal artery stenosis: experience and comparative results between surgery and angioplasty. Transpl Int 1990;3:137–140.

354. Tang S, Tso WK, Li JH, et al. Clinical outcome following percutaneous transluminal angioplasty for transplant renal artery stenoses. Transplant Proc 2000;32:1889–1891.

355. Rundback JH, Rizvi A, Tomasula J. Percutaneous treatment of transplant renal artery stenosis: techniques and results. Tech Vasc Interv Radiol 1999;2:91–97.

356. Sankari BR, Geisinger M, Zlech M, et al. Posttransplant renal artery stenosis: impact of therapy on long-term kidney function and blood pressure. J Urol 1996;155:1860–1864.

357. Lo CT, Cheng IK, Tso WK, et al. Percutaneous transluminal angioplasty for transplant renal artery stenosis. Transplant Proc 1996;28:1468–1469.

358. Thomas CP, Riad H, Johnson BF, et al. Percutaneous transluminal angioplasty in transplant renal arterial stenoses: a long-term follow-up. Transpl Int 1992;5:129–132.

359. Fauchald P, Vatne K, Paulsen D, et al. Long-term clinical results of percutaneous transluminal angioplasty in transplant renal artery stenosis. Nephrol Dial Transplant 1992;7:256–259.

360. Bover J, Montana J, Castelao AM, et al. Percutaneous transluminal angioplasty for treatment of allograft renal artery stenosis. Transplant Proc 1992;24:94–95.

361. Matalon TAS, Thompson MJ, Patel SK, et al. Percutaneous transluminal angioplasty for transplant renal artery stenosis. J Vasc Interv Radiol 1992;3:55–58.

362. Kirst G. Wilms H, Matthias K. Transluminal angioplasty as treatment for renal transplant artery stenosis. Transplantation 1990; 50:357.

363. De Meyer M, Pirson Y, Dautrebande J, et al. Treatment of renal graft artery stenosis: comparison between surgical bypass and percutaneous transluminal angioplasty. Transplantation 1989; 47:784–788.

364. Aliabadi H, McLorie GA, Churchill BM, et al. Percutaneous transluminal angioplasty for transplant renal artery stenosis in children. J Urol 1990;143:569–573.

365. Greenstein SM, Verstandig A, McLean GK, et al. Percutaneous transluminal angioplasty. Transplantation 1987;43:29–32.

366. Reynaud A, Bedrossian J, Remy P, et al. Percutaneous transluminal angioplasty of renal transplant arterial stenoses. AJR Am J Roentgenol 1986;146:853–857.

367. Lohr JW, MacDougall ML, Chonko AM, et al. Percutaneous transluminal angioplasty in transplant renal artery stenosis: Experience and review of the literature. Am J Kidney Dis 1986; 7:363–367.

368. Curry NS, Cochran S, Barbaric ZL, et al. Interventional radiologic procedures in the renal transplant. Radiology 1984;152: 647–653.

369. Tegtmeyer CJ, Kellum CD, Ayers C. Percutaneous transluminal angioplasty of the renal arteries: results and long-term follow-up. Radiology 1984;153:77–84.

370. Gerlock AJ Jr, MacDonell RC Jr, Smith CW, et al. Renal transplant arterial stenosis: percutaneous transluminal angioplasty AJR Am J Roentgenol 1983;140:325–331.

371. Sniderman KW, Sprayregen S, Sos TA, et al. Percutaneous transluminal dilation in renal transplant arterial stenosis. Transplantation 1980;30:440–444.

372. Kuo PC, Petersen J, Semba C, et al. CO2 angiography: a technique for vascular imaging in renal allograft dysfunction. Transplantation 1996;122:652–654.

373. Spinosa DJ, Matsumoto AH, Angle JF, et al. Use of gadopentetate dimeglumine as a contrast agent for percutaneous transluminal renal angioplasty and stent placement. Kidney Int 1998;131: 503–507.

374. Sierre SD, Raynaud AC, Carreres T, et al. Treatment of recurrent transplant renal artery stenosis with metallic stents. J Vasc Interv Radiol 1998;9:639–644.

375. Sharma BK, Jain S, Bali HK, et al. A follow-up study of balloon angioplasty and de novo stenting in Takayasu arteritis. Int J Cardiol 2000;75:S145–152.

376. Cook PG, Wells IP, Marshall AJ. Case report: renovascular hypertension in Takayasu's disease treated by percutaneous transluminal angioplasty. Clin Radiol 1986;37:583–584.

377. Dong ZJ, Li S, Lu X. Percutaneous transluminal angioplasty for renovascular hypertension in arteritis: experience in China. Radiology 1987;162:477–479.

378. Sharma S, Saxena A, Talwar KK, et al. Renal artery stenosis caused by nonspecific arteritis (Takayasu's disease): results of treatment with percutaneous transluminal angioplasty. AJR Am J Roentgenol 1992;158:417–422.

379. Fava MP, Foradori GB, Garcia CB, et al. Percutaneous transluminal angioplasty in patients with Takayasu arteritis: five-year experience. J Vasc Interv Radiol 1993;4:649–652.

380. Savage BJ, Gupta RK, Angle JF, et al. Takayasu arteritis presenting as a pulmonary-renal syndrome. Am J Med Sci 2003;5:275–281.

381. Tyagi S, Singh B, Kaul UA, et al. Balloon angioplasty for renovascular hypertension in Takayasu's arteritis. Am Heart J 1993;125: 1386.

382. Sharma S, Gupta H, Saena A, et al. Results of renal angioplasty in nonspecific aortoarteritis (Takayasu's disease). J Vasc Interv Radiol 1998;9:429–435.

383. Dev V, Shrivastava S, Rajani M. Percutaneous transluminal angioplasty in Takayasu' arteritis: persistent benefit over two years. Am Heart J 1990;120:222–224.

384. Giordano JM. Surgical treatment of Takayasu's arteritis. Int J Cardiol 2000;75:S123–128.

385. Greene JF Jr, Fitzwater JE, Burgess J. Arterial lesions associated with neurofibromatosis. Am J Clin Pathol 1974;62:481–487.

386. Baxi R Epstein HY, Abitbol C. Percutaneous transluminal renal artery angioplasty in hypertension associated with neurofibromatosis. Radiology 1988;139:583–584.

387. Gardiner GA Jr Freedman AM, Shlansky-Goldberg R. Percutaneous transluminal angioplasty: delayed response in neurofibromatosis. Radiology 1988;169:79–80.

388. Millan VG, McGauley J, Kopelman RI, et al. Percutaneous transluminal renal angioplasty in nonatherosclerotic renovascular hypertension: long-term results. Hypertension 1985;7:668–674.

389. Lund G, Siaiko A, Castaneda-Zuniga, et al. Percutaneous transluminal angioplasty for treatment of renal artery stenosis in children. Eur Radiol 1984;4:254–257.

390. Guzzetta PC, Ptter BM, Ruley EJ, et al. Renovascular hypertension in children: current concepts in evaluation and treatment. J Pediatr Surg 1989;24:1236–1240.

391. Green TJ, Mauro MA. SIR 2003 Film Panel Case 4: Neurofibromatosis. J Vasc Interv Radiol 2003;14:663–666.

Endovascular Interventions for Acute and Chronic Mesenteric Ischemia

22

Daniel A. Leung, Alan H. Matsumoto, Klaus D. Hagspiel,
J. Fritz Angle, David J. Spinosa

Gradual and progressive stenosis of one or more of the major mesenteric arteries is generally well-tolerated, but when intestinal blood flow is inadequate to support functional demands, mesenteric ischemia may ensue. Patients with chronic mesenteric ischemia (CMI) classically present with intestinal angina and weight loss, but occasionally, the symptoms are less clear and the diagnosis is overlooked. Generally, bowel viability is preserved with CMI because of the abundant collateral circulation that exists among mesenteric vessels. Nonetheless, a delay in revascularization may precipitate a fatal sequence of events as visceral ischemia progresses to bowel infarction.

Similarly, an abrupt decrease in blood flow to the gut may lead to acute mesenteric ischemia (AMI) and immediately threaten bowel viability. Patients with AMI classically present with abdominal pain out of proportion to abdominal tenderness. Despite improvements in the diagnosis and treatment of AMI, mortality rates remain high. The management goal in AMI is centered on prompt recognition of the condition, identification of its cause, and expedient initiation of therapy to prevent and minimize the amount of bowel infarction.

Most patients with AMI and CMI require transcatheter or noninvasive angiographic assessment, and many are potential candidates for endovascular treatment. However, AMI and CMI differ distinctly in their clinical presentation and etiology as well as in the various treatment strategies. Therefore, in this chapter, the two disease entities will be discussed separately with a focus on the endovascular treatment options for both.

ACUTE MESENTERIC ISCHEMIA (AMI)

With traditional methods of diagnosing and treating AMI, death rates greater than 70% have been reported (1–3). Use of a more aggressive approach to treating AMI has reduced the mortality to about 50% or less, depending on the etiology (4,5). Early diagnosis of AMI requires a high index of clinical suspicion and more liberal use of catheter angiography. Angiographic evaluation should initially include a lateral abdominal aortogram to assess the patency of the proximal mesenteric vessels. If the proximal SMA has no hemodynamically significant stenosis, a selective superior mesenteric arteriogram should be performed to evaluate the status of the branch arteries and superior mesenteric vein. With occlusion of the SMA, selective injection of the celiac and inferior mesenteric arteries may be necessary to assess the adequacy of collateral circulation and the age of the SMA occlusion. Unfortunately, correlating symptoms of mesenteric ischemia with the extent of vascular obstruction is not always straightforward.

Because of the acuity of the presentation, other noninvasive vascular imaging techniques such as magnetic resonance angiography (MRA) and duplex ultrasound do not play an important role in the workup of patients with suspected AMI. Computed tomography (CT) can be useful because of the ability to obtain information about the patency of the SMA and SMV, as well as bowel viability. CT findings of intestinal ischemia or infarction include bowel dilation, wall-thickening, abnormal enhancement, and intramural or portal venous gas (6). With the advent of multidetector row scanning, CT angiography can now provide detailed assessment of both arterial and venous anatomy, as well as bowel and other intra-abdominal organs, and will undoubtedly gain increasing importance as a diagnostic tool (7). Nevertheless, because of its superior definition of vascular structures and the ability to administer therapy in the same setting, catheter angiography remains the mainstay in the diagnosis of AMI.

The four major causes of AMI are SMA embolism, nonocclusive mesenteric ischemia (NOMI), SMA thrombosis, and mesenteric venous thrombosis. A small percentage of cases of AMI are related to vasculitides, trauma, dissection of the aorta, volvulus, intussusceptions, hernias, adhesions, drugs (cocaine), cholesterol emboli, and intestinal obstruction.

SMA Embolus

An acute embolus to the SMA is the most common cause of AMI and accounts for 40–50% of cases (2). Patients with an SMA embolus usually have a history of cardiac disease and present with a dramatic clinical picture characterized by the precipitous onset of severe abdominal pain and the sudden onset of diarrhea (sometimes bloody). Approximately 20% of patients will have a simultaneous peripheral arterial embolus and about one third will have a history of a prior embolic event (2,8).

Angiographic findings of an acute embolus include the presence of a filling defect outlined by contrast (frequently at arterial branch points), occlusion with a convex meniscus, and occlusion more than 3 cm beyond the origin of the SMA, usually just distal to the middle colic and first jejunal branches (Figure 22–1).

In most cases, immediate surgery is indicated. Revascularization is performed using standard balloon embolectomy catheters in the operating room. Intraoperative thrombolytic therapy has been used in cases of incompletely removed thrombus or diffuse distal emboli. Following revascularization, nonviable segments of bowel are removed. If portions of bowel are of questionable viability, surgical reexploration is performed within 24 hours.

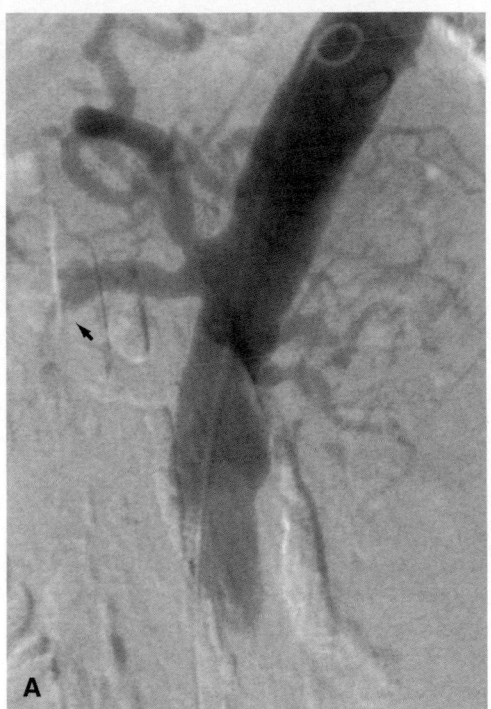

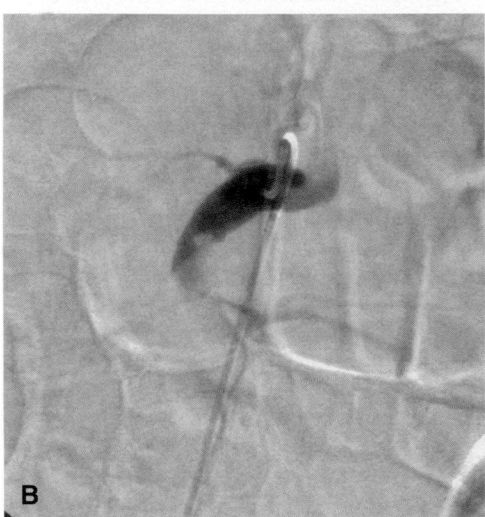

Figure 22–1 A 73-year-old patient with atrial fibrillation presents with the acute onset of severe abdominal pain out of proportion to abdominal tenderness. **A.** Lateral aortogram shows a common trunk of the celiac artery and superior mesenteric artery, with an abrupt cutoff of the latter (*arrow*). **B.** Selective superior mesenteric angiogram demonstrates a proximal embolic occlusion.

Mesenteric arterial vasoconstriction often develops in association with an SMA embolus and may persist and compromise intestinal perfusion even after removal of the arterial obstruction. Because of this persistent vasoconstriction, Dr. Boley and his colleagues have advocated liberal use of catheter-directed intra-arterial papaverine infusion (1,2). Because 90% of papaverine is metabolized on first pass through the liver, the rate of systemic hypotension and cardiac arrhythmias related to its use is low. However, the patient's cardiovascular rhythm and vital signs should be monitored closely. Precipitation within the infusate has been reported when papaverine is mixed with heparin, lactated Ringer's, thrombolytic agents, or ioxaglate contrast (Hexabrix).

Following placement of a catheter in the SMA, a 45–60 mg bolus of papaverine is given and an infusion is started at 0.5–1 mg per minute. The infusion catheter is sutured in place, and the patient is taken for operative revascularization. The papaverine infusion is usually terminated when the remaining portions of bowel have been determined to be viable and the patient's cardiovascular status has been optimized, or when a repeat arteriogram excludes persistent mesenteric vasoconstriction. Systemic anticoagulation is initiated as soon as possible to reduce the incidence of recurrent embolic events.

Because bowel ischemia can progress rapidly to bowel infarction, there are few indications for transcatheter fibrinolytic therapy for acute mesenteric arterial emboli. Yet, thrombolytic therapy may be used cautiously in patients with short vascular occlusions and adequate distal intestinal collateral circulation. Most cases involving the successful use of thrombolytic agents have been in hemodynamically stable patients without signs of bowel infarction (9,10).

The exact role of thrombolysis in the treatment of acute mesenteric ischemia secondary to an embolus should be evaluated on a case-by-case basis. It appears that thrombolytic agents can be used in a very select group of patients who do not have peritoneal signs or an elevated lactic acid level. If thrombolytic therapy is instituted, direct intrathrombus infusion is recommended. However, with reestablishment of flow, sudden release of ischemic byproducts into the systemic circulation can lead to ARDS, multiple organ failure, and death.

Nonocclusive Mesenteric Ischemia (NOMI)

Nonocclusive mesenteric vasoconstriction is responsible for 20–30% of cases of AMI (2) and carries a particularly high mortality rate (5). Splanchnic vasoconstriction usually results from a period of systemic hypotension. The vasoconstriction persists even after the cause for hypotension has been corrected. Some drugs, such as digitalis and dopamine, predispose a patient to developing nonocclusive mesenteric vasoconstriction.

Angiographic findings of NOMI include diffuse arterial vasospasm, impaired filling of distal arterial branches, markedly diminished arterial flow with reflux of contrast from the SMA into the aorta, extremely delayed or incomplete filling of the mesenteric veins, and a marked improvement in mesenteric perfusion following administration of 45–60 mg of papaverine into the SMA (Figure 22–2).

In the absence of intestinal infarction, NOMI is best treated without surgery and stabilization of the patient's cardiovascular status. Following a bolus dose of papaverine, an infusion is instituted via a catheter placed in the

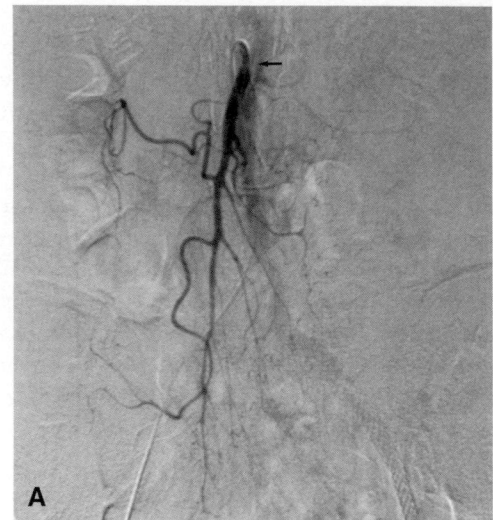

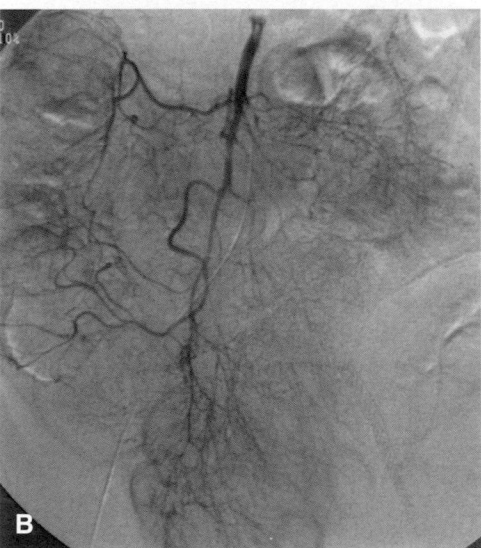

Figure 22–2 A 71-year-old patient with hypertensive cardiomyopathy and recent myocardial infarction is referred for evaluation of acute abdominal pain. **A.** Selective superior mesenteric angiogram shows no focal obstructive lesion, but there is severe pruning of the distal mesenteric branches and poor capillary and venous filling. **B.** A second superior mesenteric angiogram obtained after 24 hours of resuscitation and continuous papaverine infusion via the SMA demonstrates a dramatic improvement in arterial filling bowel perfusion. Note the reflux of contrast into the aorta on the first angiogram (*arrow in A*), which has resolved after the intra-arterial papaverine infusion.

SMA. The infusion is continued for approximately 24 hours. If the patient becomes asymptomatic, the infusion is changed to normal saline for 1–2 hours. Repeat angiography is performed whenever there are any concerns. When clinical symptoms or angiographic findings persist, the papaverine infusion is continued until all signs and symptoms of mesenteric ischemia have resolved. Nonocclusive mesenteric vasoconstriction usually resolves in 1–2 days, as long as the precipitating event has been corrected and the cardiovascular status optimized. If peritoneal signs develop, an exploratory laparotomy is performed to assess bowel viability. Papaverine infusion is continued throughout the surgical and immediate postoperative period to maximize bowel perfusion.

Acute Thrombosis

Acute mesenteric arterial thrombosis usually occurs in patients with an underlying atherosclerotic lesion. A history of intestinal angina may be elicited in up to 50% of cases (2). In contrast to the abrupt onset of symptoms associated with an embolus to the SMA, abdominal pain resulting from acute mesenteric arterial thrombosis may be more insidious.

Angiographic findings reflect the more chronic nature of the obstruction with demonstration of collateral vessels reconstituting distal SMA branches in many cases. The SMA is typically occluded within 1–2 cm of its origin, while an intraluminal filling defect or defined meniscus is usually lacking (11).

In the presence of peritoneal signs, the patient should undergo exploratory laporotomy and aortomesenteric bypass grafting or a thromboendarterectomy. Preoperative papaverine infusion is used whenever possible, but is usually not feasible because of the proximal location of the occlusion. The primary goal in acute SMA thrombosis is to reestablish flow to the SMA as quickly as possible. Following revascularization, nonviable portions of bowel are removed. A second-look operation is usually performed within 24 hours. Postoperative vasodilator infusion should be weighed against the risks of catheterizing a vessel on which surgery has been recently performed.

In the absence of peritoneal signs, endovascular revascularization has been performed using thrombolytic therapy and balloon dilatation (9). An acute deterioration in chronic ischemic symptoms suggests the presence of fresh clot superimposed on a chronic atherosclerotic lesion. A thrombolytic infusion into the occlusion will therefore minimize the chance for distal embolization of acute thrombotic material. Following unmasking of the underlying lesion with thrombolysis, balloon dilatation should be performed. Use of a vascular stent will likely improve the results in the treatment of total occlusions and may reduce the risk of distal embolization. If the patient develops peritoneal signs during the course of an endovascular intervention, the procedure should be completed as quickly as possible and the patient should undergo surgical exploration.

The current role for endovascular therapy for acute mesenteric arterial thrombosis is not well-defined. Patients on steroids or narcotic analgesics or those with an altered mental status may be difficult to evaluate for peritoneal irritation. In this patient population, the lactic acid level may be a better predictor for the presence of infarcted bowel. In the presence of peritoneal signs or a moderately elevated lactic acid level, surgical exploration is recommended. If peritoneal signs are absent and the lactic acid level is normal, endovascular intervention may be undertaken in specific cases. The risks of thrombolysis and balloon dilatation/stenting in a patient with AMI should be weighed against the risks of surgery. Keep in mind, mortality associated with surgery for AMI approaches 50% (2,5).

Mesenteric Venous Thrombosis

Mesenteric venous thrombosis accounts for less than 5% of all cases of AMI. The most common conditions associated with mesenteric venous thrombosis are portal hypertension, a hypercoagulable state, trauma, abdominal inflammatory disease, oral contraceptives, and prior surgery on the portal venous system (12). With acute mesenteric venous thrombosis and inadequate venous collateral formation, intestinal mucosa edema will develop and arterial hypoperfusion results.

The angiographic findings of mesenteric venous thrombosis include increased arterial resistance to flow; vasospasm of the mesenteric arteries with persistence of the arterial phase; prolonged and intense mucosal staining of the bowel wall; and lack of opacification of the mesenteric veins or identification of thrombus within the mesenteric vein, portal vein, or both.

Initial therapeutic efforts should be directed toward stabilizing the patient's cardiovascular status with adequate volume replacement to make up for losses of fluid into the intestinal lumen. Immediate operation with resection of nonviable bowel is required in patients with peritoneal signs, because, without surgical intervention, mortality rates approach 100% (2,12).

Although several authors have advocated venous thrombectomy, animal studies have documented that thrombectomy more than two hours after venous occlusion does not improve the overall prognosis (13). Following resection of necrotic bowel segments, recurrent thrombosis of uninvolved segments of bowel occurs in up to 29% of patients (14). Therefore, preoperative and postoperative anticoagulation are highly recommended. If mesenteric arterial vasoconstriction is documented, infusion of intra-arterial papaverine may also be useful.

In the absence of peritoneal signs or extensive submucosal hemorrhage, mesenteric venous thrombosis has been treated successfully using systemic, transarterial, or direct infusion of thrombolytic agents (15–17). With direct access into the mesenteric venous system via the transhepatic (Figure 22–3) or transjugular approach, mechanical thrombectomy, thrombolysis, PTA, and stenting have been reported with documented success (18). Attempts at endovascular revascularization should be tempered with the knowledge that patients with minimal clinical findings related to mesenteric venous occlusion usually do quite well with anticoagulation and supportive care alone. Most of these patients will require long-term anticoagulation.

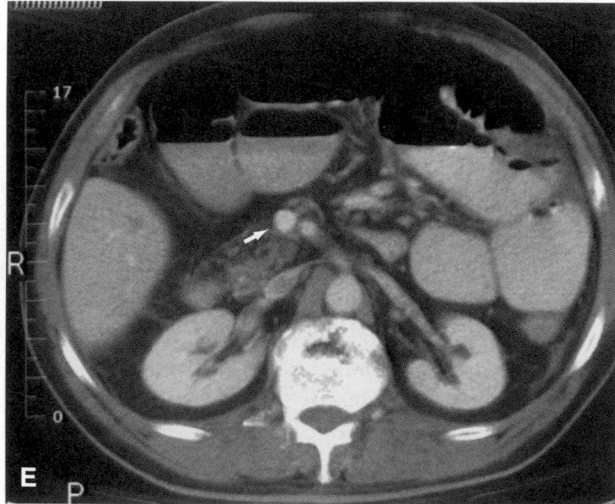

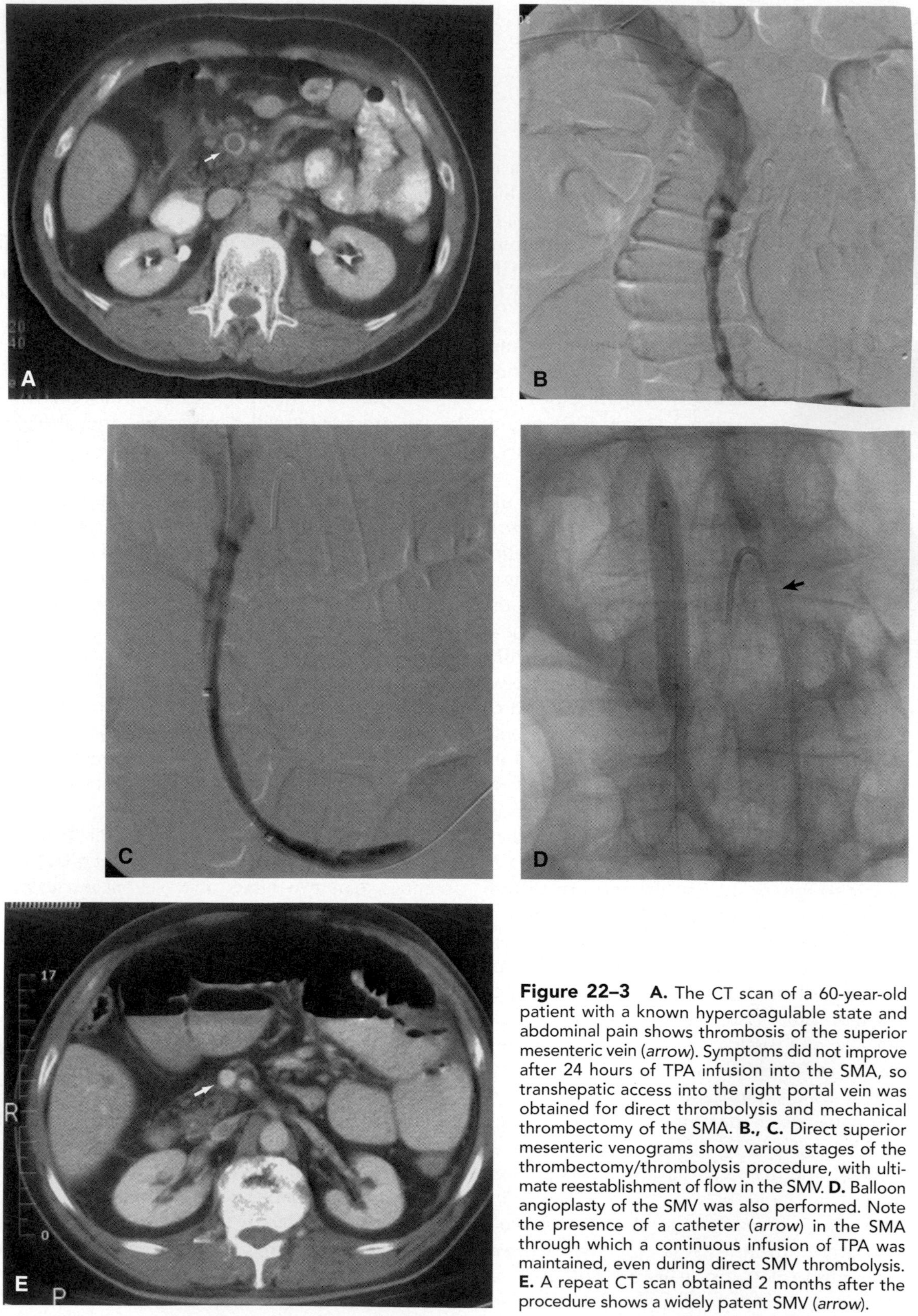

Figure 22–3   A. The CT scan of a 60-year-old patient with a known hypercoagulable state and abdominal pain shows thrombosis of the superior mesenteric vein (*arrow*). Symptoms did not improve after 24 hours of TPA infusion into the SMA, so transhepatic access into the right portal vein was obtained for direct thrombolysis and mechanical thrombectomy of the SMA. **B., C.** Direct superior mesenteric venograms show various stages of the thrombectomy/thrombolysis procedure, with ultimate reestablishment of flow in the SMV. **D.** Balloon angioplasty of the SMV was also performed. Note the presence of a catheter (*arrow*) in the SMA through which a continuous infusion of TPA was maintained, even during direct SMV thrombolysis. **E.** A repeat CT scan obtained 2 months after the procedure shows a widely patent SMV (*arrow*).

Aortic Dissection

About 5% of patients develop mesenteric ischemia as a complication related to an aortic dissection. The operative mortality in these patients approaches 90% (19). Recently, endovascular techniques have been used to treat mesenteric ischemia in the setting of an aortic dissection (20,21).

Mesenteric ischemia can result when the dissection flap extends directly into the SMA, resulting in compromised perfusion to the bowel. Dake et al. used stents to reapproximate the dissection flap against the vessel wall and reestablish adequate blood flow to the bowel (21). Balloon PTA alone usually is ineffective because elastic recoil of the flap occurs when the balloon is deflated (Figure 22–4).

With an aortic dissection, the true lumen usually communicates with the false lumen via multiple fenestrations in the dissection flap. Although the blood flow and pressure in the true lumen usually exceed that in the false lumen, occasionally the opposite occurs. Mesenteric ischemia may develop when the pressure and flow in the aortic lumen (either true or false) that supplies the SMA is not enough to meet the physiological demands of the small bowel. Inadequate exchange of flow between the two lumens occurs as a result of the absence of a distal dissection "reentry" site, insufficient fenestrations in the dissection flap, or compression of one lumen by the other lumen. Creation of de novo fenestrations and enlarging naturally occurring fenestrations has been performed by inflating PTA balloons (8–20 mm diameters) directly across the dissection flap (20,21). Percutaneous fenestration usually is performed using fluoroscopic and intravascular ultrasound guidance. Angiography and intra-arterial pressure measurements should be obtained from both lumens to define the anatomy and hemodynamics before balloon fenestration. Because the septum may be fibrous and thick, particularly with more chronic dissections, the back end of a 0.018–inch guide wire, a 21-gauge transseptal needle, or a Rosch-Uchida needle (Cook, Inc.) have been used to traverse the dissection flap. Hemodynamic pressures in both aortic channels are monitored to assess the results and to determine whether additional fenestrations are needed.

Summary of Acute Mesenteric Ischemia

Patients suspected of having AMI should undergo prompt diagnostic cathetered angiography. Once the diagnosis of AMI is confirmed, intra-arterial papaverine (whenever possible) should be infused before, during, and after surgery. The goal of therapy is to minimize the amount of bowel infarction. In the absence of peritoneal signs, catheter-directed thrombolysis, possibly with PTA/stenting, can be used in specific cases of acute emboli, arterial thrombosis, and mesenteric venous thrombosis. The risks of bleeding from infarcted bowel and distal embolization of partially lysed clot, as well as the time required for an effective endovascular intervention should be weighed in the decision process. Following thrombolysis of an acute arterial thrombosis, the underlying stenotic lesion should be treated with PTA/stenting. In patients with a small volume of nonocclusive arterial clot or mesenteric venous thrombosis and minimal or no symptoms, anticoagulation and supportive therapy may be adequate. Mechanical thrombectomy (in conjunction with thrombolysis, PTA, and/or stenting) is a consideration in patients with moderate symptoms resulting from mesenteric venous thrombosis, as long as bowel infarction or moderate to severe lactic acidosis is not present. In patients with mesenteric ischemia related to an aortic dissection, innovative techniques involving the use of intravascular ultrasound, balloon fenestration, and vascular stents have shown promise.

CHRONIC MESENTERIC ISCHEMIA (CMI)

Despite the relatively frequent involvement of the abdominal aorta and mesenteric arteries with atherosclerosis, CMI is relatively uncommon. The rarity of CMI is related to the rich mesenteric collateral circulation. Classical teaching has been that occlusive disease must involve at least two of the three main visceral arteries in order to produce symptoms. However, it is now fairly well accepted that obstruction of one, two, or any combination of the three vessels can result in CMI, and symptoms often do not correlate with the severity of angiographic findings.

The classic symptom of CMI is intestinal angina, or postprandial abdominal pain. The pain usually occurs within the first hour of food intake and lasts 1–2 hours. Many patients also suffer from weight loss because of food avoidance. Other symptoms include nausea, vomiting, and diarrhea, which are neither common nor specific for this disease entity.

Atherosclerosis is by far the most common cause of occlusive mesenteric vascular disease. However, other etiologies, such as fibromuscular dysplasia and vasculitides also have been implicated as causes of CMI. Intimal hyperplasia, usually seen at surgical anastomoses, can lead to narrowing of bypass grafts to mesenteric vessels, resulting in recurrent intestinal ischemia.

Diagnostic Evaluation

The definitive diagnostic test for the evaluation of patients suspected of having CMI is conventional catheter angiography. Angiography begins with biplane abdominal aortography. The lateral view provides the most information about obstructions at the origins of the visceral vessels—the most common site of atherosclerotic lesions. Depending on the results of aortography, selective catheterization of one or more of the mesenteric branches may be required. Often,

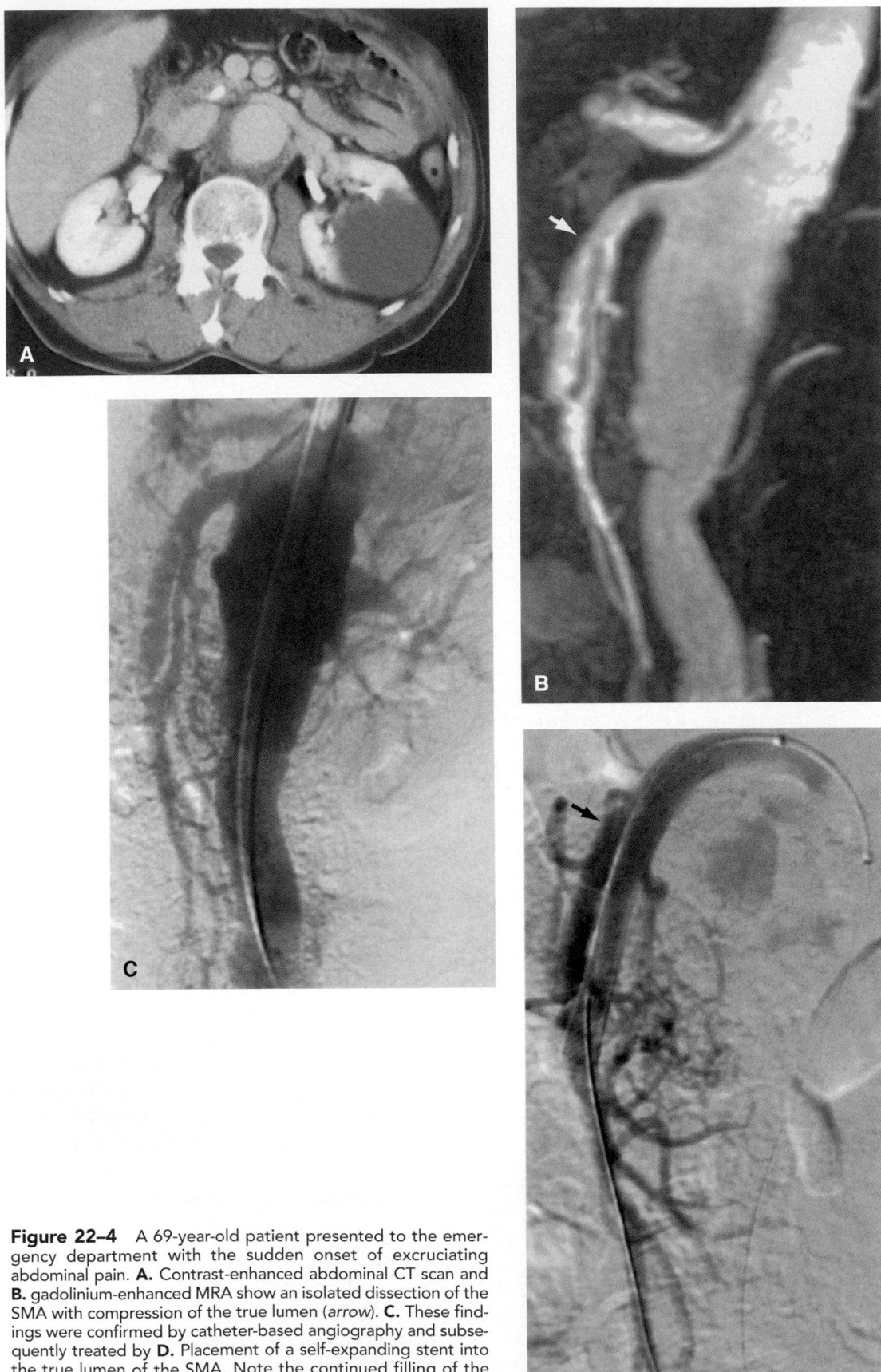

Figure 22–4   A 69-year-old patient presented to the emergency department with the sudden onset of excruciating abdominal pain. **A.** Contrast-enhanced abdominal CT scan and **B.** gadolinium-enhanced MRA show an isolated dissection of the SMA with compression of the true lumen (*arrow*). **C.** These findings were confirmed by catheter-based angiography and subsequently treated by **D.** Placement of a self-expanding stent into the true lumen of the SMA. Note the continued filling of the false lumen (*arrowhead*). The patient's symptoms resolved after stent placement.

angiography is supplemented with translesion pressure measurements whenever there is doubt about the hemodynamic significance of a stenotic lesion. Lesions are considered significant when narrowing of the cross-sectional area of the artery is equal to or greater than 70%. Stenoses are also considered significant when the cross-sectional narrowing is 50–70% and is associated with a peak-to-peak systolic pressure gradient of greater than 20 mm Hg. Lesions of less than 50% are usually not flow limiting. Translesion pressure gradient measurements can also be useful to guide endovascular interventions, such as in the need to place a stent following angioplasty.

Though catheter angiography remains the gold standard for diagnosing CMI, recent advances in noninvasive imaging techniques have had a major impact on the workup of these patients. Today, patients suspected of having CMI initially undergo a noninvasive screening test. Angiography is reserved for patients with equivocal noninvasive findings or when surgical or percutaneous revascularization is being considered. Noninvasive diagnostic tests include duplex sonography, computed tomography angiography (CTA), and magnetic resonance angiography (MRA).

Of these, duplex sonography is the most widely available and least expensive screening test. Although duplex is the only noninvasive technique that provides hemodynamic information, significant limitations hamper it. Diagnostic studies are often difficult to obtain because of patient habitus, shadowing from bowel gas, and aortic pulsatility (22,23). In addition, operator dependence and the lack of uniform criteria for the diagnosis of hemodynamically significant stenoses limit the reproducibility of sonographic examinations. Blebea and colleagues compared the use of contrast-enhanced duplex ultrasound to duplex ultrasound alone for the evaluation of mesenteric arteries in 17 patients with symptoms of chronic mesenteric ischemia (23). Including the aorta, the study consisted of 68 vessels. Duplex ultrasound alone identified 38 of 48 normal vessels (79% accuracy), and ultrasound with contrast identified 44 of 48 normal vessels (90% accuracy). Duplex ultrasound alone identified 5 of 11 stenoses ≥50% and 6 of 9 occlusions (45% and 67% accuracy, respectively). The use of contrast-enhanced ultrasound improved the diagnosis of stenoses ≥50% to 7 of 11 (78% accuracy) but did not alter the detection rate of vessel occlusions. Although the ultrasound studies were performed by experienced sonographers, 12 of 68 vessels were not visualized with duplex alone, and 3 of 68 vessels were not visualized with contrast-enhanced ultrasound. Despite the small sample size in this report, contrast-enhanced ultrasound appears to improve the visualization of mesenteric arteries and may improve the diagnosis of mesenteric arterial stenosis. However, contrast-enhanced ultrasound is not widely used, and the results of this study reemphasize the current problems that exist with duplex sonography in evaluating the visceral arteries.

CT has been used in evaluating the abdominal aorta, renal arteries, and mesenteric arteries. With the advent of multidetector row CT, routine studies can be performed much faster and with thinner collimation than with single-detector CT. The consequent improvement in temporal and spatial resolution has had a dramatic impact on the quality of CT angiograms. Rapid scanning eliminates respiratory motion artifact and enables imaging during both arterial and venous enhancement phases. Narrow beam collimation (0.5–1 mm) reduces volume averaging and improves visualization of small vessel branches. A direct comparison of CTA and catheter-based angiography for the evaluation of the mesenteric arteries has not been reported. However, CTA compares favorably with catheter angiography for the evaluation of renal artery stenosis (24,25). Additionally, CT allows for the evaluation of secondary signs of bowel ischemia, such as bowel wall thickening, submucosal hemorrhage, abnormal enhancement, mesenteric stranding, or pneumotosis. Water may be used as a low-attenuation oral contrast agent without limiting the evaluation of mesenteric arteries (26,27). CT angiography has the distinct advantage over MRA of being able to evaluate the patency of metallic stents, which is useful in patients with recurrent disease following intravascular stenting (Figure 22–5).

Unlike CTA, MRA allows for noninvasive imaging without the administration of nephrotoxic contrast agents or exposure to radiation. The advent of ultra-fast gradient systems in modern MR scanners and their application to gadolinium-enhanced MRA have enabled high-resolution breath-hold imaging and have transformed the technique into a robust and reliable diagnostic tool for evaluating the mesenteric vasculature. Indeed, gadolinium-enhanced MRA must be considered the noninvasive diagnostic test of choice for patients with suspected atherosclerotic narrowing of the main visceral arteries. The spatial resolution is still inferior to conventional angiography and does not allow reliable evaluation of the distal branch vessels. However, because the large majority of atherosclerotic lesions involve the origins of the vessels from the aorta, MRA is a very useful technique for diagnosing CMI. Moreover, many patients who have isolated involvement of distal branch vessels are not candidates for revascularization. Several reports have validated the efficacy of gadolinium-enhanced MRA in the diagnosis of disease of the proximal mesenteric vessels, with a sensitivity and specificity exceeding 90% (28, 29). Carlos et al. reported the interobserver variability in the evaluation of CMI with gadolinium enhanced MRA utilizing catheter-based angiography as the gold standard (30). Two readers, blinded to the results of catheter-based angiography, reviewed gadolinium-enhanced MRAs in 26 patients. The relative sensitivity and specificity compared well to catheter angiography with a cumulative accuracy of 0.98 with a 95% confidence interval of 0.91–1.0 for lesions equal to or greater than 75%, and 0.94 with a 95% confidence interval of 0.84–0.98 for lesions ranging from 50% to 75%.

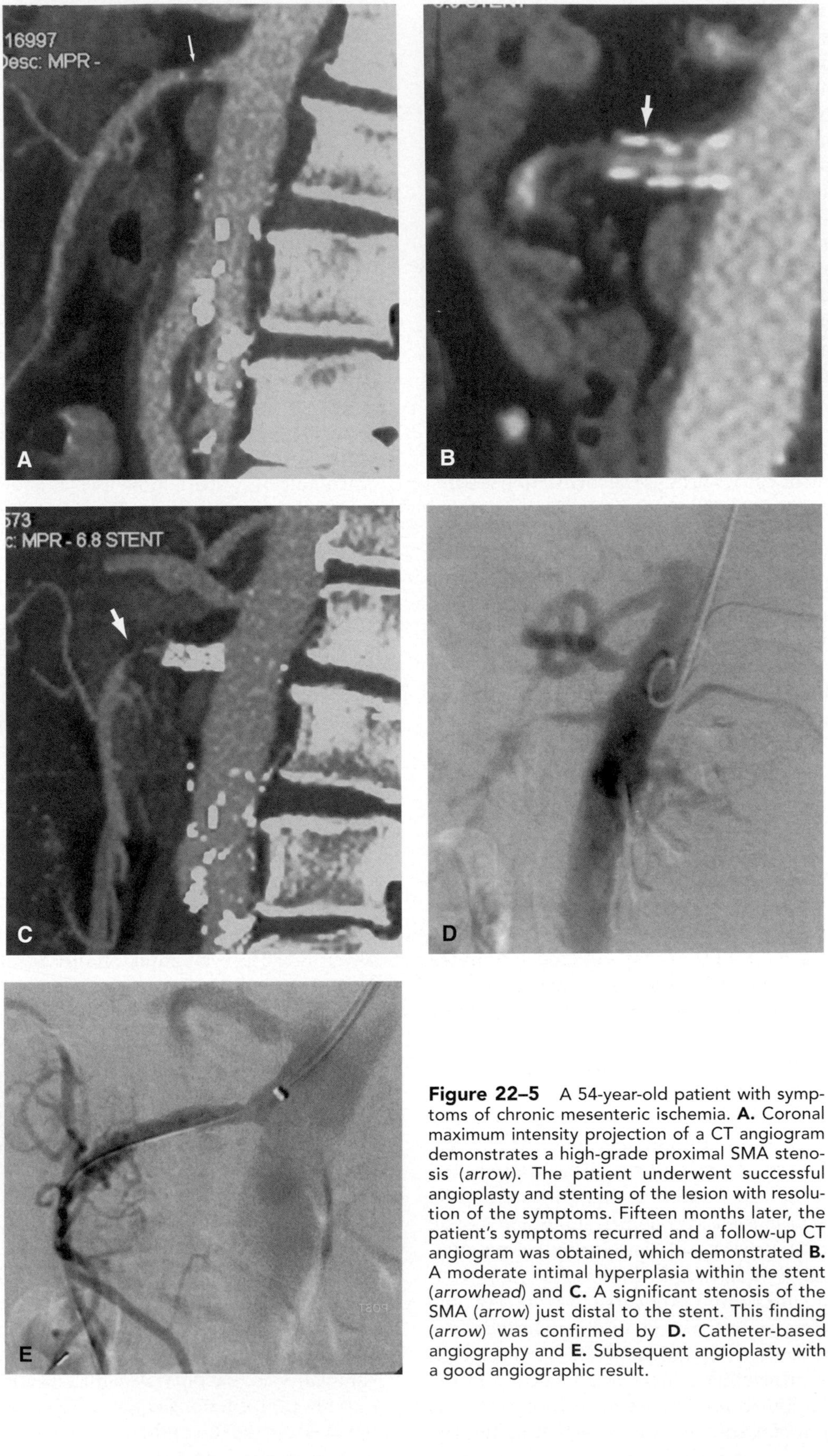

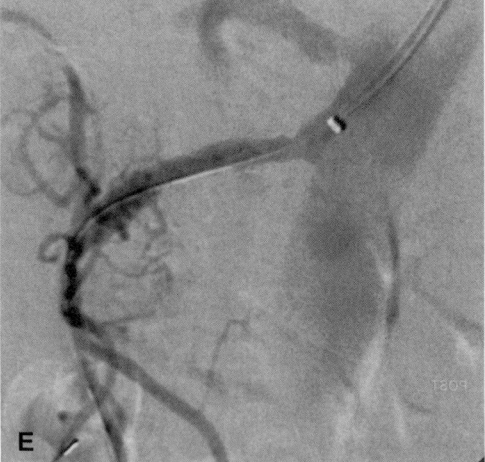

Figure 22–5 A 54-year-old patient with symptoms of chronic mesenteric ischemia. **A.** Coronal maximum intensity projection of a CT angiogram demonstrates a high-grade proximal SMA stenosis (*arrow*). The patient underwent successful angioplasty and stenting of the lesion with resolution of the symptoms. Fifteen months later, the patient's symptoms recurred and a follow-up CT angiogram was obtained, which demonstrated **B.** A moderate intimal hyperplasia within the stent (*arrowhead*) and **C.** A significant stenosis of the SMA (*arrow*) just distal to the stent. This finding (*arrow*) was confirmed by **D.** Catheter-based angiography and **E.** Subsequent angioplasty with a good angiographic result.

Perhaps the most powerful feature of gadolinium-enhanced MRA is the ability to postprocess the three-dimensional data set, enabling the unfolding of tortuous anatomy, facilitating the profiling of vessel origins, and generating images with a remarkable resemblance to digital subtraction angiography (Figure 22–6).

Treatment

Patients with signs and symptoms consistent with intestinal angina who have a hemodynamically significant stenosis in one or more of the mesenteric arteries should undergo revascularization. The goals of revascularization are to relieve symptoms, improve nutritional status, and prevent intestinal infarction. Surgery has been the traditional approach to CMI. The nature of the surgical procedure is determined by the surgeon's experience, the anatomic distribution of the disease, and the institutional bias, but usually it consists of transaortic endarterectomy or aortomesenteric grafting (Figure 22–6). Reported overall technical success rates are 90–98%, with long-term clinical success rates of 61–100%. Morbidity ranges from 13 to 54%, with a 30-day mortality of 0–8% (31–35). Surgery for CMI classically involves revascularization of multiple mesenteric vessels. The rationale for this approach is to establish as much independent circulation as possible should one of the grafts fail. The celiac and superior mesenteric arteries are the most commonly revascularized vessels. However, Foley and coworkers recently showed comparable results for revascularization of the SMA alone in patients who had additional visceral arteries available for bypass grafting and suggest that "complete" revascularization is unnecessary (36).

Improvements in balloon catheters, guide wires, and stent technology have allowed for endovascular therapy to have an increasing role in the treatment of patients with CMI. Recent data suggest that complication and mortality rates associated with PTA and stent placement can be minimized, and survival and clinical success rates comparable to surgical revascularization can be achieved (37–39) In addition, endovascular procedures rarely compromise subsequent surgical intervention in cases of technical or clinical failure. Treatment of chronic mesenteric arterial occlusions is technically more challenging than that of stenotic lesions and is typically reserved for surgical revascularization. However, short chronic occlusions can be successfully treated percutaneously (9,39,40), especially with the availability of intravascular stents (Figure 22–7).

Recently, Kasirajan et al. reported on a comparative study of surgical revascularization versus percutaneous angioplasty and stenting for the treatment of CMI (41). In this series, 28 patients were treated over a 3.5-year period with angioplasty alone (18%) or angioplasty and stenting (82%). Results were compared with a previously published series of 85 patients treated with surgical revascularization. Statistical comparison showed no significant difference between the two groups with respect to morbidity, death, and recurrent stenosis. However, the PTA/stenting group had a significantly higher incidence of recurrent symptoms. Based on these findings, the authors concluded that surgical revascularization should be offered preferentially to patients with CMI who are surgical candidates. Apart from the fundamentally questionable validity of a nonrandomized controlled comparison in this context, a mortality rate of 10.7%, length of hospital stay of 5 days, and symptomatic recurrence rate of 28% at 1 year for patients undergoing endovascular treatment seem excessive, and the results do not compare favorably with other studies of endovascular treatment for CMI. Nonetheless, this is one of very few studies that has attempted to compare surgery to endovascular therapy for CMI, and it is a useful series for the results of the endovascular treatment arm alone. In addition, the recommendation of surgical revascularization as the treatment of choice in patients deemed fit for surgery has been echoed by other investigators (35).

Prophylactic PTA of asymptomatic visceral artery stenosis remains controversial because of the adequacy of collateral arterial flow. However, the development of mesenteric ischemia after reconstructive abdominal aortic surgery is associated with a high mortality rate (42,43). Therefore, prophylactic treatment of compromised visceral arterial circulation may be indicated in preparation for more complex surgical repair of the abdominal aorta. In a long-term follow-up series (38), the authors studied four patients who were treated with mesenteric PTA for this indication. Two of these patients had significant disease of the SMA, IMA, abdominal aorta, and the common and internal iliac arteries. The SMA was balloon dilated in both patients because of concern about the development of mesenteric ischemia following an aortobifemoral bypass graft. The third patient had 100% occlusion of the SMA, 90% stenosis of the celiac, and 10% stenosis of the IMA, as well as a large abdominal aortic aneurysm. The patient underwent prophylactic PTA of the celiac artery. The abdominal aortic aneurysm was repaired surgically without sequelae. The fourth patient developed complete occlusion at the site of an ostial IMA stenosis following PTA of the abdominal aorta. Balloon dilatation of the IMA was performed to reestablish flow in the IMA distribution. None of these four patients developed signs or symptoms of mesenteric ischemia during a follow-up period ranging from 7 to 73 months.

Mesenteric PTA in patients with symptoms atypical for CMI or with nonostial stenosis of the celiac artery appears to be less effective. Extrinsic compression of the celiac artery resulting from the median arcuate ligament (MAL) does not respond favorably to PTA. The placement of a balloon-expandable stent may lead to collapse or distortion of the stent resulting from extrinsic compression and, possibly, abrupt occlusion of the artery. In addition, symptoms secondary to MAL compression may be related to pressure on the celiac ganglion. Therefore, surgical therapy remains

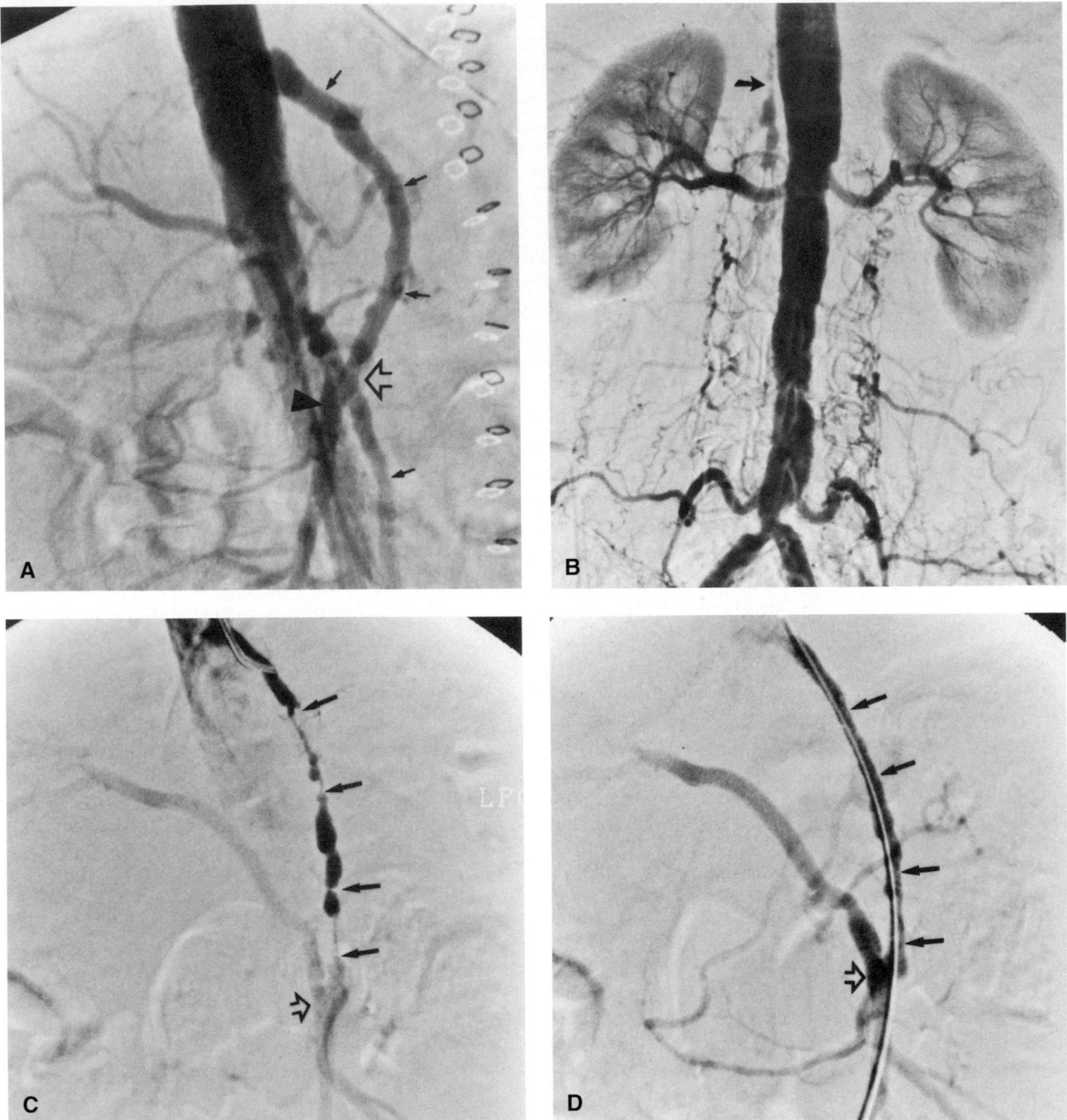

Figure 22–6 A 61-year-old woman with postprandial abdominal pain and weight loss had a diagnostic arteriogram that revealed complete occlusion of the celiac artery, SMA, and IMA with reconstitution of these vessels via internal iliac artery collaterals. **A.** The patient underwent bypass surgery and a postoperative arteriogram shows the side-to-side anastomosis (*open arrow*) between the venous bypass graft (*small arrows*) and the SMA (*arrowhead*) with extention of the graft to the IMA in an end-to-side fashion. She was asymptomatic for 12 months. **B.** The patient presented 15 months after her bypass surgery with a 3-month history of recurrent symptoms, a 10-pound weight loss, and an abdominal bruit. An aortogram revealed diffuse disease of the bypass graft (*arrow*) with no antegrade flow into the SMA or IMA. The internal iliac arteries reconsitituted the mesenteric circulation via collaterals. **C.** Selective catheterization of the venous bypass graft demonstrates diffuse disease of the venous conduit (*closed arrows*) to the level of the side-to-side anastomosis with the SMA (*open arrow*). **D.** After PTA with a 5-mm-diameter balloon, the venous bypass graft is widely patent (*closed arrows*) and the anastomosis to the SMA (*open arrow*) has a satisfactory appearance. The patient's symptoms resolved and she remained asymptomatic for 8 weeks of follow-up.

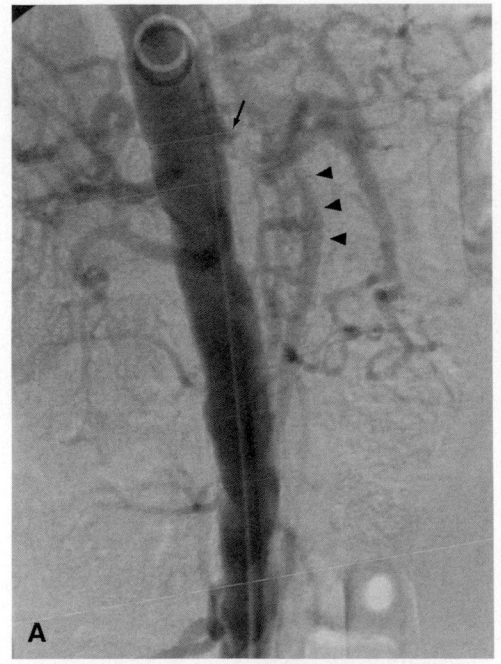

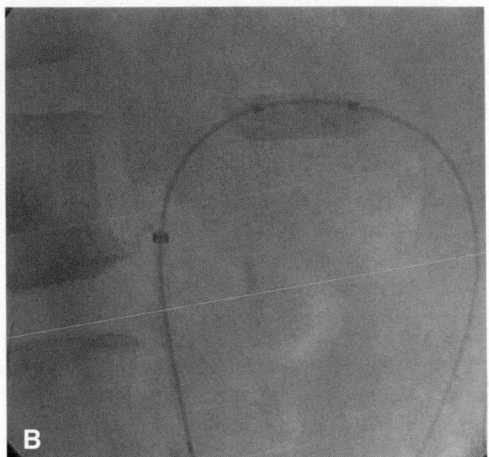

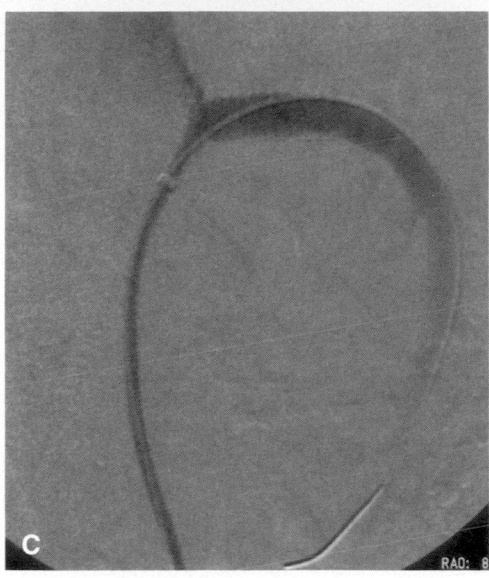

Figure 22–7   A 57-year-old patient presents with intestinal angina. **A.** Lateral aortogram demonstrates proximal occlusion of the SMA, with filling of a small stump at the origin (*arrow*) and reconstitution approximately 3 cm distally (*arrowheads*). Note the high-grade ostial IMA stenosis. **B., C.** The SMA occlusion was successfully crossed and stented with an excellent angiographic result.

the treatment of choice for patients with MAL syndrome (44) (Figure 22–8). Finally, occult abdominal or retroperitoneal malignancies may mimic the symptoms of CMI. Therefore, an immediate technical or clinical failure of endovascular treatment for mesenteric artery stenosis should raise the suspicion of extrinsic compression or an occult malignancy.

Endovascular Techniques

Technical Considerations

Continuous improvements have been made to the technique of visceral artery PTA and stenting since its inception, and changes will likely continue as the technology matures.

The technical aspects of endovascular revascularization of the visceral arteries do not differ substantially from those of the renal arteries. The average size of the celiac and superior mesenteric arteries is slightly larger than that of renal arteries. Therefore, it is recommended that the operator use a 0.035-inch guide wire platform for the procedure, similar to an iliac artery intervention, because of the likelihood of requiring balloon and stent sizes up to 7 or 8 mm. When treating the IMA, which is usually a smaller caliber vessel, a 0.014 or 0.018–inch guide wire platform may be preferable because of the reduced chance of complications that include vessel trauma or thromboembolic phenomena. Although guide wire "purchase" in mesenteric arteries is often better than in the renal arteries, the chance is greater of requiring a brachial approach because of the sharp angulation of the

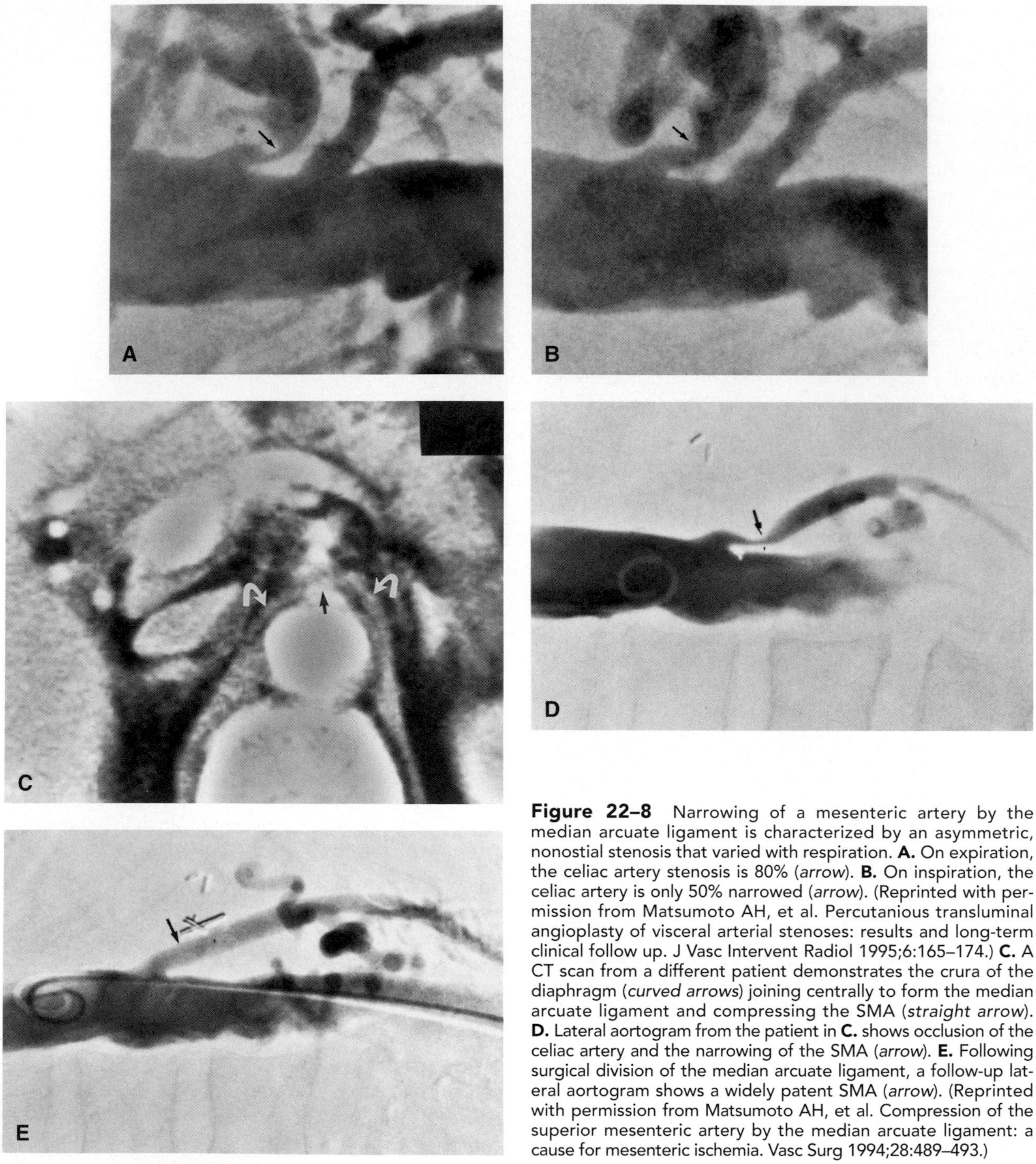

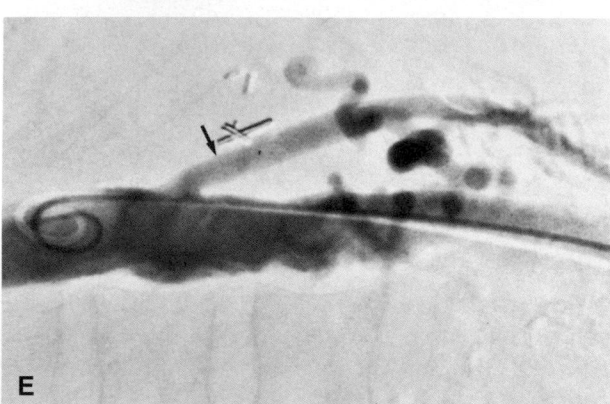

Figure 22–8 Narrowing of a mesenteric artery by the median arcuate ligament is characterized by an asymmetric, nonostial stenosis that varied with respiration. **A.** On expiration, the celiac artery stenosis is 80% (*arrow*). **B.** On inspiration, the celiac artery is only 50% narrowed (*arrow*). (Reprinted with permission from Matsumoto AH, et al. Percutanious transluminal angioplasty of visceral arterial stenoses: results and long-term clinical follow up. J Vasc Intervent Radiol 1995;6:165–174.) **C.** A CT scan from a different patient demonstrates the crura of the diaphragm (*curved arrows*) joining centrally to form the median arcuate ligament and compressing the SMA (*straight arrow*). **D.** Lateral aortogram from the patient in **C.** shows occlusion of the celiac artery and the narrowing of the SMA (*arrow*). **E.** Following surgical division of the median arcuate ligament, a follow-up lateral aortogram shows a widely patent SMA (*arrow*). (Reprinted with permission from Matsumoto AH, et al. Compression of the superior mesenteric artery by the median arcuate ligament: a cause for mesenteric ischemia. Vasc Surg 1994;28:489–493.)

vessel origin, particularly in patients who have experienced severe weight loss. Indeed, in the published series of patients mentioned earlier, the brachial artery approach was more common than the femoral artery approach. Nonetheless, with the improved flexibility and trackability of modern catheter and stent systems, a higher proportion of the patients can now be treated via the femoral approach, which will spare patients the risks of a brachial artery puncture. The impact of new endovascular technologies, including distal embolic protection devices, cutting balloons, and drug-eluting stents, is, at the present time, unexplored with regard to mesenteric arterial interventions, but it will likely mirror that of renovascular interventions.

Results

Percutaneous transluminal angioplasty (PTA) of atherosclerotic stenosis in mesenteric arteries was first described in

1980 (45). Since then, the literature has consisted predominantly of small series and case reports (37–41,46–59). A meta-analysis of the 10 largest published series on mesenteric PTA (107 total patients) reveals a mean initial technical success rate (per patient) of 84%. Excluding the technical failures, the mean initial clinical success rate was 95%, with long-term primary and secondary clinical success rates of 75% and 90%, respectively. The morbidity rate was 7%, with a mortality rate of 4%. Mean follow-up varied between nine and 28 months (37).

The largest published series of endovascular treatment for CMI consists of 47 vessels in 33 patients who were treated over an 18-year period (38). The patient population consisted of 12 men and 21 women whose ages ranged from 40 to 89 years (mean age of 63 years). Risk factors for atherosclerosis included tobacco use (52%), hypertension (58%), coronary artery disease (52%), and diabetes (9%). Eighty-eight percent of the patients presented with the classic symptoms of postprandial abdominal pain. Seventy percent of patients presented with weight loss ranging from 6 to 80 pounds (median of 28 pounds). A "fear of food" was elicited in 49% of the patients. Forty-nine percent of the 33 patients (16) had endoscopy, CT, or biopsy results consistent with intestinal ischemia. Twenty-one patients underwent PTA alone in 32 vessels, and 12 patients underwent PTA and stenting in 15 vessels. Etiologies of the stenoses were atherosclerosis in 22 (67%), fibromuscular dysplasia in one (3%), intimal hyperplasia in a surgical bypass graft in three (9%), and median arcuate ligament in combination with atherosclerosis or fibromuscular dysplasia in seven patients (21%). No attempts were made to treat total arterial occlusions in this series.

The initial technical success rate for PTA was 81% (per vessel) and 100% for PTA and stenting (per vessel). The primary clinical success rate per patient was 82% (29 of 33 patients) for complete resolution of symptoms and 6% (2 of 33 patients) for partial, but significant, improvement in symptoms. Four immediate clinical failures were encountered (12%). Two of the patients who were considered immediate clinical failures subsequently were found to have malignancies (pancreatic carcinoma and adenocarcinoma with metastasis to the porta hepatis). These malignancies were believed to be responsible for their symptoms of abdominal pain and weight loss. Both patients were treated before 1986, when CT scans were not obtained routinely as part of the initial evaluation. A third patient underwent a technically successful PTA of the celiac artery, with untreated total occlusions of the SMA and IMA. The patient experienced incomplete resolution of symptoms and subsequently underwent aortobifemoral bypass grafting for distal aortic and iliac occlusive disease. At the time of surgery, an IMA endarterectomy was also performed, and the patient's symptoms were completely resolved. The fourth immediate clinical failure occurred in a patient with complete occlusion of the celiac and inferior mesenteric arteries. An SMA stenosis, with characteristic appearance of median arcuate ligament compression, was treated with PTA without significant improvement in the stenosis. The patient underwent surgical release of the MAL with complete resolution of symptoms.

Follow-up data were available in all 29 patients who experienced an initial clinical benefit for the procedure. The mean duration of clinical follow-up was 38 months, with a range of 1 to 123 months. The median duration of follow-up was 25 months. Angiographic follow-up was obtained in 15 of the 29 patients (52%), at a mean of 20 months (1 to 99 months). Three patients were eventually lost to follow-up, but all three had a minimum follow-up of at least 20 months (a range of 20 to 35 months). All three of these patients were asymptomatic at the time of being lost to follow-up. Eight of the 29 patients died 2–117 months (mean of 46 months) after their procedure.

Of the 29 patients who experienced an initial clinical benefit from the procedure, five developed recurrent symptoms between 5 and 19 months. Four patients underwent repeat PTA with clinical improvement for a primary assisted success rate of 97% (28 of 29 patients). The fifth patient initially was treated with PTA for a 90% atherosclerotic stenosis of the celiac artery with superimposed MAL compression of the celiac artery. The procedure was a technical failure because of a 50% residual stenosis secondary to persistent MAL compression of the celiac artery. However, the patient's clinical symptoms did not resolve. Nineteen months after the procedure, the patient presented with recurrent symptoms and underwent surgical repair.

Including the patient encounters for the treatment of recurrent stenoses, 39 procedures were performed. Five (13%) major complications occurred; three were access site thromboses and two were hematomas that required further treatment. No episodes of acute mesenteric ischemia developed secondary to any of the procedures. The 30-day mortality rate was 0% (0 in 39 patient encounters).

In the 39 patient procedures, 34 brachial and 24 femoral accesses were used. Only one of the femoral access sites (4.2%) was associated with a major complication, and four of the 34 brachial punctures (11.8%) were associated with a major complication. In the 24 procedures in which PTA alone was used, four access site complications (19%) occurred. Three of these complications occurred during the era in which large balloon catheters (7 French to 8 French catheter shafts) were used. In the 15 procedures in which PTA and stenting were performed, only one major access site complication (6.7%) occurred.

Fifty-eight vessels were treated in the 39 patient encounters. With the initial 33 procedures, the celiac artery was treated 14 times, SMA 21 times, IMA nine times, and bypass grafts three times. For recurrent stenoses, 11 vessels were retreated in four patients (two patients were retreated once and two patients were retreated twice). The celiac artery, SMA, and IMA were retreated five times, five times, and one time, respectively. When evaluating the primary clinical success rate by the number of vessels initially treated,

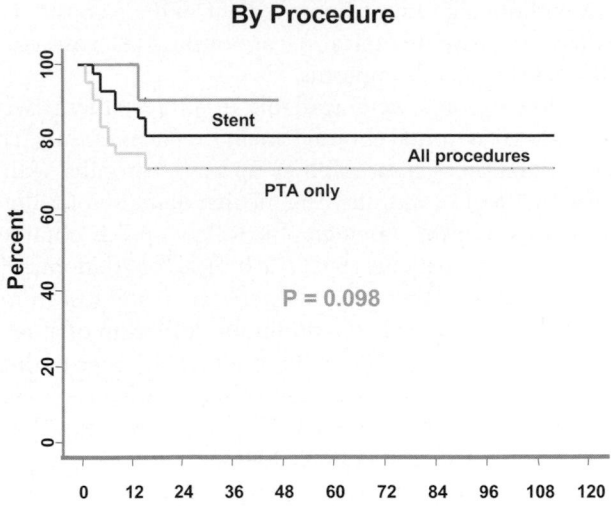

Figure 22–9   Primary long-term clinical success by procedure. (Reprinted with permission from Matsumoto AH, Angle JF, Spinosa DJ, et al. Percutaneous transluminal angioplasty and stenting in the treatment of chronic mesenteric ischemia: results and long-term follow-up. J Am Coll Surg 2002;194:22–31.)

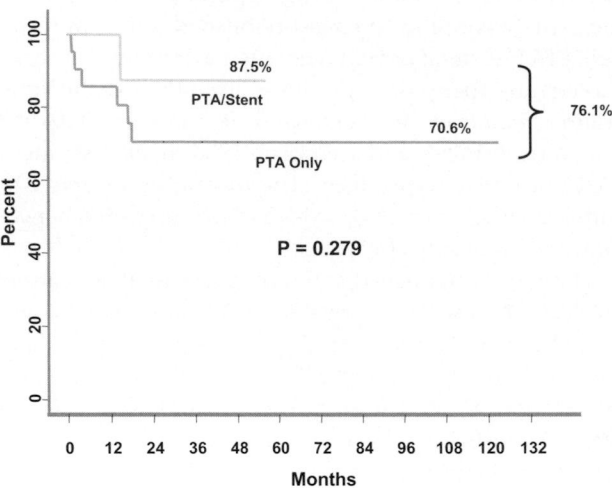

Figure 22–10   Survival by procedure. (Reprinted with permission from Matsumoto AH, Angle JF, Spinosa DJ, et al. Percutaneous transluminal angioplasty and stenting in the treatment of chronic mesenteric ischemia: results and long-term follow-up. J Am Coll Surg 2002;194:22–31.)

no statistical difference existed between patients who had more than one vessel treated. When evaluating the primary success rate by whether or not the SMA was treated, no statistically significant difference was seen.

In the 12 patients in whom stents were used during the initial procedure, 16 stents were placed in 15 vessels. The primary technical success rate was 100%, and the primary clinical success rate was 100%. The mean follow-up period for patients who had a stent placed was 15 months (a range of 1–48 months). Recurrent symptoms occurred in one patient secondary to in-stent restenosis at 14 months. The restenosis was treated successfully with PTA.

When comparing the primary clinical success rate of those patients who underwent PTA alone versus those patients who underwent PTA in addition to stenting, no statistical difference in the primary long-term clinical success appeared (Figure 22–9).

The 5-year survival rate for the 29 patients was 76.1%. In the 21 patients who underwent PTA alone, 5-year survival was 70.6%. In the patients who underwent PTA and stenting, the longest follow-up was 48 months. Based on Life Table Analysis, the 5-year survival rate for patients treated with stents was 87.5%. The difference in survival between patients who underwent PTA alone versus PTA and stenting was not statistically significant (Figure 22–10). When evaluating survival based on whether one vessel or more than one vessel was treated, no statistical difference existed. When comparing whether survival was affected by intervention on the SMA, no statistical difference was seen ($p = 0.654$).

Sheeran et al. reported on the treatment of 12 patients with 10 focal atherosclerotic stenoses and 3 chronic occlusions with stent placement (40). Vessels treated included

9 SMA, 3 celiac, and 1 aorto-SMA bypass graft. The initial technical success reported was 92% (12 of 13 vessels). The one technical failure occurred because of rupture of the angioplasty balloon while deploying a balloon-expandable stent. The stent was recaptured and deployed in the iliac artery. Despite a residual pressure gradient after PTA, the patient reported improved symptoms at 6 month follow-up. Primary stent placement was used for calcified ostial stenoses, chronic occlusions, and high-grade eccentric stenoses in eight of 13 stent placements. Patients underwent secondary stent placement for residual stenosis of more than 30%, a significant residual pressure gradient, and flow-limiting dissections after PTA. Of the 12 patients, short-term mortality (<30 day) was reported in one patient secondary to bowel ischemia. This patient presented with acute worsening of chronic abdominal symptoms but was deemed a nonsurgical candidate and underwent a technically successful stent placement in the SMA. No minor or major technical complications were encountered, and no complications associated with puncture site hematoma, acute vessel occlusion, or distal embolization existed.

Surgical revascularization remains the mainstay of treatment for complete mesenteric arterial occlusions. However, Sheeran et al. reported on the treatment of three patients (two SMA and one aorto-SMA bypass graft) with chronic occlusions using PTA and stent placement. All three patients remained asymptomatic at 13 to 38 months of follow-up (40).

The largest reported series of patients who underwent visceral artery stenting was published recently by Sharafuddin and coworkers and includes 25 consecutive patients, 21 of whom were treated for CMI. Twenty-one balloon-expandable and seven self-expanding stents were used. The authors reported a high technical success rate (96%), with primary and primary-assisted clinical benefit of 85% and 91%, respectively (39). Based on the favorable results and low complication rates compared with the known morbidity and mortality of surgical therapy, the authors recommended a selective primary endovascular approach for the management of occlusive mesenteric disease, an approach that has been advocated by other investigators (60).

SUMMARY

Because of the extensive collateral circulation in the mesenteric bed, the prevalence of CMI in the general population is relatively low. Clinical studies comparing surgical and endovascular techniques in the treatment of mesenteric ischemia are lacking. Also, most surgical and endovascular series are relatively small. However, endovascular therapy represents an effective alternative to surgery, with overall favorable morbidity and mortality rates and comparable clinical benefit. Although the value of endovascular therapy for patients at high risk for an operation is undisputed, the use of endovascular therapy in good surgical candidates is more debatable. Nonetheless, based on the experience of Matsumoto, Sharafuddin, Steinmetz (37,39,60), and others, a primary endovascular approach in the management of occlusive mesenteric disease may be justifiable. Recurrent disease after PTA/stenting can be retreated successfully by endovascular means, reserving surgical repair for immediate and delayed failures not amenable to endovascular therapy. For complete arterial occlusions, surgical revascularization remains the mainstay of therapy, but with the availability of stents, patients at relatively high risk for surgery may benefit from endovascular revascularization. Lastly, an immediate technical or clinical failure of mesenteric artery PTA/stenting that is not related to a technical complication should raise the concern for underlying vascular compression by the median arcuate ligament or an occult malignancy.

REFERENCES

1. Boley SJ, Sprayregen SS, Veith FJ. An aggressive roentgenologic and surgical approach to mesenteric ischemia. Surg Annu 1973; 5:355.
2. Kaleya RN, Sammartano RJ, Boley SJ. Aggressive approach to acute mesenteric ischemia. Surg Clin North Am 1992;72:157–182.
3. Heys SD, Brittenden J, Crofts TJ. Acute mesenteric ischaemia: the continuing difficulty in early diagnosis. Postgrad Med J 1993; 69:48–51.
4. Batellier J, Kieny R. Superior mesenteric artery embolism: eighty-two cases. Ann Vasc Surg 1990;4:112–116.
5. Park WM, Gloviczki P, Cherry KJ Jr, et al. Contemporary management of acute mesenteric ischemia: factors associated with survival. J Vasc Surg 2002;35:445–452.
6. Lee R, Tung HK, Tung PH, et al. CT in acute mesenteric ischaemia. Clin Radiol 2003;58:279–287.
7. Kirkpatrick ID, Kroeker MA, Greenberg HM. Biphasic CT with mesenteric CT angiography in the evaluation of acute mesenteric ischemia: initial experience. Radiology 2003;291:91–99.
8. McKinsey JF, Gewertz BL. Acute mesenteric ischemia. Surg Clin North Am 1997;77:307–318.
9. Simonetti G, Lupattelli L, Urigo F, et al. [Interventional radiology in the treatment of acute and chronic mesenteric ischemia.] Radiol Med (Torino) 1992;84:98–105.
10. Vujic I, Stanley J, Gobien RP. Treatment of acute embolus of the SMA by topical infusion of streptokinase. Cardiovasc Intervent Radiol 1984;7:94–96.
11. Clark RA, Gallant TE. Acute mesenteric ischemia: angiographic spectrum. AJR Am J Roentgenol 1984;142:555–562.
12. Grendell, JH, Ockner RK. Mesenteric venous thrombosis. Gastroenterology 1982;82:358–372.
13. Freidenberg MJ, et al. Superior mesenteric arteriography in experimental mesenteric venous thrombosis. Radiology 1965; 85:38–45.
14. Abdu RA, Zakhour BJ, Dallis DJ. Mesenteric venous thrombosis—1911–1984. Surgery 1987;101:383–388.
15. Nemcek AAJ, Vogelzang RL. Interventional management of acute mesenteric ischemia. In: Strandness DE, van Breda A, eds. Vascular Diseases: Surgical and Interventional Management. New York: Churchill Livingstone, 1994:785–793.
16. Yankes Jr, Uglietta JP, Grant J, et al. Percutaneous transhepatic recanalization and thrombolysis of the superior mesenteric vein. AJR Am J Roentgenol 1988;151:289–290.
17. Rivitz SM, Geller SC, Hahn C, et al. Treatment of acute mesenteric venous thrombosis with transjugular intramesenteric urokinase infusion. J Vasc Interv Radiol 1995;6:219–228.
18. McManimon S, et al. Mesenteric venous thrombosis. Tech Vasc Interv Radiol 1998;1:209–215.
19. Fann JI, Sarris GE, Mitchell RS, et al. Treatment of patients with aortic dissection presenting with peripheral vascular complications. Ann Surg 1990;212:705–713.
20. Williams DM, Brothers TE, Messina SM. Relief of mesenteric ischemia in type III aortic dissection with percutaneous fenestration of the aortic system. Radiology 1990;174:450–452.
21. Dake MD, Semba CP, Kee ST. Endovascular stents and stent-grafts in the management of thoracic aortic dissections and aneurysms. In: Matsumoto AH, eds. Noncardiac Thoracic Interventions, Baltimore: Williams and Wilkins, 1997:223–254.
22. Miralles M, Cairols M, Cotillas J et al. Value of Doppler parameters in the diagnosis of renal artery stenosis. J Vasc Surg 1996; 23:428–435.
23. Blebea J, Volteas N, Neumyer M, et al. Contrast enhanced duplex ultrasound imaging of the mesenteric arteries. Ann Vasc Surg 2002;16:77–83.
24. Bergi JP, Elkohen M, Deklunder G, et al. Helical CT angiography compared with arteriography in the detection of renal artery stenosis. AJR Am J Roentgenol 1996;167:495–501.
25. Rubin GD, Dake MD, Napel, et al. Spiral CT of renal artery stenosis: comparison of three-dimensional rendering techniques. Radiology 1994;190:181–189.
26. Horton KM, Fishman EK. Multidetector row CT of mesenteric ischemia: can it be done? Radiographics 2001;21:1463–1473.
27. Laghi A, Iannaccone R, Catalano C, et al. Multislice spiral computed tomography of mesenteric arteries. Lancet 2001;358: 638–639.
28. Meaney JF, Prince MR, Nostrant TT, et al. Gadolinium-enhanced MR angiography of visceral arteries in patients with suspected chronic mesenteric ischemia. J Magn Reson Imaging 1997;71: 171–176.
29. Baden JG, Racy DJ, Grist TM. Contrast-enhanced three-dimensional magnetic resonance angiography of the mesenteric vasculature. J Magn Reson Imaging 1999;10:369–375.
30. Carlos RC, Stanley JC, Stafford-Johnson D, et al. Interobserver variability in the evaluation of chronic mesenteric ischemia with gadolinium-enhanced MR angiography. Acad Radiol 2001;8: 879–887.
31. Rapp JH, Reilly LM, Qvarfordt PG et al. Durablity of endarterectomy and antegrade grafts in the treatment of chronic visceral ischemia. J Vasc Surg 1986;3:799–806.
32. Rheudasil JM, Stewart MT, Schellack JV, et al. Surgical treatment of chronic mesenteric arterial insufficiency. J Vasc Surg 1988;8: 495–500.
33. Calderon M, Reul GJ, Gregoric ID, et al. Long-term results of surgical management of symptomatic chronic intestinal ischemia. J Cardiovasc Surg 1992;33:723–728.

34. Mateo RB, O'Hara PJ, Hertzer NR, et al. Elective surgical treatment of symptomatic chronic mesenteric occlusive disease: early results and late outcomes. J Vasc Surg 1999;29:821–832.

35. Park WM, Cherry KJ Jr, Chua HK, et al. Current results of open revascularization for chronic mesenteric ischemia: a standard for comparison. J Vasc Surg 2002;35:853–859.

36. Foley MI, Moneta GI, Abou-Zamzam AM, et al. Revascularization of the superior mesenteric artery alone for treatment of intestinal ischemia. J Vasc Surg 2000;32:37–47.

37. Matsumoto AH, Tegtmeyer CJ, Fitzcharles EK, et al. Percutaneous transluminal angioplasty of visceral arterial stenoses: results and long-term clinical follow-up. J Vasc Interv Radiol 1995;6:165–174.

38. Matsumoto AH, Angle JF, Spinosa DJ, et al. Percutaneous transluminal angioplasty and stenting in the treatment of chronic mesenteric ischemia: results and long-term follow-up. J Am Coll Surg 2002;194:22–31.

39. Sharafuddin MJ, Olson CH, Sun SL. Endovascular treatment of celiac and mesenteric arteries stenoses: applications and results. J Vasc Surg 2003;38:692–698.

40. Sheeran SR, Murphy TP, Khwaja A, et al. Stent placement for treatment of mesenteric artery stenosis or occlusions. J Vasc Interv Radiol 1999;10:861–867.

41. Kasirajan K, O'Hara PJ, Gray BH, et al. Chronic mesenteric ischemia: open surgery versus percutaneous angioplasty and stenting. J Vasc Surg 2001;33:63–71.

42. Gonzalez LL, Jaffe MS. Mesenteric arterial insufficiency following abdominal aortic resection. Arch Surg 1966;93:10–20.

43. Rogers DM, Thompson JE, Garrett WV, et al. Mesenteric vascular problems: a 26-year experience. Ann Surg 1982;195:554–565.

44. Tribble CG, Harman PK, Mentzer RM Jr. Celiac artery compression syndrome: report of a case and review of the current opinion. J Vasc Surg 1986;20:120–129.

45. Furrer J, Grüntzig A, Kugelmeier J, et al. Treatment of abdominal angina with percutaneous dilatation of an arteria mesenterica superior stenosis. Preliminary communication. Cardovasc Intervent Radiol 1980;3:43–44.

46. Uflacker R, Goldany MA. Resolution of mesenteric angina with percutaneous transluminal angioplasty of a superior mesenteric artery stenosis using a balloon catheter. Gastrointest Radiol 1980; 5:367–369.

47. Novelline RA. Percutaneous transluminal angioplasty: Newer applications. AJR Am J Roentgenol 1980;135:983–988.

48. Golden DA, et al. Percutaneous angioplasty in the treatment of abdominal angina. AJR Am J Roentgenol 1982;139:247–249.

49. Roberts L, Wertman DA, Mills SR, et al. Transluminal angioplasty of the superior mesenteric artery: an alternative to surgical revascularization. AJR Am J Roentgenol 1983;141:1039–1042.

50. Wilms G, Baert Al. Transluminal angioplasty of superior mesenteric artery and celiac trunk. Ann Radiol (Paris) 1986;29:535–538.

51. Levy PJ, Haskell L, Gordon RL. Percutaneous transluminal angioplasty of splanchnic arteries: an alternative method to elective revascularisation in chronic visceral ischaemia. Eur J Radiol 1987;7:239–242.

52. Howd A, Loose H, Chamberlain J. Transluminal angioipasty in the treatment of mesenteric vein graft stenosis. Cardiovasc Intervent Radiol 1987;10:43–45.

53. McShane MD, Proctor A, Spencer P, et al. Mesenteric angioplasty for chronic intestinal ischaemia. Eur J Vasc Surg 1992;6:333–336.

54. Crotch-Harvey MA, Gould DA, Green AT. Case report: percutaneous transluminal angioplasty of the inferior mesenteric artery in the treatment of chronic mesenteric ischaemia. Clin Radiol 1992;46:408–409.

55. Warnock NG, Gaines PA, Beard JD, et al. Treatment of intestinal angina by percutaneous transluminal angioplasty of a superior mesenteric artery occlusion. Clin Radiol 1992;45:18–19.

56. Sniderman KW. Transluminal angioplasty in the management of chronic intestinal ischemia. In: Strandness DE, van Breda A, eds. Vascular Diseases: Surgical and Interventional Therapy. New York: Churchill Livingstone, 1994:803–809.

57. Hallisey MJ, Deschaine J, Illescas FF, et al. Angioplasty for the treatment of visceral ischemia. J Vasc Interv Radiol 1995;6:785–791.

58. Rose SC, Quigley TM, Raker EJ. Revascularization for chronic mesenteric ischemia: comparison of operative arterial bypass grafting and percutaneous transluminal angioplasty. J Vasc Interv Radiol 1995;6:339–349.

59. Allen RC, Martin GH, Rees CR, et al. Mesenteric angioplasty in the treatment of chronic intestinal ischemia. J Vasc Surg 1996; 24:415–423.

60. Steinmetz E, Tatou E, Favier-Blavoux C, et al. Endovascular treatment as first choice in chronic intestinal ischemia. Ann Vasc Surg. 2002;16:693–699.

Endovascular Stent Grafts for Treatment of Thoracic Aortic Diseases

23

David S. Wang, Michael D. Dake

The traditional management of thoracic aortic diseases is open surgical graft replacement of the diseased aortic segment, requiring thoracotomy and aortic cross-clamping (1–3). Despite advances in surgical technique, anesthetic management, and postoperative care over the last 30–40 years, the morbidity and mortality associated with conventional surgical repair remains substantial, partly because of a patient population that is often elderly and harbors multiple comorbidities (1,2,4–7). The advent and evolution of endovascular stent-graft technology herald the potential benefits of a promising, less-invasive, therapeutic alternative to conventional surgical repair for treatment of various thoracic aortic diseases.

The concept of transluminally placed endovascular stent grafts was pioneered by Dotter in 1969 (8) and was subsequently studied in animal models of abdominal aortic aneurysm (AAA) and acute aortic dissection (9–17). The first successful clinical use of stent grafts was reported by Parodi, Palmaz, and Barone in 1991 for exclusion of AAAs (18). Indeed, the development of stent grafts for repair of AAAs has led the way in the clinical application of endovascular aortic therapy. Studies reported to date have demonstrated that the endovascular approach to AAA repair relative to conventional surgery results in reduced 30-day morbidity; comparable

30-day and 1-year survival rates; decreased length of hospital stay; earlier return to preoperative levels of activity; and lower complication rates (19–23). Currently, the United States Food and Drug Administration (FDA) has approved four commercially developed devices for treatment of AAAs. Even though long-term data remain pending (24), estimates suggest that half of all AAAs will be repaired using the endovascular approach in the future (23,25). These experiences have spurred the exploration of stent grafts for use in the thoracic aorta (26,27), subclavian artery (28–31), iliac arteries (32–34), popliteal arteries (35), arteriovenous fistulas (36,37), and peripheral occlusive diseases (38,39).

Following closely on the heels of early clinical experiences with stent grafting of the abdominal aorta, adaptation of this technology for the descending thoracic aorta was initiated in 1992 for the management of descending thoracic aortic aneurysm (TAA) (26). Since these initial feasibility and safety studies for TAA, a rapidly growing number of applications have been reported for a wide spectrum of thoracic aortic diseases. These include acute and chronic dissection (27,40,41), penetrating atherosclerotic ulcer (PAU) (42–44), traumatic injury (45–47), mycotic aneurysm (48,49), aortobronchial fistula (50–51), aneurysm after coarctation repair (52), and rupture (53,54).

This chapter explores the use of endovascular stent grafts for the management of diseases of the descending thoracic aorta. To begin, devices and technical considerations are discussed. This is followed by a review of clinical experiences with endovascular management of various thoracic aortic pathologies. Although the cumulative experience with thoracic stent-graft repair is limited, studies to date have demonstrated promising preliminary results, supporting further evaluation of this technology.

DEVICES

Initial clinical experiences with stent grafting of the thoracic aorta employed first-generation, homemade devices. Although several commercially developed stent grafts for the abdominal aorta have been designed, tested, and approved for clinical use in the United States and abroad, device development for the thoracic aorta has lagged behind that of its infrarenal counterpart. To date, no thoracic endografts have been approved by the FDA. However, three are available outside the United States that are currently undergoing clinical trials for FDA approval. These are the TAG, or Thoracic Excluder (W. L. Gore & Associates); the Talent (AVE/Medtronic, Inc.); and the Zenith TX2 (Cook, Inc.) (Figure 23–1). Much more experience with the first two devices has been accumulated. There are several other existing devices that are less widely distributed, and many new thoracic endografts are in development.

First-Generation Devices

Detailed discussion of the various first-generation, homemade devices is only of modest historical interest. Suffice it to say, most of these prototypical prostheses were self-expanding and based on a combination of polyester graft with a modified type of Gianturco Z stent. Most delivery systems were large (24 French to 27 French), relatively rigid, and difficult to deploy precisely because of a marked frictional resistance encountered during withdrawal of the outer device-containing sheath. Detailed descriptions of individual systems, components, fabrication processes, and deployment techniques are provided elsewhere (26,55,56).

Commercially Developed Devices

The current designs of these three commercially manufactured devices represent modified versions of each, featuring considerable improvements over the initial designs. In general, the current versions incorporate considerable improvements in ease of use, durability, and reliability. The individual benefits of these new iterations are discussed in detail in the following section.

The Gore TAG

Device Description

Gore's TAG is composed of a self-expanding nitinol stent lined with polytetrafluoroethylene (PTFE) graft material. The first version of this device, the TAG Excluder, is lined with an ultra-thin wall PTFE graft with a 30 μm internodal distance similar to the pore size of conventional PTFE vascular grafts. The new TAG uses a different proprietary multilayer composition that is more durable and scratch-resistant than the prior graft material in preclinical in vitro comparison tests. Grafts are available in a range of diameters between 26 and 40 mm and a selection of lengths between 7.5 and 40 cm.

The ends of this prosthesis have a scalloped contour to enhance graft contact with the aortic wall over a wide range of aortic tortuosities and angulations. The scalloped projections are covered with PTFE, and their length is directly proportional to the diameter of the graft. The device is very flexible radially and longitudinally. The TAG Excluder has two S-shaped stabilization wires anchored 180 degrees apart that span the length of the device. These wires are designed to stabilize the implant and prevent any longitudinal compression during deployment. The current version is without these stabilization wires; rather, the new graft material is engineered to perform the same function as that provided by the longitudinal wires.

The device has a novel delivery system. Before deployment, the graft is compressed axially onto the end of the delivery catheter and constrained by a PTFE corset laced with PTFE suture. This suture, often described as a ripcord that unravels the endograft when pulled, runs the length of the catheter and attaches to a deployment knob at the opposite end. The size of the delivery system and compatible introducer sheaths vary according to the diameter of the device and scale over a range of 20 French to 24 French.

To deliver the device, the appropriately sized 30 cm-long introducer sheath is advanced over a guide wire to

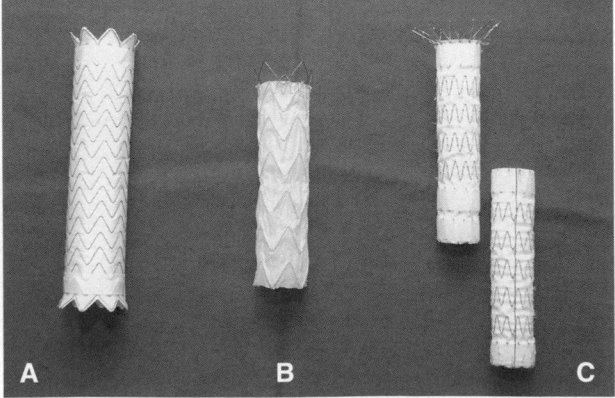

Figure 23–1 Current thoracic stent grafts undergoing U.S. clinical trials. **A.** The Gore TAG device is composed of polytetrafluoroethylene graft material and nitinol stent forms. **B.** The Medtronic Talent thoracic graft is fabricated from nitinol and polyester graft. **C.** Cook's TX2 Zenith device is a two-component endograft with stainless steel stent bodies and polyester graft material.

the infrarenal aorta. Alternatively, in certain situations, the catheter delivery system may be introduced over the guide wire without the use of a sheath. In either case, the device catheter is tracked over the wire until it reaches the selected target.

After final positioning is completed, the device is deployed with a pull of the knob adjacent to the catheter hub. As the knob is smoothly retracted, the attached suture is withdrawn. Opening of the corset occurs initially in the middle, then proceeds toward both ends simultaneously; instantaneous expansion of the underlying, self-expanding stent graft ensues similarly. This deployment pattern is intended to limit distal migration during deployment. After deployment, a catheter (TAG Thoracic Excluder Balloon Catheter) with a multilobed silicone balloon mounted on its leading end is used to smooth and seat the stent graft against the aortic wall.

The procedure is complete when the desired position of the graft is achieved. However, if the device is poorly positioned or is not fully expanded and a perigraft leak is present, supplemental maneuvers can be performed, including placing additional stent grafts or gently expanding the balloon over the segment of incomplete expansion.

Clinical Experience

The TAG Excluder was the first thoracic stent-graft device to initiate clinical testing in the United States. The trial was a prospective, nonrandomized study conducted at 17 sites with device deployment in 142 patients (57). Successful implantation of the device was achieved in 139 patients, and freedom from death and aneurysm death at 2 years were rated at 75% and 97%, respectively. Two perioperative deaths were the result of strokes. More alarmingly, fractures of the longitudinally oriented wires were observed after implantation in 18 patients. Worldwide, the frequency of wire fracture occurred in 10–30% of the implants and appeared to be related to the length of time since implantation, tortuosity of the device once implanted, and the presence of overlapping endografts. As a result of these stent fractures, Gore voluntarily withdrew the product from the global market, suspending sales in February 2001. Sales of the revised TAG device, without the stabilization wires, began in March 2004.

The Medtronic Talent

Device Description

Medtronic's Talent prosthesis is similar in design to the Talent abdominal endograft and is composed of sinusoidal nitinol stent elements sandwiched between thin layers of Dacron fabric. The individual stent forms are secured in place with oversewn sutures to prevent migration; however, they are not connected to one another and segments of unsupported graft are interposed between stents. This design allows independent stent motion and confers a degree of longitudinal flexibility. Similar to the TAG Excluder device, the Talent utilizes two longitudinal wires to provide stabilization and columnar support. The Talent stent graft is available in a wide range of diameters and lengths. In addition, custom fabrication of a prosthesis based on an individual patient's anatomy is possible within three weeks.

A unique aspect of the device is its uncovered proximal margin with broadbased nitinol wire scallops. The wide, uncovered interstices may be placed across the origin of the left subclavian artery in cases in which a short proximal neck of between 10 and 20 mm exists. In this setting, placement of the uncovered stent across the left subclavian artery helps to optimally orient the graft, stabilize its position, and, during deployment, secure precise targeting of the graft material at the distal subclavian margin.

The device is packaged in a more straightforward delivery system. The delivery catheter has a flexible, conical tip for improved trackability and maneuverability. An integrated balloon set back from the tip is used for smoothing the graft material and promoting adequate stent expansion after deployment. The prosthesis is collapsed over the distal segment of the delivery catheter and maintained in this packed configuration by an overlying transparent sheath. Proximal to the loaded stent graft is a blunt metal stopper that functions as a brace to maintain the device position as the constraining sheath is withdrawn. The delivery profile for Talent is between 22 French and 27 French depending on the diameter and length of the device.

The stent graft is usually positioned 1–3 cm proximal to the desired landing zone to mitigate against an inadvertent downstream drift during deployment. The overlying sheath is then withdrawn slowly. As the initial uncovered stent elements cantilever open, gentle retraction of the device is applied until the exact desired position of the proximal graft margin is obtained. After the device is fully deployed, the balloon may be withdrawn and, when necessary, expanded within the proximal segments to fully expand the prosthesis.

Clinical Experience

In November 2003, Medtronic began patient enrollment for its Phase II study. The results are pending as of this writing, but several centers have reported their preliminary individual experiences with the Talent prosthesis in the treatment of various thoracic aortic diseases (40,58–60). In a study by Criado et al (60) that analyzed their 6-year experience with the Talent stent-graft system exclusively used in 125 patients, successful implantation was achieved in 123 patients. Among the 51 patients with aortic dissection, the false lumen became completely thrombosed after endovascular treatment in 74% of patients. Thirty-day mortality was 4.8%, and mortality with a mean follow-up of 35 months was 6.4% ($n = 8$). Of these deaths, five were unrelated to the device or aortic disease, and two were the result of unknown causes. Twelve patients (9.6%) demonstrated an endoleak at 30 days, and five patients developed symptoms of spinal cord ischemia.

The Cook Zenith TX2

Device Description

Cook's Zenith TX2 thoracic endograft is a two-component device; its predecessor, the TX1, is a single-piece device sold exclusively outside the United States. The TX2 is made with Dacron fabric of standard thickness and stainless steel Gianturco Z stents. It incorporates a distal, uncovered stent-body in conjunction with graft material extending to the proximal margin of the endograft. Furthermore, fixation barbs are employed around the proximal aspect (pointing distally) and distal extent (pointing proximally).

The modular design of the TX2 endograft requires that the two components—a proximal and a distal piece—are placed in each case, irrespective of the length of the disease to be treated. The intent of this concept is to confer increased flexibility upon the endograft and to allow for optimal accommodation to any conformational changes that may occur long-term.

Clinical Experience

Although the Zenith TX2 is approved for commercial distribution in Canada, Australia, and Asia, reports on its use in the literature are sparse. Clinical trials in the United States began in April of 2004.

Device Comparison

When selecting for the appropriate device, the particular disease process and anatomy may recommend one over another. The marked flexibility of the TAG Excluder device and its delivery system as well as its smaller introduction profile make it better suited for patients with severely angled aortic anatomy or iliofemoral conduit arteries that are small, calcified, or tortuous. In cases in which a short proximal neck between the left subclavian artery and the diseased aorta (<15 mm) is present, the Talent device may be preferred because its leading stent segment is uncovered. In terms of ease of use, the Medtronic device has some advantages. The maximum graft length available is 20 cm compared with 13 cm for a noncustom Talent device. In combination with its simple and straightforward deployment, this makes it more efficient to extend the treatment zone.

In the treatment of aortic dissection, the relative radial force exerted by the prosthesis may be a consideration. In the acute setting, the lower hoop strength of the TAG Excluder may allow adequate coverage of the entry site without causing an iatrogenic secondary tear in the thin, fragile dissection flap. Regarding this, reports suggest that the relatively rigid leading bare metal proximal segment of the Talent device can injure the aortic wall adjacent to the entry tear and create a retrograde type A dissection. On the other hand, the greater radial force of the Talent prosthesis may be beneficial in cases of chronic dissection in which greater force is needed to displace a thick and resistant dissection septum.

TECHNICAL CONSIDERATIONS

Preoperative Evaluation

In case intraoperative complications arise and conversion to open intervention is needed, preoperative evaluation for endovascular repair is performed in the same way as it is for surgical replacement. Evaluation begins with careful assessment of cardiopulmonary and renal reserves, existing comorbidities, and overall procedural risks. To fully characterize the lesion and assess the patient's suitability for endovascular repair, thorough preprocedural imaging is of prime importance. Considerations include the presence of normal segments of native aorta that can serve as proximal and distal fixation sites for the device (the so-called "landing zone" or "neck"), the relationship between the lesion and significant aortic branches, the overall tortuousity of the aorta, and the availability of suitable access sites. Detailed preoperative evaluation can be obtained using spiral CT or MRI. Optimally, preprocedural assessment is enhanced by three-dimensional reconstructions and angiography. Catheter-based angiography remains the gold standard for getting an overall sense of the anatomic suitability of lesions and access vessels. Measurements and dimensions derived from imaging data are used to select the appropriate diameter and length of device needed. In general, endovascular stents are oversized by 10–20% of the aortic diameter to provide sufficient radial force for adequate fixation.

In the case of stent grafting for treatment of aortic dissection, precise localization of the proximal entry tear is a key factor. CT angiography, MRI, and transesophageal echocardiography (TEE) can be used for this purpose; however, CT angiography is most common. In addition, because of the idiosyncratic morphologic manifestations of aortic dissections, the optimal method for selecting the correct prosthesis diameter is a common issue. Because the true lumen is a fraction of the overall transaortic diameter and is rarely cylindrical in shape, choosing the correct device dimension presents a unique challenge. Most practitioners base their selection on more than one measurement. Perhaps, the most compelling is the diameter of the nondissected aorta immediately proximal to the entry tear. This is a good estimate of the original size of the proximal involved segment before dissection. This measurement, in addition to an oversize factor of 20% to ensure secure anchoring and a tight circumferential seal, is the approximation of device size most frequently used in current practice. If retrograde proximal extension of the dissection from the entry site occurs, other planning steps must be taken. These include calculating the mean true lumen diameter from measurements of the maximum and minimum true lumen dimensions and selecting an arbitrary diameter that corresponds to a value larger than the true lumen but less than the overall aortic diameter.

Deployment

The implant procedure is performed in the operating room or angiographic suite with fluoroscopy. Use of high-quality fluoroscopic equipment is essential to ensure accurate placement of the device. Digital image acquisition, playback, and "roadmapping" guidance capabilities are minimum requirements. TEE and intravascular ultrasound (IVUS) can help with deployment accuracy. A blood-recycling cell salvage system and cardiopulmonary bypass capability should be available. The procedure generally is performed with the patient intubated and under general anesthesia, although regional and local anesthesia techniques have been used. A review of appropriate anesthesia for endovascular stent-graft placement is found in Lippmann et al. (61). The patient is prepared and draped in the same way as for a left thoracotomy in case of open conversion. Depending on the anatomy of the patient, possible vascular access sites include the femoral artery, iliac artery, and infrarenal aorta. The femoral artery is the most common access site. A more in-depth discussion of access will follow later in this chapter.

After arterial access is obtained, the patient is heparinized and the stent-graft device is introduced and advanced over a guide wire under fluoroscopic guidance. To minimize the forward force encountered by the endovascular graft during deployment, the patient's arterial blood pressure may be lowered routinely to a mean of 60 to 80 mm Hg using an intravenous solution of sodium nitroprusside. Following graft expansion, the blood pressure is allowed to normalize.

To enhance deployment precision, some groups use adenosine to induce transient cardiac asystole (62). However, concerns regarding device malpositioning and migration during deployment apply more to early balloon-expandable stent-graft systems (63). With the current use of self-expandable devices, the need for such maneuvers is diminishing.

Use of multiple prostheses is common. When more than one endoprosthesis of the same diameter is needed, the distal device generally should be placed first. When more than one device of differing diameters is required, the smaller device is deployed first, irrespective of relative location. The larger diameter device is subsequently placed coaxially with an overlap to enhance the interference seal between the grafts.

After deployment, a postprocedure angiogram is performed to assess adequacy of repair. If no additional procedures are necessary, all deployment devices are removed and the arterial access site is repaired. Protamine sulfate is given for heparin reversal.

Postoperative Evaluation

Patients usually spend the first 12–24 hours after the procedure in the intensive care unit until they are extubated and become hemodynamically stable. No postprocedural anticoagulation is administered. Before discharge, patients should undergo additional imaging evaluation and undergo a repeat CT examination 6 months after placement, then yearly thereafter (Figure 23–2). Follow-up imaging should evaluate for device failures, changes in lesion morphology, and endoleaks. If one or more endoleak is noted on the initial follow-up imaging study, another exam at 1–3 months is prudent, unless earlier reintervention is warranted.

Endoleak is defined by the persistence of blood flow outside the lumen of the endoluminal graft but within the aneurysm sac (64,65). They represent evidence of incomplete exclusion of the aneurysm from the circulation and are associated with persistent or recurrent aneurysmal sac pressurization that can cause progressive expansion and rupture (66–68). Endoleaks are classified according to their site of origin (Table 23–1) and time of occurrence relative to the operative procedure. An endoleak first observed within 30 days of deployment is defined as a "primary endoleak;" one detected thereafter is termed a "secondary endoleak" (65). Lastly, the related term "endotension" is used when aneurysm enlargement occurs after endovascular repair in the absence of a detectable endoleak and is sometimes referred to as a type IV endoleak (64,69,70). If an endoleak is suspected, additional workup with angiography is recommended. Endotension is best evaluated by MR angiography (71).

Many patients experience a postimplantation syndrome that is characterized by fever, leukocytosis, and elevated C-reactive protein in the absence of signs of bacteremia or graft infection (72). Usually, this resolves in 4–7 days and is thought to be a foreign body reaction to the graft material.

APPLICATIONS

The emergence of endoluminal stent grafting as an alternative treatment modality is being explored for a number of diseases involving the thoracic aorta. This section examines the current clinical experiences with endovascular treatment of specific thoracic aortic lesions. To establish a baseline comparison and context, the epidemiology, etiology, and natural history as well as outcomes of traditional

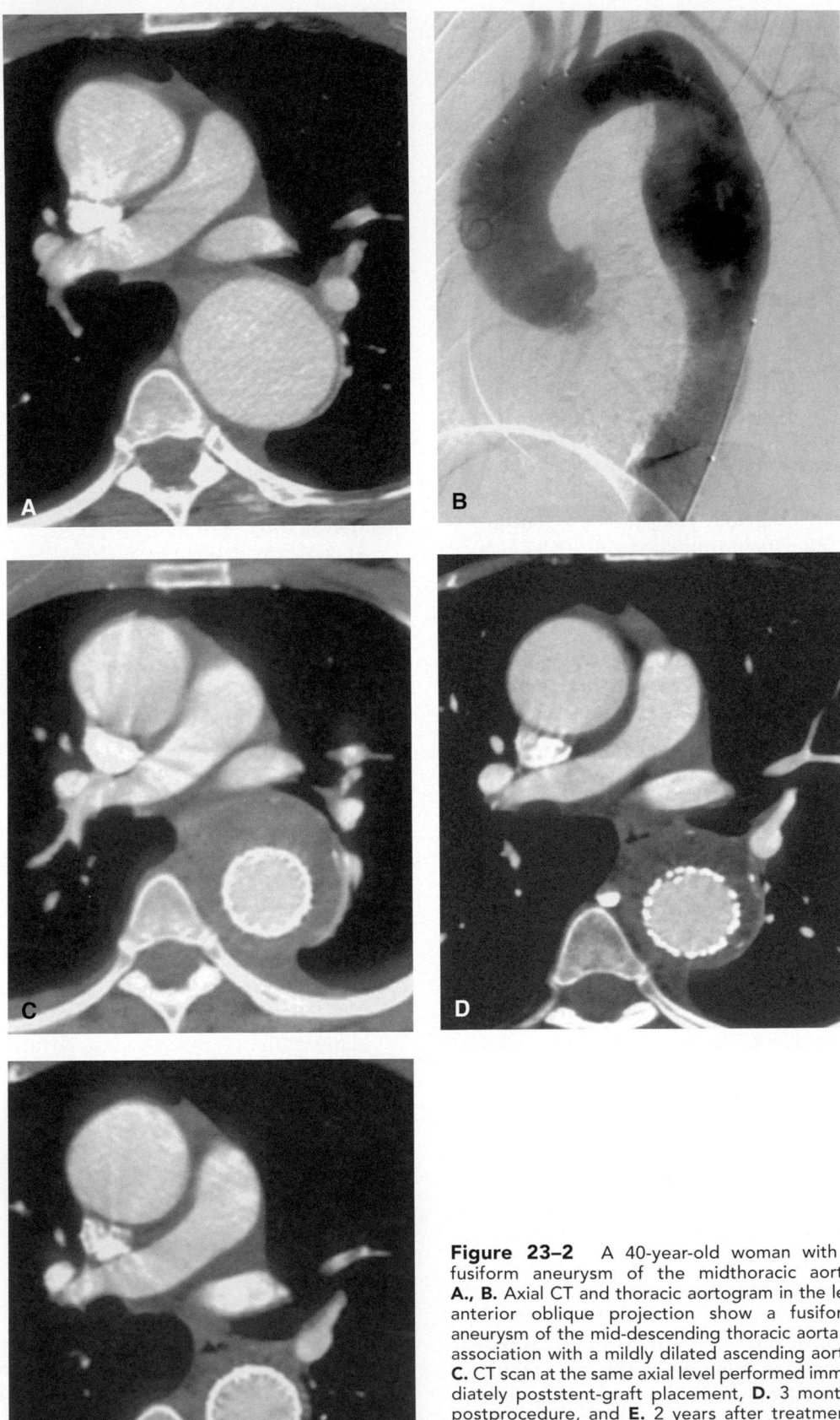

Figure 23–2 A 40-year-old woman with a fusiform aneurysm of the midthoracic aorta. **A., B.** Axial CT and thoracic aortogram in the left anterior oblique projection show a fusiform aneurysm of the mid-descending thoracic aorta in association with a mildly dilated ascending aorta. **C.** CT scan at the same axial level performed immediately poststent-graft placement, **D.** 3 months postprocedure, and **E.** 2 years after treatment. Demonstrate thrombosis of the aneurysm sac surrounding a patent stent graft. An obvious progressive decrease in the diameter of the aneurysm is evident. Of note, during the same interval, no increase has been seen in the diameter of the ascending aorta.

TABLE 23-1
ENDOLEAK CLASSIFICATION

Type I	Perigraft leak, result of incompetent seal at either the proximal or distal attachment site
Type II	Non–graft-related retrograde flow from collateral branches
Type III	Fabric graft tear, poor modular seal, or modular disconnection
Type IV	Fabric graft wall porosity

treatment modalities will be presented first. It should be noted that the development of thoracic stent-graft technology for clinical application remains in its adolescent stages and, therefore, the current state of literature consists mostly of studies with small and midsize samplings and near-term to midterm follow-up. Although early results are encouraging, the long-term effectiveness and durability of endovascular stent grafts remain under investigation.

Thoracic Aortic Aneurysm

Background

True TAA is defined as an abnormal dilation, 50% over the normal diameter, of the thoracic aorta that undergoes progressive expansion and includes all three layers of the vessel wall (intima, media, and adventitia) (73). Normal diameter of the thoracic aorta is less than 4.0 cm for the ascending and less than 3.0 cm for the descending portions. The incidence of TAA ranges from 5.9 to 10.4 per 100,000 person-years (74–76). Although occurring less often than AAAs, its incidence is increasing presumably because of increases in life expectancy and the availability of improved diagnostic modalities (76). Furthermore, according to a recent population-based study, 51% of TAA patients are female, in contrast to AAAs for which the majority is male (76).

Aneurysms can be classified by location and etiology. Up to 25% of all aortic aneurysms are located in the thoracic aorta and, of these, 40–50% are located in the descending portion (75,77). Notably, 20–25% of patients with a thoracic aneurysm also have an aneurysm in the abdominal aorta (78–80), emphasizing the importance of thorough examination of the entire aorta upon diagnosis. Furthermore, patients with aneurysms frequently have significant coexisting medical conditions including hypertension, coronary artery disease, chronic obstructive pulmonary disease, congestive heart failure, and cerebrovascular disease (5,77,81,82).

A broad spectrum of etiologies exists for TAA, but most are histologically characterized by fragmentation and degeneration of elastic fibers within the medial layer (83). A more advanced form of medial degeneration, termed cystic medial necrosis (CMN), also involves smooth muscle cell loss and interstitial accumulation of basophilic ground substance and is found mostly in aneurysms of the ascending thoracic aorta (83,84). Further studies on aortic aneurysms have suggested that loss of structural integrity of the adventitia, in particular, is necessary for aneurysm formation because the adventitia functions to mechanically maintain the aortic outer diameter (85).

The etiology of TAA is correlated with location. Atherosclerosis has long been believed to be the predominant cause of aneurysms in the descending thoracic aorta and the abdominal aorta (83,86). Aneurysm formation may represent a late degenerative stage of aortic atherosclerosis (87,88); therefore, such aneurysms are also classified as "degenerative" (65). Significant controversy exists, however, over whether atherosclerosis is actually an underlying cause or merely an associated disease process (83,87,89,90). Other etiologies of aneurysms of the descending thoracic aorta include chronic type B dissection, infectious and inflammatory aortitides, trauma, and CMN (83). Aneurysms of the ascending thoracic aorta, in contrast, are more commonly caused by chronic type A dissection and CMN associated with Marfan's or Ehlers-Danlos syndrome. Less common causes include poststenotic dilatation from aortic stenosis, infectious and inflammatory aortitides, trauma, and surgical correction of aortic coarctation (83,91). Infectious and inflammatory aortitides includes syphilis, mycotic conditions, Takayasu's arteritis, and Behcet's disease. In addition, Coady et al. demonstrated familial patterns of TAA development among patients without collagen vascular deficiency syndromes (89), providing evidence that genetic factors contribute to the development of this disease. Indeed, major loci for familial TAA have been mapped to 5q13–14 (termed the TAAD1 locus) and 3p24–25 (TAAD2) (92,93).

Aneurysms may be fusiform (concentric radial dilatation) or saccular (eccentric radial dilatation) in morphology. The majority of TAAs are fusiform in configuration with half distributed in the descending thoracic aorta and the other half in the ascending thoracic aorta or transverse arch. Saccular aneurysms are less common and are mostly located in the ascending thoracic aorta and transverse arch.

TAA is often diagnosed incidentally. Approximately 50% of patients with descending TAA are free of symptoms when the initial diagnosis is made because thoracic aneurysms rarely produce symptoms until progressive growth causes compression of adjacent structures or rupture (5,79,94). Depending on the location of the aneurysm, patients may present with vague chest, back, flank, or abdominal pain that may increase in severity as the aneurysm enlarges. Hoarseness from compression of the left recurrent laryngeal nerve, hemidiaphragmatic paralysis resulting from compression of the phrenic nerve, tracheal deviation, persistent cough, and other respiratory symptoms are sometimes seen with ascending and arch thoracic aneurysms (80,82,95).

The natural history of aneurysms, as governed by LaPlace's law, is one of progressive expansion, thinning of the aortic wall, and eventual rupture—a usually lethal outcome (2,83,94,96). In a Swedish study by Johansson et al. the overall mortality rate associated with ruptured TAAs was 97%, despite 41% of their patients reaching the hospital alive (97). Authors describing the natural history of untreated TAA estimate 5-year survival rates of 13–56% (75,76,79,86,96,98), with more recent studies reporting rates around 50% (76,98). Rupture was responsible for 29–68% of the mortality in these cases (75,79,96,99). Coexisting cardiovascular disease also contributes to mortality and is the second most common cause of death.

Studies of both AAA and TAA have demonstrated clearly that the most important determinant of rupture is the size of the aneurysm (76,98,100–104). The Yale Center for Thoracic Aortic Disease documented among 370 TAAs the median aneurysm size at the time of rupture or dissection to be 59 mm for ascending and 72 mm for descending aneurysms (102). Indeed, thoracic aneurysms with a diameter exceeding 60 mm have been found to demonstrate a significant increase in risk of rupture (76,102,105). The Yale group reported that the odds ratio for rupture of TAAs greater than 60 mm was increased 27-fold compared to those in the range of 40–49 mm (102). In similar analyses, certain patient subsets were found to have a higher risk of rupture—those with collagen vascular deficiency syndromes and those with chronic dissection along with TAA (75,96,106). In one study, 5-year survival of 7% was observed for aneurysm patients with dissection compared to 19.2% for those without dissection (75). Other proposed but less established risk factors for rupture include smoking, age, and presence of chronic obstructive pulmonary disease (COPD) (99,104).

Using data from prospective evaluation of the natural risk of rupture in descending TAA patients, Juvonen et al. generated the following mathematical model that allows the calculation of the probability of rupture (λ) based on various risk factors (104):

$$\text{Ln } \lambda = -21.055 + 0.093 \text{ (age/years)} + 0.841 \text{ (pain)}$$
$$+ 18.22 \text{ (COPD)} + 0.643 \text{ (diameter}_{\text{descending aorta}}/\text{cm)}$$
$$+ 0.405 \text{(diameter}_{\text{abdominal aorta}}/\text{cm)}$$

Pain and COPD = 1, if present, and 0, if absent or not reported. Age refers to the time of the most recent scan. The probability of rupture within 1 year = $1-e^{-\lambda}$ (365). Surgical repair is recommended when the calculated risk of rupture within 1 year exceeds the anticipated operative risk.

Conventional Therapy

The risk of eventual rupture mandates consideration for elective surgical treatment in all individuals who are suitable candidates for operation. Operative repair is recommended for any TAA that causes symptoms—regardless of size, whether it exceeds two times the transverse diameter of an adjacent normal-caliber aortic segment, or is 60 mm in diameter or larger. A more aggressive approach is recommended for smaller aneurysms that demonstrate evidence of acceleration in the rate of enlargement. The expected growth rate of most TAAs is 0.1–0.3 cm per year (99,102). The Yale group, based on analysis of 1600 TAA and dissection patients, recommends intervention for the ascending aorta at 55 mm and for the descending thoracic aorta at 65 mm (103). Earlier intervention is warranted at 50 mm for patients with a collagen vascular deficiency syndrome or chronic dissection (103,107,108). Those with smaller, asymptomatic TAA should be followed with serial CT or MRI scans at 6- to 12-month intervals.

Conventional operative repair of TAA involves median sternotomy, left thoracotomy, or both (depending on the extent and location of the aneurysm); establishment of proximal and distal vascular control; resection of the diseased aortic segment; and prosthetic graft interposition (109) (Figure 23–3). Unlike surgical repair of AAAs, thoracic aneurysm repair often requires cardiopulmonary bypass and specific methods to address end-organ protection in order to obtain vascular control (110). The published 30-day mortality following elective surgical repair of TAA is in the region of 5–15% (4,5,80,111–116), with an associated actuarial survival at 5 and 10 years of 70–79% and 40–49%, respectively (5,80,117). In-hospital mortality rates for emergency operations of TAA are significantly greater and can reach as high as 50% (5,79,118). Interestingly, mortality outcomes for elective surgical repair of ascending aneurysms have proved more favorable compared to that of descending aneurysms (5,103,119).

Hospital mortality associated with elective surgery of TAA has improved significantly in recent years, but considerable morbidity remains. Major complications associated with open repair include paraplegia or paraparesis resulting from intraoperative or postoperative spinal cord ischemia, respiratory insufficiency, renal insufficiency secondary to hypoperfusion or distal embolization, and stroke. The risk of spinal cord ischemia ranges from 5 to 25% (114–116, 120–125), despite many varied adjunctive procedures to preserve spinal cord perfusion (126–133). In a series of 1,509 TAA patients who underwent open repair, paraparesis or paraplegia developed in 16%, and kidney failure occurred in 18% with 9% requiring dialysis (122).

Endovascular Treatment

Aneurysm is the most common lesion of the thoracic aorta requiring surgical treatment, and descending TAA is currently the application with the greatest cumulative clinical experience of stent grafting with an estimated

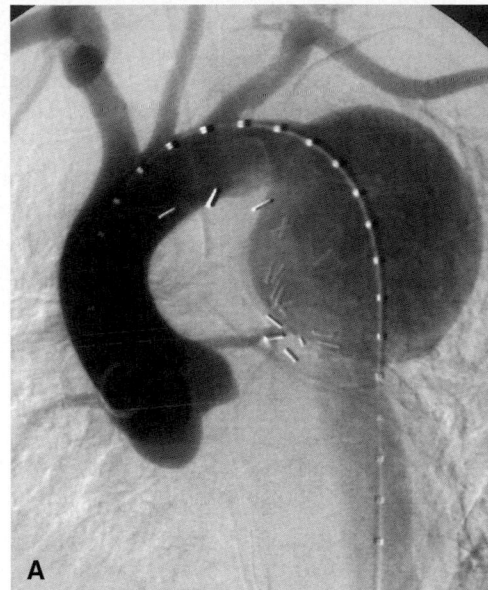

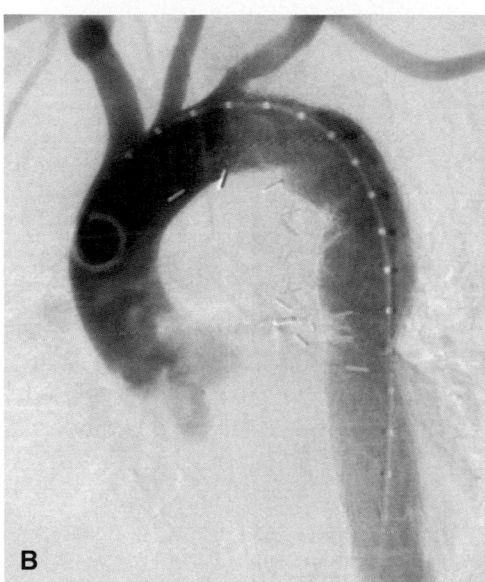

Figure 23–3 Anastomotic aneurysm following open repair of a traumatic aortic injury 30 years earlier. **A.** Aortogram performed in a left anterior oblique projection shows a large saccular aneurysm of the proximal descending thoracic aorta in a 49-year-old man who underwent an open interposition graft repair of an aortic injury when he was an adolescent. Multiple surgical clips are evident. **B.** After stent-graft placement in a position bridging the aneurysm, a thoracic aortogram demonstrates a good result without residual filling of the aneurysm sac.

candidates, patient selection for endovascular repair is currently limited to individuals deemed at high operative risk who have permissible anatomic features. Current anatomic requirements are listed in Table 23–2. As additional clinical experience with this therapeutic approach is accumulated with operable patients, indications will likely expand. The following section provides a review of the current literature on stent grafting of descending TAA and highlights studies with larger sample sizes and longer follow-up while observing overall trends.

Clinical Experience

The literature on endovascular therapy of descending TAA consists mostly of small to midsize case series from individual

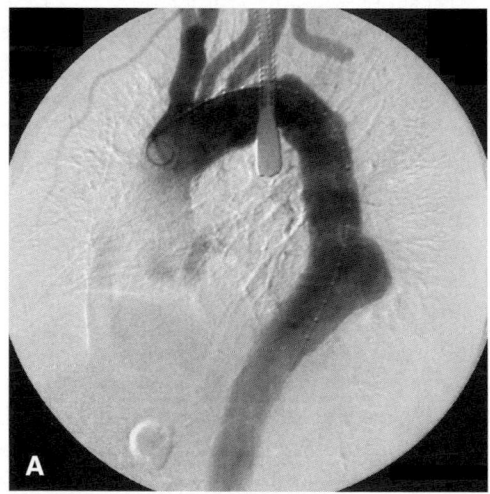

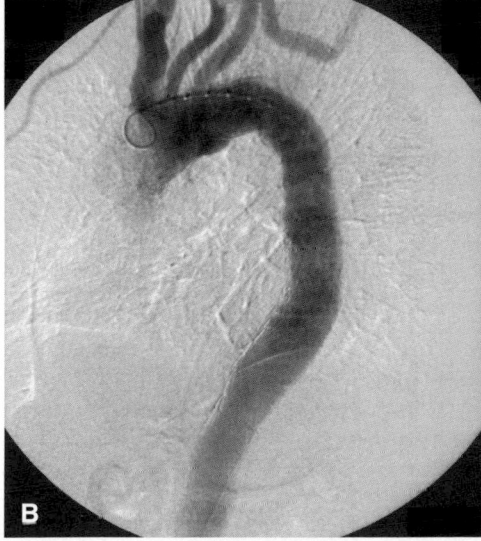

Figure 23–4 Descending thoracic aortic aneurysm. **A.** A 69-year-old man with degenerative aneurysm of the descending thoracic aorta. Thoracic aortogram in the left anterior oblique projection demonstrates a lobular aneurysm involving the mid and distal segments of the descending aorta. **B.** Thoracic aortogram following endograft placement reveals a successful treatment of the lesion without evidence of contrast media filling the aneurysm.

5,000 implements worldwide to date (Figure 23–4). The goal of endovascular repair is to provide durable exclusion of the aneurysm sac from aortic flow, thereby decreasing sac pressure, allowing for thrombosis formation, and eventually leading to a stabilization or decrease in the aneurysm's transverse diameter.

As initial studies demonstrated feasibility and safety in cohorts of patients who were mostly high-risk surgical

TABLE 23-2

ANATOMIC REQUIREMENTS FOR TAA STENT-GRAFT PLACEMENT

1. A proximal neck at least 15–25 mm from the origin of the left subclavian artery
2. A distal neck at least 15–25 mm proximal to the origin of the celiac artery
3. Absence of severe tortuosity, calcification, or atherosclerotic plaque burden involving both the aortic and pelvic vasculature
4. Transverse diameter of the proximal and distal neck within the range of available devices to accommodate appropriately

institutions. Mid-term to long-term data are just beginning to surface. Several available studies have reported aggregated clinical outcomes across a variety of distinct aortic diseases for various prosthetic designs, elective and emergent situations, or both making comparison of clinical experiences specific for this disease and for particular devices problematic. Published studies on endovascular stent grafting of mixed thoracic aortic diseases are summarized in Table 23-3; those specific to descending TAAs are summarized in Table 23-4.

At the First International Summit on Thoracic Aortic Endografting in March 2001, representative groups, with series greater than 40 patients (range 40–260) and limited to non–dissection-associated TAA, presented data on operative mortality rates between 0 and 4%, technically successful device deployments in 98–100%, and aneurysm thrombosis achieved in 90–100% (166–170). In terms of neurologic complications, paraplegia was found in 0–1.6% and stroke occurred in 0–2.8%. Conversion to open surgical repair was necessary in 0–4%, and late endoleaks were noted in 2–3%. The collective experiences of the UK and EUROSTAR Thoracic Stenting Registries, perhaps the largest multicenter series at this time, reported similar results (165). Among 217 TAA patients, half of whom were deemed high risk for open surgery, successful aneurysm exclusion was achieved in 83%, 30-day mortality was 8.5%, and paraplegia occurred in 3.5%.

While prospective randomized controlled trials comparing concurrent patients treated with either surgical repair or stent grafting are commencing (171), a few studies have compared endovascular results to anatomically similar open surgery historic controls (58,156). As part of a Phase II clinical study, Najibi et al. deployed the Gore Excluder in 19 TAA patients who were candidates for open repair and compared their clinical experiences with a historic nonrandomized cohort of 10 patients who had undergone open repair prior to the availability of thoracic stent grafts (156). Endograft deployment was successful in 95% of cases, and 78.9% demonstrated a decrease in aneurysm diameter at one month. The 1-year survival rate was 89.5% in the endovascular group and 70% in the

open surgery group. As expected, mean hospital stay (6.2 days versus 16.3 days) and length of intervention (155 minutes versus 256 minutes) were significantly less among those treated endovascularly. Paraplegia did not occur in either group. Similarly, Ehrlich et al. found decreased 30-day mortality (10% versus 31%), mean hospital stay (6 days versus 10 days), and mean intervention time (150 minutes versus 325 minutes) among the endovascular treatment group, but also demonstrated decreased paraplegia rates with stent grafting (0% versus 12%) (58). Despite these results, lack of randomized controlled trial data precludes true comparisons between results achieved after conventional therapy and the endovascular alternative.

The longest follow-up data on stent grafting of TAAs are entering the mid-term to long-term and are based on continued monitoring of patient cohorts from preliminary feasibility studies that employed crude, first-generation, homemade devices. The short-term results of these studies were satisfactory despite early design issues and a high-risk patient population, prompting further evaluation of this technology (226,55,155). Between 1992 and 1997, the Stanford University Medical Center carried out a prospective observational study of 103 patients who underwent endovascular treatment of aneurysms of the descending thoracic aorta. In general, patients in the study were older and of higher surgical risk than their conventional repair counterparts, who were also treated at Stanford. In fact, 60% of the patient cohort were judged to be unsuitable candidates for open repair (55,172). All devices deployed were homemade (Dacron over Gianturco Z stent endoskeleton). Reports on the outcomes of these patients have come periodically (26,55,56,173–175). The short-term outcomes of this series included: complete aneurysm thrombosis achieved in 84%, perioperative mortality of 9%, paraplegia/paraparesis in 3%, stroke in 7%, and primary endoleak of 24% (55). While perioperative mortality and paraplegia/paraparesis rates are comparable to those of contemporary surgical series (4,5,80,111–115), the incidence of stroke is disappointingly high but likely secondary to manipulation of stiff and large introducers and delivery sheaths, required of the admittedly primitive first-generation devices, within the aortic arch. Most of these early deaths resulted from unrelated causes, such as cancer and pulmonary embolism.

This patient cohort was recently revisited with a mean follow-up of 4.5 years (maximal of 10 years) (173). Among all patients, actuarial survival estimates 1, 5, and 8 years after stent-graft placement were 82%, 49%, and 27%, respectively. Upon examining the inoperable and operable patients separately, operative patients had a significantly better life expectancy than those who were unsuitable for open repair (93% versus 74% at 1 year and 78% versus 31% at 5 years). Late survival for inoperable patients was bleak, but most died of coexisting diseases. Among all late deaths

SUMMARY DATA ON STUDIES OF ENDOVASCULAR TREATMENT OF VARIOUS THORACIC AORTIC DISEASES

Reference	N	Mean Follow-up (Months)	Devices	Technical Success	30-day Mortality	Long-term Survival (Time)	Paraplegia	Endoleak
Taylor et al. (2001)	37: 18 degenerative aneurysm, 5 pseudoaneurysm, 4 acute dissection, 4 transection, 3 aneurysm related to surgery for coarctation, 2 chronic dissection, 1 traumatic dissection	17.5	Excluder, AneuRx, Vanguard, Stenford	97.3%	8.1%	NA	0%	NA
White et al. (2001)	26: 17 TAA, 9 chronic dissection	9	AneuRx	96.2%	3.8%	42.3% (mean = 9 months)	4%	NA
Won et al. (2001)	23: 11 aneurysm, 12 chronic dissection type B	25.1	Homemade	91.3%	0%	91% (cumulative 1 yr)	0%	NA
Buffolo et al. (2002)	191: 120 dissection type B, 61 TAA, 6 penetrating ulcer or IMH, 4 trauma	NA	Homemade	91.1%	10%	87.4% (actuarial survival ~68 months)	0%	NA
Cambria et al. (2002)	28: 18 degenerative aneurysm, 4 chronic dissection, 3 pseudoaneurysm, 1 trauma, 2 anastomotic aneurysm, 2 IMH, 1 aneurysm related to surgery for coarctation	17.8	Homemade, Excluder	96.4%	3.6%	86% (mean = 17.8 months)	0%	21.4%
Criado et al. (2002)	47: 31 TAA, 16 dissection type B	18	Talent	95.7%	2.1%	87.3% (mean = 18 months)	0%	10.6%
Lepore et al. (2002)	43: 16 dissection, 14 degenerative aneurysm, 7 contained rupture, 3 mycotic aneurysm, 2 posttraumatic aneurysm, 1 aneurysm of anomalous right subclavian artery	19	Excluder, Talent, AneuRx, Hemobahn	100%	7%	83% (mean = 19 months)	7%	16.3%

(continued)

TABLE 23-3
(continued)

Reference	N	Mean Follow-up (Months)	Devices	Technical Success	30-day Mortality	Long-term Survival (Time)	Paraplegia	Endoleak
Thompson et al. (2002)	46: 23 degenerative aneurysm, 14 dissection, 3 aortobronchial fistula, 3 pseudoanerysm, 2 traumatic rupture, 1 ruptured ulcer	8.5	Excluder	100%	4.3%	6.5% (mean = 8.5 months)	0%	4.3%
Bell et al. (2003)	67: 36 degenerative aneurysm, 8 infectious aneurysm, 8 chronic dissection, 6 acute dissection, 5 aneurysm related to surgery for coarctation, 3 transection, 1 vasculitis	17	Excluder, Talent, AneuRx, Endofit, Cook, Stentor, Vanguard	100%, 89.6% complete exclusion	7.5%	83.6% (mean = 17 months)	4.5%	14.9%
Ellozy et al. (2003)	84: 51 degenerative aneurysm, 5 traumatic pseudoaneurysm, 13 para-anastomotic aneurysm, 9 dissection, 2 mycotic aneurysm, 4 penetrating ulcer	15	TAG, Talent	90.5%, 82% complete exclusion	6%	67% (mean = 40 months)	4%	13%
Fattori et al. (2003)	70: 18 degenerative aneurysm, 22 dissection, 21 traumatic, 6 penetrating ulcer, 2 suture detachment, 1 pseudoaneurysm	25	Excluder, Talent	97.1%	3%	92.3% (mean = 25 months)	0%	14.3%
Gerber et al. (2003)	17: 5 degenerative aneurysm, 3 dissection type B, 1 IMH, 1 pseudoaneurysm	18.6	Excluder, Talent, Vanguard	76.5%	5.9%	NA	6%	35.3%
Grabenwoger et al. (2003)	19: 11 acute dissection type B, 6 penetrating ulcer, 2 traumatic aneurysm	17.2	Excluder, Talent	100%	0%	94.7% (17.2 months)	5.3%	NA
Lambrechts et al. (2003)	26: 12 degenerative aneurysm, 11 dissection type B, 3 traumatic rupture	8	Excluder, Talent, AneuRx	100%	0%	84.6% (mean = 8 months)	0%	11.5%

(continued)

TABLE 23-3
(continued)

Reference	N	Mean Follow-up (Months)	Devices	Technical Success	30-day Mortality	Long-term Survival (Time)	Paraplegia	Endoleak
Lamme et al. (2003)	21: 8 degenerative aneurysm, 6 pseudoaneurysm, 4 traumatic rupture, 2 mycotic aneurysm, 1 ruptured aneurysm	24	TAG, Talent, AneuRx	NA	0%	95.2% (mean = 24 months)	4.8%	9.5%
Matravers et al. (2003)	24: 11 degenerative aneurysm, 9 dissection type B, 3 penetrating ulcer, 1 traumatic pseudoaneurysm	11	Excluder, Talent, AneuRx	83%	8.3%	79.2% (mean = 11 months)	0%	48%
Orend et al. (2003)	74: 34 degenerative aneurysm, 6 posttraumatic aneurysm, 14 dissection type B with aneurysm, 12 transection from blunt trauma, 5 thoracoabdominal aneurysm, 2 aneurysm related to surgery for coarctation, 1 aortobronchial fistula	22	Excluder, Talent, Corvita, Vanguard, Stenford	100%	9.5%	83.8% (mean = 22 months)	2.7%	21.6%
Steinmetz et al. (2004)	41: 24 degenerative aneurysm, 8 IMH, 6 dissection type B, 3 traumatic aneurysm	9.8	Talent	92.7%	0%	NA	0%	7.3%
Rodriguez et al. (2004)	20*: 113 degenerative aneurysm, 45 dissection type B, 18 pseudoaneurysm, 12 PAU, 5 aortobronchial fistula, 5 traumatic transection, 2 embolization	2 to 48	Excluder, Talent, Endomed	NA	5.4%	NA	2%	9%
Ishida et al. (2004)	40: 26 degenerative aneurysm, 7 dissection with aneurysm, 3 traumatic aneurysm, 2 mycotic aneurysm, 1 anastomotic aneurysm, 1 penetrating ulcer	16.7	Homemade	97.5%	2.5%	84.2% (1 yr), 84.2% (2 yr)	3%	30%

TABLE 23–4
SUMMARY DATA ON STUDIES OF ENDOVASCULAR TREATMENT OF THORACIC AORTIC ANEURYSMS

Reference	N	Mean Follow-up (Months)	Devices	Technical Success	30-day Mortality	Long-term Survival (Time)	Paraplegia	Endoleak
Ehrlich et al. (1998)	10	NA	Talent	80% complete thrombosis	10%	NA	0%	20%
Cartes-Zumelzu et al. (2000)	32	16	Excluder, Talent	90.6%	9.4%	90.6% (32 mth)	3.1%	15.4%
Grabenwoger et al. (2000)	21	NA	Talent, Prograft	100%	9.5%	NA	0%	14.3%
Greenberg et al. (2000)	25	15.4	Homemade	NA	20% (12.5% for elective, 33% for emergent)	NA	12%	12%
Temudom et al. (2000)	14	5.5	Homemade, Vanguard, Excluder	78.6%	14.3%	NA	7.1%	14.3%
Najibi et al. (2000)	24	12	Excluder, Talent	94.7%	5.3%	89.5% (1 yr)	0%	0%
Heijmen et al. (2002)	28	21	Talent, AneuRx, Excluder	96.4%	0%	96.4% (mean = 21 mth)	0%	28.6%
Schoder et al. (2003)	28	22.7	Excluder	100%, 89.3% complete exclusion	0%	96.1% (1 yr), 80.2% (3 yr)	0%	25%
Marin et al. (2003)	94	15.4	Excluder, Talent	85.1%	NA	NA	NA	24%
Lepore et al. (2003)	21	12	Excluder, Talent	100%	9.5%	76.2% (1 yr)	4.8%	19%
Sunder-Plassman et al. (2003)	45	21	Corvita, Stenford, Vanguard, AneuRx, Talent, Excluder	NA	6.7%	NA	2.2%	22.2%
Ouriel et al. (2003)	31	6	Excluder, Talent, Other commercial	NA	12.9%	81.6% (1 yr)	6.5%	32.3%
Bergeron et al. (2003)	33	24	Excluder, Talent	NA	9.1%	75.8% (mean = 24 mth)	0%	0%
Czerny et al. (2003)	54	38	Excluder, Talent	94.4%	9.3%	63% (3 yr event free)	0%	27.8%
Makaroun et al. (2004)	142	29.6	TAG	97.9%	1.5%	75% (2 yr freedom from death)	3.5%	8.8%
Bell et al. (2004)	217	NA	Other commercial	83% complete exclusion	8.5%	NA	3.5%	NA

(beyond 30 days from deployment), 5.4% resulted from TAA rupture, 5.4% resulted from aortoesophageal or aortobronchial fistula formation, and 12.5% resulted from unknown causes. Interestingly, late ruptures occurred exclusively in patients with documented endoleaks. Nineteen patients (18%) developed a new type I or type III endoleak during follow-up (proximal type I in 9, distal type I in 8, proximal and distal type I leaks in 2, and type III in 1). It must be emphasized that the results achieved with the use of crude and cumbersome first-generation thoracic stent grafts do not represent the outcomes that potentially can be attained by using current, commercially manufactured devices. The results from this study, therefore, should be viewed as a baseline "worst case" scenario.

Indeed, significant improvements in adverse outcomes have been achieved with commercially manufactured devices. Czerny and colleagues were one of the first groups to begin deployment of the Talent and Excluder devices, and they recently reported encouraging results with mean follow-up of 3.2 years (maximal of 6 years) (164). Thirtyday mortality was 3.7%, while survival given mean followup was 92.6%. No adverse neurological events were encountered, but four secondary endoleaks were seen for both type I and type III.

General Trends

With the considerable worldwide experience that has been accumulated in evaluating this treatment modality for descending TAAs, a consensual pattern of outcomes is emerging that defines a shared reality (Table 23–4). To begin, the periprocedural mortality among TAA-specific studies of elective endovascular repair ranges from 0 to 14%, and the 5-year actuarial survival for high-risk operable patients in the SUMC study was 78% (63,156,157,160–163,165,173), both of which fall within the range of that associated with open repair (4,5,80,111–115). When viewed in the context of the specific patient populations employed (usually operable, but high-risk surgical candidates), these results suggest that perioperative mortality and 5-year survival rates will tend to shift favorably as this treatment modality is studied in good or average surgical candidates. This will be especially true as devices and their delivery systems continue to evolve and experience in deployment accumulates (176). As expected, many centers have reported that early deaths and early complications occurred more often during their initial year of thoracic stent grafting (55,164).

However, given that the sobering life expectancy results for the inoperable cohort in the study came mostly from death caused by other coexisting diseases, it is unlikely that improvements in stent-graft device technology and deployment technique will benefit such patients. Although there was no control group for direct comparison, the survival benefit derived from stent-graft placement was probably minimal and not enough to justify the associated risks. Furthermore, stent grafting does not enhance quality of life

in asymptomatic patients, so its use for palliative purposes is questionable. A study based on the large EUROSTAR AAA multicenter registry found that the 1-year cumulative survival for patients unfit for surgery was a bleak 20% (177). These findings raise the important philosophical question of whether endovascular treatment should be withheld in inoperable patients with asymptomatic aneurysms.

In terms of major morbidities, paraplegia is considered the Achilles heel of endovascular treatment because reimplantation of intercostal arteries is technically not feasible. Because of the absence of aortic cross-clamping and reperfusion, endovascular repair was expected to be associated with lower incidences of spinal cord ischemia compared to conventional therapy (154,155,178). Indeed, experiences to date have substantiated this expectation—most studies report spinal cord ischemic complication rates of 0–4% (55,58,154,156–158,160,161,163–165). Delayed presentation of paraplegia, 12 hours to 28 days after stent-graft deployment, has been reported, emphasizing the need for vigilant postoperative monitoring for neurologic complications (157). Several risk factors for spinal cord ischemia have been identified: previous or concurrent abdominal aortic repair (179), increased overall length of aneurysm being excluded (155), and perioperative hypotension (180). Although the incidence of spinal cord ischemic complications appears to be reduced with the endovascular approach, cerebrospinal fluid (CSF) drainage and a number of other protective measures have been proposed to further decrease the occurrence of this devastating complication. These are further reviewed in the Specific Considerations section.

The development of endoleaks is the most common failure mode of stent-graft implantation for aneurysm exclusion, and it remains a key issue for endovascular treatment of both thoracic and abdominal aortic aneurysms. The presence of endoleaks prevents substantial decrease in aneurysm size (68). Although a wide range of early and late endoleak rates have been reported for stent grafting of TAAs, there is clear indication that endoleaks in general, irrespective of specific type, occur less frequently after TAA versus AAA repair (181). In this regard, when observed, TAA endoleaks tend to be type I attachment-site endoleaks, whereas most endoleaks observed after repair of AAA are of the type II variety—reversal of flow in aortic branch vessels that then empty into the aneurysm sac (68). Although type II endoleaks via intercostals or bronchial arteries have been reported after TAA therapy (157–159,164), the incidence is very low. The reason for this difference is unknown. A general consensus exists on the need to expeditiously treat type I and III endoleaks because they represent direct communications between the aneurysm sac and arterial blood under systemic pressures and are associated with an increased risk of rupture (182,183). These leaks can be treated using embolization coils, angioplasty balloons, endovascular graft extensions or cuffs, or even open repair (184,185). In contrast, type II endoleaks are generally benign, and repair is reserved until aneurysm growth occurs (182).

Intuitively, poor landing zone morphology plays a significant role in attachment-site endoleak formation. Landing zones that are short, large diameter, angulated, ulcerated, conical-shaped, and thrombus containing are not conducive to constructing a seal between the stent graft and native vessel. Improvements in device designs for stronger fixation and more rigid patient selection based on appropriate landing zone anatomy should reduce the rate of early and late type I endoleaks. Delayed endoleak formation, however, may also be related to the dynamic nature of degenerative aneurysms. Particularly in patients with diffuse disease, the lesion may progress proximally, distally, or both over time, leading to slow dilatation of the landing zones. Device migration after stent-graft kinking has been another proposed cause of late endoleak formation (668). This phenomenon has been observed primarily with first-generation devices; stent-graft migration rarely has been reported with commercially manufactured devices.

Findings from AAA and TAA studies highlight the basic tenet that stent-graft placement in inappropriate anatomical substrate leads to poor outcomes. Anatomic challenges remain the most important basis for endovascular treatment failure. Arterial access sites and landing zones are particularly important. Given the greater proportion of female patients (in which smaller iliac arteries are the norm) (76) and the larger delivery systems necessary to accommodate the larger diameter of the thoracic aorta, arterial access poses a more significant challenge for endovascular repair of TAA versus AAA. Arterial access complications can be minimized with careful preoperative assessment of the pelvic vessels and development of an appropriate operative plan accordingly. The common femoral artery is the most common site of vascular access, while the iliac artery and abdominal aorta by retroperitoneal exposure are alternative routes. Accessory conduits may facilitate device passage in access vessels with excessive tortuosity, calcification, and occlusive disease. Balloon angioplasty or endoluminal balloon endarterectomy can be employed in patients with focal stenotic lesions. More novel methods include antegrade access through the carotid artery (186) and directly through a small incision made in the aortic arch (187–189). In patients with multiple aneurysms involving the descending thoracic and abdominal aorta or descending thoracic aorta and aortic arch, thoracic stent-graft placement can be combined with open abdominal aneurysm repair (190–194) or the elephant trunk method (195,196), respectively. Hybrid open and endovascular procedures are discussed later.

Regarding landing zones, proximal and distal aneurysm necks must be at least 15–25 mm in length to ensure adequate wall contact for graft fixation and a tight circumferential seal. Recently, exceptions are developing as more proximal descending TAAs are being treated endovascularly.

In this regard, the precise inclusion criteria for neck length are device specific and may depend on individual aortic arch and aneurysm morphologies. Cases in which the distance between the proximal aneurysm origin and left subclavian artery is too short require the landing zone to be lengthened by prophylactic left subclavian to left carotid artery transposition or bypass graft placement. Such maneuvers were employed in 43% of patients in one series (154) and will be discussed in more detail later in this chapter.

Recently, this approach has given way to a trend toward intentional coverage with expectant management in which secondary revascularization is performed when related symptoms, such as left hand or arm ischemia and subclavian steal syndrome, develop. Isolated case reports of inadvertent coverage of the left subclavian origin with a stent graft that resulted in no associated complications (197) led to subsequent studies investigating this approach (198–200). Early results of this revised algorithm suggest that it is safe as long as there is no obstruction of the right vertebral or carotid artery and the left internal mammary artery is not used as a coronary bypass conduit (198–200). This may be explained by the rich, potential, collateral blood supply to the arm, most naturally via retrograde left vertebral flow, which is commonly referred to as the subclavian steal phenomenon. The long-term effects of this approach, however, remain unknown.

In contrast, no easy management strategies exist to deal with an inadequate distal neck above the celiac artery. Intentional stent-graft coverage of the celiac axis is not advised given the potential for hepatic and visceral ischemia. It is difficult to predict whether a coexisting normal superior mesenteric artery can provide sufficient collateral supply. In addition, embolic occlusion of celiac branches with resultant ischemia and, in some cases, tissue necrosis has been implicated as the cause of complications following stent-graft extension across the celiac origin. Of note, without adjunctive transcatheter occlusion of the proximal celiac trunk, a prominent collateral supply may also become a source of retrograde endoleak from the celiac axis.

Although there is reasonable consensus regarding the anatomic requirements for endovascular repair of descending TAAs, the clinical context to which this less invasive treatment option should be applied remains a work in progress and often controversial. Despite the theoretic advantages offered by the endovascular approach, the treatment modality must be viewed in the context of life expectancy and risks. The accumulating mid-term to long-term experience with TAA stent-graft repair in a mostly high-risk patient population has demonstrated survival rates at least comparable to those of open repair, while the risk of morbidities, particularly paraplegia, seems to be reduced. The rapid advances in thoracic stent-graft technology is expected to translate to further outcome improvements in the future, but the long-term durability, benefits, and risks of these devices are currently unknown. With the resolution of these issues pending, the current recommendation is to employ the endovascular approach to TAA repair in high surgical risk, elderly patients who have focal anatomic lesions associated with small, minimally angulated, and cylindrical proximal and distal landing zones of sufficient length. The applicability of this technique to younger, lower risk patients in whom conventional repair can be accomplished with low morbidity and mortality remains to be defined. Data from prospective randomized controlled trials are anxiously awaited.

Aortic Dissection

Background

Aortic dissection occurs when flowing blood enters the aortic wall through a disruption in the intimal lining and cleaves a longitudinal plane within the medial layer. Propagation of this delamination process can progress in variable lengths in a proximal and/or distal direction from the entry tear (with isolated antegrade progression being the more common pattern). As the process extends, a dissection flap or septum consisting of the cleaved lamellar layer of intima and partial thickness of media is created and partitions the original intima-lined lumen ("true" lumen) from a newly formed intramural channel ("false" lumen). This process may lead to additional disruptions in the intimal flap, producing exit or entry sites for flow between the dual lumens. Dissection propagation can also obstruct flow into aortic branch vessels, compromising downstream perfusion and causing distal ischemia. This is termed malperfusion syndrome. Potentially involving the coronaries to iliac arteries, aortic branch vessel compromise occurs by two mechanisms: static obstruction, in which the aortic dissection flap extends directly into an aortic branch, or dynamic obstruction, in which the dissection flap prolapses over the ostium of the branch vessel or collapses the true lumen of the aorta above it (201). The eventual trajectory of flap progression results in a unique morphology for each case; thus, idiosyncratic anatomic relationships are formed between the flap, true lumen, false lumen, and the aortic branch vessels that are involved.

With an incidence of 2.6–3.5 per 100,000 person-years (75,202,203), aortic dissection is considered the most common aortic catastrophe, occurring two to three times more frequently than AAA rupture (204–206). It tends to affect males more frequently with a male-to-female ratio ranging from 2:1 to 5:1 (83,207–210). In a report from the International Registry of Acute Aortic Dissection (IRAD), 63 was the average age among 464 aortic dissection patients (207). Patients with dissections involving the ascending aorta tended to present at a younger age (50–55 years old) than those with dissections of the descending aorta (60–70 years old) (205,207,211,212).

The vast majority of aortic dissections originate in one of two locations: the lateral wall of the ascending aorta within a few centimeters of the aortic valve or in the descending aorta just distal to the site of insertion of the ligamentum arteriosum. These regions presumably are subjected to the greatest hemodynamic stress (213). Anatomically, aortic dissections are classified under two systems. Under the DeBakey system, type I dissection begins in the proximal aorta and involves both the ascending and descending thoracic aorta, type II is confined to the ascending aorta, and type III is confined to the descending aorta (214). Under the Stanford system, type A aortic dissection involves the ascending aorta, whereas type B dissection does not (215). The more simple Stanford system has proved popular as the presence of ascending aortic involvement is associated with well-established prognostic implications and therapeutic considerations. Approximately 60–70% of aortic dissections are type A (204,207). Aortic dissections are also classified according to duration. In general, dissections that are present for less than 2 weeks are considered acute, while those greater than 2 weeks are chronic. At 2 weeks, mortality curves of untreated aortic dissections begin to plateau (209). A review of aortic dissection patients evaluated at the Mayo Clinic found one-third to be chronic at diagnosis (211).

Although the etiology of aortic dissection is not well-defined and the precise initiating event remains unclear, several predisposing factors have been identified (216). As seen with aortic aneurysms, conditions that cause medial degeneration and, in turn, decrease aortic wall integrity and cohesiveness increase the risk of dissection. Patients with inherited connective tissue disorders, such as Marfan's syndrome and Ehlers-Danlos syndrome, display vascular CMN and are at high risk for aortic dissection. Such patients tend to present at a younger age and with lesions involving the ascending aorta (217–219). In an IRAD study, Marfan's syndrome was present in half of those 40 years old and under (220). Necropsy studies have demonstrated, however, that medial degeneration is neither the predominant histological pattern of these lesions nor a prerequisite for dissection formation (221). Other congenital predispositions to dissection include Turner's syndrome (222–224), Noonan's syndrome (225), aortic coarctation (221,226), and bicuspid aortic valve (227,228). In the absence of congenital risk factors, systemic hypertension—found in 70–80% of all dissection patients—is the most important predisposing factor (207–211,221,229). The incidence of coexisting hypertension is higher in type B dissections (70% versus 36%) (207,209,221). By placing a greater mechanical strain on the arterial wall, hypertension may accelerate the normal medial degeneration associated with aging. The potential causative role of hypertension is underlined by the near exclusive occurrence of pulmonary artery dissection in the setting of pulmonary hypertension (230). Other less common acquired risk factors include giant cell aortitis (231,232), cocaine-use (233–237), and deceleration and iatrogenic trauma (238–241). Also, a controversial association exists between pregnancy and dissection in young women (241–245).

The cardinal feature of acute aortic dissection is severe chest or back pain (sometimes both) that is sharp, ripping, or tearing in nature and is almost always abrupt in onset (207,246,247). Patients with type A dissections more frequently experience anterior chest pain, whereas patients with type B dissections tend to experience back and abdominal pain (207). Chronic dissection, in contrast, is usually painless and without symptoms (211). At least one third of acute aortic dissection patients are complicated by manifestations secondary to aortic branch occlusion, proximal extension to the aortic root, and leakage to surrounding structures (248,249). Such complications include acute aortic regurgitation, myocardial ischemia or infarction, cardiac tamponade, stroke, syncope, pulse deficits, visceral ischemia, limb ischemia, and renal failure (207,248).

The natural history of acute aortic dissection is particularly poor for type A dissections; the mortality rate for untreated type A dissection approximates 1–2% per hour during the first 24 hours after symptom onset and reaches 80% by 2 weeks (206,209,250). Type B dissections, however, are less lethal and are associated with a better prognosis (207,215,251,252). Common causes of death include aortic rupture, severe aortic regurgitation, and end-organ compromise secondary to major branch vessel obstruction (203,207,209). Chronic aortic dissection is also associated with a high incidence of rupture with a 5-year survival of 10–15% (250). Progression to aneurysmal dilatation is common in chronic phase dissections. In a 20-year follow-up of operated survivors of aortic dissection (DeBakey et al.), the development of and subsequent rupture of aortic aneurysms was shown to be the leading cause of late deaths (208).

With improvements in diagnostic imaging modalities, two radiologic and pathologic variants of aortic dissection have been recently recognized and diagnosed with increasing frequency: intramural hematoma (IMH) and PAU (216,253–259). When associated with acute symptoms, these pathologic entities are often grouped together under the general classification termed "acute aortic syndrome." It is estimated that 5–17% of diagnosed aortic dissections may actually be IMH or PAU (216,260,261). IMH, considered a precursor of classic dissection, is characterized by blood in the aortic wall without an intimal disruption and is thought to originate from rupture of the vaso vasorum (216,262). PAU is defined by an ulceration of aortic atherosclerotic plaque that penetrates the internal elastic lamina, intima, media, and possibly the adventitia (254,255,263). Compared to classic aortic dissection, IMH and PAU tend to be found in older patients with a history of hypertension and are more likely to be located in the descending thoracic

aorta (43% in IMH and 90% in PAU) (216,255,264,265). Both entities can progress to frank dissection, rupture, or aneurysm formation (254,257,263,266–268). IMH tends to behave in a similiar way as classic aortic dissection. Like type A dissection, type A IMH is associated with a greater risk of adverse progression (269). In contrast, PAU rarely progresses to classic dissection; rather, it forms aneurysms more frequently (up to 50%) (255).

Conventional Therapy

A critical event in the evaluation of patients with suspected aortic dissection is the determination of whether the ascending aorta is involved. Therapeutic strategy hinges on whether type A or B dissection is present. In general, acute type A dissections are considered surgical emergencies, while uncomplicated type B dissections are treated medically (270). Regardless of dissection location, however, all patients in whom a strong suspicion of aortic dissection exists should be placed immediately on antihypertensive therapy to limit dissection progression (271,272).

Acute Type B Dissection

Patients with acute type B dissection are at lower risk of early death from complications and tend to be older and of higher surgical risk. A large retrospective series of uncomplicated type B dissection patients from Duke and Stanford suggested equivalent outcome with medical and surgical treatment (281). Consequently, the preferred treatment for most patients has been medical, in the form of aggressive antihypertensive treatment predominantly with beta-blockers. Surgical intevention is generally reserved for those who develop complications, such as rupture, dissection progression, aneurysmal growth, refractory hypertension, intractable pain, and malperfusion syndromes from aortic branch vessel obstruction (274,282,283). Underlying connective tissue disease should also prompt consideration for early operative repair (7,284). An IRAD study of the outcomes of this complication-specific approach revealed in-house mortality rates of 11% and 31% for medical and surgical treatment groups, respectively (207). Surgical treatment is also associated with significant morbidity, particularly paraplegia (7–36%) (4,285–287). However, it is important to note that because medical therapy alone does not stop blood flow to the false lumen, 20–50% of patients who survive the acute phase develop aneurysmal dilatation of the false lumen within 1–5 years after onset (213,252,288).

Acute Type A Dissection

Given the associated high risk of sudden death resulting from aortic rupture, aortic regurgitation, cardiac tamponade, or myocardial infarction, type A dissection mandates expeditious diagnosis and emergent operative intervention

(273,274). Surgical therapy involves excision of the intimal tear, removal of the most diseased segment of aorta, obliteration of the false channel, reconstitution of the aorta directly or with the interposition of a synthetic graft, and, when necessary, restoration of aortic valve competence (273). In a review of 547 type A dissections in the IRAD, the in-hospital mortality was 27% for patients treated surgically and 56% for those treated medically (275). The associated survival benefit of surgical intervention remained in patients who were more than 70 years old (276).

A small subset of type A dissections exists in which the entry tear is in the descending aorta and propagation occurs up to the ascending aorta in a retrograde manner (retrograde type A). The incidence of this subtype ranges from 10 to 27% among DeBakey type III dissections and from 4 to 20% among Stanford type A dissections (7,215,277–279). Though contoversial, emergent surgical treatment is still recommended for this subtype, even though it poses a difficult dilemma (7,277–280). Excision of the entry tear and replacement of both the ascending aorta and aortic arch is associated with high mortality and morbidity. On the other hand, graft replacement of only the ascending aorta retains the primary entry tear and consequently the postoperative risk of rupture (278,279).

Chronic Dissection

By definition, patients with chronic dissection have survived the acute phase of high mortality. In-hospital survival rates of such patients have approximated 90%, independent of whether they were managed surgically or medically (289). Medical therapy, therefore, is recommended for patients with both type A and type B chronic dissection, with surgery reserved for those who develop an aneurysm or rupture (290,291).

Malperfusion Syndrome

Aortic dissection is complicated by malperfusion syndromes that result from aortic branch vessel obstruction in 30–50% of patients (292,293). Such cases are associated with a particularly poor prognosis; those complicated by mesenteric and renal ischemia have surgical mortality rates of up to 87% and 70%, respectively (292–295). In type A dissection, aortic branch vessel obstruction is usually corrected concomitantly with surgical management for dissection (292). In type B dissection, complication with malperfusion syndrome is an indication for surgical intervention and treatment options include fenestration of the intimal flap, replacement of the diseased aorta, and establishment of bypasses to the ischemic vessels (295).

IMH and PAU

The treatment paradigm for IMH parallels the approach in classical aortic dissection (264,296). A meta-analysis review of 11 IMH studies found cumulative mortality for type A IMH to be 24% for those treated surgically, 47% for those treated medically, and 34% overall; mortality for type B IMH was 14% overall with little difference between surgical (15%) and medical (13%) treatment groups (297). At present, no consensus therapeutic strategy for PAU exists, although a more aggressive surgical approach—independent of location—is being increasingly considered, especially in symptomatic patients (254,266,298). The Yale Center for Thoracic Aortic Disease has identified a 40% rupture rate among PAU patients managed medically (254,266). At a minimum, PAU patients with complications should undergo surgical treatment (299).

Endovascular Treatment

Aortic dissection is the second most common investigational application of thoracic stent-graft technology. The concept of endovascular stent-graft repair of aortic dissection is predicated on successful placement of the device over the primary entry tear to obliterate blood flow into the false lumen (Figure 23–5). The intent is to mimic the effect of successful operative repair with isolation of the false lumen from the circulation and redirection of blood flow into the true lumen. As demonstrated in experimental models of dissection, coverage of the primary entry tear is the optimal method of relieving true lumen collapse, and it promotes thrombosis of the false lumen concomitantly (300). Interestingly, dissections with naturally thrombosed false lumen are associated with improved prognosis (277,301,302). False lumen patency, in contrast, contributes to progressive aortic dilatation and is a predictor of late mortality (303). In the typical type B dissection case, progressive thrombosis proceeds distally, irrespective of the location of the primary intimal disruption (304). The tempo of false lumen thrombosis is variable and influenced by several factors, such as the size of the false lumen and amount of residual false lumen flow via uncovered additional tears. Over time, the false lumen thrombus consolidates and the dissection lumen itself resolves. Besides such gains in aortic remodeling, this endovascular surrogate for open surgery confers two additional benefits: reversal of downstream branch vessel ischemia (particularly in patients with dynamic obstruction) and protection against thoracic false lumen aneurysm formation. Reversal of dynamic obstruction occurs expeditiously after stent-graft placement (27).

Clinical evaluations of stent grafts for the treatment of complicated and uncomplicated acute type B dissection, retrograde type A dissection, and chronic dissection with false lumen aneurysm formation are ongoing at a growing number of institutions worldwide. Applications, however, are limited to dissections with entry tears distal to the left subclavian artery. Initial results are encouraging. Unfortunately, as is the case with TAA, the literature

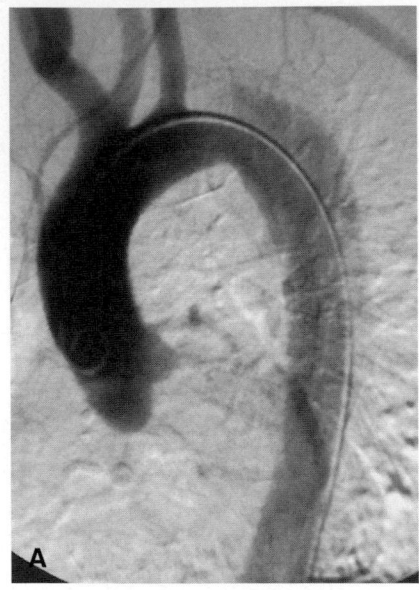
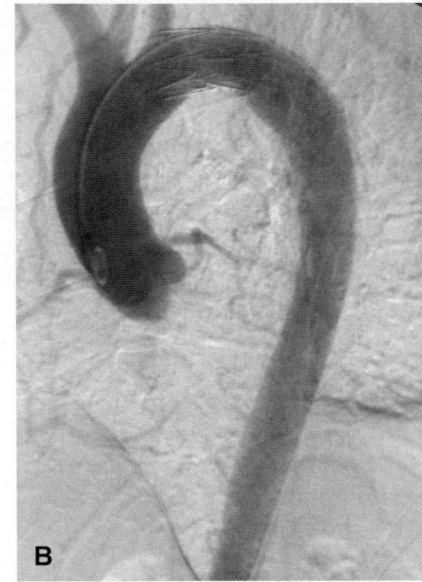
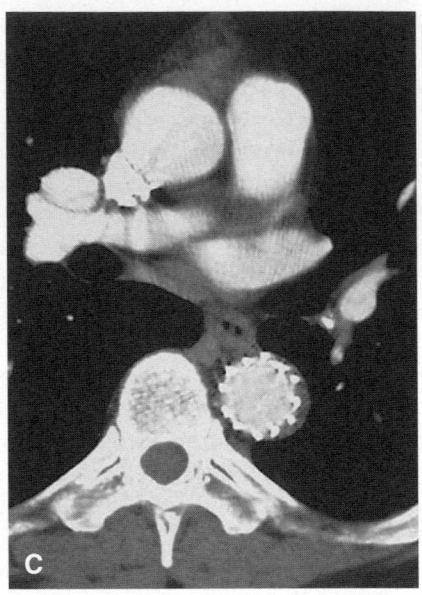

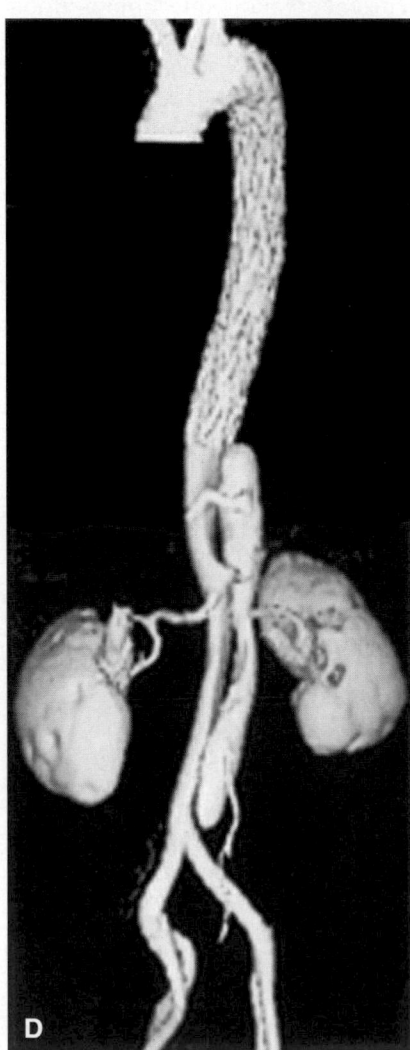
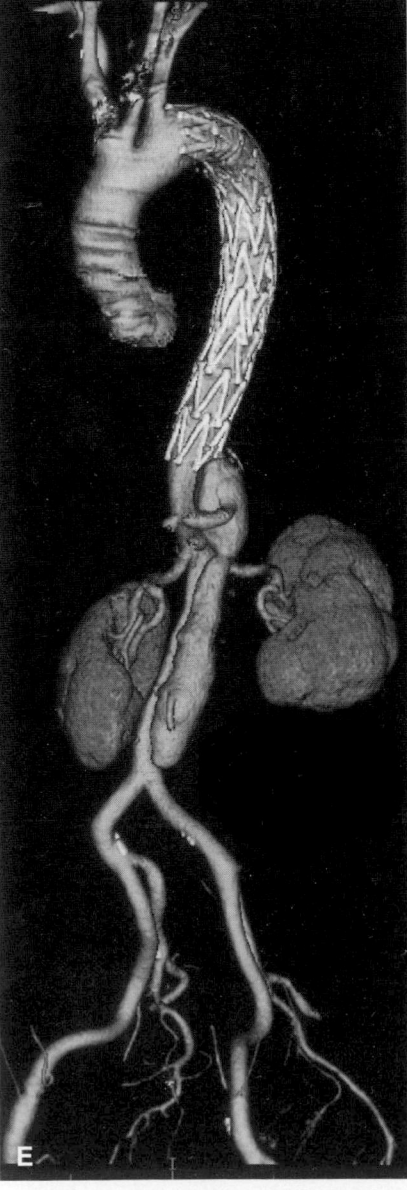

Figure 23–5 Acute type B aortic dissection. **A.** A 44-year-old man with acute back pain and new onset hypertension. Thoracic aortogram in an oblique projection demonstrates an entry tear distal to the left subclavian artery with filling of both true and false lumens. **B.** After stent-graft placement over the primary entry tear, the false lumen is no longer opacified and the true lumen is enlarged. **C., D.** Axial CT at the level of the mid-descending aorta and three-dimensional reconstruction of the CT data set performed 20 months after the endograft procedure show not only thrombosis of the thoracic aortic false lumen but its virtual disappearance. Persistent isolated patency of the false lumen in the abdominal aorta occurs via fenestrations in the dissection septum at the level of the celiac, left renal, and inferior mesenteric arteries, all of which arise from the false lumen. **E.** Similar three-dimensional rendering performed 7.5 years following stent-graft placement confirms a stable appearance without interval evolution. The persistently patent false lumen in the abdomen has not enlarged, and the stented thoracic aorta is unchanged.

for aortic dissection often mixes outcomes from applications in different clinical contexts in terms of age of dissection, extent of disease, and presence of complications. Nonetheless, valuable lessons from this early experience have served to fuel progress in the understanding of the disease process as well as its management by less invasive means. Table 23–5 summarizes the published results of studies on endovascular stent grafting for aortic dissections. In the next section, a review of clinical experiences within specific categories of acute dissection is provided, and an overview of aggregate results, trends, and challenges follows.

Acute Type B Dissection

Although there is general consensus that acute type B dissection should be managed medically and surgical treatment should be reserved for cases with complications (270), the intermediate-term and long-term outcome resulting from this treatment paradigm remains unsatisfactory. The mortality rate among patients treated medically alone ranges from 11 to 20% (205,207,283); furthermore, such patients are at continued long-term risk of aneurysm formation and rupture (213,252,288). Mortality among type B patients treated surgically ranges from 30 to 35% and is significantly worse for those complicated by end-organ ischemia (7,207,289,292).

A recent study investigated the use of thoracic stent grafts among 15 complicated acute type B and four retrograde type A dissection patients at Stanford University and Mie University School of Medicine in Japan (Figure 23–6) (27). Eleven of these patients exhibited symptomatic branch vessel obstruction. The primary entry tear was sealed in 95% of cases with associated complete and partial thrombosis of the thoracic false lumen in 79% and 21% of patients, respectively. In all cases, true lumen expansion occurred immediately, but no aneurysmal expansion or rupture appeared on follow-up. More impressively, follow-up imaging found complete false lumen resolution and no residual evidence of dissection in six cases. Thirty-day mortality was 16% with no additional deaths during mean follow-up of 13 months. Hutschala et al. explored the use of stent grafts in a cohort of acute type B patients who were without indications for surgery and found similar outcomes (309). In light of these results, a prospective, multicenter, randomized, controlled clinical study—the INSTEAD trial (Investigation of stent grafts in patients with type B aortic dissection)—is underway to compare the 1-year outcome of type B aortic dissection treated by stent-graft placement with conventional antihypertensive therapy (316).

Acute Type A Dissection

Significant controversy remains over the proper treatment for patients who have acute type A dissection and an entry tear in the descending aorta. Kato and colleagues treated 10 retrograde type A patients (none of whom showed evidence of cardiac tamponade or severe aortic regurgitation) using endovascular stent grafts (307,317). Entry closure and complete thrombosis of the false lumen of the ascending and the descending aorta were achieved in all patients. During mean follow-up of 20 months, all patients were alive and without rupture or aneurysm formation.

Chronic Dissection

Application of endoluminal stent grafts in the setting of chronic dissection was initially met with skepticism given the anatomic and hemodynamic complexity of such lesions (172). The thick and fibrotic nature of a chronic dissection flap may limit true lumen expansion after device placement. Additionally, multiple fenestrations between the true and false lumens often exist and may hinder false lumen thrombosis. A number of groups, however, have achieved good results with stent-graft treatment of chronic dissections (310,313,318,319).

Nienaber et al. prospectively evaluated stent-graft treatment in 12 patients with chronic type B dissection and compared the results with 12 matched surgical controls (40). Proximal entry closure and complete thrombosis of the false lumen at three months was achieved in all patients. Stent-graft treatment resulted in no mortality or morbidity, while surgical treatment resulted in four deaths and five adverse events. At 3 months, complete thrombosis of the false lumen was achieved in all patients with clear evidence of true lumen expansion and false lumen shrinkage. A similar study by Kato et al. also demonstrated favorable aortic remodeling (41). However, in a second study by the same group that evaluated chronic and acute dissections, complete false lumen thrombosis was documented in all patients, but complete obliteration of the false lumen was found in only 38.5% of the chronic dissection patients versus 70% of the acute dissection patients (mean follow-up of 27 months) (313).

Malperfusion Syndrome

Endovascular stent-graft treatment of aortic dissections offers the additional benefit of relieving dynamic branch vessel obstruction. In a Dake et al. study of acute dissection patients (27), 11 presented with symptomatic branch vessel obstruction involving 38 infradiaphragmatic vascular beds. Of these beds, 22 were obstructed exclusively by a dynamic process, 15 by both dynamic and static mechanisms, and one by static obstruction alone. After stent-graft placement, all 22 of the branch vessels with exclusively dynamic obstruction and six of the 15 arteries with combined dynamic and static involvement were immediately reperfused. Adjunctive endovascular procedures were used to relieve persistent ischemia in the remaining obstructed cases.

Briefly, two other endovascular techniques can be used to relieve branch obstruction. Endovascular placement of an uncovered stent in the true lumen of the obstructed

TABLE 23-5

SUMMARY DATA ON STUDIES OF ENDOVASCULAR TREATMENT OF AORTIC DISSECTIONS

Reference	N	Mean Follow-up (Months)	Devices	Sealing of Primary Entry Tear	Thrombosis of False Lumen	30-day Mortality	Long-term Survival (Time)	Paraplegia
Dake (1999)	19: 4 acute retrograde type A, 15 acute type B (11 with symptomatic compromise of branch vessels)	13	Homemade	94.7%	78.9% complete, 21.1% partial	15.8%	84.2% (mean = 13 mth)	0%
Nienaber et al. (1999)	12 chronic type B (12 matched surgical controls)	12	Talent	100%	100% complete	0% stent-graft, 8.7% surgical	100% for endovascular, 66.7% for surgical (12 mth)	0%
Czermak et al. (2000)	7 type B: 5 acute, 2 chronic	14	Talent, Vanguard	85.7%	85.7%	0%	85.7% (mean = 14 mth)	0%
Hausegger et al. (2001)	5 acute type B uncomplicated	13.4	Talent	100%	100% complete	0%	100% (mean 13.4 mth)	0%
Kato et al. (2001)	15 chronic: 14 type B, 1 type A	24	Homemade	100%	100% complete	0%	100% (mean 24 mth)	0%
Kato et al. (2001)	10 type A retrograde (7 acute, 3 chronic)	20	Homemade	100%	100% complete	0%	100% (mean 20 mth)	0%
Sailer et al. (2001)	7 acute and chronic type B, 4 PAU	8.5	Excluder, Talent, Vanguard	100%	63.6% complete, 27.3% partial	0%	100% (mean 8.5 mth)	0%
Hutschala et al. (2002)	9 acute type B uncomplicated	3	Excluder, Talent	100%	22.2% complete, 77.8% partial	0%	100% (mean 3 mth)	11%

(continued)

436

TABLE 23-5
(continued)

Reference	N	Mean Follow-up (Months)	Devices	Sealing of Primary Entry Tear	Thrombosis of False Lumen	30-day Mortality	Long-term Survival (Time)	Paraplegia
Kato et al. (2002)	38: 10 acute type A, 14 acute type B, 14 chronic type B	27	Homemade	NA	NA	5.3%	92% acute, 100% chronic (1 yr)	3%
Palma et al. (2002)	7C: 35 acute type B, 23 chronic type B, 6 IMH, 6 PAU	29	Homemade	92.9%	NA	5.7%	91.4% (mean 29 mth)	0%
Shim et al. (2002)	15 type B	31.5	Homemade	93.3%	66.7% complete	6.7%	86.7% (mean = 31.5 mth)	NA
Shimono et al. (2002)	37: 16 acute complicated (9 type A retrograde, 7 type B), 8 acute type B uncomplicated, 13 chronic type B	24.5	Homemade	100%	94.4% complete or partial	2.7% overall, 6.3% acute complicated	97.3% overall (actuarial survival 2 yr), 93.8% acute complicated, 100% acute uncomplicated, 100% chronic	NA
Lonn et al. (2003)	20: 14 acute type B, 4 chronic type B, 2 chronic type A	13	Excluder, Talent, Hemobahn	100%	90%	15%	85% (mean = 13 mth)	5%
Lopera et al. (2003)	10 type B complicated: 4 acute, 6 chronic	20	Homemade	90%	60% complete, 30% partial	0%	90% (mean = 20 mth)	NA
Bell et al. (2004)	115	NA	Commercial	82%	NA	6.9%	NA	0.9%
Nienaber et al. (2004)	105: 87 type B, 18 type A	32.4	NA	100%	NA	2.9%	89.5% (mean 32.4 mth)	0%

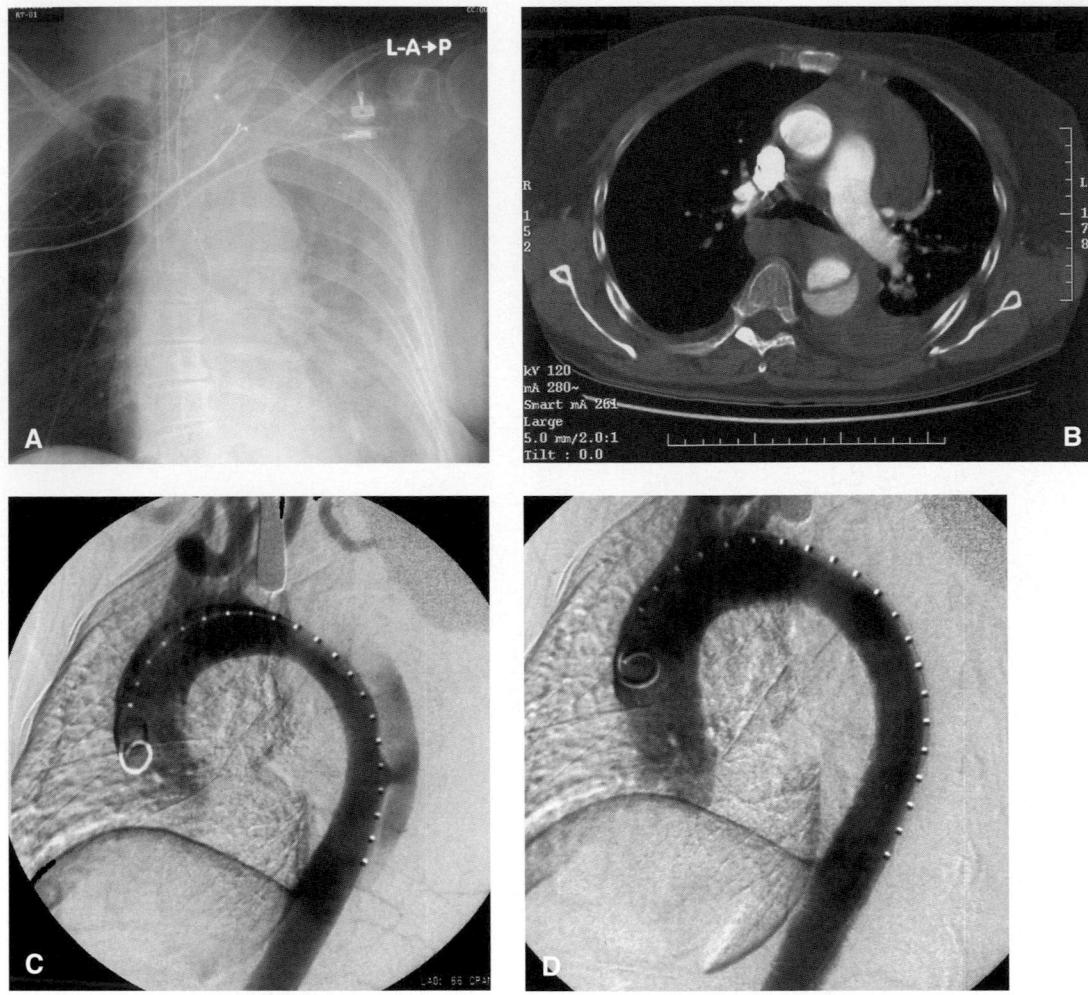

Figure 23–6   Acute type B dissection with aortic rupture. **A.** Frontal radiograph of a 74-year-old woman who experienced chest pain while gardening. Abnormal opacification of the left hemithorax is obvious. **B.** CT scan at the level of the mid-descending thoracic aorta demonstrates abnormal mediastinal hemorrhage and pleural fluid associated with type B aortic dissection. The anterior true lumen is separated from the posterior false lumen by the aortic dissection flap. The ascending aorta is without evidence of dissection. **C.** Thoracic aortogram identifies a type B aortic dissection with flow into the false lumen through a primary entry tear at the level of the mid-descending aorta. Opacification of the false lumen is evident. **D.** After stent-graft deployment across the entry tear with coverage from the left subclavian artery to the distal third of the descending aorta, a thoracic aortogram demonstrates obliteration of the entry tear communication without contrast media filling the false lumen.

branch vessel can attenuate static obstruction (320,321). Percutaneous balloon fenestration can be used to mitigate dynamic obstructions by creating an artificial tear in the dissection flap, allowing communication between true and false lumens (322). In this procedure, the intimal flap is usually first punctured using a needle, crossed with a guide wire, then opened with a balloon. Although the early results of these endovascular treatments appear encouraging (320–323), the long-term outcomes are unknown.

IMH and PAU

Efforts to extend application of endovascular stent-graft technology to aortic dissection variants have focused predominantly on PAU (42,43,324,325). Because PAU is usually focal and almost always in the descending aorta, it is an ideal anatomic target for endovascular stent-graft repair (Figure 23–7) (298). To minimize the risk of paraplegia, a short device could be used to locally seal and stabilize the lesion.

In a meta-analysis of 54 patients accumulated from 13 studies, complete sealing of the ulcer was achieved in 94%, neurologic complications occurred in 6%, and in-hospital mortality was 5% (326). A recently studied cohort of 26 symptomatic type B PAU patients (half of whom were deemed inoperable) was treated by endovascular repair (43). The primary success rate was 92%, and perioperative mortality was 12% with no cases of paraplegia. At 1 and 5 years, survival estimates were 81% and 65%, respectively.

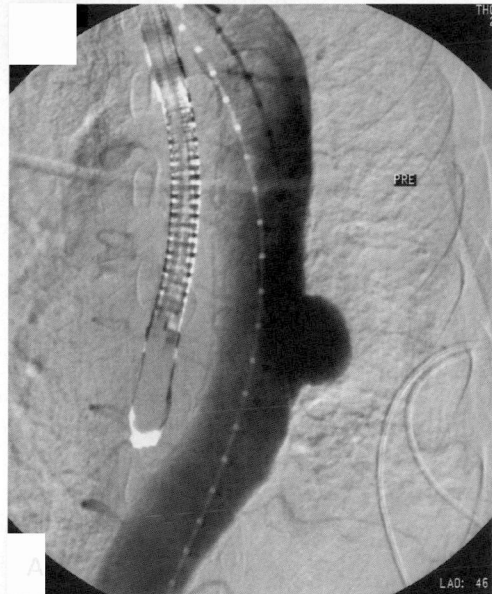

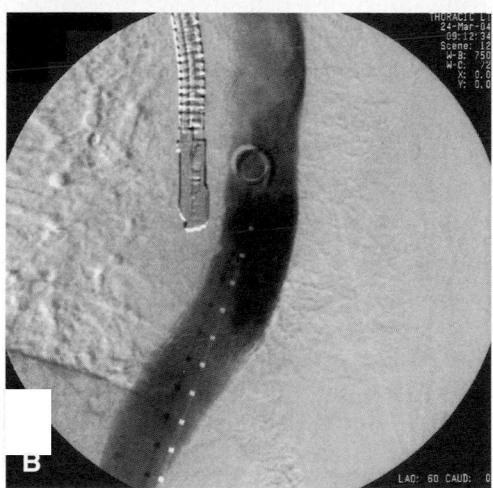

Figure 23–7 Symptomatic giant aortic ulcer. **A.** A 78-year-old man with isolated large ulcer involving the mid-to-distal descending thoracic aorta. This aortogram was obtained after he was admitted through the emergency department with acute back pain. **B.** Thoracic aortogram following stent-graft deployment over the ulcer demonstrates a good result without contrast media filling of the ulcer crater.

General Trends

Upon review of the literature across the multiple subtypes of aortic dissection (Table 23–5), closure of the primary entry tear was successful in 85–100% of cases. Because most primary entry tears in the descending aorta begin immediately distal to the left subclavian artery, adequate proximal anchoring of the device may be difficult. In several studies, anatomical selection criterion for minimum distance between entry tear and subclavian artery origin was set at 5 mm (40,307,310). Intentional coverage of the left subclavian origin with expectant management was commonly used in these studies (306). Alternatively, a device with a proximal segment consisting of a bare stent can be placed across the left subclavian artery to effectively

maximize the length of graft contact with the aortic wall before the tear. However, in other settings in which a retrograde proximal extension of the dissection from the tear to the subclavian artery appears, it may be necessary to place the graft over the branch with its leading margin between the left carotid and subclavian arteries. In addition to carefully monitoring the patient postprocedure for ischemic symptoms referable to the covered left subclavian, it is important to carefully image the thoracic aorta to exclude persistent perfusion of the false lumen via retrograde subclavian flow around the device.

In parallel, successful entry tear coverage induced complete or partial thoracic false lumen thrombosis in 85–100% of patients, even in the settings of chronic and retrograde type A dissections. Partial thrombosis of the false lumen can still be advantageous and can protect the false lumen from enlarging over time because systemic blood pressure is no longer directly transmitted through the primary entry tear. The age of the disease process may play a role in the degree of false lumen thrombosis; it has been found to be most pronounced in those dissections treated within 6 months of presentation (304). True lumen expansion and partial or full false lumen resolution was noted in several studies (27,40,312,313).

Whereas false lumen thrombosis was consistently observed at the level of the implanted stent graft, thrombosis distal to the device and particularly in abdominal false lumens was less common. Uncovered portions of a dissection flap are believed to oscillate with retrograde flow through distal flap disruptions, preventing false lumen thrombosis. This holds implications regarding device length. Most investigators implant stent grafts that are clearly longer than needed to seal the entry tear, usually in the range of 10–15 cm long. This added length confers an appearance to the aortic morphology after implantation that is more normal anatomically, especially in the arch, than that observed after placement of a short device focally over the entry tear. In addition, the longer device promotes a more rapid tempo of thrombus formation within the proximal false lumen. Given that aortic rupture is a cause of death after device implantation (27), acceleration of false lumen thrombosis may improve mortality outcomes. However, extension of stent-graft coverage into the distal one third of the descending thoracic aorta increases the risk of spinal cord ischemia. It has thus been suggested that distal extension with bare stents may provide the structural stability needed to promote false lumen thrombosis without sacrificing intercostal flow.

The development of endovascular stent-graft technology and its application as an alternative management strategy to medical therapy and open surgical intervention of patients with aortic dissection is an exciting and potentially valuable advance. Improved treatment options are desired because conventional therapies for aortic dissection and its attendant complications are often associated with significant failure rates, result in substantial morbidity and mortality, or do little to reduce the risk of aneurysm formation. This section has reviewed the current clinical experience with stent-graft placement for treatment of complicated and uncomplicated acute type B dissection, retrograde type A dissection, chronic dissection, and PAU. It is imperative to first appreciate the wide array of clinical, anatomic, and temporal manifestations within the umbrella pathology of aortic dissection. Evaluation of the role of endoluminal stent-graft technology must be performed within the context of each of these subgroups through rigorous, prospective-controlled investigations and compared against respective standard treatment. Although this evaluation poses a much more significant challenge, the encouraging early results highlighted here underscore the potential for stent-graft therapy to supplant conventional—and often suboptimal—treatment paradigms and to provide patients with a less invasive therapeutic alternative that may concomitantly achieve gains in survival.

Thoracic Aortic Injury

Background

Blunt traumatic injury to the thoracic aorta results in a transverse tear in the aortic wall of varying depth; the extent of damage ranges from a partial tear in the intima to complete transection. Traumatic aortic disruption (TAD) is uncommon but catastrophic. Approximately 80–90% of patients, particularly those with complete transection, die before reaching the hospital (327–329). Of those who survive to reach medical attention, up to 40% die within the first 24 hours because of aortic rupture or other serious injuries (330). Rapid diagnosis and treatment is, therefore, essential.

Most lesions are generated by sudden deceleration injuries such as frontal-impact motor vehicle collisions (which account for up to 18% of motor vehicle-related deaths) (331,332), falls from great height, or injuries caused by explosions (333). The dominant pathophysiologic mechanism of TAD is sudden deceleration with creation of a shear force between a relatively mobile part of the thoracic aorta and an adjacent fixed segment (334). The thoracic aorta is relatively immobile at the ligamentum arteriosum, the atrial attachment of the pulmonary veins and vena cava, and the diaphragm. Consequently, the aortic isthmus is the most common location of injury (50–71%), followed by the ascending aorta (18%) and the distal aorta (14%) (328).

TAD patients are typically young and present with severe coexisting head, chest, abdominal, and orthopedic injuries. Clinical manifestations of TAD are often deceptively meager and may be masked by a clinical picture of polytraumatism. The most common TAD symptom is interscapular or retrosternal pain, but unlike nontraumatic aortic dissection, it is present in only 25% of patients (335).

In 1–2% of cases, the injury is not diagnosed initially and the patient survives long enough to develop a chronic traumatic false aneurysm (328). The temporal definition of chronic varies in the literature between 36 hours and 3 months (45,336–340). Unlike typical degenerative aneurysms, these are usually localized, calcified, saccular in morphology, and located just distal to the left subclavian artery (341). Like most chronic aortic diseases, chronic traumatic pseudoaneurysms are at risk of continual expansion and eventual rupture. In a study of 413 chronic traumatic pseudoaneurysm patients, 42% developed signs or symptoms of expansion within 5 years (338). Of those who were not treated operatively, 33% died of rupture or other complications.

Conventional Therapy

The standard treatment for TAD is early open surgical repair with an interposition graft through a left thoracotomy with either passive or active cardiopulmonary bypass (342). TAD patients commonly present with multiple complex nonaortic injuries that can render conventional open repair difficult. For example, use of systemic heparin may aggravate associated neurologic, visceral, or orthopedic injuries. Additionally, up to 20% patients have thoracic or cervical spine injuries that make proper positioning difficult (331). In cases in which prompt repair is not feasible, several authors have advocated initial hypotensive and negative inotropic therapy with surgical treatment delayed for instances in which patients become more stable (343–347). Although this treatment approach has been shown to improve outcomes (343,345), surgical repair overall continues to be associated with high rates of mortality and morbidity. According to contemporary studies, the operative mortality rate after open operation ranges from 8 to 33%, and the risk of paraplegia can reach 26% (339,348–352).

Surgical intervention is also standard therapy for chronic traumatic pseudoaneurysm patients who have symptoms or demonstrate aortic expansion (336–339). Open repair for chronic traumatic pseudoaneurysm is associated with a mortality rate of 4–17% and a risk of paraplegia between 1 and 5% (338,349).

Endovascular Treatment

Aortic endografting is an attractive repair strategy for TAD because of its minimally invasive characteristics and the avoidance of anticoagulation and circulation assistance. In addition, stent-graft placement may be particularly useful in the setting of polytrauma because it can be performed with little delay after the management of another life-threatening lesion and applied during the acute phase without the risk of destabilizing patients. In return, TAD presents a favorable anatomic target for stent-graft exclusion given its focal nature and proclivity to being located in the proximal descending aorta (Figure 23–8).

The current clinical experience of endovascular stent grafting for treatment of TAD is limited, with fewer than 200 total implements worldwide. Most published studies consist of small cohorts of fewer than 15 patients. The results of 19 studies are summarized in Table 23–6. Upon review of these preliminary studies in aggregate, the

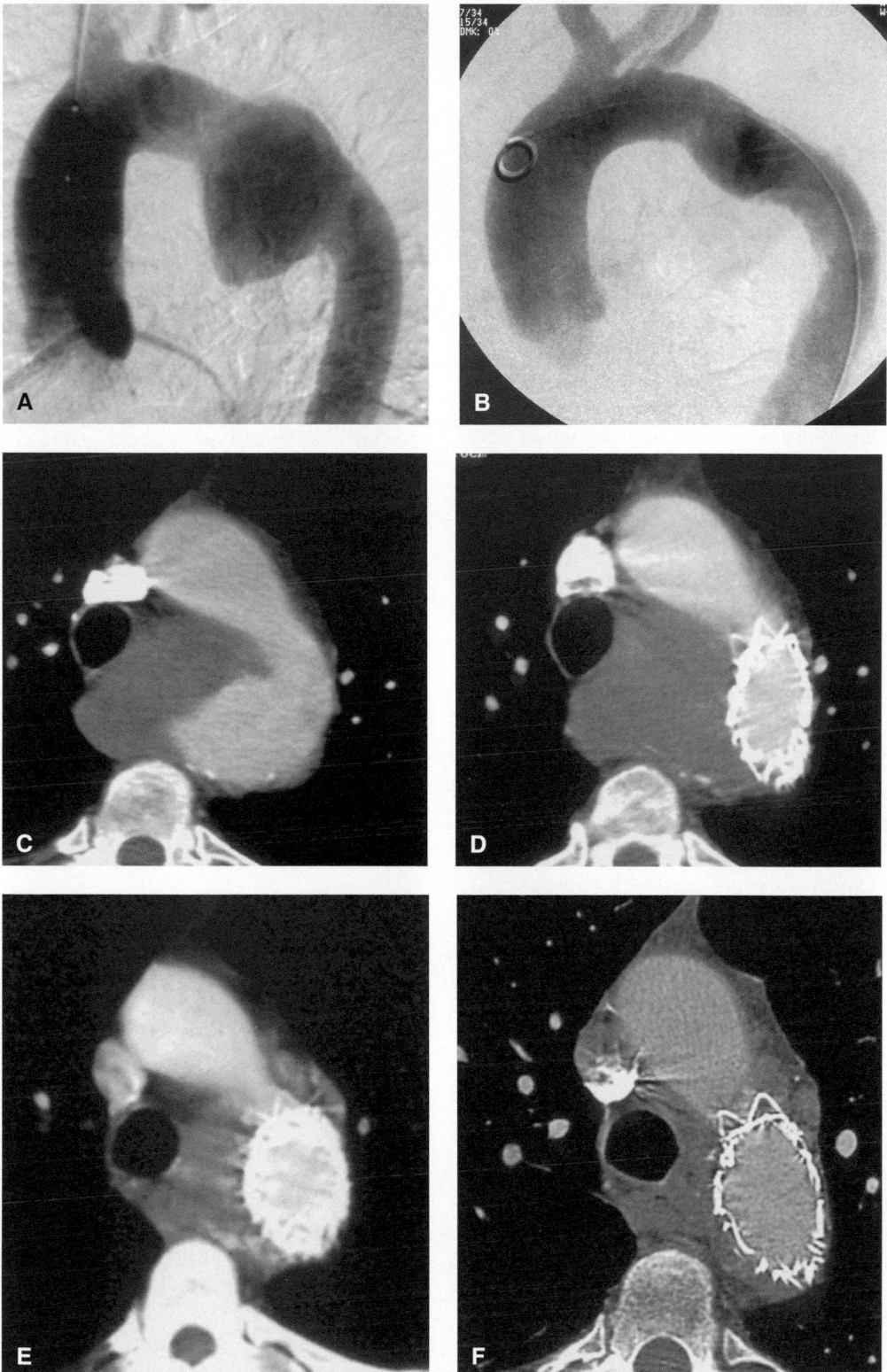

Figure 23–8 A 54-year-old man with chronic traumatic aneurysm of the transverse arch. **A.** Thoracic aortogram reveals a large aneursym of the proximal descending aorta. **B.** A similar left anterior oblique projection of the aortic arch after stent-graft deployment demonstrates good position of the stent graft with no filling of the aneurysm sac. Axial CT images at the level of the transverse arch and proximal descending aorta performed prior to endovascular management. **C.** Immediately prior to hospital discharge after stent-graft placement, **D.** at 1-year follow-up, **E.**, and 3 years after the procedure, **F.** These scans, comparing the appearance of the aneurysm over time, demonstrate persistent thrombosis of the aneurysm sac with a progressive decrease in the diameter of the traumatic lesion.

outcomes of stent-graft therapy compare favorably relative to conventional treatment. The use of endovascular stent grafting in these studies was associated with a technical success rate of 99%, a mortality rate of 5.5%, a postoperative paralysis rate of 0%, and an endoleak rate of 8.2%. Of the 10 deaths, all but three were primarily the result of comorbid injuries. One patient died of hemorrhagic shock secondary to an undetected incomplete proximal seal (353). A second died of delayed rupture from an undetected ascending aorta lesion (354).

To date, no cases of paraplegia have been reported. This is likely because the proximal location of such lesions and the need to cover only a small portion of the thoracic aorta, sparing most intercostals and lumbar arteries that supply the spinal cord.

The majority of endoleaks observed in these studies were proximal perigraft leaks. Proximal sealing may be more difficult in this setting because patients tend to be younger and with a tighter radius of curvature into the arch. Furthermore, because TAD usually begins at the aortic isthmus, a proximal landing zone greater than 15 mm in length distal to the left subclavian artery is rarely encountered. Intentional coverage of the left subclavian artery with expectant management was the more common approach in these studies and, as seen with aortic dissection, also was well-tolerated in this setting (Figure 23–9).

STRATEGIES TO EXPAND STENT-GRAFT APPLICABILITY

The cumulative worldwide experience with endovascular stent-graft treatment of abdominal and thoracic aortic diseases has highlighted not only its great potential as an advance in treatment but also its limitations in terms of complications, anatomical restrictions, and high-risk clinical settings. Various strategies are being explored to address these limitations and may potentially permit stent-grafting in settings that would have otherwise precluded use of this less invasive approach. In this section, methods to minimize complications, such as spinal cord ischemia, will be discussed, and innovative approaches to extend the application of stent grafts to lesions involving branches of the aortic arch or abdominal aorta will be presented. The conclusion addresses the potential of applying stent graft technology to aortic rupture—the most feared sequelae shared by a range of thoracic aortic conditions.

Complication Prevention

Adjunctive Measures for Spinal Cord Protection

Cerebrospinal fluid (CSF) drainage has emerged as a potential protective measure to reduce the incidence of spinal cord ischemia in open and endovascular procedures

(126,368). Regarding mechanisms, a decrease in intrathecal pressure is thought to promote spinal cord artery perfusion (369). This adjunctive procedure was found to reduce neurological deficit in a randomized study of open repair (370), and it was also successfully used to reverse delayed neurological deficit following endovascular TAA exclusion (371). Thus, some groups advocate use of CSF drainage in patients treated endovascularly for thoracic aortic lesions specifically in those with concurrent or previous abdominal aortic repair (368). Others have developed methods to identify patients at high risk for spinal cord ischemia. Ishimaru and colleagues at Tokyo University Medical School monitor evoked spinal cord potentials during temporary interruption of the intercostal arteries by a specially designed retrievable occlusive device (372).

Overcoming Anatomical Limitations

Proximal Lesions

This chapter thus far has focused on thoracic aortic lesions distal to the left subclavian artery origin. As discussed, it is common for lesions of the descending thoracic aorta to be located within the proximal neck length necessary for adequate device fixation. This has been commonly managed by intentional coverage with expectant management (373). However, when the lesion involves the left subclavian artery or is located more proximally in the transverse arch or even the ascending aorta, adjunctive procedures are needed (374).

Bypass and Transposition Procedures
When the left subclavian artery origin is involved in the actual lesion, reflux endoleak is a significant concern. Left subclavian to left carotid artery transposition, bypass graft placement with proximal ligation, or simple coil embolization of the proximal left subclavian artery should be performed before stent-graft deployment. The left common carotid artery origin may also become involved and in such cases, unlike with the subclavian artery, intentional graft coverage is not appropriate. Disconnection and revascularization of the left common carotid artery through crossover carotid-to-carotid bypass at the time of the left subclavian artery operation is recommended (374).

Elephant Trunk Technique
In patients with diffuse thoracic aortic disease involving the ascending aorta, transverse arch, and descending thoracic aorta, the elephant trunk technique (375,376), a two-staged procedure, can be used to reconstruct most or all of the thoracic aorta (377). In the first stage, total ascending aorta and transverse arch repair is performed via a median sternotomy and an excess portion of the graft, the elephant trunk, is left dangling within the lumen of the diseased

TABLE 23–6
SUMMARY DATA ON STUDIES OF ENDOVASCULAR TREATMENT OF TRAUMATIC AORTIC DISRUPTIONS

Reference	N	Mean Follow-up (Months)	Devices	Technical Success	Deaths	Paraplegia	Endoleak
Kato et al. (1997)	10	15	Homemade	100%	0	0	1
Rousseau et al. (1999)	9	11.6	Talent, MinTec	100%	0	0	0
Ruchat et al. (2001)	4	11	Talent	100%	0	0	0
Bortone et al. (2002)	6	14.8	Excluder, Talent	100%	0	0	0
Czermak et al. (2002)	6	17.4	Excluder, Talent	83.3%	0	0	1
Fattori et al. (2002)	19	20	Excluder, Talent	100%	0	0	1
Fujikawa et al. (2002)	6	(0–36)	Homemade	100%	1	0	0
Lachat et al. (2002)	12	17	Excluder, Talent, Homemade	100%	1	0	2
Thompson et al. (2002)	5	20.2	Excluder	100%	0	0	0
Orend et al. (2002)	11	14	Excluder, Talent	100%	1	0	2
Daenen et al. (2002)	7	9	Excluder, Talent	100%	1	0	0
Karmy-Jones et al. (2003)	11	(2–24)	Homemade, Talent, AneuRx, Ancure	100%	3	0	4
Marty-Ane et al. (2003)	9	(4–20)	Excluder, Talent	100%	0	0	1
Orford et al. (2003)	9	21	Homemade, Cook-Zenith	100%	1	0	0
Demers et al. (2004)	15	55	Excluder, Homemade	100%	1	0	2
Dunham et al. (2004)	16	10.7	Talent, AneuRx, Ancure	100%	1	0	0
Kato et al. (2004)	6	6	Homemade	100%	0	0	1
Ott et al. (2004)	6 (vs. 12 surgical)	24	Talent	100%	0 (2 surgical)	0 (2 surgical)	0
Richeux et al. (2004)	16	32	Excluder, Talent	100%	0	0	NA
Total	183			99.1%	5.5%	0%	8.2%

443

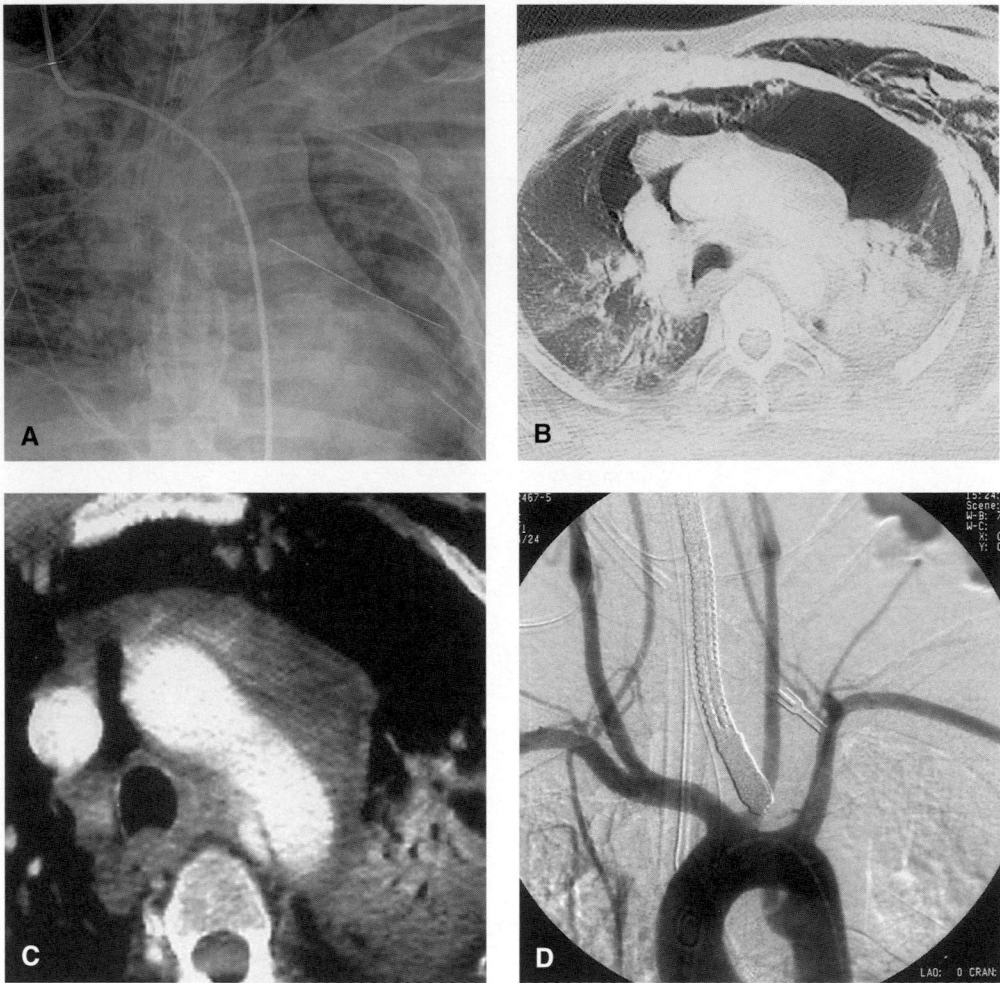

Figure 23–9 Acute traumatic injury of the thoracic aorta following a motorcycle accident. Frontal chest radiograph **A.** and axial CT scan **B.** of a 60-year-old man after motorcycle accident show a shift of mediastinal structures from left to right, pulmonary contusions, bilateral pneumothoraces, multiple displaced rib fractures, and subcutaneous emphysema. **C.** CT image at the level of proximal descending thoracic aorta demonstrates a pseudoaneurysm and associated large mediastinal hematoma. **D., E.** PA and LAO thoracic aortograms show an obvious pseudoaneurysm associated with an injury at the aortic isthmus.

proximal descending aorta. In the second stage, usually 2–3 months later, the descending thoracic aorta is repaired via left thoracotomy. Because of the dangling elephant trunk, the second stage is greatly facilitated because it is no longer necessary to obtain exposure of the proximal descending thoracic aorta and distal arch. A few centers have reported successful deployment of thoracic stent grafts in place of the second stage of a traditional elephant trunk procedure (195,377,378). Here, the proximal end of the stent graft is inserted within the previously inserted elephant trunk extension (Figure 23–10).

Distal Lesions

Approximately 5% of patients with AAA also have a descending TAA (379); 20–25% of patients with descending TAA also have AAA (78–80). Patients with aortic disease of the thoracic and the abdominal aorta present a formidable challenge. Traditional management includes simultaneous or sequential open repair through separate incisions. Both methods result in poor outcomes (78,380).

Combined Endovascular and Open Repair

In an effort to decrease the cumulative risk associated with thoracotomy and laparotomy, 18 patients at Stanford were treated simultaneously with conventional abdominal aortic replacement and endovascular stent-graft placement into the descending thoracic aorta (190). One patient died perioperatively, but the actuarial survival rate was 92% at 1 year. All remaining patients demonstrated complete exclusion of the aneurysm, and half experienced shrinkage of the aneurysm sac. Although the long-term results of such an approach are unknown, this hybrid open and endovascular

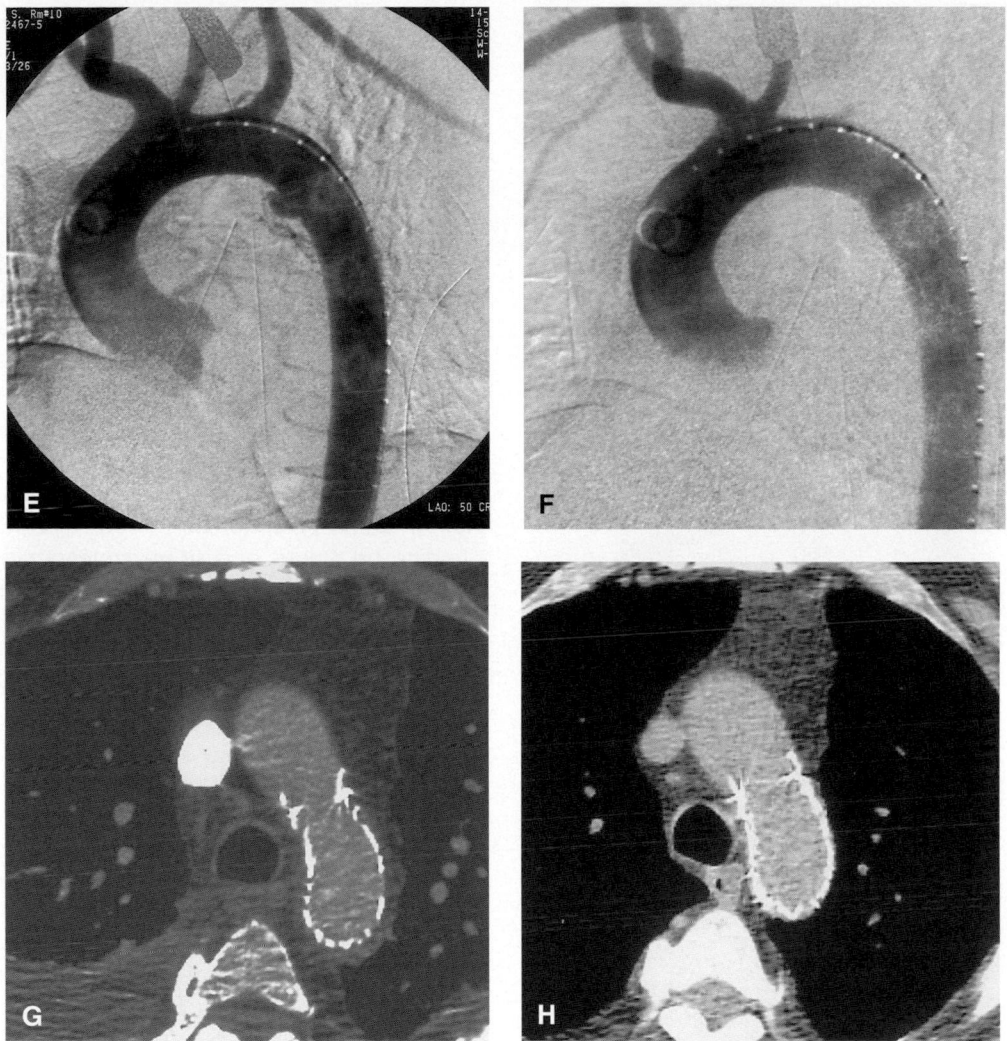

Figure 23–9 *(continued)*   **F.** LAO thoracic aortogram after stent-graft placement demonstrates a good result without residual abnormality. Given the proximity of the pseudoaneurysm to the left subclavian artery, the stent graft was intentionally placed across the ostium of the subclavian artery. Perfusion of the left arm is provided via retrograde flow in the left vertebral artery. Subsequently, the patient recovered uneventfully without systems. Axial CT scans immediately prior to hospital discharge **G.** and 9 months after the procedure **H.** demonstrate no pseudoaneurysm and progressive resolution of mediastinal blood.

treatment for multilevel disease seems promising and warrants further investigation. Since this study, a few case reports have explored the use of endovascular stent-graft treatment for aortic disease at both levels (381,382).

Device-Based Strategies

An inadequate proximal or distal implantation site commonly renders endovascular repair unsuitable. Efforts to preserve aortic branch flow and extend sealing zones in endoluminal repair of thoracic and abdominal aortic lesions have led to the development of fenestrated and branched devices. Although early devices were made to accommodate flow into the renal and superior mesenteric arteries in AAA stent-graft repair, these device-based solutions can be readily adapted for thoracic endografts.

Fenestrated Stent Grafts

Use of fenestrations in the stent-graft body to maintain perfusion to the renal arteries in AAA repair was first described in 1996 (383) and was later developed by Australian groups led by Anderson and Lawrence-Brown (384–386). The basic design involves the custom creation of holes in the proximal part of the fabric of the device to mirror the location and size of ostia of renal and visceral arteries. Precise preoperative imaging and measurements are necessary for accurate placement of the fenestrations. In terms of implantation technique, the prosthesis is first partially deployed to allow for longitudinal and rotational manipulation of the endograft for exact positioning of the fenestrations with their respective ostia using previously placed radiopaque markers. Catheterization of renal vessels is then carried out from

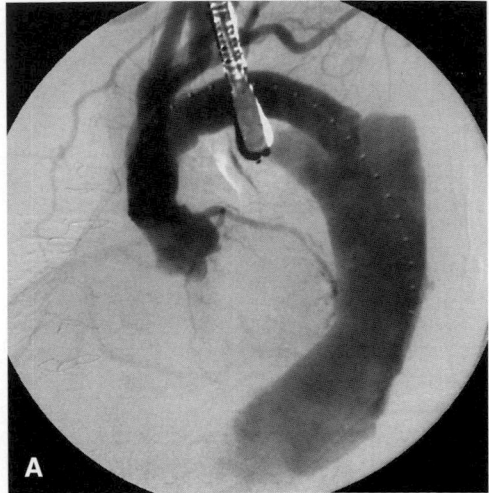

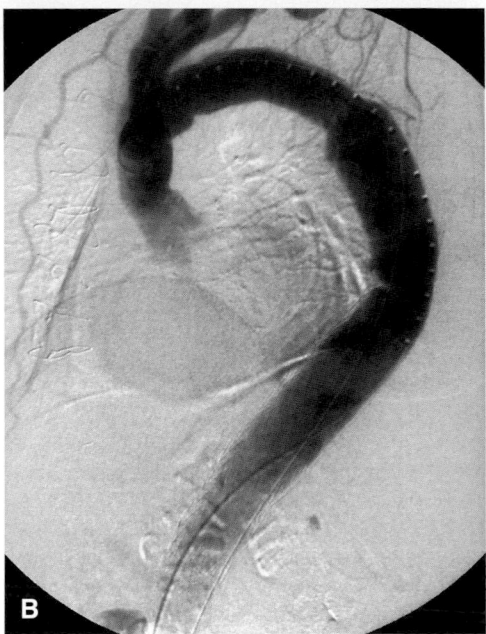

Figure 23–10 Second phase of a staged thoracic aneurysm repair utilizing an aortic stent graft following an open elephant trunk procedure with ascending aortic replacement. **A.** A 73-year-old woman with total thoracic aneurysm returns for second-stage repair of the descending thoracic aorta. Four weeks earlier, she underwent open repair of the ascending aorta, aortic arch, and creation of an elephant trunk anchored just beyond the left subclavian artery and placed within the descending component of the aneurysm. A left anterior oblique thoracic aortogram shows the elephant trunk within the arch and proximal descending aorta surrounded by a large aneurysm. **B.** Thoracic aortogram following placement of two thoracic stent grafts. The first was deployed well within the elephant trunk while the distal device overlapped within the first and extended to the distal aneurysm neck at the celiac artery. Good circumferential sealing of the devices is noted without residual filling of the aneurysm sac.

within the graft lumen, and angioplasty balloons are positioned and partially inflated in the renal artery ostia to act as railings for accurate alignment of the graft fenestrations. The device is then fully deployed. To stabilize the graft-renal ostium junction and improve fixation of the device overall,

modified bare stents are often deployed with two thirds of the stent in the renal artery and the rest in the graft lumen. Further, because simple apposition of the fenestration to the ostium poses a risk for endoleak, the aortic end of the renal stent is often flared using balloons to rivet the fabric against the aortic wall.

Greenberg et al. (387) and Verhoeven et al. (388) used fenestrated stent grafts for treatment of AAAs in 32 and 18 patients, respectively. The combined results of these two studies showed only one death (2%) and one type I endoleak (2%) occurring within 30 days of device implantation. Of the 129 total target vessels treated, impaired blood flow was detected in seven vessels (5.4%). In the Greenberg study, aneurysmal sac shrinkage was observed in 76% of patients at 12 months.

In light of these encouraging results in AAA repair, adaptation of this technique for thoracic diseases seems feasible. To date, no reports of customized fenestrated stent grafts to preserve flow to the left subclavian artery have been completed, although stent grafts with partial, U-shaped fenestrations (389), also called scallop-edged grafts, and complete proximal uncovered regions, such as the Talent device, have been employed with successful branch perfusion maintenance.

Branched Stent Grafts

Inoue and colleagues were the first to design branched stent grafts to accommodate flow to renal and visceral branches as well as to aortic arch vessels (390–394). These devices are constructed using Dacron polyester fabric supported by multiple rings of nickel titanium wire, and branches are incorporated into the main body of the device. Thoracic devices with one branch for the left subclavian artery and three branches for all three arch vessels have been made and deployed in patients (391). To place the branched graft section within the left subclavian artery, a gooseneck snare wire inserted percutaneously through the left brachial artery is used to catch and pull back on a traction wire previously attached to the tip of the branched graft section. Although short-term data using these devices demonstrated feasibility and acceptable outcomes (391), it is readily apparent that the associated implantation technique is highly complex. Successful deployment requires a level of technical skill that will be difficult to replicate.

Chuter et al. conceived alternative branched devices using a modular rather than unibody system for treatment of thoracoabdominal and arch aortic lesions (395–399). In the thoracic version (395,398), the prosthesis contains a bifurcated proximal component and a tubular distal component. The proximal component is shaped like an upside down "Y" with a long narrow innominate limb and a short, wide aortic limb. Before stent-graft implantation, carotid to carotid bypass and left subclavian to left carotid transposition are performed. Device deployment involves delivery of the collapsed proximal component through the right carotid artery and innominate artery followed by release of the device with the innominate limb in the innominate artery and the aortic limb in the aortic arch. This is followed by retrograde delivery of the distal component and deployment into the aortic limb of the previously placed module.

Intraoperative Fenestration

Successful use of fenestrated and branched stent grafts requires careful preoperative planning, precise graft manufacturing, and considerable technical expertise. Furthermore, the need for custom manufacturing of these devices limits its widespread application. McWilliams et al. investigated the use of intraoperative fenestration to maintain branch perfusion (400,401). They reported clinical application of this highly experimental technique in one patient with a thoracic stent graft covering the left subclavian artery (401). In this case, graft fenestration was made through the left subclavian artery via a supraclavicular incision using the reverse end of a stiff guide wire. The fenestration was then further dilated using serial cutting balloons and stented. Six-month follow-up imaging showed no endoleak and a patent subclavian artery.

Aortic Rupture

The natural history of nearly every thoracic aortic disease is eventual progression to rupture, a catastrophic event. Aortic rupture, whether because of aneurysm, dissection, or trauma, is associated with a community-based mortality of 80–90% (5,83,350,402–405). One of the main objectives of surgical and endovascular stent-graft treatment of thoracic aortic lesions is to prevent progression to rupture. Rupture itself has recently been a proposed indication for endovascular therapy (Figure 23–11). Stanford University Medical Center treated 23 patients with aortic rupture resulting from a range of etiologies (8 acute trauma, 7 dissection, and 8 other) using the Gore TAG stent graft. Survival with mean follow-up of 10.2 months was 78% with no cases of paraplegia, open conversion, or need for dialysis. These preliminary results underscore the potential for expanding the application of thoracic stent-graft technology to this high-risk clinical setting.

SUMMARY

The recent development of endovascular stent-graft technology and its application as an alternative therapy to open surgical treatment of patients with various thoracic aortic diseases is an exciting and potentially valuable advance. The exact role that this less invasive treatment option will play remains to be defined as studies continue to accumulate long-term data and experience and as devices and techniques continue to evolve. Rather than replacing open surgical treatment, endoluminal stent grafting will likely play a complementary role and add a

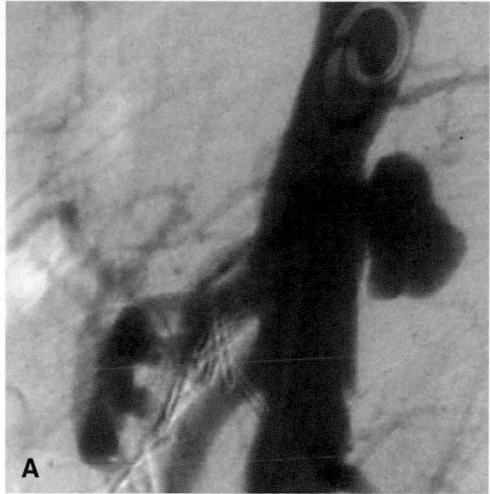

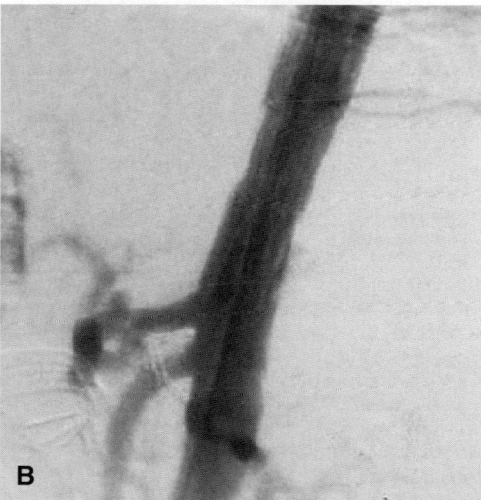

Figure 23–11 A 22–year-old woman with acute pseudoaneurysm of the aorta at the level of the celiac trunk after a gun shot injury. **A.** A lateral aortogram demonstrates a polypoid pseudoaneurysm of the aorta projecting posteriorly just above the celiac artery. **B.** Lateral aortogram performed immediately after stent-graft placement shows successful coverage of the pseudoaneurysm with preservation of flow to the celiac artery.

less invasive option to the medical armamentarium for treatment of thoracic aortic diseases. It is clear that the limitations of both treatment approaches are distinct. What is considered high risk for surgery is defined by clinical parameters in terms of existing comorbidities and physiologic reserve, yet contraindications for endovascular stent-graft treatment are more defined by anatomical constraints. In this regard, each may fulfill the treatment gaps left open by the other.

REFERENCES

1. DeBakey ME, McCollum CH, Graham JM. Surgical treatment of aneurysms of the descending thoracic aorta: long-term results in 500 patients. J Cardiovasc Surg (Torino) 1978;19:571–576.

2. Kouchoukos NT, Dougenis D. Surgery of the thoracic aorta. N Engl J Med 1997;336:1876–1888.

3. Greenberg R, Khwaja J, Haulon S, et al. Aortic dissections: new perspectives and treatment paradigms. Eur J Vasc Endovasc Surg 2003;26:579–586.

4. Svensson LG, Crawford ES, Hess KR, et al. Variables predictive of outcome in 832 patients undergoing repairs of the descending thoracic aorta. Chest 1993;104:1248–1253.

5. Moreno-Cabral CE, Miller DC, Mitchell RS, et al. Degenerative and atherosclerotic aneurysms of the thoracic aorta. Determinants of early and late surgical outcome. J Thorac Cardiovasc Surg 1984; 88:1020–1032.

6. Fann JI, Smith JA, Miller DC, et al. Surgical management of aortic dissection during a 30-year period. Circulation 1995;92(Suppl): II113–121.

7. Miller DC, Mitchell RS, Oyer PE, et al. Independent determinants of operative mortality for patients with aortic dissections. Circulation 1984(3 Pt 2);70:I153–164.

8. Dotter CT. Transluminally placed coilspring endarterial tube grafts. Long-term patency in canine popliteal artery. Invest Radiol 1969;4:329–332.

9. Balko A, Piasecki GJ, Shah DM, et al. Transfemoral placement of intraluminal polyurethane prosthesis for abdominal aortic aneurysm. J Surg Res 1986;40:305–309.

10. Chuter TA, Green RM, Ouriel K, et al. Transfemoral endovascular aortic graft placement. J Vasc Surg 1993;18:185–195; discussion 195–187.

11. Laborde JC, Parodi JC, Clem MF, et al. Intraluminal bypass of abdominal aortic aneurysm: feasibility study. Radiology 1992; 184:185–190.

12. Lawrence DD, Jr., Charnsangavej C, Wright KC, et al. Percutaneous endovascular graft: experimental evaluation. Radiology 1987;163: 357–360.

13. Mirich D, Wright KC, Wallace S, et al. Percutaneously placed endovascular grafts for aortic aneurysms: feasibility study. Radiology 1989;170:1033–1037.

14. Palmaz JC, Sibbitt RR, Tio FO, et al. Expandable intraluminal vascular graft: a feasibility study. Surgery 1986;99:199–205.

15. Palmaz JC, Tio FO, Laborde JC, et al. Use of stents covered with polytetrafluoroethylene in experimental abdominal aortic aneurysm. J Vasc Interv Radiol 1995;6:879–885.

16. Yoshioka T, Wright KC, Wallace S, et al. Self-expanding endovascular graft: an experimental study in dogs. AJR Am J Roentgenol 1988;151:673–676.

17. Moon MR, Dake MD, Pelc LR, et al. Intravascular stenting of acute experimental type B dissections. J Surg Res 1993;54:381–388.

18. Parodi JC, Palmaz JC, Barone HD. Transfemoral intraluminal graft implantation for abdominal aortic aneurysms. Ann Vasc Surg 1991;5:491–499.

19. Dattilo JB, Brewster DC, Fan CM, et al. Clinical failures of endovascular abdominal aortic aneurysm repair: incidence, causes, and management. J Vasc Surg 2002;35:1137–1144.

20. Finlayson SR, Birkmeyer JD, Fillinger MF, et al. Should endovascular surgery lower the threshold for repair of abdominal aortic aneurysms? J Vasc Surg 1999;29:973–985.

21. Hill BB, Wolf YG, Lee WA, et al. Open versus endovascular AAA repair in patients who are morphological candidates for endovascular treatment. J Endovasc Ther 2002;9:255–261.

22. Howell MH, Strickman N, Mortazavi A, et al. Preliminary results of endovascular abdominal aortic aneurysm exclusion with the AneuRx stent graft. J Am Coll Cardiol 2001;38:1040–1046.

23. Rutherford RB, Krupski WC. Current status of open versus endovascular stent-graft repair of abdominal aortic aneurysm. J Vasc Surg 2004;39:1129–1139.

24. LREAR Steering Committee. Lifeline Registry of Endovascular Aneurysm Repair: Registry data report. J Vasc Surg 2002;35: 616–620.

25. Bush RL, Lin PH, Lumsden AB. Endovascular management of abdominal aortic aneurysms. J Cardiovasc Surg (Torino) 2003;44: 527–534.

26. Dake MD, Miller DC, Semba CP, et al. Transluminal placement of endovascular stent grafts for the treatment of descending thoracic aortic aneurysms. N Engl J Med 1994;331:1729–1734.

27. Dake MD, Kato N, Mitchell RS, et al. Endovascular stent-graft placement for the treatment of acute aortic dissection. N Engl J Med 1999;340:1546–1552.

28. May J, White G, Waugh R, et al. Transluminal placement of a prosthetic graft-stent device for treatment of subclavian artery aneurysm. J Vasc Surg 1993;18:1056–1059.

29. Szeimies U, Kueffer G, Stoeckelhuber B, et al. Successful exclusion of subclavian aneurysms with covered nitinol stents. Cardiovasc Intervent Radiol 1998;21:246–249.

30. Hilfiker PR, Razavi MK, Kee ST, et al. Stent-graft therapy for subclavian artery aneurysms and fistulas: single-center midterm results. J Vasc Interv Radiol 2000;11:578–584.

31. Schoder M, Cejna M, Holzenbein T, et al. Elective and emergent endovascular treatment of subclavian artery aneurysms and injuries. J Endovasc Ther 2003;10:58–65.

32. Marin ML, Veith FJ, Lyon RT, et al. Transfemoral endovascular repair of iliac artery aneurysms. Am J Surg 1995;170:179–182.

33. Razavi MK, Dake MD, Semba CP, et al. Percutaneous endoluminal placement of stent grafts for the treatment of isolated iliac artery aneurysms. Radiology 1995;197:801–804.

34. Dorros G, Cohn JM, Jaff MR. Percutaneous endovascular stent-graft repair of iliac artery aneurysms. J Endovasc Surg 1997;4: 370–375.

35. Marin ML, Veith FJ, Panetta TF, et al. Transfemoral endoluminal stented graft repair of a popliteal artery aneurysm. J Vasc Surg 1994;19:754–757.

36. Marin ML, Veith FJ, Panetta TF, et al. Percutaneous transfemoral insertion of a stented graft to repair a traumatic femoral arteriovenous fistula. J Vasc Surg 1993;18:299–302.

37. Tielliu IF, Verhoeven EL, Prins TR, et al. Stent-graft repair of a recurrent popliteal arteriovenous fistula. J Endovasc Ther 2002;9:375–378.

38. Cragg AH, Dake MD. Percutaneous femoropopliteal graft placement. Radiology 1993;187:643–648.

39. Sanchez LA, Marin ML, Veith FJ, et al. Placement of endovascular stented grafts via remote access sites: a new approach to the treatment of failed aortoiliofemoral reconstructions. Ann Vasc Surg 1995;9:1–8.

40. Nienaber CA, Fattori R, Lund G, et al. Nonsurgical reconstruction of thoracic aortic dissection by stent-graft placement. N Engl J Med 1999;340:1539–1545.

41. Kato N, Hirano T, Shimono T, et al. Treatment of chronic aortic dissection by transluminal endovascular stent-graft placement: preliminary results. J Vasc Interv Radiol 2001;12:835–840.

42. Brittenden J, McBride K, McInnes G, et al. The use of endovascular stents in the treatment of penetrating ulcers of the thoracic aorta. J Vasc Surg 1999;30:946–949.

43. Demers P, Miller DC, Mitchell RS, et al. Stent-graft repair of penetrating atherosclerotic ulcers in the descending thoracic aorta: midterm results. Ann Thorac Surg 2004;77:81–86.

44. Eggebrecht H, Baumgart D, Schmermund A, et al. Endovascular stent-graft repair for penetrating atherosclerotic ulcer of the descending aorta. Am J Cardiol 2003;91:1150–1153.

45. Kato N, Dake MD, Miller DC, et al. Traumatic thoracic aortic aneurysm: treatment with endovascular stent grafts. Radiology 1997;205:657–662.

46. Demers P, Miller C, Scott Mitchell R, et al. Chronic traumatic aneurysms of the descending thoracic aorta: midterm results of endovascular repair using first and second-generation stent grafts. Eur J Cardiothorac Surg 2004;25:394–400.

47. Ott MC, Stewart TC, Lawlor DK, et al. Management of blunt thoracic aortic injuries: endovascular stents versus open repair. J Trauma 2004;56:565–570.

48. Semba CP, Sakai T, Slonim SM, et al. Mycotic aneurysms of the thoracic aorta: repair with use of endovascular stent grafts. J Vasc Interv Radiol 1998;9:33–40.

49. Nishimoto M, Hasegawa S, Asada K, et al. Stent-graft placement for mycotic aneurysm of the thoracic aorta: report of a case. Circ J 2004;68:88–90.

50. Bockler D, Schumacher H, Schwarzbach M, et al. Endoluminal stent-graft repair of aortobronchial fistulas: bridging or definitive long-term solution? J Endovasc Ther 2004;11:41–48.

51. Thompson CS, Ramaiah VG, Rodriquez-Lopez JA, et al. Endoluminal stent graft repair of aortobronchial fistulas. J Vasc Surg 2002;35:387–391.

52. Ince H, Petzsch M, Rehders T, et al. Percutaneous endovascular repair of aneurysm after previous coarctation surgery. Circulation 2003;108:2967–2970.

53. Scheinert D, Krankenberg H, Schmidt A, et al. Endoluminal stent-graft placement for acute rupture of the descending thoracic aorta. Eur Heart J 2004;25:694–700.

54. Kato N, Hirano T, Ishida M, et al. Acute and contained rupture of the descending thoracic aorta: treatment with endovascular stent grafts. J Vasc Surg 2003;37:100–105.

55. Dake MD, Miller DC, Mitchell RS, et al. The "first generation" of endovascular stent grafts for patients with aneurysms of the descending thoracic aorta. J Thorac Cardiovasc Surg 1998;116: 689–703; discussion 703–684.

56. Mitchell RS, Dake MD, Sembra CP, et al. Endovascular stent-graft repair of thoracic aortic aneurysms. J Thorac Cardiovasc Surg 1996;111:1054–1062.

57. Makaroun MS, Dillavou ED, Kee ST, et al. Endovascular treatment of thoracic aortic aneurysms: results of the Phase II multi-center trial of the GORE TAG thoracic endoprosthesis. Presented at the Society for Vascular Surgery Annual Meeting, Anaheim, CA, USA, 2004.

58. Ehrlich M, Grabenwoeger M, Cartes-Zumelzu F, et al. Endovascular stent graft repair for aneurysms on the descending thoracic aorta. Ann Thorac Surg 1998;66:19–24; discussion 24–15.

59. Fattori R, Napoli G, Lovato L, et al. Descending thoracic aortic diseases: stent-graft repair. Radiology 2003;229:176–183.

60. Criado FJ, McKendrick C, Monaghan K, et al. The talent thoracic stent graft: A 6-year experience. Supplement to Endovascular Today; 2003:6–9.

61. Lippmann M, Lingam K, Rubin S, et al. Anesthesia for endovascular repair of abdominal and thoracic aortic aneurysms: a review article. J Cardiovasc Surg (Torino) 2003;44:443–451.

62. Dorros G, Cohn JM. Adenosine-induced transient cardiac asystole enhances precise deployment of stent grafts in the thoracic or abdominal aorta. J Endovasc Surg 1996;3:270–272.

63. Temudom T, D'Ayala M, Marin ML, et al. Endovascular grafts in the treatment of thoracic aortic aneurysms and pseudoaneurysms. Ann Vasc Surg 2000;14:230–238.

64. White GH, Yu W, May J. Endoleak—a proposed new terminology to describe incomplete aneurysm exclusion by an endoluminal graft. J Endovasc Surg 1996;3:124–125.

65. Chaikof EL, Blankensteijn JD, Harris PL, et al. Reporting standards for endovascular aortic aneurysm repair. J Vasc Surg 2002;35:1048–1060.

66. Alric P, Hinchliffe RJ, Wenham PW, et al. Lessons learned from the long-term follow-up of a first-generation aortic stent graft. J Vasc Surg 2003;37:367–373.

67. Harris PL, Vallabhaneni SR, Desgranges P, et al. Incidence and risk factors of late rupture, conversion, and death after endovascular repair of infrarenal aortic aneurysms: the EUROSTAR experience. European Collaborators on Stent/graft techniques for aortic aneurysm repair. J Vasc Surg 2000;32:739–749.

68. Resch T, Koul B, Dias NV, et al. Changes in aneurysm morphology and stent-graft configuration after endovascular repair of aneurysms of the descending thoracic aorta. J Thorac Cardiovasc Surg 2001;122:47–52.

69. Gilling-Smith GL, Martin J, Sudhindran S, et al. Freedom from endoleak after endovascular aneurysm repair does not equal treatment success. Eur J Vasc Endovasc Surg 2000;19:421–425.

70. White GH, May J. How should endotension be defined? History of a concept and evolution of a new term. J Endovasc Ther 2000;7: 435–438; discussion 439–440.

71. Cesare ED, Giordano AV, Cerone G, et al. Comparative evaluation of TEE, conventional MRI, and contrast-enhanced 3D breath-hold MRA in the postoperative follow-up of dissecting aneurysms. Int J Card Imaging 2000;16:135–147.

72. Blum U, Voshage G, Lammer J, et al. Endoluminal stent grafts for infrarenal abdominal aortic aneurysms. N Engl J Med 1997; 336:13–20.

73. Johnston KW, Rutherford RB, Tilson MD, et al. Suggested standards for reporting on arterial aneurysms. Subcommittee on Reporting Standards for Arterial Aneurysms, Ad Hoc Committee on Reporting Standards, Society for Vascular Surgery, and North American Chapter, International Society for Cardiovascular Surgery. J Vasc Surg 1991;13:452–458.

74. Bettmann MA, Dake MD, Hopkins LN, et al. Atherosclerotic vascular disease conference: Writing Group VI: revascularization. Circulation 2004;109:2643–2650.

75. Bickerstaff LK, Pairolero PC, Hollier LH, et al. Thoracic aortic aneurysms: a population-based study. Surgery 1982;92:1103–1108.

76. Clouse WD, Hallett JW Jr, Schaff HV, et al. Improved prognosis of thoracic aortic aneurysms: a population-based study. JAMA 1998;280:1926–1929.

77. Pressler V, McNamara JJ. Thoracic aortic aneurysm: natural history and treatment. J Thorac Cardiovasc Surg 1980;79:489–498.

78. Crawford ES, Cohen ES. Aortic aneurysm: a multifocal disease. Arch Surg 1982;117:1393–1400.

79. Pressler V, McNamara JJ. Aneurysm of the thoracic aorta. Review of 260 cases. J Thorac Cardiovasc Surg 1985;89:50–54.

80. DeBakey ME, McCollum CH, Graham JM. Surgical treatment of aneurysms of the descending thoracic aorta: long-term results in 500 patients. J Cardiovasc Surg 1978;19:571–576.

81. Griepp RB, Ergin MA, Galla JD, et al. Natural history of descending thoracic and thoracoabdominal aneurysms. Ann Thorac Surg 1999;67:1927–1930; discussion 1953–1928.

82. McNamara JJ, Pressler VM. Natural history of arteriosclerotic thoracic aortic aneurysms. Ann Thorac Surg 1978;26:468–473.

83. Coady MA, Rizzo JA, Goldstein LJ, et al. Natural history, pathogenesis, and etiology of thoracic aortic aneurysms and dissections. Cardiol Clin 1999;17:615–635; vii.

84. Hasham SN, Guo DC, Milewicz DM. Genetic basis of thoracic aortic aneurysms and dissections. Curr Opin Cardiol 2002;17: 677–683.

85. White JV, Scovell SD. Etiology of abdominal aortic aneurysms: the structural basis for aneurysm formation. In: Calligaro KD, Dougherty MJ, Hollier LH, eds. Diagnosis and Treatment of Aortic and Peripheral Arterial Aneurysms. Philadelphia: WB Saunders, 1999.

86. Joyce JW, Fairbairn JF, Kincaid OW, et al. Aneurysms of the thoracic aorta. A clinical study with special reference to prognosis. Circulation 1964;29:176–181.

87. Reed D, Reed C, Stemmermann G, et al. Are aortic aneurysms caused by atherosclerosis? Circulation 1992;85:205–211.

88. Zarins CK, Glagov S, Vesselinovitch D, et al. Aneurysm formation in experimental atherosclerosis: relationship to plaque evolution. J Vasc Surg 1990;12:246–256.

89. Coady MA, Davies RR, Roberts M, et al. Familial patterns of thoracic aortic aneurysms. Arch Surg 1999;134:361–367.

90. Tilson MD. Atherosclerosis and aneurysm disease. J Vasc Surg 1990;12:371–372.

91. von Kodolitsch Y, Aydin MA, Koschyk DH, et al. Predictors of aneurysmal formation after surgical correction of aortic coarctation. J Am Coll Cardiol 2002;39:617–624.

92. Guo D, Hasham S, Kuang SQ, et al. Familial thoracic aortic aneurysms and dissections: genetic heterogeneity with a major locus mapping to 5q13–14. Circulation 2001;103:2461–2468.

93. Hasham SN, Willing MC, Guo DC, et al. Mapping a locus for familial thoracic aortic aneurysms and dissections (TAAD2) to 3p24–25. Circulation 2003;107:3184–3190.

94. Najafi H, Javid H, Hunter JA, et al. An update of treatment of aneurysms of the descending thoracic aorta. World J Surg 1980;4:553–561.

95. Cooke JC, Cambria RP. Simultaneous tracheobronchial and esophageal obstruction caused by a descending thoracic aneurysm. J Vasc Surg 1993;18:90–94.

96. Crawford ES, DeNatale RW. Thoracoabdominal aortic aneurysm: observations regarding the natural course of the disease. J Vasc Surg 1986;3:578–582.

97. Johansson G, Markstrom U, Swedenborg J. Ruptured thoracic aortic aneurysms: a study of incidence and mortality rates. J Vasc Surg 1995;21:985–988.

98. Davies RR, Goldstein LJ, Coady MA, et al. Yearly rupture or dissection rates for thoracic aortic aneurysms: simple prediction based on size. Ann Thorac Surg 2002;73:17–27; discussion 27–18.

99. Dapunt OE, Galla JD, Sadeghi AM, et al. The natural history of thoracic aortic aneurysms. J Thorac Cardiovasc Surg 1994;107: 1323–1332; discussion 1332–1323.

100. Szilagyi DE, Smith RF, DeRusso FJ, et al. Contribution of abdominal aortic aneurysmectomy to prolongation of life. Ann Surg 1966;164:678–699.

101. Cronenwett JL. Variables that affect the expansion rate and rupture of abdominal aortic aneurysms. Ann N Y Acad Sci 1996; 800:56–67.

102. Coady MA, Rizzo JA, Hammond GL, et al. Surgical intervention criteria for thoracic aortic aneurysms: a study of growth rates and complications. Ann Thorac Surg 1999;67:1922–1926; discussion 1953–1928.

103. Elefteriades JA. Natural history of thoracic aortic aneurysms: indications for surgery and surgical versus nonsurgical risks. Ann Thorac Surg 2002;74:S1877–1880; discussion S1892–1878.

104. Juvonen T, Ergin MA, Galla JD, et al. Prospective study of the natural history of thoracic aortic aneurysms. Ann Thorac Surg 1997;63:1533–1545.

105. Perko MJ, Norgaard M, Herzog TM, et al. Unoperated aortic aneurysm: a survey of 170 patients. Ann Thorac Surg 1995;59:1204–1209.

106. Finkbohner R, Johnston D, Crawford ES, et al. Marfan syndrome. Long-term survival and complications after aortic aneurysm repair. Circulation 1995;91:728–733.

107. Coselli JS, de Figueiredo LF. Natural history of descending and thoracoabdominal aortic aneurysms. J Card Surg 1997(Suppl II);12:285–289; discussion 289–291.

108. Crawford ES, Hess KR, Cohen ES, et al. Ruptured aneurysm of the descending thoracic and thoracoabdominal aorta. Analysis according to size and treatment. Ann Surg 1991;213:417–425; discussion 425–416.

109. Fann JI. Descending thoracic and thoracoabdominal aortic aneurysms. Coron Artery Dis 2002;13:93–102.

110. Jacobs MJ, Eijsman L, Meylaerts SA, et al. Reduced renal failure following thoracoabdominal aortic aneurysm repair by selective perfusion. Eur J Cardiothorac Surg 1998;14:201–205.

111. Borst HG, Jurmann M, Buhner B, et al. Risk of replacement of descending aorta with a standardized left heart bypass technique. J Thorac Cardiovasc Surg 1994;107:126–132; discussion 123–132.

112. Coselli JS, Plestis KA, La Francesca S, et al. Results of contemporary surgical treatment of descending thoracic aortic aneurysms: experience in 198 patients. Ann Vasc Surg 1996;10:131–137.

113. Verdant A. Descending thoracic aortic aneurysms: surgical treatment with the Gott shunt. Can J Surg 1992;35:493–496.

114. Livesay JJ, Cooley DA, Ventemiglia RA, et al. Surgical experience in descending thoracic aneurysmectomy with and without adjuncts to avoid ischemia. Ann Thorac Surg 1985;39:37–46.

115. Hollier LH, Symmonds JB, Pairolero PC, et al. Thoracoabdominal aortic aneurysm repair. Analysis of postoperative morbidity. Arch Surg 1988;123:871–875.

116. Cambria RP, Clouse WD, Davison JK, et al. Thoracoabdominal aneurysm repair: results with 337 operations performed over a 15-year interval. Ann Surg 2002;236:471–479; discussion 479.

117. Hilgenberg AD, Rainer WG, Sadler TR Jr. Aneurysm of the descending thoracic aorta: replacement with the use of a shunt or bypass. J Thorac Cardiovasc Surg 1981;81:818–824.

118. Mastroroberto P, Chello M. Emergency thoracoabdominal aortic aneurysm repair: clinical outcome. J Thorac Cardiovasc Surg 1999;118:477–481; discussion 481–472.

119. Liddicoat JE, Bekassy SM, Rubio PA, et al. Ascending aortic aneurysms. Review of 100 consecutive cases. Circulation 1975;52:I202–209.

120. Verdant A, Cossette R, Page A, et al. Aneurysms of the descending thoracic aorta: three hundred sixty-six consecutive cases resected without paraplegia. J Vasc Surg 1995;21:385–390; discussion 390–381.

121. Rectenwald JE, Huber TS, Martin TD, et al. Functional outcome after thoracoabdominal aortic aneurysm repair. J Vasc Surg 2002;35:640–647.

122. Svensson LG, Crawford ES, Hess KR, et al. Experience with 1509 patients undergoing thoracoabdominal aortic operations. J Vasc Surg 1993;17:357–368; discussion 368–370.

123. LeMaire SA, Miller CC III, Conklin LD, et al. Estimating group mortality and paraplegia rates after thoracoabdominal aortic aneurysm repair. Ann Thorac Surg 2003;75:508–513.

124. Panneton JM, Hollier LH. Dissecting descending thoracic and thoracoabdominal aortic aneurysms: Part II. Ann Vasc Surg 1995;9:596–605.

125. Panneton JM, Hollier LH. Nondissecting thoracoabdominal aortic aneurysms: Part I. Ann Vasc Surg 1995;9:503–514.

126. Cina CS, Abouzahr L, Arena GO, et al. Cerebrospinal fluid drainage to prevent paraplegia during thoracic and thoracoabdominal aortic aneurysm surgery: a systematic review and meta-analysis. J Vasc Surg 2004;40:36–44.

127. Crawford ES, Svensson LG, Hess KR, et al. A prospective randomized study of cerebrospinal fluid drainage to prevent paraplegia after high-risk surgery on the thoracoabdominal aorta. J Vasc Surg 1991;13:36–45; discussion 45–36.

128. Svensson LG. An approach to spinal cord protection during descending or thoracoabdominal aortic repairs. Ann Thorac Surg 1999;67:1935–1936; discussion 1953–1938.

129. Svensson LG, Hess KR, D'Agostino RS, et al. Reduction of neurologic injury after high-risk thoracoabdominal aortic operation. Ann Thorac Surg 1998;66:132–138.

130. Kouchoukos NT, Masetti P, Murphy SF. Hypothermic cardiopulmonary bypass and circulatory arrest in the management of extensive thoracic and thoracoabdominal aortic aneurysms. Semin Thorac Cardiovasc Surg 2003;15:333–339.

131. Ross SD, Kron IL, Parrino PE, et al. Preservation of intercostal arteries during thoracoabdominal aortic aneurysm surgery: a retrospective study. J Thorac Cardiovasc Surg 1999;118:17–25.

132. Hamilton IN, Jr., Hollier LH. Adjunctive therapy for spinal cord protection during thoracoabdominal aortic aneurysm repair. Semin Thorac Cardiovasc Surg 1998;10:35–39.

133. Laschinger JC, Izumoto H, Kouchoukos NT. Evolving concepts in prevention of spinal cord injury during operations on the descending thoracic and thoracoabdominal aorta. Ann Thorac Surg 1987;44:667–674.

134. Taylor PR, Gaines PA, McGuinness CL, et al. Thoracic aortic stent grafts—early experience from two centres using commercially available devices. Eur J Vasc Endovasc Surg 2001;22:70–76.

135. White RA, Donayre CE, Walot I, et al. Endovascular exclusion of descending thoracic aortic aneurysms and chronic dissections: Initial clinical results with the AneuRx device. J Vasc Surg 2001;33:927–934.

136. Won JY, Lee DY, Shim WH, et al. Elective endovascular treatment of descending thoracic aortic aneurysms and chronic dissections with stent grafts. J Vasc Interv Radiol 2001;12:575–582.

137. Buffolo E, da Fonseca JH, de Souza JA, et al. Revolutionary treatment of aneurysms and dissections of descending aorta: the endovascular approach. Ann Thorac Surg 2002;74:S1815–1817; discussion S1825–1832.

138. Cambria RP, Brewster DC, Lauterbach SR, et al. Evolving experience with thoracic aortic stent-graft repair. J Vasc Surg 2002;35:1129–1136.

139. Criado FJ, Clark NS, Barnatan MF. Stent-graft repair in the aortic arch and descending thoracic aorta: a 4-year experience. J Vasc Surg 2002;36:1121–1128.

140. Lepore V, Lonn L, Delle M, et al. Endograft therapy for diseases of the descending thoracic aorta: results in 43 high-risk patients. J Endovasc Ther 2002;9:829–837.

141. Thompson CS, Gaxotte VD, Rodriguez JA, et al. Endoluminal stent grafting of the thoracic aorta: initial experience with the Gore Excluder. J Vasc Surg 2002;35:1163–1170.

142. Bell RE, Taylor PR, Aukett M, et al. Midterm results for second-generation thoracic stent grafts. Brit J Surg 2003;90:811–817.

143. Ellozy SH, Carroccio A, Minor M, et al. Challenges of endovascular tube graft repair of thoracic aortic aneurysm: midterm follow-up and lessons learned. J Vasc Surg 2003;38:676–683.

144. Gerber M, Immer FF, Do DD, et al. Endovascular stent-grafting for diseases of the descending thoracic aorta. Swiss Med Wkly 2003;133:44–51.

145. Grabenwoger M, Fleck T, Czerny M, et al. Endovascular stent-graft placement in patients with acute thoracic aortic syndromes. Eur J Cardiothorac Surg 2003;23:788–793; discussion 793.

146. Lambrechts D, Casselman F, Schroeyers P, et al. Endovascular treatment of the descending thoracic aorta. Eur J Vasc Endovasc Surg 2003;26:437–444.

147. Lamme B, de Jonge IC, Reekers JA, et al. Endovascular treatment of thoracic aortic pathology: feasibility and midterm results. Eur J Vasc Endovasc Surg 2003;25:532–539.

148. Matravers P, Morgan R, Belli A. The use of stent grafts for the treatment of aneurysms and dissections of the thoracic aorta: a single centre experience. Eur J Vasc Endovasc Surg 2003;26:587–595.

149. Orend KH, Scharrer-Pamler R, Kapfer X, et al. Endovascular treatment in diseases of the descending thoracic aorta: 6-year results of a single center. J Vasc Surg 2003;37:91–99.

150. Steinmetz OK, Tse LW, MacKenzie KS, et al. Four-year experience with the Talent endovascular stent-graft for repair of thoracic aortic lesions. J Endovasc Ther 2004;11:I37. Abstract.

151. Rodriguez JA, Olsen D, Ramaiah V, et al. Application of endograft to treat thoracic aorta pathologies: Signe center experience. Presented at the Society for Vascular Surgery Annual Meeting, Anaheim, CA, USA, 2004.

152. Ishida M, Kato N, Hirano T, et al. Endovascular stent-graft treatment for thoracic aortic aneurysms: short- to midterm results. J Vasc Interv Radiol 2004;15:361–367.

153. Cartes-Zumelzu F, Lammer J, Kretschmer G, et al. Endovascular repair of thoracic aortic aneurysms. Semin Interv Cardiol 2000;5: 53–57.

154. Grabenwoger M, Hutschala D, Ehrlich MP, et al. Thoracic aortic aneurysms: treatment with endovascular self-expandable stent grafts. Ann Thorac Surg 2000;69:441–445.

155. Greenberg R, Resch T, Nyman U, et al. Endovascular repair of descending thoracic aortic aneurysms: an early experience with intermediate-term follow-up. J Vasc Surg 2000;31:147–156.

156. Najibi S, Terramani TT, Weiss VJ, et al. Endoluminal versus open treatment of descending thoracic aortic aneurysms. J Vasc Surg 2002;36:732–737.

157. Heijmen RH, Deblier IG, Moll FL, et al. Endovascular stent grafting for descending thoracic aortic aneurysms. Eur J Cardiothorac Surg 2002;21:5–9.

158. Schoder M, Cartes-Zumelzu F, Grabenwoger M, et al. Elective endovascular stent-graft repair of atherosclerotic thoracic aortic aneurysms: clinical results and midterm follow-up. AJR Am J Roentgenol 2003;180:709–715.

159. Marin ML, Hollier LH, Ellozy SH, et al. Endovascular stent graft repair of abdominal and thoracic aortic aneurysms: a ten-year experience with 817 patients. Ann Surg 2003;238:586–593; discussion 593–585.

160. Lepore V, Lonn L, Delle M, et al. Treatment of descending thoracic aneurysms by endovascular stent grafting. J Card Surg 2003;18:436–443.

161. Sunder-Plassmann L, Scharrer-Pamler R, Liewald F, et al. Endovascular exclusion of thoracic aortic aneurysms: midterm results of elective treatment and in contained rupture. J Card Surg 2003;18:367–374.

162. Ouriel K, Greenberg RK. Endovascular treatment of thoracic aortic aneurysms. J Card Surg 2003;18:455–463.

163. Bergeron P, De Chaumaray T, Gay J, et al. Endovascular treatment of thoracic aortic aneurysms. J Cardiovasc Surg (Torino) 2003;44:349–361.

164. Czerny M, Cejna M, Hutschala D, et al. Stent-graft placement in atherosclerotic descending thoracic aortic aneurysms: midterm results. J Endovasc Ther 2004;11:26–32.

165. Bell RE, Buth J, Taylor PR, et al. UK and EUROSTAR thoracic stenting registries: combined experience [Abstract]. J Endovasc Ther 2004;11:I6.

166. Dake MD. The advent of thoracic aortic endografting. Presented at the First International Summit on Thoracic Aorta Endografting, Tokyo, Japan, 2001.

167. Ehrlich MP. Thoracic aorta endografting: the Austrian experience. Presented at the First International Summit on Thoracic Aorta Endografting, Tokyo, Japan, 2001.

168. Fattori R. Endovascular treatment of the thoracic aorta. Presented at the First International Summit on Thoracic Aorta Endografting, Tokyo, Japan, 2001.

169. Ishimaru S. Thoracic aorta grafting: the reliable treatment option. Presented at the First International Summit on Thoracic Aorta Endografting, Tokyo, Japan, 2001.

170. Lauterjung L. Endovascular stent grafting for the thoracic aorta. Presented at the First International Summit on Thoracic Aorta Endografting, Tokyo, Japan, 2001.

171. Medtronic. Medtronic begins Talent thoracic stent graft study in the United States. November 10, 2003.

172. Fann JI, Miller DC. Endovascular treatment of descending thoracic aortic aneurysms and dissections. Surg Clin North Am 1999;79:551–574.

173. Demers P, Miller DC, Mitchell RS, et al. Midterm results of endovascular repair of descending thoracic aortic aneurysms with first-generation stent grafts. J Thorac Cardiovasc Surg 2004;127:664–673.

174. Mitchell RS, Miller DC, Dake MD, et al. Thoracic aortic aneurysm repair with an endovascular stent graft: the "first generation." Ann Thorac Surg 1999;67:1971–1974; discussion 1979–1980.

175. Semba CP, Mitchell RS, Miller DC, et al. Thoracic aortic aneurysm repair with endovascular stent grafts. Vasc Med 1997;2:98–103.

176. Laheij RJ, van Marrewijk CJ, Buth J, et al. The influence of team experience on outcomes of endovascular stenting of abdominal aortic aneurysms. Eur J Vasc Endovasc Surg 2002;24:128–133.

177. Laheij RJ, van Marrewijk CJ. Endovascular stenting of abdominal aortic aneurysm in patients unfit for elective open surgery. Eurostar group. EUROpean collaborators registry on Stent-graft Techniques for abdominal aortic Aneurysm Repair. Lancet 2000;356:832.

178. Bortone AS, Schena S, Mannatrizio G, et al. Endovascular stent-graft treatment for diseases of the descending thoracic aorta. Eur J Cardiothorac Surg 2001;20:514–519.

179. Mitchell RS. Endovascular stent graft repair of thoracic aortic aneurysms. Semin Thorac Cardiovasc Surg 1997;9:257–268.

180. Gravereaux EC, Faries PL, Burks JA, et al. Risk of spinal cord ischemia after endograft repair of thoracic aortic aneurysms. J Vasc Surg 2001;34:997–1003.

181. Thurnher SA, Grabenwoger M. Endovascular treatment of thoracic aortic aneurysms: a review. Eur Radiol 2002;12:1370–1387.

182. Baum RA, Stavropoulos SW, Fairman RM, et al. Endoleaks after endovascular repair of abdominal aortic aneurysms. J Vasc Interv Radiol 2003;14:1111–1117.

183. Buth J, Harris PL, van Marrewijk C, et al. The significance and management of different types of endoleaks. Semin Vasc Surg 2003;16:95–102.

184. Kato N, Semba CP, Dake MD. Embolization of perigraft leaks after endovascular stent-graft treatment of aortic aneurysms. J Vasc Interv Radiol 1996;7:805–811.

185. Chuter TA, Faruqi RM, Sawhney R, et al. Endoleak after endovascular repair of abdominal aortic aneurysm. J Vasc Surg 2001;34: 98–105.

186. Estes JM, Halin N, Kwoun M, et al. The carotid artery as alternative access for endoluminal aortic aneurysm repair. J Vasc Surg 2001;33:650–653.

187. Sueda T, Orihashi K, Okada K, et al. Fate of aneurysms of the distal arch and proximal descending thoracic aorta after transaortic endovascular stent-grafting. Ann Thorac Surg 2003;76:84–89; discussion 89.

188. Sueda T, Watari M, Okada K, et al. Endovascular stent-grafting through the aortic arch: an alternative approach for distal arch aortic aneurysm. Ann Thorac Surg 2000;70:1251–1254.

189. Sueda T, Watari M, Orihashi K, et al. Endovascular stent-grafting via the aortic arch for distal arch aneurysm: an alternative of endovascular stent grafting in a complicated case. Ann Thorac Cardiovasc Surg 1999;5:206–208.

190. Moon MR, Mitchell RS, Dake MD, et al. Simultaneous abdominal aortic replacement and thoracic stent-graft placement for multilevel aortic disease. J Vasc Surg 1997;25:332–340.

191. Buth J, Penn O, Tielbeek A, et al. Combined approach to stent-graft treatment of an aortic arch aneurysm. J Endovasc Surg 1998; 5:329–332.

192. Quinones-Baldrich WJ. Descending thoracic and thoracoabdominal aortic aneurysm repair: 15-year results using a uniform approach. Ann Vasc Surg 2004;18:335–342

193. Quinones-Baldrich WJ, Panetta TF, Vescera CL, et al. Repair of type IV thoracoabdominal aneurysm with a combined endovascular and surgical approach. J Vasc Surg 1999;30:555–560.

194. Yoshida H, Izumi Y, Magishi K, et al. [Simultaneous abdominal aortic replacement and thoracic stent-graft placement for multiple aortic aneurysms: report of a case]. Kyobu Geka 2000;53:734–737.

195. Fann JI, Dake MD, Semba CP, et al. Endovascular stent grafting after arch aneurysm repair using the "elephant trunk." Ann Thorac Surg 1995;60:1102–1105.

196. Miyamoto S, Hadama T, Anai H, et al. Stented elephant trunk method for multiple thoracic aneurysms. Ann Thorac Surg 2001;71:705–707.

197. Hausegger KA, Oberwalder P, Tiesenhausen K, et al. Intentional left subclavian artery occlusion by thoracic aortic stent grafts without surgical transposition. J Endovasc Ther 2001;8:472–476.

198. Tiesenhausen K, Hausegger KA, Oberwalder P, et al. Left subclavian artery management in endovascular repair of thoracic aortic aneurysms and aortic dissections. J Card Surg 2003;18:429–435.

199. Gorich J, Asquan Y, Seifarth H, et al. Initial experience with intentional stent-graft coverage of the subclavian artery during endovascular thoracic aortic repairs. J Endovasc Ther 2002;9(Suppl II): 39–43.

200. Burks JA, Jr., Faries PL, Gravereaux EC, et al. Endovascular repair of thoracic aortic aneurysms: stent-graft fixation across the aortic arch vessels. Ann Vasc Surg 2002;16:24–28.

201. Williams DM, Lee DY, Hamilton BH, et al. The dissected aorta: part III. Anatomy and radiologic diagnosis of branch-vessel compromise. Radiology 1997;203:37–44.

202. Clouse WD, Hallett JW Jr, Schaff HV, et al. Acute aortic dissection: population-based incidence compared with degenerative aortic aneurysm rupture. Mayo Clin Proc 2004;79:176–180.

203. Meszaros I, Morocz J, Szlavi J, et al. Epidemiology and clinico-pathology of aortic dissection. Chest 2000;117:1271–1278.

204. Sorensen HR, Olsen H. Ruptured and dissecting aneurysms of the aorta. Incidence and prospects of surgery. Acta Chir Scand 1964;128:644–650.

205. Wheat MW Jr. Acute dissecting aneurysms of the aorta: diagnosis and treatment—1979. Am Heart J 1980;99:373–387.

206. Anagnostopoulos CE, Prabhakar MJ, Kittle CF. Aortic dissections and dissecting aneurysms. Am J Cardiol 1972;30:263–273.

207. Hagan PG, Nienaber CA, Isselbacher EM, et al. The International Registry of Acute Aortic Dissection (IRAD): new insights into an old disease. JAMA 2000;283:897–903.

208. DeBakey ME, McCollum CH, Crawford ES, et al. Dissection and dissecting aneurysms of the aorta: twenty-year follow-up of five hundred twenty-seven patients treated surgically. Surgery 1982;92:1118–1134.

209. Hirst AE Jr, Johns VJ Jr, Kime SW Jr. Dissecting aneurysm of the aorta: a review of 505 cases. Medicine (Baltimore) 1958;37: 217–279.

210. Wilson SK, Hutchins GM. Aortic dissecting aneurysms: causative factors in 204 subjects. Arch Pathol Lab Med 1982;106:175–180.

211. Spittell PC, Spittell JA Jr, Joyce JW, et al. Clinical features and differential diagnosis of aortic dissection: experience with 236 cases (1980 through 1990). Mayo Clin Proc 1993;68:642–651.

212. Roberts WC. Aortic dissection: anatomy, consequences, and causes. Am Heart J 1981;101:195–214.

213. Wheat MW Jr. Acute dissection of the aorta. Cardiovasc Clin 1987;17:241–262.

214. DeBakey ME, Beall AC Jr, Cooley DA, et al. Dissecting aneurysms of the aorta. Surg Clin North Am 1966;46:1045–1055.

215. Daily PO, Trueblood HW, Stinson EB, et al. Management of acute aortic dissections. Ann Thorac Surg 1970;10:237–247.

216. Coady MA, Rizzo JA, Elefteriades JA. Pathologic variants of thoracic aortic dissections. Penetrating atherosclerotic ulcers and intramural hematomas. Cardiol Clin 1999;17:637–657.

217. Roberts WC, Honig HS. The spectrum of cardiovascular disease in the Marfan syndrome: a clinico-morphologic study of 18 necropsy patients and comparison to 151 previously reported necropsy patients. Am Heart J 1982;104:115–135.

218. Smith JA, Fann JI, Miller DC, et al. Surgical management of aortic dissection in patients with the Marfan syndrome. Circulation 1994;90:II235–242.

219. Stolle CA, Pyeritz RE, Myers JC, et al. Synthesis of an altered type III procollagen in a patient with type IV Ehlers-Danlos syndrome. A structural change in the alpha 1(III) chain which makes the protein more susceptible to proteinases. J Biol Chem 1985;260:1937–1944.

220. Januzzi JL, Isselbacher EM, Fattori R, et al. Characterizing the young patient with aortic dissection: results from the International Registry of Aortic Dissection (IRAD). J Am Coll Cardiol 2004;43:665–669.

221. Larson EW, Edwards WD. Risk factors for aortic dissection: a necropsy study of 161 cases. Am J Cardiol 1984;53:849–855.

222. Birdsall M, Kennedy S. The risk of aortic dissection in women with Turner syndrome. Hum Reprod 1996;11:1587.

223. Clement CI, Brereton J, Clifton-Bligh P. Aortic dissection in Turner syndrome. Med J Aust 2004;180:584.

224. Rubin K. Aortic dissection and rupture in Turner syndrome. J Pediatr 1993;122:670.

225. Shachter N, Perloff JK, Mulder DG. Aortic dissection in Noonan's syndrome (46 XY turner). Am J Cardiol 1984;54:464–465.

226. Moodie DS. Aortic dissection and coarctation. Curr Opin Cardiol 1990;5:649–654.

227. Edwards WD, Leaf DS, Edwards JE. Dissecting aortic aneurysm associated with congenital bicuspid aortic valve. Circulation 1978;57:1022–1025.

228. Roberts CS, Roberts WC. Dissection of the aorta associated with congenital malformation of the aortic valve. J Am Coll Cardiol 1991;17:712–716.

229. Roberts WC. The hypertensive diseases. Evidence that systemic hypertension is a greater risk factor to the development of other cardiovascular diseases than previously suspected. Am J Med 1975;59:523–532.

230. Steurer J, Jenni R, Medici TC, et al. Dissecting aneurysm of the pulmonary artery with pulmonary hypertension. Am Rev Respir Dis 1990;142:1219–1221.

231. Ginsburg R. Aortic aneurysm and dissection in giant cell arteritis. Ann Intern Med 1996;124:615.

232. Liu G, Shupak R, Chiu BK. Aortic dissection in giant-cell arteritis. Semin Arthritis Rheum 1995;25:160–171.

233. Fisher A, Holroyd BR. Cocaine-associated dissection of the thoracic aorta. J Emerg Med 1992;10:723–727.

234. Perron AD, Gibbs M. Thoracic aortic dissection secondary to crack cocaine ingestion. Am J Emerg Med 1997;15:507–509.

235. Hsue PY, Salinas CL, Bolger AF, et al. Acute aortic dissection related to crack cocaine. Circulation 2002;105:1592–1595.

236. Eagle KA, Isselbacher EM, DeSanctis RW. Cocaine-related aortic dissection in perspective. Circulation 2002;105:1529–1530.

237. Rashid J, Eisenberg MJ, Topol EJ. Cocaine-induced aortic dissection. Am Heart J 1996;132:1301–1304.

238. Januzzi JL, Sabatine MS, Eagle KA, et al. Iatrogenic aortic dissection. Am J Cardiol 2002;89:623–626.

239. Rogers FB, Osler TM, Shackford SR. Aortic dissection after trauma: case report and review of the literature. J Trauma 1996;41: 906–908.

240. Still RJ, Hilgenberg AD, Akins CW, et al. Intraoperative aortic dissection. Ann Thorac Surg 1992;53:374–379; discussion 380.

241. Nienaber CA, Eagle KA. Aortic dissection: new frontiers in diagnosis and management: Part I: from etiology to diagnostic strategies. Circulation 2003;108:628–635.

242. Mandel W, Evans EW, Walford RL. Dissecting aortic aneurysm during pregnancy. N Engl J Med 1954;251:1059–1061.

243. Cavanzo FJ, Taylor HB. Effect of pregnancy on the human aorta and its relationship to dissecting aneurysms. Am J Obstet Gynecol 1969;105:567–568.

244. Schnitker MA, Major MC, Bayer CA. Dissecting aneurysm of the aorta in young individuals, particularly in association with pregnancy: With report of a case. Ann Intern Med 1944;20:486–511.

245. Immer FF, Bansi AG, Immer-Bansi AS, et al. Aortic dissection in pregnancy: analysis of risk factors and outcome. Ann Thorac Surg 2003;76:309–314.

246. Klompas M. Does this patient have an acute thoracic aortic dissection? JAMA 2002;287:2262–2272.

247. von Kodolitsch Y, Schwartz AG, Nienaber CA. Clinical prediction of acute aortic dissection. Arch Intern Med 2000;160:2977–2982.

248. Khan IA, Nair CK. Clinical, diagnostic, and management perspectives of aortic dissection. Chest 2002;122:311–328.

249. Oderich GS, Panneton JM. Acute aortic dissection with side branch vessel occlusion: open surgical options. Semin Vasc Surg 2002;15:89–96.

250. Lindsay J Jr, Hurst JW. Clinical features and prognosis in dissecting aneurysm of the aorta. A re-appraisal. Circulation 1967;35: 880–888.

251. Nienaber CA, Eagle KA. Aortic dissection: new frontiers in diagnosis and management: Part II: therapeutic management and follow-up. Circulation 2003;108:772–778.

252. Doroghazi RM, Slater EE, DeSanctis RW, et al. Long-term survival of patients with treated aortic dissection. J Am Coll Cardiol 1984;3:1026–1034.

253. Dake MD. Aortic intramural haematoma: current therapeutic strategy. Heart 2004;90:375–378.

254. Coady MA, Rizzo JA, Hammond GL, et al. Penetrating ulcer of the thoracic aorta: what is it? How do we recognize it? How do

we manage it? J Vasc Surg 1998;27:1006–1015; discussion 1015–1006.

255. Harris JA, Bis KG, Glover JL, et al. Penetrating atherosclerotic ulcers of the aorta. J Vasc Surg 1994;19:90–98; discussion 98–99.

256. Lui RC, Menkis AH, McKenzie FN. Aortic dissection without intimal rupture: diagnosis and management. Ann Thorac Surg 1992; 53:886–888.

257. Nienaber CA, Richartz BM, Rehders T, et al. Aortic intramural haematoma: natural history and predictive factors for complications. Heart 2004;90:372–374.

258. Nienaber CA, Sievers HH. Intramural hematoma in acute aortic syndrome: more than one variant of dissection? Circulation 2002;106:284–285.

259. Song JK, Kim HS, Kang DH, et al. Different clinical features of aortic intramural hematoma versus dissection involving the ascending aorta. J Am Coll Cardiol 2001;37:1604–1610.

260. Bolognesi R, Manca C, Tsialtas D, et al. Aortic intramural hematoma: an increasingly recognized aortic disease. Cardiology 1998;89:178–183.

261. Lansman SL, McCullough JN, Nguyen KH, et al. Subtypes of acute aortic dissection. Ann Thorac Surg 1999;67:1975–1978; discussion 1979–1980.

262. Gore I. Pathogenesis of dissecting aneurysm of the aorta. AMA Arch Pathol 1952;53:142–153.

263. Stanson AW, Kazmier FJ, Hollier LH, et al. Penetrating atherosclerotic ulcers of the thoracic aorta: natural history and clinicopathologic correlations. Ann Vasc Surg 1986;1:15–23.

264. Nienaber CA, von Kodolitsch Y, Petersen B, et al. Intramural hemorrhage of the thoracic aorta. Diagnostic and therapeutic implications. Circulation 1995;92:1465–1472.

265. Maraj R, Rerkpattanapipat P, Jacobs LE, et al. Meta-analysis of 143 reported cases of aortic intramural hematoma. Am J Cardiol 2000;86:664–668.

266. Tittle SL, Lynch RJ, Cole PE, et al. Midterm follow-up of penetrating ulcer and intramural hematoma of the aorta. J Thorac Cardiovasc Surg 2002;123:1051–1059.

267. Ganaha F, Miller DC, Sugimoto K, et al. Prognosis of aortic intramural hematoma with and without penetrating atherosclerotic ulcer: a clinical and radiological analysis. Circulation 2002;106: 342–348.

268. Sueyoshi E, Matsuoka Y, Sakamoto I, et al. Fate of intramural hematoma of the aorta: CT evaluation. J Comput Assist Tomogr 1997;21:931–938.

269. von Kodolitsch Y, Csosz SK, Koschyk DH, et al. Intramural hematoma of the aorta: predictors of progression to dissection and rupture. Circulation 2003;107:1158–1163.

270. Erbel R, Alfonso F, Boileau C, et al. Diagnosis and management of aortic dissection. Eur Heart J 2001;22:1642–1681.

271. Wheat MW Jr, Palmer RF, Bartley TD, et al. Treatment of dissecting aneurysms of the aorta without surgery. J Thorac Cardiovasc Surg 1965;50:364–373.

272. Wheat MW Jr. Current status of medical therapy of acute dissecting aneurysms of the aorta. World J Surg 1980;4:563–569.

273. Miller DC, Stinson EB, Oyer PE, et al. Operative treatment of aortic dissections. Experience with 125 patients over a sixteen-year period. J Thorac Cardiovasc Surg 1979;78:365–382.

274. Masuda Y, Yamada Z, Morooka N, et al. Prognosis of patients with medically treated aortic dissections. Circulation 1991;84: III7–13.

275. Mehta RH, Suzuki T, Hagan PG, et al. Predicting death in patients with acute type A aortic dissection. Circulation 2002;105:200–206.

276. Mehta RH, O'Gara PT, Bossone E, et al. Acute type A aortic dissection in the elderly: clinical characteristics, management, and outcomes in the current era. J Am Coll Cardiol 2002;40:685–692.

277. Erbel R, Oelert H, Meyer J, et al. Effect of medical and surgical therapy on aortic dissection evaluated by transesophageal echocardiography. Implications for prognosis and therapy. The European Cooperative Study Group on Echocardiography. Circulation 1993;87:1604–1615.

278. Kazui T, Tamiya Y, Tanaka T, et al. Extended aortic replacement for acute type A dissection with the tear in the descending aorta. J Thorac Cardiovasc Surg 1996;112:973–978.

279. Lansman SL, Galla JD, Schor JS, et al. Subtypes of acute aortic dissection. J Card Surg 1994;9:729–733.

280. von Segesser LK, Killer I, Ziswiler M, et al. Dissection of the descending thoracic aorta extending into the ascending aorta.

A therapeutic challenge. J Thorac Cardiovasc Surg 1994;108: 755–761.

281. Glower DD, Fann JI, Speier RH, et al. Comparison of medical and surgical therapy for uncomplicated descending aortic dissection. Circulation 1990;82(Suppl IV):39–46.

282. Fann JI, Miller DC. Aortic dissection. Ann Vasc Surg 1995;9: 311–323.

283. Elefteriades JA, Hartleroad J, Gusberg RJ, et al. Long-term experience with descending aortic dissection: the complication-specific approach. Ann Thorac Surg 1992;53:11–20; discussion 20–11.

284. Schor JS, Yerlioglu ME, Galla JD, et al. Selective management of acute type B aortic dissection: long-term follow-up. Ann Thorac Surg 1996;61:1339–1341.

285. Svensson LG, Crawford ES, Hess KR, et al. Dissection of the aorta and dissecting aortic aneurysms. Improving early and long-term surgical results. Circulation 1990;82(Suppl IV):24–38.

286. Miller DC. The continuing dilemma concerning medical versus surgical management of patients with acute type B dissections. Semin Thorac Cardiovasc Surg 1993;5:33–46.

287. Neya K, Omoto R, Kyo S, et al. Outcome of Stanford type B acute aortic dissection. Circulation 1992;86:II1–7.

288. Richter GM, Allenberg JR, Schumacher H, et al. Aortic dissection—when operative treatment, when endoluminal therapy? Radiologe 2001;41:660–667.

289. Crawford ES, Svensson LG, Coselli JS, et al. Aortic dissection and dissecting aortic aneurysms. Ann Surg 1988;208:254–273.

290. Juvonen T, Ergin MA, Galla JD, et al. Risk factors for rupture of chronic type B dissections. J Thorac Cardiovasc Surg 1999;117: 776–786.

291. Kato M, Bai H, Sato K, et al. Determining surgical indications for acute type B dissection based on enlargement of aortic diameter during the chronic phase. Circulation 1995;92:II107–112.

292. Cambria RP, Brewster DC, Gertler J, et al. Vascular complications associated with spontaneous aortic dissection. J Vasc Surg 1988; 7:199–209.

293. Fann JI, Sarris GE, Mitchell RS, et al. Treatment of patients with aortic dissection presenting with peripheral vascular complications. Ann Surg 1990;212:705–713.

294. Borst HG, Laas J, Heinemann M. Type A aortic dissection: diagnosis and management of malperfusion phenomena. Semin Thorac Cardiovasc Surg 1991;3:238–241.

295. Heinemann MK, Buehner B, Schaefers HJ, et al. Malperfusion of the thoracoabdominal vasculature in aortic dissection. J Card Surg 1994;9:748–755; discussion 755–747.

296. Robbins RC, McManus RP, Mitchell RS, et al. Management of patients with intramural hematoma of the thoracic aorta. Circulation 1993;88:II1–10.

297. Sawhney NS, DeMaria AN, Blanchard DG. Aortic intramural hematoma: an increasingly recognized and potentially fatal entity. Chest 2001;120:1340–1346.

298. Eggebrecht H, Baumgart D, Herold U, et al. Multiple penetrating atherosclerotic ulcers of the abdominal aorta: treatment by endovascular stent-graft placement. Heart Dis 2001;85:526.

299. Braverman AC. Penetrating atherosclerotic ulcers of the aorta. Curr Opin Cardiol 1994;9:591–597.

300. Chung JW, Elkins C, Sakai T, et al. True-lumen collapse in aortic dissection: part II. Evaluation of treatment methods in phantoms with pulsatile flow. Radiology 2000;214:99–106.

301. Ergin MA, Phillips RA, Galla JD, et al. Significance of distal false lumen after type A dissection repair. Ann Thorac Surg 1994;57: 820–824; discussion 825.

302. Williams DM, Andrews JC, Marx MV, et al. Creation of reentry tears in aortic dissection by means of percutaneous balloon fenestration: gross anatomic and histologic considerations. J Vasc Interv Radiol 1993;4:75–83.

303. Bernard Y, Zimmermann H, Chocron S, et al. False lumen patency as a predictor of late outcome in aortic dissection. Am J Cardiol 2001;87:1378–1382.

304. Kato M, Matsuda T, Kaneko M, et al. Outcomes of stent-graft treatment of false lumen in aortic dissection. Circulation 1998;98: II305–311; discussion II311–302.

305. Czermak BV, Waldenberger P, Fraedrich G, et al. Treatment of Stanford type B aortic dissection with stent grafts: preliminary results. Radiology 2000;217:544–550.

306. Hausegger KA, Tiesenhausen K, Schedlbauer P, et al. Treatment of acute aortic type B dissection with stent grafts. Cardiovasc Intervent Radiol 2001;24:306–312.

307. Kato N, Shimono T, Hirano T, et al. Transluminal placement of endovascular stent grafts for the treatment of type A aortic dissection with an entry tear in the descending thoracic aorta. J Vasc Surg 2001;34:1023–1028.

308. Sailer J, Peloschek P, Rand T, et al. Endovascular treatment of aortic type B dissection and penetrating ulcer using commercially available stent grafts. AJR Am J Roentgenol 2001;177:1365–1369.

309. Hutschala D, Fleck T, Czerny M, et al. Endoluminal stent-graft placement in patients with acute aortic dissection type B. Eur J Cardiothorac Surg 2002;21:964–969.

310. Kato N, Shimono T, Hirano T, et al. Midterm results of stent-graft repair of acute and chronic aortic dissection with descending tear: the complication-specific approach. J Thorac Cardiovasc Surg 2002;124:306–312.

311. Palma JH, de Souza JA, Rodrigues Alves CM, et al. Self-expandable aortic stent grafts for treatment of descending aortic dissections. Ann Thorac Surg 2002;73:1138–1141; discussion 1141–1132.

312. Shim WH, Koo BK, Yoon YS, et al. Treatment of thoracic aortic dissection with stent grafts: midterm results. J Endovasc Ther 2002;9:817–821.

313. Shimono T, Kato N, Yasuda F, et al. Transluminal stent-graft placements for the treatments of acute onset and chronic aortic dissections. Circulation 2002;106:I241–247.

314. Lonn L, Delle M, Falkenberg M, et al. Endovascular treatment of type B thoracic aortic dissections. J Card Surg 2003;18:539–544.

315. Lopera J, Patino JH, Urbina C, et al. Endovascular treatment of complicated type B aortic dissection with stent grafts: midterm results. J Vasc Interv Radiol 2003;14:195–203.

316. Nienaber CA, Rehders TK, Fratz S, et al. Stent-graft intervention for type B aortic dissection: Update of European trail results [Abstract]. J Endovasc Ther 2004;11:I29.

317. Shimono T, Kato N, Tokui T, et al. Endovascular stent-graft repair for acute type A aortic dissection with an intimal tear in the descending aorta. J Thorac Cardiovasc Surg 1998;116:171–173.

318. Nienaber CA, Ince H, Petzsch M, et al. Endovascular treatment of acute aortic syndrome. Supplement to Endovascular Today 2003:12–15.

319. Kato N, Hirano T, Shimono T, et al. Treatment of chronic type B aortic dissection with endovascular stent-graft placement. Cardiovasc Intervent Radiol 2000;23:60–62.

320. Slonim SM, Miller DC, Mitchell RS, et al. Percutaneous balloon fenestration and stenting for life-threatening ischemic complications in patients with acute aortic dissection. J Thorac Cardiovasc Surg 1999;117:1118–1126.

321. Slonim SM, Nyman U, Semba CP, et al. Aortic dissection: percutaneous management of ischemic complications with endovascular stents and balloon fenestration. J Vasc Surg 1996;23:241–251; discussion 251–243.

322. Williams DM, Lee DY, Hamilton BH, et al. The dissected aorta: percutaneous treatment of ischemic complications—principles and results. J Vasc Interv Radiol 1997;8:605–625.

323. Chavan A, Hausmann D, Dresler C, et al. Intravascular ultrasound-guided percutaneous fenestration of the intimal flap in the dissected aorta. Circulation 1997;96:2124–2127.

324. Kos X, Bouchard L, Otal P, et al. Stent-graft treatment of penetrating thoracic aortic ulcers. J Endovasc Ther 2002;9(Suppl II):25–31.

325. Murgo S, Dussaussois L, Golzarian J, et al. Penetrating atherosclerotic ulcer of the descending thoracic aorta: treatment by endovascular stent-graft. Cardiovasc Intervent Radiol 1998;21:454–458.

326. Eggebrecht H, Baumgart D, Schmermund A, et al. Penetrating atherosclerotic ulcer of the aorta: treatment by endovascular stent-graft placement. Curr Opin Cardiol 2003;18:431–435.

327. Strassmann G. Traumatic rupture of the aorta. Am Heart J 1947;33:508–515.

328. Parmley LF, Mattingly TW, Manion WC, et al. Nonpenetrating traumatic injury of the aorta. Circulation 1958;17:1086–1101.

329. Demetriades D, Theodorou D, Murray J, et al. Mortality and prognostic factors in penetrating injuries of the aorta. J Trauma 1996;40:761–763.

330. Jamieson WR, Janusz MT, Gudas VM, et al. Traumatic rupture of the thoracic aorta: third decade of experience. Am J Surg 2002;183:571–575.

331. Williams JS, Graff JA, Uku JM, et al. Aortic injury in vehicular trauma. Ann Thorac Surg 1994;57:726–730.

332. Greendyke RM. Traumatic rupture of aorta: special reference to automobile accidents. JAMA 1966;195:527–530.

333. Hunt JP, Baker CC, Lentz CW, et al. Thoracic aorta injuries: management and outcome of 144 patients. J Trauma 1996;40:547–555; discussion 555–546.

334. Richens D, Field M, Neale M, et al. The mechanism of injury in blunt traumatic rupture of the aorta. Eur J Cardiothorac Surg 2002;21:288–293.

335. Eckstein M, Henderson S, Markovchick V. Thorax. In: Marx JA, ed. Rosen's Emergency Medicine: Concepts and Clinical Practice. 5th Ed. St. Louis, MO: Mosby, 2002: 381–414.

336. McCollum CH, Graham JM, Noon GP, et al. Chronic traumatic aneurysms of the thoracic aorta: an analysis of 50 patients. J Trauma 1979;19:248–252.

337. Katsumata T, Shinfeld A, Westaby S. Operation for chronic traumatic aortic aneurysm: when and how? Ann Thorac Surg 1998;66:774–778.

338. Finkelmeier BA, Mentzer RM Jr, Kaiser DL, et al. Chronic traumatic thoracic aneurysm. Influence of operative treatment on natural history: an analysis of reported cases, 1950–1980. J Thorac Cardiovasc Surg 1982;84:257–266.

339. Bacharach JM, Garratt KN, Rooke TW. Chronic traumatic thoracic aneurysm: report of two cases with the question of timing for surgical intervention. J Vasc Surg 1993;17:780–783.

340. Rousseau H, Soula P, Perreault P, et al. Delayed treatment of traumatic rupture of the thoracic aorta with endoluminal covered stent. Circulation 1999;99:498–504.

341. Bennett DE, Cherry JK. The natural history of traumatic aneurysms of the aorta. Surgery 1967;61:516–523.

342. Nagy K, Fabian T, Rodman G, et al. Guidelines for the diagnosis and management of blunt aortic injury: an EAST Practice Management Guidelines Work Group. J Trauma 2000;48:1128–1143.

343. Maggisano R, Nathens A, Alexandrova NA, et al. Traumatic rupture of the thoracic aorta: should one always operate immediately? Ann Vasc Surg 1995;9:44–52.

344. Kipfer B, Leupi F, Schuepbach P, et al. Acute traumatic rupture of the thoracic aorta: immediate or delayed surgical repair? Eur J Cardiothorac Surg 1994;8:30–33.

345. Pate JW, Fabian TC, Walker W. Traumatic rupture of the aortic isthmus: an emergency? World J Surg 1995;19:119–125; discussion 125–116.

346. Galli R, Pacini D, Di Bartolomeo R, et al. Surgical indications and timing of repair of traumatic ruptures of the thoracic aorta. Ann Thorac Surg 1998;65:461–464.

347. Symbas PN, Sherman AJ, Silver JM, et al. Traumatic rupture of the aorta: immediate or delayed repair? Ann Surg 2002;235:796–802.

348. Jahromi AS, Kazemi K, Safar HA, et al. Traumatic rupture of the thoracic aorta: cohort study and systematic review. J Vasc Surg 2001;34:1029–1034.

349. von Oppell UO, Dunne TT, De Groot MK, et al. Traumatic aortic rupture: twenty-year meta-analysis of mortality and risk of paraplegia. Ann Thorac Surg 1994;58:585–593.

350. Fabian TC, Richardson JD, Croce MA, et al. Prospective study of blunt aortic injury: Multicenter trial of the American Association for the Surgery of Trauma. J Trauma 1997;42:374–380; discussion 380–373.

351. Turney SZ. Blunt trauma of the thoracic aorta and its branches. Semin Thorac Cardiovasc Surg 1992;4:209–216.

352. Cowley RA, Turney SZ, Hankins JR, et al. Rupture of thoracic aorta caused by blunt trauma. A fifteen-year experience. J Thorac Cardiovasc Surg 1990;100:652–660; discussion 660–651.

353. Lachat M, Pfammatter T, Witzke H, et al. Acute traumatic aortic rupture: early stent-graft repair. Eur J Cardiothorac Surg 2002;21:959–963.

354. Fujikawa T, Yukioka T, Ishimaru S, et al. Endovascular stent grafting for the treatment of blunt thoracic aortic injury. J Trauma 2001;50:223–229.

355. Ruchat P, Capasso P, Chollet-Rivier M, et al. Endovascular treatment of aortic rupture by blunt chest trauma. J Cardiovasc Surg (Torino) 2001;42:77–81.

356. Bortone AS, Schena S, D'Agostino D, et al. Immediate versus delayed endovascular treatment of posttraumatic aortic pseudoaneurysms and type B dissections: retrospective analysis and premises to the upcoming European trial. Circulation 2002;106: I234–240.

357. Czermak BV, Waldenberger P, Perkmann R, et al. Placement of endovascular stent grafts for emergency treatment of acute disease of the descending thoracic aorta. AJR Am J Roentgenol 2002;179:337–345.

358. Fattori R, Napoli G, Lovato L, et al. Indications for, timing of, and results of catheter-based treatment of traumatic injury to the aorta. AJR Am J Roentgenol 2002;179:603–609.

359. Thompson CS, Rodriguez JA, Ramaiah VG, et al. Acute traumatic rupture of the thoracic aorta treated with endoluminal stent grafts. J Trauma 2002;52:1173–1177.

360. Orend KH, Pamler R, Kapfer X, et al. Endovascular repair of traumatic descending aortic transection. J Endovasc Ther 2002;9: 573–578.

361. Daenen G, Maleux G, Daenens K, et al. Thoracic aorta endoprosthesis: the final countdown for open surgery after traumatic aortic rupture? Ann Vasc Surg 2003;17:185–191.

362. Karmy-Jones R, Hoffer E, Meissner MH, et al. Endovascular stent grafts and aortic rupture: a case series. J Trauma 2003;55:805–810.

363. Marty-Ane CH, Berthet JP, Branchereau P, et al. Endovascular repair for acute traumatic rupture of the thoracic aorta. Ann Thorac Surg 2003;75:1803–1807.

364. Orford VP, Atkinson NR, Thomson K, et al. Blunt traumatic aortic transection: the endovascular experience. Ann Thorac Surg 2003;75:106–111; discussion 111–102.

365. Dunham MB, Zygun D, Petrasek P, et al. Endovascular stent grafts for acute blunt aortic injury. J Trauma 2004;56:1173–1178.

366. Kato M, Yatsu S, Sato H, et al. Endovascular stent-graft treatment for blunt aortic injury. Circ J 2004;68:553–557.

367. Richeux L, Dambrin C, Marcheix B, et al. [Towards a new management of acute traumatic aortic ruptures]. J Radiol 2004;85:101–106.

368. Carroccio A, Marin ML, Ellozy S, et al. Pathophysiology of paraplegia following endovascular thoracic aortic aneurysm repair. J Card Surg 2003;18:359–366.

369. Coselli JS, LeMaire SA, Schmittling ZC, et al. Cerebrospinal fluid drainage in thoracoabdominal aortic surgery. Semin Vasc Surg 2000;13:308–314.

370. Coselli JS, Lemaire SA, Koksoy C, et al. Cerebrospinal fluid drainage reduces paraplegia after thoracoabdominal aortic aneurysm repair: results of a randomized clinical trial. J Vasc Surg 2002;35:631–639.

371. Tiesenhausen K, Amann W, Koch G, et al. Cerebrospinal fluid drainage to reverse paraplegia after endovascular thoracic aortic aneurysm repair. J Endovasc Ther 2000;7:132–135.

372. Ishimaru S, Kawaguchi S, Koizumi N, et al. Preliminary report on prediction of spinal cord ischemia in endovascular stent-graft repair of thoracic aortic aneurysm by retrievable stent graft. J Thorac Cardiovasc Surg 1998;115:811–818.

373. Dake MD. Endovascular stent-graft management of thoracic aortic diseases. Eur J Radiol 2001;39:42–49.

374. Criado FJ, Barnatan MF, Rizk Y, et al. Technical strategies to expand stent-graft applicability in the aortic arch and proximal descending thoracic aorta. J Endovasc Ther 2002;9(Suppl II): 32–38.

375. Borst HG. The elephant trunk operation in complex aortic disease. Curr Opin Cardiol 1999;14:427–431.

376. Heinemann MK, Buehner B, Jurmann MJ, et al. Use of the "elephant trunk technique" in aortic surgery. Ann Thorac Surg 1995;60:2–6; discussion 7.

377. Svensson LG, Kim KH, Blackstone EH, et al. Elephant trunk procedure: newer indications and uses. Ann Thorac Surg 2004;78: 109–116.

378. Yano H, Ishimaru S, Kawaguchi S, et al. Endovascular stent grafting of the descending thoracic aorta after arch repair in acute type A dissection. Ann Thorac Surg 2002;73:288–291.

379. Urdaneta E, Wright B, Wright IS. Re-opening the case of the abdominal aortic aneurysm. Circulation 1956;13:754–768.

380. Crawford ES, Crawford JL, Safi HJ, et al. Thoracoabdominal aortic aneurysms: preoperative and intraoperative factors determining immediate and long-term results of operations in 605 patients. J Vasc Surg 1986;3:389–404.

381. Palma JH, Miranda F, Gasques AR, et al. Treatment of thoracoabdominal aneurysm with self-expandable aortic stent grafts. Ann Thorac Surg 2002;74:1685–1687.

382. White RA, Donayre C, Walot I, et al. Regression of a descending thoracoabdominal aortic dissection following staged deployment of thoracic and abdominal aortic endografts. J Endovasc Ther 2002;9(Suppl II):92–97.

383. Park JH, Chung JW, Choo IW, et al. Fenestrated stent grafts for preserving visceral arterial branches in the treatment of abdominal aortic aneurysms: preliminary experience. J Vasc Interv Radiol 1996;7:819–823.

384. Anderson JL, Berce M, Hartley DE. Endoluminal aortic grafting with renal and superior mesenteric artery incorporation by graft fenestration. J Endovasc Ther 2001;8:3–15.

385. Browne TF, Hartley D, Purchas S, et al. A fenestrated covered suprarenal aortic stent. Eur J Vasc Endovasc Surg 1999;18:445–449.

386. Stanley BM, Semmens JB, Lawrence-Brown MM, et al. Fenestration in endovascular grafts for aortic aneurysm repair: new horizons for preserving blood flow in branch vessels. J Endovasc Ther 2001;8:16–24.

387. Greenberg RK, Haulon S, O'Neill S, et al. Primary endovascular repair of juxtarenal aneurysms with fenestrated endovascular grafting. Eur J Vasc Endovasc Surg 2004;27:484–491.

388. Verhoeven EL, Prins TR, Tielliu IF, et al. Treatment of short-necked infrarenal aortic aneurysms with fenestrated stent grafts: short-term results. Eur J Vasc Endovasc Surg 2004;27:477–483.

389. Kruger AJ, Holden AH, Hill AA. Endoluminal repair of a thoracic arch aneurysm using a scallop-edged stent-graft. J Endovasc Ther 2003;10:936–939.

390. Hosokawa H, Iwase T, Sato M, et al. Successful endovascular repair of juxtarenal and suprarenal aortic aneurysms with a branched stent graft. J Vasc Surg 2001;33:1087–1092.

391. Inoue K, Hosokawa H, Iwase T, et al. Aortic arch reconstruction by transluminally placed endovascular branched stent graft. Circulation 1999;100:II316–321.

392. Inoue K, Iwase T, Sato M, et al. Clinical application of transluminal endovascular graft placement for aortic aneurysms. Ann Thorac Surg 1997;63:522–528.

393. Inoue K, Iwase T, Sato M, et al. Transluminal endovascular branched graft placement for a pseudoaneurysm: reconstruction of the descending thoracic aorta including the celiac axis. J Thorac Cardiovasc Surg 1997;114:859–861.

394. Inoue K, Sato M, Iwase T, et al. Clinical endovascular placement of branched graft for type B aortic dissection. J Thorac Cardiovasc Surg 1996;112:1111–1113.

395. Chuter TA, Buck DG, Schneider DB, et al. Development of a branched stent-graft for endovascular repair of aortic arch aneurysms. J Endovasc Ther 2003;10:940–945.

396. Chuter TA, Gordon RL, Reilly LM, et al. An endovascular system for thoracoabdominal aortic aneurysm repair. J Endovasc Ther 2001;8:25–33.

397. Chuter TA, Gordon RL, Reilly LM, et al. Multi-branched stent-graft for type III thoracoabdominal aortic aneurysm. J Vasc Interv Radiol 2001;12:391–392.

398. Chuter TA, Schneider DB, Reilly LM, et al. Modular branched stent graft for endovascular repair of aortic arch aneurysm and dissection. J Vasc Surg 2003;38:859–863.

399. Schneider DB, Curry TK, Reilly LM, et al. Branched endovascular repair of aortic arch aneurysm with a modular stent-graft system. J Vasc Surg 2003;38:855.

400. McWilliams RG, Fearn SJ, Harris PL, et al. Retrograde fenestration of endoluminal grafts from target vessels: feasibility, technique, and potential usage. J Endovasc Ther 2003;10:946–952.

401. McWilliams RG, Murphy M, Hartley D, et al. In situ stent-graft fenestration to preserve the left subclavian artery. J Endovasc Ther 2004;11:170–174.

402. Johansson G, Swedenborg J. Little impact of elective surgery on the incidence and mortality of ruptured aortic aneurysms. Eur J Vasc Surg 1994;8:489–493.

403. Auer J, Berent R, Eber B. Aortic dissection: incidence, natural history, and impact of surgery. J Clin Basic Cardiol 2000;3:151–154.

404. Heller JA, Weinberg A, Arons R, et al. Two decades of abdominal aortic aneurysm repair: have we made any progress? J Vasc Surg 2000;32:1091–1100.

405. Kantonen I, Lepantalo M, Brommels M, et al. Mortality in ruptured abdominal aortic aneurysms. The Finnvasc Study Group. Eur J Vasc Endovasc Surg 1999;17:208–212.

Endovascular Repair of Abdominal Aortic Aneurysms

24

Richard A. Baum, Roy K. Greenberg

More than a decade ago, endovascular aneurysm repair (EVAR) was first introduced clinically (1). Since that time, an explosion of interest by physicians, patients, and the medical device industry has taken place. Presently, approximately 15,000 patients have undergone this procedure in the United States, with 25,000 worldwide. In 2004, more than 8,000 implantations occurred in the United States.

Like the introduction of any new evolving technology, advances have been made in a step-by-step manner. Overall, the current status of EVAR continues to be exceptionally robust and promising. The introduction of new devices allows more patients to qualify for this procedure, and this number continues to expand. Today's devices are smaller, better tapered, and more durable. This is quite a change from the initial 24 French non-tapered devices that were used a decade ago.

This chapter will review the background of abdominal aortic aneurismal disease and examine the prerequisite anatomy currently needed in endovascular aneurysm repair. Also, the differences among devices and the basic deployment sequences involved are described. Finally, the chapter explores the follow-up and surveillance of patients after endovascular aneurysm repair, including when and how secondary interventions are to be performed.

It is our hope that the basic concepts introduced here will have applicability in the future, even though the actual devices may change.

EPIDEMIOLOGY OF ABDOMINAL AORTIC ANEURYSMS

Dissections and aneurysmal disease of the aorta are serious medical problems associated with significant morbidity and mortality. Abdominal aneurysms, the most common manifestation of aortic aneurysmal disease, were responsible for 16,000 deaths in 2000 (2) and represent the tenth leading cause of death in men 65–74 years old. In the year 2000, more than 30,000 open surgical repairs were performed for abdominal aneurysms in the United States. When the medical and societal burdens of abdominal aneurysms are coupled with aneurysms of the thoracic aorta, aortic branches, and aortic dissections, the magnitude of the problem dramatically increases.

Multicenter reports on conventional (open surgical) treatments for infrarenal aortic aneurysms define a mortality rate of 3–6% and a significant incidence of morbidities, including myocardial infarction, renal failure, pulmonary failure, amputation, graft-related complications, and ischemic complications of the mesenteric and lower extremity circulation (3–5). Endovascular aneurysm repair is now commonly used to treat patients with amenable anatomy (6). The justification for the use of such a technique relates to observed short-term diminished morbidity, in contrast to open surgery; however, the long-term results of such treatments remain under scrutiny (7–9).

TRADITIONAL ABDOMINAL AORTIC ANEURYSM REPAIR

Open surgery for aortic aneurysms was originally described in the 1960s. Although the technique has been modified, the basics remain the same and the procedure has proved effective at preventing long-term aortic rupture. The open procedure can be performed via a transabdominal or retroperitoneal approach to expose the aorta above and below the diseased segment. The patient is anticoagulated, the aorta clamped proximally and distally, and an interposing graft placed by suturing the fabric to healthy aorta. The position of the proximal clamp is critical in terms of defining

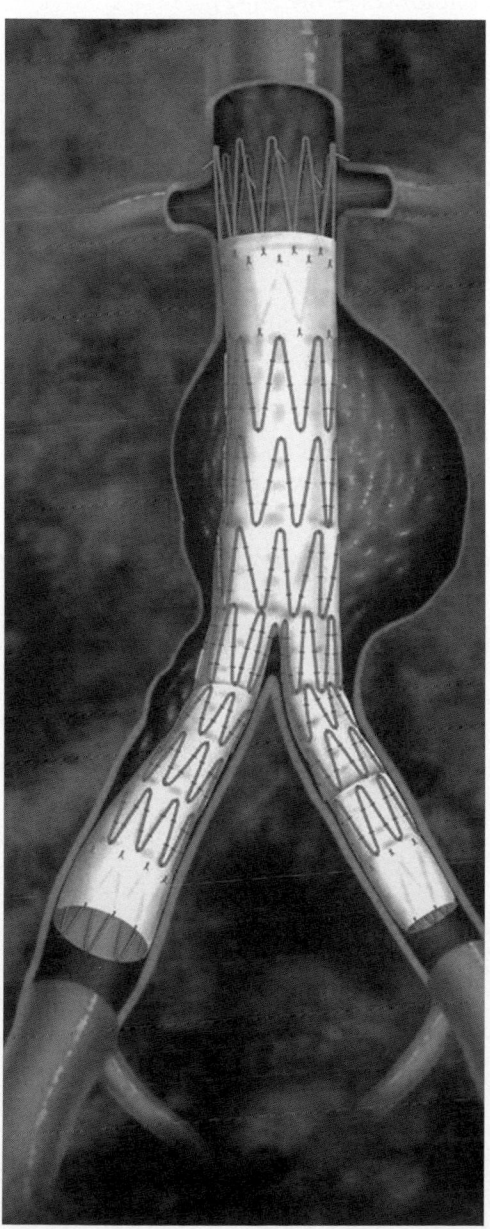

Figure 24–1 Schematic drawing of endovascular aneurysm repair (EVAR). A Zenith endograft is seen excluding an abdominal aortic aneurysm.

TABLE 24–1		
CLINICAL APPROACH TO PATIENTS WITH ABDOMINAL AORTIC ANEURYSMAL DISEASE		
	Low-Risk Physiology	**High-Risk Physiology**
Low-Risk Anatomy	Open Surgery or EVAR (remaining question)	EVAR
High-Risk Anatomy	Open Surgery	EVAR (if possible)

the complexity of the repair. Clamps can be placed in the infrarenal, suprarenal, supraceliac, or thoracic aortic positions. As a general rule, the more proximal the required clamp, the higher the expected complication rate. The same concept relates to the need to incorporate visceral vessels. For example, an aneurysm that requires only one renal reimplantation is much simpler than one that requires the visceral vessels to be reinserted into the repair. Even for conventional infrarenal aneurysms, when clamps are placed below the renal arteries, the mortality remains significantly higher than for similar anatomies treated with an endovascular graft (10).

Overall, the choice of endovascular or open surgery is not a simple one, and it relates to the complexity of the anatomy involved and the overall health and life expectancy of the patient (11–15) (Figure 24–1). Patients with anatomic features that make device deployment difficult, such as short angulated proximal necks, are defined as high risk. Patients with various comorbidities, such as coronary artery disease and COPD, are defined as having high-risk physiology (Table 24–1).

Obviously, when a patient is "sick" and the anatomy is "complex," a higher threshold for advocating treatment and repair is recommended. In the absence of acute growth or symptoms, high-risk physiology patients are rarely treated unless their aneurysm significantly exceeds the 5.5 cm threshold that has been defined by the two small aneurysm trials (16,17). Whether or not aneurysms smaller than 5.5 cm should be treated with an endovascular approach is now the subject of much debate, and prospective randomized trials are ongoing (13,18–23).

PREOPERATIVE EVALUATION FOR PATIENTS UNDERGOING ENDOVASCULAR ANEURYSM REPAIR

It cannot be emphasized enough that careful patient selection and preoperative imaging are critical to procedural success. Several questions arise that need to be answered before a patient is ready for endovascular aneurysm repair:

Does the patient have an aneurysm large enough that it needs to be repaired?

As described earlier, the exact size required of an aneurysm to be repaired is still being debated. An aneurysm of 5.5 cm is believed by most to require correction either by surgical or endovascular repair—provided that the patient has a life expectancy greater than 2–5 years were the aneurysm successfully corrected. This number is based on earlier studies comparing operative risk to rupture risk. Five and a half centimeters is the crossover point at which the risk of rupture is greater than the risk of traditional surgery. Trying to apply this concept to endovascular repair is difficult because the risk of mortality following endovascular repair may be less than that of open surgery. In light of this, some have concluded that aneurysm-related death rates will be lower if smaller aneurysms are repaired with EVAR as opposed to waiting for growth. Others argue that because the risk of rupture is so low in small aneurysms (less than 5 cm), the anatomy should be left alone and watched.

Is the patient a good candidate for endovascular repair?

Preoperative evaluation for a patient undergoing EVAR should include an extensive investigation of the patient's vascular anatomy from the celiac axis to the femoral bifurcation. This is best accomplished with thin-slice, dynamically enhanced computer tomography (CTA). Anatomic information displayed in 3D on CT makes it superior to 2D projectional contrast angiography. Although the exact CT imaging protocols are equipment dependent, all scans must be performed using dynamic contrast enhancement with 2–3 mm slice thickness. The one potential drawback with CTA is in providing length measurements that are required for device planning. Counting CT slices to provide these types of measurements can be misleading because of vessel tortuosity (24,25). This can cause measurements to be shorter than the actual longitudinal vessel segment. Any modern workstation can overcome this limitation by reconstructing the images into a 3D model. Centerline length measurements can be easily obtained using workstation software. Preoperative angiography, which was once standard, is now rarely performed in experienced centers and should be reserved for problem-solving or when the CT scan cannot answer specific questions. Preoperative dynamically enhanced magnetic resonance angiography (MRA) sometimes can be useful, particularly in those patients with renal insufficiency (26,27). In these patients, the use of iodinated water soluble contrast material should be avoided.

Complex Anatomy

Certain anatomic features may make undergoing endovascular aneurysm repair (28) difficult for some patients. When deciding whether or not a patient is a good candidate for EVAR, several distinct locations in the infrarenal aorta and iliofemoral vessels must be closely examined (29).

The aortic neck is a normal segment of aorta and is defined as the distance of this segment from the lowest renal artery to the beginning of the aneurysm sac. This distance is typically described as a centerline measurement in centimeters.

Traditional endografts require at least some length of normal infrarenal aorta for the fixation of the proximal attachment. The minimal aortic neck length required for proper fixation depends on the device used and the experience of the operator. Necks less than 1.5 centimeters limit the margin for deployment error and reduce the fixation and sealing zone to questionable levels (30–32).

The angle of the aortic neck is also an important consideration when evaluating patients for endografts. Angles of greater that 45 degrees may create difficulties with respect to endograft alignment within the proximal neck (particularly relating to renal artery preservation) and introduction or delivery system challenges, and they provide additional stress upon implant materials that were not intended for marked tortuosity (Figure 24–2).

The shape of the aortic neck is another factor that is essential in patient selection. Trapezoidal or conical necks that enlarge distally can be especially challenging (Figure 24–3). Similarly, thrombus or atheromatous debris within the neck is indicative of disease and potential instability (33) (Figure 24–4). In the absence of an adequate proximal neck, the device fixation systems may not provide enough stability to prevent downward migration, resulting in the endoprosthesis sliding into the aneurysm sac. Devices with suprarenal fixation and barbs may be of benefit here; however, the need for placing fixation and sealing zones into a healthy, stable aorta cannot be overemphasized (29,30,32–39).

Iliofemoral anatomy is another important consideration in determining whether a patient is able to undergo endovascular

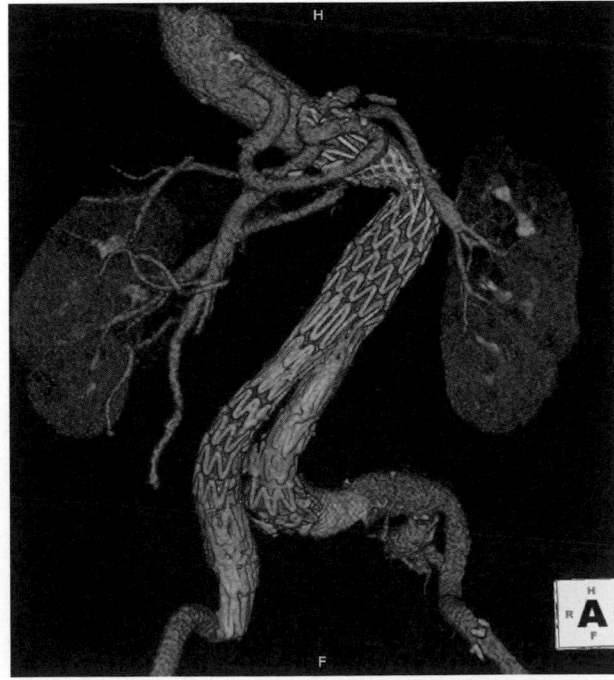

Figure 24–2 Complex anatomy. A reconstruction from a spiral CTA shows a fenestrated endograft in a patient with complex anatomy.

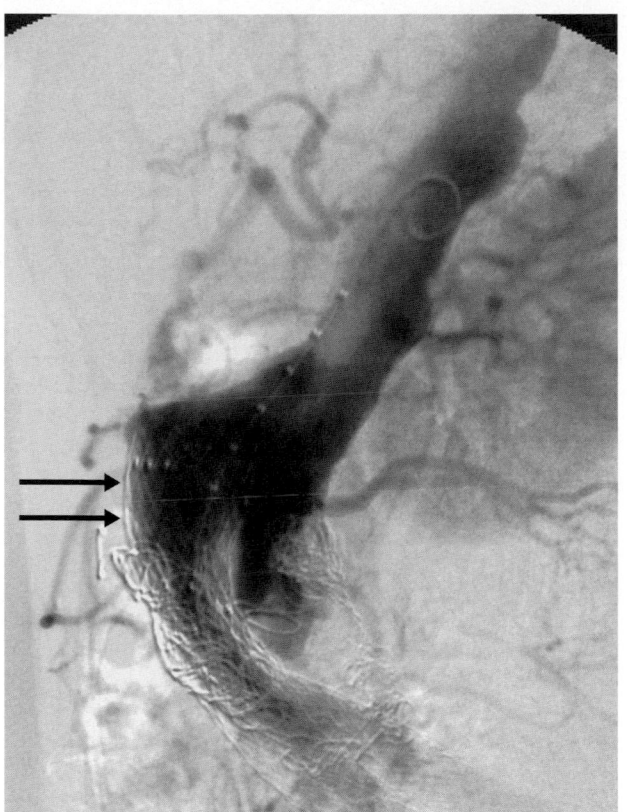

Figure 24–3 Trapezoidal aortic neck. A lateral angiogram shows a trapezoidal aortic neck and an endograft that has fallen into the aneurysm sac (*arrows*).

aneurysm repair. These vessels must be large and straight enough in diameter to allow devices to be passed in a retrograde direction (40). The minimal sizes of these vessels are device specific, and they depend on the amount of calcification and tortuosity (Figures 24–5 and 24–6). Eight millimeters is large enough for modern devices, although this number will certainly decrease in the future. In patients with iliofemoral anatomy that is too small, calcified, or torturous, an iliac conduit can be created through a retroperitoneal incision (whereby a prosthetic graft 8–10 mm in diameter is sewn directly onto the common iliac artery) (41). Access to the aneurysm through this graft is then established, allowing the main body of the device to be introduced without any traversal of the femoral or external iliac arteries. At the completion of the case, the distal end of this graft can be ligated or sewn to the femoral artery, creating an iliofemoral bypass.

It is not infrequent that the extent of aneurismal disease extends beyond the iliac bifurcation. In these patients, the common iliac artery is too large to create a good seal and the endograft limb must be extended into the external iliac artery. Consequently, the proximal internal iliac artery remains in continuity with the aneurysm sac. Retrograde flow in this vessel will cause a direct communication from the systemic circulation to the aneurysm sac. It is therefore important to occlude flow in the proximal internal iliac artery before extending the endograft limb into the external iliac artery. This is accomplished by preoperative internal iliac artery embolization (42–47). It is important to

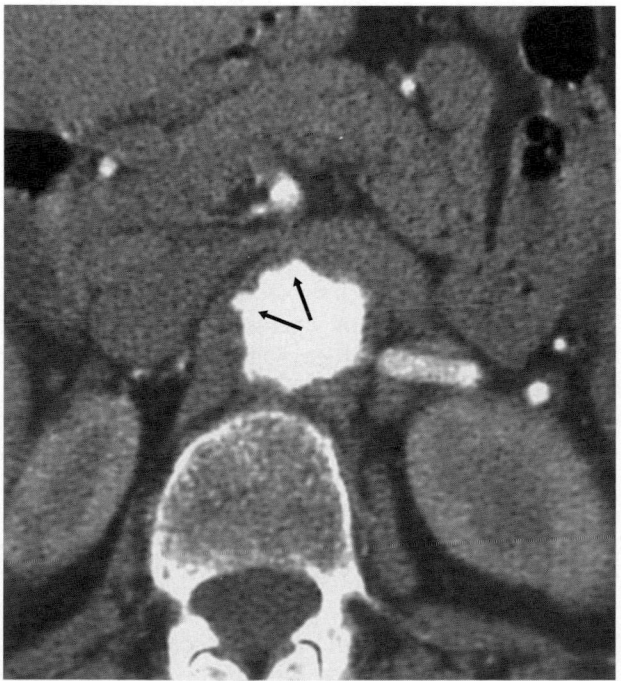

Figure 24–4 Ulcerated aortic neck. A single slice from a dynamic CT angiogram shows irregularity and ulceration of the aortic neck (*arrows*).

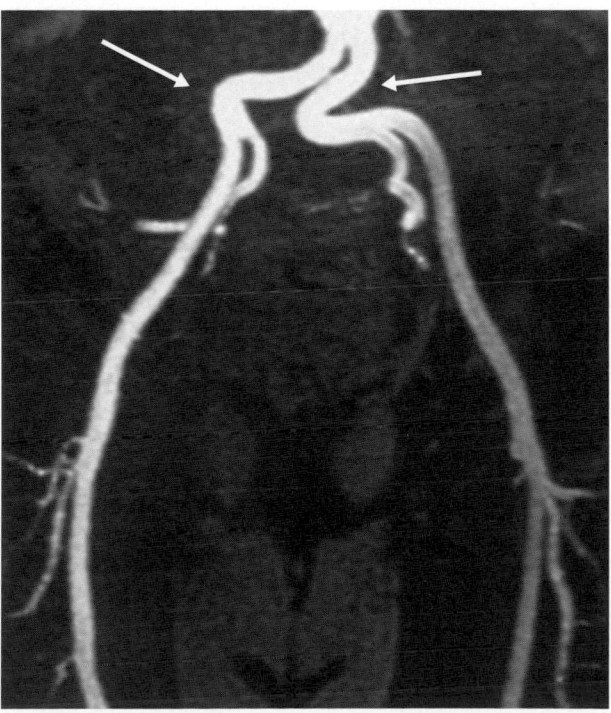

Figure 24–5 Tortuous iliac arteries. A dynamically enhanced magnetic resonance angiogram shows tortuosity of the iliac arteries.

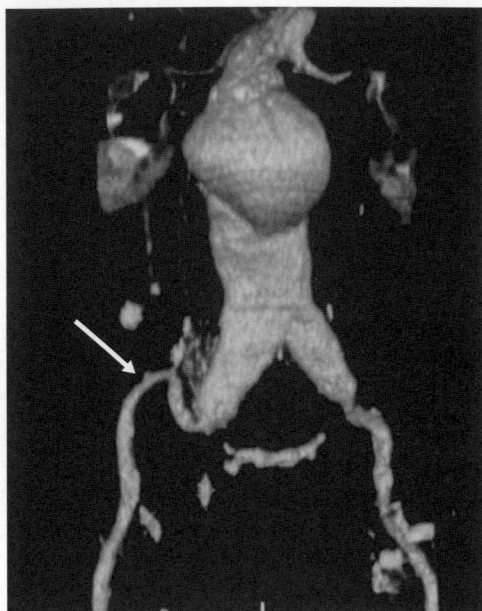

Figure 24–6 Complex anatomy. A surface-rendered CT angiogram shows poor iliofemoral anatomy (*arrow*) and an angled proximal neck.

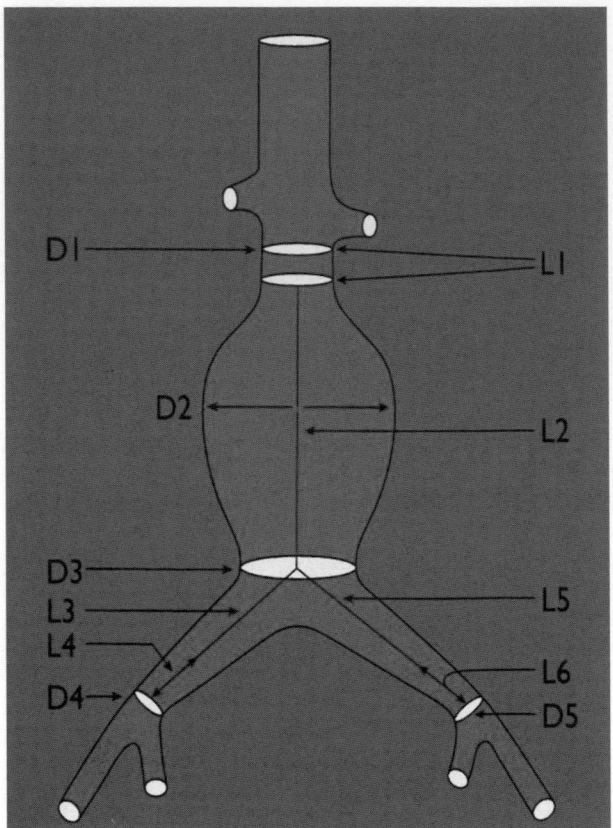

Figure 24–7 Standard measurements needed to design a modular endograft. A series of diameter (D) and length (L) measurements are obtained to choose pieces that fit together in vivo to construct an endograft.

embolize the proximal internal iliac trunk and maintain continuity between the anterior and posterior divisions of the internal iliac arteries, whenever possible. These vessels play an important role in the collateral circulation of the pelvis and lower extremity.

Which is the best device to repair the aneurysm?

Device selection depends on availability and a thorough knowledge of each device. For example, some devices may provide more secure proximal fixation and would therefore be useful in patients with short aortic necks. Other devices may have a lower profile allowing them to be placed through narrow, calcified, or torturous iliac arteries. Others may provide fixation in larger aortic necks (48,49). At the present time, the perfect endograft does not exist. All current endografts have advantages and disadvantages. A skilled operator will use this information to match a specific graft type and design to an individual patient. Newer endografts have expanded the number of patients who qualify for this procedure (31,50–53).

What size and endograft configuration is needed?

Current endografts are modular in nature. As a result, each device component is individually selected to fit properly with other components inside the patients' aneurysm. Proper preoperative endograft sizing is critical for a successful aneurysm repair. Components are selected from a series of diameter and length measurements and deployed in sequence using various locking mechanisms to attach them to the other pieces (Figure 24–7). Fixation and sealing of the endograft remain paramount to successful aneurysm treatment. Adequate fixation will ensure that the endograft will not succumb over time to the hemodynamic forces that continuously provide caudal traction. Sealing prevents blood from leaking around the endograft that would allow the aneurysm sac to remain pressurized.

PROCEDURAL CONSIDERATIONS

Patients are usually admitted to the hospital on the morning of the procedure. Endografts have successfully been implanted with the use of several different anesthesia methods (54–61). The choice of general, epidural, or local anesthesia depends on the patient's clinical status, the device used, and the experience of the team (54).

Access to the vascular system is usually achieved from the femoral arteries either by femoral cutdown or percutaneous puncture. Closure devices have been successfully used to repair large arterial punctures and allow cases to be performed percutaneously that otherwise would have required cutdown and arteriotomy (62,63).

Using the Seldinger technique, sheaths and endografts are advanced into the aneurysm and secured in place. The exact deployment sequence depends on the graft used. A series of intraoperative angiograms followed by endograft component deployment is the typical sequence. It is critical that operators become completely familiar with the deployment sequence and components of the particular device they are using. It is also important to learn various troubleshooting maneuvers that are unique to each type of endograft (64).

Completion angiography with a pigtail catheter positioned just above the proximal anastomosis is performed to ensure successful aneurysm exclusion and no systemic flow within the aneurysm sac. When performing completion angiography, it is important to examine both the proximal and distal anastomoses for endoleaks. When an endoleak is present, images at high frame rates may be obtained so that the direction of flow into the aneurysm sac can be studied. Another useful technique for determining the source of an intraoperative endoleak is to observe the direction of flow in the aortic branch arteries (lumbar and IMA). If flow in the lumbar artery is in a retrograde direction, a collateral endoleak is present (type II). If flow is in an antegrade direction, a type I endoleak is present and further evaluation of the attachment sites must be performed.

FOLLOW-UP AND SURVEILLANCE

Accurate abdominal aortic imaging is not only required for planning and placement but is also crucial for the follow-up of patients undergoing endovascular treatment of abdominal aortic aneurysms.

During the preoperative period, spiral computed tomography, gadolinium-enhanced MR angiography, Doppler ultrasound, and conventional contrast angiography help determine the patients who are candidates for endovascular aneurysm repair. These same modalities are also used to design the size and type of graft to be utilized. Intraoperatively, contrast angiography and possibly intravascular ultrasound are employed to ensure proper graft deployment and to determine whether the aneurysm sac has been isolated from the systemic circulation.

Postoperative imaging and surveillance also plays an important role in maintaining long-term patency. This is not drastically different from patients who have undergone traditional surgical repair. Given that patients presenting with an infrarenal aneurysm are at a higher risk for the later development of more proximal aneurysms, most physicians advocate lifelong follow-up for all aneurysm patients. The number of follow-up imaging studies in patients treated with EVAR is greater than after open repair to ensure that the endograft has not migrated and that the aneurysm sac has not increased in size and continues to be excluded from the systemic circulation. This is most often accomplished using dynamic spiral CT angiography.

Although quick and noninvasive, the use of spiral CT to follow stent graft patients has its drawbacks. Intravenous contrast administration in recently postoperative patients, many of whom have baseline renal insufficiency, is not ideal. Compounding this is the large contrast load the patient receives during stent graft deployment and potential

problems related to suprarenal fixation of these devices, which may leave bare springs across both renal artery orifices. For these reasons, other postoperative imaging methods have been attempted.

Magnetic resonance angiography has proved useful in evaluating the vascular system in several disease states and, in some cases, has eliminated the need for conventional contrast angiography. Multiplanar imaging, along with lack of nephrotoxicity, makes this an attractive method for evaluating postoperative stent graft patients. At times, this can be challenging because metallic exoskeletons and fixation devices can make MRA imaging of postoperative stent graft patients difficult.

Plain radiographs and duplex Doppler ultrasound can also be used for the evaluation of the postoperative EVAR patient.

Aneurysm Sac Shrinkage

The goal of both traditional and endovascular repair of abdominal aortic aneurysms is to prevent rupture. The physiologic response of the aneurysm sac to an endograft is a complex and poorly understood process. Many variables exist that determine whether an aneurysm will shrink after EVAR. Some of these include endoleaks (65), graft type, initial aneurysm size, wall calcification, thrombus, number of branch vessels, infection, graft configuration, smoking, hypertension, pulse pressure, and anticoagulation. Whether it is desirable for an aneurysm to decrease in size following EVAR is the subject of some debate. It remains critical for the physician to be assured that by treating the aneurysm, the natural history of aneurismal disease, namely growth and rupture, has been reversed. Therefore, a shrinking aneurysm (Figure 24–8) clearly provides evidence in this regard—a nongrowing aneurysm does less so—and an aneurysm increasing in size, regardless of the cause, gives rise to great concern.

ENDOLEAKS

As with traditional repair, the goal of EVAR is to protect the aneurysm sac from the systemic circulation, thus preventing continued expansion and eventual rupture. Unlike traditional repair, approximately one third of patients will develop flow around the device and into the aneurysm sac (endoleaks) (Figure 24–9). Surveillance CT scans are required at regular intervals to confirm continued successful exclusion of the aneurysm sac from the systemic circulation. Endoleaks are defined as "the persistence of blood flow outside the lumen of the endoluminal graft but within an aneurysm sac or adjacent vascular segment being treated by the graft" (66–69). To better understand this phenomenon, a classification system has evolved in which endoleaks are organized into four categories based on their source (Table 24–2). It is important to remember that regardless of the type, all endoleaks transmit systemic pressure into the aneurysm sac (70,71).

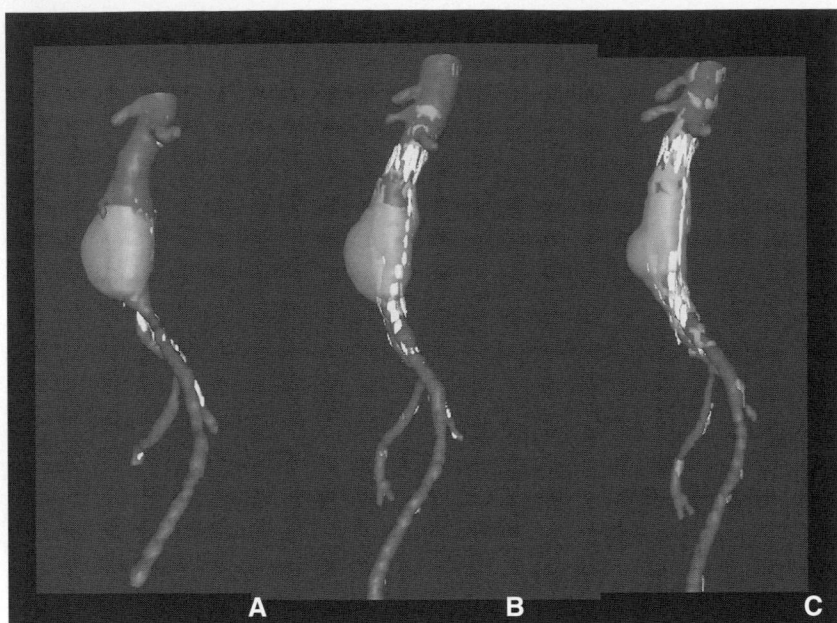

Figure 24–8 Decreasing size of aneurysm following EVAR. **A.** Prior to endovascular repair. **B.** Twelve months following repair. **C.** Twenty-four months following repair.

Type I Endoleak

If flow into the aneurysm sac originates from around a stent graft attachment site (proximally or distally), it is called type I. This represents a failure of the stent graft to seal along the native arterial wall, creating a direct communication with the systemic arterial circulation (Figure 24–10). This type of endoleak is rare, occurring in 3–5% of patients. Balloons, stents, and extender cuffs are used for securing the malfunctioning segment to the arterial wall. Continued aortic neck dilatation after EVAR has been widely observed (34,35,39,72–78). This is a potential source of proximal type I endoleaks.

Type II Endoleak

This is the most common type of endoleak, and it occurs when reversal of flow in aortic branch vessels empties into the aneurysm. Type II endoleaks occur when blood flow takes a circuitous route traveling through aortic branches proximal or distal to the endovascular repair through anastomotic connections into vessels with a direct communication with the aneurysm sac. Blood then travels in a retrograde direction in these vessels, eventually emptying into the sac behind the stent graft (Figure 24–11). These vessels, before aortic exclusion via the stent graft, carried blood from the aorta to nutrient beds of lower resistance. When their native ostia resides within the excluded aneurysm sac, the flow dynamics change, resulting in flow reversal. This does not occur following traditional surgical repairs as these vessels are ligated from within the opened aneurysm sac. Typical culprits include the inferior mesenteric and lumbar arteries. This

type of endoleak occurs in approximately 20% of patients and is a problem unique to endovascular aneurysm repair (79,80).

Much has been learned in recent years regarding the characteristics of collateral endoleaks. It is now understood that two distinct morphologic types of collateral (type II)

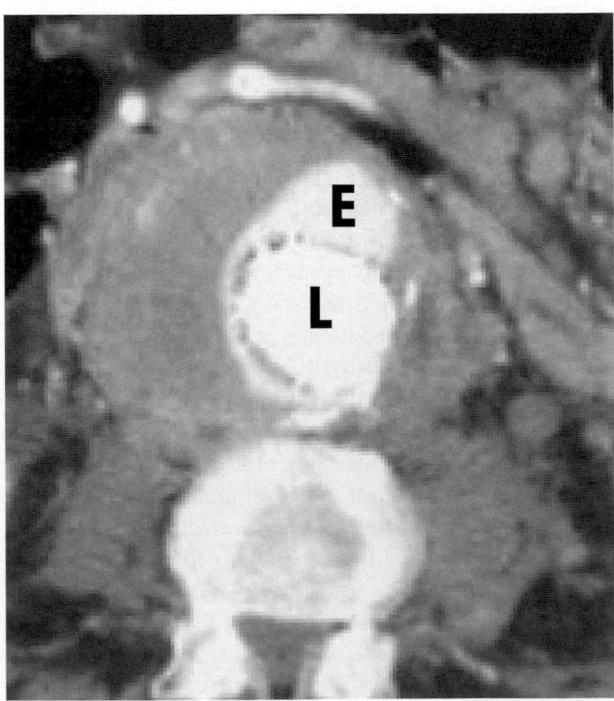

Figure 24–9 A single axial slice from a dynamic CT angiogram shows a large endoleak (E) in the aneurysm sac outside the stent graft lumen (L).

TABLE 24–2
TYPES, ETIOLOGY, AND TREATMENT OF ENDOLEAKS

Type	Etiology	Treatment
1	Attachment Site	PTA, Balloons, Stents
2	Collaterals	Embolization
3	Graft Failure	Graft Repair
4	Pourosity	No Treatment Needed

endoleaks exist. This has important implications in the way patients with these types of endoleaks are treated. In the first type, flow travels in a retrograde direction through a single aortic branch vessel into the aneurysm sac. Blood flow then enters the endoleak cavity during systole and exits the cavity during diastole. There is a single ingress and egress channel for the endoleak. Flow in the endoleak cavity itself is slow and turbulent. This type of collateral endoleak is described as "simple." It is important to distinguish this type of endoleak from others because it likely has a more benign course (Figure 24–12).

The second type of collateral endoleak has "complex" anatomy. This type of endoleak has flow through one aortic

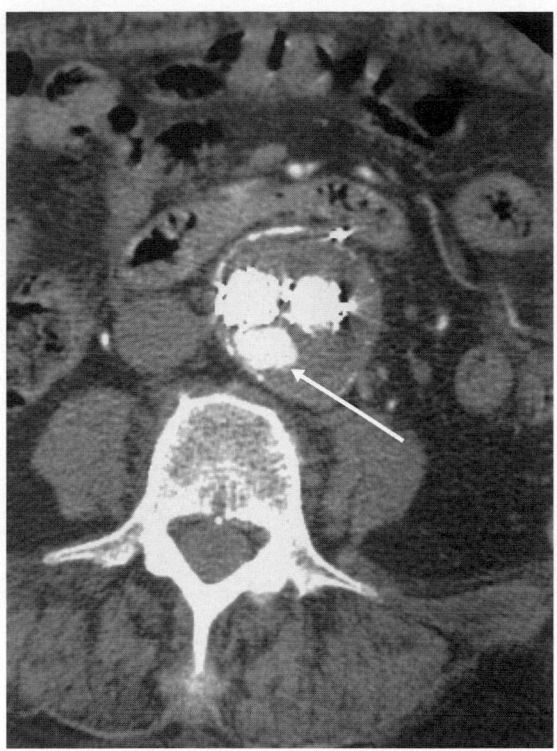

Figure 24–11 Type II endoleak. An axial slice from a dynamic CT angiogram shows a posterior type II endoleak (*arrow*). It is difficult to determine the origin of an endoleak on the basis of CTA alone.

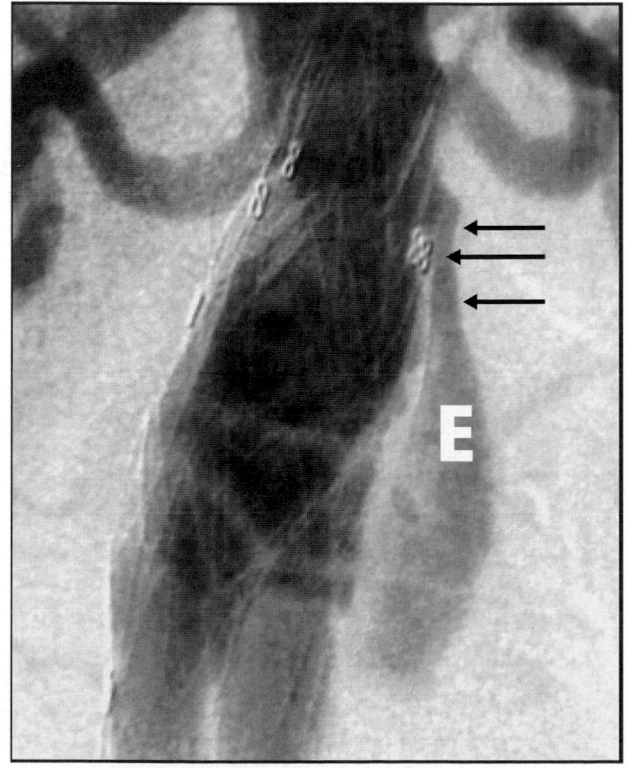

Figure 24–10 Type I endoleak. An angiogram in the anterior-posterior projection shows contrast entering the aneurysm sac (*arrows*) around the proximal anastomosis. This represents a proximal type I endoleak.

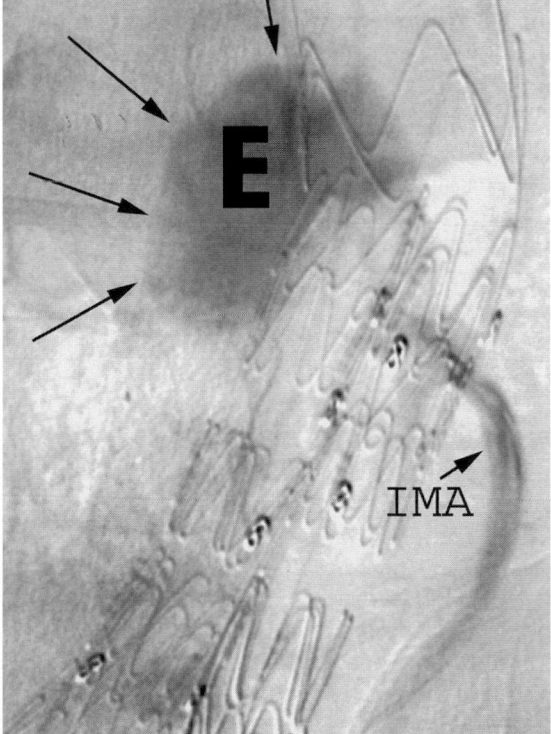

Figure 24–12 Type II endoleak (simple type). An injection in the inferior mesenteric artery (IMA) shows retrograde flow and filling of an aneurysm sac (E). There are no other egress vessels, therefore making this a "simple type" collateral endoleak.

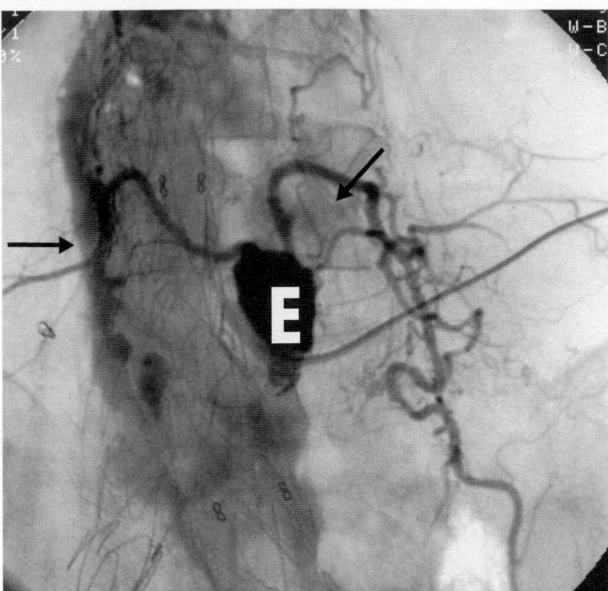

Figure 24–13 Type II endoleak (complex type). A translumbar endoleak angiogram shows the endoleak cavity (E) and several egress lumbar arteries making this a "complex"-type collateral endoleak. It is unlikely that this type of endoleak will spontaneously thrombose.

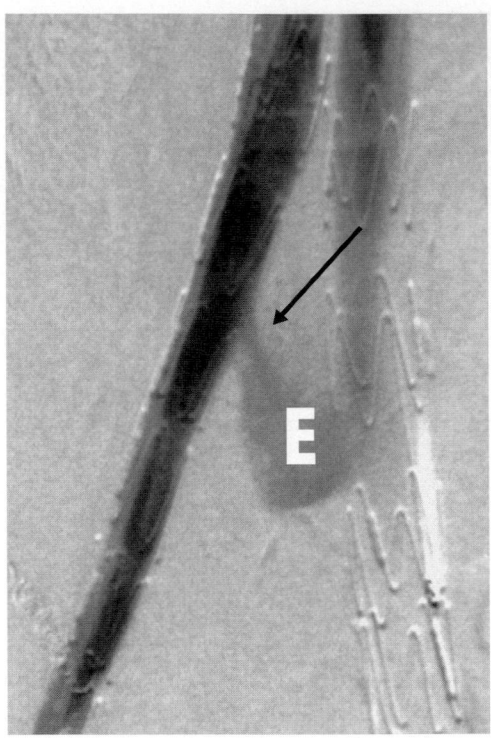

Figure 24–14 Type III endoleak. A contrast angiogram shows a jet of contrast coming from a hole in the endograft limb (*arrow*) and filling an endoleak.

branch vessel into the aneurysm sac and endoleak cavity and out through another aortic branch. Flow is therefore directly through the aneurysm sac having multiple potential ingress and egress channels (Figure 24–13).

Although both types of endoleaks contain systemic pressure, it is likely that the physiology associated with each type of collateral endoleak is quite different. The flow in the simple type of collateral endoleaks is similar to a pseudoaneurysm. Flow swirls in the cavity and exits through the same site it entered. As with a small number of pseudoaneurysms, some believe that many simple collateral endoleaks will eventually thrombose. If true, this could explain why some endoleaks thrombose spontaneously while others continue to grow and enlarge. Taken one step further, the question arises: Why do some patients with endoleaks have continued aneurysm enlargement and others have their aneurysm sacs shrink?

In contrast, complex type II endoleaks have flow through multiple branches into the leak and multiple vessels exiting the leak. These endoleaks are extremely dynamic structures constantly recruiting vascular feeders and remodeling the endoleak cavity. These endoleaks behave like arterial-venous malformations. Flow in these endoleaks is torrential, and it has been postulated that these leaks do not thrombose over time and may cause aneurysm sac enlargement with the potential for future rupture (81–101).

Type III Endoleaks

These occur when a mechanical problem with the stent graft itself exists. Holes, fractures, and separations fall into this

category (Figure 24–14). Repetitive stresses are placed on the grafts from arterial pulsations. In addition, as the aneurysm sac shrinks over time, additional forces are applied to the grafts that can cause failure. Although this type of leak is rare today, it will become more prevalent as implanted stent grafts begin to age and long-term follow-up is accrued on these patients. Type III endoleaks are repaired by correcting the mechanical defect using extension pieces but, in severe cases, may require removal of the endograft (102–105).

Type IV Endoleaks

These leaks occur through the fabric wall of the stent graft because of increased porosity. They are identified at the time of implantation when patients are fully anticoagulated and require no specific intervention except for normalization of the coagulation profile (Figure 24–15).

It is critical to properly identify and classify endoleaks given that the significance and treatment options are so different. Dynamic CT angiography is a sensitive method for identifying the presence or absence of endoleak. It cannot, however, distinguish between types. This is because endoleaks are classified based on the source of the leak, and CT imaging cannot determine the direction of flow within the leak. If, for example, an endoleak cavity is seen communicating with a lumbar artery on CTA, determining the direction of flow in the leak is impossible. The best and most reliable way to determine endoleak etiology is with a dedicated endoleak

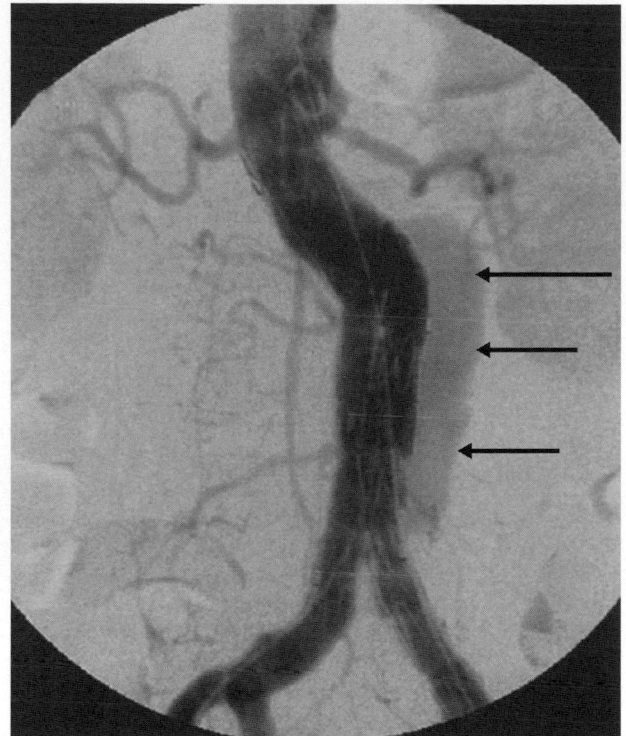

Figure 24–15 Type IV endoleak. A "blush" of contrast is seen filling the aneurysm sac on this intraoperative angiogram (*arrows*). No treatment was needed, and the patient did not have an endoleak on the 30-day CT scan.

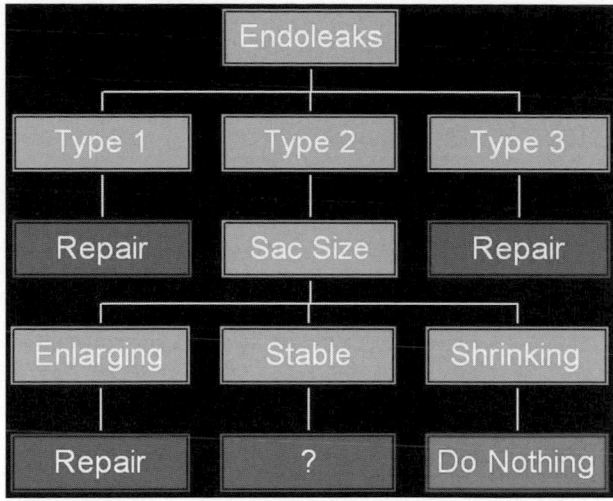

Figure 24–16 Endoleak treatment algorithm type I and 3 endoleaks are repaired as soon as they are diagnosed. Type II endoleaks are repaired if present for longer that 6 months. Consideration should also be given to the status of the aneurysm sac size. The treatment of type II endoleaks in the presence of a stable aneurysm sac (not shrinking or enlarging) remains controversial.

angiogram (Table 24–3). Some have also advocated prolonged injections up to 60 seconds to better demonstrate collateral endoleaks (98).

When and how to treat endoleaks?

There has been much discussion about how and when to treat endoleak patients (106). The significance of endoleaks depends on the type and chronicity of the leak. Patients typically get CT angiography 30 days after endovascular aneurysm repair. If an endoleak is present, then a repeat

CTA is performed 6 months later. If the endoleak is still present, it should be repaired because an endoleak present at 6 months is very unlikely to thrombose (Figure 24–16). The type of treatment depends on the category of the endoleak. This can only be accurately determined from a dedicated endoleak angiogram. It is useful to perform this angiogram at a separate time so that a treatment plan can be formulated.

The treatment of types I and III endoleaks are straightforward and involve separating the systemic circulation from the aneurysm sac. The management of type II endoleaks can be complicated by vascular and endograft anatomy. It has been shown that the embolization of feeding vessels to the endoleak is not effective in providing a durable repair. The embolization of an inferior mesenteric artery (IMA), for

TABLE 24–3
STANDARD ANGIOGRAPHIC ENDOLEAK EVALUATION

Run No.	Location	Projection	Catheter	Injection Rate (cc)	Injection Duration (Seconds)	To Check
1	PAS	AP	Pigtail	25	1	Proximal Attachment Site
2	PAS	Lateral	Pigtail	25	1	Proximal Attachment Site
3	Intragraft	45 degrees LAO	Pigtail	8	3	Graft and Distal Attachment
4	Intragraft	45 degrees RAO	Pigtail	8	3	Graft, Distal Attachment, Lumbar Collaterals
5	SMA	10 degrees LAO	Simons 1	7	5	SMA-IMA Collaterals

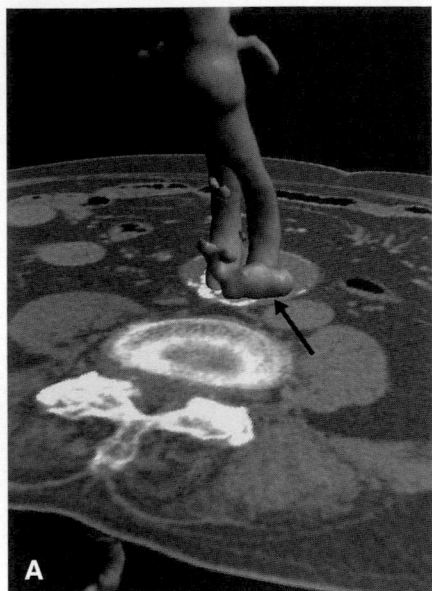 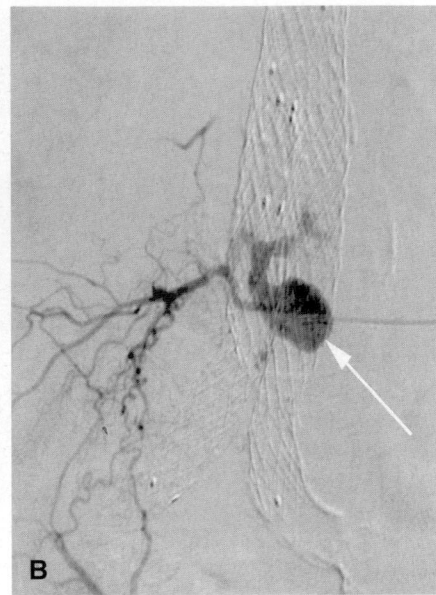 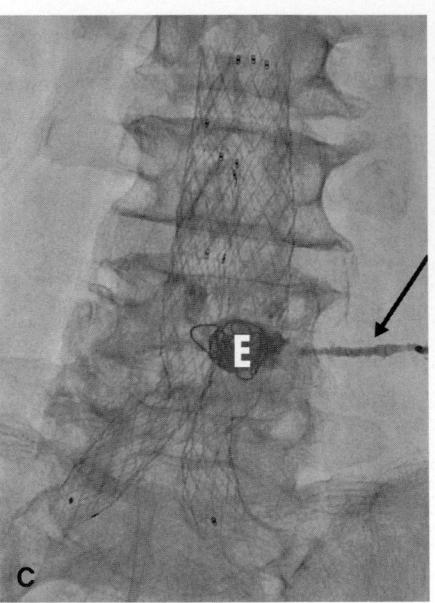

Figure 24–17 Translumbar endoleak embolization. **A., B.** Three-dimensional reconstruction of a dynamic CT angiogram shows a large posterior endoleak (*arrow*). **C.** A translumbar endoleak embolization is performed using coils and glue. A trail of glue is seen "sealing" the aneurysm sac (*arrow*).

example, will not provide a durable repair of an IMA to lumbar endoleak. Endoleaks are dynamic structures and occluding a single inflow vessel will lead to the redistribution of flow from other aortic branch vessels. Lumbar arteries that once served as egress from an IMA endoleak will become ingress after the IMA is embolized. In many respects, endoleaks resemble arterial-venous malformations (AVM). Embolizing a feeding vessel to an AVM has been shown to be ineffective. To effectively treat the malformation, the nidus must be destroyed (83). This central area is where the connection of feeding and draining vessels occurs. The same concept applies to type II endoleaks. To effectively treat these leaks, the central endoleak cavity needs to be thrombosed. Once this occurs, the various feeding and draining vessels to the endoleak cavity will also thrombose back to their origins. To facilitate easy access to the endoleak cavity, the technique of translumbar endoleak embolization has been developed (82) (Figure 24–17).

Translumbar endoleak embolization is performed with the patient in a prone position on a fluoroscopy table (some have also performed this procedure using CT). The location of the endoleak is first referenced to bony anatomic landmarks and to radiopaque markers on the endograft (82). The patient is given antibiotics, and the aneurysm sac is entered using a standard translumbar needle. The needle is guided fluoroscopically from a puncture site approximately one hand-width from midline. The puncture can be done from either left or right translumbar approach. In many cases, a right translumbar approach will need to traverse the inferior vena cava on the way into the aneurysm sac. It is sometimes useful to aim for the vertebral body. Once the

needle in contact with the vertebral body, it can be backed away and angled more laterally for entering the aneurysm sac. The advantage of this technique is that it helps avoid the transverse processes that can block access to the aneurysm sac.

Entry into the sac can usually be felt as a slight pop. It is a similar feeling to entering a calcified femoral artery. Once the needle is within the aneurysm sac, it should be advanced slowly into the endoleak cavity. Rotating the C arm to the lateral position is very helpful in preventing the advancing needle from traveling too far anterior and exiting the aneurysm sac. The inner stylet should be occasionally withdrawn to determine proper positioning. Entry into the endoleak cavity is signaled by the brisk systemic pressure return of arterial blood through the end of the needle. A small length of connecting tubing is attached to a syringe of contrast and an endoleak angiogram is performed using a hand injection of 5–10 mL. This maps the feeding and draining vessels. It is important to remember that these vessels are not the target of embolotherapy. They will thrombose on their own once the central endoleak cavity is obliterated.

Embolization of the endoleak cavity is performed with a combination of coils and glue. Coil embolization is performed to slow flow, and glue is injected because it typically travels into areas beyond the coils. Care must be taken so that the catheter delivering the glue is not glued in place in the aneurysm sac. This is done by withdrawing the catheter slowly as the glue is dispensed into the endoleak cavity. Some have also used glue to "seal" the way out of the aneurysm sac.

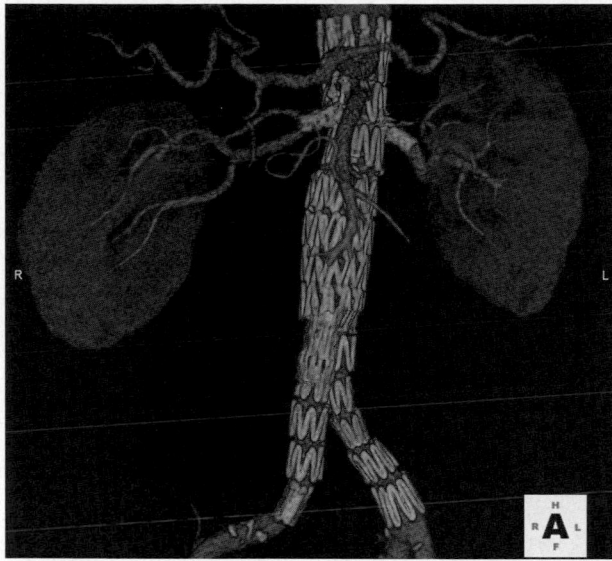

Figure 24–18 Fenestrated aortic endograft. The future probably includes the routine use of fenestrated endografts to extend fixation above the renal arteries. A surface-rendered reconstruction from a CT angiogram shows a fenestrated endograft with components extending into both renal arteries and the SMA.

LIMB KINKING

Endograft limbs in tortuous iliac artery anatomy can lead to narrowing or kinking. In addition, longitudinal foreshortening of the aneurysm sac is common after EVAR. This causes the angle of the common iliac artery takeoff to increase and can also lead to kinked limbs. Patients typically present with increasing claudication and, in some cases, critical limb ischemia. Treatment is straightforward and involves supporting the narrowed limb with stents, additional stent graft limbs, or both. Rapid diagnosis of kinked limbs is important to avoid progression to limb thrombosis. In cases of thromboses, a combination of thrombectomy and thrombolysis is typically required to remove the large clot burden that is present. Once flow is restored, the limbs can then be supported with stents (107–109).

SUMMARY

Endovascular aneurysm repair has permanently changed the way aneurysm patients are diagnosed and treated. There is still much to learn about the long-term durability, but one thing is for certain—EVAR is here to stay. With continued improvements, these devices will be available to an increasing number of patients (Figure 24–18).

REFERENCES

1. Parodi JC, Palmaz JC, Barone HD. Transfemoral intraluminal graft implantation for abdominal aortic aneurysms. Ann Vasc Surg 1991;5(6):491–499.
2. Minino AM, Arias E, Kochanek KD, et al. Deaths: final data for 2000. Natl Vital Stat Rep 2002;50(15):1–119.
3. Johnston KW, Scobie TK. Multicenter prospective study of non-ruptured abdominal aortic aneurysms. Part I. Population and operative management. J Vasc Surg 1988;7(1):69–81.
4. Johnston KW. Multicenter prospective study of nonruptured abdominal aortic aneurysm. Part II. Variables predicting morbidity and mortality. J Vasc Surg 1989;9(3):437–447.
5. Hallett JW Jr, Marshall DM, Petterson TM, et al. Graft-related complications after abdominal aortic aneurysm repair: reassurance from a 36-year population-based experience. J Vasc Surg 1997;25(2):277–284; discussion 285–286.
6. Blum U, Voshage G, Lammer J, et al. Endoluminal stent-grafts for infrarenal abdominal aortic aneurysms [see comments]. N Engl J Med 1997;336(1):13–20.
7. Greenberg RK, Chuter TA, Sternbergh WC III, et al. Zenith AAA endovascular graft: intermediate-term results of the US multicenter trial. J Vasc Surg 2004;39(6):1209–1218.
8. Matsumura JS, Brewster DC, Makaroun MS, et al. A multicenter controlled clinical trial of open versus endovascular treatment of abdominal aortic aneurysm. J Vasc Surg 2003;37(2):262–71.
9. Arko FR, Hill BB, Olcott C, et al. Endovascular repair reduces early and late morbidity compared to open surgery for abdominal aortic aneurysm. J Endovasc Ther 2002;9(6):711–718.
10. Greenhalgh RM, Brown LC, Kwong GP, et al. Comparison of endovascular aneurysm repair with open repair in patients with abdominal aortic aneurysm (EVAR trial 1), 30-day operative mortality results: randomised controlled trial. Lancet 2004;364(9437):843–848.
11. Bertrand M, Godet G, Koskas F, et al. Endovascular treatment of abdominal aortic aneurysms: is there a benefit regarding postoperative outcome? Eur J Anaesthesiol 2001;18(4):245–250.
12. May J. Long-term outcome after aortic endovascular repair: the Sydney experience. Semin Vasc Surg 2003;16(2):123–128.
13. Zarins CK, Heikkinen MA, Lee ES, et al. Short- and long-term outcome following endovascular aneurysm repair. How does it compare to open surgery? J Cardiovasc Surg (Torino) 2004;45(4):321–333.
14. Biebl M, Lau LL, Hakaim AG, et al. Midterm outcome of endovascular abdominal aortic aneurysm repair in octogenarians: a single institution's experience. J Vasc Surg 2004;40(3):435–442.
15. Parodi JC. Long-term outcome after aortic endovascular repair: the Buenos Aires experience. Semin Vasc Surg 2003;16(2):113–122.
16. Lederle FA, Wilson SE, Johnson GR, et al. Design of the abdominal aortic Aneurysm Detection and Management Study. ADAM VA Cooperative Study Group. J Vasc Surg 1994;20(2):296–303.
17. Schermerhorn ML, Cronenwett JL. The UK small aneurysm trial. J Vasc Surg 2001;33(2):443.
18. Hua HT, Cambria RP, Chuang SK, et al. Early outcomes of endovascular versus open abdominal aortic aneurysm repair in the National Surgical Quality Improvement Program—Private Sector (NSQIP-PS). J Vasc Surg 2005;41(3):382–389.
19. Zeebregts CJ, Geelkerken RH, van der Palen J, et al. Outcome of abdominal aortic aneurysm repair in the era of endovascular treatment. Br J Surg 2004;91(5):563–568.
20. Ouriel K, Clair DG, Greenberg RK, et al. Endovascular repair of abdominal aortic aneurysms: device-specific outcome. J Vasc Surg 2003;37(5):991–998.
21. Walschot LH, Laheij RJ, Verbeek AL. Outcome after endovascular abdominal aortic aneurysm repair: a meta-analysis. J Endovasc Ther 2002;9(1):82–89.
22. Ligush J Jr, Pearce JD, Edwards MS, et al. Analysis of medical risk factors and outcomes in patients undergoing open versus endovascular abdominal aortic aneurysm repair. J Vasc Surg 2002;36(3):492–499.
23. Thomas SM, Gaines PA, Beard JD, Vascular Surgical Society of Great Britain and Ireland; British Society of Interventional Radiology. Short-term (30-day) outcome of endovascular treatment of abdominal aortic aneurism: results from the prospective Registry of Endovascular Treatment of Abdominal Aortic Aneurism (RETA). Eur J Vasc Endovasc Surg 2001;21(1):57–64.
24. Armon MP, Whitaker SC, Gregson RH, et al. Spiral CT angiography versus aortography in the assessment of aortoiliac length in patients undergoing endovascular abdominal aortic aneurysm repair. J Endovasc Surg 1998;5(3):222–227.

25. Broeders IA, Blankensteijn JD, Olree M, et al. Preoperative sizing of grafts for transfemoral endovascular aneurysm management: a prospective comparative study of spiral CT angiography, arteriography, and conventional CT imaging. J Endovasc Surg 1997;4(3):252–261.

26. Lutz AM, Willmann JK, Pfammatter T, et al. Evaluation of aortoiliac aneurysm before endovascular repair: comparison of contrast-enhanced magnetic resonance angiography with multidetector row computed tomographic angiography with an automated analysis software tool. J Vasc Surg 2003;37(3):619–627.

27. Neschis DG, Velazquez OC, Baum RA, et al. The role of magnetic resonance angiography for endoprosthetic design. J Vasc Surg 2001;33(3):488–494.

28. Greenberg RK, Clair D, Srivastava S, et al. Should patients with challenging anatomy be offered endovascular aneurysm repair? J Vasc Surg 2003;38(5):990–996.

29. Dillavou ED, Muluk SC, Rhee RY, et al. Does hostile neck anatomy preclude successful endovascular aortic aneurysm repair? J Vasc Surg 2003;38(4):657–663.

30. Greenberg R, Fairman R, Srivastava S, et al. Endovascular grafting in patients with short proximal necks: an analysis of short-term results. Cardiovascular Surg 2000;8(5):350–4.

31. Verhoeven EL, Prins TR, Tielliu IF, et al. Treatment of short-necked infrarenal aortic aneurysms with fenestrated stent-grafts: short-term results. Eur J Vasc Endovasc Surg 2004;27(5):477–483.

32. Hovsepian DM, Hein AN, Pilgram TK, et al. Endovascular abdominal aortic aneurysm repair in 144 patients: correlation of aneurysm size, proximal aortic neck length, and procedure-related complications. J Vasc Interv Radiol 2001;12(12):1373–1382.

33. Gitlitz DB, Ramaswami G, Kaplan D, et al. Endovascular stent grafting in the presence of aortic neck filling defects: early clinical experience. J Vasc Surg 2001;33(2):340–344.

34. Badran MF, Gould DA, Raza I, et al. Aneurysm neck diameter after endovascular repair of abdominal aortic aneurysms. J Vasc Interv Radiol 2002;13(9 Pt 1):887–892.

35. Cao P, Verzini F, Parlani G, et al. Predictive factors and clinical consequences of proximal aortic neck dilatation in 230 patients undergoing abdominal aorta aneurysm repair with self-expandable stent-grafts. J Vasc Surg 2003;37(6):1200–1205.

36. Filis KA, Arko FR, Rubin GD, et al. Three-dimensional CT evaluation for endovascular abdominal aortic aneurysm repair. Quantitative assessment of the infrarenal aortic neck. Acta Chir Belg 2003;103(1):81–86.

37. Ingle H, Fishwick G, Thompson MM, et al. Endovascular repair of wide neck AAA—preliminary report on feasibility and complications. Eur J Vasc Endovasc Surg 2002;24(2):123–127.

38. Sternbergh WC III, Carter G, York JW, et al. Aortic neck angulation predicts adverse outcome with endovascular abdominal aortic aneurysm repair. J Vasc Surg 2002;35(3):482–486.

39. Sternbergh WC III, Money SR, Greenberg RK, et al. Influence of endograft oversizing on device migration, endoleak, aneurysm shrinkage, and aortic neck dilation: results from the Zenith Multicenter Trial. J Vasc Surg 2004;39(1):20–26.

40. Timaran CH, Lipsitz EC, Veith FJ, et al. Endovascular aortic aneurysm repair with the zenith endograft in patients with ectatic iliac arteries. Ann Vasc Surg 2005;19(2):161–166.

41. Abu-Ghaida AM, Clair DG, Greenberg RK, et al. Broadening the applicability of endovascular aneurysm repair: the use of iliac conduits. J Vasc Surg 2002;36(1):111–117.

42. Criado FJ, Wilson EP, Velazquez OC, et al. Safety of coil embolization of the internal iliac artery in endovascular grafting of abdominal aortic aneurysms. J Vasc Surg 2000;32(4):684–688.

43. Cynamon J, Marin ML, Veith FJ, et al. Endovascular repair of an internal iliac artery aneurysm with use of a stented graft and embolization coils. J Vasc Interv Radiol 1995;6(4):509–512.

44. Cynamon J, Lerer D, Veith FJ, et al. Hypogastric artery coil embolization prior to endoluminal repair of aneurysms and fistulas: buttock claudication, a recognized but possibly preventable complication. J Vasc Interv Radiol 2000;11(5):573–577.

45. Halloul Z, Burger T, Grote R, et al. Sequential coil embolization of bilateral internal iliac artery aneurysms prior to endovascular abdominal aortic aneurysm repair. J Endovasc Ther 2001;8(1):87–92.

46. Lin PH, Bush RL, Chaikof EL, et al. A prospective evaluation of hypogastric artery embolization in endovascular aortoiliac aneurysm repair. J Vasc Surg 2002;36(3):500–506.

47. Tefera G, Turnipseed WD, Carr SC, et al. Is coil embolization of hypogastric artery necessary during endovascular treatment of aortoiliac aneurysms? Ann Vasc Surg 2004;18(2):143–146.

48. Greenberg RK, Haulon S, O'Neill S, et al. Primary endovascular repair of juxtarenal aneurysms with fenestrated endovascular grafting. Eur J Vasc Endovasc Surg 2004;27(5):484–491.

49. Greenberg RK, Haulon S, Lyden SP, et al. Endovascular management of juxtarenal aneurysms with fenestrated endovascular grafting. J Vasc Surg 2004;39(2):279–287.

50. Verhoeven EL, Zeebregts CJ, Kapma MR, et al. Fenestrated and branched endovascular techniques for thoraco-abdominal aneurysm repair. J Cardiovasc Surg (Torino) 2005;46(2):131–140.

51. Stanley BM, Semmens JB, Lawrence-Brown MM, et al. Fenestration in endovascular grafts for aortic aneurysm repair: new horizons for preserving blood flow in branch vessels. J Endovasc Ther 2001;8(1):16–24.

52. Macierewicz JA, Jameel MM, Whitaker SC, et al. Endovascular repair of perisplanchnic abdominal aortic aneurysm with visceral vessel transposition. J Endovasc Ther 2000;7(5):410–414.

53. Park JH, Chung JW, Choo IW, et al. Fenestrated stent-grafts for preserving visceral arterial branches in the treatment of abdominal aortic aneurysms: preliminary experience. Vasc Interv Radiol 1996;7(6):819–823.

54. Parra JR, Crabtree T, McLafferty RB, et al. Anesthesia technique and outcomes of endovascular aneurysm repair. Ann Vasc Surg 2005;19(1):123–129.

55. Aadahl P, Lundbom J, Hatlinghus S, et al. Regional anesthesia for endovascular treatment of abdominal aortic aneurysms. J Endovasc Surg 1997;4(1):56–61.

56. De Virgilio C, Romero L, Donayre C, et al. Endovascular abdominal aortic aneurysm repair with general versus local anesthesia: a comparison of cardiopulmonary morbidity and mortality rates. J Vasc Surg 2002;36(5):988–991.

57. Cao P, Zannetti S, Parlani G, et al. Epidural anesthesia reduces length of hospitalization after endoluminal abdominal aortic aneurysm repair. J Vasc Surg 1999;30(4):651–657.

58. Lachat M, Pfammatter T, Turina M. Transfemoral endografting of thoracic aortic aneurysm under local anesthesia: a simple, safe and fast track procedure. Vasa 1999;28(3):204–206.

59. Lachat ML. Regarding "Feasibility of endovascular repair of abdominal aortic aneurysms with local anesthesia with intravenous sedation." J Vasc Surg 2000;31(2):415.

60. Lachat M, Pfammatter T, Bernard E, et al. Successful endovascular repair of a leaking abdominal aortic aneurysm under local anesthesia. Swiss Surg 2001;7(2):86–89.

61. Leotta L, Merlo M, Bitossi G, et al. Mid-term results of endovascular repair for abdominal aortic aneurysm, with loco-regional anesthesia, in high-risk patients. Minerva Cardioangiol 2001;49(1):23–29.

62. Teh LG, Sieunarine K, van Schie G, et al. Use of the percutaneous vascular surgery device for closure of femoral access sites during endovascular aneurysm repair: lessons from our experience. Eur J Vasc Endovasc Surg 2001;22(5):418–423.

63. Haas PC, Krajcer Z, Diethrich EB. Closure of large percutaneous access sites using the Prostar XL Percutaneous Vascular Surgery device. J Endovasc Surg 1999;6(2):168–170.

64. Chuter TA, Reilly LM, Kerlan RK, et al. Endovascular repair of abdominal aortic aneurysm: getting out of trouble. Cardiovasc Surg 1998;6(3):232–239.

65. Ermis C, Kramer S, Tomczak R, et al. Does successful embolization of endoleaks lead to aneurysm sac shrinkage? J Endovasc Ther 2000;7(6):441–445.

66. White GH, Yu W, May J. Endoleak—a proposed new terminology to describe incomplete aneurysm exclusion by an endoluminal graft. J Endovasc Surg 1996;3(1):124–125.

67. White GH, May J, Waugh RC, et al. Type I and type II endoleaks: a more useful classification for reporting results of endoluminal AAA repair [letter]. J Endovasc Surg 1998;5(2):189–191.

68. White GH, May J, Waugh RC, et al. Type III and type IV endoleak: toward a complete definition of blood flow in the sac after endoluminal AAA repair. J Endovasc Surg 1998;5(4):305–309.

69. White GH, Yu W, May J, et al. Endoleak as a complication of endoluminal grafting of abdominal aortic aneurysms: classification, incidence, diagnosis, and management. J Endovasc Surg 1997;4(2):152–168.

70. Baum RA, Carpenter JP, Tuite CM, et al. Diagnosis and treatment of inferior mesenteric artery associated endoleaks after endovascular repair of abdominal aortic aneurysms. Radiology 2000;215(2): 409–413.

71. Baum RA, Carpenter JP, Cope C, et al. Aneurysm sac pressure measurements after endovascular repair of abdominal aortic aneurysms. J Endovasc Surg 2001;33(1):32–41.

72. Makaroun MS, Deaton DH. Is proximal aortic neck dilatation after endovascular aneurysm exclusion a cause for concern? J Vasc Surg 2001;33(Suppl II):S39–S45.

73. Napoli V, Sardella SG, Bargellini I, et al. Evaluation of the proximal aortic neck enlargement following endovascular repair of abdominal aortic aneurysm: 3-years experience. Eur Radiol 2003; 13(8):1962–1971.

74. Sonesson B, Malina M, Ivancev K, et al. Dilatation of the infrarenal aneurysm neck after endovascular exclusion of abdominal aortic aneurysm. J Endovasc Surg 1998;5(3):195–200.

75. Walker SR, Macierewicz J, Elmarasy NM, et al. A prospective study to assess changes in proximal aortic neck dimensions after endovascular repair of abdominal aortic aneurysms. J Vasc Surg 1999;29(4):625–630.

76. Walker SR, Macierewicz J, Whitaker SC, et al. Vascular surgical society of Great Britain and Ireland: changes in proximal aortic neck dimensions following endovascular repair of abdominal aortic aneurysm. Br J Surg 1999;86(5):697.

77. Wever JJ, de Nie AJ, Blankensteijn JD, et al. Dilatation of the proximal neck of infrarenal aortic aneurysms after endovascular AAA repair. Eur J Vasc Endovasc Surg 2000;19(2):197–201.

78. May J. The ins and outs of the excluded abdominal aortic aneurysm: decreasing diameters and dilating necks. J Endovasc Surg 1997;4(1):31–32.

79. Baum RA, Carpenter JP, Stavropoulous SW, et al. Diagnosis and management of type 2 endoleaks after endovascular aneurysm repair. Tech Vasc Interv Radiol 2001;4(4):222–226.

80. Baum RA, Stavropoulos SW, Fairman RM, et al. Endoleaks after endovascular repair of abdominal aortic aneurysm. J Vasc Interv Radiol 2003;14(9 Pt 1):1111–1117.

81. Arko FR, Rubin GD, Johnson BL, et al. Type–II endoleaks following endovascular AAA repair: preoperative predictors and long-term effects. J Endovasc Ther 2001;8(5):503–510.

82. Baum RA, Cope C, Fairman RM, et al. Translumbar embolization of type 2 endoleaks after endovascular repair of abdominal aortic aneurysms. J Vasc Interv Radiol 2001;12(1):111–116.

83. Baum RA, Carpenter JP, Golden MA, et al. Treatment of type 2 endoleaks after endovascular repair of abdominal aortic aneurysms: comparison of transarterial and translumbar techniques. J Vasc Surg 2002;35(1):23–29.

84. Bargellini I, Napoli V, Petruzzi P, et al. Type II lumbar endoleaks: hemodynamic differentiation by contrast-enhanced ultrasound scanning and influence on aneurysm enlargement after endovascular aneurysm repair. J Vasc Surg 2005;41(1):10–18.

85. Steinmetz E, Rubin BG, Sanchez LA, et al. Type II endoleak after endovascular abdominal aortic aneurysm repair: a conservative approach with selective intervention is safe and cost-effective. J Vasc Surg 2004;39(2):306–313.

86. Schmid R, Gurke L, Aschwanden M, et al. CT-guided percutaneous embolization of a lumbar artery maintaining a type II endoleak. J Endovasc Ther 2002;9(2):198–202.

87. Sampaio SM, Panneton JM, Mozes GI, et al. Aneurysm sac thrombus load predicts type II endoleaks after endovascular aneurysm repair. Ann Vasc Surg In press, 2005.

88. Rial R, Serrano FF, Vega M, et al. Treatment of type II endoleaks after endovascular repair of abdominal aortic aneurysms: translumbar puncture and injection of thrombin into the aneurysm sac. Eur J Vasc Endovasc Surg 2004;27(3):333–335.

89. Parry DJ, Kessel DO, Robertson I, et al. Type II endoleaks: predictable, preventable, and sometimes treatable? J Vasc Surg 2002; 36(1):105–110.

90. Maldonado TS, Gagne PJ. Controversies in the management of type II "branch" endoleaks following endovascular abdominal aortic aneurysm repair. Vasc Endovascular Surg 2003;37(1):1–12.

91. Martin ML, Dolmatch BL, Fry PD, et al. Treatment of type II endoleaks with Onyx. J Vasc Interv Radiol 2001;12(5):629–632.

92. Parent FN, Meier GH, Godziachvili V, et al. The incidence and natural history of type I and II endoleak: a 5-year follow-up assessment with color duplex ultrasound scan. J Vasc Surg 2002; 35(3):474–481.

93. Krueger K, Zaehringer M, Gawenda M, et al. Successful treatment of a type-II endoleak with percutaneous CT-guided thrombin injection in a patient after endovascular abdominal aortic aneurysm repair. Eur Radiol 2003;13(7):1748–1749.

94. Haulon S, Tyazi A, Willoteaux S, et al. Embolization of type II endoleaks after aortic stent-graft implantation: technique and immediate results. J Vasc Surg 2001;34(4):600–605.

95. Hansen CJ, Kim B, Aziz I, et al. Late-onset type II endoleaks and the incidence of secondary intervention. Ann Vasc Surg 2004; 18(1):26–31.

96. Hinchliffe RJ, Singh-Ranger R, Whitaker SC, et al. Type II endoleak: transperitoneal sacotomy and ligation of side branch endoleaks responsible for aneurysm sac expansion. J Endovasc Ther 2002; 9(4):539–542.

97. Gorich J, Rilinger N, Sokiranski R, et al. Embolization of type II endoleaks fed by the inferior mesenteric artery: using the superior mesenteric artery approach. J Endovasc Ther 2000;7(4):297–301.

98. Faries PL, Briggs VL, Bernheim J, et al. Increased recognition of type II endoleaks using a modified intraoperative angiographic protocol: implications for intermittent endoleak and aneurysm expansion. Ann Vasc Surg 2003;17(6):608–614.

99. Carpenter JP. Regarding: "The incidence and natural history of type I and II endoleak: a 5-year follow-up assessment with color duplex ultrasound scan." J Vasc Surg 2002;35(3):595–597.

100. Bonvini R, Alerci M, Antonucci F, et al. Preoperative embolization of collateral side branches: a valid means to reduce type II endoleaks after endovascular AAA repair. J Endovasc Ther 2003; 10(2):227–232.

101. Eliason JL, Guzman RJ, Passman MA, et al. Infected endovascular graft secondary to coil embolization of endoleak: a demonstration of the importance of operative sterility. Ann Vasc Surg 2002;16(5):562–565.

102. Joseph G, Rajendiran G, Aggarwal S, et al. Successful treatment of type I and type III primary endoleaks and a femoral pseudoaneurysm using Passager stent grafts following endoluminal repair of an abdominal aortic aneurysm. Indian Heart J 2000; 52(2):218–220.

103. Teutelink A, van der Laan MJ, Milner R, et al. Fabric tears as a new cause of type III endoleak with Ancure endograft. J Vasc Surg 2003;38(4):843–846.

104. Teruya TH, Ayerdi J, Solis MM, et al. Treatment of type III endoleak with an aortouniiliac stent graft. Ann Vasc Surg 2003;17(2):123–128.

105. Powell A, Benenati JF, Becker GJ, et al. Postoperative management: type I and III endoleaks. Tech Vasc Interv Radiol 2001;4(4):227–231.

106. Veith FJ, Baum RA, Ohki T, et al. Nature and significance of endoleaks and endotension: summary of opinions expressed at an international conference. J Vasc Surg 2002;35(5):1029–1035.

107. Alerci M, Wyttenbach R, Bogen M, et al. Endovascular treatment of proximal bilateral iliac limb dislocation and kinking following endovascular abdominal aortic aneurysm repair. Cardiovasc Intervent Radiol In press, 2005.

108. Baum RA, Shetty SK, Carpenter JP, et al. Limb kinking in supported and unsupported abdominal aortic stent grafts. J Vasc Interv Radiol 2000;11(9):1165–1171.

109. Boyle JR, Thompson MM, Clode-Baker EG, et al. Torsion and kinking of unsupported aortic endografts: treatment by endovascular intervention. J Endovasc Surg 1998;5(3):216–221.

Percutaneous Coronary Intervention and Related Techniques

25

Sameer Rohatgi, Howard C. Herrmann,
John W. Hirshfeld, Jr.

HISTORY OF CORONARY ANGIOPLASTY

The first coronary angioplasty, performed in 1977 by Andreas Gruentzig at the Kantonspital in Zurich, Switzerland, was the culmination of a decade of creative research directed toward that goal (1). Gruentzig had carefully studied the work of Dotter and Judkins, which had received relatively little attention (2). He realized that Dotter's coaxial catheter technique had fundamental shortcomings that limited its efficacy in the peripheral circulation and precluded any attempt to apply it to the coronary circulation. He identified two major problems that needed to be solved to enhance angioplasty in general and to extend it to the coronary circulation: (1) the catheters needed to be miniaturized and the dilation diameter needed to be considerably larger than the catheter shaft diameter and (2) entirely new techniques were needed to manipulate catheters within the coronary circulation.

To overcome these obstacles, Gruentzig and associates (3) formulated two fundamental concepts that have had far-reaching implications for all interventional radiological procedures: (1) Balloon dilation became the solution to miniaturization and the disparity between catheter shaft diameter and dilation diameter, and (2) the coaxial guide catheter-balloon catheter system provided a means of leading the relatively flexible small balloon catheter to the coronary circulation and provided the axial supporting force needed to advance it into the coronary vessels. This system

was later enhanced greatly by the development of the steerable movable guide wire.

Initially, coronary angioplasty was believed to have relatively limited clinical applicability. In the early years after its introduction, articles were written anticipating that coronary angioplasty would be applicable to a maximum of 5% of the population of patients with coronary artery disease (4). These early opinions failed to appreciate the overwhelming attractiveness of a coronary revascularization procedure that did not require thoracotomy. This spawned a prodigious effort on the part of industry and physicians to refine the instrumentation used for coronary angioplasty and to develop techniques to address more complex situations.

The earliest compendium of the results of coronary angioplasty was the National Heart, Lung, and Blood Institute (NHLBI) Percutaneous Transluminal Coronary Angioplasty (PTCA) Registry, which represented procedures performed with crude, early-generation equipment by skilled and experienced diagnostic catheterizing personnel who were learning the techniques of angioplasty "on the job." It demonstrated an acute procedure success rate of only 59% and a major complication rate of 18% (5). This modest success rate was achieved in procedures that by current standards would be considered easy and straightforward. Today's exacting standards for operator training and greatly refined radiologic and catheter equipment have yielded acute procedure success rates ranging between 90–95% with major complication rates of less than 3% (6).

In response to the striking improvement in the success rate of coronary angioplasty, there has also been a dramatic increase in the number of procedures. The American Heart Association estimated that more than 1,000,000 coronary angioplasty procedures were performed in the United States in 2003 (7). Thus, in the United States, coronary angioplasty is now a widely used technique for coronary revascularization and is performed at a frequency exceeding that of coronary bypass surgery.

DIFFERENCES BETWEEN CORONARY ANGIOPLASTY AND ANGIOPLASTY IN OTHER VESSELS

Coronary Artery Dimensions and Accessibility

Coronary angioplasty and angioplasty in other vascular beds necessitate the use of specific instrumentation, techniques, and monitoring practices, but there are differences between the two. Coronary arteries range in diameter from 2.0–4.0 mm. Their small dimensions make thrombosis more likely, and angioplasty-induced dissections are more likely to cause acute occlusion. Their small size also makes restenosis more likely. Also, because the coronary arteries are remote from vascular access sites, a large family of instruments and techniques is required to reach target sites within the coronary circulation.

Myocardial Metabolic Rate

The working myocardium, supplied by the coronary circulation, has one of the highest metabolic rates in the body and has limited on-site energy and substrate stores (8). Consequently, the heart can tolerate only brief periods of coronary flow disruption (generally 1–2 minutes). In addition, the heart must support the circulation during the angioplasty procedure. The contractile performance of myocardium deteriorates after less than 1 minute of coronary occlusion (9). Thus, any ischemia caused by a coronary angioplasty procedure must be brief, and its severity must be minimized so that the heart can continue to function while the procedure is performed. Myocardial necrosis begins within 30 minutes of interruption of coronary blood flow (10). In the event of an angioplasty-induced complete occlusion of a target artery, prompt restoration of flow is essential to prevent myocardial infarction. If the myocardium affected by such an occlusion is an important fraction of the patient's total functioning myocardium, the depression of cardiac contractile performance will cause circulatory deterioration leading to cardiogenic shock. Consequently, the safe performance of interventional cardiac procedures requires that the operator be able to recognize and treat myocardial

ischemia and its consequences and also be familiar with the therapeutic agents and devices necessary to support the circulation of a patient who is experiencing an acute myocardial ischemic episode. In addition, as discussed in the next section, current patient safety requires the prompt on-site availability of cardiac surgery to restore coronary blood flow in circumstances that cannot be salvaged by angioplasty techniques.

Monitoring Requirements

Patients undergoing coronary angioplasty have provocable and possibly unstable myocardial ischemia and many have impaired left ventricular contractile function. The overall stress of the procedure, including the administration of a possibly large volume of x-ray contrast agent, may aggravate the patient's condition, particularly when there is extensive coronary disease and impaired left ventricular function. Furthermore, the angioplasty process provokes episodes of myocardial ischemia because the balloon, and at times the guide catheter, transiently occlude the target artery. Consequently, extensive physiologic monitoring is essential for safe, successful coronary angioplasty. Many intraprocedural conduct decisions are based on information about the patient's current condition derived from the monitoring information.

Hemodynamic Monitoring

Proper hemodynamic monitoring enables the operator to recognize and react to impending problems before they become clinically evident. The basics of hemodynamic monitoring begin with the continuous monitoring of aortic pressure. This is accomplished by monitoring the pressure at the tip of the guide catheter. This information discloses not only the patient's systemic arterial pressure but also the degree to which the guide catheter is obstructing the coronary orifice. Guide catheter obstruction of the proximal portion of the target artery may cause ischemic deterioration of cardiac performance and circulatory collapse. Circulatory deterioration must be recognized before circulatory collapse occurs. In addition, in patients who have impaired cardiac performance (seriously reduced left ventricular ejection fraction), concurrent monitoring of pulmonary artery pressure or pulmonary capillary wedge pressure discloses any changes in the patient's circulatory condition that may result from the multiple stresses of the procedure. Central venous access, generally by the femoral route, should be considered because, if needed, it makes possible the prompt insertion of a temporary pacemaker or a right heart catheter.

Electrocardiographic Monitoring

Continuous electrocardiographic monitoring has two purposes: (1) the traditional monitoring of cardiac rhythm and conduction and (2) recognition of myocardial ischemia caused by the procedure. Consequently, the electrocardiographic monitoring should include ECG leads that reflect the zone of myocardium supplied by the target artery. In general, this would include lead V2 for the left anterior descending artery, lead II for the right coronary artery, and lead I for the circumflex artery.

Coagulation Status Monitoring

Because a fresh angioplasty site is denuded of endothelial cells, adequate anticoagulation during the procedure is essential to prevent thrombosis at this site. Anticoagulation choices currently include unfractionated heparin and low molecular-weight heparin; both antithrombin III inhibitors; and bivalirudin, a direct thrombin inhibitor. Because individual patients differ in their dose-response characteristics to unfractionated heparin, real-time monitoring of the degree of anticoagulation is essential. The most frequently used system is the automated measurement of the activated clotting time (ACT) (11), which is essentially an accelerated Lee-White clotting time. Typical values for the conduct of coronary angioplasty are an ACT of 250–350 seconds. These values should be maintained up to the completion of the procedure. Low molecular-weight heparin and bivalirudin have predictable bioavailability and can be dosed based on weight, obviating the need for monitoring.

Requirement for Cardiac Surgical Backup

There are complications of coronary angioplasty that can only be salvaged by emergent cardiac surgery. These include coronary occlusion at the angioplasty site, coronary perforation resulting in cardiac tamponade, and proximal coronary occlusion—generally caused by guide catheter-induced dissection. Because of the serious nature of these complications and because of the rapidity with which serious consequences occur, coronary angioplasty has been performed only in settings in which immediate transfer to a cardiac operating room was possible. Indeed, the emergent surgery rates for angioplasties performed in the 1980s and early 1990s approached 5%. The development and refinement of coronary stents has permitted the catheter-based treatment of many but not all of these complications. As a result, current emergent surgery rates have decreased to 0.5–1.0% (12). The declining frequency of emergent cardiac surgery has fueled a movement advocating the spread of coronary angioplasty to facilities without on-site surgery. This movement has not been endorsed by the American College of Cardiology, the American Heart Association, or the Society for Cardiovascular Angiography and Interventions whose published guidelines recommend the performance of elective coronary angioplasty only in a setting in which immediate access to emergent cardiac surgery is available (13). Accomplishing emergent cardiac

surgery effectively requires the rapid response of a skilled team of cardiovascular surgeons, anesthesiologists, and nurses. Executing this kind of response is particularly demanding when the patient has circulatory instability resulting from the coronary occlusion. Thus, the safe performance of coronary angioplasty requires the immediate availability of such a team and the necessary supporting physical facilities within the institution in which coronary angioplasty is performed.

Prompt surgical revascularization is impossible in patients who have had previous cardiac surgery because pericardial adhesions preclude rapid thoracotomy and establishment of cardiopulmonary bypass. If a patient who has been operated on previously develops an acute occlusion, it is unlikely that revascularization can be accomplished in less than 2 hours and, thus, significant myocardial necrosis is likely to occur. In such circumstances, the emergent institution of percutaneous cardiopulmonary bypass minimizes myocardial metabolic rate—which will protect ischemic myocardium—and stabilizes the systemic circulation, which may be lifesaving.

Radiologic Equipment

In coronary angioplasty, as in any interventional radiologic procedure, excellent image quality is essential. The need to resolve fine details of coronary lesion structure and to be able to visualize small instruments in moving vessels in real time has prompted an active effort to enhance the video presentation of fluorographic images. Digital image acquisition and image processing matured during the decade of the 1990s. The first decade of the new millennium has seen the development of flat-panel radiograph image detectors that provide a direct digital video signal obviating the need for the image intensifier and video camera combination.

PERCUTANEOUS CORONARY INTERVENTION

Instrumentation

From the beginning, Gruentzig realized that the complexities of reaching the coronary arteries and manipulating catheters within them meant that coronary angioplasty could not be accomplished with a single catheter. He, therefore, developed a coaxial catheter system consisting of an outer guide catheter to deliver the dilating catheter system to the coronary orifice and an inner balloon-bearing dilating catheter that could be manipulated into position within the stenosis to be dilated. Since then, there have been innumerable advances and refinement made to the instruments for percutaneous coronary interventions, which this section cannot fully cover. Instead, an overview of basic design principals is presented.

Guide Catheters

The guide catheter serves four basic functions:

1. To lead the dilating catheter to the appropriate coronary or graft orifice (Gruentzig's original German designation was *Furungskatheter*, which means "leading catheter.")
2. To inject contrast agent into the target coronary artery to aid in positioning of the dilating catheter
3. To provide the axial force (or "backup support") needed to advance the dilating catheter against resistance into the coronary artery system and across the target stenosis
4. To monitor systemic arterial pressure using an external pressure transducer

Most guide catheter tip curve designs are derived from the standard Judkins and Amplatz coronary angiographic curves, generally with some relaxation of the acuteness of the bends to facilitate passing equipment through them. Most guide catheters also incorporate a soft, or atraumatic, tip to minimize guide catheter-induced coronary orifice trauma. Some catheters are also constructed with side holes that are 2–3 cm proximal to the tip to enable blood flow into the coronary vessel in the event that the guide catheter tip obstructs the coronary orifice. The current minimum acceptable guide catheter lumen diameter is 1.42 mm. Guide catheters with this lumen diameter have been fabricated with 5 French external diameters; 6 French guide diameters are most commonly used. Guides are also available in 7 and 8 French sizes for circumstances in which the need exists to improve visibility when injecting contrast or to provide a large sufficient lumen dimension to deliver multiple wires, balloons, and even multiple stents.

Selection of the appropriate guide catheter is critical. The ideal guide catheter aligns coaxially with the proximal portion of the target vessel without obstructing it and braces sufficiently against other parts of the aortic root to provide the axial support needed to advance the dilating catheter to the target site. Axial support is particularly important when advancing stent-delivery balloon catheters and stents through tortuous vessels and tight stenoses.

There are no absolute rules for guide catheter selection. Judkins left curves are often optimal for the left anterior descending artery and frequently are satisfactory for the left circumflex artery. Amplatz left curves frequently provide more selective engagement and better axial support but are more difficult to manipulate and more likely to traumatize the proximal left coronary artery. The XB curve family also works effectively in many left coronary anatomic situations. Although Judkins right curves often work successfully for the right coronary artery, there are substantial variations of the right coronary orifice location and direction of its proximal course. These variations, together with variations in the shape, diameter, and length of the ascending aorta, require many different right coronary curves.

Amplatz right and left curves, multipurpose A and B curves, and hockey stick curves are among the curves that may be useful in specific situations for the right coronary artery. The orifice location and proximal course of saphenous vein grafts also vary considerably. Most of the curves that are useful for the right coronary artery are also useful for saphenous vein grafts. Several specialized curves for vein grafts have also been designed. The internal mammary artery is generally best engaged with curves specifically designed for that purpose.

In some centers, the preferred approach for both diagnostic and coronary intervention is from the radial or brachial approach. This approach is also necessary in some patients who have peripheral vascular disease and cannot be accessed from the femoral approach. The Amplatz curves, and occasionally Judkins curves, may be used successfully from the brachial or radial approach. The advantage of these approaches, include patient comfort with the ability to sit up or walk immediately after the procedure. While 6 French catheters can be comfortably used from this approach, larger French catheters can increase vascular complications.

Guide Wires

The original fixed balloon dilatation catheters contained a short segment of guide wire attached to the tip for steerability. This design allowed little control over the tip and ensured an inability to change the guide tip shape during procedures. This design was quickly replaced with the moveable guide wire system design that contained a long and steerable guide wire that moved independently over which a balloon dilation catheter, stent, or other equipment could be placed.

The basic guide wire design consists of a solid core that has a progressive taper at the distal end that is then covered by a Teflon-coated stainless steel spring coil with a soft distal segment without a central core. The tip of the guide wire is often made of a more radiopaque material such as platinum or tungsten for improved visibility and has the ability to be shaped by the operator. The standard guide wire diameter is 0.014 inch, although 0.009–0.021-inch designs are available. There are many different guide wire designs. Different stiffness of the shaft of the wire from floppy to super stiff are available depending on the desired support. In addition, different tip designs are available with a shorter segment of spring coil distal to the solid core or a stiffer tip for increased pushability that may be necessary for crossing chronic total occlusions. There is also a family of plastic covered guide wires with a hydrophilic coating allowing navigation of extremely tortuous vessels.

Coronary Balloon Catheters

The ideal coronary balloon angioplasty catheter has four attributes: (1) a small shaft diameter to minimize guide catheter lumen diameter requirements; (2) a small deflated balloon profile to facilitate crossing tight stenoses; (3) shaft flexibility for negotiating tortuous vascular segments ("trackability"); and (4) shaft axial stiffness, allowing the catheter to be advanced against resistance ("pushability"). Achieving the optimal combination of these properties in the quest for superior performance requires several complex engineering tradeoffs. This has led to the development of many creative designs that employ innovative materials. The typical range of inflated balloon diameters used for native coronary arteries is 1.5–4.0 mm. Most commonly used coronary angioplasty catheters have shaft diameters and deflated balloon profiles of less than 1 mm. Balloon catheters also come in a range of lengths from 6.0 mm to greater than 30.0 mm.

The original fixed-wire balloon catheters had a short 2–5 cm malleable fixed wire attached to the tip. Although the wire could not be moved with respect to the catheter, a curve could be imparted to the wire tip and the entire unit could be steerable. This design was quickly replaced with over-the-wire catheters that have an inner lumen that reaches to the catheter tip, through which a movable, steerable guide wire is placed. This wire is moved and steered independently of the catheter, and one can exchange balloon catheters without having to recross the stenosis. Although fixed-wire catheters do not allow this maneuver, their smaller shaft and deflated balloon diameters may enhance their ability to cross very tight stenoses.

There are two types of over-the-wire catheters: (1) standard catheters in which the wire passes through the entire length of the catheter shaft and exits at the hub, and (2) monorail or rapid exchange catheters in which the wire only passes through the distal 20 cm of the catheter and along the side of the more proximal portion of the dilatation catheter within the guide catheter. Monorail systems have the advantage of allowing the balloon to be controlled by a single operator without needing to use an exchange-length guide wire.

One controversial characteristic is the optimal degree of balloon compliance; that is, the degree to which the balloon expands as its cavity pressure increases. Arguments for noncompliant balloons center on the reliability and stability of inflated balloon dimensions over a large range of inflation pressures (12). However, there is no convincing demonstration that this property enhances procedure safety or efficacy (13). Arguments for compliant balloons emphasize that the ability to increase the balloon dimension in a controlled manner by increasing pressure facilitates optimal dilation.

Finally, balloons are also rated with respect to three inflation pressure-related properties. The nominal pressure is the pressure at which the balloon reaches its labeled diameter. The rated burst pressure is the pressure below which 99.9% of these balloons will not rupture, while the mean burst pressure is the pressure at which 50% of balloons will rupture.

Coronary Stents

Stenting consists of deployment of an expandable endovascular prosthesis at an angioplasty site. Stenting was developed initially to solve two dilemmas of coronary angioplasty: inadequate lumen enlargement of the target site and acute occlusion resulting from dissection flaps. More recently, stenting has acquired the additional attribute of a platform to accomplish local drug delivery to attenuate restenosis. Virtually all coronary stents in current use are based on slotted tube designs and are fabricated from 316L stainless steel.

The Palmaz-Schatz stent received FDA approval in 1994. It is a slotted stainless steel tube that is 15 mm in length and is furnished crimped to an angioplasty balloon catheter inside a retractable sheath. Early clinical research with the Palmaz-Schatz stent demonstrated its ability to improve the acute outcome (in terms of lumen dimensions) of coronary angioplasty (14), to salvage failed conventional angioplasties (15), and to reduce restenosis after angioplasty (16,17). These attributes firmly established stenting as an adjunct to balloon coronary angioplasty. The principal limitations of the Palmaz-Schatz stent were a large delivery profile and a lack of flexibility that impeded delivery in tortuous vessels.

The poor deliverability of the Palmaz-Schatz stent spawned the development of many competing designs that featured smaller delivery profiles and had enhanced flexibility while preserving radial strength. There are two categories of current stent designs. Closed cell designs have uniform size of cells on both the convex and concave side (BxVelocity, Cordis) while open cell designs have larger-sized cells on the convex side and smaller cells on the concave side (Express Stent, Boston Scientific). All currently available stents can be delivered through conventional 6 French coronary guide catheters and are compatible with conventional 0.014-inch angioplasty guide wires.

As a result of improved acute results and a modest reduction in restenosis, stents promptly became firmly established as the standard for coronary angioplasty. However, the efficacy of stenting with bare metal stents was undermined by in-stent restenosis, which occurred, by angiographic definition, in 30–40% of stent deployments and was severe enough to require repeat revascularization in 20% (16,17). In-stent restenosis presents a serious therapeutic challenge because it responds poorly to repeated intervention and often led to a requirement for coronary bypass surgery. Thus, research and development focused on ways to prevent restenosis.

Drug-eluting stents are the current strategy to reduce the frequency of restenosis. They consist of a conventional metal stent coated with a drug-binding polymer impregnated with a cytostatic drug. Following stent deployment, the drug is eluted into the adjacent vessel wall at a controlled rate making it available locally in a therapeutic concentration without achieving significant systemic levels. The drug is ideally delivered over the requisite time period that the restenosis process operates. Two coronary drug-eluting stents are currently FDA approved—the Cypher stent (Cordis) that elutes sirolimus and the Taxus stent (Boston Scientific) that elutes paclitaxel. Drug-eluting stents will be discussed in more detail later in this chapter.

TECHNIQUE

Pharmacology

An angioplasty site is denuded of endothelial cells and has tears that expose the subendothelial vascular matrix to the lumen. Consequently, it is extremely prothrombotic. In addition, coronary angioplasty is frequently performed in the setting of an unstable cardiac ischemic syndrome, which is caused by plaque degeneration that leads to thrombus formation on the lesion surface. Anticoagulation and adequate platelet inhibition significantly reduce the risk of periprocedure site thrombosis and possibly of distal embolization of thrombotic material.

Anticoagulation strategies include antithrombin III inhibition through unfractionated heparin or low molecular weight heparin and direct thrombin inhibitors, such as bivalirudin. Antiplatelet therapies include treatment with cyclooxygenase inhibitors, thienopyridines, and intravenous platelet glycoprotein IIb/IIIa inhibitors.

Unfractionated heparin is generally used in a dose sufficient to elevate the ACT to >250 seconds when used without IIb/IIIa inhibition. Lower achieved ACTs (200–250 seconds) are employed when concomitant IIb/IIIa inhibitors are used.

Low molecular-weight heparin's principal activity is against factor Xa rather than against thrombin, and it does not affect the ACT in a dose-dependent manner. Because of more consistent bioavailability than unfractionated heparin, it is considered to have more predictable dose response characteristics and, accordingly, is labeled for use without monitoring. Early studies have shown that use of the low molecular-weight heparin, enoxaparin, in low-risk to moderate-risk patients, lowered the number of ischemic events without increasing the risk of major bleeding (18). In a more recent study, enoxaparin showed no advantage over heparin for ischemic events in high-risk patients and, additionally, showed an increased risk of major bleeding (19).

Bivalirudin is a direct thrombin inhibitor that has some antiplatelet activity. It also has a predictable dose response and is FDA labeled for use without monitoring. In low-risk to moderate-risk patients, bivalirudin with provisional glycoprotein IIb/IIIa use has been shown to be equivalent to heparin with planned glycoprotein IIb/IIIa use (20).

Antiplatelet therapy is the cornerstone for the treatment of coronary disease. Antiplatelet therapy includes cyclooxygenase inhibitors such as aspirin, thienopyridines such as ticlopidine and clopidogrel, and intravenous glycoprotein IIb/IIIa inhibitors such as abciximab, eptifibatide, and tirofiban.

It is clearly established that preprocedure aspirin therapy is essential (21). Both retrospective analyses and prospective studies have shown that the acute thrombotic complication rate is considerably greater in patients who are not pretreated with aspirin. Fragmentary data from a retrospective study suggested that the combination of aspirin and dipyridamole confers an even lower risk of acute thrombosis, but this has not been confirmed by a prospective trial (22).

Subsequent work has identified an important additional benefit of dual antiplatelet therapy. Dual antiplatelet therapy, with a combination of aspirin and a thienopyridine, provides incremental protection against acute thrombotic events and the risk of late stent thrombosis. The high subacute thrombosis rate, particularly in the setting of emergent use, was greatly ameliorated by dual antiplatelet therapy with aspirin and ticlopidine as compared with aspirin alone or the combination of aspirin and warfarin (23). Subsequently, chronic ticlopidine therapy was found to have an important risk of a thrombotic thrombocytopenic purpura syndrome and a 1% risk of neutropenia (24). This led to further studies that showed ticlopidine could be safely stopped 2 weeks after placement of a bare metal stent with little risk of late stent thrombosis (25).

Clopidogrel, another thienopyridine, has been shown to be equivalent to ticlopidine in the prevention of late stent thrombosis. Additionally, clopidogrel has a much safer profile without risk of neutropenia and a significantly lower risk of thrombotic thrombocytopenic purpura. Based on these studies, clopidogrel is now the preferred thienopyridine used in conjunction with aspirin for at least 2–4 weeks after bare metal stent placement and 3–6 months after drug-eluting stent implantation (26–28).

Recently, glycoprotein IIb/IIIa inhibitors have been used to block the final common pathway of platelet aggregation. The first to be developed, abciximab, is a mouse antibody that binds to the IIb/IIIa integrin thereby inactivating it. Abciximab has an extremely avid binding constant and, when available in stochiometric quantities, will occupy and inactivate virtually all the expressed glycoprotein IIb/IIIa integrins. Although its binding constant is very avid, it slowly dissociates from the integrin. Thus, to maintain a high level of IIb/IIIa blockade, it is necessary to administer a low dose continuous infusion of the drug. Abciximab was initially studied in the setting of patients with unstable angina (29) and in higher-risk patients (30). These studies showed lower rates of thrombotic complications; however, it came at the cost of higher rates of bleeding complications. Additional studies decreased bleeding complications by reducing the heparin dose (31). While these initial studies consisted of primarily balloon angioplasty interventions, abciximab in the setting of stenting has also been shown to be beneficial (32). Additionally, two small molecule IIb/IIIa inhibitors, eptifabitide (33) and tirofiban (34) have been shown to decrease thrombotic complications in the setting of coronary stenting. The exact role of these drugs in all coronary interventional procedures remains a subject of debate. They clearly decrease the risk of periprocedural coronary ischemic complications in the highest-risk subgroup of patients with unstable ischemic syndromes. However, their incremental benefit in lower-risk patients with stable coronary disease is negligible or, at most, modest (35).

Radiologic Projections

Accurate delineation of the target stenosis and of the relevant coronary anatomy proximal and distal to it is essential for executing coronary angioplasty successfully. Ideally, the target stenosis should be imaged in two mutually perpendicular radiologic projections. This is not always feasible given the variable geometry and configuration of an individual patient's coronary anatomy. The selected projections should place the stenosis as parallel to the image plane as possible; separate the stenosis from other adjacent opacified vessels; and clearly identify the origin of branches proximal and distal to the target stenosis and, in particular, their relationship to the target stenosis.

Procedure

Once it has been determined that a lesion needs to be treated, current treatment includes planned stenting. Stenting can be performed indirectly with a predilation or directly.

Prior to the introduction and wide adoption of coronary stents there were many sophisticated nuances concerning the optimal execution of balloon angioplasty. These have been largely replaced by the use of balloon angioplasty as a technique to predilate a stenosis to facilitate stent delivery and deployment. Balloon predilation should minimize vascular injury to minimize the amount of intimal trauma and minimize the risk of creating a dissection flap before stent deployment. Typical balloon predilation parameters are a 2.0–2.5 mm inflated diameter and a balloon length just sufficient to cover the tightest portion of the stenosis.

Baseline coronary angiograms are performed in projections selected according to the criteria outlined earlier. Digital road maps of these angiograms are selected for display to guide the operator in crossing the stenosis with the guide wire and positioning the balloon catheter. The guide wire is then advanced across the stenosis and passed as far distally in the vessel as possible (Figure 25–1 A and B). The balloon catheter is advanced over the wire, centered within the target stenosis, then inflated to dilate the stenosis (Figure 25–1 C). Occlusion of the vessel by the balloon catheter will produce a variable degree of myocardial ischemia, depending upon the size of the distribution of the target vessel and the extent of development of intercoronary collaterals. Consequently, predilation balloon inflation should be brief—just long enough to predilate the stenosis. Once the dilation has been completed, the balloon catheter is deflated and withdrawn into the guide catheter and follow-up angiography is performed to assess the effect of the dilation (Figure 25–1 D). This angiogram is used to evaluate the degree of stenosis reduction and the presence or absence of a dissection flap or thrombus. Following completion of predilation, a stent of appropriate length and diameter is selected, delivered over the same guide wire to the target site, and deployed (Figure 25–1 E and F). The deployed stent diameter should ensure that all portions of the stent achieve satisfactory contact with the vascular wall. The decision that the procedure is completed is based on the operator's assessment of the degree of stenosis relief and his or her judgment of the presence or absence of dissections at the proximal and distal edges of the stent (Figure 25–1 G).

Alternatively, it is often feasible to deliver a stent directly to a target site without predilation. "Direct stenting," when feasible, is likely a superior strategy to stenting following predilation provided that the stent can be delivered, accurately positioned, and appropriately expanded. Direct stenting has the advantage that only the segment stented is exposed to angioplasty trauma, theoretically reducing the risk of restenosis.

When deploying a bare metal stent, the shortest possible length that will cover the target site should be chosen. This is to minimize the length of stented vessel thereby minimizing the length of vessel at risk for restenosis. Three aspects of stent deployment are critical to success: (1) Accurate positioning is essential because a stent cannot be repositioned once it is deployed. It is undesirable to place a stent across a major side branch, and such positioning should be avoided whenever possible. (2) Uniform stent expansion with complete vessel wall contact is important to achieve a satisfactory hydraulic result and to minimize the risk of stent thrombosis. (3) The development of any filling defect within a freshly deployed stent signifies the development of thrombus and identifies the patient as being at significant risk for subsequent thrombotic occlusion of the vessel.

For bare metal stenting, the final expanded size of the stent should be between 100% and 110% of the diameter of the vessel adjacent to the stenosis. This is because it is highly likely that there will be an important degree of neointimal growth within the stent. Slightly oversizing the stent provides additional dimension to accommodate the neointimal growth. This principle is likely not as important for drug-eluting stents because, in most circumstances, the degree of neointimal growth is minimal. However, for drug-eluting stents, there is relatively little neointimal growth and it is even more important to be certain that the stent is sufficiently expanded to accomplish complete vascular wall contact and reduce the risk of subacute stent thrombosis.

If the stent is visibly incompletely expanded or if there is a concern for incomplete apposition of the stent, postdilation can be performed via delivery of a balloon over the same guide wire. Postdilation is generally performed with a noncompliant balloon, so that for the same balloon diameter, a greater degree of force can be applied. It is important to ensure that the postdilatation balloon is within the

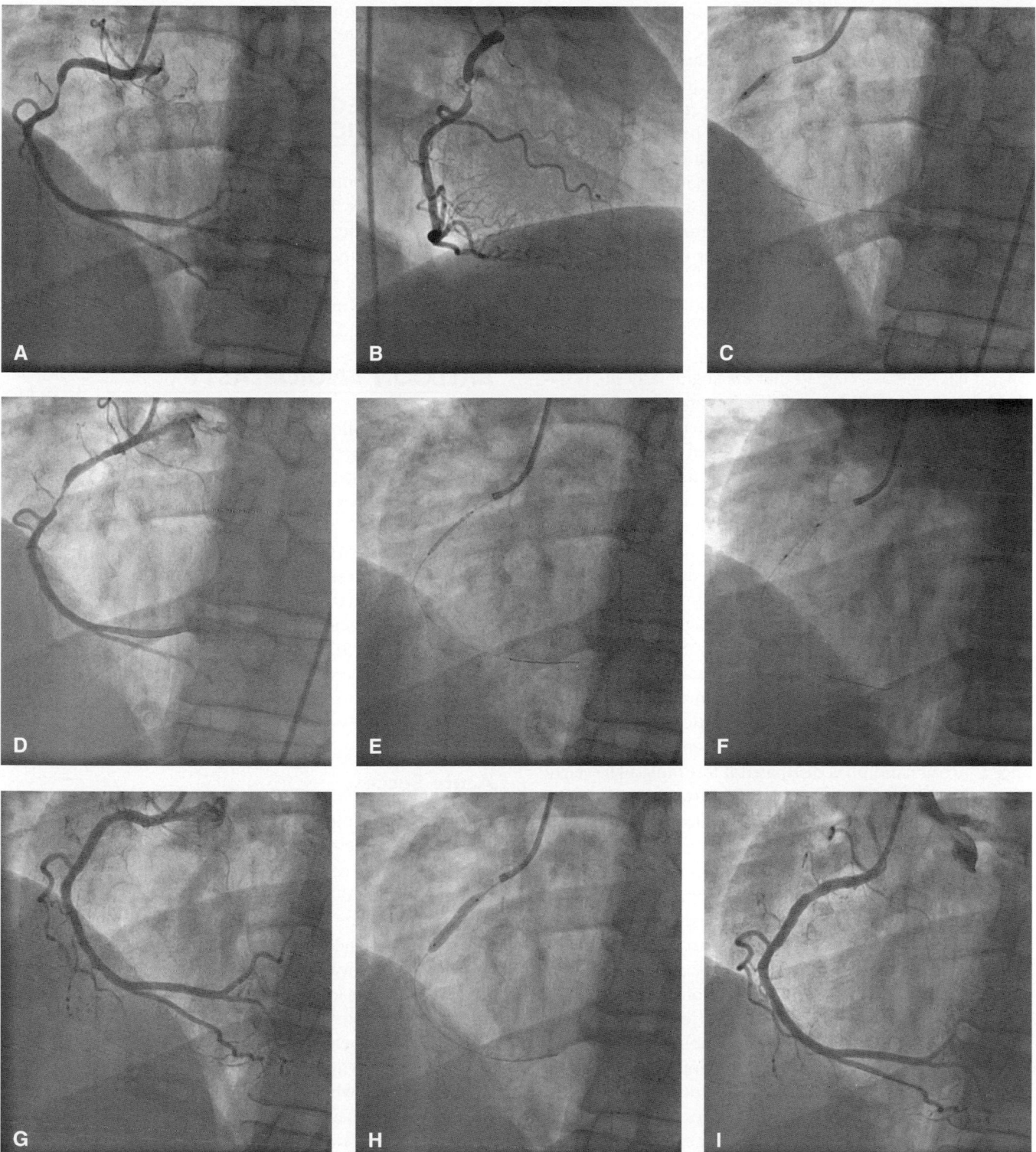

Figure 25–1 Angiograms illustrating the sequential steps of conventional percutaneous coronary intervention. **A.** Baseline angiogram in the left anterior oblique projection. **B.** Baseline angiogram in the right anterior oblique projection showing 80–90% stenosis of the midright coronary artery. **C.** Image after passage of a coronary guide wire across the stenosis and predilatation of the lesion showing complete expansion of the balloon. **D.** Angiogram in the left anterior oblique projection after predilatation showing recoil of the lesion with no obvious dissection flaps. **E.** Image showing position of coronary stent across the original lesion also covering the area of predilatation. **F.** Image showing stent inflation. **G.** Angiogram poststent deployment showing slight underexpansion in the midstent with no evidence for either proximal or distal edge dissection. **H.** Image showing positioning of a postdilatation balloon within the stent, being sure not to injure unstented artery. **I.** Final angiography showing complete stent expansion and no edge dissection.

stented segment so that the stent edges are not traumatized (Figure 25-1 H and I).

Intravascular ultrasound (IVUS) is an additional tool that can be used for the diagnosis and treatment of coronary artery disease. These devices can be inserted through a 6 French guide over a standard 0.014-inch guide wire. Applications for IVUS include diagnostic in determining the degree of stenosis of ambiguous angiographic lesions; elucidation of the cause of angiographic filling defects such as thrombus, or dissection; assistance in choosing stent diameter and stent length; and assurance of circumferential stent apposition to the vessel wall.

Postprocedure Care

Once it has been ascertained that the angioplasty site is stable, the patient is transferred from the catheterization laboratory to the cardiac care unit. The heparinization is not reversed, and the vascular sheaths are left in place unless a vascular access site closure device is used. Intravenous IIb/IIIa inhibitors, if used during the procedure, are continued by intravenous infusion for 12–18 hours postprocedure. On arrival in the cardiac care unit, a 12-lead ECG is recorded to assess whether any periprocedural changes have occurred and to serve as a baseline for monitoring.

The current standard of care is overnight postprocedure monitoring in the hospital on telemetry. Some institutions are examining the safety and utility of same-day discharge following vascular access site closure with a closure device. If a closure device was not utilized, vascular sheaths are removed when the ACT <160–180 if heparin was used or once anticoagulation has dissipated if low molecular-weight heparin or bivalirudin was used. If intravenous II/b/IIIa inhibitors are used, an infusion is continued for 12–18 hours postprocedure and a platelet count should be checked 4 hours after its initiation to check for thrombocytopenia.

In addition to treatment of the coronary lesion, attention should be given to treatment of the underlying atherosclerotic process. While this will be tailored for the individual patient, there are some basic guidelines. Aspirin is recommended for life for all patients with coronary disease. Dual antiplatelet therapy is not necessary after balloon angioplasty alone. However, after placement of a stent, a thienopyridine—either ticlopidine or clopidogrel—should be used. For bare metal stents, dual antiplatelet therapy should be continued for at least 2–4 weeks, while for drug-eluting stents, dual antiplatelet therapy should be continued for 3–6 months depending on the drug used because of delayed endothelialization. Virtually all patients with coronary artery disease will benefit from lipid lowering tailored to their particular lipoprotein disorder. For the majority of such patients, a statin will be appropriate. Other patients will benefit from combination lipid lowering therapy. In the appropriate setting, β-blocker therapy and angiotensin-converting enzyme inhibition should be considered, and for diabetics, aggressive glycemic control should be initiated.

Patients with coronary disease should continue to have regular follow-up with their internist and cardiologist.

PERCUTANEOUS CORONARY INTERVENTION RESULTS

Virtually all of contemporary coronary intervention involves stent deployment. The stents used are increasingly likely to be drug-eluting stents. Although stenting has become the dominant coronary interventional technique, it is important to understand the other complementary coronary interventional techniques as well.

BALLOON ANGIOPLASTY

Conventional balloon angioplasty is a controlled injury to the target site. Success requires an optimal degree of lesion stretching. Failure to achieve a satisfactory increase in lumen dimension is associated with a high frequency of inadequate acute results and a high probability of restenosis (36). Vascular tissue is inherently elastic and recoils after dilation. This presents the angiographer with a dilemma: whereas inadequate dilation or excessive lesion elasticity will cause dilation failure because of elastic recoil of the dilated site, overdilation may create a dissection flap that can cause acute occlusion (37). The concept of stenting was developed both to oppose elastic recoil and to "scaffold" dissection flaps away from the vascular lumen.

Acute Success

The standard definition of acute success is reduction of the target site's diameter stenosis to less than 50% without any cardiac ischemic complications. Using this definition, current reported success rates range between 90–95% (38,39).

Success rates are heavily influenced by case selection and operator experience and skill. The principal case selection variable is the location and geometric complexity of the stenosis. Stenoses located distal to highly tortuous coronary artery segments may be difficult to reach because of substantial friction between the tortuous vascular segment and both the guide wire and the balloon catheter. This issue is most significant when the vessel is also rigid because of the presence of extensive, calcified, nonocclusive atheroma. A classification of stenosis complexity has been developed (40). In the past, correlations existed between increasing complexity and decreasing success rate (41). However, equipment and technique refinement have modified the relationships between lesion complexity and success rate. This is principally because stents solve many problems that occur following balloon angioplasty of complex lesions. The total occlusion remains the greatest technical challenge to coronary interventional work yielding the lowest success rates (30–60%), chiefly because of problems crossing the stenosis with a guide wire (42,43). Consequently, the prevalence of the total occlusions in any series of procedures has an important impact on the success rate.

Causes of Early Failure and Acute Complications

Causes of early coronary angioplasty failure can be divided into five groups:

1. Failure to cross with the guide wire (most common in tortuous vessels, geometrically complex stenoses, and total occlusions)
2. Failure to cross a successfully wired stenosis with the balloon or, more likely, a stent delivery system (generally caused by excessive stenosis severity and hardness but also by proximal tortuosity)
3. Failure of balloon inflation to dilate the stenosis successfully (usually caused by excessive stenosis hardness but occasionally by excessive stenosis elasticity)
4. Abrupt vessel closure after a successfully executed dilation (usually caused by dissection, thrombosis, or both, and occasionally by vascular spasm; it has been largely eliminated by the replacement of balloon angioplasty with stenting)
5. Injury of the orifice of the target vessel by the guide catheter

The most severe complications of early angioplasty failure are consequences of myocardial ischemia caused by acute closure of the angioplasty site or guide catheter-induced injury to the target vessel orifice. The severity of ischemia, its clinical importance, and the appropriate response to it are determined by the size of the perfusion territory of the target vessel, the presence of intercoronary collaterals, and the extent and severity of other coronary artery disease. Ischemic complications of coronary angioplasty are reported in 4–8% of procedures (44,45).

There are three potential responses to an acute ischemic complication: (1) restoration of flow through a catheter-based technique, (2) emergent aortocoronary bypass surgery, or (3) conservative nonrevascularization therapy. The most appropriate response to a particular ischemic complication is determined by the overall clinical context in which it occurs. Considerations in selecting the optimal response include the severity of the ischemia and the suitability of the patient for the various alternative treatments. In the 1980s and 1990s, emergency coronary artery bypass surgery frequency ranged between 3% and 5% (46). Principally because of the ability of stenting to solve many ischemic problems, the current frequency of truly emergent bypass surgery has decreased to 0.5%–1.0% in reported series (47). Unless it is carried out with great rapidity, emergent bypass surgery, although potentially lifesaving, has a limited ability to ameliorate the extent of myocardial necrosis. Both the operative mortality and the perioperative myocardial infarction

rate are much greater for emergent bypass surgery conducted to salvage failed coronary angioplasty than for elective bypass surgery (48). In circumstances of severe ischemia because of acute occlusion of a proximal vessel, initiation of percutaneous bypass in the catheterization laboratory can be lifesaving.

Most other clinically important early complications of coronary angioplasty are related to vascular access. These include (1) bleeding and hematoma formation and (2) pseudoaneurysm and arteriovenous fistula formation (49). The tendency to develop these problems is enhanced by the relatively large catheters needed for vascular access and the aggressive anticoagulation frequently required in the early postangioplasty period.

Late Results

During its first 25 years, the major shortcoming of coronary angioplasty was a substantial restenosis frequency. Using the criterion of a 50% diameter stenosis at least 3 months after the procedure, reported angiographic coronary restenosis rates for conventional balloon angioplasty range between 30% and 45% (36,50,51). The predominant cause of restenosis is neointimal proliferation, in which media-derived smooth muscle cells proliferate and migrate into the intimal layer of the vessel, reducing the diameter of the lumen (52). The cause of this process is not understood. Current concepts regard it as a nonspecific response to the physical trauma of the angioplasty process, which, unfortunately, causes the deposition of tissue that occupies space in the vascular lumen, reducing its dimension (53).

Although the mechanism of restenosis is not known, its frequency, time course, and correlates of its development have been extensively characterized. So-called clinical restenosis rates are less than "angiographic restenosis rates" because a certain fraction of stenoses that are restenotic by angiographic criteria do not cause sufficient myocardial ischemia to provoke clinical symptoms (54). Nobuyoshi et al. (55) showed in serial angiographic studies that the process continues for approximately 4 months after the angioplasty procedure and stabilizes.

Several correlates of restenosis probability have been identified. Most describe the lesion and the quality of the angioplasty result rather than the characteristics of the patient (although some series have reported a greater frequency of restenosis in diabetic patients). Variables that correlate with increased restenosis likelihood include (36,56):

1. Decreasing normal vessel lumen diameter
2. Decreasing stenosis lumen diameter and increasing percent stenosis
3. Increasing stenosis length
4. Increasing stenosis geometric complexity
5. Stenosis located in the left anterior descending artery
6. Stenosis located in saphenous vein grafts

7. Increasing residual stenosis severity following angioplasty
8. Previous restenosis at the angioplasty site

A common theme for many of these variables is the amount of room for the deposition of neointimal proliferative tissue and the aggressiveness with which the process occurs. Thus, it is not surprising that restenosis is more common in small vessels with severe long stenoses in which a poor increase in lumen dimension is achieved. This also explains the apparently greater frequency of restenosis in the coronary vascular bed than in other beds in which the vessels have larger diameters.

The entire restenosis knowledge base described here has been rendered somewhat anachronistic by drug-eluting stents. These devices have successfully reduced the average thickness of neointimal growth to 100 microns or less, reducing angiographic restenosis to the 5% range regardless of baseline vessel and lesion characteristics.

Total Occlusions

Total occlusions represent a major obstacle to both the short- and long-term success of coronary angioplasty. Acute procedure success rates are lower than for angioplasty of patent vessels because of difficulties in passing guide wires across the total occlusion. The success rates for recent total occlusions (80%) are greater than for occlusions known to be present for at least 3 months (40–60%) (57). Multiple guide wires have been developed in an effort to aid in crossing total occlusions. Most are based on a combination of hydrophilic coatings and increasing degrees of stiffness. Perforation is the principal risk of attempting to cross occlusions with such wires.

BARE METAL CORONARY STENTING

All of the currently available designs perform well acutely, and reported delivery success rates are greater than 90% (15,58,59). Bare metal stents are being progressively superseded by drug-eluting stents.

The principal short-term problem of stenting is subacute thrombosis, which, depending on the stent used, the circumstances of deployment and concomitant pharmacologic therapy occurs in 0.5–1.6% of patients within the first 14 days, with a maximal incidence on the fifth day after stent deployment (14,15,58–60). Subacute thrombosis is a catastrophic event that generally presents as an ST-elevation myocardial infarction. It is frequently not associated with prodromal symptoms, thus the patient and physician have no warning that enables them to anticipate the problem.

Before the recognition of the value of dual antiplatelet therapy, subacute thrombosis was distressingly common. The STARS (STent Anti-thrombotic Regimen Study) trial (23) established the value of dual antiplatelet therapy with aspirin and a thienopyridine drug. Dual antiplatelet therapy is essential in all patients who have had a coronary stent deployed, and it has reduced the frequency of subacute thrombosis to less than 1%. The risk of subacute thrombosis in bare metal stents becomes negligible 14 days following stent deployment. However, drug-eluting stents carry an ongoing subacute thrombosis risk that persists for at least 3–6 months, making dual antiplatelet therapy essential for at least that period.

The most important facet of late performance is the impact of stenting on restenosis. The restenosis rate following bare metal stenting with the Palmaz-Schatz stent has been examined in two prospective randomized trials (16,17). Both studies showed that, compared to conventional balloon angioplasty, stenting provides a larger lumen diameter acutely. At 6-month follow-up angiography, the average amount of lumen dimension lost is greater in stented lesions than in lesions treated with conventional balloon angioplasty. However, because the dimension achieved acutely is considerably greater, the net effect of stenting is a slightly greater lumen diameter compared to balloon angioplasty at 6-month angiographic follow-up. In the Stent Restenosis Study, stented lesions had a mean minimal lumen diameter at follow-up of 1.75 (± 0.60 mm), whereas lesions treated with conventional balloon angioplasty had a mean minimal lumen diameter of 1.55 (± 0.56 mm). There was a statistically significantly lower binary restenosis rate (29.1 versus 42.7%) in the stented group (16).

DRUG-ELUTING STENTS

Drug-eluting stents have dramatically reduced restenosis rates by reducing the thickness of neointimal growth. In the SIRIUS trial that compared sirolimus-eluting stents to bare metal stents, the angiographic late loss within stents 6 months following stent deployment was 1.0 (± 0.7 mm) for bare metal stents, yielding a binary restenosis rate of 35% that was virtually identical to the results of the initial trials that compared bare metal stents to balloon angioplasty. For sirolimus-eluting stents, the mean angiographic late loss within stents was 0.17 (± 0.45 mm), yielding a restenosis rate of 3.2%. Sirolimus-eluting stents had a late loss in the adjacent unstented segments of 0.24 (± 0.47 mm). Thus, the overall restenosis rate considering the aggregate of the stented segment and its immediately adjacent unstented coronary segments was 8.9%—a dramatic decrease from the 36.3% overall restenosis rate for bare metal stents (61).

Similar results have been reported for paclitaxel-eluting stents, although the late loss associated with paclitaxel is slightly greater than with sirolimus. In the TAXUS-IV trial, the mean angiographic late loss within stents for paclitaxel-eluting stents was 0.39 (± 0.50 mm) compared to 0.92 (± 0.58 mm) for the comparison bare metal stents. The binary restenosis rate in the paclitaxel-eluting stents was

7.9% compared to 26% in the bare metal stent group (62,63). Thus, both stent platforms are highly effective at attenuating the restenosis process. Consequently, bare metal stenting is decreasing in frequency in the United States except for vessels with reference diameters greater than 4 mm (for which drug-eluting stents are currently not available).

RELATED TECHNIQUES

Coronary Brachytherapy

Before the development of drug-eluting stents, bare metal stents had a significant clinical restenosis rate (16,17). Pharmacologic therapies for the prevention of restenosis after percutaneous coronary intervention had with limited success (64). In November 2000, the Food and Drug Administration granted approval of devices that deliver intracoronary brachytherapy for the treatment of in-stent restenosis. The concept was that delivery of an appropriate amount of radiation to the target site would inhibit neointimal proliferation. Animal studies demonstrated 18–24 gray to be the optimal delivered dose to the target vessel. Intracoronary brachytherapy involves the placement of a "ribbon" containing radioactive seeds within the coronary artery at the site of the stenosis for a short period of time after percutaneous revascularization. The specific activity of these sources is quite large in order to deliver the necessary dose in a practically useful time period. Both β-radiation and γ-radiation radioactive sources are FDA approved. β radiation proved to be quite easy to manage because of the short mean free path of β particles in tissue. Because γ radiation has greater tissue penetration and very high photon energy, conventional shielding for diagnostic radiograph affords inadequate protection requiring that catheterization laboratories be reconfigured to reduce personnel exposure. Trials using γ radiation (65–67) and β radiation (68) to treat in-stent restenosis showed significantly lower repeat restenosis rates of 17–32% when compared to repeat restenosis rates of 50–60% with angioplasty alone. Recently similar results have been shown with using drug-eluting stents for the treatment of in-stent restenosis (69). Because of both the decreased prevalence of restenosis with drug-eluting stents and the difficult with logistics of performing brachytherapy, coronary brachytherapy has been largely abandoned.

Plaque Modification

The term *atherectomy* encompasses several systems that mechanically destroy, and in some cases remove, atheromatous plaque. These have been developed in an attempt to improve the results obtained with balloon angioplasty. In theory, removal of obstructing atheroma in a coronary artery should provide a better relief of the stenosis, greater

predictability of the result, fewer complications (such as dissection), and a lower rate of restenosis than is achieved with conventional balloon angioplasty.

Rotational Atherectomy

The Rotablator (Boston Scientific) is a mechanical ablation device that consists of diamond chips embedded in an abrasive brass burr (in diameters of 1.0–3.0 mm) welded to a flexible driveshaft that tracks over a 0.009-inch guide wire. The burr is rotated by a turbine at 150,000–190,000 rpm and is designed to grind the atheroma into small particles (<5 μm). This device has an advantage over other atherectomy devices in that it is more flexible; can be used with standard 9 French guiding catheters (in smaller burr sizes); and appears to cut even calcified lesions, leaving smooth lumen borders (70). In the large multicenter registry, procedural success was approximately 95%, and major complications included death (1%), emergency surgery (2%), Q-wave and non–Q-wave myocardial infarction (1% and 5%, respectively), and a restenosis rate of 50%. The overall results differ from those of conventional PTCA in that the rate of non–Q-wave infarction is higher, possibly because of embolization of particulate matter (71). However, rotational atherectomy has not been shown to reduce restenosis rates either in de novo lesions (72) or in in-stent restenotic lesions (73). The principal niche for rotational atherectomy is as a means of weakening a very hard and calcified stenosis so that it will respond better to balloon dilation and stent delivery. In highly selected circumstances, rotational atherectomy makes it possible to dilate stenoses that would otherwise be too hard to expand with balloon inflation.

Directional Atherectomy

The Simpson AtheroCath (DVI, Inc.) was developed in an effort to excise and retrieve slices of atheroma. It is a catheter-based system with a cylindrical steel cutting blade housed at the distal tip of a rigid cylinder. The cylinder has a 5-mm or 10-mm cutting window occupying 25% of its circumference, with a compliant balloon on the opposite side. The tip of the catheter is a flexible nosecone that facilitates advancement of the device across an obstruction and stores excised fragments of tissue for retrieval and pathologic analysis. The cutter is connected to a handheld disposable motor drive that rotates it at 2,000 rpm. The entire device tracks over a standard 0.014-inch PTCA guide wire.

Although the immediate improvement in lumen diameter achieved by atherectomy (5–15% residual stenosis) is frequently better than that achieved with balloon angioplasty (30–40%) (74), long-term results have shown no advantage in terms of restenosis rates compared to balloon angioplasty. The Coronary Angioplasty Versus Excisional Atherectomy Trial (CAVEAT) compared the rates of restenosis after atherectomy with balloon angioplasty (75). CAVEAT patients receiving DCA had higher composite rates of acute complications (11 versus 5%, $p = <0.001$) but only slightly lower rates of angiographic restenosis at 6 months (50 versus 57%, $p = 0.06$) (75). Consequently, directional atherectomy has been largely abandoned.

Fractional Flow Reserve

Coronary angiography provides an anatomic assessment of a coronary lesion. However, its ability to determine the physiologic significance of a coronary stenosis is based on inference by estimating the percent diameter stenosis or the actual stenosis lumen dimension. As a consequence, lesions of ambiguous severity are common. The physiologic impact of a stenosis is determined by its effect on the ability of the coronary vessel to transmit a flow increasing response to a vasodilatory stimulus (such as increased myocardial metabolic rate). This may be expressed as the coronary flow reserve, which is the ratio of the resting coronary flow rate to the peak achievable coronary flow rate. Normal coronary flow reserve is between three and five. Measurement of coronary flow is feasible but technically cumbersome, requiring catheters with Doppler transducers at their tips or coronary sinus thermodilution. Fluid dynamic theory demonstrates that the coronary flow reserve can be inferred from the transstenotic pressure gradient (76). The transstenotic pressure gradient is easily measured using a 0.014-inch angioplasty guide wire that has a miniature pressure transducer mounted on its tip. The transducer is passed across the stenosis of interest, and the pressure gradient between the coronary orifice (measured from the guide catheter) and the distal site is recorded. Maximal coronary microvascular vasodilation may be provoked via injection of intracoronary adenosine. The pressure proximal and distal to the stenosis is measured during the period of peak coronary vasodilatation. The ratio of the distal pressure to the proximal pressure is termed the *fractional flow reserve* (FFR) and is an indirect measure of coronary flow reserve. An FFR of 0.75 or less indicates that the stenosis is sufficiently severe to cause ischemia and that it merits treatment (77). Thus, coronary fractional flow determination constitutes an excellent simple technique for evaluating ambiguously severe stenoses.

CLINICAL IMPLICATIONS OF PERCUTANEOUS CORONARY INTERVENTION

Acute Myocardial Infarction and Unstable Angina

The value of early restoration of flow through the occluded infarct artery in acute myocardial infarction is well established. Although this has been accomplished most commonly by systemic thrombolysis, direct angioplasty of the

infarct artery is also an excellent strategy. Although success rates are lower than for elective angioplasty of stable lesions, direct angioplasty, when performed by highly experienced, skilled operators, achieves a greater vessel patency rate than systemic thrombolysis (85% versus 70%) (78). With the use of stents, patency rates >90% can be achieved and the need for target vessel revascularization is decreased from 17% to 7.7% (79). In addition to providing a greater frequency of flow restoration, direct infarct angioplasty is associated with a smaller frequency of bleeding complications (particularly marked for intracranial bleeding) compared to systemic thrombolysis. Direct angioplasty also provides a lower infarct vessel reocclusion rate than does systemic thrombolysis.

When performed at facilities that are organized to provide an extremely prompt response, direct angioplasty also compares favorably with systemic thrombolysis in terms of the time from presentation to the establishment of reperfusion. However, because of the extreme demands for operator experience and skill and for timely responsiveness, the general applicability of this strategy has not been determined. For patients who present with acute myocardial infarction complicated by cardiogenic shock, early revascularization has been shown to improve long-term survival (80).

The success rate of coronary angioplasty in patients with unstable angina is lower than that for patients with stable angina, primarily because of more frequent thrombotic complications (81,82). Controversy had existed as to whether such patients should be treated for a period of time with aggressive antithrombotic therapy before angioplasty. However, with improved antithrombotic therapy, including glycoprotein IIb/IIIa use and increased use of stents, early percutaneous coronary intervention has been shown to be preferred to conservative therapy in the treatment of unstable angina (83).

Comparison of PTCA with Coronary Bypass Surgery in Multivessel Disease

The ultimate goal of coronary angioplasty is to provide a level of efficacy in coronary revascularization that is comparable or possibly superior to that achieved by coronary bypass grafting. Once balloon coronary angioplasty matured as a technique, it was natural to compare it to coronary bypass surgery. Historically, the efficacy of coronary angioplasty has been limited by its inability to revascularize completely occluded vessels and its high frequency of late failure because of restenosis. The risk of having at least one angioplasty site restenose increases with the number of sites treated. Consequently, the initial role of coronary angioplasty was largely confined to symptomatic single vessel coronary disease where it presented a logical alternative because of the relatively less severe nature of the disease and the lower restenosis risk than that for multivessel disease.

The role of angioplasty in the treatment of single-vessel coronary artery disease that is sufficiently severe to warrant revascularization is clearly established. As angioplasty technique matured, it was natural to explore the potential of coronary angioplasty to provide suitable revascularization in patients with multivessel coronary disease that was anatomically suitable for either angioplasty or coronary bypass surgery.

In the 1980s, balloon angioplasty was compared to coronary bypass surgery in four trials that enrolled patients. The Bypass Angioplasty Revascularization Investigation (BARI) was an NIH-funded randomized comparison of PTCA and CABG as treatment for patients with multivessel disease and severe angina or ischemia (84). The German Angioplasty Bypass Investigation (GABI) randomly compared PTCA and CABG in 358 patients at eight centers with coronary disease in at least two major coronary vessels (85). The Revascularization in Treatment of Angina trial (RITA) enrolled more than 1,000 patients randomized between coronary angioplasty and bypass surgery at 16 British hospitals (86). The Emory Angioplasty Versus Surgery Trial (EAST) was a single-center study that randomized 700 patients suitable for both multivessel PTCA and CABG between the two treatment strategies (87). Each of these trials found similar survival rates and similar degrees of angina relief comparing the angioplasty and the bypass surgery groups at varying durations of late follow-up. However, in all four studies, patients randomized to an initial treatment strategy of angioplasty had a substantially higher frequency of need for repeat revascularization procedures during follow-up. Thus, these studies indicated that angioplasty can provide revascularization with efficacy comparably effective to bypass surgery but that its efficacy is undermined by the high frequency of restenosis.

The advent of bare metal stenting led to a revisiting of the comparison of angioplasty to bypass surgery. The most prominent trial is the ARTS-I (Arterial Revascularization Therapy Study). It randomized 1,202 patients to multivessel angioplasty (2.7 lesions per patient) versus bypass surgery. The frequencies of death, myocardial infarction, and stroke during follow-up were comparable in the two groups. The coronary stent group had a substantially greater frequency of requiring repeat revascularization (17% versus 4%) (88). The ARTS-I stent group revascularization rate represented a substantial improvement compared to the previous balloon angioplasty trials. This was because of a combination of improved acute procedure efficacy and reduced late restenosis. However, the restenosis rate was still sufficient to cause a substantially greater requirement for revascularization in the stent group.

More recently, the ARTS-I trial has been replicated with a registry group (ARTS-II registry) of 607 patients similar to the ARTS-I cohort who were treated with sirolimus-eluting stents. In this registry, the frequency of death, myocardial infarction, and stroke was less than in the ARTS-I bypass surgery group, and the repeat surgery rate in the ARTS-II registry had decreased to 7.4%, which was still greater than the rate in the ARTS-I surgery group but considerably closer.

SUMMARY

These observations have led to the conclusion that angioplasty with drug-eluting stents now provides a highly durable revascularization strategy for those patients with coronary disease who are anatomically suitable. As a result, coronary angioplasty has become a viable alternative for revascularization in patients with multiple coronary stenoses who, previously, would have been selected for bypass surgery. Future research in the clinical application of coronary angioplasty should focus on case selection strategies. If coronary angioplasty with drug-eluting stents continues to succeed, it will be natural to examine the extension of the technique to higher-risk and lower-risk populations encompassing patients who are asymptomatic as well as those with advanced coronary disease, including left main and only remaining patent vessel circumstances.

REFERENCES

1. Gruntzig AR, Senning A, Siegenthaler WE. Nonoperative dilatation of coronary-artery stenosis: percutaneous transluminal coronary angioplasty. N Engl J Med 1979;301(2):61–68.
2. Dotter CT, Judkins MP. Transluminal treatment of arteriosclerotic obstruction. Description of a new technic and a preliminary report of its application. Circulation 1964;30:654–670.
3. Gruntzig AR, Turina MI, Schneider JA. Experimental percutaneous dilatation of coronary artery stenosis. Circulation 1976;54:81.
4. Berger SM, Gorfinkel HJ. Candidates for transluminal coronary angioplasty. Am J Cardiol 1981;48(4):810.
5. Holmes DR Jr, Holubkov R, Vlietstra RE, et al. Comparison of complications during percutaneous transluminal coronary angioplasty from 1977 to 1981 and from 1985 to 1986: the National Heart, Lung, and Blood Institute Percutaneous Transluminal Coronary Angioplasty Registry. J Am Coll Cardiol 1988;12(5):1149–1155.
6. Ellis SG, Cowley MJ, Whitlow PL, et al. Prospective case-control comparison of percutaneous transluminal coronary revascularization in patients with multivessel disease treated in 1986–1987 versus 1991: improved in-hospital and 12-month results. Multivessel Angioplasty Prognosis Study (MAPS) Group. J Am Coll Cardiol 1995;25(5):1137–1142.
7. Heart and Stroke Facts: American Heart Association—2003.
8. Graham TPJ, Covell JW, Sonenblick EH, et al. Control of myocardial oxygen consumption: relative influence of contractile state and tension development. J Clin Invest 1968;47.375.
9. Vatner SF. Correlation between acute reductions in myocardial blood flow and function in conscious dogs. Circ Res 1980;47(2):201–207.
10. Jennings RB, Reimer KA, Hill ML, et al. Total ischemia in dog hearts, in vitro. 1. Comparison of high-energy phosphate production, utilization, and depletion and of adenine nucleotide catabolism in total ischemia in vitro vs. severe ischemia in vivo. Circ Res 1981;49(4):892–900.
11. Dougherty KG, Gaos CM, Bush HS, et al. Activated clotting times and activated partial thromboplastin times in patients undergoing coronary angioplasty who receive bolus doses of heparin. Cathet Cardiovasc Diagn 1992;26(4):260–263.
12. McGrath PD, Malenka DJ, Wennberg DE, et al. Changing outcomes in percutaneous coronary interventions: a study of 34,752 procedures in northern New England—1990 to 1997. Northern New England Cardiovascular Disease Study Group. J Am Coll Cardiol 1999;34(3):674–680.
13. Smith SC, Jr., Dove JT, Jacobs AK, et al. ACC/AHA guidelines for percutaneous coronary intervention (revision of the 1993 PTCA guidelines)—executive summary: a report of the American College of Cardiology/American Heart Association task force on practice

guidelines (Committee to revise the 1993 guidelines for percutaneous transluminal coronary angioplasty) endorsed by the Society for Cardiac Angiography and Interventions. Circulation 2001;103(24): 3019–3041.

14. Schatz RA, Baim DS, Leon M, et al. Clinical experience with the Palmaz-Schatz coronary stent. Initial results of a multicenter study. Circulation 1991;83(1):148–161.

15. Herrmann HC, Buchbinder M, Clemen MW, et al. Emergent use of balloon-expandable coronary artery stenting for failed percutaneous transluminal coronary angioplasty. Circulation 1992; 86(3):812–819.

16. Fischman DL, Leon MB, Baim DS, et al. A randomized comparison of coronary-stent placement and balloon angioplasty in the treatment of coronary artery disease. Stent Restenosis Study Investigators. N Engl J Med 1994;331(8):496–501.

17. Serruys PW, de Jaegere P, Kiemeneij F, et al. A comparison of balloon-expandable stent implantation with balloon angioplasty in patients with coronary artery disease. Benestent Study Group. N Engl J Med 1994;331(8):489–495.

18. Cohen M, Demers C, Gurfinkel EP, et al. Low-molecular-weight heparins in non–ST-segment elevation ischemia: the ESSENCE trial. Efficacy and safety of subcutaneous enoxaparin versus intravenous unfractionated heparin in non–Q-wave coronary events. Am J Cardiol 1998;82:19L–24L.

19. Ferguson JJ, Califf RM, Antman EM, et al. Enoxaparin versus unfractionated heparin in high-risk patients with non–ST-segment elevation acute coronary syndromes managed with an intended early invasive strategy: primary results of the SYNERGY randomized trial. JAMA 2004;292(1):45–54.

20. Lincoff AM, Bittl JA, Harrington RA, et al. Bivalirudin and provisional glycoprotein IIb/IIIa blockade compared with heparin and planned glycoprotein IIb/IIIa blockade during percutaneous coronary intervention: REPLACE-2 randomized trial. JAMA 2003;289(7):853–863.

21. Schwartz L, Bourassa MG, Lesperance J, et al. Aspirin and dipyridamole in the prevention of restenosis after percutaneous transluminal coronary angioplasty. N Engl J Med 1988;318(26): 1714–1719.

22. Barnathan ES, Schwartz JS, Taylor L, et al. Aspirin and dipyridamole in the prevention of acute coronary thrombosis complicating coronary angioplasty. Circulation 1987;76(1):125–134.

23. Leon MB, Baim DS, Popma JJ, et al. A clinical trial comparing three antithrombotic-drug regimens after coronary-artery stenting. Stent Anticoagulation Restenosis Study Investigators. N Engl J Med 1998;339(23):1665–1671.

24. Bennett CL, Weinberg PD, Rozenberg-Ben-Dror K, et al. Thrombotic thrombocytopenic purpura associated with ticlopidine. A review of 60 cases. Ann Intern Med 1998;128(7):541–544.

25. Berger PB, Bell MR, Hasdai D, et al. Safety and efficacy of ticlopidine for only 2 weeks after successful intracoronary stent placement. Circulation 1999;99(2):248–253.

26. Berger PB, Bell MR, Rihal CS, et al. Clopidogrel versus ticlopidine after intracoronary stent placement. J Am Coll Cardiol 1999; 34(7):1891–1894.

27. Moussa I, Oetgen M, Roubin G, et al. Effectiveness of clopidogrel and aspirin versus ticlopidine and aspirin in preventing stent thrombosis after coronary stent implantation. Circulation 1999; 99(18):2364–2366.

28. Muller C, Buttner HJ, Petersen J, et al. A randomized comparison of clopidogrel and aspirin versus ticlopidine and aspirin after the placement of coronary-artery stents. Circulation 2000; 101(6):590–593.

29. Randomised placebo-controlled trial of abciximab before and during coronary intervention in refractory unstable angina: the CAPTURE Study. Lancet 1997;349(9063):1429–1435.

30. Use of a monoclonal antibody directed against the platelet glycoprotein IIb/IIIa receptor in high-risk coronary angioplasty. The EPIC Investigation. N Engl J Med 1994;330(14):956–961.

31. Platelet glycoprotein IIb/IIIa receptor blockade and low-dose heparin during percutaneous coronary revascularization. The EPILOG Investigators. N Engl J Med 1997;336(24):1689–1696.

32. Randomised placebo-controlled and balloon-angioplasty-controlled trial to assess safety of coronary stenting with use of platelet glycoprotein-IIb/IIIa blockade. The EPISTENT Investigators. Evaluation of Platelet IIb/IIIa Inhibitor for Stenting. Lancet 1998;352(9122): 87–92.

33. Novel dosing regimen of eptifibatide in planned coronary stent implantation (ESPRIT): a randomised, placebo-controlled trial. Lancet 2000;356:2037–2044.

34. Effects of platelet glycoprotein IIb/IIIa blockade with tirofiban on adverse cardiac events in patients with unstable angina or acute myocardial infarction undergoing coronary angioplasty. The RESTORE Investigators. Randomized Efficacy Study of Tirofiban for Outcomes and REstenosis. Circulation 1997;96(5): 1445–1453.

35. Topol EJ, Mark DB, Lincoff AM, et al. Outcomes at 1 year and economic implications of platelet glycoprotein IIb/IIIa blockade in patients undergoing coronary stenting: results from a multicentre randomised trial. EPISTENT Investigators. Evaluation of Platelet IIb/IIIa Inhibitor for Stenting. Lancet 1999;354:2019–2024.

36. Leimgruber PP, Roubin GS, Hollman J, et al. Restenosis after successful coronary angioplasty in patients with single-vessel disease. Circulation 1986;73(4):710–717.

37. Roubin GS, Douglas JS Jr, King SB III, et al. Influence of balloon size on initial success, acute complications, and restenosis after percutaneous transluminal coronary angioplasty. A prospective randomized study. Circulation 1988;78(3):557–565.

38. Myler RK, Shaw RE, Stertzer SH, et al. Lesion morphology and coronary angioplasty: current experience and analysis. J Am Coll Cardiol 1992;19(7):1641–1652.

39. Kahn JK, Hartzler GO. Frequency and causes of failure with contemporary balloon coronary angioplasty and implications for new technologies. Am J Cardiol 1990;66(10):858–860.

40. Ryan TJ, Faxon DP, Gunnar RM, et al. Guidelines for percutaneous transluminal coronary angioplasty. A report of the American College of Cardiology/American Heart Association Task Force on Assessment of Diagnostic and Therapeutic Cardiovascular Procedures (Subcommittee on Percutaneous Transluminal Coronary Angioplasty). Circulation 1988;78(2): 486–502.

41. Ellis SG, Vandormael MG, Cowley MJ, et al. Coronary morphologic and clinical determinants of procedural outcome with angioplasty for multivessel coronary disease. Implications for patient selection. Multivessel Angioplasty Prognosis Study Group. Circulation 1990;82(4):1193–1202.

42. Bell MR, Berger PB, Bresnahan JF, et al. Initial and long-term outcome of 354 patients after coronary balloon angioplasty of total coronary artery occlusions. Circulation 1992;85(3):1003–1011.

43. Ivanhoe RJ, Weintraub WS, Douglas JS Jr, et al. Percutaneous transluminal coronary angioplasty of chronic total occlusions. Primary success, restenosis, and long-term clinical follow-up. Circulation 1992;85(1):106–115.

44. Lincoff AM, Popma JJ, Ellis SG, et al. Abrupt vessel closure complicating coronary angioplasty: clinical, angiographic and therapeutic profile. J Am Coll Cardiol 1992;19(5):926–935.

45. Kuntz RE, Piana R, Pomerantz RM, et al. Changing incidence and management of abrupt closure following coronary intervention in the new device era. Cathet Cardiovasc Diagn 1992;27(3): 183–190.

46. Talley JD, Weintraub WS, Roubin GS, et al. Failed elective percutaneous transluminal coronary angioplasty requiring coronary artery bypass surgery. In-hospital and late clinical outcome at 5 years. Circulation 1990;82(4):1203–1213.

47. Lotfi M, Mackie K, Dzavik V, Seidelin PH. Impact of delays to cardiac surgery after failed angioplasty and stenting. J Am Coll Cardiol 2004;43(3):337–342.

48. Craver JM, Weintraub WS, Jones EL, et al. Emergency coronary artery bypass surgery for failed percutaneous coronary angioplasty. A 10-year experience. Ann Surg 1992;215(5):425–433; discussion 433–424.

49. Wyman RM, Safian RD, Portway V, et al. Current complications of diagnostic and therapeutic cardiac catheterization. J Am Coll Cardiol 1988;12(6):1400–1406.

50. Beatt KJ, Serruys PW, Hugenholtz PG. Restenosis after coronary angioplasty: new standards for clinical studies. J Am Coll Cardiol 1990;15(2):491–498.

51. Hirshfeld JW Jr, Schwartz JS, Jugo R, et al. Restenosis after coronary angioplasty: a multivariate statistical model to relate lesion and procedure variables to restenosis. The M-HEART Investigators. J Am Coll Cardiol 1991;18(3):647–656.

52. Forrester JS, Fishbein M, Helfant R, et al. A paradigm for restenosis based on cell biology: clues for the development of new preventive therapies. J Am Coll Cardiol 1991;17(3):758–769.

53. Libby P, Schwartz D, Brogi E, et al. A cascade model for restenosis. A special case of atherosclerosis progression. Circulation 1992;86:III47–52.

54. Popma JJ, van den Berg EK, Dehmer GJ. Long-term outcome of patients with asymptomatic restenosis after percutaneous transluminal coronary angioplasty. Am J Cardiol 1988;62(17): 1298–1299.

55. Nobuyoshi M, Kimura T, Nosaka H, et al. Restenosis after successful percutaneous transluminal coronary angioplasty: serial angiographic follow-up of 229 patients. J Am Coll Cardiol 1988; 12(3):616–623.

56. Teirstein PS, Hoover CA, Ligon RW, et al. Repeat coronary angioplasty: efficacy of a third angioplasty for a second restenosis. J Am Coll Cardiol 1989;13(2):291–296.

57. DiSciascio G, Vetrovec GW, Cowley MJ, et al. Early and late outcome of percutaneous transluminal coronary angioplasty for subacute and chronic total coronary occlusion. Am Heart J 1986; 111(5):833–839.

58. Roubin GS, Cannon AD, Agrawal SK, et al. Intracoronary stenting for acute and threatened closure complicating percutaneous transluminal coronary angioplasty. Circulation 1992;85(3):916–927.

59. Sigwart U, Puel J, Mirkovitch V, et al. Intravascular stents to prevent occlusion and restenosis after transluminal angioplasty. N Engl J Med 1987;316(12):701–706.

60. Strecker EP, Liermann D, Barth KH, et al. Expandable tubular stents for treatment of arterial occlusive diseases: experimental and clinical results. Work in progress. Radiology 1990;175(1):97–102.

61. Moses JW, Leon MB, Popma JJ, et al. Sirolimus-eluting stents versus standard stents in patients with stenosis in a native coronary artery. N Engl J Med 2003;349(14):1315–1323.

62. Stone GW, Ellis SG, Cox DA, et al. A polymer-based, paclitaxel-eluting stent in patients with coronary artery disease. N Engl J Med 2004;350(3):221–231.

63. Stone GW, Ellis SG, Cox DA, et al. One-year clinical results with the slow-release, polymer-based, paclitaxel-eluting TAXUS stent: the TAXUS-IV trial. Circulation 2004;109(16):1942–1947.

64. Frishman WH, Chiu R, Landzberg BR, et al. Medical therapies for the prevention of restenosis after percutaneous coronary interventions. Curr Probl Cardiol 1998;23(10):534–635.

65. Teirstein PS, Massullo V, Jani S, et al. Catheter-based radiotherapy to inhibit restenosis after coronary stenting. N Engl J Med 1997;336(24):1697–1703.

66. Waksman R, White RL, Chan RC, et al. Intracoronary gamma-radiation therapy after angioplasty inhibits recurrence in patients with in-stent restenosis. Circulation 2000;101(18):2165–2171.

67. Leon MB, Teirstein PS, Moses JW, et al. Localized intracoronary gamma-radiation therapy to inhibit the recurrence of restenosis after stenting. N Engl J Med 2001;344(4):250–256.

68. Raizner AE, Oesterle SN, Waksman R, et al. Inhibition of restenosis with beta-emitting radiotherapy: Report of the Proliferation Reduction with Vascular Energy Trial (PREVENT). Circulation 2000;102(9):951–958.

69. Kastrati A, Mehilli J, von Beckerath N, et al. Sirolimus-eluting stent or paclitaxel-eluting stent versus balloon angioplasty for prevention of recurrences in patients with coronary in-stent restenosis: a randomized controlled trial. JAMA 2005;293(2):165–171.

70. Mintz GS, Potkin BN, Keren G, et al. Intravascular ultrasound evaluation of the effect of rotational atherectomy in obstructive atherosclerotic coronary artery disease. Circulation 1992;86(5): 1383–1393.

71. Bertrand ME, Lablanche JM, Leroy F, et al. Percutaneous transluminal coronary rotary ablation with Rotablator (European experience). Am J Cardiol 1992;69(5):470–474.

72. Whitlow PL, Bass TA, Kipperman RM, et al. Results of the study to determine rotablator and transluminal angioplasty strategy (STRATAS). Am J Cardiol 2001;87(6):699–705.

73. Dietz U, Rupprecht HJ, de Belder MA, et al. Angiographic analysis of the angioplasty versus rotational atherectomy for the treatment of diffuse in-stent restenosis trial (ARTIST). Am J Cardiol 2002;90(8):843–847.

74. Hillis LD. Efficacy and safety of coronary balloon angioplasty and directional atherectomy. Circulation 1990;82(1):305–307.

75. Topol EJ, Leya F, Pinkerton CA, et al. A comparison of directional atherectomy with coronary angioplasty in patients with coronary artery disease. The CAVEAT Study Group. N Engl J Med 1993;329(4):221–227.

76. Pijls NH, van Son JA, Kirkeeide RL, et al. Experimental basis of determining maximum coronary, myocardial, and collateral blood flow by pressure measurements for assessing functional stenosis severity before and after percutaneous transluminal coronary angioplasty. Circulation 1993;87(4):1354–1367.

77. de Bruyne B, Bartunek J, Sys SU, et al. Simultaneous coronary pressure and flow velocity measurements in humans. Feasibility, reproducibility, and hemodynamic dependence of coronary flow velocity reserve, hyperemic flow versus pressure slope index, and fractional flow reserve. Circulation 1996;94(8):1842–1849.

78. Grines CL, Browne KF, Marco J, et al. A comparison of immediate angioplasty with thrombolytic therapy for acute myocardial infarction. The Primary Angioplasty in Myocardial Infarction Study Group. N Engl J Med 1993;328(10):673–679.

79. Grines CL, Cox DA, Stone GW, et al. Coronary angioplasty with or without stent implantation for acute myocardial infarction. Stent Primary Angioplasty in Myocardial Infarction Study Group. N Engl J Med 1999;341(26):1949–1956.

80. Hochman JS, Sleeper LA, Webb JG, et al. Early revascularization in acute myocardial infarction complicated by cardiogenic shock. SHOCK Investigators. Should we emergently revascularize occluded coronaries for cardiogenic shock. N Engl J Med 1999;341(9):625–634.

81. Laskey MA, Deutsch E, Hirshfeld JW Jr, et al. Influence of heparin therapy on percutaneous transluminal coronary angioplasty outcome in patients with coronary arterial thrombus. Am J Cardiol 1990;65(3):179–182.

82. Laskey MA, Deutsch E, Barnathan E, et al. Influence of heparin therapy on percutaneous transluminal coronary angioplasty outcome in unstable angina pectoris. Am J Cardiol 1990;65(22): 1425–1429.

83. Cannon CP, Weintraub WS, Demopoulos LA, et al. Invasive versus conservative strategies in unstable angina and non–Q-wave myocardial infarction following treatment with tirofiban: rationale and study design of the international TACTICS-TIMI 18 Trial. Treat angina with Aggrastat and determine cost of therapy with an invasive or conservative strategy. Thrombolysis in myocardial infarction. Am J Cardiol 1998;82(6):731–736.

84. Comparison of coronary bypass surgery with angioplasty in patients with multivessel disease. The Bypass Angioplasty Revascularization Investigation (BARI) Investigators. N Engl J Med 1996;335(4):217–225.

85. Hamm CW, Reimers J, Ischinger T, et al. A randomized study of coronary angioplasty compared with bypass surgery in patients with symptomatic multivessel coronary disease. German Angioplasty Bypass Surgery Investigation (GABI). N Engl J Med 1994; 331(16):1037–1043.

86. Coronary angioplasty versus coronary artery bypass surgery: the Randomized Intervention Treatment of Angina (RITA) trial. Lancet 1993;341:573–580.

87. King SB III, Lembo NJ, Weintraub WS, et al. A randomized trial comparing coronary angioplasty with coronary bypass surgery. Emory Angioplasty versus Surgery Trial (EAST). N Engl J Med 1994;331(16):1044–1050.

88. Serruys PW, Unger F, Sousa JE, et al. Comparison of coronary-artery bypass surgery and stenting for the treatment of multivessel disease. N Engl J Med 2001;344(15):1117–1124.

Interventional Radiology of the Gastrointestinal System

V

Arteriographic Diagnosis and Treatment of Gastrointestinal Bleeding

26

Stanley Baum

The beginning of interventional radiology can be traced to the introduction of selective arteriography for the diagnosis and treatment of gastrointestinal bleeding.

Since its introduction in 1963, selective arteriography has become established as an accurate, safe, and important technique for the diagnosis and treatment of gastrointestinal bleeding (1–3). When this procedure was initially introduced, it was used exclusively for diagnosis. The selective arterial infusion of vasoconstricting drugs through the same catheter used to identify the bleeding site was a natural outgrowth of diagnostic arteriography. This progression from a diagnostic to a therapeutic application

of the angiographic catheter heralded the beginning of interventional radiology (4).

To use angiography effectively in the emergency management of gastrointestinal bleeding, one must perform it rapidly and efficiently. Well-trained personnel must be available on short notice, 24 hours per day, 7 days per week. The indications as well as the limitations of angiography for acute gastrointestinal bleeding must be well understood by both the radiologist and the attending clinician. About 75% of patients requiring hospitalization for gastrointestinal bleeding can be managed conservatively with sedation, bed rest, and replacement of blood volume

(5). These patients are obviously not candidates for emergency angiography. Transcatheter therapy is most useful in patients in whom bleeding does not respond to conservative treatment or in those who are poor surgical risks.

BLEEDING SITE LOCALIZATION

Although angiography is only one of several methods available for locating sources of gastrointestinal bleeding, it has become an important and commonly used clinical tool (6–12). The procedure may be performed on severely ill patients and requires little patient cooperation. The angiographic criteria of bleeding are straightforward, and the examination requires little special preparation and can be performed despite the presence of large amounts of blood in the gastrointestinal tract.

For successful visualization, however, the patient must be bleeding at a rate of at least 0.5 mL per minute. The major limitation of the technique relates to the intermittent nature of gastrointestinal bleeding, which can result in a negative study if the bleeding has temporarily stopped at the time of the injection (13). Another serious limitation has been the inability of a selective arteriogram to demonstrate venous bleeding. This is also a problem if the patients studied are bleeding massively from esophageal varices.

Experimental gastrointestinal hemorrhage has recently been demonstrated with contrast-enhanced magnetic resonance imaging (MRI) (14–16) as well as computed tomography (17–19). Prior endoscopy can also be of great help to the angiographer. Even if the endoscopist cannot be certain exactly where the bleeding is coming from, the identification of the region of bleeding, such as the duodenum or stomach, is of value in guiding catheterization of the appropriate vessel. If the bleeding is observed coming from esophageal varices, initial therapy is directed toward intravenous vasopressin infusion rather than early angiography. Unfortunately, an accurate endoscopic diagnosis is not always possible because direct visualization is made difficult by active bleeding and blood in the gastrointestinal tract.

The intravenous administration of radionuclides has proved to be a valuable diagnostic technique for demonstrating active bleeding prior to angiography. This technique is totally noninvasive, simple, and capable of visualizing both arterial and venous bleeding at rates as low as 0.1 mL per minute. The isotope procedure is performed with an intravenous injection of technetium-99m (^{99m}Tc) sulfur colloid, a liver-scanning agent (20). As the isotope reaches the bleeding site, a small amount extravasates. With each additional circulation, more of the isotope leaks into the gut. As activity in the vascular system is removed by the liver and spleen, a difference is quickly reached between the bleeding site and the background (Figures 26–1 and 26–2). The extravasated isotope within the gut can usually be demonstrated in the first

5–10 minutes following the injection. If sites of bleeding cannot be identified on the early scan, the examination is continued so as to identify activity that moves away from the hepatic or splenic flexure. Such an area may be obscured at first by the activity in the overlying spleen and liver, but as continued peristalsis moves the isotope along the gastrointestinal tract, it becomes visible. The technique is frequently used as a screening procedure and enables better selection of patients to be studied by angiography.

With an alternate isotopic technique using tagged red blood cells, bleeding does not have to be occurring at the time of the injection. The tagged red cells are injected, and the scans are taken at 1-minute intervals for 1 hour. If the scans are negative, the patient can be sent back to the floor and scans repeated when clinically indicated (21–24).

If bleeding occurs, the tagged red cells extravasate into the gastrointestinal tract and can be detected on repeated scans. The disadvantage of this technique is that bleeding may occur in one place, but because the labeled red cells can travel in a retrograde or antegrade fashion, the scan may show the activity in a more distal or proximal site.

The value of emergency barium examinations in patients with severe gastrointestinal bleeding is limited. Large amounts of blood in the gut make upper gastrointestinal barium studies difficult to interpret except in the presence

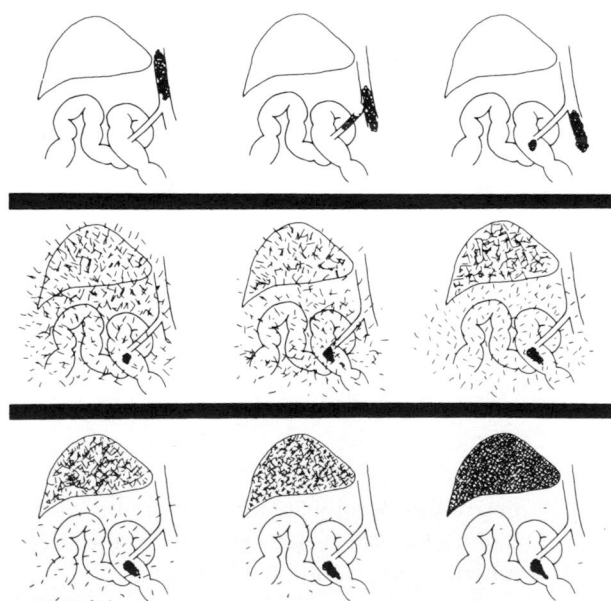

Figure 26–1 ^{99m}Tc sulfur colloid scan for the detection of gastrointestinal bleeding. After the injection of ^{99m}Tc sulfur colloid into a patient who is actively bleeding, the radioactive agent is cleared by the liver, and only a fraction of the injected material will extravasate at the bleeding site. This process is repeated each time the blood circulates, adding another, but smaller, fraction to the material already at the site of the hemorrhage. Immediately after the intravenous administration of the radioactive agent, the background activity decreases exponentially, and the activity at the bleeding site increases exponentially.

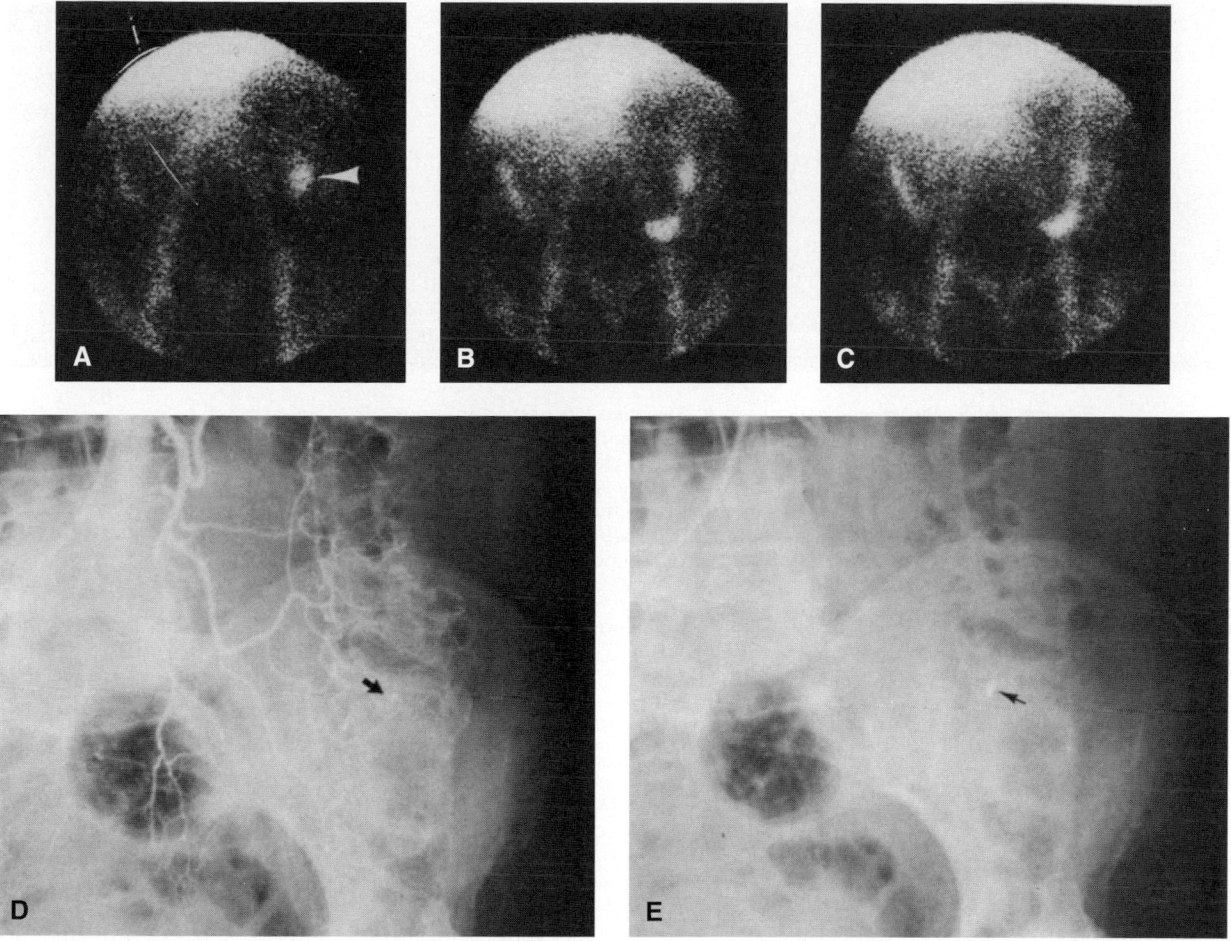

Figure 26–2 Bleeding diverticulum demonstrated with a ^{99m}Tc sulfur colloid scan. **A.** Ten minutes after the injection of 10 mCi intravenously, an area of abnormal activity is seen in the left iliac fossa (*arrow*). **B., C.** Scans obtained 15 and 30 minutes later demonstrate movement of activity in the lumen of the bowel. The activity outlines a configuration of the descending and proximal sigmoid colons. **D.** Twenty minutes after the isotope scan, an inferior mesenteric arteriogram was obtained that demonstrates an area of extravasation (*arrow*) in the descending colon superimposed on the iliac fossa. **E.** A late film obtained during inferior mesenteric arteriography shows persistence of extravasated contrast material in the descending colon (*arrow*). The patient was successfully treated by a vasopressin infusion. Before discharge, a barium examination showed the arteriographic abnormality to correspond to a colonic diverticulum.

of very large and obvious lesions. Barium enemas are even more limited because of fecal material in the unprepared bowel. If the barium examination is positive, there is no assurance that the detected pathologic processes (e.g., duodenal ulcers, esophageal varices, or colonic diverticular disease) are responsible for the current bleeding episode (25,26). In addition, the presence of barium in the gastrointestinal tract precludes the possibility of a subsequent angiographic examination and also interferes with direct endoscopic visualization.

More recently, a technique that utilizes wireless capsule endoscopy has been useful for detecting obscure sites of gastrointestinal bleeding. Because it is safe and painless, some investigators suggest that it should become the initial diagnostic choice for patients with obscure GI bleeding (27,28).

ANGIOGRAPHIC APPEARANCE OF BLEEDING

When bleeding is first detected during the arterial phase of a selective arteriogram, it typically appears as a localized puddle of contrast material. As the filming continues, the bleeding becomes increasingly obvious and persists after all the intravascular contrast has washed out. In the presence of very brisk bleeding, one may see excellent opacification of the mucosa of the gastrointestinal tract. Small amounts of extravasation appear as localized flecks, which occasionally outline either an ulcer crater (Figure 26–3) or a colonic diverticulum (Figure 26–4). If the lumen of the gastrointestinal tract is filled with blood clots, extravasated contrast material will occasionally appear tubular in configuration and resemble a venous structure

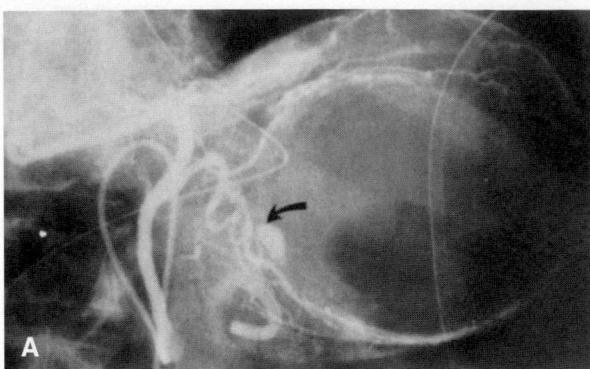
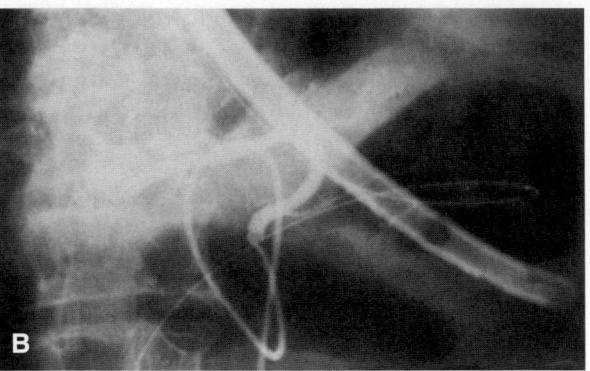

Figure 26–3 Bleeding gastric ulcer. **A.** Selective left gastric arteriography demonstrates a common left hepatic–left gastric trunk and active bleeding (*arrow*) from a fundal branch of the left gastric artery. **B.** Repeat left gastric arteriography during the infusion of vasopressin demonstrates marked vasoconstriction of the left gastric artery without any evidence of continued bleeding. The left hepatic artery branch appears unaffected by the vasopressin. This impression is in keeping with experimental evidence that although vasopressin causes initial vasoconstriction of the hepatic artery, it does not maintain the vasoconstriction during an infusion. It is generally assumed, therefore, that it is safe to infuse the hepatic artery selectively in patients with normal liver function.

(29). This "pseudovein" (Figure 26–5) is easily distinguished from a vascular malformation because the extravasated contrast persists well beyond the venous phase of the arteriogram.

PITFALLS IN THE ANGIOGRAPHIC DIAGNOSIS OF BLEEDING

The intermittent nature of bleeding in some patients can result in a negative angiographic study if during the injection the bleeding has ceased. Some angiographers have attempted to provoke bleeding in these cases (30,31); however, the author's own experience with both heparin and vasodilators such as tolazoline hydrochloride (Priscoline) has not been successful. The author has found the isotope technique helpful in selecting those patients who are actively bleeding, and its use has reduced the number of negative arteriograms.

Venous bleeding is almost never demonstrated angiographically, and the diagnosis of esophageal variceal bleeding is made on angiography only indirectly by demonstrating

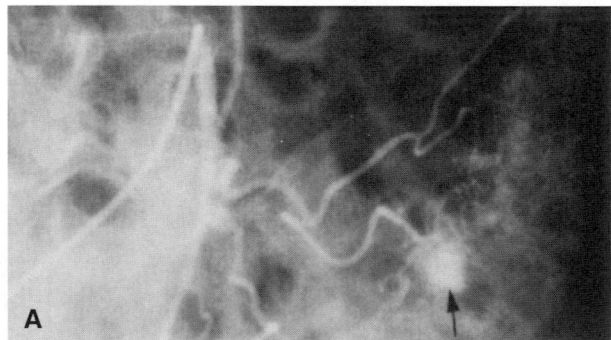
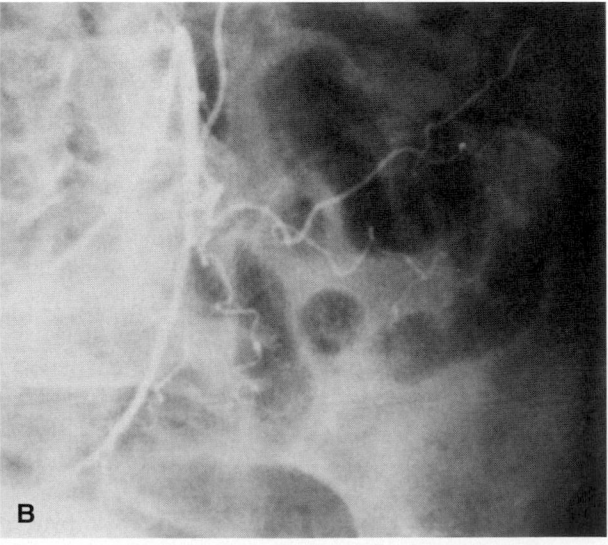

Figure 26–4 Bleeding diverticulum in the descending colon outlined with extravasated contrast material. **A.** Arterial phase of a selective inferior mesenteric arteriogram shows extravasation of contrast material (*arrow*) in the midportion of the descending colon. The extravasated contrast appears to outline the diverticulum itself. **B.** During the infusion of vasopressin at 0.2 unit per minute into the inferior mesenteric artery, a repeat arteriogram demonstrates peripheral vasoconstriction of the arterial branches and cessation of the bleeding. After the patient was weaned from the vasopressin, the bleeding did not recur, and the patient was discharged without surgery.

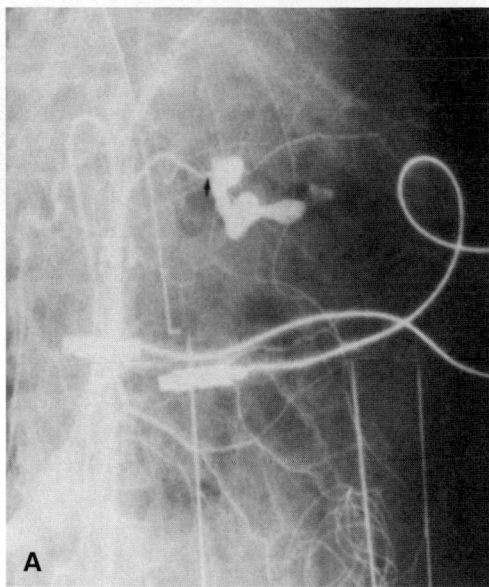

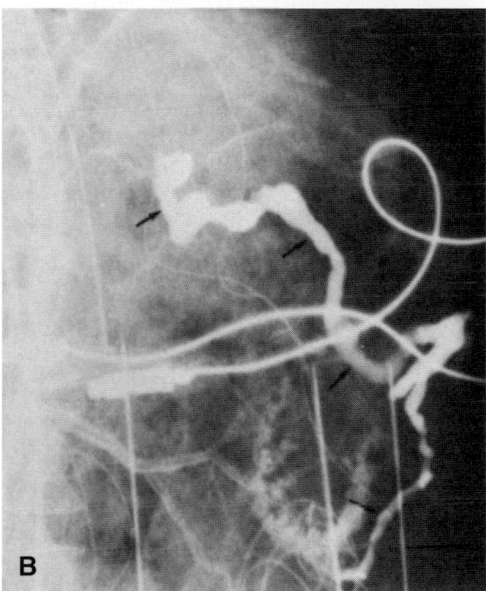

Figure 26–5 Pseudovein appearance of extravasated contrast material. **A.** Selective left gastric arteriography performed on a patient with an actively bleeding stress ulcer in the fundus of the stomach demonstrates extravasation from a branch of the left gastric artery (*arrow*). **B.** A film obtained during the capillary phase of the study demonstrates the extravasated contrast material (*arrows*) puddled between clots within a dilated, blood-filled stomach. Although the appearance of the contrast material is that of a vascular structure, this should not be confused with either an arterial or a venous malformation.

portal hypertension and excluding all other potential arterial and/or mucosal sites of bleeding.

False-Negative Examination

Occasionally in a patient actively bleeding from an arterial and/or a capillary site, the arteriogram will not demonstrate an area of extravasation. This is usually the result of injecting the wrong vessel. If clinical or endoscopic evidence exists of upper gastrointestinal bleeding, a complete examination must include opacification of the left gastric, gastroduodenal, pancreaticoduodenal, and splenic arteries. In the absence of a gastrojejunostomy, the history of having vomited blood generally indicates that the bleeding is coming from some portion of the gastrointestinal tract proximal to the ligament of Treitz. The history of having passed bright red blood per rectum, however, does not preclude the patient's having a bleeding site in the upper gastrointestinal tract. Examination of the vasculature of the stomach and duodenum should also be carried out if a negative superior and inferior mesenteric arteriogram is obtained in a patient presenting with lower gastrointestinal hemorrhage.

False-Positive Examination

False-positive diagnoses will occasionally be made when normal parenchymal blushes are confused with extravasation. One of the most commonly made errors is the superimposition of a densely opacified left adrenal gland on the gastric fundus (Figure 26–6). This often occurs when the inferior phrenic arteries originate either as branches of or adjacent to the left gastric artery or celiac axis. The arteriographic parenchymal blush of the adrenal gland resembles a railroad track, being linear in appearance with a radiolucency in the center.

Another instance of a false-positive examination can occur in some patients in whom selective left gastric arteriography demonstrates a marked increase in the size and number of vessels supplying the gastric fundus accompanied by an intense mucosal stain. Although this appearance is similar to that seen in hemorrhagic gastritis, unless one can identify actual points of extravasation the diagnosis of bleeding gastritis should not be made. The hyperemic appearance can be caused by vigorous lavaging of the stomach prior to arteriography in an attempt to stop the bleeding. It must also be remembered that patients bleeding from other causes such as duodenal ulcers or Mallory-Weiss tears of the stomach will frequently have gastritis (Figure 26–7).

Even after a site of extravasation is identified on the arteriogram, errors can occur in knowing exactly where the bleeding site is within the gastrointestinal tract. In the anteroposterior projection of a superior mesenteric arteriogram, extravasation from a bleeding duodenal ulcer that is being supplied from the inferior pancreaticoduodenal artery may seem to originate in the transverse colon (Figure 26–8). The surgeon will therefore be misled unless the angiographer is certain as to the site of extravasation. All doubt can be resolved by repeating the superior mesenteric arteriography with the patient in a right posterior oblique position. Another common error is confusing a prepyloric ulcer that is actively bleeding with a duodenal ulcer. This can also be resolved by repeating the injection with the patient in a left posterior oblique position.

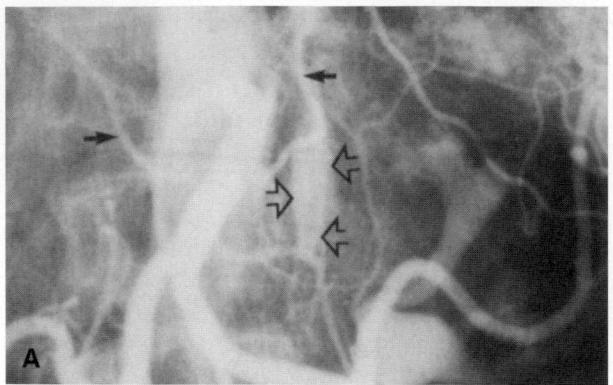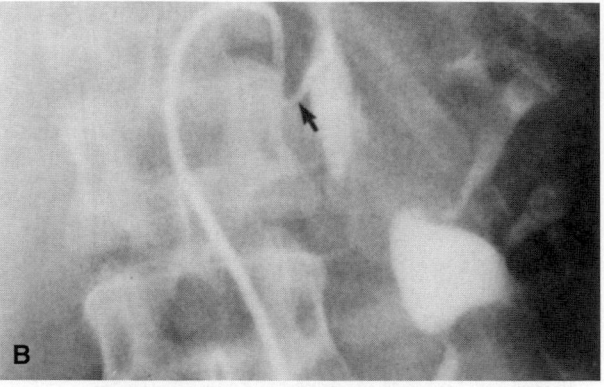

Figure 26–6   Left adrenal gland opacification simulating extravasation. **A.** Selective celiac arteriography performed on a patient studied for upper gastrointestinal bleeding demonstrates large phrenic arteries coming off as early branches of the celiac axis (*solid arrows*). During the arterial phase of the examination, opacification of the left adrenal gland appears (*open arrows*) as a result of adrenal branches from the inferior phrenic artery. There is no evidence on the celiac arteriogram of arterial extravasation. **B.** Intense opacification of the left adrenal gland persists well after the venous phase of the examination and is superimposed on the lesser curvature aspect of the fundus of the stomach. The fact that the tip of the catheter is partially wedged in the left inferior phrenic artery probably accounts for the intense opacification of the adrenal gland and the poor washout of the phrenic artery (*arrow*). The patient did not have any angiographic evidence of arterial or mucosal bleeding.

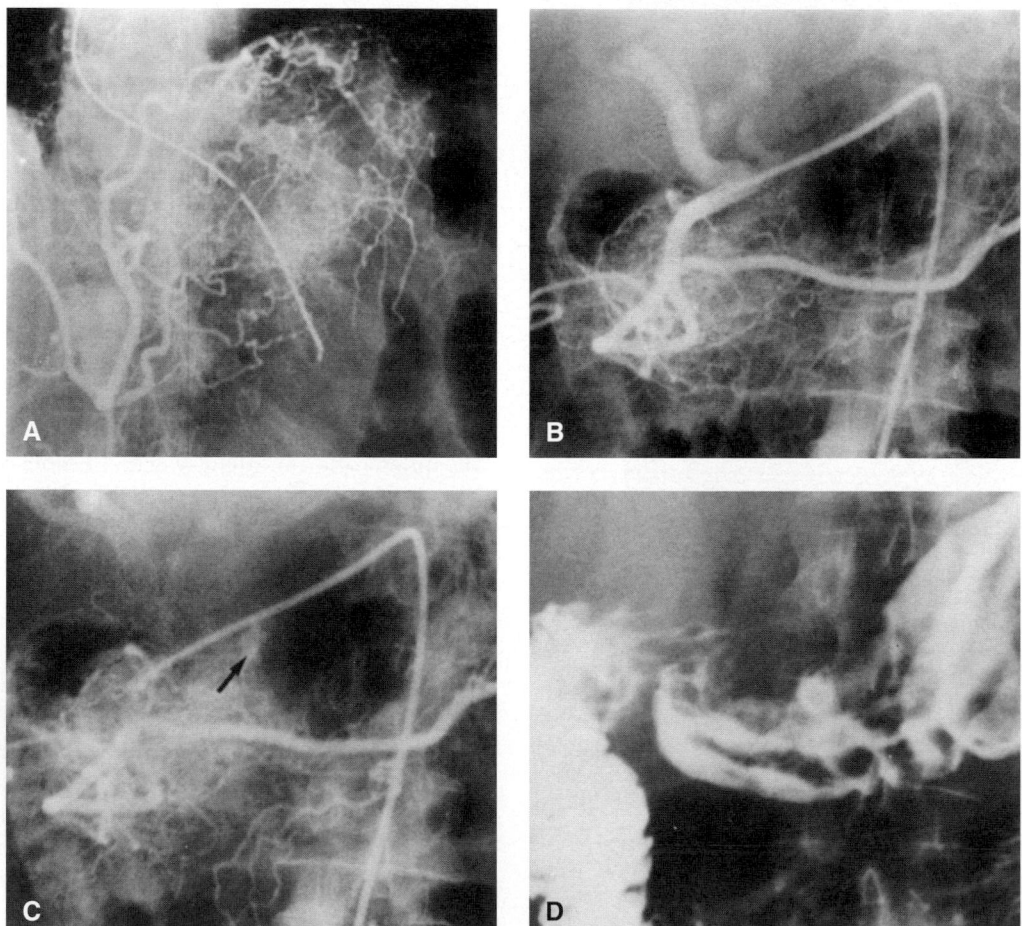

Figure 26–7   Fundal gastritis and actively bleeding lesser curvature peptic ulcer in a patient presenting with massive upper gastrointestinal bleeding. **A.** Selective left gastric arteriography demonstrates marked hypervascularity in the gastric fundus without any evidence of discrete extravasation. The angiographic appearance is that of gastritis. **B.** Early phase of a selective gastroduodenal arteriogram. **C.** Late arterial phase of the gastroduodenal arteriogram demonstrates extravasation of contrast material (*arrow*) at the site of an antral ulcer that was seen on a prior upper gastrointestinal series. This bleeding was controlled by infusing vasopressin into the gastroduodenal artery. **D.** Upper gastrointestinal series performed 2 weeks earlier demonstrates a lesser curvature ulcer.

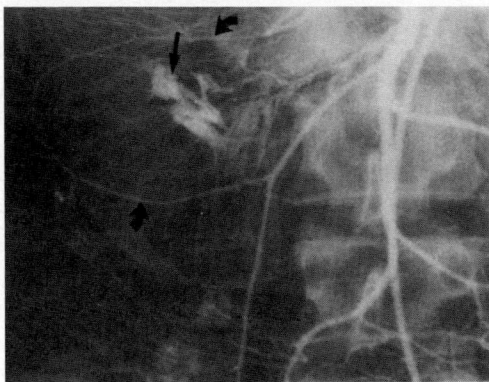

Figure 26–8   Bleeding duodenal ulcer that can be easily confused with bleeding in the proximal transverse colon, seen in an elderly man who presented with bright red rectal bleeding without any history of having vomited blood. Superior mesenteric arteriography demonstrates right-upper-quadrant extravasation (*straight arrow*) surrounded by the right colic (*lower curved arrow*) and the middle colic (*upper curved arrow*) arteries. In view of the clinical history and the proximity of the colic vessels, this duodenal bleed, which actually derived its blood supply from the inferior pancreaticoduodenal artery, could easily be taken for a bleeding lesion in the proximal transverse colon.

The Precise Localization of Small Bowel Bleeding

During superior mesenteric arteriography it is usually very difficult to be sure which loop of small bowel is bleeding. Athanasoulis and other investigators have successfully demonstrated the pathologic segment of bleeding in the small bowel by subselectively catheterizing the specific superior mesenteric arterial branch involved immediately prior to the laparotomy (32,33). After the small bowel has been surgically exposed, methylene blue or Evans blue is injected into the catheter, resulting in a transient staining of the abnormal bowel. If the patient is actively bleeding at the time of the surgery, the isotopic scanning technique developed by Alavi et al. (20) can be used intraoperatively to localize the bleeding site in the small bowel. A technique that places platinum coils at the time of angiography has also been described (34).

ANGIOGRAPHIC TECHNIQUES FOR THE CONTROL OF GASTROINTESTINAL BLEEDING

After angiography has demonstrated a bleeding site, the catheter can be used to diminish flow and thereby control bleeding. This can be accomplished by mechanically obstructing the lumen of the bleeding vessel with embolic material (35–37). If this is not possible because the catheter cannot be advanced distal enough or if the bleeding is diffuse, as occurs in hemorrhagic gastritis, the infusion of a vasoconstrictor into the vessel supplying the bleeding point can be effective in achieving hemostasis.

Pharmacologic Infusion

Selective arterial embolization is effective and safe in controlling gastrointestinal bleeding when the catheter can be positioned close to the bleeding vessel. If arterial embolization is not possible or if the bleeding is diffuse, vasopressin has been shown to be a safe and reliable vasoconstrictor. The vasopressin used for this purpose is an aqueous solution of the pressor principle of the posterior pituitary gland and is relatively free of oxytocic principle. It causes contraction of the smooth muscles of the gastrointestinal tract as well as the vascular bed. These effects are not antagonized by adrenergic blocking agents or prevented by vascular denervation. The antidiuretic properties of vasopressin are important and well known (38).

Since its introduction, vasopressin has been the preferred drug for transcatheter infusion therapy of gastrointestinal bleeding because of its significant and sustained reduction in splanchnic blood flow (6–9). More recently, the prostaglandins have been investigated but to date have been untried in any large clinical series (39). Other vasoconstrictors such as norepinephrine were previously evaluated, but because they do not have sustained actions, they have never become popular for this form of therapy.

Vasopressin's action is direct and immediate. A repeat arteriogram obtained 20 minutes after the infusion is begun will accurately determine the effectiveness of the therapy. Also, the dose of vasopressin can be modified so as to produce various degrees of vasoconstriction and thereby cause a more controlled and reversible ischemia than that of mechanical embolic therapy.

The selective infusion of vasopressin into a bleeding splanchnic vessel at the dose of 0.2 unit per minute is generally sufficient to stop gastrointestinal arterial or mucosal bleeding. Extensive experimental and clinical experience with this method has shown it to be safe when used in the gastrointestinal tract with little danger of significant organ ischemia. Even direct infusions into the hepatic (40,41) or splenic artery are well tolerated, so infusion of the celiac axis is a viable alternative when more subselective catheterization of the left gastric artery is not technically possible.

The use of vasopressin is particularly successful in gastric mucosal bleeding when the left gastric artery is selectively infused. If the bleeding is coming from the small or large bowel, the selective infusion of the main superior or inferior mesenteric artery is generally sufficient, obviating subselective catheterization of the specific branch supplying the diseased segment.

Vasopressin diluted in either saline or 5% dextrose and water is usually infused at a constant rate of 0.2 unit per minute for 20 minutes. A repeat arteriogram is obtained to evaluate the success of the therapy. If no further bleeding is demonstrated on the subsequent arteriogram, the infusion is continued at 0.2 unit per minute. If bleeding persists, however, the infusion can be increased to 0.4 unit per minute for another 20 minutes, followed by a repeat arteriogram.

Failure to control the bleeding using 0.4 unit per minute indicates that the bleeding is unlikely to be controlled by vasopressin and that alternative methods of therapy should be considered. The angiogram obtained 20 minutes after the start of the infusion is analyzed to be sure that (1) moderate reduction in caliber of the infused vessels has occurred with preservation of good forward flow into the capillary and venous phases, (2) there is still filling of branches in the area of the bleeding point, and (3) there is no further extravasation.

If all these criteria are met, a pressure dressing is applied around the catheter entry site, and the patient can be sent back to the intensive care unit for careful monitoring. If there is no clinical evidence of recurrent bleeding, the initial infusion rate is continued for 12–24 hours and then reduced by 50% for an additional 24 hours. The vasopressin infusion can then be stopped, but the catheter is generally kept in place and its patency maintained by the infusion of either normal saline or dextrose and water for another 12 hours. If the patient remains clinically stable, the catheter can then be removed. If bleeding recurs as the vasoconstrictor dose is being tapered, a return to the initial dose rate usually controls it.

Because vasopressin is also a coronary artery vasoconstrictor, older patients may have nitroglycerin administered sublingually, intravenously, or, more commonly, by a skin patch (42–46).

The intra-arterial infusion of vasopressin at the doses described should be well tolerated by most patients. After initial abdominal cramping, which may last for 15–30 minutes, the infusion should be pain free. If the patient complains of continuous abdominal pain during the course of the treatment, the infusion should be stopped and the patient reexamined. Pain may be a result of the catheter tip wedging into a small mesenteric arterial branch or the catheter having slipped into the abdominal aorta.

ROLE OF ANGIOGRAPHY IN THE MANAGEMENT OF ESOPHAGEAL VARICEAL BLEEDING

Before its intra-arterial use for gastrointestinal bleeding, vasopressin was injected intravenously in fairly large doses (20 units over 20 minutes) in an attempt to reduce portal pressure during the treatment of variceal bleeding (47). Although bleeding esophageal varices cannot be constricted by direct infusion of pharmacologic agents, vasopressin is a potent splanchnic vasoconstrictor that causes a significant reduction in mesenteric blood flow and, consequently, portal pressure. Because a relatively large dose of vasopressin given intravenously can be associated with side effects, including decreased cardiac output and coronary artery vasoconstriction, the selective mesenteric artery infusion of vasopressin appeared to be an attractive alternative when it

was first introduced in 1971 (48). This technique of continuously infusing the superior mesenteric artery with doses of vasopressin at 0.2 unit per minute was highly effective in controlling variceal bleeding and could be maintained for long periods of time without the development of tachyphylaxis. It was less efficacious in controlling bleeding in patients with advanced cirrhosis (49), probably because of the increased arterialization of the portal system from the hepatic artery in patients with severe liver disease. In 1973, Barr et al. (50) showed that vasopressin, infused intravenously at the same low dose rates used in the superior mesenteric artery, reduces portal pressure by 40–50%. The systemic side effects with the low-dose intravenous infusions are about the same as those with the intra-arterial infusion. Johnson et al. (51) reported a randomized clinical study confirming that the systemic infusions of vasopressin at low dose rates were as effective as intra-arterial infusions at the same rate in controlling variceal bleeding. Therefore, there appears to be no advantage to the selective intra-arterial infusion of vasopressin into the superior mesenteric artery in the treatment of bleeding esophageal varices.

The administration of propanolol to lower the portosystemic gradient has been used as a medical therapy for the control of variceal bleeding (52). Controlled trials have also shown the benefit of long-standing beta blockade for the prophylaxis of variceal bleeding in patients with portal hypertension (53–55). Further techniques, including endoscopic, surgical, and transjugular intrahepatic portosystemic shunt (TIPS) for the treatment of bleeding esophageal varices, are described in detail in Chapter 31.

The percutaneous transhepatic approach to the portal vein was popularized in 1974 by Lunderquist (56,57). This technique gives direct access to the portal vein and its tributaries. In the absence of marked ascites the procedure is not technically difficult, and the risk of bleeding from the point of entry is negligible. The more common complication involved in this study is the formation of thrombi in the portal vein as a result of the introduction of the catheter (58,59). After the catheter has been introduced into the portal vein, the coronary vein can generally be selectively catheterized without too much difficulty. Various embolic materials can then be introduced into the coronary gastric veins to interrupt flow to the varices rapidly and to thereby control the bleeding (Figure 26–9) (60).

Unfortunately, follow-up studies have shown that varices become patent within 1–4 weeks, and permanent occlusion seldom results (61). Control of the bleeding by this technique is generally temporary and allows the patient to be stabilized and prepared for elective surgery. Various materials have been used for occlusion of the coronary veins, including gelatin sponges (Gelfoam), steel coils, balloons, and even bucrylate. At the present time, transhepatic variceal embolization is seldom used unless it is combined with transjugular intrahepatic portosystemic shunts.

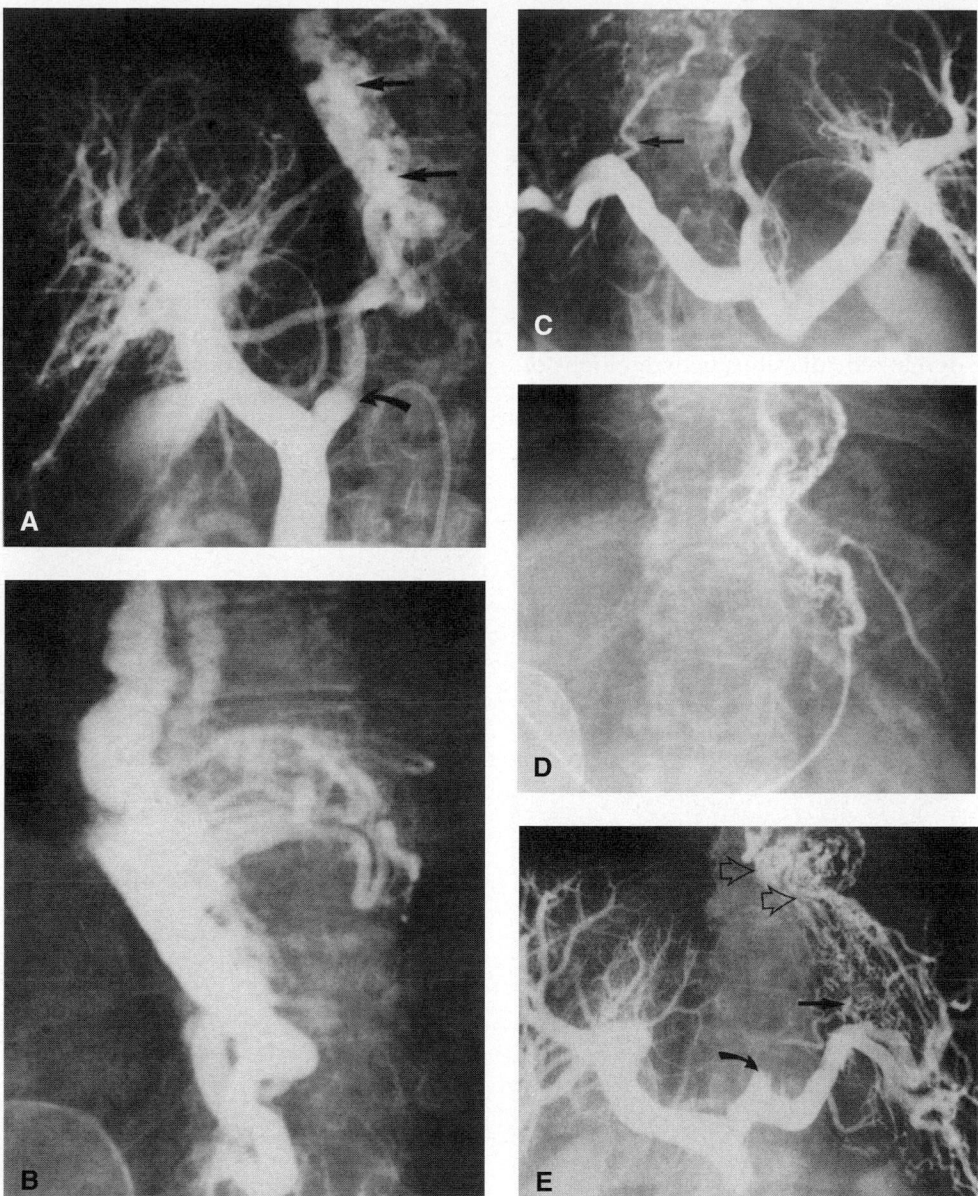

Figure 26–9   Bleeding esophageal varices treated by percutaneous transhepatic catheterization of the portal vein and embolization of the coronary veins. **A.** Direct portography following percutaneous catheterization of the portal vein demonstrates a large coronary vein (*curved arrow*) supplying large gastric and esophageal varices (*straight arrows*). **B.** Selective catheterization of the coronary vein defines with greater clarity the large gastric and esophageal varices. **C.** Following embolization of the coronary vein with Gelfoam, repeat direct portography demonstrates occlusion of the coronary vein. However, there is now filling of a short gastric vein (*arrow*) that appears to be supplying the gastric varices. **D.** Selective catheterization of the short gastric vein demonstrates that it is, indeed, feeding the gastric and esophageal varices. This vessel was embolized with Gelfoam. After embolization of the coronary and short gastric veins, the patient stopped bleeding. **E.** Repeat direct portography performed several days later when the patient's bleeding recurred demonstrates that the coronary vein (*curved arrow*) has remained occluded, as has the short gastric vein (*straight arrow*). Large gastric and esophageal varices (*open arrows*) are now being supplied by multiple gastric veins originating from the splenic vein in the area of the hilus of the spleen.

BLEEDING MESENTERIC VARICES

On the parietal surface of the gut, extremely small, delicate venous communications join the portal branches of the mesenteric vein to the systemic venous channels in the retroperitoneum and abdominal wall. Most varices from portal hypertension occur in the esophagus, rectum, and umbilicus. Some patients, however, have intestinal varices as a result of dilatation of these preexisting intestinal branches—particularly patients who have had previous surgery and have developed adhesions between loops of bowel and the abdominal wall. In patients with portal hypertension, the varices may become exceedingly large

and capable of bleeding in a manner similar to that of esophageal varices (62,63).

Varicosities may also grow across adhesions in the pelvis, allowing for decompression of the portal vein by the gonadal systemic veins. The pelvic adhesions may be the result of either inflammatory disease or previous surgery (Figure 26–10). Localized varicosities involving the superior mesenteric vein and its branches can occur secondary to pancreatitis or neoplasms of the pancreas that invade the superior mesenteric vein or to neoplasms of the gastrointestinal tract that secondarily occlude mesenteric veins (Figure 26–11). Intestinal varices have been seen as a result of the extensive desmoplastic reaction that occurs in the root of the mesentery secondary to carcinoid tumors (64,65).

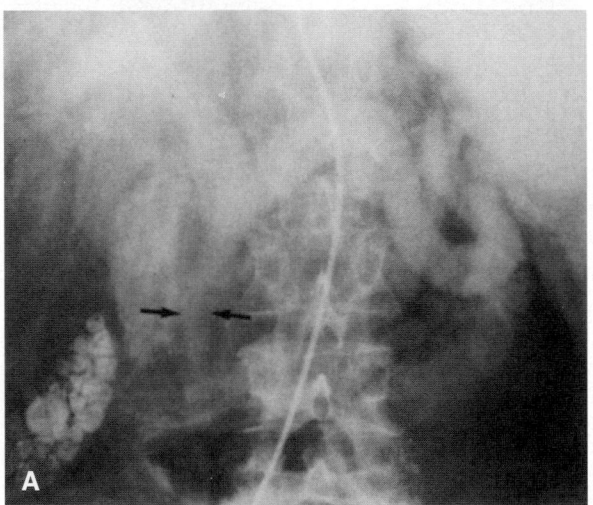

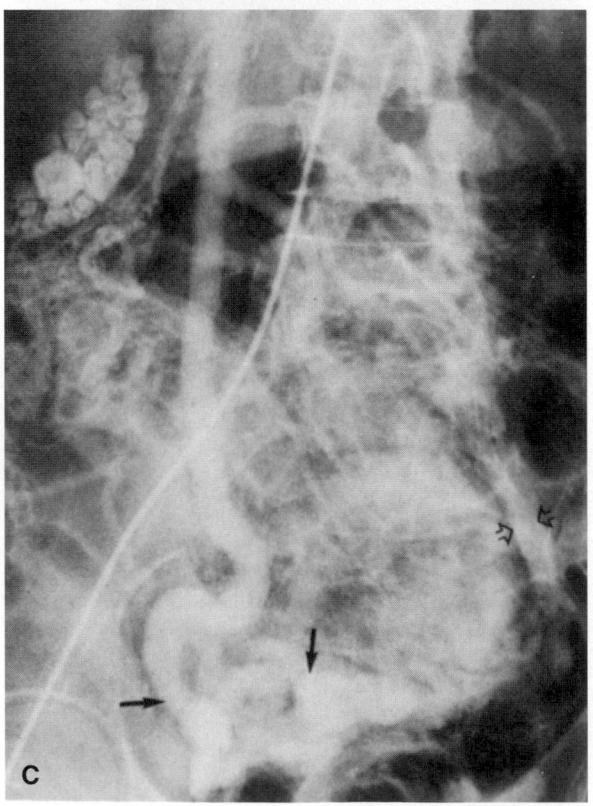

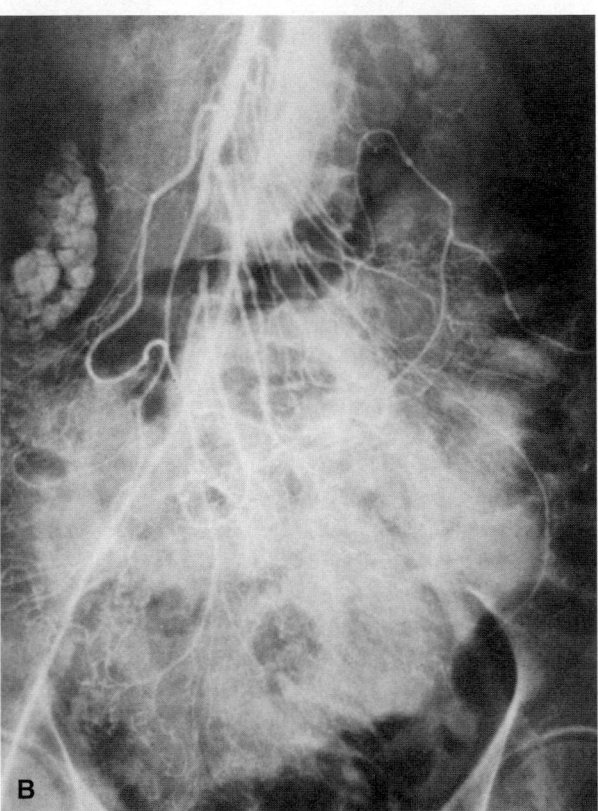

Figure 26–10 Bleeding mesenteric varices in a 68-year-old woman with cirrhosis referred for mesenteric arteriography because of lower gastrointestinal bleeding. **A.** The venous phase of the selective splenic arteriogram demonstrates patency of the splenic and portal veins. There is retrograde filling of the superior mesenteric vein (*arrows*). **B.** A selective superior mesenteric arteriogram fails to demonstrate evidence of an arterial or mucosal bleeding site. **C.** During the venous phase of the superior mesenteric arteriogram, retrograde flow is seen in the superior mesenteric vein draining into large pelvic varicosities (*solid arrows*). The pelvic varices decompress the mesenteric vein by the left gonadal vein (*open arrows*). The patient had had pelvic surgery many years earlier. After this examination, the patient was re-explored, and at surgery, adhesions containing large varicosities were seen extending between the pelvic organs and the ileal loops of the small bowel. In the resected specimen of the ileum, one of the large mucosal veins was bleeding as a result of an overlying area of mucosal ulceration.

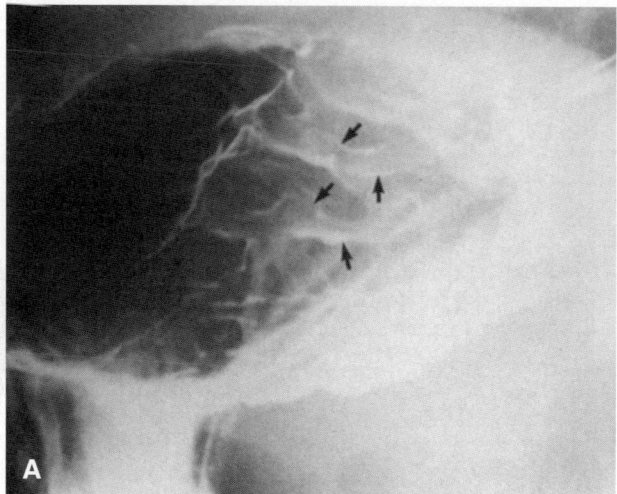

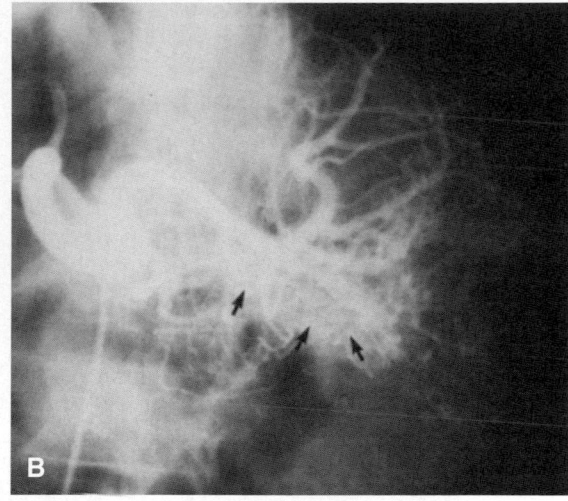

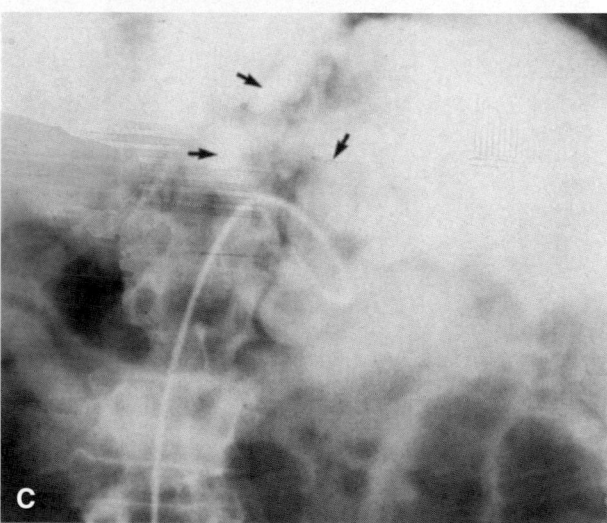

Figure 26–11   A 66-year-old man presented with a history of hematemesis. **A.** An upper gastrointestinal series with the patient in a steep right posterior oblique position demonstrates gastric varices (*arrows*) without any evidence of esophageal varices. This picture suggested splenic vein obstruction; the patient was referred for angiography. **B.** Selective splenic arteriography demonstrates tumor vessels in the distal portion of the pancreas extending into the hilus of the spleen (*arrows*). **C.** In the venous phase of the splenic arteriogram, multiple gastric varices (*arrows*) are seen draining into a patent portal vein. The patient had had a left nephrectomy 15 years earlier for a renal cell carcinoma, and the tumor disclosed in the tail of the pancreas on the present examination was renal cell carcinoma metastatic to the pancreas, causing splenic vein occlusion and gastric varices.

ARTERIAL EMBOLIZATION

Arterial embolization is performed by positioning the arterial catheter as close as possible to the site of extravasation and carefully injecting embolic material to block the artery. The very rich collateral arterial supply to the gastrointestinal tract usually protects these organs from significant ischemia and infarction after embolization of the bleeding vessel (Figure 26–12).

This method is usually successful in stopping the bleeding; however, therapeutic failures may arise when bleeding takes place in an area that has a dual arterial blood supply (66). The occlusion of only one limb of such a vascular arcade may result in failure to control bleeding because the abnormal segment continues to be supplied by a second arterial limb (Figure 26–13). Successful control, therefore, may require individual treatment of each limb, whether by vasopressin infusion or occlusion (Figure 26–14). A control arteriogram is essential to confirm cessation of previously demonstrated bleeding. If a dual blood supply exists, it may be necessary to embolize both sides of an arcade.

Examples of vascular arcades that may be significant in the angiographic management of bleeding include (1) middle colic–left colic artery anastomosis at the splenic flexure of the colon, (2) superior pancreaticoduodenal–inferior pancreaticoduodenal arterial arcades in the duodenum, (3) left gastric–right gastric arcade along the lesser curvature of the stomach, and (4) right gastroepiploic–left gastroepiploic arterial communications along the greater curvature of the stomach.

Various embolic materials have been tried in a search for a safe, effective, and simple agent (67) (see Chapter 10). Gelfoam, a slowly absorbed gelatin sponge, is the most widely used embolic material in the treatment of gastrointestinal bleeding (68). Although autologous blood clot has the advantage of providing very small emboli that lodge peripherally and thereby lessen the chance of collateral bleeding, this form of control tends to be only temporary because of lysis of the clot, generally within 12–14 hours (69,70). Clots that are pretreated with thrombin, aminocaproic acid, or oxidized cellulose (Oxcel) persist for a longer time. Ivalon particles provide

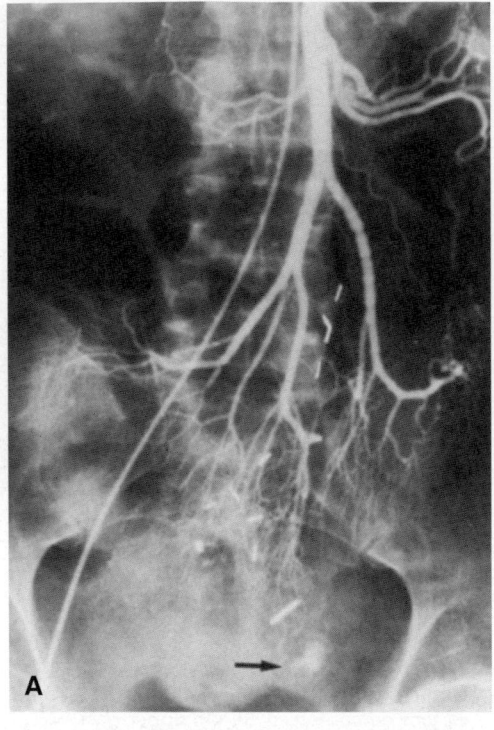

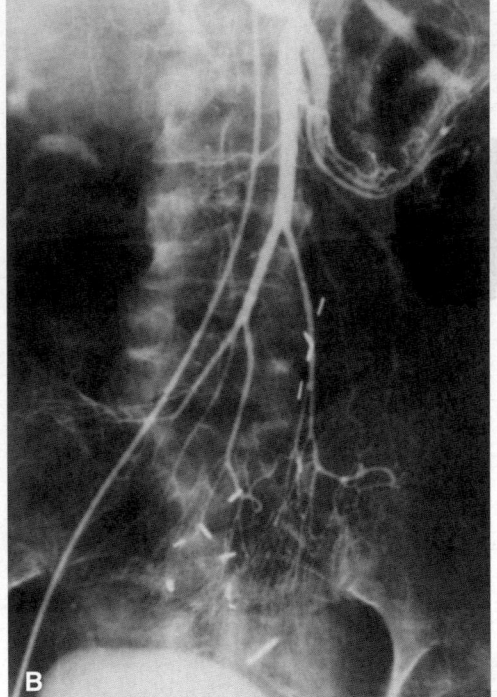

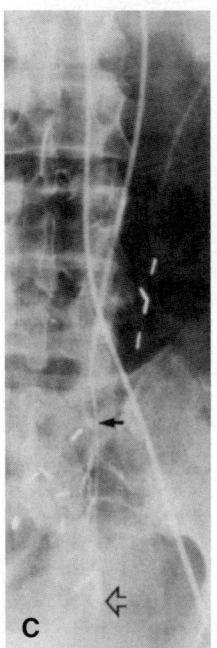

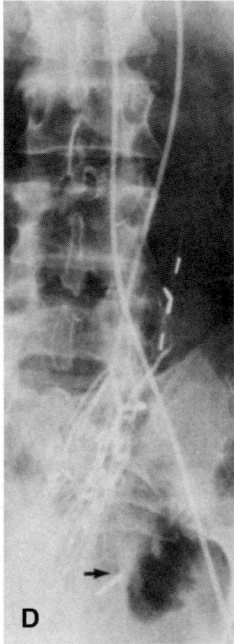

Figure 26–12   Bleeding ileitis in a patient with a long-standing history of ileitis and multiple surgical procedures, referred to angiography because of lower gastrointestinal bleeding. Because the pelvic ileal loops were bound together by multiple adhesions, the patient was a poor surgical candidate. **A.** Selective superior mesenteric arteriography demonstrates extravasation of contrast material (*arrow*) from one of the pelvic ileal branches. **B.** Bleeding was controlled by the infusion of 0.2 unit of vasopressin per minute into the superior mesenteric artery. There was, however, great difficulty in weaning the patient from the vasopressin, and each time the dose was reduced, the bleeding recurred. **C.** Because of the desire of the clinicians to avoid surgery, selective embolization of the bleeding vessel was attempted. The catheter was advanced into the small jejunal artery (*solid arrow*) supplying the bleeding site, and a small hand injection of contrast material once again shows extravasation (*open arrow*). **D.** After embolization with a small Gelfoam plug, the bleeding was controlled, and repeat arteriography with the catheter partially withdrawn shows very selective occlusion of the small ileal branch (*arrow*). The patient did not rebleed and was discharged from the hospital without having to undergo an operation.

even longer-lasting occlusions but are more difficult to use (71–74).

Rapidly setting tissue adhesives such as isobutyl 2-cyanoacrylate (bucrylate) produce long-term occlusion (75–77). These rapidly setting glues are liquid monomers that undergo rapid polymerization and solidification when they come in contact with charged ions in the blood. They are difficult to use and must be administered through a coaxial catheter system.

Double-lumen balloon-tipped catheters can be used for the temporary control of gastrointestinal bleeding (78,79). They can also be of great value with injection of embolic material, preventing possible reflux of emboli to more distant sites (80). Small, detachable balloons are at present under clinical trial (81). These devices have some advantage in that they are flow directed and can be retrieved and their position altered if they are not producing the desired effect. They give the angiographer much more control in

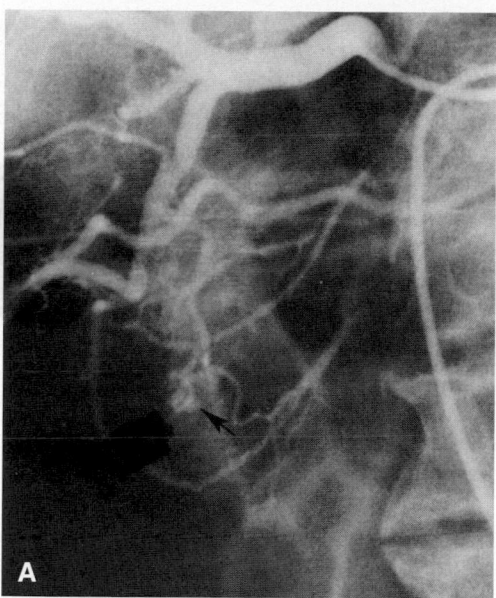 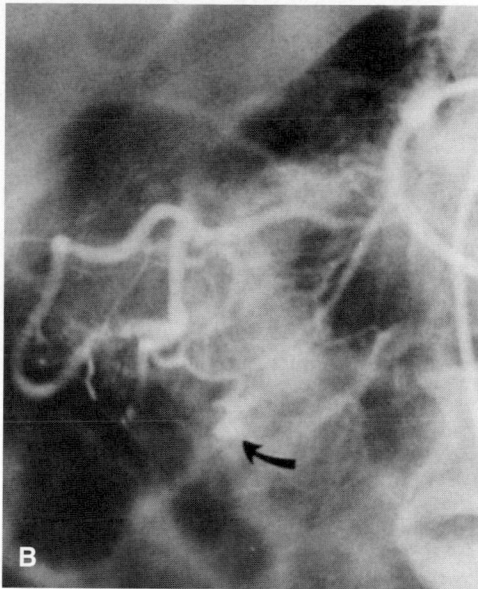

Figure 26–13 Dual blood supply of a bleeding duodenal ulcer. **A.** After selective hepatic arteriography, extravasation in the duodenum (*arrow*) can be identified as coming from a small branch of the superior pancreaticoduodenal artery. **B.** Selective inferior pancreaticoduodenal arteriography demonstrates the same point of extravasation (*arrow*). In cases like these, infusions into both superior and inferior pancreaticoduodenal arteries may be necessary if angiographic control is attempted.

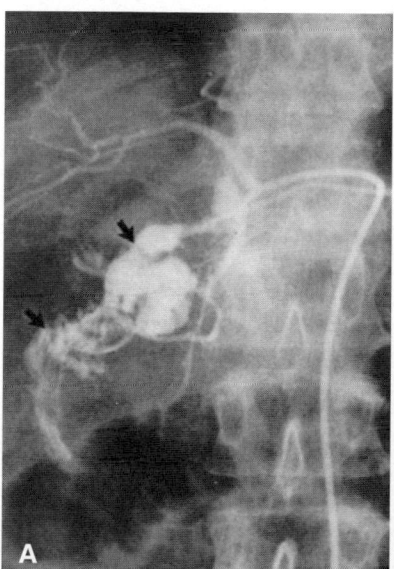 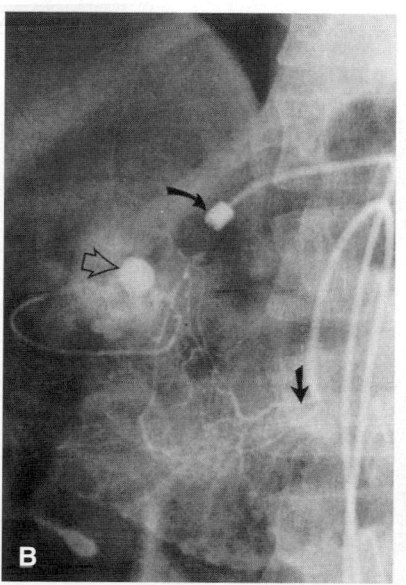 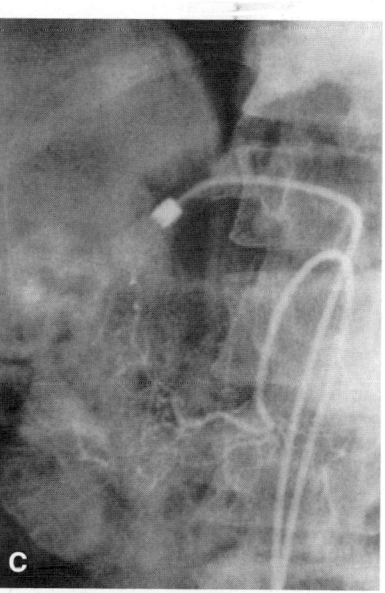

Figure 26–14 Bleeding duodenal ulcer controlled by angiographically treating both limbs of an arcade. **A.** Selective gastroduodenal arteriogram demonstrates massive extravasation of contrast material (*arrows*) into the duodenum from a branch of the superior pancreaticoduodenal artery. **B.** A balloon catheter (*curved arrow*) was placed through the angiographic catheter and is occluding the gastroduodenal artery. A second catheter was placed in the inferior pancreaticoduodenal branch of the superior mesenteric artery (*straight arrow*), and on injection of this vessel, bleeding is once again demonstrated in the duodenal ulcer (*open arrow*). **C.** Embolization of the inferior pancreaticoduodenal artery with small Gelfoam plugs successfully interrupted the inferior pancreaticoduodenal arcade, and the bleeding was controlled.

occluding a vessel, and the danger of inadvertent occlusion, always associated with emboli, is thereby eliminated. One disadvantage of balloon-tipped catheters is that they occlude bleeding vessels much more proximally than do injected embolic materials. Because of the hemodynamics of bleeding in the presence of a rich collateral blood flow, distal occlusion is a desirable feature.

Wool- or nylon-tufted stainless steel coils have been successful in permanently occluding large vessels where Gelfoam emboli are not suitable. Although the original Gianturco coils (82) had to be delivered through a relatively large Teflon catheter, smaller coils are now available that can be delivered through smaller, more versatile catheters (Figure 26–15); thus, their field of application is extended.

ANGIOGRAPHIC CONTROL OF GASTROINTESTINAL HEMORRHAGE FROM SPECIFIC ARTERIAL SITES

Esophageal Bleeding

Esophageal tumors, esophagitis, and hiatus hernia rarely cause massive bleeding. When this does occur, however, angiography is able to demonstrate the bleeding site if the bleeding segment of the esophagus derives its blood supply from branches of the left gastric artery (Figure 26–16). Bleeding of the upper and middle portions of the esophagus generally cannot be angiographically demonstrated because

of the difficulty associated with catheterizing the appropriate vessels. If the bleeding site can be identified angiographically, selective arterial embolization or the selective arterial infusion of vasopressin almost always controls the bleeding. Mallory-Weiss tears at the cardioesophageal junction as well as bleeding esophagitis are readily responsive to vasopressin infusions (Figure 26–17) and embolic therapy.

Gastric Mucosal Hemorrhage

Acute ulcerations of the stomach and duodenum are frequently the cause of significant gastrointestinal bleeding. These ulcerations may be part of any of the following conditions: (1) stress ulcerations, (2) drug- or alcohol-induced gastritis, (3) idiopathic gastritis, (4) curling ulcers seen in burn patients, and (5) uremia.

These lesions are being seen less frequently than in the past because of the aggressive use of histamine H_2-receptor antagonists by surgeons and gastroenterologists. When gastric acidity is decreased, patients are less prone to develop mucosal ulcerations. When ulcerations do occur, they tend to be acute and multiple and may be the cause of massive gastrointestinal bleeding.

Patients who develop ulcerations of the gastrointestinal tract following severe physiologic stress usually have ulcers in the stomach, but in some cases they extend up to the esophagus or into the duodenum. The second and third portions of the duodenum may be another site of mucosal ulcerations, and in some patients these may be the only

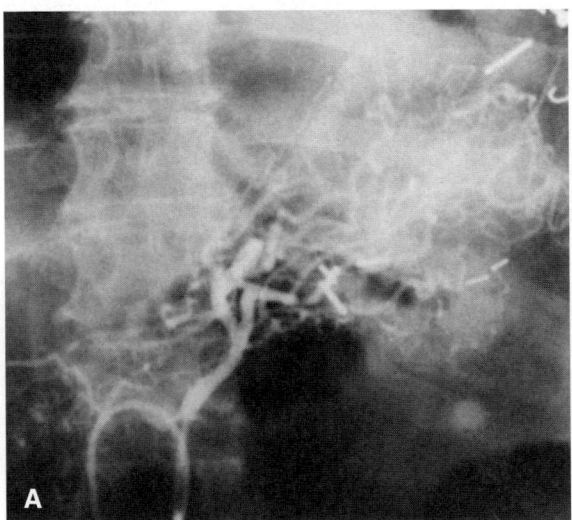 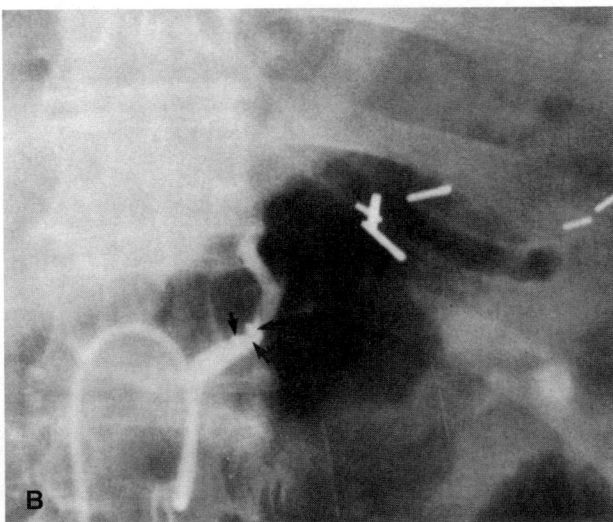

Figure 26–15   Hemorrhagic gastritis treated with Gelfoam embolization and proximal occlusion of the left gastric artery with a nylon-tufted steel coil. **A.** The patient was referred for angiography because of upper gastrointestinal bleeding following pancreatic surgery. Selective left gastric arteriography demonstrates a marked hyperemia involving the entire upper portion of the stomach consistent with the diagnosis of hemorrhagic gastritis. Oozing around the catheter site in the groin made it impossible to maintain a continuous infusion of vasopressin, and embolization techniques were therefore resorted to. **B.** Gelfoam pellets were embolized into the left gastric artery, and the proximal portion of the left gastric artery was occluded by inserting a nylon-tufted Gianturco coil (*arrows*).

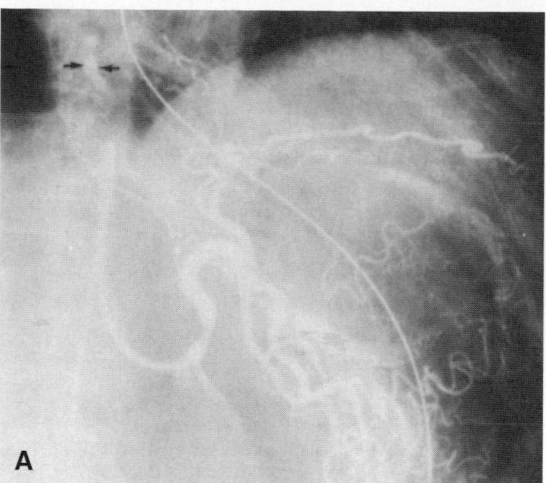
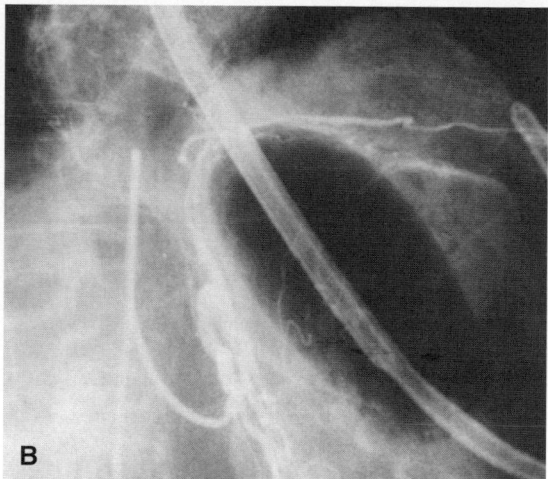

Figure 26–16 A 91-year-old man with a long history of a hiatal hernia was referred for arteriography because of massive hematemesis. **A.** A selective left gastric arteriogram demonstrates arterial extravasation in the distal esophagus (*arrows*). In addition, there is marked hyperemia of the entire stomach, consistent with a gastritis. **B.** Selective left gastric arteriography during infusion of 0.2 unit per minute of vasopressin shows vasoconstriction of the peripheral branches of the left gastric artery and cessation of the bleeding in the distal esophagus. The bleeding was controlled in this patient, and surgery was not required.

ulcers that are actively bleeding (Figure 26–18). For reasons that are not completely understood, the ulcers in the second and third portions of the duodenum are seen more often in patients who have had recent cardiac surgery and who are receiving digitalis (83).

The angiographic appearance of bleeding stress ulceration may be that of massive extravasation in an otherwise normal-appearing stomach (Figure 26–3) or duodenum. The bleeding of gastritis, on the other hand, may appear as multiple areas of extravasation in a vascular bed that is diffusely hyperemic (Figure 26–19) (6).

Because the therapy in all these lesions is directed toward achieving hemostasis, superselective intra-arterial embolization or infusion of vasopressin is a highly attractive alternative

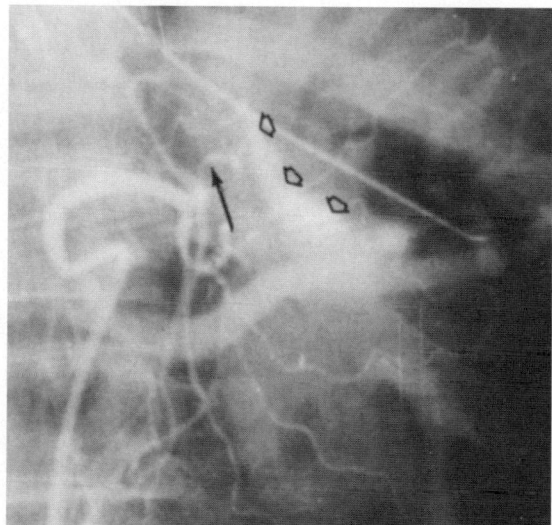
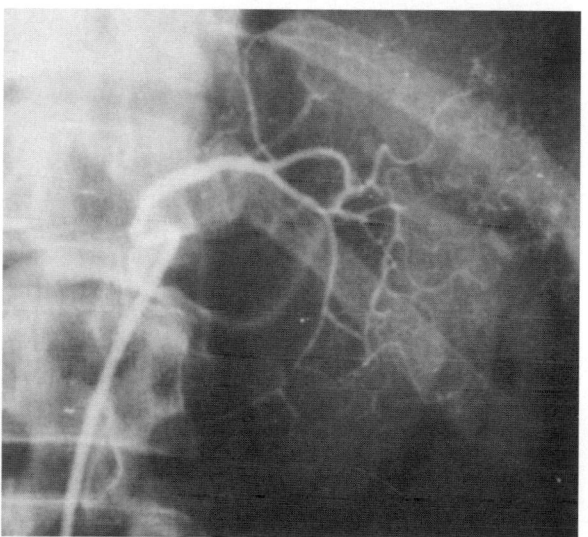

Figure 26–17 Bleeding Mallory-Weiss tear at the cardioesophageal junction controlled by the infusion of vasopressin into the left gastric artery. **A.** Selective left gastric arteriography demonstrates extravasation of contrast material from a branch of the left gastric artery (*solid arrow*) into the stomach (*open arrows*). **B.** During the infusion of 0.2 unit per minute of vasopressin, repeat arteriogram shows opacification of the left gastric artery and its branches without any further evidence of extravasation. The patient had an uneventful recovery with no recurrences of hemorrhage. (Reprinted with permission from Baum S, Nusbaum M. The control of gastrointestinal hemorrhage by selective mesenteric arterial infusion of vasopressin. Radiology 1971;98:497.)

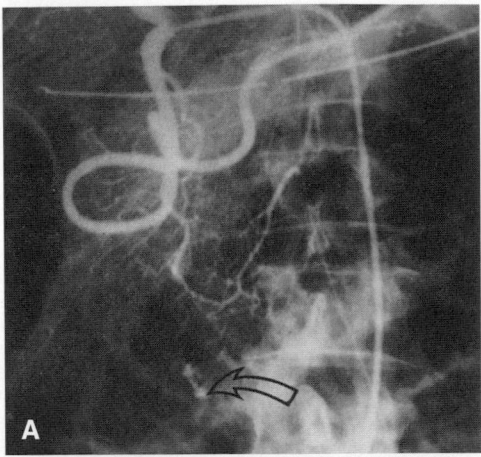

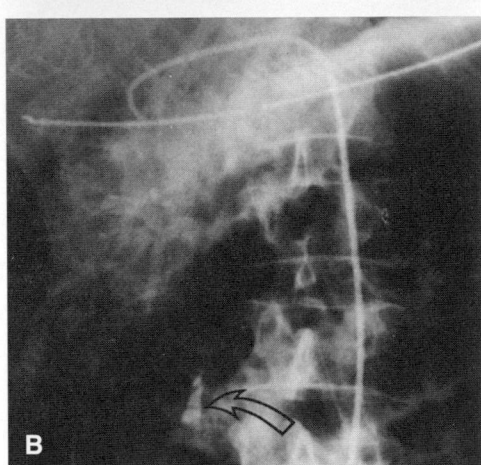

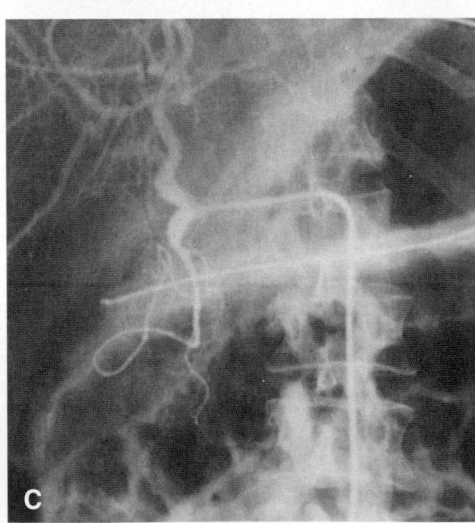

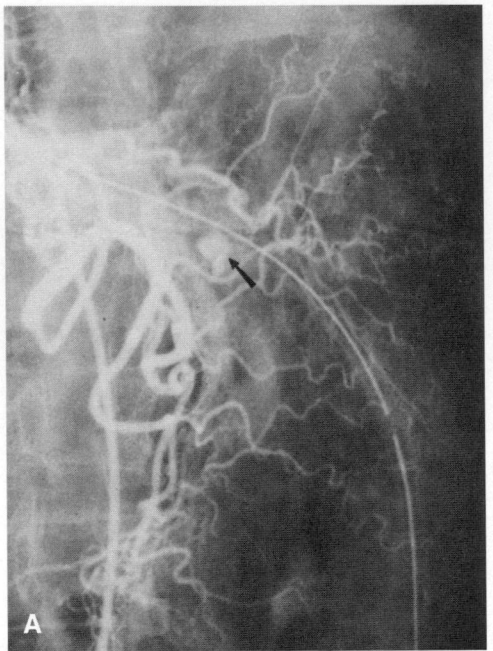

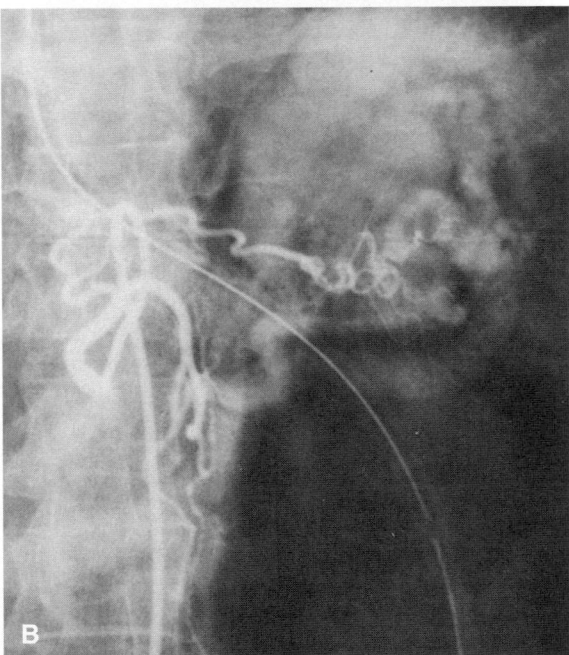

Figure 26–18   Bleeding stress ulcer at the junction of the second and third portions of the duodenum. **A.** Selective gastroduodenal arteriogram of a patient presenting with massive upper gastrointestinal bleeding 4 days after aortic valve replacement demonstrates arterial bleeding at the junction of the second and third portions of the duodenum (*arrow*). **B.** During the late capillary phase of the study, persistent contrast material remains (*arrow*), outlining mucosal folds. **C.** Control of the bleeding stress ulcer was obtained by the infusion of 0.2 unit of vasopressin per minute into the gastroduodenal artery. Repeat arteriography shows peripheral vasoconstriction without any evidence of extravasation. The patient had no further clinical evidence of bleeding from this site.

Figure 26–19   Bleeding hemorrhagic gastritis in a 60-year-old woman who had had multiple surgical procedures for regional enteritis. Postoperatively, the patient began to bleed massively from the gastrointestinal tract. Endoscopy showed several ulcers in the gastric fundus. **A.** Selective left gastric arteriography demonstrates extravasation from a branch of the left gastric artery (*arrow*). **B.** Repeat left gastric arteriography during the infusion of 0.2 unit per minute of vasopressin shows constriction of peripheral arterial branches without further evidence of extravasation. The infusion was continued for 2 days, and the bleeding was clinically controlled.

to surgery when patients do not stop bleeding on medical therapy. Despite the theory that stress ulceration is ischemic in origin, experience has been that stress ulcers as well as ulcerations associated with gastritis heal following arterial embolization or during the infusion of vasopressin, and rebleeding usually does not occur. The selective infusion of vasopressin into the left gastric artery has been reported to control bleeding of this sort in more than 80% of cases (84–86). Of this group, about 15% of patients have recurrent bleeding after the initial control, and these patients are suitable candidates for repeat treatment.

Peptic Ulceration of the Stomach and Duodenum

Bleeding that results from an erosion into a small branch vessel can generally be controlled by arterial embolization or vasopressin infusion of the left gastric, gastroduodenal, or superior pancreaticoduodenal arteries. If there is erosion into a main vessel such as a gastroduodenal artery, vasopressin

infusion has usually been unsuccessful (87,88), and in this setting, embolization of the bleeding vessel may be the only way to achieve hemostasis (Figures 26–20 through 26–22) (69).

In most peptic ulcer patients, angiography is only a temporary measure to control bleeding and is clearly not the definitive form of therapy. Surgery is still required to deal with the basic problem and prevent recurrence of the disease. Excessive time should not, therefore, be spent on the angiographic procedure unless the patient is unsuitable for surgery. The introduction of histamine antagonists such as cimetidine for the treatment of peptic ulcer disease has caused a reevaluation of the indications for surgery (89). The angiographic control of bleeding coupled with cimetidine therapy may, in fact, provide the definitive answer in some patients.

Anastomotic Ulcers

Selective mesenteric arteriography can be used to demonstrate bleeding from an anastomotic ulcer at the site of gastrojejunostomy (90,91). The bleeding site is usually

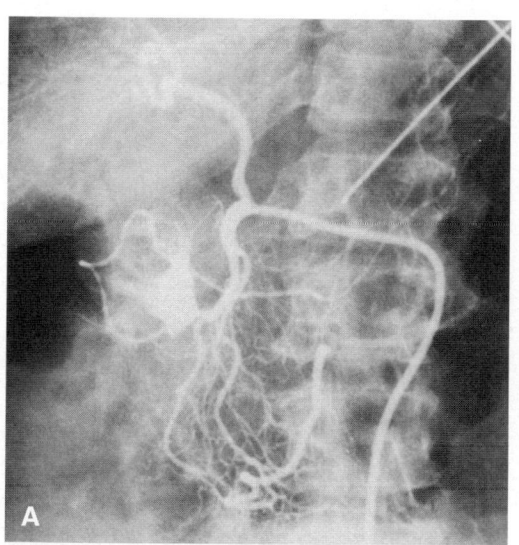

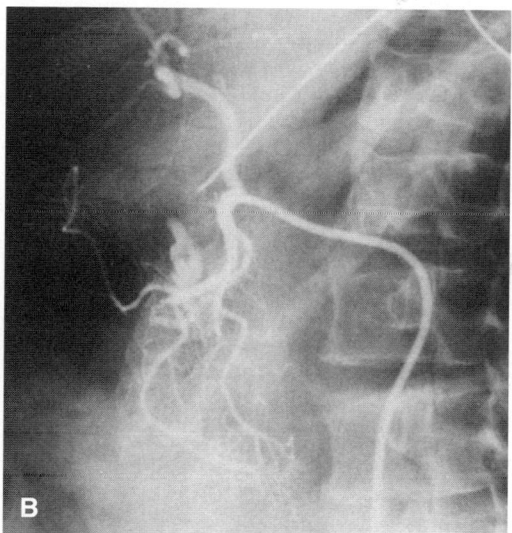

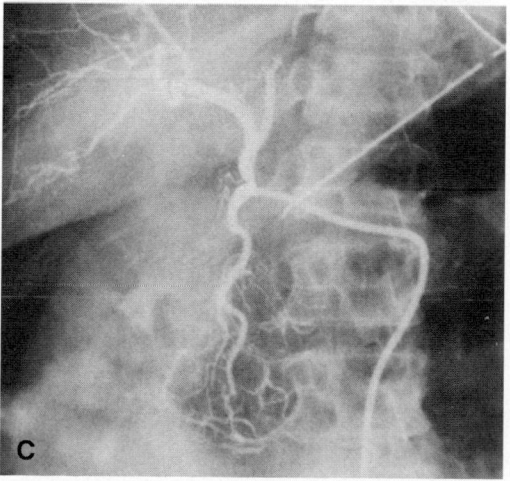

Figure 26–20 Actively bleeding duodenal ulcer controlled by the selective embolization of a small amount of autologous blood clot. **A.** Arterial phase of a selective gastroduodenal arteriogram shows massive extravasation from a branch of the superior pancreaticoduodenal artery. **B.** Infusion of 0.4 unit per minute of vasopressin was unable to stop the bleeding clinically, and on the repeat arteriogram, continued extravasation can be seen. **C.** Several strands of autologous clot were embolized into both the anterior and the posterior pancreaticoduodenal arcades, thereby disrupting the normal collateralization from the inferior pancreaticoduodenal artery. In addition, the superior pancreaticoduodenal artery was occluded. The bleeding stopped clinically, and a repeat arteriogram failed to show any evidence of extravasation.

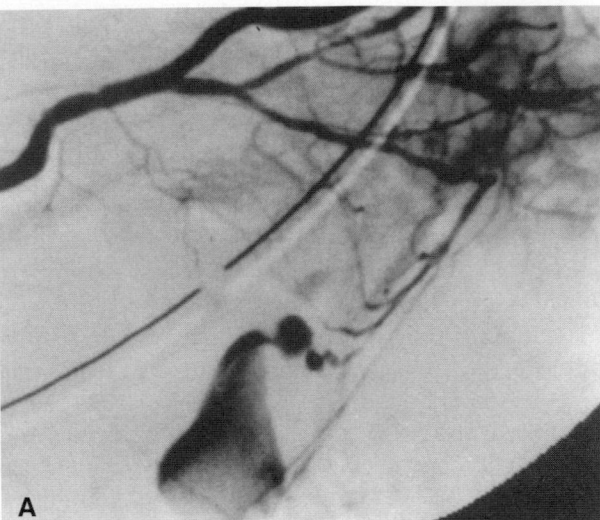
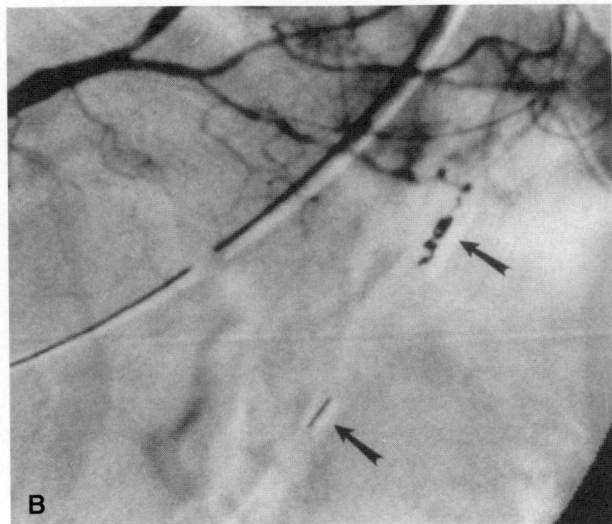

Figure 26–21   Upper gastrointestinal bleeding from a greater curvature ulcer. The patient had undergone previous surgery, and the gastroduodenal artery was ligated. **A.** Selective splenic arteriogram shows massive contrast extravasation from the left gastroepiploic artery. **B.** Splenic arteriogram after embolization fails to demonstrate any extravasation. A microcatheter was used to deposit microcoils (*arrows*) in the gastroepiploic artery proximal and distal to the bleeding site. The bleeding stopped and did not recur.

supplied by a jejunal branch of the superior mesenteric artery (Figure 26–23) and can frequently be controlled by infusing vasopressin into the superior mesenteric artery. After gastric surgery, many collateral vessels are ligated, possibly making embolic therapy dangerous. In addition, embolization requires subselective catheterization of the appropriate feeding vessel, which is difficult to accomplish in this particular group of patients.

Postoperative Hemorrhage

Bleeding caused by indwelling tubes or slipped ligatures can often be definitively controlled by vasopressin infusion or embolic therapy, thus avoiding the inconvenience and hazard of reexploration and major abdominal surgery (92,93). Further, since most of the patients do not have an underlying disease responsible for the bleeding, the therapy is directed only at controlling the hemorrhage. This method of treatment has also proved helpful after hemorrhage from endoscopic biopsies during colonoscopy (Figure 26–24).

Diverticular Bleeding

The complication of bleeding has been reported to occur in about 10–30% of patients with colonic diverticulosis (94,95). In most patients the blood loss is small, and the bleeding stops when the patient is put at rest. Persistent severe diverticular bleeding, however, may require emergency operative treatment. Because this is a disease of the

elderly, emergency colectomy carries extremely high morbidity and mortality rates (96).

Establishing the diagnosis of hemorrhage from colonic diverticula by nonarteriographic techniques is difficult and is usually done by exclusion. Emergency mesenteric arteriography during the time of the actual bleeding episode is by far the best method for accurate localization of the bleeding site. The only other nonangiographic technique that has proved of significant value is radionuclide scanning with ^{99m}Tc sulfur colloid (Figure 26–1) or Tc-99m red blood cell (15,97).

Mesenteric arteriography can localize the site of bleeding to the right or left colon (Figures 26–25 and 26–26). Bleeding demonstrated angiographically is found more commonly in the ascending and transverse colon. In one series, 75% of patients with massive diverticular bleeding had the bleeding site localized to the right of the splenic flexure (98,99).

Once the extravasation of contrast material has been demonstrated, superselective embolization after advancing the catheter into the bleeding artery or the selective infusion of vasopressin into the superior or inferior mesenteric artery is successful in controlling the bleeding in approximately 80–90% of the patients treated (100–103). After the bleeding is controlled and the catheter removed, management of the patients remains controversial. If bleeding recurs, it usually does so within the first week after the angiographic treatment. The long-term follow-up of patients treated by vasopressin infusion suggests that after the first week, these patients are probably no more likely to

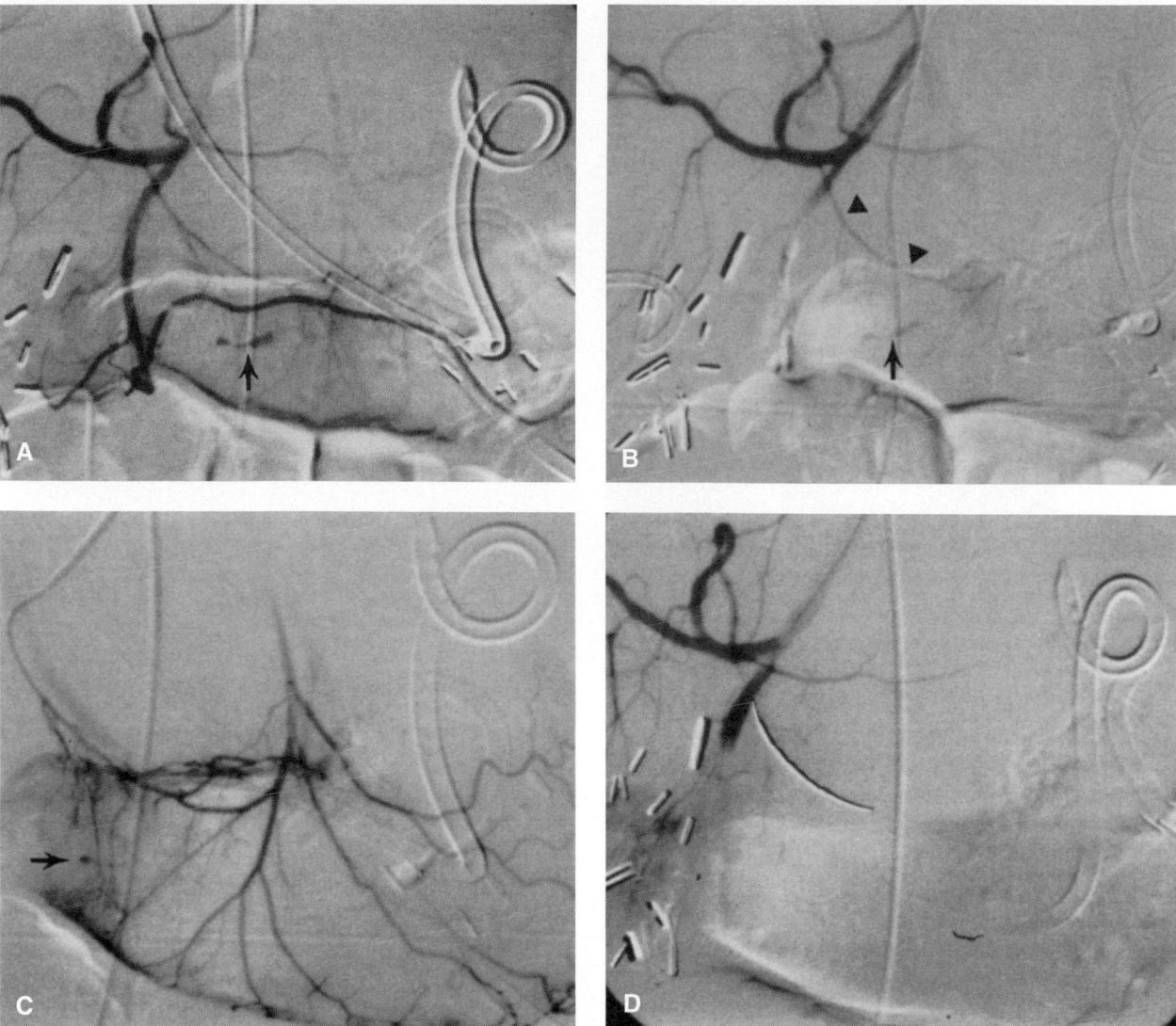

Figure 26–22 Upper gastrointestinal bleeding from a prepyloric ulcer. **A.** Selective gastroduodenal arteriogram shows a bleeding site adjacent to the right gastroepiploic artery (*arrow*). **B.** Gastroduodenal arteriogram after embolization of the gastroduodenal artery with Gelfoam shows persistent extravasation of contrast (*arrow*) from branches of the right gastric artery (*arrowheads*). **C.** Superselective right gastric arteriogram via a 3 French catheter shows the bleeding site (*arrow*) and anastomosis to the left gastric artery. **D.** After embolization of the right gastric artery proximal and distal to branches feeding the bleeding site, a gastroduodenal arteriogram shows no further bleeding.

experience recurrent bleeding than those with diverticular bleeding that resolves spontaneously. If, however, it is decided to operate on a patient either because of rebleeding or as prophylaxis, a segmental colonic resection based on the precise localization of the bleeding point can be performed rather than a subtotal colectomy or "blind" hemicolectomy. The initial angiographic catheter control of the bleeding episode makes high-risk emergency surgical intervention unnecessary. It allows for preparation of the patient and elective surgery under more favorable circumstances. The placement of microcoils at the exact site of the bleeding vessel may also be successful in stopping

the bleeding and thus avoiding emergency surgery (Figures 26–27 and 26–28). Another technique that has recently been described is the intentional induction of vasospasm in the bleeding vessel with the use of superselective catheterization (104).

Inflammatory Bowel Disease

Rectal bleeding may at times be the first manifestation of colitis. Some patients are, therefore, referred for emergency arteriography, and the diagnosis of bleeding colitis is first made by the angiographer (Figure 26–29). The infusion of

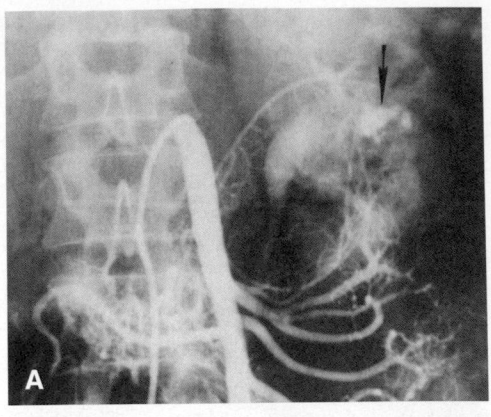
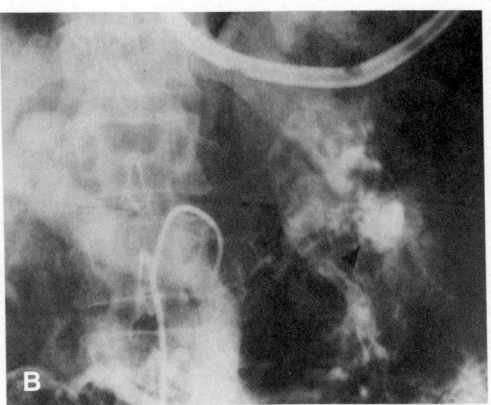
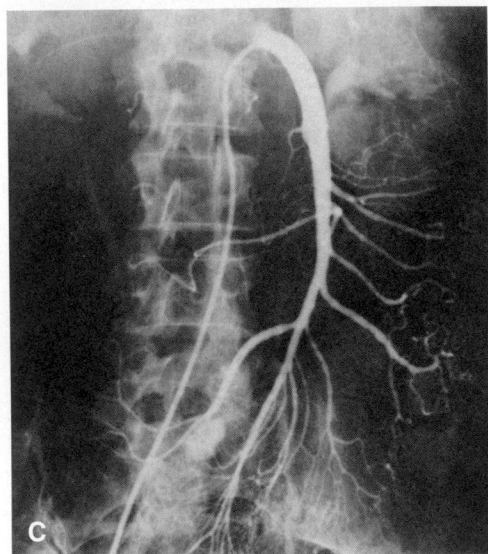

Figure 26–23 Bleeding anastomotic ulcer at the site of a Billroth II anastomosis. **A.** Selective superior mesenteric arteriography demonstrates extravasation of contrast material (*arrow*) from a jejunal branch at the site of the gastrojejunostomy. **B.** Venous phase of the examination shows persistence of contrast material within the jejunum (*arrowhead*). **C.** Control of the bleeding was achieved by infusion of 0.2 unit per minute of vasopressin into the superior mesenteric artery.

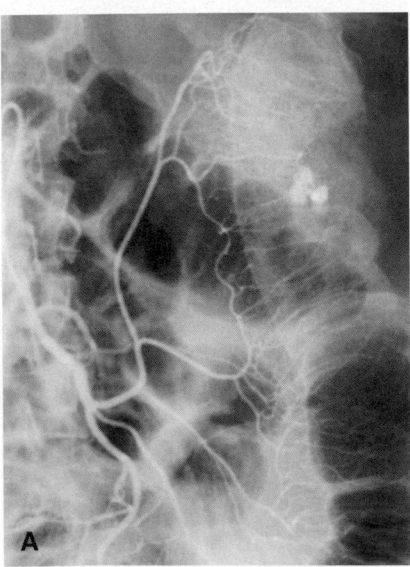
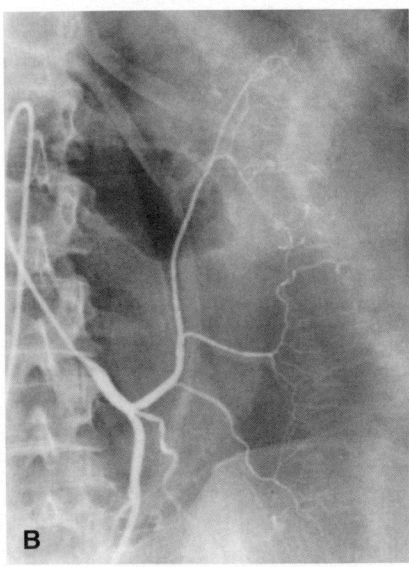

Figure 26–24 Lower gastrointestinal bleeding following the colonoscopic removal of a polyp from the descending colon. **A.** Arterial phase of a selective inferior mesenteric arteriogram demonstrates bleeding from a branch of the left colic artery at the site of the previous polypectomy. **B.** Repeat inferior mesenteric arteriogram 20 minutes after the beginning of an infusion of vasopressin at 0.2 unit per minute. Bleeding can no longer be identified and did not recur. The infusion was continued at the same rate for 12 hours and decreased to 0.1 unit per minute for another 12 hours. The patient was discharged from the hospital without surgery.

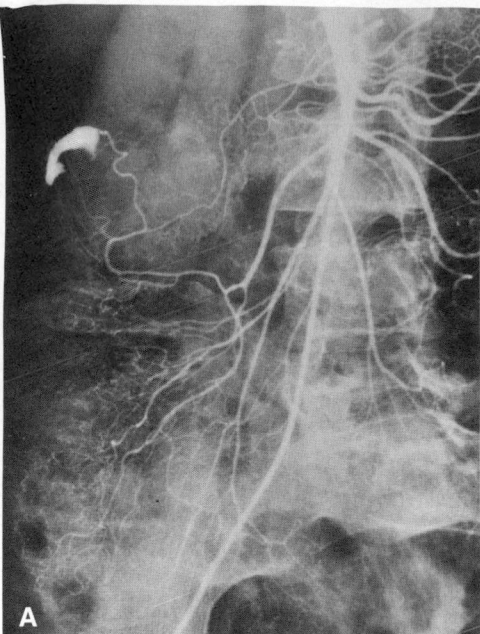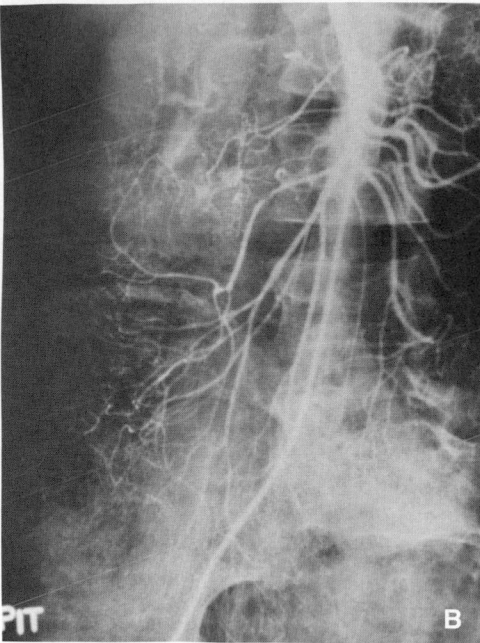

Figure 26–25   Bleeding diverticulum in the hepatic flexure in an 80-year-old man presenting with massive lower gastrointestinal bleeding. **A.** Selective superior mesenteric arteriogram shows extravasation of contrast material from a branch of the right colic artery in the area of the hepatic flexure. **B.** Repeat selective superior mesenteric arteriogram during infusion of 0.2 unit per minute of vasopressin shows complete cessation of the bleeding. The patient was infused with vasopressin for 72 hours at decreasing doses, and the catheter was removed at the end of the third day. Bleeding did not recur, and the patient was discharged from the hospital without surgery.

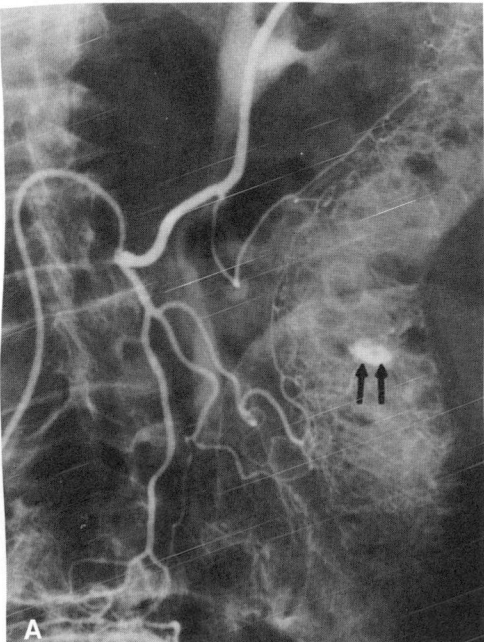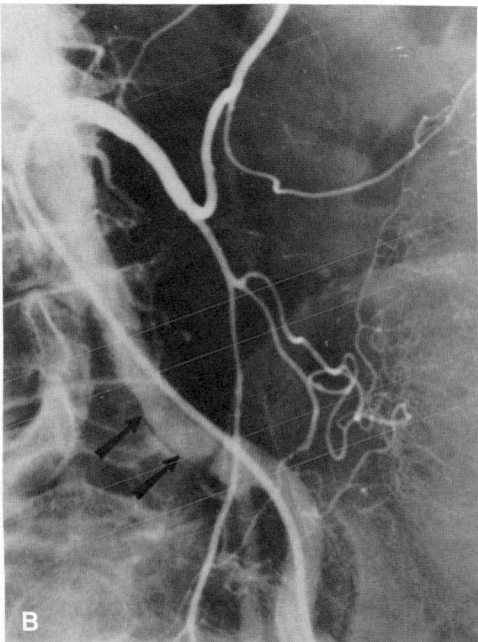

Figure 26–26   Bleeding diverticulum in the descending colon in a 73-year-old man with lower gastrointestinal hemorrhage. **A.** Selective inferior mesenteric arteriography shows extravasation of contrast material in the sigmoid colon (*arrows*). **B.** Repeat arteriogram during infusion of 0.2 unit per minute of vasopressin into the inferior mesenteric artery shows no further extravasation. Note the constriction of the peripheral vessels and reflux into the aorta and iliac vessels (*arrows*), confirming the increase in peripheral resistance. (Reprinted with permission from Baum S, Rösch J, Dotter CT, et al. Selective mesenteric arterial infusions in the management of massive diverticular hemorrhage. N Engl J Med 1973;288:1269.)

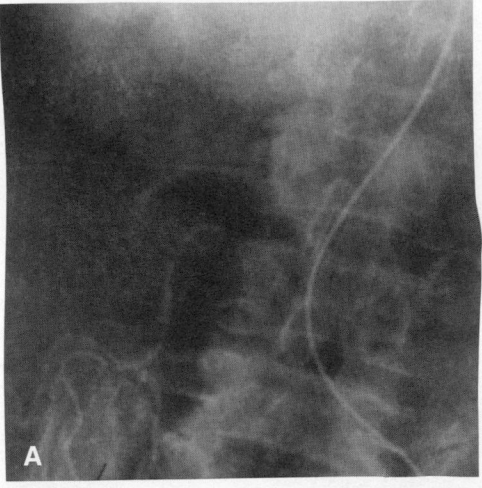
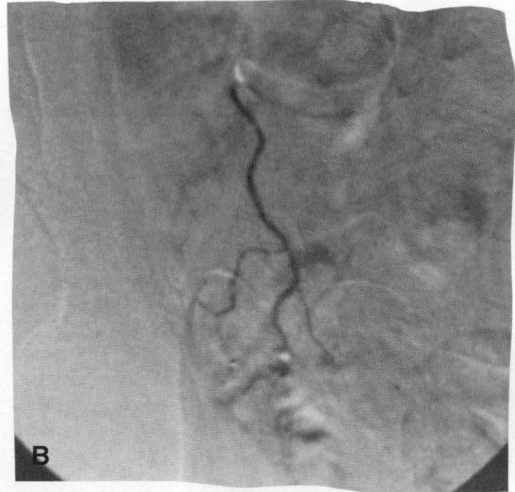
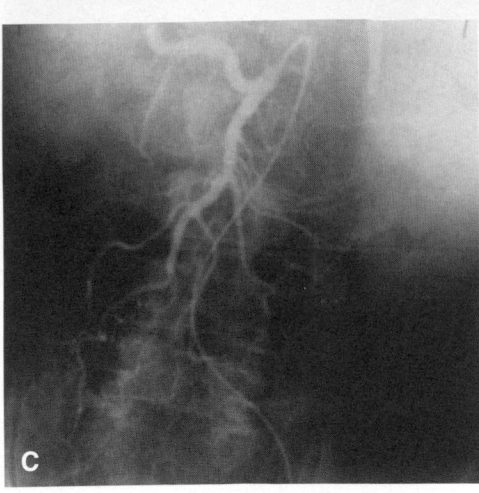

Figure 26–27 Bleeding diverticulum in the right colon in an elderly man presenting with massive lower gastrointestinal bleeding. The bleeding was controlled with selective embolization. **A.** Selective superior mesenteric arteriography shows the bleeding site in the right colon (*arrow*). **B.** Because of preexisting coronary artery disease, the bleeding site was controlled by selective embolization with coils rather than vasopression infusion. **C.** Repeat mesenteric arteriogram after embolization fails to demonstrate any further bleeding.

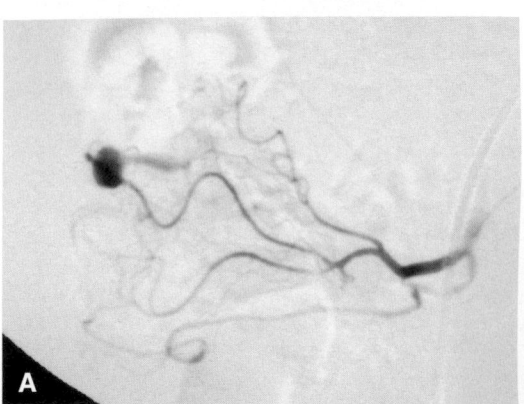
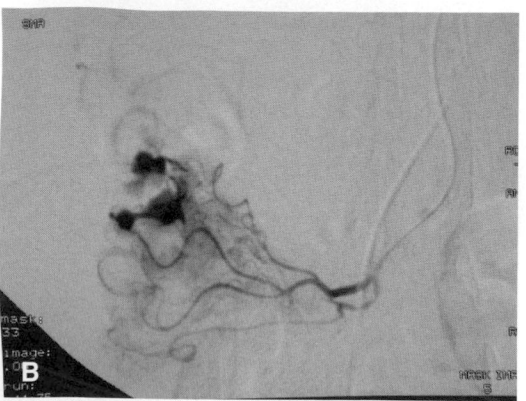
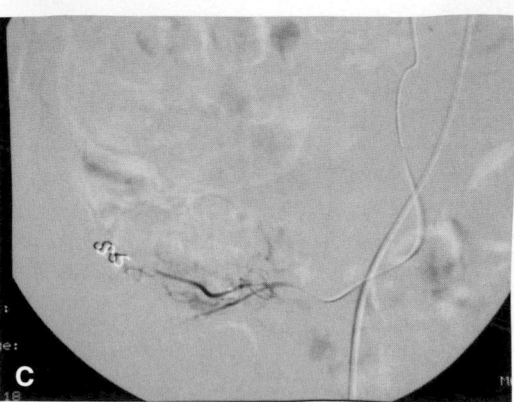

Figure 26–28 Cecal diverticulum in a 50-year-old man treated by embolization with microcoils. **A.** Superselective injection into a branch of the ileocecal artery demonstrates massive extravasation of contrast material. **B.** Several seconds later, the extravasation extends into the cecum. **C.** Extravasation stops after the microcoils are deposited in the bleeding vessel.

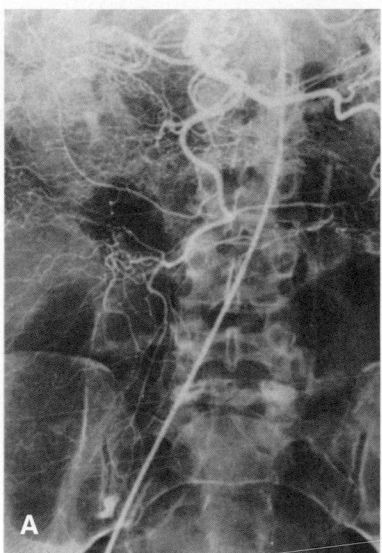 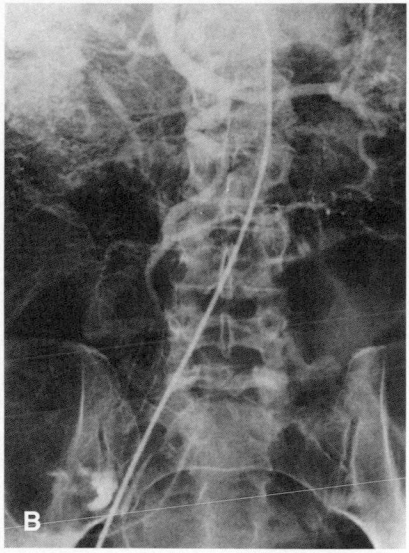 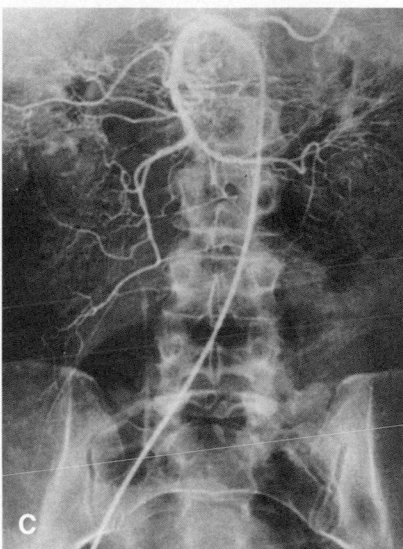

Figure 26–29   Chronic ulcerative colitis with massive lower gastrointestinal bleeding. **A.** Selective superior mesenteric arteriogram shows extravasation from a cecal branch of the ileocecal artery. **B.** The extravasated contrast material persists well into the venous phase of the arteriogram. **C.** Bleeding stopped during the infusion into the superior mesenteric artery of 0.2 unit per minute of vasopressin. Control of the acute bleeding episode allowed the patient to be adequately prepared and to have a successful elective right colectomy several weeks later.

vasopressin in cases of actively bleeding colitis can quickly arrest the bleeding, thereby converting an emergency colectomy to an elective one that allows for much better patient preparation.

Angiodysplasia

Vascular ectasia or angiodysplasia of the colon is a frequent cause of bleeding in elderly patients who have either chronic low-grade or intermittent acute lower gastrointestinal bleeding. The lesions tend to be very small and localized in the cecum, ascending colon, and proximal transverse colon. Although they generally cannot be detected by barium studies, they can be seen on selective arteriography and on colonoscopy. The surgeon almost never finds these lesions at laparotomy, and the pathologist has difficulty demonstrating them unless guided by preliminary specimen injections.

The clinical manifestation of colonic vascular ectasia or angiodysplasia is usually assumed to be intermittent low-grade lower gastrointestinal bleeding (105,106). Nevertheless, in at least one series of 34 patients, half the cases presented with acute episodes of massive rectal bleeding (107). In most of these patients, the stool became guaiac-negative between episodes of hemorrhage.

It is difficult to assess the incidence of colonic angiodysplasia among various age groups. The first description of the entity was probably recorded in 1839 (108). In 1976, Bently collected 234 cases from the literature and added 110 cases from the Mayo Clinic files (109). These reports, however, include a variety of vascular abnormalities of the

intestines, such as congenital arteriovenous malformations and/or vascular neoplasms. Since 1960, when Margulis et al. (110) introduced operative angiography as a tool in the search for gastrointestinal bleeding sites, and 1965, when Baum et al. (111) introduced selective angiography for the preoperative localization of bleeding sites, the unusual character of colonic angiodysplasia has been recognized. These lesions have been reported in many patients with otherwise unexplained gastrointestinal hemorrhage. In one study performed on autopsy specimens, colonic angiodysplasia was demonstrated in 2% of asymptomatic elderly patients (112).

Because colonic angiodysplasia may coexist with other lesions of the gastrointestinal tract, conventional x-ray barium examinations and colonoscopy assume great diagnostic importance. Other pathologic conditions must be excluded before a right colectomy is undertaken. Most patients with angiodysplasia are not studied during periods of active bleeding because the hemorrhage from this condition tends to be more episodic than continuous. Therefore, specific localization of a bleeding site, shown by the extravasation of contrast material, is the exception rather than the rule. Because the surgeon can neither see nor palpate the colonic angiodysplasia, the decision to resect the ascending and proximal transverse colon is generally made on the basis of preoperative colonoscopy or angiographic findings. There have been some reports of being able to detect these lesions by preoperative multidetector CT scans (113,114). Pathologic identification of the lesions in the resected specimen is difficult; lesions are small and focal, and serial sections of the entire specimen are not practical. Hence, injection of the right colic artery with silicone rubber is helpful because this material causes the vessels to remain distended during the tissue fixation. Pathologically, angiodysplasia appears as a conglomeration of vascular spaces, often multiple and often coalescent, with adjacent arteries and veins standing out against the homogeneous surface of the normal colonic mucosa. Histologically, the dilated vascular spaces correspond to thin-walled clusters of veins in the submucosa and mucosa.

Angiographically, an increased number of small arteries is seen during the arterial phase of the arteriogram. In the capillary phase of the study, an accumulation of contrast material appears in the vascular spaces associated with an intense opacification of the bowel wall. The veins draining the lesion are identified early in the examination and paradoxically seem to persist late into the venous phase (Figures 26–30 and 26–31).

The etiology of these angiodysplasias is obscure. It is generally assumed that they are acquired because they are

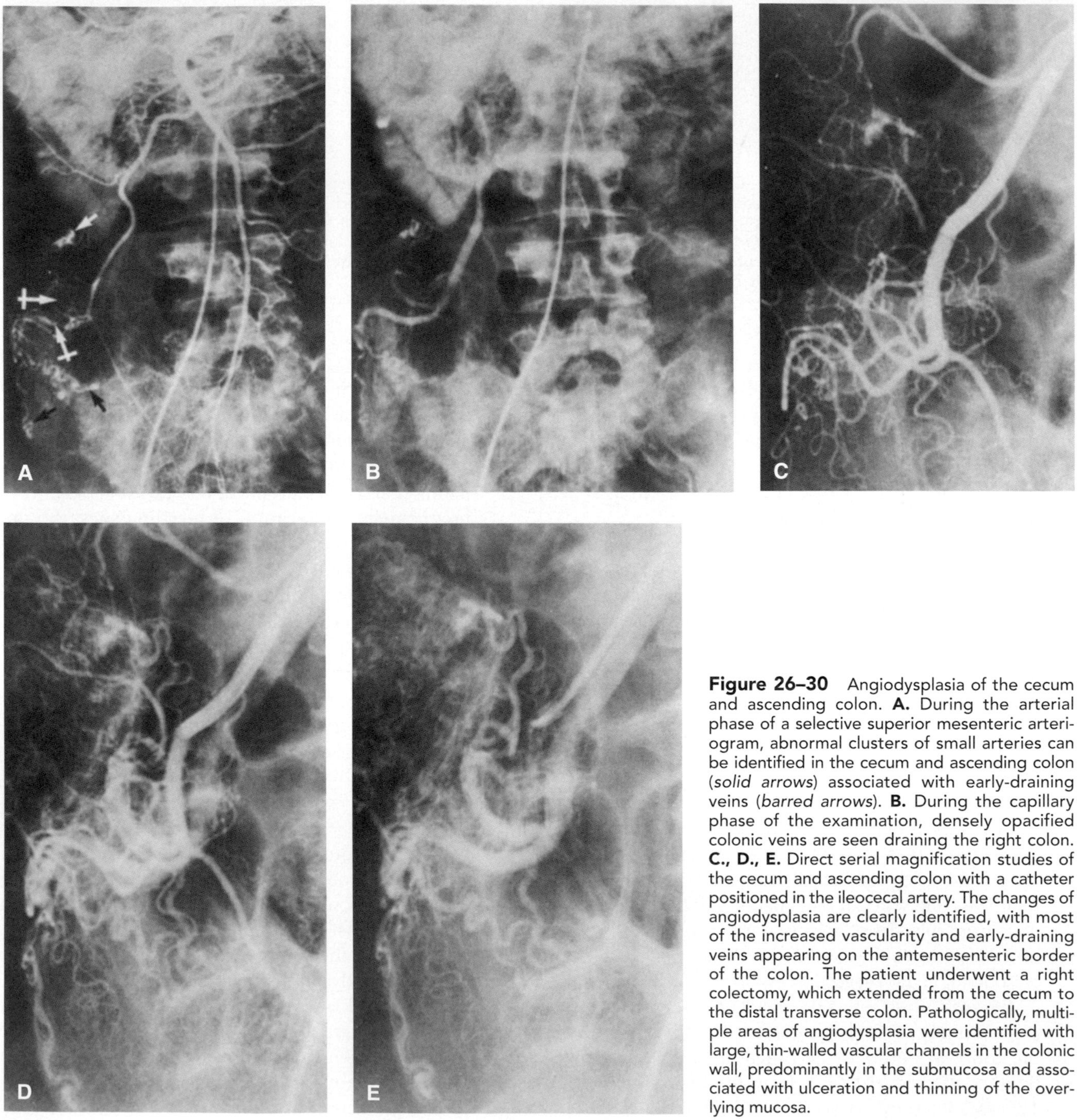

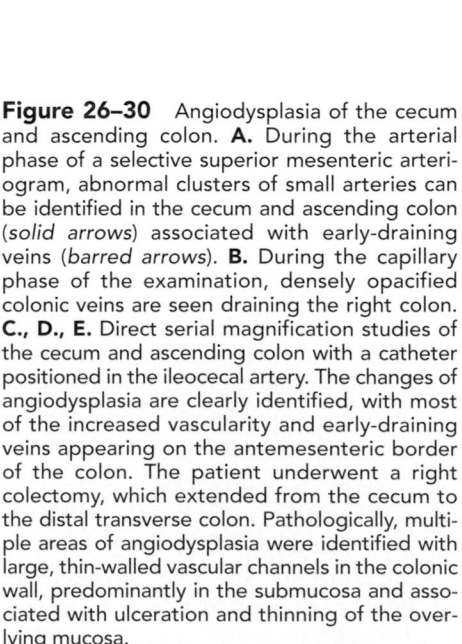

Figure 26–30 Angiodysplasia of the cecum and ascending colon. **A.** During the arterial phase of a selective superior mesenteric arteriogram, abnormal clusters of small arteries can be identified in the cecum and ascending colon (*solid arrows*) associated with early-draining veins (*barred arrows*). **B.** During the capillary phase of the examination, densely opacified colonic veins are seen draining the right colon. **C., D., E.** Direct serial magnification studies of the cecum and ascending colon with a catheter positioned in the ileocecal artery. The changes of angiodysplasia are clearly identified, with most of the increased vascularity and early-draining veins appearing on the antemesenteric border of the colon. The patient underwent a right colectomy, which extended from the cecum to the distal transverse colon. Pathologically, multiple areas of angiodysplasia were identified with large, thin-walled vascular channels in the colonic wall, predominantly in the submucosa and associated with ulceration and thinning of the overlying mucosa.

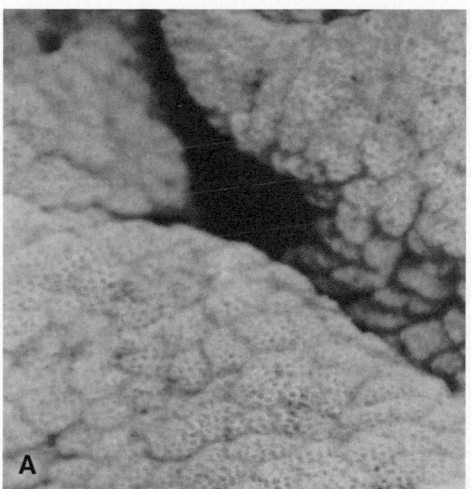
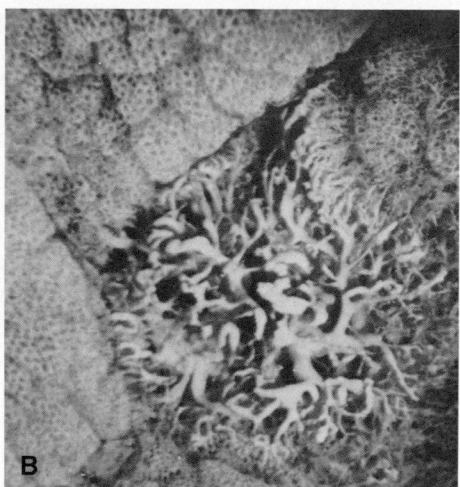
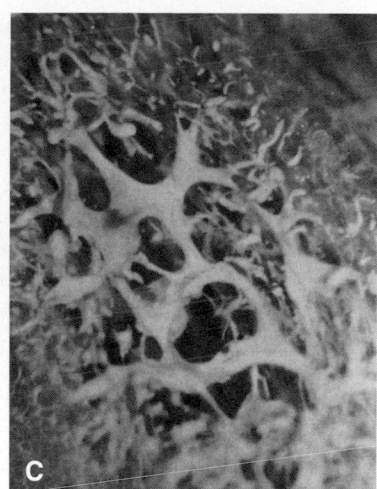
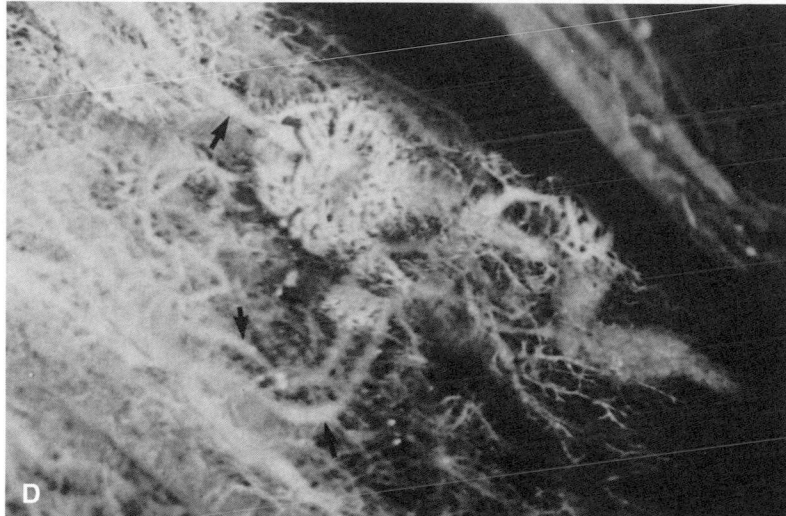

Figure 26–31 Microvascular anatomy of angiodysplasia of the cecum and ascending colon on pathologic specimens. **A.** Photograph (X40) of normal colonic mucosa viewed with a dissecting microscope after silicone rubber injection into right colic and ileocolic arteries and tissue clearing using absolute alcohol followed by methyl salicylate. **B., C., D.** Specimens of colonic angiodysplasia as viewed under the dissecting microscope following the tissue-clearing technique. The angiodysplasias appear as clusters of tortuous and dilated vessels against a homogeneous background of normal colonic mucosa. Histologically, these vessels are primarily venules extending from the submucosa into the mucosa. Occasionally, as in **(D)** (*arrows*), the feeding arteries and draining veins can be identified.

not seen in children. Some investigators consider the lesions to be related to a chronic form of ischemic bowel disease that results in poor mucosal perfusion associated with submucosal arterial venous shunting (81). Other authors have compared them to localized varicosities within the submucosa (115), and some feel that they are degenerative in nature (116,117). An association has also been noted between angiodysplasia and aortic valve disease (81,118). Pathologically, angiodysplasias look like they have developed as a result of increased angiogenesis. It is known that the basement membrane of the gastrointestinal tract produces an antiangiogenesis factor (119). An attractive hypothesis regarding their etiology is that with aging, the basement membrane of the colonic wall is damaged and no longer produces the protective antiangiogenesis factor. The increased diameter of the right colon and the resultant higher pressure in the wall as a result of peristalsis could result in shearing of the basement membrane and would explain the propensity of angiodysplasia for the cecum and ascending colon.

Neoplasms

When bleeding occurs from a neoplasm of the gastrointestinal tract or from an invading contiguous tumor, the bleeding site may be demonstrated angiographically (120). Vasopressin infusions have not been successful in controlling such bleeding because the tumor vessels themselves do not appear to respond to vasoconstrictors. If the bleeding is life threatening and surgical intervention is contraindicated, embolization techniques may be employed. Wallace and Goldstein have reported a series of patients with gastrointestinal bleeding secondary to tumors who were successfully handled in this manner (121).

COMPLICATIONS

Catheter-Related Problems

The risks involved in arteriography are low and are well documented (122). Thrombosis at the puncture site is clearly the most common complication and occurs in about 0.1% of studies. Patients studied because of gastrointestinal bleeding seem to have altered coagulability and are less likely to form thrombus around the catheter. Although many studies have shown that a catheter in the vascular system rapidly becomes coated with a fibrin sheath, catheters have been left in place during vasopressin infusion therapy for as long as 7 days without evidence of thromboembolic disease. Mild oozing in the groin and around the catheter may occur. When the catheter is removed, care should be taken not to exert excessive pressure at the puncture site because this may cause the fibrin sheath, which is almost always around the catheter, to be stripped and left behind in the femoral artery. Manual compression of the artery after removal of the catheter nearly always stops the bleeding, although pressure may have to be applied for up to 2 hours.

Problems Related to the Vasopressin Infusion

Almost all patients complain of abdominal cramps when vasopressin is initially infused into the celiac or superior or inferior mesenteric arteries. The pain generally subsides within the first 10–15 minutes of the infusion and should not recur. It usually has been assumed that the discomfort experienced at first is caused by contraction of the bowel itself and the increased peristalsis. Often patients will evacuate as a sequel to the abdominal cramping. If the catheter tip changes position during the time of infusion and becomes lodged in a small jejunal or colic branch, localized bowel ischemia may result. Persistent severe abdominal cramps suggest ischemia, and the position of the catheter should be checked by repeat arteriography.

Although the dose of vasopressin that is infused intraarterially is quite small, the systemic antidiuretic effect almost always occurs after several hours of continuous infusion. Urinary output and electrolytes must be monitored carefully. Water retention and electrolyte imbalance should be treated by diuretics and suitable electrolyte infusions and not by alteration of the rate or dose of infusion of vasopressin.

Rarely, idiosyncratic reactions to the vasopressin are encountered, and the drug has to be discontinued. Sometimes patients exhibit a marked peripheral vasoconstriction in their extremities, which may have a mottled appearance. Occasionally this is troublesome enough so that the drug has to be discontinued. At the recommended dose rates, reduction in cardiac output is not a frequent problem, but this may depend on the individual cardiac status of the patient. As mentioned earlier, sublingual, intravenous, or, more commonly, a skin patch of nitroglycerin may be used during the vasopressin infusion to prevent coronary artery vasoconstriction.

Problems Related to Embolization Techniques

After embolic material is discharged from the catheter tip, the emboli cannot be retrieved. The final position of an embolus cannot be precisely determined before it is injected, and therefore balance between hemostasis and end-organ ischemia is difficult to control. Embolic therapy is much less controllable than pharmacologic infusions, which can be stopped, slowed, or increased. Complications that have occurred with the use of particulate emboli include end-organ necrosis (76) and reflux of embolic material from the selected artery with final embolization to unwanted sites. Embolic reflux can be prevented by using a balloon catheter; this is inflated proximally in the artery, as emboli are delivered distally through the lumen of the catheter (80).

After Gelfoam embolization, patients may experience a transient rise in temperature to about 39°C (102°F), which may persist for 24–36 hours before subsiding spontaneously. Blood cultures in these patients are sterile, and white cell counts tend to be normal.

REFERENCES

1. Nusbaum M, Baum S. Radiographic demonstration of unknown sites of gastrointestinal bleeding. Surg Forum 1963;13:374.
2. Baum S, Stein GN, Nusbaum M, et al. Selective arteriography in the diagnosis of hemorrhage in the gastrointestinal tract. Radiol Clin North Am 1969;7:131.
3. Baum S, Nusbaum M, Clearfield HR, et al. Angiography in the diagnosis of gastrointestinal bleeding. Arch Intern Med 1967;119:16.
4. Baum S. The radiologist intervenes. N Engl J Med 1980;302:1141.
5. Welch CE, Hedberg S. Gastrointestinal hemorrhage: I. General considerations of diagnosis and therapy. Adv Surg 1973;7:95.
6. Athanasoulis CA, Waltman AC, Novelline RA, et al. Angiography: its contribution to the emergency management of gastrointestinal hemorrhage. Radiol Clin North Am 1976;14:265.
7. Conn HO, Ramsby GR, Storer EH. Selective intraarterial vasopressin in the treatment of upper gastrointestinal hemorrhage. Gastroenterology 1972;63:634.
8. Rösch J, Gray RK, Grollman JH, et al. Selective arterial drug infusions in the treatment of acute gastrointestinal bleeding. Gastroenterology 1970;59:341.
9. Baum S, Athanasoulis CA, Waltman AC, et al. Angiographic diagnosis and control of gastrointestinal bleeding. In: Hardy JD, Zollinger RM, eds. Advances in Surgery. Chicago: Year Book, 1973:149.
10. Shapiro MJ. The role of the radiologist in the management of gastrointestinal bleeding. Gastroenterol Clin North Am 1994;23:123–181.
11. Shapiro M, Simon D. Angiography in massive UGI bleeding—would you believe better than endoscopy? Am J Gastroenterol 1991;86:1090–1091.
12. Zuckerman DA, Bocchini TP, Birnbaum EH. Massive hemorrhage in the lower gastrointestinal tract in adults: diagnostic imaging and intervention. AJR Am J Roentgenol 1993;161:703–711.
13. Sos TA, Lee JG, Wixson D, et al. Intermittent bleeding from minute to minute in acute massive gastrointestinal hemorrhage: arteriographic demonstration. AJR Am J Roentgenol 1978;131:1015.
14. Gupta H, Weissleder R, Bogdanov AA Jr, et al. Experimental gastrointestinal hemorrhage: detection with contrast-enhanced MR imaging and scintigraphy. Radiology 1995;196:239–244.
15. Hilfiker PR, Weishaupt D, Kacl GM, et al. Comparison of three dimensional magnetic resonance imaging in conjunction with a blood pool contrast agent and nuclear scintigraphy for the detection

of experimentally induced gastrointestinal bleeding. Gut 1999;45:581–587.

16. Chan FP, Chhor CM. Active lower gastrointestinal hemorrhage diagnosed by magnetic resonance angiography: case report. Abdom Imaging 2003;28:637–639.

17. Ernst O, Bulois P, Saint-Drenant S, et al. Helical CT in acute lower gastrointestinal bleeding. Eur Radiol 2003;13:114–117.

18. Penner RM, Owen RJ, Williams CN. Diagnosis of a bleeding Dieulafoy lesion on computed tomography and its subsequent embolization. Can J Gastroenterol 2004;18:525–527.

19. Yoshikawa K, Yamaguti T, Nakamura M, et al. The role of dual-phase enhanced helical computed tomography in difficult intestinal bleeding. J Clin Gastroenterol 2000;31:83–84.

20. Alavi A, Dann RW, Baum S, et al. Scintigraphic detection of acute gastrointestinal bleeding. Radiology 1977;124:753.

21. Bentley DE, Richardson JD. The role of tagged red blood cell imaging in the localization of gastrointestinal bleeding. Arch Surg 1991;126:821–824.

22. Orecchia PM, Hensley EK, McDonald PT, et al. Localization of lower gastrointestinal hemorrhage: experience with red blood cells labeled in vitro with technetium Tc-99m. Arch Surg 1985;120:621–624.

23. Dolezal J, Vizd'a J, Bures J. Detection of acute gastrointestinal bleeding by means of technetium-99m in vivo labelled red blood cells. Nucl Med Rev Cent East Eur 2002;5:151–154.

24. Orellana P, Vial I, Prieto C, et al. 99mTc red blood cell scintigraphy for the assessment of active gastrointestinal bleeding. Rev Med Chil 1998;126:413–418.

25. Conn HO, Brodoff M. Emergency esophagoscopy in the diagnosis of upper gastrointestinal hemorrhage. Gastroenterology 1964;47:505.

26. McCray RS, Martin F, Amir-Ahmadi H, et al. Erroneous diagnosis of hemorrhage from esophageal varices. Am J Dig Dis 1969;14:755.

27. Voderholzer WA, Ortner M, Rogalla P, et al. Diagnostic yield of wireless capsule enteroscopy in comparison with computed tomography enteroclysis. Endoscopy 2003;35:1009–1014.

28. Ge ZZ, Hu YB, Xiao SD. Capsule endoscopy and push enteroscopy in the diagnosis of obscure gastrointestinal bleeding. Chin Med J (Engl) 2004;117:1045–1049.

29. Ring EJ, Athanasoulis CA, Waltman AC, et al. The pseudovein: an angiographic appearance of arterial hemorrhage. J Can Assoc Radiol 1973;24:242.

30. Ryan JM, Key SM, Dumbleton SA, et al. Nonlocalized lower gastrointestinal bleeding: provocative bleeding studies with intraarterial tPA, heparin, and tolazoline. J Vasc Interv Radiol 2001;12:1273–1277.

31. Mernagh JR, O'Donovan N, Somers S, et al. Use of heparin in the investigation of obscure gastrointestinal bleeding. Can Assoc Radiol J 2001;52:232–235.

32. Athanasoulis CA. Therapeutic applications of angiography. N Engl J Med 1980;302:1117.

33. Remzi FH, Dietz DW, Unal E, et al. Combined use of preoperative provocative angiography and highly selective methylene blue injection to localize an occult small-bowel bleeding site in a patient with Crohn's disease: report of a case. Dis Colon Rectum 2003;46:260–263.

34. Schmidt SP, Boskind JF, Smith DC, et al. Angiographic localization of small bowel angiodysplasia with use of platinum coils. J Vasc Interv Radiol 1993;4:737–739.

35. Duszak RL, Soulen MC, Shlansky-Goldberg RD, et al. Transcatheter embolization in nonvariceal upper gastrointestinal hemorrhage: laboratory, clinical, and angiographic factors contributing to success. Radiology 1995;197(Suppl):416.

36. Ljungdahl M, Eriksson LG, Nyman R, et al. Arterial embolization can often substitute surgery in bleeding ulcer. When endoscopic hemostasis is not successful an alternative emergency treatment is needed. Lakartidningen 2004;101:768–772.

37. Alibert S, Sassenou I, Heyries L, et al. Hematochezia due to jejunal diverticula and treated by arterial embolization. Gastroenterol Clin Biol 2003;27:648–650.

38. Goodman LS, Gilman A, eds. The Pharmacological Basis of Therapeutics. 5th Ed. New York: Macmillan, 1975:855.

39. Scarpignato C, Pelosini I. Somatostatin for upper gastrointestinal hemorrhage and pancreatic surgery. A review of its pharmacology and safety. Digestion 1999;60(Suppl):1–16.

40. Barr JW, Lakin RC, Rösch J. Vasopressin and hepatic artery: effect of selective celiac infusion of vasopressin on the hepatic artery flow. Invest Radiol 1975;10:200.

41. Simmons JT, Baum S, Sheehan BA, et al. The effects of vasopressin on hepatic artery blood flow. Radiology 1977;124:637.

42. Tsai YT, Lay CS, Lai KH, et al. Controlled trial of vasopressin plus nitroglycerin vs. vasopressin alone in the treatment of bleeding esophageal varices. Hepatology 1986;6:406–409.

43. Gimson AE, Westaby D, Hegarty J, et al. A randomized trial of vasopressin and vasopressin plus nitroglycerin in the control of acute variceal hemorrhage. Hepatology 1986;6:410–413.

44. Conn HO. Vasopressin and nitroglycerin in the treatment of bleeding varices: the bottom line. Hepatology 1986;6:523–525.

45. Sirinek KR, Adcock DK, Levine BA. Simultaneous infusion of nitroglycerin and nitroprusside to offset adverse effects of vasopressin during portosystemic shunting. Am J Surg 1989;157:33–37.

46. Bosch J, Groszmann RJ, Garcia-Pagan JC, et al. Association of transdermal nitroglycerin to vasopressin infusion in the treatment of variceal hemorrhage: a placebo-controlled clinical trial. Hepatology 1989;10:962–968.

47. Shaldon S, Sherlock S. The use of vasopressin (Pitressin) in the control of bleeding of oesophageal varices. Lancet 1960;2:222.

48. Baum S, Nusbaum M. The control of gastrointestinal hemorrhage by selective mesenteric arterial infusion of vasopressin. Radiology 1971;98:497.

49. Conn HO, Ramsby GR, Stover EH, et al. Intraarterial vasopressin in the treatment of upper gastrointestinal hemorrhage: prospective controlled clinical trial. Gastroenterology 1975;68:211.

50. Barr JW, Lakin RC, Rösch J. Similarity of arterial and intravenous vasopressin on portal and systemic hemodynamics. Gastroenterology 1975;69:13.

51. Johnson WC, Widrich WC, Ansell JE, et al. Control of bleeding varices by vasopressin: a prospective radiological study. Ann Surg 1977;186:369.

52. LeBrec D, Nouel O, Corbic M, et al. Propanolol, a medical treatment for portal hypertension. Lancet 1980;2:180–182.

53. Lebrec D. Current status and future goals of pharmacologic reduction of portal hypertension. Am J Surg 1990;160:12–25.

54. Greig JD, Garden OJ, Carter DC. Prophylactic treatment of patients with esophageal varices: is it ever indicated? World J Surg 1994;18:176–184.

55. Pagliaro L, D'Amico G, Sorensen TI, et al. Prevention of first bleeding in cirrhosis: a meta-analysis of randomized trials of nonsurgical treatment. Ann Intern Med 1992;117:59–70.

56. Lunderquist A, Vang J. Transhepatic catheterization and obliteration of the coronary vein in patients with portal hypertension and esophageal varices. N Engl J Med 1974;291:646.

57. Lunderquist A, Vang J. Sclerosing injection of esophageal varices through transhepatic selective catheterization of the gastric coronary vein: a preliminary report. Acta Radiol 1974;15:546.

58. L'Hermine C, Chastanet P, Delemazure O, et al. Percutaneous transhepatic embolization of gastroesophageal varices: results in 400 patients. Am J Roentgenol 1989;152:755–760.

59. Sos T. Transhepatic portal venous embolization of varices: pros and cons. Radiology 1983;148:569–570.

60. Pereiras R, Viamonte M Jr, Russell E, LePage J, White P, Hutson D. New techniques for interruption of gastroesophageal venous blood flow. Radiology 1977;124:313.

61. Lunderquist A, Simert G, Tylén U, et al. Follow-up of patients with portal hypertension and esophageal varices treated with percutaneous obliteration of gastric coronary vein. Radiology 1977;122:59.

62. Moncure AC, Waltman AC, Vander Salm TJ, et al. Gastrointestinal hemorrhage from adhesion-related mesenteric varices. Ann Surg 1976;183:24.

63. Naef M, Holzinger F, Glattli A, et al. Massive gastrointestinal bleeding from colonic varices in a patient with portal hypertension. Dig Surg 1998;15:709–712.

64. Case Records of the Massachusetts General Hospital. Weekly clinicopathological exercises. Case 1-1973. N Engl J Med 1973;288:36.

65. Miao YM, Catnach SM, Barrison IG, et al. Colonic variceal bleeding in a patient with mesenteric venous obstruction due to an ileal carcinoid tumour. Eur J Gastroenterol Hepatol 1996;8:1133–1135.

66. Ring EJ, Oleaga JA, Freiman D, et al. Pitfalls in the angiographic management of hemorrhage: hemodynamic considerations. AJR Am J Roentgenol 1977;129:1007.

67. White RI Jr, Strandberg JV, Gross GS, et al. Therapeutic embolization with long-term occluding agents and their effect on embolized tissues. Radiology 1977;125:677.

68. Reuter RS, Chuang VP, Bree RL. Selective arterial embolization for control of massive upper gastrointestinal bleeding. AJR Am J Roentgenol 1975;125:119.

69. Eisenberg H, Steer ML. The nonoperative treatment of massive pyloroduodenal hemorrhage by retracted autologous clot embolization. Surgery 1976;79:414.

70. Bookstein JJ, Closta EM, Foley D, et al. Transcatheter hemostasis of gastrointestinal bleeding using modified autogenous clot. Radiology 1974;113:277.

71. Tadavarthy SM, Moller JH, Amplatz K. Polyvinyl alcohol (Ivalon)—a new embolic material. AJR Am J Roentgenol 1975;125:609.

72. Castaneda-Zuniga WR, Sanchez R, Amplatz K. Experimental observations on short- and long-term effects of arterial occlusion with Ivalon. Radiology 1978;126:783.

73. Lang EV, Picus D, Marx MV, et al. Massive upper gastrointestinal hemorrhage with normal findings on arteriography: value of prophylactic embolization of the left gastric artery. AJR Am J Roentgenol 1992;158:547–549.

74. Sharma S, Kothari SS, Rajani M, et al. Life-threatening arterial haemorrhage: results of treatment by transcatheter embolization using home-made steel coils. Clin Radiol 1994;49:252–255.

75. Dotter CT, Goldman ML, Rösch J. Instant selective arterial occlusion with isobutyl 2-cyanoacrylate. Radiology 1975;114:227.

76. Goldman ML, Freeney PC, Tallman JM, et al. Transcatheter vascular occlusion therapy with isobutyl 2-cyanoacrylate (bucrylate) for control of massive upper-gastrointestinal bleeding. Radiology 1978;129:41.

77. Kish JW, Katz MD, Marx MV, et al. N-butyl cyanoacrylate embolization for control of acute arterial hemorrhage. J Vasc Interv Radiol 2004;15:689–695.

78. Wholey MH. The technology of balloon catheters in interventional angiography. Radiology 1977;125:671.

79. Dotter CT, Rösch J, Lakin PC, et al. Injectable flow-guided coaxial catheters for selective angiography and controlled vascular occlusion. Radiology 1972;104:421.

80. Greenfield AJ, Athanasoulis CA, Waltman AC, et al. Prevention of embolic reflux using balloon catheters. AJR Am J Roentgenol 1978;131:651.

81. White RI Jr, Ursic TA, Kaufman SL, et al. Therapeutic embolization with detachable balloons: physical factors influencing permanent occlusion. Radiology 1978;126:521.

82. Gianturco C, Anderson JH, Wallace S. Mechanical devices for arterial occlusion. AJR Am J Roentgenol 1975;124:428.

83. Baum S, Ward S, Nusbaum M. Stress bleeding from the mid-duodenum: an often unrecognized source of gastrointestinal hemorrhage. Radiology 1970;95:595.

84. Athanasoulis CA, Baum S, Waltman AC, et al. Control of acute gastric mucosal hemorrhage: intra-arterial infusion of posterior pituitary extract. N Engl J Med 1974;290:597.

85. Ljungdahl M, Eriksson LG, Nyman R, et al. Arterial embolisation in management of massive bleeding from gastric and duodenal ulcers. Eur J Surg 2002;168:384–390.

86. Hamlin JA, Petersen B, Keller FS, et al. Angiographic evaluation and management of nonvariceal upper gastrointestinal bleeding. Gastrointest Endosc Clin N Am 1997;7:703–716.

87. Waltman AC, Greenfield AJ, Novelline RA, et al. Pyloroduodenal bleeding and intraarterial vasopressin: clinical results. AJR Am J Roentgenol 1979;133:643.

88. Sherman LM, Shenoy SS, Cerra FB. Selective intraarterial vasopressin: clinical efficacy and complications. Ann Surg 1979;189:298.

89. Fordtran JS, Grossman MI. Third symposium on histamine H2-receptor antagonists: clinical results with cimetidine. Gastroenterology 1978;74:339.

90. Rosenbaum A, Siegelman S, Sprayregen S. The bleeding marginal ulcer: catheterization diagnosis and therapy. AJR Am J Roentgenol 1975;125:812.

91. Oglevie SB, Smith DC, Mera SS. Bleeding marginal ulcers: angiographic evaluation. Radiology 1990;174:943–944.

92. Athanasoulis CA, Waltman AC, Ring EJ, et al. Angiographic management of post-operative bleeding. Radiology 1974;113:37.

93. Nicholson T, Travis S, Ettles D, et al. Hepatic artery angiography and embolization for hemobilia following laparoscopic cholecystectomy. Cardiovasc Intervent Radiol 1999;22:20–24.

94. Behringer GE, Albright NL. Diverticular disease of the colon: a frequent cause of rectal bleeding. Am J Surg 1973;125:419.

95. Welch CE, Hedberg S. Gastrointestinal hemorrhage. In: Hardy JD, Zollinger RM, eds. Advances in Surgery. Chicago: Year Book, 1973;95.

96. Rigg M, Ewing MR. Current attitudes on diverticulitis with particular reference to colonic bleeding. Arch Surg 1966;92:321.

97. O'Neill BB, Gosnell JE, Lull RJ, et al. Cinematic nuclear scintigraphy reliably directs surgical intervention for patients with gastrointestinal bleeding. Arch Surg 2000;135:1076–1081; discussion 1081–1082.

98. Casarella WJ, Kanter IE, Seaman WB. Right-sided colonic diverticula as a cause of acute rectal hemorrhage. N Engl J Med 1972;286:450.

99. Athanasoulis CA, Baum S, Rösch J, et al. Mesenteric arterial infusions of vasopressin for hemorrhage from colonic diverticulosis. Am J Surg 1975;129:212.

100. Baum S, Rösch J, Dotter CT, et al. Selective mesenteric arterial infusions in the management of massive diverticular hemorrhage. N Engl J Med 1973;288:1269.

101. Gady JS, Reynolds H, Blum A. Selective arterial embolization for control of lower gastrointestinal bleeding: recommendations for a clinical management pathway. Curr Surg 2003;60:344–347.

102. Burgess AN, Evans PM. Lower gastrointestinal haemorrhage and superselective angiographic embolization. ANZ J Surg 2004;74:635–638.

103. DeBarros J, Rosas L, Cohen J, et al. The changing paradigm for the treatment of colonic hemorrhage: superselective angiographic embolization. Dis Colon Rectum 2002;45:802–808.

104. Cynamon J, Atar E, Steiner A, et al. Catheter-induced vasospasm in the treatment of acute lower gastrointestinal bleeding. J Vasc Interv Radiol 2003;14:211–216.

105. Jakab F, Balazs M, Faller J, et al. Gastrointestinal angiodysplasia. Acta Chir Hung 1991;32:57–68.

106. Lau WY, Chu KW, Yuen WK, et al. Bleeding angiodysplasia of the gastrointestinal tract. Aust NZ J Surg 1992;62:344–349.

107. Baum S, Athanasoulis CA, Waltman AC, et al. Angiodysplasia of the right colon: a cause of gastrointestinal bleeding. AJR Am J Roentgenol 1977;129:789.

108. Phillips B. Letter to the editor. London Med Gaz 1839;1:514.

109. Bently PG. The bleeding caecal angioma: a diagnostic problem. Br J Surg 1976;63:455.

110. Margulis AR, Heinbecker P, Bernard HR. Operative mesenteric arteriography in the search for the site in unexplained gastrointestinal hemorrhage. Surgery 1960;48:534.

111. Baum S, Nusbaum MH, Blakemore SW. The preoperative radiographic demonstration of intra-abdominal bleeding from undetermined sites by percutaneous selective celiac and superior mesenteric arteriography. Surgery 1965;58:797.

112. Baer JW, Ryan S. Analysis of cecal vasculature in the search for vascular malformations. AJR Am J Roentgenol 1976;126:394.

113. Junquera F, Quiroga S, Saperas E, et al. Accuracy of helical computed tomographic angiography for the diagnosis of colonic angiodysplasia. Gastroenterology 2000;119:293–299.

114. Ettorre GC, Francioso G, Garribba AP, et al. Helical CT angiography in gastrointestinal bleeding of obscure origin. AJR Am J Roentgenol 1997;168:727–731.

115. Boley SJ, Sammartano RS, Adams A, et al. On the nature and etiology of vascular ectasia of the colon: degenerative lesions of aging. Gastroenterology 1977;72:650.

116. Foutch PG. Colonic angiodysplasia. Gastroenterologist 1997;5: 148–156.
117. Dodda G, Trotman BW. Gastrointestinal angiodysplasia. J Assoc Acad Minor Phys 1997;8:16–19.
118. Ikuta T, Shibata T, Hirai H, et al. Small-intestinal bleeding from angiodysplasia after aortic valve replacement. J Heart Valve Dis 2003;12:458–460.
119. Judah Folkman, *personal communication*, 2000.
120. Rösch J, Steckel RJ. Selective angiography of the abdominal viscera. In: Hanafee WN, ed. Selective Angiography. Baltimore: Williams & Wilkins, 1972:17.
121. Wallace S, Goldstein HM. Intra-vascular occlusive therapy. Postgrad Med 1976;59:141.
122. Sigstedt B, Lunderquist A. Complications of angiographic examinations. AJR Am J Roentgenol 1978;130:455.

Interventional Therapies for Hepatic Malignancy

27

Michael J. Pentecost

The management of the patient with unresectable hepatic malignancy, whether primary or metastatic, represents one of the most difficult problems in cancer care. The interests of interventional radiologists have centered on regional therapies for a group of unresectable tumors that are typically confined to the liver—hepatocellular carcinoma and metastases from colorectal carcinoma, ocular melanoma, and carcinoid and islet cell tumors. Because of the association with chronic hepatitis B in Asia, hepatocellular carcinoma is the most common fatal malignancy worldwide. Colorectal carcinoma claims 57,000 American lives annually; about half of these patients succumb to liver metastases long after the primary malignancy has been resected successfully. Ocular melanoma and carcinoid and islet cell tumors are much less common malignancies; all share a propensity to metastasize exclusively to the liver, where they are notoriously resistant to systemic chemotherapy.

Overall, the results of treating liver tumors with systemic chemotherapy have been disappointing. After 3 decades, even with the addition of oxaliplatin and irinotecan, most trials of 5-fluorouracil in the treatment of colorectal liver metastases still show response rates in the range of 20% (1). Similarly poor results (20–30% response rates) have been reported with hepatocellular carcinoma, and for the most part, systemic chemotherapy has been abandoned as a treatment option in these patients (2).

The studies of Clarkson and Sullivan (3,4) opened the door to several regional therapies for hepatic malignancies—in these instances, it was the hepatic artery infusion of antineoplastic agents via surgically or percutaneously placed catheters. The aim of these therapies was twofold: to deliver a higher concentration of drug directly to the tumor and to reduce toxicity by lowering the systemic level of agent. Over the past 3 decades, several novel treatments have come about in the wake of these reports, including the embolization of liver tumors with particulate agents (5), the isolation of hepatic blood flow during massive infusion of chemotherapy (6), the concurrent use of hyperthermia and intra-arterial chemotherapy (7), the direct percutaneous instillation of agents such as ethanol and acetic acid (8,9), portal vein infusion of chemotherapeutic agents (10), and the injection of radioactive particles into the hepatic artery (11). Currently, the greatest enthusiasm centers on two regional therapies: intra-arterial infusion/embolization and radiofrequency ablation.

REGIONAL ARTERIAL INFUSION AND EMBOLIZATION

The simultaneous infusion of particulate and chemotherapeutic agents is called *chemoembolization*. The rationale for this combination has been to provoke tumor ischemia and simultaneously increase the dwell time of the drug. Since the original experiences were described in the early 1980s (12–14), myriad different agents in various combinations have been investigated in the management of hepatocellular carcinoma and liver metastases.

PHYSIOLOGIC BASIS

Several fortuitous circumstances permit regional hepatic artery infusions to be applied safely and effectively: the dual blood supply of the liver, the blood supply of tumors by the hepatic artery, and the ease of percutaneous catheterization of the hepatic artery.

The liver has a dual blood supply. Depending on body position, satiety, and other factors, the portal vein supplies about three fourths and the hepatic artery one fourth of hepatic circulation. This dual circulation allows for occlusion of either vessel without infarction. There have now been decades of experience in surgical and radiologic practice confirming the safety of intentional ligation or embolization of the hepatic artery or portal vein in the management of liver trauma and neoplasia.

Recent experiments have increased the understanding of these circulations. The previously held notion of the liver as a passive recipient of blood flow has been challenged. Lautt et al. observed the ability of the liver to vary oxygen extraction from the portal circulation in the face of a decline in flow in, or occlusion of, the hepatic artery (15). Using color Doppler sonography, Ralls described the reversibility of portal flow between hepatopetal (toward the liver) and hepatofugal (away from the liver) in patients with cirrhosis (16). Further, hepatofugal and hepatopetal flow in different branches of the portal vein have been demonstrated in the same patient. Even in patients with chronic hepatitis, cirrhosis, and hepatocellular carcinoma, this reciprocal, autoregulated flow allows hepatofugal flow in the portal vein to revert to hepatopetal in the face of hepatic artery embolization.

The supply of primary and metastatic liver tumors by the hepatic artery was originally described in studies using injection techniques and anatomic sectioning (17,18). These observations have been confirmed in a number of physiologic studies. Sigurdson et al., with direct observation in surgery, infused fluorodeoxyuridine (FUDR) into the hepatic artery or portal vein before biopsy of liver metastases (19). When radiolabeling techniques were used for assay, significantly higher levels of FUDR were found in specimens where the hepatic artery was injected than where the portal vein was infused. In a study using nitrogen-labeled amino acids, a greater nutrient supply to tumors was observed when the hepatic artery, rather than the portal vein, was injected (20).

The dual circulation of the liver and the arterial supply of tumors would be moot points if selective and superselective catheterization of the hepatic artery could not be achieved expeditiously. Lubricious coating materials and microcatheters permit coaxial placement of catheters in the hepatic artery beyond branches to the intestine and gallbladder, even in the face of aberrant circulation or parasitized collateral vessels.

CHEMOTHERAPEUTIC AND EMBOLIC AGENTS

Many pharmacologic agents have been used for hepatic artery infusion (Table 27–1). Most, though not all, are agents that have some demonstrable activity at levels achievable during systemic infusion, including 5-FU, FUDR, doxorubicin, bleomycin, cyclophosphamide, vincristine, mitomycin, and streptozotocin. The most frequently used drugs for chemoembolization are doxorubicin, cisplatin, and mitomycin.

Most agents used for regional infusion have two characteristics. First, when infused into the hepatic artery, the drug must be rapidly cleared by the liver (high "first-pass" clearance); this accounts for the 100- to 400-fold difference in concentration between the liver and systemic circulation of drugs such as 5-fluorouracil and FUDR (21). Without such clearance, the hepatic artery and systemic levels would be similar and no advantage would be conferred by regional treatment. Second, the drug must be more effective at higher doses (for example, it would have a steep dose-response curve). If the agent worked only in the dose range achieved with systemic infusion, there would be no point in directly injecting the hepatic artery. Added benefit is gained in that regional infusions result in lower systemic levels of drug and, therefore, less toxicity.

A number of embolic agents have been used to treat liver tumors (Table 27–2). The agents are categorized broadly into *mechanical* and *particulate* (further subdivided into *permanent* and *temporary*). Mechanical agents such as coils, differing little from proximal surgical ligation of a vessel, have little role in the primary management of liver tumors. The ischemic effect of such agents is, at best, fleeting because collateral flow develops quickly around the point of occlusion (22). Mechanical coils are used intentionally to occlude vessels ("coil blockade") so that the

---

TABLE 27–1

CYTOTOXIC AGENTS FOR HEPATIC ARTERY INFUSION AND CHEMOEMBOLIZATION

Bleomycin	Epirubicin	Bacille Calmette-Guérin
Carboplatinum	Mitomycin	Cisplatin
Doxorubicin	Mitomycin C	Cyclophosphamide
5-fluorouracil	Nitrogen mustard	Ethanol
Floxuridine	Phenylalanine mustard	Ifosfamide
Methotrexate	Streptozotocin	Interferon
Mitoxantrone	Vinblastine	Interleukin
SMANCS	Vincristine	Tumor necrosis factor
	Vindesine	

TABLE 27–2

EMBOLIC AGENTS USED FOR EMBOLIZATION AND CHEMOEMBOLIZATION

Collagen	^{131}ILipiodol	Gelfoam
Ethylcellulose microspheres	Gianturco coils	Platinum microcoils
Lipiodol	Glass microspheres	Starch microspheres
Polyvinyl alcohol	Liposomes	

chemotherapeutic agent or particles will not perfuse a non-target circulation. Examples include embolization of the gastroduodenal artery when the left hepatic artery arises from the common hepatic artery and surgical ligation of the left hepatic artery before placement of a catheter in the right hepatic artery—so that the left lobe is perfused by intrahepatic collaterals.

In the cancer patient, the most experience has been accumulated with the embolic agents Gelfoam, polyvinyl alcohol, and Lipiodol. Gelfoam is a temporary agent made from gelatin surgical sponge. Experiments in animals demonstrate arterial recanalization after 2–6 weeks. Recanalization time in humans is less clear and, given the dwell time of chemotherapeutic agents, probably irrelevant. Polyvinyl alcohol particles, which range in size from 150–1,000 μm, are also a frequent agent in chemoembolization. Proponents of embolization alone (to be distinguished from chemoembolization) advocate polyvinyl alcohol particles because of their ability to provide permanent occlusion. Of course, with the angiogenesis and parasitization of flow that accompanies hepatic malignancies, no embolic agent is truly permanent.

No controlled clinical trial has evaluated embolization or chemoembolization with the only variable being different particles. Therefore, any advantage of one agent over another is only conjecture. Some animal experiments demonstrate an inverse relationship between the tissue concentration of cisplatin and the size of accompanying embolic particle (23).

Lipiodol is an oily agent that has been used for diagnostic imaging studies of the liver. There is now physiologic evidence to support the combination of Lipiodol and embolic particles in addition to chemotherapeutic agents as the appropriate mixture for chemoembolization. Kan et al. (24,25), using in vivo microscopy, observed arterioportal shunting of Lipiodol in liver tumors in animals; that is, blood (or Lipiodol) flowed from arteriole to portal venule before entering the tumor bed. Lipiodol was then washed away by incoming higher-pressure arterial flow. The authors posited that the washout of drug and Lipiodol would be delayed by the addition of embolic particles, which would obstruct arterial flow. This would sandwich the liver tumors between Lipiodol in the portal vein and Gelfoam or polyvinyl alcohol in the hepatic arteries while bathing them

TABLE 27-3

TUMOR NECROSIS: HISTOLOGIC COMPARISON BETWEEN OILY EMBOLIZATION AND CHEMOEMBOLIZATION

Agent	Complete Necrosis, Main Tumor (%)	Necrosis, Daughter Nodule (%)
Oil	0	0
Oil + doxorubicin	13	6
Oil + doxorubicin + Gelfoam	83	53

Adapted from Takayasu K, Shima Y, Muramatsu Y, et al. Hepatocellular carcinoma: treatment with intraarterial iodized oil with and without chemotherapeutic agents. Radiology 1987;162:345–351.

in the chemotherapeutic agent; the occlusion of both arterial and portal vessels would interrupt the reciprocal flow to tumors between these two circulations. Two clinical studies support the notion of the synergistic effect of both agents. Takayasu et al. (26) (Table 27–3) observed significantly greater necrosis when both embolic agents were used than when oil alone or oil with doxorubicin was used. Similarly, Nakamura et al. (27) (Table 27–4) described longer survival rates when Lipiodol, Gelfoam, and doxorubicin were used compared to Gelfoam and doxorubicin alone.

PATIENT SELECTION

Regional palliative therapies of liver tumors are predicated on two assumptions. First, the tumor, whether primary or metastatic, should be confined to the liver. One of the premises of regional infusions is the higher concentration of chemotherapeutic agent in the involved organ with a corresponding lower systemic level. Occasional exception is made

TABLE 27-4

CUMULATIVE SURVIVAL RATE IN HEPATOCELLULAR CARCINOMA: THE EFFECT OF ADDING OIL TO THE CHEMOEMBOLIC INFUSION

Agent	6 Months (%)	1 Year (%)	2 Years (%)	3 Years (%)
Doxorubicin + Gelfoam	67	45	16	4
Doxorubicin + Gelfoam + Lipiodol	82	54	33	18

Adapted from Nakamura H, Hashimoto T, Oi H, et al. Transcatheter oily chemoembolization of hepatocellular carcinoma. Radiology 1989;170: 783–786.

TABLE 27-5

FACTORS INFLUENCING RESPONSE OR SURVIVAL IN PATIENTS TREATED WITH HEPATIC CHEMOEMBOLIZATION

Encephalopathy	Elevated bilirubin, SGOT, SGPT
Cirrhosis	Serum albumin
Ascites	Portal vein invasion
Size of tumor	Oil retention
Grade (Edmondson and Steiner)	Change in alpha-fetoprotein
Biliary obstruction	

when extrahepatic tumor burden is minimal or the response uneven, such as when pulmonary lesions are responding to systemic chemotherapy but liver tumors are not.

Second, the liver tumors should be unresectable. The aim of surgical therapy is curative, not palliative as with regional infusions; indeed, newer techniques permit resection of extensive primary and metastatic tumors. Combining better surgical techniques, more accurate preoperative staging, and new chemotherapeutic approaches has led to steady progress in the management of colorectal liver metastases. Currently, the generally accepted notion is that one in five patients presenting with liver metastases will be resectable and that, after 5 years, one in three of these will be alive and free of disease (28,29).

Liver transplantation also has been offered to patients with primary tumors; in a carefully selected group, survival rates as high as 75% have been reported (2,30). The patients most likely to benefit from the regional therapies for hepatic malignancy are those in the earlier stages of disease. Numerous factors affecting response or survival have been investigated (Table 27-5). Predictably, patients with normal liver function do better than those with ascites, portal vein invasion, encephalopathy, jaundice, and hypoalbuminemia. Patients with even mild biliary obstruction are at particular risk for lobar infarction after chemoembolization, probably because of alteration in portal flow in the hepatic sinusoids in the presence of bile duct obstruction. With a lesser tumor burden, the response with chemoembolization is more beneficial and the postembolization syndrome less severe.

TECHNIQUE

A precise definition of the hepatic arterial supply is essential for safe and effective use of the regional vascular therapies. There are several common variations in the arterial supply of the liver. The right hepatic artery is a branch of the superior mesenteric artery in about 15% of patients, and the left hepatic artery is a branch of the left gastric artery in about 25%. The gastroduodenal artery, the right

gastric artery, the duodenal branches of the proper hepatic artery, and the cystic arteries all must be identified to avoid nontarget embolization. In patients with hypervascular liver tumors, reversal of flow is frequent in the gastroduodenal artery (with filling via inferior pancreaticoduodenal branches of the superior mesenteric artery).

As noted earlier, regional vascular treatments depend on the dual or backup circulation of the liver by the portal vein. Because the hepatic artery is to be embolized intentionally, confirmation of portal vein patency is essential. This can be accomplished with superior mesenteric or splenic artery angiography (Figure 27-1). This is particularly important in patients with hepatocellular carcinoma, in whom portal vein occlusion can occur in up to 39% (31). Even in the presence of portal vein thrombus, hepatic chemoembolization can be performed safely if collateral flow is adequate (Figure 27-2) (32). Because cirrhosis and hepatocellular carcinoma coexist frequently in patients with chronic hepatitis, the portal circulation should also be assessed for hepatofugal flow.

Once the arterial supply of the liver is mapped out and portal vein patency is established, catheterization of the hepatic arteries is undertaken. With the new lubricious coatings, this usually can be accomplished with 5.0–5.5 French catheters. Should these efforts be unsuccessful, microcatheters (2–3 French) can be placed coaxially into nearly any vessel supplying the liver—whether native circulation or parasitized collateral (Figure 27-3). Coaxial catheterization techniques are also helpful when the upper abdominal tumor mass results in distortion or occlusion of native visceral vessels, particularly the celiac axis (Figure 27-4).

With repeated chemoembolizations, the blood supply of the liver must be reassessed continuously because different flow patterns will emerge over time. This is especially true when repeated embolizations result in obliteration of the native hepatic arteries (Figure 27-5). Experience has shown that collateral vessels such as the inferior phrenic, adrenal, intercostal, and internal mammary arteries can be embolized safely. On occasion, the development of unusual collateral circulation ("culprit vessels") can cause the paradoxical appearance of growing and responding tumors in the same patient (Figure 27-6).

Frequently, vessels supplying the intestinal viscera are immediately adjacent to the hepatic arteries—such as the left hepatic artery (a branch of the left gastric artery), the right gastric artery (a branch of the proper or left hepatic artery), or the left hepatic off the common hepatic artery (Figures 27-7, 27-8, and 27-9). This proximity may prevent stable catheterization of the target vessel without placing intestinal tissue at risk. In such cases, "coil blockade," or the intentional mechanical occlusion of the arteries supplying normal organs, can be undertaken (Figure 27-7); collateral circulation from distant sites will sustain these tissues while the mechanical coils prevent nontarget embolization (Figure 27-8).

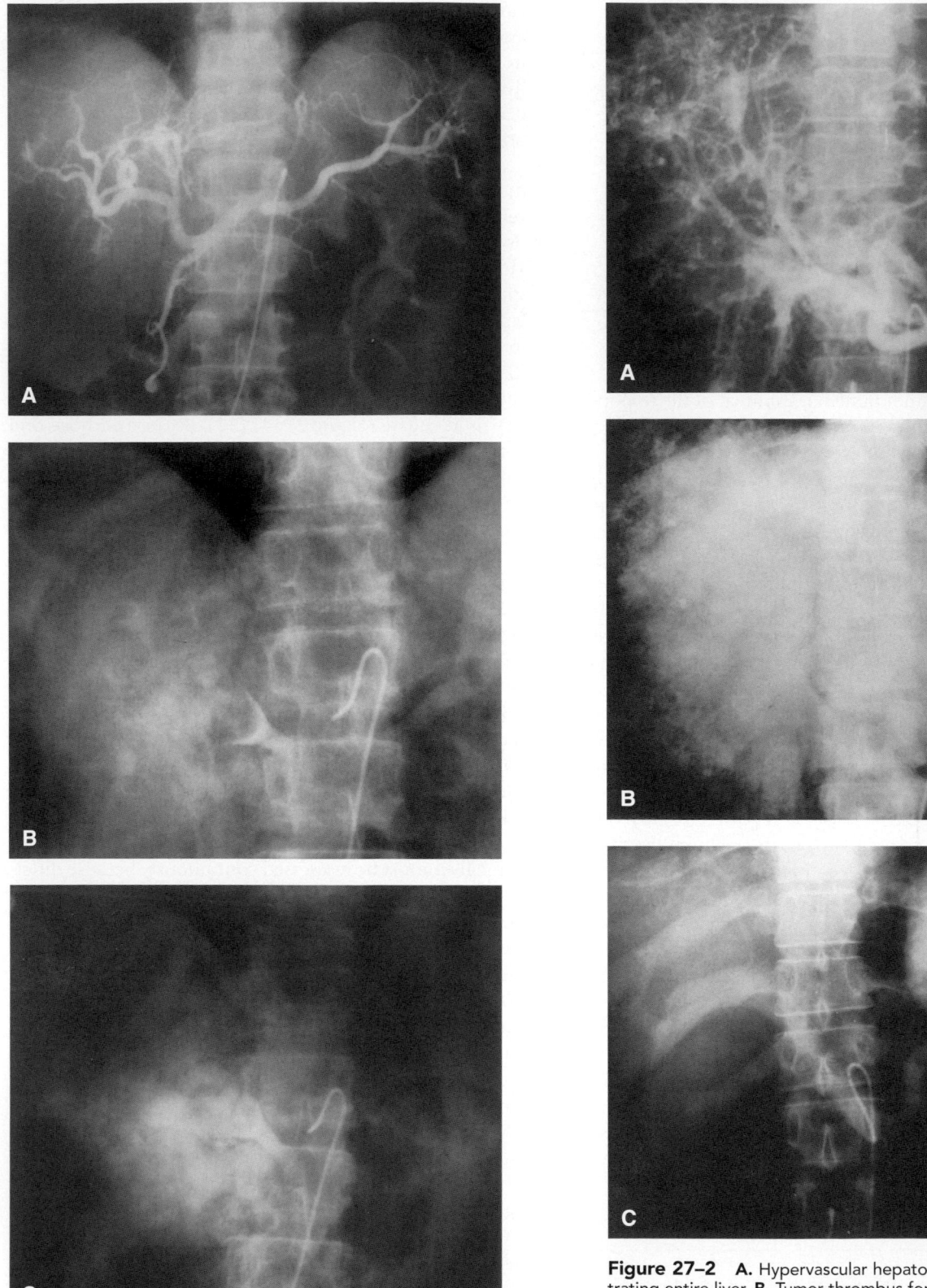

Figure 27–1 **A.** Celiac angiography in patient with cirrhosis and hepatocellular carcinoma. **B., C.** Large tumor thrombus filling and distending the portal vein in the liver hilum. Note the minimal opacification of the liver, mostly the inferior right lobe, from collateral flow.

Figure 27–2 **A.** Hypervascular hepatocellular carcinoma infiltrating entire liver. **B.** Tumor thrombus forms a cast of the portal vein on delayed images. Nonetheless, extensive flow around the thrombus permitted safe chemoembolization. **C.** Recanalization of the portal vein as tumor thrombus regresses with therapy.

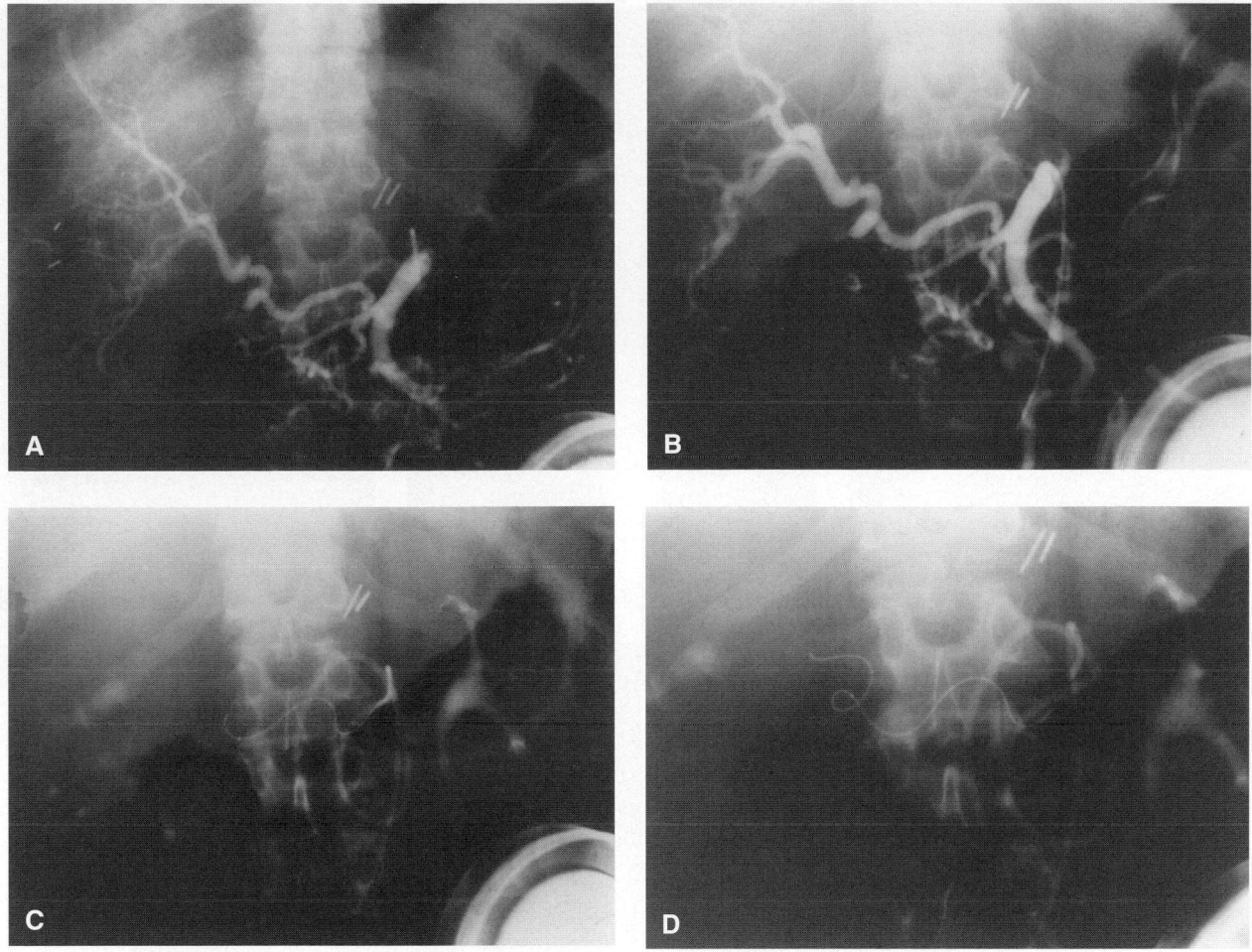

Figure 27-3   A. Patient with metastatic ocular melanoma and occlusion of the hepatic artery by a surgically implanted pump (*reservoir in left lower quadrant*). Arterial supply of the liver is by a collateral branch of the superior mesenteric artery. **B.** Narrowing at the origin of the collateral branch prevents safe catheterization with a 5.0–5.5 French catheter. **C.** A Simmons catheter in the superior mesenteric artery acts as a guide for the microcatheter. **D.** Successful placement in the hepatic artery distal to intestinal branches.

Frequently, severe pain accompanies these procedures, which is possibly the result of stretching of the capsule or embolization of the gallbladder. Effective analgesia with celiac ganglion block and intra-arterial lidocaine has been described (33,34). Chemoembolization can cause sepsis and hepatic abscess, although routine antibiotic coverage has reduced this risk significantly (35).

RESULTS

The results of regional treatments for unresectable liver tumors can be evaluated on the basis of relief of symptoms, shrinkage of tumors or response rate, and prolongation of survival. Embolization and chemoembolization are used infrequently for symptomatic relief. In the early stages of development, durable response rates are the standard by which treatments are compared. In liver cancer, such response rates are judged by cross-sectional imaging examinations, although the accuracy of these modalities has been questioned (36). After some treatments, clear-cut liquefication of tumor is visible on CT; however, because of the nature of surrounding hepatic parenchyma, the tumor mass may not decrease in size. Prospective studies comparing prolongation of survival are few in number and available mostly for common tumors such as hepatocellular carcinoma and colorectal metastases.

HEPATOCELLULAR CARCINOMA

Hepatocellular carcinoma is relatively resistant to systemic chemotherapy, with response rates rarely above 30% (2). Hepatic artery chemotherapy infusions have also met with disappointing results. Embolization and chemoembolization have been used widely, particularly in Asia and Europe,

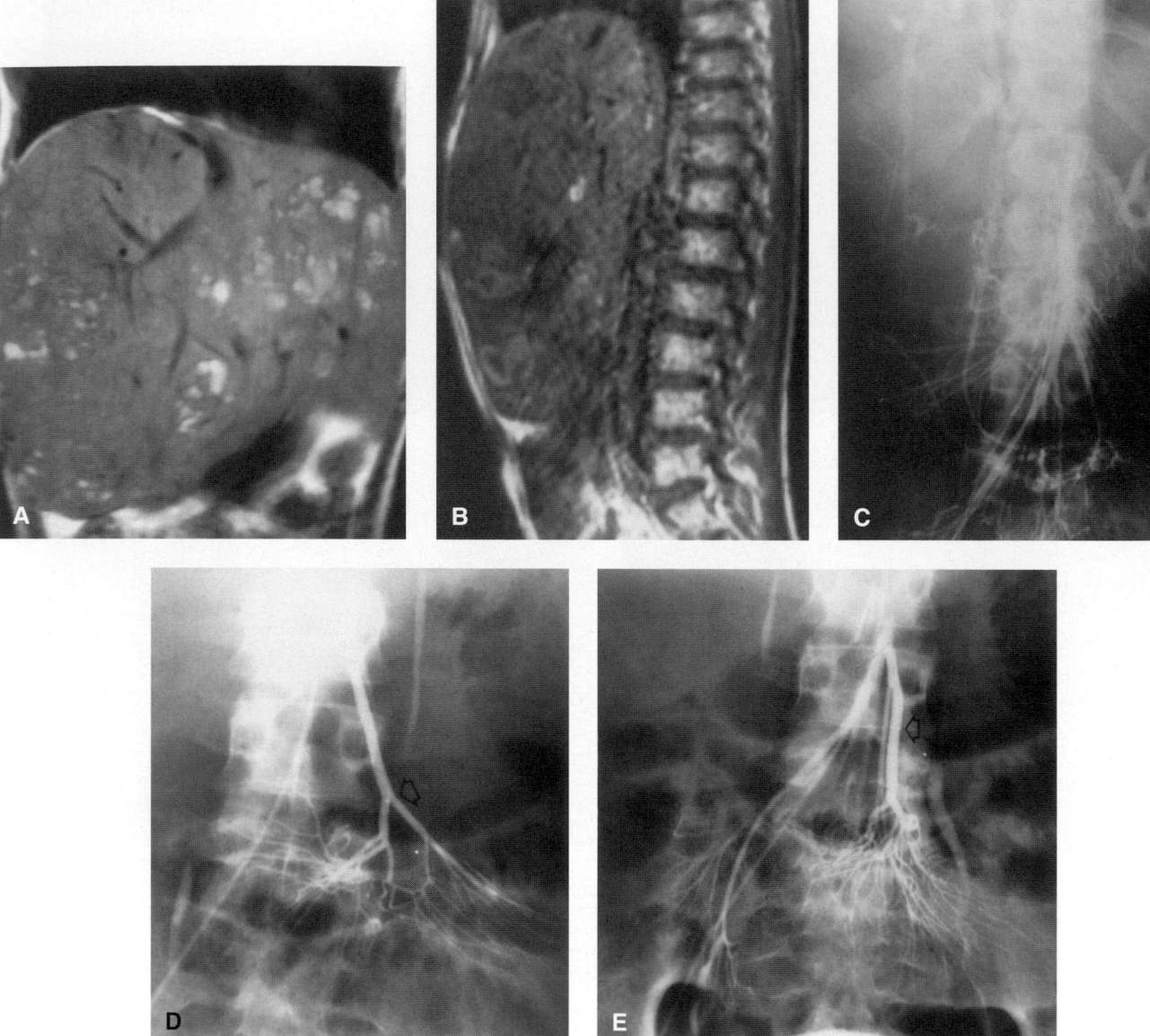

Figure 27–4 **A.**, **B.** Coronal and sagittal MR images demonstrating a large hepatocellular carcinoma filling the upper abdomen of a 15-year-old boy. **C.** Occlusion of the celiac axis by the tumor mass (opacification of celiac vessels during superior mesenteric artery injection). **D., E., F.** Sequential angiography of superior mesenteric artery branches with microcatheter (*arrows*) in an attempt to locate a collateral route to the celiac axis. **G., H.** Successful catheterization via the inferior pancreaticoduodenal arcade. **I.** Proper hepatic artery placement of the tip of a microcatheter (*arrow*). **J.** Marked shrinkage of the tumor after repeated chemoembolizations.

and a large body of data has been accumulated (37–47). With chemoembolization, response rates from 22 to 75% (Table 27–6) have been reported in the larger clinical series. In uncontrolled clinical trials, survival has ranged from 24 to 88% at 1 year, 4 to 64% at 2 years, and 12 to 51% at 3 years (Table 27–7).

Lin et al. evaluated embolization, embolization and systemic chemotherapy, and systemic chemotherapy alone in three groups of patients (48). Survival with the first two was similar (with both significantly better than chemotherapy alone). Four controlled studies have compared chemoembolization to conservative or supportive therapy (Table 27–8). In each, survival was longer in the treatment arm. However, in the most rigorous and recent study, this survival benefit was not significant (49).

A meta-analysis of 18 randomized trials of chemoembolization has been compiled recently (50,51–57). In the five most rigorously constructed trials, chemoembolization was found to significantly improve the 2-year survival compared to less aggressive treatments. Further, in the 2,500

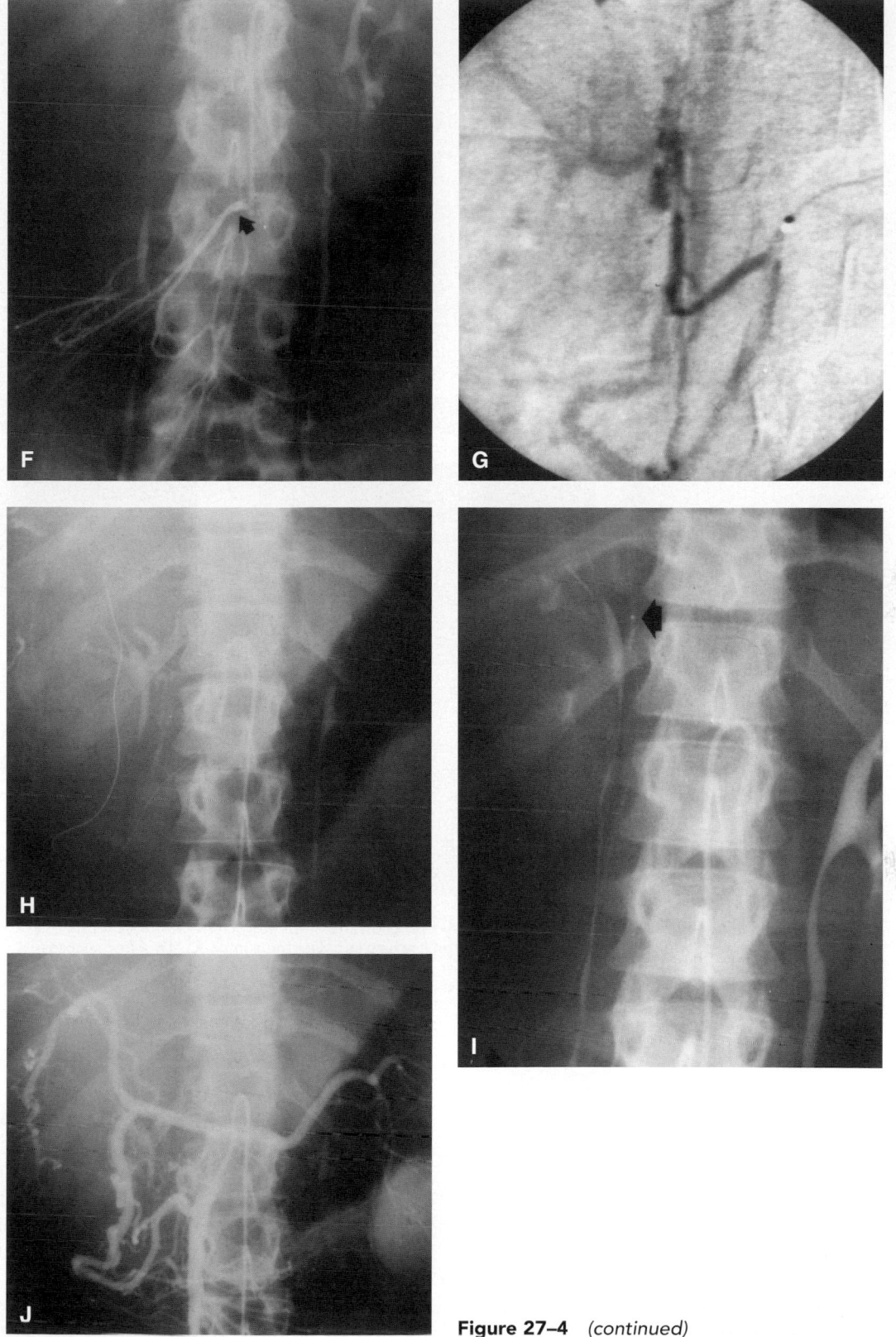

Figure 27–4 *(continued)*

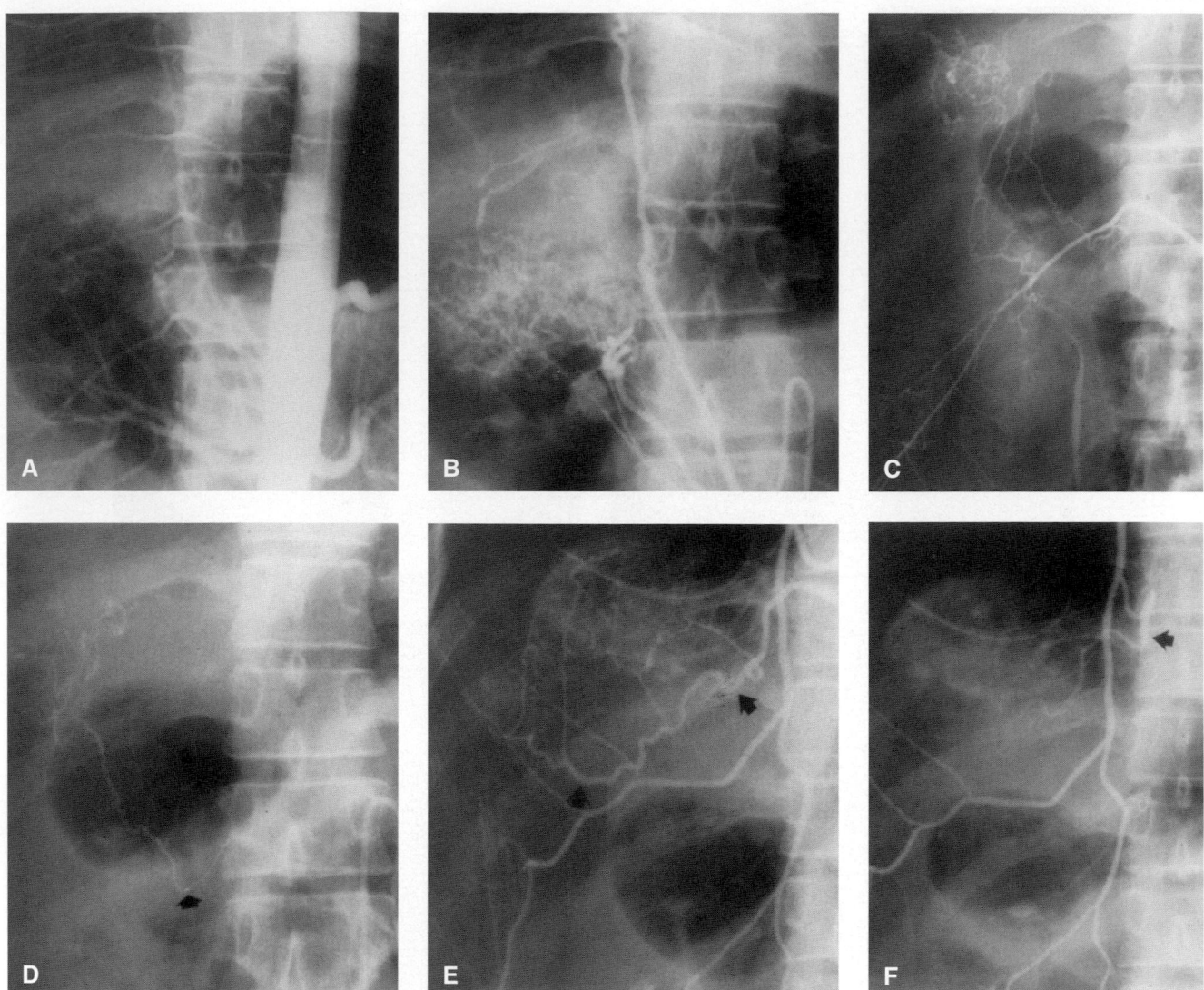

Figure 27–5 **A., B.** Absence of hepatic artery branches after repeated chemoembolization. The superior adrenal branch of the right inferior phrenic artery supplies the tumor. **C., D.** After successful embolization of the adrenal branch, the tumor parasitizes flow from the intercostal artery (*arrow, D*), which is treated. **E., F.** The next affected vessel is the right internal mammary artery (*arrows; pre-embolization and postembolization views*).

patients in all trials, the partial response rate was 27%, and the complete response rate was 6%.

Ethanol, delivered intravascularly and by direct intratumoral injection, has been studied recently, both alone and in concert with transcatheter embolization (58,59). The theory behind combining these therapies is that embolization will be more effective against the periphery of the tumor while ethanol will directly fix the tissues in the center. Encouraged by the results of this combination therapy, investigators have treated patients with small (<5 cm) hepatocellular carcinomas with percutaneous ethanol injection alone. Livraghi et al. reported treating 746 patients with ethanol injection. They observed a 5-year survival rate in 47% of patients with Child's A cirrhosis and tumors smaller than 5 cm (60).

COLORECTAL HEPATIC METASTASES

For those with colorectal hepatic metastases, the response rate with systemic chemotherapy is poor (1). Until recently, many patients in whom systemic therapy failed became candidates for one of the regional infusion treatment protocols, typically 5-FU or FUDR.

Using surgically placed infusion pumps, early prospective but uncontrolled trials reported response rates roughly double those of systemic therapy (40% versus 20%) with two reporting rates up to 90% (61,62). Five large trials evaluating intra-arterial versus systemic treatment (two permitting crossover between the treatment arms and three not) have been reported recently (Table 27–9) (63–66). As with

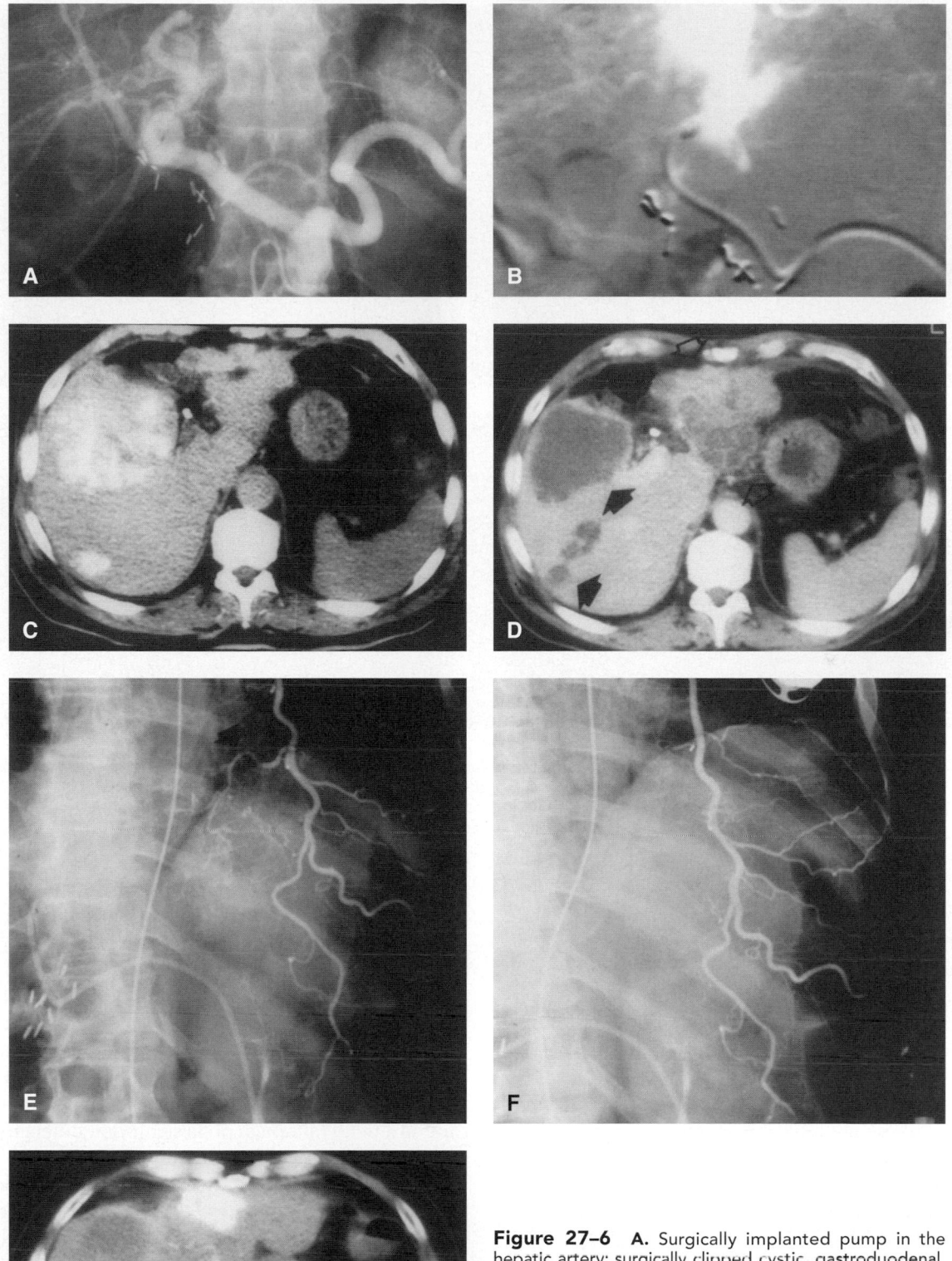

Figure 27–6 **A.** Surgically implanted pump in the hepatic artery; surgically clipped cystic, gastroduodenal, and right gastric arteries. **B.** The catheter has migrated into the left hepatic artery; note the extravasation of contrast into the left lobe of the liver. **C.** After chemoembolization, there is deposition of embolic material and contrast into the right lobe of the tumor. **D.** Follow-up CT scan reveals shrinkage of the right-lobe tumor (*closed black arrows*) yet marked progression of left-lobe disease (*open arrow*). **E., F.** The "culprit vessel" is the left internal mammary artery (*preembolization and postembolization views*). **G.** CT scan after embolization with dense staining of the tumor.

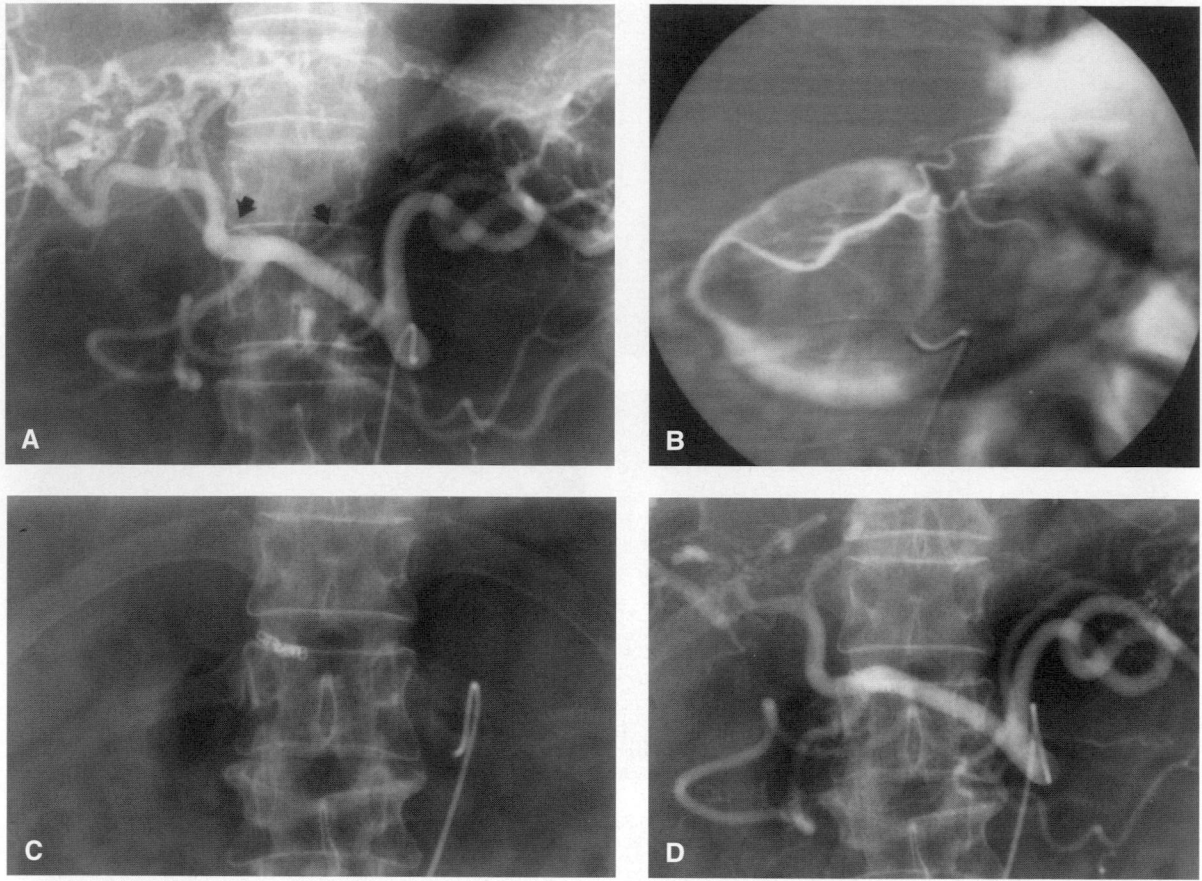

Figure 27–7 **A.** Prominent right gastric artery (*arrows*) at trifurcation of the proper hepatic artery into right, middle, and left hepatic branches. **B.** Selective injection into the right gastric artery with a coaxially placed microcatheter. **C., D.** "Coil blockade" of the right gastric artery to prevent nontarget embolization by reflux of chemoembolic particles.

earlier reports, these trials described responses to systemic treatment of 9–21% and regional therapy of 42–62%. Despite such a difference, no survival benefit was demonstrated in the reports by Chang, Martin, and Rougier. Survival benefit could not be assessed in the studies that allowed nonresponders in the systemic arm to cross over to regional treatment.

Explanations for this lack of survival benefit included a high complication rate from infusate pumps, local toxicity from the infusion, and inappropriate selection of the drug for infusion. Complications and local toxicity were high; Kemeny et al. described ulcer disease (because of nontarget, unintentional intestinal infusion of chemotherapy) in 17% of patients and biliary sclerosis (because of FUDR toxicity) in 8% (69). Hohn et al. noted catheter-related complications of 13% and biliary toxicity of 52% (65). Many of these nontarget intestinal infusions were the result of catheter migration, pericatheter spasm, and thrombosis, which altered the dynamics of flow to the tumors over time (Figures 27–6 and 27–10). Thus, the clear-cut response difference with regional infusion was offset by the morbidity of catheter insertion and

maintenance. Such morbidity and complications can be expected, whether the catheters are placed surgically or radiologically (68).

Given the refractory nature of catheter-related problems, investigators have concentrated on modifying the dose of FUDR and adding other agents to reduce toxicity. Kemeny et al. (69), in an attempt to reduce the toxicity of intra-arterial FUDR, alternated steroid treatment with chemotherapy and found a trend (although not a significant difference) toward increased survival with this new treatment.

Several reports have described favorable results with chemoembolization. Lorenz et al. (70) observed responses in 4 of 11 patients treated with degradable starch microspheres and mitomycin C. Hunt et al. conducted a randomized evaluation of supportive management, embolization, and chemoembolization with 5-FU and starch microspheres (71). They identified a trend toward prolonged survival in patients with less than 50% liver involvement. Martinelli et al. reported responses in 25% of patients undergoing embolization or chemoembolization, all of whom had failed systemic chemotherapy (72). Another

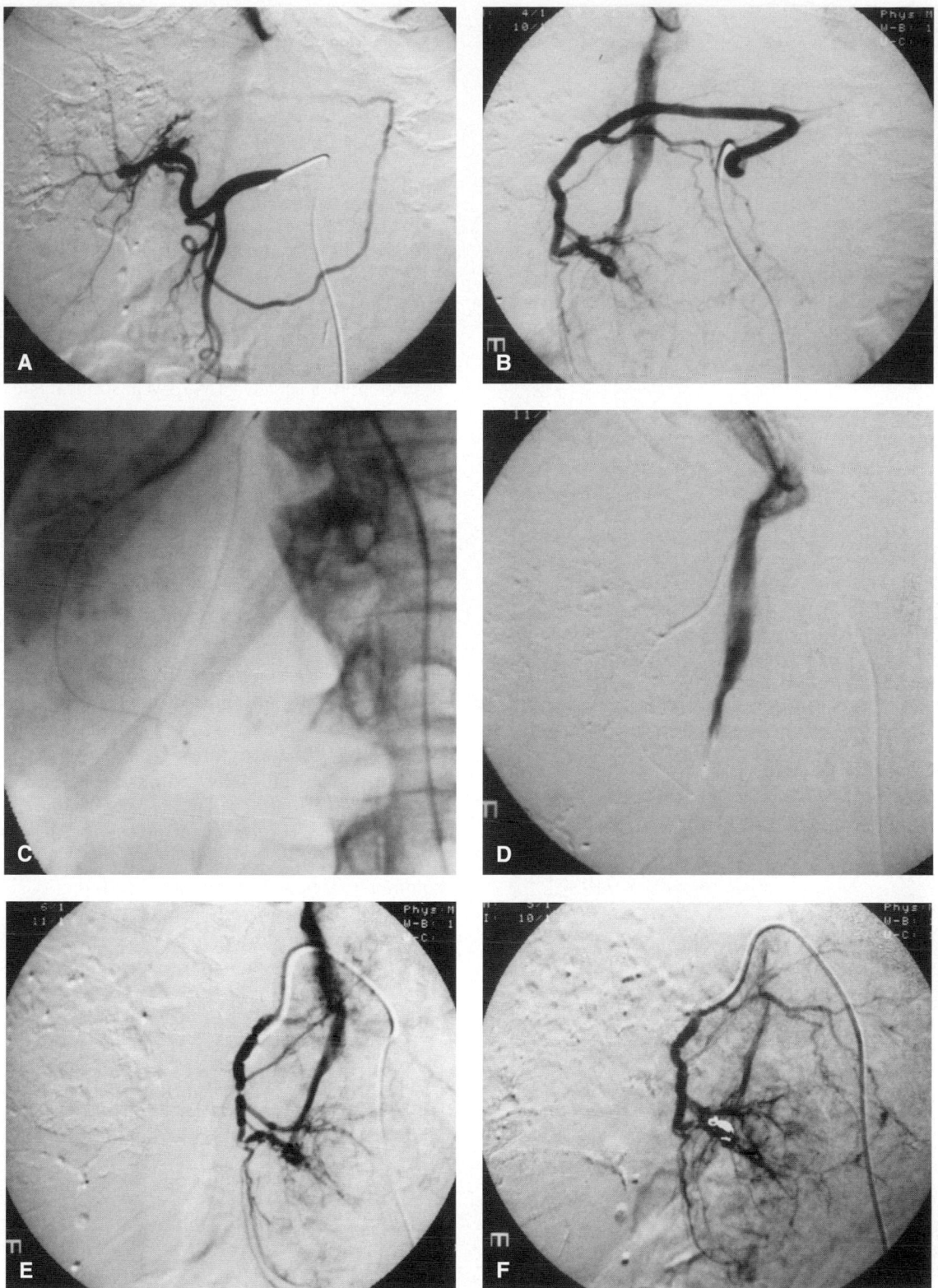

Figure 27–8   **A., B.** Common and left gastric artery injections demonstrating a hypervascular liver tumor and fistula from the left hepatic artery to the inferior vena cava (presumably from a previous biopsy). During common hepatic injection, note the gastroepiploic-to-left-gastric collateral flow caused by the siphon effect of the fistula. **C., D.** Coaxial placement of a microcatheter and guide wire via a Simmons guiding catheter through the fistula and injection of contrast into the vena cava. **E., F.** Selective left hepatic artery injection before and after coil embolization (or "coil blockade") to prevent left-to-right shunting during chemoembolization.

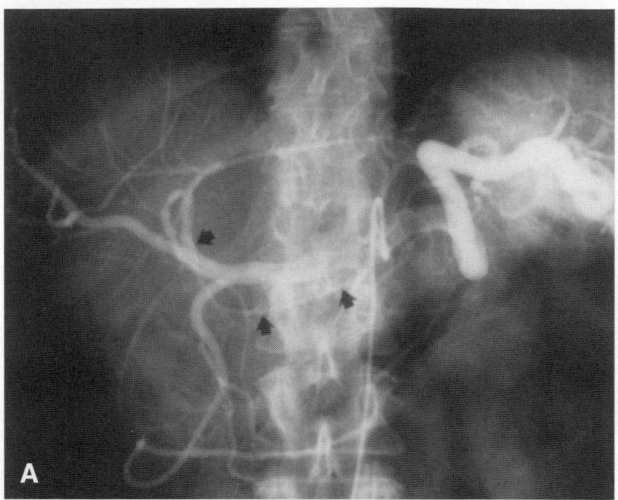

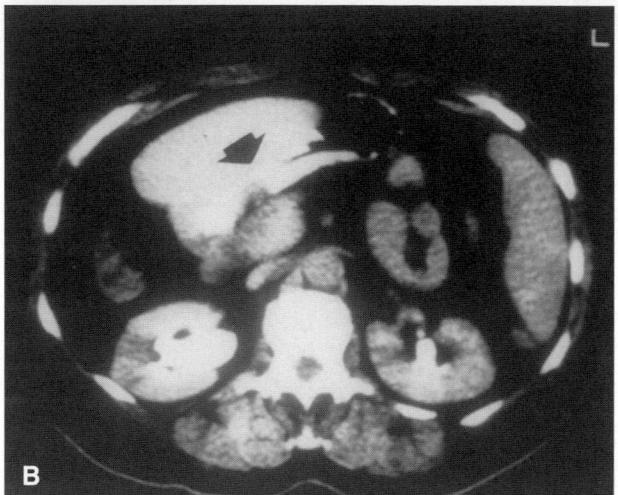

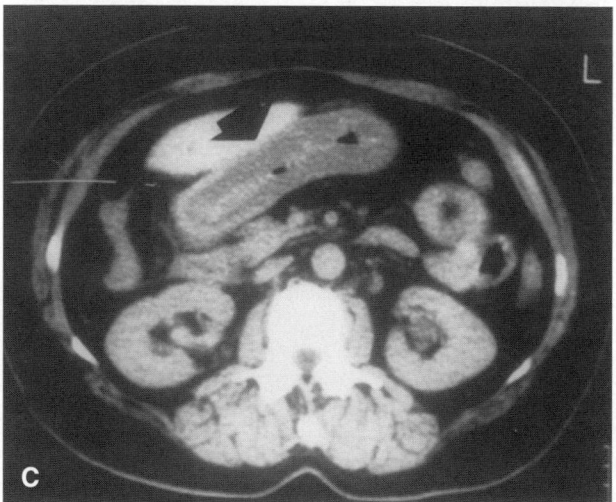

Figure 27–9 A. Prominent right gastric artery (*arrow*) mistaken for a branch of the left hepatic artery. **B.** Deposition of embolic material (*arrow*) in gastric antrum is shown on CT scan immediately after the procedure. **C.** Marked thickening (*arrow*) of gastric wall 2 days later.

TABLE 27–6

HEPATOCELLULAR CARCINOMA: RESPONSE RATES WITH CHEMOEMBOLIZATION IN LARGE CLINICAL SERIES

Study	No. of Patients	Response Rate (complete + partial) (%)
Yamada, 1983 (37)	120	75
Yamada, 1990 (38)	739	75
Yamashita, 1990 (39)	85	22
Bismuth, 1992 (40)	291	27

recent report observed a 15% 3-year survival rate in patients treated with chemoembolization (73). The mean survival from initiation of intra-arterial treatment is usually 18 months.

In the Northwestern experience, Tellez described a 63% response rate with a median survival of 29 months after diagnosis of metastatic disease (74).

CARCINOID AND ISLET CELL TUMORS

The management of patients with carcinoid and islet cell carcinoma is among the most difficult in cancer care. These tumors—known collectively as apudomas (amine precursor undergoing decarboxylation)—can secrete serotonin, insulin, gastrin, glucagon, adrenocorticotropic hormone (ACTH), somatostatin, and many other hormones. Typically, systemic manifestations such as the carcinoid syndrome begin as the primary tumor becomes large or, even more commonly, as hepatic metastases develop.

The carcinoid syndrome is rare; the largest clinical series describes less than 100 patients (75). The largest experience with radiologic management is 18–25 patients (76,77).

TABLE 27–7

HEPATOCELLULAR CARCINOMA: CUMULATIVE SURVIVAL RATES WITH CHEMOEMBOLIZATION

Study	6 Months (%)	1 Year (%)	2 Years (%)	3 Years (%)
Yamada, 1983 (37)		44	29	15
Ohnishi, 1984 (41)	65	24		
Yamada, 1990 (38)		51	24	12
Yamashita, 1990 (39)	70	32	4	
Beppu, 1991 (42)		81	64	51
Ikeda, 1991 (43)		77	55	41
Nakao, 1991 (44)		88	57	42
Taguchi, 1992 (45)		54	33	18
Park, 1993* (46)		75	56	40
Nakamura, 1994 (47)		56	33	18

*Recurrent tumors after partial hepatectomy.

TABLE 27-8

RESULTS OF CONTROLLED TRIALS COMPARING CHEMOEMBOLIZATION AND CONSERVATIVE THERAPY FOR HEPATOCELLULAR CARCINOMA

Study	1 Year (%)		2 Years (%)	
	Control	Chemoembolization	Control	Chemoembolization
Pelletier, 1990 (51)	31	24		
Vetter, 1991 (52)	0	59		30
Bronowicki, 1994 (53)	18	64	6	38
Trinchet, 1995 (49)	44	62	26	38

Most therapies concentrate initially on symptomatic management because most of these tumors have an indolent course (the median survival rate for those patients with liver metastases was 3 years; in the Mayo Clinic series, 30% survived 5 years, and 1 patient was alive 41 years after diagnosis) (78). Initially, pharmacologic treatment focuses on the agonist to the particular hormone, such as somatostatin analogues in the carcinoid syndrome and H_2 blockers in the Zollinger-Ellison syndrome. Later, systemic chemotherapeutic agents such as streptozotocin, 5-FU, and doxorubicin are used. The results with these agents are usually short-lived. The reported response rates with a single agent are typically 30–40%, and with multiple agents, 50–60%. The fleeting duration of these responses has led some investigators to skip systemic chemotherapy alone in favor of a combination treatment with embolization (79).

Transcatheter embolization alone has been used in the management of carcinoid and islet cell tumors. After using Gelfoam, polyvinyl alcohol, and steel coils, Mitty et al. reported a 72% objective response rate (such as decreased serum levels of serotonin or tryptophan; decreased urinary excretion of 5-hydroxyindoleacetic acid, indoleacetic acid, or tryptamine) in 18 patients with the carcinoid syndrome; 94% of patients experienced symptomatic relief (76). Carrasco et al. described responses in 80% of 25 patients undergoing transcatheter embolization for carcinoid

hepatic metastases (77). Marlink et al. reported partial or complete responses in 7 of 10 patients and symptomatic improvement in all patients treated with particulate embolization alone (79).

Moertel observed a 90% success rate in the treatment of carcinoid and islet cell tumors with a combination of systemic chemotherapy (5-FU and streptozotocin) and transcatheter embolization. These responses were also quite durable—24 months for carcinoid and 18 months for islet cell (78). In another study of transcatheter embolization alone, Ajani et al. described partial remission in 22 patients who had islet cell tumor metastatic to the liver (80). In contrast to embolization alone, chemoembolization has been described as successful in controlling symptoms in 79–90% of patients (81–84).

OCULAR MELANOMA

Ocular melanoma is quite uncommon, affecting about 2,000 Americans annually. The tumor has the unusual tendency of spreading only to the liver, where it is notoriously resistant to systemic chemotherapy (response rates of 4–5%) (85). Mavligit et al. described successful treatment in 14 of 30 patients with a median survival of 11 months (in contrast to the usual 2–6 months) (86). In a recent study comparing chemoembolization to arterial infusion,

TABLE 27-9

SYSTEMIC VERSUS INTRA-ARTERIAL CHEMOTHERAPY FOR COLORECTAL HEPATIC METASTASES: RESULTS OF RANDOMIZED TRIALS

Study	Intraarterial (%)	Systemic (%)	GI Complications (%)	Biliary Complications (%)	Survival Benefit*
Kemeny, 1987 (64)	50	20	25	19	Crossover
Chang, 1987 (63)	62	12	21	33	N.S.
Hohn, 1989 (65)	42	10	0	52	Crossover
Martin, 1990 (66)	48	21	13	26	N.S.
Rougier, 1992 (67)	43	9	25	37	N.S.

* N.S. = not significant; crossover = crossover permitted, survival benefit could not be evaluated.

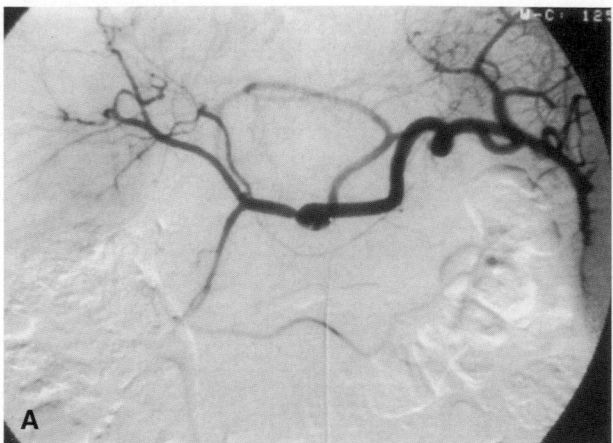

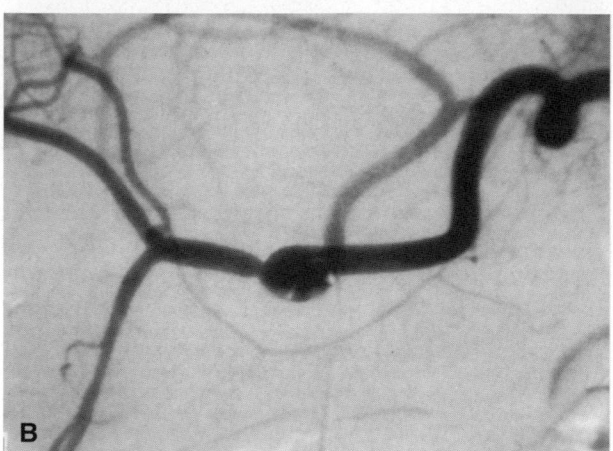

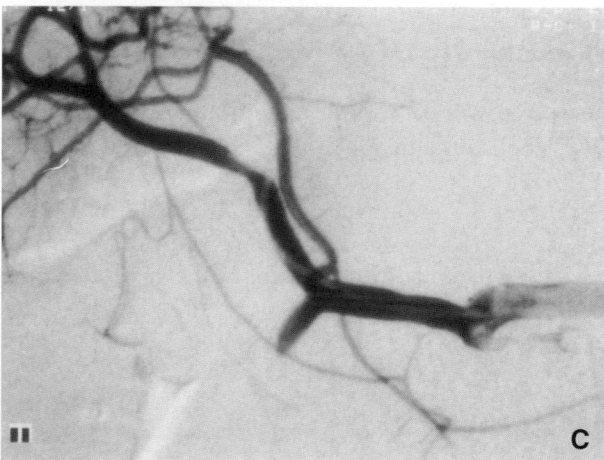

Figure 27–10 **A.** Preliminary celiac angiography demonstrates the left hepatic artery as a branch of the left gastric artery as well as a prominent right gastric artery; otherwise, there is unremarkable hepatic circulation and no evidence of aberrant intestinal circulation. **B.** Magnified view of the celiac circulation. **C.** Because of spasm at the catheter tip, repeat hepatic angiography was performed. A branch of the right hepatic artery to the intestine is unexpectedly present. Had selective right hepatic angiography not been performed, inexplicable nontarget embolization would have resulted.

Agarwala found that of 10 patients in the former group, seven (70%) responded or had disease stabilization (87).

COMPLICATIONS

Significant complications are described in patients undergoing embolization or chemoembolization (Table 27–10). These include intestinal ischemia, cholecystitis, infection, and hepatic insufficiency. With appropriate antibiotics, the rate of liver abscess has been lowered to 2% (35). Postembolization syndrome is so common that it is expected. Some complications, such as nontarget intestinal embolization, are preventable with meticulous technique. The studies of Martin, Chang, and Rougier have demonstrated that, for the higher response rates of regional treatments to be translated into survival benefit, complications must be minimized (63,66,67).

RADIOFREQUENCY ABLATION

The radiofrequency ablation of liver tumors, first described in 1994, has been the subject of considerable excitement among radiologists, surgeons, oncologists, and hepatologists. The underlying principle is the local creation of heat, via a percutaneously or surgically placed probe, that destroys tumor tissue while insulating and sparing adjacent normal liver (88). Though heat can be generated feasibly

TABLE 27–10
COMPLICATIONS OF CHEMOEMBOLIZATION

Complication	Range (%)
Common	
Ascites	4–20
Cholecystitis	1–11
Death	1–2
Encephalopathy	1–3
GI hemorrhage	1–3
Hepatic abscess	2–5
Intestinal infarction	1–3
Postembolization syndrome	40–90
Renal failure	1–10
Rupture	1–2
Septicemia	1–3
Uncommon	
Variceal bleeding	
Hemoperitoneum	
Tumor lysis syndrome	
Pancreatitis	
Pleural effusion	
Hepatic infarction	
Bile duct necrosis	
Intrahepatic aneurysm	

from sources such as laser, high-intensity ultrasound, and microwave energy, the most experience has been gained with radiofrequency energy. In this technique, using probes as small as 15-gauge to 17-gauge needles, alternating current causes tissue coagulation by frictional heating. Tumor tissue is ablated as temperatures reach 50–100°C, and yet, noncancerous tissue as close as 0.5 cm away is spared.

The enthusiasm for radiofrequency ablation (RFA) is understandable for several reasons. For one, RFA can be performed percutaneously, surgically, or laparoscopically and, therefore, is a complement to resection and embolization. RFA seems to be tolerated better by patients than other radiological interventions such as chemoembolization. Specifically, infarction and infection, the bugaboos of chemoembolization, are not hazards of RFA. Unlike intra-arterial treatments in which the feeding vessels inevitably occlude after repeated embolization, RFA can be repeated numerous times. RFA can also complement chemoembolization in some patients (Figure 27–11).

RFA has been applied in similar settings to chemoembolization, namely in patients who are not candidates for surgical resection, have no extrahepatic disease, and have limited tumor burden. Limited tumor burden generally means masses smaller than 3.5–4.0 cm because uniform heat diffusion is problematic in larger lesions. Specific indications have included patients with small hepatocellular carcinomas (often in a setting of cirrhosis), colorectal liver metastases, and neuroendocrine tumors that have spread to the liver and are causing symptoms.

Regional ablations, whether with heat, cold, or chemicals such as alcohol and acetic acid, are aggressive therapies and, not surprisingly, they effectively destroy tumor tissue. Most of the published trials describe results as responses, a combination of the traditional classification of partial and complete responses. These response rates generally fall into the 85–95% range (89–96). Chemoembolization, by comparison, has a complete and partial response rate of about 40%.

As impressive as 85–95% response rates are, they are no substitute for controlled trials comparing RFA to systemic chemotherapy, resection, and other interventional therapies. Indeed, in these limited studies, survival and disease-free intervals with RFA have not meant surgery. While treating patients with hepatocellular carcinoma and cirrhosis, Vivarelli and colleagues found 1- and 3-year disease-free survival rates of 79% and 50% in those undergoing surgery versus 60% and 20% in the RFA cohort (97). In patients undergoing resection for colorectal liver metastases, Abdalla found a 4-year survival rate of 65% compared to 22% in those treated with RFA (98).

The largest series of complications from RFA reported six deaths in 2,320 patients (0.3%) from sepsis, hemorrhage,

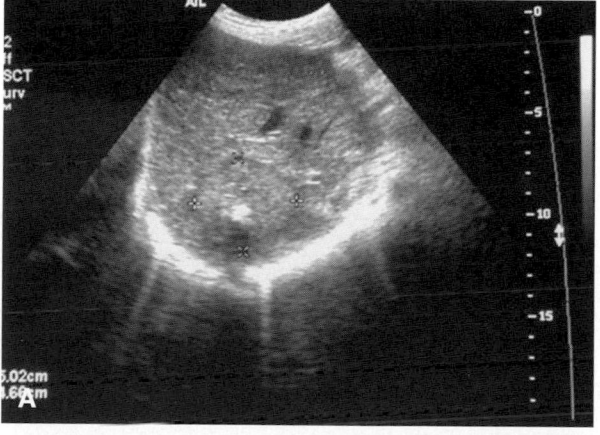

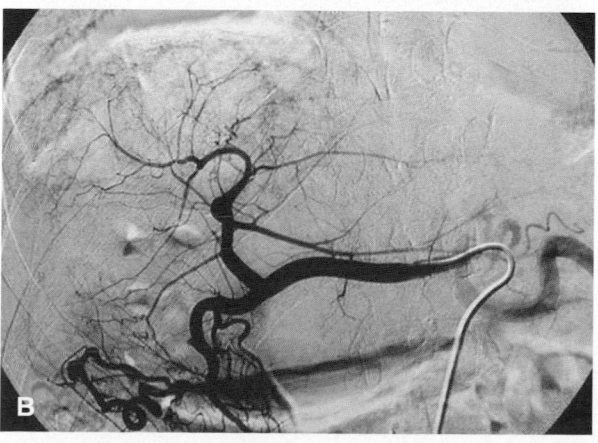

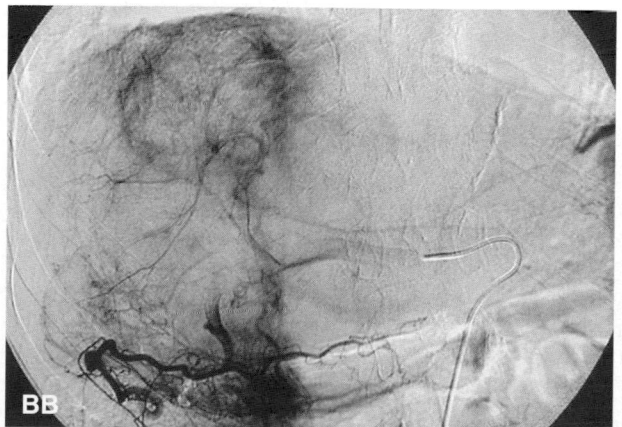

Figure 27–11   A. An 81-year-old man with hepatic metastasis from colorectal cancer. **B.** Hepatic angiography reveals hyperemic border of large right lobe lesion.

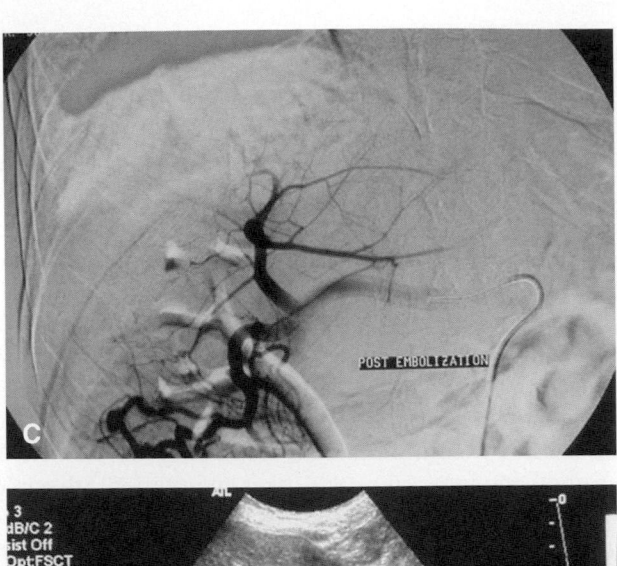

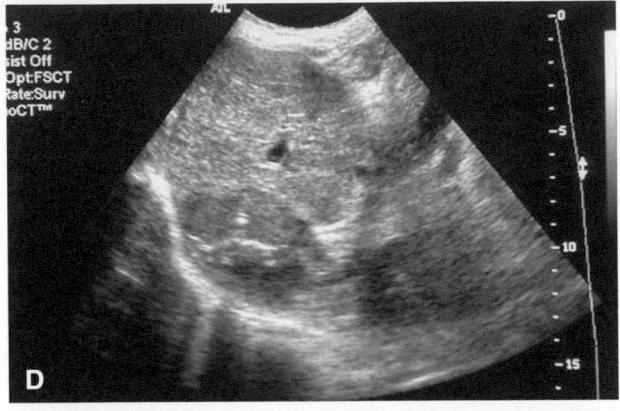

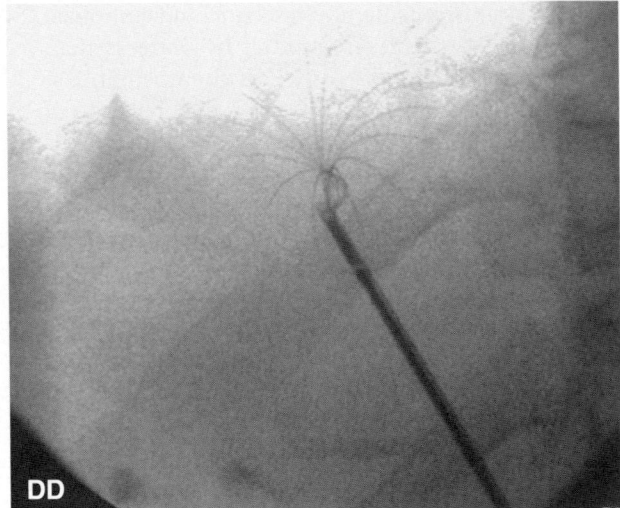

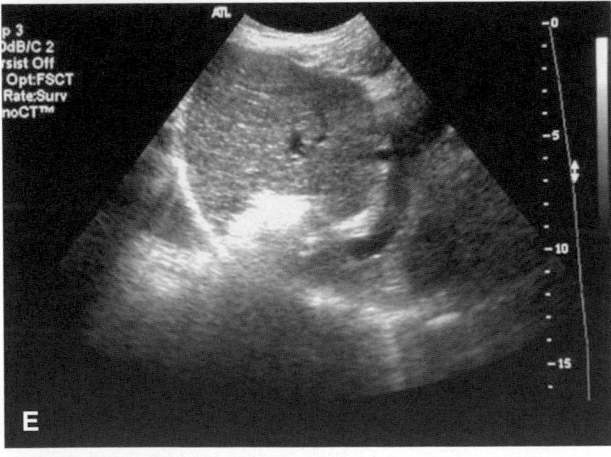

Figure 27–11 *(continued)*   **C.** After embolization. **D.** Radiofrequency (RF) ablation of right lobe lesion after embolization. **E.** Ultrasound immediately after RF ablation.

and intestinal perforation (99). Major complications were identified in 50 patients (2.2%) including perforation, needle track seeding, hemorrhage, and liver abscess. By comparison, a meta-analysis of results from chemoembolization identified complications in 5.6% of subjects (50). Because of the local application of heat, some relatively unique complications have been described. These include portal vein thrombosis, biloma, biliary fistula, localized bile duct strictures, skin burns, and thermal injuries to the intestine (100,101). In addition to hepatic lesions, RFA has been used in kidney and lung tumors as well as osteoid osteomas.

SUMMARY

Interest in percutaneous regional therapies for unresectable hepatic tumors has grown as technical developments have made their applications feasible and clinical experience has improved their safety and utility. This interest has been fueled by continued disappointments in systemic therapies and the lack of demonstrable survival benefit with therapies delivered by surgically implanted pumps. Large prospective studies may establish the effectiveness of these therapies as appropriate treatment of primary and metastatic liver cancer. Recently reported experiences justify cautious optimism as such trials evolve.

REFERENCES

1. Braun AH, Achterrath W, Wilke H, et al. New systemic frontline treatment for metastatic colorectal carcinoma. Cancer 2004;100: 1558–1577.
2. Johnson PJ. Hepatocellular carcinoma: is current therapy really altering outcome? Gut 2002;51:459–462.
3. Clarkson B, Young C, Dierick W, et al. Effects of continuous hepatic artery infusion of antimetabolites on primary and metastatic cancer of the liver. Cancer 1962;15:472–488.
4. Sullivan RD, Norcross JW, Watkins E. Chemotherapy of metastatic liver cancer by prolonged hepatic-artery infusion. N Engl J Med 1964;270:321–327.
5. Chuang VP, Wallace S. Hepatic artery embolization in the treatment of hepatic neoplasms. Radiology 1981;140:51–58.
6. Behesti MV, Denny DF, Glickman MG, et al. Percutaneous isolated liver perfusion for treatment of hepatic malignancy: preliminary report. J Vasc Interv Radiol 1992;3:453–458.
7. Hamazoe R, Murakami A, Hirooka Y, et al. A phase II pilot study of the combined application of hyperthermia and intra-hepato-arterial chemotherapy using cisplatinum and 5-fluorouracil. J Surg Oncol 1991;48:127–132.
8. Livraghi T, Bolondi L, Lazzaroni S, et al. Percutaneous ethanol injection of hepatocellular carcinoma in cirrhosis: a study in 207 patients. Cancer 1992;69:925–929.
9. Ohnishi K, Ohyama N, Ito S, et al. Small hepatocellular carcinoma: treatment with US-guided intratumoral injection of acetic acid. Radiology 1994;193:747–752.
10. Tsujitani S, Watanabe A, Kakeji Y, et al. Hepatic recurrence not prevented with low-dosage, long-term, intraportal 5-FU infusion after resection of colorectal liver metastasis. Eur J Surg Oncol 1991;17:526–529.
11. Order S, Stillwagon GB, Klein J, et al. Iodine 131 antiferritin, a new treatment modality in hepatoma: a Radiation Therapy Oncology Group study. J Clin Oncol 1985;3:1573–1582.
12. Kato T, Nemoto R, Mori H, et al. Arterial chemoembolization with microencapsulated anticancer drug. JAMA 1981;245:1123–1127.
13. Chuang VP, Wallace S, Soo C, et al. Therapeutic Ivalon embolization of hepatic tumors. AJR Am J Roentgenol 1982;138:289–294.
14. Clouse ME, Lee RGL, Duszlak EJ, et al. Peripheral hepatic artery embolization for primary and secondary hepatic neoplasms. Radiology 1983;147:407–411.
15. Lautt WW, Greenway CV. Conceptual review of the hepatic vascular bed. Hepatology 1987;7:952–963.
16. Ralls PW. Doppler sonography of the hepatic artery and portal venous system. AJR Am J Roentgenol 1990;155:517–525.
17. Breedis C, Young G. Blood supply of neoplasms of the liver. Am J Pathol 1954;30:969–985.
18. Healy JE. Vascular patterns in human metastatic liver tumors. Surg Gynecol Obstet 1965;120:1187–1193.
19. Sigurdson ER, Ridge JA, Kemeny N, et al. Tumor and liver drug uptake following hepatic artery and portal vein infusion. J Clin Oncol 1987;5:1836–1840.
20. Ridge JR, Bading JA, Gelbard AS, et al. Perfusion of colorectal hepatic metastases: relative distribution of flow from the hepatic artery and portal vein. Cancer 1987;59:1547–1553.
21. Ensminger W, Gyves J. Regional chemotherapy of neoplastic diseases. Pharmacol Ther 1983;21:277–293.
22. Martin JK, Moertel CG, Adson MA, et al. Surgical treatment of functioning metastatic carcinoid tumors. Arch Surg 1983;118:537–542.
23. Sternlicht M, Sales SF, Daniels JR, et al. Renal cisplatin chemoembolization with Angiostat, Gelfoam, and Ethiodol in the rabbit: renal platinum distributions. Radiology 1989;170:1073–1075.
24. Kan Z, Sato M, Ivancev K, et al. Distribution and effect of iodized poppyseed oil in the liver after hepatic artery embolization: experimental study in several animal species. Radiology 1993;186: 861–866.
25. Kan Z, Ivancev K, Lunderquist A, et al. In vivo microscopy of hepatic tumors in animal models: a dynamic investigation of blood supply to hepatic metastases. Radiology 1993;187:621–626.
26. Takayasu K, Shima Y, Muramatsu Y, et al. Hepatocellular carcinoma: treatment with intra-arterial iodized oil with and without chemotherapeutic agents. Radiology 1987;162:345–351.
27. Nakamura H, Hashimoto T, Oi H, et al. Transcatheter oily chemoembolization of hepatocellular carcinoma. Radiology 1989; 170:783–786.
28. Poston GJ. Surgical strategies for colorectal liver metastases. Surgical Oncology 2004;13:125–136.
29. Hughes K, Scheele J, Sugarbaker PH. Surgery for colorectal cancer metastatic to the liver. Surg Clin North Am 1989;69:340–359.
30. Haug CE, Jenkins RL, Rohrer RJ, et al. Liver transplantation for primary hepatic cancer. Transplantation 1992;53:376–382.
31. Lai CL, Lam KC, Wong KP, et al. Clinical features of hepatocellular carcinoma: review of 211 patients in Hong Kong. Cancer 1981; 47:2746–2755.
32. Pentecost MJ, Daniels JR, Teitelbaum GP, et al. Hepatic chemoembolization: safety with portal vein thrombosis. J Vasc Interv Radiol 1993;4:347–351.
33. Coldwell DM, Lopez KA. Regional anesthesia for hepatic arterial embolization. Radiology 1989;172:1039–1040.
34. Molgaard CP, Teitelbaum GP, Pentecost MJ, et al. Intra-arterial administration of lidocaine for analgesia in hepatic chemoembolization. J Vasc Interv Radiol 1990;1:81–85.
35. Reed RA, Teitelbaum GP, Daniels JR, et al. Prevalence of infection following hepatic chemoembolization with cross-linked collagen with administration of prophylactic antibiotics. J Vasc Interv Radiol 1994;5:367–371.
36. Venook AP, Stagg RJ, Lewis BJ, et al. Chemoembolization for hepatocellular carcinoma. J Clin Oncol 1990;8:1108–1114.
37. Yamada R, Sato M, Kawabata M, et al. Hepatic artery embolization in 120 patients with unresectable hepatoma. Radiology 1983; 148:397–401.
38. Yamada R, Kishi K, Sonomura T, et al. Transcatheter arterial embolization in unresectable hepatocellular carcinoma. Cardiovasc Intervent Radiol 1990;13:135–139.
39. Yamashita Y, Takahashi M, Koga Y, et al. Prognostic factors in liver metastases after transcatheter arterial embolization or arterial infusion. Acta Radiol 1990;31:269–274.
40. Bismuth H, Morino M, Sherlock D, et al. Primary treatment of hepatocellular carcinoma by arterial chemoembolization. Am J Surg 1992;163:387–394.
41. Ohnishi K, Tsuchiya S, Nakayama T, et al. Arterial chemoembolization of hepatocellular carcinoma with mitomycin C microcapsules. Radiology 1984;152:51–55.
42. Beppu T, Ohara C, Yamaguchi Y, et al. A new approach to chemoembolization for unresectable hepatocellular carcinoma using aclarubicin microspheres in combination with cisplatin suspended in iodized oil. Cancer 1991;68:2555–2560.
43. Ikeda K, Kumada H, Saitoh S, et al. Effect of repeated transcatheter arterial embolization on the survival time in patients with hepatocellular carcinoma: an analysis by the Cox proportional hazard model. Cancer 1991;68:2150–2154.
44. Nakao N, Kamino K, Miura K, et al. Recurrent hepatocellular carcinoma after partial hepatectomy: value of treatment with transcatheter arterial chemoembolization. AJR Am J Roentgenol 1991;156:1177–1179.
45. Taguchi T, Nakamura H. Chemoembolization therapy for hepatocellular carcinoma in Japan. J Infusional Chemo 1992;2:124–127.
46. Park JH, Han JK, Chung JW, et al. Postoperative recurrence of hepatocellular carcinoma: results of transcatheter arterial chemoembolization. Cardiovasc Intervent Radiol 1993;16:21–24.
47. Nakamura H, Mitani T, Murakami T, et al. Five-year survival after transcatheter chemoembolization for hepatocellular carcinoma. Cancer Chemother Pharmacol 1994;33(Suppl):89–92.
48. Lin D, Liaw Y, Lee T, et al. Hepatic arterial embolization in patients with unresectable hepatocellular carcinoma: a randomized controlled trial. Gastroenterology 1988;94:453–456.
49. Trinchet JC, Rached AA, Mathieu D, et al. A comparison of lipiodol chemoembolization and conservative treatment for unresectable hepatocellular carcinoma. Groupe d'Etude et de Traitement du Carcinome Hepatocellulaire. N Engl J Med 1995;332:1256–1261.
50. Camma C, Schepis F, Orlando A, et al. Transarterial chemoembolization for unresectable hepatocellular carcinoma: meta-analysis of randomized controlled trials. Radiology 2002;224:47–54.
51. Pelletier G, Roche A, Ink O, et al. A randomized trial of hepatic arterial chemoembolization in patients with unresectable hepatocellular carcinoma. J Hepatol 1990;11:181–184.

52. Vetter D, Wenger JJ, Bergier JM, et al. Transcatheter oily chemoembolization in the management of advanced hepatocellular carcinoma in cirrhosis: results of a western comparative study in 60 patients. Hepatology 1991;13:427–433.

53. Bronowicki JP, Vetter D, Dumas F, et al. Transcatheter oily chemoembolization for hepatocellular carcinoma: a 4-year study of 127 French patients. Cancer 1994;74:16–24.

54. Pelletier G, Ducreaux M, Gay F, et al. Treatment of unresectable hepatocellular carcinoma: results of a multicenter randomized trial. J Hepatology 1998;29:129–134.

55. Bruix J, Llovet JM, Castellis A, et al. Transarterial embolization versus symptomatic treatment in patients with advanced hepatocellular carcinoma: results of a randomized, controlled trial is a single institution. Hepatology 1998;27:1578–1583.

56. Llovet JM, Real MI, Montana X, et al. Arterial embolization or chemoembolisation versus symptomatic treatment in patients with unresectable hepatocellular carcinoma: a randomised controlled trial. Lancet 2002;359:1734–1739.

57. Lo CM, Ngan H, Tso WK, et al. Randomized controlled trial of transarterial lipiodol chemoembolization for unresectable hepatocellular carcinoma. Hepatology 2002;35:1164–1171.

58. Yamakado K, Hirano T, Kato N, et al. Hepatocellular carcinoma: treatment with a combination of transcatheter arterial chemoembolization and transportal ethanol injection. Radiology 1994;193:75–80.

59. Lencioni R, Vignali C, Caramella D, et al. Transcatheter arterial embolization followed by percutaneous ethanol injection in the treatment of hepatocellular carcinoma. Cardiovasc Intervent Radiol 1994;17:70–75.

60. Livraghi T, Giorgio A, Marin G, et al. Hepatocellular carcinoma and cirrhosis in 746 patients: long-term results of percutaneous ethanol injection. Radiology 1995;197:101–108.

61. Balch CM, Urist MM, Soong SJ, et al. A prospective phase II clinical trial of continuous FUDR regional chemotherapy for colorectal metastases to the liver using a totally implantable drug infusion pump. Ann Surg 1983;198:567–573.

62. Niederhuber JE, Ensminger W, Gyves J, et al. Regional chemotherapy of colorectal cancer metastatic to liver. Cancer 1984;53:1336–1343.

63. Chang AE, Schneider PD, Sugarbaker PH, et al. A prospective randomized trial of regional versus systemic continuous 5-fluorodeoxyuridine chemotherapy in the treatment of colorectal liver metastases. Ann Surg 1987;206:685–693.

64. Kemeny N, Daly J, Reichman B, et al. Intrahepatic or systemic infusion of fluorodeoxyuridine in patients with liver metastases from colorectal carcinoma. Ann Intern Med 1987;107:459–465.

65. Hohn DC, Stagg RJ, Friedman MA. A randomized trial of continuous intravenous versus hepatic intra-arterial floxuridine in patients with colorectal cancer metastatic to the liver: the Northern California Oncology Group Trial. J Clin Oncol 1989;7:1646–1654.

66. Martin JK, O'Connell MJ, Wieand HS, et al. Intra-arterial floxuridine vs. systemic fluorouracil for hepatic metastases from colorectal cancer. Arch Surg 1990;125:1022–1027.

67. Rougier P, Laplanche A, Huguier M, et al. Hepatic arterial infusion of floxuridine in patients with liver metastases from colorectal carcinoma: long-term results of a prospective randomized trial. J Clin Oncol 1992;10:1112–1118.

68. Yoshikawa M, Ebara M, Nakano T, et al. Percutaneous transaxillary catheter insertion for hepatic artery infusion chemotherapy. AJR Am J Roentgenol 1992;158:885–886.

69. Kemeny N, Seiter K, Neidzwiecki D, et al. A randomized trial of intrahepatic infusion of fluorodeoxyuridine with dexamethasone versus fluorodeoxyuridine alone in the treatment of metastatic disease colorectal cancer. Cancer 1992;69:327–334.

70. Lorenz M, Herrmann G, Kirkow-Reimann M. Temporary chemoembolization of colorectal liver metastases with degradable starch microspheres. Eur J Surg Oncol 1989;15:453–462.

71. Hunt TM, Flowerdew ADS, Birch SJ, et al. Prospective randomized controlled trial of hepatic arterial embolization or infusion chemotherapy with 5-fluorouracil and degradable starch microspheres for colorectal liver metastases. Br J Surg 1990;77:779–782.

72. Martinelli DJ, Wadler S, Bakal CW, et al. Utility of embolization or chemoembolization as second-line treatment in patients with advanced or recurrent colorectal carcinoma. Cancer 1994;74:1706–1712.

73. Lang EK, Brown CB Jr. Colorectal metastases to the liver: selective chemoembolization. Radiology 1993;189:417–422.

74. Tellez C, Benson AB, Lyster MT, et al. Phase II trial of chemoembolization for the treatment of metastatic colorectal carcinoma to the liver and review of the literature. Cancer 1998;82:1250–1259.

75. Davis Z, Moertel CG, McIlrath DC. The malignant carcinoid syndrome. Surg Gynecol Obstet 1973;137:628–644.

76. Mitty HA, Warner RRP, Newman LH, et al. Control of carcinoid syndrome with hepatic artery embolization. Radiology 1985;155:623–626.

77. Carrasco CH, Charnsangavej C, Ajani JA, et al. The carcinoid syndrome: palliation by hepatic artery embolization. AJR Am J Roentgenol 1986;147:149–154.

78. Moertel CG. Karnofsky memorial lecture. An odyssey in the land of small tumors. J Clin Oncol 1987;5:1503–1522.

79. Marlink RG, Lokich JJ, Robins JR, et al. Hepatic arterial embolization for metastatic hormone-secreting tumors. Cancer 1990;65:2227–2232.

80. Ajani JA, Carrasco CH, Charnsangavej C, et al. Islet cell tumors metastatic to the liver: effective palliation by sequential hepatic artery embolization. Ann Intern Med 1988;108:340–344.

81. Rivera E, Ajani JA. Doxorubicin, streptozocin, and 5-fluorouracil chemotherapy for patients with metastatic islet-cell carcinoma. Am J Clin Oncol 1998;21:36–38.

82. Kim YH, Ajani JA, Carrasco CH, et al. Selective hepatic arterial chemoembolization for liver metastases in patients with carcinoid tumor or islet cell carcinoma. Cancer Invest 1999;17:474–478.

83. Ruszniewski P, Malka D. Hepatic arterial chemoembolization in the management of advanced digestive endocrine tumors. Digestion 2000;62:79–83.

84. Dominguez S, Denys A, Madeira I, et al. Hepatic arterial chemoembolization with streptozotocin in patients with metastatic digestive endocrine tumours. Eur J Gastroenterol Hepatol 2000;12:151–157.

85. Feldman ED, Pingpank JF, Alexander HR. Regional treatment options for patients with ocular melanoma metastatic to the liver. Ann Surg Oncol 2004;11:290–297.

86. Mavligit GM, Charnsangavej C, Carrasco CH, et al. Regression of ocular melanoma metastatic to the liver after hepatic arterial chemoembolization with cisplatin and polyvinyl sponge. JAMA 1988;260:974–976.

87. Agarwala SS, Panikkar R, Kirkwood JM. Phase I/II randomized trial of intrahepatic arterial infusion chemotherapy with cisplatin and chemoembolization with cisplatin and polyvinyl sponge in patients with ocular melanoma metastatic to the liver. Melanoma Res 2004;14:217–222.

88. Goldberg SN, Gazelle GS, Mueller PR. Thermal ablation therapy for focal malignancy: a unified approach to underlying principles, techniques, and diagnostic imaging guidance. AJR Am J Roentgenol 2000;174:323–331.

89. Curley SA, Izzo F, Delrio P, et al. Radiofrequency ablation of unresectable primary and metastatic heparic malignancies: results in 123 patients. Ann Surg 1999;230:1–8.

90. Goldberg SN, Gazelle GS, Compton CC, et al. Treatment of intrahepatic malignancy with radiofrequency ablation: radiologic-pathologic correlation. Cancer 2000;88:2452–2463.

91. Livraghi T, Goldberg SN, Lazzaroni S, et al. Hepatocellular carcinoma: radiofrequency ablation of medium and large lesions. Radiology 2000;214:761–768.

92. Mazzaferro V, Battiston C, Perrone S, et al. Radiofrequency ablation of small hepatocellular carcinoma in cirrhotic patients awaiting liver transplantation: a prospective study. Ann Surg 2004;240:900–909.

93. Poon RT, Ng KK, Lam CM, et al. Effectiveness of radiofrequency ablation for hepatocellular carcinoma larger than 3 cm in diameter. Arch Surg 2004;139:281–287.

94. de Baere T, Elias D, Dromain C, et al. Radiofrequency ablation of 100 hepatic metastases with a mean follow-up of more than one year. AJR Am J Roentgenol 2000;175:1619–1625.

95. Curley SA, Izzo F, Ellis LM, et al. Radiofrequency ablation of hepatocellular cancer in 110 patients with cirrhosis. Ann Surg 2000;232:381–391.

96. Tateishi R, Shiina S, Teratani T, et al. Percutaneous radiofrequency ablation for hepatocellular carcinoma. Cancer 2005; 103:1201–1209.

97. Vivarelli EW, Holck PS, Levy AE, et al. Surgical resection versus percutaneous radiofrequency ablation in the treatment of hepatocellular carcinoma in the cirrhotic liver. Ann Surg 2004;240:102–107.

98. Abdalla EK, Vauthey JN, Ellis LM, et al. Recurrence and outcomes following hepatic resection, radiofrequency ablation, and combined resection/ablation for colorectal liver metastases. Ann Surg 2004;239:818–825.

99. Livraghi T, Solbiati L, Meloni MF, et al. Treatment of focal liver tumors with percutaneous radiofrequency ablation: complications encountered in a multicenter study. Radiology 2003;226: 441–451.

100. Curley SA, Marra P, Beaty K, et al. Early and late complications after radiofrequency ablation of malignant liver tumors in 608 patients. Ann Surg 2004;239:450–458.

101. de Baere T, Risse O, Kuoch V, et al. Adverse events during radiofrequency treatment of 582 hepatic tumors. AJR Am J Roentgenol 2003;181:695–700.

Benign Biliary Obstruction

28

Roy L. Gordon

Stenosis or obstruction of the bile ducts can be caused by many different entities, which may lead to similar and overlapping clinical presentations (1). Benign biliary obstruction is a much different entity when compared to malignant obstruction (see Chapter 29). The two outstanding differences are that the most common cause of benign obstruction is previous surgery and that the treatment chosen must reestablish internal bile flow for a patient with otherwise normal life expectancy. Radiology plays a key role both in the diagnosis and in the treatment of benign biliary obstruction.

This chapter focuses on these postsurgical lesions and on those of sclerosing cholangitis, which are the most frequent types of obstruction encountered by the interventional radiologist. The spectrum of other benign causes of biliary obstruction is outlined in Table 28–1. A complete consideration of these other causes is beyond the scope of this chapter, but the table provides key references. Obstructions associated with bile duct stones or liver transplantation are covered in Chapters 36 and 30, respectively.

Numerous papers have substantiated the predominant causative role of biliary surgery in the etiology of benign strictures (2,3). In 1971, Warren et al. reviewed 958 patients treated at the Lahey Clinic for benign biliary obstructions (2). Previous biliary surgery was responsible for the stricture in 918 patients, gastric surgery in nine, and pancreatic surgery in two. The remaining 29 obstructions were not a result of previous surgery.

Laparoscopic cholecystectomy has largely replaced open cholecystectomy. The laparoscopic technique has many advantages over open surgery, and, as a result, more people undergo cholecystectomy today than before laparoscopic removal was available. Laparoscopy does result in a higher rate of bile duct injuries. When this increased number of operations is coupled with the higher rate of bile duct injuries, it is easy to understand the higher incidence of benign biliary injuries and obstructions that are currently seen.

In 1989, at the beginning of the laparoscopic cholecystectomy era, Roslyn analyzed a random sample of 42,474 patients undergoing open cholecystectomy. This represented about 8% of all patients undergoing cholecystectomy in the United States in a 12-month period. The incidence of bile duct injuries was 0.2%, with an overall mortality rate of 0.17%. The mortality rate was 0.03% in patients younger than 65 years of age and 0.5% in those older than 65 (4). This rate of bile duct injury of one in 500 patients for open cholecystectomy is widely accepted. There is less agreement on the true rate of bile duct injuries after laparoscopic cholecystectomy despite the publication of numerous studies.

An analysis published in 1993 of a national survey of 77,604 cases of laparoscopic cholecystectomy found bile duct injuries in about six of 1,000 cases (0.6%) (5). The authors of that study suggested that this rate of incidence was likely to decrease as surgeons gained more experience with laparoscopic cholecystectomy. Some decrease has occurred since that time, but more recent publications are still finding bile duct injury rates of 0.14% to 0.5% for laparoscopic cholecystectomy compared with 0.2% for open surgery (6,7,8).

An extensive literature deals with the types of bile duct injury, the types of surgical repair, and the results of these repairs (2–17). In general, the higher or closer to the porta hepatis the injury is, the more difficult is the repair. Better results are achieved with lower lesions. The level of

CAUSES OF BENIGN BILIARY OBSTRUCTION

Postsurgical stricture (1)
Traumatic stricture
Post-liver transplantation: rejection of ischemia (2,3)
Papillary stenosis
Duodenal diverticulum
Biliary atresia
Choledochal cyst (4)
Hepatic cyst, polycystic liver
Sclerosing cholangitis (5)
Oriental cholengiohepatitis (6)
Cholangitis following chemotherapy (7)
AIDS-related cholangitis (8)
Parasitic infection: *Clonorchis sinensis*, (9) *Fasciola hepatica*,
   Ascaris lumbricoides, *Echinococcus* (10,11)
Tuberculosis
Sarcoidosis
Acute and chronic pancreatitis (12)
Impacted biliary calculus
Mirizzi syndrome (13)

obstruction is described in the Bismuth classification (18). Type 1 is a low stricture of the common hepatic duct with the hepatic duct stump longer than 2 cm. Type 2 is a mid stricture of the common hepatic duct with the hepatic duct stump shorter than 2 cm (Figure 28–1). Type 3 is a high or a hilar structure without any hepatic duct but with an intact confluence of right and left hepatic ducts (Figure 28–2). Type 4 is obliteration of the hilar confluence with separation of the right and left hepatic ducts. Type 5 is injury to a right aberrant hepatic duct with or without concomitant injury to the common duct (Figure 28–3). With the advent of laparoscopic cholecystectomy, injuries

have tended to be more complex (9). Repair is usually performed by construction of a Roux loop that is anastomosed to the remaining bile duct, although other operations are sometimes performed (1).

The outcome of surgical repair depends on many factors other than the level of injury. Better results are achieved if the injury is recognized immediately, if ductal anatomy is completely delineated by preoperative cholangiography, if good percutaneous drainage is instituted, and if the repair is carried out by an experienced surgeon working on non-inflamed tissues. Results are less good if diagnosis is delayed and if the patient's condition is complicated by cholangitis or periductal infection. The presence of cirrhosis or portal hypertension makes the surgery more difficult and the outcome less satisfactory. Stricture recurrence develops in 10–30% of patients after initial surgical repair. Important aspects of surgical repair concern long-term durability and quality of life survey (16,17). The group from Johns Hopkins reported on the repairs in 156 patients. The group had a mean follow-up of 57.5 months in 142 patients, and 90.8% of the patients were considered to have a successful outcome without the need for follow-up invasive, diagnostic, or therapeutic interventional procedures. The report cautions that long-term results are still not available. Of interest both to the treated patient in terms of quality of life and to the treating interventional radiology team is that postoperative stenting was used for longer than 9 months in 89 patients (62.7%), 4–9 months in 30 patients (20%), and less than 4 months in 23 patients (16%) (15).

Repair of recurrent strictures is even more difficult. Subsequent recurrence following a second repair occurs in 22% of patients, even in the most experienced hands (12). Postoperative morbidity is high, with at least one in 10 patients having one or more major nonfatal complications (1).

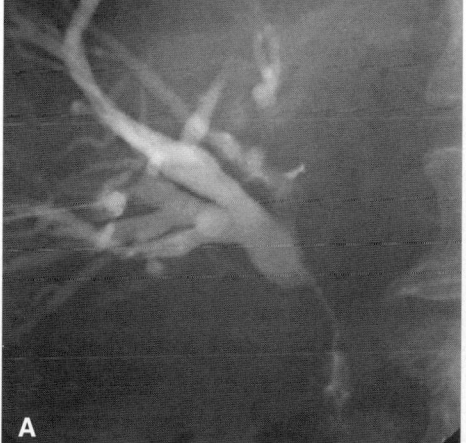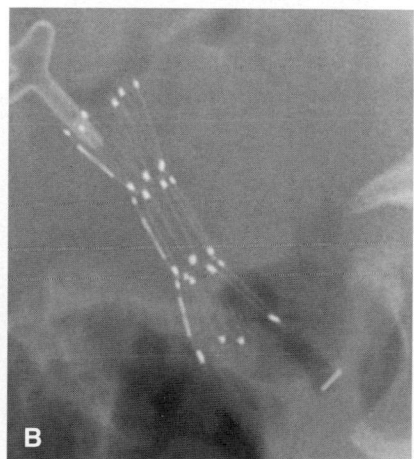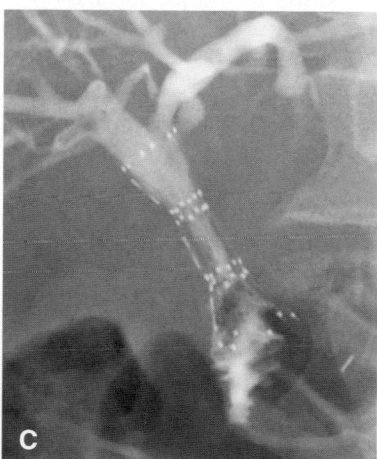

Figure 28–1 **A.** Cholangiogram of a 53-year-old man with a Bismuth type 2 biliary stricture of the common hepatic duct. A Whipple operation had been performed 2 years earlier because of a small ampullary tumor. **B.** A plain film showing three-segment, 8-mm diameter Gianturco stent with "flared" proximal and distal ends for greater stability. **C.** The cholangiogram shows that the stent is in stable position with good drainage into the Roux loop.

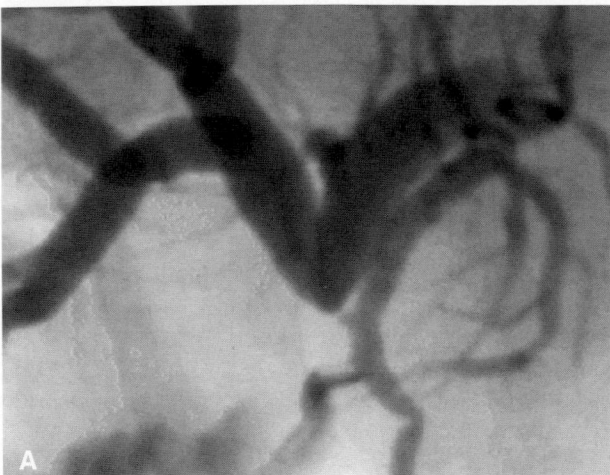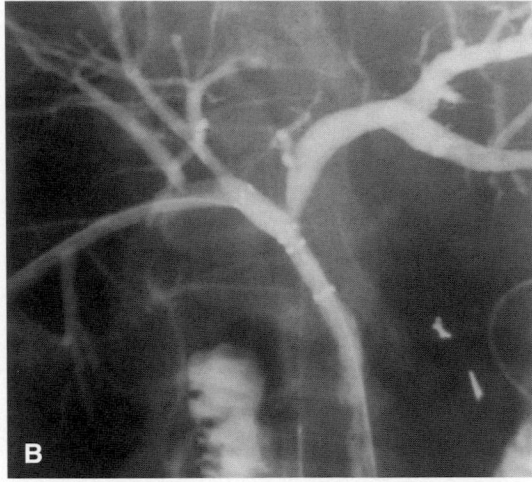

Figure 28–2   A. Cholangiogram of an 80-year-old woman with a complete biliary obstruction of Bismuth type 3. **B.** Because of her age, a Gianturco 8-mm stent with two segments was placed by the percutaneous transhepatic route, with excellent results.

From these statistics, it is clear that the surgery of bile duct lesions presents a formidable challenge, with high rates of recurrence and significant morbidity. Surgery is the treatment of choice for benign biliary strictures. Interventional techniques such as percutaneous drainage are frequently used as an adjunct to biliary repair. The development of percutaneous balloon dilatation techniques and placement of endoprostheses has provided a valuable treatment alternative when patients are unsuitable for surgery or when nonoperative techniques are chosen after surgical failure.

IMAGING PROCEDURES

Radiology has an important role in the diagnostic workup of patients before surgical repair. Ultrasound is an excellent and noninvasive technique for demonstrating ductal dilatation above a stricture or obstruction. A general idea of the level of the lesion may be obtained, but in most cases, a more detailed demonstration of the ductal anatomy is required. Ultrasound is of value in demonstrating other intra-abdominal fluid collections or hepatic lesions. Intrahepatic ductal dilatation may be absent in spite of biliary obstruction in patients with conditions such as sclerosing cholangitis or with hard, diseased livers such as in advanced cirrhosis. The ultrasound examination may reveal important information on the patency of the hepatic arteries and the portal veins, and the presence of venous or arterial collaterals.

In 2003, Alves et al. reported on angiographic studies performed on 55 patients with postcholecystectomy bile duct injuries. They found a vascular injury in 47% of the patients; the most frequent were right-sided hepatic artery disruptions (36%). However, they found no difference in the outcome of

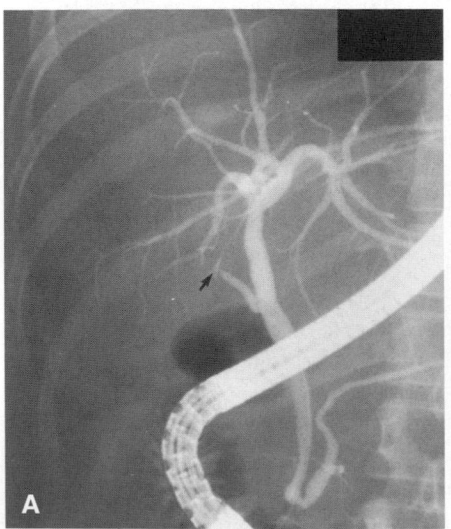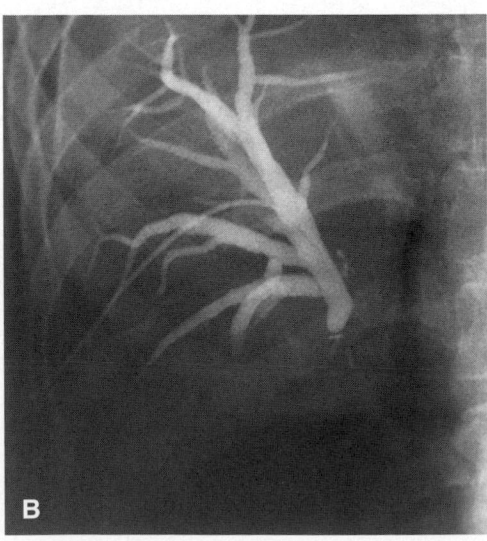

Figure 28–3   A. Cholangiogram of a 42-year-old woman suffering from intermittent bouts of cholangitis following open cholecystectomy for stone disease. On ERCP a clip (*arrow*) is noted on the aberrant right hepatic duct, Bismuth type 5. Note that too few ducts are seen in the right lobe. **B.** Percutaneous transhepatic cholangiography delineates the clipped-off ductal system of the right lobe.

the repairs in patients with or without vascular injury (19). Routine angiography is not commonly used.

Computed tomography (CT) provides general information on ductal dilatation, liver masses, fluid collections, and vascular anatomy. Normal intravenous contrast agents do not opacify the bile ducts, but recent work has used the older intravenous contrast agents such as cholographin to opacify the bile ducts. This technique depends on secretion of the cholographin into the bile ducts, which is not reliable in the face of biliary obstruction or impaired liver function but which may be useful in selected cases (20). It is sometimes helpful to perform a CT scan after a percutaneous cholangiogram or a tube cholangiogram to see whether the liver has areas with isolated ducts that appear nonopacified.

Isotope scanning using hepatic imino diacetic acid (HIDA) provides some functional assessment in cases of incomplete strictures and in the postoperative evaluation of biliary anastomoses. It is a sensitive and specific test for leakage of bile from a damaged biliary tree (21).

Advances are occurring in magnetic resonance imaging, termed magnetic resonance cholangiography (MRC), and are providing excellent noninvasive imaging of the complete biliary tree. This technique is progressing rapidly, and its full impact on the future management of biliary obstruction is evolving (22,23).

Many surgeons, at present, are most familiar and comfortable with and rely on invasive cholangiography both to delineate anatomy and then to allow ductal intubation and drainage. Complete and accurate demonstration of the bile duct obstruction and of the bile ducts above and below the lesion is a key element in the management of bile duct stenoses and obstructions. This will usually require opacification of the bile ducts by percutaneous transhepatic cholangiography (PTC), endoscopic retrograde cholangiopancreatography (ERCP), or injection of contrast through any indwelling catheters such as T tubes (24,25).

All branches of the biliary tree should be outlined, with particular care taken to show the confluence of the main right and left ducts at the liver hilus; the level, completeness, and nature of the obstructing lesions; and the status of the extrahepatic bile duct below the stricture. Ducts draining all the areas of the liver should be seen. Intraductal filling defects such as stones should be noted, as should any intrahepatic or extrahepatic narrowings or dilatations. Leaks from the biliary tree should also be identified.

Injection of large volumes of contrast material can lead to overfilling of the ducts. If these obstructed ducts are filled with stagnant infected bile, overdistention may force bacteria or toxins into the bloodstream with resultant sepsis. It is difficult to quantify what constitutes overfilling, but the author has found it safest to use the smallest volume of contrast consistent with obtaining a satisfactory cholangiogram. After a period of drainage, more extensive cholangiograms can be performed if necessary. Use of a tilting table, cradle, and C arm are helpful in achieving good ductal delineation without overfilling the system. Alternatively, rolling the patient into suitable oblique or prone positions may achieve the same result.

The least invasive route for contrast injection into the biliary tree is via a preexisting T tube or other surgical drainage tube. This may allow adequate delineation of the biliary tree. In the absence of such tubes, ERCP is the next choice of access route for contrast cholangiography and is often satisfactory, provided that the biliary stricture is not complete. Adequate filling of the intrahepatic ducts above the narrowing may require the use of an occlusion balloon, especially when there is a sphincterotomy or duct-to-bowel anastomosis. Suitable oblique radiographs are almost always required. In three situations, ERCP is of very limited value.

1. If there is a complete obstruction of the bile duct, retrograde injection via ERCP will show only the distal duct. The intrahepatic duct system above the obstruction will require delineation by PTC.
2. Complex hilar lesions are sometimes difficult to evaluate adequately by ERCP.
3. After surgery, such as a Roux-en-Y or Billroth II partial gastrectomy, access to the bile duct by ERCP may be impossible.

When the preceding approaches do not provide adequate information, PTC with a fine needle is used. PTC is often the key examination in the complete evaluation of the ductal system in patients with benign biliary obstruction. It is an effective technique, with success rates in the range of 97–100% and a low incidence of serious complications (24,25,28,29). In a multi-institutional survey of 2,006 PTCs, the complication rate was 3.4% (sepsis, 1.4%; bile leakage, 1.45%; intraperitoneal hemorrhage, 0.35%; and death 0.20%) (24). In studies from a single institute experienced in biliary work, a negligible complication rate was recorded, which is in keeping with the author's experience (28). Complete delineation of the ductal system may require separate punctures of individual but noncommunicating segments of the biliary tree. Among the great advantages of PTC compared with ERCP are that it is readily available in most centers, does not require special equipment, and is effective and safe. As with the other techniques, overfilling must be avoided, and prophylactic antibiotic coverage is usually indicated.

The diagnostic studies should enable one to classify the lesion according to Bismuth types. The choice of treatment and outcome are influenced by the level of obstruction (11,12,18). It is of critical importance that the complete biliary tree be opacified. Patients in Bismuth groups 4 and 5 may have isolated segments that may be missed on ERCP or PTC (Figure 28–3). To avoid this problem, cholangiograms should be obtained in the left posterior oblique (LPO) projection, which is the best projection to show the whole liver and to identify parts of the liver that appear to lack opacified bile ducts. The standard semiprone position in which ERCP is routinely performed yields a right posterior oblique

(RPO) projection cholangiogram. This often superimposes the right and left lobes of the liver and tends to hide areas of the liver without ducts. Repeated passes with a fine needle should be made into these apparently duct-deficient areas to opacify isolated segments (Figure 28–3). Correlation with cross-sectional imaging studies may alert one to nonopacified segments.

TREATMENT

Nonoperative techniques of percutaneous biliary draining and stenting and similar endoscopic techniques have become established as the methods of choice for treatment of inoperable malignant biliary disease (30). However, treatment of benign biliary strictures is different from the palliative, short-term therapy that is so successfully provided by these nonoperative techniques in malignant disease. Patients with benign strictures are often young to middle-aged with a normal life expectancy. Consequently, the leak or stricture treatment should be durable. Studies evaluating and comparing the various treatment options should have follow-up commensurate with the projected life expectancy of the patient and should ideally extend beyond 10 years. For benign lesions, surgical repair is generally preferred when possible because of better durability of the surgical repair.

The treatment options include surgery and the more recently developed nonoperative approaches. In many cases, both traditional surgical methods of repair and non-operative techniques will be needed and used in a complementary fashion. An important element in treatment is to institute good percutaneous drainage of all fluid collections such as bilomas or abscesses. Drainage is guided by ultrasound or CT and is needed to reduce inflammation and allow healing. Many patients will have percutaneous fluid drains and biliary stents for variable periods of time that are typically managed by interventional radiology. Radiology is frequently involved in the team approach in managing benign biliary problems. In the next section, the individual nonsurgical techniques of dilation and stenting are considered.

These nonsurgical techniques are based on the retrograde endoscopic route (31) or on the percutaneous transhepatic route (32,33). In some additional cases, an existing tube or puncture of a Roux or Hutson loop can be used (34,35). The nonsurgical techniques allow dilatation of the stricture by tapered bougie or dilatation balloon. The dilated stricture may then be temporarily stented or left without a stent. Repeated dilatations may be performed. Patients are usually treated under local anesthetic with intravenous sedation. Frequently, much of the therapy can be undertaken on an outpatient basis. Studies published in 1986 with 73 patients and in 1987 with 74 patients show early success of 67% with percutaneous dilatation of biliary strictures (32,36). The studies highlight the potential of dilatation therapy for benign lesions.

Unfortunately, strictures may recur, even after repeated dilatation. Although dilatation may be satisfactory in the short term, proof of long-term cure has not yet been accumulated in large, well-controlled series. Indwelling internal stents (endoprostheses) are immune to the stricture recurrence associated with dilatation, but their usefulness is limited because all currently available plastic stents become occluded over time (37). Expandable metallic stents are widely available but have proved disappointing in their ability to provide long-term prolonged patency.

DILATATION

Early reports showing the feasibility of percutaneous biliary dilatation using balloon dilation catheters include those of Burhenne (1975) (38) via a T-tube tract and of Molnar and Stockum (1978) (39) via the transhepatic route. Since then, various authors have published their experiences in dilating benign biliary strictures (32,36,38–44). Review of this literature unfortunately does not produce an entirely coherent picture because of variation in stricture type, treatment, and follow-up. The method of dilatation used by radiologists is almost always balloon catheter. Some workers perform multiple inflations, and others use prolonged inflations; the author and many others simply inflate the balloon once or twice until any waist disappears, believing that all that is required is to rupture the fibrous bands of the stricture. No published data are available showing an advantage of one dilatation technique over another, and this appears to be a question of little real importance. The balloon size should match the estimated caliber of the duct on either side of the stricture and is usually in the 4- to 8-mm range. Duct rupture is most unusual with correctly sized balloons even though high pressures (up to 16 atm) are not infrequently needed to dilate the stricture. Progress in balloon manufacture now provides balloons that can be used at up to 20 atmospheres in pressure. Stricture dilatation can be very painful, and adequate sedation and pain control are important. Some authors advocate the use of general anesthesia in selected cases.

Management following dilatation varies from center to center. Some centers favor prolonged stenting after dilatation to try to avoid restenosis (Figure 28–4) (36). They suggest that the stent acts as a scaffold, allowing healing to occur in a mature, stable, and nonstenosed form. This view echoes the arguments of surgeons such as Warren et al. (2) and Pitt et al. (13) in favor of stenting. Others believe stenting has no advantage and may, in fact, be harmful by stimulating further fibrosis (12). Long-term stenting has an increased rate of infectious complication and has an increased rate of morbidity. Williams et al. reported on dilatation of benign biliary strictures in 74 patients with stenting for 4–6 months (36). Complications related to long-term indwelling stents were common and included tube plugging or dislodgment in 29 patients, intraductal stones in nine patients, stricture extension in five patients, and right portal vein thrombosis in one patient. Citron et al., who stented for 3–6 months (with an average of 20 weeks), noted that on average, patients required a total of 17 days in the hospital after dilatation at various times (44). Mueller et al., in their report dealing with 73 patients from four different centers, discussed the controversial question of long-term stenting but did not provide data that were helpful in resolving the issue (32).

The author's approach has been to inflate the balloon once or twice to efface any balloon waist. A drainage catheter, of 10–12 French and occasionally 14 French, is left across the stricture for 6 weeks and then exchanged for

a new self-retaining catheter positioned in the biliary tree above the stricture. If contrast flows through the dilated stricture, the tube is capped externally, and the patient is followed up 2 or 3 weeks later. The tube is removed after this test period if the dilated stricture remains widely patent. If restenosis occurs during the test period, repeat dilatation is performed, and the patient is followed for a similar period. Dilatation is considered unsuccessful after two attempts (12).

The initial results of balloon dilatation are good, with immediate success in the range of 67–87%. Mueller et al. had a 67% patency rate in 73 patients followed up for a

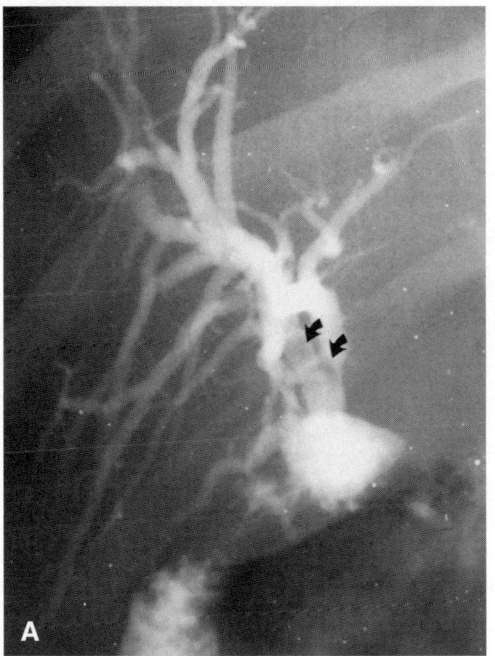

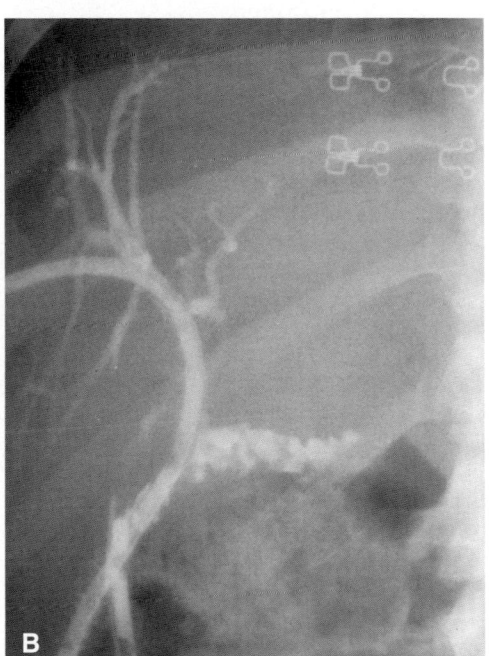

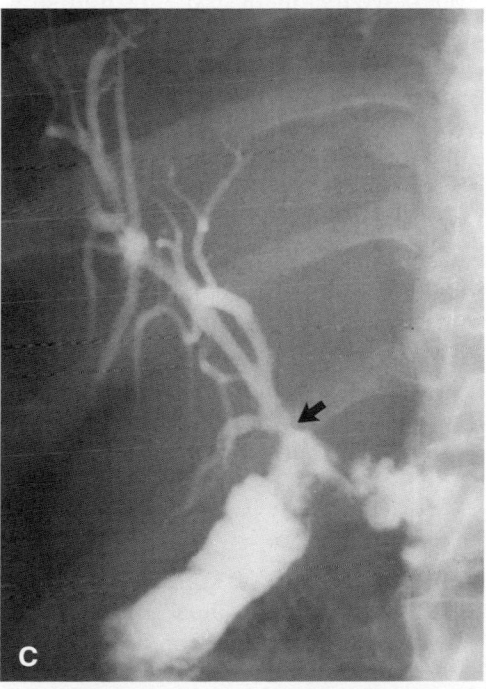

Figure 28–4 **A.** Cholangiogram of a 60-year-old woman who underwent open cholecystectomy with damage to an aberrant right hepatic duct. This was repaired at the time of injury by anastomosing the right duct to a Roux loop. Eight years later the patient suffered from intermittent attacks of cholangitis, and a PTC showed the right ductal system to be dilated and partially obstructed by stones (*arrows*) above a narrow biliary–enteric anastomosis. **B.** The stenosis underwent successful dilatation with a 6-mm balloon. The stones were pushed into the loop and the anastomosis stented with a 14 French Silastic catheter for 6 weeks. **C.** The anastomosis (*arrow*) is widely patent and remained so for 4 years until the patient died from colon cancer.

minimum of 36 months (32). They divided their strictures into three groups: 44 patients with anastomotic strictures (choledochojejunostomy or hepaticojejunostomy), 28 patients in an ill-defined group described as "iatrogenic" (presumably bile duct strictures other than those at a biliary–enteric anastomosis), and 17 patients with sclerosing cholangitis. The 36-month patency rates were 67, 76, and 42%, respectively. However, 25 patients (34%) had recurrent strictures, 16 treated by repeated dilatations and nine treated by surgery. It is unclear whether these authors' 36-month patency rate refers to primary patency or is an assisted-patency rate that includes those patients treated by repeated dilatations.

The large series of 74 patients with benign biliary obstruction carefully reported by Williams et al. is instructive to consider in detail (36). Their population does not include sclerosing cholangitis. Initially, successful balloon dilatation was performed in 74 patients, but it is not stated whether there were any unsuccessful attempts. Forty-nine patients had strictures of a biliary–enteric anastomosis. Forty of these patients had their stenting tubes removed, and nine retained their stents. Of these 40 patients, 27 (67%) had to undergo redilatations before the stents could be removed. After stenting for an average of 8.8 months, 29 of 40 strictures (72.5%) were considered to have been successfully dilated. The other group comprised 25 patients with ductal strictures, and these responded better to dilatation. Twenty-four had their stenting tubes removed, and one patient remained stented. Ten of 24 patients (42%) required redilatation before the stents could be removed. After an average of 4.7 months of stenting, 21 of 24 patients (87%) were considered successfully treated. For the whole group, the success rate was 67.5% (50 of 74 patients). Follow-up ranged from 1 to 58 months (with a mean of 28 months). Sixty percent of patients (actual numbers are not stated) were without stents at a 24-month follow-up, and 38% at 36 months or longer. Strictures recurred after stent removal in 14 of 64 patients (22%). These posttreatment failures occurred at 1–36 months (with a mean of 13.8 months and median of 8 months), but 13 of 14 were successfully treated by repeat dilatations involving additional periods of stenting averaging 9.6 months. This important series proves that benign strictures can be treated in the short term but that they recur frequently. Aggressive management with prolonged stenting and frequent redilatations is essential but results in significant morbidity. Hospitalization time averaged 10 days. Complication rates in both the acute procedure-related category and in the chronic catheter-related category were not insignificant. There is no clear consensus in the literature on whether lesions of the bile duct or those at a biliary–enteric anastomosis respond better to dilatation.

Randomized prospective trials comparing balloon dilatation and surgical repair of strictures are not available, but in 1989, Pitt et al. compared the results of these two techniques in a single institution (13). They studied 25 patients who were repaired using a Roux loop and compared them with 20 patients treated by balloon dilatation. The two groups were considered similar in many parameters that might have influenced outcome. The authors summarized their findings as follows.

"Twenty-five patients underwent surgical repair with Roux-en-Y choledocho- or hepatico-jejunostomy with postoperative transhepatic stenting for a mean of 13.8 ± 1.3 months. Twenty patients had balloon dilatation a mean of 3.9 times and were stented transhepatically for a mean of 13.3 ± 2.0 months. Mean length of follow-up was 57 ± 7 and 59 ± 6 months for surgery and balloon dilatation, respectively. No patients died after any of the procedures. The same definition of a successful outcome was applied to both groups and was achieved in 88% of the surgical and in 55% of the balloon dilatation patients ($p < 0.02$). Significant hemobilia occurred more often with balloon dilatation (20% vs. 4%, $p < 0.02$). The total hospital stay and cost of balloon dilatation was [*sic*] not significantly different from surgery" (13).

Although Pitt et al. concluded that surgery was preferable, they pointed out the value of dilatation for high-risk patients or those unwilling to undergo further surgery. In both groups, patients had the inconvenience of stents for more than 13 months, and the study again illustrates the problems involved in adequately treating benign biliary strictures.

Although nonoperative dilatation is not indicated in patients who are candidates for surgical repair, it represents an important treatment option for patients in whom surgical repair is not possible for anatomic reasons, for patients at high surgical risk, for patients with portal hypertension, and for patients unwilling to undergo further surgery. Dilatation is of particular value in patients of advanced age or in those with serious concomitant disease, when the possibility of late recurrence is of less concern. The choice of treatment should, when possible, take into account the current results achieved by operative compared with nonoperative treatment in the institute in which the patient will be treated, rather than by reference to published data from other centers of excellence. Because of the complexity of managing biliary strictures, patients are best referred to centers where both surgery and nonoperative interventions are performed by experienced experts in biliary disease (45). Modern management of bile duct strictures benefits from the combined use of surgical and nonoperative techniques. The surgical group at UCLA noted a change in their treatment strategies in the period 1953 through 1990 (14). As nonoperative dilatation became available, it was used to correct recurrent anastomotic strictures.

An example of a combined surgical and radiological approach is that of Hutson, Russell, and colleagues, who cooperated in developing a transjejunal access route to the biliary tree to allow for periodic balloon dilatations of the biliary ducts. A Roux-en-Y loop was constructed and anastomosed to the extrahepatic bile duct. The afferent limb was attached to the abdominal wall, and access to this limb was originally through a surgically created stoma (34). In later patients, the limb was closed but marked with clips at the site of attachment to the abdominal wall to facilitate percutaneous puncture. This technique provided simple access for periodic bile duct dilatations (35). In some patients, percutaneous access to a suitably located Roux loop is possible, even if a Hutson loop has not been intentionally constructed (46).

ENDOPROSTHESES

To address the problems of stricture recurrence and the morbidity of chronic indwelling stent catheters, indwelling endoprostheses have been developed. These devices are implanted across the lesion, percutaneously or endoscopically. An endoprosthesis must either remain patent for a long time or be easily exchangeable if it is to offer an advantage over balloon dilatation. Endoprostheses must meet the usual biocompatibility standards, must be safe and easy to insert, and must resist migration. A 12 French plastic endoprosthesis works well for a period of months but in time will occlude and may migrate, particularly when placed across a biliary–enteric anastomosis (37). In patients with normal anatomy, stents can be exchanged endoscopically on a routine basis at intervals of about 3 months. This will usually avoid the problems caused by a blocked endoprosthesis. However, such management places considerable burden and expense on the patient and should be considered only in the absence of any better alternative. A further modification of this approach is to sequentially place multiple stents across the biliary stricture. Balloon dilatation is performed initially with placement of one stent, followed by a second stent and, if possible, by a third stent by the endoscopic route at 12-week intervals. Some 12 months after initial stent placement, all stents are removed. The theory is that occlusion of all the stents is less likely to occur and more effective dilatation is maintained. A number of centers have advocated this approach. In 2002, Draganov et al. published a retrospective review of their results with this technique in 29 cases of benign biliary stricture. They concluded that favorable results could be expected in patients with postoperative strictures of the low Bismuth type 1. They had a mean follow-up of 48 months and low morbidity. This approach may be an alternative to surgery in selected patients. It is not suited to patients with chronic pancreatitis or high strictures in the porta hepatis of the Bismuth type 3 (47,48).

Many strictures are at biliary–enteric anastomoses that cannot be reached by the endoscopic route. In these patients, it is almost always possible to place an endoprosthesis via the percutaneous transhepatic route. However, placement of an indwelling plastic endoprosthesis via this route is only a temporary measure because of inevitable clogging of the endoprosthesis. The need for routine percutaneous transhepatic exchanges, although technically feasible, renders the repeated percutaneous replacement of a plastic endoprosthesis an unsuitable means of long-term treatment of benign strictures. In those few patients with no other treatment options, a permanent transhepatic internal–external biliary catheter can be used. This catheter can be changed easily over a guide wire at regular intervals. This is a simple outpatient procedure and much less difficult for the patient than undergoing repeated percutaneous punctures. The obvious downside of this approach is that the patient lives with a permanent drainage catheter with all its attendant problems of inconvenience, pain, infection, and limitations in lifestyle. Wherever possible, when such an internal–external arrangement is needed, the catheter is much better tolerated when a left or anterior subcostal entry site is used rather than a right intercostal approach. The constant irritation caused by respiration is less, and with the anterior placement, the tube is easier to see and manage by the patient.

EXPANDABLE METALLIC STENTS

The development of expandable metallic stents has provided a new form of implantable endoprosthesis. These stents have the advantage that they can be inserted percutaneously or endoscopically using small-caliber introducers (6–12 French). Once in position, the stents expand to diameters as large as 12 mm. It was hoped that the large bore of these metallic stents would render the metallic stent more resistant to clogging than the small-bore plastic endoprostheses and consequently provide a good treatment option in dealing with benign biliary strictures. This promise has unfortunately not yet materialized, and it must be strongly emphasized that all metallic stents become occluded over time. They do remain patent for longer periods than plastic endoprostheses, but they are not suitable as a frontline method of choice for treating benign conditions, despite their widespread effective use in palliating malignant biliary obstructions.

In 1985, Carrasco et al. published the results of the first experimental use of the Gianturco stent in the extra hepatic bile ducts of dogs, with encouraging results (49). In 1988, Uchida et al. described modifications to the Gianturco stent achieved by adding circumferential monofilament nylon sutures to limit stent expansion and to allow linking of Gianturco stent chains together (50). These modifications gave extra length and flexibility without sacrificing resistance to compressibility (Figure 28–5).

A study published in 1989 by Irving et al. summarized the early clinical experience of five hospitals in four European countries using the Gianturco stent (51). Eleven patients with benign biliary strictures were stented after failure of prior treatment with balloon dilatation or surgical reconstruction. Eight patients had good results and were without jaundice, pruritus, or infection during follow-up of 6–21 months. One patient in this group died of carcinoma of the bronchus 4 months after stenting but was asymptomatic from a biliary standpoint. Of the remaining three patients, one had early stent migration and underwent bypass surgery with stent removal, one had stent migration at 4–5 months, and one had stent occlusion from

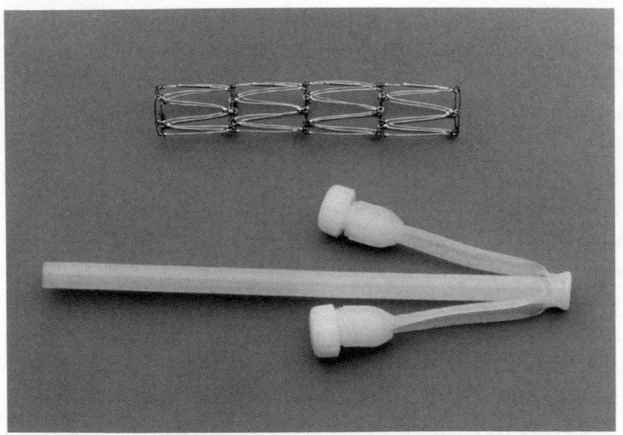

Figure 28–5 A Gianturco stent of 10 mm in diameter with four linked segments. The peel-away introducer is shown below the stent.

epithelial proliferation within the stent after 10 months. This work and similar work by Coons (52) showed the utility of the Gianturco stents in the short-term treatment of benign biliary strictures and led to further clinical use.

In 1990, Rossi et al. published their results using the modified Gianturco stent in 17 patients with benign biliary strictures who had failed repeated previous attempts at surgical correction and dilatation (53). Fourteen of their 17 patients were free of symptoms at an average of 8 months' (range 4–12 months) follow-up. These workers continued to follow their patients for an average of 37 months (range 30–41 months), adding one patient stented with a Wallstent (33). Ten of 18 patients (55.5%) were asymptomatic, although in one patient a stent had migrated into the bowel 6 months after placement. Recurrent symptoms occurred in five patients (27.7%). Stent obstruction occurred in three of these patients after 4, 13, and 22 months, respectively. Stent migration resulted in restenosis in one patient, and papillary stenosis caused obstruction in the fifth patient. Three patients died. One patient with Hodgkin's disease died 9 months after stent placement. The stent was patent, but there was intrahepatic narrowing from sclerosing cholangitis. A second patient died at 6 months with recurrent jaundice, cholangitis, secondary sclerosing cholangitis, liver failure, and occluded stent. The final patient died with peritoneal spread from a gastric carcinoma resected 10 years previously, but with no sign of bile stasis.

In 1992, Coons summarized his experience with the modified Gianturco-Rösch stent in 54 patients with benign lesions (54). Eleven had sclerosing cholangitis, leaving a group of 43 patients with benign strictures who had failed previous treatment. The number of patients who were symptom free was two at more than 4 years; two at more than 3 years; eight at more than 2 years; 10 at more than 1 year; and 21 at less than 1 year. The overall occlusion rate for the 43 patients was 7%. For the 22 followed more than 1 year, the occlusion rate was 13%, and for the four followed more than 3 years, it was 25%. For these longer follow-ups, the

numbers of patients are too small to draw statistically relevant conclusions.

In 1996, Hausegger et al. published their results using the Wallstent to treat benign biliary obstruction in 20 patients and concluded that "results of stent placement for treatment of benign biliary strictures are not encouraging." They had a heterogeneous population, including seven with chronic pancreatitis, 10 with postsurgical strictures, two with fibrous papillary stenosis, and one with sclerosing cholangitis. Median primary patency was only 32 months ± 8.7 (55).

In 1997, Bonnel et al. reported on their results using the Gianturco stent to treat 25 patients with postoperative biliary strictures, whom they followed for a mean of 55 months (range of 9–84 months). Eight patients had stenosis of the common bile duct, which recurred in seven patients at an average of 23 months (range of 7–41 months) after stent placement. This clearly demonstrates that the Gianturco stent is a poor treatment choice for this group. In the remaining group of 17, the patients had already undergone repair by hepaticojejunostomy and presented with stricturing of the anastomosis. Here treatment with the Gianturco stent was much more effective, resulting in a patent anastomosis in 16 of 17 patients at an average of 56 months (range of 9–84 months). However, no less than seven of these patients had recurrent bouts of cholangitis despite the patent stent. This type of ascending cholangitis is also observed after successful hepaticojejunostomy with a widely patent anastomosis (56).

A sober and realistic paper by Gabelmann et al. in 2001 followed 12 patients with benign biliary stricture treated by Palmaz, Accuflex, or Wallstents. The primary patency rate decreased from 75% at 12 months to 25% after 36 months. The researchers pointed out that metallic stents were no longer in use as a primary choic, but were used only as a last resort. Although primary patency was poor, the researchers focused on the possibilities of restoring secondary patency with adjunctive interventions in these patients without better options (57).

A few workers have focused on the reaction of the bile ducts to implanted metallic stents to better understand their function. Vorwerk et al. studied the patency of Wallstents placed across experimentally induced benign stenoses in the common bile ducts of 12 dogs (58). They used silicone-coated Wallstents in three dogs. In two dogs, the coated Wallstents occluded at 3 and 4 months. In one dog, the stent migrated to the bowel within 4 weeks, leaving the common bile duct stenosed. The authors quoted personal communication with H. Rousseau and C. Zollikofer, who always had early migration of coated Wallstents, and they concluded, despite the small numbers, that silicone-coated Wallstents should not be used in clinical applications. However, Alvarado et al. studied 18 dogs using Palmaz stents coated with silicone rubber or segmented polyether-polyurethane and noted no instances of stent migration (59). Vorwerk suggested that the inflexible, rigid nature of the Palmaz stent may have prevented the migration.

In the 10 animals with noncoated Wallstents in Vorwerk's studies, all animals showed significant wall thickening within the stent during the 15- to 24-month follow-up. The thickening was mucosal hyperplasia, with soft, fingerlike hyperplasia protruding through the stent interspaces initially. This led to morphologic high-grade narrowing of the stent lumen but did not result in functional obstruction to bile flow. The mucosal hyperplasia increased within the first year after implantation but leveled off during longer follow-up periods. The hyperplasia was histologically related to stent position within the mucosal or superficial submucosal layer. Once the stent entered deeper into the bile duct wall, mucosal thickening decreased. In the early study by Carrasco et al. using Gianturco stents with shorter follow-up (4–23 weeks), complete stent incorporation, as described above, was not seen (49). There was mucosal hyperplasia with some pressure necrosis and sloughing, and only partial incorporation.

In their clinical study, Maccioni et al. concluded that the main cause of late stent occlusion was tissue ingrowth (33). Biopsy specimens collected through a cholangioscope or by intraductal brushing showed hyperplastic epithelium and/or granulation tissue within the stent. CT studies of asymptomatic patients showed a lining of soft tissue density inside the stent of various degrees at different levels without significant changes at subsequent follow-ups, suggesting the presence of reactive, hyperplastic tissue. Maccioni and colleagues believe that tissue ingrowth reaches a certain extent and then stabilizes without completely occluding the stent, thus allowing an unimpeded flow of bile through the stented stricture. The large final diameter of the stent, some six times wider than the common bile duct, easily accommodates this hyperplasia. They could not exclude the possibility that sludge was imaged by the CT scans rather than hyperplasia. Work on stent development continues, and areas of interest include stents that can be removed (60), bio-absorbable stents (61), covered stents (62), and drug-eluting stents or coated stents (63).

INDICATIONS FOR STENTING

The author's approach has been to use metallic stents only after all surgical options have been exhausted and after resolute attempts at balloon dilatation have failed. The Gianturco stent appears to provide reasonable palliation in some patients treated over the currently available follow-up. Some patients are now asymptomatic as long as 5 years after stenting. A number of others have returned with cholangitis and stone formation (Figure 28–6). Reintervention from a percutaneous transhepatic approach has allowed for stone removal and clearing of the ducts, thus prolonging secondary patency. In a small number of cases, a highly localized stenosis has recurred within the stent at the same location as the treated stricture (Figure 28–7). The author has empirically treated these recurrences by placing a coaxial Wallstent or Palmaz stent within the narrowed Gianturco stent.

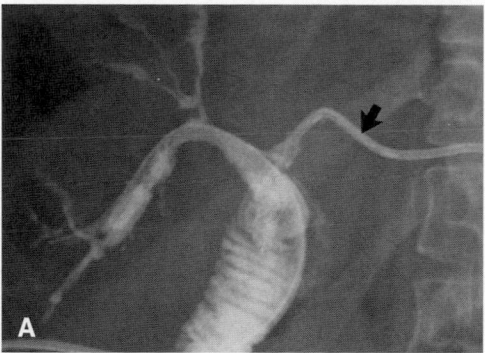

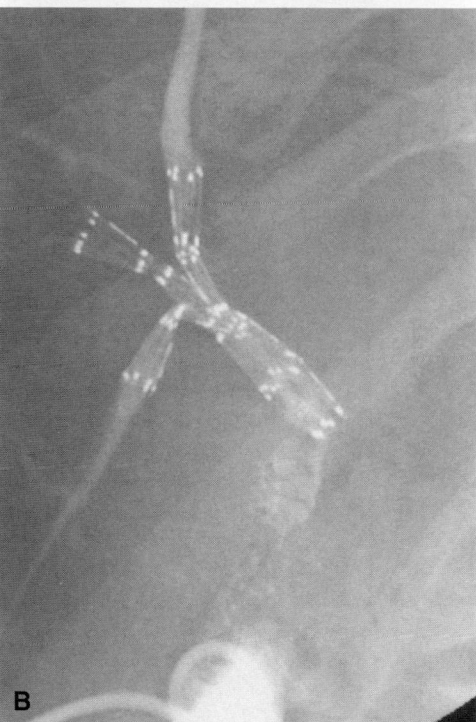

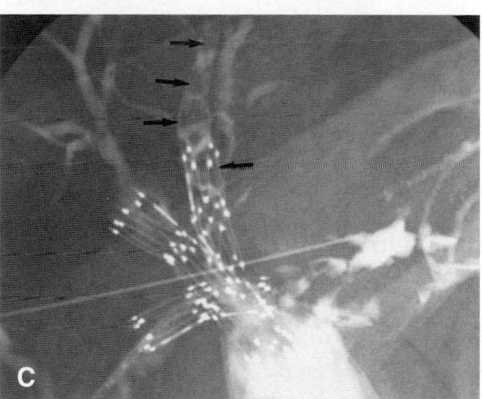

Figure 28–6 **A.** Cholangiogram of a 54-year-old woman with sclerosing cholangitis and a Roux loop. The right-sided ducts show severe narrowing. There is one percutaneous catheter inserted via the Roux loop into the right-sided bile ducts. A separate percutaneous transhepatic catheter (*arrow*) drains the left ducts. Repeated balloon dilatations provided only transient clinical improvement. **B.** The right-sided ducts have been stented with multiple Gianturco stents, leading to marked clinical improvement. **C.** Six months later, the patient's clinical situation deteriorated, and a PTC showed blocked stents with numerous stones (*arrows*).

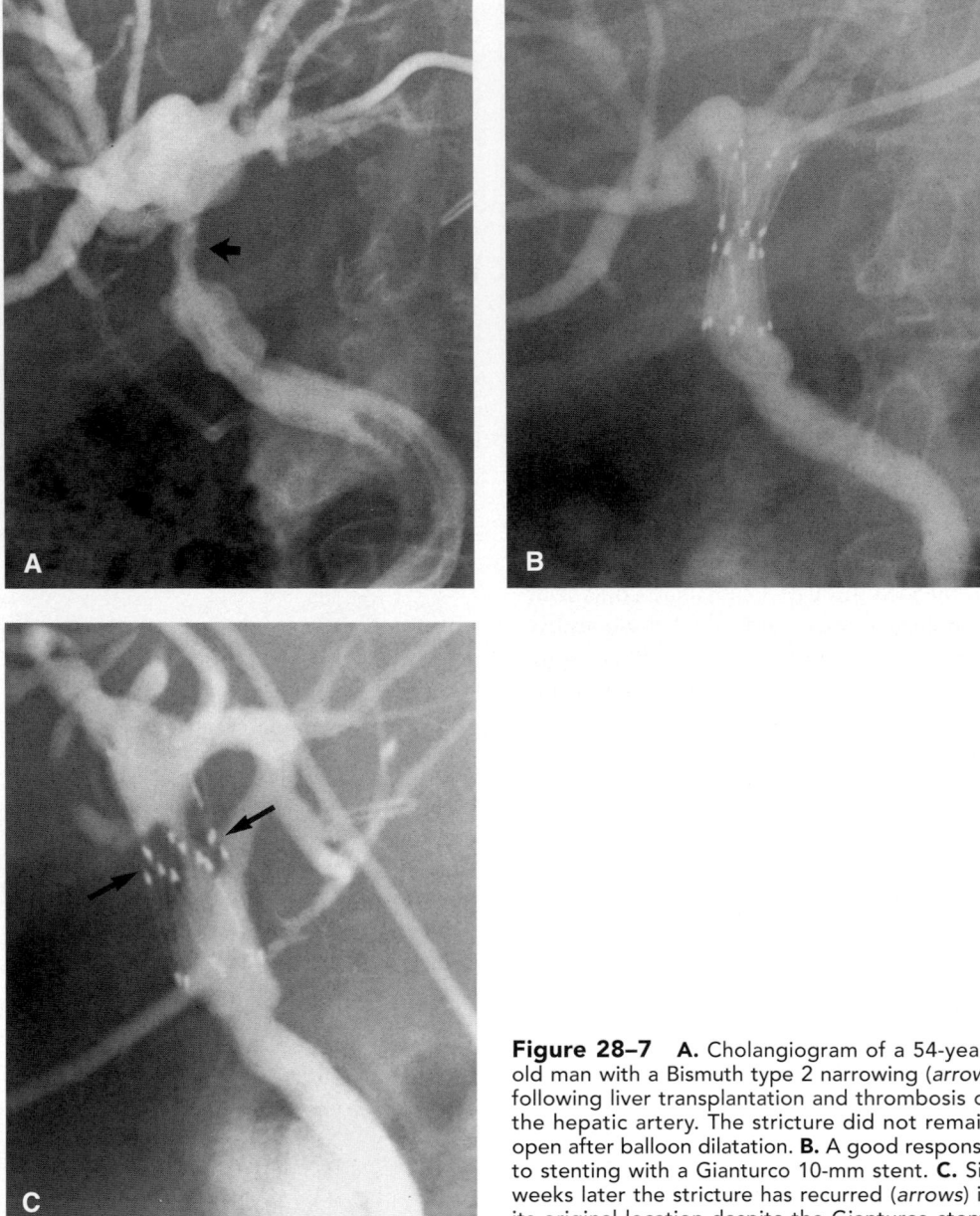

Figure 28–7 **A.** Cholangiogram of a 54-year-old man with a Bismuth type 2 narrowing (*arrow*) following liver transplantation and thrombosis of the hepatic artery. The stricture did not remain open after balloon dilatation. **B.** A good response to stenting with a Gianturco 10-mm stent. **C.** Six weeks later the stricture has recurred (*arrows*) in its original location despite the Gianturco stent.

TECHNIQUE

The author's preference for stenting benign lesions is to use the modified Gianturco-Rösch stent. Most experience in benign lesions has been published with this stent. It is easier to place accurately than the Wallstent because it is much more radiopaque and does not shorten. Many other balloon-expandable or self-expandable metallic stents are available. There is little published data to aid in choosing a stent for benign lesions. It is probably most reasonable to use the stent with which one is most familiar, which is easiest to see well, and which is easiest to position accurately. The shortest stent that can cover the stenosis is likely to provide the best results. Gianturco stents are available in diameters of 8, 10, or 12 mm. They are made

up of individual units 15 mm long that can be linked in flexible chains containing one to five units (Figure 28–5). The Gianturco stent covers a smaller circumferential area of the duct mucosa than the Wallstent, which appears to be an advantage in benign lesions, where the stent is required only as a scaffold to prevent stricture formation.

Placement can be performed via a percutaneous transhepatic approach or via an existing T tube. The lesion is crossed using standard techniques, and care is taken to carefully define the upper and lower margins of the stricture. A catheter placed over the wire, with contrast injected through a side-arm adapter, can be helpful at this stage. Accurate delineation is important for selecting the correct stent length and diameter and for positioning the stent. The delivery system, consisting of a sheath with injection side port, radiopaque distal marker, and tapered dilator, is passed over the wire and across the stricture. The dilator is removed, and the small peel-away introducer is loaded on the back end of the wire, followed by the stent (Figure 28–5). Care must be taken that the wire passes cleanly through the stent lumen and does not pass through one of the struts of the stent. The stent is carefully loaded into the introducer by manual compression. The introducer and stent are fed through the valve on the external end of the delivery sheath. A blunt-ended pusher then goes over the wire and pushes the stent to the delivery site within the sheath. The introducer is peeled away and, with the stent maintained in the predetermined position with the pusher, the sheath is drawn back, releasing the stent. In most cases, the stent will dilate on its own.

A self-retaining catheter is positioned through the stent or in the biliary tree above the stent for check cholangiography the following day. The selection of stent diameter is based on the size of the bile ducts. Single-segment stents are not used because of their marked tendency to migrate. Modified stents with small hooks were once developed and tested in an attempt to prevent migration, but the hooks made the stents difficult to employ, and the devices were abandoned. Instead, if there is a short-segment stricture, the author places a double stent, with the junction between the stents centered at the narrowest part of the lesion. In some cases, to try to secure a more stable position for the stent, some of the nylon suture links of the leading and/or trailing edges of the stent are cut. On delivery, these wings flare out, holding the stent more securely in place (Figures 28–1B and 28–1C). When crossing through a Gianturco stent with a wire, it is important not to inadvertently pass through a side strut or to displace the stent. For this reason, the original wire is removed only when it is clear that no further manipulations are required. If it is necessary to recross a stent, a 3-mm J wire can be helpful.

SUMMARY OF THE ROLE OF RADIOLOGY AS PART OF THE TEAM TREATING BENIGN BILIARY LESIONS

Radiology is very important in the management of benign biliary lesions in three distinct areas:

1. Diagnosis and delineation of the problem as described above in the section on imaging procedures, specifically in showing ductal anatomy, bile leaks, and fluid collections. This may involve both invasive and noninvasive techniques.
2. Providing percutaneous drainage of intra-abdominal fluid collections and of bile ducts. Often, patients are in suboptimal condition following bile duct injury. The ultimate treatment of choice will be surgical repair, but an important intermediate step is to drain all fluid collections and tide the patient over the presenting condition. Percutaneous biliary drains may be needed to control bile leakage or to provide bile drainage in

cases of obstruction. The combination of fluid/abscess drainage combined with biliary drainage will often allow the patient to be discharged home and recover while awaiting elective surgical repair of the bile duct problem. In the author's institution, surgeons often find the percutaneous biliary drainage catheter of assistance in identifying the biliary structures at the time of surgical repair. The transhepatic catheter is often utilized as a postoperative stent. In some cases, biliary dilatation will be attempted as a first line of therapy.
3. Providing ongoing monitoring and adjustment of tubes that are placed both surgically and percutaneously.

PRIMARY SCLEROSING CHOLANGITIS

Primary sclerosing cholangitis (PSC) is characterized by a cholangiographic picture of multiple diffusely located strictures of intra- and extrahepatic bile ducts. The cause of the syndrome is unknown, but inflammatory bowel disease is present in about two-thirds of patients with PSC. Ulcerative colitis is the main type of bowel disease, with Crohn disease accounting for only about 7% of cases (range of 1.5–13.0%). Men are afflicted most commonly, with a male–female ratio greater than 2:1 (64,65).

Initial presentation occurs between 25 and 45 years of age, and more than two thirds of patients are under 45 years of age when diagnosed. Typically, the clinical picture is of a gradual onset of progressive fatigue and pruritus, followed by jaundice in a younger male who has inflammatory bowel disease. The syndrome is progressive, following an unpredictable time course from chronic fibrosing inflammation of the bile ducts, to cirrhosis, portal hypertension, liver failure, and death.

Diagnosis

Diagnosis is usually based on cholangiographic findings by endoscopic retrograde cholangiopancreatography (ERCP) or percutaneous transhepatic cholangiography (PTC). MacCarty et al. described the cholangiographic appearance in 86 patients with PSC (66). The most common findings were diffuse, multifocal strictures involving both the intra- and extrahepatic biliary ducts. In 20% of patients, only the intrahepatic and proximal extrahepatic ducts were involved, and the distal common bile duct was spared. The cystic duct was considered abnormal in 18% of 60 patients. However, the spiral valves and complicated anatomic course of the cystic duct make this assessment difficult. The pancreatic ducts were abnormal in 8% of 40 patients, but this may be only a coincidental finding. Strictures were typically short (1–2 cm) and annular, alternating with normal or minimally dilated segments, giving a beaded appearance. In more advanced disease, long, confluent strictures were seen. Very short (1- to 2-mm) bandlike strictures were noted in 18 patients (21%), most often in the extrahepatic ducts. In nine patients, these strictures were associated with outpouchings resembling diverticula, which often protruded between adjacent strictures. In 14 patients, similar outpouchings were seen without band strictures. Thirty-eight patients (44%) demonstrated mural irregularities that gave a "shaggy" appearance. These varied from a fine "brush border" to coarse filing defects with a frankly nodular appearance and were seen more frequently in the extrahepatic (40%) than in the intrahepatic ducts. Focal dilatation of ductal segments between strictures was relatively frequent (42%), but diffuse dilatation of the biliary tree was infrequent.

The incidence of cholangiocarcinoma in patients with PSC has been reported as 4–9% in a number of studies (64,67,68). A much higher incidence, 30–40%, is found at autopsy of patients dying of PSC (64), and study of excised livers of patients undergoing liver transplantation for PSC shows an incidence of 9–33% (64). Diagnosis of cholangiocarcinoma in patients with PSC is difficult. A sudden, unexplained deterioration in clinical condition with rapidly deepening jaundice, weight loss, and abdominal discomfort may suggest cholangiocarcinoma. On the cholangiogram, marked and rapidly progressive ductal dilatation seen on consecutive studies is suggestive of cholangiocarcinoma. A polypoid mass may rarely be seen (46). Cytologic examination of material obtained by brushing the lumen of the duct has a disappointingly low sensitivity, as does percutaneous biopsy, although specificity is good, about 100%, if cells are obtained. CT misses the diagnosis in about 50% of cases and is of greater value in more advanced cases where a mass lesion, metastatic invasion of lymph nodes, or liver metastases may be demonstrated (64).

Treatment

The cause of PSC is unknown, and no specific treatment has proved to be effective. Management is, therefore, directed at ameliorating the consequences of bile duct narrowing and obstruction using endoscopic, radiological, or surgical techniques. Because PSC is a progressive disease, it is thought that deterioration in liver function may be aggravated or accelerated by backpressure from dominant strictures and any intraductal debris that may be present. It is hoped that reduction of this obstruction may halt, delay, or even reverse progression to cirrhosis and liver failure (69,70). Relief of jaundice, pruritus, and cholangitis by the use of periodic dilatation and antibiotics is of symptomatic value to the patient even if the progression of the disease course is not altered. In patients with end-stage cirrhosis, the benefit of arduous dilatation treatments to the patient's well-being must be carefully considered and possibly abandoned.

Endoscopic Treatment

In most patients, PSC is diagnosed by ERCP. Dominant strictures can be dilated using standard endoscopic techniques with over-the-wire bougies or dilatation balloon catheters. Dominant strictures in the extrahepatic ducts can usually be dilated successfully by endoscopists (69,70). When dominant strictures within the intrahepatic ducts require dilatation, radiologists have often been able to assist their endoscopic colleagues by manipulating a torqueable guide wire, such as the Terumo guide wire, through intrahepatic strictures (45).

Some endoscopists perform a sphincterotomy to allow for easier manipulation of instruments during dilatation and subsequent passage of stone debris. As in the case of stricture dilatation in most parts of the body, there is considerable debate and uncertainty over the value of leaving indwelling stents in the narrowed duct after dilatation. The author's clinical experience with PSC suggests that, wherever possible, plastic stents should not be used (71). With the characteristically narrow ducts found in PSC, plastic endoprostheses tend to hinder drainage by obturating the whole ductal lumen, compromising drainage from side branches and leading to infection and possible exacerbation of the PSC. If stents are used, they should be removed or exchanged after 2–3 months, before they become occluded.

The results of endoscopic management are generally positive, but the published series are somewhat limited by the size of the patient group and the length of follow-up. In 1991, Johnson et al. reported on 35 patients with PSC treated by endoscopic dilatation, with an average follow-up of 24 months (72). Mean serum bilirubin decreased from 10 to 4 mg/dL in the 19 patients who presented with jaundice. There was a significant decrease in the number of episodes of cholangitis and in the need for hospitalization. The radiographic evaluation, which assigned numerical scores to pre- and postdilatation strictures seen on the cholangiogram, also showed a significant improvement. Eleven patients were stented. Complications were hemorrhage requiring transfusion following sphincterotomy in one patient and pancreatitis requiring hospitalization in another.

Cotton and Nickl at Duke University reported on a 3-year experience with 20 patients with symptomatic PSC whom they treated endoscopically (69). They failed to dilate the dominant stricture in three patients, treated three others with nasal biliary drainage and lavage, and treated one by successfully removing a stone. The remaining 13 were dilated successfully, and in six of these, indwelling endoprostheses were used. The authors' cautious summary was: "Mean follow-up is so far only 17 months, but more patients have improved clinically and biochemically than have deteriorated" (69).

Percutaneous Radiological Management

Access to the biliary tree can be achieved by the established percutaneous transhepatic route, by percutaneous puncture of a subcutaneously located bowel loop in patients with a choledochojejunostomy and Roux-en-Y (35,71) or by way of a surgically placed T tube or U tube.

An experienced radiologist can usually establish percutaneous transhepatic access, but it is more difficult to cannulate the nondilated and strictured ducts found in PSC than it is in other types of obstructive jaundice, which typically have dilated ducts. After access is achieved, manipulation within the biliary tree can also be difficult because of the multiple strictures.

In 1985, May et al. reported on their experience in balloon-dilating dominant strictures in 14 patients (73). Access was by percutaneous transhepatic puncture in nine patients and via a surgically placed T tube in five. They achieved initial success in all 14 patients. Their follow-up was 12–34 months (with a mean of 16 months). Before dilatation, bacterial cholangitis occurred at 9.3 ± 5.8 episodes per year but decreased significantly after dilatation to 0.5 ± 0.9 episodes per year. Total serum bilirubin decreased significantly from 11.5 ± 9.5 mg/dL before dilatation to 1.8 ± 0.12 mg/dL after dilatation in the four patients who had jaundice less than 6 months before dilatation. In the five patients who had jaundice longer than 6 months, no significant change in bilirubin occurred after dilatation. Recurrence of the dominant stricture recurred at 6–18 months in three patients. Five patients had complications, which were bacteremia and cholangitis requiring hospitalization. Four of five patients who showed no symptomatic response died of liver failure.

Skolkin et al. reported on percutaneous balloon cholangioplasty in 14 patients with PSC in 1989 (74). Access was by transhepatic puncture in 12 patients and via a T tube in the remaining two patients. They had one failed attempt at transhepatic drainage. Although initial success was achieved in 14 of 15 patients, the researchers reported that PTC, drainage, and cholangioplasty were often technically challenging. Attempts at leaving stents in place for 6 months were successful in only four of 14 patients because of septic cholangitis and poor tolerance of the tubes. They had a mean follow-up of 18–19 months (range of 1–42). Thirteen of 14 patients experienced varying degrees of clinical improvement. Pruritus resolved or decreased in seven of seven patients. Malaise and pain were more difficult to assess because of the contribution of the indwelling stent to this symptom complex. The researchers reported only general trends for biochemical response because of the small number of patients and varied patient condition before treatment. Complications included frequent fevers, cholangitis, and sepsis, one arterial hemorrhage requiring embolization, three instances of pleural effusion as a result of high tube placement across the pleural space, one subphrenic abscess, and one subcutaneous abscess. Both abscesses were drained percutaneously.

On the basis of this reported experience and the author's own experience, an endoscopic approach is recommended when possible. When balloon dilatation is performed transhepatically or via a T tube, the dilatation is completed without stenting, and an effort is made to remove all tubes from the biliary tree as soon as possible (71). The same

principles apply when the approach is retrograde via a percutaneous puncture of the Roux loop. A self-retaining catheter retained in the loop allows for subsequent access to the biliary tree without the infectious complications of an indwelling tube in the biliary tree. All manipulations are performed under antibiotic cover.

The availability of expandable metallic stents has provided additional ways of treating the strictures of PSC. In a few patients who did not respond to periodic dilatations of dominant strictures and who were not yet candidates for liver transplantation, the author has implanted Gianturco stents. Multiple stents can provide an extensive intraductal scaffold to maintain patency, as shown in Figure 28–8. Obviously, these stents do not represent a permanent treatment option but may be useful as a temporary measure to delay the need for liver transplantation. The author's experience so far is favorable but is too limited at this time to offer any firm data.

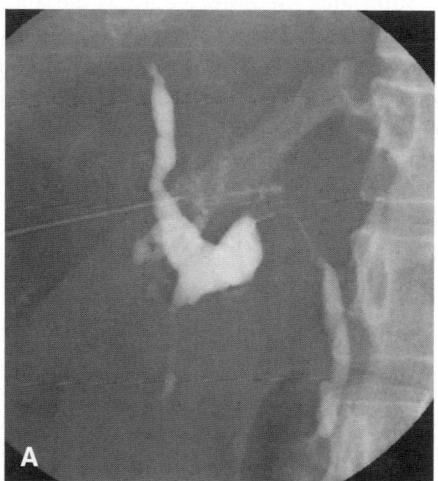

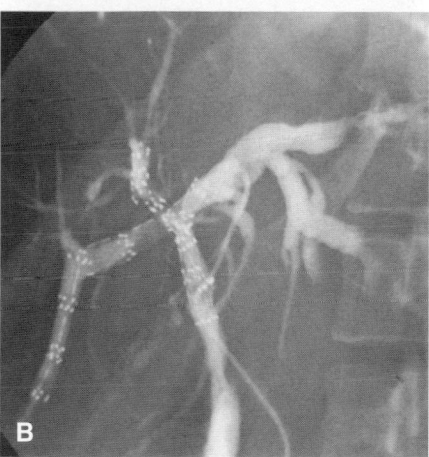

Figure 28–8 **A.** Cholangiogram of a 34-year-old woman with sclerosing cholangitis and ulcerative colitis. The PTC shows a few irregular dilated ducts on the right, no filling of ducts on the left, and tight stricturing of the common hepatic duct. **B.** Multiple Gianturco stents have been placed to keep open the main intrahepatic ducts, with excellent clinical results. Follow-up at 6 months shows maintenance of good health.

Surgical Treatment

Biliary surgery for the treatment of strictures in PSC has largely been replaced by the nonoperative techniques described above (75). Although surgeons at Johns Hopkins have advocated resection of the extrahepatic biliary tree, operative intrahepatic dilatation, and hepaticoenteric or choledochoenteric anastomosis with long-term indwelling Silastic stents, there seems to be little support for such an aggressive approach (75). Periodic dilatations can be achieved much more easily by nonoperative techniques, and the burden and morbidity of indwelling transhepatic tubes can be avoided. Moreover, subsequent liver transplantation is made more difficult by previous biliary surgery of this type.

Anastomosis of the extrahepatic bile duct to a Roux-en-Y loop, with one part tacked up to the abdominal wall, allows for percutaneous puncture and cannulation of the loop (35). From the loop, radiologists can gain retrograde access to the biliary tree to dilate dominant strictures. This approach eliminates the transhepatic route and the need for indwelling catheters. The loop leading to the ducts should be short and straight for easy percutaneous manipulation. However, increased endoscopic expertise in stricture dilatation and the problems with subsequent liver transplantation have also rendered this technique of only occasional value.

The most important operative procedure for PSC is liver transplantation, which is the treatment of choice for patients with end-stage liver disease (76). Bass outlines the current indications for transplantation in PSC as patients with (1) complications of portal hypertension; (2) impaired synthetic function of the liver; and (3) severe or worsening cholestasis and cirrhosis on biopsies or recurrent cholangitis refractory to medical or interventional management (64). The results of liver transplantation for PSC are 3- to 4-year survival rates of 85–88%. In PSC, the donor duct is anastomosed to a Roux-en-Y loop rather than to the stump of the recipient's common duct, which may be narrow and is always suspect as a site of recurrent PSC. Unfortunately, recent surveys have shown that intrahepatic and nonanastomotic extrahepatic biliary strictures are significantly more common in patients who have undergone liver transplantation for PSC than in patients who receive allografts for other end-stage liver diseases (26,77). Strictures of the choledochojejunostomy anastomosis occur with equal frequency in both groups. Sheng et al. from Pittsburgh compared 100 transplant patients with PSC to a control group of 543 patients who received choledochojejunostomy biliary anastomoses transplanted for non-PSC liver failure (77). In the PSC group, intrahepatic strictures were found in 27% of patients, compared with 13% in the control group, a significant difference. Nonanastomotic extrahepatic strictures were also significantly more frequent: 6% compared with 2%. Anastomotic strictures were 18% to 15%, which

was not statistically significant. The long-term implications of these findings have not yet been resolved.

AIDS-RELATED CHOLANGIOPATHY

Some patients with AIDS have been described as suffering from biliary tract abnormalities. It is important that radiologists be familiar with this recently recognized type of biliary obstruction. Cello found a typical presentation of severe right upper quadrant abdominal pain, spiking fevers, markedly elevated serum alkaline phosphatase levels, or any combination of the three findings (78). In a study of 26 patients, 20 patients (77%) had markedly abnormal cholangiograms at ERCP. Cello recognized four patterns of disease at ERCP: sclerosing cholangitis and papillary stenosis (10 patients); only papillary stenosis (three patients); only sclerosing cholangitis (four patients); and long, extrahepatic bile duct strictures (three patients).

Only short-lived, beneficial responses followed endoscopic sphincterotomy. At present, patients suffering from AIDS have a limited life expectancy. Endoprostheses may, therefore, be of benefit to them until a specific treatment for AIDS is developed (79).

REFERENCES

1. Blumgart LH, Jarnigan WR. Benign biliary strictures. In: Blumgart LH, Fong Y, eds. Surgery of the Liver and Biliary Tract. Philadelphia: WB Saunders, 2000.
2. Warren KW, Mountain JC, Midell AI. Management of strictures of the biliary tract. Surg Clin North Am 1971;51:711–731.
3. Blumgart LH, Kelley CJ, Benjamin IS. Benign bile duct stricture following cholecystectomy: critical factors in management. Br J Surg 1984;71:836–843.
4. Roslyn JJ, Binns GS, Hughes EF, et al. Open cholecystectomy. A contemporary analysis of 42,474 patients. Ann Surg 193; 218: 129–137.
5. Deziel DJ, Millikan KW, Economou SG, et al. Complications of laparoscopic cholecystectomy: a national survey of 4,292 hospitals and an analysis of 77,604 cases. Am J Surg 1993;165:9–14.
6. Wherry DC, Marohn MR, Malanoski MP, et al. An external audit of laparoscopic cholecystectomy in the steady state performed in medical treatment facilities of the Department of Defense. Ann Surg 1996;224:145–154.
7. Adamsen S, Hansen OH, Funch-Jensen P, et al. Bile duct injury during laparoscopic cholecystectomy: a prospective nationwide series. J Am Coll Surg 1997;184:571–578.
8. Way LW, Stewart L, Gantert W, et al. Causes and prevention of laparoscopic bile duct injuries: Analysis of 252 cases from a human factors and cognitive psychology perspective. Ann Surg 2003;237:460–469.
9. Stewart L, Way LW. Bile duct injuries during laparoscopic cholecystectomy. Arch Surg 1995;130:1123.
10. Rossi RL, Schirmer WJ, Braasch JW, et al. Laparoscopic bile duct injuries: risk factors, recognition, and repair. Arch Surg 1992; 127: 596–602.
11. Pitt HA, Miyamoto T, Parapatis SK, et al. Factors influencing outcome in patients with postoperative biliary strictures. Am J Surg 1982;144:14–21.
12. Pellegrini CA, Thomas MJ, Way LW. Recurrent biliary stricture: patterns of recurrence and outcome of surgical therapy. Am J Surg 1984;147:175–180.

13. Pitt HA, Kaufman SL, Coleman J, et al. Benign postoperative biliary strictures. Ann Surg 1989;210:417–425.
14. Millis JM, Tompkins RK, Zinner MJ, et al. Management of bile duct strictures: an evolving strategy. Arch Surg 1992;127 : 1077–1084.
15. Lillemoe KD, Melton GB, Cameron JL, et al. Postoperative bile duct strictures: management and outcomes in the 1990s. Ann Surg 2000;232:430–441.
16. Melton GB, Lillemoe KD, Cameron JL, et al. Major bile duct injuries associated with laparoscopic cholecystectomy. Effect of surgical repair on quality of life. Ann Surg 2002;235:888–895.
17. Boerma D, Rauws EA, Keulemans YC, et al. Impaired quality of life 5 years after bile duct injury during laparoscopic cholecystectomy. A prospective analysis. Ann Surg 2001;234:750–757.
18. Bismuth H. Postoperative strictures of the bile duct. In: Blumgart LH, ed. The Biliary Tract. Clinical Surgery International, vol 5. Edinburgh: Churchill Livingstone, 1982.
19. Alves A, Farges O, Nicolet J, et al. Incidence and consequence of an hepatic artery injury in patients with postcholecystectomy bile duct injuries. Ann Surg 2003;238:93–96.
20. Yeh BM, Breiman RS, Taouli B, et al. Biliary tract depiction in living potential liver donors: Comparison of conventional MR cholangiography, mangafodipir trisodium excretory MR cholangiography, and multidetector CT cholangiography—initial experience. Radiology 2004;230:645–651.
21. Gelman R, Alexander MS, Zucker KA, et al. The use of radionuclide imaging in the evaluation of suspected biliary damage during laparoscopic cholecystectomy. Gastrointest Radiol 1991;16: 201–204.
22. Courbiere M, Pilleul F, Henry L, et al. Value of magnetic resonance cholangiography in benign and malignant biliary stenosis: comparative study with direct cholangiography. J Comput Assist Tomogr 2003;27:315–320.
23. Romagnuolo J, Bardou M, Rahme E, et al. Magnetic resonance cholangiopancreatography: a meta-analysis of test performance in suspected biliary disease. Ann Intern Med 2003;139:547–557.
24. Harbin WP, Mueller PR, Ferrucci JT. Transhepatic cholangiography: complications and use patterns of the fine-needle technique: a multi-institutional survey. Radiology 1980;135:15–22.
25. Ferrucci JT, Wittenberg J, Sarno RA, et al. Fine needle transhepatic cholangiography: a new approach to obstructive jaundice. Am J Roentgenol 1976;127:403–407.
26. Letourneau JG, Day DL, Hunter DW, et al. Biliary complications after liver transplantation in patients with preexisting sclerosing cholangitis. Radiology 1988;167:349–351.
27. Colonna JO, Shaked A, Gomes AS, et al. Biliary strictures complicating liver transplantation. Ann Surg 1992;216:344–352.
28. Pereiras R, Chiprut RO, Greenwald RA, et al. Percutaneous transhepatic cholangiography with the "skinny" needle. A rapid, simple, and accurate method in the diagnosis of cholestasis. Ann Intern Med 1977;86:562–568.
29. Mueller PR, Harbin WP, Ferrucci JT, et al. Fine-needle transhepatic cholangiography: reflections after 450 cases. AJR Am J Roentgenol 1981;136:85–90.
30. Gordon RL, Ring EJ, LaBerge JM, et al. Malignant biliary obstruction: treatment with expandable metallic stents—follow-up of 50 consecutive patients. Radiology 1992;182:697–701.
31. Foerster EC, Hoepffner N, Domschke W. Bridging of benign choledochal stenoses by endoscopic retrograde implantation of mesh stents. Endoscopy 1991;23:133–135.
32. Mueller PR, van Sonnenberg E, Ferrucci JT, et al. Biliary stricture dilatation: multicenter review of clinical management in 73 patients. Radiology 1986;160:17–22.
33. Maccioni F, Rossi M, Salvatori FM, et al. Metallic stents in benign biliary strictures: three-year follow-up. Cardiovasc Intervent Radiol 1992;15:360–366.
34. Hutson DG, Russell E, Schiff E, et al. Balloon dilatation of biliary strictures through a choledochojejuno-cutaneous fistula. Ann Surg 1984;199:637–647.
35. McPherson SJ, Gibson RN, Collier NA, et al. Percutaneous transjejunal biliary intervention: 10-year experience with access via Roux-en-Y loops. Radiology 1998;206:665–672.
36. Williams HJ, Bender CE, May GR. Benign postoperative biliary strictures: dilation with fluoroscopic guidance. Radiology 1987; 163:629–634.
37. Mueller PR, Ferrucci JT, Teplick SK, et al. Biliary stent endoprosthesis: analysis of complications in 113 patients. Radiology 1985;156:637–639.
38. Burhenne HJ. Dilatation of biliary tract strictures: a new roentgenologic technique. Radiol Clin 1975;44:153–159.
39. Molnar W, Stockum AE. Transhepatic dilatation of choledochoenterostomy strictures. Radiology 1978;129:59–64.
40. Salomonowitz E, Castaneda-Zuniga WR, Lund G, et al. Balloon dilatation of benign biliary strictures. Radiology 1984;151:613–616.
41. Gallagher DJ, Kadir S, Kaufman SL, et al. Nonoperative management of benign postoperative biliary strictures. Radiology 1985;156:625–629.
42. Moore AV, Illescas FF, Mills SR, et al. Percutaneous dilation of benign biliary strictures. Radiology 1987;163:625–628.
43. Trambert JJ, Bron KM, Zajko AB, et al. Percutaneous transhepatic balloon dilatation of benign biliary strictures. AJR Am J Roentgenol 1987;149:945–948.
44. Citron SJ, Martin LG. Benign biliary strictures: treatment with percutaneous cholangioplasty. Radiology 1991;178:339–341.
45. Gordon RL, Ring EJ. Combined radiologic and retrograde endoscopic and biliary interventions. Radiol Clin North Am 1990;28: 1289–1295.
46. Maroney TP, Ring EJ. Percutaneous transjejunal catheterization of Roux-en-Y biliary-jejunal anastomoses. Radiology 1987; 164: 151–153.
47. Draganov P, Hoffman B, Marsh W, et al. Long-term outcome in patients with benign biliary strictures treated endoscopically with multiple stents. Gastrointest Endosc 2002;55:680 686.
48. Bergman JJ, Burgemeister L, Bruno MJ, et al. Long-term follow-up after biliary stent placement for postoperative bile duct stenosis. Gastrointest Endosc 2001;54:154–161.
49. Carrasco CH, Wallace S, Charnsangavej C, et al. Expandable biliary endoprothesis: an experimental study. AJR Am J Roentgenol 1985;145:1279–1281.
50. Uchida BT, Putnam JS, Rösch J. Modifications of Gianturco expandable wire stents. AJR Am J Roentgenol 1988;150: 1185–1187.
51. Irving JD, Adam A, Dick R, et al. Gianturco expandable metallic biliary stents: results of a European clinical trial. Radiology 1989;172:321–326.
52. Coons HG. Self-expanding stainless steel biliary stents. Radiology 1989;170:979–983.
53. Rossi P, Bezzi M, Salvatori FM, et al. Recurrent benign biliary strictures: management with self-expanding metallic stents. Radiology 1990;175:661–665.
54. Coons H. Metallic stents for the treatment of biliary obstruction: a report of 100 cases. Cardiovasc Intervent Radiol 1992;15: 367–374.
55. Hausegger KA, Kugler C, Uggowitzer M, et al. Benign biliary obstruction: Is treatment with the Wallstent advisable? Radiology 1996;200:437–441.
56. Bonnel DH, Liguory CL, Lefebvre JF, et al. Placement of metallic stents for treatment of postoperative biliary strictures: Long-term outcome in 25 patients. AJR Am J Roentgenol 1997;169: 1517–1522.
57. Gabelmann A, Hamid H, Brambs H, et al. Metallic stents in benign biliary strictures: Long-term effectiveness and interventional management of stent occlusion. AJR Am J Roentgenol 2001;177:813–817.
58. Vorwerk D, Kissinger G, Handt S, et al. Long-term patency of Wallstent endoprostheses in benign biliary obstructions: experimental results. J Vasc Intervent Radiol 1993;4:625–634.
59. Alvarado R, Palmaz JC, Garcia OJ, et al. Evaluation of polymer-coated balloon-expandable stents in bile ducts. Radiology 1989; 170:975–978.
60. Petersen BD, Timmermans HA, Uchida BT, et al. Treatment of refractory benign biliary stenoses in liver transplant patients by placement and retrieval of a temporary stent-graft: work in progress. J Vasc Interv Radiol 2000;11:919–929.
61. Ginsberg G, Cope C, Shah J, et al. In vivo evaluation of a new bioabsorbable self-expanding biliary stent. Gastrointest Endosc 2003;58:777–784.
62. Schoder M, Rossi P, Uflacker R, et al. Malignant biliary obstruction: treatment with ePTFE-FEP- covered endoprostheses initial

technical and clinical experiences in a multicenter trial. Radiology 2002;225:35–42.

63. Kalinowski M, Alfke H, Kleb B, et al. Paclitaxel inhibits proliferation of cell lines responsible for metal stent obstruction: possible topical application in malignant bile duct obstructions. Invest Radiol 2002;37:399–404.

64. Mahadevan U, Bass NM. Sclerosing cholangitis. In: Feldman M, Friedman LS, Sleisenger MH, eds. Sleisenger and Fordtran's Gastrointestinal and Liver Disease. 7th Ed. Philadelphia: WB Saunders, 2002.

65. Levy C, Lindor KD. Current management of primary biliary cirrhosis and primary sclerosing cholangitis. J Hepatol 2003;38:524–537.

66. MacCarty RL, LaRusso NF, Wiesner RH, et al. Primary sclerosing cholangitis: findings on cholangiography and pancreatography. Radiology 1983;149:39–44.

67. MacCarty RL, LaRusso NF, May GR, et al. Cholangiocarcinoma complicating primary sclerosing cholangitis: cholangiographic appearances. Radiology 1985;156:43–46.

68. Stiehl A. Primary sclerosing cholangitis: neoplastic potential in bile ducts, colon and the pancreas? J Hepatol 2002;36:433–434.

69. Cotton PB, Nickl N. Endoscopic and radiologic approaches to therapy in primary sclerosing cholangitis. Semin Liver Dis 1991;11:40–48.

70. Schrumpf E, Boberg KM. Endoscopic treatment for primary sclerosing cholangitis? J Hepatol 2002;36:278–279.

71. Kerlan RK, LaBerge JM, Goldberg HI, et al. Interventional radiologic management of sclerosing cholangitis. AJR Am J Roentgenol 1986;147:1002–1006.

72. Johnson GK, Geenen JE, Venu RP, et al. Endoscopic treatment of biliary tract strictures in sclerosing cholangitis: a larger series and recommendations for treatment. Gastrointest Endosc 1991;37:38–43.

73. May GR, Bender CE, LaRusso NF, et al. Nonoperative dilatation of dominant strictures in primary sclerosing cholangitis. AJR Am J Roentgenol 1985;145:1061–1064.

74. Skolkin MD, Alspaugh JP, Casarella WJ, et al. Sclerosing cholangitis: palliation with percutaneous cholangioplasty. Radiology 1989;170:199–206.

75. Lillemoe KD, Pitt HA, Cameron JL. Primary sclerosing cholangitis. Surg Clin North Am 1990;70:1381–1402.

76. Langnas AN, Grazi GL, Stratta RJ, et al. Primary sclerosing cholangitis: the emerging role for liver transplantation. Am J Gastroenterol 1990;85:1136–1141.

77. Sheng R, Zajko AB, Campbell WL, et al. Biliary strictures in hepatic transplants: prevalence and types in patients with primary sclerosing cholangitis vs. those with other liver disease. AJR Am J Roentgenol 1993;161:297–300.

78. Cello JP. Acquired immunodeficiency syndrome cholangiopathy: spectrum of disease. Am J Med 1989;86:539–546.

79. Enns R. AIDS cholangiopathy: "an endangered disease". Am J of Gastroenterology 2003;98:2111–2112.

Malignant Obstruction of the Hepatobiliary System

29

**Anthony C. Venbrux, Elizabeth A. Ignacio, Amy P. Soltes,
Stanley B. Washington**

The percutaneous management of patients with malignant hepatobiliary obstruction continues to evolve. If the patient is deemed surgically unresectable and quality-of-life issues are of primary concern, the placement of biliary endoprostheses in the hepatobiliary system provides a minimally invasive image-guided therapeutic option. This option provides patients freedom from external biliary drainage catheters. Although gastroenterologists provide excellent care in applying endoscopically directed endoprostheses for those patients with distal common bile duct obstruction, extensive lesions involving the hilum (i.e., biliary bifurcation) are often inadequately managed using endoscopic techniques.

Patients with hilar lesions can be managed by creating unilateral or bilateral transhepatic tracts followed by fluoroscopically guided placement of biliary endoprostheses, although this procedure is more invasive. The trend is to use self-expanding metallic stents (endoprostheses) because the transhepatic tract is smaller in diameter relative to the larger caliber of the plastic stents used for palliation. After placement of biliary endoprostheses, the external biliary drainage catheters may be removed, freeing the patient from the issues associated with chronic external drainage catheters (flushing the catheters, changing the dressings, risk of skin and biliary infections, etc.). The purpose of this chapter is (1) to outline the technique of percutaneous transhepatic biliary drainage, (2)

to discuss the application of self-expanding metallic biliary endoprostheses in patients with malignant biliary obstruction, and (3) to review indications, contraindications, complications, and the current literature.

The etiology of hepatobiliary obstruction includes (1) pancreatic carcinoma; (2) primary malignancy arising from the bile duct epithelium (e.g., cholangiocarcinoma); and (3) metastatic disease to the bile ducts or to adjacent tissues (e.g., metastatic disease to lymph nodes in the hilum of the liver that causes central [hilar] biliary obstruction). In general, patients with pancreatic carcinoma who are deemed unresectable have a limited life expectancy, and thus the use of biliary endoprostheses for palliation is a reasonable therapeutic option. As all biliary endoprostheses occlude over time, patients with expected longer-term survival (e.g., patients with cholangiocarcinoma) may be treated initially with internal/external biliary drainage catheters and later with endoprostheses as the disease progresses. Because biliary endoprostheses cannot be easily removed once in place, such endoluminal devices should be reserved for those patients with limited life expectancy. Biliary endoprostheses of the self-expanding metallic variety *should not* be used in patients with benign biliary strictures. In such instances, the stent struts eventually become embedded in the bile duct epithelium and are generally impossible to remove. Should a patient with benign biliary disease receiving a metallic endoprosthesis require eventual biliary reconstructive surgery, the previously stented benign disease and the surgical resection thereafter may be more extensive than originally planned. In such instances, the use of nonmetallic stents (e.g., plastic endoprostheses) may be a reasonable alternative for those patients who cannot be managed with external drainage catheters and periodic catheter exchanges.

DEMOGRAPHICS OF MALIGNANT BILIARY OBSTRUCTION

Pancreatic cancer, otherwise known as pancreatic adenocarcinoma, is the fourth leading cause of cancer deaths in both men and women in the United States (1). Only about 10% of patients are found to have tumors that are surgically resectable (2). As mentioned earlier, distal common bile duct obstruction due to pancreatic carcinoma may be managed endoscopically or percutaneously. If the distal common bile duct obstruction cannot be crossed under endoscopic guidance, the patient is sent to the interventional radiology suite for transhepatic drainage. Because 70% of adenocarcinomas of the pancreas arise in the head, neck, and uncinate process, many of these patients, if surgically unresectable, are well served with either endoscopic or transhepatic palliative placement of biliary endoprostheses.

The majority of cholangiocarcinomas are extrahepatic. Approximately 10% of cholangiocarcinomas are intrahepatic (3). Cholangiocarcinoma involving the hilar region frequently results in bilateral (i.e., right and left) biliary ductal obstruction. If the patient is deemed surgically unresectable, bilateral percutaneous transhepatic cholangiography and bilateral biliary drainage are frequently required. These are followed by placement of biliary endoprostheses when the patient's disease has progressed and the patient's life expectancy is limited (6 months to a year). Cholangiocarcinoma tends to be slow growing, whereas pancreatic carcinoma tends to progress rapidly. Associated conditions that increase incidence of cholangiocarcinoma include (1) primary sclerosing cholangitis; (2) Caroli disease; (3) choledochal cysts; (4) thorium dioxide exposure; and (5) parasitic infestation (4,5).

Cholelithiasis has been seen in up to one third of patients with cholangiocarcinoma. However, although there is a strong positive correlation between gallstones and gallbladder carcinoma, a definite cause-and-effect relationship has not been established for cholangiocarcinoma (6).

Growth patterns of cholangiocarcinoma are either infiltrating-scirrhous, nodular, or papillary. The infiltrating-scirrhous type is the most common and characteristically presents as a focal biliary stricture, often without evidence of a mass. Differentiation from benign causes of biliary stricture is made more difficult by the fact that the malignant cells may be difficult or impossible to detect in the midst of an extensive desmoplastic reaction that these neoplasms tend to incite (7–10).

EVALUATION OF PATIENTS WITH MALIGNANT DISEASE OF THE HEPATOBILIARY SYSTEM

Workup of patients with suspected hepatobiliary malignancy often begins with clinical evaluation, laboratory analysis, and cross-sectional imaging studies. The patient may be initially seen by a family physician, internist, gastroenterologist, hepatologist, or surgeon.

The role of the radiologist in the management of patients with hepatobiliary malignancy includes the following:

1. Performing and interpreting cross-sectional imaging studies to preoperatively stage the patient. At the author's institution, initial imaging usually consists of computed tomography (CT). Less frequently, ultrasonography is used. Magnetic resonance imaging (MRI) with magnetic resonance cholangiopancreatography (MRCP) is now used in many centers to assist in evaluating liver and/or biliary anatomy.
2. Further defining biliary anatomy using the technique of percutaneous transhepatic cholangiography (PTC).
3. Providing percutaneous biliary drainage (PBD).
4. Improving the metabolic status of the patient (e.g., decreasing the total bilirubin and relieving obstruction in the setting of infection).
5. In patients where cross-sectional imaging is equivocal, performing an arteriogram to further define the anatomy (i.e., variant anatomy) and help clarify the issue of vascular encasement by tumor (11).

THE TECHNIQUE OF PERCUTANEOUS TRANSHEPATIC CHOLANGIOGRAPHY (PTC) AND PERCUTANEOUS BILIARY DRAINAGE (PBD)

The technique of PTC/PBD is well described (11–14). For the PTC/PBD procedure, a right midaxillary or a left subxyphoid approach (or both) may be used. The suitability of the initial PTC puncture site for subsequent biliary drainage is determined by several factors. These include (1) the general location of the puncture site within the biliary tree (i.e., peripherally or centrally); (2) the angle formed by the junction of the needle and the specific duct entered; and (3) the therapeutic objectives of future biliary interventions. After the diagnostic PTC is performed using a 21- to 23-gauge "skinny needle" (Chiba needle or trocar needle), a percutaneous biliary drainage (PBD) is performed.

Technique of PBD

If the initial "skinny needle" puncture site into the biliary system is anatomically favorable, conversion of the "skinny needle" ductal puncture site into a larger-caliber, more "secure" access is possible using a wire and sheath-dilator-cannula (i.e., a coaxial system). If the initial percutaneous puncture is unfavorable for access (Figures 29–1 and 29–2), a second puncture is made after duct opacification with contrast (i.e., after PTC) (Figure 29–3), and access is achieved with a "one stick" coaxial kit (Figure 29–4). If possible, advancement of a guide wire into the duodenum (i.e., across the obstruction) is preferable (Figure 29–5). This may require several sessions in the interventional suite, especially if the patient is bacteremic or septic. In such cases, initial external drainage alone is sufficient, with a return once the patient's biliary system is decompressed and the patient is clinically improved. Eventual placement of an 8–10F multi–side-hole locking pigtail catheter across the obstruction is standard at the authors' institution (Figure 29–6). Initial decompression to an externally draining bile collection bag and continued intravenous antibiotic therapy is essential. Once the patient's serum bilirubin has decreased and the patient is clinically improved, the drainage catheter(s) may be capped, allowing bile to drain into the duodenum.

If the obstruction extends to the level of the biliary bifurcation, bilateral (i.e., right [midaxillary] and left [subxyphoid]) drainages may be required. Occasionally (e.g., in extensive cholangiocarcinoma), two right and one left biliary drainage catheters are required.

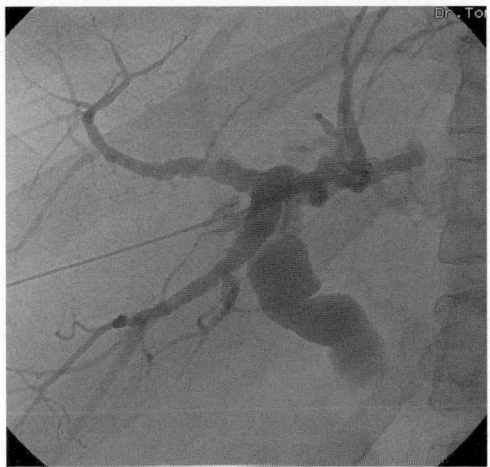

Figure 29–2 AP digital spot image documenting a "skinny needle" (Chiba needle or trocar needle) being withdrawn as dilute contrast is instilled. The needle tip opacifies the bile ducts. A sample of bile has been aspirated and sent to the laboratory for Gram's stain, culture, and sensitivity. Note that in this patient, the entry site into the biliary system is adequate to define anatomy (i.e., percutaneous transhepatic cholangiogram [PTC]) but is too central for percutaneous transhepatic biliary drainage (PBD or PTBD). A central drainage site increases the risk of vascular injury (e.g., to the hepatic artery and other vascular sites).

Placement of Biliary Endoprostheses

With the patient's biliary system decompressed, placement of biliary endoprostheses is technically feasible from the transhepatic approach if the patient is deemed surgically unresectable and requires palliative therapy. If the obstruction is at the bifurcation of the main right and left biliary ducts (e.g., pancreatic carcinoma with metastatic nodes in the hilum of the liver), setting the stage by

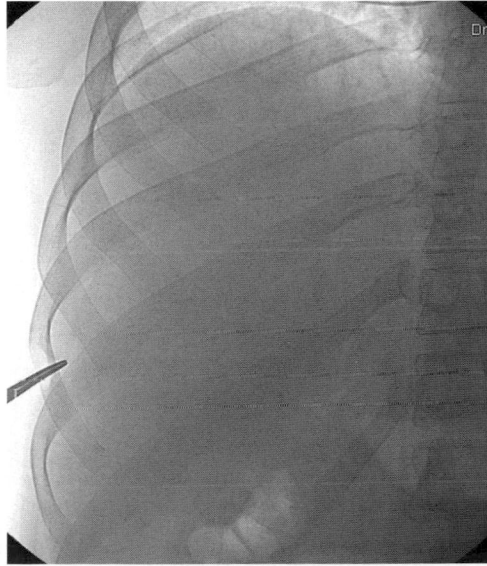

Figure 29–1 Antero-posterior (AP) digital spot image indicating the planned percutaneous access site from a right midaxillary approach. The tip of a hemostat marks the proposed entry. Care is taken to avoid puncturing either the lung or the hepatic flexure of the colon. The access should be just over the cephalic edge of a rib so as to avoid potential injury to the neurovascular bundle.

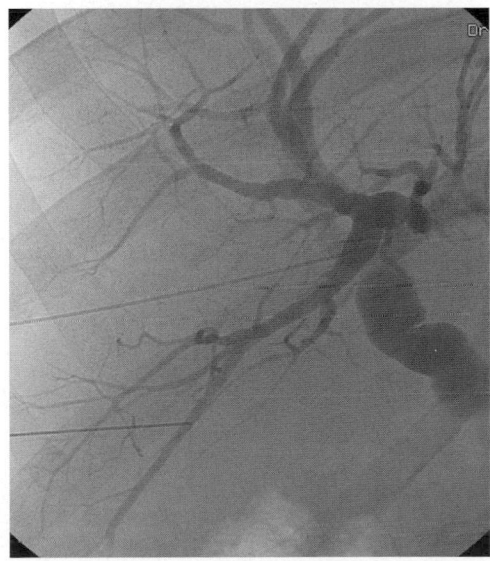

Figure 29–3 AP digital spot image showing placement of a second "skinny needle." The tip has been advanced under fluoroscopic guidance into a more peripheral location.

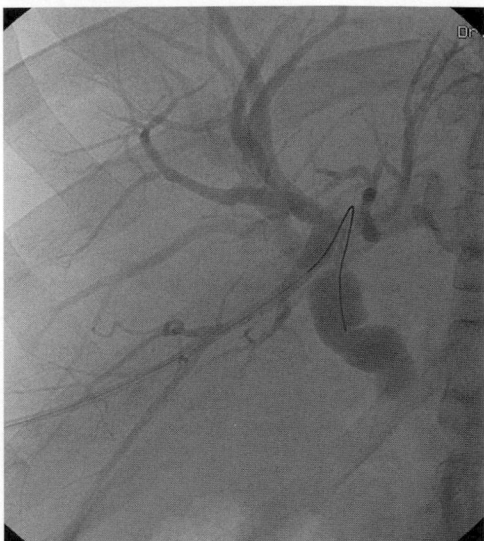

Figure 29–4 A Jeffrey's set, consisting of a stiff cannula-dilator-sheath assembly, has been advanced into the peripheral right bile duct over a 0.018 inch in diameter guide wire.

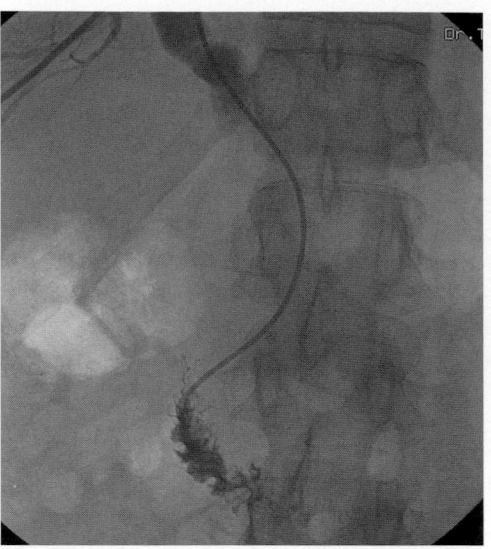

Figure 29–6 AP digital spot film (final cholangiogram) shows the completed right-sided biliary drainage catheter in place. The catheter contains multiple side holes, which facilitate biliary drainage above and below the level of extrahepatic biliary obstruction. Having completed the PBD (or PTBD), the percutaneous access may then serve as the means for placement of a biliary endoprosthesis.

accomplishing percutaneous biliary drainage (one, two, or three catheters) is required before placing the metallic endoprosthesis (Figure 29–7). In such patients with extensive hilar obstruction, endoscopic placement of a metallic or plastic endoprosthesis may not be optimal to provide bilateral drainage because of high intrahepatic location of the lesions. Thus, the authors prefer the percutaneous transhepatic approach for endoprosthesis placement. As mentioned earlier, biliary endoprostheses may be either

plastic or metallic. Most investigators feel that the metallic biliary endoprostheses are advantageous for the following reasons:

1. The metallic biliary stents used for palliation of malignant biliary obstruction caused by pancreatic carcinoma are generally placed through a smaller percutaneous transhepatic tract than plastic endoprostheses are.

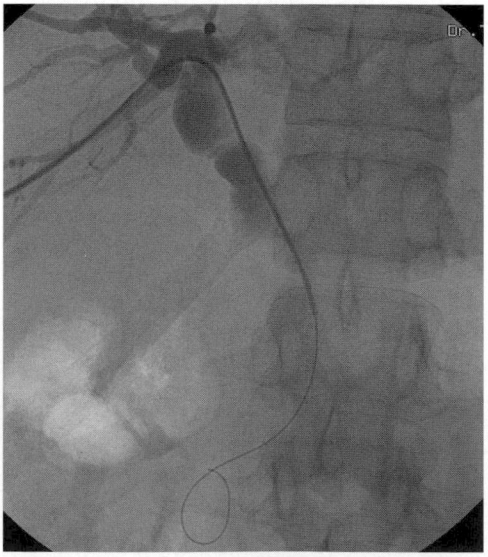

Figure 29–5 AP digital spot film documenting use of a hydrophilic-coated angled tip 5 French catheter (Glide-cath, Terumo, Meditech). The catheter tip has been advanced through the 6.5F sheath of the Jeffrey's set (Cook, Inc.). With a hydrophilic-coated catheter and a torqueable guide wire, the tumor causing this patient's biliary obstruction was crossed. The guide wire now enters the small bowel, and the 5 French catheter is advanced into the duodenum (*not shown*).

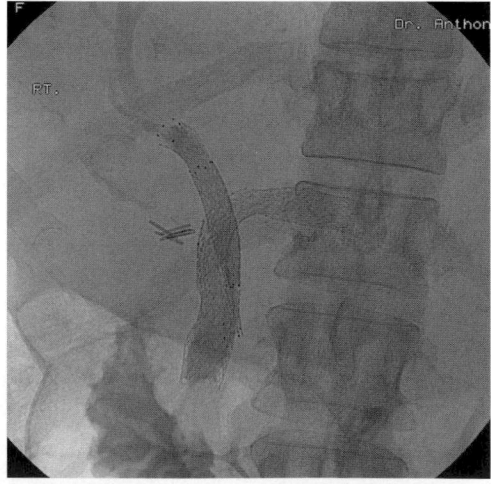

Figure 29–7 AP digital spot film after placement of overlapping bilateral 10-mm-diameter biliary endoprosthesis (Smart Nitinol Stent). The external biliary drainage catheters have been removed after the final cholangiogram. (This patient required separate right (i.e., midaxillary) and left (i.e., subxyphoid) percutaneous biliary drainage procedures.) Placement of biliary endoprotheses may be accomplished in a single step if there is no significant bleeding during the PTC/PBD procedures. Because of eventual endoprosthesis occlusion, such devices are used for palliation in patients with unresectable malignant disease and limited life expectancy (e.g., 6 months to 1 year).

2. There is controversy in the medical literature, but in general, it is felt that metallic biliary endoprostheses have a better long-term patency than plastic endoprostheses.
3. The metallic endoprostheses may be placed in a single-step procedure (i.e., PTC followed by PBD and endoprostheses placement in those patients deemed nonsurgical candidates).

Disadvantages of metallic endoprostheses include the following:

1. Their cost is considerable (at least 10 times that of plastic endoprostheses).
2. They cannot be removed except through a major surgical resection.
3. In the setting where metallic endoprostheses occlude, repeat percutaneous or endoscopic drainage is required.

A partial list of commercially approved metallic biliary endoprostheses is provided below. Those approved by the U.S. Food and Drug Administration for palliation of malignant biliary obstruction include the following:

1. Self-expanding open mesh stents. Examples include the following:
   a. Gianturco Z-stent (Cook Inc., Bloomington, IN)
   b. Luminexx Biliary Stent (Bard Peripheral Vascular, Tempe, AZ)
   c. Protégé GPS (EV3, Plymouth, MN)
   d. Smart Stent (Cordis Corporation, Miami, FL)
   e. Symphony (Boston Scientific, Natick, MA)
   f. Wallstent (Boston Scientific-Schneider Inc, Minneapolis, MN)

2. Balloon-expandable open mesh stents. Examples include the following:
   a. Express Biliary LD (Boston Scientific, Natick, MA)
   b. Omni Flex Biliary (Angio Dynamics Inc, Queensbury, NY)
   c. Palmaz and Palmaz Genesis (Cordis Corporation, Miami, FL)

3. Self-expanding covered stents: An example includes the following:
   a. Viabil (W. L. Gore Associates, Flagstaff, AZ)

In general, metallic endoprostheses require a 7F–9F access, whereas the less expensive but larger caliber plastic endoprostheses generally require a 10F–14F transhepatic tract. In the case of placement of a plastic endoprostheses, tract dilatation may be associated with considerable patient discomfort and risk of hemobilia.

If no hemobilia is noted after PTC/PBD, the metallic endoprosthesis may be placed in a single step, thus offsetting the increased cost of the device. In contrast, plastic endoprosthesis placement from a percutaneous transhepatic approach generally requires multiple steps (i.e., PTC/PBD), tube tract maturation, tract dilatation, and endoprosthesis placement. Multiple steps add to the overall cost and to the potential patient discomfort and risk.

The advantages of palliative placement of an endoprosthesis in the setting of unresectable malignant biliary obstruction include the following:

1. Restoration of bile flow into the duodenum with its associated improved metabolic effects
2. Conversion of an internal–external biliary drainage catheter (stent) into a self-contained intraductal device, eliminating the external component of the tube and the daily care required for a conventional internal–external biliary drainage catheter (i.e., the endoprosthesis offers the patient the advantage of enhanced quality of life because the patient is no longer burdened with a catheter that requires maintenance).

The disadvantages of an endoprosthesis for palliation include the following:

1. Premature endoprosthesis occlusion with the associated complications (e.g., recurrent jaundice, possible sepsis, etc.)
2. Possible dislodgment of the device
3. Increased cost of the device (potentially offset by a reduced hospitalization time if the endoprosthesis is placed in a single step)

A bare metal biliary endoprosthesis (stent) cannot be exchanged either endoscopically or transhepatically. Should premature occlusion occur (or should the patient outlive the patency rate of the stent), a repeat PBD is necessary, either with placement of a new endoprosthesis inside the old one or placement of an internal–external biliary drainage catheter. Occasionally, a patient with an occluded endoprosthesis undergoes endoscopic placement of a new endoprosthesis through the occluded metallic stent. However, if the cause of endoprosthesis occlusion is tumor overgrowth at the upper end of the stent, the level of obstruction may be beyond the reach of the endoscopic cannula. A repeat percutaneous transhepatic approach with drainage will then be required.

COMPLICATIONS OF PERCUTANEOUS TRANSHEPATIC CHOLANGIOGRAPHY (PTC) AND PERCUTANEOUS BILIARY DRAINAGE (PBD)

Major and minor complications are associated with PTC/PBD. Major complications include hemobilia requiring blood transfusion and cholangitis/sepsis (15,16). Hemobilia occurs in 2.6–9% of patients undergoing PTC/PBD (17). Major bleeding, however, is rarely a cause of death in patients undergoing percutaneous transhepatic biliary interventions.

The management of hemobilia includes an initial cholangiogram to assess whether or not the vascular system opacifies. If the patient experiences venous bleeding (dark blood that is nonpulsatile), treatment by tube upsizing to tamponade the injured vein is generally all that is necessary. Should the patient develop pulsatile bright red blood from the tube or from the tube tract during biliary catheter exchange, the patient must be consented for emergent hepatic arteriography and possible transcatheter embolization. During arterial embolization procedures, it is important to bridge the bleeding site (i.e., begin embolization just distal to the injured hepatic arterial vessel and continue embolization proximally until the injured site is crossed). In such instances, this limited transcatheter embolization is analogous to surgical ligation of a pseudoaneurysm or fistula (i.e., distal and proximal ligation is necessary to trap or bridge the injured artery). Once successful arterial embolization has been performed, the percutaneous entry site of the transhepatic tube tract need not be changed (i.e., does not need to be moved to a different location).

Fever and chills may occur in 5–26% of patients undergoing biliary drainage. Four to twelve percent of patients develop frank septicemia. Cholangitis may occur in as many as 50% of patients with long-term biliary drainage catheters.

Other complications associated with PTC/PBD include inadvertent puncture of other structures, which may include the colon, gallbladder, and so on.

CLINICAL RESULTS USING PALLIATIVE ENDOPROSTHESES

Multiple studies have been published describing the use of open mesh metallic and plastic endoprostheses. In general, clinical results using percutaneously placed transhepatic biliary endoprostheses as palliation for malignant biliary obstruction have varied results (18, 19). In a large series of 334 patients published by Lammer, the results since 1982 of transhepatic placement of endoprostheses are reported. Of the 334 patients in this series, 320 had malignant biliary obstruction. Plastic endoprostheses were placed transhepatically in 297 patients and metallic endoprostheses in 37 patients. Of the 297 patients receiving plastic endoprostheses, malignancy was the cause of obstruction. Premature occlusion of plastic endoprostheses was noted in 25 of 297 patients (8.4%).

Recent advances included the application of covered biliary endoprostheses in an attempt to improve long-term patency. These are now commercially available. Stent coverings include polyurethane (20) and polytetrafluoroethylene (PTFE) (21,22). The long-term patency of such covered stents for management of patients with malignant hepatobiliary disease is still under active investigation because covered stents are a relatively recent addition to the interventional and endoscopic armamentarium.

Whether the sphincter of Oddi should be rendered incompetent (i.e., stented) in the setting of malignant biliary disease is still an area of debate. In theory, if the sphincter of Oddi is maintained, reflux of enteric contents into the biliary system is prevented. Whether this truly improves long-term patency is the topic of discussion. In general, in patients with large, clinically aggressive tumors, the trend is to "overstent" (i.e., use multiple stents to accommodate eventual tumor growth and extension and perhapsreduce the requirement for repeated interventions at a later date). However, no large-scale clinical trials addressing this question have been completed.

SUMMARY

The management of patients with malignant hepatobiliary obstruction is often challenging for the endoscopist, interventional radiologist, and surgeon. The long-term patency of either plastic or metallic endoprostheses is limited. Advantages of placing metallic endoprostheses include the ability to deploy such devices in a single step (at the time of the PTC/PBD). In contrast, plastic endoprostheses are generally of a larger caliber and require transhepatic tract maturation prior to placement of the endoprostheses. Although metallic stents are generally approximately 10 to 15 times more expensive than plastic endoprostheses, most investigators prefer such devices for palliation because of the ability to place them during the initial biliary drainage procedure. The role of the interventional radiologist in the management of patients with malignant hepatobiliary disease continues to expand. The goal of providing a patient who has unresectable malignant biliary obstruction with freedom from daily catheter maintenance is, in the authors' opinion, an important adjuvant to medical and surgical therapies.

ACKNOWLEDGMENTS

The authors wish to express their thanks to Melissa Wubbold, Dana Murphy, and Shundra Dinkins for their technical expertise in the preparation of this manuscript.

REFERENCES

1. Greenlee RT, Murray T, Bolden S, et al. Cancer statistics 2000. CA Cancer J Clin 2000; 50:7–33.
2. DiMagno EP, Malagelada JR, Taylor WF, et al. A prospective comparison of current diagnostic tests for pancreatic cancer. N Engl J Med 1977; 297:737–742.
3. Craig GR, Peters RL, Edmonson HA. Tumors of the liver and intrahepatic bile ducts. In: Atlas of Tumor Pathology (2nd series). Washington, DC: Armed Forces Institute of Pathology, 1989.
4. Zimmerman A. Tumours of the bile duct: pathological aspects. In: Blumgart LH, ed. Surgery of the Liver and Biliary Tract. Edinburgh: Churchill Livingstone, 1994:925–940.

5. Yoshida H, Itai Y, Minami M, et al. Biliary malignancies occurring in choledochal cysts. Radiology 1989;173:389–392.
6. Yeo CJ, Venbrux AC, Thuluvath PJ. Cholangiocarcinoma. In: Pitt HA, Carr-Locke DL, Ferrucci JT, eds. Hepatobiliary and Pancreatic Disease: The Team Approach to Management. Boston: Little, Brown, 1995:305–318.
7. Meyer DG, Weinstein BJ. Klatskin tumors of the bile ducts: sonographic appearance. Radiology 1983;148:803–804.
8. Subramanyan BR, Raghavendra BN, Balthazar EJ, et al. Ultrasonic features of cholangiocarcinoma. J Ultrasound Med 1984; 3: 405–408.
9. Schnur MJ, Hoffman JC, Koenigsberg M. Ultrasonic demonstration of intraductal biliary neoplasms. J Clin Ultrasound 1982;10:246–248.
10. Dachman A. Primary biliary neoplasia. In: Friedman A, Dachman A, eds. Radiology of the Liver, Biliary Tract, and Pancreas. St. Louis: Mosby, 1994:611–632.
11. Venbrux AC. Pancreatic carcinoma: percutaneous treatment. In: Cameron JL, ed. Pancreatic Cancer: American Cancer Society Atlas of Clinical Oncology. London: ; BC Decker, Inc., 2001: 203–214.
12. Venbrux AC, Osterman FA Jr. Percutaneous management of benign biliary strictures. In: Semba CP, Katzen BT, eds. Techniques in Vascular and Interventional Radiology, vol. 4, no.3. Philadelphia: WB Saunders, 2001:141–146.
13. Morgan RA, Adam AN. Malignant biliary disease: percutaneous interventions. In: Semba CP, Katzen BT, eds. Techniques in Vascular and Interventional Radiology, vol. 4, no.3. Philadelphia: WB Saunders, 2001:147–152.
14. Kim HS, Lund GB, Venbrux AC. Advanced percutaneous transhepatic biliary access. In: Semba CP, Katzen BT, eds. Techniques in Vascular and Interventional Radiology, vol. 4, no.3. Philadelphia: WB Saunders, 2001:153–171.
15. Yee CAN, Ho CS. Complications of percutaneous biliary drainage: benign vs malignant diseases. AJR Am J Roentgenol 1987;148: 1207–1209.
16. Oikarinen H, Leinonen S, Karttunen A, et al. Patency and complications of percutaneously inserted metallic stents in malignant biliary obstruction. J Vasc Interv Radiol 1999;10:1387–1393.
17. Venbrux AC, Osterman FA Jr. Percutaneous management of benign biliary strictures. Semin Intervent Radiol 1996;13:207–214.
18. Lammer J. Biliary endoprotheses: plastic versus metal stents. Radiol Clin North Am 1990;28:1211–1222.
19. Gordon RL, Ring EJ, LaBerge JM, et al. Malignant biliary obstruction: treatment with expandable metal stents—follow-up of 50 consecutive patients. Radiology 1992;182:697–701.
20. Isayama H, Komatsu Y, Tsujino T, et al. Polyurethane-covered metal stent for management of distal malignant biliary obstruction. Gastrintest Endosc 2002;55:366–370.
21. Bezzi M, Zolovkins A, Cantisani V, et al. New ePTFE/FEP-covered stent in the palliative treatment of malignant biliary obstruction. J Vasc Interv Radiol 2002;13:581–589.
22. Schoder M, Rossi P, Uflacker R, et al. Malignant biliary obstruction: treatment with ePTFE-FEP-covered endoprotheses initial technical and clinical experiences in a multicenter trial. Radiology 2002;225:35–42.

Liver Transplantation

Associated Interventions

Robert K. Kerlan Jr., Jeanne M. LaBerge

Liver transplantation has become a common alternative for managing patients with progressive liver failure and selected patients with hepatocellular carcinoma. Though initially the 1-year survival rate in patients undergoing orthotopic liver transplantation (OLT) was 50–60%, refinements in surgical technique, improved immunosuppressive agents, and the evolution of interventional radiology has allowed 1-year survival rates to approach 85% (1).

Until recently, orthotopic cadaveric organs provided the only donor source. Often, the donor organ can be split, with the right lobe or right lobe and medial segment of the left lobe being donated to an adult and the left lateral segment given to a child. However, despite such utilization, there remains a critical shortage of donor organs when compared with the number of patients on the liver transplant waiting list. This shortage of organs stimulated the development of using right and left hepatic lobes from living donors with matching ABO blood types for urgent transplantation.

As with any complex surgical procedure, complications following orthotopic liver transplantation are not infrequent and occur in the acute postoperative period as well as months to years later. These complications may be symptomatic or detected by surveillance laboratory and imaging studies.

This chapter reviews pertinent features of liver transplantation relevant to the interventional radiologist.

SURGICAL ANATOMY

Appropriate management of complications is predicated on a thorough understanding of the surgical anatomy (2). There are significant differences in the postsurgical anatomy depending on whether a whole cadaveric liver has been used or a right or left lobe from either cadaveric or living donor origin has been used.

Whole Liver

The whole liver transplant requires five anastomoses: (1) suprahepatic inferior vena cava (IVC), (2) infrahepatic IVC, (3) portal venous, (4) hepatic arterial, and (5) bile duct.

Suprahepatic IVC

The suprahepatic IVC anastomosis is created first and is usually performed in an end-to-end fashion. If there is a marked mismatch in size between the donor and recipient, the suprahepatic cava may be attached in "piggyback" fashion, attaching the dorsal aspect of the donor organ to the ventral aspect of the recipient's upper cava. Moreover, this type of anastomosis creates less physiologic stress on the recipient as inferior vena caval blood flow can be more or less maintained (depending upon clamp positioning) during the transplant operation.

Factors that make the suprahepatic caval anastomosis more difficult include patients being transplanted for Budd-Chiari syndrome and patients who have previously undergone transjugular intrahepatic portosystemic shunt (TIPS) placement.

Patients who are being transplanted for Budd-Chiari syndrome may have a small IVC or may have a suprahepatic cava containing webs or thrombus. In some circumstances, the anatomic alteration can be so severe that transplantation is not possible.

Patients who have undergone prior transjugular intrahepatic portosystemic shunt placement (TIPS) may have the stent protruding into the suprahepatic IVC, making placement of a vascular clamp in this location difficult. If it is not possible to place this vascular clamp from the transabdominal approach, a midline sternotomy may be required to gain control of the caval–atrial junction. The protruding TIPS may also cause stenosis of the suprahepatic cava, making the creation of the suprahepatic caval anastomosis more difficult.

Stenosis of the suprahepatic caval anastomosis caused by either postsurgical scarring, technically poor anastomosis, kinking, or torsion leads to inferior vena caval and hepatic venous outflow obstruction. Symptoms associated with this complication include ascites, lower extremity edema, and allograft dysfunction.

Infrahepatic IVC

The second anastomosis is the infrahepatic IVC. Because of the improved exposure and ability to mobilize an appropriate length of recipient cava, the infrahepatic anastomosis is usually not problematic. The anastomosis is created end to end. Stenosis of this anastomosis is rare, but such a stenosis potentially can lead to lower extremity edema or IVC thrombosis.

Obviously, if a piggyback anstomosis is created, an infrahepatic inferior vena caval anastomosis is not required.

Portal Vein

The third anastomosis is the portal vein. This anastomosis is most commonly created end to end from the recipient portal vein 2–5 centimeters beyond the confluence of the splenic vein (SV) and superior mesenteric vein (SMV). If the recipient's native portal vein is small or thrombosed, it may be necessary to extend a jump graft to the SV–SMV confluence. The jump graft is usually constructed from the cadaveric donor iliac vein.

Stenosis of the portal venous anastomosis leads to prehepatic portal hypertension with the usual complications of ascites, bleeding, and hypersplenism. A severe stenosis of the portal vein anastomosis can also lead to portal vein thrombosis and allograft dysfunction.

Hepatic Artery

Many types of hepatic arterial anastomoses can be created, reflecting the variability of hepatic arterial anatomy in both the donor and recipient. In most cases, the celiac artery is harvested at its origin during donor explantation. The left gastric, splenic, gastroduodenal, and small pancreatic branches are oversewn, and the celiac stump is anastomosed end to end to the recipient's proper hepatic artery just beyond the origin of the recipient's gastroduodenal artery. This excess length of allograft artery allows creation of a tension-free anastomosis, which is less prone to stenosis. However, the excessive length of artery may also lead to redundancy and tortuosity, complicating postoperative superselective catheterization.

An accessory left hepatic artery from the left gastric artery can be incorporated without difficulty by ligating the left gastric artery beyond the take-off of the hepatic vessel rather than at its origin. Accessory right hepatic arteries taking origin from the superior mesenteric artery (SMA) can be reimplanted into the stump of the donor splenic artery.

If the recipient hepatic artery is small and unsuitable for vascular reconstruction, or if a preexisting celiac artery stenosis or occlusion is present, a jump graft can be placed from the abdominal aorta to the donor hepatic artery. This jump graft is usually made of synthetic material (polytetrafluoroethylene [PTFE] or Dacron).

Stenosis of the hepatic artery (HA) anastomosis usually leads to allograft dysfunction. Hepatic artery thrombosis (HAT) may be precipitated by an underlying stenosis or occur de novo. The hepatic artery supplies the bile duct. The bile duct has been rendered devoid of collateral arterial supply during donor hepatectomy, and arterial insufficiency typically leads to nonanastomotic biliary strictures and potentially diffuse biliary ductal infarction. Hepatic artery thrombosis may lead to irretrievable allograft damage and necessitate retransplantation.

Bile Duct

The fifth and final anastomosis created in whole-liver orthotopic liver transplantation is the bile duct. Two types of biliary anastomoses are used (Figure 30–1): (1) choledochocholedochostomy (CDCD) and (2) choledochojejunostomy (CDJ).

The choledochocholedochostomy (Figure 30–1A) is an end-to-end anastomosis of the donor common bile duct to the recipient common bile duct. The CDCD is the preferred biliary anastomosis for several reasons. These reasons include preservation of sphincteric function, avoidance of bowel surgery in a patient who will be immunosuppressed, and maintenance of anatomic relationships, which allows retrograde cholangiography and stent placement if a postoperative biliary complication develops.

The CDCD anastomosis may be performed over a T tube. If a T tube is placed, postoperative bile production can be monitored, and the biliary tree can be easily investigated by T-tube cholangiography. However, because of complications associated with T-tube placement as well as biliary leakage following tube removal, many centers have abandoned routine T-tube placement during the creation of CDCD anastomosis.

If a patient has a diseased or small extrahepatic bile duct, it may not be possible to create a CDCD anastomosis. These patients include those with primary sclerosing cholangitis most pediatric patients, and all pediatric patients with biliary atresia. Moreover, if there is a substantial donor–recipient duct size mismatch, a CDCD anastomsis may not be the most attractive option.

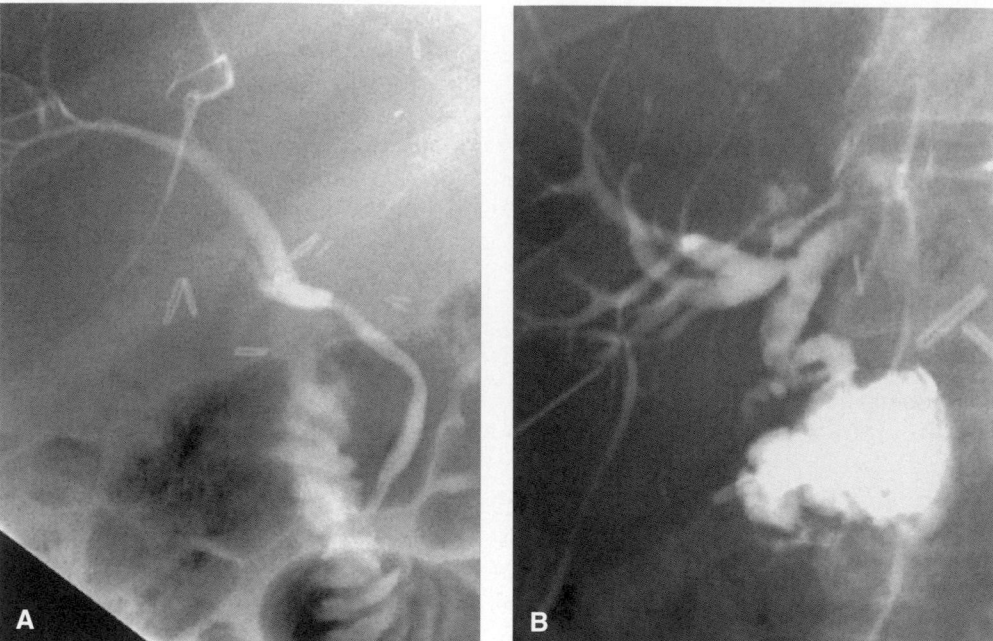

Figure 30–1 Normal orthotopic liver transplant biliary anatomy. **A.** Choledochocholedochostomy is the preferred biliary anastomosis, in which the donor common bile duct is joined to the recipient common bile duct. **B.** Choledochojejunostomy is performed when a choledochocholedochostomy is not feasible. With this anatomy, the donor common bile duct is anastomosed to the side of a Roux loop of the recipient jejunum.

When a CDCD anastomosis is not feasible, a choledochojejunostomy (Figure 30–1B) is performed. This anastomosis is created by attaching the end of the common bile duct to the side of a loop of jejunum that is pulled up to the region of the porta hepatis in a Roux-en-Y configuration. This maneuver requires surgical closure of the free end of the jejunal loop adjacent to the biliary anastomosis as well as a distal jejunojejunostomy to maintain continuity of the alimentary tract. The biliary anastomosis to the bowel can be created obliquely extending into the side of the common bile duct, creating a large anastomotic channel. The CDJ anastomosis can also be constructed over a bridging tube that can be fixed with resorbable sutures and pass spontaneously into the bowel several weeks following the procedure. Alternatively, this stent can be brought externally through the abdominal wall if the jejunal loop is adfixed appropriately. However, most centers create the CDJ anstomosis without a bridging stent.

Complications related to the biliary anastomosis include bile leak and obstruction caused by stricture formation.

Split Liver

Split-liver transplantation is becoming increasingly common. Cadaveric livers can be split, with the left lobe going to a child and the right lobe going to an adult. Moreover, split-liver transplantation can be performed using livers from living donors when urgent transplantation is necessary.

Living donor liver transplantation was first applied in the late 1980s as a technique for pediatric transplantation, in which a parent donated the left lobe to a child. This approach to pediatric liver transplantation was quite successful and was soon applied as a technique for adult transplantation. Unfortunately, living donor left lobe transplantation was much less successful in adults because the transplanted liver volume was often insufficient to meet the demands of the adult recipient. As an alternative, transplantation of the donor right lobe was introduced in the mid 1990s, and preliminary results with this approach have been so favorable that it has become the standard surgical technique for adult-to-adult liver transplantation (3).

Though the technique of split-liver and living donor transplantation differs significantly from whole liver transplantion, the order of anastomosis creation remains the same. Though the donor inferior vena cava may be used with the right lobe in split-liver transplantation, it is obviously not taken with living donor donation. When the IVC is not included in the allograft, the hepatic vein or veins must be anastomosed to the recipient's hepatic veins or hepatic sinus. Problems with this anastomosis include stenosis secondary to fibrosis or torsion leading to outflow obstruction. Outflow obstruction creates Budd-Chiari pathophysiology with the attendant problems of hepatic dysfunction and ascites (Figure 30–2).

When the allograft does not contain the donor inferior vena cava, an infrahepatic caval anastomosis is unnecessary because the recipient's native IVC is left intact.

The portal vein anastomosis is more difficult with split-liver transplantation because significant size mismatch of the donor right or left portal vein to the recipient main portal

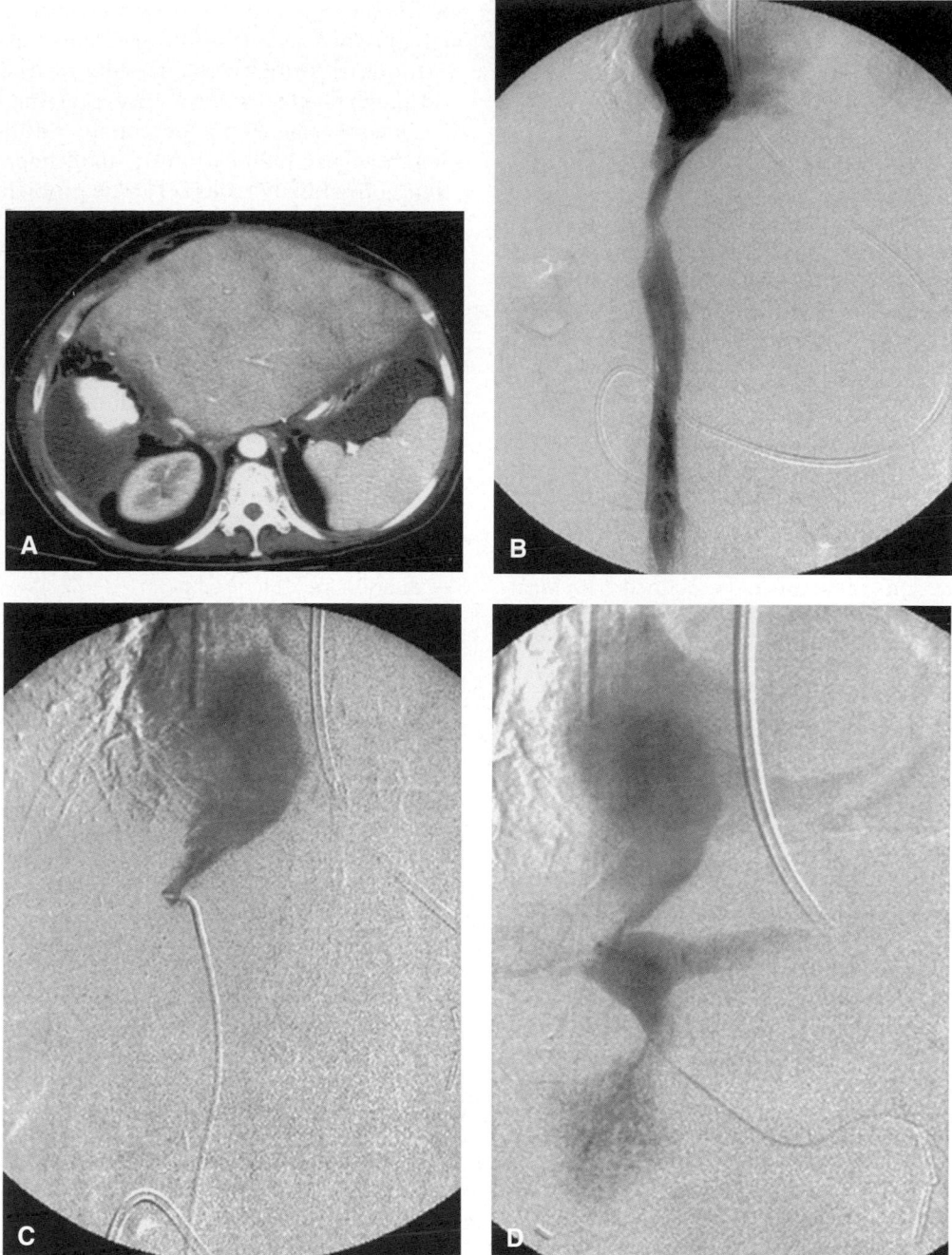

Figure 30–2 A 65-year-old woman developed abdominal distension and ascites 2 months after left lobe split-liver transplantation. **A.** Abdominal CT reveals ascites and an enlarged left lobe with absent opacification of the left hepatic vein. **B.** Transfemoral inferior vena cavagram is normal. **C.** Direct catheterization of the left hepatic vein from IVC could not be performed. **D.** Transhepatic hepatic venography demonstrates stenosis or torsion of hepatic vein at the anastomosis with the IVC.

vein is commonly encountered. This size mismatch may make the surgical anastomosis more difficult, resulting in a stenosis. Moreover, the size mismatch makes postoperative assessment with duplex ultrasound more difficult because turbulence and increased velocity may simulate the appearance of a stenosis. When a true stenosis develops, problems related to portal hypertension may be observed.

The biliary anastomosis in the split-liver transplant can be more technically challenging compared with whole liver transplantation because only a short segment of donor right (or left) hepatic duct may be available to use. With living donor transplantation, not causing harm to the donor is of paramount importance. Therefore, the biliary duct is severed at a safe distance from the common hepatic duct to avoid stricture formation in the donor. As a result, the segment of hepatic duct available for anastomosis is often short, making creation of a tension-free anastomosis difficult. Moreover, variations in donor biliary anatomy may necessitate the creation of more than one biliary anastomosis. Some anatomic situations, such as a right segmental duct draining into the left duct, may require ligation of duct rather than a biliary anastomosis.

Most commonly, the split-liver biliary anastomosis is established via a Roux-en-Y jejunal anastomosis. In some patients, it is feasible to create an anastomosis to the recipient's extrahepatic bile duct. Both biliary obstruction and bile leak are encountered with problematic biliary reconstructions.

LIVING DONOR EVALUATION

The best method of preoperative anatomic evaluation of the living hepatic donor remains to be defined. The ideal technique would clearly delineate the hepatic arteries, portal veins, hepatic veins, bile ducts, and hepatic parenchyma without requiring contrast media or ionizing radiation. Although magnetic resonance imaging with Magnetic Resonance Angiography potentially fulfills some of these requirements, delineation of small hepatic arteries and diminutive biliary radicles can be problematic. Therefore, in many centers, living donor evaluation is performed with computed tomographic angiography (CTA) coupled with computed tomographic cholangiography (CTC). CTC is performed by obtaining highly collimated axial CT images following the intravenous injection of meglumine iodipamide (Cholografin, Bracco Diagnostics) (Figure 30–3). Three-dimensional reconstructions are then performed to clearly elucidate the biliary anatomy. Though a more detailed biliary evaluation would be advantageous, the risks of retrograde cholangiography are considered to be excessive for routine evaluation of the healthy living donor. Specific anatomic features pertinent to living donor evaluation are described next.

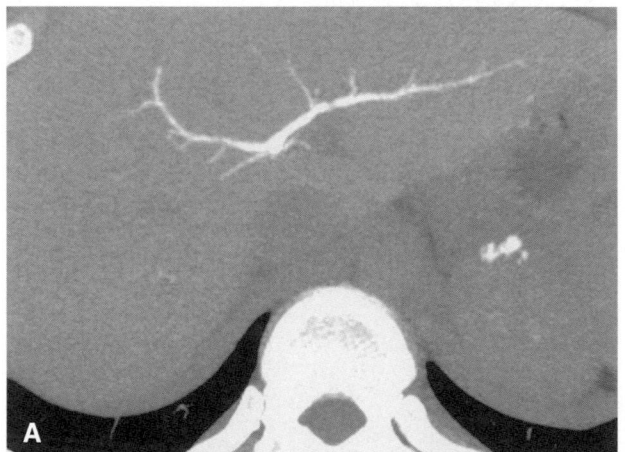

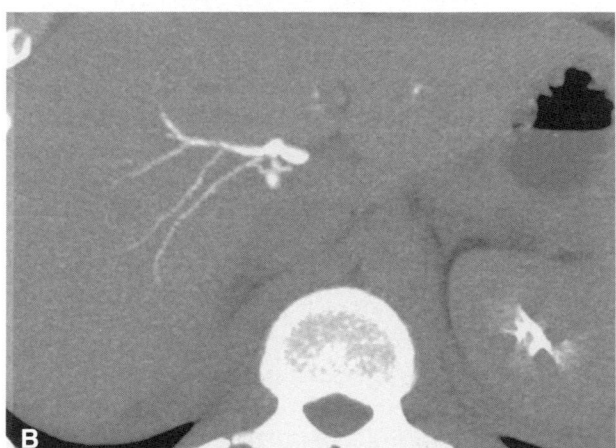

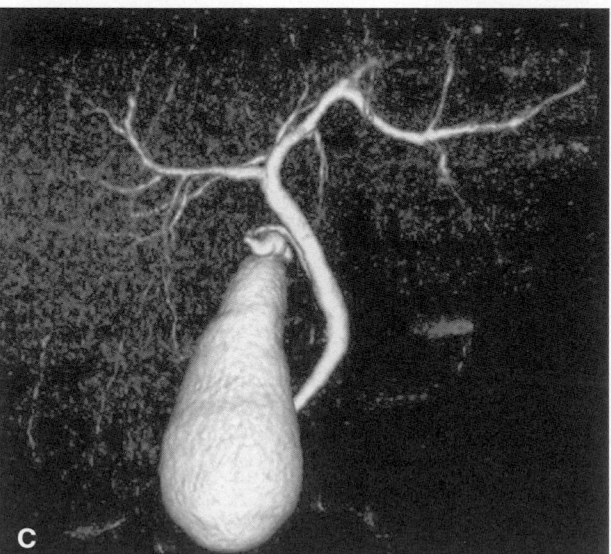

Figure 30–3 Computed tomographic cholangiography was performed in a potential living donor. **A., B.** Axial CT images acquired after the intravenous administration of meglumine iodipamide (Cholografin, Bracco Diagnostics) show conspicuous opacification of biliary ducts. **C.** Three-dimensional reconstruction in this case demonstrates anomalous insertion of the right posterior duct into the left duct. Images courtesy of Ben Yeh, M.D., University of California, San Francisco.

Hepatic Veins

The right hepatic vein is the longest vein in the liver; it divides the anterior from the posterior segments of the right lobe and is single in about 94% of patients (4). The middle hepatic vein divides the right and left lobes of the liver and forms a common trunk with the left hepatic vein in about 85% of patients (5). When right lobe transplant is being contemplated, large accessory right hepatic veins should be noted as they may complicate the donor lobectomy and require a separate anastomosis to the recipient's inferior vena cava. The other abnormality to be aware of is the small right hepatic vein. In this circumstance, the middle hepatic vein can provide essentially the sole drainage from the anterior segment of the right lobe of the liver. In some centers, this anatomy is considered a contraindication to right lobe donation (6).

If lateral segment harvest for pediatric liver transplantation is being planned, identification of the segment III vein is necessary because this vein occasionally drains into the middle hepatic vein. When this anatomic variation is encountered, a separate anastomosis of this vein into the inferior vena cava may be necessary.

Portal Veins

The conventional anatomy of the portal vein is bifurcation of the main portal vein into the right and left portal veins and subsequent bifurcation of the right portal vein into the right anterior and right posterior segmental branches. In 10–15% of cases, the portal vein trifurcates into these principle branches. Other common variations include origination of the right anterior segmental portal vein from the left portal vein and the right posterior portal vein taking origin from the main portal vein prior to its bifurcation. A rare variation is absence of the left portal vein. In this variation, the main portal vein enters the liver, ascends cranially, and then turns left, crossing the umbilical fissure to enter the lateral segment of the left lobe.

When the right lobe is harvested, trifurcations of the portal vein may require two separate venous anastomoses unless a venoplasty can be used to fuse the branches into a single orifice. If the right anterior segmental vein is draining into the left portal vein, the anterior segmental vein is usually ligated, which normally does not lead to allograft dysfunction. Absence of the left portal vein in the hilum is an absolute contraindication to right lobe donation, although left lateral segment donation is still feasible by using an intraparenchymal access to the vein. In this circumstance, the aberrant vein is isolated as it enters the lateral segment, and then a jump graft is extended from the recipient's portal vein to the donor vessel (7).

Hepatic Arteries

The anatomic variations of the hepatic arterial system are well recognized. Approximately 55% of the population has conventional anatomy in which the left and right hepatic arteries take origin from the proper hepatic artery (8). The two most common variations are origin of a left hepatic artery from the left gastric artery, seen in 25% of the patient population, and origin of a right hepatic artery from the superior mesenteric artery, observed in 17% of patients. Accessory right hepatic arteries are also not infrequently observed taking origin from the common hepatic artery proximal to the origin of the gastroduodenal or from the celiac trunk. Unusual variations include origin of the entire hepatic blood supply from the superior mesenteric artery, directly from the aorta, or, rarely, from the left gastric artery.

The presence of aberrant blood vessels significantly complicates living donor transplants as substantially shorter arteries require reconstruction and anastomosis. As a general rule, an attempt is made to preserve all arteries supplying the allograft. Therefore, a thorough depiction of the arterial anatomy can facilitate preoperative planning and diminish operative time.

The arterial supply to segment IV is of particular concern in living donor transplantation. Though segment IV usually derives arterial supply via branches of the left hepatic artery, not uncommonly the supply originates from branches of the right. When this anomaly is detected, the right hepatic artery should be severed beyond the origin of this vessel to diminish the chances of a postoperative bile leak in the donor (9).

A dual blood supply to the lateral segment of the left lobe (branches from both the proper hepatic and left gastric) has been considered a contraindication to living donation of the lateral segment for pediatric transplantation (10). However, many groups will use microsurgical arterial reconstructive techniques and accept donors with this anatomy (11).

Bile Ducts

As with the arterial circulation, numerous variations of biliary anatomy are present with so-called normal anatomy being present in only 57% of patients (12). Normal anatomy is considered to be a right hepatic duct bifurcating into left and right hepatic ducts with the right duct subsequently bifurcating into anterior and posterior segmental ducts. A trifurcation of the common hepatic duct into left, right anterior segmental, and right posterior segmental ducts is observed in 12%. Other common variations include origin of the right anterior or posterior segmental ducts from either the common hepatic duct or left hepatic duct. Rarely, the right posterior segmental duct will join the cystic duct prior to entry into the extrahepatic bile duct.

Accurate assessment of the biliary anatomy is critical in living donor transplantation because a biliary injury potentially has great significance to the donor. Despite the preoperative minimally invasive imaging, intra-operative cholangiography is usually performed prior to initiation of the donor lobectomy. The most common challenge is dealing with a right segmental duct entering the left ductal system. If this anatomic variation is not recognized, a postoperative bile leak may develop in both the recipient and the donor. When identified preoperatively, surgical plans to either create a separate Roux-en-Y anastomosis or perform ligation of the duct on the cut surface of the donor lobe can be made.

Unrecognized anomalous drainage of the segment IV duct into the right hepatic ductal system can also lead to a bile leak in both the recipient and the donor.

COMPLICATIONS IN LIVER DONORS

Right hepatectomy is a major surgical procedure, and ethicists have expressed concern about the risks of this procedure to the normal adult volunteer (13). To date, the risks to liver donors have not been precisely quantified because the technique for right lobe transplantation is evolving and because the reporting of donor complications has not been comprehensive. Of greatest concern is the risk of death to the donor. According to Surman (14), by August 2002, eight donor deaths had been reported worldwide after live donor transplantation. Three deaths occurred in the United States, with two in association with right lobe transplantation. More recently, Pomfret (15) estimated that the mortality of right lobe liver donors is about 0.3%.

Postoperative complications occur in up to 35% of donors (15). Most complications are attributable to major abdominal surgery, and these include wound infection, bowel obstruction, and pulmonary complications. Biliary complications are seen in 5–13% of right lobe donors but in only 2–4% of left lobe donors (16–18). Bile leak from the cut edge of the liver is the most common biliary complication, and it can usually be managed conservatively with surgical drains. Image-guided percutaneous biloma drainage may be necessary. Biliary stricture has been reported in 1.5% of right lobe donors. Stricture occurs at the stump of the ligated right lobe duct and has been successfully treated by endoscopic dilatation but may require reoperation and Roux revision.

PRETRANSPLANT HEPATIC ARTERIAL CHEMOEMBOLIZATION

In patients who have suspected or documented hepatocellular carcinoma and who are undergoing transplantation, hepatic arterial chemoembolization is often performed immediately prior to the surgery. In theory, during the mobilization of explantation, viable tumor cells may be dislodged into the circulation, promoting either postoperative tumor recurrence within the liver or extrahepatically. Though a therapeutic benefit has not been unequivocally demonstrated, several studies document the safety of this approach (19–21). The technique of chemoembolization is discussed elsewhere.

NONVASCULAR COMPLICATIONS

Biliary Complications

The biliary tract has been referred to as the "Achilles heel" of liver transplantation (22). Problems with the surgical anastomosis between the donor biliary tract and the recipient may lead to a wide variety of clinical problems (Figure 30–4). Moreover, the biliary system is sensitive to ischemia and may be damaged either by prolonged preservation prior to transplantation or by problems with hepatic arterial flow.

Despite refinements in surgical technique, biliary complications continue to be observed in 15–20% of allograft recipients (23). Two types of biliary complications are encountered: leak and obstruction.

Bile Leaks

Bile leaks usually occur early in the postoperative period and originate from three sources: the biliary anastomosis, the T-tube entry site (in patients who have had T tubes placed), or the cut surface of the liver (in patients with split or reduced-sized allografts).

In a patient with a CDCD anastomosis performed over a T tube, seepage through the T-tube choledochostomy is the most common cause of a bile leak (24). This type of leak is usually identified on routine postoperative T-tube cholangiography. The initial treatment is to open the T tube to gravity drainage, which is curative in up to 60% of patients (25). If this treatment is unsuccessful, endoscopic sphincterotomy may be useful.

Bile leaks may also develop following removal of the T tube, 3–6 months following the transplant operation. Immunosuppression may prevent the formation of a connective tissue tract, allowing bile to drain freely into the peritoneal cavity. Retrograde stent placement or percutaneous transhepatic drainage coupled with percutaneous drainage of the biloma controls the leak in most patients. However, up to one-third of these patients require operative intervention with surgical revision for closure (26).

Because of the aforementioned problems related to T tubes, some centers have elected to perform the CDCD anastomosis without T-tube insertion. In a study by Randall et al. (27), a group of 59 patients who had T tubes placed were compared with 51 patients who had CDCD anastomoses without T tubes. This comparison revealed no difference in biliary complication rates or survival.

Bile leaks that occur at the anastomotic site are much more difficult to manage conservatively. Though either retrograde stenting or PTBD is potentially useful in controlling the leak, surgical revision is necessary in a substantial percentage of patients. In the authors' institution, a short trial of either PTBD or retrograde stent placement is often attempted, but surgical revision is performed if the perforation does not rapidly seal (Figure 30–5).

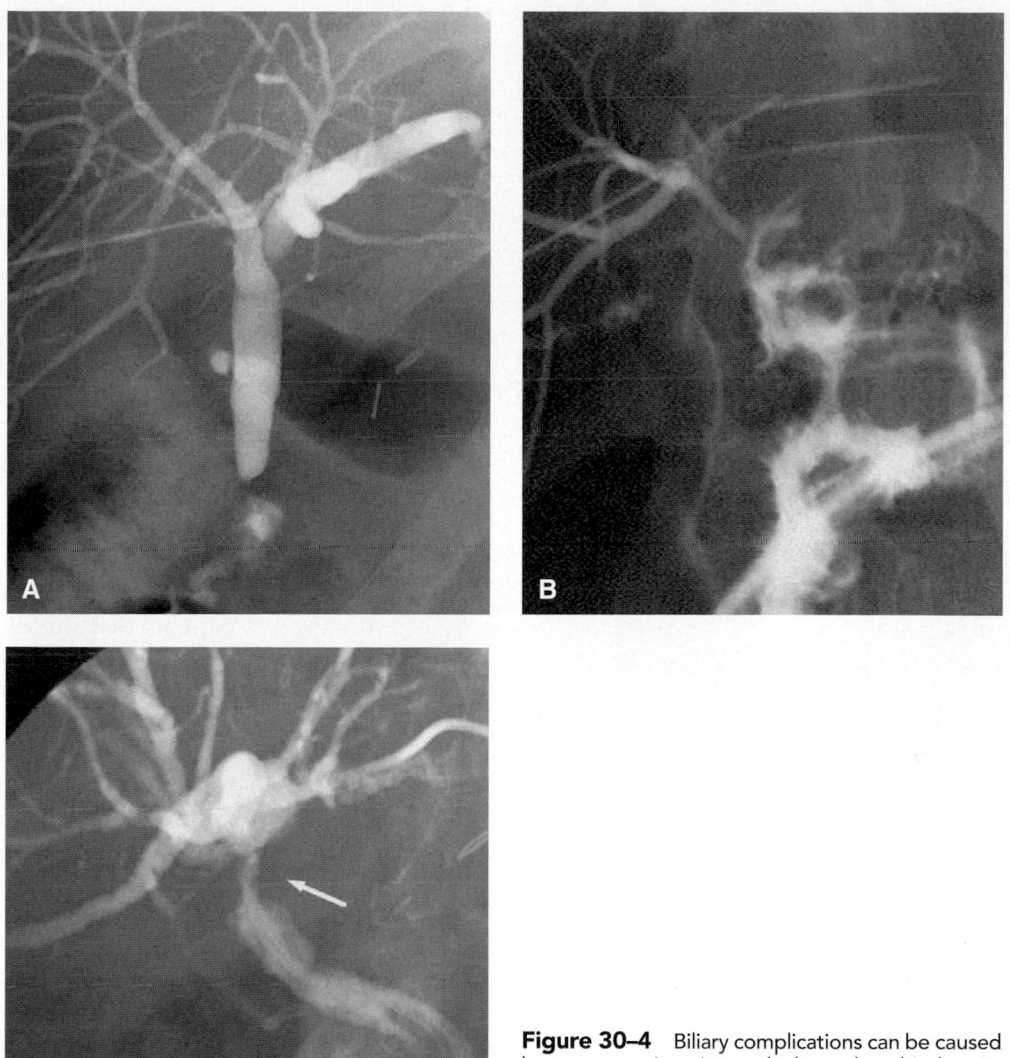

Figure 30–4   Biliary complications can be caused by anastomotic stricture, leak, or ductal ischemia. **A.** This patient developed a tight stricture at the Roux anastomosis. **B.** An early biliary leak is seen here at the Roux anastomosis. **C.** This patient developed a hilar biliary stricture (*arrow*) secondary to ischemia from hepatic artery occlusion.

Biliary Obstruction

Some degree of biliary obstruction following orthotopic liver transplantation is encountered in 10–20% of patients (28). The most common problem is a stricture at the biliary anastomosis. Biliary obstruction related to occluded or malpositioned T tubes may also be encountered.

Additional causes of biliary obstruction include nonanastomotic strictures, mucocele of the cystic duct remnant, dysfunction of the sphincter of Oddi, as well as blockage of the duct with stones or necrotic debris.

The clinical presentation of biliary obstruction can be nonspecific, particularly when one considers that the transplant patient has many potential etiologies of fever, elevated liver function tests, and leukocytosis. Noninvasive evaluations for potential obstruction with ultrasound

(US), computed tomography (CT), and magnetic resonance imaging (MRI) may be difficult because a significant number of patients will not have ductal dilatation (29). Therefore, direct cholangiography is often necessary to exclude or confirm the diagnosis. In a patient with a T tube in place, T-tube cholangiography is the indicated study. In a patient with a CDCD anastomosis without a T tube, endoscopic retrograde cholangiography is usually performed. In a patient with a CDJ anastomosis, percutaneous transhepatic cholangiography (PTC) is required.

When a stenosis of a CDCD anastomosis is identified in the early postoperative period, it may merely represent edema and/or inflammatory reaction at the anastomotic site. In this circumstance, a short period (2–6 weeks) of endoscopic stenting may be curative. If endoscopic cannulation cannot be achieved, a transhepatic internal–external biliary

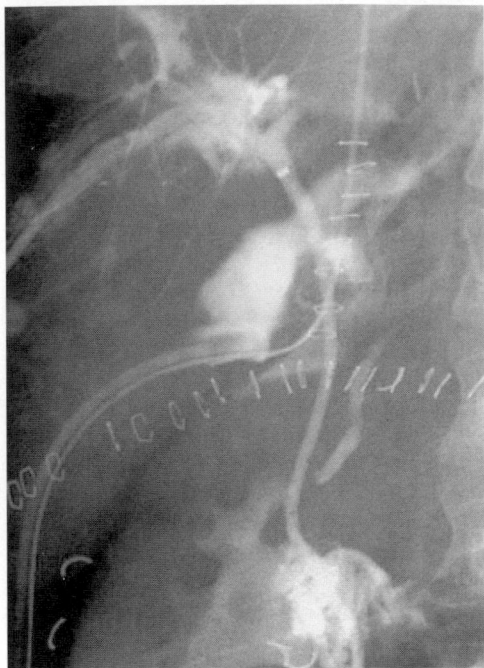

Figure 30–5 Management of biliary leak. This patient presented with pain and fever after OLT and was noted to have a CDCD anastomotic leak. The patient was treated nonoperatively with biliary diversion via a percutaneous biliary drainage and exchange of surgical biloma drain.

an internal–external biliary drainage tube for a period of 4–6 weeks can be an effective treatment. Using this technique with balloons ranging from 7 mm to 14 mm in diameter, Zajko et al. (30) reported a 73% success rate at 2 years and a 66% success rate at 6 years in a series of 56 patients with anastomotic strictures.

When balloon dilatation of an anastomotic stricture fails in a patient who is considered to be a poor surgical risk, placement of a Gianturco-Rösch Z stent has been performed (Figure 30–6). Unfortunately, the rate of recurrent stenosis and formation of obstructing debris in the biliary tree is extremely high, and most centers have abandoned this therapeutic alternative (Figure 30–7). Moreover, it should be noted that stent placement can potentially preclude or complicate definitive surgical repair. To circumvent this problem, the concept of retrievable stent-graft placement was put forth by Petersen et al. (31). In this series, Gianturco-Rösch Z stents were covered with expanded polytetrafluoroethylene (ePTFE) and inserted for a period of 2–9 months. All patients had the stents successfully retrieved. Five of six patients with anastomotic strictures (two CDCD, four CDJ) had successful outcomes during the 6- to 20-month follow-up period.

Nonanastomotic strictures may also be encountered related to hepatic artery thrombosis, prolonged cold preservation times, acute or chronic rejection, and cytomegalovirus infection. In addition, 5–20% of patients undergoing transplantation for primary sclerosing cholangitis develop recurrent intrahepatic biliary strictures (32). Because there are no surgical options other than retransplantation for this group of patients, balloon dilatation with or without stent placement has formed the mainstay of clinical management (Figure 30–8). In the aforementioned study by Zajko et al.

drainage tube should be placed. However, if the stenosis persists or recurs, surgical revision to a CDJ is often the most efficient and durable solution.

As an alternative to surgical reconstruction, percutaneous transhepatic dilatation followed by the placement of

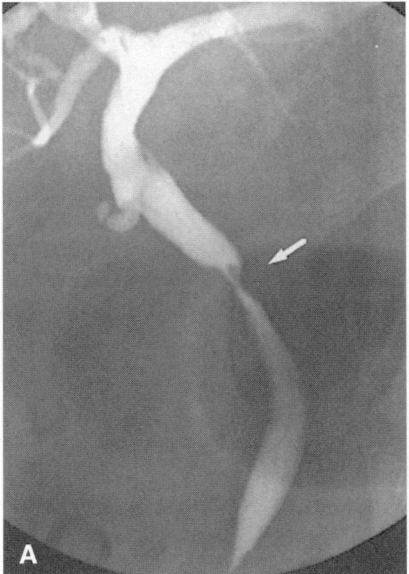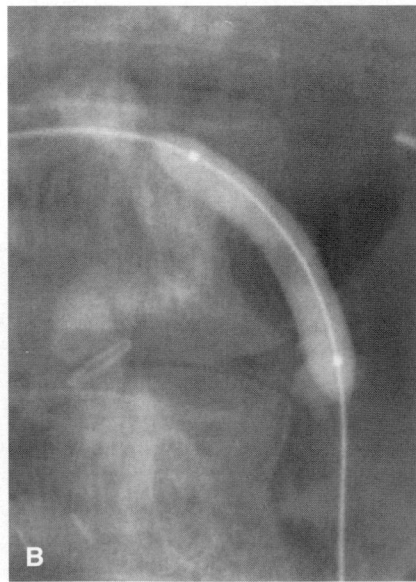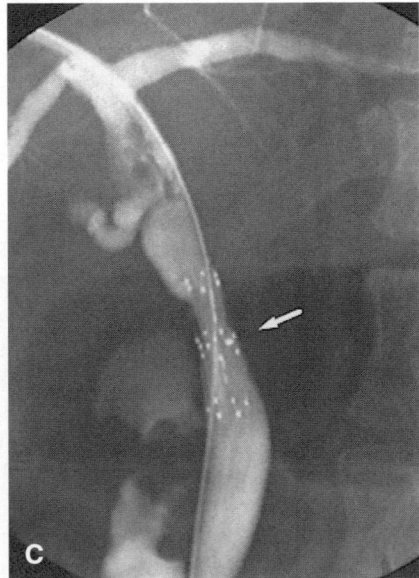

Figure 30–6 Management of biliary stricture with biliary stent. **A.** PTC demonstrates a duct-to-duct anastomotic stricture. **B.** Balloon dilatation was attempted but did not result in a durable improvement in patency. **C.** A recurrent stricture was treated with a Gianturco stent.

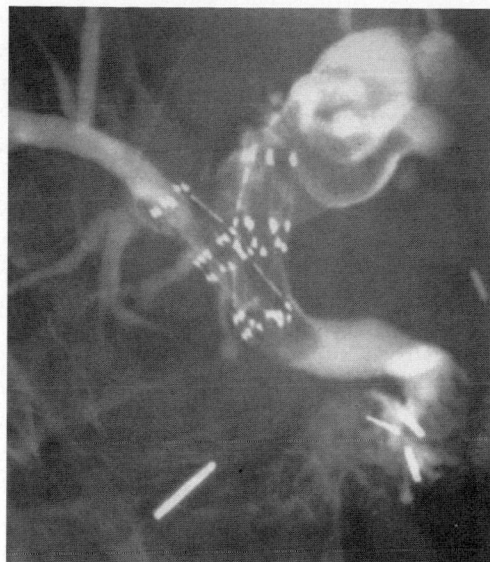

Figure 30–7 Complications of biliary stenting. This patient developed cholangitis 1 year after placement of intrahepatic Gianturco stents. Stones and sludge are filling the obstructed left duct, giving the appearance of a large filling defect.

(30), a 94% success rate at 2 years and 84% success rate at 5 years were reported using balloon dilatation in a group of 16 patients with nonanastomotic strictures.

Stents have been used in the management of nonanastomotic strictures that fail to respond to balloon dilatation because therapeutic alternatives may be limited. Although the immediate result is often gratifying, there is a tendency for stents to serve as nidus of stone and debris formation. The long-term durability of stents in these patients has not been thoroughly evaluated, and stents should be considered only when other therapeutic alternatives, including prolonged tube drainage, have been exhausted.

In a patient who has had the biliary anastomosis performed with the placement of a T tube, the tube may become occluded with debris or the limb displaced, leading to biliary obstruction. It is often possible to rectify T-tube problems using interventional radiologic techniques. However, as transplant patients form mature tracts at a much slower rate compared with patients who are not immunosuppressed, simple replacement is sometimes not possible. If access is lost during attempted revision of a T tube, it may be necessary to perform an additional transhepatic or retrograde procedure to ensure adequate biliary drainage.

Mucocele of the donor cystic duct remnant is an unusual but well-recognized cause of biliary obstruction (33). Though percutaneous aspiration of a cystic duct mucocele may provide temporary relief of obstruction, a surgical revision is usually required for definitive therapy.

Dysfunction of the sphincter of Oddi in a patient with a CDCD anastomosis can also inhibit the flow of bile. Though the etiology of this disorder is not clearly defined, its occurrence is well recognized. An endoscopically guided sphincterotomy is curative.

Obstruction of the bile duct by stones, sludge, or necrotic debris may also be encountered. Stones may be encountered in any patient with biliary obstruction, but the presence of necrotic debris usually indicates a prolonged cold preservation injury, rejection, or hepatic arterial insufficiency. Stones and debris generally can be treated with percutaneous transhepatic or endoscopic retrograde techniques, including basket retrieval and balloon

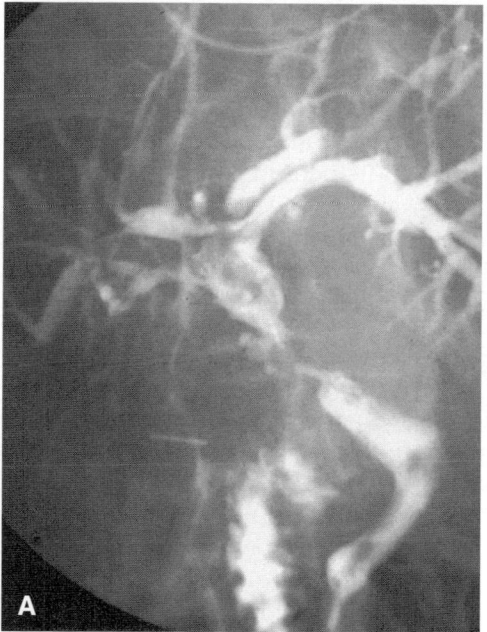

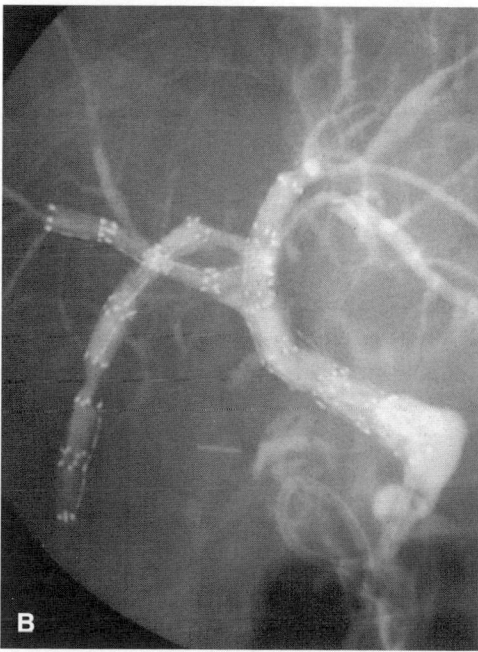

Figure 30–8 Intrahepatic stents. This 70-year-old man who had undergone prior OLT developed ischemia in his second transplant. **A.** The right ducts are strictured, and there is a filling defect in the hilum. **B.** Because there were no other therapeutic alternatives, the intrahepatic ducts were reconstructed using Gianturco stents.

sweeping. However, unless the underlying etiology is addressed, recurrent obstruction from newly formed material is likely to occur.

Management of Postoperative Fluid Collections

Sterile Fluid Collections

Postoperative fluid collections are frequently observed following orthotopic liver transplantation. The majority of these collections are not infected (34). However, image-guided aspiration may be necessary to confirm that a collection is not contaminated with bacteria. Some patients develop postoperative ascites requiring blind or image-guided paracentesis to maximize patient comfort and ventilatory status. The performance of these procedures is identical to that in the nontransplant population. As a general rule, tubes should not be placed into sterile postoperative fluid collections because of the risk of causing bacterial contamination and infection.

Abscess

Patients undergoing orthotopic liver transplantation are more prone to infected postoperative fluid collections than most patients for several reasons. Liver transplantation is technically complex, requiring prolonged operative times and raising the chance of contamination. Anastomoses are created to the biliary tree, and the bile may be colonized with bacterial organisms. In patients requiring choledochojejunostomy, the bowel anastomoses may leak. Many patients have ascites that may become sequestered and contaminated. Portal hypertension leads to splenomegaly and neutropenia that predispose the patient to bacterial infection. Finally, transplant patients are immunosuppressed, increasing the liklihood of a postoperative infectious complication.

Management of postoperative abscesses in the transplant patient is identical to that of the nontransplant patient, with image-guided percutaneous drainage for accessible collections in the majority of patients. One particularly common area of postoperative abscess in the liver transplant patient is the right subphrenic space. Fluid is commonly encountered in this location because of donor–recipient size and shape variation. The right subphrenic space offers unique challenges for percutaneous drainage because of its location. Often a choice must be made between a transhepatic approach, potentially leading to damage of the allograft, and a transpleural approach, which may potentially contaminate the pleural space.

Overall, percutaneous drainage of postoperative infected fluid collections in the liver transplant patient carries a high success and low complication rate (35). However, durable resolution of the abscess depends on the underlying cause. Infected fluid collections containing bile

should be further evaluated with retrograde or antegrade cholangiography to assess the presence of bile duct obstruction or leak. Moreover, patency of the hepatic artery should be confirmed in all patients with a bilious postoperative collection. Kaplan et al. (36) reported percutaneous drainage in 15 patients with hepatic artery occlusion. Eleven patients required retransplantation, and four patients were managed for more than 30 months with indwelling drainage catheters.

Hematoma

Hematomas are common following orthotopic liver transplantation. Transplant patients are often coagulapathic because of hepatic dysfunction and thrombocytopenia caused by splenic sequestration. Moreover, underlying portal hypertension makes the surgical dissection difficult with extensive venous collaterals throughout the peritoneum and retroperitoneum. Hematomas may occur anywhere but are most common in the subhepatic space. A definitive diagnosis of hematoma can often be made with computed tomography, where the appearance and density may be characteristic. Small, uninfected hematomas should be observed. Unfortunately, in the patient with fever and/or leukocytosis, percutaneous aspiration of the hematoma may be necessary to confirm or exclude the presence of infection. In general, infected hematomas cannot be completely evacuated through percutaneous drainage tubes, and operative evacuation is warranted when symptomatic. In patients who are poor operative risks, insertion of large-bore drainage tubes (20 French or larger) may lead to resolution, but prolonged drainage is often required (37). Some investigators recommend instillation of intracavitary fibrinolytics to dissolve the hematoma (38). However, insufficient numbers of patients have been reported to validate this therapeutic strategy.

VASCULAR COMPLICATIONS

Hepatic Arterial Complications

Arterial complications include hepatic artery stenosis (HAS), hepatic artery thrombosis (HAT), and arterial hemorrhage with pseudoaneurysm formation.

Hepatic artery stenosis has been reported to occur in up to 12% of transplant recipients (39,40). HAS usually occurs at the site of arterial anastomosis and may be secondary to intimal hyperplasia, kinking caused by arterial redundancy, or poor surgical technique.

Symptoms related to hepatic arterial stenosis include nonanastomotic biliary stricture formation, biliary obstruction caused by sludge or necrotic debris generated by biliary endothelial sloughing, or insidious graft dysfunction. Cholangiographic abnormalities are present in 60% (41) of patients with significant hepatic artery stenosis, and the median time to diagnosis following transplantation is 100 days (42).

When the diagnosis of symptomatic hepatic artery stenosis is made, percutaneous transluminal angioplasty appears to be the appropriate therapeutic alternative. Several studies have documented the safety of this procedure in small numbers of patients (43–45). Mondragoon et al. (46) reported improvement in liver function tests in seven transplant patients treated with balloon angioplasty. Two of the seven patients eventually required retransplantation. In a series of 21 patients reported by Orons et al. (47), balloon angioplasty of hepatic artery stenosis was established to be safe and durable; however, most patients who presented with significant alterations in their liver function tests eventually required retransplantation.

If recurrent hepatic artery stenosis develops following an initially successful PTA, redilatation may be performed. Raby et al. (45) reported two patients who did well following repeated dilatation and speculated that a second dilatation may be more durable than the initial PTA.

In patients with stenoses that fail to respond or recur following balloon angioplasty, percutaneous hepatic arterial stents may be considered. Unfortunately, only case reports (48–51) are available, and long-term follow-up in a significant number of patients is lacking. However, both balloon-expandable and self-expandable stents have been used safely, with patency up to 25 months having been reported.

Hepatic artery stenosis can progress to hepatic artery thrombosis. Moreover, thrombosis can occur without a significant underlying stenosis. This complication is observed in 2–8% of adult liver transplantations (52–57). In a recent series of 1,192 consecutive transplants reported by Stange et al. (58), HAT was observed in 2.5% of transplant patients. Hepatic artery thrombosis is the second leading cause of allograft failure in the immediate postoperative period, with primary nonfunction being the leading cause. HAT is even more common in the pediatric transplant patient, being observed in 10–25% of patients younger than 2 years (59). HAT does not appear to be more common in vascular jump grafts from the aorta compared with more direct arterial anastomoses (60) unless the flow falls below 400 mL/minute. If the flow through the graft falls below that level, it is five times more likely to thrombose than a graft with flows above 400 mL/minute (61).

Hepatic artery thrombosis presents in a variety of ways, including recurrent bacteremia, delayed bile leak, and hepatic failure within 2 months of transplantation. In general, the risk of hepatic failure from HAT is greater when it occurs within 2 weeks of transplantation. In some patients, hepatic artery thrombosis is completely asymptomatic.

Diagnosis of hepatic artery thrombosis is usually suggested by ultrasound (62) and confirmed with arteriography, computed tomographic angiography (CTA) (63,64), or Magnetic Resonance Angiography (MRA) (65).

Therapy for HAT is largely dictated by the physiologic impact of the thrombosis and ranges from observation to urgent retransplantation. When significant hepatic compromise is present, intervention is warranted. The traditional intervention has been surgical thrombectomy coupled with anastomotic revision (66,67). Though the success in salvaging the graft ranges only between 20 and 40%, the transient reperfusion may allow the patient's condition to stabilize prior to retransplantation. Surgical thrombectomy followed by aortohepatic arterial graft placement is associated with an 82% survival rate in asymptomatic patients but only a 40% survival rate in patients experiencing symptoms (68).

Interventional radiologic options include fibrinolytic therapy or pharmacomechanical thrombectomy coupled with angioplasty with or without stent placement. Unfortunately, only scattered case reports (69–72) are available documenting the results of this therapeutic strategy, making selection of this therapeutic alternative in the individual patient difficult. When HAT occurs within the acute postoperative period, the possibility of inducing intra-abdominal bleeding must be considered. However, withholding therapy also carries with it a significant risk of biliary necrosis and allograft failure.

The final arterial complication is pseudoaneurysm formation. Pseudoaneurysm formation is a rare complication that is most often encountered at the arterial anastomosis. Pseudoaneurysms have also been reported at the stump of the donor gastroduodenal artery (73). Technical failure is the most common cause. Infection can also be a contributing factor in the formation of a mycotic pseudoaneurysm (74). Intrahepatic pseudoaneurysms of hepatic arterial branches may be secondary to biopsy or percutaneous biliary interventions.

Extrahepatic pseudoaneurysms may rupture, leading to intraperitoneal bleeding, gastrointestinal bleeding, or hemobilia. When the bleeding is brisk, hypotension and death (75) can occur; therefore, detection of pseudoaneurysms is of critical importance. Most of these aneurysms are incidentally detected during routine surveillance sonography (76). On sonography, an enlarged sonolucent area is present that is round to ovoid in shape with arterial flow on Doppler evaluation. A variable amount of thrombus may be seen surrounding or layered within the confines of the pseudoaneurysm. Psuedoaneurysms may also be detected on contrast enhanced computed tomography (CT) or magnetic resonance imaging (MRI).

Extrahepatic pseudoaneurysms generally require surgical exploration and repair. However, in patients who are poor surgical risks, a variety of endovascular and percutaneous options are available. Embolization of extrahepatic pseudoaneurysms has been described (77,78), but these series were not in transplant patients, where maintaining patency of the hepatic artery is of critical importance. Madariaga et al. (79) reported seven transplant patients with hepatic artery pseudoaneurysms treated either with hepatic artery ligation or hepatic artery embolization 10–70 days following transplantation. Of these seven patients, four survived, and one developed significant biliary strictures.

Theoretically, percutaneous insertion of a hepatic artery stent graft would appear to be a reasonable therapeutic alternative for a transplant patient with an uninfected pseudoaneurysm. A stent graft should seal the arterial defect and maintain arterial flow to the allograft. Percutaneous insertion of a hepatic artery stent graft has been described (80) in a patient with cholangiocarcinoma and a hepatic artery pseudoaneurysm, but not in a transplant patient. With the greater flexibility of commercially available stent grafts, the technique would appear feasible in a transplant patient, depending upon the degree of postsurgical hepatic arterial redundancy.

Percutaneous thrombin injection is another potential nonoperative therapy that has been used to treat an extrahepatic hepatic artery pseudoaneurysm in a transplant patient. Patel et al. (81) described a patient with chronic infection who developed a 3-cm pseudoaneurysm at the arterial anastomosis. Under sonographic guidance, 4,000 units of bovine thrombin were slowly injected, successfully occluding the aneurysm and maintaining patency of the subjacent hepatic artery. The aneurysm remained occluded, and the hepatic artery remained patent at a 6-month follow-up sonogram. It should be noted that the thrombin dose used in this patient is somewhat higher compared with the doses usually reported for occlusion of femoral arterial pseudoaneurysms (500–1,000 units).

Intrahepatic pseudoaneurysms can be asymptomatic, or they can be the source of significant hemorrhage. Both hemobilia and hemoperitoneum may result from pseudoaneurysms of this type. Hemoperitoneum develops if a tract (usually from an instigating needle) extends from the pseudoaneurysm through the hepatic capsule. As these aneurysms may be quite small, they will often be missed on routine surveillance ultrasonography. Angiography may be required to make the diagnosis and is the appropriate diagnostic test when bleeding complicates a biopsy or percutaneous biliary intervention. When a symptomatic intrahepatic pseudoaneurysm is identified, superselective embolization is the most appropriate therapeutic alternative (Figure 30–9). Occlusion of the artery on both sides of the arterial defect should be performed when possible to avoid continued bleeding from collateral perfusion. If superselective catheterization is not possible, sonographically guided percutaneous thrombin injection may also be used to treat intrahepatic false aneurysms.

Portal Vein Complications

As mentioned above, the portal venous anastomosis is usually accomplished with an end-to-end anastomosis of the extrahepatic donor portal vein to the extrahepatic portal vein of the recipient. If the recipient has a diminutive or thrombosed portal vein, a jump graft is usually created using donor common iliac vein between the allograft and the recipient's infrapancreatic superior mesenteric vein (82). When split-liver transplantation is performed, the anastomosis must be established to the right or left portal veins. Portal vein complications include portal vein stenosis and portal vein thrombosis.

Both stenosis and thrombosis can be caused by multiple factors, including a technically poor anastomosis, as well as torsion, tension, or venous redundancy induced by the geometric relationship of the allograft to the donor's portal vein. The use of venovenous bypass shunt catheters during the transplant operation can cause endothelial damage leading to portal vein occlusion. In some patients, hypercoagulable states may be related to the thrombosis. Moreover, patients with jump grafts to circumvent preexisting portal vein thrombosis appear to be at higher risk for venous occlusion.

Portal vein thrombosis is less common than hepatic artery thrombosis, being observed in 1–3% of patients (83). Clinical manifestations depend on when the thrombosis occurs with respect to transplantation. Occlusion within 1 month generally leads to problems with hepatic function, ranging from asymptomatic enzyme elevation to hepatic failure. When thrombosis occurs at a time remote from transplantation, sequelae of portal hypertension dominate the clinical picture, including variceal bleeding, ascites, and hepatic encephalopathy (84,85).

The diagnosis of portal vein stenosis or portal vein thrombosis can be made without difficulty on ultrasonography with duplex Doppler, computed tomography, magnetic resonance imaging, or arterial portography. Most often, the diagnosis is made on routine posttransplant surveillance ultrasound. On occasion, the diagnosis of portal vein stenosis is not straightforward because size mismatch may cause the anastomosis to appear somewhat narrowed and because turbulent flow may make Doppler analysis difficult (86).

In general, symptomatic portal vein stenosis requires treatment (87). The initial therapeutic intervention is usually balloon dilatation with or without stent placement (88–90). Balloon dilatation of the portal vein is usually performed from the percutaneous transhepatic approach although the transjugular-transhepatic route could also be utilized. Stents, usually of the self-expanding type, are inserted when balloon dilatation fails to create a nonstenotic lumen or when a stenosis recurs following balloon dilatation (Figure 30–10).

No substantial series of patients has been reported in the literature to document the long-term durability of balloon dilatation with stent placement in the adult population. However, in a series of 25 pediatric patients who underwent transplantation of the left lateral segment of a living donor, Funaki et al. (91) reported a 76% success rate with a mean follow-up of 46 months. In this series, a heterogeneous group of patients with both portal vein stenosis and portal vein thrombosis were treated. In the six patients who were immediate technical failures, a thrombosed portal vein

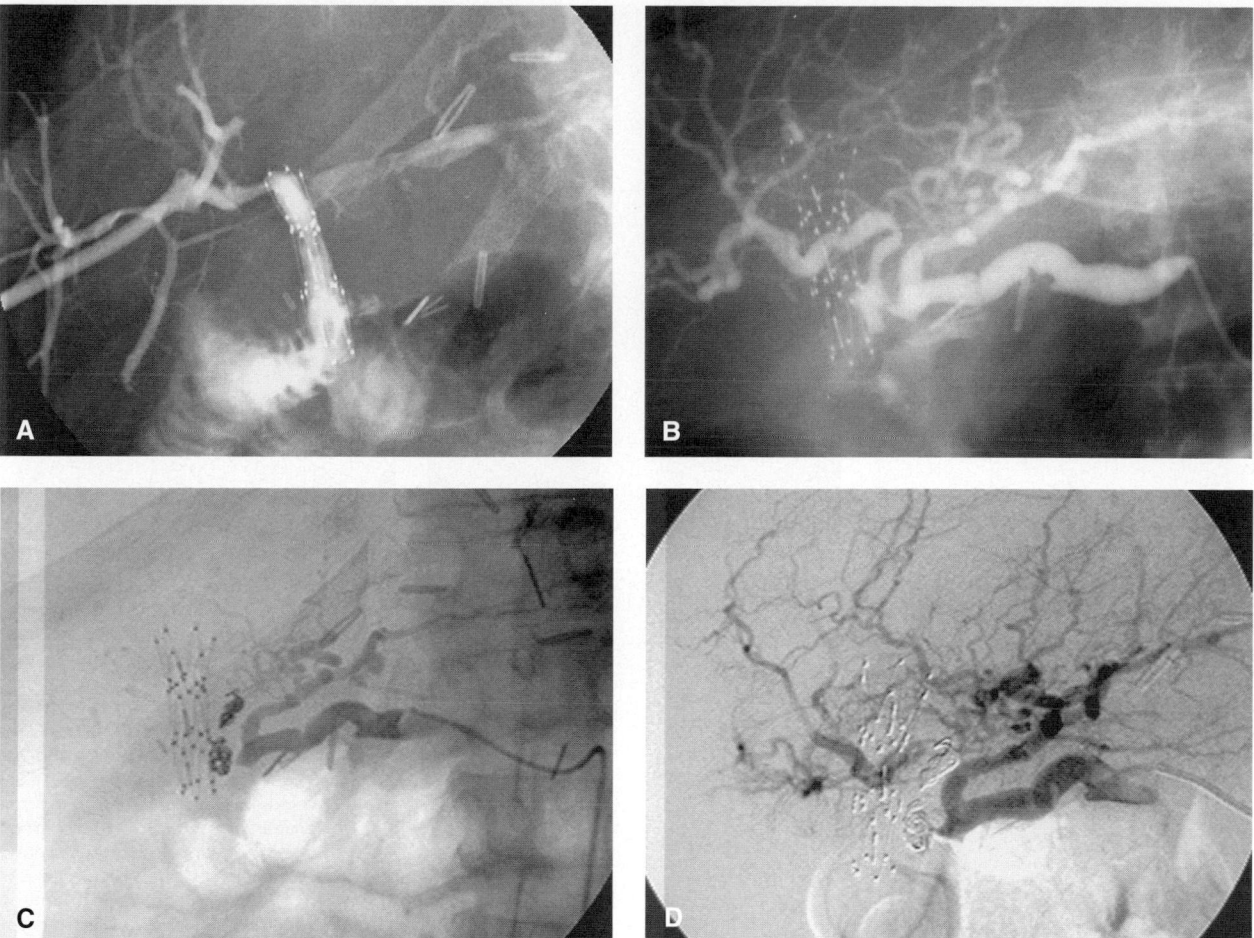

Figure 30–9 A 70-year-old woman with cryptogenic cirrhosis underwent OLT. **A.** The patient developed a stricture at the Roux anastomosis that was treated with a Gianturco stent. **B.** One year after stent placement, the patient developed upper gastrointestinal (GI) tract bleeding. Selective hepatic arteriogram showed a pseudoaneurysm adjacent to the stent. **C.** The right hepatic artery was embolized with microcoils to occlude the pseudoaneurysm, and the patient's bleeding resolved. **D.** Postembolization angiogram shows perfusion of the right lobe via intrahepatic collaterals.

could not be successfully traversed with a guide wire. Of the 19 patients who underwent technically uneventful balloon dilatation, five patients required immediate stent placement to treat elastic recoil at the site of dilatation. Of the remaining 14 patients, seven had a durable result from the balloon angioplasty with a mean follow-up of 36.7 months. The remaining seven patients developed recurrent stenoses at a mean time of 6.3 months following the initial dilatation and required stents to be placed. In the aggregate group of 12 patients who received portal venous stents, no recurrent stenoses or thromboses developed during a mean follow-up period of 47 months.

Acute posttransplant portal vein thrombosis associated with hepatic dysfunction can be extremely serious and usually requires treatment (92). The treatment options are surgical thrombectomy (59), venous bypass (93), retransplantation, or percutaneous intervention. Percutaneous interventions include regional fibrinolytic therapy (94) or mechanical

thrombectomy (95) followed by balloon dilatation and stent placement. At least five successful cases using this strategy have been reported, with significant long-term durability ranging from 1 month (96) to 4.5 years (88). Percutaneous thrombolytic therapy and stent placement with restoration of patency has also been described in a portal vein jump-graft conduit (97). Despite these encouraging results, it should be noted that percutaneous techniques are not uniformly successful in re-establishing portal vein patency, and the procedure carries a risk of hemorrhage and rethrombosis (98).

As an alternative approach, placement of a transjugular intrahepatic portosystemic shunt (TIPS) with local thrombolysis has been performed to treat early portal vein thrombosis following transplantation (99). This approach would appear to be an excellent way to prevent complications of portal hypertension but may not be effective in increasing hepatic perfusion because the portal venous flow may be shunted into the systemic circulation.

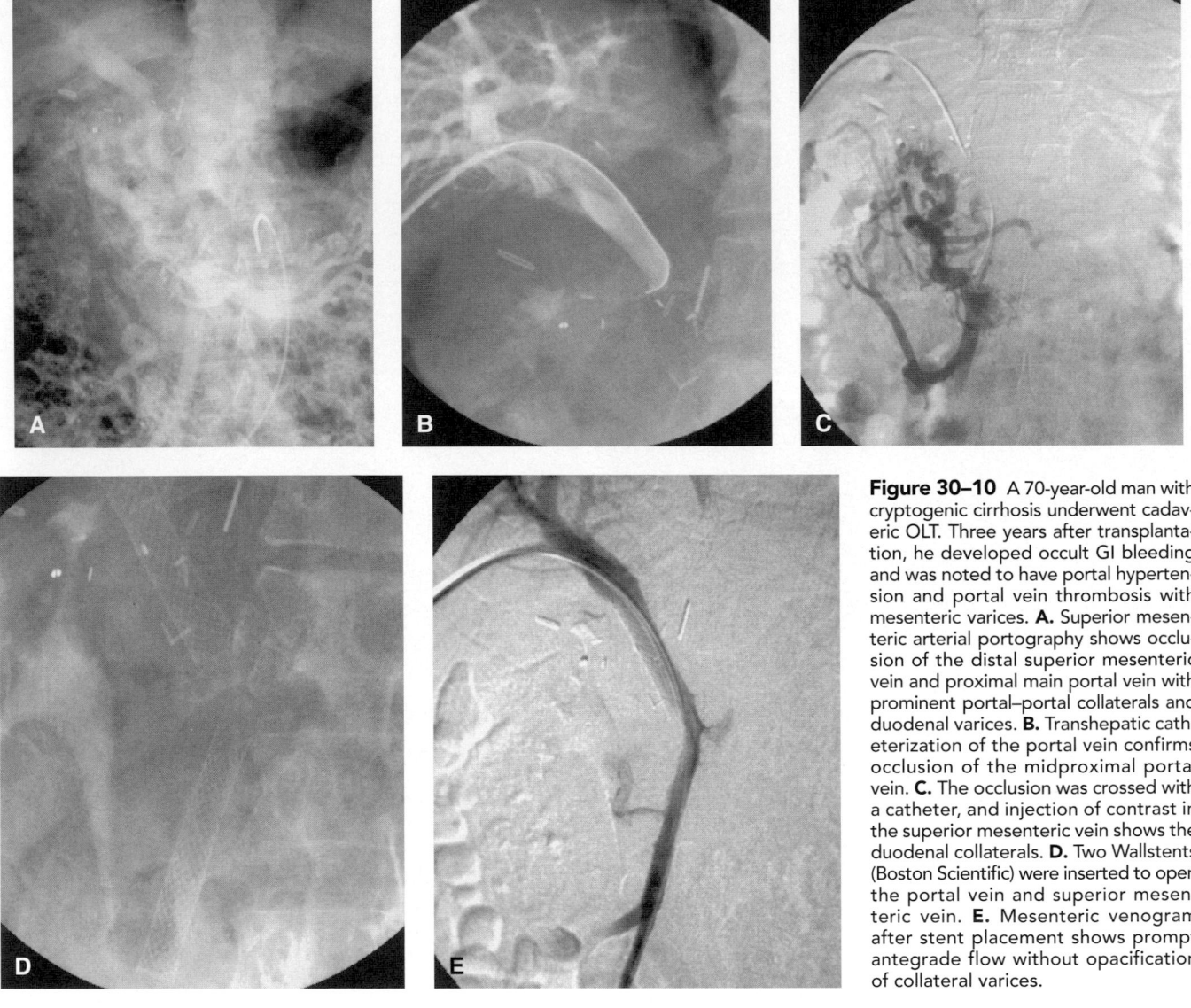

Figure 30–10 A 70-year-old man with cryptogenic cirrhosis underwent cadaveric OLT. Three years after transplantation, he developed occult GI bleeding and was noted to have portal hypertension and portal vein thrombosis with mesenteric varices. **A.** Superior mesenteric arterial portography shows occlusion of the distal superior mesenteric vein and proximal main portal vein with prominent portal–portal collaterals and duodenal varices. **B.** Transhepatic catheterization of the portal vein confirms occlusion of the midproximal portal vein. **C.** The occlusion was crossed with a catheter, and injection of contrast in the superior mesenteric vein shows the duodenal collaterals. **D.** Two Wallstents (Boston Scientific) were inserted to open the portal vein and superior mesenteric vein. **E.** Mesenteric venogram after stent placement shows prompt antegrade flow without opacification of collateral varices.

Hepatic Veins and Inferior Vena Caval Complications

As previously discussed, the inferior vena caval anastomosis can be constructed in two ways. The traditional method has been the creation of end-to-end anastomoses in the suprahepatic and infrahepatic IVC. The alternative method is to use the piggyback technique, in which the hepatic veins of the recipient are surgically conjoined to create a single outflow vessel, which is then anastomosed to the donor suprahepatic IVC. When a TIPS is present or when extending into the inferior vena cava or the recipient's hepatic veins is unsuitable, the dorsal wall of the allograft cava can be opened and anastomosed to the ventral wall of the recipient cava (100). In most variations of the piggyback technique, the caudal aspect of the donor IVC is ligated. The piggyback technique maintains at least partial flow through the recipi-

ent's IVC during the transplant procedure, avoiding the necessity of venovenous bypass and simplifying anesthetic management of bloodpressure.

The systemic venous anastomoses with split-liver and living donor transplantation are generally made end to end with the right or left hepatic veins, depending upon the nature of the allograft. Controversy exists regarding the fate of the donor's middle hepatic vein when the right lobe is transplanted. The decision is usually based upon the size of the donor and recipient in conjunction with the specific hepatic venous anatomy. Both graft survival and complications in the living donor appear comparable whether the middle hepatic vein is incorporated in the allograft or left with the donor's remnant liver (101).

Problems with the systemic venous anastomoses are unusual and are observed in fewer than 1% of patients undergoing transplantation (102). Stenoses and thromboses are almost invariably related to the anastomoses. Patients with obstruction of the suprahepatic caval anastomoses present with clinical features typical of the Budd-Chiari syndrome, including ascites and a variable degree of hepatic dysfunction (103). Lower extremity edema may or may not be present.

Stenoses of the infrahepatic inferior vena caval anastomoses in patients undergoing traditional end-to-end caval reconstructions present solely with lower extremity edema (104). Extrinsic pressure on the inferior vena cava from a hematoma or other large fluid collection may also cause outflow obstruction and lead to similar pathophysiology.

Diagnosis of a hepatic vein or caval stenosis can be difficult and may be missed by routine sonographic surveillance unless is the clinical presentation engenders a high index of suspicion. The diagnosis may also be suggested by contrast-enhanced CT or MRI, although confirmatory venography with pressure measurements is often needed to confirm the diagnosis.

When a symptomatic systemic venous stenosis is detected, transluminal angioplasty is usually the preferred therapeutic intervention. If angioplasty is unsuccessful because of elastic rebound or recurrence, stent placement may be necessary. Self-expanding stents appear to be a better choice for caval stenoses, whereas either self-expanding or balloon-expandable stents can be used for hepatic vein stenoses. Care must be taken not to extend stents into the right atrium because arrhythmias and atrial perforation may ensue.

Zajko et al. (89) reported six IVC stenoses treated with balloon angioplasty. Initial technical results were good, and all six patients experienced symptomatic relief, including resolution of ascites. However, three of the six patients required repeated balloon dilatations for recurrent stenoses. Raby et al. (45) reported recurrent stenosis in one of three patients dilated for IVC stenosis. The higher recurrence rate of stenoses in the IVC compared with portal venous dilatations may reflect torsion or other geometric issues of the caval anastomoses.

The recurrent stenoses data following stent placement is somewhat better compared with simple balloon dilatation. In a group of patients refractory to balloon dilatation, Borsa et al. (105) reported placement of 10 stents into six patients with five of six patients maintaining primary patency during a mean follow-up period of 11 months. One patient developed recurrent stenosis at 3 weeks and was successfully restented.

Weeks et al. (106) reported nine patients with symptomatic IVC and hepatic vein stenoses following liver transplantation. In this series, patients were primarily managed with the placement of Gianturco stents. Technical success was achieved in all nine patients with clinical success in eight of nine patients. No recurrent stenoses were observed during the average follow-up period of 491 days. A similar high success rate was noted by Simo et al. (107) in three patients using double-barrel Gianturco stents. However, problems with stent movement were encountered in two of the three patients.

Complete thrombosis of the inferior vena cava has also been managed with endovascular techniques. Orons et al. (108) used catheter-directed thrombolysis to successfully remove the thrombus and uncover a severe retrohepatic caval stenosis. The stenosis was then addressed using balloon angioplasty, followed by placement of a self-expanding stent. The patient remained asymptomatic with no evidence of recurrent IVC stenosis at 20-month follow-up.

Isolated hepatic vein stenoses are unusual in patients who receive a whole-liver allograft. In these patients, no surgical anastomosis is created through the hepatic vein when conventional end-to-end anastomosis is used. When a piggyback technique is employed, a stenosis can develop at the donor caval-to-recipient hepatic vein confluence anastomosis. Sze et al. (109) reported two patients who were successfully treated using expandable metallic stents with primary patency at 3- and 39-month follow-up.

In split-liver transplant or living donor recipients, isolated hepatic vein stenoses may be encountered at the surgical anastomosis (Figure 30–11). Egawa et al. (110) reported five patients who underwent successful PTA of anastomotic hepatic venous stenoses with maintenance of patency as assessed by follow-up Doppler sonography at 3–7 months following the procedure.

TRANSJUGULAR BIOPSY IN THE POSTTRANSPLANT PATIENT

Transjugular liver biopsy is a useful technique in which histologic specimens of the liver are obtained without, in most cases, violating the hepatic capsule. When the hepatic capsule is not punctured, the chance of postbiopsy bleeding is presumably reduced. It is particularly useful in patients with ascites or coagulopathy, who may be at increased risk for bleeding complications. The transjugular biopsy system developed by Colapinto and Blendis (111) has given way in most centers to spring-loaded automated biopsy devices ranging from 18-gauge to 20-gauge (112). Prudent clinical judgment must be used in deciding when the freshly created caval anastomosis is healed enough to allow the passage of these relatively stiff instruments from the jugular vein into the hepatic vein and hepatic parenchyma. However, the procedure appears to be relatively safe, even in the early posttransplant period. Azoulay et al. (113) reported 124 transjugular liver biopsies in 105 transplant recipients within 30 days of the transplant operation. In this group, 89% had standard end-to-end caval anastomoses, and the remaining 11% had piggyback caval–caval anatomy. An 87% technical success rate was observed with an adequate specimen rate of 86%. Clinical management was influenced by the biopsy result in 65% of patients. No complications were reported in this series, although bleeding and inadvertent puncture of the kidney (114) have been documented with this technique. An overall complication rate of 2.4%, including three intraperitoneal hemorrhages, one of which was fatal, was observed in a series of 371 patients reported by Smith et al. (115).

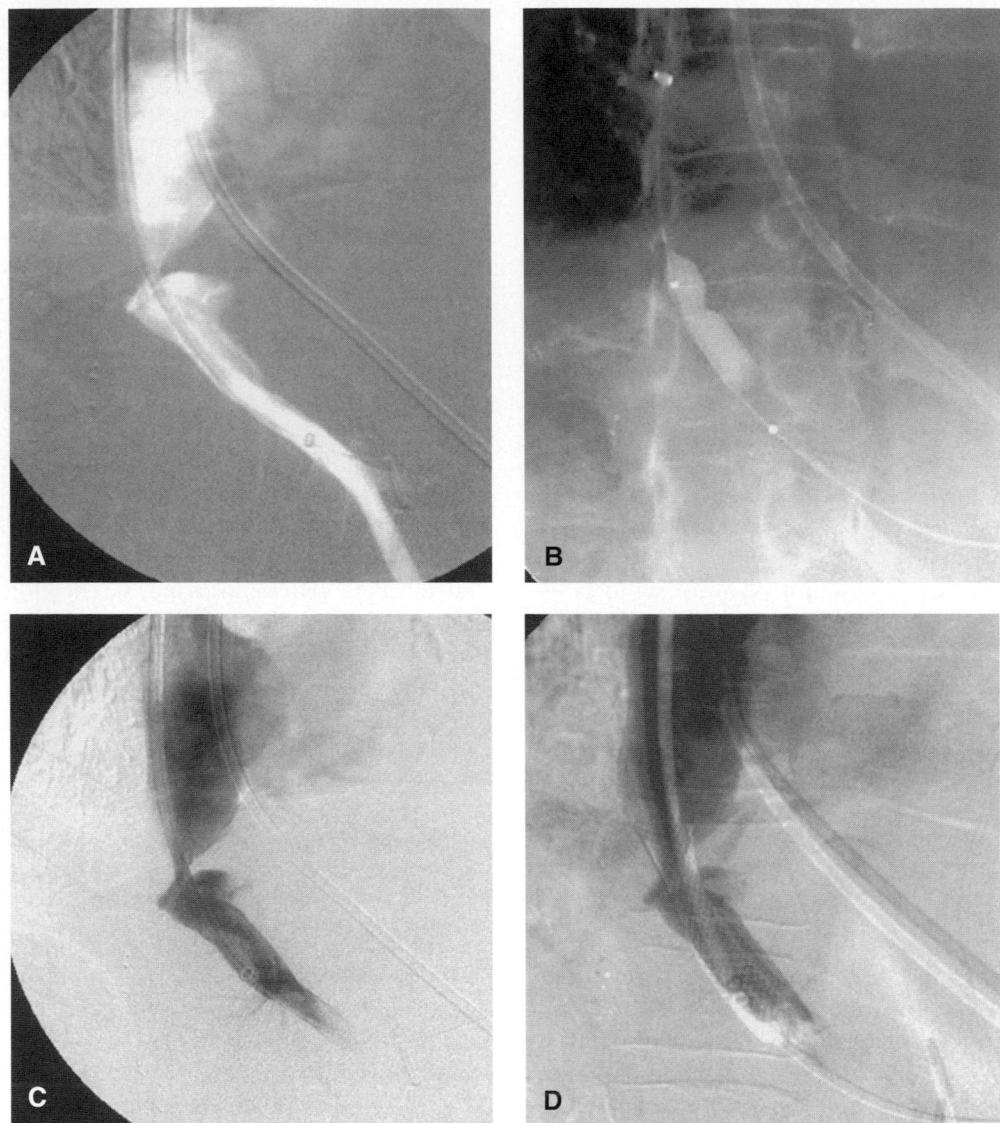

Figure 30–11 This patient developed ascites 2 months after left-lobe liver transplantation. Imaging revealed HV obstruction (see diagnostic images Figure 30–2). She was treated using endovascular techniques. **A.** A 9F transjugular sheath was placed into the left hepatic vein. **B.** The stenosis was dilated with a 10-mm balloon. **C.** Angioplasty alone was not effective in relieving the obstruction. **D.** A 12- × 40-mm Wallstent (Boston Scientific) was placed across the stenosis with immediate resolution of obstruction and reduction of pressure gradient.

TIPS IN THE TRANSPLANT PATIENT

Transjugular intrahepatic portosystemic shunt (TIPS) placement has become an integral part of managing patients with complications of portal hypertension. When clinically warranted, TIPS can be used both before and after orthotopic liver transplantation.

TIPS Prior to OLT

TIPS is a potentially lifesaving intervention in patients with uncontrollable variceal hemorrhage and intractable ascites. In salvaging patients of this nature, TIPS serves as a bridge to transplantation. Moreover, early in the TIPS experience it was hoped that TIPS placement would decompress varices and facilitate the transplant operation. Unfortunately, several studies (116,117) have shown that pretransplant TIPS placement fails to shorten operative time, reduce intraoperative blood loss, or diminish postoperative complications. Moreover, concerns have been raised that the presence of a TIPS potentially complicates the transplant operation. Khan et al. (118) analyzed 21 patients with TIPS who underwent liver transplantation and compared this group with 131 patients without TIPS undergoing the same procedure. No difference in length of hospital stay or graft survival was observed. Similar results confirming the absence of a deleterious effect of TIPS placement on orthotopic liver transplantation was reported by Chui et al. (119).

Although no increase in surgical morbidity or mortality was observed in the TIPS patients, distal extension into the portal vein was noted, requiring the stent to be cut and removed in piecemeal fashion or peeled en bloc from the portal vein wall. A stent displaced into the inferior vena cava required removal by simple traction during explantation of the native liver.

Despite these studies, numerous case reports of complications created by the presence of the TIPS during transplantation have appeared. Hutchins et al. (120) reported a case requiring a significant modification of the portal vein anastomosis because of an embedded stent that extended well into the portal vein. Rumi et al. (121) reported a case of a TIPS stent that embolized to the left pulmonary artery during the transplant operation. In this case, the stent was removed by endovascular techniques following the transplantation. Wilson et al. (122) reported three patients in which the liver transplant operation was prolonged due to malpositioned TIPS stents. In this series, problems were encountered in both the portal venous and inferior vena caval anastomoses. Suffice it to say that although trans-plantation is often performed following TIPS, a malpositioned TIPS can adversely affect the operative procedure, and every effort should be made not to extend stents far into the extrahepatic portal vein or inferior vena cava.

TIPS after OLT

TIPS may also be necessary if complications of portal hypertension develop following orthotopic liver transplantation (Figure 30–12). The procedure can be performed in a fashion identical to that in the nontransplant patient. Amesur et al. (123) reported performing TIPS in 12 transplant patients 6 months to 13 years after surgery. In this series, no technical problems were encountered. In contrast, Lerut et al. (124) reported two of eight TIPS as technically difficult because of piggyback inferior vena caval anastomoses. Moreover, these authors suggested that close immunosuppression monitoring following TIPS in the transplant patient was warranted because of modified metabolization of cyclosporine and perhaps tacrolimus, which may bypass the liver through the shunt.

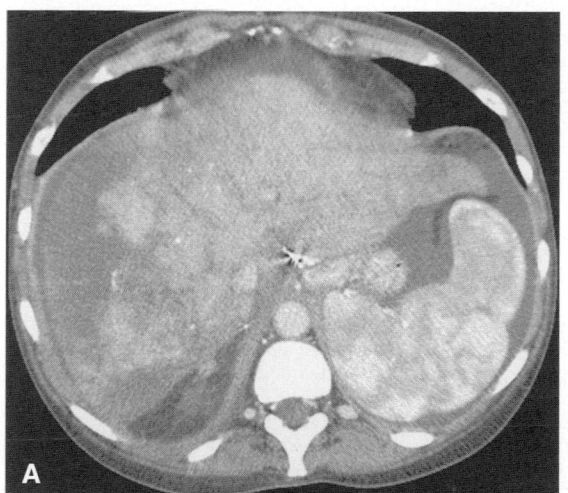

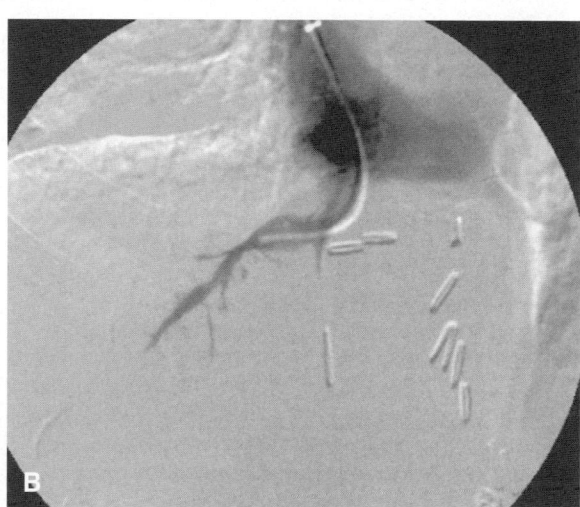

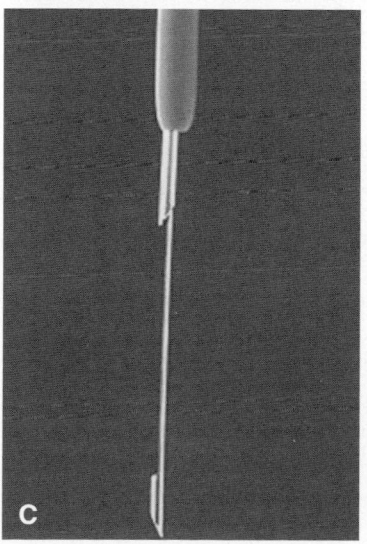

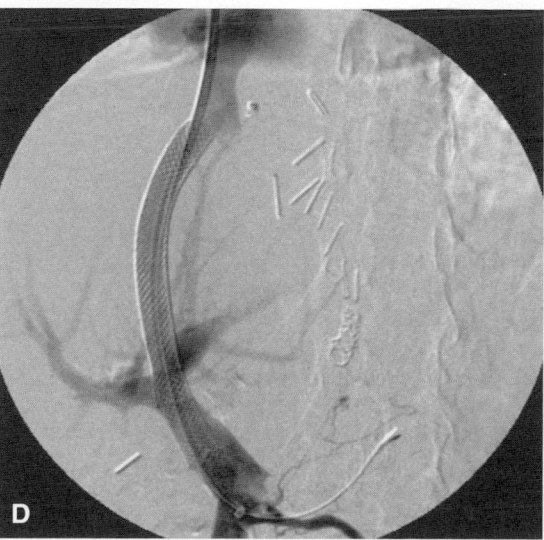

Figure 30–12 A 52-year-old woman underwent OLT for Budd-Chiari syndrome. Three years later she developed recurrent ascites. **A.** Contrast-enhanced CT was suggestive of recurrent Budd-Chiari syndrome. **B.** Transjugular hepatic venography supported this diagnosis. The right hepatic vein is small, and the tributary veins are attenuated. **C.** Transjugular liver biopsy was performed with an 18-gauge core biopsy needle. Adequate specimens were obtained, and analysis revealed centrolobular necrosis. **D.** TIPS was performed, and the patient's ascites resolved.

SUMMARY

Advances in diagnostic imaging and interventional radiologic techniques have clearly complemented advances in surgical technique and immunosuppressive therapy, reducing morbidity and mortality of orthotopic liver transplantation. Catheter techniques have been developed to treat vascular and nonvascular complications following orthotopic liver transplantation that heretofore required an open surgical procedure. Advances in imaging have allowed minimally invasive evaluation of living donors, potentially reducing complications following lobectomy in these individuals.

REFERENCES

1. United Network for Organ Sharing, Organ Procurement and Transplantation Network data page. Available at http://www.unos.org. Accessed October 2003.
2. Kato T, Levi D, Nery JR, et al. Operative procedures. In: Maddrey WC, Schiff ER, Sorrell MF, eds. Transplantation of the Liver. Philadelphia: Lippincott Williams and Wilkins, 2001:47–64.
3. Trotter JF, Wachs M, Everson GT, et al. Adult-to-adult transplantation of the right hepatic lobe from a living donor. N Engl J Med 2002;346:1074–1082.
4. Nakamura S, Tsuzuki T. Surgical anatomy of the hepatic veins and inferior vena cava. Surg Gynecol Obstet 1981;152:43–50.
5. Delattre J, Avisse C, Flament JB. Anatomic basis of hepatic surgery. Surg Clin North Am 1989;69:179–192.
6. Reichert PR, Renz JF. Anatomical variations hampering the use of right lobe in living donor transplantation. Liver Transpl 2001; 7: 86–94.
7. Mitchell A, Mirza D, De Ville de Goyet J, et al. Absence of the left portal vein: a difficulty for reduction of liver grafts? Transplantation 2000;69:1731–1732.
8. Michels NA. Newer anatomy of the liver and its variant blood supply and collateral circulation. Am J Surg 1966;112:337–347.
9. Deshpande RR, Heaton ND, Rela M. Surgical anatomy of segmental liver transplantation. Br J Surg 2002;89:1078–1088.
10. Broelsch CE, Whitington PF, Emond JC, et al. Living transplantation in children from living related donors. Surgical techniques and results. Ann Surg 1991;214:428–437.
11. Sugawara Y, Makuuchi M: Technical advances in living-related liver transplantation. J Hepatobiliary Pancreat Surg 199;6:245–253.
12. Smadja C, Blumgart LH. The biliary tract and the anatomy of biliary exposure. In: Blumgart LH, ed. Surgery of the Liver and Biliary Tract, vol. 1, 2nd Ed. Edinburgh: Churchill Livingston, 1994:11–24.
13. Surman OS. The ethics of partial-liver donation. N Engl J Med 2002;346:1038.
14. Surman OS. Transplantation of the right hepatic lobe. N Engl J Med 2002;347:618.
15. Pomfret EA. Early and late complications in the right-lobe adult living donor. Liver Transpl 2003;19:S45–S49.
16. Pasher A, Sauer IM, Walter M, et al. Donor evaluation, donor risks, donor outcome, and donor quality of life in adult–adult living donor liver transplantation. Liver Transpl 2003;8:829–837.
17. Ito T, Kiuchi T, Egawa H, et al. Surgery-related morbidity in living donors of right-lobe graft: lessons from the first 200 cases. Transplantation 2003;76:158–163.
18. Umeshita K, Fujiwara K, Kiyosawa K, et al. Operative morbidity of living liver donors in Japan. Lancet 2003;362:687–690.
19. Venook AP, Ferrell LD, Roberts JP, et al. Liver transplantation for hepatocellular carcinoma: results with preoperative chemoembolization. Liver Transpl Surg 1995;1:242–248.
20. Graziadei IW, Sandmueller H, Waldenberger P, et al. Chemoembolization followed by liver transplantation for hepatocellular carcinoma impedes tumor progression while on the waiting list and leads to excellent outcome. Liver Transpl 2003;9: 557–563.
21. Richard HM III, Silberzweig JE, Mitty HA, et al. Hepatic arterial complications in liver transplant recipients treated with pre-transplantation chemoembolization for hepatocellular carcinoma. Radiology 2000;214:775–779.
22. Starzl TE, Ishikawa M, Putnam CW, et al. Progress in and deterrents to orthotopic liver transplantation, with special reference to survival, resistance to hyperacute rejection, and biliary duct reconstruction. Transplant Proc 1974;6:129–139.
23. Lerut J, Gordon RD, Iwatsuki S, et al. Biliary tract complications in human orthotopic liver transplantation. Transplantation 1987;43:47–51.
24. Zajko AB, Campbell WL, Bron KM, et al. Diagnostic and interventional radiology in liver transplantation. Gastroenterol Clin North Am 1988;17:105–143.
25. Sheng R, Sammon JK, Zajko AB, et al. Bile leak after hepatic transplantation: cholangiographic features, prevalence, and clinical outcome. Radiology 1994;192:413–416.
26. Ward EM, Wiesner RH, Hughes RW, et al. Persistent bile leak after liver transplantation: biloma drainage and endoscopic retrograde cholangiopancreatographic sphincterotomy. Radiology 1991;179:719–720.
27. Randall HB, Wachs ME, Somberg KA, et al. The use of T tube after orthotopic liver transplantation. Transplantation 1996;61:258–261.
28. Lebeau G, Yamaga K, Marsh AV, et al. Analysis of surgical complications after 397 hepatic transplantations. Surg Gynecol Obstet 1990;170:317–322.
29. Zemel G, Zajko AB, Skolnick ML, et al. The role of sonography and hepatic cholangiography in the diagnosis of biliary complications after liver transplantation. Am J Roentgenol 1988;151:943–946.
30. Zajko AB, Sheng R, Zetti GM, et al. Transhepatic balloon dilation of biliary strictures in liver transplant patients: a 10-year experience. J Vasc Interv Radiol 1995;6:79–83.
31. Petersen B, Timmermans HA, Uchida BT, et al. Treatment of refractory benign biliary stenoses in liver transplant patients by placement and retrieval of a temporary stent-graft: work in progress. J Vasc Interv Radiol 2000;11:919–929.
32. Graziadei IW. Recurrence of primary sclerosing cholangitis after liver transplantation. Liver Transpl 2002;8:575–581.
33. Zajko AB, Bennett M, Campbell WL, et al. Mucocele of the cystic duct remnant in eight liver transplant recipients: findings at cholangiography, CT and US. Radiology 1990;177:691–693.
34. Dupuy D, Costello P, Lewis D, et al. Abdominal CT findings after liver transplantation in 66 patients. Am J Roentgenol 1991; 156: 1167–1170.
35. Cheng YF, Chen YS, Huang TL, et al. Interventional radiologic procedures in liver transplantation. Transpl Int 2001;14:223–229.
36. Kaplan SB, Zajko AB, Koneru B. Hepatic bilomas due to hepatic artery thrombosis in liver transplant recipients: percutaneous drainage and clinical outcome. Radiology 1990;174:1031–1035.
37. Garcia-Vila J, Saiz-Paches V, Domenech-Iglesias MA, et al. Infected intraabdominal hematomas: percutaneous drainage. Abdom Imaging 1993;18:313–317.
38. Griebling TL, Chang PJ, Loening SA, et al. Percutaneous thrombolysis of an infected retroperitoneal hematoma with urokinase. J Urol 1995;154:1477.
39. Wozney P, Zajko AB, Bron K, et al. Vascular complications after liver transplantation: a 5-year experience. Am J Roentgenol 1986; 147:657–663.
40. Bechstein WO, Blumhardt G, Ringe B, et al. Surgical complications in 200 consecutive liver transplants. Transplant Proc 1987; 19: 3830–3831.
41. Orons PD, Sheng R, Zajko AB. Hepatic artery stenosis in liver transplant recipients: prevalence and cholangiographic appearance of associated biliary complications. Am J Roentgenol 1995;165:1145–1149.
42. Abbasoglu O, Levy MF, Vodapally MS, et al. Hepatic artery stenosis after liver transplantation—incidence, presentation, treatment, and long-term outcome. Transplantation 1997;63:250–255.
43. Castaneda F, So SK, Hunter DW, et al. Reversible hepatic transplant ischemia: case report and review of the literature. Cardiovasc Intervent Radiol 1990;13:88–90.

44. Abad J, Hidalgo EG, Cantarero JM, et al. Hepatic artery anastomotic stenosis after transplantation: treatment with percutaneous transluminal angioplasty. Radiology 1989;171:661–662.

45. Raby N, Karani J, Thomas S, et al. Stenosis of vascular anastomoses after hepatic transplantation: treatment with balloon angioplasty. Am J Roentgenol 1991;157:167–171.

46. Mondragoon RS, Karani JB, Heaton ND, et al. The use of percutaneous transluminal angioplasty in hepatic artery stenosis after transplantation. Transplantation 1994;57:228–231.

47. Orons PD, Zajko AB, Bron KM, et al. Hepatic artery angioplasty after liver transplantation: experience in 21 allografts. J Vasc Interv Radiol 1995;6:523–529.

48. Vorwerk D, Gunter R, Klever P, et al. Angioplasty and stent placement for treatment of hepatic artery thrombosis following liver transplantation. J Vasc Interv Radiol 1994;5:309–311.

49. Karatzas T, Lykaki-Karatzas E, Webb M, et al. Vascular complications, treatment, and outcome following orthotopic liver transplantation. Transplant Proc 1997;29:2853–2855.

50. Stein M, Rudich SM, Riegler JL, et al. Dissection of an iliac artery conduit to liver allograft: treatment with an endovascular stent. Liver Transpl Surg 1999;5:252–254.

51. Cotroneo AR, Di Stasi C, Cina A, et al. Stent placement in four patients with hepatic artery stenosis or thrombosis after liver transplantation. J Vasc Interv Radiol 2002;13:619–623.

52. Lerut JP, Gordon RD, Iwatsuki S, et al. Human orthotopic liver transplantation: surgical aspects in 393 consecutive grafts. Transplant Proc 1988;20:603–606.

53. Langnas AN, Marujp W, Stratta RJ, et al. Vascular complications after liver transplantation. Am J Surg 1991;161:76–83.

54. Marujo WC, Langnas AN, Wood RP, et al. Vascular complications following liver transplantation: outcome and role of urgent revascularization. Transplant Proc 1991;23:1484–1486.

55. Wozney P, Zajko AB, Bron KM, et al. Vascular complications after liver transplantation: a 5-year experience. Am J Roentgenol 1986;147:657–663.

56. Tzakis AG, Gordon RD, Shaw BW, et al. Clinical presentation of hepatic artery thrombosis after liver transplantation in the cyclosporine era. Transplantation 1985;40:667–671.

57. Valente JF, Alonso MH, Weber FL, et al. Late hepatic artery thrombosis in liver allograft recipients is associated with intrahepatic biliary necrosis. Transplantation 1996;61:61–65.

58. Stange BJ, Glanemann M, Nuessler NC, et al. Hepatic artery thrombosis after adult liver transplantation. Liver Transpl 2003;9:612–620.

59. Everson GT, Kam I. Immediate postoperative care. In: Maddrey WC, Schiff ER, Sorrell MF, eds. Transplantation of the Liver. Philadelphia: Lippincott Williams and Wilkins, 2001:141.

60. Muiesan P, Rela M, Nodari F, et al. Use of infrarenal conduits for arterial revascularization in orthotopic liver transplantation. Liver Transpl Surg 1998;4:232–235.

61. Abbasoglu O, Levy MF, Testa G, et al. Does intraoperative hepatic artery flow predict arterial complications after liver transplantation? Transplantation 1998;66:598–601.

62. Hall TR, McDiarmid SV, Grant EG, et al. False negative duplex Doppler studies in children with hepatic artery thrombosis after liver transplantation. Am J Roentgenol 1990;154:573–575.

63. Vogl TJ, Hanninen EL, Bechstein WO, et al. Biphasic spiral computed tomography versus digital subtraction angiography for evaluation of arterial thrombosis after orthotopic liver transplantation. Invest Radiol 1998;33:136–140.

64. Quiroga S, Sebastia C, Margarit C, et al. Complications of orthotopic liver transplantation: spectrum of findings with helical CT. Radiographics 2001;21:1085–1102.

65. Stafford-Johnson DB, Hamilton BH, Dong Q, et al. Vascular complications of liver transplantation: evaluation with gadolinium-enhanced MR angiography. Radiology 1998;207:153–160.

66. Marujo WC, Langnas AN, Wood RP, et al. Vascular complications following orthotopic liver transplantation: outcome and the role of urgent revascularization. Transplant Proc 1991;23:1484–1486.

67. Langnas AN, Marujo W, Stratta RJ, et al. Hepatic allograft rescue following arterial thrombosis: role of urgent revascularization. Transplantation 1991;51:86–90.

68. Sheiner PA, Varma CV, Guarrera JV, et al. Selective revascularization of hepatic artery thromboses after liver transplantation improves patient and graft survival. Transplantation 1997;64:1295–1299.

69. Hidalgo EG, Abad J, Cantarero JM, et al. High dose intraarterial urokinase for the treatment of hepatic artery thrombosis in liver transplantation. Hepatogastroenterology 1989;36:529–532.

70. Olausson M, Backman L, Mjornstedt L, et al. Thrombectomy and in situ fibrinolysis in the treatment of acute hepatic arterial thrombosis after liver transplantation in two children. Eur J Surg 1999;165:618–620.

71. Torrasa J, Llado L, Figueras J, et al. Diagnostic and therapeutic management of hepatic artery thrombosis after liver transplantation. Transpl Proc 1999;31:2405.

72. Bjerkvik S, Vatne K, Mathisen O, et al. Percutaneous revascularization of post-operative hepatic artery thrombosis in a liver transplant. Transplantation 1995;59:1746–1748.

73. Zajko AB, Chablani V, Bron KM, et al. Gastroduodenal artery mycotic pseudoaneurysm: an unusual cause of lower gastrointestinal bleeding following liver transplantation. Transplantation 1988;45:990–991.

74. Lowell JA, Coopersmith CM, Shenoy S, et al. Unusual presentations of nonmycotic hepatic artery pseudoaneurysms after liver transplantation. Liver Transpl Surg 1999;5:200–203.

75. Hesselink EL, Sloof MJH, Schuur KH, et al. Consequences of hepatic artery pathology after orthotopic liver transplantation. Transplant Proc 1987;19:2476–2477.

76. Tobben PJ, Zajko AB, Sumkin JH, et al. Pseudoaneurysms complicating organ transplantation: roles of CT, duplex sonography, and angiography. Radiology 1988;169:65–70.

77. Reber PU, Baer HU, Patel AG, et al. Superselective microcoil embolization: treatment of choice in high-risk patients with extrahepatic pseudoaneurysms of the hepatic arteries. J Am Coll Surg 1998;186:325–330.

78. Yamakado K, Nakatsuka A, Tanaka N, et al. Transcatheter arterial embolization of ruptured pseudoaneurysms with coils and n-butyl cyanoacrylate. J Vasc Interv Radiol 2000;11:66–72.

79. Madariaga J, Zajko AB, Tzoracoleftherakis E, et al. Hepatic artery pseudoaneurysm ligation after orthotopic liver transplantation—a report of 7 cases. Transplantation 1992;54:824–828.

80. Paci E, Antico E, Candelari R, et al. Pseudoaneurysm of the common hepatic artery: treatment with a stent graft. Cardiovasc Interv Radiol 2000;23:472–474.

81. Patel JV, Weston MJ, Kessel DO, et al. Hepatic artery pseudoaneurysm after liver transplantation: treatment with percutaneous thrombin injection. Transplantation 2003;75:1755–1760.

82. Tzakis AG, Todo S, Steiber AC, et al. Venous jump grafts for liver transplantation in patients with portal vein thrombosis. Transplantation 1989;48:530–531.

83. Lerut J, Tzakis AG, Bron K, et al. Complications of venous reconstruction in human orthotopic liver transplantation. Ann Surg 1987;205:404–414.

84. Helling TS. Thrombosis and recanalization of the portal vein in liver transplantation. Transplantation 1985;40:446–448.

85. Zajko AB, Bron KM. Hepatopedal collaterals after portal vein thrombosis following liver transplantation. Cardiovasc Intervent Radiol 1986;9:46–48.

86. Glockner JF, Forauer AR. Vascular or ischemic complications after liver transplantation. Am J Roentgenol 1999;173:1055–1059.

87. Scantlebury VP, Zajko AB, Esquivel CO, et al. Successful reconstruction of late portal vein stenosis after liver transplantation. Arch Surg 1989;124:503–505.

88. Zajko AB, Bron KM, Orons PD. Vascular complications in liver transplant recipients: angiographic diagnosis and treatment. Semin Intervent Radiol 1992;9:317–322.

89. Zajko AB, Sheng R, Bron K, et al. Percutaneous transluminal angioplasty of venous anastomotic stenoses complicating liver transplantation: intermediate-term results. J Vasc Interv Radiol 1994;5:121–126.

90. McDaniel HM, Johnson M, Pescovitz MD, et al. Intraoperative placement of a Wallstent for portal vein stenosis and thrombosis after liver transplantation. Transplantation 1997;63:607–608.

91. Funaki B, Rosenblum JD, Leef JA, et al. Percutaneous treatment of portal venous stenosis in children and adolescents with segmental hepatic transplants: long-term results. Radiology 2000;215:147–151.

92. Koneru B, Tzakis AG, Bowman J III, et al. Postoperative surgical complications. Gastroenterol Clin North Am 1988;17:71–91.

93. Hashimoto K, Shimada M, Suehiro T, et al. Gore-Tex jump graft for portal vein thrombosis following living donor transplantation. Hepatogastroenterology 2003;50:1146–1148.

94. Cherukuri R, Haskal ZJ, Naji A, et al. Percutaneous thrombolysis and stent placement for the treatment of portal vein thrombosis after liver transplantation: long-term follow-up. Transplantation 1998;65:1124–1126.

95. Baccarani U, Gasparini D, Risaliti A, et al. Percutaneous mechanical fragmentation and stent placement for the treatment of early posttransplantation portal vein thrombosis. Transplantation 2001;72:1572–1582.

96. Olcott EW, Ring EJ, Roberts JP, et al. Percutaneous transhepatic portal vein angioplasty and stent placement after liver transplantation: early experience. J Vasc Interv Radiol 1990;1:17–22.

97. Bhattacharjya T, Olliff SP, Bhattacharjya S, et al. Percutaneous portal vein thrombolysis and endovascular stent for management of posttransplant portal venous conduit thrombosis. Transplantation 2000;69:2195–2198.

98. Bilbao JI, Vivas I, Elduayen B, et al. Limitations of percutaneous techniques in the treatment of portal vein thrombosis. Cardiovasc Intervent Radiol 1999;22:417–422.

99. Ciccarelli O, Goffette P, Laterre PF, et al. Transjugular intrahepatic portosystemic shunt approach and local thrombolysis for treatment of early posttransplant portal vein thrombosis. Transplantation 2001;72:159–161.

100. Kato T, Levi D, Nery JR, et al. Operative procedures. In: Maddrey WC, Schiff ER, Sorrell MF, eds. Transplantation of the Liver. Philadelphia: Lippincott Williams and Wilkins, 2001:53.

101. de Villa VH, Chen CL, Chen YS, et al. Right lobe living donor liver transplantation—addressing the middle hepatic vein controversy. Ann Surg 2003;238:275–282.

102. Nghiem H. Imaging of hepatic transplantation. Radiol Clin North Am 1998;36:429–442.

103. Zajko AB, Claus D, Clapuyt P, et al. Obstruction to hepatic venous drainage after liver transplantation: treatment with balloon angioplasty. Radiology 1989;170:763–765.

104. Rose BS, Van Aman ME, Simon DC, et al. Transluminal balloon angioplasty of infrahepatic caval anastomotic stenosis following liver transplantation: case report. Cardiovasc Intervent Radiol 1988;11:79–81.

105. Borsa JJ, Daly CP, Fonaine AB, et al. Treatment of inferior vena cava anastomotic stenoses with the Wallstent endoprosthesis after orthotopic liver transplantation. J Vasc Interv Radiol 1999;10:17–22.

106. Weeks SM, Gerber DA, Jaques PF, et al. Primary Gianturco stent placement for inferior vena cava abnormalities following liver transplantation. J Vasc Interv Radiol 2000;11:177–187.

107. Simo G, Echenagusia A, Camunez F, et al. Stenosis of the inferior vena cava after liver transplantation: treatment with Gianturco expandable metallic stents. Cardiovasc Intervent Radiol 1995;18:212–216.

108. Orons PD, Hari AK, Zajko AB, et al. Thrombolysis and endovascular stent placement for inferior vena caval thrombosis in a liver transplant recipient. Transplantation 1997;64:1357–1361.

109. Sze DY, Semba CP, Razavi MK, et al. Endovascular treatment of hepatic venous outflow obstruction after piggyback technique liver transplantation. Transplantation 1999;68:446–449.

110. Egawa H, Tanaka K, Uemoto S, et al. Relief of hepatic vein stenosis by balloon angioplasty after living-related donor liver transplantation. Clin Transplant 1993;7:306–311.

111. Colapinto RF, Blendis LM. Liver biopsy through the transjugular approach. Modification of instrumentation. Radiology 1983;148:306.

112. Choh J, Dolmatch B, Safadi R. Transjugular core liver biopsy with a 19-gauge spring-loaded cutting needle. Cardiovasc Intervent Radiol 1998;21:88–90.

113. Azoulay D, Raccuia JS, Roche B, et al. The value of early transjugular liver biopsy after liver transplantation. Transplantation 1996;15:406–409.

114. Little AF, Zajko AB, Orons PD. Transjugular liver biopsy: a prospective study in 43 patients with the Quick-Core biopsy needle. J Vasc Interv Radiol 1996;7:127–131.

115. Smith TP, Presson TL, Heneghan MA, et al. Transjugular biopsy of the liver in pediatric and adult patients using an 18-gauge automated core biopsy needle: a retrospective review of 410 consecutive procedures. Am J Roentgenol 2003;180:167–172.

116. Tripathi D, Therapondos G, Redhead DN, et al. Transjugular intrahepatic portosystemic stent-shunt and its effects on orthotopic liver transplantation. Eur J Gastroenterol Hepatol 2002;14:827–832.

117. Rosado B, Kamath PS. Transjugular intrahepatic portosystemic shunts: an update. Liver Transpl 2003;9:207–217.

118. Khan TT, Reddy KS, Johnston TD, et al. Transjugular intrahepatic portosystemic shunt migration in patients undergoing liver transplantation. Int Surg 2002;87:279–281.

119. Chui AK, Rao AR, Waugh RC, et al. Liver transplantation in patients with transjugular intrahepatic portosystemic shunts. Aust N Z Surg 2000;70:493–495.

120. Hutchins RR, Patch D, Tibballs J, et al. Liver transplantation complicated by embedded transjugular intrahepatic portosystemic shunt: a new method for portal anastomosis—a surgical salvage procedure. Liver Transpl 2000;6:237–238.

121. Rumi MN, Schumann R, Freeman RB, et al. Acute transjugular intrahepatic portosystemic shunt migration into pulmonary artery during liver transplantation. Transplantation 1999;67:1492–1494.

122. Wilson MW, Gordon RL, LaBerge JM, et al. Liver transplantation complicated by malpositioned transjugular intrahepatic portosystemic shunts. J Vasc Interv Radiol 1995;6:695–699.

123. Amesur NB, Zajko AB, Orons PD, et al. Transjugular intrahepatic portosystemic shunt in patients who have undergone liver transplantation. J Vasc Interv Radiol 1999;10:569–573.

124. Lerut JP, Goffettee P, Molle G, et al. Transjugular intrahepatic portosystemic shunt after adult transplantation: experience in eight patients. Transplantation 1999;15:379–384.

Percutaneous Management of Portal Hypertension

31

Ziv J. Haskal

The role of interventional radiologists in the management of portal hypertension is a long and innovative one. It spans management of surgically created portosystemic shunts, stand-alone therapies such as variceal sclerotherapy and embolization, and, ultimately, an endovascular replacement for the surgical shunt: the transjugular intrahepatic portosystemic shunt (TIPS). The latter, available for patients since 1988, has transformed the management of life-threatening complications of portal hypertension and, with continuing device and procedural evolution, offers the promise of definitive control of symptoms in suitable candidates.

TRANSHEPATIC VARICEAL EMBOLIZATION

Percutaneous transhepatic catheterization of the portal vein was first described in 1971 by Weichel (1). In 1974, Lunderquist and Vang published their initial results with transhepatic catheterization and occlusion of the coronary vein in patients with portal hypertension and esophageal varices (2). Numerous clinical studies followed, reporting the results of transhepatic or transjugular approaches to deliver a number of embolic agents, including autologous clot, gelfoam sponges soaked in tetradecyl sulfate, stainless steel Gianturco coils, bucrylate, and, most widely, ethanol (3–21) (Figure 31–1). The latter had the advantage of causing an intense coagulation of blood cells, disruption of vascular endothelium, and vascular thrombosis. As experience with the procedure grew, several significant problems emerged, eclipsing promising early results. First, recurrent bleeding was common, ranging from 30% to 61%. Despite transcatheter occlusion of all demonstrable coronary and short gastric veins, latent veins would enlarge or recanalize to resupply the varices. Second, the procedure led to portal vein thrombosis in 16–20% of cases because occlusion of the coronary and short gastric veins, which provided the major venous outflow in those patients, led to stagnation of portal flow.

The largest published experience with transhepatic variceal embolization was reported by L'Hermine et al. in 1989 (22–26). Four hundred patients underwent embolization over a 7-year period. Overall technical failure and complication rates were 9% and 7%, respectively. Sixty-five percent of patients had Child's class C cirrhosis, and 35% had class B. Patients were embolized with either ethanol and stainless steel coils or bucrylate. Bleeding was controlled in 83% of patients treated emergently. The 10-day survival rate was 76%, with 97 deaths from recurrent bleeding or liver failure. Recurrent bleeding occurred in 55% of patients at 6 months (38% Child's class B, 70% class C) and 81% of patients at 2 years (71% Child's class B, 90% Child's class C). Half the patients who rebled were controlled with medical therapy. At 1 year, 48% were alive, and at 5 years, 26% were alive.

These sobering results, combined with the emergence of flexible endoscopy and proven efficacy of sclerotherapy

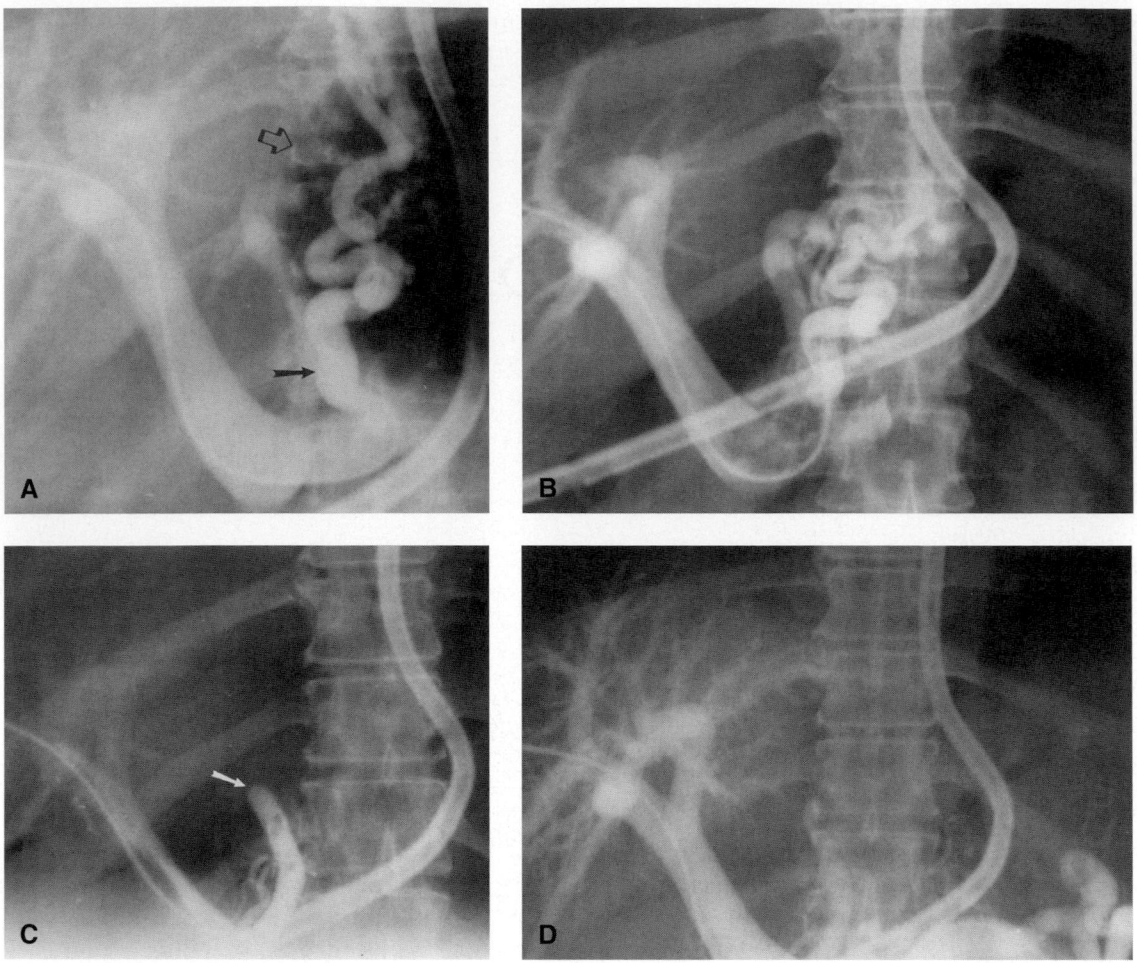

Figure 31–1 Transhepatic variceal embolization in a 43-year-old man with uncontrolled variceal bleeding. **A.** Transhepatic portography demonstrates hepatofugal filling of varices (*arrow*) despite an inflated balloon tamponade catheter (*open arrow*). **B.** The coronary vein is catheterized with a curved angiographic catheter, and contrast venography is performed. **C.** Coronary venography after embolization with absolute alcohol demonstrates successful occlusion of the vein (*arrow*). **D.** Final splenic venography demonstrates no residual variceal flow. The balloon tamponade catheter has been deflated. (Courtesy of C. Cope, M.D.)

obviated the need for transhepatic embolization in most patients. At present, the procedure has been abandoned except when performed in concert with formation of transjugular intrahepatic portosystemic shunts, treatment of residual or recurrent varices after portosystemic shunt surgery, or for control of excessive encephalopathy because of large spontaneous native shunts.

PERCUTANEOUS REVISION OF SURGICAL PORTOSYSTEMIC SHUNTS

The role of surgical shunts has waned since the dissemination of transjugular intrahepatic portosystemic shunts (TIPS). Shunts still have importance in specific scenarios, including pediatric patients, certain cases of noncirrhotic portal hypertension, chronic and extensive cavernous

transformation of the portal system (wherein nonanatomic shunts can be constructed), and cases of repeatedly failing TIPS. Once created, most shunts are prone to varying degrees of stenosis, intimal hyperplasia, and thrombosis. Most surgical shunts, excepting Rex shunts, can be readily catheterized from a femoral venous approach. This access affords several possible interventions, including balloon dilatation of stenotic shunts, recanalization of occluded shunts, and transshunt embolization of recurrent or residual varices.

Stenoses caused by intimal hyperplasia or technical factors may occasionally limit flow through small-bore surgical shunts. As with most forms of bypass grafts, balloon dilatation can improve luminal diameter, although recurrent stenosis may be frequent (23–26). Use of metallic stents to possibly lessen recurrence of stenoses and/or to establish larger lumina is well accepted (27).

Completely occluded shunts can often be recanalized by probing the anastomosis with standard coaxial angiographic catheters. Occlusive thrombus can be macerated using balloon catheters, angioplasty, and stent placements. Another approach was that reported by Cope et al., who successfully used fibrinolytic therapy to restore flow through occluded mesocaval and mesoatrial shunts (28,29). In most cases, though, the amount of thrombus within a shunt is relatively small, and the described mechanical means are both sufficient and more rapid than catheter-directed lysis.

Transshunt catheterization of the portal system can be used to embolize residual or recurrent varices. Partially decompressive surgical portosystemic shunts often leave residual flow to the varices. Some surgeons routinely request variceal embolization 1 week after creation of small-bore portocaval shunts. Postoperative transshunt embolization is less likely to cause portal vein thrombosis than transhepatic embolization alone because the shunt provides an alternate low-pressure outlet for portal flow (25,30). In addition, this may increase the percentage of nutritive flow reaching the intrahepatic portal vein. Variceal embolization is also useful in patients with selective surgical shunts. The distal splenorenal shunt disconnects the splenic–coronary–short gastric pathway responsible for variceal engorgement from the intact mesenteroportal axis and redirects its flow into the left renal vein. Over time, native portosystemic collaterals often develop between the high-pressure mesenteroportal system and lower-pressure splenorenal system, leading to recurrent varices. These varices can occasionally be treated with transfemoral catheterization of the splenorenal shunt and collateral vein embolization (13,31).

Finally, intentional coil occlusion of surgical or spontaneous portosystemic shunts has been performed to reverse severe postoperative portosystemic encephalopathy or accelerated liver failure (13,32,33).

TRANSJUGULAR INTRAHEPATIC PORTOSYSTEMIC SHUNTS (TIPS)

The concept of percutaneously creating a portosystemic shunt within the liver was envisioned by Drs. Rosch and Hanafee in 1969 during canine investigations of transjugular cholangiography (34). The procedure was replicated in humans in 1982 by Colapinto et al. (35). However, a full 20 years elapsed from postulate to the first "modern" human transjugular intrahepatic portosystemic shunt (TIPS) because of the development of the metal stent. In 1988, shunts were created in humans by Richter et al. and lined with Palmaz stents. At that time, the procedures were complex, multihour procedures involving transhepatic targeting baskets, transjugular approaches, and so on. Since then, the procedure has undergone many iterative technical improvements (36). Tens of thousands of TIPS have been performed worldwide for the treatment of complications of liver disease, and more than 1,200 relevant scientific

papers have been published in the English language alone, including numerous randomized trials. TIPS now represents a routine and mandatory option in the treatment of portal hypertension.

Technique

The prototypic TIPS is created in several steps: mapping a suitable hepatic vein, typically the dominant right hepatic vein; passing a long, curved needle from within it into the liver parenchyma until a suitable branch of the intrahepatic portal vein is punctured; passing guide wires and catheters across this liver tract into the portal system, mapping it, and performing hemodynamic assessments; dilating the tissue bridge between the portal and hepatic vein; and deploying a stent across this tract and enlarging it to a diameter that achieves the desired degree of portal (and portosystemic pressure gradient) reduction to suit the specific clinical indication (Figures 31–2 through 31–4).

Many variations exist in the instrument sets, stents, and techniques used to fashion a TIPS, although basic principles remain the same. Shunts are created using purely fluoroscopic guidance, combined external ultrasound and fluoroscopic guidance (37), fluoroscopic and intravascular ultrasound guidance (38,39), CT guidance (40,41), directly from the inferior vena cava (transcaval), through retrograde transmesenteric approaches (through minilaparotomies) (42,43), and so on. Most of the variations in technique have focused on attempts to expedite creation of the transvenous tract because this step remains the most difficult for most operators. The majority of procedures are still performed using fluoroscopic guidance alone. With experience, this approach can accomplish TIPS formation routinely in 1.5 hours or less. It can be performed under conscious sedation or general anesthesia. Elective patients are typically discharged the next morning.

Contraindications and Complications

The contraindications to creating a TIPS are partly shared with surgical portosystemic shunts and partly unique to the procedure. Heart failure, marked pulmonary hypertension, severe encephalopathy, and advanced liver disease all represent potentially absolute contraindications to TIPS either because of the inability to handle the increased cardiac work associated with the natural elevations in atrial pressures and cardiac output after a portosystemic shunt (44) or because of the poor liver reserve and inability to handle further deprivation of nutrient portal flow. Several relative contraindications to TIPS have been described, including portal system thromboses (Figure 31–5), hepatic vein thromboses (Figure 31–6), hepatic malignancies, polycystic liver disease, and biliary dilatation. Though these pose greater technical challenges, shunts have been routinely created in all these settings. Creating shunts in appropriate candidates with these conditions (e.g., palliating refractory ascites in a hepatoma patient with intraportal

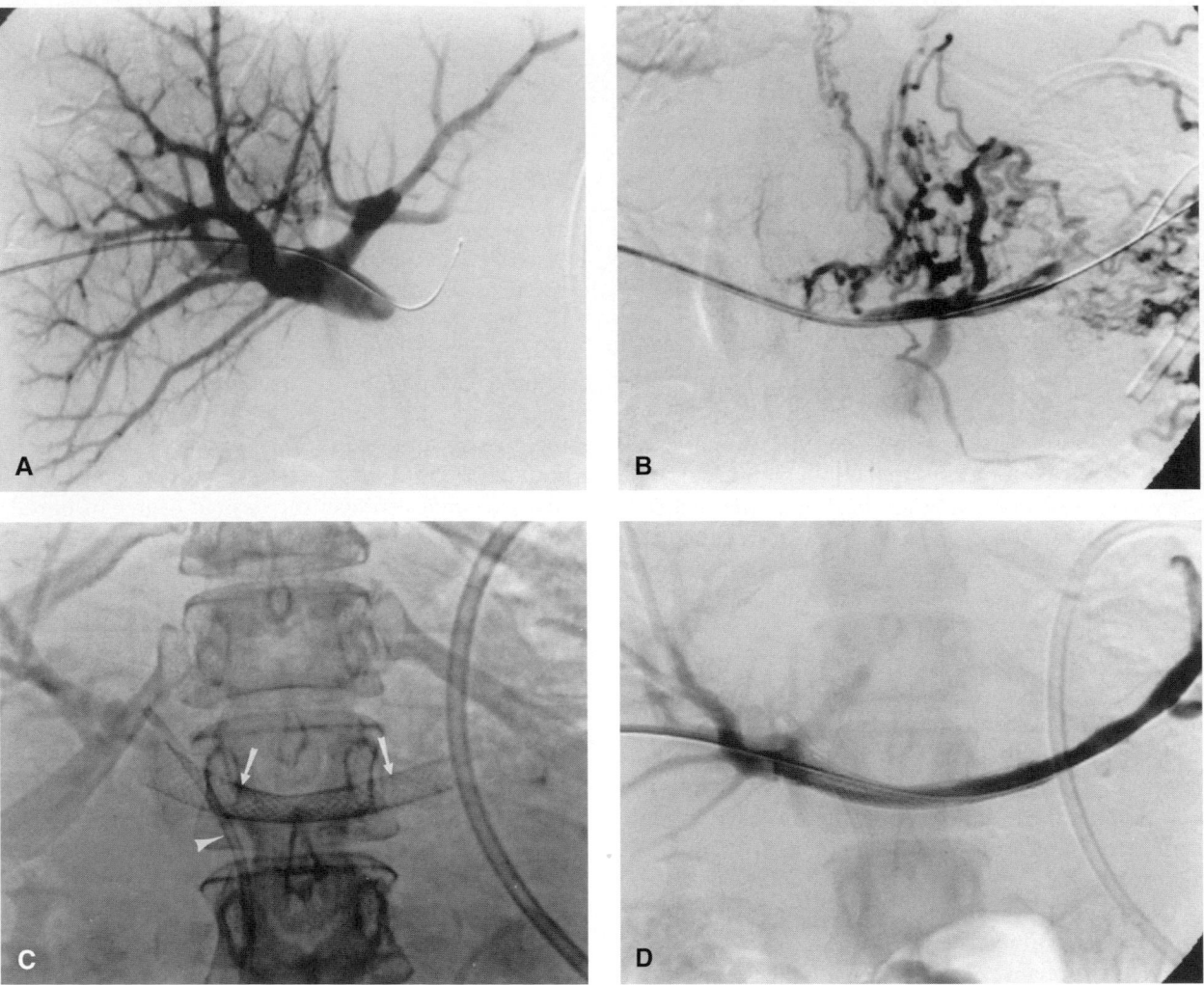

Figure 31–2 Percutaneous treatment of sinistral portal hypertension. Transhepatic recanalization of splenoportal thrombosis in a 39-year-old woman with a history of prior pancreatitis and gastric variceal bleeding. Liver biopsy was normal. **A.** Transhepatic portography demonstrates the occlusion of the mid portal vein. The intrahepatic portal vein is unremarkable. The portal pressure is 6 mm Hg. **B.** Hand-injected splenic venography demonstrates hepatofugal flow into multiple short gastric veins leading to gastric varices. The distal splenic vein, at the splenoportal confluence, is occluded. The splenic vein pressure is 17 mm Hg. **C.** A Wallstent has been deployed across the occlusion (*arrows*). A preexisting endoscopic biliary stent is visible (*arrowhead*). **D.** Splenic venography after stent placement demonstrates no residual variceal flow. The splenic and portal vein pressures measure 8 mm Hg.

thrombus) requires careful preprocedure imaging and planning. This emphasizes the necessity of preprocedure cross-sectional imaging in all but the emergent life-threatening indications, using either ultrasound, MRI, or CT. Assessment of portal vein patency and detection of hepatic masses is performed at this point.

In elective TIPS patients with impaired hepatic synthetic function (e.g., total serum bilirubin >3 mg/dL), careful consultations with referring hepatologists is important in understanding the medical necessity of the procedure (compared with alternatives) and the possibility of transplant rescue should liver function significantly deteriorate after TIPS.

The reported complications of TIPS are many, ranging from procedurally related ones to those shared by all forms of portal decompression (e.g., worsening liver function and encephalopathy). In experienced hands, procedural complications should be infrequent. A Society of Interventional Radiology TIPS Quality Improvement document described a list of the more common important complications, dividing them into major and minor severities, and described the following reported incidences for each (45):

- Major complications (3%): hemoperitoneum, 0.5%; gallbladder puncture, 1%; stent malposition, 1%; hemobilia, 2%; radiation skin burn, 0.1%; hepatic infarction, 0.5%; renal failure requiring chronic dialysis, 0.25%; hepatic artery injury, 1%

- Minor complications (4%): transient contrast-induced renal failure, 2%; encephalopathy controlled by medical therapy, 15–25%; fever, 2%; transient pulmonary edema, 1%; entry site hematoma, 2%

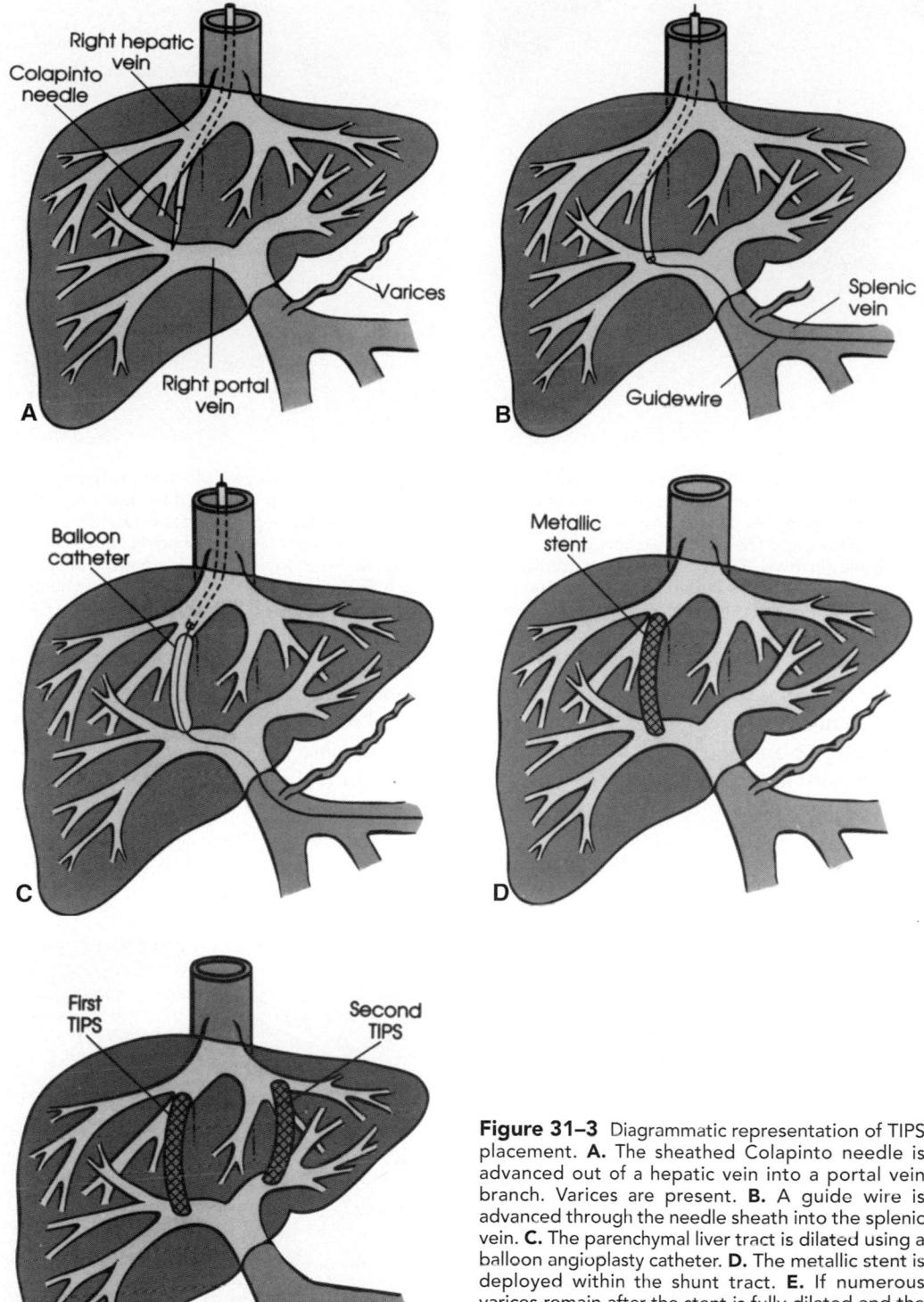

Figure 31–3 Diagrammatic representation of TIPS placement. **A.** The sheathed Colapinto needle is advanced out of a hepatic vein into a portal vein branch. Varices are present. **B.** A guide wire is advanced through the needle sheath into the splenic vein. **C.** The parenchymal liver tract is dilated using a balloon angioplasty catheter. **D.** The metallic stent is deployed within the shunt tract. **E.** If numerous varices remain after the stent is fully dilated and the portosystemic gradient remains elevated, then a second, parallel TIPS is constructed. (Reprinted with permission from Current Techniques in Interventional Radiology. Current Medicine, 1994.)

Mortality rates attributable to intraprocedural complications should not exceed 1–2%. The reported incidence of new or worsened encephalopathy ranges 15–31% and largely depends on the severity of preexisting liver disease and encephalopathy (46–48). Patients treated for refractory ascites often have higher baseline encephalopathy than those with variceal bleeding and better preserved liver function and thus may experience more encephalopathy after TIPS. In controlled trials comparing TIPS with alternative forms of therapy (large-volume paracentesis), the incidence

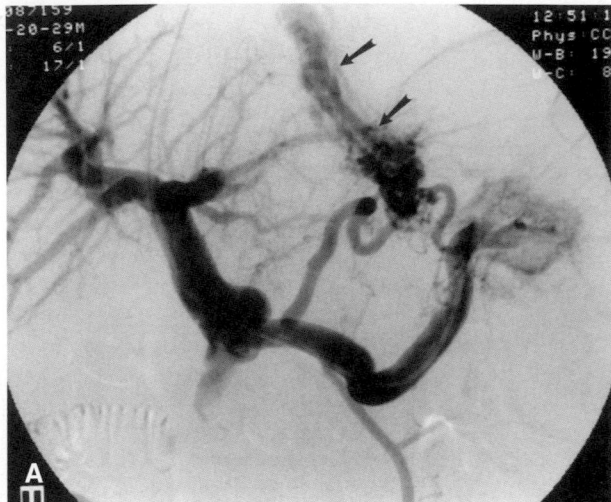
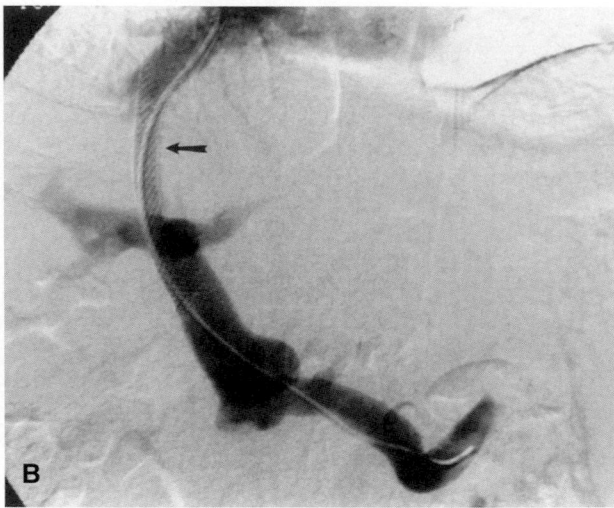

Figure 31–4   TIPS placement in a patient with a patent portal vein. A 36-year-old man presents for elective TIPS after repeated episodes of esophageal variceal hemorrhage despite three episodes of sclerotherapy. **A.** Initial transjugular splenic venography demonstrates hepatopedal portal flow with fugal flow into the coronary, short gastric, and inferior mesenteric veins. The esophageal varices are visible (*arrows*). The portosystemic gradient is 18 mm Hg. **B.** Transjugular portogram after placement of a 10-mm right hepatic-to-right portal vein TIPS (*arrow*) demonstrates flow through the shunt into the hepatic vein. There is no residual variceal flow. The portosystemic gradient is 9 mm Hg.

of encephalopathy was always greater in those who received a TIPS. Fortunately, for most patients the encephalopathy responds to standard therapy, and only rarely (~5%) must the TIPS be adjusted to control the encephalopathy. In cases of uncontrolled encephalopathy, the shunts can be intentionally narrowed or occluded using a variety of reported techniques (49–54). Caution is warranted when intentionally occluding

a shunt because doing so has been reported to initiate hepatorenal syndrome in a small number of patients (55). There is no evidence that using lactulose in all patients following a TIPS reduces the incidence of encephalopathy.

Shunt dysfunction (reported at 18–78%) (56–62) has been inaptly described as a complication of TIPS; this is no more true of TIPS than is erroneously classifying loss of

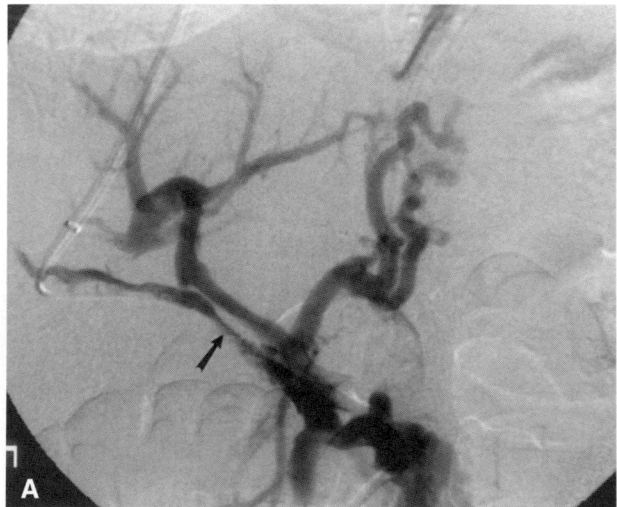
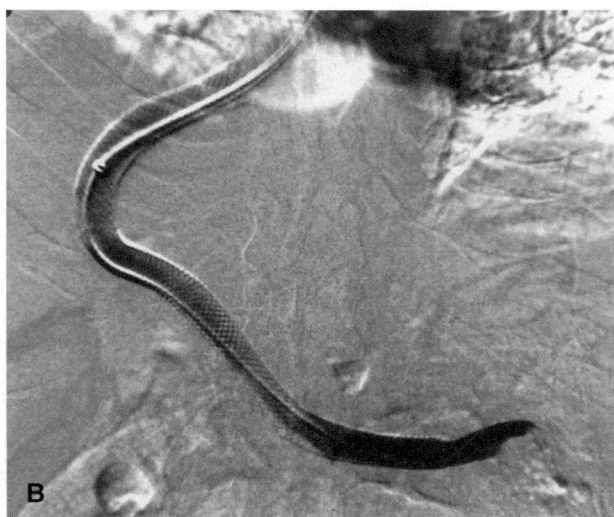

Figure 31–5   TIPS formation in the setting of distal splenic and portal vein thrombosis. A 52-year-old female with alcoholic cirrhosis and seven episodes of gastric and esophageal variceal bleeding. Preshunt sonography demonstrated no flow in the portal vein. **A.** Portography after transjugular recanalization of the chronically occluded portal vein. After balloon fragmentation of the thrombus, there is some hepatopetal flow in the portal vein (*arrow*). Hepatofugal variceal flow is present. The initial portosystemic gradient was 28 mm Hg. **B.** Splenic venography after recanalization of the splenic and portal veins and creation of a 12-mm diameter TIPS. The stents extend from the occluded splenic vein into the right hepatic vein. No variceal flow remains. The portosystemic gradient is 12 mm Hg.

patency of femoropopliteal grafts as a complication. The topic of TIPS patency is addressed in a later section in this chapter.

Indications and Results

The ability to create a portosystemic shunt through this non-operative fashion has both largely made obsolete the conventional surgical portosystemic shunt and vastly increased the indications for and use of portal decompression therapies. Suggested indications for TIPS have included acute esophageal variceal bleeding, recurrent esophageal variceal bleeding, gastric variceal bleeding, ectopic varices bleeding (e.g., intestinal, anorectal, and stomal), portal gastropathy and gastric antral vascular ectasia (GAVE), refractory ascites, hepatic hydrothorax, Budd-Chiari syndrome, hepatopulmonary syndrome, and hepatorenal syndrome.

Acute Esophageal Variceal Bleeding Refractory to Medical Treatment

Actively bleeding esophageal varices can be controlled with pharmacologic and endoscopic therapy (band ligation or sclerotherapy) in most patients. These treatments form first-line therapy. Patients who continue to bleed or who rebleed despite aggressive management become candidates for portal decompression. Most reports of emergent surgical shunting in this setting describe high mortality rates (30–77%) (63–65). Vangeli et al. pooled data from 15 reports on 509 acutely bleeding TIPS patients who failed medical therapy (66). They found the mean rate of control of acute variceal bleeding by TIPS was 93.6 ± 6.7%, with an early rebleeding rate of 12.4 ± 6.1%. Notably, the in-hospital or 6-week mortality rate was 35.8 ± 16%. Thus TIPS is quite

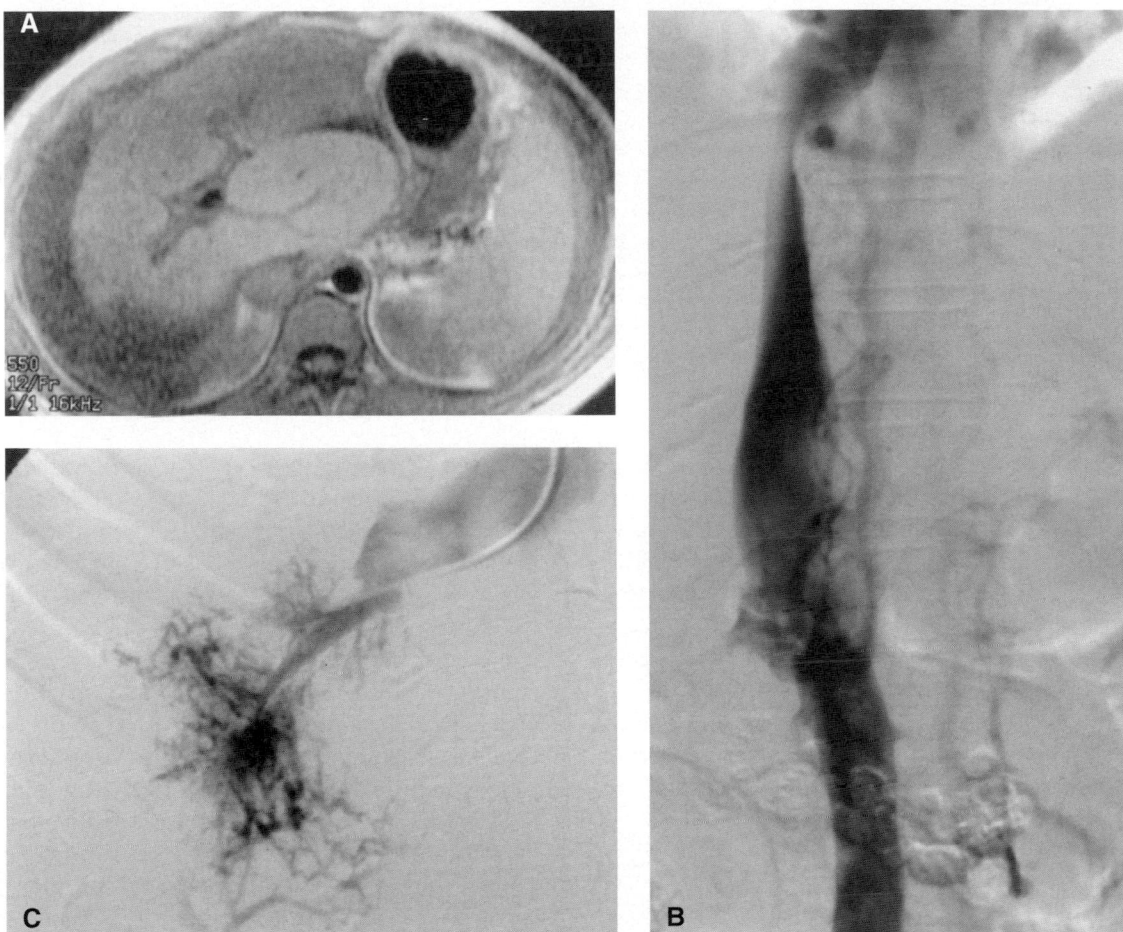

Figure 31–6 TIPS for treatment of hepatic veno-occlusive disease/Budd-Chiari syndrome. A 27-year-old woman presented with hypotension, variceal bleeding, massive ascites, hepatosplenomegaly, and lower extremity edema. Subsequent bone marrow biopsy revealed a myeloproliferative disorder. Within 1 week of TIPS placement, the patient spontaneously diuresed 16 kg of fluid; her ascites and pedal edema completely resolved. At 2-year follow-up, she was fully functional and remains free of symptoms. Her liver function is normal. **A.** Upper abdominal magnetic resonance image demonstrates marked enlargement of the caudate lobe and ascites. **B.** Inferior vena cavagram demonstrates marked narrowing of the intrahepatic cava and collateral filling of the paravertebral veins. A 28-mm Hg gradient was measured across the caval narrowing.

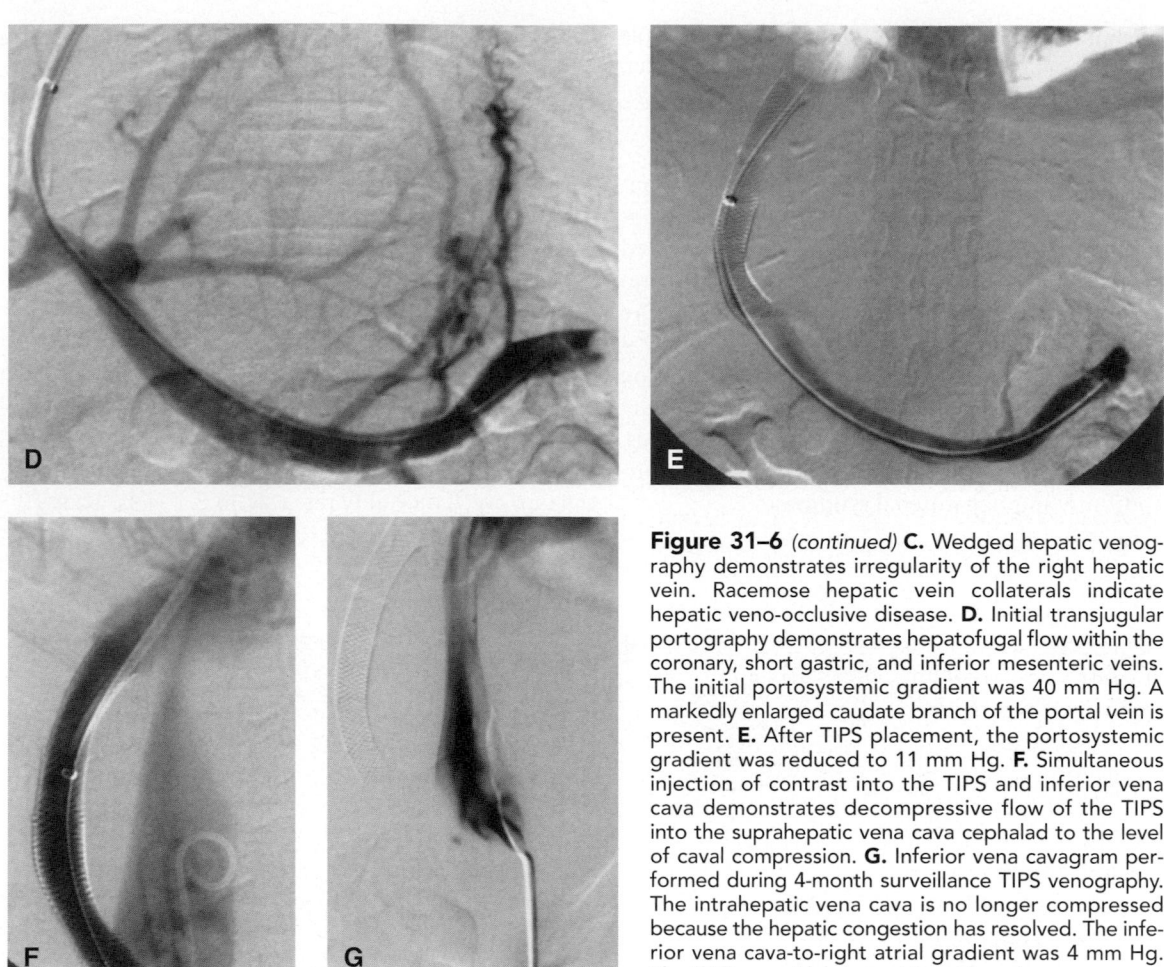

Figure 31–6 *(continued)* **C.** Wedged hepatic venography demonstrates irregularity of the right hepatic vein. Racemose hepatic vein collaterals indicate hepatic veno-occlusive disease. **D.** Initial transjugular portography demonstrates hepatofugal flow within the coronary, short gastric, and inferior mesenteric veins. The initial portosystemic gradient was 40 mm Hg. A markedly enlarged caudate branch of the portal vein is present. **E.** After TIPS placement, the portosystemic gradient was reduced to 11 mm Hg. **F.** Simultaneous injection of contrast into the TIPS and inferior vena cava demonstrates decompressive flow of the TIPS into the suprahepatic vena cava cephalad to the level of caval compression. **G.** Inferior vena cavagram performed during 4-month surveillance TIPS venography. The intrahepatic vena cava is no longer compressed because the hepatic congestion has resolved. The inferior vena cava-to-right atrial gradient was 4 mm Hg. The TIPS was widely patent (*not shown*).

effective in arresting bleeding with a low risk of rebleeding. Unfortunately, as expected mortality is quite high; approximately one third of patients die within 6 weeks of the procedure. Many reports have described prognostic variables predicting early mortality after TIPS. Significant factors include (but are not limited to) MELD scores (67–72), Child-Pugh class or score (73), pre-TIPS APACHE II scores (74–78), preprocedure total bilirubin (>3 mg/dL) (75), urgency of the procedure, and endotracheal intubation (79,80). Salvage therapy with TIPS is important in the acute setting but may not increase midterm survival in many of these critically ill patients.

Recurrent Esophageal Variceal Bleeding

Once esophageal varices have bled, the risk of rebleeding is at least 50%, and many patients who rebleed will die (81,82). Hence, a number of therapies have been used to prevent rebleeding in these patients (63). When surgical shunts were compared with endoscopic therapy, rebleeding rates were reduced in the surgical shunt cases, although hepatic encephalopathy was increased and mortality was unaffected (63,83,84). In meta-analyses of 376 and 811

patients, rebleeding rates for endoscopic therapies were 49.8% and 46.6% versus 12.4% and 18.9% for TIPS, respectively (63,84). As TIPS is a partially decompressive portosystemic shunt, the expectation has been that similar findings would be reported when TIPS was compared with alternative forms of therapy. More than 10 randomized trials have compared TIPS with endoscopic treatment of varices (mostly sclerotherapy) (56–62,85–87). These trials vary widely in inclusion criteria, including severity of liver disease, number of prior bleeding episodes, severity of (and preexisting therapies for) encephalopathy, and timing of randomization. Nevertheless, all trials focused on secondary prevention of variceal bleeding. Not surprisingly, as with surgery, the rate of variceal rebleeding was lower with TIPS, although encephalopathy was higher. The median rebleeding rate in nine trials was 16% for TIPS and 44% for endoscopic therapies. The cost of treating these patients with a TIPS was greater than endoscopic therapy in one report (88). Survival was rarely improved (85), emphasizing the progressive nature of advanced liver disease and the need for these patients to be under the cooperative care of hepatologists, interventional radiologists, and transplant surgeons who are focused on potential liver transplantation.

It is clear that both TIPS and surgical shunts are the most effective methods for the prevention of rebleeding. One trial has been published in which TIPS was compared with an H-graft surgically placed shunt (89,90). The patients were not randomized but were studied as pairs, that is, one receiving a surgical shunt and the second a TIPS. Selection criteria, reporting biases, and operator experience flaw the study and limit the ability to generalize its results. The frequency of rebleeding was 16% in the TIPS group and 3% in the surgical group. The patients undergoing TIPS required frequent interventions to maintain TIPS patency. In numerous cases, failing TIPS could not be restored to patency—an event that would be deemed extraordinary with current practice. Thirty-day and total mortality were 15% versus 20% and 43% versus 30% in the TIPS and surgery groups, respectively. Another randomized, controlled trial comparing TIPS with distal splenorenal shunts is approaching completion.

No evidence supports the use of TIPS for primary prophylaxis of variceal bleeding, that is, at initial diagnosis of varices but prior to any bleeding. Until controlled trials, primary prophylaxis is achieved with medical therapy and, rarely, endoscopic means.

TIPS has also been compared with pharmacologic therapy in a small number of patients. In one series of 91 patients, the risk of rebleeding during 2 years of follow-up was 39% in those who received pharmacologic therapy and 13% in those receiving a TIPS (91). Encephalopathy developed in 14% of those receiving drugs and 38% of TIPS patients. Child-Pugh class improved in 72% of the drug group but in only 45% of the TIPS group. The 2-year probability of survival was the same in both groups, 72%. The cost of therapy for those receiving a TIPS was twice that of the pharmacologic group (91). Of note is that in some of the trials, the patients were medical failures, whereas in others, they had a single bleed before being randomized.

Gastric Varices

The efficacy of TIPS in the control of bleeding from gastric varices has been reported in a number of small series. In none of the trials were the patients randomized to alternative therapies, and in most, the TIPS was performed because of refractory bleeding. In some series, the initial portosystemic gradient in patients with gastric varices was lower than those with esophageal varices, whereas in other series, no differences were seen (92–96). In these small series, TIPS was equally effective in controlling bleeding from gastric as well as esophageal varices. Controlled trials comparing surgical shunts or glue in the treatment of these patients would help to better define the role of TIPS in the management of patients with bleeding from gastric varices. In the author's opinion, TIPS is an important tool in the control of gastric variceal bleeding, although the final portosystemic gradient required to achieve variceal decompression may be lower than that required for esophageal

variceal bleeding, and embolization of the varices also may be required.

In recent years, Asian researchers have reported increasing use of balloon-occluded retrograde transvenous obliteration (BRTO) for treatment of fundal varices (97–101). The left renal vein and outflow of the gastric varices (often normally decompressing through a spleno–gastro–renal pathway) are catheterized. An occlusion balloon is inflated within the portosystemic collateral, and a sclerosing agent is infused. One 20-patient trial comparing endoscopic sclerotherapy to transvenous obliteration reported results similar to endoscopic therapy with less transvenous sclerosant used. In another, 1-year follow-up endoscopies revealed variceal decrease or disappearance in 81%. Some authors have suggested that portal perfusion can be improved by occlusion of competing splenorenal shunts in such patients (102).

Ectopic Varices

Duodenal, intestinal, stomal, and anorectal varices are uncommon when compared with esophageal and gastric varices and, as such, are unlikely to be evaluated in a randomized trial comparing TIPS with alternative treatments (103–119). Few alternative therapies exist (once medical management has failed) short of surgical shunts or resection of affected bowel segments. As varices in these settings represent spontaneous portosystemic collateral pathways that become manifest in response to portal hypertension, it is not surprising that these varices can respond well to TIPS.

It is worth emphasizing the difficulty of diagnosing intestinal varices. There are no reports validating the role of CT or MRI in this setting. This emphasizes the need for diagnostic visceral angiography in patients with liver disease and unexplained lower gastrointestinal bleeding, even in the absence of active bleeding. Careful attention to the venous phase will demonstrate the presence of varices, often at the sites of adhesions related to prior surgeries. These varices may decompress into more unusual channels, such as the gonadal or ovarian veins. Capsule endoscopy may also be useful in establishing the diagnosis.

Portal Hypertensive Gastropathy (PHG) and Gastric Antral Vascular Ectasia (GAVE)

These two entities are distinct yet can both co-exist or be difficult to distinguish during endoscopy. The mucosa in PHG can show a mosaiclike pattern, usually within the fundus or body of the stomach. GAVE is characterized by linear or diffuse red patches within the antrum. PHG is limited to patients with portal hypertension, whereas GAVE can be seen in a variety of conditions (120). Several series have examined the effect of TIPS on PHG and GAVE (121–126). In one report, 75% of patients with severe PHG showed both endoscopic improvement and a decrease in the need for transfusions (126). In another series, 9 of 10 patients showed endoscopic improvement in PHG following TIPS (127). In the author's experience, TIPS is useful in controlling blood loss due to portal gastropathy or its similar manifestations within the duodenum or small bowel. In contrast, bleeding from GAVE in patients with cirrhosis was unaffected by TIPS. At present, GAVE is not an indication for TIPS. It is best treated with endoscopic ablation, using either argon plasma coagulation, lasers, or heater probes. For patients with severe recurrent bleeding or uncontrollable acute bleeding from GAVE, an antrectomy with Billroth I anastomosis may be needed.

Refractory Ascites

In the early 1990s the lead indication for TIPS was variceal bleeding. As experience has grown, and, perhaps, endoscopic therapies have evolved, refractory ascites has become the leading indication for TIPS at many transplant centers. Ascites is considered refractory to medical treatment when it is unresponsive to or intolerant of sodium restriction and high doses of diuretics (400 mg/day spironolactone and 160 gm/day furosemide) (128). Once refractory ascites develops, the patient has a poor prognosis, with approximately 50% of the patients dead within 12 months (129). While far fewer randomized trials comparing TIPS with paracentesis exist, compared to those for variceal bleeding, conclusions can still be drawn. TIPS can clearly reduce the incidence of cirrhotic ascites and reduce the need for diuretic use and large-volume paracentesis (LVP). Pooling the data from four controlled trials encompassing 264 patients, the mean improvement in ascites was 57.8% for TIPS, compared with 19% for LVP (130–133). The number of paracentesis procedures was lower in the TIPS group. Improvements in creatinine clearance and reduced diuretic requirements were described in survivors. Encephalopathy was somewhat greater in the TIPS groups, 34.0 ± 19.8%, compared with the LVP groups, 18.5 ± 12.0%. Somewhat surprisingly, there was no difference in the quality of life between the two groups in one of the studies (132). Cost effectiveness was not examined in any of the studies. A transplant-free survival benefit for TIPS was seen in one trial (131) but not in another (132). Overall survival was not improved in the NASTRA trial, although a 6-month mean survival difference was seen in the TIPS patients—arguably notable in a patient population in whom survival without transplant is typically limited.

One recent prospective study randomized patients with refractory ascites to TIPS and pleuroperitoneal (Denver) shunts (134). Primary median shunt patencies were similar (TIPS, 4.4 months; Denver, 4.0 months), although assisted patencies were 31 months for TIPS, compared with 13 months for the Denver shunts. Survival in the TIPS groups was also longer, 28.7 months versus 16 months. These findings favor the use of TIPS in refractory ascites patients who can tolerate portal decompression.

The technical challenges of creating a TIPS in patients with refractory ascites may be greater as the liver and donor hepatic veins are more shrunken than in typical variceal bleeding patients. Technical tricks in these settings include the use of carbon dioxide wedged portography to visualize the portal system, reduced iodinated contrast volumes, exaggerated curves upon the portal access needles, vein exit sites that lie more dorsal and closer to the junction with the inferior vena cava, and the use of transmesenteric techniques or intravascular ultrasound guidance for transcaval shunt construction.

Refractory Hepatic Hydrothorax

Hepatic hydrothorax can develop in patients with cirrhotic ascites when diaphragmatic pores allow fluid to pass between the peritoneal and pleural spaces. In most patients the defect is in the diaphragm that overlies the dome of the liver. Hepatic hydrothorax is estimated to occur in approximately 5% of cirrhotics and may be found in the presence or absence of concomitant ascites. In a series of small studies, the effect of TIPS has been relatively uniform, with resolution of the hepatic hydrothorax or a decrease in the need for thoracentesis (135–142). Because alternatives are few for these patients (e.g., pleuroperitoneal shunts), TIPS provides important first-line care when diuresis fails.

Hepatorenal Syndrome (HRS)

Hepatorenal syndrome (HRS) is a feared complication of liver disease whose development often brings a poor prognosis. It exists in two forms. Type 1 is a rapidly progressive form (2 weeks) of renal failure, whereas type 2 hepatorenal syndrome brings a more insidious onset of renal failure. The prognosis for patients with type 1 HRS is significantly worse than for those with type 2 hepatorenal syndrome (143,144). TIPS has been used in a number of patients with HRS, yielding reports of improved glomerular filtration rates, renal plasma flow, and urine sodium handling and drops in serum creatinine and plasma aldosterone (145–152). Whereas survival in type 1 HRS after TIPS appears improved compared with historical expectations, none of the trials was randomized, and no comparative survival benefits have been shown. In one series, only 20% of the patients with type 1 HRS were alive 1 year after TIPS insertion, whereas with type 2 HRS approximately 45% were alive after 1 year (145,152). In the four controlled trials in which TIPS was compared with LVP in the control of refractory cirrhotic ascites discussed above, there was no consistent improvement in renal function with TIPS compared with LVP. although one did find a reduced incidence of HRS in those receiving a TIPS (132). Pre-TIPS bilirubin levels were predictive of survival in these patients as well (152). TIPS needs to be compared with other therapies, such as terlipressin, before its widespread role in the treatment of the HRS is determined (153).

Budd-Chiari Syndrome (BCS)

Budd-Chiari syndrome (BCS) results from blockage of exit of the blood from the liver, resulting from either hepatic vein thrombosis or obstruction of the inferior vena cava (154,155). Liver injury, fibrosis, and cirrhosis result from unremitting hepatic congestion, a condition unmitigated by anticoagulation. Surgical shunts have long proved useful in preventing or stabilizing liver disease in BCS patients, although their prothrombotic tendencies and caval compression have required more extensive surgeries, including mesoatrial shunts. Accordingly, it is logical that TIPS could afford the same benefits in properly selected BCS patients. While numerous case series (156–174) have described the beneficial use of TIPS in acute and chronic BCS, no long-term or prospective controlled trials have compared TIPS with medical or surgical therapies. Reports of greater need for reinterventions have been reported in BCS patients undergoing TIPS (168,175), likely related to underlying hypercoagulability or anatomic issues related to the TIPS. Indeed, it must be noted that TIPS construction in BCS patients can be significantly more demanding that in cirrhotic patients. In BCS patients, the liver is swollen in both posteroanterior and cephalocaudal dimensions (the opposite of the often shrunken liver seen in ascites patients), the liver parenchyma may be "soft" (making it easier to disrupt with needle passes), and extensive hepatic vein collateral may provide near-continuous confusing return of blood into the puncture needle during its slow withdrawal during TIPS formation. The underlying prothrombotic tendencies may require heavy doses of anticoagulant to prevent acute thrombosis of bare stents. Finally, in the absence of hepatic vein remnants, the shunt must be constructed from the vena cava, raising the risk of inadvertent right atrial or intraperitoneal puncture. In the author's decade-long experience of treating acute and chronic BCS patients with TIPS, these technical challenges have proved significant and warrant adjustments in conventional techniques, including the use of adjunctive imaging such as external ultrasound, coaxial fine-needle systems, percutaneous cholangiography-type injections of contrast (for portal localization), and antiplatelet agents. With these modifications, however, shunts can be constructed safely and expeditiously (Figure 31–6). In the author's experience, only one BCS patient in 10 years treated with TIPS has undergone liver transplantation—a patient with preexisting established Child's class C cirrhosis. Annual biopsies of these patients have shown regression of sinusoidal congestion after TIPS and absence of developing fibrosis (176).

Shunt Patency

As TIPS use spread in the early 1990s, it became clear that stenoses and occlusions developed frequently, placing patients at risk of potentially serious or life-threatening recurrent complications (Figure 31–7). Numerous studies described the phenomenon and rates of TIPS dysfunction, ranging 18–78% (56–58,60,61,86,87,177). Undoubtedly, these variations reflect sampling intervals and relative accuracies of surveillance techniques. Most physicians have utilized Doppler sonography to assess shunt patency (178–199). Indeed, many early reports described high accuracies, although these retrospective case series suffered from inconsistent patency standards, lack of gold-standard comparisons with catheter venography, and, arguably, lack of clinically relevant definitions of patency. Further, some larger later studies were flawed because sonographic criteria of shunt dysfunction were used to trigger gold-standard venography, but when sonography suggested no shunt dysfunction, patency was assumed without venographic proof (192,200). Sonography is, by nature, limited in its ability to characterize degrees of relevant shunt patency because minimum lumen diameter and percent diameter stenosis alone are surrogates for TIPS patency. Maintenance of a low portosystemic pressure gradient is the goal—a measure that inconsistently follows percent diameter stenosis (201).

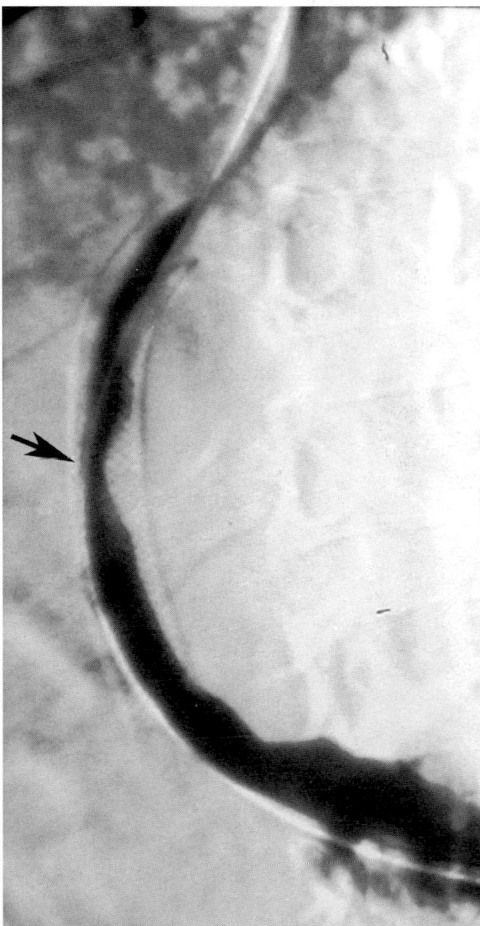

Figure 31–7 Six-month venography of a TIPS created with a Wallstent demonstrates diffuse intrastent and outflow hepatic vein stenosis.

One prospective study compared 151 Doppler sonograms with TIPS venograms and assessments of portal pressure. Using a success or failure definition of a portosystemic gradient of < or ≥15 mm Hg, respectively, sonography provided a sensitivity and specificity of only 86% and 48%, respectively (191). Thus, an abnormal Doppler ultrasound is predictive of occlusion or stenosis whereas a normal ultrasound does not exclude TIPS dysfunction (191,196,202–205). The best indicator of TIPS dysfunction is a recurrence of the problem for which the TIPS was originally inserted, either variceal bleeding, hepatic hydrothorax, or ascites. If recurrent varices are identified by upper endoscopy, the TIPS is most likely insufficient. Documentation of patency can be achieved with certainty only by recatheterization of the shunt, venography, and hemodynamic assessments. Interestingly, though, as device developments improve primary shunt patency and physician confidence increases, sonography may become increasingly useful, because absolute accuracy will be less necessary.

The histopathology of TIPS thrombosis and stenosis has been characterized (206–213). In 1991, LaBerge first described the histology of TIPS in seven patients who had undergone liver transplantation (208). At 4 days after TIPS, fresh clot adhered to the mesh of the Wallstents lining the tracts. By 3 weeks, the shunt lumen was lined with a 400–600 µm-thick layer of pseudointimal tissue. At 3 months, the stents were enveloped within a layer of dense collagen. Analyses have also been performed of the histopathologic response of humans and swine to TIPS creation (214). Human livers from necropsy and liver transplantation containing TIPS that had been in place 10–1,089 days were evaluated using a variety of histologic stains, including hematoxylin and eosin, trichrome, and immunohistochemical stains for smooth muscle cell actin, high-molecular-weight cytokeratins, and factor VIII. The parenchymal tracts of the shunts were lined with circumferential layers of myofibroblasts and collagen matrix. The

cells appeared to originate from the liver surface (by proliferating nuclear cell antibody studies) and grew to entirely encapsulate the stents. The shunt lumina were lined with a single cell layer that stained positive for factor VIII, indicating that neoendothelia had formed.

In 1993, LaBerge expanded upon her initial findings in a small series of TIPS patients with stenotic and occluded shunts (207). Based upon bile staining seen in several occluded shunts, the authors proposed that the inflammatory effect of biliary leakage into the shunt lumen might have contributed to thrombus accumulation and shunt occlusion. Several clinical case reports reporting biliary fistulae and shunt occlusions followed (210,215–217). In 1996, Saxon et al. reported a comparative study of 13 swine TIPS and 21 human TIPS, in which they proposed that macroscopic leaks of bile contributed to loss of shunt patency in a large proportion of their swine and human TIPS (209). Jalan provided further support of the bile leak theory by describing stenotic TIPS biopsies that revealed bile incorporation within thrombus (218). In three cases, major bile duct transection was closely related to shunt stenosis.

In the author's experience, bile leaks have played a visible and potent role in rapid and recurrent shunt thrombosis in a prominent but small portion of human patients with stenotic or occluded TIPS. Bile-to-TIPS fistulae were implicated in shunt thrombosis within hours of TIPS creation and as late as 2.5 years after TIPS. Sanyal et al. characterized the histology of 35 shunts, finding that smooth muscle cell proliferation was found in both stenotic and nonstenotic TIPS, independent of the gross morphology or presence of biliary fistulae within the shunts (206).

An experiment by Teng et al. sheds light on the role of bile in acute shunt thrombosis (212). In culturing smooth muscle cells with bile, serum and bile, and serum alone, they found that bile was a powerful inhibitor of smooth muscle cell proliferation. These findings suggest that TIPS failure associated with bile leaks is probably caused by the thrombogenic effect of bile combined with its inhibitory effect upon endothelialization and healing of the TIPS tract. Thus bile plays a prominent, partial role in the mechanism of TIPS stenosis. In cases of rapid and recurring stenosis, bile duct transection may be the prime mover, whereas in other cases, the proliferative fibroblast layers may simply represent a healing response to the massive local liver injury that occurs with stretching and tearing of liver parenchyma during tract angioplasty and stent placement. As fibroblasts are scattered throughout the liver, it is not surprising that they proliferate in response to shunt creation.

The outflow hepatic vein represents a separate site of shunt stenosis (177). In one prospective study of TIPS, all hepatic veins shrank an average of 50% in diameter in response to TIPS, accounting for the flow-limiting lesions in most cases (219). Typically, this process begins 3–6 months after the shunt creation. The proliferating smooth muscle cells that narrow the hepatic vein are identical and

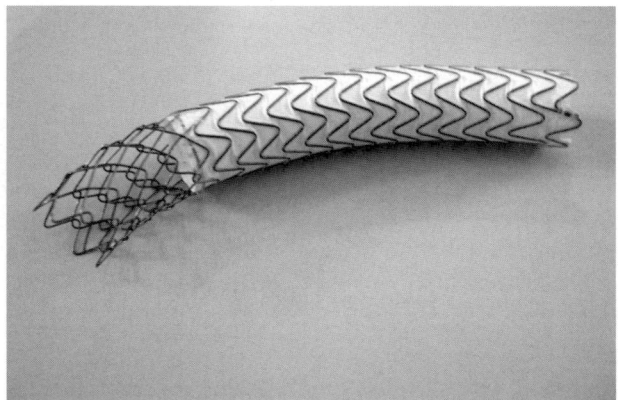

Figure 31–8 Viatorr (W. L. Gore) TIPS endosprosthesis is an expanded polytetrafluorethylene-lined stent graft designed for TIPS applications. The leading 2-cm-long bare end is placed within the patent portal vein. The graft-bearing portion lines the parenchymal tract and outflow hepatic vein.

continuous with those that line the parenchymal tract (206,213). This intimal hyperplasia mimics the standard biologic response seen at many surgical graft anastomoses, including dialysis access grafts, coronary bypasses, or lower extremity bypass grafts. Bile leaks have no apparent role in the remote hepatic vein stenosis in TIPS—the latter is likely related phenomena implicated in intimal hyperplasia elsewhere, including shear stress (220,221). Anticoagulation might not be expected to affect secondary hepatic vein stenosis resulting from intimal hyperplasia, but it might reduce early shunt thrombosis related to bile or other unknown local or systemic factors. Sauer et al. evaluated this question by randomizing 49 patients with variceal bleeding to prophylactic anticoagulation after TIPS (222). During the 3 months of post-TIPS anticoagulation, five shunt occlusions developed in the control group, with none in the treatment group. During subsequent months of follow-up, there was no difference in the rate of shunt stenosis between the two groups. It is unknown whether any of the occlusions were related to bile leaks. Siegerstetter et al. randomized 84 patients to receive standard heparin treatment or a combination of trapidil, a drug with anti-platelet-derived growth factor (PDGF) activity, and ticlopidine, a platelet aggregation inhibitor (223). These findings suggest that the incidence of hepatic vein stenosis could be reduced by combined inhibition of platelet aggregation and PDGF activity. Certainly it is clear that TIPS failure occurs at multiple sites and for multiple reasons. Treatments intended to prolong shunt patency must address all causes.

Improving TIPS Patency: The Use of Stent Grafts

Research into improving TIPS patency has moved in many directions, including brachytherapy (single doses with afterloaders and fractionated doses via "hot" stents), external-beam irradiation, oral medications (e.g., anticoagulants, antiplatelet agents), and local delivery of antiproliferative drugs into the TIPS tract. Most investigations, however, have been directed toward combining porous stent skeletons with biocompatible graft materials. TIPS stent grafts have proved to be the next step in TIPS evolution and the ones that will affect the day-to-day management of TIPS.

The porcine model is well suited to TIPS formation and device testing because shunt formation is achieved using the identical techniques and equipment used in humans, and the porcine pathologic response is similar to that seen in human TIPS, that is, fibroblast proliferation and extracellular matrix deposition within the parenchymal tract, followed by hepatic vein stenoses at a later stage (224). Unlike humans, however, the model provides a highly accelerated rate of shunt stenosis, typically occurring within 2–4 weeks of TIPS formation (Figures 31–6, 31–7). Fortunately, porcine TIPS stenoses develop in the absence of portal hypertension—an advantage, because inducing durable portal hypertension in pigs has proved extremely difficult (225,226).

A variety of graft materials and coatings have been studied in both swine and human TIPS in an attempt to prolong TIPS patency, including silicone, polytetrafluoroethylene (PTFE), and polyethylene terephthalate (PET), composite polyurethane-coated Dacron-covered stents, and polycarbonate urethane covered stents. Swine TIPS lined with expanded PTFE (ePTFE) have shown marked improvements in shunt patency when compared with bare stent controls. In 1995, Nishimine et al. published the first animal investigation evaluating the efficacy of covered stents for TIPS (224). They compared the results of 13 swine TIPS lined with bare stents with 13 swine TIPS lined with handmade PTFE stent grafts. At 4 weeks, one control TIPS was patent (8%), whereas 9 of 13 (69%) of the PTFE stent grafts demonstrated a stenosis of less than 50%. By 3 months, six of the 13 stent grafts remained patent (defined as <50% shunt stenosis). In five cases, hepatic vein stenoses contributed to loss of graft patency. In 1997, these results were expanded upon using an encapsulated, ePTFE stent graft designed specifically for TIPS (227). Eight TIPS were created in eight pigs by using this stent graft. All but one shunt were patent at 1-, 3-, 4-, and 5-month explant and venography. In contrast, the Wallstent control group developed occlusions or stenoses of 45–85% within 4 weeks. The observed histologic responses mimicked those of humans. One year later, similar results were reported using a different experimental nitinol stent lined with ultrathin ePTFE (W. L. Gore & Associates). At follow-up ranging 30–60 days, the mean stenosis within the graft group was 16% compared with 59% in the control group (228). This stent graft was subsequently redesigned to further reduce its permeability to bile and cells; it served as the basis for the current Viatorr device (W. L. Gore & Associates). In controlled trials using this stent graft for porcine shunt creation and revision of stenotic TIPS, mean luminal shunt stenosis seen at 60 and 90 days proved lower still.

Other graft materials have failed to show the improvements of PTFE. Tanihata et al. found near-uniform early shunt thrombosis in 14 swine TIPS lined with silicone-covered Wallstents (229). Otal et al. reported high occlusion rates in swine TIPS lined with prototype PET-covered nitinol stent grafts (230). Haskal and Brennecke noted no improvement in patency with PET-covered Wallstents (Wallgrafts) compared with bare stents, with mean stenoses of 53% and 45%, respectively (231). In both series, the PET incited a reaction typical of polyester vascular implants, including diffuse penetration and paving of the grafts by fibroblasts and collagen matrix. The porosity of polyester grafts is much higher than that of PTFE, allowing transgraft tissue growth, a phenomenon that may limit the success of such grafts in humans. Presumably, the fabric would fail as a bile barrier because of its gross permeability.

In 1998, Bloch et al. reported the use of a polyurethane-coated, Dacron-covered spiral Z stent graft in six young swine. At 3 weeks, 5 of 6 shunts were occluded. At 6 weeks, all were occluded. Histology reportedly demonstrated a marked foreign body reaction with superimposed thrombosis (232). Haskal and Brennecke evaluated polycarbonate urethane stent grafts of porous and nonporous formulations for TIPS (233). Akin to the PET grafts, the porous graft-lined samples showed marked inflammation with diffuse fibroblast proliferation through the lumina. In contrast, the nonporous devices elicited little pseudointimal hyperplasia within the lumen, yielding a mean maximum percent stenosis of 26% at 8 weeks. Of note, however, were 2 of 7 (28%) shunt thromboses.

These experimental findings suggest that the exclusionary effect of a biocompatible graft is one of the most important in a TIPS application. The findings also support the concept that the stimulus for myofibroblast proliferation originates within the liver parenchyma rather than the bloodstream because the tissue collar develops on the outer surface of the grafts, at the liver surface.

Saxon et al. published the results of an important pilot study evaluating stent grafts for revisions of TIPS stenoses and occlusions (234). Six patients with an initial mean primary TIPS patency of 50 days (range, 9–100 days) had their TIPS lined with a modified Z-stent endoskeleton supporting a 4-mm Gore PTFE graft (W. L. Gore & Associates) that had been dilated to 14 mm in diameter. Once delivered, the PTFE was sandwiched against the shunt lumen with a standard Wallstent. Three patients had initially demonstrable biliary fistulae. Of five surviving patients, three remained patent at a mean venographic follow-up of 315 days. One shunt occluded, and one became stenotic because of graft misplacement. The authors concluded that PTFE-covered stent grafts were effective for revision of TIPS in patients with tract stenosis and occlusion.

Ferral et al. reported use of a modified Cragg Endopro System I stent graft (Mintec), a polyester fabric-coated nitinol stent, for creation of TIPS in 13 patients (235). Using unspecified sonographic criteria, one shunt was deemed stenotic at an unspecified follow-up interval, while two shunts were found occluded at 2- and 3-month follow-up. While performance of shunt venography, the gold-standard exam for evaluating the degree of shunt stenosis, was described as having been performed, the results of these portograms were not; this technical note focused largely upon the acute and short-term results of the devices in a TIPS application. A small series later described repeated acute shunt thrombosis in patients who had TIPS lined with PET-covered Wallstents, all of which were successfully salvaged using PTFE stent grafts (236). Why polyester stent grafts incite thrombosis in de novo TIPS in contrast to their desirable properties in arterial applications is unclear. Whether they are equally thrombotic in revision TIPS applications is also unknown.

Expanding on the promising results with animal and pilot studies with PTFE, numerous case reports and series reporting patency improvements when homemade PTFE TIPS stent grafts appeared (38,236–241). In 2000, the Viatorr

TIPS endoprosthesis (W. L. Gore & Associates) became available in Europe (Figure 31–8). Since then, several thousand TIPS stent grafts have been implanted for de novo or revision applications and reports of outcome are rapidly appearing in publication (242–250). In one series typifying the results described in other retrospective Viatorr series, Hausegger et al. reported primary patencies of 87% and 80% at 6 and 12 months, respectively, using sonographic or venographic criteria (247). Notably, the mean initial post-TIPS patency of 6 mm Hg was almost unchanged in those patients undergoing 6-month venography—arguably one of the most critical endpoints in shunt function. In a retrospective case-matched series of bare stent TIPS versus stent grafts, Angermayr et al. reported statistically significant survival improvements in patients receiving PTFE grafts (244).

In 1999, the multicenter U.S. pivotal randomized trial comparing de novo TIPS created with the Wallstent and Viatorr was begun. This trial was completed in 2004, after enrolling 253 patients. As such, it represents the largest randomized, controlled trial in TIPS to date. While final study data has not been published, several data can be shared by the principal investigator (Z. Haskal). At 6-month venography, percent diameter TIPS stenosis was significantly lower in the Viatorr group (16% versus 42%, $p < 0.001$) (Figures 31–9, 31–10). For perspective, a 40% stenosis within a 10-mm TIPS (as was created in the majority of enrollees) reduces the effective shunt lumen to 6 mm, yielding a percent flow reduction of greater than 80%. A 16%-mm reduction in a 10-mm Viatorr TIPS represents a 0.8-mm thickness of luminal tissue lining the shunts, arguably representing

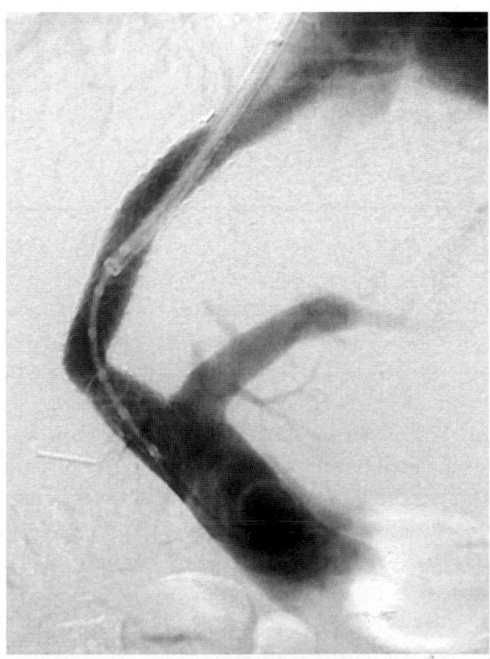

Figure 31–9 Nine-month portal venogram of a TIPS lined with the Viatorr stent graft demonstrates no evidence of shunt stenosis.

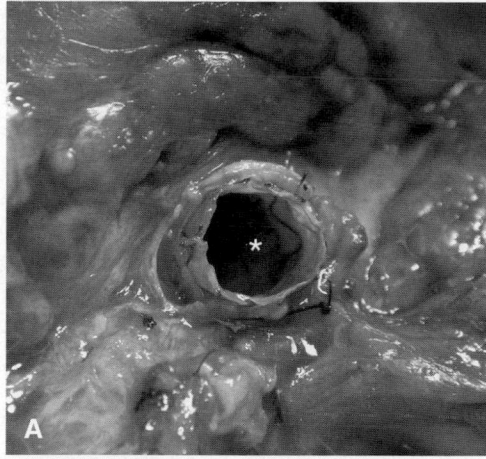

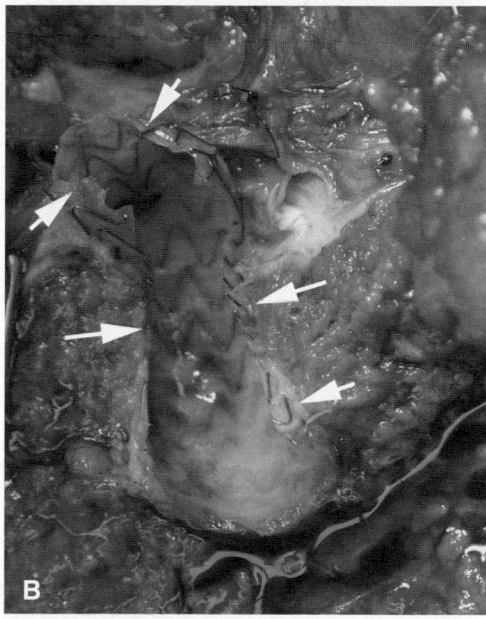

Figure 31–10 Fourteen-month explant of a Viatorr-lined TIPS at liver transplantation. **A.** Cross-sectional view of the hepatic vein end demonstrates a widely patent lumen (*asterisk*). **B.** Clamshell view of the shunt (*arrows*) demonstrates a thin, glistening layer of tissue on the interior of the patent shunt.

desirable graft incorporation. Portosystemic gradients were also significantly higher in the Wallstent group at 6 months, compared with similar initial postprocedure gradient endpoints. There was only one Viatorr patency loss resulting from diameter stenosis (DS) greater than 50%, occurring in an unstented hepatic vein. In contrast, 11 Wallstent patency losses occurred, a 10-fold greater incidence. By Kaplan Meyer analysis, time to reinterventions was also significantly shorter in the Wallstent group (p = 0.007). Encephalopathy and serious adverse events were not significantly different between the groups. These results and the additional ones that will emerge from this trial (and other prospective PTFE TIPS graft trials) indicate a dramatic and inarguable improvement in primary TIPS patency and a reduction in the need for subsequent invasive interventions

and vigilant patency surveillance. As such, TIPS stent grafts mark a major step in TIPS evolution, by providing the out-of-the-gate durability lacking in bare stents. Studies comparing TIPS, endoscopic therapies, and surgery may bear repetition, and controlled trials of smaller caliber may prove useful in select populations by minimizing the negative effects of portal decompression on liver perfusion.

REFERENCES

1. Weichel KL. Tekniken vid perkutan transhepatisk portapunton (PTP). Nord Med 1971; 86:912–913.
2. Lunderquist A, Vang J. Transhepatic catheterization and obliteration of the coronary vein in patients with portal hypertension and esophageal varices. N Engl J Med 1974;291:646–649.
3. Lunderquist A, Borjesson B, Owman T, Bengmark S. Isobutyl 2-cyanoacrylate (bucrylate) in obliteration of gastric coronary vein and esophageal varices. AJR Am J Roentgenol 1978; 130:1-6.
4. Uflacker R. Percutaneous transhepatic obliteration of gastroesophageal varices using absolute alcohol. Radiology 1983;148: 621–625.
5. Widrich WC, Srinivasan M, Johnson WC. Transhepatic embolisation of gastroesophageal varices: analysis of results in 190 patients. Semin Intervent Radiol 1988;5:76–84.
6. Sos TA. Transhepatic portal venous embolization of varices: pros and cons. Radiology 1983;148:569–570.
7. Vinel JP, Scotto JM, Levade M, et al. Embolization of esophageal varices by the transjugular route in severe digestive hemorrhage in cirrhotic patients. Prospective study of 83 patients. Gastroenterol Clin Biol 1985;9:814–818.
8. Menu Y, Gayet B, Nahum H. Bleeding duodenal varices: diagnosis and treatment by percutaneous portography and transcatheter embolization. Gastrointest Radiol 1987;12:111–113.
9. Ozaki CK, Hansen M, Kadir S. Transhepatic embolization of superior mesenteric varices in portal hypertension. Surgery 1989;105: 446–448.
10. Samaraweera RN, Feldman L, Widrich WC, et al. Stomal varices: percutaneous transhepatic embolization. Radiology 1989;170 : 779–782.
11. Benner KG, Keeffe EB, Keller FS, et al. Clinical outcome after percutaneous transhepatic obliteration of esophageal varices. Gastroenterology 1983;85:146–153.
12. Bengmark S, Borjesson B, Hoevels J, et al. Obliteration of esophageal varices by PTP: a follow-up of 43 patients. Ann Surg 1979;190:549–554.
13. Widrich WC, Robbins AH, Nabseth DC. Transhepatic embolization of varices. Cardiovasc Intervent Radiol 1980;3:298–303.
14. Keller FS, Dotter CT, Rosch J. Percutaneous transhepatic obliteration of gastroesophageal varices: some technical aspects. Radiology 1978;129:327–332.
15. Widrich WC, Johnson WC, Robbins AH, et al. Esophagogastric variceal hemorrhage: its treatment by percutaneous transephatic coronary vein occlusion. Arch Surg 1978;113:1331–1338.
16. Viamonte M Jr, Pereiras R, Russell E, et al. Transhepatic obliteration of gastroesophageal varices: results in acute and nonacute bleeders. AJR Am J Roentgenol 1977;129:237–241.
17. Ellman BA, Curry TS 3rd, Glotzbach RE, et al. Systemic embolization as a complication of transhepatic venography. Radiology 1981;141:67–71.
18. Johnson WC, Nabseth DC, Widrich WC, et al. Bleeding esophageal varices: treatment with vasopressin, transhepatic embolization and selective splenorenal shunting. Ann Surg 1982;195:393–400.
19. Terabayashi H, Ohnishi K, Tsunoda T, et al. Prospective controlled trial of elective endoscopic sclerotherapy in comparison with percutaneous transhepatic obliteration of esophageal varices in patients with nonalcoholic cirrhosis. Gastroenterology 1987;93: 1205–1209.
20. Funaro AH, Ring EJ, Freiman DB, et al. Transhepatic obliteration of esophageal varices using the stainless steel coil. AJR Am J Roentgenol 1979;133:1123–1125.

21. Durham JD, Kumpe DA, Van Stiegmann G, et al. Direct catheterization of the mesenteric vein: combined surgical and radiologic approach to the treatment of variceal hemorrhage. Radiology 1990;177:229–233.
22. L'Hermine C, Chastanet P, Delemazure O, et al. Percutaneous transhepatic embolization of gastroesophageal varices: results in 400 patients. Am J Roentgenol 1989;152:755–760.
23. Cope C. Dilatation of mesocaval shunts. Ann Radiol 1986;29:178–180.
24. Grosso M, Spalluto F, Rossato D, et al.. Percutaneous unblocking of porto-systemic shunts. Personal experience with 11 cases. Radiol Med 1990;80:334–338.
25. Ruff RJ, Chuang VP, Alspaugh JP, et al. Percutaneous vascular intervention after surgical shunting for portal hypertension. Radiology 1987;164:469–474.
26. Soyer P, Levesque M, Zeitoun G. Treatment of mesocaval shunt stenosis with a metallic stent. AJR Am J Roentgenol 1992;158:1251–1253.
27. Hausegger KA, Klein GE, Fluckiger F, et al. Stenosis of a surgical portosystemic shunt—treatment with angioplasty and placement of a Wallstent. Cardiovasc Intervent Radiol 1993;16:243–244.
28. Cope C. Balloon dilatation of closed mesocaval shunts. AJR Am J Roentgenol 1980;135:989–993.
29. Savader SJ, Venbrux AC, Klein AS, et al. Percutaneous intervention in portosystemic shunts in Budd-Chiari syndrome. J Vasc Interv Radiol 1991;2:489–495.
30. Coldwell DM, Moore AD, Ben-Menachem Y, et al. Bleeding gastroesophageal varices: gastric vein embolization after partial portal decompression. Radiology 1991;178:249–251.
31. Henderson JM, Gong-Liang J, Galloway J, et al. Portaprival collaterals following distal splenorenal shunt. Incidence, magnitude and associated portal perfusion changes. J Hepatol 1985;1:649–661.
32. Uflacker R, d'Albuquerque LA, de Oliveira e Silva A, et al. Embolization to reverse severe recurrent hepatic encephalopathy. Arq Gastroenterol 1988;25:21–25.
33. Uflacker R, de Oliveira e Silva A, d'Albuquerque LA, et al. Chronic portosystemic encephalopathy: embolization of portosystemic shunts. Radiology 1987;165:721–725.
34. Rosch J, Hanafee WN, Snow H. Transjugular portal venography and radiologic portacaval shunt: an experimental study. Radiology 1969;92:1112–1114.
35. Colapinto RF, Stronell RD, Gildiner M, et al. Formation of intrahepatic portosystemic shunts using a balloon dilatation catheter: preliminary clinical experience. AJR Am J Roentgenol 1983;140:709–714.
36. Richter GM, Palmaz JC, Noldge G, et al. The transjugular intrahepatic portosystemic stent-shunt. A new nonsurgical percutaneous method. Radiologe 1989;29:406–411.
37. Roeren T, Richter GM, Limberg B, et al. Ultrasound guided puncture of the portal vein in transjugular intrahepatic portasystemic stent shunt (TIPSS). Radiologe 1996;36:677–682.
38. Petersen B, Uchida BT, Timmermans H, et al. Intravascular US-guided direct intrahepatic portacaval shunt with a PTFE-covered stent-graft: feasibility study in swine and initial clinical results. J Vasc Interv Radiol 2001;12:475–486.
39. Petersen B. Intravascular ultrasound-guided direct intrahepatic portacaval shunt: description of technique and technical refinements. J Vasc Interv Radiol 2003;14:21–32.
40. Bloch R, Fontaine A, Borsa J, et al. CT-guided transfemoral portacaval shunt creation. Cardiovasc Intervent Radiol 2001;24:106–110.
41. Quinn SF, Sheley RC, Semonsen KG. Creation of a portal vein to inferior vena cava shunt using CT guidance and a covered endovascular stent. AJR Am J Roentgenol 1997;169:1159–1160.
42. Rozenblit G, Del Guercio LR. Combined transmesenteric and transjugular approach for intrahepatic portosystemic shunt placement. J Vasc Interv Radiol 1993;4:661–666.
43. Rozenblit G, DelGuercio LR, Savino JA, et al. Transmesenteric-transfemoral method of intrahepatic portosystemic shunt placement with minilaparotomy. J Vasc Interv Radiol 1996;7:499–506.
44. Azoulay D, Castaing D, Dennison A, et al. Transjugular intrahepatic portosystemic shunt worsens the hyperdynamic circulatory state of the cirrhotic patient: preliminary report of a prospective study. Hepatology 1994;19:129–132.
45. Haskal ZJ, Martin L, Cardella JF, et al. Quality improvement guidelines for transjugular intrahepatic portosystemic shunts.
SCVIR Standards of Practice Committee. J Vasc Interv Radiol 2001;12:131–136.
46. Jalan R, Elton RA, Redhead DN, et al. Analysis of prognostic variables in the prediction of mortality, shunt failure, variceal rebleeding and encephalopathy following the transjugular intrahepatic portosystemic stent-shunt for variceal haemorrhage. J Hepatol 1995;23:123–128.
47. Sanyal AJ, Freedman AM, Shiffman ML, et al. Portosystemic encephalopathy after transjugular intrahepatic portosystemic shunt: results of a prospective controlled study. Hepatology 1994;20:46–55.
48. Somberg KA, Riegler JL, LaBerge JM, et al. Hepatic encephalopathy after transjugular intrahepatic portosystemic shunts: incidence and risk-factors. Am J Gastroenterol 1995;90:549–555.
49. Haskal ZJ, Middlebrook MR. Creation of a stenotic stent to reduce flow through a transjugular intrahepatic portosystemic shunt. J Vasc Interv Radiol 1994;5:827–830.
50. Brophy D, Haskal ZJ. Simpler ways to deliver the stenotic stent for reducing TIPS flow. J Vasc Interv Radiol 1998;9:1032–1033.
51. Hauenstein KH, Haag K, Ochs A, et al. The reducing stent: treatment for transjugular intrahepatic portosystemic shunt-induced refractory hepatic encephalopathy and liver failure. Radiology 1995;194:175–179.
52. Kerlan RK Jr., LaBerge JM, Baker EL, et al. Successful reversal of hepatic encephalopathy with intentional occlusion of transjugular intrahepatic portosystemic shunts. J Vasc Interv Radiol 1995; 6:917–921.
53. Haskal ZJ, Cope C, Soulen MC, et al. Intentional reversible thrombosis of transjugular intrahepatic portosystemic shunts. Radiology 1995;195:485–488.
54. Forauer AR, McLean GK. Transjugular intrahepatic portosystemic shunt constraining stent for the treatment of refractory postprocedural encephalopathy: a simple design utilizing a Palmaz stent and Wallstent. J Vasc Interv Radiol 1998;9:443–446.
55. Paz-Fumagalli R, Crain MR, Mewissen MW, Varma RR. Fatal hemodynamic consequences of therapeutic closure of a transjugular intrahepatic portosystemic shunt. J Vasc Interv Radiol 1994;5:831–834.
56. Jalan R, Forrest EH, Stanley AJ, et al. A randomized trial comparing transjugular intrahepatic portosystemic stent-shunt with variceal band ligation in the prevention of rebleeding from esophageal varices. Hepatology 1997;26:1115–1122.
57. Cello JP, Ring EJ, Olcott EW, et al. Endoscopic sclerotherapy compared with percutaneous transjugular intrahepatic portosystemic shunt after initial sclerotherapy in patients with acute variceal hemorrhage. A randomized, controlled trial. Ann Intern Med 1997;126:858–865.
58. Sanyal AJ, Freedman AM, Luketic VA, et al. Transjugular intrahepatic portosystemic shunts compared with endoscopic sclerotherapy for the prevention of recurrent variceal hemorrhage. A randomized, controlled trial. Ann Intern Med 1997;126:849–857.
59. Sauer P, Theilmann L, Stremmel W, Benz C, Richter GM, Stiehl A. Transjugular intrahepatic portosystemic stent shunt versus sclerotherapy plus propranolol for variceal rebleeding. Gastroenterology 1997;113:1623–1631.
60. Cabrera J, Maynar M, Granados R, et al. Transjugular intrahepatic portosystemic shunt versus sclerotherapy in the elective treatment of variceal hemorrhage. Gastroenterology 1996;110:832–839.
61. Garcia-Villarreal L, Martinez-Lagares F, Sierra A, et al. Transjugular intrahepatic portosystemic shunt versus endoscopic sclerotherapy for the prevention of variceal rebleeding after recent variceal hemorrhage. Hepatology 1999;29:27–32.
62. Merli M, Salerno F, Riggio O, et al. Transjugular intrahepatic portosystemic shunt versus endoscopic sclerotherapy for the prevention of variceal bleeding in cirrhosis: a randomized multicenter trial. Gruppo Italiano Studio TIPS (G.I.S.T.). Hepatology 1998;27:48–53.
63. D'Amico G, Pagliaro L, Bosch J. The treatment of portal hypertension: a meta-analytic review. Hepatology 1995;22:332–354.
64. Sarfeh IJ, Carter JA, Welch HF. Analysis of operative mortality after portal decompressive procedures in cirrhotic patients. Am J Surg 1980;140:306–311.
65. Sarfeh IJ, Rypins EB. The emergency portacaval H graft in alcoholic cirrhotic patients: influence of shunt diameter on clinical outcome. Am J Surg 1986;152:290–293.

66. Vangeli M, Patch D, Burroughs AK. Salvage tips for uncontrolled variceal bleeding. J Hepatol 2002;37:703–704.

67. Schepke M, Roth F, Fimmers R, et al. Comparison of MELD, Child-Pugh, and Emory model for the prediction of survival in patients undergoing transjugular intrahepatic portosystemic shunting. Am J Gastroenterol 2003;98:1167–1174.

68. Salerno F, Merli M, Cazzaniga M, et al. MELD score is better than Child-Pugh score in predicting 3-month survival of patients undergoing transjugular intrahepatic portosystemic shunt. J Hepatol 2002;36:494–500.

69. Rosado B, Kamath PS. Transjugular intrahepatic portosystemic shunts: an update. Liver Transpl 2003;9:207–217.

70. Kamath PS, Wiesner RH, Malinchoc M, et al. A model to predict survival in patients with end-stage liver disease. Hepatology 2001;33:464–470.

71. Angermayr B, Cejna M, Karnel F, et al. Child-Pugh versus MELD score in predicting survival in patients undergoing transjugular intrahepatic portosystemic shunt. Gut 2003;52:879–885.

72. Alessandria C, Gaia S, Marzano A, et al. Application of the model for end-stage liver disease score for transjugular intrahepatic portosystemic shunt in cirrhotic patients with refractory ascites and renal impairment. Eur J Gastroenterol Hepatol 2004;16:607–612.

73. LaBerge JM, Somberg KA, Lake JR, et al. Two-year outcome following transjugular intrahepatic portosystemic shunt for variceal bleeding: results in 90 patients. Gastroenterology 1995;108:1143–1151.

74. Rubin RA, Haskal ZJ, O'Brien CB, et al. Transjugular intrahepatic portosystemic shunting: decreased survival for patients with high APACHE II scores. Am J Gastroenterol 1995;90:556–563.

75. Rajan DK, Haskal ZJ, Clark TW. Serum bilirubin and early mortality after transjugular intrahepatic portosystemic shunts: results of a multivariate analysis. J Vasc Interv Radiol 2002;13:155–161.

76. Brensing KA, Raab P, Textor J, et al. Prospective evaluation of a clinical score for 60-day mortality after transjugular intrahepatic portosystemic stent-shunt: Bonn TIPSS early mortality analysis. Eur J Gastroenterol Hepatol 2002;14:723–731.

77. Aggarwal A, Ong JP, Younossi ZM, et al. Predictors of mortality and resource utilization in cirrhotic patients admitted to the medical ICU. Chest 2001;119:1489–1497.

78. LaBerge JM, Ring EJ, Gordon RL, et al. Creation of transjugular intrahepatic portosystemic shunt (TIPS) with the Wallstent endoprosthesis: results in 100 patients. Radiology 1993;187:413–420.

79. Chalasani N, Clark WS, Martin LG, et al. Determinants of mortality in patients with advanced cirrhosis after transjugular intrahepatic portosystemic shunting. Gastroenterology 2000;118:138–144.

80. Patch D, Nikolopoulou V, McCormick A, et al. Factors related to early mortality after transjugular intrahepatic portosystemic shunt for failed endoscopic therapy in acute variceal bleeding. J Hepatol 1998;28:454–460.

81. Chalasani N, Kahi C, Francois F, et al. Improved patient survival after acute variceal bleeding: a multicenter, cohort study. Am J Gastroenterol 2003;98:653–659.

82. Sharara AI, Rockey DC. Gastroesophageal variceal hemorrhage. N Engl J Med 2001;345:669–681.

83. Boyer TD, Henderson JM. Portal hypertension and bleeding esophageal varices. In: Zakim D, Boyer TD, eds. Hepatology: A textbook of liver disease. 4th Ed. Philadelphia: W.B. Saunders, 2002:581–629.

84. Papatheodoridis GV, Goulis J, Leandro G, et al. Transjugular intrahepatic portosystemic shunt compared with endoscopic treatment for prevention of variceal rebleeding: A meta-analysis. Hepatology 1999;30:612–622.

85. Pomier-Layrargues G, Villeneuve JP, Deschenes M, et al. Transjugular intrahepatic portosystemic shunt (TIPS) versus endoscopic variceal ligation in the prevention of variceal rebleeding in patients with cirrhosis: a randomised trial. Gut 2001;48:390–396.

86. Rossle M, Deibert P, Haag K, et al. Randomised trial of transjugular-intrahepatic-portosystemic shunt versus endoscopy plus propranolol for prevention of variceal rebleeding. Lancet 1997;349:1043–1049.

87. Sauer P, Hansmann J, Richter GM, et al. Endoscopic variceal ligation plus propranolol vs. transjugular intrahepatic portosystemic stent shunt: a long-term randomized trial. Endoscopy 2002;34:690–697.

88. Meddi P, Merli M, Lionetti R, et al. Cost analysis for the prevention of variceal rebleeding: a comparison between transjugular intrahepatic portosystemic shunt and endoscopic sclerotherapy in a selected group of Italian cirrhotic patients. Hepatology 1999;29:1074–1077.

89. Rosemurgy AS, Serafini FM, Zweibel BR, et al. Transjugular intrahepatic portosystemic shunt vs. small-diameter prosthetic H-graft portacaval shunt: extended follow-up of an expanded randomized prospective trial. J Gastrointest Surg 2000;4:589–597.

90. Rosemurgy AS 2nd, Goode SE, Camps M. The effect of small-diameter H-graft portacaval shunts on portal blood flow. Am J Surg 1996;171:154–156; discussion 156–157.

91. Escorsell A, Banares R, Garcia-Pagan JC, et al. TIPS versus drug therapy in preventing variceal rebleeding in advanced cirrhosis: a randomized controlled trial. Hepatology 2002;35:385–392.

92. Chau TN, Patch D, Chan YW, et al. "Salvage" transjugular intrahepatic portosystemic shunts: gastric fundal compared with esophageal variceal bleeding. Gastroenterology 1998;114:981–987.

93. Barange K, Peron JM, Imani K, et al. Transjugular intrahepatic portosystemic shunt in the treatment of refractory bleeding from ruptured gastric varices. Hepatology 1999;30:1139–1143.

94. Rees CJ, Nylander DL, Thompson NP, et al. Do gastric and oesophageal varices bleed at different portal pressures and is TIPS an effective treatment? Liver 2000;20:253–256.

95. Tripathi D, Therapondos G, Jackson E, et al. The role of the transjugular intrahepatic portosystemic stent shunt (TIPSS) in the management of bleeding gastric varices: clinical and haemodynamic correlations. Gut 2002;51:270–274.

96. Chikamori F, Kuniyoshi N, Shibuya S, et al. Correlation between endoscopic and angiographic findings in patients with esophageal and isolated gastric varices. Dig Surg 2001;18:176–181.

97. Choi YH, Yoon CJ, Park JH, et al. Balloon-occluded retrograde transvenous obliteration for gastric variceal bleeding: its feasibility compared with transjugular intrahepatic portosystemic shunt. Korean J Radiol 2003;4:109–116.

98. Ibukuro K, Mori K, Tsukiyama T, et al. Balloon-occluded retrograde transvenous obliteration of gastric varix draining via the left inferior phrenic vein into the left hepatic vein. Cardiovasc Intervent Radiol 1999;22:415–417.

99. Kim ES, Park SY, Kwon KT, et al. The clinical usefulness of balloon occluded retrograde transvenous obliteration in gastric variceal bleeding. Taehan Kan Hakhoe Chi 2003;9:315–323.

100. Kiyosue H, Mori H, Matsumoto S, et al. Transcatheter obliteration of gastric varices: Part 2. Strategy and techniques based on hemodynamic features. Radiographics 2003;23:921–937; discussion 937.

101. Kiyosue H, Mori H, Matsumoto S, et al. Transcatheter obliteration of gastric varices. Part 1. Anatomic classification. Radiographics 2003;23:911–920.

102. Baik GH, Kim DJ, Lee HG, et al. Therapeutic efficacy of balloon-occluded retrograde transvenous obliteration in the treatment of gastric varices in cirrhotic patients with gastrorenal shunt. Korean J Gastroenterol 2004;43:196–203.

103. Bernstein D, Yrizarry J, Reddy KR, et al. Transjugular intrahepatic portosystemic shunt in the treatment of intermittently bleeding stomal varices. Am J Gastroenterol 1996;91:2237–2238.

104. Johnson PA, Laurin J. Transjugular portosystemic shunt for treatment of bleeding stomal varices. Dig Dis Sci 1997;42:440–442.

105. Kishimoto K, Hara A, Arita T, et al. Stomal varices: treatment by percutaneous transhepatic coil embolization. Cardiovasc Intervent Radiol 1999;22:523–525.

106. Labori KJ, Carlsen E. Treatment of bleeding peristomal varices. Eur J Surg 2002;168:654–656.

107. Lashley DB, Saxon RR, Fuchs EF, et al. Bleeding ileal conduit stomal varices: diagnosis and management using transjugular transhepatic angiography and embolization. Urology 1997;50: 612–614.

108. Lagier E, Rousseau H, Maquin P, et al. Treatment of bleeding stomal varices using transjugular intrahepatic portosystemic shunt. J Pediatr Gastroenterol Nutr 1994;18:501–503.

109. Shibata D, Brophy DP, Gordon FD, et al. Transjugular intrahepatic portosystemic shunt for treatment of bleeding ectopic varices with portal hypertension. Dis Colon Rectum 1999;42:1581–1585.

110. Toumeh KK, Girardot JD, Choo IW, et al. Percutaneous transhepatic embolization as treatment for bleeding ileostomy varices. Cardiovasc Intervent Radiol 1995;18:179–182.

111. Weinberg GD, Matalon TA, Brunner MC, et al. Bleeding stomal varices: treatment with a transjugular intrahepatic portosystemic shunt in two pediatric patients. J Vasc Interv Radiol 1995;6:233–236.

112. Wong RC, Berg CL. Portal hypertensive stomapathy: a newly described entity and its successful treatment by placement of a transjugular intrahepatic portosystemic shunt. Am J Gastroenterol 1997;92:1056–1057.

113. Haskal ZJ, Scott M, Rubin RA, et al. Intestinal varices: treatment with the transjugular intrahepatic portosystemic shunt. Radiology 1994;191:183–187.

114. Wilson SE, Stone RT, Christie JP, et al. Massive lower gastrointestinal bleeding from intestinal varices. Arch Surg 1979;114:1158–1161.

115. Demirel H, Pieterman H, Lameris JS, et al. Transjugular embolization of the inferior mesenteric vein for bleeding anorectal varices after unsuccessful transjugular intrahepatic portosystemic shunt. Am J Gastroenterol 1997;92:1226–1227.

116. Fantin AC, Zala G, Risti B, et al. Bleeding anorectal varices: successful treatment with transjugular intrahepatic portosystemic shunting (TIPS). Gut 1996;38:932–935.

117. Godil A, McCracken JD. Rectal variceal bleeding treated by transjugular intrahepatic portosystemic shunt. Potentials and pitfalls. J Clin Gastroenterol 1997;25:460–462.

118. Katz JA, Rubin RA, Cope C, et al. Recurrent bleeding from anorectal varices: successful treatment with a transjugular intrahepatic portosystemic shunt. Am J Gastroenterol 1993;88:1104–1107.

119. Ory G, Spahr L, Megevand JM, et al. The long-term efficacy of the intrahepatic portosystemic shunt (TIPS) for the treatment of bleeding anorectal varices in cirrhosis. A case report and review of the literature. Digestion 2001;64:261–264.

120. Burak KW, Lee SS, Beck PL. Portal hypertensive gastropathy and gastric antral vascular ectasia (GAVE) syndrome. Gut 2001;49:866–872.

121. Dagher L, Burroughs A. Variceal bleeding and portal hypertensive gastropathy. Eur J Gastroenterol Hepatol 2001;13:81–88.

122. Garcia N, Sanyal AJ. Portal hypertensive gastropathy and gastric antral vascular ectasia. Curr Treat Options Gastroenterol 2001;4:163–171.

123. Mezawa S, Homma H, Ohta H, et al. Effect of transjugular intrahepatic portosystemic shunt formation on portal hypertensive gastropathy and gastric circulation. Am J Gastroenterol 2001;96:1155–1159.

124. Panes J, Pique JM. Therapeutic options for bleeding portal hypertensive gastropathy. J Gastroenterol Hepatol 1998;13:977–979.

125. Sarin SK, Agarwal SR. Gastric varices and portal hypertensive gastropathy. Clin Liver Dis 2001;5:727–767,x.

126. Kamath PS, Lacerda M, Ahlquist DA, McKusick MA, Andrews JC, Nagorney DA. Gastric mucosal responses to intrahepatic portosystemic shunting in patients with cirrhosis. Gastroenterology 2000;118:905–911.

127. Urata J, Yamashita Y, Tsuchigame T, et al. The effects of transjugular intrahepatic portosystemic shunt on portal hypertensive gastropathy. J Gastroenterol Hepatol 1998;13:1061–1067.

128. Runyon BA. Management of adult patients with ascites due to cirrhosis. Hepatology 2004;39:841–856.

129. Gines P, Cardenas A, Arroyo V, Rodes J. Management of cirrhosis and ascites. N Engl J Med 2004;350:1646–1654.

130. Lebrec D, Giuily N, Hadengue A, et al. Transjugular intrahepatic portosystemic shunts: comparison with paracentesis in patients with cirrhosis and refractory ascites: a randomized trial. French Group of Clinicians and a Group of Biologists. J Hepatol 1996;25:135–144.

131. Rossle M, Ochs A, Gulberg V, et al. A comparison of paracentesis and transjugular intrahepatic portosystemic shunting in patients with ascites. N Engl J Med 2000;342:1701–1707.

132. Sanyal AJ, Genning C, Reddy KR, et al. The North American Study for the Treatment of Refractory Ascites. Gastroenterology 2003;124:634–641.

133. Gines P, Uriz J, Calahorra B, et al. Transjugular intrahepatic portosystemic shunting versus paracentesis plus albumin for refractory ascites in cirrhosis. Gastroenterology 2002;123:1839–1847.

134. Rosemurgy AS, Zervos EE, Clark WC, et al. TIPS versus peritoneovenous shunt in the treatment of medically intractable ascites: a prospective randomized trial. Ann Surg 2004;239:883–889; discussion 889–891.

135. Siegerstetter V, Deibert P, Ochs A, et al. Treatment of refractory hepatic hydrothorax with transjugular intrahepatic portosystemic shunt: long-term results in 40 patients. Eur J Gastroenterol Hepatol 2001;13:529–534.

136. Gordon FD, Anastopoulos HT, Crenshaw W, et al. The successful treatment of symptomatic, refractory hepatic hydrothorax with transjugular intrahepatic portosystemic shunt. Hepatology 1997;25:1366–1369.

137. Haskal ZJ, Zuckerman J. Resolution of hepatic hydrothorax after transjugular intrahepatic portosystemic shunt (TIPS) placement. Chest 1994;106:1293–1295.

138. Lazaridis KN, Frank JW, Krowka MJ, et al. Hepatic hydrothorax: pathogenesis, diagnosis, and management. Am J Med 1999;107:262–267.

139. Spencer EB, Cohen DT, Darcy MD. Safety and efficacy of transjugular intrahepatic portosystemic shunt creation for the treatment of hepatic hydrothorax. J Vasc Interv Radiol 2002;13:385–390.

140. Strauss RM, Boyer TD. Hepatic hydrothorax. Semin Liver Dis 1997;17:227–232.

141. Degawa M, Hamasaki K, Yano K, et al. Refractory hepatic hydrothorax treated with transjugular intrahepatic portosystemic shunt. J Gastroenterol 1999;34:128–131.

142. Cardenas A, Kelleher T, Chopra S. Hepatic hydrothorax. Aliment Pharmacol Ther 2004;20:271–279.

143. Gines P, Guevara M, Arroyo V, et al. Hepatorenal syndrome. Lancet 2003;362:1819–1827.

144. Runyon BA. Historical aspects of treatment of patients with cirrhosis and ascites. Semin Liver Dis 1997;17:163–173.

145. Brensing KA, Textor J, Strunk H, et al. Transjugular intrahepatic portosystemic stent-shunt for hepatorenal syndrome. Lancet 1997;349:697–698.

146. Cardenas A, Arroyo V. Hepatorenal syndrome. Ann Hepatol 2003;2:23–29.

147. Guevara M, Gines P, Bandi JC, et al. Transjugular intrahepatic portosystemic shunt in hepatorenal syndrome: effects on renal function and vasoactive systems. Hepatology 1998;28:416–422.

148. Jalan R, Forrest EH, Redhead DN, et al. Reduction in renal blood flow following acute increase in the portal pressure: evidence for the existence of a hepatorenal reflex in man? Gut 1997;40:664–670.

149. Lerut J, Goffette P, Laterre PF, et al. Sequential treatment of hepatorenal syndrome and posthepatic cirrhosis by intrahepatic portosystemic shunt (TIPSS) and liver transplantation. Hepatogastroenterology 1995;42:985–987.

150. Sturgis TM. Hepatorenal syndrome: resolution after transjugular intrahepatic portosystemic shunt. J Clin Gastroenterol 1995;20:241–243.

151. Wong F, Pantea L, Sniderman K. Midodrine, octreotide, albumin, and TIPS in selected patients with cirrhosis and type 1 hepatorenal syndrome. Hepatology 2004;40:55–64.

152. Brensing KA, Textor J, Perz J, et al. Long term outcome after transjugular intrahepatic portosystemic stent-shunt in non-transplant cirrhotics with hepatorenal syndrome: a phase II study. Gut 2000;47:288–295.

153. Ortega R, Gines P, Uriz J, et al. Terlipressin therapy with and without albumin for patients with hepatorenal syndrome: results of a prospective, nonrandomized study. Hepatology 2002;36:941–948.

154. Valla DC. The diagnosis and management of the Budd-Chiari syndrome: consensus and controversies. Hepatology 2003;38:793–803.

155. Okuda K, Kage M, Shrestha SM. Proposal of a new nomenclature for Budd-Chiari syndrome: hepatic vein thrombosis versus thrombosis of the inferior vena cava at its hepatic portion. Hepatology 1998;28:1191–1198.

156. Perello A, Garcia-Pagan JC, Gilabert R, et al. TIPS is a useful long-term derivative therapy for patients with Budd-Chiari syndrome uncontrolled by medical therapy. Hepatology 2002;35:132–139.

157. Mancuso A, Fung K, Mela M, et al. TIPS for acute and chronic Budd-Chiari syndrome: a single-centre experience. J Hepatol 2003;38:751–754.

158. Ochs A, Sellinger M, Haag K, et al. Transjugular intrahepatic portosystemic stent-shunt (TIPS) in the treatment of Budd-Chiari syndrome. J Hepatol 1993;18:217–225.

159. Peltzer MY, Ring EJ, LaBerge JM, et al. Treatment of Budd-Chiari syndrome with a transjugular intrahepatic portosystemic shunt. J Vasc Interv Radiol 1993;4:263–267.

160. Rogopoulos A, Gavelli A, Sakai H, et al. Transjugular intrahepatic portosystemic shunt for Budd-Chiari syndrome after failure of surgical shunting. Arch Surg 1995;130:227–228.

161. Richard HM 3rd, Cooper JM, Ahn J, et al. Transjugular intrahepatic portosystemic shunts in the management of Budd-Chiari syndrome in the liver transplant patient with intractable ascites: anatomic considerations. J Vasc Interv Radiol 1998;9:137–140.

162. Strunk HM, Textor J, Brensing KA, et al. Acute Budd-Chiari syndrome: treatment with transjugular intrahepatic portosystemic shunt. Cardiovasc Intervent Radiol 1997;20:311–313.

163. Nicoll A, Fitt G, Angus P, et al. Budd-Chiari syndrome: intractable ascites managed by a trans-hepatic portacaval shunt. Australas Radiol 1997;41:169–172.

164. Kuo PC, Johnson LB, Hastings G, et al. Fulminant hepatic failure from the Budd-Chiari syndrome. A bridge to transplantation with transjugular intrahepatic portosystemic shunt. Transplantation 1996;62:294–296.

165. Hastings GS, O'Connor DK, Pais SO. Transjugular intrahepatic portosystemic shunt placement as a bridge to liver transplantation in fulminant Budd-Chiari syndrome [letter]. J Vasc Interv Radiol 1996;7:616.

166. Uhl MD, Roth DB, Riely CA. Transjugular intrahepatic portosystemic shunt (TIPS) for Budd-Chiari syndrome. Dig Dis Sci 1996;41:1494–1499.

167. Blum U, Rossle M, Haag K, et al. Budd-Chiari syndrome: technical, hemodynamic, and clinical results of treatment with transjugular intrahepatic portosystemic shunt. Radiology 1995;197:805–811.

168. Ryu RK, Durham JD, Krysl J, et al. Role of TIPS as a bridge to hepatic transplantation in Budd-Chiari syndrome. J Vasc Interv Radiol 1999;10:799–805.

169. Avenhaus W, Ullerich H, Menzel J, et al. Budd-Chiari syndrome in a patient with factor V Leiden—successful treatment by TIPSS placement followed by liver transplantation. Z Gastroenterol 1999;37:277–281.

170. Sanyal AJ. Budd-Chiari syndrome: is TIPS tops? [editorial; comment]. Am J Gastroenterol 1999;94:559–561.

171. Brunerova L, Bartakova H, Jankovska M, et al. The Budd-Chiari syndrome in a patient with primary thrombocythemia treated with interferon alfa and transjugular portosystemic shunt. Cas Lek Cesk 2004;143:198–201.

172. Rossle M, Olschewski M, Siegerstetter V, et al. The Budd-Chiari syndrome: outcome after treatment with the transjugular intrahepatic portosystemic shunt. Surgery 2004;135:394–403.

173. Das HS, Punamiya S, Kalokhe S, et al. Budd-Chiari syndrome treated with transjugular intrahepatic portosystemic shunt. J Assoc Physicians India 2003;51:309–310.

174. Blokzijl H, de Knegt RJ. Long-term effect of treatment of acute Budd-Chiari syndrome with a transjugular intrahepatic portosytemic shunt. Hepatology 2002;35:1551–1552.

175. Cejna M, Peck-Radosavljevic M, Schoder M, et al. Repeat interventions for maintenance of transjugular intrahepatic portosystemic shunt function in patients with Budd-Chiari syndrome. J Vasc Interv Radiol 2002;13:193–199.

176. Cura MA, Haskal ZJ, Lefkowitch J, et al. Control of Budd Chiari syndrome using TIPS: clinicopathologic findings using stent-grafts and Wallstents [abstract]. Phoenix, AZ: Society of Interventional Radiology Annual Meeting, 2004.

177. Saxon RS, Ross PL, Mendel-Hartvig J, et al. Transjugular intrahepatic portosystemic shunt patency and the importance of stenosis location in the development of recurrent symptoms. Radiology 1998;207:683–693.

178. Bodner G, Peer S, Fries D, et al. Color and pulsed Doppler ultrasound findings in normally functioning transjugular intrahepatic portosystemic shunts. Eur J Ultrasound 2000;12:131–136.

179. Wachsberg RH. Doppler ultrasound evaluation of transjugular intrahepatic portosystemic shunt function: pitfalls and artifacts. Ultrasound Q 2003;19:139–148.

180. Ferguson JM, Jalan R, Redhead DN, et al. The role of duplex and colour Doppler ultrasound in the follow-up evaluation of transjugular intrahepatic portosystemic stent shunt (TIPSS). Br J Radiol 1995;68:587–589.

181. Longo JM, Bilbao JI, Rousseau HP, et al. Color doppler ultrasound guidance in transjugular placement of intrahepatic portosystemic shunts. Radiology 1992;184:281–284.

182. Chong WK, Malisch TA, Mazer MJ, et al. Transjugular intrahepatic portosystemic shunt: US assessment with maximum flow velocity. Radiology 1993;189:789–793.

183. Ferral H, Foshager MC, Bjarnason H, et al. Early sonographic evaluation of the transjugular intrahepatic portosystemic shunt (TIPS). Cardiovasc Intervent Radiol 1993;16:275–279.

184. Foshager MC, Ferral H, Finlay DE, et al. Color Doppler sonography of transjugular intrahepatic portosystemic shunts (TIPS). Am J Roentgenol 1994;163:105–111.

185. Ralls PW, Egan RT, Katz MD, et al. Color Doppler sonography to evaluate transjugular intrahepatic portacaval stent shunt. J Ultrasound Med 1993;12:487–489.

186. Surratt RS, Middleton WD, Darcy MD, et al. Morphologic and hemodynamic findings at sonography before and after creation of a transjugular intrahepatic portosystemic shunt. Am J Roentgenol 1993;160:627–630.

187. Talavera A, Artaza T, Gomez R, et al. Usefulness of Doppler sonography in monitoring transjugular intrahepatic portosystemic shunts. J Clin Ultrasound 1994;22:137–140.

188. Lind CD, Malisch TW, Chong WK, et al. Incidence of shunt occlusion or stenosis following transjugular intrahepatic portosystemic shunt placement. Gastroenterology 1994;106:1277–1283.

189. Foshager M, Ferral H, Nazarian G, et al. Duplex sonography after transjugular intrahepatic portosystemic shunts (TIPS): normal hemodynamic findings and efficacy in predicting shunt patency and stenosis. Am J Roentgenol 1995;165:1–7.

190. Dodd GD 3rd, Zajko AB, Orons PD, et al. Detection of transjugular intrahepatic portosystemic shunt dysfunction: value of duplex Doppler sonography. AJR Am J Roentgenol 1995;164:1119–1124.

191. Haskal ZJ, Carroll JW, Jacobs JE, et al. Sonography of transjugular intrahepatic portosystemic shunts: detection of elevated portosystemic gradients and loss of shunt function. J Vasc Interv Radiol 1997;8:549–556.

192. Kanterman RY, Darcy MD, Middleton WD, et al. Doppler sonography findings associated with transjugular intrahepatic portosystemic shunt malfunction. AJR Am J Roentgenol 1997;168:467–472.

193. Kimura M, Sato M, Kawai N, et al. Efficacy of Doppler ultrasonography for assessment of transjugular intrahepatic portosystemic shunt patency. Cardiovasc Intervent Radiol 1996;19:397–400.

194. Feldstein VA, Patel MD. Doppler ultrasonography of transjugular intrahepatic portosystemic shunts. West J Med 1996;165:56–57.

195. Chong WK, Mazer MJ. Doppler velocity criteria for transjugular intrahepatic portosystemic shunt (TIPS) stenosis [letter; comment]. AJR Am J Roentgenol 1996;166:215–216.

196. Murphy TP, Beecham RP, Kim HM, et al. Long-term follow-up after TIPS: use of Doppler velocity criteria for detecting elevation of the portosystemic gradient. J Vasc Interv Radiol 1998;9:275–281.

197. Menzel J. Duplex ultrasonography of TIPS: how useful is it? [letter]. Gastroenterology 1999;116:1272–1273.

198. Zizka J, Elias P, Krajina A, et al. Value of Doppler sonography in revealing transjugular intrahepatic portosystemic shunt malfunction: a 5-year experience in 216 patients. AJR Am J Roentgenol 2000;175:141–148.

199. Benito A, Bilbao J, Hernandez T, et al. Doppler ultrasound for TIPS: does it work? Abdom Imaging 2004;29:45–52.

200. Feldstein V, Patel M, LaBerge J. Transjugular intrahepatic portosystemic shunt: accuracy of Doppler US in determination of patency and detection of stenoses. Radiology 1996;201:141–147.

201. Haskal ZJ, Rees CR, Ring EJ, et al. Reporting standards for transjugular intrahepatic portosystemic shunts. Technology Assessment Committee of the SCVIR. J Vasc Interv Radiol 1997;8:289–297; erratum in: J Vasc Interv Radiol 1997;8:493.

202. Eloubeidi M, Trotter JF, Rockey DC. Ultrasonography or venography for the diagnosis of TIPS malfunction? Gastroenterology 1998;115:1604; author reply 1605–1606.

203. LaBerge J, Feldstein VA. Ultrasound surveillance of tips—why bother? Hepatology 1998;28:1433–1434.

204. Owens CA, Bartolone C, Warner DL, et al. The inaccuracy of duplex ultrasonography in predicting patency of transjugular intrahepatic portosystemic shunts. Gastroenterology 1998;114:975–980.

205. Menzel J. Duplex ultrasonography of TIPS: how useful is it? Gastroenterology 1999;116:1272–1273.

206. Sanyal AJ, Contos MJ, Yager D, et al. Development of pseudointima and stenosis after transjugular intrahepatic portasystemic shunts: characterization of cell phenotype and function. Hepatology 1998;28:22–32.

207. LaBerge JM, Ferrel LD, Ring EJ, et al. Histopathologic study of stenotic and occluded transjugular intrahepatic portosystemic shunts. J Vasc Interv Radiol 1993;4:779–786.

208. LaBerge JM, Ferrell LD, Ring EJ, et al. Histopathologic study of transjugular intrahepatic portosystemic shunts. J Vasc Interv Radiol 1991;2:549–556.

209. Saxon RR, Mendel-Hartvig J, Corless CL, et al. Bile duct injury as a major cause of stenosis and occlusion in transjugular intrahepatic portosystemic shunts: comparative histopathologic analysis in humans and swine. J Vasc Interv Radiol 1996;7:487–497.

210. Terayama N, Matsui O, Kadoya M, et al. Transjugular intrahepatic portosystemic shunt: histologic and immunohistochemical study of autopsy cases. Cardiovasc Intervent Radiol 1997;20:457–461.

211. Ducoin H, El-Khoury J, Rousseau H, et al. Histopathologic analysis of transjugular intrahepatic portosystemic shunts. Hepatology 1997;25:1064–1069.

212. Teng GJ, Bettmann MA, Hoopes PJ, et al. Transjugular intrahepatic portosystemic shunt: effect of bile leak on smooth muscle cell proliferation. Radiology 1998;208:799–805.

213. Sanyal AJ, Mirshahi F. Endothelial cells lining transjugular intrahepatic portasystemic shunts originate in hepatic sinusoids: implications for pseudointimal hyperplasia. Hepatology 1999;29:710–718.

214. Haskal ZJ, Lehr S, Furth EE, et al. Histopathologic analysis of the biologic response to transjugular intrahepatic portosystemic shunts (TIPS) and proposal of a pathogenetic model. Radiology 1996;202(P):140.

215. Cohen GS, Young HY, Ball DS. Stent-graft as treatment for TIPS-biliary fistula. J Vasc Interv Radiol 1996;7:665–668.

216. Stout LC, Lyon RE, Murray NG, et al. Pseudointimal biliary epithelial proliferation and Zahn's infarct associated with a 6 1/2-month-old transjugular intrahepatic portosystemic shunt. Am J Gastroenterol 1995;90:126–130.

217. Mallery S, Freeman ML, Peine CJ, et al. Biliary-shunt fistula following transjugular intrahepatic portosystemic shunt placement. Gastroenterology 1996;111:1353–1357.

218. Jalan R, Redhead DN, Allan PL, et al. Prospective evaluation of haematological alterations following the transjugular intrahepatic portosystemic stent-shunt (TIPSS). Eur J Gastroenterol Hepatol 1996;8:381–385.

219. Haskal ZJ, Pentecost MJ, Soulen MC, et al. Transjugular intrahepatic portosystemic shunt stenosis and revision: early and midterm results. Am J Roentgenol 1994;163:439–444.

220. Mattsson EJ, Kohler TR, Vergel SM, et al. Increased blood flow induces regression of intimal hyperplasia. Arterioscler Thromb Vasc Biol 1997;17:2245–2249.

221. Zarins CK, Zatina MA, Giddens DP, et al. Shear stress regulation of artery lumen diameter in experimental atherogenesis. J Vasc Surg 1987;5:413–420.

222. Sauer P, Theilmann L, Herrmann S, et al. Phenprocoumon for prevention of shunt occlusion after transjugular intrahepatic portosystemic stent shunt: a randomized trial. Hepatology 1996;24:1433–1436.

223. Siegerstetter V, Huber M, Ochs A, et al. Platelet aggregation and platelet-derived growth factor inhibition for prevention of insufficiency of the transjugular intrahepatic portosystemic shunt: a randomized study comparing trapidil plus ticlopidine with heparin treatment. Hepatology 1999;29:33–38.

224. Nishimine K, Saxon RR, Kichikawa K, et al. Improved transjugular intrahepatic portosystemic shunt patency with PTFE-covered stent-grafts: experimental results in swine. Radiology 1995;196:341–347.

225. Kichikawa K, Saxon RR, Nishimine K, et al. Experimental TIPS with spiral Z-stents in swine with and without induced portal hypertension. Cardiovasc Intervent Radiol 1997;20:197–203.

226. Pavcnik D, Saxon RR, Kubota Y, et al. Attempted induction of chronic portal venous hypertension with polyvinyl alcohol particles in swine. J Vasc Interv Radiol 1997;8:123–128.

227. Haskal ZJ, Davis A, McAllister A, et al. PTFE-encapsulated endovascular stent-graft for transjugular intrahepatic portosystemic shunts: experimental evaluation. Radiology 1997;205:682–688.

228. Haskal Z, Zaetta J. Comparison of a novel ePTFE-based endovascular stent-graft versus the Wallstent for de novo transjugular intrahepatic portosystemic shunts formation in a porcine model [abstract]. Radiology 1998;209:519.

229. Tanihata H, Saxon RR, Kubota Y, et al. Transjugular intrahepatic portosystemic shunt with silicone-covered Wallstents: results in a swine model. Radiology 1997;205:181–184.

230. Otal P, Rousseau H, Vinel JP, et al. High occlusion rate in experimental transjugular intrahepatic portosystemic shunt created with a Dacron-covered nitinol stent. J Vasc Interv Radiol 1999;10:183–188.

231. Haskal ZJ, Brennecke LH. Transjugular intrahepatic portosystemic shunts formed with polyethylene terephthalate-covered stents: experimental evaluation in pigs. Radiology 1999;213:853–859.

232. Bloch R, Pavcnik D, Uchida BT, et al. Polyurethane-coated Dacron-covered stent-grafts for TIPS: results in swine. Cardiovasc Intervent Radiol 1998;21:497–500.

233. Haskal ZJ, Brennecke LJ. Porous and nonporous polycarbonate urethane stent-grafts for TIPS formation: biologic responses. J Vasc Interv Radiol 1999;10:1255–1263.

234. Saxon RR, Timmermans HA, Uchida BT, et al. Stent-grafts for revision of TIPS stenoses and occlusions: a clinical pilot study. J Vasc Interv Radiol 1997;8:539–548.

235. Ferral H, Aleantara-Peraza A, Kimura Y, et al. Creation of transjugular intrahepatic portosystemic shunts with use of the Cragg Endopro System I. J Vasc Interv Radiol 1998;9:283–287.

236. Haskal ZJ, Weintraub JL, Susman J. Recurrent TIPS thrombosis after polyethylene stent-graft use and salvage with polytetrafluoroethylene stent-grafts. J Vasc Interv Radiol 2002;13:1255–1259.

237. Andrews RT, Saxon RR, Bloch RD, et al. Stent-grafts for de novo TIPS: technique and early results. J Vasc Interv Radiol 1999;10:1371–1378.

238. DiSalle RS, Dolmatch BL. Treatment of TIPS stenosis with ePTFE graft-covered stents. Cardiovasc Intervent Radiol 1998;21:172–175.

239. Haskal ZJ. Improved patency of transjugular intrahepatic portosystemic shunts in humans: creation and revision with PTFE stent-grafts. Radiology 1999;213:759–766.

240. Sze DY, Vestring T, Liddell RP, et al. Recurrent TIPS failure associated with biliary fistulae: treatment with PTFE-covered stents. Cardiovasc Intervent Radiol 1999;22:298–304.

241. LaBerge JM, Kerlan RK. Liver infarction following TIPS with a PTFE-covered stent: is the covering the cause? Hepatology 2003;38:778–779; author reply 779.

242. Cejna M, Peck-Radosavljevic M, Thurnher SA, et al. Creation of transjugular intrahepatic portosystemic shunts with stent-grafts: initial experiences with a polytetrafluoroethylene-covered nitinol endoprosthesis. Radiology 2001;221:437–446.

243. Cejna M, Peck-Radosavljevic M, Thurnher S, et al. ePTFE-covered stent-grafts for revision of obstructed transjugular intrahepatic portosystemic shunt. Cardiovasc Intervent Radiol 2002;25 : 365–372.

244. Angermayr B, Cejna M, Koenig F, et al. Survival in patients undergoing transjugular intrahepatic portosystemic shunt: ePTFE-covered stentgrafts versus bare stents. Hepatology 2003;38: 1043–1050.

245. Hausegger KA, Portugaller H, Macri NP, et al. Covered stents in transjugular intrahepatic portosystemic shunt: healing response to nonporous ePTFE covered stent grafts with and without intraluminal irradiation. Eur Radiol 2003;13:1549–1558.

246. Angeloni S, Merli M, Salvatori FM, et al. Polytetrafluoroethylene-covered stent grafts for TIPS procedure: 1-year patency and clinical results. Am J Gastroenterol 2004;99:280–285.

247. Hausegger KA, Karnel F, Georgieva B, et al. Transjugular intrahepatic portosystemic shunt creation with the Viatorr expanded polytetrafluoroethylene-covered stent-graft. J Vasc Interv Radiol 2004;15:239–248.

248. Maleux G, Pirenne J, Vaninbroukx J, et al. Are TIPS stent-grafts a contraindication for future liver transplantation? Cardiovasc Intervent Radiol 2004;27:140–142.

249. Maleux G, Nevens F, Wilmer A, et al. Early and long-term clinical and radiological follow-up results of expanded-polytetrafluoroethylene-covered stent-grafts for transjugular intrahepatic portosystemic shunt procedures. Eur Radiol 2004;14:1842–1850.

250. Rossi P, Salvatori FM, Fanelli F, et al. Polytetrafluoroethylene-covered nitinol stent-graft for transjugular intrahepatic portosystemic shunt creation: 3-year experience. Radiology 2004;231:820–830.

Percutaneous Gastrostomy and Gastrojejunostomy

32

Daniel B. Brown, Daniel Picus

Direct enteral feeding can be given by a variety of techniques. Tube feedings by the nasogastric, orogastric, or nasojejunal route are simple. However, these tubes are uncomfortable for the patient and are poorly tolerated for long-term nutrition. Additionally, nasojejunal tubes, because of their long length and relatively small caliber, frequently clog and require replacement. For long-term enteral nutrition, direct gastrostomy or gastrojejunostomy tubes are the most straightforward and best method available (1,2).

Currently, a variety of different techniques are available for the placement of gastrostomy and gastrojejunostomy tubes. Each of these uses a different guidance method. Surgical gastrostomy is performed through a laparotomy incision and uses direct visualization of the stomach for catheter placement. This technique has been available for more than 100 years. Surgical gastrostomy requires an abdominal incision and therefore is usually performed under general anesthesia. Because of this, this technique can be associated with significant morbidity and expense (3,4).

Less invasive methods for gastrostomy placement have become the standard of practice. Percutaneous endoscopic gastrostomy (PEG) uses endoscopic guidance to direct a needle and then a catheter into the stomach in either an antegrade or retrograde fashion. Percutaneous gastrostomy, as performed by interventional radiologists, uses fluoroscopic guidance and standard Seldinger technique to percutaneously place a feeding tube into the stomach and, if necessary, direct it into the jejunum. Because percutaneous gastrostomy does not require either a surgical incision or endoscopy, it rarely requires significant amounts of intravenous (IV) sedation and is the least invasive method for direct placement of catheters into either the stomach or the jejunum.

This chapter reviews the indications for and techniques of percutaneous fluoroscopically guided gastrostomy and gastrojejunostomy. It also reviews the results of and complications with these techniques and compares them to those obtained with both the surgical and endoscopic gastrostomy techniques.

INDICATIONS

The most common indication for percutaneous gastrostomy and gastrojejunostomy is long-term nutritional support in adults and children (1,5–14). Such patients include those unable to swallow because of esophageal obstruction secondary to head and neck cancer, or central nervous system diseases, including strokes and organic brain syndrome. Another group of patients is that group predisposed to aspiration with advanced neurologic diseases, including amyotrophic lateral sclerosis, multiple sclerosis, and muscular dystrophy. Finally, more unusual indications include enteral nutrition in patients with esophageal perforation, advanced malignancy, or unusual psychiatric problems such as anorexia nervosa or severe depression (5,6,8,15)

Intestinal decompression is a less common but excellent indication for percutaneous gastrostomy (5,8,15–19).

For patients who require long-term decompression, a gastrostomy tube is much more comfortable than a nasogastric tube. Additionally, gravity drainage through a gastrostomy tube is usually sufficient for decompression, while nasogastric decompression requires mechanical suction (16). The most common indication for decompressive gastrostomy in the authors' practice is in patients with bowel obstruction from peritoneal carcinomatosis secondary to gynecological malignancies. Decompressive gastrostomy can also be of value in patients with postoperative anastomotic obstructions and diabetic gastroparesis.

Gastrostomy Versus Gastrojejunostomy

Whenever possible, the authors prefer to place a gastrostomy rather than a gastrojejunostomy tube. Technically, gastrostomy tube placement is much simpler, requiring much less manipulation than gastrojejunostomy placement. Additionally, gastrojejunostomy tubes are longer than gastrostomy tubes without an increase in caliber. This results in more frequent clogging for gastrojejunostomy tubes, necessitating more frequent tube changes (20). Finally, with gastrostomy tube feedings, the function of the stomach is preserved, and therefore, almost any type of diet can be used. Gastrojejunostomy tubes bypass the stomach, delivering feedings directly into the jejunum. Gastrojejunostomy feedings therefore require a more expensive elemental diet as well as the use of an infusion pump with slower, more prolonged infusions to avoid dumping syndrome.

We reserve gastrojejunostomy tube placement for patients with either poor gastric emptying or those at high risk for gastroesophageal reflux (21–22). Poor gastric emptying is seen in patients with diabetic gastroparesis or partial gastric outlet obstruction. Significant gastroesophageal reflux can accompany a wide variety of neurologic problems. However, pulmonary aspiration in these patients is more often a result of problems with swallowing rather than reflux (20).

One clear advantage of the percutaneous technique over other techniques for enteral tube placement is the ability to easily convert from a gastrostomy tube to a gastrojejunostomy tube if problems develop (23,24). The authors generally wait 7–10 days for the percutaneous tract to mature before converting a gastrostomy tube to a gastrojejunostomy catheter (23,25).

CONTRAINDICATIONS

There are few absolute contraindications to percutaneous gastrostomy tube placement. The most important absolute contraindication is the lack of a safe access route to the stomach. The colon rarely can block access to the stomach. While the authors routinely place gastrostomy catheters through the transverse mesocolon, occasionally they are unable to access the stomach because of overlying transverse colon. Insufflation of the stomach almost always pushes the transverse colon inferiorly, allowing safe access to the stomach. If the colon is still in the way, then overnight placement of either a nasogastric tube or rectal tube may allow sufficient colonic decompression to allow a safe access route. Small bowel rarely lies anterior to the stomach. Simple rotational fluoroscopy is extremely useful in these cases and almost always shows small bowel to lie posterior to the stomach.

Relative contraindications to percutaneous gastrostomy include coagulopathy, gastric varices, ascites, and gastric carcinoma. Coagulopathy is usually correctable with appropriate blood products or vitamin K. In patients with ascites, preprocedural paracentesis and the use of T-fasteners may prevent ascitic fluid leakage around the catheter (see below) (17,19). Placement of a percutaneous gastrostomy tube through a gastric carcinoma may result in bleeding and failure of tract maturation. Therefore, in patients with gastric or peritoneal malignancy, a preprocedural computerized tomographic (CT) scan may be helpful in allowing selection of an appropriate window for gastrostomy tube placement.

The authors do not consider partial gastrectomy to be a contraindication to gastrostomy tube placement (26). The previous surgical procedure may even make percutaneous gastrostomy easier because of the adhesions that develop between the stomach and abdominal wall. However, placement of a percutaneous gastrostomy tube in a patient with a previous partial gastrectomy may require modifications in the standard technique, including more frequent insufflation of the stomach, use of compound angles with C-arm fluoroscopy, and use of a longer needle.

TECHNIQUE

A variety of techniques are used for percutaneous gastrostomy and gastrojejunostomy (1,5–9,11,23,27–29). The standard approach to these procedures is described next, followed by a discussion of several modifications to those procedures.

Percutaneous Gastrostomy

Figure 32–1 illustrates a percutaneous gastrostomy. Patients should have nothing by mouth or nasogastric tube beginning the night before the examination. A nasogastric tube is placed before the patient arrives in the radiology department. The evening before tube placement, CT contrast is injected into the tube in patients scheduled for tube placement for feeding. By the next day, this contrast typically is in the colon, so the operator can avoid puncturing the viscus. Preferably, this nasogastric tube is placed to suction for 2 to 3 hours before the procedure, especially if the gastrostomy is planned for decompression. If a nasogastric tube placement is unsuccessful, a 5 French angiographic catheter can usually be placed under fluoroscopic guidance in the interventional radiology suite.

Intravenous sedation, when necessary, can be given during the procedure (e.g., fentanyl citrate, midazolam, etc.). Intravenous sedation is usually required for gastrostomy tube placement in children but is rarely needed in adults.

Fluoroscopy is used to evaluate the abdomen before selecting a skin entry site. It is critical to avoid puncturing overlying transverse colon. Additionally, the access must be below the costal margin. Usually, an appropriate site is easily identified in the upper abdomen to the left of midline. This skin site is then prepared in a sterile fashion.

Before air insufflation, glucagon (1 mg IV push) is routinely administered to decrease gastric peristalsis and emptying. Generally, 250–400 cc of air is sufficient to bring the anterior wall of the stomach to the anterior abdominal wall, separate the anterior and posterior gastric walls, and force the transverse colon inferiorly. Fluoroscopic guidance is used to monitor the appropriate volume of gastric distention. Distention of the stomach is critical to provide an appropriate counterforce to the passage of the needle, dilators, and gastrostomy catheter.

A site is selected over the midbody of the stomach. It is important to avoid the greater and lesser curvatures of the stomach to prevent puncture of the gastroepiploic and gastric artery arcades. Lidocaine is used to anesthetize both the skin and the peritoneum. For routine percutaneous gastrostomy placement, the authors use a standard kit modified to their specifications (Mallinckrodt Institute Gastrostomy Set, Cook, Inc.). This kit contains everything necessary for percutaneous gastrostomy placement, including the needle, guide wire, dilators, and catheter (5).

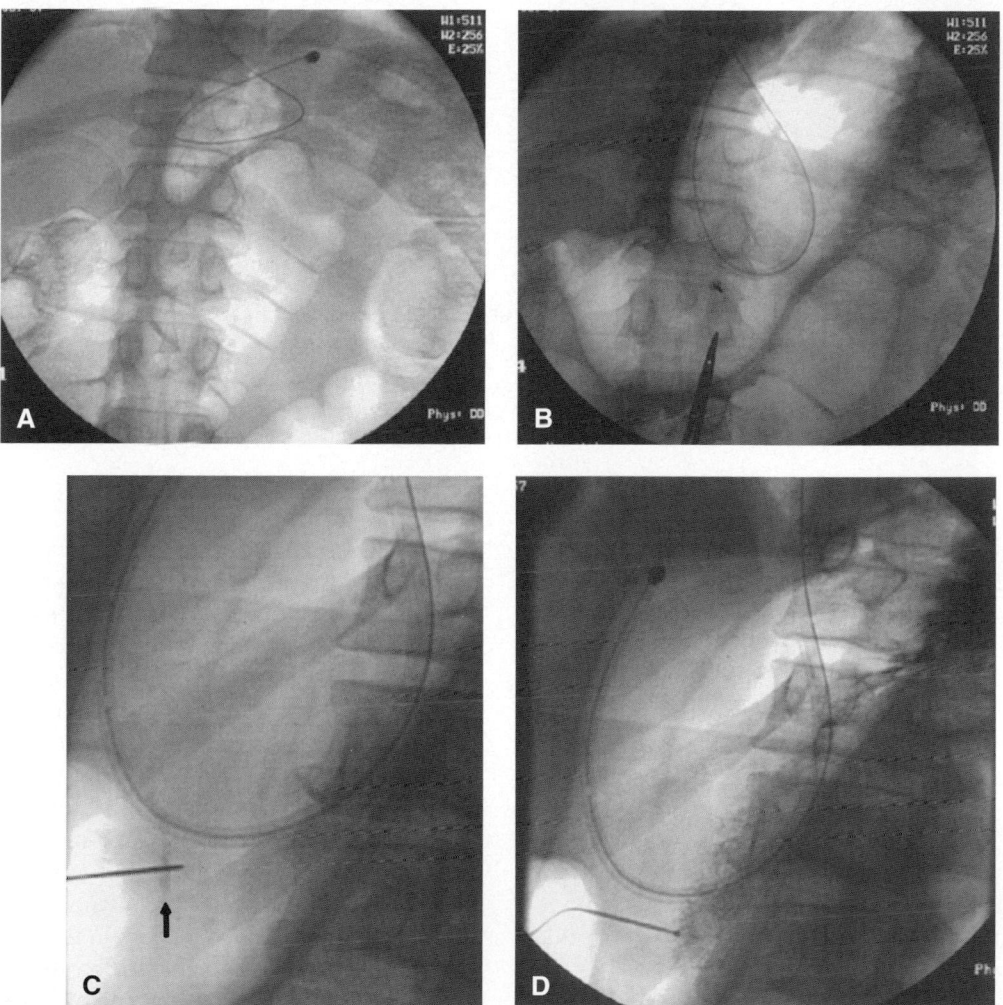

Figure 32–1 Percutaneous gastrostomy tube placement—technique. **A.** Initial fluoroscopy demonstrates a decompressed stomach with the colon occupying much of the left mid- and upper abdomen. **B.** Following air insufflation, the colon is pushed inferiorly. The access needle is localized midway between the greater and lesser curvatures. **C.** The image intensifier is rotated into a left anterior oblique position to allow gastric puncture without radiation exposure to the operator's hands. Note the tenting of the anterior gastric wall (*arrow*). **D.** After aspirating air, contrast is injected into the stomach to confirm appropriate positioning.

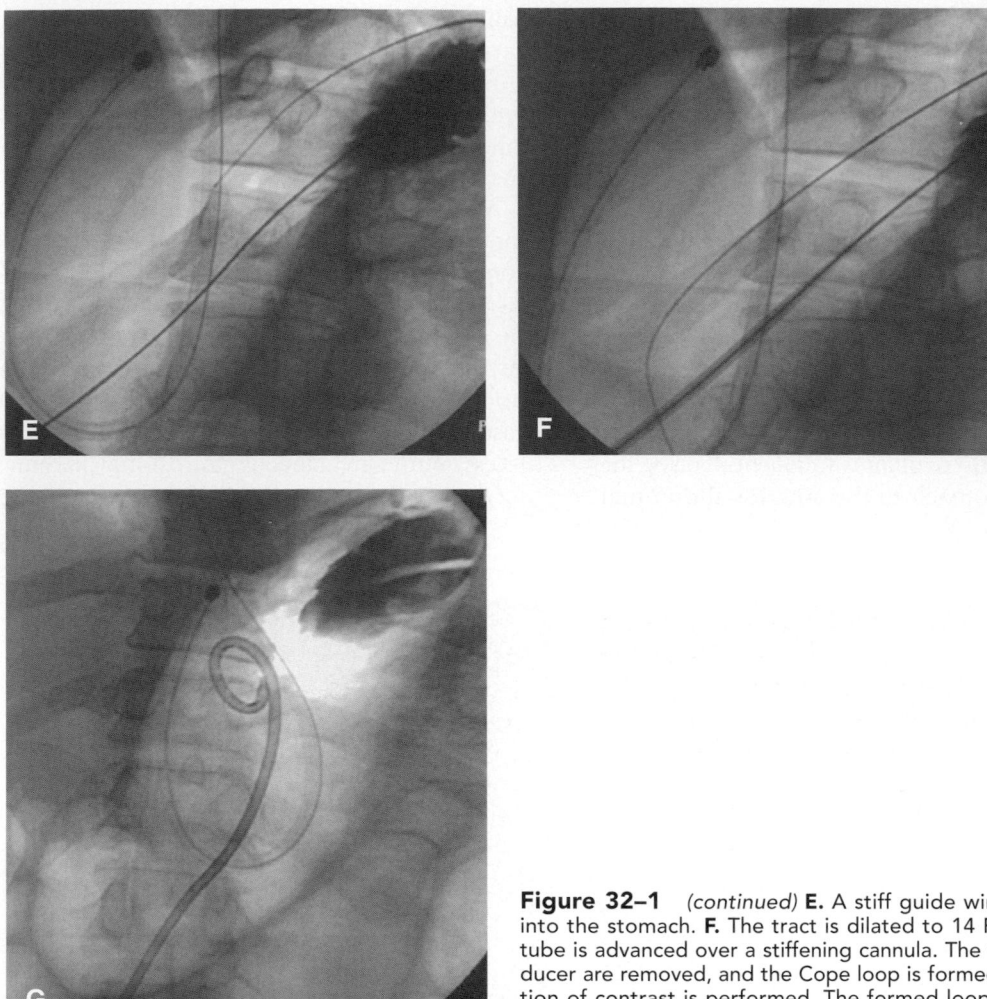

Figure 32–1 *(continued)* **E.** A stiff guide wire is advanced into the stomach. **F.** The tract is dilated to 14 French. **G.** The tube is advanced over a stiffening cannula. The wire and introducer are removed, and the Cope loop is formed. A final injection of contrast is performed. The formed loop should rotate freely in the gastric lumen.

A 7.5-cm 18-gauge Teflon sheathed needle is directed vertically into the stomach under fluoroscopic guidance. Frequently, tenting of the anterior wall of the stomach is observed under fluoroscopy, ensuring an intragastric location of the needle tip. The metal stylet is removed, and air is aspirated. Contrast injection should outline rugal folds as the contrast flows freely away from the tip of the Teflon sheath. If the tip of the sheath is in the retroperitoneum, the contrast will extravasate into the retroperitoneal tissue in a typical pattern. Intraperitoneal position is obvious as the contrast outlines the peritoneal space. If the sheathed needle is not positioned appropriately, it is either advanced or withdrawn so that it lies within the stomach.

Once the intragastric position of the Teflon sheath is confirmed, a 0.038-inch Amplatz extra-stiff guide wire is coiled within the fundus of the stomach. The tract is then dilated in two steps to 14 French. As the dilators are advanced into the stomach, it is important to fluoroscopically observe tenting of the anterior wall of the stomach. Often, additional air must be added to the stomach to provide appropriate counterforce.

It is absolutely critical to confirm that each dilator adequately passes through the anterior wall of the stomach into the gastric lumen. The stomach tends to back away from the dilator. Often, a forceful twisting thrust is necessary to enter the gastric lumen.

Different authors use a variety of percutaneous gastrostomy catheters. All require some type of retention device. The authors prefer a modified pigtail catheter. This 14 French gastrostomy catheter has extra large side-holes, as well as a standard Cope loop retention mechanism. The catheter is placed with the use of a flexible stiffening cannula. To prevent partial extragastric/intraperitoneal placement, it is important to be certain that the catheter is well positioned into the stomach before forming the Cope loop. Proper intragastric placement is confirmed by contrast injection. The authors do not pull the catheter back against the anterior wall of the stomach. This is not necessary for gastrostomy tract maturation. Pulling the tube back too forcefully risks that one of the side-holes in the pigtail portion may be pulled into the peritoneal cavity, leading to peritonitis.

The authors prefer to secure the catheter in place with a single O-Prolene suture. It is important to secure the catheter to the anterior abdominal wall. If the catheter is not adequately secured, it may be carried by peristalsis into the duodenum. This can lead to diarrhea and abdominal cramping during feeds. Long-term positioning in this location can lead to duodenal perforation and/or obstruction.

The catheter is initially placed to external drainage overnight. The patient is seen the next morning, and if the abdominal exam is benign, feedings may begin.

Percutaneous Gastrojejunostomy

Figure 32–2 illustrates a percutaneous gastrojejunostomy. The initial steps outlined in the previous section (to the point of puncture site selection) are similar for percutaneous gastrojejunostomy placement. Passage of a catheter through the stomach into the jejunum is facilitated by directing the puncture downhill toward the pylorus. Therefore, it is advantageous to select an entry site slightly higher on the body of the stomach, with the needle angled toward the antrum.

Because of the additional manipulations necessary to access the jejunum, the authors routinely place two to four T-fasteners prior to accessing the stomach (Figure 32–2). The stomach is accessed between the T-fasteners. After passage of a guide wire via the access needle, an angled catheter and guide wire are used in combination to gain access to the ligament of Treitz. A variety of tip configurations may be useful to facilitate passage through the pylorus. The authors routinely use an angled multipurpose configuration. Also useful may be a headhunter or Cobra catheter. Either a floppy-tipped wire (e.g., Bentson) or a hydrophilic angled wire (e.g., Terumo wire) is used in combination with the catheter to access the jejunum.

Once the catheter is manipulated into the jejunum, the tract is dilated over a stiff wire, and a peel-away sheath is placed. The use of a peel-away sheath decreases the resistance to catheter passage through the abdominal wall, allowing easier placement of the catheter into the jejunum. Additionally, the authors prefer to use a large, nontapered-endhole gastrojejunostomy catheter because these nontapered catheters are less prone to plugging. Because these catheters are not tapered to the guide wire, they require placement through a peel-away sheath.

Standard gastrojejunostomy tubes have either a Cope loop or friction-lock Malecot retention mechanism (Figure 32–3A). The tip of the gastrojejunostomy catheter is placed in the proximal jejunum distal to the ligament of Treitz. The retention mechanism is formed in the stomach after the peel away sheath is removed. The tip of the single lumen gastrojejunostomy catheter is not tapered to limit obstruction (Figure 32–3B).

In contrast to gastrostomy tube placement, feeding through the gastrojejunostomy catheters begins immediately after the procedure. Because these tubes are prone to plugging, they should be irrigated liberally with water after each use.

Procedural Modifications

A variety of alternative catheters are available for both percutaneous gastrostomy and gastrojejunostomy tube placement. Some authors prefer Foley balloon catheters for percutaneous gastrostomy. The authors have found the complication rate with Foley catheters with an immature tract to be significantly higher than that with Cope loop catheters and prefer not to use Foley catheters (5,30).

Occasionally, patients will require gastric decompression as well as jejunal feedings. For this purpose, the authors use a double-lumen gastrojejunostomy tube. For this tube to adequately decompress the stomach, the gastric port must be in the fundus of the stomach. Therefore, this catheter must be looped in the fundus of the stomach before passing into the jejunum (Figure 32–4). This can be done either during the initial access procedure or after access into the jejunum is obtained.

Several authors have described a variety of devices to simulate surgical apposition of the stomach to the anterior abdominal wall. These devices are called T-fasteners or suture anchor devices (Figure 32–5) (7,31–34). These T-fasteners are placed with a large-bore needle (16 or 18 gauge) either as a single fixation point or at the corners of a triangle with the gastrostomy tube placed in the middle. Advocates of this technique believe it encourages adequate tract maturation as well as minimizes leakage of gastric contents into the peritoneal cavity. However, many series report no such problems with percutaneous gastrostomy and gastrojejunostomy; even though T-fasteners were not used routinely. Some authors feel that routine use of T-fasteners may actually be disadvantageous (35,36). The increased number of punctures necessary to place these devices may increase the risk of bleeding during the procedure. Additionally, the suture may lead to an increased infection rate. Published data comparing the techniques for simple gastrostomy placement is limited (34) The authors prefer to use T-fasteners for selected indications in which it may be more important to assure apposition between the stomach and the anterior abdominal wall. Examples include patients with ascites, uncooperative patients, patients with poor healing (e.g., resulting from steroid therapy), and patients in whom extensive manipulations will be necessary (e.g., gastrojejunostomy tube placement).

Placement of a percutaneous gastrostomy tube in a patient with partial gastrectomy may require modifications of the standard technique (27). Often, the adhesions that form between the stomach and the anterior abdominal wall following gastric surgery are advantageous for percutaneous placement. However, because the gastric remnant is small and the pylorus is absent, frequent insufflation of air during the procedure may be necessary to keep the stomach distended. Additionally, the gastric remnant may lie high

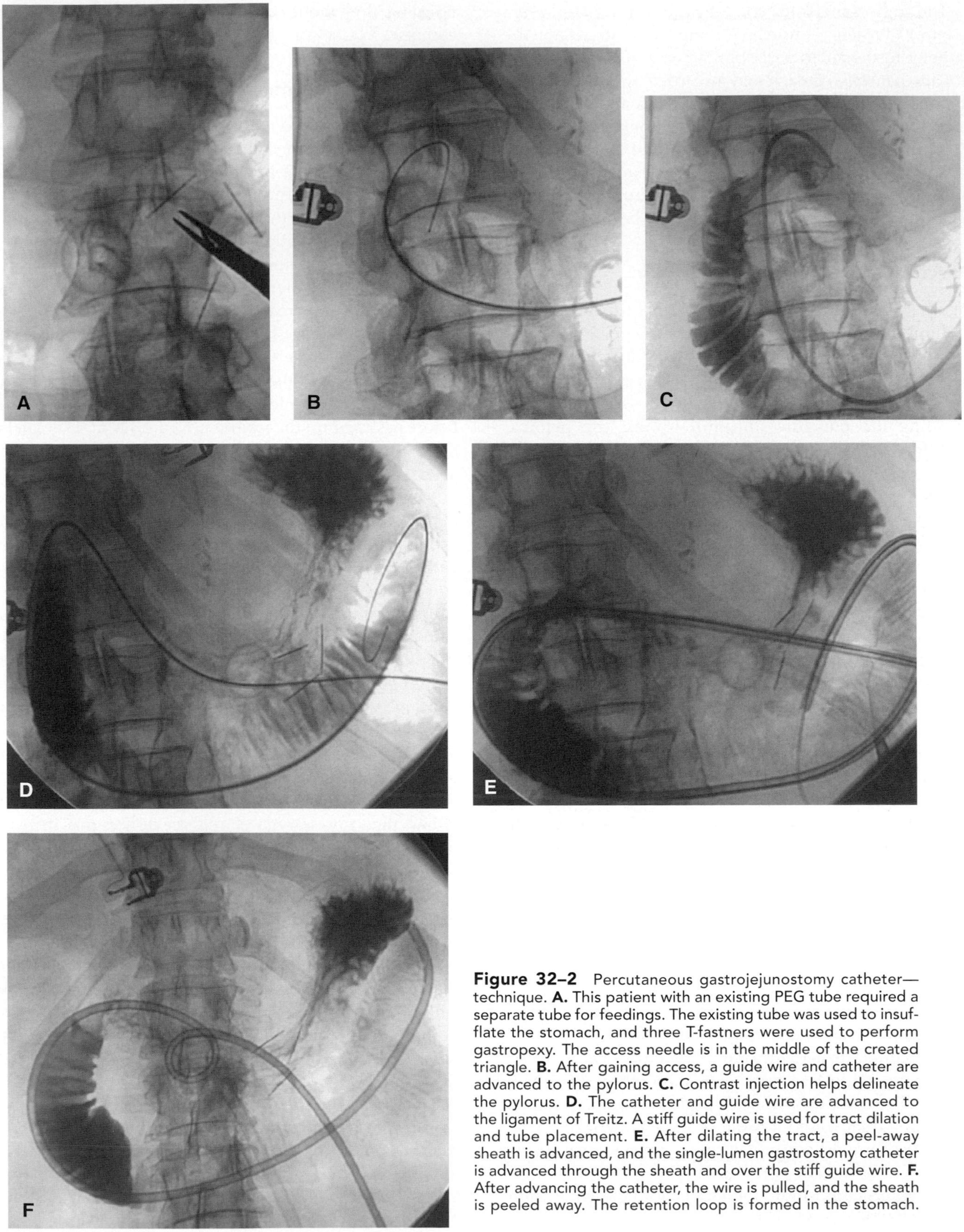

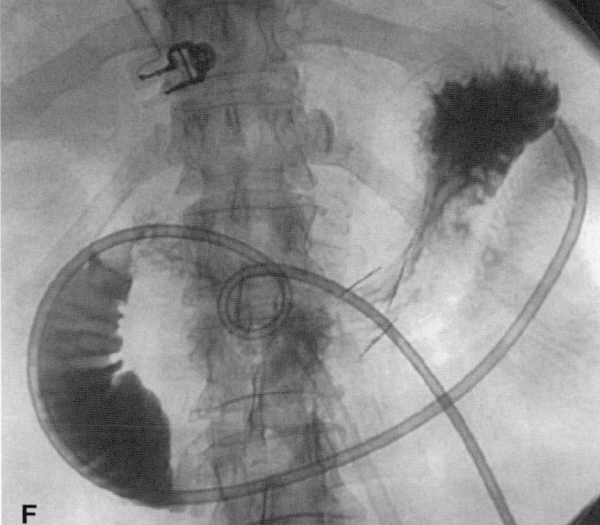

Figure 32–2 Percutaneous gastrojejunostomy catheter—technique. **A.** This patient with an existing PEG tube required a separate tube for feedings. The existing tube was used to insufflate the stomach, and three T-fastners were used to perform gastropexy. The access needle is in the middle of the created triangle. **B.** After gaining access, a guide wire and catheter are advanced to the pylorus. **C.** Contrast injection helps delineate the pylorus. **D.** The catheter and guide wire are advanced to the ligament of Treitz. A stiff guide wire is used for tract dilation and tube placement. **E.** After dilating the tract, a peel-away sheath is advanced, and the single-lumen gastrostomy catheter is advanced through the sheath and over the stiff guide wire. **F.** After advancing the catheter, the wire is pulled, and the sheath is peeled away. The retention loop is formed in the stomach.

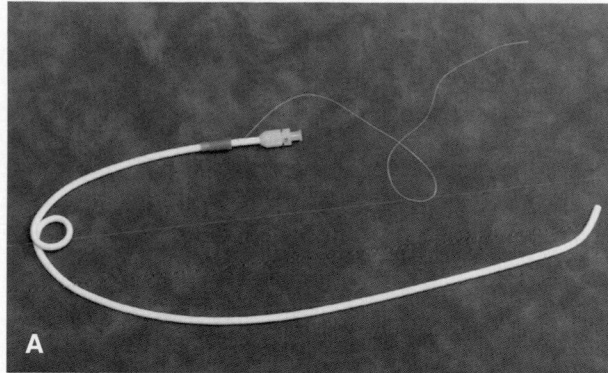

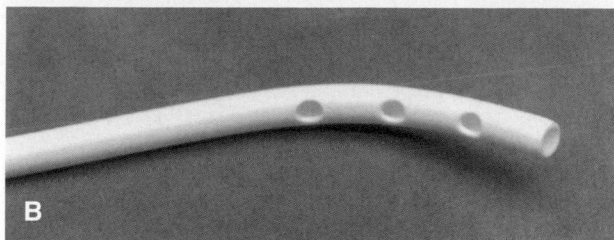

Figure 32–3 The Carey-Alzate Coons Single Lumen Gastrojejunostomy Catheter (Cook Inc.). **A.** The retention loop is proximal and forms in the stomach. **B.** The catheter tip is nontapered, requiring passage through a peel-away sheath. This design limits tube clogging.

underneath the costal margin, and complex angulation may be necessary to direct the needle into the stomach. Such complex angulation is facilitated by the use of C-arm fluoroscopy. Finally, a relatively long tract may be needed to access the stomach—particularly in a subcostal location. This may require the use of a longer (15–30 cm) needle.

When a standard nasogastric tube cannot be placed, it is usually possible to manipulate a 5 French catheter into the stomach using standard guide wire techniques and fluoro-

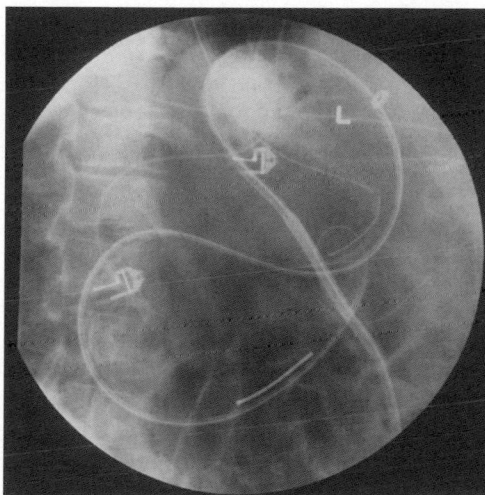

Figure 32–4 Double lumen gastrojejunostomy catheter. Contrast has been injected through the gastrostomy port into the gastric fundus. The feeding lumen extends into the proximal jejunum.

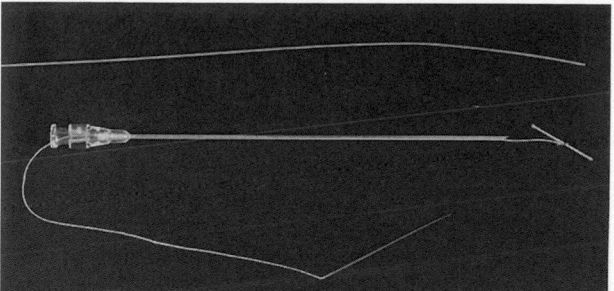

Figure 32–5 The Cope suture anchor (Cook Inc.). Initially, the anchor is within the needle housing. After the needle has been inserted into the stomach, the guide wire is coaxially advanced to extrude the anchor. The needle is then removed, and the suture is sewn to the skin.

scopic guidance. Occasionally, however, even this is not possible in patients with high-grade esophageal obstructions. In these patients, if a gastric air collection can be seen with fluoroscopy, the stomach can be entered directly with a 22-gauge needle (14). This 22-gauge needle can then be used for air insufflation as described above. In these patients, it may be helpful to place a T-fastener because access to the stomach may be tenuous.

Placement of PEG-type tubes using fluoroscopic techniques alone can be performed (Figure 32–6). These tubes are frequently 20–24 French rather than the 14–16 French tubes typically placed during fluoroscopic gastrostomy. Some referring clinicians prefer larger-bore access. Also, the deformable mushroom button on some kits makes the tubes more difficult for neurologically impaired patients to pull out. A 5 French orogastric catheter is used to distend the stomach. After puncturing the stomach with an 18-gauge needle, a short sheath is used to advance a gooseneck snare. A wire is passed through the orogastric tube, snared, and pulled through the abdominal puncture site. The gastrostomy tube is loaded at the oral end of the through-and-through wire and pushed over the wire until the leading edge of its dilator is identified at the abdominal wall. The dilator is then pulled until the mushroom bumper fits snugly against the anterior gastric wall. The guide wire is removed, and the tube is trimmed appropriately. Success in clinical trials ranges 97–100% with complications comparable to standard fluoroscopic gastrostomy (37–39). Complications of note using this technique include skin infection from passage of the tube via the oral mucosa. Prophylactic antibiotics, which are standard prior to PEG tube placement, are recommended (40,41).

Occasionally, CT guidance is necessary to direct percutaneous gastric access. CT guidance is particularly useful in patients with gastric malignancies or abdominal masses that require careful gastric access (42). The authors prefer to either mark an appropriate access route on the abdominal wall or place a needle into the stomach under CT guidance and then transfer the patient to the fluoroscopy suite for the completion of the procedure. The use of fluoroscopy is extremely

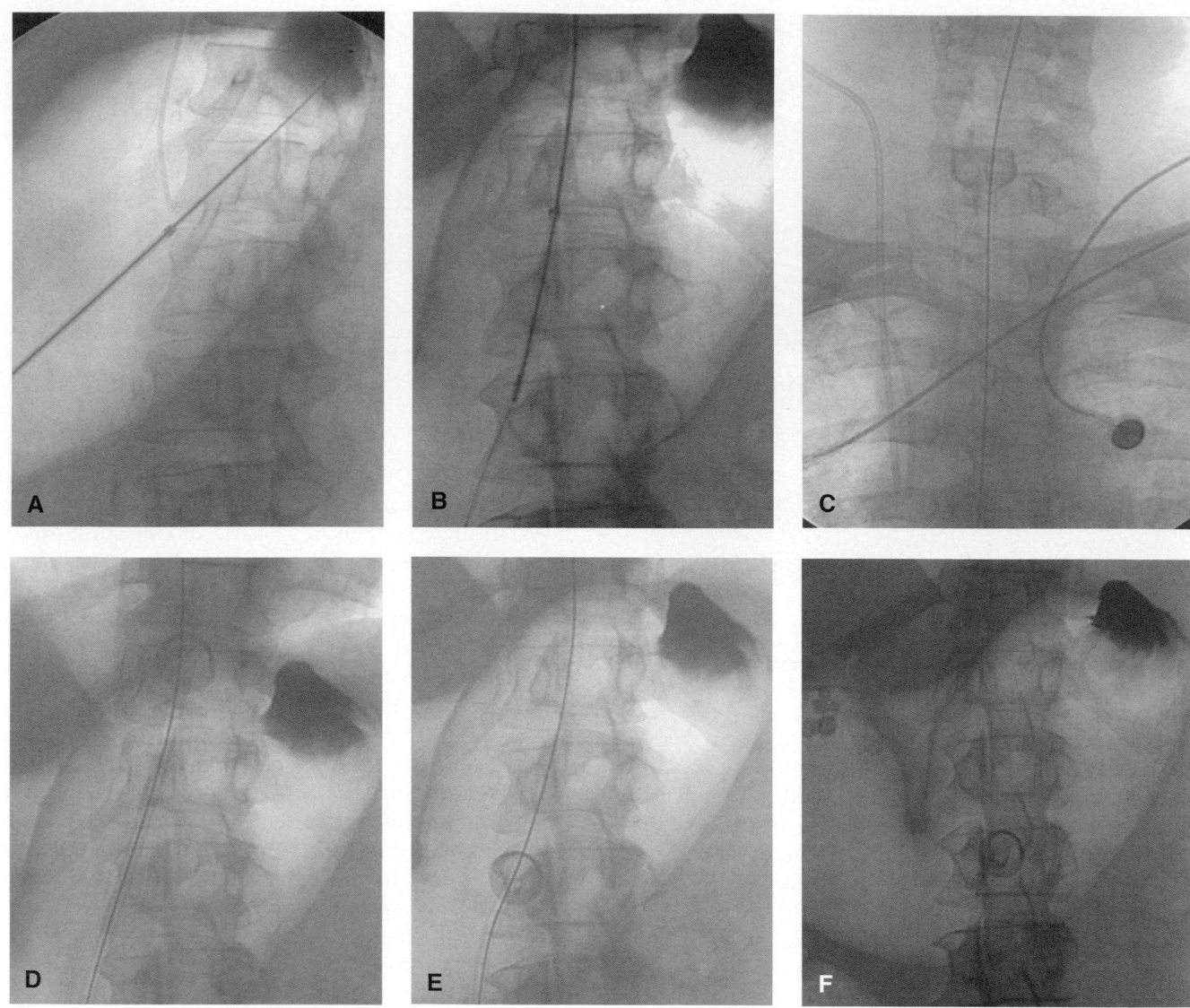

Figure 32–6 Pull gastrostomy—technique. **A.** An orogastric tube is placed, and the stomach is distended with air. Puncture is made as with a typical gastrostomy. A sheath is then advanced over the guide wire. **B.** A 240-cm guide wire is snared via the gastric sheath and pulled out the sheath, providing through-and-through access. **C.** The pull gastrostomy catheter is pushed from above while tension is maintained at both ends of the wire. **D.** As the retention bumper approaches the stomach, the tapered end of the gastrostomy catheter will reach the stomach. Pulling on this end of the tube helps seat the retention bumper against the anterior gastric wall. **E.** The retention device is pulled against the gastric wall. **F.** The wire is removed.

helpful to ensure that both the dilators and the gastrostomy catheter are appropriately positioned in the stomach.

The presence of ascites presents a particular challenge for percutaneous gastric access. The authors routinely use ultrasound to evaluate all patients with ascites before gastrostomy tube placement. Occasionally, a window can be found to the stomach where no ascites is present. If this is not possible, a percutaneous peritoneal catheter can be placed to withdraw ascitic fluid to optimize apposition of the anterior gastric wall with the anterior abdominal wall. T-fasteners may also be helpful to draw the wall of the stomach to the anterior abdominal wall and decrease ascitic fluid leakage following gastrostomy tube placement (17–19).

Management

To minimize complications, it is essential that the interventional radiologist take care of the short-term and long-term management of gastrostomy tube patients. Immediately following the procedure, the percutaneous gastrostomy catheter is left to external drainage. This allows assessment of postprocedural bleeding as well as decreases short-term gastric distention after tube placement. The patient is visited the next morning, and if the patient is afebrile with a benign abdominal exam, feedings may begin. Gastric feedings are begun initially at a slow rate to see how the patient tolerates them. Additionally, it is important to check for residuals before each feeding. If the patient has a large amount of residual intragastric material, the subsequent feedings should be held. In the authors' experience, most major complications occur within 3 days of gastrostomy tube placement (M. E. Hicks, *unpublished data*). Therefore, the routine is to see these patients on a daily basis for at least 3 days following the procedure.

If the patient develops large residuals or symptoms of reflux, he or she should be fed in a semierect position and kept in this position for at least 30 minutes after feeding. If large residuals continue to be a problem or the patient develops signs or symptoms of aspiration, the gastrostomy tube can be converted to a gastrojejunostomy catheter.

Long-term management is important as well. All patients and their caregivers should receive a gastrostomy care sheet (Table 32–1). They should be instructed to contact the radiologist directly with any difficulties or questions. The authors do not perform routine gastrostomy tube changes. However, catheter changes are frequently required 4–6 months after placement because of tube malfunctions. This is easily done as an outpatient procedure using fluoroscopic guidance.

If gastrostomy tube removal is indicated, it is important to be certain the percutaneous tract is mature before tube removal. Tract maturation usually occurs 1–3 weeks following tube placement (25). If integrity of the tract is a concern, contrast may be injected into the tract while a guide wire is left in the stomach to preserve access.

Gastrostomy Button Placement

A variety of skin-level gastrostomy devices are available from different manufacturers (e.g., Bard, Inc., Kimberly Clark, Inc.) (Figure 32–7). The main advantage of these skin-level devices is that they are less intrusive than a standard gastrostomy catheter and may be more cost effective in the long term (43–44). This may be particularly important in an ambulatory patient, a child, or patients receiving physical therapy. A patient's self-image may be improved with the use of these skin-level devices.

The authors generally wait 2–3 months after the initial gastrostomy tube placement before attempting placement of a gastrostomy button. The percutaneous tract must be well healed prior to manipulation. The authors use button devices that are 18 or 24 French in size. Because the gastrostomy tube may not be that large, the tract usually must be dilated before button placement. Alternatively, albeit uncommonly, this may be done by placing gastrostomy catheters of increasingly larger sizes at scheduled intervals.

Prior to button placement, it is critically important to accurately measure the length of the percutaneous tract to the stomach (45). Percutaneous gastrostomy tracts tend to be longer than surgical tracts. This obviously requires the use of a longer device for button placement in patients with percutaneous gastrostomy tubes. Additionally, if the button is too long, it will move in and out at the skin site. Such excessive movement can stimulate exuberant granulation tissue.

It is preferred to place buttons under fluoroscopic guidance with a guide wire protecting the tract. If the device cannot be advanced into the stomach for any reason, a gastrostomy catheter can be easily replaced over the guide wire. Fluoroscopic guidance is helpful to be certain that the button is appropriately placed within the gastric lumen. Once the button is in place, injection of contrast should be performed to document appropriate position.

The authors prefer buttons with a balloon type of retention mechanism (Mic-Key, Kimberly Clark, Inc.). These balloon buttons are lower-profile devices and therefore easier to place. Surgeons more commonly place buttons

TABLE 32–1

HOW TO CARE FOR THE FEEDING TUBE (GASTROSTOMY TUBE)

Each patient, family, or caregiver is provided with a tube care sheet. The sheet includes specific directions on dressing changes, feedings, and a number to call with any questions or problems.

I. Dressing changes—every 1–2 days.
    A. Clean around tube with hydrogen peroxide.
    B. Dress with gauze pads and tape. Position tube so that it does not kink.
II. Showers—no tub baths.
    A. Cover dressing with a double layer of plastic wrap, and tape edges.
    B. Remove plastic wrap and change dressing after you shower.
III. Activities—no specific restrictions.
IV. Feedings.
    A. Use water to flush the tube after each feeding.
    B. Use liquid forms of medication if possible.
    C. Ask your doctor or nurse to provide you with specific information about feedings or medications.
V. Problems with the tube. Please call the appropriate number listed for any of the following problems.
    A. Leakage of feedings around the tube.
    B. Signs of infection such as swelling, tenderness, redness, or drainage of pus around the tube.
    C. If the tube falls out completely, call <u>immediately</u>. The tube usually can be easily replaced if it is done within 24 hours from the time it fell out. Waiting longer could mean that a separate new tube will have to be placed.
VI. Call us anytime if the tube plugs up or if you have any questions or problems regarding the tube.

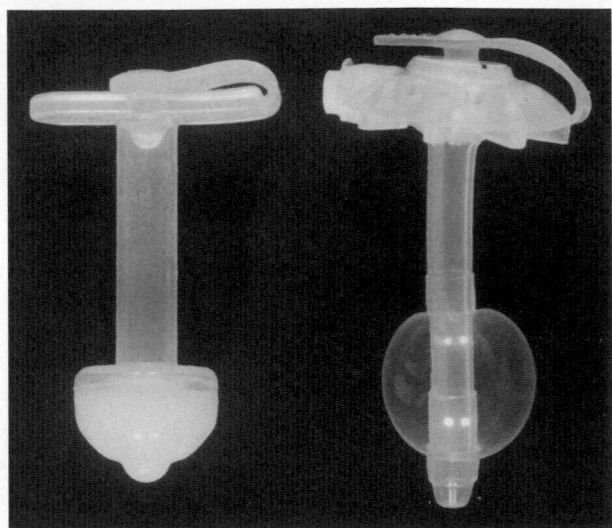

Figure 32–7 Gastric buttons. Bard button (*left*) and the Mic-Key button (*right*). Note the balloon retention device on the Mic-Key button.

with a mushroom-type of retention device. These devices are slightly less expensive but often require considerable force to advance into the tract.

All buttons have a one-way valve in the lumen to prevent reflux of gastric contents after feeding. These valves will eventually fail. Patients and their caregivers should be given instructions to return for button replacement when the device begins to leak. In the case of balloon buttons, the caregivers themselves often are able to replace the button when it malfunctions.

RESULTS

Percutaneous gastrostomy is a procedure associated with a high technical success rate. Most authors report technical success rates ranging 98–100% (1,5–8,13–14). Failure usually results from lack of a safe access route—most commonly caused by overlying transverse colon. Other causes for technical failure include massive ascites, gastric cancer, peritoneal carcinomatosis, an intrathoracic stomach, large overlying open abdominal incisions, and previous gastric surgery.

Occasionally, access to the stomach is lost during attempts at tract dilatation. In most cases, this should not result in technical failure (34). If access can be promptly established through a new puncture, significant complications usually do not occur.

COMPLICATIONS

Most authors report a relatively low rate of major and minor complications associated with percutaneous gastrostomy.

Pooling the data from several large series of gastrostomy and gastrojejunostomy tube placements (3,125 patients) demonstrates a 2.2% major and a 5.9% minor complication rate (1,5–8,13–14). Various authors classify complications differently. Also, most series include different patient populations. In general terms, however, most series of endoscopic or surgical gastrostomy tube placements report minor complications ranging 5–10% and major complications ranging 3–10% (1,3,46–48).

As more surgeons become familiar with PEG tube placement, it is likely that open gastrostomy will be reserved for situations in which patients undergo laparotomy for a simultaneous procedure (4,49). Comparison of the complication rate resulting from percutaneous gastrostomy and that seen with endoscopic gastrostomy is limited but suggests that the percutaneous method has greater success, takes less time to perform, and requires less sedation (21,50,51). The most common minor complication associated with percutaneous gastrostomy tube placement is skin site infection (1,5,10). Early peristomal infection usually occurs 3–5 days following tube placement. These infections can almost always be treated with local skin care, but occasionally antibiotics are required.

Another minor tube site problem is fluid leakage around the catheter. Fluid leakage around a gastrostomy catheter usually represents ascitic fluid. Such an ascitic fluid leak can become a difficult management problem and is best treated by trying to decrease the amount of ascites and placing T-fastners at the time of gastrostomy. If necessary, a purse-string suture around the skin entry site can be placed for several days. Feedings can leak out through the tract if the catheter erodes a larger hole through the skin. Feeding can be differentiated from ascites by placing food coloring in the patient's feedings.

Other late minor tube complications include tube malfunction as well as displacement of the gastrostomy catheter. In patients with a mature gastrostomy tract, such problems are easily managed by simply changing to a new tube. However, if the tube falls out and the tract closes prior to replacing the catheter, a new access may be required.

The most serious major complication associated with percutaneous gastrostomy tube placement is peritonitis. Frequently, patients requiring gastrostomy tube placement are severely debilitated. Peritonitis in these elderly, debilitated patients can result in major morbidity and even death. Peritonitis associated with percutaneous gastrostomy is extremely unusual. When it does occur, it usually results from tube displacement in a patient with an immature tract. This displacement may be subtle, resulting from a single side-hole of the catheter that pulls back into the peritoneal cavity. Perforation of the stomach or duodenum also can result in peritonitis. Frank perforation can occur from erosion by the tip of the gastrostomy catheter (5). In patients in whom peritonitis is suspected, tube feedings should be held. Either fluoroscopically guided contrast injection or computed tomography with contrast injected into the tube can be performed for further evaluation. Patients with peritonitis usually require immediate operative intervention.

Significant bleeding associated with percutaneous gastrostomy is rare but most often related to an underlying coagulopathy. Once the coagulopathy is corrected, the bleeding should stop. If patients continue to bleed through the gastrostomy catheter, than gastritis or gastric ulceration should be suspected. These usually can be treated with medical therapy but may require endoscopy for diagnosis.

Aspiration pneumonia can occur from reflux of gastric feedings. The use of food coloring in the feedings can be helpful to differentiate aspiration pneumonia secondary to reflux of feedings from pneumonia resulting from other causes. If the patient develops symptoms of aspiration, consideration should be given to converting the gastrostomy tube to a gastrojejunostomy catheter.

Pneumoperitoneum is frequently seen following percutaneous gastrostomy and is not considered a complication (52). Free air in the peritoneum following the procedure is not clinically significant unless it is increasing in volume or associated with signs of peritoneal irritation.

ADVANTAGES AND DISADVANTAGES OF VARIOUS APPROACHES

Surgical gastrostomy has little advantage over the less-invasive techniques unless it is done at the time of another major surgical procedure. Surgical gastrostomy requires a laparotomy incision to expose the stomach and, therefore, usually requires general anesthesia. This introduces additional morbidity to the procedure (3,53). Additionally, the performance of gastrostomy in the operating room is more expensive than either endoscopic or radiological placement (53,54). There have been several reports of laparoscopic placement of gastrostomy tubes (55,56). The utility of this procedure is questionable and far from proved. It is more invasive and expensive than either the endoscopic or fluoroscopic alternative. There appears to be little indication for laparoscopic gastrostomy unless it is done in conjunction with another laparoscopic procedure.

The endoscopic technique can be performed at the bedside in critically ill patients who are unable to come to the radiology department. The endoscopic technique also allows endoscopic inspection of the esophagus and stomach in patients in whom such an examination is indicated. However, the endoscopic technique has several distinct disadvantages when compared with fluoroscopically guided gastrostomy tube placement. Because it requires upper endoscopy, significantly more sedation is needed for the endoscopic technique than for the fluoroscopic technique (51). The endoscopic technique also requires two operators and carries the risk of respiratory distress and aspiration during introduction of the endoscope (47,57). In patients with esophageal obstruction, it may be difficult or

even impossible to pass the endoscope into the stomach; however, using fluoroscopy, in these patients it is almost always possible to place a 5 French catheter to insufflate the stomach. Finally, most endoscopically placed gastrostomy catheters have a bumper in the stomach. This requires repeat endoscopy for tube changes.

Fluoroscopically guided gastrostomy tube placement is the least invasive of the three alternatives. Because it does not require the use of either the operating room or endoscopy, it is also the least expensive of the three alternatives. In most patients, percutaneous gastrostomy requires minimal to no sedation, and because it uses direct fluoroscopic control, there is little risk of placing the tube through the colon or small bowel. Fluoroscopically guided gastrostomy can be performed rapidly by one operator. Additionally, with standard guide wire and catheter techniques, it is usually a simple matter to place a catheter into the jejunum at the time of initial gastrostomy tube placement. A percutaneous gastrostomy usually can be easily converted to a gastrojejunostomy if problems with aspiration develop. The same cannot be said for surgical or endoscopic access (23).

SUMMARY

Percutaneous fluoroscopically guided gastrostomy and gastrojejunostomy provide safe, effective, and economical access to the intestinal tract for either enteral nutrition or decompression. The technique is useful in patients of all ages and in almost all clinical circumstances. The skills required for this procedure are identical to those in common use by interventional radiologists for all types of drainage and organ access procedures. This technique should be a standard part of all interventional radiology practices.

REFERENCES

1. Ho C-S, Yeung EY. Percutaneous gastrostomy and transgastric jejunostomy. AJR Am J Roentgenol 1992;158:251–257.
2. Park RH, Allison MC, Lang J, et al. Randomised comparison of percutaneous endoscopic gastrostomy and nasogastric tube feeding in patients with persisting neurological dysphagia. Br Med J 1992;304:1406–1409.
3. Shellito PC, Malt RA. Tube gastrostomy. Techniques and complications. Ann Surg 1985;201:180–185.
4. Dwyer KM, Watts DD, Thurber JS, et al. Percutaneous endoscopic gastrostomy: the preferred method of elective feeding tube placement in trauma patients. J Trauma 2002;52:26–32.
5. Hicks ME, Surratt RS, Picus D, et al. Fluoroscopically guided percutaneous gastrostomy and gastroenterostomy: analysis of 158 consecutive cases. AJR A J Roentgenol 1990;154:725–728.
6. Halkier BK, Ho C-S, Yee ACN. Percutaneous feeding gastrostomy with the Seldinger technique: review of 252 patients. Radiology 1989;171:359–362.
7. Saini S, Mueller PR, Gaa J, et al. Percutaneous gastrostomy with gastropexy: experience in 125 patients. AJR Am J Roentgenol 1990;154:1003–1006.
8. O'Keeffe F, Carrasco CH, Charnsangavej C, et al. Percutaneous drainage and feeding gastrostomies in 100 patients. Radiology 1989;172:341–343.

9. vanSonnenberg E, Wittich GR, Cabrera OA, et al. Percutaneous gastrostomy and gastroenterostomy: 2. clinical experience. AJR Am J Roentgenol 1986;146:581–586.

10. Malden ES, Hicks ME, Picus D, et al. Fluoroscopically guided percutaneous gastrostomy in children. J Vasc Interv Radiol 1992;3: 673–677.

11. Towbin RB, Ball WS, Bissett GS. Percutaneous gastrostomy and percutaneous gastrojejunostomy in children: antegrade approach. Radiology 1988;168:473–476.

12. Ho C-S, Yee CN, McPherson R. Complications of surgical and percutaneous nonendoscopic gastrostomy: review of 233 patients. Gastroenterology 1988;95:1206–1210.

13. Dewald CL, Hiette PO, Sewall LE, et al. Percutaneous gastrostomy and gastrojejunostomy with gastropexy: experience in 701 procedures. Radiology 1999;211:651–656.

14. de Baere T, Chapot R, Kuoch V, et al. Percutaneous gastrostomy with fluoroscopic guidance: single-center experience in 500 consecutive cancer patients. Radiology 1999;210:651–654.

15. Wills JS, Oglesby JT. Percutaneous gastrostomy. Radiology 1988;167:41–43.

16. Picus D, Marx MV, Weyman PJ. Chronic intestinal obstruction: value of percutaneous gastrostomy tube placement. AJR Am J Roentgenol 1988;150:295–297.

17. Lee MJ, Saini S, Brink JA, et al. Malignant small bowel obstruction and ascites: not a contraindication to percutaneous gastrostomy. Clin Radiol 1991;44:332–334.

18. Herman LL, Hoskins WJ, Shike M. Percutaneous endoscopic gastrostomy for decompression of the stomach and small bowel. Gastrointest Endosc 1992;38:314–318.

19. Ryan JM, Hahn PF, Mueller PR. Performing radiologic gastrostomy or gastrojejunostomy in patients with malignant ascites. AJR Am J Roentgenol 1998;171:1003–1006.

20. Hoffer EK, Cosgrove JM, Levin DQ, et al. Radiologic gastrojejunostomy and percutaneous endoscopic gastrostomy: a prospective, randomized comparison. J Vasc Interv Radiol 1999;10:413–420.

21. Olson DL, Krubsack AJ, Stewart ET. Percutaneous enteral alimentation: gastrostomy versus gastrojejunostomy. Radiology 1993;187:105–108.

22. Gray RR, St. Louis EL, Grosman H. Percutaneous gastrostomy and gastro-jejunostomy. Br J Radiol 1987;60:1067–1070.

23. Lu DS, Mueller PR, Lee MJ, et al. Gastrostomy conversion to transgastric jejunostomy: technical problems, causes of failure, and proposed solutions in 63 patients. Radiology 1993;187:679–683.

24. Mathus-Vliegen LM, Koning H. Percutaneous endoscopic gastrostomy and gastrojejunostomy: a critical reappraisal of patient selection, tube function and the feasibility of nutritional support during extended follow-up. Gastrointest Endosc 1999;50:746–754.

25. vanSonnenberg E, Wittich GR, Brown LK, et al. Percutaneous gastrostomy and gastroenterostomy: techniques derived from laboratory evaluation. AJR Am J Roentgenol 1986;146:577–580.

26. Stevens SD, Picus D, Hicks ME, et al. Percutaneous gastrostomy and gastrojejunostomy after gastric surgery. J Vasc Interv Radiol 1992;3:679–683.

27. Giuliano AW, Yoon HC, Lomis NN, Miller FJ. Fluoroscopically guided percutaneous placement of large-bore gastrostomy and gastrojejunostomy tubes: review of 109 cases. J Vasc Interv Radiol 2000;11:239–246.

28. Gehman KE, Elliott JA, Inculet RI. Percutaneous gastrojejunostomy with a modified Cope loop catheter. AJR Am J Roentgenol 1990;155:79–80.

29. Alzate GD, Coons HG, Elliott J, et al. Percutaneous gastrostomy for jejunal feeding: a new technique. AJR Am J Roentgenol 1986;147:822–825.

30. O'Keefe KP, Dula DJ, Varano V. Duodenal obstruction by a nondeflating Foley catheter gastrostomy tube. Ann Emerg Med 1990;19: 1454–1457.

31. Wills JS, Oglesby JT. Controlled percutaneous gastrostomy: nylon T-fastener for fixation of the anterior gastric wall. Radiology 1986;160:278.

32. Brown AS, Mueller PR, Ferrucci JT. Controlled percutaneous gastrostomy: nylon T-fastener for fixation of the anterior gastric wall. Radiology 1986;158:543–545.

33. Cope C. Suture anchor for visceral drainage. AJR Am J Roentgenol 1986;146:160–161.

34. Thornton FJ, Fotheringham T, Haslam PJ, et al. Percutaneous radiologic gastrostomy with and without T-fastener gastropexy: a randomized comparison study. Cardiovasc Interv Radiol 2002;25: 467–471.

35. Moote DJ, Ho C-S, Felice V. Fluoroscopically guided percutaneous gastrostomy: is gastric fixation necessary? Can Assoc Radiol J 1991;42:113–118.

36. Deutsch LS, Kannegieter L, Vanson DT, et al. Simplified percutaneous gastrostomy. Radiology 1992;184:181–183.

37. Clark JA, Pugash RA, Pantalone RR. Radiologic peroral gastrostomy. J Vasc Interv Radiol 1999;10:927–932.

38. Funaki B, Peirce R, Lorenz J, et al. Comparison of balloon- and mushroom-retained large-bore gastrostomy catheters. AJR Am J Roentgenol 2001;177:359–362.

39. Cahill RM, Kaye RD, Fitz CR, et al. "Push-pull" gastrostomy: a new technique for percutaneous gastrostomy tube insertion in the neonate and young infant. Pediatr Radiol 2001;31:550–554.

40. Ahmad I, Mouncher A, Abdoolah A, et al. Antibiotic prophylaxis for percutaneous endoscopic gastrostomy—a prospective, randomised, double-blind trial. Aliment Pharmacol Ther 2003;18: 209–215.

41. Panigrahi H, Shreeve DR, Tan WC, et al. Role of antibiotic prophylaxis for wound infection in percutaneous endoscopic gastrostomy (PEG): result of a prospective double-blind randomized trial. J Hosp Infect 2002;50:312–315.

42. Sanchez RB, vanSonnenberg E, D'Agostino HB, et al. CT guidance for percutaneous gastrostomy and gastroenterostomy. Radiology 1992;184:201–205.

43. Malki TA, Langer JC, Thompson V, et al. A prospective evaluation of the button gastrostomy in children. Can J Surg 1991;34: 247–250.

44. Gauderer MW, Olsen MM, Stellato TA, et al. Feeding gastrostomy button: experience and recommendations. J Pediatr Surg 1988;23: 24–28.

45. McQuaid KR, Little TE. Two fatal complications related to gastrostomy "button" placement. Gastrointest Endosc 1992;38:601–603.

46. Rogers DA, Bowden TA. Gastrostomy: operative or nonoperative? Surg Clin North Am 1992;72:515–524.

47. Larson DE, Burton DD, Schroeder KW, et al. Percutaneous endoscopic gastrostomy. Indications, success, complications and mortality in 314 consecutive patients. Gastroenterology 1987;93:48–52.

48. Ponsky JL, Gauderer WL, Stellato TA. Percutaneous endoscopic gastrostomy. A review of 150 cases. Arch Surg 1983;118:913–914.

49. Lowe JB, Page CP, Schwesinger WH, et al. Percutaneous endoscopic gastrostomy tube placement in a surgical training program. Am J Surg 1997;174:627–628.

50. Barkmeier JM, Trerotola SO, Wiebke EA. Percutaneous radiologic, surgical endoscopic, and percutaneous endoscopic gastrostomy/gastrojejunostomy: comparative study and cost analysis. Cardiovasc Interv Radiol 1998;21:324–328.

51. Wollman B, D'Agostino HB. Percutaneous radiologic and endoscopic gastrostomy: a 3-year institutional analysis of procedure performance. AJR Am J Roentgenol 1997;169:1551–1553.

52. Wojtowycz MM, Arata JA, Micklos TJ, et al. CT findings after uncomplicated percutaneous gastrostomy. AJR Am J Roentgenol 1988;151:307–309.

53. Grant JP. Comparison of percutaneous endoscopic gastrostomy with Stamm gastrostomy. Ann Surg 1988;207:598–603.

54. Stiegmann GV, Goff JS, Silas D, et al. Endoscopic versus operative gastrostomy: final results of a prospective randomized trial. Gastrointest Endosc 1990;36:1–5.

55. Morris JB, Mullen JL, Yu JC, et al. Laparoscopic guided jejunostomy. Surgery 1992;112:92–96.

56. Duh QY, Way LW. Laparoscopic gastrostomy using T-fasteners as retractors and anchors. Surg Endosc 1993;7:60–63.

57. Gibson SE, Wenig BL, Watkins JL. Complications of percutaneous endoscopic gastrostomy in head and neck cancer patients. Ann Otol Rhinol Laryngol 1992;101:46–50.

Interventional Radiology of the Lacrimal System

33

Ho-Young Song, Deok Hee Lee, Sung-Gwon Kang

ANATOMY AND PATHOPHYSIOLOGY

The lacrimal drainage system (Figure 33-1) includes the superior and inferior puncta, superior and inferior canaliculi, common canaliculus, lacrimal sac, and nasolacrimal duct (1,2). The canaliculi are about 1 mm in diameter and 8 mm long, and the lacrimal sac is 12-15 mm in vertical length. The nasolacrimal duct extends from the inferior portion of the lacrimal sac through the nasolacrimal canal and opens into the inferior meatus of the nasal cavity. The nasolacrimal duct is approximately 18 mm long and angulates 15 degrees posteriorly and 5 degrees slightly inward. An obstruction in the lacrimal drainage system leads to insufficient drainage of tears into the inferior meatus. As a result, the tears fall over the lid margin onto the cheek, a condition that is termed epiphora (3,4). Epiphora is common in ophthalmological practice, and it is an annoying disability because patients have to frequently dab the tears with a tissue or handkerchief (2). Furthermore, chronic dacryocystitis and an eczematous condition of the lids can be produced. Dacryolithiasis is associated with 10-30% of chronic dacryocystitis cases (5-7) and may cause recurrent dacryocystitis and symptomatic nasolacrimal obstruction (8).

Although there are many causes of acquired lacrimal outflow obstructions, such as trauma or infection, the majority of cases are a result of idiopathic inflammation and scarring of the nasolacrimal duct (3). Congenital obstruction of the lacrimal drainage system is a relatively common clinical problem, affecting as many as 20% of all infants (9). The most common form of congenital obstruction is caused by a persistent layer of lacrimal and nasal epithelial cells at the level of the valve of Hasner (10,11). Except in infants, in whom the cause is usually congenital obstruction, epiphora rarely resolves spontaneously.

CONVENTIONAL THERAPIES

Historically, external dacryocystorhinostomy (DCR) has been the standard treatment for acquired obstructions below the common canaliculus with success rates of 89-95% in primary repairs (12-16). The invasive surgical procedure usually requires general anesthesia and leaves a permanent facial scar (17-20). Although complications of DCR are uncommon, they can include a hyperthrophic facial scar and regrowth of mucous membrane over the nasolacrimal opening (17). In some institutes, physicians perform endonasal endoscopic DCR with or without a laser to avoid the facial scar. However, the reported success rates are not as high as those of external DCR (18).

The conventional methods for treating acquired canalicular obstructions have included both invasive surgical procedures, such as conjunctival DCR (C-DCR) with

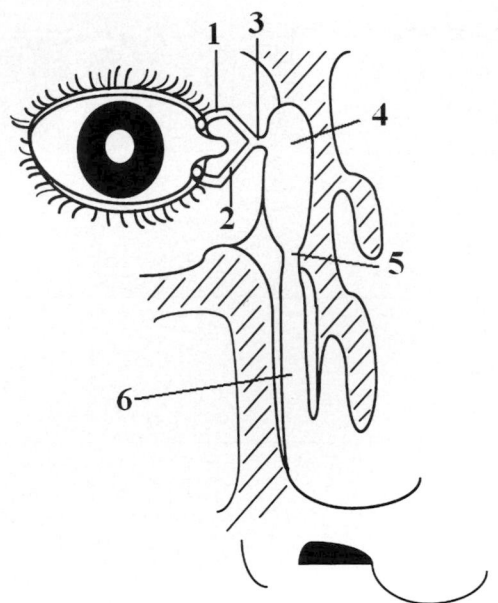

Figure 33–1 Anatomy of the lacrimal drainage system. **1.** Superior canaliculus. **2.** Inferior canaliculus. **3.** Common canaliculus. **4.** Lacrimal sac. **5.** Junction between the lacrimal sac and the nasolacrimal duct. **6.** Nasolacrimal duct.

permanent bypass tube placement (19–24), and nonsurgical procedures, such as probing and temporary silicone tube placement (25–28). In C-DCR, a conventional DCR is performed and a tract is made from the conjunctival surface to the internal anastomosis, creating a continuous tract from the conjunctiva to the nasal cavity. A bypass tube is permanently inserted into the tract. The reported success rate has varied from 57– 98% (19,21–23). Rose and Welham (21) reported that during a 23-year follow-up after C-DCR with the Lester Jones bypass tube in 326 eyes of 310 patients with canalicular obstruction, replacement of the bypass tube was needed in 44% of the cases because of spontaneous loss of the tubes. Steinsapir et al. (22) reviewed 79 C-DCR cases performed over a 16-year period in 75 patients and reported the following complication rates: 51% extrusion, 23% obstruction, 9% medial migration, 9% malposition, 7% granuloma formation, 4% hypermobility of the tube, and 3% infection. Although probing is used in the treatment of congenital stenosis of the lacrimal system, it is usually ineffective after the age of 2 years (17). Repeated probing of a canalicular obstruction with successively larger Bowman probes is potentially traumatic (23,24). The temporary placement of a silicone tube without DCR has not met with widespread acceptance or universal success, probably because the manipulation of probes down the narrow, bony canal of the nasolacrimal duct leads to further fibrosis and aggravates the obstruction (19).

A variety of treatments have been described for congenital obstruction of the lacrimal drainage system, including local massage, probing, silicone intubation, and DCR

(11,29–33). Congenital obstruction responds well to conservative treatment and to probing if performed in the first year of life (11); after 24 months of age, probing fails in as many as 67% of cases (29). For infants who are not candidates for probing, silicone intubation can be used as an effective alternative. However, complications such as slitting of the canaliculi and early removal of the tube by the child may occur (31–33).

In 1965, Jones (34) described 30 cases of dacryoliths that he had experienced for 39 months. Approximately 70% of the cases had partial obstruction at the nasolacrimal duct. In incomplete obstruction of the nasolacrimal duct, dacryoliths could spontaneously pass through the nasolacrimal duct into the nasal cavity (6) or could be removed by nonsurgical techniques such as massaging over the lacrimal sac and/or saline irrigation of the canaliculus under pressure (34). In complete obstruction of the nasolacrimal duct, surgical removal of the dacryolith along with DCR was necessary.

INTERVENTIONAL THERAPIES

The landmark study of Becker and Berry (12) in 1989 opened the door to several interventional therapies for obstructions of the lacrimal drainage system. They introduced a 3- to 4-mm angioplasty balloon catheter through the canaliculus in an antegrade approach. In 1990, Munk et al. (35) introduced a 3- to 4-mm angioplasty balloon catheter through the inferior opening of the nasolacrimal duct in a retrograde approach, which is considered safer than the antegrade approach (36). In the wake of these reports, the next decade saw the development of several novel treatments for congenital and acquired obstructions of the lacrimal drainage system, including balloon dilatation (36–48), stent placement (49–61), stent removal (58,62), and stone removal (38,61). This chapter reviews techniques, clinical applications, results, and problems of the interventional procedures performed over the past decade.

TECHNIQUES AND RESULTS

Balloon Dilatation

A variety of instruments and techniques for balloon dilatation have been described (36–46). The authors' techniques include subtraction dacryocystography (Figure 33–2) to evaluate the lacrimal system before balloon dilatation. To evaluate drainage of the whole system, including canaliculi, it is important to place the needle tip in the middle of the inferior or superior canaliculus rather than in the lacrimal sac. For local anesthesia and decongestion of the nasal mucosa, a nasal pack is placed for 3–5 minutes in the inferior nasal meatus using 2–3

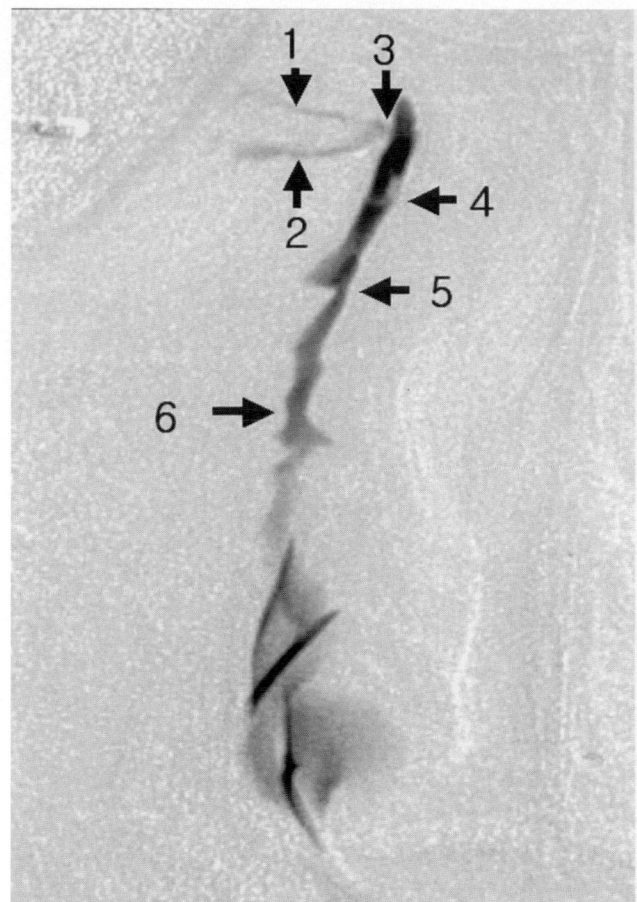

Figure 33–2   Normal right subtraction dacryocystogram. **1.** Superior canaliculus. **2.** Inferior canaliculus. **3.** Common canaliculus. **4.** Lacrimal sac. **5.** Junction between the lacrimal sac and the nasolacrimal duct. **6.** Nasolacrimal duct.

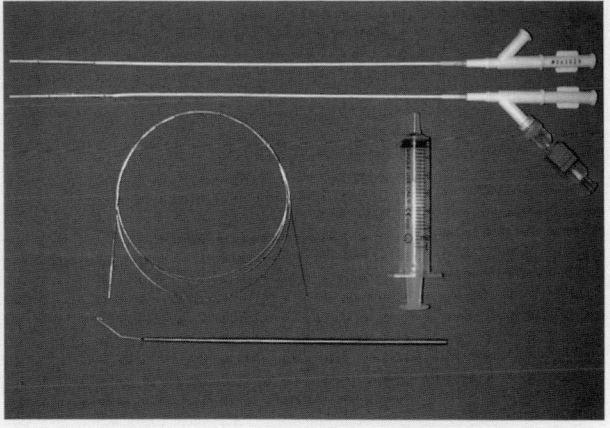

Figure 33–3   Devices for lacrimal balloon dilatation. **Top to bottom:** a 3-mm balloon catheter, a 4-mm balloon catheter, an 0.018-inch ball-tipped guide wire (*right*), a syringe (*left*), and a hook.

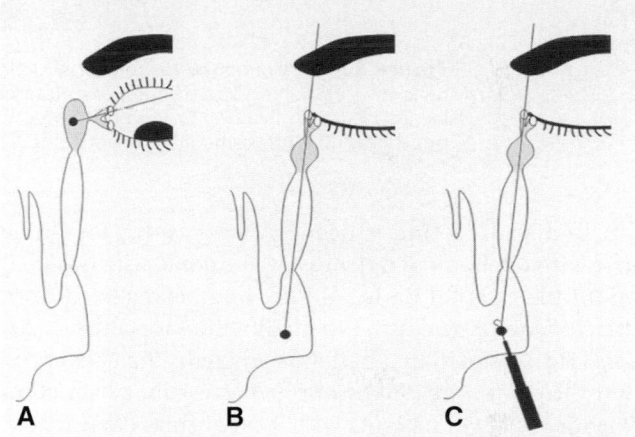

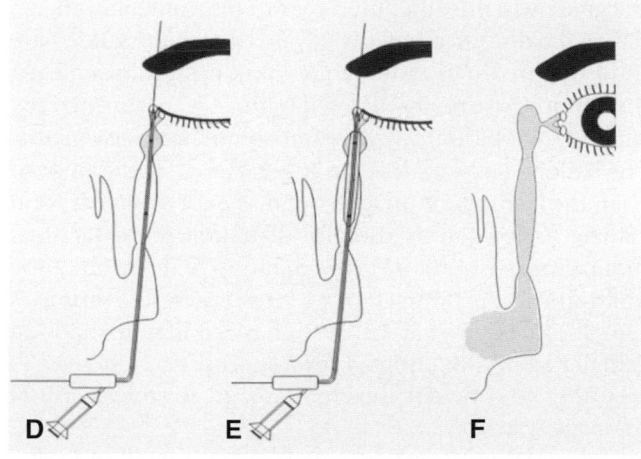

Figure 33–4   Technical steps in lacrimal balloon dilatation. **A.** Introduction of a guide wire through the punctum into the lacrimal sac. **B.** Negotiation of the guide wire through the obstruction into the inferior meatus of the nasal cavity. **C.** Grasping the distal end of the guide wire with the use of a hook. **D.** Introduction of a deflated balloon catheter over the guide wire until its end passes through the obstruction. **E.** Inflation of the balloon catheter using water-soluble contrast media. **F.** Dacryocystography performed after balloon dilatation.

cotton pledgets moistened with equal parts of cocaine hydrochloride (10%) and epinephrine (1:100,000). Topical anesthesia of the eyes is accomplished with 0.5 % proparacaine, and an infratrochlear nerve block over the medial canthal and lacrimal sac areas is accomplished with 2% lidocaine.

The superior punctum is dilated using a punctal dilator when necessary. Because the ampulla portions of the lacrimal systems are oriented vertically for about 2 mm, a guide wire (Figure 33–3) is first introduced vertically into the punctum and then rotated 90 degrees horizontally to conform to the bend in the first portion of the superior canaliculus. In patients with incomplete obstructions of the lacrimal drainage system, an 0.014-inch flexible guide wire can be used to negotiate the obstruction (37,38). In patients with complete obstructions, an 0.018-inch ball-tipped guide wire is useful for opening the complete obstruction (36,39). A hook (Cook) is placed in the nasal cavity under fluoroscopic guidance and aimed laterally toward the inferior meatus to grasp the guide wire (Figure 33–4). When the tip of the hook touches the guide wire, soft metallic contact is

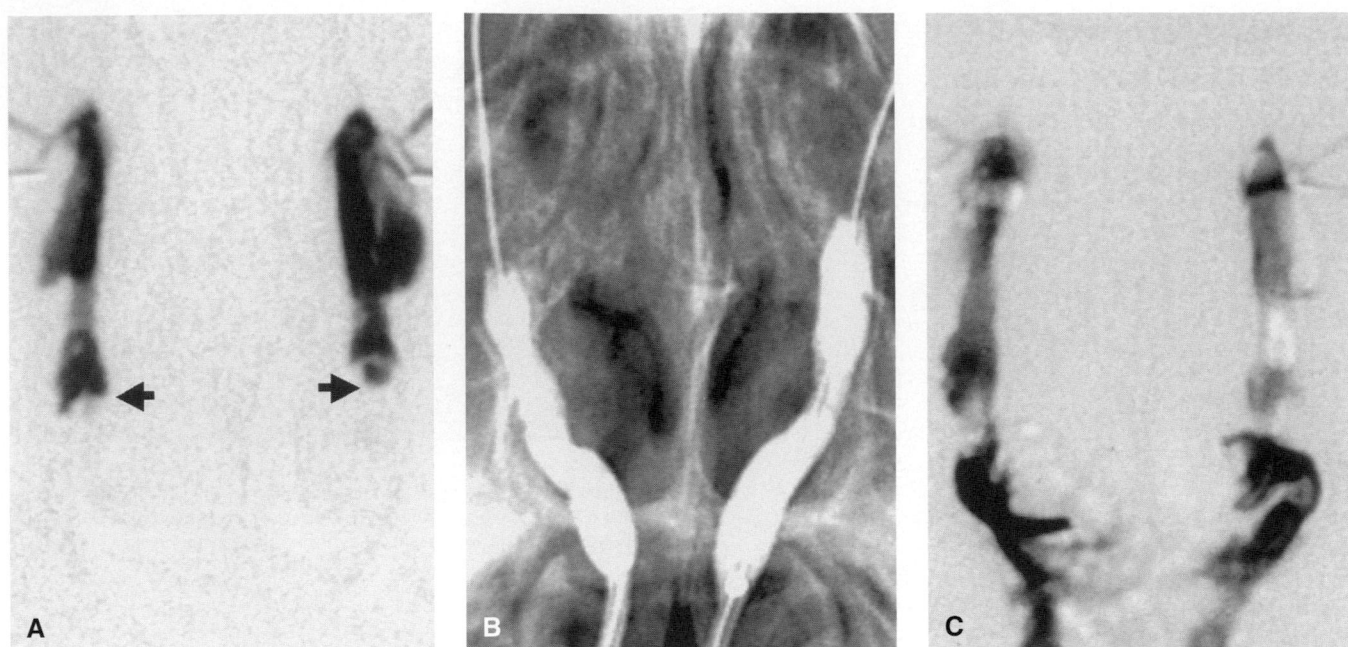

Figure 33–5 Congenital bilateral obstructions. **A.** Subtraction dacryocystogram obtained before balloon dilatation reveals bilateral complete obstructions (*arrows*) at the distal portion of the nasolacrimal duct. **B.** Bilateral balloon dilatation. **C.** Postdilatation subtraction dacryocystogram reveals good flow of contrast medium on both sides.

felt, and a soft sound is heard. After grasping the guide wire with the hook or a hemostat, the guide wire is pulled out of the external naris, and the hook is removed from the guide wire by cutting the ball with wire-cutting scissors (Storz). A deflated balloon catheter is then advanced over the guide wire and positioned across the obstruction (Figure 33–5). In patients with a canalicular obstruction, a 3F tapered dilator (Cook) is passed retrogradely over the guide wire through the superior punctum, and then a deflated balloon catheter is advanced over the guide wire until the proximal radiopaque mark passes through the punctum (Figure 33–6). Dilatation is performed by inflating the balloon with water-soluble contrast media. The balloon catheter and the guide wire are then removed from the lacrimal drainage system. A 3- or 4-mm balloon catheter is commonly used for dilatation of the lacrimal drainage system (40–43). The duration of inflation of the balloon catheter ranges from 20 seconds to 5 minutes (35–50). Janssen et al. (37) emphasized that the balloon catheter should be inflated for a short period, such as 30 seconds, to prevent severe damage to the lacrimal drainage system.

Several large series performed since the work of Becker and Berry (12) have attested to the efficacy of lacrimal balloon dilatation (Table 33–1). Technical success rates have ranged from 89–95% (12,35–50), and no major complications have been reported. A majority of the patients express mild pain during the inflation of the balloon and complain of slightly blood-tinged nasal discharge for 1–72 hours after the procedure. Ilgit et al. (45) reported a 69%

initial improvement rate of epiphora in 80 eyes, while Janssen et al. (48) reported a 96% initial improvement rate and an 84% 1-year improvement rate in 100 eyes. The largest series documenting clinical results of balloon dilatation was reported in 2001 by Lee et al. (42), involving 430 eyes of 350 patients. In the series, the technical success rate was 95%, and the overall improvement rates were 57% initially. The improvement rates were 48% at 2 months, 39% at 1 year, and 37% at 5 years.

A problem in comparing the results from these studies is the variety of treatment techniques and methods used. Therefore, different factors, such as patient selection, negotiation technique, balloon diameter, balloon inflation time, and length of the follow-up period, may be contributing to the results. For example, a low initial success rate may be attributable to the making of a false tract resulting from the use of a ball-tipped guide wire (Figure 33–7). Using a soft-tipped guide wire is believed to be less traumatic than using a ball-tipped guide wire (37,42). However, cannulation of the whole system with a soft-tipped guide wire is a difficult and time-consuming procedure in the lesions with complete obstruction. As many authors have already described, initial and long-term improvement rates have been greatest in the cases of lesions with obstructions of the nasolacrimal duct.

Becker et al. (46) reported a 95% initial improvement rate of epiphora in 61 eyes with congenital obstructions of the lacrimal drainage system. Cho et al. (40) performed balloon dilatation in 20 eyes of 16 patients with obstructions of the lacrimal drainage system (age range, 12–78 months;

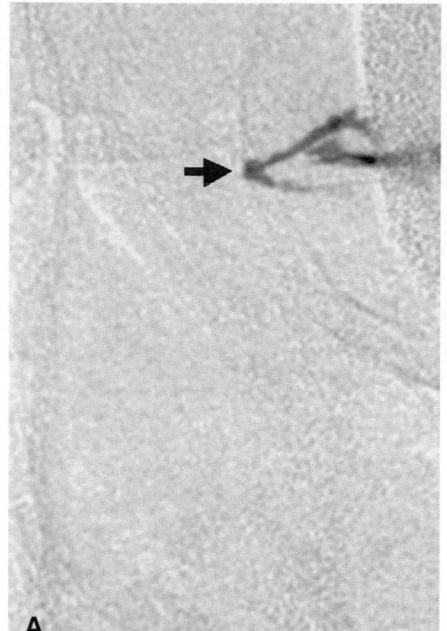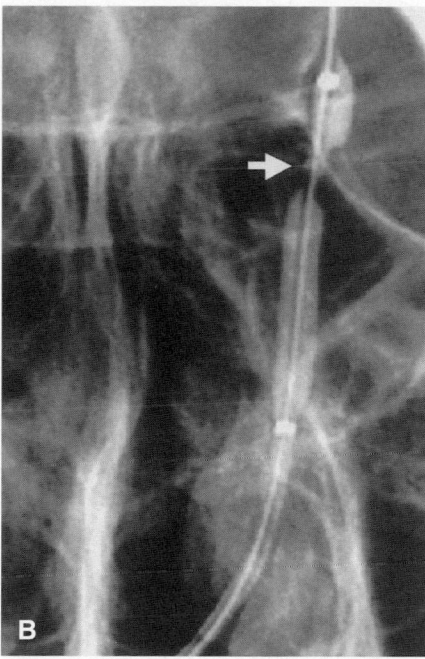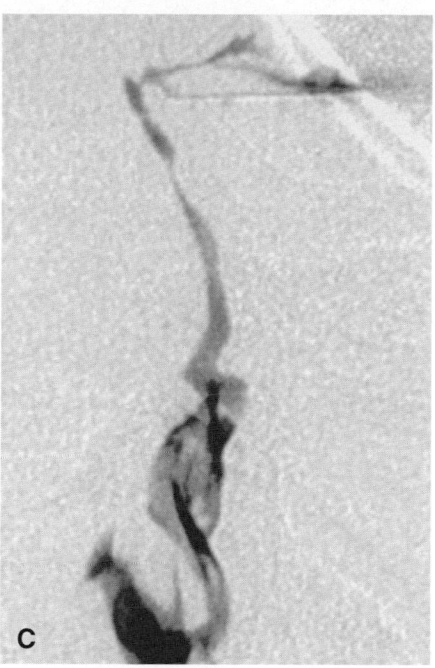

Figure 33–6 **A.** Subtraction dacryocystogram obtained before balloon dilatation reveals a complete obstruction (*arrow*) at the left common canaliculus. **B.** Plain radiograph obtained during balloon dilatation shows a waist deformity of the balloon at the canaliculus (*arrow*). A 3-year follow-up dacryocystogram reveals a patent lacrimal system.

mean, 33 months). The technical success rate and initial improvement rate were both 95%. No patients showed recurrence during the mean follow-up of 2 years. Balloon dilatation should be considered for children in whom local massage or probing fails, regardless of their age (63).

Stent Placement

The techniques for providing local anesthesia of the eyes and nasal mucosa and for introducing the guide wire through the punctum into the inferior meatus of the nasal cavity as well as the trapping of the ball-tipped guide wire out of the naris are the same as for balloon dilatation. A stent is implanted using a stent set (Figure 33–8), comprising a stent, a 6.3F introducer set (a dilator, a sheath, a stent loader, and a pusher catheter), a hook, and a dacryocystography needle (51). Under fluoroscopic guidance, a 6.3F sheath with a dilator from the stent set is passed retrogradely over the guide wire and advanced across the lesion until the proximal tip of the dilator is lying in the dilated lacrimal sac (Figure 33–9). To place the tip of the sheath properly in the lacrimal sac, the

TABLE 33–1

RESULTS OF BALLOON DILATATION

	Becker et al. (46)	Lee et al. (42)	Janssen et al. (48)	Berkefeld et al. (47)	Ilgit et al. (45)
No. of lacrimal systems	61	430	100	85	80
Cause of obstructions	Congenital	Both	Acquired*	Acquired	Acquired
Location of obstructions	Subcanalicular	All	Subcanalicular	Subcanalicular	All
Diameter of balloons (mm)	2–3	2–5	3	3	2–4
Balloon inflation time (minutes)	2	2–5	0.5	1–2	5
Major complications	No	No	No	No	No
Technical success rate (%)	100	95	NA	73	81
Initial improvement rate (%)	95	57	96	76	69
Range of follow-up (months)	4–10	1–69	5–48	NA	6–18
1-year improvement rate (%)	NA	39	84	72	NA
5-year improvement rate (%)	NA	37	NA	NA	NA

Note: NA, not applicable; Both, congenital and acquired causes; All, canalicular and subcanalicular locations.
* The causes of obstructions were acquired in 99 lacrimal systems and congenital in the remaining one lacrimal system.

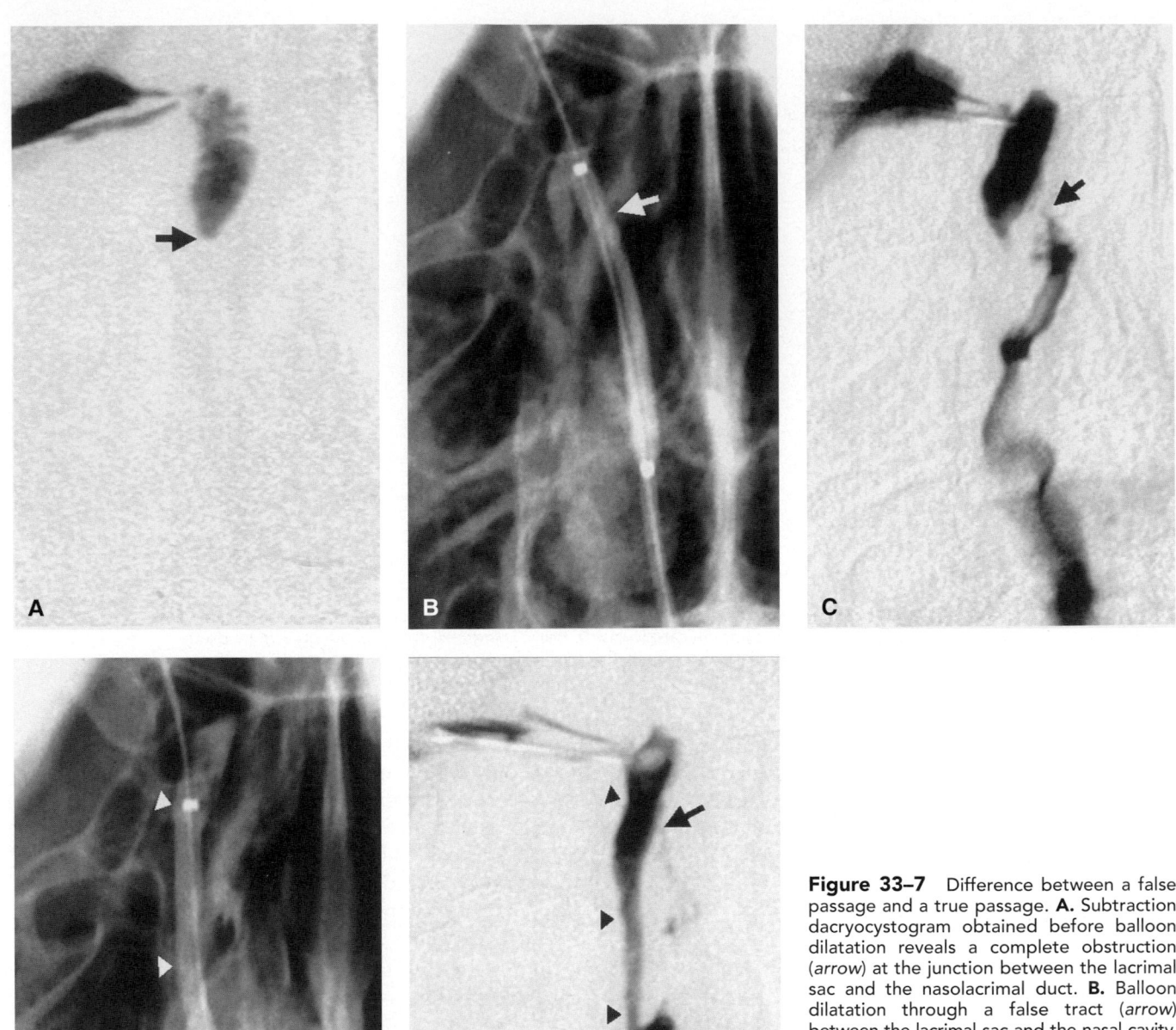

Figure 33–7 Difference between a false passage and a true passage. **A.** Subtraction dacryocystogram obtained before balloon dilatation reveals a complete obstruction (*arrow*) at the junction between the lacrimal sac and the nasolacrimal duct. **B.** Balloon dilatation through a false tract (*arrow*) between the lacrimal sac and the nasal cavity. **C.** Postdilatation dacryocystogram shows the direct flow (*arrow*) of contrast medium from the lacrimal sac into the nasal cavity, as in the case of a dacryocystorhinostomy. **D.** Repeat balloon dilatation through the right tract at the same sitting. Note the location of the balloon catheter (*arrowheads*). **E.** Postdilatation dacryocystogram reveals good flow of contrast medium through the right tract (*arrowheads*) into the nasal cavity as well as little flow through the false tract (*arrow*).

sheath is advanced approximately 3 mm into it while the dilator is withdrawn from the sheath. After the dilator is removed from the sheath, a stent is introduced over the guide wire into the sheath with the help of a stent loader and is advanced by using a pusher catheter until the tip of the stent is located at the sheath tip. The pusher catheter is held in place while the sheath is withdrawn.

This frees the stent, allowing the tip of the stent to expand and lie within the dilated lacrimal sac and the body of the stent to lie within the nasolacrimal duct, slightly protruding into the inferior meatus of the nasal cavity. After the stent is released from the sheath, the sheath containing the pusher catheter is pulled out inferiorly, and the guide wire is pulled out superiorly. During

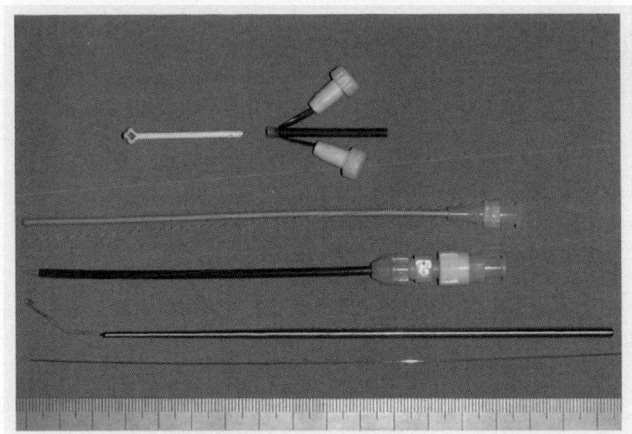

Figure 33–8   Top to bottom: a polyurethane stent (*left*) and a stent loader (*right*), a pusher catheter, and a 6F sheath containing a dilator, a hook, and a ball-tipped guide wire.

patients experience slightly blood-stained nasal discharge for 1–48 hours after the procedure, but this disappears spontaneously. Most patients with canalicular stent placement report a foreign-body sensation when they blink or move their eyes for 1–10 days after stent placement, after which the sensation disappears spontaneously. There have been no reports of major procedural complications. However, placement of bare expandable metallic stents has not come to be regarded as the therapeutic model because of the high frequency of blockage of the metallic stents by granulation tissue and because the stents could not be removed without surgery (49,51,53). Although covered metallic stents are retrievable, their long-term patency rates are discouraging (55).

The largest series documenting clinical results of polyurethane stent placement was reported in 2002 by Kang et al. (59), who reported on treatment results in 727 lacrimal systems of 588 patients with epiphora resulting from obstruction of the lacrimal system (Figure 33–10). In this series, the overall technical failure rate was 4%, and complications included blood-stained nasal discharge, headaches, infection, pain, extravasation, and false passage. The 7-day patency rate was 91% but fell to 12% at 3 years and 5% at 5 years. The causes of recurrence were obstruction of the stent by mucoid materials or granulation tissue. In patients with recurrence, the lacrimal system was irrigated with saline. When the obstructed stent was not recanalized by saline irrigation, the stent was removed from the lacrimal system.

In 2000, Janssen et al. (60) performed temporary stent placement—supported by local and systemic antibiotics—in 10 cases with a lacrimal abscess resulting from chronic or subacute dacryocystitis. All cases involved active inflammation

placement of a canalicular stent, the stent is advanced with a pusher catheter until the tip of the stent is located in the superior canaliculus, 2–3 mm from the superior punctum (52).

Three types of stents have been used in the treatment of obstruction of the lacrimal drainage system: bare expandable metallic stents (53,54), covered expandable metallic stents (55), and plastic stents (51,52,55–59,62,63). The technical failure rate has been reported to be higher in patients with traumatic obstruction than in those with idiopathic obstruction (49,57). The initial results with these techniques appear promising, with short-term success rates approaching 97% in most series. The majority of

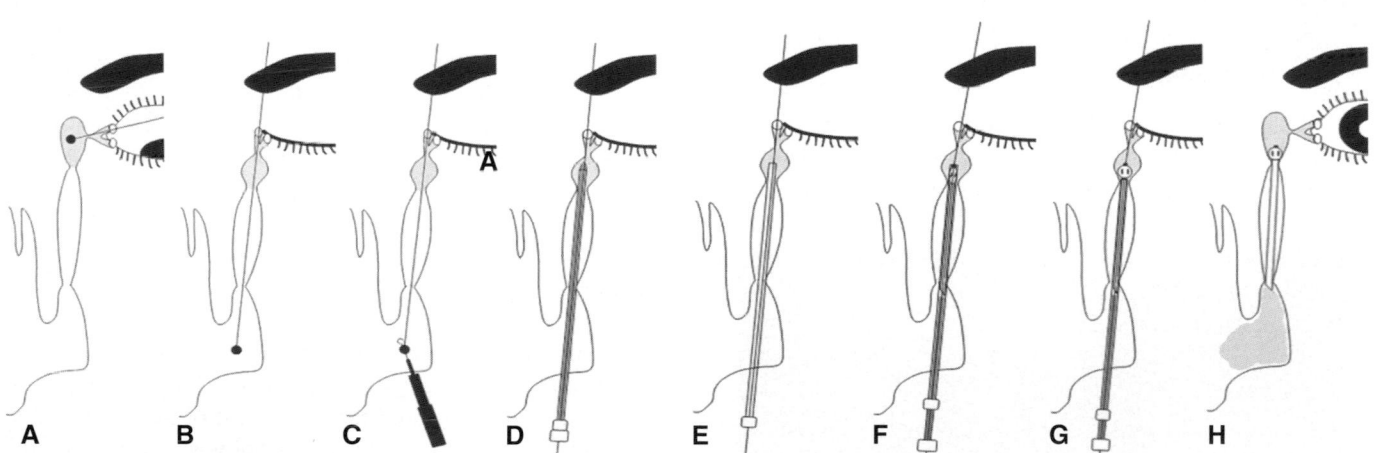

A   B   C   D   E   F   G   H

Figure 33–9   Technical steps in lacrimal stent placement. **A.** Introduction of a guide wire through the punctum into the lacrimal sac. **B.** Negotiation of the guide wire through the obstruction into the inferior meatus of the nasal cavity. **C.** Grasping the distal end of the guide wire with a hook. **D.** Introduction of a dilator and sheath over the guide wire until the end of the sheath passes through the obstruction. **E.** Removal of the dilator from the sheath. **F.** Introduction of a stent over the guide wire into the sheath with the aid of a stent loader. **G.** Withdrawal of the sheath over the pusher catheter. **H.** Dacryocystography performed after stent placement.

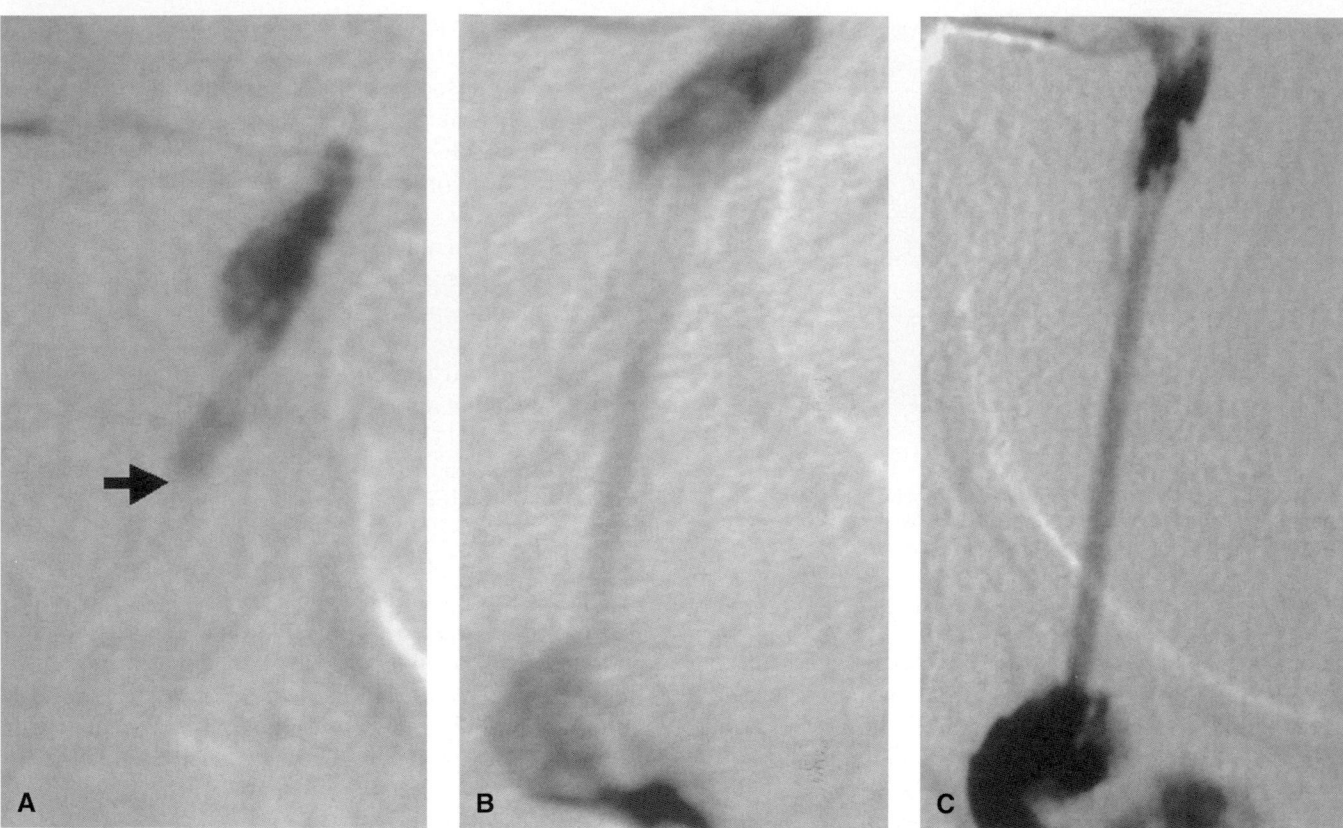

Figure 33–10 **A.** Subtraction dacryocystogram obtained before stent placement reveals a complete obstruction (*arrow*) at the right nasolacrimal duct. **B.** Postprocedure subtraction dacryocystogram reveals a good flow of contrast media through the stent into the inferior meatus of the nasal cavity. **C.** A 5-year follow-up dacryocystogram reveals patency of the stent.

with pus in the swollen lacrimal sac. Stent removal after several weeks resulted in abscess cure in all cases with no further epiphora.

Stent Removal

A stent can be removed from the nose either by using a hemostat under headlight or nasal-endoscope guidance or by using a stent-retrieval hook under fluoroscopic guidance

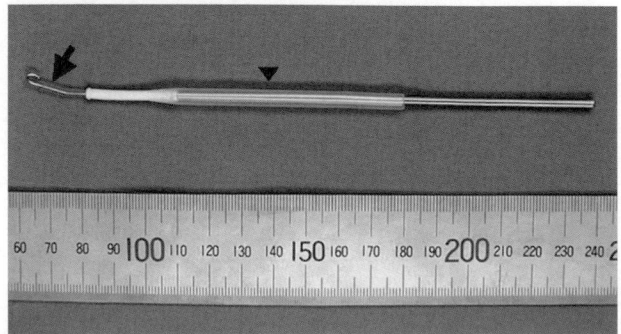

Figure 33–11 Photograph of a lacrimal stent-retrieval hook. Arrow indicates hook part, and arrowhead indicates pusher part.

(58,62). The lacrimal system is then irrigated with saline through the punctum to wash out possible blood clots and mucoid material. The stent-retrieval hook (Figure 33–11) consists of an inner hook and an outer pusher (58,62). To remove the stent, the hook is placed in the nasal cavity and is aimed laterally toward the inferior meatus to grasp the distal end of the stent (Fig. 33–12), after which the sheath is pushed to fully grasp it. After removing the stent, dacryocystography is performed through the punctum to verify the patency of the lacrimal system.

Kim et al. (62) attempted to remove the stent from the nose in 267 cases using a stent-retrieval hook. The procedure failed in only 8 (2%) of the 267 cases; failure was a result of tight growth of granulation tissue into the stent in seven cases and inaccessibility of the hook to the distal tip of the stent in the remaining case. Seven of the eight stents were removed by an otorhinolaryngologist using a hemostat under nasal-endoscope guidance, and the other was removed by an ophthalmologist during a DCR. Mucoid material was present in 89 of the removed stents, with granulation tissue (Figure 33–13) in the remaining 170 stents. The granulation tissue consisted of abundant mononuclear lymphocytes and some plasma cells, suggesting chronic

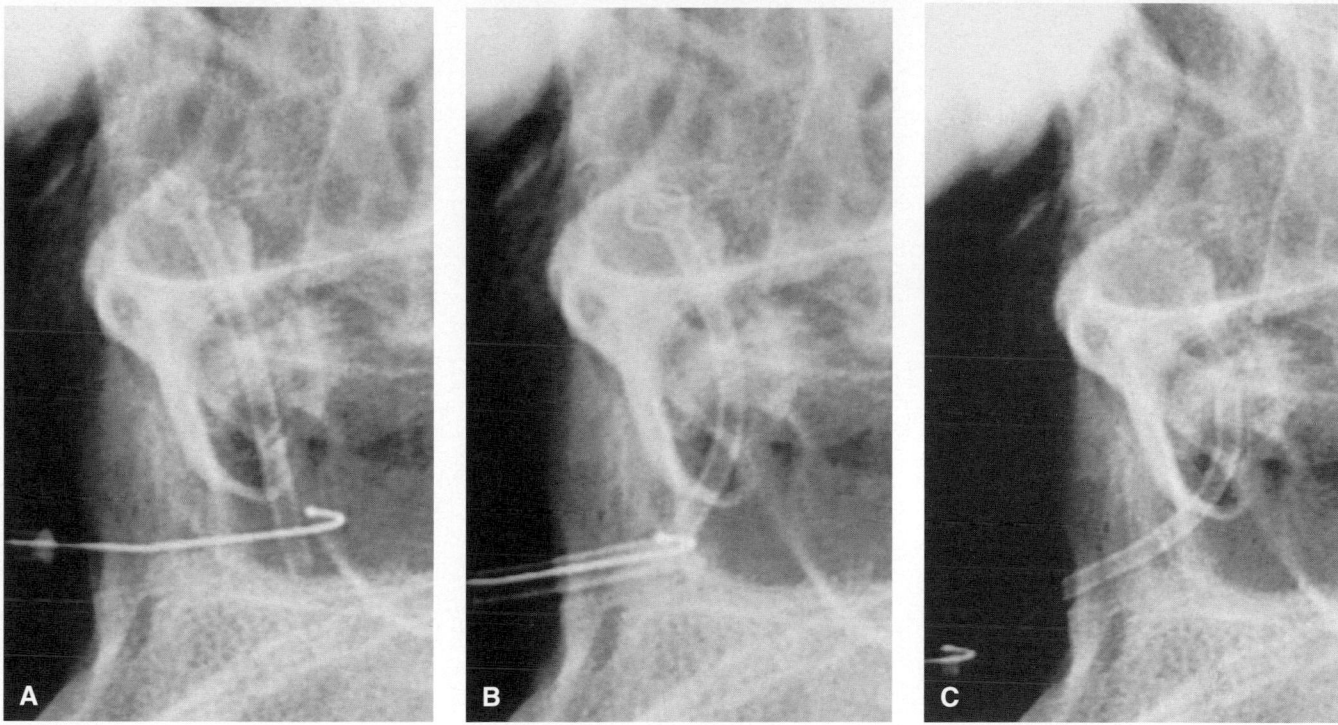

Figure 33–12   Technical steps in lacrimal stent removal. **A.** Introduction of a retrieval hook into the inferior meatus of the nasal cavity. **B.** Grasping the distal end of the stent by pushing the outer pusher over the inner hook. **C.** Pulling the stent out of the nasal cavity.

inflammation. There was also a proliferation of endothelial cells and capillaries. During removal of the stent, 10% of the cases in whom the stent was lengthened reported severe pain. Epistaxis occurred in six cases and was controlled by a nasal pack. After stent removal, 51% of the cases showed patency of the lacrimal system on a 7-day follow-up dacryocystogram, and 33% of the cases maintained the patency on a 1-year follow-up dacryocystography.

Stone Removal

Wilhelm et al. (38) performed balloon dilatation to widen the nasolacrimal duct obstructions and to fragment dacryoliths and then irrigated the lacrimal drainage system with saline through the lacrimal punctum. In patients with incomplete dacryolith washout, Wilhelm et al. aspirated the fragmented dacryoliths through a 6.3F sheath introduced into the nasolacrimal duct. They also used a gooseneck snare to remove the dacryoliths.

Wilhelm et al. (38) attempted to remove dacryoliths in 10 patients with severe epiphora caused by partial (n = 8) or complete (n = 2) obstruction of the lacrimal drainage system. The procedure was technically successful in all patients. During the mean follow-up period of 6 months (range, 3–18 months), five patients showed complete resolution of epiphora, and the remaining five patients showed partial resolution. Dacryoliths may break into fragments

during stent placement (61), and these fragmented dacryoliths may pass through the stent into the pharynx while irrigating the lacrimal system (Figure 33–14).

SUMMARY

Advances in interventional techniques for the lacrimal drainage system have expanded our armamentarium for the easy treatment of epiphora. Clearly, the interventional procedures are relatively simple, safe, and cost effective: They result in no facial scars and few problems with bleeding, and patients need less postoperative care. For children with congenital obstruction of the lacrimal drainage system, balloon dilatation is probably the treatment of choice. Although the initial success rate of balloon dacryocystoplasty is relatively low in acquired obstructions, a long-term success can be expected when the initial treatment is successful. Initial excellent results of stent placement can be obtained in patients with complete obstructions of the lacrimal drainage system, but the long-term results are not as encouraging. Fluoroscopic removal of dacryoliths and temporary stent placement for a lacrimal abscess are novel techniques in the field of interventional radiology of the lacrimal drainage system. Studies with longer follow-up periods might establish the effectiveness of the new techniques as appropriate treatment methods.

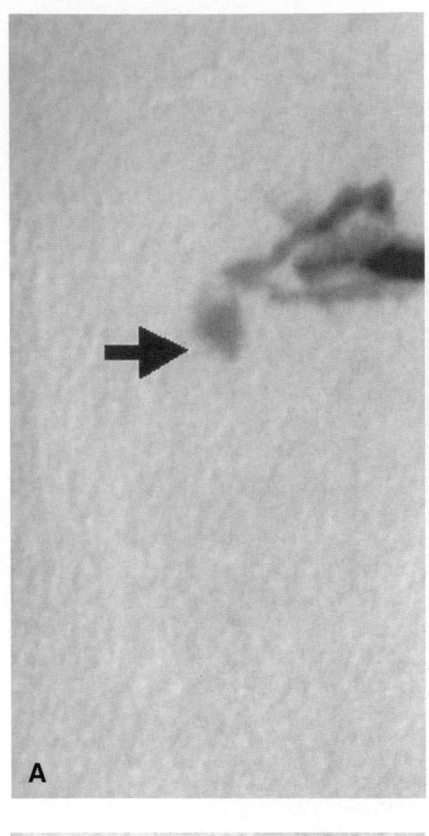

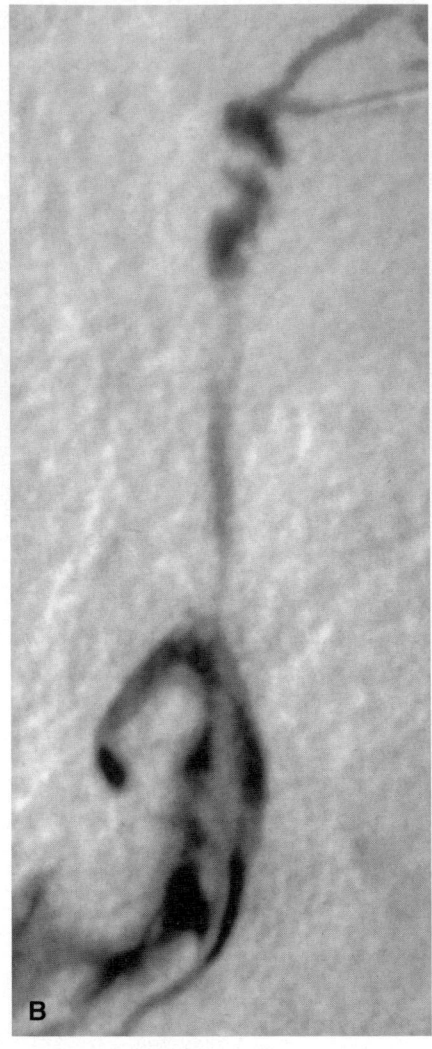

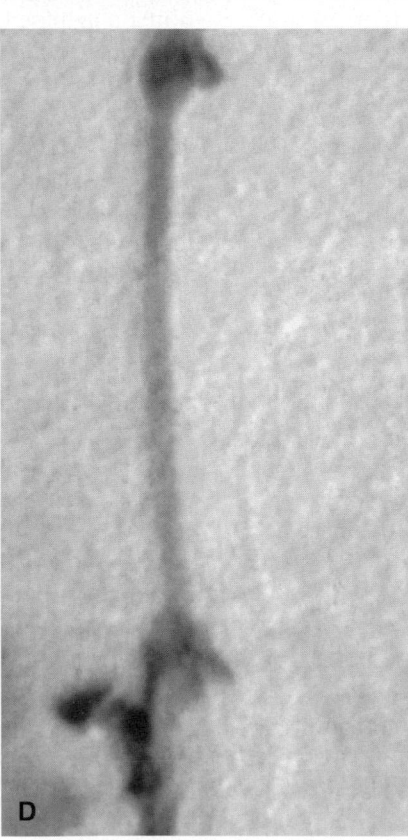

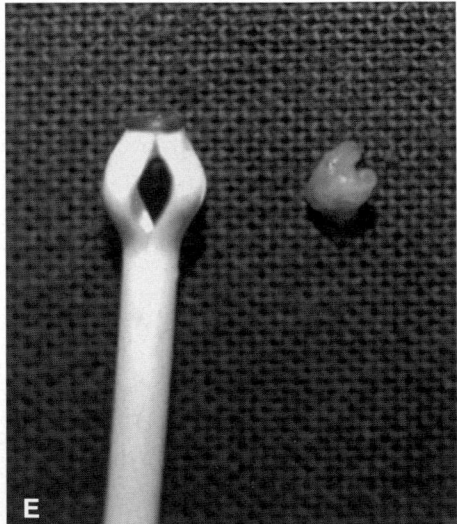

Figure 33–13 **A.** Left subtraction dacryocystogram reveals complete obstruction (*arrow*) at the lacrimal sac. **B.** One-week follow-up dacryocystogram reveals good flow of contrast media through the stent into the inferior meatus of the nasal cavity. **C.** Two-month follow-up dacryocystogram reveals a filling defect (*arrow*) at the upper end of the stent. **D.** Dacryocystogram obtained immediately after removal of the occluded stent shows a patent lacrimal system. **E.** Photograph of the removed stent and tissue removed from the end of the removed stent.

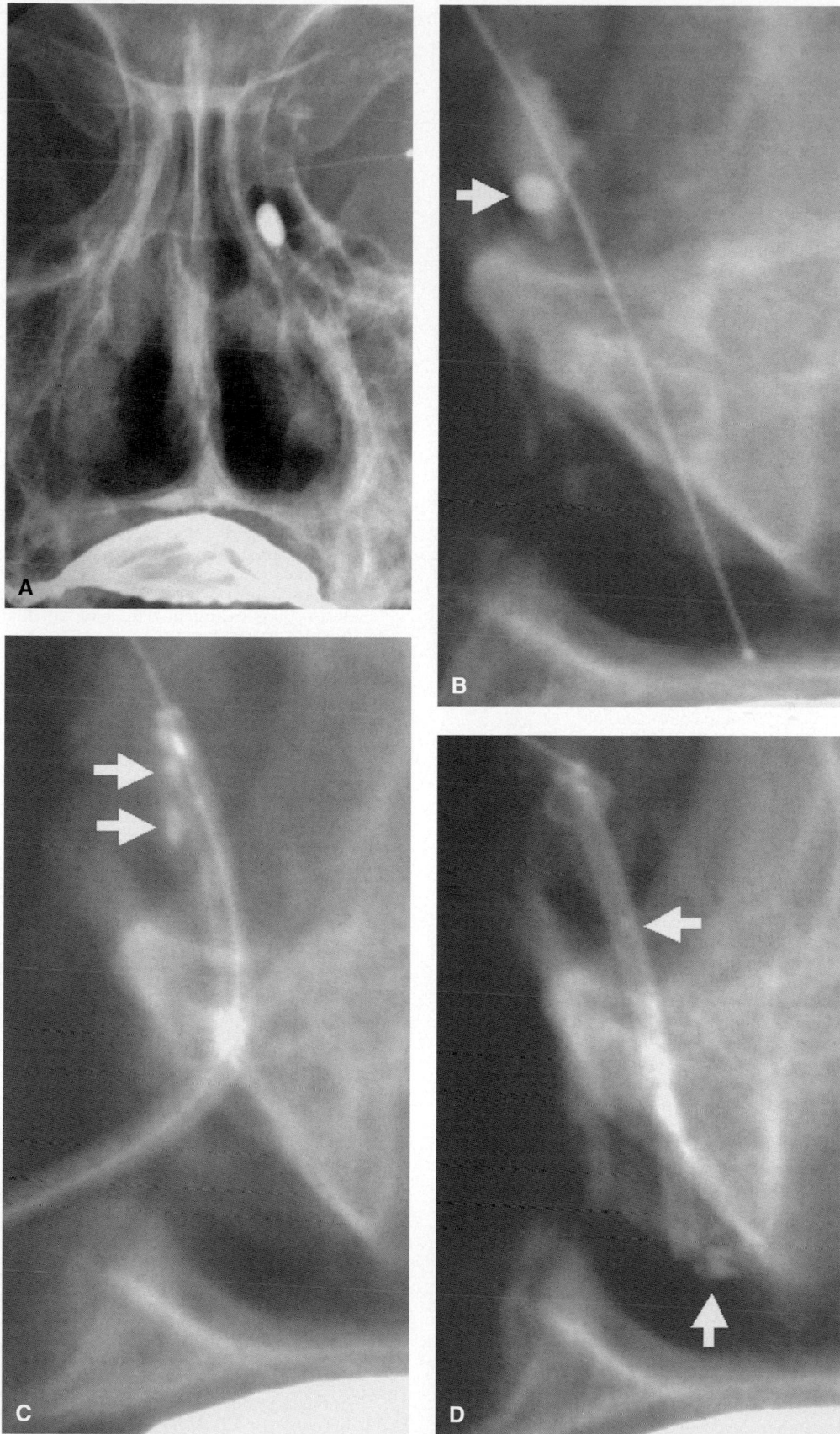

Figure 33–14 **A.** Plain radiogram shows a radiopaque stone on the left lacrimal sac area. **B.** Lateral plain radiogram obtained after insertion of a ball-tipped guide wire through the contrast-media-filled lacrimal sac into the inferior meatus of the nasal cavity shows the stone (*arrow*). **C.** Lateral plain radiogram obtained after insertion of a sheath with a dilator shows fragmented stones (*arrows*). **D.** Lateral plain radiogram obtained during irrigation with saline after stent placement shows fragmented stones (*arrows*) flowing through the stent into the nasal cavity.

REFERENCES

1. McCord CD. The lacrimal drainage system. In: Duane TD, Jager EA, eds. Clinical Ophthalmology, vol 4. New York: Harper & Row, 1985:1–24.
2. Duke-Elder S. System of Ophthalmology: The Ocular Adnexa, vol 13. London: Henry Kimpton, 1974:675–693.
3. Linberg JV, McCormick SA. Primary acquired nasolacrimal duct obstruction: a clinicopathologic report and biopsy technique. Ophthalmology 1986;93:1055–1063.
4. Traquair HM. Chronic dacryocystitis: its causation and treatment. Arch Ophthalmol 1941;26:165–180.
5. Berlin AJ, Rath R, Rich L. Lacrimal system dacryoliths. Ophthal Surg 1980;11:435–436.
6. Maltzman BA, Favetta JR. Dacryolithiasis. Ann Ophthalmol 1979;11:473–475.
7. Wilkins RB, Pressly JP. Diagnosis and incidence of lacrimal calculi. Ophthalmic Surg 1980;11:787–789.
8. Baratz KH, Bartley GB, Campbell RJ, et al. An eyelash nidus for dacryoliths of the lacrimal excretory and secretory systems. Am J Ophthalmol 1991;111:624–627.
9. MacEwen CJ, Young JDH. Epiphora during the first year of life. Eye 1991;5:596–600.
10. Dusse H, Müler KM, Kroll P. Radiological and histological findings of the lacrimal passages of newborns. Arch Ophthalmol 1980;98:528–532.
11. Kushner BJ. Congenital nasolacrimal system obstruction. Arch Ophthalmol 1982;100:597–600.
12. Becker BB, Berry FD. Balloon catheter dilatation in lacrimal surgery. Ophthalmic Surg 1989;20:193–198.
13. Massaro BM, Gonnering RS, Harris GJ. Endonasal laser dacryocystorhinostomy. Arch Ophthalmol 1990;108:1172–1176.
14. Welham RAN, Henderson P. Failed dacryocystorhinostomy. Trans Am Acad Ophthalmol Otolaryngol 1974;78:824–828.
15. Blaylock WK, Moore CA, Linberg JV. Anterior ethmoid anatomy facilitates dacryocystorhinostomy. Arch Ophthalmol 1990;108:1774–1777.
16. Dresner SC. Outpatient dacryocystorhinostomy and anesthesia techniques. In: Linberg JV, ed. Lacrimal Surgery. New York: Churchill-Livingstone, 1988:143–149.
17. Thornton SP. Nasolacrimal duct reconstruction with the nasolacrimal duct prosthesis: an alternative to standard dacryocystorhinostomy. Ann Ophthalmol 1977;9:1575–1582.
18. Massaro BM, Gonnering RS, Harris GJ. Endonasal laser dacryocystorhinostomy. Arch Ophthalmol 1990;108:1172–1176.
19. Katowitz JA. Silicone tubing in canalicular obstructions. A preliminary report. Arch Ophthalmol 1974;91:459–462.
20. Griffith TP. Polythene tubes in canaliculus surgery. Br J Ophthalmol 1963;47:203–210.
21. Rose GE, Welham RA. Jones' lacrimal canalicular bypass tubes: twenty-five years' experience. Eye 1991;5:13–19.
22. Steinsapir KD, Glatt HJ, Putterman AM. A 16-year study of conjunctival dacryocystorhinostomy. Am J Ophthalmol 1990;109:387–393.
23. Huggert A. The treatment of stenosis of the lacrimal canaliculi. Acta Ophth 1959;37:355–358.
24. Quickert MH, Dryden RM. Probes for intubation in lacrimal drainage. Trans Am Acad Ophthalmol Otolaryngol 1970;74:431–433.
25. Keith CG. Intubation of the lacrimal passages. Am J Ophth 1968;65:70–74.
26. Pashby RC, Rathbun JE. Silicone tube intubation of the lacrimal drainage system. Arch Ophthalmol 1979;97:1318–1322.
27. Veloudios A, Harvey JJ, Philippon M. Long-term placement of silastic nasolacrimal tubes. Ophthalmic Surg 1991;22:225–227.
28. Lauring L. Silicone intubation of the lacrimal system: pitfalls, problems and complications. Ann Ophthamol 1976;8:489–498.
29. Katowitz JA, Welsh MG. Timing of initial probing and irrigation in congenital nasolacrimal duct obstruction. Ophthalmology 1987;94:698–705.
30. Migliori ME, Putterman AM. Silicone intubation for treatment of congenital nasolacrimal duct obstruction: successful results removing the tubes after six weeks. Ophthalmology 1988;95:792–795.
31. Dortzbach RK, France TD, Kushner BJ, et al. Silicone intubation for obstruction of the nasolacrimal duct in children. Am J Ophthalmol 1982;94:585–590.
32. Leone CR, Van Gemert JV. The success rate of silicone intubation in congenital nasolacrimal duct obstruction. Ophthalmic Surg 1990;21:90–92.
33. Kraft SP, Crawford JS. Silicone tube intubation in disorders of the lacrimal system in children. Am J Ophthalmol 1982;94:290–299.
34. Jones LT. Tear-sac foreign bodies. Am J Ophthalmol 1965;60:111–113.
35. Munk PL, Lin DTC, Morris DC. Epiphora: treatment by means of dacryocystoplasty with balloon dilation of the nasolacrimal drainage apparatus. Radiology 1990;177:687–690.
36. Song HY, Ahn HS, Park CK, et al. Complete obstruction of the nasolacrimal system. Part I. Treatment with balloon dilatation. Radiology 1993;186:367–371.
37. Janssen AG, Mansour K, Krabbe GJ, et al. Dacryocystoplasty: treatment of epiphora by means of balloon dilation of the obstructed nasolacrimal duct system. Radiology 1994;193:453–456.
38. Wilhelm KE, Hofer U, Textor HJ, et al. Dacryoliths: nonsurgical fluoroscopically guided treatment during dacryocystoplasty. Radiology 1999;212:365–370.
39. Lee JM, Song HY, Han YM, et al. Balloon dacryocystoplasty: results in the treatment of complete and partial obstructions of the nasolacrimal system. Radiology 1994;192:503–508.
40. Cho YS, Song HY, Ko GY, et al. Congenital lacrimal system obstruction: treatment with balloon dilation. J Vasc Interv Radiol 2000;11:1319–1324.
41. Ko GY, Lee DH, Ahn HS, et al. Balloon catheter dilation in common canalicular obstruction of the lacrimal system: safety and long-term effectiveness. Radiology 2000;214:781–786.
42. Lee DH, Song HY, Ahn HS, et al. Balloon dacryocystoplasty: results and factors influencing outcome in 350 patients. J Vasc Interv Radiol 2001;12:500–506.
43. Song HY, Lee CH, Park SS, et al. Lacrimal canaliculus obstruction: safety and effectiveness of balloon dilation. J Vasc Interv Radiol 1996;7:929–934.
44. Becker BB, Berry FD. Balloon catheter dilatation in pediatric patients. Ophthalmic Surg 1991;22:750–752.
45. Ilgit ET, Yuksel D, Unal M, et al. Transluminal balloon dilatation of the lacrimal drainage system for the treatment of epiphora. AJR Am J Roentgenol 1995;165:1517–1524.
46. Becker BB, Berry FD, Koller H. Balloon catheter dilatation for treatment of congenital nasolacrimal duct obstruction. Am J Ophthalmol 1996;121:304–309.
47. Berkefeld J, Kirchner J, Müller HM, et al. Balloon dacryocystoplasty: indications and contraindications. Radiology 1997;205:785–790.
48. Janssen AG, Mansour K, Bos JJ. Obstructed nasolacrimal duct system in epiphora: long-term results of dacryocystoplasty by means of balloon dilation. Radiology 1997;205:791–796.
49. Song HY. Interventional techniques in the lacrimal system. In: Castaneda-Zuniga, Tadavarthy SM, Qian Z, et al., eds. Interventional Radiology, vol 2. Baltimore: Williams & Wilkins, 1997:1679–1690.
50. Song HY, Yoon HK, Sung KB. Lacrimal balloon dilatation and stent placement. In: Han MC, Park JH, eds. Interventional Radiology. Seoul, Korea: Ilchokak, 1999:727–733.
51. Song HY, Jin YH, Kim JH, et al. Nonsurgical placement of a nasolacrimal polyurethane stent. Radiology 1995;194:233–237.
52. Song HY, Lee CH, Park SS, et al. Lacrimal canaliculus obstruction: nonsurgical treatment with a newly designed polyurethane stent. Radiology 1996;199:280–282.
53. Song HY, Ahn HS, Park CK, et al. Complete obstruction of the nasolacrimal system. Part II. Treatment with expandable metallic stents. Radiology 1993;186:372–376.
54. Ilgit ET, Yuksel D, Unal M, et al. Treatment of recurrent nasolacrimal duct obstructions with balloon-expandable metallic stents: results of early experience. AJNR Am J Neuroradiol 1996;17:657–663.
55. Ko GY, Song HY, Seo TS, et al. Obstruction of the lacrimal system: treatment with a covered, retrievable, expandable nitinol stent versus a lacrimal polyurethane stent. Radiology 2003;227:270–276.

56. Song HY, Jin YH, Kim JH, et al. Nasolacrimal duct obstruction treated nonsurgically with use of plastic stents. Radiology 1994;190:535–539.

57. Song HY, Jin YH, Kim JH, et al. Nonsurgical placement of a nasolacrimal polyurethane stent: long-term effectiveness. Radiology 1996;200:759–763.

58. Song HY, Lee DH, Kim JH, et al. Lacrimal system obstruction treated with lacrimal polyurethane stents: outcome of removal of occluded stents. Radiology 1998;208:689–694.

59. Kang SG, Song HY, Lee DH, et al. Nonsurgically placed nasolacrimal stents for epiphora: long-term results and factors favoring stent patency. J Vasc Interv Radiol 2002;13:293–300.

60. Janssen AG, Mansour K, Bos JJ, et al. Abscess of the lacrimal sac due to chronic or subacute dacryocystitis: treatment with temporary stent placement in the nasolacrimal duct. Radiology 2000; 215:300–304.

61. Song HY, Jin YH, Lee HK, et al. Nonoperative management of dacryolithiasis. J Vasc Interv Radiol 1995;6:647–650.

62. Kim HS, Song HY, Kim TH, et al. Use of a lacrimal stent retrieval hook in the removal of occluded plastic and expandable metallic lacrimal stents. J Vasc Interv Radiol 2000;11:762–766.

63. Song HY, Lee DH, Ahn HS, et al. Intervention in the lacrimal drainage system. Cardiovasc Intervent Radiol 2002;25:165–170.

Esophageal Stent Placement

34

Ho-Young Song, Hyun Ki Yoon, Kyu-Bo Sung

PRINCIPLES AND BACKGROUND

The worldwide variation in the incidence of carcinoma of the esophagus is greater than that of other tumors (1). Dysphagia and weight loss are seen in more than 90% of patients. Dysphagia does not occur until the lumen is narrowed to one-half to one-third of its original size. Other initial symptoms can also include odynophagia, hoarseness, cough, and glossopharyngeal neuralgia (2,3).

Treatment can be divided broadly into curative and palliative. Curative surgery with or without radiation therapy involves a subtotal or total esophagectomy. However, approximately 60% of all patients with esophageal carcinoma presenting with dysphagia have extensive tumors that are not amenable to surgical resection (4–6).

The best method of palliation in patients with dysphagia caused by nonresectable esophageal neoplasms remains controversial. Surgical bypass procedures using the stomach, colon, or jejunum often produce unsatisfactory results with considerable mortality (7). Radiotherapy is effective in 60–80% of the patients treated in this way, but abatement of symptoms is apparent only after 4–6 weeks (6–8), during which time the patient needs to be nourished for that period. Furthermore, radiotherapy is followed by dysphagia in more than 25% of cases, usually because of a fibrotic cicatrical narrowing (9). The use of Nd:YAG (neodymium yttrium aluminum garnet) laser treatment is limited by its high cost, the requirement of frequent treatment sessions, and the frequency of tumor recurrence (10). In addition, submucosal or extrinsic compressing lesions are inaccessible to treatment by the Nd:YAG laser (11).

Esophageal intubation is an attractively simple and rapid method for palliation of dysphagia caused by malignant neoplasms (7).

The potential benefits of stent placement in esophageal carcinoma were anticipated by Symonds in 1885, who used a tube made of boxwood and ivory (12). For its fixation, the tube relied on strings that emerged through the nostrils and were tied behind the ears. Since the introduction of the esophageal tube, many types of nonexpendable esophageal prostheses inserted surgically or endoscopically have been described (5,6,13–25). Such prostheses were pushed through (pulsion) the stricture from above, usually via the peroral route, or pulled through (traction) the stricture from below, via a high gastrostomy. Traction techniques required laparotomy and gastrostomy, which increased the morbidity and mortality. These disadvantages were avoided with the introduction of peroral pulsion techniques (7). However, despite these efforts, esophageal stent placement continued to be plagued by a high morbidity and mortality as well as by a limited effectiveness in the relief of dysphagia (6,19). Recently, fluoroscopic or endoscopic placement of a covered or bare expandable metallic stent increasingly is being used for the treatment of malignant (11,26–50) and benign esophageal strictures (51–54), because this type of stent is thought to overcome the considerable mortality and morbidity as well as the limited effectiveness in the relief of dysphagia associated with the conventional esophageal prostheses. This chapter covers techniques, clinical applications, results, and problems associated with esophageal metallic stent placement.

PATIENT SELECTION

Permanent or temporary esophageal stent placement is indicated in the following types of patient who have dysphagia to soft or liquid diet because of esophageal strictures:

1. Patients with unresectable or inoperable esophagogastric neoplasms
2. Patients with resectable esophageal neoplasms who reject surgery
3. Patients who need nourishment before surgery or chemoradiation therapy
4. Patients with esophagorespiratory fistula (ERF) resulting from a malignant tumor
5. Patients with a benign stricture refractory to balloon dilation

Removal of placed stents is indicated in the following types of patient (49,54,55):

1. Patients with complications after stent placement such as severe pain, stent migration, or stent deformity
2. Patients with stent placement for the purpose of nourishment before surgery or chemoradiation therapy
3. Patients with a benign stricture who undergo temporary stent placement

There are no absolute contraindications. However, the following are considered relative contraindications for esophageal stent placement:

1. Uncontrollable bleeding diathesis
2. Severely ill patients with a very limited life expectancy
3. Severe vocal cord palsy
4. Multiple obstructive lesions of the small bowel, such as peritoneal seedings

TECHNIQUES

Stent Placement

Several bare or covered expandable metallic stents have been used in the treatment of esophageal strictures, including the covered Gianturco-Rösch Z stent (Cook Europe), the covered Gianturco Z stent (Cook Europe), the Dua Z stent (Wilson Cook Medical), the covered Song esophageal endoprosthesis (Sooho Medi-Tech), the covered Choo stent (Sooho Medi-Tech), the bare Ultraflex stent (Boston Scientific), the covered Ultraflex stent (Microvasive Endoscopy/Boston Scientific), the bare Wallstent (Medinvent), the partially covered Wallstent (Schneider), the partially covered Flamingo stent (Microinvasive/Boston Scientific), the bare EsophaCoil (InStent), and the Niti-S esophageal covered stent (Taewoong Medical). Various stent delivery systems are used, and they range in diameter from 18 French to 38 French.

Several instruments and techniques for stent placement have been addressed (26–50). The techniques have included local anesthesia of the pharynx with an aerosol lidocaine spray. Under fluoroscopic guidance, a small amount of contrast medium is swallowed for opacification of the narrowed esophageal lumen. The location of the stricture is marked on the patient's skin under fluoroscopic control. With the patient in the left anterior oblique or supine position and during extension of the neck, a 0.035-inch stiff-type guide wire (Radiofocus M, Terumo) is inserted, with or without the help of an angiographic catheter, through the mouth across the stricture into the distal esophagus or stomach. A graduate sizing catheter (Cook) is passed over the guide wire to measure the length of stricture, after which this catheter is removed, with the guide wire left in place. A stent delivery system with a stent inside, whose proximal part is lubricated with jelly, is passed over the guide wire into the esophagus and advanced until the distal tip of the stent reaches beyond the stricture (Figure 34–1). In cases of strictures that are too tight to accommodate the stent delivery system, balloon dilation is needed first. The introducing sheath is withdrawn slowly over the pusher in a continuous motion, which frees the stent and allows it to lie within the stricture and expand. The delivery system and guide wire are then removed. Esophagography can be performed immediately or 1 day after stent placement to verify the position and patency of the stent and to detect any esophageal perforation. Patients are allowed a liquid diet initially, followed by

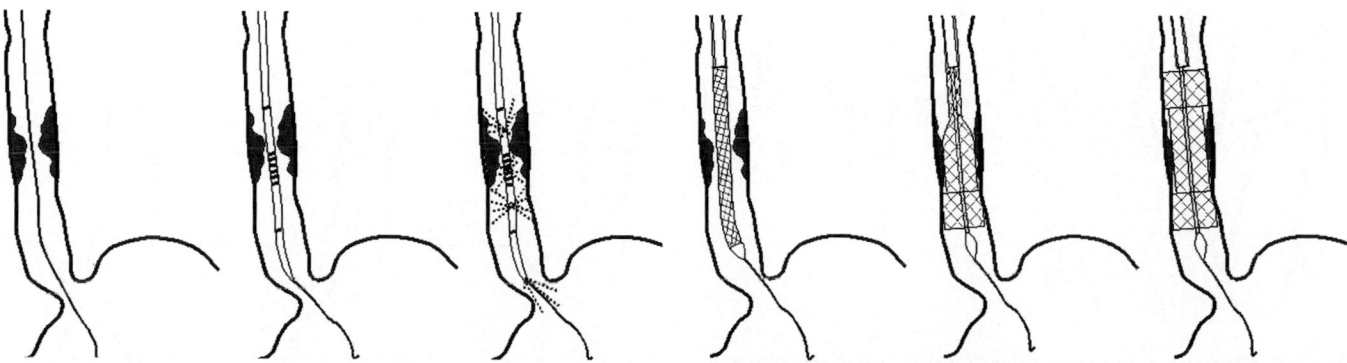

Figure 34–1 Technical steps in esophageal stent placement.

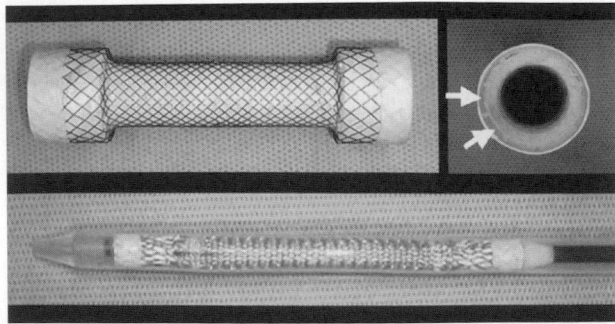

Figure 34–2 Top to bottom: a lateral view of a PTFE-covered retrievable nitinol stent (*right*), a top view of the stent showing draw-strings (*arrows*), and a stent delivery system (guiding olive tip, compressed stent, sheath, pusher catheter).

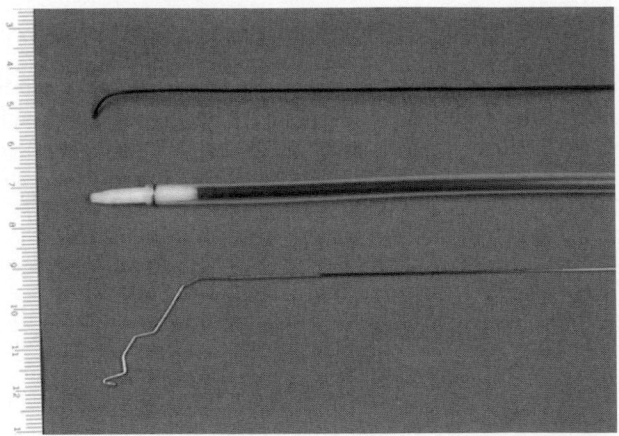

Figure 34–4 Top to bottom: a guide wire, a dilator with sheath, and a hook.

a diet of soft solids. Patients in whom the stent straddled the distal esophageal sphincter are advised to sleep in a semi-erect position to minimize the reflux and aspiration of gastric contents.

Stent Removal

The Niti-S esophageal covered stent (Taewoong Medical) has two nylon drawstrings at its upper inner margin (Figure 34–2). To make a retrievable stent, a loop of nylon was hooked inside each bend of the proximal stent and secured by suture (34,49,54). Other nylon threads (draw-strings) were passed through each of the nylon loops to make a larger loop of nylon filling the circumference of the inside of the proximal stent (Figure 34–3). The resulting loop was strung with a thread. The retrieval set consists of a 10 French retrieval hook catheter, a 10 French dilator and a 13 French sheath (Figure 34–4).

After topical anesthesia of the pharynx with an aerosol spray, a 0.035-inch stiff type guide wire (Radiofocus M, Terumo) is introduced through the mouth and across the stent into the distal esophagus or stomach. A sheath with a

dilator is passed down over the guide wire into the proximal stent lumen. After the guide wire and the dilator are removed from the sheath, a hook catheter is introduced into the sheath and advanced until its metal part passes through the sheath into the stent lumen. The sheath with the hook catheter is then pulled out of the stent so that its metal part hooks onto the nylon thread. When this happens, the hook catheter is withdrawn through the sheath to collapse the proximal stent when it reaches the sheath tip. The sheath, hook catheter, and stent are then pulled out of the esophagus (Figure 34–5).

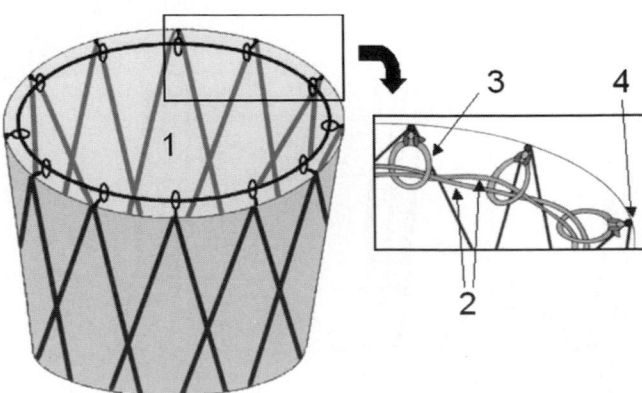

Figure 34–3 Diagrams show drawstrings attached to the upper inner margin of the stent. 1 = central lumen, 2 = drawstrings, 3 = nylon loop, 4 = upper margin of the wire.

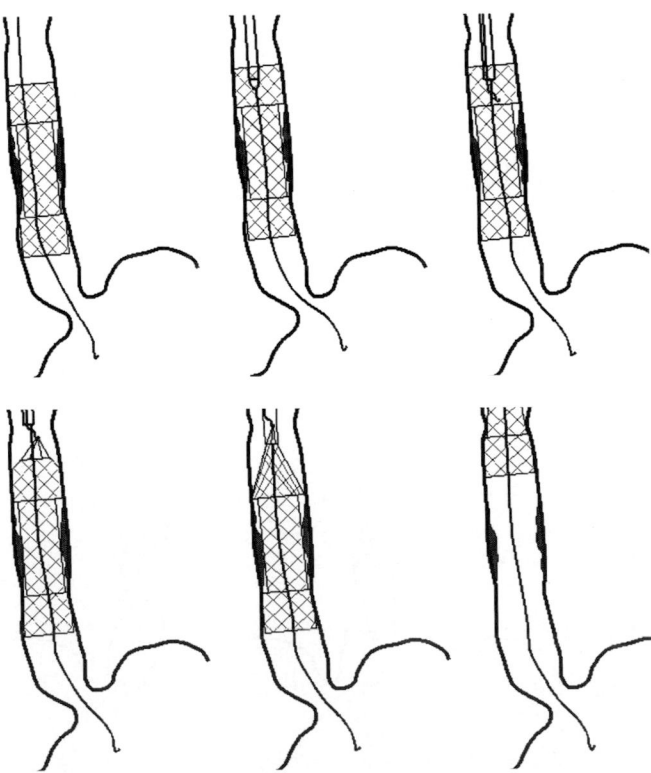

Figure 34–5 Technical steps in stent removal.

RESULTS

Malignant Esophageal Strictures

In cases of malignant esophageal strictures with dysphagia, placement of expandable metallic stents is better tolerated and safer than placement of plastic tubes because expandable stents can be delivered in compressed form using a small-diameter device. They also provide excellent relief from dysphagia and less frequent blockage by food because their luminal diameter is greater than that of the plastic tubes used (29,36–38).

Overall success rates of 96–100% have been reported in studies involving 9–153 patients (27–50). Adam et al. (37) reported that improvements in dysphagia scores at 1 month after stent placement were the same for covered and bare stents in a randomized prospective trial. Covered stents have the disadvantage of stent migration, which reportedly leads to a recurrence of dysphagia in 5–32% of patients. On the other hand, bare esophageal stents have relatively low migration rates (0–3%) as a result of fixation of the stent wires within the tumor (32,37,38). However, bare stents are not suitable for the treatment of ERFs. In addition, progressive tumor ingrowth through the openings between the wire filaments of bare stents tends to cause progressive dysphagia (Figure 34–6). Covered stents were placed in 61 patients with ERF resulting from esophageal or bronchogenic carcinoma (55). The stent completely sealed off the fistula in 49 (80%) of 61 patients such that they had no further aspiration symptoms, which indicates initial clinical success; however, the fistula reopened in 17 (35%) of these 49 patients. The survival period in patients with initial clinical success for ERF was significantly longer than in those patients with initial clinical failure (15.1 versus 6.2 weeks, $p < 0.05$).

In Song et al., removal of the placed stent was needed in 15 of 108 patients (14%) with malignant esophageal strictures because of complications (49). The stent was removed 2 days to 16 weeks (mean of 4 weeks) after stent placement because of severe pain ($n = 7$), stent migration ($n = 6$), and stent deformity ($n = 2$). Removal of the stent was well-tolerated in all patients. Stent placement with no radiation therapy caused fewer complications than stent placement with concurrent radiation therapy ($p = 0.005$ and $p < 0.001$, respectively). However, the survival period was significantly longer in patients with stent placement and concurrent radiation therapy than in patients with stent placement with no concurrent radiation therapy ($p = 0.034$). The conclusion is that temporary placement (Figure 34–7) of a covered retrievable stent for 3–4 weeks with concurrent radiation therapy for malignant esophageal strictures is more effective than permanent stent placement at reducing delayed complications and related reinterventions (49,50).

Benign Esophageal Strictures

In some institutes, covered stents and bare stents have been used in patients with benign strictures refractory to balloon dilation (51–53). The long-term results of permanent placement of covered or bare stents have been considered discouraging because of the high reported rates (40–100%) of late complications caused by stent migration or the formation of new stricture. Although bare stents tend not to migrate, nonsurgical removal of bare stents is difficult because of mucosal hyperplasia through the openings between the wire filaments.

Song et al. (54) placed retrievable expandable stents in 25 patients with benign esophageal strictures. After stent placement, all patients could ingest solid food (Figure 34–8). One patient passed a stent via the rectum, and another patient regurgitated a stent. In the remaining 23 patients, the placed stents were removed 1–8 weeks after placement. After stent removal or migration, all patients could ingest solid food. During the mean follow-up period of 13 (range of 2–25) months after stent removal or migration, 12 of 25 patients maintained improvement of dysphagia and needed no further treatment.

COMPLICATIONS AND MANAGEMENT

Esophageal Perforation or Fistula Formation

The rate of esophageal perforation or delayed ERF associated with placement of an expandable stent has been reported to be 0–7% (25–63). The perforation can occur during the process of stent placement by the formation of a false passage through or below the strictures, and after stent placement, delayed perforation from pressure necrosis can occur. Delayed ERF can be managed by additional stent replacement (29,55).

Bleeding

Massive bleeding after stent placement has been reported to be 0–19% (25–63). Any penetration of the aorta or other mediastinal vessels leads to a massive and fatal hematemesis (9). The chance of massive bleeding is higher in patients who undergo radiation therapy after stent placement than in patients who do not undergo radiation therapy after stent placement (29).

Stent Migration

Stent migration rates of 4–14% have been reported (25–63). Migration is more common in covered stents than in bare stents. Migration is also more common in benign strictures as well as in soft and eccentric malignant strictures, especially when the strictures are in the esophagogastric junction (29). Stent removal in patients with stent migration seems not to be urgent, not only because the migrated stent can pass through the rectum, but also because it can remain for a long time in the stomach without causing symptoms (29,37,53). However, some authors have reported that a migrated stent causes complications that include pain, ulcer, and obstruction (31,37).

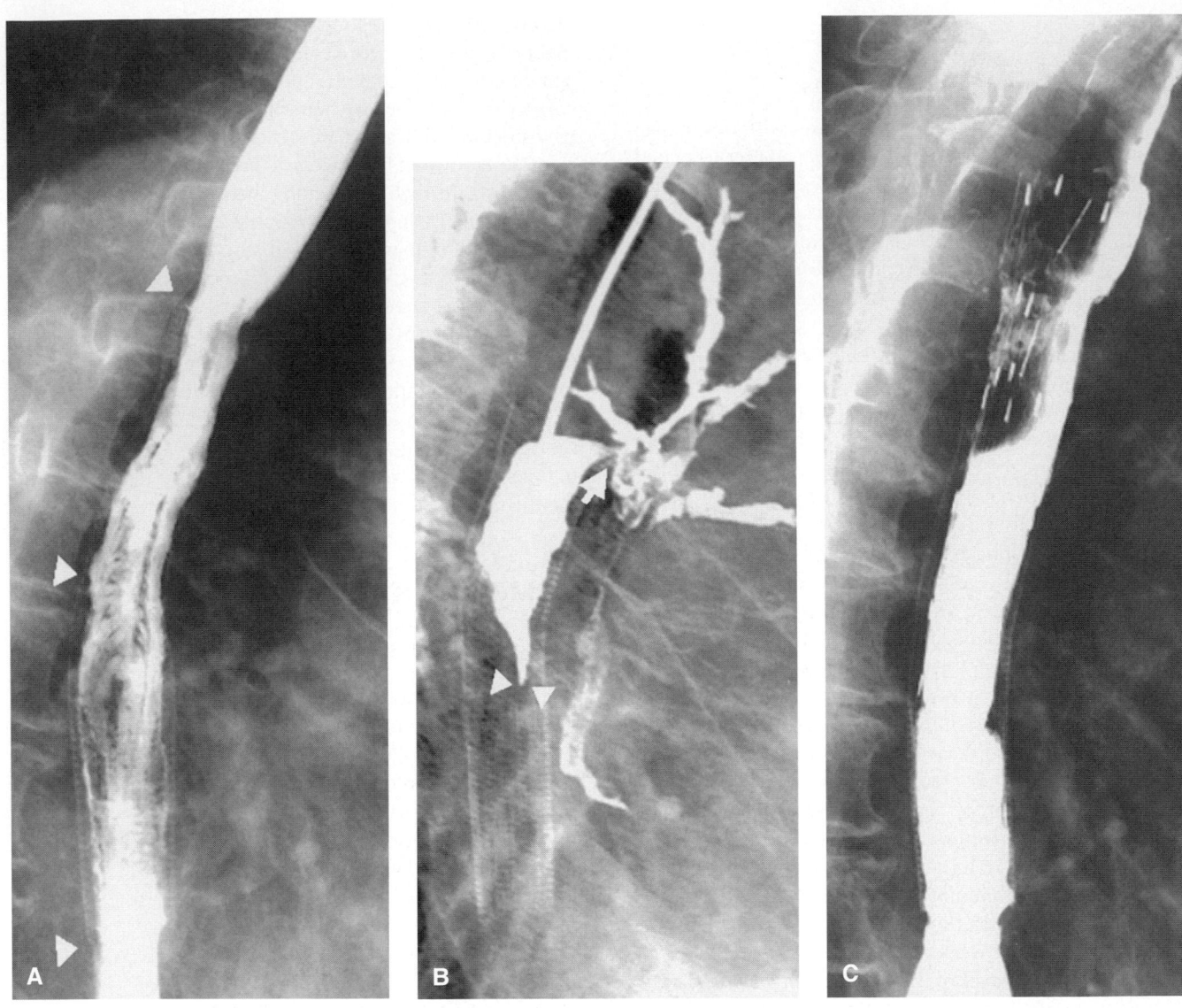

Figure 34–6 A. Esophagogram obtained just after placement of a bare Ultraflex stent (*arrowheads*) shows good flow of contrast medium. **B.** Esophagogram obtained 3 months later shows complete obstruction (*arrowheads*) of the stent as a result of tumor ingrowth and an esophagobronchial fistula (*arrow*). **C.** Esophagogram obtained after placement of a covered Z stent overlapping the bare stent.

Tumor Ingrowth, Overgrowth, or Food Impaction

Blockage of the expandable stents can occur by tumor ingrowth, tumor overgrowth, and food impaction (3– 36%). Growth of the tumor may occlude the proximal or distal end of the stent. This can be easily managed by the addition of another stent (Figure 34–9) that overlaps the end of the first stent. An impacted food bolus can be displaced into the stomach using a balloon catheter or an endoscope (29).

Granulation Tissue Formation

The rate of granulation-tissue formation after stent placement for a malignant stricture has been reported to be 0–13% (25–49). This can be easily managed by the addition

of another stent that overlaps the end of the first stent in patients with stent placement for a malignant stricture. The formation of granulation tissue is more common in patients with stent placement for a benign stricture (54). In patients with granulation-tissue formation after stent placement, it is necessary to remove the stent not only because this improves the condition but also because granulated tissue eventually causes recurrence of dysphagia (Figures 34–10 and 34–11).

Tracheal Compression

The rate of tracheobronchial compression after esophageal stent placement has been reported to be 0–6% (25–63). In some institutes, aggravation of dyspnea was rare in patients with esophageal stent placement as long as the mass does

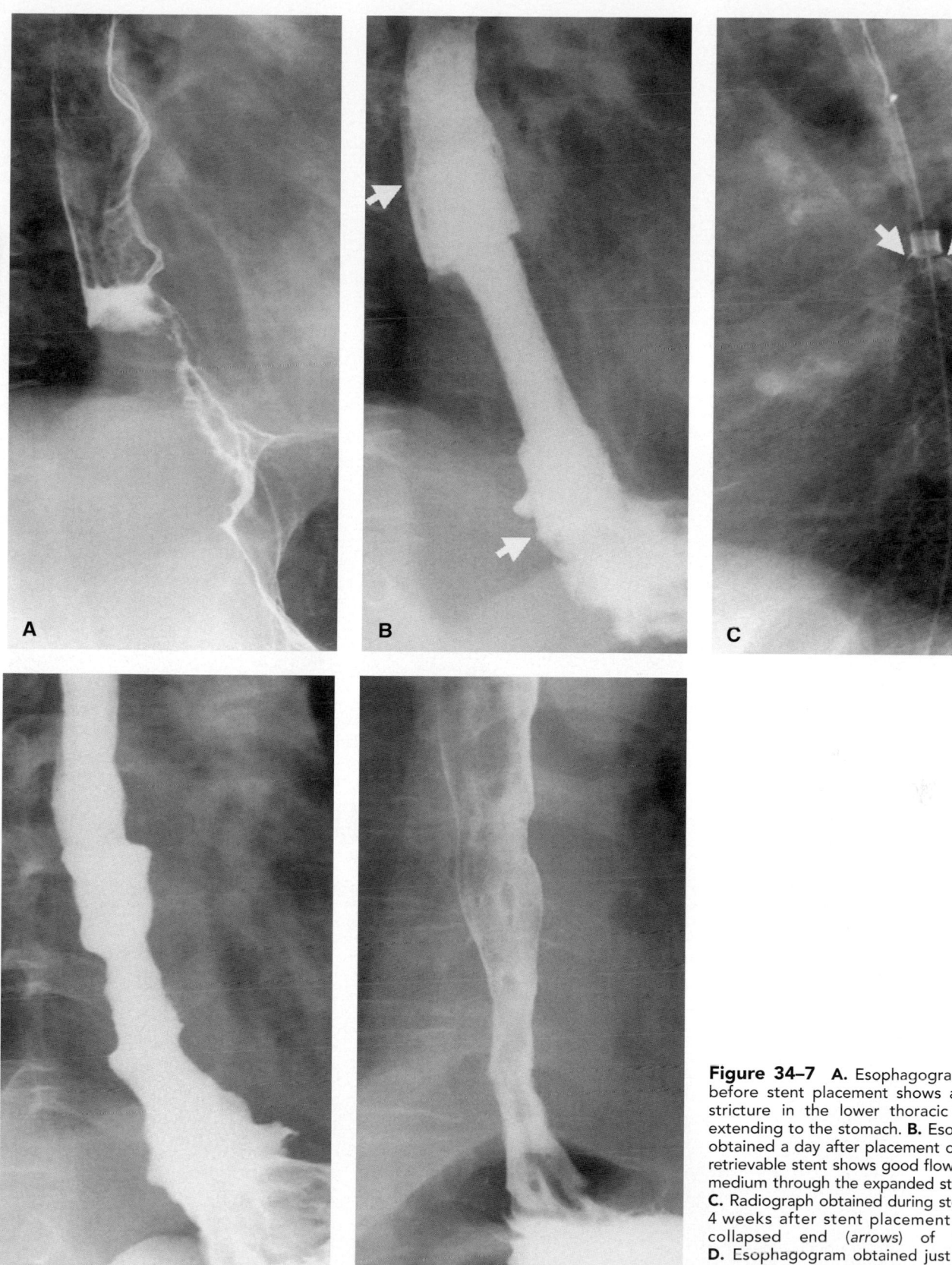

Figure 34–7 **A.** Esophagogram obtained before stent placement shows a malignant stricture in the lower thoracic esophagus extending to the stomach. **B.** Esophagogram obtained a day after placement of a covered retrievable stent shows good flow of contrast medium through the expanded stent (*arrows*) **C.** Radiograph obtained during stent removal 4 weeks after stent placement shows the collapsed end (*arrows*) of the stent. **D.** Esophagogram obtained just after stent removal shows improvement of the stricture. **E.** Esophagogram obtained 4 weeks after stent removal shows maintained improvement.

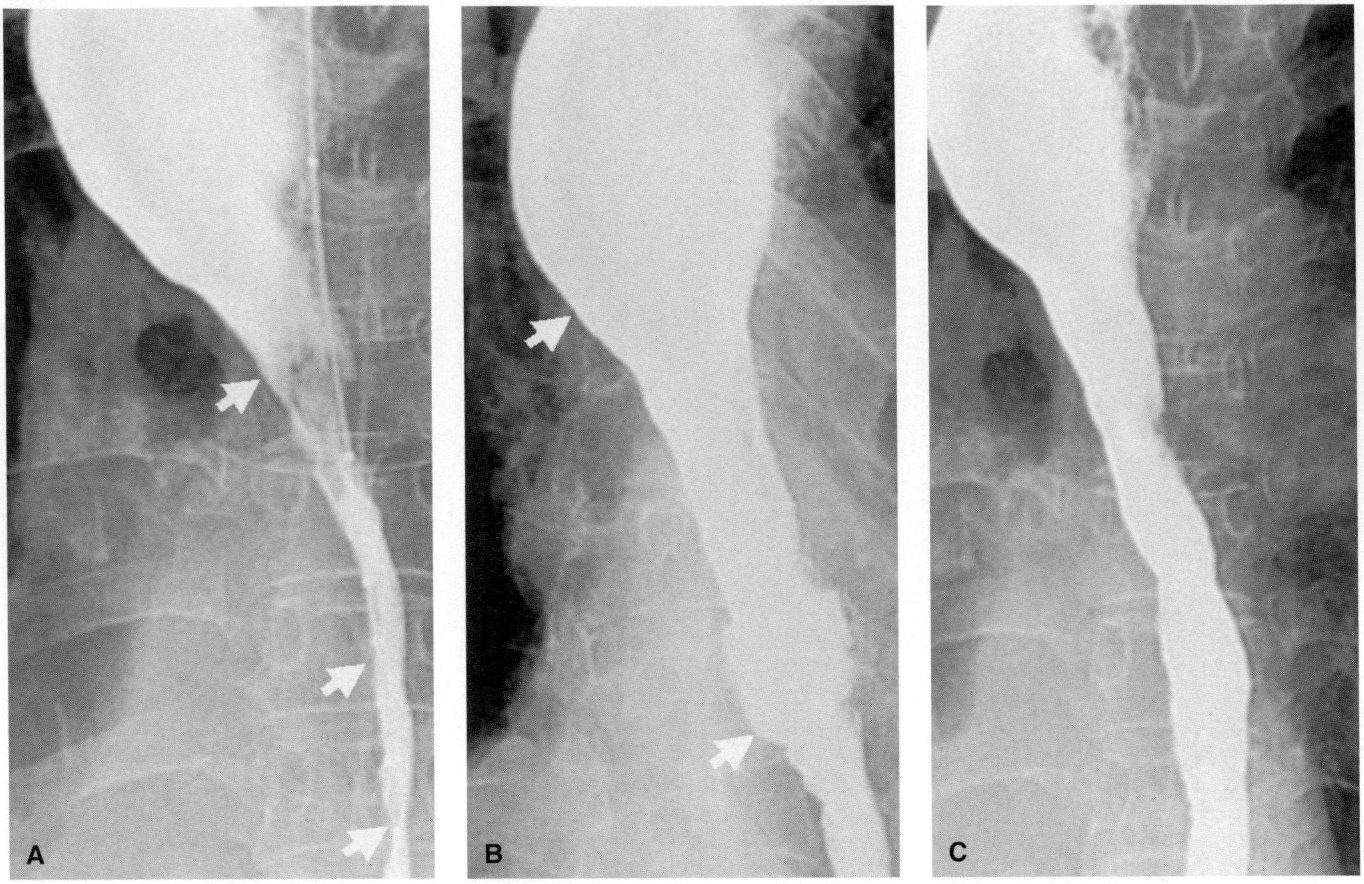

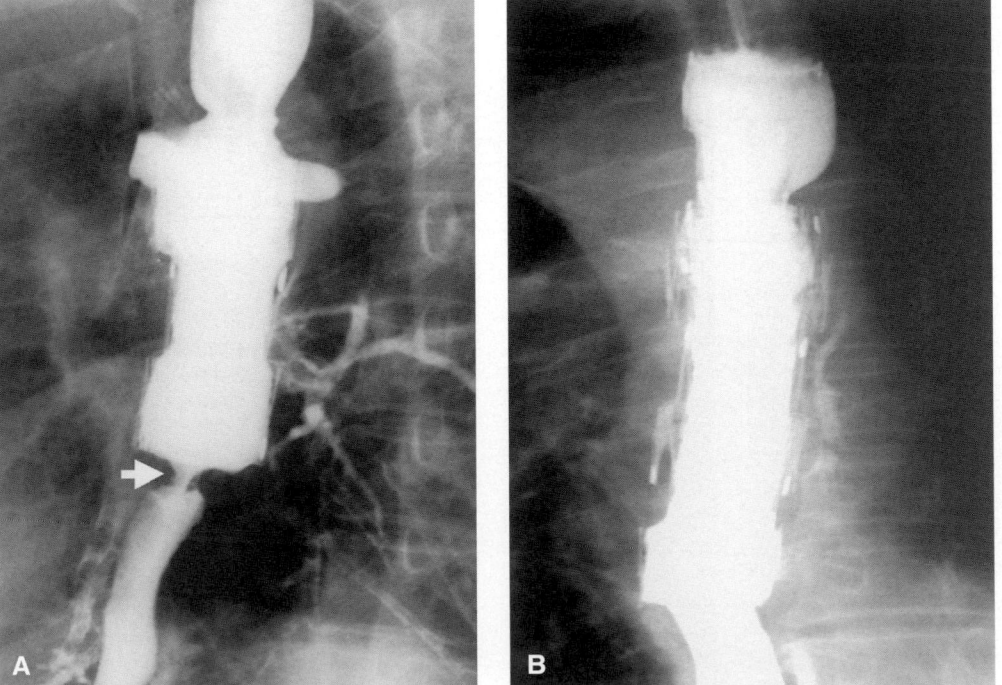

Figure 34–8 A. Esophagogram obtained before stent placement shows a diffuse corrosive stricture (*arrows*). **B.** Esophagogram obtained 8 weeks after placement of a covered retrievable stent shows good flow of contrast medium through the expanded stent (*arrows*) **C.** Radiograph obtained 1 year after stent removal shows improvement of the stricture.

Figure 34–9 A. Esophagogram obtained 6 months after stent placement of a covered Z stent shows a stricture (*arrow*) distal to the stent resulting from tumor overgrowth. **B.** Esophagogram obtained 1 day after placement of a second covered Z stent longer than the first stent shows closure of the fistula.

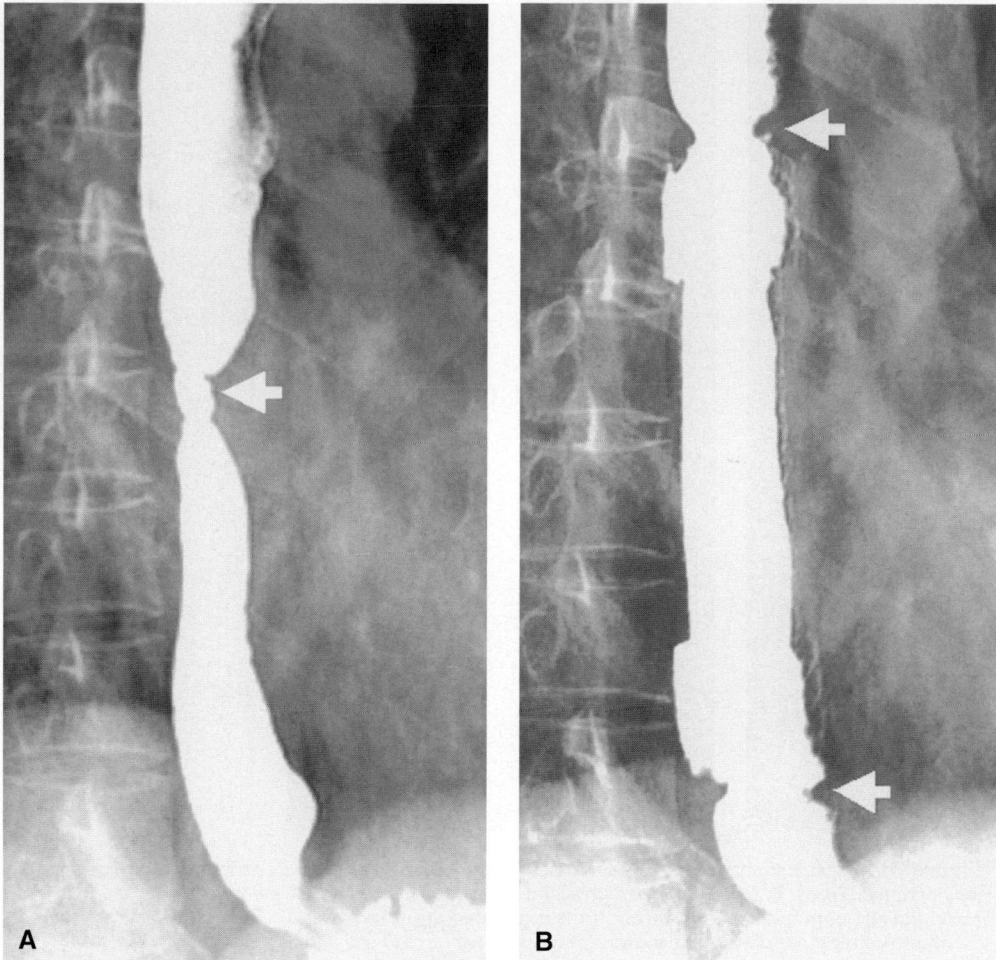

Figure 34–10 A. Esophagogram obtained before stent placement shows a corrosive stricture (*arrow*) in the lower thoracic esophagus. **B.** Esophagogram obtained 2 weeks after placement of a covered retrievable stent shows formation of new strictures (*arrows*) above and below the stent.

not extend to the tracheobronchial tree. Tracheobronchial compression after esophageal stent placement can be managed by either tracheobronchial stent placement (55) or removal of the esophageal stent.

Reflux

Gastroesophageal reflux is a problem in patients who have a stent in the lower one third of the esophagus bridging the gastroesophageal junction. The symptoms can be relieved with the use of antacids, by sleeping with the head of the bed raised approximately 30 degrees, and by avoiding large meals before going to bed. Gastroesophageal reflux can be prevented with the use antireflux stents (39–41).

Reopening of ERF

The reopening rate ranges from 0–35% (25–63). The causes of reopening include stent occlusion often because of tumor overgrowth or ingrowth, food impaction, or granulation tissue

formation, stent migration, funnel phenomenon, and stent-covering disruption (27,30,55–58,60). These conditions can be managed by additional stent replacement, saline irrigation, injection of tissue glue in the peri-stent space, or tracheobronchial stent placement (29,55,60).

Miscellaneous Complications

A metallic stent placed in patients with cervical esophageal stricture can cause a foreign body sensation in the throat (29). Other complications include mucosal prolapse into the stent and aspiration pneumonia in patients with stent placement in the esophagogastric junction.

SUMMARY

The use of covered stents and bare stents is useful in patients with malignant esophageal strictures. The main problem with bare stents, however, is that they are not useful in the

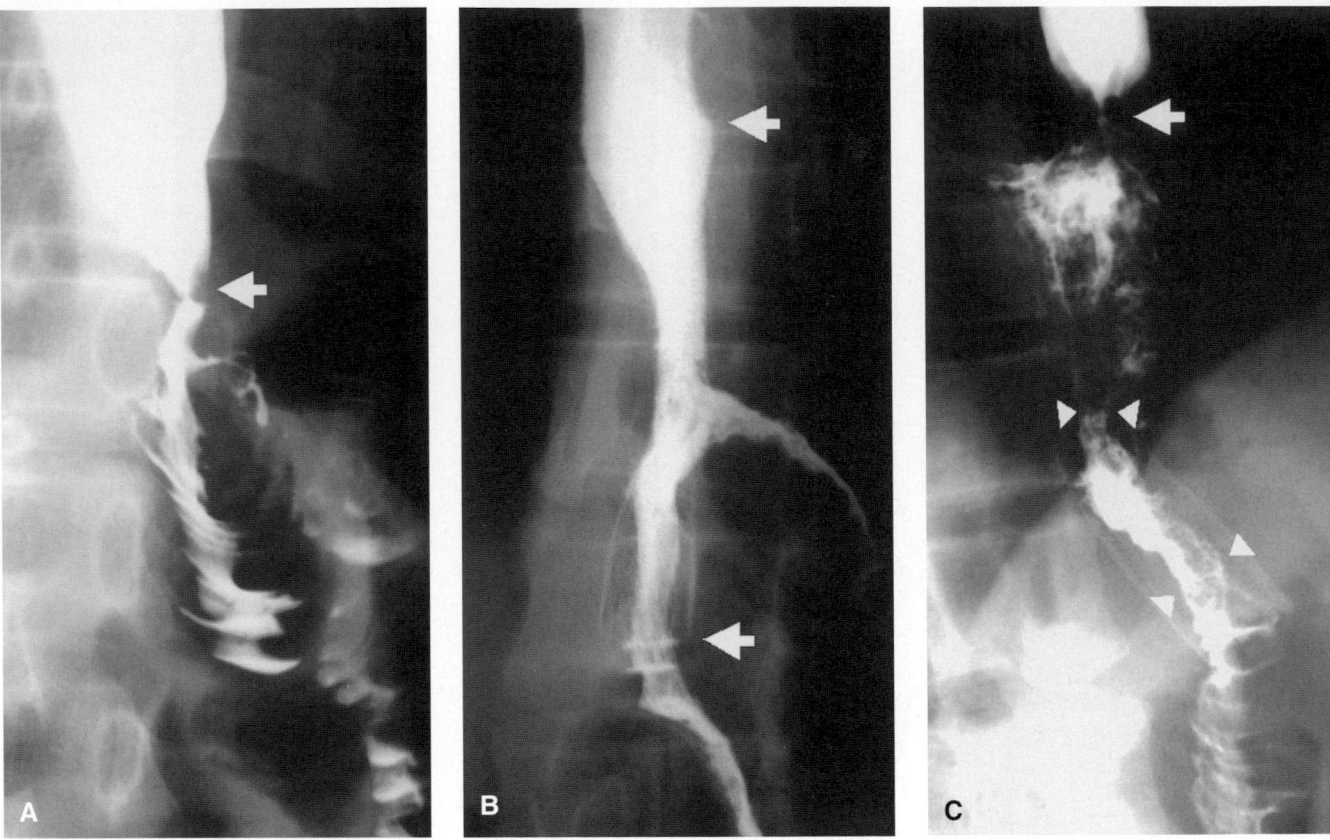

Figure 34–11 A. Esophagogram obtained before stent placement shows a stricture at the esophago-jejunostomy (*arrow*). **B.** Esophagogram obtained 1 day after placement of a bare Ultraflex stent shows good flow of contrast medium through the expanded stent (*arrows*). **C.** Esophagogram obtained 12 months after stent placement shows strictures above (*arrow*) and within (*arrowheads*) the stent.

treatment of ERF. In addition, bare stents are not suitable for temporary placement in the treatment of benign strictures because nonsurgical removal of the stents is very difficult. By using covered retrievable expandable stents temporarily, indications for stent placement are extended to patients with benign esophageal strictures refractory to balloon dilation.

Stents placed in patients with malignant esophageal strictures need to be removed in 14% of cases because of complications. In patients with stent placement for malignant ERF, close follow-up must ensue not only because the reopening rate is rather high (35%), but also because the reopening can be treated. Patients with radiation therapy after stent placement experience more complications than other groups. Therefore, temporary placement of a covered retrievable expandable stent for 3–4 weeks with concurrent radiation therapy for malignant esophageal strictures warrants further investigation.

REFERENCES

1. Rosenberg JC, Franklin R, Steiger Z. Squamous cell carcinoma of the thoracic esophagus: an interdisciplinary approach. Curr Probl Cancer 1981;5:1–52.
2. Rosenberg JC, Schwade JG, Vaitkevicius VK. Cancer of the esophagus. In: DeVita VT, Hellman S, Rosenberg SA, eds. Cancer: Principles and Practice of Oncology. Philadelphia: JB Lippincott 1982;499.
3. Moertel CG. The esophagus. In: Holland JF, Prei E, eds. Cancer Medicine. 2nd Ed. Philadelphia: Lea & Febiger 1982;1753.
4. Earlam R, Cunha-Melo JR. Oesophageal squamous carcinoma. A critical review of surgery. Br J Surg 1980;67:381–390.
5. Saunders NR. The celestin tube in the palliation of carcinoma of the esophagus and cardia. Br J Surg 1979;66:419–421.
6. Ogilvie AL, Dronfield MW, Ferguson R, et al. Palliative intubation of oesophagogastric neoplasms at fiberoptic endoscopy. Gut 1982:23:1060–1067.
7. Angorn IB, Haffejee AA. Endoesophageal intubation for palliation in obstructing esophageal carcinoma. In: Manning TA, ed. Interventional Trends in General Thoracic Surgery, vol 4. St. Louis: Mosby, Delarue, and Eschapasse, 1988:410–419.
8. Caspers R, Welvaart K, Verkes R, et al. The effect of radiotherapy on dysphagia and survival in patients with esophageal cancer. Radiother Oncol 1988;12:15–23.
9. Earlam R, Cunha-Melo JR. Malignant esophageal strictures: a review of techniques for palliative intubation. Br J Surg 1982; 69:61–68.
10. Fleischer D, Sivak M. Endoscopic Nd:YAG laser therapy as palliation for esophagogastric cancer. Parameters affecting initial outcome. Gastroenterology 1985;89:827–831.
11. Schaer J, Katon RM, Ivancev K, et al. Treatment of malignant esophageal obstruction with silicone-coated metallic self-expanding stents. Gastrointest Endosc 1992;38:7–11.
12. Symonds CJ. A case of malignant stricture of the oesophagus illustrating the use of a new form of oesophageal catheter. Trans Chir Soc Lond 1885;18:155–158.
13. Souttar HS. A method of intubating the oesophagus for malignant stricture. Br Med J 1924;1:782–783.
14. Celestin LR. Permanent intubation in inoperable cancer of the oesophagus and cardia. A new tube. Ann R Coll Surg Engl 1959:25: 165–170.
15. Girardet RE, Randell HJ, Whear MS. Palliative intubation in the management of esophageal carcinoma. Ann Thorac Surg 1974; 18:417–430.

16. Den Hartog Jager FCA, Bartelsman JFWM, et al. Palliative treatment of obstructing esophagogastric malignancy by endoscopic positioning of a plastic prosthesis. Gastroenterology 1979;77:1008–1014.

17. Hankins JR, Cole FN, Saffu A, et al. Palliation of esophageal carcinoma with intraluminal tubes: experience with 30 patients. Ann Thorac Surg 1979;18:226–229.

18. Lishman AH, Dellipiani AW, Delvlin HB. The insertion of oesophagogastric tubes in malignant oesophageal strictures: endoscopy or surgery? Br J Surg 1980;67:257–259.

19. Haynes JW, Miller PR, Steiger Z, et al. Celestin tube use: radiographic manifestations of associated complications. Radiology 1984;150:41–44.

20. Valbuena J. Endoscopic palliative treatment of esophageal and cardial cancer: a new antireflux prosthesis. A study of 40 cases. Cancer 1984;53:993–998.

21. Ghazi A, Nussbaum M. A new approach to the management of malignant esophageal obstruction and esophagorespiratory fistula. Ann Thorac Surg 1986;41:531–534.

22. Frimberger E. Expanding spiral—a new type of prosthesis for the palliative treatment of malignant esophageal stenoses. Endoscopy 1983;15:213–214.

23. Loizou LA, Rampton D, Bown SG. Treatment of malignant strictures of the cervical esophagus by endoscopic intubation using modified endoprostheses. Gastrointest Endosc 1992;38:158–164.

24. Liakakos TK, Ohri SK, Townsend ER, et al. Palliative intubation for dysphagia in patients with carcinoma of the esophagus. Ann Thorac Surg 1992;53:460–463.

25. Sarr MG, Harper PH, Kettlewell MGW. Peroral pulsion intubation of malignant esophageal strictures using a fiberoptic technique. Am Surg 1984;50:437–440.

26. Song HY, Choi KC, Cho BH, et al. Esophagogastric neoplasms: palliation with a modified Gianturco stent. Radiology 1991;180:349–354.

27. Miyayama S, Matsui O, Kadoya M, et al. Malignant esophageal stricture and fistula: palliative treatment with polyurethane-covered Gianturco stent. J Vasc Interv Radiol 1995;6:243–248.

28. Watkinson AF, Ellul J, Entwisle K, et al. Esophageal carcinoma: initial results of palliative treatment with covered self-expanding endoprostheses. Radiology 1995;195:821–827.

29. Song HY, Do YS, Han YM, et al. Covered expandable esophageal metallic stent tubes: experiences in 119 patients. Radiology 1994;193:689–695.

30. Han YM, Song HY, Lee JM, et al. Esophagorespiratory fistulae due to esophageal carcinoma: palliation with a covered Gianturco stent. Radiology 1996;199:65–70.

31. Knyrim K, Wagner HJ, Bethge N, et al. A controlled trial of an expansile metal stent for palliation of esophageal obstruction due to inoperable cancer. N Engl J Med 1993;329:1302–1307.

32. Acunas B, Rozanes I, Akpinar S, et al. Palliation of malignant esophageal strictures with self-expanding nitinol stents: drawbacks and complications. Radiology 1996;199:648–652.

33. Do YS, Song HY, Lee BH, et al. Esophagorespiratory fistula associated with esophageal cancer: treatment with a Gianturco stent tube. Radiology 1993;187:673–677.

34. Song HY, Park SI, Jung HY, et al. Benign and malignant esophageal strictures: treatment with a polyurethane-covered retrievable expandable metallic stent. Radiology 1997;203:747–752.

35. Rozanes I, Akpinar S, Tunaci A, et al. Palliation of malignant esophageal strictures with self-expanding nitinol stents: drawbacks and complications. Radiology 1996;199:648–652.

36. Saxon RR. Morrison KE, Lakin PC, et al. Malignant esophageal obstruction and esophagorespiratory fistula: palliation with a polyurethane-covered Z-stent. Radiology 1997;202:349–354.

37. Adam A, Ellul J, Watkinson AF, et al. Palliation of inoperable esophageal carcinoma: a prospective randomized trial of laser therapy and stent placement. Radiology 1997;202:344–348.

38. Cwikiel W, Tranberg KG, Cwikiel M, et al. Malignant dysphagia: palliation with esophageal stents—long-term results in 100 patients. Radiology 1998;207:513–518.

39. Do YS, Choo SW, Suh SW, et al. Malignant esophagogastric junction obstruction: palliative treatment with an antireflux valve stent. J Vasc Interv Radiol 2001;12:647–651.

40. Dua KS, Kozarek R, Kim J, et al. Self-expanding metal esophageal stent with anti-reflux mechanism. Gastrointest Endosc 2001;53:603–613.

41. Laasch HU, Marriott A, Wilbraham L, et al. Effectiveness of open versus antireflux stents for palliation of distal esophageal carcinoma and prevention of symptomatic gastroesophageal reflux. Radiology 2002;225:359–365.

42. Wengrower D, Fiorini A, Valero J, et al. EsophaCoil: long-term results in 81 patients. Gastrointest Endosc 1998;48:376–382.

43. Olsen E, Thyregaard R, Kill J. EsophaCoil expanding metal stent in the management of patients with nonresectable malignant esophageal or cardiac neoplasm: a prospective study. Endoscopy 1999;31:417–420.

44. Bartelsman JEW, Bruno MJ, Jensema AI, et al. Palliation of patients with esophagogastric neoplasms by insertion of a covered expandable modified Gianturco-Z endoprosthesis: experiences in 153 patients. Gastrointest Endosc 2000;51:134–138.

45. Siersema PD, Hop WCJ, van Blankenstein M, et al. A new design metal stent (Flamingo stent) for palliation of malignant dysphagia: a prospective study. Gastrointest Endosc 2000;51:139–145.

46. Siersema PD, Hop WCJ, van Blankenstein M, et al. A comparison of 3 types of covered metal stents for the palliation of patients with dysphagia caused by esophagogastric carcinoma: a prospective, randomized study. Gastrointest Endosc 2001;54:145–153.

47. Mayoral W, Fleisher D, Calcedo J, et al. Nonmalignant obstruction is a common problem with metal stents in the treatment of esophageal cancer. Gastrointest Endosc 2000;51:556–559.

48. Ell C, May A. Self-expanding metal stents for palliation of stenosing tumors of the esophagus and cardia. A critical review. Endoscopy 1997;29:392–398.

49. Song HY, Lee DH, Seo TS, et al. Retrievable covered nitinol stents: experiences in 108 patients with malignant esophageal strictures. J Vasc Interv Radiol 2002;13:285–292.

50. Tan BS, Kennedy C, Morgan R, et al. Using uncovered metallic endoprostheses to treat recurrent benign esophageal strictures. AJR Am J Roentgenol 1997;169:1281–1284.

51. Cwikiel W, Willen R, Stridbeck H, et al. Self-expanding stent in the treatment of benign esophageal strictures: experimental study in pigs and presentation of clinical cases. Radiology 1993;187:667–671.

52. Song HY, Park SI, Do YS, et al. Expandable metallic stent placement in patients with benign esophageal strictures: results of long-term follow-up. Radiology 1997;203:131–136.

53. Song HY, Jung HY, Park SI, et al. Covered retrievable expandable nitinol stents in patients with benign esophageal strictures: initial experience. Radiology 2000;217:551–557.

54. Shin JH, Song HY. Esophagorespiratory fistula: long-term results of palliation with covered expandable metallic stents in 61 patients. Radiology 2004;232:252–259.

55. Saxon RR, Barton RE, Katon RM, et al. Treatment of malignant esophagorespiratory fistulas with silicone-covered metallic Z stents. J Vasc Interv Radiol 1995;6:237–242.

56. Morgan RA, Ellul JP, Denton ER, et al. Malignant esophageal fistulas and perforations: management with plastic-covered metallic endoprostheses. Radiology 1997;204:527–532.

57. Wu WC, Katon RM, Saxon RR, et al. Silicone covered self-expanding metallic stents for the palliation of malignant esophageal obstruction and esophagorespiratory fistulas: experience in 32 patients and a review of the literature. Gastrointest Endosc 1994;40:22–33.

58. Tomaselli F, Maier A, Sankin O, et al. Successful endoscopical sealing of malignant esophageotracheal fistulae by using a covered self-expandable stenting system. Eur J Cardiothorac Surg 2001;20:734–738.

59. Wang MQ, Sze DY, Wang ZP, et al. Delayed complications after esophageal stent placement for treatment of malignant esophageal obstructions and esophagorespiratory fistulas. J Vasc Interv Radiol 2001;12:465–474.

60. Kozarek RA, Raltz S, Brugge WR, et al. Prospective multicenter trial of esophageal Z-stent placement for malignant dysphagia and tracheoesophageal fistula. Gastrointest Endosc 1996;44:562–567.

61. May A, Ell C. Palliative treatment of malignant esophagorespiratory fistulas with Gianturco-Z stents: A prospective clinical trial and review of the literature on covered metal stents. Am J Gastroenterol 1998;93:532–535.

62. Grundy A, Glees JP. Aorto-oesophageal fistula: a complication of oesophageal stenting. Br J Radiol. 1997;70:846–849.

63. Shin JH, Ko GY, Yoon HK, et al. Temporary stent placement during radiation therapy in patients with malignant esophageal strictures: initial experience. Radiology 2002;225(P): 162.

Colonic Stenting

35

Manuel Maynar, Miguel A. de Gregorio, Antonio Mainar, Eloy Tejero, Wilfrido R. Castañeda-Zuñiga

Colorectal cancer is an important social and health problem. Nearly one million new cases of colorectal cancer are diagnosed worldwide each year, the result of which is half a million deaths. In Europe and the United States, 300,000 new cases of colorectal cancer are detected every year (1,2). Seven to twenty-nine percent of these cases have complete or partial obstruction of the large bowel at the time of presentation (3,4). The traditional management of acute intestinal obstruction resulting from colorectal cancer is surgical (5), which commonly requires an emergency procedure involving high-risk patients with an unprepared colon. Typically, these patients end up having a surgical colostomy performed to allow cleansing of the bowel and staging of the disease (6,7). Emergency surgical resection of colon cancer in a patient with an unprepared bowel is associated with high morbidity and mortality (8). The surgical mortality rate decreases from 15–20% to 0.9–6% when patients with colon cancer undergo elective surgery (9). Colon cancer patients who present with acute obstruction of the large bowel have a 5-year survival rate of less than 20%—a far poorer prognosis than patients who present without obstruction (10). In spite of the increasing popularity of primary resection and anastomosis, only 40% of the left-sided colonic obstructions secondary to carcinoma can be treated with intraoperative lavage and subtotal colectomy (11). The rest of the patients will need a colostomy, which can be temporary or permanent depending on the stage of the disease—with the concomitant impact on the patient's quality of life (12).

METALLIC STENTS: GENERAL CONCEPTS

Self-expandable metallic stents increasingly are being used for the palliative management of malignant stenoses and obstructions of the gastrointestinal tract. Metallic stents have made it possible to reestablish luminal continuity in patients with malignant obstruction of the biliary tree, esophagus, gastric outlet, and small and large bowel who have a high surgical risk (13). Dohmoto and colleagues first used colonic metallic stents in 1990 (14). Metallic endoprostheses have been used as palliative treatment to manage acute malignant occlusion of the colon (15–17). In 1994, Tejero et al. described the use of stents as a "bridge to surgery" in two patients with colorectal malignant obstruction. Five days poststent insertion and following cleansing of the bowel and staging of the disease, both patients were subjected to an elective surgical resection with primary colorectal anastomosis (18). The placement of a metallic stent across an obstructed segment is an effective therapeutic alternative for primary palliation in patients with malignant acute or chronic inoperable colorectal obstruction (19,20). A few reports in the literature describe the placement of metallic stents in patients with benign colorectal strictures (21,22). Other nonsurgical treatments have been used for the same purpose, including balloon dilatation, endoscopic laser ablation, and decompression tubes (23), with limited effectiveness.

Metallic stent placement has proved to be an effective palliative alternative to surgery in nonresectable colon cancer (24–26) and is an effective method for the nonsurgical decompression of the obstructed left-sided colon, avoiding the need for emergency colostomy (18).

Indications and Contraindications

The placement of metallic stents across obstructive bowel lesions is an effective nonsurgical alternative for reestablishing luminal patency (25,26). The main indications for endoluminal metallic stent placement in the colon and rectum are the following:

1. Temporary decompression in patients presenting with acute bowel obstruction as a "bridge" to an elective, single-stage surgical resection
2. Long-term palliation in patients with an unresectable colon carcinoma
3. Long-term decompression in patients with colonic obstruction caused by extrinsic compression by metastasis from prostate, gynecologic, or other cancer
4. Long-term decompression in patients with benign colonic strictures secondary to postsurgical scarring or postradiation fibrosis
5. Temporary decompression in patients with large bowel obstruction resulting from diverticulitis to allow stabilization of the process and elective surgical resection
6. As temporizing treatment in patients with ileocolic, colovesical, or colocutaneous fistulae (19,20,27–33,15)

The only absolute contraindication for this procedure is clinical (or radiologic) evidence of acute perforation or infection of the colon. Relative contraindications include: long segment colonic tumors, lesions that are too proximal or too distal in the colon, and in patients with a tortuous, elongated colon (23,27,34).

METALLIC STENT TECHNOLOGY

Several commercially available metallic stents have been used for the endoluminal management of colonic obstruction. Most of the current stents in use are made of nitinol or stainless steel. They are self-expandable and cylindrical in shape, with diameters of 20–24 mm and lengths that vary between 40 mm and 100 mm.

The current generation of stents continues to be modified and improved. The ideal device should include the following features:

1. High expansion ratio
2. High flexibility and adaptability
3. Large diameter (25 mm or more)
4. Mechanical stability (no migration)
5. Adequate radial expandable force (dumb-bell shape)
6. Prevention of restenosis resulting from tumor ingrowths
7. Prevention of restenosis resulting from hyperplasia
8. Small and flexible delivery system
9. Biodegradable or readily removable stent for benign strictures
10. Lack of interference during imaging and tumor staging
11. Nonferromagnetic

Stent selection should be based on the location of the tumor (distal or proximal), size of the lesion, method of guidance, and the presence or absence of tortuosity of the colon distal to the lesion. With a few exceptions, the Wallstent enteral endoprosthesis has proved to be adaptable to all of the variables.

The different types of metallic stents include the Ultraflex Stent System (Microvasive-Boston Scientific), the Wallstent Uni Endoprosthesis (Microvasive-Boston Scientific) (Figure 35–1), the Colonic Z Stent (Cook Europe) (Figure 35–2), the Memotherm colorectal stent (Bard Inc), the Wallstent enteral endoprosthesis (Microvasive-Boston Scientific) (Figure 35–3), the Choostent stent (Life Europe), the Colonic stent (TecnoStent), and the EsophaCoil stent (InStent) (35–39).

The most commonly used device is the Wallstent, in any of its variants. This self-expandable stent is made of a nonferromagnetic alloy, and its advantages include the small delivery system, adequate flexibility, and large diameter. The main disadvantage of this stent is the sharp ends of the stent resulting from the presence of free filaments (40). Some authors have used a flexible partially covered stent with polytetrafluroethylene (PTFE) or translucent polyurethane. The principal disadvantage of this design is the high rate of migration (38,41,42).

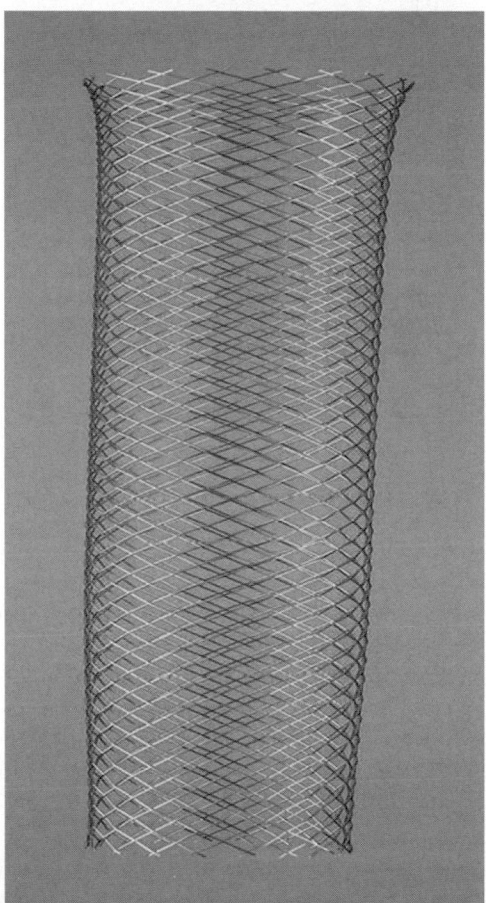

Figure 35–1 Photograph of an enteral Wallstent. This enteral endoprosthesis is a self-expandable metallic stent designed for colonic use and is made of monofilament wire with a diameter of 18–22 mm and is available in lengths of 6 and 9 cm. (Courtesy of Medi-Tech-Boston Scientific).

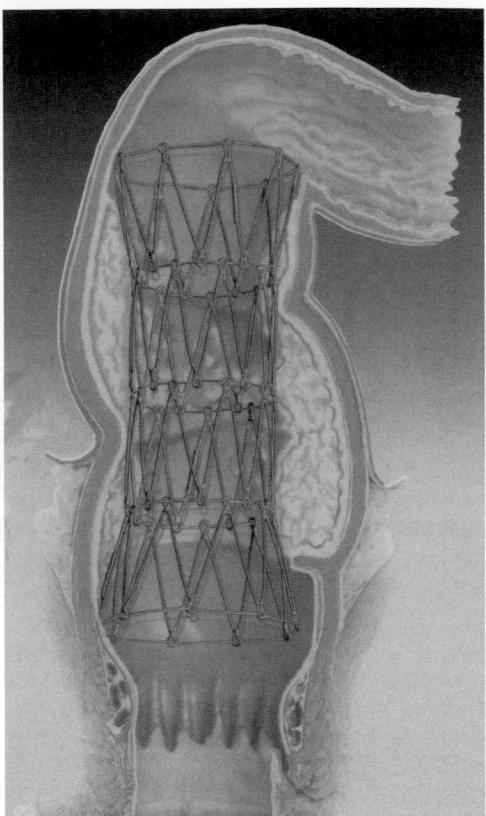

Figure 35–2 Photograph of a colonic Z stent. This colonic endoprosthesis Z stent is a self-expandable metallic stent with a flared end diameter of 35 mm and a shaft diameter of 25 mm. It is available in lengths of 4 and 12 cm. (Courtesy of Cook Europe).

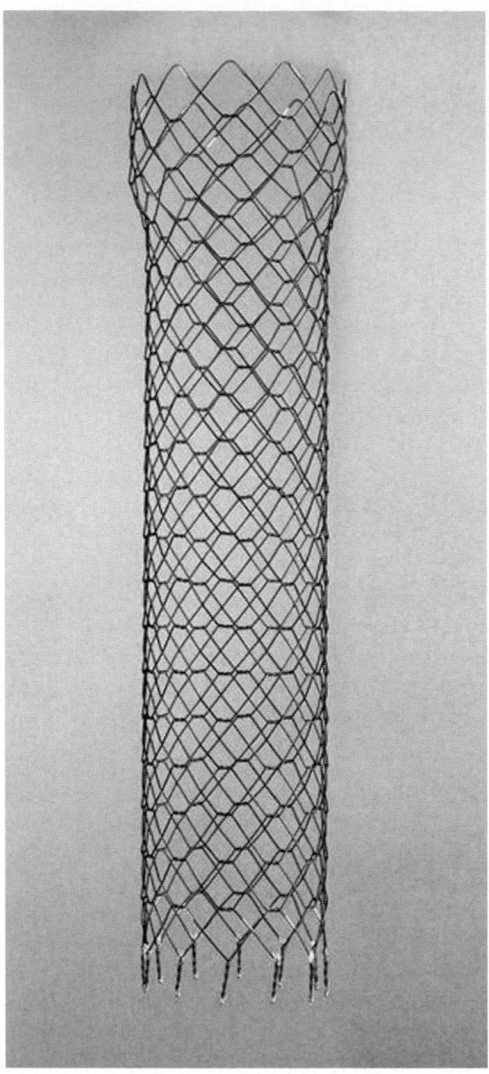

Figure 35–3 Photograph of a Wallstent Precision. This endoprosthesis is a self-expandable metallic stent with a flared end diameter of 30 mm and a shaft diameter of 25 mm. It is available in lengths of 6 and 12 cm. The Precision delivery system is 16 French. (Courtesy of Microvasive-Boston Scientific).

TECHNICAL CONSIDERATIONS

Stent deployment in the colon can be achieved under fluoroscopic and colonoscopic guidance alone or using a combined approach (fluoroscopy and colonoscopy). In the distal sigmoid colon and rectum, deployment can be performed under fluoroscopic or endoscopic guidance alone (23,24,28,43,44). Because of the redundant course of more proximal portions of the colon, especially when associated with a tortuous sigmoid segment, some authors (23,27) prefer the combined use of fluoroscopy and endoscopy for stent placement in the descending colon. Endoscopy is frequently used to cross colonic strictures and place stents, although this is not strictly necessary. Other authors, however, consider fluoroscopy, an absolute requirement for stent placement (20,28,34,35,45).

Distal bowel cleansing may be desirable to facilitate endoscopic stenting, although full cleansing is not always possible. Moreover, oral bowel preparation is contraindicated because of the risk of perforation in an obstructed system.

The procedure does not require general anesthesia. In noncooperative patients—those with high levels of anxiety—or in those in whom colonoscopy is going to be used for stent deployment, sedation with midazolam and analgesia is used.

A water-soluble contrast enema should be performed before stent placement to identify the location, length, and caliber of the obstructing lesion. The enema is also useful for determining the best position to display the lesion in a plane perpendicular to the radiograph (27). In the gastroenterology literature, endoscopy has been reported as being mandatory for the diagnosis and management of intestinal obstructions (43,46). In the fluoroscopy-guided procedure, with the patient in either a supine or lateral decubitus position, a high-torque angiographic catheter or guiding catheter is advanced over a 0.035-inch angled hydrophilic stiff guide wire (Radiofocus, Terumo) that is used to traverse the obstructed segment under fluoroscopic guidance. If an excessively tortuous or redundant rectosigmoid region is encountered, the use of a 0.035-inch Lunderquist extra stiff guide wire (Cook Europe) is recommended to facilitate the progression of the angiographic catheter to the level of the obstruction (18–20,28).

The obstruction is crossed with the help of the catheter/guide wire combination. As soon as the catheter is passed proximal to the obstructed site, water-soluble contrast medium is injected through the catheter to document the characteristics and length of the obstruction and to rule out the possibility of perforation. Radiopaque markers can then be placed on the surface to identify the two ends of the obstructed segment. An appropriately sized stent and delivery system are chosen based on the information obtained from the contrast examination. A 0.038-inch Amplatz super stiff guide wire is introduced through the catheter to a position proximal to the obstructed segment. After the catheter is withdrawn, the delivery system is advanced over the super stiff guide wire and is positioned at the level of the obstructed segment (Figure 35–4). The stent should be long enough not only to cover the entire obstructed segment but also to extend beyond the proximal and distal margins of the lesion by at least 1–2 cm. If stent coverage is inadequate, an additional stent can be deployed to completely cover the lesion and its margins.

Several types of self-expanding metallic stents can be used. Although desirable, particularly in cases of benign strictures, covered stents are not used because they tend to migrate more easily. Choo et al. reported a 50% migration rate with the use of two different types of covered stents in 20 patients (42). The combined use of endoscopy and fluoroscopy can facilitate the catheterization of the distal

segment of the colon in patients with proximal colonic lesions (high descending colon and transverse colon) and in those patients who have marked colonic angulations. In patients with severely angulated colonic segments, there has been successful use of a 10–12 French, 40-cm long introducer sheath (47) in combination with two guide wires and a catheter: a hydrophilic guide wire with a catheter to manipulate across the obstruction and a Lunderquist super stiff guide wire to stiffen the system. The presence of the introducer sheath facilitates the manipulations of the catheter/guide wire combination, by preventing looping of the guide wire in the dilated, tortuous colon. Additional advantages of the introducer sheath include allowing biopsy of the lesion, allowing introduction of contrast medium alongside the catheter/guide wire combination to evaluate the anatomy and to estimate the length of the lesion, and facilitating stent deployment (Figure 35–5).

In palliative cases in which crossing the site of obstruction through a retrograde approach is not possible, the antegrade placement of colonic stents through a cecostomy or colostomy is a feasible alternative (48–50). In two nonsurgical patients, with obstruction in the transverse colon and marked tortuosity of the colon, stents were deployed through a percutaneous colostomy and cecostomy respectively (49) (Figure 35–6).

After stent deployment, additional balloon dilation is not recommended because it is associated with a high risk of perforation. Because of the nature of self-expansion, stents are allowed to slowly expand over time. The peristaltic movements of the colon after decompression may facilitate full expansion.

A water soluble enema examination is performed immediately after stent placement to check for patency and leakage (51,52). A CT performed with oral contrast, a water soluble enema, or both can be done to assess patency and to correct positioning, although this is commonly not needed.

The ends of the stent should not be covered with colonic folds. If this happens, the position of the stent should be adjusted immediately after deployment. Some have suggested a low-residue diet and mineral oil to prevent stent occlusion by impacted fecal material. After the procedure is completed, the patient's vital signs are monitored and serial electrolyte measurements are obtained until they return to normal values. Twenty-four hours after stent placement, a plain radiograph of the abdomen is obtained to evaluate the position of the stent, to check for stent migration or perforation, and to assess changes in the radiographic appearance of the obstruction (Figure 35–7). During patient recovery, staging of the malignancy is undertaken in order to determine resectability and surgical risk. Tumor staging is achieved by computed tomography or ultrasound of the abdomen. If the patient recovers satisfactorily the preoperative assessment can be carried out on an outpatient basis.

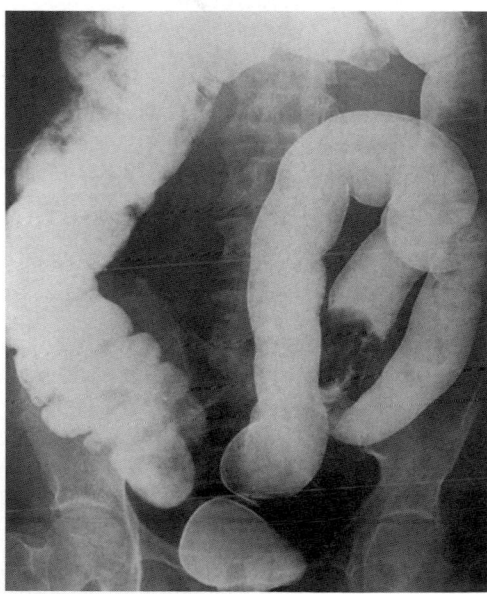

Figure 35–4 A water-soluble contrast enema should be performed before stent placement to identify the location, length, and caliber of the obstructing lesion. The enema is also useful to determine the best position in which to place the patient to display the lesion in a plane perpendicular to the x-ray beam.

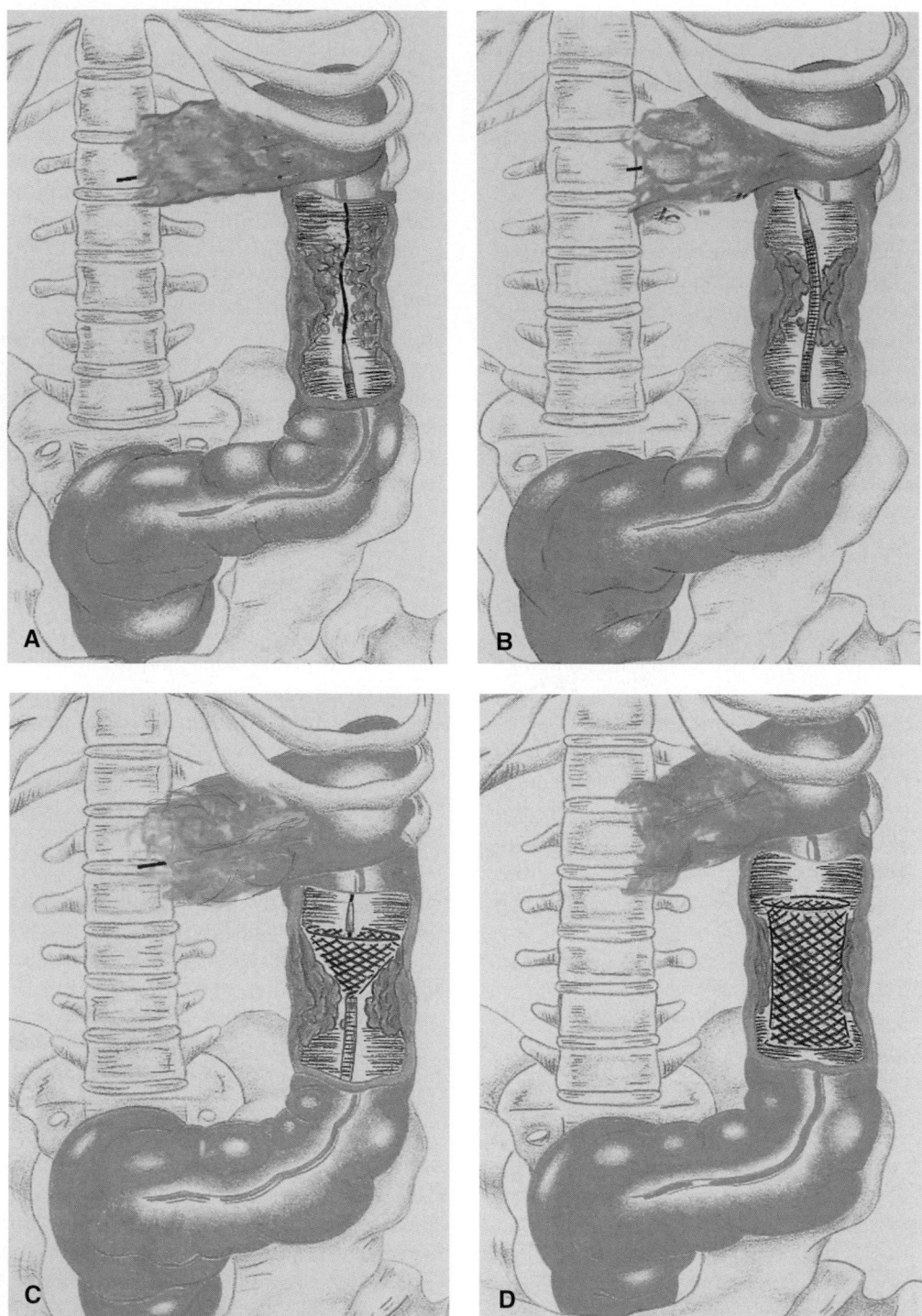

Figure 35–5 Schematic drawings of fluoroscopic placement of a colonic stent showing the stent deployment technique. **A.** Neoplasia within the descending colon. The guide wire has crossed the area of obstruction. **B.** Stent partially deployed in the area of malignant obstruction. The delivery system can be seen. **C.** Stent totally deployed and partially expanded. **D.** Radiographic control with stent totally expanded.

Patients with unresectable disease or who have diffuse metastasis and receive a stent as palliation are instructed after discharge to contact the managing team in the event of clinical deterioration. Periodically, the patient is seen in the clinic to ensure stability. Follow-up radiography should be undertaken when the patient develops obstructive symptoms or peritoneal signs. During physical examinations (digital rectal examination, for example) and at surgery in patients who are candidates for resection, special consideration should be given to the presence of

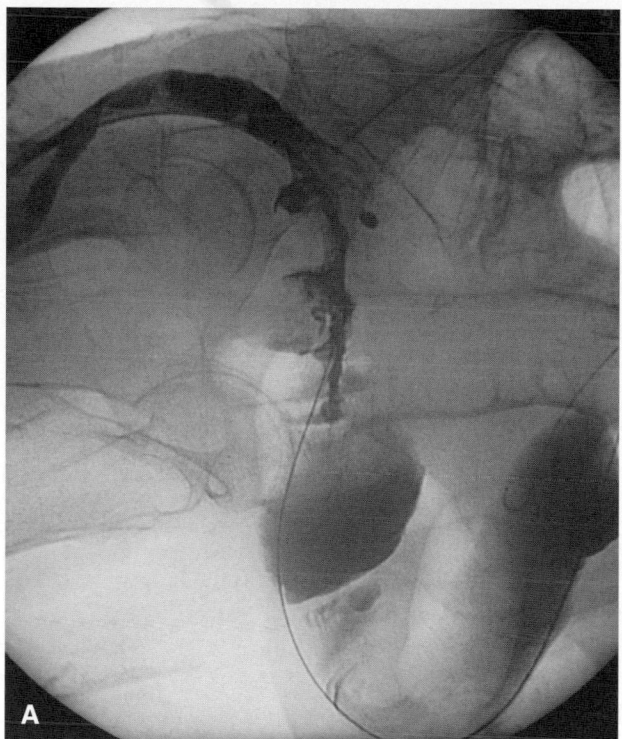

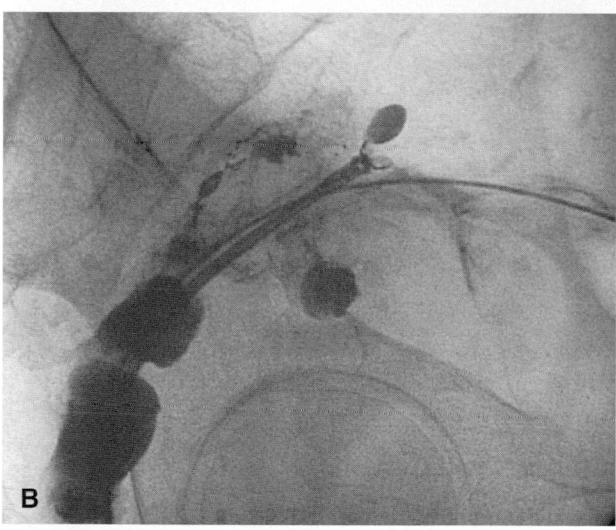

Figure 35-6   Utilization of a 10 French introducer sheath to facilitate the technique. **A.** Introduction of contrast through the sheath to determine the morphology and extension of the lesion keeping a guide wire distal to it. **B.** Obtaining a biopsy sample with forceps through the sheath and guide wire distal to the lesion for safety purposes.

a metallic stent to avoid injury to the examining physician (40).

Fluoroscopic Guidance Versus Endoscopic Guidance

The placement of colorectal stents has been carried out with endoscopic guidance, fluoroscopy guidance, or a combined technique. Both methods have advantages and disadvantages. Stent placement in the proximal colonic segment benefits from the combined endoscopic/fluoroscopic assistance (Figure 35-8), whereas fluoroscopic guidance is adequate for lesions in the distal descending colon, sigmoid, and rectum and is associated with tolerable radiation doses (27,53,54). With both techniques, the effectiveness and the technical success rate are similar in experienced hands. According to Binkert et al., endoscopic assistance reduces radiation dose but increases the cost and requires sedation in all patients (53).

To compare both methods of guidance—November 1999 to December 2002— De Gregorio et al. carried out a prospective, nonrandomized study analyzing the feasibility of the procedure and the technical success of stent implantation, procedure time, and radiation dose using fluoroscopy alone and fluoroscopy assisted by endoscopy (55). The interventional radiologist without previous formal training used the endoscope. A total of 25 stents were implanted in 26 patients; 13 in each group (15 men and 11 women). There was a technical failure using the combined technique in one patient with stenosis at the rectosigmoid level. The mean age was 58.7 (range 42–82 years), and the lesions were located as follows: two in the rectum, 16 in the sigmoid colon, six in the proximal descending colon, and two in the proximal transverse colon.

The mean distance from the anus to the lesion was 23.69 cm (a range of 11–35 cm) for the fluoroscopy group and of 30.8 cm (a range of 10–63 cm) in the combined technique group. The mean fluoroscopy time and radiation dose for the procedure were 19.76 minutes (a range of 12–45 minutes) and 2,763.6 dGy/cm^2 (a range of 1,026–6,789 dGy/cm^2) for the fluoroscopy group and 15.0 minutes (a range of 15–35 minutes) and 2,250 dGy/cm^2 (a range of 1,362–4,523 dGy/cm^2) for the combined technique group.

RESULTS

Technical success in deploying the stents with fluoroscopic, endoscopic, or combined guidance is obtained in 88–100 % of patients (27). Stent insertion permits rapid symptomatic resolution of the obstruction, providing time to stabilize the patient and to stage the disease. (2,18–27). Clinical success (improvement of obstructive symptoms) has been reported in 80–92% of patients (27,35,45,46). In a systematic review of the published data (1990–2000) by Khot et al. (56) totaling 598 patients with colonic stents, the technical success was 92%, and the clinical success was 88%. Palliation was achieved in 302 of 336 cases (90%). In 223 of 262 (85%) surgical candidates, the stent was an effective "bridge" to surgery. There were three deaths (1%). Perforation occurred in 22 patients (4%). Stent migration was reported in 54 (10%) of 551 technically successful cases. The rate of stent re-obstruction was 10% (52 of 525) with re-obstruction occurring, mainly in the palliative group. In the same study,

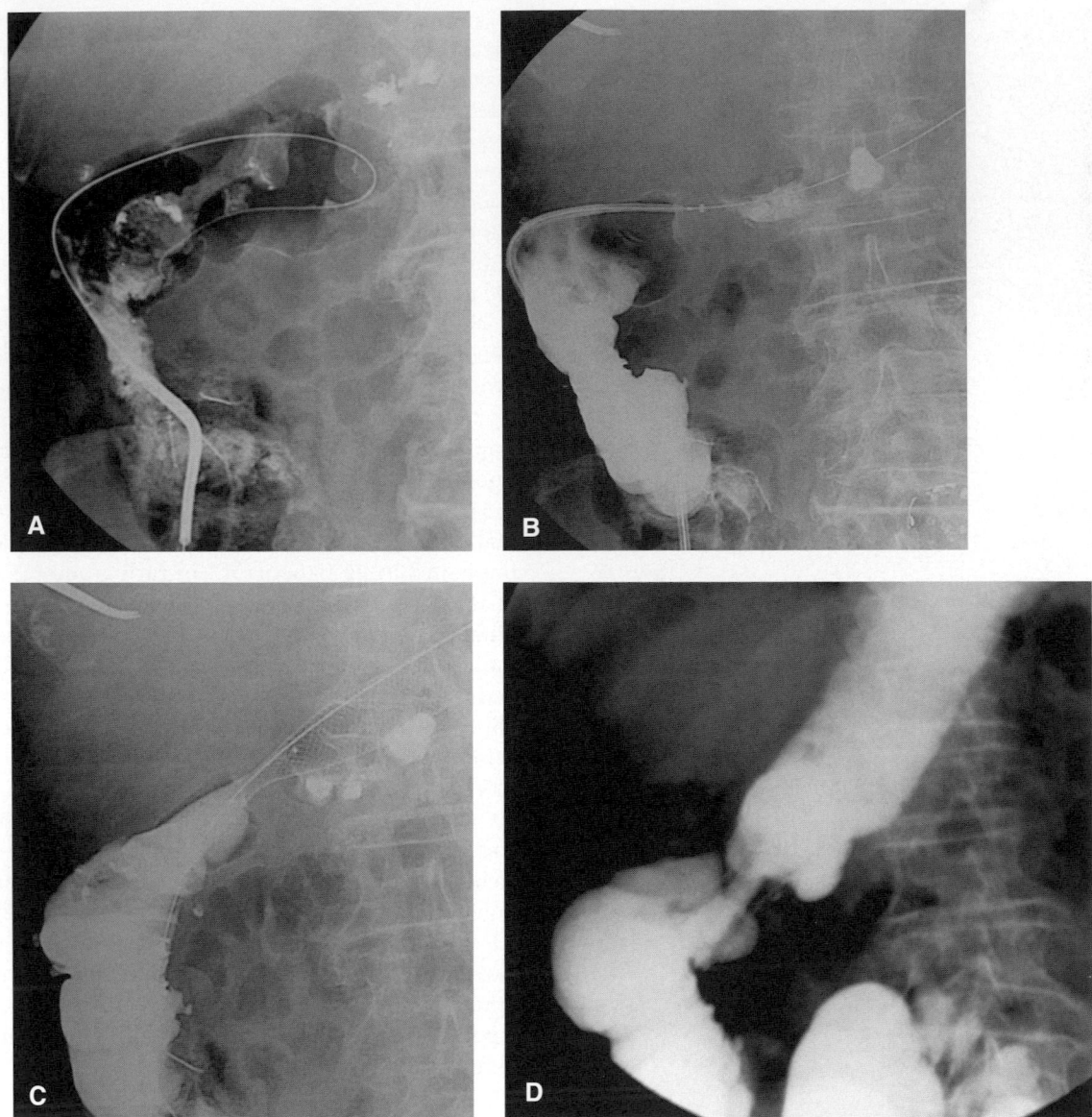

Figure 35–7 Antegrade approach for the deployment of a colonic stent. **A.** Guide wire in the area of malignant obstruction with access through a percutaneous cecostomy. **B.** Guide wire crossing the area of malignant obstruction. **C.** Delivery system introduction carrying the stent through a 10 French sheath placed in the cecostomy. Stent fully open. **D.** Water enema control 3 months after stent placement.

technical failure was reported in 47 of 598 (8%) patients. The main causes included inability to cross the stenosis with a guide wire in 36 patients, inadequate positioning in four patients, and perforation in two patients.

Beltran (57) compared two groups of patients with carcinoma of the left colon. One hundred patients were included in this study, equally distributed between both groups. Group A included patients with tumors on the left colon, obstructive symptoms, and a colonic stent implanted before surgery. Patients in Group B had left-sided colon malignancy but no obstruction, and they underwent elective surgical intervention. In this study, no significant differences were observed between either group in terms of morbidity (50.5% versus 45%), mortality (3.5%

versus 2.8%), recurrence (3.5% versus 8.4%), and survival at 3 years (76% versus 66%).

Saida et al. (58) retrospectively evaluated the long-term prognosis of expandable metallic stent insertion compared with emergency surgery without stent in 84 patients. Forty of the patients underwent emergency operations, and 44 had stent insertion followed by elective surgery. The postoperative complications were significantly less common in the stent group, and there was no significant difference in the long-term prognosis (5 years was 44% versus 40%).

Martinez et al., in a study of 72 patients, compared the use of self-expandable stents before elective surgery (study group) and conventional emergency surgery (control

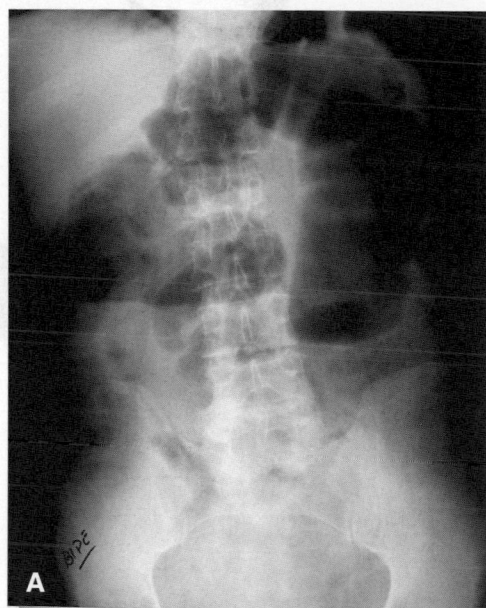

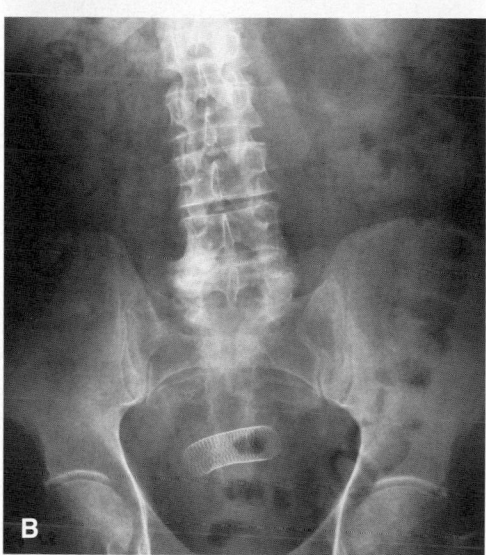

Figure 35–8   A. Single view of the abdomen showing significant abdominal distention with dilatation of the colon proximal to the site of obstruction. **B.** Radiographic control 24 hours postimplantation of the stent. Resolution of the obstructive pattern.

group) for the treatment of malignant left-sided colorectal obstructions. They concluded that placement of colonic stents prevented 94% of unnecessary surgical interventions and 84.6% of colostomies. Total hospitalization stay, intensive care unit stay and complications were significantly lower in the study group than in the control group (59).

Stent insertion carried out by an experienced team of interventional radiologist and endoscopist averages 60–75 minutes (28,53). The stent insertion failed to achieve adequate decompression in 10% of patients. This failure has been attributed to difficulty in crossing the stenosis, incorrect

positioning of the stent, blockage by stool or barium, mucosal prolapse, and the presence of an additional proximal synchronous tumor (2,52,53). It has been pointed out by some (2,60) that distal lesions are more common and theoretically easier to stent than lesions in the proximal colon.

Ahmad and Mee (2) reported that inflammatory changes and possible infection in the colon around the implanted stent could prove difficult and could complicate the surgery. In one institution, 259 consecutive patients with large intestinal obstruction from colon carcinoma were treated from January 1994 to December 2002. Barium enema located the lesions in the sigmoid colon (121 patients), descending colon (66 patients), rectosigmoid junction (43 patients), splenic angle (17), and transverse colon (12 patients). Patient selection criteria for transanal stent insertion included malignant obstruction in the left hemicolon. The stent used most often was the Wallstent (Boston Scientific) measuring 22 mm in diameter and with lengths 66–100 mm. The criteria for successful stent placement were relief of colonic obstruction, allowing preoperative bowel preparation, and successful palliation for those patients not eligible for surgery.

Colonic obstruction resolved in 234 (90.3%) patients. Bowel movements occurred within the first 24 hours in 210 (89.7%) patients and after 24 hours in 24 (10.2%) patients. Bowel preparation was followed by colonic resection and primary anastomosis in 166 (70.9%) patients. Palliative decompression was achieved in 68 (29.5%) patients who attained a mean survival of 8.2 months (range 0.4–17 months) after stent insertion. Colostomy was performed in 25 (9.6%) patients in whom colonic obstruction persisted because of an inability to place the stent (20 patients) and in five patients despite stent placement.

COMPLICATIONS

Minor complications of stent placement, including mild to moderate rectal bleeding, transient anorectal pain, temporary incontinence, and fecal impaction are common in many reports (60). A review of the literature showed complication rates varying from 0% to 30% (24,46). More severe life threatening complications also have been described, including procedure related deaths. In a review by Khot et al., three of 598 (1%) patients died from colon perforation and unsuccessful decompression (30). Perforation occurred in 22 of 598 (3.6%) patients. There was a higher incidence of perforation in the pre-stent balloon dilatation group (10%). Stent migration occurred in 54 of 551 patients (9.8%). Stent migration usually occurred after an average of 3 days. Obstruction after successful initial stent decompression occurred in 52 of 525 patients (9.9%). This phenomenon was related to tumor ingrowths in 32 patients, stent migration in seven patients, and fecal impaction in 13 patients.

Mild to moderate low gastrointestinal bleeding occurred in 24 patients and major bleeding in three patients (4.5% total). Minor abdominal or rectal pain was described in 31 of 598 patients (5.1%).

In a long-term study by Saida et al., (58) comparing surgery without preoperative stenting versus surgery following stent decompression (bridge to surgery) for the treatment of obstructive colorectal cancer, the postoperative complications were significantly less common in the stent group: wound infection was 14% versus 2% and anastomotic leakage was 11% versus 3%.

Colonic perforation, stent migration, and stent occlusion are the main complications encountered with stent placement. Perforation has been reported in 0–16% of cases (25,26). Scurtu et al. (61) reported a higher incidence of colonic perforations after the deployment of self-expandable stents with endoscopic guidance (83%). Stent migration has been reported to occur in up to 40 % of cases (27). Stent migration is more common following the use of small diameter stents, short stents, deployment of stents in minimally stenotic colonic lesions, and covered stents.

Restenosis has been reported in up to 25% of cases and is usually the result of tumor ingrowths through the open interstices of the stent (36–42) (Figure 35–9). Other complications described are related to specific stent design, including stent fracture followed by obstruction and colonic perforation (62) (Figure 35–10). Complications have occurred in 46 of 259 patients (17.7%), and they included self-limiting rectal bleeding in 13 patients (5%), stent migration in 15 patients (5.7%), stent defecation in four patients (1.5%), symptomatic colonic perforation in five patients (1.9%), and restenosis resulting from tumor ingrowths on nine patients (3.4%).

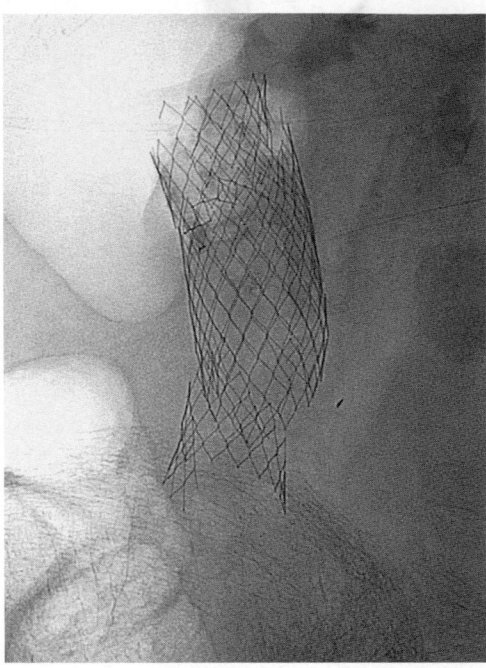

Figure 35–10 Rupture of a stent. A 76-year-old patient diagnosed and treated for colon carcinoma 7 years prior. Placement of stent across a left colon lesion. Stent was implanted without complications (Memotherm 25 x 80 mm). Thirty months after the procedure, the patient presented with new intestinal obstruction. Abdominal exam shows rupture of the stent. A new stent was implanted without incident (Wallstent 24 x 70 mm). (Images provided by Dr. J. Urbano).

COST EFFECTIVENESS

Although stents are an added cost, the procedure is cost-effective, because a two-stage emergency surgery (colostomy and resection) can be avoided in patients presenting with acute bowel obstruction. Furthermore, surgery is prevented in those with advanced disease (63). Sufficient justifications for the added cost of the stent (53) include the fact that the shorter the hospitalization, fewer surgical procedures will be needed, and a decrease in time spent in the intensive care unit will result. Osman et al. estimated that the cost of palliative treatment with colon stenting was less than half that of surgical decompression, £1,445 versus £3,205 respectively (64). Osman also estimated an overall reduction in total expenditures of 12% in the preoperative stenting group versus those who have a two-stage surgical procedure, £5,035 versus £5,720 respectively.

Binkert et al. carried out a retrospective study comparing the total cost in two groups of patients: one group treated with preoperative stents (12 patients) versus a second group treated by surgical alone (11 patients) (53). They reported savings of up to 20% for the first group. The decrease in cost was attributed mainly to the shorter hospital stay. It is necessary to remark that besides the psychological benefit to the patient provided by avoiding the need for a colostomy, there is an added economic benefit because these patients can be integrated more rapidly into the work force (65,66).

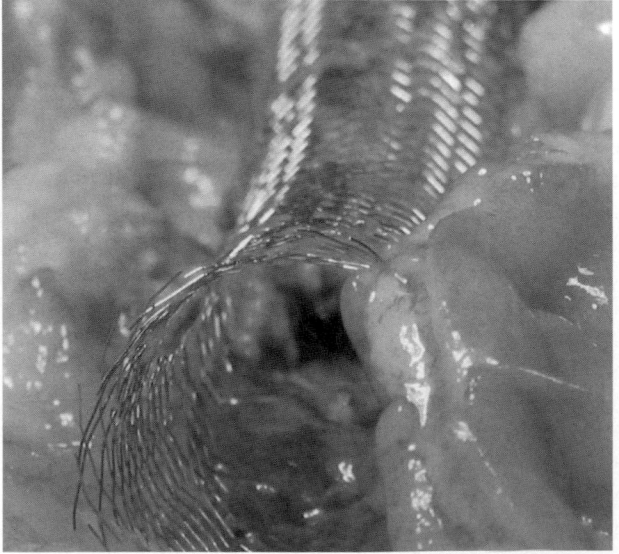

Figure 35–9 Surgical specimen from colectomy performed 7 days after stent implantation. Minimal tumoral growth through the stent with narrowing of the lumen is noted. The patient remained asymptomatic during the time the stent was in place.

RADIATION DOSE

The radiation exposure to the patient and to the operator when the procedure is carried out under fluoroscopic guidance is a very important issue. One group measured the duration of the procedure and fluoroscopy time and estimated the total radiation dose (dGy/cm^2) in 12 patients. The average procedure time was 57.3 minutes, and fluoroscopy time was 20.9 minutes. Mean total dose was 3,593 dGy/cm^2 (67). It has been reported that the transanal placement of metallic stents performed in a combined fashion with endoscopic assistance may decrease fluoroscopy time (68).

PROCEDURE LIMITATIONS

Stents should not be inserted across distal rectal tumors because they can cause severe tenesmus or fecal incontinence (69). Although studies with large series of patients exist, there are no randomized prospective studies comparing preoperative stents with standard surgical treatment in patients with potentially resectable primary colorectal carcinoma and obstruction (70). There are a few studies comparing the effectiveness, complications, and cost benefit of the treatment of obstructive colorectal cancer using the traditional surgical treatment versus surgery preceded by placement of a decompressing stent, and none of these studies is randomized (58,59,69).

SUMMARY

There is agreement that management of the obstructed colon by means of stent placement is a safe and effective technique before definitive surgical treatment of the tumor. Colonic stent placement is also useful as a palliative treatment for the patient with obstructive carcinoma of the left colon who is not a surgical candidate or who are unresectable (71). Currently, the Wallstent enteral constitutes the device of choice for the treatment of malignant colonic obstruction. This assertion is supported by the published results and the low incidence of complications. It is necessary, however, to continue research and development efforts to improve the current devices. Goals of the new developments should include prevention of tumor ingrowths, migration, and better profile. These should also include more flexible delivery systems for improving technical success and for decreasing the complexity of the procedure. Finally, there is a need for prospective randomized studies to confirm the results from published series.

REFERENCES

1. Boyle P, Leon M. Epidemiology of colorectal cancer. Br Med Bull 2002;64:1–25.
2. Ahmad T, Mee AS. Expandable metal stents in malignant colorectal obstruction. Br Med J 2000;321:584–585.
3. Dean GT, Krukowski Z, Irwin S. Malignant obstruction of the left colon. Br J Surg 1994;81:1270–1276.
4. Boyle P. Some recent developments in the epidemiology of colorectal cancer. In: Bleiberg H, Rougier P, Wilke HJ, eds. Management of Colorectal Cancer. St. Louis: Mosby 1998:19–34.
5. Duxbury M, Brodribb A, Oppong F, et al. Management of colorectal cancer: variations in practice in one hospital. Eur J Surg Oncol 2003;29:400–402.
6. Law W, Chu KW, Ho J, et al. Self-expandable metallic stent in the treatment of colonic obstruction caused by advanced malignancies. Dis Colon Rectum 2000;43:1522–1527.
7. Griffith R. Prospective medical obstacles to surgery. Cancer 1992;70:1333–1341.
8. Smothers L, Hynan L, Fleming J, et al. Emergency surgery for colon carcinoma. Dis Colon Rectum 2003;46:24–30.
9. Witzig J, Morel P, Erne M, et al. [Surgery of digestive system cancers in patients over 80 years of age]. Helv Chir Acta 1993;59:767–769.
10. Ohman U. Prognosis in patients with obstructing colorectal carcinoma. Am J Surg 1982;143:742–747.
11. Brillari P, Aurello P, de Angelis R, et al. Management and survival of patients affected with obstructive colorectal cancer. Int Surg 1992;7:251–255.
12. Nugent K, Daniels P, Stewart B, et al. Quality of life in stoma patients. Dis Colon Rectum 1999;42:1569–1574.
13. Mergener K, Kozarek R. Stenting of the gastrointestinal tract. Dig Dis Sci 2002;20:173–181.
14. Dohmoto M, Rupp K, Hohlbach G. [Endoscopically implanted prosthesis in rectal carcinoma]. Dtsch Med Wochenschr 1990;115:915.
15. Cwikiel W, Andren-Sandberg A. Malignant stricture with colovesical fistula: stent insertion in the colon. Radiology 1993;186:363–364.
16. Keen R, Orsay CP. Rectosigmoid stent for obstructing colonic neoplasms. Dis Colon Rectum 1992;35:912–913.
17. Itabashi M, Humano K, Kameoka S, et al. Self-expanding stainless steel stent application in rectosigmoid stricture. Dis Colon Rectum 1993;36:508–511.
18. Tejero E, Mainar A, Fernandez L, et al. New procedure for the treatment of colorectal neoplastic obstructions. Dis Colon Rectum 1994;37:1158–1159.
19. De Gregorio MA, Mainar A, Tejero E, et al. Acute colorectal obstruction: stent placement for palliative treatment: results of a multicenter study. Radiology 1998;209:117–120.
20. Paul L, Pinto I, Fernandez R, et al. Palliative treatment of malignant colorectal strictures with metallic stents. Cardiovasc Intervent Radiol 1999;22:29–36.
21. Lo SK. Metallic stenting for colorectal obstruction. Gastrointest Endosc Clin N Am. 1999;9:459–478.
22. Seo TS, Song HY, Sung KB, et al. Benign colorectal stricture: treatment with a retrievable expandable nitinol stent. Cardiovasc Intervent Radiol 2003;26:181–183.
23. Zollikofer C, Jost R, Schonh E, et al. Gastrointestinal stenting. Eur Radiol 2000;10:1158–1159.
24. Aviv RI, Shyamalan G, Watkinson A, et al. Radiological palliation of malignant colonic obstruction. Clin Radiol 2002;57:347–351.
25. Rey J, Romanczyk T, Greef M. Metal stents for palliation of rectal carcinoma: a preliminary report of 12 patients. Endoscopy 1995;27:501–504.
26. Spinelli P, Dal Fante M, Manchini A. Rectal metal stents for palliation of colorectal malignant stenosis. Bilgebung 1993;60(Suppl) 1:48–50.
27. Mauro M, Koehler R, Baron T. Advances in gastrointestinal intervention: the treatment of gastroduodenal and colorectal obstructions with metallic stents. Radiology 2000;215:659–669.
28. Mainar A, Tejero E, Maynar M, et al. Colorectal obstruction: treatment with metallic stents. Radiology 1996;198:761–764.
29. Law W, Choi H, Chu K, et al. Radiation stricture of rectosigmoid treated with self-expanding metallic stent. Surg Endosc 2002;16:1106–1107.
30. Miyayama S, Matsui O, Kifune K, et al. Malignant colonic obstruction due to extrinsic tumor: palliative treatment with a self-expanding nitinol stents. AJR Am J Roentgenol 2000;175:1631–1637.
31. Dormann J, Deppe H, Wigginghaus B. Self-expanding metallic stents for continuous dilatation of benign stenoses in gastrointestinal

tract—first results of long-term follow-up in interim stent application in pyloric and colonic obstruction. Z Gastroenterol 2001;39:957–960.

32. Friedland S, Hallenbeck J, Soetikno R. Stenting the sigmoid colon in a terminally ill patient with prostate cancer. J Palliat Med 2001;4:153–156.

33. Carter J, Valmadre S, Dalrymple C, et al. Management of large bowel obstruction in advanced ovarian cancer with intraluminal stents. Gynecol Oncol 2002;84:176–179.

34. De Gregorio MA, Mainar A, D'Agostino H, et al. Transanal metallic stents for malignant colonic obstructions in 126 patients. J Vasc Interv Radiol 1999;10(Suppl):219.

35. Mainar A, De Gregorio MA, Tejero E, et al. Acute colorectal obstruction: treatment with self-expandable metallic stents before scheduled surgery—results of a multicenter study. Radiology 1999;210:65–69.

36. Mischima R, Sawada S, Tanigawa N, et al. Expandable metallic stent treatment for malignant colorectal strictures. Cardiovasc Intervent Radiol 1999;22:155–158.

37. Akle CA. Endoprostheses for colonic strictures. Br J Surg 1998;85: 310–314.

38. Song HY. Malignant gastric outlet obstruction: treatment by means of coaxial placement of uncovered and covered expandable nitinol stents. J Vasc Interv Radiol 2002;13:275–283.

39. Canon CL, Baron TH, Morgan DE, et al. Treatment of colonic obstruction with expandable metal stents: radiologic features. AJR Am J Roentgenol 1997;168:199–205.

40. Lopera J, Ferral H, Wholey M, et al. Treatment of colonic obstruction with metallic stent: indications, technique, and complications. AJR Am J Roentgenol 1997;169:1285–1290.

41. A damsen S, Holm J, Meisner S, et al. [Endoscopic treatment of colorectal obstruction with self-expandable metal endoprosthesis]. Ugeskr Laeger 2000;162:1560–1563.

42. Choo I, Do Y, Suh S, et al. Malignant colorectal obstruction: treatment with a flexible covered stent. Radiology 1998;206:415–421.

43. Dite P, Lata J, Novotny I. Intestinal obstruction and perforation: the role of the gastroenterologist. Dig Dis 2003;21:63–67.

44. Keymling M. Colorectal stenting. Endoscopy 2003;35:234–238.

45. Camuñez F, Echenagusia A, Simo G, et al. Malignant colorectal obstruction treated by means of self-expanding metallic stents: effectiveness before surgery and in palliation. Radiology 2000;216: 492–497.

46. Ely C, Arregui M. The use of enteral stents in colonic and gastric outlet obstruction. Surg Endosc 2003;17:89–94.

47. De Gregorio MA, Mainar A, Tejero E, et al. Use of an introducer sheath for colonic stent placement. Eur Radiol 2002;12:2250–2252.

48. Velling TE, Hall L, Brennan F. Colonic stent placement facilitated by percutaneous cecostomy and antegrade enema. AJR Am J Roentgenol 2000;175:119–120.

49. Gimeno MJ, Alfonso ER, Herrera M, et al. Palliative treatment of malignant stenoses of transverse colon by autoexpandable metallic stent through percutaneous cecostomy or colostomy. Cardiovasc Intervent Radiol 2002;25(Suppl):208.

50. Gomez H, Paul I, Pinto I, et al. Placement of a colonic stent by percutaneous colostomy in a case of malignant stenosis. Cardiovasc Intervent Radiol 2001;24:67–69.

51. Saida Y, Sumiyama Y, Nagao J, et al. Stent endoprosthesis for obstructing colorectal cancers. Dis Colon Rectum 1996;39:552–555.

52. Baron T, Dean P, Yates M, et al. Expandable metal stents for the treatment of colonic obstruction: techniques and outcomes: Gastrointest Endosc 1998;47:227–286.

53. Binkert C, Lederman H, Jost R, et al. Acute colonic obstruction: clinical aspects and cost effectiveness of preoperative and palliative treatment with self-expanding metallic stents. A preliminary report. Radiology 1998;206:199–204.

54. Ben Soussan E, Savoye G, Hochain P, et al. Expandable metal stent in palliative treatment of malignant colorectal stricture: a report of 17 consecutive patients. Gastroenterol Clin Biol 2001; 25:463–467.

55. De Gregorio MA, D'Agostino H, Gimeno MJ, et al. Transanal colonic stent implantation under fluoroscopy alone and under fluoroscopy and endoscopy. A comparative study. Intervencionismo 2003;5:103–111.

56. Khot U, Lang A, Murali K, et al. Systematic review of the efficacy and safety of colorectal stents. Br J Surg 2002;89:1096–1102.

57. Beltran JM. Left obstructive colonic carcinoma. Comparative study of short and middle term results after a new therapeutic procedure based in self-expanding metallic stents placement [doctoral thesis]. Universidad de Zaragoza, Spain. June 2003.

58. Saida Y, Sumiyama Y, Nagao J, et al. Long-term prognosis of preoperative "bridge to surgery" expandable metallic stent insertion for obstructive colorectal cancer: comparison with emergency operation. Dis Colon Rectum 2003;46:44–49.

59. Martinez-Santos C, Lobato R, Fradejas JM, et al. Self-expandable stent before elective surgery vs. emergency surgery for the treatment of malignant colorectal obstructions: comparison of primary anastomosis and morbidity rates. Dis Colon Rectum 2002;45:401–406.

60. Harris G, Senagore A, Lavery I, et al. The management of neoplastic colorectal obstruction with colonic endoluminal stenting devices. Am J Surg 2001;181:499–506.

61. Scurtu R, Barrier A, Andre T, et al. [Self-expandable metallic stent for palliative treatment of colorectal malignant obstructions: risk of perforation]. Ann Chir 2003;128:359–363.

62. Odurny A. Colonic anastomotic stenoses and Memotherm stent fracture: a report of three cases. Cardiovasc Intervent Radiol 2001; 24:336–339.

63. Targownik LE, Spiegel BM, Sack J, et al. Colonic stent vs. emergency surgery for management of acute left-sided malignant colonic obstruction: a decision analysis. Gastrointest Endosc 2004;60:865–874.

64. Osman H, Rashid H, Sathananthan N, et al. The cost effectiveness of self-expanding metal stents in the management of malignant left sided bowel obstruction. Colorectal Dis 2000;2:233–237.

65. Sprangers M, Taal B, Aaronson N, et al. Quality of life in colorectal cancer. Dis Colon Rectum 1995;38:361–369.

66. Londono-Schimmer E, Leong A, Philips R. Life table analysis of stoma complications following colostomy. Dis Colon Rectum 1994;37:916–920.

67. De Gregorio MA, Mainar A, Gimeno MJ, et al. Radiation exposure during metallic stent placement for the treatment of malignant colonic obstruction: experience with 12 patients. Cardiovas Intervent Radiol 2001;24:S189.

68. Gimeno MJ, Medrano J, Alfonso ER, et al. Utility of fluoroscopy combined with endoscopy in the treatment of malignant colorectal stenosis with metallic stents. Cardiovasc Intervent Radiol 2002;25:S203.

69. Turegano-Fuentes F, Echenagusia-Belda A, Simo-Muerza A, et al. Transanal self-expanding metal stents as an alternative to palliative colostomy in selected patients with malignant obstruction of the left colon. Br J Surg 1998;85: 232–235.

70. Baron T. Expandable metal stents for the treatment of cancerous obstruction of the gastrointestinal tract. N Engl J Med 2001; 3441:681–1687.

71. Maynar M, Qian Z. Current status of the expandable metallic stent for the treatment of colorectal obstruction. Cardiovasc Intervent Radiol 2001;21(Suppl):114–116.

Percutaneous Management of Biliary Calculi

36

Aalpen A. Patel, S. William Stavropoulos, Constantin Cope

Although it is estimated that more than 20 million people in the United States have gallstones and that 1–2% of new cases develop each year, the majority of cases are asymptomatic. The prevalence of stones is influenced by race, sex, age, and a diversity of ethnic and cultural backgrounds (1).

The most common symptom of cholelithiasis is biliary colic (2). The syndrome of biliary colic is caused by intermittent obstruction of the cystic duct by one or more gallstones. Inflammation of the gallbladder is not required with the obstruction. With biliary colic, the pain is visceral in origin and, therefore, poorly localized (3). Typically, the patient experiences episodes of epigastric or right upper quadrant pain (4). The pain may last from 15 minutes to 2–3 hours. Bloating, dyspepsia, and nausea are not specific for making the diagnosis (5). Mild symptoms ascribed to gallstones are believed to occur in 1–2% of this population over a 20-year period, but significant disease requiring intervention is estimated to occur in only 1% over 20 years (6). Because the complications and morbidity of gallstones in the asymptomatic population are minimal, treatment is based on the presentation of severe gallbladder colic or on the complications of cholelithiasis, such as cholecystitis, pancreatitis, occlusion, or stricture of bile ducts. In the past 2 decades, alternatives to traditional cholecystectomy have been introduced, including oral and contact litholysis, extracorporeal shock wave lithotripsy (ESWL), and percutaneous cholecystolithotomy, in an effort to provide procedures that

are safer and better tolerated than surgery, especially in older, more fragile patients and those with limited life expectancy. Laparoscopic cholecystectomy has nearly replaced open cholecystectomy and has supplanted the need for percutaneous procedures in otherwise healthy ambulatory patients.

Retained stones within the bile ducts can be managed safely by extraction through a postcholecystectomy T-tube tract, by percutaneous transhepatic catheterization, by endoscopic retrograde cholangiopancreatographic techniques, or by a combination of these techniques with ESWL or litholysis. Gallstones can be divided into two major types on the basis of their composition: (1) cholesterol stones (80% of all stones) that contain more than 50% cholesterol monohydrate, with calcium salts and mucin accounting for the balance; and (2) pigment stones that contain primarily calcium bilirubinate, smaller amounts of other calcium salts, and some cholesterol. Pigment stones may be classified into *black* stones, which are often found in association with hemolysis, cirrhosis, and old age, and softer, more fatty *brown* stones, which are found primarily in bile ducts and associated with strictures, bile stasis, and infection.

Ten to fifteen percent of gallstones are radiopaque on plain film. In the study of 110 patients by Trotman et al. (7), two-thirds of the grossly calcified stones were pigment, and the rest were cholesterol. Conversely, 15% of radiolucent stones are made of pigment. Large, densely calcified stones tend to be very hard and difficult to break up with stone baskets and even, at times, with lithotripters (8). Because stones can form over the long term around retained sutures, metal clips, and catheter fragments or prosthetic stents, it is important to remove all such foreign bodies from the biliary system when possible.

PATIENT PREPARATION

All patients with symptomatic stone disease should have their coagulation, basic liver, pancreatic, and kidney function profiles tested. Those scheduled for transhepatic or transcholecystic stone extraction should be hospitalized. Postcholecystectomy patients with T tubes and retained stones may be scheduled for extraction through the mature sinus track as outpatients or in short-stay units. A broad-spectrum antibiotic is administered intravenously usually within 2–4 hours of the procedure. If the patient is considered to be an unusually high risk for sepsis because of old age, debility, or previous instrumentation, a second antibiotic (such as an aminoglycocide) may be added for synergy. Most percutaneous stone extraction procedures can be performed comfortably under conscious sedation. However, this requires that the patient avoid oral intake for the previous 6 hours. If it is anticipated that the procedure will be unusually painful (as in dilatation of biliary strictures) or will be prolonged (as in extraction of multiple large stones), epidural anesthesia may be useful. In the hands of an experienced anesthesiologist, epidural anesthesia is well-tolerated in patients with coexisting severe cardiac or pulmonary disease (9).

PERCUTANEOUS MANAGEMENT OF BILE DUCT STONES

The earliest attempts to manage calculi through a postoperative T-tube tract were either too hazardous (using ether or chloroform to dissolve cholesterol stones) or too unpredictable (using plain or heparinized saline irrigation). Large red rubber drains were also used to dilate the sphincter and allow the passage of small calculi. The first consistently successful stone extraction technique was introduced by Mazzariello (10), who used specially designed, low-profile, curved forceps inserted through the predilated T-tube tract to break up and retrieve ductal stones. However, this traumatic procedure was replaced by more efficacious and less painful basket retrieval techniques.

Many useful techniques are now available to retrieve stones from the biliary tree. Some of the common methods are described below. Most of these techniques have common features. Percutaneous access to the biliary tree can be established through a T-tube tract or through a transhepatic or transjejunal approach. Once access is obtained, the ducts may be evaluated with cholangiogram, direct cholangioscopy, or both for presence of stones. Once discovered, the stones may be retrieved or advanced into the gastrointestinal tract. When stones are too big, several methods may be used to perform lithotripsy. A more detail discussion of these methods follows.

Stone Extraction Through a T-Tube Tract

Ten to fifteen percent of patients in the United States who are undergoing cholecystectomy for cholecystolithiasis have coexisting, common duct stones (11). Most of these stones have originated from the gallbladder by passing through the cystic duct as small calculi. Larger common duct stones can be diagnosed by ultrasound imaging and may be removed by retrograde endoscopy before or after surgery. However, small stones can pass into the bile ducts during surgery and may be missed by intraoperative cholangiography. This is especially true when the stones have migrated into the intrahepatic ducts or when the ducts have become partially filled with air or blood clots. If retained stones are not identified on the postoperative T-tube cholangiogram, the patient may present later with biliary obstruction.

When retained stones are identified on a postoperative T-tube cholangiogram, the patient is required to return for stone extraction 5–6 weeks later. This allows sufficient time for the intraperitoneal tract to mature. The T tube is then removed over a guide wire. Through the T-tube tract, a selective 5 French catheter and a wire are advanced in the direction of the stone-bearing duct. Because stones usually are easier to handle and are less prone to retrograde migration when they are in the distal common bile duct, the intrahepatic and extrahepatic calculi should be maneuvered down to that level. This usually can be accomplished by either flushing saline through a small coaxial catheter inserted past the stone or by passing a small compliant balloon catheter beyond the stone and pulling it down after inflating the balloon to the size of the duct. A variety of stone baskets measuring 15–25 mm may be used for trapping, retrieving, or fragmenting stones up to 12–15 mm in diameter (Figure 36–1). Stones in the 6-mm range can be retrieved through the T-tube tract. Hard stones that are 8–10 mm in diameter can also be extracted by this route when the tract is predilated to that size and a large sheath is inserted to prevent the mature T-tube tract membrane disruption. To capture stones, it is necessary to use short clockwise and counterclockwise movements and a basket that is wider in diameter than the stone to allow for easy stone entrapment between the wire struts. During extraction, the basket should be pulled back wide open with the stone lodged in its distal cone. If the basket is closed to secure the stone better, the calculus may either be extruded back into the duct or crushed into smaller fragments.

For many years, interventionalists preferred to extract stones through the T-tube tract rather than to push them into the duodenum, fearing sepsis, acute pancreatitis, or future duct strictures—complications reported both by surgeons

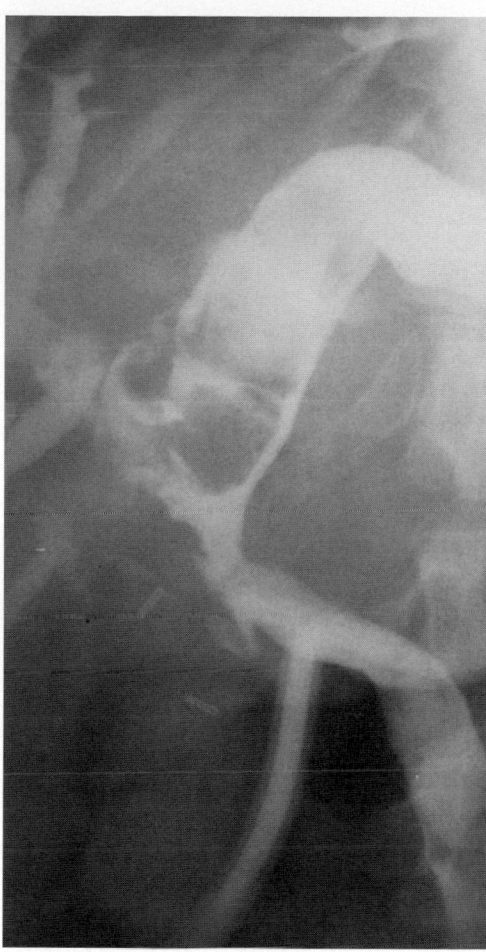

Figure 36–1 Extraction of giant biliary stones. A 24 French cannula was inserted into a T-tube tract after gradual dilatation over several days. The stones were then fragmented with a large four-wire basket, and pieces were retrieved by the basket-balloon occlusion technique. Today, the stones would be fragmented by EHL through a 14–16 French sheath.

(for example, after intraoperative sphincter dilatation with rigid Bakes dilators) and by gastroenterologists (such as after retrograde sphincterotomy) (12,13). By contrast, interventional radiologists have found that dilatation of the sphincter with angioplasty balloons leads to fewer clinical complications (14,15). The discrepancy in complication rate between sphincter dilatation and sphincterotomy may be because of the fact that catheterization of the ampulla from above is inherently easier and less traumatic than by the retrograde route and does not involve accidental entry into the pancreatic duct. In addition, Minami et al. (16) reported better preservation of sphincter function with sphincteroplasty when compared to sphincterotomy. Better drainage is obtained with large percutaneous catheters, which can be accurately positioned, monitored, and easily exchanged if occluded. Elevations of serum amylase have been noted after transhepatic biliary drainage, but these are usually transient and only occasionally associated with signs of overt short-lived pancreatitis (17). There appear to

be no contraindications to sphincteroplasty from above except for the presence of a duodenal diverticulum, which could be ruptured by balloon dilatation, with complicating peritonitis.

One of the disadvantages associated with basketing is that stones may break up into small fragments, escape into intrahepatic ducts, and be difficult to identify and retrieve. Many interventionalists prefer to use the alternative techniques that allow direct expulsion of stones and stone fragments from the bile duct into the duodenum (Figure 36–2) (18). A 12 French or 14 French sheath with a check-flow valve and irrigating side arm is introduced into the T-tube tract to permit opacification of the biliary system and the introduction of various devices. After a floppy-tipped guide wire or a Glidewire (Medi-Tech) is passed into the duodenum, sphincteroplasty is performed (with an angioplasty balloon inflated to the size of the largest retained stone but not greater than the diameter of the common duct). After all the stones are directed into the distal duct by irrigation or with a compliant balloon, an occlusion balloon catheter is inserted over the guide wire through the T-tube tract, inflated to the diameter of the common duct, and advanced over the guide wire into the duodenum. This maneuver is repeated until all stones are advanced into the bowel. When stones are large and hard, they first may be fragmented using a stone-crushing device, such as the Soehendra lithotriptor (Wilson Cook) (Figure 36–3) (8). It consists of a stiff 12 French helical steel spring-guiding catheter that can be threaded over the basket leader wire and a powerful windlass-type handle. In contrast to a plastic catheter, the metal spring-reinforced guiding sheath will not accordion as increasing pull pressure is exerted on the stone-bearing basket. Furthermore, the device either will fragment the stone or break the basket wires. In either case, the basket will not be trapped irreversibly around a large unbroken stone. Because it is easy for a stone fragment to escape into intrahepatic ducts during the course of these maneuvers, an occlusion balloon or a guide wire may be placed above the cystic duct to prevent retrograde stone migration or to allow the introduction of a catheter for irrigation. In more complicated cases in which the calculi are large, multiple, or lodged intrahepatically, the extraction may take several visits. A silastic or articulated T tube (Cook, Inc.) (19) is easy to reinsert atraumatically for drainage or for maintaining access to the tract between treatments. The success rate for percutaneous extraction of postoperative retained stones is more than 90%, with failures resulting from impacted or large intrahepatic stones. Patients with sclerosing cholangitis, recurrent pyogenic cholangitis, Caroli disease, and longstanding large retained stones pose special procedural problems because of recurrent bouts of sepsis and duct stricture (20–22). Although 72–94% of these patients can be rendered stone-free over a period of years with the use of several interventional techniques (see below), the best long-term results are obtained through a multidisciplinary team approach (23).

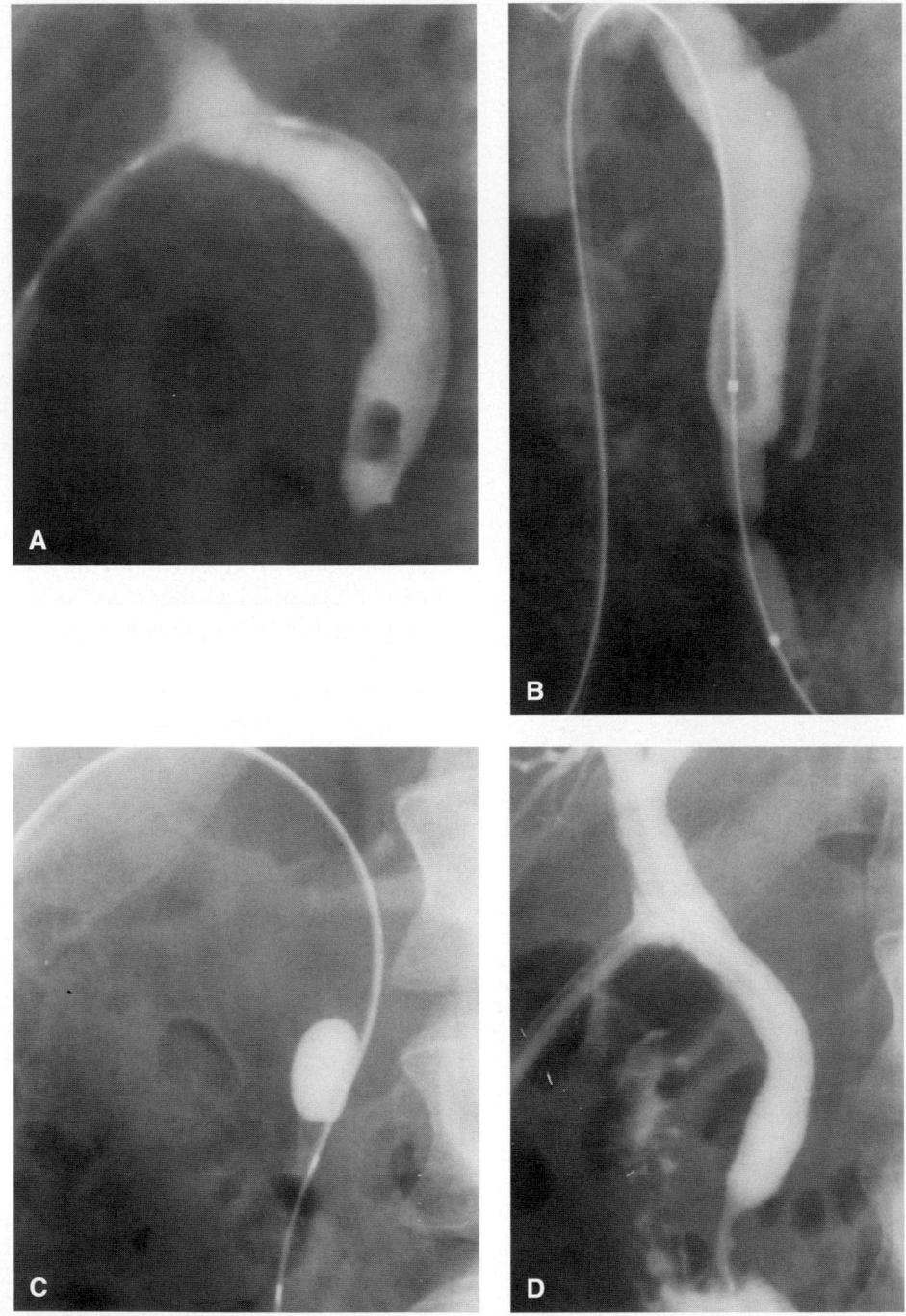

Figure 36–2 Technique for expelling bile duct stones into bowel. **A.** Calculus in the distal common bile duct and poor flow of contrast medium into the duodenum suggest papillary stenosis. **B.** Sphincteroplasty is performed with a 6-mm angioplasty balloon. **C.** The stone is pushed into the bowel with an occlusion balloon. A T tube is reinserted percutaneously. **D.** Forty-eight hours later, the bile ducts are free of stones and contrast medium flows freely through the ampulla.

TRANSHEPATIC CHOLEDOCHOLITHOTOMY

Although most common duct stones are thought to have originally arisen from the gallbladder, stones can arise de novo in the bile ducts when there is bile stasis or infection.

Clinically, this problem arises in patients with benign or malignant strictures, sclerosing cholangitis, and recurrent pyogenic cholangitis. Such patients may present with abdominal pain, fever, and borderline liver function tests with transient elevations of serum alkaline phosphatase and bilirubin resulting from intermittent stone obstruction of

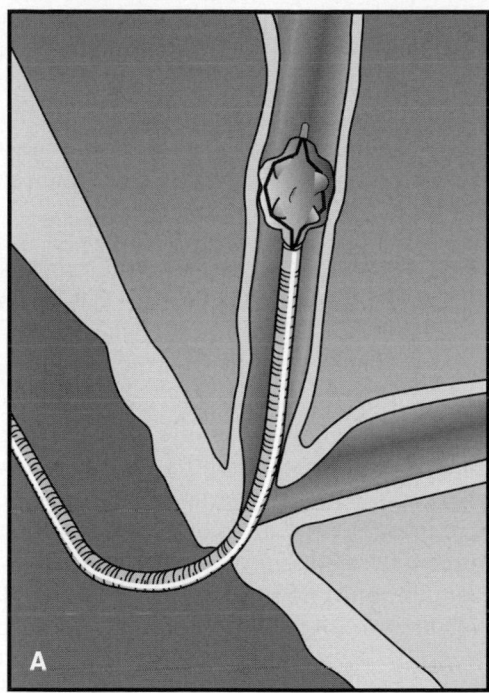 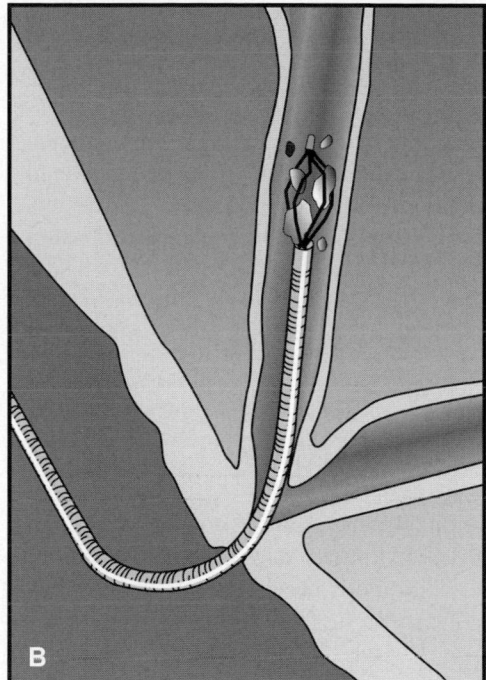

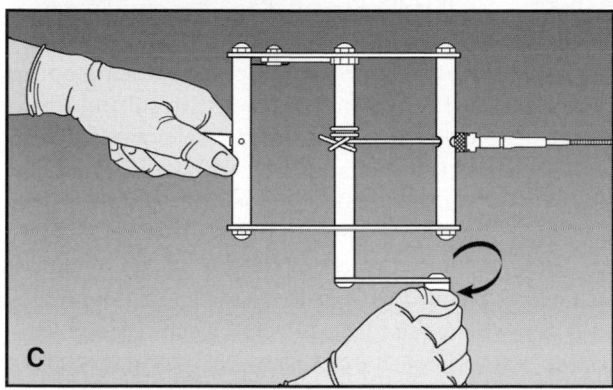

Figure 36–3 **A., B.** The illustration demonstrates capture and fragmentation of the stone from an endoscopic approach. A similar maneuver can be performed for percutaneous approaches. (Courtesy of Cook, Inc.) **C.** This is the handle that attaches to the basket. Rotating it grants mechanical advantage over fragmentation by manual maneuvers.

bile ducts. The diagnosis is then confirmed by retrograde endoscopic cholangiography, and the stones are extracted after sphincterotomy. If an endoscopist is unable to catheterize the common bile duct because of anomalies, stricture, or a choledochoenterostomy (24), the patient should be managed by the transhepatic route. A preoperative ultrasound, CT, or MRI examination of the liver to determine the presence and site of ductal dilatation is useful for choosing the preferred hepatic lobe to access. In some cases, the intrahepatic ducts are not dilated, and it may be difficult to obtain a diagnostic cholangiogram. Once the presence of calculi is documented, a 21- or 22-gauge needle is used to access the duct of interest. A 0.018-inch guide wire is advanced through the needle, maneuvered into the common bile duct, and exchanged for a standard 0.035-inch guide wire over an intermediary exchange dilator (Cope Introduction System, Cook, Inc.; Accustick system Medi-Tech; or Jeffery set, Cook, Inc.). Following this, an appropriate catheter and

guide wire may be manipulated through the distal duct and bowel. It would be traumatic to extract large calculi through the transhepatic tract. Therefore, a technique that will allow expulsion of stones or stone fragments through the duct into the duodenum must be used. As previously described, sphincteroplasty may be performed by dilating the papillary sphincter. Then, the stones may be expelled into the duodenum with an occlusion balloon. If the stones are very large, they are first fragmented by the Soehendra lithotriptor (Wilson Cook), by an electrohydraulic lithotripter, or by a laser lithotripter under transhepatic fluoroscopic or endoscopic control. Small stone fragments located in intrahepatic radicles usually can be flushed or maneuvered down into the common bile duct with a selective catheter or a balloon before expulsion into the duodenum. When stones have been cleared, a 10 French Cope locking-loop or Malecot-type drain is inserted into the common bile duct for external drainage until liver function tests have returned to normal and the associated bacteremia has been controlled. The catheter is then capped for internal drainage to ensure that there is unobstructed flow of bile into the duodenum. If the patient remains asymptomatic for 3–6 weeks and there is no distal duct obstruction or retained stones by cholangiography, the drain is removed. Note should be made however, if the patient is infected when initial drainage is performed, the patient should be allowed to recover from the infection with biliary drainage and antibiotics before undergoing the stone removal procedure. Significant manipulation in an infected patient may lead to sepsis and death.

TRANSJEJUNAL CHOLEDOCHOLITHOTOMY

Patients who have undergone choledochojejunostomy for tumor, bile duct stricture, trauma, sclerosing cholangitis, or recurrent pyogenic cholangitis are subject to anastomotic strictures with secondary stone formation. Although these stones often can be managed by a standard transhepatic technique, it is often more efficacious to extract them from a transjejunal retrograde approach through a choledochojejunostomy, especially when dealing with diseases associated with recurrent calculi and duct strictures affecting both hepatic lobes. The advantage of this approach is that it allows free access to each hepatic duct with only one catheter entry site and permits monitoring and treatment of long-term recurrent disease without the trauma associated with repeated transhepatic catheterization. Even if the Roux-en-Y loop has not been tacked to the anterior abdominal wall or furnished with a Hutson ostomy because of its anterior position, the enteric loop usually is easily accessible to needle puncture and catheterization (25). It can be punctured with a skinny needle after preliminary opacification by percutaneous transhepatic cholangiography or sometimes by an upper gastrointestinal series. The loop may also be accessed under ultrasound or computed tomographic (CT) guidance. To ensure that the colon is not punctured accidentally, the hepatic flexure can be preopacified by having the patient take an oral contrast agent the evening before the procedure. Once the small bowel lumen has been located, a metal anchoring device (Gastric anchor, Cook, Inc.) may be used for jejunopexy before catheter insertion. This serves two purposes: First, it allows the drain to be easily reinserted if it falls out accidentally before a peritoneal track is well-formed, and, second, it provides a useful radiopaque target for recatheterizing the bowel loop at a future date if the choledochoenteric anastomosis needs to be redilated or if stones recur. Once a selective catheter has been inserted into the jejunal loop, it is easy to locate and catheterize the hepatic ducts because of their close proximity to the enterostomy site. The anastomotic strictures are then balloon-dilated, and the stones are extracted into the bowel by a combination of techniques involving irrigation, basket snaring, or retrieval with occlusion balloons, with or without endoscopy. In patients with chronic recurrent stones and strictures, it is possible to provide convenient long-term access to the bile ducts for outpatient endoscopic and radiologic procedures through a well-functioning Hutson loop ostomy; however, this entry site can be associated with a 15% complication rate (26).

COMPLICATED STONE EXTRACTION

When stones are mobile, few in number, smaller than the common duct in size and easily maneuvered into the CBD, it is relatively simple and safe to extract retained duct stones by standard basket and balloon techniques. However, when numerous large stones, adherent calculi, recurrent sepsis, and coexisting bile duct strictures are present, treatment becomes more complex and may require multiple staged treatments over days or months. Communication and close association between the interventionalist and a surgeon is essential to provide the patient with, if necessary, better routes of access or with tailored segmental hepatectomy in advanced disease. The successful management of stone disease must involve the proper control of infection and attempts at eradicating significant strictures. Sepsis resulting from cholangitis and coexisting intrahepatic abscesses are first treated with antibiotics and by percutaneous drainage. Once infection is controlled, it is essential to dilate all major strictures adequately to prevent the recurrent cycle of bile stasis/infection/stone formation/stricture. Such benign strictures may be treated with balloon dilatation and prolonged stenting with large silastic catheters. Overall, benign stricture patency rates approach that of surgical intervention. (27). Stricture resulting from lithiasis, periductal encasement, chronic pancreatitis, choledochoenterostomies, sclerosing cholangitis, and recurrent pyogenic cholangiohepatitis require constant vigilance, frequent redilatations, and even catheters for life. (28,29). There is little role for metal stent placement in benign stricture management, and it should be considered only in extreme circumstances (30). The following instruments and techniques, singly or in combination, may need to be used in these difficult cases.

Fogarty Balloon Catheters

Intrahepatic calculi may be found lodged within an ampullary dilatation at a duct confluence. It may not be possible to extract the calculus either with a retrieval basket (because it cannot be sufficiently opened because of the relative stenosis of the efferent main bile duct) or with an occlusion balloon (because the calculus will be extruded into a side duct when it is pulled back). If the calculus is soft, it can be retrieved by blocking one afferent duct within a 2 or 3 French Fogarty balloon and using another similar-size balloon to pull back the stone.

Larger Angioplasty Balloon Catheters

Although there is a natural reluctance to overdilate the ampulla for fear of destroying the terminal sphincter mechanism or tearing the duct, it can be done safely as long as the balloon diameter does not exceed the common duct diameter and there is no duodenal diverticulum. In the presence of giant duct stones and proportionately enlarged common bile ducts, dilating the ampulla to 15 mm is possible and, if necessary, even to 20 mm with no complications or gross loss of sphincter competence on evaluation of upper gastrointestinal series (14,15). However, this is rarely necessary if the stones first can be fractured with intracorporeal or extracorporeal lithotripsy (Figure 36–4).

Litholytic Agents

Litholytic agents are merely of historical interest and are rarely used today. Monooctanoin is the only agent approved for human use in the United States. Although methyl tert-butyl ether (MTBE) is a better solvent of cholesterol stones, it has not achieved widespread application because of its potential toxicity and the difficulties associated with its administration. Monooctanoin is administered through a T-tube tract or a transhepatic drain over 3–10 days at a rate of 3–5 mL/hr. A second drain should be inserted for venting during the infusion to prevent pressure buildup and systemic absorption of the drug (31). The majority of cholesterol stones that respond to this agent will become softer or shrink in size and will become more amenable to being crushed with baskets. Only about 30% will be dissolved completely. This agent is used to facilitate breaking up of large, hard stones only when other modalities have failed. Side effects include diarrhea, nausea, and vomiting, and, if the infusion rate is too high, the patient may develop biliary colic, chills, hypotension, or even pulmonary edema (32).

Electrohydraulic Lithotripsy

In this procedure, a high-voltage generator creates a series of sparks at the tip of a flexible bipolar electrode that can generate hydraulic shocks of sufficient energy to fragment most calculi (33). Flexible catheter electrodes are available in sizes varying from 1.6 French to 9 French. The 1.6 French and 3 French probes can be passed through the instrument channel of small flexible endoscopes under 4 mm or through the hollow stem of some retrieval baskets. This makes them ideally suited for use in smaller intrahepatic ducts. The best results are obtained by using irrigating solution made up of one-sixth normal saline and by having the electrode tip directly facing the stone at 1–2 mm from its surface. Because serious bleeding and perforation can occur if the electrode were accidentally to come close to or to make contact with the wall of the duct, it is safer to steer and monitor the position of the electrode tip under endoscopic control (Figure 36–5). If it is not possible to pass an endoscope into the stone-bearing duct because of excessive angulation, strictures, or space-occupying giant stones, an over-the-guide wire type of Segura basket (Medi-Tech), which allows in-line insertion of an EHL electrode, can be used to capture and fragment the calculus. Some large calcified stones may not break, even when the larger and more powerful 9 French EHL electrode is used. On these rare occasions, the stones may be fragmented with laser lithotripsy. Giant stones that cannot be fragmented may be managed with long-term catheter drainage or, eventually, segmental hepatectomy or liver transplant if the patient can be prepared to tolerate major surgery.

Extracorporeal Shock Wave Lithotripsy (ESWL)

It is sometimes difficult to remove or break up large stones greater than 15–20 mm, especially when they are located intrahepatically. As a calculus grows in size over the years, the duct in which it is contained also locally expands to form a sac. Because the efferent duct of this sac remains of normal caliber or narrows further because of stricture formation, it becomes impossible for the larger stone to pass spontaneously. It is also difficult to introduce and deploy baskets around the stone because of the marked disparity in diameter between the stone-containing sac and the smaller draining intrahepatic duct. Similarly, severe duct angulation, strictures, and lack of maneuvering space around the stone can limit the use of EHL or laser under endoscopic control. When these percutaneous techniques fail and surgery is contraindicated because of coexisting risks or illnesses, ESWL has been shown to be safe and efficacious (34).

Because ESWL is performed mostly with units that require centering the shock waves under fluoroscopic control, the common bile duct must have a catheter in good position for opacification of the stones. This is performed either through an endoscopic nasobiliary catheter or a percutaneous transhepatic or T-tube tract catheter. Preliminary sphincteroplasty must be performed to allow passage of stone fragments. During ESWL the patient must be immobilized with general or epidural anesthesia so that the treatment can be carried out with the patient in the best position for fragmenting the stones safely and efficiently. The patient should be on antibiotic coverage until stone clearance has been achieved. Since ESWL was first described in 1986 for the management of choledocholithiasis, it has been found to be an important method for treating large, irretrievable stones, with a fragmentation rate of more than 90% after one or two sessions (34). Despite successful fragmentation of these stones in situ, their constituent fragments greater than 6 mm in diameter usually will not pass spontaneously. In fact, supplemental percutaneous or endoscopic extraction procedures must be performed in as many as 96% of patients to achieve complete stone clearance. Complications of ESWL include hemobilia, ileus, pancreatitis, biliary sepsis, hematuria, and abdominal pain, with a 0.9% 30-day mortality rate. Contraindications to performing ESWL include vascular aneurysms, calcified

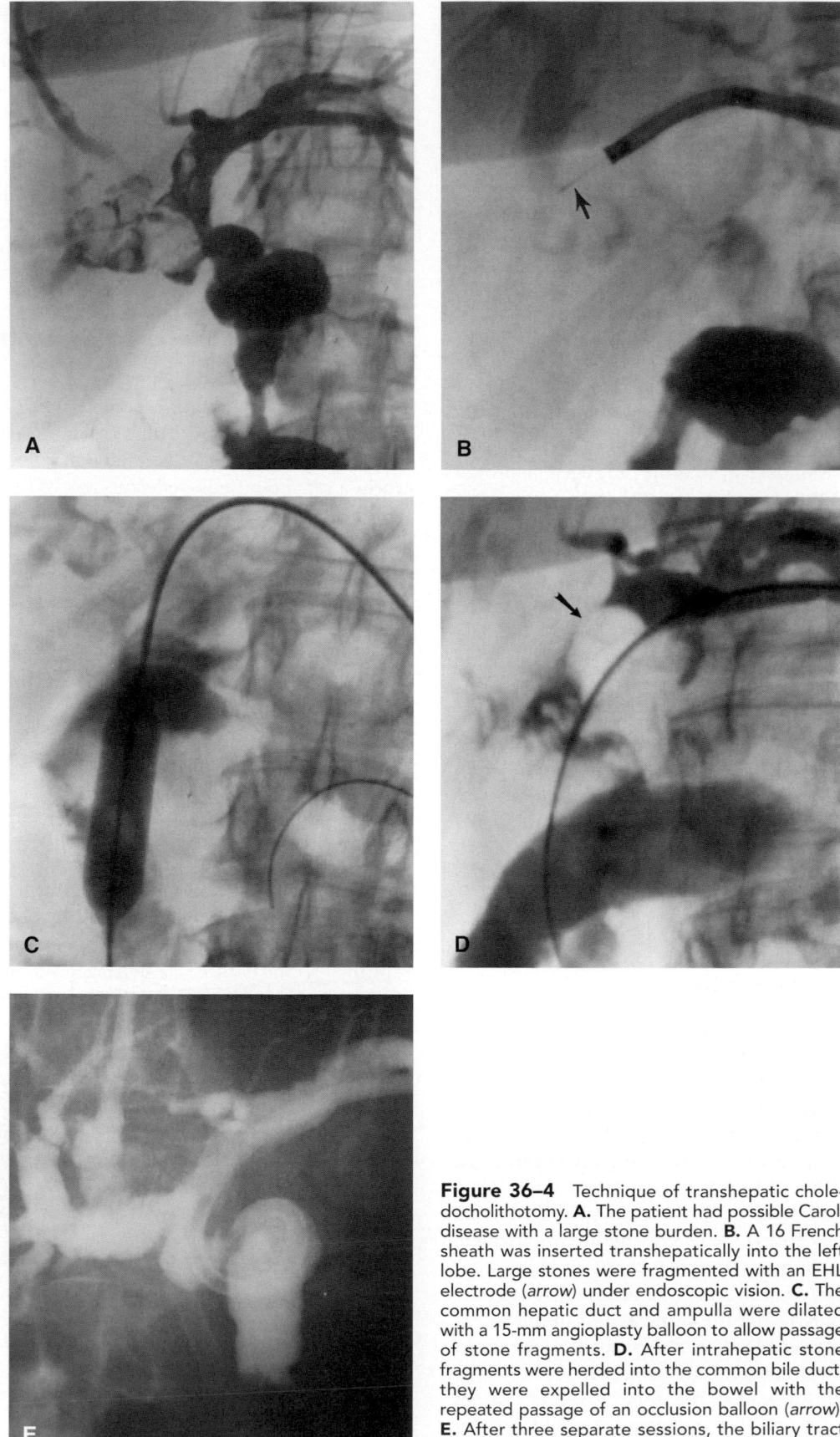

Figure 36–4   Technique of transhepatic chole-docholithotomy. **A.** The patient had possible Caroli disease with a large stone burden. **B.** A 16 French sheath was inserted transhepatically into the left lobe. Large stones were fragmented with an EHL electrode (*arrow*) under endoscopic vision. **C.** The common hepatic duct and ampulla were dilated with a 15-mm angioplasty balloon to allow passage of stone fragments. **D.** After intrahepatic stone fragments were herded into the common bile duct, they were expelled into the bowel with the repeated passage of an occlusion balloon (*arrow*). **E.** After three separate sessions, the biliary tract was clear of retained stones.

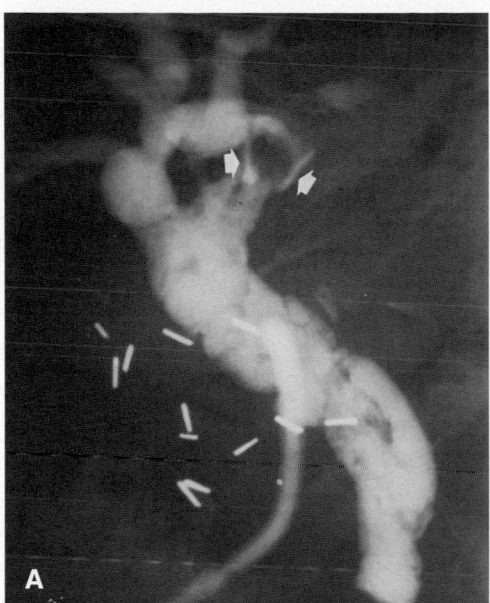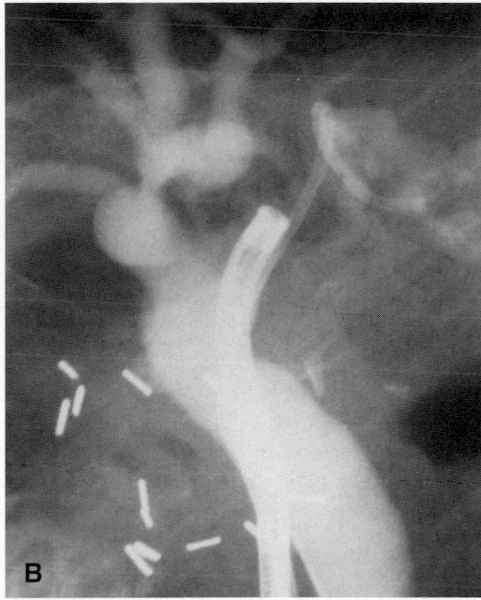

Figure 36–5 Removal of stone trapped in the left duct. **A.** A 1-cm stone could not be snared or retrieved with a balloon catheter. Note that the stone is larger in diameter than the efferent duct (*arrows*). **B.** A 6 French loop catheter locked distal to the stone was pulled to bring the stone into view of the endoscope so that it could be fragmented by EHL.

vessels, uncorrectable coagulopathy, pacemakers, and inability to focus the shock wave beam safely.

Percutaneous Cholangioscopy

The use of cholangioscopy through percutaneous and surgical drain tracts has become increasingly common with small diameter flexible endoscopes (now available in 3–5 mm sizes). These scopes have instrument channels, tip deflection capability, and matching light sources and recording capabilities, making them ideal for percutaneous exploration of the biliary tree and retained stone management. Although surgeons are also able to extract stones by endoscopy through T-tube tracts or by laparoscopic techniques, many patients are still being referred to the interventional radiologist for removal of small missed stones or for complicated cases that require the combination of fluoroscopy and cholangioscopy.

An increasing number of interventional radiologists with a busy full-time practice have a cholangioscope available to them (35,36), which can be invaluable for visualizing, biopsying, and managing lesions that are difficult to reach or to treat solely by radiographic means (Figure 36–6). Percutaneous endoscopy is useful for distinguishing stone from tumor, clot, or sludge; for finding the opening of unopacified intrahepatic ducts; for biopsying suspicious ductal lesions; and for extracting and fragmenting stones under direct vision with Fogarty balloons, stone baskets, laser, or EHL. Harris et al. reported a 96% initial clearance rate for stone burden (37). A 3–5 mm endoscope can be passed through a properly dilated T-tube tract for management of

large calculi within the common bile or hepatic ducts. The patient should receive a broad-spectrum antibiotic before any type of complex endoscopic procedure. To obtain a clear field of view, bile ducts must be kept slightly distended by

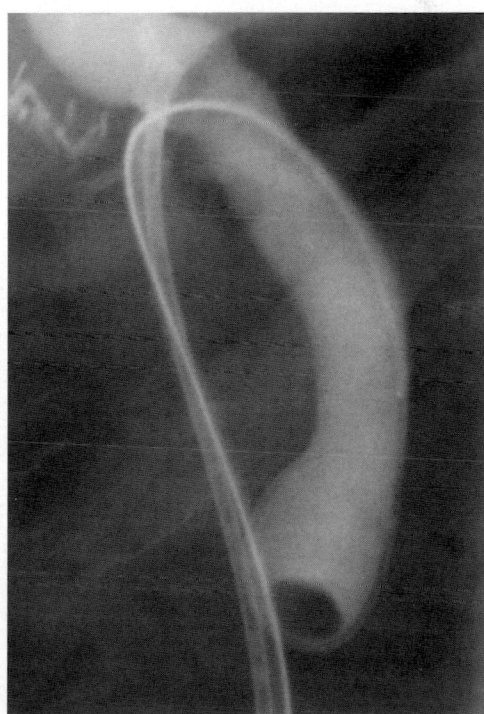

Figure 36–6 Pseudocalculus of the common bile duct. Stone disease was ruled out by flexible endoscopy, and balloon sphincteroplasty was performed to dilate the papillary stricture.

being flushed with saline through the irrigation channel either by hand or from a bag suspended 15–20 cm above the level of the common bile duct. Adherent large blood clots should be removed by being flushed through catheters or by suction. It is important that free egress of the fluid occur through the common duct or through a transhepatic catheter introduction sheath to prevent undue pressure elevation, which will lead to sepsis or leakage of contaminated fluid into the peritoneal cavity.

The tip of the endoscope should always be advanced under direct vision and be angled so that it faces the long axis of the duct. The endoscope is directed toward the suspected calculi by endoscopically following a previously placed guide wire and, if necessary, occasionally confirming its course by fluoroscopy.

The small flexible endoscopes used in these procedures are delicate and expensive. The internal quartz fibers used for viewing and illumination can be fractured easily when the instrument is hyperflexed during clinical endoscopy or when it is being cleaned and sterilized.

MORBIDITY AND MORTALITY IN TREATING CHOLEDOCHOLITHIASIS

The complication rate associated with the percutaneous management of choledocholithiasis depends on many factors. These include:

1. Size, consistency, number, and intrahepatic or extra-hepatic location of stones
2. Presence of recurring cholangitis, intrahepatic abscesses, or both
3. Preprocedural endoscopic or surgical complications
4. Coexisting medical risks associated with old age, advanced cardiopulmonary disease, stroke, and other conditions
5. Degree of technical complexity required for stone extraction
6. Need for a percutaneous transhepatic or transjejunal approach
7. Presence of sclerosing cholangitis or recurrent pyogenic cholangiohepatitis

The morbidity rate for simple postoperative stone extraction through a T-tube tract is less than 5% (20). However, in patients with multiple large or intrahepatic calculi, longer and more traumatic intraductal manipulations can lead to sepsis, hemobilia, and pancreatitis, all of which usually respond to conservative management. The T-tube tract can rupture if it is overdilated too quickly or if the operator attempts to extract a large, hard stone through a small tract.

Compared to the morbidity associated with stone extraction via a T-tube tract, there is potentially a higher morbidity when this is performed via a transhepatic approach because of the additional complications that can occur from the creation of a new transhepatic tract (38). In patients with

malignant duct obstruction, the immediate morbidity of percutaneous biliary drainage seen in studies of more than 100 patients varies between 5–22%. Potential serious complications include severe hemobilia (requiring blood transfusion, hepatic arterial embolization, or surgery), intrahepatic or subphrenic abscesses, pneumothorax, pleural effusion, peritonitis, and cholangitis with septic shock. Multiple other series report an overall complication rate for transhepatic stone extraction with cholangioscopic assistance to range between 14.5–22% (39–41).

PERCUTANEOUS CHOLECYSTOLITHOTOMY (PCCL)

Interventional procedures for PCCL include direct percutaneous extraction of stones and removal of stone fragments after stone fragmentation and contact dissolution with a litholytic agent, which, as mentioned earlier, is rarely used (42). At this time, PCCL plays a very small role because of the advent of laparoscopic cholecystectomy (LC), which is the accepted treatment for management of symptomatic gallstones (43). PCCL should be viewed as an option of last resort. The contraindications to PCCL include gangrenous gallbladder with possible perforation, severely contracted gallbladder with no measurable lumen, large diffusely calcified stones greater than 3–4 cm, porcelain gallbladder, uncorrectable coagulation disorder, and severe allergy to iodinated contrast media.

OVERVIEW OF TECHNIQUES

In this section, direct percutaneous extraction of stones and removal of stone fragments after internal stone fragmentation will be discussed. Cholecystostomy techniques are discussed in more detail in Chapter 37. Depending on the size of stones and fragments in the gallbladder, the diameter of the cholecystostomy tract that is required for their extraction may vary from 16 French to as large as 30 French. An access to the gallbladder may be obtained through a transhepatic route or transperitoneal route. If a transhepatic route is chosen, one should consider the risk of causing severe hemorrhage from an arterial or liver laceration (45). Picus et al. (46) accessed the gallbladder in one step via the transhepatic route by traversing the thin sliver of liver that overlies the body of the gallbladder and dilating the tract coaxially to insert an introducer sheath no larger than 18 French. Others who prefer this route dilate the transhepatic tract stepwise over a few weeks or longer (after a percutaneous cholecystostomy is performed to address the acute component of the disease) (47,48). The transhepatic route may prevent peritoneal leakage of bile without having to perform temporary cholecystopexy. Some prefer to use the direct approach to the gallbladder fundus via a subhepatic transperitoneal route, in line with the long axis of the gallbladder (49–54).

The advantage of this approach is that it does not require complex retrograde catheter and endoscope maneuvers for reaching and retrieving calculi.

With either approach, complications can be minimized when cholecystostomy is performed to address the cholecystitis first. Once, the acute cholecystitis has resolved, the tract should be dilated over time to accept the instruments that will be used to perform lithotripsy and stone extraction. The basic interventions for PCCL used by various authors are the same but vary in detail depending on the approach and technique used to cannulate the gallbladder, the type of instrumentation preferred to break up and retrieve stones, the preferential use of endoscopy versus fluoroscopy (or a combination of both), the follow-up, and the timing of drain tube removal.

PREFERRED INTERVENTIONAL METHODS FOR PCCL

Review of preoperative imaging is essential to determine the relationship of the gallbladder to the liver and colon. If preoperative imaging is not available, the relationship can be assessed with ultrasound. It is also useful to have the right hepatic flexure opacified at the time of gallbladder puncture so that the needle can be guided more safely past the large bowel under both fluoroscopic and ultrasound control. The gallbladder fundus is punctured with a trocar needle under ultrasound guidance. A stiff guide wire is then coiled in the gallbladder. The cholecystostomy tract is dilated sequentially and a drainage catheter is placed. After the acute cholecystitis has resolved, the tract is dilated gradually to the usually required size of 16 French to 30 French. Techniques for dilating the cholecystostomy tract include the use of serial or coaxial dilators and the use of angioplasty balloon catheters. The gallbladder wall in chronic cholelithiasis is often thickened and leathery. Therefore, tract dilatation may be difficult and can be unsuccessful in 5.3–9.0% of cases. Wall invagination or complete loss of access because of partial decompression of the gallbladder lumen and displacement of guide wires into the peritoneal cavity are additional problems encountered (46–56). These problems can be minimized by the insertion of a removable T-anchor (Cook, Inc.) through the initial cholecystostomy needle into the lumen of the gallbladder to perform a temporary cholecystopexy (57). A transitionless introducer sheath (Cook, Inc.) may also facilitate entry into such a fibrotic gallbladder because of its stepless profile (58). It is also important to keep the gallbladder slightly distended with fluid during dilatation. A safety wire may be inserted into the tract outside the sheath and advanced to the neck of the gallbladder. In addition, a 5 French catheter or locking-loop catheter may be inserted in parallel through a separate puncture to function as an irrigation port for opacifying the gallbladder, for directing calculi toward the basket, or for flushing stone fragments out through the large cannula.

Once a large cholecystostomy tract has been established, the operator may choose from a wide variety of instruments for stone extraction. The three most useful are Dormia baskets, nitinol baskets with an instrument channel and the Soehendra kit (Cook, Inc.) (59), and crushing and triradiate forceps (Figure 36–7). Large stones greater than 15 mm are best broken up by EHL or laser lithotripsy. Stone fragments and small calculi can be flushed out by irrigation or extracted with Malecot catheters, which are passed repeatedly in and out of the gallbladder with suction. Once the gallbladder is cleared of stones, a 16 French to 18 French Foley catheter is inserted into the gallbladder for gravity drainage. The next day, the patient is reevaluated with cholangiography and cholecystoscopy for extraction of any residual stones from the gallbladder, cystic duct, or common bile duct. Small movable stones that have migrated into the cystic duct usually are simple to extract with small baskets or balloons. The management of larger stones, which may be impacted in the cystic duct, can be difficult because of the tortuosity and narrow caliber of the duct. The cystic duct is first catheterized and the stone bypassed with the combination of a catheter and a Glidewire (Medi-Tech). This will allow the insertion of an extra stiff guide wire and a 7 French catheter, which will cause straightening of the cystic duct and will simplify the insertion of instruments. If the duct can be dilated sufficiently to insert a small flexible endoscope, the stone can be pulverized with EHL and removed (Figure 36–8).

If the T anchor has been used, it should be removed at this time because removing it after 10–20 days will be difficult because of tissue ingrowth (50). The patients are discharged on average in 1–3 days after stone extraction. The Foley catheter is allowed to drain externally to a bag for 10–15 days, and it is then clamped for a week. If, after clamping, there is leakage of bile around the drain indicating cystic duct or common bile duct obstruction, the gallbladder is reevaluated with both cholangiography and endoscopy. The Foley catheter is reinserted after treatment of residual stones and is kept on external drainage for another 1–2 weeks. The test clamping cycle is repeated until tube occlusion is tolerated. It is important to perform cholangiography and cholecystoscopy prior to the drain removal because small retained stones may be overlooked easily by cholangiography (50,54). If there is continued leakage around the Foley catheter, it is important to rule out common bile duct obstruction by stones or papillary stenosis. Both of these conditions can be treated through the cystic duct with balloon catheters, as previously described in the section on choledocholithotomy. Drain catheters usually can be removed when a "tractogram" shows a mature tract without intraperitoneal leakage.

Subsequently, patients are followed-up in the interventional radiology clinic at regular intervals for stone recurrence both clinically and by ultrasonography. Some patients are placed on oral ursodeoxycholic acid therapy for several months to dissolve residual cholesterol particles, which may act as foci for recurrent stones (54,61).

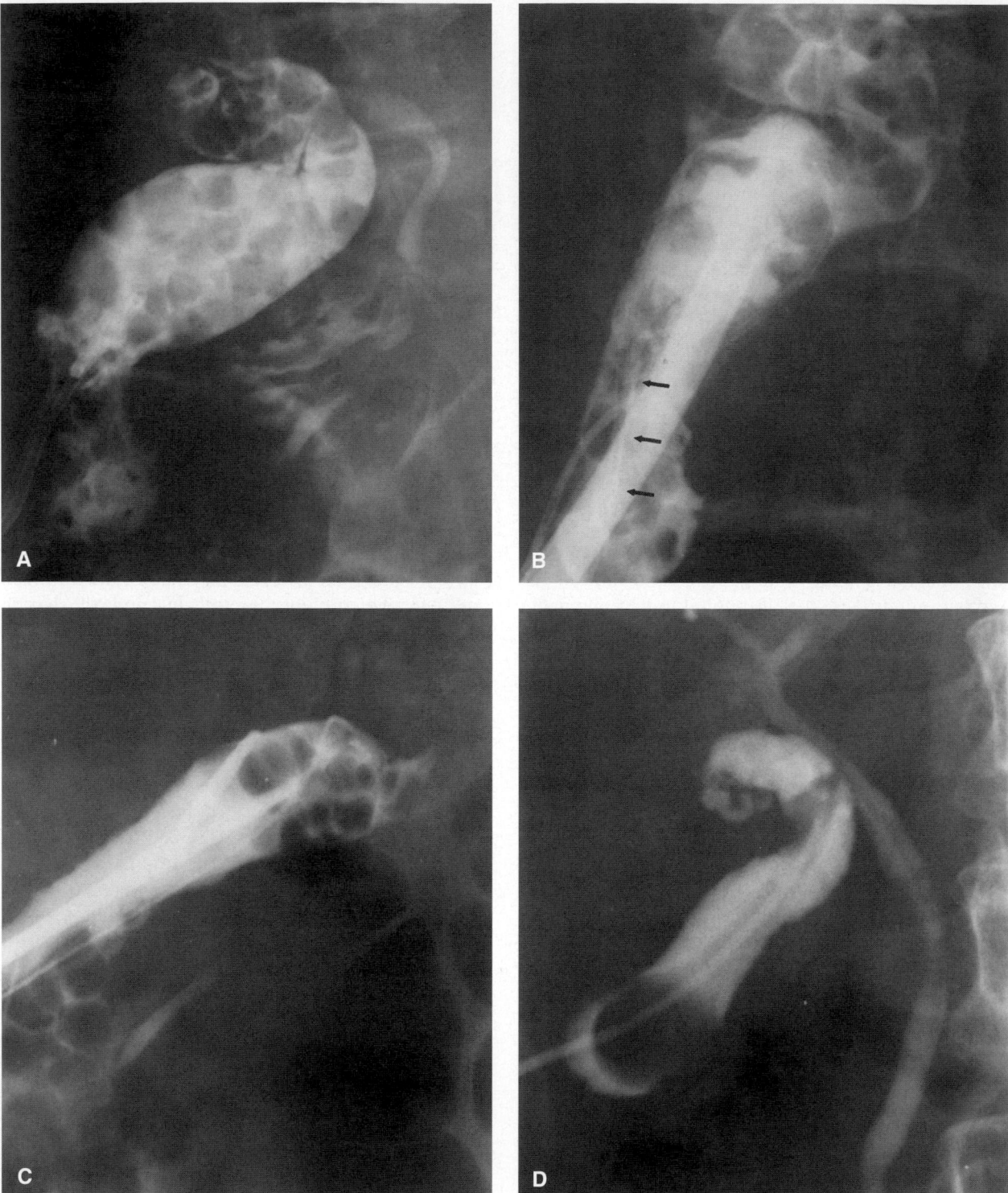

Figure 36–7   PCCL techniques. **A.** Opacification of a long, sinuous gallbladder full of noncalcified stones. **B.** A 24 French introducing sheath was inserted into the gallbladder after percutaneous coaxial balloon dilatation of a second cholecystostomy tract. A removable anchor (*arrows*) was used to prevent invagination of the floating gallbladder. **C.** The stones were removed with crushing forceps. **D.** The gallbladder was cleared of all stones after two sessions. A Foley catheter is in place for external drainage.

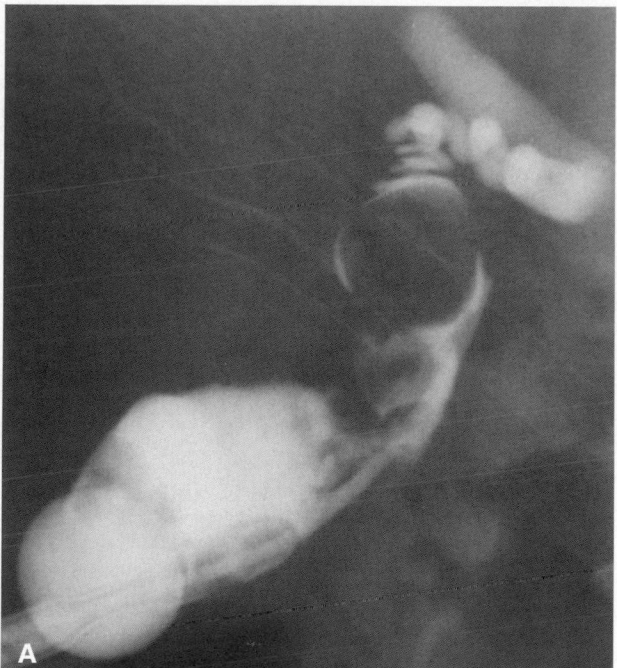 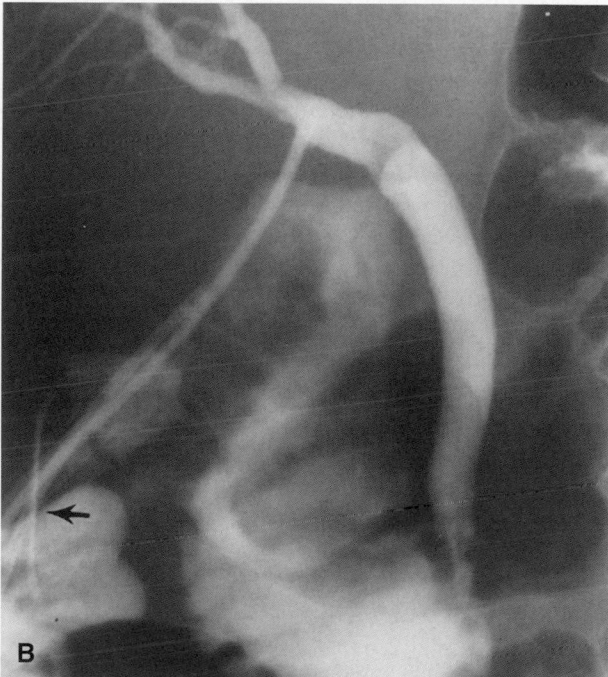

Figure 36–8   Removal of impacted infundibular stone. **A.** This elderly patient was admitted for acute calculous cholecystitis. After 2 weeks of percutaneous external drainage, about 20 calculi were extracted from the gallbladder. Because of the excessive angulation of the gallbladder, the infundibular stone could not be brought into view endoscopically. **B.** After transcystic catheterization of the common bile duct, the gallbladder axis was straightened with an extra stiff guide wire. The stone could now be endoscoped easily and fragmented with EHL. Note the retaining gallbladder anchor (*arrow*).

GALLSTONE DISSOLUTION THERAPY

As previously mentioned, two contact solvents have been used clinically for gallstone therapy. They are of historical interest only and are rarely used. Monooctanoin is a relatively poor, rarely used cholesterol solvent that requires long-term infusion. Methyl tert-butyl ether, or MTBE, (61), unlike diethyl ether, is liquid at body temperature and is 50 times more potent than monooctanoin. It can dissolve pure cholesterol stones, irrespective of size and number, usually within a day. Larger stones of more uncertain composition may take 2–3 days to completely or partially dissolve. The administration of MTBE is safe when it can be confined within the lumen of the gallbladder. Local extravasation along the tube tract can cause peritonitis or liver necrosis. If it reaches the duodenum in sufficient quantities, it can cause erosions with gastrointestinal bleeding, and its absorption into the bloodstream can lead to untoward sedation and hemolysis. Supplemental procedures may be needed for extraction of insoluble residues (62). MTBE is not approved for general use by the FDA and can only be administered to patients on a compassionate basis.

Gallbladder ESWL

ESWL of the gallbladder is rarely used before PCCL and will not be discussed further.

Results with PCCL

Because of the advent and success of laparoscopic cholecystectomy (LC) in replacing noninvasive or percutaneous gallstone extraction, the greatest activity and experience with PCCL have occurred from 1985 to 1992. The rate of failure or difficulty in accessing the gallbladder with a large introduction sheath could be as high as 27% in early studies (55,56) but has varied between only 3–7% in the larger series (44,46,48,49,52,55,56). Catheterization of the gallbladder, when successful, led to an immediate stone clearance rate of more than 90%. The causes of post-PCCL retained stones were related to inadequate endoscopic inspection before the cholecystostomy drain was removed, (44,50) either because the stones could not be extracted from difficult positions within the cystic duct or because they were too large to break up. It should be emphasized that small retained stones can be missed easily on cholecystography. Most of the time, flexible endoscopy can evaluate the entire gallbladder at the time of the cholecystostomy drain removal, preventing missed stones (59).

The PCCL morbidity has been 9–12% in the largest series. The types of complications seen were related to:

1. The use of general anesthesia—myocardial infarction, respiratory problems, ileus, deep venous thrombosis (53)
2. Vasovagal reaction (50)

3. Cholecystostomy technique—inability to dilate chole-cystostomy tract fully, with resulting peritonitis (46,52,55,56), colon puncture with fistula (52,53), or hepatic or gallbladder hemorrhage (62)
4. Problems during stone extraction—loss of tract, gallbladder wall perforation, missed retained calculi requiring a second procedure or other forms of surgery (48,49,54)
5. Post-PCCL bile leakage—immature peritoneal tract, subphrenic collection, or leaky transhepatic tract (46,52,54).

Except for problems involving loss of or unsuccessful access to the gallbladder that necessitated emergency cholecystectomy, most complications resolved by conservative management with antibiotics, fluid replacement, supplemental peritoneal drainage, or recatheterization of the gallbladder. It is important to note that none of these reported complications is associated with bile duct laceration. Picus et al. (46) found the 30-day mortality to be 3%, mostly because of severe coexisting illnesses. One death directly related to PCCL was described in a debilitated patient on steroids who succumbed after laparotomy for unsuspected transhepatic tract bile leak 3 days after removal of the cholecystostomy drain, which had been in place for 29 days.

The main objection to PCCL has to do with failure to remove a diseased organ that may be subject to stone recurrence (63) and a low incidence of carcinoma (64). Data on long-term stone recurrence are available from series of subjects who have had surgical cholecystolithotomy (65,66) or who were observed after clearance of gallstones following oral bile administration. Reports of gallstone recurrence range widely from 20–50% over 2–20 years (65,66). Villanova et al. (67) showed that more than 50% of patients were found to be free of recurrence at 5 years, and 30% had remained stone free by the 11-year observation point.

When PCCL was introduced, it was thought that the minimal procedural trauma to the gallbladder, combined with endoscopic stone clearance and adjuvant ursodeoxycholic acid therapy, would lead to markedly delayed stone recurrence. However, two studies, (44,60) have demonstrated that retained stone fragments could be missed by rigid endoscopy and that ursodeoxycholic acid did not, as predicted by Villanova, prevent stone formation in the older age group being treated (60). Discounting the cases with retained stones (because flexible scopes allow better visualization), others found a recurrent stone incidence of about 4% and 22% over a mean period of 14 months and 26 months, respectively. In the group described by McDermott et al. (60), 25% died of unrelated causes during the 3-year period of observation. Patients with recurrent stones had normal gallbladder ejection fractions and were generally asymptomatic. Among the three patients who had recurrent right upper quadrant pain, only one had recurrent calculi. These results suggest that recurrent gallstones appear in the second and third year after PCCL and are generally asymptomatic. Hence, in patients who are at high risk, who are elderly, or who have limited life expectancy, PCCL may be useful and relatively safe.

PCCL is an option of last resort, and LC remains the standard of care. However, if the patient is not an operative candidate, PCCL is an available option for managing symptomatic gallstone disease in elderly and critically ill patients with a limited life expectancy.

REFERENCES

1. Way LW, Pelligrini CA, eds. Surgery of the Gallbladder and Bile Ducts. Philadelphia: WB Saunders, 1987.
2. Berger MY, van der Velden JJ, Lijmer JG, et al. Abdominal symptoms: do they predict gallstones? A systematic review. Scand J Gastroenterol 2000;35:70–76.
3. Middelfart HV, Jensen P, Hojgaard L, et al. Pain patterns after distension of the gallbladder in patients with acute cholecystitis. Scand J Gastroenterol 1998;33:982.
4. Fenster LF, Lonborg R, Thirlby RC, et al. What symptoms does cholecystectomy cure? Insights from an outcomes measurement project and review of the literature. Am J Surg 1995;169:533.
5. Diehl AK, Sugarek NJ, Todd KH. Clinical evaluation for gallstone disease: usefulness of symptoms and signs of diagnosis. Am J Med 1990;89:29–33.
6. Gracie WA, Ransohoff DF. The natural history of silent gallstones. N Engl J Med 1982;307:798–800.
7. Trotman BW, Petrella EJ, Soloway RD, et al. Evaluation of radiographic lucency or opaqueness of gallstones as a means of identifying cholesterol or pigment stones. Gastroenterology 1975;68:1563–1566.
8. Binmoeller KF, Bruckner M, Thonke F, et al. Treatment of difficult bile duct stones using mechanical, electrohydraulic, and extracorporeal shock wave lithotripsy. Endoscopy 1993;25:201–206.
9. Harshfield DL, Teplick SK, Brandon JC. Pain control during interventional biliary procedures: epidural anesthesia vs. IV sedation. AJR Am J Roentgenol 1993;161:1057–1059.
10. Mazzariello R. Review of 220 cases of residual bile calculi treated without reoperation: an eight-year study. Surgery 1973;73:299–330.
11. Madden JL. Common duct stones: their origin and surgical management. Surg Clin North Am 1973;53:1095–1100.
12. Siddique I, Mohan K, Khajah A, et al. Sphincterotomy in patients with gallstones, elevated LFTs, and a normal CBD on ERCP. Hepatogastroenterology 2003;50(53):1242–1245.
13. Vandervoort J, Soetikno RM, Tham TC, et al. Risk factors for complications after performance of ERCP. Gastrointest Endosc 2002;56(5):652–656.
14. Berkman WA, Bishop AF, Palagallo GL, et al. Percutaneous dilatation of the distal common bile duct and ampulla of Vater for removal of calculi. Radiology 1988;167:453–455.
15. Gil S, de la Iglesia P, Verdú JF, et al. Effectiveness and safety of balloon dilation of the papilla and the use of an occlusion balloon for clearance of bile duct calculi. AJR Am J Roentgenol 2000;174:1455–1460.
16. Minami A, Nakatsu T, Uchida N, et al. Papillary dilation vs. sphincterotomy in endoscopic removal of bile duct stones. A randomized trial with manometric function. Dig Dis Sci 1995;40(12):2550–2554.
17. Savader SJ, Venbrux AC, Robbins AK, et al. Pancreatic response to percutaneous biliary drainage: a prospective study. Radiology 1991;178:343–346.
18. Meranze SG, Stein EJ, Burke DR, et al. Removal of common bile duct stones with angiographic occlusion balloons. AJR Am J Roentgenol 1986;146:383–385.
19. Cope C, Gensburg RS. Drainage of bile ducts with an articulated T-tube. J Vasc Interv Radiol 1990;1:113–116.
20. Burhenne HJ. Percutaneous extraction of retained biliary tract stones: 661 patients. AJR Am J Roentgenol 1980;134:888–898.
21. Choi BI, Han JK, Han MC. Percutaneous removal of retained intrahepatic stones utilizing a combination of techniques with emphasis on a preshaped angulated catheter: review of 170 patients. Eur J Radiol 1992;2:199–203.

22. Jeng KS, Yang FS, Ohta I, et al. Dilatation of intrahepatic strictures in patients with hepatolithiasis. World J Surg 1990;14:587–593.
23. Pitt HA, Venbrux AC, Coleman JA, et al. Intrahepatic stones: the transhepatic team approach. Ann Surg 1994;219:527–537.
24. Cotton PB. Endoscopic management of bile duct stones (apples and oranges). Gut 1984;25:587–597.
25. Maroney TP, Ring EJ. Percutaneous transjejunal catheterization of Roux-en Y biliary-jejunal anastomoses. Radiology 1987;164:151–153.
26. Fan ST, Mok F, Zheng SS, et al. Appraisal of hepaticocutaneous jejunostomy in the management of hepatolithiasis. Am J Surg 1993;165:332–335.
27. Laasch HU, Martin DF. Management of benign biliary strictures. Cardiovasc Intervent Radiol 2002;25:457–466.
28. Citron SJ, Martin LG. Benign biliary strictures: treatment with percutaneous cholangioplasty. 1991;178:339–341.
29. Gibson RN, Adam A, Yeung E, et al. Percutaneous techniques in benign hilar and intrahepatic strictures. J Intervent Radiol 1988;3:125–130.
30. Lopez RR, Cosenza CA, Lois J, et al. Long-term results of metallic stents for benign biliary strictures. Arch Surg 2001;136:664–669.
31. Haskin P, Teplick SK. Percutaneous management of biliary stones. Semin Intervent Radiol 1985;2:81–96.
32. Hine LK, Arrowsmith JB, Gallo-Torres HE. Monooctanoin-associated pulmonary edema. Am J Gastroenterol 1988;83:1128–1131.
33. Picus D. Intracorporeal biliary lithotripsy. Radiol Clin North Am 1990;28:1241–1249.
34. Sauerbruch T, Stern M. Fragmentation of bile duct stones by extracorporeal shock waves: a new approach to biliary calculi after failure of routine endoscopic measures. Gastroenterology 1989;96:146–152.
35. Venbrux AC, Robbins KV, Savader SJ, et al. Endoscopy as an adjuvant to biliary radiologic intervention. Radiology 1991;180:355–361.
36. Cope C. Needle endoscopy in special procedures. Radiology 1988;168:353–358.
37. Harris, VJ, Sherman S, Trerotola SO, et al. Complex biliary stones: treatment with a small choledochoscope and laser lithotripsy. Radiology 1996;199(1):71–77.
38. Clements WD, Diamond T, McCrory DC, et al. Biliary drainage in obstructive jaundice: experimental and clinical aspects. Br J Surg 1993;80:834–842.
39. Cheung MT, Wai SH, Kwok PCH. Percutaneous transhepatic choledochoscopic removal of intrahepatic stones. Br J Surg 2003;90(11):1409–1415.
40. Jan YY, Chen MF. Percutaneous transhepatic cholangioscopic lithotomy for hepatolithiasis: long-term results. Gastrointest Endosc 1995;42:1–5.
41. Ponchon T, Genin G, Mitchell R, et al. Method, indications, and results of percutaneous choledochoscopy: a series of 161 procedures. Ann Surg 1996;223:26–36.
42. Fache JS. Transcholecystic intervention. Radiol Clin North Am 1990;28:1157–1169.
43. Airan M, Appel M, Berci G, et al. Retrospective and prospective multi-institutional laparoscopic cholecystectomy study organized by the Society of American Gastrointestinal Endoscopic Surgeons. Surg Endosc 1992;6:169–178.
44. Cheslyn-Curtis S, Gillams AR, Russell RCG, et al. Selection, management, and early outcome of 113 patients with symptomatic gallstones treated by percutaneous cholecystolithotomy. Gut 1992;33:1253–1259.
45. Savader SJ, Trerotola SO, Merine DS, et al. Hemobilia after percutaneous transhepatic biliary drainage: treatment with transcatheter embolotherapy. J Vasc Interv Radiol 1992;3:345–352.
46. Picus D, Hicks ME, Darcy MD, et al. Percutaneous cholecystolithotomy: analysis of results and complications in 58 consecutive patients. Radiology 1992;183:779–784.
47. Kerlan RK, LaBerge JM, Ring EJ. Percutaneous cholecystolithotomy: preliminary experience. Radiology 1985;157:653–656.
48. Akiyama H, Okazaki T, Takashima I, et al. Percutaneous treatments for biliary diseases. Radiology 1990;176:25–30.
49. Hruby W, Stackl W, Urban M, et al. Percutaneous endoscopic cholecystolithotripsy. Work in progress. Radiology 1989;173:477–479.
50. Cope C, Burke DR, Meranze SG. Percutaneous extraction of gallstones in 20 patients. Radiology 1990;176:19–24.
51. Griffith DP, Gleeson MJ, Appel MF, et al. Percutaneous cholecystolithotomy: a minimally invasive alternative to cholecystectomy and to shock wave lithotripsy. Arch Surg 1990;125:1114–1118.
52. Chiverton SG, Inglis JA, Hudd C, et al. Percutaneous cholecystostomy: the first 60 patients. Br Med J 1990;300:1310–1312.
53. van Heerden JA, Segura JW, LeRoy AJ, et al. Early experience with percutaneous cholecystostomy. Mayo Clin Proc 1991;66:1005–1009.
54. Gillams A, Curtis SC, Donald J, et al. Technical considerations in 113 percutaneous cholecystolithotomies. Radiology 1992;183:163–166.
55. Hwang MH, Mo LR, Chen GD, et al. Percutaneous transhepatic cholecystic ultrasonic lithotripsy. Gastrointest Endosc 1987;33:301–302.
56. Hwang MH, Tsai CC, Mo LR, et al. Percutaneous choledochoscopic biliary tract stone removal: experience in 645 consecutive patients. Eur J Radiol 1993;17:184–190.
57. Cope C. Percutaneous subhepatic cholecystostomy with removable anchor. AJR Am J Roentgenol 1988;151:1129–1132.
58. Cope C. Improved catheter introducer with recessed sheath. AJR Am J Roentgenol 1989;152:1346–1347.
59. Cope C. Novel nitinol basket instrument for percutaneous cholecystolithotomy. AJR Am J Roentgenol 1990;155:515–516.
60. McDermott VG, Arger P, Cope C. Gallstone recurrence and gallbladder function following percutaneous cholecystolithotomy. J Vasc Interv Radiol 1994;5:473–478.
61. van Sonnenberg E, Casola G, Varney RP, et al. Gallbladder and bile duct stones: percutaneous therapy with primary MTBE dissolution and mechanical methods. Radiology 1988;169:505–509.
62. Larsen TB, Gothlin JH, Jensen D, et al. Ultrasonically and fluoroscopically guided therapeutic percutaneous catheter drainage of the gallbladder. Gastrointest Radiol 1988;13:37–40.
63. Bass EB, Steinberg EP, Pitt HA, et al. Cost-effectiveness of extracorporeal shock wave lithotripsy versus cholecystectomy for symptomatic gallstones. Gastroenterology 1991;101:189–199.
64. So CB, Gibney RG, Scudamore CH. Carcinoma of the gallbladder: a risk associated with gallbladder-preserving treatments for cholelithiasis. Radiology 1990;174:127–130.
65. Norrby S, Shonebeck J. Long-term results with cholecystolithotomy. Acta Chir Scand 1970;136:711–713.
66. Gibney RG, Chow K, So CB, et al. Gallstone recurrence after cholecystostomy. AJR Am J Roentgenol 1989;153:287–289.
67. Villanova N, Bazzoli F, Taroni F, et al. Gallstone recurrence after successful oral bile acid treatment. Gastroenterology 1989;97:726–731.

Percutaneous Cholecystostomy

37

S. William Stavropoulos, Aalpen A. Patel, Constantin Cope

Percutaneous trocar decompression of the gallbladder was recorded as far back as 1743 and became used clinically by the end of the 19th century (1). Diagnostic cholecystography by direct percutaneous puncture was first performed in 1922, but it was soon replaced by oral cholecystography (2). Before the advent of antibiotics and the benefits of localizing imaging techniques, percutaneous cholecystostomy (PC) was associated with a high risk of serious or fatal peritonitis resulting from leakage of infected bile, and consequently was usually performed by surgeons only as an emergency diagnostic or decompression procedure before scheduled surgery.

Percutaneous transhepatic cholangiography (PTC) was introduced to provide a more accurate depiction of the biliary tree than was obtainable by oral cholecystography (3). The procedure was further refined and rendered safer by Okuda and his colleagues at Chiba University through the use of smaller-gauge 0.7-mm needles, which were introduced via a right intercostal approach (4). Accidental puncture of the gallbladder was not uncommon during PTC. This was regarded as a potentially serious complication, despite the fact that it usually did not lead to biliary peritonitis if the operator aspirated most of the bile before removing the needle or, in cases of common bile duct obstruction, left a smaller catheter in place for external drainage until the patient had surgery (5). Wannagat demonstrated the potential safety of needle puncture of the gallbladder by performing under laparoscopic-controlled, direct-needle cholecystography in 2,115 patients with only one patient developing biliary peritonitis (6).

Despite the initial fears that percutaneous needle puncture or catheterization of the gallbladder would lead to an unacceptable morbidity, an increasing number of published reports began to appear, starting in 1979, which demonstrated that PC was generally safe when performed under ultrasound guidance with fine needles and catheters (7,8). Today's techniques for PC have become fairly standardized and are being applied to a wide variety of clinical diagnostic and therapeutic procedures.

ANATOMIC CONSIDERATIONS

The gallbladder is a thin-walled, pear-shaped viscus with a capacity of 50–70 mL of bile. It has a remarkable potential for expansion to very large volumes in the face of bile duct obstruction. It lays inferoposteriorly in a fossa of the right hepatic lobe in line with the anatomic division of the liver into right and left lobes. The peritoneum completely covers the sides and posterior surfaces of the body and neck of the gallbladder as well as its fundus, which usually protrudes just beyond the liver edge. The anterior wall of the gallbladder is connected to the liver by fibroareolar tissue to form the bare area, which is quite variable in extent and difficult to recognize by ultrasound examination. Except in unusual congenital anomalies, the anterior relationship of the fundus and body of the normal-sized gallbladder to the liver and anterior abdominal wall is fairly constant. The interventional radiologist should be aware that occasionally the gallbladder may be covered by colon, may be freely movable when anchored by only a mesenteric attachment, or may be located completely within the liver parenchyma (9). The normal gallbladder position and its relationship to other abdominal viscera also may be significantly altered by tumor, hepatomegaly, and hepatic lobe atrophy (10). It is important to appreciate these anatomic variants by prior imaging to find the optimal window for safe cholecystostomy.

PERCUTANEOUS CHOLECYSTOSTOMY

Patients scheduled to undergo percutaneous cholecystostomy should have a detailed history and physical examination; baseline studies of serum bilirubin, amylase, lipase, and alkaline phosphatase; CBC; and a normal or correctable coagulation profile. Because bile in diseased gallbladders is commonly infected, a broad-spectrum antibiotic should be administered 1–4 hours before the diagnostic contrast study or the interventional procedure and continued for another 12 hours or longer in the presence of cholecystitis or cholangitis (11). When available, ultrasound (US) or computed tomography (CT) exams of the abdomen should be reviewed before PC to help in planning the approach to the gallbladder.

Percutaneous cholecystostomy can often be done under local anesthesia with intravenous sedation administered for pain control. If the gallbladder is enlarged or tense and protrudes below the liver, it can be directly punctured transhepatically or subhepatically under real-time ultrasound monitoring with a catheter sheath needle or trocar. Various types of over-the-needle sheaths are commercially available that can be deployed into a locking Cope loop drain with multiple side holes (12). These provide good drainage and largely diminish the chance of accidental removal with resulting biliary peritonitis (Figure 37–1). Although the one-step trocar technique is useful for emergency bedside use and, theoretically, may prevent intraperitoneal bile spillage, it is not always a benign procedure, especially when the gallbladder is not distended or when its wall is chronically thickened (12–15). Under these conditions, the gallbladder may become displaced, invaginated, or perforated and further decompressed. When it is difficult to penetrate, additional fruitless attempts to enter the gallbladder with the large trocar may lead to liver laceration or perforation of the neighboring bowel. In patients with chronic cholecystolithiasis without distended gallbladders, it may therefore be safer initially to insert a removable anchoring device (Figure 37–2) through a coaxial 22-gauge/ 17-gauge needle introducer so that the operator can fixate the fibrotic gallbladder. This precautionary step may prevent loss of the cholecystostomy track or frustrating invagination

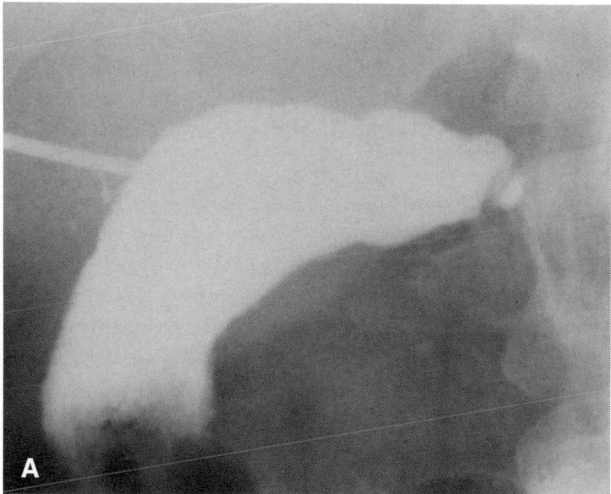

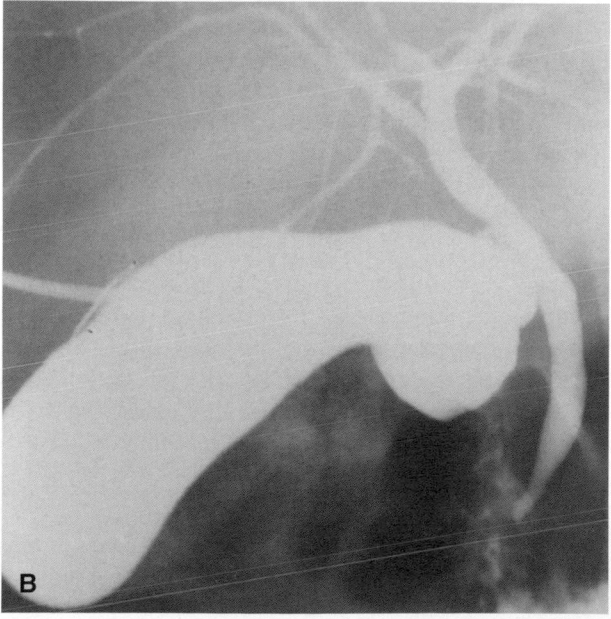

Figure 37–2 PC for acalculous cholecystitis. **A.** A locking-loop catheter has been inserted subhepatically into the gallbladder with an anchor. Note occlusion of the cystic duct. **B.** After 48 hours, there is good drainage into the common bile duct and duodenum. The retaining anchor is visible.

Figure 37–1 An 8 French Cope locking-loop catheter for percutaneous gallbladder drainage.

of the gallbladder wall during the insertion of the cholecystostomy drain (16).

Because of the inherent risks of the one-step trocar technique to access the gallbladder, the Seldinger technique is generally the preferred method for PC. This is accomplished by initially puncturing the gallbladder with a needle under real-time US guidance (13–15). The transhepatic route is preferred when using small needles or catheters because there is less hazard of puncturing the colon and a better likelihood of the liver tamponading the cholecystostomy tract, especially when it passes through the bare area of the gallbladder. In addition, accessing the gallbladder through a transhepatic route causes it to be in a more stable position with less chance that the needle, catheter, or both will push away the gallbladder. Immediately after access to the gallbladder has been obtained, 5 mL of bile is aspirated for analysis and culture. If an 18- or 19-gauge needle is used to access the gallbladder, a 0.035-inch diameter wire can be used to exchange the needle for a dilator, then an 8 French or 10 French locking loop drain can be placed. Alternatively, a 21- or 22-gauge needle can be used for initial US-guided gallbladder access. If a small-diameter needle is used, the needle is exchanged over a 0.018-inch guide wire for a coaxial dilator/sheath assembly. A 0.035 wire can then be placed through the outer portion of the coaxial catheter. The intrahepatic tract can then be dilated, and an 8 French or 10 French locking loop drain can be placed. A commonly used system for access with a 21-gauge needle is the AccuStick II system (Boston Scientific). All exchanges should be done under fluoroscopic guidance to ensure that access to the gallbladder has not been lost. The locking loop catheter can then be secured in place and the gallbladder decompressed. During the procedure, a small amount of contrast may be used to confirm placement in the gallbladder. However, care must be taken not to distend the gallbladder because of the risk of causing sepsis. The catheter can then be placed to gravity drainage. These catheters should be capped only when patency of the cystic duct is confirmed with a contrast injection. This can be done days after initial PC, after the patient has had a chance to recover from the acute event.

Because it may take 2–6 weeks for a transhepatic or subhepatic cholecystostomy tract to form, especially in older, chronically debilitated patients, premature removal of the drainage catheter may lead to gallbladder leakage and peritonitis. For this reason, the operator should check the tract for maturity over a safety guide wire by opacifying it with contrast medium before removing the drain.

BILE SAMPLING

Simple diagnostic procedures of the gallbladder are performed with 21- to 22-gauge needles and are useful for chemical, cellular, and bacteriologic analysis (17). In patients with possible cholecystitis, bile aspirates should be sent to the laboratory for Gram stain, white blood cell count, and bacterial culture. If the bile is light yellow and perfectly clear, the needle may be removed, after as much bile as possible has been aspirated. If the clinical concern for cholecystitis remains high, a 6–8 French Cope-type locking loop drain (Cook, Inc.) may then be inserted as discussed earlier.

CHOLECYSTOCHOLANGIOGRAPHY

In patients with high serum alkaline phosphatase levels and moderate or intermittent elevation of serum bilirubin resulting from possible tumor or stones, percutaneous cholecystocholangiography is a very useful procedure for evaluating the biliary tract for incipient partial obstruction, especially when the intrahepatic bile ducts are insufficiently dilated to be easily punctured transhepatically (Figure 37–3). Once the needle or catheter has been used to empty the gallbladder of bile, contrast medium is injected slowly while the patient is appropriately positioned for optimal opacification of all the major intrahepatic and extrahepatic ducts. Intrahepatic bile duct obstructions may at times be difficult to demonstrate when there is preferential flow of contrast medium into the duodenum. Intravenous administration of 1–2 mg of morphine may, by constricting the sphincter of Oddi, help to retain contrast and lead to better intrahepatic filling.

OBSTRUCTIVE JAUNDICE

In certain patients with complete obstruction of the distal common bile duct, it is not uncommon to find that the intrahepatic ducts are not as proportionally dilated as the

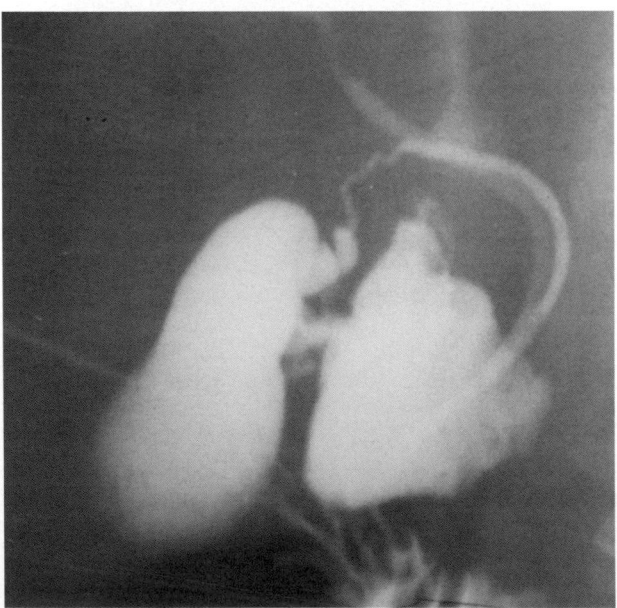

Figure 37–3 Normal transhepatic cholecystocholangiography. A 23-gauge Teflon-sheathed needle was used to opacify the gallbladder and bile ducts in a patient with low-grade bilirubinemia.

gallbladder and the extrahepatic ducts. In fact, intrahepatic ducts may at times remain normal in size or dilated only slightly in the face of a moderately to markedly distended gallbladder. In the presence of minimally enlarged intrahepatic ducts, transhepatic cholangiography and percutaneous transhepatic biliary catheterization may result in a prolonged, frustrating, painful procedure that sometimes may lead to sepsis and may have to be aborted. Under these conditions, the enlarged gallbladder can become a much easier alternative target for percutaneous drainage (18). The gallbladder drain can be used either on a temporary basis for decompressing the biliary system before surgery or for opacifying the intrahepatic ducts so that they can then be punctured more accurately and catheterized under fluoroscopic guidance (Figure 37–4). In the latter case, the cholecystostomy catheter is, of course, not removed until transhepatic biliary drainage has been firmly established. Patients with biliary sepsis following unsuccessful endoscopic biliary catheterization or partial common duct obstruction are especially good candidates for drainage from the gallbladder because they often do not have dilated intrahepatic ducts.

ACUTE CHOLECYSTITIS

The primary treatment for acute cholecystitis in ambulatory patients is cholecystectomy. Emergency surgery in some elderly and frail patients with severe cardiopulmonary disease, however, can be hazardous. Under these conditions, PC may be performed as a temporizing measure until the patient can be stabilized and be given a more complete clinical evaluation (19–21). Sometime later, when the acute cholecystitis has resolved, the patient may be considered for cholecystectomy or for percutaneous stone extraction. Acute cholecystitis in pregnancy represents another condition for which surgery may be hazardous because it may lead to fetal loss. Allmendinger et al. (22) reported two such cases in which PC was performed successfully in pregnant patients using ultrasound guidance.

In hospitalized, critically ill patients and especially in those with multiple system disorders after major surgery or trauma, acute cholecystitis is a potentially lethal complication that can go unrecognized. Right upper quadrant pain, fever, leukocytosis, and a palpable gallbladder can be difficult to elicit or differentiate from other organ system diseases. Other tests, such as ultrasonography and hepatobiliary scanning, are unreliable in diagnosing acute cholecystitis in severely sick and bedridden patients (23,24). These patients usually are too ill to undergo cholecsytectomy (25). In comparison, PC is a safe technique for managing these difficult cases (20,21,26,27). The advantages of the percutaneous method over surgery include increased safety, the need for only local anesthesia with little to no sedation, and less risk to the patient if the diagnosis of acute cholecystitis is in error (28).

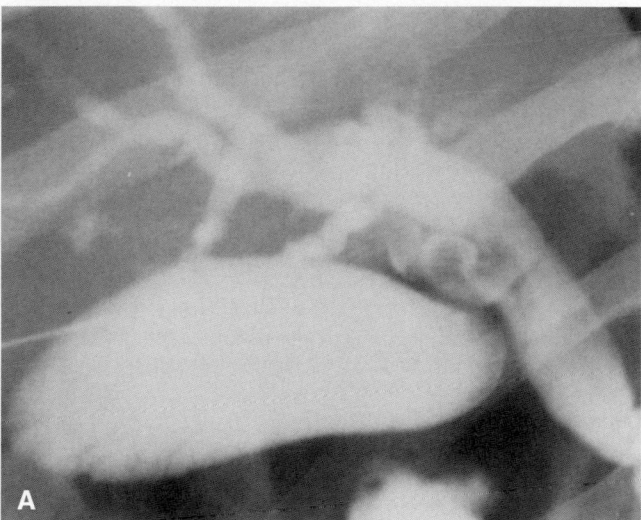

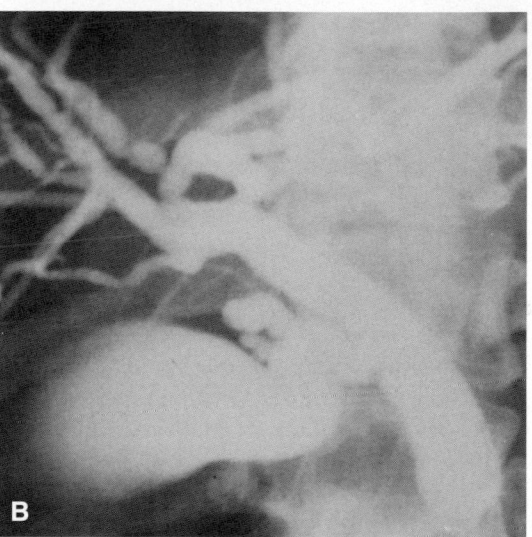

Figure 37–4 Transcholecystic opacification of intrahepatic bile ducts to assist transhepatic biliary puncture. **A.** After six unsuccessful transhepatic biliary duct punctures, the 22-gauge needle was inserted into the gallbladder. The common bile duct and gallbladder are dilated because of a distal malignant stricture, but there is a dearth of enlarged intrahepatic ducts in the dorsocaudal hepatic lobe where initial punctures were made. **B.** Opacification of ducts allowed for prompt insertion of a transhepatic biliary drain. Note that there is no gallbladder leakage after removal of the skinny needle.

Originally, it was believed that the diagnosis of acute cholecystitis could be made by examining aspirated bile for bacteria and the presence of pus and awaiting a positive culture (23). However, with increased experience, McGahan and Lindfors showed that the sensitivity of bile examination is below 50%, most probably because the bile has been rendered sterile by potent antibiotics or else the cholecystitis is not primarily the result of an infectious process (29). A negative aspirate of gallbladder bile does not, therefore, exclude the diagnosis of acute cholecystitis. Today, acute cholecystitis usually is diagnosed, even when the bile is not infected, by observing the patient on continued gallbladder drainage for defervescence of fever, normalization of white blood cell count, and marked clinical improvement over a period of 48 hours (Figure 37–2). If there is no obvious improvement in clinical signs, a cholangiogram is performed to document patency of the cystic duct. Bile duct strictures may also give rise to sepsis and may be treated by dilatation and more selective drainage through the cystic duct. Gross empyema of the gallbladder rapidly can be fatal; however, with early diagnosis and prompt adequate percutaneous drainage, survival rates are high. All patients who are treated or evaluated for cholecystitis by catheter

technique should be considered for immediate cholecystectomy if they develop increasing right upper abdominal pain or peritoneal signs, which can be indicative of a gangrenous or perforated gallbladder (19).

Some patients present with pericholecystic collections by imaging and yet have minimal or no peritoneal signs and little evidence of sepsis, suggesting that they may have a walled-off infection (30). Such patients can be managed successfully by simultaneous percutaneous drainage of the gallbladder and of the perforation abscess (Figure 37–5). Subsequently, the patient may undergo cholecystectomy on an elective basis.

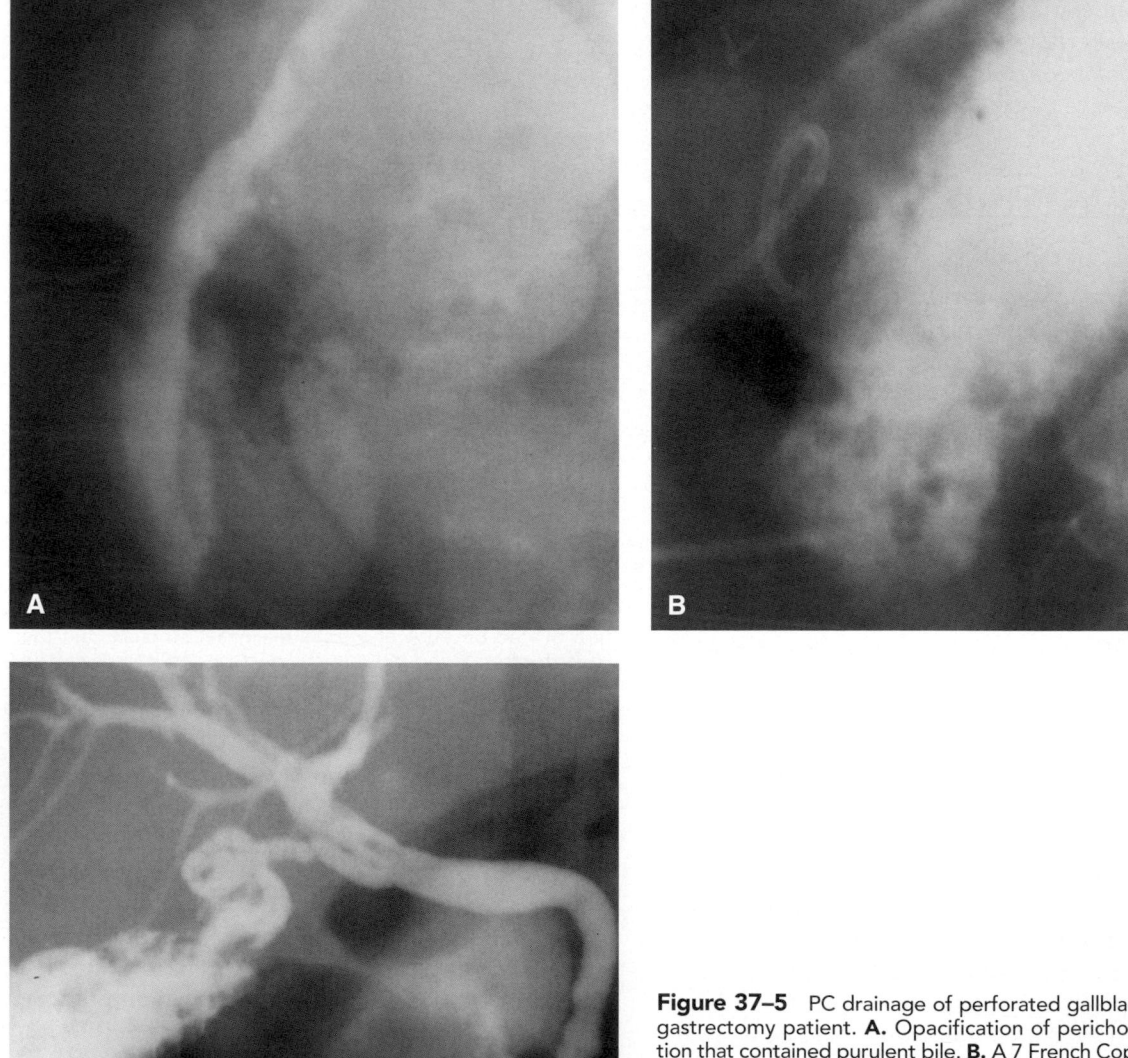

Figure 37–5 PC drainage of perforated gallbladder in a postgastrectomy patient. **A.** Opacification of pericholecystic collection that contained purulent bile. **B.** A 7 French Cope locking-loop drain was inserted in the collection. Opacification of the gallbladder demonstrates multiple gallstones and no drainage through the cystic duct. **C.** Two days later, there is good drainage of the gallbladder into the common bile duct, and the bile is clear. Stones were successfully extracted percutaneously after 10 days, and cholecystectomy was performed 4 months later.

CYSTIC DUCT CATHETERIZATION

Once acute cholecystitis has subsided, and after an adequate period of time on percutaneous drainage, cholecystography may demonstrate unsuspected disease in the cystic duct or major bile ducts, such as benign and malignant strictures or retained calculi, which can be amenable to interventional treatment. In the past, it was believed that normal or moderately dilated cystic ducts could not be traversed from the gallbladder because of the difficulty in passing a catheter past the valves of Heister. With increasing experience and the introduction of hydrophilic catheters and guide wires, however, it is possible today to access the common bile duct in most cases if the cystic duct is patent. The cholecystostomy drain is first removed and replaced with a 7–8 French catheter-introducing sheath positioned with its tip against the opening of the cystic duct to prevent coaxial catheters from coiling within the gallbladder lumen. A 5 French cobra-shaped catheter is passed through the sheath and gently advanced as far as possible into the cystic duct. A guide wire then probes the cystic duct, while at the same time, the catheter is advanced as the guide wire moves forward. Once the guide wire reaches the common duct, the cystic duct will straighten out immediately, making it easy for the catheter to subsequently be maneuvered toward the liver or the duodenum.

The practical clinical usefulness of reaching the common bile duct from the gallbladder includes possibilities for balloon-dilating duct strictures, inserting internal-external drains or stents in patients with pancreatic malignancies, and expelling retained stones (31). If the angle of the cystic duct at its junction with the common duct is not too acute, the common hepatic ducts and their intrahepatic branches may also be catheterized for selective drainage, dilatation, and dislodgment of calculi.

ENDOSCOPY

Following PC, it may be difficult to differentiate sludge from small stones contained within sludge. Calculi adherent to the wall, particularly in the chronically diseased gallbladder, can be confused with cholesterol or inflammatory polyps and adenomas. After percutaneous cholecystolithotomy, it may not be possible to visualize small, retained stone fragments by cholecystography or to distinguish clots from stones. Endoscopy of the gallbladder is a much more accurate way of identifying small calculi and clearing them out. Likewise, the endoscopic recognition of premalignant or malignant tumors can lead to a prompt curative resection. Obviously, it is very important not to leave any stone behind, because retained stone fragments may subsequently grow in size, cause new stone formation, or serve as foci of infection (32). Rigid or flexible endoscopes less than 4 mm in diameter can be readily introduced into the gallbladder through the cholecystostomy tract for inspection, evaluation for retained stones, and, if necessary, biopsy of suspicious mucosal lesions.

BILE PERITONITIS

Bile leakage leading to clinically symptomatic peritonitis is a feared complication of both percutaneous transhepatic biliary drainage and PC. Some patients undergoing percutaneous biliary procedures may develop massive biliary ascites with no immediate ill effects, whereas in others, a minor bile leakage may lead to serious biliary peritonitis (33). Obviously, the role of bacterial infection is paramount in the development of this complication. It has been shown in rats that bile injected intraperitoneally produces no adverse effects; however, when the bile is mixed with an inoculum of *Escherichia coli*, the combination gives rise to a much higher mortality rate than when *E. coli* alone is administered (34). Leakage of infected bile can be minimized with the use of small needles and catheters and with replacement of the gallbladder bile immediately after entry with sterile saline or dilute contrast medium. Preprocedural, wide-spectrum antibiotics should be administered before percutaneous gallbladder interventional procedures are undertaken.

OTHER COMPLICATIONS

In addition to the potential for biliary peritonitis, complicated bile leakage may also occur days or weeks later if the drainage catheter gets removed inadvertently or displaced into the peritoneal cavity or when the drain is extracted prematurely (35). It should be remembered that a mature cholecystostomy tract may take 4–6 weeks to develop in elderly debilitated patients and 2–3 months or longer in patients who are immunocompromised. Other reported complications of PC include hemobilia, severe vasovagal reactions, pneumothorax, intraperitoneal hemorrhage, and sepsis (13).

Although only minor complications are described in series dealing with simple diagnostic PC using only fine needles and catheters, reviews of larger studies that include interventional procedures indicate that major complications requiring surgery, transfusions, or vascular pressor therapy can reach values as high as 5.6–8.7% (13,36,37). Such morbidity is often because of a diseased gallbladder wall, the use of larger trocars and drains, or the presence of severe concurrent illness or multisystem failure. The procedure-related mortality rate caused by hemorrhage, gallbladder perforation, and sepsis is less than 2% and (as discussed earlier) is often related to patients' comorbid medical conditions.

SUMMARY

Percutaneous cholecystostomy is a safe procedure for diagnostic bacteriologic and contrast studies. When it is used as an access route for interventional procedures, it is well-tolerated and has been found to be especially useful for managing patients with multiple risk factors, either as a temporizing measure or as a definitive treatment.

REFERENCES

1. Glenn F, Grafe WR Jr. Historical events in biliary tract surgery. Arch Surg 1966;93:848–855.
2. Burckhardt H, Muller W. Versuche über die punktion der Gallenbläse und ihre Röntgendarstellung. Dtsch Z Chir 1921; 162:168–171.
3. Glenn F, Evans JA, Mujahed Z, et al. Percutaneous transhepatic cholangiography. Ann Surg 1962;156:451–462.
4. Okuda K, Tanikawa K, Emura T, et al. Nonsurgical, percutaneous transhepatic cholangiography—diagnostic significance in medical problems of the liver. Am J Dig Dis 1974;19:21–36.
5. DeMasi CJ, Akdamar K, Sparks RA, et al. Puncture of the gallbladder during percutaneous transhepatic cholangiography. JAMA 1967;201:225–228.
6. Wannagat L. [Laparoscopic cholangiography]. Radiologe 1973; 13:26–34.
7. Elyaderani M, Gabriele O. Percutaneous cholecystostomy and cholangiography in patients with obstructive jaundice. Radiology 1979;130:601–602.
8. Shaver RW, Hawkins IF Jr, Soong J. Percutaneous cholecystostomy. AJR Am J Roentgenol 1982;138:1133–1136.
9. Chuang VP. The aberrant gallbladder: angiographic and radioisotopic considerations. AJR Am J Roentgenol 1976;127:417–421.
10. Gore RM, Ghahremani GG, Joseph AE, et al. Acquired malposition of the colon and gallbladder in patients with cirrhosis: CT findings and clinical implications. Radiology 1989;171:739–742.
11. Farnell MB, van Heerden A, Beart RW. Elective cholecystectomy: the role of biliary bacteriology and administration of antibiotics. Arch Surg 1981;116:537–540.
12. McGahan JP. A new catheter design for percutaneous cholecystostomy. Radiology 1988;166:49–52.
13. Teplick SK, Brandon JC, Wolferth CC, et al. Percutaneous interventional gallbladder procedures: personal experience and literature review. Gastrointest Radiol 1990;15:133–136.
14. Sosna J, Copel L, Kane RA, et al. Ultrasound-guided percutaneous cholecystostomy: update on technique and clinical applications. Surg Technol Int. 2003;11:135–139.
15. Akhan O, Akinci D, Ozmen MN. Percutaneous cholecystostomy. Eur J Radiol 2002;43:229–236.
16. Cope C. Percutaneous subhepatic cholecystostomy with removable anchor. AJR Am J Roentgenol 1988;151:1129–1132.
17. Swobodnik W, Hagert N, Janowitz P, et al. Diagnostic fine-needle puncture of the gallbladder with US guidance. Radiology 1991; 178:755–758.
18. van Sonnenberg E. The benefits of percutaneous cholecystostomy for decompression of selected cases of obstructive jaundice. Radiology 1990;176:15–18.
19. Werbel GB, Nahrwold DL, Joehl RL, et al. Percutaneous cholecystostomy in the diagnosis and treatment of acute cholecystitis in the high-risk patient. Arch Surg 1989;124:782–786.
20. Bryne MF, Suhocki P, Mitchell RM, et al. Percutaneous cholecystostomy in patients with acute cholecystitis: experience of 45 patients at a US referral center. J Am Coll Surg 2003;197:206–211.
21. Berman M, Nudelman IL, Fuko Z, et al. Percutaneous transhepatic cholecystostomy: effective treatment of acute cholecystitis in high risk patients. Isr Med Assoc J 2002;4:331–333.
22. Allmendinger N, Hallisey MJ, Ohki SK, et al. Percutaneous cholecystostomy treatment of acute cholecystitis in pregnancy. Obstet Gynecol 1995;86:653–654.
23. McGahan JP, Walter JP. Diagnostic percutaneous aspiration of the gallbladder. Radiology 1985;155:619–622.
24. Lee MJ, Saini S, Brink JA. Treatment of critically ill patients with sepsis of unknown cause: value of percutaneous cholecystostomy. AJR Am J Roentgenol 1991;156:1163–1166.
25. Glenn F. Cholecystostomy in the high risk patient with biliary tract disease. Ann Surg 1977;185:185–191.
26. Teplick SK, Brandon JC, Wolferth CC. Percutaneous interventional gallbladder procedures: personal experience and literature review. Gastrointest Radiol 1990;15:133–136.
27. Davis CA, Landercasper J, Gundersen LH, et al. Effective use of percutaneous cholecystostomy in high-risk surgical patients: techniques, tube management, and results. Arch Surg 1999;134: 727–731.
28. Herbel GB, Nahrwold DL, Voehl RJ, et al. Percutaneous cholecystostomy in the diagnosis and treatment of acute cholecystitis in the high-risk patient. Arch Surg 1989;124:782–785.
29. McGahan JP, Lindfors KK. Acute cholecystitis: diagnostic accuracy of percutaneous aspiration of the gallbladder. Radiology 1988;167:669–671.
30. van Sonnenberg E, D'Agostino HB, Casola G, et al. Gallbladder perforation and bile leakage: percutaneous treatment. Radiology 1991;178:687–689.
31. Dawson SL, Girard MJ, Saini S, et al. Placement of a metallic biliary endoprosthesis via cholecystostomy. AJR Am J Roentgenol 1991;157:4911–4913.
32. Cope C, Burke DR, Meranze SG. Percutaneous extraction of gallstones in 20 patients. Radiology 1990;176:19–24.
33. Taormina V, McLean GK. Chronic bile peritonitis with progressive bile ascites: a complication of percutaneous biliary drainage. Cardiovasc Intervent Radiol 1985;8:103–105.
34. Andersson R, Tranberg KG, Bengmark S. Roles of bile and bacteria in biliary peritonitis. Br J Surg 1990;77:36–39.
35. Hawkins IF Jr. Percutaneous cholecystostomy. Semin Intervent Radiol 1985;2:97–103.
36. Takahashi T, Tada S, Ida M, et al. Complications of percutaneous transhepatic gallbladder drainage. Radiology 1993;189P:307.
37. van Sonnenberg E, D'Agostino HB, Goodacre BW, et al. Percutaneous gallbladder puncture and cholecystostomy: results, complications, and caveats for safety. Radiology 1992;183: 167–170.

Interventional Radiology of the Genitourinary System

VI

Nephroureteral Obstruction

38

Parvati Ramchandani

Radiologically directed percutaneous interventional procedures are applicable in the management of urinary tract obstructions that result from virtually any cause. This chapter addresses percutaneous nephrostomy (PCN), ureteral stenting and dilation, and interventions in obstructed renal transplants.

PERCUTANEOUS NEPHROSTOMY (PCN)

From the first descriptions in the mid-1950s (1,2), PCN has evolved to become the cornerstone of interventional procedures in the urinary tract. Radiologists perform the majority of upper urinary tract decompressions, nearly 74% (3), and urologists typically perform the remainder. Urologist-initiated renal access is often a prelude to stone removal (percutaneous nephrostolithotomy, or PCNL), but the availability of C-arm fluoroscopy units in operating rooms and ultrasound machines in urology departments allows urologists to perform PCN for decompression of the collecting systems as well (4–7). PCN has established itself as a safe and effective

alternative to surgical nephrostomies, which it has almost completely supplanted.

Although initially developed as a technique to drain obstructed urinary tracts, PCN now is increasingly used to provide access to the collecting system. Thus, it is often just the first step in performing various other interventional procedures in the kidney and ureter. The indications for PCN vary depending on the referral patterns and the patient population in an individual institution and include the following:

1. *To rapidly relieve urinary obstruction, whether acute or long-standing.* PCN is most often requested in patients after imaging studies demonstrate hydroureteronephrosis. These studies may also indicate the etiology as well as the anatomic level of the obstruction. In a recent series of patients with renal impairment resulting from ureteral obstruction (8,9), noncontrast CT was found to be the best imaging modality for identifying calculus causes of obstruction, while magnetic resonance urography (MRU) was superior for identifying noncalculus causes of obstruction. In patients with normal renal function,

contrast-enhanced CT can identify the presence and cause of hydronephrosis in nearly all cases (10). MRU is particularly helpful in delineating the anatomy in patients with urinary diversion to bowel conduits (11). In one series (12), urinary obstruction was related to calculus disease in 26% of patients and malignancy in 61%. Carcinoma of the bladder, cervix, and colon were the most common primaries in the patients with malignancies and urinary obstruction.

It is important to attempt or at least to consider the retrograde approach for renal drainage before resorting to the percutaneous route; the latter should ideally be reserved for patients in whom retrograde attempts are either unsuccessful or not feasible (13).

2. *To gain access to the collecting system for therapeutic and diagnostic procedures.* This application of PCN is the most frequent indication for the procedure in many institutions (14,15), particularly where the urologists are active in endourologic therapy.

Examples of such procedures include: the treatment of renal or ureteral calculi such as stone fragmentation, removal, or chemolysis (Figure 38–1); ureteral interventions such as stricture dilation or stent placement; retrieval of foreign bodies such as fractured stent

fragments; nephroscopic surgery such as endopyelotomy for ureteropelvic junction (UPJ) obstruction; and brush biopsy or percutaneous therapy of urothelial tumors (Figures 38–2 and 38–3). Interventions can often be done at the same sitting as the PCN when the procedure is not complicated by excessive bleeding and no infection exists.

3. *Urinary diversion to allow closure of a ureteral fistula or a dehiscent urinary tract anastomosis.* In most cases, PCN drainage alone is unsuccessful in totally diverting the urine output from the kidney, and the addition of either ureteral stenting or ureteral occlusion (the latter in patients with intractable vesicovaginal fistulas) is required. In Farrell's large series of patients (12), urinary fistulae were the most common nonobstructive indication for PCN placement; this series did not include patients undergoing PCN for removal of stones. Urine diversion by PCN alone has been used with some success to treat patients with intractable hemorrhagic cystitis (16).

4. *To assess residual function in a chronically obstructed kidney that appears to be either nonfunctioning or poorly functioning.* Temporary renal drainage by PCN may allow assessment of residual recoverable function so that one

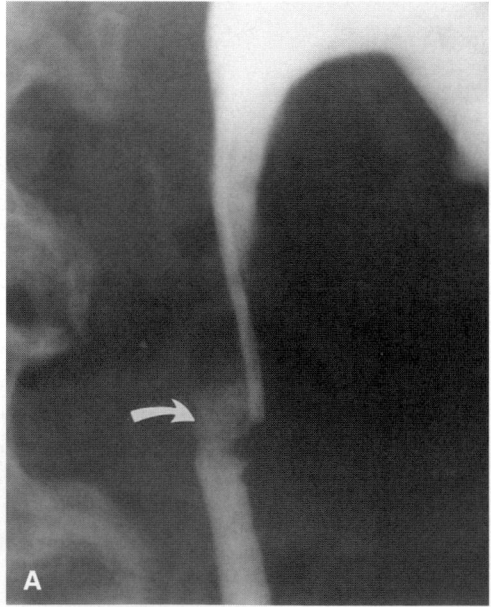
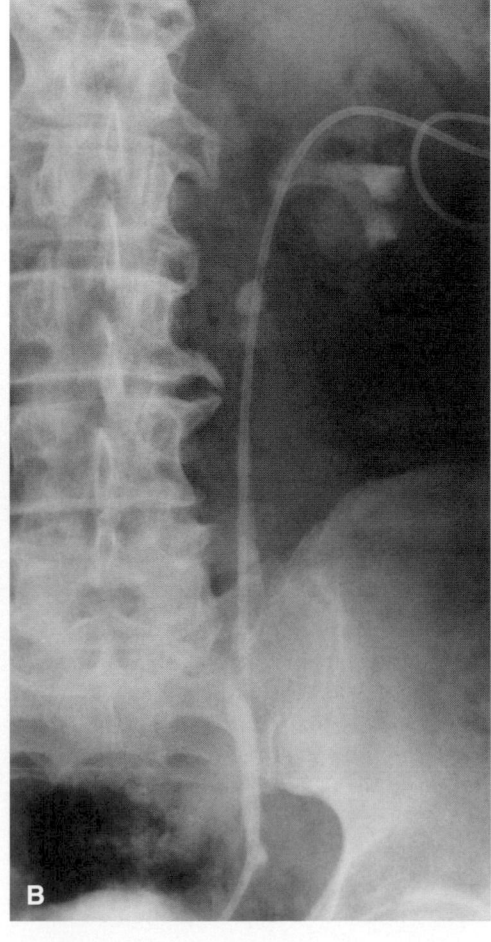

Figure 38–1 Percutaneous nephrostomy (PCN) for obstructing proximal ureteral calculus. Extracorporeal shock wave lithotripsy had failed to fragment the stone. **A.** Obstructing proximal ureteral calculus (*arrow*). **B.** A 5 French catheter was negotiated past the calculus, but the stone could not be trapped within a basket because it was embedded in the wall. It was removed ureteroscopically.

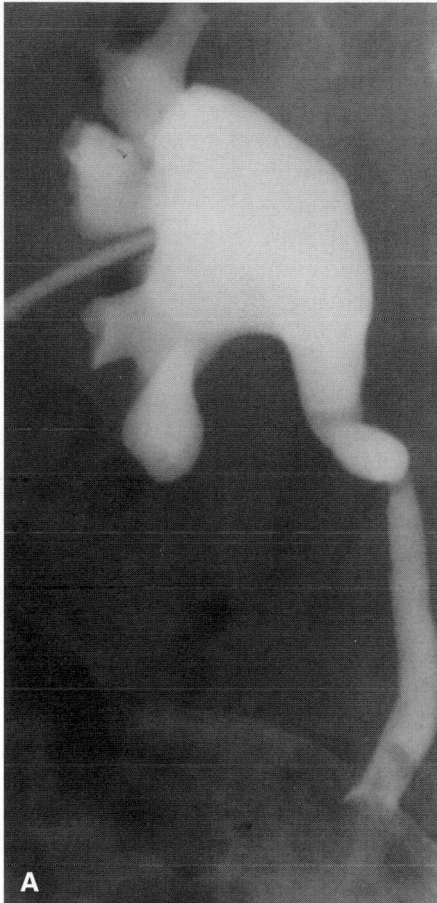
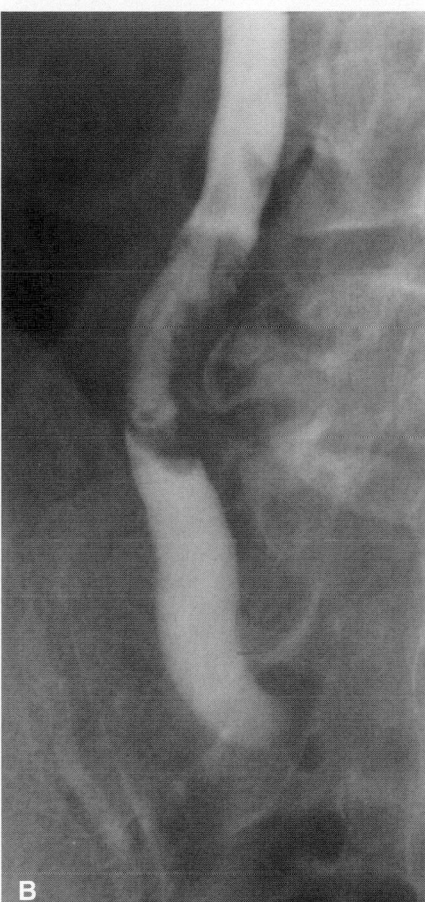

Figure 38–2 PCN for right renal obstruction in a patient with a history of bladder cancer. **A.** Contrast injection in the right collecting system shows moderate hydronephrosis and a filling defect in the right distal lumbar ureter. **B.** Selective contrast injection into the ureter demonstrates to better advantage the large and irregular filling defect in the right ureter. Subsequent brush biopsy via the nephrostomy tract confirmed transitional cell carcinoma recurrence in the ureter.

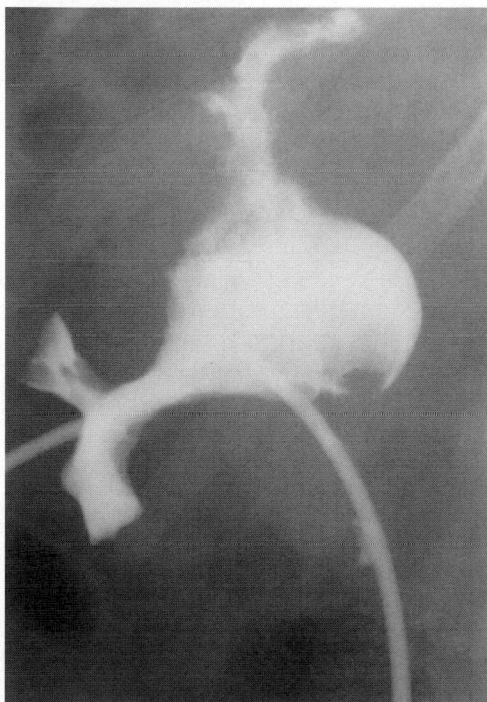

Figure 38–3 Percutaneous nephrostomy for obstructing transitional cell carcinoma in renal pelvis of solitary kidney. The patient underwent nephroscopic resection of the tumor, which was managed with a nephroureteral drainage catheter.

can determine whether a kidney is worth salvaging. Kidneys that contribute 15–20% of overall renal function after relief of obstruction usually are deemed to be worth salvaging. A substantial increase in renal plasma flow within 10 days after decompression of an obstructed kidney is a reliable predictor of recovering renal function. The presence of renal parenchymal atrophy on computed tomography (CT) or renal ultrasonography does not always portend a poor potential for functional recovery after a PCN. However, in patients with bilateral obstruction resulting from an underlying malignancy, imaging can help determine the kidney that is less obstructed; when unilateral PCN is performed in such patients, drainage of the less affected kidney may be more effective in restoring renal function to baseline.

TECHNIQUE

Preprocedural Evaluation

Preprocedural evaluation in patients being considered for PCN includes a clinical history to identify a potential bleeder as well as routine laboratory tests of coagulation and renal function (17–20). Although laboratory coagulation screening is widespread among radiologists, the surgical and medical literature does not support this practice (17,21,22). The radiology literature has advocates who subscribe to both views; routine testing of all patients undergoing invasive procedures is advised by some (20,23), while others may not postpone an emergent PCN to wait for laboratory results (24). Some authorities believe it is sufficient to carefully question the patient for bleeding history and for known liver disease, renal failure, and use of antiplatelet drugs and anticoagulants (25).

Correction of abnormal coagulation is needed when the international normalized ratio (INR)—the standardized reporting of prothrombin time—and activated partial thromboplastin time (PTT) are more than 1.5 times above the normal range (21). Fresh frozen plasma (FFP) will correct congenital factor deficiency and acquired coagulopathy. The corrective effect lasts only 6 hours, so the procedure has to be appropriately timed with the FFP infusion. When patients are on heparin, discontinuing the infusion and waiting 2–3 hours to perform the procedure are often sufficient, because heparin has a half-life of 60 minutes (longer in patients with liver disease) (21), but activated coagulation time can be checked whenever there is clinical concern. Abnormalities related to warfarin can be corrected with vitamin K1 or FFP administration (21).

If the patient is taking aspirin or other drugs known to interfere with platelet function, such as nonsteroidal anti-inflammatory drugs or newer betalactam antibiotics (21), a planned elective procedure either can be postponed for 3–10 days after the last dose of aspirin or the bleeding time can be used as a guide and the procedure delayed if the bleeding time exceeds the upper range of normal (19). Most interventionalists do not postpone invasive procedures in patients who have taken aspirin (17). Platelet transfusion will correct drug-induced prolongation of the bleeding time, if needed.

Farrell et al. reported that platelet counts <100,000/dL (12) were a significant risk factor for bleeding and were associated with a higher transfusion rate after PCN. However, platelet counts <50,000/dL is a safe value for most patients (21).

Septicemia is less common with genitourinary interventions than with biliary procedures, but the risk of periprocedural sepsis is increased in the elderly; in diabetics; and in patients with indwelling catheters, stones, ureterointestinal anastomosis, or the clinical presence of infection. Septic shock can occur in as many as 7% of patients with pyonephrosis (26–28). The organisms that commonly infect the genitourinary tract are gram-negative rods and include E. coli, Proteus, Klebsiella, and enterococcus. Antibiotic prophylaxis ideally should be based on culture results. In patients with obstruction and overt clinical infection in whom a specific organism has not yet been identified, broad-spectrum antibiotics active against the common urinary pathogens is prudent. Some options are aminoglycosides, such as gentamycin, in conjunction with ampicillin or cefazolin, or ceftriaxone (29). Antibiotics are best administered immediately before or less than 2 hours before the procedure (29); if given more than 3 hours

before the procedure, incidence of adverse infectious events increases fivefold (30). Antibiotic therapy should be continued until satisfactory renal drainage is assured to avoid postprocedural bacteremia caused by entry of organisms into the bloodstream (18,29,31). Cochran et al. (18) reported that prophylactic antibiotics were beneficial in decreasing the development of sepsis in both high-risk patients, including those with struvite stones, diabetes, urinary tract obstruction, indwelling catheters, previous manipulation, or instrumentation of the urinary tract, and in patients with a low risk for developing sepsis. They recommended that the antibiotics be administered in such a way that maximum blood levels would be attained during the procedure and that the antibiotics be continued for 24–48 hours in low-risk groups and for 48–72 hours in high-risk groups.

PCNs are often performed as an inpatient procedure. When performed on an outpatient basis, 12–25% of patients may require admission to the hospital after the procedure because of complications, such as bleeding or sepsis (25). Patients who may not be suitable candidates for outpatient PCN include those with hypertension, untreated urinary tract infection, coagulopathy, and staghorn calculi (18,25). Outpatient PCN has also been performed successfully in children and adolescents with no tube- or procedure-related problems (32).

Periprocedural Monitoring

Continuous electrocardiogram monitoring during the procedure is advisable. Large-bore and secure intravenous access should be established routinely before the procedure so that intravenous sedation and analgesia can be administered during the procedure and intravenous access is readily available when other medications need to be administered. Intravenous sedation combined with local anesthesia is sufficient to keep most patients comfortable; such patients require transcutaneous oximetry. Epidural anesthesia can be used in patients with renal calculi who are to undergo stone removal through the nephrostomy track either on the same day or on the following day; in these cases, a flexible epidural catheter is placed in the epidural space through which local anesthetic agents can be instilled. This serves to keep patients comfortable for both the PCN and the subsequent track dilatation and percutaneous nephrostolithotomy.

Procedure

The patient is positioned in either a prone or prone oblique position with the ipsilateral side elevated 20–30 degrees. The procedure can be performed with the patient in a supine oblique position if he or she cannot lie prone. CT guidance is particularly helpful in this circumstance, allowing completion of the procedure in 81% of patients in one series in which a hybrid CT-fluoroscopy unit was used (33);

initial puncture was performed with CT guidance and the subsequent manipulations for catheter placement were performed with fluoroscopic guidance.

The collecting system can be localized with fluoroscopy or ultrasound (US) guidance (Figure 38–4). When the collecting system is moderately or severely dilated, US guidance is successful in aiding entry into the collecting system in 85–95% of patients; conversely, in mildly dilated collecting systems, the success rate may be as low as 50% (34). If renal function is poor (the usual case with obstruction) or if contrast cannot be administered, US guidance is the preferred way to localize the collecting system because, in part, it can provide a precise measurement of the depth of the pelvocaliceal system and also can direct the puncture into the optimal calix. Real-time ultrasound (either a portable scanner or a unit housed in the fluoroscopy suite) and a transducer-mounted needle guide can facilitate the procedure. The needle can be observed as it is advanced from the skin into the kidney. The transducer is covered with a sterile sleeve, and the needle tip is followed with real-time scanning as it enters the retroperitoneum, kidney, and the collecting system (Figure 38–4).

Fluoroscopic guidance is used to enter the collecting system when a previous urographic study is available for guidance, when an opaque caliceal calculus can serve as the target for puncture, or when the collecting system can be opacified with contrast (either by excretion after intravenous administration or by means of a retrograde catheter). Once the collecting system has been entered, the remainder of the procedure is performed with fluoroscopic guidance although there are reports of using sonography alone for the entire procedure (35). Blind punctures of the kidney using anatomic landmarks, such as the "lumbar notch" (6,36), are apt to require multiple punctures for optimal entry in as many as 40% of cases and should be measures of last resort in modern radiology departments in which the availability of ultrasound can facilitate appropriate and safe puncture of the collecting system with the fewest number of sticks.

As mentioned earlier, CT-controlled fluoroscopy has been used to allow PCN placement with the patient in a supine or supine oblique position (33,37). CT has been used to perform the entire procedure (37) or only for the initial needle placement with fluoroscopic guidance being used for the catheter placement itself (33). Preprocedural CT or MR scanning is necessary and highly recommended in patients with aberrant anatomy, such as severe scoliosis or congenital abnormalities, so that the relationship of the kidney to the liver, spleen, colon, gallbladder, and pleural space can be determined (Figure 38–5).

Puncturing the collecting system in patients who do not have collecting system dilation can be difficult. When intravenous (IV) contrast can be administered, fluoroscopic guidance is used for the procedure. However, when IV contrast cannot be given, such as in patients with renal failure resulting from obstruction but no detectable dilation of the collecting system (38) or in patients in whom intravenous contrast cannot be administered, ultrasound guidance has been used after IV administration of a diuretic agent (39). MR-guided PCN has also been described in the nondilated porcine urinary tract (40,41).

Numerous techniques have been described for PCN placement (12,23,36,42–45), and all entail imaging and puncturing the collecting system, dilating the tract, and placing a catheter. Planning the puncture site is the most crucial step in the procedure because a poorly placed puncture can make the track dilation technically arduous and fraught with complications.

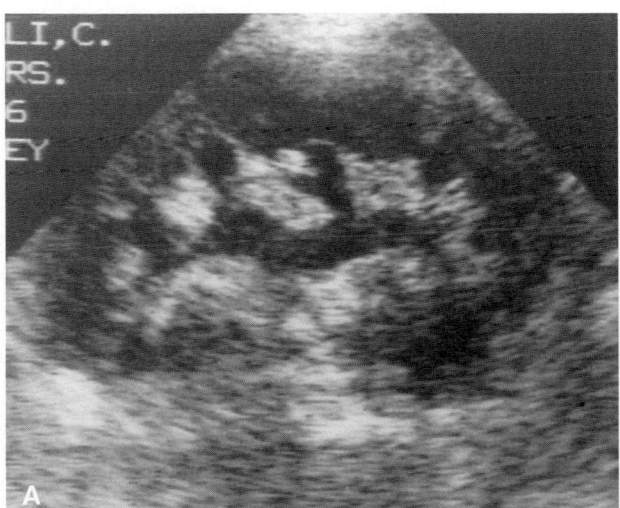 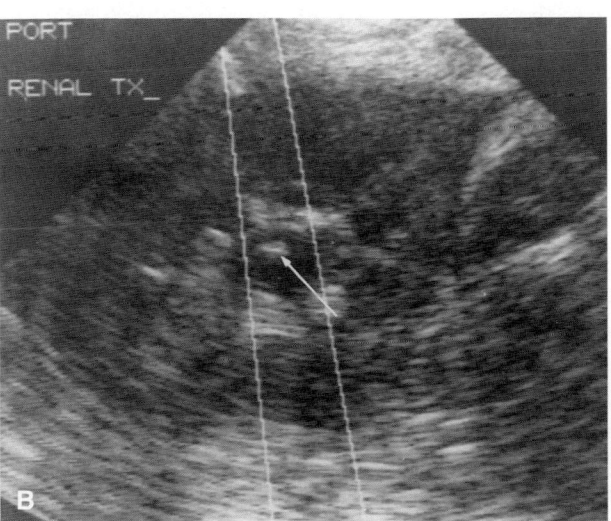

Figure 38–4   Ultrasound guidance for nephrostomy placement. **A.** Ultrasonogram of a renal transplant demonstrates hydronephrosis. **B.** Electronic lines define the track into the collecting system. The needle tip is visualized as an echogenic focus (*arrow*).

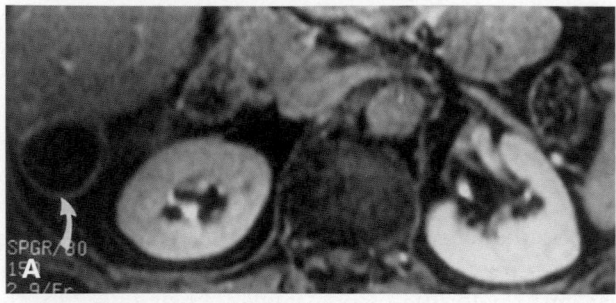

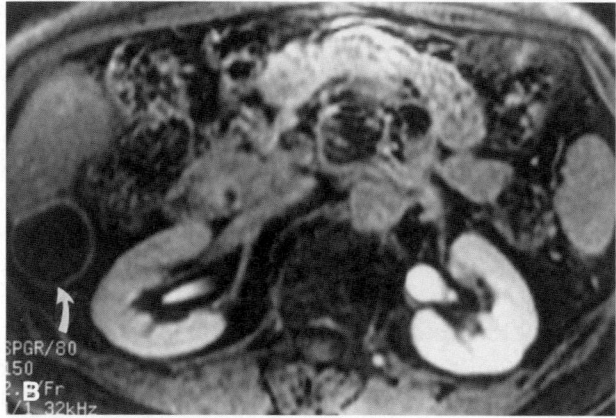

Figure 38–5 MRI demonstration of relationship of spleen and gallbladder to kidneys. Higher section **A.** and lower section **B.** demonstrate the proximity of the spleen and distended gallbladder (*arrow*) to the kidneys. Both organs are likely to be entered inadvertently by a puncture that is too far lateral beyond the posterior axillary line.

The skin puncture site is chosen so that the catheter enters the flank in the posterior axillary line, approximately 5–7 fingerbreadths lateral to the midline and just lateral to the erector spinae muscle below the twelfth rib. The track should course subcostally, well below the inferior margin of the twelfth rib. This placement minimizes the chances of injury to the intercostal artery and decreases the chances of intercostal nerve irritation, which can be very painful. If the intercostal space between the eleventh and twelfth ribs is used, care should be taken to stay close to the superior aspect of the twelfth rib to avoid the neurovascular bundle. The puncture should be advanced at an angle of approximately 30–45 degrees and should traverse the renal parenchyma before entering a posteriorly directed calix. This approach results in an oblique (posterolateral) nephrostomy tract that passes lateral to the paraspinous muscles (and medial and posterior to the peritoneum and colon) and enters the renal parenchyma at the relatively avascular posterolateral plane of the kidney (Brödel line), minimizing the risk of entering the large vessels in the renal hilum. The avascular plane of Brödel is in the zone where the renal artery divides into major ventral and dorsal branches and lies at the junction of the anterior two thirds and posterior one third of the kidney, just posterior to the lateral convex border of the kidney. The posterior calyces point to this plane and can be identified as the more medially positioned

calices; air introduced into the collecting system accumulates in the posterior calyces in the prone position, while contrast outlines the dependent anterior calyces (36). Such a track is not only safer but also more likely to be comfortable for a patient in the supine recumbent position. Also, the risk of catheter kinking is minimized. All nephrostomy catheters should traverse the renal parenchyma before entering the collecting system so that the parenchyma can provide a secure seal around the catheter.

If PCN is being performed for drainage alone, virtually any posterior calyx can be suitable for access, although an interpolar or lower polar posterior calyx is usually chosen. However, when PCN is to be followed by ureteral stent insertion, an interpolar caliceal entry is preferable so that the vector of pushing forces can be directed toward the ureteropelvic junction. Access through the upper pole calices may be required in patients with stones, in which case an intercostal tract may be needed.

Once the puncture site is chosen, local anesthesia is administered liberally into the skin site and throughout the proposed track to the level of the renal fascia. Several puncture sets using coaxial needles, sheaths, or both are commercially available for the procedure. After localization, the collecting system is initially punctured with thin-walled, flexible, 21- or 22-gauge needles. A sample of urine is withdrawn and sent for culture, if necessary. A small amount of contrast is then injected to confirm the needle position and to determine the caliceal entry site. In a dilated and obstructed collecting system, an attempt should be made to decompress the collecting system before contrast injection. Care should be taken to inject a volume of contrast that is less than the volume of urine aspirated to avoid overdistention and possible sepsis. The purpose of contrast injection is merely to confirm the position of the needle. If the initial entry point into the collecting system is not optimal, a second puncture is performed into the desired calix with either a second 21-gauge needle (the first needle is not removed to avoid decompression of the collecting system through the needle site and to provide a route for continuing opacification) or an 18-gauge trocar stylet needle. In patients undergoing nephrostomy for subsequent stone removal, puncture with 18-gauge needles may be preferable because such larger-gauge needles are less flexible and thus easier to direct into the desired calyx. Puncture of the renal infundibula or pelvis should be avoided because of a high risk of injury to the interlobar vessels and the major segmental branches of the renal artery and vein. Sampaio and associates found that punctures through the caliceal fornix were highly unlikely to cause renal arterial injury, whereas infundibular punctures lacerated interlobar or segmental arteries in 23% of cases, and direct renal pelvic punctures caused injury to a large retropelvic vessel in 33% of cases (46).

If a 21-gauge needle has been used for the puncture, the commercially available introducer sets are used to eventually place a 0.038-inch (0.87-mm) guide wire into the collecting system. If an 18-gauge needle has been used, the

0.038-inch guide wire can be directly advanced through the needle. The nephrostomy track is then dilated with fascial dilators to one size larger than the intended nephrostomy catheter, then a nephrostomy catheter is placed. A self-retaining catheter is preferable, which may be of a pigtail, accordion, Malecot, or Foley type. A "self-retaining" loop-type catheter (Cope loop catheter) is used in most cases and is less prone to being inadvertently withdrawn than Malecot and Foley catheters. Initially, even these catheters are best secured to the skin with a suture to prevent accidental withdrawal. With well-developed nephrostomy tracks, skin sutures are rarely necessary. The tubes are held to the skin with either gauze and adhesive tape or clear "breathable" skin dressing. The self-retaining loop catheters are also available with a hydrophilic coating, which theoretically should facilitate catheter insertion. However, with proper tract selection and guide wire use, the placement of nephrostomy catheters in most cases is straightforward.

Contraindications

Contraindications have to be considered in the context of the potential risks and benefits for each individual patient. The only absolute contraindication is the presence of an uncorrectable bleeding disorder; however, if the bleeding diathesis is the result of a coagulopathy caused by urosepsis, urinary drainage will be necessary before the bleeding abnormality can be corrected. If there are severe electrolyte changes because of the obstructive uropathy, such as hyperkalemia with serum potassium levels above 7 mEq/L, emergency hemodialysis, ion exchange therapy, or both should be considered before PCN to quickly correct the electrolyte abnormalities, because the cardioplegia associated with hyperkalemia can be refractory to all therapy.

Results

A PCN catheter can be successfully placed in 98–99% of patients with obstructed dilated kidneys and allows for immediate renal decompression. (12,24,47,48,49). In nondilated systems or in complex stone cases, 85–90% success has been reported (42). Success rates are lower, in the range of 91–92%, when sonography alone is used for the procedure (35,50).

Lee et al. (24) analyzed the outcomes of emergency nephrostomies performed by radiologists who had different levels of experience; all operators performed a minimum of 10 PCNs a year. Although the operators successfully placed drainage catheters on an emergent basis, mean procedure and fluoroscopy times were significantly longer for the more inexperienced radiologists—fluoroscopy and procedure times were 2 minutes/25 minutes for experienced operators and 10 minutes/42 minutes for inexperienced operators. Furthermore, 20–33% of the procedures performed by inexperienced operators were repeated the next day because of catheter dislodgment or malposition. Lewis et al. (51) found that proportionately more complications occurred when the

procedures were performed after regular working hours rather than during regular working hours (5.7% versus 1.8%). Lee et al. (24) also found that emergency PCNs by less experienced radiologists resulted in higher rates of postprocedure sepsis and transfusions. These are potentially worrisome findings because many patients experiencing the procedure after hours are sicker and have more complications than those undergoing elective procedures. Availability of radiologists experienced in performing PCNs and availability of other critical support staff on a 24/7 basis varies across institutions, but there is consensus that in the ideal situation, appropriate staff and equipment are available to provide the same high level of care after hours as during regular daytime hours (23,52).

When obstruction is complicated by urosepsis or azotemia, the response to renal decompression is marked and often immediate with fever and flank pain improving in 24–48 hours after PCN drainage (53). In one series (54), PCN decreased the mortality from gram-negative septicemia from 40% to 8% in patients with urinary obstruction complicated by infection. When obstruction and infection are because of ureteral calculi, retrograde ureteral catheterization and PCN are equally effective in relieving the obstruction and infection; neither technique is superior to the other in promoting rapid drainage or clinical defervescence (55). Although pyonephrosis mandates emergent drainage, percutaneous manipulations themselves can readily precipitate septicemia (manifested as shaking, chills, and fever) in these patients. It is important to treat these patients with intravenous antibiotics before the attempted PCN. In addition, forceful opacification of the collecting system to visualize the site and the cause of obstruction should be deferred until the collecting system has been adequately decompressed for 24–48 hours and the patient is afebrile (Figure 38-6). The addition of contrast to an already distended, infected system may force bacteria into the peripapillary veins and induce urosepsis (28,54). In patients with fungal urinary infections, topical antibiotics can be infused directly into the kidneys whenever systemic toxicity prevents one from achieving effective therapeutic levels by parenteral administration; in addition, obstructing fungus balls can be extracted through the nephrostomy track (56).

In patients with azotemia secondary to obstruction, PCN provides rapid amelioration of impending renal failure with return of renal function to normal or near normal levels (57). In one series (58), renal function normalized in 66% of patients in 15 days and improved enough to obviate dialysis in 28%; mean number of days needed for normalization of renal function was 7.7 ± 4.1 days. Patients with benign causes of obstruction or gynecologic malignancies showed the best improvement, while older patients and those with prostate cancer showed the least improvement in their renal function. PCN can be a temporizing measure to improve or at least preserve renal function, while other therapies such as radiation or chemotherapy are given time to reverse the underlying obstruction. PCN drainage may also

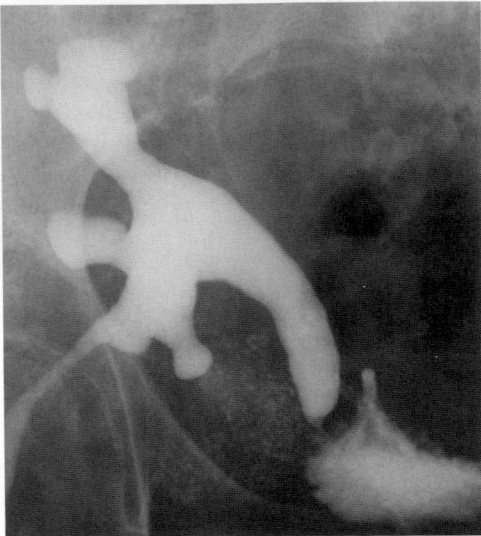

Figure 38–6 Overly vigorous nephrostogram in a renal transplant with a distal ureteral stricture. There is retrograde opacification of the collecting ducts in the upper and lower poles. This degree of overdistention can result in sepsis.

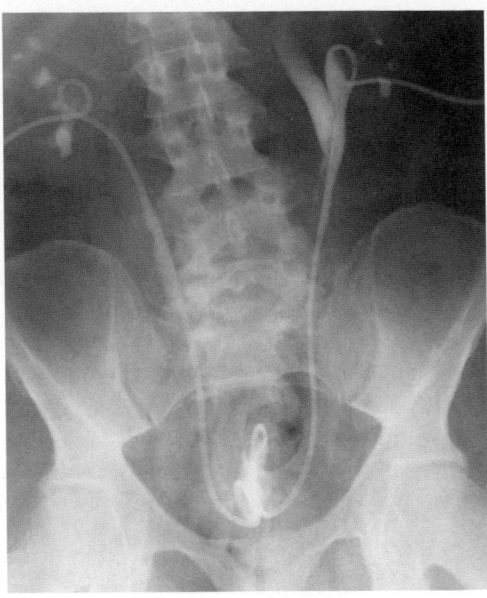

Figure 38–7 Bilateral nephroureteral catheters in a 40-year-old man with advanced prostate cancer. The proximal loops of the catheters are self-retaining (Cope loops). Although malignant ureteral obstruction is usually well-managed with a unilateral nephrostomy, bilateral drainage catheters were placed, in view of the patient's age.

be required to optimize renal function before definitive surgery or to allow the administration of nephrotoxic drugs, such as cisplatin.

In patients with malignancies, the ureters can be obstructed by contiguous involvement or extrinsic compression. The need for external nephrostomy drainage is often permanent in such patients because ureteral stents often fail to drain adequately in patients with extrinsic obstruction (59,60). The physical and financial burdens posed by the presence of a drainage catheter have to be weighed against the benefit of extending life for a few months (61). Even with careful patient selection, 32% of patients are unable to achieve any improvement in the quality of life after percutaneous nephrostomy (62). Long-term survival after palliative diversion for malignant ureteral obstruction is poor, with only 25% of patients alive at 1 year in one series (63), while patients with ureteral obstruction secondary to bladder cancer had a mean survival of 4.9 months (range 1–14 months) in another series (64). When a PCN is performed in these circumstances, only unilateral drainage is usually required and bilateral nephrostomy confers no benefit (58,65). As a group, patients with hormone-responsive prostate carcinoma tend to live longer than those with hormone-resistant prostate cancer or other pelvic malignancies (66). Bilateral drainage may be a preferable option in these patients, particularly when the patient is young (Figure 38–7), so that maximum renal function can be preserved. Our approach in patients with bilateral obstruction resulting from malignancies is similar to others (23); the symptomatic side is initially drained, if there is one, or the kidney that appears to have more preserved renal parenchyma as gauged by cross-sectional imaging is drained. The contralateral kidney is drained only when there is suspected infection or when unilateral drainage

does not improve renal function enough to administer the necessary chemotherapy.

Complications

The standards of practice document by the Society of Cardiovascular and Interventional Radiology (SCIR) and an American College of Radiology (ACR) Practice Guideline for the performance of PCN provide guidelines and thresholds for complications associated with PCN (67,68) The overall serious complication rate of PCN is low, with a mortality of 0.2% compared to a surgical mortality of 6.0% (12,45).

Complications related to percutaneous nephrostomy can be divided into major procedure-related complications (4–6% incidence) (12,45,47,48) and minor complications (10–28% incidence). Major complications include hemorrhage and sepsis.

Hemorrhage requiring transfusion or other therapy is a complication in 1.0–2.4% of patients (12,47,48,69) and is related to renal arterial pseudoaneurysms or arteriovenous fistulas resulting from laceration of lobar arteries (Figure 38–8). In one series (70), using small-needle access systems (21- or 22-gauge needles) was found to be no safer than using 18-gauge needle systems. However, avoiding puncture of the anteromedial renal vessels by accessing the kidney through its relatively avascular posterolateral aspect, or "Brödel line," may decrease the incidence of this complication (71). Most hemorrhage associated with nephrostomy placement is transient and self-limited; it is not uncommon to have pink or slightly bloody urine drainage for several days after a nephrostomy, and this is not considered a complication. If the urine is

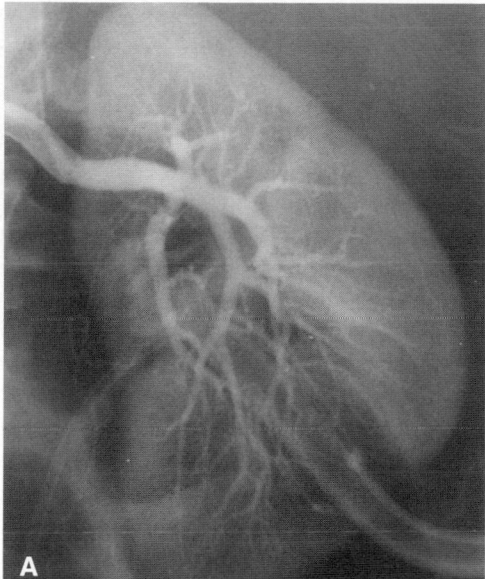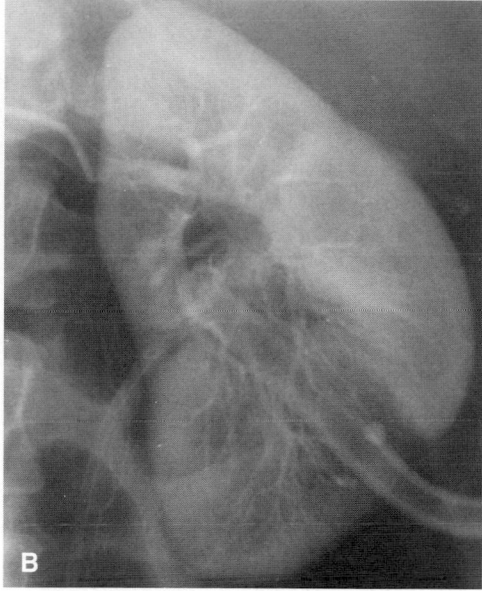

Figure 38–8 Pseudoaneurysm following percutaneous stone removal. **A.** Early phase and **B.** late phase films from a selective renal arteriogram demonstrate a pseudoaneurysm in the nephrostomy track. In a patient with suspected vascular injury, if the study is negative with the nephrostomy catheter in place, the injection should be repeated after removing the catheter over a guide wire to counteract the possible tamponading effects of the nephrostomy catheter.

grossly bloody or large clots are seen on the nephrostogram, repeated irrigation, such as with cold saline or placement of a slightly larger catheter of at least 2 French or larger to tamponade the bleeding vessel, is usually effective in controlling the bleeding (Figure 38–9). Serious vascular trauma is suspected when the urine continues to be grossly bloody after 3–5 days, when new intrapelvic clots are observed on nephrostograms, or when a significant drop in the hematocrit occurs. If the drop in the hematocrit is out of proportion to the urine blood loss, a retroperitoneal hematoma should be suspected and a CT scan obtained (Figure 38–10). Unsuspected retroperitoneal hematomas not requiring treatment have been reported in 13% of patients on CT scans performed after nephrostomy tube placement (72). Angiography and possible arterial embolization should be considered in patients who have significant continuous or recurrent bleeding for longer than 4–5 days after PCN placement (69). If the initial angiogram fails to show a source of bleeding, the study should be repeated immediately after the drainage catheter is removed over a guide wire so that the tamponading effect of the catheter is relieved and the bleeding site can be angiographically localized (Figure 38–8) (73). Although unusual, development of a perirenal hematoma has been described after removal of a nephrostomy catheter that had been in place for 3 months (74).

The incidence of sepsis after nephrostomy tube placement has been reported as 1.4–21.0% (12,18,47,48,54). This wide variance is likely a result of the differing definitions of sepsis in different series. Cochran et al. (18) considered fever and shaking chills to be signs of sepsis and noted them in 21% of patients. Lee et al. (48) defined sepsis as

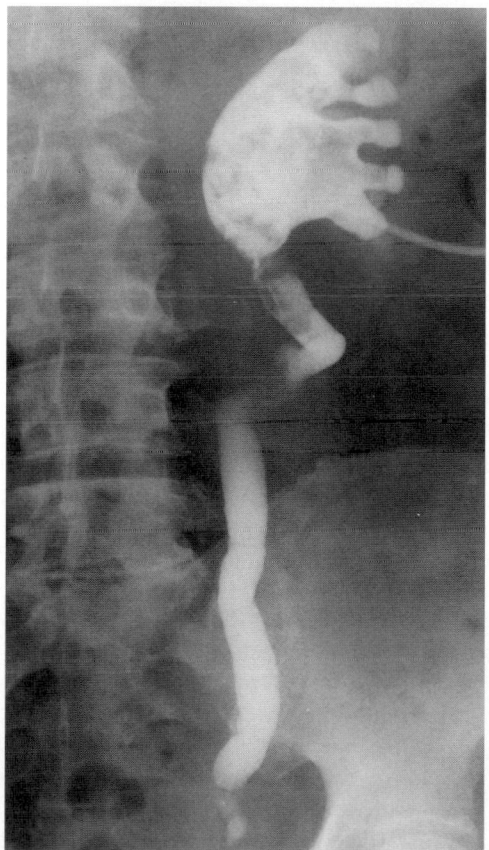

Figure 38–9 Large blood clots are seen as filling defects in the opacified collecting system. The patient was clinically stable and the urine cleared within a week after the procedure.

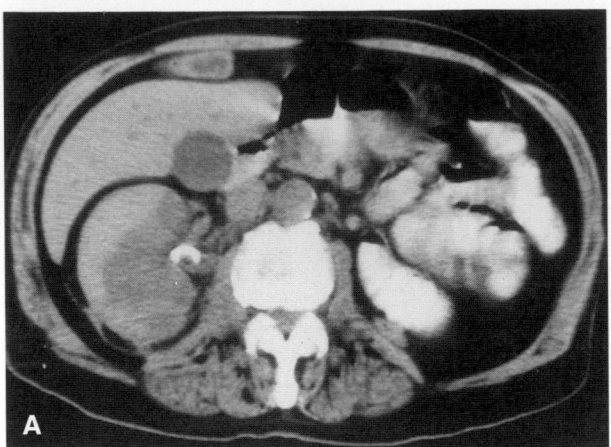

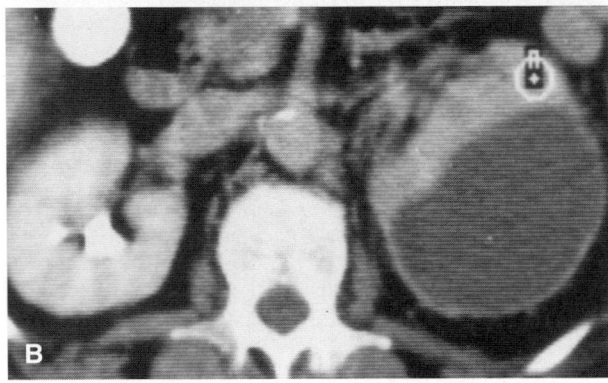

Figure 38–10 Subcapsular hematomas following PCN in two different patients. **A.** Unenhanced CT scan. The hematoma is denser than the renal parenchyma. **B.** On contrast-enhanced CT, the hematoma appears to be of low attenuation compared to the enhancing renal parenchyma.

fever above 101°F (38.4°C) with shaking chills and noted its occurrence in less than 3.6% of patients who underwent emergent drainage. All 160 patients in their series developed a transient increase in body temperature, which usually lasted less than 6 hours. Farrell et al. (12) reported that 1.3% of their patients required observation in the intensive care unit for sepsis or hypotension. Fifteen percent of patients undergoing nephrostomy drainage for pyonephrosis developed postprocedure fever, and 7% developed septic shock (28), despite the use of aminoglycoside prophylaxis. The use of antibiotic-bonded nephrostomy catheters appears to have no influence on the overall incidence of infective complications associated with nephrostomy drainage (75).

Air embolism has been reported in patients in whom air was injected through a retrograde catheter (pneumopyelogram) to visualize the collecting system (76,77). Embolism can occur before percutaneous puncture of the kidney with distension of the collecting system (76) alone or when air is injected into the collecting system after it has already been punctured (77). One option to avoid this complication is to use CO_2 rather than air as a negative contrast in the collecting system.

Inadvertent injury of adjacent organs is uncommon, with no such complications in a series of 160 emergent procedures (24) and only one pneumothorax in Farrell's series of 454 patients (12). Puncture of the gastrointestinal tract is a rare complication. The colon may lie posterior or posterolateral to the kidney and can be entered during a PCN (78–80). Retrorenal position of the colon is more common in patients who are thin and have little retrorenal fat, have colonic dilation, or have abnormal anatomy such as marked kyphosis or scoliosis (78). The colon was behind the medial two thirds of the kidney in 4.7% of prone patients at the level of the lower poles and behind the lateral one third of the kidney in 10% of patients in one report (81). When safe access is in doubt, preprocedure CT to delineate the anatomy is prudent.

Transcolonic nephrostomy track was seen in 2/1,000 cases of percutaneous nephrostolithotomy in one series (78). The complication can often be managed conservatively, with drainage of both the kidney and the colon by separate catheters until the nephrocolic fistula heals (78,79).

Duodenal injury is a rare complication (82). A renoduodenal fistula has been reported in a patient with xanthogranulomatous pyelonephritis who underwent PCN (83). Inadvertent puncture of the spleen can cause severe hemorrhage or even a splenic abscess in patients with infected urine (84).

An intercostal approach (often required for access to the upper poles of the kidneys) causes more thoracic complications than a subcostal puncture (85). In expiration, a posterior intercostal approach between the eleventh and twelfth ribs poses little risk of injury to the spleen and liver (81), but the lungs remain vulnerable to puncture in many patients. The right lung is in the path of the needle in 29%, and the left lung is in the path in 14% of patients in expiration. During maximal inspiration, the lung would be in the needle path in most patients in whom an intercostal puncture is performed. Other thoracic complications include pleural effusion, pneumonia, atelectasis, hydrothorax, and pneumothorax.

Minor complications that may occur are catheter dislodgment and urine extravasation. Catheter dislodgment in the early period postplacement occurs in less than 1% of patients, but it increases to 11–30% in the subsequent months (4,12,24). Dislodgment is more common in obese patients (23) and in disoriented patients. CT has been used in the evaluation of malpositioned PCN catheters and in the repositioning of such catheters (86); reportedly, a CT nephrostogram in such cases allows accurate assessment of the position of the catheter relative to the pelvicaliceal system and adjacent organs. Dislodgment in the first week after placement often necessitates a fresh track. Renal pelvic perforation is unusual in a routine PCN performed for drainage of an obstructed collecting system and is more likely to occur in patients with large staghorn stones. It is usually a self-limiting complication. On occasion, a perforated renal pelvis may not heal, despite prolonged nephrostomy drainage, and may necessitate surgical repair (51). Iatrogenic intussusception of the ureter can occur when the loop of a self-retaining nephrostomy catheter is reformed within the ureter rather than the renal pelvis (87); the tension on the thread can cause the tip of the catheter to lodge in the ureter and intussuscept the ureter as the catheter is withdrawn into the renal pelvis.

Nephrostomy tube placement is considered a low radiation dose procedure (88) with peak skin doses usually less than 1 Gy, although exposure can be higher in as many as 12% of cases (89,90). This is an important consideration in pregnant patients who present with obstruction and require percutaneous drainage (91).

Follow-Up

Most PCN drainage catheters are replaced every 3–4 months on an outpatient basis (Figure 38–11); an interval longer than 3 months is frequently associated with tube blockage (23). Replacement of blocked nephrostomy tubes can pose a

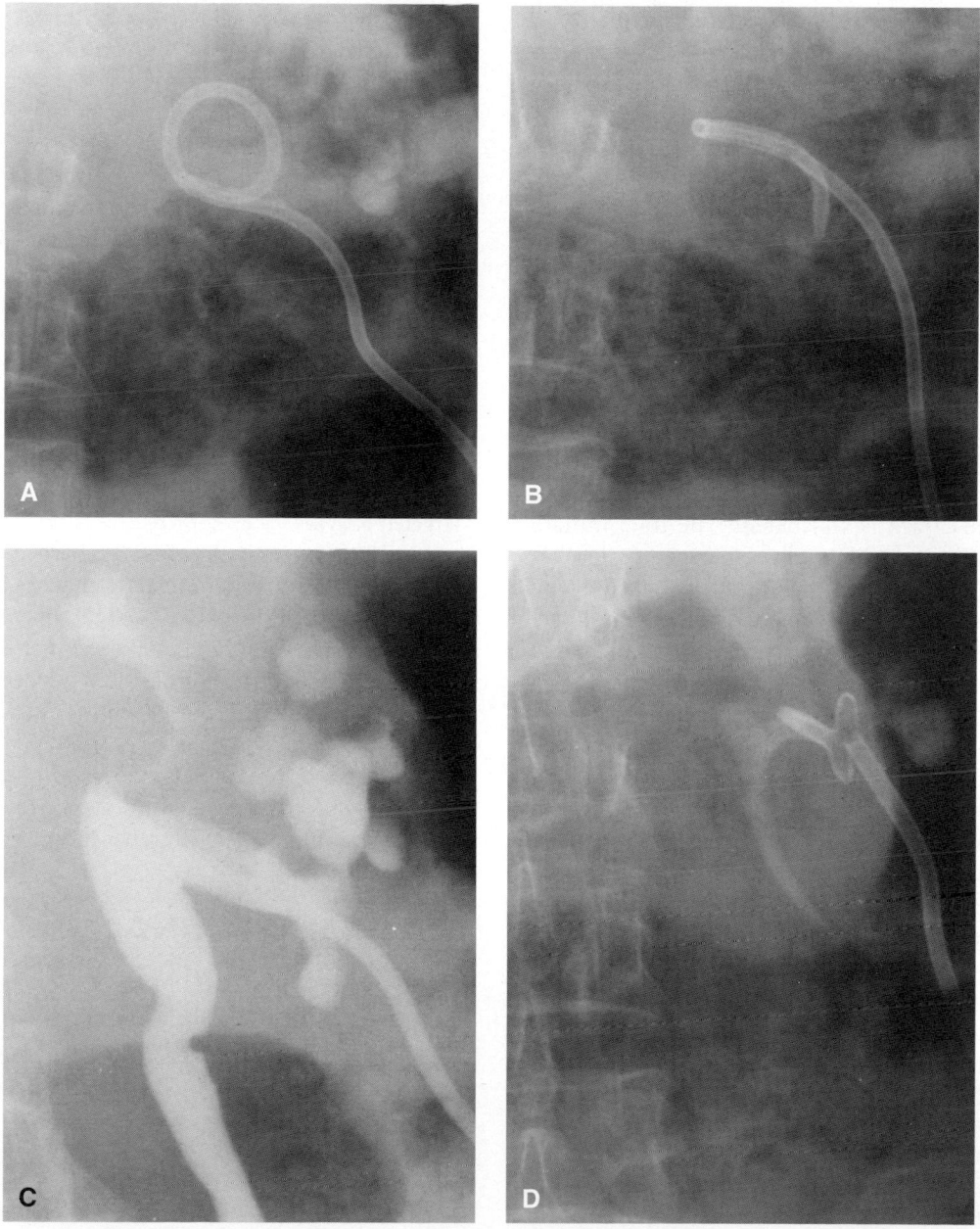

Figure 38–11 Patient with a chronic nephrostomy catheter placed for ureteral stricture and severe flank pain. **A.** Well-formed Cope loop within the renal pelvis immediately after a routine catheter change. **B., C.** Two days later, the loop has retracted into the lower pole infundibulum, causing the flank discomfort. Catheter retraction into an infundibulum is an extremely common event, and most patients are asymptomatic with it. **D.** A Malecot nephrostomy catheter was replaced because there is no foolproof method of ensuring that the catheter loop will remain within the renal pelvis. The Malecot catheter distended the infundibulum less, and the patient's flank pain resolved.

challenge because intraluminal encrustation may prevent passage of a guide wire. Maneuvers that may be useful in such a situation include advancing a sheath over the nephrostomy catheter (the sheath is selected to be slightly larger than the nephrostomy catheter, such as a 9 French sheath for an 8.3 French nephrostomy catheter) until the tip of the sheath is within the collecting system and withdrawing the nephrostomy catheter through it (92). A parallel guide wire method has also been described to replace blocked tubes (92) as well as puncture of the occluded catheter within the pelvocaliceal system with an 18-gauge needle (93). Hydrophilic guide wires can often be negotiated successfully through an encrusted catheter that does not allow the passage of a standard Teflon-coated guide wire. If the encrustations trap the retention string, the loop on the self-retaining catheters may not open, and the catheter may have to be withdrawn in a loop configuration through a large sheath. Care should be taken not to break the string, because retained nephrostomy catheter thread can serve as a nidus for stone formation (94). With Malecot catheters, tissue occasionally may grow through the wings of the catheter and make them resistant to removal (95). Stewart et al. believe that when nephrostomy tube drainage is required for longer than a few weeks, Malecot-type winged catheters should not be used to avoid this complication (95).

When the catheters are extruded completely, the first step is to inject contrast medium into the skin opening to determine whether the track is still patent. The tract initially should not be infiltrated with local anesthetic to avoid creating a false tract (23). Failure to define a track into the renal pelvis usually indicates that the catheter has been dislodged for more than 48 hours and may necessitate a fresh nephrostomy. If the track can be opacified, an 8 French pediatric feeding tube or a 4 French angiographic sheath can usually be negotiated through the track over a straight or angled-tip guide wire. Hydrophilic guide wires are extremely useful when the track is particularly tortuous. An alternative approach proposed by some urologists is to use a rigid ureteroscope to recannulate the nephrostomy track after catheter dislodgment (96) with the purported advantage being the ability to perform the entire replacement in the urology suite. In an occasional patient who is disoriented or confused, accidental tube dislodgment can become a frequent occurrence. A U-shaped nephrostomy tube may be a consideration in such cases.

The presence of a nephrostomy tube invariably causes bacteriuria, candiduria, or pyuria within 9 weeks of initial nephrostomy tube drainage; prophylactic antibiotics in patients with PCN tubes do not prevent bacteriuria; rather, they can cause the emergence of organisms that are resistant to the antibiotics being administered (97). Antibiotic prophylaxis is unnecessary in routine catheter exchanges when the catheters have been draining adequately and, in fact, fail to prevent bacteremia (97,98). Cronan et al. found that asymptomatic bacteremia occurred in 11% of routine tube changes and that preprocedural antibiotics were unsuccessful in preventing bacteremia. This has implications for patients at risk for endocarditis, in whom routine tube changes should be preceded by antibiotic therapy with the aim of eradicating bacteriuria. Antibiotics should be chosen for activity against the organisms isolated in the urine, and after bacteriuria has been eliminated, an antibiotic regimen recommended in the American Heart Association guidelines for genitourinary procedures should be administered in conjunction with an elective nephrostomy tube change (97,98). In patients who are not at risk for endocarditis, antibiotic prophylaxis before elective tube change should be considered only in the event the catheter is occluded, when urine drainage has been suboptimal (indicating impending catheter occlusion), or when the patient is febrile (in which case the antibiotics should be continued for 24–48 hours). Defervescence of fever usually occurs when free drainage is established (18).

Catheter flushing at home between tube changes, whether by visiting nurses or the patient, does little to favorably influence the incidence of tube encrustation in most patients. In patients with rapid tube encrustation, a high fluid intake is the best way to keep catheters open.

An unusual complication that may be seen in patients who undergo extracorporeal shock wave lithotripsy (ESWL) of a renal calculus with a PCN catheter in place is damage to the catheter, causing it to bulge in an aneurysm-like configuration (99). The catheter damage may be related to poorly targeted ESWL.

Nephrostograms in patients who have long-term nephrostomy catheters often demonstrate changes of pyelitis cystica (Figure 38–12), probably related to chronic irritation. When renal CT scans are performed after catheter removal, surprisingly few morphologic changes are evident; Hruby and Marberger (100) reported slight capsular fibrosis at the puncture site in 22% of patients, slight perirenal scarring in 28%, a 1-cm cortical scar at the puncture site in one patient, and no signs of loss of renal function. Thus, PCNs produce no significant late effect on renal morphology or function.

URETERAL STENTING

Ureteral intubation is an essential component in the management of patients with nephroureteral obstruction or urinary fistulas, in patients undergoing open ureteral surgery, and if there is obstruction after previous ESWL.

Stent Materials

The ideal ureteral stent has the following characteristics: is easy to insert, retrieve, and therefore, to change; is biocompatible and resistant to encrustation, infection, and occlusion; is biodurable and thus remains chemically stable in urine and resists breakage; is easy to manipulate, requiring low-surface friction, radiopacity, and resistance to buckling during insertion; is resistant to migration; has

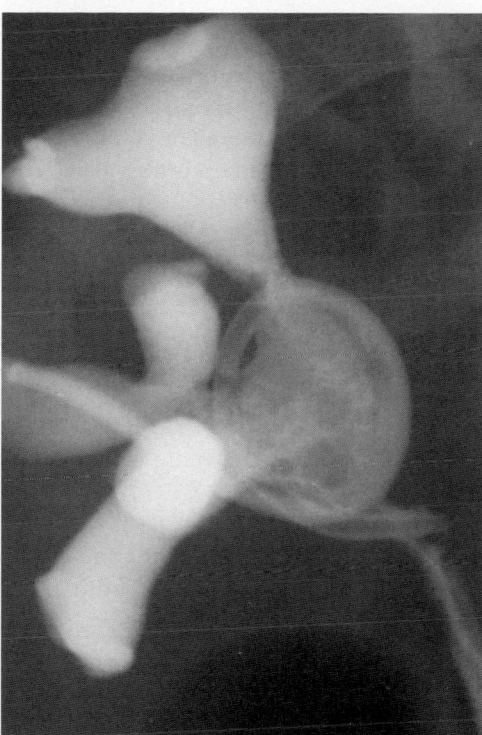

Figure 38–12 Pyelitis cystica in a patient with nephrostomy catheter drainage for 6 years. These changes can occur as early as a few weeks after catheter placement. The multiple filling defects represent submucosal cysts.

good flow characteristics so that urine flow can be effectively restored and maintained in both intramural and extramural obstruction; and is comfortable for the patient. A number of materials have been used in the quest to produce an ideal ureteral stent, but there is no such ideal material available (101–104) that satisfies all the above-mentioned criteria.

Initially, ureteral stents were made of polyethylene and polyurethane and were widely used by radiologists because the stent design and stiffness permitted insertion over a standard guide wire, making percutaneous antegrade placement feasible. Polyethylene is a waxlike polymer that was used extensively to fabricate stents but becomes brittle in urine. Reports of stent fractures in patients whose polyethylene stents were left indwelling beyond the maximum recommended 6-month period (104–108) led to its being phased out in favor of polyurethane stents. Polyurethane is a generic class of condensation polymers that are derived from poly-isocyanate and a polyol (104), which are highly versatile and inexpensive materials and thus are popular for stent manufacture. However, pure polyurethane is a stiff and rubbery material. Marx et al. (109) evaluated stents within canine ureters and found that polyurethane stents caused epithelial erosions and ulcers in all cases, whereas other stent materials rarely did so. Mardis et al. (104) speculate that the poor biocompatibility of polyurethane may be related to its irregular surface, best demonstrated by electron microscopy.

Urinary stents are currently made of blends of synthetic polymers such as polyurethane, silicone, and blends of other materials. Polyurethane alone, besides its disadvantages discussed above, is also a relatively rigid and uncomfortable material for stents. However, its combination with other materials makes it more comfortable (101,102). Ureteral stents made of silicone, C-Flex, and Percuflex are also in wide clinical use and are offered by many manufacturers. Silicone stents are the gold standard with respect to tissue compatibility and their inert nature. Silicone stents retain their softness, flexibility, and elasticity often more than 10 years after placement, which is an advantage. Silicone's disadvantages include inherently low tensile strength that limits the inner diameter of the stents, as well as the size of the side holes, and reduces the functional efficacy of the stent; a high coefficient of surface friction that hampers stent insertion and requires placement through a peel-away sheath; and weak coil strength that allows the pigtail configuration of the coiled ends of the stent to straighten easily, making the stents prone to spontaneous migration. Silicone is also poorly radiopaque, making fluoroscopic monitoring during insertion difficult. For these reasons, silicone is not the preferred choice of material for stents, particularly indwelling ureteral stents. Currently, silicone stents usually are placed intra-operatively.

Percuflex is a proprietary and biocompatible olefinic copolymer material from Boston Scientific Corporation (Medi-Tech, Microvasive) that has high tensile strength (and therefore, the largest available inner lumen for a given outside diameter); an intrinsic low coefficient of friction that facilitates stent placement; and long-term bio-durability with resistance to fracture and migration (110). Although the manufacturer recommends replacing the stents every 6 months, Rackson et al. (110) found that the Percuflex stents remained patent for a mean period of 10 months. Of all currently available stent materials, Percuflex may represent one of the most balanced materials.

C-Flex is a proprietary silicone-modified copolymer (Consolidated Polymer Technologies) that was designed to be urine-compatible. Although not as strong as Percuflex or polyurethane, the material has sufficient tensile strength to allow good flow rates and coil strength. The stents resist both migration and fracture (111), are less rigid than polyurethane stents, and demonstrate an overall patency of 80%. The external surface of the stent is slippery, a property that enhances resistance to stent encrustation and makes stent placement easier.

To summarize, at the current time, stents made of C-Flex and Percuflex appear to confer the most advantages with regard to patency, flexibility, resistance to migration, good urine flow rates, and resistance to fracturing. The manufacturers recommend stent exchange at intervals of 3–6 months, although in certain clinical situations, including terminal malignancy, stent replacement can be deferred for a longer period if the stent is functioning well. Coating stents with hydrogels—hydrophilic polymer that allows water to be trapped in the chemical structure—appears to improve bio-compatibility by reducing frictional irritation and encrustation (102,105).

Endoureteral implantation of self-expanding metal stents was a natural offshoot of experience with metal stent use in the biliary tract and urethra. The stents have been used primarily in patients with malignant ureteral obstruction (112–115) as an alternative to conventional double pigtail ureteral stents, with the hope that ureteral patency could be maintained for a longer period without the need for stent exchange. The potential incorporation of the stent into the ureteric wall with covering by urothelium should theoretically avoid calcium encrustation, infection, and risk of migration. However, hyperplasia of the urothelium leading to stent occlusion, encrustation, and hematuria has been reported with Wallstent (Medinrent) (112–114), and the role of metal stents in the treatment of ureteral obstruction continues to evolve. Because the biocompatibility of metallic devices in the urinary tract is unknown, as are the effects of the corrosive action of urine and extracellular fluids on the metal, researchers have been reluctant to use metal stents in ureteral obstruction that results from benign disease (103,116–118).

Recently, metal stents made of nickel-titanium alloy (nitinol) have been used. Kulkarni et al. (119) reported on a thermoexpandable, shape-memory alloy Memokath 051 ureteral stent (developed by engineers and doctors in Copenhagen, Denmark) that was placed in patients with malignant and benign ureteral strictures. They reported no encrustation or epithelial hyperplasia with a mean follow-up of 19.3 months. The stents can also be removed many weeks after placement by cooling them to 10°C.

There is keen interest in using biodegradable materials to obviate the necessity of stent removal in patients who require temporary stenting (102,120). Variation in the time to degradation is one of the problems with these materials. Under investigation for use in long-term stenting are pH-sensitive stents that dissolve when the urine is alkalinized with oral bicarbonate administration (121).

Technique

Ureteral stents can be inserted in one of three ways (Figure 38–13), including: (1) percutaneously (antegrade), (2) per urethral (retrograde), and (3) transconduit (retrograde). The transconduit approach will be discussed in Chapter 41 (Interventions in Urinary Diversions). In difficult cases, a combined approach may be required. Regardless of the route used for insertion, ureteral stent placement provides the benefits of urine drainage and diversion without the inconvenience of a drainage bag with its attendant cosmetic problems and the risk of inadvertent dislodgment. When the urinary bladder is markedly contracted or diseased (as with neoplastic invasion, radiation cystitis, or tuberculosis) or in patients with incontinence, drainage via a percutaneous nephrostomy is preferable to ureteral stenting.

Antegrade Ureteral Stenting

When retrograde insertion fails or is not possible, percutaneous antegrade stent insertion is performed. Antegrade ureteral stenting requires percutaneous access to the collecting system, preferably through an interpolar or upper pole calix because this approach allows the pushing forces to be directed toward the ureteropelvic junction. A guide wire is then maneuvered across the ureteral obstruction using a combination of preshaped catheters (for example, a cobra or multipurpose catheter) and guide wires. Hydrophilic-coated guide wires ("glidewires") are particularly helpful in crossing tight strictures. The use of transrenal Teflon sheaths (peel-away or non–peel-away) also facilitates the placement of stents by preventing buckling in the subcutaneous tissues and in the renal pelvis (108,122,123) because the stent encounters high resistance in the area of a tight stricture. In difficult cases, a guide wire can be passed antegrade through the urethra so that it can be grasped at both ends and the stent can be advanced by pushing and pulling (124,125). If the urine draining from the nephrostomy is bloody or infected, stent placement should be deferred until the urine clears.

Two kinds of ureteral stents can be inserted in an antegrade fashion: (1) an internal stent, such as a double-J or double-pigtail, or (2) an external, or nephroureteral, stent. External-internal stents (nephroureteral stents) are introduced percutaneously and advanced into the urinary bladder or bowel (Figure 38–13). A segment of the stent remains protruding from the flank and is capped externally to allow antegrade urine drainage. Side holes at the level of the renal pelvis allow urine to drain distally through the stent. External stents are exchanged with ease percutaneously and can be irrigated to maintain patency. External stents are used in patients in whom the stent placement is only for a short period, such as after stone removal or ureteral dilation. They are also indicated in patients in whom retrograde stent exchange would be difficult because of bladder disease or distortion or because of neurologic or orthopedic problems that make cystoscopy challenging.

Completely internalized ureteral stents do not protrude from the flank, an obvious cosmetic and nursing advantage. A period of external drainage through a PCN for 2–7 days, before attempted ureteral stent placement, was the convention when the procedure first became widely used, but it is no longer necessary in most cases (62,126,127). A nephrostomy tube is left in for 24–48 hours after stent placement so that antegrade pyelography can be performed to confirm stent patency before the nephrostomy catheter is removed (Figure 38–14). It is important to use fluoroscopic guidance when removing the nephrostomy catheter to prevent inadvertent extraction of a double-pigtail ureteral stent that may be trapped by the nephrostomy catheter (128). If the urine is bloody, nephrostomy catheter drainage should be maintained until the urine clears. Recently, Patel et al. (127) reported on their experience in 41 patients in whom ureteral

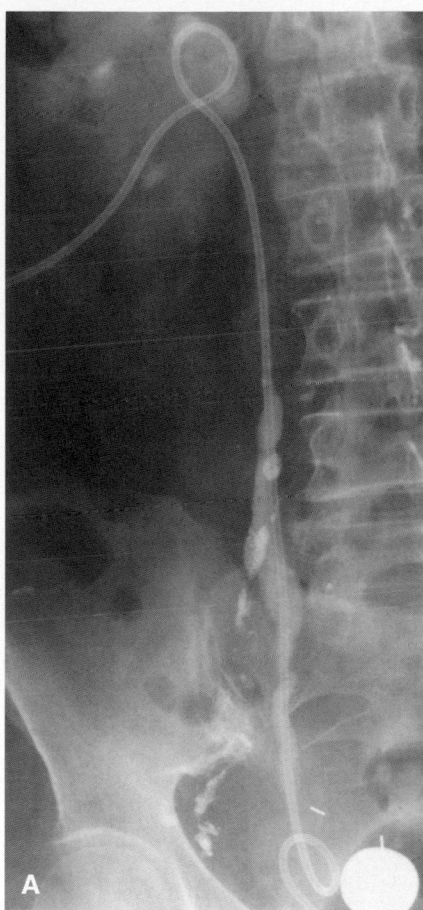
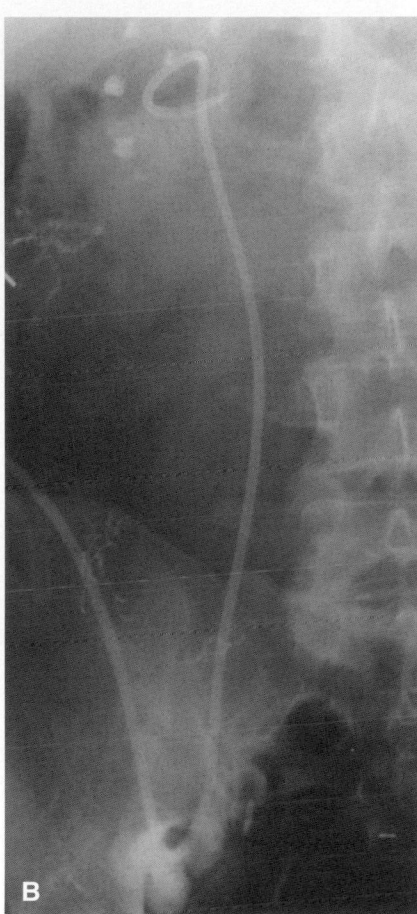

Figure 38–13 Ureteral stents. **A.** Nephroureteral catheter placed in an antegrade fashion. **B.** Transconduit retrograde placement of a nephrostomy catheter through an ileal conduit. The catheter loops up distally to exit through the urostomy stoma.

stents were placed without a postprocedural nephrostomy tube. Exclusion criteria included suspected pyonephrosis, coagulopathy, and emergency cases. After stent placement, they performed a nephrostogram, and a nephrostomy tube was not placed whenever there was contrast flow into the bladder, blood clot filling less than half the renal pelvis, and no bleeding around a wire left in the track after stent placement. The procedure was technically successful in 36 of 41 patients (88%) and clinically successful in 34 of 41 (83%) patients; two patients became septic and required repeat nephrostomy tube insertion. Based on their experience, Patel and associates also recommend that patients with genitourinary tract surgery or recent instrumentation, such as a failed attempt at retrograde stent insertion, should have nephrostomy tubes left in postprocedure for drainage because such patients have a predisposition to infection (127).

Per Urethral (Retrograde) Ureteral Stenting

For access to the kidneys or ureters, the retrograde route is a familiar one for most urologists. When the endoscopic retrograde approach is unsuccessful in placing a stent or a guide wire, a percutaneous nephrostomy is usually performed followed by stent placement (Figure 38–15). However, an unsuccessful or incomplete retrograde procedure can often

be completed successfully with fluoroscopy and the use of guide wires and catheters (129,130).

Primary retrograde catheterization of the ureter without cystoscopic assistance has been reported (131–133). The procedure was successful in 70% of cases in a small series (131), with patients requiring only mild intravenous sedation and with fluoroscopy times averaging less than 3 minutes. The trigone is identified by cystography, and the ureteral orifice is cannulated using a combination of angled-tip glidewires and angled hockey-stick catheters. Replacement of ureteral stents using fluoroscopic control (as opposed to cystoscopy) has been reported with successful exchange in 97% of cases (134,135). The bladder end of the stent is grasped with a snare or lasso, withdrawn through the urethra, and replaced over a guide wire using standard technique. The technique is easiest in female patients, although it has been used in a few male patients.

Choosing the Correct Length of Ureteral Stent

Ureteral stents of the correct length will ensure patient comfort, trouble-free drainage, and prevention of irritative voiding symptoms. Ureteral stents are available in lengths ranging from 20 to 28 cm—a greater range of shorter stents is also available for renal transplant patients—and a specific

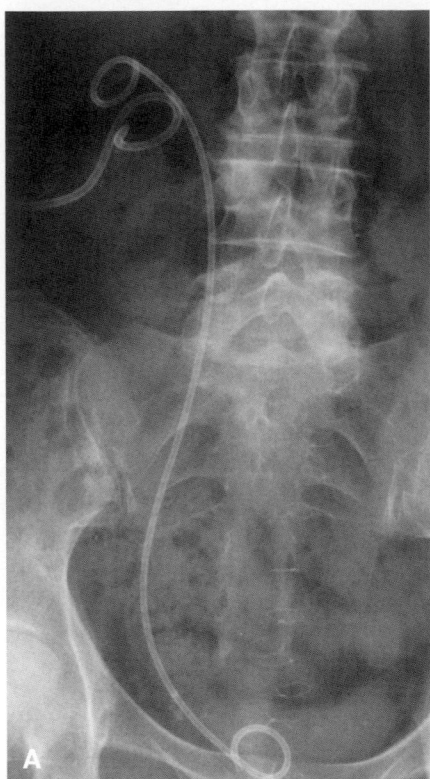
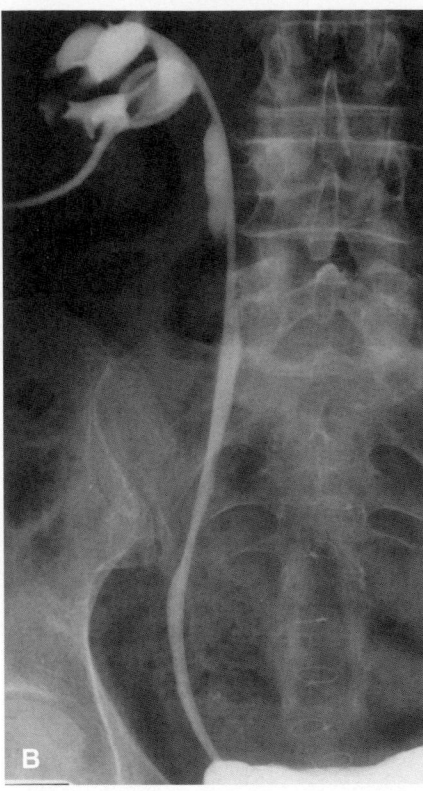

Figure 38–14 Internalized double-pigtail ureteral stent. **A.** A nephrostomy catheter is left in place for continuing access after the procedure. **B.** Contrast injection through the nephrostomy catheter the next day confirms satisfactory stent function with contrast draining rapidly into the urinary bladder (and no blood clots in the collecting system). The nephrostomy catheter was removed under fluoroscopic guidance.

length has to be chosen for each patient. Multilength or flexible-length ureteral stents are also available; they are made of a softer polymer that allows the pigtail to unfurl to the proper length, but these stents are less stable in position and positioning the pigtails properly can be difficult (136).

In a correctly positioned stent, the proximal pigtail should be formed within the renal pelvis, and the distal pigtail should project beyond the vesicoureteral junction (VUJ). Stents that are too short will retract into the ureter when the proximal pigtail forms in the renal pelvis, complicating stent retrieval. An overly long stent will be redundant within the bladder and may cause irritative voiding symptoms.

A few techniques have been tried to estimate stent length accurately (122,136). In the kinked-bent wire technique, an attempt is made to directly measure ureteral length by kinking a wire when it is just beyond the VUJ in the urinary bladder then kinking it again after withdrawing it into the renal pelvis. Patel et al. found that this technique overestimated the ureteral length in 83% of patients (127). These authors found that the patient height was the most reliable method to estimate stent length, with patients <5 ft/10 inches receiving 22-cm long stents, 5 ft/10 inches–6 ft/4 inches receiving 24-cm long stents, and patients >6 ft/4 inches getting 26-cm long stents. Other authors have also reported using patient height as a guide for stent length (136,137).

Other methods to estimate ureteral length include using an endocatheter ruler and calculating ureteral length from a previous imaging study, such as an intravenous urogram (138,139).

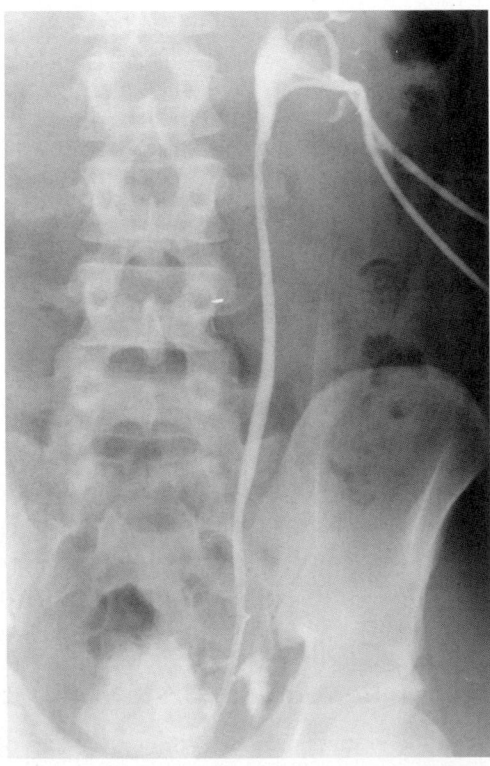

Figure 38–15 Antegrade ureteral stent placement for distal ureteral perforation that occurred during ureteroscopic stone extraction. Cystoscopically assisted retrograde placement of a ureteral stent was unsuccessful. The patient eventually developed a stricture at the site of perforation that was treated successfully with balloon dilation.

Results and Complications

Antegrade ureteral stenting is successful in 88–96% of cases. More than 80% of obstructed ureters can be stented successfully without the need for previous nephrostomy (126,127,129). Failure of placement usually is related to marked ureteral angulation or encasement by tumor or fibrosis. Technical failures can be minimized by placing the nephrostomy in a favorable calix to provide the best vector for stent advancement, liberally using transrenal sheaths as a buttress, and using appropriately stiff guide wires. Passing the wire through the urethra to gain control over both ends of the wire is also helpful in particularly difficult cases (108). Partial ureteral obstruction, where a guide wire can be passed across the stricture, does not necessarily equate to an easier attempt at stenting (126).

When stenting cannot be accomplished at the initial sitting, attempts following nephrostomy drainage for a few days are often successful because of a decrease in ureteral tortuosity, edema related to ureteral obstruction, or both. In Patel's series (127), of 5 of 41 patients who could not be stented initially because of tight strictures, 4 of 5 eventually were stented successfully. In the same series, all patients who underwent a two-step procedure—nephrostomy drainage for some duration followed by stenting—were stented successfully. The complication rate was slightly higher in the one-step patient group (6%), compared to the two-step group (2%). Complications consisted primarily of sepsis, and the one-step procedure was found to be significantly less expensive.

Ureteral stenting may not be as effective in relieving the obstruction caused by extrinsic obstruction related to malignancies as it is in relieving intrinsic obstruction resulting from intrinsic causes such as stones and strictures (140). Yossepowitch et al. reported that initial success at retrograde stenting was 94% for intrinsic disease and 73% for extrinsic disease and, at 3 months postplacement, stents functioned in all patients with intrinsic disease but only in 56.4% of patients with extrinsic obstruction. These authors also found that stent diameter did not correlate with successful drainage. Docimo et al. (60) also noted a 45% rate of stent failure in patients with extrinsic obstruction. Chung et al. reported similar results and noted stent failure in 40% of patients with extrinsic ureteral compression by malignant disease (141). The etiology for the impaired stent function in extrinsic obstruction is not completely clear. It is believed that urine drainage in a stented ureter is primarily the result of ureteral peristalsis, which causes urine to flow around the stent. With extrinsic ureteral compression, the tumor encasement affects the muscular activity and, hence, the ureteral peristalsis of the ureter, preventing ureteral distension, which is necessary to maintain flow around the stent (142). In some patients in whom 7 French internalized ureteral stents fail to drain adequately, 10 French nephroureteral catheters will often be effective in allowing antegrade urine drainage and obviating a bag.

There is also a report of successful drainage with the placement of two ureteral stents when a single ureteral stent had failed (143); two 7 French stents or a combination of 8 and 6 French stents were used, flank pain and hydronephrosis was alleviated, and the patients reported no discomfort associated with the presence of two stents.

The results with permanent indwelling metal stents are still evolving (112–119,144–148). In a few small series (147), high patency rates have been reported. In other series, however, primary patency has ranged from 31% (114) to 16% (148). As mentioned earlier, the metal stents made of thermoexpandable shape-memory alloy Memokath 051 ureteral stent may have a better patency rate and may experience fewer problems with epithelial overgrowth (119).

There are other situations where stents may not function well or may be poorly tolerated. Such patients may be better served by PCN drainage. Patients with large pelvic tumors that compress the bladder or who have high intraluminal pressures within the bladder (as with bladder outlet obstruction) may not drain well antegrade. Patients with small, irritable bladders, as with tuberculous cystitis, or who may be following radiation or chemotherapy may not tolerate the presence of a stent within the bladder. Further, in patients with incontinence or fistulae, supravesical urinary diversion is preferable (122).

In patients with impassable ureteral strictures, novel approaches have been explored. Cornud et al. (149) created a neotract between the ureter and bladder using electrocautery, and Lang and others (150,151) used a perforating guide wire to create a ureteroneocystostomy. Fistulas to the alimentary tract were a serious (and fatal) complication in Cornud's series (149). Mishra et al. (152) reported on inadvertent catheterization of a uretero rectal fistula in a patient with a rectal stump and advanced colon cancer; a double-pigtail stent was placed through and served to keep the obstructed kidney decompressed. Bilbao et al. (153) described direct translumbar puncture of the ureter with subsequent stent placement in patients in whom ureteral laceration or rigid ureteral kinking prevented stent placement. The interested reader is referred to the original source for details regarding the technique. Extra-anatomic ureteral replacement with a subcutaneous, silicone-PTFE prosthesis has also been reported (154).

The single most frequent complication encountered is occlusion of stents resulting from encrustation, which is an unpredictable phenomenon and depends on the degree of crystalloid supersaturation in the urine. The stent serves as a nidus for crystal deposition and the longer the stent is in, the higher the prevalence of complications. Sixty-eight percent of stents that were indwelling for 9 weeks were found to be obstructed with mucus and microcalculi when they were removed (155,156). El-Faqih et al. (157) found that in patients in whom stents were placed for treatment of urinary stones, there was minimal morbidity when the indwelling time was 6 weeks or less, and encrustation was present in 9.2% of stents retrieved before 6 weeks, 47.5% of stents at 6–12 weeks, and 76.3% after 12 weeks. Therefore, all patients should be encouraged to maintain a high fluid intake after stent placement to dilute the urine, and routine follow-up should be mandatory. Any infections should be treated aggressively.

Evaluation to confirm that the stent is functioning optimally and is patent can sometimes be difficult. Flank pain may occur with both functioning and nonfunctioning stents and is not a useful clinical parameter to monitor stent function. With unilateral obstruction, blood chemistry does not reflect the status of the stented collecting system when contralateral renal function is normal. Imaging studies that are employed include cystography, excretory urography, or radionuclide urography. Many, though not all, patent stents will reflux at voiding cystourethrography. Diuretic renography is reportedly the most sensitive test in evaluating stent patency (158). Pyelocaliectasis often persists even after relief of obstruction with a ureteral stent, and the upper urinary tract may remain abnormal in appearance. Thus, imaging may be unhelpful in predicting obstructed stents in patients. Intrarenal Doppler sonography can be used to distinguish between patency and obstruction. Platt et al. (159) reported that obstructed stents were associated with increased mean resistive indices (0.78), whereas patent stents were associated with a resistive index of less than 0.70. Assessment of jets in the urinary bladder with color Doppler ultrasonography has also been used (160) to evaluate stent patency.

Stents should be changed every 3–6 months, whether cystoscopically by urologists or in a retrograde per urethral fashion by radiologists; the physician placing the stent bears the responsibility to make the patient aware of the necessity of follow-up and monitoring. Severe encrustation on indwelling ureteral stents tends to be at the renal or bladder ends, and this propensity has been attributed to ureteral peristalsis, "wiping" clean the ureteral portion of the stent (161). A "twinkling" artifact may be seen in encrusted stents on color Doppler sonography (162). Minimally encrusted stents may be removed without event. but more severe encrustation can be complicated to treat and often may require ESWL in combination with endoscopic techniques (163–166).

Proximal stent migration can lead to perforation of the renal pelvis or calyces (167), which can result in a urinoma or even catastrophic exsanguination because of erosion of the stent tip into a renal vessel. Stents that have migrated into the kidney above a lower ureteral stricture or anastomosis can be extracted through a nephrostomy track under fluoroscopic guidance (Figure 38–16). A second approach is to use ureteroscopy to reposition the caudal end of the stent within the bladder. A stent that is positioned too far cephalad (so that the distal end is no longer within the urinary

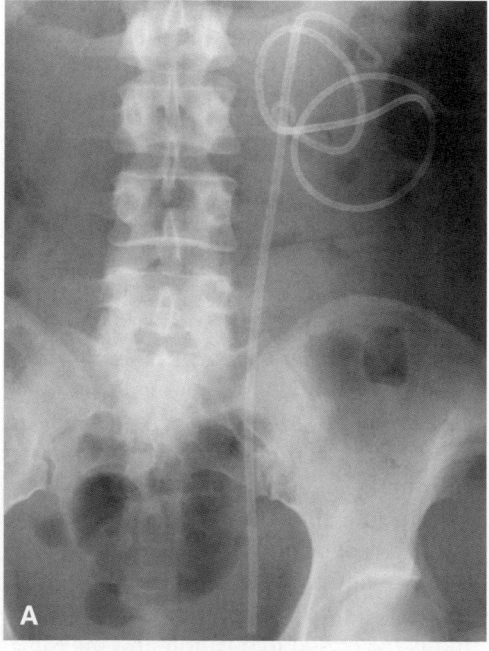

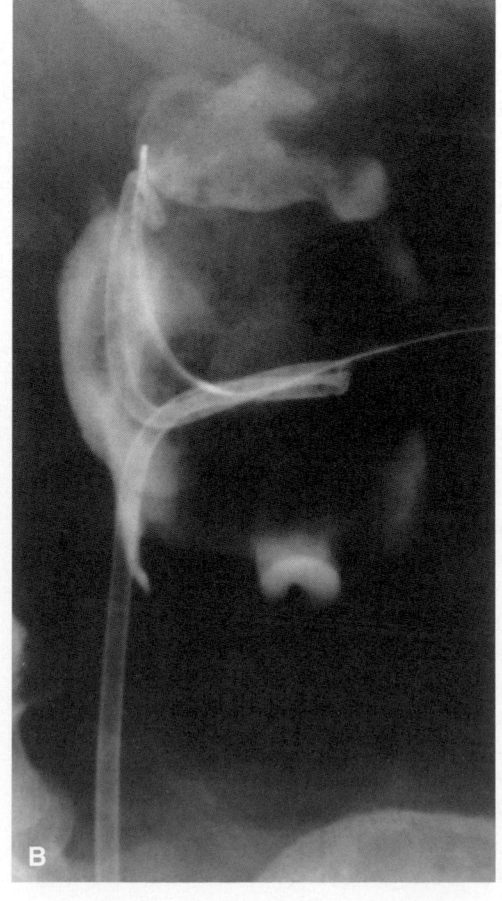

Figure 38–16 Malpositioned left ureteral stent. This complication usually is related to poor positioning of the stent at the time of placement rather than to retraction. **A.** The distal end of the stent is within the distal ureter and not the urinary bladder. **B.** Through the nephrostomy track, the stent was snared with a tip-deflecting guide wire and removed through the nephrostomy track. Another option would have been ureteroscopic repositioning of the distal end within the urinary bladder.

bladder) is usually related to placement of too short a stent rather than to cephalad migration (168). Fractured stents are best approached with a combined percutaneous-endoscopic technique. Although the stent fragments can be removed percutaneously, the fragments tend to be brittle and to refracture into smaller pieces when they are grasped with forceps or baskets. Therefore, removal under endoscopic guidance is most likely to result in complete extraction (107). Distal migration is more common than proximal migration and may be a result of inappropriate positioning.

Fistulas between the iliac artery and the ureter have been reported in patients with pelvic surgery, irradiation, and indwelling ureteral stents (169–171). The primary predisposing factor is compromise of the vascular supply of the ureter with a fistula occurring where the ureter crosses the iliac artery. Underlying abnormalities of the iliac artery, including aneurysm, are an additional risk factor. Prompt diagnosis requires an awareness of the condition, selective or subselective arterial injections in multiple projections, and provocative maneuvers such as stent removal or manipulation during angiography when the angiogram is being performed in a quiescent period. Unsuspected and undiagnosed ureteroarterial fistulas are associated with 52% mortality, whereas a correct preoperative diagnosis allows 89% of patients to be successfully discharged from the hospital (172).

A vexing complication with an indwelling stent is discomfort in the flank or pelvis that can range from mild to severe. A long intravesical segment can cause significant dysuria and bladder spasms resulting from irritation of the trigone and may necessitate removal of the stent. However, even an appropriately placed stent can cause irritative bladder symptoms. Most patients can be managed with antispasmodics and hydration. Flank pain may be worse during voiding, but some patients complain of flank discomfort even in the nonvoiding state. Intolerance to ureteral stents is neither material nor design-specific. Pryor et al. (173) found no significant differences in patient symptoms in an analysis of stents made of polyurethane, silicone, Silitek, and C-Flex. In cases of extreme discomfort, changing to a different stent can sometimes ameliorate the patient's symptoms. When significant symptoms exist, an abdominal radiograph is often helpful in assuring that the stent remains well-positioned.

Stents are associated with microscopic hematuria in the majority of patients. Gross hematuria and pyuria may also be seen.

URETERAL STRICTURE DILATION

The management of ureteral strictures has been altered dramatically by the introduction and refinement of interventional and endourologic techniques. Iatrogenic causes predominate in the development of ureteral strictures. Gynecologic and general surgical procedures are widely considered to be common causes of ureteral trauma and stricture formation, but endourologic procedures, such as ureteroscopy and ureterolithotomy, that facilitate less invasive management of many conditions may paradoxically cause ureteral injury (Figure 38–15) (174–176). A 1–11% incidence of stricture formation has been reported after upper tract endoscopy (177). Selzman et al. (178) found that urologic, gynecologic, and general surgical procedures accounted for 42%, 34%, and 24% of ureteral injuries respectively; of the urological injuries, 21% occurred during open procedures and 79% during endoscopic procedures, with stone removal being the most common.

Urologic procedures implicated in ureteral stricture formation include transurethral resections, radical prostatectomy (Figure 38–17), ureteral meatotomy, traumatic ureteral catheterization, ureteroneocystostomy, and renal transplantation. Gynecologic procedures associated with strictures include hysterectomies for benign or malignant disease, cesarean sections, and tubal ligations; Selzman et al. (178) found that radical abdominal hysterectomy accounted for most of the gynecologic injuries in their series. Surgical procedures that may cause ureteral trauma and stricture formation are abdominal aortic aneurysm repair, bowel resection, and pelvic exenterations. Selzman et al. (178) found that colorectal surgery and abdominal aortic surgery accounted for most of the ureteral injuries during general surgery, and these injuries were transections in 62% of cases.

Ureteral strictures can also develop in patients with chronic calculous disease as well as after penetrating abdominal trauma, particularly high-velocity gunshot wounds. Urinary extravasation and ureteral ischemia may contribute to scar formation in these cases and in postoperative strictures. Chronic inflammatory diseases, such as tuberculosis and schistosomiasis, can also cause strictures. Ureteroenteral anastomotic strictures associated with urinary diversion are considered in Chapter 41.

With malignant strictures, the goal of treatment is to provide drainage (percutaneous or internal) so that renal function can be improved. Chronic stenting is often an appropriate (and most reasonable option) for these patients. For benign strictures, stenting alone is not the optimal therapy, and attempts are made to relieve the obstruction, with balloon dilation often being the initial mode of therapy. When successful, balloon dilation obviates the use of chronic indwelling stents and additional open surgery.

Ureteral dilation can be performed through either an antegrade or retrograde approach or a combination of the two. The antegrade approach is the preferred route for several reasons. Many strictures that may be impassable by a retrograde approach can be negotiated in an antegrade fashion (Figure 38–18). More importantly, once dilation and stenting have been completed, the remaining nephrostomy tube can be used to assess the results of the dilation as well as to perform urodynamic tests, such as the Whitaker test, for more physiologic evaluation. The only disadvantage of the antegrade route is the invasiveness of establishing a percutaneous access track.

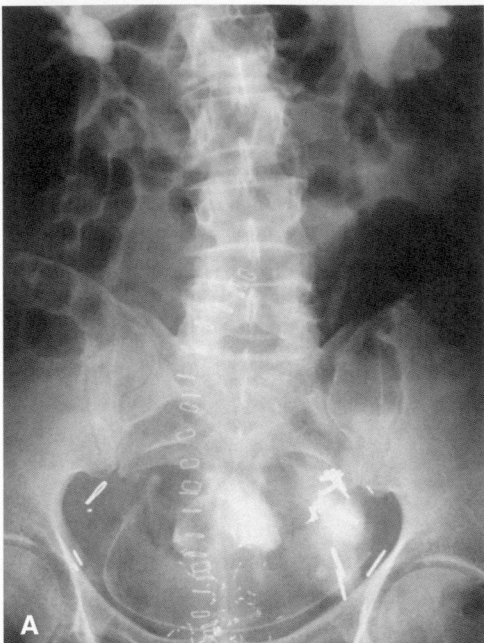

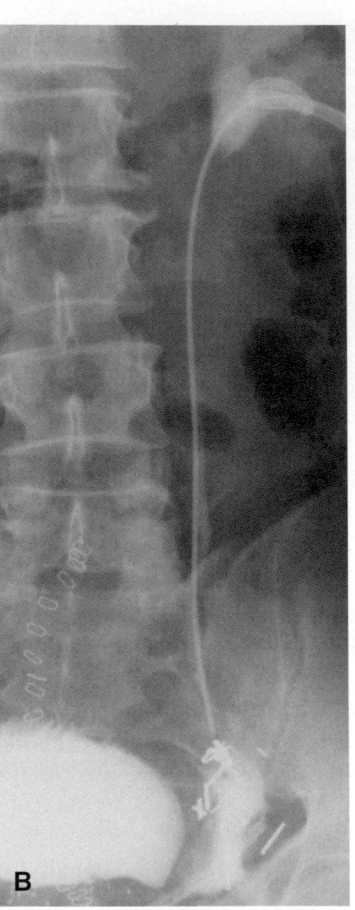

Figure 38–17 Left ureteral transection during radical prostatectomy. **A.** Intravenous urogram 2 days after surgery demonstrates contrast extravasation on the left side. **B.** A nephrostomy was performed. Attempts at traversing the transected ureteral segment with a guide wire were unsuccessful. The patient underwent ureteral reimplantation. The ureteral catheter was positioned as far distal as possible in the ureter to facilitate identification at surgery.

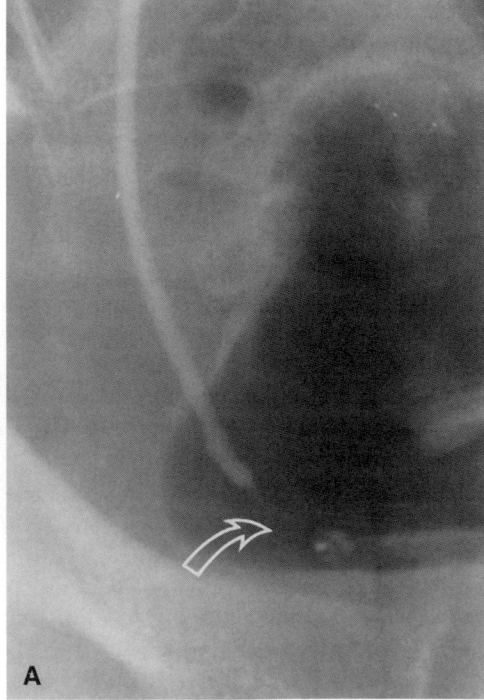

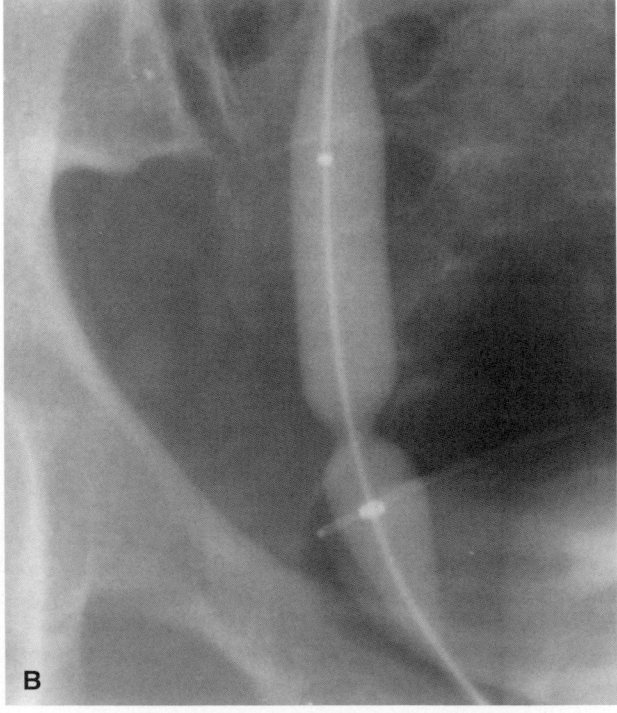

Figure 38–18 **A.** Distal ureteral stricture that developed after hysterectomy and radiation therapy for cervical cancer. The stricture (*arrow*) could not be crossed by the retrograde approach at cystoscopy. **B.** Balloon dilation with deformity at the site of the stricture. The stricture could not be dilated, despite maximal inflation of a high-pressure balloon. Patient underwent ureteral reimplanatation.

The retrograde approach is the least invasive method of management. Access can be gained by either cystoscopy or ureteroscopy and a retrograde catheter inserted, which can then be exchanged for guide wires and balloon dilators.

For dilation, reinforced high-pressure balloon catheters are used. A "waist" deformity is seen in the balloon on initial inflation and should disappear with continued or subsequent inflations. There is no consensus in the literature regarding the most effective method of dilation, whether it be the optimal size of balloon or the inflation period. In experimental studies (179), twofold dilation of the ureter was well-tolerated, but threefold dilation produced changes ranging from hydronephrosis to complete rupture. Inflated balloon diameters in published reports range between 4 and 10 mm, number of inflation cycles from 1 to 10, and the duration of inflation from 30 seconds to 10 minutes (177) to as long as 1–16 hours in various series. Similarly, there is no uniformity regarding the number of inflations that should be performed. The various technical approaches have been summarized in reviews by Meretyk et al. and Chang et al. (180–182).

After dilation, there is no consensus regarding the necessity for stenting. Some leave in stents for several days to several months; others avoid stenting altogether. Laboratory studies of ureteral healing demonstrate reepithelialization in 7–10 days and muscular healing in 6–8 weeks. Thus, 6 weeks of postprocedural stenting appears prudent because the stent serves as a scaffold for organized reepithelialization and smooth muscle growth (183). In published reports, stent sizes vary between 6 French to 16 French and stenting duration varies from 2 days to 12 weeks (177). The ultimate outcome may depend more on the nature and etiology of the stricture rather than on the technical nuances of dilation.

When performing balloon dilation through the preferred antegrade route and after dilation, a ureteral stent is placed (7–10 French native ureters, 6–8 French transplanted ureters) and left in place for at least 6 weeks to allow muscular healing while the ureteral caliber is maintained. Nephroureteral stents (external-internal stents) are preferred; they are initially left to gravity drainage and can then be capped. The patient is asked to uncap the tube in the event of flank pain, fever, or drainage around the catheter. The stent is exchanged for a nephrostomy catheter at the end of 6–8 weeks. The efficacy of the dilation can then be assessed by nephrostograms and urodynamic studies before catheter removal. The tube can be safely removed when the opening pressures are low (less than 14 cm of water), the renal pelvic residual volumes are low, and the stricture itself appears to be anatomically improved, with satisfactory flow through the previously strictured segment. If the studies demonstrate a recurrent stricture, a second attempt at redilation is usually made. Subsequent failures are managed with either open surgical repair or chronic stenting, depending on the circumstance.

When balloon dilation is apparently successful, follow-up intravenous urography or renal scans is performed at 1, 6, and 12 months and periodically as indicated—to check on the continuing patency of the ureter (184).

As mentioned previously, percutaneous ureteroneocystostomy and direct percutaneous ureteral puncture are other techniques that have been used in the management of impassable ureteral strictures (149–151). Electrocautery and rotational atherolytic devices have also been used to recanalize occluded ureters and stenotic ureteropelvic junctions (185–187), but their efficacy remains unproved.

Results

The response of strictures to balloon dilation is influenced by factors that include the etiology of the stricture, the length and location of the stricture, the duration of time that the stricture has been present, and the presence of ischemia or dense fibrosis (as in patients who have undergone radical extirpative surgery or have had radiation therapy). The relatively nonischemic strictures associated with endourologic surgery appear to respond better than do ischemic strictures.

Overall, 50% of all benign strictures respond favorably to one attempt at balloon dilation. Lang and Glorioso (188) reported that 91% of strictures less than 3 months old responded to dilation, compared to 53% of strictures that were treated more than 3 months later. In the presence of ischemia or fibrosis, only 21% of strictures were dilated successfully, whereas 70% of strictures not associated with vascular compromise responded. In a small series, Kim et al. (189) found that balloon dilation and stenting were successful in dilating tuberculous strictures in 75% of cases with good long-term results. Bilharzial strictures also respond to endourologic management, with the longer strictures requiring endoureterotomy (190). Chang et al. (182) reported 100% success in dilating strictures less than 1.5 cm in length, and O'Brien et al. (191) reported no difference in the outcomes whether the interval between ureteral injury and dilation was short or long. They reported 65% overall success in dilating benign ureteral strictures. Kwak et al. (192) found that multiple dilations were of no benefit in prolonging or maintaining ureteral patency.

Strictures related to ureterolithotomy, ureteral endoscopy, and gynecologic surgery responded in 100%, 71%, and 62% of cases, respectively, in Van Arsdalen and Banner's series (176). However, strictures associated with radical hysterectomy or retroperitoneal fibrosis responded poorly, 33 and 0%, respectively.

Endoscopic incision is advocated for treatment of most ureteral strictures. An antegrade, retrograde, or combined approach can be used. Cutting devices in use are a cold knife, electrocautery, lasers, and the Acucise cutting balloon catheter (177). Endoureterotomy success rates range from 55 to 85% for benign ureteral strictures (180,185).

Balloon dilation and stenting have been used to treat ureteropelvic junction obstruction (UPJO) primarily as an alternative to pyeloplasty and in secondary obstruction following pyeloplasty. The reported success rate varies from

64% to 86% (184,193–195). In the series reported by Snow et al. (193), resolution of the waist in an inflated balloon was accompanied by a successful outcome in 75% of cases, whereas persistence of the waist was associated with success in only 43% of cases. Balloon dilation has been nearly completely superseded by endopyelotomy, which may be more effective in treating UPJO. Reported success varies from 32% to 67% (196–198) with a higher success rate of 74% in treating secondary UPJ obstruction, which are obstructions occurring after a pyeloplasty, and 65% in treating primary UPJO (196). After dilation, the renal component of the stent placed across the UPJ should be 12–14 French in size so that wide-caliber regeneration of the UPJ can occur. Such stents taper to a 5–7 French ureteral segment.

OBSTRUCTED RENAL TRANSPLANTS

Urologic complications occur in 2–10% of renal transplant recipients, with ureteral complications and leaks accounting for the majority (199–201).

Actuarial data predict that the rate of posttransplant ureteral stenosis is 9.7% at 5 years (199). Ureteric strictures can be related to one or more of the following: postoperative urine leak with periureteral fibrosis, ureteral ischemia with resultant necrosis, selective ureteral rejection, and surgical technique used to harvest the ureter as well as to create the ureteroneocystostomy (UNC) (202–204). Ureteric obstruction because of intraluminal pathology such as a blood clot, fungus ball, or calculus is less common, as is extrinsic compression by the spermatic cord. The most common site of obstruction is at the distal ureter, near the UNC site (199,204–206), likely because of the surgical manipulations required to create the surgical anastomosis. Strictures in the proximal and middle ureter are more likely to be ischemic in nature. Urinary obstruction is a likely suspect when serum creatinine levels increase, urinary output is poor, or renal ultrasonography or radioisotope renal scan suggests hydronephrosis.

Transplant ureteral leaks are also most frequent at the UNC site and usually present in the second or third postoperative week—almost always within 5–6 weeks of transplantation (204,205). Leaks are usually the result of ureteral necrosis resulting from rejection or vascular insufficiency; extensive dissection during donor nephrectomy can jeopardize the ureteral blood supply because the ureteral vessels run in the renal hilus and periureteral soft tissue. Urinary leaks are reportedly more common in living donors than with cadaveric kidneys because more dissection is required to harvest a kidney from a living donor (207). Urinary extravasation predisposes to infection and sepsis in these immune-compromised patients and, therefore, prompt diagnosis and management is very important. Other complications that can affect renal transplants are renal artery stenosis and perirenal fluid collections, which can occur in the early or late postoperative periods.

Technique for Percutaneous Urinary Interventions in Renal Transplants

The standard preprocedural preparations for a PCN are instituted. When planning the percutaneous puncture, it is important to avoid entry into the peritoneum by staying lateral to the lateral border of the transplant and the skin sutures; transperitoneal punctures are more likely when an upper polar access is used and when the puncture is medial to the skin incision. Real-time ultrasound is useful in directing puncture into an anterolateral calix with a minimal number of sticks.

Although ultrasound is quite sensitive in detecting hydronephrosis, mild nonobstructive fullness of the transplant collecting system is not infrequent. Some believe that this may be related to denervation of renal transplants. Another cause for mild dilation of the collecting system is reflux through the UNC. Therefore, antegrade pyelography plays a crucial role in confirming the status of the transplant collecting system in patients with suspected obstruction or leak; the procedure confirms the presence of obstruction or leak, helps to localize the site of obstruction or leak, and assists in establishing an etiology, when possible (Figure 38–19).

Antegrade pyelography is performed using standard technique, as in nontransplant nephrostomies. When a stricture or occlusion is found, balloon dilation followed by

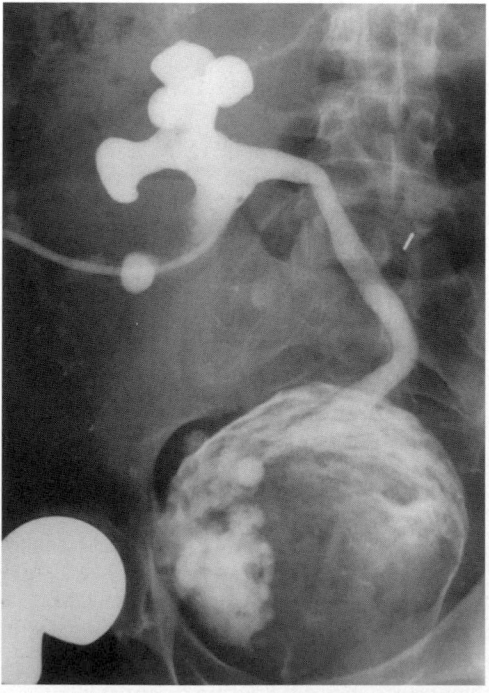

Figure 38–19   Obstruction resulting from large clots in the urinary bladder in a renal transplant patient with hemorrhagic cystitis. There is no ureteral stricture. Antegrade pyelography is of great value in transplant patient population in confirming the presence and level of obstruction.

stenting (205) or stenting alone (201,204) are treatment options. Bhagat et al. (204) used a 4-mm balloon to facilitate placement of a stent in selected patients and used 6–10 French double-pigtail ureteral stents in all patients; the distance between the pigtails was customized for each patient and varied between 8 and 10 cm. Fontaine et al. (205) balloon dilated all strictures with 5–8-mm balloons before nephroureteral stent placement. Pappas et al. (201) reported on 13 patients, of whom 8 had distal obstruction and 4 had UPJ or proximal ureteral obstruction; these authors dilated the stricture in only 7–12 patients (58%) before placement of 24-cm long double-pigtail ureteral stents in all 12 patients. The stents were left in place for a mean duration of 15 months. One preference of Kim et al. (206) is to balloon dilate all ureteral strictures with 6–10-mm high-pressure balloons (17 atm) before stenting with a nephroureteral catheter; some use commercially available, special-order catheters (Cook, Inc.) that are 8–10 French in diameter with

an 8–10-cm distance between the two pigtails. Only the proximal pigtail is self-retaining, as is the case with nephroureteral catheters used for ureteral stenting in native nontransplant urinary tracts. Internalized stents reportedly have fewer infection complications because there is no external catheter, but percutaneous access (Figure 38–20) is lost, obviating radiologic evaluation of the strictured segment. Stents were left indwelling without interval change for a mean duration of 15 months in one series (201) and up to 2 years in another series (204), without evidence of obstruction.

Surgical management of ureteral obstructions is required when the stricture cannot be traversed with a wire, the stricture does not respond to balloon dilation and stenting, or the radiographic findings strongly suggest extrinsic compression by vascular structures or the spermatic cord (Figure 38–21). In these cases, the nephrostomy serves as a diagnostic tool as well as a temporizing measure to improve renal function preoperatively. Graft survival appears to be higher in patients

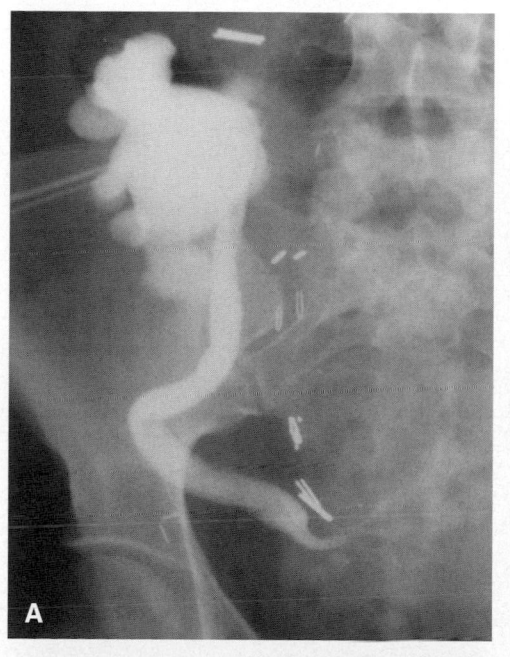
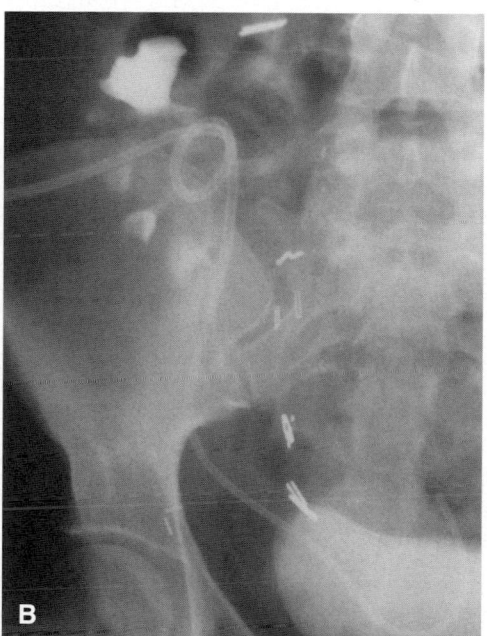
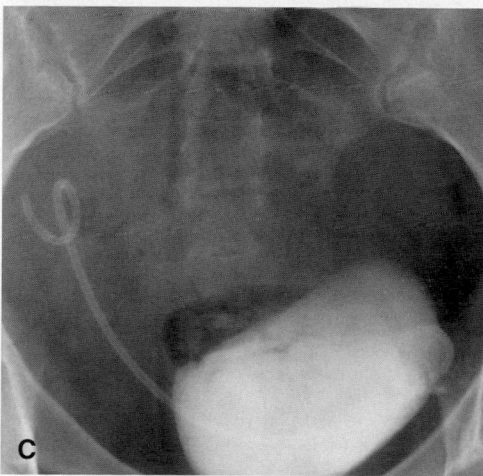

Figure 38–20 A. Ureteral stricture at ureteroneo-cystostomy site following renal transplant. **B.** Nephroastogram demonstrates hydronephrosis and stricture at the ureteroneocystostomy site that was balloon-dilated. **C.** A nephroureteral catheter was initially placed after dilation and followed by an internalized stent. The latter was removed cystoscopically after 8 weeks.

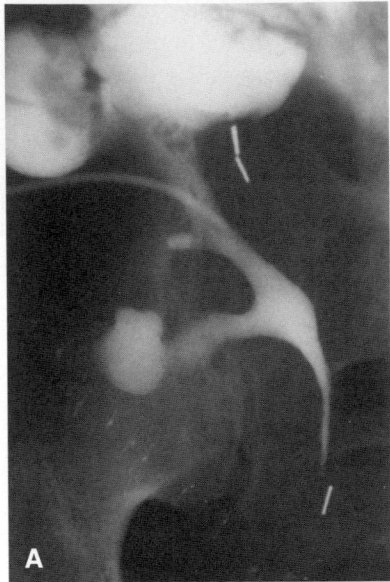
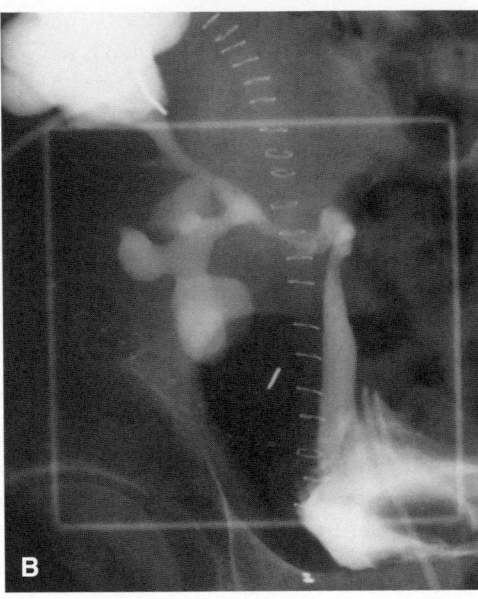

Figure 38–21 Midureteral stricture in renal transplant 16 years after the transplant. **A.** Antegrade nephrostogram demonstrates a high-grade stricture in the ureter that could not be traversed with a guide wire. Note the contrast leakage from the dilated upper pole calix resulting from spontaneous rupture of the calyx. **B.** The patient underwent ureteroureterostomy (native ureter anastomosed to transplant ureter proximal to stricture). Postoperative nephrostogram demonstrates good contrast flow through the ureteral anastomotic site into the urinary bladder.

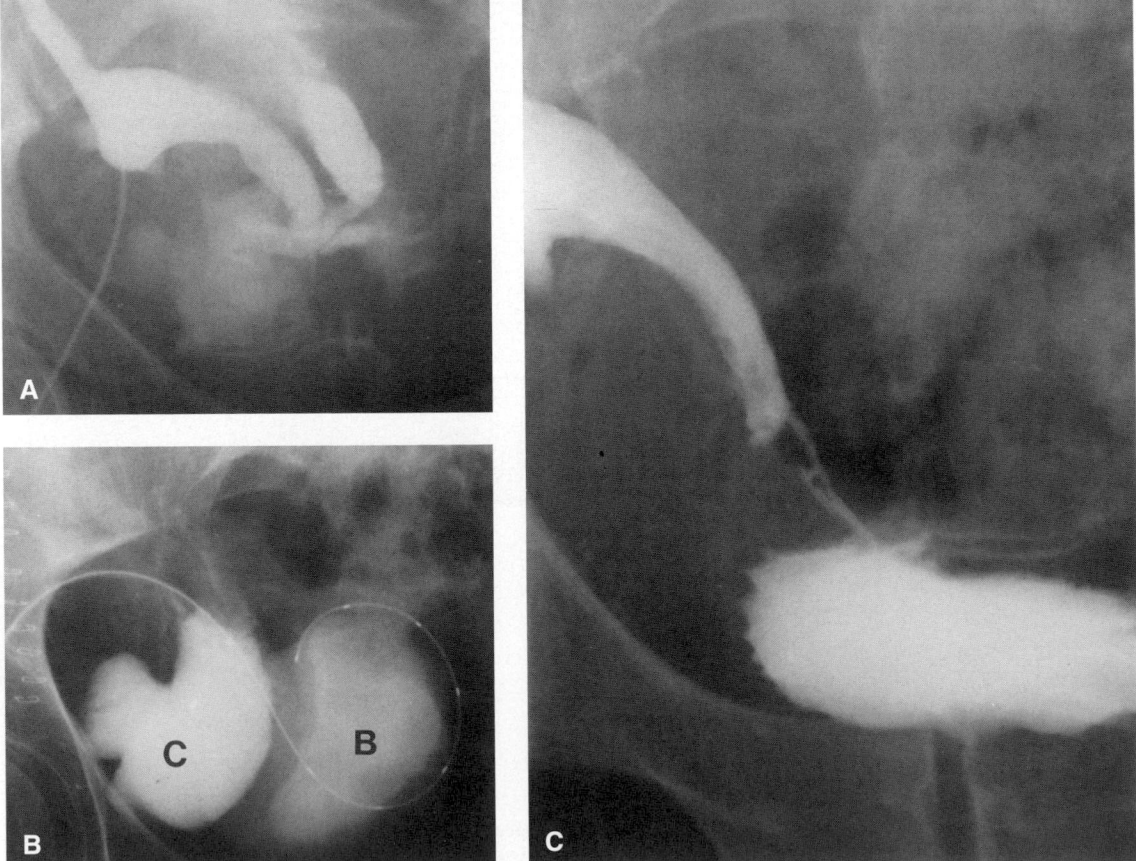

Figure 38–22 Dehiscence at ureteroneocystostomy site. **A.** Antegrade pyelogram demonstrates marked extravasation at ureteral anastomotic site with no contrast entering the urinary bladder. **B.** A guide wire was successfully advanced into the bladder and a stent was placed: (C) extravasated contrast and (B) bladder. **C.** Two months later, a high-grade stricture is seen in the distal ureter that was unresponsive to balloon dilation.

treated with ureteral stent placement as opposed to surgery (208).

Balloon dilation of transplant ureteral strictures has been reported to be effective in 40–78% of patients (201,204,206–212). Initial technical success in dilating the stricture does not translate into long-term success. Failure of balloon dilation becomes evident usually within weeks of the stent removal; Streem and colleagues (210) found that every failure presents within 12 months of dilation. Strictures that present early—within 3 months of surgery, for example—have been reported by some to respond better to balloon dilation and stenting (204–206), but other series have not shown this result (206). Early strictures reportedly respond in 62–100% of cases and late strictures (less than 3 months) respond in 16–66% of cases (211). Endoureterotomy, which involves incision of the stricture, has also been used for UNC strictures (212,213); the results and indications for endoureterotomy are still evolving with the reported series consisting of only a few patients each. Prolonged ureteral stenting alone may be effective in treating transplant ureteral strictures (201,204). Bhagat et al. (204) reported that 69% (18 of 26) of early obstructions and 33% (5 of 15) late obstructions (overall success rate of 57%—25 of 44 patients) responded to a stenting period of an average of 75 days, and the failures were treated with either surgery or chronic stent placement. Pappas et al. (201) reported that 75% of their cases responded successfully.

Strictures that develop at the ureteroneocystostomy site appear to respond better to balloon dilation than strictures at other sites in the ureter (Figure 38–20) (205). This may be related to the ischemic nature of strictures in the proximal and middle ureter, whereas strictures at the ureteral anastomotic site are related to either errors in surgical technique (particularly for strictures that present in the early postoperative period) or to periureteral fibrosis in the later period. Strictures sometimes developing in association with dehiscence at the ureteroneocystostomy site are generally resistant to balloon dilation and require surgery for definitive therapy (Figure 38–22).

Ureteral leaks also occur most frequently at the UNC; Bhagat et al. (204) reported that 80% of leaks were at the UNC, and 50% of leaks were associated with stenoses. Ureteral stenting is effective in promoting healing and resolution of the leak in 59–80% of cases (204,205). If ureteral leak persists, surgical repair is usually required. With large leaks, cannulating the ureter distal to the leak may be problematic because the guide wire tends to pass out through the ureteral rent.

The only complication unique to the transplant nephrostomy is intraperitoneal leak of contrast resulting from inadvertent puncture of the peritoneum (204). This problem usually resolves spontaneously without event. Because the patients are immunocompromised, special vigilance is required to avoid precipitating septicemia when percutaneous interventions are performed. Minor urinary tract infections reportedly can occur in as many as 38% of patients after the procedure (205).

REFERENCES

1. Goodwin WE, Casey WC, Woolf W. Percutaneous trocar (needle) nephrostomy in hydronephrosis. JAMA 1955;157:891–894.
2. Fowler JS, Meares EM Jr, Goldin AR. Percutaneous nephrostomy: techniques, indications, and results. Urology 1975;6:428.
3. Levin DC, Flanders SJ, Spettell CM, et al. Participation by radiologists and other specialists in percutaneous vascular and nonvascular interventions: findings from a seven-state database. Radiology 1995;196:51–54.
4. Mahaffey KG, Bolton DM, Stoller ML. Urologist directed percutaneous nephrostomy tube placement. J Urol 1994;152:1973–1976.
5. Smith, AD. Editorial: Percutaneous punctures-is this the endourologist's turf? J Urol 1994;152:1982–1983.
6. Chien GW, Bellman GC. Blind percutaneous renal access. J Endourology 2002;16:93–95.
7. Pearle MS. Editorial comment. J Endourology 2002;16:96.
8. Shokeir AA, El-Diasty T, Eassa W, et al. Diagnosis of ureteral obstruction in patients with compromised renal function: the role of noninvasive imaging modalities. J Urol 2004;171:2303–2306.
9. Shokeir AA, El-Diasty T, Eassa W, et al. Diagnosis of noncalcareous hydronephrosis: role of magnetic resonance urography and noncontrast computed tomography. Urology 2004;63:225–229.
10. El-Ghar MEA, Shokheir AA, El-Diasty T, et al. Contrast enhanced spiral computerized tomography in patients with chronic obstructive uropathy and normal serum creatinine: a single session for anatomical and functional assessment. J Urol 2004;172:985–988.
11. Zielonko J, Studniarek M, Markuszewski M. MR urography of obstructive uropathy: diagnostic value of the method in selected clinical groups. Eur Radiol 2003;13:802–809.
12. Farrell TA, Hicks MS. A review of radiologically guided percutaneous nephrostomies in 303 patients. J Vasc Interv Radiol 1997;8:769–774.
13. Banner MP, Ramchandani P, Pollack HM. Interventional procedures in the upper urinary tract. Cardiovasc Intervent Radiol 1991;14:267–284.
14. Fritzsche P. Antegrade pyelography: therapeutic applications. Radiol Clin North Am 1986;24:573–586.
15. Barbaric ZL. Percutaneous nephrostomy for urinary tract obstruction. AJR Am J Roentgenol 1984;143:803–809.
16. Zagoria RJ, Hodge RG, Dyer RB, et al. Percutaneous nephrostomy for treatment of intractable hemorrhagic cystitis. J Urol 1993;149:1449–1451.
17. Silverman SG, Mueller PR, Pfister RC. Hemostatic evaluation before abdominal interventions: an overview and proposal. AJR Am J Roentgenol 1990;154:233–238.
18. Cochran ST, Barbaric ZL, Lee JJ, et al. Percutaneous nephrostomy tube placement: an outpatient procedure. Radiology 1991;179:843–847.
19. Rapaport SI. Assessing hemostatic function before abdominal interventions. AJR Am J Roentgenol 1990;154:239–240.
20. Ferral H, Stackhouse DJ, Bjarnason H, et al. Complications of percutaneous nephrostomy tube placement. Semin Intervent Radiol 1994;11:198–206.
21. Payne CS. A primer on patient management problems in interventional radiology. AJR Am J Roentgenol 1998;170:1169–1176.
22. Rohrer MJ, Michelotti MC, Nahrwold DL. A prospective evaluation of the efficacy of preoperative coagulation testing. Ann Surg 1988;208:554–557.
23. Millward SF. Percutaneous nephrostomy: a practical approach. J Vasc Interv Radiol. 2000;11:955–964.
24. Lee WJ, Mond DJ, Patel M, et al. Emergency percutaneous nephrostomy: technical success based on level of operator experience. J Vasc Interv Radiol 1994;5:327–330.
25. Gray RR, So BC, McLoughlin RF, et al. Outpatient percutaneous nephrostomy. Radiology 1996;198:85–88.
26. McDermott VG, Schuster MG, Smith TP. Antibiotic prophylaxis in vascular and interventional radiology. AJR Am J Roentgenol 1997;169:31–38.

27. Larsen E, Gasser T, Madsen P. Antibiotic prophylaxis in urologic surgery. Urol Clin North Am 1986;13:591–604.

28. Yoder IC, Pfister RC, Lindfors KK, et al. Pyonephrosis: imaging and intervention. AJR Am J Roentgenol 1983;141:735–740.

29. Ryan MJ, Ryan BM, Smith TP. Antibiotic prophylaxis in interventional radiology. J Vasc Interv Radiol 2004;15:547–556.

30. Classen DC, Evans RS, Pestonik SL. The timing of prophylactic administration of antibiotics and the risk of surgical wound infection. N Engl J Med 1992;326:281–286.

31. Spies JB, Rosen RJ, Lebowitz AS. Antibiotic prophylaxis in vascular and interventional radiology: a rational approach. Radiology 1988;166:381–387.

32. Hogan MJ, Coley BD, Jayanthi VR, et al. Percutaneous nephrostomy in children and adolescents: outpatient management. Radiology 2001;218:207–210.

33. Barbaric ZL, Hall T, Cochran ST, et al. Percutaneous nephrostomy: placement under CT and fluoroscopy guidance. AJR Am J Roentgenol 1997;169:151–155.

34. Ozden E, Yaman O, Soygur T, et al. Sonography-guided percutaneous nephrostomy: success rates according to the grade of hydronephrosis. J of Ankara Med School 2002;24(2):69–72.

35. von der Recke P, Nielsen MB, Pedersen JF. Complications of ultrasound-guided nephrostomy: a 5-year experience. Acta Radiol 1994;35:452–454.

36. Dyer RB, Regan JD, Kavanagh PV, et al. Percutaneous nephrostomy with extensions of the technique: step by step. Radiographics 2002;22:503–525.

37. LeMaitre L, Mestdagh P, Marecaux-Delomez J, et al. Percutaneous nephrostomy: placement under laser guidance and real-time CT fluoroscopy. Eur Radiol 2000;10:892–895.

38. Naidich JB, Rackson ME, Mossey RT, et al. Nondilated obstructive uropathy: percutaneous nephrostomy performed to reverse renal failure. Radiology 1986;160:653–657.

39. Gupta S, Gulati M, Suri S. Ultrasound-guided percutaneous nephrostomy in nondilated pelvicaliceal systems. J Clin Ultrasound 1998;26(3):177–179.

40. Nolte-Ernsting CCA, Bucker A, Neuerburg JM, et al. MR imaging-guided percutaneous nephrostomy and use of MR-compatible catheters in the nondilated porcine urinary tract. J Vasc Interv Radiol 1999;10:1305–1314.

41. Merkle EM, Hashim M, Wendt M, et al. MR-guided percutaneous nephrostomy of the nondilated upper urinary tract in a porcine model. AJR Am J Roentgenol 1999;172:1221–1225.

42. Reznek RH, Talner LB. Percutaneous nephrostomy. Radiol Clin North Am 1984;22:393–406.

43. Newhouse JH, Pfister RC. Percutaneous catheterization of the kidney and perinephric space: trocar technique. Urol Radiol 1981;2:157–164.

44. Hawkins IF Jr, Hunter P, Leal G, et al. Retrograde nephrostomy for stone removal—combined cystoscopic/percutaneous technique. AJR Am J Roentgenol 1984;143:299–304.

45. Stables DP. Percutaneous nephrostomy: techniques, indications, and results. Urol Clin North Am 1982;9:15–29.

46. Sampaio FJB, Zanier JFC, Aragao AHM, et al. Intrarenal access: three-dimensional anatomical study. J Urol 1992;148:1769–1773.

47. Stables DP, Ginsberg NJ, Johnson ML. Percutaneous nephrostomy: a series and review of the literature. AJR Am J Roentgenol 1978;130:75–82.

48. Lee WJ, Patel U, Patel S, et al. Emergency percutaneous nephrostomy: results and complications. J Vasc Interv Radiol 1994;5:135–139.

49. Leroy AJ. Percutaneous nephrostomy: techniques and instrumentation. In: Pollack HM, ed. Clinical Urography. Philadelphia: Saunders, 1990:2726.

50. Gupta S, Gulati M, Uday Shankar K, et al. Percutaneous nephrostomy with real time sonographic guidance. Acta Radiol 1997;38:454–457.

51. Lewis S, Patel U. Major complications after percutaneous nephrostomy—lessons from a department audit. Clin Radiol 2001;59:171–179.

52. Riddell AM, Charig MJ. A survey of current practice in out of hours percutaneous nephrostomy insertion in the United Kingdom. Clin Radiol 2002;57:1067–1069.

53. Camunez F, Echenagusia A, Prieto ML, et al. Percutaneous nephrostomy in pyonephrosis. Urol Radiol 1989;11:77–81.

54. Lang EK, Price ET. Redefinitions of indications for percutaneous nephrostomy. Radiology 1983;147:419–426.

55. Pearle MS, Pierce HL, Miller GL, et al. Optimal method of urgent decompression of the collecting system for obstruction and infection due to ureteral calculi. J Urol 1996;160:1260–1264.

56. Bell AD, Rose SC, Starr NK, et al. Percutaneous nephrostomy for nonoperative management of fungal urinary tract infections. J Vasc Interv Radiol 1993;4:311–315.

57. Gadducci A, Madrigali A, Facchini V, et al. Percutaneous nephrostomy in patients with advanced or recurrent cervical cancer. Clin Exp Obstet Gynecol 1994;21:71–73.

58. Pappas P, Stravodimos KG, Mitropoulos D, et al. Role of percutaneous urinary diversion in malignant and benign obstructive uropathy. J Endourol 2000;14:401–405.

59. Feng MI, Bellman GC, Shapiro CE. Management of ureteral obstruction secondary to pelvic malignancies. J Endourol 1999;13(7):521–524.

60. Docimo SG, Dewolf WC. High failure rate of indwelling ureteral stents in patients with extrinsic obstruction: experience at 2 institutions. J Urol 1989;142:277–279.

61. Shekarriz B, Shekarriz H, Upadhyay J, et al. Outcome of palliative urinary diversion in the treatment of advanced malignancies. Cancer 1999;85:998–1003.

62. Hoe JWM, Tung KH, Tan EC. Re-evaluation of indications for percutaneous nephrostomy and interventional uroradiological procedures in pelvic malignancy. Br J Radiol 1993;71:469–472.

63. Markowitz DM, Wong KT, Laffey KJ, et al. Maintaining quality of life after palliative diversion for malignant ureteral obstruction. Urol Radiol 1989;11:129–132.

64. Ekici S, Sahin A, Ozen H. Percutaneous nephrostomy in the management of malignant ureteral obstruction secondary to bladder cancer. J Endourol 2001;15(8):827–829.

65. Chapman ME, Reid JH. Use of percutaneous nephrostomy in malignant ureteric obstruction. Br J Radiol 1991;64:318–320.

66. Dowling RA, Carrasco CH, Babaian RJ. Percutaneous urinary diversion in patients with hormone refractory prostate cancer. Urology 1991;37:89–91.

67. Ramchandani P, Cardella JF, Grassi CJ, et al. Quality improvement guidelines for percutaneous nephrostomy. J Vasc Interv Radiol 2001;12:1247–1251.

68. Ramchandani P, Lewis CA, Bakal C, et al. ACR practice guidelines for the performance of percutaneous nephrostomy. Effective 1/1/02, pp 335–343.

69. Cope C, Zeit RM. Pseudoaneurysms after nephrostomy. AJR Am J Roentgenol 1982;139:255–261.

70. Clark TW, Abraham RJ, Flemming BK. Is routine micropuncture access necessary for percutaneous nephrostomy?: a randomized trial. Can Assoc Radiol J 2002;53:87–91.

71. Zagoria RJ, Dyer RB. Dos and don'ts of percutaneous nephrostomy. Acad Radiol 1999;6:370–377.

72. Cronan JJ, Dorfman GS, Amis ES, et al. Retroperitoneal hemorrhage after percutaneous nephrostomy. AJR Am J Roentgenol 1985;144:801–803.

73. Routh WD, Tatum CM, Lawdahl RB, et al. Tube tamponade: potential pitfall in angiography of arterial hemorrhage associated with percutaneous drainage catheters. Radiology 1990;174:945–949.

74. Merine D, Fishman EK. Perirenal hematoma following catheter removal—an unusual complication of percutaneous nephrostomy. Clin Imaging 1989;13:74–76.

75. Nosher JL, Ericksen AS, Trooskin SZ, et al. Antibiotic-bonded nephrostomy catheters for percutaneous nephrostomies. Cardiovasc Intervent Radiol 1990;13:102–106.

76. Varkarakis J, Su Li-Ming, Hsu THS. Air embolism from pneumopyelography. J Urol 2003;169:267.

77. Cadeddu JA, Arrindell D, Moore RG. Near fatal air embolism during percutaneous nephrostomy placement. J Urol 1997;158:1519.

78. Leroy AJ, Williams HJ Jr, Bender CE, et al. Colon perforation following percutaneous nephrostomy and renal calculus removal. Radiology 1985;155:83–85.

79. Miller G, Summa J. Transcolonic placement of a percutaneous nephrostomy tube: recognition and treatment. J Vasc Interv Radiol 1997;8:401–403.

80. Vallancien G, Capdeville R, Veillon B, et al. Colonic perforation during nephrolithotomy. J Urol 1985;134:1185–1187.

81. Hopper KD, Yakes WF. The posterior intercostal approach for percutaneous renal procedures: risk of puncturing the lung, spleen, and liver as determined by CT. AJR Am J Roentgenol 1990;154:115–117.

82. Lopes Neto ACL, Tobias-Machado M, Juliana RV, et al. Duodenal damage complicating percutaneous access to kidney. Sao Paulo Med J 2000;118:116–117.

83. Morris DB, Siegelbaum MH, Pollack HM, et al. Renoduodenal fistula in a patient with chronic nephrostomy drainage: a case report. J Urol 1991;146:835–837.

84. Reinberg Y, Moore LS, Lange PH. Splenic abscess as a complication of percutaneous nephrostomy. Urology 1989;34:274–276.

85. Picus D, Weyman PJ, Clayman RV, et al. Intercostal space nephrostomy for percutaneous stone removal. AJR Am J Roentgenol 1986;147:393–397.

86. Jones CD, McGahan JP. Computed tomographic evaluation and guided correction of malpositioned nephrostomy catheters. Abdom Imaging 1999;24:422–425.

87. Liu DM, Torreggiani WC, Rowley VA. Hydrostatic reduction of iatrogenic intussusception of the ureter secondary to percutaneous nephrostomy catheter exchange. J Vasc Interv Radiol 2000;11:1076–1078.

88. Marx VM. The radiation dose in interventional radiology study: knowledge brings responsibility. J Vasc Interv Radiol 2003;14:947–951.

89. Miller DL, Balter S, Cole PE, et al. Radiation doses in interventional radiology procedures: the RAD-IR study: part I—overall measurement of dose. J Vasc Interv Radiol 2003;14:711–727.

90. Miller DL, Balter S, Cole PE, et al. Radiation doses in interventional radiology procedures: the RAD-IR study: part II—skin dose. J Vasc Interv Radiol 2003;14:977–990.

91. Trewhella M, Reis B, Gillespie A, et al. Percutaneous nephrostomy to relieve renal tract obstruction in pregnancy. Br J Radiol 1991;64:471–472.

92. Pollack HM, Banner MP. Replacing blocked or dislodged percutaneous nephrostomy and ureteral stent catheters. Radiology 1982;145:203–205.

93. Cazenave FL, Glass-Royal MC, Barth KH. Exchange of an obstructed loop nephrostomy catheter: technical note. Cardiovasc Intervent Radiol 1990;13:327–328.

94. Ahn J, Trost DW, Topham SL, et al. Retained nephrostomy thread providing a nidus for atypical renal calcification. Br J Radiol 1997;70:309–310.

95. Stewart LH, Kernohan RM, Loughridge WG. Nephrostomy tubes resistant to removal. Br J Urol 1992;70:213–214.

96. Vaccaro JA, Davis R, Hansberry K. Replacement of nephrostomy tube using ureteroscopes. J Urol 1993;149:334.

97. Cronan JJ, Marcello A, Horn DL, et al. Antibiotics and nephrostomy tube care: preliminary observations: part I—bacteriuria. Radiology 1989;172:1041–1042.

98. Cronan JJ, Horn DL, Marcello A, et al. Antibiotics and nephrostomy tube care: preliminary observations: part II—bacteremia. Radiology 1989;172:1043–1045.

99. Orme R, Scott-Cook H, Farrar DJ. 'Aneurysm' of nephrostomy catheter complicating extracorporeal shock-wave lithotripsy. Clin Radiol 1999;54:408–410.

100. Hruby W, Marberger M. Late sequelae of percutaneous nephrostomy. Radiology 1984;152:383–385.

101. Beiko DT, Knudsen BE, Denstedt JD. Advances in ureteral stent design. J Endourol 2003;17:195–199.

102. Chew BH, Knudsen BE, Denstedt JD. Advances in ureteral stent design and construction. Contemp Urol 2004;10:16–20.

103. Holmes SAV, Kirby RS, Whitfield HN. Urinary tract prostheses and their biocompatibility. Br J Urol 1993;71:378–383.

104. Mardis HK, Kroeger RM, Morton JJ, et al. Comparative evaluation of materials used for internal ureteral stents. J Endourol 1993;7:105–115.

105. Mardis HK, Kroeger RM. Ureteral stents: materials. Urol Clin North Am 1988;15:471.

106. El-Faqih SR, Shamsuddin AB, Chakrabarti A, et al. Polyurethane internal ureteral stents in treatment of stone patients: morbidity related to indwelling times. J Urol 1991;146:1487–1491.

107. Leroy AJ, Williams HJ, Segura JW, et al. Indwelling ureteral stents: percutaneous management of complications. Radiology 1986;158:219–222.

108. Mitty HA, Dan SJ, Train JS. Antegrade ureteral stents: technical and catheter related problems with polyethylene and polyurethane. Radiology 1987;165:439–443.

109. Marx M, Bettman MA, Bridges S, et al. The effects of various indwelling ureteral catheter materials on the normal canine ureter. J Urol 1988;139:180.

110. Rackson ME, Mitty HA, Lossef SV, et al. Biocompatible copolymer ureteral stent: maintenance of patency beyond 6 months. AJR Am J Roentgenol1 989;153:783–784.

111. Cardella JF, Castañeda-Zuniga WR, Hunter DW, et al. Urine-compatible polymer for long-term ureteral stenting. Radiology 1986;161:313–318.

112. Pauer W, Lugmayr H. Metallic Wallstents: a new therapy for extrinsic ureteral obstruction. J Urol 1992;148:281–284.

113. Lugmayr H, Pauer W. Self-expanding metal stents for palliative treatment of malignant ureteral obstruction. AJR Am J Roentgenol 1992;159:1091–1094.

114. Lugmayr H, Pauer W. Wallstents for the treatment of extrinsic malignant ureteral obstruction: midterm results. Radiology 1996;198:105–108.

115. Flueckiger F, Lammer J, Klein GE, et al. Malignant ureteral obstruction: preliminary results of treatment with metallic self-expandable stents. Radiology 1993;186:169–173.

116. van Sonnenberg E, D'Agostino HB, O'Laoide R, et al. Malignant ureteral obstruction: treatment with metal stents—technique, results and observations with percutaneous intraluminal US. Radiology 1994;191:765–768.

117. Cussenot O, Bassi S, Desgrandchamps F, et al. Outcomes of non–self-expandable metal prostheses in strictured human ureter: suggestions for future developments. J Endourol 1993;7:205–209.

118. Desgrandchamps F, Cussenot O, Cochand-Priollet B, et al. Strecker stent as ureteral stent: experimental study. J Endourol 1992;6:433–437.

119. Kulkarni R, Bellamy E. Nickel-titanium shape memory alloy Memokath 051 ureteral stent for managing long-term ureteral obstruction: 4-year experience. J Urol 2001;166:1750–1754.

120. Lingeman JE, Preminger GM, Berger Y, et al. Use of a temporary ureteral drainage stent after uncomplicated ureteroscopy: results from a phase II clinical trial. J Urol 2003;169:1682–1688.

121. Schlick RW, Plantz K. In vitro results with special plastics for biodegradable endourethral stents. J Endourol 1998;12:451–455.

122. Dyer RB, Chen MY, Zagoria RJ, et al. Complications of ureteral stent placement. Radiographics 2002;22:1005–1022.

123. Lee MJ, Lu DS, Papanicolaou N, et al. Antegrade ureteral stents: proposed solutions to technically difficult problems. Radiology 1993;189(P):371.

124. Mitty HA. Ureteral stenting facilitated by antegrade transurethral passage of guide wire. AJR Am J Roentgenol 1984;142:831–832.

125. D'Souza R, Tait P, Thomson RW, et al. Case report: an alternative approach to stenting the ureter. Br J Radiol 1993;66:460–461.

126. Watson GMT, Patel U. Primary antegrade ureteric stenting: prospective experience and cost-effectiveness analysis in 50 ureters. Clin Radiol 2001;56:568–574.

127. Patel U, Abubacker MZ. Ureteral stent placement without postprocedural nephrostomy tube: experience in 41 patients. Radiology 2004;230:435–442.

128. Greenstein A, Shoval Y, Chen J, et al. Incidental extraction of double pigtail catheter during nephrostomy removal. Urol Radiol 1989;11:121–122.

129. Seymour H, Patel U. Ureteral stenting: current status. Semin Intervent Radiol 2000;17:351–366.

130. Amendola MA, Banner MP, Pollack HM, et al. Fluoroscopically guided pyeloureteral interventions by using a perurethral transvesical approach. AJR Am J Roentgenol 1989;152:97–102.

131. Babel SG, Winterkorn KG. Retrograde catheterization of the ureter without cystoscopic assistance: preliminary experience. Radiology 1993;187:547–549.

132. Huang TY, Perkins T, Mader G. Retrograde placement of internal double-J ureteral stents by using cystographic guidance. AJR Am J Roentgenol 1994;163:371–372.

133. Babel SG, Winterkorn KG. Primary retrograde placement of ureteral stents by radiologists. AJR Am J Roentgenol 1995;164:1555.

134. deBaere T, Denys A, Pappas P, et al. Ureteral stents: exchange under fluoroscopic control as an effective alternative to cystoscopy. Radiology 1994;190:887–889.

135. Yedlicka JW, Aizpuru R, Hunter DW, et al. Retrograde replacement of internal double-J ureteral stents. AJR Am J Roentgenol 1991; 156:1007–1009.

136. Pilcher JM, Patel U. Choosing the correct length of ureteric stent: a formula based on the patient's height compared with direct ureteric measurement. Clin Radiol 2002;57:59–62.

137. Eiley DM, McDougall EM, Smith AD. Techniques for stenting the normal and obstructed ureter. J Endourol 1997;11:419–429.

138. Herrera M, Brawerman S. The endocatheter ruler: a useful new device. AJR Am J Roentgenol 1982;139:828–829.

139. Wills MI, Gilbert HW, Chadwick DJ, et al. Which ureteric stent length? Br J Urol 1991;68:440.

140. Yossepowitch O, Lifshitz DA, Dekel Y, et al. Predicting the success of retrograde stenting for managing ureteral obstruction. J Urol 2001;166:1746–1749.

141. Chung SY, Stein RJ, Landsittel D, et al. 15-year experience with the management of extrinsic ureteral obstruction with indwelling ureteral stents. J Urol 2004;172:592–595.

142. Fine H, Gordon RL, Lebensart PD. Extracorporeal shock-wave lithotripsy and stents: fluoroscopic observations and a hypothesis on the mechanisms of stent function. Urol Radiol 1989;11:37.

143. Rotaru P, Yohannes P, Alexianu M, et al. Management of malignant extrinsic compression of the ureter by simultaneous placement of two ipsilateral ureteral stents. J Endourol 2001;15:979–983.

144. Lang EK, Irwin RJ, Lopez-Martinez RA, et al. Placement of metallic stents in ureters obstructed by carcinoma of the cervix to maintain renal function in patients undergoing long-term chemotherapy. AJR Am J Roentgenol 1998;171:1595–1599.

145. Diaz-Lucas EF, Martinez-Torres JL, Mena JF, et al. Self-expanding Wallstent endoprosthesis for malignant ureteral obstruction. J Endourol 1997;11:441–447.

146. Ahmed M, Bishop MC, Bates CP, et al. Metal mesh stents for ureteral obstruction caused by hormone-resistant carcinoma of the prostate. J Endourol 1999;13:221–224.

147. Slavis SA, Wilson RW, Jones RJ, et al. Long-term results of permanent indwelling Wallstents for benign midureteral strictures. J Endourol 2000;14:577–581.

148. Pollak JS, Rosenblatt MM, Egglin TK, et al. Treatment of ureteral obstructions with the Wallstent endoprosthesis: preliminary results. J Vasc Interv Radiol 1995;6:417–425.

149. Cornud FE, Casanova JP, Bonnel DH, et al. Impassable ureteral strictures: management with percutaneous ureteroneocystostomy. Radiology 1991;180:451–454.

150. Lang EK. Percutaneous ureterocystostomy and ureteroneocystostomy. AJR Am J Roentgenol 1988;150:1065–1068.

151. Rosdy E. Percutaneous transrenal ureteroneocystostomy. J Endourol 1999;13:369–372.

152. Mishra VC, Rao AR, Desai AR, et al. A unique extra-anatomic urinary diversion. J Endourol 2004;18:57–58.

153. Bilbao JI, Longo JM, Martin-Palance A, et al. Direct percutaneous ureteral approach for the treatment of ureteral stenosis or obstruction. J Vasc Interv Radiol 1992;3:553–555.

154. Jabbour ME, Desgrandchamps F, Angelescu E, et al. Percutaneous implantation of subcutaneous prosthetic ureters: long-term outcome. J Endourol 2001;15:611–614.

155. Thomas R. Indwelling ureteral stents: impact of material and shape on patient comfort. J Endourol 1993;7:137–140.

156. Ramsay JWA, Crocker RP, Ball AJ, et al. Urothelial reaction to ureteric intubation: a clinical study. Br J Urol 1987;60:504.

157. El-Faqih SR, Shamsuddin AB, Chakrabarti A, et al. Polyurethane internal ureteral stents in treatment of stone patients: morbidity related to indwelling times. J Urol 1991;146:1487–1491.

158. Fox CW Jr, Vaccaro JA, Kiesling FJ Jr, et al. Determination of indwelling ureteral stent patency: comparison of standard contrast and nuclear cystography and Lasix renography. Urology 1994;43:442–445.

159. Platt JR, Ellis JH, Rubin JM. Assessment of internal ureteral stent patency in patients with pyelocaliectases: value of renal duplex sonography. AJR Am J Roentgenol 1993;161:87–90.

160. Haferkamp A, Brkovic D, Wiesel M, et al. Role of color-coded Doppler sonography in the assessment of internal ureteral stent patency. J Endourol 1999;13:199–203.

161. Singh I, Gupta MP, Hemal AK et al. Severely encrusted polyurethane ureteral stents: management and analysis of potential risk factors. Urology 2001;58:526–531.

162. Trillaud H, Pariente J-L, Rabie A, et al. Detection of encrusted indwelling ureteral stents using a twinkling artifact revealed on color Doppler sonography. AJR Am J Roentgenol 2001;176: 1446–1448.

163. Bukkapatnam R, Seigne J, Helal M. 1-step removal of encrusted retained ureteral stents. J Urol 2003;170:1111–1114.

164. Lam JS, Gupta M. Tips and tricks for the management of retained ureteral stents. J Endourol 2002;16:733–741.

165. Monga M, Klein E, Castañeda-Zuniga WR, et al. The forgotten indwelling ureteral stent: a urological dilemma. J Urol 1995; 153:1817–1819.

166. Somers WJ. Management of forgotten or retained indwelling ureteral stents. Urology 1996;47:431–435.

167. Salazar JE, Johnson JB, Scott RL. Perforation of renal pelvis by internal ureteral stents. AJR Am J Roentgenol 1984;143:816–818.

168. Slaton JW, Kropp KA. Proximal ureteral stent migration: an avoidable complication. J Urol 1996;155:58–61.

169. Quillin SP, Darcy MD, Picus D. Angiographic evaluation and therapy of ureteroarterial fistulas. AJR Am J Roentgenol 1994;162: 873–878.

170. Vandersteen DR, Saxon RR, Fuchs E, et al. Diagnosis and management of ureteroiliac artery fistula: value of provocative arteriography followed by common iliac artery embolization and extra-anatomic arterial bypass grafting. J Urol 1997;158:754–758.

171. Batter SJ, McGovern FJ, Cambria RP. Ureteroarterial fistula: case report and review of the literature. Urology 1996;48:481–489.

172. Keller FS, Barton RE, Routh WD, et al. Gross hematuria in two patients with ureteral ileal conduits and double-J stents. J Vasc Interv Radiol 1990;1:69–79.

173. Pryor JL, Langley MJ, Jenkins AD. Comparison of symptom characteristics of indwelling ureteral catheters. J Urol 1991;145:719.

174. Netto NR, Ferreira U, Lemos GC, et al. Endourological management of ureteral strictures. J Urol 1990;144:631.

175. Kramolowsky EV, Tucker RD, Nelson CMK. Management of benign ureteral strictures: open surgical repair or endoscopic dilation. J Urol 1989;141:285.

176. Van Arsdalen KN, Banner MP. The management of ureteral and anastomotic strictures. Prog Urol 1992;6:420–432.

177. Hafez KS, Wolf JS. Update on minimally invasive management of ureteral strictures. J Endourol 2003;17:453–464.

178. Selzman AA, Spirnak JP. Iatrogenic ureteral injuries: a 20-year experience in treating 165 injuries. J Urol 1996;155:878–881.

179. Selmy G, Hassovna M, Begin LR, et al. Effect of balloon dilation of ureter on upper tract dynamics and ureteral wall morphology. J Endourol 1993;7:211–219.

180. Meretyk S, Albala DM, Clayman RV, et al. Endoureterotomy for treatment of ureteral strictures. J Urol 1992;147:1502.

181. Meretyk S, Albala DM, Kavoussi LR, et al. Endosurgery: non-calculus applications in the upper urinary tract. In: Clayman RU, ed. Monographs in Urology. Florida: Medical Directions, 1991:68–89.

182. Chang R, Marshall FF, Mitchell S. Percutaneous management of benign ureteral strictures and fistulas. J Urol 1987;137:1126.

183. Lee CK, Smith AD. Role of stents in open ureteral surgery. J Endourol 1993;7:141–144.

184. Beckmann CF, Roth RA, Bihrle W. Dilatation of benign ureteral strictures. Radiology 1989;172:437–441.

185. Chandhoke PS, Clayman RV, Stome AM, et al. Endopyelotomy and endoureterotomy with the Acucise ureteral cutting balloon device: preliminary experience. J Endourol 1993;7:45–51.

186. Cardella JF, Hunter DW, Castañeda-Zuniga WR, et al. Electrolysis for recanalization of urinary collecting system obstructions: a percutaneous approach. Radiology 1985;155:87–90.

187. Uflacker R, Wholey MH. A new low-speed rotational atherolytic device for ureteral recanalization. AJR Am J Roentgenol 1988; 151:1157–1158.

188. Lang EK, Glorioso LW III. Antegrade transluminal dilatation of benign ureteral strictures: long-term results. AJR Am J Roentgenol 1988;150:131–134.

189. Kim SH, Yoon HK, Park JH, et al. Tuberculous stricture of the urinary tract: antegrade balloon dilation and ureteral stenting. Abdom Imaging 1993;18:186–190.

190. El Abd SA, El Sharaby MD, El Shaer AF, et al. Long-term results of endourological and percutaneous management of ureteral strictures in bilharzial patients. J Endourol 1996;10:35–43.

191. O'Brien WM, Maxted WC, Pahira JJ. Ureteral stricture: experience with 31 cases. J Urol 1988;140:737.
192. Kwak S, Leef JA, Rosenblum JD. Percutaneous balloon catheter dilation of benign ureteral strictures: effect of multiple dilation procedures on long-term patency. AJR Am J Roentgenol 1995; 165:97–100.
193. Snow TM, Wells IP, Hammonds JC. Balloon rupture and stenting for pelviureteric junction obstruction: abolition of waisting is a prognostic marker. Clin Radiol 1994;49:708–710.
194. Gerber GS, Lyon ES. Endopyelotomy: patient selection, results and complications. Urology 1994;43:2–10.
195. McClinton S, Steyn JH, Hussey JK. Retrograde balloon dilatation for pelviureteric junction obstruction. Br J Urol 1993;71:152–155.
196. Knudsen BE, Cook AJ, Watterson JD, et al. Percutaneous antegrade endopyelotomy: long term results from one institution. Urology 2004;63:230–234.
197. Albani JM, Yost AJ, Streem SB. Ureteropelvic junction obstruction: determining durability of endourological interventions. J Urol 2004;171:579–582.
198. Sofras F, Livadas K, Alivizatos G, et al. Retrograde acucise endopyelotomy: Is it worth the cost? J Endourol 2004;18:466–468.
199. Kinnaert P, Hall M, Janssen F, et al. Ureteral stenosis after kidney transplantation: true incidence and long-term follow-up after surgical correction. J Urol 1985;133:17.
200. Makisalo H, Eklund B, Salmela K, et al. Urological complications after 2,084 consecutive kidney transplantations. Transplant Proc 1997;29:152–153.
201. Pappas P, Giannopoulos A, Stravodimos KG, et al. Obstructive uropathy in the transplanted kidney: definitive management with percutaneous nephrostomy and prolonged ureteral stenting. J Endourol 2001;15:719–723.
202. Thrasher JB, Temple DR, Spees EK. Extravesical versus Leadbetter-Politano ureteroneocystostomy: a comparison of urological complications in 320 renal transplants. J Urol 1990;144:1105–1109.
203. Swierzewski SJ III, Konnak JW, Ellis JH. Treatment of renal transplant ureteral complications by percutaneous techniques. J Urol 1993;149:986–987.
204. Bhagat VJ, Gordon RL, Osorio RW, et al. Ureteral obstructions and leaks after renal transplantation: outcome of percutaneous antegrade ureteral stent placement in 44 patients. Radiology 1998; 209:159–167.
205. Fontaine AB, Nijjar A, Rangaraj R. Update on the use of percutaneous nephrostomy/balloon dilation for the treatment of renal transplant leak/obstruction. J Vasc Interv Radiol 1997;8:649–653.
206. Kim JC, Banner MP, Ramchandani P, et al. Balloon dilation of ureteral strictures after renal transplantation. Radiology 1993; 186:717–722.
207. Waltzer WC, Frischer Z, Shabtai M, et al. Early aggressive management for the prevention of renal allograft loss and patient mortality following major urologic complications. Clin Transplant 1992; 6:318–322.
208. Kashi SH, Lodge JPA, Giles GR, et al. Ureteric complications of renal transplantation. Br J Radiol 1992;70:139–143.
209. Voegeli ER, Crummy AB, McDermott JC, et al. Percutaneous dilation of ureteral strictures in renal transplant patients. Radiology 1988;169:185–188.
210. Streem SB, Novick AC, Steinmuller DR, et al. Long-term efficacy of ureteral dilation for transplant ureteral stenosis. J Urol 1988;140: 32–35.
211. Yong AA, Ball ST, Pelling MX, et al. Management of ureteral strictures in renal transplants by antegrade balloon dilatation and temporary internal stenting. Cardiovasc Intervent Radiol 1999;22: 385–388.
212. Erturk E, Burzon DT, Waldman D. Treatment of transplant ureteral stenosis with endoureterotomy. J Urol 1999;161:412–414.
213. Bhayani SB, Landman J, Slotoroff C, et al. Transplant ureter stricture: Acucise endoureterotomy and balloon dilation are effective. J Endourol 2003;17:19–22.

Renal Calculus Disease

39

Parvati Ramchandani

Although the first percutaneous nephrostomy for stone removal was performed in 1975 (1), open surgery was the treatment of choice for patients with symptomatic stones in the kidneys and proximal ureters until the early 1980s. In the ensuing decades, advances in percutaneous management of stone disease were paralleled by concurrent refinements in shock wave lithotripsy (SWL) and ureteroscopy—all three techniques have had a significant impact on the management of upper urinary tract stone disease. Percutaneous management of urinary tract calculi is currently limited to patients who are not candidates for SWL or ureteroscopy. Percutaneous techniques are also used to salvage SWL or ureteroscopic failures. Open surgical procedures for stone disease are currently performed in only 1–2% of cases (2,3).

PERCUTANEOUS STONE REMOVAL

Indications

Percutaneous methods of stone removal have indisputable advantages compared to open surgical techniques; however, the widespread worldwide availability of SWL, its efficacy, and its relative noninvasiveness compared to percutaneous nephrostolithotomy (PCNL) make it the treatment of choice for most renal and ureteral calculi. Lately, the role of ureteroscopy in stone treatment is also being reassessed because of the introduction of second- and third-generation SWL machines that appear to be less effective in stone fragmentation than the original unmodified Dornier HM3 SWL machine (2). The availability of these many different treatment options has resulted in some controversy and confusion over the indications for each of the management options (4). The American Urological Association has published suggested guidelines for the treatment of stones (5,6).

In many situations, percutaneous stone removal is the primary procedure of choice. Table 39–1 lists the current indications in which percutaneous techniques are considered the first line of treatment. In all of these clinical situations, SWL suffers from certain disadvantages and is less effective than PCNL in complete stone removal. These indications are discussed below.

Stone Size

In patients with large calculi, SWL has a poor chance of complete success, a high probability of requiring adjunctive therapy, and a significant incidence of complications. As the size of stones increases to more than 2–3 cm, the fragmentation efficiency with SWL decreases, necessitating numerous SWL attempts before complete breakup occurs (7,8). Correspondingly, stone-free rates drop and the number of ancillary procedures required to aid the passage of calculus particles increases (7,9). Some calculi that are 3 cm or larger, but are of low radiographic density (such as stones composed of struvite or apatite), may respond to numerous SWL treatments. But for most large stones, including staghorn calculi, SWL is not the treatment of choice. With stones larger than 2.5–3.0 cm, only 30–35% may be rendered stone free with SWL, compared to 70–90% of those treated with PCNL (10). Furthermore, 60–75% of patients with stones greater than 2.5 cm in size treated with SWL require additional procedures, such as repeat SWL, PCNL, ureteroscopy, percutaneous nephrostomy, or stone manipulation, compared to 30% of patients treated primarily with PCNL (7). Roth et al. reported that only 38% of patients with stones larger than 3 cm were treated successfully with SWL monotherapy; additional SWL increased success to 43% and subsequent percutaneous procedures raised the success rate to only 64% (11). In the same series, initial PCNL of these large calculi was successful in 83% of patients with adjunctive therapy, such as SWL, increasing the overall success rate to 90%.

There is also a direct correlation between the size of the stone being treated with SWL and the subsequent

TABLE 39-1

INDICATIONS FOR PERCUTANEOUS THERAPY FOR STONE DISEASE

- Large stones (>2–2.5 cm)
- Staghorn calculi
- Stone + urinary obstruction or compromised urine drainage (includes stones in dependent calices and in caliceal diverticula)
- Cystine calculi
- Abnormal body habitus
- Symptomatic stones during pregnancy
- Certain removal of all calculous material important
- Stones for which other treatment modalities have failed

accumulation of stone fragments, or *steinstrassen,* in the distal ureter. Fedullo et al. (12) reported that the prevalence of steinstrassen was 17% when the calculi being treated were smaller than 10 mm, 26% when stones were 10–19 mm, 61% when stones were 20–29 mm, and 57% when stones were 30 mm or larger in size (Figure 39–1). Therefore, it appears prudent to treat stones greater than 2.5 cm in size with PCNL, while recognizing that the urologist's personal preference, the stone composition, the availability of personnel skilled in interventional techniques, and the patient's size are additional factors that influence the mode of therapy finally adopted. It should be noted that a single stone larger than 25–30 mm is of a different significance than

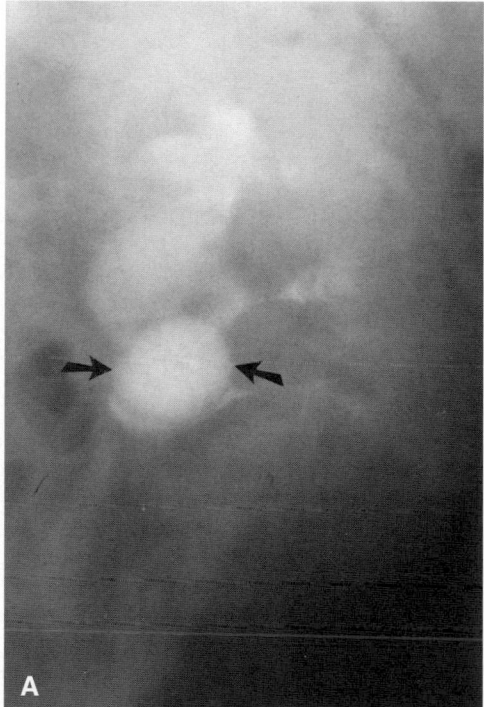
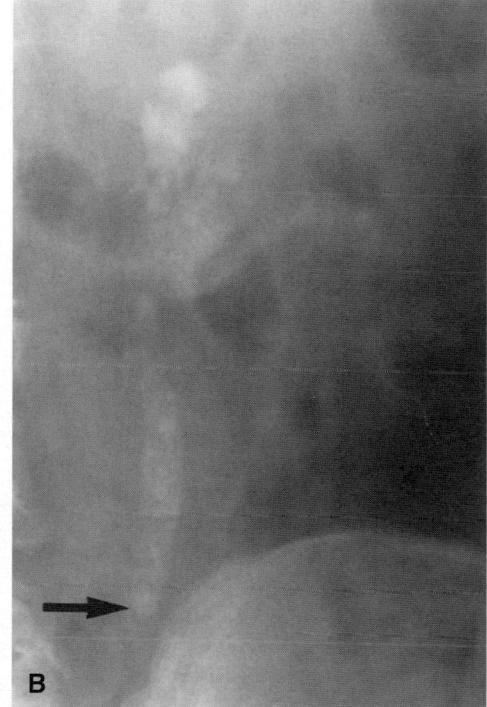

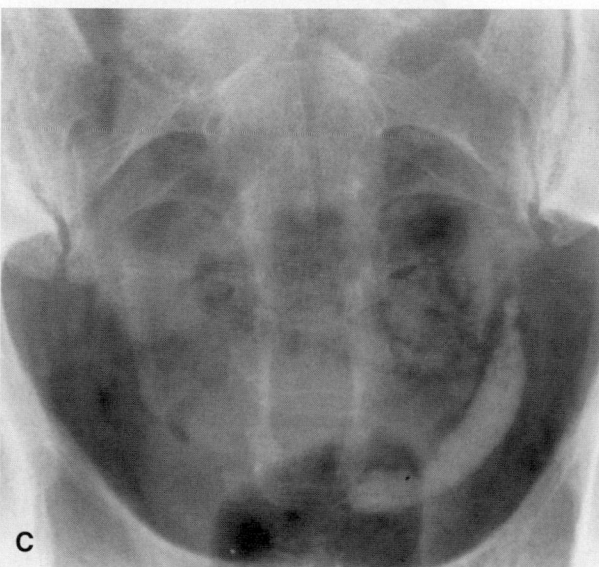

Figure 39–1 Extracorporeal shock wave lithotripsy (1SWL) of left renal calculus. **A.** Image from an intravenous urogram demonstrates a 2.5-cm calculus in the left renal pelvis (*arrows*) with upper pole hydronephrosis. The stone is at the upper limits of the ideal size for SWL. **B.** After SWL, stone fragments (steinstrassen) are seen in the pelvicaliceal system and proximal ureter. Note the large lead fragment (*arrow*) that impedes the passage of other smaller calculus fragments. **C.** A few days later, the column of steinstrassen moved spontaneously to the distal ureter. Although many patients can pass the calculus fragments, this patient required ureteroscopic extraction of the lead fragment preceded by ureteral meatotomy.

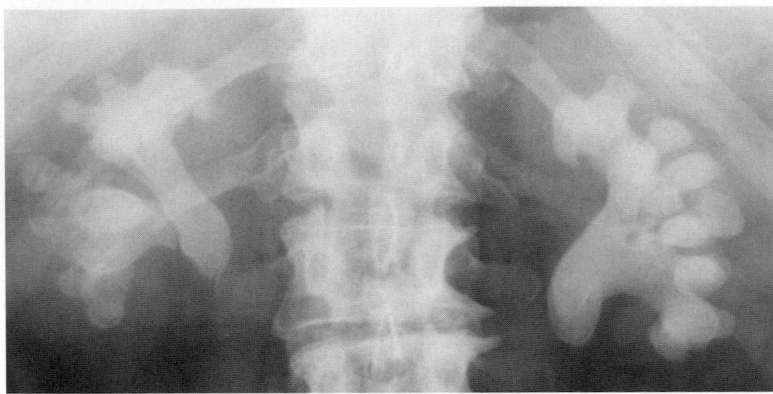

Figure 39–2 Bilateral staghorn calculi. Note the laminations in the stones, indicating that they represent infection stones. Percutaneous nephrostolithotomy (PCNL) for debulking followed by SWL was performed on both sides to render the patient stone free.

several stones that are each 5 mm in diameter; the former is initially better managed with percutaneous techniques, whereas SWL is better for many smaller stones that are scattered throughout the collecting system and, therefore, are less accessible to percutaneous techniques. Although each stone may easily be targeted for SWL, the presence of numerous stones does decrease the efficiency of SWL and the stone-free rate as compared to a single small stone.

Staghorn Calculi

Staghorn calculi are most commonly composed of struvite and are associated with recurrent urinary tract infections. Complete stone removal is essential in these patients because failure to do so allows persistence of infection and the eventual regrowth of the stone (Figure 39–2). Other stones that occasionally may have a staghorn configuration are cystine stones (Figure 39–3), uric acid stones, and, rarely, calcium oxalate monohydrate stones. Staghorn calculi can range in size from a surface area of less than 250 mm^2 to more than 5,000 mm^2; more than 60% of staghorn calculi treated by Lingeman et al. (9) ranged between 500 mm^2 to 1,500 mm^2.

Although the treatment of staghorn calculi has varied with treatment philosophies ranging from monotherapy with SWL or PCNL alone to a varying combination of the two modalities, a consensus has been reached that the primary approach to these stones should be by PCNL. Branched staghorn stones that fill most of the collecting system pose special problems because stones may be located deep in infundibula and calices that may be difficult to reach from the initial percutaneous tract or tracts. The most efficacious method for treating such staghorn calculi is the so-called *sandwich* technique (13–15). PCNL is initially used to rapidly remove large volumes of easily accessible stone with ultrasonic or electrohydraulic lithotripsy ("debulking"). If infundibulocaliceal fragments are inaccessible from the nephrostomy tract when using the usual endourological techniques, SWL is used to break up the small volumes of remaining stones, followed by PCNL to remove the residual fragments. Some advocate a second percutaneous procedure to remove the stone gravel because stone fragments have a tendency to remain in dilated collecting systems for prolonged periods while others allow

the stone fragments to pass spontaneously after adjunctive SWL (16,17). PCNL followed by SWL and second-look nephroscopy, if necessary, have been shown to be the most cost-effective method for treating staghorn calculi (18).

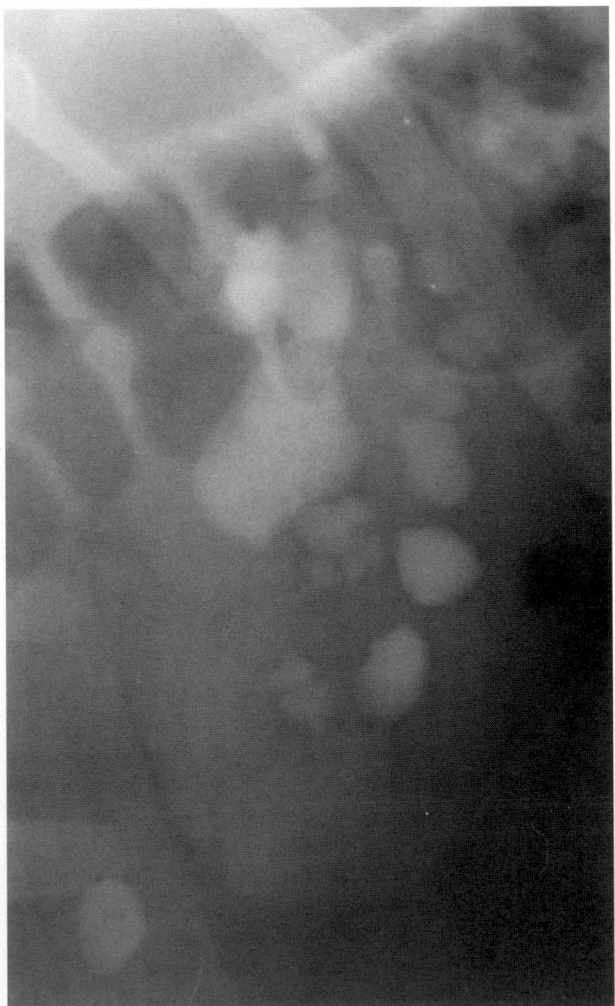

Figure 39–3 Cystine staghorn stone with additional proximal ureteral calculus in a 19-year-old woman. The homogeneous, smooth ("ground glass") opacity of the stone suggests its composition. These stones respond poorly to SWL but fragment readily with ultrasonic lithotripsy, making PCNL the treatment of choice.

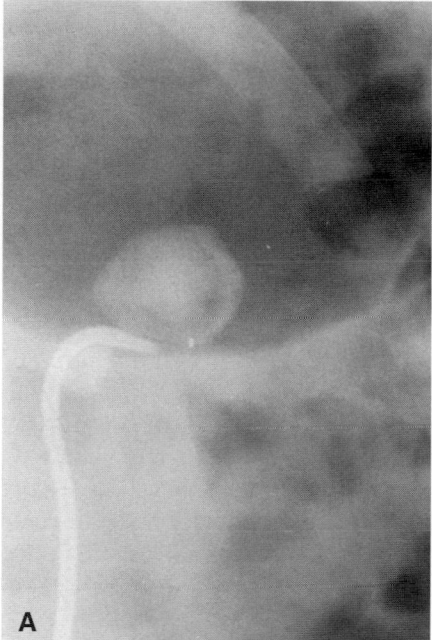 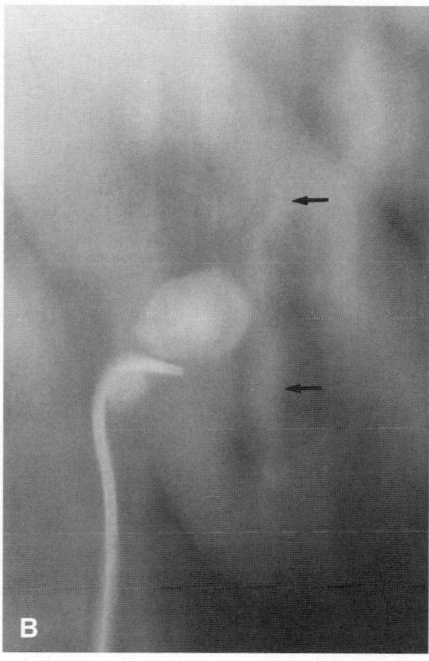 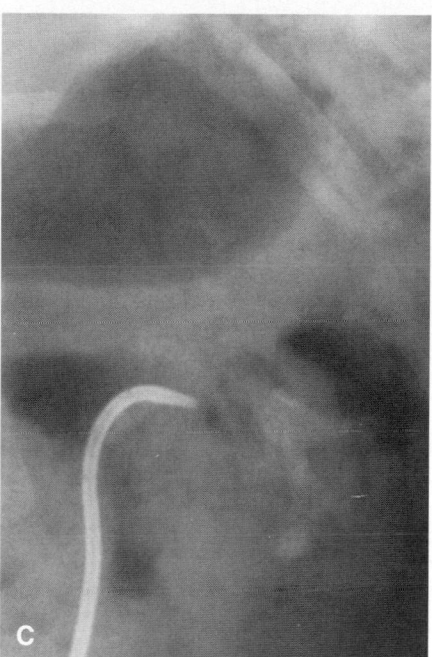

Figure 39–4   Staghorn calculus treated with SWL. **A.** Plain film demonstrates a laminated calculus in the renal pelvis. **B.** Tomography demonstrates the faintly opaque caliceal and infundibular components of the stone (*arrows*) that could not be appreciated on the plain film. **C.** After SWL, calculus fragments are seen to coat the collecting system, with a denser concentration in the lower pole infundibula and calices. The lower pole is the most common site for residual fragments to accumulate.

Martin et al. (19) reported that in their 97 patients with complete staghorn stones, 46% were treated with one session of PCNL alone, 40% in two stages (PCNL in addition to SWL), 10% in three stages, and 4% in four stages. Patients treated in one or two stages were more likely to be stone free than those treated in three or four stages.

In patients with partial staghorn calculi, monotherapy with SWL is an option (Figure 39–4). Lingeman (9) reported that patients who had staghorn calculi less than 500 mm^2 in size and with no dilatation of the collecting system could be made stone free in more than 90% of cases with SWL alone. They cautioned, however, that such small-volume staghorn calculi are uncommon and, in fact, made up only 3% of the staghorn stones treated in their series. An additional indication for SWL monotherapy of staghorn calculi is the presence of a partial or complete staghorn calculus in a nondilated collecting system (17) (Figure 39–4). It is recommended that SWL be performed with an indwelling ureteral catheter in such cases. Lingeman's series (9) showed that when all staghorn calculi were considered, stones treated with SWL monotherapy tended to be smaller—with a mean surface area of 693 mm^2 (a range of 161–5,907 mm^2)—compared to stones treated with initial PCNL, which tended to be larger—with a mean surface area of 1,378 mm^2 (a range of 302–6,028 mm^2). Furthermore, ancillary procedures to facilitate the passage of stone fragments were required much more frequently in patients undergoing SWL monotherapy than in those being treated with PCNL alone or PCNL with SWL (30.5% versus 3.4%, respectively).

In another series (20), SWL monotherapy of complete staghorn calculi, without stents, had a reported stone-free rate of 44% at 6 months. With incomplete staghorn calculi, SWL monotherapy without ureteral stents resulted in a stone-free rate of 48% at 6 months. In patients with indwelling ureteral stents, the results were appreciably better, with a stone-free rate of 85%.

When staghorn calculi are considered a group, reported stone-free rates for PCNL alone vary from 71% to 86% (21,22), compared to 84.2% for PCNL with or without SWL (9). Even though the addition of SWL at first glance appears to confer no advantage over PCNL alone as far as the stone-free success rate is concerned, the combination of the two procedures minimizes or eliminates the need for multiple renal accesses as well as for secondary endourologic procedures. The latter advantage simplifies the otherwise technically arduous goal of complete stone removal in extensive bulky staghorn calculi and also decreases the risks inherent in establishing multiple access tracks. Only a few staghorn calculi require the addition of SWL to PCNL. During initial PCNL, efforts should be made to remove as much stone material as possible; when residual stone material is unavoidable, efforts should be directed toward removing enough stone material so that the residual stone burden is less than 2.0–2.5 cm in diameter (and thus can be treated more effectively with SWL).

To summarize, the effectiveness of SWL monotherapy in treating staghorn stones is directly proportional to the stone burden (23), with stone-free rates of 91.7% for staghorn

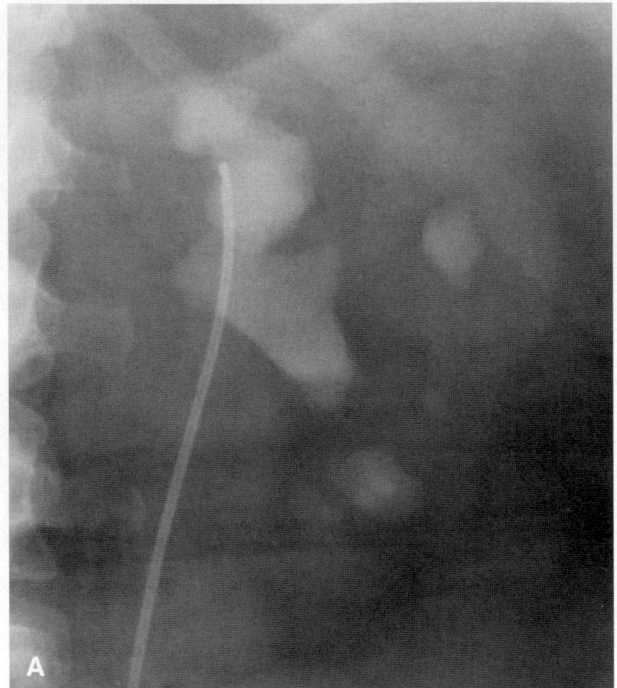

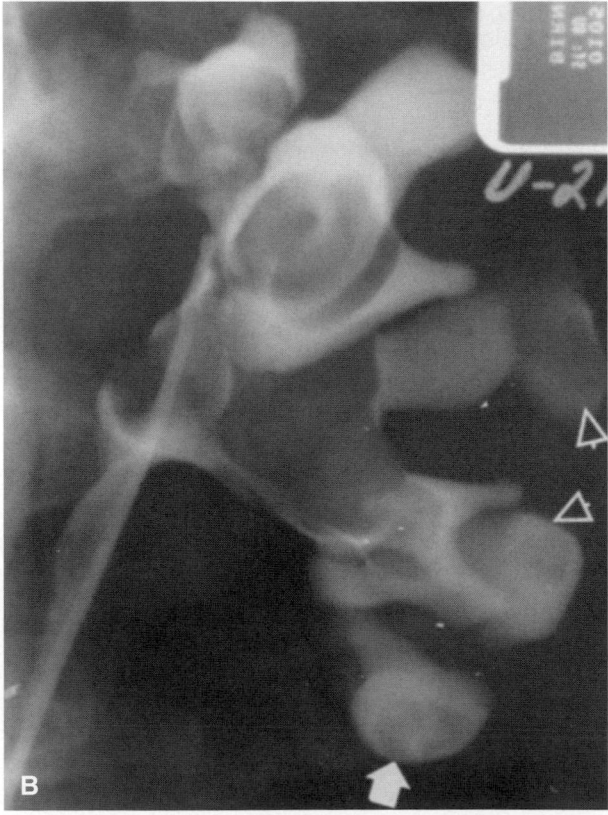

Figure 39–5   Staghorn calculus with multiple detached caliceal fragments. **A.** Plain film and **B.** retrograde pyelogram demonstrate a staghorn calculus with discontinuous caliceal fragments in interpolar and lower pole calices. The collecting system is hydronephrotic, making PCNL the therapy of choice. After access was gained through the medial lower pole calix (*arrow in B*), the renal pelvis and upper and lower pole components of the stone were removed. SWL was used to fragment the calculi in the interpolar and lateral lower pole calix (*arrowheads in B*).

stones that are smaller than 500 mm^2 and 51.2% for larger stones (24). In contrast, the efficacy of PCNL is excellent independent of stone size until extremely large staghorn calculi (>2,500 mm^2) are treated, with stone-free rates of approximately 85% (Figure 39–5). In addition, with SWL monotherapy, achieving the final stone-free rate can take a year or more.

Urinary Obstruction and Compromised Urinary Drainage

Urinary stasis can predispose to calculus formation. The most common examples of stones in association with obstruction are in ureteropelvic junction (UPJ) obstruction (Figures 39–6 and 39–7) and caliceal diverticula. Other examples are stones in dilated lower pole calices (Figure 39–7), malrotated kidneys, ectopic kidneys, horseshoe kidneys, and obstruction caused by renal cysts or other renal masses. Changes in ureteral caliber or course because of congenital anomalies (such as retrocaval ureter or crossed ectopia) or previous surgery (such as ureterolithotomy or ureteral reimplantation) and chronic obstruction with resultant tortuosity or retroperitoneal processes (retroperitoneal fibrosis or tumors) can also impede ureteral drainage.

Although SWL can successfully break up the symptomatic calculi in these situations, the fragments are unlikely to be able to successfully pass even when the stone debris is adequately fragmented (25). A study (26) that compared SWL for stones in abnormal and normal urinary tracts found that although fragmentation rates were similar for the two groups, clearance rates of fragments were significantly different (78% versus 56%). PCNL is often preferred to shock wave lithotripsy in these situations because the percutaneous removal of the calculi circumvents the anatomic abnormalities that prevent stone passage. Absolute stone-free rates with SWL in patients with renal anomalies, such as horseshoe kidneys and pelvic kidneys, average 62% (27), with many patients requiring numerous SWL treatments as well as additional procedures, including PCNL and ureteroscopy, to render them stone free. A recent multicenter study reported that primary PCNL in patients with horseshoe kidneys had an 87.5% success rate in making patients stone free, but major complications were reported in 9% of patients in this series (28). The availability of small-caliber, flexible, actively deflectable ureteroscopes and holmium laser lithotripsy—an effective lithotrite to vaporize and fragment stones—has positioned ureteroscopy as an effective alternative to PCNL and SWL in treating stones in anomalous kidneys with a reported stone-free rate of 75% in one small series (27).

Calculi that occur in transplanted kidneys can be treated effectively with PCNL (29,30). Percutaneous dilation of the track may be difficult because of perirenal fibrosis that may occur in some patients, but the approach is otherwise similar to that used in native kidneys.

In patients with UPJ obstruction, PCNL is often combined with an endopyelotomy. Briefly, incisions are made

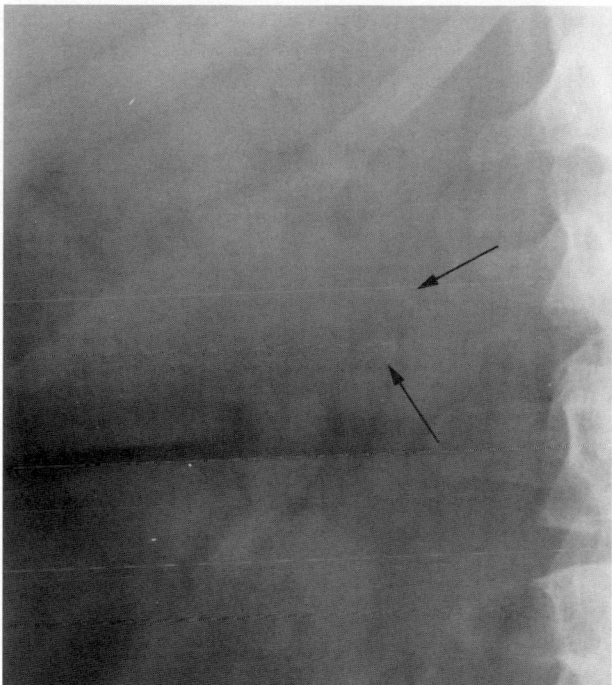
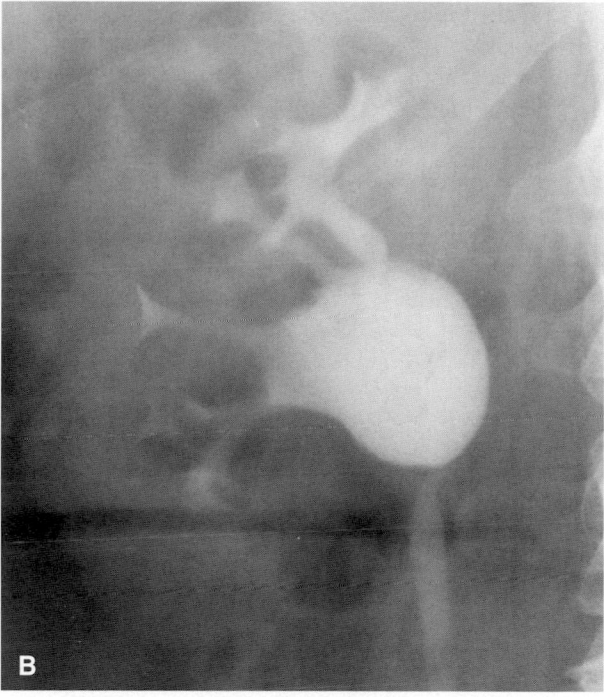

Figure 39–6 Small uric acid calculi in a patient with congenital ureteropelvic junction (UPJ) narrowing. **A.** Plain film demonstrates very faintly opaque calculi in the right renal pelvis (*arrows*). **B.** Urogram demonstrates a prominent extrarenal pelvis with poor funneling of the ureteropelvic junction (UPJ). The calculi are obscured by the densely opacified renal pelvis. The calculi would respond well to SWL—because they are small and composed of uric acid—but the fragments are unlikely to pass in toto. The patient underwent PCNL.

along the posterior and lateral margins of the UPJ, with the incisions extending through the ureteral wall into the periureteric fat. Such an approach avoids the vascular structures that are usually located anteriorly and medially. After

the procedure, the ureter is stented for 6–8 weeks with a large-bore stent. The reported success for relief of obstruction varies from 64% to 86% (31). When an endopyelotomy is planned, PCNL access through a posterior interpolar calix

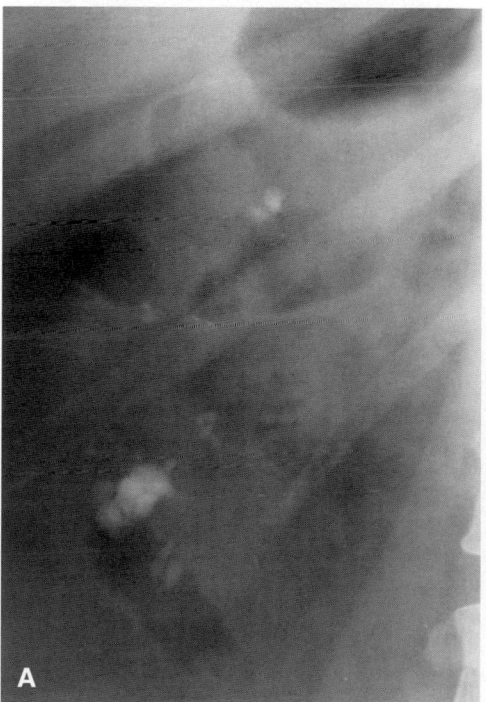
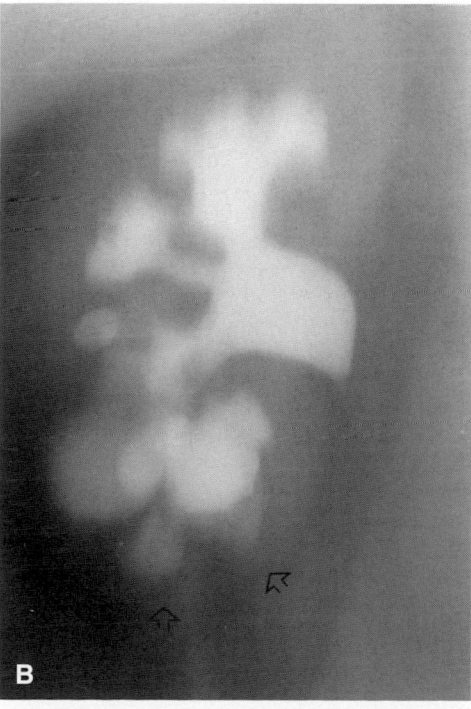

Figure 39–7 Renal calculi in conjunction with lower pole hydronephrosis and UPJ narrowing. **A.** Plain film demonstrates multiple calculi with the largest in the lower pole. The patient had undergone SWL in the past and had a long history of stone disease. **B.** Tomogram after contrast administration shows selective hydronephrosis in the lower pole with marked parenchymal atrophy (*arrowheads outline cortical margin*). There is also narrowing of the right UPJ. The patient underwent PCNL through the stone-bearing lower pole calix. Other lower pole calculi were flushed out during stone removal.

or upper polar calix provides the most direct and straight access to the UPJ.

Calculi occur in about 40% of caliceal diverticula. Usually, they are asymptomatic and are of little clinical significance. However, they may be associated with flank pain, chronic urinary tract infections, or both (32). Open surgery with either marsupialization or excision of the diverticulum and fulguration or closure of the narrow neck is highly successful. Occasional patients may also be treated with partial or, rarely, total nephrectomy.

SWL of stones within caliceal diverticula may alleviate symptoms temporarily. However, SWL does not address the underlying stasis within the diverticulum, the narrow neck of which can prevent adequate passage of calculus fragments that consequently remain in situ within the diverticulum (Figure 39–8). Not surprisingly, the results of SWL are poor, and stone-free rates of only 20–25% have been reported (33–35) with SWL. Curiously, relief of symptoms can occur even when the patient is not rendered stone free; residual fragments eventually do grow and become symptomatic

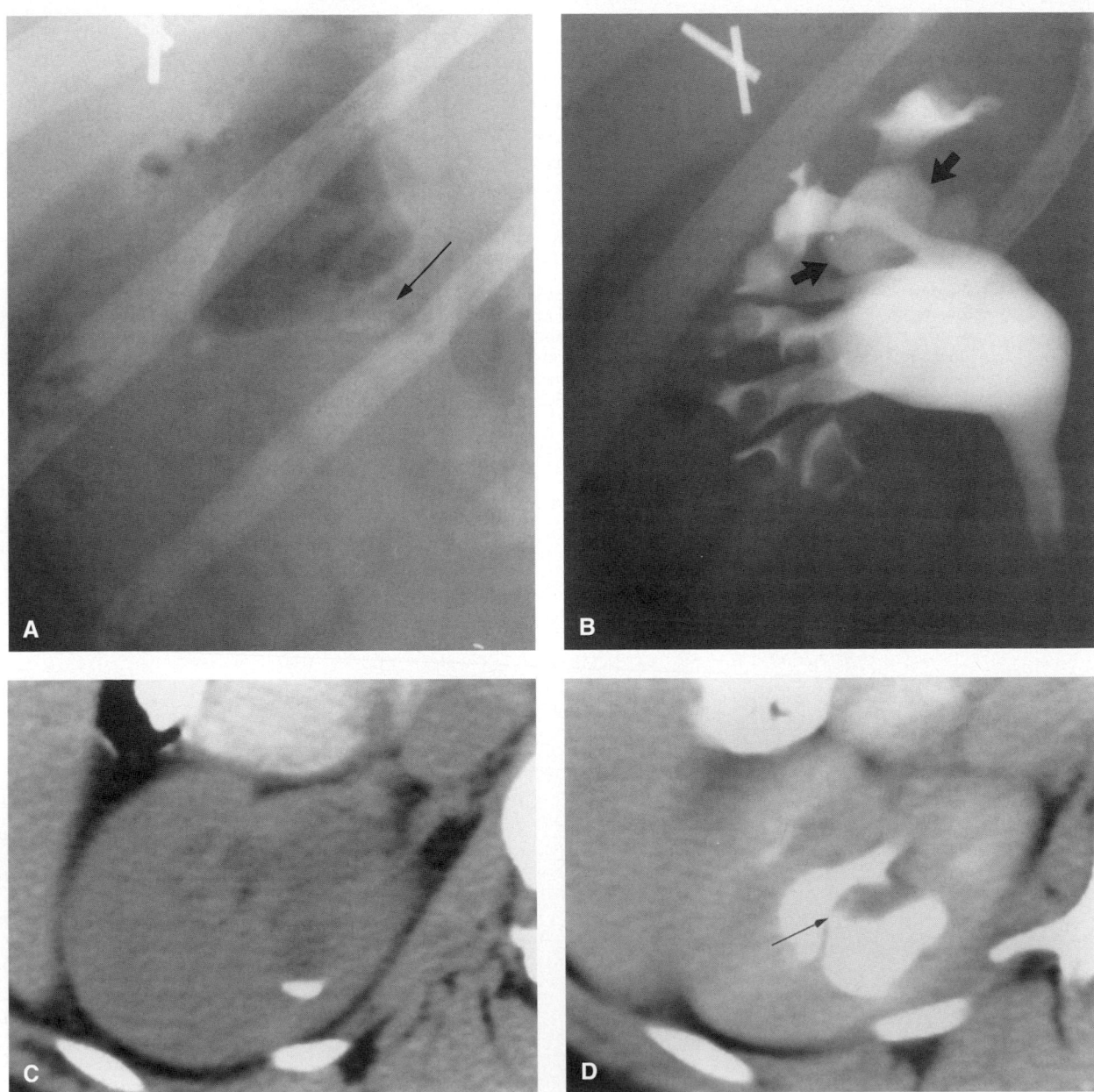

Figure 39–8   Calculus in caliceal diverticulum. **A.** Plain film and **B.** urogram demonstrate calculi (*arrow in A*) in a caliceal diverticulum (*arrows in B*). The calculus had been treated previously with SWL, but the patient remained symptomatic. **C.** Unenhanced CT scan demonstrates layering of the calculus fragments. **D.** After contrast administration, the diverticulum fills with contrast through a narrow neck (*arrow*). CT confirmed that the diverticulum could be safely accessed percutaneously.

again. Moreover, 65% of patients with caliceal diverticula and urinary tract infections continue to have persistent infection after SWL (36).

For these reasons, percutaneous procedures are advocated (37–40) as the safe and effective alternative for the management of symptomatic caliceal diverticular calculi. Retrograde ureteroscopic techniques (41), as well as a combined technique using both retrograde flexible ureteroscopy and simultaneous caliceal puncture (30), have also been used.

The percutaneous technique consists of direct puncture of the symptomatic diverticulum (37–40) followed by tract dilation to 24–34 French and nephroscopic stone extraction. Subsequently, either the neck of the diverticulum is dilated to 18–34 French to enlarge its connection to the collecting system or the diverticular cavity is obliterated by electrocoagulation. Direct puncture into the diverticulum offers the advantage that a rigid nephroscope can be used for the procedure, and calculus extraction can be accomplished without accessing the diverticular neck should it prove to be difficult. Wire placement across the neck of the diverticulum is often easiest after the calculus has been removed nephroscopically.

The treatment of stones within anteriorly positioned diverticula can be technically challenging. Direct puncture of these diverticula results in an acute angle such that the neck of the diverticulum cannot be negotiated with either an endoscope or a guide wire. Therefore, the neck of these diverticula cannot be dilated, although the stone within the diverticulum can be extracted, after which the diverticulum can be fulgurated (36). Whenever direct puncture of the symptomatic diverticulum is technically unfeasible, the diverticulum may be approached indirectly via a puncture of a distant calix, dilation of the diverticular neck, then a flushing of the stones into the collecting system for extraction (37). Lang has described the creation of a new communication between the renal pelvis and a caliceal diverticulum or obstructed calix ("percutaneous infundibuloplasty") in cases in which the infundibulum is stenotic and impassable (42). The neoinfundibulum reportedly remained patent in 67% of the patients for 2–7 years.

Percutaneous techniques result in a stone-free rate of 95–100% (37–40) with obliteration of the diverticulum in 80% of patients and a marked decrease in size in the remaining 20% (38). These results are far superior to those obtainable by SWL and justify the use of PCNL as a preferred treatment, despite its greater invasiveness.

In an effort to overcome the shortcomings of percutaneous techniques in treating anterior caliceal diverticula, as well as small-volume symptomatic diverticula, Grasso et al. (32) described the use of retrograde, actively deflectable, flexible ureteroscopy in four patients. This was combined with simultaneous percutaneous puncture in patients with a caliceal diverticular stone burden greater than 1 cm. The technique was successful in all four patients, and symptoms resolved. When a standard retrograde approach was employed, Fuchs et al. described great difficulty in entering the necks of lower pole diverticula (43), all of which then had to be treated percutaneously. Further, 23% of patients in whom a retrograde approach to a caliceal diverticulum was used required a second retrograde or percutaneous approach. Another concern with using the retrograde approach is the creation of ureteral strictures because of the extended procedural time required to find the neck of the diverticulum in a retrograde fashion (38,44). It should be noted that Grasso et al. (32) reported that procedural times for flexible retrograde ureteroscopy averaged only 2.5 hours, and they believe it to represent a more efficient technique than standard retrograde ureteroscopy.

The clearance of stone fragments from the dependent calices—the lower pole of the kidneys—is variable, unpredictable, and problematic after SWL. When stones occur in association with lower pole hydronephrosis, the clearance of fragments can be expected to further diminish (Figure 39–7). Lingeman et al. (45) reported stone-free rates of 90% for PCNL versus 59% for SWL and also noted that results of SWL correlated inversely with the stone burden treated, whereas the results of PCNL were independent of the stone burden. The results reported by Lingeman et al. were also substantiated by a meta-analysis of other series that reported stratified data for lower pole stone treatment with SWL and PCNL (45). The stone-free rate for SWL of lower pole calculi overall was 60%, compared to 90% for PCNL; patients with stones smaller than 1 cm in size had a stone-free rate of 74% for SWL, compared to 100% for PCNL. With stones that were 1–2 cm in size or larger than 2 cm, stone-free rates with SWL were 56% and 33%, compared to 89% and 94%, respectively, for PCNL. Albala et al. (46) reported that with stones smaller than 1 cm in the lower poles, retreatment or auxiliary procedures were needed in 36% (15/42) after SWL compared with 11% (4/38) undergoing PCNL.

When the stone burden is small and located in a nondilated collecting system, stone fragments are more likely to be propelled and expelled out of the lower dependent calices by the coaptation of the nondilated calices and infundibula during normal peristalsis (45) (Figure 39–9). Coaptation of the calices and infundibula is less likely in hydronephrotic collecting systems in which peristalsis is often diminished or absent. There is a tendency for the fragments of lower pole calculi to remain within the dependent calices after SWL (Figure 39–10), and these retained stone particles in the lower pole can serve as a nidus for stone growth. Stone recurrence rates in the lower pole following SWL range from 22% to 58% (47,48).

The American Urologic Association Clinical Guidelines Panel review (45) suggests that an increasing percentage of stones currently being treated with SWL are located in the lower pole. Two percent of the treated stones in 1984 were in the lower pole, compared to 48% in 1991. There has been a corresponding decrease in the incidence of renal pelvic calculi treated with SWL during the same period, from 87% to 26%. Gerber et al. (49) reported that despite the poor

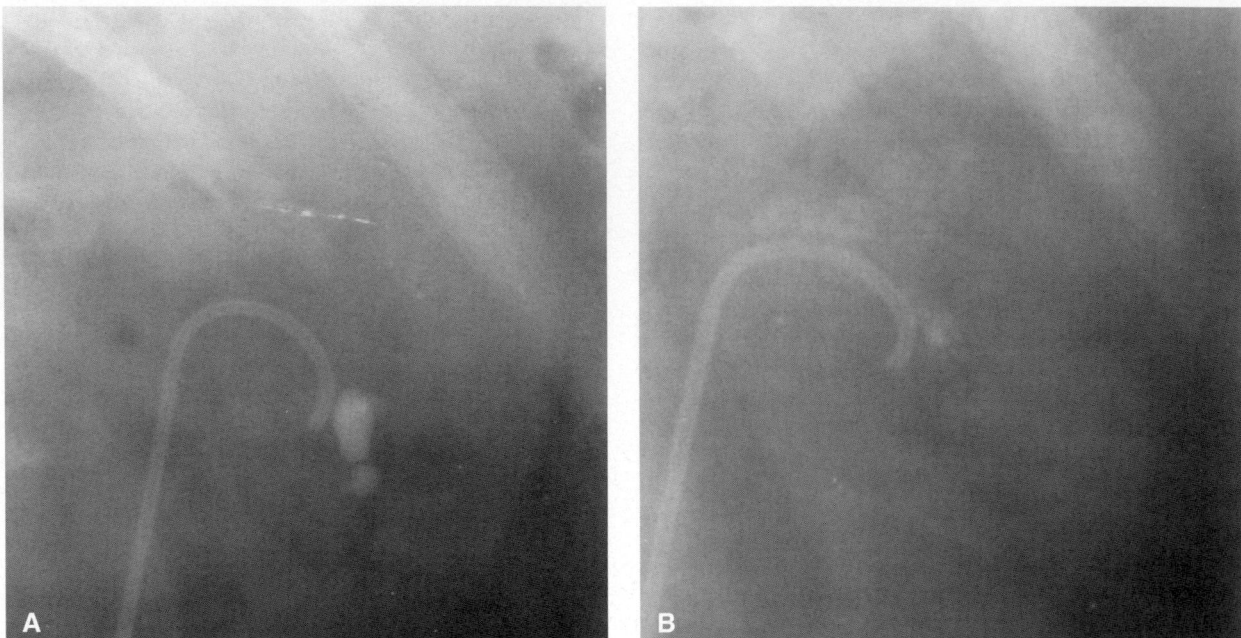

Figure 39–9 Small lower pole calculi in a nondilated collecting system, treated with SWL. **A.** Plain film before SWL demonstrates small lower pole calculi. The ureteral stent was placed for an obstruction because of migration of a calculus into the ureter; the stone was displaced back into the kidney during stent placement. **B.** After SWL, fragments are dispersed in the renal pelvis and lower pole. The patient was rendered stone free by SWL.

published results for treating lower pole stones less than 2 cm with SWL, 21% of urologists in their survey still preferred and recommended SWL over PCNL, while 65% of urologists treated 1–2 cm lower pole stones with SWL despite stone-free rates of just 41–56% (45,50,51). Thus, although SWL continues to be the preferred initial therapy for lower pole stones by many urologists, the proven success and efficacy of PCNL in treating these calculi would argue

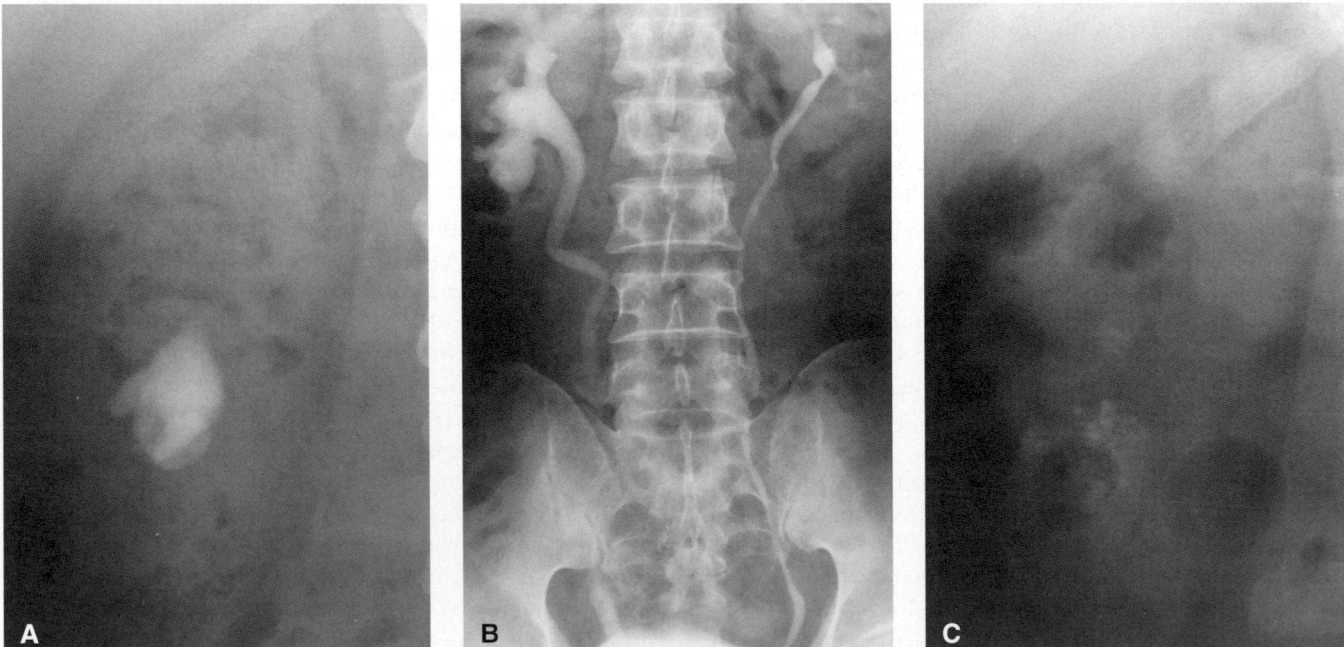

Figure 39–10 Lower pole calculus treated with SWL. **A.** Plain film and **B.** urogram demonstrate a large lower pole calculus with hydronephrosis of the lower pole calices. **C.** After SWL, a plain radiograph demonstrates that fragments remain in the lower pole and fail to clear. The patient developed a recurrent lower pole stone within a short time.

for PCNL being the therapeutic modality of choice. It remains unclear whether caliceal and infundibular anatomy can be predictive of lower pole stone clearance. Some factors that may be influential are the lower infundibular length-to-diameter ratio, overall infundibular diameter, and the number of minor calyces (50,51).

PCNL has been successfully applied in the treatment of calculus disease in anomalous kidneys, including crossed-fused renal ectopia (52), horseshoe kidneys (53), and pelvic kidneys (54,55). These complicated cases call for extensive preprocedural planning. With pelvic kidneys, laparoscopy in conjunction with retrograde (54) and antegrade nephrostomy (55) has been used by some. A posterior approach to a pelvic kidney reportedly led to femoral neuropathy in one patient (56); the authors speculated that direct trauma occurred to the dorsal divisions of the lumbar plexus (which form the femoral nerve) lying along the psoas muscle.

Stone Composition

The composition of a given calculus is critical when one is deciding on the best method of management. Certain calculi are readily fragmented by ultrasonic lithotripsy but are refractory to SWL, such as cystine calculi, making PCNL the treatment of choice. On the other hand, uric acid calculi respond well to SWL but not to ultrasonic lithotripsy.

Calculi composed of cystine fragment unreliably with SWL, and they require a greater number of treatments and total number of shocks compared to other calculi (57). Because many of these patients are plagued with numerous stone events that have required multiple previous interventions—and this can be anticipated again—, a trial of SWL for stones smaller than 2 cm in size is reasonable. Rough, spiculated cystine stones that have recently formed respond better to SWL than do homogeneous, smooth, long-standing stones (58). High-power machines such as the HM3 also appear to be more effective. For stones larger than 2 cm, proceeding directly to PCNL is the best option (Figure 39-3). All stone material must be removed at the time of the percutaneous procedure to ensure that the patient will remain stone free.

Medical treatment (acetyl cysteine) has been unreliable in removing residual fragments (59), but its efficacy can be improved by infusing the drugs through percutaneously placed catheters. Because cystine calculi characteristically break into chunks with SWL, further pulverization requires additional SWL sessions, percutaneous extraction, and ultrasonic lithotripsy or chemical dissolution.

Stones composed of calcium oxalate dihydrate and struvite break up well with SWL or any other form of power lithotripsy, whereas stones composed either partially or completely of calcium oxalate monohydrate do not respond well to SWL. With these stones, the volume of the stone is the main determinant of the most desirable mode of therapy.

Anatomic Abnormalities and Abnormal Body Habitus

A misshapen body habitus such as that caused by scoliosis or, more commonly, morbid obesity may make SWL unfeasible because the patients cannot be positioned so that the stone is in the focal point of the machine. PCNL may also be technically demanding in these patients, but it carries fewer risks than open surgery. A preprocedural CT scan is helpful in such patients to evaluate the anatomy and plan an access route that avoids bowel and other viscera (60) (Figure 39-11).

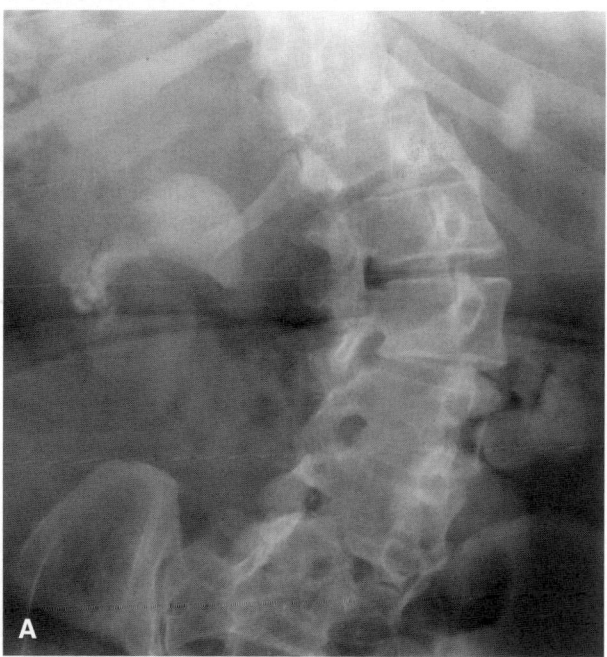

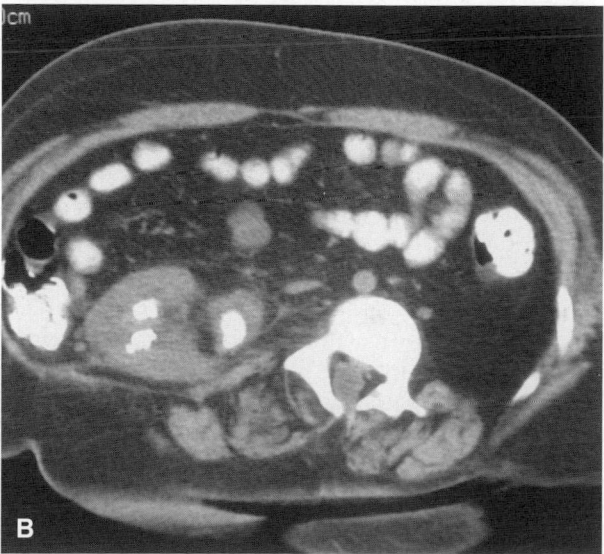

Figure 39-11 Renal calculi in a patient with scoliosis and myelomeningocele. **A.** Plain film demonstrates right staghorn calculus, left renal calculus, marked scoliosis, and spinal dysraphism. **B.** CT scan demonstrates that access to the lower pole of the right kidney can be achieved safely. The patient underwent successful PCNL.

Certainty of Final Results

When the presence of residual fragments and the attendant uncertainties related to their passage are unacceptable to the patient for psychological or occupational reasons, such as with airline pilots as the classic example, PCNL is an optimal option because of its superior 95–98% stone-free rate.

Symptomatic Stones during Pregnancy

Renal colic affects 1 in 1,500 pregnancies, usually during the second and third trimesters. Many believe stones may be more frequent in multiparous women than in primiparous patients, although there is no universal agreement on this (61). Symptomatic stones are usually located in the midureter or distal ureter with flank pain, microhematuria, and urosepsis being the common presenting symptoms. The diagnosis can be confirmed by a limited intravenous urogram (IVU), sonography, or noncontrast CT scan. IVU and sonography may be challenging to interpret in pregnant patients because of the difficulty in differentiating upper tract dilation resulting from progressive hydronephrosis of pregnancy (a common and expected change) from upper tract dilation resulting from obstruction by a stone (62,63).

Conservative treatment consisting of analgesia and hydration is effective in most patients, and the renal calculi pass spontaneously in 75% of patients (64). More aggressive therapy is required in patients with refractory pain, sepsis, renal insufficiency (particularly in cases of a solitary kidney), and colic-induced preterm labor.

Therapeutic interventions during pregnancy are restricted to drainage of the affected collecting system by either a ureteral stent placed in a retrograde fashion or a percutaneous nephrostomy (Figure 39–12). Ureteral stents can be placed with local anesthesia and are usually tolerated well during pregnancy (65,66). Endoluminal ultrasound has been used to place a ureteral stent (67), thus avoiding the potential risks of radiation exposure. Wolf et al. (67) used a 20-MHz transducer (through a 6.2 French catheter) for stent placement in a 27-week gravid patient. If stent placement fails, percutaneous nephrostomy is performed. The necessity for periodic stent changes during pregnancy is controversial. Some authors believe that there is accelerated stent encrustation during pregnancy (68) and that stents should be changed every 8–12 weeks to avoid this complication (66). Others are of the opinion that stents may be left in place for 3–9 months without a change being necessary (65,69).

SWL, as well as ultrasonic and laser lithotripsy, are contraindicated during pregnancy. Other definitive therapy for the calculus is best postponed until 6 weeks postpartum. PCNL, ureteroscopic stone extraction, and open surgery (pyelolithotomy or ureterolithotomy) have been performed during pregnancy (65), and general anesthesia can be administered safely during pregnancy (70). Because

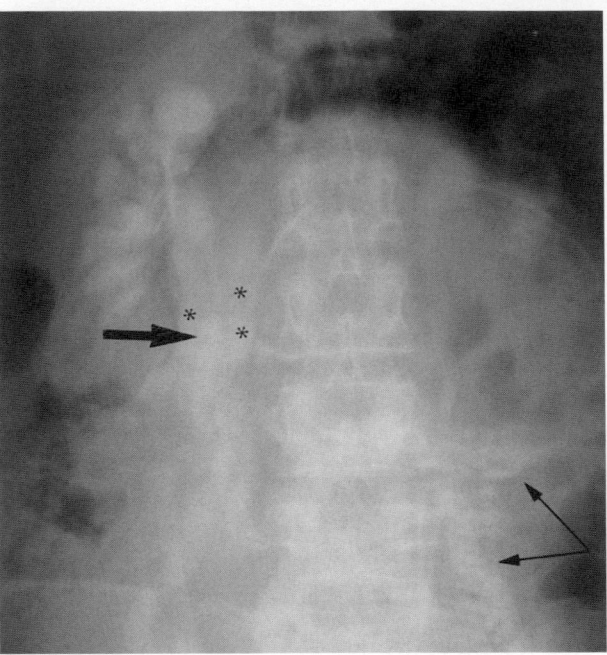

Figure 39–12   Obstructing ureteral calculus in pregnant patient. Urogram demonstrates contrast extravasation in the retroperitoneum (*asterisks*) because of a proximal ureteral calculus (*large arrow*). Note the fetal skull and skeleton (*long arrows*). A percutaneous nephrostomy was performed for drainage. The patient passed the calculus spontaneously when she was postpartum.

radiologic monitoring during ureteroscopy is not essential and can be eliminated, it is preferred over PCNL whenever stone extraction is deemed necessary (71).

Technique

Two primary components in the percutaneous therapy of upper urinary tract calculi are the establishment of an access tract and the removal of the actual stone itself. The technical details of the procedure cannot be addressed here but have been described previously (72–74).

Access to the upper urinary tract can be obtained either percutaneously or in a retrograde fashion. The percutaneous route is used most frequently to approach renal and upper ureteral calculi. Although a team approach is advocated by and practiced in many institutions (75), many endourologists believe that the nephrostomy track placement is rightfully performed by the urologist (9,76–79), preferably in the operating room. However, Bird et al. (4) found that only 11% of urologists performing PCNL created the access themselves.

Accurate access is the essential underpinning of a successful PCNL; a well-placed access track can simplify a complex procedure, and conversely, a poorly placed track may make removal of even the most accessible of calculi impossible. Fluoroscopic control is usually preferred for the procedure, especially if the calculi are radiopaque. CT is useful in preprocedural planning in patients with aberrant anatomy so that the liver, spleen, colon, and pleural space can be avoided by the proposed track (60,80) (Figure 39–11).

If the calculus is located in a calix or diverticulum, access should be obtained through that particular calix or diverticulum. For large-volume calculi, a lower pole or interpolar caliceal puncture through a subcostal approach offers the advantages of avoiding the pleura while being certain to clear the dependent lower pole calices of calculi. Stone-free rate of more than 95% can be achieved using a subcostal approach (72). An intercostal puncture may be performed to access an upper pole calix, usually to extract upper pole staghorn calculi, for concurrent endopyelotomy (although the latter usually can be successfully accomplished via a posterior interpolar access), and in patients with a large stone burden (81–86).

Narasimham et al. (81) used an intercostal approach in 24% of their cases. In two of the three patients, with access above the eleventh rib, thoracic complications requiring treatment—hydrothorax or pneumothorax—occurred. The authors recorded no clinically significant complications in cases in which the puncture was below the eleventh rib and into a middle or lower calix. Fuchs et al. (82) used an intercostal approach in 30% of their patients, of whom 5% had a major thoracic complication. The authors of both series (81,82) recommend that access above the eleventh rib be avoided. Hopper et al. (87) performed CT on prone patients to estimate the risks associated with a puncture between the tenth and eleventh ribs and found that an eleventh or twelfth rib intercostal approach would puncture the right lung in 14% of patients (and the left lung in 29% of patients in expiration), and the risk of puncturing the liver and spleen was minimal in full expiration. However, the risk to the lungs was considered prohibitive with a tenth or eleventh intercostal approach, regardless of the degree of respiration. Munver et al. (86) used a supracostal approach in 33% of their cases (27% of tracks above the eleventh rib and 73% above the twelfth rib) and reported complications in 34% of supra eleventh rib procedures and 9.7% incidence in supra twelfth rib procedures. Intrathoracic complications were 16-fold greater in supra eleventh rib access when compared to supra twelfth rib and 46-fold greater than subcostal access (intrathoracic complications in 23.1% of supra eleventh rib access versus 1.4% of supra twelfth rib and 0.5% of subcostal access). Complications include introperative hydrothorax/hemothorax, nephropleural fistula, and pneumothorax. Seven of eight intrathoracic complications occurred in supracostal cases in Munver's series (86). Kekre et al. reported 10% thoracic complications (85).

Puncture of the desired calix can be performed with either a skinny 21-gauge or 22-gauge needle (with conversion to a larger guide wire using commercially available introducer systems) or directly with an 18-gauge needle. The rigidity of the latter needle facilitates precise placement into the targeted calix, a task that can be more difficult with the flexible 21-gauge needles. In most cases in which the calculus is radiopaque (and can therefore serve as a target for puncture),

contrast opacification of the collecting system before puncture is unnecessary, as long as a previous intravenous urogram or retrograde pyelogram is available to evaluate the anatomy of the pyelocaliceal system. If the calculi are faintly opaque or the collecting system is not dilated, placement of a retrograde catheter before the puncture is invaluable and allows both opacification and distension of the collecting system. Local anesthesia and intravenous sedation are generally sufficient for establishing the track. Occasionally, when the stone removal is to follow immediately afterward, epidural anesthesia has been used for both the percutaneous nephrostomy and the subsequent track dilation and stone removal. PCNL is customarily performed in the prone position but has also been performed in a lateral decubitus position (88) and the supine position in patients who are unable to lie prone (89,90).

The technique for access in a retrograde fashion is briefly described here (91,92). Using a transurethral retrograde route, a catheter is placed coaxially over a wire into the exact calix picked for puncture. A sharp wire or needle is then passed through the catheter under fluoroscopic control, through the calix, kidney, and flank, and out the skin. The wire is captured at the skin, and dilation is performed as outlined when a track is established percutaneously. The purported advantage of this technique is a greater degree of control over track placement and the ability to perform it in a standard cystoscopy suite (7). However, this technique of access has not gained popularity because it is technically arduous and, in fact, may not be as precise as a percutaneously placed track.

After the puncture is made, a 0.038-inch guide wire is placed into the collecting system and maneuvered into the ureter. Depending on the circumstances unique to the institution, track dilation may be performed at the same sitting, in the radiology suite, or in the operating room immediately after the nephrostomy (72,93) with the urologists extracting the calculus under nephroscopic guidance. At the author's institution, a 6 French ureteral access catheter is placed with its tip in the midureter after the nephrostomy is performed (Figure 39–13). An additional nephrostomy catheter is placed to drain the collecting system only in cases of obstruction. Subsequent track dilation and stone extraction are performed by the urologists in the operating room, usually on the following day. Experience has proved that tracts can be dilated acutely to 24–30 French with no adverse effects; this approach considerably shortens hospitalization and physician time (93). In most cases, bleeding associated with the track dilation does not hamper visibility enough to require postponing the procedure.

Track dilation is a painful procedure and requires that the patient be under either general anesthesia (preferably) or regional anesthesia. The dilation can be performed with tapered-tip fascial dilators of 10–30 French size or high-pressure track balloons measuring 10 cm in length and 10 mm in width when inflated. Secure placement of a sturdy super stiff guide wire from the flank into the urinary bladder

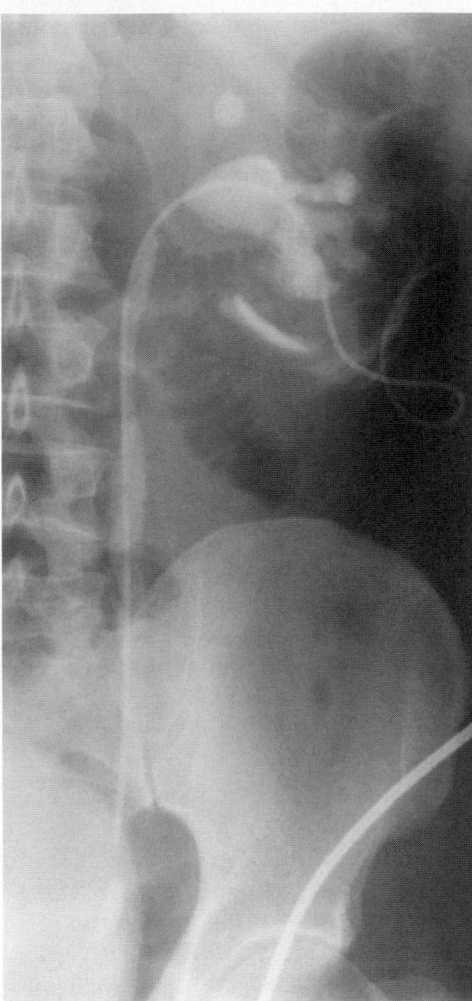

Figure 39–13   Ureteral access catheter placed percutaneously in a patient with a large left staghorn calculus. Because the collecting system was not obstructed, a separate nephrostomy catheter was not placed. Note that access is through the lower pole.

is essential to prevent inadvertent withdrawal of the guide wire from the collecting system, which will cause either loss of access or perforation of the collecting system. Track dilation should be performed under fluoroscopic monitoring, with care being taken to avoid perforation of the medial aspect of the renal pelvis when the stiff dilators are advanced.

Depending on the size and complexity of the stone, several access tracts may be necessary to remove the stone in its entirety (94,95). The addition of SWL to PCNL can reduce the number of tracks required, with SWL being used to fragment the residual stone and the fragments being extracted through the existing nephrostomy track. Simultaneous bilateral PCNL has been described for bilateral staghorn calculi (96–98), with no significant difference in the results or complication rate as compared to unilateral PCNL.

Small calculi can be extracted directly through the sheath using forceps or a basket. For larger calculi, some form of lithotripsy is used to break the stone into smaller fragments. Ultrasonic lithotripsy is frequently used—the vibrating probe breaks up the calculus and the fragments

are aspirated through the hollow probe (Figure 39–14). For particularly hard stones, electrohydraulic lithotripsy or laser is used. Flexible nephroscopy is valuable in identifying and breaking up caliceal and ureteral fragments.

After the procedure, the collecting system is inspected to ensure a stone-free state. It is standard practice to leave in a ureteral catheter and a large bore nephrostomy tube (20–24 French Malecot catheters or Foley catheters) after the procedure to provide reliable drainage of urine, to tamponade the track and allow the renal puncture to heal, and to permit access to the collecting system in the event additional procedures are required. The nephrostomy catheter is removed in 48 hours to 1 week, after a nephrostogram demonstrates no leaks from the collecting system or residual stones (7). The routine placement of nephrostomy tubes after an uncomplicated PCNL with complete calculus clearance is increasingly being questioned because of the discomfort associated with the presence of a large bore nephrostomy tube (99,100). In one series (101), 30 patients were randomized to receive a standard (20 French) nephrostomy drainage catheter, small bore (9 French) nephrostomy drainage catheter, or no nephrostomy drainage. All patients with no postprocedural nephrostomy drainage catheters had antegrade placement of a 6 French double-J stent for 4 weeks. All three groups had similar duration of hematuria and decrease in hematocrit postprocedure, but analgesics requirements were the highest in the large catheter group and the lowest in the no-catheter group, and the tubeless group also had the shortest hospital stay and the smallest amount of postoperative percutaneous site urine leak. Totally tubeless PCNL has also been reported as a safe and effective procedure (102); exclusion criteria for a tubeless approach are more than two percutaneous accesses, significant perforation of the collecting system, a large residual stone burden, significant postoperative bleeding, ureteral obstruction, and renal anomaly. To promote hemostasis after percutaneous surgery, particularly when large bore nephrostomy tubes are not left in after the procedure, materials such as fibrin sealant, tissue adhesive, and gelatin matrix have been injected into the nephrostomy tract to promote hemostasis. Cauterization of the access tract has also been performed for the same reason (103–106).

Contraindications

An uncorrected bleeding diathesis is the only absolute contraindication. The procedure should not be performed if a stone-bearing kidney is uninfected and nonfunctioning. A relative contraindication is the inability to establish a safe access track.

Complications

Bleeding

Significant arterial bleeding occurs in 0.5–1.5% of patients (107). Stoller et al. (108) reported an average blood loss of 2.8 g/dL hemoglobin for an uncomplicated one-stage,

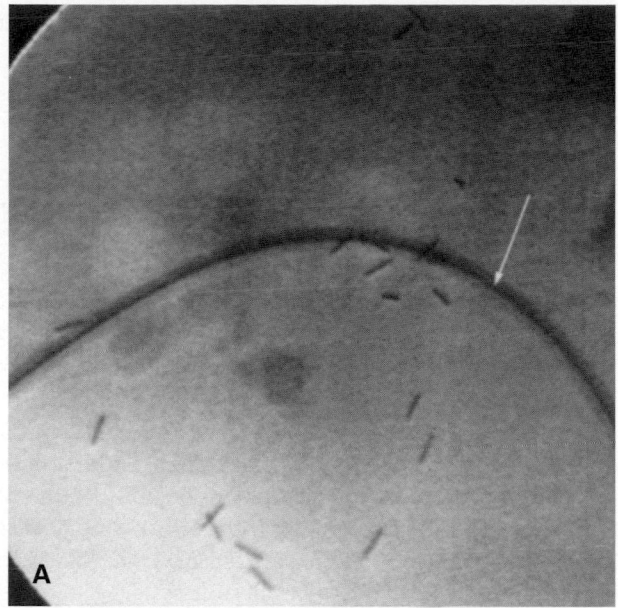

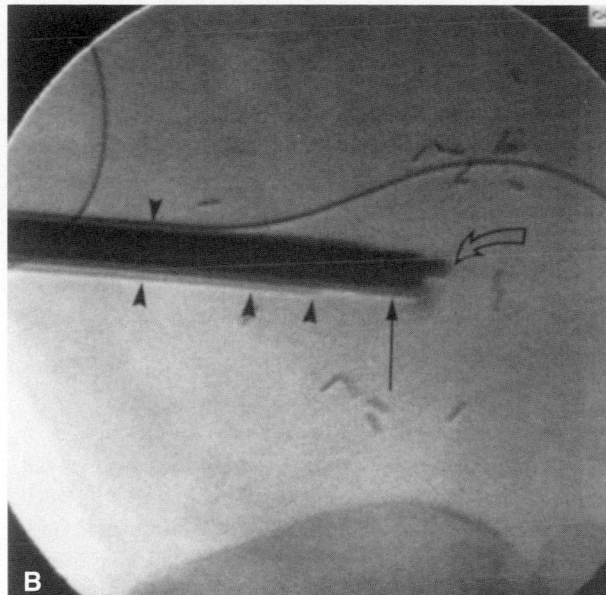

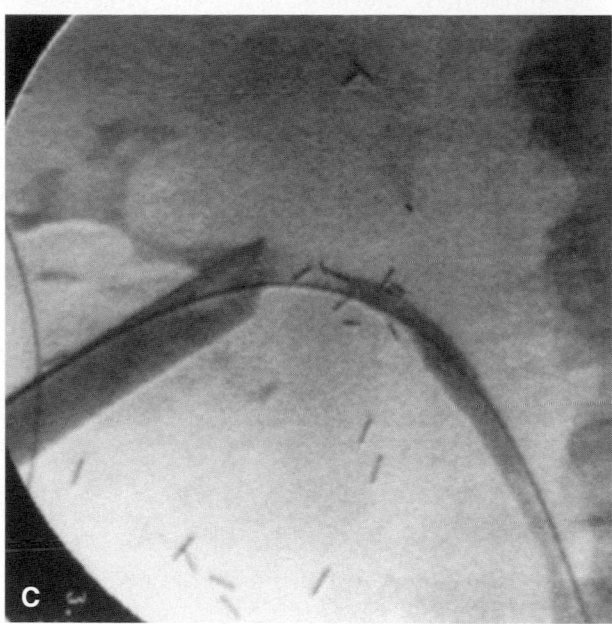

Figure 39–14 Stone removal. **A.** Intraoperative spot film before track dilation demonstrates a staghorn calculus in a patient who had previous open surgery for stone disease. A guide wire is in place within the ureteral access catheter (*arrow*). **B.** After track dilation, a 30 French sheath (*arrowheads*) was placed. Note the nephroscope (*long arrow*) and ultrasonic lithotripsy probe (*open arrow*). Most of the stone has been removed. The safety guide wire is visible outside the sheath. **C.** After stone removal, contrast injection demonstrates no extravasation. A Malecot catheter and straight ureteral catheter were placed.

single-puncture PCNL. A twofold increase in blood loss occurred in complicated staghorn calculi—requiring numerous punctures—and in cases with renal pelvic perforation. Total blood loss was not affected by the presence of hypertension, the type of fascial dilation, previous open surgery, or SWL. Interestingly, mature nephrostomy tracks bled half as frequently as fresh tracks. Davidoff et al. (109) reported that in their experience, balloon dilation of the track was associated with less renal hemorrhage and lower transfusion rates than track dilation performed with sequential Amplatz dilators.

Vascular injury during the placement of the access track or track dilation can lead to pseudoaneurysms, arteriovenous fistulas, perinephric hematomas, and loss of functional parenchyma (110). Initial puncture into a calix rather than an infundibulum or the renal pelvis is preferable, and

it is the least likely to cause major vascular injury. If excessive bleeding occurs during or after PCNL, then the nephrostomy tube may be clamped to tamponade the track and the collecting system. If that fails, a larger nephrostomy catheter may be placed that will tamponade the track better and allow blood clots, as well as residual calculus fragments, to pass. Forced diuresis by means of intravenous mannitol administration and vigorous hydration may help by causing the kidney to swell within its capsule and thus tamponade (108). Selective angiography and embolization should be considered whenever these measures fail (111,112).

Injury to Adjacent Organs

The colon can be nicked whenever it is positioned posterior to the kidney. In one series, CT scanning showed that the ascending colon was more posterior than the mid-right kidney in 39.4% at the level of the lower pole, and the descending colon was more posterior in 30.6% at the level of the left lower pole (113). Furthermore, in 75% of patients, the colon moved more posteriorly in the prone position. The colonic injury may not be obvious until the postprocedure nephrostogram demonstrates colonic filling with contrast. If the nick is small, the injuries can be managed conservatively by drainage of the kidneys with a double-pigtail ureteral stent placed from below, pulling the nephrostomy tube into the colon, and leaving it as drainage to act as a colostomy tube. The track usually seals in a few days (114). If a more serious injury occurs, open repair may be required (115).

Injury to the duodenum is uncommon and occurs when the large-bore dilators perforate the medial aspect of the right renal pelvis and enter the duodenum during track dilation. Conservative management with nasogastric tube drainage reportedly has been effective (7). Injury to the liver and spleen is uncommon, and especially so when puncture is performed in full expiration.

Pleural and lung injuries have been discussed previously. The injury is usually recognized when the nephrostogram is done. A chest tube may be required whenever a large amount of pleural fluid accumulates.

Candidemia

Segura (7) described candidemia in four patients who underwent stone removal. All patients had an indwelling nephrostomy tube and had been on antibiotics. There was overgrowth of candida in the urinary tract related to the presence of the tube and the antibiotic administration. The urine of such patients should be sterilized before stone removal is attempted.

Sepsis

PCNL is considered a clean-contaminated procedure in patients with sterile urine preoperatively, and although the need for prophylactic antibiotics is unclear, a short course of antibiotics is often administered in all patients. A rise in temperature is common after stone removal; postoperative bacteremia and pyrexia have been reported in up to 34% and 74% of patients, respectively (116,117). A 2% rate of bacteremia after percutaneous surgery (with antibiotic prophylaxis) is perhaps the most reflective of current procedures (117). In a series (117) that evaluated antibiotic administration regimens, no difference was found in infectious complications such as bacteremia and bacteriuria between a single dose of antibiotics administered immediately before procedure and treatment doses administered until removal of nephrostomy catheter after the stone treatment. In the same series (117), postoperative fever was reported in 21% of patients and bacteremia in 2.4%; the most important factors affecting postoperative fever were the duration of surgery and the amount of irrigant fluid used, but these same factors did not affect postoperative bacteriuria or bacteremia.

Perforation

During the process of stone removal, the renal pelvis can be perforated by a sharp fragment of stone or by one of the instruments (such as the ultrasound probe) in as many as 10% of cases (118). Most such perforations heal within 12–24 hours as long as good urine drainage is maintained. Serial nephrostograms will show that even sizable renal pelvic and ureteral lacerations heal in a few days without stricture formation.

A calculus can extrude through a urothelial tear (Figure 39–15). If the calculus is not recognized at endoscopy, it will usually become obvious on postprocedural radiographs, and antegrade or retrograde contrast injections may sometimes be necessary for confirmation (119). Extruded calculi will be closely related to the collecting system and ureter, yet be outside these structures on different projections. Renal pelvic extrusions should be treated with nephrostomy drainage, whereas ureteral tears should be treated with stenting for a few weeks. In the absence of infection, extrusion of calculus material into the perinephric and periureteral tissues appears to be of no clinical consequence (119). Thus, aggressive attempts to retrieve the extruded stones are not advised because persistent attempts to remove the stone can increase the degree of ureteral injury. Extraureteral infected stones are also initially managed by placement of a ureteral stent and a course of intravenous drugs (118), with close follow-up to monitor for complications such as a retroperitoneal abscess. Ureteral perforation with retroperitoneal stone expulsion has been reported in 0.5–2.3% of ureteroscopic cases (118).

Entrapped Nephrostomy Tube

Malecot tubes are often placed after PCNL to allow residual fragments to drain. If the renal pelvis is small and intrarenal, tissue bridges can grow through the wings of the Malecot tube, making it resistant to removal (120–122). Therefore, it is unwise to place a Malecot type of nephrostomy catheter for more than 2–3 weeks in patients with small, intrarenal pelves. Nephroscopy is usually required to incise the anchoring tissue bridges. Forceful removal of the catheter is unwise because it may result in incomplete removal or significant renal injury.

EXTRACORPOREAL SHOCK WAVE LITHOTRIPSY (SWL)

SWL was one of the most significant advances in modern urologic history. The success of the original Dornier HM3 lithotripter was greatly appealing to both physicians and patients, with SWL being the preferred initial treatment for

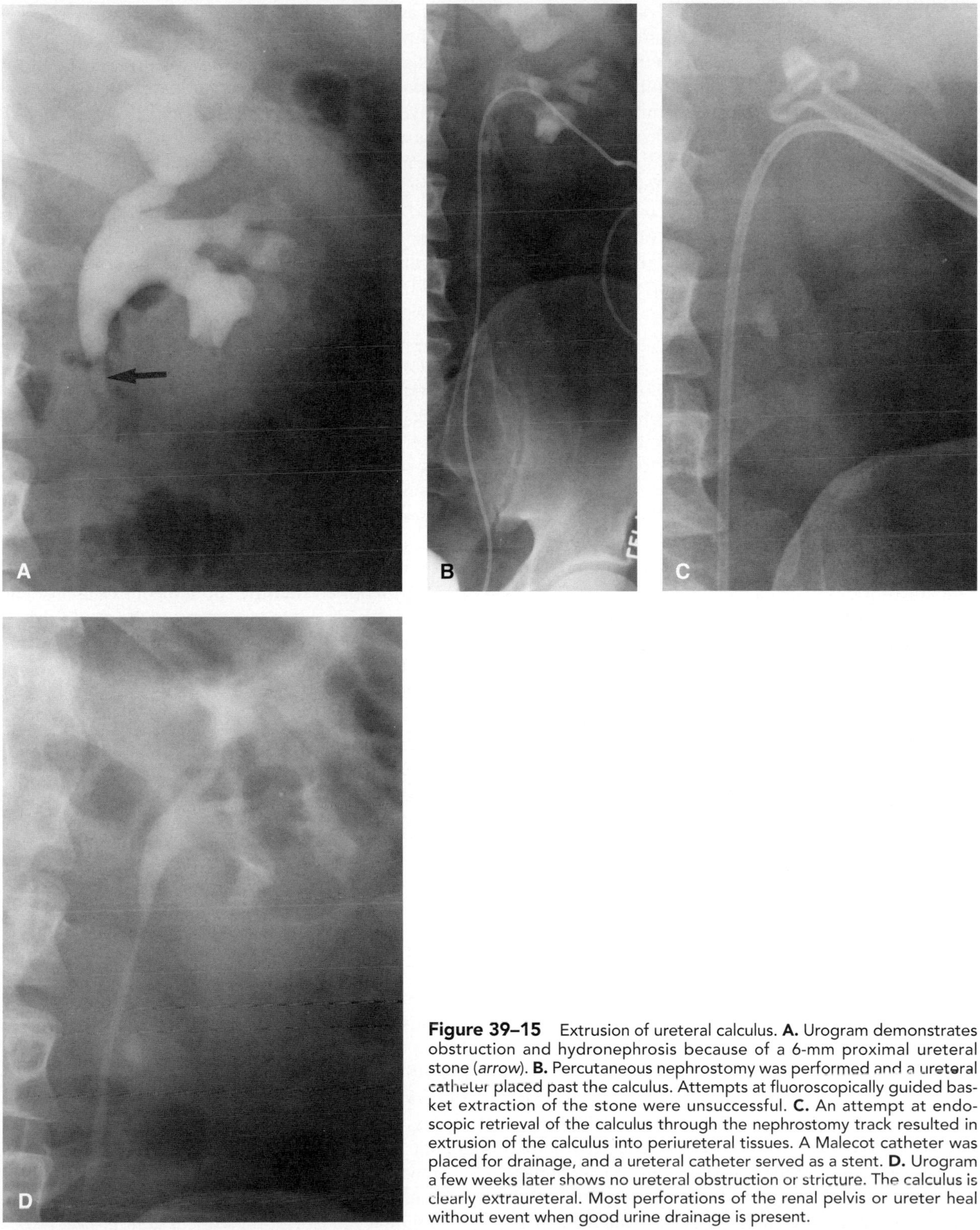

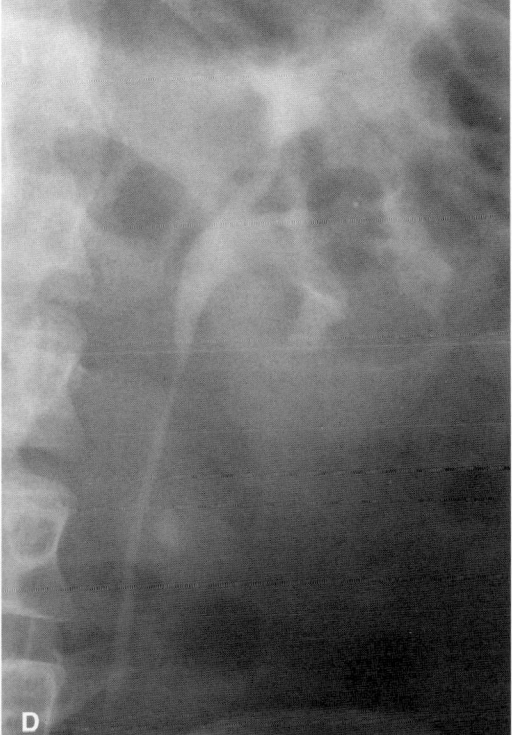

Figure 39–15 Extrusion of ureteral calculus. **A.** Urogram demonstrates obstruction and hydronephrosis because of a 6-mm proximal ureteral stone (*arrow*). **B.** Percutaneous nephrostomy was performed and a ureteral catheter placed past the calculus. Attempts at fluoroscopically guided basket extraction of the stone were unsuccessful. **C.** An attempt at endoscopic retrieval of the calculus through the nephrostomy track resulted in extrusion of the calculus into periureteral tissues. A Malecot catheter was placed for drainage, and a ureteral catheter served as a stent. **D.** Urogram a few weeks later shows no ureteral obstruction or stricture. The calculus is clearly extraureteral. Most perforations of the renal pelvis or ureter heal without event when good urine drainage is present.

80–90% of calculi. Reports suggested stone-free rates of about 70% for a broad range of stone patients and rates of more than 90% in selected series of small renal pelvic or upper ureteral stones. About 97% of stones were effectively fragmented with one SWL treatment, and an additional

2% with a second treatment (123–125). However, the introduction of second-generation and third-generation SWL machines in the last decade has raised concerns because these newer machines appear to be less effective in stone fragmentation than the original unmodified Dornier

HM3 SWL machine (2,126,127). The newer machines have a smaller focal zone that, in theory, should hit the stone harder while sparing the renal tissues from trauma. In reality, newer machines have been disappointingly less effective in breaking up stones while causing more side effects such as perinephric hematomas (128). Wu et al. (129) recently reported a success rate of only 61% for impacted upper ureteral stones as compared to 91% for ureteroscopy. PCNL has a reported 100% success rate for removal of large (>1.5 cm) impacted upper ureteral stones (130), although the procedure is more invasive than SWL and may have a higher complication rate than ureteroscopy.

Principles

The basic premise of SWL is that kidney stones will break up when exposed to a series of relatively low energy shock waves. A shock wave is produced by an electric spark in water then is made to focus on the kidney stone by an ellipsoid reflector. The shock waves can be produced by a spark gap, piezoelectricity, electromagnetic shock wave generation, or a microexplosive technique. The original Dornier HM3 lithotripter (Dornier Company) uses the spark gap technique for shock wave generation.

The shock waves are transmitted to the kidney either through a water bath into which the patient is immersed or through a fluid-filled cushion coupled to the patient's body. The trend is toward eliminating the cumbersome water bath and instead using more compact coupling devices and lower-power shock waves to allow for therapy with little or no anesthesia.

In most instances, the stones are localized with biplane fluoroscopy. For localizing nonopaque or poorly opaque stones, contrast instillation is a necessity and requires the placement of ureteral catheters. Some lithotripters use ultrasound to localize calculi (131). However, ultrasound limits the effectiveness of these machines in treating ureteral calculi because such calculi often cannot be identified accurately. Some machines have both fluoroscopy and ultrasound (124) available for stone localization.

Results

A stone-free state should be the most important yardstick for any therapy addressing urinary calculi. However, the widespread application of SWL and the inevitable generation of fragments by shock wave therapy have led some to adopt the phrase "clinically insignificant residual fragments." There is great confusion and controversy over the size of fragment that can be deemed clinically insignificant. Some investigators believe that stone fragments 4 mm or less in size are insignificant because they have about an 85% chance of spontaneously passing (7,124). However, because calculi of this size can cause both ureteral obstruction and symptoms as they pass down the ureter, others believe that the goal of any therapy for stone disease should be to achieve a stone-free state.

To assess whether or not a patient is stone-free, it is best to allow sufficient time for the fragments to pass. Most investigators believe that when fragments are still present at 3 months, they are unlikely to pass (124) and thus bode poorly for recurrent stone disease. Residual stone fragments are associated with a twofold to threefold increase in the incidence of stone recurrence within 2 years of treatment (17–22% versus 7% when the patient was stone-free). Persistent stone fragments in patients who have a history of urinary tract infections cause a 10-fold increase in recurrent urinary tract infections (84% versus 6% when stone-free) (132).

Treatment results are influenced by many factors (133,134), including stone size, stone location, stone composition, efficacy and quality of stone disintegration, urinary tract anatomy, and metabolic stone management.

The choice of therapy as it pertains to stone size has been discussed previously. Stone-free success is influenced greatly by the stone size, with stones that are 1 cm or less in size representing the ideal for SWL (Figure 39–16). Riehle (133,134) reported a stone-free rate of 87% for stones that were 1–2 cm in size, and Graff et al. (135) reported that with stones 1.5 cm or less in size, 85% were stone-free at 3 months. Khaitan et al. (136) reported that the spontaneous clearance rate was highest for residual stone fragments in the renal pelvis—53% of fragments in the renal pelvis cleared while fragments retained in the calyces went on to become clinically significant. These authors also noted that stone clearance continued up to 12 months after SWL although maximum clearance was in the first six months after SWL.

For stones more than 2.5–3.0 cm in size, PCNL is the preferred treatment in the United States. When large stones are treated with SWL monotherapy, many urologists place an indwelling double-pigtail ureteral stent to facilitate the passage of stone fragments and to ensure that the kidney remains unobstructed.

Stone location affects treatment results. Primary ureteral stones rarely (17%) have residual fragments after treatment, with most of the fragments accumulating in the lower calices. In most series reporting on SWL, the lower calices are the most common site for fragment retention (Figures 39–4, 39–10, and 39–16). The relative efficacies of SWL and PCNL in treating lower pole calculi have been discussed previously. Stone-free rates for patients with calculi in the lower calices are less than 60%, compared to 75–80% for stones in the middle and upper calices.

In patients with metabolically active stone disease, fragmentation of a solitary stone into numerous fragments creates multiple niduses for subsequent stone growth (137,138). In these patients, vigorous treatment of the underlying metabolic abnormality is clearly of prime importance in achieving a long-term stone-free state.

The presence of multiple stones decreases the efficacy of SWL and the stone-free rate. In one study, the stone-free rate in patients with four or more stones dropped to 30%. For comparison, in the same study, the stone-free rate was 82%

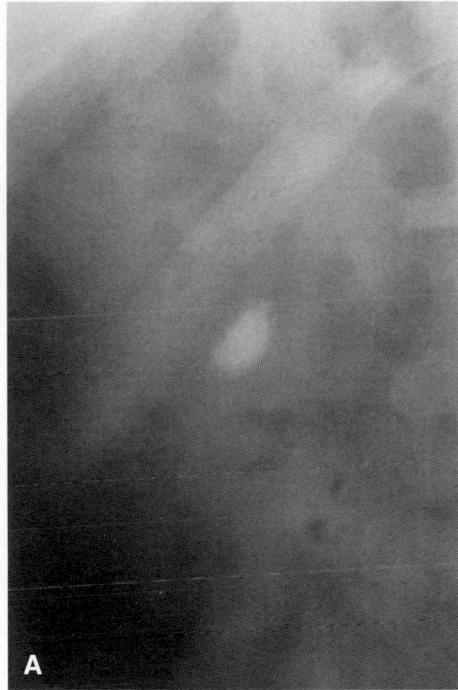 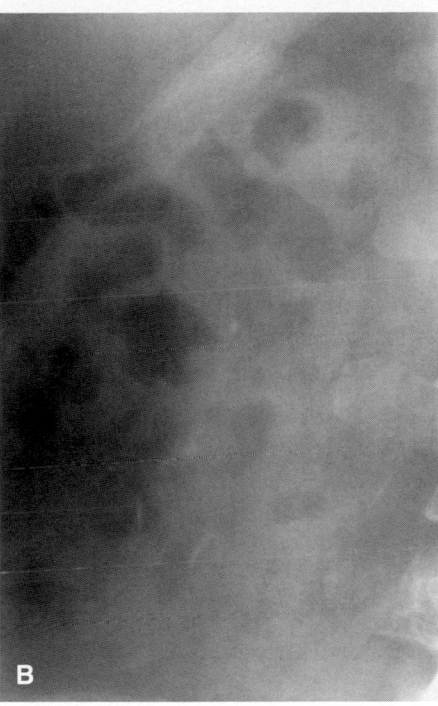

Figure 39–16 Satisfactory results with SWL. **A.** Plain film before SWL demonstrates a 1.5-cm spiculated calcium dihydrate stone in the renal pelvis. **B.** After SWL, only tiny fragments coat the lower pole calices. Fragments can be eliminated completely in a few days or a few weeks. If fragments are still present 3 months after SWL, they are unlikely to pass.

for single stones smaller than 1 cm in size and 53% for 2- to 3-cm stones) (139).

The effect of stone composition on SWL efficacy has been mentioned previously. Calcium oxalate dihydrate, struvite, and uric acid stones fragment easily with SWL. Cystine stones, calcium oxalate monohydrate, hydroxyapatite, and brushite stones are more resistant to fragmentation with SWL and thus more likely to produce large fragments that may require repeat SWL or endourologic procedures for removal. Density of stones as measured by Hounsfield units on CT has been used in an effort to predict the efficacy of ESWL. Pareek et al. (140) reported that patients who were stone free after SWL had mean HU values of 577 ± 182.5, while residual stones remained when HU values of the calculi were 910 ± 190.

Obese patients present special problems. For the Dornier HM3 lithotripter, the weight limit is 130 kg. With other machines (although there is no set weight limit), the ability to image and effectively fragment the stone is compromised in obese patients because the stone may be difficult to position in the focal range. Pareek et al. (141) reported that SWL was unsuccessful in fragmenting upper urinary calculi in patients with a body mass index (BMI) greater than 30.

Contraindications

The accumulation of clinical experience with SWL and the availability of advanced lithotripters have greatly minimized the number of absolute and relative contraindications to SWL. At present, only pregnancy and uncontrolled or uncorrectable coagulopathic conditions are considered the absolute contraindications to SWL. Uncorrected bleeding disorders

predispose to intraparenchymal or subcapsular hematomas when SWL is employed. Therefore, hematologic abnormalities should be corrected before SWL. Anticoagulants, anti-inflammatory drugs, and aspirin should be discontinued before the procedure. Several patients with hemophilia have been successfully treated (142).

Shortly after its introduction, SWL was believed to be contraindicated in a few clinical situations (discussed below). Clinical experience has proved that SWL can be performed safely in these patients.

Renal arterial aneurysms and aortic aneurysms in proximity to a stone that required treatment were previously regarded as relative contraindications to SWL. However, SWL can be performed safely in such patients without incurring an increased risk of rupture (143,144) and should be considered the treatment of choice when these patients have stones that require treatment and that are suitable for SWL. Calcification of the renal artery or aorta adjacent to a symptomatic stone is not a contraindication to SWL because the shock wave energy does not affect arterial calcifications (17). Similarly, vascular clips in the vicinity of treatment are of no consequence (145).

Patients with cardiac pacemakers can be treated safely with SWL. Such patients should be monitored by a cardiologist so that, when necessary, a temporary transvenous pacemaker can be inserted or a pacemaker reprogrammed if it malfunctions as a result of the shock waves (145–148). The standard HM3 lithotripter had traditionally been used with general or epidural anesthesia, which made SWL a relative contraindication in patients who were at high risk for anesthesia complications. This is no longer a significant factor in most patients because intravenous sedation can be used successfully to treat patients, even with the HM3 lithotripters (149). It was hoped that with the newer lithotripters, less anesthesia may be required because the shock waves are less powerful (124), but this has not proved to be the case (150).

A relative contraindication is the coexistence of calculi with obstruction, such as ureteral strictures and ureteropelvic junction obstruction, as discussed previously in the section on PCNL. Ureteral obstruction distal to a stone can be managed with ureteral stents or catheters.

Active urinary tract infections require treatment before, during, and after SWL. Similarly, patients with struvite stones should have their urine cultured and be treated with antibiotics before SWL.

Complications

SWL is well-tolerated by most patients, and major complications are rare. The complications can be divided into several categories:

1. Complications related to the effects of the shock waves on the kidney and adjacent organs
2. Residual stone fragments
3. Complications related to ureteral obstruction because of the passage of stone fragments
4. Anesthetic and cardiac complications

Mechanical Effects of Shock Waves

Renal Parenchymal Damage

The number of shock waves that the kidney can tolerate safely at a given kilovoltage is unknown. Shock wave-induced renal parenchymal damage does not cause a measurable reduction in renal function, as judged by serum creatinine and creatinine clearance or excretory urography. There is a transient increase in urinary excretion of enzymes that are specific markers for renal injury, such as gamma-glutamyltransferase, beta-galactosidase, and N-acetyl-beta-glucosaminidase (151,152). Some immediate decrease in renal plasma flow has been reported in 30% of kidneys treated with SWL (153), but no abnormalities were seen on 131I-hippurate scans done 4 years after SWL (154).

Hematuria for the first 24 hours is extremely common. This reaction is believed to be related to trauma to the renal parenchyma and not to injury to the urothelium by the calculus fragments.

Clinically significant subcapsular or perinephric hematomas have been reported in 0.5–2.5% of patients and represent the most common, serious extrarenal complication (155,156). CT is the best modality with which to evaluate these complications (Figure 39–17). CT demonstrates (157) perinephric soft tissue stranding and fascial thickening in 70% of patients, subcapsular hematomas in 15%, and intrarenal contusions in 4%. Resolution of the hematomas was seen in scans done several months later.

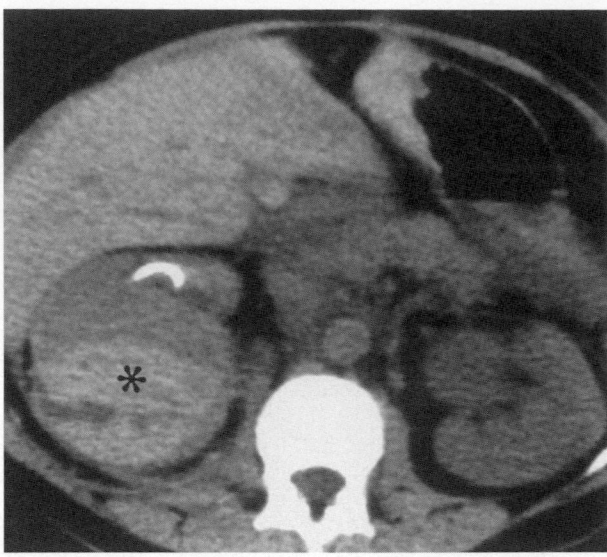

Figure 39–17   Unenhanced CT scan demonstrates a high-density subcapsular hematoma on the posterior aspect of the right kidney (*asterisk*) after SWL. Note the proximal end of the ureteral stent in the renal pelvis.

Similarly, MRI shows swelling of the kidney and fluid in the perinephric, subcapsular, and intraparenchymal regions (158,159), with changes reverting to normal in 3 months. MRI demonstrates abnormalities in 85% of patients (160) treated with SWL; they consist of loss of the corticomedullary junction in 52% of patients, intrarenal hemorrhage in 18%, and perinephric changes in 64%. Lower-power piezoelectric lithotripters, in contrast, cause demonstrable morphologic changes in only 5% of patients (such as edema in the perinephric space). This suggests that lower-power, piezoelectric lithotripters with small focal range may induce less acute renal parenchymal damage than higher-power electrohydraulic lithotripters (161), even though the former require a larger number of shocks to be equally effective in stone fragmentation.

Injury to Adjacent Organs

Damage to neighboring organs is not unexpected after renal SWL. Sporadic cases of pancreatitis (138), bowel hematomas (intramural and mucosal), and transient gastrointestinal erosions with mucosal bleeding have been reported. Colonic ileus is a frequent but transient occurrence after SWL and usually resolves in 24–48 hours. Small bowel perforation after SWL for a ureteral stone has been reported (162).

Pulmonary hemorrhage because of lung damage may be seen whenever the lower lung is included in the high shock wave energy field. This usually occurs with aberrant anatomy such as in myelodysplastic infants and in children. Gallstones have been inadvertently shattered during renal SWL.

Iliac vein and iliac arterial thrombosis have been reported after SWL of lower ureteral calculi. Cutaneous bruising can occur at the shock wave entry site.

Hypertension after Lithotripsy

The occurrence of SWL-associated hypertension is a source of debate and controversy. Initial reports suggested the new onset of hypertension one or more years after SWL. Subsequent large series suggest that there is no increased incidence of hypertension after SWL (163).

Ureteral Obstruction

Ureteral colic, obstruction, or urosepsis can result from the passage of calculus fragments into the ureter. The fragments can line up in the ureter, simulating the appearance of a cobblestoned street and are referred to as *steinstrasse*. This complication occurs in 1–6% of cases, depending on the lithotripter used, and intervention is required in 6–35% of cases (12,164). Frequently, a larger lead fragment is responsible for the obstruction and the subsequent piling up of fragments proximally. Steinstrasse occurs 72–75% of the time in the distal ureter (12,164), 18% in the proximal ureter, and 6% in the midureter. In Sulaiman's series (164), with stones greater than 1 cm in size, no cases of steinstrasse occurred while stones of 10–19 mm were associated with steinstrasse in 4%, stones

20–29 mm in 14% and less than 30 mm in 30%. Fragments can often pass spontaneously, and interventions are reserved for patients with pain, total obstruction (particularly of a solitary kidney), urosepsis, and failure to pass fragments (Figure 39-18). It is not uncommon for patients to be asymptomatic despite urinary obstruction and impaired renal function—the obstruction being diagnosed on a routine post-SWL urogram. When intervention is required, ureteroscopic removal of the lead fragment, ureteral meatotomy, or ureteroscopic lithotripsy followed by stenting is helpful. Another option is to drain the kidney by means of a percutaneous nephrostomy and allow the fragments to pass spontaneously, which they often do. For large steinstrasse (greater than one-third ureteral length), a combined percutaneous and ureteroscopic approach may be required. Upper ureteral steinstrasse may also be treated by repeat SWL to the "lead" fragment.

Prophylactic ureteral stenting is often used before SWL to prevent ureteral obstruction when large stones are being treated. Until recently, it was generally believed that ureteral stents increased the speed of stone fragment passage while reducing the incidence of colic. It appears that stents are useful for preventing obstruction and sepsis after lithotripsy but do not necessarily facilitate the passage of

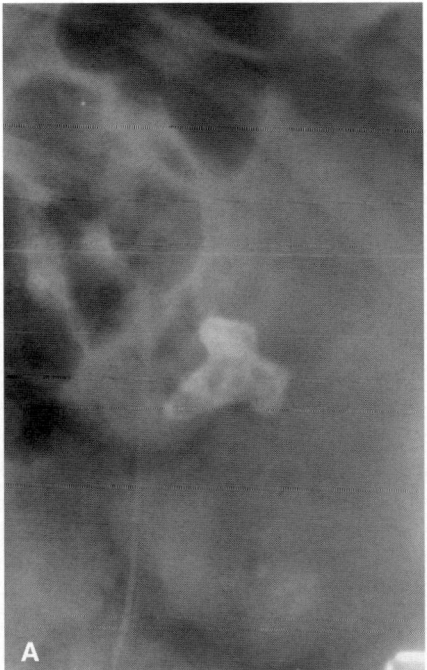
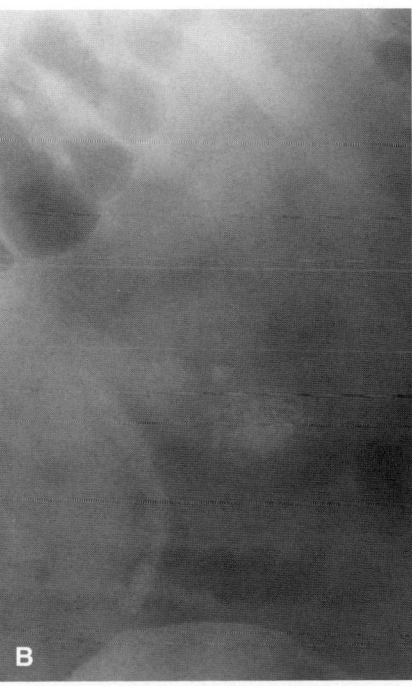
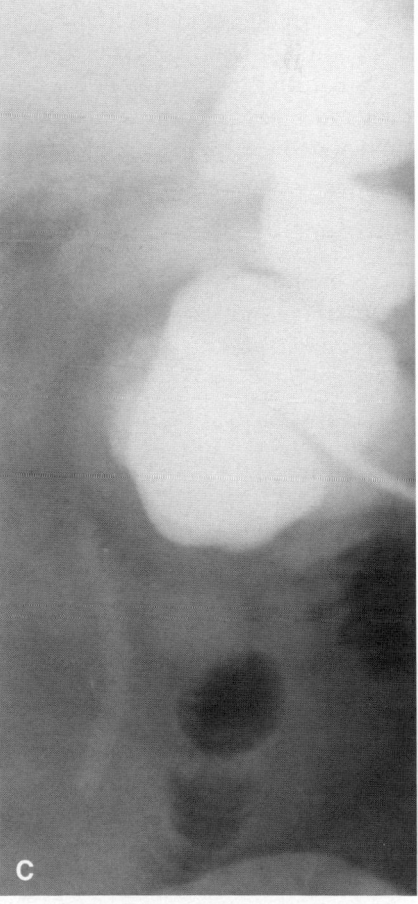

Figure 39–18 Obstructing steinstrasse after SWL. **A.** Plain radiograph shows a partial left staghorn calculus in a patient with a solitary kidney. The patient was treated with SWL. **B.** One week later, the serum creatinine level was found to be markedly elevated to 17 mg. The patient was asymptomatic. Radiograph demonstrates ureteral steinstrasse and residual lower pole fragments. **C.** An emergent percutaneous nephrostomy was performed for renal decompression. The ureteral fragments eventually cleared spontaneously.

stone fragments (165). Sulaiman et al. found that ureteral stents did not affect the occurrence of steinstrasse for stones greater than 15 mm in size, but for stones larger than 15 mm, 15% of patients with stents developed steinstrasse compared to 28% of patients without stents (164).

Sepsis

The range of patients who develop septic complications after SWL is 0–1.5% (11). Aggressive treatment of urinary tract infections before SWL can reduce the incidence of this complication. In addition, patients with large infection stones (staghorn stones) should be treated with ureteral stenting or percutaneous nephrostomy after, or preferably before, SWL to prevent the large volume of fragments from precipitating a urinary obstruction. Rarely, lithotripsy of an infected stone can lead to the development of a perinephric abscess (166).

Cardiac and Anesthetic Complications

Anesthetic complications are self-evident. The effect of the shock waves on the myocardium can provoke arrhythmias, especially at high treatment voltages. Prevention of arrhythmias can be done through use of a gating system so that shock waves discharge only during the refractory period of the heart, following the R wave (11) and preventing aberrant electrical stimulation. Ventricular dysrhythmias may be seen in 6% of patients without a previous history of arrythmias (148).

Body warming because of immersion in the water bath of the HM3 unit can cause vasodilation, central blood pooling, and cardiac stress in patients with severe heart disease. Focal damage to a nephrostomy catheter because of ESWL has been reported (167).

Treatment of Ureteral Calculi

Management of ureteral calculi is determined largely by their location and size (6). Up to 98% of stones that are smaller than 5 mm in diameter will pass spontaneously.

Proximal Ureteral Calculi

Stones in the upper ureter can be treated by SWL either in situ in the ureter or after displacement into the kidney (by forceful retrograde injection of saline or contrast or sometimes by simple advancement of a retrograde catheter). The success rate of fragmentation is 82–96% (2) and is reportedly higher, with stone-free rates approaching 100%, when upper ureteral stones are pushed into the kidney and treated with SW (135,168,169). In contrast, in situ therapy is successful in 60–85% of cases. In situ SWL of ureteral calculi generally requires a higher kilovoltage and more shock waves than for kidney stones. With the newer lithotriptors, success rates are lower; Wu et al. (129) recently reported a success rate of only 61% for impacted upper ureteral stones as compared to 91% for ureteroscopy.

Upper and midureteral calculi can also be approached in a percutaneous, antegrade fashion. In one series (170), 35 of 37 proximal ureteral calculi and 20 of 20 midureteral calculi were removed successfully by flexible nephroscopy. The stones were removed under direct vision, basketed under fluoroscopy, or fragmented with ultrasonic or electrohydraulic lithotripsy and removed. Maheshwari et al. (130) reported 100% success rate for removal of large (>1.5 cm) impacted upper ureteral stones with PCNL.

Midureteral and Distal Ureteral Calculi

When ureteral stones overlie the pelvic bones, SWL has to be performed in the prone position so that the shock waves do not have to traverse the pelvic bones. The prone position can also be used to treat some horseshoe kidneys, pelvic kidneys (171,172), and calculi in the distal ureter or at the ureterovesical junction.

The optimal therapy for lower ureteral calculi is the subject of considerable debate and controversy, centered primarily on whether ureteroscopy or SWL is the better modality. Transurethral ureteroscopy is a natural extension of ureteroscopic techniques and increasingly is being used by urologists for both diagnostic and therapeutic purposes, largely because of the current availability of smaller, more flexible ureteroscopes that can be maneuvered easily even into the proximal and midureter. In contrast, rigid ureteroscopes are difficult to advance past the iliac vessel crossing and are therefore limited in their application on a routine basis (except for calculi lodged at the ureterovesical junction). In the United States, ureteroscopic removal of distal ureteral calculi is favored, whereas European urologists more often use SWL in these patients. Ureteroscopy has a higher initial success rate than SWL in the treatment of distal ureteral stones, with reported success rates of greater than 95%. However, ureteroscopy is more invasive, has a higher complication rate (primarily ureteral avulsion or perforation and ureteral stricture formation because of trauma caused by the ureteroscope or the stone fragmentation device (173), and is extremely operator dependent. The success of ureteroscopic stone retrieval decreases the higher the stone is in the ureter; reported success rates are 38% for upper ureteral calculi, 50% for stones in the midureter, and 96% for the distal ureter (174). The converse is true for SWL. Hendrikx et al. (175) reported that stone-free rate following SWL for miduretal and distal ureteral stones was 51% compared to stone-free rate of 91% following ureteroscopy. In the same report, stones that were smaller than 11 mm had poorer results as compared to stones larger than 11 mm in size— 75% versus 85% for smaller stones with ureteroscopy and 17% versus 73% for SWL.

Small stones that are less than 5 mm in diameter are removed under direct ureteroscopic guidance with baskets or instruments. It is important to note that the very small working channel (2–4 French) of flexible ureteroscopes limits the size of the instruments that can be used for stone extraction. Larger stones (>5 mm) are often difficult to grasp with small baskets or forceps and require fragmentation with direct contact fragmentation devices (pulsed dye laser lithotripsy or electrohydraulic lithotripsy) for successful stone removal. Blind passage of cystoscopically guided baskets into the ureter in a retrograde fashion is rare today because of the availability of ureteroscopy (Figure 39–19).

The necessity for placement of ureteral stents when treating ureteral calculi with SWL is also controversial, with many authors believing that ureteral stones can be treated just as successfully without stents bypassing the stone. When a stent is placed past a stone, it allows urine to surround the calculus and thus creates a fluid-filled expansion chamber around the stone. This is believed to facilitate stone fragmentation by allowing the disintegrated outer fragments to fall away while the shock waves disintegrate the core of the calculus. Previous reports had suggested that only 78% of ureteral calculi treated in situ without a stent were completely disintegrated, compared to 90% of stones when bypass stent placement was possible (176). Dretler et al. (177) reported 60% successful disintegration in situ without a stent and 100% after stent placement. However, other

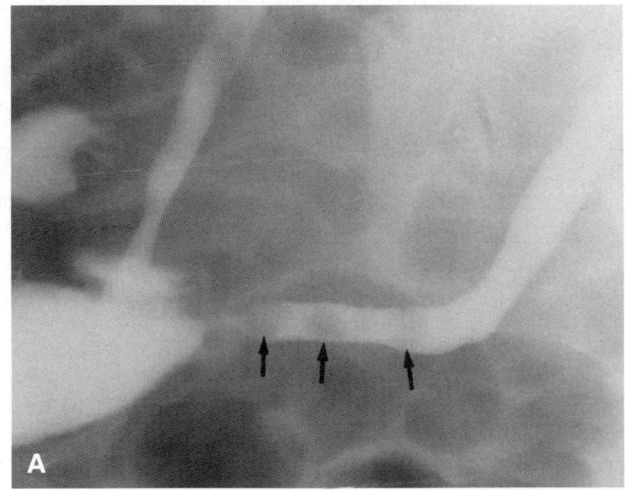

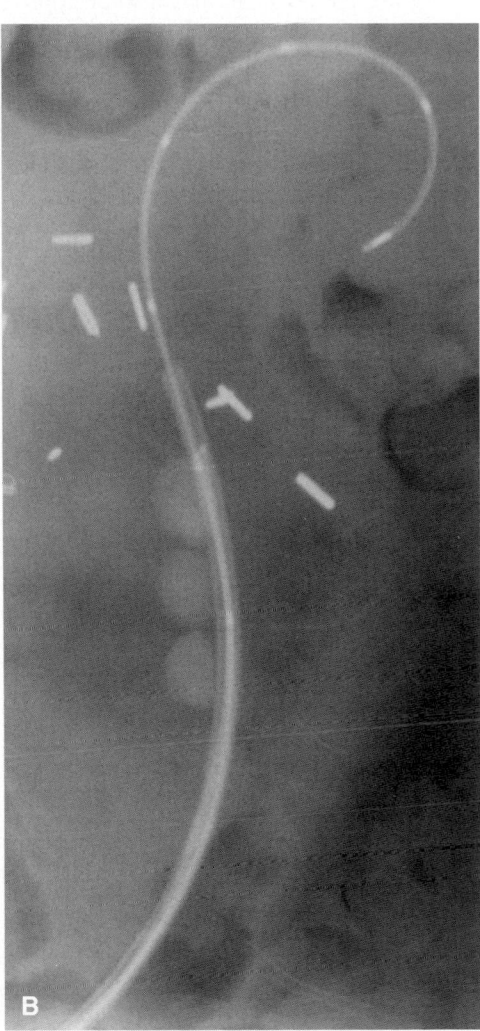

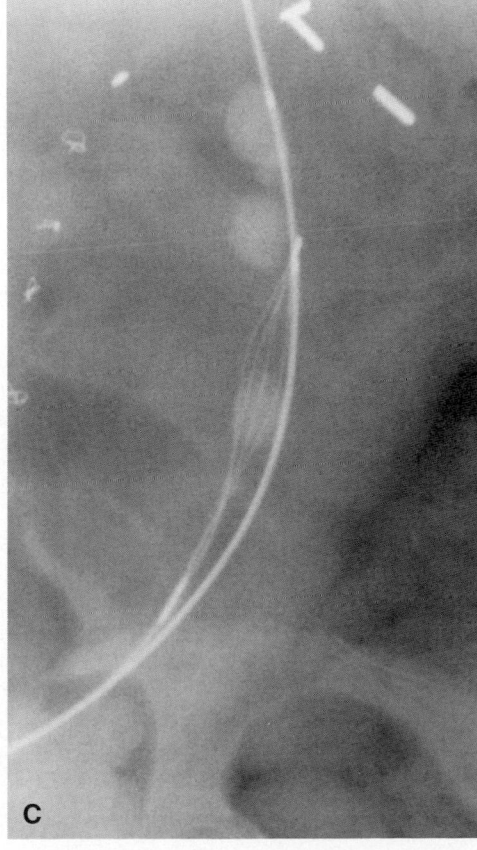

Figure 39–19 Distal ureteral calculi in a patient with ileal conduit urinary diversion. **A.** Loopogram demonstrates three calculi (*arrows*) in the left ureter, just proximal to the ureteroileal anastomosis. **B.** Sheath and guide wire placed proximal to the calculi. **C.** The calculi were removed by being basketed under fluoroscopy. Diverted ureters are difficult to approach by ureteroscopy but can be catheterized easily with fluoroscopic guidance when the ureteroileal anastomoses are not strictured.

reports (178,179) suggest that ureteral calculi can be fragmented successfully without stent placement with high rates of success—77% after one treatment and 97% overall. The Clinical Guidelines Panel summary of the American Urological Association (6) does not support the routine use of stents for SWL of ureteral stones.

SUMMARY

SWL is the treatment of choice for upper ureteral calculi and has higher success rates when the stone can be pushed back into the kidney. These calculi may also be approached in a percutaneous, antegrade fashion. In the midureter, most authors favor ureteroscopic extraction of calculi or retrograde displacement of the calculus into the kidney followed by SWL. SWL with the patient prone is yet another option. For distal ureteral stones, ureteroscopic extraction is probably the technique of choice (180) because of its high initial success rate, the rare need for secondary treatments and postureteroscopic interventions, and the low complication rate of ureteroscopy in the distal ureter. However, the treatment of choice for distal ureteral calculi has not been universally chosen, and there are many institutional and individual variations.

Ureterolithotomy for stone removal is unusual because there are so many other viable treatment options. Rarely, stones that are impacted or embedded in the ureter may require open surgical removal. SWL has been used successfully to fragment stones that were entrapped within stone baskets (181) and also to fragment calculus encrustations on indwelling ureteral stents, thus permitting their removal (182).

REFERENCES

1. Fernstrom I, Johannson B. Percutaneous pyelolithotomy: a new extraction technique. Scand J Urol Nephrol 1976;10:257.
2. Kerbl K, Rehman J, Landman J, et al. Current management of urolithiasis: progress or regress? J Endourol 2002;16:281–288.
3. Segura JW. Surgical management of urinary calculi. Semin Nephrol 1990;10:53–63.
4. Bird VG, Fallon B, Winfield HN. Practice patterns in the treatment of large renal stones. J Endourol 2003;17:355–363.
5. Segura JW, Preminger GM, Assimos DG, et al. Nephrolithiasis Clinical Guidelines Panel summary report on the management of staghorn calculi. The American Urological Association Nephrolithiasis Clinical Guidelines Panel. J Urol 1994;151: 1648–1651.
6. Segura JW, Preminger GM, Assimos DG, et al. Ureteral Stones Clinical Guidelines Panel summary report on the management of ureteral calculi. The American Urological Association. J Urol 1997;158:1951–1921.
7. Segura JW. Percutaneous nephrolithotomy: technique, indications, and complications. AUA Update Series 1993;12:154–159.
8. Lingeman JE, Zafar FS. Lithotripsy systems. In: Smith AD, ed. Smith's Textbook of Endourology. St. Louis: Quality Medical Publishing, 1996:553–589.
9. Lingeman JE. Staghorn. Stones: the continued challenge. AUA Update Series 1993;12:146–151.
10. Al-Kohlany KM, Shokeir AA, Mosbah A, et al. Treatment of complete staghorn stones: a prospective randomized comparison of open surgery versus percutaneous nephrolithotomy. J Urol 2005;173:469–473.
11. Roth RA, Beckmann CF. Complications of extracorporeal shock wave lithotripsy and percutaneous nephrolithotomy. Urol Clin North Am 1988;15:155.
12. Fedullo LM, Pollack HM, Banner MP, et al. The development of steinstrassen after ESWL: frequency, natural history, and radiologic management. AJR Am J Roentgenol 1988;151:1145–1147.
13. Streem SB, Lammert G. Long-term efficacy of combination therapy for struvite staghorn calculi. J Urol 1992;147:563.
14. Schulze H, Hertle L, Kutlar A, et al. Critical evaluation of treatment of staghorn calculi by percutaneous nephrolithotomy and ESWL. J Urol 1989;141:822–825.
15. Streem SB, Yost A, Dolmatch B, et al. Combination "sandwich" therapy for extensive renal calculi in 100 consecutive patients: immediate, long-term and stratified results from a 10-year experience. J Urol 1997;158:342–345.
16. Miller K, Bachor R, Sauter T, et al. Percutaneous nephrolithotomy/ESWL versus stent/ESWL for large stones and staghorn calculi: what have we learned? J Endourol 1989;3:287.
17. Chaussy CG, Fuchs GJ. Current state and future developments of noninvasive treatment of human urinary stones with extracorporeal shock wave lithotripsy. J Urol 1989;141:782.
18. Chandhoke PS. Cost-effectiveness of different treatment options for staghorn calculi. J Urol 1996;156:1567–1571.
19. Martin X, Tajra LC, Gelet A, et al. Complete staghorn stones: percutaneous approach using one or more multiple accesses. J Endourol 1999;13:367–368.
20. Constantinides C, Recker F, Jaegar P, et al. Extracorporeal shock wave lithotripsy as monotherapy of staghorn renal calculi: 3 years' experience. J Urol 1989;142:1415.
21. Chibber PJ. Percutaneous nephrolithotomy for large and staghorn calculi. J Endourol 1993;7:293–295.
22. Patterson DE, Segura JW, LeRoy AJ. Long-term follow-up of patients treated by percutaneous ultrasonic lithotripsy for struvite staghorn calculi. J Endourol 1987;1:777.
23. Vandeursen H, Baert L. Extracorporeal shock wave lithotripsy monotherapy for staghorn stones with the second generation lithotripters. J Urol 1990;143:252.
24. Lingeman JE, Coury TA, Newman DM, et al. Comparison of results and morbidity of percutaneous nephrostolithotomy and extracorporeal shock wave lithotripsy. J Urol 1987;138:485.
25. Kirkali Z, Esen AA, Mungan MU. Effectiveness of extracorporeal shock wave lithotripsy in the management of stone bearing horseshoe kidneys. J Endourol 1996;10:13–15.
26. Demirkesen O, Yaycioglu O, Onal B, et al. Extracorporeal shockwave lithotripsy for stones in abnormal urinary tracts: analysis of results and comparison with normal urinary tracts. J Endourol 2001;15:681–685.
27. Weizer AZ, Springhart WP, Ekeruo WO, et al. Ureteroscopic management of renal calculi in anomalous kidneys. Urology 2005; 65:265–269.
28. Raj GV, Auge BK, Weizer AZ, et al. Percutaneous management of calculi within horseshoe kidneys. J Urol 2003;170:48–51.
29. Francesca F, Felipetto R, Mosca F, et al. Percutaneous nephrolithotomy of transplanted kidneys. J Endourol 2002;16:225–227.
30. Lu HF, Shekarriz B, Stoller M. Donor-gifted allograft urolithiasis: early percutaneous management. Urology 2002;59:25–27.
31. Gerber GS, Lyon ES. Endopyelotomy: patient selection, results, and complications. Urology 1994;43:2–10.
32. Grasso M, Lang G, Loisides P, et al. Endoscopic management of the symptomatic caliceal diverticular calculus. J Urol 1995;153: 1878–1881.
33. Psihramis KE, Dretler SP. Extracorporeal shock wave lithotripsy of caliceal diverticula calculi. J Urol 1987;138:707–711.
34. Ritchie AWS, Parr NJ, Moussa SA, et al. Lithotripsy for calculi in caliceal diverticula? Br J Urol 1990;66:6–8.
35. Hendrikx AJM, Bierkens AF, Bos R, et al. Treatment of stones in caliceal diverticula: extracorporeal shock wave lithotripsy versus percutaneous nephrolitholapaxy. Br J Urol 1992;70:478–482.
36. Streem SB, Yost A. Treatment of caliceal diverticular calculi with extracorporeal shock-wave lithotripsy: patient selection and extended follow-up. J Urol 1992;148:1043–1046.

37. Ellis JH, Patterson SK, Sonda LP, et al. Stones and infection in renal caliceal diverticula: treatment with percutaneous procedures. AJR Am J Roentgenol 1991;156:995–1000.

38. Bellman GC, Silverstein JI, Blickensderfer S, et al. Technique and follow-up of percutaneous management of caliceal diverticula. Urology 1993;42:21–25.

39. Donnellan SM, Harewood LS, Wenn DR. Percutaneous management of caliceal diverticular calculi: technique and outcome. J Endourol 1999;13:83–88.

40. Auge BK, Munver R, Kourambas J, et al. Endoscopic management of symptomatic caliceal diverticula: a retrospective comparison of percutaneous nephrolithotripsy and ureteroscopy. J Endourol 2002;16:557–563.

41. Pang K, David R, Fuchs GJ. Treatment of stones in caliceal diverticula using retrograde endoscopic approach: critical assessment after 2 years [Abstract]. J Endourol 1992;6(Suppl): F–15.

42. Lang EK. Percutaneous infundibuloplasty: management of caliceal diverticula and infundibular stenosis. Radiology 1991;181: 871–877.

43. Fuchs AM, David RD, Fuchs GJ. Treatment of stones in caliceal diverticuli using retrograde endoscopic approach. J Endourol 1990;4:109.

44. Meretyk I, Meretyk S, Clayman RV. Endopyelotomy: comparison of ureteroscopic retrograde and antegrade techniques. J Urol 1992;148:775–783.

45. Lingeman JE, Siegel YI, Steele B, et al. Management of lower pole nephrolithiasis: a critical analysis. J Urol 1994;151:663–667.

46. Albala DM, Assimos DG, Clayman RV, et al. Lower pole I: a prospective randomized trial of extracorporeal shock wave lithotripsy and percutaneous nephrostolithotomy for lower pole nephrolithiasis—Initial results. J Urol 2001;166:2072–2080.

47. Graff J, Diederichs W, Schulze H. Long-term follow-up in 1,003 extracorporeal shock wave lithotripsy patients. J Urol 1988; 140:479.

48. McCullough DL. Extracorporeal shock wave lithotripsy and residual stone fragments in lower calices: letter to the editor. J Urol 1989;141:140.

49. Gerber GS. Management of lower-pole caliceal stones. J Endourol 2003;17:501–503.

50. Sumino Y, Mimata H, Tasaki Y, et al. Predictors of lower pole stone clearance after extracorporeal shock wave lithotripsy. J Urol 2002;168:1344–1347.

51. Sorensen CM, Chandhoke PS. Is lower pole caliceal anatomy predictive of extracorporeal shock wave lithotripsy success for primary lower pole kidney stones? J Urol 2002;168:2377–2382.

52. Siegel YI, Lingeman JE. Percutaneous transilial access for stone removal in crossed fused renal ectopia. Urology 1993;42:82–85.

53. Segura JW, Patterson DE, LeRoy AJ, et al. Percutaneous removal of kidney stones: review of 1,000 cases. J Urol 1985;134:1077–1081.

54. Lee CK, Smith AD. Percutaneous transperitoneal approach to the pelvic kidney for endourologic removal of calculus: three cases with two successes. J Endourol 1992;6:133–135.

55. Toth C, Holman E, Pasztor I, et al. Laparoscopically controlled and assisted percutaneous transperitoneal nephrolithotomy in a pelvic dystopic kidney. J Endourol 1993;7:303–305.

56. Monga M, Castañeda-Zuñiga WR, Thomas R. Femoral neuropathy following percutaneous nephrolithotomy of a pelvic kidney. Urology 1995;45:1059–1061.

57. Hockley NM, Lingeman JE, Hutchinson CL. Relative efficacy of extracorporeal shock wave lithotripsy and percutaneous nephrostolithotomy in the management of cystine calculi. J Endourol 1989;3:273.

58. Motola JA, Smith AD. Therapeutic options for the management of upper tract calculi. Urol Clin North Am 1990;17:191.

59. Knoll LD, Segura JW, Patterson DE. Long-term follow-up in patients with cystine urinary calculi treated by percutaneous ultrasonic lithotripsy. J Urol 1988;140:246.

60. Matlaga BR, Shah OD, Zagoria RJ, et al. Computerized tomography guided access for percutaneous nephrolithotomy. J Urol 2003;170:45–47.

61. Horowitz E, Schmidt JD. Renal calculi in pregnancy. Clin Obstet Gynecol 1985;28:324–338.

62. MacNeily AE, Goldenberg SL, Allen GJ, et al. Sonographic visualization of the ureter in pregnancy. J Urol 1991;146:298–301.

63. Loughlin KR. Management of urologic problems during pregnancy. Urology 1994;44:159.

64. Cass AS, Smith CS, Gleich P. Management of urinary calculi in pregnancy. Urology 1986;28:370–372.

65. Drago JR, Rohner TJ, Chez RA. Management of urinary calculi in pregnancy. Urology 1982;20:578–581.

66. Loughlin KR, Bailey RB Jr. Internal ureteral stents for conservative management of ureteral calculi during pregnancy. N Engl J Med 1986;315:1647–1649.

67. Wolf MC, Hallander JB, Salisz JA, et al. A new technique for ureteral stent placement during pregnancy using endoluminal ultrasound. Surg Obstet Gynecol 1992;175:575–576.

68. Goldfarb RA, Neerhut GJ, Lederer E. Management of acute hydronephrosis of pregnancy by ureteral stenting: risk of stone formation. J Urol 1989;141:921–922.

69. Spirnak JP, Resnick MI. Stone formation as a complication of indwelling ureteral stents: a report of 5 cases. J Urol 1985;134: 349–351.

70. Shnider SM, Webster GM. Maternal and fetal hazards of surgery during pregnancy. Am J Obstet Gynecol 1965;92:891–900.

71. Watterson JD, Girvan AR, Beiko DT, et al. Ureteroscopy and holmium: YAG laser lithotripsy: an emerging definitive management strategy for symtpmatic ureteral calculi in pregnancy. Urology 2002;60:383–387.

72. Bush WH, Brannen GE, Burnett LL, et al. Ultrasonic renal lithotripsy: single-stage percutaneous technique and adjuvant radiological procedures. Radiology 1984;152:387–390.

73. LeRoy AJ, May GR, Segura JW, et al. Percutaneous ultrasonic lithotripsy. Radiol Clin North Am 1984;22:427–432.

74. Lingeman JE, Smith LH, Woods JR, et al. Percutaneous procedures. In: Urinary Calculi: ESWL, Endourology, and Medical Therapy. Philadelphia: Lea & Febiger, 1989:322–359.

75. Feagins BA, Preminger GM. Options in stone management. In: Stein BS, ed. Clinical Urologic Practice. New York: Norton, 1995:523.

76. Mahaffey KG, Bolton DM, Stoller ML. Urologist-directed percutaneous nephrostomy tube placement. J Urol 1994;152:1973–1976.

77. Smith AD. Percutaneous punctures—is this the endourologist's turf? J Urol 1994;152:1982–1983.

78. Chien GW, Bellman GC. Blind percutaneous renal access. J Endourology 2002;16:93–95.

79. Pearle MS. Editorial comment. J Endourology 2002;16:96.

80. Ng CS, Herts BR, Streem SB. Percutaneous access to upper pole renal stones: role of prone 3-dimensional computerized tomography in inspiratory and expiratory phases. J Urol 2005;173: 124–126.

81. Narasimham DL, Jacobsson B, Vijayan P, et al. Percutaneous nephrolithotomy through an intercostal approach. Acta Radiol 1991;32:162–165.

82. Fuchs EF, Forsyth MJ. Supercostal approach for percutaneous ultrasonic lithotripsy. Urol Clin North Am 1990;17:99–102.

83. Wong C, Leveillee RJ. Single upper-pole percutaneous access for treatment of > or = 5-cm complex branched staghorn calculi: is shockwave lithotripsy necessary? J Endouro 2002:16:477–481.

84. Golijanin D, Katz R, Verstandig A, et al. The supracostal percutaneous nephrostomy for treatment of staghorn and complex kidney stones. J Endourol 1998;12:403–405.

85. Kekre NS, Gopalakrishnan GG, Gupta GG, et al. Supracostal approach in percutaneous nephrolithotomy: experience with 102 cases. J Endourol 2001;15:789–791.

86. Munver R, Delvecchio FC, Newman GE, et al. Critical analysis of supracostal access for percutaneous renal surgery. J Urol 2001;166: 1242–1246.

87. Hopper KD, Yakes WF. The posterior intercostal approach for percutaneous renal procedures: risk of puncturing the lung, spleen and liver as determined by CT. AJR Am J Roentgenol 1990;154: 115–117.

88. Gofrit ON, Shapiro A, Donchin Y, et al. Lateral decubitus position for percutaneous nephrolithotripsy in the morbidly obese or kyphotic patient. J Endourol 2002;16:383–386.

89. Shoma AM, Eraky I, El-Kenawy MR, et al. Percutaneous nephrolithotomy in the supine position: technical aspects and functional outcome compared with the prone position. Urology 2002;60:388–392.

90. Ng MT, Sun WH, Cheng CW, et al. Supine position is safe and effective for percutaneous nephrolithotomy. J Endourol 2004; 18:469–474.

91. Hosking DH. Retrograde nephrostomy: experience with two techniques. J Urol 1986;135:1146.

92. Hunter PT, Hawkins IF, Finlayson B, et al. Hawkins-Hunter retrograde transcutaneous nephrostomy: a new technique. Urology 1983;23:583–587.

93. LeRoy AJ, May GR, Segura JW, et al. Rapid dilatation of percutaneous nephrostomy tracks. AJR Am J Roentgenol 1984;142: 355–357.

94. Lang EK, Glorioso LW. Multiple percutaneous access routes to multiple calculi, calculi in caliceal diverticula, and staghorn calculi. Radiology 1986;158:211–214.

95. Mercado S, Hunter DW, Castañeda-Zuñiga WR. The double puncture: an effective percutaneous technique for removing complex, multiple renal calculi. Radiology 1986;158:207–209.

96. Regan JS, Shang Lam H, Lingeman JE. Simultaneous bilateral percutaneous nephrolithotomy. J Endourol 1992;6:245–247.

97. Maheshwari PN, Andankar M, Hegde S, et al. Bilateral single-session percutaneous nephrolithotomy: a feasible and safe treatment. J Endourol 2000;14:285–287.

98. Holman E, Salah MA, Coth C. Comparison of 150 simultaneous bilateral and 300 unilateral percutaneous nephrolithotomies. J Endourol 2002;16:33–36.

99. Limb J, Bellman GC. Tubeless percutaneous renal surgery: review of first 112 patients. Urology 2002;59:527.

100. Pietrow PK, Auge BK, Lallas CD, et al. Pain after percutaneous nephrolithotomy: impact of nephrostomy tube size. J Endourol 2003;17:411–414.

101. Desai MR, Kukreja RA, Desai MM, et al. A prospective randomized comparison of type of nephrostomy drainage following percutaneous nephrostolithotomy: large bore versus small bore versus tubeless. J Urol 2004;172:565–567.

102. Aghamir SMK, Hosseini SR, Gooran S. Totally tubeless percutaneous nephrolithotomy. J Endourol 2004;18:647–648.

103. Noller MW, Baughman SM, Morey AF, et al. Fibrin sealant enables tubeless percutaneous stone surgery. J Urol 2004;172:166–169.

104. Soler M, Greenstein A, Chen J, et al. Immediate closure of nephrostomy tube wounds using a tissue adhesive: a novel approach following percutaneous endourological procedures. J Urol 2003;169: 2034–2036.

105. Lee DI, Uribe C, Eichel L, et al. Sealing percutaneous nephrolithotomy traces with gelatin matriX hemostatic sealant: initial clinical use. J Urol 2004;171:571–578.

106. Jou YC, Cheng MC, Sheen JH, et al. Cauterization of access tract for nephrostomy tube-free percutaneous nephrolithotomy. J Endourol 2004;18:547–549.

107. Patterson DE, Segura JW, LeRoy AJ, et al. The etiology and treatment of delayed bleeding following percutaneous lithotripsy. J Urol 1985;133:447.

108. Stoller ML, Wolf JS, St Lezin MA. Estimated blood loss and transfusion rates associated with percutaneous nephrolithotomy. J Urol 1994;152:1977–1981.

109. Davidoff R, Bellman GC. Influence of technique of percutaneous tract creation on incidence of renal hemorrhage. J Urol 1997;157: 1229–1231.

110. Clayman RV, Surya V, Hunter D, et al. Renal vascular complications associated with the percutaneous removal of renal calculi. J Urol 1984;132:228.

111. Kernohan RM, Johnston LC, Donaldson RA. Bleeding following percutaneous nephrolithotomy resulting in loss of the kidney. Br J Urol 1990;65:657.

112. Kalash SS, Young JD Jr. Serious complications associated with percutaneous nephrolithotomy. Urology 1987;29:290.

113. Hopper KD, Sherman JL, Williams MD, et al. The variable anteroposterior position of the retroperitoneal colon to the kidneys. Invest Radiol 1987;22:298–302.

114. LeRoy AJ, Williams HJ, Bender CE, et al. Colon perforation following percutaneous nephrostomy and renal calculus removal. Radiology 1985;155:83–85.

115. Vallancien G, Capdeville R, Veillon B, et al. Colonic perforation during percutaneous nephrolithotomy: case report. J Urol 1985; 134:1185.

116. Rao PN, Dube AD, Weightman NC, et al. Prediction of septicemia following endourological manipulation for stones in the upper urinary tract. J Urol 1991;146:955–960.

117. Dogan HS, Sahin AS, Cetinkaya Y, et al. Antibiotic prophylaxis in percutaneous nephrolithotomy: prospective study in 81 patients. J Endourol 2002;16:649–653.

118. Evans CP, Stoller ML. The fate of the iatrogenic retroperitoneal stone. J Urol 1993;150:827–829.

119. Verstandig AG, Banner MP, VanArsdalen KN, et al. Upper urinary tract calculi: extrusion into perinephric and periureteric tissues during percutaneous management. Radiology 1986;158:215–218.

120. Sardina JI, Bolton DM, Stoller ML. Entrapped Malecot nephrostomy tube: etiology and management. J Urol 1995;153: 1882–1883.

121. Stewart LH, Kernohan RM, Loughbridge WG. Nephrostomy tubes resistant to removal. Br J Urol 1992;70:213.

122. Koolpe HA, Lord B. Eccentric nephroscopy for the incarcerated nephrostomy. Urol Radiol 1990;12:96.

123. Lingeman JE, Newman D, Mertz JHO, et al. Extracorporeal shock wave lithotripsy: the Methodist Hospital of Indiana experience. J Urol 1986;135:1134.

124. McCullough DL. Extracorporeal shock wave lithotripsy. In: Walsh PC, Retik AB, Stamey TA, et al, eds. Campbell's Urology. Philadelphia: Saunders, 1992:2157–2182.

125. Chaussy CG, Fuchs GJ. Extracorporeal shock wave lithotripsy (ESWL) for the treatment of upper urinary tract stones. In: Gillenwater JY, Grayhack JT, Howards ST, et al, eds. Adult and Pediatric Urology. Chicago: Year Book, 1987.

126. Lingeman JE. Editorial: Extracorporeal shock wave lithotripsy—what happened? J Urol 2003;169:63.

127. Lingeman JE. Stone treatments: current trends and future possibilities. J Urol 2004;172:1774.

128. Dhar N, Yost A, Streem SB. The incidence of and a multivariate analysis of risk factors associated with subcapsular hematoma formation following electromagnetic shock wave lithotripsy. J Urol 2004;17:495.

129. Wu CF, Shee JJ, Lin WY, et al. Comparison between extracorporeal shock wave lithotripsy and semirigid ureterorenoscope with holmium: YAG laser lithotripsy for treating large proximal ureteral stones. J Urol 2004;172:1899–1902.

130. Maheshwari PN, Oswal AT, Andankar M, et al. Is antegrade ureteroscopy better than retrograde ureteroscopy for impacted large upper ureteral calculi? J Endourology 1999;13:441.

131. Virgili G, Mearini E, Micali S, et al. Extracorporeal piezoelectric shockwave lithotripsy of ureteral stones: are second generation lithotripters obsolete? J Endourology 1999;13:543–547.

132. Clayman RV, McClennan BL, Garvin TJ, et al. An electromagnetic acoustic shock wave unit for extracorporeal lithotripsy. J Endourol 1989;3:307.

133. Riehle RA, Naslund EB, Fair W, et al. Impact of shock wave lithotripsy on upper urinary tract calculi. Urology 1986;28:261.

134. Riehle RA, Naslund EB. Patient management and results after ESWL. In: Riehle RA, Newman DM, eds. Principles of Extracorporeal Shock Wave Lithotripsy. New York: Churchill- Livingstone, 1989: 121.

135. Graff J, Pastor J, Funke PJ, et al. Extracorporeal shock wave lithotripsy for ureteral stones: a retrospective analysis of 417 cases. J Urol 1988;139:513.

136. Khaitan A, Gupta NP, Hemal AK, et al. Post-ESWL, clinically insignificant residual stones: reality or myth? Urology 2002;59: 20–24.

137. Segura JW. Role of percutaneous procedures in the management of renal calculi. Urol Clin North Am 1990;17:207.

138. Fine JK, Pak CYC, Preminger GM. Residual fragments following ESWL—the role of medical management. J Urol 1992;2:79.

139. Drach GW, Dretler S, Fair W, et al. Report of the United States cooperative study of extracorporeal shock wave lithotripsy. J Urol 1986;135:1127.

140. Pareek G, Armenakas NA, Fracchia JA. Hounsfield units on computerized tomography predict stone-free rates after extracorporeal shock wave lithotripsy. J Urol 2003;169:1679–1681.

141. Pareek G, Armenakas NA, Panagopoulos G, et al. Extracorporeal shock wave lithotripsy success based on body mass index and Hounsfield units. Urology 2004;65:33–36.

142. Christensen JG, McCullough DL, Cline WA Sr. Extracorporeal shock wave lithotripsy in hemophiliac patient. Urology 1989; 33:424.

143. Deliveliotis CH, Kostakopoulos A, Stavropoulos E, et al. Extracorporeal shock wave lithotripsy in 5 patients with aortic aneurysm. J Urol 1995;154:1671–1672.

144. Thomas R, Cherry R, Neal DW Jr. The use of extracorporeal shock wave lithotripsy in patients with aortic aneurysms. J Urol 1991; 146:409.

145. Abber JD, Langberg J, Mueller SC, et al. Cardiovascular pathology and extracorporeal shock wave lithotripsy. J Urol 1988;140:408.

146. Asroff SW, Kingston TE, Stein BS. Extracorporeal shock wave lithotripsy in patient with cardiac pacemaker in an abdominal location: case report and review of the literature. J Endourol 1993;7:189–192.

147. Drach GW, Weber C, Donovan JM. Treatment of pacemaker patients with extracorporeal shock wave lithotripsy: experience from 2 continents. J Urol 1990;143:895.

148. Zanetti G, Ostini F, Montanari E, et al. Cardiac dysrhythmias induced by extracorporeal shock wave lithotripsy. J Endourol 1999;13:409–412.

149. Petterson B, Tiselius HG, Anderson A, et al. Evaluation of extracorporeal shock wave lithotripsy without anesthesia using a Dornier HM3 lithotripster without technical modification. J Urol 1989;142:1189.

150. Sorensen C, Chandhoke P, Moore M, et al. Comparison of intravenous sedation versus general anesthesia on the efficacy of the Doli 50 lithotripter. J Urol 2002;168:35.

151. Assimos DG, Boyce WH, Gurr EG, et al. Selective elevation of urinary enzyme levels after extracorporeal shock wave lithotripsy. J Urol 1989;142:687.

152. Graber SF, Danuser H, Hochreiter WW, et al. A prospective randomized trial comparing 2 lithotriptors for stone disintegration and induced renal trauma. J Urol 2003;169:54–57.

153. Kaude JV, Williams CM, Millner MR, et al. Renal morphology and function immediately after extracorporeal shock wave lithotripsy. AJR Am J Roentgenol 1985;145:305.

154. Chaussy CG, Fuchs GJ. Extracorporeal shock wave lithotripsy. Monogr Urol 1987;4:80.

155. Krysiewicz S. Complications of renal extracorporeal shock wave lithotripsy reviewed. Urol Radiol 1992;13:139–145.

156. Papanicolaou N, Stafford SA, Pfister RC, et al. Significant renal hemorrhage following extracorporeal shock wave lithotripsy: imaging and clinical features. Radiology 1987;163:661–664.

157. Rubin JI, Arger PH, Pollack HM. Kidney changes after extracorporeal shock wave lithotripsy: CT evaluation. Radiology 1987;162:21.

158. Baumgartner BR, Dickey KW, Ambrose SS, et al. Kidney changes after extracorporeal shock wave lithotripsy: appearance on MR imaging. Radiology 1987;163:531.

159. Dyer RB, Karstaedt N, McCullough DL, et al. Magnetic resonance imaging evaluation of immediate and intermediate changes in kidneys treated with extracorporeal shock wave lithotripsy. J Lithotripsy Stone Dis 1990;2:302.

160. Knapp PM, Scott JW. Magnetic resonance imaging following extracorporeal shock wave lithotripsy with the Dornier HM3 lithotripter. J Urol 1987;132:287A.

161. Wilson WT, Miller G, Morris JS, et al. Morphologic renal changes following piezoelectric and spark gap lithotripsy. In: Lingeman JE, Newman DM, eds. Shock Wave Lithotripsy II: Urinary and Biliary. New York: Plenum, 1989.

162. Netto NR, Ikonomidis JA, Longo JA, et al. Small-bowel perforation after shock wave lithotripsy. J Endourol 2003;17:719–720.

163. Lingeman JE, Newman DM, Mosbaugh PG, et al. The risk of hypertension following various forms of treatment for urolithiasis. J Urol 1989;141:241A.

164. Sulaiman MN, Buchholz NP, Clark PB. The role of ureteral stent placement in the prevention of steinstrasse. J Endourol 1999;13: 151–155.

165. Banner MP. Extracorporeal shock wave lithotripsy: selection of patients and long-term complications. Radiol Clin North Am 1991;29:543–556.

166. Karamalegos AZ, Diokno AC, Moylan DF. Formation of perinephric abscess following extracorporeal shock wave lithotripsy. Urology 1989;34:277.

167. Orme R, Scott-Cook H, Farrar DJ. "Aneurysm" of nephrostomy catheter complicating extracorporeal shock wave lithotripsy. Clin Radiol 1999;54:408–410.

168. Lingeman JE, Shirrell WL, Newman DM, et al. Management of upper ureteral calculi with extracorporeal shock wave lithotripsy. J Urol 1987;138:720.

169. Fuchs GJ, Chaussy CG, Stenzl A. Current management concepts in the treatment of ureteral stones. J Endourol 1988;2:107.

170. Kahn RI. Endourological treatment of ureteral calculi. J Urol 1986;135:239–243.

171. Locke DR, Newman RC, Sternbock GS, et al. Extracorporeal shock wave lithotripsy in horseshoe kidneys. Urology 1990;35:407.

172. Jenkins AD, Gillenwater JY. Extracorporeal shock wave lithotripsy in the prone position: treatment of stones in the distal ureter or anomalous kidney. J Urol 1988;139:911.

173. Kramolowsky EV. Complications of ureteroscopy. Semin Urol 1989;7:39–42.

174. Kostakopoulos A, Sofras F, Karayiannis A, et al. Ureterolithotripsy: report of 1,000 cases. Br J Urol 1989;63:243.

175. Hendrikx AJ, Strijbos WE, de Knijff DW, et al. Treatment for extended mid- and distal ureteral stones: SWL or ureteroscopy? Results of a multicenter study. J Endourol 1999;13:727–733.

176. Lingeman JE, Smith LH, Woods JR, et al. Percutaneous procedures. In: Urinary Calculi: ESWL, Endourology, and Medical Therapy. Philadelphia: Lea & Febiger, 1989:198.

177. Dretler SP, Weinstein A. A modified algorithm for the management of ureteral calculi: 100 consecutive cases. J Urol 1988;140:732–736.

178. Barr JD, Tegtmeyer CJ, Jenkins AD. In situ lithotripsy of ureteral calculi: review of 261 cases. Radiology 1990;174:103–108.

179. Becht E, Mohl V, Neisius D, et al. Treatment of prevesical ureteral calculi by extracorporeal shock wave lithotripsy. J Urol 1988; 139:916.

180. Banner MP, Van Arsdalen KN, Pollack HM. Extracorporeal shock wave lithotripsy of ureteral calculi. Radiology 1990;174:12–14.

181. Durano AC, Hanosh JJ. A new alternative for entrapped stone basket in the distal ureter. J Urol 1988;139:116.

182. Flam TA, Brochard M, Zerbib M, et al. Extracorporeal shock wave lithotripsy to remove calcified ureteral stents. Urology 1990;36:164.

The Lower Genitourinary Tract

40

Flavio Castañeda, José M. Hernandez-Graulau

In recent years, the field of medicine has witnessed a proliferation of interventional radiologic techniques and procedures, largely because of impressive technological advances and the continuous search for simpler, less invasive, and less costly procedures. These advances have reduced costs and significantly decreased the morbidity and mortality rates associated with the surgical procedures used to treat various conditions.

This technologic revolution has affected the management of lower genitourinary tract disease. Many old therapeutic techniques have been replaced, improved, or combined with surgical techniques, resulting in better outcomes. The development of transrectal ultrasound is one of these major advances. In the late 1960s, the experimental work of Watanabe et al. (1) on the diagnostic application of transrectal ultrasound set the stage for the development of high-resolution axial and sagittal imaging of the prostate. This technology has produced significant advances in the early detection and staging of prostatic cancer because its high sensitivity allows for directed biopsies of abnormal or equivocal areas. Transrectal ultrasound has also helped in the imaging of and intervention in other perineal structures, such as the seminal vesicles, bladder, and rectum.

Balloon catheter technology has also progressed from the early Gruntzig design to the current designs that provide almost limitless accessibility. This technology has allowed for access to anterior urethral strictures that were previously impassable or inaccessible by either an antegrade or a retrograde approach. This therapeutic modality is less traumatic than the use of bougies, which are sometimes impossible to advance through the more severe strictures. Special large balloons with small profiles have been developed for prostatic urethroplasty, one of the nonsurgical treatments of benign prostatic hyperplasia (BPH) (2–6).

Metal stent technology, initially used intravascularly and later applied to almost all body systems, has also been applied to the genitourinary system. *Hyperthermia*, used initially for tumor shrinking and ablation, is now being tried in humans for BPH and carcinoma. *Hypothermia*, used for carcinoma, is yielding excellent preliminary results in the prostate. Because interventional radiologists either conceptualized or developed most of these advances, they have assumed an ever-increasing role in the management of lower urinary tract disease.

THE BLADDER

The bladder is the end point of almost all upper genitourinary interventions that drain or bypass upper collecting or ureteral obstructions. It also serves as a temporary reservoir for stones or other foreign bodies that cannot be removed through the nephrostomy tracts. However, there are very few specific indications for direct bladder access.

Interventional Procedures in the Bladder

Although voiding cystourethrograms (VCUGs) are performed most satisfactorily with the use of a urethral catheter in the vast majority of patients, the suprapubic route has been advocated as a way of avoiding ascending infection and for use in patients in whom transurethral catheterization is either difficult or contraindicated (7). This is exactly the same access used in a suprapubic cystostomy for temporary or permanent bladder drainage. Percutaneous puncture is made two to three fingerbreadths above the symphysis pubis in the midline after the area is infiltrated with a local anesthetic. To enter the bladder, a 19-gauge sheathed needle (such as the Amplatz needle, Becton-Dickinson Co.) is directed 10 degrees cranially to avoid damage to the bladder neck. Once the bladder has been entered, contrast material can be injected to fill the bladder to perform the VCUG, or a straight floppy-tip guide wire can be advanced and coiled in the bladder and a 10–12 French self-retaining pigtail catheter deployed over the guide wire after dilatation of the tract if a cystostomy catheter is needed. To prevent urine leakage, taut tension is placed on the catheter until the tract matures. If longer catheters are needed, Councill catheters of the desired caliber can be placed either through peel-away sheaths or using the Councill stiffening rods.

THE URETHRA

The Male Urethra

The male urethra is a fibroelastic structure that extends from the internal urethral orifice at the vesical neck to the external urethral meatus at the tip of the glans penis. It is divided by the urogenital diaphragm into three parts: prostatic, membranous, and penile (Figure 40–1). The prostatic urethra is the widest and is about 3 cm long in normal adults. The lumen of the urethra is distensible but normally is obliterated by elastic fibers that cause apposition of its anterior and posterior walls. In prostatic lateral lobe hyperplasia, the urethral wall is changed into a wide anteroposterior fissure by encroachment of the enlarged lateral lobes on the urethra.

The urethral crest extends along the posterior floor of the urethra from its origin on the vesical trigone to its bifurcated end. The prostatic sinus is a depressed fossa on each side of the crest and has many orifices from prostatic ducts. The seminal colliculus or verumontanum is the greatest prominence of the urethral crest, and the prostatic utricle opens in its central surface. The finer, slitlike orifices of the ejaculatory ducts open beside the prostatic utricle.

The membranous urethra is the shortest, about 1.5 cm long, and passes through the urogenital diaphragm between its superior and inferior layers of fascia. This part of the urethra has no proper surrounding tissue but contains the circular fibers of the deep transverse perineal muscle, called the external urethral sphincter. This is a voluntary muscle controlled by the perineal branch of the internal pudendal nerve.

Behind the membranous urethra, close to the inferior layer of the urogenital diaphragm, lie the bulbourethral glands of Cowper, which open into the penile urethra at its bulbous part on each side.

The penile urethra is the longest segment and is surrounded by the spongy body. It is about 15 cm long when the penis is flaccid and has a right-angled curve at the penoscrotal junction. The bulbous urethra is dilated and forms the perineal curve. Openings of the bulbourethral glands of Cowper lie at its posterior wall. On the floor of the penile urethra are numerous small lacunae and mucosal glands, known as the glands of Littre. The external meatus is the narrowest part of the urethra. The preterminal urethra, next to the meatus, has a dilated lumen known as the fossa navicularis. The function of the fossa navicularis may be to convert the energy of the narrow, but faster, urinary stream in the distal urethra into a slower stream, but with higher pressure. The result is increased velocity as the stream passes through the narrow meatus; the increased velocity provides a jet for directing the stream to prevent self-contamination. The arterial supply to the urethra is derived from branches of the internal pudendal and inferior vesical arteries. Veins drain into the pudendal and perivesical plexuses. Lymphatic drainage is to the inguinal nodes and lymphatic glands along the iliac vessels.

The membranous urethra is involved in urinary incontinence and control of ejaculation of semen. The remainder of the urethra serves two different functions: one is to allow the free passage of urine during urination, and the other is to assist the expulsion of the semen during ejaculation. The glands of Littre are responsible for lubricating the urethra before ejaculation.

The male urethra can be visualized readily either by retrograde urethrography (RUG) studies or by voiding films. The delineation of its three main segments usually can be easily made radiographically (Figure 40–2).

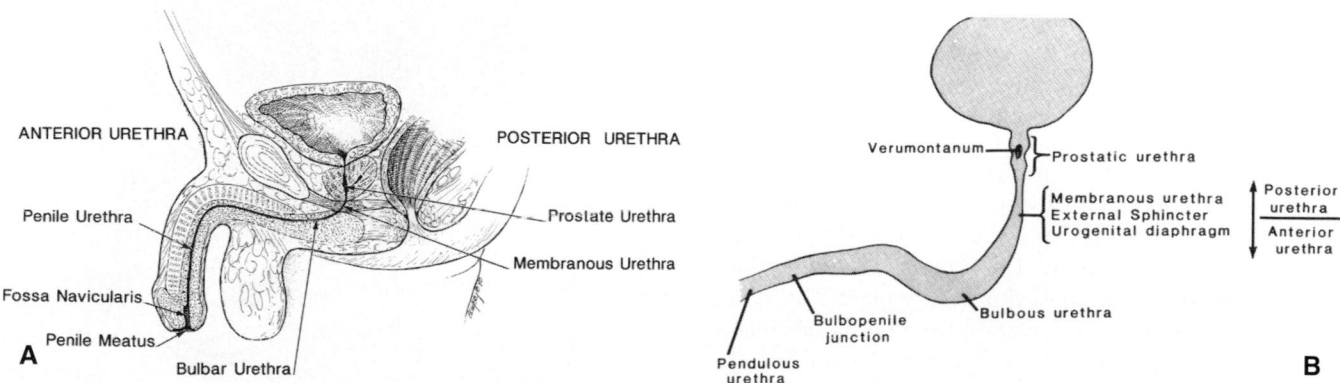

Figure 40–1 Schematic representation of the male lower genitourinary tract **A.** showing its relationships with the pelvic organs and structures and **B.** showing in more detail the different structures and portions of the urethra and bladder.

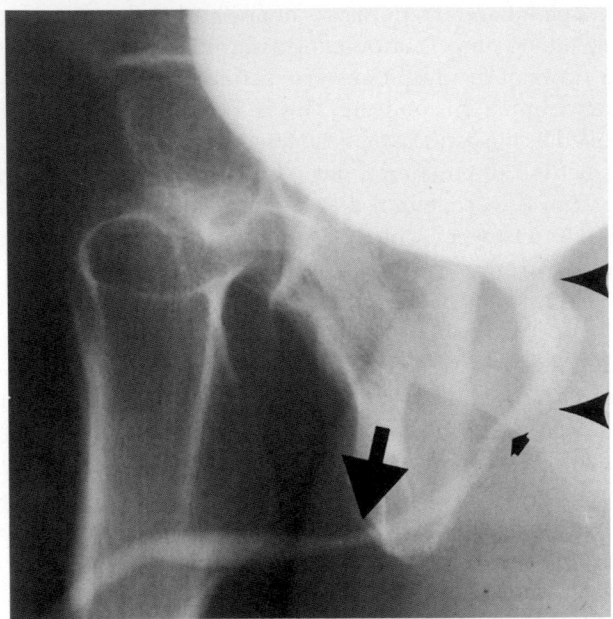

Figure 40–2   Normal voiding cystourethrogram in a male patient showing the appearance of the prostatic urethra (*arrowheads*); the location of the membranous urethra, which corresponds with the location of the external sphincter or urogenital diaphragm (*small arrow*); and, finally, the anterior or pendulous urethra (*large arrow*).

The Female Urethra

The female urethra is approximately 4–5 cm long and begins at the internal urethral orifice or vesical neck. It follows a slightly curved course downward and forward and terminates at the external urethral meatus on the roof of the vestibule.

The epithelium of the female urethra is squamous in its distal portion and transitional in its proximal segment. Numerous periurethral glands are embedded in the submucosal layer; the largest are the glands of Skene, which open just inside the meatus.

The longitudinal smooth muscle layer of the bladder neck is prolonged to encase the urethra, but at the portion that pierces the urogenital diaphragm, it is surrounded by striated sphincter muscle, as in the man. The urethra also passes through the levator ani muscle before traversing the diaphragm and is supported by bulbocavernous muscle under the diaphragm.

Because the female urethra is short and its diameter is only 6 mm, care must be taken not to damage the urethral wall in operative or interventional procedures. (The female urethra represents the entire sphyncteric mechanism for the bladder.) A distinct sphincter action is not always demonstrable in a woman. The female urethra is much more readily dilatable than that of the male. The entire female urethra receives innervation from both divisions of the autonomic nervous system and from the somatic system. Parasympathetic cholinergic nerve endings, as well as adrenergic nerve endings, especially alpha-adrenergic, are found throughout the entire length of the urethra. Somatic

fibers coming from the pudendal nerve supply the striated external sphincter in both sexes.

The radiographic anatomy of a normal female urethra is well visualized during a VCUG. Radiographically, the female urethra is a uniform, smooth, wide, tubular structure with gentle ventral curvature, adequate lumen throughout, and relative narrowing right at the meatus.

Urethral Strictures

A urethral stricture is a scar that is usually the result of tissue injury caused by urethral trauma, pelvic fracture, inflammatory disease, or neoplasia. As this scar heals, it contracts and creates fibrotic narrowing composed of dense collagen and fibroblasts. Fibrosis usually extends into the surrounding corpus spongiosum, causing spongiofibrosis. Urethral strictures can be congenital, traumatic, inflammatory, or neoplastic.

Congenital Strictures

Congenital lesions are found most commonly at the external urethral meatus, often associated with hypospadias orifices (8), but the membranous urethra and the penoscrotal junction frequently are involved. They are seen in both sexes but are more common in men.

Traumatic Strictures

Traumatic lesions are the result of tears or ruptures of the urethra caused by blows to the perineum or by pelvic fracture, or they are iatrogenic. They can occur anywhere in the anterior or the membranous urethra, but they probably are most common in the bulbomembranous portion (Figure 40–3). Chemical strictures, which are considered to be traumatic,

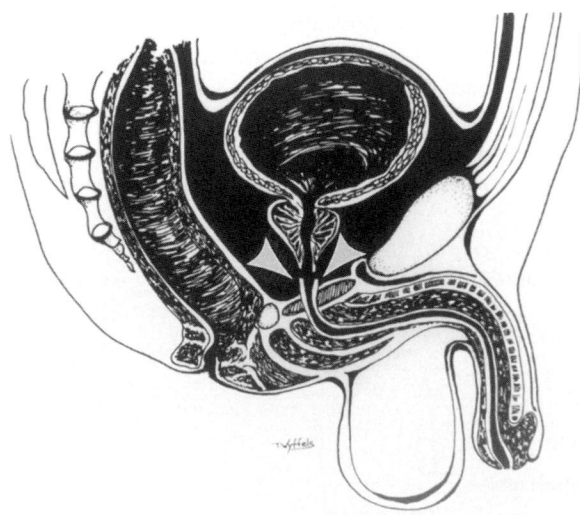

Figure 40–3   After bulbomembranous urethral ruptures (*arrowheads*), blood and urine tend to collect extraperitoneally, displacing and elevating contiguous structures.

usually occur in the anterior urethra. Iatrogenic strictures are a common form of traumatic stricture of the urethra in children and adults, secondary to instrumentation. Traumatic strictures usually develop much more rapidly than inflammatory strictures. They also tend to be dense and longer because of more ischemic necrosis.

Inflammatory Strictures

Inflammatory strictures may be caused by gonorrhea, tuberculosis, syphilis, or nonspecific infections. Although gonococcal urethritis is seldom a cause of stricture, infection remains a major cause, particularly infection from long-term use of indwelling urethral catheters. Large catheters and instruments are more likely than small ones to cause ischemia and internal trauma. Approximately 75% of inflammatory strictures occur at the bulbomembranous junction. The strictures caused by infection tend to be more diaphragmlike and short. Tuberculosis is spread from another focus, usually higher up in the urinary tract and most likely from the prostate. The urethra appears to be particularly resistant to tuberculous infection, but when these strictures occur, they are intractable and often associated with fistula formation and abscesses.

Neoplastic Strictures

Neoplastic strictures are the result of primary urethral carcinoma or are secondary from the bladder or the prostate. They may occur at any place in the urethra but are most common in the bulbomembranous area. Recurrent stricture disease of the urethra, even in the absence of hematuria, demands periodic RUG to rule out the possibility of a clinically occult urethral cancer. Transitional cell carcinoma of the urethra may be associated with a bladder cancer. This possibility must be ruled out before the urethral lesion is addressed.

Signs and Symptoms

The patient with urethral stricture usually has symptoms of bladder outlet obstruction, which are described in detail later, in the discussion of BPH. Gross observation of the urinary stream may reveal a decrease in the usual force and caliber, as well as multiple streams. Obstruction from BPH may coexist with a previously undiagnosed stricture, and the effect may be additive. Stricture occasionally may be suggested by a careful palpation of the urethra. Induration may be present, more so with posttraumatic stricture than with strictures from instrumentation or gonococcal urethritis.

Radiologic Findings

VCUGs best demonstrate dilatation behind a stricture, but RUGs best demonstrate the stricture itself. Although strictures may be diagnosed by the insertion of a cystoscope into the urethra, important information, such as length, caliber, location, and multiplicity, cannot be obtained without the use of urethrograms.

Strictures of the urethra appear as narrowed segments, which can vary in length and appearance from valvelike structures to long constrictions. Approximately 10% are multiple. The congenital type is single, usually short, and regular in appearance. The inflammatory stricture may be single or, more commonly, multiple; it may be short or long. It usually appears more irregular than either the congenital or traumatic stricture. The traumatic stricture can be single or multiple but is more commonly single. It may be long or short and is usually smooth. Neoplastic strictures are irregular and long and tend to occur with fistulous formation.

Complications

The most common complication of urethral stricture is significant lower urinary tract obstruction. Over time, the obstruction leads to characteristic changes in the bladder and upper urinary tract. These changes may be observed cystoscopically as well as radiologically. Bladder trabeculation or hypertrophy of the detrusor muscle causes the individual muscle fascicles to become prominent beneath the vesical mucosa. The interureteric ridge (Bell muscle) also participates in this process of hypertrophy, as does the bladder neck. Hypertrophy of the vesical neck causes an acute angulation between the trigone and the prostatic urethra.

Cellule formation can also be a complication of long-standing stricture disease. Extreme degrees of trabeculation allow the vesical mucosa to be pushed between the muscle fibers of the bladder wall, forming small pockets called *cellules.*

Diverticulum formation or herniation of the vesical mucosa through the detrusor muscle constitutes a bladder diverticulum. Acquired bladder diverticula contain no muscular components and are, therefore, prone to poor emptying, even if the bladder is emptied by catheterization. Because of a stasis of urine within the diverticula, they are likely to harbor infection, stones, and urothelium cancer. A diverticulum near the ureteric orifice (Hutch diverticulum) may cause vesicoureteral reflux.

Bladder calculi form most commonly as a result of outflow obstruction, residual urine, stasis, and infection. The presence of a bladder calculus is strong evidence of a long-standing bladder outflow obstruction. The most common mineral constituent of these stones in developed countries is calcium oxalate.

Patients with urethral strictures frequently accumulate residual urine. The integrity of the upper urinary tract may be jeopardized by the lower tract obstruction. With hypertrophy and thickening of the detrusor muscle, increased work is required to transport the urinary bolus from the ureter into the bladder. This process results in ureteral muscle hypertrophy, which is analogous to bladder hypertrophy. In the early stages, the condition appears, radiologically, as a mild dilatation of the distal segment, elongation, and some tortuosity of the ureter. Later, there is more marked dilatation of the entire ureter, attenuation of the ureteral wall, and marked tortuosity.

Periurethral abscess is closely related in its development to that of urinary extravasation. Periurethral abscess may cause multiple urethrocutaneous fistulas in the perineum, buttocks, and thighs.

Role of Interventional Radiology in Urethral Lesions

The urethra offers such easy access for direct endoscopic procedures that interventional radiology has only a limited role in managing lower urinary tract problems; however, such a limited role can be lifesaving on many occasions. For example, when cystoscopy is not possible because of urethral stricture, bladder contracture, malformation of the urethra, or trauma-related changes, interventional radiology may offer an alternative form of treatment. Interventional radiology of the urethra depends on gaining access by percutaneous catheter or needle and on monitoring the events by fluoroscopy, ultrasonography, or computed tomography (CT).

As mentioned above, radiologic assistance is seldom required in performing a simple transurethral catheterization; however, with a stricture or urethral trauma, when the urethral continuity has been violated, major developmental abnormalities are present, or multiple urethral false passages are present, RUG may give useful information before catheterization.

Cases of urethral trauma or disruption can be treated atraumatically by using a coaxial catheter-guide wire system under fluoroscopy after administering local anesthesia (1% lidocaine jelly; Uro-Jet, IMS Ltd.). When the transurethral route is not accessible, a transvesical approach provides good access for various interventional procedures. Percutaneous puncture is made two to three fingerbreadths above the symphysis pubis in the midline, after the area is infiltrated with a local anesthetic. To enter the bladder, a 19-gauge sheathed needle (such as the Amplatz needle) is directed 10 degrees cranially to avoid damage to the bladder neck. After the bladder has been entered, a straight floppy-tip guide wire can be advanced and coiled in the bladder. A 5–7 French curved catheter (Headhunter, hockey stick, or cobra curve) with good torque properties can then be advanced over the guide wire into the bladder for directing the guide wire into the bladder neck and subsequently into the urethra. Even with complete, hard obstructions, this can be performed without much difficulty, especially with the new hydrophilic guide wires. After the wire is out of the urethral meatus, a Councill catheter can be placed over this through-and-through wire for restoration of urethral continuity in cases of urethral trauma or disruption. This wire can provide an easy access for placing balloons to dilate difficult urethral strictures.

Balloon Dilatation of Strictures

The method used most commonly by urologists for treating urethral strictures is dilatation using different calibrated sounds. This method, although acceptable in many situations, has certain disadvantages, one of which is that the patients have to be treated at regular intervals over many years. Dilatation is a blind technique and may result in urethral trauma with formation of false passages. Also, besides the obvious discomfort, infection may complicate its course. Therefore, dilatation of urethral strictures is not usually curative, but it fractures the scar tissue of the stricture and temporarily enlarges the lumen. Dilatation of the urethra must be a process of gradual stretching because forceful disruption of this stricture area will lead to further scarring and subsequent worsening of the situation. It is not advisable to dilate a urethral stricture beyond 30 French or 10 mm in a male patient. Rather, the patient should be asked to return at weekly intervals. If dilatation is going to be an acceptable modality, the eventual interval between each visit should be 6–12 months.

Balloon dilatation has several theoretical advantages related to the radial forces of dilatation by the balloon catheter. In theory, these forces should produce less tissue trauma and scarring and fewer complications (such as urethral and periurethral perforations and false passages) compared with the longitudinal shearing forces applied by bouginage.

A baseline RUG or VCUG is performed to assess the exact location and extent of the stricture. Under fluoroscopic guidance, a guide wire is advanced through the urethra into the bladder. If the stricture is tight, angiographic techniques using different catheters and guide wires are usually successful in most cases. Once the stricture is traversed with the guide wire, and after the correct balloon has been chosen (balloons not exceeding 8–10 mm in diameter with the smallest profile possible and of adequate length), dilatation is carried out until the initial balloon waist disappears. Prolonged dilatations are avoided to prevent further ischemic damage to the urothelium and adjacent tissues. All manipulations should be performed with abundant lubricating jelly or viscous lidocaine to minimize trauma.

Preliminary results are encouraging (9,10), but reports of long-term follow-ups are lacking. Unfortunately, the consensus is that repeated dilatations are required to maintain adequate flows. However, this technique is useful, especially in tight or impassable strictures that can be converted to traversable lesions (11,12). These lesions may then be candidates for internal urethrotomy, which produces better long-term results. Bleeding and pain are the major problems caused by bougie or sound dilatation, as well as perforation of the urethral wall and creation of false passages, which are avoided by balloon dilatation.

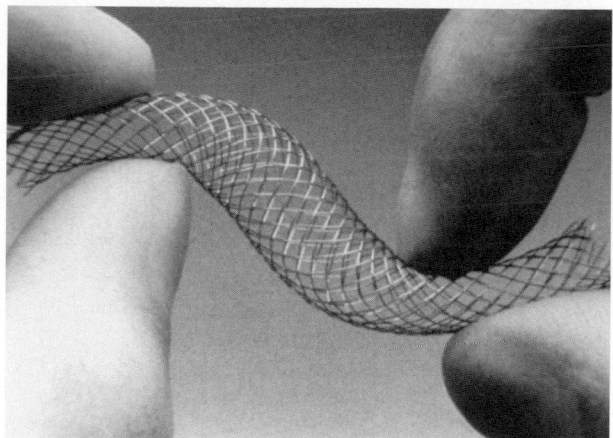

Figure 40–4 The Wallstent is a highly flexible, self-expanding metallic stent that accommodates well to the ureteral contours and has sufficient strength to keep the urethral lumen patent without causing significant discomfort.

Urethral Stents

As described above, the treatment for urethral strictures, either by surgery or by dilatation, is still far from ideal. Recurrences, difficulty in performing the urethroplasty procedures and the specialized surgical skills required, morbidity rates of the procedures, and difficult management have hampered the success of such procedures.

The search for new techniques in the treatment of this common problem is ongoing. Recent technical developments in metallic stent technology, initially developed for intravascular (13–15) and biliary (16,17) use, have precipitated its use in the urinary system for the treatment of urethral strictures (18).

The metallic stent most commonly used for this purpose is the Wallstent (Medinvent S.A.) (18), which is a self-expandable, stainless steel, woven wire tube that can be manufactured to different diameters and lengths (Figure 40–4). The stent comes loaded on a small-diameter (7 French) delivery catheter (Figure 40–5) and is constrained in its compressed form by a coaxial restraining sleeve that is pulled back while the delivery catheter is held in place across the area of the stricture (Figure 40–6). As the stent is being deployed, it expands to fit the luminal diameter, and because of the elastic properties of the mesh, it will hold against the wall of the urethra and thus will not migrate or dislodge.

It is of crucial importance to measure the desired caliber and length of the area to be stented to select the most appropriate stent. It should be noted that the deployed length of the stent is shorter than when it is loaded in its collapsed state. Long strictures can be bridged by several stents placed in tandem.

Technique

After the urethra has been catheterized and a guide wire has been placed in the bladder, the site of the stricture is

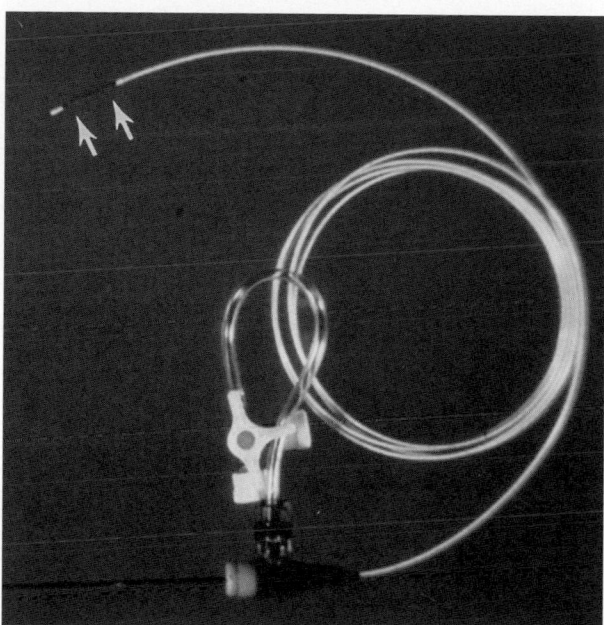

Figure 40–5 The 7 French delivery catheter and introduction system that allows an almost atraumatic placement. The arrows show the location of the compressed and restrained stent before deployment.

dilated to diameters of as much as 10 mm with complete resolution of the balloon waist, and the balloon catheter is removed. Assurance is made that the site of the stricture is well marked, and the guide wire is left in place. Over the guide wire, the stent delivery system is advanced to the desired location, taking into consideration the shortening of the stent that will occur after deployment. Once in position,

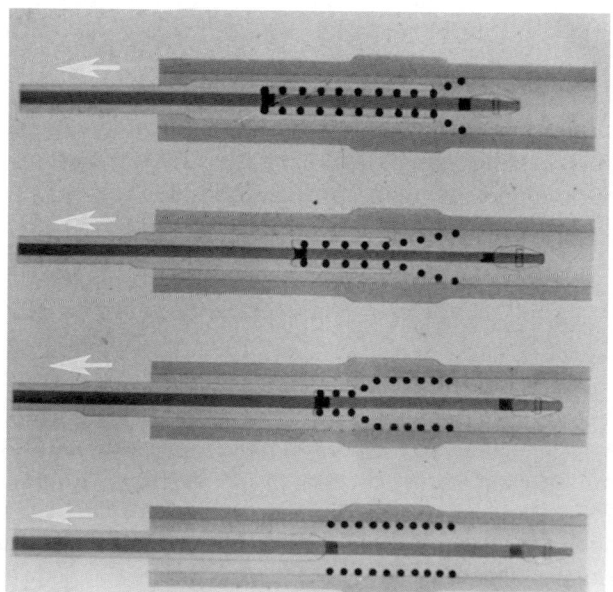

Figure 40–6 As the restraining catheter is pulled back (*arrows*) while the inner coaxial delivery catheter is held in place across the desired location, the stent is deployed, and the self-expanding device conforms to the diameter and shape of the urethra.

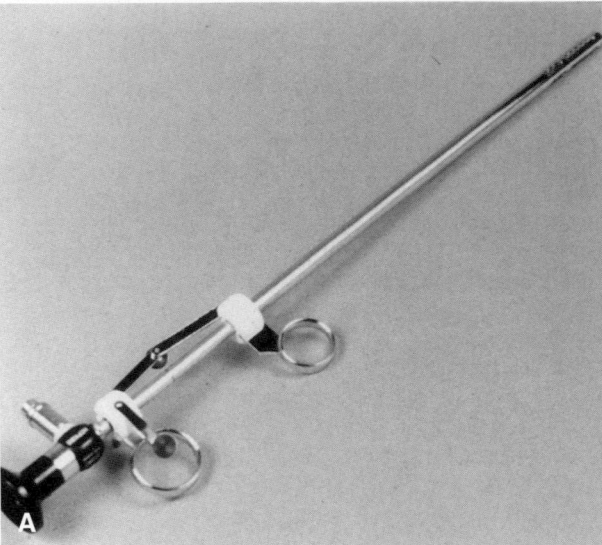
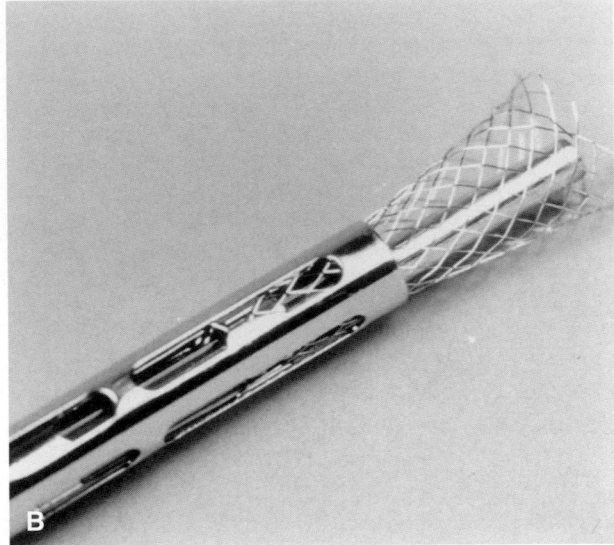

Figure 40–7   A. This endoscopic delivery tool, developed specifically for the urologist, has a 24 French diameter and incorporates some of the features of the urologic endoscopic tools. **B.** Close-up view of the distal end, with the stent partially deployed, shows its mechanism of action in better detail.

the delivery catheter is held securely in position, and the restraining catheter is then slowly pulled back to allow adequate delivery and expansion until the stent is fully deployed. If more stents are required, the same procedure is repeated until the entire length of the stricture is covered. There should be a slight overlap between the stents at the ends to avoid restenosis in these areas.

All patients are covered prophylactically with broad-spectrum antibiotics for about a week, starting the day of the procedure. There is no need to leave indwelling draining catheters either transurethrally or suprapubically because all patients are able to empty the bladder. The patient, relatives, and medical personnel are instructed to avoid retrograde catheterization in the immediate post-stenting period because it may cause dislodgment. If such catheterization becomes necessary, caution should be exercised; preferably, the procedure should be performed under fluoroscopic guidance using angiographic catheterization technique. Patients are also advised to avoid sexual intercourse for 1 month after stent placement.

A device has been developed (Figure 40–7) for cystoscopic stent placement. However, excessive bleeding after stricture dilatation may preclude successful cystoscopic operation. This does not occur when fluoroscopy is used because a guide wire is always in the lumen and the stricture location is always known from previous radiologic localization. Also, when fluoroscopy is used, the deployment systems are much smaller (7 French) than the systems specifically designed for the cystoscope (24 French). Another advantage of the small delivery system is that, when several stents are necessary, it is easier to move in and out of previously placed stents with less risk of migration or dislodgment.

Results

In all the reported cases (18), the procedure has been successful and free from complications for as long as 2 years without evidence of recurrence. The general trend has been significant improvement in the obstruction and urine flow without alteration of sexual function or ejaculation. The stents have been covered completely and incorporated by urothelium in 4–6 months. This result seems to prevent the infection and incrustations seen with other types of stents placed in the urinary system.

The most common complaint has been transient discomfort at the site of the stent, which usually resolves in 2–3 weeks. In a few patients, mild postmicturation dribbling has also been noted, and this resolves after the stent is completely covered with urothelium.

THE PROSTATE

Surgical Anatomy

The prostate is a chestnut-shaped, multilobular, glandular, fibromuscular organ that surrounds the first part of the urethra between the bladder neck and the urogenital diaphragm, or external sphincter. It is traversed throughout its length by the posterior urethra and is fixed to the pelvic floor by investments of the parietal and endopelvic fascia. Two dense condensations of the endopelvic fascia, which affixes the prostate to the pubis, are the puboprostatic ligaments. Anteriorly, the prostate is separated from the symphysis pubis by the extraperitoneal, prevesical (retropubic) space of Retzius. The prostatic venous plexus and the puboprostatic ligaments are found in this space. Posteriorly, the prostate is separated from the rectum by Denonvilliers fascia, which represents the connective tissue remaining from the obliterated peritoneal cul-de-sac between the rectum and the prostate. The prostate is covered by a firm, fibrous capsule.

Traditionally, the prostate is divided into five lobes: anterior, posterior, median, and two lateral lobes. The lateral lobes constitute the major portion of the gland. These lobes are a frequent site of benign adenomas. The posterior aspect of the prostate is traversed by the terminal portions of the vas deferens, which exit in the ejaculatory ducts and the posterior urethra. The posterior urethra, which traverses the prostate, houses a small mound on the dorsal aspect, termed the *verumontanum*. This part of the prostate is readily palpable by digital rectal examination and is a frequent site of cancer of the prostate. In the middle portion of the verumontanum is a small pit called the *utricle*. The ejaculatory ducts exit on the verumontanum. The middle lobe lies between the urethra and the ejaculatory ducts and is intermittently related to the vesical neck. Because of this anatomic relationship, even small adenomas in this lobe may obstruct the vesical outlet. The anterior lobe of the prostate is formed by approximately 13 tubules that grow out from the anterior wall of the prostatic urethra. After first becoming large and multibranched, these tubules decrease in both size and number; at birth, more than two are rarely present. Usually it is impossible to identify the anterior lobe in the gland of the adult, but occasionally it persists.

The blood supply of the prostate is primarily derived from the prostatic artery, which is derived from the inferior vesical artery. There are two main groups of arteries: a capsular group and a urethral group. Some accessory vessels to the prostate are supplied by the middle, hemorrhoidal, and internal pudendal arteries. The venous drainage of the prostate is through a prostatic plexus that joins the venous drainage of the penis in Santorini plexus and then drains into the hypogastric veins. It is important to note that the prostatic plexus connects with the prevertebral veins, also called *Batson plexus.*

The innervation of the prostate is through sympathetic fibers from L1 and L2 and from the third and fourth sacral nerves through the sacral plexus.

Prostatic lymphatics egress via vesical, hypogastric, external iliac, and sacral lymph nodes.

Zonal Anatomy

As described above, traditional concepts of prostate anatomy emphasized the lobar nature of the gland. More recently, extensive histopathologic studies have led to a description of anatomic zones of the prostate, each with a distinct histologic character (19–22).

The pioneering work of McNeal (19) and others (20–22) on the histology of the prostate has led to the concept of four major categories of tissue within the gland: the periurethral, the transitional (or preprostatic), the fibromuscular, and the

acinar glandular regions (Figure 40–8). The periurethral zone is a small region referred to by some as the *internal gland* and is composed of glands that line the urethra from the bladder neck to the verumontanum. The transitional, or preprostatic, zone is histologically similar to the glandular peripheral zone. It is typically small, situated between the anterior fibromuscular zone and the peripheral zone, and related to the preprostatic sphincter above the verumontanum. The anterior fibromuscular tissue is located anterior to the urethra along the entire craniocaudad extent of the gland. It is least prominent at the prostatic apex and widens maximally at the level of the midprostate. It has both smooth and striated muscle components.

The central glandular region lies posterior to the urethra and is broadest at the base of the gland, tapering toward the apex. It is through this region that the ejaculatory ducts course obliquely downward and anteriorly into the verumontanum in the prostatic urethra. However, the predominant glandular region in the normal prostate is the peripheral zone, which comprises approximately 75% of the acinar tissue of the prostate. It is situated primarily posterolaterally but also extends anterolaterally, especially in the more cranial aspects of the gland. The peripheral zone is somewhat funnel shaped and surrounds the central glandular tissue. It is the tissue that composes most of the prostatic apex.

The seminal vesicles are paired, saccular, elliptical organs that lie immediately cephalad to the prostate. The ejaculatory ducts join with the ampullae of the vas deferens to course through the central glandular region of the prostate to the verumontanum.

The normal anatomic regions of the prostate can be defined to a variable degree by sophisticated high-resolution imaging modalities. Axial and longitudinal transrectal sonography is capable of defining some zonal anatomy of the normal prostate (Figure 40–9) (23). The periurethral region is characterized by a slightly hypoechoic region surrounding the curvilinearly coursing urethra. The tissue of the central and peripheral glandular zones produces a medium level of echogenicity, with the two areas often not

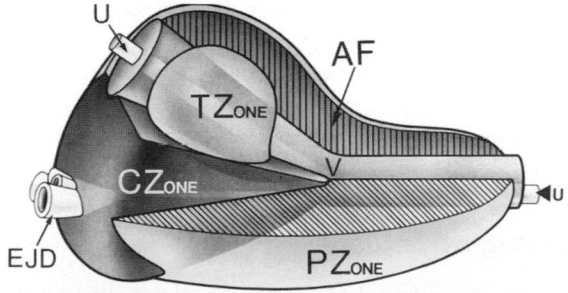

Figure 40–8   Three-dimensional schematic representation of the prostate gland with its different tissue characteristics as well as the structures coursing through its parenchyma. *AF,* anterior fibromuscular region; *C Zone,* central zone; *EJD,* ejaculatory ducts; *P Zone,* peripheral zone; *T Zone,* transitional zone; *U,* urethra.

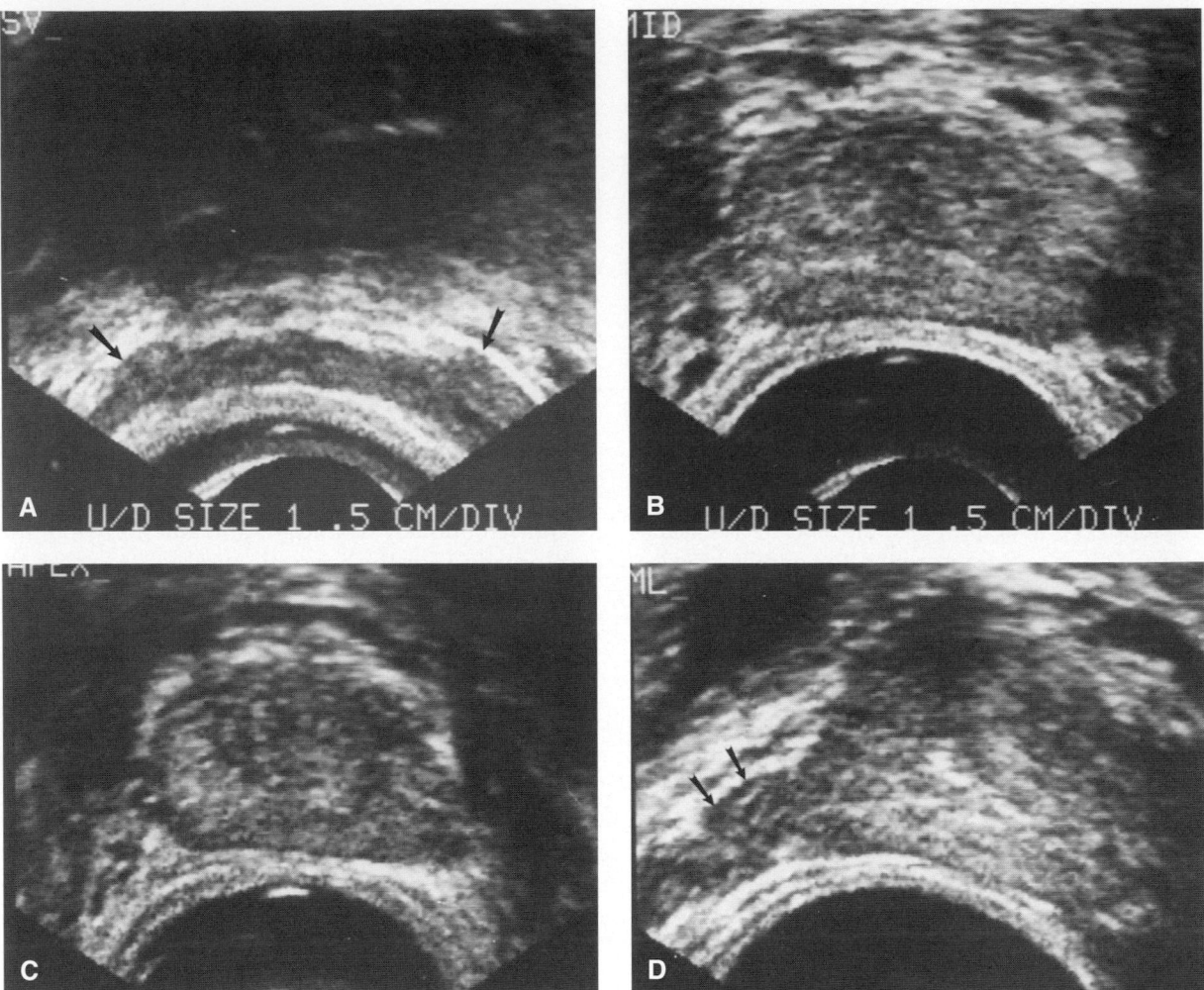

Figure 40–9   Normal anatomy of the prostate gland, shown by transrectal ultrasound using a 7.0-MHz probe. **A.** Transverse view of the seminal vesicles (*arrows*). **B.** Transverse view of midprostate showing more central and peripheral zones. **C.** Transverse view at apex also showing the peripheral zone distant from the other anatomic zones of the prostate. **D.** Longitudinal view of the right side of the prostate at the right seminal vesicle (*arrows*).

sonographically distinct. Distinction between the central regions and the peripheral acinar regions can also occasionally be made by CT. More recently, magnetic resonance imaging (MRI) with high field strengths and T_2-weighted sequences has shown improved capabilities for defining zonal prostate anatomy (Figure 40–10) (24–27). The lower signal intensity of the anterior fibromuscular region can be differentiated easily from the intermediate intensity of the central glandular region and the higher intensity of the peripheral zone.

Pathologic Anatomy

The zonal anatomy of the prostate relates directly to the pathologic processes that affect the gland (22). Histopathologic studies reveal that malignancy and inflammation principally involve the peripheral glandular zone (22). It is thought that 80% of prostate cancer arises in

the peripheral zone (Figure 40–11). However, this figure also implies that a small proportion of prostate cancer does originate in more central regions, the transitional zone and the central glandular zone. Prostatitis is also principally a process of the peripheral zone (22); however, with severe infections of the gland, inflammation extends throughout the prostate, making differentiation of the various regions by sonography difficult.

BPH primarily affects the transitional and, to a lesser extent, the periurethral zones of the gland (Figure 40–12) (22). In extreme cases, the massive enlargement of these regions compresses the central glandular tissue and displaces it posteriorly.

As described above, different disease processes selectively affect different regions of the prostate. New high-resolution imaging techniques provide noninvasive means of understanding both the normal prostate and the pathologic processes that affect it.

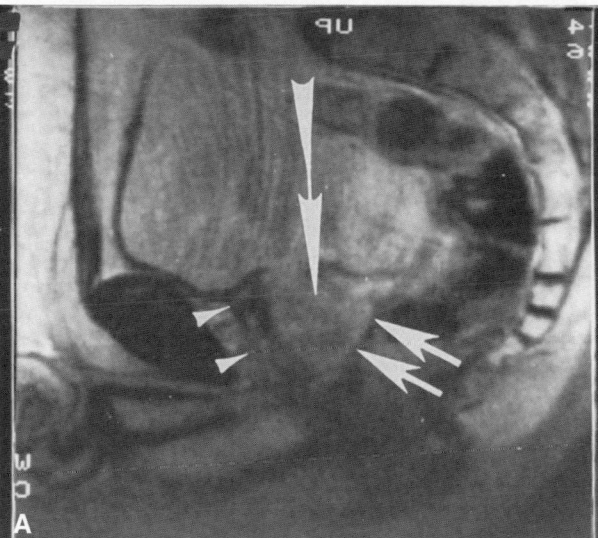
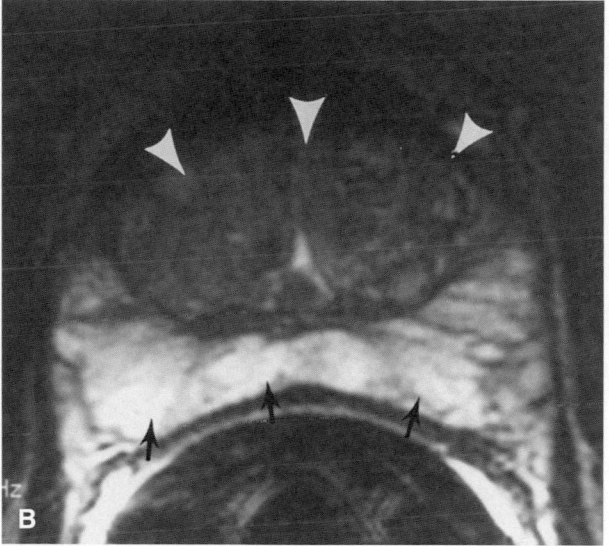

Figure 40–10   **A.** T$_2$-weighted image of the prostate performed with a pelvic multicoil array showing the different signal intensities of the different regions. The anterior fibromuscular zone (*arrowheads*) has a lower intensity than the peripheral zone (*short arrows*). The central, more adenomatous region (*long arrow*) is characterized by a more inhomogeneous midrange intensity. **B.** Transverse T$_2$-weighted image of the prostate performed with a high-resolution endorectal coil. The peripheral zone is hyperintense (*arrows*). The central gland appears hypointense with some areas of increased signal (*arrowheads*).

Examination of the Prostate

Examination of the prostate is best performed with the patient standing, bent over the examining table or bed, and supported on his elbows. An alternative and less desirable position is the lateral decubitus position, with one leg drawn up toward the abdomen. The examiner's gloved, generously lubricated index finger is inserted slowly into the rectum. The purpose of the prostatic examination is to gain information regarding prostatic size, symmetry, consistency, and motility; to assess anal tone; and to determine the presence of rectal masses. A lax anal sphincter that the patient cannot contract may indicate peripheral neuropathy.

The average prostate is about 4 cm in length and width. It is widest superiorly, at the bladder neck. As the gland enlarges, the lateral sulci become relatively deeper, and the median furrow becomes obliterated. The prostate may also elongate.

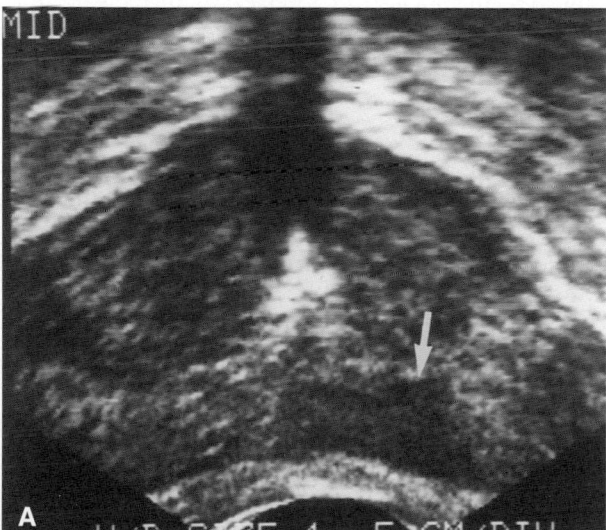
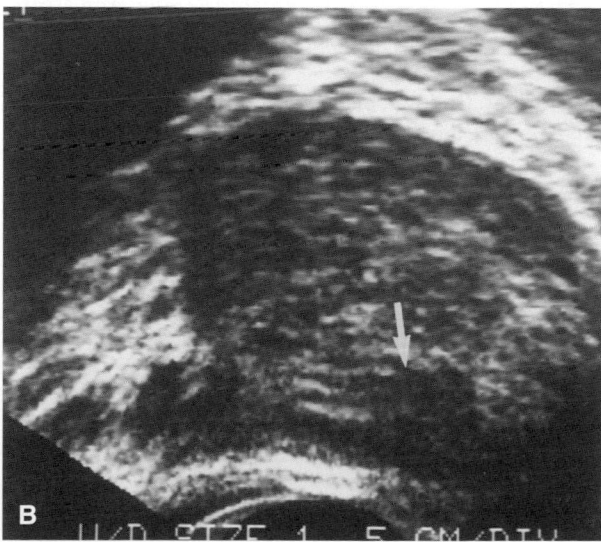

Figure 40–11   Adenocarcinoma of the prostate. Transverse view **A.** and sagittal view **B.** from transrectal ultrasound show a hypoechoic adenocarcinoma in the left peripheral zone (*arrow*). The diagnosis was proved by ultrasound-guided needle biopsy. Note the calcification and adenomatous change centrally.

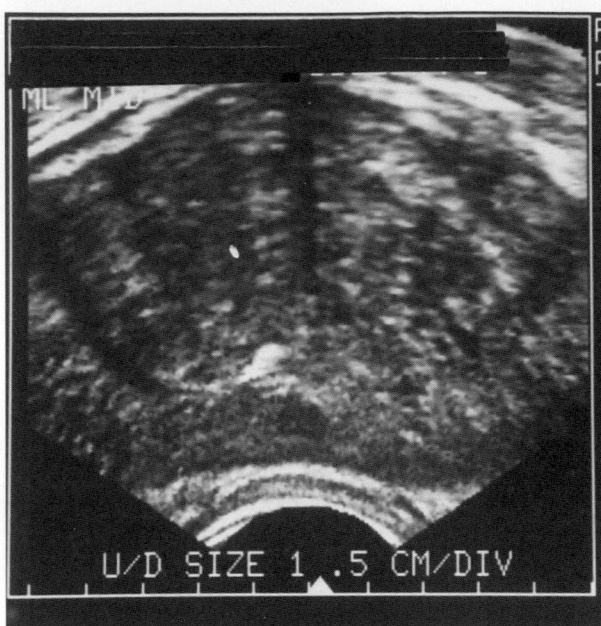

Figure 40–12 Transverse view from transrectal ultrasound shows an enlarged gland with calcification and adenomatous change in the central gland—characteristics of benign prostatic hypertrophy.

The clinical importance of clinical hyperplasia is measured by the severity of symptoms and the amount of residual urine, not by the size of the gland. Normally, the consistency of the gland is similar to that of the contracted thenar eminence of the thumb. It is rather rubbery. It may be mushy if congested (resulting from chronic infection with impaired drainage), indurated (resulting from chronic infection with or without calculi), or stony-hard (resulting from advanced carcinoma). The normal prostate has a weight of approximately 18–20 g. Any areas of induration are termed *suspicious prostate nodules* and should be biopsied.

The differential diagnosis of a prostate nodule includes prostate cancer, asymmetric benign prostatic hypertrophy, prostatic calculi, and granulomatous prostatitis. Approximately 50% of prostate nodules discovered on rectal examination prove to be carcinoma on biopsy.

Functions of the Prostate

The functions of the prostate can be summarized as follows:

1. The prostate produces approximately 1 mL of cloudy fluid daily, which is carried out in the urine.
2. The prostate is responsible for about half the semen volume of ejaculation.
3. The prostatic fluid facilitates fertilization by acting as a vehicle for spermatozoa and as an aid to semen liquefaction through the enzyme fibrinolysin.

Benign Prostatic Hyperplasia

BPH represents a nonmalignant neoplasm of the prostate. BPH as a cause of urinary dysfunction has been known for several centuries. It was mentioned in the Egyptian papyri as early as 1500 B.C. and was discussed by Hippocrates 1,000 years later. Hyperplasia describes an increase in the number of individual tissue elements, whereby the bulk of the organ is increased. Hypertrophy describes a general increase in the bulk of an organ through an increase in size, but not in number, of the individual tissue elements. BPH is a hyperplastic process because there is a net growth of the epithelial and stromal elements of the prostate. The natural history of BPH involves two phases. The first, the pathologic phase, involves two stages, microscopic and macroscopic BPH, neither of which produces clinical symptoms. Nearly all men worldwide eventually develop microscopic BPH if they live long enough. In only about half of these men, however, will microscopic BPH grow to produce a macroscopic enlargement of the gland, suggesting that additional factors are required for the progression of microscopic to macroscopic BPH.

The second, or clinical, phase involves the progression of pathologic BPH to clinical BPH, in which the patient develops symptomatic dysuria. Only about one-half of men with macroscopic BPH progress to having clinical BPH that requires therapeutic intervention. Thus, approximately 25% of all men eventually require some type of treatment for clinical BPH.

Pathogenesis

Although the pathogenesis of BPH remains unknown, it is universally accepted that a source of circulating androgens is required for the development of BPH because males castrated before puberty do not develop BPH. Regression of the prostate has also been reported after castration in adults. BPH can be produced by hormones in animal models. BPH is also associated with abnormal accumulation of the hormone dihydrotestosterone. The precise role of the testes in the pathogenesis of BPH, however, is controversial. There is no convincing evidence that alteration of serum or prostatic androgen levels are related to the development of BPH. It is important to note that there is no relation between BPH and cancer of the prostate.

Prevalence of BPH

The prevalence of BPH in the aging male population has been estimated from histologic examination of prostates obtained at autopsy. A comprehensive review of such autopsy data is described by Berry et al. (28). These data show that BPH rarely occurs in men younger than 40 years and that approximately 50% of men have histologic evidence of BPH by the age of 60 years. It is known that there is a slow increase in prostatic size from birth until puberty.

For the prostate to reach the adult size of 20–25 g, two factors are necessary: time and testes. There is a rapid increase in the size of the prostate from puberty to age 20. The size remains constant until about age 45, at which time the prostate either atrophies and progressively decreases in size or develops BPH.

Spectrum of Clinical Manifestations

The clinical manifestations of BPH are related primarily to obstruction caused by prostatic enlargement. Prostatism, the symptom complex associated with BPH, is a syndrome composed of obstructive and irritative symptoms. The obstructive symptoms include hesitancy and straining to urinate, a diminished caliber and interrupted urinary stream, and postmicturition dribbling. The irritative symptoms include urinary frequency, nocturia, dysuria, and urgency to urinate. As the severity of the obstruction progresses, bladder hypertrophy is unable to compensate for the obstruction, resulting in incomplete bladder emptying. The incomplete bladder emptying exacerbates the symptoms of prostatism and further disposes the patient to urinary tract infections. Complete urinary retention is one of the most severe sequelae of bladder outlet obstruction secondary to BPH; the other is chronic renal insufficiency. Hematuria represents the only clinically significant manifestation of BPH not related to bladder outlet obstruction.

Diagnosis of BPH

The diagnostic approach to patients suspected of having outflow obstruction should include an orderly, well-planned assessment to determine whether there is objective evidence of obstruction and, if so, the level of the obstruction and the effect on the more proximal urinary tract. The assessment should begin with a careful history and physical examination.

To facilitate the assessment of the patient's symptoms, the American Urological Association (AUA) has developed a symptom score evaluation form, and most urologists follow a simple algorithm to treat bladder outflow obstruction (Figure 40–13). Laboratory tests should include urinalysis, urine culture, complete blood count, and levels of serum creatinine, blood urea nitrogen, serum electrolytes, and prostate-specific antigen (PSA).

Indications for Intervention

The indications for surgical or nonsurgical treatment of BPH are highly variable. An absolute indication requires immediate attention. Urinary retention, recurrent urinary tract infections, renal insufficiency secondary to BPH, and/or persistent gross hematuria are generally accepted as absolute indications for treatment. Relative indications for intervention include moderate postvoid residual urine, bothersome symptoms of prostatism, and urodynamic evidence of obstruction. Cystoscopic evidence of BPH should be considered a weak indication for intervention of BPH.

The decision to intervene surgically, medically, or by interventional (minimally invasive) techniques in a man with relative indications should reflect the impact of the symptoms on his quality of life, his expectations and treatment preference, his general medical condition, and the relative effectiveness and morbidity rate of available treatment options.

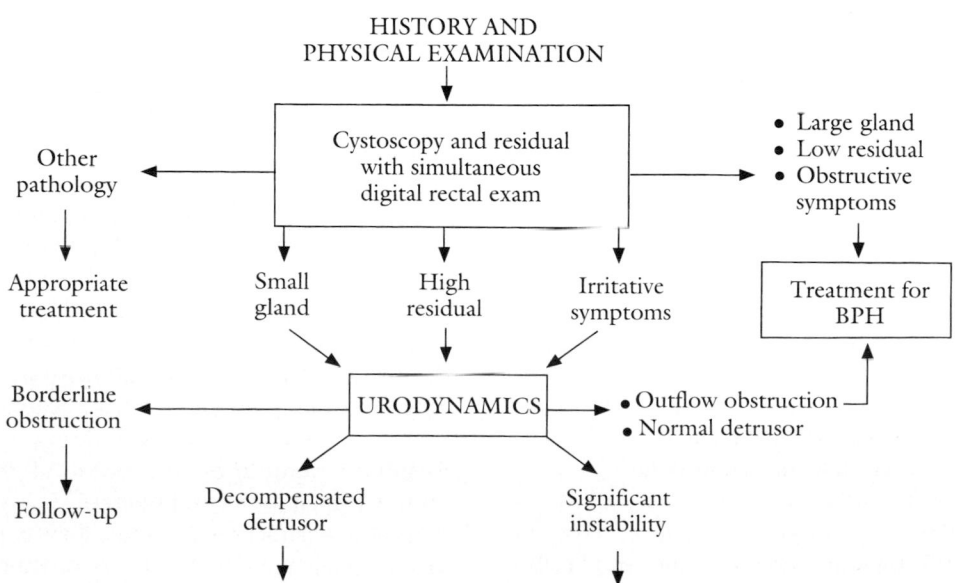

Figure 40–13   Diagnostic algorithm for bladder outflow obstruction.

Surgical Therapy: Transurethral Resection

Transurethral resection of the prostate (TURP), though still the most common operative treatment of benign prostatic hyperplasia, has steeply declined in frequency over the past decade. From 165,000 inpatient procedures in 1992, 105,000 in 1995, and 79,000 in 1998, the number of surgeries had fallen to 87,000 by 2000 (29). Although TURP has been associated with a low surgical mortality rate and a good outcome, the need to control rising medical costs has led to a reevaluation of prostatectomy with regard to the indications for therapeutic intervention and the long-term as well as short-term results. Although most patients undergoing TURP experience long-term improvement in symptoms and quality of life, short-term complications, such as clot retention, and occasional long-term complications, such as incontinence and impotence, may occur (30,31).

In the United States, mortality is adversely correlated to surgical volume (32). Mortality is also nearly two times higher in smaller hospitals and more than three times higher in non-university hospitals (33). For a given age group, a man undergoing TURP is almost three times more likely to die the same year as a man not having TURP (28). Nearly two-thirds of post-TURP deaths occur in the first 3 months after discharge (33,34). Compounding the initial risk is a 20% 8-year probability of reoperation (33). With advancing age, operative mortality may increase by almost six times (34). Age also determines postoperative ability to void, complications, and length of stay (38).

Notwithstanding the above, the overall mortality and morbidity associated with TURP have decreased over the past 3 decades (35). Better recognition and management of individual risk factors, preoperative prophylaxis, and advances in instrumentation have been responsible.

Medical Therapy

Clinical Trials with α-Blockers

The first clinical study using an α-blocker was published by Caine et al. (36). In this study, 49 patients received 10 mg of phenoxybenzamine twice a day. Administration of the drug resulted in improvement in daytime and nighttime frequency and overall symptomatic improvement. Two other studies, by Abrams et al. (37) and Brooks et al. (38), were not able to identify urodynamic or symptomatic improvement in patients receiving phenoxybenzamine. Because blockers using phenoxybenzamine have caused side effects, such as hypotension (orthostatic), nasal congestion, or absence of ejaculation, and because they have been associated with intestinal malignancy in rats, trials of several other blockers, mostly selective α₁-blockers, have been undertaken.

Results Clinical trials of α-blockers are of short duration with no long-term follow-up, and some are not placebo controlled or blinded. The number of patients is often small, and the criteria for including patients are seldom well defined. Therefore, definite conclusions are difficult to draw at this time.

Hormonal Treatment with Antiandrogens

A number of approaches have been used in the hormonal treatment of BPH. One group of antiandrogen drugs works centrally and prevents production of testosterone. Another group acts peripherally on the prostatic cell. This peripherally acting group prevents transformation of testosterone to dihydrotestosterone (5-α-reductase inhibitor) or competes for binding to the androgen receptor. Peters and Walsh (39) demonstrated a positive effect of medical castration using a centrally acting antiandrogen, a luteinizing hormone-releasing hormone (LH-RH) analogue. The prostate size regressed by approximately 25% based on ultrasound measurement. Biopsy from the prostate confirmed that regression was in the glandular tissue. There was no change in stromal tissue. Gabrilove et al. (40) describe the use of the analogue leuprolide.

These centrally working drugs have many side effects, including impotence, and drugs that do not substantially alter sexual function would be more desirable.

In a study by Stone (41) investigating flutamide, which blocks the uptake of dihydrotestosterone by the cytoplasmic androgen receptor, 84 patients were randomized into equal drug and placebo groups. Twelve patients were studied for 6 months, and 58 were studied 12 or more weeks. At 6 weeks, peak urinary values had increased by 12% in the placebo group and by 30% in the drug group. However, symptom reduction was identical in both groups. The study is not completed, but at this time, it can be concluded that antiandrogens should be taken for a prolonged period of time to achieve maximum efficacy.

Geller et al. (42) described the effect of megestrol acetate in the treatment of BPH. A total of 61 patients were randomized into placebo and megestrol acetate groups and studied over a 5-month period. Improvement in symptoms of prostatism was similar in both groups. Seventy percent of the drug-treated patients reported a reduction of libido. Sexual side effects have kept the steroidal antiandrogens, such as megestrol, from being used widely for BPH.

A large, prospective, randomized clinical trial comparing a 5-α-reductase inhibitor with a placebo is being conducted in the United States and abroad. Results of this investigation are not available, but preliminary reports suggest that the administration of synthetic α₁-reductase inhibitor causes regression of prostate size on a magnitude similar to that with LH-RH analog administration. Very few side effects, including impotence, have been reported.

Results Prevention of contraction of the smooth muscle should, from a theoretical point of view, provide the patient relief from obstruction. However, there is an important factor that has not been considered. Stereometric studies by Bartsch (43,44) and Ohrh and Bartsch (45) demonstrated that although the prostate is usually considered to be a glandular organ, it contains a large quantity of fibromuscular stroma. In normal prostates, the ratio of stroma to epithelium is 2:1, whereas in BPH it is approximately 5:1. The stroma consists of smooth muscle and intermuscular components, such as collagen. The extractability of collagen is the limiting factor in the contraction and release of the smooth muscle. The effect of the α-blockers will therefore depend on nonmuscular components. At the present time, very little is known about age-related changes in these components.

Hormonal treatment of BPH has resulted largely in regression of the epithelial component; there is no apparent effect on the stroma. It is important to keep in mind that prostate involution because of regression of the epithelial part may not necessarily decrease urethral resistance and therefore may not reduce the symptoms of prostatism. Again, BPH is characterized by more stromal than epithelial enlargement.

Interventional Therapy

Prostatic Urethroplasty

Prostatic urethroplasty with a balloon catheter is meant to be entirely an outpatient procedure, performed under topical anesthesia aided by mild intravenously administered sedation. Its morbidity is minimal (2–6,46–51), and no mortality is expected. The procedure is relatively simple in skilled hands, and few guidelines have to be followed to avoid complications such as incontinence from dilating the external urinary sphincter. This procedure should markedly reduce the cost of treatment of BPH and should lead to greater patient acceptance. It can be performed on almost any patient regardless of his medical condition.

Technique For this procedure, the patient is placed in a supine position on the table. Optimal imaging and guidance are obtained in either oblique projection. The desired oblique position can be obtained by placing a sponge wedge on either side of the patient, or, if a C-arm fluoroscopy unit is available, the tube can be rotated either way. The latter method is preferable because the patient is more comfortable in a flat, supine position.

An intravenous line is started before the procedure for the administration of antibiotics and sedatives or for emergency medication should it become necessary. Broad-spectrum prophylactic antibiotics, such as cephalosporin, ampicillin, or a combination of sulfamethoxazole and trimethoprim, are started before the procedure and continued orally for 5–7 days, after completion of the procedure.

The penis is prepared and draped as it would be for a surgical procedure. Transureteral topical 2% viscous lidocaine is applied generously in the urethra. All catheter and guide wire maneuvers are performed under fluoroscopic guidance.

A baseline RUG is performed to assess the degree of obstruction and to determine the landmarks that will be followed throughout the procedure, such as the position of the external sphincter, the length of the prostatic urethra, and the position of the bladder floor and neck. This baseline RUG is performed by advancing a 20–22 French Council catheter to the midanterior urethra or just beyond the meatus; the balloon is filled with 1 or 2 mL of dilute contrast material. This ensures snug occlusion of the urethra so that forceful injection of contrast material can be accomplished to achieve maximal distention of the anterior and posterior urethra without retrograde reflux. The catheter can be positioned at the midanterior urethra or just beyond the meatus so that the partially inflated balloon lodges in the fossa navicularis.

After the urethra has been occluded, an RUG is performed with a 60-mL catheter-tip syringe (Figure 40–14). The catheter tip ensures that the connections are snug and leakproof. The operator then determines and marks the position of the external sphincter, either by putting a small-gauge needle through the skin directed toward and overlapping the position of the external sphincter or by rotating the C arm so that the position of the external sphincter is overlapped by a known bony landmark, such as the inferior margin of the inferior pubic ramus. From this point on, the tube angle and the patient should remain as stable as possible so that the landmarks remain unchanged.

The length of the prostatic urethra is determined so that it may be dilated in its entirety. Some contrast material should be kept in the bladder to identify the bladder base

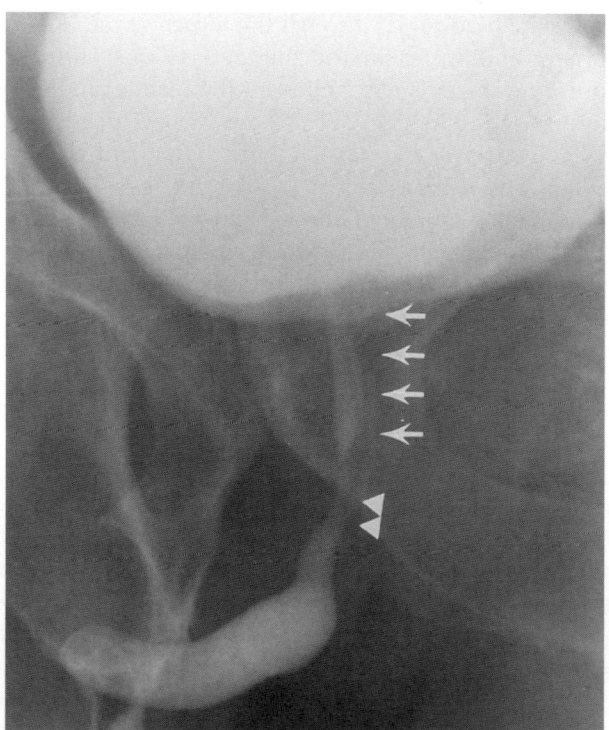

Figure 40–14 RUG showing the length and caliber of the prostatic urethra (*arrows*) as well as the location of the membranous urethra that corresponds to the external sphincter (*arrowheads*).

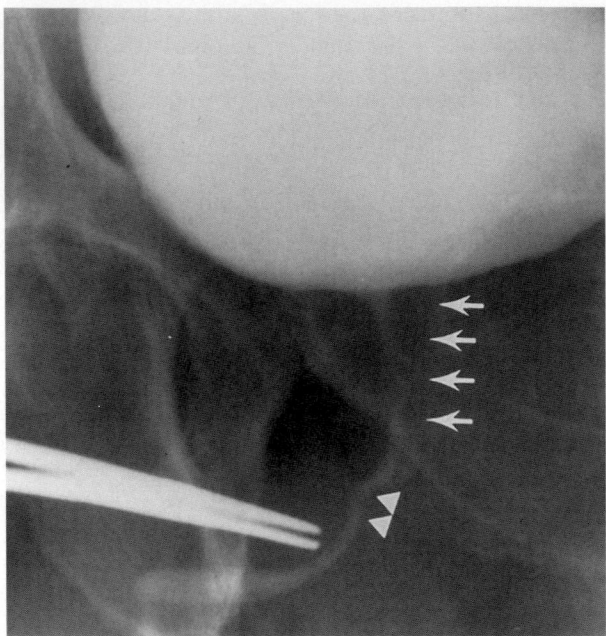

Figure 40–15   VCUG in the same patient showing the length and different morphologic appearance of the prostatic urethra (*arrows*) obtained in this dynamic study as well as the location of the external sphincter (*arrowheads*).

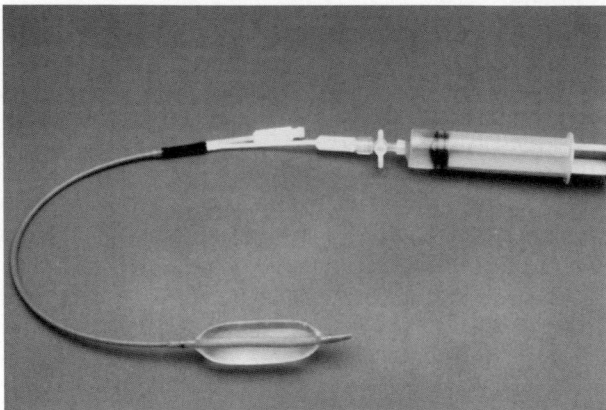

Figure 40–16   The 30-mm-diameter prostatic urethroplasty balloon catheter used by most investigators.

because this is where most of the prostatic bulk lies, and it is extremely crucial to dilate this area adequately. Once this has been accomplished, the Councill catheter balloon is deflated, and the catheter is advanced into the bladder. A guide wire is advanced through the lumen of the Councill catheter and curled in the bladder. At this point, the Councill catheter is removed from the bladder and penis. Although not essential, a VCUG can be performed on the table (Figure 40–15), especially if the patient feels like voiding. This helps to confirm the landmarks.

A generous amount of lubricant is applied to the prostatic urethroplasty balloon catheter before it is advanced over the guide wire. The catheter is advanced so that the proximal balloon marker is placed beyond the external sphincter. The authors use a balloon diameter of 30 mm (Figure 40–16) (Cook, Inc.); smaller balloons do not decrease the morbidity and might be less effective. At this point, and especially if the patient or the C-arm arc has moved, a repeat RUG can be performed using a small (6 French) pediatric feeding tube, which should be advanced *alongside* the shaft of the catheter to approximately the midanterior urethra. Compression should be applied to the penis so that the proximal urethral channel is occluded adequately and no reflux of contrast material can occur. A repeat injection of contrast material will determine the relationship of the external sphincter to the proximal balloon marker. These repeat RUGs can be performed at any time during the dilatation procedure, even when the balloon is fully inflated, to ensure that the landmarks have remained unchanged.

The balloon catheter is inflated slowly to its maximal diameter and pressure (Figure 40–17). Because the patient experiences the most discomfort during the initial inflation, adequate intravenously administered sedation should be available. More intense than the pain is the extreme urge to void, which results from the stretching of the muscle and nerve fibers of the bladder neck. Because the balloon has a strong tendency to migrate into the bladder, the place of least resistance, strong tension should be applied on the

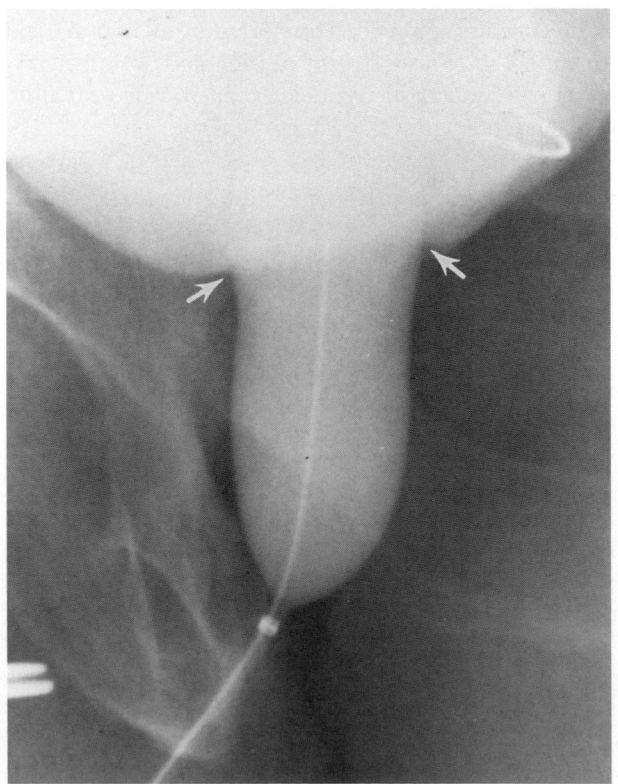

Figure 40–17   Image showing the balloon fully inflated in the prostatic urethra, including the bladder neck (*arrows*) and the entirety of the prostatic urethra.

catheter while the balloon is being inflated. If at any point the balloon has migrated into the bladder or distal in the prostatic urethra, it should be deflated and repositioned so that adequate dilatation of the entire prostatic urethra, including the apex, may be accomplished. If there is any doubt about the position of the external sphincter, a repeat RUG with the feeding tube should be performed. The balloon may appear as if it is being pulled proximal to the external sphincter and anterior urethra. However, the pelvic floor is formed by a group of muscles, tendon attachments, and soft tissues, and the external sphincter is a very strong muscular structure that most likely will not allow the balloon to go through when fully inflated. If there is any doubt, a repeat RUG will show that the relationships are still the same and it is merely the pelvic floor that is being pulled. After a few minutes of full balloon inflation, the tension required on the catheter shaft will decrease as the compliance of the prostatic and periprostatic tissues increases with the forces applied by the balloon. The balloon should be left in place for approximately 10 minutes.

In some instances the prostatic urethra is so long that the balloon has to be repositioned more distally to dilate the entire urethra, including the bladder neck. If this is necessary, an extra 5–10 minutes of dilatation should be adequate.

At the completion of the dilatation, the balloon is fully deflated and removed and the guide wire left in place. During balloon catheter removal, the shaft of the catheter should be turned continuously in the same direction in which the balloon was originally folded so that the catheter collapses as much as possible, thus avoiding more trauma to the anterior urethra.

The next step is to repeat the RUG (Figure 40–18) to assess the results. The same 20–22 French Councill catheter is advanced *alongside* the guide wire to the midanterior urethra. Again, the Councill catheter balloon is partially inflated with 1–2 mL of dilute contrast material to ensure snug occlusion of the urethra. (Note: If the Councill catheter is advanced *over* the guide wire, the seal between the syringe and the injecting port of the Councill catheter will be faulty, allowing leakage of contrast material and precluding a good, forceful injection to distend the anterior and posterior urethra adequately.) The RUG is performed in an oblique projection to evaluate the prostatic urethra. If no significant dilatation has been obtained, repeat dilatation will be necessary. Increased incidence of hematuria or complications because of repeat dilatations have not been described. Again, a VCUG can be obtained on the table (Figure 40–19), although this is not mandatory.

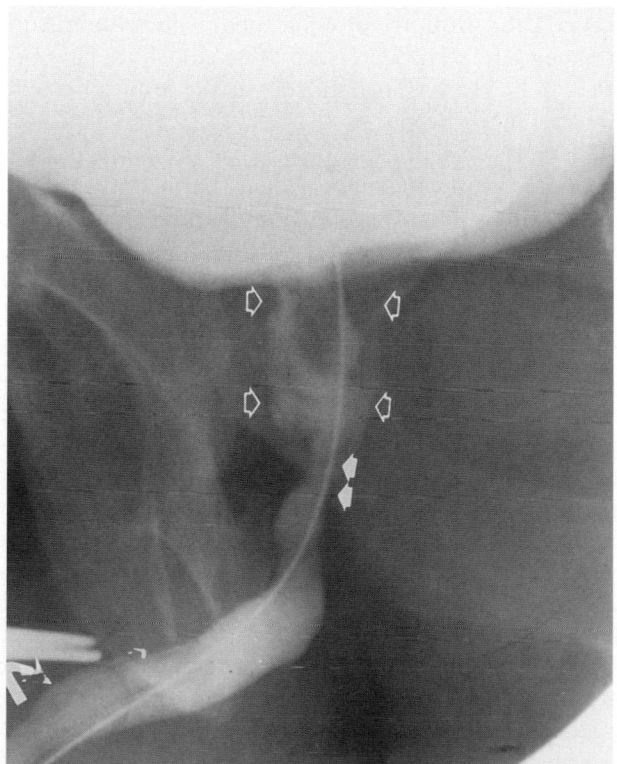

Figure 40–18 RUG immediately after balloon dilatation while the guide wire is still in place and curling in the bladder. Note the significant increase in the prostatic urethra caliber (*open arrows*) after dilatation and the intactness of the external sphincter (*solid arrows*). The Councill catheter balloon has been partially inflated to ensure snug occlusion of the urethra for the adequate performance of the RUG (*curved arrow*).

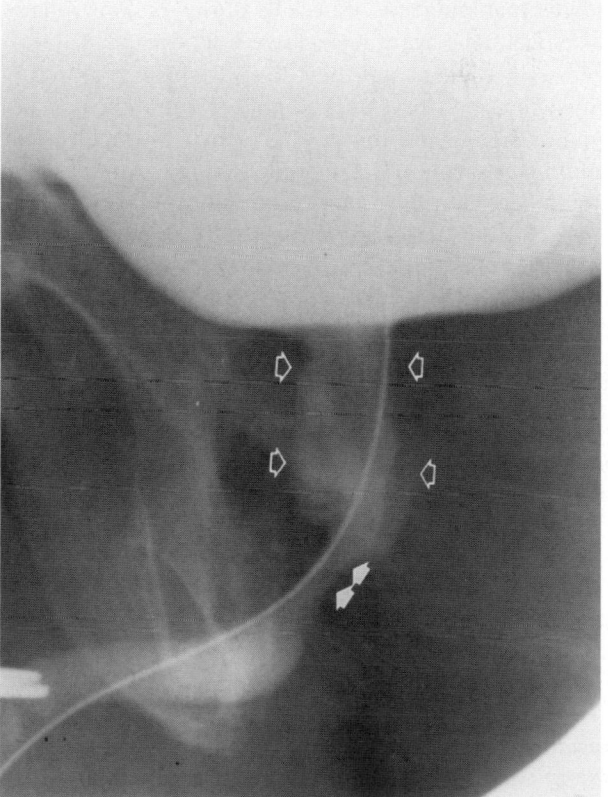

Figure 40–19 VCUG obtained immediately after balloon dilatation while the guide wire is still in place. Again, note the significantly increased prostatic urethra caliber (*open arrows*) as well as the intactness and preservation of the external sphincter (*solid arrows*).

To verify that the prostatic commissures have been disrupted, the RUG is repeated in a straight anteroposterior projection. This radiographic impression will show a much narrower prostatic urethra than the oblique projection because the anterior and posterior commissures have been disrupted, allowing an increase in the anteroposterior caliber but not in the transverse diameter because of the opposing prostatic lobes. The increase in the anteroposterior caliber by disruption of the prostatic commissures, plus the stretching of the prostatic capsule, is enough to allow the creation of a larger lumen so that the bladder outlet resistance decreases.

If the dilatation is adequate, the partially inflated Councill catheter balloon is deflated and removed to be advanced later *over* the guide wire into the bladder. At this point, the guide wire is removed, and the 5-mL Councill catheter balloon is inflated with 20 mL of very dilute contrast material or saline. The balloon usually will not rupture at this volume because it is made of latex, which is very distensible. Tension on the catheter from the inflated balloon will prevent it from falling into the traumatized prostatic fossa, which might produce significant discomfort and bleeding after the local anesthesia has worn off.

The bladder is irrigated vigorously, and all blood and clots are removed. The catheter should be left in place, with slight tension applied to the end to decrease the amount of subsequent hematuria. Most of the hematuria occurs during catheter manipulations, especially during balloon inflation. The hematuria may seem excessive, but once the bladder has been well irrigated and the clots have been removed, the urine will usually have only a light red tint. If the hematuria remains significant, the 20–22 French Councill catheter should be exchanged over a guide wire for a larger one, perhaps 26–30 French, so that the small capillary bleeding is tamponaded. Continuous tension at the end of the catheter should also help to decrease the hematuria, which should be minimal by 24 hours.

The patient is instructed to be relatively sedentary the rest of the day so that the hematuria does not recur or continue. In most instances, the Councill catheter is removed the following morning. The patient's bladder is fully filled before catheter removal. The patient is instructed to void after removal to ensure that he can void and will not go into retention at home. In a few instances, a patient has developed delayed retention and required recatheterization. This has occurred in patients with very large prostates in whom the superimposed edema has resulted in retention. If this situation seems likely, the drainage catheter should be left for longer periods of time (48–72 hours).

Results As more procedures are performed and longer follow-ups are available, it has become clear that the procedure is not for everyone; but when the indications are followed and the patients are carefully selected, satisfactory results should occur in approximately 75–85% of cases (47–49,51–59). These results have been fairly consistent among the different published series, even in those in which patient selection has been suboptimal. Improvement is noted on both the obstructive and irritative symptoms. An approximately 50% improvement in average and peak uroflows, a 75% increase in average uroflow volumes, and a 300% average decrease in postvoid residuals have been noted after prostatic urethroplasty in a nonrandomized, nonselective study (59).

All the studies that made special note of the presence of an enlarged middle lobe have reported a significant decrease in the success rate (57,59,60). Therefore, this group of patients should be carefully screened and excluded if possible, especially if other options are available for these patients.

Patients with bladder dyssynergic problems, large residuals, or atony are also not good candidates because adequate detrusor function is required for emptying of bladder contents and, therefore, the relief of prostatism and associated complications. This group of patients probably would not benefit from other procedures, such as TURP, either.

Complications Although prostatic urethroplasty with a balloon catheter is an easy procedure to perform, certain guidelines must be followed to avoid complications such as damage to the external sphincter with resulting incontinence. All postdilatation manipulations over a guide wire must be done under fluoroscopic or direct vision to avoid the creation of false passages that could result in a perineal abscess(es) (61), bleeding, or further trauma to the already lacerated and disrupted prostatic urethra and commissures. In none of the studies in which these guidelines have been strictly followed has incontinence as the result of external sphincter injury been seen.

There has been one case of a perineal abscess that developed after a difficult blind bladder recatheterization in a patient with a significantly enlarged prostate and previous retention who was confined to catheter drainage before balloon urethroplasty and who remained in retention after catheter removal. As previously stated, this type of complication can easily be avoided if the guidelines are followed.

There have been no significant long-term complications. Prolonged hematuria requiring hospital admission is seen in approximately 4% of cases (47,49,59) and is associated mainly with concomitant coagulopathy or severe hypertension. In none of the reported series has this complication required a blood transfusion; it can be managed by catheter traction and bladder irrigations in approximately 24 hours.

Urinary retention is another possible complication that is rarely seen, usually in patients with very large prostates, in whom the slightest amount of edema tips the patient into retention. This complication is managed by careful recatheterization and drainage for 48–72 hours.

If the procedural guidelines are followed, if proper antibiotic coverage is given before and after the procedure, if coagulopathies are corrected or foreseen before the procedure, if prostatic size is taken into consideration, and if prolonged catheterization is used prophylactically, the procedure should be free of complications.

TABLE 40–1

CHARACTERISTICS OF THE PROSTATE AND REQUIREMENTS FOR BEST RESULTS OF BALLOON DILATATION

Bilobar prostatic enlargement
Prostatic size less than 50 g
Prostatic urethral length between 2.5 and 4.5 cm
Moderate symptoms of prostatism
Adequate detrusor function

Summary Prostatic urethroplasty is a relatively new procedure for which data are still being gathered, but so far it has been shown to provide symptomatic improvement in 75–85% of a carefully selected group of patients (Tables 40–1 and 40–2). It is meant to be an outpatient procedure performed under local anesthesia and intravenously administered sedation and therefore should decrease medical costs significantly.

The higher recurrence rate, compared with that of TURP, is a real issue and should be weighed against the higher morbidity rate and side effects associated with TURP in relatively healthy patients, although it probably should not be an issue in high-risk patients.

Prostatic Stents

Four stents have found the most clinical applications in Europe: the double-helix or Fabian stent, the Wallstent (Medinvent) tubular mesh stent, the balloon-expandable titanium stent, and the double Malecot intraurethral plastic stent. All these devices can be placed with cystoscopic or fluoroscopic guidance. The procedure is similar to the ones described above. Cystoscopy or radiographic studies are performed to determine anatomic landmarks, to measure the length of the prostatic urethra, and to exclude other abnormalities. The patients receive antibiotics for about a week. The introduction and placement of the device are monitored

TABLE 40–2

ABSOLUTE AND RELATIVE CONTRAINDICATIONS FOR THE PERFORMANCE OF BALLOON DILATATION OF THE PROSTATE

Absolute Contraindications

Localized prostatic malignancy
Obstructing median lobe
Decompensated detrusor
Very large prostate (>60–70 g)

Relative Contraindications

Multiple large prostatic calculi
Chronic bacterial prostatitis
High residual urine (>50% of total bladder capacity)
Urethral strictures

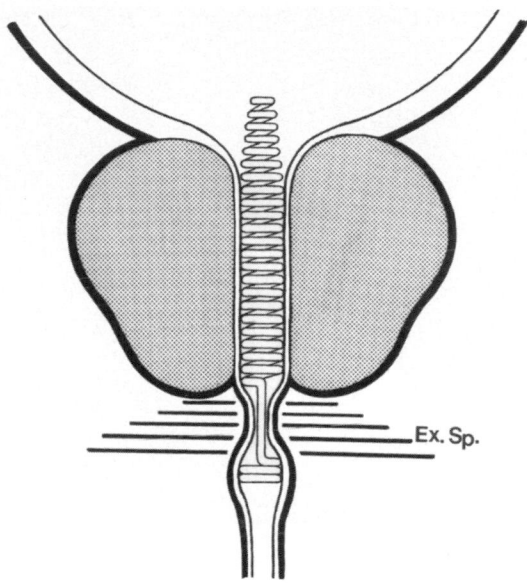

Figure 40–20 Diagrammatic presentation of the Fabian stent and anatomic relationships. *Ex.Sp.*, external sphincter.

closely for correct deployment. The patients are also instructed to avoid retrograde urethral catheterizations.

Double-Helix or Fabian Stent This intraurethral prosthesis (Figure 40–20) (Uromed, Kurt Drews) is made of stainless steel and consists of three parts: a body formed by spiral loops very close to one another that will remain in the prostatic urethra and include the bladder neck; a neck, 2 cm long, that will remain in the membranous urethra; and a head formed by two spiral loops that should remain in the bulbous urethra. Four lengths are available: 45, 55, 65, and 75 mm; the size is selected according to the prostatic urethral length plus 1 cm so that the proximal portion of the body surpasses the cervical adenomatous border.

The prosthesis can be placed under fluoroscopic, sonographic, or cystoscopic guidance with subsequent radiographic confirmation. The new prostheses are gold-plated to reduce contact allergy and incrustation. They can be removed, if desired, for repositioning. Because of the tight winding of the coils, there is no incorporation of the stent by urothelium. For this reason, it was originally recommended that the stent be changed yearly; however, follow-up studies have reported patients with no infections, incrustations, or stent migration for close to 2 years (62–66).

Wallstent or Tubular Wire Mesh This stent has been discussed under urethral stents. Its advantage is that, because of the spaces between the mesh, the stent is completely incorporated into the adjacent tissues within 4–6 months, and infectious incrustation or migration is therefore avoided. The proximal portion of the placed stent should avoid the external sphincter to preclude incontinence or irritation but should include the bladder neck (67).

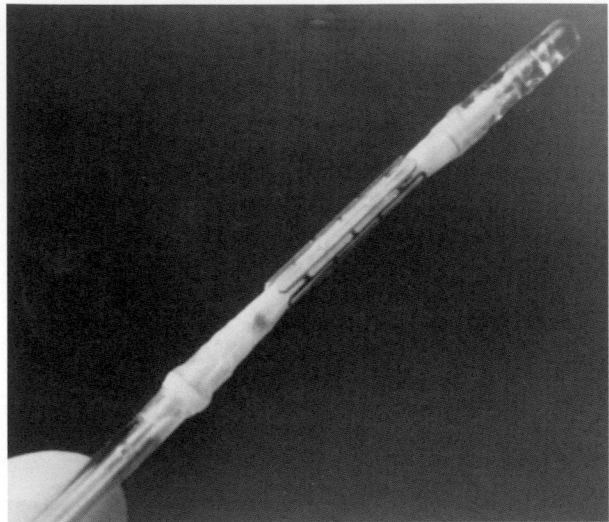

Figure 40–21 Titanium prostatic stent crimped over the deployment balloon catheter.

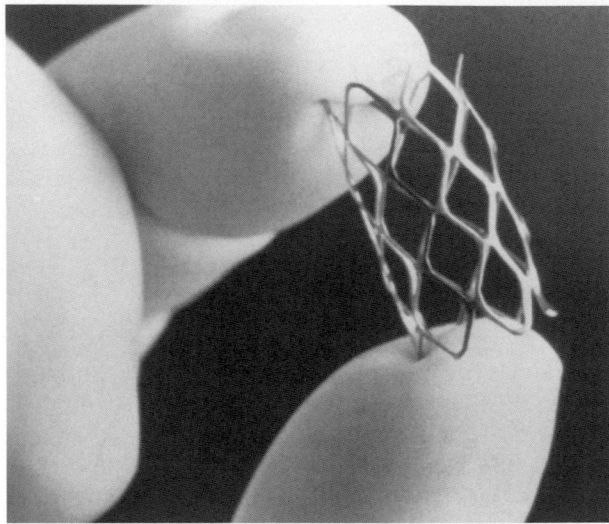

Figure 40–22 Appearance of the fully expanded titanium stent, which resembles the Palmaz vascular stent.

Balloon-Expandable Titanium Stent This stent (68) comes collapsed and mounted over a high-pressure balloon (Figure 40–21) that deploys it to its full diameter; therefore, secondary dilatations are not needed (Figure 40–22). It is available in several lengths, from 22 to 58 mm.

The insertion is simple and similar to the techniques previously mentioned. This stent also becomes incorporated into the urethral and periurethral tissues.

Double Malecot Plastic Urethral Stent This stent (Angiomed) is made of a plastic polymer (Figure 40–23A)

and comes in special kits (Figure 40-23B) for cystoscopic or fluoroscopic placement. The stent consists of a larger intravesical "basket" that localizes to the bladder neck and a smaller basket that localizes just proximal to the verumontanum and proximal to the external sphincter. These baskets are bridged by a 16 French catheter of various lengths, depending on the prostatic urethral length. The distal end of the catheter has a suture that allows withdrawal and repositioning and is removed after the procedure is completed. Like other plastic stents or drainage catheters elsewhere in the urinary system, this stent requires periodic changes.

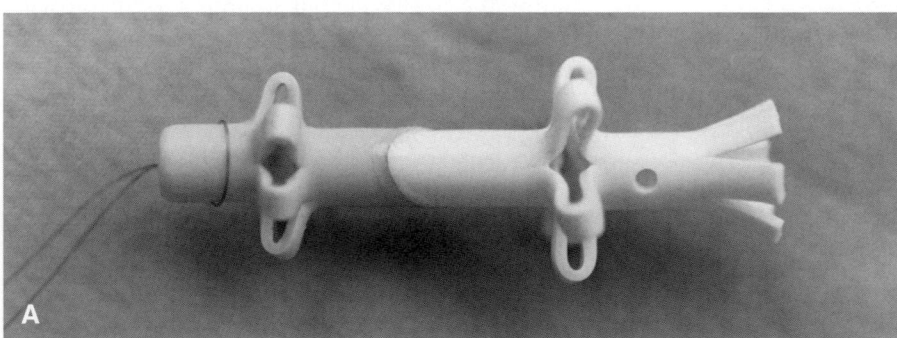

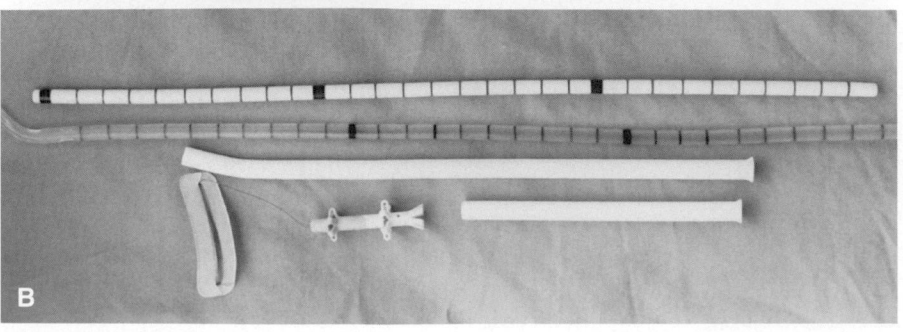

Figure 40–23 **A.** Cone-down magnified view of the double Malecot prostatic urethral stent. **B.** Components of the deployment kit.

Memotherm Stent The Memotherm stent, made of nickel titanium alloy (nitinol) has been in use since 1993 in patients considered to be at high risks for surgery. Nitinol has proved to be a useful component in stent manufacturing, and this device can be deployed endoscopically. With body heat, the device expands to 42F, permitting repeated cystoscopy in patients with bladder tumors or stone disease, a distinct advantage over some other stents. An analysis of 123 patients found initial benefit in 95% (69). Over time, stent migration occurred in 10%, and uroepithelial hyperplasia resulted in recurrent obstruction in 15%. Stent removal because of intractable dysuria, urgency, or infections was necessary in fewer than 2% of patients.

Summary Temporary prostate stents inserted under local anesthesia offer a useful alternative for the short-term relief of urinary retention and prostate symptoms in patients who have limited life expectancy or who are awaiting prostate surgery. Because of problems with incrustation and infection, the stents cannot be left in place for a long period of time and must be changed. If long-term results confirm the early successes with these devices, permanent prostate stents, such as the Wallstent and Palmaz stents, which are known to be incorporated by epithelium (Figure 40–24) while holding open the prostatic urethra, will offer a simple and effective alternative to prostate surgery for many patients.

Prostatic Hyperthermia

Hyperthermia is the central elevation of tissue temperature. The concept that hyperthermia has some curative benefits has been known for millennia. This idea developed from the observation that after a high fever, many ailments resolved or improved. In 1866, Busch (70) published the first scientific report of the complete regression of a histologically proven sarcoma after a bout of erysipelas with high fever. In 1877, Bruns (71) reported the complete cure of a patient terminally ill with multiple recurrent melanomas after erysipelas. In 1893, Coley (72) reported a series of patients with advanced cancer who were either cured or significantly improved by accidental or deliberate exposure to erysipelas. Many other reports followed, with similar results after natural exposure or injection of filtered extracts of highly pyrogenic toxins (73,74). By the same principle, others reported cure or significant improvement after deliberate hyperthermia exposure locally or of the whole body (73,75–84). It is well known that some bacteria and viruses adapted to body temperatures find it difficult to proliferate at temperatures only a few degrees higher.

In the past few years, interest has been revived in the effects of hyperthermia on biologic systems, particularly for the treatment of cancer. Investigations have focused on hyperthermia as the sole treatment or combined with radiotherapy, with or without cytotoxic drugs.

Hyperthermia alone has the capacity to kill cells selectively. Temperatures from 42°C–45°C cause selective death of tumor cells (85). One of the factors that make cancer cells more susceptible than normal cells is the defective heat dissipation by neoplastic tissue resulting from the poor blood supply and decreased vasodilatation capacity of the neovascular bed in response to the thermal load. Other factors known to influence tumor cell sensitivity to heat include nutritional factors, pH, and O_2 concentration, all of which are also related to tumor perfusion (86–88). These effects are potentiated by both radiation and chemotherapy.

Hyperthermia may be applied externally or interstitially. External techniques include radiofrequency current fields, ultrasound, and microwave. Interstitial techniques include radiofrequency current between implanted electrodes, microwave heating with needle-shaped implanted antennas, implanted ferromagnetic seeds or needles heated by radiofrequency magnetic induction, hot water circulated through implanted hollow tubes, and conductive heating catheters (89–94). This expanding knowledge of hyperthermia benefits has motivated its use in almost every system and organ in the body, including the prostate. Hyperthermia has been used for both malignant tumors and BPH (95–102). There are two basic delivery methods of hyperthermia: transrectally, as used by Servadio and others (93,99,101,103), Yerushalmi et al. (95,100), and Mendecki et al. (96); and transurethrally, as used by Astrahan et al. (102). All these techniques have used temperatures in the range of 42°C–46°C and require a prolonged series of treatments, ranging from 6 to 18. The preferred course for best results is 12–15 treatments. The treatments are 1 hour each, one or two times per week. The reported early clinical results are encouraging, although most lack objective documentation, such as uroflow, urodynamic, and prostate volumetric data before and after treatments.

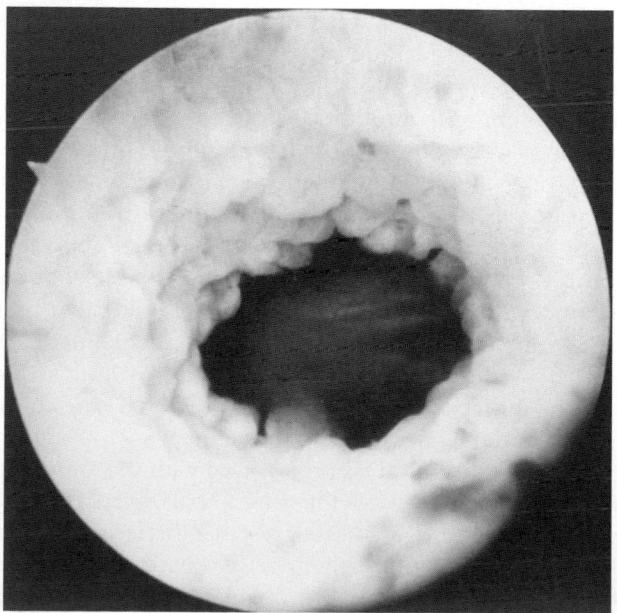

Figure 40–24 Cystoscopic follow-up 6 months after prostatic urethral Wallstent placement. The extrudent and overgrown urothelium through the stent mesh gives the typical cobblestone appearance while keeping the prostatic urethral caliber wide open.

It is the authors' opinion that this protracted course of treatments will not replace either completely or in specific instances the conventional mode of BPH therapy. To compete with transurethral resection, a procedure would have to be safer, less expensive, less involved, and accomplished in a single treatment on an outpatient basis.

With these premises as background, the authors' research has completely changed the previously established clinical and experimental protocols. The goal of this therapy is to produce central prostatic tissue ablation (Figure 40–25), with subsequent debulking (Figure 40–26) of the periurethral adenomatous tissue, by a retrograde transurethral approach that uses much higher temperatures—in the range of 80°C–90°C—for a single exposure period ranging from 15 to 60 minutes.

The current prototype is a 7 French, computer-controlled, heat-emitting catheter that has been used only in experimental animals. With this catheter, the depth and amount of tissue to be ablated and subsequently debulked from the central periurethral adenoma can be adequately controlled.

Histopathologic findings have shown coagulative necrosis that extended to different depths, depending on the treatment and length of exposures used. After treatment and complete resolution of the initial inflammatory response, reepithelialization, widening of the prostatic urethra, atrophy of the periurethral prostatic tissue glands, maintenance of the normal architecture of the periurethral prostatic tissue glands, and maintenance of the normal architecture of the periurethral connective tissue were seen on subsequent follow-ups.

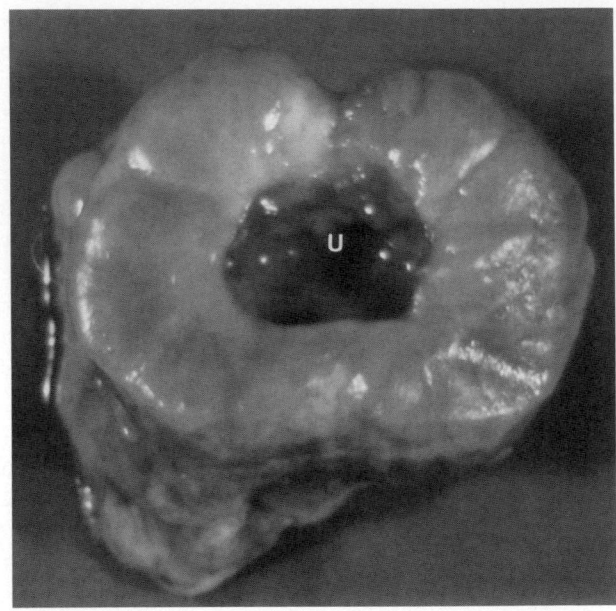

Figure 40–26   One-month posttreatment gross prostatic specimen transversely sectioned showing the much larger central prostatic urethral lumen once the necrosed tissue has sloughed off. *U*, urethral channel.

With this technique, it is possible to ablate periurethral prostatic tissue completely with resultant debulking. Experimentally, this produces a large central lumen in the bladder outlet obstruction caused by central adenomatous tissue (Figure 40–27). This limited resection of a central channel has been proposed by some urologists (104) in high-risk patients in an effort to limit the intervention. The technique suggested here accomplishes the goal in a single treatment, and because it is easy to control and selectively ablate the desired amount of periurethral tissue, the chances of complications are diminished. The authors doubt that other complications, such as strictures, would develop because of the normal appearance of the regenerated tissues. Because the major nerve networks are more toward the periphery, impotence, another condition that might be of concern, probably will not occur if the ablation is deep enough only to open a reasonable channel. This procedure may be performed on an outpatient basis because there is no bleeding or need for external drainage. The necrosed tissue sloughs off gradually, without sequelae. The procedure would require regional anesthesia because of the higher temperatures used.

Some of the clinical issues involved with this procedure will be resolved only when the clinical trial begins. However, experimental animal studies suggest that this technique may be a nonsurgical, minimally invasive way of debulking the central prostatic adenoma. The ongoing clinical series using low temperatures have not produced results comparable to those of transurethral resection of the prostate, the standard mode of BPH treatment. Although the proposed high-temperature debulking of the periurethral central

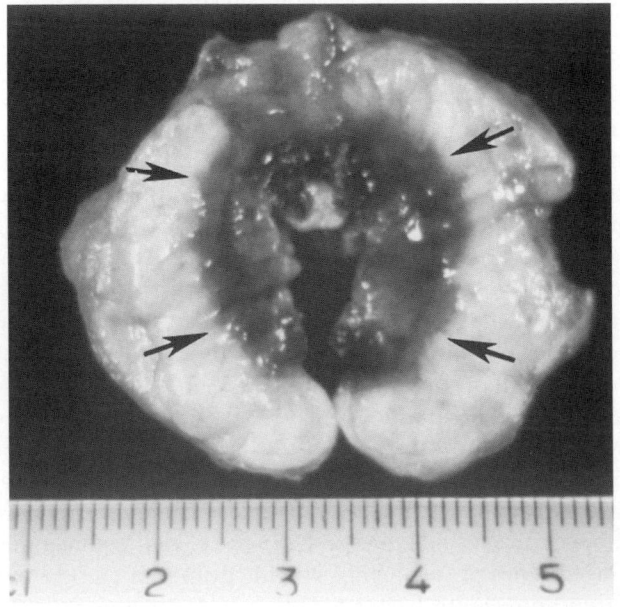

Figure 40–25   Transverse microscopic section of the prostate at its midportion showing the clear-cut demarcation between the area of acute coagulative necrosis (*arrows*) and the healthy surrounding peripheral prostatic tissue after exposure to conductive hyperthermia at 95°C.

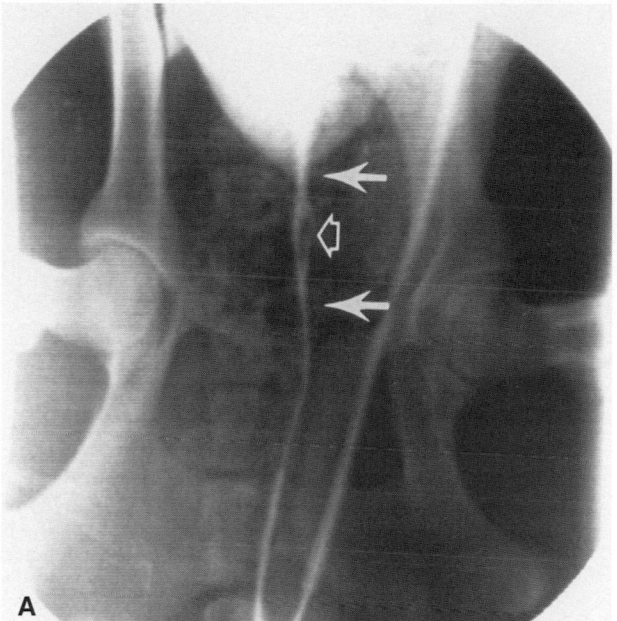

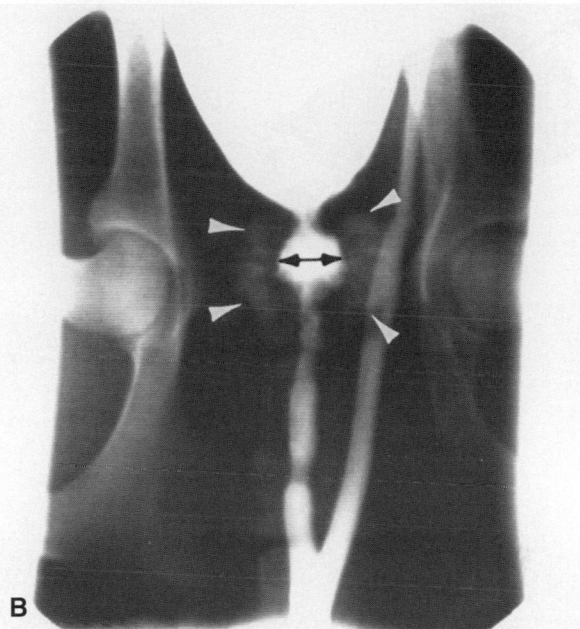

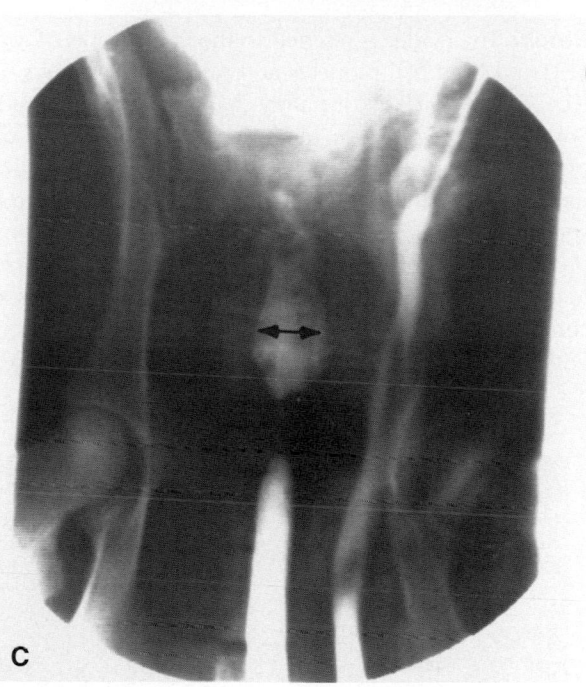

Figure 40–27 **A.** Baseline RUG of male canine showing the length of the prostatic urethra (*solid arrows*) and the location of the verumontanum (*open arrow*). **B.** Two weeks after prostatic conductive hyperthermia, there is a much larger prostatic urethral lumen (*double black arrow*) as compared with baseline. At this time, there is still evidence of generalized prostatic swelling, as evidenced by the contra reflux into the periphery of the prostatic glands (*arrowheads*). **C.** After 1 month there is further increase of the central prostatic urethral channel (*double black arrow*) from further tissue sloughing.

adenoma has not reached the clinical stage, it has many theoretical advantages over previous methods.

Prostatic Biopsy

Sonography-guided transrectal prostatic biopsy is usually performed as an outpatient procedure. The medical history is reviewed, and a physical examination is performed. Biopsy is contraindicated in patients who have coagulopathy, who are on anticoagulant therapy, or who have acute prostatitis.

Sedation is not required except in patients with severe anxiety or pain. Because the biopsy will be performed through the rectal wall and in order to prevent infectious complications, a broad-spectrum antibiotic is given immediately before and for 3–5 days after the procedure. Local anesthesia is achieved with topical intrarectal 2% lidocaine jelly or 1% lidocaine (Xylocaine, Astra Pharmaceutical) injected through a fine needle into the rectal wall. Sonographic artifacts related to air or feces in the rectum are minimized by a preprocedural cleansing enema. The patient is scanned in the left lateral decubitus knee–chest position. Having the patient maintain a partially distended urinary bladder aids in imaging the base of the prostate.

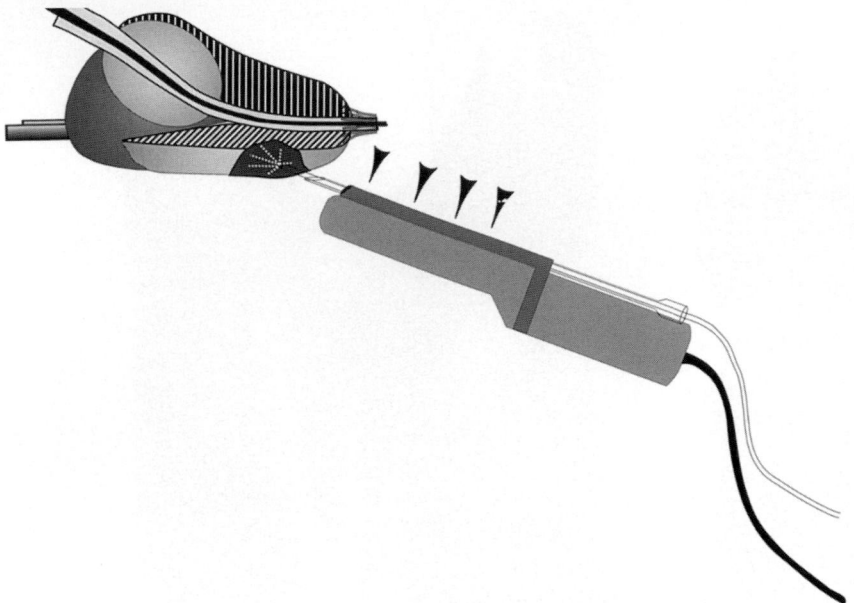

Figure 40–28 Diagram highlighting the biopsy channel of needle (*arrowheads*) for the accurate performance of prostatic biopsies done through the transrectal prostatic ultrasound probe.

Biplanar imaging of the prostate is performed with a high-frequency transducer (5–7 MHz). The probe should have a needle channel and an electronic targeting guide for precise transrectal needle positioning (Figure 40–28). A condom is placed over each probe to decrease the risks of contamination and infection. An acoustic window is provided by interfacing water in the protecting condom between the transducer and the rectal wall.

After application of local anesthesia in the periprostatic tissues, an 18-gauge needle is advanced through the biopsy channel of the linear-array probe. The biopsy needle is placed in an automatic spring-loaded biopsy gun (Biopty, Bard Urologic). The needle is advanced under continuous direct sonographic guidance so that the echogenic tip is placed adjacent to, but not at, the area to be biopsied. (One must be aware that no sample is obtained from the 5 mm of tissue immediately adjacent to the needle tip.) The biopsy gun is fired, sampling the tissue of interest with a histologic core. The biopsy tract can be seen sonographically as an echogenic line within the prostatic parenchyma (Figure 40–29).

Typically, the authors obtain two to three histologic cores from the area with abnormal sonographic features and an additional sample of sonographically normal contralateral prostatic lobe as a control biopsy. It is desirable to include the prostatic capsule and, if possible, a sample of the adjacent seminal vesicle in the biopsy specimen. The cores are submerged in formaldehyde for analysis.

After the procedure, the patient is briefly reexamined to rule out formation of periprostatic fluid collections, suggesting hemorrhage. Vital signs are compared with the values obtained before the biopsy. Only a few patients complain of pain during or after the procedure and are usually discharged, requiring only the antibiotic therapy and conditional analgesics.

Results The reader is referred to the latest works of McNeal (19) and Lee (24), pioneers and primary researchers of this technology, which is constantly changing and being updated. Sonography offers the most sensitive evaluation of the prostate, with predictive values equivalent to those of the digital rectal examination (DRE). The use of DRE and prostate-specific antigen (PSA) results further increases the positive predictive value of transrectal ultrasound (TRUS), which may help in the management of TRUS-positive small lesions. The currently accepted "standard of care" for early detection, the DRE, must be expanded to include the use of TRUS and PSA.

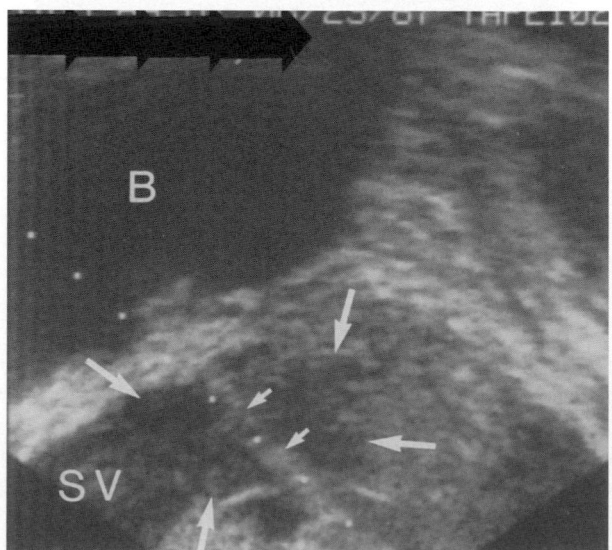

Figure 40–29 Longitudinal transrectal ultrasound image of the prostate showing a large hypoechoic nodule (*long white arrows*) in the base of the prostate extending into the seminal vesicles (*SV*), suspicious for a carcinoma. The needle (*short white arrows*) is noted sampling the center of the suspicious nodule. *B,* bladder.

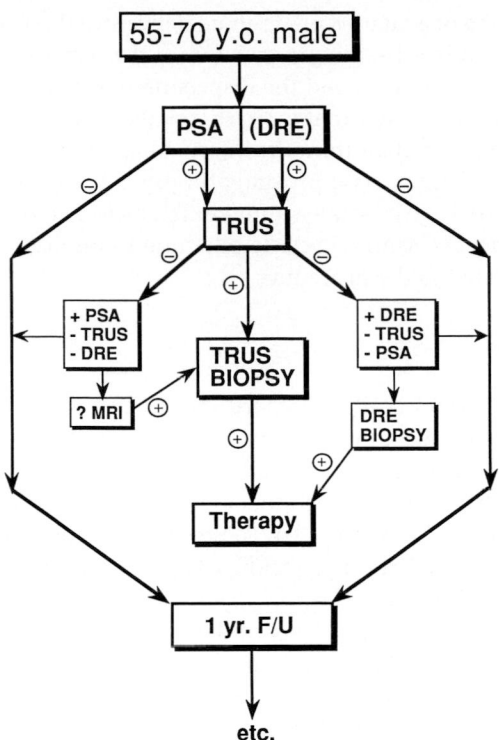

Figure 40–30 Prostate cancer screening algorithm showing the sequence of events according to the results obtained on digital rectal examination (*DRE*), prostate-specific antigen (*PSA*) levels, and transrectal ultrasound (*TRUS*) imaging.

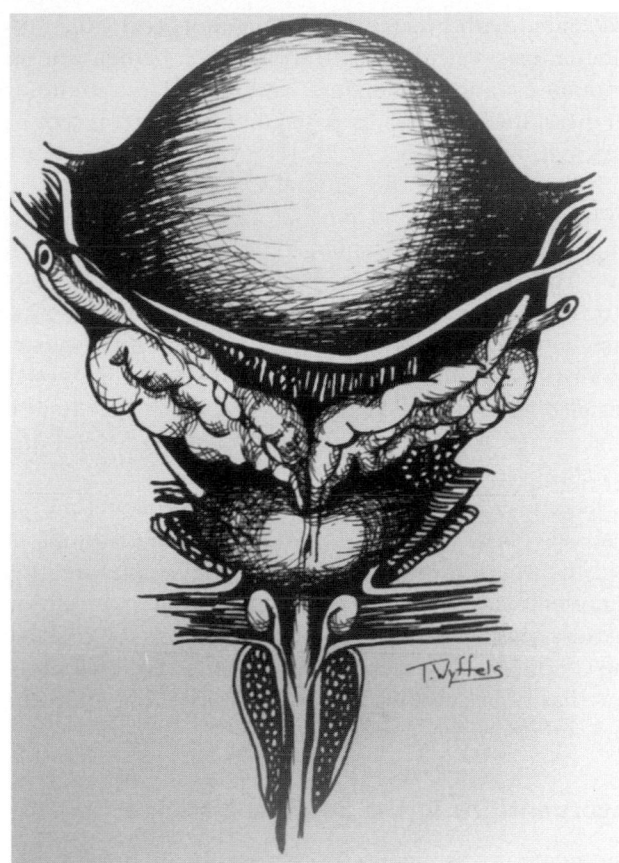

Figure 40–31 Diagram showing the relationship and location of the seminal vesicles and the pelvic floor.

The current lack of definitive data should not prevent the cost-effective use of appropriate technology in the early detection of prostate cancer. Littrup and Lee (105) have devised a clinical algorithm for efficacious patient care (Figure 40–30), which, if followed, should increase early cancer detection.

THE SEMINAL VESICLES AND EJACULATORY DUCTS

Surgical Anatomy

The seminal vesicles (Figure 40–31) are two sacculated and contorted tubes between the posterior surface of the bladder and the rectum. Each vesicle is about 5 cm long and is somewhat pyramidal in form, the base being directed backward, upward, and laterally. Each seminal vesicle consists of a single tube coiled upon itself and giving off several irregular diverticula; the separate coils, as well as the diverticula, are connected together by fibrous tissue. The tube has a diameter of 3–4 mm, and its length, when uncoiled, varies from 10 to 15 cm. It ends above in a cul-de-sac; its lower extremity becomes constricted into a narrow, straight duct that joins with the corresponding deferential duct to form the ejaculatory duct. The arteries supplying the seminal vesicles are derived from the inferior vesical and middle

rectal arteries. The veins and lymph vessels accompany the arteries. The nerves are derived from the pelvic plexuses.

The ejaculatory ducts, one on each side of the median plane, are formed by the union of the duct of a seminal vesicle with a terminal part of a different duct and are nearly 2 cm long. They arise at the base of the prostate, run anteroinferiorly between the median and right (or left) lobes, pass along the sides of the prostatic utricle, and end on the colliculus seminalis in a slitlike orifice on or just within the margins of the opening of the utricle. The ducts diminish in size and also converge toward their termination.

The spermatic cord is composed of arteries, veins, link vessels, nerves, and the deferential duct, connected together by areolar tissue. The arteries of the spermatic cord are the testicular, cremasteric, and deferential. The nerves are the genital branch of the genitofemoral nerve, the cremasteric nerve, and the testicular plexus of the sympathetic nerve, joined by filaments from the pelvic plexus that accompany the deferential artery.

Important Affections of the Seminal Vesicles

Important affections of the seminal vesicles include nonspecific seminal vesiculitis or seminal vesicle inflammation, which is usually a secondary inflammatory process associated with prostatitis (106); gonococcal vesiculitis; tuberculosis; calculi; calcification; cysts; benign tumors; primary carcinoma; sarcoma; and secondary carcinoma. Of these, the only one discussed in this chapter is seminal vesicle inflammation.

Inflammation of the seminal vesicle in the absence of an inflamed prostate is unusual, but it may occur. Ultrasonography may show enlarged, echogenic seminal vesicles. This appearance is best appreciated by endorectal ultrasonography, which may also demonstrate seminal vesicle or ejaculatory duct calculi (107). CT demonstration of cystic dilatation of an inflamed seminal vesicle has also been reported (108,109). It is very important to treat seminal vesiculitis because it may lead to seminal vesicle abscess (106).

In general, inflammatory conditions of the prostate and seminal vesicles are usually diagnosed by clinical symptoms and the physical examination. Imaging studies are often complementary and may guide appropriate intervention. Because seminal vesiculitis and prostatitis can be challenging conditions to treat clinically, an interventional procedure has been developed that can be beneficial in treating these inflammatory processes.

Interventions in the Seminal Vesicles

Candidates for seminal vesicle aspiration and injection are patients with chronic prostatitis unresponsive to standard medical therapy in whom seminal vesiculitis is suspected. Patients with bleeding disorders or acute prostatitis are excluded. After cleansing enemas, a standard biplanar transrectal ultrasound examination of the seminal vesicles is performed with the patient in the left lateral decubitus knee–chest position. The probe needs to have a channel and electronic guidance for direct transrectal needle puncture. This channel is also used to administer local anesthesia and as a port for the transrectal diagnostic aspiration or therapeutic injection of the seminal vesicles.

After sonographic evaluation of the size and internal sonographic pattern of the seminal vesicles, the lateral aspect or more distended portion of the seminal vesicles is localized. Local anesthesia is accomplished with a 22-gauge needle and 1% lidocaine. The seminal vesicles are then punctured with an 18-gauge needle under continuous sonographic monitoring. Accurate positioning of the needle is verified with imaging of the echogenic needle tip in the seminal vesicles and by the aspiration of seminal vesicle fluid. Thick secretions often do not permit the easy acquisition of a fluid sample despite an accurate needle position. It is then necessary to inject 1–2 mL of sterile nonbacteriostatic saline before again attempting aspiration. Fluid samples are submitted for aerobic, anaerobic, chlamydial, and ureaplasmal cultures.

After diagnostic aspiration of the seminal vesicles, the needle can be reinserted for therapeutic injection. Each seminal vesicle is injected with 2 mL of 1% lidocaine and

20–40 mg of gentamycin. Accurate delivery of these drugs is confirmed by observing expansion of the seminal vesicles during the injection and the dispersion of small echogenic foci within the seminal vesicles, related to movement of microbubbles of air from the injected material.

As with transrectal prostatic biopsy, a broad-spectrum antibiotic is given orally immediately before and for 3–5 days after the seminal vesicle puncture to minimize infection related to the procedure.

Results

The only series available reports the results of seminal vesicle aspirations and injections performed in 19 men of ages 28–70 years (mean, 44.5 years) with symptoms of chronic prostatitis unresponsive to therapy for periods ranging 1–40 years (mean, 11 years) (110). These patients underwent seminal vesicle aspiration, injection, or both for suspected seminal vesiculitis.

The sonographic pattern of the seminal vesicles is variable. Normally, the seminal vesicles display a homogeneous low level of echogenicity in comparison with the adjacent prostatic parenchyma (Figure 40–32). Although the seminal vesicles appeared normal in some patients in this series, diffuse cystic changes or inhomogeneous increased echogenicity within the glands were also seen. The seminal vesicles were enlarged in 11 of the patients; some degree of asymmetry was frequently noted.

Aspiration yielded material for microbiologic culture in 18 of 23 attempts (12 bilateral, 6 unilateral; 78%), and 15 of those aspirates yielded positive cultures. Except for

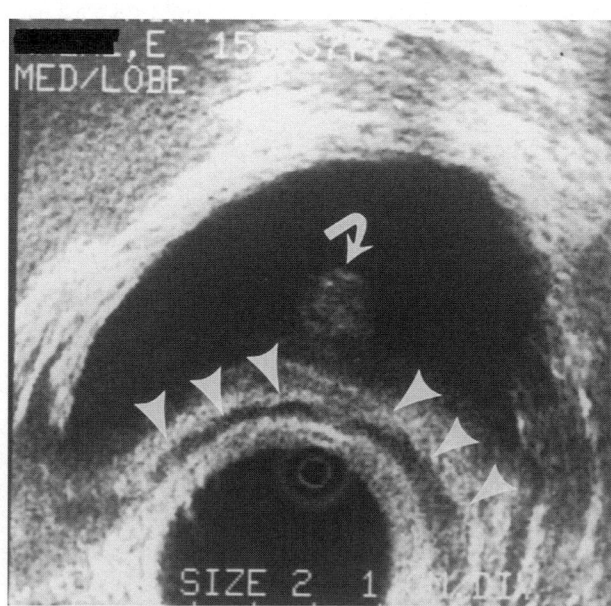

Figure 40–32 Transverse transrectal ultrasound image of the seminal vesicles (*arrowheads*) showing their normal characteristic hypoechogenicity. Incidentally noted is the presence of a prostatic middle zone protruding and elevating the bladder floor (*curved arrow*).

two instances, all positive cultures revealed multiple bacteria, including both aerobes and anaerobes. *Pseudomonas paucimobilis* was cultured in the two aspirates showing a single organism. No cases of *Chlamydia* or ureaplasma were found.

A total of 21 seminal vesicle injections were performed in 18 patients; all but one were bilateral. Temporary relief of symptoms (range, 2 days–6 months) was reported in association with 10 procedures (48%), and no change was seen following the other 9 (43%). Adequate follow-up was not available in the remaining cases.

Summary

Transrectal sonography provides a means of directly imaging the seminal vesicles and also of localizing those structures for direct puncture. Diagnostic aspiration and therapeutic injection of the seminal vesicles are technically easy procedures that may reflect new areas of clinical application of transrectal sonography, providing a potentially powerful tool for evaluating infectious processes of the seminal vesicles.

The temporary relief of symptoms after therapeutic seminal vesicle injection in patients with chronic prostatitis may reflect a contribution by seminal vesiculitis to the clinical manifestations classically ascribed to chronic prostatic infection. In this setting, therapeutic seminal vesicle injection may represent a means of treating seminal vesiculitis; however, more long-term follow-up is necessary to evaluate the role of this procedure.

THE SCROTUM

Surgical Anatomy

The scrotum is a cutaneous and fibromuscular contractile sac containing the testes and the lower parts of the spermatic cords. It is dependent below the pubic symphysis, in front of the upper parts of the thighs. It is divided on its surface into right and left halves by a cutaneous ridge or raphe, which is continued ventrally to the inferior surface of the penis and dorsally along the middle line of the perineum to the anus; the left usually descends a little more than the right, in correspondence with the greater length of the left spermatic cord. The raphe indicates the bilateral origin of the scrotum from the genital swellings. The scrotum consists of the skin and the dartos muscle, together with the external spermatic, cremasteric, and internal spermatic fascia, already described in connection with the spermatic cord. The inner surface of the internal spermatic fascia is loosely attached to the parietal layer of the tunica vaginalis.

The arteries supplying the scrotum are the external pudendal branches of the femoral artery, the scrotal branches of the femoral cutaneous nerve. The anterior third of the scrotum is supplied mainly from the first lumbar segment of the spinal cord (through the ilioinguinal and genitofemoral nerves), whereas the posterior two thirds are supplied mainly from the third sacral segment (through the perineal and posterior femoral cutaneous nerves).

The Scrotum and the Role of Ultrasonography in Interventional Techniques

High-resolution, high-frequency ultrasound images of the scrotum have assumed a significant role in the evaluation of both acute and chronic scrotal lesions. This safe and rapid technique produces information that is complementary to the clinical history and examination and to physiologic studies such as radioisotope scanning or Doppler ultrasonography. Successful images can be obtained with dynamic or static scanning and can be performed using either contact scanning of the scrotum or a water bath, to permit the transducer to stand off from the scrotum. Frequencies between 7.5 and 20 MHz are generally employed.

The testes are identified sonographically as homogeneously echogenic structures. The lobes of the testes cannot be defined sonographically. The head, body, and tail of the epididymis can be identified as contiguous with the testes. This structure is at least as brightly reflected as the testes. The multiple, individual layers of the scrotal skin are generally seen as a single echogenic band; differences in skin thickness between the two sides are an important sonographic finding. Among the small structures that are frequently seen are the normal veins of the pampiniform plexus, as well as the appendix of the testis or epididymis, which may be identified as a punctate echogenic focus.

Although interventional techniques in the scrotum using ultrasonography are limited, they can be important in the evaluation of patients with hydrocele. Aspirations of hydroceles are not commonly performed; however, this procedure may be the treatment of choice in patients who refuse surgical treatment or in patients with multiple medical problems who are not candidates for surgical drainage. It can also be used in the evaluation of patients with hydrocele secondary to an underlying lesion, to provide a better physical examination of the testicle.

The technique is rather simple. The authors prefer to use a 22-gauge needle attached to a 10-mL syringe. The scrotal skin is cleaned with either Betadine or alcohol. The skin is penetrated with a needle in the most dependent part of the scrotum, without injuring the testicle itself or the epididymis. This can obviously be accomplished under ultrasound guidance (Figure 40–33).

In the past, the use of sclerosing agents such as tetracycline has been advocated for the treatment of recurrent hydrocele. However, this technique is rarely used in today's practice.

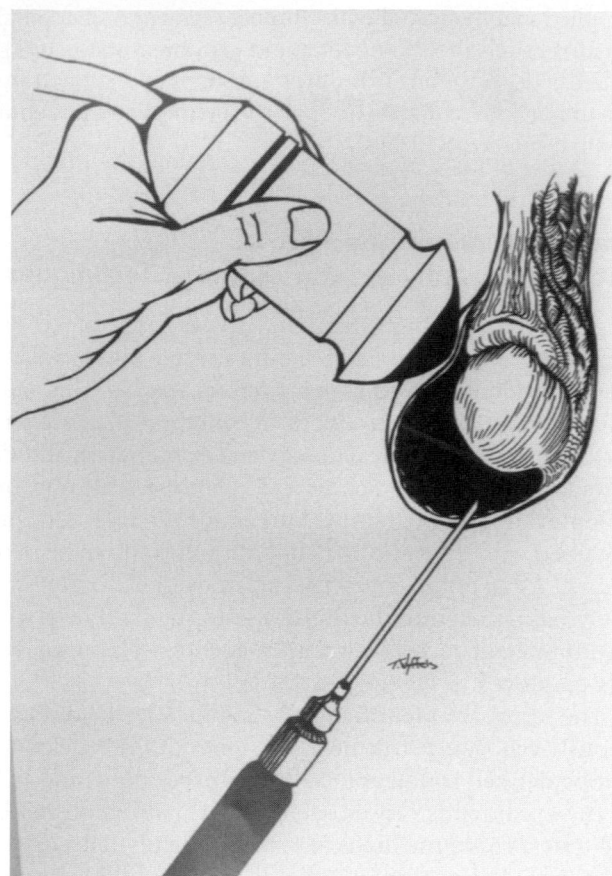

Figure 40–33   Diagram showing the technique for real-time ultrasound-guided hydrocele diagnostic puncture and drainage.

REFERENCES

1. Watanabe H, Kato H, Kato T, et al. Diagnostic application of ultrasonotomography to the prostate. Nippon Hinyokika Gakkai Zasshi 1968;59:273–279.
2. Castaneda F, Lund G, Larson BW, et al. Prostatic urethra: experimental dilation in dogs. Radiology 1987;163:649–654.
3. Castaneda F, Johnson S, Hulbert J, et al. Urethroplasty with balloon catheter in prostatic hypertrophy. AJR Am J Roentgenol 1987;149:313–314.
4. Castaneda F, Reddy P, Wasserman N, et al. Benign prostatic hypertrophy: retrograde transurethral dilation of the prostatic urethra in humans. Work in progress. Radiology 1987;163:649–654.
5. Castaneda F, Reddy P, Hulbert J, et al. Retrograde prostatic urethroplasty with balloon catheter. Semin Intervent Radiol 1987;4:115–121.
6. Castaneda F, Isorna S, Hulbert J, et al. The importance of separation of prostatic lobes in relief of prostatic obstruction by balloon catheter urethroplasty: studies in dogs and humans. AJR Am J Roentgenol 1989;153:1301–1304.
7. Amis ES, Pfister RC, Yoder IC. Interventional radiology of the adult bladder and urethra. Semin Roentgenol 1983;18:322.
8. Lattimer JK. Similar urogenital anomalies in identical twins. Am J Dis Child 1944;67:199–200.
9. Mohammed SH, Wirima J. Balloon catheter dilatation of urethral strictures. AJR Am J Roentgenol 1988;150:327–330.
10. Russinovich NA, Lloyd LK, Griggs WP, et al. Balloon dilatation of urethral strictures. Urol Radiol 1980;2:33–37.
11. Hare WS, McOmish D, Nunn IN. Percutaneous transvesical antegrade passage of urethral strictures. Urol Radiol 1981;3:107–112.
12. Scales FE, Katzen BT, van Breda A, et al. Impassable urethral strictures: percutaneous transvesical catheterization and balloon dilatation. Radiology 1985;157:59–61.
13. Palmaz JC, Richter GM, Noeldge G, et al. Intraluminal stents in atherosclerotic iliac artery stenosis: preliminary report of a multicenter study. Radiology 1988;168:727–731.
14. Sigwart U, Puel J, Mirkovitch V, et al. Intravascular stents to prevent occlusion and restenosis after transluminal angioplasty. N Engl J Med 1987;316:701–706.
15. Rousseau H, Puel J, Joffre F, et al. Self-expanding endovascular prosthesis: an experimental study. Radiology 1987;164:709–714.
16. Coons H. Self-expanding stainless steel biliary stents. Radiology 1989;170:979–983.
17. Irving JD, Adam A, Dick R, et al. Gianturco expandable metallic biliary stents: results of a European clinical trial. Radiology 1989;172:321–326.
18. Milroy E, Chapple C, Eldin A, et al. A new stent for the treatment of urethral strictures: preliminary report. Br J Urol 1989;63:392–396.
19. McNeal JE, Bostwick DG, Kindrachuk RA, et al. Patterns of progression in prostate cancer. Lancet 1986;1:60–63.
20. Kaufman JJ, Schultz JI. Needle biopsy of the prostate: a re-evaluation. J Urol 1962;87:164–168.
21. Golimbu M, Morales P, Al-Askari SA, et al. CAT scanning in staging of prostatic cancer. Urology 1981;18:305–308.
22. Pollack HM. Clinical imaging of prostatic carcinoma. Prog Clin Biol Res 1987;239:643–657.
23. Watanabe H. Historical perspectives on the use of transrectal sonography of the prostate. Prog Clin Biol Res 1987;237:5–13.
24. Lee F, Gray JM, McLeary RD, et al. Transrectal ultrasound in the diagnosis of prostate cancer: location, echogenicity, histopathology, and staging. Prostate 1985;7:117–129.
25. Rifkin MD, Friedland GW, Shortliffe L. Prostatic evaluation by transrectal endosonography: detection of carcinoma. Radiology 1986;158:85–90.
26. Griffiths GJ, Clements R, Jones DR, et al. The ultrasound appearances of prostatic cancer with histological correlation. Clin Radiol 1987;38:219–227.
27. Lee F. Transrectal ultrasound in the diagnosis, staging, guided needle biopsy, and screening for prostatic cancer. Prog Clin Biol Res 1987;237:73–109.
28. Berry SJ, Coffey DS, Walsh PC, et al. The development of human benign prostatic hyperplasia with age. J Urol 1984;132:474–479.
29. Wei JT, Calhoun EA, Jacobsen SJ. Benign prostatic hyperplasia. In: Litwin MS, Saigal CS, eds. Urologic Diseases in America. U.S. Department of Health and Human Services, Public Health Service, National Institutes of Health, National Institute of Diabetes and Digestive and Kidney Diseases. Washington: U.S. Government Publishing Office, 2004. Available at: http://kidney.niddk.nih.gov/statistics/uda/benign_prostatic_hyperplasia. Accessed April 29, 2005.
30. Bruskewitz RC, Larsen EH, Madsen PO, et al. 3-year followup of urinary symptoms after transurethral resection of the prostate. J Urol 1986;136:613–615.
31. Fowler FJ Jr, Wennberg JE, Timothy RP, et al. Symptom status and quality of life following prostatectomy. JAMA 1988;259:3018–3022.
32. Riley G, Lubitz J. Outcomes of surgery among the Medicare aged: surgical volume and mortality. Health Care Finance Rev 1985;7:37–47.
33. Wennberg JE, Roos N, Sola L, et al. Use of claims data systems to evaluate health care outcomes: mortality and re-operation following prostatectomy. JAMA 1987;257:933–936.
34. Lubitz J, Riley G, Newton M. Outcomes of surgery among the Medicare aged: mortality after surgery. Health Care Finance Rev 1985;6:103–105.
35. Mebust WK, Holtgrewe HL, Cockett AT, et al. Transurethral prostatectomy: immediate and postoperative complications. A cooperative study of 13 participating institutions evaluating 3,885 patients. J Urol 1989;141:243–247.
36. Caine M, Perlberg S, Meretyk S. A placebo-controlled double-blind study of the effect of phenoxybenzamine in benign prostatic obstruction. Br J Urol 1978;50:551.
37. Abrams PH, Shah PJ, Stone R, et al. Bladder outflow obstruction treated with phenoxybenzamine. Br J Urol 1982;54:527.

38. Brooks ME, Sidi AA, Hanani Y, et al. Ineffectiveness of phenoxy-benzamine in treatment of benign prostatic hypertrophy: a controlled study. Urology 1983;21:474–478.

39. Peters CA, Walsh PC. The effect of nafarelin acetate, a luteinizing-hormone-releasing hormone agonist, on benign prostatic hyperplasia. N Engl J Med 1987;317:599.

40. Gabrilove JL, Levine AC, Kirschenbaum A, et al. Effect of long-acting gonadotropin-releasing hormone analog (leuprolide) therapy on prostatic size and symptoms in 15 men with benign prostatic hypertrophy. J Clin Endocrinol Metab 1989;68:461.

41. Stone N. Flutamide in the treatment of benign prostatic hypertrophy. Urology 1989;34(Suppl):64.

42. Geller J, Nelson CG, Albert JD, et al. Effects of megestrol acetate on uroflow rates in patients with benign prostatic hypertrophy. Urology 1979;14:467.

43. Bartsch D. Electron microscopic stereological analysis of the normal human prostate and of benign prostatic hyperplasia. J Urol 1979;122:481.

44. Bartsch D. Light microscopic stereological analysis of the normal human prostate and of benign prostatic hyperplasia. J Urol 1979;122:487.

45. Ohrh P, Bartsch D. Human benign prostatic hyperplasia: stroma disease. New prospective by quantitative morphology. Urology 1980;16:625.

46. Klein L, Lemming B. Balloon dilatation for prostatic obstruction: long-term follow-up. Urology 1989;33:198–201.

47. Goldenberg L, Perez-Marrero R, Lee L, et al. Endoscopic balloon dilation of the prostate: early experience. J Urol 1990;144:83–88.

48. Dowd JB, Smith JJ 3rd. Balloon dilatation of the prostate. Urol Clin North Am 1990;17:671–677.

49. Daughtry JD, Rodan BA, Bean WJ. Balloon dilation of prostatic urethra. Urology 1990;36:203–209.

50. Grado G, Larson T, McKee G. Urethral dilation in prostatic malignancies for obstructive uropathy secondary to radiation-induced edema. Presented at the Radiological Society of North America, Chicago, IL, 1990.

51. Lopatin W, Martynik M, Hickey DP, et al. Retrograde transurethral balloon dilation of prostate: innovative management of abacterial chronic prostatitis and prostatodynia. Urology 1990;36:508–510.

52. Abrams P, Lewis P, Gillatt D, et al. Balloon dilatation in BPH under endoscopic control. Presented at meeting of the American Urological Association, Dallas, TX, 1989.

53. Hernandez-Graulau J, Goldberg H, Choudhury M, et al. Transurethral prostate divulsion for treatment of benign hyperplasia: New York Medical College preliminary report. Presented at meeting of the American Urological Association, Dallas, TX, 1989.

54. Klein LA, Perez-Marrero R, Bowers GW, et al. Balloon dilatation of the prostate: a multicenter study with one-year follow-up. Presented at meeting of the American Urological Association, Dallas, TX, 1989.

55. McCullough DL, Herrera M, Harrison LH, et al. Transurethral balloon dilatation of the prostate (TUBDP)—alternative to transurethral resection of the prostate. Presented at meeting of the American Urological Association, Dallas, TX, 1989.

56. Perez-Marrero RA, Emerson L. Urodynamic changes after prostatic balloon dilatation for outflow tract obstruction. Presented at meeting of the American Urological Association, Dallas, TX, 1989.

57. Reddy PK. Role of balloon dilation in the treatment of benign prostatic hyperplasia. Prostate 1990(Suppl);3:39–48.

58. Wasserman NF, Reddy PK, Zhang G, et al. Experimental treatment of benign prostatic hyperplasia with transurethral balloon dilation of the prostate: preliminary study in 73 humans. Radiology 1990;177:485–494.

59. Winfield HN, Castaneda F, Richardson K. Transurethral balloon dilation: University of Iowa experience. In: Castaneda F, Smith A, Castaneda-Zuniga W, eds. Therapeutic Alternatives in the Management of Benign Prostatic Hyperplasia. New York: Thieme, 1993:65–103.

60. Machan L, Gill KP, Abel P, et al. Prostatic urethroplasty: results at the Royal Postgraduate Medical School. Semin Intervent Radiol 1989;6:65–71.

61. Castaneda F, Hulbert JC, Letourneau JG, et al. Perineal abscess after prostatic urethroplasty with balloon catheter: report of a case. Radiology 1990;174:49–50.

62. Vicente J, Chechile G, Salvador J, et al. Long-term follow-up of patients with intraurethral prostheses. Semin Intervent Radiol 1989;6:82–89.

63. Reuter JH, Oettinger M. Las primeras experiencias con la espiral de acero en lugar del cateter permanente. Arch Esp Urol 1986;39:65–68.

64. Fabian KM. Der intraprostatische, partielle katheter (urologische spirale). Urologe 1980;19:236–238.

65. Fabricius PG, Matz M, Zepnick H. Die endourethralspiraleeine alternative zum daverkatheter? Arztl Fortbild (Jena) 1983;77:482–485.

66. Yachia D, Lask D, Rabinson S. Self-retaining intraurethral stent: an alternative to long-term indwelling catheters or surgery in the treatment of prostatism. AJR Am J Roentgenol 1990;154:111–113.

67. Milroy E. Self-expandable metallic prostatic urethral stents. In: Castaneda F, Smith A, Castaneda-Zuniga W, eds. Therapeutic Alternatives in the Management of Benign Prostatic Hyperplasia. New York: Thieme, in press.

68. Gesenberg A, Sintermann R. Management of benign prostatic hyperplasia in high risk patients: long-term experience with the Memotherm stent. J Urol 1998; 160:72–76.

69. Perez-Marrero R, Emerson LE. Balloon expandable titanium prostatic urethral stents. In: Castaneda F, Smith A, Castaneda-Zuniga W, eds. Therapeutic Alternatives in the Management of Benign Prostatic Hyperplasia. New York: Thieme, 1993:145–150.

70. Busch W. Ober den Einfluss welchen Heftigere Erysipeln Zuweilen auf Organisierte Neubildugen Ausuben. Verh Naurh Preuss Rhein Westphal 1866;23:28–30.

71. Bruns P. Die heilwirkung des Erysipels auf Geschwulste. Beitr Klin Chir 1877;3:443–466.

72. Coley WB. The treatment of malignant tumors by repeated inoculations of erysipelas—with a report of ten original cases. Am J Med Sci 1893;105:487–511.

73. Rohdenburg GL. Fluctuations in the growth of malignant tumors in man, with special reference to spontaneous recession. J Cancer Res 1918;3:193–225.

74. Nauts HC, Fowler GA, Bogatko FH. A review of the influence of bacterial infections and bacterial products (Coley's toxin) on malignant tumors in men. Acta Med Scand (Suppl) 1953;267:1–103.

75. Westermark F. Ober die Behandlung des Ulcerirenden Cervixcarcinomas. Mittel Konstanter Warme. Zentralbl Gynaekol 1898:1335–1339.

76. Gottschalk S. Zur Behandlung des Ulcerirenden inoperablen Cervixcarcinomas. Zentralbl Gynaekol 1899:79–80.

77. Vidal E. Travaux de la Deuxieme Conference Internationale pour l'Etude du Cancer. Paris, 1911:160.

78. Percy JF. Heat in the treatment of carcinomas of the uterus. Surg Gynecol Obstet 1916;22.77–79.

79. Goetz O. Ortliche Homogene Oberwarmung Gesunder und Kranker Gliedmassen. Dtsch Z Chir 1932;234:577–589.

80. Warren SL. Preliminary study of the effect of artificial fever upon hopeless tumor cases. AJR Am J Roentgenol 1935;33:75-87.

81. Woodhall B, Prickrill KL, Georgiade NG, et al. Effect of hyperthermia upon cancer chemotherapy—application to external cancer of head and face structures. Ann Surg 1960;151:750–759.

82. Crile G Jr. Selective destruction of cancers after exposure to heat. Ann Surg 1962;156:404–407.

83. Shingleton WW, Bryan FA, O'Quinn WL. Selective heating and cooling of tissue in cancer chemotherapy. Ann Surg 1962;156:408–416.

84. Kirsch R, Schmidt D. Erste Experimentelle and Klinische Erfahrungen mit der Gaszkorper-Extrem-Hyperthermie. In: Doerr W, Linder F, Wagner G, eds. Aktuelle Probleme aus dem Gebiet der Cancerologie. Heidelberg: Springer-Verlag, 1966:53–70.

85. Cavaliere R, Ciocatto EC, Giovanella BC, et al. Selective heat sensitivity of cancer cells. Biochemical and clinical studies. Cancer 1967;20:1351–1381.

86. Bicher HI, Hetzel FW, Sandhu TS, et al. Effects of hyperthermia on normal and tumor microenvironment. Radiology 1980;137:523–530.

87. Song CW, Kang MS, Rhee JG, et al. The effect of hyperthermia on vascular function, pH, and cell survival. Radiology 1980;137:795–803.

88. Emami B, Song CW. Physiological mechanisms in hyperthermia: a review. Int J Radiat Oncol Biol Phys 1984;10:289–295.

89. Astrahan MA, Norman A. A localized current field hyperthermia system for use with 192-iridium interstitial implants. Med Phys 1982;9:419–424.

90. Samaras GM. Intracranial microwave hyperthermia: heat induction and temperature control. IEEE Trans Biomed Eng 1984;31:63–69.

91. Strohbehn JW, Trembly BS, Douple EB. Blood flow effects on the temperature distributions from an invasive microwave antenna array used in cancer therapy. IEEE Trans Biomed Eng 1982;29:649–661.

92. Lyons BE, Britt RH, Strohbehn JW. Localized hyperthermia in the treatment of malignant brain tumors using an interstitial microwave antenna array. IEEE Trans Biomed Eng 1984;31:53–62.

93. Stauffer PR, Cetas TC, Jones RC. Magnetic induction heating of ferromagnetic implants for inducing localized hyperthermia in deep seated tumors. IEEE Trans Biomed Eng 1984;31:235–251.

94. Brezovich IA, Atkinson WJ, Lilly MB. Local hyperthermia with interstitial techniques. Cancer Res 1984;44 (Suppl):4752s–4756s.

95. Yerushalmi A. Localized, non-invasive deep microwave hyperthermia for the treatment of prostatic tumors: the first 5 years. Recent Results Cancer Res 1988;107:140–146.

96. Mendecki J, Friedenthal E, Botstein C, et al. Microwave applicators for localized hyperthermia treatment of cancer of the prostate. Int J Radiat Oncol Biol Phys 1980;6:1583–1588.

97. Kaver I, Ware JL, Koontz WW Jr. The effect of hyperthermia on human prostatic carcinoma cell lines: evaluation in vitro. J Urol 1989;141:1025–1027.

98. Lindner A, Golomb J, Siegel Y, et al. Local hyperthermia of the prostate gland for the treatment of benign prostatic hypertrophy and urinary retention: a preliminary report. Br J Urol 1987;60:567–571.

99. Servadio C, Leib Z, Lev A. Diseases of the prostate treated by local microwave hyperthermia. Urology 1987;30:97–99.

100. Yerushalmi A, Fishelovitz Y, Singer D, et al. Localized deep microwave hyperthermia in the treatment of poor operative risk patients with benign prostatic hyperplasia. J Urol 1985;133:873–886.

101. Servadio C, Leib Z, Lev A. Further observations on the use of local hyperthermia for the treatment of diseases of the prostate in man. Eur Urol 1986;12:38–40.

102. Astrahan MA, Sapozink MD, Cohen D, et al. Microwave applicator for transurethral hyperthermia of benign prostatic hyperplasia. Int J Hyperthermia 1989;5:283–296.

103. Leib Z, Rothem A, Lev A, et al. Histopathological observations in the canine prostate treated by local microwave hyperthermia. Prostate 1986;8:93–102.

104. Blandy JP. The history and current problems of prostatic obstruction. In: Blandy JP, Lytton BJ, eds. The Prostate. Chicago: Butterworths, 1986:17–18.

105. Littrup PJ, Lee F. Screening for prostate cancer: state of the art. Semin Intervent Radiol 1989;6:10–19.

106. Lee SB, Lee F, Solomon MH, et al. Seminal vesicle abscess: diagnosis by transrectal ultrasound. J Clin Ultrasound 1986;14:546.

107. Littrup PJ, Lee F, McLeary RD, et al. Transrectal US of the seminal vesicles and ejaculatory ducts: clinical correlation. Radiology 1988;168:625.

108. Patel PS, Wilbur AC. Cystic seminal vesiculitis: CT demonstration. J Comput Assist Tomogr 1987;11:1103.

109. Rifkin MD. Ultrasound of the Prostate. New York: Raven, 1988.

110. Llerena J, Letourneau JG. Other prostatic interventions: seminal vesicles. Semin Intervent Radiol 1989;6:102–107.

Interventions in Urinary Diversions

41

Parvati Ramchandani

Urinary diversion is performed in patients who have undergone cystectomy and in those with dysfunctional or nonfunctioning urinary bladders. The technique has evolved from the surgical creation of cutaneous fistulas such as nephrostomy, pyelostomy, or ureterostomy for urinary drainage to the use of the intestinal tract to divert and reconstruct the urinary tract (1).

Ureterosigmoidostomy was the most common form of urinary drainage into the bowel until the early 1950s. In this procedure, the ureters are anastomosed to an intact sigmoid colon that is in continuity with the fecal stream. The frequent occurrence of complications such as pyelonephritis, upper urinary tract deterioration, and colon carcinoma at the site of the ureteral anastomosis led to decreasing enthusiasm for this form of urinary diversion (2,3). However, patients with this form of urinary diversion are still seen occasionally in current clinical practice (4) (Figure 41–1).

Currently, ureters are implanted into bowel segments that are isolated from the intestinal and fecal streams. Two primary forms of such urinary diversion are the ileal conduit and the continent urinary diversions.

Ileal conduits, also referred to as ileal loop, ureteroileostomy, and Bricker loop, were introduced by Bricker in 1950 (5) and are an important form of permanent supravesical urinary drainage. A 15–25-cm loop of distal small bowel is isolated, and its proximal end is brought to the lower abdominal wall as a stoma while the distal end (the "butt" end) is closed. The ureters are anastomosed in an end-to-side fashion to the isolated ileal segment, a technique that permits free retrograde reflux of ileal segment contents (urine admixed with mucus) into the ureters (Figure 41–2). Ileal conduits are relatively easy to construct and are the gold standard by which all urinary diversions

are judged. However, the necessity for an external appliance on the stoma to collect the urine and a significant rate of long-term complications, including reflux-induced deterioration in renal function, led to the development of alternative procedures.

Continent urinary diversions are low pressure, large capacity reservoirs constructed from small bowel alone or from a combination of small and large bowel. They drain through either a continent abdominal wall stoma—cutaneous, or the urethra—orthotopic (6,7) (Figure 41–3). With cutaneous reservoirs, the stoma is placed at or below the umbilicus, and the patient self-catheterizes every 3–4 hours. Patients with orthotopic pouches void by abdominal straining. The many variations in surgical technique and radiologic imaging are not discussed in this chapter, but they are addressed in numerous reviews on the subject (8–13). Patients have accepted the cutaneous and orthotopic continent diversions enthusiastically because these procedures obviate the use of an external urine collection device. The long-term results and effects on renal function with continent diversions remain a subject of study (14); reports suggest that the detrimental effects on renal function with orthotopic reservoirs may be less than with ileal conduit diversions (7,15).

COMPLICATIONS OF URINARY DIVERSION

Complications such as metabolic alterations, urinary tract infections, and alterations in renal function and morphology are not considered in this chapter; however, interventional procedures for complications associated with ileal

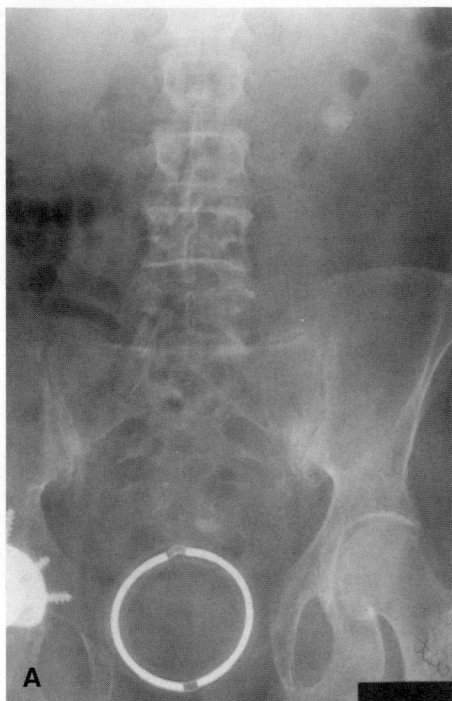

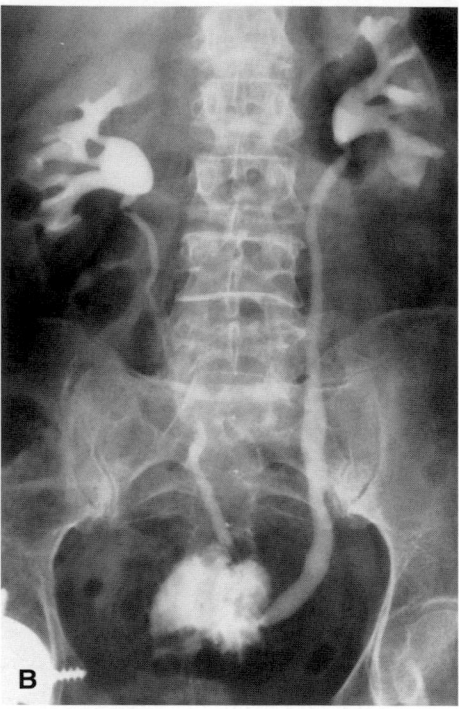

Figure 41–1 Ureterosigmoidostomy in a patient with bladder exstrophy. **A.** Plain film demonstrates calculus in lower pole of left kidney and in distal left ureter. There is a vaginal pessary with a radiopaque ring in place for prolapse unrelated to the urinary diversion. **B.** Intravenous urogram (IVU) demonstrates ureteral insertion into sigmoid colon. The renal and ureteral calculi were removed percutaneously (*not illustrated*).

conduit urinary diversions and continent diversions are addressed. These will be discussed together because of their similarities.

Early complications that occur fewer than 30 days postoperatively can be separated into two main groups: general postoperative complications and complications related to the urinary pouch or the ureteral-pouch anastomotic site. General complications include those related to the wound and collections in the cystectomy bed, such as hematomas and abscesses. The management of them is similar to that of collections at other sites (16,17).

Urinary extravasation is the most common urologic complication in the early postoperative period and may be seen in 17–30% of patients (18,19). Leakage usually occurs at one or more of the suture lines and may be from the urinary pouch or ileal conduit, the ureteroenteric anastomosis, or the ureteral-pouch anastomosis. Patients may present with abdominal pain, prolonged ileus, decreasing urine output from the reservoir or ileal conduit, or increased drainage from surgical drains in the operative site. Definitive diagnosis is made by contrast study of the ileal conduit or reservoir (Figure 41–4). Evaluation of fluid drainage from

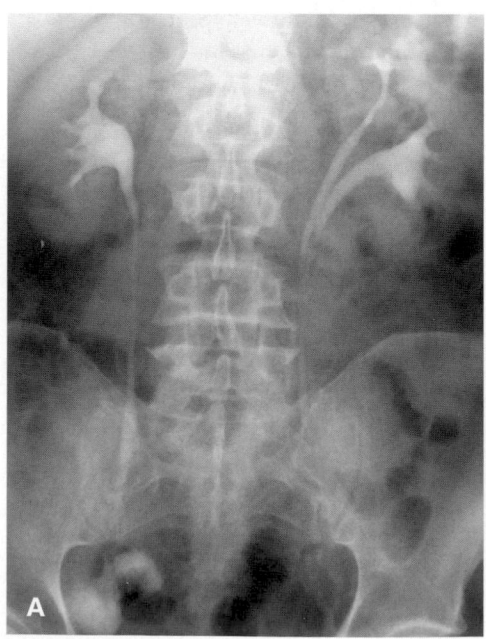

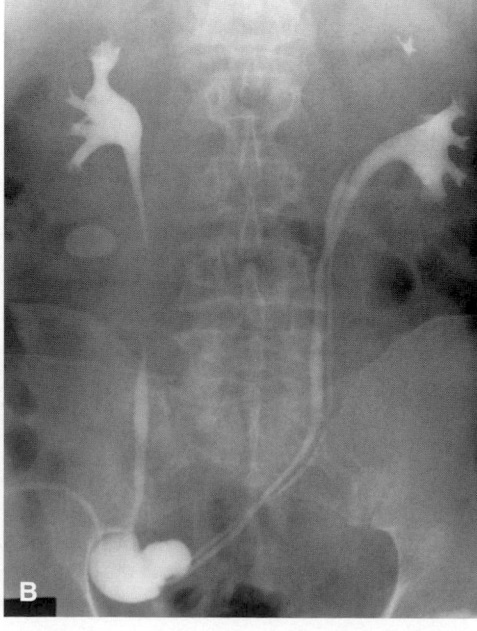

Figure 41–2 Urinary diversion to an ileal conduit. **A.** IVU and ileal conduit injection (loopogram) demonstrate the expected normal appearance. **B.** There is free bilateral reflux into the ureters and collecting systems on the loopogram.

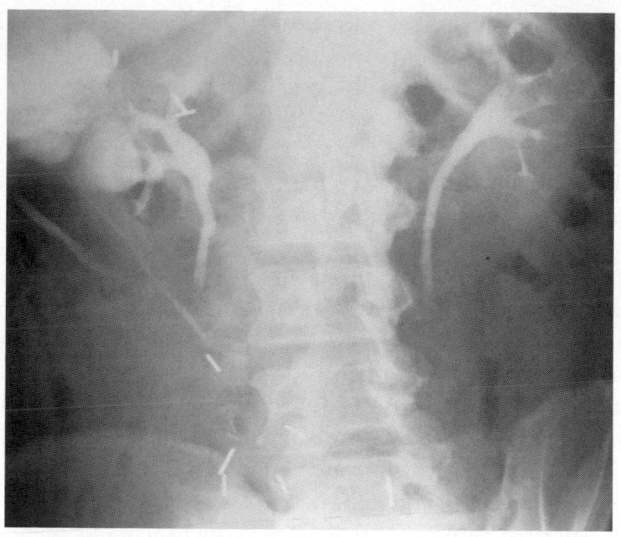

Figure 41–3 Continent urinary diversion, normal appearance. Cutaneous diversion (Indiana pouch) with ureters draining into a colonic pouch in the right upper abdomen.

surgical drains for blood urea nitrogen (BUN) and creatinine is also sensitive in diagnosing a urinary leak. Most patients can be treated successfully with continued catheter drainage of the urinary pouch and with placement of a drainage catheter extraluminally at the leak site (19,20). Close proximity of Jackson-Pratt (JP) drains to the anastomosis sometimes can cause persistent leakage because of the suction created by these large bore drains. In such cases, replacement of the large bore JP drains with smaller pigtail drainage catheters at a greater distance from the anastomosis can be very helpful (19).

Extravasation at the ureteroileal or ureteroenteric anastomosis is clinically indistinguishable from leaks emanating from the conduit or reservoir. The diagnosis usually is made by contrast studies of the ureteral stents left in postoperatively—a common surgical practice for both ureteroileostomies and continent diversions (Figure 41–5), or by an intravenous urogram (IVU) or CT scan with imaging in the excretory phase. Most such

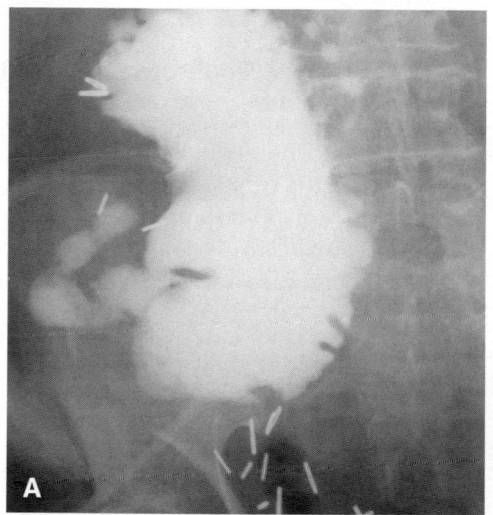

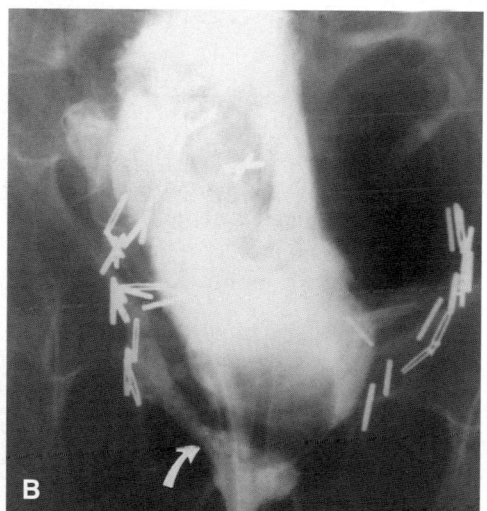

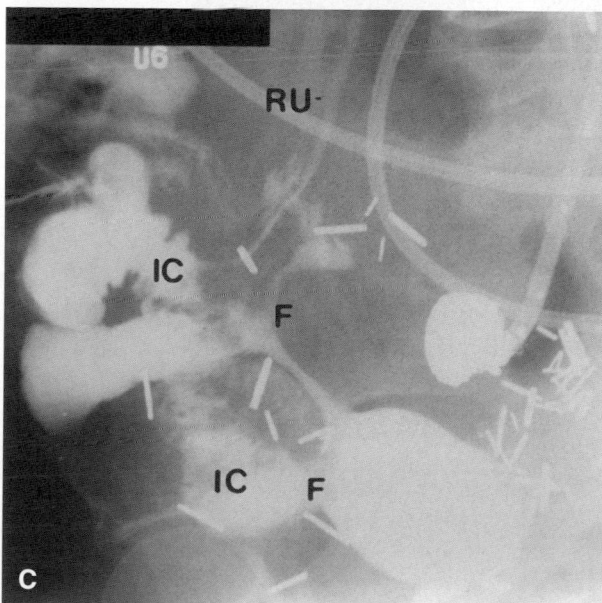

Figure 41–4 Contrast studies of urinary pouches. **A.** Normal appearance of an Indiana pouch. Contrast was injected through a catheter left in the pouch postoperatively. **B.** Extravasation from anastomosis of orthotopic pouch to urethra (*arrow*), successfully managed with prolonged Foley catheter drainage of pouch. **C.** Enteroenteral fistulas after ureteroileostomy. IC, ileal conduit; RU, right ureter; F, fistulas.

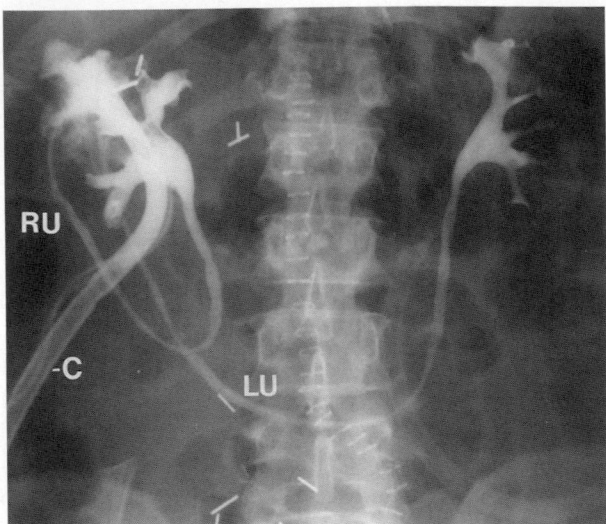

Figure 41–5 Normal contrast study performed through ureteral stents in a patient with an Indiana pouch. No extravasation is seen. (RU) right ureter; (LU) left ureter; (C) drainage catheter in pouch.

leaks will heal spontaneously if the ureteral stents are left in place until complete healing occurs. Percutaneous nephrostomy and ureteral stenting are required when leaks develop after the stents have been removed. Anastomotic leaks appear to be more prevalent in highly irradiated ileal conduit patients, probably because of radiation injury to the distal ureters in patients with pelvic neoplasms (21). A higher rate of extravasation has been reported in patients with ileal conduits than with continent diversions (21).

Occasionally, extravasation at the anastomosis is related to actual detachment of the ureter.

Minor, and occasionally large degrees of extravasation at the ureteroenteral anastomotic site, can often be successfully treated with ureteral stenting with no untoward sequelae (22). However, extravasation can predispose to later stricture formation in the ureter or at the ureteroenteral anastomosis (23).

Late complications, defined as those occurring 30 days or more after surgery, may be related to the ureteroenteral anastomosis and to the ileal conduit or continent bowel reservoir. It is important to emphasize that significant complications that may affect renal function adversely may develop silently and may not be apparent clinically (Figure 41–6). Periodic radiologic evaluation of these patients is therefore mandatory, with the first postoperative sonogram being obtained at 3 months to assess for hydronephrosis and subsequent studies being performed annually if the patient remains asymptomatic (20,23,24). A baseline IVU is performed at 3 months if the patient's renal function is normal and at regular intervals thereafter to monitor the upper urinary tract for recurrence of urothelial tumor.

Ureteroenteral Anastomotic Strictures

Strictures at the anastomosis of the ureter to the pouch or conduit are often benign. However, benign obstructive stricturing at the ureteroenteral anastomosis is the most significant surgical complication of urinary diversions because it can result in impairment of renal function. Reportedly, it occurs in 4–30% of patients (25–27). One

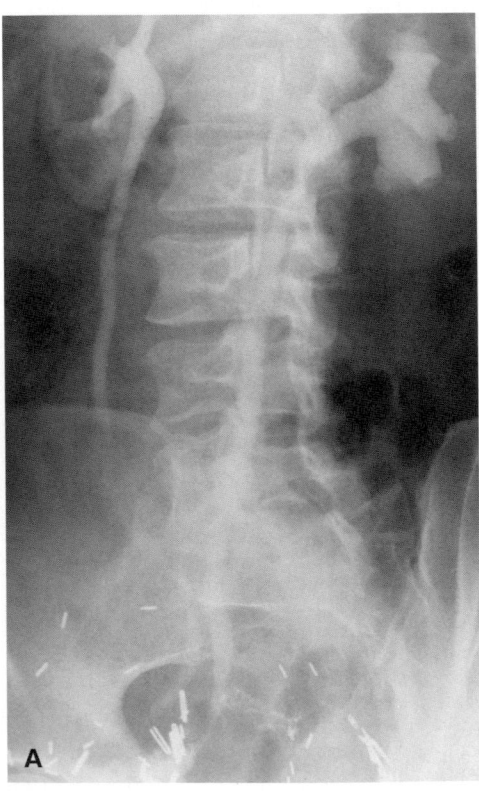
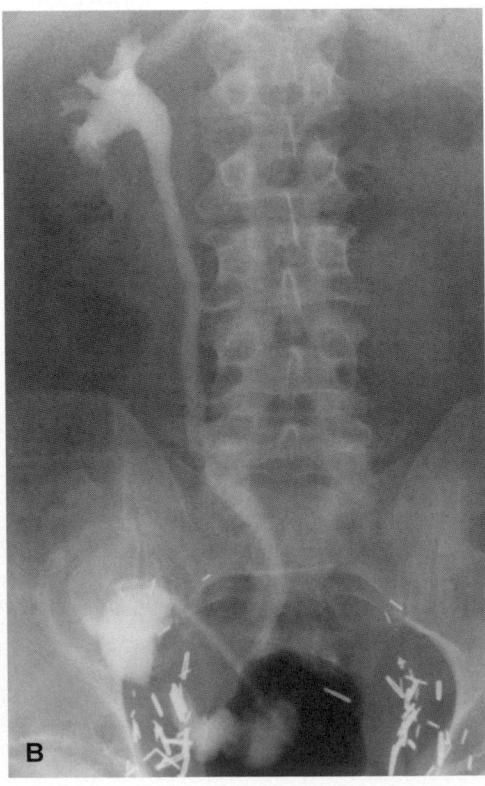

Figure 41–6 Ureteroileal anastomotic stricture. **A.** IVU demonstrates left hydronephrosis and stricture at ureteroileal anastomotic site. **B.** Loopogram demonstrates no reflux through the stenotic left anastomosis and ready reflux on the right side.

study that compared complications in the different forms of urinary diversion reported the incidence of ureteroenteric strictures in ileal conduits to be 6.5%, compared to 10.0% in the continent reservoir group and 13.6% in patients who underwent ureterosigmoidostomy (26). The predisposing factors are ischemic necrosis and subsequent fibrosis and stricture resulting from excessive mobilization and skeletonization of the ureter. Preoperative radiation therapy appears to have a compounding effect. Extravasation at the anastomosis may progress to scarring and, subsequently, to a stricture; rarely, recurrent tumor in the ureter may present with obstruction. Stenoses tend to be more prevalent on the left side, probably because of the necessity for high mobilization of the left ureter (to ensure a gradual course to the right), which often requires the middle ureteric artery to be sacrificed (28). Rarely, ureteral obstruction can be the result of extrinsic compression by a crossing vessel or to compression at the site at which the left ureter is brought through the sigmoid mesocolon into the peritoneal cavity to be anastomosed to the ileal conduit. Strictures can predispose patients to urinary infections, stone formation, and loss of renal function, which can often be clinically silent.

Surgical revision of anastomotic strictures is fraught with technical difficulty because of fibrotic adhesions from prior surgery and frequently, from prior radiation therapy. Nonoperative interventional therapy has been embraced as an alternative, but results to date have been disappointing and not equivalent to those of surgical repair. However, the lower morbidity of interventional techniques and the ability to perform open repair whenever interventional procedures fail justify the continuing primary application of interventional and endourologic procedures.

The diagnosis of an anastomotic stricture is made when an intravenous urogram, renal ultrasound, or CT scan demonstrates progressive hydronephrosis or a loopogram demonstrates absence of ureteral reflux in a patient in whom the diagnosis of a stricture is being entertained (Figure 41–6). Although highly sensitive, ultrasound examination in this situation demonstrates a specificity of only 50% because of the high prevalence of dilated collecting systems that are not obstructed in patients with ureteroileostomies (29). Both antegrade and retrograde studies are performed in an attempt to define the site, length, degree of narrowing, and possible etiology of the stricture. Brush biopsies are performed whenever there is a concern that the stricture may be malignant. There is consensus that malignant obstruction is best treated by ureteral stenting and drainage. With benign strictures, as previously mentioned, the frequency and severity of complications associated with repeat surgery for repair of the strictures have led to the acceptance of percutaneous interventions as the primary modality of treatment.

Ureteroenteral anastomotic strictures are best cannulated through a combined antegrade and retrograde approach (30). Nonrefluxing strictured anastomoses are difficult to catheterize in a transconduit fashion—success occurs in only 14–56% of patients (31,32). Continent diversions, whether cutaneous or orthotopic, are treated by the antegrade route.

The retrograde route usually is successful in catheterizing patent ureteroileal anastomoses in 85–100% of patients (31–34) (Figure 41–7). Patients with patent ureteroenteral anastomosis require the procedure to drain partially obstructing ureteral strictures, to extract renal or ureteral calculi (in patients who would otherwise require a

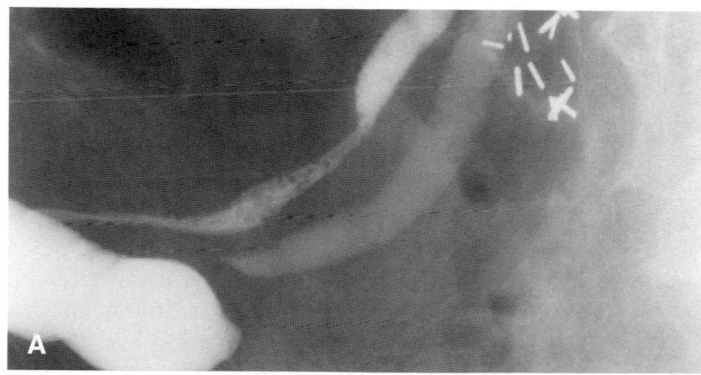

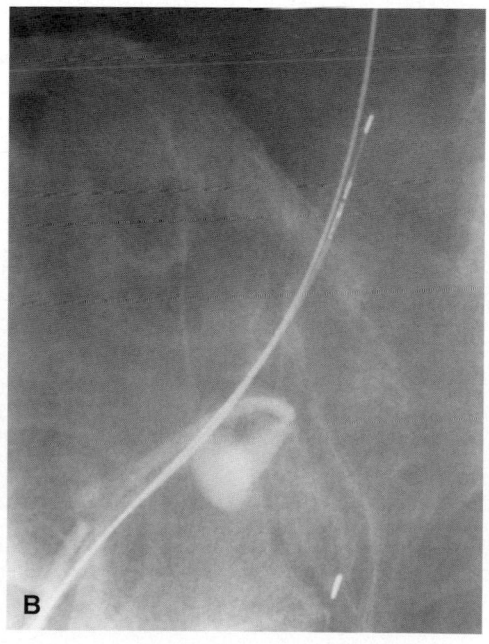

Figure 41–7   A. Patent ureteroenteral anastomosis with bilateral reflux. Multiple filling defects were seen in the distal portion of the right ureter, which was catheterized easily in a retrograde fashion **B.** for brush biopsy to rule out tumor recurrence of transitional cell carcinoma. Filling defects proved to be the result of ureteritis cystica and not tumor recurrence.

percutaneous nephrostomy), and for brush biopsies of filling defects in the collecting systems. Endoscopy of an ileal conduit is not always successful in identifying or catheterizing the ureteroenteral anastomosis. Retrograde ureteroscopy has been reported to be successful in 10 of 13 patients with orthotopic ileal neobladder urinary diversion in one series (35).

The radiologic management of a ureteroenteral anastomotic in an ileal conduit urinary diversion stricture consists of performing a percutaneous nephrostomy; maneuvering a guide wire down the ureter, across the anastomotic stricture, through the ileal conduit, and out the stoma; then advancing a balloon catheter to the site of the stricture. High-pressure, reinforced balloons of 8–10 mm in diameter and 4–10 cm in length are preferable. As with balloon dilation of other benign ureteral strictures, there is no consensus on the size of the balloon, the ideal period of balloon inflation, the necessity or desirability of repeated inflations, and, lastly, the size of the catheter used to stent the newly dilated anastomosis. The ureteral stent placement following the balloon dilation is performed in a retrograde transconduit fashion through the ileal conduit. The stent should have a large lumen with side holes only in the renal pelvis, and it should be long enough to extend beyond the stoma into the ileostomy drainage bag (Figure 41–8). The standard-length 25-cm nephrostomy catheter is not long enough to protrude through the stoma into the drainage bag. Use of 8–10 French all-purpose locking loop catheters of 40–50 cm in length is recommended. Side holes along the shaft of the catheter should be avoided because intestinal mucus can reflux into the renal pelvis and predispose to occlusion of drainage holes

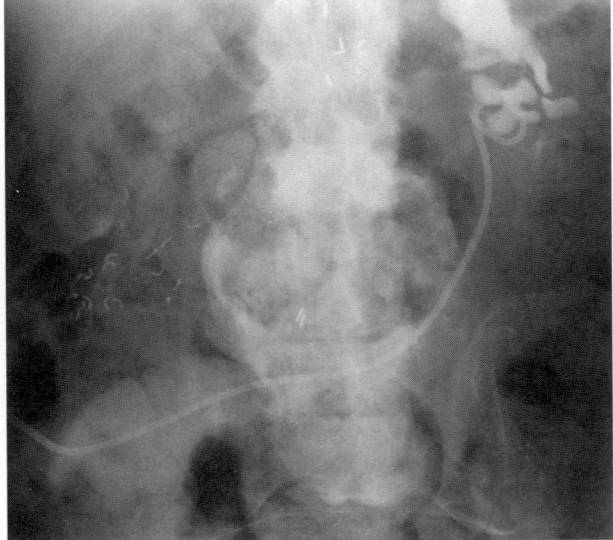

Figure 41–8   Placement of a drainage catheter in a retrograde, transconduit fashion through an ileal loop. The distal end of the catheter drains into a bag attached to the stoma.

(33,36). Thus, the standard double pigtail ureteral stent, with one pigtail in the renal collecting system and the other end within the conduit, is not appropriate for drainage in patients with urinary diversions to the bowel. Some studies (37) have reported no problems with catheter occlusion even with side holes positioned within the conduit. The catheter is left in place for roughly 6 weeks, after which a nephrostogram is performed. If the stricture appears persistent, a second attempt at balloon dilation is made. Because of the high recurrence rate of ureteral strictures after apparently successful balloon dilation, close follow-up is essential to detect stricture recurrence before renal function deteriorates.

With continent diversions, a large-bore, self-retaining, single pigtail catheter is placed through the nephrostomy site with the pigtail end in the pouch. Then, the catheter is capped externally. This catheter merely stents open the newly dilated segment. An additional nephrostomy catheter is placed to drain the kidney. Placing a stent that can allow mucus from the pouch to reflux into the renal collecting system is not prudent because the stent can be occluded easily and may even cause sepsis (36).

The long-term results of balloon dilation of ureteroenteral anastomotic strictures are poor, indicating that the strictures are resistant to nonoperative therapy. Shapiro et al. (38) reported a patency rate of only 30% at 6 months and 16% at 1 year. Similarly, Chang and Kramolowsky (39,40) reported patency rates of 20–38% at 1 year. Kwak et al. (37) reported a 9-month success rate of 18% for continuing patency of balloon-dilated anastomotic strictures. They found that multiple dilations were of no benefit in maintaining ureteral patency. Overall, the average success rate in many series is 29% at 14 months (41).

The addition of endoscopic electroincision of the stricture to balloon dilation may improve patency rates to 42–71% (36,42,43), with average follow-up of 16–28 months. Wolf et al. (44) used electrocautery and Acucise cutting balloon and reported success rates of 72%, 51%, and 32% at 1, 2, and 3 years, respectively; right-sided strictures had a better outcome with 68% of strictures improved at 3 years versus 17% of left-sided strictures. The authors also found no correlation between successful treatment and stricture length or stricture diameter, but they did report a higher success rate with the use of stents of 12 French or larger with a stenting period longer than 4 weeks, and with treatment of strictures within 24 months after the inciting event. Holmium laser endoureterotomy (45) has a reported success rate of 57–83% for right-sided strictures and 38% for left-sided strictures. Injury to the iliac artery has been reported with endoureterotomy (46). Cornud et al. (47) reported that incision of strictures had an actuarial 3-year patency rate of 62%. The authors also found that strictures associated with a continent neobladder responded more favorably than did the ureteroileal strictures.

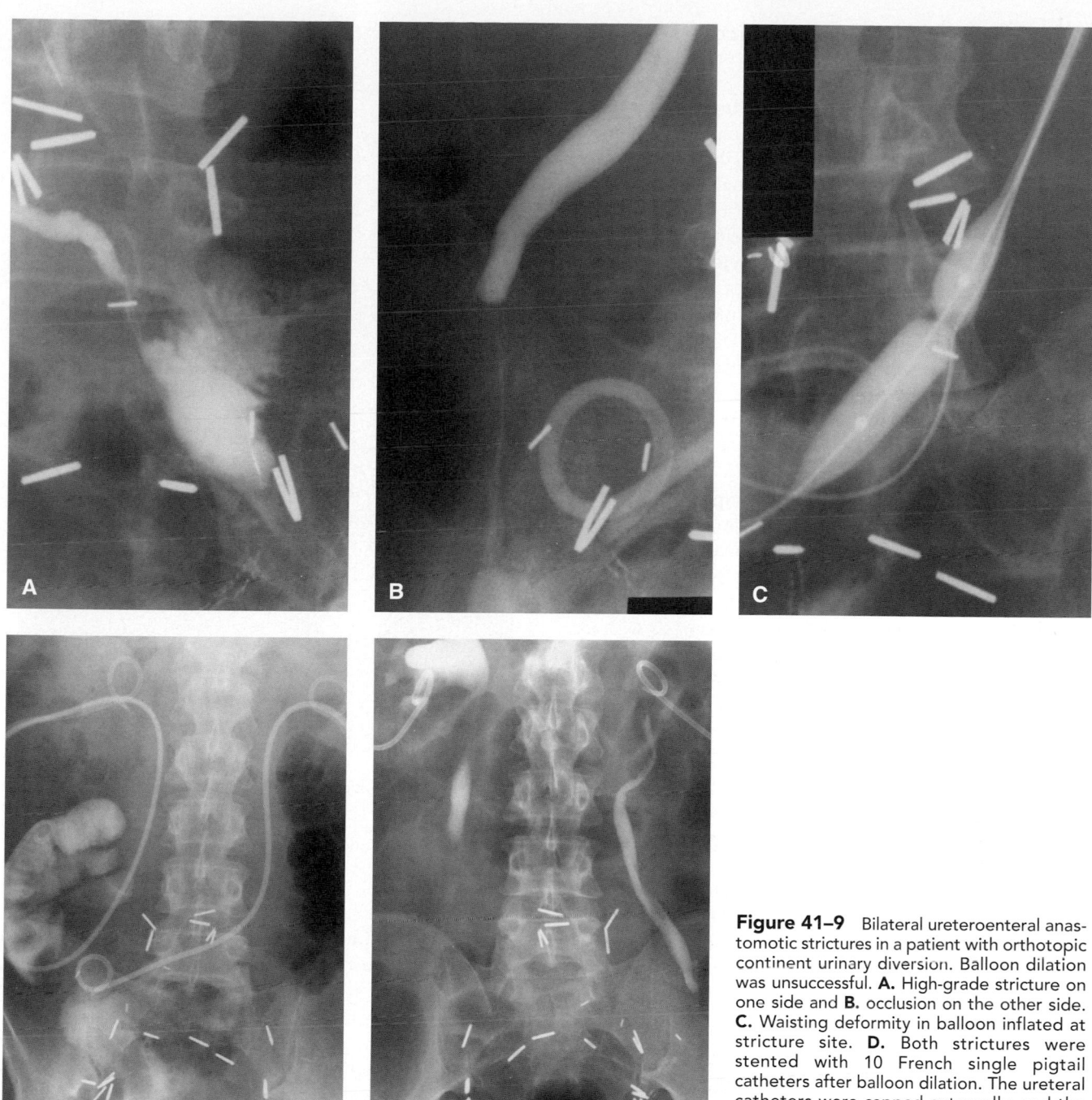

Figure 41-9 Bilateral ureteroenteral anastomotic strictures in a patient with orthotopic continent urinary diversion. Balloon dilation was unsuccessful. **A.** High-grade stricture on one side and **B.** occlusion on the other side. **C.** Waisting deformity in balloon inflated at stricture site. **D.** Both strictures were stented with 10 French single pigtail catheters after balloon dilation. The ureteral catheters were capped externally, and the kidneys were drained by nephrostomy catheters. **E.** Nephrostogram 1 week after ureteral stent removal shows no passage of contrast into the urinary pouch. The patient underwent successful surgical repair.

Metal stents have also been used to treat anastomotic strictures. To date, the reported series are small. Pollak et al. (48) reported that metallic stents (Wallstent endoprostheses) are ineffective in keeping benign ureteroileal strictures patent. Only one of six stents remained patent at 11 months; the remainder showed occlusions resulting from hyperplastic tissue growth within the stent. Other series report 100% patency at 10 months and 22 months (49,50). The role of metal stents in the management of these patients continues to evolve, and judgment must be deferred until larger cohorts of patients have been treated.

Ureteroenteral Anastomotic Strictures in Continent Diversions

Rates of ureteral obstruction vary depending on the type of pouch and ureteral anastomosis, with a reported 3% incidence for Kock reservoirs (51) and a 10% incidence for the modified Indiana pouch (52). Wilson et al. (52) reported dismal results with combined therapy of balloon dilation and incision of strictures. The failure rate of percutaneous therapy was 83%, whereas subsequent ureteral reimplantation was successful in 91%. They also reported an increased risk for stricture complications in patients who received preoperative radiation therapy, whereas Frazier et al. (26) reported no increase in the risk of long-term complications with radiation therapy. Strictures that develop in patients with orthotopic neobladders appear to respond more favorably than do those in ileal conduits or cutaneous continent diversions (47).

A few technical points need to be emphasized at this juncture. The antegrade route is the safest and most practical approach for stricture dilation because there is no reported experience regarding the feasibility and safety of cannulating nonrefluxing ureterocolonic anastomoses. After dilation, an 8–10 French stent is placed across the anastomosis with its distal end in the colonic pouch and the proximal end obturated to prevent intrarenal reflux of mucus. In addition, a nephrostomy catheter is placed within the renal pelvis to facilitate drainage of the kidney. There are no reports regarding the effect of balloon dilation on the antireflux properties of the anastomosis, but the experience of some operators indicates no significant ureteral reflux when the balloon dilation is successful. After a 6- to 8-week period of stenting, the ureteral stent is removed, and the effects of balloon dilation are assessed by a nephrostogram performed via the remaining nephrostomy catheter (Figure 41–9). When open surgical repair of the anastomotic stricture becomes necessary, the preoperative placement of a stent across the stricture (through a nephrostomy access) is helpful because it facilitates identification of the ureter (52).

Complications Related to the Conduit

Ileal Conduit

Patients with ureteroileostomies may develop parastomal hernias, volvulus of the conduit (usually because of an excessively long ileal segment), fistulas (often enteroenteric), and conduit malfunction. In addition, stenoses and calculi can form in the conduit (Figure 41–10). Interventional procedures have no significant role in managing conduit-related complications other than for calculi. The stenoses are characterized histologically by a chronic inflammatory reaction in the mucosa and submucosa, and such stenoses respond poorly to balloon dilation. Conduit stenoses can occur at the level of the stoma, the fascia, or the ileal segment itself (Figures 41–10 and 41–11).

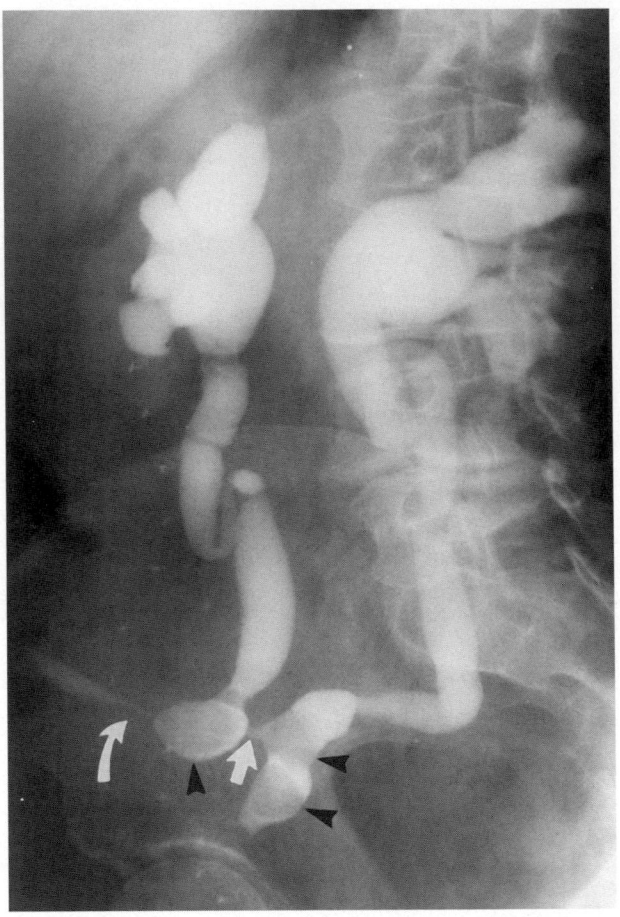

Figure 41–10   Multiple stenotic segments (*arrows*) in ileal conduit with stones (*arrowheads*) seen as filling defects in the opacified conduit. Note the bilateral hydronephrosis. Conduit stenoses respond poorly to balloon dilation and generally require surgical revision.

Stones in a conduit usually occur in relation to strictures within the conduit or on exposed metallic staples (53). The incidence of staple-related calculi is 3–7%, with the stones forming in the first 3 postoperative years. Most calculi usually can be managed by the use of endoscopically directed electrohydraulic lithotripsy, whereas the stenoses require surgical revision. When calculi develop within the ureters, they can be approached through the ileal conduit in a retrograde fashion (Figure 41–12), whereas renal calculi require a percutaneous approach or extracorporeal shock wave lithotripsy, depending on stone and patient characteristics (Figure 41–13). Sutures and staples can migrate to the renal pelvis and serve as a nidus for calculous formation (54).

Iliac arterioureteral fistula is a potentially lethal complication and is seen in patients with prolonged ureteral catheterization and ureteral ileal urinary diversion. Often, there is a history of previous radiation therapy. The constant pulsation of an iliac artery transmitted to a firm stent within a compromised ureter can produce pressure necrosis where the ureter crosses the iliac artery (55,56). Patients

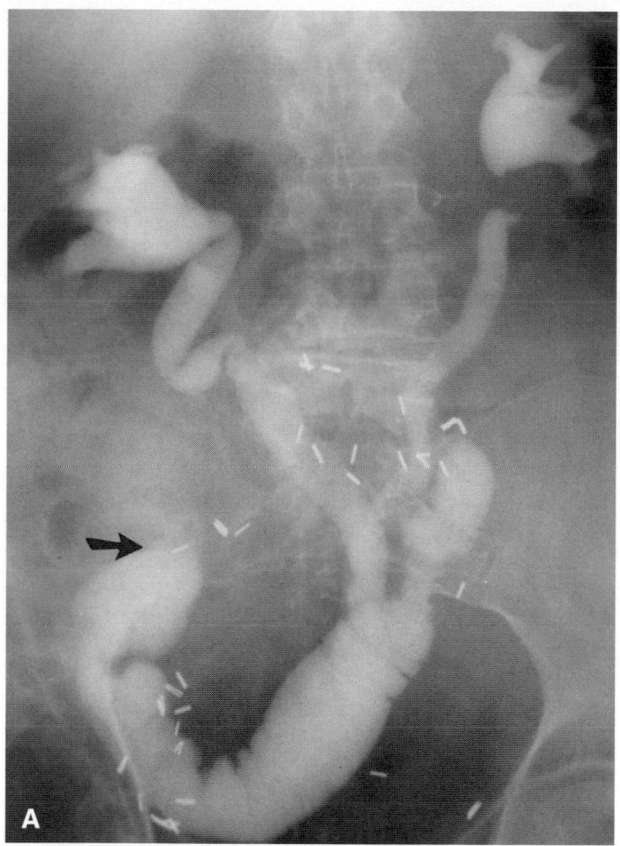

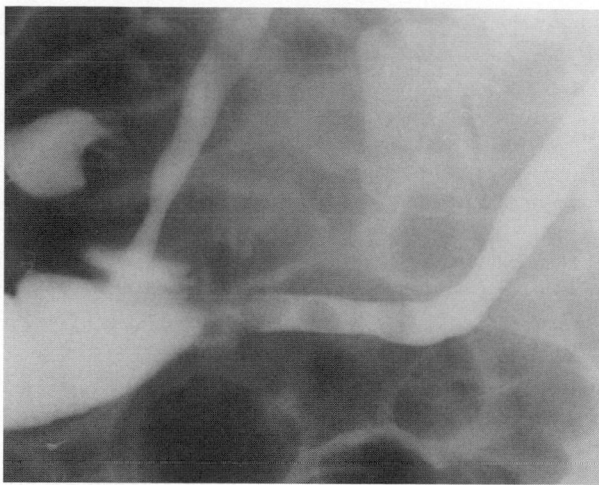

Figure 41–12 Loopogram demonstrating multiple calculi in distal left ureter. Calculi are seen as filling defects (*arrows*) in the opacified ureter. They were removed in a transconduit retrograde fashion with a basket.

may present with life threatening hematuria or prolonged intermittent urinary tract bleeding. Correct preoperative diagnosis usually has a happy outcome, while an undiagnosed iliac arterioureteral fistula is associated with a high mortality rate.

CONTINENT DIVERSIONS

Most interventional procedures related to the reservoir in continent urinary diversion are for the management of calculi. Kock pouches appear to be particularly vulnerable to this complication because of the use of metallic staples that act as a foreign-body nidus (57). The reported incidence varies from 3–33%. Urolithiasis has not been a problem with the Indiana pouch (52). Most stones can be treated successfully by endoscopic stone removal. Extracorporeal shock wave lithotripsy has a more peripheral role for these calculi (57). Endoscopy may be performed either through the stoma (and the efferent limb) or by establishing a percutaneous track into the neobladder (58). Also, staples exposed on the mucosal surface can serve as a nidus for stone formation in continent diversions (59); these sutures and metallic staples can migrate to the renal pelvis in a retrograde fashion and simulate urothelial neoplasm (60).

If the stoma or the efferent limb of a cutaneous continent diversion becomes stenotic, fluoroscopy and standard interventional techniques may be used to negotiate the stenotic limb for placing a drainage catheter into the pouch. If these attempts fail, percutaneous puncture of the pouch may be performed using ultrasound or fluoroscopic guidance—if contrast can be instilled into the pouch through the stoma.

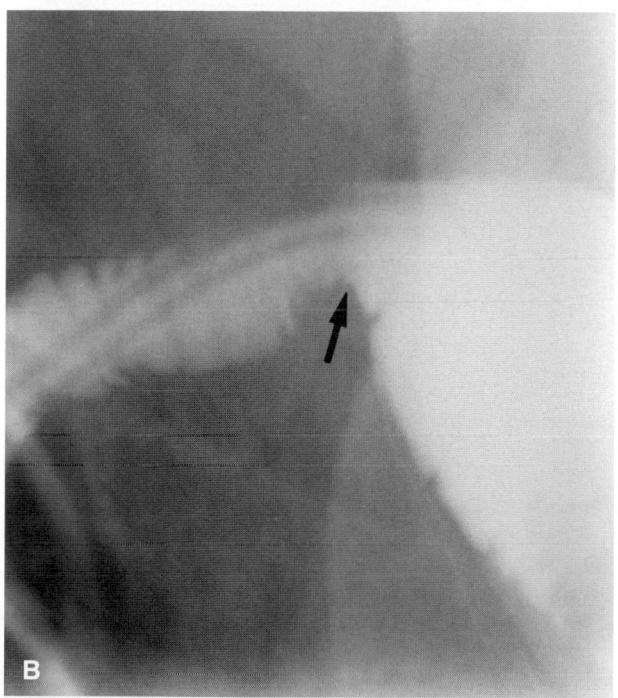

Figure 41–11 Stenosis at fascial level causing obstruction of ileal conduit. **A.** Loopogram demonstrates dilation of conduit proximal to fascial stenosis (*arrow*). **B.** The conduit distal to the stenosis (*arrow*) is of smaller caliber.

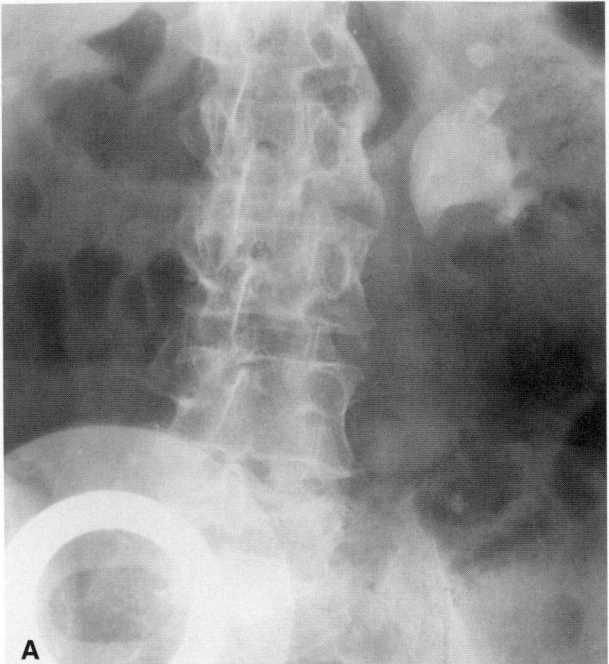

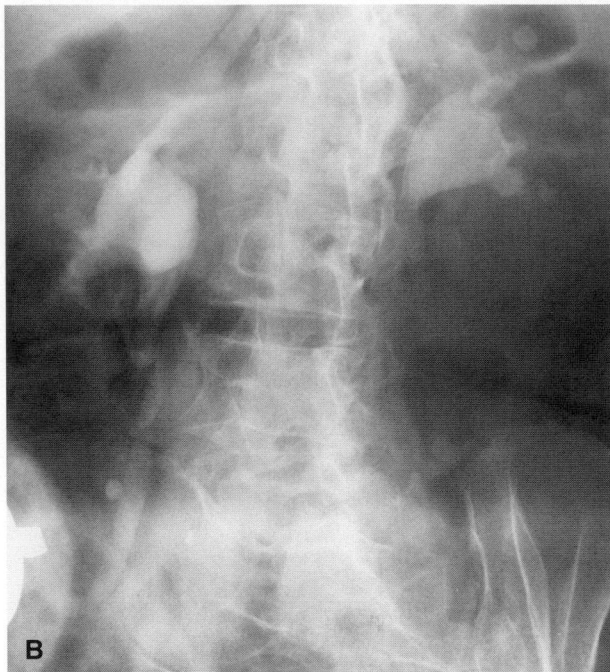

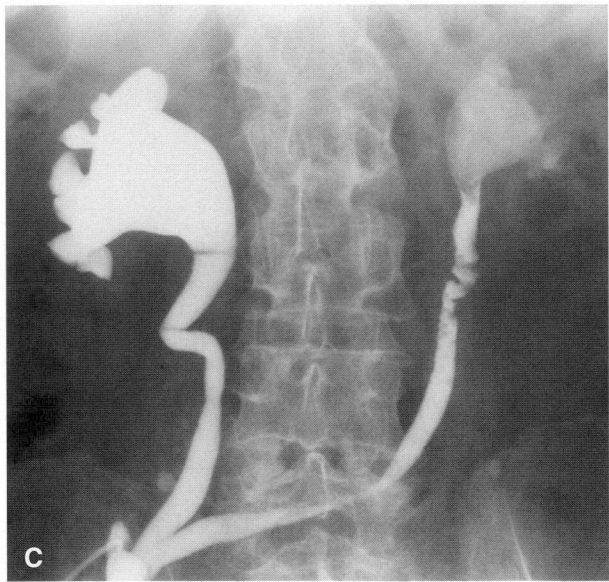

Figure 41–13 Staghorn calculus in patient with ileal conduit urinary diversion. **A.** Plain film and **B.** IVU demonstrate a large left staghorn calculus. **C.** Loopogram demonstrates no stricture at the ureteroenteral anastomosis. The patient was treated with percutaneous stone removal.

REFERENCES

1. Rosen MA, Roth DR, Gonzales ET. Current indications for cutaneous ureterostomy. Urology 1994;43:92–96.
2. Clarke BG, Leadbetter WF. Ureterosigmoidostomy: collective results in 2,897 reported cases. J Urol 1955;73:999–1008.
3. Sooriyaarachchi GS, Johnson RO, Carbone PP. Neoplasms of the large bowel following ureterosigmoidostomy. Arch Surg 1977; 112:1174–1177.
4. Sakhuja V, Das T, Malik N, et al. A 55-year follow-up of a patient with bilateral ureterosigmoidostomy. J Urol 1992;147:1104–1106.
5. Bricker EM. Bladder substitution after pelvic evisceration. Surg Clin North Am 1950;30:1511–1521.
6. Middleton AW Jr, Hendren WH. Ileal conduits in children at the Massachusetts General Hospital from 1955 to 1970. J Urol 1976;115:591.
7. Madersbacher S, Schmidt J, Eberle JM, et al. Long-term outcome of ileal conduit diversion. J Urol 2003;169–985–990.
8. Amis ES, Newhouse JH, Olsson CA. Continent urinary diversions: review of current surgical procedures and radiologic imaging. Radiology 1988;168:395–401.
9. Goldwasser B, Webster GD. Continent urinary diversion. J Urol 1985;134:227–236.
10. Spring DB, Deshon GE. Radiology of vesical and supravesical urinary diversions. In: Pollack HM, ed. Clinical Urography. Philadelphia: WB Saunders, 1990:296–310.
11. Keogan MT, Carr L, McDermott VG, et al. Continent urinary diversion procedures: radiographic appearances and potential complications. AJR Am J Roentgenol 1997;169:173–178.
12. Heaney MD, Francis IR, Cohan RH, et al. Orthotopic neobladder reconstruction: findings on excretory urography and CT. AJR Am J Roentgenol 1999;172:1213–1220.

13. Sung DJ, Cho SB, Kim YH, et al. Imaging of the various continent urinary diversions after cystectomy. J Comput Assist Tomogr 2004;28:299–310.

14. Holmes DG, Thrasher JB, Park GY, et al. Long-term complications related to the modified Indiana pouch. Urology 2002;60:603–606.

15. Thoeny HC, Sonnenschein MJ, Madersbacher S, et al. Is ileal orthotopic bladder substitution with an afferent tubular segment detrimental to the upper urinary tract in the long term? J Urol 2002;168:2030.

16. Lee JKT, McClennan BL, Stanley RJ, et al. Use of CT in evaluation of postcystectomy patients. AJR Am J Roentgenol 1981;136:483–487.

17. Spring DB, Moss AA. Computed tomography of ideal loop urinary diversion in adults. J Comput Assist Tomogr 1984;8:866–870.

18. Ralls PW, Barakos JA, Skinner DG, et al. Imaging of the Kock continent ileal urinary reservoir. Radiology 1986;161:477–483.

19. Bodner L, Nosher JL, Siegel R, et al. The role of interventional radiology in the management of intra- and extra-peritoneal leakage in patients who have undergone continent urinary diversion. Cardiovasc Intervent Radiol 1997;20:274–279.

20. Rowland RG. Monitoring the silent complications of continent urinary diversion. Contemp Urol 1995;7:17–27.

21. Ahlering TE, Weinberg AC, Razor B. A comparative study of the ileal conduit, Kock pouch, and modified Indiana pouch. J Urol 1989;142:1193–1196.

22. Bettmann MA, Murray PD, Perlmutt LM, et al. Ureteroileal anastomotic leaks: percutaneous treatment. Radiology 1983;148:95–100.

23. Banner MP, Pollack HM, Bonavita JA, et al. The radiology of urinary diversions. Radiographics 1984;4:885–913.

24. Fichtner J. Follow- up after urinary diversion. Urol Int 1999;63:40–45.

25. Schmidt JD, Hawtrey CE, Flocks RH, et al. Complications, results, and problems of ileal conduit diversions. J Urol 1973;109:210–216.

26. Frazier HA, Robertson JE, Paulson DF. Complications of radical cystectomy and urinary diversion: a retrospective review of 675 cases in 2 decades. J Urol 1992;148:1401–1405.

27. Gburek BM, Lieber MM, Blute ML. Comparison of Studer ileal neobladder and ileal conduit urinary diversion with respect to perioperative outcome and late complications. J Urol 1998;160:721–723.

28. Vandenbroucke F, Van Poppel H, Vandeursen H, et al. Surgical versus endoscopic treatment of nonmalignant ureteroileal anastomotic strictures. Br J Urol 1993;71:408–412.

29. Cronan JJ, Amis ES, Scola FH, et al. Renal obstruction in patients with ileal loops: US evaluation. Radiology 1986;158:647–648.

30. Delvecchio FC, Kuo RL, Iselin CE, et al. Combined antegrade and retrograde endoscopic approach for the management of urinary-diversion associated pathology. J Endourol 2000;14:251–256.

31. Zaleski GX, Funaki B, Newmark G. Placement of retrograde nephroureteral stents through ileal conduits. AJR Am J Roentgenol 1998;170:1275–1278.

32. Drake MJ, Cowan NC. Fluoroscopy-guided retrograde ureteral stent insertion in patients with a ureteroileal urinary conduit: method and results. J Urol 2002;167:2049–2051.

33. Tal R, Bachar GN, Belenky A. External-internal nephroureteroileal stents in patients with an ileal conduit: long-term results. Urology 2004;63:438–441.

34. Banner MP, Amendola MA, Pollack HM. Anastomosed ureters: fluoroscopically guided transconduit retrograde catheterization. Radiology 1989;170:45–49.

35. Nelson CP, Wolf JS, Montie JE, et al. Retrograde ureteroscopy in patients with orthotopic ileal neobladder urinary diversion. J Urol 2003;170:107–110.

36. Van Arsdalen KN, Banner MP. The management of ureteral and anastomotic strictures. Probl Urol 1992;6:420–432.

37. Kwak S, Leef JA, Rosenblum JD. Percutaneous balloon catheter dilation of benign ureteral strictures: effect of multiple dilation procedures on long-term patency. AJR Am J Roentgenol 1995;165:97–100.

38. Shapiro MJ, Banner MP, Amendola MA, et al. Balloon catheter dilation of ureteroenteric strictures: long-term results. Radiology 1988;168:385–387.

39. Chang R, Marshall FF, Mitchell S. Percutaneous management of benign ureteral strictures and fistulas. J Urol 1987;1237:1126–1131.

40. Kramolowsky EV, Clayman RV, Weyman PJ. Endourological management of ureteroileal anastomotic strictures: is it effective? J Urol 1987;137:390–394.

41. Hafez KS, Wolf JS. Update on minimally invasive management of ureteral strictures.J Endourol 2003;17:453–464.

42. Kramolowsky EV, Clayman RV, Weyman PJ. Management of ureterointestinal anastomotic strictures: comparison of open surgical and endourological repair. J Urol 1988;139:1195–1198.

43. Cornud F, Mendelsberg M, Chretien Y, et al. Fluoroscopically guided percutaneous transrenal incision of ureterointestinal anastomotic strictures. J Urol 1992;147:578–581.

44. Wolf JS Jr, Elashry OM, Clayman RV. Long-term results of endoureterotomy for benign ureteral and ureteroenteric strictures. J Urol 1997;158:759–764.

45. Laven BA, O'Connor RC, Steinberg GD, et al. Long-term results of antegrade endoureterotomy using the holmium laser in patients with ureterointestinal strictures. Urology 2001;58:924–929.

46. Roth S, Schmidt C, Weyand M, et al. Nearly fatal injury of iliac artery after inaccurate incision of ureterointestinal stricture in orthotopic neobladder. J Urol 1996;155:640–641.

47. Cornud F, Chretien Y, Helenon O, et al. Percutaneous incision of stenotic ureteroenteric anastomosis with a cutting balloon catheter: long-term results. Radiology 2000;214:358–362

48. Pollak JS, Rosenblatt MM, Egglin TK, et al. Treatment of ureteral obstructions with the Wallstent endoprosthesis: preliminary results. J Vasc Intervent Radiol 1995;6:417–425.

49. Rapp DE, Laven BA, Steinberg GD, et al. Percutaneous placement of permanent metal stents for treatment of ureteroanastomotic strictures. J Endourol 2004;18:677–681.

50. Palascak P, Bouchareb M, Zachoval R, et al. Treatment of benign ureterointestinal anastomotic strictures with permanent ureteral Wallstent after Camey and Wallace urinary diversion: long-term follow-up. J Endourol 2001;15:575–580.

51. Freeman JA, Skinner DG. Orthotopic urinary diversion. Contemp Urol 1995;6:29–41.

52. Wilson TG, Moreno JG, Weinberg A, et al. Late complications of the modified Indiana pouch. J Urol 1994;151:331–334.

53. Brenner DO, Johnson DE. Ileal conduit calculi from stapler anastomosis: a long-term complication? Urology 1985;26:537–540.

54. McCarthy P, Cheung L, Hanno P, et al. Metallic staples refluxing to the upper urinary tract: a source of renal calculi in patients with ileal conduit urinary diversion. Br J Radiol 1991;64:467–469.

55. Babel SG, McDermott JC, Goldrath DE, et al. Case report and review of the literature: ureteroarterial fistula after balloon dilation and stent placement. J Vasc Interv Radiol 19883:135–138.

56. Keller FS, Barton RE, Routh WD, et al. Gross hematuria in two patients with ureteral-ileal conduits and double-J stents. J Vasc Interv Radiol 1990;1:69–79.

57. Young PR, Weinreth JL. Endoscopic management of calculi in Kock pouch continent urinary diversion. Probl Urol 1992;6:392–398.

58. Faerber GJ, Wan J, Bloom DA, et al. Percutaneous extraction of calculi from continent augmentation cystoplasty. J Endourol 1992;6:417–419.

59. Gronau E, Pannek J. Reflux of a staple after Kock pouch urinary diversion: a nidus for renal stone formation. J Endourol 2004;18:481–482.

60. Klotz LH, Egeldie RB, Herschorn S. Migrating suture masquerading as a renal pelvic carcinoma: an unusual complication of the Kock pouch. Urol Radiol 1989;11:100–101.

Renal Cysts and Urinomas

42

Michael Darcy

RENAL CYSTS

Appropriate management of renal cysts first requires an understanding of the different types of renal cysts. Most common is the simple cortical cyst, which is a cavity lined by a single layer of benign cuboidal epithelium. Simple cysts account for 80–85% of all space-occupying lesions in the kidneys (1). Cysts are extremely common in adults. Autopsy studies have shown that more than half of patients more than 50 years of age have renal cysts. Simple cysts are rare in pediatric patients, with an incidence of 0.22–0.55% (2,3). However, the incidence of simple cysts has been documented to be much higher (8%) in children with acquired immunodeficiency syndrome (AIDS) and may be a manifestation of HIV-related nephropathy (4). Although the etiology of simple cysts is unclear, the age distribution indicates that they are acquired lesions. Pathologic studies have shown that cysts start as dilatations or diverticulum of the tubules in the nephron, and it has been postulated that they may result from focal infarcts or inflammation (5,6). Cysts detach from the tubule when they reach 2 mm in diameter.

Parapelvic cysts are another type of cyst amenable to interventional therapy. Parapelvic cysts account for 5% of all renal cysts in adults but are rare in children (7). These cysts arise in the parenchyma adjacent to the renal sinus and extend into the sinus. They may not be surrounded by renal parenchyma, as are simple cortical cysts, but their etiology is probably similar. The major difference in their management is that, with parapelvic cysts, one must pay close attention to avoid damaging adjacent vessels or the collecting system. *Parapelvic* cysts need to be distinguished from *peripelvic* cysts, which are small, multiple confluent cysts that arise primarily in the renal sinus. These may arise

either from a congenital embryologic remnant or from acquired lymphatic obstruction, and they rarely cause symptoms requiring treatment (8). Typically, they can be distinguished at ultrasound by the presence of multiple linear sepations extending to the renal hilum (9).

Multilocular renal cysts are rare, benign, unilateral, solitary, multiloculated cysts (10). Although studies indicate that these cysts have no potential for malignant transformation, they should be explored surgically because of the difficulty in differentiating them from cystic neoplasms (11,12). Cysts occurring in polycystic kidneys or multicystic dysplastic kidneys also usually are not treated with interventional techniques except when specific complications develop such as infection or pain from intracyst hemorrhage. Distinguishing the actual cyst that is causing the symptoms can be difficult. Comparison to older cross-sectional imaging studies is vital for finding changes in cyst density, internal structure, size, or contrast enhancement. Infection or intracyst hemorrhage can lead to increases in cyst size and density. Enhancement of the cyst wall on computed tomography (CT) may indicate cyst infection. [111]Indium-labeled leukocyte scans have also been used to help determine the cyst that might be infected (13). MRI may help distinguish infected cysts by gandolinium enhancement of the infected cyst wall and internal septations (14).

Cyst Symptoms and Diagnosis

Natural history studies have shown that cysts do not increase rapidly in size as the patient ages; rather, the number of cysts tends to increase (2,15). A study of 45 patients over 6 years showed an average diameter increase of only 2.8 mm per year (16). Also, because most cysts never cause symptoms, the mere presence of a cyst does not mandate intervention. However, cysts may cause significant symptoms, with pain being the most common problem. Pain probably results from distention of the renal capsule but may also be a secondary effect because of obstruction of the collecting system. Parapelvic cysts may obstruct the ureter or low pelvis (Figure 42–1), whereas peripheral cortical cysts can obstruct infundibuli or calices. Cysts cause some degree of collecting system obstruction in 2.5–16.0% of

cases (7,8). Hypertension is another reported result of the compressive effects of cysts. In a comparison of patients with cysts to age matched controls, the patients with cysts had significantly higher blood pressure (17). Compression of the surrounding parenchyma can induce a hyperreninemic state, and drainage of cysts has been shown to cure hyperreninemic hypertension in some cases (18).

Infection of cysts occurs in 2.5% of cases (19). This can result from either hematogenous spread of bacteria or from local extension of pyelonephritis. In addition to pain, patients generally present with elevated white blood cell counts and fever. Pain caused by infected cysts can be severe enough to mimic an acute abdomen (19). Infected cysts are managed initially the same as an abscess—by percutaneous drainage and IV antibiotics.

Cyst rupture can be a source of significant pain. Rupture can occur after intracyst hemorrhage or infection increases the pressure within the cyst. Alternatively, rupture can be caused by blunt trauma (20). Hematuria is seen in 64–84% of patients with cyst rupture and relates to the cyst rupturing into an adjacent calyx (21). Less often, cysts may rupture through the renal capsule, causing a perirenal urinoma or hemorrhage (22,23). Drainage of the perirenal collection may be required to relieve pain, compression, or infection. In cases of perirenal hemorrhage, it is important to exclude the presence of a tumor because tumors are a more common cause of spontaneous perirenal hemorrhage (22).

Before attempting interventional obliteration of cysts, it is important to determine that the lesion is not a malignancy. Four percent of renal cell carcinomas are cystic. Simple cysts and renal cell carcinomas have been found to coexist in the same kidney in 2–3% of cases, although carcinoma arising within the cyst itself is rare (24–28). Differentiation of benign simple cysts from cystic malignancy can be straightforward when classic imaging findings are present. Ultrasound relies on the identification of a thin-walled cavity containing fluid of low echogenicity with good through-transmission and no internal echoes. The cyst wall should be regular with no mass effects. Fine, strand-like septations may be present but should be less than 1 mm thick and have no associated solid-mass component. Parapelvic lesions should also be interrogated with duplex ultrasound to exclude a vascular mass, such as an aneurysm or vascular malformation (29,30). Similarly, CT should demonstrate a thin-walled, fluid-filled cyst with no internal mass or wall irregularity. Cyst fluid should be of low attenuation (in the range of 0–20 HU). Hyperdense benign cysts have been described with fluid attenuation in the range of 60–100 HU (possibly resulting from previous intracyst hemorrhage) (1,31,32). These should meet all the other criteria for a simple cyst. Complex cysts require further investigation, usually exploration. A study of 32 complex cysts (including Bosniak category I–IV) managed with surgical exploration yielded malignancy in 41% of cases (33), but in another series limited to Bosniak category II and III cysts, only 19% proved to be malignant at exploration (34).

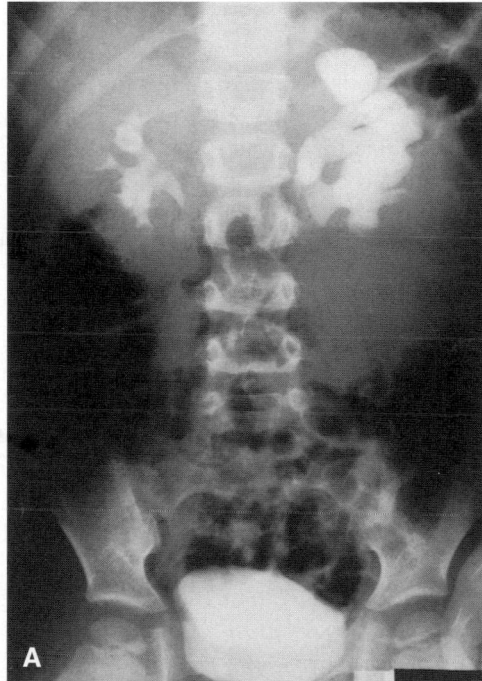

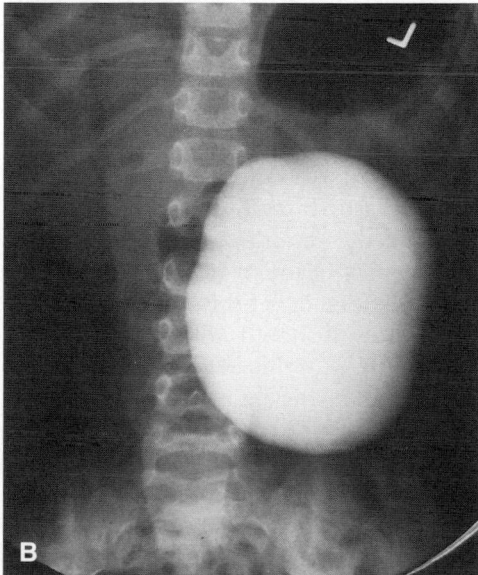

Figure 42–1 **A.** Intravenous pyelogram in a 5-year-old child shows obstruction of the left ureteral pelvic junction. **B.** Cystogram shows the large cyst causing the obstruction. Drainage of this cyst resolved the obstructive uropathy.

There is controversy about the diagnostic value of calcium within a lesion. Bosniak (35) believed that the type of calcification is important and that a small amount of thin, smooth calcification in a cyst wall is acceptable. However, he also has stated that there is no specific number of millimeters of calcium that is allowable before classifying the lesion as a Bosniak category III lesion (36). Although central, thick, or irregular calcification is certainly the most suggestive of malignancy, approximately 20% of peripherally calcified lesions are malignant (37). In polycystic kidneys, this is an even less helpful distinguishing point because calcification can be seen in up to 75% of cysts (31). Contrast enhancement of the cyst wall is another sign suggestive of malignancy. Infected cysts may also enhance, but clinical symptoms and white blood cell count should distinguish these lesions from malignancies.

Ultrasound and CT are generally believed to be more than 90% accurate at distinguishing simple benign cysts from other processes, such as cystic malignancies (15, 38–40). There are rare reported cases of malignancies that appeared to be benign cysts by all standard ultrasound or CT criteria. There has also been a case report of a simple cyst that transitioned over 3 years into a lesion with septation and wall thickening and proved to be a carcinoma (41). Results with MRI have been varied. In one older study (40), MRI was not able to distinguish between carcinoma and cysts with hemorrhage in 32% of cases. However, more recent findings of mural irregularity and intense enhancement on MRI have shown high correlation with the presence of malignancy (42).

Cyst Puncture and Aspiration

For renal masses that are still indeterminate after cross-sectional imaging, cyst puncture with aspiration cytology and contrast cystography can be a useful adjunct. Preparation for cyst puncture requires precautions similar to those taken before other interventional procedures. Bleeding history and clotting parameters, as well as platelet count, need to be checked. Inquiry must be made about the patient's contrast allergy history and any other medical conditions that could be exacerbated by the procedure.

The skin entry point for cyst puncture should be chosen similar to a nephrostomy access. For most cortical cysts, the puncture should be started around the lateral border of the major erector muscles of the back. A more lateral entry point increases the risk of hitting nontarget organs such as colon, liver, or spleen. A more medial entry point is acceptable when there is no plan to leave a drainage tube in place, but a medial entry for a drainage catheter is not advised. Patients experience discomfort because the catheter goes through more muscle mass and makes it more difficult to avoid lying on the tube in this location. For parapelvic cyst, a more medial entry point may be warranted because entering along the lateral border of the erector muscles may cause the tract to skim through the renal parenchyma. Cyst puncture generally is guided by ultrasound, although fluoroscopy may also be used when iodinated contrast has been given and the cyst is large enough to distort the collecting system or to cause a defect in the nephrogram. CT is rarely needed to guide cyst puncture except when trying to hit a very small cyst or in obese patients in whom there is poor ultrasound penetration. CT guidance is also helpful when it is necessary to puncture one specific cyst in a patient with polycystic disease. A 21- or 22-gauge needle is generally sufficient for aspiration and a cystogram. When catheter drainage is planned, use of an 18-gauge needle may facilitate the procedure because 18-gauge needles will accept a larger 0.035–0.038 inch guide wire. Thus, one can avoid using a less stiff 0.018-inch guide wire as well as the extra step of using a transition dilator to introduce the larger guide wire.

The cyst should be punctured as atraumatically as possible to decrease bleeding into the cyst. The fluid in a benign simple cyst should be clear or slightly yellowish. A small amount of blood in the fluid that clears during the drainage indicates a traumatic tap. Bloody fluid that does not become more serous is suggestive of a tumor (43,44), although cystic malignancies may contain clear fluid (26). The aspirated fluid should be sent for cytologic evaluation, which in some series has shown good sensitivity for malignancy (25). However, others have indicated that a negative cytology does not exclude malignancy (27,45). In fact, Kleist et al. (45) found that cytology failed to detect malignant cells in 9 of 11 cystic malignancies that they studied. Some also recommend analyzing the aspirated fluid for lipid content, which in cystic malignancies is approximately five times higher than that seen in benign cysts (45). However, both false-positive and false-negative lipid analyses are possible (26).

A cystogram should be performed after the cyst fluid is aspirated. This may be done using a single contrast technique in which the cyst fluid is replaced with dilute contrast. Contrast must be diluted to avoid obscuring details of the cyst wall. Double contrast techniques have also been described (44) in which 50% of the aspirated volume of the cyst is replaced with air and 25% of the volume is replaced by contrast. The cyst walls in a simple benign cyst should be perfectly smooth. Any irregularity of the wall raises the possibility of tumor (Figure 42–2). Internal septations or lobulations may be seen in up to 19% of cases (46), but the cyst wall should still be smooth in these situations. Interpretation of the cystogram may be more difficult when incomplete distention of the cyst leads to some cyst wall irregularity. A similar pitfall can occur when prior cyst rupture leads to partial collapse, lending an irregular appearance to the wall. Organized or adherent thrombus from prior hemorrhage may also mimic malignancy. With the combination of cyst fluid analysis and cystogram, the accuracy of cyst aspiration for exclusion of malignancy has been reported to be around 95–98% (1,47). The accuracy of these techniques decreases in the setting of hemorrhagic cysts or highly septated cysts.

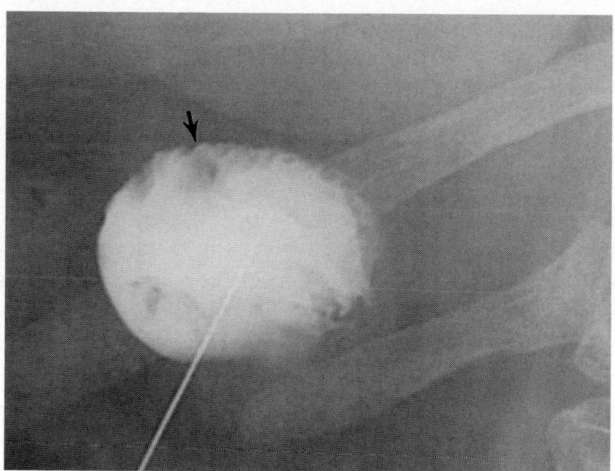

Figure 42–2 Cyst puncture shows a mass (*arrow*) protruding from the cephalad aspect of the cyst. Pathology confirmed this to be a renal cell carcinoma.

Cyst aspiration may also be used to determine whether a cyst is infected. If infected, cyst drainage is valuable because some antibiotics do not penetrate into cyst fluid even when the cyst wall is inflamed (48). Other indications for drainage include when the cyst causes pain, urinary obstruction, or hypertension. Cyst drainage may be used either to initiate therapy or as a diagnostic trial to see whether it eliminates the symptoms.

Simple needle aspiration of cysts is a safe procedure. Major complications are uncommon and occur in only 0.75–3.00% of cases (49,50). The most common complication is perirenal hemorrhage, which occurs in 0.18–0.30% of cases when 20- to 22-gauge needles are used. Other reported complications include pneumothorax, arteriovenous fistula, infection, urinoma formation, and inadvertent puncture of adjacent bowel. Pneumothorax occurs most frequently with punctures of upper pole cysts, particularly in the left kidney. Aside from these immediate procedural complications, the only long-term problem that has been noted is tumor seeding along the tract after aspiration of a cystic malignancy. However, this is a rare complication, with only a few case reports in the literature (38,51). The problem with simple aspiration is the high recurrence rate, because the epithelium of cysts can rapidly produce more fluid and refill the cyst (52). Recurrence of renal cysts after simple aspiration occurs in anywhere from 30% to 100% of cases in the series reported (53–56).

Sclerosis of Cysts

Simple catheter drainage is rarely used, and the likelihood of success is low because of the active secretion of cyst fluid. To decrease the incidence of cyst recurrence, sclerosis is used to destroy the secreting epithelial cells lining the cyst. Although sclerosis may be performed via the aspirating needle, sclerotherapy generally can be performed more safely

and effectively after placement of a catheter within the cyst. Use of a catheter has several advantages. With the catheter in place, it is possible to get delayed cystograms after initial drainage, allowing one to detect communications with the collecting system that were not apparent at the time of initial drainage (Figure 42–3). Subsequent cystograms allow monitoring of the collapse of the cyst cavity and determination of the volume of sclerosant needed. Monitoring the volume of cyst drainage helps gauge the adequacy of sclerosis. The fibrous tract that forms around a drainage catheter is also beneficial because sclerosant leaking from the cyst will drain along the tract as opposed to extravasating freely into the perirenal space. Before placing a catheter, it is important to determine whether the catheter material is stable in alcohol to avoid damaging the catheter's structural integrity. Both trocar and Seldinger techniques can be used to place catheters within renal cysts. Although the Seldinger technique is probably most common, passing the catheter through the nondistended cyst wall can still be difficult if the cyst decompresses into the perirenal space during exchanges.

After catheter placement in the cyst, a thorough cystogram is done to ensure that there is no communication with the collecting system. Of cysts that partially or completely rupture, 52% rupture into the caliceal system. These communications may partially seal, allowing the cyst to redistend but still maintain communication with the collecting system (21). It is important to identify such connections to avoid introducing a sclerosing agent into the collecting system. If the cyst is infected, it should be drained until the infection clears before sclerosis is initiated. Sclerosis of an infected cyst theoretically could lead to loculation of infected material.

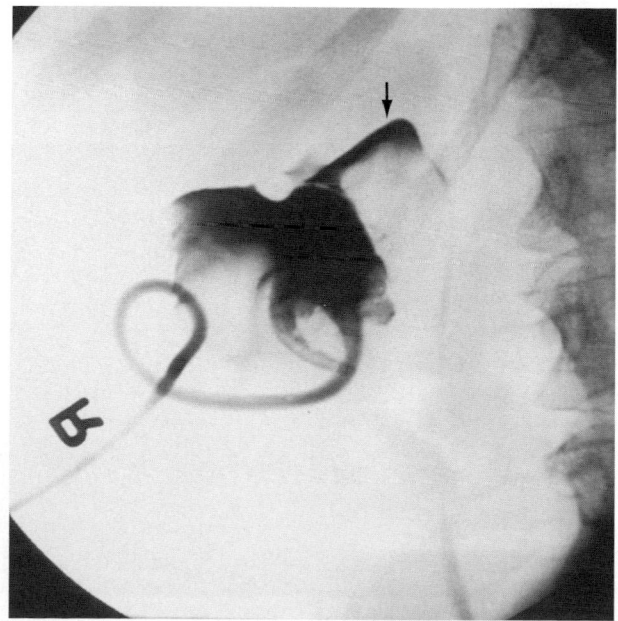

Figure 42–3 A cystogram performed several days after percutaneous drainage shows communication with the collecting system (*arrow*). No communication was seen at the time of initial drainage.

After complete drainage of the cyst fluid, replacement with contrast allows estimates to be made about the cyst volume to determine the amount of sclerosant to use. Extravasation of contrast along the catheter into the perirenal space should be noted. If this occurs freely without overdistention of the cyst, it is advisable to continue catheter drainage until a fibrous tract forms around the catheter. The volume of sclerosant used should approximate 25–50% of the volume of the cyst estimated by the injection of contrast.

Multiple agents have been used to sclerose cysts, including glucose, phenol, pantopaque, tetracycline, bismuth, Betadine, and cyanoacrylate glue (3,55,57–61). Absolute alcohol is currently the most commonly used sclerosant. Bean (56) showed experimentally that although the cyst wall epithelium becomes nonviable after 1–3 minutes of exposure to alcohol, it takes approximately 4–12 hours for alcohol to penetrate the cyst capsule. Thus, this agent can safely defunctionalize the secreting cells of the cyst without affecting adjacent renal parenchyma. Alcohol also has the advantages of being inexpensive and readily available. Some advocate Betadine, which also is inexpensive and readily available, because it is less toxic than ethanol (60,62).

Once alcohol is instilled, the patient should be turned at intervals onto each side and into both prone and supine positions to expose all portions of the cyst wall to the alcohol. Midway through the sclerosis session, the alcohol typically is aspirated and replaced with a fresh aliquot. The alcohol is left in the cyst for 15–20 minutes, and the catheter is then placed back to drainage. Often, repeat sclerosis is done in subsequent sessions until the drainage from the cyst becomes negligible. The optimal frequency of sclerosis has not been determined. Sometimes, cysts with high output may need to be sclerosed daily, and in some cases, patients with chronic drainage can be taught to perform the sclerosis at home. Other sclerosis regimens have been advocated. Two series (63,64) that utilized daily sclerosis for only 2 and 3 days respectively reported complete cyst resolution in 84% and 97% of cases. Single-session drainage and sclerosis with ethanol has been reported in one series of 32 patients (65), but this appears to be less effective because the cyst resolution was seen in only 22%. Similarly Kim et al. (61) attempted single-session sclerosis using N-butyl cyanoacrylate instilled into cysts through a needle without catheter placement. Although success was claimed in 81% of cysts, the cyst only had to decrease to less than 50% of the original diameter to be considered a successful sclerosis. When attempting to sclerose giant cysts, it is important to recognize that the cyst walls may adhere to themselves and form separate loculated compartments (Figure 42–4). This may require manipulation of the catheter into the loculations or even placement of an additional drainage catheter.

Although cyst sclerosis commonly can cause some pain or fever, significant complications are infrequent. Bean (56) reported microscopic hematuria in 2 of 29 patients (6.9%) but no major complications. Gelet et al.(59), on the other hand, reported infectious-type complications in 2 of 10 patients (20%) after Betadine sclerosis. One patient developed sepsis after the procedure, and one patient developed delayed infection of a residual cyst cavity 3 months after sclerosis. The more typical incidence of infectious complication is 0–0.5% (56,66). No other major complications have been described for peripheral cysts. Sclerosis of parapelvic cysts carries the additional theoretic risk of damage to adjacent hilar structures. Ureteral pelvic obstruction caused by sclerosis-induced fibrosis has been described (66).

The effectiveness of sclerotherapy appears to vary with the sclerosing agent used. Series in which tetracycline or ethanol were used have reported a high degree of technical success with minimal recurrences (Figure 42–5) (3,54,56,67). Bean

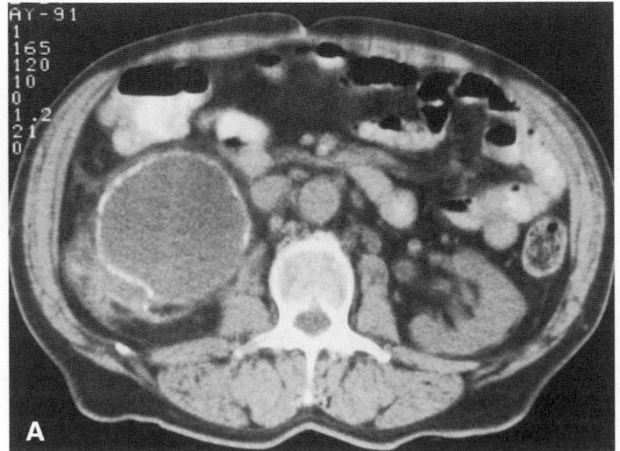 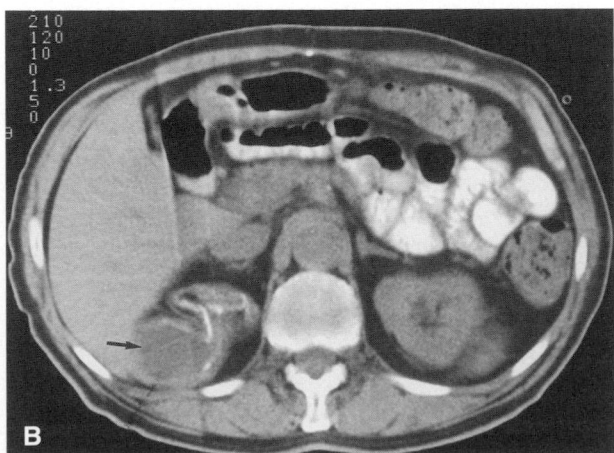

Figure 42–4 **A.** CT scan shows a large cyst in a dysplastic right kidney. Drainage and sclerosis were planned because of the patient's right flank pain. **B.** CT performed because of fever after several sclerotherapy sessions shows that a portion of the cyst has become loculated (*arrow*) as the cyst walls collapsed together. This loculation required placement of an additional drainage catheter.

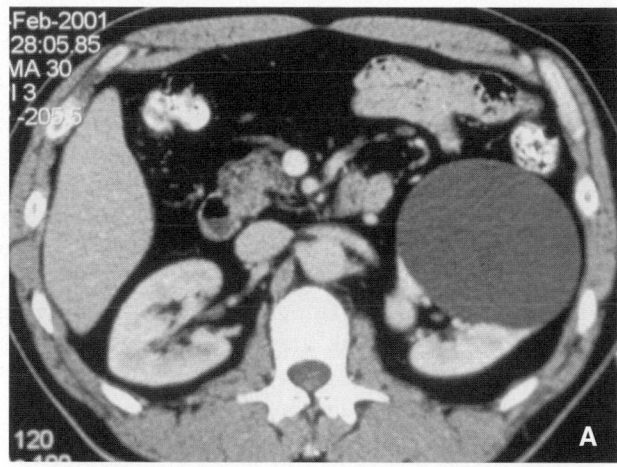

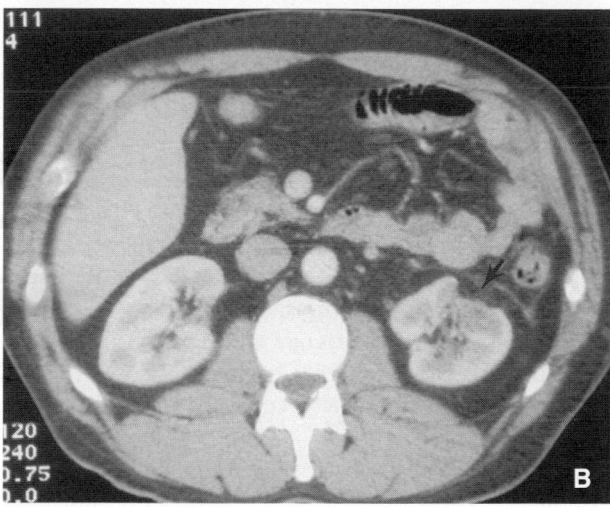

Figure 42–5 **A.** Large left cyst that was causing flank pain. **B.** After drainage and sclerosis, a 6-month follow-up CT scan shows complete resolution of the cyst with only mild scarring (*arrow*) at the cyst site.

noted one recurrence in 34 cysts (2.9%), and it occurred in a patient with a giant cyst and an initial volume of approximately 2 liters (56). Other series using Betadine, pantopaque, bismuth, or other agents to attempt sclerosis have shown incomplete obliteration of cyst cavities in 25–56% of cases (55,57,59,60).

Surgical Therapy of Cysts

Surgery has been proposed as a better way of managing cysts because it can eliminate the cyst in one step rather than requiring return visits for sclerosis, it allows for direct inspection of the cyst to exclude malignancy with greater confidence, and surgical specimens of the cyst wall can be obtained for pathologic examination. Although a normal appearance at surgical inspection should exclude malignancy, there has been at least one case reported in which disseminated renal cell carcinoma developed shortly after laparoscopic decortication of what appeared to be a simple cyst (68).

Open surgical cyst unroofing is associated with a morbidity of 8–16%, and the average hospital stay can be up to 9 days for this procedure (50,69). This approach has been supplanted largely by laparoscopic unroofing, which is much less invasive (69–72). Laparoscopic unroofing is done through a transperitoneal or retroperitoneal approach depending on cyst location. After identification of the cyst laparoscopically, the procedure involves aspiration of cyst fluid, which is then sent for cytology; resection of the cyst wall, sent for pathology; visual inspection of the remaining cyst wall; resection of any masses, submitted for frozen section; and fulguration of the base of the cyst.

Parapelvic cysts are more difficult to manage laparoscopically as evidenced by longer operative time, greater blood loss, and longer hospital stays compared to peripheral cysts (73). While urologists advocate that sclerosis is dangerous in the parapelvic region, laparoscopic techniques also may be complicated by laceration or stricture of the renal pelvis or ureter. In the renal hilum, adjacent major arteries and veins may limit the resection of the cyst wall and distinguishing the cyst from the renal vein may be difficult enough to require the use of a laparoscopic ultrasound (74).

Another surgical alternative is to marsupialize the cyst into the collecting system. This can be combined with fulguration of the cyst wall to cause the cavity to close through scarring (Figure 42–6). Although this can be done via a retrograde ureteroscopic approach (47), the more common access is via a percutaneous tract into the cyst (75). This requires placement of a 24–30 French sheath to provide access large enough for the endoscope. Rather than marsupializing the cyst into the collecting system, this percutaneous technique may be used to unroof the cyst into the retroperitoneum by resecting part of the cyst wall after pulling back the sheath (76).

Despite the more invasive nature of endourologic management, complete cyst obliteration may not be possible in all cases. In one series (59), complete obliteration was achieved in only 60% of cysts even though cyst-related symptoms initially resolved in all cases. In Hoenig's study (74), only 75% of patients achieved resolution of their symptoms. Recurrence rates range from 3% (with no recurrent symptoms) to 17% symptomatic recurrence (59,73). Complication rates range from 13–33% (71,73) and include complications such as ureteral stricture, diaphragm injury, ileus, and large retroperitoneal hematoma.

The success rates of surgical therapy and cyst sclerosis are fairly comparable; however, sclerosis has multiple advantages. Sclerotherapy can be incorporated easily as an extension of an initial diagnostic procedure. Catheter placement and sclerosis can be performed with local anesthesia unlike surgical techniques that require general anesthesia. Lack of operating room fee or anesthesia charge makes percutaneous sclerotherapy less costly. Sclerosis can be accomplished through a single 8–10 French catheter, which is considerably smaller than the

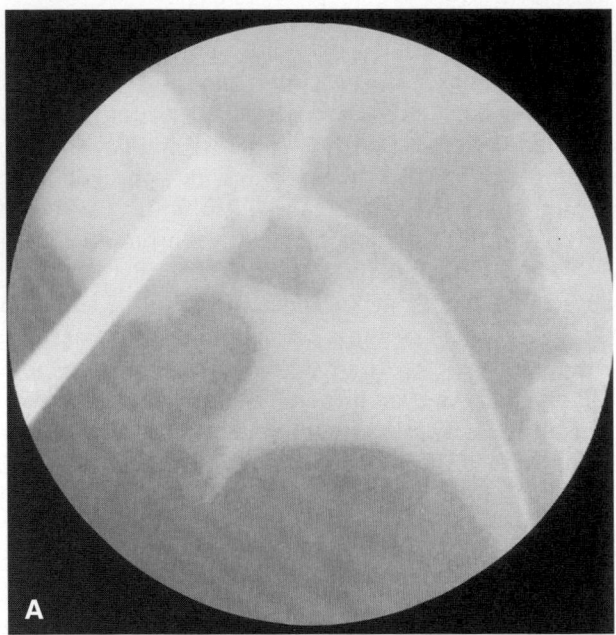

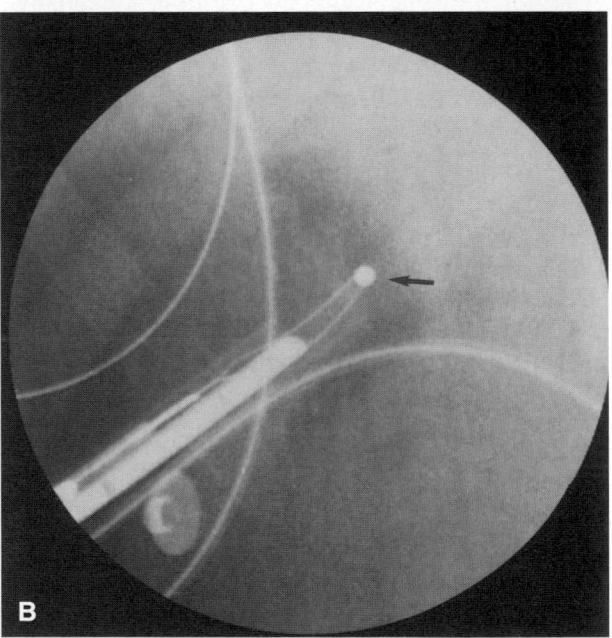

Figure 42–6 A. Endoscopic marsupialization of a cyst into the collecting system. A sheath was placed percutaneously into the cyst, and an endoscope with a cutting electrode was used to create a communication into the collecting system. **B.** The lining of the cyst is then endoscopically fulgurated using a roller-ball electrode (*arrow*) to devitalize the cyst lining and to cause the cyst to close through scarring.

size of an endourologic sheath. When treated laparoscopically, four small incisions are required for the various ports used for visualization and manipulation. Further proof of the increased complexity of laparoscopic therapy is the fact that operative time averages 187–338 minutes (73,74), which is much longer than percutaneous catheter drainage. Thus, interventional techniques are less complex and less invasive.

URINOMAS

Urinomas are caused by several different conditions and may arise from obstruction of the ureter or collecting system with subsequent forniceal rupture. This can occur in neonates because of obstruction from posterior urethral valves (77–79) or in adults because of calculi or malignancy-related ureteral obstruction (80,81). Rarely, a urinoma may be the presenting symptom of a pelvic malignancy (82). Urinomas also may occur secondary to rupture of cortical cysts, leading to communication between the collecting system and the perirenal space. Urinomas are a common occurrence after renal transplants. Ureteral leak in conjunction with ureteral obstruction accounts for 95% of transplant urologic complications (83,84). The cause of a peritransplant urinoma may be suspected based on the time of presentation. A leak that occurs within the first week after transplant is most likely because of a technical error with dehiscence of the neoureterocystotomy. After the first week, ischemia of the ureter with perforation is more likely.

Blunt or penetrating trauma may cause urinomas by direct disruption of the pelvis or ureter or in a delayed fashion by parenchymal necrosis and degeneration of nonviable tissue. Despite the fact that urinomas in this setting typically are perinephric, trauma can lead to subcapsular urine collections (85), though rarely. Surprisingly, traumatic disruptions of the pelvis or ureter often go unrecognized initially (86). Surgical trauma to the ureter also may lead to urinoma formation (Figure 42–7). Pelvic or abdominal operations are implicated most often, but other operations, such as spine surgery, can cause ureteral injury (87). Finally, minimally invasive procedures are another potential source for urinomas. Urinomas have been reported after percutaneous nephrostomy, stone basketing, cystoscopy, transurethral prostate resection, and extracorporeal shock wave lithotripsy (88–92).

The symptoms that lead to the discovery of urinomas are related most often to the mass and pressure effects. Distention of the perinephric space or displacement of adjacent organs may lead to pain. Pain may also result secondarily from hydronephrosis because of ureteral obstruction. In pediatric cases, the mass effect from urinomas can put pressure on the diaphragm, leading to pulmonary compression and even respiratory distress (77,79,93). As mentioned, the mass effect may lead to ureteral obstruction (Figure 42–8), which may be manifested by rising creatinine levels or decreased urine output. In patients recently postrenal transplant, urine may track to and leak out of the surgical incision rather than form a retroperitoneal collection. When urinomas become infected, the patient may present with fever or an elevated white blood cell count.

Urinoma Diagnosis

Both CT and ultrasound can detect urinomas accurately when the urine forms a well-defined collection. However,

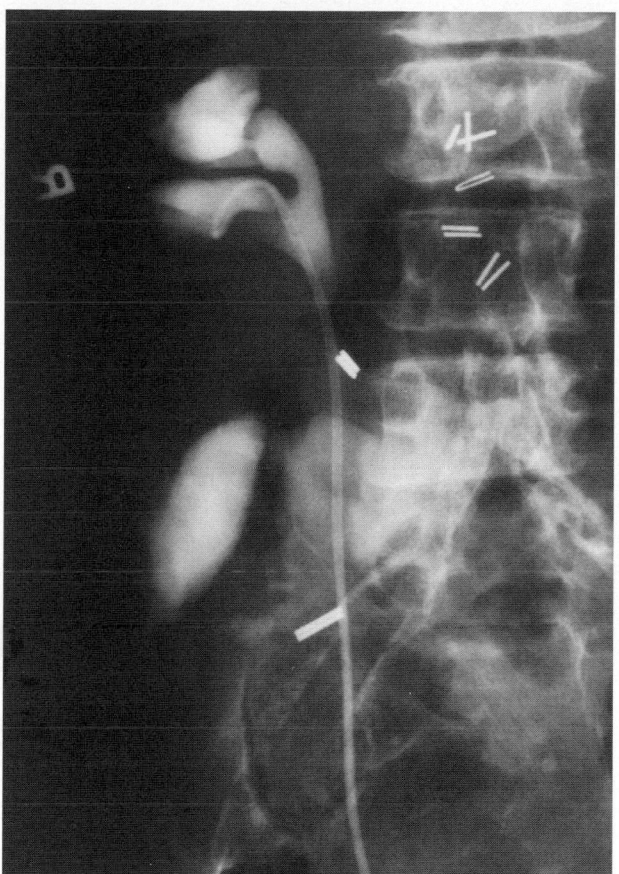

Figure 42–7 Iatrogenic urinoma caused by ureteral injury during aortobifemoral bypass graft surgery. Contrast is seen to extravasate from the midureter. The urinoma was treated successfully by internal stenting.

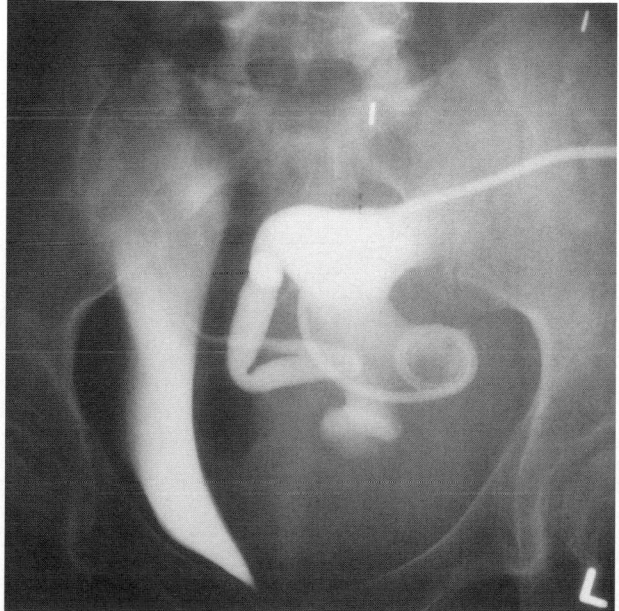

Figure 42–8 Transplant nephrostogram showing compression of the bladder as well as distal ureteral obstruction caused by a large urinoma. In addition to the nephrostomy, a drainage catheter into the urinoma was required to relieve the distal ureteral obstruction.

these studies may be negative in renal transplants when the urine leaks out the incision rather than collecting locally around the kidney. The volume of urine leakage may also be small enough that the surrounding tissues can resorb the urine readily. Thus, a defined urinoma collection may not be seen in 23–33% of renal transplants in which there is a ureteral leak (94,95). The other pitfall of ultrasound and CT is their specificity. Although fluid may be detected, it is generally not possible to distinguish a urinoma from a lymphocele, which is more commonly seen after transplants. Nuclear scintigraphy has been proposed as a more sensitive method of detecting urine extravasation; however, in two series, scintigraphy failed to detect urinary leak in 50–67% of cases (94,95). This most likely was because of decreased renal function and masking of a leak by overlying bladder.

Antegrade nephrostograms can be useful in the diagnosis of urinomas. This study can allow assessment of the location of a urinary leak, which in turn makes it easier to plan the appropriate therapy. Renal transplants are the only population in which the accuracy of antegrade nephrostograms has been assessed. In these patients, a leak may not be detected in 17–43% of cases (94,95). False-negative studies often are because of the coexistence of ureteral obstruction. Although antegrade nephrostograms may be performed with a high degree of technical success, the procedure tends to be more difficult in patients with active urinary leak because the collecting system may be decompressed. Nevertheless, significant complications are uncommon (95,96). Self-limited minor hematuria usually is the only sequela seen.

Because of the problems with noninvasive diagnosis, needle aspiration plays an important role in the diagnosis of urinomas. Aspiration of the fluid and analysis of the cell counts and creatinine level can definitively distinguish between urinoma and other fluid collections. Aspiration also may be diagnostically useful to obtain material for culture, particularly for peritransplant urinomas, which may be infected 60% of the time (97). In addition, these patients may not manifest normal signs of infection because of their immunosuppressive therapy. Aspiration generally can be performed with a 22- or 21-gauge needle passed under CT or ultrasound guidance. In most cases, unobstructed access to the collection can be found easily.

Urinoma Therapy

The main therapy for a urinoma should be tailored to treat the underlying problem that led to the urinoma. When the urinoma has resulted from obstruction, the obstructing lesion (whether it is posterior ureteral valves or a ureteral stone) must be addressed. In the case of malignant obstructions, percutaneous nephrostomy, ureteral stenting, or both should be provided to relieve the obstruction. Iatrogenic urinary leaks should be treated with decompression of the collecting system or stenting to divert the urine past the leak point. This diversion must be maintained until the breach in the urothelium heals. The same principle applies to leaks resulting from trauma. After trauma, additional therapy may be needed when tissue necrosis leads to nonhealing of the disrupted collecting system and prolonged urinary leakage. Surgical removal of devitalized tissue has been used in the past, but a less invasive approach involves arterial embolization of the renal parenchyma that is supplying the leak. Selective embolization may also preserve more renal parenchyma than the surgical option. Microcoils have been the embolic agent used in several reports (98,99), but ethanol may be a better embolic agent for destroying the functioning parenchyma and stopping urine production (Figure 42–9).

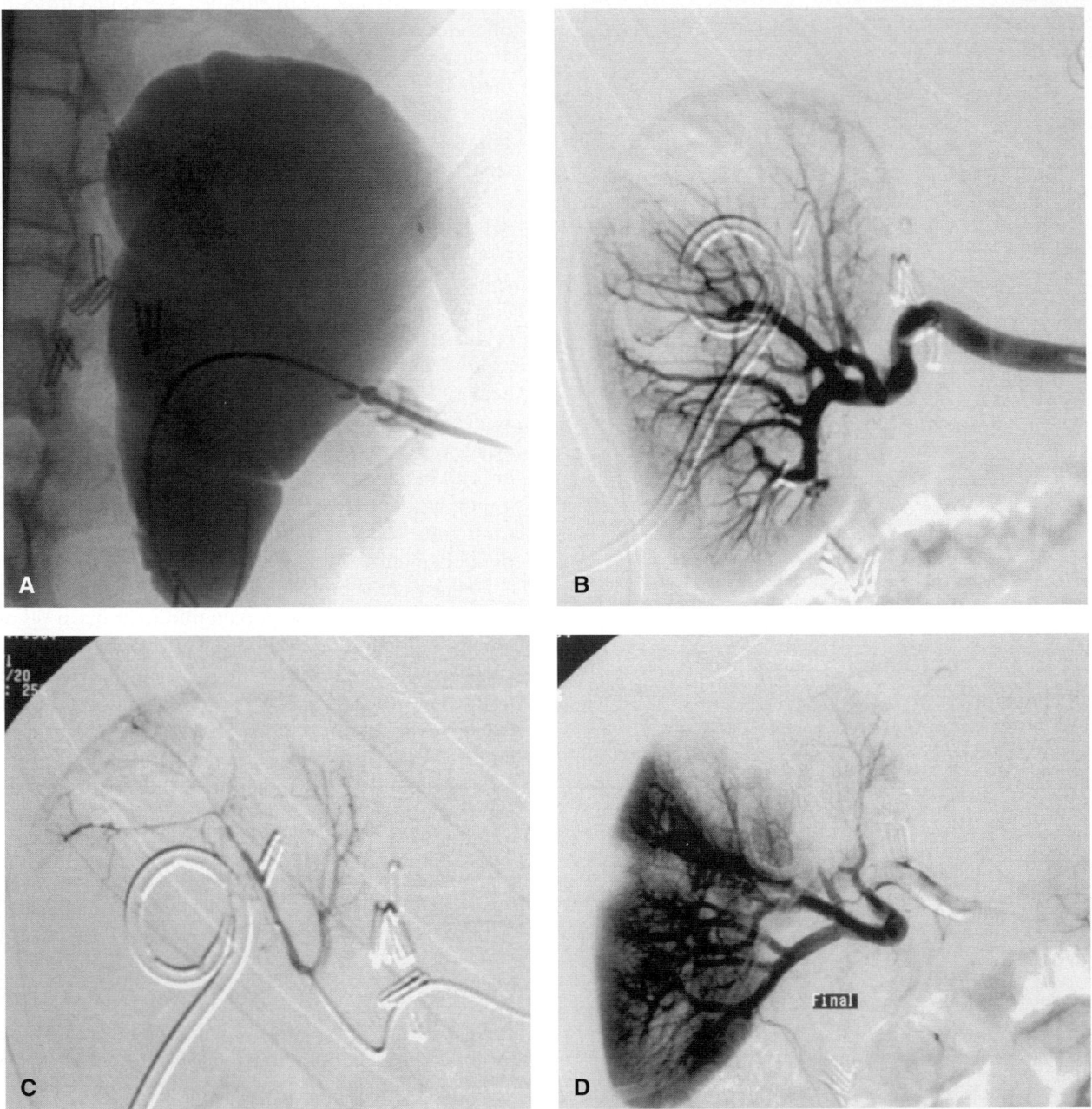

Figure 42–9 A. Young female with a large urinoma postresection of a duplicated collecting system obstructed upper pole component. This image was obtained at the time of catheter drainage of the urinoma. **B.** Despite long-term drainage (longer than 9 months), surgical fulguration of the surface, and internal stenting, urine output from the catheter remained high. It was decided to embolize the parenchyma that was supplying the leak. Initial renal arteriogram shows branches draped around a hypovascular upper portion of the kidney. **C.** Selective catheterization of the branches likely supplying the surgical bed. Ethanol was injected to obliterate this section of kidney. **D.** Postembolization arteriogram shows a devascularized upper segment of the kidney. Output from the urinoma drain became negligible by the next day.

Finally, transplant-related urinomas should be managed first by drainage of the collecting system to decrease the amount of urine flow to the urinary leak. An internal-external ureteral stent may be used to divert urine further away from the leak, which most often arises from the distal ureter. A ureteral stent has the additional advantage of helping to hold open the ureteral obstruction, which is a frequent concomitant condition. When percutaneous methods are used, ureteral transplant leaks will seal in 54–100% of cases, although sometimes prolonged stenting is required (100–102).

Drainage of urinomas often takes a secondary role compared to definitive treatment of the underlying problem. In fact, when the primary problem is corrected, urinomas may spontaneously resolve and not require drainage. However, when the urinoma is large, drainage helps resolve the symptoms more quickly. Urinoma drainage is definitely indicated when the urinoma causes significant discomfort or compressive effects, such as obstruction of the ureter in a renal transplant or respiratory compromise in pediatric urinomas. Infection of the urinoma is also an indication for drainage. Even when definitive surgical therapy is ultimately required to treat the urinary leak, preoperative drainage of infected urinomas can help stabilize the patient and allow for the institution of appropriate antibiotics.

Before a urinoma is drained, the patient should undergo a typical preintervention evaluation starting with a history and physical examination. Coagulation factors and platelet count may be assessed, although in the absence of bleeding history coagulation studies are not good predictors of bleeding complications. Assessment with CT or ultrasound is essential in choosing a safe access and avoiding perforation of adjacent structures, such as the bowel or kidney. Cross-sectional imaging may reveal extension of the urinoma into unusual places, including the chest or mediastinum, which may alter the approach to the drainage procedure. Antibiotic coverage is indicated whenever any fever or elevation of the leukocyte count is present. In most cases, renal transplants should receive predrainage antibiotics because of the high incidence of urinoma infection in this population (97).

Urinomas can be simply aspirated through a needle, which may suffice as long as the underlying problem is addressed sufficiently (81,103). Catheter drainage has several advantages. Generally, more complete drainage can be obtained, and having the catheter in place allows the degree of urine leak to be monitored. This monitoring reveals the adequacy of the therapy for the underlying problem. In addition, visual inspection of the fluid possibly may not determine the nature of the fluid collection and whether it is infected. Placement of a catheter maintains access into the collection until the fluid analysis is complete.

Urinomas can be drained with a high degree of technical success and low morbidity. They are generally superficial enough that access can be obtained without risk of puncture to adjacent structures. Because significant septations or loculations are not common and urine is not viscous, a single small-bore catheter will suffice to drain most urinomas. Although urinoma drainage has been described in several papers, no larger series have detailed the technical success rate. No failed drainages have been reported, and no significant complications related to urinoma drainage have been described. This is not surprising, because the path of the drainage catheter usually only crosses some subcutaneous fat and minimal abdominal musculature. Theoretically, if the urinoma is infected, bacteremia could result. This should be prevented with use of prophylactic preprocedural antibiotics and through avoidance of vigorous contrast injections until adequate drainage has occurred

SUMMARY

Although urinomas and renal cysts vary significantly in their incidence and etiologies, each condition can benefit diagnostically and therapeutically from interventional radiologic techniques.

REFERENCES

1. Lang EK. Renal cyst puncture studies. Urol Clin North Am 1987; 14(1):91–102.
2. McHugh K, Stringer DA, Hebert D, et al. Simple renal cysts in children: diagnosis and follow-up with US. Radiology 1991; 178(2):383–385.
3. Reiner I, Donnell S, Jones M, et al. Percutaneous sclerotherapy for simple renal cysts in children. Br J Radiol 1992;65(771):281–282.
4. Zinn HL, Rosberger ST, Haller JO, et al. Simple renal cysts in children with AIDS. Pediatr Radiol 1997;27(10):827–828.
5. Mosli H, MacDonald P, Schillinger J. Caliceal diverticula developing into simple renal cyst. J Urol 1986;136(3):658–661.
6. Grantham JJ. Pathogenesis of renal cyst expansion: opportunities for therapy. Am J Kidney Dis 1994;23(2):210–218.
7. Patel K, Caro PA, Chatten J. Parapelvic renal cyst causing UPJ obstruction. Investigation by IVP, ultrasound, and CT. Pediatr Radiol 1988;19(1):2–5.
8. Amis ES Jr, Cronan JJ. The renal sinus: an imaging review and proposed nomenclature for sinus cysts. J Urol 1988;139(6): 1151–1159.
9. Patel U, Huntley L, Kellett MJ. Sonographic features of renal obstruction mimicked by peripelvic cysts. Clin Radiol 1994; 49(7):481–484.
10. Egerdie RB, Buckspan MB, Klotz PG, et al. Bilateral multilocular renal cysts. J Urol 1986;135(2):346–348.
11. Castillo OA, Boyle ET Jr, Kramer SA. Multilocular cysts of kidney. A study of 29 patients and review of literature. Urology 1991;37(2): 156–162.
12. Morgan C, Greenberg ML. Multilocular renal cyst: a diagnostic pitfall on fine-needle aspiration cytology: case report. Diagn Cytopathol 1995;13(1):66–70.
13. Fortner A, Taylor A Jr, Alazraki N, et al. Advantage of indium-111 leukocytes over ultrasound in imaging an infected renal cyst. J Nucl Med 1986;27(7):1147–1149.
14. Chicoskie C, Chaoui A, Kuligowska E, et al. MRI isolation of infected renal cyst in autosomal dominant polycystic kidney disease. Clin Imaging 2001;25(2):114–117.
15. Dalton D, Neiman H, Grayhack JT. The natural history of simple renal cysts: a preliminary study. J Urol 1986;135(5):905–908.
16. Terada N, Ichioka K, Matsuta Y, et al. The natural history of simple renal cysts. J Urol 2002;167(1):21–23.
17. Pedersen JF, Emamian SA, Nielsen MB. Significant association between simple renal cysts and arterial blood pressure. Br J Urol 1997;79(5):688–691.

18. Pearl M, Klein S. Simple renal cyst and hypertension. Ann Radiol (Paris) 1986;29(3-4):421-423.
19. de Lichtenberg MH, Nielsen OS. Infected renal cyst simulating acute abdomen. Case report. Acta Chir Scand 1989;155(2):135.
20. Hughes CR, Stewart PF Jr, Breckenridge JW. Renal cyst rupture following blunt abdominal trauma: case report. J Trauma 1995; 38(1):28-29.
21. Papanicolaou N, Pfister RC, Yoder IC. Spontaneous and traumatic rupture of renal cysts: diagnosis and outcome. Radiology 1986;160(1):99-103.
22. Davis JM III, McLaughlin AP. Spontaneous renal hemorrhage due to cyst rupture: CT findings. AJR Am J Roentgenol 1987; 148(4):763-764.
23. Blakeley CJ, Thiagalingham N. Spontaneous retroperitoneal haemorrhage from a renal cyst: an unusual cause of haemorrhagic shock. Emerg Med J 2003;20(4):388.
24. Emmett JL, Levine SR, Woolner LB. Co-existence of renal cyst and tumor: incidence in 1,007 cases. Br J Urol 1963;35:403-410.
25. Lang EK. The differential diagnosis of renal cysts and tumors. Cyst puncture, aspiration, and analysis of cyst content for fat as diagnostic criteria for renal cysts. Radiology 1966;87(5):883-888.
26. Lang EK. Co-existence of cyst and tumor in the same kidney. Radiology 1971;101(1):7-16.
27. Ljungberg B, Holmberg G, Sjodin JG, et al. Renal cell carcinoma in a renal cyst: a case report and review of the literature. J Urol 1990;143(4):797-799.
28. Hayakawa M, Hatano T, Tsuji A, et al. Patients with renal cysts associated with renal cell carcinoma and the clinical implications of cyst puncture: a study of 223 cases. Urology 1996;47(5):643-646.
29. Mishal J, Lebovici O, Bregman L, et al. Huge renal arteriovenous malformation mimicking simple parapelvic cyst. Clin Imaging 2000;24(3):166-168.
30. Kwon HS, Shin SJ, Yun SN, et al. Renal artery aneurysm manifested as parapelvic cyst on abdominal sonography. Nephron 1996;74(1):229.
31. Meziane MA, Fishman EK, Goldman SM, et al. Computed tomography of high-density renal cysts in adult polycystic kidney disease. J Comput Assist Tomogr 1986;10(5):767-770.
32. Coleman BG, Arger PH, Mintz MC, et al. Hyperdense renal masses: a computed tomographic dilemma. AJR Am J Roentgenol 1984;143(2):291-294.
33. Cloix P, Martin X, Pangaud C, et al. Surgical management of complex renal cysts: a series of 32 cases. J Urol 1996;156(1):28-30.
34. Limb J, Santiago L, Kaswick J, et al. Laparoscopic evaluation of indeterminate renal cysts: long-term follow-up. J Endourol 2002;16(2):79-82.
35. Bosniak MA. The current radiological approach to renal cysts. Radiology 1986;158(1):1-10.
36. Bosniak MA. The use of the Bosniak classification system for renal cysts and cystic tumors. J Urol 1997;157(5):1852-1853.
37. Weyman PJ, McClennan BL, Lee JK, et al. CT of calcified renal masses. AJR Am J Roentgenol 1982;138(6):1095-1099.
38. Clayman RV, Surya V, Miller RP, et al. Pursuit of the renal mass: is ultrasound enough? Am J Med 1984;77(2):218-223.
39. McClennan BL, Stanley RJ, Melson GL, et al. CT of the renal cyst: is cyst aspiration necessary? AJR Am J Roentgenol 1979;133(4): 671-675.
40. Marotti M, Hricak H, Fritzsche P, et al. Complex and simple renal cysts: comparative evaluation with MR imaging. Radiology 1987; 162(3):679-684.
41. Bowers DL, Ikeguchi EF, Sawczuk IS. Transition from renal cyst to a renal carcinoma detected by ultrasonography. Br J Urol 1997; 80(3):495-496.
42. Balci NC, Semelka RC, Patt RH, et al. Complex renal cysts: findings on MR imaging. AJR Am J Roentgenol 1999;172(6):1495-1500.
43. Newhouse JH, Pfister RC. Renal cyst puncture. In: Anthasoulis CA, Pfister RC, Greene RE, Roberson GH, eds. Interventional Radiology. Philadelphia: WB Saunders, 1982:409-425.
44. Sandler CM. Renal cyst puncture and percutaneous drainage of perirenal fluid. In: Kadir S, ed. Current Practice of Interventional Radiology. Philadelphia: Decker, 1991:662-668.
45. Kleist H, Jonsson O, Lundstam S, et al. Quantitative lipid analysis in the differential diagnosis of cystic renal lesions. Br J Urol 1982;54(5):441-445.
46. Amis ES Jr, Cronan JJ, Yoder IC, et al. Renal cysts: curios and caveats. Urol Radiol 1982;4(4):199-209.
47. Kavoussi LR, Clayman RV, Mikkelsen DJ, et al. Ureteronephroscopic marsupialization of obstructing peripelvic renal cyst. J Urol 1991;146(2):411-414.
48. Ohkawa M, Motoi I, Hirano S, et al. Biochemical and pharmacodynamic studies of simple renal cyst fluids in relation to infection. Nephron 1991;59(1):80-83.
49. Lang EK. Renal cyst puncture and aspiration: a survey of complications. AJR Am J Roentgenol 1977;128(5):723-727.
50. Zelch J, Lalli AF, Stewart BH, et al. Complications of renal cyst exploration versus renal mass aspiration. Urology 1976;7(3): 244-247.
51. von Schreeb T, Arner O, Skovsted G, et al. Renal adenocarcinoma: is there a risk of spreading tumour cells in diagnostic puncture? Scand J Urol Nephrol 1967;1(3):270-276.
52. Jacobsson L, Lindqvist B, Michaelson G, et al. Fluid turnover in renal cysts. Acta Med Scand 1977;202(4):327-329.
53. Wahlqvist L, Grumstedt B. Therapeutic effect of percutaneous puncture of simple renal cyst. Follow-up investigation of 50 patients. Acta Chir Scand 1966;132(4):340-347.
54. Ozgur S, Cetin S, Ilker Y. Percutaneous renal cyst aspiration and treatment with alcohol. Int Urol Nephrol 1988;20(5):481-484.
55. Holmberg G, Hietala SO. Treatment of simple renal cysts by percutaneous puncture and instillation of bismuth-phosphate. Scand J Urol Nephrol 1989;23(3):207-212.
56. Bean WJ. Renal cysts: treatment with alcohol. Radiology 1981; 138(2):329-331.
57. Raskin MM, Poole DO, Roen SA, et al. Percutaneous management of renal cysts: results of a four-year study. Radiology 1975; 115(3):551-553.
58. Pfister RC, Schaffer D. Percutaneous ablation of renal cysts. AJR Am J Roentgenol 1979;132:1031.
59. Gelet A, Sanseverino R, Martin X, et al. Percutaneous treatment of benign renal cysts. Eur Urol 1990;18(4):248-252.
60. Phelan M, Zajko A, Hrebinko RL. Preliminary results of percutaneous treatment of renal cysts with povidone-iodine sclerosis. Urology 1999;53(4):816-817.
61. Kim SH, Moon MW, Lee HJ, et al. Renal cyst ablation with n-butyl cyanoacrylate and iodized oil in symptomatic patients with autosomal dominant polycystic kidney disease: preliminary report. Radiology 2003;226(2):573-576.
62. Peyromaure M, Debre B, Flam TA. Sclerotherapy of a giant renal cyst with povidone-iodine. J Urol 2002;168(6):2525.
63. Fontana D, Porpiglia F, Morra I, et al. Treatment of simple renal cysts by percutaneous drainage with three repeated alcohol injection. Urology 1999;53(5):904-907.
64. Delakas D, Karyotis I, Loumbakis P, et al. Long-term results after percutaneous minimally invasive procedure treatment of symptomatic simple renal cysts. Int Urol Nephrol 2001;32(3):321-326.
65. Paananen I, Hellstrom P, Leinonen S, et al. Treatment of renal cysts with single-session percutaneous drainage and ethanol sclerotherapy: long-term outcome. Urology 2001;57(1):30-33.
66. Camacho MF, Bondhus MJ, Carrion HM, et al. Ureteropelvic junction obstruction resulting from percutaneous cyst puncture and intracystic isophendylate injection: an unusual complications. J Urol 1980;124(5):713-714.
67. van der Ent CK, van Dalen A, Enterman JH. Antibiotic sclerotherapy for renal cysts. Rofo 1989;150(3):339-341.
68. Meng MV, Grossfeld GD, Stoller ML. Renal carcinoma after laparoscopic cyst decortication. J Urol 2002;167(3):1396.
69. Nieh PT, Bihrle W III. Laparoscopic marsupialization of massive renal cyst. J Urol 1993;150(1):171-173.
70. Morgan C Jr, Rader D. Laparoscopic unroofing of a renal cyst. J Urol 1992;148(6):1835-1836.
71. Hulbert JC. Laparoscopic management of renal cystic disease. Semin Urol 1992;10(4):239-241.
72. Amar AD, Das S. Surgical management of benign renal cysts causing obstruction of renal pelvis. Urology 1984;24(5):429-433.
73. Roberts WW, Bluebond-Langner R, Boyle KE, et al. Laparoscopic ablation of symptomatic parenchymal and peripelvic renal cysts. Urology 2001;58(2):165-169.
74. Hoenig DM, McDougall EM, Shalhav AL, et al. Laparoscopic ablation of peripelvic renal cysts. J Urol 1997;158(4):1345-1348.

75. Hulbert JC, Hunter D, Young AT, et al. Percutaneous intrarenal marsupialization of a perirenal cystic collection—endocystolysis. J Urol 1988;139(5):1039–1041.

76. Kang Y, Noble C, Gupta M. Percutaneous resection of renal cysts. J Endourol 2001;15(7):735–738; discussion 738–739.

77. Feinstein KA, Fernbach SK. Septated urinomas in the neonate. AJR Am J Roentgenol 1987;149(5):997–1000.

78. Fernbach SK, Feinstein KA, Zaontz MR. Urinoma formation in posterior urethral valves: relationship to later renal function. Pediatr Radiol 1990;20(7):543–545.

79. Connor JP, Hensle TW, Berdon W, et al. Contained neonatal urinoma: management and functional results. J Urol 1988;140(5 Pt 2):1319–1322.

80. McClinton S, Richmond P, Steyn JH. Spontaneous extravasation and urinoma formation secondary to cervical carcinoma. Br J Urol 1989;64(1):100–101.

81. Spurlock JW, Burke TW, Dunn NP, et al. Calyceal rupture with perirenal urinoma in a patient with cervical carcinoma. Obstet Gynecol 1987;70(3 Pt 2):511–513.

82. Cormio G, Cormio L, Di Gesu' G, et al. Calyceal rupture and perirenal urinoma as a presenting sign of recurrent ovarian cancer. Gynecol Oncol 2001;83(2):415–417.

83. Mundy AR, Podesta ML, Bewick M, et al. The urological complications of 1,000 renal transplants. Br J Urol 1981;53(5):397–402.

84. Loughlin KR, Tilney NL, Richie JP. Urologic complications in 718 renal transplant patients. Surgery 1984;95(3):297–302.

85. Matlaga BR, Veys JA, Jung F, et al. Subcapsular urinoma: an unusual form of page kidney in a high school wrestler. J Urol 2002;168(2):672.

86. Boone TB, Gilling PJ, Husmann DA. Ureteropelvic junction disruption following blunt abdominal trauma. J Urol 1993;150(1):33–36.

87. Flynn DE, Caroline DF, Gembala RB, et al. Urinoma secondary to surgical spinal fusion: radiologic diagnosis and treatment. Abdom Imaging 1993;18(3):292–294.

88. Braf ZF, Morag B, Many M. Spontaneous peripelvic extravasation of urine after transurethral resection of bladder tumor. Urology 1983;21(2):182–184.

89. Alkibay T, Karaoglan U, Gundogdu S, et al. An unusual complication of extracorporeal shock wave lithotripsy: urinoma due to rupture of the renal pelvis. Int Urol Nephrol 1992;24(1):11–14.

90. Portela LA, Patel SK, Callahan DH. Pararenal pseudocyst (urinoma) as complication of percutaneous nephrostomy. Urology 1979;13(5):570–571.

91. Rajendran LJ, Rao MS, Bapna BC, et al. Peripelvic extravasation and formation of perinephric urinoma after cystoscopy. Urology 1980;16(2):199–201.

92. Thompson IM, Ross G Jr, Ezzard J, et al. Experiences with 16 cases of pararenal pseudocyst. J Urol 1976;116(3):289–292.

93. Hoffer FA, Winters WD, Retik AB, et al. Urinoma drainage for neonatal respiratory insufficiency. Pediatr Radiol 1990;20(4):270–271.

94. Cullmann HJ, Prosinger M. Necrosis of the allograft ureter—evaluation of different examination methods in early diagnosis. Urol Int 1990;45(3):164–169.

95. Smith TP, Hunter DW, Letourneau JG, et al. Urine leaks after renal transplantation: value of percutaneous pyelography and drainage for diagnosis and treatment. AJR Am J Roentgenol 1988;151(3):511–3.

96. Turner AG, Howlett KA, Eban R, et al. The role of anterograde pyelography in the transplant kidney. J Urol 1980;123(6):812–814.

97. Kinnaert P, Hall M, Janssen F, et al. Ureteral stenosis after kidney transplantation: true incidence and long-term follow-up after surgical correction. J Urol 1985;133(1):17–20.

98. Horikami K, Matsuoka Y, Nagaoki K, et al. Treatment of post-traumatic urinoma by means of selective arterial embolization. J Vasc Interv Radiol 1997;8(2):221–224.

99. Pinto IT, Chimeno PC. Treatment of a urinoma and a post-traumatic pseudoaneurysm using selective arterial embolization. Cardiovasc Intervent Radiol 1998;21(6):506–508.

100. Darcy MD. Radiologic diagnosis and management of urologic complications of renal transplantation. Semin Intervent Radiol 1992;9:246–255.

101. Lieberman RP, Glass NR, Crummy AB, et al. Nonoperative percutaneous management of urinary fistulas and strictures in renal transplantation. Surg Gynecol Obstet 1982;155(5):667–672.

102. Matalon TA, Thompson MJ, Patel SK, et al. Percutaneous treatment of urine leaks in renal transplantation patients. Radiology 1990;174(3 Pt 2):1049–1051.

103. Lang EK, Glorioso L III. Management of urinomas by percutaneous drainage procedures. Radiol Clin North Am 1986;24(4):551–559.

Perspectives on Varicocele Management

43

Richard Shlansky-Goldberg, Jeffery Adam Solomon

The expression "The more things change, the more they stay the same" is exemplified by the study of varicoceles. In the years since publication of the previous version of this chapter in the late 1990s, controversy regarding the impact of varicocele on fertility has remained. Although most retrospective studies support the concept that varicoceles decrease fertility in some men, several studies and reviews continue to fuel suspicion about the potential association between the two (1). Until well-controlled prospective trials are conducted, debate will continue.

HISTORY

The relationship between semen and male infertility has been recognized since the 18th century; however, it was not until the late 19th century that the effect of varicoceles on seminal parameters was demonstrated (2). Barwell, in 1885, reported his experience with the "subcutaneous wire loop" ligation of 100 varicoceles (3). Bennett, in 1889, reported improvement in semen quality in a patient with bilateral varicoceles "after one side had been cured" by surgery (4). Not until the early 1950s in Britain, when Tulloch reported the production of sperm after varicocele ligation in a previously azoospermic male resulting in a pregnancy, did the implication that varicocele might cause infertility become apparent (5). In 1962, Charny was the first in the United States to publicize the effects of varicocele on fertility (6). Finally, MacLeod studied the semen analyses from 200 men with varicoceles because of the developing reports of improvement in semen characteristics after surgical ligation (7). He defined the "stress pattern," which is an increased number of immature cells and tapered forms with decreased motility with or without a decrease in concentration, confirming the

effect of varicoceles on sperm quality. Although this pattern may be seen with other conditions, including congenital adrenal hyperplasia, alcohol abuse, and aftermath of a febrile or viral episode, it is best known for its association with varicocele. Iaccarino and Lima et al. published the first reports, in 1977 and 1978 respectively, of percutaneous therapy for the correction of varicoceles with a sclerosing agent (8,9).

Percutaneous treatment of varicocele for infertility has become very popular as a primary treatment or as an adjuvant to failed surgery (10,11). Other indications for varicocele correction include pain and swelling (12), in addition to testicular atrophy in the pediatric or adolescent population (13,14). Boys with varicocele are at significant risk for testicular atrophy (15). Although debate continues about when to correct a varicocele in a pediatric patient, studies suggest that there is a clear benefit to the treatment of adolescent varicocele with the ultimate goal to prevent infertility (16).

DEFINITION AND INCIDENCE

A varicocele is an abnormal venous dilatation of the *pampiniform plexus*, which may extend from the spermatic veins to the level of the left renal vein or inferior vena cava. Rarely, the varicocele can also be associated with dilated intratesticular veins or subcutaneous varices (17,18). The incidence of varicocele in healthy males is 8–23%. The left side is involved in 70–100% of cases, and isolated right-side involvement occurs in 0–9% of cases. Both sides are involved in 0–23% of cases (19–22). Gat et al. considers varicocele a bilateral disease in patients being treated for infertility (23,24). In a prospective analysis, Gat and associates found that approximately 80% of patients in the study had bilateral disease when using methods of evaluation. The incidence of varicocele rises at the onset of puberty and is 16.2% at the ages of 10–19 (20). Varicocele is considered to be an important factor in infertility in approximately 21–41% of infertile males who visit infertility clinics, with 20–25% of these men seeking percutaneous or surgical correction (19–21,25).

ANATOMY

Venous drainage of the testicle is by several routes (Figure 43–1). The spermatic venous plexus, also called

the pampiniform plexus, is formed by multiple venous sinuses that are dilated and tortuous, with an approximate diameter of 5 mm (26). Opposite the head of the femur, the veins coalesce and unite to form the internal spermatic vein, which is the major draining route (26). With conventional anatomy, the internal spermatic vein drains into the left renal vein on the left and into the infrarenal inferior vena cava on the right (27) (Figure 43–2). In a left-sided vena cava, the left spermatic vein drains directly into the vena cava (28). There are three additional routes of venous drainage from the scrotum and testicle: the external pudendal, vasal, and cremasteric veins (26,29). The external

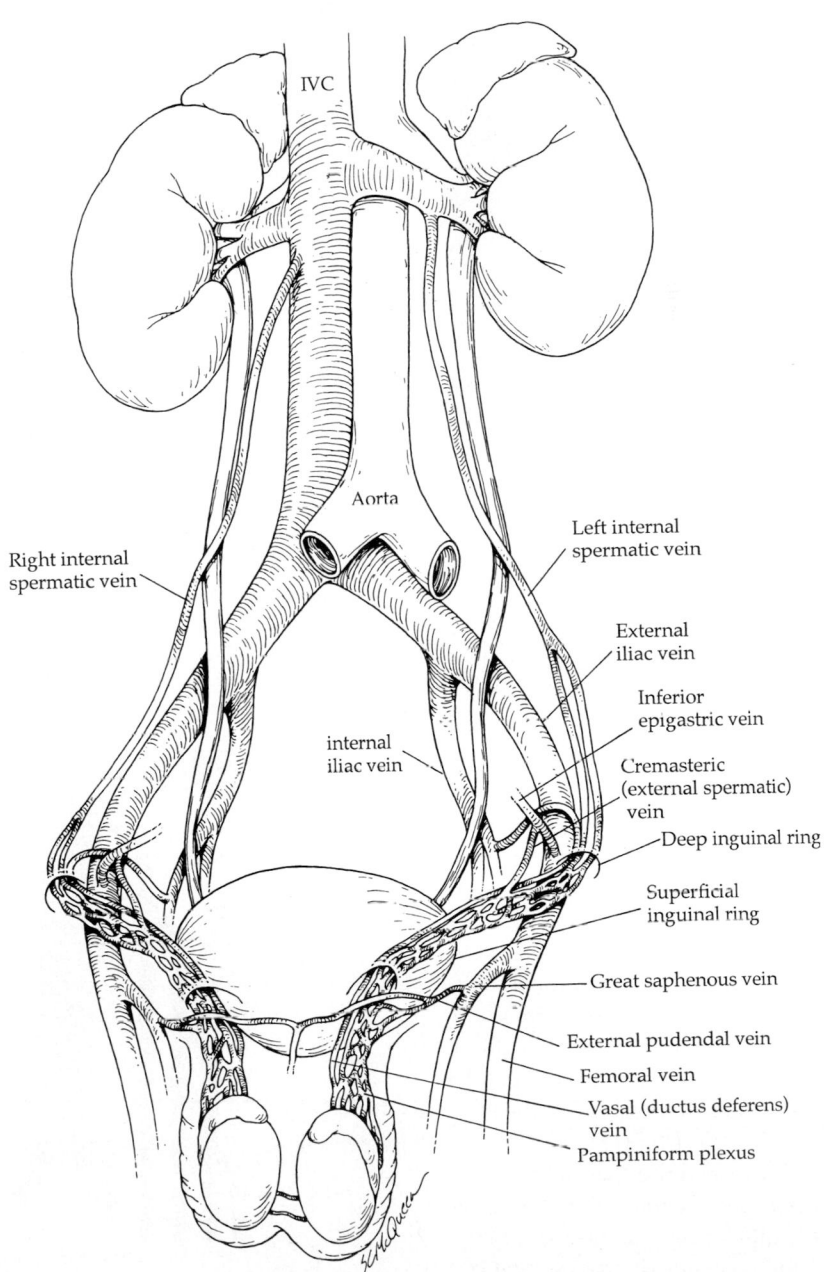

Figure 43–1 Classic gonadal venous drainage for both the right and left testicles. The main drainage of the testicle involves several veins that originate from the pampiniform plexus as the spermatic, cremasteric, pudendal, and vasal veins. The left gonadal vein enters the left renal vein, while the right renal vein enters the inferior vena cava below the right renal vein.

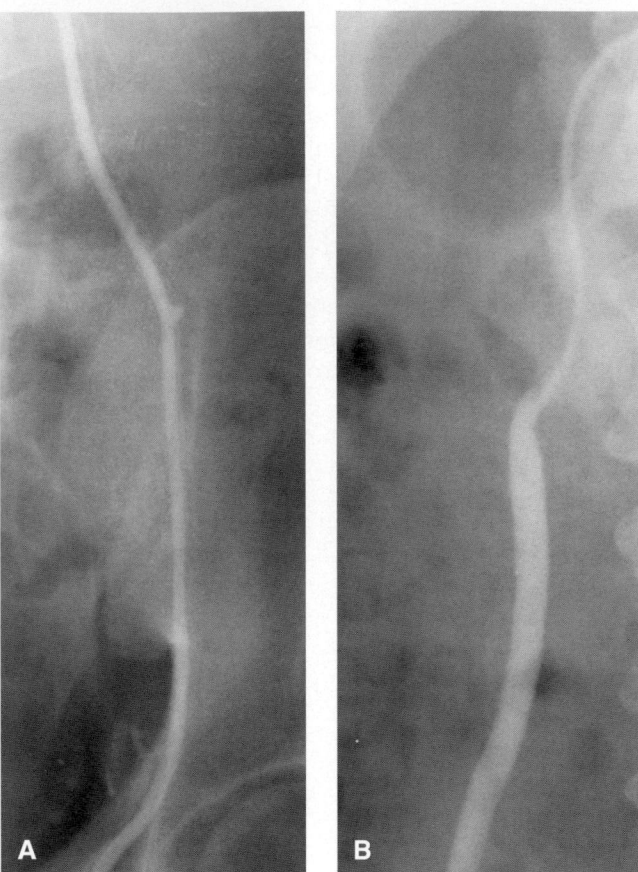

Figure 43–2 Typical spermatic venogram associated with varicocele demonstrating reflux of contrast without evidence of valves. **A.** Left gonadal venogram. **B.** Right gonadal venogram with a Simmons 3 catheter.

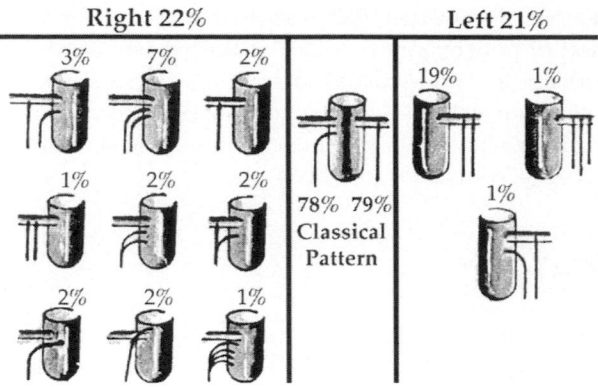

Figure 43–3 Anatomic variation in the termination of the right and left gonadal veins with the percentages of each variation as seen in 200 gonadal veins. The classic pattern of a single left spermatic vein entering the left renal vein is seen in 79% of cases, and a single right spermatic vein entering into the inferior vena cava below the right renal vein is seen in 78% of cases as determined by Lechter et al. (27).

pudendal vein, also named the superficial external pudendal vein, originates from the plexus at the level of the inferior pubic ramus and travels superiolaterally to terminate in the long saphenous vein that drains into the femoral vein. The vasal vein, also named the ductus deferens vein, is a small vessel that arises near the testis and passes upward to join into the internal iliac vein via the inferior or superior vesical. The cremasteric vein, also called the external spermatic vein, arises at the level of the superior pubic ramus, passes laterally and superiorly to anastomose to the external iliac vein via the inferior epigastric vein. Although typically involving the internal spermatic vein, the cremasteric vein may also be involved in the formation of the varicocele (30). After embolization or ligation, the external pudendal vein most often provides the major drainage from the scrotum followed by the cremasteric vein (26,31).

Several investigators have described the spermatic venous anatomy using postmortem specimens or venography. Unfortunately, considerable differences exist in the description of venous collaterals, the existence of cross-scrotal collaterals, and venous valves (26,27,29,32–36). Lechter et al. analyzed 200 spermatic veins from 100 cadavers and found that the classic pattern was present 78% of the time on the right and 79% of the time on the left (27) (Figure 43–3).

The spermatic vein may terminate in the right renal vein in 8% of cases. Double or multiple terminations may be found in 16% of cases on the right and rarely may enter above the right renal vein. On the left, a double system goes to the renal vein in 19%, a triple system in 1%, and rarely its accessing branches may also enter the inferior vena cava left (27) (Figure 43–3).

Analysis of the spermatic vein trunks usually demonstrates one to six trunks originating in the lower one third as they ascend, merging to form fewer trunks in the upper third of the spermatic vein (27). In some cases, one trunk in the lower third ascends into multiple veins (27) (Figures 43–4 and 43–5).

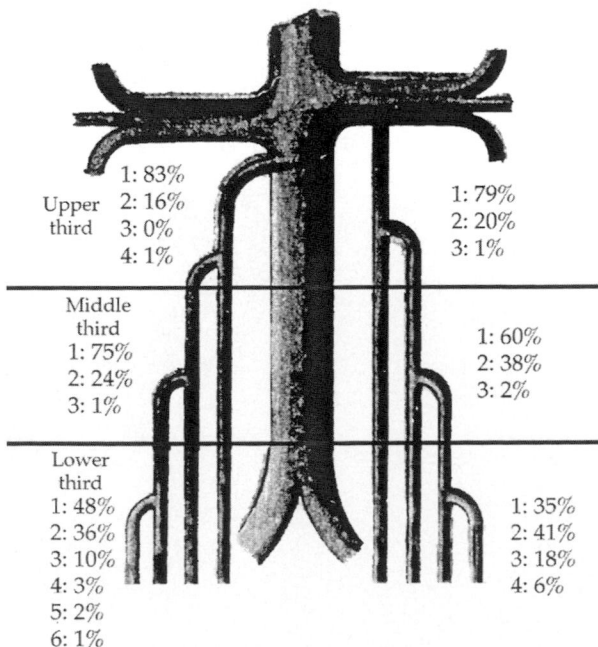

Figure 43–4 Number of venous trunks as they ascend from the pampiniform plexus, with the percentage seen in 200 gonadal veins as determined by Lechter et al. (27).

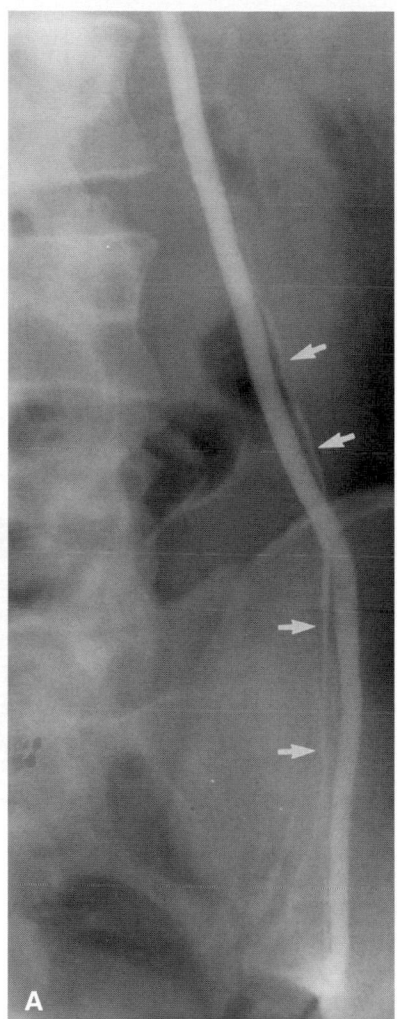

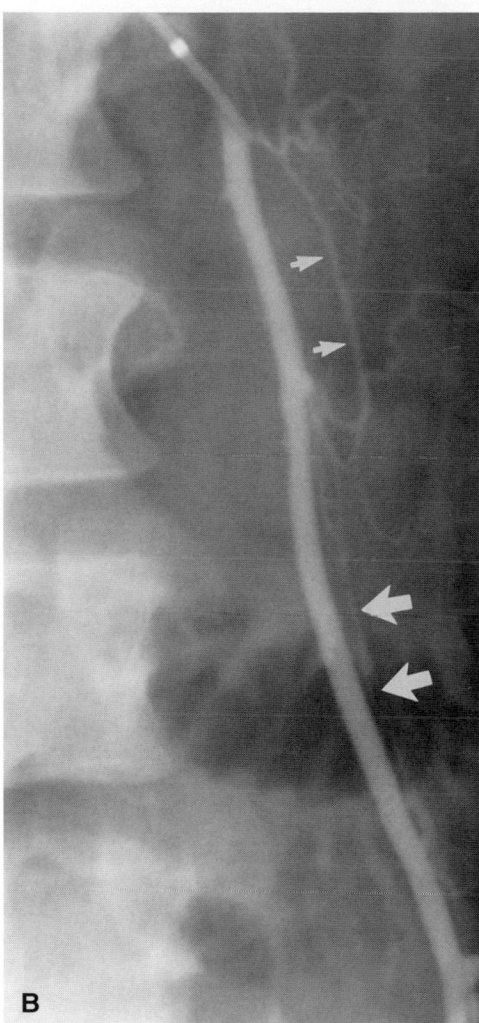

Figure 43–5 Two left gonadal venograms demonstrating multiple venous trunks. **A.** Two venous trunks with one large and an additional smaller parallel trunk (*white arrows*). **B.** Several small trunks, one in the cephalad portion of the vein (*small arrows*) and additional ones in the inferior portion (*large arrows*).

The number of valves distributed along the course of the spermatic vein may be 0–3, with some investigators finding more veins valvulated on the left and others finding more on the right (27,36) (Figure 43–6). Analysis by still other investigators has demonstrated no valves at all, including Wishahi, who failed to find valves in a postmortem review of 40 men (35).

Collateral vessels around the spermatic vein create anastomoses to the systemic circulation at the cremasteric, pudendal, vasal, retroperitoneal, ureteral, peritoneal, renal,

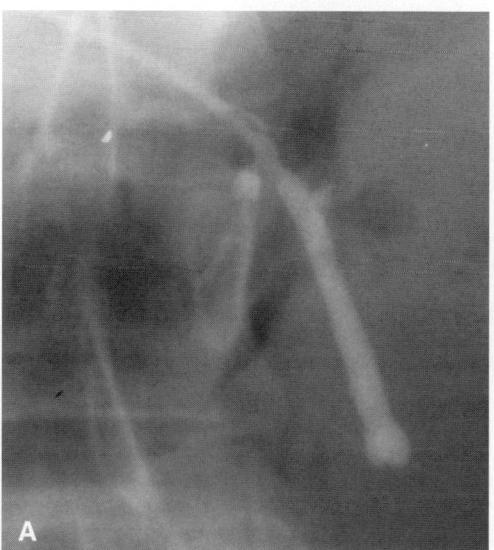

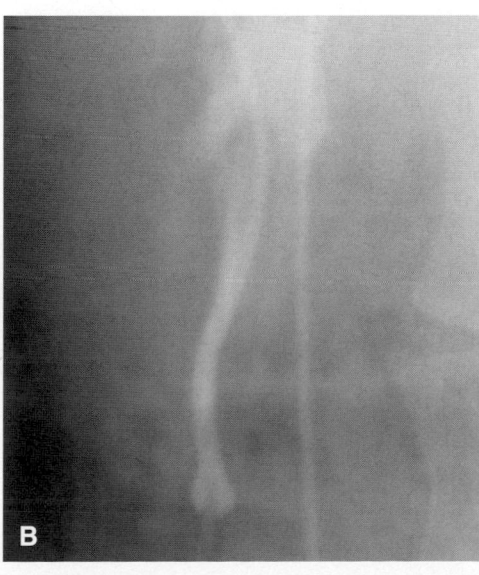

Figure 43–6 Normal competent venous valves. **A.** Left spermatic vein with valve near entrance into left renal vein. **B.** Right spermatic vein with valve near entrance into inferior vena cava.

right testicular, and adrenal veins, in addition to the IVC and portal system through the splenic, superior mesenteric, and sigmoid colonic veins (26,27,32,34,35) (Figures 43–7, 43–8, and 43–9). Lechter et al. found that 67% of the left side veins and 49% of the right side veins demonstrated collaterals, with those in the upper third of the vein coming from Gerota's fascia and the lower third coming from the retroperitoneum (27). Examining autopsy specimens, Wishahi noted

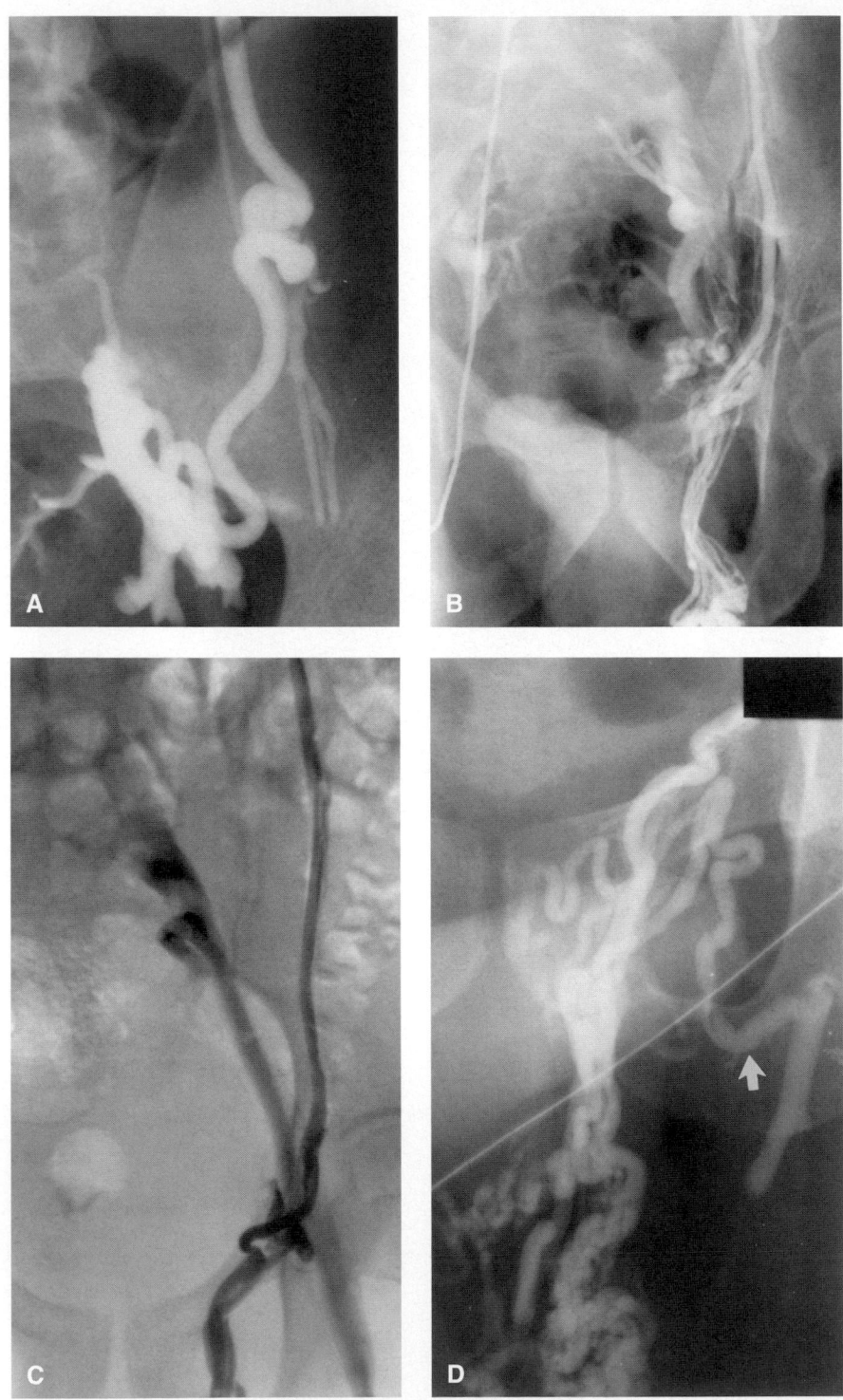

Figure 43–7 Venograms demonstrating communication to the systemic circulation. **A.** Left spermatic vein injection demonstrating filling of the internal iliac artery without filling of the varicocele. **B.** Left spermatic venogram demonstrating filling of the varicocele, which communicates with the internal iliac artery most likely through the vasal veins. Note cross-sacral venous collaterals. **C.** Left spermatic venogram demonstrating filling of the varicocele and the left external iliac vein, probably via the cremasteric or pudendal veins. **D.** Left spermatic venogram demonstrating filling of the greater saphenous vein via the external pudendal (*arrow*).

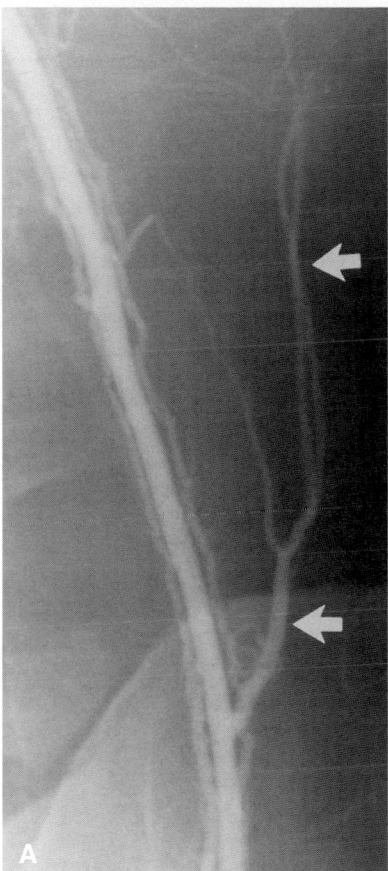
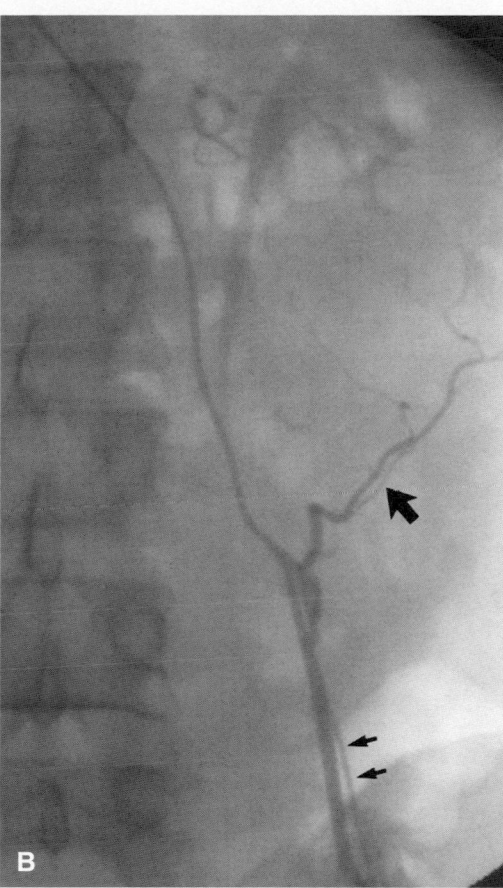

Figure 43–8 Left spermatic venograms demonstrating retroperitoneal collaterals. These have the appearance of the medial and lateral divisions as described by Wishahi (35). **A.** Left spermatic vein with major medial division and smaller lateral division (*arrows*), which probably communicates with the retroperitoneum and the renal capsule. Note the smaller parallel venous trunks. **B.** Left spermatic venogram demonstrating another example of retroperitoneal collaterals (*large arrows*) with a small parallel trunk in the caudal portion of the vein (*small arrows*).

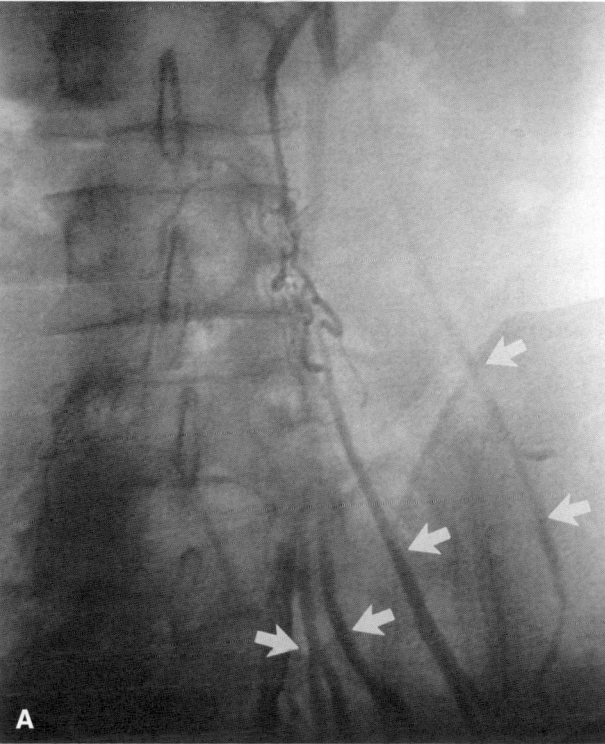
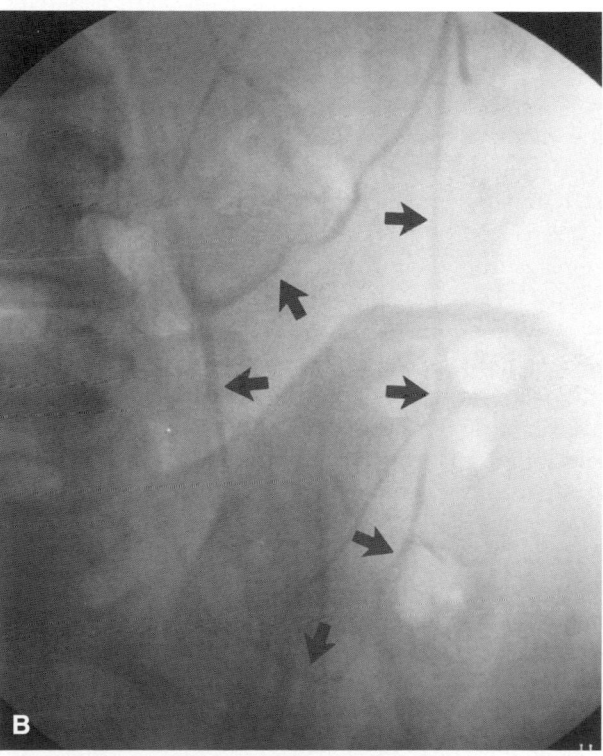

Figure 43–9 Left spermatic venogram demonstrating communication with portal circulation. **A.** Venogram demonstrates filling of superior mesenteric vein branches (*arrows*). **B.** Venogram demonstrates filling of the colonic vein branches (*arrows*) from the inferior mesenteric vein.

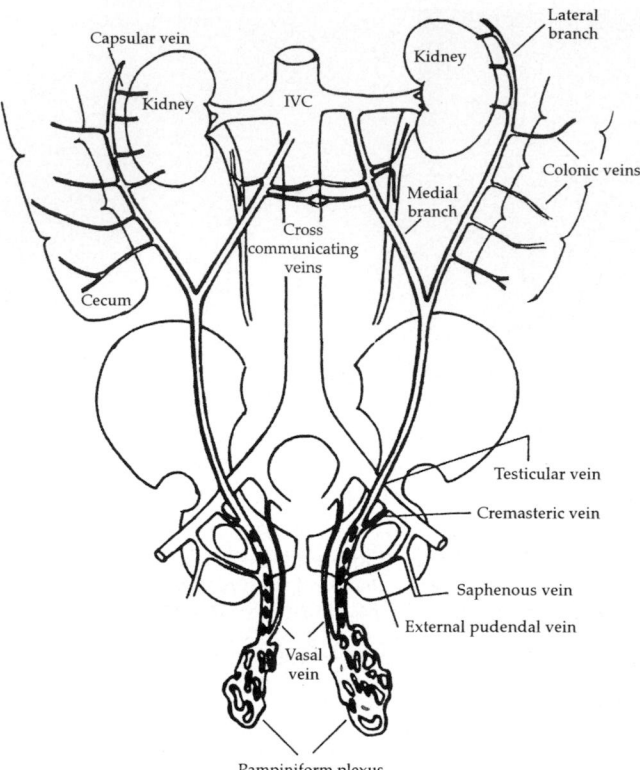

Figure 43–10 Anatomy of the left and right gonadal vein as described by Wishahi (34). Note the presence of the medial and lateral branches in addition to portal venous and systemic collaterals. (Modified with permission from Wishahi MM. Anatomy of the venous drainage of the human testis: testicular vein cast, microdissection, and radiographic demonstration. A new anatomical concept. Eur Urol 1991;20:154–160.)

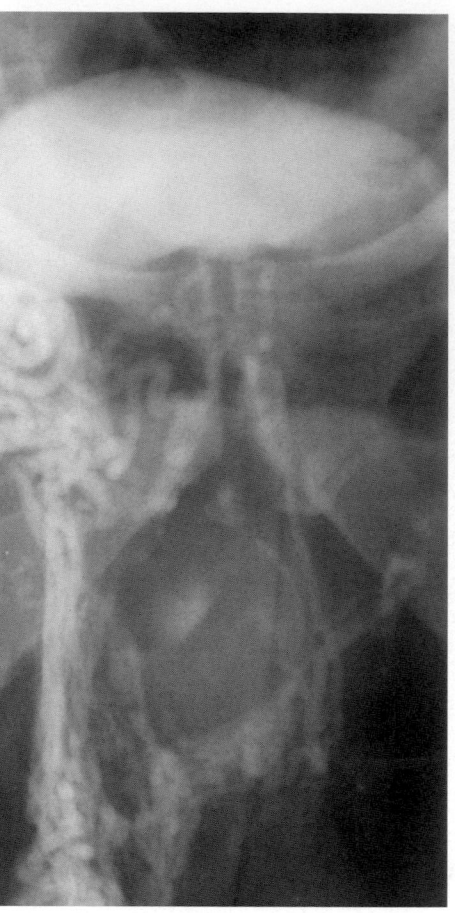

Figure 43–11 Left spermatic venogram demonstrating filling of the varicocele and cross-scrotal and pelvic collaterals.

that the spermatic vein divided at L4 into medial and lateral divisions (Figure 43–10). The medial division was the largest, terminating in the left renal vein on the left and the inferior vena cava on the right. At the level of L3, multiple veins emerge from the medial division to anastomose with the veins of the bladder, ureter, and pelvis of the kidney. The lateral division terminates in the perinephric fat. Multiple veins extend from the lateral division toward the lateral border of the kidney to join the renal capsular vessels and the colonic veins of the portal system (35) (Figure 43–8). Wishahi found no cross-communication between left and right systems in the scrotal, retropubic, or pelvic areas on venography but did find cadaver evidence of communication at the L3 level between the medial spermatic vein divisions in 55% of cases. Others have demonstrated scrotal cross-collaterals (37) (Figure 43–11). Sofikitis et al. found the gonadal vein to bifurcate into medial and lateral divisions, as described by Wishahi, in only 45% of cases, with cross-lumbar collaterals occurring in 4% of specimens (32).

Many of these collaterals or divisions cause bypassing anastomoses that create aberrantly fed varicoceles, as described by Marsman in 17–19% of patients, making successful percutaneous embolization more difficult with a

lower technical success rate (38) (Figure 43–12). Typically, these high parallel or renal collaterals cause recurrences for patients treated with embolization, and mid-vessels and low vessels cause recurrences for patients treated with surgical ligation (39,40). Other causes of recurrence were because of transscrotal collaterals (39). The surgical recurrences may be treated easily by embolization, while embolization recurrences are more difficult to successfully re-treat (41).

PATHOPHYSIOLOGY

Varicoceles may be primary or secondary. Secondary causes of varicocele are from compression of the veins draining the pampiniform plexus because of pelvic and abdominal tumors, such as lymphoma, metastasis from renal cell adenocarcinoma, and cecal carcinoma. These cases may present as an isolated right varicocele (42–44). Cases of rupture of an aortic aneurysm into the renal vein causing left-sided varicocele and compression by a false aneurysm from an aortic graft causing a right varicocele have also been described (45,46). Another cause of solitary or predominately right-sided varicocele is situ inversus (47).

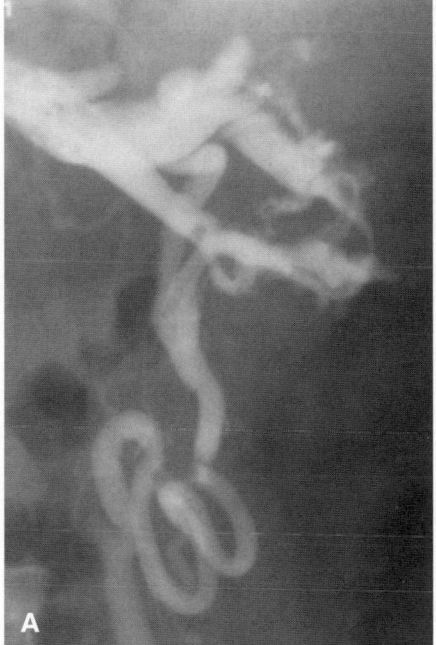 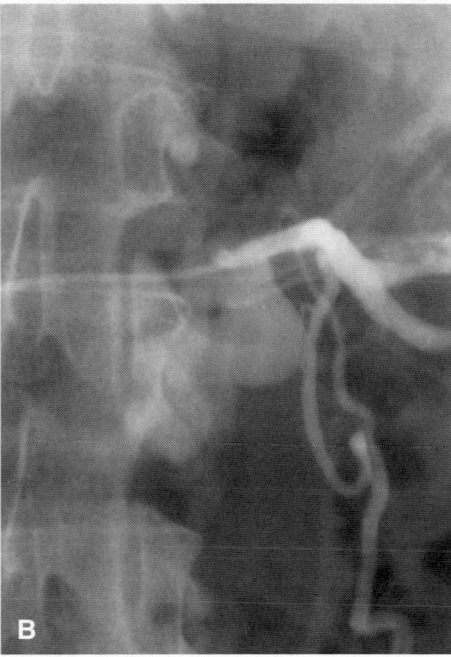 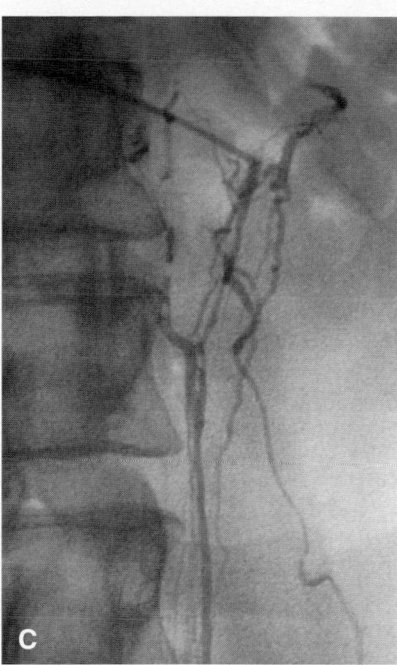

Figure 43–12 Left spermatic venograms demonstrating tortuous vessels with a serpiginous course and bypassing anastomoses, making embolization difficult. **A.** Two vessels entering into different branches of the renal vein. **B.** Another example of two vessels entering the renal vein with one entering the main renal vein and the other entering a branch. **C.** Venogram demonstrating multiple collaterals extending into the renal vein.

Most varicoceles, especially those associated with infertility, are primary. Several hypotheses exist to explain the etiology of primary varicoceles. One is that there is a lack of venous valves in the spermatic vein or an abnormality of the vein that transmits hydrostatic pressure from the inferior vena cava (48). This hypothesis alone cannot explain the cause of varicocele, because individuals without varicocele may lack valves. In addition, valvular incompetence may be secondary to the internal spermatic vein dilatation rather than the cause of the dilatation (49).

Another suspected cause of varicocele is the "nutcracker phenomenon" (50). This theory maintains that the left renal vein is compressed between the aorta and superior mesenteric artery, particularly when a patient is erect, causing increased pressure in the gonadal vein that results in the dilatation. Other causes of left renal vein compression are also possible (50). This phenomenon includes not only renal vein compression but also compression of the iliac vein by the iliac artery, the so-called "lower nutcracker" (51). Several studies have supported this theory using anatomic and pressure measurements (50,52–55). Other theories concerning the etiology of varicocele suspect that it may be because of anatomic differences between the left and right renal veins. The left spermatic vein is longer and enters the left renal vein at a right angle, across from the orifice of the adrenal vein, possibly causing turbulence and valvular dysfunction (49). Another theory, disproved by Sayfan et al., suggested a defect in the cremaster muscles with diminished

tension of the fasciomuscular tube of the spermatic cord, resulting in decreased venous return and venous congestion, the so called "cremasteric pump mechanism" (56–58).

ETIOLOGY OF INFERTILITY

Several theories have postulated the effect varicoceles have on testicular function, and more than one theory may be correct. The two most plausible hypotheses are elevated testicular temperatures and reflux of toxic metabolites that cause testicular dysfunction and infertility.

Many investigators believe that the varicocele causes increased scrotal temperature, possibly by interfering with the normal counter-current heat exchange (6,19). Elevated testicular temperature is known to have an adverse effect on spermatogenesis (59). In experimental animal models, Kay et al. and Saypol et al. demonstrated that there is an increase in blood flow and temperature within the scrotum associated with varicoceles (60,61). Normal scrotal temperature is lower than body core temperature, with the difference between core body temperature and scrotal temperature being smaller in men with varicoceles (62). Several studies have demonstrated higher scrotal temperatures in patients with varicocele (8,59,62,63). The average temperature is $0.3\,^{\circ}\mathrm{C}$ higher on the side with the varicocele compared to the normal side, with the greatest difference obtained with the patient standing (59). Using a device to lower testicular temperatures in men with varicocele has resulted in improvement in semen quality, resulting in pregnancies (64).

Reflux of renal and adrenal metabolites has also been hypothesized as a cause of testicular dysfunction. The compounds reach the testicles by backflow into the spermatic vein from the renal vein and by venous crossover to the contralateral testis. A few investigators have reported catecholamine concentrations in patients with varicoceles to be higher than patients without (65,66). Others found cortisol and renin levels not to be different (65,67). Charny and Baum in 1968 found no significant difference in adrenal steroid concentrations from peripheral blood samples, compared to spermatic vein samples in patients with varicocele (68). At present, no data suggest that prostaglandins PGE_2 and $PGF_{2\alpha}$ produced in the kidneys reflux into the gonadal vein to cause impaired spermatogenesis resulting from vasoconstriction and inhibition of luteinizing hormone (62,69). Higher levels of PGE_2 and $PGF_{2\alpha}$ have been found in the gonadal vein of varicocele patients than in peripheral blood and phospholipase A2 levels in semen decrease after varicocele correction (62).

Another etiology includes an alteration in the hypothalamic-pituitary-gonadal axis (70), in which Hudson describes a population of varicocele patients whose gonadotropin response to gonadotropin-releasing hormone and prolactin response to thyrotropin-releasing hormone to be excessive. These patients had improvement in their semen after correction. Hudson suggests that there is an abnormality in the pantesticular hormone synthesis and spermatogenesis in some men with varicocele that, after correction, undergoes some improvement (70). Other explanations for the abnormality in spermatogenesis include Leydig cell dysfunction and hypoxia that results from venous stasis, in addition to alterations in the thickness of intratesticular blood vessels because of changes in nutrient transfer and edema (71–75). More recently, reactive oxygen species have been called into suspicion (76).

DIAGNOSIS

Varicoceles generally are diagnosed by palpation, then they are graded. A varicocele is considered to be grade 1 or small when it is palpable with a Valsalva maneuver. A moderate varicocele or grade 2 is present when it is palpable without a Valsalva maneuver. A grade 3 or larger is visible without palpation (77).

Subclinical varicoceles are those that cannot be palpated, but the patient is infertile and there is an abnormal semen analysis including the demonstration of "stress-forms" that are consistent with a varicocele (77). Usually, this is diagnosed by duplex Doppler ultrasound. Subclinical varicoceles are those that cannot be palpated, but the patient is infertile and there is an abnormal semen analysis including the demonstration of "stress-forms" that are consistent with

a varicocele (77). Usually, this is diagnosed by duplex and color Doppler ultrasound (Figure 43–13). Other methods of diagnosis include thermography, radionuclide scrotal imaging, and magnetic resonance imaging (MRI) in addition to spermatic venography (Figure 43–14).

Conventional duplex scanning with a high-resolution, dedicated, small-parts transducer (5–10 MHz) is used to diagnose varicocele by demonstrating a dilated pampiniform plexus greater than 2–3 mm, while color Doppler allows demonstration of venous reflux into the varicosity (78). Performing a Valsalva maneuver in the supine and erect positions aids the diagnosis of a small varicocele. Petros et al. demonstrated that ultrasound can detect 93% of the venographically evident, subclinical varicoceles when compared to physical examination, which only detected 71% (79–81). Sonographic criteria of venous dilatation has a sensitivity of 92.2%, specificity of 100%, and an accuracy of 92.7% when compared to thermography for the diagnosis of varicocele (82). Sigmund et al. described two different types of hemodynamic patterns in varicoceles as determined by bidirectional Doppler flow studies and confirmed by venography, called stop-type and shunt-type varicoceles (83) (Figure 43–15). The stop-type varicocele refluxes only into the spermatic vein. The shunt-type first refluxes into the spermatic vein then has physiologic retrograde and orthograde flow in the cremasteric, the deferential veins, or both, thus providing a shunt or venous bypass (83). The pathophysiology is explained by incompetence of the venous valves in the region of the pampiniform plexus and the communicating veins. The shunt-type was more frequent and believed to be a precondition for medium and large varices.

Spermatic venography, first described by Ahlberg in 1966, is generally considered the gold standard for demonstrating reflux into the gonadal vein (84,85). One concern about the diagnosis of varicocele by venography is that the diagnosis of venous reflux is made under conditions of variable injection pressure and catheter-tip placement, which may be beyond or be disruptive to the valves and may not represent normal physiologic conditions (11). In addition, injecting into the renal vein may also not represent true physiologic conditions under which the patient may reflux into the spermatic vein, especially when the patient is not fully erect.

Although the size of varicoceles can be graded, investigators originally believed that this parameter did not influence the improvement seen after varicocele correction, and a subclinical varicocele could impact infertility as much as a grade 3 (86). Marsman demonstrated that the venographic differences between clinical and subclinical varicoceles was in the degree of reflux (86), and he classified the degree of reflux into grades 0–5, with grade 0 representing no reflux and 1–5 representing reflux into the upper lumbar, lower lumbar, upper pelvic, lower pelvic, or inguinal portion of the spermatic veins, respectively. Other classification systems deal with the venographic findings of varicocele and their collaterals. Porst et al. established a classification based on five venographic patterns (Types I–V) (87). Some types were

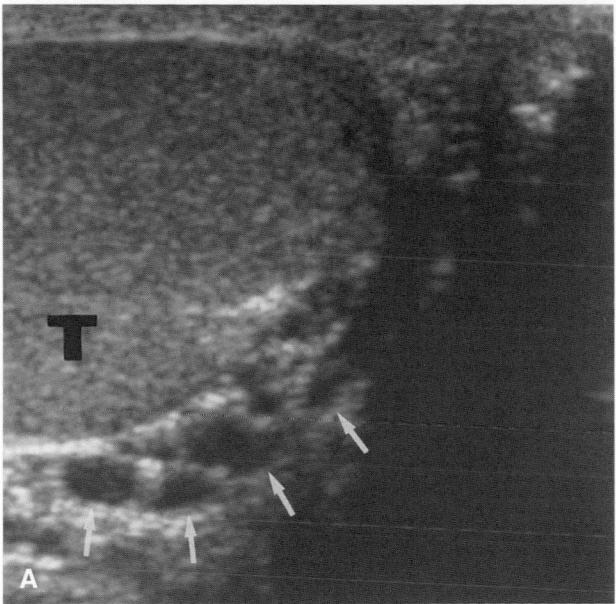

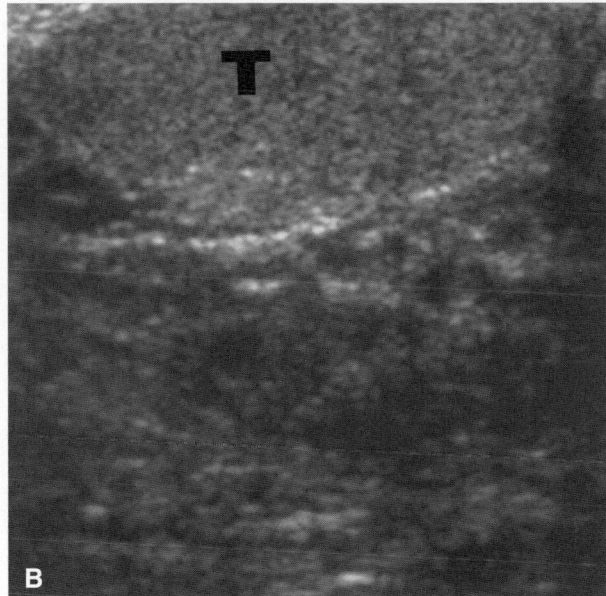

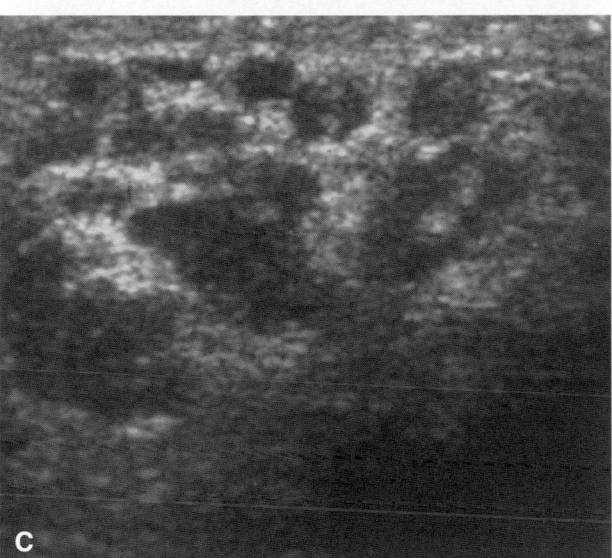

Figure 43–13 Duplex ultrasound demonstrating varicoceles. **A.** A moderate-sized varicocele seen with hypoechoic tubular structures (*arrows*) behind the testicle (T), representing veins of the dilated pampiniform plexus. **B.** A large-sized varicocele behind the testicle (T) filling most of the scrotum. **C.** Another view of the varicocele seen in B demonstrating the large hypoechoic varicosities.

more frequent than others and easier to embolize percutaneously with sclerotherapy (Figure 43–16). More recently, this lack of association with size has been called into question with the general belief that the subclinical varicoceles do not cause infertility (76).

SURGICAL CORRECTION

Before the advent of percutaneous therapy, surgical correction of varicocele was the main treatment option. There are three major surgical procedures currently performed that vary by the level at which the spermatic vein is ligated. These are called the retroperitoneal, inguinal, or subinguinal approach (Figure 43–17). The modified Palomo procedure, or retroperitoneal approach, involves an incision approximately

3 cm medial and 5–6 cm below the anterior portion of the iliac crest (88). This allows access to the retroperitoneal space to ligate one or more of the branches of the internal spermatic veins immediately superior to the inguinal ring (43,77). A lower retroperitoneal approach, the Ivanissevich procedure, is carried out through an inguinal incision to ligate the internal spermatic vein or its tributaries at the level of the internal ring (43,77,89). More recently, Marmar et al. described a subinguinal approach requiring microdissection at the external inguinal ring, thus requiring only a subcutaneous incision without disturbing fascial planes (90). This technique is performed with local anesthesia on an outpatient basis and requires only a few days of recovery time. The recovery time for inguinal or retroperitoneal approaches is generally longer, with patients returning to work within a few days and to full activity in 3–4 weeks (43).

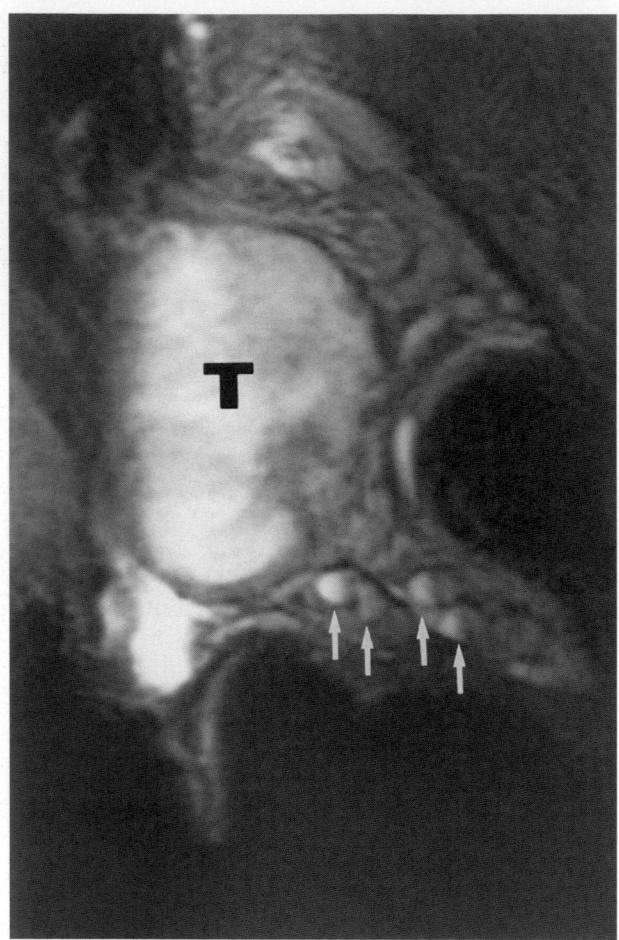

Figure 43–14 Sagittal MRI (TR/TE: 5,000/150 m/sec) of the scrotum demonstrating high intensity testicle (T) with dilated veins (*arrows*) of the pampiniform plexus. Note the slow flow within the varicocele, causing a "hematocrit effect."

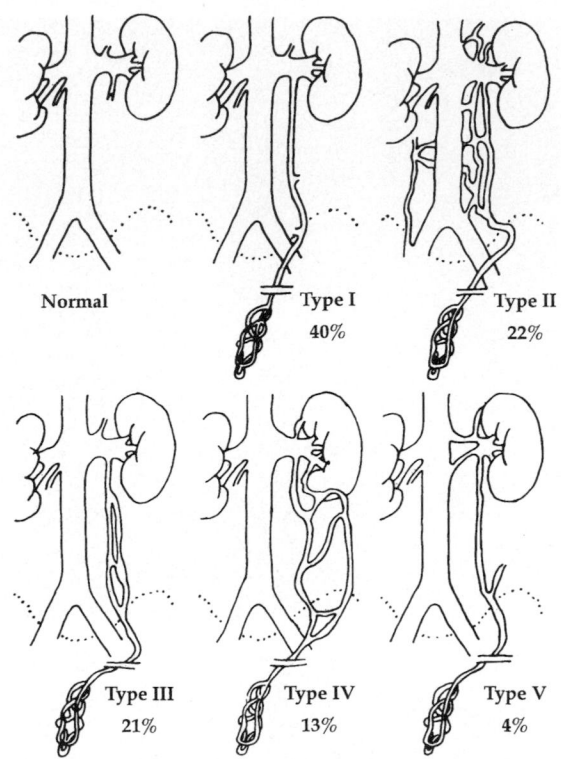

Figure 43–16 Venographic classification of the course of the left renal vein with percentages in their study population of 259 left-sided varicoceles as described by Porst et al. (87). *Type I*: Single renal vein without valves—the most common type. *Type II*: Collateral retroperitoneal vessels to ascending lumbar vein or retroaortal to caval vein. *Type III*: Duplicated internal spermatic vein with cross-connecting vessels. *Type IV*: Collaterals to renal or capsular veins. *Type V*: Retroaortic bifurcated renal vein. (Reprinted with permission from Porst H, Bahren W, Lenz M, et al. Percutaneous sclerotherapy of varicoceles—an alternative to conventional surgical methods. Br J Urol 1984;56:73–78.)

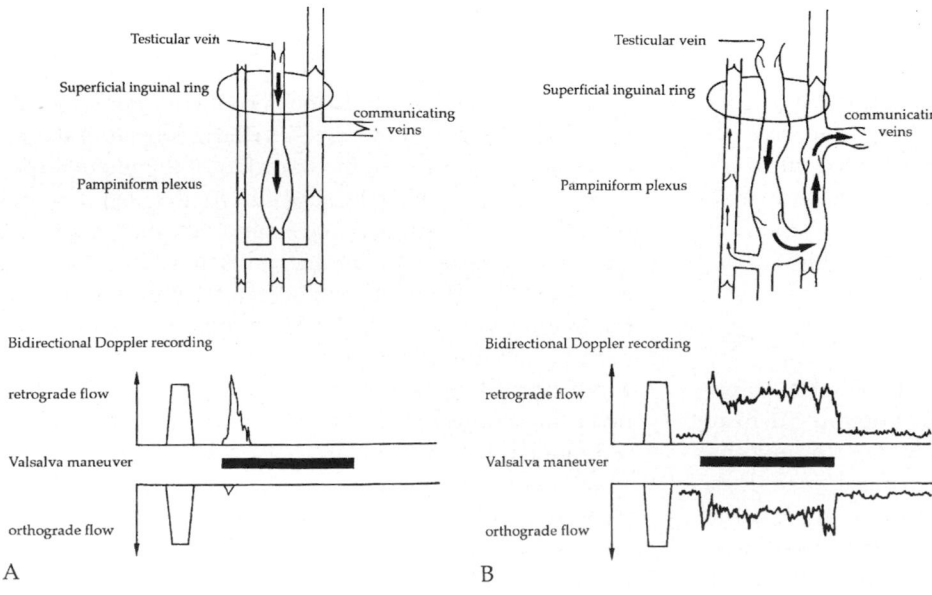

Figure 43–15 Schematic diagram of stop-type and shunt-type varicocele demonstrating reflux (*arrows*) with bidirectional Doppler recording below each diagram as described by Sigmund et al. (83). **A.** In the stop-type, reflux is stopped by competent valves within the pampiniform plexus above the level of the communicating veins (vasal and cremasteric veins) causing spermatic vein dilatation. **B.** In the shunt-type, because of absent or incompetent valves within the pampiniform plexus, blood flow is shunted to the communication veins, causing bidirectional blood flow that increases with Valsalva as demonstrated by Doppler.

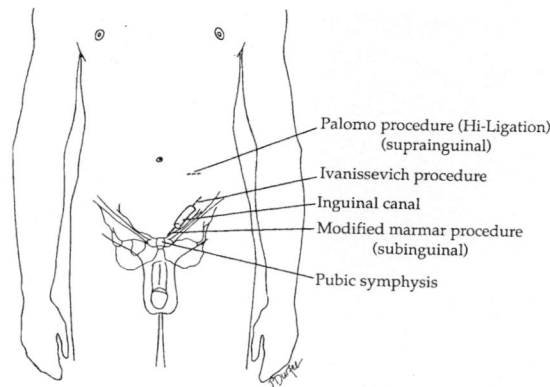

Figure 43–17 Schematic drawing demonstrating location of incisions for the three types of surgical corrections for varicocele. (Reprinted with permission from La Nasa JA Jr, Lewis RW. Varicocele and its surgical management. Urol Clin North Am 1987; 14:127–136.)

The main principle of surgery is to interrupt the dilated spermatic vein with preservation of the testicular artery and lymphatics to prevent testicular atrophy and formation of a hydrocele (Figure 43–18). Newer techniques include the use of laparoscopic varicocelectomy, particularly in the adolescent population (91) and the use of antegrade sclerotherapy (92–95). Surgery for varicocele treatment generally carries a low morbidity with the usual complications associated with

any operation, including hematoma and wound infections. In a review of varicocelectomy in 986 men, Dubin et al. reported a rate of hematoma, infection, and hydrocele of 1%, 0.7%, and 3% respectively (96). The pregnancy rates and semen improvement rates reported from various surgical papers have varied from 0–63% and 0–92%, respectively (96,97). Surgical studies generally report pregnancy rates and semen analysis improvements rather than recurrence rates. Of the studies that report recurrences, the rate is 0–37%, which is higher than the percutaneous rate (58,96,98,99). Although the recurrence rate for surgery tends to be higher than the percutaneous rate, many urologists advocate percutaneous therapy only for surgical failures because they believe that the technical success rate for surgery is higher than percutaneous embolization (100).

Some surgeons advocate the use of venography during surgical ligation of the gonadal vein to better isolate the spermatic vein and its tributaries, particularly in the pediatric patient, while others use a sclerosing agent during their surgical procedure (101–104). Venography performed after ligation has demonstrated several routes of recurrence. After high ligation of left varicocele, Morag et al. studied 40 patients because of recurrence or persistence. More than 50% of the patients still demonstrated a left varicocele, while additional patients demonstrated a right varicocele (10). There were three patterns of persistent varicocele filling after surgical ligation. The first was filling of the

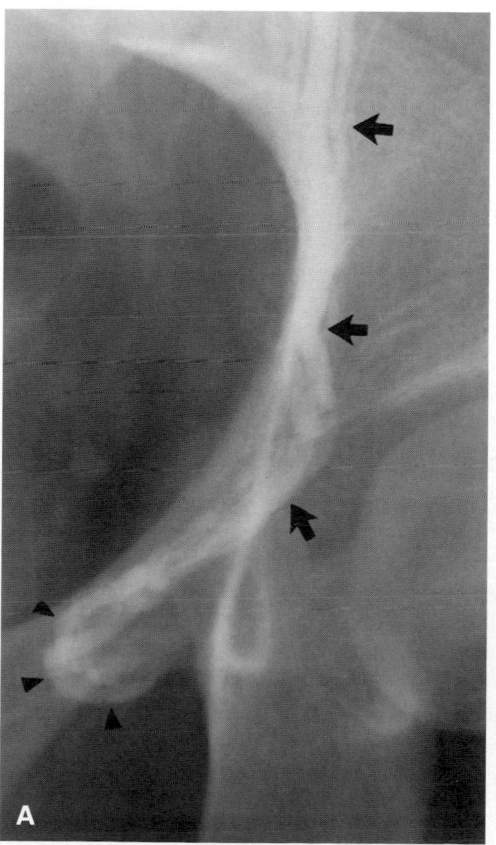
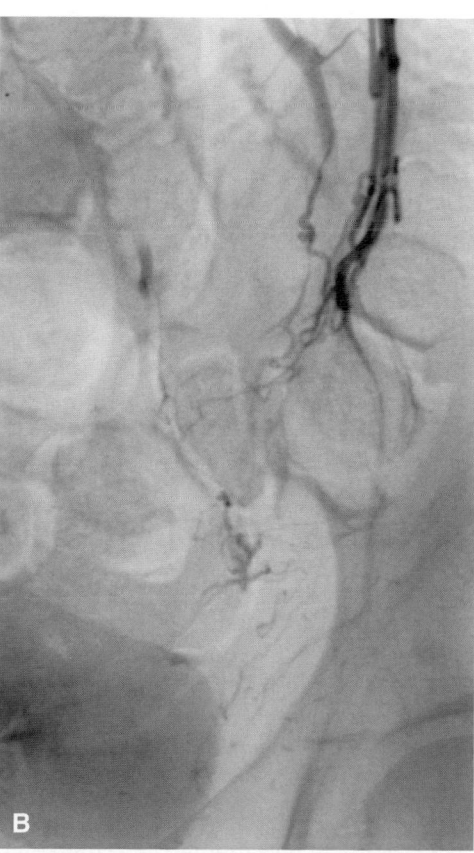

Figure 43–18 Left spermatic venogram after surgical ligation. **A.** Venogram demonstrates the spermatic vein (*arrows*) filling just below the femoral head where it terminates abruptly (*arrowheads*), consistent with surgical ligation. **B.** Left spermatic venogram demonstrating filling of gonadal vein that terminates relatively high in the pelvis with the filling of a few very small collaterals.

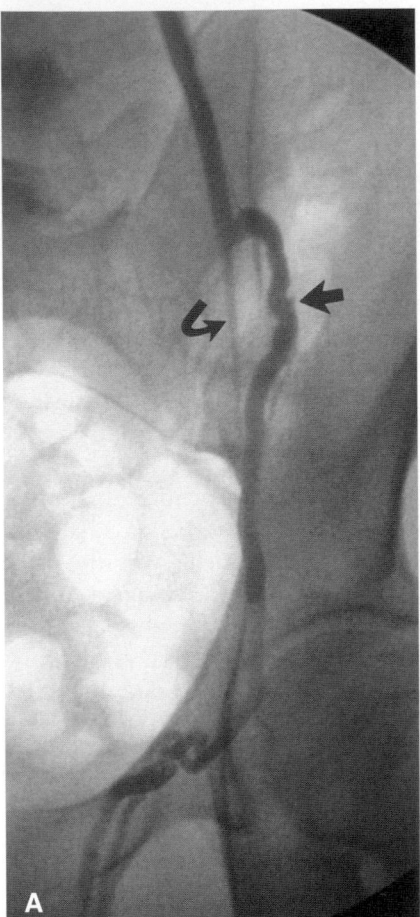 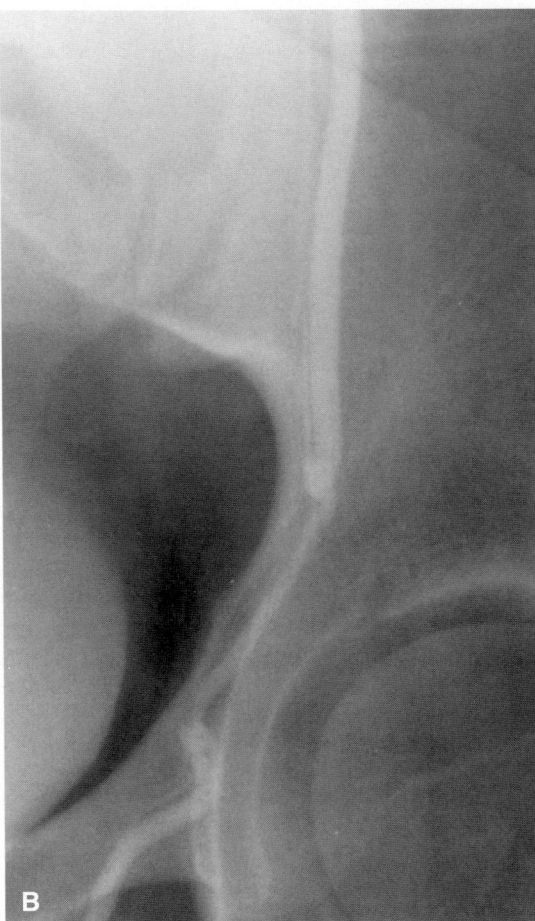

Figure 43-19 Venogram demonstrating recurrence after surgical ligation because of collateral vessels. **A.** Left spermatic venogram reveals a large collateral vein (*arrow*) that bypasses the site of surgical ligation (*curved arrow*). **B.** Smaller collateral vein bypasses the site of surgical ligation.

varicocele via collateral veins bypassing the site of ligation (Figure 43-19). The second pattern was by a large additional branch of the spermatic vein that was not ligated (Figure 43-20). The third pattern of varicocele filling was by direct filling resulting from ligature slippage or misidentification of the spermatic vein (Figure 43-21). Kaufman et al. studied five patients after surgery with varicocele recurrence, all of whom had collaterals that were not ligated (40). Some recurrences may also be because of cross-filling from an undetected right varicocele (10,40). Both authors treated recurrences with embolotherapy (10,40).

PERCUTANEOUS EMBOLIZATION

Typically, percutaneous embolization is performed as an outpatient procedure with intravenous conscious sedation and analgesia, unless the patient has a severe bleeding diathesis or previous life-threatening reaction to contrast (41). Initial reports in the 1970s used sclerosing agents followed by the use of metal coils (9,105,106). Today, the transjugular approach that was described originally by Formanek et al. in 1981 is used because of the simplicity and safety of gaining access into the gonadal vein (Figure 43-22) (107).

Morag et al. reported a greater success rate for right gonadal vein occlusion via the jugular versus femoral vein access—89% versus 62.5%, respectively (108). Kuroiwa et al. reported a greater success rate with the basilic vein compared to the femoral vein access (109). More recently, several authors have reported the use of guiding catheters or coaxial systems using the transfemoral approach as an aid to performing embolizations with balloons or coils (110-113).

Varicocele embolization is performed at several levels along the internal spermatic vein because of the variations in collaterals. Unembolized communications with large collaterals may result in immediate failure with little improvement, while small collaterals may increase in size with time, resulting in a recurrence. Fobbe et al. evaluated the success of treatment with regard to location of occlusion of the gonadal vein with the use of a sclerosing agent (114). They had a 68% technical success rate, determined 3 months after treatment, when the occlusion was performed in the cranial portion of the vein, as opposed to an 82% success rate when the vein was occluded at the caudal extent near the inguinal ring, thus eliminating many of the collateral vessels.

One approach to varicocele embolization involves giving the patient IV sedation, such as midazolam HCl and fentanyl citrate with nifedipine (10 mg) sublingually, to

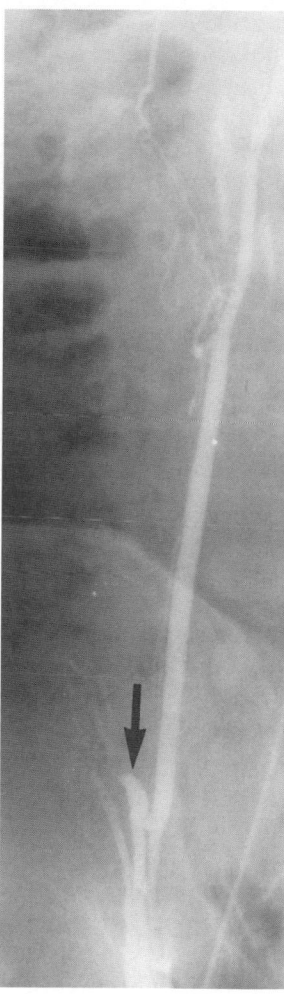

Figure 43–20   Right spermatic venogram demonstrating main large gonadal vein remains after surgical ligation. Remnant of parallel double vein that was ligated is seen low in the pelvis.

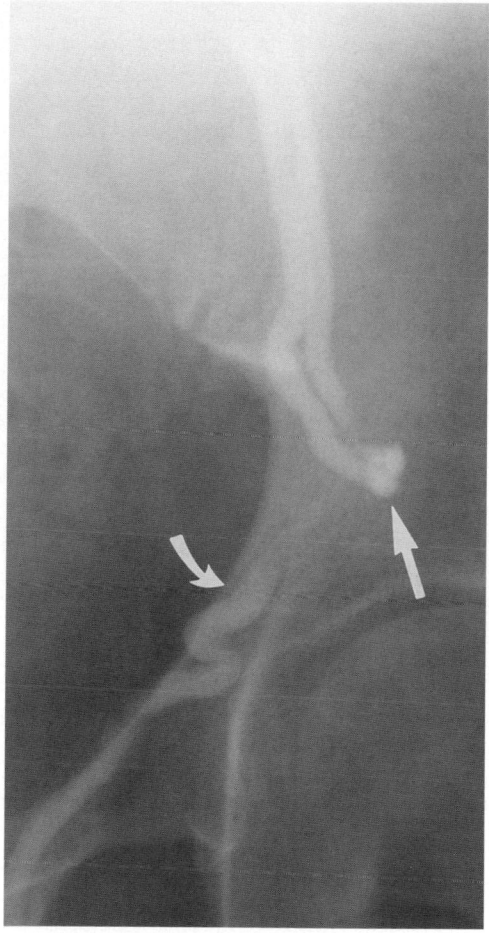

Figure 43–21   Left spermatic venogram during hard Valsalva maneuver in a weightlifter who had a recurrence after surgical ligation. Surgical ligation site is identified by termination of the vein (*arrow*); however, contrast is still able to pass through ligation site (*curved arrow*).

reduce potential venous spasm in the gonadal vein. Then, a 401 microvascular set (Cook, Inc.) with a 21-gauge needle is used to puncture the internal jugular, exchanging up to a 0.038-inch guide wire to gain access to the inferior vena cava. A long 30-cm, 6 French sheath (Medi-Tech) is introduced, through which a 5.5 French H1H (Cook Inc.) or 5 French Bernstein catheter (Medi-Tech) catheterizes the renal veins, usually with the aid of an angled Glidewire (Terumo). If the right common femoral vein approach is used, a 5 French straight catheter (Cook Inc.) with a tip-deflecting wire (Cook Inc.) is used to access the left gonadal vein, and a 5.5 French Simmons 3 catheter (Cook Inc.) is used for the right gonadal vein. A newer technique utilizes a guiding catheter rather than a tip-deflecting wire (113).

The patient is placed in reversed Trendelenburg position, and a left renal venogram is performed to search for reflux into the gonadal vein. The left gonadal vein is catheterized, and a gonadal venogram is performed to search for reflux and filling of systemic and portal collaterals. Care is taken to minimize exposure of the testicles by shielding or adequately

collimating. Direct filming of the varicocele is not necessary and increases the radiation dose to the gonads. The catheter is advanced to the region of the inguinal canal, thereby avoiding imaging over the scrotum. Use of 5-mm and 8-mm Gianturco coils (Cook Inc.) is recommended (because of their ease of placement and low cost) while attempting to block all collaterals that could result in a recurrence. Great care must be taken to avoid deployment of a coil partially into the renal vein or sizing the coil too small in diameter, especially when the vein is in spasm, which might result in coil migration to the lungs. If spasm is encountered, 1 mL aliquots of nitroglycerin (100 μg/mL) can be given to reverse it.

After embolization of the left gonadal vein, an attempt is made to selectively catheterize the right gonadal vein. If competent, no embolization is performed. If incompetent, embolization is performed as with the left renal vein. The patient is discharged 4–6 hours after the procedure. The patient is told to refrain from physical activity for 24 hours. Postprocedure symptoms include testicular and back pain

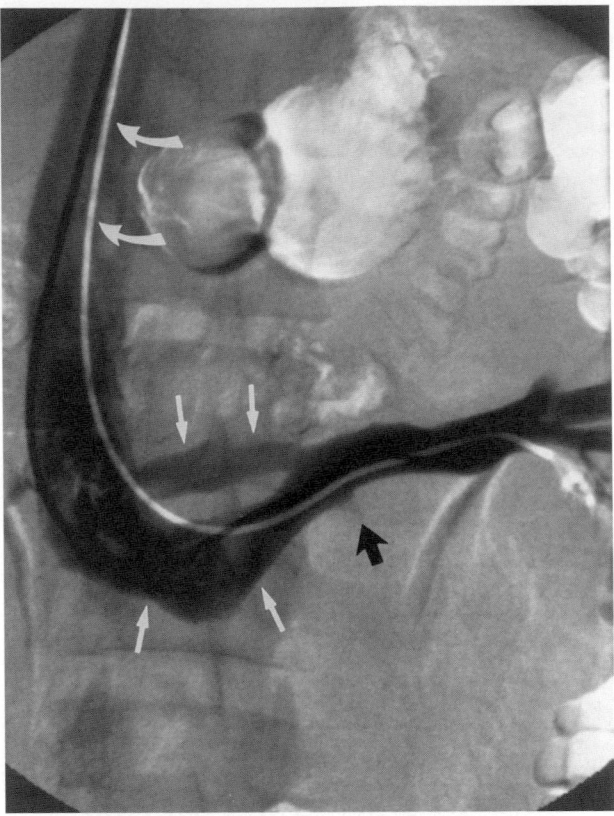

Figure 43–22 Left renal venogram performed from the right internal jugular approach. Catheterization of the gonadal vein is facilitated by the ability to advance the catheter (*curved white arrows*) in one direction deep into the spermatic vein. Appearance of double catheters is from subtraction artifact. Note circumaortic renal vein (*white straight arrows*) is demonstrated with competent valve (*black arrow*) preventing reflux into the left gonadal vein.

and possibly low-grade fever, which can be treated with nonsteroidal anti-inflammatories.

Numerous published studies have reported on the use of different agents, and even multiple agents, for embolization. Technical success rates can be given for correction of the varicocele, but they can vary depending on the imaging modality used to detect the recurrences. In reviewing their 11-year experience using various types of embolic agents, including balloons, coils, and different sclerosing agents, Zuckerman et al. did not find a statistical difference in the type of embolic agent used (115). The technical failure rate was 4.3%. Reasons for their failure included: (1) an inability to cannulate the left gonadal vein or to pass through a partially competent valve; (2) too many collaterals; (3) origin of the vein from upper pole of the kidney at too acute an angle; (4) a balloon or catheter that was too large for the gonadal vein, stenotic vein, or circumaortic renal vein; (5) spasm of the gonadal vein; and (6) bradycardia (Figures 43–12 and 43–23). Although the left spermatic vein is embolized most often, solitary right embolizations are performed for several reasons. In a report by Shuman et al., 10 of 227 patients had only a right varicocele embolized. One patient had a solitary right varicocele, six had an accompanying left varicocele but competent left valves, and three had recurrent varicoceles with previously successful left embolizations (116).

Initial experience with percutaneous embolization involved the use of sclerosing agents (Figure 43–24). Several milliliters of the agent are injected usually with an occlusion balloon in the gonadal vein. One agent used in multiple studies is Varikocid (Combustinwerk), which is sodium morrhuate (55 mg/mL) and benzyl alcohol (20 mg/mL)

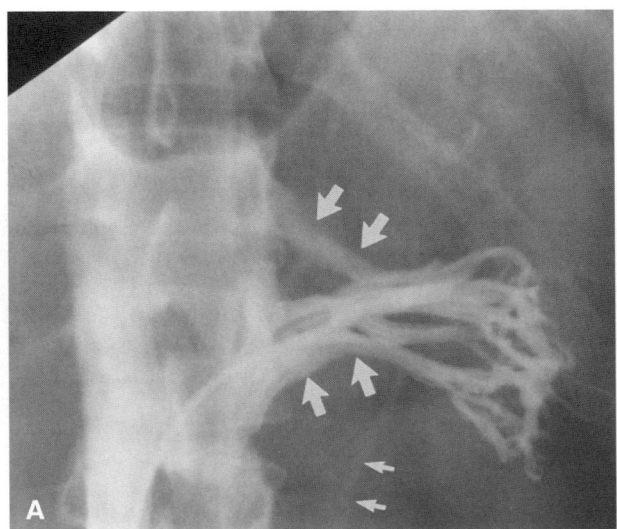

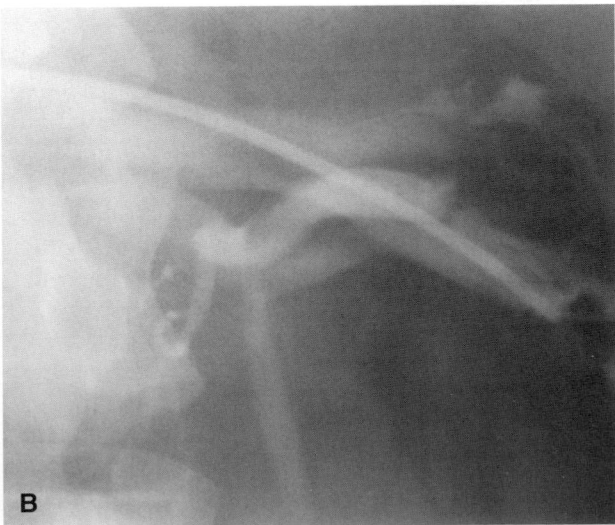

Figure 43–23 Left renal venograms demonstrating renal vein variants that may make catheterization of the renal vein difficult. **A.** Venogram revealing circumaortic renal vein (*large arrows*). Note faint reflux into left spermatic vein (*small arrows*). **B.** Venogram demonstrating two veins with the catheter in the upper vein and the spermatic vein entering into the lower vein along with possible bypassing collaterals.

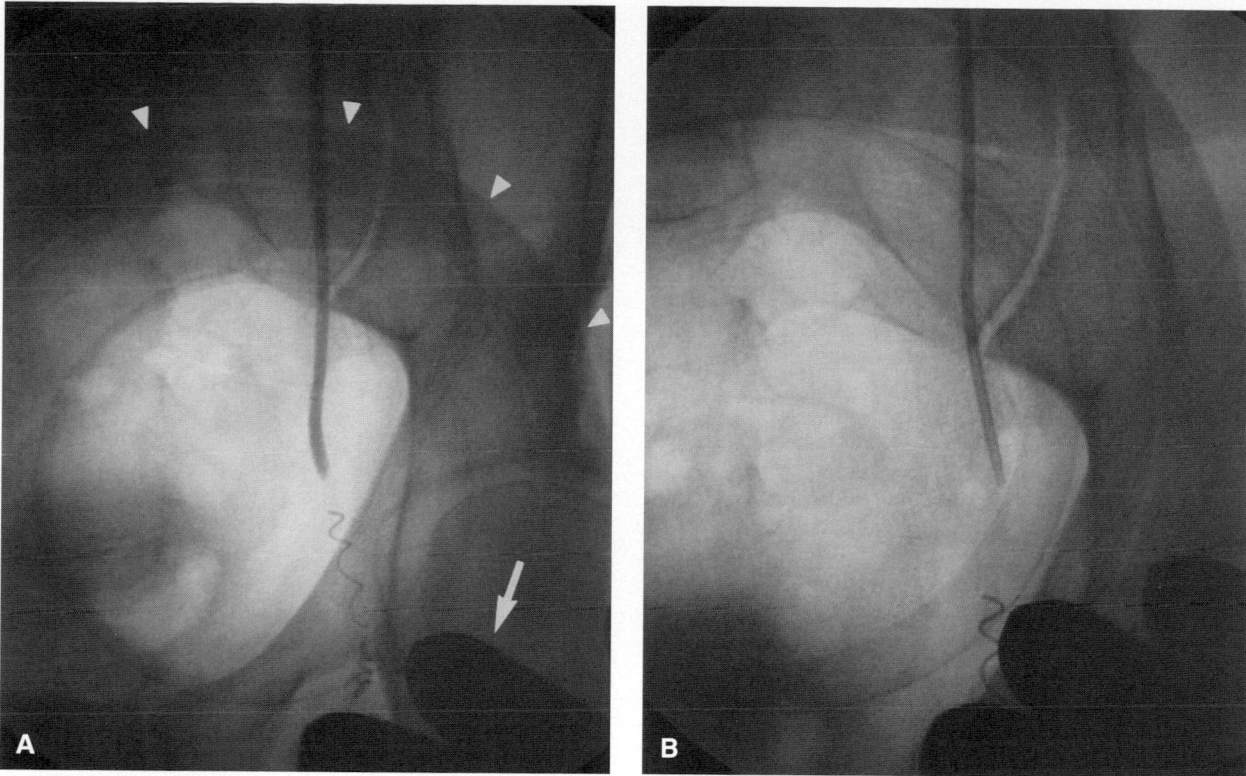

Figure 43-24 Embolization of left gonadal vein with ethanol. **A.** Left spermatic venogram demonstrating contrast injection terminating in pelvis. A coil is placed in the lower portion of the vein to prevent reflux into the pampiniform plexus. Note circular compression device (*arrowheads*) and shielded hand (*arrow*) pressing abdomen at inguinal ligament to prevent reflux into the scrotum. **B.** Ethanol is injected to clear contrast from vein.

(87,114,117–120). Another agent used less frequently is polydocanol (Aethoxysclerol, Kreussler Co.), which is Hydroxypolyaethoxydodecanol (119,121–124). Other agents include hypertonic glucose (70–80%) with monoethanolamine and absolute ethanol (122). Typically, the sclerosing agent is injected and allowed to remain in contact with the vein for several minutes. Manual compression at the inguinal canal may be performed to prevent reflux into the scrotum. Complications associated with a sclerosing agent usually result from flow of the sclerosing agent into the pampiniform plexus, which can lead to painful scrotal swelling, phlebitis, and testicular damage, with possible temporary depressions of sperm count or testicular atrophy. A plastic compression device has been used by some investigators to prevent sclerosant from flowing into the scrotum (125).

Investigators have used Gianturco steel coils ranging in sizes of 3, 5, 8, and 12 mm because of their low cost, safety, and ability to be placed easily in multiple locations (106,108,109,126–128) (Figure 43–25). Some authors have implicated coils in producing chronic inflammation resulting in pain, which can be a particular problem in young patients (128,129). Retrieval of incorrectly placed coils from the lung has been reported by Chomyn et al. (130). Newer complex coil designs using platinum may

also be used. Although more expensive, these coils have the advantage of producing less MR artifact. This can be a concern for an older patient who may need additional cross-sectional imaging for other reasons.

Other investigators advocate the use of detachable silicone balloons through a guiding sheath. These include a mini-balloon (Becton-Dickinson) and a detachable silicone balloon (Interventional Therapeutic). Though such balloons are no longer available for sale in the United States, proponents of their use claim that they can be optimally positioned in the internal spermatic vein because the balloon can be inflated and contrast infused to visualize potential collaterals before permanent deployment (129,131,132) (Figure 43–26). In addition, there is no need for superselective catheterization of the gonadal vein because a guiding sheath is used and test occlusions can be performed before detachment of the balloons (129). Shuman et al. published a series of right internal spermatic vein embolizations with balloon occlusions that demonstrated an 89% success rate with only an 11% technical failure rate (116). Other benefits include the use of a single device to obstruct the whole vein rather than using multiple coils and a sclerosing agent that can be trapped below the balloon if desired (132). Makita et al. report the use of a guide wire-directed balloon that they believe aids in the delivery of the balloon, compared

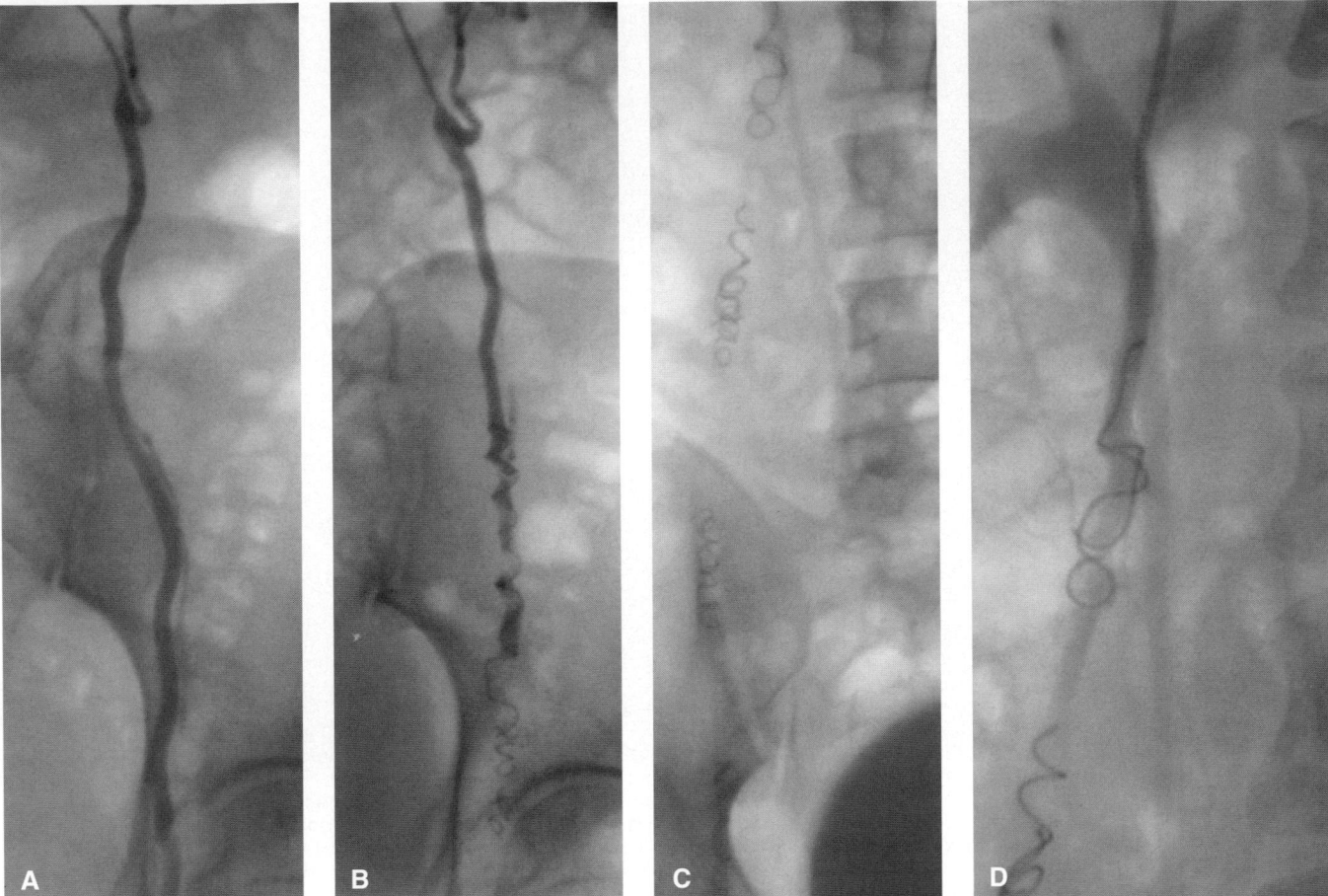

Figure 43–25   Spermatic venogram demonstrating the use of coils. **A.** Left spermatic venogram performed before embolization. Note collateral vessel in lower one third of the vein. **B.** Venogram after placement of multiple 5-mm and 8-mm coils. The larger coils are placed more cephalad in the vein to prevent possible migration of the smaller coils. No flow to the varicocele exists. The collateral vein does not fill because the coils are positioned across their communication with the main vein. **C.** Plain film of right abdomen demonstrating coils placed within the right gonadal vein. **D.** Venogram of patient (C) demonstrating occlusion of vein high in the abdomen.

to conventional flow-directed balloons (133). The problems with balloons include cost, availability, and the possibility that they may become dislocated or deflated, resulting in embolization to the lungs (129,132).

Other agents used for percutaneous embolization have included hot iodinated contrast medium and isobutyl-2-cyanoacrylate (Bucrylate, Ethicon Inc.). Smith et al. reported the use of hot contrast to obliterate varicoceles (134) and has suggested that the advantage of hot contrast as opposed to mechanical devices is that it is readily available and creates no additional expense. Also, it has the advantage of creating an occlusion of both the main channel and collateral vessels, similar to sclerotherapy. Thrombosis of the gonadal veins by injection of hot contrast (average 25.8 mL on the left and 21.4 mL on the right) resulted in a pregnancy rate of 40.5% with only minor complications. Other mechanical types of agents have included compressed Ivalon plugs (Scientific Apparatus Shop), which are polyvinyl alcohol sponges that expand to obstruct the vein, and spiderlons (Scientific

Apparatus Shop), which are combinations of Ivalon plugs attached to spidercoils to provide occlusion (107).

RESULTS OF PERCUTANEOUS VARICOCELE CORRECTION

Technical success of percutaneous embolization ranges from 50–100%, with a recurrence rate of 2–12 % (100,115,135). The etiology of recurrences after embolization is similar to that of surgical recurrences, as previously discussed, and usually is related to the enlargement of small collateral vessels that were not originally embolized. Kaufman et al. reported an 11% rate of recurrence when the spermatic vein was embolized at the L3 or L4 level and recommended that embolization be performed in the inguinal portion of the vein below the level of the collaterals (40).

Complications are generally minor, except for nontarget embolization to the lungs with embolic agents, although

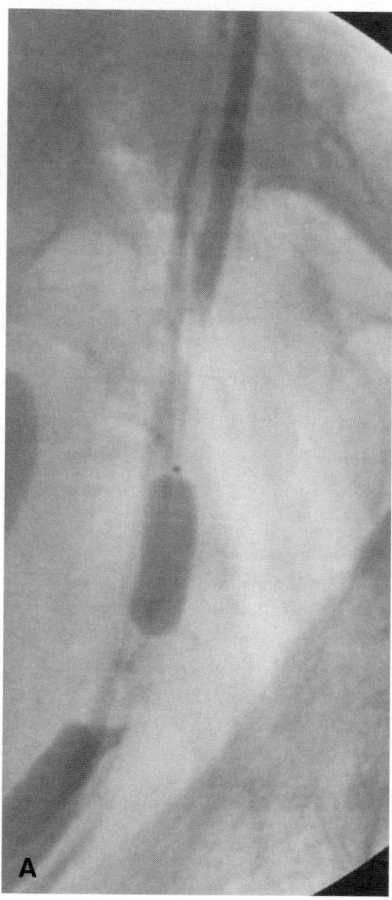
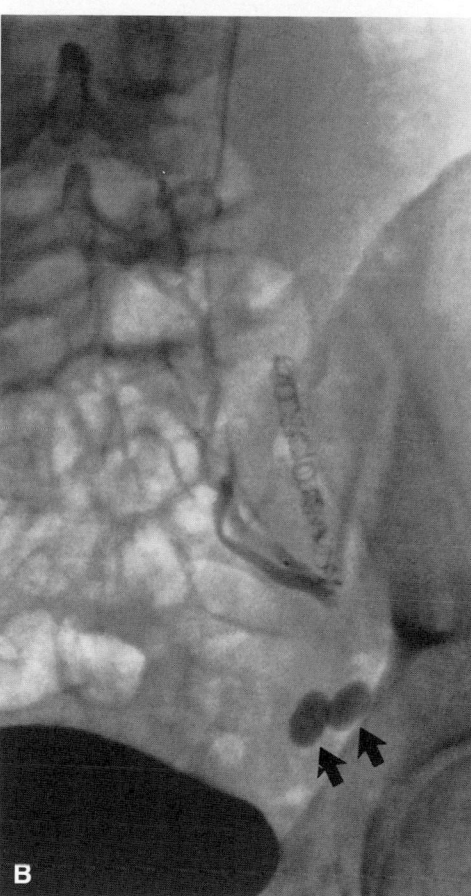

Figure 43–26 Embolization performed with detachable balloons. **A.** Balloon placed low in the left spermatic vein. Contrast injection demonstrates occlusion of main vein before detachment. Another balloon is seen lower in the pelvis. **B.** Two balloons (*arrows*) are present low in the pelvis with coils above the balloons.

these usually are asymptomatic. Minor complications include extravasation of contrast, contrast reactions, testicular thrombophlebitis from sclerosing agents, pain, venous spasm, and complications associated with the venous puncture (Figure 43–27). Rates of these complications range from 1–30% (100,115,135). Radiation exposure has been reported to be low, with Walsh et al. reporting a mean testicular dose of 26 mrad with shielding, while Weissbach et al. reported a rate of 1,350 mrad without (128,131). More recently, Pieri reported a rate of 18 mSv using a transbrachial approach with retrograde varicocele sclerosis, whereas the doses for plain abdominal radiographs and urography was 1.31 mSv and 4.6 mSv, respectively (136).

SEMEN ANALYSIS

Semen analysis is critical in the evaluation of the infertile male. As previously described, MacLeod introduced the concept of stress pattern defined as greater than 15% of tapered forms (7,137). Other characteristics include immature cells of the germinal line, especially spermatids and severe oligospermia (7,137). Although first described with varicocele, this pattern is not pathognomonic for varicocele and may be seen in infertile males without varicocele

because of other causes (100). Seminal parameters studied for infertility, evaluated prevaricocele and postvaricocele correction, include sperm density, motility, and morphology. The reports of multiple studies, including surgical and percutaneous techniques, have demonstrated improvement in density, motility, and morphology that ranged from no significant change to a dramatic improvement in the various parameters (138). Schlesinger et al. performed an extensive review of treatment outcomes after varicocelectomy to determine the efficacy of treatment (138). Although the results vary, they concluded that varicocelectomy does improve sperm density. The improvement is more pronounced when initial densities are greater than 10 million/mL. In addition, they describe a "ceiling effect" with less response when the preprocedure sperm density is greater than 40 million/mL. In spite of anecdotal reports of improvement in azoospermia patients, varicocele correction for these patients is not widely supported.

Motility and morphology may improve significantly after correction when associated with a rise in density. Isolated improvements in motility or morphology may occur, but generally there must be a significant improvement in density. The conclusion, then, is that despite occasional studies asserting that varicocele correction does not improve fertility, most of the literature supports the efficacy of correction

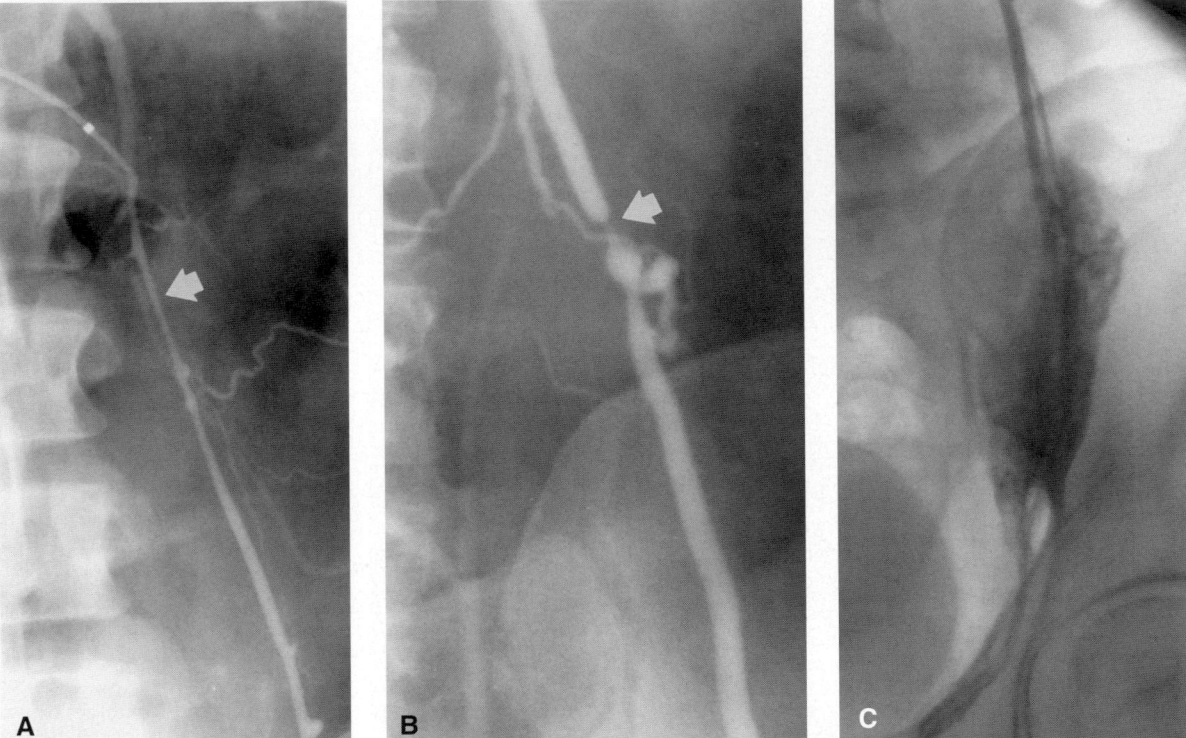

Figure 43–27 Complications associated with varicocele embolization. **A.** Left gonadal venogram demonstrating venous spasm. The cephalad portion of the gonadal vein is narrowed (*arrow*) compared to the caudal portion, making catheterization more difficult. **B.** Left spermatic venogram demonstrating focal narrowing because of spasm (*arrow*). **C.** Left spermatic venogram demonstrating extravasation of contrast in the lower portion of the vein.

in improving fertility. Improvement in semen quality ranges from 24–84% after surgical correction and 27–78% after percutaneous embolization (100,115,120,121,139,140).

PREGNANCY RATES

The most important outcome variable to assessing the efficacy of spermatic embolization for fertility is the pregnancy rate. There is, however, considerable difficulty in reviewing studies that are not well-controlled because fertility and pregnancy are multifactorial with both males and females undergoing therapy. In addition, the percutaneously treated population of men is heterogenous, with different size varicoceles; some are already fertile and others are treated for recurrences after previous surgery. Until the pathophysiology of varicoceles is understood and prospective randomized controlled studies are performed, no definitive conclusions can be drawn about whether treatment is truly beneficial, even though most of the evidence supports varicocele correction as an aid to infertility. Pregnancy rates after varicocele correction vary from 0% to as high as 70% (100,115, 138,141–143). Comhaire et al. evaluated the factors affecting the probability of pregnancy embolization with Bucrylate. Fifty and one-half percent of couples achieved

pregnancy, with a constant probability of conception of 3.9% per cycle determined by life-table analysis. The factors found to predict success for pregnancy from varicocele embolization were the coincidence of other disease in the man or woman interfering with fertility, serum follicle-stimulating hormone concentration, total testicular volume, and pretreatment semen quality, with the probability of conception ranging from 8–80% (144). For all members in the study by Zuckerman et al., the average time to pregnancy after percutaneous occlusion was 17 months ± 15.8 months, while the time was shorter for individuals who were treated only with embolization (115). The reported improvement in pregnancy rate because of surgical ligation or percutaneous embolization is similar, with few prospective studies to compare the two techniques (43). Some studies suggest that there is a difference in pregnancy outcome from surgery compared to percutaneous techniques, while others show no difference (122,138,145–147). Nieschlag et al. and Yavetz et al. performed randomized prospective studies comparing surgery to embolization (145,146). Although neither demonstrated an advantage of percutaneous embolization over surgery in improving pregnancy rates, both demonstrated greater patient acceptance with shorter hospital stays and less discomfort with embolization (145,146) (Figure 43–28).

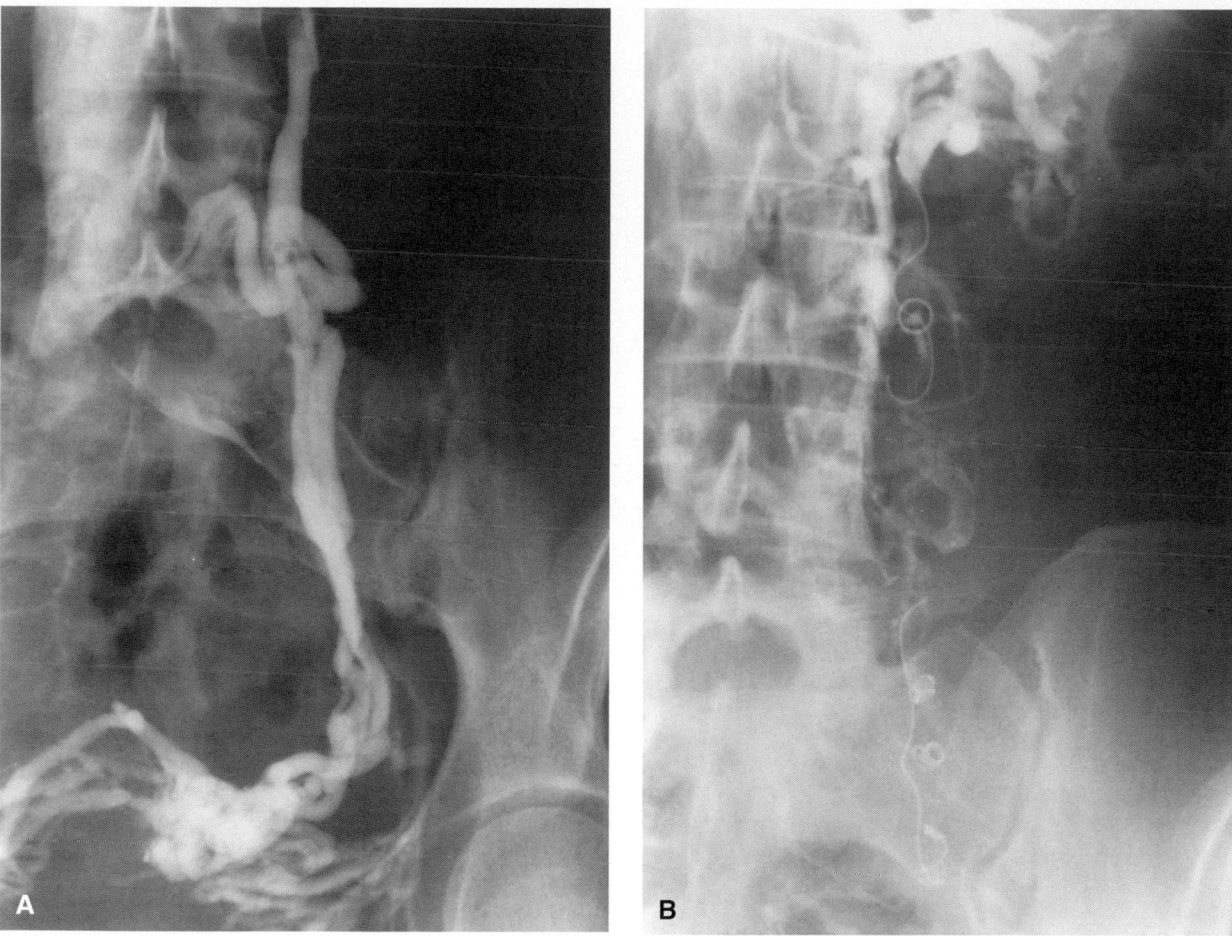

Figure 43–28 Gonadal venogram performed in a woman with pelvic pain, resulting from venous congestion, treated with embolization. **A.** Left gonadal venogram demonstrating reflux into the gonadal vein and cross-pelvic collateral filling consistent with an ovarian varicocele. **B.** Successful treatment with percutaneous embolization of the ovarian varicocele.

More recent prospective controlled studies have been performed with limited success. In a Cochrane Database of Systemic Reviews in 2001, Evers et al. evaluated the literature for randomized trials dealing with the impact of surgery or embolization on the pregnancy rate of infertile couples. Six studies met inclusive criteria; however, one was an extension of a previously published study, leaving five for the analysis. One trial by Madgar (148), previously discussed in this chapter, reported a statistically significant improvement in pregnancy rate. None of the other four studies showed individually a significant effect on pregnancy rates of varicocele treatment over no treatment (142,149,150) or over counseling only (151,152). The combined RR (Relative Risk; random effects method) of the five studies is 1.06 (95% CI 0.57–1.94), the Peto OR (Odds Ratio) is 1.15 (95% CI 0.73–1.83). Evers et al. concluded that there was insufficient evidence that the treatment of varicocele in men, from couples with otherwise unexplained subfertility, improves the couple's spontaneous pregnancy chances.

In a follow-up report for 2003, Evers and Collins added two more studies to their meta-analysis, neither of which demonstrated benefit. From seven studies, they identified 61 pregnancies among 281 treated couples and 50 pregnancies among 259 controls. The overall relative benefit of treatment was 1.01 (95% CI 0.73–1.40) by the fixed effects model and 1.04 (0.62–1.75) by the random effects model. They concluded that varicocele repair does not seem to be an effective treatment for male or unexplained subfertility and might even hurt fertility stating that "routinely treating varicoceles in men from subfertile couples seems ill-advised, especially if undertaken outside the context of a properly done randomised control trial." (153).

In commentary to these two reviews, Templeton was concerned that a large WHO trial that remains unpublished in only abstract form was left out of their review. Marmar commented that the conclusion of this meta-analysis by Evers was regrettable because the data in this meta-analysis was questionable (154). In addition, Sandlow commented that although these studies were chosen because of their status as randomized clinical trials, no evaluation of the methods was performed. On review, one study evaluated only subclinical varicocele; three others had methodological problems and Madgar's study did show sizeable benefit. In addition, given the amount of nonrandomized evidence that supports improvement as demonstrated by Shlesinger's meta-analysis discussed earlier, it is difficult to attribute these findings to chance. Sandlow (1) concluded:

> Despite conflicting evidence from both randomized and nonrandomized trials, clinical experience still favors the surgical treatment of clinical varicoceles in men with infertility. In addition, even though some of these reviewed studies have flaws, the findings "raise the valid point of why most men with varicoceles are fertile, as well as why some infertile men with varicocele do not improve after repair." However, it is incumbent on fertility specialists to design and recruit participants (or patients) in randomized, properly controlled trials to reach a definitive conclusion.

Current recommendations published in 2004 by the Male Infertility Best Practice Policy Committee of the American Urological Association (AUA) and the Practice Committee of the American Society for Reproductive Medicine (ASRM) support the treatment of varicocele for infertility. These recommendations are outlined in Table 43–1.

TREATMENT OF VARICOCELE IN THE ERA OF ASSISTED REPRODUCTIVE TECHNOLOGY (ART)

Given the availability of the ART, including intracytoplasmic sperm injection (ICSI), in vitro fetilization (IVF), and intrauterine insemination (IUI), is there a need for varicocele repair? Several authors have reviewed this issue, including Cayan et al., who found that a significant proportion of their patients were able to undergo less sophisticated ART or obviate the need for it following repair (155). Varicocele repair

---

TABLE 43–1

2004 RECOMMENDATIONS OF THE MALE INFERTILITY BEST PRACTICE POLICY COMMITTEE OF THE AMERICAN UROLOGICAL ASSOCIATION (AUA) AND THE PRACTICE COMMITTEE OF THE AMERICAN SOCIETY FOR REPRODUCTIVE MEDICINE (ASRM)

Detection

Routine evaluation of infertile men with varicoceles should include a medical and reproductive history, a physical examination, and a minimum of two semen analyses. Imaging studies are not indicated for the standard evaluation unless physical exam is inconclusive.

Indications for Treatment

When all of the following are present, varicocele treatment should be offered to the male partner of a couple attempting to conceive: (1) A varicocele is palpable; (2) The couple has documented infertility; (3) The female has normal fertility or potentially correctable infertility; and (4) The male partner has one or more abnormal semen parameters or sperm function test results. Adult men with a palpable varicocele and abnormal semen analyses but are not currently attempting to conceive should also be offered varicocele repair. Young men who have a varicocele and normal semen analyses should be followed-up with semen analyses every 1–2 years. Adolescents with a varicocele and who have objective evidence of reduced ipsilateral testicular size should be offered varicocele repair. Adolescents who have a varicocele but normal ipsilateral testicular size should be offered follow-up monitoring with annual objective measurements of testicular size, semen analyses, or both.

Varicocele Treatment, Intrauterine Insemination, and In Vitro Fertilization (IVF)/Intracytoplasmic Sperm Injection (ICSI)

Varicocele repair may be considered as the primary treatment option when a man with varicocele has suboptimal semen quality and a normal female partner. IVF with or without ICSI may be considered the primary treatment option when an independent need exists for such techniques to treat a female factor, regardless of the presence of varicocele and suboptimal semen quality.

Two Options for Varicocele Treatment—Surgery Versus Percutaneous Embolization

The treating physician's experience and expertise, as well as the available options, should determine the choice of varicocele treatment.

Results of Varicocele Treatment

Despite the absence of definitive studies on the fertility outcome of varicocele repair, varicocele treatment should be considered an option for appropriate infertile couples because varicocele repair improves semen parameters in most men, varicocele treatment can improve fertility, and its risks are small.

Follow-up

Persistence or recurrence of a varicocele may be treated by surgical ligation or percutaneous embolization of the refluxing veins. After treatment of a varicocele, semen analysis should be done at approximately 3-month intervals for at least 1 year or until pregnancy occurs.
Reprinted with permission from the Male Infertility Best Practice Policy Committee of the American Urological Association and the Practice Committee of the American Society for Reproductive Medicine. Report on varicocele and infertility. Fertil Steril 2004;82(Suppl I):S142–S145.

may also prevent further deterioration of semen sample that would require more invasive ART in the future (156). In addition, Penson evaluated the cost-effectiveness of four treatment strategies for varicocele related infertility: (1) observation, (2) surgical varicocele repair followed by IVF if unsuccessful, (3) IUI followed by IVF if unsuccessful, and (4) immediate IVF. They found that immediate IVF was more costly and less effective than varicocele repair followed by IVF or IUI followed by IVF (157). Given the earlier discussion, even though a couple may be undergoing ART, for those men with varicocele, repair is prudent to optimize semen parameters for current or potential future pregnancies.

SUMMARY

Percutaneous embolization of varicocele remains a straight-forward procedure that is both enjoyable and rewarding to interventional radiologists. It represents a minimally invasive therapy for patients with painful varicocele, adolescent testicular atrophy, and infertility. The percutaneous procedure gives hope to many infertile couples and provides a therapy requiring less recovery and morbidity than the standard surgical techniques. The most difficult part remains in drawing conclusions as to its definite utility in patients with infertility. Despite the enormous data in favor of the therapeutic benefit and the extremely limited number of prospective evaluations, controversy will remain until more well-controlled randomized trials are performed.

ACKNOWLEDGMENTS

I would like to thank many of my colleagues for their contributions to the text and illustrations: Constantin Cope MD, Michael C. Soulen MD, Harvey Nisenbaum MD, Evan Siegelman MD, Scott Savader MD, and Lindsay Machan MD.

REFERENCES

1. Sandlow J. Pathogenesis and treatment of varicoceles. BMJ 2004; 328:967–968. Erratum appears in BMJ 2004;328:1486.
2. Zorgniotti AW. The spermatozoa count. A short history. Urology 1975;5:672–673.
3. Barwell R. One hundred cases of varicocele treated by subcutaneous wire loop. Lancet 1885;1:978.
4. Bennett W. Varicocele: particularly with reference to its radical cure. Lancet 1889;1:261–265.
5. Tulloch W. Consideration of sterility factors in the light of subsequent pregnancies: Subfertility in the male. Trans Obstet Soc (Edinburgh) 1952;59:29–34.
6. Charny C. Effect of varicocele on fertility. Results of varicocelectomy. Fertil Steril 1962;13:47–56.
7. MacLeod J. Seminal cytology in the presence of varicocele. Fertil Steril 1965;16:735–757.
8. Iaccarino V. Trattamento conservativo del varicocele: flebografia selectiva escleroterapia delle vene goandiche. Riv Radiol 1977; 17:107–117.
9. Lima S, Castro M, Costa O. A new method for the treatment of varicocele. Andrologia 1978;10:103–106.
10. Morag B, Rubinstein ZJ, Madgar I, et al. The role of spermatic venography after surgical high ligation of the left spermatic veins: diagnosis and percutaneous occlusion. Urol Radiol 1985;7: 32–34.
11. Demas BE, Hricak H, McClure RD. Varicoceles. Radiologic diagnosis and treatment. Radiol Clin North Am 1991;29:619–627.
12. Peterson AC, Lance RS, Ruiz HE. Outcomes of varicocele ligation done for pain. J Urol 1998;159:1565–1567.
13. Kass EJ. The adolescent varicocele: treatment and outcome. Curr Urol Rep 2002;3:100–106.
14. Greenfield SP, Seville P, Wan J. Experience with varicoceles in children and young adults. J Urol 2002;168:1684–1688; discussion 1688.
15. Thomas JC, Elder JS. Testicular growth arrest and adolescent varicocele: does varicocele size make a difference? J Urol 2002;168: 1689–1691; discussion 1691.
16. Kubal A, Nagler HM, Zahalsky M, et al. The adolescent varicocele: diagnostic and treatment patterns of pediatricians. A public health concern? J Urol 2004;171:411–413.
17. Weiss AJ, Kellman GM, Middleton WD, et al. Intratesticular varicocele: sonographic findings in two patients. AJR Am J Roentgenol 1992;158:1061–1063.
18. Van der Sluiszen PL, Leguit P, Sanders FB. Subcutaneous varices of the scrotum: a possible presentation of varicocele. Eur J Radiol 1990;10:198–200.
19. Turner T. Varicocele: still an enigma. J Urol 1983;129:695–699.
20. Steeno O, Knops J, Declerck L, et al. Prevention of fertility disorders by detection and treatment of varicocele at school and college age. Andrologia 1976;8:47–53.
21. Comhaire F. Varicocele infertility: an enigma. Int J Androl 1983; 6:401–404.
22. Meacham RB, Townsend RR, Rademacher D, et al. The incidence of varicoceles in the general population when evaluated by physical examination, grayscale sonography, and color Doppler sonography. J Urol 1994;151:1535–1538.
23. Gat Y, Bachar GN, Zukerman Z, et al. Varicocele: a bilateral disease. Fertil Steril 2004;81:424–429.
24. Gat Y, Bachar GN, Zukerman Z, et al. Physical examination may miss the diagnosis of bilateral varicocele: a comparative study of 4 diagnostic modalities. J Urol 2004;172:1414–1417.
25. Gorelick JI, Goldstein M. Loss of fertility in men with varicocele. Fertil Steril 1993;59:613–616.
26. Wishahi MM. Anatomy of the spermatic venous plexus (pampiniform plexus) in men with and without varicocele: intraoperative venographic study. J Urol 1992;147:1285–1289.
27. Lechter A, Lopez G, Martinez C, et al. Anatomy of the gonadal veins: a reappraisal. Surgery 1991;109:735–739.
28. Wilms G, Oyen R, Baert AL. Left spermatic vein in left-sided vena cava. Cardiovasc Intervent Radiol 1987;10:258–260.
29. Turner TT, Howards SS. The venous anatomy of experimental left varicocele: comparison with naturally occurring left varicocele in the human. Fertil Steril 1994;62:869–875.
30. Hill J, Green N. Varicocele: a review of radiological and anatomical features in relation to surgical treatment. Br J Surg 1977;64: 747–752.
31. Hill J, Hirsh A, Pryor J, et al. Changes in the appearance of venography after ligation of a varicocele. J Anat 1982;135:47–52.
32. Sofikitis N, Dritsas K, Miyagawa I, et al. Anatomical characteristics of the left testicular venous system in man. Arch Androl 1993;30:79–85.
33. Shafik A, Moftah A, Olfat S, et al. Testicular veins: anatomy and role in varicocelogenesis and other pathologic conditions. Urology 1990;35:175–182.
34. Wishahi MM. Anatomy of the venous drainage of the human testis: testicular vein cast, microdissection, and radiographic demonstration. A new anatomical concept. Eur Urol 1991;20: 154–160.
35. Wishahi MM. Detailed anatomy of the internal spermatic vein and the ovarian vein. Human cadaver study and operative spermatic venography: clinical aspects. J Urol 1991;145:780–784.
36. Ahlberg N, Bartley O, Chidekel N, et al. Right and left gonadal veins: an anatomical and statistical study. Acta Radiol 1966;4: 593–601.
37. Erturk E, Sheinfeld J, Cockett AT. Male infertility due to communicating bilateral varicoceles. Urology 1984;24:390–391.

38. Marsman JW. The aberrantly fed varicocele: frequency, venographic appearance, and results of transcatheter embolization. AJR Am J Roentgenol 1995;164:649–657.

39. Murray RR Jr, Mitchell SE, Kadir S, et al. Comparison of recurrent varicocele anatomy following surgery and percutaneous balloon occlusion. J Urol 1986;135:286–289.

40. Kaufman S, Kadir S, Barth K, et al. Mechanisms of recurrent varicocele after balloon occlusion or surgical ligation of the internal spermatic vein. Radiology 1983;147:435–440.

41. Halden W, White RI Jr. Outpatient embolotherapy of varicocele. Urol Clin North Am 1987;14:137–144.

42. Roy CR, Wilson T, Raife M, et al. Varicocele as the presenting sign of an abdominal mass. J Urol 1989;141:597–599.

43. Thomas AJ Jr, Geisinger MA. Current management of varicoceles. Urol Clin North Am 1990;17:893–907.

44. Shaji S, Steele C, Qasim A, et al. Right testicular varicocele: an unusual presentation of cecal adenocarcinoma. Am J Gastroenterol 2003;98:701–703.

45. Corlett MP, Gwynn BR, Hamer JD. Right-sided varicocele caused by false aneurysm from aortic graft. Br J Urol 1992;70:204–205.

46. Linsell JC, Rowe PH, Owen WJ. Rupture of an aortic aneurysm into the renal vein presenting as a left-sided varicocele. Case report. Acta Chir Scand 1987;153:477–478.

47. Wilms G, Oyen R, Casselman J, et al. Solitary or predominantly right-sided varicocele: a possible sign of situs inversus. Urol Radiol 1988;9:243–246.

48. Kohler E. On the etiology of varicocele. J Urol 1967;97:741–742.

49. Verstoppen G, Steeno O. Varicocele and the pathogenesis of the associated subfertility. A review of the various theories. III: Theories concerning the deleterious effects of varicocele on fertility. Andrologia 1977;9:133–140.

50. Mali WP, Oei HY, Arndt JW, et al. Hemodynamics of the varicocele. Part II. Correlation among the results of renocaval pressure measurements, varicocele scintigraphy, and phlebography. J Urol 1986;135:489–493.

51. Bomalaski MD, Mills JL, Argueso LR, et al. Iliac vein compression syndrome: an unusual cause of varicocele. J Vasc Surg 1993;18:1064–1068.

52. Kim SH, Park JH, Han MC, et al. Embolization of the internal spermatic vein in varicocele: significance of venous pressure. Cardiovasc Intervent Radiol 1992;15:102–106;discussion 106–107.

53. Carl P, Stark L, Ouzoun N, et al. Venous pressure in idiopathic varicocele. Eur Urol 1993;24:214–220.

54. Mali WP, Oei HY, Arndt JW, et al. Hemodynamics of the varicocele. Part I. Correlation among the clinical, phlebographic ,and scintigraphic findings. J Urol 1986;135:483–488.

55. Sayfan J, Halevy A, Oland J, et al. Varicocele and left renal vein compression. Fertil Steril 1984;41:411–417.

56. Shafik A, Khalil A, Saleh M. The fasciomuscular tube of the spermatic cord: A study of its surgical anatomy and relation to varicocele. A new concept for the pathogenesis of varicocele. Br J Urol 1972;44:147–151.

57. Shafik A. The cremasteric muscle: role in varicocelogenesis and in thermoregulatory function of the testicle. Invest Urol 1973;11:92–94.

58. Sayfan J, Halevy A, Shperber Y, et al. The role of the spermatic cord layers in the development of varicoceles. J Urol 1985;133:223–224.

59. Zorgniotti A, MacLeod J. Studies in temperature, human semen quality, and varicocele. Fertil Steril 1973;24:854–863.

60. Kay R, Alexander N, Baugham W. Induced varicoceles in rhesus monkeys. Fertil Steril 1979;31:195–199.

61. Saypol D, Howards S, Turner T, et al. Influence of surgically induced varicocele on testicular blood flow, temperature, and histology in adult rats and dogs. J Clin Invest 1981;68:39–45.

62. Takihara H, Sakatoku J, Cockett AT. The pathophysiology of varicocele in male infertility. Fertil Steril 1991;55:861–868.

63. Ali JI, Weaver DJ, Weinstein SH, et al. Scrotal temperature and semen quality in men with and without varicocele. Arch Androl 1990;24:215–219.

64. Zorgniotti AW, Sealfon AI. Scrotal hypothermia: new therapy for poor semen. Urology 1984;23:439–441.

65. Comhaire F, Vermeulen A. Varicocele sterility: cortisol and catecholamines. Fertil Steril 1974;25:88–95.

66. Cohen M, Plaine L, Brown J. The role of internal spermatic vein plasma catecholamine determinations in subfertile men with varicoceles. Fertil Steril 1975;26:1243–1249.

67. Lindholmer C, Thulin L, Eliasson R. Concentrations of cortisol and renin in the internal spermatic vein of men with varicocele. Andrologia 1973;5:21–22.

68. Charny C, Baum S. Varicocele and infertility. JAMA 1968;204:75–78.

69. Ito H, Fuse H, Minagawa H, et al. Internal spermatic vein prostaglandins in varicocele patients. Fertil Steril 1982;37:218–222.

70. Hudson RW, Perez-Marrero RA, Crawford VA, et al. Hormonal parameters of men with varicoceles before and after varicocelectomy. Fertil Steril 1985;43:905–910.

71. Rodriguez-Rigau L, Weiss D, et al. A possible mechanism for the detrimental effect of varicocele on testicular function in man. Fertil Steril 1978;30:577–585.

72. Donohue R, Brown J. Blood gases and pH determinations in the internal spermatic veins of subfertile men with varicocele. Fertil Steril 1969;20:365–369.

73. Chakraborty J, Hikim AK, Jhunjhunwala J. Stagnation of blood in the microcirculatory vessels in the testes of men with varicocele. J Androl 1985;6:117–126.

74. Spera G, Alei G, Coia L, et al. Histological lesions in the testis of infertile men with varicocele. Arch Androl 1979;2:335–339.

75. Sharpe RM. Paracrine control of the testis. Clin Endocrinol Metab 1986;15:185–207.

76. Nagler HM. Varicocele: where, why and, if so, how? J Urol 2004;172:1239–1240.

77. La Nasa JA Jr, Lewis RW. Varicocele and its surgical management. Urol Clin North Am 1987;14:127–136.

78. Kim ED, Lipshultz LI. Role of ultrasound in the assessment of male infertility. J Clin Ultrasound 1996;24:437–453.

79. Geatti O, Gasparini D, Shapiro B. A comparison of scintigraphy, thermography, ultrasound, and phlebography in grading of clinical varicocele. J Nucl Med 1991;32:2092–2097.

80. Aydos K, Baltaci S, Salih M, et al. Use of color Doppler sonography in the evaluation of varicoceles. Eur Urol 1993;24:221–225.

81. Petros JA, Andriole GL, Middleton WD, et al. Correlation of testicular color Doppler ultrasonography, physical examination, and venography in the detection of left varicoceles in men with infertility. J Urol 1991;145:785–788.

82. Hamm B, Fobbe F, Sorensen R, et al. Varicoceles: combined sonography and thermography in diagnosis and posttherapeutic evaluation. Radiology 1986;160:419–424.

83. Sigmund G, Gall H, Bahren W. Stop-type and shunt-type varicoceles: venographic findings. Radiology 1987;163:105–110.

84. Ahlberg N, Bartley O, Chidekel N, et al. Phlebography in varicocele scroti. Acta Radiol Diagn (Stockh) 1966;4:517–528.

85. Comhaire F, Kunnen M. Selective retrograde venography of the internal spermatic vein: a conclusive approach to the diagnosis of varicocele. Andrologia 1976;8:11–24.

86. Marsman JW. Clinical versus subclinical varicocele: venographic findings and improvement of fertility after embolization. Radiology 1985;155:635–638.

87. Porst H, Bahren W, Lenz M, et al. Percutaneous sclerotherapy of varicoceles—an alternative to conventional surgical methods. Br J Urol 1984;56:73–78.

88. Palomo A. Radical cure of varicocele by a new technique. J Urol 1949;61:604–607.

89. Ivanissevich O. Left varicocele due to reflux: Experience with 4,470 operative cases in 42 years. J Int Coll Surg 1960;24:742–756.

90. Marmar JL, DeBenedictis TJ, Praiss D. The management of varicoceles by microdissection of the spermatic cord at the external inguinal ring. Fertil Steril 1985;43:583–588.

91. Franco I. Laparoscopic varicocelectomy in the adolescent male. Curr Urol Rep 2004;5:132–136.

92. Minucci S, Mazzoni G, Gallina A, et al. Evolution in varicocele sclerosing treatment: the ante/retrograde (A/R) approach. Arch Ital Urol Androl 2004;76:29–33.

93. Sautter T, Sulser T, Suter S, et al. Treatment of varicocele: a prospective randomized comparison of laparoscopy versus antegrade sclerotherapy. Eur Urol 2002;41:398–400.

94. Mazzoni G, Minucci S, Gentile V. Recurrent varicocele: role of antegrade sclerotherapy as first choice treatment. Eur Urol 2002;41:614–618; discussion 618.

95. Ficarra V, Sarti A, Novara G, et al. Antegrade scrotal sclerotherapy and varicocele. Asian J Androl 2002;4:221–224.

96. Dubin L, Amelar RD. Varicocelectomy: twenty-five years of experience. Int J Fertil 1988;33:226–228,231–235. Review.

97. Mordel N, Mor-Yosef S, Margalioth EJ, et al. Spermatic vein ligation as treatment for male infertility. Justification by postoperative semen improvement and pregnancy rates. J Reprod Med 1990;35:123–127.

98. Comhaire F, Kunnen M, Nahoum C. Radiologic anatomy of the internal spermatic vein(s) in 200 retrograde venograms. Int J Androl 1981;4:379.

99. Mozes M, Bogokowsky H, Antebi E. Surgical treatment of varicocele. J Int Coll Surg 1965;44:44.

100. Pryor JL, Howards SS. Varicocele. Urol Clin North Am 1987;14:499–513.

101. Levitt S, Gill B, Katlowitz N, et al. Routine intraoperative postligation venography in the treatment of the pediatric varicocele. J Urol 1987;137:716–718.

102. Zaontz MR, Firlit CF. Use of venography as an aid in varicocelectomy. J Urol 1987;138:1041–1042.

103. Hart RR, Rushton HG, Belman AB. Intraoperative spermatic venography during varicocele surgery in adolescents. J Urol 1992;148:1514–1516.

104. Tauber R, Johnsen N. Antegrade scrotal sclerotherapy for the treatment of varicocele: technique and late results. J Urol 1994;151:386–390.

105. Riedl P. [Selective phlebography and catheter-sclerosation of the spermatic vein in primary varicocele. An angiographic-anatomical and clinical study (author's transl)]. Wein Klin Wochenschr Suppl 1979;91:3–20.

106. Thelen M, Weissbach L, Franken T. [The treatment of idiopathic varicoceles by transfemoral spiral occlusion of the left testicular vein (author's transl)]. Rofo 1979;131:24–29.

107. Formanek A, Rusnak B, Zollikofer C, et al. Embolization of the spermatic vein for treatment of infertility: a new approach. Radiology 1981;139:315–321.

108. Morag B, Rubinstein ZJ, Goldwasser B, et al. Percutaneous venography and occlusion in the management of spermatic varicoceles. AJR Am J Roentgenol 1984;143:635–640.

109. Kuroiwa T, Hasuo K, Yasumori K, et al. Transcatheter embolization of testicular vein for varicocele testis. Acta Radiol 1991;32:311–314.

110. Berkman WA, Price RB, Wheatley JK, et al. Varicoceles: a coaxial coil occlusion system. Radiology 1984;151:73–77.

111. Berger T, Sorensen R. Varicoceles: distal occlusion with coaxial catheter system. Radiology 1987;162:271.

112. Takeyama M, Honjoh M, Kodama M, et al. Testicular steroids in spermatic and peripheral veins after single injection of hCG in patients with varicocele. Arch Androl 1990;24:207–213.

113. Trerotola SO, Venbrux AC, Savader SJ, et al. Guiding catheter for varicocele embolization. J Vasc Interv Radiol 1993;4:433–434.

114. Fobbe F, Hamm B, Sorensen R, et al. Percutaneous transluminal treatment of varicoceles: where to occlude the internal spermatic vein. AJR Am J Roentgenol 1987;149:983–987.

115. Zuckerman AM, Mitchell SE, Venbrux AC, et al. Percutaneous varicocele occlusion: long-term follow-up. J Vasc Interv Radiol 1994;5:315–319.

116. Shuman L, White RI Jr, Mitchell SE, et al. Right-sided varicocele: technique and clinical results of balloon embolotherapy from the femoral approach. Radiology 1986;158:787–791.

117. Seyferth W, Jecht E, Zeitler E. Percutaneous sclerotherapy of varicocele. Radiology 1981;139:335–340.

118. Sigmund G, Bahren W, Gall H, et al. Idiopathic varicoceles: feasibility of percutaneous sclerotherapy. Radiology 1987;164:161–168.

119. Pisco JM, Basto I, Batista AM, et al. Percutaneous sclerotherapy of varicocele. Acta Med Port 1992;5:477–481.

120. Bach D, Bahren W, Gall H, et al. Late results after sclerotherapy of varicocele. Eur Urol 1988;14:115–119.

121. Riedl P, Kumpan W, Maier U, et al. Long-term results after sclerotherapy of the spermatic vein in patients with varicocele. Cardiovasc Intervent Radiol 1985;8:46–49.

122. Belgrano E, Puppo P, Quattrini S, et al. The role of venography and sclerotherapy in the management of varicocele. Eur Urol 1984;10:124–129.

123. Salgarello G, Cagossi M, Salgarello TL, et al. Transvenous sclerotherapy of the gonadal veins for treatment of varicocele: long-term results. Angiology 1990;41:427–431.

124. Di Bisceglie C, Fornengo R, Grosso M, et al. Follow-up of varicocele treated with percutaneous retrograde sclerotherapy: technical, clinical and seminal aspects. J Endocrinol Invest 2003;26:1059–1064.

125. Hunter DW, Bildsoe MC, Amplatz K. Aid for safer sclerotherapy of the internal spermatic vein. Radiology 1989;173:282.

126. Pochaczevsky R, Lee WJ, Mallett E. Management of male infertility: roles of contact thermography, spermatic venography, and embolization. AJR Am J Roentgenol 1986;147:97–102.

127. Rooney MS, Gray RR. Varicocele embolization through competent internal spermatic veins. Can Assoc Radiol J 1992;43:431–435.

128. Weissbach L, Thelen M, Adolphs H. Treatment of idiopathic varicoceles by transfemoral testicular vein occlusion. J Urol 1981;126:354–356.

129. White R, Kaufman S, Barth K, et al. Occlusion of varicoceles with detachable balloons. Radiology 1981;327–334.

130. Chomyn JJ, Craven WM, Groves BM, et al. Percutaneous removal of a Gianturco coil from the pulmonary artery with use of flexible intravascular forceps. J Vasc Interv Radiol 1991;2:105–106.

131. Walsh P, White R. Balloon occlusion of the internal spermatic vein for the treatment of varicoceles. JAMA 1981;246:1701–1702.

132. Pollak JS, Egglin TK, Rosenblatt MM, et al. Clinical results of transvenous systemic embolotherapy with a neuroradiologic detachable balloon. Radiology 1994;191:477–482.

133. Makita K, Furui S, Tsuchiya K, et al. Guide wire-directed detachable balloon: clinical application in treatment of varicoceles. Radiology 1992;183:575–577.

134. Smith TP, Hunter DW, Cragg AH, et al. Spermatic vein embolization with hot contrast material: fertility results. Radiology 1988;168:137–139.

135. Reyes BL, Trerotola SO, Venbrux AC, et al. Percutaneous embolotherapy of adolescent varicocele: results and long-term follow-up. J Vasc Interv Radiol 1994;5:131–134.

136. Pieri S, Agresti P, Morucci M, et al. Analysis of radiation doses in the percutaneous treatment of varicocele in adolescents. Radiol Med (Torino) 2003;105:500–510.

137. MacLeod J. Further observations on the role of varicocele in human infertility. Fertil Steril 1969;20:545–563.

138. Schlesinger MH, Wilets IF, Nagler HM. Treatment outcome after varicocelectomy. A critical analysis. Urol Clin North Am 1994;21:517–529.

139. Braedel HU, Steffens J, Ziegler M, et al. Outpatient sclerotherapy of idiopathic left-sided varicocele in children and adults. Br J Urol 1990;65:536–540.

140. Trombetta C, Liguori G, Bucci S, et al. Percutaneous treatment of varicocele. Urol Int 2003;70:113–118.

141. Vermeulen A, Vandeweghe M. Improved fertility after varicocele correction: fact or fiction? Fertil Steril 1984;42:249–256.

142. Breznik R, Vlaisavljevic V, Borko E. Treatment of varicocele and male fertility. Arch Androl 1993;30:157–160.

143. Nabi G, Asterlings S, Greene DR, et al. Percutaneous embolization of varicoceles: outcomes and correlation of semen improvement with pregnancy. Urology 2004;63:359–363.

144. Comhaire FH, Kunnen M. Factors affecting the probability of conception after treatment of subfertile men with varicocele by transcatheter embolization with Bucrylate. Fertil Steril 1985;43:781–786.

145. Nieschlag E, Behre HM, Schlingheider A, et al. Surgical ligation vs. angiographic embolization of the vena spermatica: a prospective randomized study for the treatment of varicocele-related infertility. Andrologia 1993;25:233–237.

146. Yavetz H, Levy R, Papo J, et al. Efficacy of varicocele embolization versus ligation of the left internal spermatic vein for improvement of sperm quality. Int J Androl 1992;15:338–344.

147. Parsch EM, Schill WB, Erlinger C, et al. Semen parameters and conception rates after surgical treatment and sclerotherapy of varicocele. Andrologia 1990;22:275–278.

148. Madgar I, Weissenberg R, Lunenfeld B, et al. Controlled trial of high spermatic vein ligation for varicocele in infertile men. Fertil Steril 1995;63:120–124.

149. Yamamoto M, Hibi H, Hirata Y, et al. Effect of varicocelectomy on sperm parameters and pregnancy rate in patients with subclinical

varicocele: a randomized prospective controlled study. J Urol 1996;155:1636–1638.

150. Nilsson S, Edvinsson A, Nilsson B. Improvement of semen and pregnancy rate after ligation and division of the internal spermatic vein: fact or fiction? Br J Urol 1979;51:591–596.

151. Nieschlag E, Hertle L, Fischedick A, et al. Update on treatment of varicocele: counseling as effective as occlusion of the vena spermatica. Hum Reprod 1998;13:2147–2150.

152. Nieschlag E, Hertle L, Fischedick A, et al. Treatment of varicocele: counseling as effective as occlusion of the vena spermatica. Hum Reprod 1995;10:347–353.

153. Evers JL, Collins JA. Assessment of efficacy of varicocele repair for male subfertility: a systematic review. Lancet 2003;361:1849–1852. Review.

154. Marmar J, Benoff S. New scientific information related to varicoceles. J Urol 2003;170:2371–2373.

155. Cayan S, Erdemir F, Ozbey I, et al. Can varicocelectomy significantly change the way couples use assisted reproductive technologies? J Urol 2002;167:1749–1752.

156. Tanahatoe SJ, Maas WM, Hompes PG, et al. Influence of varicocele embolization on the choice of infertility treatment. Fertil Steril 2004;81:1679–1683.

157. Penson DF, Paltiel AD, Krumholz HM, et al. The cost-effectiveness of treatment for varicocele related infertility. J Urol 2002;168:2490–2494.

158. Male Infertility Best Practice Policy Committee of the American Urological Association and the Practice Committee of the American Society for Reproductive Medicine. Report on varicocele and infertility. Fertil Steril 2004;82(Suppl I):S142–S145.

Uterine Fibroid Embolization

44

James B. Spies

For generations, the mainstay of therapy for uterine fibroids has been hysterectomy. In the early 1990s, interest grew among patients for alternatives that would be effective for symptom control, but that would spare the uterus. Myomectomy had long been the primary uterine-sparing therapy for fibroids, but it remained a major operative procedure, with significant bleeding risk (1). The desire for less-invasive therapies grew.

At about the same time, Drs. Ravina and Merland of the Hospital Lariboisière in Paris, France, were evaluating the use of preoperative embolization of the uterus to reduce blood loss during myomectomy. They were surprised when some patients had their symptoms resolve while awaiting surgery. They followed the progress of 16 such patients and reported this experience in 1995 (2). This was the first report in the English language medical literature of uterine embolization as a sole therapy for managing symptoms from uterine fibroids.

That report of uterine embolization led Drs. McLucas and Goodwin at UCLA to evaluate this treatment. They published their initial results in 1997 (3), creating considerable interest among the lay press and other investigators in the United States. These early reports led to subsequent investigations by others, resulting in the ultimate acceptance of uterine fibroid embolization (UFE) as a therapy for fibroids.

Uterine embolization is now offered in hundreds of hospitals across the world, and there is growing interest in the treatment among both interventionalists and gynecologists. With such widespread interest, a review of the procedure is needed for practicing physicians, and this chapter is intended to serve as an introduction for them. It summarizes the indications, technique, pitfalls, complications, and outcome from therapy. Before discussing UFE, however, some background on fibroids will be helpful to place this therapy in context.

UTERINE FIBROIDS

Uterine fibroids, also called myomas or leiomyomas, are benign muscular tumors and are the most common tumors of the female reproductive tract (4). Forty percent of women still menstruating beyond the age of 50 years have fibroids (1). In the United States, 30% of women will have had a hysterectomy by age 60, and 60% of these will be for fibroids (5). The cost to the health care system is enormous, with annual expenditures for hysterectomy for fibroids alone at $2 billion (6). A number of factors predispose to the development of fibroids, including African-American ethnicity, early menarche, and high body mass index (7).

Both hysterectomy and myomectomy have been mainstays of the surgical management of fibroids, along with a variety of medical therapies. These include oral contraceptives, oral and intramuscular progesterones, and gonadotropin-releasing hormone agonists. Despite the frequency of fibroids and the severe symptoms they cause, relatively little innovation in their management had occurred until the 1990s. Since then, hysteroscopic and laparascopic skills have advanced, allowing less invasive approaches for fibroid removal in some patients. However, for many women, hysterectomy and myomectomy remain the primary therapeutic options offered, and it is in the context of these more invasive therapies that UFE has become accepted as the primary minimally invasive approach to this condition.

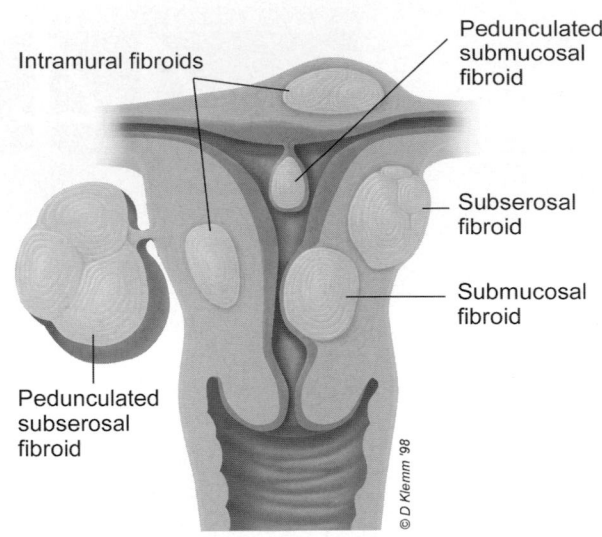

Figure 44–1 Illustration of different anatomic locations of fibroids.

Fibroids are named according to their position in the uterus, as shown in Figure 44–1. The three primary types are submucosal, intramural, and serosal, with the position of the center of the fibroid dictating the name. Both submucosal and serosal fibroids may be pedunculated, and the degree to which they are attached to the body of the uterus is often a factor in determining whether UFE is the best therapeutic choice. Fibroids may also be transmural, extending from the serosal surface of the uterus to the endometrial surface. Rarely, they may also arise in the broad ligament, and the role of embolization in this rare subset of fibroids is unknown.

Symptoms associated with fibroids generally relate to their position in the uterus, with heavy menstrual bleeding occurring most commonly in uteri where fibroids distort the endometrial surface (submucosal and intramural). Bulk symptoms, such as pressure, heaviness, pain, or urinary symptoms, relate more to the overall size of the uterus. Uterine enlargement is most commonly because of intramural and serosal fibroids and depends on their individual size and number. Pedunculated serosal fibroids also are likely to cause pressure symptoms by compressing adjacent organs, such as the rectum, or they may extend into the flank and cause localized symptoms related to their size and position.

PATIENT SELECTION FOR UTERINE FIBROID EMBOLIZATION

As with all medical therapies, the effectiveness and safety of uterine embolization will be enhanced by the proper assessment and selection of patients before therapy. Not only does the diagnosis of fibroids need to be confirmed, but also the symptoms that the patient is having should correspond to the size and position of the fibroids. In addition, other likely causes of symptoms and even important asymptomatic

pathology should be excluded. These efforts are facilitated greatly by a routine protocol for preprocedure assessment.

Preprocedure Interview

The most important part of the preprocedure assessment is the medical history, because 25% of women develop fibroids during their lives, yet only 10–20% of these women have symptoms. Therefore, only a minority of women ever requires treatment. The most common symptoms associated with fibroids are heavy menstrual bleeding, pelvic pressure, bloating, pain, and urinary symptoms, which are discussed in greater detail below.

Heavy Menstrual Bleeding

The most common symptom associated with fibroids is abnormal bleeding, which typically presents as heavy menstrual bleeding. Anemia is a common side effect. As the severity of bleeding increases, clot passage with the menstrual period commonly occurs. As these clots pass, they may cause severe menstrual cramping.

To determine whether heavy menstrual bleeding is present, a standard menstrual history is obtained. Most patients with bleeding that is heavy enough to cause anemia will have 2 or 3 heavy days of bleeding with pad or tampon change every 2 hours or less for at least 2 or more of those days. Patients may also relate accidental soiling of clothes, furniture, and the like. Even with heavy bleeding, many women are able to maintain a normal blood count with regular use of iron supplements. For this reason, anemia should not be a prerequisite for diagnosing heavy bleeding.

The mechanism by which fibroids cause abnormal bleeding is not known with certainty. Fibroids are believed to alter muscular contraction of the uterus, which may prevent the uterus from controlling the degree of bleeding during a patient's period. In addition, fibroids have been shown to compress veins in the wall of the uterus, resulting in dilation of the veins within the endometrium. This has been postulated as a primary mechanism of heavy bleeding (8).

Heavy menstrual bleeding usually is caused by submucosal fibroids or intramural fibroids that distort the endometrial lining of the uterus. Small intramural fibroids or subserosal fibroids do not cause abnormal bleeding.

There are many other potential causes of heavy menstrual bleeding, so a careful gynecologic history and physical examination are important parts of the evaluation of a patient experiencing heavy bleeding. The fact that a patient has fibroids does not mean that the fibroids are the cause of abnormal bleeding. Possible etiologies include endometrial hyperplasia, endometrial polyps, adenomyosis, and even uterine cancer. These conditions often will present with metrorrhagia or irregular bleeding pattern. If the bleeding is more frequent than every 21 days (inter-period bleeding) or lasts longer than 10 days, then endometrial hyperplasia, polyps, or other nonfibroid causes become likely alternatives to fibroids. In this circumstance, endometrial sampling (endometrial biopsy or D&C with hysteroscopy) may be performed. In most cases, endometrial biopsy is adequate.

This discussion highlights the importance of assessing the patient in the context of the differential diagnosis to ensure that the proper condition is being treated and emphasizes the necessity of consultation with a gynecologist in cases in which there is doubt.

Pelvic Pain, Pressure, and Bloating

Pelvic pain caused by fibroids is relatively uncommon. On rare occasions, a fibroid may suddenly degenerate, which is a painful process that may last several days or weeks. This type of severe pain is unusual. Patients may also report increasingly severe menstrual cramps with the growth of their fibroids.

Severe or burning pain at the time of a menstrual cycle is perhaps caused more commonly by other conditions, such as endometriosis. If an unusual or atypical pattern of pain is present, laparoscopy may be indicated to exclude other etiologies for the pain before concluding that fibroids are the cause.

When fibroids cause symptoms related to the pressure they exert on other structures, it is most commonly a sensation of pressure or discomfort in the pelvis. This may feel like heaviness, bloating, a dull ache, or mild tenderness of the fibroids themselves. The discomfort may be greater with exercise, while bending over, or during sexual intercourse, and the symptoms often are worse just before and during the menstrual period. As fibroids grow, they may cause referred pain in the back, flank, or legs.

Urinary and Rectal Symptoms

Pressure on the urinary system also may be caused by fibroids. Typically, this results in urinary frequency, urgency, nocturia, and, infrequently, incontinence or urinary retention. Occasionally, an enlarged uterus may press on the ureters and cause asymptomatic hydronephrosis. Fibroids may also cause rectal pain or pressure, although this usually occurs when a pedunculated serosal fibroid compresses directly on the rectosigmoid area.

Fibroids and Fertility

Infertility, repeated miscarriage, and complicated pregnancies often have been suggested as being caused by fibroids. Data do suggest that complicated pregnancies are more likely to occur in those women with fibroids (9), but the statistical evidence for infertility is lacking (4). Some researchers have suggested that the presence of fibroids may predispose a patient to miscarriage, but again, firm statistical evidence to support this possibility is not yet available. There have been studies in infertile women in whom the only identifiable cause is the presence of fibroids. These studies have shown

that after myomectomy, 40–60% of previously infertile women have been able to become pregnant (10).

However, because large studies have not been completed and infertility may have many causes, it is imprudent to assume that fibroids are a potential cause without careful investigation for other etiologies. Given the lack of data on the effect of UFE on fertility, infertile patients should be approached cautiously and the procedure should be performed only in infertile women seeking to become pregnant in whom myomectomy is likely to have a poorer outcome. Additional discussion about the possible impact of uterine embolization on pregnancy is found later in this chapter.

Preprocedure Gynecologic Evaluation

Every patient should be evaluated by a gynecologist prior to UFE, preferably within 3 months of therapy, to assess the patient's overall gynecologic health, including ensuring that a Pap smear is negative. In those cases in which atypical symptoms are present or the pattern of bleeding is unusual, additional gynecologic evaluation may be needed. Each patient will also benefit from a formal opinion about the need for therapy and the available gynecologic options.

For all these reasons, a cooperative relationship with gynecologists and interventionalists is important. For appropriate selection of patients for UFE and other fibroid therapies, both specialties need to contribute their skills. As most interventionalists performing UFE soon realize, some patients are best treated by medical or surgical therapies and the relationship with gynecologists is reciprocal.

Preprocedure Imaging

The diagnosis of fibroids should be confirmed with preprocedure imaging, which will more precisely define the size and location of the fibroids. The position of the larger fibroids should be correlated with the symptoms that the patient is experiencing. At this time, the standard methods of preprocedure imaging are ultrasound (US) and magnetic resonance imaging MRI.

MRI is preferred by many for several reasons. First, it gives greater anatomic detail of the location and size of the fibroids when compared to ultrasound. The measurements obtained are not as operator-dependent as those obtained with ultrasound. Second, ultrasound often has difficulty penetrating through very large uteri, and the ovaries may not be identified. In nearly all cases, the ovaries can be seen with MRI. Third, the internal architecture of the fibroids is more readily apparent with MRI; specifically, MRI makes it possible to determine whether a fibroid has already degenerated. With the use of contrast, the enhancement pattern of the fibroids and the surrounding uterus can be evaluated easily. If a fibroid is avascular before treatment, embolization will not provide any additional benefit. Finally, MRI is more sensitive and specific for the presence of adenomyosis (11,12) (Figure 44–2).

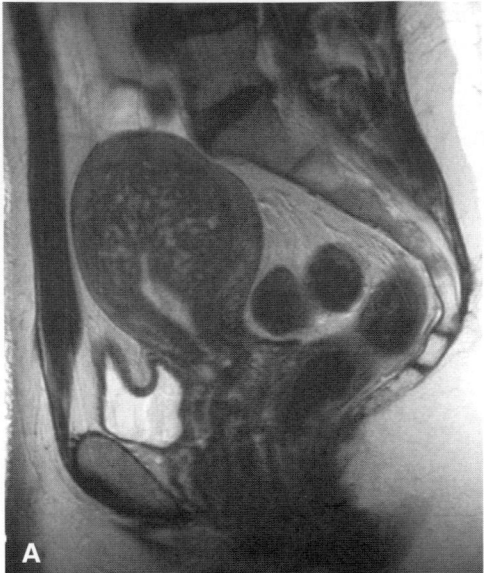
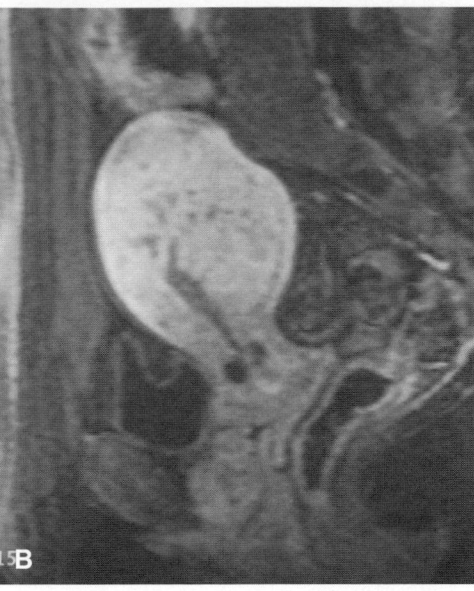

Figure 44–2 Adenomyosis. **A.** T$_2$-weighted sagittal MRI image of the pelvis demonstrating extensive thickening of the junctional zone compatible with adenomyosis. **B.** T$_1$-weighted sagittal contrast-enhanced image demonstrating uniform enhancement of both the normal myometrium and the areas of adenomyosis. This patient had a 7-year diagnosis of fibroids before this study.

Omary et al. investigated the effect of magnetic resonance imaging on the decisions related to uterine embolization and demonstrated that diagnostic certainty increased with MRI (13). In that study, the initial diagnosis was changed in 11% of cases because of the MRI study, and the clinical management changed in 22% of patients. Many potential protocols exist for MR imaging of the pelvis, including breath-hold orthogonal single shot fast spin echo (Haste; Siemens) and T$_1$-weighted spoiled gradient echo sequences obtained at 30 seconds, 60 seconds, and 90 seconds after the dynamic infusion of intravenous gadolinium (14).

Patient Selection

After the workup is completed, the decision remains: Should this patient be offered UFE or should she have a different therapy? To date, very little objective study has occurred regarding the comparative outcomes of the various therapies, and thus, few data exist upon which to base a sound decision (15). Until those data are available, clinical experience must be the guide.

The first decision is whether the patient's symptoms warrant therapy. Presuming that the symptoms are the result of fibroids, are they severe enough to affect the daily life and activities of the patient? Many patients will present with a diagnosis of fibroids and a recommendation by a gynecologist to have a hysterectomy. This recommendation may be given even in the absence of symptoms. The patient may then seek an alternative therapy, such as UFE. Many only need reassurance that no therapy is necessary, or at least not currently. The only circumstances in which therapy is indicated in asymptomatic patients are those in which there is hydronephrosis, a uterine mass that appears to represent a sarcoma, and when fertility problems are directly referable to the fibroids or massive uterine enlargement is a factor.

The same logic may be applied when the symptoms are mild. When bleeding is increased only mildly, medical therapies, such as nonsteroidal anti-inflammatory medications, birth control pills, or progesterone agents, may be effective. Bulk-related therapies do not respond well to medical therapies and, generally, UFE or surgery is the only practical approach. However, the patient should be reassured that treatment can wait until symptoms become more severe. It should be remembered that results are measured in symptom improvement, and minimal symptoms will result in minimal benefit.

Given sufficient symptoms to treat, most patients are candidates for UFE. The patients who might be better served by other therapies include those with pedunculated submucosal fibroids, pedunculated dominant serosal fibroids, and massively enlarged uteri. Pedunculated submucosal fibroids that are completely intracavitary may be amenable to hysteroscopic resection (Figure 44–3). This is a simple outpatient procedure with excellent results in experienced hands, although the procedure often requires pretreatment with a gonadotropin-releasing hormone agonist for 3 months to devascularize the fibroid and reduce its size. Also, large (>4 cm) fibroids may not be easily resectable. UFE certainly works in this group, but it should be reserved for those circumstances in which hysteroscopic resection has failed or the patient has refused.

Submucosal fibroids that have a significant intramural component (or conversely, intramural fibroids with a substantial submuscosal component) are not well-managed by hysteroscopy because significant portions may be left in to regrow. Although symptoms are often temporarily improved, recurrence is very likely. In this circumstance, UFE may be very effective. The decision on therapy relies on quality imaging during the initial assessment.

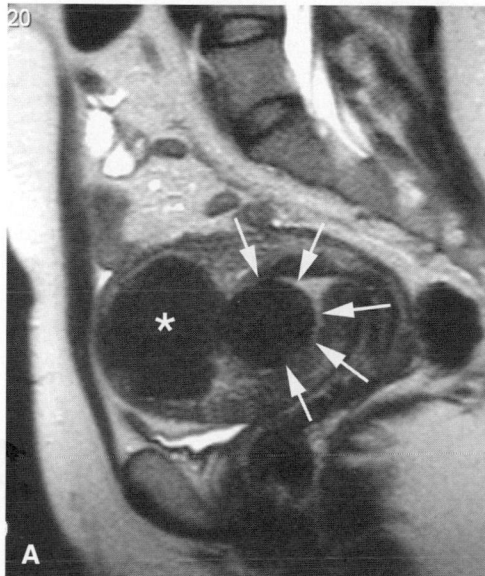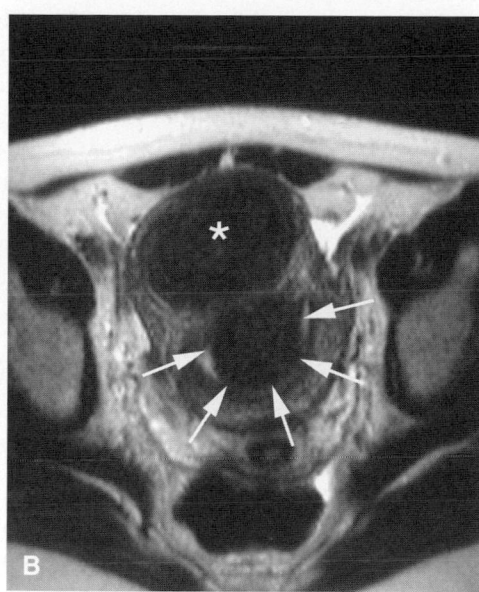

Figure 44–3 Pedunculated submucosal fibroid. **A.** Sagittal T$_2$-weighted MRI image of the pelvis demonstrating an intramural fibroid (*asterisk*) and a pedunculated submucosal fibroid (*arrows*) almost completely within the endometrial cavity. **B.** Axial image of the same patient confirming the intracavitary position of the submucosal fibroid (*arrows*).

Large pedunculated subserosal fibroids that are the dominant or sole fibroid usually are referred for myomectomy (Figure 44–4). UFE may work, but there have been concerns that these may have parasitized blood supply from other pelvic vessels and may prevent complete infarction. In at least one case in France (16), a pedunculated subserosal fibroid sloughed into the abdominal cavity and became infected. There are other published reports of adhesion formation with this type of fibroid, leading in a few cases to bowel obstruction (17). These fibroids are also easily accessible by surgery and until more data on the behavior of this group of fibroids after UFE are developed, myomectomy may be preferred.

Finally, patients with a massively enlarged uterus (greater than 22–24 cm in length) may be recommended for hysterectomy. This recommendation is based on experience showing that very large uteri shrink more slowly and even with a 50% reduction in volume, a very large uterus will remain. Patients with this enlargement may become disappointed when their uterus does not return to a more normal size. Some anecdotal reports show that some patients with massive uterus have had persistent pain for months after embolization, and some concern exists that very large uteri may be more likely to become infected. No published data confirm this, but some physicians have made the admittedly arbitrary judgment to refer this group for surgery.

It is clearly important to be certain that the symptoms patients experience are related to fibroids. Some patients with trivial fibroids and symptoms unrelated to these fibroids have been referred for uterine embolization. These patients must be triaged appropriately to avoid a treatment failure because of misdiagnosis.

Other contraindications include patients with indeterminate endometrial abnormalities (Figure 44–5) or adnexal masses. Similarly, postmenopausal bleeding in a patient with fibroids is rarely due to the fibroids, and thus, endometrial sampling is necessary. While this list is not exhaustive, it provides a sense of the type of circumstances that indicate additional evaluation by a gynecologist.

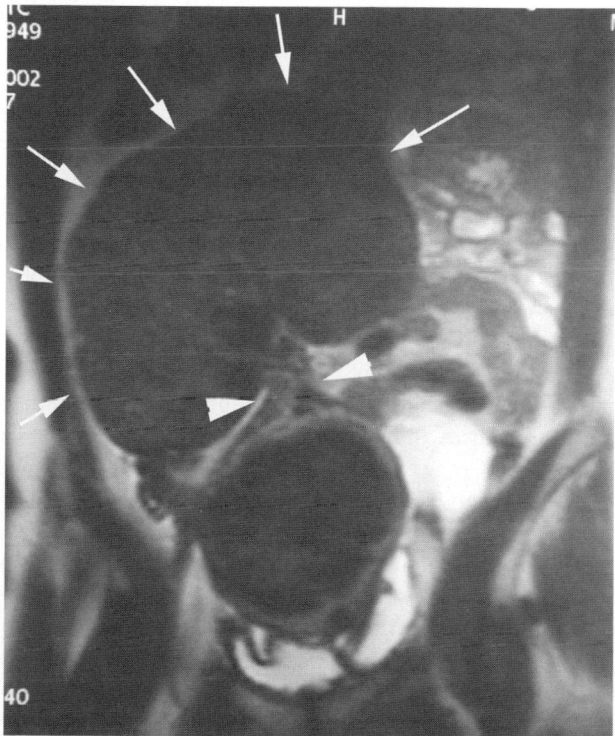

Figure 44–4 Large pedunculated serosal fibroid. A coronal pelvic MRI study demonstrating a massive fibroid projecting from the right uterine fundus (*arrows*). It is attached to the uterus by a narrow stalk (*between arrowheads*).

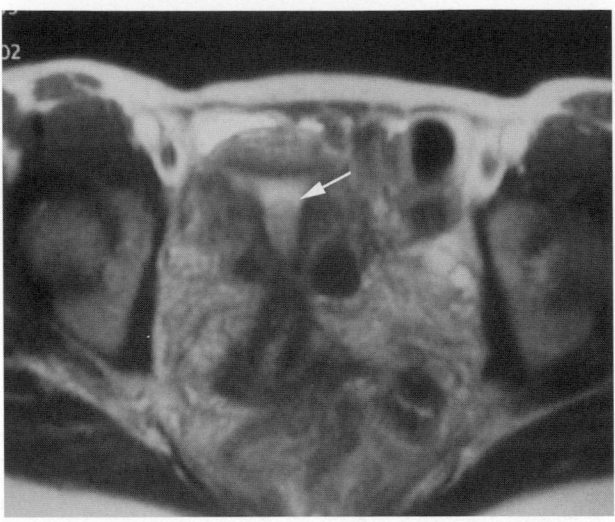

Figure 44–5 Endometrial polyp, axial T$_2$-weighted MRI image. A poorly-defined, rounded, soft tissue mass is seen in the endometrium (*arrow*), which is not clearly a fibroid. Hysteroscopy demonstrated it to be an endometrial polyp.

All of these recommendations are general in nature, and exceptions will occur. Each patient must be evaluated individually. For this reason, a cooperative relationship with referring gynecologists is valuable. With appropriate collaboration, patients will obtain the best therapy and the best outcome.

TECHNIQUE OF UTERINE FIBROID EMBOLIZATION

UFE requires the selective catheterization of the uterine arteries and injection of the embolic material to occlude fibroid arterial supply. The initial challenge, then, is to enter the uterine artery successfully.

In many cases, this is a simple matter. The first step is to obtain a roadmap (or "fluorofade" image) that best demonstrates the origin of the uterine artery. Without a clear depiction of the origin, catheterization will usually be more difficult. To start, the contralateral oblique view is usually used. For example, for the left hypogastric artery, one would use the right anterior oblique view for the initial roadmap. If the vessel origin is not well-demonstrated, then the ipsilateral oblique view often will reveal the exact origin of the vessel. Often, the origin of the right uterine artery is seen best in the ipsilateral (right anterior) oblique. The ipsilateral oblique view also helps in visualizing the uterine arteries with a high origin on either side.

Once an adequate view of the origin has been obtained, an angiographic wire (or microwire) can be advanced into the uterine artery and a catheter advanced over it. If the vessel is large and not too tortuous, a 4 French or 5 French catheter may be used, although if it causes spasm, then a microcatheter should be used coaxially and the outer catheter retracted into the hypogastric artery. In many cases, a microcatheter is used to avoid or resolve spasm. The catheter is advanced to the major medial turn of the vessel and is placed in the proximal portion of the transverse segment of the uterine artery.

Most practitioners use a single catheter to treat both uterine arteries—first one then the other. The first vessel usually entered is the one opposite the puncture site. To enter the ipsilateral uterine artery, a Waltman loop is often used (18). During UFE, a Waltman loop may be created in the following manner: With the catheter tip in the opposite hypogastric artery, a stiff angiographic wire (or the stiff end of a standard angiographic wire) is advanced to the level of the aortic bifurcation. With the wire held in place, the catheter is advanced at the groin and twisted to create a gentle bend in the lower aorta. With continued advancement, the bend begins to ascend in the aorta, dragging the tip of the catheter with it. Once the tip of the catheter clears the aortic bifurcation, the catheter can then be withdrawn at the groin to guide the catheter tip into the ipsilateral hypogastric artery and uterine artery. Once in place, the loop can be reduced by continual withdrawal at the groin until the excess catheter forming the loop has been withdrawn. Shlansky-Goldberg and Cope described an easy alternative technique for loop creation using a suture technique (19).

An alternative is to use a two-catheter approach—one from each common femoral artery. This has the advantage of allowing simultaneous embolization, which reduces the fluoroscopy dose dramatically (20). It does have the disadvantage of a second femoral puncture.

The Difficult Catheterization

Within minutes of attempting to catheterize the uterine artery, the degree of difficulty will become clear. Most experienced operators will be able to succeed within 2–3 minutes of fluoroscopy. Once this does not occur, the most important next step is to obtain a roadmap image that best shows the origin of the vessel. Trial and error with various angles of the gantry may be needed. Steep oblique views may help where shallow obliques fail. For very small vessels, one level of magnification may help, although the routine use of magnification is discouraged because it will nearly double the fluoroscopy dose.

With an adequate view of the vessel origin, the reason for the difficulty usually becomes clear. Angulation of the origin of the vessel is perhaps the most common problem (Figure 44–6). Sometimes, this difficulty may be overcome by advancement of the catheter past the uterine artery and slow retraction of it during slow injection of contrast. The catheter tip will, on occasion, spring into the origin of the vessel. This method often works when the uterine vessel has a diameter greater than the catheter. Once the origin of the vessel is engaged, then the microcatheter usually can be advanced into the vessel.

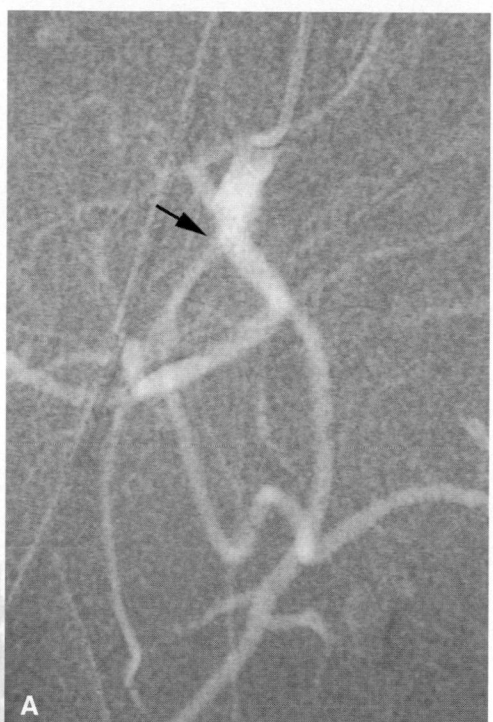
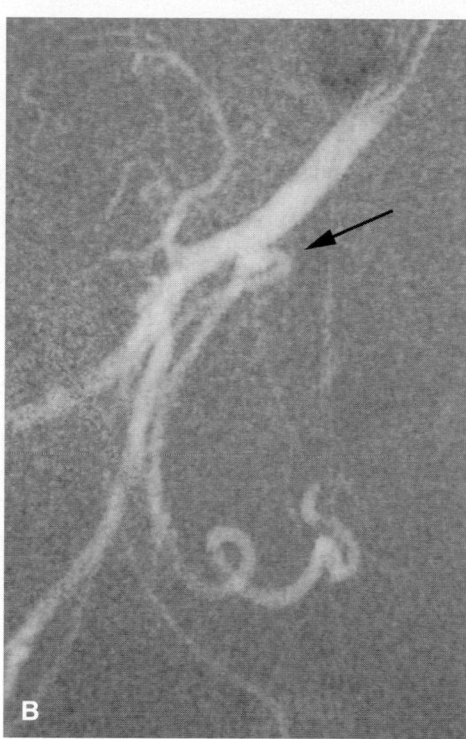

Figure 44–6 **A.** Initial attempt to catheterize the uterine artery failed with this view (*arrow*). **B.** Severely angulated origin of the artery is clear on the opposite oblique roadmap image.

When the uterine artery is smaller than the catheter, the method just described usually will not work. However, it will allow placement of the catheter near the origin of the uterine artery. In this case, the vessel can be approached with a microcatheter and microwire passed coaxially.

Several types of microcatheters are available for use, depending on operator preference and the situation. For some very small or tortuous vessels, a nonbraided catheter may be preferred. In situations in which a small vessel arises from a large artery, a stiffer, braided style microcatheter to give support when trying to pass the wire into the uterine artery may be more useful. On occasion, steam has been used to shape a microcatheter or even a 5 French catheter. Because each patient exhibits a different pattern of branching, standard curves may not meet the need in every case.

A wide variety of microwires are available that may be used as well, but for the average operator, three or perhaps four different types will meet nearly any need. These should be shaped to aid in selective passage into the vessel.

When these methods do not work, change some component of the system. Use a Waltman loop to better position the catheter tip or try a contralateral approach whenever ipsilateral fails. A Waltman loop may be very effective on the contralateral side, even though typically it is used only on an ipsilateral approach. Try switching from a cobra curve catheter to a simple angled tip straight catheter. This removes any frictional force that may be exerted on the secondary curve of the catheter by the small pelvic vessels. Try several different microcatheter and microwire combinations in succession until one appears to be successful.

Penetration into Vessel: How Far Is Too Far?

Embolization should be avoided until the catheter tip is securely within the uterine artery so that embolic material does not reflux into other vessels. Ideally, the catheter is passed several centimeters into the uterine artery. However, on many occasions, severe vessel tortuosity prevents catheter passage for more than a centimeter without spasm. Spasm usually occurs when the catheter distorts the natural curves of the artery. Thus, a location is chosen that is the best compromise between ideal and achievable. With embolization, the forward flow in the vessel initially may be sufficient to prevent reflux, but as the embolization progresses, the forward flow in the vessel slows and in nearly all cases, a small amount of retrograde flow of contrast, embolic material, or both may occur. When several centimeters of vessel are available to contain the retrograde flow, the risk of misembolization is low. But when the catheter is barely in the vessel, there is a shorter buffer segment and great care should be taken to avoid even minimal reflux. Nonselective embolization of the anterior division vessels should never be performed; it is not known how frequently this might result in clinical misembolization in this young, healthy population, and effective surgical alternatives do exist in the case of a failed catheterization.

The group at UCLA has stressed the potential importance of placement of the catheter tip beyond the cervicovaginal branch of the uterine artery to avoid misembolization into it (21). The concern has been the potential for sexual dysfunction related to possible ischemic injury to the paracervical plexus. At this time, it is not known whether this is a cause of sexual dysfunction. In addition, it may be technically difficult to advance the catheter past that branch routinely. The uterine artery is often very tortuous, and distal passage of the catheter usually results in spasm, which may impede embolization. Therefore, when the uterine artery can be catheterized beyond the cervicovaginal branch without extensive manipulation, it may add an additional margin of safety. If it cannot, then embolization can proceed, with an endpoint of sluggish forward flow in the uterine artery (discussed next); in most of these cases, this method leaves the cervicovaginal branch patent at the end of the procedure.

Embolization Technique

The method of embolization is straightforward, although the technique has evolved over time. Early in the experience with embolization, the typical endpoint of embolization was complete occlusion of the uterine artery with use of either an angiographic coil or a gelatin sponge plug as an adjunct (3). In recent years, a subtotal occlusion of the uterine artery has been demonstrated to be effective (22,23), and embolization is now commonly performed without supplemental embolics.

There are two endpoints of embolization in current use. The first is embolization until the occurrence of stasis or near stasis in the uterine artery. Typically, this endpoint correlates with complete occlusion of all the major branches of the uterine artery and is best achieved with polyvinyl alcohol particles. The second common endpoint is associated with trisacryl gelatin microspheres, in which the embolic material is slowly injected and carried by arterial flow to the vessels feeding the fibroids until the forward flow slows to sluggishness within the uterine artery. This corresponds to an angiographic image in which the fibroid feeding branches are distally occluded, but the uterine arteries and the proximal portions of its branches are patent, sometimes called the "pruned tree" appearance (23).

The choice of embolic material has received less study in comparative studies, but a recent study comparing polyvinyl alcohol particles and trisacryl gelatin microspheres demonstrated that when the endpoints were used as described, both materials were equally effective at infarcting fibroids (24). This study also showed no other differences between the two embolics in terms of periprocedural pain or other aspects of recovery.

Regardless of the embolic material used or the endpoint employed, it is important to wait a few minutes at the conclusion of embolization to be sure there is not early recanalization, which may allow for continued perfusion of the fibroids. This subject is discussed in the section on the failed procedure.

PERIPROCEDURE PATIENT MANAGEMENT

Before beginning a UFE practice, a clear plan for patient evaluation and management is essential. This should include a consultation with the patient ahead of time, with an evaluation that leads to a determination that the patient is a candidate for treatment. Once that judgment is made, it is important that the risks, benefits, and alternatives to UFE be explained to the patient. Patients also need to be informed of the character of the recovery after treatment. Detailed written discharge instructions help in this process and can be given to the patient before admission for treatment. The better the patient is informed, the fewer the problems that will occur in follow-up.

While UFE is a minimally invasive procedure, recovery period continues for 7–10 days. Just as important as the procedure, the appropriate management of that recovery is necessary for a successful outcome. Most patients will have moderate to intense pain for 2–6 hours after the procedure, which may be accompanied by nausea. While this resolves over several hours, most patients will develop recurrent moderate cramps 1–2 days after treatment, along with a flu-like syndrome characterized by malaise, loss of appetite, muscles aches, and low-grade nausea. About one third will have fever. With proper planning, these side effects can be anticipated and easily managed.

The scope of this chapter does not permit a detailed discussion of management strategies. In brief, the pain after UFE is quite variable, so developing a standard protocol to ensure relief of the patient's pain is important. Nearly all physicians performing UFE regularly use a combination of nonsteroidal anti-inflammatories and narcotics for the first several days after the procedure. In most cases, the pain that occurs is most severe the day of the procedure. Intravenous patient-controlled analgesia (PCA), narcotics, or epidural (or spinal) analgesia are used while the patient is in the hospital. In some practices, ketoprofen 30 mg is given every 6 hours intravenously, beginning at the conclusion of the procedure, combined with a morphine PCA pump. In other centers, fentanyl or hydromorphone PCA pumps are the routine. Because each institution has its own standard protocols, the hospital anesthesia service should be consulted before a UFE program is begun. In some hospitals, the anesthesia service must be consulted before a PCA pump can be ordered. These arrangements need to be made before the procedure. The pain after UFE can be intense, and it may begin immediately. It is important that no delay occur in addressing it. As an alternative to overnight hospital stay, Siskin et al. (25) have developed a detailed protocol for the outpatient management of pain after UFE that allows discharge after 6–8 hours for most patients.

Nausea is also common in the first hours after embolization. Parenteral antiemetics, such as ondansetron or promethazine, are often required and are commonly used prophylactically. A common protocol is ondansetron 4 mg intravenously at the end of the procedure and one additional dose 6 hours later. If this does not control nausea, additional doses may be given in 4 mg increments.

Regardless of whether a patient stays in the hospital overnight or is discharged the same day, the symptoms over the first week will also need active management. Most UFE providers use a combination of oral nonsteroidal anti-inflammatory agents, oral narcotics, and antiemetics. One regimen is to prescribe ibuprofen (Motrin 800 mg every 6 hours for 4 days, then as needed), oxycodone with acetaminophen (Percocet 5/325, 1 or 2 every 3–4 hours as needed for pain) and an antiemetic (promethazine 25 mg orally every 4–6 hours or ondansetron 4 mg every 6 hours as needed). There are many different acceptable protocols for postprocedure management. Choose one and, with experience, alter it to meet patients' needs. Actively monitor the success of the regimen and adjust it as needed. Proper management of postprocedure symptoms is a key part of the long-term tolerability and acceptance of this procedure.

OUTCOME FROM EMBOLIZATION

Since the inception of uterine embolization, there have been many reports regarding its outcome, both from the perspective of symptom control and imaging outcome. Beyond these standard measures, there has been interest in other measures of outcome, such as menstrual charts and changes in health-related quality of life. Finally, efforts are currently underway to assess outcome as it compares to other fibroid therapies.

Early Reports

The first report by Ravina in 1995 (2) detailed the outcome in 16 patients who were treated using polyvinyl alcohol particles. With a mean follow-up of 20 months, symptoms resolved in 11 of 16. Three patients had partial improvement, and the residual heavy bleeding was subsequently controlled with progestins. There were two failures: one that required hysterectomy 6 weeks after the procedure and another that required myomectomy 6 months after the procedure.

Using a technique similar to that of Ravina's group, Goodwin et al. had similar outcomes (3). Of 11 patients, the dominant symptom was noticeably improved in eight of them. In one patient, only unilateral embolization was done. There was one symptomatic failure. This patient developed endometritis and pyometrium within 3 weeks of the procedure that required hysterectomy. The eleventh patient was lost to follow-up. On imaging follow-up, the mean decrease in uterine volume was 40%, and dominant fibroid volume decreased 60–65% at 3-month follow-up. Other small early series (26,27) reported positive outcomes. These successes encouraged others to study the procedure in larger numbers of patients.

Larger Case Series

Between 1998 and 2003, 11 case series of 50 patients or larger have been published (16,28–37), and the results of these are summarized in Table 44–1.

This experience demonstrates that symptoms are improved in the large majority of patients. Between 81% and 94% of patients experience improvement in their menorrhagia. For the bulk-related symptoms caused by fibroids, which include pelvic pain, pressure, and bloating, as well as urinary frequency, 64–96% of patients have improvement. The variability in outcome relates in part to the means of assessment of outcome. In most of these series, the symptom follow-up was obtained via questionnaire, with patients rating their symptom change. The duration of follow-up varied from 6–29 months, although no long-term studies have been conducted on a large number of patients or have been published as of this writing. Thus, the rate at which patients will have recurrent symptoms, will develop new fibroids, or will need a hysterectomy in the long term is not known.

Imaging Outcome

One follow-up MRI or ultrasound examination is routinely done in most centers at 3–6 months after embolization. This has been the basis of most of the reports of uterine and fibroid volume decrease after embolization. These findings are summarized in Table 44–1, with volume reductions ranging from 20–73% depending on the interval of imaging after embolization. This has been one measure of outcome success, with the implication that greater shrinkage is likely to indicate a more successful outcome.

Unfortunately, the degree to which the fibroid shrinks does not appear to correlate with outcome. In the largest analysis of the impact of baseline and short-term imaging outcome, there was no clear association between symptom improvement and degree of shrinkage (38). The study did indicate that larger dominant leiomyoma volume was associated with smaller percent reduction in volume at 3 months ($p = 0.03$). Submucosal leiomyoma location was associated with a greater volume reduction at 3 months ($p = 0.02$), but it did not persist at 12 months ($p = 0.09$). After adjusting for other variables, odds of improved bleeding and bulk-related symptoms were not higher for leiomyoma volume change or location.

Not only does the degree of shrinkage not predict symptom improvement in the short run, it is unlikely to predict the long-term outcome. Complete infarction of all the

TABLE 44–1

EVIDENCE TABLE ON UTERINE ARTERY EMBOLIZATION FOR FIBROIDS

Peer-Reviewed Published Case Series (2,126 Patients in Total) Inclusion Criteria: Series Including a Minimum of 50 Patients (Excluding Duplicate Reports)

Reference	# of Patients	Duration of Follow-Up (mean)	Menorrhagia % Improved	Pressure/Pain % Improved	Mean Fibroid Volume Reduction	Reported Complications (Number)
Hutchins et al. (1999)	305	12 months	86% @ 3 months 85% @ 6 months 92% @ 12 months	64% @ 3 months 77% @ 6 months 92% @ 12 months	-	Puncture site hematoma (4) Hysterectomy (1) Readmission for pain (2)
Goodwin et al. (1999)	60	16.3 months	81%	93%	48.8%	Hysterectomy for infection (1)
Ravina et al. (1999)	188	29 months	90%	-	50–100% in 87% of patients at 6 months	Fibroid expulsion (6) Hysterectomy (1) for uterine necrosis and bowel obstruction
Pelage et al. (2000)	76	-	94%	-	20% @ 2 months 52% @ 6 months	Hysterectomy for infection (1) Amenorrhea (4) Fibroid passage (4)
Brunneau et al. (2000)	58	12 months	90% @ 3 months 92% @ 6 months 93% @ 1 year	-	23% @ 3 months 43% @ 6 months 51% @ 1 year	External iliac artery dissection (1) Hysterectomies (0)
McLucas et al. (2001)	167	6 months	82% @ 6 months	-	49% @ 6 months 52% @ 12 months	Fibroid passage (5%) Hysterectomy for infection (1)
Andersen et al. (2001)	62	6 months	96%	70%	68% @ 6 months	Fibroid expulsion (2) Endometritis (1) Hysterectomy (0)
Spies et al. (2001)	200	21 months	86% @ 3 months 88% @ 6 months 90% @ 1 year	93% @ 3 months 93% @ 6 months 91% @ 1 year	42% @ 3 months 60% @ 1 year	Hysterectomies (0) Endometrial infection (2) Fibroid expulsion (1) Pulmonary embolus (1), DVT (1)
Walker et al. (2002)	400	16.7 months	84%	79%	73% @ mean of 9.7 months	Hysterectomies (3 for infection), Amenorrhea (7%) Fibroid expulsion/ hysteroscopy (3.5%)
Pron et al. (2003)	550	8.9 months (median)	83%	77%	42% @ 3 months	-

fibroids in general results in excellent long-term outcomes with no recurrence of fibroids at 3 years in most cases (39) (Figure 44–7). The question of the frequency of recurrence of fibroids (either fibroids not completely treated or new fibroids) is not yet clear, but there is evidence that incomplete fibroid infarction does result in regrowth over time with recurrence of symptoms. This can be predicted using MRI with contrast enhancement. Even with short-term symptomatic improvement, the presence of persisting viable fibroid tissue on MRI is likely to lead to early recurrence. This is discussed further in the next section.

Partial infarction without any continued growth 3 months after therapy may indicate a partial technical failure. On the other hand, if there is continued growth of portions of the fibroid even with partial infarction, it may mean that the "fibroid" was in fact a leiomyosarcoma, for which surgery is the standard therapy.

Health–Related Quality of Life After UFE

A broader assessment of health status and outcome from therapy is possible using a quality of life questionnaire. This type of questionnaire assesses overall health status and addresses broad categories such as general health perception, mental status, bodily pain, vitality, emotional status, self-image, and sexual functioning. An early pilot study using a fibroid-specific quality of life questionnaire to assess outcome from fibroid embolization has been published (40). It demonstrated statistically significant improvement in all the general health scales at month 3 and month 6, with marked improvement in general health perception, comparative health perception, physical functioning, energy, mental health, sexual functioning, and self-image. There were corresponding decreases in the three measures of restricted activity: difficulty with activity, pain, and health distress. All the

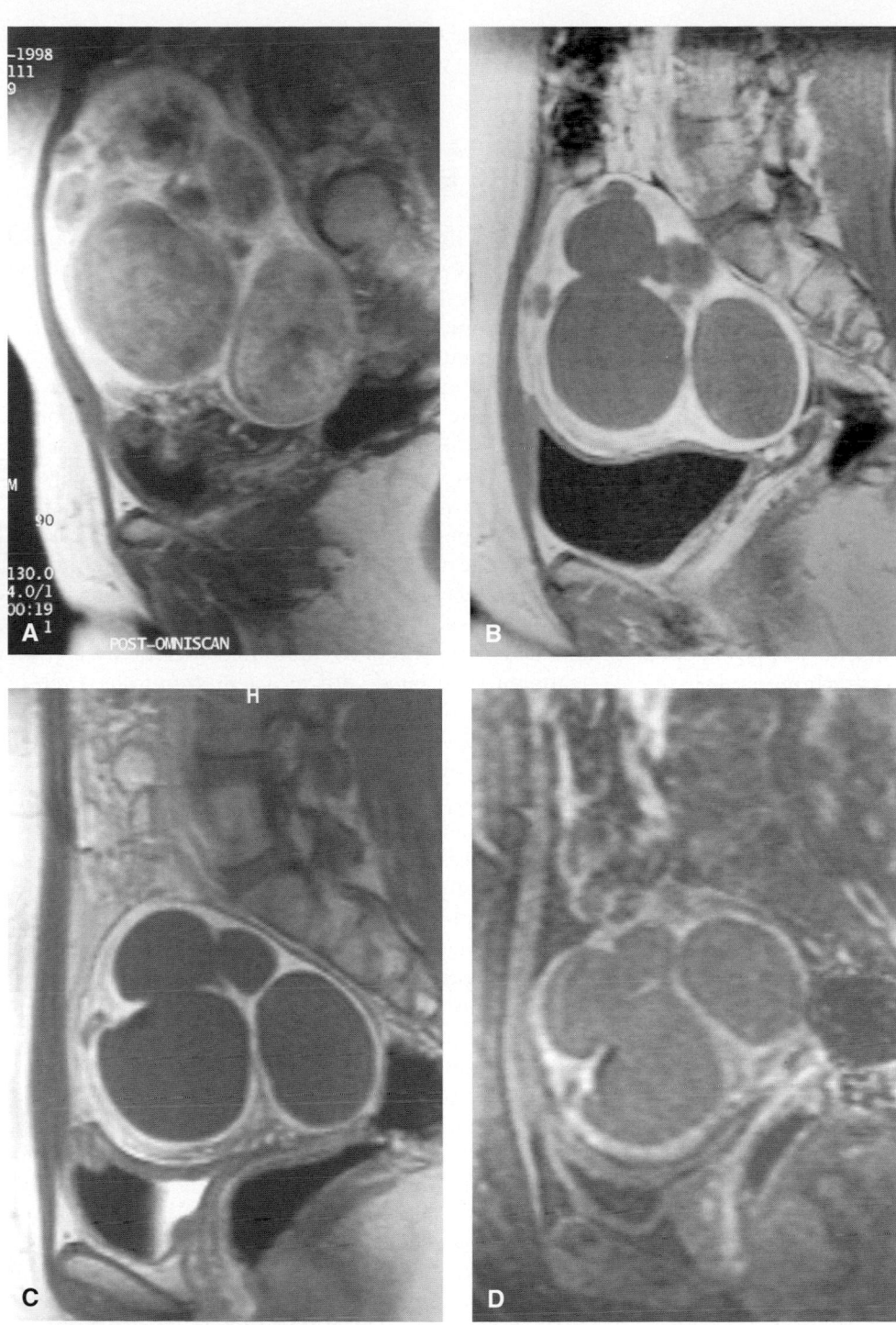

Figure 44–7 Series of sagittal T_1-weighted contrast-enhanced images of the pelvis before and after embolization. **A.** Preembolization image showing enhancing fibroids. **B.** Image 3 months after embolization, revealing no enhancement of the fibroids. **C., D.** Images at 1 year and 3 years after treatment, demonstrating continued decrease in the fibroid volume.

symptom specific measures significantly improved by month 3, and all but one (backaches) improved by month 6. These findings suggest that health-related quality of life is substantially improved by UFE.

Other studies have confirmed the positive impact of embolization on health status. In a comparative study of the outcome of uterine embolization and hysterectomy, one measure of outcome was the SF-12, a 12-question general health-related quality of life questionnaire. Even this relatively insensitive instrument showed substantial improvements in the mental and physical summary scores, with no difference detected between the two therapies (41).

Other Measures of Symptom Change

Beyond quality-of-life changes, several measures focus on other outcomes, primarily menstrual bleeding and pelvic pain. The methods used include menorrhagia questionnaires (42) and pictorial blood loss assessment charts (43). When these instruments have been used, they have shown that menstrual bleeding and pelvic pain are significantly improved (41) after embolization.

Fibroid Therapies: How Do They Compare?

To date, few studies have compared outcomes between embolization and other standard therapies. None can yet be considered definitive in determining the relative short- or long-term outcome. Among the first was the retrospective review of two small groups of patients by Broder and Goodwin (44). Fifty-nine patients underwent embolization, and 30 patients had abdominal myomectomy. The patient groups were identified retrospectively with a minimum of 3 years since therapy and, as a result, the groups were not comparable at baseline, with the embolization patients on average older and having greater severity of fibroid disease. The key finding of that study was that this group of myomectomy patients was significantly less likely to have subsequent fibroid interventions (3% versus 29%, $p = 0.004$), suggesting that myomectomy was more durable. In another small study of similar retrospective design, Razavi and coworkers found nearly opposite outcomes, with embolization patients much more likely to be improved in terms of menorrhagia (92% versus 64%, $p < 0.05$) and pelvic mass effect (91% versus 76%, $p < 0.05$) (45). These authors also found that in myomectomy patients, there were higher complication rates, longer use of postoperative narcotics, and longer hospitalization and recovery times.

Both of these studies share similar flaws. Both identified the cohorts that were compared months or years after therapy. Baseline variables were not controlled, and even the indications for therapy may have been different. For these reasons, conclusions favoring one or the other of the therapies cannot be relied upon based on these studies.

There has been one single randomized comparison published (46). It was also a very small study (40 UFE patients, 20 hysterectomy), and its power analysis was based on length of stay. Not surprisingly, the length of stay was shorter for UFE. Six months after therapy, 31 of 36 embolization patients had improved bleeding, with three failures undergoing hysterectomy. Again, the data available currently are too few to provide conclusions.

Two larger prospective comparative studies have been completed, although neither was a randomized design. The first, comparing uterine embolization to hysterectomy, was a prospective study of the outcome using the same outcome measures (41). The study reported on 102 embolization patients and 50 hysterectomy patients. Both groups had similar short-term outcomes on nonbleeding symptoms, although hysterectomy had an advantage for controlling pelvic pain 12 months after therapy ($p = 0.021$). Most complications were minor, but the frequency of complications after embolization was half that of hysterectomy (50% versus 27.5%, $p = 0.01$). The other completed prospective study compared the outcome from myomectomy and

embolization. As of this writing, the results of that study are not published nor have they been presented.

TECHNICAL CHALLENGES IN UTERINE EMBOLIZATION

While a very high proportion of patients will be improved after UFE, 10–15% of patients will not improve after embolization. There are several potential reasons.

First, technical failure may occur, with failure to catheterize the uterine artery on one side or both sides. In most cases, unless the contribution of one uterine artery to the fibroids is tiny, the likely result is that at least a portion of the fibroids will not infarct and the procedure will not succeed long-term. Cited earlier, the long-term imaging outcome was carefully evaluated using contrast MRI 3 months and 3 years postprocedure, and from this analysis, it was clear that short-term recurrence of symptoms and fibroid growth is likely to recur unless all of the fibroids infarct (39). In each of the cases in which the dominant fibroid did not infarct, regrowth of the fibroid occurred by 3 years after treatment, associated with recurrent symptoms. Even in instances when the uterine volume decreases and the dominant fibroid shrinks, recurrence can be predicted when fibroids do not infarct. Failure of catheterization and thus nonembolization of one side is likely to result in the failure of fibroid infarction.

Another reason for failure is reperfusion of the fibroids after apparently successful embolization of the blood supply. This may result from redistribution of the embolic particles after final embolization images are obtained. One strategy to counter this is to wait at least 5 minutes after embolization to reevaluate uterine flow after complete embolization has been "completed." In about 10–20% of cases, additional embolization is needed to occlude flow that has become reestablished in the interval.

This phenomenon of a false endpoint can be exacerbated by arterial spasm. Most commonly, this is because of angular distortion of the vessel by the catheter. Often, this is most prominent when the catheter traverses a kink or a severely angulated segment of the vessel. This type of spasm often does not respond to antispasm medications, such as papaverine or nitroglycerin. This may be because the source of the spasm is at a vessel kink several centimeters proximal to the tip of the catheter where the medication is delivered intra-arterially. Often exchanging the 4 French or 5 French catheter for a soft microcatheter or repositioning the catheter can relieve the spasm.

Finally, parasitization of vascular supply from other sources may result in failure. The most common source is the ovarian artery, which may supply the fibroids in up to 5% of cases. As mentioned earlier, there are documented instances of a fibroid not completely infarcting because of blood vessels in the same distribution originating from the ovarian arteries (Figure 44–8). Whether ovarian embolization

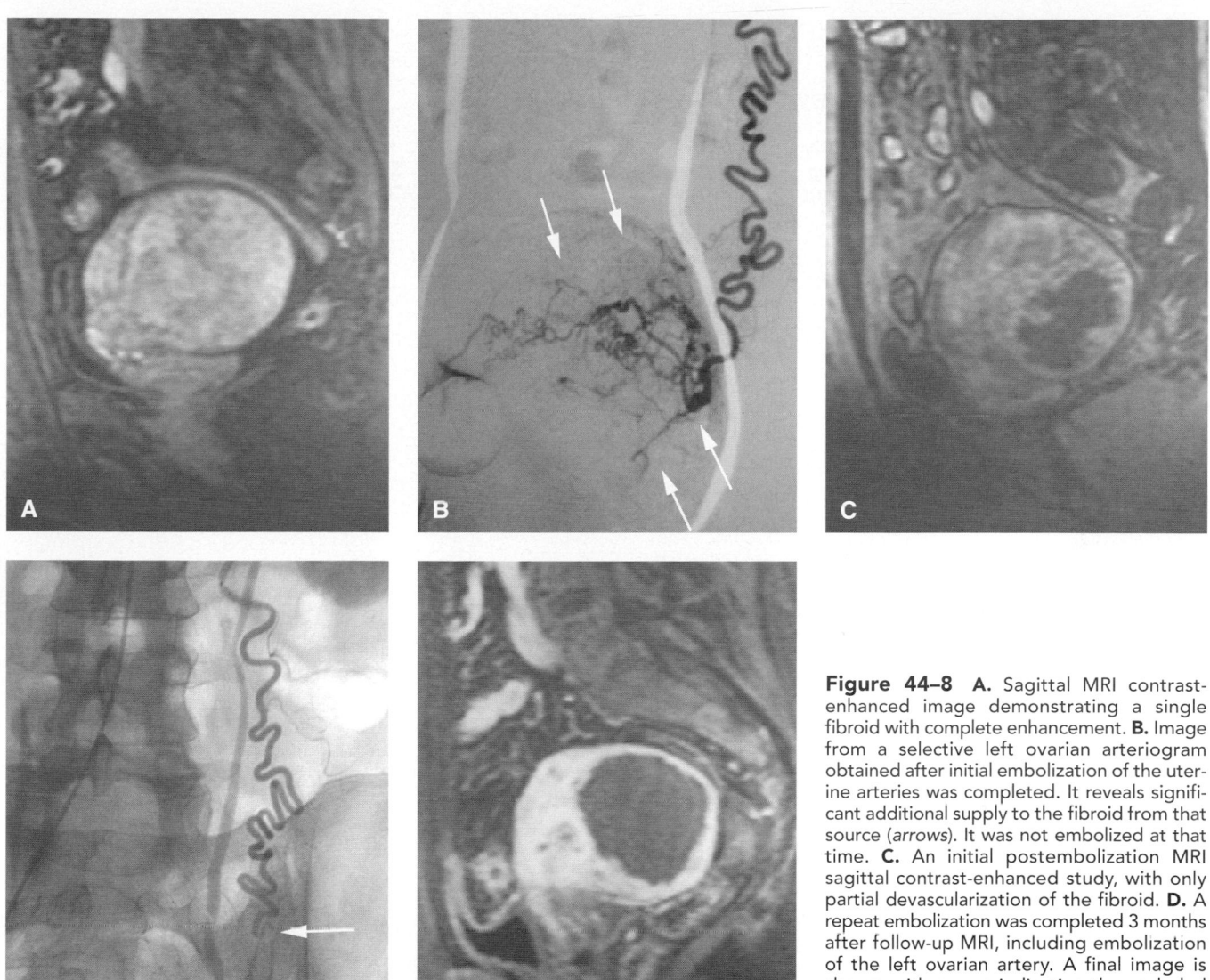

Figure 44–8 A. Sagittal MRI contrast-enhanced image demonstrating a single fibroid with complete enhancement. **B.** Image from a selective left ovarian arteriogram obtained after initial embolization of the uterine arteries was completed. It reveals significant additional supply to the fibroid from that source (*arrows*). It was not embolized at that time. **C.** An initial postembolization MRI sagittal contrast-enhanced study, with only partial devascularization of the fibroid. **D.** A repeat embolization was completed 3 months after follow-up MRI, including embolization of the left ovarian artery. A final image is shown, with arrows indicating the occluded distal part of the ovarian artery. **E.** Final MRI study demonstrating completion of the fibroid devascularization as a result of the ovarian embolization.

can result in successful infarction of the fibroids is a subject of ongoing discussion among researchers in this area, and the most effective method of ovarian embolization is uncertain. There is some evidence that supplemental embolization of the ovarian arteries can be effective in completing the infarction of fibroids (47).

COMPLICATIONS

To date, UFE has been remarkably safe, with few serious complications. However, as experience with the procedure has grown, several complications have been identified, and some can be quite serious. Three deaths have been reported as a result of UFE (48–50), and one additional unpublished

death resulting from pulmonary embolus (51). The potential for such tragic outcomes underscores the need for recognition and prompt management of complications.

For convenience, the complications from UFE may be divided into several categories, including arteriographic complications, allergic and other adverse drug reactions, misembolization, fibroid expulsion (with or without associated endometritis), uterine infection or injury, and thromboembolic complications. Relatively little information exists about the incidence of complications, although one summary of complications in a large group of patients has been published (52). Table 44–2 provides a summary of the complications from that study. Three additional large case series have been conducted from which the relative frequency of complications can be inferred (28,33,53).

TABLE 44–2

SUMMARY OF COMPLICATIONS BY TYPE AND SCVIR CLASS*

Complication	N (% of Study Experiencing Complication)*	95% Confidence Interval	SCVIR Class A	SCVIR Class B	SCVIR Class C	SCVIR Class D	SCVIR Class E	SCVIR Class F
None	358 (90%)	86.1%, 92.3%						
Allergic reaction/rash	10 (2.5%)	1.2%, 4.5%	0	10	0	0	0	0
Leiomyoma passage	10 (2.5%)	1.2%, 4.5%	0	1	6	3	0	0
Recurrent/prolonged pain	5 (1.25%)	0.4%, 2.9%	0	1	4	0	0	0
Urinary tract infection	4 (1%)	0.3%, 2.5%	0	4	0	0	0	0
Endometritis	2 (0.5%)	0.1%, 1.8%	0	0	2	0	0	0
Femoral nerve injury	3 (.75%)	0.2%, 2.2%	0	3	0	0	0	0
Vessel injury	2 (0.5%)	0.1%, 1.8%	0	2	0	0	0	0
Urinary retention	2 (0.5%)	0.1%, 1.8%	0	2	0	0	0	0
Vaginal discharge	1 (0.25%)	0.0%, 1.4%	0	1	0	0	0	0
Hematoma	1 (0.25%)	0.0%, 1.4%	1	0	0	0	0	0
Deep venous thrombosis	1 (0.25%)	0.0%, 1.4%	0	1	0	0	0	0
Drug reaction	1 (0.25%)	0.0%, 1.4%	0	1	0	0	0	0
Thrush	1 (0.25%)	0.0%, 1.4%	0	1	0	0	0	0
C. difficile infection	1 (0.25%)	0.0%, 1.4%	0	1	0	0	0	0
IV phlebitis	1 (0.25%)	0.0%, 1.4%	0	1	0	0	0	0
Arterial thrombosis	1 (0.25%)	0.0%, 1.4%	0	0	0	1	0	0
Pulmonary embolism	1 (0.25%)	0.0%, 1.4%	0	0	0	1	0	0
Total	47		1	29	12	5	0	0

* Forty-seven complications occurred in 42 patients.
Reprinted with permission from Spies J, Spector A, Roth A, et al. Complications after uterine artery embolization for leiomyomas. Obstet Gynecol 2002;100:873–880.

Arteriographic Complications

Perhaps because UFE usually is performed on women in their 30s and 40s, arteriographic complications are very unusual and usually are directly related to the puncture site. Hematoma may be the most common complication in this group, although its exact incidence is not known. In part, this reflects the lack of consensus about the definition of hematoma. However, it is rare that a patient might require prolonged hospitalization or operative intervention for hematoma.

More serious puncture site complications occur even more rarely. There have been reports of arterial dissection or perforation during embolization (53) and arterial thrombosis (52). It appears that this type of injury occurs in less than 1% of patients.

Allergic and Drug Reactions

While difficult to anticipate and avoid, allergic reactions to medications, as well as intolerances and adverse reactions to other drugs are relatively common in this patient population. Of the complications requiring some therapy, this class is the most common, occurring in nearly 2.5% of patients (52). Similar experience was noted in the Ontario Trial (53). The most common manifestation was periprocedural urticaria. Because most patients will have received a number of medications before, during, and immediately after the procedure, it is often difficult to determine the identity of the offending agent. There are also occasional patients who develop a rash several days to a week after the procedure. This may present as a raised red rash on the trunk or extremities, which may be confluent in areas and papular in others and is usually pruritic. Because the presentation is often a week or more after the procedure, the etiology is unclear in these cases. Most patients are not taking narcotics at that stage and may be taking no medication at all. Some speculate that it may have represented a cutaneous manifestation of a foreign body reaction or an "allergic" reaction to the embolic material. In all cases to date, a short course of oral diphenhydramine or corticosteroids have controlled these reactions.

Nausea and epigastric pain secondary to gastritis related to the use of nonsteroidal anti-inflammatories does occasionally occur. There has been one report of upper gastrointestinal bleeding secondary to persistent vomiting (54).

The routine use of prophylactic antibiotics is common, but it has the potential to cause complications. There have been two confirmed cases of *Clostridium difficile* infections reported after just one preprocedure dose of antibiotics (52), raising a question about the benign nature of antibiotic prophylaxis. These are the only reports to date.

Misembolization

Although the complication of misembolization is always feared with any embolization procedure, it has rarely occurred after UFE. For one to occur to another part of the pelvis, particles would have to reflux into another branch. There has been a report of transient labial ischemic ulcer after UFE, which resolved in several days with conservative management (55). As of 2003, there have been no other published episodes of a clinically significant misembolization (except perhaps the ovary), but there is anecdotal evidence of sciatic nerve injury and at least one case of distal ureteral stricture resulting from UFE.

Amenorrhea, in most cases presumably caused by ovarian dysfunction, may occur after uterine embolization (3,32,33,54,56), and its incidence ranges from 2–15% of cases. Most cases of amenorrhea have occurred in women over the age of 45. In only one series has the incidence been reported higher than 5% (56). The authors of that report investigated the potential cause and demonstrated that ovarian vessels do become occluded after embolization in the majority of cases, at least when polyvinyl alcohol particles were used to complete stasis (57). These imaging findings have been confirmed in at least one case, in which embolic material was discovered in ovarian vessels (58). The potential effect on ovarian function is discussed further in the section on uterine embolization.

As a final note, not all cases of amenorrhea are because of ovarian injury; there are at least two reports of amenorrhea resulting from endometrial atrophy, believed to be because of excessive myometrial ischemia (56,59). In one of the cases, small size PVA (150–250 μ) was used and may have caused excessive deep myometrial injury.

Fibroid Expulsion

Perhaps the most common complication requiring additional gynecologic intervention is fibroid expulsion, often associated with either bleeding or infection (30,33, 52,60,61). When a fibroid is completely expelled after embolization, some have viewed this as a desirable event and not a complication. If a fibroid is passing, there usually is significant cramping pain, and an infection or unusual bleeding can occur. Because this is an uncontrolled event with an unpredictable outcome, it has to be considered an adverse event. In approximately 3% of patients, either a dilatation and curettage (D&C), hysteroscopic resection, or short hospitalization has been necessary for fibroid expulsion (52). Two patients (0.2%) required hysterectomy for complications of fibroid passage.

Given the potential severity of the secondary complications of fibroid passage, these patients are monitored closely. Initially, they should have a pelvic examination to determine whether the cervix is open or to determine whether there is extruding tissue. Both of these findings suggest that an infection is likely to develop unless the fibroid is removed. The pelvic examination also will allow the physician to determine whether there is uterine tenderness or pain with cervical motion, which would indicate more generalized infection of the uterus. A complete blood count and vital signs are obtained when an infection or heavy bleeding is present. Fevers that first arise more than 10 days after the procedure may be considered suspicious for infection. Cervical cultures are usually done, although empiric therapy for both gram-negative organisms and anaerobes is suggested.

Patients who appear toxic should be admitted and treated with intravenous antibiotics. Inpatient management is indicated for those with heavy bleeding and severe pain. In these patients, an MRI of the pelvis to assess the status of the uterine cavity and the fibroids is very helpful. Often, the migration of the fibroid into the uterine cavity and toward the lower uterine segment is evident, confirming the diagnosis (Figure 44–9). After initiation of antibiotics, the patient usually is observed for a brief time (up to 48 hours). If the fibroid does not spontaneously pass within 48 hours of onset of symptoms, early intervention by a gynecologist with D&C or hysteroscopic resection of intracavitary fibroids has been useful.

Complications Leading to Hysterectomy after Embolization

While a minor endometrial infection may be controlled with oral or intravenous antibiotics, left unchecked it might progress to pyometritis, uterine rupture, or sepsis (3,33,48,50). Hysterectomy may be the inevitable consequence of uncontrolled infection and thus early intervention is important. Similarly, off-cycle and severe bleeding may occur during fibroid passage. While reembolization may be possible, its efficacy in this circumstance is not known. If bleeding is not controlled, hysterectomy may be needed.

Although rare, severe ischemic uterine injury without generalized uterine infection has been reported (25). While the published literature is sparse on uterine injuries after UFE, a few patients have required hysterectomy for persistent severe pain after uterine embolization (62). The etiology of the pain is not clear, but it appears to be persisting ischemia of the normal myometrium, and this has been confirmed on pathologic examination.

In all cases in which concern about myometrial injury or pyometrium is present, MRI may clarify the diagnosis. If the MRI were to show evidence of diffuse uterine abnormality suggesting infection and the patient were septic and not responding to initial resuscitation, then emergency hysterectomy would be indicated.

Rare late complications have led to hysterectomy as well. These include ischemic uterine rupture 3 months after embolization (63), uterine necrosis requiring hysterectomy 2 months after embolization (64), vesicouterine fistula developing after embolization (65), and adhesion formation leading to bowel obstruction (17). Although rare, these cases highlight the need to consider a uterine injury when atypical symptoms present weeks or months after embolization.

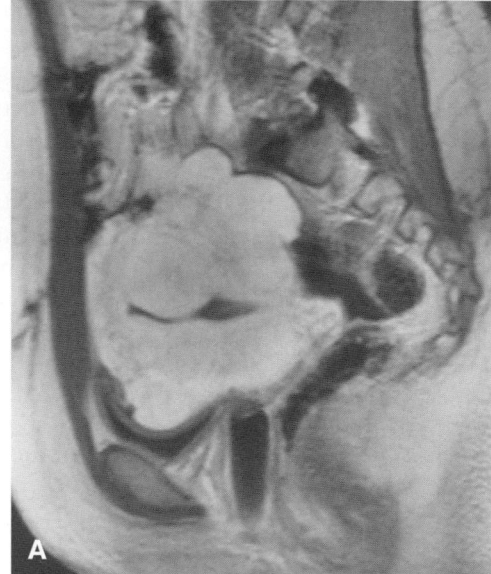

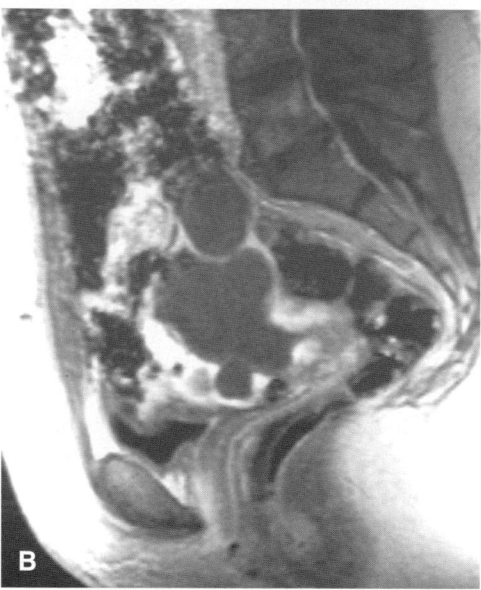

Figure 44–9 **A.** Sagittal contrast-enhanced MRI image revealing several enhancing fibroids. **B.** Two months after emoblization, patient developed 3 days of cramping pain, with follow-up MRI revealing all fibroids devascularized, but with migration into lower uterine segment compatible with impending fibroid passage.

Thromboembolic Complications

Deep venous thrombosis, pulmonary embolus, and thrombosis of the arterial puncture site have been reported as complications of UFE, including the two deaths mentioned earlier (49,51,52). As with many operative interventions, UFE results in tissue injury that can activate the clotting cascade. In a study that measured several prothrombotic factors before and after embolization (66), there was clearly an increase that suggested moderate transient hypercoagulability. While the factors increased, it was to a lesser extent than those seen in many surgical procedures, and the extent

of the clinical risk relative to surgery appears low. Only three patients in 400 developed clinically detectable thrombus (one DVT, one PE, and one arterial thrombosis) in the largest series of complications to date (52).

There are known predisposing factors to thromboembolic disease. In the population undergoing UFE, the use of birth control pills and other exogenous hormones is a known risk factor for the development of venous thrombus, but the benefit of stopping hormones to reduce perioperative risk is unclear (67,68). Any attempt to routinely discontinue oral contraceptives before embolization will need to be begun 4–6 weeks prior to the procedure to ensure normalization of clotting factors, and it must be weighed against the risk of an unwanted pregnancy in the interim.

Regardless of predisposing factors, some measures may reduce the risk of thrombosis. Early ambulation after UFE may decrease the chance of deep vein thrombosis. Automated venous compression devices after UFE have been used in patients who may be at increased risk, including those patients on hormones.

Vigilance is the key to detecting venous thromboembolic disease. Symptoms suggesting either arterial or venous thrombus need immediate evaluation and appropriate management.

PREGNANCY AFTER UTERINE EMBOLIZATION

The long-term effect that UFE may have on a woman's ability to have a child is not known. It may reduce chances of becoming pregnant for some women, but in others, it may be just as likely that the chances will increase.

Fertility may be affected by UFE in a number of ways. During the procedure, some of the flow in the uterine arteries is decreased at least temporarily. It is uncertain what effect this will have on the ability to become pregnant. It appears that in most patients, the arteries reopen to the normal portions of the uterus after UFE, and it is rare for a permanent injury to the uterus to occur. However, uterine wall defects have been described (69,70), and this may weaken the wall and potentially interfere with implantation of a fetus. This appears to be more likely with large fibroids that span the entire wall of the uterus. However, fibroids compress the normal uterine tissue adjacent to them, and as they shrink, normal tissue usually is restored to a more normal configuration. For any individual, it is difficult to predict whether the uterus will be weakened to the point where there might be a problem during labor. At the time pregnancy is confirmed, a sonogram should be performed to assess the site of implantation relative to the residual fibroid tissue and the overall integrity of the uterine wall.

Several published studies have evaluated the potential impact of UFE on ovarian function. In an early study, the

Georgetown group measured basal (third day of menstrual cycle) follicle stimulating hormone (FSH) in a group of women before and after embolization (71). FSH levels are an indirect measure of ovarian reserve and commonly used in infertility practice as a predictor of successful in vitro fertilization. Among the 35 women in the study under the age of 45, there was no permanent change in FSH. None of the women in that study had cessation of menstrual periods. A second study by Ahmad and coworkers (72) found similar results. However, Tulandi did see a trend toward an increase in FSH levels and suggested that there may be a subclinical effect on ovarian function (73). All of these studies were completed early in the experience of UFE. It may be that the current trend toward less extensive embolization may result in less impact on ovarian flow, but this awaits further study.

Published Data on Pregnancy after Uterine Embolization

Thus far, more than 100 patients worldwide have become pregnant after this procedure. There have been two papers summarizing pregnancy after UFE. In Ravina's study, among 184 women who had uterine embolization, 12 unexpected pregnancies occurred during the follow-up period (74). The average age of this group of patients was 36. There were five miscarriages (in three women) among the 12 pregnancies. There were seven deliveries—four by cesarean. There was one twin pregnancy. There was one fetal death from an infection during delivery. The mother in this case had AIDS and had a serious streptococcal infection at the time of the delivery. The other seven infants were normal. In McLucas's study (75), 52 women under the age of 40 stated an interest in pregnancy. Of these, there were 17 pregnancies in 14 patients, for a 33% pregnancy rate. There were 10 term pregnancies, five miscarriages, and two ongoing pregnancies at the time of publication. Both of these studies are small and are not of sufficient size to determine overall fertility rates.

Goldberg et al. summarized 50 pregnancies reported after uterine embolization (76). Thirty-seven of these were in patients embolized for fibroids. In this subset, the authors noted a 32% miscarriage rate, 65% cesarean rate, 9% small for gestational age, and a 22% malposition rate. They also noted that these rates of pregnancy-related problems are well above the rates among the general population, and they infer that embolization was the cause of these complications. While this may be true, it is perhaps even more likely that the presence of fibroids is the cause of these complications (9). The Goldberg study is also flawed because it summarizes published case reports without regard to other potential causes of pregnancy-related complications, such as prior myomectomy. Further, the patients summarized here are among the first patients treated with embolization, and the techniques have improved markedly over time. Clearly, this study does not provide definitive answers regarding pregnancy after UFE, and additional study is needed.

At this time, there is insufficient information to predict the percentage of women who will be able to become pregnant after UFE. It is very likely that the chance of pregnancy will depend on the extent of the fibroids. Those patients with extensive fibroids are probably less likely to become pregnant than others, whether they have UFE, myomectomy, or no therapy at all. In the absence of more definitive data, each patient's treatment will need to be carefully considered, and UFE recommended for those patients in whom other more established therapies have failed or are likely to reduce fertility even further.

FUTURE DIRECTIONS

While remarkable growth has occurred in our knowledge of UFE since its introduction in the mid-1990s, unanswered questions remain. The key issues are the relative effectiveness of UFE compared to other therapies, whether there are subsets of patients best treated with one or another of the available treatments, what the long-term recurrence rates will be, and which therapy is best for patients who wish to become pregnant.

In meeting the research challenge, the Cardiovascular and Interventional Radiology Research and Education Fund (CIRREF) has sponsored several key initiatives. As the first to provide the means to measure and compare outcomes for embolization, the organization sponsored the development of a fibroid-specific quality of life questionnaire (77). This 37-item questionnaire provides a symptoms and quality of life score and can be used to compare patients at a given point in time or to follow the status of a group of patients over time.

This questionnaire has been one of the prime outcome tools for the FIBROID registry, the second major research initiative of CIRREF. This prospective registry was created to determine the short-term and long-term outcomes from embolization. Managed by the Duke Clinical Research Institute, more than 85 participating sites, including 28 core sites contributed to the registry and now more than 3,100 patients are enrolled and being followed. With this huge dataset, it is hoped that the registry will answer the questions asked earlier, as well as some of the questions about subsequent pregnancies after UFE.

SUMMARY

Uterine embolization for fibroids appears to be effective, both in terms of symptom control and also in improving health-related quality of life. Complications are infrequent and usually minor, and serious complications are rare. The preliminary data comparing this therapy to others show a similar level of effectiveness, although more definitive comparative studies are needed. With the outcomes that have been observed after treatment, this has become an accepted treatment for those women with symptomatic fibroids.

REFERENCES

1. Buttram V, Reiter R. Uterine leiomyomata; etiology, symptomatology, and management. Fertil Steril 1981;36:433–445.
2. Ravina J, Herbreteau D, Ciraru-Vigneron N, et al. Arterial embolisation to treat uterine myomata. Lancet 1995;346:671–672.
3. Goodwin S, Vedantham S, McLucas B, et al. Preliminary experience with uterine artery embolization for uterine fibroids. J Vasc Interv Radiol 1997;8:517–526.
4. Stewart EA. Uterine fibroids. Lancet 2001;357:293–298.
5. Management of Uterine Fibroids. Summary, Evidence Report/Technology Assessment: Number 34. AHRQ Publication No. 01-E051, January 2001. Agency for Healthcare Research and Quality, Rockville, MD. Available at: http://www.ahrq.gov/clinic/epcsums/utersumm.htm. Accessed November 15, 2003.
6. Zhao SZ, Wong JM, Arguelles LM. Hospitalization costs associated with leiomyoma. Clin Ther 1999;21:563–75.
7. Faerstien E, Szklo M, Rosenshein N. Risk factors for uterine leiomyoma: a practice-based case-control study. I. African-American heritage, reproductive history, body size, and smoking. Am J Epidemiol 2001;153:1–10.
8. Farrer-Brown G, Beilby JO, Tarbit MH. Venous changes in the endometrium of myomatous uteri. Obstet Gynecol 1971;38:743–751.
9. Coronado G, Marshall L, Schwartz S. Complications in pregnancy, labor, and delivery with uterine leiomyomas: a population-based study. Obstet Gynecol 2000;95:764–769.
10. Vercellini P, Maddalena S, De Giorgi O, et al. Abdominal myomectomy for infertility: a comprehensive review. Hum Reprod 1998;13:873–879.
11. Ascher S, Arnold L, Schruefer J. Adenomyosis: prospective comparison of MR imaging and transvaginal sonography. Radiology 1994;190:803–806.
12. Bazot M, Cortez A, Darai E. Ultrasonography compared with magnetic resonance imaging for the diagnosis of adenomyosis: correlation with histopathology. Hum Reprod 2001;16:2427–2433.
13. Omary R, Vasireddy S, Chrisman H, et al. The effect of pelvic MR imaging on the diagnosis and treatment of women with presumed symptomatic uterine fibroids. J Vasc Interv Radiol 2002;13:1149–1153.
14. Jha R, Ascher S, Imaoka I, et al. Symptomatic fibroleiomyomata: MR imaging of the uterus before and after uterine arterial embolization. Radiology 2000;217:228–235.
15. Myers E, Barber M, Gustilo-Ashby T, et al. Management of uterine leiomyomata: what do we really know? Obstet Gynecol 2002;100:8–17.
16. Ravina J, Ciraru-Vigneron N, Aymard A, et al. Uterine artery embolisation for fibroid disease: results of a 6 year study. Min Invas Ther Allied Technol 1999;8:441–447.
17. Payne J, Haney A. Serious complications of uterine artery embolization for conservative treatment of fibroids. Fertil Steril 2003;79:128–130.
18. Waltman A, Courey W, Athanasoulis C, et al. Technique for left gastric artery catheterization. Radiology 1973;109:732–734.
19. Shlansky-Goldberg R, Cope C. A new twist on the Waltman loop for uterine artery embolization for fibroids. J Vasc Interv Radiol 2001;12:997–1000.
20. Nikolic B, Spies JB, Campbell L, et al. Uterine artery embolization: reduced radiation with refined technique. J Vasc Interv Radiol 2001;12:39–44.
21. Lai A, Goodwin S, Bonilla S, et al. Sexual dysfunction after uterine artery embolization. J Vasc Interv Radiol 2000;11:755–758.
22. Banovac F, Ascher S, Jones D, et al. MR imaging outcome after uterine artery embolization for leiomyomata using trisacryl gelatin microspheres. J Vasc Interv Radiol 2002;13:681–687.
23. Spies J, Benenati J, Worthington-Kirsch R, et al. Initial experience with use of trisacryl gelatin microspheres for uterine artery embolization for leiomyomata. J Vasc Interv Radiol 2001;12:1059–1063.
24. Spies J, Allison S, Sterbis K, et al. Choice of embolic material for uterine embolization: results of a randomized trial. J Vasc Interv Radiol 2004;15:793–800.
25. Siskin G, Stainken B, Dowling K, et al. Outpatient uterine artery embolization for symptomatic uterine fibroids: experience in 49 patients. J Vasc Interv Radiol 2000;11:305–311.
26. Bradley E, Reidy J, Forman R, et al. Transcatheter uterine artery embolisation to treat large uterine fibroids. Br J Obstet Gynaecol 1998;105:235–240.
27. Burn P, McCall J, Chinn R, et al. Embolization of uterine fibroids. Br J Radiol 1999;72:159–161.
28. Hutchins FL, Worthington-Kirsch R, Berkowitz RP. Selective uterine artery embolization as primary treatment for symptomatic leiomyomata uteri. J Am Assoc Gynecol Laparosc 1999;6:279–284.
29. Katsumori T, Nakajima K, Tokuhiro M. Gadolinium-enhanced MR imaging in the evaluation of uterine fibroids treated with uterine artery embolization. AJR Am j Roentgenol 2001;177:303–307.
30. Pelage J, Le Dref O, Soyer P, et al. Fibroid-related menorrhagia: treatment with superselective embolization of the uterine arteries and midterm follow-up. Radiology 2000;215:428–431.
31. Pron G, Bennett J, Common A, et al. The Ontario Uterine Fibroid Embolization Trial. Part 2. Uterine fibroid reduction and symptom relief after uterine artery embolization for fibroids. Fertil Steril 2003;79:120–127.
32. Spies J, Ascher SA, Roth AR, et al. Uterine artery embolization for leiomyomata. Obstet Gynecol 2001;98:29–34.
33. Walker WJ, Pelage J. Uterine artery embolisation for symptomatic fibroids: clinical results in 400 women with imaging follow-up. Br J Obstet Gynaecol 2002;109:1262–1272.
34. Goodwin S, McLucas B, Lee M, et al. Uterine artery embolization for the treatment of uterine leiomyomata: midterm results. J Vasc Interv Radiol 1999;10:1159–1165.
35. Brunereau L, Herbreteau D, Gallas S, et al. Uterine artery embolization in the primary treatment of uterine leiomyomas: technical features and prospective follow-up with clinical and sonographic examination in 58 patients. AJR Am J Roentgenol 2000;175:1267–1272.
36. Andersen PE, Lund N, Justesen P, et al. Uterine artery embolization for symptomatic uterine fibroids: initial success and short-term results. Acta Radiol 2001;42:234–238.
37. McLucas B, Adler L, Perella R. Uterine fibroid embolization: nonsurgical treatment for symptomatic fibroids. J Am Coll Surg 2001;192:95–105.
38. Spies JB, Roth, AR, Jha RC, et al. Uterine artery embolization for leiomyomata: factors associated with successful symptomatic and imaging outcome. Radiology 2002;222:45–52.
39. Pelage J, Guaou N, Jha RC, et al. Uterine fibroid tumors: long-term MR imaging outcome after embolization. Radiology. 2004;230:803–809.
40. Spies J, Warren E, Mathias S, et al. Uterine fibroid embolization: measurement of health-related quality of life before and after therapy. J Vasc Interv Radiol 1999;10:1293–1303.
41. Spies JB, Cooper J, Worthington-Kirsch RM, et al. Outcome of uterine embolization and hysterectomy for leiomyomas: results of a multicenter study. Am J Obstet Gynecol 2004;191:22–31.
42. Ruta DA, Garratt AM, Chadha YC, et al. Assessment of patients with menorrhagia: how valid is a structured clinical history as a measure of health status? Qual Life Res 1995;4:33–40.
43. Higham J, O'Brien P, Shaw R. Assessment of menstrual blood loss using a pictorial chart. Br J Obstet Gynaecol 1990;97:734–739.
44. Broder M, Goodwin S, Chen G, et al. Comparison of long-term outcomes of myomectomy and uterine artery embolization. Obstet Gynecol 2002;100:864–868.
45. Razavi M, Hwang GL, Jahed A, et al. Abdominal myomectomy versus uterine fibroid embolization in the treatment of symptomatic uterine leiomyomas. AJR Am J Roentgenol 2003;180:1571–1575.
46. Pinto I, Chimeno P, Romo A, et al. Uterine fibroids: uterine artery embolization versus abdominal hysterectomy for treatment—a prospective, randomized, and controlled clinical trial. Radiology 2003;226:425–431.
47. Barth MM, Spies JB. Ovarian embolization supplementing uterine embolization for leiomyomata. J Vasc Interv Radiol 2003;14:1177–1182.

48. Vashisht A, Studd J, Carey A, et al. Fatal septicaemia after fibroid embolisation. Lancet 1999;354:307–308.
49. Lanocita R, Frigerio L, Patelli G, et al. A fatal complication of percutaneous transcatheter embolization for treatment of uterine fibroids [Abstract]. Presented at the 11th annual meeting of SMIT/CIMIT, Boston, 1999.
50. de Blok S, de Vries C, Prinssen HM, et al. Fatal sepsis after uterine artery embolization with microspheres. J Vasc Interv Radiol 2003;14:779–783.
51. Landow W. Deaths after uterine embolization. In: 2001. Spies J, Warren E, Mathias S, Walsh S, Roth A, Pentecost M. Uterine Fibroid Embolization. Personal Communication. Wendy Landow, SIR Foundation 2001.
52. Spies J, Spector A, Roth A, et al. Complications after uterine artery embolization for leiomyomas. Obstet Gynecol 2002;100: 873–880.
53. Pron G, Bennett J, Common A, et al. Technical results and effects of operator experience on uterine artery embolization for fibroids: the Ontario Uterine Fibroid Embolization Trial. J Vasc Interv Radiol 2003;14:545–554.
54. Worthington-Kirsch R, Popky G, Hutchins F. Uterine arterial embolization for the management of leiomyomas: quality-of-life assessment and clinical response. Radiology 1998;208:625–629.
55. Yeagley T, Goldberg J, Klein T, et al. Labial necrosis after uterine artery embolization for leiomyomata. Obstet Gynecol 2002;100: 881–882.
56. Chrisman H, Saker M, Ryu R, et al. The impact of uterine fibroid embolization on resumption of menses and ovarian function. J Vasc Interv Radiol 2000;11:699–703.
57. Ryu R, Chrisman H, Omary R, et al. The vascular impact of uterine artery embolization: prospective sonographic assessment of ovarian arterial circulation. J Vasc Interv Radiol 2001;12:1071–1074.
58. Payne J, Robboy S, Haney A. Embolic microspheres within ovarian arterial vasculature after uterine artery embolization. Obstet Gynecol 2002;100:883–886.
59. Tropeano G, Litwicka K, Di Stasi C, et al. Permanent amenorrhea associated with endometrial atrophy after uterine artery embolization for symptomatic uterine fibroids. Fertil Steril 2003;79: 132–135.
60. Berkowitz R, Hutchins F, Worthington-Kirsch R. Vaginal expulsion of submucosal fibroids after uterine artery embolization: a report of three cases. J Reprod Med 1999;44:373–376.
61. Abbara S, Spies J, Scialli A, et al. Transcervical expulsion of a fibroid as a result of uterine artery embolization for leiomyomata. J Vasc Interv Radiol 1999;10:409–411.
62. Pron G, Mocarski E, Cohen M, et al. Hysterectomy for complications after uterine artery embolization for leiomyoma: results of a Canadian multicenter clinical trial. J Am Assoc Gynecol Laparosc 2003;10:99–106.
63. Shashoua A, Stringer N, Pearlman J, et al. Ischemic uterine rupture and hysterectomy 3 months after uterine artery embolization. J Am Assoc Gynecol Laparosc 2002;9:217–220.
64. Godfrey C, Zbella E. Uterine necrosis after uterine artery embolization for leiomyoma. Obstet Gynecol 2001;98:950–952.
65. Sultana C, Goldberg J, Aizenman L, et al. Vesicouterine fistula after uterine artery embolization: a case report. Am J Obstet Gynecol 2002;187:1726–1727.
66. Nikolic B, Kessler C, Jacobs H, et al. Changes in blood coagulation markers associated with uterine artery embolization for leiomyomata. J Vasc Interv Radiol 2003;14:1147–1153.
67. Sue-Ling H, Hughes L. Should the pill be stopped preoperatively? Br Med J 1988;296:447–448.
68. Oakes J, Hahn P, Lillicrap D, et al. A survery of recommendations by gynecologists in Canada regarding oral contraceptive use in the perioperative period. Am J Obstet Gynecol 2002; 187:1539–1543.
69. De Iaco P, Muzzupapa G, Golfieri R, et al. A uterine wall defect after uterine embolization for symptomatic myomas. Fertil Steril 2002;77:176–178.
70. De Iaco P, Golfieri R, Ghi T, et al. Uterine fistula induced by hysteroscopic resection of an embolized migrated fibroid: a rare complication after embolization of uterine fibroids. Fertil Steril 2001;75:818–820.
71. Spies J, Roth A, Gonsalves S, et al. Ovarian function after uterine artery embolization: assessment using serum follicle-stimulating hormone assay. J Vasc Interv Radiol 2001;12:437–442.
72. Ahmad A, Qadan L, Hassan N, et al. Uterine artery embolization treatment of uterine fibroids: effect on ovarian function in younger women. J Vasc Interv Radiol 2002;13:1017–1020.
73. Tulandi T, Sammour A, Valenti D, et al. Ovarian reserve after uterine artery embolization for leiomyomata. Fertil Steril 2002;78: 197–198.
74. Ravina J, Vigneron N, Aymard A, et al. Pregnancy after embolization of uterine myoma: report of 12 cases. Fertil Steril 2000;73: 1241–1243.
75. McLucas B, Goodwin S, Adler L, et al. Pregnancy following uterine fibroid embolization. Int J Gynaecol Obstet 2001;74:1–7.
76. Goldberg J, Pereira L, Berghella V. Pregnancy after uterine artery embolization. Obstet Gynecol 2002;100:869–872.
77. Spies J, Coyne K, Guaou Guaou N. The UFS-QOL, a new disease-specific symptom and health-related quality of life questionnaire for leiomyomata. Obstet and Gynec 2002;99: 290–300.

Obstetric Hemorrhage

45

Filip Banovac

Obstetric hemorrhage is a major cause of maternal morbidity and mortality. In the United States, postpartum hemorrhage (PPH) ranks among the top three causes of maternal death (1). PPH is defined as bleeding of 500 mL or more following a vaginal delivery and 1,000 mL or more following a cesarean section. Because it is difficult to determine the amount of blood lost during vaginal bleeding, a more quantitative definition of PPH specifies a 10% hematocrit drop between admission and the postpartum period or the clinical need for a transfusion (2).

The first line of treatment for PPH includes conservative measures such as laceration repair, uterine packing, correction of coagulopathies, and administration of uterotonic medications. When these measures have failed, health care providers have tried surgical ligation of the arterial supply to the uterus or hysterectomy with associated loss of fertility.

In the last 25 years, a new angiographic approach for treatment of PPH has emerged. Angiographic evaluation and embolization for PPH has been established to be safe and effective (3–7). In addition to its high technical success rate, the primary advantage of the angiographic approach is preservation of fertility.

ETIOLOGY AND CLINICAL PRESENTATION OF OBSTETRIC HEMORRHAGE

Postpartum hemorrhage can be categorized into early or delayed onset. Early PPH occurs during the first 24 hours after delivery, and late PPH occurs more than 24 hours but less than 6 weeks after delivery. Early PPH is most often because of uterine atony (8,9), although genital tract lacerations can also cause significant bleeding in the early postpartum period (10). Delayed PPH usually is a result of retained placental fragments.

Other causes of obstetric hemorrhage include arteriovenous malformations (AVM), invading trophoblastic tissue, and complications related to evacuation of ectopic pregnancies. AVMs infrequently cause PPH. The acquired AVM can result from instrumentation in the peripartum period or from invading trophoblastic tissue. AVMs can be seen after uterine curettage for miscarriages, removal of an intrauterine device, or as a result of gestational trophoblastic disease (11,12). This latter problem is likewise an uncommon cause of hemorrhage. Cervical and abdominal ectopic pregnancies are frequently difficult to evacuate surgically and thus are occasionally associated with significant hemorrhage.

Early PPH occurs in the immediate postpartum period after vaginal or cesarean deliveries. Although the amount of bleeding can be significant, the patient is still under close supervision of the obstetric team and thus management can start immediately. This management usually involves immediate clinical evaluation. Manual pressure can be applied to the atonic uterus, the uterus can be packed, and lacerations can be identified and repaired. Women with PPH are frequently coagulopathic at time of presentation (9). Therefore, attempts to correct the coagulopathy may be initiated. If these efforts fail, traditional management approaches include surgical ligation of the arterial supply to the uterus and hysterectomy as a lifesaving measure. Angiographic treatments (discussed in detail later in this chapter) are now gaining wider acceptance.

In the cases of delayed (or secondary) PPH, bleeding most frequently occurs between 8–14 days after delivery and usually is because of retained placental fragments or genital tract lacerations. At the time of delayed PPH, most women have been discharged already and readmission is required for further management. Initial management of delayed PPH starts with a careful clinical examination, administration of uterotonic drugs, repair of lacerations, and curettage. However, if these measures fail, angiographic evaluation and embolization remain an option.

Intrapartum and postpartum hemorrhage are sometimes encountered in certain high-risk patient populations; namely, patients with placentation abnormalities such as placenta previa, accreta, increta, or percreta. This population is at higher risk of bleeding during and after the delivery. The most common abnormality is placenta previa, in which the placenta covers the internal cervical os. Placenta accreta, increta, and percreta involve a spectrum of abnormalities describing degrees of abnormal attachment of the placenta to the uterine wall. Placenta accreta entails invasion of chorionic villi to the level of the myometrium, increta involves invasion into the myometrium, and percreta includes extension of the placenta through the myometrium and the serosal surface of the uterus. Surgical management of these problems is difficult, and radiological diagnosis of them is of great value for appropriate management during and after the delivery. This chapter presents some angiographic strategies that can be useful in the management of placentation abnormalities.

Finally, obstetric hemorrhage occurs with higher incidence in the operative management of ectopic pregnancies. Advances in ultrasonography and serologic testing for beta chorionic gonadotropin have greatly decreased the incidence of hemorrhage associated with ectopic pregnancies because early diagnosis has become possible. These advances have allowed for medical management with chemotherapeutic agents such as methotrexate. Nonetheless, operative management is still necessary in abdominal pregnancies and occasionally in cervical pregnancies, with increased risk of hemorrhage in both. Interventional radiologists can play an important role in preoperative evaluation and treatment of these entities.

TECHNIQUES AND STRATEGIES

The management of various disease entities that result in obstetric hemorrhage shares some essential angiographic principles and interventional techniques. However, approaches differ based on the clinical situation. Therefore, the management of PPH, placentation abnormalities, ectopic pregnancies, AVMs, and gestational trophoblastic disease has a few unique technical features and clinical management strategies that deserve separate attention.

EARLY POSTPARTUM HEMORRHAGE

Initial management includes a clinical evaluation with volume replacement and a transfusion when necessary. A bimanual examination should be performed, and the genital tract should be evaluated for lacerations. Suturing of lacerations, uterine massage, vaginal packing, and administration of uterotonic drugs is the next line of treatment.

Historically, the surgical approach to persistent and massive PPH involved an emergent hysterectomy. Other surgical options to avoid hysterectomy, such as uterine artery ligation and internal iliac artery ligation, were available for women who wished to preserve their fertility. However, internal iliac artery ligation remains technically challenging and is successful in only 42% of cases (13). This poor success rate may result from distal reconstitution of the internal iliac arteries in the setting of a markedly hypervascular postpartum uterus (14). If ligation fails to control the bleeding, hysterectomy after failed ligation carries a higher morbidity rate than hysterectomy alone (13).

More recently, angiographic techniques have become available to treat PPH (Table 45–1). Brown et al. first reported uterine artery embolization for intractable postpartum hemorrhage in 1979 (15); these were followed shortly thereafter by Pais et al. in 1980 (14). Interestingly, embolization technique has remained largely unchanged from these initial reports. Direct puncture of the common femoral artery is performed, and a cobra-shaped catheter or a reverse curve catheter, such as a Roberts Uterine Catheter (Cook, Inc.), is directed into the anterior division of internal iliac arteries for selective angiograms. When the source of bleeding can be identified, selective catheterization is performed, and small gelfoam (Upjohn) cubes suspended in a contrast slurry are delivered until antegrade flow in the vessel stops. Gelfoam is the agent of choice because it causes a temporary occlusion with recanalization of blood flow in 2–4 weeks.

The exact source of bleeding usually can be identified with selective angiography. Detected extravasation rates in the literature vary from 33% (9) to 100% (16). Some authors have noted that the uterine artery is the most frequent source of postpartum hemorrhage (9), whereas others report that the vaginal artery is the most common source (6). Nonetheless, when the source of bleeding cannot be identified, empiric embolization of the anterior division of the internal iliac arteries is carried out with gelfoam pledgets or slurry. In one report, the ovarian artery was the sole source of postpartum hemorrhage after hysterectomy failed to control the blood loss. Consequently, the authors advocated a more thorough angiographic evaluation and subsequent embolization (17). From a technical standpoint, it is prudent to perform abdominal and pelvic aortography to look for aberrant or collateral supply to the uterus (Figure 45–1).

Coil embolization for PPH alone is not advocated. The bleeding from the extensive collateral circulation of the genital tract and the need for selective embolization of the bleeding branches were recognized in very early reports about PPH (14,18). The failure of coil embolization was well-illustrated in an early report by Minck et al. in which initial coil placement into the internal iliac artery seemed to

TABLE 45–1

UTERINE ARTERY EMBOLIZATION FOR TREATMENT OF POSTPARTUM HEMORRHAGE

Authors	Number	Embolic Material	Artery Embolized	Complications
Brown et al. (1979)	1	gelfoam	internal pudental	none
Pais et al. (1980)	1	coil, gelfoam	internal iliacs	uterine perforation, fever
Heffner et al. (1985)	3	gelfoam	not specified	none
Rosenthal et al. (1985)	2	coil	internal iliac	failed embolization, wound infection
Greenwood et al. (1987)	6	gelfoam, coil	internal iliac (anterior descending), uterine, fourth lumbar, middle sacral, medial femoral circumflex	transient buttock ischemia, external iliac perforation
Feinberg et al. (1987)	1	gelfoam, coil	internal iliac	none
Shweni et al. (1987)	4	gelfoam	not specified	none
Chin et al. (1989)	2	gelfoam, coil	internal pudental, internal iliac, uterine	fever
Yamashita et al. (1991)	6	gelfoam	anterior division of internal iliac, pudental	fever
Bakri and Linjawi (1992)	3	gelfoam, coils	not specified	femoral hematoma
Gilbert et al. (1992)	6	gelfoam	bilateral internal iliac	none
Mitty et al. (1993)	7	gelfoam, coil	internal pudental, uterine	none
Abbas et al. (1994)	1	gelfoam, coil PVA	internal iliac, uterine	readmission, fever, vaginal bleeding, abdominal hematoma, septic shock
Joseph et al. (1994)	2	gelfoam, coil	internal iliac, pudental	none
Yamashita et al. (1994)	15	gelfoam, coil	anterior division of internal iliac, pudental, uterine, obturator	none
Merland et al. (1996)	16	gelfoam, PVA	uterine	none
Dubois et al. (1997)	2	gelfoam	internal iliac	none
Stancato-Pasik et al. (1997)	12	gelfoam	uterine, internal pudental	none
Hsu and Wan (1998)	2	gelfoam	anterior division of internal iliac	none
Pelage et al. (1998)	27	gelfoam, PVA	internal iliac	repeat embolization, hysterectomy
Hansch et al. (1999)	5	gelfoam, coil, PVA	anterior division of internal iliac, uterine	none
Pelage et al. (1999)	14	gelfoam n-butyl-2-cyanoacrylate	uterine	none

(Modified with permission from Badawy SZ, Etman A, Singh M, et al. Uterine artery embolization: the role in obstetrics and gynecology. Clin Imaging 2001;25:288–295.)

stop the hemorrhage. However, bleeding recurred and repeat angiography was necessary. Collateral branches, such as the medial circumflex artery from the profunda femoris and branches from the inferior epigastric artery, reconstituted the distal supply and bleeding continued. Only after selective gelfoam embolization of these collateral branches did the hemorrhage finally stop (18). As the body of literature on embolization for obstetric hemorrhage has developed in subsequent years, particle embolization, most commonly with gelfoam, has shown itself to be a superior technique (Figure 45–2).

The next technical consideration is whether to perform unilateral or bilateral embolization of the internal iliac arteries, uterine arteries, or both. Both approaches have been widely reported. Although selective unilateral embolization can achieve hemostasis in some patients, the rich vascular supply of the uterus and the genital tract predisposes patients to bleeding from branches originating in the contralateral

internal iliac artery. Reports of eventual hysterectomy after failed embolization because of persistent bleeding from the branches of the contralateral internal iliac artery have illustrated the need for thorough angiography and the importance of searching for other sources of bleeding after unilateral embolization is performed (19). Because no definitive prospective studies have evaluated the comparative efficacy of unilateral and bilateral embolization for PPH, the technique is left up to the discretion of the operator.

Angiographic methods for embolization of obstetric hemorrhage are usually not very technically challenging. However, sporadic technical problems or difficult clinical situations have been reported. For example, vasospasm of the uterine arteries can preclude selective catheterization (6,9). However, use of vasodilators can allow for more selective catheterization (6) and eventual embolization. Embolic particle reflux can occur in severely hemodynamically compromised patients; in one report, considerable

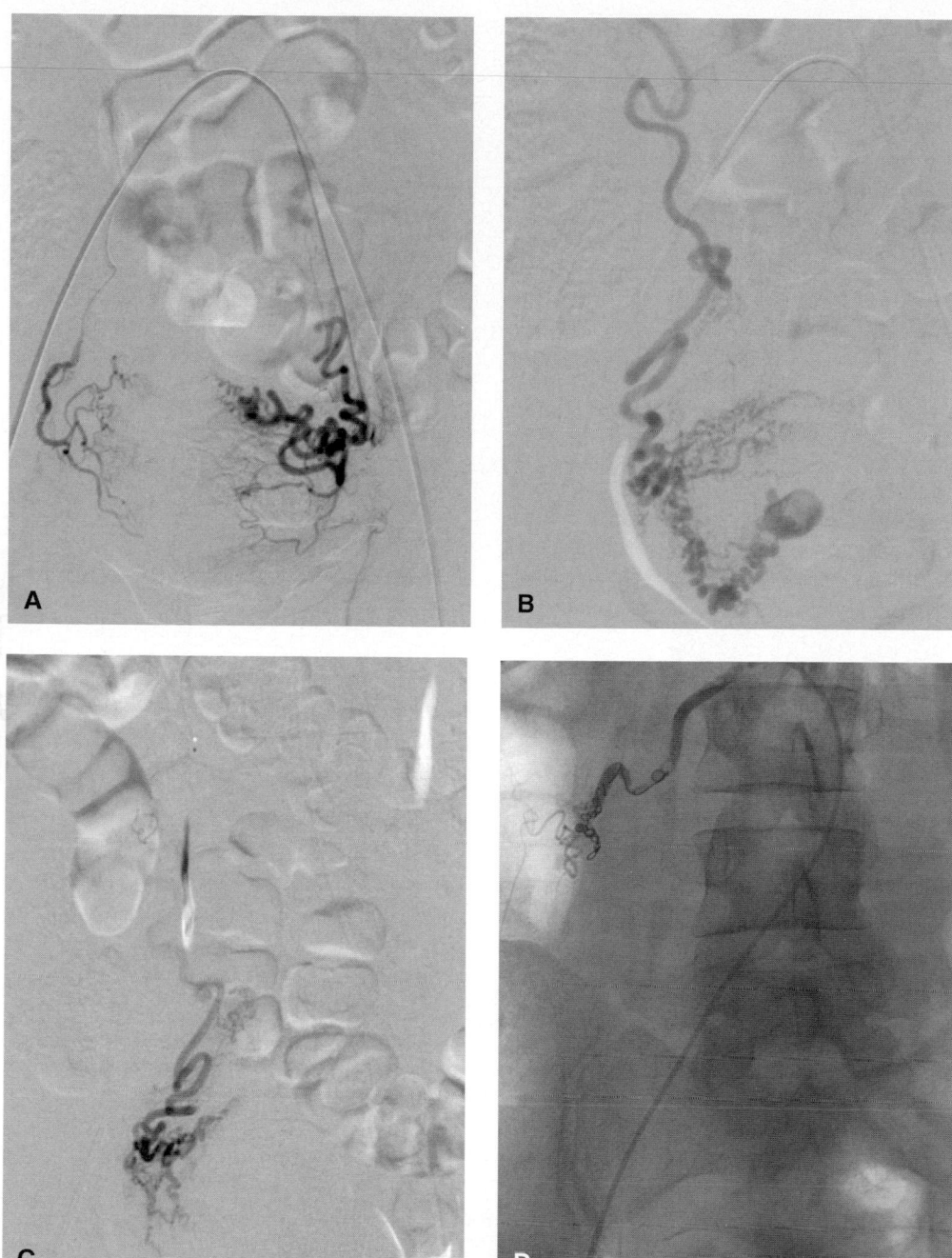

Figure 45–1 A 33-year-old woman at 3 weeks postpartum with intermittent vaginal bleeding. **A.** Selective uterine artery arteriograms using simultaneous injections through catheters placed via left and right common femoral approach fail to demonstrate any active extravasation. **B.** More thorough search for the source of bleeding resulted in a selective arteriogram of the right ovarian artery that demonstrated a pseudoaneurism. **C.** Gelfoam slurry embolization of the right ovarian artery through a coaxially placed microcatheter successfully amputated the flow to the distal branches that were supplying the pseudoaneurism. **D.** Shortly after the procedure, the hemorrhage continued and patient was brought back to the interventional radiology suite for microcoil embolization. Coils were deposited into the right ovarian artery, effectively arresting antegrade flow.

vasospasm was encountered with little antegrade flow in the internal iliac arteries. Gelfoam refluxed, and eventual embolization with isobutyl-2-cyanoacrylate glue had to be performed to control the hemorrhage (20). However, the glue should not be the embolic agent of choice for PPH. Other angiographic techniques aimed at controlling PPH have been reported. Selective catheterization and direct infusion of vasopressin into the bleeding vessel have controlled the bleeding (21), but no prospective series were ever performed to evaluate the efficacy of vasopressin infusion to control PPH.

DELAYED POSTPARTUM HEMORRHAGE

The technical approaches to angiography and embolization for delayed or late PPH are the same as those for early PPH. Secondary PPH is caused predominantly by genital tract lacerations and retained placental fragments with or without endometritis. If the bleeding persists after curettage or primary repair of lacerations, embolization is an alternative to surgical ligation or hysterectomy (22,23). A unilateral femoral approach is used for initial angiography, and a cobra-shaped catheter is used to select the contralateral

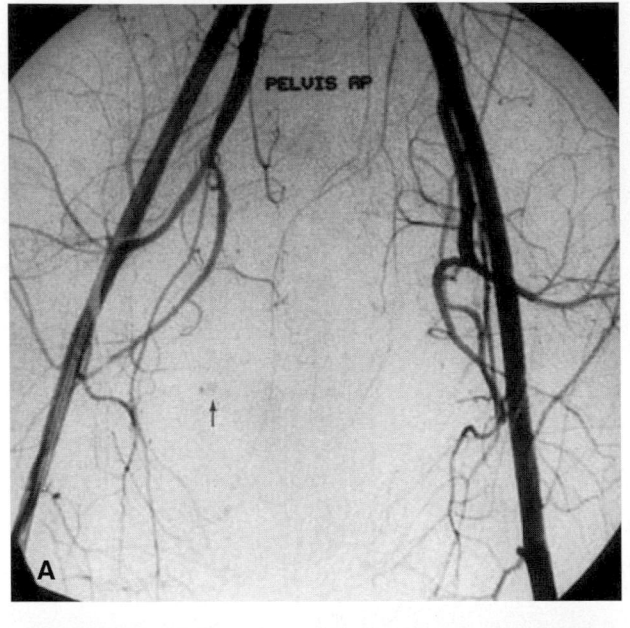

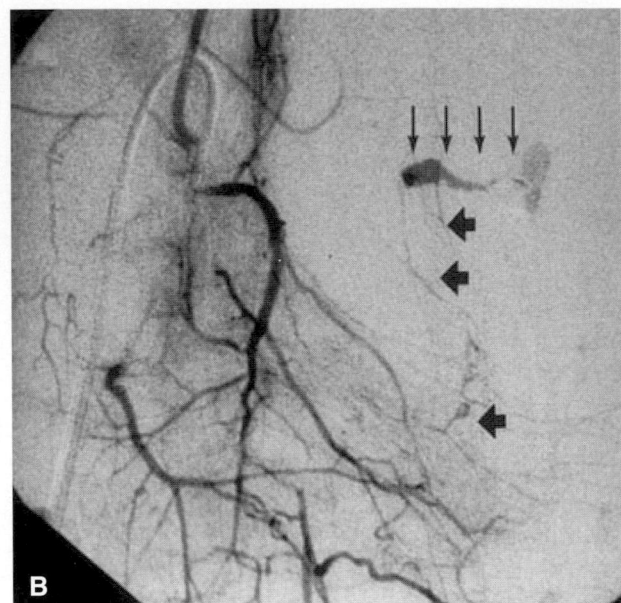

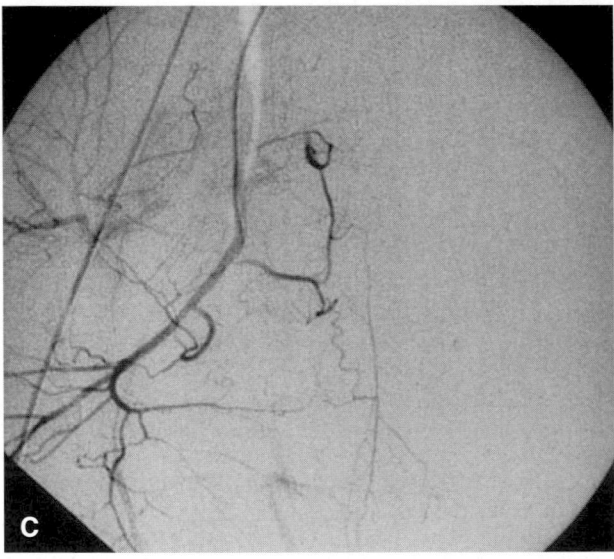

Figure 45–2 A. Nonselective pelvic arteriography indefinitely demonstrated the pseudoaneurism (*short arrow*) at the right side of the pelvis. **B.** Selective right internal iliac artery injection showed the pseudoaneurism (*long arrows*) that was supplied by the small collateral branches (*large arrows*). **C.** Postembolization angiogram clearly displayed total closure of the small collateral feeders as well as the pseudoaneurism. (Reprinted with permission from Cantasdemir et al. Arch Gynecol Obstet 2002; 267:104–106.)

internal iliac and uterine arteries (22,23). The ipsilateral internal iliac and uterine arteries are also selectively catheterized. Most authors primarily have used gelfoam pledgets for embolization. Pelage et al. selectively catheterized and embolized the uterine arteries in most cases, while Feinberg et al. reported gelfoam and coil embolization of internal iliac arteries (23,24).

EMBOLIZATION FOR ECTOPIC PREGNANCY AND GESTATIONAL TROPHOBLASTIC DISEASE

Initial diagnosis of ectopic pregnancy by clinical suspicion, ultrasound visualization, and elevated β-hCG levels usually results in medical or surgical treatment early enough that major hemorrhagic complications are avoided. Occasionally,

however, hemorrhage does occur and necessitates additional treatment.

Many groups have reported successful arterial embolization to control the bleeding related to abdominal ectopic pregnancies (3,4,25–27). Likewise, preoperative embolization of cervical ectopic pregnancies has successfully reduced operative blood loss (28,29).

The most common strategy is to embolize the ectopic pregnancy before surgical removal. Using standard angiographic techniques, vascular supply to the pregnancy is determined and selective gelfoam embolization is performed. Badawy et al. reviewed 11 reports totaling 21 cases of arterial embolization for cervical and abdominal pregnancies between 1988 and 1997 and reported a 100% success rate in controlling the bleeding (11). Occasionally, hemorrhage ensues after operative removal of the abdominal pregnancy; in these cases, selective embolization to the placental remnant is performed (30). Complications associated with embolization of abdominal pregnancies are rare but have included bowel infarct, abscess formation, and bowel perforation (3,4).

Gestational trophoblastic disease also entails considerable bleeding risk because of the extensive arteriovenous network created by the invasive trophoblastic tissue. Successful embolization of severe hemorrhage associated with invasive trophoblastic tissue, followed by the more conventional chemotherapeutic treatment, has been reported to result in (31) complete remission of the trophoblast.

EMBOLIZATION FOR PLACENTATION ABNORMALITIES: ACCRETA, INCRETA, PERCRETA

Placentation abnormalities present a formidable clinical challenge for the obstetrician. Abnormal placentation usually goes undiagnosed until after delivery, when physicians cannot remove the placenta and hemorrhage ensues. Abnormal placentation is the most common cause of hysterectomy in obstetric care (32). Placenta percreta, in which the ingrowth extends through the uterine myometrium and beyond the serosal surface of the uterus, is the most problematic because uterine rupture and hemorrhage can occur. In a comprehensive review of placenta previa and placenta accreta, Miller et al. quantified the amount of blood loss during cesarean hysterectomy associated with placenta accreta in a group of 62 patients. Estimated blood loss exceeded 2,000 mL in 41 patients; 5,000 mL in nine patients; 10,000 mL in four patients; and 20,000 mL in two patients (33).

Several management algorithms have been proposed. Cesarean delivery is performed most often in this clinical setting. Angiographic options include catheterization either before or after delivery. Predelivery catheterization involves arterial access of the axillary artery (4). In this approach, operative delivery and sterile preparation of the lower abdomen and pelvis make femoral access difficult. The fetus is shielded with lead during catheter positioning. After delivery, catheters are already in place, in case bleeding occurs and embolization becomes necessary. If arterial access was not obtained preoperatively and hemorrhage occurs after delivery, femoral access can be performed before embolization. Mitty et al. described the value of prophylactic angiography in the prepartum period in high-risk patients with placenta accreta and abdominal pregnancy. The authors subsequently embolized and controlled the bleeding in those patients who could not be managed by conservative means (4). Implications for fertility are also favorable. Embolization in the postpartum period in the case of placenta percreta with bladder invasion allowed removal of the placenta 12 days later, with resumption of periods and normal bladder function (34).

Two groups have suggested a modification of the preoperative catheterization approach. Dubois et al. (35) and

Weeks et al. (36) temporarily occluded the anterior division of the internal iliac arteries with occlusion balloons. Weeks and colleagues used femoral arterial access while Dubois et al. used axillary arterial access. This latter approach is advocated when the catheters are placed before the delivery. The technique involves preoperative placement of balloon occlusion catheters in the internal iliac arteries. The balloons are left deflated throughout the delivery, and the catheters and sheaths are flushed with a heparinized saline infusion (36). The balloons are inflated immediately after operative delivery, while the patient is still in the operating room (Figure 45–3). This allows adequate time to better control the hemorrhage surgically. Alternatively, embolization can be performed. Dubois et al. embolized the anterior division of the internal iliac arteries before eventual hysterectomy by injecting gelfoam particles through the end-hole of the occlusion catheter. Alternatively, a 3 French microcatheter can be inserted through the end-hole of the occlusion balloon catheter to select the uterine arteries and embolize them with sterile gelfoam (37). Most authors report acceptable blood losses and good clinical outcomes. However, some authors question the value of prophylactic balloon placement before delivery. Using a similar balloon occlusion technique, they failed to demonstrate any benefit in prevention of postpartum hemorrhage in a small, prospective cohort study (38). Therefore, the benefit of this technique has yet to be determined.

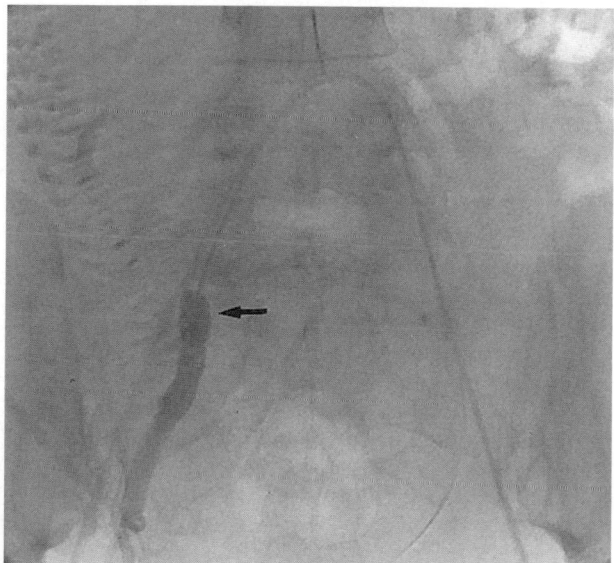

Figure 45–3 A 27-year-old woman at 34 weeks gestation with placenta parcreta who had pelvic angiography before cesarean section delivery and anticipated hysterectomy. Balloon occlusion of the anterior division of the right internal iliac artery via a left common femoral artery approach was performed. Injection of contrast material with the balloon inflated (*arrow*) demonstrates stagnant flow. Balloon was inflated after delivery to successfully reduce the blood loss during hysterectomy. (Reprinted with permission from Weeks SM, Stroud TH, Sandhu J, et al. Temporary balloon occlusion of the internal iliac arteries for control of hemorrhage during cesarean hysterectomy in a patient with placenta previa and placenta increta. J Vasc Interv Radiol 2000;11:622–624.)

EMBOLIZATION FOR ARTERIOVENOUS MALFORMATIONS

AVMs are rarely seen in the postpartum period and are a rare cause of postpartum hemorrhage. They can be congenital or acquired (11). Congenital AVMs can cause uterine bleeding but fall outside the scope of obstetric hemorrhage because they are not a result of the peripartum process. Acquired AVMs usually are caused by instrumentation after the delivery, such as uterine curettage for placental remnants or after cesarean delivery. Acquired AVMs can also occur as a complication of invading gestational trophoblastic disease (11,12). Usually, diagnosis is made by arteriography after exclusion of other more common causes of uterine bleeding. Occasionally, hysteroscopic visualization

of a pulsatile mass in the uterine cavity can also establish the diagnosis. Regardless of etiology, the technical approach to treatment is similar. The AVM can be embolized with particulate embolic material, such as gelfoam or PVA, until arterial supply to the malformation is occluded (Figure 45–4). Several groups described successful treatment of AVMs with selective arterial embolization (39,40). Selective catheterization of the supplying artery is desirable, but when selective embolization is not possible, the internal iliac artery and its branches can be embolized (39). In a rather comprehensive review of arterial embolization for AVMs, Badawy et al. reported 94% success rates in controlling the bleeding (11). Preservation of fertility is one of the main advantages that embolization for AVMs has over more definitive surgical options such as hysterectomy.

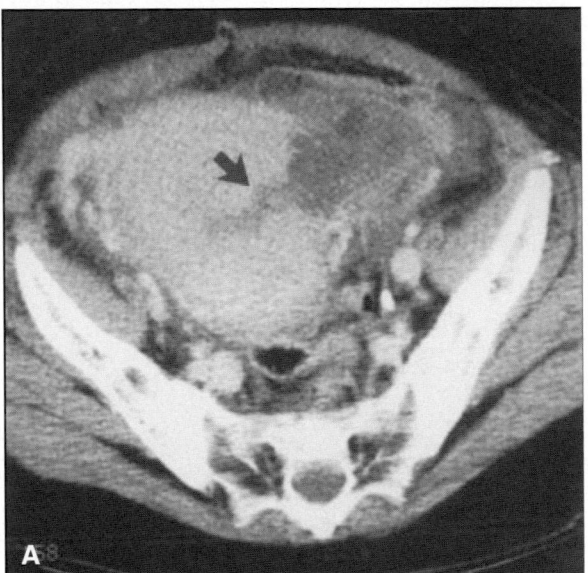

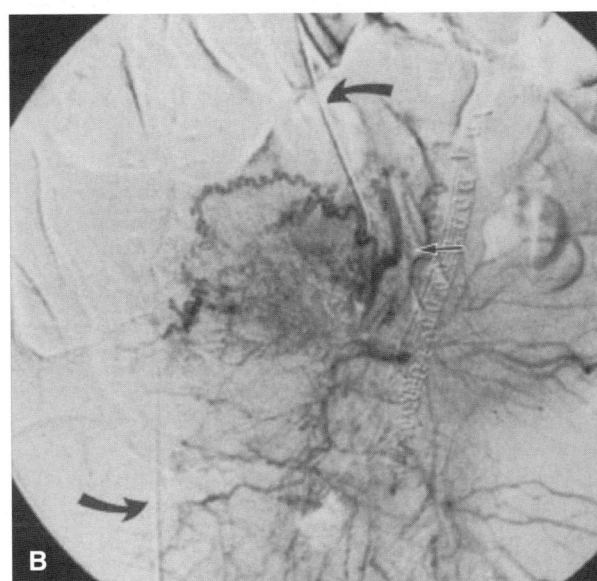

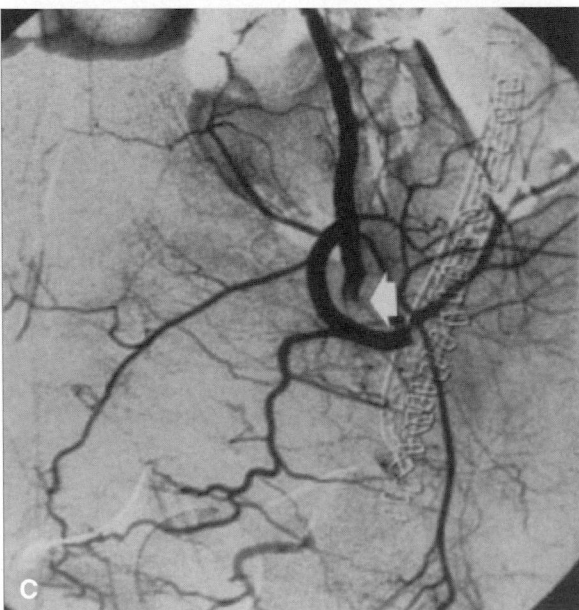

Figure 45–4 A 43-year-old woman 2 days after cesarean delivery who, because of religious beliefs, refused blood transfusion. **A.** CT scan shows uterine dehiscence (*arrow*) and free fluid in the pelvis. **B.** Late arterial phase pelvic angiogram shows early draining vein (*straight arrow*), consistent with abnormal arteriovenous malformation. Catheter (*curved arrow*) is coming from right femoral access. **C.** Left internal iliac angiogram shows good result after gelfoam embolization. Note truncated internal iliac artery (*arrow*). Patient's hematocrit level stabilized. (Reprinted with permission from Velling et al., AJR Am J Roentgenol, 2000, 175:1273–1278 © American Roentgen Ray Society.)

EFFECTS OF EMBOLIZATION ON FERTILITY

Embolization for PPH, regardless of etiology, deprives the uterus of its blood supply to some degree. Ischemic injury to the uterus after embolization is extremely rare. However, the future fertility of patients who undergo embolization is of interest to obstetricians and interventional radiologists alike. Consequently, several groups have evaluated fertility after embolization for PPH. Overall, the implications are favorable. Normal resumption of menses (7,10,26,41) as well as normal pregnancies have been reported by numerous authors (7,22,26,42,43).

Although no large prospective studies have been done, several case series have been reported. Boulleret et al. conducted a long-term follow-up in 23 patients: 91% resumed regular menstrual cycles, and 8.7% had dysmenorrhea. New pregnancy occurred in 13% (44). Stancato-Pasik et al. found that 11 of the 12 women in their group (92%) resumed normal menses within 2–5 months after embolization. There were no complications related to embolotherapy. The follow-up period was 1–6 years. All three patients who wished to conceive gave birth to full-term, healthy newborns (26). Similar results were reported by Ornan et al. All of their patients who desired further pregnancies were able to conceive after embolization for PPH (45).

However, some groups encountered recurrent PPH in patients who were embolized for PPH during previous deliveries (7,46). It is unclear whether these were isolated incidents or whether the rates of PPH in these groups are actually increased. To this date, no prospective trials have been published to determine the incidence of PPH in those women who had embolizations for PPH in previous deliveries.

The effects of embolization on fetal development in subsequent pregnancies have been reported only sporadically. Most authors report normal pregnancies after embolization for PPH, followed by normal deliveries of healthy children. However, some difficult pregnancies with unfavorable outcomes have been noted. In one such case, embolization of the bilateral internal iliac arteries with coils and gelfoam was prompted by an AVM. The patient later experienced a complicated twin pregnancy with in utero death of one of the twins at 18 weeks gestation and preeclampsia that occurred at 26 weeks (47). It is not clear whether embolization was a contributable cause of complicated pregnancy in this case.

COMPLICATIONS OF EMBOLIZATION FOR POSTPARTUM HEMORRHAGE

Complications of angiography and embolization for PPH are few. Pais et al., in 1980, addressed initial concerns about uterine ischemia with embolic particles early in the evolution of this procedure (14). The authors looked at the hysterectomy specimen of a patient who had bilateral embolization of the internal iliac arteries, and their histological study did not reveal any characteristics of ischemia. Much later, ischemic uterine necrosis was reported when small (150–250 μm) polyvinyl alcohol particles (PVA) were used along with gelatin sponge pledgets (48). Small PVA particles cause very distal embolization and can place the uterus at risk.

Technical complications are rare during embolization for PPH. Usually, the patients are young and healthy and free of vascular disease. These circumstances simplify catheterization and angiography from a technical standpoint. Additionally, in the peripartum period, the uterus and related arterial supply have a high flow state; therefore, undesired reflux of embolic particles is not usually a concern.

Eventually, the body of literature on embolization for PPH expanded, and the procedure was established as safe. Badawy et al. reviewed 22 publications totaling 138 cases of postpartum hemorrhage treated by arterial embolization between 1979 and 1999 and reported a clinical success rate of 94.9% for stopping the bleeding (11). Only seven cases in their review required hysterectomy because of failed embolization. They also summarized the complications, which included external iliac perforation (3), transient fever (10,49), transient buttock ischemia (3), paravaginal abscess, transient foot ischemia, groin hematoma, pelvic abscess, abdominal wall abscess, bladder gangrene, and several cases of repeat embolization. Transient buttock and lower extremity parasthesia were also reported in more recent studies and were usually self-limited (7). Rarely, embolization does fail, and hysterectomy is needed to stop the bleeding (9).

MANAGEMENT OF HEMORRHAGE IN OTHER ORGAN SYSTEMS DURING PREGNANCY

Occasionally, the hemodynamic and hormonal changes associated with pregnancy predispose other organs to bleeding. For example, cavernous hemangioma of the liver with spontaneous hemorrhage has been reported and successfully treated with selective arterial embolization (50). Similarly, pregnancy-related adrenal hemorrhage (51) and liver rupture (52) have also been effectively treated with embolization. In most cases, selective angiography is required. Embolization with gelfoam particles stops the bleeding and causes only a temporary occlusion of the bleeding vessels.

SUMMARY

Selective arterial embolization for intractable PPH has proven safe and effective. The obstetric and gynecologic literature now urges practitioners to use the services of interventional radiologists to perform embolization in the event that conservative treatment measures fail. In fact, the literature advocates embolization over surgical intervention (53,54).

Embolization for PPH has many advantages over surgical options. Embolization avoids morbidity in patients who usually are poor surgical candidates because of anemia and coagulopathies. Hysterectomy precludes future fertility while surgical ligation of the internal iliac vessels carries high failure rates and precludes angiographic access in the case that embolization becomes necessary. On the other hand, embolization does not preclude surgical ligation or hysterectomy should surgical approaches become necessary. In the hands of a trained interventional radiologist, embolization is technically achievable without major difficulties and it quickly restores hemostasis. Modern strategies allow angiographic techniques to serve as an adjunct in management of ectopic pregnancies and placentation abnormalities. Interventional radiologists and obstetricians should become familiar with the angiographic options in treatment of PPH.

REFERENCES

1. Kaunitz AM, Hughes JM, Grimes DA, et al. Causes of maternal mortality in the United States. Obstet Gynecol 1985;65:605–612.
2. Combs CA, Murphy EL, Laros RK Jr. Factors associated with postpartum hemorrhage with vaginal birth. Obstet Gynecol 1991; 77:69–76.
3. Greenwood LH, Glickman MG, Schwartz PE, et al. Obstetric and nonmalignant gynecologic bleeding: treatment with angiographic embolization. Radiology 1987;164:155–159.
4. Mitty HA, Sterling KM, Alvarez M, et al. Obstetric hemorrhage: prophylactic and emergency arterial catheterization and embolotherapy. Radiology 1993;188:183–187.
5. Gilbert WM, Moore TR, Resnik R, et al. Angiographic embolization in the management of hemorrhagic complications of pregnancy. Am J Obstet Gynecol 1992;166:493–497.
6. Deux JF, Bazot M, Le Blanche AF, et al. Is selective embolization of uterine arteries a safe alternative to hysterectomy in patients with postpartum hemorrhage? AJR Am J Roentgenol 2001;177: 145–149.
7. Chung JW, Jeong HJ, Joh JH, et al. Percutaneous transcatheter angiographic embolization in the management of obstetric hemorrhage. J Reprod Med 2003;48:268–276.
8. Dildy GA III. Postpartum hemorrhage: new management options. Clin Obstet Gynecol 2002;45:330–344.
9. Pelage JP, Le Dref O, Mateo J, et al. Life-threatening primary postpartum hemorrhage: treatment with emergency selective arterial embolization. Radiology 1998;208:359–362.
10. Yamashita Y, Takahashi M, Ito M, et al. Transcatheter arterial embolization in the management of postpartum hemorrhage due to genital tract injury. Obstet Gynecol 1991;77:160–163.
11. Badawy SZ, Etman A, Singh M, et al. Uterine artery embolization: the role in obstetrics and gynecology. Clin Imaging 2001;25: 288–295.
12. Kelly SM, Belli AM, Campbell S. Arteriovenous malformation of the uterus associated with secondary postpartum hemorrhage. Ultrasound Obstet Gynecol 2003;21:602–605.
13. Clark SL, Phelan JP, Yeh SY, et al. Hypogastric artery ligation for obstetric hemorrhage. Obstet Gynecol 1985;66:353–356.
14. Pais SO, Glickman M, Schwartz P, et al. Embolization of pelvic arteries for control of postpartum hemorrhage. Obstet Gynecol 1980;55:754–758.
15. Brown BJ, Heaston DK, Poulson AM, et al. Uncontrollable postpartum bleeding: a new approach to hemostasis through angiographic arterial embolization. Obstet Gynecol 1979;54: 361–365.
16. Yamashita Y, Harada M, Yamamoto H, et al. Transcatheter arterial embolization of obstetric and gynaecological bleeding: efficacy and clinical outcome. Br J Radiol 1994;67:530–534.
17. Oei PL, Chua S, Tan L, et al. Arterial embolization for bleeding following hysterectomy for intractable postpartum hemorrhage. Int J Gynaecol Obstet 1998;62:83–86.
18. Minck RN, Palestrant A, Cherny WB. Successful management of postpartum vaginal hemorrhage by angiographic embolization. Ariz Med 1984;41:537–538.
19. Rosenthal DM, Colapinto R. Angiographic arterial embolization in the management of postoperative vaginal hemorrhage. Am J Obstet Gynecol 1985;151:227–231.
20. Walker WJ. Case report: successful internal iliac artery embolisation with glue in a case of massive obstetric haemorrhage. Clin Radiol 1996;51:442–444.
21. Magrina JF, Moffat RE, Masterson BJ, et al. Selective arterial infusion of Pitressin for the control of puerperal hemorrhage after hypogastric artery ligation. Obstet Gynecol 1981;58:646–648.
22. Pelage JP, Le Dref O, Jacob D, et al. Selective arterial embolization of the uterine arteries in the management of intractable postpartum hemorrhage. Acta Obstet Gynecol Scand 1999;78:698–703.
23. Pelage JP, Soyer P, Repiquet D, et al. Secondary postpartum hemorrhage: treatment with selective arterial embolization. Radiology 1999;212:385–389.
24. Feinberg BB, Resnik E, Hurt WG, et al. Angiographic embolization in the management of late postpartum hemorrhage. A case report. J Reprod Med 1987;32:929–931.
25. Kerr A, Trambert J, Mikhail M, et al. Preoperative transcatheter embolization of abdominal pregnancy: report of three cases. J Vasc Interv Radiol 1993;4:733–735.
26. Stancato-Pasik A, Mitty HA, Richard HM III, et al. Obstetric embolotherapy: effect on menses and pregnancy. Radiology 1997; 204:791–793.
27. Cardosi RJ, Nackley AC, Londono J, et al. Embolization for advanced abdominal pregnancy with a retained placenta. A case report. J Reprod Med 2002;47:861–863.
28. Lobel SM, Meyerovitz MF, Benson CC, et al. Preoperative angiographic uterine artery embolization in the management of cervical pregnancy. Obstet Gynecol 1990;76:938–941.
29. Suzumori N, Katano K, Sato T, et al. Conservative treatment by angiographic artery embolization of an 11-week cervical pregnancy after a period of heavy bleeding. Fertil Steril 2003;80:617–619.
30. Martin JN Jr, Ridgway LE III, Connors JJ, et al. Angiographic arterial embolization and computed tomography-directed drainage for the management of hemorrhage and infection with abdominal pregnancy. Obstet Gynecol 1990;76:941–945.
31. Pearl ML, Braga CA. Percutaneous transcatheter embolization for control of life-threatening pelvic hemorrhage from gestational trophoblastic disease. Obstet Gynecol 1992;80:571–574.
32. Zorlu CG, Turan C, Isik AZ, et al. Emergency hysterectomy in modern obstetric practice. Changing clinical perspective in time. Acta Obstet Gynecol Scand 1998;77:186–190.
33. Miller DA, Chollet JA, Goodwin TM. Clinical risk factors for placenta previa-placenta accreta. Am J Obstet Gynecol 1997;177: 210–214.
34. Descargues G, Clavier E, Lemercier E, et al. Placenta percreta with bladder invasion managed by arterial embolization and manual removal after cesarean. Obstet Gynecol 2000;96:840.
35. Dubois J, Garel L, Grignon A, et al. Placenta percreta: balloon occlusion and embolization of the internal iliac arteries to reduce intraoperative blood losses. Am J Obstet Gynecol 1997;176: 723–726.
36. Weeks SM, Stroud TH, Sandhu J, et al. Temporary balloon occlusion of the internal iliac arteries for control of hemorrhage during cesarean hysterectomy in a patient with placenta previa and placenta increta. J Vasc Interv Radiol 2000;11:622–624.
37. Hansch E, Chitkara U, McAlpine J, et al. Pelvic arterial embolization for control of obstetric hemorrhage: a five-year experience. Am J Obstet Gynecol 1999;180:1454–1460.
38. Levine AB, Kuhlman K, Bonn J. Placenta accreta: comparison of cases managed with and without pelvic artery balloon catheters. J Matern Fetal Med 1999;8:173–176.
39. Lim AK, Agarwal R, Seckl MJ, et al. Embolization of bleeding residual uterine vascular malformations in patients with treated gestational trophoblastic tumors. Radiology 2002;222: 640–644.
40. Garner EI, Meyerovitz M, Goldstein DP, et al. Successful term pregnancy after selective arterial embolization of symptomatic arteriovenous malformation in the setting of gestational trophoblastic tumor. Gynecol Oncol 2003;88:69–72.

41. Descargues G, Mauger Tinlot F, et al. Menses, fertility, and pregnancy after arterial embolization for the control of postpartum haemorrhage. Hum Reprod 2004;19:339–343.

42. Wang H, Garmel S. Successful term pregnancy after bilateral uterine artery embolization for postpartum hemorrhage. Obstet Gynecol 2003;102:603–604.

43. Casele HL, Laifer SA. Successful pregnancy after bilateral hypogastric artery ligation. A case report. J Reprod Med 1997;42:306–308.

44. Boulleret C, Chahid T, Gallot D, et al. Hypogastric arterial selective and superselective embolization for severe postpartum hemorrhage: a retrospective review of 36 cases. Cardiovasc Intervent Radiol 2004;27:344–348.

45. Ornan D, White R, Pollak J, et al. Pelvic embolization for intractable postpartum hemorrhage: long-term follow-up and implications for fertility. Obstet Gynecol 2003;102:904–910.

46. Salomon LJ, deTayrac R, Castaigne-Meary V, et al. Fertility and pregnancy outcome following pelvic arterial embolization for severe post-partum haemorrhage. A cohort study. Hum Reprod 2003;18:849–852.

47. Abbas FM, Currie JL, Mitchell S, et al. Selective vascular embolization in benign gynecologic conditions. J Reprod Med 1994;39:492–496.

48. Cottier JP, Fignon A, Tranquart F, et al. Uterine necrosis after arterial embolization for postpartum hemorrhage. Obstet Gynecol 2002;100:1074–1077.

49. Chin HG, Scott DR, Resnik R, et al. Angiographic embolization of intractable puerperal hematomas. Am J Obstet Gynecol 1989; 160:434–438.

50. Graham E, Cohen AW, Soulen M, et al. Symptomatic liver hemangioma with intra-tumor hemorrhage treated by angiography and embolization during pregnancy. Obstet Gynecol 1993; 81:813–816.

51. Christie J, Batool I, Moss J, et al. Adrenal artery rupture in pregnancy. BJOG 2004;111:185–187.

52. Herbert WN, Brenner WE. Improving survival with liver rupture complicating pregnancy. Am J Obstet Gynecol 1982;142:530–534.

53. Tourne G, Collet F, Seffert P, et al. Place of embolization of the uterine arteries in the management of post-partum haemorrhage: a study of 12 cases. Eur J Obstet Gynecol Reprod Biol 2003;110:29–34.

54. Merland JJ, Houdart E, Herbreteau D, et al. Place of emergency arterial embolisation in obstetric haemorrhage about 16 personal cases. Eur J Obstet Gynecol Reprod Biol 1996;65:141–143.

55. Heffner LJ, Mennuti MT, Rudoff JC, et al. Primary management of postpartum vulvovaginal hematomas by angiographic embolization. Am J Perinatol 1985;2:204–207.

56. Shweni PM, Bishop BB, Hansen JN, et al. Severe secondary postpartum haemorrhage after caesarean section. S Afr Med J 1987; 72:617–619.

57. Bakri YN, Linjawi T. Angiographic embolization for control of pelvic genital tract hemorrhage. Report of 14 cases. Acta Obstet Gynecol Scand 1992;71:17–21.

58. Joseph JF, Mernoff D, Donovan J, et al. Percutaneous angiographic arterial embolization for gynecologic and obstetric pelvic hemorrhage. A report of three cases. J Reprod Med 1994; 39:915–920.

59. Hsu YR, Wan YL. Successful management of intractable puerperal hematoma and severe postpartum hemorrhage with DIC through transcatheter arterial embolization—two cases. Acta Obstet Gynecol Scand 1998;77:129–131.

Pelvic Venous Incompetence

46

Pelvic Congestion Syndrome

Anthony C. Venbrux

ETIOLOGY

Pelvic pain in women has numerous etiologies. Pain may result from pathologic conditions related to the uterus, fallopian tubes, or ovaries, and the vascular, urinary tract, gastrointestinal, musculoskeletal, and nervous systems (1). Disease states affecting these organ systems may be classified broadly as congenital or acquired. Vascular etiologies causing pelvic pain in women may be arterial or venous (including arteriovenous malformations and ovarian and pelvic varices). This chapter focuses on nonsurgical treatment of venous abnormalities.

DEMOGRAPHICS

Estimates are that 150,000–200,000 women in the United States have varicose veins in the pelvis (2). The presence of pelvic venous incompetence in women is not always associated with pelvic pain nor is there an association with decreased fertility. In contrast, the analogous condition in males (scrotal varicocele) is associated with a decreased fertility rate.

DEFINITION OF TERMS

Although approximately 15% of all women have ovarian and internal iliac varices, only some of these women have the clinical picture of pelvic pain (2,3). The presence of ovarian and pelvic varices may be associated with a group of symptoms referred to as pelvic pain syndrome or pelvic congestion syndrome. Some authors contend that these terms carry unwanted psychiatric connotations and recommend that this condition be termed *pelvic venous incompetence*, or PVI, a term that is more anatomically accurate and less pejorative.

The term *ovarian varices* refers to varicosities visualized after contrast is injected into the ovarian veins. The term *pelvic varices* is defined as varicosities visualized when contrast is injected into the internal iliac veins. *Chronic pelvic pain* is defined as noncyclic pain that has a duration of more than 6 months (4).

Although venous catheterization with contrast injection, such as venography, confirms the presence of varices and allows treatment, including transcatheter embolotherapy, it is invasive. Before venous catheterization, noninvasive imaging is useful to screen for the presence or absence of pelvic venous disease.

Clinical Features of the Patient with Ovarian and Pelvic Varices

A woman with pelvic venous incompetence may complain of the following:

1. Pain that is described as a "heaviness," "pelvic fullness," "throbbing"
2. Pain that is worse in the upright position (standing or sitting) and is generally relieved when lying supine

3. Pain that is made worse with intercourse or increases in severity around the time of the menstrual cycle

Pain may also intensify during pregnancy or in the postpartum interval. Ovarian and internal iliac varices may be seen concurrently with varices in the buttocks, lower extremities, and vulvovaginal regions (5,6).

Clinical Approach to the Patient with Pelvic Pain

Recognizing the diverse etiologies of pelvic pain, a multidisciplinary approach to the patient presenting with suspected pelvic venous incompetence is important. A team consisting of several health care specialties is helpful: gynecology, gastroenterology, physical therapy, regional anesthesia, interventional radiology, neurology, orthopedic surgery, general surgery, psychiatry, and social services. A close working relationship with such a multidisciplinary team helps avoid unnecessary duplication of services, including physical examinations, laboratory data, imaging studies, invasive procedures, and the like.

IMAGING IN PELVIC VENOUS INCOMPETENCE (PELVIC CONGESTION SYNDROME)

Historically, several techniques and imaging modalities have been combined to evaluate women with suspected ovarian and pelvic varices (7–9). These include:

1. Ultrasonography performed either transabdominally or transvaginally (7)
2. Vulvar phlebography that includes the injection of contrast media into vulvar varices after surgical exposure of a vein or percutaneous venous puncture
3. Transuterine venography—an outpatient procedure in which the patient is placed in a lithotomy position and a specially designed cannula with a needle is placed through the cervix into the myometrium. Hyaluronidase and iodinated contrast material are then injected, and pelvic images are acquired over time, usually at 20–40 seconds after injection.
4. Selective ovarian and internal iliac venography (1)

Ideally, when ultrasound (US) is used, a patient with suspected ovarian and internal iliac varices should theoretically be evaluated in the supine and upright positions. This is not always technically possible, and patients with pelvic venous incompetence may have "normal" upright (or supine) pelvic ultrasound scans. The use of Doppler studies during pelvic sonography can confirm that tubular structures identified are dilated veins showing nonpulsatile flow. Audible Doppler signals may further characterize the venous flow within the larger tubular structures.

Other cross-sectional imaging modalities, including computed tomography (CT) or magnetic resonance imaging (MRI), are generally used to rule out other pathologic conditions such as tumors and uterine leiomyomata.

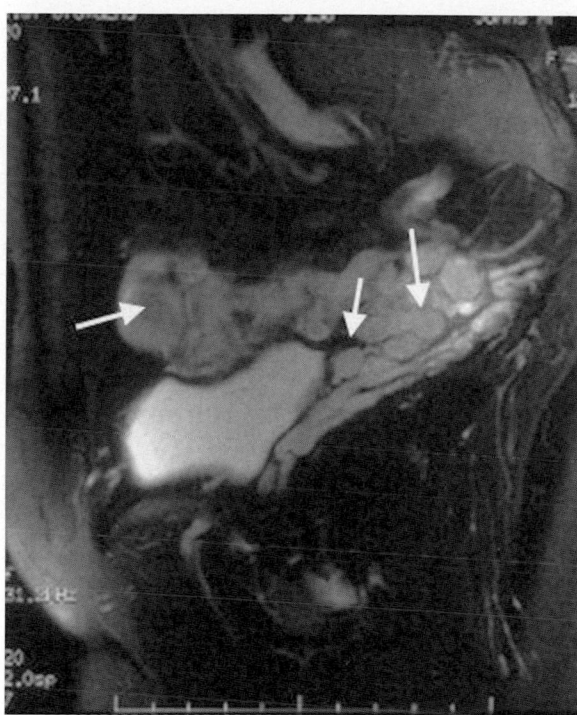

Figure 46–1 A T_2-weighted parasagittal MR image of the pelvis in a 46-year-old woman documents pelvic varices (*arrows*).

The technique of pelvic MRI with attention directed to venous anatomy (Figure 46–1) is the noninvasive imaging modality of choice. The MRI, when performed correctly, is extremely sensitive at picking up not only ovarian and pelvic varices but other potential pathologic conditions in the pelvis and abdomen as well. When a high clinical suspicion for ovarian and pelvic varices exists and imaging studies are equivocal or "negative," the next step may become diagnostic venography with "the intent to treat varices."

PITFALLS OF CROSS-SECTIONAL IMAGING AND LAPAROSCOPIC EVALUATION OF THE PELVIS

A woman presenting with chronic pelvic pain undergoes a physical examination and a cross-sectional imaging study. As mentioned earlier, the latter may include a transabdominal or endovaginal ultrasound (US), a computed tomography (CT) scan, or a magnetic resonance imaging (MRI) scan. Because such procedures are performed with the patient in the supine position, ovarian and pelvic varices may be overlooked. In the supine position, distention of venous structures is generally less the result of reduced hydrostatic pressure with resultant venous decompression. In men, the situation is clinically similar. The analogous male condition, a varicocele, may not be clinically detected in instances where the patient is examined in the supine position. Only in the upright position do the scrotal varicosities become clinically evident and generally palpable. The similar venous anatomy of ovarian and pelvic varices compared with the male varicocele lends support to the observation that ovarian and pelvic varices may be entirely overlooked using conventional supine cross-sectional imaging studies.

It is generally believed that direct endoscopic visualization of the structures in the female pelvis during laparoscopy should confirm the suspected diagnosis of pelvic venous incompetence. However, false-negative evaluations also occur because the patient is frequently placed in a Trendelenburg position—body inclined with head down—and during laparoscopic evaluation the peritoneal cavity is insufflated with carbon dioxide. The high intraperitoneal pressure created by the carbon dioxide may optimize endoscopic visualization of the uterus, fallopian tubes, ovaries, and other pelvic organs, but it may significantly compress the pliable, thin-walled venous structures (varices).

ANATOMY OF OVARIAN AND INTERNAL ILIAC VARICES

The normal venous drainage of the pelvis is through the common iliac, external iliac, internal iliac, and ovarian veins (10). The internal iliac veins have visceral and parietal branches. The visceral branches of the internal iliac vein consist of:

- Vesical plexus
- Vaginal plexus
- Uterine plexus
- Rectal branches
- Labial, clitoral, and inferior rectal veins

The internal iliac vein visceral branches intercommunicate. Parietal branches of the internal iliac vein include:

- Iliolumbar veins
- Superior and inferior gluteal veins
- Sacral venous plexus
- Obturator veins

The last named group may drain wholly or partly into the internal or external iliac venous system.

The left ovarian vein originates in the pelvis and courses cephalad to empty into the left renal vein. The right ovarian vein similarly originates in the right pelvis and courses cephalad. In most patients, it empties into the inferior vena cava just inferior to the right renal vein. Multiple trunks may be identified bilaterally. On the left, the gonadal vein and the inferior mesenteric vein may communicate, which has significant implications for embolization, particularly when sclerosing agents are used. This communication could potentially lead to complications if a liquid sclerosant—a liquid embolic agent, for example—is inadvertently refluxed into the inferior mesenteric circulation, such as inadvertent thrombosis of left colonic veins or the portal vein. Similar anatomic venous communications on the left are seen in men.

Ahlberg et al. investigated the left and right gonadal veins in 84 autopsy cases—30 men and 54 women. Valves were absent more often in men than in women, and both sexes lacked valves more frequently on the left than on the right side. Autopsy studies further revealed that women more often than men had incompetent valves and wider veins on both the right and left sides. The latter changes were attributed to past pregnancies (10).

Some authors report that pelvic venous incompetence is present only when the diameter of the ovarian vein is larger than 10 mm. This traditional view has been questioned recently. The diameter of the ovarian vein does not seem to correlate with the presence or absence of pelvic venous incompetence. Contrast venography has shown that internal iliac varices frequently communicate with ovarian varices. Because of this, the ovarian vein trunks per se may not be enlarged, despite the presence of pelvic venous incompetence and documentation on cross-sectional imaging studies, such as MRI.

To summarize, communications may exist between venous systems—from the left ovarian vein to the left colon or between the left or right ovarian veins and the internal iliac veins. Transpelvic collaterals, arising from the ovarian veins, the internal iliac veins, or a combination of these, also provide venous communication between the right and left sides of the pelvis. Thus, a defined ovarian vein diameter does not determine the presence or absence of pelvic venous incompetence.

In cases involving a strong clinical suspicion for the presence of ovarian and pelvic varices, the vessels can be injected even when a "competent" ovarian vein valve is found. This primary valve is often close to the outflow of the ovarian vein (for example, near the IVC on the right side and near the left renal vein on the left side). In other words, the valve or valves may need to be transgressed to achieve complete ovarian venography. Should varices then be found, embolization may proceed immediately.

General Considerations for Contrast Venography and Embolotherapy in Women with Pelvic Venous Incompetence

The technique of contrast venography is well-described (11–15). Optimal visualization is based on selective catheterization of the left and right ovarian and internal iliac veins using specially configured catheters followed by contrast injections. Balloon occlusion venography is used to confirm the presence of internal iliac varices. In contrast, the ovarian venograms often require the use of coaxial selective catheters but not the use of balloon occlusion catheters. Such contrast studies will confirm the presence of ovarian and pelvic varices and provide the means for minimally invasive image-guided therapy, such as transcatheter embolization. Sequential balloon occlusion venography of both internal iliac veins is performed because of the rapid venous outflow from the pelvis. With the occlusion balloon inflated, contrast may be injected retrograde, optimizing opacification of internal iliac varices.

When possible, the patient should undergo selective catheterization of the left and right ovarian and internal iliac veins in the supine and semi-erect positions. These positions attempt to mimic anatomic venous caliber changes described in the supine and upright positions, such as increased pooling of contrast in varices when the patient is upright. This is not always possible because of table configurations in the interventional suite, nor is it safe to do when the patient is sedated. The technique for transcatheter embolization is similar to that described for men. One limitation includes the inability to reduce gonadal radiation exposure adequately (shielding of the ovaries is not technically possible). Therefore, fluoroscopy and spot films must be kept to a minimum.

Specifics of the Embolization Technique

The ovarian veins may be selected from a femoral or a jugular approach; the femoral approach is preferable for some because of room configurations, including the position of the image intensifier relative to the position of the patient and the fluoroscopic monitors. A 7 French femoral venous sheath is placed and a 7 French guiding catheter with a Hopkins curve ("Hopkins hook") shape (Cordis Endovascular) is used to select the left renal vein. This guiding catheter, when advanced forward into the left renal vein, engages or selects the orifice of the left ovarian vein. Once seated, a 5 French coaxially directed hydrophilic-coated catheter is advanced over a guide wire approximately to the level of the sacroiliac joint and into the pelvic ovarian vein plexus. Hand injections of contrast are then performed, providing a rough estimate of the sclerosant volume required for embolization (Figure 46–2). A slurry of gelfoam (Pharmacia and Upjohn) and 5% sodium morrhuate (American Regent Laboratories) is injected based on the previously injected volume of contrast. One recommended approach is to reduce the volume of gelfoam/sodium morrhuate slurry by 1–2 cc during sclerotherapy (embolization) to reduce the risk of reflux of the mixture into the central venous system. After an interval of 5–10 minutes, the approximate time for venous thrombosis, the main left ovarian vein is coiled.

From the inferior vena cava, the right ovarian vein is then selectively catheterized with a more acutely angled hook-shaped guiding catheter (Figures 46–3, 46–4, and 46–5). This Simmons I or II guiding catheter may be made in the interventional suite by careful heat shaping of the left-sided Hopkins hook-guiding catheter. A hydrophilic-coated 5 French coaxillary directed catheter is also advanced through this guiding catheter. Should a 5 French Simmons I or II catheter be used to select the right ovarian vein, a microcatheter is generally used and advanced coaxially over a fine-caliber guide wire into the right pelvis. Right ovarian venography is performed, and the same gelfoam/sodium morrhuate mixture is then injected, followed by occlusion of the right ovarian vein trunk or trunks with embolic spring coils.

Having embolized left and right ovarian varices, attention is directed next to the internal iliac veins (Figures 46–6 and 46–7). To adequately treat the internal iliac varices, a

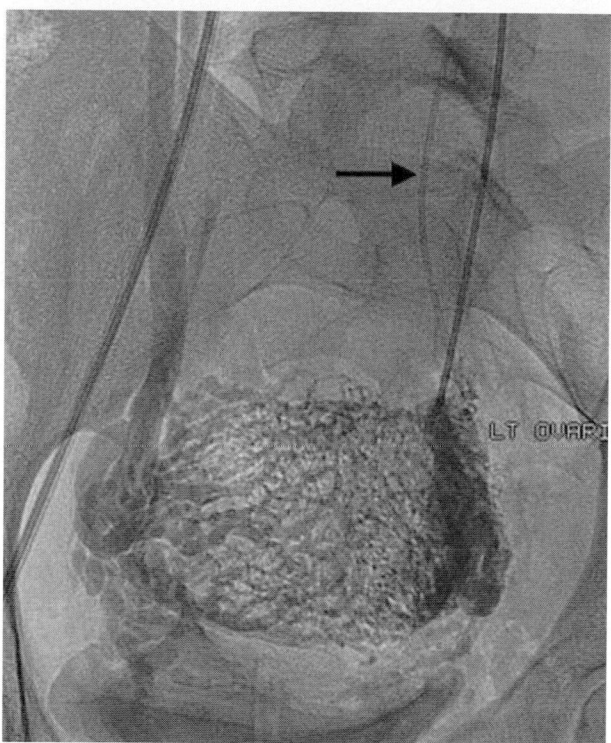

Figure 46–2 Anteroposterior digital spot film obtained during left ovarian venography (hand injection of iodinated contrast) in a 30-year-old woman with chronic pelvic pain and left ureteral colic. The patient had a double-J ureteral stent placed earlier for left flank pain (*arrow*). Contrast refluxes across the midline and opacifies the contralateral (*right*) ovarian varices and ovarian vein trunk.

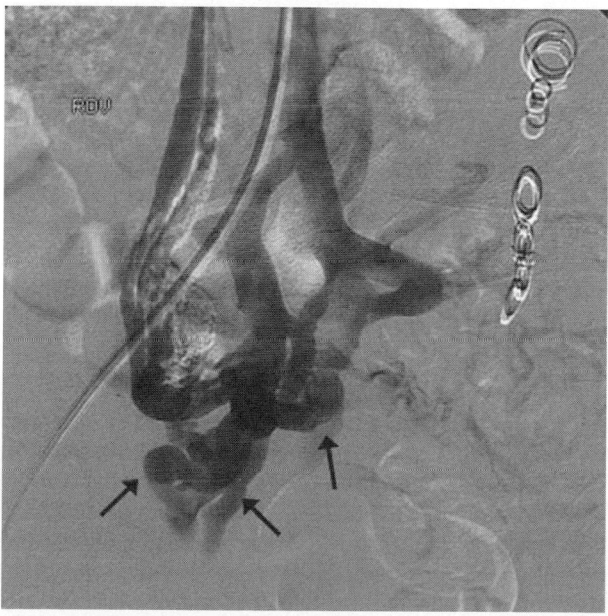

Figure 46–3 A 60-year-old woman with chronic pelvic pain and pelvic varices on MRI (*not shown*). Left anterior oblique digital spot film obtained during selective catheterization of the right ovarian vein. Note the reflux into the internal iliac vein with associated pelvic sidewall varices (*arrows*). The left ovarian vein had been embolized previously at an outside institution.

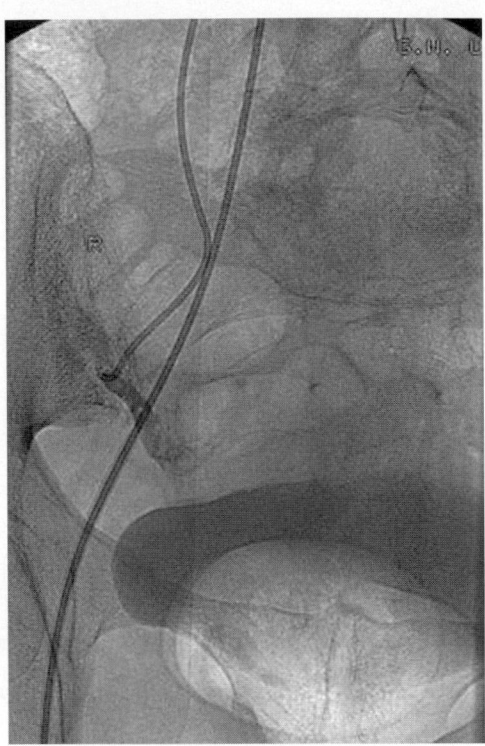

Figure 46–4 Left anterior oblique digital spot film obtained after embolization of the right ovarian vein with a slurry of gelfoam and sodium morrhuate (sclerosing agent). The same patient is shown in Figure 46–3.

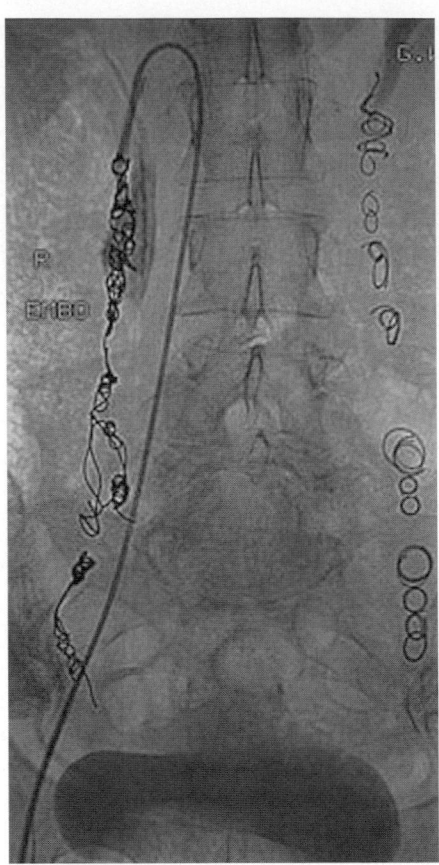

Figure 46–5 Anteroposterior (AP) digital subtraction spot film after sclerotherapy and coil embolization of the right ovarian varices. The same patient is shown in Figures 46–3 and 46–4.

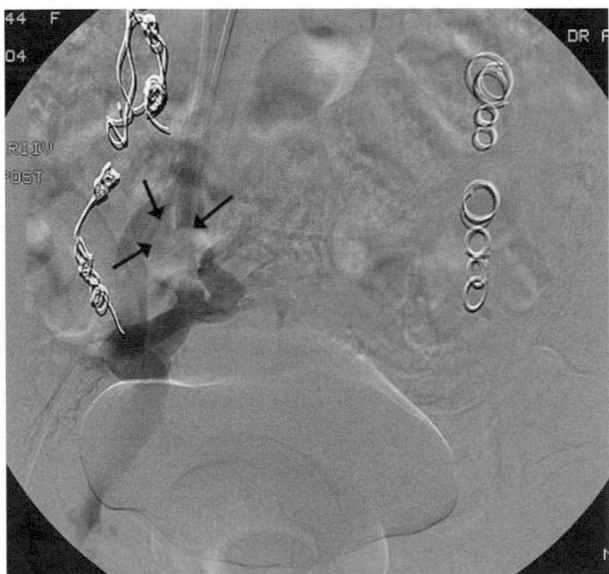

Figure 46–6 Balloon occlusion digital subtraction venogram in the AP projection documents residual internal iliac varices. This patient's right and left ovarian veins had been embolized previously. Note the inflated balloon (*arrows*). The same patient is shown in Figures 46–3, 46–4, and 46–5.

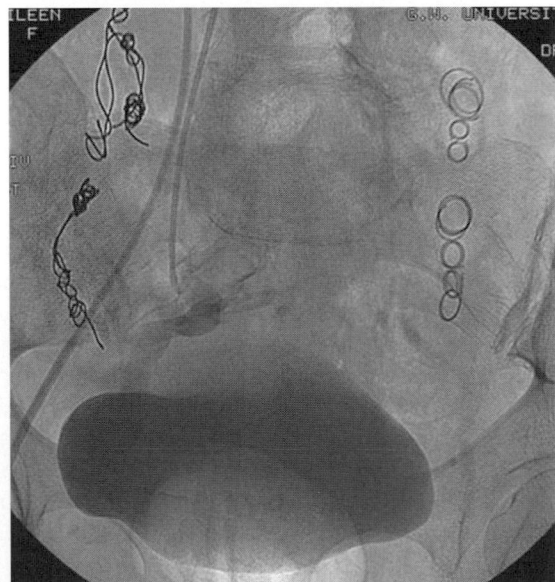

Figure 46–7 AP digital spot film after embolization of the right internal iliac varices. A gentle contrast injection confirms thrombosis. Care must be taken to avoid vigorous injections and avoid refluxing the gelfoam/sodium morrhuate slurry and thrombus into the iliac and central venous systems. The same patient is shown in Figures 46–3, 46–4, 46–5, and 46–6.

larger caliber occlusion balloon catheter (perhaps 11.5 mm in diameter) is used to achieve stasis during sclerotherapy. As in ovarian varices embolization, the slurry of gelfoam and 5% sodium morrhuate is useful. The volume of gelfoam/sodium morrhuate slurry used is again estimated based on the volume of injected contrast required to achieve opacification of the internal iliac venous plexus varices. Again, a slightly reduced volume of the thick embolic agent (slurry or "pudding") is injected. The balloon remains inflated for about 10 minutes to reduce the dilutional effects of returning pelvic venous blood flow. Coils tend to be used infrequently in the internal iliac vein tributaries because of the risk of potential embolization to the pulmonary circulation.

The ovarian and internal iliac varices embolization procedure may be staged or performed in a single session. In some cases, such as when the patient lives nearby, transcatheter embolotherapy of the right and left ovarian veins may be performed, the patient is given time to recover, and embolotherapy of the internal iliac varices follows in 3–6 weeks. This sequential approach is based on the patient's pain tolerance and practical time constraints.

POSTPROCEDURE CARE

In general, after sclerotherapy of the ovarian varices, patients experience considerable pain. For this reason, the patient is generally admitted for access to a patient-controlled anesthesia (PCA) intravenous narcotic pump. The patient is observed overnight, and on the following morning, the PCA pump is discontinued. The patient is then given a trial of several hours of oral narcotics (if needed), and if pain relief is adequate, he or she is discharged by midday.

When pelvic pain after embolization of ovarian varices is less severe, anti-inflammatory drugs administered orally or intravenously may be used. In contrast to the intense pain of sclerotherapy of ovarian varices, sclerotherapy of internal iliac varices is associated with far less pain. Thus, if staged, this second procedure may be performed on an outpatient basis. After completion of both embolization procedures, the patient is contacted and may later be seen in clinic.

Patients are discharged with prescriptions for oral antibiotics, antiemetics, and analgesics. Use of oral narcotics is discouraged, and the patient is switched to oral nonsteroidal anti-inflammatory agents as quickly as possible, such as ibuprofen. Because the time interval for pain relief experienced after both embolization procedures varies, the author has noted a wide range of clinical improvement from several days to several months (unpublished data).

RESULTS IN THE LITERATURE

In 1984, Rundqvist et al. (16) described a surgical technique of treatment for pelvic varicosities by extraperitoneal resection of the left ovarian vein. A case report by Edwards et al. (15) in 1993 described successful treatment of a patient with PVI by bilateral ovarian vein embolization using transcatheter embolotherapy. A 40-year-old woman with a 2-year history of chronic pelvic pain, dyspareunia, and dysmenorrhea remained asymptomatic after embolotherapy at 6 month follow-up. After treatment, her menstrual cycle became regular and she no longer complained of dysmenorrhea. Follow-up venography 1 month after transcatheter embolotherapy demonstrated complete occlusion of both ovarian veins. Internal iliac venography showed no evidence of reflux into the ovarian venous plexus.

Capasso et al. (12) described a series of 19 patients treated with ovarian vein embolization for pelvic pain associated with ovarian varices. The treatments consisted of 13 unilateral embolizations, six bilateral embolizations, and five treated recurrences (30 procedures total). The embolizations were performed with enbucrilate, steel coils, or a combination of these. Complete relief of pain was achieved in 11 patients (57.9%), and partial relief was achieved in three patients (15.8%). Five patients (26.3%) had persistent pain. Dyspareunia was suggested as a poor prognostic factor, which occurred in all eight patients with partial or no pain relief compared with two of 11 patients experiencing complete relief of pain. Follow-up, consisting of clinical and Doppler duplex evaluation, averaged 15.4 months. Three of four patients "not using an accepted contraceptive method" became pregnant following treatment. At publication, two had given birth without complications. According to Capasso and colleagues, eight of 10 patients undergoing ovarian and pelvic varices embolization achieved a statistically significant decrease in pain as measured by a visual analog scale (VAS) at follow-up of 3.0–31.5 weeks (12).

Venbrux et al. (11) published an initial study of 56 patients (with mean age of 32.3 years) treated for chronic pelvic pain using the transcatheter embolotherapy techniques described in this chapter. The authors found percutaneous transcatheter embolotherapy of ovarian and pelvic varices to be technically successful in 56 of 56 patients (100%); three patients developed recurrent varices, two of whom were treated with repeat transcatheter embolotherapy. Two patients, early in the experience, had complications in which coils placed in the internal iliac veins embolized to the pulmonary circulation—the coils were snared without clinical sequelae. On the VAS, the mean baseline pain level was 7.8 (a range of 3.2–9.8; $n = 56$); at 3-month follow-up, it was 4.2 (a range of 0.0–7.2; $n = 56$); at 6 months, 3.8 (a range of 0.0–6.7; $n = 41$); and at 12 months, 2.7 (a range of 0.0–6.9, $n = 32$). Differences were significant ($p < 0.001$) between baseline pain levels and those at all follow-up intervals (3, 6, and 12 months). The mean decrease in VAS was 5.1 (a 65% decrease). The clinical follow-up in this series ranged between 6 months and 38 months; the mean was 22.1 months. Regarding the impact of embolization on menstruation, all 24 patients responding to questionnaires indicated no change in menstrual cycle.

ANTICIPATED SUCCESS RATES AND COMPLICATIONS OF THERAPY

Estimates, based on pooled data from the medical literature, indicate that 50–80% of women with chronic pelvic pain and having documented ovarian and pelvic varices who undergo treatment, including the surgical or minimally invasive techniques described earlier, will experience some measure of pain relief, which is defined as a reduction in the quantity of pain medications required or a reduction of pelvic pain. As mentioned previously, VAS has been useful for tracking levels of chronic pain (17,18).

Complications are primarily those associated with any invasive contrast study and those of transcatheter embolotherapy. These include, but are not limited to, thrombosis at the percutaneous puncture site (such as the femoral or jugular veins) with associated pain, swelling, and pulmonary embolism risk, which is rare; contrast reaction; and inadvertent loss of a coil with migration to the lung. Fortunately, the latter situation is generally treatable using a transcatheter loop snare to retrieve the device.

The long-term effects of ovarian and pelvic varices embolization on fertility are not known; this is an area of ongoing clinical investigation. Additionally, whether bilateral embolization should be performed when right and left ovarian veins are found to be incompetent, as opposed to treating only one side, is similarly unclear.

SUMMARY

The minimally invasive approach to the management of chronic pelvic pain continues to evolve. When pain is associated with the presence of extensive ovarian and internal iliac varices, well-described techniques of transcatheter embolotherapy may provide significant relief. Unfortunately, many patients are referred after extensive surgical procedures, such as after numerous laparoscopic evaluations (including hysterectomy). Thus, the ability to sort out the potential etiologies of chronic pelvic pain is challenging.

Pelvic venous incompetence is rarely caused by internal iliac varices alone; however, it has been found in a limited number of patients after initial embolization of only the ovarian veins. In other words, embolization of the ovarian veins alone does not necessarily eliminate potential additional sources of varices arising from the internal iliac system. Though the two systems freely communicate (unlike in males), some authors believe that aggressive therapy of both ovarian and internal iliac veins is necessary to achieve the most durable results.

Currently, most imaging studies and laparoscopy are limited because of patient positioning—the decompression of varices in the supine position. Although minimally invasive, contrast venography provides an opportunity to proceed immediately with treatment. As mentioned earlier in the chapter, the long-term effects of embolization

of ovarian and internal iliac varices are unknown, but initial series indicate no significant deleterious effect on the menstrual cycle. Durability of the transcatheter procedure and impact on fertility are areas of ongoing clinical investigation.

Acknowledgments

The author wishes to express his thanks to Melissa Wubbold, Shundra Dinkins, and Toni Acfalle for their expertise in the preparation of this manuscript.

REFERENCES

1. Venbrux AC, Lambert DL. Ovarian and pelvic varices in the female patient. In: Savader SJ, Trerotola SO, eds. Venous Interventional Radiology, New York: Thieme Medical Publishers; Inc., 2000: 210–216.
2. Machan L, Vogelzang R. Interventional radiologic diagnosis and embolization of ovarian varicoceles in the treatment of chronic pelvic pain. The Female Patient 1997;22:25–28.
3. Edlundh KO. Pelvic varicosities in women: a preliminary report. Acta Obstet Gynecol Scand 1964;43:399.
4. Robinson, JC. Chronic pelvic pain. Curr Opin Obstet Gynecol 1993;5:740–713.
5. Beard RW, Reginald PW, Wadsworth J. Clinical features of women with chronic lower abdominal pain and pelvic congestion. Br J Obstet Gynaecol 1988;95:153–161.
6. Hobbs JT. The pelvic congestion syndrome. Br J Hosp Med 1990; 43:200–206.
7. Giacchetto C, Cotroneo GB, Marincolo F, et al. Ovarian varicocele: ultrasonic and phlebographic evaluation. J Clin Ultrasound 1990;18:551–555.
8. Chidekel N. Female pelvic veins demonstrated by selective renal phlebography with particular reference to pelvic varicosities. Acta Radiol 1968;7:193–211.
9. Kennedy A, Hemmingway A. Radiology of ovarian varices. Br J Hosp Med 1990;44:38–43.
10. Ahlberg NE, Bartley O, Chidekel N. Right and left gonadal veins: an anatomical and statistical study. Acta Radiol Diagn (Stockh) 1966;4:593–601.
11. Venbrux AC, Chang AH, Kim HS, et al. Pelvic congestion syndrome (pelvic venous incompetence): impact of ovarian and internal iliac vein embolotherapy on menstrual cycle and chronic pelvic pain. J Vasc Interv Radiol 2002;13:171–178.
12. Capasso P, Simons C, Trotteur G, et al. Treatment of symptomatic pelvic varices by ovarian vein embolization. Cardiovasc Intervent Radiol 1997;20:107–111.
13. Tarazov PG, Prozorovskij KV, Ryzhkov VK. Pelvic pain syndrome caused by ovarian varices: treatment by transcatheter embolization. Acta Radiol 1997;38:1023–1025.
14. Sichlau MJ, Yao JST, Vogelzang RL. Transcatheter embolotherapy for the treatment of pelvic congestion syndrome. Obstet Gynecol 1994;83:892–896.
15. Edwards RD, Robertson IR, MacLean AB, et al. Case report: pelvic pain syndrome—successful treatment of a case by ovarian vein embolization. Clin Radiol 1993;47:429–431.
16. Rundqvist E, Sondhohn LE, Larrson G. Treatment of pelvic varicosities with extraperitoneal resection of the left ovarian vein. Ann Chir Gynaecol 1984;73:399–441.
17. Grossman SA, Sheidler VR, McGuire DB, et al. A comparison of the Hopkins Pain Rating Instrument with standard visual analog and verbal descriptor scales in patients with cancer pain. J Pain Symptom Manage 1992;7:196–203.
18. Lambert DL, Venbrux AC. Visual analog scale for use in assessing levels of pelvic pain before and after ovarian vein embolization for the treatment of pelvic congestion syndrome. J Vasc Interv Radiol 1999;10(Suppl):249.

Interventional Radiology of the Central Nervous System

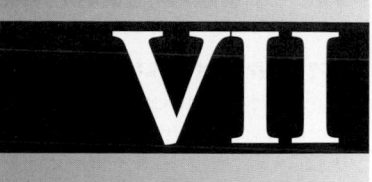

VII

Revascularization in the

47

Central Nervous System

Robert W. Hurst

Because of the widespread prevalence of cerebrovascular disease, ischemic brain damage represents an immense medical problem that has individual and public health consequences. Recent developments in interventional neuroradiology have made possible the revascularization of regions of the central nervous system (CNS) that have been or may become deprived of adequate blood flow. Revascularization procedures encompass various methods for restoring and increasing blood flow in CNS ischemia. These procedures permit possible salvage of CNS tissue and function in the face of ischemia. With these techniques, the potential exists to prevent or ameliorate a significant portion of damage resulting from acute cerebral infarction, the most common neurologic disease and the third leading cause of mortality in the developed world.

Throughout the last decade of the 20th century, revascularization procedures including intra-arterial thrombolysis for acute stroke and pharmacological dilation or balloon angioplasty of symptomatic intracranial vasospasm have come into widespread use and have been responsible for reversal of acute neurologic deficits in large numbers of patients. In addition, increasing evidence and experience with angioplasty and stenting for atherosclerotic disease of extracranial vessels indicates that these procedures are finding greater use in effective prevention of ischemic stroke.

INTRA-ARTERIAL THROMBOLYTIC THERAPY FOR TREATMENT OF ACUTE STROKE

The term *stroke* refers to a sudden onset, nonconvulsive, neurologic deficit of cerebrovascular origin. Etiologies of stroke include a heterogenous group of cerebrovascular disorders ranging from ischemia to intracranial hemorrhage. Ischemic stroke is by far the most common type and can be divided into the more common large vessel occlusive disease and small vessel disease or lacunar stroke. Eighty to ninety percent of ischemic strokes result from atherothrombotic or thromboembolic events with occlusion of "large" vessels, which are those exceeding 1 mm in diameter (1). Most often, emboli originate from the extracranial carotid arteries or the heart. In patients studied angiographically within 6 hours of ischemic stroke onset, an occlusive vascular lesion correlating to the clinical deficit has been found in more than 75% (2,3). The need for rapid, effective treatment in ischemic stroke is highlighted by the frequently dismal outcome of affected patients when managed conservatively.

Despite recent improvement in short-term survival rates, which is largely because of improved supportive care, more than 15% of patients admitted to a hospital with ischemic stroke will die within 30 days. More than 80% of patients with stroke secondary to acute occlusion of the middle cerebral artery will die or will manifest severe persistent neurologic deficits 3 months after the ictus (4). The long-term prognosis for return to normal life is also poor because even 1 year later, fewer than half of the patients suffering major ischemic stroke will be able to live independently (5).

Pathophysiology

Understanding basic pathophysiology of embolic infarction is essential to developing a meaningful appreciation of potential benefits, complications, and contraindications to intra-arterial thrombolytic therapy in the treatment of stroke.

Acute occlusion of an artery supplying CNS tissue results in ischemic injury to the tissue supplied by the vessel. Experimental studies of focal ischemia suggest that the severity of injury depends both on the time and completeness of the ischemic insult. At least two critical thresholds of blood flow exist as cerebral blood flow declines from normal values of approximately 50 mL/100 gm per minute. By the time blood flows that are below 15–17 mL/100 g/min are reached, neurologic deficits are present, which reflect failure of normal neuronal function. Although neuronal electrical activity has ceased, cell viability can be maintained, at least temporarily. Neuronal activity and neurologic deficits may be restored to normal with increases in blood flow. As flow rates decrease further—below about 10 mL/100 gm per minute—failure of ion pumps and other cell mechanisms occur with disruption of the cell membrane and relatively rapid onset of irreversible infarction or cell death.

The area of ischemic brain receiving blood flow between the two thresholds—the upper threshold of electrical failure and the lower threshold of pump failure and cell death—represents a zone of injured but potentially viable tissue that surrounds the most severely affected region of irreversible ischemic damage. This area, known as the "ischemic penumbra," is often capable of functional recovery following restoration of blood flow (6).

Clinical studies in humans with embolic stroke have confirmed the existence of an ischemic penumbra. The studies also suggest that a finite interval exists following vascular occlusion after which ischemic damage is most likely irreversible. Chances for return of function within the ischemic penumbra are therefore greater with earlier reperfusion (7).

Clinical studies and experience confirm that both the degree and duration of ischemia are important in determining the amount of neurologic damage. Even severe ischemia may be reversible after a short duration while infarction may develop in less severely ischemic areas whenever the duration of ischemia is prolonged. As the time from onset of ischemia increases, more brain tissue is transformed from potentially salvageable ischemic penumbra into irreversible infarction (8,9).

Multiple clinical features of the embolic episode in addition to the time of occlusion are important in determining the severity and amount of ischemic damage. The site and completeness of occlusion as well as the availability of collateral flow also directly affect the degree of ischemia and consequently, the amount of salvageable penumbra (7,10,11). In the anterior circulation, emboli most commonly occlude the middle cerebral artery (MCA), a vessel whose distribution has limited effective collateral supply. Proximal MCA occlusion often blocks the territory of the lenticulostriate arteries, a region with even more limited collateral availability. Because severe ischemia results, irreversible injury tends to occur relatively early (12). In the vertebrobasilar circulation, multiple potential collaterals often permit longer viability of marginally perfused tissue after embolic occlusion.

Embolic occlusion of a vessel is often followed by fragmentation of the embolus and distal migration. In addition, physiological fibrinolytic mechanisms act to lyse the obstructing clot. Although more than 90% of embolic occlusions eventually show angiographic reopening, fewer than 20% recanalize within 24 hours of stroke onset (1,13). Spontaneous recanalization within the substantially shorter interval needed to preserve cerebral tissue and restore function is even less common (14,15). The speed and extent of physiological mechanisms of clot lysis are therefore unpredictable and often do not permit reperfusion within sufficient time to prevent infarction. Intra-arterial infusion of thrombolytic agent dissolves obstructing clots and accelerates reopening of the vessel in an effort to salvage ischemic but still viable tissue.

With lysis or distal migration of the embolus, reperfusion may expose a recently ischemic or infarcted area to the force of arterial blood pressure. Distension and congestion of the capillary bed follows with possible extravasation of red cells into ischemic areas, a phenomenon known as *hemorrhagic transformation*. The occurrence of red cell extravasation is related to the volume of tissue affected as well as the extent and severity of ischemic damage. This change represents hemorrhagic transformation of a "bland" ischemic infarct into a hemorrhagic infarct. In most embolic occlusions, hemorrhagic transformation is mild with only microscopic or petechial hemorrhage into part of the infarcted area. Some degree of hemorrhagic infarction is common and is reported in 10–43% of patients in CT studies of embolic infarction (16–20). Frequently seen in patients who are clinically stable or improving, the clinical significance of hemorrhagic transformation is usually minimal.

When larger amounts of bleeding occur into an area of infarction, frank parenchymal hemorrhage may occur. Virtually always associated with clinical deterioration, parenchymal hemorrhage represents homogeneous clot with mass effect that may displace, damage, or destroy the involved area as well as adjacent brain. Clinically significant parenchymal hemorrhage following untreated ischemic stroke is fortunately uncommon with an incidence of less than 5% (20). While risk factors predisposing to this condition are not fully understood, parenchymal hemorrhage appears more commonly in patients who have been treated with thrombolysis.

The time course of hemorrhagic transformation has important therapeutic implications. Spontaneous hemorrhagic transformation in the anterior circulation is uncommon before 6 hours postocclusion and is identified in only 5% of cardioembolic strokes within the first 24 hours. Most instances occur even later with nearly one-quarter occurring at greater than 1 week after the ictus (21). The usual delay in occurrence of hemorrhagic transformation implies the existence of a therapeutic window during which vessel reopening may be accomplished with an acceptably low chance of clinically significant hemorrhage into the ischemic area.

Any therapy designed to reperfuse ischemic CNS tissue also has the potential for causing or worsening hemorrhage into the ischemic area. The result may be clinically insignificant hemorrhagic transformation or less often, parenchymal hemorrhage. In each case, the risk of clinically significant hemorrhage must be balanced against the potential for regaining CNS function. Successful early thrombolytic recanalization has actually been shown to decrease the amount of hemorrhagic transformation compared to patients not undergoing recanalization (22).

In cases of stroke caused by thromboembolic occlusion of vessels supplying the central nervous system, acute treatment with intra-arterial thrombolysis is therefore based on the premise that timely reopening of vessels with consequent restoration of blood flow to the affected regions may result in significant resolution of neurologic deficits. With individual patients, making the decision to use thrombolytic agents to reverse cerebral ischemic deficits is predicated on three key assumptions: (1) that a viable region of "ischemic penumbra" is present and capable of restored function with reperfusion, (2) that thrombolytic agents can effectively recanalize the vessels supplying the area, and (3) that the associated risk of hemorrhage associated with thrombolysis is outweighed by the potential benefit of restored perfusion.

The first investigation into the use of thrombolytic agents for the treatment of acute stroke was reported in 1958 (23). Later trials during the pre-CT scan era were hampered by an inability to diagnose the cause of acute neurologic deficit before intravenous thrombolytic treatment. In these early studies, limited angiographic diagnosis of vessel occlusion and infrequent follow-up angiography impaired accurate diagnosis of vascular

pathology and vessel reopening. With the introduction of CT scanning, diagnosis was improved, particularly with regard to the exclusion of intracranial hemorrhage. Nevertheless, early studies of intravenous use of thrombolytic agents resulted in systemic fibrinolytic effects and discouraging numbers of hemorrhagic complications (24).

The situation changed in 1995 when the results of the first randomized prospective trial showing a statistically significant benefit of treatment in ischemic stroke were published. The NINDS Trial demonstrated that administration of intravenous tPA resulted in a 30% relative increase in the likelihood of minimal or no residual disability compared to patients given placebo. All patients received treatment within 3 hours of ischemic stroke onset. The clinical benefits remained statistically significant despite a nearly 10-fold increase in the intracranial hemorrhage rate in the treated group (25). Later studies have shown that thrombolytic treatment for acute ischemic stroke appears to be cost effective as well as clinically beneficial (26).

Intravenous administration of tPA is currently recommended as a first-line therapy of ischemic stroke for patients who meet several criteria for its administration. Nevertheless, many concerns have been expressed in the literature regarding both the use of intravenous thrombolysis in stroke without vascular imaging and its suitability for occlusions of particular locations within the cerebrovascular system. Specifically, occlusions of the proximal internal carotid artery, proximal middle cerebral artery, or basilar artery may respond poorly, if at all, to recanalization attempts with intravenous thrombolysis.

The intra-arterial injection of thrombolytic agent has been found to be useful in the treatment of vascular disease involving both peripheral and coronary circulations. However, the application of intra-arterial thrombolysis to the central nervous system (CNS) lagged behind. By the 1980s, advances in superselective arterial catheterization made possible the local infusion of thrombolytic agent directly into occluded vessels of the CNS. This technique permitted the use of smaller amounts of thrombolytic medication, minimizing systemic effects. An additional benefit of the intra-arterial route was suggested by angiographic studies indicating that stagnation of flow proximal to an occlusion might prevent delivery of thrombolytic agent to the blockage unless the agent was infused locally into the obstructed vessel. Several studies began to appear in the literature reporting successful reopening of occluded CNS vessels with good resolution of deficits and minimal hemorrhagic complications (22,27,28).

The first randomized prospective trial of intra-arterial thrombolytic agents in acute stroke was reported in 1999 (29). PROACT II (Prolyse in Acute Cerebral Thromboembolism II) enrolled 180 patients with acute ischemic stroke of less than 6 hours' duration caused by angiographically proven occlusion of the proximal MCA (M_1 or M_2). All patients were without hemorrhage or major early infarction on CT and were randomized to receive IA r-proUK plus heparin or heparin only. The study found that despite an increased frequency of early symptomatic intracranial hemorrhage affecting 10% of r-proUK patients and 2% of control patients, IA treatment significantly improved clinical outcome at 90 days. Forty percent of IA patients had slight or no neurologic disability at 90 days (modified Rankin score of 2 or less), while only 25% of control patients had modified Rankin of 2 or less (p = 0.04). The recanalization rate was 66% for the r-proUK group and 18% for the control group (p <0.001).

Current data support consideration of IA therapy for M_1 and M_2 occlusions when administered within 6 hours of onset of the deficit. In acute vertebrobasilar occlusions, IA thrombolysis is the only lifesaving therapy that has demonstrated benefit with regard to mortality and outcome, although randomized trials have not been conducted (30,31).

Before treating with intra-arterial thrombolytic agents, accurate diagnosis of the etiology of the neurologic deficit and evaluation of potential contraindications are necessary.

Pretreatment Evaluation

Guidelines for acute intra-arterial fibrinolytic therapy in stroke must focus primarily on rapid and thorough neurologic evaluation to select, appropriate patients. Patients most likely to benefit include those with severe acute onset of neurologic deficits secondary to thromboembolic occlusion. Exclusion of intracranial hemorrhage is paramount and can be accomplished without difficulty using CT scan. Patients with stroke secondary to lacunar infarction, global hypoperfusion, or diffuse intracranial vascular disease have no large vessel occlusive lesion and have not been shown to benefit from intra-arterial thrombolysis. Clinical differentiation of these potential causes for stroke may be challenging and may require expert neurologic consultation and frequently angiographic evaluation.

Careful history and physical examination are necessary to exclude potential contraindications to thrombolytic therapy. Any condition predisposing to an increased risk of hemorrhage must be actively sought and may exclude patients from consideration. Examples of potential contraindications include intracranial aneurysm, arteriovenous malformation, recent surgery, or biopsy. Other systemic conditions, such as ulcer disease, diverticulosis, coagulation defect, uncontrolled hypertension, or conditions associated with an expected shortened survival (such as malignancy, hepatic disease, or coma) may also exclude thrombolytic therapy. Evaluation of baseline coagulation parameters, including PT, PTT, and platelet count, is performed.

The need to ensure the presence of potentially viable "ischemic penumbra" introduces the concept of a time window within which thrombolysis is most likely to be successful. In the anterior circulation, a time window of 6 hours following the onset of the clinical deficit is commonly used. Although few data support rigid adherence to a specific time window, later therapy may be less effective in restoring function and may also expose the patient to an increased risk of hemorrhagic transformation of a previously infarcted area.

In the vertebrobasilar circulation, safety and effectiveness of thrombolysis after intervals of occlusion longer than 6 hours have been demonstrated—although not proven with randomized trials. With basilar occlusion, additional sources of collateral circulation may delay irreversible clinical deterioration and minimize potential for hemorrhagic transformation. In addition, the devastating and frequently fatal outcome of acute vertebrobasilar occlusion often justifies the potentially higher risk associated with later treatment. Intra-arterial thrombolytic treatment at up to 24 hours in patients with partial deficits of brainstem function has been reported to result in good resolution of clinical deficits. Several clinical features of vertebrobasilar ischemia portend a poor outcome however and represent contraindications to thrombolysis. These include coma lasting more than 6 hours, decerebration, and angiographic evidence of chronic occlusion (28).

An unenhanced CT scan is obtained before starting thrombolytic treatment. CT evidence of intracranial hemorrhage represents a contraindication to the use of thrombolytic agents. Large hypodense infarcts and mass effect on CT have been found to predict the development of later hemorrhagic transformation or parenchymal hemorrhage (16,19,20). While uncommon within the first hours of embolic stroke, these imaging findings also represent relative contraindications to the use of thrombolytic therapy.

MR imaging has not been shown to be able to exclude hyperacute hemorrhage with sufficient confidence to proceed with fibrinolytic therapy on the basis of MRI alone. MR angiography may detect the abrupt vessel cutoff that suggests embolic occlusion, but it does not eliminate the need for angiography and often delays the initiation of therapy. Consequently, at many institutions, MRI is not routinely incorporated into the evaluation of patients being considered for urgent intracranial thrombolytic therapy.

At present, conventional angiography represents not only the means for delivery of therapy but also the diagnostic method of choice for confirming and localizing the site of vessel occlusion. A high-resolution digital angiography unit with roadmapping capability is essential for identification of the lesion and navigation within intracranial vessels. The transfemoral approach is used. Injection of the symptomatic vessel distribution is performed including appropriate oblique views when necessary to confirm occlusion as the etiology of the clinical deficit and to localize the site of vessel occlusion (Figure 47–1). Diagnostic angiography of other vessel distributions may also be necessary. Evaluation of the contralateral carotid, for example, may be important to demonstrate cross filling of the intracranial circulation, especially in cases of complete carotid occlusion.

Pharmacologic agents useful for thrombolysis in the CNS—urokinase (UK) and tissue plasminogen activator (tPA)—have been widely studied for use in peripheral and

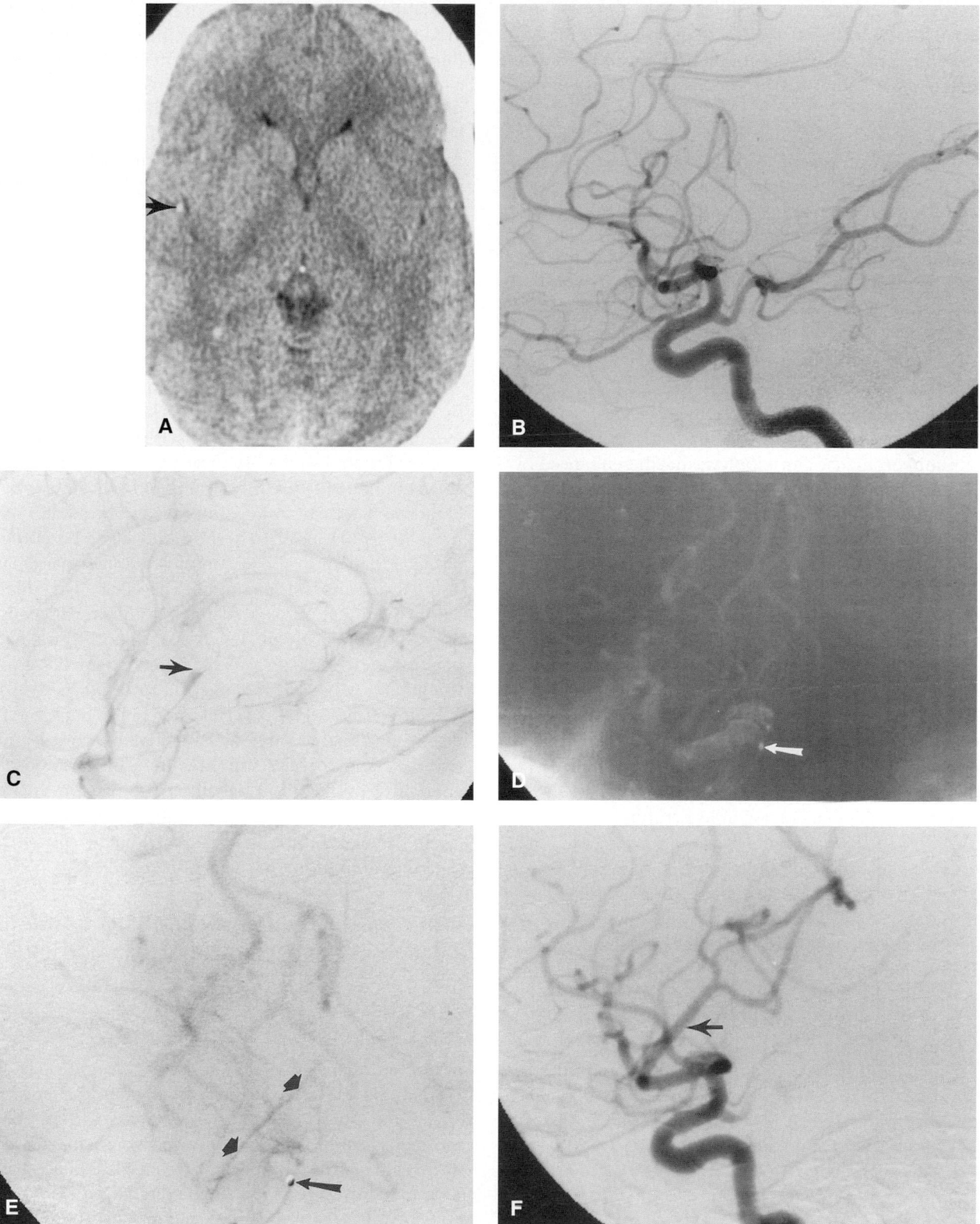

Figure 47–1 A. A 28-year-old female with new onset left hemiparesis, left sensory deficits, and left hemianopsia. CT scan 3 hours after onset of neurologic deficit shows hyperdensity in right sylvian fissure compatible with embolus within a branch of the MCA (*arrow*). **B.** Lateral right internal carotid artery injection (early arterial phase) demonstrates no filling of inferior trunk of right MCA. **C.** Venous phase shows gradual filling of the inferior trunk of the right MCA with abrupt meniscus cutoff at the site of the embolic occlusion (*arrow*). **D., E.** Unsubtracted and subtracted film of selective right MCA injection shows filling of obstructed branch (*arrowheads*) before superselective catheterization and urokinase infusion (*arrow shows catheter tip*). **F.** Right internal carotid injection after thrombolysis shows filling of the previously occluded branch (*arrow*). Patient made full recovery. Evaluation showed cardiac source of embolus.

coronary circulations. All clinically available thrombolytic agents act by enhancing conversion of plasminogen to plasmin, a serine protease that degrades fibrin and fibrinogen and factors II, Va, and VIIIa. Thrombolytic effects are comparable for both agents, but there are differences in relative clot selectivity, plasma half-life, dose, and cost. A complete comparison of the characteristics of these and other agents is beyond the scope of this chapter, but readers are encouraged to consult other chapters in this volume as well as additional resources for more detailed coverage of this topic.

Patients are placed under general anesthesia before intra-arterial intracranial thrombolysis. This eliminates the ability to follow the neurologic examination, but it enhances patient safety by ensuring immobility and permits rapid initiation of management should intracranial hemorrhage occur during the procedure.

After angiographic localization of the occlusion, selective catheterization of the occluded vessel is accomplished through use of a microcatheter. Thrombolysis may be enhanced by several microcatheter and guide wire techniques that have proved useful. The microcatheter is placed within the occluded vessel as closely as possible to the site of obstruction, and infusion of thrombolytic agent is started (Figure 47–2). In the event that infusion just proximal to the obstruction fails to lyse the blockage, the catheter tip may be embedded in the obstruction and infusion continued. In some cases, gentle advancement of a flexible guide wire and catheter past the embolus may be possible with initial injection of agent distal to the clot. The catheter is then withdrawn through the clot while continued injection perfuses the clot itself with thrombolytic agent. Infusion is continued into and proximal to the obstruction. Reported rates of urokinase infusion have varied from 2,000 to more than 13,000 units per minute with total doses of up to 1,000,000 units. Doses of tPA up to 20 mg have also been reported. Infusion is terminated when recanalization occurs or after 2 hours of infusion (27,32,33) (Figure 47–3).

Heparinization is instituted during the angiogram following the arterial puncture. Depending on the etiology of the occlusion and the completeness of reopening, heparinization may be continued postprocedure for a short period (2–3 days) or more commonly, stopped at the end of the procedure. Long-term therapy with anticoagulants or antiplatelet agents is based on the etiology of the obstructive lesion and the potential for recurrence. Follow-up values of PT, PTT, fibrinogen, and platelet counts are checked.

Results

Although current information indicates a major role for IA thrombolysis in the management of acute stroke, its ultimate place will be known with complete certainty only after larger clinical trials have been conducted (34). The only randomized prospective study of intra-arterial infusion of thrombolytic agent, PROACT II (mentioned earlier), suggested that the procedure is safe and effective (29).

The Emergency Management of Stroke (EMS) Bridging Trial evaluated the feasibility of initial treatment with IV thrombolysis followed by IA treatment (35). The study was a randomized trial with 35 patients receiving either IV tPA or placebo followed by IA tPA. A significant improvement in recanalization of the occluded vessels was demonstrated in the combined treatment group, which had 83% reopening of the occluded vessel as opposed to only 55% reopening in the control group. Despite the improved reopening in the treated group, no improvement in clinical outcome was demonstrated in this small study.

The potential for benefit in posterior circulation events is even more striking. As noted earlier, the devastating outcome of acute vertebrobasilar occlusion has been amply demonstrated with untreated mortality in the range of 70–100% (28). Significant survival benefits have been shown for acute occlusions. In Hacke et al., nearly 70% of patents in the study whose vessels were recanalized survived compared to a 13% survival rate in patients treated conventionally (28). Other studies of IA thrombolysis have demonstrated substantially improved survival rates ranging from 40–87% (36,37). These studies suggest a potentially immense benefit in this group of ischemic strokes, particularly because most studies to date have included patients in whom treatment was started at relatively long intervals after onset of the neurologic deficit. Continued efforts to institute therapy as early as possible following the onset of neurologic deficit would be expected to result in even fewer complications and more significant clinical benefit (33,38).

Nevertheless, it must be kept in mind that however impressive, the angiographic results are not nearly as important an endpoint as the clinical benefits resulting from treatment. Studies such as PROACT II have confirmed the clinical benefit of intra-arterial thrombolytic treatment under specific conditions; however, additional data are required.

Intracranial Angioplasty and Pharmacologic Dilation in Postsubarachnoid Hemorrhage

Vasospasm

Intracranial aneurysm rupture is responsible for nearly 80% of nontraumatic subarachnoid hemorrhages (SAH). In the United States, aneurysmal subarachnoid hemorrhage affects more than 26,000 patients per year with estimates of mortality as high as 50–65%. The prognosis for survivors of aneurysmal subarachnoid hemorrhage is equally grim. Of those patients well enough to be discharged from the hospital, nearly two thirds never regain the quality of life experienced before rupture (1). After aneurysm rupture, the risk of recurrent rupture is high in untreated cases, up to 2% per day for the first 2 weeks, with mortality of up to 60% associated with rebleeding. Modern techniques including coil embolization and microneurosurgery usually permit closure of ruptured aneurysms thereby minimizing rebleeding as a cause of significant morbidity. Currently, the leading

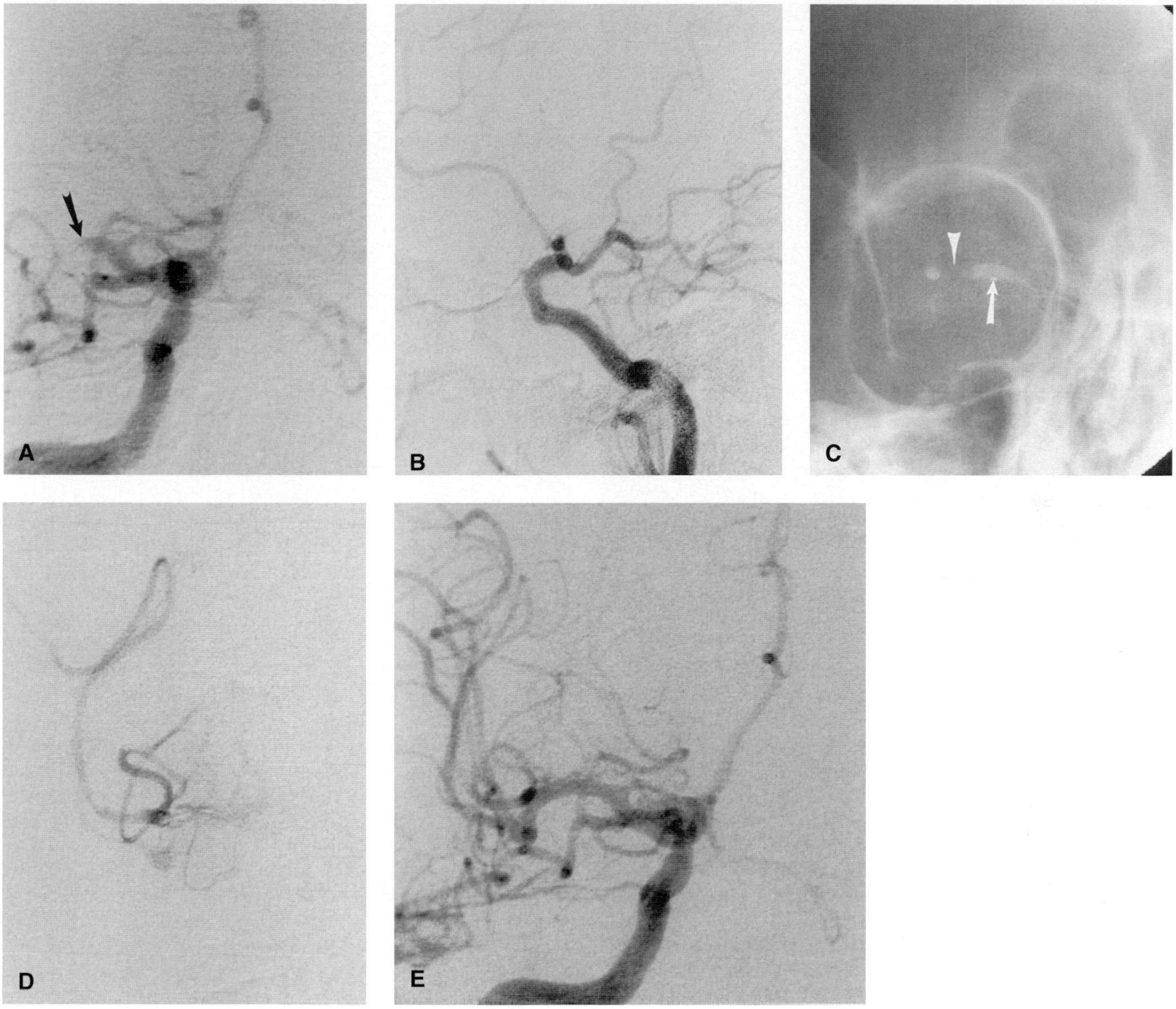

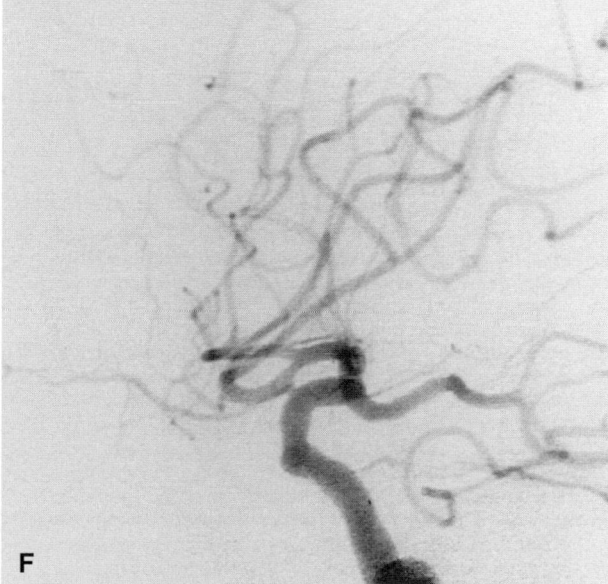

Figure 47–2 **A., B.** Anteroposterior and lateral views demonstrate acute right MCA occlusion (*arrow*). **C.** Unsubtracted view with microcatheter tip (*arrow*) adjacent to embolus (*arrowhead*). No distal filling of distal MCA branches occurs. **D.** Anteroposterior subtracted view after lysis of the embolus shows filling of distal branches of the MCA. **E., F.** Anteroposterior and lateral views of right internal carotid artery (RICA) injection after urokinase infusion demonstrating reperfusion of distal MCA branches.

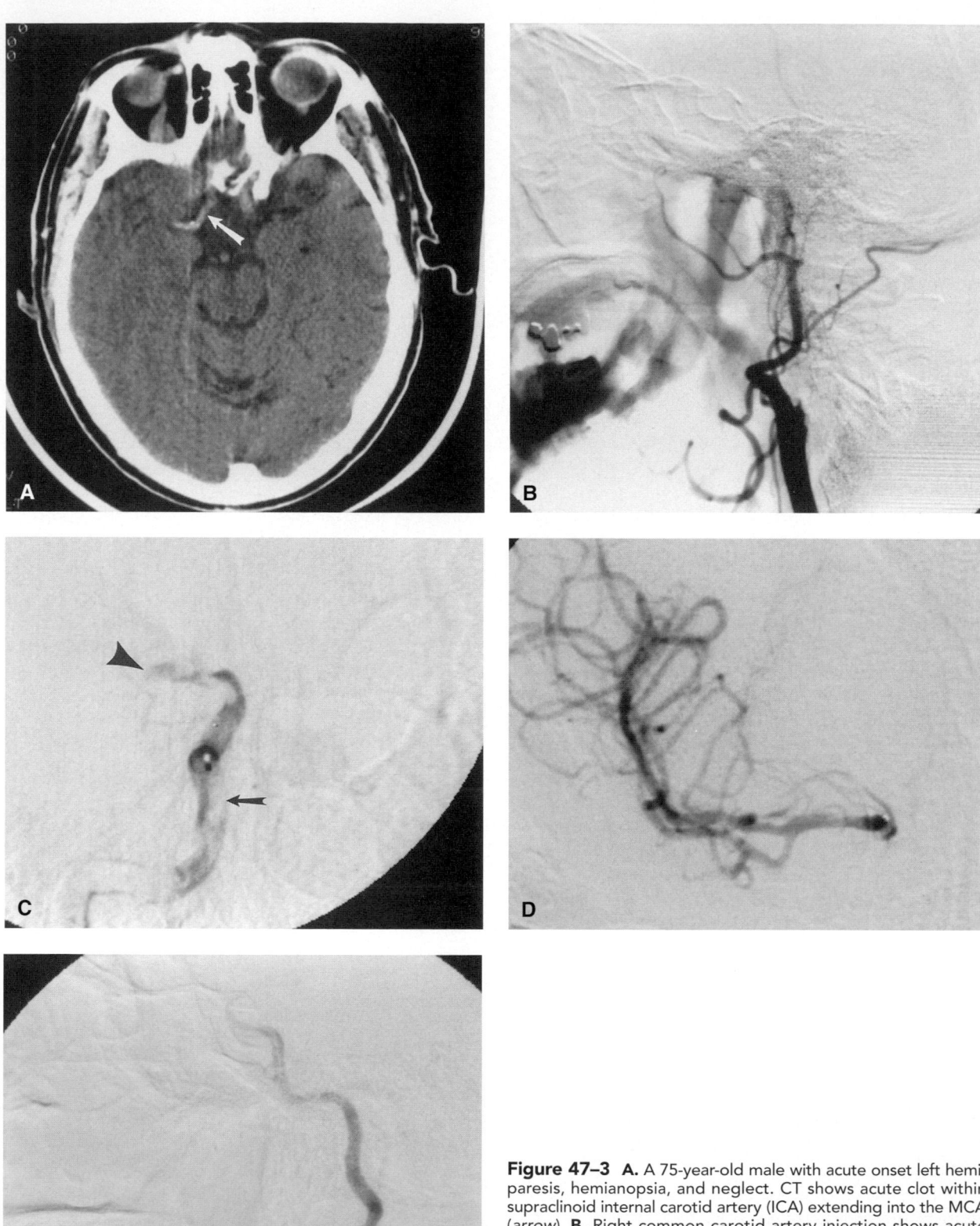

Figure 47–3 A. A 75-year-old male with acute onset left hemiparesis, hemianopsia, and neglect. CT shows acute clot within supraclinoid internal carotid artery (ICA) extending into the MCA (*arrow*). **B.** Right common carotid artery injection shows acute occlusion of the RICA. **C.** Anteroposterior angiogram with microcatheter in cavernous ICA during thrombolysis. Considerable residual clot remains within the ICA (*arrow*) with complete obstruction distally (*arrowhead*). **D.** Anteroposterior angiogram during thrombolysis after opening of middle and anterior cerebral arteries. **E.** Proximal ICA injection following thrombolysis shows tight atherosclerotic stenosis at the origin of the reopened ICA (*arrow shows catheter tip*). Patient improved neurologically during the thrombolysis procedure. Endarterectomy was performed, and there were no neurologic deficits 24 hours later.

contributor to both morbidity and mortality in patients surviving aneurysmal subarachnoid hemorrhage is delayed ischemic damage caused by intracranial vasospasm.

Although incompletely understood, the pathophysiology of postsubarachnoid hemorrhage vasospasm is initiated by the presence of blood in the subarachnoid space. Vasoactive substances resulting from the presence of subarachnoid blood act on the vessel wall to cause abnormal contraction of vascular smooth muscle and narrowing of luminal diameter. Evidence has implicated several substances, including oxyhemoglobin released from erythrocytes in the subarachnoid space, as potential spasmogens that engender this contraction (39). The narrowed vessel lumen decreases delivery of blood to the cerebral parenchyma with consequent ischemia and infarction.

Over time, a spectrum of morphologic change develops in the vessel wall. Histological findings include the occurrence within days of intimal and medial swelling. By 1–6 weeks, intimal proliferation and myonecrosis are present with associated luminal narrowing. Medial fibrosis and enlargement of luminal diameter have been found to develop after 3–6 months. The arteriopathic response of the cerebral arteries following exposure to subarachnoid blood appears to be both time and dose dependent (40).

Estimates of the incidence of angiographically visible vasospasm following subarachnoid hemorrhage (SAH) range as high as 76%. Less frequent, but more important clinically, is the incidence of symptomatic vasospasm giving rise to ischemic deficits. Delayed ischemic deficits resulting from vasospasm are reported with a frequency of about 30% from major referral centers. Clinically significant vasospasm that results in delayed ischemic deficit is therefore not equivalent to angiographic vasospasm. At present, treatment modalities are directed only toward those patients who manifest symptoms of cerebral ischemia.

Clinically symptomatic vasospasm usually presents between the fourth and twelfth day following subarachnoid hemorrhage. Most often heralded by headache, the development of symptomatic vasospasm is also associated with impairment of consciousness, often accompanied by the appearance of focal neurologic signs. Progression of the signs and symptoms of clinical vasospasm is usually rapid, peaking within hours of onset.

The focal neurologic features of symptomatic vasospasm reflect not only the anatomy of the involved vascular territories but also the adequacy of potential collateral routes and cerebral autoregulatory capacity. Thus, vasospasm of intracranial vessels is often far more extensive than is suggested by the focal neurologic deficits. The clinical localization of a vascular territory responsible for a given deficit is important however, because it permits therapy to be directed toward the areas affected by the most clinically significant ischemia. Involvement of the MCA results in hemiparesis often with aphasia or contralateral neglect depending on whether the dominant or nondominant hemisphere is involved. If unilateral, anterior cerebral artery (ACA) involvement results in

contralateral leg weakness. Commonly occurring bilaterally after rupture of anterior communicating aneurysms, ACA spasm may cause diplegia in company with abulia, mutism, akinesia, incontinence, and other evidence of impairment of frontal lobe function. Posterior cerebral artery (PCA) spasm may manifest hemianopsia in addition to obtundation, bilateral ptosis, and memory deficits suggesting rostral basilar artery embolism. With involvement of posterior fossa vasculature, deficits referable to the brainstem are often the most prominent clinical features. Dysconjugate gaze and skew deviation may occur, often accompanied by coma. Autonomic derangements may be prominent and may include alterations of blood pressure, temperature, and respiration (41).

The amount of blood present on early CT scanning is the most accurate predictor of a high risk of subsequent vasospasm. Localized clot surrounding a vessel or a layer of blood greater than 1 mm thick are features that have been suggested to indicate a particularly high risk (Figure 47–4). The distribution and severity of vasospasm have been found to correlate not only with the clot distribution on CT scans but also with the amount of blood within the subarachnoid space (42–45).

The availability of transcranial Doppler (TCD) ultrasonography provides a means of noninvasive evaluation of flow velocities within the major intracranial arteries at the base of the brain. When constant flow is maintained, narrowing of the vessel lumen with the onset of vasospasm results in a proportional increase in flow velocity.

Daily serial assessment of flow velocities with TCD typically is performed in patients after subarachnoid hemorrhage. With the development of vasospasm, increasing flow velocities are seen. Because increased flow velocities on TCD precede the development of clinical ischemic deficits, identification of high-risk patients is often possible before the development of clinically significant vasospasm. Because of limited collateral networks supplying the territory of the middle cerebral arteries (MCA), close correlation is often found between the amount of MCA narrowing angiographically and increases in flow velocities measured by TCD. Normal blood flow velocities in the proximal MCA range between 30–80 cm/sec with a mean of 62 cm/sec. Velocities greater than 120 cm/sec usually correlate with angiographically visible spasm, while velocities greater than 200 cm/sec usually reflect severe spasm with greater than 50% vessel narrowing. Increased velocities may also be found in the supraclinoid internal carotid artery, ACA, PCA, and basilar arteries if involved by vasospasm.

Several features and indexes that include TCD have been used to identify those patients likely to develop clinical vasospasm. Rapid increases in TCD velocities on or before the fifth day posthemorrhage, for example, suggest patients at high risk of developing subsequent infarction. The early identification of high risk patients permits close observation and rapid institution of therapy as soon as clinical signs of vasospasm develop (45,46).

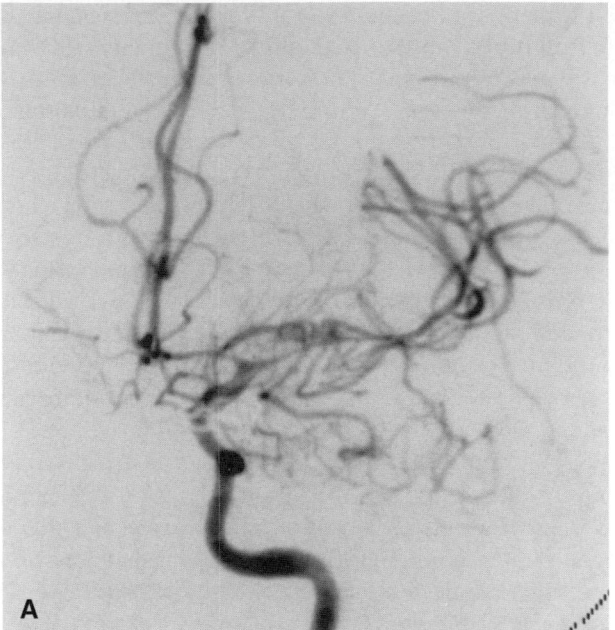

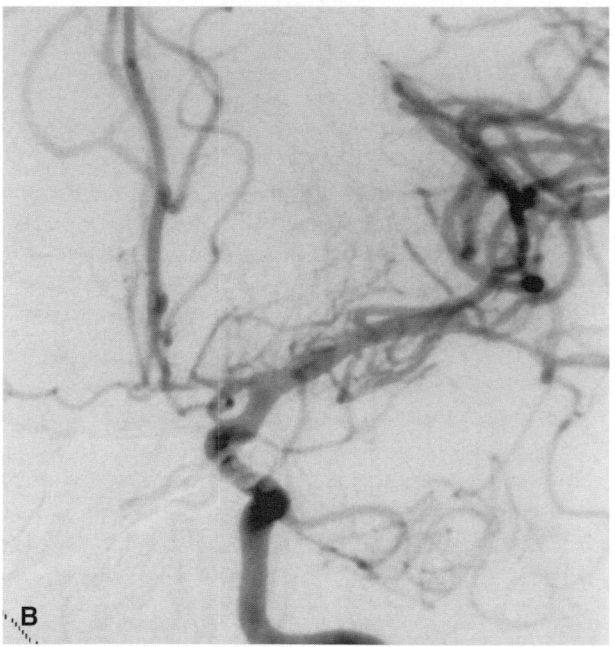

Figure 47–4 A. Anteroposterior left ICA injection with diffuse spasm in 40-year-old female with new onset aphasia and right hemiparesis 2 days after aneurysm clipping. **B.** After angioplasty of the left MCA, there is improved filling of MCA and distal branches.

Medical Treatment of Postsubarachnoid Hemorrhage (SAH) Vasospasm

Reversal of ischemic neurologic deficits secondary to vasospasm was first documented in 1967 following therapy with induced hypertension (47). In 1976, Kosnik and Hunt reversed vasospasm-associated neurologic deficits in 6 of 7 patients using a combination of induced hypertension and volume expansion (48). Later studies confirmed the usefulness of volume expansion and pharmacologically

induced hypertension to increase perfusion to ischemic areas in the face of impaired autoregulation. Fluid status is monitored via a swan-ganz catheter, and pressor agents are added whenever neurologic deficits persist in the face of volume expansion. Reversal of neurologic deterioration may be seen in more than 80% of patients so treated. Reasons for failure of therapy include preexisting infarct, rebleeding, or inability to induce hypertension. Complications have included rebleeding from unclipped aneurysm, pulmonary edema, hyponatremia, coagulopathy, and myocardial infaction. Conversion of bland into hemorrhagic infarcts has not been reported with mean blood pressures in the range of 150 mm (49).

Studies have confirmed the usefulness of the calcium-channel blocking medication such as nimodipine in ameliorating the effects of vasospasm-induced ischemia (50). Calcium antagonists have been shown in several studies to significantly reduce the proportion of ischemic neurologic deficits to improve overall outcome within 3 months of aneurysmal subarachnoid hemorrhage (SAH) (51). Patients are started at a dose of 60 mg q 4 hours within 96 hours of SAH.

Current vasospasm management protocols include treatment with calcium channel blockers as well as presurgical supportive measures. Following aneurysm closure, volume expansion and induced hypertension may be instituted in the event that clinical spasm occurs. Failure of maximal medical treatment to resolve vasospasm-induced ischemic deficits should prompt early consideration of interventional neuroradiologic therapy.

Interventional Neuroradiologic Treatment

In addition to medical management using hypertensive and hypervolemic therapy, revascularization techniques have assumed a significant role in the treatment of delayed ischemic deficits caused by postsubarachnoid hemorrhage vasospasm.

Angioplasty of vasospastic intracranial vessels with an inflatable intravascular balloon catheter results in mechanical dilation of the vessel lumen with concomitant increase in blood flow. First reported in 1984 by Zubkov, several series have confirmed the clinical usefulness of intracranial angioplasty in the treatment of selected patients with symptomatic vasospasm (52–55).

Vasospasm-induced neurologic deficits that persist in the face of maximal medical therapy constitute the major indication for interventional neuroradiologic treatment of vasospasm. To maximize the risk-benefit ratio, patients are selected to ensure that the procedure is performed only when necessary in patients most likely to benefit. Patients benefiting most are those symptomatic with new onset neurologic deficits following SAH. Ideally, a trial of maximal medical therapy has failed to reverse the deficits. Abnormal flow velocities on TCD are virtually always present, and they confirm the etiology of the deficits before angiography. Recent CT scanning must be available to exclude the most common differential causes for new onset deficits in this clinical setting, including rehemorrhage, hydrocephalus, and established cerebral infarction.

As with any treatment for cerebral ischemic deficit, angioplasty should be performed as soon as possible after the onset of symptoms. Most significant recovery is usually seen following treatment instituted within 6–12 hours after deficit although recovery may occur following later angioplasty.

Angiography is performed via a transfemoral approach on a high-resolution digital angiography unit with roadmapping capability. General anesthesia is used whenever possible because patient motion, a significant problem with patients having impaired consciousness, interferes with visualization and increases the risk of the procedure. An initial limited angiogram is performed to confirm the presence and extent of vasospasm, its severity, and sources of collateral circulation, as well as to exclude residual aneurysm. In patients whose aneurysms have been secured by either clipping or coiling, heparin is used during the procedure.

Intracranial arteries involved by vasospasm demonstrate smooth angiographic narrowing. Distal widening of a vessel or the presence of a branch with a diameter greater than the parent vessel also indicates a high probability of involvement by vasospasm. Irregular discontinuous areas of spasm may be seen, and on occasion, a more beaded appearance is present. With severe spasm, slowing of flow through the involved vessel distributions may occur and prolonged filming sequences are required. Spasm may involve only a localized area adjacent to the aneurysm or be distributed diffusely and extensively throughout the intracranial circulation (56).

Comparison with prior angiograms is very useful for determining the extent of vasospastic narrowing in an individual vessel. Previously present intracranial atherosclerotic disease, as well as areas of vessel hypoplasia, should be identified. Hypoplasia of one A_1 segment is particularly common in patients with aneurysms of the anterior communicating artery complex and must be excluded before angioplasty of this segment is attempted.

Intracranial dilation using angioplasty or pharmacologic means is performed only in vessel distributions not harboring an unclipped, previously ruptured aneurysm. Increasing blood flow through an unprotected aneurysm may result in hemorrhage with potentially fatal consequences.

Several types of microballoon are available for intracranial angioplasty. Silicone balloon catheters are generally best. These devices have a low inflation pressure, and they elongate within the vessel lumen, thereby minimizing the risk of vessel rupture. It is important to properly select the size of the balloon to avoid overdilation of the vessel that may lead to rupture. Inflation of the balloon without a wire in place permits leakage of contrast from the distal opening of the balloon, creating a calibrated leak balloon catheter. This technique exerts transient low pressure on the vessel wall with each inflation. Immediate deflation occurs through the distal leak in the balloon. Balloon catheters may also be inflated with a guide wire in place to increase stability in the vessel.

The technique of angioplasty for intracranial vasospasm reflects the underlying pathology of the vessel wall. The mechanism of dilation in vasospasm is believed to be stretching and disruption of connective tissue that abnormally proliferates in the vessel wall in response to subarachnoid blood. This mechanism of vessel dilation is in marked contrast to the mechanism of angioplasty of vessels affected by atherosclerosis. In atherosclerotic disease, high intraluminal pressure is needed to fracture intraluminal plaque and dilate the vessel. As noted earlier, in vasospasm, only transient low dilation pressures are necessary to accomplish angioplasty. High pressures or overdilation of intracranial vessels are dangerous and should be avoided.

Following intracranial angioplasty for vasospasm, no angiographic evidence of dissection or anatomic disruption of the vessel wall should be present (Figures 47–5 and 47–6). Restoration of normal luminal diameter and configuration is

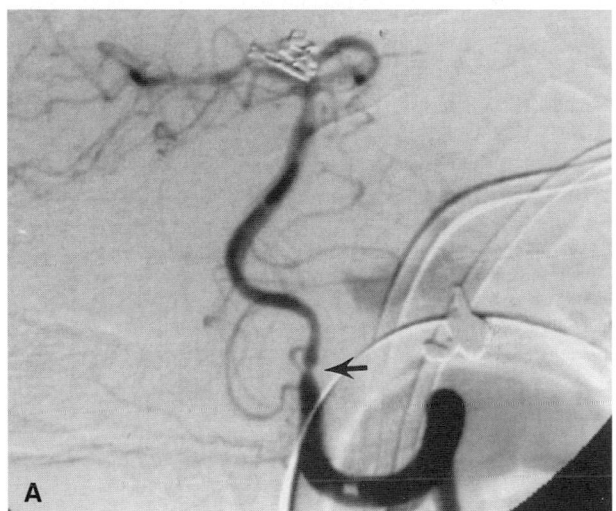

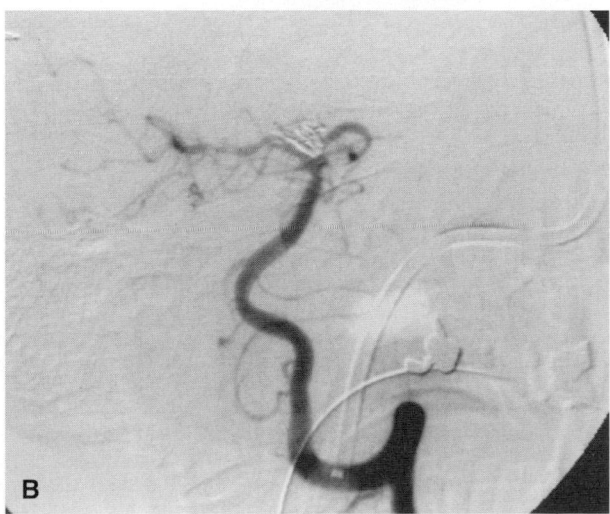

Figure 47–5 A. A 64-year-old male with new onset cranial nerve deficits and decreased level of consciousness 2 days after clipping of basilar tip aneurysm. Left vertebral artery injection shows spasm of the intracranial vertebral artery (*arrow*) and proximal basilar artery. **B.** After angioplasty, there is return of normal caliber.

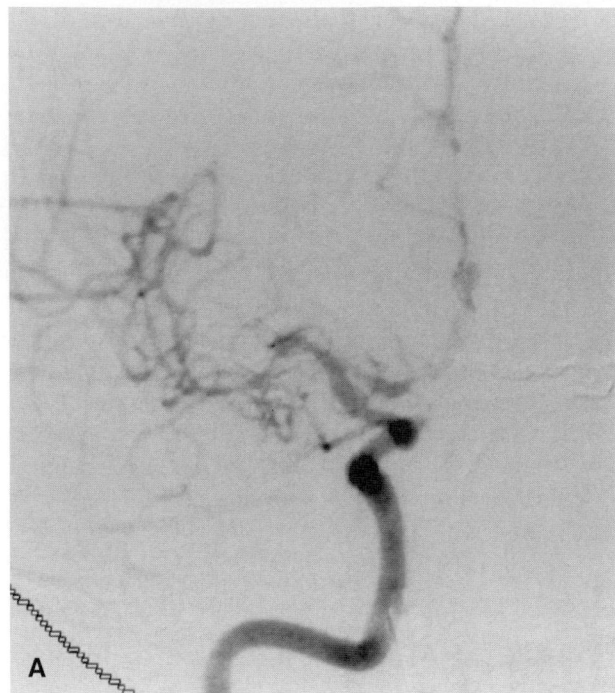

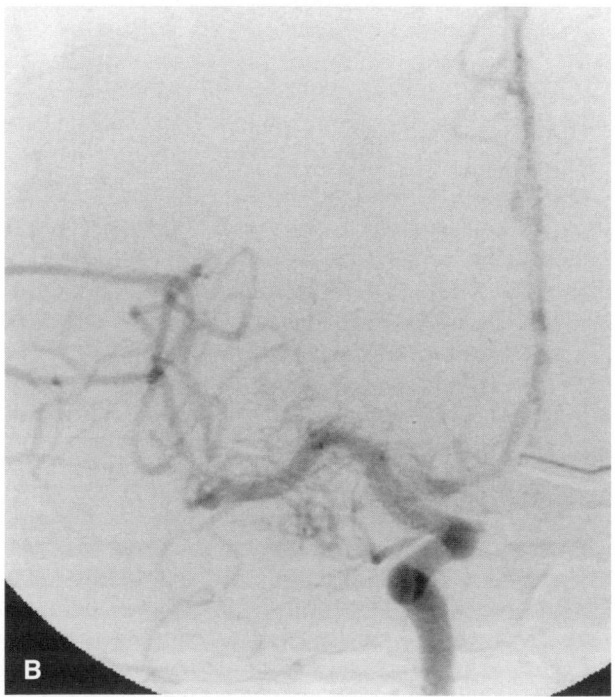

Figure 47–6 **A.** A 45-year-old female with new onset left upper extremity and left facial paresis 4 days after clipping of an anterior communicating artery aneurysm. Anteroposterior right internal carotid artery (RICA) injection shows diffuse spasm. **B.** After angioplasty, there is dilation of A_1 and M_1 segments with improved filling of distal branches.

seen throughout the treated portion of the vessel. Following treatment by angioplasty, no recurrence of vasospasm has been observed in treated segments of the vessel (57).

Intracranial angioplasty is performed in involved vessel distributions responsible for clinical deficits. Dilation using angioplasty is limited to the larger intracranial vessels including the supraclinoid ICA, intracranial vertebral arteries, basilar artery, and proximal segments of anterior, middle, and posterior cerebral arteries. Attempts to angioplasty more distal segments incur a high risk of vessel rupture with currently available balloon catheters. Angioplasty in the immediate vicinity of an aneurysm clip is also to be avoided because of the potential for clip dislodgement and the possibility of angiographically invisible wall defects that might predispose to rupture (58).

Postangioplasty, angiographic evaluation is performed to ensure that all segments of the involved vessel distribution amenable to angioplasty have been dilated. This requires filming of the vessel in anteroposterior (AP) and lateral views. Any residual segments involved by vasospasm are then dilated. Following angioplasty of proximal vessels, improved filling of the more distal portions of the distribution is usually observed.

Reported results of intracranial angioplasty indicate that significant clinical improvement may be expected in the majority of patients treated (59–61).

While generally safe, complications, including rare vessel rupture, have been reported, particularly when more distal portions of vessels are treated (53–55).

Following angioplasty, patients are monitored in the intensive care unit and hypertensive hypervolemic therapy is continued as required. Follow-up TCD is performed to confirm decreased flow velocity after dilation. Recurrent increases in flow velocity seen on follow-up TCD studies may indicate the development of new areas of spasm in previously uninvolved portions of the vessel (62).

In some cases, vasospasm involves arterial branches that cannot be selectively catheterized or more distal branches in which angioplasty is unsafe. Under these circumstances, intra-arterial infusion of vasodilating medication may be performed. Several studies have documented the effectiveness and safety of intra-arterial papaverine infusion for the treatment of vasospasm following subarachnoid hemorrhage (63,64). Selective infusion is performed directly into the involved vessel through a microcatheter (Figure 47–7). Three hundred milligrams of papaverine in 100 cc of normal saline is typically infused over 20 minutes to 1 hour. Results indicate a 65–90% success rate in dilating arterial distributions involved by vasospasm. Transient increases in heart rate, ICP, and respiratory rate may occur however during the infusion. Vital sign alterations are usually reversed by a decrease in the rate or by stoppage of the infusion. Unlike intracranial angioplasty, the effects of papaverine infusion are not necessarily permanent, and recurrent symptomatic vasospasm may develop in treated vessel distributions that require retreatment (65).

Interventional neuroradiologic treatment offers significant benefit to many patients with intracranial vasospasm who fail to respond to medical treatment. These patients would otherwise be expected to sustain severe neurologic deficits that in many cases would result in permanent disability. Early consideration and application of these methods is important for the optimal management of appropriately

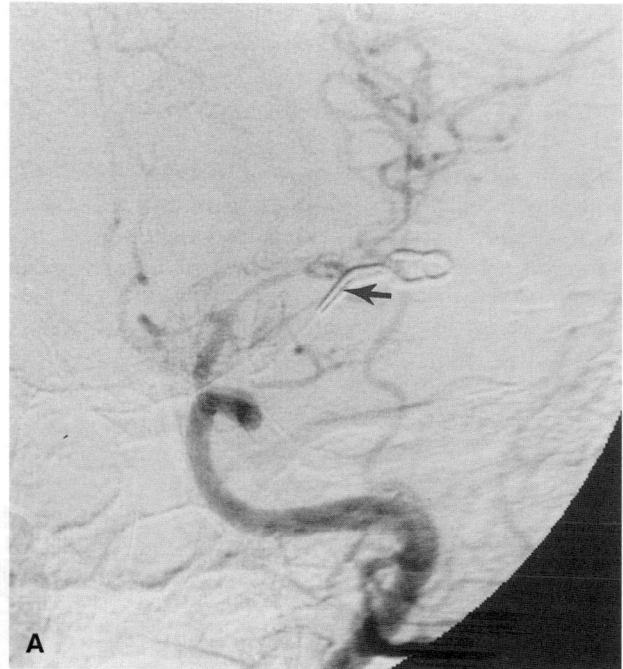

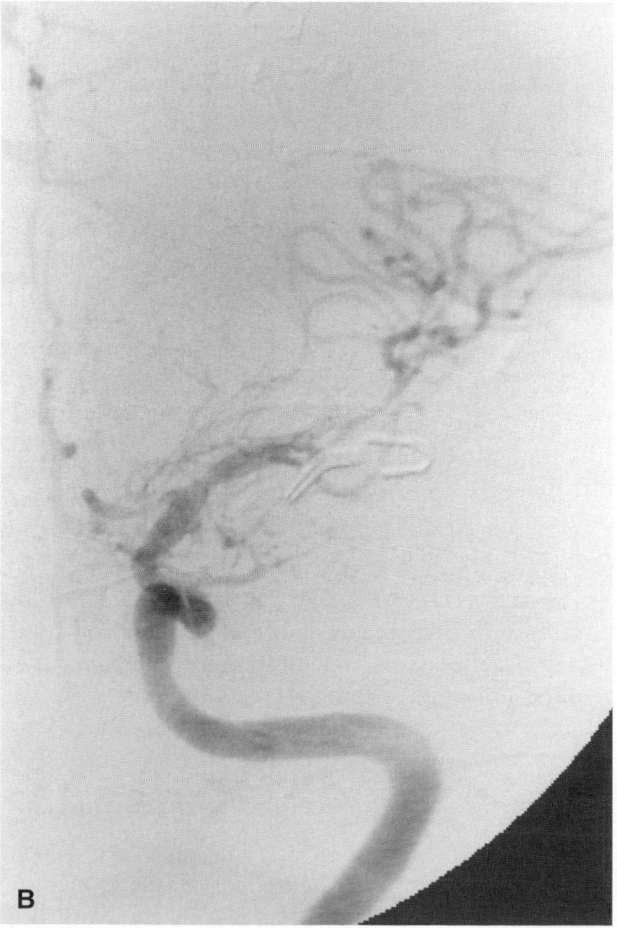

Figure 47–7 A. A 38-year-old female with new onset right hemi-paresis and aphasia 7 days after subarachnoid hemorrhage (SAH) and 6 days after clipping of a left MCA bifurcation aneurysm. Anteroposterior left internal carotid injection shows diffuse spasm involving ACA and MCA distributions (*arrow shows clip*). **B.** After angioplasty of the M₁ segment proximal to the clip followed by papaverine infusion into distal branches, there is improved filling.

selected patients with postsubarachnoid hemorrhage vasospasm.

CAROTID ARTERY ANGIOPLASTY

Atherosclerotic narrowing of the internal carotid lumen has a low incidence in the general population that increases with advancing age. In asymptomatic patients above 65 years of age, the incidence of carotid stenosis measuring ≥50% is approximately 8% (66). In patients presenting with stroke or transient ischemic attack (TIA), however, the incidence of stenosis is much higher—in the range of 30–60% (67). The clear association between atherosclerosis of the internal carotid artery (ICA) and ischemic stroke has been recognized for many years. Consequently, the anatomic correction of atherosclerotic internal carotid stenosis has long been of interest for the prevention of stroke.

Attempts to prevent stroke in the setting of ICA athero-sclerosis have focused on both medical treatment involving antiplatelet agents and anatomic correction of the carotid artery stenosis. The proven usefulness and low risk of antiplatelet therapy have made medical treatment a univer-sal component of effective preventive stroke treatment. Therefore, the potential benefit of any type of anatomic cor-rection of atherosclerotic involvement of the arterial lumen must be evaluated in addition to the benefit provided by medical treatment alone.

The two major techniques presently available for the anatomic correction of atherosclerosis of the ICA include carotid endarterectomy (CEA) and carotid angioplasty and stent placement (CAS).

At the time of this writing, several large studies support CEA as the standard technique for anatomic correction of atherosclerotic narrowing of the internal carotid artery when preventive treatment is necessary (68). The appropriate ther-apy in an individual case is, however, not a simple decision, and several caveats exist. When operators with specific levels of experience and competency with low complication rates perform CEA, the procedure has been shown conclusively to benefit patients who meet stringent clinical criteria.

The successes and shortfalls that characterize the devel-opment and current state of CEA for stroke prevention hold crucial lessons for the development and application of carotid angioplasty. To better understand the evolving role of carotid angioplasty in the prevention of stroke caused by carotid disease, it is necessary to have a good understanding of the development, its translation into clinical practice, and the current state of surgical treatment for carotid ather-osclerosis using CEA.

Carotid Endarterectomy

The history of CEA for stroke prevention began in the early 1950s. At that time, the operation was perceived as useful, and it rapidly acquired acceptance by the surgical commu-nity. By the mid-1980s, more than 100,000 CEAs were being performed in the United States every year. Nevertheless, considerable controversy continued to surround the treatment of carotid stenosis with CEA nearly 30 years after its inception. Two randomized trials published in the early 1980s that compared CEA with medical management failed to demonstrate benefit of surgical treatment (69,70). The Joint Study of Extracranial Arterial Occlusion reporting in 1970 found no benefit of CEA for prevention of stroke, and it reported an 11.4% mortality and morbidity associated with the procedure (69). A second trial also failed to show benefit and was terminated early because of a perioperative stroke-death rate of 25% (70). Despite the failure of randomized studies to demonstrate benefit, CEA remained popular in the United States because of the clinical impression many referring physicians and surgeons had that the operation was beneficial. By 1987, more than a million CEAs had been performed in the United States, and its frequency was increasing rapidly.

The existence of even moderately effective medical treatment makes the potential benefit of CEA for stroke prevention very dependent on the complication rate associated with the procedure. In fact, American Heart Association guidelines for CEA indicate that in *symptomatic* patients, the procedure is indicated only when it can be performed with a surgical complication rate of ≤6%. In *asymptomatic* patients, the acceptable complication rate is much smaller (≤3%) (71). Otherwise, the benefit of endarterectomy compared to medical treatment alone decreases significantly. This means that as complication rates associated with the procedure rise above these levels, more strokes actually result from the surgical therapy than will be prevented in the respective patient populations.

By the late 1980s, the disparity between the rising clinical practice of CEA and the lack of support for the operation in the medical literature had resulted in calls for more formal evaluation of the specific situations in which CEA might be useful for stroke prevention. These resulted in the North American Symptomatic Carotid Endarterectomy Trial, or the NASCET study (68).

The NASCET study evaluated the role of CEA in the treatment of symptomatic atherosclerotic carotid stenosis. The study incorporated several design features that differed from previous studies but ensured the validity of NASCET's conclusions:

1. NASCET ensured appropriate patient selection by requiring input from neurologists before enrollment and calling for follow-up on each patient. Patients had to be symptomatic with transient ischemic attack (TIA) or nondisabling stroke referable to the diseased artery within 120 days before patient's entry into study.
2. NASCET documented the severity of stenosis using specific NASCET critieria for angiographic measurement.
3. NASCET ensured that surgeons participating in the study had verified levels of experience and technical skill.

In the NASCET study, symptomatic patients were randomized into two groups: Members of one group were treated medically with aspirin only; members of a second group were treated with surgery and aspirin. The groups were stratified by the severity of stenosis.

The initial NASCET results, reported in 1991, showed that in the group with 70–99% stenosis, a statistically significant benefit to surgery existed. At a mean follow-up of 24 months:

- The rate of ipsilateral stroke and death in the medically treated group was 26%.
- The rate of ipsilateral stroke and death in the surgically treated group was 9%.
- The absolute benefit in the surgical group was 17%.

In other words, the initial NASCET data indicated that about six operations were necessary to prevent one stroke of *any* severity over 2 years in the symptomatic population with high-grade carotid stenosis when the NASCET criteria are met.

Of much more importance for stroke preventive treatment is its ability to prevent severe or debilitating strokes, the major reason for exposing patients to risks of preventive therapy. With respect to this critical aspect, NASCET also confirmed a statistically significant benefit in the surgical group.

At 2 years, the rate of major or fatal ipsilateral stroke in the medical group was 13.1%, while the rate in the surgical group was only 2.5%, giving an absolute benefit of 10.1% in the surgical group. That is, it requires approximately 10 carotid endarterectomies to prevent one severe stroke in this patient population.

NASCET had a surgical complication rate of 5.8% for any stroke or death; a surgical complication rate of 2.1% for severe stroke and death; and a surgical mortality rate of 0.6%. The initial NASCET results therefore confirmed that stroke preventive benefit from CEA was statistically significant. This was shown to be true however, only when the conditions of the study were met, or

When

- Patients were <80 years of age and had neurologic symptoms of TIA, transient monocular blindness, or nondisabling stroke referable to the appropriate arterial distribution within the past 4 months;

And

- Patients had angiographically documented high-grade atherosclerotic stenosis of the internal carotid artery;

And

- Patients had none of the exclusion criteria including organ failure or cancer that may likely cause death within 5 years; a large infarct of either hemisphere; neurologic syndrome x (sx) attributable to nonatherosclerotic disease such as seizure, aneurysm, tumor, or FMD; a cardiac disorder that is likely to be associated with embolic symptoms; prior CEA;

And

- Patients were evaluated by a neurologist and surgeon, both of whom agree on the appropriateness of the surgical treatment;

And

- Patients were operated on by surgeons having verified experience and technical expertise;

Then

- Patients showed a benefit from CEA, provided that the perioperative complication rate was sufficiently low.

That is, NASCET showed benefit under specifically restricted conditions that must be applied to both the individual patient and individual surgeon by an unbiased evaluation that includes a neurologist capable of such an evaluation. The NASCET results must be considered achievable when the procedure is performed under optimal conditions with objective neurologic evaluation and surgical competence.

Limiting the applicability of NASCET's initial conclusions to the symptomatic patient was also an important restriction of the study's results. The difference in prognosis between patients who are symptomatic with carotid stenosis and those who are asymptomatic is important: Symptomatic patients have a 13–16% annual risk of stroke, while those who are asymptomatic have an annual risk of only 2–2.5% (72). In addition, 45% of strokes in patients with asymptomatic stenosis are attributable to lacunar disease or cardiogenic emboli, pathophysiology that would not be expected to be influenced by correction of carotid stenosis. Therefore, the risks of treating asymptomatic patients must be lower, <3% by the AHA criteria—although there are data to suggest even lower levels are required (73)—to make the treatment beneficial in comparison with medical therapy.

Other studies attempted to show that the benefit of CEA extended to asymptomatic patients. Despite the failure of several prospective randomized studies to show a benefit of CEA in asymptomatic patients, the Asymptomatic Carotid Artery Study (ACAS) reported its results in 1995. The specifics of the study are interesting both in what they demonstrated and in what they failed to confirm:

- ACAS was a prospective randomized multicenter trial of CEA in patients with asymptomatic carotid stenosis of >60%. Exclusion criteria for ACAS were stringent and similar to those of NASCET. Of 42,000 patients screened for the study, less than 4% (1,662 of 42,000) met inclusion criteria and were randomized. Participating surgeons were also carefully screened, and 29% of those applying for participation in the study were excluded for failing to meet acceptable complication rates (74). In addition, a neurologist and surgeon were required to jointly evaluate each patient and give approval for randomization.
- Results showed that the medically treated group had a cumulative risk of any ipsilateral stroke or death over

5 years of 11% versus a 5.1% risk for the surgical group (i.e., a rate of 2% per year that was reduced to 1% per year in the surgical group). The perioperative complication rate reported in the ACAS study was quite low at 2.3%. Periprocedural mortality was also low at 0.1%.

The ACAS results confirmed a statistically significant benefit in reduction of any stroke or death, but the absolute risk reduction was small, with a reduction of risk from approximately 2% annually to 1% annually—the surgical group outcome was actually worse until after the first year. In comparison with the effects of CEA in symptomatic patients in the NASCET study, the results in the asymptomatic group would require approximately 50 operations to prevent one stroke of any severity over 2 years versus six operations to prevent one stroke of any severity in 2 years for the NASCET population of symptomatic patients. Lastly, but perhaps most importantly, there was no significant reduction of major stroke and death demonstrated in the ACAS population.

Considerable controversy continues to surround the application of CEA in asymptomatic patients (73). Following the publication of ACAS, the Canadian Stroke Consortium stated that carotid endarterectomy in asymptomatic patients could not be recommended despite the results of the ACAS study. They cited a lack of evidence that any disabling strokes are prevented by such operations and their concerns that the results of studies on asymptomatic patients were not generalizable to the overall population (75). Their concerns regarding generalizability revolved around the high standards required of the participating surgeons and the low complication rates achieved in the study.

Other authors, including those of a meta-analysis of randomized controlled trials, reached similar conclusions and also recommended against the routine application of CEA in the asymptomatic population (76). Despite these concerns and the limited benefits demonstrated by ACAS, the study is often enthusiastically embraced as being supportive of the performance of CEA on asymptomatic patients.

These points emphasize the need for caution regarding procedural treatment of carotid stenosis in most asymptomatic patients. The main purpose of preventive treatment, with its exposure of patients to attendant risk, is to prevent severe or disabling stroke. This outcome has not been demonstrated convincingly in the asymptomatic patient population.

Even more important is the often unstated but nevertheless implicit assumption that results reported in large studies can be generalized to the overall population and that the results achieved in these studies can be translated into clinical practice. How do these data, obtained from large and carefully supervised studies, compare with the results from actual clinical practice of CEA?

Certainly, the effect of the randomized trials on the numbers of CEAs performed was immediate. The frequency and rate of CEA showed prompt increases following publication of clinical trial results. The total number of procedures performed on Medicare patients more than doubled from 46,571 in 1989 to 108,275 in 1996 (77).

Unfortunately, considerable data indicate that the outcome of CEA in actual clinical practice often differs considerably from that of the randomized multicenter studies so much that many patients would be better treated medically. Evidence from several studies indicates that much higher complication rates occur in actual practice than in the recommended levels or levels found to be achievable in large randomized studies. One review of published CEA studies found complication rates exceeding 6% in 7 of the 14 studies published after the publication of NASCET (78).

A study reviewing mortality rates of Medicare CEAs—the majority of CEA patients in the United States—indicated that as late as 1996, the mortality rate for CEA among Medicare beneficiaries was nearly 2% (77). This is more than three times the mortality of the NASCET study, which showed a mortality rate of 0.6%. Because the NASCET results were obtained for a population of entirely symptomatic patients, they should therefore approximate the upper limit of acceptable mortality and morbidity values. While morbidity data were not studied in this report, the fact that in the NASCET trial the ratio of deaths to strokes was approximately 1:9 raises serious questions regarding the overall complication rate of CEA in clinical practice.

Data from the Healthcare Cost and Utilization Project found an in-hospital mortality rate of 1.2% associated with CEA, twice the mortality achieved in NASCET. Again, morbidity data were not available. Mortality increased with increasing age, from 0.9% in those younger than 65 years to 1.7% in those aged 75 and older. Mortality was also found to be markedly higher when CEA was performed as a secondary procedure (6.1%) or with any surgical complication (5.9%) (79).

Additional study of Medicare claims data found that the combined mortality and stroke rates for Medicare CEA in the United States were between 5% and 11%, a figure made even more significant by the fact that more than half of these patients were likely asymptomatic (80). Currently, most CEAs in the United States are performed on asymptomatic patients (81).

Evidence of similar, unacceptably high CEA complication rates was documented in a study of the Ontario Carotid Endarterectomy Registry. In this population of 6,038 patients, perioperative stroke and death rates were 7.3% for symptomatic patients and 4.7% for asymptomatic patients (82). Rates exceeded recommended levels for both patient populations and were similar for both male and female patients.

Another recent prospective study reviewed the practice of CEA at an academic medical center with close follow-up of patients by neurologists (83). The authors documented a 30-day 4.5% mortality rate and a 30-day stroke or death rate of 11.4%. They confirmed that with close prospective neurologic follow-up, the complication rate of CEA was

much higher than those reported in controlled clinical trials. Their results further supported the contention that the generalizability of results from clinical trials was often very limited. The authors concluded that local audits of complication rates are necessary to establish the risk-benefit ratios for individual hospitals and surgeons.

Kresowik et al. reviewed Medicare records of 10,561 CEA procedures in 10 different states to determine indications, care processes, and outcomes. Seventy-two percent of the patients were either asymptomatic or had symptoms described as "nonspecific." They found large variations in utilization rates of CEA among states as well as in combined event rates (30-day stroke or death). Event rates in asymptomatic patients, for example, ranged from 2.3% to 6.7%. They concluded that the striking variation among states indicated considerable room for improvement in the utilization, care processes, and outcomes of CEA and recommended that surgeons performing CEA participate in outcome assessment and adopt standardized protocols (84). Amazingly, in 6 of the 10 states reviewed in this large study, the procedure was actually found to be more often harmful than beneficial, with more strokes occurring than would have been expected without the procedure (85).

Outcome data therefore indicate that the results of large randomized clinical trials for stroke prevention often are not generalized effectively to the clinical practice of CEA. What are the differences in the performance of CEA in actual practice that underlie the striking differences in outcome compared to outcomes achieved in large clinical trials? Major differences include failure to objectively evaluate patients before CEA, leading to inappropriate performance of the operation and high complication rates; failure of surgeons and referring physicians to monitor complication rates associated with the procedure; and performance of CEA by surgeons with little experience and/or in hospitals with low volumes of CEAs.

Lack of Objective Patient Evaluation

A critical component of all randomized prospective studies evaluating the usefulness of CEA has been neurologic evaluation of the patients studied. The neurologist serves as an objective source of neurologic evaluation and follow-up and in all randomized studies is an integral part of the decision to operate or treat medically. Is input by a neurologist obtained in actual clinical practice as was the case in the studies on which CEA practice is supposedly based? Is neurologic input essential in patient selection and does it have an impact on reported complication rates? These questions are addressed in several studies:

One study found that only 55% of primary care physicians surveyed indicated that they would consult a patient's neurologist with what they diagnosed as a carotid TIA. The danger of this practice is highlighted by data indicating that 81% of TIA diagnoses made by primary care physicians could not be confirmed by a stroke neurologist (86). This suggests that patients with asymptomatic carotid disease often are incorrectly believed to have a symptomatic lesion in the carotid artery and be treated accordingly. An additional study concluded that the preoperative evaluation of patients with suspected carotid disease is often performed by the same physician performing the procedure without independent input or even examination by a neurologist (87). That the lack of objective neurologic consultation in the decision to perform CEA is detrimental has also been confirmed in several studies.

Rothwell, in a review of 51 published studies of CEA, found that reported complication rates varied widely depending on whether the patients were evaluated by a neurologist. Studies in which surgeons individually reported on their own patients reported relatively low mean perioperative combined stroke and death rates averaging 2.3%. In contrast, studies in which a neurologist evaluated the patients found complication rates more than three times higher, averaging 7.7% and exceeding the acceptable AHA complication rates. The authors concluded that in the absence of neurologist involvement, neurologic complications of CEA were not diagnosed and not reported (78).

These problems assume even more significance in view of the fact that the number of CEAs continues to increase, and the operation is being performed increasingly on asymptomatic patients. Proper patient selection is also exceedingly important in the asymptomatic patient population. This was highlighted in a study that evaluated 144 asymptomatic patients who had been excluded from participating in the Asymptomatic Carotid Artery Study (ACAS) because they met exclusion criteria as determined by the medical consultant/neurologist. ACAS, as with all major randomized trials, required that the neurologist *and* the surgeon agree on the appropriateness of the procedure. While the patients who were not eligible for ACAS actually had a lower average stenosis, they were more likely to have coronary artery disease, pulmonary disease, or renal disease. Despite the lack of agreement by the neurologist/consultant, these patients underwent CEA without being enrolled in ACAS. Their CEAs were performed at the same institution by the same group of surgeons during the same time frame as the ACAS study was being conducted (88).

Perioperative complication rates in this group of 144 patients included a combined stroke-death rate of 6.7% (stroke rate of 2.5% and mortality rate of 4.2%). This rate exceeded that recommended by the AHA for effective stroke prevention even in symptomatic patients. In addition, the patients suffered a rate of myocardial infarction of 6.7%. In other words, these patients, in whom objective neurologic evaluation and medical consultation had recommended against CEA, had nearly a 14% rate of serious complications for the treatment of an asymptomatic condition. This should be compared with the 2.3% stroke-death rate reported in the ACAS study in which the consultant recommendation and exclusion criteria were followed. The

authors concluded that their results "reinforced the value of joint evaluation by medical and surgical specialists in patient selection for this procedure (88)."

Clearly, a lack of objective neurologic evaluation in patients under consideration for CEA increases the risk of inappropriate procedures and the risk of complications should such procedures be performed. In addition, little or no monitoring of actual CEA complication rates seems to be the rule. In a nationwide study, only 15% of physicians knew the actual CEA complication rate at the hospital at which they practice or refer patients. Only 50% of neurologists and 60% of surgeons reported that they were familiar with these rates (89). In another study, only 50% of surgery residency programs indicated that they systematically monitored CEA complication rates and were able to report specific rates at their institutions (87).

Complication rates in clinical practice are, therefore, difficult to ascertain and are often not monitored. In addition, complications other than stroke and death are not reported as endpoints of studies and are, therefore, often not considered in the risk-benefit equation. Nevertheless, data indicate that the frequency of uniquely surgical complications is considerable. NASCET, for example, reported 7.6% cranial nerve complications, 5.5% wound hematoma, 3.4% wound infection, and cardiac complications totaling 3.9% (MI, CHF, arrhythmia, and others) for a rate of 20.4% of these nonendpoint complications, virtually all of which are related to the operative procedure. Other large studies have reported significant nonneurologic complication rates (particularly cardiac) at 6.7–8.9% (88).

Large randomized trials of CEA recognized the association of surgical excellence and outcome. They emphasized the importance of training, skill, and experience and demanded minimum standards for participating centers and surgeons. NASCET required demonstrated mortality and morbidity rates of less than 6% for the prior 50 CEAs. ACAS required demonstrated mortality and morbidity rates of less than 3% for asymptomatic patients and <5% for all patients for 50 CEAs. Surgeons were required to perform more than 12 CEAs per year.

Recent data indicate that actual performance of CEA is too often done by surgeons or at institutions that fail to meet standards that would be required for participation in randomized trials. A large study evaluated carotid endarterectomy in California and New York and in the Canadian province of Ontario (90). The authors confirmed a dramatic resurgence in the rates of the procedure from 1989 to 1995 following the publication of favorable clinical studies. They found however, that these increased rates were not associated with proportionally greater numbers of referrals of patients to hospitals with low mortality rates. In addition, mortality rates at many hospitals were substantially higher than rates reported in NASCET and ACAS. Although during the period from 1990 to 1995 an increasing number of surgeons performed CEA, the authors confirmed relatively low volumes by many CEA surgeons. For example, half of CEA surgeons in New York performed five or fewer procedures per year, and only 27% performed more than 15 cases per year. The authors concluded that the absence of selective referral of patients to centers with the lowest mortality rates raised questions about whether the benefits of carotid endarterectomy in the general population are similar to those demonstrated in the clinical trials.

Recent data regarding mortality and morbidity of CEA surgeons in Pennsylvania also found that low surgical volume predicted a bad outcome rate. Surgeons performing low volumes of CEA were common with 23% performing fewer than two CEAs per year and nearly half doing fewer than the 12 per year that was required for ACAS participation. Less than 4% of Pennsylvania CEA surgeons performed more than 50 CEAs per year (91). Therefore, anatomic correction of carotid stenosis with CEA has been shown in carefully conducted trials to confer lasting benefits in selected patients, but CEA as it is presently practiced in North America differs substantially from that validated by randomized prospective studies. In fact, data indicate that the actual state of CEA performance today often fails to meet even the minimum mortality and morbidity standards set by the AHA for symptomatic patients. Major differences exist in terms of evaluation procedures followed, patients treated, surgeons treating, and most importantly, complication rates. As shown by the studies just mentioned, these discrepancies undoubtedly are detrimental to the overall effectiveness of CEA as it is currently practiced for the prevention of stroke. For many patients undergoing CEA, this raises significant concerns about its beneficial effects.

These comments are not meant to discourage the application of CEA under appropriate circumstances. In fact, CEA remains the objective standard for anatomic correction of carotid stenosis against which other treatments, including carotid angioplasty and stenting, must be validated. Nevertheless, the considerable shortfalls and failures that currently characterize the actual clinical application of CEA provide important lessons that must be incorporated into the evaluation and application of carotid angioplasty if it is to provide effective preventive treatment of stroke.

Carotid Angioplasty

Carotid angioplasty has a considerably shorter history than CEA—it was first performed in 1980. Despite widespread application of angioplasty for correction of arterial stenosis throughout the peripheral and coronary circulation, the application of the procedure in the carotid artery was delayed because of concern for ischemic complications affecting the CNS.

There is ample reason for concern because performing a procedure on the carotid artery is, in effect, performing a procedure on the brain, which is an organ less tolerant of ischemia and the effect of emboli than any other. Potential effects of ischemia from even small emboli are significant.

This potential danger is illustrated by the number of proximally originating CNS arteries that can be occluded by emboli that are less than 1 mm in diameter and that may give rise to debilitating neurologic deficits. Such vessels include the ophthalmic artery, the anterior choroidal artery, and perforating arteries originating from the anterior and middle cerebral arteries.

In addition, the initial presentation of devastating neurologic deficits, including aphasia and other higher cortical deficits, is often subtle and enhances the risk posed by the vulnerable configuration of the cerebrovascular anatomy. Because any type of nonclinical monitoring is ineffective at detecting neurologic deficits, this means that careful clinical neurologic examination by competent personnel must be conducted throughout the procedure.

Consequently, physicians performing carotid angioplasty should be prepared to clinically identify and treat the most likely and potentially devastating complication—intracranial emboli—using intra-arterial thrombolysis or other endovascular treatment when necessary.

That the procedure is not benign when performed without high levels of training and safeguards is illustrated by the first reported randomized study comparing the results of CEA with carotid angioplasty. This study randomized 23 patients to CEA or carotid angioplasty. The carotid angioplasties were performed by an operator who had "more than 5,000 peripheral angioplasties to his experience." Of the seven patients randomized to angioplasty, five suffered complications. The results caused premature termination of the study and the conclusion by the authors that angioplasty was too dangerous for preventive treatment of stroke (92). Subsequent correspondence to the journal emphasized that regardless of the experience of the operator in performing angioplasty in the peripheral or coronary circulations, safety considerations are unacceptable without documented experience with intervention in the carotid artery (93).

While this early small study might be dismissed as not relevant for overall practice, the lessons of excessive carotid angioplasty complication rates and their potential to eliminate benefits for stroke prevention should raise concern. The concern is underlined by another trial of angioplasty and stenting, the Wallstent trial, which was also stopped prematurely because of a 12.2% ipsilateral stroke rate at 1 year (94).

In addition, the publication of the Carotid and Vertebral Artery Transluminal Angioplasty Study (CAVATAS) further reinforces the need for caution in the application of carotid angioplasty (95). CAVATAS compared CEA to carotid angioplasty with or without stenting. Five hundred four patients with carotid stenosis were randomly assigned to either carotid angioplasty ($n = 251$) or CEA ($n = 253$) in a multicenter trial. Minimal specific training was required for operators performing angioplasty within the trial, and CEAs were performed by surgeons credentialed at each participating institution. Twenty-six percent of the endovascular group were stented, the rest received angioplasty alone. The study found no significant differences between endovascular treatment and angioplasty treatment. However, outcomes for both treatments were poor, with rates of stroke lasting more than 7 days or death of 10% for endovascular treatment and 9.9% for CEA. These results exceed the recommended AHA outcomes for stroke preventive treatment. Had surgical outcomes not been so poor, the study would likely have been stopped early (96). Unfortunately, as seen by the data on CEA earlier, the CEA results reported in CAVATAS likely mirror those in actual clinical practice.

Because only a minority of CAVATAS patients (26%) who underwent angioplasty was stented, the results are not directly comparable to randomized carotid angioplasty and stent trials currently underway. Nevertheless, available data reinforce the fact that when not properly performed, carotid angioplasty with or without stent placement has the potential to cause excessive complications and to expend immense sums of money with little benefit for stroke prevention and the potential for doing considerable harm.

Similar to the experience of CEA, it is likely that carotid angioplasty and stenting will be found most effective when strict standards of practice, training, and experience are applied. The specific aspects of the procedure are currently under development and evaluation in a number of large randomized studies. Current information suggests the following:

Technique

Careful history and neurologic examination are essential. Although criteria vary for patient enrollment into randomized studies, patients with symptomatic disease at high risk for stroke who are also at high risk for CEA might be expected to receive the most benefit. During randomized trials, neurologic consultation is required although the experience with CEA supports the importance of objective neurologic evaluation and follow-up in clinical practice outside of trails.

The medical component of treatment remains crucial for procedural success. Patients undergoing carotid angioplasty and stenting (CAS) are generally placed on antiplatelet therapy with two medications, usually aspirin and clopidogrel, for at least 48 hours before the procedure. In cases of urgent treatment in patients not currently on treatment, a loading dose of clopidogrel may be administered.

Maximizing the medical component of treatment in conjunction with CAS remains an active area of research, and several additional medications are currently under evaluation. Attempts to decrease the frequency of ischemic events with the use of abciximab, a platelet glycoprotein IIb/IIIa receptor inhibitor, have not initially shown success, and in addition, increased numbers of intracranial hemorrhages have occurred (97).

Proper angiographic equipment is essential for safe and efficient performance of the procedure. Biplane fluoroscopic equipment facilitates multiple views of the extracranial and intracranial vasculature while minimizing contrast use. Subtracted fluoroscopy aids in precise location of the lesion and becomes a critical requirement should intra-arterial thrombolysis become necessary.

A diagnostic angiogram is first performed to identify the lesion and to exclude significant distal carotid or intracranial disease. Examination of the contralateral side should also be available including the intracranial vasculature and collateral routes involving the Circle of Willis.

An 80–90 cm 5 French to 7 French sheath is placed into the common carotid artery. The sheath provides stability for the angioplasty, particularly in the face of proximal arterial tortuosity and aortic arch disease. In addition, a sheath of appropriate size permits simple exchange of catheters and guide wires and permits good visualization of even the intracranial vasculature with contrast injection.

At the time of catheterization of the common carotid artery, heparin is given in sufficient dose to raise the ACT to 300–350 seconds.

Depending on the device used, the lesion is crossed with a 0.014–0.018-inch wire followed by a balloon catheter. Frequently, predilation of high-grade stenosis, usually to 3 or 4 mm, is necessary before stent placement. Predilation may also be necessary before placement of those cerebral protection devices currently available (Figure 47–8).

Cerebral protection devices are designed to decrease the rate of neurologic complications by preventing emboli from reaching the intracranial vasculature. Initial studies used a nondetachable balloon placed distally in the cervical internal carotid artery before dilation of carotid stenosis (98). Newer devices consist of expandable mesh or nets designed to trap emboli while permitting uninterrupted blood flow through the vessel. The devices are often incorporated onto an exchange-length guide wire (99). The distal tip of the wire, on which the device is mounted, is placed distal to the lesion. Following deployment of the device, dilation and stent placement are performed using the guide wire. After dilation and stenting, the device is withdrawn, removing any emboli released from the lesion. The role of cerebral protection devices remains under investigation, and the use of these devices has been incorporated into several carotid stent trials.

Preliminary data indicate that the use of cerebral protection devices may decrease the incidence of embolic neurologic deficits associated with CA (100). Nevertheless, currently available devices are often limited in their usefulness by their relatively high profile that may require predilation to permit placement distal to the stenotic lesion. In addition, the relative stiffness of currently available devices may cause spasm or even dissection of the vessel, especially in tortuous carotid arteries.

Dilation of the area of stenosis using an angioplasty balloon is performed while maintaining wire access across the lesion. The angioplasty balloon is removed, and the stent is deployed. Relatively slow inflation and deflation of the balloon has been suggested to minimize the production of emboli.

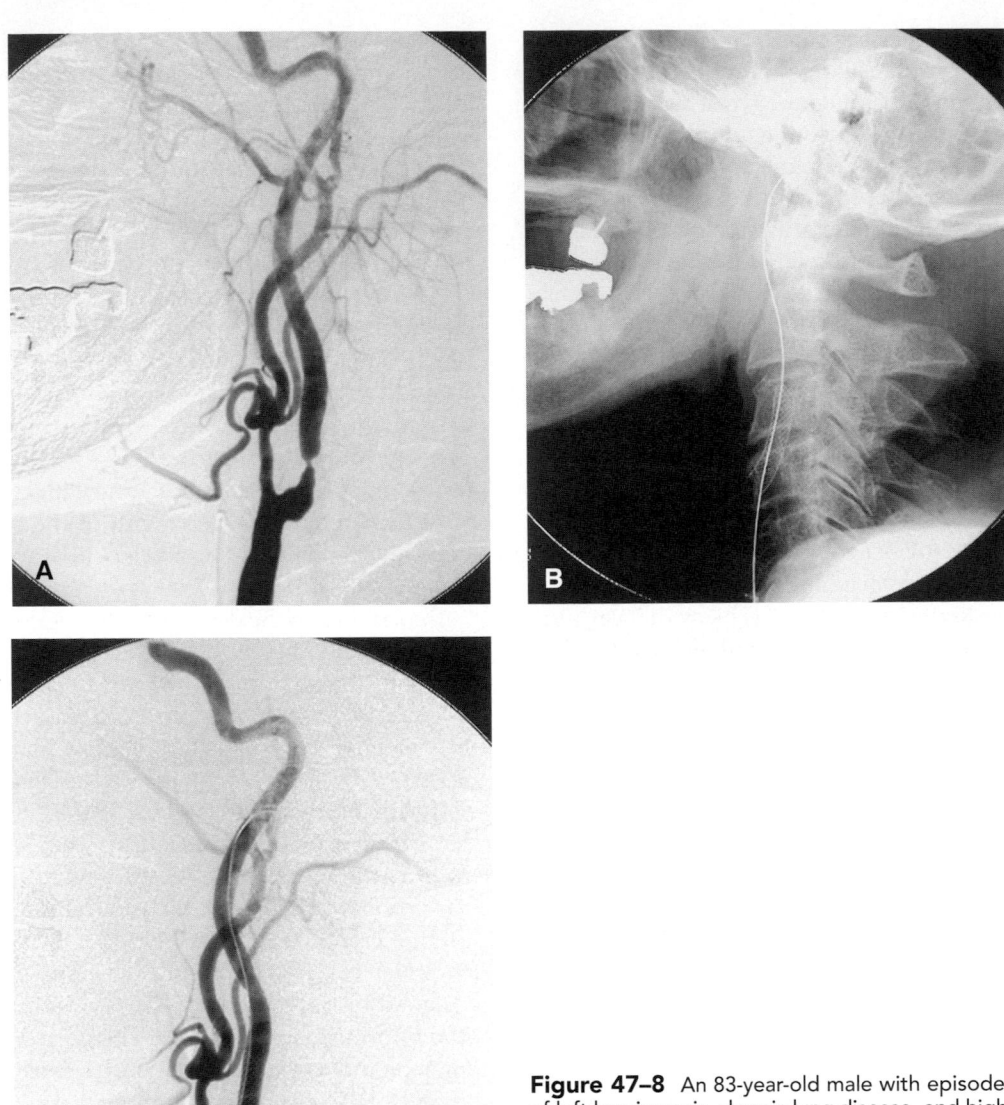

Figure 47–8 An 83-year-old male with episodes of left hemiparesis, chronic lung disease, and high-grade right internal carotid artery (RICA) stenosis. **A.** Lateral view of the right common carotid artery demonstrates high-grade stenosis involving the proximal RICA. **B.** After crossing the lesion and predilating to 3 mm, a self-expanding stent is deployed. **C.** Poststent angiogram demonstrates restoration of lumen diameter.

Stents usually used for carotid angioplasty are of the self-expanding type. The distal end of the stent is placed just distal to the diseased area, and the device is deployed proximally, often with the crossing of the common carotid bifurcation with the proximal end of the stent within the distal common carotid artery. Covering the origin of the external carotid artery by the stent has not been shown to cause detrimental effects. Currently available stents come in several sizes, with some tapering from a smaller distal to a larger proximal diameter for best fit across the common carotid bifurcation.

Following stent placement, poststent dilation is usually performed. High pressures are to be avoided, and the balloon should be inflated and deflated slowly to minimize emboli. Care is taken to ensure that the balloon remains within the stent to prevent dissection of the vessel distal to the stent.

After stent placement, angiography is performed to visualize both the stented area and the intracranial vasculature. The intracranial vessels are examined carefully for delay in filling, vessel cutoffs, or parenchymal staining that might indicate intracranial emboli. Neurologic examination at frequent intervals throughout the procedure is essential. Any delay in detection of neurologic deficits can minimize or eliminate treatment options and contribute to permanent neurologic morbidity. The development of any new neurologic deficit requires immediate angiographic evaluation of the extracranial carotid artery as well as the intracranial circulation. After the procedure, the sheath is removed and the patient is closely observed for neurologic changes before being discharged.

Because patients undergoing carotid angioplasty and stenting often have coexisting vascular disease, the type and duration of posttreatment antiplatelet therapy must be individualized. Treatment with two antiplatelet medications usually is maintained for at least several months, after which a single medication may be adequate.

Results and Recommendations

Carotid angioplasty continues to benefit from rapid advances in the design and manufacture of endovascular devices. This means that devices considered for routine use undergo modification or replacement within relatively short time frames. Although the process is designed to enhance the effectiveness, ease, and safety of the procedure, the rapid pace of changes in device design makes evaluation difficult. The evolving technology makes carotid angioplasty a "moving target" in terms of the current best devices and techniques available.

In addition, it is evident from the earlier discussion that relatively small differences in both periprocedural and long-term outcome can have a major impact on the conclusion that a procedural treatment is useful for stroke prevention. Because CAS must be compared to CEA, large numbers of procedures must be studied in order to discern a benefit of one in comparison to the other. The effect is particularly evident on attempts to determine the long-term effects of CAS, and it has created problems in the design of large studies that typically extend over a period of years.

These considerations mean that the indications for carotid angioplasty are currently under development, although available data indicate potentially significant benefit for a number of patient groups. Although no multicenter prospective randomized comparison studies of CAS have been completed, early partial results as well as data from single center studies are becoming increasingly available and provide valuable information on which to base clinical management of patients.

In one of the earliest large studies, Theron et al. reported a total of 259 angioplasties over a 12-year period. Ninety-three were performed during a 5-year period (1990–1995) with relatively uniform technique and stent placement in 65 patients. In this latter group, a 2% complication rate with a 4% restenosis rate was reported by this experienced group (101). More recently, Kao et al. reported on CAS in 118 patients with a mean age of 72.8 years, with 129 narrowed carotid arteries. The mean pretreatment diameter stenosis was 85% and final residual diameter stenosis 14%. The periprocedural stroke and death rate was 4.2%, and the restenosis rate was 3.1% (102).

Several studies have attempted to evaluate safety and efficacy of carotid angioplasty and stenting (CAS) in patient populations, with conditions associated with increased risk of complications from CEA. Patients include those with medical comorbidity, prior carotid endarterectomy, or carotid stenosis associated with cervical irradiation (Figure 47–9). Yadav et al. studied 107 high-risk patients with prior CEA and medical comorbidity. Rates of all stroke or death were 7.9%; the ipsilateral major stroke/death rate was 1.6%. At 6 months, the investigators found a 4.9% rate of asymptomatic restenosis (103).

Shawl also reported on carotid artery stenting (CAS) in 299, predominantly high-risk patients, 70% of whom would have been excluded from the major trials of CEA. Risk factors included unstable angina, previous ipsilateral CEA, contralateral carotid occlusion, and other severe comorbid illnesses. Twenty-five percent of the patients were aged 80 years or more. Within 30 days post-CAS, there were two (0.6%) major and seven (2.3%) minor strokes. At a mean follow-up period of 26 ± 13 months, 2.7% had asymptomatic restenosis. The authors concluded that CAS can be performed even in high-risk patients with reasonable complication rates and low rates of restenosis (104).

Alric et al. studied 21 patients, 4 with radiation-induced carotid stenoses and 17 with postsurgical restenoses. They reported technical success in 91%. No complications were encountered in the periprocedural period, and no neurologic events were observed during a mean follow-up of 16.6 months (105). Bonaldi also treated 71 patients with cervical carotid bifurcation stenoses by angioplasty, stenting, or both. The stenosis was atherosclerotic in 61 cases, postsurgical or postradiation in 10 cases. Complications included three minor strokes with complete regression of neurologic deficits (4.2%) and one major stroke (1.4%). At follow-up of at least 1 year for 50 patients, the authors reported restenosis of less than 50% occurred in four (8%) (106).

Ross reported on 33 patients who had 35 procedures for recurrent carotid stenosis, 11 of whom were symptomatic and 24 asymptomatic. The 30-day major stroke rate was 2.4%, and the overall 30-day stroke and transient ischemic attack (TIA) rate was 7.3%. While these rates would be considered excessive for primary treatment of a predominantly asymptomatic population, the increased risk of CEA in patients with restenosis as noted earlier, further highlights CAS as a potentially useful option in this patient population (107).

As experience with CAS grows, studies of restenosis become increasingly important. Rates have been reported (above) in conjuction with a number of studies and appear reasonable. In a large single-center experience which specifically addressed restenosis after carotid stent placement, Willfort-Ehringer et al. found a 3% restenosis rate at 1 year in 303 arteries treated with self-expanding stents. They found that restenosis could most often be treated safely by additional angioplasty (108).

As noted above, the use of cerebral protection devices to prevent emboli to intracranial vessels is an attractive technique with the potential to decrease complications from

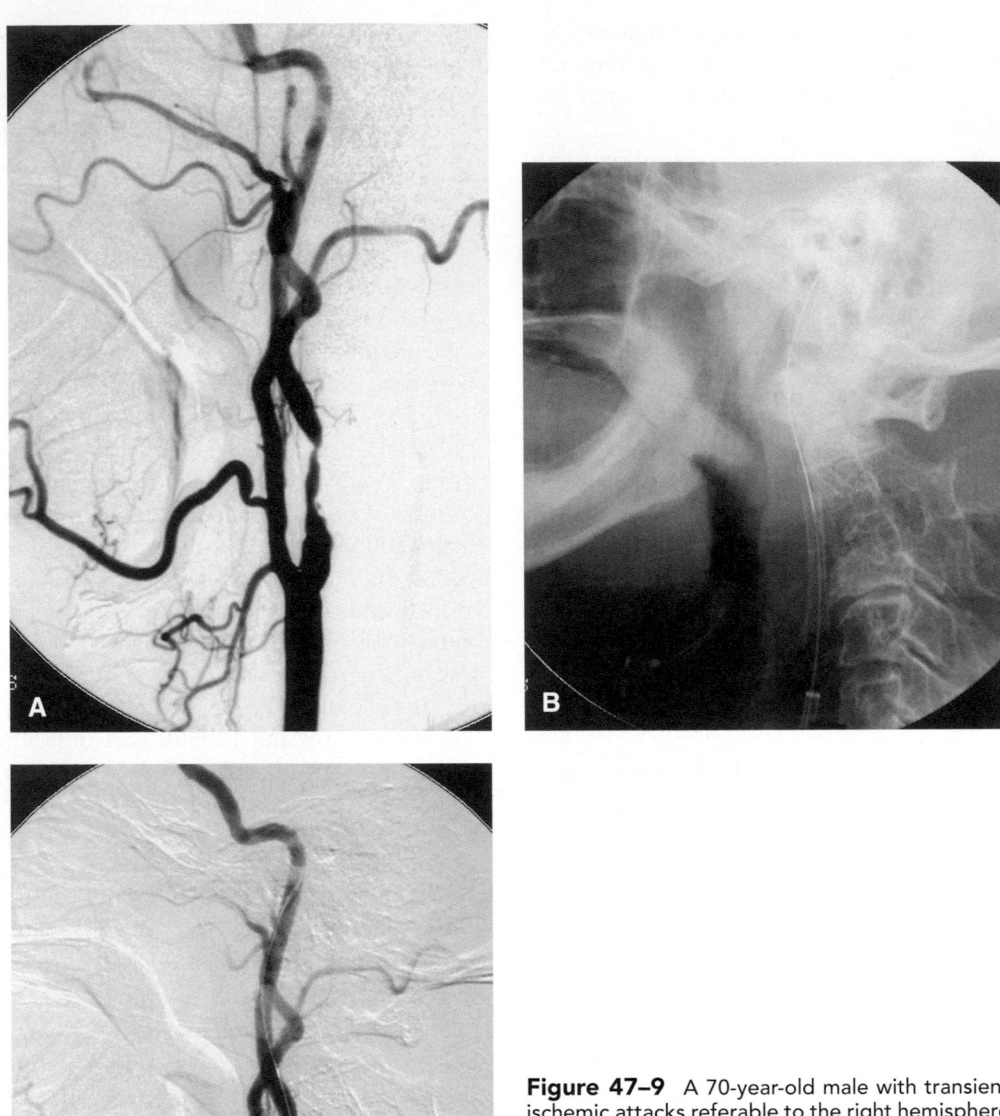

Figure 47–9 A 70-year-old male with transient ischemic attacks referable to the right hemisphere who is status quo after radiation therapy of the neck for squamous cell carcinoma more than 15 years ago. **A.** Lateral view of the right common carotid artery injection demonstrates irregular segmental narrowing of the internal carotid artery just distal to the carotid bulb. **B.** Unsubtracted lateral view after stent placement. **C.** Poststent angiogram of the right common carotid artery showing reopening of lumen.

CAS. Much information regarding performance of cerebral protection devices is currently under evaluation in large multicenter trials, the results of which are not currently available. Nevertheless, data from single center experiences and reviews suggest the potential benefit of these devices. Kastrup et al. looked at comparative outcomes of CAS with and without the use of cerebral protection devices. They systematically reviewed published studies reporting on the incidence of minor stroke, major stroke, or death within 30 days after CAS. A total of 2,537 procedures without protection devices and 896 procedures with protection devices were reviewed. They found that reported combined stroke and death rates in both symptomatic and asymptomatic patients was 1.8% in patients treated with cerebral protection devices compared with 5.5% in patients treated without cerebral protection devices. They noted that the improved outcome was primarily because of a decrease in minor strokes, which were reported in 3.7% without cerebral protection versus 0.5% with cerebral protection and the incidence of major strokes that occurred in 1.1% without cerebral protection versus 0.3% with cerebral protection. Death rates were almost identical at 0.8%. They concluded that the use of cerebral protection devices appears to reduce thromboembolic complications during CAS (100).

Guimaraens et al. reported 194 carotid stenting procedures in 164 patients with the use of cerebral protection devices. Ninety-two percent of patients were symptomatic. These authors reported a morbidity rate of 1.03% and mortality rate of 1.9% (109).

Perioperative results of 307 patients randomized in the Stenting and Angioplasty with Protection in Patients at High Risk for Endarterectomy (SAPPHIRE) Trial have been presented although not published (110). Perioperative stroke and death rates were 4.4% for patients treated with carotid angioplasty and stenting and 7.3% for those undergoing CEA. When only asymptomatic patients were considered, however, a stroke and death rate of 5.8% for carotid angioplasty and stenting was found, while that for CEA was 6.1%. Although not statistically significant, both of the latter values exceed recommended levels for treatment of patients with asymptomatic carotid disease (110).

Preliminary results of studies on carotid angioplasty and stent placement indicate that complication rates within acceptable ranges for effective stroke prevention are likely achievable, at least for patients who have symptomatic carotid disease. Nevertheless, the lessons learned from the development of CEA must be applied in the evaluation of all patients for stroke preventive treatment, including CAS. These lessons include:

- The difference in prognosis, treatment implications, and acceptable complication rates between symptomatic and asymptomatic carotid stenosis
- The importance of appropriately low complication rates to the benefits of the procedure
- The necessity for neurologic consultation in all patients to select the population most likely to benefit and to determine outcomes
- The importance of knowing complication rates of the individual institutions and physicians involved in the treatment

Carotid angioplasty is a logical and promising technique currently under development, study, and increasing clinical application for the anatomic correction of atherosclerotic stenosis of the internal carotid artery to prevent stroke. The ongoing evaluation of carotid angioplasty supports a significant role for the procedure in the preventive treatment of stroke resulting from carotid atherosclerosis. Data currently available suggest that carotid angioplasty will be useful in many patients, particularly those who are not ideal surgical candidates for the preventive treatment of stroke because of ICA stenosis. At the present time, carotid stenting should be restricted to patients involved in clinical trials and to high-risk candidates for carotid endarterectomy. Such patients include those with medical comorbidities, previous neck surgeries or radiation, restenosis after endarterectomy, or other technical contraindications for surgery (111). A full evaluation of the role of CAS will require additional study to determine the optimal patient population, to select the safest and most efficacious techniques, and to determine the value of the procedure's contribution to actual stroke prevention.

SUMMARY

Interventional neuroradiologic procedures including thrombolysis, angioplasty, and pharmacologic vasodilation have been shown to be of immense benefit in preventing the development of ischemic stroke and restoring blood flow to ischemic regions of the CNS. While still evolving, these procedures promise continued expansion of therapeutic alternatives in areas of therapy that have, in the past, been extremely limited.

REFERENCES

1. Mohr JP, Caplan LR, Melski JW, et al. The Harvard cooperative stroke registry: A prospective registry. Neurology 1978;28:754–762.
2. Fieschi C, Argentino C, Lenzi GL, et al. Clinical and instrumental evaluation of patients with ischemic stroke within the first six hours. J Neurol Sci 1989;91:311–321.
3. Sloan MA. Thrombolysis and stroke. Past and future. Arch Neurol 1987;44:748–768.
4. Saito I, Segawa H, Shiokawa Y, et al. Middle cerebral artery occlusion: correlation of computed tomography and angiography with clinical outcome. Stroke 1987;18:863–868.
5. Coull B, Briley D. Outcome and rehabilitation in ischemic stroke. In: Awad I, ed. Cerebrovascular Occlusive Disease and Brain Ischemia. Illinois: AANS Publications Committee, 1992:265–280.
6. Astrup J, Siesjo BK, Symon L. Thresholds in cerebral ischemia–the ischemic penumbra. Stroke 1981;12:723–725.
7. Olsen TS, Larsen B, Herning M, et al. Blood flow and vascular reactivity in collaterally perfused brain tissue. Evidence of an ischemic penumbra in patients with acute stroke. Stroke 1983;14:332–341.
8. Jones TH, Morawetz RB, Crowell RM, et al. Thresholds of focal cerebral ischemia in awake monkeys. J Neurosurg 1981;54:773–782.
9. Weinstein PR, Anderson GG, Telles DA. Neurological deficit and cerebral infarction after temporary middle cerebral artery occlusion in unanesthetized cats. Stroke 1986;17:318–24.
10. Baird AE, Donnan GA, Austin MC, et al. Early reperfusion in the "spectacular shrinking deficit" demonstrated by single-photon emission computed tomography. Neurology. 1995;45:1335–1339.
11. Marchal G, Serrati C, Rioux P, et al. PET imaging of cerebral perfusion and oxygen consumption in acute ischaemic stroke: relation to outcome. Lancet 1993;341:925–927.
12. Theron J, Courtheoux P, Casasco A, et al. Local intra-arterial fibrinolysis in the carotid territory. AJNR Am J Neuroradiol 1989;10:753–765.
13. Teal PA, Pessin MS. Hemorrhagic transformation. The spectrum of ischemia-related brain hemorrhage. Neurosurg Clin N Am 1992;3:601–610.
14. Liebeskind A, Chinichian A, Schechter MM. The moving embolus seed during serial cerebral angiography. Stroke 1971;2:440–443.
15. Dalal PM, Shah PM, Sheth SC, et al. Cerebral embolism. angiographic observations on spontaneous clot lysis. Lancet 1965;42:61–64.
16. Lodder J. CT-detected hemorrhagic infarction: relation with the size of the infarct and the presence of midline shift. Acta Neurol Scand 1984;70:329–335.
17. Okada Y, Yamaguchi T, Minematsu K, et al. Hemorrhagic transformation in cerebral embolism. Stroke 1989;20:598–603.
18. Pessin MS, del Zoppo GJ, Estol CJ. Thrombolytic agents in the treatment of stroke. Clin Neuropharmacol 1990;13:271–289.
19. Weisberg LA. Nonseptic cardiogenic cerebral embolic stroke: clinical-CT correlations. Neurology 1985;35:896–869.
20. Hornig C, Dorndorf W, Agnoli A. Hemorrhagic cerebral infarction: a prospective study. Stroke 1986;17:174–185.
21. Levine S, Brott T. Thrombolytic therapy in cerebrovascular disorders. Prog Cardiovasc Dis 1992;34:235–262.
22. Mori E, Tabuchi M, Yoshida T, et al. Intracarotid urokinase with thromboembolic occlusion of the middle cerebral artery. Stroke 1988;19:802–812.

23. Sussman B, Fitch T. Thrombolysis with fibrinolysin in cerebral arterial occlusion. JAMA 1958;167:1705–1709.

24. Meyer JS, Gilroy J, Barnhart MI, et al. Anticoagulants plus streptokinase therapy in progressive stroke. JAMA 1964;189:373.

25. Tissue plasminogen activator for acute ischemic stroke. The National Institute of Neurological Disorders and Stroke rt-PA Stroke Study Group. N Engl J Med 1995;333:1581–1587.

26. Fagan SC, Morgenstern LB, Petitta A, et al. Cost-effectiveness of tissue plasminogen activator for acute ischemic stroke. NINDS rt-PA Stroke Study Group. Neurology 1998;50:883–890.

27. del Zoppo GJ, Ferbert A, Otis S, et al. Local intra-arterial fibrinolytic therapy in acute carotid territory stroke. A pilot study. Stroke 1988;19:307–313.

28. Hacke W, Zeumer H, Ferbert A, et al. Intra-arterial thrombolytic therapy improves outcome in patients with acute vertebrobasilar occlusive disease. Stroke 1988;19:1216–1222.

29. Furlan A, Higashida R, Wechsler L, et al. Intra-arterial prourokinase for acute ischemic stroke. The PROACT II study: a randomized controlled trial. Prolyse in Acute Cerebral Thromboembolism. JAMA 1999;282:2003–2011.

30. Saver JL. Intra-arterial thrombolysis. Neurology 2001;57(Suppl II):S58–S60.

31. Schellinger PD, Fiebach JB, Mohr A, et al. Thrombolytic therapy for ischemic stroke—a review. Part II—Intra-arterial thrombolysis, vertebrobasilar stroke, phase IV trials, and stroke imaging. Crit Care Med 2001;29:1819–1825.

32. Jungreis C, Wechsler L, Horton J. Intracranial thrombolysis via a catheter embedded in the clot. Stroke 1989;20:1578–1580.

33. Zeumer H, Freitag HJ, Grzyska U, et al. Local intra-arterial fibrinolysis in acute vertebrobasilar occlusion. Technical developments and recent results. Neuroradiology 1989;31:336–340.

34. Wardlaw JM, Warlow CP. Thrombolysis in acute ischemic stroke: does it work? Stroke 1992;23:1826–1839.

35. Lewandowski CA, Frankel M, Tomsick TA, et al. Combined intravenous and intra-arterial r-TPA versus intra-arterial therapy of acute ischemic stroke: Emergency Management of Stroke (EMS) Bridging Trial. Stroke 1999;30:2598–25605.

36. Egan R. Efficacy of intra-arterial thrombolysis of basilar artery stroke. J Stroke Cereb Vas Dis 1999;8:22–27.

37. Becker KJ, Monsein LH, Ulatowski J, et al. Intra-arterial thrombolysis in vertebrobasilar occlusion. AJNR Am J Neuroradiol 1996;17:255–262.

38. Harper GD, Haigh RA, Potter JF, et al. Factors delaying hospital admission after stroke in Leicestershire. Stroke 1992;23:835–838.

39. Findlay JM, Macdonald RL, Weir BK. Current concepts of pathophysiology and management of cerebral vasospasm following aneurysmal subarachnoid hemorrhage. Cerebrovasc Brain Metab Rev 1991;3:336–361.

40. Mayberg MR, Okada T, Bark DH. Morphologic changes in cerebral arteries after subarachnoid hemorrhage. Neurosurg Clin N Am 1990;1:417–432.

41. Barker FG II, Heros RC. Clinical aspects of vasospasm. Neurosurg Clin N Am 1990;1:277–288.

42. Kistler JP, Crowell RM, Davis KR, et al. The relation of cerebral vasospasm to the extent and location of subarachnoid blood visualized by CT scan: a prospective study. Neurology 1983;33:424–436.

43. Adams HP Jr, Kassell NF, Torner JC, et al. Predicting cerebral ischemia after aneurysmal subarachnoid hemorrhage: influences of clinical condition, CT results, and antifibrinolytic therapy. A report of the Cooperative Aneurysm Study. Neurology 1987;37:1586–1591.

44. Claassen J, Bernardini GL, Kreiter K, et al. Effect of cisternal and ventricular blood on risk of delayed cerebral ischemia after subarachnoid hemorrhage: the Fisher scale revisited. Stroke 2001;32:2012–2020.

45. Qureshi AI, Suarez JI, Bhardwaj A, et al. Early predictors of outcome in patients receiving hypervolemic and hypertensive therapy for symptomatic vasospasm after subarachnoid hemorrhage. Crit Care Med 2000;28:824–829.

46. Soustiel JF, Shik V, Shreiber R, et al. Basilar vasospasm diagnosis: investigation of a modified "Lindegaard Index" based on imaging studies and blood velocity measurements of the basilar artery. Stroke 2002;33:72–77.

47. Farhat SM, Schneider RC. Observations on the effect of systemic blood pressure on intracranial circulation in patients with cerebrovascular insufficiency. J Neurosurg 1967;27:441–445.

48. Kosnik EJ, Hunt WE. Postoperative hypertension in the management of patients with intracranial arterial aneurysms. J Neurosurg 1976;45:148–154.

49. Kassell NF, Peerless SJ, Durward QJ, et al. Treatment of ischemic deficits from vasospasm with intravascular volume expansion and induced arterial hypertension. Neurosurgery 1982;11:337–343.

50. Grotta JC. Clinical aspects of the use of calcium antagonists in cerebrovascular disease. Clin Neuropharmacol 1991;14:373–390.

51. Feigin VL, Rinkel GJ, Algra A, et al. Calcium antagonists in patients with aneurysmal subarachnoid hemorrhage: a systematic review. Neurology 1998;50:876–883.

52. Zubkov Y, Nikiforov B, Shustin V. Balloon catheter technique for dilation of constricted cerebral arteries after aneurysmal subarachnoid hemorrhage. Acta Neurochirurgica 1984;70:65–69.

53. Newell D, Eskridge J, Mayberg M. Angioplasty for the treatment of symptomatic vasospasm following subarachnoid hemorrhage. Neurosurgery 1989;71:654–660.

54. Higashida RT, Halbach VV, Cahan LD, et al. Transluminal angioplasty for treatment of intracranial arterial vasospasm. J Neurosurg 1989;71(Pt 1):648–653.

55. Higashida RT, Halbach VV, Dowd CF, et al. Intravascular balloon dilatation therapy for intracranial arterial vasospasm: patient selection, technique, and clinical results. Neurosurg Rev 1992;15:89–95.

56. Niizuma H, Kwak R, Otabe K, et al. Angiography study of cerebral vasospasm following the rupture of intracranial aneurysms: Part II. Relation between the site of aneurysm and the occurrence of the vasospasm. Surg Neurol 1979;11:263–267.

57. Yamamoto Y, Smith R, Bernanke D. Mechanism of action of balloon angioplasty in cerebral vasospasm. Neurosurgery 1992;30:1–6.

58. Linskey ME, Horton JA, Rao GR, et al. Fatal rupture of the intracranial carotid artery during transluminal angioplasty for vasospasm induced by subarachnoid hemorrhage. Case report. J Neurosurg 1991;74:985–990.

59. Firlik AD, Kaufmann AM, Jungreis CA, et al. Effect of transluminal angioplasty on cerebral blood flow in the management of symptomatic vasospasm following aneurysmal subarachnoid hemorrhage. J Neurosurg 1997;86:830–839.

60. Song JK, Elliott JP, Eskridge JM. Neuroradiologic diagnosis and treatment of vasospasm. Neuroimaging Clin N Am 1997;7:819–835.

61. Eskridge JM, McAuliffe W, Song JK, et al. Balloon angioplasty for the treatment of vasospasm: results of first 50 cases. Neurosurgery 1998;42:510–516; discussion 516–517.

62. Hurst RW, Schnee C, Raps EC, et al. Role of transcranial Doppler in neuroradiological treatment of intracranial vasospasm. Stroke 1993;24:299–303.

63. Numaguchi Y, Zoarski GH, Intra-arterial papaverine treatment for cerebral vasospasm: our experience and review of the literature. Neurol Med Chir (Tokyo) 1998;38:189–195.

64. Polin RS, Hansen CA, German P, et al. Intra-arterially administered papaverine for the treatment of symptomatic cerebral vasospasm. Neurosurgery 1998;42:1256–1264; discussion 1264–1267.

65. Liu JK, Tenner MS, Oestreich HM, et al., Reversal of radiographically impending stroke with multiple intra-arterial papaverine infusions in severe diffuse cerebral vasospasm induced by subarachnoid hemorrhage. Acta Neurochir (Wien) 2001;143:1249–1255; discussion 1256.

66. Fine-Edelstein JS, Wolf PA, O'Leary DH, et al. Precursors of extracranial carotid atherosclerosis in the Framingham Study. Neurology 1994;44:1046–1050.

67. Hankey GJ, Warlow CP. Symptomatic carotid ischaemic events: safest and most cost effective way of selecting patients for angiography, before carotid endarterectomy. Br Med J 1990;300:1485–1491.

68. Beneficial effect of carotid endarterectomy in symptomatic patients with high-grade carotid stenosis. North American Symptomatic Carotid Endarterectomy Trial Collaborators. N Engl J Med 1991;325:445–453.

69. Fields WS, Maslenikov V, Meyer JS, et al. Joint study of extracranial arterial occlusion. V. Progress report of prognosis following surgery or nonsurgical treatment for transient cerebral ischemic attacks and cervical carotid artery lesions. JAMA 1970;211:1993–2003.

70. Shaw DA, Venables GS, Cartlidge NE, et al. Carotid endarterectomy in patients with transient cerebral ischaemia. J Neurol Sci 1984;64:45–53.

71. Biller J, Feinberg WM, Castaldo JE, et al. Guidelines for carotid endarterectomy: a statement for healthcare professionals from a special writing group of the Stroke Council, American Heart Association. Stroke 1998;29:554–562.

72. Inzitari D, Eliasziw M, Gates P, et al. The causes and risk of stroke in patients with asymptomatic internal-carotid-artery stenosis. North American Symptomatic Carotid Endarterectomy Trial Collaborators. N Engl J Med 2000;342:1693–1700.

73. Chaturvedi S, Halliday A. Concerns regarding carotid endarterectomy guidelines. Stroke 1998;29:1475–1476.

74. Moore WS, Vescera CL, Robertson JT, et al. Selection process for surgeons in the Asymptomatic Carotid Atherosclerosis Study. Stroke 1991;22:1353–1357.

75. Perry JR, Szalai JP, Norris JW. Consensus against both endarterectomy and routine screening for asymptomatic carotid artery stenosis. Canadian Stroke Consortium. Arch Neurol 1997;54:25–28.

76. Benavente O, Moher, D, Pham B. Carotid endarterectomy for asymptomatic carotid stenosis: a meta-analysis. Br Med J 1998; 317:1477–1480.

77. Hsia DC, Moscoe LM, Krushat WM. Epidemiology of carotid endarterectomy among Medicare beneficiaries: 1985–1996 update. Stroke 1998;29:346–350.

78. Rothwell PM, Slattery J, Warlow CP. A systematic review of the risks of stroke and death due to endarterectomy for symptomatic carotid stenosis. Stroke 1996;27:260–265.

79. Lanska DJ, Kryscio RJ. In-hospital mortality following carotid endarterectomy. Neurology 1998;51:440–447.

80. Dyken ML. Controversies in stroke: past and present. The Willis Lecture. Stroke 1993;24:1251–1258.

81. Barnett HJ, Eliasziw M, Meldrum HE, et al. Do the facts and figures warrant a 10-fold increase in the performance of carotid endarterectomy on asymptomatic patients? Neurology 1996;46: 603–608.

82. Kapral MK, Wang H, Austin PC, et al. Sex differences in carotid endarterectomy outcomes: results from the Ontario Carotid Endarterectomy Registry. Stroke 2003;34:1120–1125.

83. Chaturvedi S, Aggarwal R, Murugappan A. Results of carotid endarterectomy with prospective neurologist follow-up. Neurology 2000;55:769–772.

84. Kresowik TF, Bratzler D, Karp HR, et al. Multistate utilization, processes, and outcomes of carotid endarterectomy. J Vasc Surg 2001;33:227–234; discussion 234–235.

85. Barnett HJ. Decision-making for carotid endarterectomy. The trials are only the start. Can J Neurol Sci 2002;29:302–304.

86. Ferro JM, Pinto AN, Falcao I, et al. Diagnosis of stroke by the nonneurologist. A validation study. Stroke 1998;29:1106–1109.

87. Chaturvedi S, Hachinski V. Does the neurologist add value to the carotid endarterectomy patient? Neurology 1998;50:610–613.

88. Marcinczyk MJ, Nicholas GG, Reed JF III. Asymptomatic carotid endarterectomy. Patient and surgeon selection. Stroke 1997;28: 291–296.

89. Goldstein LB, Bonito AJ, Matchar DB, et al. US national survey of physician practices for the secondary and tertiary prevention of ischemic stroke. Medical therapy in patients with carotid artery stenosis. Stroke 1996;27:1473–1478.

90. Tu JV, Hannan EL, Anderson GM, et al. The fall and rise of carotid endarterectomy in the United States and Canada. N Engl J Med 1998;339:1441–1447.

91. O'Neill L, Lanska DJ, Hartz A. Surgeon characteristics associated with mortality and morbidity following carotid endarterectomy. Neurology 2000;55:773–781.

92. Naylor AR, Bolia A, Abbott RJ, et al. Randomized study of carotid angioplasty and stenting versus carotid endarterectomy: a stopped trial. J Vasc Surg 1998;28:326–334.

93. Hobson RW II. Regarding "Randomized study of carotid angioplasty and stenting versus carotid endarterectomy: a stopped trial." J Vasc Surg 2000;31:622–624.

94. Alberts M. Results of a multicenter prospective randomized trial of carotid artery stenting versus carotid endarterectomy [Abstract]. Stroke 2001;32:325.

95. No authors given. Endovascular treatment and carotid surgery are similarly effective for preventing stroke in people with carotid stenosis, but endovascular treatment has more adverse effects. Evidence-based cardiovascular medicine 2001. Abstracted from CAVATAS investigators, endovascular versus surgical treatment in patients with carotid stenosis in the Carotid and Vertebral Artery Transluminal Angioplasty study (CAVATAS): a randomized trial. Lancet 2001;357:1729–1737.

96. Spence D, Eliasziw M. Endarterectomy or angioplasty for treatment of carotid stenosis? Lancet 2001;357:1722–1723.

97. Qureshi AI, Suri MF, Ali Z, et al. Carotid angioplasty and stent placement: a prospective analysis of perioperative complications and impact of intravenously administered abciximab. Neurosurgery 2002;50:466–473; discussion 473–475.

98. Theron J, Courtheoux P, Alachkar F, et al. New triple coaxial catheter system for carotid angioplasty with cerebral protection. AJNR Am J Neuroradiol 1990;11:869–874; discussion 875–877.

99. Fasseas P, Orford JL, Denktas AE, et al. Distal protection devices during percutaneous coronary and carotid interventions. Curr Control Trials Cardiovasc Med 2001;2:286–291.

100. Kastrup A, Groschel K, Krapf H, et al. Early outcome of carotid angioplasty and stenting with and without cerebral protection devices: a systematic review of the literature. Stroke. 2003;34: 813–819.

101. Theron JG, Payelle GG, Coskun O, et al. Carotid artery stenosis: treatment with protected balloon angioplasty and stent placement. Radiology 1996;201:627–636.

102. Kao HL, Lin LY, Lu CJ, et al. Long-term results of elective stenting for severe carotid artery stenosis in Taiwan. Cardiology 2002;97: 89–93.

103. Yadav JS, Roubin GS, Iyer S, et al. Elective stenting of the extracranial carotid arteries. Circulation 1997;95:376–381.

104. Shawl FA. Carotid artery stenting: acute and long-term results. Curr Opin Cardiol 2002;17:671–676.

105. Alric P, Branchereau P, Berthet JP, et al. Carotid artery stenting for stenosis following revascularization or cervical irradiation. J Endovasc Ther 2002;9:14–19.

106. Bonaldi, G. Angioplasty and stenting of the cervical carotid bifurcation: report of a 4-year series. Neuroradiology 2002;44:164–174.

107. Ross CB, Naslund TC, Ranval TJ. Carotid stent-assisted angioplasty: the newest addition to the surgeons' armamentarium in the management of carotid occlusive disease. Am Surg 2002;68:967–975; discussion 975–977.

108. Willfort-Ehringer A, Ahmadi R, Gschwandtner ME, et al. Single-center experience with carotid stent restenosis. J Endovasc Ther 2002;9:299–307.

109. Guimaraens L, Sola MT, Matali A, et al. Carotid angioplasty with cerebral protection and stenting: report of 164 patients (194 carotid percutaneous transluminal angioplasties). Cerebrovasc Dis 2002;13:114–119.

110. Yadav J. Stenting and angioplasty with protection in patients at high risk for endarterectomy (SAPPHIRE) Trial. Presented: Chicago, IL: American Heart Association Scientific Sessions 2002.

111. Mukherjee D, Yadav JS. Percutaneous treatment for carotid stenosis. Cardiol Clin 2002;20:589–597.

Endovascular Therapy of Cerebral Arteriovenous Malformations

48

Tony P. Smith

A cerebral arteriovenous malformation (AVM) is a life-threatening entity profoundly affecting patients and their families. The diagnosis of arteriovenous malformations (AVMs) is tied to imaging, and treatment involves a multidisciplinary approach, including, but rarely limited to, endovascular techniques. This chapter provides a basis for understanding cerebral AVMs and discusses the role of endovascular therapy in their treatment.

As with AVMs elsewhere in the body, a cerebral AVM is an abnormal shunting between arterial inflow and venous outflow without a normal capillary network. Radiographically, two major types of shunts are possible: *plexiform nidus*, which represents a collection of small vessels with arteriovenous shunting and is most often seen in parenchymal arteriovenous malformations; and *fistula(s)*, which represents single-hole communications between an artery and vein. Although this classification is often used when describing an AVM, in practice, there is often a mixture of these two types. Cerebral AVMs may also be anatomically divided into three types: *dural*, *pial*, or *mixed*, depending on topography and blood supply, although only pial types are discussed in this chapter. A number of classification systems have been devised for cerebral AVMs based on clinical factors, mostly for therapeutic purposes. Of these classification schemes, clearly the most widely used is that of Spetzler and Martin (1) (Table 48–1), where the surgical resectability is based on point values ranging 1–5, which correlate with location, size, and venous drainage patterns of the AVM. Further refinements in this grading scheme have also been published (2).

Cerebral arteriovenous malformations are believed to be at least in part congenital, although probably too small to be identified in utero (3,4). Autopsy numbers have suggested the prevalence of cerebral AVMs to be as great as 0.5%, but most now agree those numbers appear to be inflated (5,6). Berman et al. (7) found the number to be approximately 0.01%. Al-Shahi and Warlow (8) systematically reviewed the literature regarding frequency and clinical course of AVMs. Although the methods of most studies were flawed, they found the incidence to be approximately 1/100,000 with equal frequency between sexes. At the time of detection, approximately 15% of patients are asymptomatic, 20% present with seizures, and approximately 65% present with intracranial hemorrhage. Headache as the presenting symptom in the absence of neurological symptoms is rare (0.3%). The authors estimate the long-term crude annual fatality rate to be 1–1.5%; the annual risk of first-occurrence hemorrhage from an unruptured AVM is approximately 2%; but the risk of rehemorrhage may be as high as 18% in the first year (8).

DIAGNOSIS

Cross-sectional imaging including CT, MRI, and MRA are essential in fully evaluating the AVM and surrounding cerebral structures. After an acute hemorrhage, an AVM may not be demonstrated angiographically, may be displaced, or may be separated by the adjacent hematoma (9). Therefore, such additional imaging studies are even more critical. Eloquent

TABLE 48–1

SPETZLER-MARTIN (1) GRADING OF ARTERIOVENOUS MALFORMATIONS FOR PREDICATION OF NEUROLOGICAL COMPLICATIONS OF SURGERY

Graded Feature	Points
Size of the Nidus	
Small (<3 cm)	1
Medium (3–5 cm)	2
Large (>6 cm)	3
Eloquence of Brain	
Noneloquent	0
Eloquent	1
Pattern of Venous Drainage	
Superficial only	0
Deep	1

Arteriovenous malformation grade (1–5) equals total number of points. A grade 1 AVM would be small, located in a noneloquent area of the brain, and have superficial venous drainage only. Conversely, a grade 5 AVM would be large, located in an eloquent portion of the brain, and have deep venous drainage.

brain tissue around the AVM can be evaluated using functional MR imaging, which may be useful prior to therapy.

High-quality, rapid-sequence cerebral angiography is essential in embolotherapy planning for AVMs. Biplane angiographic evaluation is ideal, and image acquisition rates must be very high in order to delineate AVM characteristics in high-flow states. Angiographic evaluation must include the size and location of the nidus, the location and number of feeding arteries, the amount of flow through the lesion, including the presence of fistulas, the eloquence of the surrounding brain, the presence of aneurysms, the patterns of venous drainage, and the accessibility for treatment.

The risks of hemorrhage from a cerebral AVM may be suggested by angiography and include the *size and location of the malformation,* the presence of *aneurysms,* and the *pattern and integrity of venous drainage* (10). The risks of hemorrhage based on the angiographic size of the nidus are still controversial. Reports have stated that small AVMs (<3 cm) have a near five-times increased risk for hemorrhage (11), others found that larger AVMs (>5 cm) have a greater propensity to bleed (12–14), and still others noted little difference in the rate of hemorrhage based on size (10,15).

Two types of AVM-related aneurysms are differentiated in most reports based on location: aneurysms within the AVM nidus (nidus aneurysms) and aneurysms on the feeding vessels to the AVM (feeding artery aneurysms) (Figure 48–1A). There is little controversy regarding the increased risks of hemorrhage and the presence of aneurysms (16). However, there is controversy regarding the location of aneurysms and their correlation with hemorrhage (17–19). Meisel et al. (20)

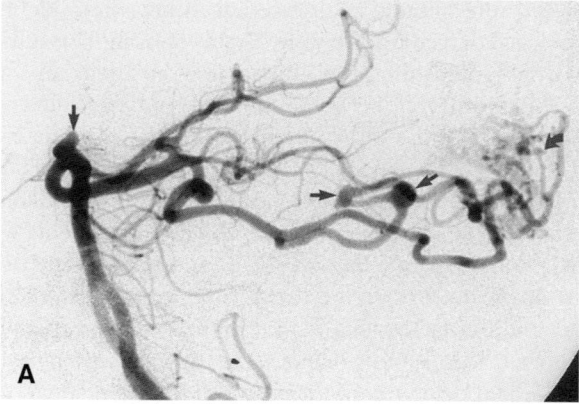

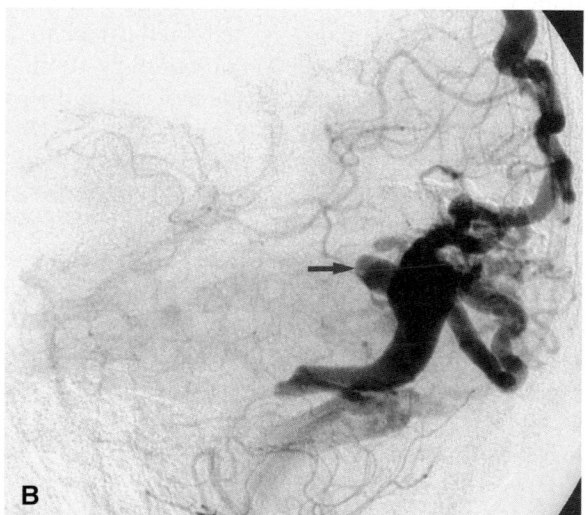

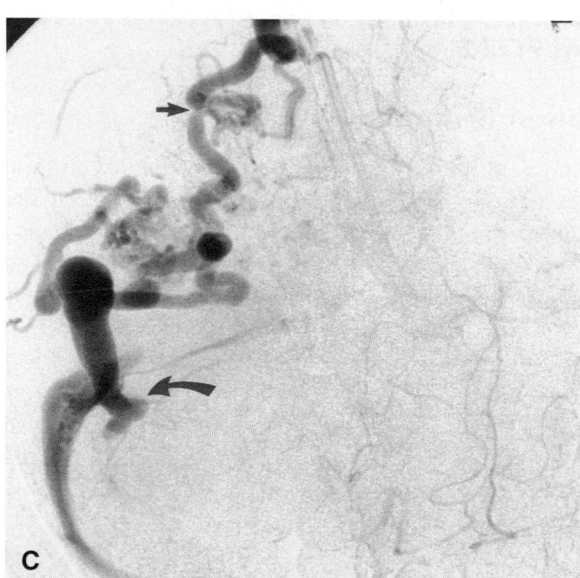

Figure 48–1 Right occipital AVM. **A.** Lateral view of left vertebral angiography shows at least three feeding artery aneurysms (*arrows*) as well as at least one nidus aneurysm (*curved arrow*). **B.** Later image from the same angiogram demonstrates a severe restrictive venous pattern with varices (*arrow*). **C.** Frontal view of the same left vertebral angiogram obtained using biplane imaging confirms a venous restrictive pattern with areas of venous narrowing (*arrow*) and occlusion (*curved arrow*). The AVM was successfully embolized, and surgical resection was complete.

analyzed 662 patients with cerebral AVMs where 305 had either nidal or feeding artery aneurysms or both. The authors performed targeted embolotherapy for the aneurysms and found that feeding artery aneurysms were not associated with rehemorrhage but intranidal aneurysms were. Alternatively, Staf et al. (21) analyzed 463 consecutive, prospectively enrolled patients from the Columbia AVM Databank, and arterial aneurysms were found in 117 (25%) patients with AVMs. No significant effect was seen for intranidal and unrelated aneurysms; however, the attributable risk of feeding artery aneurysms for incident hemorrhage in patients with AVM was 6%, suggesting that feeding artery aneurysms are an independent determinant for increased risk of incident AVM hemorrhage.

AVM hemorrhage is also related to the pattern and integrity of venous drainage. Venous outflow restriction refers to alteration in the normal pattern of venous drainage, with areas of stenosis and/or occlusion (Figure 48–1B, C). Vinuela et al. (22) suggested a relationship between an increased incidence of intracranial bleeding and impaired venous outflow, particularly for deep-seated cerebral AVMs, and others have confirmed a statistical correlation between severely impaired venous drainage and the risk of cerebral hemorrhage (23,24). Finally, regarding the pattern of venous drainage, there is also a recognized correlation between hemorrhage and the presence of a small number of draining veins, particularly when only a single vein is present (23,25) as well as the presence of deep venous drainage (26).

EMBOLOTHERAPY OF ARTERIOVENOUS MALFORMATIONS

Tools of Endovascular Therapy

A variety of guiding catheters, microcatheters, and guide wires as well as embolic agents are necessary, particularly for more difficult situations. One should not undertake the endovascular treatment of cerebral AVMs without an adequate inventory of interventional supplies. Placement of the guiding catheter or sheath into the carotid or vertebral artery for embolotherapy is of critical importance to the success of the procedure. Once the guiding catheter is placed in a stable location, microcatheter placement is then undertaken. It is obvious that using high-quality biplane fluoroscopy equipped with the most recent accessories enhances neurointerventional procedures.

Microcatheters

Embolotherapy of cerebral AVMs is performed exclusively with microcatheters. There are two basic designs of microcatheters: those that are primarily placed over a guide wire, and those whose placement is dependent on flow. Over-the-wire catheters can be accurately guided into small vessels feeding the AVM by using shapeable guide wires that can be accurately maneuvered into even small vessels. Such catheter-wire combinations, however, tend to cause headache in the awake patient and have the reputation of being more prone to vessel perforation. These catheters, however, can be placed into vessels with slow blood flow and have larger lumens that can accommodate larger-sized embolic agents such as particles and coils.

Flow-directed catheters are composed of soft, flexible material distally and are very small, which allows them to be carried with high blood flow distally into even small vessels or to the nidus of the AVM. Flow-directed microcatheters are by and large used to treat only arteriovenous malformations. They can be placed painlessly and have a decreased risk of vessel perforation when compared with their over-the-wire counterparts. However, the resulting small lumen allows use of only small embolic agents and mostly liquids. Recently, however, hydrophilic coatings for catheters and wires as well as improved catheter and wire technologies have made it possible to combine the two techniques. Smaller guide wires can be placed through flow-directed catheters to help guide them into appropriate vessels when flow alone does not suffice, and larger lumens in these catheters allow for the use of limited larger embolic agents, including small particles.

Embolic Agents

Because of a number of anatomical factors, including tortuous feeding vessels, associated aneurysms, and large, fistulous arteriovenous communications, the endovascular treatment of cerebral AVMs requires a thorough understanding and the availability of a variety of embolic agents. There are four main groups of such agents: particles, coils, balloons, and liquids, and all except detachable balloons are commonly used in the endovascular treatment of AVMs.

Particulate agents consist mostly of either polyvinyl alcohol sponge (PVA) or gelatin spheres. These agents are most often used through over-the-wire catheters, although some of the smallest agents can be successfully placed through flow-directed catheters if the mixture is kept relatively dilute. Particles are advantageous because they tend to occlude proximal to the nidus of the AVM, allowing the draining veins to remain patent (Figure 48–2A, B). However, such proximal occlusion permits the formation of collateral blood supply to the AVM nidus, making particulate embolotherapy a nonpermanent option only. There are also concerns regarding recanalization around traditional PVA, but these concerns have lessened with the newer polymers and spherical PVA particles. Purdy et al. (27) reviewed 108 embolized and surgically resected AVMs and concluded that PVA for distal occlusion and microcoils for proximal occlusion appeared to result in fewer complications when compared with other embolic agents.

A number of types of coils are available for the treatment of AVMs, including controlled release and pushable platinum coils. These types of coils are most often used to

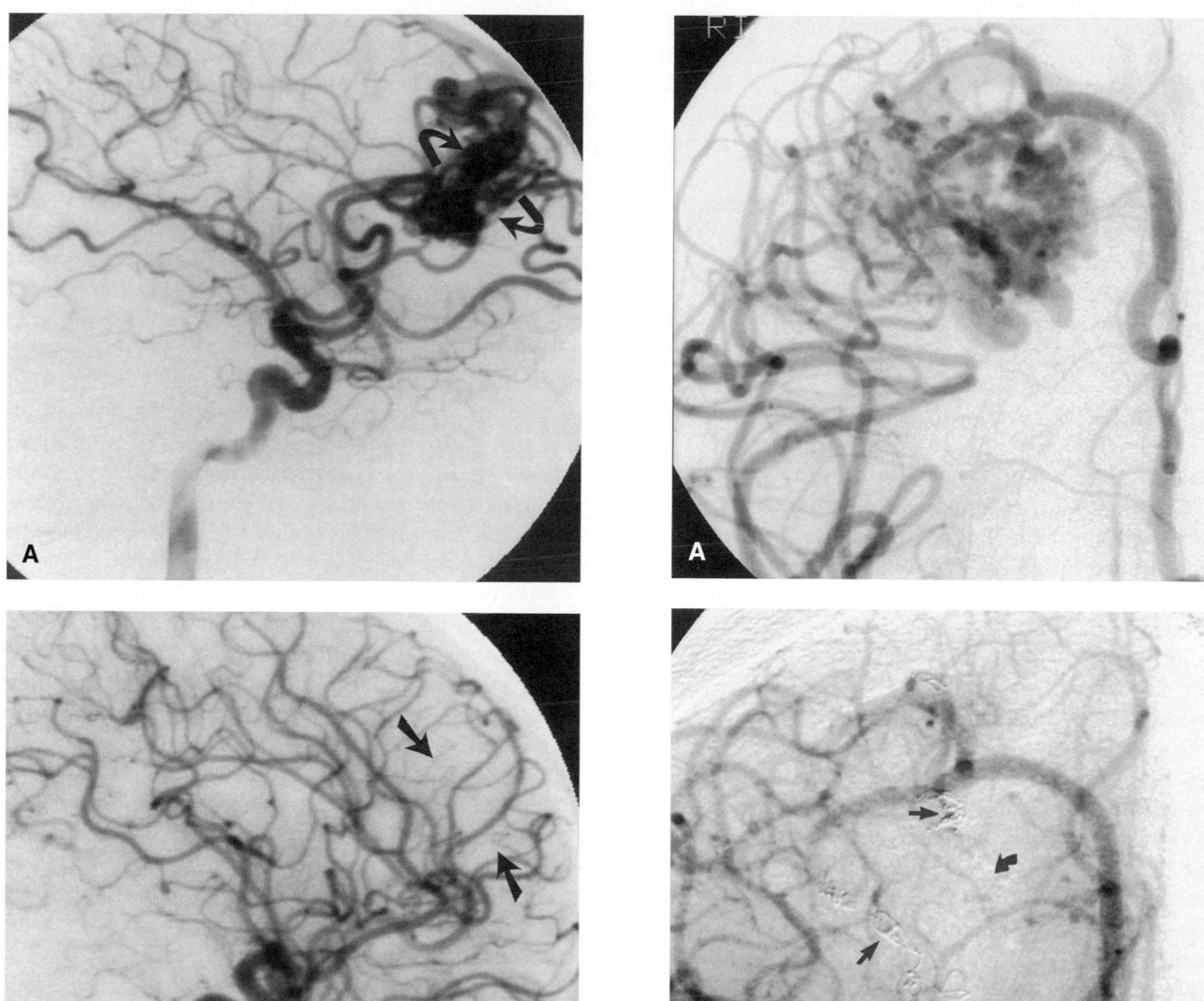

Figure 48–2 Lateral internal carotid angiograms of a frontal AVM. **A.** Preembolization AVM (*arrows*). **B.** After embolization with PVA sponge particles, there is virtually no filling of the AVM (*arrows*). The patient underwent complete surgical resection of the AVM.

Figure 48–3 Right frontal AVM pre- and postembolization. **A.** Frontal view of right internal carotid artery angiography prior to embolization demonstrates a large AVM supplied by the anterior and middle cerebral arteries. **B.** Frontal view of right internal carotid artery angiography postembolization and prior to surgical resection. This AVM had a number of fistulas that required liquid, coils (*arrows*), NBCA (*curved arrow*) as well as PVA and hand-cut pieces of silk suture. The lesion was completely resected, and the patient remained neurologically intact throughout.

treat fistulous connections or feeding artery aneurysms. Another coil variety consists of very small, fine platinum coils (Berenstein Liquid Coil Occlusion Device, Boston Scientific Target), which can be injected through small catheters, including flow-directed varieties, and are carried via blood flow distally in an attempt to treat larger arteriovenous fistulas. These coils are used almost exclusively for the treatment of AVMs and have the advantage of being radiopaque (Figure 48–3A, B). The same mechanical occlusion can be achieved by injecting small hand-cut

pieces of silk suture (4-0 for flow-directed catheters). Song et al. (28) reviewed the use of silk suture as an embolic agent in 230 consecutive preoperative AVM embolization procedures in 70 patients and found silk sutures to be an effective and relatively safe embolic agent. Although inexpensive, silk suture is not without problems. Devikis et al. (29) found the inflammatory response to silk may explain its effectiveness in producing vascular occlusion. However, a fulminate vasculitis theoretically can predispose a patient to delayed hemorrhage. Other problems with silk include the pressure required to inject the agent and the inability to determine the final site of deposition of the silk because it is radiolucent.

Liquid embolics are worldwide the most popular agents used for the endovascular treatment of cerebral AVMs. Liquid agents have the advantage of being easily injected through small microcatheter lumens as long as the liquid is of low viscosity. A liquid can potentially penetrate deeply into the AVM nidus. The greatest disadvantage of liquid agents is occlusion of the venous outflow of the AVM if the agent passes through the nidus, particularly where there are larger fistulous connections (Figure 48–3B). Occlusion of the venous outflow of the AVM prior to complete arterial occlusion, assuming such complete occlusion is even possible, can result in hemorrhage. Cyanoacrylates (glues) are the most commonly used embolic agents. In the past, isobutyl-2-cyanoacrylate (IBCA) was used but has largely been replaced by N-butyl-2-cyanoacrylate (NBCA), which is available in the United States (Trufill Liquid Embolic System, Cordis Neurovascular, Inc.). NBCA is a clear, free-flowing liquid that polymerizes into a solid material via an anionic mechanism upon contact with an ionic solution such as blood. To add radiopacity and decrease the polymerization time, the NBCA is mixed with ethiodized oil in a ratio based on where, anatomically, the interventionist wishes the eventual location of the solid agent to be (Figure 48–3B). An ethiodized oil-to-NBCA ratio of 3:1 to 2:1 is recommend by the manufacturer for intranidal injections and a 2:1 to 1:1 ratio for feeding vessel occlusion (Trufill Liquid Embolic System package insert). One must, however, understand that the use of cyanoacrylates requires experience, and such ratios are to be used only as a general framework. Catheters need to be flushed with a 5% dextrose solution to prevent premature polymerization of the cyanoacrylate in the microcatheter. Gluing the microcatheter to the blood vessel is a legitimate concern, particularly in the past, but this has recently been avoided for the most part by using hydrophilic microcatheters to which the glue will not easily adhere. NBCA is considered a permanent embolic agent in that recanalization of the vessel is rare. As with particles, however, if the nidus is not obliterated, collateral vascularity can form.

Other liquid agents have been used to treat cerebral AVMs. Absolute alcohol has a sclerosing effect on the vascular tissues, leading to intimal denudation and eventual thrombosis. Its effect on the vessel results in a permanent occlusion (30). Unfortunately, any liquid sclerosing agent is difficult to control as it courses through the AVM into the venous system and may not be effective in a high-flow circumstance, where contact time with the vessel surface is minimized. Ethanol has also been shown to be quite toxic to cerebral tissues. However, some promising results have been produced using alcohol in the hands of interventionists

experienced with the nuances of such an agent (30). Copolymer agents have been tested, chiefly ethylene vinyl alcohol (Onyx, MicroTheurapeutics, Inc.) (31). Such agents have the advantage of being liquid and becoming solidified following injection but are nonadhesive, decreasing the risks of catheter adhesion problems and theoretically being more malleable agents during surgical resection (32).

Deciding which agents are best for a particular patient requires assessment of the features of the AVM by an experienced interventionist taking into account the goals for embolotherapy. Wallace et al. (33) compared the safety and effectiveness of embolotherapy between an earlier population of patients using PVA with their late series using NBCA and found the latter to have lower complication rates in their single center. Although the study was fraught with a number of problems, the results prompted the authors to suggest a prospective clinical trial comparing the two. Such a trial was carried out for the U.S. Food and Drug Administration's approval of NBCA for intravascular use (34). The purpose of this study was to verify the effectiveness and safety of an NBCA/tantalum powder/ethiodized oil mixture compared with conventional treatment (PVA) for preoperative embolization of cerebral AVMs. One hundred four patients at 13 centers were prospectively randomized to undergo preoperative embolization using the NBCA mixture or PVA. The reduction of AVM dimensions and the mean number of vessels embolized was similar in the two groups. No differences were detected in surgical resection time, number of patients who required transfusion, volume and number of transfusion units, or type and volume of fluid replacement. The study concluded that NBCA and PVA were equivalent preoperative embolic agents.

Provocative Testing

After subselective angiography via the microcatheter and before AVM embolization, provocative testing can be used in an attempt to predict any functional loss from vessel occlusion. Provocative testing is performed by injecting a short-acting barbiturate, sodium amobarbital (Amytal Sodium, Eli Lilly & Co.), superselectively at the site of proposed embolization (35). This test is a selective version of the intracarotid Wada and Rasmussen test (36) for lateralization of cerebral speech dominance. The dose of sodium amobarbital varies according to vessel size and flow and is usually in the range of 25–50 mg per vessel. The sodium amobarbital is injected at the same rate as blood flow, and a neurological examination is performed. Often, the neurological examination is also combined with electroencephalography (EEG) (37,38). EEG alone is utilized when neurological testing is not possible, as in the patient who is under general anesthesia. Two percent (cardiac) lidocaine is often used as a provocative agent extracranially and may be indicated intracranially as well. Fitzsimmons et al. (39) found lidocaine detected clinically significant neurological deficits that amobarbital alone did not in a small number of patients. The authors believed this likely was a result of the pharmacodynamic differences between the two agents and concluded the use of lidocaine with amobarbital for superselective provocative testing in patients with cerebral AVMs may improve the sensitivity and predictive value of provocative testing.

In theory, provocative testing with liquid agents represents the expected result of distal embolization with liquid agents. Larger particles may not penetrate to small vessels, and more proximal vessel occlusive agents may, therefore, result in what appears to be a false-positive test. Functional imaging continues to improve and may become the most reliable method of predicting neurological deficits from embolization and from subsequent surgery.

THE GOALS OF EMBOLOTHERAPY FOR CEREBRAL ARTERIOVENOUS MALFORMATIONS

Spontaneous and complete regression of cerebral AVMs have been reported but are quite rare (40,41). Schwartz et al. (40) reported three cases and found 59 reported in the literature up to the year 2002. These authors believed regression requires a hemodynamic change compromising or closing the limited, usually single venous drainage. Hemorrhage may contribute to such closure but may, in fact, be associated with the resulting venous hypertension from outflow closure. The largest of the reported series is that of Patel et al. (42), who found 28 cases of spontaneous obliteration in a series of 2,162 patients with pial arteriovenous malformations. Interestingly, more than half their cases had exclusively superficial venous drainage.

Once treatment has been decided on, the role of AVM embolotherapy can be divided into adjunctive or sole treatment modalities as follows: preoperative; preradiosurgery; curative; palliative.

Preoperative

The role of embolotherapy as an adjunct to surgery is to diminish the arteriovenous shunting and to embolize arterial feeders that are difficult to access surgically. A relatively large number of studies have been published on the results of embolization preoperatively since the initial case by Luessenhop and Spence in 1960 (43). Preoperative embolization has been reported to empirically decrease operative blood loss and may make large, previously unresectable AVMs surgical candidates (44). Jafar et al. (45) reported on a comparison of two groups receiving surgery for AVMs, with one receiving preoperative embolization. The embolized group had significantly larger AVMs (3.9 cm versus 2.3 cm), but there was no statistical difference between groups for operative times or blood losses. DeMerritt et al. (46) compared 30 patients who underwent surgery and embolization with 41 patients who underwent

surgery only. Both groups were categorized by Spetzler-Martin grade and evaluated using the Glasgow Outcome Scale at various intervals. The arteriovenous malformations in the surgery and embolization group had a larger average greatest diameter. No significant difference in the preoperative or immediate postoperative (less than 24 hours) Glasgow Outcome Scale was identified between the two groups. At 1 week after surgery, the surgery and embolization group displayed a significantly better outcome evaluation, and the long-term evaluation continued to favor the surgery and embolization patients. Wong et al. (47) reported on 21 patients who underwent complete surgical excision of their AVMs. Eight patients had preoperative embolization with NBCA prior to surgical excision of their AVMs. Thirteen patients had excision of their AVMs without preoperative embolization, and these were used as the control group. Statistically significant reduction in blood loss occurred in Spetzler-Martin grade 3 and 4 AVMs but not in grade 1 and 2 AVMs undergoing preoperative embolization with NBCA. Operative time was reduced in grade 3 and 4 AVMs but not in grade 1 and 2 AVMs, although this was not statistically significant. Vinuela et al. (48) reported on 101 patients who underwent surgical resection of their AVMs after embolization. Fifty-seven of these malformations were greater than 5 cm in diameter. Ninety patients were embolized with liquid adhesives, six with PVA alone and 28 with a combination of PVA, microfibrillar collagen, and 30% ethanol. Complete surgical removal and subsequent cure were reported in 97 patients (96%). The authors reported 12 complications (12%) and a single death (1%). Vinuela (49) updated his series with 283 patients, 270 of whom were embolized with liquid adhesives either alone or in combination with other agents. There were 131 cases of surgical removal, with complete excision in 127 cases (97%). Higashida et al. (50) treated 100 patients with a combination of surgery and embolization, resulting in complete obliteration of the AVM in 99 patients (99%). The researchers used PVA particles in combination with larger hand-cut pieces of PVA, silk suture, detachable balloons, and platinum microcoils for larger shunts. There were 12 transient neurological deficits (12%), three permanent neurological deficits (3%), and a single death (1%), which resulted from intracranial hemorrhage.

Embolotherapy reportedly can allow large AVMs to be treated surgically (51). Spetzler et al. (52) reported on 20 patients with giant AVMs (>6 cm) embolized preoperatively with PVA particles. Complete surgical excision was achieved in 18 of these patients (90%). However, long operative times were still necessary for excision. It should, however, be clear that when one is applying embolotherapy to a very large AVM, whether the lesion actually reaches a state where surgical resection is a reasonable option may not be known until after multiple embolization sessions. This type of lesion should be approached as if it is also being treated palliatively if the angioarchitecture even after embolization does not permit safe surgical resection. For surgical series, the postoperative complications of perioperative edema and/or hemorrhage have correlated positively with preoperative angiographic steal, the diameters of the feeding vessels, and the recruitment of perforating vessels (53). As with staged surgical resection, only a portion of larger AVMs should be embolized in a single session.

Preradiosurgery

Radiation therapy induces phenotypic and biochemical alterations in cells of the vessel wall, which triggers an increased thrombogenicity and intimal hyperplasia, resulting in a gradual vascular lumen obliteration (54). A review of the more widely used forms of radiotherapy shows that the incidence of hemorrhage during the first 2 years after treatment is not different from that in the observed natural history of AVMs (55). Therefore, the vascular changes secondary to radiation may not completely confer protection until at least 2 years after treatment or when the AVM is completely obliterated.

Embolization has two main goals as an adjunct to radiosurgery: to decrease the size of the AVM volume and slow its rate of blood flow, and to protect areas that are at high risk of bleeding while awaiting the effects of radiosurgery. Because of the ability to concentrate the higher doses of radiation to smaller areas, smaller AVMs respond much better to radiation therapy than larger lesions. To decrease the size of the AVM nidus, vessels that supply the periphery of the lesion should be targeted to decrease the volume for treatment. Embolizing the center of the AVM does not necessarily decrease the volume for radiation therapy. Although it has not been definitely proved that embolotherapy provides protection from hemorrhage while the radiation-induced vascular changes develop, most interventionists attempt to target areas of greatest concern such as aneurysms. Most centers use permanent agents for embolization because the areas embolized may not be subjected to radiation and the radiation effects are quite delayed, as noted above (56). Liquid adhesives have been used by most centers, often in combination with coils, although particles have been used successfully with little recanalization (57,58).

Incomplete treatment of AVMs, especially larger ones, is common with radiosurgery (59). Henkes et al. (60) published their results of 300 endovascular procedures in 64 patients who were subselectively embolized prior to radiosurgery. A size reduction in AVM between 10% and 95% (average 63%) was achieved by embolotherapy, but complete nidus obliteration was achieved in only 14 patients following radiation. These authors also presented a review of 11 published series consisting of 752 patients who had combined radiosurgical and endovascular treatment of AVMs with much the same results. The largest of those series were that of Steiner et al. (61) (214 patients), who had complete obliteration of the AVM in 8%, and Gobin (62) (125 patients), who fared somewhat better with 33%.

Although both studies were hampered by a poor rate of angiographic follow-up, one can see how embolotherapy of intracranial AVMs may have a role following radiosurgery to assist in the management of unresponsive or incompletely responsive lesions (63).

Curative and Palliative Embolotherapy

Embolotherapy as a stand-alone procedure is most often undertaken in hopes of a cure or more likely for palliation when surgery and radiosurgery are not possible. AVMs have the greatest chance of cure when they consist of an isolated fistula, which is uncommon in parenchymal AVMs (Figure 48-4A, B). For nidus AVMs, curative embolotherapy is limited almost exclusively to small AVMs, which, of course, are the ones that are also amenable to surgery or radiation.

Intracerebral direct arteriovenous connections without an associated nidus are relatively rare but are one situation where the malformation has a high potential for cure by endovascular means alone. They consist of one or more major arteries emptying directly into a large vein, often a varix. Halbach et al. (64) reported five fistulas out of 320 AVMs. Lownie et al. (65) presented the experiences of two institutions (14 cases) as well as a literature review (35 cases) for a total of 48 patients. The clinical presentation ranged from hemorrhage, mass effect, and seizures to congestive heart failure in large fistulas. The endovascular treatment of fistulas involves interruption of the fistulous site. Transarterial occlusion is usually accomplished using balloons or platinum coils. Treatment is based on positioning the embolic material at the fistulous connection. Of 14 patients in their institution, Lownie et al. (65) treated five patients with fistulas using balloons, with excellent results in four. Halbach et al. (64) treated five patients using balloons or coils and silk suture. Surgical intervention was necessary in only one of their cases because of embolic occlusion of an arterial feeder proximal to the fistula site.

In general, AVMs with a defined nidus are rarely cured by endovascular means as a sole therapy (66). Vinuela (49) reported his series with 283 patients, 270 of whom were embolized with liquid adhesives either alone or in combination with other agents. He achieved complete cures in only 20 cases (7%), and in all these cases the AVMs were small (<3 cm in diameter). Fournier et al. (67) reported on 33 patients who were treated with liquid adhesives alone and followed with angiography at 2 years, with clinical follow-up at 2–6 years. A morphologic cure was obtained in seven (21%) of these patients; however, three of these were single-hole fistulas. Two patients had delayed bleeding from subtotal occlusion. However, some do report better results. Using almost exclusively NBCA, Valavanis and Yasargil (68) had a 40% cure rate, and Wikholm et al. (69) had a 13% cure rate from embolization as a stand-alone procedure.

The indications for palliative treatment are usually based on size, location, and patient symptoms. The symptoms may range from hemorrhage to mass effect and vascular

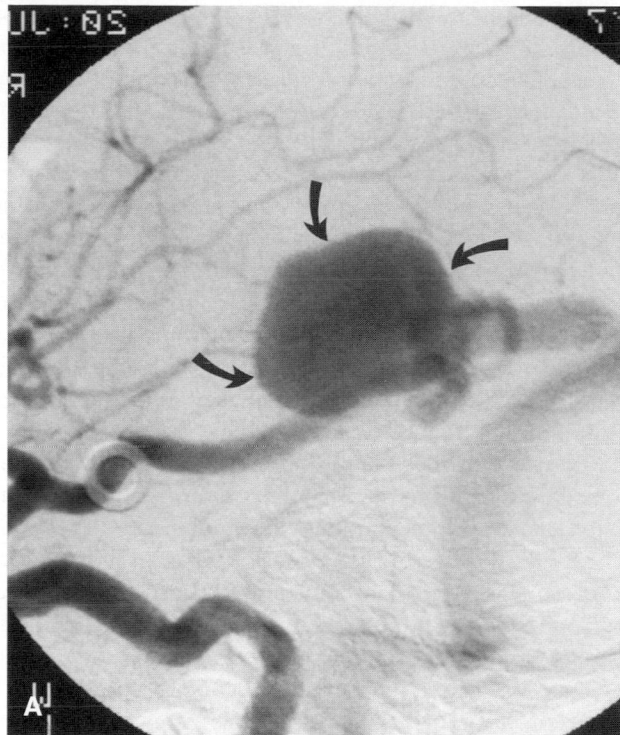

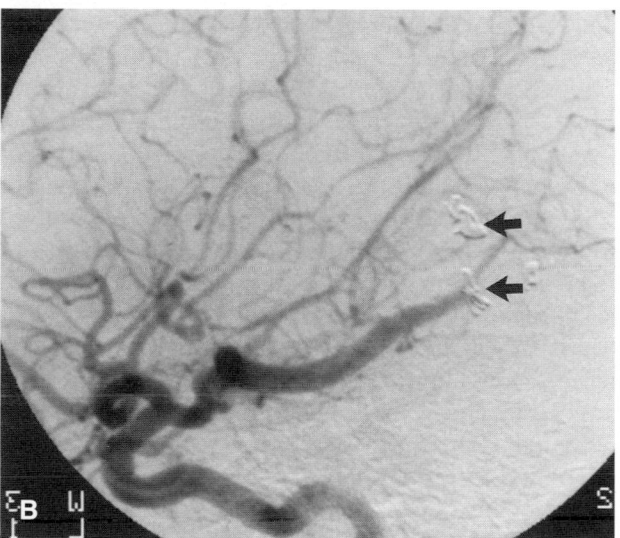

Figure 48–4 Direct arteriovenous fistula. **A.** Direct fistula with large varix (*arrows*). **B.** After embolization with coils, there is nonfilling of the fistula (*arrows*). This type of single-hole arteriovenous fistula can be completely cured by intravascular embolization techniques.

steal from the surrounding normal brain. When a patient presents with hemorrhage, embolotherapy is usually directed at suspicious areas such as aneurysms in hope of preventing a second hemorrhagic episode. More diffuse symptoms such as seizure activity and motor and/or sensory deficits are more difficult to target. Embolization has been shown to produce significant clinical improvement in a number of these cases, but the exact mechanism for improvement is still unknown. Vascular steal may account for these symptoms, but this hypothesis is still somewhat

controversial (70–72). It has been questioned whether palliative partial embolotherapy produces better results than medical therapy alone (73), and some have even reported that partial treatment may worsen the natural progression of cerebral AVMs (74). Kwon et al. (73) reviewed 16 patients who were treated medically and 11 patients who received partial embolization. Twenty-five percent (four cases) of patients in the medical group and 46% (five cases) of patients in the embolization group suffered from hemorrhage during the follow-up period. In addition, complications related to embolization occurred in three cases, prompting the authors to conclude that palliative partial embolization of intracranial AVMs, in all probability, does not produce better clinical results than medical treatment. Use of embolotherapy as the sole treatment when trying to palliate a patient's symptoms should be undertaken with caution, and the decision to proceed should be based on the individual patient in light of the anatomy and clinical presentation. However, Meisel et al. (75) reported that partial targeted embolization with NBCA reduced the long-term risk of hemorrhage by 24–78% compared with studies giving the natural history of AVMs. The risk reduction was apparent 1–2 years after the treatment. In this series, embolization was focused to suspicious areas such as intranidal aneurysms or fistulas. There are reports of feeding artery aneurysms decreasing in size following treatment of the AVM. Piotin et al. (16) in their review found that aneurysms arising on distal feeding arteries near the nidus had a high probability of regressing with substantial or curative AVM therapy.

Almost all series use permanent agents for stand-alone embolotherapy, most notably NBCA. Sorimachi et al. (76) embolized 36 AVMs with PVA particles alone and achieved complete obliteration of the nidus immediately after embolization in five patients, and 80–99% obliteration was attained in 12. Angiographic follow-up examinations were performed 1 week to 60 months (mean of 7 months) after embolization in 31 patients and showed an increase in nidal size in 15 (29%) and a decrease in seven (14%). In 28 of the 51 angiograms obtained more than 1 month after follow-up, 12 (43%) showed AVM enlargement. In four (80%) of five cases of complete obliteration, the nidus reappeared on follow-up angiograms. The authors concluded that embolization with PVA particles can produce significant initial volume reduction in the AVM nidus, but recanalization is not uncommon.

ARTERIOVENOUS MALFORMATIONS IN CHILDREN

The manifestation of parenchymal cerebral AVMs in childhood is quite rare, and the course is somewhat different than in the adult. D'Aliberti et al. (77) reported on 19 consecutive children with cerebral arteriovenous malformations over a 14-year period and compared these patients with a series of 120 consecutive adult patients with the same pathology, managed during the same period, and found that children seem to harbor smaller and simpler lesions than adults. Furthermore, despite a more severe clinical presentation, children appeared to fare better than adults. However, Millar et al. (78) reviewed a 10-year experience with 56 children who presented to their institution for treatment of cerebral AVMs. The symptoms at the time of presentation varied somewhat from adults whereas, even though hemorrhage was responsible for 50%, seizures and hydrocephalus accounted for 36% and congestive heart failure (CHF) for 18%. Regarding the latter, morbidity and mortality associated with cerebral AVMs is high when associated with congestive heart failure, with an overall mortality of 20%.

Treatment principles and options are like of those of the adult. Hoh et al. (79) retrospectively reviewed 40 consecutive pediatric patients with AVMs and found that like adults, a combined multimodality approach of surgery, radiosurgery, and embolization in managing AVMs in pediatric patients can improve outcomes and minimize morbidity and mortality. Radiosurgery is an acceptable treatment for small AVMs in children and adolescents in whom a higher obliteration rate can be achieved with lower risks of interval hemorrhage compared with the reported results in the general population (80). As in the adult, embolotherapy plays a definite role and may be especially useful in the infant presenting with CHF. Hladky et al. (81) reviewed their experience with cerebral AVMs in 62 patients where most patients underwent surgical resection following embolotherapy. Fifty patients had a satisfactory outcome based on the Glasgow Outcome Scale, although four died.

A prominent type of arteriovenous malformation of the fistulous type is the vein of Galen malformation (VGAM). It is rare, occurring in less than 1 of 2,500 deliveries, and anatomically represents the persistence of the embryologic prosencephalic vein of Markowski, which drains only the arteriovenous shunt and does not drain normal brain tissue (82). The true vein of Galen fails to develop. In addition, there is retention of fetal anatomic features and frequent occlusions of the dural sinuses of the posterior fossa with associated anomalies of venous drainage.

Treatment in these patients depends on their clinical condition. If they can be stabilized medically, treatment may be deferred until there has been interval somatic growth and the vascular systems are easier to access. However, acute clinical deterioration may necessitate more urgent intervention, particularly in cases of severe and uncontrollable CHF, acute hydrocephalus, or deterioration in the patient's neurological status (83). Definitive treatment requires interruption of the arteriovenous shunt. Surgical therapy for this condition has been universally poor in the neonatal period (84). Ciricillo et al. (85) reported on 13 neonates in which all five treated surgically died in the perioperative period, whereas six of eight (75%) treated with endovascular techniques survived.

Based on the relatively poor surgical results, embolotherapy has become the treatment of choice for VGAMs.

Embolization can be performed from either the arterial or venous route and should be performed with permanent agents. Embolotherapy usually begins with occlusion of the arterial feeding vessels (Figure 48–5). The initial goal of embolotherapy, particularly in the infant, is to improve the patient's clinical condition, particularly regarding preservation of neurological tissue and abating congestive cardiac symptoms. It is obviously advantageous if a complete cure can be achieved in the first sitting, but this is rare. The most practical initial goal is to embolize the largest feeding arteries and to manage the patient medically until more stable or even after a period of somatic growth. As with all patients, it is critical to individualize the therapy to a particular patient regarding when to intervene and to what degree.

Regarding embolotherapy for VGAM via the arterial route, larger fistulous sites may be occluded using a number of agents such as balloons, silk suture, coils, or cyanoacrylate. Arterial embolization of the largest feeder(s) should be performed initially, and embolization should occur at the fistula site if possible. For coiling, coil sizing is important, and mechanical or electrolytically detachable coils are preferred to prevent losing the coil into the venous outflow. A combination of agents may also be useful, particularly cyanoacrylate after initial coiling, which allows the glue to adhere to the coils and provides complete and permanent occlusion of the feeding vessel. A complete cure is possible after arterial embolization alone, depending on the anatomical configuration of the VGAM, most importantly the number and accessibility of the feeding vessels (86). However, complete obliteration often requires a transvenous approach to occlude the venous aspect of the malformation.

The transvenous route can be femoral or jugular or via a retrograde catheterization from the torcula (87,88) (Figure 48–6). The transtorcular approach allows direct access to the dilated venous structure. The choice of transfemoral versus transtorcular approach depends on the size of the fistulous flow and the venous anatomy. The placement of large numbers of coils and/or the frequent association of venous anomalies must be a consideration for the route chosen. Transvenous embolization should begin at the fistulous portions and continue posteriorly. Because by definition VGAMs do not drain normal brain, the entire vein can be occluded. The transvenous route usually uses coils but may also involve use of other agents, particularly cyanoacrylate.

The results of VGAM embolotherapy are guarded, but one must keep in mind the course of the untreated disease process and the difficulties encountered during embolotherapy in this difficult group of patients (89,90). In addition, as with many series of this type, there are significant reporting inconsistencies (91). Garcia-Monaco et al. (89) reported on 39 cases of embolization in which 26 patients (67%) were either normal or had mild manifestations (stable macrocephaly or asymptomatic cardiomegaly) after embolotherapy. Lylyk et al. (92) treated 28 patients with VGAM using a combination of transfemoral and transarterial approaches

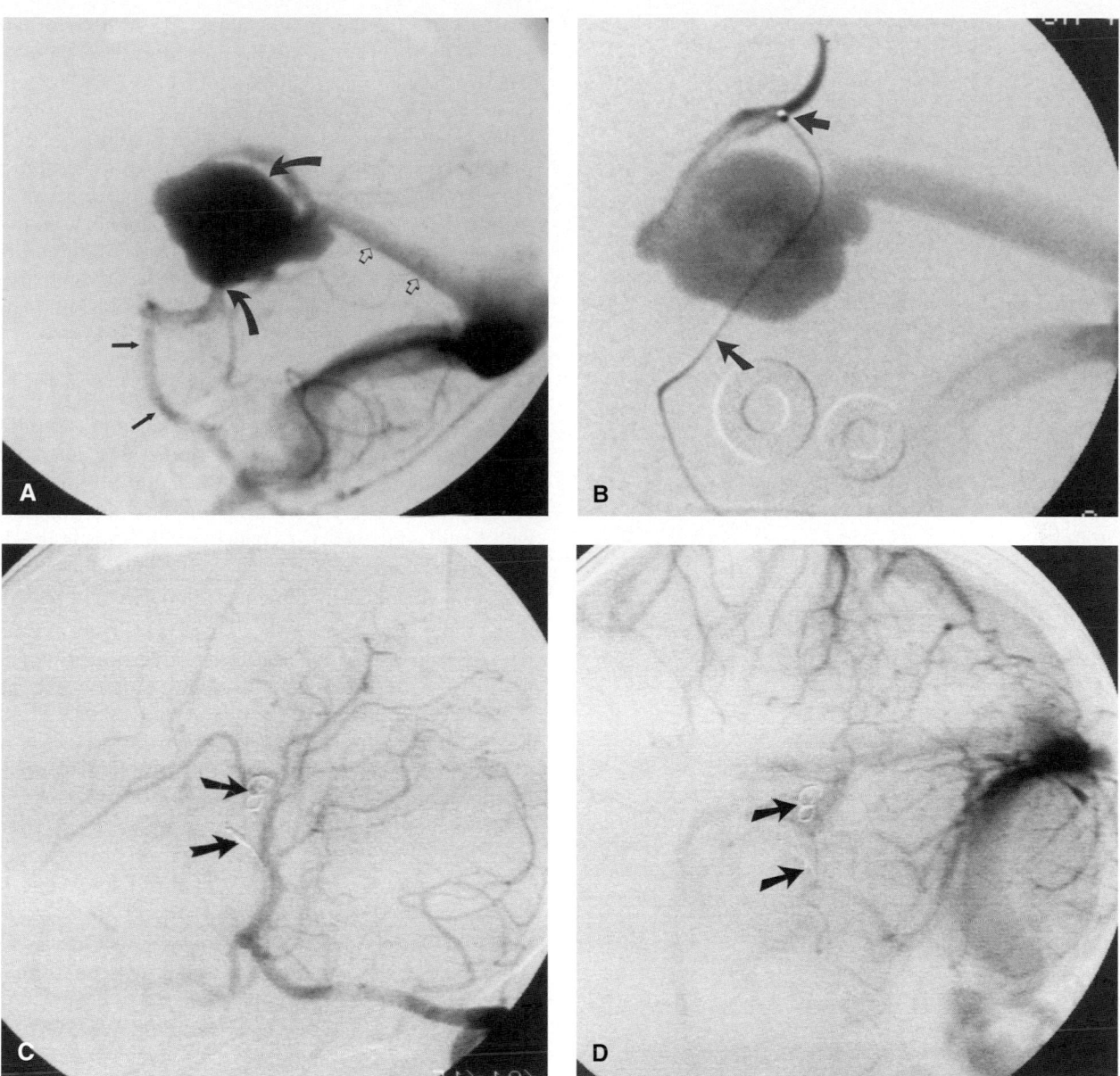

Figure 48–5 Vein of Galen malformation. **A.** Vertebral artery injection shows a large vein of Galen malformation (*curved arrows*) draining into the straight sinus (*open arrows*). Supply is from the posterior circulation via the basilar artery (*arrows*). **B.** Transarterial catheter (*arrows*) placed selectively into the posterior lateral choroidal artery for arterial embolization with coils. **C.** Frontal view of the left vertebral artery after embolization. The malformation is completely embolized by the coils (*arrows*). **D.** Lateral view of the left vertebral artery (venous phase) after embolization with coils (*arrows*). The malformation is completely embolized. The patient was completely cured.

with an immediate improvement in the patient's clinical status in 23 (82%) patients and good long-term clinical outcomes in 17 patients (61%). There were five deaths (18%) in this series. Jones et al. (93) evaluated and treated 13 children for VGAM, eight of which presented as neonates with CHF. Two of the eight patients presenting during the neonatal period achieved normal or near-normal outcomes, one experienced significant impairment, and the other five died. Their experience confirmed that children with VGAM presenting during the neonatal period have a generally worse prognosis than do those presenting later in childhood.

Lasjaunias et al. (86) presented 43 patients with VGAM, 34 of whom were embolized transarterially with cyanoacrylates. Forty-seven percent of the children had a completely occluded lesion at follow-up angiography, and 53% were found to be completely normal or to have only mild cardiac failure that could be treated medically or moderate macrocephaly without neurological symptoms or mental retardation. The overall mortality (embolized and nonembolized groups) in the neonatal children was 28%. These results compared favorably with surgical or other techniques of arterial occlusion as well as transvenous embolization.

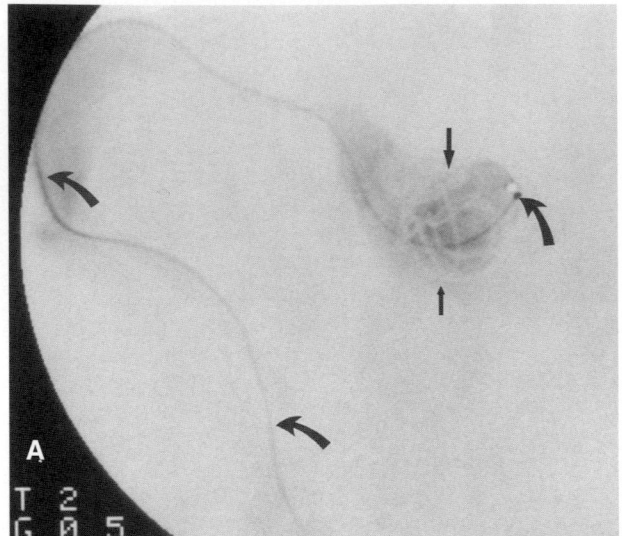

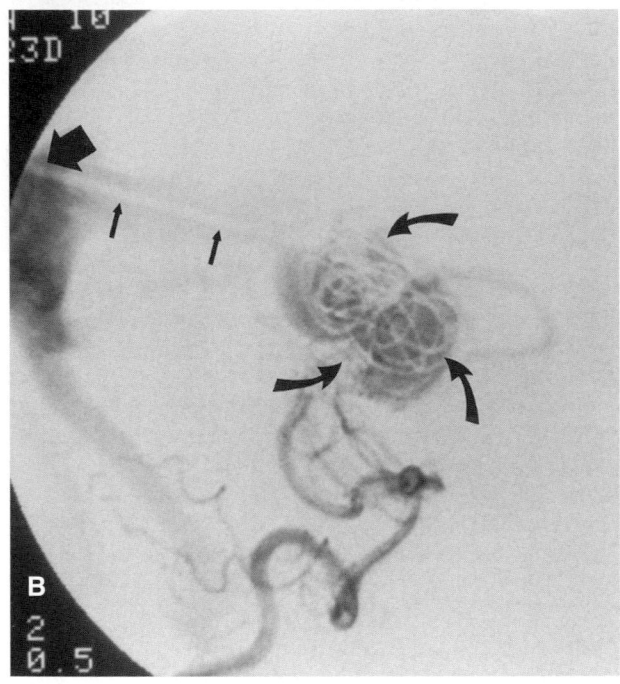

Figure 48–6 Vein of Galen malformation. **A.** Transvenous approach. Note the catheter through the venous sinus system (*curved arrows*) into the malformation, where coils (*straight arrows*) have been placed. **B.** Transtorcular approach. A sheath (*small arrows*) has been placed through a surgical exposure of the torcula (*large arrow*). Coils have been placed into the malformation (*curved arrows*).

COMPLICATIONS AND POSTEMBOLIZATION CARE

The success of embolotherapy and avoidance of complications vary with the experience of the interventional team. The location of the AVM, its size, and whether it has previously bled are regarded as important factors in considering patients for therapy. In addition, the goal of embolotherapy is crucial. If one is attempting to cure the AVM or if embolotherapy is the only viable option, then one may have to be more aggressive in the therapeutic approach. Although this may increase the success rates of the procedure, it will also surely increase the complications. Wikholm et al. (69), in reporting their 13% cure rate in 150 consecutive patients treated with NBCA embolization, also reported a mortality of 1.3% and a morbidity of 33%. However, Valavanis and Yasargil (68) reported a mortality and a permanent morbidity of 1.3% each in their study of 387 consecutive patients, even in light of their 40% cure rate from embolization alone. Frizzel and Fisher (94) reviewed 32 series of 1,246 patients who underwent embolization of brain AVMs. Although there was obviously a great deal of variability in the reporting of data, they found the cure rate to be 4–5%. Permanent morbidity was 8–9%, with death in 1–2% over an interval of 35 years.

Location of the AVMs is certainly a factor in complication rates, although none of the larger studies have attempted to define the location of the AVM in relationship to success or complications (95). Vinuela et al. (96) reported embolization with liquid adhesives of 16 patients with AVMs in the dominant hemisphere. Although early complications were common (50%), only three patients (19%) had mild permanent deficits at 6 months. However, Hartman et al. (97) prospectively evaluated 233 patients undergoing one or more embolotherapy sessions and found that no morphological characteristics of the AVM predicted treatment complications. New posttreatment neurological deficits were associated with increasing patient age, absence of a pretreatment neurological deficit, and the number of embolotherapy sessions.

After embolization therapy, the two most dreaded delayed consequences are hemorrhage and ischemia. Delayed hemorrhage of an AVM is most likely the result of changes in the hemodynamics after embolotherapy. The patient is particularly at risk if the venous outflow to the AVM is occluded without complete arterial occlusion. Postembolization edema is also believed to be produced by a combination of sudden removal of the AVM sump effect and a lack of regional vascular autoregulation of the surrounding normal brain (normal perfusion pressure breakthrough phenomenon) (98). This same phenomenon can also lead to hemorrhage.

Delayed ischemia is most often a result of arterial or venous thrombosis that may continue to occur after embolization (99). Retrograde arterial thrombosis has been shown to occur after surgical removal of AVMs and has been correlated in a small series with advanced patient age, large AVM size, and markedly dilated and elongated arterial feeding arteries (100). These data are also applicable to patients after embolotherapy.

REFERENCES

1. Spetzler RF, Martin NA. A proposed grading system for arteriovenous malformations. J Neurosurg 1986;65:484–489.
2. Lawton MT. Spetzler-Martin Grade III arteriovenous malformations: surgical results and a modification of the grading scale. Neurosurgery 2003;52:740–749.

3. Mullan S, Mojtahedi DL, Johnson DL, et al. Embryological basis of some aspects of cerebral vascular fistulas and malformations. J Neurosurg 1996;85:1–8.

4. Lasjaunias P. A revised concept of the congenital nature of cerebral arteriovenous malformations. Intervent Neuroradiol 1997; 3:275–281.

5. ApSimon HT, Reef H, Phadke RV, et al. A population-based study of brain arteriovenous malformation: long-term treatment outcomes. Stroke 2002;33:2794–2800.

6. Al-Shahi R, Bhattacharya JJ, Currie DG, et al. Prospective, population-based detection of intracranial vascular malformations in adults: the Scottish Intracranial Vascular Malformation Study (SIVMS). Stroke 2003;34:1163–1169.

7. Berman MF, Sciacca RR, Pile-Spellman J, et al. The epidemiology of brain arteriovenous malformations. Neurosurgery 2000;47: 389–397.

8. Al-Shahi R, Warlow C. A systematic review of the frequency and prognosis of arteriovenous malformations of the brain in adults. Brain 2001;124:1900–1926.

9. Wilson CB, Hoi Sang U, Domingue J. Microsurgical treatment of intracranial vascular malformations. J Neurosurg 1979;51: 446–454.

10. Crawford PM, West CR, Chadwick DW. Arteriovenous malformations of the brain: natural history in unoperated patients. J Neurol Neurosurg Psychiatry 1986;49:1–10.

11. Graf CJ, Perret GE, Torner JC. Bleeding from cerebral arteriovenous malformations as part of their natural history. J Neurosurg 1983;58:331–337.

12. Pollock BE, Flickinger JC, Lunsford LD, et al. Factors that predict the bleeding risk of cerebral arteriovenous malformations. Stroke 1996;27:1–6.

13. Karlsson B, Lindquist C, Johansson A, et al. Annual risk for the first hemorrhage from untreated cerebral arteriovenous malformations. Minim Invasive Neurosurg 1997;40:40–46.

14. Stefani MA, Porter PJ, terBrugge KG, et al. Large and deep brain arteriovenous malformations are associated with risk of future hemorrhage. Stroke 2002;33:1220–1224.

15. Hofmeister C, Stapf C, Hartmann A, et al. Demographic, morphological, and clinical characteristics of 1289 patients with brain arteriovenous malformation. Stroke 2000;31:1307–1310.

16. Piotin M, Ross IB, Weill A, et al. Intracranial arterial aneurysms associated with arteriovenous malformations: endovascular treatment. Radiology 2001;220:506–513.

17. Brown RD, Wiebers DO, Forbes GS. Unruptured intracranial aneurysms and arteriovenous malformations: frequency of intracranial hemorrhage and relationship of lesions. J Neurosurg 1990;73:859–863.

18. Marks MP, Lane B, Steinberg GK, et al. Intranidal aneurysms in cerebral arteriovenous malformations: evaluation and endovascular treatment. Radiology 1992;183:355–360.

19. Redekop G, TerBrugge K, Montanera W, et al. Arterial aneurysms associated with cerebral arteriovenous malformations: classification, incidence, and risk of hemorrhage. J Neurosurg 1998;89: 539–546.

20. Meisel HJ, Mansmann U, Alvarez H, et al. Cerebral arteriovenous malformations and associated aneurysms: analysis of 305 cases from a series of 662 patients. Neurosurgery 2000;46:793–800.

21. Stapf C, Mohr JP, Pile-Spellman J, et al. Concurrent arterial aneurysms in brain arteriovenous malformations with haemorrhagic presentation. J Neurol Neurosurg Psychiatry 2002;73: 294–298.

22. Vinuela F, Nombela L, Roach MR, et al. Stenotic and occlusive disease of the venous drainage system of deep brain AVMs. J Neurosurg 1985;63:180–184.

23. Miyasaka Y, Yada K, Ohwada T, et al. An analysis of the venous drainage system as a factor in hemorrhage from arteriovenous malformations. J Neurosurg 1992;76:239–243.

24. Mansmann U, Meisel J, Brock M, et al. Factors associated with intracranial hemorrhage in cases of cerebral arteriovenous malformation. Neurosurgery 2000;46:272–279.

25. Marks MP, Lane B, Steinberg GK, et al. Hemorrhage in intracerebral arteriovenous malformations: angiographic determinants. Radiology 1990;176:807–813.

26. Mast H, Young WL, Koennecke HC, et al. Risk of spontaneous haemorrhage after diagnosis of cerebral arteriovenous malformation. Lancet 1997;350:1065–1068.

27. Purdy PD, Batjer HH, Risser RC, et al. Arteriovenous malformations of the brain: choosing embolic materials to enhance safety and ease of excision. J Neurosurg 1992;77:217–222.

28. Song JK, Eskridge JM, Chung EC, et al. Preoperative embolization of cerebral arteriovenous malformations with silk sutures: analysis and clinical correlation of complications revealed on computerized tomography scanning. J Neurosurg 2000;92:955–960.

29. Deveikis JP, Manz HJ, Luessenhop AJ, et al. A clinical and neuropathologic study of silk suture as an embolic agent for brain arteriovenous malformations. AJNR Am J Neuroradiol 1994;15: 263–271.

30. Yakes WF, Krauth L, Ecklund J, et al. Ethanol endovascular management of brain arteriovenous malformations: initial results. Neurosurgery 1997;40:1145–1152.

31. Jajan R, Murayama Y, Gobin YP, et al. Embolization of arteriovenous malformations with Onyx: clinicopathological experience in 23 patients. Neurosurgery 2001;48:984–997.

32. Duffner F, Ritz R, Bornemann A, et al. Combined therapy of cerebral arteriovenous malformations: histological differences between a non-adhesive liquid embolic agent and n-butyl 2-cyanoacrylate (NBCA). Clin Neuropathol 2002;21:13–17.

33. Wallace RC, Flom RA, Khayata MH, et al. The safety and effectiveness of brain arteriovenous malformation embolization using acrylic and particles: the experiences of a single institution. Neurosurgery 1995;36:606–618.

34. n-BCA Trial Investigators. N-butyl cyanoacrylate embolization of cerebral arteriovenous malformations: results of a prospective, randomized, multi-center trial. AJNR Am J Neuroradiol 2002;23:748–755.

35. Peters KR, Quisling RG, Gilmore R, et al. Intraarterial use of sodium methohexital for provocative testing during brain embolotherapy. AJNR Am J Neuroradiol 1993;14:171–174.

36. Wada J, Rasmussen T. Intracarotid injection of sodium Amytal for the lateralization of cerebral speech dominance: experimental and clinical observations. J Neurosurg 1960;17:266–282.

37. Rauch RA, Vinuela F, Dion J, et al. Preembolization functional evaluation in brain arteriovenous malformations: the superselective Amytal test. AJNR Am J Neuroradiol 1992;13:303–308.

38. Rauch RA, Vinuela F, Dion J, et al. Preembolization functional evaluation in brain arteriovenous malformations: the ability of superselective Amytal test to predict neurologic dysfunction before embolization. AJNR Am J Neuroradiol 1992;13:309–314.

39. Fitzsimmons BF, Marshall RS, Pile-Spellman J, et al. Neurobehavioral differences in superselective Wada testing with amobarbital versus lidocaine. AJNR Am J Neuroradiol 2003;24:1456–1460.

40. Schwartz ED, Hurst RW, Sinson G, et al. Complete regression of intracranial arteriovenous malformations. Surg Neurol 2002;58: 139–147.

41. Lee SK, Vilela P, Willinsky R, et al. Spontaneous regression of cerebral arteriovenous malformations: clinical and angiographic analysis with review of the literature. Neuroradiology 2002;44: 11–16.

42. Patel MC, Hodgson TJ, Kemeny AA, et al. Spontaneous obliteration of pial arteriovenous malformations: a review of 27 cases. AJNR Am J Neuroradiol 22:531–536.

43. Luessenhop AJ, Spence WT. Artificial embolization of cerebral arteries: report of use in a case of arteriovenous malformation. JAMA 1960;172:1153–1155.

44. Pelz DM, Fox AJ, Vinuela F, et al. Preoperative embolization of brain AVMs with isobutyl-2 cyanoacrylate. AJNR Am J Neuroradiol 1988;9:757–764.

45. Jafar JJ, Davis AJ, Berenstein A, et al. The effect of embolization with N-butyl cyanoacrylate prior to surgical resection of cerebral arteriovenous malformations. J Neurosurg 1993;78:60–69.

46. DeMeritt JS, Pile-Spellman J, Mast H, et al. Outcome analysis of preoperative embolization with N-butyl cyanoacrylate in cerebral arteriovenous malformations. AJNR Am J Neuroradiol 1995;16: 1801–1807.

47. Wong SH, Tan J, Yeo TT, et al. Surgical excision of intracranial arteriovenous malformations after preoperative embolisation with N-butylcyanoacrylate. Ann Acad Med Singapore 1997;26:475–480.

48. Vinuela F, Dion JE, Duckwiler G, et al. Combined endovascular embolization and surgery in the management of cerebral arteriovenous malformations: experience with 101 cases. J Neurosurg 1991; 75:856–864.

49. Vinuela F. Functional evaluation and embolization of intracranial arteriovenous malformations. In: Vinuela F, Halbach VV, Dion JE, eds. Interventional Neuroradiology: Endovascular Therapy of the Central Nervous System. New York: Raven, 1992;77–86.

50. Higashida RT, Hieshima GB, Halbach VV. Advances in the treatment of complex cerebrovascular disorders by interventional neurovascular techniques. Circulation 1991;83(Suppl I):196–206.

51. Chang SD, Marcellus ML, Marks MP, et al. Multimodality treatment of giant intracranial arteriovenous malformations. Neurosurgery 2003;53:1–11.

52. Spetzler RF, Martin NA, Carter LP, et al. Surgical management of large AVMs by staged embolization and operative excision. J Neurosurg 1987;67:17–28.

53. Batjer HH, Devous MD, Seibert GB, et al. Intracranial arteriovenous malformation: relationship between clinical factors and surgical complications. Neurosurgery 1989;24:75–79.

54. O'Connor MM, Mayberg MR. Effects of radiation on cerebral vasculature: a review. Neurosurgery 2000;46:138–151.

55. Ogilvy CS. Radiation therapy for arteriovenous malformations: a review. Neurosurgery 1990;26:725–735.

56. Miyachi S, Negoro M, Okamoto T, et al. Embolisation of cerebral arteriovenous malformations to assure successful subsequent radiosurgery. J Clin Neurosci 2000;7(Suppl 1):82–85.

57. Dawson RC, Tarr RW, Hecht ST, et al. Treatment of arteriovenous malformations of the brain with combined embolization and stereotactic radiosurgery: results after 1 and 2 years. AJNR Am J Neuroradiol 1990;11:857–864.

58. Mathis JA, Barr JD, Horton JA, et al. The efficacy of particulate embolization combined with stereotactic radiosurgery for treatment of large arteriovenous malformations of the brain. AJNR Am J Neuroradiol 1995;16:299–306.

59. Steiner L, Lindquist C, Adler JR, et al. Clinical outcome of radiosurgery for cerebral arteriovenous malformations. J Neurosurg 1992;77:1–8.

60. Henkes H, Nahser H-C, Berg-Dammer E, et al. Endovascular therapy of brain AVMs prior to radiosurgery. Neurol Res 1998; 20:479–492.

61. Steiner L, Prasad D, Lindquist C, et al. Gamma knife surgery in vascular, neoplastic, and functional disorders of the nervous system. In: Schmidek HH, Sweet WH, eds. Operative Neurosurgical Techniques: Indications, Methods, and Results. 3rd Ed. Philadelphia: W.B. Saunders, 1995:667–694.

62. Gobin Y, Laurent A, Merienne L, et al. Treatment of brain arteriovenous malformations by embolization and radiosurgery. J Neurosurg 1996;85:19–28.

63. Marks MP, Lane B, Steinberg GK, et al. Endovascular treatment of cerebral arteriovenous malformations following radiosurgery. AJNR Am J Neuroradiol 1993;14:297–303.

64. Halbach VV, Higashida RT, Hieshima GB, et al. Transarterial occlusion of solitary intracerebral arteriovenous fistulas. AJNR Am J Neuroradiol 1989;10:747–752.

65. Lownie SP, Duckwiler GR, Fox AJ, et al. Endovascular therapy of nongalenic cerebral arteriovenous fistulas. In: Vinuela F, ed. Interventional Neuroradiology: Endovascular Therapy of the Central Nervous System. New York: Raven, 1992;87–106.

66. Wilson CB, Hieshima GB, Higashida RT, et al. Interventional radiologic adjuncts in cerebrovascular surgery. Clin Neurosurg 1989;37:332–352.

67. Fournier D, TerBrugge KG, Willinsky R, et al. Endovascular treatment of intracerebral arteriovenous malformations: experience in 49 cases. J Neurosurg 1991;75:228–233.

68. Valavanis A, Yasargil MG. The endovascular treatment of brain arteriovenous malformations. Adv Tech Stand Neurosurg 1998;24: 131–214.

69. Wikholm G, Lundqvist C, Svendsen P. Embolization of cerebral arteriovenous malformations: Part I—Technique, morphology, and complications. Neurosurgery 1996;39:448–459.

70. Wade JPH. Neurological deficit from an inoperable arteriovenous malformation: an indication for therapeutic embolization? Arch Neurol 1986;43:508–509.

71. Morgan M, Winder M. Haemodynamics of arteriovenous malformations of the brain and consequences of resection: a review. J Clin Neuroscience 2001;8:216–224.

72. Taylor CL, Selman WR, Ratcheson RA. Steal affecting the central nervous system. Neurosurgery 2002;50:679–689.

73. Kwon OK, Han DH, Han MH, Chung YS. Palliatively treated cerebral arteriovenous malformations: follow-up results. J Clin Neurosci 2000;7(Suppl 1):69–72.

74. Han PP, Ponce FA, Spetzler RF. Intention-to-treat analysis of Spetzler-Martin grades IV and V arteriovenous malformations: natural history and treatment paradigm. J Neurosurg 2003;98:3–7.

75. Meisel HJ, Mansmann U, Alvarez H, et al. Effect of partial targeted N-butyl-cyano-acrylate embolization in brain AVM. Acta Neurochir (Vienna) 2002;144:879–888.

76. Sorimachi T, Koike T, Takeuchi S, et al. Embolization of cerebral arteriovenous malformations achieved with polyvinyl alcohol particles: angiographic reappearance and complications. AJNR Am J Neuroradiol 1999;20:1323–1328.

77. D'Aliberti G, Talamonti G, Versari PP, et al. Comparison of pediatric and adult cerebral arteriovenous malformations. J Neurosurg Sci 1997;4:331–336.

78. Millar C, Bissonnette B, Humphreys RP. Cerebral arteriovenous malformations in children. Can J Anesth 1994;41(4):321–331.

79. Hoh BL, Ogilvy CS, Butler WE, et al. Multimodality treatment of nongalenic arteriovenous malformations in pediatric patients. Neurosurgery 2000;47:346–358.

80. Shin M, Kawamoto S, Kurita H, et al. Retrospective analysis of a 10-year experience of stereotactic radio surgery for arteriovenous malformations in children and adolescents. J Neurosurg 2002; 97:779–784.

81. Hladky JP, Lejeune JP, Blond S, et al. Cerebral arteriovenous malformations in children: report on 62 cases. Childs Nerv Syst 1994;10:328–333.

82. Raybaud CA, Strother CM, Hald JK. Aneurysms of the vein of Galen: embryonic considerations and anatomical features relating to the pathogenesis of the malformation. Neuroradiology 1989;31:109–128.

83. Frawley GP, Dargaville PA, Mitchell PJ, et al. Clinical course and medical management of neonates with severe cardiac failure related to vein of Galen malformation. Arch Dis Child Fetal Neonatal Ed 2002;87:F144–F149.

84. Johnston IH, Whittle IR, Besser M, et al. Vein of Galen malformation: diagnosis and management. Neurosurgery 1987;20: 747–758.

85. Ciricillo SF, Edwards MSB, Schmidt KG, et al. Interventional neuroradiological management of vein of Galen malformations in the neonate. Neurosurgery 1990;27:22–28.

86. Lasjaunias P, Garcia-Monaco R, Rodesch G, et al. Vein of Galen malformation. Endovascular management of 43 cases. Childs Nerv Syst 1991;7:360–367.

87. Mickle JP, Quisling RG. The transtorcular embolization of vein of Galen aneurysms. J Neurosurg 1986;64:731–735.

88. Dowd CF, Halbach VV, Barnwell SL, et al. Transfemoral venous embolization of vein of Galen malformations. AJNR Am J Neuroradiol 1990;11:643–648.

89. Garcia-Monaco R, Lasjaunias P, Berenstein A. Therapeutic management of vein of Galen aneurysmal malformations. In: Vinuela F, Halbach VV, Dion JE, eds. Interventional Neuroradiology: Endovascular Therapy of the Central Nervous System. New York: Raven, 1992:113–127.

90. Mitchell PJ, Rosenfeld JV, Dargaville P, et al. Endovascular management of vein of Galen aneurysmal malformations presenting in the neonatal period. AJNR Am J Neuroradiol 2001;22:1403–1409.

91. Lasjaunias P, Hui F, Zerah M, et al. Cerebral arteriovenous malformations in children. Management of 179 consecutive cases and review of the literature. Childs Nerv Syst 1995;11:66–79.

92. Lylyk P, Vinuela F, Dion JE, et al. Therapeutic alternatives for vein of Galen vascular malformations. J Neurosurg 1993;78:438–445.

93. Jones BV, Ball WS, Tomsick TA, et al. Vein of Galen aneurysmal malformation: diagnosis and treatment of 13 children with extended clinical follow-up. AJNR Am J Neuroradiol 2002;23: 1717–1724.

94. Frizzel RT, Fisher WS 3rd. Cure, morbidity, and mortality associated with embolizations of brain arteriovenous malformations: a review of 1246 patients in 32 series over a 35-year period. Neurosurgery 1995;37:1031–1040.

95. Liu HM, Wang YH, Chen YF, et al. Endovascular treatment of brain-stem arteriovenous malformations: safety and efficacy. Neuroradiology 2003;45:644–649.

96. Vinuela FV, Debrun GM, Fox AJ, et al. Dominant-hemisphere arteriovenous malformations: therapeutic embolization with isobutyl-2-cyanoacrylate. AJNR Am J Neuroradiol 1983;4:959–966.

97. Hartman A, Pile-Spellman J, Stapf C, et al. Risk of endovascular treatment of brain arteriovenous malformations. Stroke 2002;33:1816–1820.

98. Spetzler RF, Wilson CB, Weinstein P, et al. Normal perfusion breakthrough theory. In: Congress of Neurological Surgeons, eds. Clinical Surgery. Baltimore: Williams & Wilkins, 1978:651–672.

99. Duckwiler GR, Dion JE, Vinuela F, et al. Delayed venous occlusion following embolotherapy of vascular malformations in the brain. AJNR Am J Neuroradiol 1992;13:1571–1579.

100. Miyasaka Y, Yada K, Ohwada T, et al. Retrograde thrombosis of feeding arteries after removal of arteriovenous malformations. J Neurosurg 1990;72:540–545.

Intracranial Aneurysm Therapy

Michael J. Alexander

Early endovascular therapy for cerebral aneurysms in the 1970s involved either deliberate parent artery occlusion or endosaccular therapy with silicone balloons innovated by Serbinenko (1), and subsequently others (2–4), as an alternative to open surgical treatment in high-risk patients. In 1990, this treatment paradigm changed with the development of engineered bare platinum coils (Guglielmi Detachable Coils) that allowed for controlled, graduated endosaccular embolization of cerebral aneurysms, which were considered high risk for surgical treatment (5–7). By 1995, the Food and Drug Administration approved GDC coils for cerebral aneurysm treatment in the United States, which has led to the widespread application of this therapy to ruptured and unruptured cerebral aneurysms.

Early small, single-center experiences have demonstrated the relative safety of aneurysm coil embolization compared to surgical clipping. A prospective, randomized trial by Vanninen et al. (8) of 111 patients with ruptured small neck aneurysms compared results of coiled aneurysms to clipped aneurysms. This study showed a slightly lower mortality rate with coiling, although overall short-term outcome between the two groups was not significantly different. From a technical standpoint, the postprocedural angiogram results of the posterior circulation aneurysms were better in the coiling group. Technical results with the anterior circulation aneurysms were better in the surgery group. This study did suggest that coil embolization could be competitive as a therapy for ruptured aneurysms with comparable morbidity and mortality data.

In a single-center trial reported by Raftopoulos et al. (9), an intention-to-treat analysis was performed in a group of 103 patients with 132 aneurysms. In the study, 64 aneurysms were prospectively assigned to endovascular treatment; the rest were assigned to surgical treatment. The outcome analysis of patients following treatment did not show a significant difference in the percentage of patients with good or favorable outcomes, although the surgical group overall did slightly better with 93.9% of patients experiencing good outcome in the surgical arm and 86.7% of patients with good outcome in the endovascular arm. Although the competing therapies were essentially comparable in results, the endovascular group had a relatively high complication rate with serious complications of thromboembolic events and arterial perforations comprising 9.4% of the study group.

Larger prospective trials have demonstrated the safety of coil embolization compared to open surgery for cerebral aneurysms. The International Study of Unruptured Intracranial Aneurysms (ISUIA) trial was a prospective nonrandomized trial evaluating patients with unruptured cerebral aneurysms (10). In the two study arms, patients were enrolled in treatment or observation groups, and the treatment arm consisted of surgery or coil embolization. The results from this study indicated lower morbidity and mortality in the coil embolization group (451 patients) compared to the surgical group (1,917 patients), particularly in posterior circulation aneurysms. The International Subarachnoid Aneurysm trial (ISAT) was a prospective, randomized, multi-institutional trial comparing surgical clipping with endovascular coiling for ruptured cerebral aneurysms that were judged amenable to either treatment arm (11). A total of 2,143 patients were enrolled in this trial, which was stopped early by the study advisory committee because a statistically significant lower morbidity was seen in the patients treated with endovascular therapy. This study showed a statistically significant reduction in death and dependency at 1-year follow-up in the embolized patients, with a 6.9% absolute risk reduction, judged by the modified Rankin scores of the patients. The question that the study has not answered with the current follow-up concerns the durability of the coil embolization procedure and whether the improved clinical results seen in the first year carry into long-term follow-up. Specifically, is the subsequent rehemorrhage rate in the coiled aneurysms significant? Longer-term follow-up will be necessary to make this assessment.

The management of intracranial aneurysms by endovascular therapy is a high–acuity-level treatment. In fact, proper treatment can be lifesaving in the case of ruptured aneurysms or preventive (of future stroke or death) in the case of unruptured aneurysms.

As an alternative to surgical treatment, endovascular therapy is less invasive; however, the potential complications of intervention include thromboembolic stroke, aneurysm or vessel perforation leading to cerebral hemorrhage, arterial dissection, and retroperitoneal hematoma, all of which are potentially severely disabling or fatal. Therefore, an experienced neurointerventionalist is needed for such therapy. Thorough counseling of the patients and their families is needed as well.

Most interventions for intracranial aneurysm therapy mandate general anesthesia, except in certain circumstances. Because a few millimeters of microcatheter movement in a cerebral aneurysm may perforate the vessel, general anesthesia is generally considered the safest management. Also, most embolization procedures for intracranial aneurysm therapy are performed with lowest risk under systemic anticoagulation. Procedural thromboembolic events are among the most common problems with aneurysm embolization; therefore, careful consideration of the anticoagulation regimen and monitoring of the treatment is advised.

SACCULAR ANEURYSMS

Saccular, or berry type, aneurysms are aneurysms that anatomically and angiographically have a well-defined neck. These are the ideal aneurysms for endovascular coiling, provided there are no significant branch arteries or perforators coming out of the aneurysm dome or neck. These aneurysms may have a small neck, which typically means a neck of fewer than 4 mm with a dome to neck ratio of 2:1 or higher; or the aneurysms may have a wide neck, which is typically a neck of greater than or equal to 4 mm with a dome to neck ratio of less than 2:1. Three-dimensional rotational angiography can help identify the best angle of the image intensifier for the embolization working view. When a working view that clearly defines the aneurysm neck from the parent artery and branch arteries cannot be obtained, then embolization is more risky and may not be the preferred treatment option. An inadequate working view is most common at the middle cerebral artery bifurcation or trifurcation and the anterior

communicating artery locations, respectively, because the orientation of the branch arteries may obscure a clean view of the aneurysm neck, particularly when the neck is wide.

ENDOSACCULAR EMBOLIZATION THERAPY

Embolization Materials

The goal of endosaccular embolization therapy is to fill the aneurysm with embolization material as completely as possible to promote thrombosis and healing of the aneurysm sac or to redirect flow from the aneurysm sac into the parent artery.

Bare Platinum Coils

The Guglielmi detachable coil (GDC) was the first bare platinum coil approved for human use in cerebral aneurysm embolization. This coil has gone through modifications over the years to provide different coil sizes, shapes, and degrees of softness or firmness to adapt to the different situations in cerebral aneurysm embolization. Other interventional companies have followed with their iterations of bare platinum or nitinol coils. Typically, the initial step in primary aneurysm embolization is providing an outer framework or basket circumferentially within the aneurysm and across the aneurysm neck. Subsequently, the basket is filled with progressively smaller and softer coils until the entire aneurysm is filled. With standard bare platinum coils, the average packing density of coils within the aneurysm is only approximately 20–40%. The remainder of the aneurysm fills with thrombus (Figure 49–1). Despite the fact that a relatively low percentage of the aneurysm is filled with coils, the aneurysm frequently appears angiographically obliterated at the end of the embolization. Particularly for large or giant aneurysms or aneurysms with a wide neck, there is a relatively high long-term recanalization rate with bare platinum coils (12–15). Pathologic studies have shown that thrombus does develop within the aneurysm with the use of bare platinum coils; however, there is little healing response, particularly at the aneurysm neck (16).

Polymer-Enhanced Coils

Because the long-term recanalization rate for bare platinum coils has been somewhat problematic, several types of polymer-enhanced coils have been developed. The goal of this technology is to have the polymer initiate a stronger healing response resulting from its bioactive properties or to have the activated polymer improve the packing density and filling capability of the coils. In 2002, Boston Scientific introduced the first polymer-coated coils for clinical use in cerebral aneurysms. The development of polyglycolic poly-lactic acid copolymer-coated coils has been an attempt to

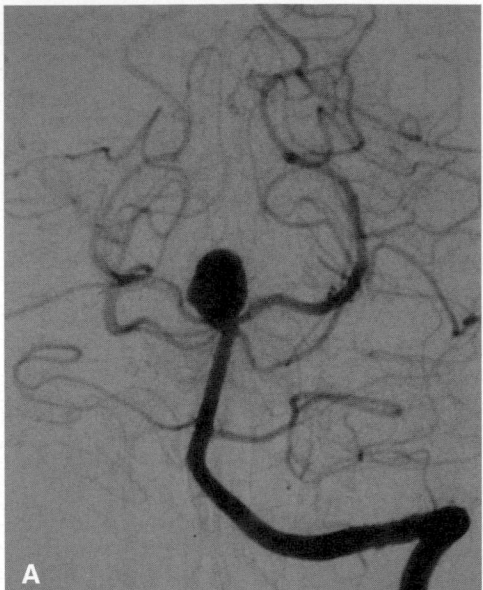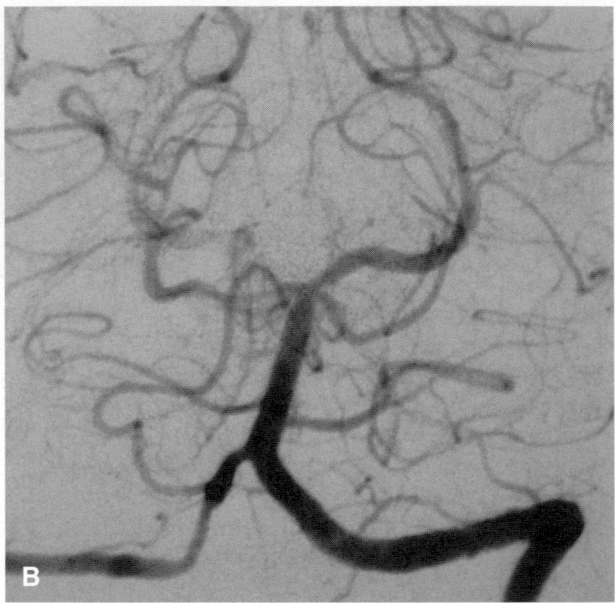

Figure 49–1 A. Townes view digital subtraction vertebral artery angiogram demonstrating ruptured basilar tip aneurysm before treatment, and **B.** immediately following treatment by coil embolization without adjunctive balloon or stent assistance. Complete occlusion is obtained with no evidence of contrast entering the aneurysm and with preservation of both P1 segments.

augment the body's own healing response, promote increased healing across the aneurysm neck, and reduce the long-term regrowth and rerupture rate (17). This coil was later paralleled by Micrus with a polymer-enhanced platinum coil with the polymer at its core.

Microvention later introduced a different concept in polymer-coated coils in which platinum coils are coated with a volume-expanding hydrogel coating designed to increase the packing density within cerebral aneurysms in a time-dependent fashion (18). Once the coated coils are introduced into the bloodstream, they begin to expand within several minutes once they are positioned securely in the aneurysm. Naturally, if additional time is required to position the coil adequately, the coil must be removed before expansion.

Liquid Polymer Embolization

A novel approach to endosaccular aneurysm embolization involves developing quickly polymerizing liquid polymers to fill 100% of the aneurysm with embolic material. This strategy relies more on flow diversion than on aneurysm thrombosis. With balloon-assisted technology, the polymer is slowly injected into the aneurysm to entirely fill the aneurysm. The balloon is deflated intermittently between polymer injections to allow for cerebral perfusion. In addition to getting a higher percentage volume filling with the liquid polymer, another advantage of liquid polymer embolization is that the polymer can conform to irregularly shaped aneurysms or very wide necks (Figure 49–2). The Cerebral Aneurysm Multicenter European Onyx (CAMEO) trial was a prospective study to evaluate a quickly polymerizing, nonadhesive ethylene vinyl alcohol copolymer—Onyx

(Micro Therapeutics Inc.)—for intracranial aneurysms (19). The midterm angiographic analysis in these patients, many of whom had giant or very complex aneurysms, showed complete aneurysm occlusion in 79% of the cases, subtotal occlusion in 13% of patients, and incomplete occlusion in 8%. These early angiographic data also, however, showed an inadvertent delayed parent artery occlusion in 9 of 71 patients (13%) with angiographic follow-up at 12 months. Not all of these occlusions were symptomatic, but it remained a setback for the trial.

ADJUNCTIVE TECHNOLOGIES FOR ENDOSACCULAR EMBOLIZATION

In situations in which the aneurysm has a wide neck, endosaccular embolization is still a viable option with the adjunctive use of balloon-assisted technology or stent assistance.

Balloon-Assisted Technology

Particularly as the very first few coils and very last few coils are being placed within an aneurysm with a wide neck, the propensity for the coil to herniate into the parent artery is high. By temporarily inflating a highly compliant balloon in the parent artery during coil delivery, the coil mass may be remodeled to keep the coils within the aneurysm. This strategy, reported by Moret and others (20,21), uses a very compliant balloon, sized closely with the parent artery size, to remodel the coils as they are inserted into the aneurysm. As more coils are delivered into the sac of the aneurysm,

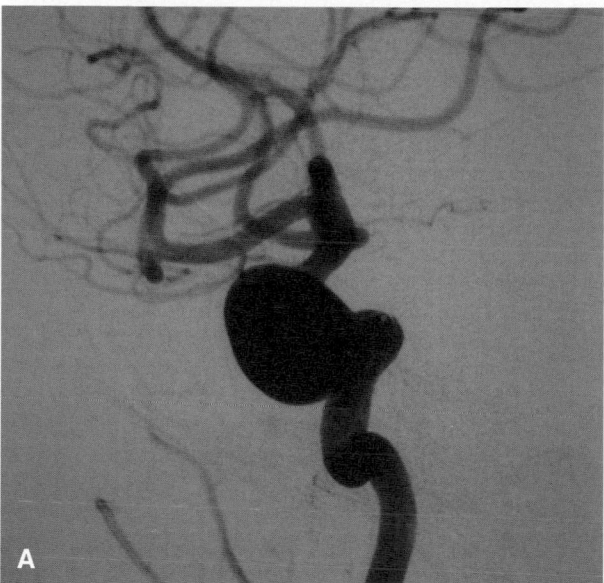
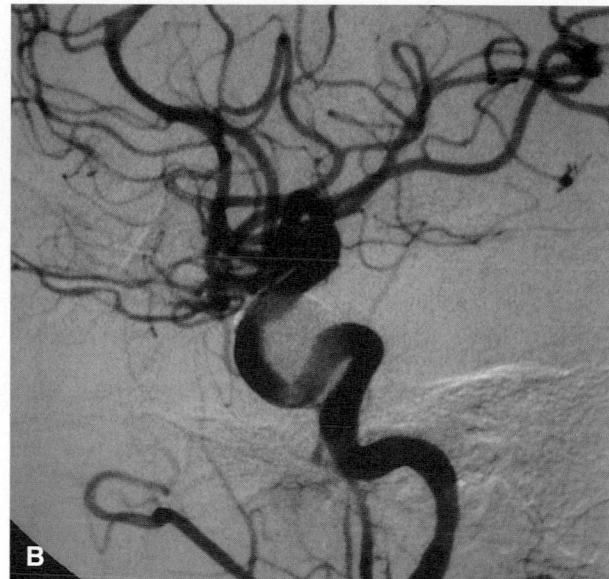

Figure 49–2 **A.** Lateral view digital subtraction carotid artery angiogram showing a giant, partially thrombosed, symptomatic, wide-neck, cavernous carotid aneurysm. **B.** The same view after balloon-assisted embolization of the complex aneurysm with a rapidly polymerizing liquid embolic agent, showing reconstruction of the arterial wall at the neck and complete occlusion of the aneurysm with preservation of the internal carotid artery.

there is complexity of the intertwining coils that leads to more coil stability. During the temporary inflation of the compliant balloon during coil delivery, the coils are remodeled to conform at the aneurysm neck to the curvature of the artery inner luminal diameter. Great care must still be used in this technique, because as the balloon is deflated, there still may be some risk of coil herniation in the parent artery if there is not enough support. In such cases, stent-assisted technology may be needed. The technique of balloon remodeling requires either the use of a large shuttle catheter to position both the balloon and microcatheter through a single access catheter or the use of bifemoral access with two guiding catheters to position the balloon and microcatheter independently.

Stent-Assisted Technology

In aneurysms in which the neck is too wide for standard embolization or balloon-assisted technology, stent-assisted embolization is a good option.

Previously, coronary stents were employed to embolize these tough aneurysms by bridging the neck with the stent struts. Unfortunately, coronary stents are typically stainless steel-based and very stiff for use in the brain. They do not track well into the brain and were extraordinarily difficult to use with aneurysms on a curve.

The development of self-expanding nitinol stents that were specifically designed for treatment of aneurysms with a wide neck has expanded the types of aneurysms that can be treated by endovascular therapy (22–24). These nitinol stents are much more flexible and have a much better capacity for tracking through the intracranial arteries than coronary

stents. Even when the dome to neck ratio is 1:1 or lower, it is sometimes possible to embolize the aneurysm with stent assistance (Figure 49–3). Stent assistance may allow for a higher packing density of coils within the aneurysm, particularly at the neck, and may, in some cases, redirect flow within the parent artery so that there is less flow into the aneurysm and more laminar flow in the parent vessel (25).

Crossing perforator arteries or branch arteries has not been an issue for the ultra-thin nitinol stent for aneurysms. These vessels appear to remain patent, even though they are "jailed" by the stent. The long-term evaluation of these stents will need to be analyzed, though the midterm results look very promising. They do not appear to have the pronounced late lumen loss seen in coronary stents for cerebral atherosclerotic disease. In a review of more than 100 intracranial nitinol stents for aneurysm embolization with a mean follow-up of 12.1 months, there was an overall patency rate of 98% (25).

FUSIFORM ANEURYSMS

Fusiform aneurysms are anatomically poorly defined aneurysms. Because the artery is circumferentially involved, primary endosaccular embolization is often not possible, even though parent artery occlusion may be warranted. Evolving stent technology can play a role in this pathologic condition.

Parent Artery Occlusion

For large or giant aneurysms and fusiform-type aneurysms, embolization of the aneurysm or surgical clipping of the

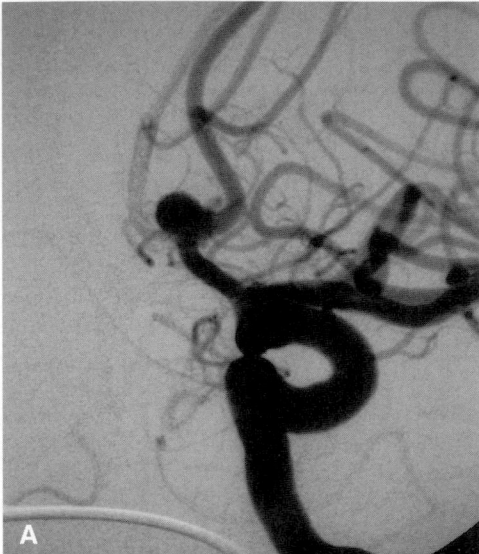
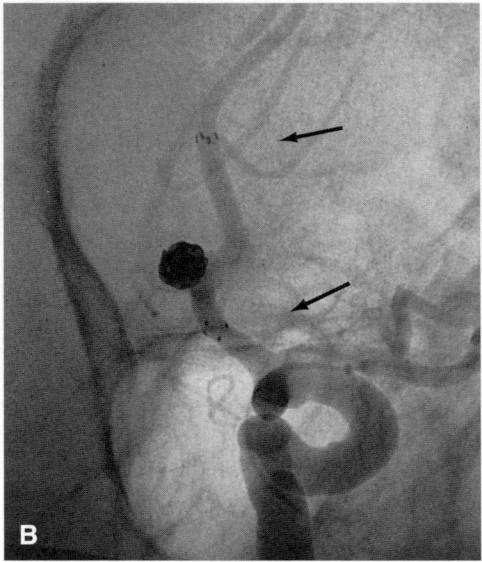

Figure 49–3 A. Slightly oblique anteroposterior (AP) view of a left carotid angiogram that shows a relatively small ruptured A1-A2 junction aneurysm with a wide neck. The aneurysm is coiled with stent assistance, using a flexible self-expanding nitinol stent. **B.** The stent struts are not seen on the radiograph at this magnification; however, the proximal and distal ends of the stent have radiopaque markers (*arrows*).

aneurysm may not be feasible, even with stent assistance. In such cases, proximal parent artery occlusion may be considered. Parent artery occlusion by endovascular methods (coil or balloon occlusion) is based historically on the surgical precedent of Hunterian ligation for aneurysms (26). The presumption is that occlusion of the parent artery proximally will redirect blood flow toward collateral arteries and away from the aneurysm, leading to aneurysm thrombosis. Naturally, if the collateral arteries continue to fill the aneurysm, then thrombosis may not occur. Therefore, the collateral circulation must be assessed carefully before a commitment is made about permanent artery occlusion. The assessment of collateral circulation typically involves a three or four vessel cerebral angiogram with Matas testing. The Matas test assesses the patency of the anterior communicating artery by manually compressing the ipsilateral carotid artery in the neck while injecting contrast into the contralateral carotid artery (27). This serves not only to determine the existence of the anterior communicating artery collaterals, but the rapidity with which the ipsilateral anterior circulation fills, with respect to the contralateral circulation. Once the angiographic anatomy is determined, a functional test is usually needed to confirm that permanent occlusion of the artery will not lead to cerebral ischemia and stroke following the procedure. A temporary balloon-test occlusion is performed in conjunction with intraprocedural neurologic testing and correlated cerebral blood flow (CBF) or functional testing (Figure 49–4). CBF testing during the balloon-test occlusion can be performed using SPECT (99m Tc-HMPAO) scanning, CT perfusion testing, or transcranial Doppler

ultrasound. Functional testing may incorporate intraprocedural EEG monitoring (28–30).

Even with proper testing and adequate embolization planning, the risk of thromboembolic or ischemic stroke is higher in patients with deliberate parent artery occlusion compared to standard endosaccular coil embolization because of the stasis in flow (31–32). Generally, patients are kept on a heparin drip overnight with a goal PTT of 55–70 following occlusion, and their systolic blood pressure is kept at 110–120% of their baseline blood pressure

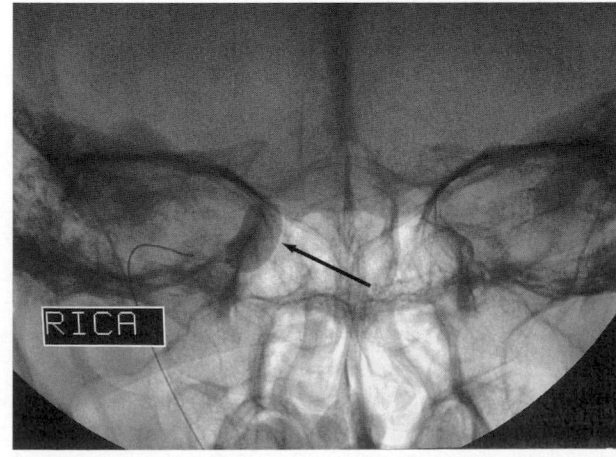

Figure 49–4 AP radiograph during a temporary balloon test occlusion of the right internal carotid artery. The very compliant balloon is inflated in the cavernous segment of the internal carotid artery (*arrow*) during functional testing of the patient.

for 24 hours to promote collateral blood flow. After the first 24 hours, the patient is often placed on aspirin or other antiplatelet therapy.

In addition to proximal permanent parent artery occlusion for large, giant, or fusiform aneurysms, permanent parent artery segmental occlusion is also used as a treatment modality for some mycotic aneurysms. The primary treatment for incidentally diagnosed unruptured mycotic aneurysms in the setting of subacute bacterial endocarditis or other infectious primary disease is intravenous antibiotics. However, when a mycotic aneurysm ruptures or has demonstrated growth radiographically while on intravenous antibiotic therapy, surgical or endovascular treatment is warranted. These aneurysms are typically in distal branches and are not usually saccular. Therefore, endosaccular coil embolization is often not possible. In these cases, the segmental occlusion of the parent artery by either coils or a rapidly polymerizing, high-concentration glue, such as N-butyl cyanoacrylate, can be performed. By occluding the artery only over the small segment that the mycotic aneurysm arises from, pial collateral vessels may supply the distal artery via retrograde flow. Again, the use of anticoagulants such as heparin or direct thrombin inhibitors such as lepirudin, following the deliberate artery occlusion, may be warranted for a short period to prevent distal thromboembolic occlusion and infarction. The clinical and angiographic situation must determine this management.

Covered Stent Therapy

In fusiform aneurysms that have too wide of a neck for embolization with stent assistance, or involve the artery circumferentially, or involve pseudoaneurysms that have no true aneurysm wall, innovative strategies must be used. This is particularly true when the patient fails a balloon-test occlusion and parent artery sacrifice is not a treatment

option. In such cases, the parent artery may be preserved or reconstructed with a stent graft that obliterates the aneurysm or pseudoaneurysm but maintains parent artery blood flow. A stent graft usually has a standard stent as its base but is covered with an impervious material, such as an expanded polytetrafluoroethylene (ePTFE) polymer (Figure 49–5).

Alexander et al. (33) were the first to describe the use of a self-expanding stent graft for a cerebral aneurysm. In this report, the Symbiot stent (Boston Scientific) was used to treat a traumatic carotid pseudoaneurysm. This stent graft used an ePTFE covering on a nitinol self-expanding stent. Less flexible, stainless steel-based covered stents have been reported for extracranial and intracranial aneurysms and pseudoaneurysms of the neurovasculature. The Jostent (Jomed) is a balloon-expandable stainless steel-covered stent with ePTFE that was designed originally for coronary artery perforation treatment, but it has been used by numerous investigators for treatment of aneurysms of the carotid and vertebral arteries (34–37). Patients treated with stent grafts in the neurovasculature usually are treated with an antiplatelet medication such as clopidogrel following the procedure for at least 6 weeks, if not longer, to reduce the risk of acute or subacute stent-graft thrombosis.

These and other stent grafts are primarily limited to treat aneurysms near the skull base. It is presumed that placement of this type of stent graft in the more distal vasculature would result in the occlusion of significant perforator arteries, which could result in infarctions.

SUMMARY

The technology involved in the endovascular treatment of cerebral aneurysms has quickly grown over the past 15 years, and it continues to evolve at a rapid pace. In 2004, the number of cerebral aneurysms addressed in the United States and treated by endovascular therapy surpassed the number of aneurysms surgically clipped for the first time. Efforts to increase coil-packing density, to redirect flow with flexible stents, and to develop more bioactive and biocompatible materials have improved the long-term results of embolization and have made treatment safer for patients with cerebral aneurysms.

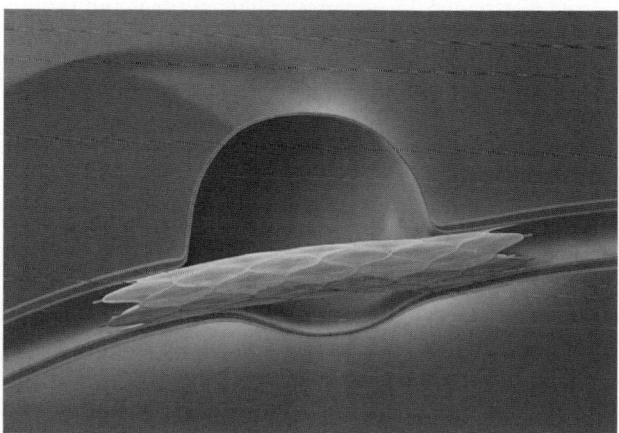

Figure 49–5 Schematic of a giant fusiform aneurysm treated by a covered, self-expanding stent graft that occludes the aneurysm but preserves the parent artery. Because the aneurysm involves the artery circumferentially, traditional coils and bare stents are not a viable treatment option.

REFERENCES

1. Serbinenko FA. Balloon catheterization and occlusion of major cerebral vessels. J Neurosurg 1974;41:125–145.
2. Aymard A, Merland JJ, Gobin PY.[Endovascular treatment of intracranial aneurysms: techniques and results. Report of 130 cases.] Agressologie 1990 May;31:265–267. French.
3. Fox AJ, Vinuela F, Pelz DM, et al. Use of detachable balloons for proximal artery occlusion in the treatment of unclippable cerebral aneurysms. J Neurosurg 1987;66:40–46.
4. Higashida RT, Halbach VV, Dormandy BS, et al. Endovascular treatment of intracranial aneurysms with a new silicone microballoon device: technical considerations and indications for therapy. Radiology 1990;174:687–691.

5. Guglielmi G, Vinuela F, Sepetka I, et al. Electrothrombosis of saccular aneurysms via endovascular approach. Part I: electrochemical basis, technique, and experimental results. J Neurosurg 1991;75:1–7.

6. Guglielmi G, Vinuela F, Dion J, et al. Electrothrombosis of saccular aneurysms via endovascular approach. Part II: preliminary clinical experience. J Neurosurg 1991;75:8–14.

7. Guglielmi G, Vinuela F, Duckwiler G, et al. Endovascular treatment of posterior circulation aneurysms by electrothrombosis using electrically detachable coils. J Neurosurg 1992;77:515–524.

8. Vanninen R, Koivisto T, Saari T, et al. Ruptured intracranial aneurysms: acute endovascular treatment with electrolytically detachable coils—a prospective randomized study. Radiology 1999;211:325–336.

9. Raftopoulos C, Mathurin P, Boscherini D, et al. Prospective analysis of aneurysm treatment in a series of 103 consecutive patients when endovascular embolization is considered the first option. J Neurosurg 2000;93:175–182.

10. Wiebers DO, Whisnant JP, Huston J III, et al. Unruptured intracranial aneurysms: natural history, clinical outcome, and risks of surgical and endovascular treatment. Lancet 2003;363:103–110.

11. Molyneux A, Kerr R, Stratton I, et al. International Subarachnoid Aneurysm Trial (ISAT) Collaborative Group. Lancet 2002;360: 1267–1274.

12. Murayama Y, Nien YL, Duckwiler G, et al. Guglielmi detachable coil embolization of cerebral aneurysms: 11 years' experience. J Neurosurg 2003;98:959–966.

13. Henkes H, Fischer S, Weber W, et al. Endovascular coil occlusion of 1811 intracranial aneurysms: early angiographic and clinic results. Neurosurgery 2004;54:268–280.

14. Raymond J, Guilbert F, Weill A. Long-term angiographic recurrence after selective endovascular treatment of aneurysms with detachable coils. Stroke 2003;34:1398–1403.

15. Sluzewski M, van Rooij WJ, Slob MJ, et al. Relation between aneurysm volume, packing, and compaction in 145 cerebral aneurysms treated with coils. Radiology 2004;231:653–658.

16. Molyneux AJ, Ellison DW, Morris J, et al. Histological findings in giant aneurysms treated with Guglielmi detachable coils. Report of two cases with autopsy correlation. J Neurosurg 1995;83:129–132.

17. Murayama Y, Tateshima S, Gonzalez NR, et al. Matrix and bioabsorbable polymeric coils accelerate healing of intracranial aneurysms: long-term experimental study. Stroke 2003;34: 2031–2037.

18. Cloft HJ, Kallmes DF. Aneurysm packing with HydroCoil embolic system versus platinum coils: initial clinical experience.AJNR Am J Neuroradiol 2004;25:60–62.

19. Molyneux AJ, Cekirge S, Saatci I, et al. Cerebral aneurysm multicenter European Onyx (CAMEO) trial: results of a prospective observational study in 20 European centers. AJNR Am J Neuroradiol 2004;25:39–51.

20. Moret J, Cognard C, Weill A, et al. Reconstruction technique in the treatment of wide-neck intracranial aneurysms: long-term angiographic and clinical results. Apropos of 56 cases. J Neuroradiol 1997;24:30–44.

21. Levy DI, Ku A. Balloon-assisted coil placement in wide-necked aneurysms. Technical note. 1997;86:724–727.

22. Benitez RP, Silva MT, Klem J, et al. Endovascular occlusion of wide-necked aneurysms with a new intracranial microstent (Neuroform) and detachable coils. Neurosurgery 2004;54: 1359–1367.

23. Fiorella D, Albuquerque FC, Han P, et al. Preliminary experience using the Neuroform stent for the treatment of cerebral aneurysms. Neurosurgery 2004;54:6–16.

24. Howington JU, Hanel RA, Harringan MR, et al. The Neuroform stent, the first microcatheter-delivered stent for use in the intracranial circulation. Neurosurgery 2004;54:2–5.

25. Alexander MJ, Zaidat OO, Tolbert M. Clinical outcome and technical feasibility of intracranial aneurysm therapy using Neuroform stent-assisted coil embolization [Abstract]. J Neurosurg 2005; 102:A421.

26. Miller JD, Jawad K, Jennett B. Safety of carotid ligation and its role in the management of intracranial aneurysms. J Neurol Neurosurg Psychiatry 1977;40:64–72.

27. Matas R. Testing the efficiency of the collateral circulation as a preliminary to the occlusion of the great surgical arteries. Ann Surg 1911;53:1–43.

28. Erba SM, Horton JA, Latchaw RE, et al. Balloon test occlusion of the internal carotid artery with stable xenon/CT cerebral blood flow imaging. AJNR Am J Neuroradiol 1988;9:533–538.

29. Eckard DA, Purdy PD, Bonte FJ. Temporary balloon occlusion of the carotid artery combined with brain blood flow imaging as a test to predict tolerance prior to permanent carotid sacrifice. AJNR Am J Neuroradiol 1992;13:1565–1569.

30. Morioka T, Matsushima T, Fujii K, et al. Balloon test occlusion of the internal carotid artery with monitoring of compressed spectral arrays (CSAs) of electroencephalogram. Acta Neurochir 1989;101:29–34.

31. Nishioka H. Report on the cooperative study of intracranial aneurysms and subarachnoid hemorrhage: results of the treatment of intracranial aneurysms by occlusion of the carotid artery in the neck. J Neurosurg 1966;25:660–682.

32. Higashida RT, Halbach VV, Dowd C, et al. Endovascular detachable balloon embolization therapy of cavernous carotid artery aneurysms: results in 87 cases. J Neurosurg 1990;72:857–863.

33. Alexander MJ, Smith TP, Tucci DL.Treatment of an iatrogenic petrous carotid artery pseudoaneurysm with a Symbiot covered stent: technical case report. Neurosurgery 2002;50:658–662.

34. Saatci I, Cekirge HS, Ozturk MH, et al. Treatment of internal carotid artery aneurysms with a covered stent: experience in 24 patients with mid-term follow-up results. AJNR Am J Neuroradiol 2004;25:1742–1749.

35. Blasco J, Macho JM, Burrel M, et al. Endovascular treatment of a giant intracranial aneurysm with a stent graft. J Vasc Interv Radiol 2004;15:1145–1149.

36. Felber S, Henkes H, Weber W, et al. Treatment of extracranial and intracranial aneurysms and arteriovenous fistulae using stent grafts. Neurosurgery 2004;55:631–639.

37. Burbelko MA, Dzyak LA, Zorin NA, et al. Stent-graft placement for wide-neck aneurysm of the vertebrobasilar junction. AJNR Am J Neuroradiol 2004;25:608–610.

Neuroendovascular Therapy of Intracranial, Extra-Axial Lesions

50

Jason Allen, Tibor Becske, Peter Kim Nelson

The development of therapeutic endovascular procedures for the treatment of central nervous system (CNS) and maxillofacial lesions has been facilitated by improvements in angiographic methods, microcatheter technology, and embolic agents, as well as by advancements in the understanding of the functional vascular anatomy of the head and neck (1–6). To be successful, the endovascular management of CNS and maxillofacial lesions must involve a multidisciplinary approach to the unique clinical needs of each patient. Neuroradiologists performing endovascular therapies should be skilled in the use of microcatheters and embolic agents. They must also have a thorough understanding of the pathologic entities and specific neurovascular anatomy involved in each case. Regardless of the technique employed, however, the ultimate degree of success in treatment is strongly dependent on appropriate patient selection and the precise definition of therapeutic goals.

Intracranial, extra-axial lesions amenable to endovascular therapy can be divided into two categories: (1) vascular disorders, including traumatic lesions resulting in vessel injury and vasculopathies affecting dural vessels or the extradural internal carotid artery (ICA), and (2) neoplasms of the dura and calvarium. Therapeutic procedures directed toward lesions of the head and neck are best performed under general anesthesia, except when patient cooperation, as in carotid or vertebral occlusion or cranial nerve testing, is required (2).

In most cases, it is possible to perform the angiographic workup and embolization in one session. Preoperative planning based on information provided by CT and MRI studies (Figures 50–2, 50–4, 50–5, and 50–6) generally facilitates this process. The diagnostic angiogram should follow a specific protocol and must delineate the arterial supply to a target lesion, to its angioarchitecture, and to its vascular compartmentalization (Figures 50–5 and 50–6), as well as to the regional collateral circulation, potential arterioarterial anastomoses with critical vascular territories, vascular supplies to cranial nerves, and/or cutaneous tissues, whichever is relevant to the specific case. In addition, the prevailing cortical or dural venous drainage and any alterations in the normal cerebrofacial venous system should be defined.

Although various preshaped catheters are used in diagnostic angiography, embolizations often require special guiding catheters that permit the coaxial introduction of microcatheters of various sizes during the superselective phase of angiography and embolization. For neurointerventional procedures requiring catheterization of distal branches arising from the external carotid artery, variable-stiffness microcatheters (7) employing a selection of specially designed guide wires are preferred because of their improved ability to negotiate tortuous distal vascular segments previously regarded as inaccessible even during slow-flow states. From a technical perspective, four principal factors determine the success of embolization: (1) the intrinsic complexity of a specific lesion, (2) the accessibility of its vascular supply, (3) the technical quality and selectivity of the superselective catheterization, and (4) the choice of embolic material (8).

FUNCTIONAL EMBOLIZATION

Selective catheterization of the distal vascular supply to a lesion presents obvious advantages because it improves the effectiveness of embolization while reducing complications resulting from nonselective embolization of normal tissues (2). The level to which a catheter may be advanced, however, is limited theoretically by the inner diameter of the artery in question relative to the outer diameter of the microcatheter, ignoring additional problems related to vessel tortuosity that increase resistance to catheter motion and promote kinking. Furthermore, attempts at deploying microcatheters distally within branches of the external carotid artery are often frustrated by the development of vasospasm or vessel injury during the catheterization. The reduction of antegrade flow beyond the distal tip of the catheter during vasospasm impedes the flow-assisted deposition of particulate agents into the vascular bed of a more distally located lesion. In certain situations, flow arrest may be desirable in achieving reversal of flow through critical anastomoses or in establishing a stagnant conduit through which liquid embolic agents may be more effectively delivered to a distal target site, thereby establishing an effective embolization point closer to the desired target than is achievable with a microcatheter alone (9,10). However, with particulate agents such as gelfoam powder or polyvinyl alcohol (PVA), free-flow embolization from a more proximal catheter position may be preferable because the emboli are better carried into the selected target by an unimpeded bloodstream. Unfortunately, embolizations from proximal catheter positions are often confounded by the wider distribution of emboli into a more extensive vascular territory that includes the lesion in question as well as normal tissues.

During embolization, normal tissues are placed at risk—depending on the specific anatomic disposition—by virtue of their vascularization directly from a branch continuation of the parent artery supplying a given lesion or through anastomotic connections with vessels supplying the lesion (Figure 50–3H and I; Figure 50–5H). Either of these conditions may necessitate some precautions to ensure safe embolization. The most obvious precaution requires advancement of the microcatheter selectively into distal vessels directly vascularizing the lesion. If this is not possible because multiple small feeding vessels are supplying a lesion or because the distal branches irrigating a lesion cannot be catheterized atraumatically, the parent artery may be temporarily occluded with an inflatable balloon distal to the origin of the target vessels. The lesion is then embolized with microparticles from a proximal position. Parent vessel occlusion is designed to protect the normal tissues distal to the occluded segment while preserving free-flow embolization into the lesion. This assumes adequate collateral supply to the protected vascular territory. In the extreme example, the protected vascular territory may be the brain, as in cavernous sinus or clival lesions supplied by the inferolateral C4 or meningohypophyseal C5 (Fischer classification) segments of the internal carotid artery (11). These lesions may be embolized with microparticles after temporary balloon occlusion of the distal supracavernous segment, assuming adequate collateral circulation at the level of the circle of Willis. Moreover, in this specific instance, to avoid embolization of microparticles into the cerebral vasculature, multiple aspirations and exchange rinsing of the occluded carotid segment with heparinized saline should be done before balloon deflation (12). Alternatively, in cases in which tumor involvement of the petrous or cavernous segments of the internal carotid artery has been implicated by axial imaging studies, temporary occlusion of the internal carotid artery may be converted to permanent occlusion, if collateral supply to the affected brain hemisphere is adequate.

Under conditions in which anastomoses have been shown between the supply to a lesion and a critical vascular territory, it may be possible to occlude the anastomotic channel with a coil or strip of gelfoam before embolizing the primary arterial feeder. When the anastomotic connection is too small to be catheterized, embolization of the lesion may be attempted using flow reversal across the anastomosis (2). The desired reversal of flow occurs when the arterial pressure differential across the anastomosis results in the flow of blood from the region of concern, such as the orbit, into the channel supplying the target lesion, thereby protecting the normal tissues. Reversal of flow across an anastomosis of concern may be established by inducing a state of flow arrest within the main pedicle supplying a lesion proximal to the anastomosis, either by wedging the microcatheter or, in selected cases, by using a proximal occlusion balloon. Under ideal conditions, flow reversal may enable early stage embolization with ultrasmall microparticles or liquid adhesives under circumstances in which the unprotected antegrade penetration of normal vascular territories through critical anastomoses would not be tolerated. For cases in which microparticles are used under flow arrest conditions, change to a particulate size larger than the anastomotic channels during the later stages of the procedure may become necessary as reflux becomes more likely. To reduce the risk of the procedure, the larger particulate sizes find utility during embolizations of meningeal vessels suspected of supplying cranial nerves and other critical anastomoses, as well as in embolizations involving transosseus branches arising from scalp vessels to avoid necrosis in cutaneous territories.

Another adaptation of functional embolization may be employed in cases in which anastomoses between divisions of the external carotid artery (ECA) and internal carotid artery (ICA) are in hemodynamic balance in supplying a dural lesion. This condition exists for lesions dually supplied by the inferolateral trunk (ILT) of the internal carotid artery and dural branches of the accessory meningeal artery, middle meningeal artery, and artery of the foramen rotundum

(Figure 50–3A and C). Cavernous segment temporary balloon occlusion of the ICA across the origin of the ILT may permit embolization of the lesion from one of the above-mentioned ECA branches, thereby exploiting the anatomic anastomoses between these meningeal vessels and the temporarily occluded ILT.

Alternatively, in situations in which flow arrest within a supplying ECA branch is achieved by way of a wedged microcatheter, a lesion supplied by meningeal arteries that are anastomosing with dural branches of the ICA may be embolized using the inflow from the ICA to carry particles introduced by way of the ECA axis into the target vascular territory. This essentially exploits a condition of flow–arrest-induced reversal of flow through the specific local ICA-ECA anastomosis (Figure 50–5). Under these conditions, however, extreme caution must be exercised in avoiding transanastomotic embolization into the ICA.

EMBOLIC AGENTS

The choice of embolic agent depends on the goal of the procedure, the selectivity accomplished during catheterization, the vascular anatomy, and the pathologic entity (2,3,13). The following are commonly used embolic materials for embolization of extra-axial lesions.

Polyvinyl Alcohol (PVA) Foam

PVA is a nonabsorbable, biocompatible sponge material. Particulate forms useful in the embolization of extra-axial lesions vary in size from 45 to 500 μm in diameter and are easily injected through an appropriately sized microcatheter. As a general rule, microparticles are preferred to fluid materials for the preoperative embolization of extra-axial tumors. They are easier and safer to use and, when employed in dilute suspensions, can reach the intratumoral vasculature where they obstruct small arteries.

Gelfoam

Gelfoam represents an alternative to microparticulate PVA embolization. It is available in powder form with particles ranging in size from 40–60 μm in diameter. Because of their smaller size, gelfoam microparticles are carried more distally into the microvasculature, promoting more complete embolic occlusion of a vascular bed. However, the smaller size increases the possibility of inadvertent embolization through dangerous anastomoses or the development of cranial nerve palsy when embolization is performed too proximally. For this reason, the larger PVA particulate sizes are preferred in embolizations of meningeal vessels that are also supplying cranial nerves or are coupled with cutaneous arteries (2,14).

Large strips of gelfoam sponge can be used for proximal occlusion of feeding vessels in a manner analogous to the deposition of metallic coils. Although this approach is not advocated for the primary embolization of arterial pedicles involved in the supply to dural-based lesions, such strips may be used advantageously to protect vascular territories in which the deposition of microparticles is undesirable. They may also be used to affect an endovascular ligation of an artery after traumatic vascular injury or to control a major arterial pedicle after microparticulate embolization of a more distally placed lesion.

N-Butyl Cyanoacrylate (n-BCA)

N-BCA (15) is a low-viscosity liquid that polymerizes rapidly after coming in contact with the electrolytic environment of the blood. The polymerization time may be delayed by dilution of the n-BCA in oil-based iodinated contrast materials, such as lipiodol or ethiodol, or by acidifying the admixture with glacial acetic acid so that a deposition target distal to the site of injection can be reached before final polymerization of the glue. Tantalum powder may be added for increased opacification and viscosity, depending on the lesion in question and the rate of blood flow through the embolized pedicle. Although of considerable use in the embolizations of dural arteriovenous malformations, n-BCA generally is less preferable to microparticles for the embolization of extra-axial tumors. Its use should be carefully controlled to avoid inadvertent embolization through dangerous anastomoses or penetration into normal vascular territories, where it may cause ischemia or necrosis of vital tissues. Skill with the use of such agents is also important to avoid gluing the catheter tip within the arterial lumen.

Ethanol

The potent sclerosing effect and relatively benign metabolism of ethanol make it an effective embolic material. As with other liquid agents, however, if it is inadvertently introduced into a normal vascular territory, serious complications related to the necrosis of normal tissues may result (2).

Coils

Metallic coils are supplied in a variety of lengths and configurations and may contain materials such as cotton or Dacron to promote thrombosis. They are easily introduced through size-matched microcatheters with the assistance of a guide wire/coil pusher. As with gelfoam strips, they may be used to protect normal vascular territories and provide endovascular ligation of traumatized vessels or pedicles previously embolized with microparticles. Where precise controlled deployment of a coil is necessary, various families of detachable platinum aneruysm coils without polymer or hydrogel coating (such as Guglielmi detachable coils) or with polymer or hydrogel coating (such as Matrix-GDC or Hydrocoils) have become more widely used for nonaneurysmal applications.

ANATOMIC CONSIDERATIONS

Extra-axial lesions may be subdivided into distinct locations by virtue of their characteristic vascular supply—the calvareal convexity, the falx cerebri, the floor of the anterior cranial fossa, the sphenoid wings, the cavernous sinus and parasellar regions, the tentorium cerebelli and adjacent dural sinuses, or the posterior fossa, including the cerebellar convexity, the cerebellar pontine angle, and the foramen magnum (13).

Lesions of the Convexity

Extra-axial lesions of the convexity and parasagittal surfaces of the skull vault predictably derive their vascular supply from branches of the middle meningeal or anterior ethmoidal arteries. The middle meningeal artery (MMA) most frequently originates from the ipsilateral internal maxillary artery (IMA) and enters the skull base through the foramen spinosum. It subsequently gives rise to several important branches vascularizing the dura of the skull base and middle cranial fossa before reaching the convexity. Although variable in their predominance, several branches are commonly recognized as supplying the cranial convexity. Anterior and posterior frontal branches may supply the frontal and anterior parietal regions of the convexity, originating most commonly from the continuation of the MMA through the foramen spinosum or, more infrequently, from the ophthalmic or the intraorbital lacrimal artery by way of a recurrent course through the superior orbital fissure (Figure 50–1). A parieto-occipital trunk may be identified as supplying the meninges of the posterior parietal and occipital regions of the supratentorial convexity. A petrosquamosal trunk is usually seen coursing within a groove defined by the petrous and squamous portions of the temporal bone. In addition to supplying the meninges throughout this region, this trunk gives tentorial branches to the basal edge of the tentorium cerebelli and may be used instead of the petrosal branch of the MMA to more safely embolize lesions involving the petrous ridge and petroclinoid region, thereby decreasing the likelihood of iatrogenic seventh cranial nerve palsy.

Two considerations must be addressed in the angiographic workup and embolization of lesions involving the parasagittal region. First, in addition to the ipsilateral meningeal vascular supply, potential contribution from the corresponding contralateral middle meningeal branches must be evaluated. The participation of contralateral supply occurs because of anastomoses along the extent of the superior sagittal sinus. The frontal parasagittal region may also include supply from the artery of the falx cerebri, which arises from the anterior ethmoidal arteries. Proper preembolization and postembolization angiographic evaluation of these lesions includes thorough assessment of the possible ipsilateral as well as contralateral middle meningeal supplies. A second consideration of importance concerns convexity and parasagittal lesions arising anteriorly along the frontal convexity. This area may derive vascular supply from meningeal branches of the anterior ethmoidal arteries and requires angiographic evaluation of potential contribution from the ophthalmic arteries.

The dural structures of the middle cranial fossa receive arterial branches from sphenoidal and middle cranial fossa divisions of the MMA. Embolization in this territory should avoid potential intervascular communications between these branches of the MMA and the cavernous internal carotid artery by way of anastomoses between the recurrent tentorial artery and the inferolateral or meningohypophyseal trunks and the orbit by way of meningolacrimal or meningo-ophthalmic anastomoses.

Lesions Involving the Falx Cerebri

Lesions arising from the falx cerebri are supplied by distal branches of the MMA that reach the midline and participate in the vascularization of the superior sagittal sinus and the falx cerebri. These vessels anastomose among themselves and potentially with their corresponding contralateral arteries as well as with transosseous branches arising from the superficial temporal artery. Lesions affecting the falx cerebri anteriorly may also be expected to receive supply from the artery of the falx cerebri, which, as previously mentioned, may arise from anterior ethmoidal branches of the ophthalmic artery. As with lesions of the convexity, in those cases in which transosseous supply from scalp vessels can be demonstrated, embolization must take into consideration maintenance of continued viable vascularization of the affected scalp. Infrequently, facial lesions may receive direct supply from the meningeal branches of the callosomarginal, pericallosal, and posterior cerebral arteries.

Lesions of the Anterior Cranial Base

Lesions involving the floor of the anterior cranial fossa can be subdivided into lateral and medial groups. Those involving the supraorbital regions are generally vascularized by anterior frontal branches of the MMA and meningeal branches of the ophthalmic artery. Conversely, midline lesions are supplied most often by meningeal branches of the anterior and posterior ethmoidal arteries that participate in a rich anastomotic network to supply the floor of the anterior cranial fossa throughout the midline. In addition to the expected anastomoses with corresponding contralateral ethmoidal arteries, the posterior ethmoidal arteries anastomose with meningeal branches of the internal carotid artery as well as with medially directed branches arising from the sphenoidal and frontal divisions of the MMA. Complete angiographic study of these lesions requires thorough selective angiographic evaluation of the internal carotid artery, the sphenopalatine artery, and the

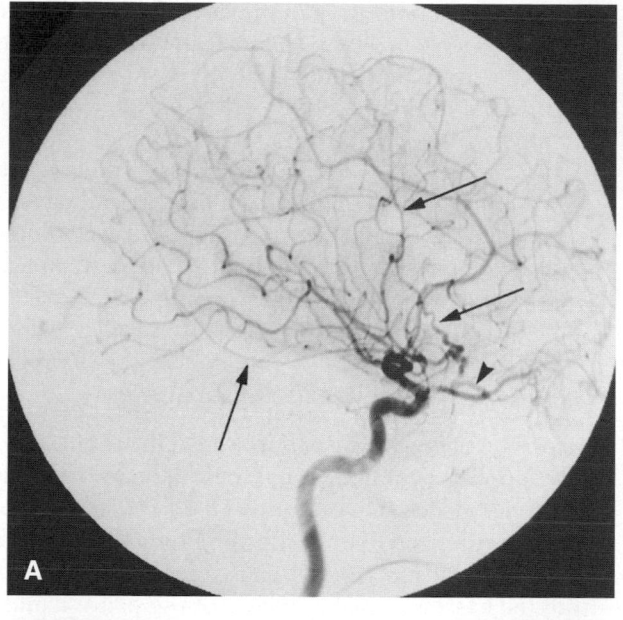

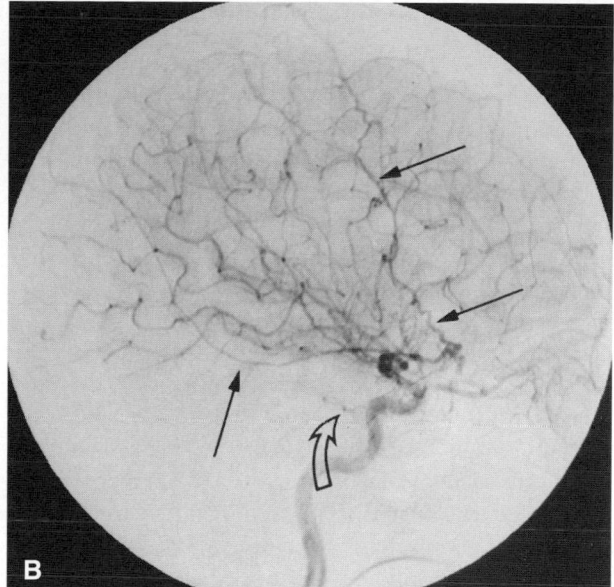

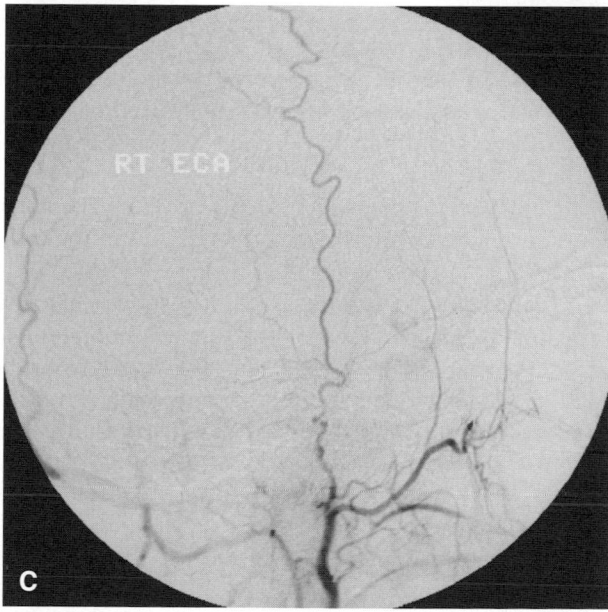

Figure 50–1 Anatomic variation of the dural blood supply. Lateral digital subtraction angiographic (DSA) images from a right internal carotid angiogram, **A.** middle and **B.** late arterial phase. The right middle meningeal artery (*arrows*) originates from the intraorbital right ophthalmic artery by way of a recurrent meningeal segment (*arrowhead*, A). The petrous territory of the right middle meningeal artery is supplied directly by way of the posterior branch of the inferolateral trunk (*open curved arrow*, B) arising from the cavernous segment of the right internal carotid artery. **C.** An accompanying right external carotid angiogram confirms the absence of a middle meningeal segment proximal to the foramen spinosum.

MMA. The study should specifically address potential anastomoses among dural vessels originating from the horizontal segment of the carotid-cavernous artery, the ophthalmic artery, and distal branches of the sphenopalatine and middle meningeal arteries. Additionally, because these lesions occur near the midline, attention must be paid to the possibility of bilateral vascular supply when embolization is being performed and evaluated.

For both classes of lesions, attention must be directed during embolization to the anastomosis with the ophthalmic artery that directly supplies the anterior and posterior ethmoidal arteries and may communicate with the sphenoidal division of the MMA via a recurrent meningeal branch arising from the second portion (lateral division) of the intraorbital ophthalmic artery.

Greater Sphenoid Wing Lesions

The vascular supply to lesions involving the greater wing of the sphenoid is often provided by sphenoidal branches of the MMA directly or by way of a recurrent meningeal vessel arising from the ophthalmic artery. Before embolization, attention must be directed toward the possibility of a dominant meningo-ophthalmic supply to the orbit or a less readily identifiable anastomosis between the middle meningeal and ophthalmic arteries occurring either across the superior orbital fissure or via the Hyrtl canal. In subtle cases, the demonstration of these anastomoses often requires superselective angiography and may not be fully disclosed by less selective angiography of the external or internal carotid arteries.

Lesions Involving the Cavernous Sinus and Parasellar Region

The vascular supply to the parasellar region, including the posterior clinoid, cavernous sinus, and petroclinoid ligament, is often complex because of extensive regional anastomoses between meningeal branches of the internal carotid, middle meningeal, and accessory meningeal arteries, and also because of contribution from the distal internal maxillary artery via the artery of the foramen rotundum. As mentioned previously, the ophthalmic artery may participate indirectly via a tentorial branch of the recurrent meningeal artery. From the perspective of angiographic workup and embolization, these lesions may be divided conceptually into two groups: (1) an anterolateral group, arising from the orbital apex and lateral cavernous sinus and (2) a posterior group, including the posterior cavernous sinus, petroclinoid ligament, and dorsum sellae.

The meningeal supply to anterior division lesions may be considered to reflect the hemodynamic balance between branches arising from the horizontal (C4) segment (Fischer classification) (11) of the cavernous internal carotid artery, most notably the inferolateral trunk (ILT) and meningeal branches of the internal maxillary artery. This latter group includes cavernous and recurrent tentorial branches of the MMA, cavernous meningeal branches of the accessory meningeal artery, and the artery of the foramen rotundum (Figure 50–3C). As expected, embolization of these meningeal arteries should be preceded by superselective angiographic analysis to prevent inadvertent embolization into the internal carotid artery or possible damage to the orbit or regional cranial nerves.

The supply to posterior division lesions is derived primarily from medial and lateral clival branches arising from the C5 segment of the internal carotid artery and their potential anastomotic connections with branches of the ascending pharyngeal and middle meningeal arteries (Figure 50–5). These most notably include the ascending clival and inferior petrosal arcades, derived from the hypoglossal and jugular divisions of the ascending pharyngeal artery, respectively; the posterior cavernous branches of the MMA; and the basal tentorial arcade supplied by the petrosal and the petrosquamosal branches of the MMA.

Three critical points should be considered before embolization of lesions involving this territory is performed:

1. The vascular supply to the intrapetrous facial nerve should be determined. This may come primarily from the petrous branch of the MMA. For this reason, petroclinoid lesions supplied by the basal tentorial arcade should be embolized preferentially from the petrosquamosal branch of the MMA, thereby avoiding the proximal petrosal artery.
2. Potential contributions from the contralateral internal carotid and ascending pharyngeal arteries via transclival anastomoses should be evaluated, particularly in lesions involving the dorsum sellae.
3. Because embolization of upper clival and petroclinoid lesions may involve the hypoglossal or jugular division of the ascending pharyngeal artery, attention must be directed to the possibility of iatrogenic lower cranial neuropathy when using n-BCA, ethanol, or gelfoam microparticles. Midline lesions requiring aggressive embolization of supplies from both ascending pharyngeal arteries should be performed as a staged procedure on different days, specifically to avoid development of bilateral hypoglossal nerve deficits.

Lesions of the Tentorium Cerebelli

Lesions involving the tentorium cerebelli are characteristically supplied by the marginal tentorial and basal tentorial arteries, depending on location. The basal insertion of the tentorium cerebelli is supplied by a vascular arcade paralleling the superior petrosal sinus. It receives supply from the basal tentorial branches of the petrosal and petrosquamosal divisions of the MMA and, potentially, from the lateral clival branch of the ICA. Infratentorial supply may also be derived from the transmastoid branch of the occipital artery, as well as from meningeal contributions from the ascending pharyngeal, vertebral, or posterior inferior cerebellar arteries.

Extra-axial lesions arising from the free margin of the tentorium cerebelli typically receive supply from the marginal tentorial branch of the meningohypophyseal trunk (Fischer C5 branch of the ICA) (11). Additional sources may include the inferolateral trunk via its superior division and a recurrent tentorial arcade variably supplied by branches of the middle meningeal and accessory meningeal arteries, as well as recurrent meningeal collaterals arising from the ophthalmic artery. Anatomically, this arcade follows the lesser wing of the sphenoid, curving posteriorly along the free margin of the tentorium. Because vessels supplying this arcade also participate in the vascular supply of cranial nerves III to VI, attention must be directed to the potential for cranial nerve deficits during embolization. Provocative testing with lidocaine may be of some benefit before devascularization of these lesions (16).

Lesions of the Posterior Fossa

Extra-axial lesions occurring in the posterior fossa may be grossly classified as convexity, cerebellar pontine angle, and foramen magnum or lower clival lesions. Depending on location, the sources of vascular supply usually originate from meningeal branches of the ascending pharyngeal, occipital, and vertebral arteries as well as from posterior fossa branches of the MMA. For lesions of the cerebellar pontine angle, the middle meningeal supply is primarily derived from branches contributing to the basal tentorial arcade. Lesions arising from the cerebellar pontine angle, depending on the specific hemodynamic balance, may also be expected to derive vascular supply from meningeal vessels arising from the transmastoid branch of the occipital artery, the subarcuate branch of the anterior inferior cerebellar artery, and the jugular division of the ascending pharyngeal artery. Lesions arising over the cerebellar convexities are supplied more characteristically by dural branches of the transmastoid artery, which participates in anastomotic balance with posterior meningeal branches of the vertebral artery. Lesions occurring more closely to the transverse sinus, or midline, may also receive supply from the artery of the falx cerebelli—variably arising from the occipital artery, the vertebral artery, or the posterior inferior cerebellar artery (PICA). There may also be a transosseous contribution from the occipital arteries at the level of the torcular herophili. In all cases, connection with the vertebral arteries via meningeal anastomoses must be considered before embolization to avert possible vertebrobasilar crisis.

Lesions involving the foramen magnum are typically vascularized from the hypoglossal division of the ascending pharyngeal artery (APA) and meningeal branches of the vertebral arteries. Embolizations involving this territory must consider the potential supply to cranial nerve XII derived from the hypoglossal division of the APA, in addition to the anastomoses of this vessel, over the odontoid arch arcade, with the vertebral artery at the C3 neuroforamen. Moreover, anastomoses between branches of the occipital artery and the ipsilateral vertebral artery exist throughout the upper cervical spaces (Figure 50–5H), permitting accidental vertebrobasilar embolization during procedures involving the occipital artery.

DURAL ARTERIOVENOUS FISTULAE

Pathologic Lesions

Approximately 10–15% of all clinically apparent intracranial arteriovenous malformations (AVMs) are of the dural type (17). These lesions are characterized by discrete AV fistulas involving the intracranial venous sinuses or dural veins. Although the etiologies of most dural arteriovenous fistulas (DAVFs) remain unknown, there is evidence that fistula formation is preceded in some instances by trauma resulting in skull fracture, sinus thrombosis, or outlet venous stenoses increasing antegrade downstream outflow impedance of the involved dural venous sinus (18–20). In cases related to preexisting sinus thrombosis, it has been postulated that during recanalization a pathologic fistula develops, possibly from degenerative changes involving a normal physiologically regulated arteriovenous shunt or from the triggering of a latent congenital dural AV shunt that ultimately progresses to a clinically and angiographically apparent syndrome (21,22). The disease, with the exception of those shunts localizing to the posterior fossa, is more prevalent in women and usually is diagnosed in patients between the ages of 30 and 80 years (23).

DAVFs are typically classified by location of the involved sinus or shunt (2,4) as well as by the pattern of venous drainage (24–27). The latter scheme allows the subdivision of DAVFs into five types found to correlate with clinical symptomatology (26). Type I DAVFs are characterized by a degree arteriovenous shunting not exceeding the involved venous sinus segment's antegrade outflow capacity, resulting in exclusive ipsilateral extracranial drainage of the shunt. Type II DAVFs exhibit a degree of AV shunting exceeding the capacity of antegrade outflow from the involved sinus resulting in retrograde venous drainage into the adjacent sinus segments (type IIa), cortical veins (type IIb) or both (type IIa/b). Types III and IV DAVFs drain directly into cortical veins, either with (type IV) or without (type III) venous ectasia. Type V DAVFs are typically localized to the tentorium or dural coverings of the posterior fossa and are further characterized by drainage inferiorly into the intrathecal spinal veins. Types II and higher DAVFs are associated with a more aggressive natural history and are generally treated when feasible because of the increased risk of symptomatic presentation.

Clinical Features of DAVFs

The clinical features associated with DAVFs generally depend on the location of the lesion, the extent of the AV shunting, and associated abnormalities of venous drainage (4,26,28,29) (Figures 50–2 and 50–3). Symptoms may be indistinguishable from those associated with pial brain arteriovenous malformations and may include headache, diplopia (double vision), blurred vision, or neurologic dysfunction (30). Focal neurologic deficits and seizures may develop in relation to disturbances in regional cortical venous drainage resulting from the redirection of venous flow from the shunt into pial veins, potentially congesting venous territory remote from the site of the dural shunt (31) (Figure 50–2B and C). In patients with severe compromise of the deep venous drainage of the brain or with diffuse intracranial hypertension resulting from the obstruction of both sigmoid sinuses, the clinical presentation may include dementia (2,32). Closure of the arteriovenous shunts may successfully reverse this state only when there are adequate residual venous channels available for the normal venous drainage of the brain (32). More rarely, cranial neuropathy or unilateral visual phenomena may arise secondary to arterial steal without evidence of associated venous hypertension (4,28). Focal symptomatology may worsen or change because of the redirection of venous outflow from a DAVF (28,31). For example, progressive thrombosis and occlusion of the inferior and superior petrosal sinuses may be associated with worsening of signs in a patient with a cavernous sinus DAVF draining anteriorly through the ipsilateral ophthalmic veins. Whenever contralateral drainage is available, the venous sinus hypertension may be transmitted to the contralateral cavernous sinus, leading to development of bilateral orbital symptomatology.

The signs and symptoms of increased intracranial pressure occasionally complicate cases of DAVFs (33). In certain instances, this can be attributed to diminished cerebral spinal

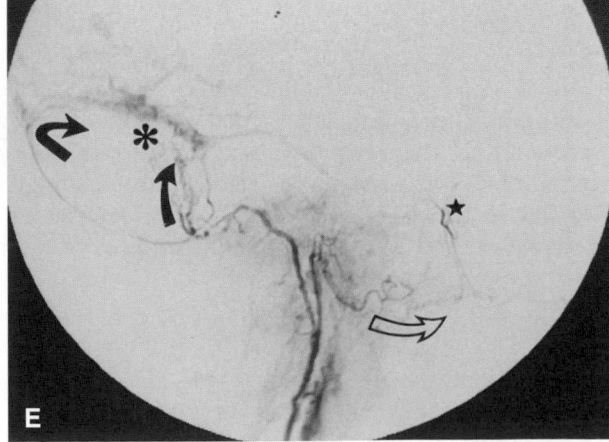

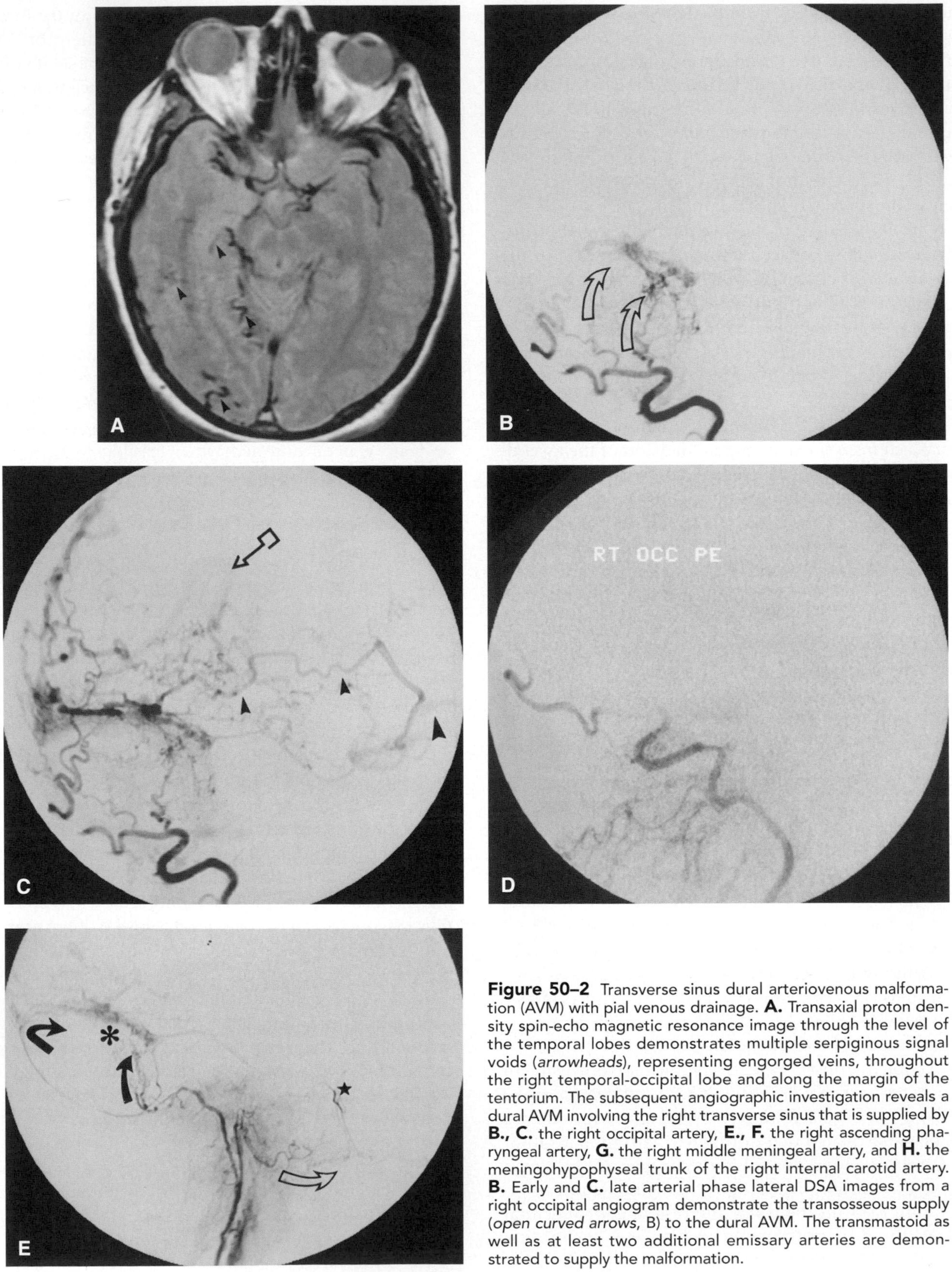

Figure 50–2 Transverse sinus dural arteriovenous malformation (AVM) with pial venous drainage. **A.** Transaxial proton density spin-echo magnetic resonance image through the level of the temporal lobes demonstrates multiple serpiginous signal voids (*arrowheads*), representing engorged veins, throughout the right temporal-occipital lobe and along the margin of the tentorium. The subsequent angiographic investigation reveals a dural AVM involving the right transverse sinus that is supplied by **B., C.** the right occipital artery, **E., F.** the right ascending pharyngeal artery, **G.** the right middle meningeal artery, and **H.** the meningohypophyseal trunk of the right internal carotid artery. **B.** Early and **C.** late arterial phase lateral DSA images from a right occipital angiogram demonstrate the transosseous supply (*open curved arrows*, B) to the dural AVM. The transmastoid as well as at least two additional emissary arteries are demonstrated to supply the malformation.

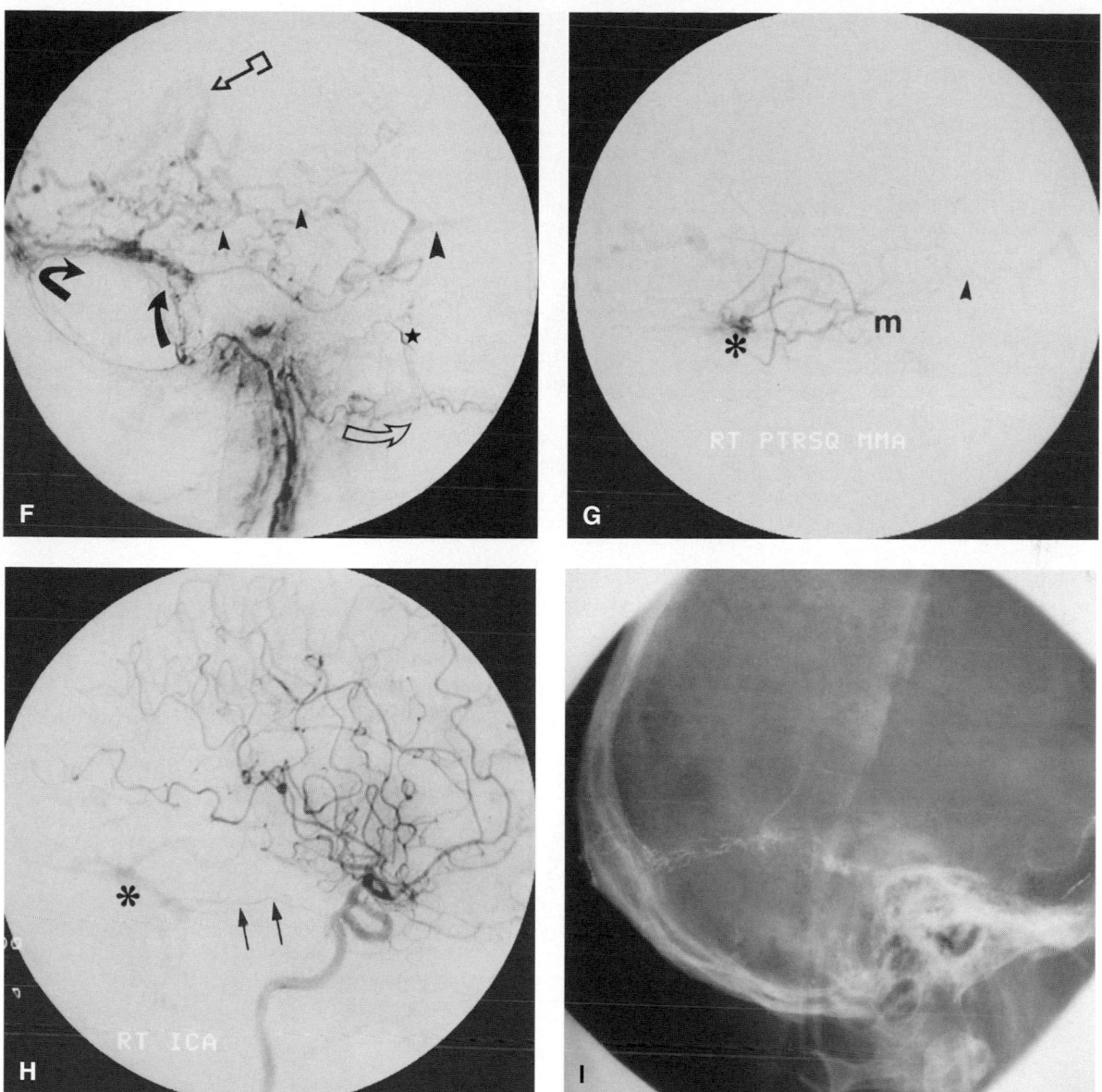

Figure 50–2 (*continued*)   **C.** The late arterial phase image reveals the extensive venous congestion of the deep and superficial veins draining the right temporal and occipital lobes. The patient's symptoms of proptosis and scleral injection correlated with the anteriorly directed venous drainage through the right vein of Labbé (*small arrowheads*, C) and the superficial sylvian system toward the right cavernous sinus and, ultimately, into the right ophthalmic veins (*large arrowhead*, C). The late arterial phase image also reveals opacification of the vein of Galen, confirming drainage into the deep venous system (*open straight arrow*, C). The right sigmoid sinus is occluded. **D.** Midarterial-phase lateral angiogram of the right occipital artery after selective embolization with a combination of NBCA and PVA, which abolished supply to the shunt from this axis. **E.** Early and **F.** late arterial phase lateral DSA images from a right ascending pharyngeal angiogram. The shunt (*asterisk*, E) is supplied primarily by meningeal collaterals arising from the jugular division (*solid curved arrow*) of the neuromeningeal trunk and a posterior meningeal branch (*solid acutely curved arrow*), in this case arising from the ascending pharyngeal artery. Note the cortical venous drainage (*small arrowheads*, F) reproducing the pattern demonstrated previously in the right occipital angiogram. Again, note the anterior drainage toward the ophthalmic veins (*large arrowhead*, F) and vein of Galen (*open straight arrow*, F). Incidentally seen is retrograde opacification of the descending palatine artery (*star*) by way of anastomotic connection with the middle pharyngeal branch of the ascending pharyngeal artery through the soft palate (*open curved arrow*). **G.** Midarterial-phase lateral DSA image from a superselective angiogram within the right middle meningeal artery. The superselective angiogram is performed through a microcatheter (*m*) located within the petrosquamosal branch of the right middle meningeal artery and discloses the contribution of these vessels to the shunt (*asterisk*). Note the superficial cortical venous drainage over the surface of the right temporal lobe (*arrowhead*), as seen on the previous right occipital and ascending pharyngeal angiograms. **H.** Late arterial phase lateral DSA image from a right internal carotid angiogram documents the contribution of the meningohypophyseal trunk (*straight arrows*) to the transverse sinus dural AVM (*asterisk*). **I.** A lateral plain film of the skull demonstrates the radiopaque NBCA cast.

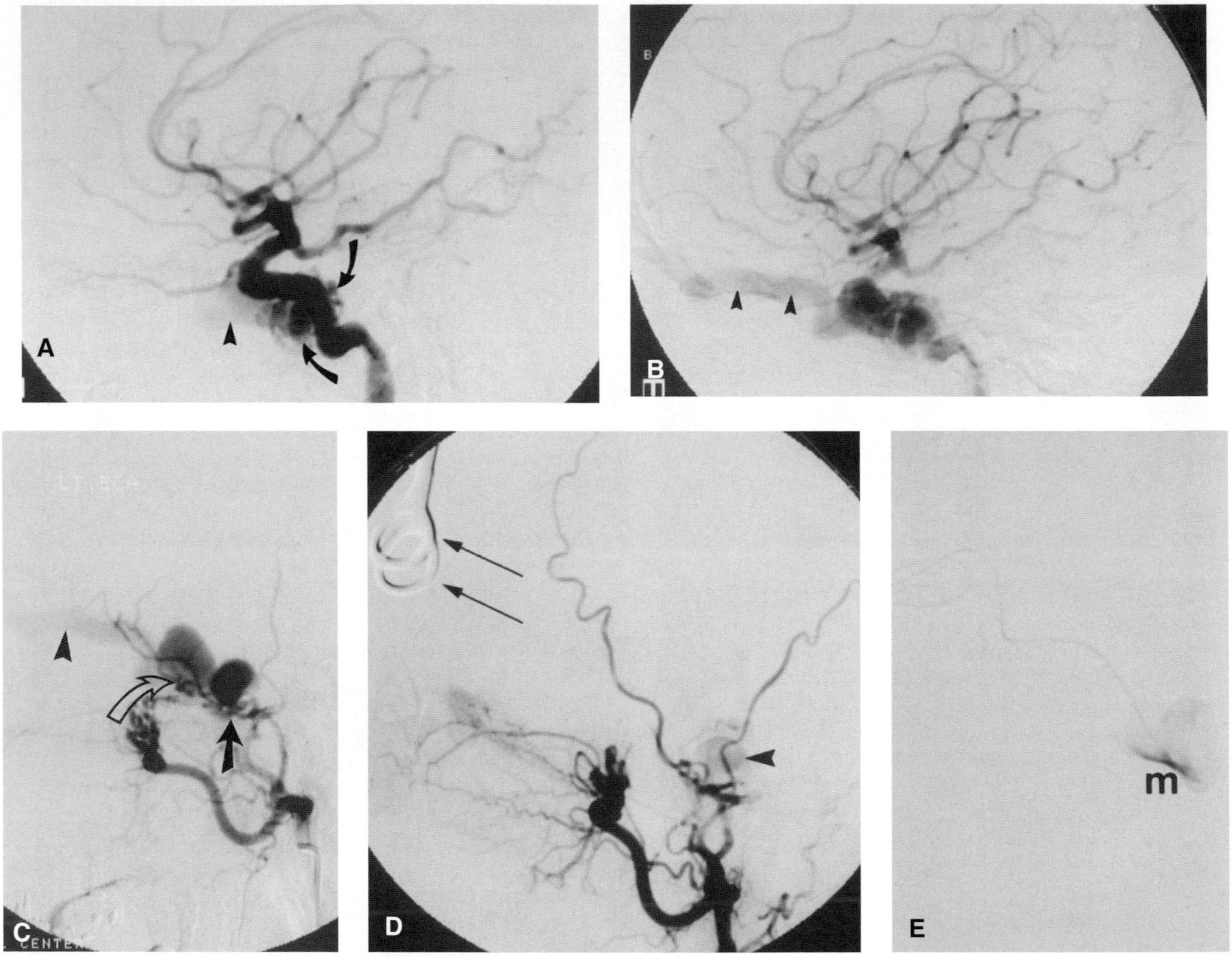

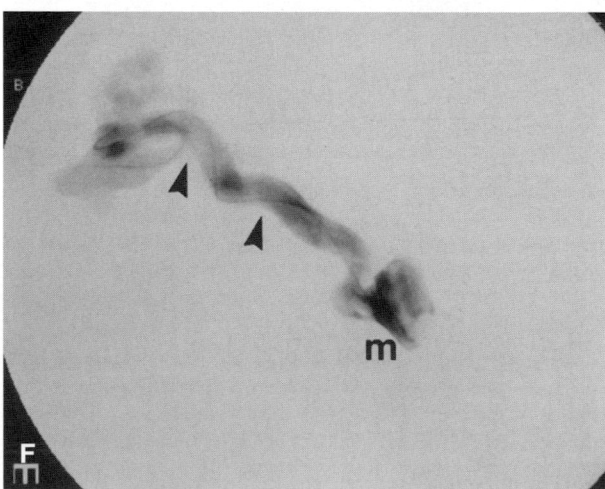

Figure 50-3 Dural AVM involving the left cavernous sinus. **A.** Early and **B.** late arterial phase lateral DSA images from a left internal carotid angiogram. The dural AVM receives supply from the left carotid-cavernous segment primarily by way of an enlarged inferolateral trunk (*solid curved arrows*, A). Note that the entire venous drainage of the AVM is conducted anteriorly through the left cavernous sinus into an enlarged superior ophthalmic vein (*arrowheads*). **C.** Early arterial phase lateral DSA image from a left external carotid angiogram discloses the external carotid contribution to the shunt by way of the artery of the foramen rotundum (*open curved arrow*) and cavernous branches of the left middle meningeal artery (*solid straight arrow*). Visible again is the exclusive drainage of the cavernous sinus malformation into the left superior ophthalmic vein (*arrowhead*).

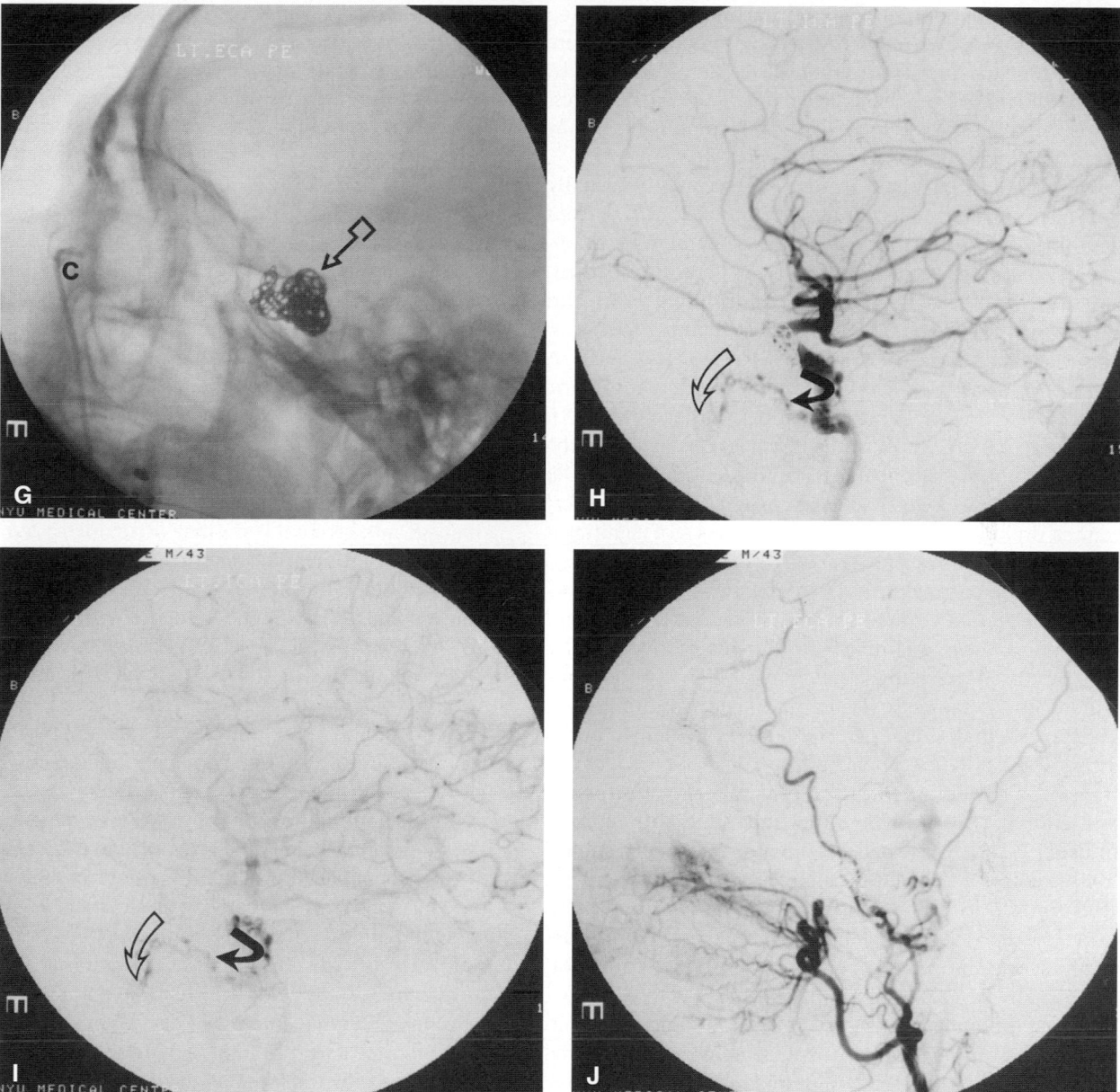

Figure 50–3 (*continued*) **D.** Midarterial-phase lateral DSA image from a left external carotid angiogram after a compressive maneuver to obstruct the left superior ophthalmic vein at the orbital margin. The external compression is employed to assess the potential for diversion of the shunt drainage into cortical veins once the ophthalmic outlet is occluded. The compressive device is evident as a metallic subtraction artifact (*straight arrows*) and, when applied, results in the marked reduction of AV shunting, confirming the feasibility of a venous approach. The minimal persistent shunting suggested by the slight opacification of the cavernous sinus in this angiogram (*arrowhead*) results from incomplete occlusion of the left superior ophthalmic outlet and was noted not to drain by an alternate route. **E., F.** Serial digital subtraction venogram performed through a microcatheter (*m*) positioned within the left cavernous sinus. The microcatheter has been introduced into the left cavernous sinus by way of retrograde catheterization through the left superior ophthalmic vein (*arrowheads*) after advancement of a guiding catheter into the distal left fascial vein. **G.** Lateral unsubtracted image documenting the deposition of metallic coils within the left cavernous sinus (*open arrow*). The position of the guiding catheter (c) within the distal left fascial vein is demonstrated. **H.** Early and **I.** late arterial phase lateral DSA images from the postembolization left internal carotid angiogram. Note the obliteration of arteriovenous shunting. The metallic coils within the left cavernous sinus are evident as a subtraction artifact projecting over the distal cavernous segment of the left internal carotid artery. Note the retrograde opacification of the artery of the foramen rotundum (*open curved arrow*) by way of anastomoses with the prominent inferolateral trunk (*solid acutely curved arrow*). These highly developed anastomoses persist after the shunt is eliminated, and they illustrate the potential danger of cerebral embolic events during transarterial embolizations of external carotid branches that anastomose with meningeal branches of the internal carotid artery. **J.** Midarterial-phase lateral DSA image from the postembolization left external carotid angiogram illustrates complete obliteration of the left cavernous sinus dural shunt by transvenous embolization.

fluid (CSF) absorption through the arachnoid villi resulting from the transmission of increased venous pressure throughout the superior sagittal sinus (30). Alternatively, obstruction of the cerebral aqueduct secondary to compression of the mesencephalon by an ectatic draining vein may occur, leading to obstructive hydrocephalus.

Moreover, aneurysmal venous ectasia may unusually cause symptomatic mechanical compression of adjacent neurologic structures, most commonly in dural AVMs draining into pial veins of the posterior fossa (33). This is particularly true for type IV DAVFs, which frequently present with clinical symptoms related to mass effect resulting from pronounced venous ectasia (26).

Approximately 20–33% of patients with symptomatic DAVFs present with an intracranial hemorrhage (4,34,35). This is encountered most frequently in lesions involving the floor of the anterior cranial fossa or the tentorium cerebelli; however, it may occur in any case associated with cortical venous drainage, particularly in the presence of significant cerebral venous ectasia (36).

As alluded to previously, DAVFs commonly involve specific sites related to the intracranial venous sinuses and dural veins. From a clinicoanatomic perspective, fistulas may be classified as those involving the cavernous sinus (Figure 50–3), transverse (Figure 50–2) and sigmoid sinuses, superior sagittal sinus, petrosal sinus, torcular, tentorial incisura, and anterior cranial base.

Approximately one third to one half of symptomatic intracranial DAVFs involve the transverse and sigmoid sinuses (26,37). These patients often present with a subjective bruit as the first clinical manifestation. The tinnitus is synchronized to arterial pulsations and results from turbulence associated with the shunting of blood into the sigmoid or transverse sinuses. Auscultation over the retroauricular area usually reveals the pulsatile bruit. As with the other DAVFs, additional neurologic symptoms and findings generally depend on the pattern of venous drainage encountered in the individual patient. Symptoms may include chronic signs of increased intracranial pressure potentially leading to papilledema (38) and optic atrophy in addition to disturbances related to balance and hearing. In progressive cases, associated with obstruction of the ipsilateral jugular outflow (Figure 50–2), redirected venous drainage into pial veins of the posterior fossa may result in brain stem or cerebellar dysfunction as well as posterior fossa hemorrhage. Rerouting of drainage into the supratentorial cortical venous compartment may be associated with the development of focal neurologic deficit or seizures as well as increased risk of intracranial hemorrhage.

DAVFs of the cavernous sinus (CSDAVFs) (Figure 50–3) generally are associated with signs and symptoms related to the orbit that fluctuate depending on alterations in the orbital venous outflow that develop secondary to thrombosis and changes in head position (39–41). Patients typically present with the gradual onset of focal or diffuse chronic eye redness distinguishable from uveitis in that close inspection

will reveal dilated tortuous conjunctival and epibulbar vessels that exhibit an acute angulation near the ocular limbus (42). These lesions are often associated with an elevation of episcleral venous pressure leading to a persistent rise in intraocular pressure in the affected eye, potentially resulting in the development of glaucoma (43,44). If both cavernous sinuses become involved in the venous drainage secondary to a change in the ipsilateral venous outflow of the affected cavernous sinus, the ocular findings may become bilateral. The patient may complain of pulsatile tinnitus, and in 25% of cases, a bruit can be auscultated over the orbit (40,41). Cranial neuropathies, most commonly involving the sixth nerve, frequently lead to ocular motor dysfunction, which also may be exacerbated by orbital venous congestion and proptosis (39,45). More important to the planning of embolization are the hypoxic ischemic retinal changes that develop in approximately 15% of patients (40). Rarely, if thrombosis in the cavernous sinus is extensive, abnormal drainage into cerebral veins may occur, increasing the likelihood of an intracranial hemorrhage or venous infarction. Unfortunately, frequently cited classification schemes of intracranial DAVFs (25,26) are deficient in their handling of CSDAVFs because of the lack of explicit consideration given to ophthalmic venous drainage and the clinical consequences of orbital venous congestion. Despite the lack of a coherent classification scheme for CSDAVFs, the implications of venous outflow from the lesion are similar to DAVFs at other locations and the analysis of venous drainage is important in understanding the pathophysiology of the disease at this site. Stiebel-Kalish et al. (46) reported an excellent and thorough study of the clinical manifestations in 85 patients with CSDAVF relative to their angiographic characteristics. In this study, the clinical symptoms found in patients with CSDAVFs were related to the abnormal venous drainage and could be predicted by analysis of the aberrant venous drainage patterns. Interestingly, central nervous system symptoms or dysfunction were found in 7 (8%) of these patients, attesting to the potential seriousness of cortical venous drainage even among patients with CSDAVF.

DAVFs involving the superior sagittal sinus (47), tentorial incisura (48), petrosal sinuses (49), and anterior cranial base (50–52) occur less frequently than DAVFs involving the transverse, sigmoid (53), or cavernous sinuses (39). In these lesions, symptoms typically depend on the route of abnormal venous drainage and associated pattern of venous hypertension and may include dysphasia, hemiparesis, hemisensory deficits, and abnormal visual phenomena. Several specific features deserve particular attention:

1. Dural fistulas involving the floor of the anterior cranial fossa are usually associated with drainage into ectatic parasagittal cortical veins and often present with intracranial hemorrhage (50,52). Moreover, these patients may exhibit unilateral visual loss secondary to arterial steal from the ophthalmic circulation into ethmoidal and recurrent meningeal supplies to the shunt (50).

2. DAVFs of the petrosal sinuses or tentorial incisura may occasionally drain inferiorly into perimedullary veins of the spinal cord (type V), resulting in progressive myelopathy similar to that encountered in spinal dural AVMs (15,54). Assuming the venous sinus drainage of the brain is otherwise unimpaired, these symptoms usually respond well to endovascular or surgical closure of the shunt.

Neuroimaging of Intracranial DAVFs

Recent advances in computed tomography (CT) and magnetic resonance imaging (MRI) have significantly contributed to the initial diagnostic evaluation of patients with suspected DAVFs (55). While routine conventional head CT and brain MRI are frequently diagnostically equivocal; dilated or thrombosed venous structures suggesting the presence of the lesion may be identified, particularly in patients with DAVFs associated with cortical venous drainage (Figure 50–2A). In patients presenting with intracranial hemorrhage, obvious findings are evident in both CT and MRI studies. Focal or generalized atrophy of the brain, possibly accompanied by hydrocephalus, are nonspecific secondary findings that may be appreciated. The chronic enlargement of meningeal branches of the external carotid or carotid-cavernous artery may be demonstrated by imaging studies. Despite the presence of secondary signs that suggest the presence of a DAVF, conventional MRI alone is generally unsuccessful in defining the exact site of fistualization (56).

The advent of computed tomographic angiography (CTA) and magnetic resonance angiography (MRA) has provided more power to the noninvasive screening of patients with suspected DAVFs. In addition to providing anatomic details, these modalities may be coupled with perfusion studies to evaluate the effect of a DAVF on regional blood flow.

MRA may be performed using a three-dimensional time-of-flight (3D TOF) technique (55,57) or MR digital subtraction angiography (MR DSA) (57,58). The presence of multiple high-intensity curvilinear or nodular structures adjacent to a sinus, in conjunction with high-intensity foci within the sinus is considered suspicious for a DAVF; however, the technique still suffers from a high false-positive rate, with as many as 14% of otherwise healthy patients incorrectly identified as possibly harboring a DAVF by 3D TOF MRA (57). Although the current spatial resolution of MR DSA is less than 3D TOF MRA, the benefit of MR DSA would be related to the temporal resolution of the technique and the ability to depict flow within cortical veins, which is particularly important in those patients with retrograde flow from a DAVF. Despite the advances in CTA and MRA, conventional digital subtraction angiography remains paramount in the diagnosis and pre-treatment analysis of intracranial DAVFs.

The angiographic evaluation usually includes selective studies of the internal and external carotid arteries bilaterally as well as of both vertebral arteries when evaluating lesions of the posterior fossa or tentorium (2). The pretherapeutic examination must be tailored to the clinically suspected location of the fistula and must disclose the entire arterial supply as well as any anastomoses between the supplying vessels and arterial distributions to the orbit, brain, or cranial nerves. This usually requires superselective arterial catheterization and angiography before the use of embolic materials. The venous anatomy must be studied with respect to the pattern of drainage from the fistula, and the adequacy of normal venous drainage of the brain must be assessed.

Therapeutic Approaches to DAVFs

An understanding of the natural history of the disease, the treatment options, and the risks and benefits of those therapies is important in the development of a treatment plan. Although spontaneous resolution of clinical signs related to DAVFs has been reported (59), most notably in patients with cavernous sinus lesions, most symptomatic DAVFs require some form of treatment. This is most urgent in those fistulas accompanied by cortical venous drainage and venous ectasias. The goals of therapy should be tailored to each individual patient and may include relief from symptoms or complete occlusion of the DAVF (2). The efficacy and safety of the treatment must be considered in conjunction with the patient's presentation and prognosis.

Carotid-Jugular Compression

Patients with Djindjian type I transverse or sigmoid sinus DAVFs or with fistulas of the cavernous sinus with otherwise normal ophthalmologic examinations may be treated conservatively. Intermittent manual compression of the carotid artery may be effective in eliminating DAVFs involving the ipsilateral cavernous sinus in patients with mild findings and no evidence of carotid vascular disease or other contraindications to carotid compression (39,40). The ipsilateral carotid artery is compressed, using the contralateral hand, for approximately 5 minutes every waking hour for 1–3 days. If this is tolerated, the compression time is increased to 10–15 minutes of compression per waking hour. The compression, when performed properly, produces concomitant partial obstruction of the ipsilateral carotid artery and jugular vein. This results in the transient reduction of arteriovenous shunting by decreasing arterial inflow while simultaneously increasing the outlet venous pressure, thereby promoting spontaneous thrombosis within the nidus. When applied to highly motivated patients with cavernous sinus DAVFs, it is approximately 30–40% effective in eliminating the shunt (39,40).

Embolization

The development of improved superselective angiographic catheter systems and embolic agents has increased the role of interventional neuroradiology in the management of these lesions, both primarily and preoperatively. Two strategies (transvenous or transarterial) have been employed, depending upon the location and complexity of the lesion as well as its vascular features. Transvenous embolization with metallic coils or detachable balloons has been advocated in the treatment of DAVFs involving the transverse, sigmoid (53), or cavernous sinus (60–62). The technique involves a transfemoral or intraoperative approach to the affected venous sinus (Figure 50–3). Several features are critical in appropriate patient selection for this method of treatment:

1. The segment of sinus to be occluded must be in proximity to the fistula and receive its entire venous drainage.
2. The sinus to be occluded should not be essential to the normal venous drainage of the brain. In this connection, the cerebral venous drainage must be evaluated thoroughly before embolization to determine the potential alternate pathways for cerebral venous outflow.
3. The target sinus must be completely occluded throughout the involved segment to avoid diversion of the fistula drainage into pial veins after embolization by way of a trapped sinus segment.

Recent modifications in transarterial embolization techniques suggest that this approach may be equal or superior to the transvenous approach in appropriately selected patients (63). Transarterial deposition of liquid polymer may have several advantages over the transvenous approach in the treatment of DAVFs. Access via the transvenous technique is frequently limited by venous access problems such as thrombosed or stenotic dural sinuses, which is avoided using a transarterial approach. The latter technique is also not limited by high-grade lesions that directly drain into cortical veins. In addition, transarterial delivery of liquid polymer provides definite occlusion of the fistula site, reducing the likelihood of diversion of shunt flow into alternative venous pathways that may lead to increased risk of intraparenchymal hemorrhage (25,64–66). Also, fistula site closure does not necessarily require the sacrifice of a venous pathway that may be draining normal brain parenchyma, as may occur with a transvenous approach. There have been reports of the development of de novo DAVFs at independent intracranial sites after apparent complete treatment through a transvenous approach (67–71). These de novo DAVFs may arise from venous hypertension-induced angiogenesis secondary to occlusion of major dural sinuses during transvenous coil embolization (72,73), which is avoided using a transarterial approach.

The transarterial technique requires selective catheterization of individual feeding vessels (2,34,39,63,74) (Figure 50–2), followed by superselective angiography to evaluate the vascular supply to the fistula, particularly with respect to potential anastomosis with the orbit or cerebral vasculature. It is important to understand that such anastomoses may not be demonstrable on the initial angiograms; however, they may become manifest as alterations in flow within the target vascular territory occur during embolization. For ease of catheterization, guide wire-directed microcatheters are typically employed in the microcatheterization of those meningeal branches supplying such lesions. The embolic agents employed through a transarterial approach are usually liquid cyanoacrylate (n-BCA), polyvinyl alcohol foam (PVA), or ethanol. Ideally, liquid acrylic agent delivered close to the shunt under wedged-microcatheter induced flow arrest conditions presents the best opportunity for embolotherapy cure of the lesion because it enables permeation of the collateral complex supplying the fistula and the immediate venous receptacle, permanently occluding the shunt. This degree of permeation is not possible when using particulate agents that characteristically lodge within supplying arterioles at a point proximal to microcollateral networks in the vicinity of the fistula, which following particulate embolization may reestablish flow through the shunt complex.

Nevertheless, PVA may find use in several situations. First, the initial use of PVA in embolizing the less favorable arterial supplies to a multipedicle fistula may facilitate more complete subsequent embolization of the fistula site with liquid cyanoacrylate through a safer conduit. The embolization of competing supplies to the shunt with PVA in this situation permits the undiluted permeation of the fistula by the liquid embolic agent without fragmentation of the liquid stream. PVA may also be useful in reducing flow through low-velocity shunts, thereby facilitating thrombosis in these DAVFs. This may be particularly applicable in managing low flow CSDAVFs, where liquid acrylic cannot be used for issues of safety; possibly, combined with manual compression in treating lesions also supplied by cavernous segment dural branches of the ipsilateral ICA. In certain situations, partial embolization of dural fistulas may be performed in an attempt to ameliorate symptoms, such as partial embolization of a cavernous sinus DAVF to reduce intraocular pressure in a patient suffering acute deterioration of visual acuity secondary to the fistula. Partial embolization may also be advocated in patients presenting with new onset dementia or in those patients with severe tinnitus. Lastly, PVA and liquid embolic agents are used in the preoperative devascularization of dural fistulas proceeding to surgical excision (75). In this situation, particulate emboli, because of their low morbidity, are generally preferred and should be applied 1–2 days before surgery. Regardless of the embolic agent (n-NBCA or PVA), when the nidus is not obliterated because of proximal occlusion of feeding vessels, the fistula will often reconstitute by way of unembolized collaterals.

The decision about which approach and embolic agent to use in treatment of a DAVF must be tailored to each individual case with the recognition that the most effective approach for permanent DAVF treatment, particularly in high-flow shunts, may require a combination of approaches and embolic agents (63).

CAROTID-CAVERNOUS FISTULAS

Carotid-cavernous fistulas (CCFs) are acquired lesions involving an abnormal vascular communication between the cavernous portion of the internal carotid artery and the enveloping cavernous sinus. The fistula most commonly results from traumatic injury to the internal carotid artery proper or a cavernous branch and generally leads to extensive, rapid arteriovenous shunting.

In 20% of cases, the fistula develops spontaneously without a history of trauma (2,76). Specific disorders associated with vascular deficiencies can be identified in approximately 60% of such cases (76). These include Ehlers-Danlos syndrome (77), osteogenesis imperfecta (78), pseudoxanthoma elasticum, fibromuscular dysplasia (79), cavernous segment aneurysms of the carotid artery, a persistent embryologic trigeminal artery, and other nonspecific angiodysplasias. The recognition that a carotid-cavernous fistula has arisen spontaneously is essential to the proper management of the shunt and the underlying disorder.

Although the clinical signs and symptoms of CCFs may fluctuate, in general, the clinical diagnosis is not difficult to establish. The patient may complain of visual blurring, diplopia, headache, orbital pain, and a subjective bruit (2,80). After extensive trauma, however, additional injuries may complicate the diagnosis and delay treatment of the underlying fistula. Signs of orbital congestion may be noted after head trauma but may be inaccurately ascribed to local orbital damage. In addition, a small pseudoaneurysm may develop after traumatic injury to the cavernous ICA and subsequently rupture after an asymptomatic period of days to weeks. In CCFs, the congestion of orbital contents results from increased flow into the superior and inferior ophthalmic veins, which contributes to orbital venous hypertension and ultimately the elevation of intraocular pressure, chemosis, and edema throughout the eyelids (76,81). The pronounced venous congestion generally leads to proptosis with the globe displaced downward and laterally. Isolated third or sixth nerve palsies or combinations of third, fourth, and sixth nerve dysfunctions are common (41–76) and occasionally may be associated with first- and second-division trigeminal nerve sensory deficits. Trigeminal motor dysfunction is almost never attributable to the CCF, but it may be a manifestation of traumatic neuropathy acquired during the precipitating event. Likewise, traumatic cases are often associated with direct injury to the third, fourth, sensory fifth, and sixth nerves as well as with cranial neuropathies of the seventh and eighth nerves resulting from accompanying basilar skull fractures (41).

Intraocular pressure is elevated in most patients with CCFs in whom the venous drainage is conducted anteriorly from the cavernous sinus into the ophthalmic veins. This may result in the development of visual changes or, less commonly, in central retinal artery occlusion in severe untreated cases (82). These changes are typically unilateral; however, if the opposite cavernous sinus is affected because of the shunting of blood across the intercavernous coronary sinus, both eyes may exhibit signs of orbital congestion and elevated intraocular pressure. Optic neuropathy, commonly with a mild reduction in visual acuity, dyschromatopsia, an

afferent pupillary defect, and a generally constricted visual field, may occur (76). In these cases, the fundus may appear normal, suggesting a retrobulbar process, most likely related to compression of the optic nerve by a distended superior ophthalmic vein.

Diagnostic Imaging of CCFs

In patients presenting with CCF secondary to head trauma, CT is often the first imaging modality of evaluation. Enlargement of the ophthalmic veins, most often the superior division, may be demonstrated readily in axial or coronal views of the orbit by contrast-enhanced CT. Orbital congestion is easily appreciated by CT as a diffuse increase in the attenuation of orbital fat and is often associated with swelling of the extraocular muscles and lacrimal gland. The ipsilateral cavernous sinus is often dilated, resulting in the convex bulging of the lateral cavernous sinus wall. Exophthalmos may be appreciated by CT; however, it is usually more easily apparent by clinical inspection. In cases associated with cortical venous drainage, dilatation of one or more cerebral veins and/or the sphenoparietal sinus may be noted. CT often reveals other stigmata of head injury, including fractures involving the skull base or paranasal sinuses and additional intracranial lesions such as epidural, subdural, or intracerebral hematomas. Of particular importance is the detection of sphenoid sinus fracture, which, when associated with a traumatic pseudoaneurysm of the carotid-cavernous artery, places the patient at risk for catastrophic epistaxis (83). Potentially life-threatening conditions resulting from intracranial injury should be attended to before definitive treatment for the CCF is initiated. By comparison, facial and orbital fractures are probably best treated after closure of this fistula, thereby permitting a reduction in the venous congestion and associated soft tissue swelling of the orbit.

With the development and recent availability of multidetector CT scanners, CT angiography has been introduced as a relative noninvasive test for the diagnosis of CCFs (84). Although CT angiography may be performed quickly and simultaneously with a conventional CT scan routinely acquired in patients with suspected traumatic CCFs, early CTA has been limited by the significant attenuation and scatter artifacts generated by the densely ossific skull base. In addition, important characteristics such as the precise site of the fistula and flow hemodynamics cannot be assessed accurately with CT angiography. Nonetheless, further research in this area is warranted and in the near future, CT angiography, particularly when coupled with subtraction techniques and CT perfusion, will likely become a routine first-line test in the diagnostic work-up of suspected CCFs and their follow-up.

Although CT is superior to MRI in the evaluation of head trauma, MRI may demonstrate changes within the cavernous sinus and orbit suggestive of the diagnosis; in particular, flow voids corresponding to engorged compartments of the cavernous sinus containing the CCF may be evident on conventional spin-echo images (85). The widespread availability of MRI and MRA has provided noninvasive tools useful in the diagnosis and posttreatment follow-up of CCFs that avoid several of the limitations of CT angiography, including ionizing radiation, skull base bony artifacts, and the use of iodinated contrast agents (86).

Although transaxial imaging may suggest the presence of a CCF, the diagnosis is primarily confirmed by conventional angiography (87). The angiographic evaluation should include several specific objectives. First, the fistula site should be precisely identified. This is usually accomplished by rapid sequential angiography of the ipsilateral internal carotid artery and employment of frame rates between 6 and 15 frames per second. If this approach fails to disclose the precise site of the fistula, the angiogram may be repeated employing a double-lumen occlusive balloon catheter placed within the cervical internal carotid artery. Under systemic heparinization, the balloon is inflated, and contrast material is injected into the occluded ICA at a low, sustained injection rate. The dilution of the contrast column by retrograde nonopacified blood flow identifies the fistula site. As an alternative, in cases presenting with a competent ipsilateral posterior communicating artery, a vertebral angiogram with or without manual compression of the affected internal carotid artery can pinpoint the exact site of the fistula (Figure 50–4H).

Second, the anatomic competence of the circle of Willis should be thoroughly evaluated by angiography. The potential collateral arterial supply to the ipsilateral hemisphere must be identified if the shunt cannot be closed without sacrificing the involved ICA. Of additional importance is the identification of potential transsellar anastomoses with the contralateral ICA in cases employing a trapping procedure as a therapeutic solution. This is necessary to avoid the creation of a persistent shunt between the occlusion balloons supplied by the contralateral ICA.

Selective angiography of the external carotid artery must be performed to determine whether the external carotid artery provides collateral contribution to the AV shunt (Figure 50–4I). This potential contribution is usually derived from the natural collaterals of C4 and C5 segment branches (Fischer classification) (11) of the affected ICA and includes cavernous branches of the middle meningeal or accessory meningeal arteries, the artery of the foramen rotundum, and the ascending pharyngeal artery, depending on the precise location of the internal carotid injury.

The angiogram will also disclose the direction of drainage away from the cavernous sinus (Figure 50–4A, B, and C) as well as indicate the presence of partial thrombosis or aneurysmal ectasia of the cavernous sinus and draining veins.

Because of the association of CCFs with traumatic injury to the head and neck, the angiographic study should include evaluation of all cervical and intracranial vessels, including the vertebrobasilar system (Figure 50–4E). Other traumatic injuries to these vessels, including vessel dissection or AV fistulas involving the ophthalmic, internal carotid, or vertebral artery, may cause persistent symptoms after closure of the CCF and may affect the treatment strategy if known prospectively. Secondary shunts may become apparent on angiography only after the dominant CCF is occluded. Cerebral angiography may also uncover those cases of cavernous origin of the ophthalmic artery. This variation may be associated with a deficiency of collateral circulation to the distal ophthalmic artery and may argue against occlusion of the internal carotid artery at the cavernous level because of the risk of blindness.

The clinical signs and symptoms related to CCFs can usually be explained by angiographic analysis of the arterial inflow, the location of the fistula, and the venous outflow (76). Each of these factors influences the abnormal hemodynamic condition and may evolve, resulting in fluctuating symptoms. The nature and degree of dysfunction depend to some degree on the extent and location of thrombosis within the cavernous sinus and draining veins as well as on the location of the compartment of the cavernous sinus directly involved with the AV shunt.

The contralateral cavernous sinus may receive arterialized flow via the anterior and posterior limbs of the coronary venous plexus, ultimately leading to orbital congestion and cranial neuropathy on the side opposite a particular shunt (Figure 50–4C). Bilateral signs of varying severity are found in approximately 20% of cases but are usually the result of a unilateral fistula. Bilateral traumatic fistulas have been described but occur in less than 1% of cases (76).

Most CCFs come to clinical attention because of orbital congestion, which can be quite impressive, particularly when the outlet venous drainage is conducted exclusively anterior into the ophthalmic venous system. Alternatively, when the venous drainage is directed posteriorly into the petrosal sinuses, patients may have few or no orbital findings related to the CCF, and a sixth nerve paresis or a retroauricular bruit may be the only presenting sign (76). When the drainage from the cavernous sinus is conducted into the sphenoparietal sinus or the deep sylvian veins, cortical venous hypertension may result, predisposing the patient to an intracranial hemorrhage (88) or signs of increased intracranial pressure.

Cases in which the accompanying circle of Willis is incompetent may be associated with ischemic infarct in the distribution of the ipsilateral internal carotid artery secondary to complete "steal" through the fistula.

Therapeutic Approaches to CCFs

Several considerations determine the urgency of intervention in the treatment of CCFs (89,90). Although emergent embolization is required in fewer than 30% of presenting cases, spontaneous closure of the high-flow CCF is unlikely. Visual loss related to persistent glaucoma, retinopathy, optic neuropathy, or corneal ulcerations evolving to complete unilateral blindness has been reported in 26–89% of untreated patients (91,92). Moreover, in patients without severe visual loss, diplopia secondary to associated cranial neuropathies has been frequently reported as a persistent finding (76). From the standpoint of treatment, recent reviews have established the efficacy of early intervention in cases complicated by the onset of transient ischemic attacks, increased intracranial pressure, cortical venous drainage, epistaxis, and loss of vision or sudden increase in intraocular pressure uncontrolled by antiglaucoma medications (76,89,90,93).

The goal of therapy is to occlude the untoward shunt, preferably with preservation of the involved internal carotid artery. Obviously, the symptoms resulting from the CCF must be considered in relation to the patient's overall clinical status, particularly as this status relates to multisystem trauma. Moreover, with respect to the orbit, the management of intraocular pressure by temporizing

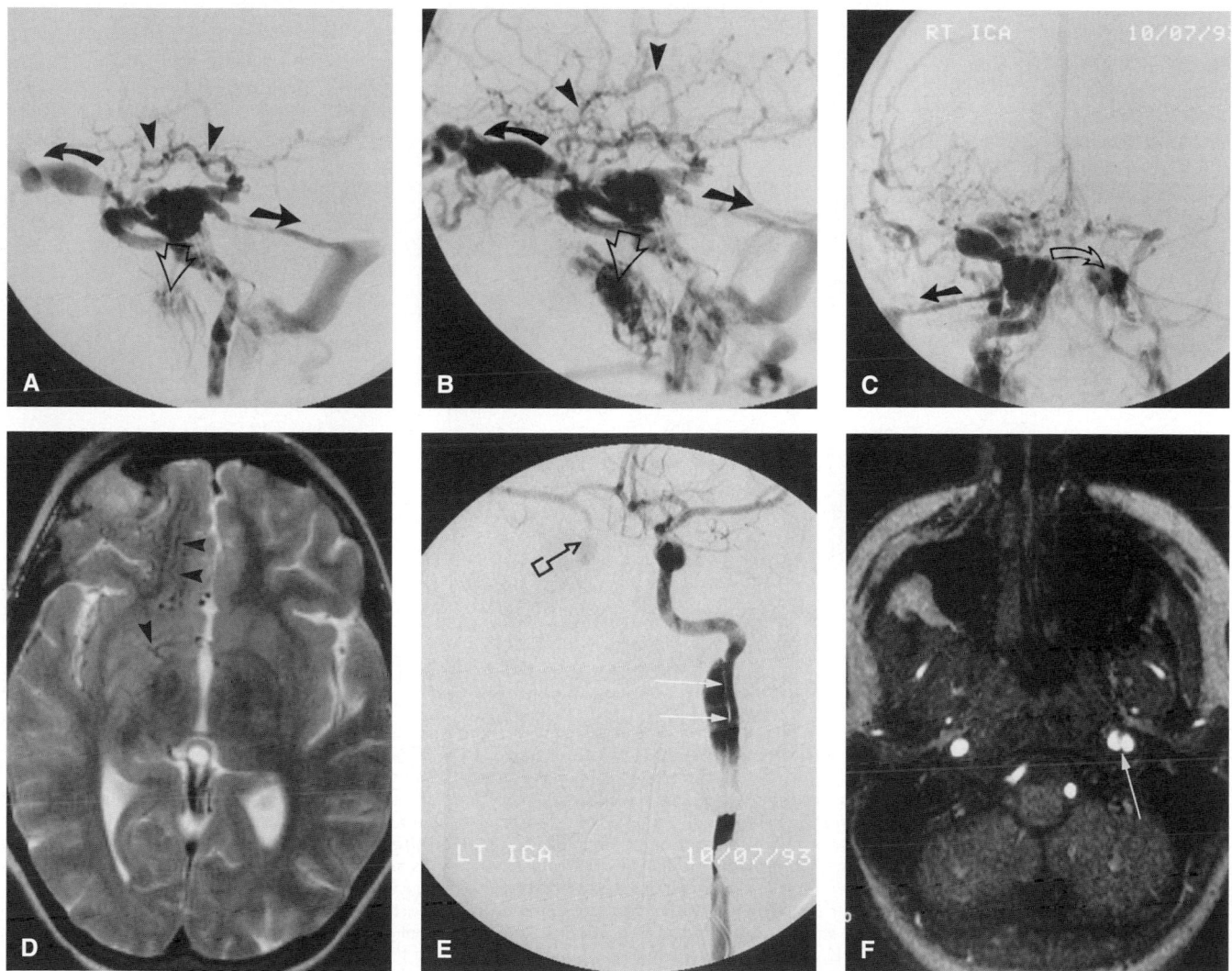

Figure 50–4 Posttraumatic right carotid-cavernous fistula. **A.** Early and **B.** late arterial phase lateral DSA images from a right internal carotid angiogram depict a high-flow right carotid-cavernous fistula (CCF). The venous drainage from the right cavernous sinus is conducted anteriorly into the superior ophthalmic vein (*solid curved arrow*), inferiorly through the foramen ovale into the pterygoid plexus of veins (*open straight arrow*), posteriorly into the superior petrosal sinus (*solid straight arrow*), and superiorly into cortical veins (*arrowheads*). Note the extensive cortical venous drainage that is conducted superficially toward the superiorsagittal sinus and into the deep venous system that empties through the vein of Galen and straight sinus. **C.** The accompanying frontal DSA image illustrates the contralateral drainage resulting in the opacification of the left cavernous sinus (*open curved arrow*). Note the posterior drainage from the right cavernous sinus into the right superior petrosal sinus (*solid straight arrow*) in the frontal projection. **D.** Transaxial T$_2$-weighted spin echo MR image demonstrates multiple serpiginous signal voids (arrowheads), reflecting engorged pial veins. **E.** Frontal DSA image illustrates an arterial dissection of the left internal carotid artery (*solid white arrows*) and retrograde opacification of the right carotid-cavernous fistula (*open straight arrow*). **F.** An accompanying transaxial gradient echo MR image through the level of the skull base shows the dissection of the left internal carotid artery along an intimal flap and accompanying pseudoaneurysm (*solid white arrow*).

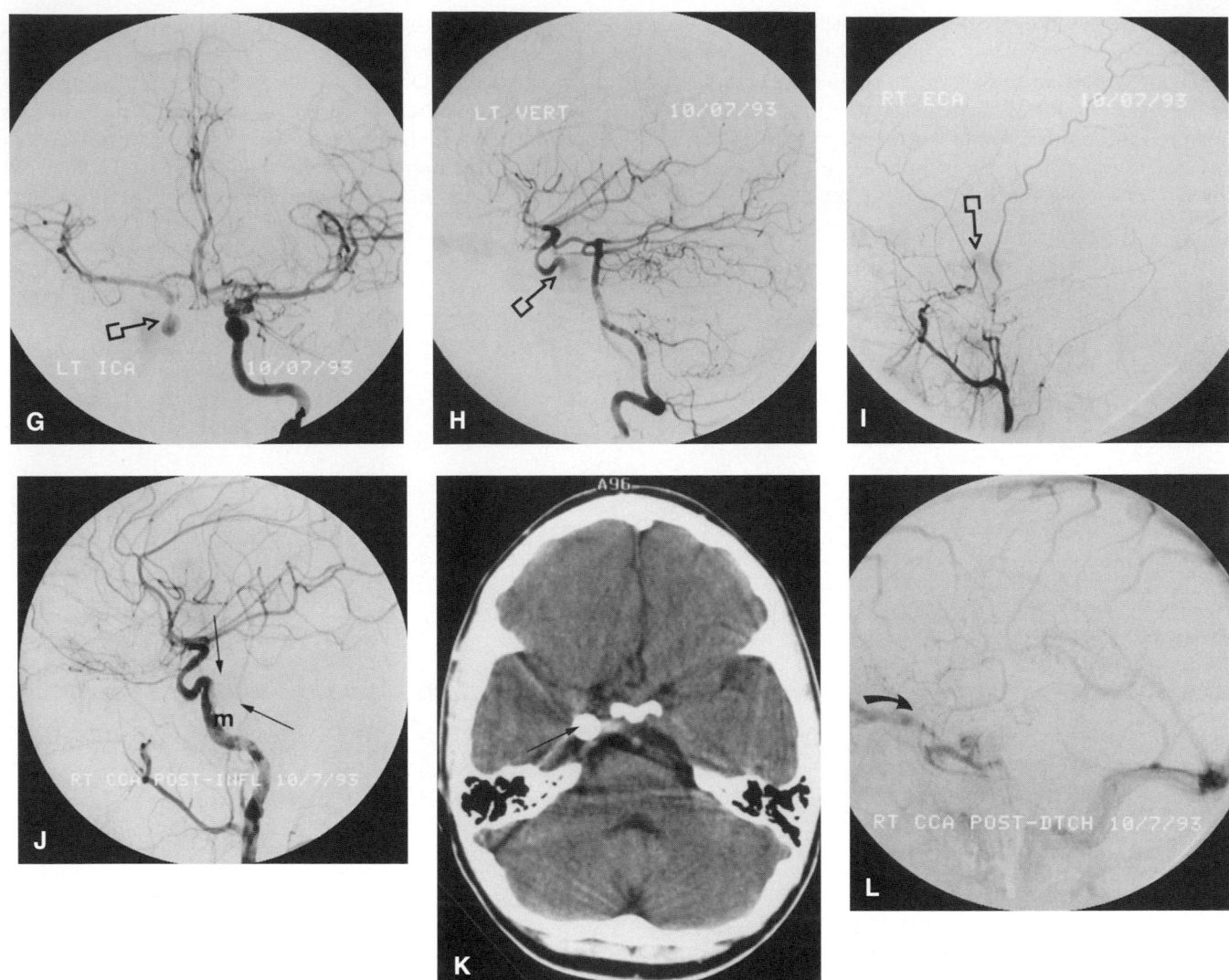

Figure 50–4 *(continued)* **G., H., I.** Retrograde opacification of the right CCF (*open straight arrow*) obtained during angiography of the left internal carotid artery (frontal DSA image, G), left vertebral artery (lateral DSA image, H), and right external carotid artery (lateral DSA image, I). The opacification of the fistula from the right external carotid artery occurs through anastomoses between the artery of the foramen rotundum and the inferolateral trunk of the left carotid-cavernous artery. **J.** Lateral midarterial-phase DSA image from a right common carotid angiogram obtained after inflation of a No. 9 latex balloon (*arrows*), which has obliterated the fistula. The inflated balloon is seen, before detachment, mounted on a microcatheter (*m*) and was previously advanced into the fistula from the arterial side. The 8 French guiding catheter is positioned within the right common carotid artery and is not visualized. Note the absence of AV shunting with restoration of antegrade sequential opacification of the right hemispheric vasculature. **K.** A postembolization transaxial CT scan through the level of the cavernous sinus depicts the contrast-inflated balloon (*arrow*). **L.** Venous phase lateral DSA image of the postembolization right internal carotid angiogram. Note the normal venous pattern of drainage and reestablishment of centripetal flow within the right superior ophthalmic vein directed toward the cavernous sinus (*curved arrow*). When this image is compared to the lateral DSA images depicted in A and B, the right superior ophthalmic vein is clearly reduced in size.

pharmacologic methods may assume importance in the preembolization period.

Neurointerventional Management of CCFs

Over the past several decades, transarterial embolization has become the accepted means of treating CCFs (2, 87,93,94). The historically standard method employs a detachable balloon mounted on a microcatheter that is introduced coaxially through a 6–8 French wide lumen guiding catheter positioned proximally within the involved internal carotid artery (Figure 50–4J). The balloon-mounted microcatheter tip is flow-guided through the lesion from the arterial side by hemodynamic conditions associated with the rapid arteriovenous shunting present. Once positioned on the venous side of the fistula, the balloon is inflated, thereby occluding the shunt, ideally without compromising the internal carotid artery. The balloon is then detached, and the microcatheter is removed. An assortment of easily mounted latex or silicone balloons is available, differing in size and shape (2,87). In general, they retain their original characteristics after multiple inflations and deflations, a feature that may be necessary in optimally positioning the balloon before detachment. In most cases, the balloon is filled with isotonic contrast to facilitate visualization during the procedure and in the postembolization follow-up. Over the course of several weeks, a latex balloon normally deflates; however, it generally provides an adequate interval of occlusion during which thrombosis of the fistula occurs. Premature deflation or change in the position of the balloon, at the time of the procedure or within 1–2 days, is usually associated with recurrence or exacerbation of symptoms coinciding with an observable change in the disposition of the balloon on plain skull film. When appropriate, treatment failure usually is followed by a second attempted transarterial closure.

If the carotid artery must be sacrificed, it is important to occlude the entire segment involved in the fistula to prevent reconstitution of the shunt through anastomoses with the ipsilateral external carotid artery, generally through C4 or C5 branches of the cavernous ICA or by way of the ophthalmic artery. Care should also be taken to avoid occlusion of the internal carotid artery proximal to the fistula, thereby allowing persistent filling of the fistula from the supraclinoid segment of the internal carotid circulation. As mentioned previously, under conditions of anticipated internal carotid sacrifice, preembolization angiography must establish the adequacy of collateral circulation through the circle of Willis.

Because of the decreasing availability of balloons, detachable coils, particularly hydrogel-coated coils, have emerged as an effective alternative agent for the treatment of CCFs (95). This technique, whether employing a transarterial-transfistula or transvenous approach, is additionally useful for cases in which the fistula cannot accommodate a balloon or for patients with reestablished CCFs in whom balloon embolization has failed because of premature partial deflation of the balloon. In addition, the use of detachable coils avoids potential hazards of balloon deployment such as premature deflation of the balloon, migration of the balloon during detachment, and venous or arterial embolization of a prematurely deflated balloon. Transarterial CCF coil embolization usually is facilitated by concomitant temporary inflation of a nondetachable balloon (analogous to balloon remodeling in the endovascular coil treatment of cerebral aneurysms) (96) or deployment of an arterial stent (97) within the cavernous segment of the carotid artery across the fistula. Either technique is useful in ensuring coil deployment within the involved cavernous sinus while protecting patency of the ICA lumen, which becomes increasingly obscured by the surrounding metallic mesh of coils within the enveloping cavernous sinus.

Various agents that induce thrombosis may be introduced directly into the cavernous sinus to effect successful closure of a CCF. When a transarterial approach cannot be performed because of traumatic vessel occlusion, vasculopathy, or a failed trapping procedure, venous access to the cavernous sinus may be considered (80,87,94,98–100). This technique involves either direct cannulation of the superior ophthalmic vein or femoral transvenous catheterization of the cavernous sinus by way of access through the inferior petrosal sinus or ophthalmic vein. Metallic coils are the preferred embolic agent by this route and should be deposited in a fashion that results in thrombosis of the cavernous sinus without diverting the drainage of the fistula into cortical veins.

After closure of the shunt, there is immediate resolution of the objective bruit, which can be used to confirm the occlusion of the CCF in the postembolization period. Recurrence of the bruit, in the absence of luminal compromise of the internal carotid artery, suggests reestablishment of the shunt even in the absence of additional symptoms. After shunt closure, elevations in intraocular pressure usually normalize within 48–72 hours (76). Other signs of orbital congestion generally resolve within days to weeks, with concomitant improvement in the associated cranial neuropathies not secondary to direct traumatic paresis.

Complications related to the embolization of CCFs are uncommon. Stroke, secondary to the premature or inadvertent deployment of embolic agents, is relatively infrequent because of the propensity of the released device to enter the fistula and lodge within the venous side (101). Cranial neuropathies that are present at the time of embolization may worsen because of the transient mass effect of the inflated balloon, which may compress cranial nerves within the cavernous sinus (102). This usually improves with the subsequent spontaneous deflation of the balloon over several weeks after treatment. The incidence of symptomatic venous pouches developing at the site of balloon deflation ranges from 2.4–21.0% (93). If symptoms persist, closure of the venous pouch with a second detachable balloon or microcoils may be contemplated. More commonly, the symptoms resolve spontaneously over several weeks to months and may be associated with shrinkage of the venous pouch as demonstrated by serial MRI following the course of the venous aneurysm.

EMBOLIZATION OF INTRACRANIAL, EXTRA-AXIAL NEOPLASMS

Neuroendovascular therapy is a useful approach to the preoperative or palliative management of extra-axial and calvarial vascular neoplasms. When coupled with contemporary microsurgical methods, selective presurgical embolization can facilitate the removal of tumor by significantly reducing intraoperative blood loss and by increasing the frequency of complete tumor resection (103–107).

Regardless of the tumor type or location, the preferred goal of tumor embolization is to devascularize the tumor capillary bed while preserving normal arterial distributions

(108). Moreover, adjunctive techniques such as permanent balloon occlusion of the internal carotid artery, when feasible, may enable more radical excision of tumors extensively involving the skull base (2).

The diagnosis of intracranial neoplasm is usually established by correlating the clinical history with transaxial imaging by CT and MRI. Formal angiography is generally reserved for those cases in which the information gained may be useful diagnostically or in planning therapeutic intervention. The angiographic evaluation should assess the arterial supply (specifically the vascular territory involved and its anatomic pattern) and the mix of dural and pial supply. Also, it should define regional arterial anastomoses and likely supplies to cranial nerves or cutaneous structures. The venous drainage of the lesion and the surrounding brain should be documented and any abnormalities pertaining to venous structures identified. Of particular importance in planning the embolization of an extra-axial tumor is the angiographic delineation of the unique vascular compartmentalization of the lesion.

Extra-axial tumors may be distinguished angiographically as monocompartmental or multicompartmental with respect to their hemodynamic composition (100,105,109). Each type of lesion may receive vascular contribution from several arterial sources, depending on the precise anatomic origin and the ultimate pattern of extension of the mass. Monocompartmental tumors may be opacified in their entirety by superselective angiography of any one of the supplying arteries (Figure 50–5). The embolization of such lesions should therefore be performed from the safest vascular approach with respect to risk to cranial nerve damage or cerebral embolization, thereby avoiding complications that may arise from a procedure conducted by way of a competing, more dangerous route. By comparison, multicompartmental tumors are composed of distinct vascular territories, each supplied by a separate arterial source (Figure 50–6). Complete devascularization of such lesions requires catheterization and embolization of several distinct supplying arteries. This implies increased risk of the procedure related to the multiplicity of potential complications unique to the separate embolizations of each vascular territory.

The therapy of choice for most extra-axial tumors is surgical removal. The introduction of surgical microtechnique and preoperative embolization has significantly improved the completeness of tumor resection while minimizing morbidity. Although a variety of extra-axial and calvarial neoplasms may satisfy specific criteria for embolic therapy, certain general principles apply to their embolization. The specific techniques employed are similar to those required in the treatment of other extra-axial lesions. Individual supplying arteries are selectively catheterized and embolized after superselective angiography to verify microcatheter position and margin of safety. Where feasible, small particulate agents such as gelfoam powder (40–60 μm) or PVA (150–250 μm) are preferred for tumor embolization. The use of small particles permits more distal penetration of the tumor vascular bed, precluding revascularization of the mass during the interval before surgery by collateral meningeal supply, and may be more effective in inducing tumor necrosis (109,110). A small aliquot of particles is diluted into contrast material and occasionally mixed with 10–30% ethanol (when performed under general anesthesia). It is then injected into the arterial feeder via the microcatheter. Strict attention is paid to avoiding extensive reflux of the embolic agent, which becomes more likely as the procedure progresses because of curtailment of antegrade runoff into the tumor vascular bed. Other particulate agents frequently used in tumor embolization include the larger sizes of PVA (250–1,000 μm), gelfoam sponge strips, and platinum fiber coils. The latter two materials find use in sealing pedicles after PVA or gelfoam powder embolization, particularly after embolizations of the MMA during which proximal occlusion is helpful in reducing bleeding from the level of the foramen spinosum during the subsequent craniotomy. As mentioned previously, gelfoam sponge strips or coils may be used to occlude potentially dangerous anastomoses before microparticulate embolization of meningiomas in certain territories.

Although the use of smaller PVA sizes is advocated for the embolization of most extra-axial tumors, the larger particulate sizes are preferred for the embolization of tumor feeders also supplying cranial nerves or other eloquent anastomoses to reduce the risk of the procedure. The larger particles may also be helpful in embolizing vessels arising from scalp arteries to avoid necrosis in territories fed by cutaneous branches.

With respect to large skull base tumors, two specific situations deserve particular attention. First, in patients in whom the cavernous sinus or carotid canal is involved by tumor and in whom the collateral circulation via the circle of Willis adequately supports the ipsilateral cerebral hemisphere, balloon occlusion of the internal carotid artery distal to the horizontal cavernous segment may be used for more effective embolization of supplies derived from cavernous or petrous branches of the ICA. Balloon occlusion of the ipsilateral internal carotid artery may also reduce the risks of pericarotid tumor removal, permitting a more radical tumor resection. Second, tumors with intradural extension, especially within the posterior fossa, are almost never amenable to complete embolization because of the variable pial supply.

Complications

When performed properly, embolization of calvarial or extra-axial masses is associated with a high degree of effectiveness and a low complication rate. Most complications pertain to cranial nerve palsies, particularly when one is embolizing skull base lesions or posterior fossa masses vascularized by the ascending pharyngeal artery or those lesions supplied by a dominant accessory meningeal artery with liquid acrylic or ethanol (2,13). In addition, facial paralysis may complicate

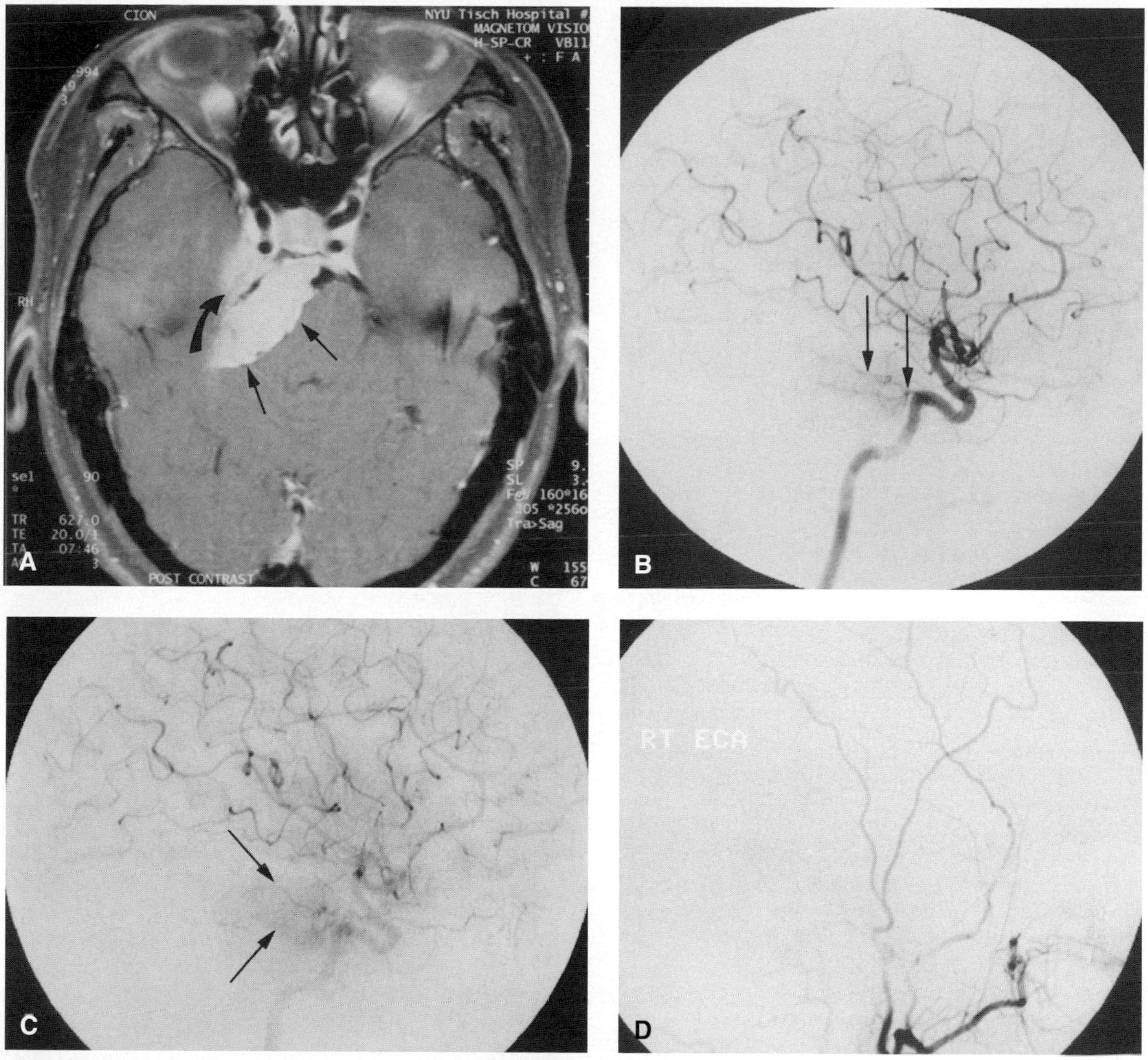

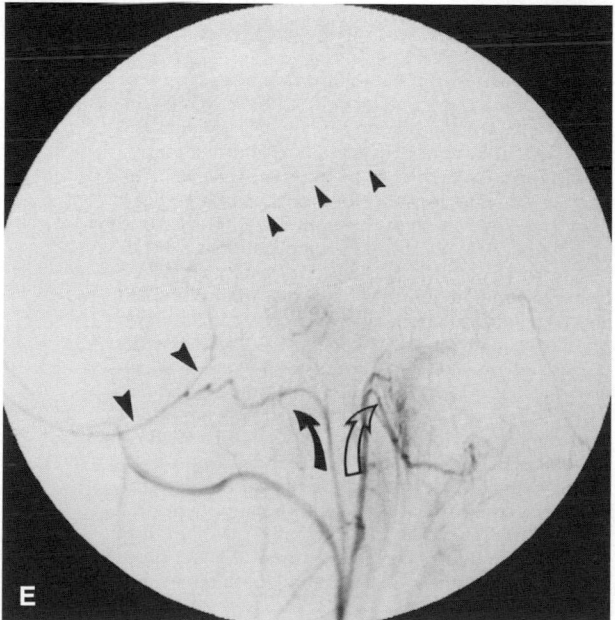

Figure 50–5 Monocompartmental right petroclival meningioma. **A.** Gadolinium-enhanced transaxial T_1-weighted MR image with fat suppression demonstrates an enhancing right petroclival tumor (*straight arrows*). The mass extends inferiorly along the clivus, displacing the brain stem toward the left and extending through Dorello's canal (*curved arrow*), possibly explaining the patient's right sixth nerve palsy. **B.** Early and **C.** late arterial phase lateral DSA image of the right internal carotid artery. Note the abnormal tumor blush developing as a result of contribution from the right internal carotid artery by way of its meningohypophyseal trunk (*arrows*). **D.** The subsequent DSA of the distal right external carotid artery failed to disclose evidence of middle or accessory meningeal contribution to the lesion, consistent with monocompartmental C5 segmental supply. **E.** Lateral DSA image of the right ascending pharyngeal artery depicts subtle supply to the lesion from the neuromeningeal trunk (*solid curved arrow*) of the ascending pharyngeal artery. Note the origin of the posterior meningeal supply to the cerebellar fossa (*large arrowheads*), which anastomoses with the right middle meningeal artery, opacifying the petrosquamosal division (*small arrowheads*). The pharyngeal division of the right ascending pharyngeal artery is also depicted (*open curved arrow*).

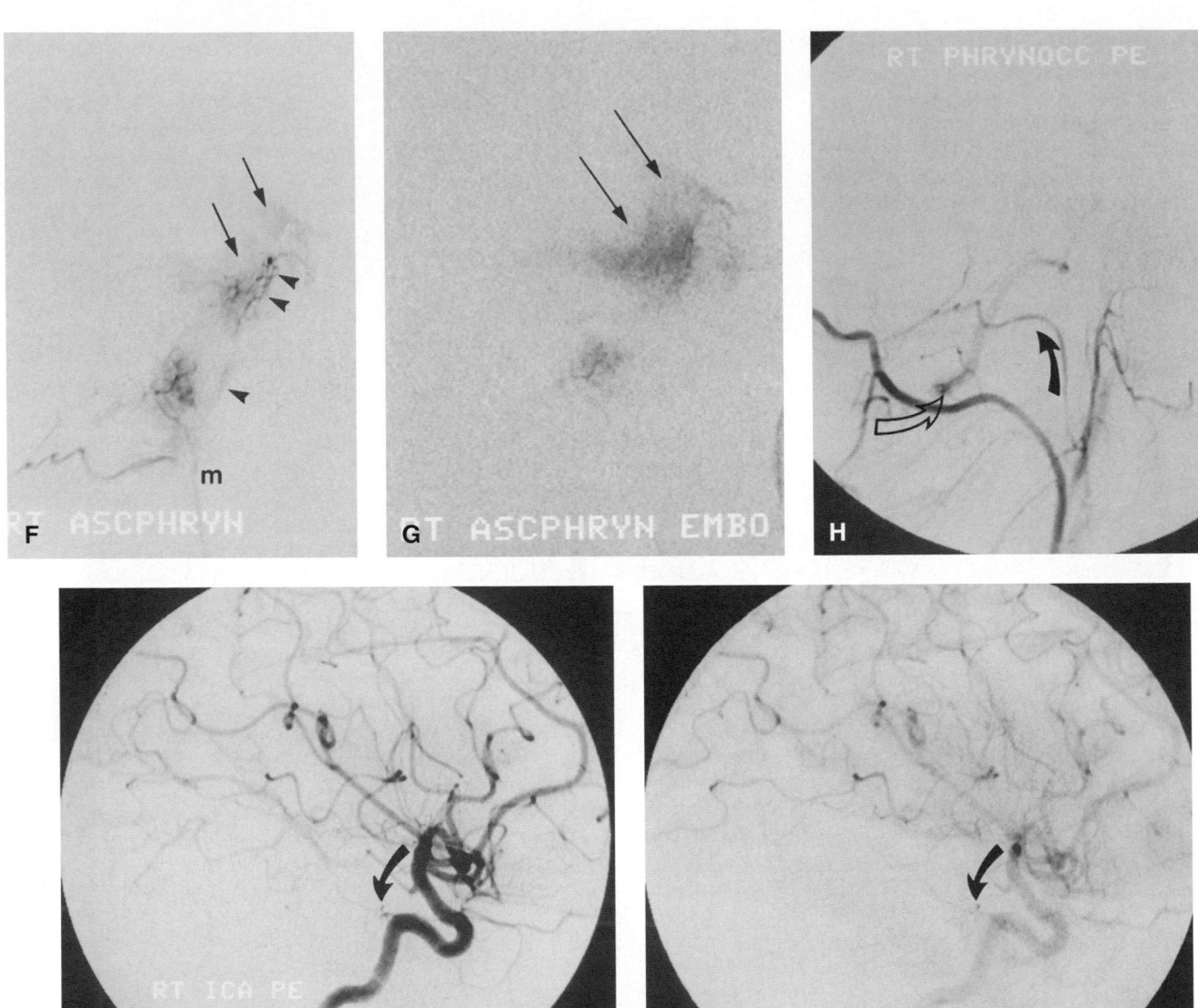

Figure 50–5 *(continued)*   **F.** Lateral superselective DSA image from the neuromeningeal trunk of the right ascending pharyngeal artery. A microcatheter (m) has been advanced to the origin of the ascending clival branches, which constitute the natural collaterals in hemodynamic balance with the clival divisions of the meningohypophyseal trunk. The subsequently obtained superselective angiogram more fully discloses the extent of the clival supply *(arrowheads)* to the mass *(arrows)*. The pattern of supply suggests a monocompartmental tumor deriving contribution from the anastomotic balance between the clival arcade and the meningohypophyseal trunk of the right cavernous carotid artery. **G.** Stagnant contrast within the meningioma *(straight arrows)* is seen during gelfoam powder embolization from the clival division of the right ascending pharyngeal artery. **H.** Postembolization lateral DSA image of the right pharyngooccipital trunk documents obliteration of the ascending pharyngeal contribution to the meningioma. The neuromeningeal trunk is preserved *(solid curved arrow)*. Note the transient opacification of the right vertebral artery by the way of C1 anastomosis with the right occipital artery *(open curved arrow)*. This finding illustrates the potential risk of vertebrobasilar embolization during procedures involving the occipital artery axis. **I.** Middle and **J.** late arterial phase lateral DSA images from the postembolization right internal carotid angiogram depict the prominent segment of the right meningohypophyseal trunk *(curved arrow)* but fail to disclose evidence of the tumor blush demonstrated in the preembolization angiogram of B and C. The single-pedicle embolization has successfully devascularized this right petroclival meningioma from the ascending pharyngeal artery without necessitating direct catheterization of the meningohypophyseal trunk of the right internal carotid artery with microparticles passing in retrograde fashion from clival feeders through the meningohypophyseal trunk. This could occur with a forceful injection of embolic agent and increases in likelihood as the preferential runoff into the tumor mass diminishes during the later stages of embolization.

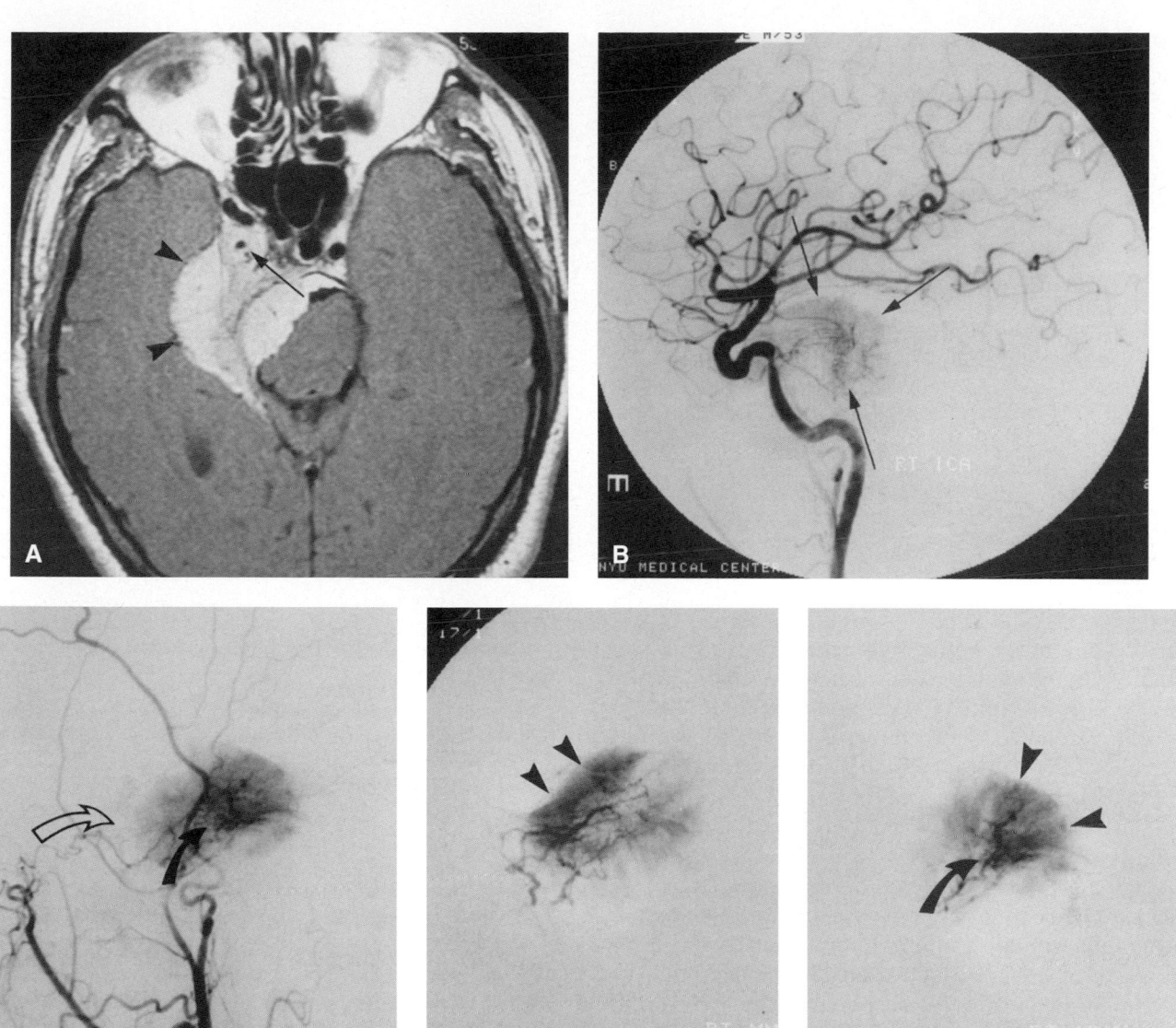

Figure 50–6 Right petroclival meningioma with supply from multiple pedicles. **A.** Gadolinium-enhanced T$_1$-weighted spin-echo MR image through the level of the cavernous sinuses depicts a right petroclival meningioma (*arrowheads*). The mass extends into the right cavernous sinus and circumferentially narrows the C5 segment of the right carotid-cavernous artery (*arrow*). **B.** Lateral midarterial-phase DSA image of the right internal carotid artery demonstrates an abnormal tumor blush (*arrows*) supplied primarily by the meningohypophyseal (C5 segment) and inferolateral (C4 segment) branches of the right internal carotid artery, consistent with a mass comprising at least two hemodynamically independent compartments. As suggested by MRI, the C5 segment of the carotid-cavernous artery is seen to be narrowed circumferentially. **C.** Lateral right external carotid artery DSA image illustrates an abnormal tumor blush developing within the anterolateral compartment of the mass. The external carotid contribution to the lesion has two components: a contribution to the posterolateral compartment derived from petrosal and cavernous branches of the right middle meningeal artery (*solid curved arrow*, C and E) and a contribution from the artery of the foramen rotundum (*open curved arrow*) that supplies the anteromedial aspect of the mass. (These separate compartmental supplies are depicted more clearly in the superselective angiograms of D–G). **D.** Frontal and **E.** lateral DSA images from the superselective right middle meningeal (*curved arrow*, E) angiogram clearly depict the segmental supply to the posterolateral compartment of the mass (*arrowheads*). The multicompartmental angiographic appearance of this lesion differs from that of the petroclival meningioma presented in Figure 50–5 and complicates the interventional approach to embolization of this specific mass. This is easily recognized from the subsequent superselective angiogram of the artery of the foramen rotundum performed after gelfoam powder embolization of the middle meningeal supply.

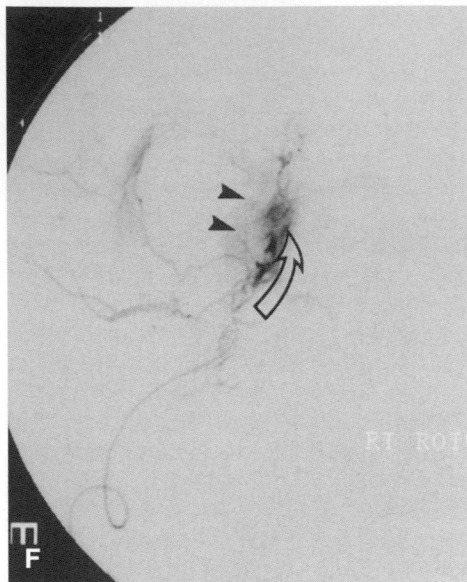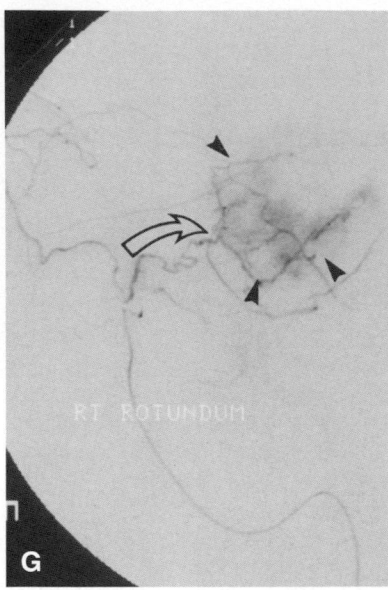

Figure 50–6 *(continued)* **F.** Frontal and **G.** lateral projections DSA images illustrate the residual supply to the cavernous portion of the meningioma (*arrowheads*, F and G) that represents the vascular territory supplied by the unembolized artery of the foramen rotundum (*open curved arrow*). The postembolization right internal carotid angiogram also showed persistent supply to the posteromedial compartment of the mass, which remains supplied by the meningohypophyseal trunk (*not shown*).

embolization involving the stylomastoid or petrosal distributions to the temporal bone. Attention should also be directed to any potential risk of cerebral embolization by way of anastomoses between meningeal branches of the ECA and ICA or vertebrobasilar circulations. Several investigators have also reported complications related to intratumoral (111), perilesional, or subarachnoid hemorrhage (112,113), in addition to acute exacerbation of mass effect secondary to postembolization swelling of the tumor (110). These complications emphasize the importance of postembolization monitoring and may necessitate emergent surgical intervention. The patient should be warned in advance of these potential complications. When liquid embolic agents are used in these vascular territories, provocative testing with intra-arterial lidocaine may be recommended.

REFERENCES

1. Dion JE. Principles and methodology. In: Vinuela F, Halbach VV, Dion JE, eds. Interventional Neuroradiology: Endovascular Therapy of the Central Nervous System. New York: Raven, 1992:1–15.
2. Lasjaunias P, Berenstein A. Surgical Neuroangiography. Vol 2: Endovascular Treatment of Craniofacial Lesions. Berlin: Springer-Verlag, 1987.
3. Valavanis A. Interventional Neuroradiology. Berlin: Springer-Verlag, 1993.
4. Lasjaunias P, Chiu M, ter Brugge K, et al. Neurological manifestations of intracranial dural arteriovenous malformations. J Neurosurg 1986;64:724–730.
5. Strother CM. Interventional neuroradiololgy. AJNR Am J Neuroradiol 2000;21:19–24.
6. Lasjaunias P, Berenstein A, ter Brugge K. Surgical Neuroangiography: Clinical Vascular Anatomy and Variations. 2nd Ed. Berlin: Springer-Verlag, 2001.
7. Berenstein A. Brachiocephalic vessels: selective and superselective catheterization. Radiology 1983;148:437–441.
8. Berenstein A, Kricheff II. Catheter and material selection for transarterial embolization: technical considerations. II. Materials. Radiology 1979;132:631–639.
9. Berenstein A, Lasjaunias P, Kricheff II. Functional anatomy of the facial vasculature in pathologic conditions and its therapeutic applications. AJNR Am J Neuroradiol 1983;5:149–153.
10. Lasjaunias P, Berenstein A, Doyon D. Normal functional anatomy of the facial artery for superselective angiography. Radiology 1979;133:631–638.
11. Fischer E. Die Lageabweichungen der vorderen Hirnarterie im Gefassbild. Zentralbl Neurochir 1938;3:300–312.
12. Theron J, Cosgrove R, Melanson D, et al. Embolization with temporary balloon occlusion of the internal carotid and vertebral arteries. Neuroradiology 1986;28:246–253.
13. Lasjaunias P, Berenstein A. Surgical Neuroangiography. Vol 1: Functional anatomy of the craniofacial arteries. Berlin: Springer-Verlag, 1987.
14. Berenstein A, Russell EJ. Gelatin sponge in therapeutic neuroradiology: a subjective review. Radiology 1981;141:145.
15. Berenstein A, Lasjaunias P. Surgical Neuroangiography. Vol 5: Endovascular treatment of spine and spinal cord lesions. Heidelberg: Springer-Verlag, 1992.
16. Horton JA, Kerber CW. Lidocaine injection in the external carotid branches: provocative test to preserve cranial nerve function in therapeutic embolization. AJNR Am J Neuroradiol 1986;7:105–108.
17. Newton TH, Cronqvist S. Involvement of dural arteries and intracranial arteriovenous malformations. Radiology 1969;93:1071–1078.
18. Chaudhary M, Sachdev VB, Cho SH, et al. Dural arteriovenous malformation of the major venous sinus—an acquired lesion. AJNR Am J Neuroradiol 1982;3:13–19.
19. Houser OW, Campbell JK, Campbell RJ, et al. Arteriovenous malformations affecting the transverse dural sinus—an acquired lesion. Mayo Clin Proc 1979;54:651–661.
20. Herman JM, Spetzler RF, Bederson JB, et al. Genesis of a dural arteriovenous malformation in a rat model. J Neurosurg 1995;83:539–545.
21. McCormick WF, Boulter TR. Vascular malformations ("angiomas") of the dura mater. J Neurosurg 1966;25:309–311.
22. Vidyasagar C. Persistent embryonic veins in the arteriovenous malformations of the dura. Acta Neurochir 1979;48:199–216.
23. Houser OW, Baker HL, Rhoton AL, et al. Dural arteriovenous malformations. Radiology 1972;105:55–64.
24. Djindjian R, Cophignon J, Theron J. Embolization by superselective arteriography from the femoral route in neuroradiology. Review of 60 cases. 1. Technique, indications, complications. Neuroradiology 1973;6:20–26.
25. Borden JA, Wu JK, Shucart WA. A proposed classification for spinal and cranial dural arteriovenous fistulous malformations and implications for treatment. J Neurosurg 1995;82:166–179.

26. Cognard C, Gobin YP, Pierot L, et al. Cerebral dural arteriovenous fistulas: clinical and angiographic correlation with a revised classification of venous drainage. Radiology 1995;194:671–680.

27. Chaloupka JC, Huddle DC. Classification of vascular malformations of the central nervous system. Neuroimaging Clin N Am 1998;8:295–321.

28. Vinuela F, Fox AJ, Pelz DM, et al. Unusual clinical manifestations of dural arteriovenous malformations. J Neurosurg 1986;64:554–558.

29. Kupersmith MJ, Berenstein A, Nelson PK, et al. Visual symptoms with dural arteriovenous malformations draining into occipital veins. Neurology 1999;52:156–62.

30. Kosnik EJ, Hunt WE, Miller DA. Dural arteriovenous malformations. J Neurosurg 1974;40:322–329.

31. Laurent A, Guimarens L, Rufenacht D, et al. Five cases of unilateral exophthalmos associated with abnormalities in the lateral sinus area. J Neuroradiol 1986;13:125–136.

32. Hurst RW, Bagley LJ, Galetta S, et al. Dementia resulting from dural arteriovenous fistulas: the pathologic findings of venous hypertensive encephalopathy. AJNR Am J Neuroradiol 1998;19:1267–1273.

33. Lamas E, Loboto RD, Esparza J. Dural posterior fossa AVM producing raised sagittal sinus pressure: case report. J Neurosurg 1977;46:804–810.

34. Halbach VV, Higashida RT, Hieshima GB, et al. Dural fistulas involving the transverse sigmoid sinuses: results of treatment in 28 patients. Radiology 1987;163:443–447.

35. Obrador S, Soto M, Silvela J. Clinical syndromes of arteriovenous malformations of the transverse-sigmoid sinus. J Neurol Neurosurg Psychiatry 1975;38:436–451.

36. Awad I, Little J, Akarawi W, et al. Intracranial dural arteriovenous malformations: factors predisposing to an aggressive neurological course. J Neurosurg 1990;72:839–850.

37. Picard L, Bracard S, Malaet J, et al. Spontaneous dural arteriovenous fistulas. Semin Intervent Radiol 1987;4:219–240.

38. Gelwan MJ, Choi IS, Berenstein A, et al. Dural arteriovenous malformations and papilledema. Neurosurgery 1988;22:1079–1084.

39. Halbach VV, Higashida RT, Hieshima GB, et al. Dural fistulas involving the cavernous sinus: results of treatment in 30 patients. Radiology 1987;163:437–442.

40. Kupersmith MJ, Berenstein A, Choi IS, et al. Management of nontraumatic vascular shunts involving the cavernous sinus. Ophthalmology 1988;95:121–130.

41. Kupersmith MJ, in collaboration with Berenstein A. Neurovascular Neuro-ophthalmology. Heidelberg: Springer-Verlag, 1993.

42. de Keizer RJW. Spontaneous carotico-cavernous fistulas. The importance of the typical limbal vascular loops for the diagnosis, the recognition of glaucoma and the uses of conservative therapy in this condition. Doc Ophthalmol 1979;46:403–412.

43. Grove AS. The dural shunt syndrome: pathophysiology and clinical course. Ophthalmology 1983;90:31–44.

44. Newton TH, Hoyt WF. Dural arteriovenous shunts in the region of the cavernous sinus. Neuroradiology 1970;1:71–81.

45. Hawke SHB, Mullie MA, Hoyt WF, et al. Painful ocular nerve palsy due to dural-cavernous sinus shunt. Arch Neurol 1989;46:1252–1255.

46. Stiebel-Kalish H, Setton A, Nimii Y, et al. Ophthalmology 2002, 109:1685–91.

47. Halbach VV, Higashida RT, Hieshima GB, et al. Treatment of dural arteriovenous malformations involving the superior sagittal sinus. AJNR Am J Neuroradiol 1988;9:337–343.

48. Halbach VV, Higashida RT, Hieshima GB, et al. Treatment of dural fistulas involving the deep cerebral venous system. AJNR Am J Neuroradiol 1989;10:393–399.

49. Barnwell SL, Halbach VV, Dowd CF, et al. Dural fistulas including the inferior petrosal sinus. AJNR Am J Neuroradiol 1990;11:511–517.

50. Halbach VV, Higashida RT, Hieshima GB, et al. Dural arteriovenous fistulas supplied by ethmoidal arteries. Neurosurgery 1990;25:816–823.

51. Ito J, Imamura H, Kobayashi K, et al. Dural arteriovenous malformations of the base of the anterior cranial fossa. Neuroradiology 1983;24:149–154.

52. Kobayashi H, Hayashi N, Noguchi Y, et al. Dural arteriovenous malformations in the anterior cranial fossa. Surg Neurol 1988;30:396–401.

53. Halbach VV, Higashida RT, Hieshima GB, et al. Transvenous embolization of dural fistulas involving the transverse sigmoid sinuses. AJNR Am J Neuroradiol 1989;10:385–392.

54. Versari PP, D'Aliberti G, Talamonti G, et al. Progressive myelopathy caused by intracranial dural arteriovenous fistula: report of 2 cases and review of the literature. Neurosurgery 1993;33(5):914–919.

55. Panasci DJ, Nelson PK. MR imaging and MR angiography in the diagnosis of dural arteriovenous fistulas. Magn Reson Imaging Clin N Am 1995;3:493–508.

56. DeMarco JK, Dillon W, Halbach VV, et al. Dural arteriovenous fistulas: evaluation with MR imaging. Radiology 1990;175:193–199.

57. Noguchi K, Melhem ER, Kanazawa T, et al. Intracranial dural arteriovenous fistulas: evaluation with combined 3D time-of-flight MR angiography and MR digital subtraction angiography. AJR Am J Roentgenol 2004;182:183–190.

58. Coley SC, Romanowski CAJ, Hodgson TJ, et al.. Dural arteriovenous fistulae: noninvasive diagnosis with dynamic MR digital subtraction angiography. AJNR Am J Neuroradiol 2002;23:404–407.

59. Luciani A, Houdart E, Mounayer C, et al. Spontaneous closure of dural arteriovenous fistulas: report of three cases and review of the literature. AJNR Am J Neuroradiol 2001;22:992–996.

60. Halbach VV, Higashida RT, Hieshima GB, et al. Transvenous embolization of dural fistulas involving the cavernous sinus. AJNR Am J Neuroradiol 1989;10:377–384.

61. Mullen S. Treatment of carotid cavernous fistulas by cavernous sinus occlusion. J Neurosurg 1979;50:131–144.

62. Takahashi A, Yoshimoto T, Kawakami K, et al. Transvenous copper wire insertion for dural arteriovenous malformations of the cavernous sinus. J Neurosurg 1989;70:751–754.

63. Nelson PK, Russell SM, Woo HH, et al. Use of a wedged microcatheter for curative transarterial embolization of complex intracranial dural arteriovenous fistulas: indications, endovascular technique, and outcome in 21 patients. J Neurosurg 2003;98:498–506.

64. Hamada Y, Goto K, Inoue T, et al. Histopathological aspects of dural arteriovenous fistulas in the transverse-sigmoid sinus region in 9 patients. Neurosurgery 1997;40:452–458.

65. Roy D, Raymond J. The role of transvenous embolization in the treatment of intracranial dural arteriovenous fistulas. Neurosurgery 1997;40:1133–1144.

66. Aihara N, Mase M, Yamada K, et al. Deterioration of ocular motor dysfunction after transvenous embolization of dural arteriovenous fistula involving the cavernous sinus. Acta Neurochir 1999;141:707–710.

67. Nakagawa H, Kubo S, Nakajima Y, et al. Shifting of dural arteriovenous malformation from the cavernous sinus to the sigmoid sinus to the transverse sinus after transvenous embolization. A case of left spontaneous carotid-cavernous sinus fistula. Surg Neurol 1992;37:30–38.

68. Yamashita K, Taki W, Nakahara I, et al. Development of sigmoid dural arteriovenous fistulas after transvenous embolization of cavernous dural arteriovenous fistulas. AJNR Am J Neuroradiol 1993;14:1106–1108.

69. Kubota Y, Ueda T, Kaku Y, et al. Development of a dural arteriovenous fistula around the jugular valve after transvenous embolization of cavernous dural arteriovenous fistula. Surg Neurol 1999;51:174–176.

70. Kiyosue H, Tanoue S, Okahara M, et al. Recurrence of dural arteriovenous fistula in another location after selective transvenous coil embolization: report of two cases. AJNR Am J Neuroradiol 2002;23:689–692.

71. Kubo M, Kuwayama N, Hirashima Y, et al. Dural arteriovenous fistulae developing at different locations after resolution of previous fistulae: report of three cases and review of the literature. AJNR Am J Neuroradiol 2002;23:787–789.

72. Terada T, Higashida RT, Halbach VV, et al. Development of acquired arteriovenous fistulas in rats due to venous hypertension. J Neurosurg 1994;80:884–889.

73. Lawton MT, Jacobowitz R, Spetzler RF. Redefined role of angiogenesis in the pathogenesis of dural arteriovenous malformations. J Neurosurg 1997;87:267–274.

74. Vinuela F, Fox AJ, Debrun GM, et al. Spontaneous carotid-cavernous fistulas: clinical, radiological, therapeutic considerations. Experience with 20 cases. J Neurosurg 1984;6:976–984.

75. Barnwell SL, Halbach VV, Higashida RT, et al. Complex dural arteriovenous fistulas: results of a new combined neurosurgical and interventional neuroradiology treatment in 16 patients. J Neurosurg 1989;7:352–358.

76. Kupersmith MJ, Berenstein A, Flamm E, et al. Neuroophthalmologic abnormalities and intravascular therapy of traumatic carotid cavernous fistulas. Ophthalmology 1986; 93:906–912.

77. Graf CJ. Spontaneous carotid-cavernous fistula: Ehlers-Danlos syndrome and related condition. Arch Neurol 1965;13:662–672.

78. de Campos JM, Ferro MO, Burzaco JA, et al. Spontaneous carotid-cavernous fistula in osteogenesis imperfecta. J Neurosurg 1982;56:590–593.

79. Kaufman HH, Lind TA, Mullen S. Spontaneous carotid-cavernous fistula with fibromuscular dysplasia. Acta Neurochir 1978;40: 123–129.

80. Klisch J, Huppertz HJ, Spetzger U, et al. Transvenous treatment of carotid cavernous and dural arteriovenous fistulae: results for 31 patients and review of the literature. Neurosurgery 2003;53: 836–856.

81. Henderson JW, Schneider RC. The ocular findings in carotid cavernous fistula in a series of 17 cases. Am J Ophthalmol 1959; 48:585–597.

82. Sanders MD, Hoyt WF. Hypoxic ocular sequelae of carotid-cavernous fistulae: study of the causes and failure before and after neurosurgical treatment in a series of 25 cases. Br J Ophthalmol 1969;53:82–97.

83. Maurer JJ, Mills M, German WJ. Triad of unilateral blindness, orbital fracture, and massive epistaxis after head trauma. J Neurosurg 1961;45:837–840.

84. Coskun O, Hamon M, Catroux G, et al. Carotid-cavernous fistulas: diagnosis with spiral CT angiography. AJNR Am J Neuroradiol 2000;21:712–716.

85. Komiyama M, Fu Y, Yagura H, et al. MR imaging of dural AV fistulas at the cavernous sinus. J Comput Assist Tomogr 1990;14: 397–401.

86. Hirai T, Korogi Y, Hamatake S, et al. Three-dimensional FISP imaging in the evaluation of carotid cavernous fistula: comparison with contrast-enhanced CT and spin-echo MR. AJNR Am J Neuroradiol 1998;19:253–259.

87. Debrun GM. Endovascular management of carotid cavernous fistulas. In: Valavanis A, ed. Interventional Neuroradiology. Berlin: Springer-Verlag, 1993:23–34.

88. Turner DM, Vangilder JC, Mojtahedi S, et al. Spontaneous intracerebral hematoma in carotid cavernous fistula. J Neurosurg 1983;59:680–686.

89. Debrun GM, Vinuela F, Fox AJ, et al. Indications for treatment and classification of 132 carotid-cavernous fistulas. Neurosurgery 1988;22:285–289.

90. Halbach VV, Hieshima GB, Higashida RT, et al. Carotid cavernous fistula: indications for urgent treatment. AJNR Am J Neuroradiol 1987;8:627–633.

91. de Schweinitz GA, Holloway TB. Pulsating Exophthalmos. Philadelphia: W.B. Saunders, 1908:11–120.

92. Palastine AG, Younge BR, Piepgras DG. Visual prognosis in carotid-cavernous fistulas. Arch Ophthalmol 1981;99:1600–1603.

93. Debrun G, Lacour P, Vinuela F. Treatment of 54 traumatic carotid-cavernous fistulas. J Neurosurg 1981;55:678–692.

94. Debrun GM, Nauta HJ, Miller NR, et al. Combining the detachable balloon technique and surgery in managing CCFs. Surg Neurol 1989;38:3–10.

95. Siniluoto T, Seppanen S, Kuurne T, et al. Transarterial embolization of a direct carotid cavernous fistula with Guglielmi detachable coils. AJNR Am J Neuroradiol 1997;18:519–523.

96. Morris PP. Balloon reconstructive technique for the treatment of a carotid cavernous fistula. AJNR Am J Neuroradiol 1999;20: 1107–1109.

97. Ahn JY, Lee B-H, Joo JY. Stent-assisted Guglielmi detachable coil embolization for the treatment of a traumatic carotid cavernous fistula. J Clin Neurosci 2003;10:96–98.

98. Halbach VV, Higashida RT, Hieshima GB, et al. Transvenous embolization of direct carotid cavernous fistulas. AJNR Am J Neuroradiol 1988;9:741–747.

99. Manelfe C, Berenstein A. Treatment of carotid cavernous fistulas by venous approach. J Neuroradiol 1980;7:13–21.

100. Moret J, Lasjaunias P. Vascular architecture of tympano-jugular glomus tumor. In: Vignaud J, Jardic C, Rosen L, eds. The Ear. Paris: Masson, 1986:289–303.

101. Barrow DL, Fleischer AS, Hoffman JC. Complications of detachable balloon technique in the treatment of traumatic intracranial arteriovenous fistulas. J Neurosurg 1982;50:396–403.

102. Kendall B. Results of treatment of arteriovenous fistulas with the Debrun technique. AJNR Am J Neuroradiol 1983;4:405–408.

103. Halbach VV, Hieshima GB, Higashida RT, et al. Endovascular therapy of head and neck tumors. In: Vinuela F, Halbach VV, Dion JE, eds. Interventional Neuroradiology: Endovascular Therapy of the Central Nervous System. New York: Raven, 1992:17–28.

104. Manelfe C, Lasjaunias P, Ruscalleda J. Preoperative embolization of intracranial meningiomas. AJNR Am J Neuroradiol 1986;7: 963–972.

105. Valavanis A. Embolization of intracranial and skull base tumors. In: Valavanis A, ed. Interventional Neuroradiology. Berlin: Springer-Verlag, 1993:63–92.

106. Wakhloo AK, Juengling FD, Delthoven VV, et al. Extended preoperative polyvinyl alcohol microembolization of intracranial meningiomas: assessment of two embolization techniques. AJNR Am J Neuroradiol 1993;14:571–582.

107. Dowd CF, Halbach VV, Higashida RT. Meningiomas: the role of preoperative angiography and embolization. Neurosurg Focus 2003;15:1–4.

108. Valavanis A. Preoperative embolization of the head and neck: indications, patient selection, goals, and precautions. AJNR Am J Neuroradiol 1986;7:943–952.

109. Masters LT, Nelson PK. Petroclival meningiomas: pre-operative angiography and embolization. Intervent Neuroradiol 1998;4: 209–21.

110. Wakhloo AK, Juengling FD, Van Velthoven V, et al. Extended preoperative polyvinyl alcohol microembolization of intracranial meningiomas: assessment of two embolization techniques. AJNR Am J Neuroradiol 1993;14:571–582.

111. Suyama T, Tamaki N, Fujiwara K, et al. Peritumoral and intratumoral hemorrhage after gelatin sponge embolization of malignant meningioma: case report. Neurosurgery 1987;21:944–946.

112. Kallmes DF, Evans AJ, Kaptain FJ, et al. Hemorrhagic complications in embolization of a meningioma: case report and review of the literature. Neuroradiology 1997;39:877–880.

113. Yu SCH, Boet R, Wong GKC, et al. Postembolization hemorrhage of a large and necrotic meningioma. AJNR Am J Neuroradiol 2004;25:506–508.

Interventional Radiology of the Thorax

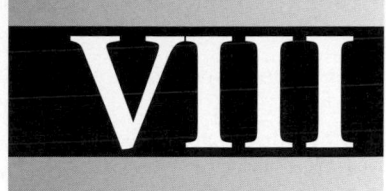

VIII

Transcatheter Bronchial Artery Embolization for Inflammation (Hemoptysis)

51

Matthew A. Mauro, Charles T. Burke, Paul F. Jaques

Massive hemoptysis, defined as 300–600 mL of blood per 24-hour period, carries a 50–85% mortality with conservative treatment and has traditionally been the principal indication for bronchial artery embolization. Asphyxiation and, less commonly, exsanguination are the usual causes of death (1). Aggressive therapeutic maneuvers are required to manage these emergencies. Surgical resection of the bleeding source is the initial treatment of choice for those patients with isolated abnormalities and adequate pulmonary reserve. However, patients with chronic lung disease and limited pulmonary reserve are often considered unacceptable surgical risks, and this group may benefit from palliative

bronchial artery embolization. In addition, there is some evidence that the surgical mortality rate may be lowered by preoperative bronchial artery embolization in those patients who are actively bleeding. It is well established that safe and rapid control of massive hemoptysis can often be obtained by therapeutic transcatheter embolization of the bronchial arteries.

More recently, moderate hemoptysis (greater than or equal to three episodes of 100 mL of blood per day within 1 week) and even mild hemoptysis (chronic or slowly increasing hemoptysis) are considered indications for transcatheter therapy (2). Recurrent nonmassive hemoptysis is particularly common in patients with cystic fibrosis, where these recurrent bleeds are debilitating and preclude routine postural drainage of other lung regions. Bronchial artery embolization for mild or moderate bouts of hemoptysis has been shown to play a valuable role in the management of this group of patients (2–4). The availability of lung transplantation has also stimulated a more aggressive approach to the management of mild to moderate hemoptysis in the cystic population.

CLINICAL CONSIDERATIONS

Severe hemoptysis most commonly present in patients with a history of chronic inflammatory lung disease. Tuberculosis with associated aspergillosis remains the most common worldwide etiology (5). In the United States, complicated pulmonary sarcoid, cystic fibrosis, and other types of bronchiectasis are the most common causes of hemoptysis that may benefit from transcatheter therapy. The chronicity of the disease is an important aspect in patient selection. It is in this clinical setting that bronchial artery hypertrophy occurs, facilitating transcatheter therapy. Without hypertrophy, bronchial artery embolization is less likely to be of benefit. In most cases, severe hemoptysis results from a systemic arterial source rather than the pulmonary circulation, and tends to be episodic. Initial management includes resuscitation, sedation, coagulation profile, chest radiograph, and early bronchoscopy. If embolotherapy is being considered, localization of the bleeding to a single lung or lobe is helpful because it will guide the angiographer to concentrate on the affected region. A review of previous and current chest radiographs and computed tomograms (if available) may also help in determining the probable site of bleeding. Bronchoscopy may localize the source of bleeding and guide the use of selective intrabronchial balloon tamponade if massive hemorrhage continues. Bronchoscopy has been shown to be of increased value when obtained early in patient management. Saumench et al. found the site of the hemorrhage in 91% of patients when bronchoscopy was performed early compared with 50% of patients when bronchoscopy was performed later in the clinical course (6). However, in a recent study by Hsiao et al., fiberoptic bronchoscopy provided additional information to radiographic studies in only three of 29 patients (7). These findings led them to conclude that bronchoscopy should be reserved for patients in whom radiographic studies fail to localize the bleeding site. Patients often experience a gurgling sensation and may be able to locate the source of bleeding themselves. If surgical treatment has been permanently or temporarily excluded, patients should undergo emergent angiography, preferably during a quiescent phase to maximize the chances of a technically successful procedure.

Patients with cystic fibrosis frequently present with a recurrent crescendo type of bleeding rather than a singular massive bleed and are more likely to have recurrent bleeds even after successful transcatheter therapy (2–4). There is a rich anastomosis between many of the mediastinal structures and the bronchial arterial circulation. Patients who have undergone previous bronchial artery embolization procedures should not be excluded from subsequent attempts at palliative embolization. Recurrent hemorrhages are secondary to recanalization of embolized vessels or hypertrophy of collateral vessels from other systemic supplies (8).

Significant bleeding of pulmonary arterial origin is rare and secondary to erosive pseudoaneurysms in association with cavitary aspergillosis, cavitary tuberculosis, or pyogenic abscesses. A pulmonary arterial source should be considered in addition to the more common systemic supply in settings of destructive lung disease. Suggestive chest radiographic findings include a necrotic cavity, a cavity closely related to a central pulmonary artery, or replacement of a cavity with a rapidly growing nodule or mass (9). A pulmonary arterial source should also be considered when bleeding continues after technically successful bronchial artery and nonbronchial systemic arterial embolization.

ANATOMY

Bronchial arteries most commonly arise from the thoracic aorta at the T3–T8 level and supply the trachea, bronchi, vagus nerve, posterior mediastinum, and esophagus. A number of anatomic variations in bronchial artery origin have been described. Cauldwell, in 1948, described four common variations: type 1—two left bronchial arteries and a single right bronchial artery (41%); type 2—single bronchial arteries bilaterally (21%); type 3—two left and two right bronchial arteries arising separately or in various combinations (21%); and type 4—a single left and two right bronchial arteries (10%) (10). In 1985, Uflacker and colleagues reported the four most frequent bronchial artery variations as single right intercostobronchial trunk with single left artery (31%), single right intercostobronchial trunk and right and left bronchial arteries sharing a common trunk (25%), single right intercostobronchial trunk and two left bronchial arteries (13%), and single right intercostobronchial trunk with separate bronchial arteries bilaterally (11%) (Figures 51–1 through 51–3). In this series, 43% of patients had common bronchial trunks (11). No left intercostobronchial trunks were identified, whereas the right bronchial arteries frequently shared origins with superior intercostal arteries. Nearly 80% of all bronchial arteries arise at the T5–T6 level. Right bronchial or intercostobronchial artery trunks typically arise from the right lateral or anterolateral surface of the descending thoracic aorta. The left bronchial arteries usually arise from the more anterior surface of the aorta or the concavity of the arch. As many as 20% of bronchial arteries have anomalous origins from sites other than the aorta, and approximately 10% originate from the concave or convex surfaces of the aortic arch. Other aberrant origins of the bronchial arteries include the subclavian, thyrocervical, internal mammary, innominate, pericardiophrenic, superior intercostal, abdominal aorta, and inferior phrenic arteries (12–14).

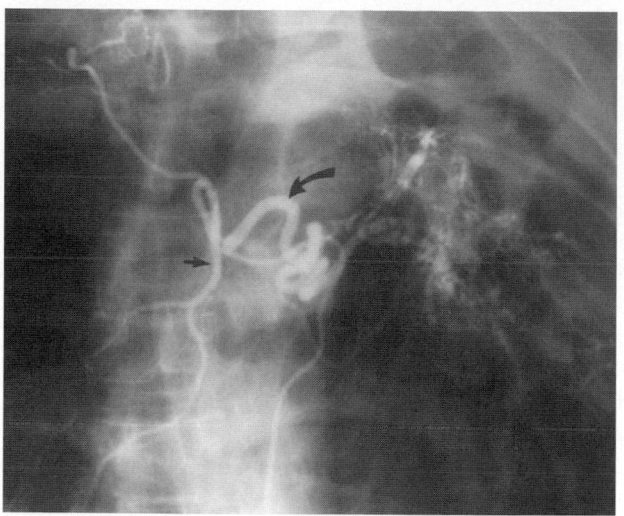

Figure 51-1   Common bronchial trunk. Left and right bronchial arteries arise from a common trunk. The right bronchial artery (*straight arrow*) appears normal, whereas the left bronchial artery (*curved arrow*) is enlarged and tortuous. Note the superior intercostal artery arising from the right bronchial artery. (From Mauro MA, Jaques PF, Morris S. Bronchial artery embolization for control of hemoptysis. Sem Intervent Radiol 1992;9:46, with permission.)

Cohen et al. reported a higher prevalence of aberrant origins of bronchial arteries (35%) among 20 patients with cystic fibrosis. In addition, they found a 10-fold higher incidence of radicular supply from the bronchial arteries (3). The authors suggest that lifelong bronchial wall inflammation causes enlargement of the existing extensive and anastomotic network that interconnects the bronchial circulation with mediastinal, head, neck, and spinal arteries.

The bronchial arteries extend along the bronchi to the level of the respiratory bronchiole, where they anastomose with the pulmonary circulation. Branches supply the vasa vasorum of the pulmonary vasculature as well as the diaphragmatic and mediastinal portions of the visceral pleural, the middle third of the esophagus, and lymph nodes. Most of the venous return occurs through the pulmonary veins by way of bronchial pulmonary anastomoses (15). There is an extensive potential anastomotic network between the bronchial arteries and other structures in the mediastinum, spine, head, and neck. These bronchial pulmonary arterial anastomoses may become prominent in the abnormal lung, reflecting either chronic inflammation or pulmonary hypertension (16,17). Transpleural systemic collateral vessels from intercostal, internal mammary, phrenic, and thyrocervical arteries as well as from branches of the axillary artery provide pulmonary bronchial supply in these situations and may be responsible for hemoptysis (17). Tanaka et al. reviewed bronchial artery drainage in patients undergoing bronchial artery embolization or chemoinfusion. They discovered four types of venous drainage: type 1—direct drainage into the pulmonary vein (42%); type 2—direct drainage into the pulmonary artery (19%); type 3—direct drainage into the pulmonary artery with retrograde flow (19%); and type 4—direct drainage into the bronchial vein (4.8%) (15).

When one is performing bronchial artery arteriography and embolization, careful consideration must be given to the arterial supply to the spinal cord. The anterior spinal artery supplies the anterior portion of the cord and runs in the ventral median sulcus. The anterior spinal artery originates from branches of the intracranial segments of the vertebral arteries and receives supply from anterior

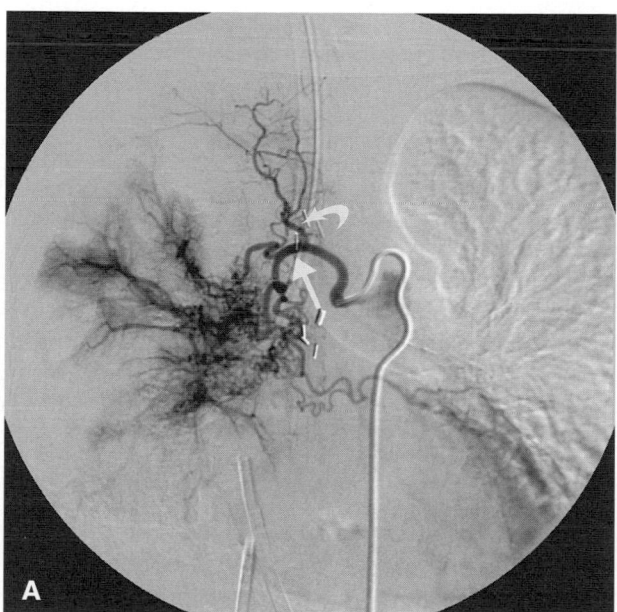
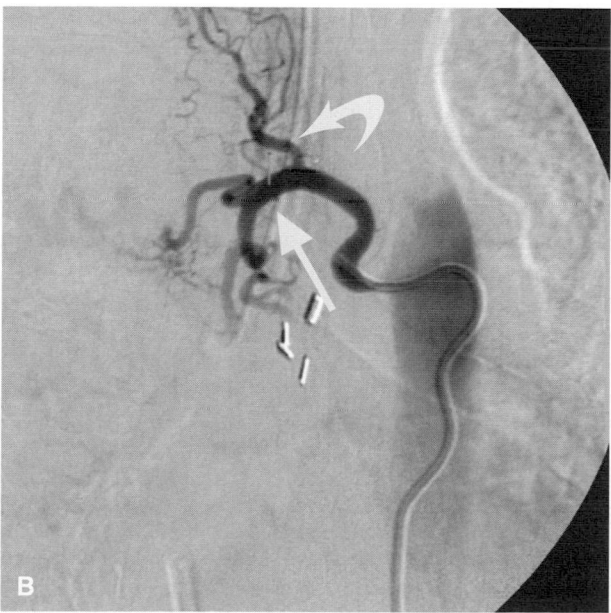

Figure 51-2   Right intercostal-bronchial trunk. **A.** The right bronchial artery (*straight arrow*) and superior intercostal artery (*curved arrow*) arise from a common trunk. **B.** Following selective embolization of the right bronchial artery (*straight arrow*), the superior intercostal artery is preserved (*curved arrow*).

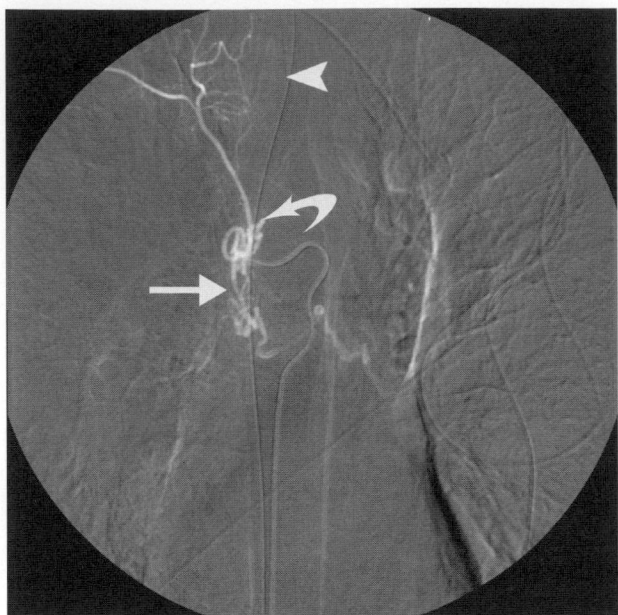

Figure 51–3 Intercostal-bronchial trunk. The left bronchial artery (*straight arrow*) and right superior intercostal artery (*curved arrow*) arise from a common trunk. Note the characteristic hairpin loop (*arrowhead*) of the spinal artery branch originating from the superior intercostal artery.

radiculomedullary branches of intercostal and lumbar arteries along its length (18). As many as six to eight contributing branches to the anterior spinal artery may exist, and each has a characteristic course resembling a hairpin loop. The largest anterior medullary branch (the artery of Adamkiewicz) has a variable origin from the T5–L5 level but is most commonly found at the T8–L1 level. In approximately 5% of the population, a right intercostobronchial artery contributes to or arises with the artery of Adamkiewicz. The right superior intercostal artery and right bronchial artery may share a common trunk and supply a branch to the anterior spinal artery (Figure 51–3). Left bronchial arteries rarely supply the anterior spinal artery. The posterior portion of the cord is supplied by a pair of posterior spinal arteries that course along the posterolateral surface of the spinal cord. These vessels are fed by posterior radicular arteries arising from intercostal and lumbar arteries and are much shorter and smaller than the anterior radiculomedullary arteries.

TECHNIQUE

Angiography

A brief neurologic examination should be performed to establish a baseline before the angiographic and embolization procedure. This will often be repeated throughout the course of the procedure to monitor the patient's neurologic status, particularly in relation to sensory and strength changes of the lower extremities. Several authors have recommended the use of somatosensory-evoked potentials to monitor ischemic spinal cord changes during the embolization procedure (19). This is cumbersome, far from routine, and in general unnecessary.

A descending thoracic aortogram can be initially performed before selective catheterization to provide a road map. If this is the first episode of hemoptysis, the involved bronchial arteries are often enlarged, and catheterization is usually straightforward. Therefore, routine thoracic aortography may not be required, and direct subselective catheterization of the bronchial arteries may be initially performed. If, however, successful catheterization of the bronchial arteries is not promptly achieved, the selective catheter can be easily replaced with a pigtail catheter to perform descending thoracic aortography.

Arterial access is most commonly achieved via common femoral artery puncture through which a sheath is inserted. An axillary or high brachial artery approach is occasionally necessary to define and embolize vessels arising from subclavian artery branches. A 5 or 6 French vascular sheath connected to an infusion system is routinely used at the authors' institution. If the patient is obese or if the iliac vessels are markedly tortuous, a long sheath is used that extends into the aorta. A variety of selected catheter curves can be used for subselective catheterization. The authors usually begin with a reverse-curve catheter: a Mikaelsson, Simmons I, or shepherd's hook. However, when there is a low aortic arch or if the bronchial artery originates from the arch, a reverse-curve catheter may fail to adequately probe the aortic wall. The apex of the reverse-curve catheter will lie partially within the transverse arch, tilting the catheter and making catheterization of more proximately located bronchial arteries impossible. In these circumstances, forward-looking catheters, such as the cobra, H1H, or RC shapes, can be used successfully. In general, 5.0 or 5.5 French catheters are initially used, reserving the larger 6.5–7.0 French catheters for a particularly tortuous vascular system where increased steerability is required.

The bronchial artery search is begun at the T5–T6 level (10). The air-filled left main stem bronchus serves as a convenient fluoroscopic landmark for this general location of bronchial artery origin. The catheter tip is initially directed laterally to anterolaterally when one is searching for the right bronchial artery or intercostobronchial trunk. A left lateral to anterolateral direction is used for left bronchial artery catheterization. Catheter occlusion of a bronchial artery, particularly a right intercostobronchial trunk, should be avoided because this may result in spinal cord ischemia if spinal artery branches are present.

Before embolization, a selective arteriogram must be performed. Bronchial arteries have characteristic branches that follow the course of the main stem bronchi toward the hila and can be easily differentiated from intercostal arteries, which have an initial cephalic course and then travel laterally along the undersurface of a rib (Figure 51–2). Coughing may be elicited during a bronchial artery injection, whereas a pure intercostal artery injection may be painful but will not initiate coughing. Nonionic contrast media should be used for all injections. The coughing response is less severe, and the risk of transverse myelitis may be lower.

Standard cut-film techniques or digital subtraction arteriography can be used when performing subselective bronchial artery injections. The injection volumes and rates must be sufficient to identify any spinal artery branches that may exist. The spinal artery can be identified by its characteristic cephalic course with a hairpin bend in the midline within the spinal canal (Figure 51–3). If there is some doubt concerning a midline branch on an anteroposterior film, an oblique film should be obtained to identify whether this branch does indeed enter the spinal canal. Tracheal and esophageal branches also originate from the bronchial artery and may appear midline on anteroposterior films but do not feature the hairpin loop. In cases of chronic inflammation, the bronchial arteries are hypertrophied and tortuous (Figures 51–1 and 51–2). Other signs include hypervascularity, systemic-to-pulmonary artery or venous shunting, and bronchial artery aneurysms. Frank contrast extravasation into a bronchus at angiography is rare (Figure 51–4) (20–25). When abnormal bronchial arteries are not identified, arch aortography and selective subclavian arteriography must be performed to search for anomalous bronchial arteries, nonbronchial systemic arterial supply, or both (18,26–28). The search for a nonbronchial systemic supply is particularly urgent in patients with recurrent bleeding after previous bronchial artery embolization, particularly if proximal coil occlusion has been performed. Vessels responsible for recurrent bleeding might include a bronchial artery not previously embolized (aberrant or nonaberrant), a recanalized bronchial artery, or nonbronchial systemic collateral vessels (Figures 51–5 and 51–6). If lower-lobe disease is present, an abdominal aortogram and examination of the inferior phrenic arteries should also be performed (Figure 51–7). If no systemic (bronchial or nonbronchial) arterial supply is identified, selective pulmonary arteriography should be performed in an attempt to identify a pulmonary arterial source such as a pseudoaneurysm or arteriovenous fistula (9,20,24,29–32).

Embolization

The goal of the embolization procedure varies, depending on whether the bleeding site has been located with some degree of reliability and whether there have been previous embolization procedures. If the site of hemorrhage is known, attention can be confined to embolization of bronchial arteries and collateral vessels supplying that area. Otherwise, bronchial artery embolization of both lungs must be attempted. In the presence of previous bronchial artery embolization, collateral pathways will require special attention, although one should remember that principal bronchial arteries embolized with Gelfoam and even coils may recanalize.

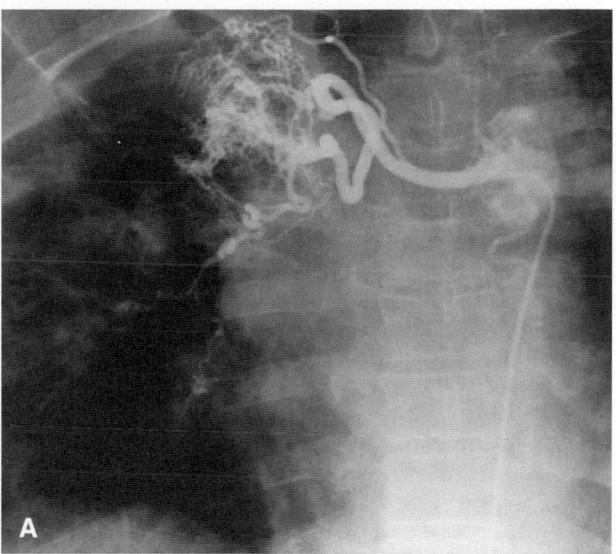

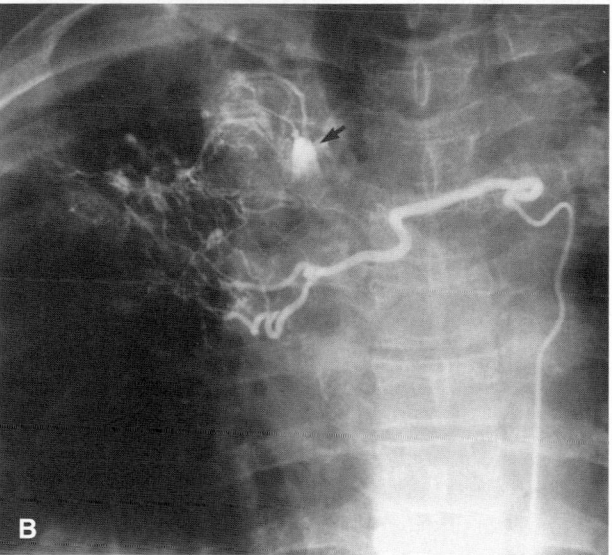

Figure 51–4 Two right bronchial arteries. **A.** Right upper bronchial arteriogram reveals hypervascularity, enlargement, and tortuosity. **B.** Right lower bronchial arteriogram shows similar hypervascularity and, in addition, an area of contrast extravasation (*arrow*). Both arteries were successfully embolized. (From Mauro MA, Jaques PF, Morris S. Bronchial artery embolization for control of hemoptysis. Sem Intervent Radiol 1992;9:48, with permission.)

When possible, any abnormal bronchial artery supplying the site(s) of hemorrhage should be embolized. The dominant feeding vessels should be embolized in all cases. It is important to realize that not all abnormal-appearing vessels need to be embolized to obtain a clinically beneficial therapeutic response. Recurrent hemorrhage at a future date, however, may be more likely to occur and occur earlier if nondominant vessels are not treated. Embolization of a bronchial artery with a documented spinal artery contribution is controversial and depends on operator experience and the risk–benefit ratio of bronchial artery embolization (that is, the clinical status of the patient) (Figure 51–3). Boushy et al. performed intra-arterial embolization in dogs and found

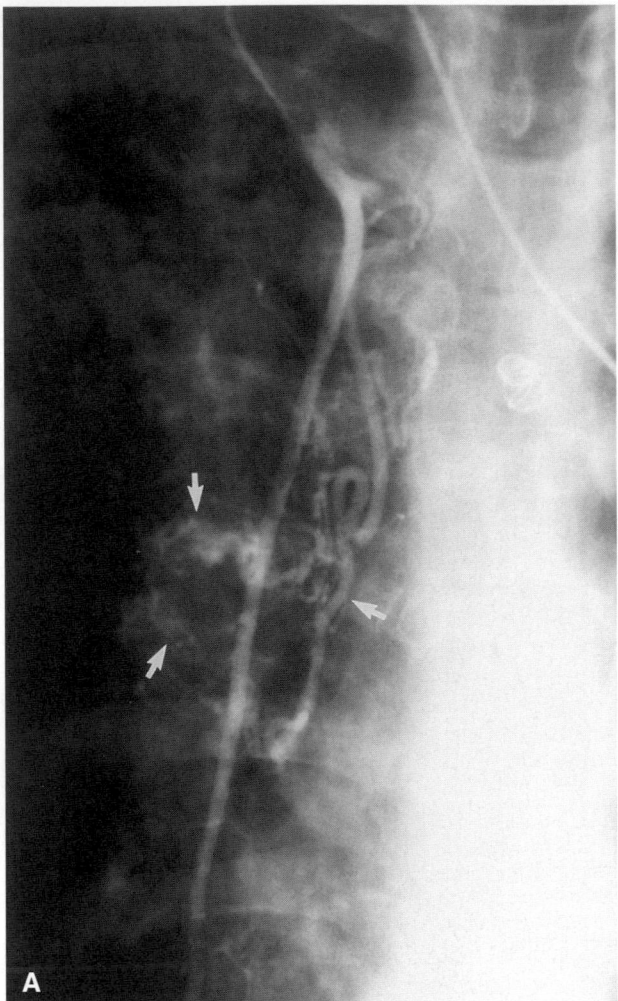

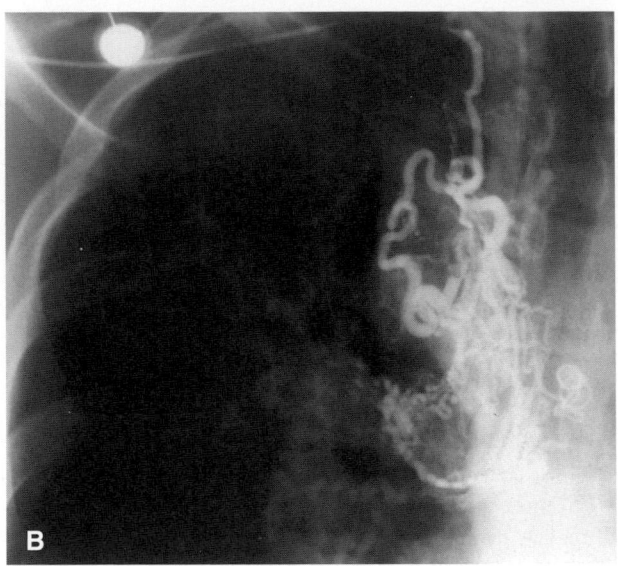

Figure 51–5 Nonbronchial systemic collaterals in a patient with recurrent hemoptysis. **A.** Right internal mammary arteriogram shows hypervascularity (*arrows*) in right hilum. **B.** Superselective injection of thyrocervical trunk branch shows massive collateral supply in a patient who had undergone previous bronchial artery embolization. (From Mauro MA, Jaques PF, Morris S. Bronchial artery embolization for control of hemoptysis. Sem Intervent Radiol 1992;9:48, with permission.)

hind limb paralysis with small (29–100 μm) microspheres and only transient weakness when larger particles (200 μm) were used (33). This suggests that particles greater than 200–250 μm are too large to enter the spinal feeders and therefore can be used for embolization (4,6,11). Clearly, a catheter position distal to the spinal artery origin is preferential and is often achievable with modern coaxial systems. Occasionally, a spinal artery branch will be identified only after partial distal embolization when the resistance of that vascular bed is elevated and smaller proximal branches are better opacified (3). Some authors have advised the use of an intra-arterial barbiturate as a provocative test in searching for an occult spinal artery contribution before bronchial artery embolization (34,35). A short-acting barbiturate, amobarbital, temporarily produces the symptoms of spinal cord ischemia when injected into a vascular bed with arterial supply to the spinal cord. Lidocaine solutions can also be used in a similar fashion. After hand injections of either of these substances, a repeat physical examination evaluating lower extremity strength is performed. When no neurologic changes are identified, one can be more comfortable that there are no significant arterial contributions to the spinal cord. Transverse

myelitis associated with this procedure has more commonly been associated with the use of ionic contrast media (36,37). Nonionic contrast agents should be routinely used.

Transcatheter embolization requires a stable catheter position. When reverse-curve catheters are used, the tip can often be advanced deeper into the vessel by simply withdrawing the catheter at the groin. Because particulate materials used for embolization require brisk forward flow of blood to be propelled distally into the vascular bed, flow occlusion by catheter wedging must be avoided.

Standard catheterization for embolization is performed with 5.0–5.5 French tapered catheters. When a stable catheter position cannot be obtained with these catheters, coaxial catheterization should be performed. Many coaxial systems are commercially available that will easily exit a 0.038-inch tapered diagnostic catheter. For routine coaxial catheterization, a dual-pressurized flush system (between the groin sheath and outer catheter and between the outer and inner catheters) may be used. For difficult or prolonged cases, a third flush between the inner catheter and micro guide wire is useful. The microcatheter should be advanced at least 1–2 cm beyond the origin of the bronchial artery to

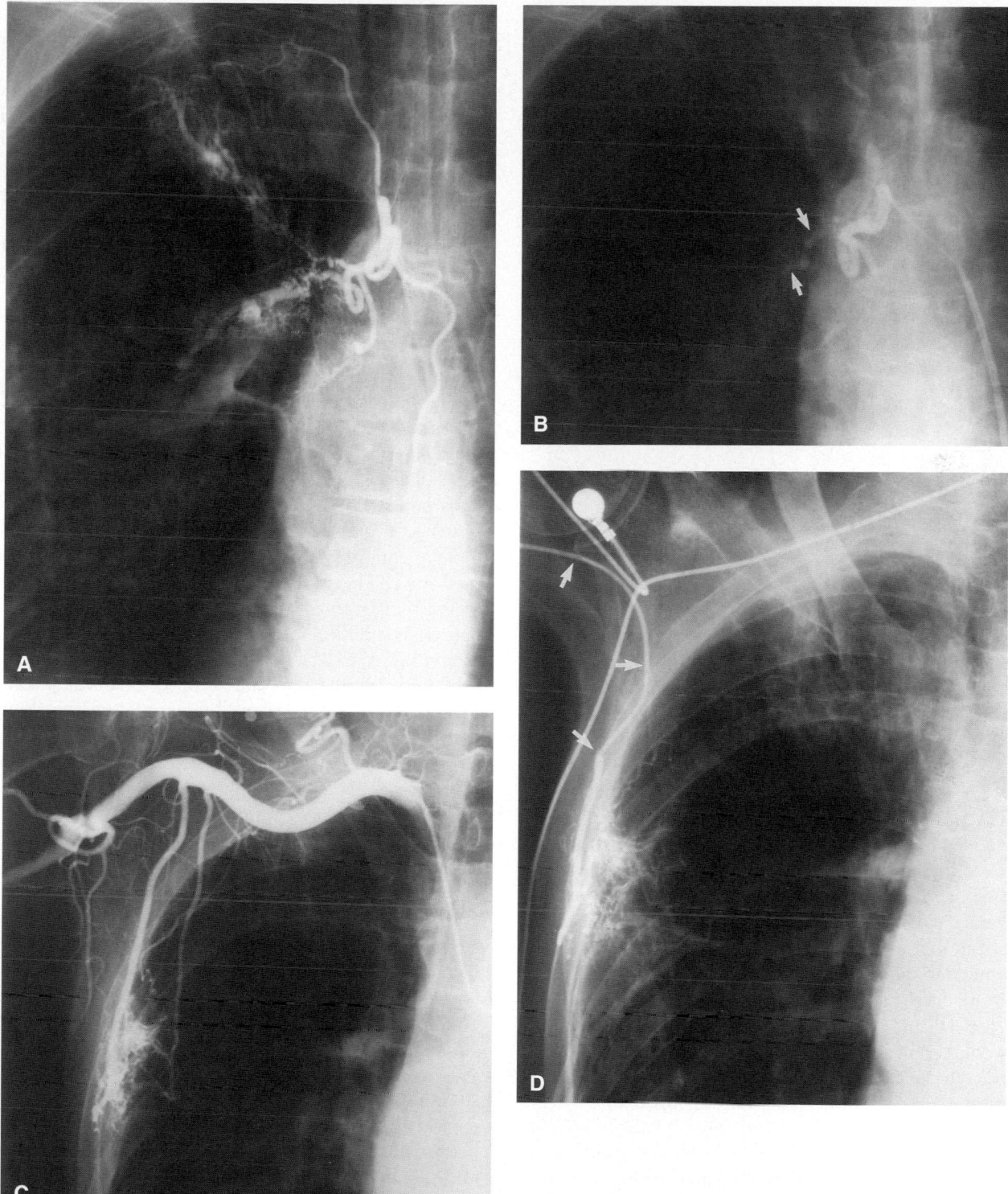

Figure 51–6   Recurrent hemoptysis in a patient with pleural disease. **A.** Right bronchial arteriogram shows hypervascularity and tortuosity. **B.** Successful embolization with a Gelfoam slurry mixture (*arrows*). Note the pleural disease along the lateral chest wall. **C.** Subclavian arteriogram 2 years later shows hypervascularity along the lateral chest wall. **D.** Selective catheterization of subscapular artery via the brachial approach (*arrows*) for embolization. (From Mauro MA, Jaques PF, Morris S. Bronchial artery embolization for control of hemoptysis. Sem Intervent Radiol 1992;9:50, with permission.)

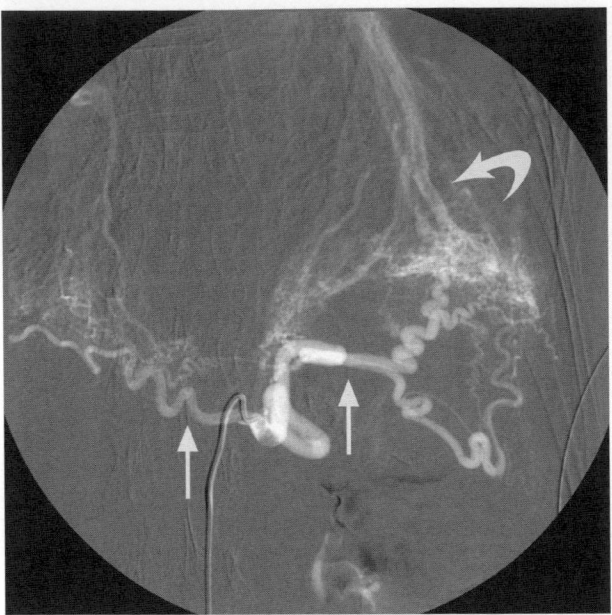

Figure 51–7 Infradiaphragmatic systemic collaterals in a patient with long history of tuberuculosis. Markedly enlarged inferior phrenic arteries (*straight arrows*) arising from a common trunk off the abdominal aorta providing collateral supply to the lung bases. Note the prominent shunting into the pulmonary vein (*curved arrow*).

be sure it is distal to any anterior radiculomedullary branches that may not be identified on initial arteriography. When present, the microcatheter should be advanced beyond the origin of the intercostal artery (in the case of an ICB trunk) or any vessel feeding the anterior spinal artery (Figure 51–3). Tanaka et al. demonstrated the value of superselective catheterization with a microcatheter (38). They documented improved hemorrhage control when using superselective as opposed to selective catheterization techniques. The authors also tended to use smaller particle sizes when performing the embolization through the microcatheter. This may also have contributed to the improved results.

Distal embolization should be performed whenever possible. If permanent proximal occlusion alone is performed, distal collateral vessels will invariably develop, and future access to the main bronchial artery may be lost. The most commonly used embolic materials for bronchial artery embolization include Gelfoam and polyvinyl alcohol (PVA) particles (3,4,8,21,23,25,39). Liquids such as ethanol or fine particles (Gelfoam powder) should be avoided because they produce highly distal embolization with occlusion of the capillary bed, leading to potential tissue infarction. Although cyanoacrylate has been used successfully, it is not recommended because it is cumbersome and requires significant operator experience (40). It will also permanently occlude the vessel, prohibiting the use of that vessel for future embolizations.

Gelfoam (gelatin sponge) is a readily available, slowly resorbable material that can be used as individual pledgets, torpedoes, or part of a slurry. For initial distal occlusion, 0.5- to 2.0-mm cubes can be used, followed by 3- to 4-mm pledgets or torpedoes for more proximal occlusion. Gelfoam pledgets are mixed with dilute contrast within a 1- or 3-mL syringe. Because the Gelfoam pledgets float within the contrast saline solution, the tip of the syringe should be pointed upward. A theoretical disadvantage of Gelfoam particles is that their resorption may lead to more rapid recanalization and recurrent bleeding (41). A Gelfoam slurry mixture composed of Gelfoam shavings, dextrose 50%, Pantopaque, and ε-aminocaproic acid may also be used and will produce a more lasting occlusion (42). This mixture is instilled in small (0.25- to 0.50-mL) amounts using a 3- or 1-mL syringe with a standard or coaxial catheter, respectively.

Polyvinyl alcohol (PVA) is the most commonly used particulate embolic material that is permanent in nature and available in several particle sizes. Particles greater than 250 μm should be used to avoid tissue ischemia or neurologic damage. PVA is available in various packaged sizes, depending on the manufacturer. Particles in the 300- to 500-μm range and 500- to 700-μm range are compatible with coaxial systems and are used routinely in the authors' practice. The more recently approved calibrated microspheres may also be used and will likely also be effective in this application. With 5 French or larger catheters, a 3- or 5-mL syringe is used for particle instillation, whereas a 1-mL syringe is preferable when using coaxial catheters or injectable wires. After the particle size is selected, the contents of the bottle are placed in a 20-mL syringe with the plunger removed. After the plunger is replaced, a solution of diluted contrast (50:50 nonionic contrast with saline) is placed into the 20-mL syringe with the PVA particles. One degasses the solution by removing the air in the syringe, placing a finger over the top, withdrawing the plunger, and shaking vigorously. After this maneuver, the solution is degassed, and particles are diffusely distributed within the 20-mL syringe, which serves as the particle reservoir. This is connected via flexible tubing to a three-way stopcock connected to the catheter and injection syringe. Before instillation, the particles are remixed with multiple in-and-out aspirations between the injection syringe and the 20-mL reservoir syringe. Because of the contrast solution, the embolization procedure can be visually monitored. Whenever there is slowing of the contrast/PVA column, the catheter should be immediately cleared of residual particulate matter with a saline injection and a formal contrast injection performed. This delivery system allows for quick, accurate, and safe delivery of PVA particles. When forward flow is markedly reduced, further embolization should be terminated. After distal embolization with small PVA particles, some authors advocate the use of Gelfoam cubes or torpedoes for more proximal embolization. These Gelfoam particles should be placed one at a time until flow all but ceases. When there is a major bronchial artery-to-pulmonary vein shunt, larger particulate particles are used initially to avoid systemic embolization.

Enormous bronchial arteries with high flow and large systemic-to-pulmonary shunts are sometimes encountered in cystic fibrosis and may require the use of coil embolization for safe and adequate occlusion (33,43). Coils should be 15–25% percent larger than the vessel diameter to avoid retrograde dislodgment, and the catheter should be well seated (44). This type of proximal coil occlusion should not be a routine practice and should be used only when other methods fail or are contraindicated or when the patient's clinical condition demands very rapid control.

COMPLICATIONS

Spinal cord infarction with transverse myelitis is the most feared complication of bronchial artery embolization, but the literature suggests that this is more a potential than a real problem (12). Transverse myelitis has been reported after diagnostic bronchial arteriography with the use of ionic hyperosmolar contrast agents (36,37). This complication should be significantly reduced by the use of nonionic contrast and the avoidance of catheter occlusions. The single reported case of paralysis after embolization for severe hemoptysis actually involved the left seventh intercostal artery and not a bronchial artery (45). Nevertheless, it is mandatory to perform preembolization angiography to identify any dominant radicular branch to the anterior spinal artery. Such a branch will usually involve a common intercostal bronchial artery anatomic variant.

Two cases of frank bronchial infarction after bronchial artery embolization have been reported, one of which was fatal (20,46). Liquid sclerosing agents (10% sodium chloride in one, ethanol in the other) were used in each case because a stable catheter position could not be obtained for a particulate embolization. The current coaxial catheter systems should overcome this difficulty, and liquid agents should be avoided. Bronchoesophageal fistulas have been reported when extremely small particulate agents were used and there was concomitant bronchial and esophageal ischemia (47,48). Chest pain and dysphagia commonly occur approximately 2–7 days after embolization procedures and are self-limiting. These are thought to occur secondary to the supply of the posterior mediastinum and esophagus by the bronchial arteries (Figure 51–8).

RESULTS

Bronchial artery embolization has been shown to be a highly effective technique for the immediate control of hemoptysis of inflammatory origin. Rabkin et al. reported the results of 306 bronchial artery embolizations in which there was immediate control of hemoptysis in 91% of patients (20). Uflacker, Rémy, and Hayakawa have published series reporting immediate control of hemoptysis in 77%, 84%, and 86% of patients, respectively (5,8,11). In a review of 63 patients, Hayakawa reported a complete remission of bleeding in 50%, partial remission in 22%, and recurrent hemoptysis in

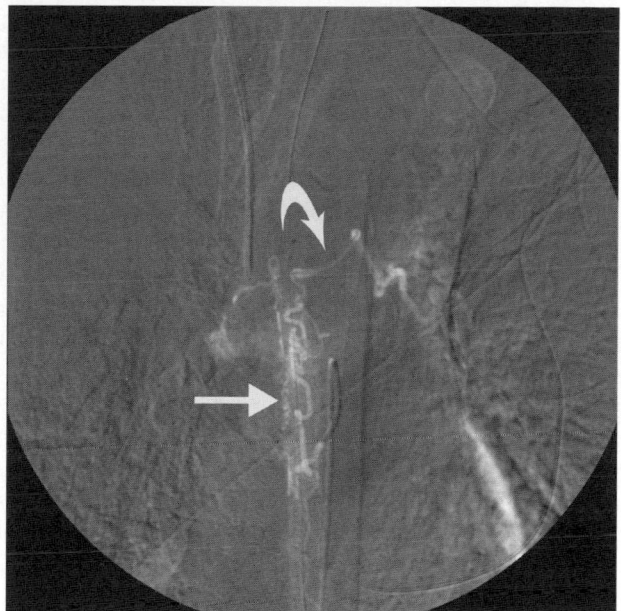

Figure 51–8 Nonbronchial systemic collaterals in a patient with cystic fibrosis and recurrent hemoptysis. Catheterization of a small branch off the aorta demonstrates enlarged esophageal collaterals (*straight arrow*) reconstituting a previously embolized left bronchial artery (*curved arrow*).

28% of patients. The recurrent bleeding rate increased to 46% after repeat embolization (8). More recently, Goh et al. published the results of a 6-year review in which they demonstrated an overall success rate of 82% (50). In 2000, Kato et al. reported nonrecurrent rates of hemoptysis after initial bronchial artery embolization of 78%, 70%, and 63% at 1, 3, and 5 years, respectively (51). For patients who underwent repeat BAE only once, the nonrecurrent rates improved to 84%, 77%, and 72% at 1, 3, and 5 years, respectively. In general, the long-term control rate of hemoptysis is approximately 70–80% and is largely determined by the natural progression of the underlying disease. Repeat embolization may be required, particularly for those younger patients with longer prognoses. Recurrent bleeding is also more commonly seen in patients with advanced pleural disease and is more difficult to control because of multiple nonbronchial systemic collateral pathways. Tamura et al. demonstrated long-term hemostasis in 70% of patients without documented pleural thickening, whereas this was achieved in only 29% of patients with significant pleural thickening (48). Therefore, pleural abnormalities negatively affect the long-term effectiveness of bronchial artery embolization (Figure 51–6).

Bronchial artery embolization may be of particular benefit in patients with cystic fibrosis. Cohen et al. reported immediate control in 19 of 20 patients with cystic fibrosis, and Fellows et al. reported immediate control in 12 of 13 patients (3,4). In 1998, Brinson reported on 13 cystic fibrosis patients undergoing 28 embolization procedures (52). Nine required only one embolotherapy session, and four required multiple sessions to control the hemorrhage during a single hospital admission. Three of the 13 patients returned with recurrent bleeds and were successfully controlled with bronchial artery embolization. The time interval between recurrent bouts of hemoptysis in this cystic fibrosis population following control with embolization averaged 20 months (range, 6–37 months). Recently, Antonelli et al. published a comparison of eight patients with cystic fibrosis treated with bronchial artery embolization compared with eight patients treated with medical therapy (53). This study confirmed that patients who underwent embolization had fewer bleeding episodes and improved quality of life. The early control of major and moderate bouts of hemoptysis is extremely important to these young patients as lung transplantation programs become more prevalent. Bronchial artery embolization does not appear to interfere with subsequent lung transplantation.

SUMMARY

Bronchial artery embolization is a well-established, worthwhile, palliative control of severe as well as recurrent mild hemoptysis secondary to inflammatory disease. Indications for embolization have expanded to include not only severe and massive bouts of hemoptysis, but also mild to chronic and intermittent episodes of hemoptysis as well. The procedure should be performed promptly when indicated, and when good embolization techniques are used, complications are infrequent.

REFERENCES

1. Wholey MH, Chamorro HA, Rao G, et al. Bronchial artery embolization for massive hemoptysis. JAMA 1976;236:2501–2504.
2. Tonkin ILD, Hanissian AS, Boulden TF, et al. Bronchial arteriography and embolotherapy for hemoptysis in patients with cystic fibrosis. Cardiovasc Intervent Radiol 1991;14:241–246.
3. Cohen AM, Doershuk CF, Stern RC. Bronchial artery embolization to control hemoptysis in cystic fibrosis. Radiology 1990; 175:401–405.
4. Fellows KE, Khaw KT, Schuster S, et al. Bronchial artery embolization in cystic fibrosis: technique and long-term results. J Pediatr 1979;95:959–963.
5. Rémy J, Arnaud A, Fardou H, et al. Treatment of hemoptysis by embolization of bronchial arteries. Radiology 1977;122:33–37.
6. Saumench J, Excarrabill J, Padró L, et al. Value of fiberoptic bronchoscopy and angiography for diagnosis of the bleeding site in hemoptysis. Ann Thorac Surg 1989;48:272–274.
7. Hsiao EI, Kirsch CM, Kagawa FT, et al. Utility of fiberoptic bronchoscopy before bronchial artery embolization for massive hemoptysis. AJR Am J Roentgenol 2001;177:861–867.
8. Hayakawa K, Tanaka F, Torizuka T, et al. Bronchial artery embolization for hemoptysis: immediate and long-term results. Cardiovasc Intervent Radiol 1992;15:154–159.
9. Rémy J, Lemaitre L, Lafitte JJ, et al. Massive hemoptysis of pulmonary arterial origin: diagnosis and treatment. AJR Am J Roentgenol 1984;143:963–969.
10. Cauldwell EW, Siekert RG, Lininger RE, et al. The bronchial arteries: an anatomic study of 150 human cadavers. Surg Gynecol Obstet 1948;86:395–412.
11. Uflacker R, Kaemmerer A, Picon PD, et al. Bronchial artery embolization in the management of hemoptysis: technical aspects and long-term results. Radiology 1985;157:637–644.
12. Tan RT, McGahan JP, Link DP, et al. Bronchial artery embolisation in management of haemoptysis. J Intervent Radiol 1991; 6:67–76.
13. McPherson S, Routh WD, Nath H, et al. Anomalous origin of bronchial arteries: potential pitfall of embolotherapy for hemoptysis. J Vasc Intervent Radiol 1990;1:86–88.
14. Cohen AM, Antoun BW, Stern RC. Left thyrocervical trunk bronchial artery supplying right lung: source of recurrent hemoptysis in cystic fibrosis. AJR Am J Roentgenol 1992;158:1131–1133.
15. Tanaka F, Hayakawa K, Satoh Y, et al. Evaluating bronchial drainage pathways in patients with lung disease using digital subtraction angiography. Invest Radiol 1993;28:434–438.
16. Roberts AC. Bronchial artery embolization therapy. J Thorac Imaging 1990;5:60–72.
17. Keller FS, Rösch J, Loflin TG, et al. Nonbronchial systemic collateral arteries: significance in percutaneous embolotherapy for hemoptysis. Radiology 1987;164:687–692.
18. Stoll JF, Bettmann MA. Bronchial artery embolization to control hemoptysis: a review. Cardiovasc Intervent Radiol 1988;11: 263–269.
19. Schrodt JF, Becker GJ, Scott JA, et al. Bronchial artery embolization: monitoring with somatosensory evoked potentials. Radiology 1987;164:135–139.
20. Rabkin JE, Astafjev V, Gothman LN, et al. Transcatheter embolization in the management of pulmonary hemorrhage. Radiology 1987;163:361–365.
21. Bookstein JJ, Moser KM, Kalafer ME, et al. The role of bronchial arteriography and therapeutic embolization in hemoptysis. Chest 1977;72:658–661.
22. Osada H, Kawada T, Ashida H, et al. Bronchial artery aneurysm. Ann Thorac Surg 1986;41:440–442.
23. Harley JD, Killien FC, Peck AG. Massive hemoptysis controlled by transcatheter embolization of the bronchial arteries. AJR Am J Roentgenol 1977;128:302–304.
24. Muthuswamy PP, Akbik F, Franklin C, et al. Management of major or massive hemoptysis in active pulmonary tuberculosis by bronchial arterial embolization. Chest 1987;92:77–82.
25. Vujic I, Pyle R, Hungerford GD, et al. Angiography and therapeutic blockade in the control of hemoptysis. Radiology 1982; 143:19–23.
26. Jardin M, Rémy J. Control of hemoptysis: systemic angiography and anastomoses of the internal mammary artery. Radiology 1988;168:377–383.
27. Parke WW, Michels NA. The nonbronchial systemic arteries of the lung. J Thorac Cardiovasc Surg 1965;49:694–707.
28. Moore LB, McWey RE, Vujic I. Massive hemoptysis: control by embolization of the thyrocervical trunk. Radiology 1986;161: 173–174.
29. Ferris EF. Pulmonary hemorrhage: vascular evaluation and interventional therapy. Chest 1981;80:710–714.
30. Rémy J, Smith M, Lemaitre L, et al. Treatment of massive hemoptysis by occlusion of a Rasmussen aneurysm. AJR Am J Roentgenol 1980;135:605–606.
31. Renie WA, Rodeheffer RJ, Mitchell S, et al. Balloon embolization of a mycotic pulmonary artery aneurysm. Am Rev Respir Dis 1982;126:1107–1110.
32. Davidoff AB, Udoff EJ, Schonfeld SA. Intraaneurysmal embolization of a pulmonary artery aneurysm for control of hemoptysis. AJR Am J Roentgenol 1984;142:1019–1020.
33. Boushy SF, Helgason AH, North LB. Occlusion of the bronchial arteries by glass microspheres. Am Rev Respir Dis 1971;103: 249–263.
34. Lois JF, Gomes AS, Smith DC, et al. Systemic-to-pulmonary collateral vessels and shunts: treatment with embolization. Radiology 1988;169:671–676.
35. Doppman JL, Girton M, Oldfield EH. Spinal WADA test. Radiology 1986;161:319–321.
36. Kardjiev V, Symeonov A, Chankov I. Etiology, pathogenesis, and prevention of spinal cord lesions in selective angiography of the bronchial and intercostal arteries. Radiology 1974;112:81–83.

37. Feigelson HH, Ravin HA. Transverse myelitis following selective bronchial arteriography. Radiology 1965;85:663–665.

38. Tanaka N, Yamakado K, Murashima S, et al. Superselective bronchial artery embolization for hemoptysis with a coaxial microcatheter system. J Vasc Interv Radiol 1997;8:65–70.

39. Matsumoto AH, Suhocki PV, Barth KH. Technical note: superselective Gelfoam embolotherapy using a highly visible small caliber catheter. Cardiovasc Intervent Radiol 1988;11:303–306.

40. van Heesch HA, Tjan GT, Lampmann LE. Treatment of haemoptysis by embolisation of the systemic arteries with isobutyl-2 cyanoacrylate: technique and long term results. J Intervent Radiol 1988;3:63–68.

41. Fairfax AJ, Ball J, Batten JC, et al. A pathological study following bronchial artery embolization for haemoptysis in cystic fibrosis. Br J Dis Chest 1980;74:345–352.

42. Mauro MA, Jaques PF. Transcatheter embolisation with a Gelfoam slurry. J Intervent Radiol 1987;2:157–159.

43. Fuhrman BP, Bass JL, Castaneda-Zuniga W, et al. Coil embolization of congenital thoracic vascular anomalies in infants and children. Circulation 1984;70:285–289.

44. Nancarrow PA, Fellows KE, Lock JE. Stability of coil emboli: an in vitro study. Cardiovasc Intervent Radiol 1987;10:226–229.

45. Vujic I, Pyle R, Parker E, et al. Control of massive hemoptysis by embolization of intercostal arteries. Radiology 1980;137:617–620.

46. Ivanick MJ, Thorwarth W, Donohue J, et al. Infarction of the left main-stem bronchus: a complication of bronchial artery embolization. AJR Am J Roentgenol 1983;141:535–537.

47. Hélénon CH, Chatel A, Bigot JM, et al. [Left esophago-bronchial fistula following bronchial artery embolization.] Nouv Presse Med 1977;6:4209.

48. Munk PL, Morris DC, Nelems B. Left main bronchial-esophageal fistula: a complication of bronchial artery embolization. Cardiovasc Intervent Radiol 1990;13:95–97.

49. Tamura S, Kodama T, Otsuka N, et al. Embolotherapy for persistent hemoptysis: the significance of pleural thickening. Cardiovasc Intervent Radiol 1993;16:85–88.

50. Goh PYT, Lin M, Teo N, et al. Embolization for hemoptysis: A six-year review. Cardiovasc Intervent Radiol 2002;25:17–25.

51. Kato A, Kudo S, Matsumoto K, et al. Bronchial artery embolization for hemoptysis due to benign diseases: Immediate and long-term results. Cardiovasc Intervent Radiol 2000;23:351–357.

52. Brinson GM, Noone PG, Mauro MA, et al. Bronchial artery embolization for the treatment of hemoptysis in patients with cystic fibrosis. Am J Respir Crit Care Med 1998;157:1951–1958.

53. Antonelli M, Midulla F, Tancredi G, et al. Bronchial artery embolization for the management of nonmassive hemoptysis in cystic fibrosis. Chest 2002;121:796–801.

Thoracic Abscesses and Malignant Pleural Effusions

52

Debra A. Gervais, Giles W. Boland, Steven L. Dawson

Management of intrathoracic abscesses and fluid collections changed dramatically with the advent of image-guided percutaneous catheter placement. Radiologic intervention in the thoracic collections is a direct extension of the principles and techniques used in abdominal intervention and developed rapidly once abdominal interventional techniques were established. The ability of ultrasound and computed tomography (CT) to detect intrathoracic disease has made possible accurate placement of drainage catheters into abscess collections. This chapter outlines the principles of percutaneous catheter drainage of thoracic fluid collections, including lung abscess, empyema, malignant effusions, and mediastinal abscess.

LUNG ABSCESS

Lung abscess is a necrotizing process in the pulmonary parenchyma that often progresses to cavitation and that is enclosed by a visceral pleural envelope. During the preantibiotic era, lung abscess carried a mortality rate of 35–70%, with fewer than half the survivors being "cured" (1). Despite advances in antibiotic therapeutic regimens, there remains a significant mortality rate approaching 30% even with aggressive therapy (2).

Lung abscesses are defined as either primary or secondary. The main predisposing factor in the development of primary lung abscess is aspiration. Primary abscesses usually arise in patients with altered states of consciousness from anesthesia, CNS-related disorders, or alcoholism. Other conditions associated with aspiration pneumonia and subsequent abscess include hiatus hernia and other esophageal conditions in which gastroesophageal reflux may occur. Another important contributing factor is poor oral and dental hygiene. Abscesses most frequently involve bronchial segments, which are dependent when the patient is in the supine or lateral decubitus position.

The bacteriology of primary lung abscess closely resembles that of aspiration pneumonia. Anaerobic organisms account for 85–90% of lung abscesses (3). Aerobic streptococci are the most common aerobic pathogens. Gram-negative rods and staphylococci are frequently cultured in nosocomially acquired infections.

Secondary lung abscess is defined as abscess formation in areas of preexisting infection or disease or as a result of hematogenous spread from a remote site. These abscesses are usually caused by secondary abscess formation in patients with preexisting aerobic pneumonias, the most important cause of which is underlying bronchial malignancy. Other predisposing factors include septic emboli, inhaled foreign bodies, bronchoesophageal fistula, emphysematous and other lung cysts, and pulmonary infarction (4). Immunocompromised hosts are susceptible to certain opportunistic infections, including tuberculosis and fungal and parasitic infections, which can lead to secondary abscess formation.

The diagnosis of lung abscess is usually made by findings of cavitary, necrotizing inflammation on conventional chest radiography in conjunction with the appropriate clinical setting. CT has become an extremely important tool for diagnosing lung abscess and in differentiating these lesions from empyema and bronchopleural fistula (5).

As many as 90% of patients with lung abscess can be treated with supportive measures, postural drainage, and antibiotics. Bronchoscopic placement of transtracheal drainage catheters may facilitate removal of pus and secretions, although reports are limited in the literature. Surgical intervention is reserved for those patients who do not respond to medical management and antibiotics. A review of the surgical series demonstrated a need for surgery in 11–21% of patients with lung abscess (4). Surgical therapy may result in bronchopleural fistula, empyema, bleeding, and spillage of pus into the tracheobronchial tree with subsequent dissemination of infection. Postoperative mortality has been reported to be 11–16% (4). Several studies have demonstrated that percutaneous radiologic catheter placement is a safe and effective alternative to surgery (2,4,5). Furthermore, quoted complication rates are lower after percutaneous drainage than after surgery, even though patients tend to be sicker in the former group.

Indications and Contraindications

The indications for catheter drainage of lung abscess are similar to those for surgical intervention, namely, sepsis that fails to respond to antibiotics and postural drainage. In addition, abscesses larger than 4 cm are generally better treated by drainage (6). When standard medical therapy is unlikely to be effective, as in bronchial obstructive lesions with an absent cough reflex, percutaneous or surgical drainage is indicated. Finally, patients requiring persistent mechanical ventilatory support usually require drainage.

Contraindications to catheter drainage include an uncorrectable bleeding diathesis and uncooperative patients, although with effective intravenous sedation, most uncooperative patients can be successfully treated. Although catheter drainage of lung abscess through normal lung is generally considered safe (2,7,8), transparenchymal drainage has led to infected bronchopleural fistulas; for this reason, whenever possible, the catheter should traverse only contiguous abnormal lung and pleura en route to the abscess (4).

Image Guidance

Initial reports of percutaneous catheter placement for lung abscess used plain radiographs and fluoroscopy for guidance (2,9,10). Fluoroscopy has the advantage of wide availability and lower cost. More recently, CT has been advocated as the primary imaging modality complemented by fluoroscopic guidance when necessary (4,11). CT allows for precise assessment of the abscess cavity and delineates the optimum transpleural route that avoids intervening normal lung. It is effective in demonstrating loculations that may require placement of more than one catheter. Fluoroscopy is more useful when real-time observation is necessary to manipulate guide wires and catheters into the abscess cavity or to reposition previously placed catheters.

Technique

Regardless of the radiologic guidance system used, initial access to the abscess cavity is obtained with a small-gauge needle, which allows for aspiration of pus for Gram stain and culture. Either the trocar or the Seldinger technique can be used for catheter placement, depending on personal preference. If the trocar technique is used with CT guidance, localization should be done with a guiding needle to reduce the risk of incorrect catheter positioning. When either fluoroscopic or CT guidance is used, the contralateral lung must not be dependent during catheter placement. Aspiration of pus into the normal lung is associated with markedly increased morbidity and mortality. As many as 22% of deaths can be attributed to aspiration of infected material into uninfected ipsilateral or contralateral lung (12). As long as the contralateral lung is not dependent, drainage can be performed with the patient supine, prone, decubitus, or in the oblique position. Consideration should also be given to how the patient will lie after catheter insertion. Because most lung abscesses are in the lower lobes, catheter placement should be via a posterior route. To avoid subsequent patient discomfort and catheter kinking, the catheter should be placed through a more lateral posterior axillary approach. Occasionally, a true posterior approach is required, and special care with catheter dressing will be necessary to prevent kinking of the catheter.

Adequate local anesthesia with infiltration of the periosteum of the adjacent rib and parietal pleura helps reduce unnecessary pain. The lung is entered using aseptic technique. Whenever a catheter is placed via an intercostal approach, the tube should be placed through the midportion of the intercostal muscle, avoiding the neurovascular bundle of the rib above and also avoiding constant rubbing of the catheter on the periosteum of the rib below. The character of the initial aspirated material dictates catheter selection. Generally, 12–16 French catheters are required because of the viscous nature of infected material found in lung abscesses.

After catheter placement, the contents of the abscess cavity should be evacuated as completely as possible. Gentle irrigation of completely walled-off cavities is then performed with normal saline to remove the more viscous pus and to help evacuate loculated areas within the abscess cavity. The catheter is secured by "flagging" the tube with cloth adhesive tape, which is then sutured to an ostomy disk (Hollister) and connected to a standard three-bottle water-seal drainage system (Pleur-evac, A4005, Deknatel). In-hospital drainage with suction at 20 cm of water is required for all patients.

An important part of the overall management is the follow-up of patients by members of the interventional radiology team. This is essential to evaluate the clinical response to drainage, to assess tube function and the amount of drainage, and to inspect the catheter insertion site for possible loosening. Goldberg et al. found catheter-related problems in 59% of patients with thoracic and abdominal percutaneous catheters. Most catheter-related problems (71%) were successfully managed at the bedside (12). If the catheter occludes, the radiologist can irrigate the catheter and the drainage system with sterile saline, which is usually sufficient to restore patency. Otherwise, the patient will need to be brought to the radiology department for further catheter assessment and manipulation.

Follow-up CT can be performed 3–5 days after catheter insertion to evaluate outcome. If the abscess cavity has collapsed, there are no undrained loculations, and the catheter drainage has decreased to less than 10 mL per day with a good associated clinical response, the catheter can be withdrawn in two stages. On the first day, the drainage system is disconnected from wall suction and placed on water seal for 12–24 hours. If no pneumothorax is present on a chest radiograph obtained the following day, the chest tube is removed, and a pressure bandage is applied. If no clinical improvement occurs after catheter insertion or if there is a deterioration in clinical status, CT is performed earlier (within 12–48 hours) to check catheter position and assess for further undrained collections or dissemination of infection.

Results and Complications

Percutaneous catheter drainage of lung abscesses is usually successful, and surgery can usually be avoided. The mean duration of drainage is approximately 10 days (4). Reasons for failure include multiloculated or poorly defined abscesses or thick-walled cavities that cannot collapse (13). Secondary lung abscesses are unlikely to resolve unless the underlying illness is treated. In these instances, the patient will require surgical resection.

Complications occur in approximately 2% of cases (11). Sepsis or bacteremia is more common if the abscess is not adequately drained. Bleeding may occur in the presence of a bleeding diathesis or from injury to adjacent vascular structures such as the intercostal or internal mammary artery.

THORACIC EMPYEMA

An empyema is an infection involving the pleural space that may result from secondary spread from pulmonary infection, thoracic trauma, a foreign body, bronchiectasis, esophageal perforation, or infradiaphragmatic disease. Light

et al. (14–16) helped define the pathophysiology of empyema, which must be understood for successful treatment. The first or exudative stage results when a focus of infection contiguous to the pleura causes an exudative pleural effusion. The fluid has normal pH and glucose levels and a mild exudate of polymorphonuclear leukocytes. Effusions at this stage may not require drainage because many spontaneously resolve with appropriate antibiotic treatment. However, once this sterile effusion is contaminated with bacteria, the glucose and pH fall, resulting in the second, or fibrinopurulent, stage. Light et al. suggest that this is chemically recognized when the pH is at or below 7, the glucose level is at or below 40 mg/dL (2.2 mmol/liter), and the LDH level is at or below 1,000 units/liter. This second-stage effusion becomes more viscous as polymorphonuclear cells and debris accumulate. Finally, in the third stage, fibrin is deposited, and an inner elastic membrane, or pleural peel, forms. Once a pleural peel forms, open thoracostomy and decortication are generally required. Although percutaneous drainage of empyema early in the third stage may be effective, the highest chance of success occurs during the second stage.

Indications and Contraindications

Any thoracentesis resulting in positive Gram stain or culture requires drainage. However, because the initial Gram stain may be inconclusive and because cultures take at least 24 hours, the decision to drain a collection is often based on Light's criteria (outlined above) in the correct clinical setting (fever, persistence of symptoms, or increasing effusion despite appropriate antibiotic therapy).

Contraindications are similar to those for all percutaneous catheter placements: uncontrollable bleeding diathesis and an uncooperative patient despite intravenous sedation.

Image Guidance

Traditionally, surgical empyema drainage was performed at the bedside using the chest radiograph as a reference. In some institutions this is still commonly practiced. However, surgical series suggest that the mortality of this technique may be as high as 5% (17), with as many as 35% of patients requiring open chest tube drainage or decortication (18). In addition, incorrect tube placement can occur in as many as 80% of blind tube thoracostomies (19), with complications including fibrothorax, bronchopleural fistula, prolonged hospitalization, and death (20,21). Therefore, image-guided catheter drainage of thoracic empyemas has become more prevalent.

For large or free-flowing empyemas, ultrasound guidance for catheter insertion is preferred. Ultrasound is highly sensitive in detecting and localizing collections and provides real-time monitoring of catheter insertion and efficacy of drainage. It also allows for immediate assessment of undrained collections. For loculated or less-accessible collections, CT is the modality of choice. CT demonstrates the wall characteristics, pleural separation, and lung compression of empyemas and can adequately distinguish them from lung abscesses, which may respond to conservative measures (22).

Fluoroscopy is now rarely used as the sole guidance system, although it may be used in combination with either ultrasound or CT for Seldinger insertion of pleural catheters or as the sole guidance method for catheter exchanges.

Technique

The patient should be seated over the side of the stretcher facing away from the radiologist. The patient is encouraged to lean forward onto a bedside table with the arms folded to provide greater access for catheter placement. If the patient cannot sit up, then he or she is positioned in the decubitus manner with the affected side up. An image-guided thoracentesis is usually performed initially on all patients, and, when the diagnosis of empyema or complicated parapneumonic effusion is confirmed according to the established criteria, a drainage catheter is inserted.

Usually, 16–24 French catheters are required. Specifically designed empyema catheters (Mueller empyema catheters, Cook, Inc.) are suitable for most collections. These catheters are designed for trocar insertion and have a stylet-cannula assembly. They have a soft, curved tip with distal side holes and are made of polyvinylchloride that is sufficiently rigid to prevent catheter compression by adjacent ribs. Occasionally, larger 24 French catheters (Thal-Quick Chest Tube, Cook, Inc.) are required for thick, purulent collections. Except for the 24 French catheters, which are inserted using Seldinger technique, the trocar technique is preferable because the Seldinger technique is more likely to introduce air and result in pneumothorax. Furthermore, with a Seldinger insertion, it is occasionally difficult to advance the catheter intercostally through the intercostal muscles and thickened pleura without buckling the guidewire or catheter.

After catheter placement, the empyema fluid is aspirated completely. The catheter is secured to the skin and connected to a water-seal pleural drainage system (Pleur-evac, Pfizer). Drainage with 20-cm water suction is essential. All patients are followed daily by members of the interventional radiology team to assess catheter function and to ensure that the catheter is securely fastened to the skin.

Usually, a CT scan is performed to assess treatment outcome, and catheters remain until fluid drainage has decreased to less than 10 mL per day. Catheters can then be removed at the bedside in a single step, without the need for progressive removal of wall suction, water seal, and follow-up chest films, as is necessary with lung abscesses.

Loculated empyemas may require multiple catheters for complete drainage. However, fibrin deposition and locule formation can make closed percutaneous drainage of empyema difficult, and until recently open surgical drainage has been the only alternative treatment. Successful and safe

use of intrapleural urokinase (Abbott) to lyse locules and improve drainage has been demonstrated (Figure 52–1) (23,24). However, recent experience in the absence of urokinase suggests that intrapleural tissue plasminogen activator (tPA) is equally successful. Generally, 4–6 mg of tPA in as much as 50 mL of 0.9% saline is placed through the catheter, which is then clamped for 30 minutes before suction is restored. If intracavitary thrombolytic therapy fails, video-assisted thoracoscopic drainage or open surgical drainage is indicated (Figure 52–2).

Results and Complications

Lee et al. reviewed the five main series in the radiologic literature and found an average success rate of 77% for percutaneous catheter drainage compared with a 35–71% success rate for conventional surgical tube thoracostomy (25). Failure occurs because of thick, viscous pus that is not amenable to drainage with standard empyema catheters. Therefore, larger 24 French catheters are used when viscous pus is encountered at thoracentesis.

Complications are uncommon and are quoted at less than 2% (25). The most significant, although fortunately rare, complication is cardiopulmonary arrest during catheter placement (26) and transient bacteremia (27).

MALIGNANT EFFUSION

Malignant pleural effusions may need to be drained for relief of symptoms. The drainage technique and use of imaging guidance is similar to that described for empyemas. However, the management differs somewhat because the goal is not treatment of infection but improvement in respiratory status. Fluid in a malignant effusion can usually be removed rapidly, and for some patients, repeat large-volume thoracentesis may be appropriate. However, for larger effusions or those that reaccumulate rapidly, chest tube drainage may be needed. Small-bore catheters placed by interventional radiologists have been shown to be as effective as large-bore surgical chest tubes for drainage of malignant effusions (28). The chest tube is placed to wall suction, and the chest tube can be removed once the drainage declines to 25–50 mL per day.

For recurrent effusions, pleurodesis may be necessary. Conventional agents for chemical pleurodesis include talc, bleomycin, and doxycycline (29–32). Doxycycline usually requires multiple applications, whereas talc and bleomycin can achieve pleurodesis with one application. For best results, pleurodesis should be attempted after daily catheter output has diminished to less than 50–75 mL per day. Ideally, no pneumothorax and little to no pleural effusion will remain so that the visceral and parietal pleural surfaces are contiguous. The inflammatory response incited by the chemical pleurodesis results in fusion of the pleural surfaces and obliteraion of the pleural space. Attempts to

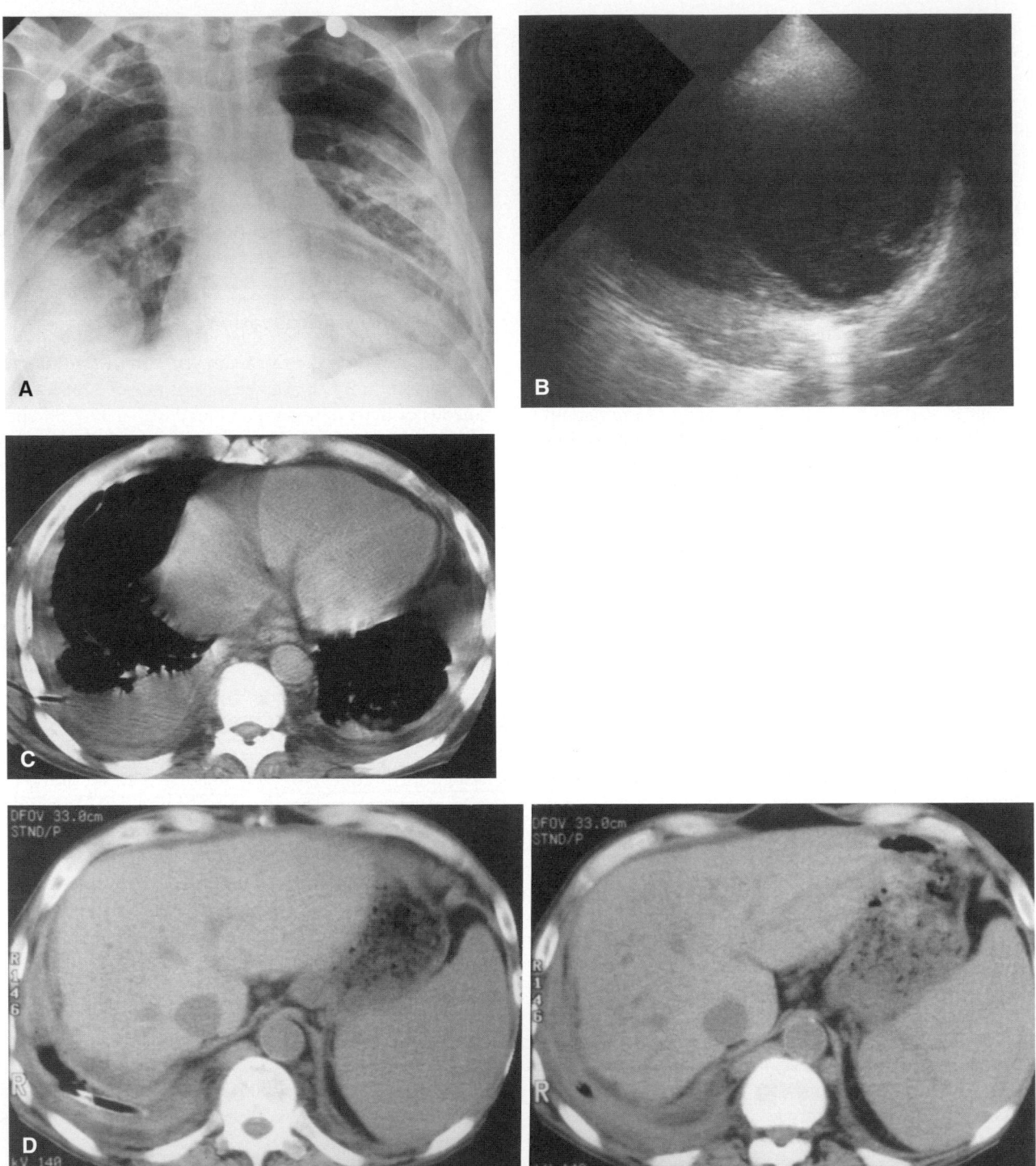

Figure 52–1   A 74-year-old man with a history of chronic lymphocytic lymphoma and prior tuber-culosis. **A.** Chest film shows a right basilar lateral pleural collection with changes of old granuloma-tous disease. **B.** Ultrasound of the right pleural collection shows loculations and low-level echoes. **C.** Ultrasound-guided chest tube placement yielded 2,000 mL of pus, but follow-up CT shows resid-ual fluid following chest tube placement. **D.** Intracavitary urokinase was used to dissolve the resid-ual debris, and follow-up CT shows complete resolution of the empyema with residual pleural thickening secondary to chronic inflammation.

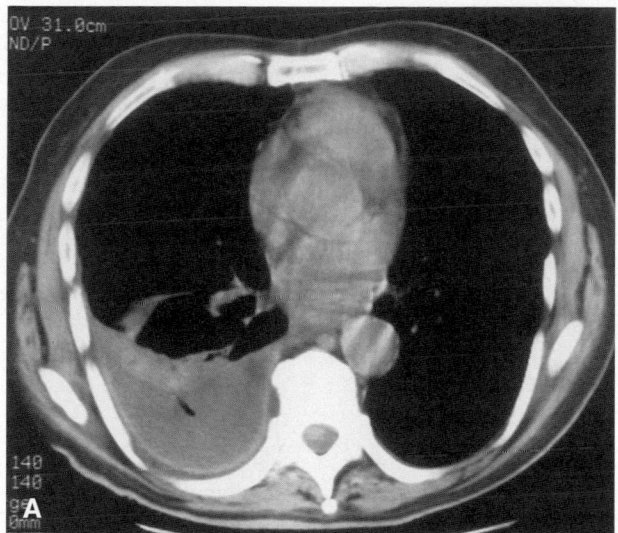

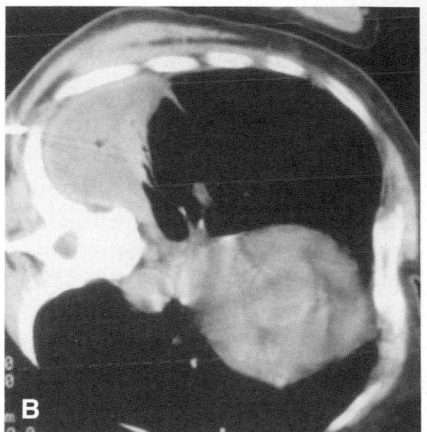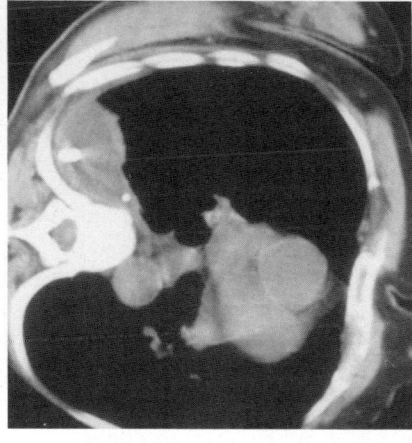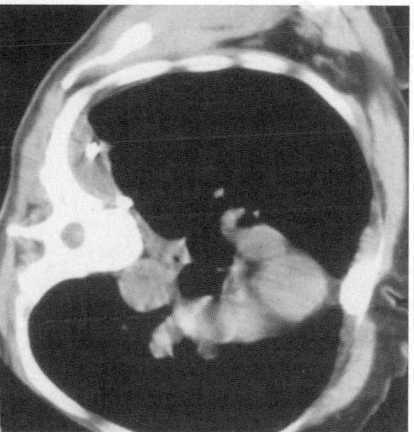

Figure 52–2 A 67-year-old man with fever and right pleural abnormality. **A.** CT scan showing a right posterior pleural collection and associated air space disease. Despite the patient's fever, drainage of the pleural collection was not attempted initially. **B.** After 2 weeks, right chest tube placement was performed using a left lateral decubitus approach. Although a 16 French catheter was placed, drainage was not successful because of the fibrinous organization of the collection (see text). The patient subsequently had surgical decortication and evacuation of the pleural collection.

perform pleurodesis with residual pleural fluid or with persistant high output can result in formation of loculated effusions, which may or may not be symptomatic.

Recently, long-term indwelling chest tubes have been possible with special tunneled catheters that can be managed on an outpatient basis (33). These tubes result in shorter hospitalizations and more rapid return to the patient's baseline function. In addition, in about 42% of patients, the indwelling catheter may result in spontaneous pleurodesis (33).

Failure of thoracentesis or chest tube drainage in malignant effusions may be related to the noncompliance of the lung related to underlying malignancy or other lung disease (34). While the fluid can be successfully removed, a pneumothorax develops because the lung is incapable of expanding to fill the thoracic cavity. In these patients, large-bore chest tubes fail to re-expand the lung, and fluid generally reaccu-

mulates to fill the cavity (34). In other patients, complex multiloculated, noninfected, malignant effusions may fail to respond to simple drainage. Recent reports suggest that intrapleural thrombolytics can result in successful drainage of effusions in these patients (35,36). Thus, intrapleural thrombolytics should be considered both in infected and malignant effusions that fail to respond to simple catheter drainage.

MEDIASTINAL ABSCESS

Mediastinal abscess formation usually occurs after esophageal perforation, which may occur either spontaneously (Boerhaave syndrome) or iatrogenically after esophageal endoscopy. Mediastinal abscess is also a well-recognized complication after median sternotomy (Figure 52–3). Patients with mediastinitis and abscess formation are usually severely

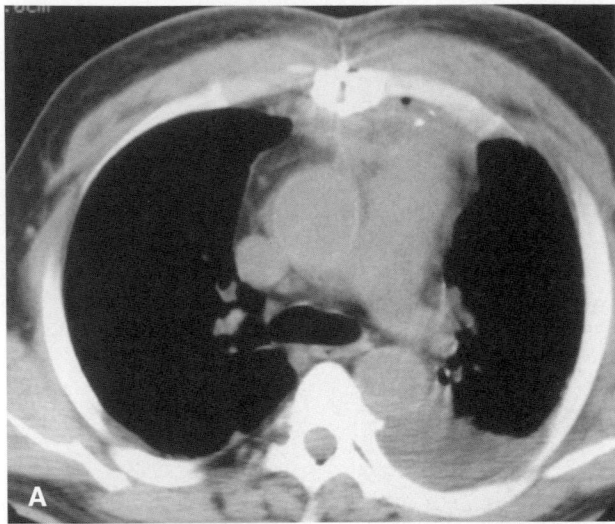

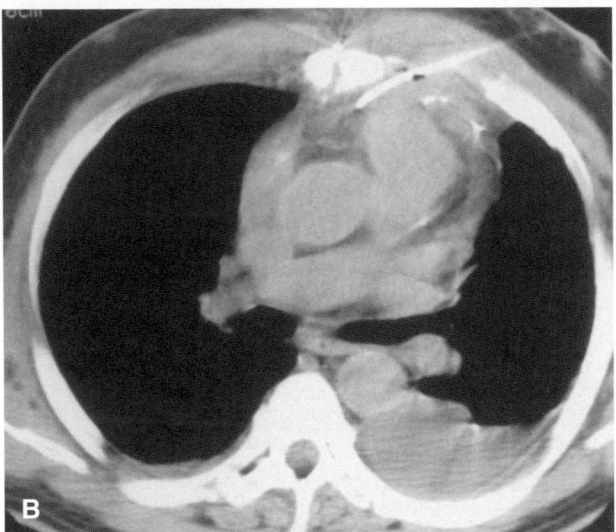

Figure 52–3 A 63-year-old man with fever for 5 days following median sternotomy and coronary artery bypass graft (CABG). **A.** CT scan shows a small retrosternal fluid collection just anterior to the main pulmonary artery, with a small bubble of air anteriorly. **B.** A left parasternal approach has been used to place an 8 French catheter into the retrosternal abscess. In retrosternal collections, thin CT slices and angling of the gantry may help to demonstrate a bone-free soft tissue window into the retrosternal mediastinum. Meticulous technique is necessary to avoid the great vessels.

ill, with a high fever, sepsis, and leukocytosis, and are often poor surgical candidates. Acute mediastinitis carries a high mortality and is considered a surgical emergency. Radiologically guided percutaneous drainage techniques are beneficial in this group of patients. Surgical repair is usually required for esophageal leaks, and percutaneous drainage permits the patient to undergo elective surgery in an improved physiologic state.

Indications and Contraindications

Percutaneous drainage of a mediastinal abscess should be considered in any severely ill patient, particularly if the collection is situated superficially. Deeply sited collections may be difficult to access and therefore require surgical drainage. Contraindications to the technique are similar to those of other radiologic percutaneous techniques and include uncorrectable bleeding diathesis and an uncooperative patient.

Image Guidance

Computed tomography (CT) is the image guidance modality of choice. CT is able to demonstrate mediastinal widening, infiltration of mediastinal fat, extent of disease, and low-density abscess collections with or without gas formation. CT is essential to delineate the relation of the abscess to vital cardiovascular and tracheobronchial structures so that catheters can be placed accurately via a safe extrapleural route.

Technique

Drainage can be performed either by an anterior or posterior approach. Regardless of which route is chosen, whenever possible, the catheter should be placed directly into the mediastinum or through the pleura without traversing normal lung. Anterior mediastinal collections are usually drained via a parasternal approach, with care taken to avoid the internal mammary artery. Posterior collections are drained paravertebrally.

The technique for CT-guided catheter placement is identical to that of catheter placement elsewhere in the chest. After initial CT scanning has localized the abscess, the precise site of entry through the skin is marked, and an initial localizing needle is inserted to a predetermined depth and location, avoiding vital organs such as the lung, heart, and great vessels. The needle should be advanced in a plane perfectly parallel to the central beam. In this way, the needle tip is clearly identified as an abrupt end to the needle with a black metallic artifact projecting beyond the needle. Angulation out of the plane of the x-ray beam will create difficulties in identifying the needle tip and multiple CT slices, and needle repositionings may be required to determine the correct angle and depth of insertion. An angled needle shaft is recognized by its tapering shape rather than an abrupt end and does not have an associated artifact. Occasionally, an oblique path to the abscess is specifically chosen to avoid vital organs. Once a satisfactory pathway has been identified, catheter placement can be performed either via a Seldinger or a trocar technique. If the abscess is relatively superficial or large, a trocar technique is preferable. However, the Seldinger technique allows for more precise catheter placement and may be necessary for deeply sited collections. The catheter size depends on the size of the abscess; small collections can be drained with 8 French catheters (Figure 52–3).

One report has suggested that periesophageal collections may be drained via a transesophageal approach under fluoroscopic guidance, particularly if there is no safe access route to the abscess (37).

Results and Complications

Percutaneous abscess drainage of mediastinal collections has been performed with similar results to percutaneous drainage of empyema and lung abscess. However, because the literature contains only limited reports (38–40), the occurrence of major complications is difficult to assess, although injury to major cardiovascular structures and the lung is possible. In addition, the position of the internal mammary artery should be considered in any percutaneous parasternal approach because injury to this structure is associated with significant hemorrhage. However, because CT guidance permits accurate assessment of the position of the internal mammary artery and other vital structures, these complications are usually avoidable.

REFERENCES

1. Estrera AS, Melvin RP, Mills LJ, et al. Primary lung abscess. J Thorac Cardiovasc Surg 1980;79:275–282.
2. Parker LA, Melton JW, Delany DJ, et al. Percutaneous small bore catheter drainage in the management of lung abscess. Chest 1987;92:213–218.
3. Pennza PT. Aspiration pneumonia, necrotizing pneumonia, and lung abscess. Emerg Med Clin North Am 1989;7:279–307.
4. van Sonnenberg E, D'Agostino HB, Casola G, et al. Lung abscess: CT guided drainage. Radiology 1991;178:347–351.
5. Lorenzo RL, Bradford BF, Black J, et al. Lung abscesses in children: diagnostic and therapeutic needle aspiration. Radiology 1985;157:79–80.
6. Bernhard WF, Malcolm JA, Wylie RH. Lung abscess: a survey of 148 cases due to aspiration. Chest 1963;43:620–630.
7. Mengoli L. Giant lung abscess treated by tube thoracostomy. J Thorac Cardiovasc Surg 1985;90:186–194.
8. Lawrence GH, Rubin SL. Management of giant lung abscess. Am J Surg 1978;136:134–139.
9. Rice TW, Ginsberg RJ, Todd TJ. Tube drainage of lung abscess. Ann Thorac Surg 1987;44:356–359.
10. Yellin A, Yellin EO, Lieberman Y. Percutaneous tube drainage: the treatment of choice for refractory lung abscess. Ann Thorac Surg 1985;39:266–270.
11. Moore AV, Zuger JH, Kelley MJ. Lung abscess: an interventional radiology perspective. Semin Intervent Radiol 1991;8:1, 36–43.
12. Goldberg MA, Mueller PR, Saini S, et al. Importance of daily rounds by the radiologist after interventional procedures of the abdomen and chest. Radiology 1991;180:767–770.
13. Kosloske AM, Ball WS Jr, Butler C, et al. Drainage of pediatric lung abscess by cough, catheter or complete resection. J Pediatr Surg 1986;21:596–600.
14. Light RW. Management of parapneumonic effusions. Chest 1976;70:325–326.
15. Light RW, Girard WM, Jenkinson SG, et al. Parapneumonic effusions. Am J Med 1980;69:507–512.
16. Light RW. Parapneumonic effusions and empyemas. Clin Chest Med 1985;6:55–61.
17. Sherman MM, Subramanian V, Berger RL. Management of thoracic empyema. Am J Surg 1977;133:474–478.
18. Varkey B, Rose HD, Kutty CP, et al. Empyema thoracis during a ten year period. Analysis of 72 cases and comparison to a previous study (1952 to 1967). Arch Intern Med 1981;141:1771–1776.
19. Stark DD, Federle MP, Goodman PC. CT and radiographic assessment of tube thoracostomy. AJR Am J Roentgenol 1983;141:253–258.
20. Maurer JR, Friedman PJ, Wing VW. Thoracostomy tube in an interlobar fissure: radiologic recognition of a potential problem. AJR Am J Roentgenol 1982;139:1155–1161.
21. Webb WR, Laberge J. Major fissure tube placement. AJR Am J Roentgenol 1983;140:1039.
22. Stark DD, Federle MP, Goodman PC, et al. Differentiating lung abscess and empyema: radiography and computed tomography. AJR Am J Roentgenol 1983;141:163–167.
23. Moulton JS, Moore PT, Mencini RA. Treatment of loculated pleural effusions with transcatheter intracavitary urokinase. AJR Am J Roentgenol 1989;153:941–945.
24. Lee KS, Im J-G, Kim YH, et al. Treatment of thoracic multiloculated empyemas with intracavitary urokinase: a prospective study. Radiology 1991;179:771–775.
25. Lee MJ, Saini S, Brink JA, et al. Interventional radiology of the pleural space: management of thoracic empyema with image-guided catheter drainage. Semin Intervent Radiol 1991;8:1, 29–35.
26. Merriam MA, Cronin JJ, Dorfman GS, et al. Radiographically guided percutaneous catheter drainage of pleural fluid collections. AJR Am J Roentgenol 1988;151:1113–1116.
27. van Sonnenberg E, Nakamoto SK, Mueller PR, et al. CT and ultrasound guided catheter drainage of empyemas after chest-tube failure. Radiology 1984;154:349–353.
28. Paruleker W, Di Primio G, Matzinger F, et al. Use of small-bore vs large-bore chest tubes for treatment of malignant pleural effusions. Chest 2001;120:19–25.
29. Marom EM, Erasmus JJ, Herndon JE 2nd, et al. Usefulness of imaging-guided catheter drainage and talc sclerotherapy in patients with metastatic gynecologic malignancies and symptomatic pleural effusions. AJR Am J Roentgenol 2002;179:105–108.
30. Ong KC, Indumathi V, Raghuram J, et al. A comparative study of pleurodesis using talc slurry and bleomycin in the management of malignant pleural effusions. Respirology 2000;5:99–103.
31. Patz EF Jr, McAdams HP, Erasmus JJ, et al. Sclerotherapy for malignant pleural effusions: a prospective randomized trial of bleomycin vs doxycycline with small-bore catheter drainage. Chest 1998;113:1305–1311.
32. Putman JB, Light RW, Rodrigueq RM, et al. A randomized comparison of indwelling pleural catheter and doxycline pleurodesis in the management of malignant pleural effusions. Cancer 1999;86:1992–1999.
33. Pollak JS, Burdge CM, Rosenblatt M, et al. Treatment of malignant pleural effusions with tunneled long-term drainage catheters. J Vasc Interv Radiol 2001;12:201–208.
34. Boland GW, Gazelle GS, Girard MJ, et al. Asymptomatic hydropneumothorax after therapeutic thoracentesis for malignant pleural effusions. AJR Am J Roentgenol 1998;170:943–946.
35. Davies CW, Traill ZC, Gleeson FV, et al. Intrapleural streptokinase in the management of malignant multiloculated pleural effusions. Chest 1999;115:729–733.
36. Gilkeson RC, Silverman P, Haaga JR. Using urokinase to treat malignant pleural effusions. AJR Am J Roentgenol 1999;173:781–783.
37. Stavas J, van Sonnenberg E, Casola G, et al. Percutaneous drainage of infected and noninfected thoracic fluid collections. J Thorac Imaging 1987;2:80–87.
38. Meranze SG, LeVeen RF, Burke DR. Transesophageal drainage of mediastinal abscesses. Radiology 1987;165:395–398.
39. Ball WS Jr, Bisset GS 3rd, Towbin RB. Percutaneous drainage of chest abscess in children. Radiology 1989;171:431–434.
40. Neff C, Lawson DW. Boerhaave syndrome: interventional radiologic management. AJR Am J Roentgenol 1985;145:819–820.

Pulmonary Arteriovenous Malformations

53

Jeffrey S. Pollak, Robert I. White, Jr.

Pulmonary arteriovenous shunts are dilated vascular channels that directly connect pulmonary arteries and veins, with no intervening capillary bed. These are most often congenital pulmonary arteriovenous malformations (PAVMs), usually in the setting of hereditary hemorrhagic telangiectasia (HHT) (1–5), although the term *PAVM* has come to encompass acquired shunts as well. Other less preferred and sometimes descriptively inaccurate terms used in the past include pulmonary arteriovenous aneurysms, pulmonary arteriovenous fistulas, pulmonary arteriovenous varices, pulmonary arteriovenous telangiectases, hemangiomas of the lung, and cavernous angiomas of the lung (6). While baseline physiological symptoms from right-to-left shunting are often well tolerated, these lesions have great potential for serious clinical complications related to paradoxical embolization and hemorrhagic rupture and so require vigorous diagnostic investigation and treatment.

Acquired pulmonary arteriovenous fistulas are less often clinically significant lesions. They are most commonly a result of cirrhosis (hepatopulmonary syndrome), with the remainder related to Glenn or Fontan shunts for cyanotic congenital heart disease, schistosomiasis, actinomycosis, hypervascular metastatic cancer, amyloidosis, Fanconi syndrome, trauma, or erosion of an aneurysm into a vein (7–12). Clinical manifestations are similar to those of congenital shunts. Treatment is generally of the underlying pathology, although directed therapy such as embolization is occasionally indicated (13–15).

HISTORY

The earliest description of PAVM was an autopsy report by Churton in 1897 (16). The association with telangiectases was recognized by Rhodes in 1938 (17). Landmark descriptions of HHT were made by Rendu in 1896, who first distinguished the presence of telangiectases and epistaxis as an entity distinct from hemophilia (18), Osler, who recognized its familial nature in 1901 (19), and Weber who further described the triad of this disorder in 1907 (20). Hanes coined the name hereditary hemorrhagic telangiectasia in 1909 (21), which is preferred over the eponym of Rendu-Osler-Weber.

HEREDITARY HEMORRHAGIC TELANGIECTASIA

Hereditary hemorrhagic telangiectasia (HHT) is a group of autosomal dominant inherited disorders in vascular development and vessel wall structure that can involve multiple organ systems. Clinically, the diagnosis is definite if three of four features are present: (a) epistaxis with recurrent, spontaneous episodes; (b) telangiectases with multiple lesions present, especially at characteristic sites such as the lips, oral cavity, fingers, and nose; (c) visceral lesions, such as gastrointestinal telangiectasia or arteriovenous malformations of the lung, liver, or central nervous system (CNS); and (d) family history of HHT involving a first-degree relative. The diagnosis is possible or suspected if two criteria are present and unlikely if fewer than two are present. Clinical confirmation of HHT can be hampered by varying symptoms and severity even within families and by increasing penetrance with age. Recently, genetic tests have become available, which should be particularly helpful in younger patients. The prevalence of HHT is probably at least 1 in 10,000, with a worldwide distribution (22–27).

The characteristic lesion of HHT is the focally dilated small vessel telangiectasis, but high-flow large vessel arteriovenous malformations (AVMs) are not uncommon. Symptoms are related to hemorrhage and shunting through these abnormal vessels. Hemostatic parameters are typically normal. Clinically evident lung involvement is almost exclusively PAVMs. Bleeding from telangiectasia of the pleura and airways is rare (28).

The HHT phenotype can result from heterozygous mutations in any of at least three different genes (29–31). The first two genes code for transmembrane proteins involved in the transforming growth factor-ß (TGF-ß) signaling system (32). HHT type 1 (HHT-1) results from various mutations in endoglin on chromosome 9q34 (33–35), and HHT-2 results from mutations in activin receptor-like kinase 1 on chromosome 12q (36,37). The third gene described as resulting in HHT is *MADH4* (also known as *SMAD4*) on chromosome 18q21.1, which codes for SMAD4 and is also one of two genes that can cause juvenile polyposis (31). This protein is a cytoplasmic mediator in the TGF-ß signaling pathway.

Reduced levels of these proteins have been hypothesized to result in vessels with impaired wall integrity that are more susceptible to dilatation and remodeling, during both development and repair after injury (29,38). HHT-1 appears to have an increased prevalence of PAVMs and possibly CNS vascular malformations than HHT-2, but these two types appear to have equal proportions of epistaxis, gastrointestinal bleeding, and symptomatic liver disease (32,37,39–44). HHT-2 is also associated with primary pulmonary hypertension in a small number of patients (45). The phenotype of the third type of HHT, associated with juvenile polyposis, has not been well described yet (31).

EPIDEMIOLOGY OF PAVM

Recent reports have found HHT in 56–97% of patients with PAVM (1–5). The real incidence is probably approximately 80% as HHT is often underdiagnosed, with 32% of patients having this diagnosis first made on a referral basis (1). The remaining patients with PAVMs are thought to have sporadic types not associated with HHT. In patients with HHT, the prevalence of PAVM is 15–35%, and it is more commonly multiple. While the prevalence is higher in HHT-1, at 29.2–41%, PAVM is still reported in 2.9–14% of other

HHT patients (32,37,39–42). PAVM appears to be slightly more common in women than men, but this is not statistically significant (46).

PATHOLOGY

Pulmonary malformations are thin-walled, endothelial-lined channels with scant surrounding connective tissue (12). They vary in size from microscopic and small telangiectatic vessels to large, macroscopic channels that can be several centimeters in diameter (47). Over 80% involve the pleura, with the remainder subpleural. Multiple PAVMs are present in as many as 58% of cases, they are bilateral in up to 42%, and they are located in the lower lobes in 55–84% (1,2,5,47). Patients with HHT more commonly have multiple PAVMs, and these patients should be assumed to have microscopic lesions in addition to any gross ones.

Initially, simple PAVMs were defined by their supply by a single enlarged feeding artery, an intervening and typically aneurysmal sac, and generally a single draining vein (1,48,49). These accounted for 80% of lesions, and complex PAVMs, having more than one feeding artery and often a complex, plexiform, septated or multichanneled connection, accounted for approximately 20%. In 1996, a more useful classification for embolization purposes was devised (49). The more frequent simple lesions (more than 80%) are now defined as having their arterial supply from a single pulmonary segment, whether this is a single artery or involves several subsegmental arteries all arising from the same segmental artery (Figure 53–1). Complex lesions have their arterial supply from more than one pulmonary segment (Figure 53–2). These account for 10–15% of PAVMs and seem to be more common in the right middle lobe and lingula (50). Simple and complex PAVMs may coexist in patients with multiple lesions. Approximately 5% of lesions in either classification are diffuse, in which varyingly sized and types of malformations extensively involve a lobe or lobes, more commonly the lower lobes (51) (Figure 53–3).

CLINICAL MANIFESTATIONS

Symptoms and signs of PAVM are a result of right-to-left shunting and the potential for rupture (Table 53–1). Manifestations are present in more than 70%, generally developing in the fourth to sixth decades, although 10% can present in childhood (1,3–5,12,29). Asymptomatic rates range from 16–47%, with higher numbers uncovered with intensive screening regimens in HHT families. PAVMs enlarge slowly over time, although pregnancy and possibly adolescence are periods of potential rapid growth and clinical deterioration, including life-threatening complications such as hemorrhage (46,52–57).

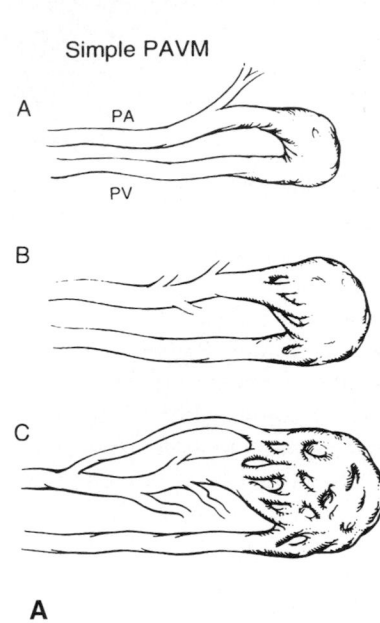

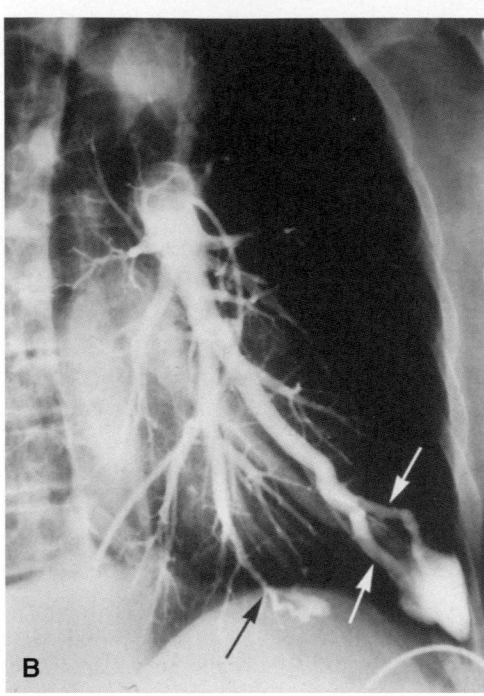

Figure 53–1   A. A simple PAVM will have its arterial supply from within a single lung segment. This may be a single feeding artery (*A*), several distal branches (*B*), or distal and proximal accessory branches (*C*). **B.** Left pulmonary angiogram showing two simple PAVMs, one with a single feeding artery in the lateral lower lobe segment (*black arrow*) and one with two distal feeding branches in the anteromedial lower lobe segment (*white arrows*). Figure 53–1A reprinted with permission from White RI Jr, Pollak JS, Wirth JA. Pulmonary arteriovenous malformations: diagnosis and transcatheter embolotherapy. J Vasc Interv Radiol 1996;7:787–804.

Older series concentrating on more severe cases had mortality rates for untreated PAVM as high as 55% (12). More recent evaluation indicates that the morbidity of untreated PAVM remains significant, with one third of untreated patients available for follow-up in one series having a neurological complication within 10 years (4).

Right-to-left shunting through PAVMs can result in arterial hypoxemia and paradoxical embolization. High-output heart failure has rarely been reported, mainly in neonates (58–60). Hypoxemia tends to be relatively well tolerated in these patients, but more than 70% will still have dyspnea and easy fatigability, which may be worse in the upright position (platypnea) because of the preponderance of PAVMs in the lung bases. Other effects include cyanosis in 9–73% (typically 34%), digital clubbing in 6–68% (typically 39%), and polycythemia in as many as 27%, although this last is often obscured by the HHT-related bleeding. A bruit or murmur may be present in 25–58%. Secondary hypertrophic osteoarthropathy has rarely been described, generally in patients with juvenile polyposis (31,61).

More than 50% of patients may present with the more serious and life-threatening complications of paradoxical embolization or hemorrhage (1,5). Although stroke or transient ischemic attack has been reported in 11–55% of patients, its prevalence is usually greater than 30% in patients having an independent neurological assessment (1,4,5,62). Seizure is reported in 5–15% and brain abscess in 5–25%. This prevalence of stroke is significantly higher than that in the general population, and stroke and brain abscess appear more likely with feeding arteries of at least 3 mm in diameter, multiple PAVMs, and diffuse PAVM (51,62,63) (Figure 53–4). Paradoxical bland or bacterial

emboli to other organs is less frequent, and thrombosis and embolization from the malformation itself is felt to rarely, if ever, be the etiology of any embolic events. Migraine headaches are also commonly associated with PAVM, occurring in 38–59% of patients (1,5,62).

Hemoptysis from PAVM is described in 4–18% of patients and hemothorax in as many as 9% (1,4,5,57). Massive bleeding occurs in as many as 8% and is of particular concern in pregnant women (46,55,56). Symptomatic worsening has been reported in 43% of women, typically after the first trimester. Possible reasons include increased blood volume, increased cardiac output, and alterations in vascular tone.

Patients with PAVM will additionally have manifestations related to other facets of coexistent HHT or, less commonly, concomitant juvenile polyposis or primary pulmonary hypertension (Table 53–1). The more serious consequences of HHT are usually bleeding with anemia, as well as the local or systemic effects of other visceral malformations. While the vascular abnormalities of HHT can affect nearly every organ, the most common manifestations are a result of involvement of the skin, nasal mucosa, lungs, CNS, gastrointestinal track, and liver. The skin telangiectases are sharply defined, 1–3 mm in diameter, red, macular or papular, blanching lesions that can be subtle. They should be carefully looked for on the face, lips, nares, oral cavity, conjunctiva, fingers, and nail beds but can also be seen on the trunk and elsewhere on the extremities (Figure 53–5). They progress with age, being present in most patients by 40 years, but skin telangiectases rarely bleed (64,65). Epistaxis is the most common symptom in HHT, affecting nearly 90% of patients by age 20–21 (42,66–68). Although less common than secondary effects from PAVM, the CNS can be primarily involved with vascular

Complex PAVM

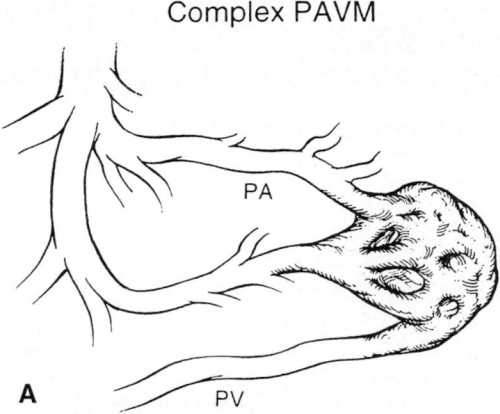

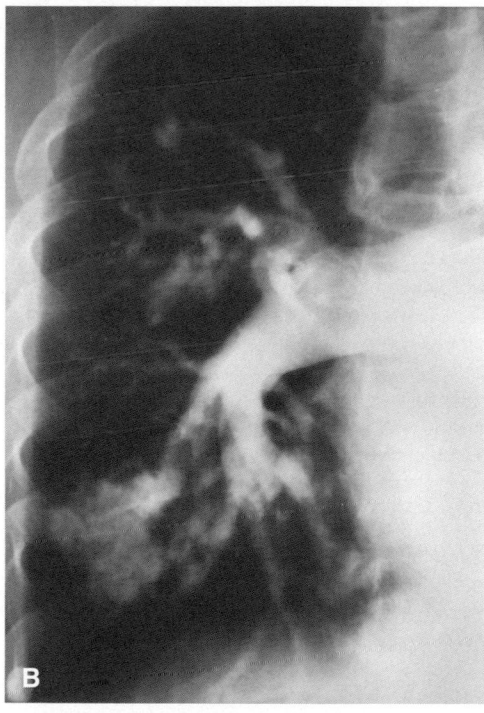

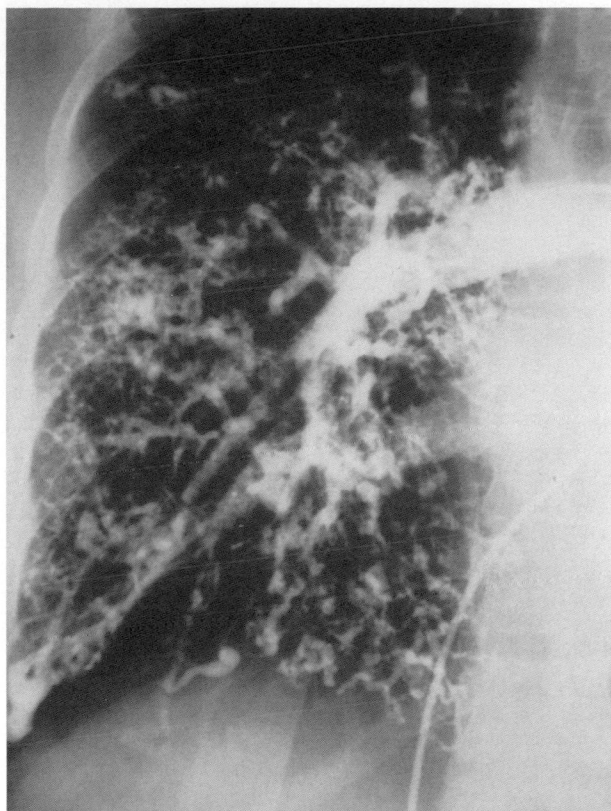

Figure 53–3 Diffuse involvement of the right lung with numerous, variously sized PAVMs well seen in the middle and lower lobes.

Figure 53–2 **A.** A complex PAVM has feeding arteries from more than one lung segment. **B.** Right pulmonary angiogram showing a complex PAVM involving the right lower lung zone, with arterial supply from several arteries from the right middle and lower lobes. Figure 53–2A reprinted with permission from White RI Jr, Pollak JS, Wirth JA. Pulmonary arteriovenous malformations: diagnosis and transcatheter embolotherapy. J Vasc Interv Radiol 1996;7:787–804.

malformations in 25–36%, which can bleed (29,69,70). Migraine headaches are often present, although these may be more related to PAVM. Gastrointestinal bleeding occurs in 11–33% of HHT patients and is principally due to telangiectases rather than AVMs (42,71–75). This bleeding typically starts after 50 years of age, often worsens with time, is difficult to manage, and is the primary cause of increased mortality in HHT patients (25). Bleeding in children should raise suspicion of juvenile polyposis, which has an increased risk of colon cancer over time (31).

While liver involvement with vascular shunts and ectatic vascular spaces has recently been found to occur in over

70% of patients via screening CT imaging, it is symptomatic in only 2.5–8% (72,76–79). Symptomatic patients may suffer from high output heart failure, portal hypertension (generally from noncirrhotic sinusoidal fibrosis with nodular hyperplasia), and/or biliary disease.

DIAGNOSTIC EVALUATION AND SCREENING

Evaluation of PAVM consists of screening to detect its presence in the high-risk HHT population and characterization of the lesion to guide treatment decisions. Diagnostic studies (Table 53–2) depend on identifying the pathophysiological effects of right-to-left shunting (pulse oximetry, arterial blood gas for oxygen tension, shunt fraction studies, and contrast echocardiography) or direct lesion imaging (chest radiography, computed tomography, magnetic resonance imaging, and pulmonary angiography) (80–86). Disadvantages of physiological studies are a lack of morphological information on the size, type, number, and location of PAVMs. These data are particularly important because a feeding artery of 3 mm or greater is considered the reasonable size for treatment to prevent significant-sized paradoxical thromboemboli—although hypoxemia

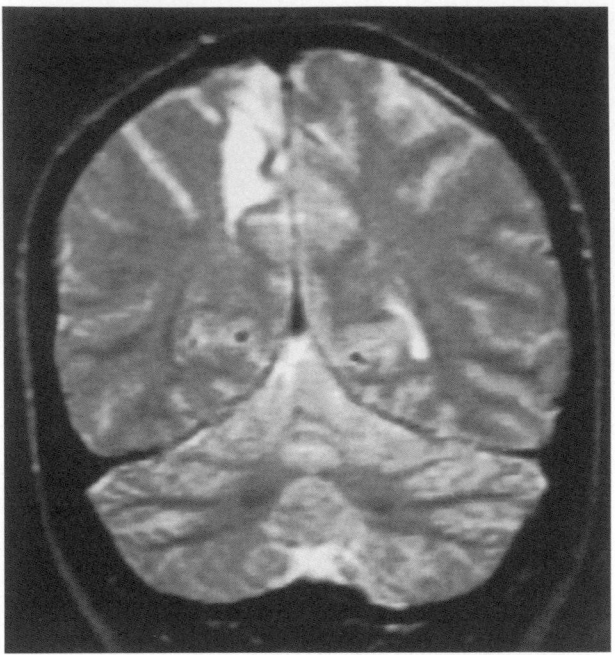

Figure 53–4 Head MRI of the patient with diffuse PAVM involvement shown in Figure 53–3, demonstrating right parietal high-signal encephalomalacia compatible with a known prior cerebral infarct.

and paradoxical bacterial embolization can still occur with numerous smaller lesions.

The classic chest radiographic finding of PAVM is a well-defined round, often lobular, soft tissue mass representing the aneurysmal communication and an enlarged feeding artery from the hilum and draining vein into the left atrium, although these channels are less frequently seen (12) (Figure 53–6). This mass may enlarge and decrease with Valsalva and Mueller maneuvers. Malformations with a complex nidus may be multilobulated and may be less well defined. Chest radiography is limited because of the relatively small size of many significant lesions and masking by normal structures, such as the diaphragms for lower lobe lesions. As many as 40% of patients may have an unrevealing study, so a negative chest radiograph should not dissuade further investigation (82,83).

Pulse oximetry can detect low oxygen saturation from right-to-left shunting in many patients with PAVM, and accuracy may be enhanced with postural changes, relying on a relative decline in the erect position because of the predilection of PAVMs for the bases. Nevertheless, its sensitivity is still at best 73%, and its specificity is limited by the presence of hypoxemia in many other diseases (83–85). Its greatest value is as a noninvasive study in young children.

A room air absolute arterial oxygen tension of less than 90–92 mm Hg has been found to be inadequate for reliably detecting PAVM and excluding other etiologies (82,83). This is also true when using an arterial oxygen tension of less than 500–600 mm Hg while breathing 100% oxygen, which is more specific for detecting right-to-left shunting.

TABLE 53–1
CLINICAL MANIFESTATIONS OF PAVM AND HHT

Pulmonary Manifestations of PAVM

Dyspnea
Fatigue
Cyanosis
Clubbing
Asymptomatic lung mass or infiltrate
Spontaneous hemoptysis or hemothorax
Polycythemia
Chest bruit or murmur

Neurological Manifestations of PAVM

Stroke or transient ischemic attack
Brain abscess
Epilepsy
Migraine headaches

HHT-related Manifestations (other than from PAVM)

Telangiectases
Recurrent epistaxis
Iron deficiency anemia
Gastrointestinal bleeding
Intracranial hemorrhage, epilepsy, and/or headache from cerebral AVM
Symptomatic liver involvement: high-output heart failure, portal hypertension with ascites and GI bleeding, and/or biliary track disease with cholestasis and cholangitis

Uncommon Other Related Conditions

Primary pulmonary hypertension
Juvenile polyposis

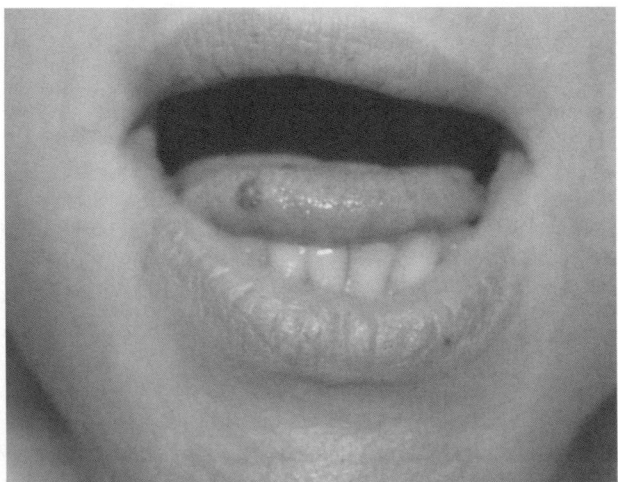

Figure 53–5 Telangiectases on the lips and tongue of a patient with HHT.

TABLE 53-2

SCREENING METHODS FOR PAVM—RESULTS OF RECENT REPORTS (80–86)

Method	Reference Study	Sensitivity	Specificity
Pulse oximetry: oxygen saturation ≤96% or decrease by ≥2% from supine to erect positioning	CE PAG	34% 53–73%	 35–90%
Arterial oxygen tension <90–92 mm Hg	PAG	67–73%	61–80%
Chest radiography	PAG	60–83%	92–100%
Pulmonary angiography	CT	61%[a]	
100% oxygen shunt fraction (>5–15%)	PAG	64–88%	71–80%
Radionuclide shunt fraction (>3.5%)	PAG	87%	61%
Helical computed tomography	PAG	97%	
Contrast echocardiography	PAG	94[b]–100%	88%[b]

[a] All the PAVMs missed by angiography but detected by CT by Remy et al. (81) had aneurysms less than 5 mm in diameter or were thrombosed. Furthermore, the sensitivity of pulmonary angiography is relatively higher than shunt fraction studies because it has been used as the reference study for them.

[b] Nanthakumar et al. (86) did not give sensitivity and specificity because they did not perform angiography on everyone, but these values can be calculated from their data.

CE, contrast echocardiography; PAG, pulmonary angiography.

Shunt fraction studies measure the flow through the shunt as a ratio to the total cardiac output. Normally, this fraction is no larger than 3–5%, as a result of drainage of poorly oxygenated blood from bronchial and thebesian veins directly into the left atrium (physiological shunt). The fraction can be measured using the 100% inspired oxygen method or less-invasive radionuclide lung perfusion scintigraphy (87). In the latter, a γ camera measures the activity of technetium-99m albumin microspheres or macroaggregates over the right kidney as an indicator of the amount of injected material having passed through PAVMs to lodge in systemic capillaries. This is compared with either the total injected dose or with the activity in normal lung capillaries plus that in systemic organs to determine the shunt fraction. Sensitivity and specificity vary as the shunt fraction used to indicate the presence of disease is increased from 3.5 to 15%, but both remain less than 90% (82–84).

Contrast (or "bubble") echocardiography relies on the passage of intravenously injected echogenic microbubbles of agitated saline or other agents from right- to left-sided cardiac chambers to diagnose right-to-left shunts. Normally, such bubbles are filtered by the pulmonary circulation. Some specificity for PAVM is gained by the delayed appearance of left-sided bubbles by three to five heartbeats as compared to within one cycle for intracardiac shunts (Figure 53–7). This study appears to have excellent sensitivity and reasonable specificity for PAVM, making it a preferred screening method for the presence of disease (86); however, it lacks the morphological information necessary to guide therapeutic decisions (88).

Computed tomography, especially helical and multidetector studies with thin, contiguous slices, offers enhanced visualization of PAVMs (81,89). These typically appear as noncalcified nodules or serpentine masses (Figure 53–8). The less constant detection of enlarged feeding and draining vessels permits a more specific diagnosis. While PAVMs enhance, so may other lesions such as vascular metastases (90), and contrast administration is not necessary. There is a lack of studies comparing CT with other modalities for screening, so its role in this regard is uncertain. Its ability to depict the number, location, and size of PAVMs, and especially the size of feeding arteries, can aid in the decision as to whether invasive treatment is needed and can permit more limited, directed catheterization at the time of embolization. Probably the most valuable current role for CT is in follow-up after treatment to assess the adequacy of occlusion. The role of MR imaging in detecting or characterizing PAVMs is not clear at this time (91–93).

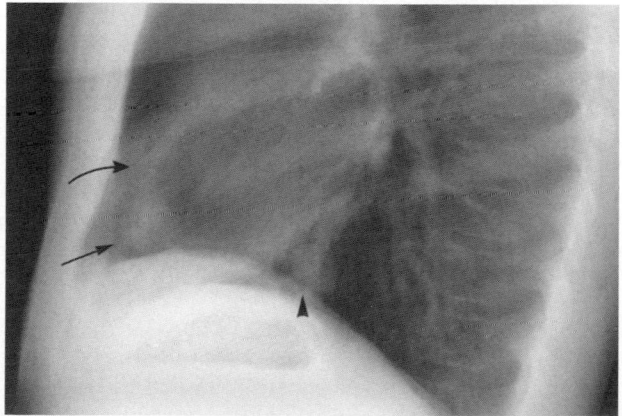

Figure 53–6 Lateral chest radiograph in a 9-year-old boy with HHT, exercise intolerance, and low oxygen saturation. Two PAVMs are seen, a rounded mass anteriorly, in the right middle lobe (*arrow*), with its feeding artery visible (*curved arrow*), and the other more posterior, in the left lower lobe (*arrowhead*).

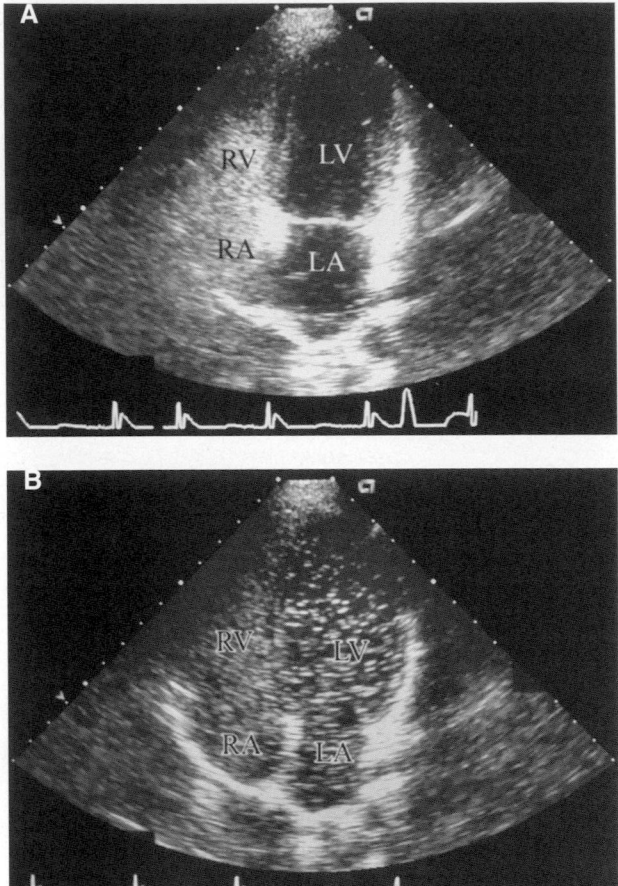

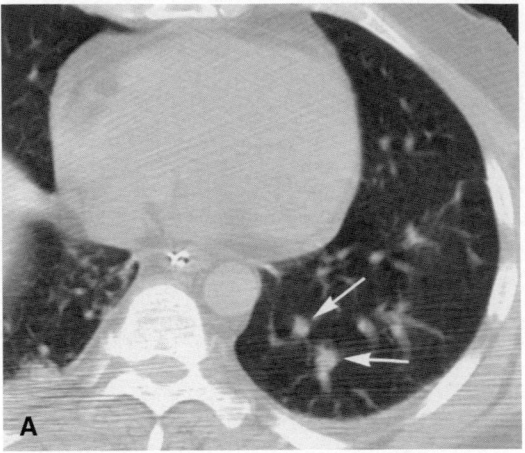

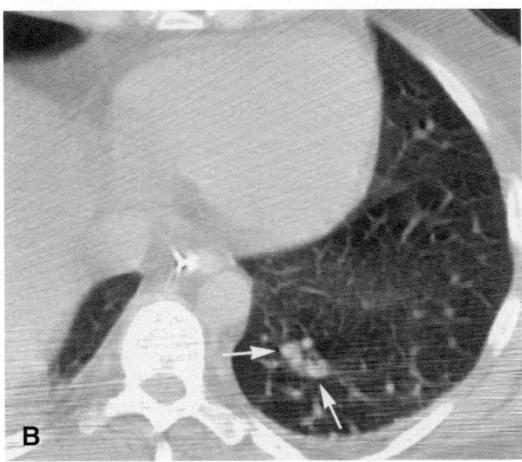

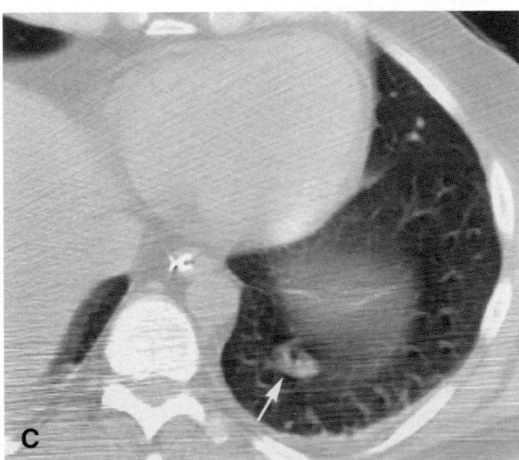

Figure 53–7 Contrast echocardiogram of a patient with PAVMs. **A.** Intravenously injected agitated saline initially producing echogenic bubbles in the right atrium (*RA*) and right ventricle (*RV*) but none in the left atrium (*LA*) or left ventricle (*LV*). **B.** After 5 seconds, the echogenic bubbles are also present in the left atrium and left ventricle, having passed through the PAVM without being filtered.

Currently, pulmonary angiography is rarely needed as a diagnostic study for the presence of PAVM, being useful only when other studies are equivocal. However, it does have a key role in further characterizing PAVMs prior to treatment (Figures 53–1 through 53–3). Although pulmonary angiography can miss lesions detected by other modalities, especially contrast echocardiography and CT scanning, these missed lesions are typically small ones that do not require directed treatment (81,83,86). The study is typically performed through a transfemoral route using standard technique to introduce a pigtail catheter into each main pulmonary artery. Particular care needs to be taken to avoid any air emboli or thrombi, including through peripheral intravenous lines, because these may embolize through a PAVM. Right heart and pulmonary artery pressures should be obtained. If pulmonary hypertension is found, it should raise the possibilities of a large hepatic AVM with left-to-right shunting or coexistent non-HHT disease (e.g., primary pulmonary hypertension) (94,95).

Figure 53–8   CT Images of a Simple Left Lower Lobe PAVM. **A., B.** Feeding and draining vessels to the PAVM (*arrows*). **C.** Aneurysmal sac of the PAVM (*arrow*).

Frontal and oblique views are obtained of each lung unless a preceding CT scan permits a more limited study. Additional projections are done as needed, including lateral views, which are often helpful for PAVMs in the right middle lobe and lingula. In addition to identifying the number and location of PAVMs, it is important to determine the origin of the arterial supply (which distinguishes simple and complex lesions) and the size and length of the feeding artery or arteries. Often the precise number of feeding arteries for a complex, and occasionally for a simple, lesion will not become apparent until selective angiograms are obtained during the embolization procedure. Diagnostic angiography can be done as an outpatient procedure unless treatment is performed at the same time, in which case the need for admission depends on the degree of embolization.

Screening Algorithm

Currently, there is broad consensus that all patients with HHT should be screened for PAVM and growing agreement for screening them for CNS malformations, probably best with MRI, both without and with contrast (a pregadolinium brain MRI helps distinguish small T2 lesions resulting from microemboli or migraine from small telangiectases or AVMs). As other organ manifestations of HHT do not tend to manifest with sudden catastrophic events, these can be evaluated and managed as clinically indicated.

A screening regimen should detect PAVM with high sensitivity and without excessive loss in specificity. Although several studies have looked at screening methods, deficiencies in these studies exist. These deficiencies include inconsistency in the performance of pulmonary angiography in patients with negative noninvasive screening studies, the questionable accuracy of pulmonary angiography as a gold standard (although missed lesions seem more likely to be small ones that do not require directed treatment), and the lack of a study comparing all screening modalities (80–86). Nevertheless, the sensitivity of studies in decreasing order appears to be contrast echocardiography, helical CT and shunt studies, pulmonary angiography, chest radiography, absolute arterial oxygen tension, and pulse oximetry (Table 53–2).

The authors' current suggested screening algorithm for asymptomatic patients with HHT starts with contrast echocardiography except for those younger than 12, in whom supine and erect pulse oximetry is performed (Figure 53–9). If these are negative, further workup is probably not necessary in adults, but repeat evaluation is warranted when a child reaches adolescence. If either is positive, a helical CT scan should be done for further evaluation, treatment planning, and as a baseline for future comparison. If a patient has manifestations of PAVM at presentation, the screening can proceed directly to a CT scan. If PAVMs with feeding arteries at least 3 mm in diameter are found, the patient should have pulmonary angiography and embolization. The need for rescreening adults with a negative initial work-up, especially women planning on pregnancy, is unclear. While the authors no longer routinely measure arterial oxygen tension or perform shunt studies, these offer added information in particular patients and play a role in some other centers' screening algorithm.

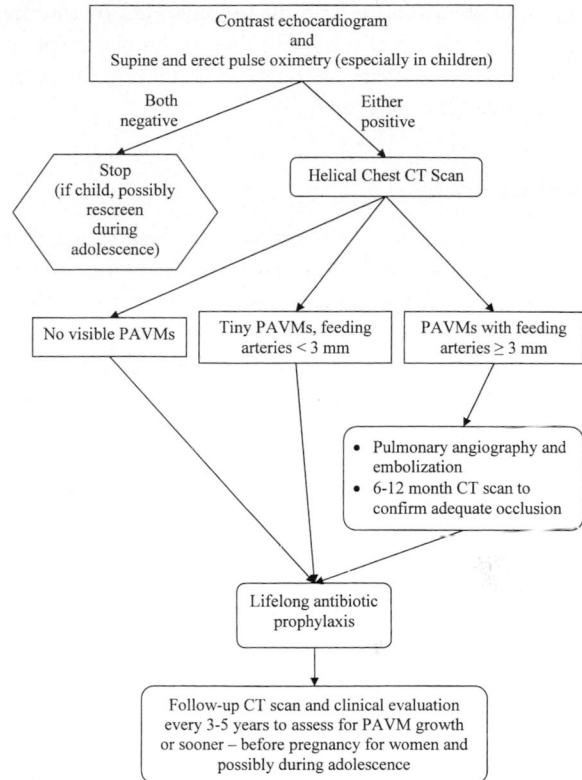

Figure 53–9 Screening and management algorithm for pulmonary arteriovenous malformations (PAVMs) in patients with HHT.

TREATMENT

Treatment of PAVM is indicated to alleviate symptoms and signs of hypoxemia and, even more importantly, to prevent the complications of paradoxical embolization and hemorrhage. All lesions with a feeding artery at least 3 mm in diameter should be occluded because this appears to be a threshold size for nearly all bland thromboemboli that could result in stroke (96). Smaller lesions may still require therapy if numerous enough to result in significant hypoxemia. Additionally, all patients with PAVMs of any size, treated or not, should receive antibiotic prophylaxis prior to dental and other invasive procedures to protect against brain abscess and other less common sites of paradoxical septic embolization.

Surgery

Pneumonectomy was the first definitive treatment for PAVM and was initially described in 1942 (97). Over time, surgery improved to more lung-conserving procedures such as segmentectomy or local excision (2,52,98). Vessel ligation can limit the loss of normal lung tissue, but this procedure is difficult and can miss accessory feeding vessels. Although mortality is generally low, 0–9% (12), surgery does have major disadvantages. These include the discomfort, risk, and recuperative period associated with thoracotomy, the loss of surrounding normal lung tissue, and the problems presented by multiple, bilateral, and growing or persistent PAVMs. Lung transplantation appears to have a very limited role, perhaps in the patient with intractable, diffuse PAVM (51,99).

Embolotherapy

Transcatheter closure of a PAVM was first reported by Porstmann in 1977 (100). Extensive experience since then has clearly shown embolotherapy to be the preferred method for treating these lesions (1,3,5, 101–103). Advantages are minimal discomfort and recuperation, a low complication rate, preservation of more normal lung tissue, and ease in treating multiple lesions at the same time as well as at later times.

Initial Steps

Depending on the amount of contrast and time required for the diagnostic pulmonary angiogram, embolotherapy may be performed on the same day or at a subsequent visit, through a contralateral femoral vein approach. A preprocedural helical CT scan indicating only one or two simple PAVMs in a single lung may permit a more tailored angiogram with immediate embolization, and a complete bilateral pulmonary angiogram and the presence of multiple, scattered, large, and complex lesions indicates the need for separate sessions. It is also recommended to try and combine the two procedures in children (especially if they require

anesthesia) and pregnant patients. Because of the occurrence of pleurisy in some patients, it is generally preferred to treat only one lung at a time if there are large PAVMs, with the patient returning in 1–2 months for treatment of contralateral disease.

The rare patient with polycythemia may require phlebotomy first to reduce the risk of pericatheter thrombus formation. As for the diagnostic study, air bubbles and clots must be avoided, both in the catheters used for the procedure and in intravenous lines. It is recommended to use air filters for intravenous lines and discontinue these as soon as possible. Patients are given low-level anticoagulation with heparin 50–80 units/kg and prophylactic antibiotic coverage with intravenous cefazolin 1 g (Kefzol, Eli Lilly and Company). Light conscious sedation is adequate and permits the patient to hold his or her breath to improve imaging and straighten out pulmonary vessels.

Selective Catheterization

A 7-5 French Lumax coaxial guiding system (Cook, Inc.) is placed through a femoral vein sheath into the pulmonary circulation (Figure 53–10). The outer multipurpose-shaped guiding catheter provides excellent support across the pulsating heart and large central pulmonary arteries as well as limited selective ability. The inner 5 French short angled catheter permits enhanced selective branch vessel catheterization. If unsuccessful, it can be rapidly exchanged through

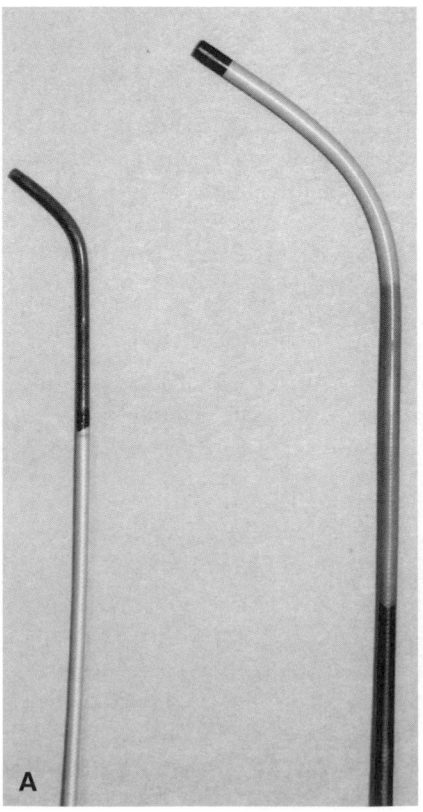
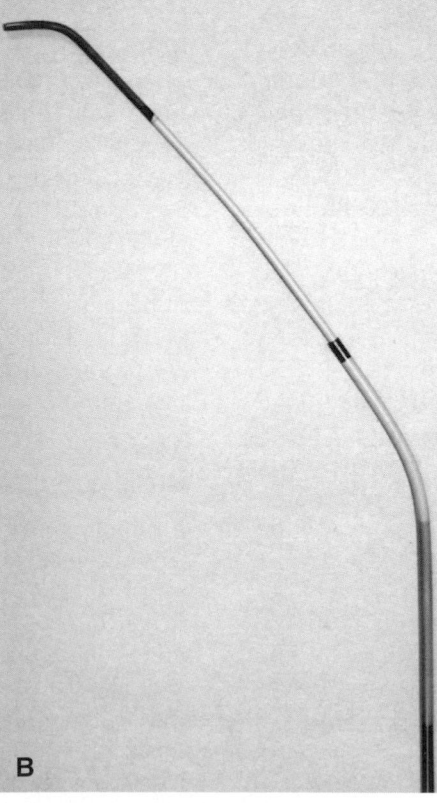

Figure 53–10 The Lumax guiding catheter system for PAVM embolization consists of an outer multipurpose-shaped 7 French guiding catheter and inner angled hydrophilic 5 French catheter. Images of the catheters separated (Figure 53–10A) and coaxial (Figure 53–10B).

the guiding catheter for a variety of 5 French catheters, including a pigtail catheter if more global angiography is desired (which is commonly done after the embolization). Selective catheterization is typically most successful using direct catheter manipulations while injecting contrast and working in the projection that best places the origin of the desired vessel in profile and separates it from adjacent vessels. Once the feeding artery is entered, the outer guiding catheter is generally able to be advanced over the inner one, providing additional support for the embolization. Selective angiography is performed to confirm proper positioning, identify the optimal projection to profile the feeding artery and its entry into the PAVM, and determine the proper site for occlusion (Figure 53–11). During this, it is important to watch for air entering the catheter during removal of any guide wires, which is prone to occur if the catheter tip is lying against a vessel wall and a vacuum is created as a wire is

retracted. This problem may be reduced by removing guide wires with the catheter hub immersed in a basin of saline. If air does enter the system, having the patient take a deep inspiration may straighten the vessel sufficiently to free the catheter tip and permit blood return. Otherwise, the catheter must be retracted until blood return occurs. Catheterization for embolization rarely requires 3 French and smaller coaxial microcatheters.

The optimal location for endoluminal occlusion is a distal segment of the feeding artery beyond the origin of any significant supply to normal lung but where the walls are still tapering or parallel. This preserves as much normal lung as possible and limits the risk that collateral flow from the bronchial circulation will develop to a hypoperfused region of lung, which in turn could result in PAVM reperfusion (104,105). As the feeding artery often dilates slightly just before entering the aneurysmal sac, it is safest to embolize

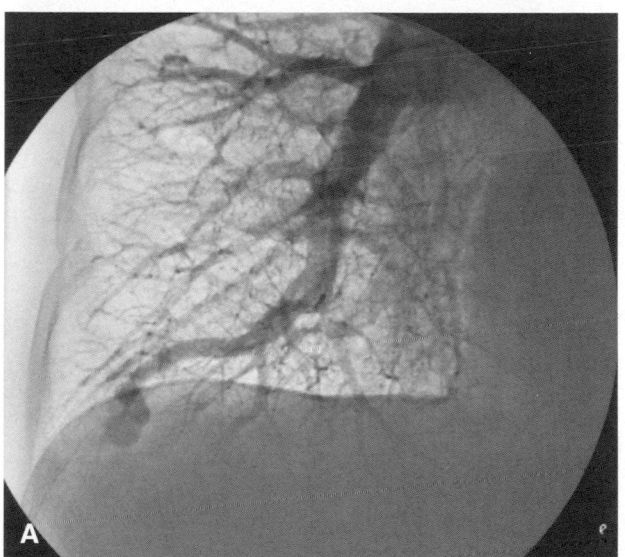

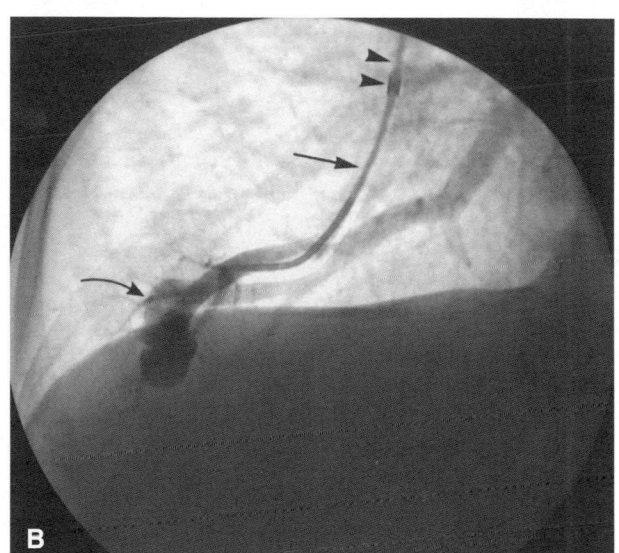

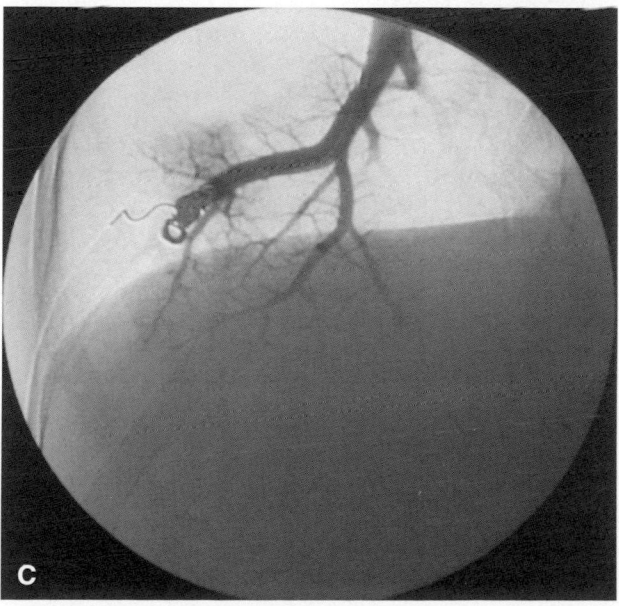

Figure 53–11 Fifty-six-year-old man with HHT, epistaxis, bleeding gastric malformations, and a simple right lower lobe PAVM. **A.** Right pulmonary angiogram demonstrating the simple PAVM in the right lower lobe. **B.** Angiography of the feeding artery to the simple PAVM after selective catheterization using the 5 French inner angled catheter (*straight arrow*) followed by advancement of the 7 French multipurpose guiding catheter (*arrowheads*). In this instance, the feeding artery has a uniform, nontapering appearance. Therefore, a small distal normal pulmonary artery branch was identified for anchoring the distal end of the first Nester coil used for embolization (*curved arrow*). **C.** Postembolization angiogram showing occlusion of the PAVM. A dense, occlusive cross-sectional plug is created by the Nester coils. The distal end of the first one is anchored in the small distal normal branch noted in B.

proximal to this, typically by 1–2 cm, to decrease the risk of device migration across the PAVM. Unlike complex systemic malformations, it is not necessary to embolize the aneurysmal sac, analogous to the nidus of a high-flow complex systemic or CNS AVM, to achieve effective occlusion.

Embolic Agents

Effective, long-term occlusion of PAVMs is best achieved by producing cross-sectional obstruction of their feeding arteries with a mechanical agent. Detachable balloons were excellent for this purpose in the past, but further development has stopped, and they are no longer available in the United States. The current preferred agents are coil emboli because of device advances, ready availability, ease of use, and greater familiarity to most interventional radiologists. Nevertheless, if desired, the Lumax guiding catheter can be used as an introducer for detachable balloons.

Although a variety of conventional 0.035- and 0.038-inch-gauge fibered coil emboli can be used, soft, highly radiopaque platinum coils such as the Nester coil (Cook, Inc.) permit easy packing ("nesting") into a tight space to give a short, dense, occlusive plug of metal (Figure 53–11C). Loosely packed coils with acute vessel thrombosis induced by their fibers do not yield a reliable long-term result (Figure 53–12). Nester coils are 14-cm-long emboli that come in diameters of 4–12 mm. The first embolus should be at least 20% larger than the diameter of the vessel. If desired, stability of the coil can be enhanced by anchoring the first few centimeters in a small, expendable side branch, with the remainder of the coil then placed in the main channel to be occluded. Although more expensive than standard Gianturco coil emboli, typically only one to three Nester coils are needed per PAVM artery.

The less radiopaque standard Gianturco stainless steel 0.038- and 0.035-inch coils (Cook, Inc.) are more rigid and have a higher degree of radial force. This interferes with dense nesting in a short space, necessitating multiple, progressively smaller-diameter coils. Additionally, it can result in pushing of the delivery catheter back during coil deployment—an issue of particular concern if the feeding artery is short. An alternative soft, platinum coil is the Tornado coil (Cook, Inc.). Finally, the Jackson Detachable Coil (Cook, Inc.) has been claimed to allow safer, more accurate, and more distal embolization of PAVMs than is possible using nondetachable coils (106). Nevertheless, nondetachable coils are quite effective and safe, with paradoxical migration in well less than 1% of placements in recent reports (50,107).

Special Situations

Short feeding arteries can present difficulties in achieving a stable catheter position. Although it may be possible to place a detachable balloon, an alternative is to use an occlusion balloon to enhance stability in the feeding artery and embolize directly through its endhole or through a coaxial

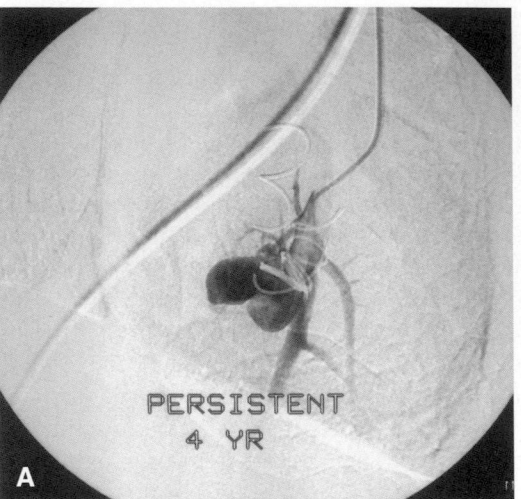

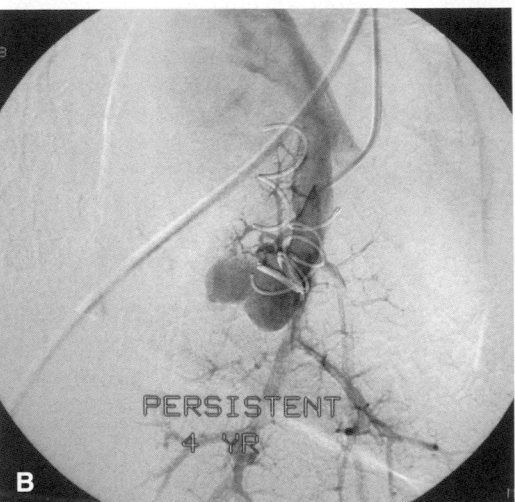

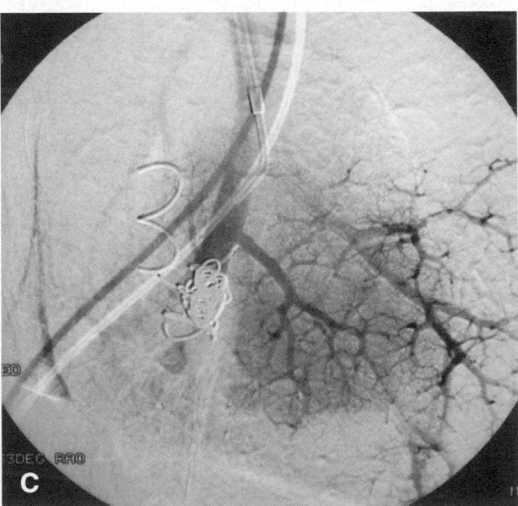

Figure 53–12 Thirty-five-year-old woman with HHT who had a large left lower lobe PAVM embolized with coils 4 years earlier and who now has recurrent decreased oxygen saturation. **A., B.** Angiography showed reperfusion through the coils, which are not tightly packed. Note that the feeding artery and draining vein of the PAVM are superimposed on these images. The separate individual coil is in another malformation. **C.** Additional coils were placed within the old ones, creating a tight, occlusive matrix.

microcatheter system. If the remaining artery is too short to embolize or if the occlusion balloon is also not sufficiently stable, the aneurysm itself can then be occluded using a coaxial microcatheter system. Intra-aneurysmal embolization should be done using softer, less-traumatic microcoils (0.018-inch gauge and thinner) (Figure 53–13). While retrievable mechanically or electrolytically detachable coils have been described for this purpose (108,109), large, non-retrievable coils are equally effective and less expensive (110,111). These should be sized to the aneurysm to prevent prolapse or flow-induced migration into the vein, and the aneurysm should be densely packed to provide a durable occlusion. If possible, at least the terminal end of the feeding artery should also be embolized.

Large, high-flow feeding arteries having diameters greater than 8 mm can result in significant drag forces on embolization agents and so risk migration. Approaches for handling this situation include an occlusion balloon to arrest flow (Figure 53–14) and anchoring of the initial portion of a coil in a distal side branch. Traditional Gianturco coils are often first placed because of their higher radial force.

Patients with diffuse PAVM generally do not have significant improvement in hypoxemia from embolization unless the area of involvement is limited and the entire region can be embolized. Nevertheless, the combined rate of stroke and brain abscess can be significantly reduced from 56% to 13% with embolization of the larger PAVM components and antibiotic prophylaxis (51).

Because of the high risk for rapid deterioration of PAVMs during pregnancy, women should be assessed and embolized prior to planned conception. If already pregnant, PAVMs can be safely embolized during the second trimester (112).

Postembolization Measures

Segmental and lobar angiography is performed after embolizing the feeding arterial supply to a PAVM to assess for an adequate occlusion and for accessory feeders, either from within a single segment for simple lesions or from an adjacent segment for complex lesions. Such feeders may only be angiographically evident after occlusion of a primary, dominant feeder (Figure 53–15). Late collateral filling of the aneurysmal

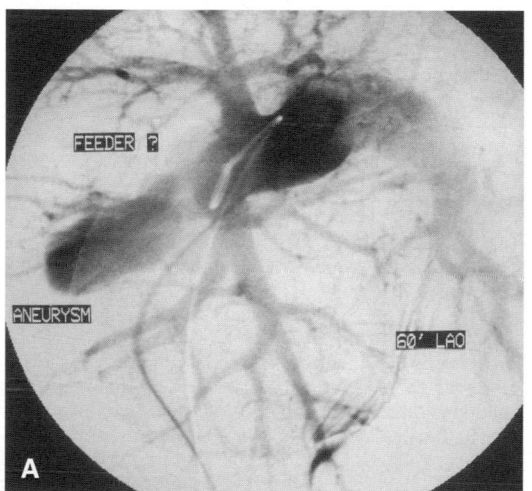

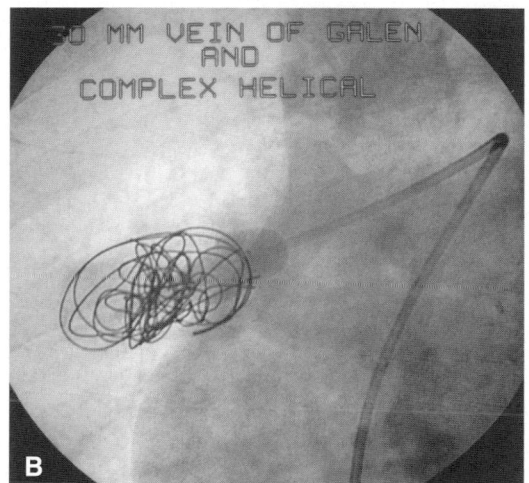

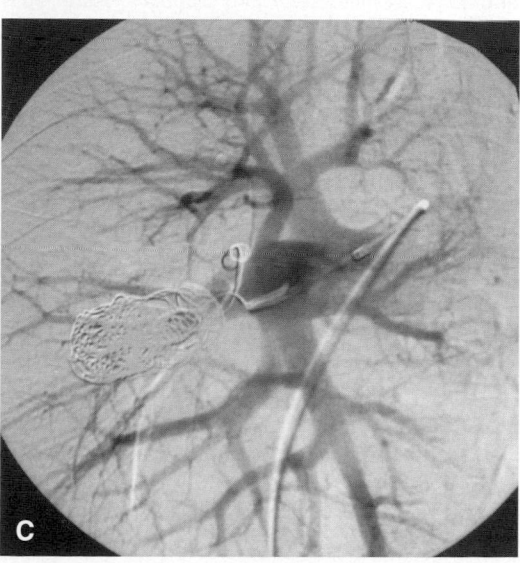

Figure 53–13 Fifty-seven-year-old woman with HHT, epistaxis, chronic hypoxemia, and a prior large right hemothorax. **A.** Right pulmonary angiography showed a large PAVM in the middle lobe with a large, short feeding artery and a large sac. **B.** An occlusion balloon was placed to achieve stability in the short feeding artery and a microcatheter advanced through this into the aneurysm. Large-diameter 0.018-inch vein of Galen and complex helical coils (Boston Scientific Corporation) were initially placed to form a matrix within the aneurysm. **C.** Further embolization was accomplished with additional 0.018 coils through the microcatheter and a few Nester coils (Cook, Inc.) through the occlusion balloon. No flow was seen through the PAVM on final right pulmonary angiography.

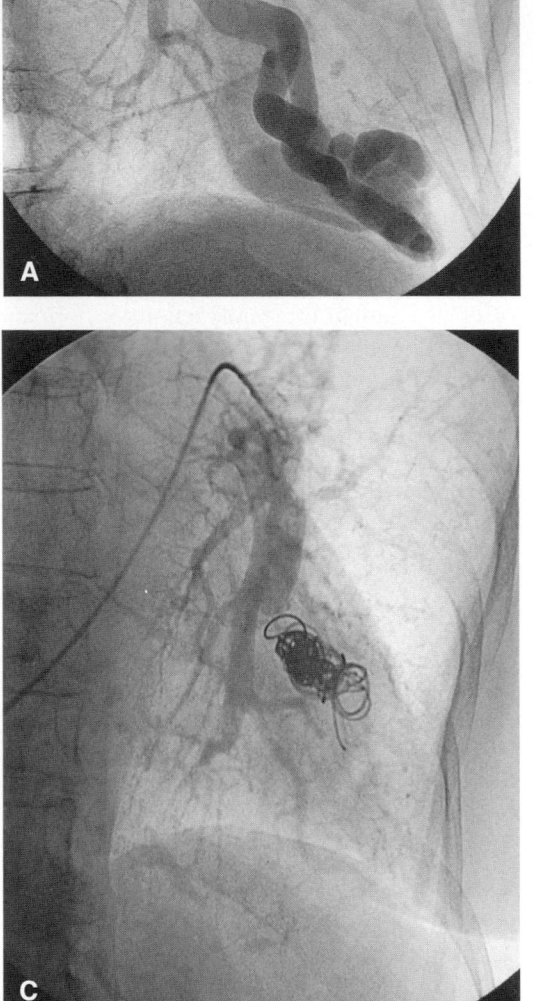

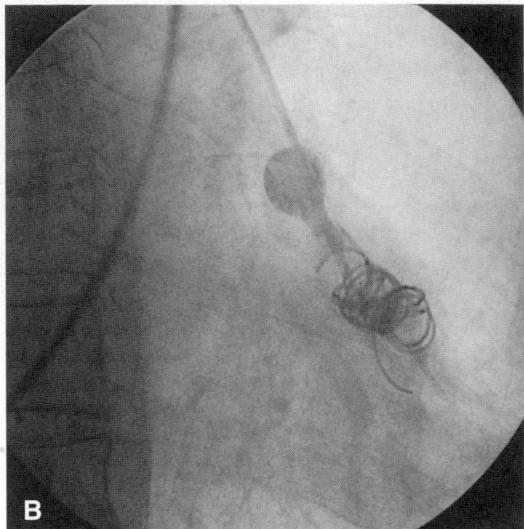

Figure 53–14 Seventy-nine-year-old woman with HHT who has dyspnea, fatigue, and hypoxemia as well as prior liver and spinal abscesses. **A.** Left pulmonary angiography shows a lower lobe PAVM with an extremely large feeding artery that divides into two large distal branches to the malformation. **B.** A 20-mm occlusion balloon catheter was placed into the feeding artery and initial stainless steel coils placed, starting with 15-mm diameter coils. **C.** Left pulmonary angiography showed successful occlusion of the feeding artery after placing additional stainless steel and platinum Nester coils, forming a dense matrix.

sac from opacified adjacent capillaries and venous channels is occasionally seen and is of no concern.

Postprocedural care consists of several hours of bed rest and removal of all intravenous lines to prevent iatrogenic paradoxical emboli through residual unoccluded PAVMs. Additionally, use of an incentive spirometer for several days, especially if a larger PAVM was occluded, may ameliorate the effects of a pleurisy that can occur several days later. A follow-up arterial blood gas measurement may be helpful in determining improvement and as a baseline for future follow-up. Patients generally stay a single night in the hospital, but they may be kept as an outpatient when undergoing straightforward embolization of smaller lesions.

Complications

Embolotherapy appears quite safe, with no mortality and rare major complications (1,3,5,49,101–103,107,113). The most common adverse event is self-limited pleuritic chest pain, often accompanied by a low-grade fever and occasionally a localized infiltrate. Three to 16% of patients will develop this within 2–4 days of the procedure, and it typically lasts 3–6 days. The etiology is thought to be thrombosis of the aneurysm and/or pulmonary infarction related to occlusion of normal pulmonary arteries. It appears to be more common after treating large PAVMs, as high as 31%, and its incidence may be reduced by appropriate distal

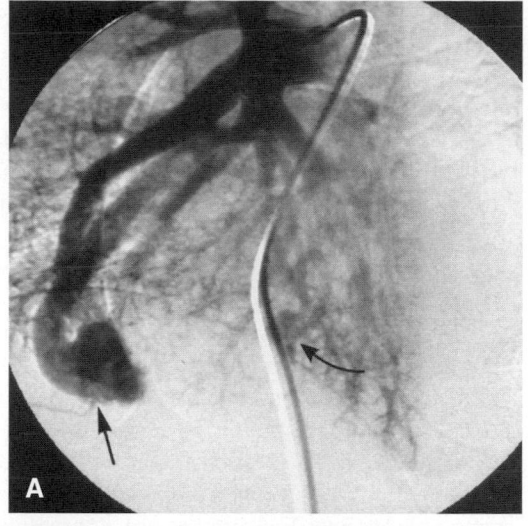
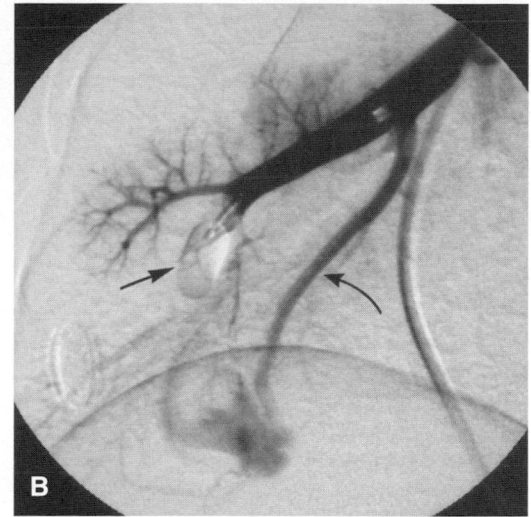
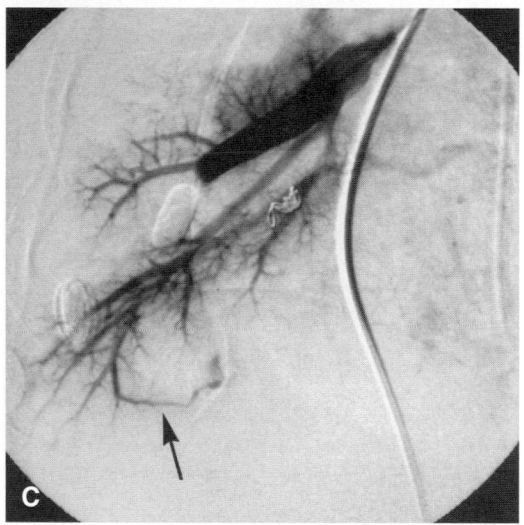

Figure 53–15 Accessory feeder uncovered after embolization of the primary feeding artery of a right middle lobe PAVM. This corresponds to the chest radiographs shown in Figure 53–6. **A.** Right posterior oblique right pulmonary angiogram showing a large middle lobe PAVM (*arrow*) and less clearly a smaller lower lobe PAVM (*curved arrow*). **B.** Angiography with a detachable balloon (*arrow*) in the large feeding artery to the right middle lobe PAVM now showed a more proximal accessory feeder (*curved arrow*). **C.** After embolization of the large feeding artery and the smaller accessory branch, a third tiny accessory vessel becomes more apparent (*arrow*).

embolization (5,102). A smaller number of patients (4–5%) may develop pleurisy with fevers and infiltrates several weeks later (50), perhaps as a result of delayed thrombosis and, less likely, infection. Pleurisy is usually well managed with nonsteroidal anti-inflammatory agents (e.g., ibuprofen). Antibiotics are occasionally indicated for the possibility of infection.

Paradoxical embolization represents the potentially most serious complication of PAVM embolotherapy. While device embolization has been reported in 0.4–2.17% of patients, major clinical effects are rare. Furthermore, this complication has basically been eliminated with the use of Nester coils and anchoring in side branches as needed. Some coils have safely been left in place, and others have been retrieved transluminally if they lodge in a critical bed (generally without complication); at least one retrieval required surgery (113). Migration of an inflated balloon or a coil to an uninvolved region of the lung is quite unusual. Late paradoxical embolization of a device has been reported with only one detachable balloon that deflated at 2 days, with no clinical

sequelae (82). A single stroke at 1 week is the only reported case suspected of being related to migration of clot from the aneurysm of an occluded PAVM (114).

Paradoxical air embolization is noted in as many as 5% of patients. The most common manifestations are angina, bradycardia, and ECG changes resulting from air entering the anteriorly located right coronary artery ostium in the supine patient. This usually resolves within minutes and can be treated with nitroglycerine, oxygen, and atropine. Less common effects are transient ischemic attack or perioral and facial paresthesias. Two reports of intraprocedural cerebrovascular accidents were of uncertain etiology but possibly resulting from air or bland thromboembolism (4,101).

Several other procedural complications have rarely been encountered. A self-limited, small amount of hemorrhage resulting from PAVM or vessel injury is typically best managed with completion of the embolization. Deep venous thrombosis is probably more likely in patients with polycythemia and those having multiple catheterizations of the same vein (1). New or worsening pulmonary hypertension is possible in patients with underlying pulmonary hypertension obscured by the low-resistance flow through the PAVMs and/or a marked left-to-right shunting, as from a coexistent liver AVM (94,95). Overall, complications appear to decrease with greater operator experience.

Results of Embolotherapy and Follow-up

Occlusion is technically successful in 88–100% of treated PAVMs and patients, although multiple catheterizations are occasionally needed (1,3–5,101–103,107). Significant improvement is seen in dyspnea, hypoxemia, and shunt fractions with the exception of patients with diffuse lesions (51). Still, the shunt fraction remains abnormal in 60–100% of patients and contrast echocardiography positive in 90% of patients because of small residual angiographically visible lesions or microscopic disease (80,101,115). Subjective improvement in exercise tolerance is generally noted by patients, but objective improvement is only occasionally documented (5,94). This may be explained by the treatment of patients with even minor or absent hypoxemic symptoms to protect against paradoxical embolization and hemorrhage.

Although long-term studies generally have less than 5 years of follow-up, the clinical improvement is sustained in the vast majority. Additionally, stroke, brain abscess, and hemorrhage are expected in less than 2% of patients (12). Groups at higher risk for late clinical morbidity are those with diffuse PAVM, women who become pregnant, and those with large PAVMs (5,51,102). This is a result of the difficulty in managing diffuse, small PAVMs with embolotherapy, growth of new lesions, and persistence or recanalization of a treated lesion.

The successfully occluded PAVM will usually have its aneurysmal sac retract and either disappear or be replaced by a small thrombosed or fibrotic remnant within 6–12 months (Figure 53–16) (102). Rarely, a larger thrombosed sac may remain. Persistence or recurrence occurs in usually no more than 6%, although it was 15% in one series considering only large feeding arteries and, anomalously, 57% in a single small series (1,3,4,102,103,105,113). Persistence or recurrence may be because of recanalization of an occluded vessel, a missed accessory branch (which can grow), collateral reperfusion from the growth or development of small pulmonary artery branches (more likely in children), and/or collateral flow distal to the site of occlusion from bronchial

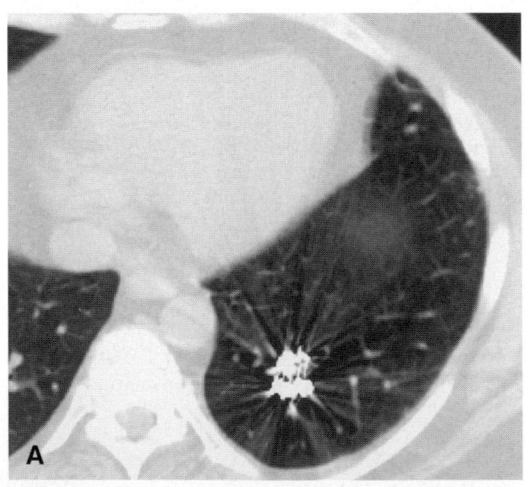
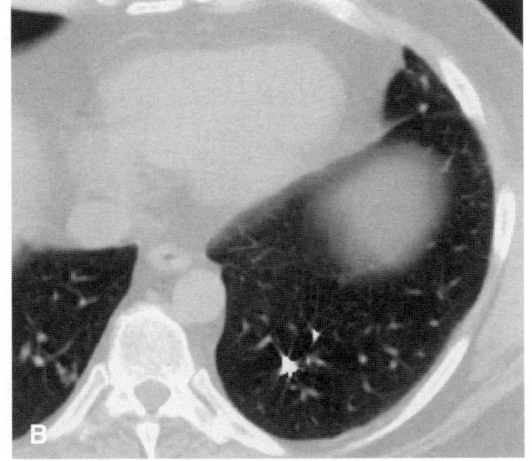
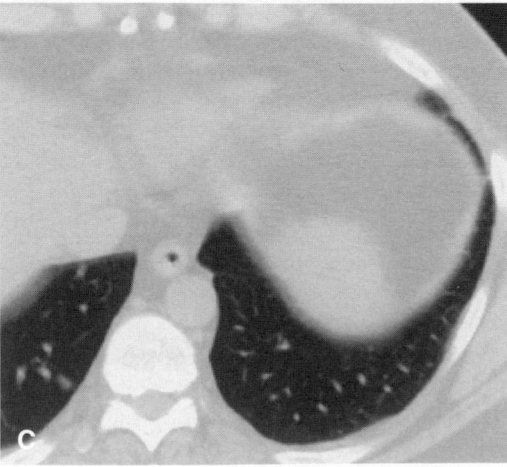

Figure 53–16. CT images 16 months after coil embolization of the simple left lower lobe PAVM shown in Figure 53–8 demonstrate the coils in the artery and disappearance of the sac.

or other systemic arteries. Repeat embolization is effective for managing all these, although it is usually needed only for significantly sized pulmonary branches. Systemic arterial collateral flow represents a small left-to-left shunt that is rarely significant as a cause hemoptysis.

Postembolization surveillance studies are needed to detect persistence or recurrence of a treated lesion at 6–12 months and then every 3–5 years to assess for enlarging, newly significant lesions. Because contrast echocardiography remains positive in most patients after embolization and because it is not a morphological study to begin with, it has little role in this regard (115). Chest radiography lacks sufficient accuracy. Oxygen shunt studies may be helpful (88), but the authors' preferred method rests primarily on helical CT scanning. The treated PAVMs are considered to have resolved if their aneurysms have completely or nearly completely involuted. If any question remains, a blood gas or shunt fraction study to look for any loss in initial improvement can give additional information. Other studies are particularly valuable in patients with multiple lesions, where the CT scan can be confusing. CT scans every 5 years are done to look for growth of small lesions to the size requiring treatment. Earlier evaluation should be considered before pregnancy and possibly in adolescents. If a woman is already pregnant, a study that avoids ionizing radiation may be more appropriate.

Other Treatment

As noted earlier, patients with PAVMs require antibiotic prophylaxis prior to invasive procedures even after embolotherapy, because of residual PAVMs, which may be microscopic (3,5,80,101,115). Although PAVMs can be a source of significant morbidity and even mortality, if a proactive approach of screening, embolotherapy, antibiotic prophylaxis, continued surveillance, and appropriate treatment of other aspects of HHT is used, nearly all patients with PAVM can be managed effectively, with alleviation of symptoms and avoidance of serious sequelae.

REFERENCES

1. White RI Jr, Lynch-Nyhan A, Terry P, et al. Pulmonary arteriovenous malformations: techniques and long-term outcome of embolotherapy. Radiology 1988;169:663–669.
2. Puskas JD, Allen MS, Moncure AC, et al. Pulmonary arteriovenous malformations: therapeutic options [see comments]. Ann Thorac Surg 1993;56:253–257; discussion 257–258.
3. Haitjema TJ, Overtoom TT, Westermann CJ, et al. Embolisation of pulmonary arteriovenous malformations: results and follow up in 32 patients [see comments]. Thorax 1995;50:719–723.
4. Swanson KL, Prakash UB, Stanson AW. Pulmonary arteriovenous fistulas: Mayo Clinic experience, 1982–1997. Mayo Clin Proc 1999;74:671–680.
5. Gupta P, Mordin C, Curtis J, et al. Pulmonary arteriovenous malformations: effect of embolization on right-to-left shunt, hypoxemia, and exercise tolerance in 66 patients. AJR Am J Roentgenol 2002;179:347–355.
6. Burke CM, Safai C, Nelson DP, et al. Pulmonary arteriovenous malformations: a critical update. Am Rev Respir Dis 1986;134:334–339.
7. Fallon MB. Hepatopulmonary syndrome: a good relationship gone bad [see comment]. Gastroenterology 2003;125:1261–1264.
8. Duncan BW, Desai S. Pulmonary arteriovenous malformations after cavopulmonary anastomosis. Ann Thorac Surg 2003;76:1759–1766.
9. Choi SH, Goo JM, Kim HC, et al. Pulmonary arteriovenous fistulas developed after chemotherapy of metastatic choriocarcinoma. AJR Am J Roentgenol 2003;181:1544–1546.
10. Kamei K, Kusumoto K, Suzuki T. Pulmonary amyloidosis with pulmonary arteriovenous fistula. Chest 1989;96:1435–1436.
11. Lundell C, Finck E. Arteriovenous fistulas originating from Rasmussen aneurysms. AJR Am J Roentgenol 1983;140:687–688.
12. Gossage JR, Kanj G. Pulmonary arteriovenous malformations. A state of the art review. Am J Respir Crit Care Med 1998;158:643–661.
13. Kerr A, Sauter D. Acquired traumatic pulmonary arteriovenous fistula: case report. J Trauma 1993;35:484–486.
14. Poterucha JJ, Krowka MJ, Dickson ER, et al. Failure of hepatopulmonary syndrome to resolve after liver transplantation and successful treatment with embolotherapy. Hepatology 1995;21:96–100.
15. Ryu JK, Oh JH. Hepatopulmonary syndrome: angiography and therapeutic embolization. Clin Imaging 2003;27:97–100.
16. Churton T. Multiple aneurysms of pulmonary artery. Br Med J 1897;1:1223.
17. Rhodes CB. Cavernous hemangiomas of lung with secondary polycythemia. JAMA 1938;110:1914–1915.
18. Rendu HJ. Épistaxis répétées chez un sujet porteur de petits angiomes cutanés et muqueux. Gaz Hôp (Paris) 1896;68:1322–1323.
19. Osler W. On a family form of recurring epistaxis, associated with multiple telangiectases of the skin and mucous membranes. Bull Johns Hopkins Hosp 1901;12:333–337.
20. Weber FP. Multiple hereditary developmental angiomata (telangiectases) of the skin and mucous membranes associated with recurring haemorrhages. Lancet 1907;2:160–162.
21. Hanes FM. Multiple hereditary telangiectases causing hemorrhage (hereditary hemorrhagic telangiectasia). Bull Johns Hopkins Hosp 1909;20:63–73.
22. Plauchu H, Bideau A. Épidémiologie et constitution d'un registre de population à propos d'une concentration géographique d'une maladie héréditaire rare. Population 1984;4:765–786.
23. Bideau A, Brunet G, Heyer E, et al. An abnormal concentration of cases of Rendu-Osler disease in the Valserine valley of the French Jura: a genealogical and demographic study. Ann Hum Biol 1992;19:233–247.
24. Guttmacher AE, McKinnon WC, et al. Hereditary hemorrhagic telangiectasia: a disorder in search of the genetics community. Am J Med Genet 1994;52(2):252–253.
25. Kjeldsen AD, Vase P, Green A. Hereditary haemorrhagic telangiectasia: a population-based study of prevalence and mortality in Danish patients. J Intern Med 1999;245:31–39.
26. Dakeishi M, Shioya T, Wada Y, et al. Genetic epidemiology of hereditary hemorrhagic telangiectasia in a local community in the northern part of Japan. Hum Mutat 2002;19:140–148.
27. Westermann CJ, Rosina AF, De Vries V, et al. The prevalence and manifestations of hereditary hemorrhagic telangiectasia in the Afro-Caribbean population of the Netherlands Antilles: a family screening. Am J Med Genet 2003;116A:324–328.
28. Robinson PJ, Phelan PD. Rendu-Osler-Weber syndrome in a 9 year old girl presenting with repeated haemoptysis. Aust Paediatr J 1989;25:248–249.
29. Shovlin CL, Letarte M. Hereditary haemorrhagic telangiectasia and pulmonary arteriovenous malformations: issues in clinical management and review of pathogenic mechanisms. Thorax 1999;54:714–729.
30. Wallace GM, Shovlin CL. A hereditary haemorrhagic telangiectasia family with pulmonary involvement is unlinked to the known HHT genes, endoglin and ALK-1. Thorax 2000;55:685–690.
31. Gallione CJ, Repetto GM, Legius E, et al. A combined syndrome of juvenile polyposis and hereditary haemorrhagic telangiectasia associated with mutations in MADH4 (SMAD4). Lancet 2004;363:852–859.

32. Jacobson BS. Hereditary hemorrhagic telangiectasia: a model for blood vessel growth and enlargement. Am J Pathol 2000;156: 737–742.

33. McDonald MT, Papenberg KA, Ghosh S, et al. A disease locus for hereditary haemorrhagic telangiectasia maps to chromosome 9q33–34. Nat Genet 1994;6:197–204.

34. Shovlin CL, Hughes JM, Tuddenham EG, et al. A gene for hereditary haemorrhagic telangiectasia maps to chromosome 9q3. Nat Genet 1994;6:205–209.

35. McAllister KA, Grogg KM, Johnson DW, et al. Endoglin, a TGF-beta binding protein of endothelial cells, is the gene for hereditary haemorrhagic telangiectasia type 1. Nat Genet 1994;8:345–351.

36. Johnson DW, Berg JN, Gallione CJ, et al. A second locus for hereditary hemorrhagic telangiectasia maps to chromosome 12. Genome Res 1995;5:21–28.

37. Johnson DW, Berg JN, Baldwin MA, et al. Mutations in the activin receptor-like kinase 1 gene in hereditary haemorrhagic telangiectasia type 2. Nat Genet 1996;13:189–195.

38. Abdalla SA, Pece-Barbara N, Vera S, et al. Analysis of ALK-1 and endoglin in newborns from families with hereditary hemorrhagic telangiectasia type 2. Hum Mol Genet 2000;9:1227–1237.

39. Berg JN, Guttmacher AE, Marchuk DA, et al. Clinical heterogeneity in hereditary haemorrhagic telangiectasia: are pulmonary arteriovenous malformations more common in families linked to endoglin? J Med Genet 1996;33:256–257.

40. Berg JN, Gallione CJ, Stenzel TT, et al. The activin receptor-like kinase 1 gene: genomic structure and mutations in hereditary hemorrhagic telangiectasia type 2. Am J Hum Genet 1997;61:60–67.

41. Shovlin CL, Hughes JM, Scott J, et al. Characterization of endoglin and identification of novel mutations in hereditary hemorrhagic telangiectasia. Am J Hum Genet 1997;61:68–79.

42. McDonald JE, Miller FJ, Hallam SE, et al. Clinical manifestations in a large hereditary hemorrhagic telangiectasia (HHT) type 2 kindred. Am J Med Genet 2000;93:320–327.

43. Abdalla SA, Geisthoff UW, Bonneau D, et al. Visceral manifestations in hereditary haemorrhagic telangiectasia type 2. J Med Genet 2003;40:494–502.

44. Berg J, Porteous M, Reinhardt D, et al. Hereditary haemorrhagic telangiectasia: a questionnaire based study to delineate the different phenotypes caused by endoglin and ALK1 mutations. J Med Genet 2003;40:585–590.

45. Trembath RC, Thomson JR, Machado RD, et al. Clinical and molecular genetic features of pulmonary hypertension in patients with hereditary hemorrhagic telangiectasia. N Engl J Med 2001;345:325–334.

46. Shovlin CL, Winstock AR, Peters AM, et al. Medical complications of pregnancy in hereditary haemorrhagic telangiectasia. Q J Med 1995;88:879–887.

47. Bosher LHJ, Blake DA, Byrd BR. An analysis of the pathologic anatomy of pulmonary arteriovenous aneurysms with particular reference to the applicability of local excision. Surgery 1959;45: 91–104.

48. White RI Jr, Mitchell SE, Barth KH, et al. Angioarchitecture of pulmonary arteriovenous malformations: an important consideration before embolotherapy. AJR Am J Roentgenol 1983;140:681–686.

49. White RI Jr, Pollak JS, Wirth JA. Pulmonary arteriovenous malformations: diagnosis and transcatheter embolotherapy. J Vasc Interv Radiol 1996;7:787–804.

50. Saluja S, Henderson KJ, White RI Jr. Embolotherapy in the bronchial and pulmonary circulations. Radiol Clin North Am 2000;38:425–448.

51. Faughnan ME, Lui YW, Wirth JA, et al. Diffuse pulmonary arteriovenous malformations: characteristics and prognosis. Chest 2000;117:31–38.

52. Dines DE, Arms RA, Bernatz PE, Gomes MR. Pulmonary arteriovenous fistulas. Mayo Clin Proc 1974;49:460–465.

53. Vase P, Holm M, Arendrup H. Pulmonary arteriovenous fistulas in hereditary hemorrhagic telangiectasia. Acta Med Scand 1985; 218:105–109.

54. Swinburne AJ, Fedullo AJ, Gangemi R, et al. Hereditary telangiectasia and multiple pulmonary arteriovenous fistulas. Clinical deterioration during pregnancy. Chest 1986;89:459–460.

55. Gammon RB, Miksa AK, Keller FS. Osler-Weber-Rendu disease and pulmonary arteriovenous fistulas. Deterioration and embolotherapy during pregnancy. Chest 1990;98:1522–1524.

56. Laroche CM, Wells F, Shneerson J. Massive hemothorax due to enlarging arteriovenous fistula in pregnancy. Chest 1992;101: 1452–1454.

57. Ference BA, Shannon TM, White RI Jr, et al. Life-threatening pulmonary hemorrhage with pulmonary arteriovenous malformations and hereditary hemorrhagic telangiectasia. Chest 1994; 106:1387–1390.

58. Allen SW, Whitfield JM, Clarke DR, et al. Pulmonary arteriovenous malformation in the newborn: a familial case. Pediatr Cardiol 1993;14:58–61.

59. Pollak Y, Katzen BT, Pollak W. High-output congestive failure in a patient with pulmonary arteriovenous malformations. Cardiol Rev 2002;10:188–192.

60. Ravasse P, Maragnes P, Petit T, et al. Total pneumonectomy as a salvage procedure for pulmonary arteriovenous malformation in a newborn: report of one case. J Pediatr Surg 2003;38:254–255.

61. Baert AL, Casteels-Van Daele M, Broeckx J, et al. Generalized juvenile polyposis with pulmonary arteriovenous malformations and hypertrophic osteoarthropathy. AJR Am J Roentgenol 1983;141:661–662.

62. Moussouttas M, Fayad P, Rosenblatt M, et al. Pulmonary arteriovenous malformations: cerebral ischemia and neurologic manifestations. Neurology 2000;55:959–964.

63. Kjeldsen AD, Oxhoj H, Andersen PE, et al. Prevalence of pulmonary arteriovenous malformations (PAVMs) and occurrence of neurological symptoms in patients with hereditary haemorrhagic telangiectasia (HHT). J Intern Med 2000;248:255–262.

64. Perry WH. Clinical spectrum of hereditary hemorrhagic telangiectasia (Osler-Weber-Rendu disease). Am J Med 1987;82: 989–997.

65. Guttmacher AE, Marchuk DA, White RI Jr. Hereditary hemorrhagic telangiectasia [see comments]. N Engl J Med 1995;333:918–924.

66. AAssar OS, Friedman CM, White RI, Jr. The natural history of epistaxis in hereditary hemorrhagic telangiectasia. Laryngoscope 1991;101:977–980.

67. Porteous ME, Burn J, Proctor SJ. Hereditary haemorrhagic telangiectasia: a clinical analysis. J Med Genet 1992;29:527–530.

68. Haitjema T, Balder W, Disch FJ, et al. Epistaxis in hereditary haemorrhagic telangiectasia. Rhinology 1996;34:176–178.

69. Roman G, Fisher M, Perl DP, et al. Neurological manifestations of hereditary hemorrhagic telangiectasia (Rendu-Osler-Weber disease): report of 2 cases and review of the literature. Ann Neurol 1978;4:130–144.

70. Maher CO, Piepgras DG, Brown RD Jr, et al. Cerebrovascular manifestations in 321 cases of hereditary hemorrhagic telangiectasia. Stroke 2001;32:877–882.

71. Vase P, Grove O. Gastrointestinal lesions in hereditary hemorrhagic telangiectasia. Gastroenterology 1986;91:1079–1083.

72. Plauchu H, de Chadarevian JP, Bideau A, et al. Age-related clinical profile of hereditary hemorrhagic telangiectasia in an epidemiologically recruited population. Am J Med Genet 1989;32:291–297.

73. Sharma VK, Howden CW. Gastrointestinal and hepatic manifestations of hereditary hemorrhagic telangiectasia. Dig Dis 1998; 16:169–174.

74. Kjeldsen AD, Kjeldsen J. Gastrointestinal bleeding in patients with hereditary hemorrhagic telangiectasia. Am J Gastroenterol 2000;95:415–418.

75. Longacre AV, Gross CP, Gallitelli M, et al. Diagnosis and management of gastrointestinal bleeding in patients with hereditary hemorrhagic telangiectasia. Am J Gastroenterol 2003;98:59–65.

76. Reilly PJ, Nostrant TT. Clinical manifestations of hereditary hemorrhagic telangiectasia. Am J Gastroenterol 1984;79:363–367.

77. Buscarini E, Buscarini L, Danesino C, et al. Hepatic vascular malformations in hereditary hemorrhagic telangiectasia: Doppler sonographic screening in a large family. J Hepatol 1997;26:111–118.

78. Garcia-Tsao G, Korzenik JR, Young L, et al. Liver disease in patients with hereditary hemorrhagic telangiectasia. N Eng J Med 2000;343:931–936.

79. Ianora AA, Memeo M, Sabba C, et al. Hereditary hemorrhagic telangiectasia: multi-detector row helical CT assessment of hepatic involvement [see comment]. Radiology 2004;230:250–259.

80. Barzilai B, Waggoner AD, Spessert C, et al. Two-dimensional contrast echocardiography in the detection and follow-up of congenital pulmonary arteriovenous malformations. Am J Cardiol 1991;68:1507–1510.

81. Remy J, Remy-Jardin M, Wattinne L, et al. Pulmonary arteriovenous malformations: evaluation with CT of the chest before and after treatment [see comments]. Radiology 1992;182:809–816.
82. Haitjema T, Disch F, Overtoom TT, et al. Screening family members of patients with hereditary hemorrhagic telangiectasia. Am J Med 1995;99:519–524.
83. Kjeldsen AD, Oxhoj H, Andersen PE, et al. Pulmonary arteriovenous malformations: screening procedures and pulmonary angiography in patients with hereditary hemorrhagic telangiectasia. Chest 1999;116:432–439.
84. Thompson RD, Jackson J, Peters AM, et al. Sensitivity and specificity of radioisotope right-left shunt measurements and pulse oximetry for the early detection of pulmonary arteriovenous malformations. Chest 1999;115:109–113.
85. Oxhoj H, Kjeldsen AD, Nielsen G. Screening for pulmonary arteriovenous malformations: contrast echocardiography versus pulse oximetry. Scand Cardiovasc J 2000;34:281–285.
86. Nanthakumar K, Graham AT, Robinson TI, et al. Contrast echocardiography for detection of pulmonary arteriovenous malformations. Am Heart J 2001;141:243–246.
87. Whyte MK, Peters AM, Hughes JM, et al. Quantification of right to left shunt at rest and during exercise in patients with pulmonary arteriovenous malformations. Thorax 1992;47:790–796.
88. Gossage JR. The role of echocardiography in screening for pulmonary arteriovenous malformations [comment]. Chest 2003;123:320–322.
89. Remy J, Remy-Jardin M, Giraud F, et al. Angioarchitecture of pulmonary arteriovenous malformations: clinical utility of three-dimensional helical CT [see comments]. Radiology 1994;191:657–664.
90. Cirimelli KM, Colletti PM, Beck S. Metastatic choriocarcinoma simulating an arteriovenous malformation on chest radiography and dynamic CT. J Comput Assist Tomogr 1988;12:317–319.
91. Khalil A, Farres MT, Mangiapan G, et al. Pulmonary arteriovenous malformations. Diagnosis by contrast-enhanced magnetic resonance angiography. Chest 2000;117:1399–1403.
92. Maki DD, Siegelman ES, Roberts DA, et al. Pulmonary arteriovenous malformations: three-dimensional gadolinium-enhanced MR angiography—initial experience. Radiology 2001;219:243–246.
93. Ohno Y, Hatabu H, Takenaka D, et al. Contrast-enhanced MR perfusion imaging and MR angiography: utility for management of pulmonary arteriovenous malformations for embolotherapy. Eur J Radiol 2002;41:136–146.
94. Pennington DW, Gold WM, Gordon RL, et al. Treatment of pulmonary arteriovenous malformations by therapeutic embolization. Rest and exercise physiology in eight patients. Am Rev Respir Dis 1992;145:1047–1051.
95. Haitjema T, ten Berg JM, Overtoom TT, et al. Unusual complications after embolization of a pulmonary arteriovenous malformation. Chest 1996;109:1401–1404.
96. Rosenblatt M, Pollak JS, Fayad PB, et al. Pulmonary arteriovenous malformations: what size should be treated to prevent embolic stroke (abstr)? Radiology 1992;185(P):134 (see also Radiology 1993;186:937 [RSNA 1992 meeting notes]).
97. Shenstone NS. Experiences with total pneumonectomy. J Thorac Surg 1942;11:405–423.
98. Dines DE, Seward JB, Bernatz PE. Pulmonary arteriovenous fistulas. Mayo Clin Proc 1983;58:176–181.
99. Reynaud-Gaubert M, Thomas P, Gaubert JY, et al. Pulmonary arteriovenous malformations: lung transplantation as a therapeutic option. Eur Respir J 1999;14:1425–1428.
100. Portsmann W. Therapeutic embolization of arteriovenous pulmonary fistula by catheter technique. In: Kelop O, ed. Current Concepts in Pediatric Radiology. Berlin: Springer, 1977;23–31.
101. Dutton JA, Jackson JE, Hughes JM, et al. Pulmonary arteriovenous malformations: results of treatment with coil embolization in 53 patients. AJR Am J Roentgenol 1995;165:1119–1125.
102. Lee DW, White RI Jr, Egglin TK, et al. Embolotherapy of large pulmonary arteriovenous malformations: long-term results. Ann Thorac Surg 1997;64:930–939; discussion 939–940.
103. Saluja S, Sitko I, Lee DW, et al. Embolotherapy of pulmonary arteriovenous malformations with detachable balloons: long-term durability and efficacy. J Vasc Interv Radiol 1999;10:883–889.
104. Wispelaere JF, Trigaux JP, Weynants P, et al. Systemic supply to a pulmonary arteriovenous malformation: potential explanation for recurrence. Cardiovasc Intervent Radiol 1996;19:285–287.
105. Sagara K, Miyazono N, Inoue H, et al. Recanalization after coil embolotherapy of pulmonary arteriovenous malformations: study of long-term outcome and mechanism for recanalization. AJR Am J Roentgenol 1998;170:727–730.
106. Coley SC, Jackson JE. Endovascular occlusion with a new mechanical detachable coil. AJR Am J Roentgenol 1998;171:1075–1079.
107. Pugash RA. Pulmonary arteriovenous malformations: overview and transcatheter embolotherapy. Can Assoc Radiol J 2001;52:92–102; quiz 74–76.
108. Takahashi K, Tanimura K, Honda M, et al. Venous sac embolization of pulmonary arteriovenous malformation: preliminary experience using interlocking detachable coils. Cardiovasc Intervent Radiol 1999;22:210–213.
109. Dinkel HP, Triller J. Pulmonary arteriovenous malformations: embolotherapy with superselective coaxial catheter placement and filling of venous sac with Guglielmi detachable coils. Radiology 2002;223:709–714.
110. Coley SC, Jackson JE. Venous sac embolization of pulmonary arteriovenous malformations in two patients. AJR Am J Roentgenol 1996;167:452–454.
111. Tal MG, Saluja S, Henderson KJ, et al. Vein of Galen technique for occluding the aneurysmal sac of pulmonary arteriovenous malformations. J Vasc Interv Radiol 2002;13:1261–1264.
112. Gershon AS, Faughnan ME, Chon KS, et al. Transcatheter embolotherapy of maternal pulmonary arteriovenous malformations during pregnancy. Chest 2001;119:470–477.
113. Remy-Jardin M, Wattinne L, Remy J. Transcatheter occlusion of pulmonary arterial circulation and collateral supply: failures, incidents, and complications [see comments]. Radiology 1991;180:699–705.
114. Mager HJ, Overtoom TT, Mauser HW, et al. Early cerebral infarction after embolotherapy of a pulmonary arteriovenous malformation. J Vasc Interv Radiol 2001;12:122–123.
115. Lee WL, Graham AF, Pugash RA, et al. Contrast echocardiography remains positive after treatment of pulmonary arteriovenous malformations [comment]. Chest 2003;123:351–358.

Management of Chylothorax

54

Constantin Cope

The development of chylothorax is a serious and often life-threatening event that requires prompt, decisive treatment if significant morbidity and mortality is to be avoided. Early attempts in the 1930s and 1940s to control this condition, which had more than a 50% mortality rate, met with little success; these included low-fat diet, readministration of chyle via intravenous, nasogastric, and rectal routes, the use of therapeutic pneumothorax, and local irradiation (1).

Following Lampson's demonstration in 1948 (2) that traumatic chylothorax could be controlled or cured by direct ligation of the thoracic duct (TD), this operation became the standard therapy for treating high-output chylothorax and had a 90% probability of correcting the problem (3,4). Open-chest TD ligation can be associated with serious complications in patients who are already debilitated from recent thoracic surgery or severe trauma and/or in whom there is delay in replacing fluid and protein losses. There was, for example, an 11.8% mortality rate in a series of 51 patients who had TD ligation performed for chylothorax complicating esophagectomy (5). Surgery can be put off in some patients with lower daily chyle output with the hope that the TD fistula will close spontaneously with intensive medical support, but this measure can be counterproductive if corrective surgery is unduly delayed in the face of progressive metabolic, nutritional, and septic complications associated with continued major loss of chylous fluid.

A minimally invasive percutaneous procedure (Figure 54–1) was recently developed that permits effective embolization of the TD fistula through the abdomen (Figure 54–1) using standard radiological catheter techniques (6,7,8,9); the author's results demonstrate that this benign procedure is curative in a high percentage of patients with chylothorax and can be used as soon as the diagnosis is made, without the need for a trial period of intensive medical treatment. (6).

ANATOMY AND FUNCTION OF THE THORACIC DUCT

The following aspects of basic anatomy and function of the thoracic duct are important because they relate to the percutaneous management of chylothorax. (Consult Chapter 76, Thoracic Duct, in *Abrams' Angiography*, 4th Ed., vol. 2 for greater details.) The cisterna chyli (CC), which represents a convenient target for transabdominal puncture and catheter access to the TD, most commonly overlies the first or second lumbar vertebra in the midline, posteromedial to the abdominal aorta. Some 95% of lymph reaching the CC is derived from the gastrointestinal tract and the liver (10). The configuration and size of the CC seen on lymphographic studies is quite variable, with diameters ranging between 2 mm to more than 16 mm (11) and an average in the author's experience of 3–6 mm (Figures 54–2 and 54–3A).

A recognizable CC may be absent in 64% of cases studied lymphangiographically (12) or in 50% at necropsy (13). When it is not developed, it is replaced by lymphatic trunks 1–2 mm in diameter or a proximal extension of the thoracic duct, which itself can be split into bifid or trifid ducts. Many patients who have undergone major abdominal surgery or trauma may be found to have major lymphatic obstruction above the L3 level, the cisterna chyli and proximal thoracic duct then being bypassed by multiple tiny lymphatic collaterals, which serve to reconstitute the central or cephalad part of the thoracic duct (6).

The TD is a 2–6-mm-wide, thin-walled valved duct that originates either from the cisterna chyli or retroperitoneal lymph trunks anywhere between the T10 and L3 levels; it ascends in the midline through the aortic hiatus between the descending aorta and the azygos vein and remains in close relationship to the dorsal aspect of the esophagus.

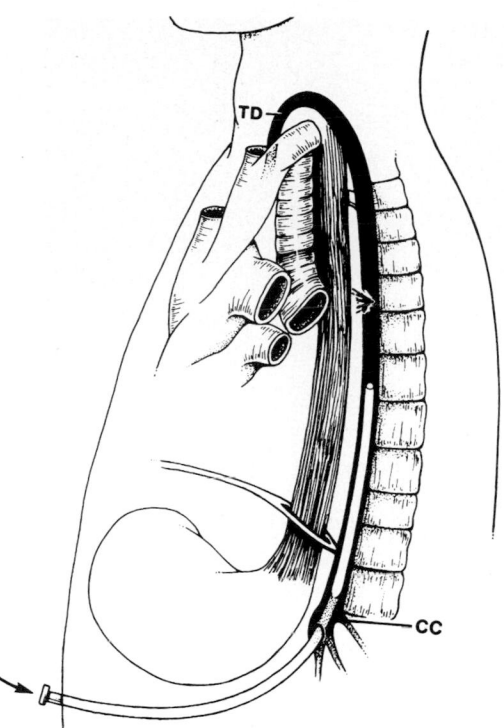

Figure 54–1 Transabdominal catheterization of the thoracic duct (TD) through the cisterna chyli (CC). Note the intimate association of the esophagus to the TD. Drawing not to scale. (Reprinted with permission from Cope C, Kaiser LR. Management of unremitting chylothorax by percutaneous embolization and blockage of retroperitoneal lymphatic vessels in 42 patients. J Vasc Interv Radiol, 2002;13:1141.)

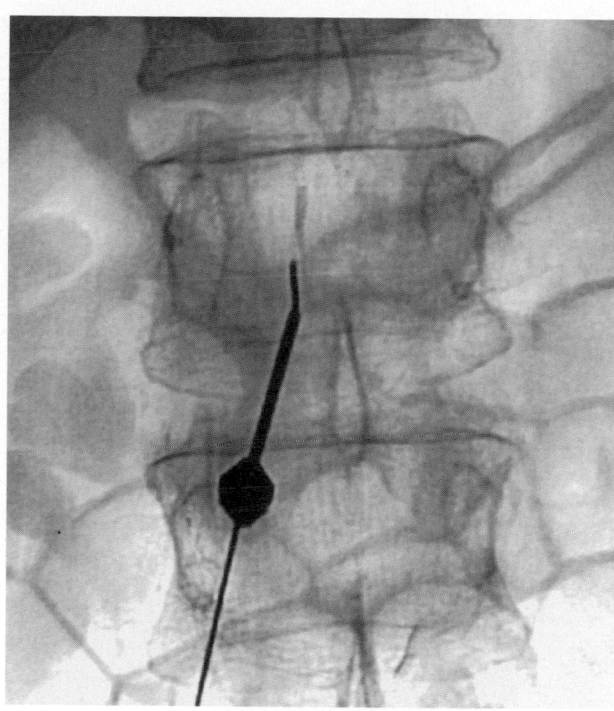

Figure 54–2 A small 1.5–2-mm-wide lymphographically opacified cisterna chyli overlying the first lumbar vertebra was successfully needled and catheterized through a stiff intraperitoneal cannula.

After swinging over from the right to the left side of the mediastinum at the T5–6 levels, it forms a supraclavicular loop before entering a large neck vein either as a single trunk or commonly via multiple trunks in a delta formation (14,15). In addition to its main anastomosis to a great neck vein, the duct has throughout its course many small branch connections to the azygos, intercostal, and small mediastinal veins, which can open up to decompress the TD when it becomes occluded.

Retrograde percutaneous catheterization of the TD through the jugular or subclavian veins is not possible because its terminal orifice is jealously guarded by semilunar valves. Although it was possible for Seeliger (16) to visualize and catheterize the lymphovenous TD opening in animals with the use of a rigid angioscope inserted through the external jugular vein, he was unable to retrogradely catheterize the duct much beyond its terminal valve.

The close association of the duct to the esophagus, aorta, and left internal mammary artery (LIMA) makes it especially vulnerable to accidental surgical lacerations when esophagectomy, aneurysm repair, and coronary artery bypass (CABG) using a LIMA are performed, respectively. Anatomical variations of the thoracic duct are common (11). In one postmortem series of more than 1,000 subjects (17), it was found that in 38% of cases, the duct was split into two or more branches that looped back to reconnect with the duct over one to six vertebral body lengths. Rare cases of more extensive doubling of the duct and of left-sided ducts have also been reported (13). Overlooking these anatomical variations by failing to find or securely ligate one or both limbs of a segmental duct loop is a common cause of failure in the surgical treatment of chylothoraces (3).

Functionally, the primary role of the TD is to deliver digestive fat, extravascular plasma proteins, and lymphocytes into the bloodstream (Table 54–1). The basal flow of chyle can increase 10-fold after a meal (18). Although the normal daily chyle output is in the range of 1.5–2.5 liters, it is not unusual to observe high chest tube outputs of more than 1.9–27 liters per day in some debilitated patients with chylothorax (19).

With continued high chyle output there is major depletion of protein and T cells, losses which are poorly tolerated because they cannot be easily replaced parenterally (20). The normal fluid pressure of the TD ranges from 10–28 cm of water; it is developed mainly through spontaneous rhythmic contractions of the proximal duct to assure intermittent chyle flow into the lower-pressured neck veins. After surgical ligation of the thoracic duct, pressures below the tie can temporarily rise to as high as 40 mm Hg (21).

CHYLOTHORAX: ETIOLOGY AND DIAGNOSIS

The incidence of posttraumatic chylothorax is in the range of 0.1–0.4%. Chylothorax arises as a result of erosion, rupture, or laceration of the thoracic duct or one of its branches with leakage of chyle into the pleural cavity. If the mediastinal pleura remains intact following TD laceration, chyle

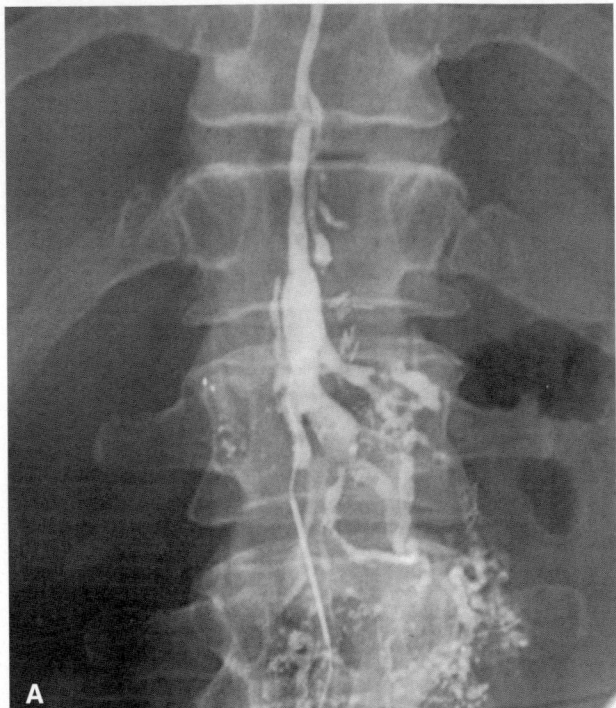

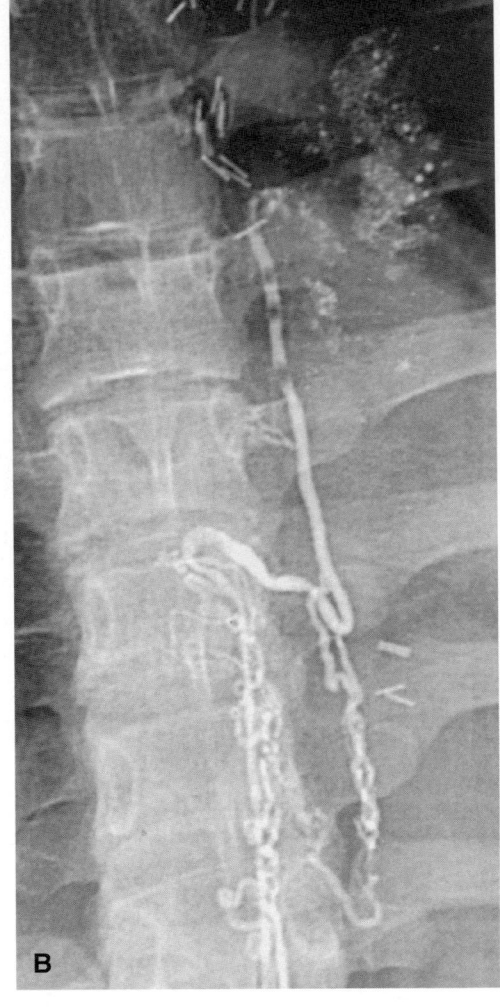

Figure 54–3 High-output chylothorax (1,200 mL/day) following resection of an upper-lobe cancer in a 39-year-old woman. **A.** Percutaneous transabdominal catheterization of a large 11-mm-wide preopacified cisterna chyli. **B.** Opacification of the TD with aqueous contrast medium shows splitting of the mid-duct with its reconstitution in the left mediastinum. There is contrast extravasation into the left pleural cavity from a traumatic fistula in the distal TD. After TD embolization, the chyle output ceased in 3 days.

accumulates locally in the mediastinum, which may initially remain asymptomatic. Chylothorax may subsequently occur after a latent period of days to weeks following the initial event if the chyloma bursts through the pleura. Once a high-output chylopleural fistula is well established, it will usually not close spontaneously. The etiology of chylothorax can be congenital, traumatic, operative, neoplastic, and miscellaneous. In a review of 191 patients with chylothorax, 72% were of nontraumatic origin, with 37% being malignancies (mostly lymphomas), 26% idiopathic, and the rest consisting of miscellaneous conditions (22).

Traumatic chylothorax found in 28% of the author's series was usually related to intrathoracic surgical procedures, esophagectomy having the highest reported incidence of more than 3%, followed by aortic surgery. Chylothorax is becoming more common following CABG as a result of injury of the terminal TD following manipulations of the adjoining left internal mammary artery.

Patients with chylothorax usually present with a history of recent onset of pleuritic pain and/or dyspnea. They demonstrate uni- or bilateral pleural effusions on chest radiographs. Some patients give a history of having undergone repeated thoracenteses over several months without having had a clear diagnosis made. The diagnosis of chylothorax (21,23) is made by examination of pleural fluid for chyle (Table 54–1). The color of the pleural fluid, which can vary from a characteristic creamy white to a nonspecific pinkish yellow, depends on the amount of fat absorbed from recent meals. A chylous effusion is characterized by a high triglyceride level of more than 110 mg/dL, the presence of chylomicra by lipoprotein electrophoresis, and a normal cholesterol titer (21). The diagnosis can be difficult to make in poorly nourished, debilitated patients who are already on total parenteral nutrition (TPN) and have normal triglyceride levels; an oral fat challenge may help make the diagnosis in these cases. Pedal lymphography is a useful procedure to determine preoperatively the presence and the site of a chyle fistula (24). It has been suggested that a conservative approach to the treatment of chylothorax may be chosen if this test fails to demonstrate chyle leakage.

TABLE 54-1
CHARACTERISTICS AND COMPOSITION OF CHYLE (21,32)

Properties	Fats	Proteins	Cells
Yellow to milky Alkaline	0.4–6 gm/dL	2–5 gm/dL	Lymphocytes: 400–6, 800/mm^3 80% T cells
Sterile Bacteriostatic	Chylomicrons Triglycerides 50–110 mg/dL Cholesterol 65–220 mg/dL	Alb/glob 3:1 Fibrinogen 50–280 mg/dL Clotting time 10–25 min	RBC: 50–600/ mm^3 Platelets: none

NONSURGICAL MANAGEMENT OF CHYLOTHORAX

When nonoperative conservative management of chylothorax is successful, in many patients chyle output can abate completely, with cure occurring within a few days. In other cases, there may be an initial significant decrease in chyle output, but complete resolution may not occur for another 2–4 weeks. Low-output fistula can, however, be well tolerated for this period of time with proper dietary measures.

Conservative medical management combined with some of the following minimally invasive procedures may render the treatment of high-output or unremitting chylothorax by open chest TD ligation unnecessary.

1. *Supportive treatment:* The management of chylothorax depends on the magnitude of daily chyle output and the clinical condition of the patient. Patients who require weekly to monthly thoracentesis can be managed on an outpatient basis with the expectation that the lympho-pleural fistula will heal on a low-fat diet consisting of medium-chain triglycerides (21). Radiation therapy can be effective in patients with lymphoma. Vasoconstrictors (25) and transjugular intrahepatic portosystemic shunts (26) have also been successfully used in a few cases. Patients with chylothoraces who fail outpatient management or have an output of more than 300 mL/day should be hospitalized for tube thoracostomy to maintain lung expansion and for institution of total TPN to decrease chyle flow and pressure within the TD.

2. *Somatostatin:* Somatostatin by intravenous infusion has been shown experimentally to decrease thoracic chyle fistula drainage; numerous anecdotal reports exist of clinical success in patients who were treated with this drug, but these successes have usually occurred in patients with low-output chylothorax who were already on TPN (27).

3. *Pleurodesis:* Pleurodesis with talc is commonly performed with some success in patients with persistent low-output chylothorax who have failed to respond to low-fat diet, multiple thoracenteses, or thoracostomy tube drainage. It should be used only in patients without sepsis and in whom the lung is capable of full expansion. It can be easily performed by instilling a slurry of 10 gm of sterile talc suspended in 250 mL of saline through the thoracostomy tube (28).

4. *Percutaneous transabdominal thoracic duct embolization:* Percutaneous antegrade TD catheter embolization by a transabdominal approach has been shown to be safe and effective in animals (29) and clinically. The technique, which is performed under local anesthesia and conscious sedation, has been described in detail previously (6). Essentially, it consists of percutaneously puncturing and catheterizing the cisterna chyli or retroperitoneal lymphatic trunks under fluoroscopy as they become opacified during pedal lymphography at the level of the first and second lumbar vertebrae (Figure 54–3A). A blunt-tipped cannula is initially inserted under local anesthesia below the xyphoid into the peritoneal cavity to serve as a stiff guide for better directional control of coaxial 22–21 gauge puncturing needles; this cannula is especially useful in patients who are obese or who have small lymphatic trunks below 2 mm in diameter (Figure 54–2); in thin patients, a "skinny" needle can be used without cannula support. Once successfully punctured, the lymph duct is catheterized over a hydromer-coated 0.018-in guide wire with a 3F microcatheter (Figures 54–3B and 54–4) or a short 4F catheter tapered to 0.018 in and stiffened with a cannula (Cook Inc.). It is important to opacify the infra- and supradiaphragmatic lymphatic channels before embolization to visualize the level of the TD fistula and to look for possible TD anomalous divisions and branches; parallel chains of small collateral lymphatics feeding the fistula from the abdomen can be easily overlooked (Figure 54–5). Occlusion of the TD is performed above the diaphragm and below the TD fistula using microcoils, microparticles, and glue in some combination. (Figures 54–3B and 54–6). Some patients with a high-output chylothorax were successfully treated by embolization, even though a chylous TD leak could not be identified by direct intraductal injection of aqueous contrast medium (Figure 54–7).

Two early cases had recurrent chylothorax resulting from TD recanalization following TD embolization with coils alone or combined with embolic particles. There have been no further failures since the author has switched to the use of glue (TruFill n-BCA; Cordis) to

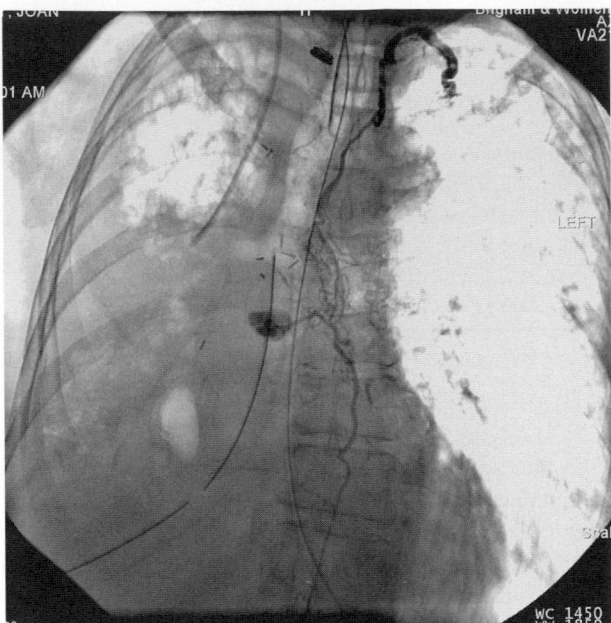

Figure 54–4 Thoracic duct leak following right lower lobe resection. Leak was successfully treated by microcoil embolization.

embolize the TD either alone or below 1–2 previously placed microcoils (Figure 54–8). As the catheter is pulled back during the injection, the glue will not only fill the TD up to the fistula level, but also can be made to flow in a

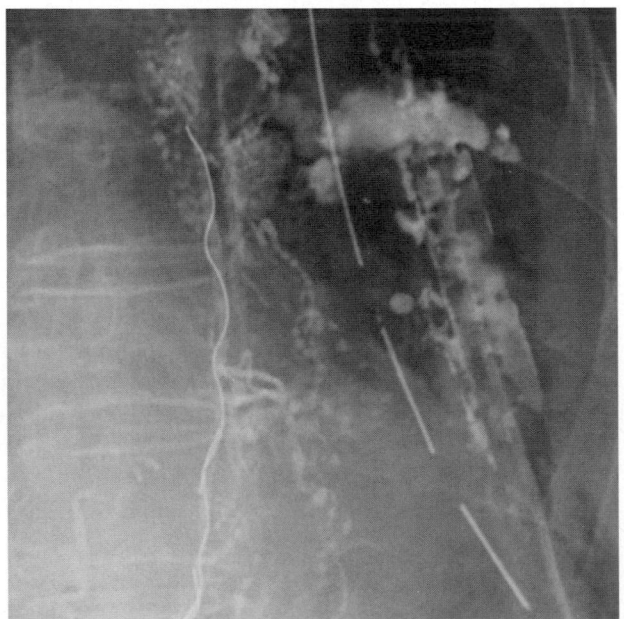

Figure 54–5 High-output chylothorax (800 mL/day) 3 weeks postthoracic aneurysm repair in a 76-year-old woman with partial embolization failure. She had failed pleurodesis. The TD was embolized with complex microcoils and 500–800 particles to accomplish stasis to the level of the large chyle leak seen overlying the chest tube. The chylothorax fluid output, however, did not resolve for more than 2 weeks because the system of lymphatic collateral vessels coursing parallel to the TD were not occluded and continued to feed the TD fistula.

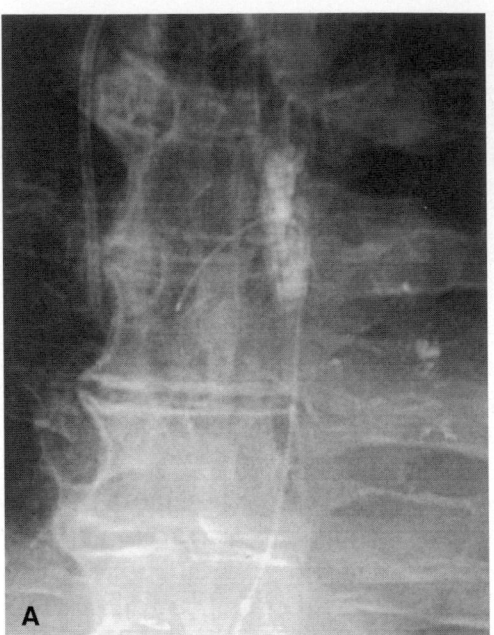

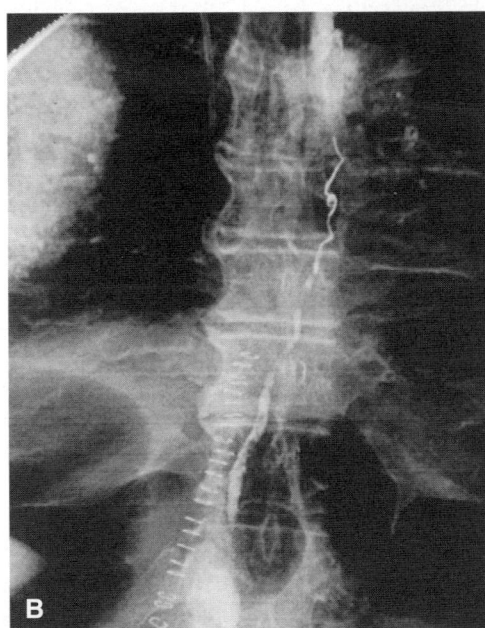

Figure 54–6 High-output right chylothorax (1,700 mL/day) 10 days following esophagectomy with gastric pull-up for cancer in a 57-year-old man. **A.** The large TD fistula is opacified and crossed by the 3 French catheter into the pleural cavity at the level of the T 5-6 thoracic vertebrae. **B.** The TD was embolized with two 5- × 50-mm complex coils and 1 mL of glue; note the contrast accumulation from the TD leak in the pleural cavity. The chest tube chyle output ceased in 2–3 days.

retrograde direction below the microcatheter insertion site; this is especially useful for occluding collateral lymph trunks that may arise below the level of the cisterna chyli and that feed the chyle fistula alone or in addition to the TD.

5. *Percutaneous transabdominal disruption of lymphatic collateral channels:* In 30% of patients in whom there was

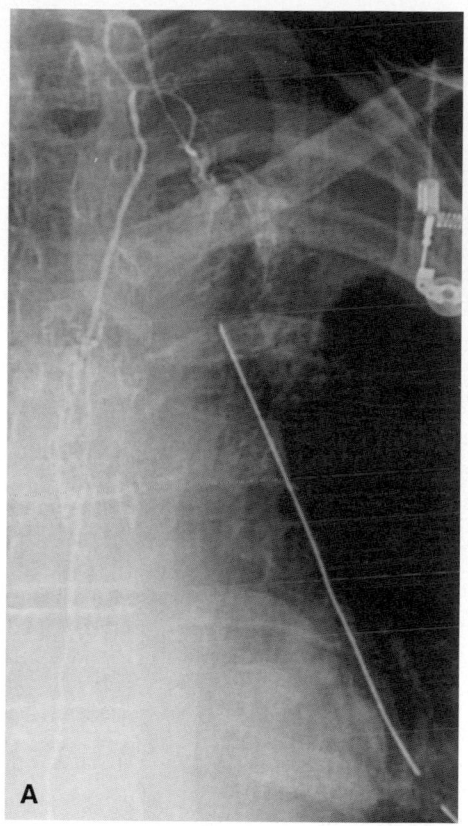

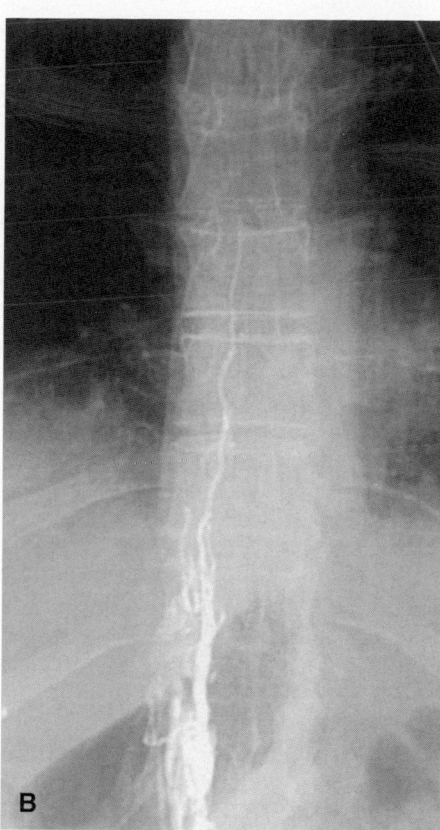

Figure 54–7 Increasing shortness of breath in the previous 4 months in a 69-year-old woman who was treated 2 years prior to admission for small-cell carcinoma with chemotherapy and x-ray therapy; chest tube output of white creamy chyle was 1,500 mL/day. **A.** There is no evidence of TD fistulous leak despite good duct catheter opacification with aqueous contrast medium. **B.** The TD was embolized with one 5- × 60-mm coil and 1 mL of glue; there was complete cessation of chyle output within 3 days.

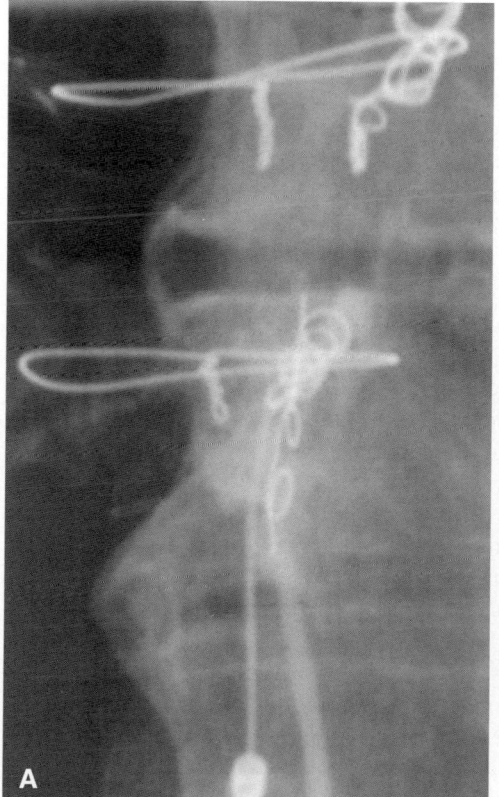

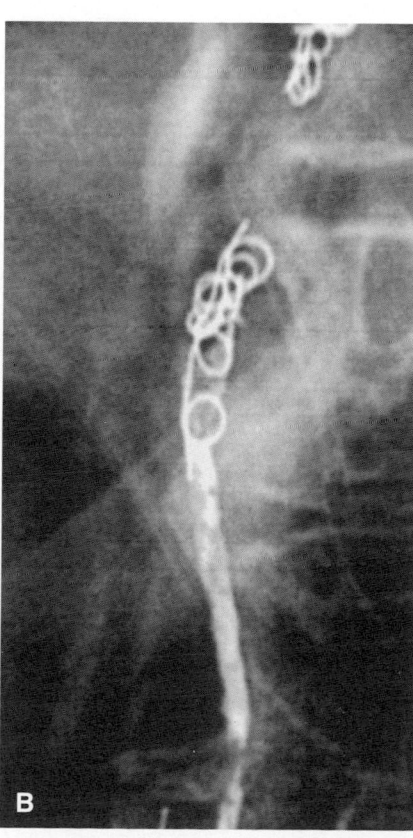

Figure 54–8 Persistent left chylothorax requiring thoracentesis at 3–4 weeks in a 61-year-old male following cardiac transplant performed 2 years prior to admission, despite two prior TD embolizations with coils and particles. **A.** Catheterization of the TD at the T12 vertebral level was performed using previously inserted coils as a target for transabdominal puncture. Antegrade flow of contrast medium was seen to pass through the recanalized coils under fluoroscopy; the proximal TD also showed retrograde opacification. **B.** There was complete TD occlusion following injection of 1 mL of glue. There was no further recurrence of the chylothorax.

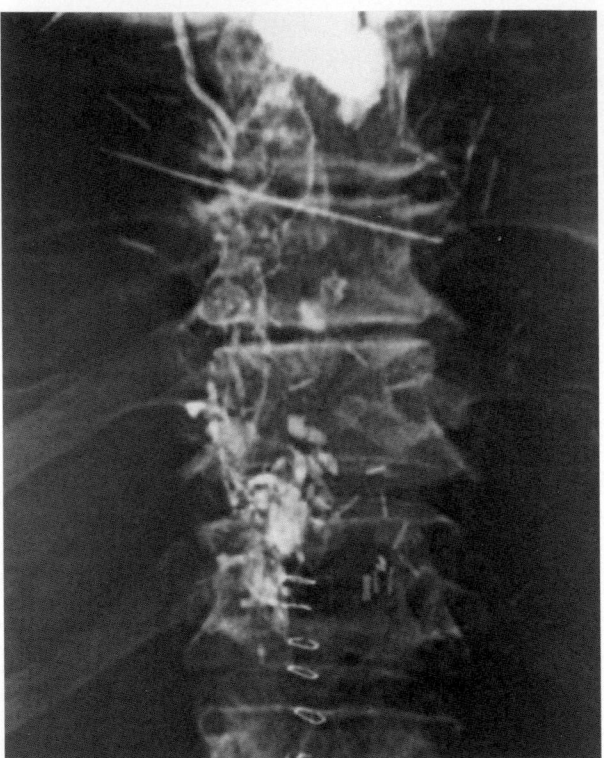

Figure 54–9 High-output bilateral chylothorax (1 L/day) following esophagectomy and subsequent ineffective TD ligation in a 60-year-old man. Lymphography demonstrates that the previously ligated TD has been replaced by small collateral lymphatic vessels that feed a site of massive contrast extravasation in the lower mediastinum. Following percutaneous needle lymphatic vessel disruption there was cessation of chyle output at 3 days from the left chest and 6 days from the right.

absence of retroperitoneal trunks large enough to be catheterized because of previous abdominal surgery or developmental anomalies, it was still possible in some cases to cure the chylothorax by needle disruption of small lymphatic channels that were feeding the TD fistula (Figure 54–9). This was performed as above through the directional peritoneal cannula with 21- or 22-gauge needles armed with a Chiba tip or Franseen multipronged point. After accurately inserting the needle tip into the opacified lymphatic channel under fluoroscopic guidance, it was repeatedly rotated back and forth to occlude, perforate, or break up the channel; this procedure was repeated to occlude other neighboring feeding lymphatic channels. This simple technique led to a 40% favorable response rate.

RESULTS

The author treated 53 patients with unremitting or high-output chylothorax who had initially been scheduled for possible thoracic duct ligation between 1998 and 2003 (Table 54–2). This technique provided a 100% prompt or

delayed cure rate in the treatment of chylothorax following pulmonary–thoracic surgery, CABG, and esophagectomy. There was, however, a lower overall 75% cure or partial cure rate in the treatment of chylothorax associated with aortic surgery, severe trauma, lymphoma, and systemic medical diseases; this resulted mostly from inability to cannulate the TD when the retroperitoneal lymphatic trunks could not be opacified because of occlusion by disease or by previous surgical eradication of retroperitoneal lymphatic channels.

There was no significant procedural morbidity as a result of percutaneous transabdominal TD embolization or retroperitoneal lymphatic vessel disruption in any treated patients, despite the possible transgression of fine needles and catheters through interposed vessels and viscera. Although leakage of chyle from retroperitoneal ducts following needle disruption or removal of catheters was expected, none of the patients developed clinically obvious chylous ascites. Of the 13 patients (24%) who failed percutaneous interventional treatment, seven (13%) underwent successful surgical TD ligation, and six (11%), who were considered inoperable, died within 1–3 weeks of surgical complications or from their primary disease.

DISCUSSION AND FUTURE DEVELOPMENTS

The author's findings indicate that percutaneous transabdominal lymphatic blockage for interventional management of high-output chylothorax is an effective procedure that can be performed safely, even in gravely ill patients. Because this procedure can be performed as soon as the diagnosis of high-output chylothorax is made, it can obviate potential severe metabolic complications that can occur when surgical TD ligation is unduly delayed because of hesitation in reoperating on patients who are severely debilitated. There exists also the possibility of even further complications when the operator fails to control the chyle fistula because of inability to isolate the duct either surgically or thoracoscopically (30) because of postoperative fibrosis, pleural adhesions, or TD anomalies.

Many interventionists have been discouraged from using this technique because of the long procedural time required to perform pedal lymphography. Other imaging modes need to be developed to simplify the procedure. The cisterna chyli can be identified by MRI when it is well developed, but unfortunately, this occurs in less than 50% of cases; when present, it can be punctured transabdominally and catheterized under fluoroscopy using the MR image as an accurate reference map without the need for lymphography (R Baum, *personal communication*, 2003). The procedure could probably also be performed in real time using an open magnet setup. It is also possible that the cisterna chyli or large lymphatic trunks could be potentially imaged and catheterized under the guidance of suitably placed ultrasound transducers in the inferior vena cava or the abdominal aorta, or within the peritoneal cavity.

TABLE 54–2

RESULTS FOLLOWING PERCUTANEOUS TRANSABDOMINAL LYMPHATIC BLOCKAGE IN 53 PATIENTS WITH CHYLOTHORAX

Chylothorax Etiology	Number of Patients	Cures by Selective TD Embolization	Cures by Lymphatic Needling	Percutaneous Rx Failures
Lung–Chest Surgery	10	9	1	0
Lobectomy, n = 7 Rib resection, n = 1 Thyroidectomy, n = 1 Node biopsy, n = 1				
Cardiac Surgery	9	4	4	1
CABG, n = 5 Transplant, n = 2 Atrial myxoma, n = 1 Pericardiectomy, n = 1				
Esophagectomy	12	9	1	2
Trauma	3	1	1	1
Aortic Surgery	5	2	0	3
Nonpenetrating	14	7	1	6
Unknown etiology, n = 4 Behcet's disease, n = 2 Sarcoidosis, n = 1 Cirrhosis, n = 1 Pleuropericardial, n = 1 Lymphoma, n = 5				
Total	**53**	**32**	**8**	**13**

SUMMARY

The management of high-output chylothorax by percutaneous transabominal technique has become in the author's institution the first line of treatment in severely debilitated patients because it is safer than surgical TD ligation and, if successful, can obviate the need for long, expensive hospital stays needed for recuperation.

REFERENCES

1. Sieczka EM, Harvey JC. Early thoracic duct ligation for post operative chylothorax. J Surg Oncol 1996;61:56–60.
2. Lampson RS. Traumatic chylothorax: a review of the literature and report of a case treated by mediastinal ligation of the thoracic duct. J Thorac Surg 1948;17:778–781.
3. Cerfolio RJ, Allen MS, Deschamps C, et al. Post operative chylothorax. J Thorac Cardiovasc Surg 1996;112:1361–1365.
4. Merrigan BA, Winter DC, O'Sullivan CO. Chylothorax. Br J Surg 1997;84:15–20.
5. Merigliano S, Molena D, Ruol A, et al. Chylothorax complicating esophagectomy for cancer: a plea for early thoracic duct ligation. J Thorac Cardiovasc Surg 2002;119:453–457.
6. Cope C, Kaiser LR. Management of unremitting chylothorax by percutaneous embolization and blockage of retroperitoneal lymphatic vessels in 42 patients. J Vasc Interv Radiol 2002;13:1139–1148.
7. Hoffer EK, Bloch RD, Mulligan MS, et al. Treatment of chylothorax by percutaneous catheterization and embolization of the thoracic duct. AJR Am J Roentgenol 2001;176:1040–1042.
8. Bonn J, Sperling D, Walinsky P, et al. Percutaneous embolization of thoracic duct injury. Circulation 2000;102:268–269.
9. Schild H, Hirner A. Percutaneous translymphatic thoracic duct embolization for treatment of chylothorax. Rofo 2001;173:580–582.
10. Shimizu K, Yoshida J, Nishimura M. Treatment strategy for chylothorax after pulmonary resection and lymph node dissection for lung cancer. J Thorac Cardiovasc Surg 2002;124:499–502.
11. Wirth W, Frommhold H. Thoracic duct and its variations. Lymphographic studies. Fortschr Geb Rontgenstr Nuclearmed 1970;112:450–459.
12. Pomerantz M, Herdt JR, Rockoff SD, et al. Evaluation of the functional anatomy of the thoracic duct by lymphangiography. J Thorac Cardiovasc Surg 1963;46:568–575.
13. Davis HK. A statistical study of the thoracic duct in man. Amer J Anat 1915;17:211–216.

14. Shimada K, Sato I. Morphological and histological analysis of the thoracic duct at the jugulo-subclavian junction in Japanese cadavers. Clin Anat 1997;10:163–167.

15. Pflug J, Calnan J. The valves of the thoracic duct at the angulus venosus. Brit J Surg 1968;55:911–916.

16. Seeliger, Witte MH, Witte CL. Thoracic duct cannulation via a transjugular endoscope (lymphoscope) in the dog. Endoscopy 1981; 13:36–39.

17. Van Pernis PA. Variations of the thoracic duct. Surgery 1949;26: 806–809.

18. Crandall LA Jr, Barker SB, Graham DG. A study of the lymph flow from a patient with thoracic duct fistula. Gastroenterology 1943;1:1040–1048.

19. Le Pimpec-Barthes F, D'Atellis N, Dujon A, et al. Chylothorax complicating pulmonary resection. Ann Thorac Surg 2002;73: 1714–1719.

20. Vallieres E, Karmy-Jones R, Wood DE. Early complications. Chylothorax. Chest Surg Clin N Am 1999;9:609–616.

21. Ross JK. A review of the surgery of the thoracic duct. Thorax 1961;16:12–21.

22. De Meester TR. The pleura. In: Sabiston DC, Spencer EC, eds. Surgery of the Chest, 4th Ed. Philadelphia: WB Saunders, 1983:873.

23. Chrobak L, Bartos V, Brzek V, et al. Coagulation properties of human thoracic duct lymph. Am J Med Sci 1967;253:69–75.

24. Sachs PB, Zelch MG, Rice TW, et al. Diagnosis and localization of laceration of the thoracic duct: usefulness of lymphangiography and CT. AJR Am J Roentgenol 1991;157:703–705.

25. Guillem P , Billeret V, Houke ML, et al. Successful management of post-esophagectomy chylothorax/chyloperitoneumby etilefrine. Dis Esophagus 1999;12:155–156.

26. Rosser BG, Poterucha JJ, McKusick MA, et al. Thoracic duct-cutaneous fistula in a patient with cirrhosis of the liver: successful treatment with a transjugular intrahepatic portosystemic shunt. Mayo Clin Proc 1996;71:793–796.

27. Buettiker V, Hug MI, Burger R, et al. Somatostatin: a new therapeutic option for the treatment of chylothorax. Intensive Care Med 2001;27:1083–1086.

28. Adler RH, Levinsky L. Persistent chylothorax. Treatment by talc pleurodesis. J Thorac Cardiovasc Surg 1978;76:859–864.

29. Cope C. Percutaneous thoracic duct cannulation: feasibility study in swine. J Vasc Interv Radiol 1995;6:559–664.

30. Wurnig PN, Hollaus PH, Ohtsuka T, et al. Thoracoscopic direct clipping of the thoracic duct for chylopericardium and chylothorax. Ann Thorac Surg 2000;70:1662–1665.

Tracheobronchial Balloon Dilatation and Stent Placement

55

Ji Hoon Shin, Gi-Young Ko, Ho-Young Song

Tracheobronchial obstruction from either benign or malignant disease produces dyspnea, stridor, and obstructive pneumonia and is occasionally life threatening as a result of suffocation. Even in the absence of parenchymal lung disease, ventilatory failure frequently occurs if the obstruction is not relieved (1). Although there are many causes of tracheobronchial obstruction, most cases result from malignant airway obstruction, in particular as a result of non–small-cell lung cancers invading the large airway.

Resection and surgical reconstruction offer the best form of definitive management of tracheobronchial obstruction; however, many patients refuse this surgery or cannot undergo such a procedure owing to anatomical limitations, metastatic disease, or overall medical condition. Even after surgical resection, treatment failure has been reported in 5–15% of cases because of anastomotic granulations, excessive tension, or devascularization (2–4). For the palliation of obstructive tracheobronchial pathology, local treatments such as balloon dilatation, laser resection, cryotherapy, electrocautery, photodynamic therapy, external-beam radiation, endobronchial brachytherapy, and endobronchial core-out have been widely utilized (1,5–8). Balloon dilatation is advocated as palliation for benign tracheobronchial stenosis. Cryotherapy, photodynamic therapy, external-beam radiation, and brachytherapy are used less because immediate results are more difficult to obtain. Laser resection, cryotherapy, electrocautery, or endobronchial core-out are not indicated for extrinsic compression or long and complicated stenoses with uncertain anatomy and high risk of bronchial rupture (9). Recently, the use of tracheobronchial stents has increased greatly because of the advantages of easy placement and prompt airway relief (5,10–14). In addition, tracheobronchial stents provide an alternative to open surgical procedures in select patients with benign tracheobronchial stenosis or obstruction, in particular those with tracheobronchial tuberculosis (15–23).

BALLOON DILATATION

General Principles

Since the first report of balloon dilatation to treat tracheobronchial stenosis by Cohen et al. (24) in 1984, several reports have described the advantages of balloon dilatation in treating airway stenosis (21,22,25–27). The balloon dilates the stenotic trachea or bronchus by stretching and expanding the bronchial wall, making balloon dilatation appropriate for treatment of cicatric annular strictures. The use of balloon dilatation has been extended to treat tracheobronchial stenoses from various causes, including postintubation tracheal stenosis, postoperative anastomotic stenosis, granulomatous stenosis (tuberculosis, histoplasmosis), radiation therapy, mediastinal fibrosis, congenital stenosis, bronchial trauma, and bronchial artery embolization (28). Fluoroscopic, nonoperative tracheobronchial balloon dilatation techniques have the following advantages: (a) General anesthesia is not needed, (b) the procedure is simple, safe, and repeatable, and (c) the procedure is easily tolerated by patients. Although there are no absolute contraindications, the following are considered relative: (a) severe bleeding diathesis, (b) tracheobronchomalacia, and (c) acute inflammation of the airway. Before balloon dilatation, the site, severity, proximal and distal extent, and characteristics of the stricture should be evaluated by means of at least conventional radiography and bronchoscopy. Recent reports show that computerized tomographic (CT) data can be reconstructed into two-dimensional (2D) reformations and three-dimensional (3D) images, including virtual bronchoscopic

renderings for evaluation of the stricture in terms of length, degree, or morphology and for preparing the appropriate size of the balloon catheter (Figure 55–1) (29,30). Exact preprocedure stricture evaluation is possible on CT scan, even in patients with high-grade airway stenoses where the bronchoscope could not pass through the lesion, as it is possible to assess distal airway patency beyond the site of stenosis. With such advances, tracheobronchography has become redundant as a preprocedure evaluation tool, although it is still highly useful during the balloon dilatation procedure (31).

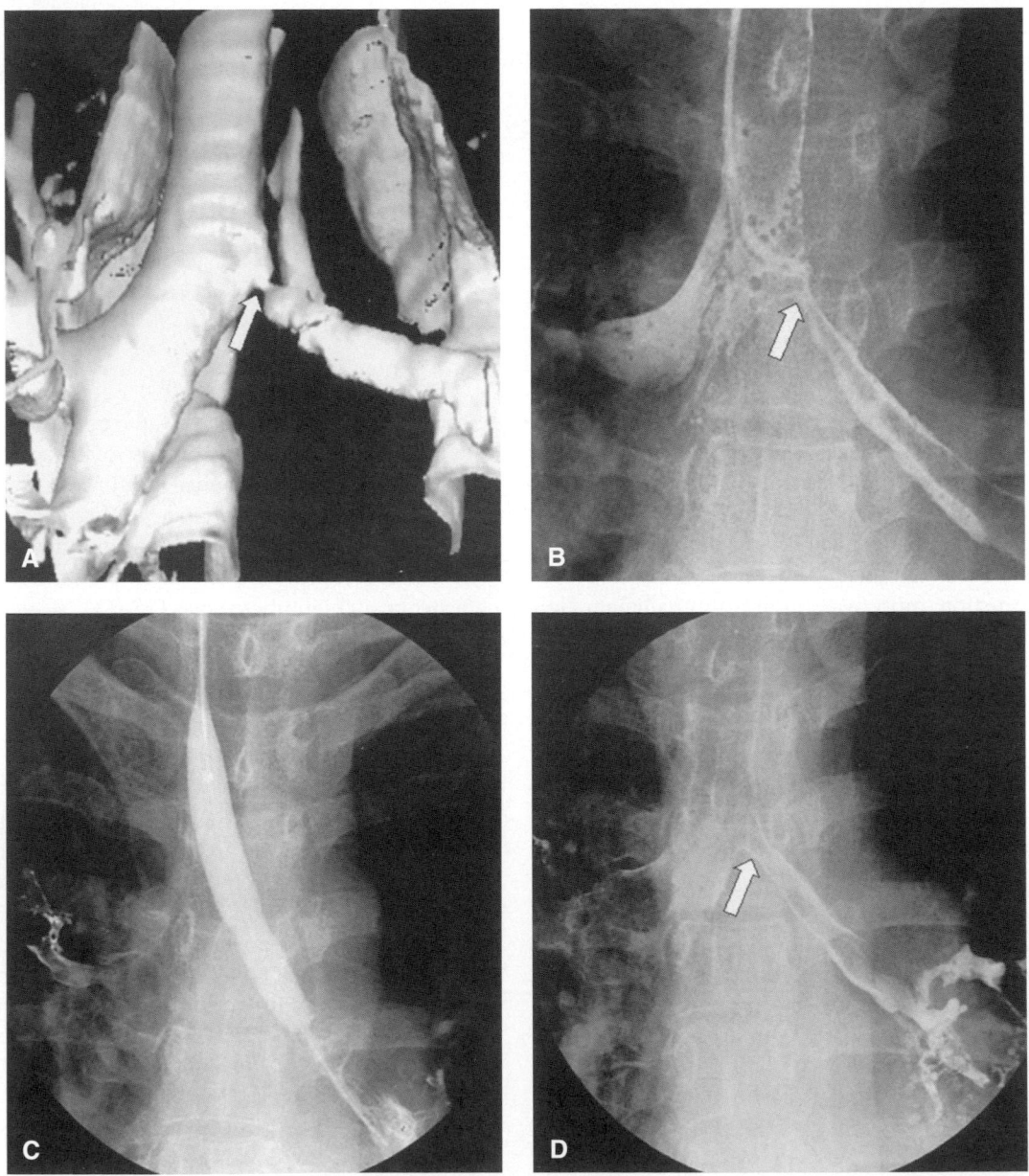

Figure 55–1 Endobronchial tuberculosis. **A., B.** A 3D-reconstructed CT image **(A)** and tracheobronchography **(B)** show a tight stenosis (*arrows*) at the orifice of the left main bronchus. **C.** The stenosis was dilated using a 10-mm balloon catheter. **D.** Immediate postprocedural tracheobronchography shows improvement of the stenosis (*arrow*).

Techniques

The authors' techniques include topical anesthesia of the pharynx and larynx using an aerosol spray 3–5 minutes before the procedure. A 0.035-inch angled exchange guide wire (Radiofocus M, Terumo) is inserted through the bronchoscope and positioned across the stenosis. (If the bronchoscope is not available, the guide wire can be inserted across the stenosis under fluoroscopic guidance.) After removing the bronchoscope, a graduated sizing catheter is passed over the guide wire to the distal part of the stricture to measure the stricture. Selective tracheobronchography using water-soluble nonionic contrast medium through the sizing catheter is performed to visualize the stricture in detail. An angioplasty balloon catheter is then passed over the guide wire to dilate the stricture. In children, 6 mm-diameter balloon catheters are used in bronchi and tracheae, whereas in adults, 10–12 mm-diameter balloon catheters are used in bronchi and 14–20 mm-diameter balloon catheters are used in tracheae. When the stenosis is too narrow for a balloon catheter larger than 10 mm in diameter to pass through, a 6 mm-diameter balloon catheter is used first to provide a passage for the larger balloon catheter. The balloon is inflated with diluted water-soluble nonionic contrast medium with inflation pressures as high as 16 atm, as determined by a pressure-gauge monitor. Selective tracheobronchography is performed to evaluate lumen dilatation after the procedure.

Results

A review of five representative studies using balloon dilatation for benign tracheobronchial stenosis shows clinical success rates of 68–100% and recurrence rates of 30–80% in 112 patients (21,22,25–27). The cause of stenosis was most commonly tuberculosis or lung posttransplantation stricture (Figure 55–1). Noninflammatory fibrous stenoses have been known to be more amenable to balloon dilatation compared with those featuring inflammation, carcinoma, calcification, external compression, or tracheobronchomalacia (25,27). It has been advocated that the fluoroscopic findings of waist formation in the balloon at the beginning of inflation and progressive or sudden disappearance of the waist indicate fibrotic stenosis and resultant clinical success (25,26). Repeated balloon dilatation may improve focal tight strictures by remodeling the tight segment.

Complications

Chest pain during dilatation, bronchospasm, atelectasis after dilatation, superficial or deep mucosal laceration, pneumomediastinum, and massive bleeding have been reported as complications associated with balloon dilatation (25,26,32). Pneumothorax or mediastinitis following bronchial laceration or rupture have not been reported, although they are theoretically possible complications. To prevent complications

resulting from overdistention of the stenosis, the diameter of the balloon must be carefully chosen according to the location of the stenosis and the diameter of the adjacent bronchus.

STENT PLACEMENT

General Principles

Endotracheal endoprostheses for benign tracheal stenosis were introduced in early 1950, and expandable metallic stents for lung cancer were introduced in mid 1980. Recent technological advances have resulted in tracheobronchial stents gaining popularity with interventional radiologists and chest physicians, particularly as stenting is effective for extraluminal lesions as well as for intraluminal lesions and offers prompt relief of acute airway distress from airway obstruction. The placement of expandable metallic stents is better tolerated and preferred to that of nonexpandable silicone stents because the former is more flexible and can be used in smaller delivery systems. Evaluation of the stricture with conventional radiography, bronchoscopy, and reconstructed CT images is the same as that for balloon dilatation (Figures 55–2 and 55–3).

Indications

Stent placement is indicated for patients with submucosal and extraluminal pathology or tracheobronchomalacia as well as for patients with intraluminal pathology (33–36). Tracheobronchomalacia is a special entity denoting a functional airway obstruction with destruction of the surrounding airway cartilage.

Table 55–1 summarizes the diverse detailed indications for tracheobronchial stent placement. In malignant pathologies, the most common indication for stent placement is bronchogenic carcinoma, which can present with extraluminal compression with or without intraluminal lesion. The most optimal situation for stent placement is in cases where an intraluminal or extraluminal tumor is obstructing the trachea or main stem bronchi without distal lobar obstruction (Figure 55–2). Tracheobronchial stenting is the only immediate treatment for unresectable extraluminal compression and can provide prompt stabilization of a threatened airway while the primary tumor is treated with chemotherapy or radiation (5,6,10–14).

Intubation is the leading cause of subsequent benign airway stenosis (Figure 55–3) (5,6,16). In some Asian countries, tuberculosis has been one of the major benign pathologies of tracheobronchial stenosis (18,22,25). Patients with postintubation stenosis undergo stent placement if they refuse surgery or if the lesion is too long for surgical reconstruction. Stent placement or balloon dilatation for anastomotic stenosis following lung transplantation or airway resection is a growing trend as these types of surgery increase

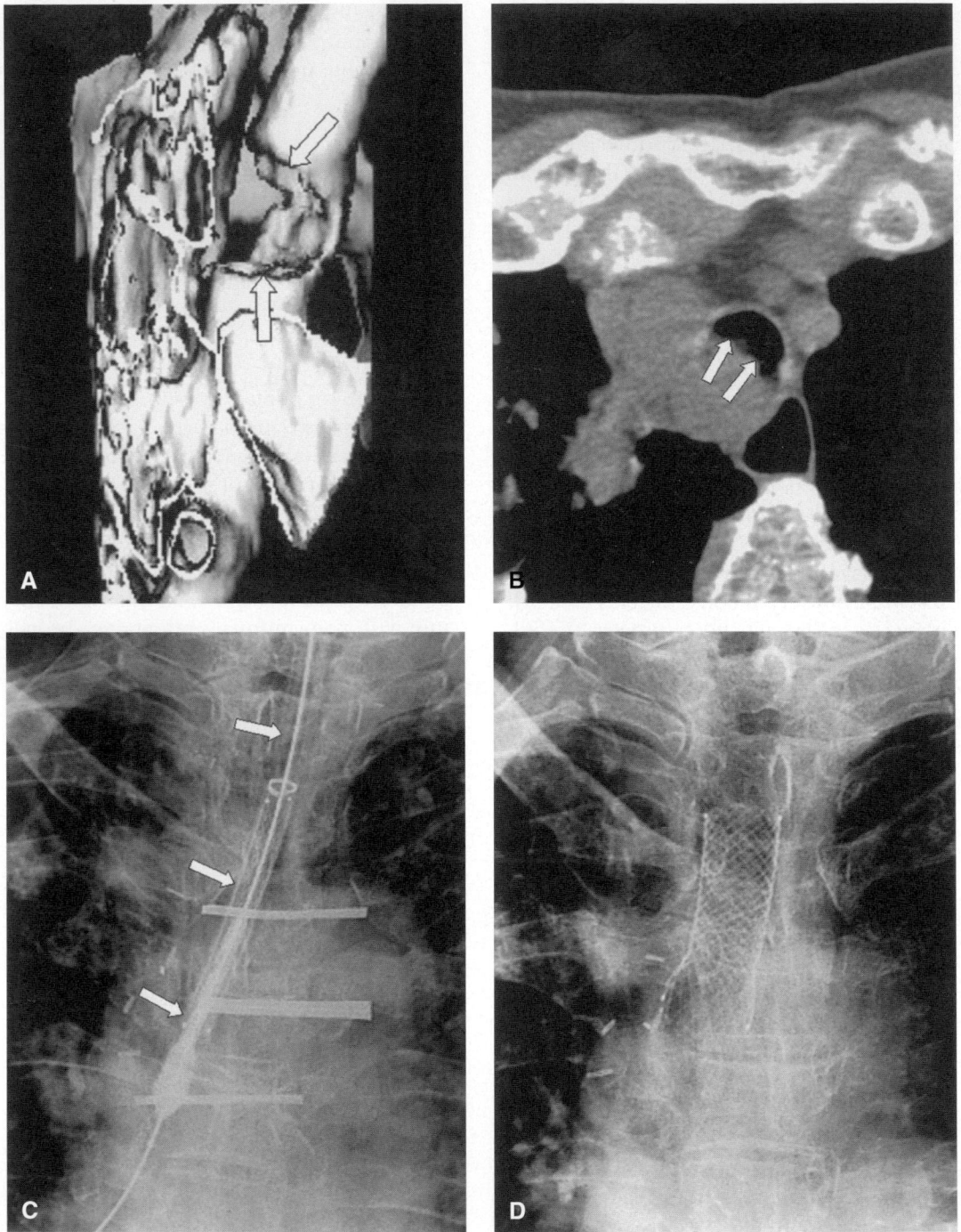

Figure 55–2 Patient with luminal narrowing of the trachea resulting from metastatic paratracheal lymphadenopathy invasion from a rectal adenocarcinoma. **A.** A 3D-reconstructed CT image shows irregular narrowing of the tracheal lumen (*arrows*). **B.** An axial CT image through the trachea shows an irregular soft tissue mass (*arrows*) protruding into the tracheal lumen. **C.** A fluoroscopic image obtained during stent placement shows a tracheal stent introducer set (*arrows*) passing over the narrow segment of the trachea. **D.** A fluoroscopic image obtained immediately after stent placement shows the stent fully expanded.

(4,19,21,29). Tracheobronchomalacia does not have a fixed stenosis but is regarded as a good indication for temporary stent placement, especially when there are multiple or long lesions or when the patient's general condition will not tolerate surgery (6,34,35). Congenital tracheal stenosis can be a good indication for expandable metallic stenting following balloon tracheoplasty where surgical management has been unsatisfactory (34,37,38).

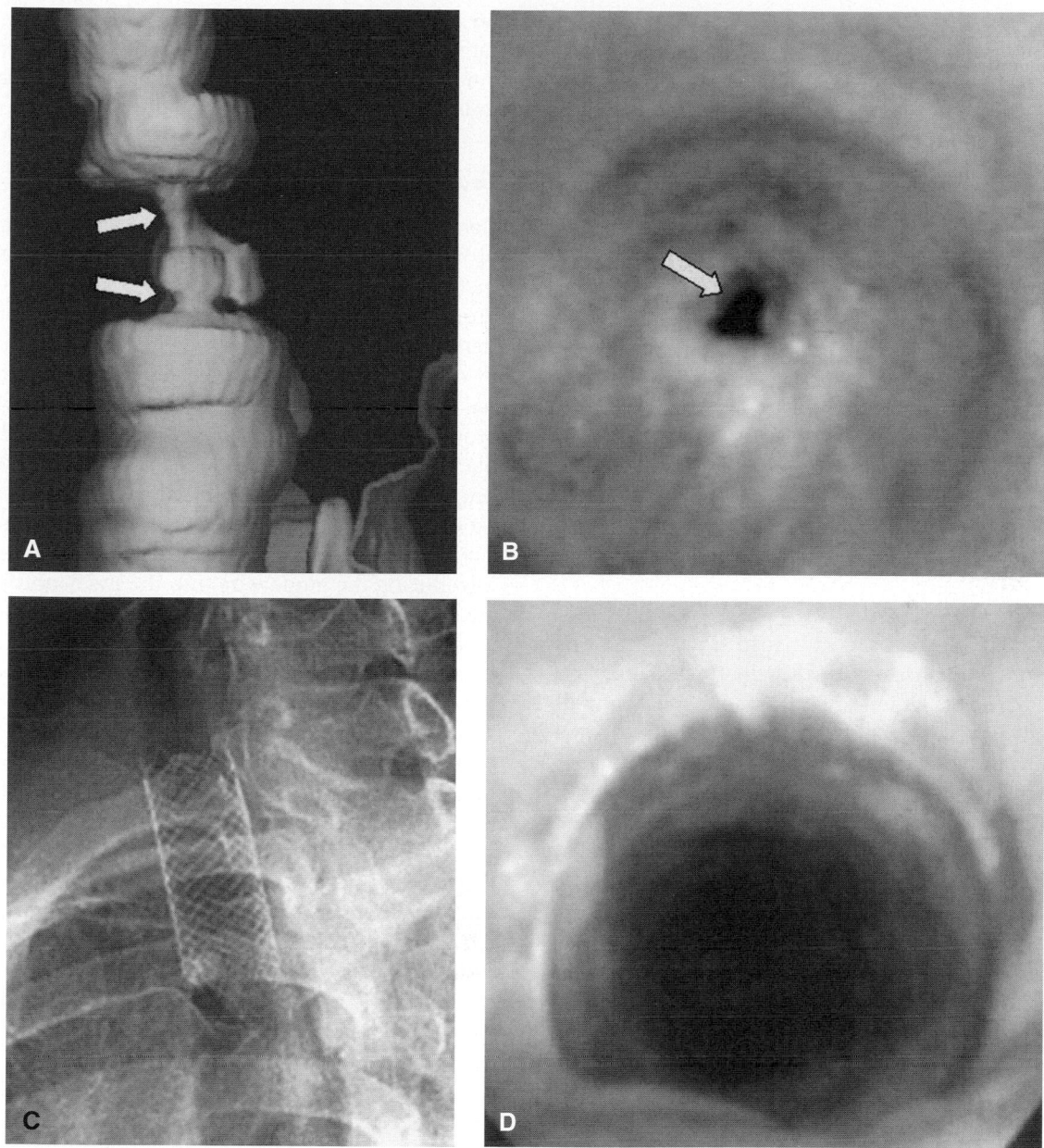

Figure 55–3 Patient with postintubation stenosis. **A., B.** A 3D-reconstructed CT image **(A)** and bronchoscopic photograph **(B)** show a short-segmental tight stenosis (*arrows*) involving the midtrachea. **C., D.** Marked lumen widening is shown by a plain radiograph **(C)** and a bronchoscopic photograph **(D)** obtained following placement of a covered expandable metallic stent.

Contraindications

There are no absolute contraindications, although the following are considered to be relative: (a) tumor with high bleeding potential, (b) severely ill patients with an extremely limited life expectancy, and (c) acute severe inflammation of the airway.

Types of Stents

At present there are basically two types of stents available—plastic and metallic. The most common plastic stent is made of silicone. Stents are inserted using a special applicator under general anesthesia and rigid bronchoscopy. Since Montgomery described the use of a T tube in 1965, a variety of silicone endotracheal stents and prostheses, such as the Dumon stent or the Freitag dynamic stent, have been described (39–41). As many as 20% of the migration incidents resulting in reocclusion have been observed using silicone stents, although repositioning or stent removal as many times as needed may be an outstanding advantage for benign tracheobronchial stenosis or for slowly growing, frequently recurring tumors (6,10,16,40,41). Also, as many as 15% of all patients with silicone stents develop clinically

TABLE 55-1

INDICATIONS FOR TRACHEOBRONCHIAL STENT PLACEMENT

Malignant	Benign
Bronchogenic carcinoma	Inflammatory
Intraluminal lesion	Tuberculosis
Extraluminal lesion	Histoplasmosis
Primary airway tumor	Postintubation stenosis
Squamous cell carcinoma	Anastomotic
Adenoid cystic carcinoma	Lung transplantation
Miscellaneous	Sleeve resection
Extraluminal malignancy	Tracheobronchomalacia
Esophageal carcinoma	Congenital tracheal stenosis
Head and neck cancer	Compression by esophageal stent
Thyroid cancer	
Airway metastases	
Renal cell carcinoma	
Colon cancer	

significant stent obstruction with inspissated secretions resulting from impairment of mucociliary clearance and impedance of the cough reflex. Furthermore, the thick wall of silicone stents results in a low internal-to-external diameter ratio such that they cannot be used in airways smaller than the main stem bronchi. To overcome the shortcomings of silicone plastic stents, uncovered or covered metallic stents used in the vascular system have also been used in tracheobronchial stenoses since the mid-1980s (11,42). The primary advantage of the expandable metallic stents is their easy delivery by means of fluoroscopy or flexible bronchoscopy under topical anesthesia and their conformability to the airway anatomy owing to their self-expanding characteristics. Two examples of self-expandable metallic stents are Wallstents made of stainless steel wire and Ultraflex stents made of a single thread of nitinol wire, and both are available in both uncovered and covered versions.

Uncovered expandable metallic stents provide advantages such as superior mucociliary clearance with resultant decreased sputum and low incidence of stent migration because of the metal lattice becoming overgrown with ciliated respiratory epithelium (33,43,44). Disadvantages of uncovered expandable metallic stents include that they are liable to produce progressive tumor ingrowth or granulation tissue through the openings between the wire filaments, they are not suitable for esophagorespiratory fistula, and they cannot be easily removed (1,5,12,33,45). There is also a potential risk of stent fracture and migration. To overcome the shortcomings of uncovered expandable metallic stents, covered expandable metallic stents are being developed (Figure 55–4) (1,13,33,44,46). Although covered expandable metallic stents may improve the long-term patency of the stent lumen, they may increase the risk of stent migration and occlusion of the upper or middle bronchi or smaller bronchi (44,47). Recently, several investigators have asserted that covered stents are definitively more advantageous than

uncovered stents because they can be removed when complications occur, such as stent migration, or when they are no longer necessary, as in patients with endobronchial tuberculosis or lymphoma following treatment (33,48).

Techniques

Generally speaking, plastic stents are inserted using rigid bronchoscopy under general anesthesia, and expandable metallic stents are inserted using fluoroscopy or flexible bronchoscopy under local anesthesia. Expandable metallic stents can be inserted using only fluoroscopic guidance and by only radiologists, with the patient under topical anesthesia. However, bronchoscopic assistance is valuable because bronchoscopic evaluation immediately before and after stent placement is important, and it is easy to insert a guide wire across the stricture into the distal portion of the trachea or bronchus through the working channel of the bronchoscope.

The techniques for providing topical anesthesia and for introducing the guide wire into the tracheobronchial tree are the same as those for balloon dilatation. After the guide wire is in place, a graduated sizing catheter is passed over the guide wire to the distal part of the stricture to measure the stricture. Selective tracheobronchography with water-soluble nonionic contrast medium through the sizing catheter is useful for marking the stricture. Subsequently, the location of the narrowed lumen can be marked on the patient's skin using radiopaque markers. With the patient in a supine position and with full extension of the neck, the delivery system, the proximal part of which is lubricated with jelly, is passed over the guide wire into the trachea and is advanced until the distal tip of the delivery system reaches beyond the stricture (Figure 55–3). When the stricture is severe, that is, when more than two thirds of the lumen is narrowed, dilatation of the stenotic portion is performed with an angioplasty balloon catheter. A stent at least 10 mm longer than the stricture is selected for placement so that its proximal and distal parts rest on the upper and lower margins of the stricture, respectively.

After stent placement, bronchoscopy is again necessary to evaluate the patency and location of the stent. Inexact stent deployment with partial obstruction of a bronchial orifice or incomplete coverage of the tumor stenosis obviously must be avoided. In such cases, the stent should be repositioned with bronchoscopic biopsy forceps, or it should be removed and its placement reattempted (5,33).

The difficulty or impossibility of stent removal has been criticized as the major drawback of expandable metallic stents. Some early investigators used forceps/rotation techniques to remove uncovered expandable metallic stents under general anesthesia (34,35), although there was a potential risk of mucosal bleeding and airway occlusion during the procedure in cases of tight welding of the stent to the tracheobronchial wall. Recently, a removal technique using a hooklike device has been reported to be highly safe and easy because the stent is completely covered and optimally designed for removal (Figure 55–4) (14,33). Stent

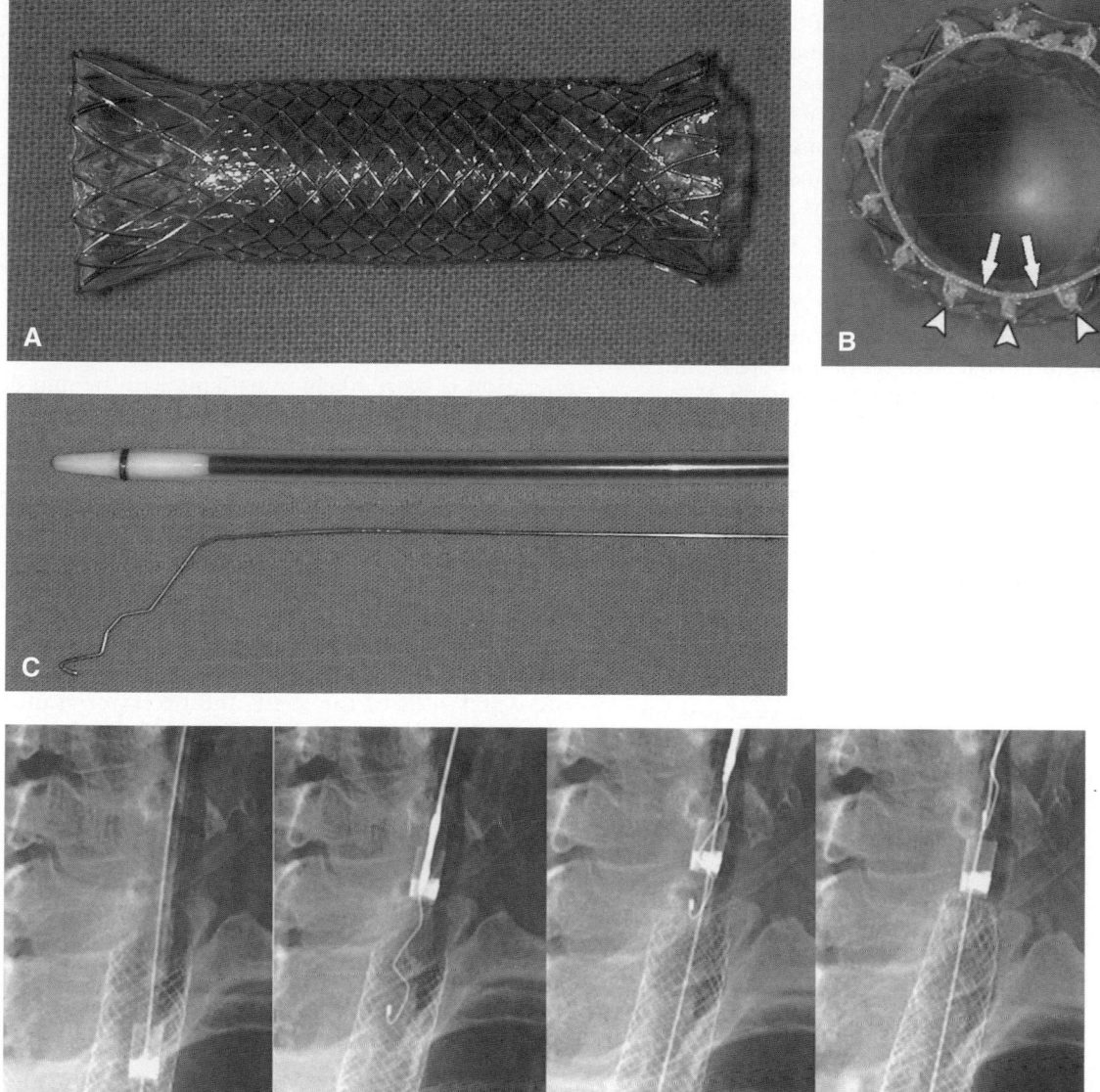

Figure 55–4   Covered retrievable expandable metallic bronchial stent. **A.** Bronchial stent flared proximally (*left*) and distally (*right*). **B.** Multiple nylon loops (*arrowheads*) are attached to the proximal inner margin of the stent, and then two nylon threads (*arrows*) are passed through each loop to form a larger drawstring. **C.** The devices for removing the stent consist of a sheath, a dilator, and a retrievable hook wire. **D.** While the hook wire withdraws the drawstring into the sheath, the proximal end of the stent is collapsed, and the entire assembly is then pulled out.

retrievability was reported to be useful when stent migration occurred or the patient's clinical status worsened after stent placement. To make the stent removable, a nylon loop is hooked inside each bend of the proximal end of the stent, and then two nylon threads are passed through each loop. For stent removal, a hook wire is introduced into the sheath and passed through it into the stent lumen. Then the sheath with the hook is pulled out of the stent so that the hook grasps the drawstring. When this occurs, the hook wire is withdrawn through the sheath to collapse the proximal

stent. The sheath, hook wire, and stent are then pulled out of the trachea (Figure 55–4).

Results

Results in Plastic Stent Placement

Several representative studies have reported on the use of silicone stents for benign tracheobronchial stenosis (2,15–17). In these studies, 163 patients (mean age, 55 years) were treated under rigid bronchoscopy and general anesthesia. Most patients had tracheal stenosis following intubation or tracheostomy. All patients had immediate symptomatic relief after stent placement with no procedure-related mortality. It would be ideal to electively remove stents from patients with benign tracheobronchial strictures after they are no longer needed because foreign material inserted into the airway will eventually cause complications such as granulation tissue formation (33,34). However, there has been much disagreement regarding the optimal time for stent removal because it is different in each case according to the cause, duration, and severity of the strictures. It is important that a tracheobronchial stent remain in place until a stricture has healed. A review of studies totaling 54 patients showed that when stents were removed 18–32 months after placement, there was no recurrence in 43 cases (80%) (2,15–17). In these studies, sputum retention was the most common complication (16%), followed by stent migration (10%) and granulation tissue formation (4%).

Several representative studies have reported on the use of silicone stents for malignant tracheobronchial stenosis, such as in lung or esophageal cancer (10,49,50). In these studies, a total of 53 patients (mean age, 66 years) were treated under rigid bronchoscopy and general anesthesia. Most patients (94%) had immediate symptomatic relief after stent placement with no procedure-related mortality. Stent migration was less than for benign stenosis and was observed in three patients (6%), and one report noted that stent removal was needed in four patients (8%) (10).

Results in Expandable Metallic Stent Placement

In benign tracheobronchial stenosis, technical success rates of 100% and clinical success rates of 88–100% have been reported in 46 patients across three representative studies using uncovered stents (18–20). The cause of stenosis was most commonly lung posttransplantation stricture or tuberculosis. Stent fracture was the most common complication, occurring in seven patients (15%), followed by granulation tissue formation (7%) and stent migration (2%). Stent removal was performed in four patients (9%) because of stent fracture or stent migration (18,19). Stent removal was difficult because the wire mesh was covered by respiratory epithelium.

In malignant tracheobronchial stenosis, technical success rates of 98–100% and clinical success rates of 82–92% have been reported in 133 patients in four representative studies; two studies used uncovered stents (11,12), and two used covered stents (13,14). As many investigators have mentioned, stent migration and sputum retention occurred much more frequently when using covered metallic stents (12–17% and 20–38%, respectively) compared with uncovered metallic stents (0% and 9%, respectively). Tumor ingrowth into the stent lumen occurred much more frequently when using uncovered metallic stents (21–23%) compared with covered metallic stents (0%) because there is no covering material between the wire mesh in uncovered metallic stents.

Complications

Tracheobronchial stents are usually well tolerated. All complications described for tracheobronchial balloon dilatations can also be encountered in tracheobronchial stent placement.

Migration of the Stent

Plastic stents (6–10% of cases) and covered expandable metallic stents (12–17%) are more likely to migrate than are uncovered expandable metallic stents (2%) because of lack of epithelialization through the wire meshes. Stent migration is more likely in patients with benign disease where there is no substantial extrinsic compression maintaining stents in place and when short stents are placed in conical stenoses. In patients with malignancy, migration can be expected after tumor shrinkage from radiation or chemotherapy.

Granulation Tissue Formation

Granulation tissue is more likely to form at the proximal and distal ends of the stent, and excessive granulation tissue can lead to obstruction of the airway. It is more common with metallic stents, especially uncovered stents (as many as 7%), than with plastic stents because metal stents are more rigid and have multiple edges, therefore causing more irritation. Such tissue can provide a reservoir for bacteria and become a source of persistent infection.

Tumor Ingrowth/Overgrowth

Uncovered expandable metallic stents do not offer protection against tumor ingrowth, which was reported to occur in as many as 53% of patients (4,5,10,12). Prevention of tumor ingrowth is considered to be the strongest indication for use of covered stents over uncovered stents in malignant tracheobronchial strictures. The incidence of tumor overgrowth at the tip of the covered metallic stent depends on the follow-up period and extent of the malignancy at the time of stent placement and has been reported to occur in 6–28% of patients (13,14). Because airway obstruction by tumor ingrowth/overgrowth can be life threatening, patients with new symptoms or radiographic findings should undergo further evaluation for diagnosis.

Sputum Retention

Plastic stents (in as many as 16% of patients) and covered expandable metallic stents (as many as 38%) are more likely to be associated with sputum retention than are uncovered expandable metallic stents (9%) because of impaired mucociliary clearance. Lack of mucociliary clearance can lead to obstruction and infection.

Stent Fracture

Although stent fracture is an uncommon complication, it may occur with metal stents in as many as 15% of cases (18–20).

Hemoptysis

Hemoptysis and possible death following stent placement have been reported to occur in 6–18% of cases using uncovered expandable metallic stents (4,5,19). It is expected that the incidence of fatal hemoptysis might be reduced in patients with covered expandable metallic stents because the wire mesh, which can erode the airway wall and lacerate major blood vessels, is covered.

SUMMARY

Balloon dilatation is a reasonable first option for restoration of the airway lumen in patients with benign strictures and may preclude the need for other interventions. Tracheobronchial stent placement provides safe, prompt, and effective management for either benign or malignant tracheobronchial strictures. Covered expandable metallic tracheobronchial stents have recently gained wider acceptance because of their ease of placement and removal, accommodation of various dimensions, and promising patency rates. The skills required for balloon dilatation and stent placement are identical to those in common use by interventional radiologists for all types of balloon dilatation and stent placement, but particular care is essential to keep the airway open during these procedures.

REFERENCES

1. Rafanan AL, Mehta AC. Stenting of the tracheobronchial tree. Radiol Clin North Am 2000;38:395–408.
2. Vergnon JM, Costes F, Polio JC. Efficacy and tolerance of a new silicone stent for the treatment of benign tracheal stenosis: preliminary results. Chest 2000;118.422–426.
3. Grillo HC, Mathisen DJ, Wain JC. Laryngotracheal resection and reconstruction for subglottic stenosis. Ann Thorac Surg 1992;53:54–63.
4. Donahue DM, Grillo HC, Wain JC, et al. Reoperative tracheal resection and reconstruction for unsuccessful repair of postintubation stenosis. J Thorac Cardiovasc Surg 1997;114:934–939.
5. Wood DE. Airway stenting. Chest Surg Clin N Am 2001;11:841–860.
6. Kim H. Stenting therapy for stenosing airway disease. Respirology 1998;3:221–228.
7. Katayama A, Konishi T, Hiraishi M, et al. A combination of laser therapy, radiation therapy, and stent placement for the palliation of complete malignant bronchial obstruction. Surg Endosc 1998;12:1419–1423.
8. Stephens KE Jr, Wood DE. Bronchoscopic management of central airway obstruction. J Thorac Cardiovasc Surg 2000;119:289–296.
9. Hautmann H, Gamarra F, Pfeifer KJ, et al. Fiberoptic bronchoscopic balloon dilatation in malignant tracheobronchial disease: indications and results. Chest 2001;120:43–49.
10. Bolliger CT, Probst R, Tschopp K, et al. Silicone stents in the management of inoperable tracheobronchial stenoses. Indications and limitations. Chest 1993;104:1653–1659.
11. Sawada S, Tanigawa N, Kobayashi M, et al. Malignant tracheobronchial obstructive lesions: treatment with Gianturco expandable metallic stents. Radiology 1993;188:205–208.
12. Miyazawa T, Yamakido M, Ikeda S, et al. Implantation of ultraflex nitinol stents in malignant tracheobronchial stenoses. Chest 2000;118:959–965.
13. Monnier P, Mudry A, Stanzel F, et al. The use of the covered Wallstent for the palliative treatment of inoperable tracheobronchial cancers. A prospective, multicenter study. Chest 1996;110:1161–1168.
14. Shin JH, Kim SW, Shim TS, et al. Malignant tracheobronchial strictures: palliation with covered retrievable expandable nitinol stent. J Vasc Interv Radiol 2003;14:1525–1534.
15. Puma F, Ragusa M, Avenia N, et al. The role of silicone stents in the treatment of cicatricial tracheal stenoses. J Thorac Cardiovasc Surg 2000;120:1064–1069.
16. Martinez-Ballarin JI, Diaz-Jimenez JP, Castro MJ, et al. Silicone stents in the management of benign tracheobronchial stenoses. Tolerance and early results in 63 patients. Chest 1996;109:626–629.
17. Schmidt B, Olze H, Borges AC, et al. Endotracheal balloon dilatation and stent implantation in benign stenoses. Ann Thorac Surg 2001;71:1630–1634.
18. Kim YS, Jeon SC, Choi CS, et al. Treatment of tracheobronchial stenosis with a self-expandable metallic stent. Korean J Radiol 1994;31:35–41.
19. Orons PD, Amesur NB, Dauber JH, et al. Balloon dilation and endobronchial stent placement for bronchial strictures after lung transplantation. J Vasc Interv Radiol 2000;11:89–99.
20. Eisner MD, Gordon RL, Webb WR, et al. Pulmonary function improves after expandable metal stent placement for benign airway obstruction. Chest 1999;115:1006–1011.
21. Carre P, Rousseau H, Lombart L, et al. Balloon dilatation and self-expanding metal Wallstent insertion. For management of bronchostenosis following lung transplantation. Chest 1994;105:343–348.
22. Lee KW, Im JG, Han JK, et al. Tuberculous stenosis of the left main bronchus: results of treatment with balloons and metallic stents. J Vasc Interv Radiol 1999;10:352–358.
23. Nashef SA, Dromer C, Velly JF, et al. Expanding wire stents in benign tracheobronchial disease: indications and complications. Ann Thorac Surg 1992;54:937–940.
24. Cohen MD, Weber TR, Rao CC. Balloon dilatation of tracheal and bronchial stenosis. AJR Am J Roentgenol 1984;142:477–478.
25. Lee KH, Ko GY, Song HY, et al. Benign tracheobronchial stenoses: long-term clinical experience with balloon dilation. J Vasc Interv Radiol 2002;13:909–914.
26. Ferretti G, Jouvan FB, Thony F, et al. Benign noninflammatory bronchial stenosis: treatment with balloon dilation. Radiology 1995;196:831–834.
27. Sheski FD, Mathur PN. Long-term results of fiberoptic bronchoscopic balloon dilation in the management of benign tracheobronchial stenosis. Chest 1998;114:796–800.
28. Nakamura K, Terada N, Ohi M, et al. Tuberculous bronchial stenosis: treatment with balloon bronchoplasty. AJR Am J Roentgenol 1991;157:1187–1188.
29. Ferretti GR, Kocier M, Calaque O, et al. Follow-up after stent insertion in the tracheobronchial tree: role of helical computed tomography in comparison with fiberoptic bronchoscopy. Eur Radiol 2003;13:1172–1178.
30. Boiselle PM, Ernst A. Recent advances in central airway imaging. Chest 2002;121:1651–1660.
31. Deutsch ES, Chidekel A, Moore JW. Management of a displaced endobronchial stent using simultaneous endoscopy and tracheobronchography. Ann Otol Rhinol Laryngol 2001;110:1165–1167.
32. Kato R, Kakizaki T, Hangai N, et al. Bronchoplastic procedures for tuberculous bronchial stenosis. J Thorac Cardiovasc Surg 1993;106:1118–1121.
33. Song HY, Shim TS, Kang SG, et al. Tracheobronchial strictures: treatment with a polyurethane-covered retrievable expandable nitinol stent—initial experience. Radiology 1999;213:905–912.

34. Filler RM, Forte V, Chait P. Tracheobronchial stenting for the treatment of airway obstruction. J Pediatr Surg 1998;33:304–311.

35. Nicolai T, Huber RM, Reiter K, et al. Metal airway stent implantation in children: follow-up of seven children. Pediatr Pulmonol 2001;31:289–296.

36. Jacobs JP, Quintessenza JA, Botero LM, et al. The role of airway stents in the management of pediatric tracheal, carinal, and bronchial disease. Eur J Cardiothorac Surg 2000;18:505–512.

37. Maeda K, Yasufuku M, Yamamoto T. A new approach to the treatment of congenital tracheal stenosis: Balloon tracheoplasty and expandable metallic stenting. J Pediatr Surg 2001;36:1646–1649.

38. Othersen HB Jr, Hebra A, Tagge EP. A new method of treatment for complete tracheal rings in an infant: endoscopic laser division and balloon dilation. J Pediatr Surg 2000;35:262–264.

39. Dumon JF. A dedicated tracheobronchial stent. Chest 1990;97: 328–332.

40. Freitag L, Eicker R, Linz B, et al. Theoretical and experimental basis for the development of a dynamic airway stent. Eur Respir J 1994;7:2038–2045.

41. Freitag L, Tekolf E, Stamatis G, et al. Clinical evaluation of a new bifurcated dynamic airway stent: a 5-year experience with 135 patients. Thorac Cardiovasc Surg 1997;45:6–12.

42. Wallace MJ, Charnsangavej C, Ogawa K, et al. Tracheobronchial tree: expandable metallic stents used in experimental and clinical applications. Work in progress. Radiology 1986;158:309–312.

43. Beer M, Wittenberg G, Sandstede J, et al. Treatment of inoperable tracheobronchial obstructive lesions with the Palmaz stent. Cardiovasc Intervent Radiol 1999;22:109–113.

44. Petersen BD, Uchida BT, Barton RE, et al. Gianturco-Rosch Z stents in tracheobronchial stenoses. J Vasc Interv Radiol 1995;6: 925–931.

45. Nakajima Y, Kurihara Y, Niimi H, et al. Efficacy and complications of the Gianturco-Z tracheobronchial stent for malignant airway stenosis. Cardiovasc Intervent Radiol 1999;22:287–292.

46. Madden BP, Datta S, Charokopos N. Experience with Ultraflex expandable metallic stents in the management of endobronchial pathology. Ann Thorac Surg 2002;73:938–944.

47. Bjarnason H, Cahill B, Klow NE, et al. Tracheobronchial metal stents: effects of covering a bronchial ostium in pigs. Acad Radiol 1999;6:586–591.

48. Schmidt B, Massenkeil G, John M, et al. Temporary tracheobronchial stenting in malignant lymphoma. Ann Thorac Surg 1999;67:1448–1450.

49. Sutedja G, Schramel F, van Kralingen K, et al. Stent placement is justifiable in end-stage patients with malignant airway tumours. Respiration 1995;62:148–150.

50. Vonk-Noordegraaf A, Postmus PE, Sutedja TG. Tracheobronchial stenting in the terminal care of cancer patients with central airways obstruction. Chest 2001;120:1811–1814.

Interventional Therapy of Pulmonary Embolism

56

Renan Uflacker

Venous thromboembolism encompasses deep venous thrombosis and pulmonary embolism (PE), and it is the third most common cardiovascular disease and a leading cause of death in the United States (1,2). The natural history of PE is incompletely characterized, and most episodes of PE go undetected (3); therefore, the true incidence of PE is not known, but it is estimated that there are more than 600,000 cases per year in the United States alone (1). Yet PE is a significant cause of morbidity and mortality in the hospitalized patient (3).

Common risk factors for development of PE are recent surgical procedures, trauma, prolonged bed rest, congestive heart failure, presence of malignancies, pregnancy, hormone therapy (including contraceptives), obesity, older age, and long-distance air traveling. Several recent reports suggest that subclinical deep venous thrombosis (DVT), also called "economy class syndrome," associated with prolonged air travel is surprisingly common, occurring in 3–10% of patients with risk factors (4). Life-threatening PE, albeit rarely, may occur in this population (4). Lapostolle et al. (5) recently established that the risk is greater on longer flights. None of the patients with PE had flown less than a distance of 2,500 km (1,554 miles). The risk of severe PE was more than 100 times higher after flights of 5,000–10,000 km and more than 400 times higher after flights longer than 10,000 km (6,214 miles), or about one case in 200,000 passengers (5).

The immediate mortality rate related to PE is less than 8% when the condition is recognized and treated correctly. Of the 70% of the patients who fail to have the diagnosis made, the mortality rate approaches 30% (1,3,6). If appropriate therapy is initiated, mortality may decrease, but the overall mortality associated with PE has not significantly changed in the past 30 years. Massive PE causes rapid increase in pulmonary arterial pressure resulting from restriction of the blood flow. Other hemodynamic changes also occur, such as vasoconstriction, pulmonary arterial hypertension, right heart congestion and failure, decrease in heart output, as well as respiratory changes, which include bronchoconstriction, increase in the death space, and decrease in pulmonary surfactant (7). If the PE episode happens in a patient with underlying cardiopulmonary disease, there will be acute ventricular dysfunction and compromised hemodynamics of the cardiopulmonary system, requiring more aggressive treatment than anticoagulation. Rapid reestablishment of pulmonary arterial flow is paramount to overcome the acute hemodynamic dysfunction and reduce the high mortality rate (8).

Pulmonary arteriography is still the gold standard in diagnosing pulmonary emboli, but several other imaging modalities have been used to diagnose PE in recent years, including ventilation perfusion lung scanning, D-Dimer, transthoracic and transesophageal echocardiography, magnetic resonance angiography, and contrast enhanced, fast multislice spiral CT (3). However, no single noninvasive test for PE is both sensitive and specific. Some tests are good for ruling in PE (e.g., helical CT), and some tests are good for ruling out PE (e.g., D-Dimer); others may be able to do both but are often inconclusive (e.g., ventilation/perfusion [V/Q] lung scanning). Choice of initial diagnostic test should take into consideration clinical assessment of the probability of PE and patient characteristics that may influence test accuracy (9). In the past decade, fast multislice spiral CT scanning revolutionized the diagnosis of PE and is becoming the standard for initial PE diagnosis, enabling quantitative assessment of acute PE severity (10), but it is still limited by the inability of patients to hold their breath, with resulting imaging degradation (11). Cardiac troponin T (cTnT) monitoring identifies the high-risk group of normotensive patients with acute severe pulmonary embolism (12). Persistent increased cTnT level (>0.01 ng/mL) in patients with PE predicts a significant risk of a complicated clinical course and fatal outcome, requiring a more aggressive treatment.

Traditional therapeutic options are anticoagulation, systemic thrombolysis, and surgical thrombectomy. More recently, multiple minimally invasive but aggressive procedures were introduced, which included catheter-directed thrombolysis, percutaneous embolectomy and embolus fragmentation techniques, pulmonary artery stent placement, or association of two or more of those techniques (2,13–16). Successful management of acute massive PE requires prompt risk stratification and decisive, early intervention (Table 56–1). At least one of the described criteria must be present to justify more aggressive treatment (12,15).

In cases of massive PE, the use of percutaneous embolectomy, catheter-directed thrombolysis, and fragmentation techniques is attractive, owing to their capacity to rapidly reestablish pulmonary blood flow, especially if systemic thrombolysis fails. The number of patients with massive PE, diagnosed by pulmonary angiography, however, is relatively small compared with the number of patients with clinically diagnosed massive PE, making it increasingly difficult to evaluate comparatively the different percutaneous techniques and devices. Despite the reduced amount of comparative information available, it may be appropriate to review the current techniques, protocols, and devices for the interventional management of massive PE, with emphasis on the percutaneous techniques.

ANTICOAGULATION

Initial intravenous administration of heparin is the therapy of choice to treat all forms of pulmonary thromboembolism. Heparin binds to and accelerates the activity of antithrombin III, prevents additional thrombus formation, and permits endogenous fibrinolytic mechanisms to lyse the clot that has already formed.

There is consensus regarding the goals of anticoagulation therapy in both DVT and pulmonary thromboembolism (PTE):

1. Immediate inhibition of the growth of thromboemboli
2. Promotion of thromboembolic resolution
3. Prevention of recurrence

Heparin achieves the first goal, encourages the second by allowing fibrinolytic dissolution to be achieved unopposed by thrombus growth, and assists in the third goal, preventing recurrence, without assurance (17). Heparin therapy, therefore, is more directed to the source of the embolism rather than to treatment of the embolus located in the pulmonary artery. If the patient survives the initial PE episode and if no treatment is initiated, there is an 18–30% chance of recurrent lethal PE (1,2,18). Anticoagulation therapy may assist in reducing recurrence of PE by reducing propagation of the venous thrombosis in the lower extremities (1,18,19). Propagation of thrombosis in the pulmonary artery, secondary to the impaction of embolus, may also be reduced by anticoagulation therapy.

In a 1960s landmark study comparing heparin with placebo, Barritt and Jordan showed that none of the 16 patients of their series had recurrent PE, with one associated death, while 52% of 19 patients receiving placebo had recurrent PE, with five fatalities (6). However, there are adverse effects related to the use of heparin, including hemorrhage, thrombocytopenia, osteoporosis, and, rarely, immunologically mediated thrombocytopenia associated with bleeding and/or thrombosis. The most common complication associated with anticoagulation with heparin is bleeding (ranging from 1.6%–14%) (20). At this time, there is no consensus regarding heparin regimens that best

TABLE 56–1

RISK STRATIFICATION AND INDICATIONS FOR AGGRESSIVE INVERVENTION TO TREAT MASSIVE PULMONARY EMBOLISM (AT LEAST ONE OF THE FOLLOWING CRITERIA MUST BE PRESENT) (2,15)

1. Arterial hypotension (<90 mm Hg systolic or drop of >40 mm Hg)
2. Cardiogenic shock with peripheral hypoperfusion and hypoxia
3. Circulatory collapse with need for cardiopulmonary resuscitation
4. Echocardiographic findings indicating right ventricular afterload stress and/or pulmonary hypertension
5. Diagnosis of precapillary pulmonary hypertension (mean PAP >20 mm Hg in presence of normal PAP occlusion pressures)
6. Widened arterial-alveolar O_2 gradient, >50 mm Hg
7. Clinically severe PE with a contraindication to anticoagulation or thrombolytic therapy

combine safety and efficacy and for how long antithrombotic therapy should be maintained. In PE, an initial large intravenous heparin bolus of 10,000–20,000 units is recommended, followed by a more standard regimen of intravenous heparin at 1,000 units per hour, 2–4 hours after the bolus (17). More recent evidence suggests that bleeding complications can be reduced with the use of low-molecular-weight heparin (LMWH) (21).

LMWHs have been recently approved in the United States for the prophylaxis of DVT after surgery (22). These fragments of unfractionated heparin bind less to proteins than regular heparin and have the advantages of greater bioavailability, more predictable dose response, longer half-life, lower complication rate, lack of need for monitoring anticoagulation (23), and association with a lower rate of heparin-associated thrombocytopenia than unfractionated heparin. Subcutaneous administration of enoxaparin and dalteparin (2,500–10,000 units/day) has been used for prevention of DVT in patients with acute medical illnesses (24) and in patients undergoing general and pelvic surgery (25). LMWHs are not approved for treatment of PE or DVT in the United States. Limited data are available on the efficacy and safety of LMWH as the initial treatment of symptomatic PE. In a randomized study including 1,021 patients, Haas (25) showed that recurrence of PE was similar between patients treated with LMWH (5.3%) and unfractionated heparin (4.9%), with comparable bleeding rates. Based on this and other studies, LMWH appeared to be as effective and safe as intravenous unfractionated heparin in patients with acute PE.

Argatroban is currently approved in the United States as an injectable heparin substitute for the prophylaxis or treatment of patients with heparin-induced thrombocytopenia (HIT). Outside the United States, it is also approved for chronic arterial obstruction, anticoagulation during hemodialysis in antithrombin III-deficient patients, and treatment of acute stroke. HIT is an uncommon immunological response that usually occurs between 5 and 14 days after initiation of heparin treatment or more rapidly for those previously exposed to heparin within the prior 3–6 months (26). The syndrome is mediated by antibodies against platelet factor 4 and heparin complexes. These complexes trigger two responses: in vivo platelet activation and endothelium activation that causes an increase in thrombin production (27). This platelet activation and resulting aggregation are a main cause of symptoms (thrombocytopenia and thrombosis) associated with this syndrome (28). Clinical symptoms of HIT can be determined by evidence of a new thromboembolic complication in rare instances or more commonly by the following clinical definition: a decrease in platelet count of more than 50% of baseline value and/or a platelet count of less than 100,000/cu mm following the initiation of heparin treatment. To date, several assays are available to confirm clinical diagnosis of HIT. Administration of Argatroban in

adults can be as much as 10.0 mcg/kg per minute until achieving the desired therapeutic range of a partial thromboplastin time (PTT) between 1.5 and 3 times baseline. This range should be checked approximately every 2 hours until the dose is adjusted, followed by daily checks throughout the treatment period.

Full anticoagulant protection with heparin should be maintained for 7–10 days. Oral anticoagulation should be started 3 or 4 days before the heparin is discontinued to allow a smooth transition between the two agents. Oral anticoagulants, warfarin 7.5–10 mg/day, or lower doses of 2–5 mg/day in smaller patients, are typically used for 3–6 months afer the initial episode of PE and following heparin treatment, targeting an International Normalized Ratio (INR) range of 2.0–3.0. A recent publication by Ridker et al. (29) demonstrated that low-intensity warfarin prophylaxis, with a targeted INR of 1.5–2.0, is superior to placebo in preventing recurrent venous thromboembolism and effective for patients requiring more than 3 months of anticoagulation therapy.

SYSTEMIC THROMBOLYSIS

Because anticoagulant therapy does not treat the pulmonary embolus itself, several trials to lyse clots with intravenous infusion of thrombolytic agents have been attempted (30,31) and showed a more rapid lysis of PE and reduction in pulmonary hypertension with improvement in perfusion lung scans when compared with heparin alone (Figure 56–1). Whether these advantages result in an improved clinical outcome and outweigh the increased risk of bleeding complications is still unknown. Sometimes there is clinical improvement without significant pulmonary artery perfusion improvement as demonstrated by the perfusion scan (Figure 56–2). The place of thrombolytic therapy in the management of PE still remains to be defined. More recent nonrandomized studies showed improvement of 1-year survival (32) and pulmonary hemodynamics (32) in patients treated with thrombolytics. A larger multicenter registry designed to investigate current management strategies in patients with major but hemodynamically stable pulmonary embolism compared thrombolytic treatment (using recombinant tissue plasminogen activator [rt-PA], streptokinase [SK], and urokinase [UK]) with heparin anticoagulation. The registry showed reduced mortality (4.7% vs. 11.1%), reduced recurrence of PE (7.7% vs. 18.7%) ($p = 0.016$) but with a higher incidence of major bleeding complications (21.9% vs. 7.8%) (33). It seems that in this registry, there is an increased bleeding complication rate with the use of thrombolytic therapy when compared with anticoagulation therapy alone for the treatment of major PE. A more recent study (33) presented a meta-analysis of 11 randomized and nonrandomized studies comparing thrombolysis

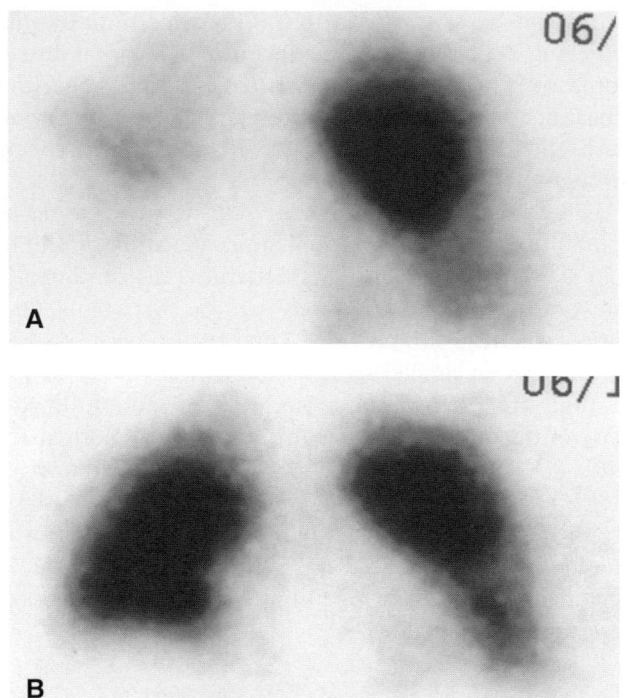

Figure 56–1 Female patient with massive pelvic vein thrombosis and pulmonary thromboembolism. **A.** Pulmonary perfusion scan showed massive occlusion of the right pulmonary artery flow and significant reduction of left lower lobe perfusion. Bilateral femoral vein infusion of urokinase at 100,000 IU/hour for 12 hours cleared the pelvic veins (*not shown*). **B.** Follow-up lung perfusion scan showed remarkable improvement 24 hours after the infusion started.

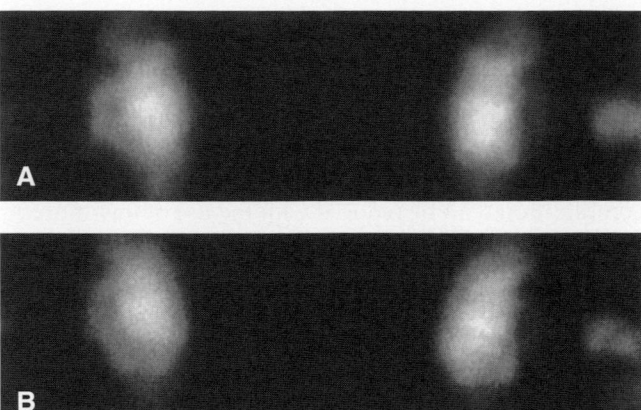

Figure 56–2 Pre- and postthrombolytic therapy lung scan showing minimal response to peripheral IV treatment with rt-PA at 100 mg over 2 hours, in association with heparin, 1,000 IU/hour in a patient with massive pulmonary embolism. Chest radiograph demonstrated right side pleural effusion (*not shown*). **A.** Pretreatment perfusion lung scan (anterior and posterior views) showed massive perfusion defects in the right lung and segmental perfusion defects in the left lung. **B.** Posttreatment lung scan (48 hours) showed mild improvement in the perfusion of the right lower lobe and left upper lobe (anterior and posterior views). Clinical improvement was observed, despite negligible perfusion improvement.

and heparin and showed a risk reduction of 41% and 40% in favor of thrombolysis, for death and recurrence, respectively. There was a major bleeding rate of 12.9% in patients receiving thrombolysis and 8.6% in patients receiving heparin (33). Another randomized study that dealt with hemodynamically stable patients with submassive PE, treated with heparin plus alteplase, compared with heparin plus placebo, showed improved clinical course and prevention of clinical deterioration that would require escalation of treatment, such as cathecolamine infusion, secondary thrombolysis, endotracheal intubation, cardiopulmonary resuscitation (CPR), surgical thrombectomy, or catheter fragmentation (34). However, the randomization schedule in this study was allowed to be broken, which generated some criticism on the validity of some of the conclusions (35). Great care should be exercised in the selection of the thrombolytic drug for treatment of massive PE because most of the available experience is with urokinase and the data are not immediately transferable to other drugs.

Proposed thrombolytic regimes for PE are as follows (36):

- Streptokinase: 250,000 IU as loading dose over 30 minutes followed by 100,000 IU/hour (31)
- Urokinase: 2,000 IU/pound loading dose over 10 minutes followed by 2,000 IU/pound per hour for 12–24 hours (36)

- rt-PA: 100 mg continuous peripheral IV infusion over 2 hours or 50 mg/2 hours plus an additional 40 mg/4 hours if necessary (36) or 100 mg IV over 7 hours (37)
- Heparin: 5,000 IU bolus followed by 1,000 IU/hour (in association with the above regimens) or weight-based heparin dosing nomogram, heparin at 100 IU/kg per hour (38)

CATHETER-DIRECTED THROMBOLYSIS

Catheter-directed thrombolytic therapy with intrapulmonary artery infusion of thrombolytic drugs is an alternative technique advocated by many authors (39–41) aiming to accelerate clot lysis and achieve more rapid reperfusion of the pulmonary circulation. The technique requires positioning of the catheter, via femoral access, wedged within the pulmonary artery clot, with injection of a bolus of thrombolytic drug followed by continuous infusion for 12–24 hours (Figure 56–3). Systemic heparinization is also used in association with thrombolytic therapy. Verstraete et al. in 1988 (37) published the results of a multicentric, comparative study between peripheral intravenous and intrapulmonary treatment of acute massive pulmonary embolism with rt-PA (100 mg over a 7-hour period) and indicated that the intrapulmonary infusion of rt-PA does not offer significant benefit over the intravenous route, it also suggested that a prolonged infusion of rt-PA over 7 hours is superior to a single infusion of 50 mg over a 2-hour period. The catheter infusion methodology described in the Verstraete study did not use any fragmentation techniques in association to thrombolytic therapy as is standard today, and this may have introduced a certain degree of bias into the conclusions. It is now known that fragmentation of a large thrombus occluding the main pulmonary artery will increase perfusion of the pulmonary vascular bed and increase the drug and/or clot contact surface, accelerating the lytic process (42). Some authors advise placement of an inferior vena caval (IVC) filter following catheter removal (13).

Proposed catheter-directed intrapulmonary thrombolytic regimens for PE are as follows (37,39–43):

- Urokinase: Infusion of 250,000 IU/hour mixed with 2,000 IU of heparin over 2 hours followed by an infusion of 100,000 IU/hour of urokinase for 12–24 hours
- rt-PA: Bolus of 10 mg followed by 20 mg/hour over 2 hours (total of 50 mg), or 100 mg over 7 hours. Or a bolus of 20 mg, followed by mechanical fragmentation and 80 mg over a period of 2 hours (total of 100 mg) (14)
- Heparin: Infusion of 1,000 IU/hour, keeping the PTT at 1.5 to 2.5 times the upper normal limits (in association with the above regimens)

Fibrinogen levels should be monitored at 4–6 hours interval, and if the level falls to less than 30–40% of the initially measured level, the infusion may have to be stopped or reduced. Fibrin degradation products and rt-PA antigens can also be measured. Association of other techniques, such as mechanical thrombus fragmentation with pulse spray, angioplasty balloon catheter, or other devices may increase the velocity of thrombolysis. It seems that the increased clot surface resulting from fragmentation is the main contributor to improved thrombolysis in such cases (Figure 56–4). On the other hand, the fragmentation of the clot, followed by peripheral dispersion of the smaller clot fragments to the peripheral branches, reduces pulmonary arterial pressure, increasing pulmonary flow. The postprocedure clinical improvement is generally noticeable in more than 90% of the patients (13), but improvements in survival and long-term pulmonary perfusion have not yet been consistently demonstrated. Although it is reasonable to assume that early reperfusion may improve long-term results, larger randomized studies will be necessary to prove this hypothesis. In a recent report, rapid clot lysis was obtained in 94% of the patients, with pronounced lysis in 66%, using rt-PA (43) (Figure 56–4).

Hemorrhagic complications are likely to be fewer with the catheter-directed thrombolysis than with the IV infusion technique, but no definitive evidence of this currently exists. However, the rate of major bleeding was 6% with catheter-directed infused rt-PA, compared with 27% and

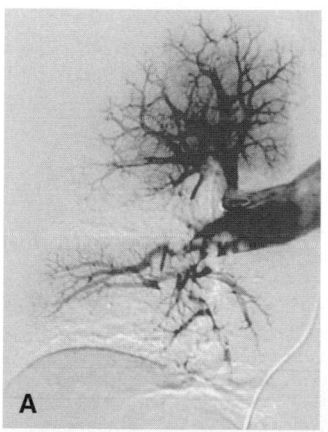 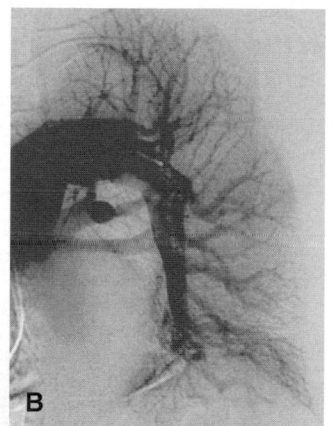 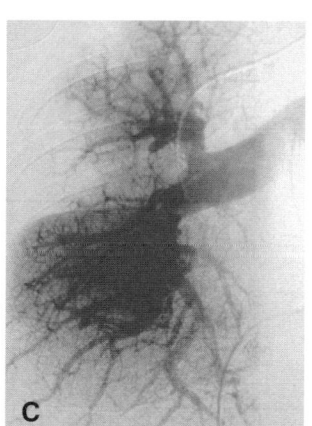 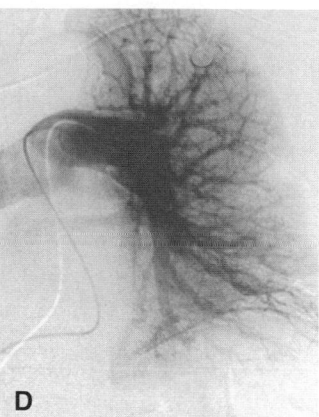

Figure 56–3 Patient with massive pulmonary embolism presented with syncope. **A.** Massive pulmonary embolism of the right pulmonary artery with a large thrombus occluding most of the artery, sparing only a portion of the right upper lobe. **B.** Left pulmonary angiogram showed large filling defect in the main left pulmonary artery. Catheter-directed thrombolytic therapy was performed. The catheter was wedged into the main thrombus in the right pulmonary artery, and urokinase was started at 100,000 IU/hour for 36 hours, with alternating catheterization of the left pulmonary artery for 12 hours. **C., D.** Posttreatment pulmonary angiography showed significant improvement of the pulmonary artery circulation in both lungs. The patient experienced dramatic recovery from the symptoms and reduction of pulmonary artery pressures. **E., F.** Pre- and posttreatment lung perfusion scans showed marked improvement of right lung perfusion. Note some improvement on the left lower lobe.

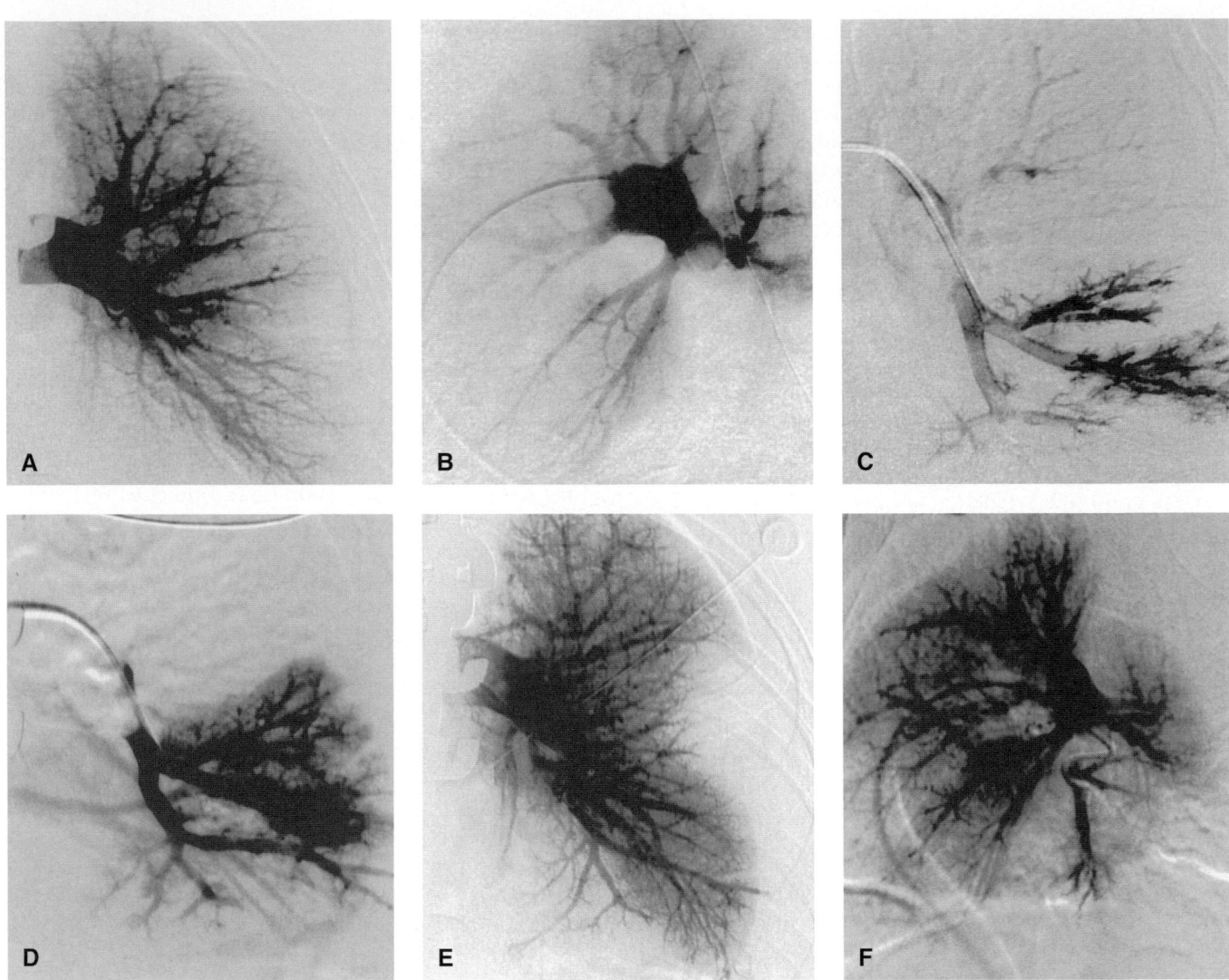

Figure 56–4 A 45-year-old female patient with lymphoma presented with chest pain and dyspnea. **A.** Left pulmonary artery angiography showed occlusion of the posterior basal segment of the left lower lobe. **B.** Lateral view of the arteriogram showed occlusion of the posterior basal segment. Note patency of the superior, anteromedial, and lateral basal segments with a wedge of the posterior basal segment missing. **C.** A straight catheter was advanced into the posterior basal segment artery, and contrast medium injection showed extensive thrombosis. The catheter was wedged, and urokinase infusion was started. **D.** Follow-up angiography, 12 hours into the treatment, showed restored patency of the peripheral branches of the posterior basal segment with persistent proximal occlusion of the posterior basal segment artery. **E., F.** Anterior and lateral view of the 24 hours follow-up angiogram showing persistent proximal occlusion and increased volume of pleural effusion, with further collapse of the superior segment and left upper lobe.

12%, respectively, for peripherally infused urokinase in phases I and II of the 1970s UPET study (30,31).

SURGICAL EMBOLECTOMY AND THROMBOENDARTERECTOMY

When pulmonary thromboembolism is massive, hemodynamic status is compromised, and cardiocirculatory shock may develop with changes that may be irreversible. Until

several years ago, if there was no response or contraindication to medical and/or thrombolytic therapy, the only treatment available was surgical thrombectomy using a sternotomy and opening of the main pulmonary artery for clot retrieval with a long forceps (Figure 56–5). Surgical therapy is now rarely considered because the results have not been encouraging. Although effective in numerous cases, surgical thrombectomy has been associated with high perioperative morbidity and mortality rates; however, more recent refinements in anesthesia and circulatory bypass technology allowed significant

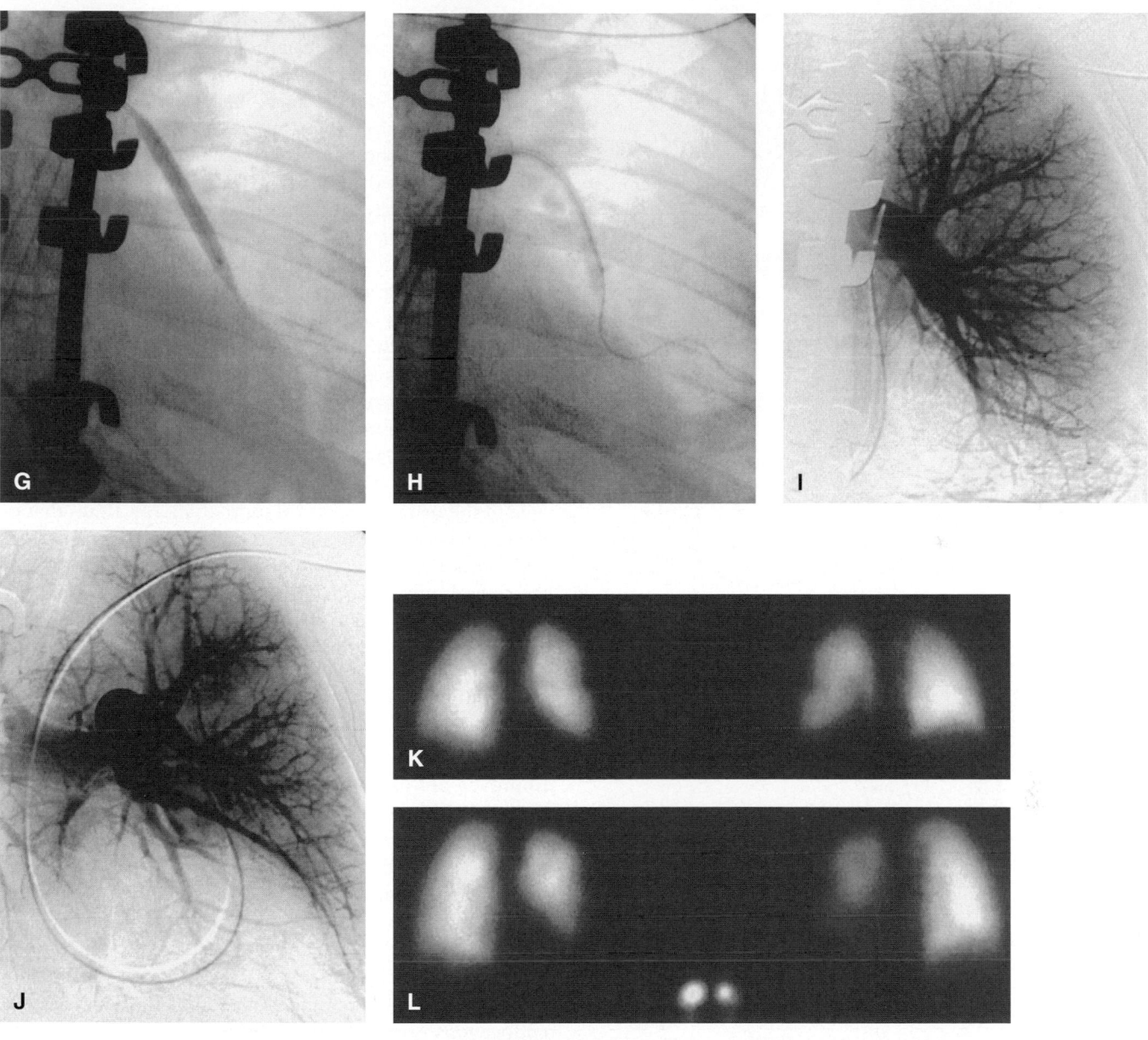

Figure 56–4 (*continued*) **G., H.** Balloon angioplasty and occlusion balloon thrombectomy was performed in the persistently occluded segment of the posterior basal segment, producing recanalization. **I., J.** Follow-up left pulmonary angiogram 1 month after treatment showed patent posterior basal segment. **K.** Pretreatment perfusion showed reduced perfusion of the left lower lobe. **L.** Posttreatment lung perfusion scan showed persistent reduced perfusion of the left lung base resulting from significant increase in pleural effusion.

improvement (44). Significant morbidity and mortality is still observed in most institutions. Operative treatment, however, may be lifesaving in patients with more than 50% obstruction of the pulmonary vascular bed, which may have an 85% mortality rate within the first 6 hours (45). Gulba et al. (46) in1994 reported on 37 consecutive patients over a period of 5 years, comparing medical treatment (IV rt-PA infusion) versus surgical embolectomy. Medical treatment was successful in 75% of the patients, with a mortality rate of 33%, and surgical treatment was successful in 85%, with a mortality rate of

23%. In this series, the data suggested that medical treatment had a higher death rate, an increased risk of major hemorrhage, and an increased recurrence rate of pulmonary embolism; however, the two nonrandomized groups of patients studied were not comparable regarding demographics, diagnostic techniques used for establishing the severity of PE, intensity of previous medical problems, and degree of adverse events, possibly creating a bias toward treating more severely afflicted patients with rt-PA infusion.

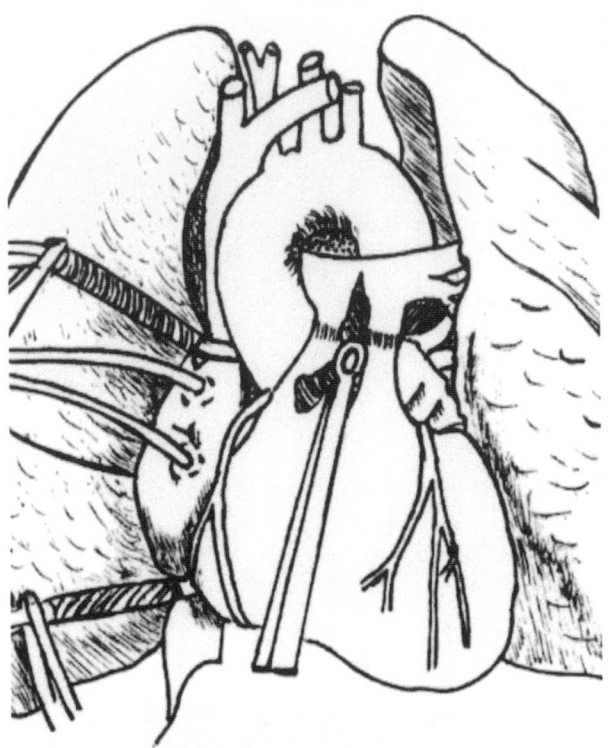

Figure 56–5 Schematic drawing of a surgical embolectomy from the main pulmonary artery with a surgical forceps. Note the circulatory bypass with catheters placed in the IVC and SVC tightened up by vascular loops.

A relatively small subset of patients with pulmonary hypertension and right heart failure secondary to chronic thromboembolic disease may also benefit from pulmonary thromboendarterectomy if selection is carefully performed. In the Jamieson series (44), mortality ranged from 5–12%, noted to be related to the learning curve, but in the surviving patients, mean pulmonary pressure decreased from 49 to 29 mm Hg, with decreased pulmonary resistance and improved cardiac output.

Venous interruption (IVC filter) preceding or following pulmonary embolectomy should always be considered in patients with extensive lower extremity venous thrombi to prevent immediate recurrent embolism in those patients on whom surgery was performed because of the inadequacy or failure of heparin therapy.

PERCUTANEOUS EMBOLECTOMY, CATHETER FRAGMENTATION, AND THROMBECTOMY

Frequently, the comorbid conditions that make patients poor thrombolysis candidates may also deem them unsuitable for an open surgical approach (47). Fortunately, when thrombolytic therapy fails or is contraindicated, the nonsurgical, less invasive option available for this group of patients with massive PE is percutaneous embolectomy and thrombectomy using some of the current thrombectomy mechanical devices. Some of these devices are not available in the United States or are still undergoing clinical trials for other applications unrelated to the treatment of PE. Some of the devices are aimed at removing clots, and others work through fragmentation, maceration, or aspiration. Extensive information on the different devices is already available. Mechanisms of action as well as experimental and clinical outcomes have been extensively discussed in the literature (48,49). Some of the techniques available do not totally eliminate the clots, but rather break down the thrombus into smaller fragments that will migrate peripherally in the pulmonary artery circulation, opening up the main pulmonary artery and improving perfusion (50). The rationale for using these devices in the pulmonary circulation is based on the rapid relief of central obstruction. The knowledge that the cross-sectional area of the distal arterioles is more than four times that of the central circulation and that the volume of the peripheral pulmonary circulatory bed is about two times that of the central pulmonary arteries suggests that the redistribution of larger central clots into the peripheral pulmonary arteries may acutely improve cardiopulmonary hemodynamics, with significant increase in total pulmonary blood flow and right ventricular function (Figure 56–6) (42,51). Although, this rationale is disputed by some (52), there is evidence of a reduction in pulmonary pressure and of improved perfusion as verified by follow-up catheterization and pulmonary perfusion studies (42,51,53).

The action of the thrombectomy devices may be facilitated in certain circumstances by softening of the thrombus mass by thrombolytic therapy, which helps speed up the debulking and fragmentation of the occlusive clots (42). Fragmentation can and should be used as a complement to thrombolytic therapy (Figure 56–4). On the other hand, fragmentation of the clot exposes fresh surfaces for endogenous urokinase and infused thrombolytic drugs to further break down the emboli (54). Furthermore, as a result of the improved flow in the previously occluded artery, the clots come into more intimate contact with the increased concentration of the infused drug. The importance of fragmentation of pulmonary emboli cannot be stressed enough.

An ideal thrombectomy device for the pulmonary artery should have the following characteristics:

- Be easy to use and position within the clots and branches of the pulmonary artery
- Have adequate steerability during the procedure or in use over the wire
- Be able to promote complete removal of clots or fragmentation into extremely small particles
- Be long enough to reach the pulmonary artery, have a low profile, and still treat a large vessel
- Have a low cost

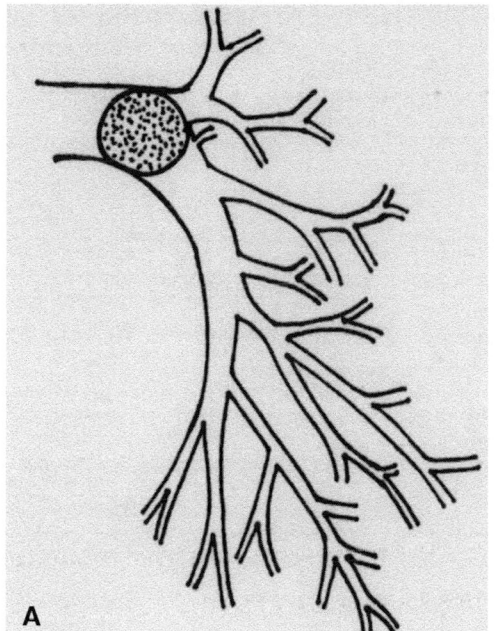
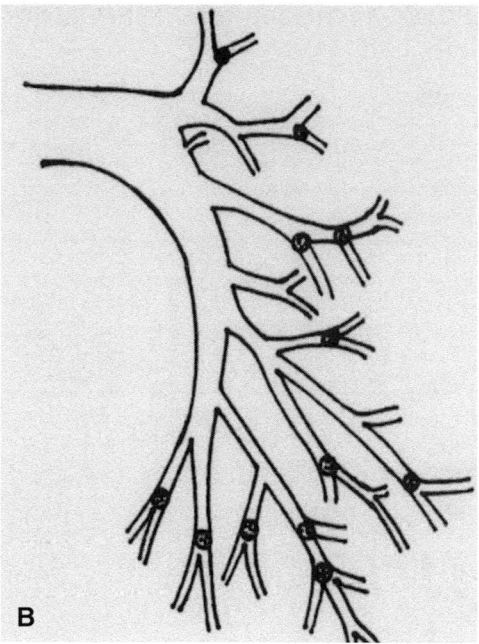

Figure 56–6 Schematic drawing demonstrating the effect of mechanical fragmentation of a total occlusive central thrombus in the pulmonary artery, **A.** before and **B.** after mechanical fragmentation and dispersion of the smaller clots into the peripheral branches of the pulmonary artery. Fragmentation and distal dispersion is likely to reduce pulmonary artery pressure and increase total pulmonary perfusion. Note that a number of peripheral branches of the pulmonary artery are open following fragmentation of the thrombus.

Following is a brief review of some of the concepts and information available for some of the percutaneous devices and techniques that are potentially useful or that have been successfully used in the treatment of massive PE (Table 56–2).

THROMBECTOMY AND EMBOLECTOMY DEVICES

Greenfield Embolectomy Device

The Greenfield embolectomy device (GED) (Boston Scientific) is a 10 French braided, steerable catheter with a 5-mm or 7-mm plastic cup at the tip. It was designed to be inserted through a venotomy via femoral or jugular veins. The GED was the first device designed for the treatment of massive pulmonary embolism and has been available for more than 30 years. By manual suction with a large syringe, the device pulls out the nonorganized clots through the venotomy or a large valveless vascular sheath (Figure 56–7). Multiple passes may be required to complete the treatment. In the hands of the inventor and developer of the device, it has been successful in extracting pulmonary thrombus in 76% of the cases, with significant reduction of the mean pulmonary artery pressure and increase in cardiac output (55). Despite hemodynamic improvement, the 30-day mortality rate was still around 30%. The device was less useful in chronic recurrent PE as a result of the organization of the thrombus, making it less likely to be removed. GED was more successful for cases of major acute PE. The same device, however, has been less successful in the hands of other investigators (56). Fracture of the extracted pulmonary

thrombus with distal embolization is still an unsolved problem of the technique, which usually requires multiple additional passes of the device and makes it more difficult to clean up the pulmonary circulation.

Balloon Angioplasty for Clot Fragmentation

Balloon angioplasty for fragmentation of pulmonary emboli has been used for several years in an attempt to produce rapid restoration of pulmonary blood flow and promote improvement of cardiac output and reduction of pulmonary pressure (42,51). Balloon fragmentation of the clots is achieved relatively rapidly, with distal dispersion of the smaller fragments. Manipulation with other, more conventional pigtail catheters and latex occlusion balloons is also useful in many cases when the clots are fresher (57,58).

Mechanical fragmentation using angioplasty balloon catheter (from 6- to 16-mm in diameter) associated with pharmacologic thrombolysis (urokinase, 80,000–100,000 IU/hour for 8–24 hours) for massive PE was recently described as highly successful, with an 87.5% recovery rate as measured by pulmonary artery pressures, blood O_2 values, and clinical outcomes (13,42) (Figure 56–8).

Kensey Dynamic Device (Trac-Wright System)

The Kensey device (Dow Corning) was the first available flexible rotating-tip catheter and the predecessor of several generations of rotational catheters. The device was made of flexible polyurethane catheter, in 5 French and 8 French sizes. At the distal tip was a high-speed rotating cam, which was driven at speeds of 5,000–100,000 rpm by a bedside direct

TABLE 56-2
TECHNIQUE AND DEVICE LISTING WITH CURRENT INFORMATION FOR THE TREATMENT OF PE

Device/Technique	Advantages	Disadvantages	Size French	Efficacy	FDA Approval/Modality	Current US Trial	Availability in United States
Anticoagulation	Reduces mortality and recurrence of PE	Does not treat existing thrombus	N/A	Effective			
Heparin	Large experience	Bleeding complications	N/A	Effective	Yes	N/A	Yes
LMWH	Reduced bleeding complications	Small experience	N/A	Presumed effective	No	Unknown	Yes
Argatroban	Alternative to heparin in HIT	Small experience	N/A	Presumed effective	No	No	Yes
Systemic Thrombolysis	Accelerates clot lysis, pulmonary reperfusion; improves pulmonary capillary blood volume	Bleeding complications; presumed less effective than local	N/A	Effective	Yes	N/A	Yes
Streptokinase	Effective	Small experience; allergic reactions			Yes	N/A	Yes
Urokinase	Effective; large experience	Currently not available			Yes	N/A	No
rt-PA	Effective	Small experience			Yes	N/A	Yes
Catheter-Directed Thrombolysis	Accelerates clot lysis and reperfusion	Bleeding complications	Small	Effective	No	No	Yes
Surgical Embolectomy	Acute reperfusion of pulmonary circulation	High morbidity and mortality	N/A	Effective	N/A	N/A	Yes
Percutaneous Embolectomy/ Thrombectomy							
Greenfield	Rapid reperfusion	Difficult manipulation; arrythmias	Large	Effective	Yes	No	Yes
Balloon angioplasty and fragmentation	Rapid reperfusion	Moderate morbidity	Small	Effective	No	No	Yes
Kensey	Potential reperfusion	High morbidity	Small	Moderate	No	No	No
Hydrolyser	Potential reperfusion	High morbidity	Small	Low	No	No	Yes
Oasis	Potential reperfusion	Low power	Small	Low	No	No	Yes
AngioJet	Potential reperfusion	Effective in peripheral branches and some central in some cases	Small	Moderate	No	No	Yes
Impeller basket	Rapid reperfusion	Limited steerability and experience	Small	Effective	No	No	No
Thrombolizer	Rapid reperfusion	Trauma to the vessel; limited experience	Small	Moderate	No	No	No
Modified impeller catheter	Rapid reperfusion	Trauma to the vessel; limited experience	Small	Moderate	No	No	No
Rotatable pigtail	Rapid reperfusion	Potential trauma	Small	Effective	No	No	No
Arrow-Trerotola	Rapid reperfusion	Potential trauma; not steerable	Small	Effective	No	No	Yes*
Amplatz (ATD)	Rapid reperfusion	Potential trauma; not over the wire	Small	Effective	No	No	Yes
Lang Device	Rapid reperfusion; homemade	Potential trauma; limited experience	Large	Effective	No	No	Yes
AMATC	Rapid reperfusion	Potential trauma	Small	Effective	No	No	No
Rotarex	Unknown	Potential trauma for small vessels	Small	Promising	No	No	No
Pulmonary Artery Stent							
Wallstent Z stent	Rapid reperfusion	Potential trauma; migration	Small	Effective	No	No	Yes

*Available in a different configuration. *LMWH*, low-molecular-weight heparin; *AMATC*, Amplatz Maceration Aspiration Thrombectomy Catheter; *ATD*, Amplatz thrombectomy device.

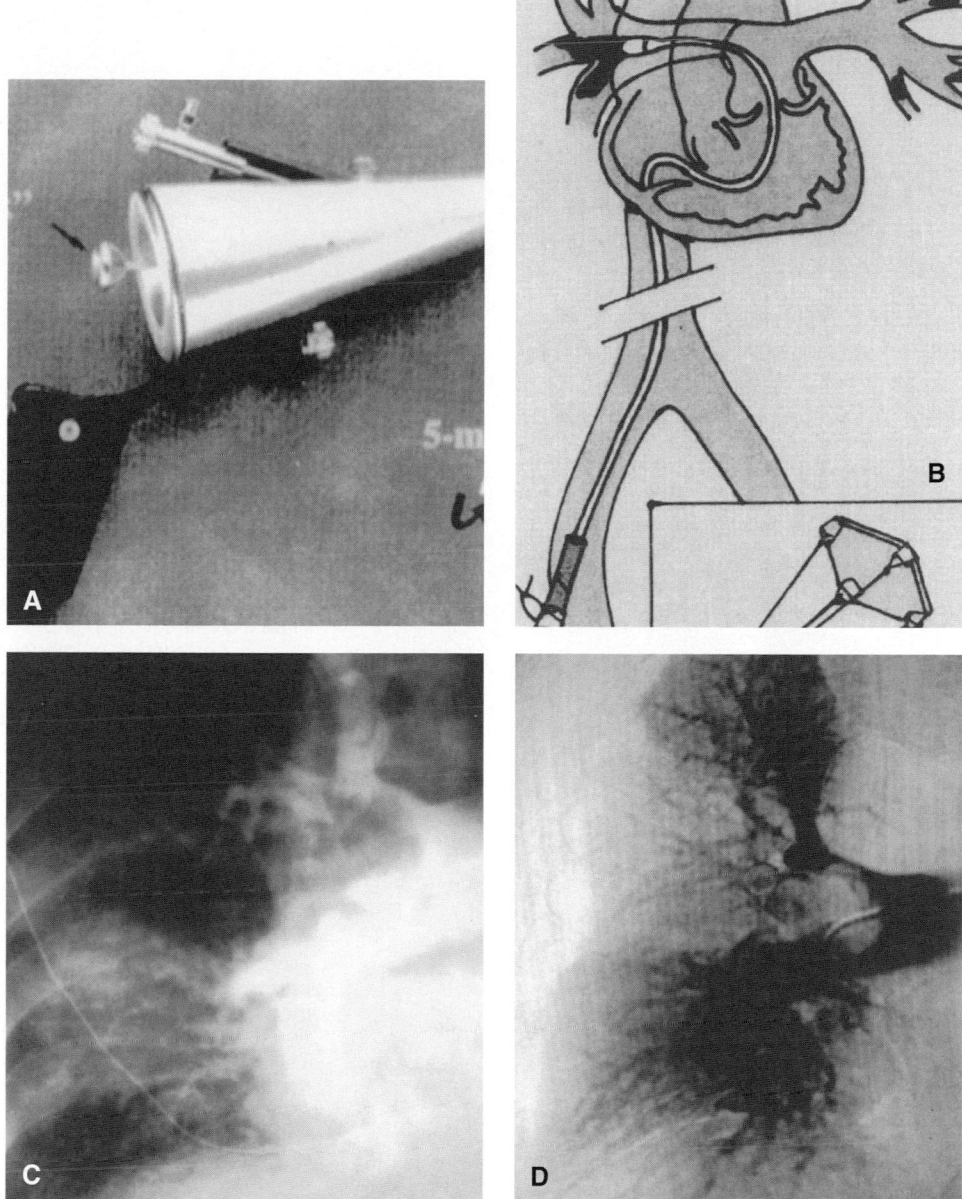

Figure 56–7   A. Greenfield embolectomy device. The 10 French steerable catheter is seen with the 7-mm cup at the tip (*curved arrow*). The large metallic handle is used to attach the catheter, and the "joystick" is used to steer the tip of the catheter (*straight arrow*). The port at the top of the handle is for suction through the lumen of the catheter. **B.** Schematic drawing of the embolectomy procedure showing the catheter inserted through the right femoral vein, passing through the right atrium and right ventricle into the pulmonary artery, sucking the thrombus with the catheter cup. **C.** Right pulmonary artery arteriogram showed massive pulmonary embolism with occlusion of the main right pulmonary artery and multiple main peripheral branches of the pulmonary artery. **D.** Postembolectomy pulmonary angiogram showed significant improvement in right pulmonary perfusion, but the major clot persisted. There was clinical improvement.

current motor. A vortex was created at the catheter tip promoting fragmentation of thrombus that comes in contact with the rotating tip (Figure 56–9). A later version of the device could be used over the wire. A number of complications, mainly related to the unprotected rotational tip, were observed, including vessel perforation, intimal dissection,

and extravasation of contrast material. The device was initially designed as an atherectomy catheter and was used quite successfully for the treatment of PE in an animal model (59). The Kensey device was approved by the FDA for atherectomy, but it is not currently available in the United States, and although it has been used for thrombectomy in a few human

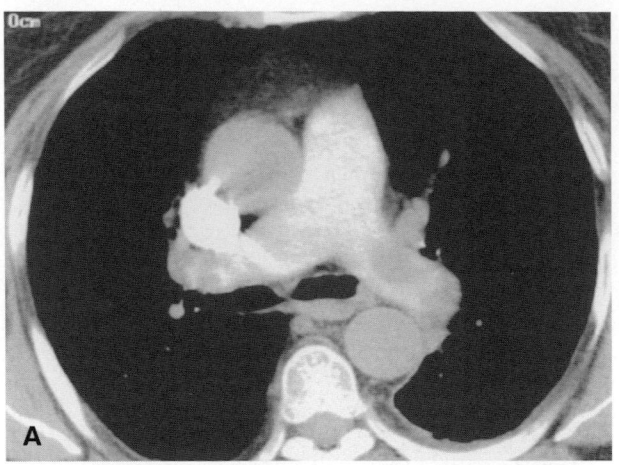

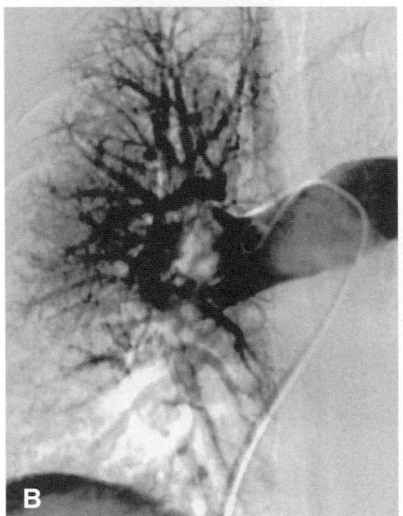

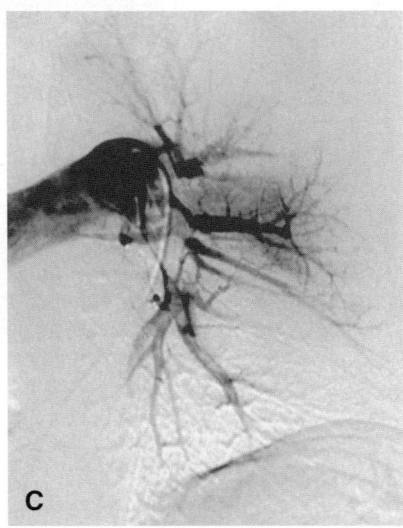

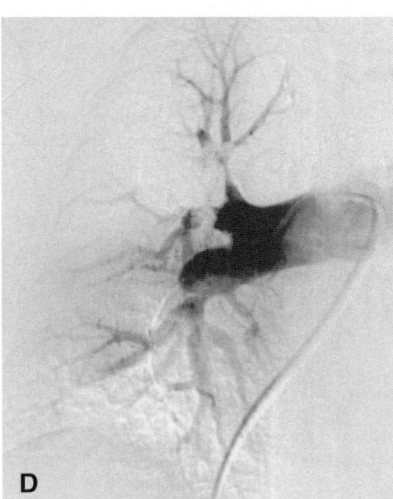

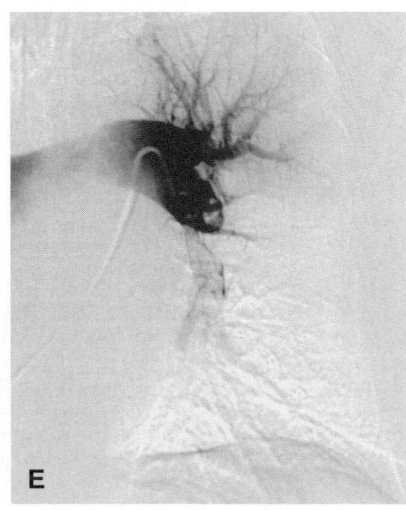

Figure 56–8 A 78-year-old female patient with chronic obstructive pulmonary disease, on home oxygen, with a history of myocardial infarction 1 month before, presented at the ER at another institution with symptoms of DVT, chest pain, shortness of breath, and congestive heart failure. The patient underwent a chest CT scan that was positive for pulmonary embolism. V/Q scan showed massive perfusion defects. The patient was transferred to the author's institution, and a pulmonary arteriogram was requested for diagnosis and possible thrombolytic treatment. **A.** CT scan of the chest showed large filling defects in both main pulmonary arteries. After being hemodynamically stabilized, the patient was transferred, and a pulmonary arteriogram was performed at the author's institution. **B.** Right pulmonary artery angiogram showed massive obstruction of the bifurcation of the right pulmonary artery. There is persistent, but reduced, perfusion of the right upper lobe and marked hypoperfusion of the right lower lobe. **C.** Left pulmonary artery angiogram showed massive embolism in the left lower lobe segment, with marked reduction in peripheral perfusion. The pulmonary artery pressure was 39 mm Hg. **D.** Follow-up right pulmonary artery angiogram after 15 hours of treatment, with urokinase at 250,000 IU/hour through the pigtail catheter wedged into the thrombus on the right side, showed marked improvement of the thrombus obstruction with some residual clots mainly occluding the right upper and middle lobe. There was improvement in the right lower lobe perfusion. **E.** Follow-up arteriogram of the left pulmonary artery showed worsening of the occlusion of the left lower lobe, probably by distal migration of the thrombus from the main branch into the more peripheral circulation. Pulmonary artery pressure was 46 mm Hg.

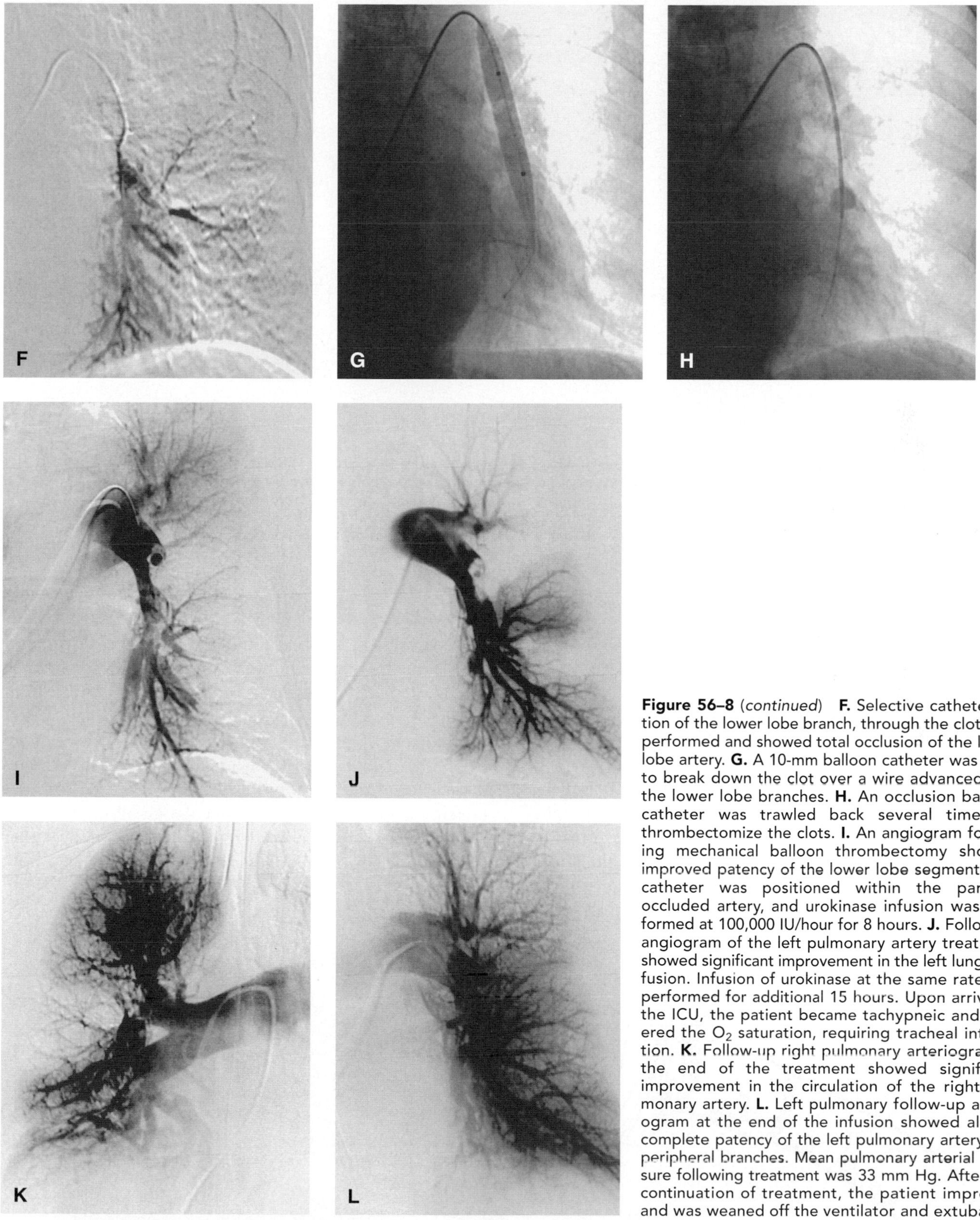

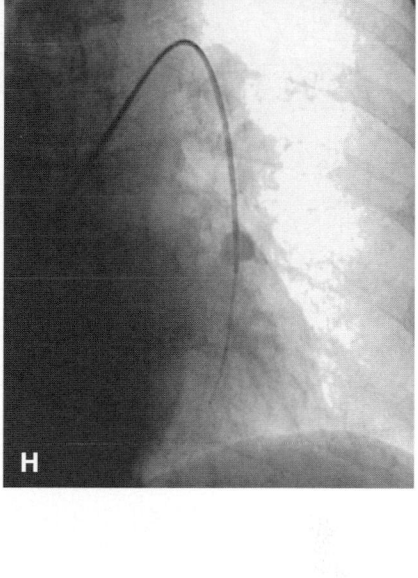

Figure 56–8 (*continued*)   **F.** Selective catheterization of the lower lobe branch, through the clot, was performed and showed total occlusion of the lower lobe artery. **G.** A 10-mm balloon catheter was used to break down the clot over a wire advanced into the lower lobe branches. **H.** An occlusion balloon catheter was trawled back several times to thrombectomize the clots. **I.** An angiogram following mechanical balloon thrombectomy showed improved patency of the lower lobe segment. The catheter was positioned within the partially occluded artery, and urokinase infusion was performed at 100,000 IU/hour for 8 hours. **J.** Follow-up angiogram of the left pulmonary artery treatment showed significant improvement in the left lung perfusion. Infusion of urokinase at the same rate was performed for additional 15 hours. Upon arrival at the ICU, the patient became tachypneic and lowered the O_2 saturation, requiring tracheal intubation. **K.** Follow-up right pulmonary arteriogram at the end of the treatment showed significant improvement in the circulation of the right pulmonary artery. **L.** Left pulmonary follow-up arteriogram at the end of the infusion showed almost complete patency of the left pulmonary artery and peripheral branches. Mean pulmonary arterial pressure following treatment was 33 mm Hg. After discontinuation of treatment, the patient improved and was weaned off the ventilator and extubated.

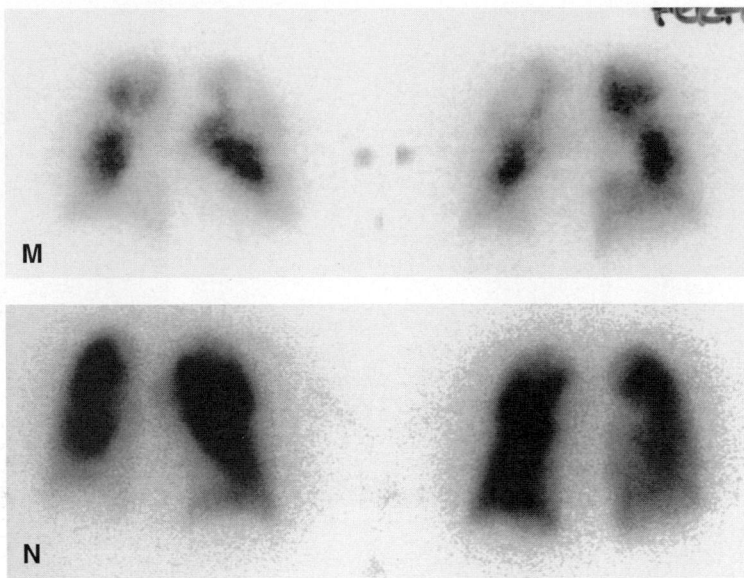

Figure 56–8 (*continued*) **M.** Pretreatment perfusion scan showed a high probability picture with multiple extensive areas of hypoperfusion, suggesting massive pulmonary embolism. **N.** Perfusion scan 3 days following thrombolytic treatment showed remarkable improvement in bilateral pulmonary perfusion. After discharge from the ICU, the patient began to show signs of acute renal failure that reversed in 5 days to normal creatinine levels. The patient was discharged home 5 days after the end of the treatment for PE.

patients with PE, that utilization, to the best of the author's knowledge, has never been reported in the literature.

Hydrodynamic Thrombectomy Catheter (Hydrolyser) and Oasis (SET) Catheter

The Hydrolyser catheter system (Cordis) is a 7 French, over-the-wire catheter, 65 or 80 cm long, with a straight but relatively flexible tube and a large side hole near the distal tip. The system has a double-lumen shaft; the larger one is dedicated to aspiration of the fragmented clots, and the smaller lumen is the injection channel with a metallic tubing looped at 180 degrees in the opposite direction to the tip of the catheter (Figure 56–10). High-velocity injection through the small lumen creates lower pressure dynamics in the larger lumen and a vortex that causes fragmentation of the clots and aspiration resulting from the pressure gradient (60). The device design allows for effective aspiration in vessels ranging from 5–9 mm in diameter. When used in larger vessels, it tends to create a tract

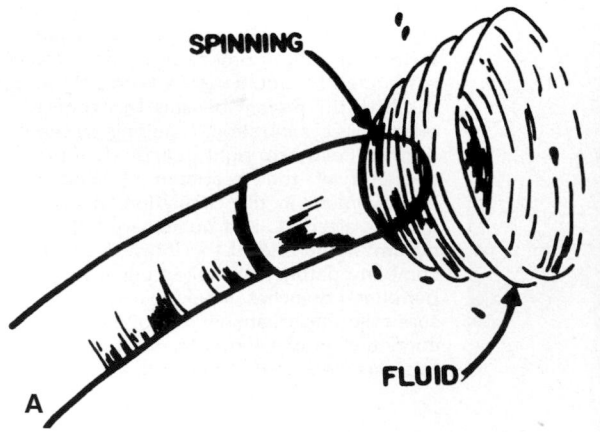
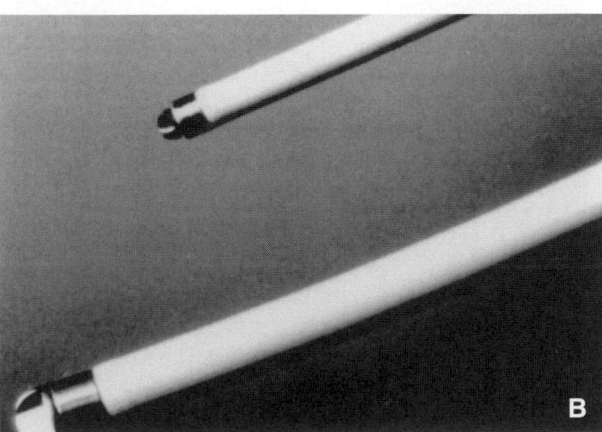

Figure 56–9 **A.** Diagrammatic illustration of the Kensey catheter, showing the high-energy vortex created by the infusate and the rotational cam. **B.** Kensey catheters in 5 French and 8 French sizes. Note at the distal end of the catheter a high-speed rotational metallic cam. In another version, the device can be used over the wire.

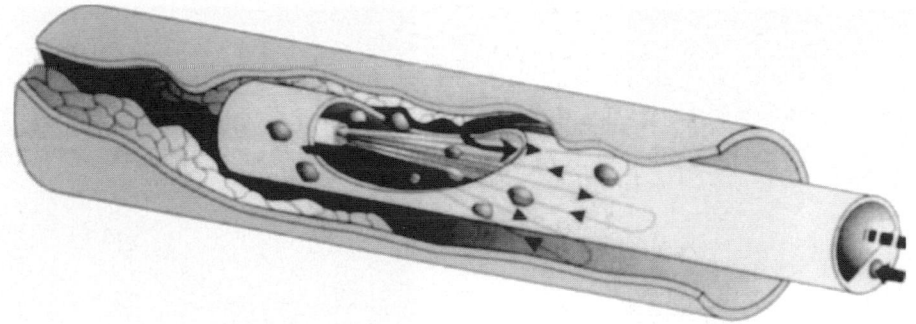

Figure 56–10 Diagram of the Hydrolyser catheter. This device is a 7 French, over-the-wire, hydrodynamic thrombectomy catheter, with a double-lumen shaft. The larger lumen is for aspiration of the fragmented clots, and the smaller lumen is for the injection channel of the high-pressure saline. The small lumen channel ends in a metallic tubing looped at 180 degrees in the opposite direction to the tip of the catheter. The high-velocity fluid passes beneath the large side hole near the tip and enters the main lumen. The velocity of the fluid creates a low-pressure dynamic in the area around the side hole, and the adjacent thrombus is fragmented, aspirated, and subsequently flushed out through the main lumen.

within the clot. For the pulmonary artery application, because of the available length, the device is used from the internal jugular vein and advanced, over a 0.025-inch guide wire, into the pulmonary artery. The rigidity of the catheter causes some difficulty in advancing through the right atrium and ventricle into the pulmonary artery. A few unreported cases performed in Europe showed no effective declotting in the central pulmonary artery. The application of the Hydrolyser in the pulmonary artery circulation seems to be limited to fresh clots and to more peripheral branches. However, a recently published case report presented a successful thrombectomy of major branches of the pulmonary artery (61). Although effective for smaller vessels, the low power of the device in the current design is a major limitation for the treatment of larger vessels. Improvements in the device may be available in the future, including longer lengths, a more powerful hydrodynamic effect achieved with the use of an additional proximal Venturi system, and a special pigtail tip for the pulmonary artery application. Those modifications, however, are not commercially available, and the efficacy has not yet been proved.

The Oasis catheter (formerly known as the shredding embolectomy thrombectomy [S.E.T.] catheter) (Boston Scientific) also works with a Venturi-based system. It creates a vortex that causes fragmentation and aspiration of the clots (48) (Figure 56–11). Because of the design, limited power, and size, it encounters limited application in larger vessels. Larger devices might be available in the future and possibly more useful for larger vessels such as the pulmonary artery.

Rheolytic Thrombectomy Catheter (AngioJet or Possis Device)

The AngioJet (Possis) is similar to the Hydrolyser and Oasis catheters in concept. It also uses the Venturi effect to perform thrombectomy, but it is different in design from the Hydrolizer and Oasis catheters. It is a double-lumen system with a diameter ranging from 4–6 French. The smaller lumen is made of a fine metal tubing that conducts the high-pressure, high-velocity stream of saline fluid. The metal tubing makes a circle (ring) at the tip of the end hole of the catheter, and the jet is oriented backward, in the direction of the main lumen of the catheter shaft, creating a low-pressure area promoting fragmentation and evacuation

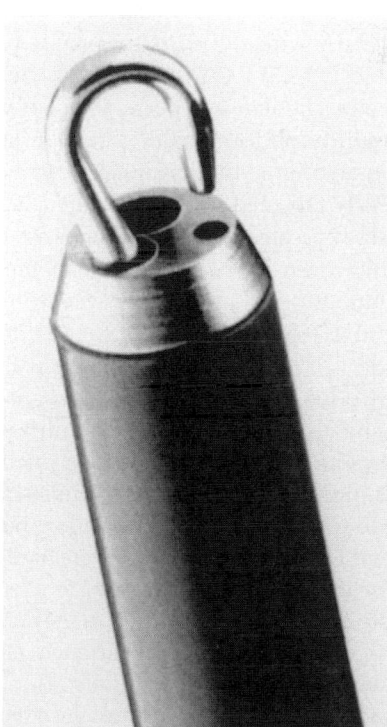

Figure 56–11 The Oasis catheter also works with a Venturi-based system. The catheter has three lumens: two smaller lumens (one for the guide wire and one for the high-pressure fluid injection) and the larger lumen for flushing the clots out via the low-pressure flow dynamics created by the high-velocity fluid jet.

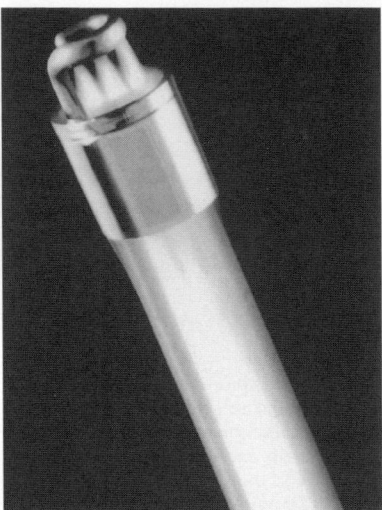

Figure 56–12 The AngioJet system works with the Venturi effect to perform thrombectomy. It has a double-lumen shaft. The smaller lumen is for injection of a high-velocity stream of saline fluid. The small lumen ends in a metal tubing ring with side holes oriented backward, in the direction of the main lumen of the catheter shaft. The low-pressure dynamics created promote fragmentation and suction of the clots. The device can be used over the wire, passed through the main lumen. The device showed here is an older design of the AngioJet, but it better shows the structure of the device.

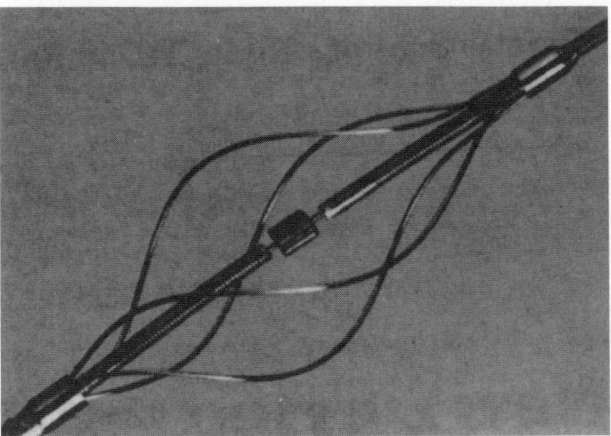

Figure 56–13 Impeller basket device depicted in a blown up view of the self-expandable metal basket. Note the small impeller in the center of the basket attached to the axis in the center of the system. The rotation of the impeller creates a vortex that pulls the clots inside the basket with subsequent fragmentation. The basket wire touches the vessel walls, protecting the wall from the impeller. The system is relatively rigid and difficult to properly position. (Reprinted with permission from Schmitz-Rode T, Vorwerk D, Günther RW, et al. Percutaneous fragmentation of pulmonary emboli in dogs with the impeller basket catheter. Cardiovasc Intervent Radiol 1993;16:234–242.)

of the clots (Figure 56–12). The newer design of the AngioJet includes side holes that provide lateral spray jets to aid in the breakdown of the clots. It also allows the simultaneous use of thrombolytic drugs. The catheter can be advanced over the wire, allowing for precise placement in the desired vessel (48,51), which is advantageous when used in the pulmonary circulation. The treatment of massive PE is a potential application for this device, and it has been used successfully in an animal model and in a number of clinical cases, as recently reported in the literature (62,63), including clots centrally located in the pulmonary artery. Koning et al. reported improvement of the pulmonary pressure in one of two patients, but the procedures were long, and large amounts of mixed saline and blood were retrieved, requiring interruption of the procedure (62). As is the case with the other hydrodynamic systems, this device is likely to be more successful in patients with fresher thrombus that is more peripherally located in the pulmonary circulation. The use of the AngioJet device in other vascular beds, such as portal vein and for TIPS shunt recanalization, has been occasionally related to the occurrence of severe bradyarrhythmia and type III heart block, possibly related to adenosine liberated from hemolyzed red cells acting on the atrioventricular node (64). Hyperkalemia causing ST segment elevations has also been described (64). Personally, the author has observed bradyarrhythmia in a neonate when using the AngioJet device in the IVC, but without ST segment elevation. To the best of the author's knowledge, this problem has not been reported during the use of the AngioJet in the pulmonary circulation.

Impeller Basket Device

The impeller basket device (Cook) is formed by a flexible wire shaft inside a 7 French catheter with a small impeller mounted on the wire and in the center of a metallic self-expandable basket. The impeller is connected through the wire to an external electric motor that may produce up to 100,000 rpm. The impeller creates a vortex inside the vessel lumen and pulls the thrombus into the basket, causing fragmentation of the clots (Figure 56–13). The basket protects the vessel wall from the rotational impeller (65). This device was designed for the treatment of PE and has been tested in animals and used in a limited number of unreported human cases, with relative success and without significant vessel wall damage. The particles obtained with the device were extremely small after only a few seconds of activation time. The device is limited in steerability and is relatively stiff. Multiple subsegmental occlusions were observed in the animal model after treating the thrombus in the main pulmonary artery (66).

Thrombolizer and Modified Impeller Catheter

The thrombolizer and the modified impeller catheter are similar devices in design and operation. The thrombolizer is an over-the-wire thrombectomy catheter consisting of an outer 8 French catheter with an inner 5 French catheter with longitudinal slits in the distal tip. The 5 French catheter is designed to rotate relative to the outer catheter. The centrifugal force created causes the flat segments of the catheter

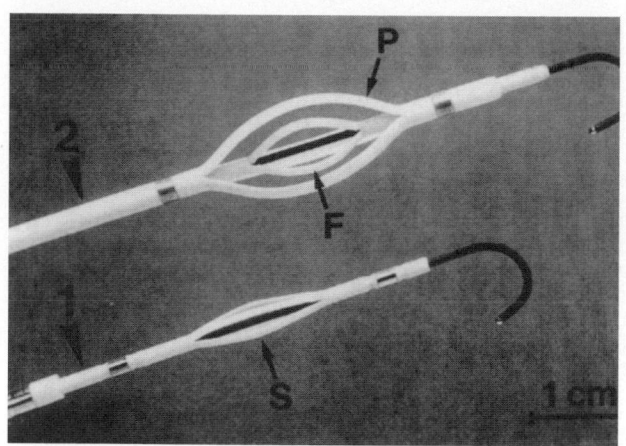

Figure 56–14 The thrombolizer and the modified impeller device (MID) are all plastic rotational devices that create a vortex within the vessel, pulling the clots and causing fragmentation. The MID (1) is placed through a guiding catheter, and the slitted catheter (S) expands like a basket as a result of the rotational movement of the catheter. Note that the basket is not protected and will scrape the vessel wall during activation. The thrombolizer (2) is a coaxial catheter system with a plastic, self-expandable basket (P), with a small rotational basket inside (F) that creates the vortex for thrombus fragmentation. Both systems work over the wire, which increases the chances for correct positioning. (Reprinted with permission from Schmitz-Rode T, Adam G, Kilbingr M, et al. Fragmentation of pulmonary emboli: in vivo experimental evaluation of two high-speed rotating catheters. Cardiovasc Intervent Radiol 1996;19:165–169.)

shaft, between the slits, to open into a basket shape, causing fragmentation of the clots. The turbine providing rotational energy to this device can produce as many as 100,000 rpm (Figure 56–14).

The impeller catheter consists of an over the wire outer 8 French Teflon catheter and an inner rotational 5 French catheter. The outer catheter has slits in the walls and is able to expand to 10 mm in diameter. The inner rotational catheter opens its basket to 5 mm in diameter, independently of the rpm applied to the system. This system rotates to high speeds of approximately 100,000 rpm, creating a strong vortex and clot fragmentation (67).

Both devices have been tried experimentally in animal models and were relatively successful in promoting fragmentation of pulmonary emboli and a decrease in pulmonary artery pressures. However, fracture of the device was observed in a few cases with the thrombolizer. Histologic evaluation of the treatment site showed significant periarterial and peribronchial hemorrhage, which was more evident in the cases in which the thrombolizer catheter was used. There are no reports of the use of these devices in humans, and it is unclear at this point whether there will be a role for clinical application of these devices.

Rotatable Pigtail Catheter

The rotatable pigtail catheter is a custom-made device using a modified high-torque 5 French pigtail catheter with a

radiopaque tip, 115 cm in length, and with 10 side holes for contrast material injection. A jugular version of the catheter is 105 cm long. There is an oval side hole, pierced in the outer aspect of the beginning of the pigtail loop in straight projection with the axis of the catheter lumen, allowing direct passage of a guide wire through the hole to act as a central axis around which the catheter rotates. The catheter is used through 90-cm-long, 5.5 French flexible sheath, and a Y fitting allows for adjustable tightening and flushing around the catheter shaft (Figure 56–15). A low-speed electrical motor may be attached to the proximal catheter hub and activated when the catheter tip is within the intrapulmonary thrombus; however, the catheter may be used manually, which is enough to break most clots. The pigtail tip of the catheter disrupts the clot into multiple smaller fragments, which migrate distally in the pulmonary circulation pushed by the pulmonary artery blood flow. The catheter may be advanced into the more peripheral branches and manually rotated to further fragment the clot. No damage to the tip of the catheter was observed in the initial experimental trials. Extensive experimental work in animal models has been done in previous years (68). The clinical application of this device is more recent, and a 1998 publication by Schmitz-Rode showed a 70% success rate in 10 patients (69) with clinical improvement and reduction of systolic and diastolic pulmonary artery pressure. The rotatable catheter can be used for diagnostic injections as well as for the thrombectomy procedure. Adjuvant thrombolytic therapy with rt-PA was utilized in addition to the mechanical thrombectomy with the rotatory catheter during the clinical trial (69). A more recent unreported update in this experience dealing with 20 patients showed a 33% recanalization rate by fragmentation alone, but a higher yield was obtained with the association of thrombolytic therapy. Mortality in this series was 20% (T. Schmitz-Rode, MD, *personal communication*, 2000).

Arrow-Trerotola Percutaneous Thrombolytic Device

The Arrow-Trerotola device (Arrow) is a low-speed rotational basket (3,000 rpm) used for thrombectomy in dialysis grafts (Figure 56–16). It scrapes the walls of the vessel and fragments the thrombus. The device was adapted for the treatment of PE in an animal model and shown to be effective in fragmenting the clots and relatively safe for treating large, acute central pulmonary emboli (70). The modified 120-cm-long device was used over a 0.025-inch guide wire and had an 8 French constraining catheter. The nitinol wire basket measures 9–15 mm in diameter when expanded. Histologically, there was moderate acute intimal injury but no evidence of pulmonary artery disruption; however, a device became entangled with the pulmonary artery wall of the animal. Mild periadvential bleeding was identified in all the animals, most commonly in the distal branches. On a longer-term follow-up, no pulmonary hypertension or

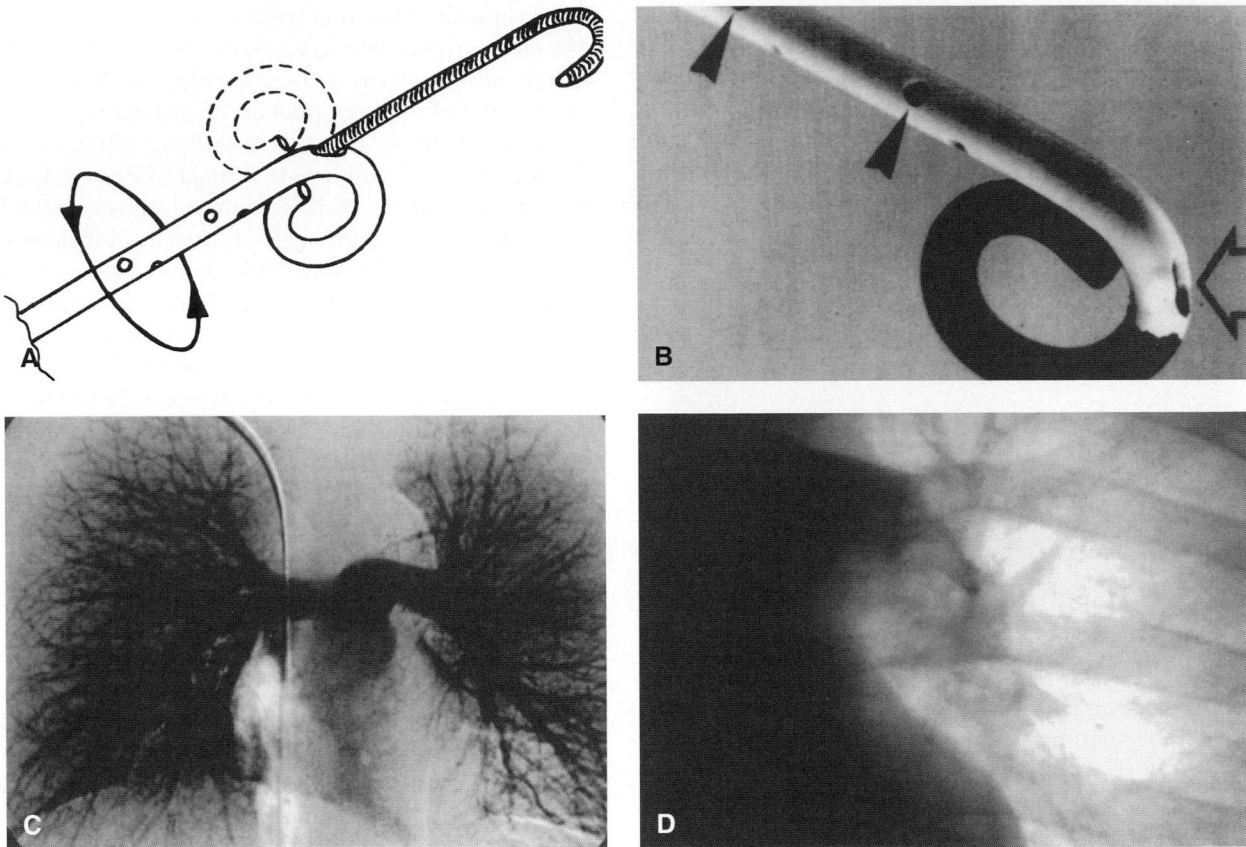

Figure 56–15 A. Schematic drawing of the pigtail rotational catheter over the stationary guide wire, passed through the distal hole, and used as a directing axis of rotation. The clots are fragmented by the mechanical action of the rotating pigtail tip. The wire also allows the catheter to be advanced or withdrawn over the wire. **B.** Tip of the rotational pigtail catheter, with a diameter of 7 mm. The oval-shaped side hole (*arrow*) allows the wire to pass out through the outer curvature of the pigtail. The side holes (*arrowhead*) are used for contrast material injection as in a regular angiographic catheter. **C.** A 36-year-old-male patient with multiple fractures in the legs and cervical spine presented with right DVT and massive PE. Pulmonary arteriogram showed complete occlusion of the left pulmonary artery. Fragmentation was performed with the pigtail rotational catheter, followed by additional thrombolysis with 70 mg of rt-PA. **D.** Control angiography 3 days after the treatment showed excellent perfusion of both pulmonary arteries. (Reprinted with permission from Schmitz-Rode T, Günther RW, Pfeffer JG, et al. Acute massive pulmonary embolism: use of a rotatable pigtail catheter for diagnosis and fragmentation therapy. Radiology 1995;197:157–162.)

histological evidence of scar formation was observed. There is only one case report in the literature demonstrating the clinical usefulness of this device (80 cm long, over the wire) for mechanical thrombectomy of massive pulmonary embolism (71) as of this writing. In that report, the device was difficult to direct into some of the vessels being treated, there was no improvement in pulmonary pressure, and large portions of clot remained untreated, although clinical improvement was observed. The Arrow-Trerotola device is potentially more useful in clots that are older and more organized, where the other devices yield decreased success; however, the safety of this device in native vessels is unproved.

Amplatz Thrombectomy Device

The Amplatz thrombectomy device (ATD, Microvena) is a 120-cm-long, 7 or 8 French reinforced polyurethane catheter with a distal metal tip (can) housing an impeller mounted on a drive shaft. The metal can has three side ports behind the impeller used for recirculation of the particles. The high speed of the impeller creates a vortex inside the vessel, pulling the clots toward the impeller, which recirculates and pulverizes the fresh clots, creating a fluid with smaller particles. The system is propelled by an air turbine that can generate as many as 150,000 rpm at a pressure of 50 psi. Infusion of saline through the catheter lubricates the shaft and cools off the system. There is a distal side port in the polyurethane catheter that allows for contrast injection to improve visualization of the clots during thrombectomy (Figure 56–17).

The access into the pulmonary artery is achieved through a 10 French, 95-cm-long guiding catheter. The guiding catheter is advanced into the clot, and the ATD is introduced through the catheter and activated at full speed. The device

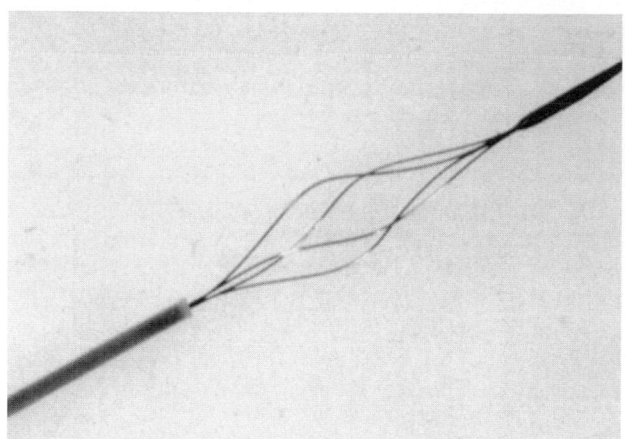

Figure 56-16 The Arrow-Trerotola percutaneous thrombolytic device is a mechanical thrombectomy system that uses a self-expandable metal basket that comes into direct contact with the clots and the vessel wall. Note a flexible silicone rubber tip to reduce chances of vessel wall perforation in this configuration. The prototype device used for pulmonary thrombectomy is used through a 5 French catheter, has a larger basket, and is placed over the wire.

should be used in a slow, back-and-forth motion. As the smaller clots migrate peripherally, the ATD and guiding catheter system are advanced to treat smaller clots. The multipurpose shape of the guiding catheter allows some degree of steerability. Pulmonary pressures should be measured before and after the thrombectomy. Initial experience with the ATD device showed clinical improvement in a limited group of patients, with reduction of the respiratory symptoms and improvement of hypotension (15) (Figures 56–18 and 56–19). One episode of hemoptysis at the end of the procedure was observed in one patient in that series, but without demonstrable arterial damage, extravasation, or dissection, and was followed by complete recovery. The complication was considered to be likely related to reperfusion of infarcted pulmonary tissue, according to previous evidence in the literature (72). One patient died at the end of the procedure, suffering a major seizure and irreversible respiratory and cardiac arrest. The ATD always causes some degree of hemolysis, which is mostly transient and has never caused renal failure in the published series for the treatment of PE and other vessels (15,73–75). A more recent report of a young patient with large-cell lymphoma and severe segmental pulmonary embolism is also available. Treatment with the Amplatz device resulted in marked improvement in the scintigraphic pulmonary perfusion follow-up (76). A number of unreported cases of massive PE had been treated by the ATD in Europe and the United States, but the result of this experience is not available in the literature for analysis. This device is known to be more effective in fresher clots and, in its current design, presents significant difficulty in steerability, requiring a guiding catheter for positioning within the pulmonary artery. Considerable modification of the design would be necessary for this device to be more effective in the pulmonary circulation. Possible improvements should include over-the-wire capability, more power, and the possibility of exposing the impeller for increased clot maceration.

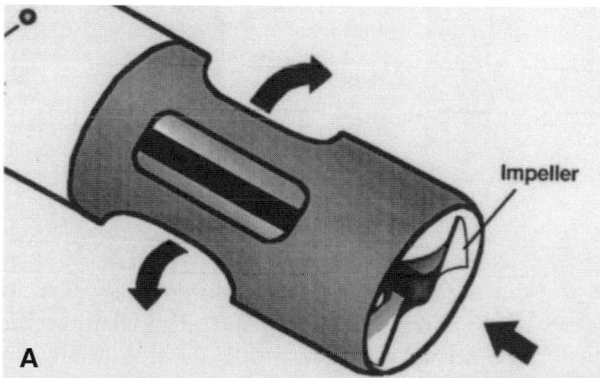

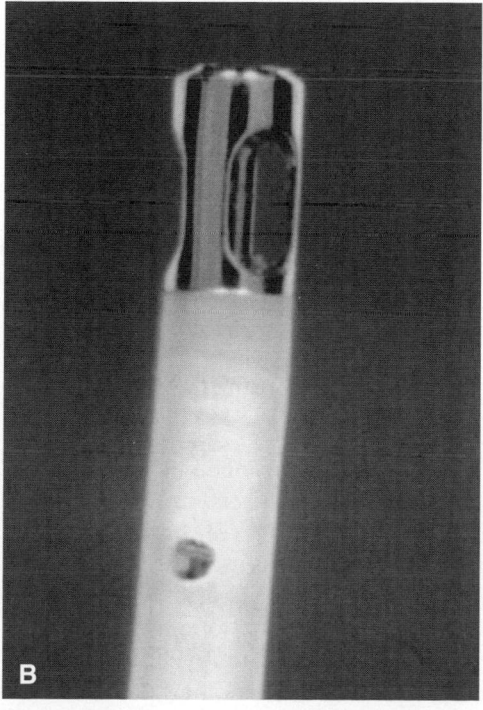

Figure 56–17 **A.** Schematic drawing of the distal tip of the 8 French ATD. A recessed impeller is driven by a drive shaft at high speed within a 5-mm metal capsule. The thrombus is aspirated, fragmented, and expelled through the side ports for further recirculation and fragmentation. **B.** Close-up view of the tip of the ATD. Note the metallic cap with the side ports. It is possible to see the drive shaft within the distal part of the cap. The two side holes are used to inject saline solution. A more recently developed device uses the helix impeller technology and is 27% more potent and 23% smaller in profile (7 French). (Reproduced with permission from Uflacker R, Strange C, Vujic I. Massive pulmonary embolism. Preliminary results of treatment with the Amplatz thrombectomy device. J Vasc Interv Radiol 1996;7:519–528.)

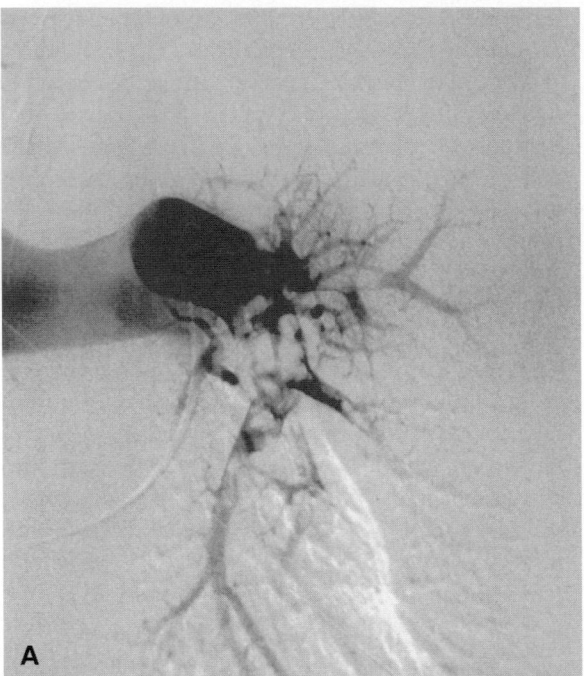

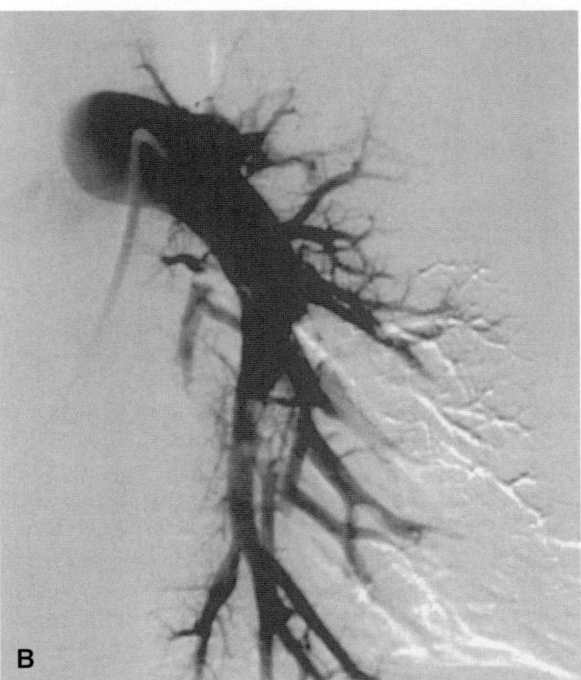

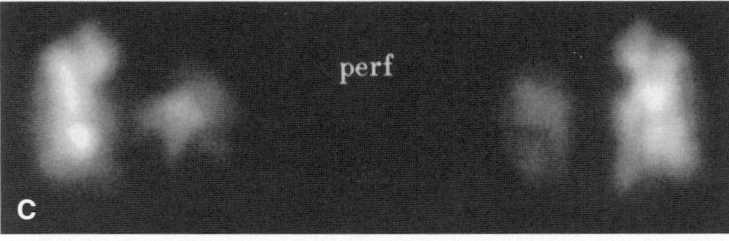

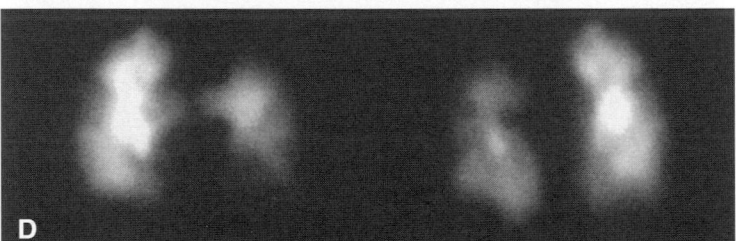

Figure 56–18 A. Pulmonary angiogram showed massive PE occluding the left main pulmonary artery. Mechanical thrombectomy was indicated in this case due to recent neurologic surgery. The ATD device was used through a 10 French guiding catheter. **B.** Postthrombectomy pulmonary arteriogram showed improved patency in the main pulmonary artery and improved lung perfusion. **C.** Initial positive perfusion scan shows bilateral PE that is massive on the left side. **D.** Follow-up perfusion scan shows improved perfusion in the left lung, mostly appreciated in the posterior view. (Reproduced with permission from Uflacker R, Strange C, Vujic I. Massive pulmonary embolism. Preliminary results of treatment with the Amplatz thrombectomy device. J Vasc Interv Radiol 1996;7:519–528.)

A 7 French, 27% more powerful device recently became available, but it has not been extensively tested in the pulmonary circulation at the time of this writing.

Lang Percutaneous Pulmonary Thrombectomy Device

The suction catheter system described by Lang et al. (77) is a homemade device that uses commercially available catheters of different sizes. A 14 French, 90-cm-long Ultratane nontapered catheter is used through a 16 French, 40-cm-long stationary sheath. The 14 French catheter is advanced over a 6 French, 97-cm-long multipurpose guiding catheter and a Rosen wire to provide the stiffness and taper necessary for advancement of the system. A peel-away sheath is used for introduction of the system into the stationary sheath (Figure 56–20). The suction catheter is used to compact, trap, and propel the clot distally, and a 50-mL syringe is used to suck the 14 French catheter as it is withdrawn. The peel-away sheath with the clots is carefully removed and flushed. The procedure is repeated as many times as necessary, and the more distal clots in smaller branches are sucked with the 6 French guiding catheter. The reported clinical experience with the technique, although successful, was small and included pretreatment of the clots with urokinase and fragmentation with a pigtail catheter or a large angioplasty balloon. Improvement in the hemodynamic and pulmonary perfusion was rapidly achieved in all three reported patients that had aging clots embolized from a distal site.

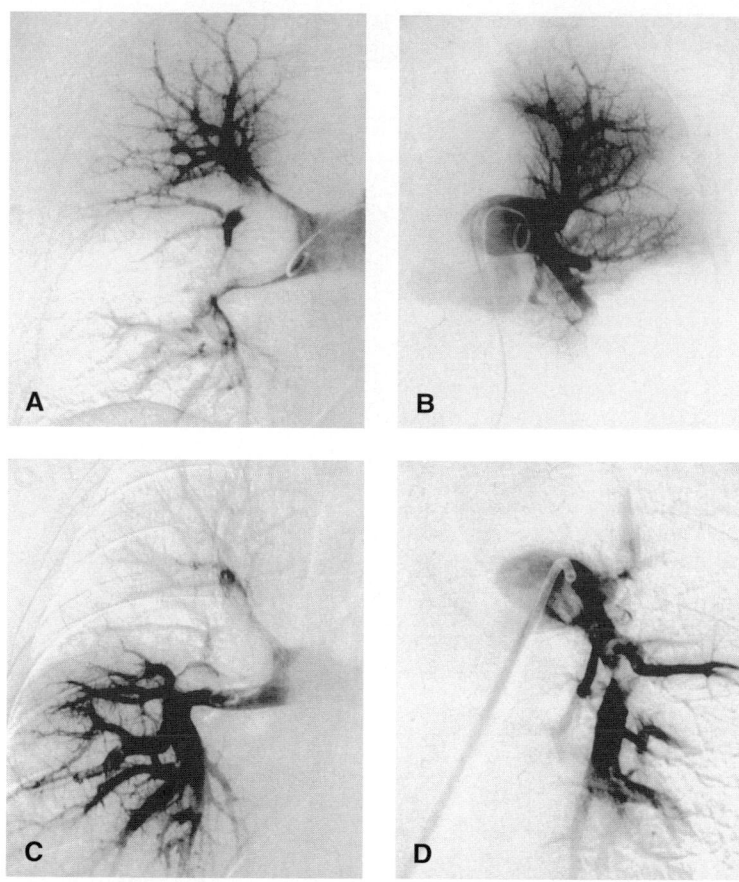

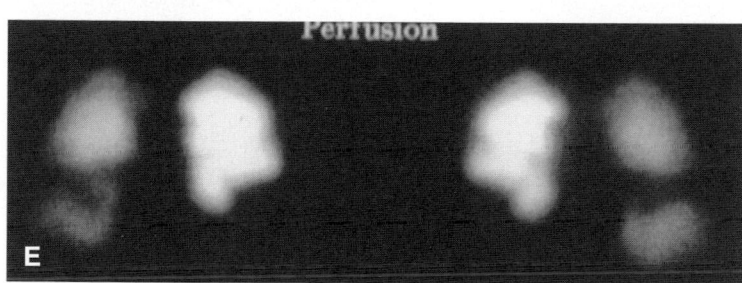

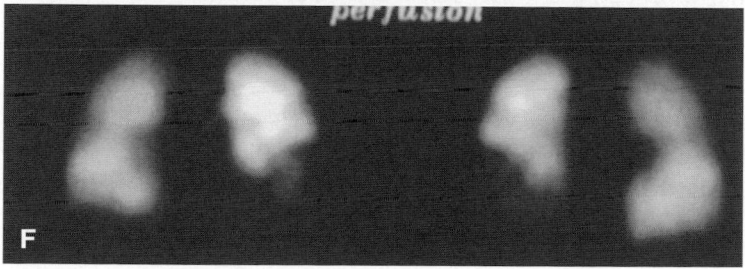

Figure 56–19 A. Pulmonary arteriogram shows massive PE in the main right pulmonary artery with severely decreased perfusion of the whole right lung. **B.** Pulmonary arteriogram shows complete obstruction of the descending left pulmonary artery and no substantial flow into the left lower lobe. The diagnostic catheter was exchanged for a 10 French guiding catheter, and the ATD was used to debulk the PE on both sides. Activation time was 8 minutes, 11 seconds. At the end of the procedure, the patient experienced hemoptysis of about 900 mL. **C.** Postthrombectomy right pulmonary arteriogram shows improved perfusion of the right lower lobe, with a large filling defect within the bifurcation of the pulmonary artery. **D.** Postthrombectomy left pulmonary arteriogram shows improved perfusion of the left lower lobe and no extravasation of contrast medium. Large filling defects remain within the left main pulmonary artery. **E.** Prethrombectomy perfusion scan shows signs of reduced perfusion in both lungs consistent with massive PE. **F.** Follow-up perfusion scan obtained 12 hours after the procedure shows improved pulmonary perfusion on both sides. (Reproduced with permission from Uflacker R, Strange C, Vujic I. Massive pulmonary embolism. Preliminary results of treatment with the Amplatz thrombectomy device. J Vasc Interv Radiol 1996;7:519–528.)

Amplatz Maceration Aspiration Thrombectomy Catheter (AMATC)

The Amplatz maceration aspiration thrombectomy catheter (AMATC) is an experimental double-lumen, 9 French aspiration catheter with a large side window close to the tip, where there is an occlusion balloon. Inside, an electrically powered basket is rotated at 5,000 rpm, at the level of the window, while manual suction is applied to the main lumen for aspiration of the clots macerated by the basket. The device can be placed over the wire, which allows for adequate guidance in more straight vessels. The device was effective in fresher thrombus, but only partial thrombectomy was achieved in older, partially organized clots. The AMATC was used in the

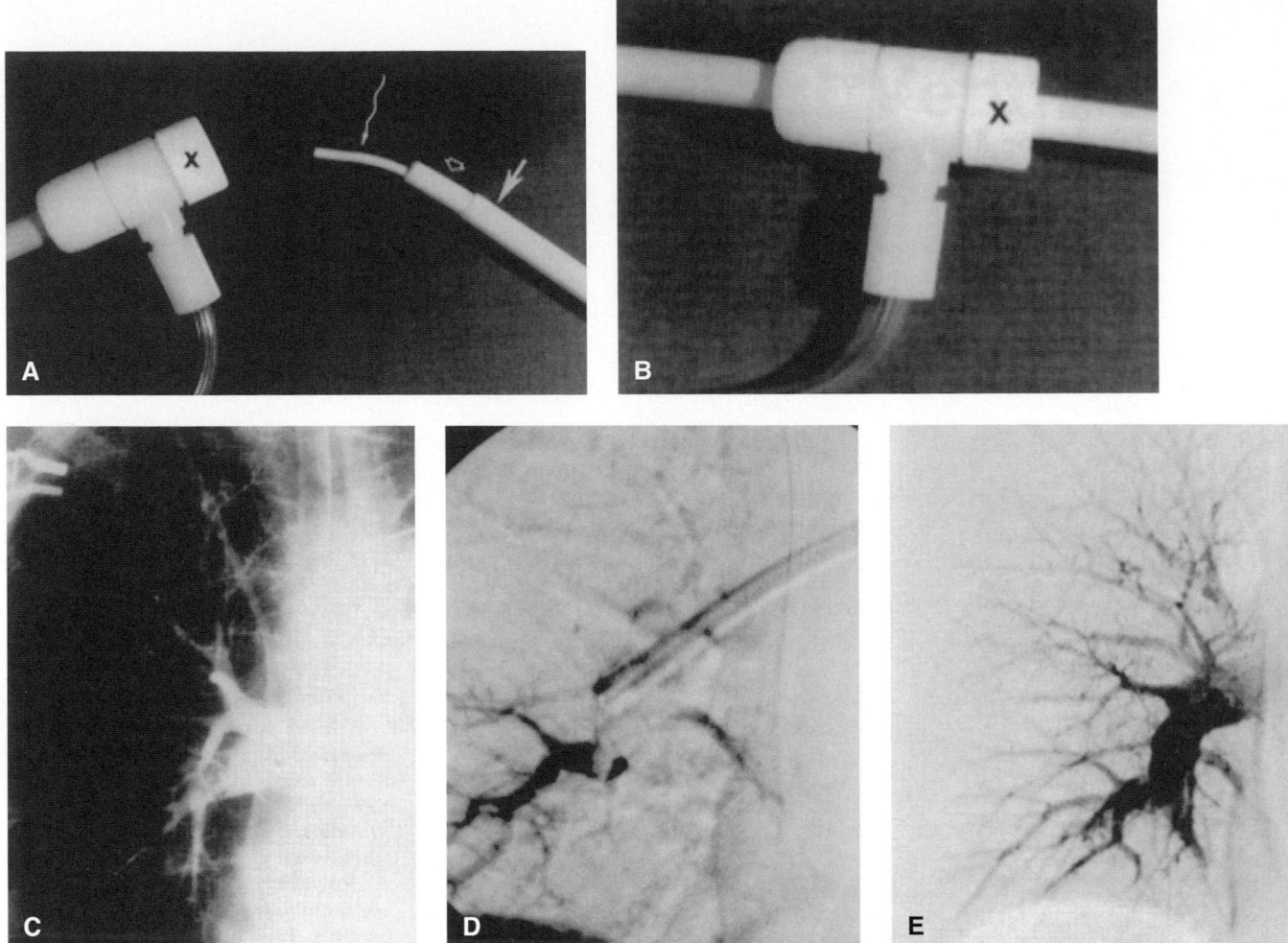

Figure 56–20 A. Suction catheter system. The 6 French guiding catheter (*wavy arrow*) is coaxially loaded into the 14 French suction catheter (*open arrow*). The 14 French peel-away sheath is piggy-backed onto the assembly (*closed arrow*). The assembly is advanced over a guide wire into the valve of the 16 French stationary sheath (X). **B.** The assembly has been introduced into the stationary sheath (X) with advancement of the 14 French peel-away sheath (*closed arrow*). The suction catheter (*open arrow*) is loaded into the peel-away sheath. **C.** Initial pulmonary arteriogram shows a large clot in the right descending pulmonary artery. **D.** Note distal migration of the clot, compacted by the tip of the suction catheter, as compared with C. **E.** Pulmonary arteriogram after clot suction. (Reproduced with permission from Lang EV, Barnhart WH, Walton DL, et al. Percutaneous pulmonary thrombectomy. J Vasc Intervent Radiol 1997;8:427–432.)

pulmonary circulation in an animal model and was effective in 60% of the cases, with minimal intimal injury. Difficulties in guidance of the device within the pulmonary artery and orientation of the side window, apparently, were responsible for the failures (49).

Rotarex Catheter

The Rotarex catheter is a new device for percutaneous mechanical removal of fresh and organized thrombi. The device has three components: the catheter, an electric motor drive, and an electronic control unit. Inside the 8 French catheter rotates a stainless steel spiral, over the wire. The catheter head consists of two cylinders that fit over each other. The outer rotating cylinder is fixed to the spiral, and the inner one is attached to the catheter shaft. Each cylinder has two oval slits. The high frequency of revolution creates a negative pressure at the catheter head, and soft and solid occlusive material is caught in the slits, cut and transported by the internal spiral to the proximal sideport, and discharged into a bag. This device has been tested in vitro and in an animal model, and experimental data suggest the use of the catheter for the treatment of obstructed vessels with a diameter as large as 8 mm in diameter (78). The device has been utilized clinically only in the peripheral arterial circulation, and significant changes will be necessary to apply the device in larger vessels such as the pulmonary arteries.

PULMONARY ARTERY STENT PLACEMENT

Although effective in most patients and lifesaving under the proper circumstances, all the techniques described above may fail or be contraindicated, leaving extremely sick patients with no viable alternative for treatment. A couple of recent reports described the use of metallic stents placed alongside organized treatment-resistant pulmonary artery emboli. Both Wallstent (79) and Gianturco Z stents (80) were used in critical situations where the patients presented with cor pulmonale, profound arterial hypoxemia, and hypotension and did not respond to thrombolytic therapy and fragmentation. The stent placement in the proximal main pulmonary arteries promoted immediate relief of the heart insufficiency, improvement of elevated pulmonary arterial pressure, and systemic hypotension. As long-term behavior of stents in the pulmonary arteries is not completely understood, the use of stents, at this time, would be advisable only when there is a real life-threatening condition requiring immediate opening of the pulmonary circulation to decrease pulmonary vascular resistance and increase pulmonary blood flow when other techniques fail.

OVERVIEW

Successful management of acute massive PE requires prompt risk stratification and decisive, early intervention (Table 56–1) (47). Typically, clinically undetected right heart failure worsens with time, causing dependence to pressors, and it may lead to unremitting cardiogenic shock. If at this point thrombolysis or surgical embolectomy is considered for treatment, the likelihood of a good outcome is slim (47). Despite adequate anticoagulation, right ventricular dysfunction is still a severe, life-threatening condition.

When high-risk PE patients are identified, adequate anticoagulation should be instituted, and the patients need to be screened for pharmacological thrombolysis. Thrombolysis offers the chance of clot removal without the risks and morbidity of surgical embolectomy; however, thrombolytic therapy is not without risks, and careful evaluation is necessary. There is increased risk of major bleeding, including the possibility of intracranial hemorrhage. However, thrombolytic therapy also offers the opportunity of dissolution of more peripheral clots in the pulmonary circulation. Verstraete et al. (37) compared the recanalization effects of intrapulmonary versus intravenous infusion of rt-PA and showed that transcatheter intrapulmonary delivery does not offer a significant benefit over the intravenous route, which resulted in a loss of interest in the technique. Despite this controversy regarding the efficacy of peripheral versus intrapulmonary thrombolytic therapy, recent experimental evidence in vitro and in vivo (81) suggests that when there is a massive pulmonary occlusion by an embolus, a vortex forms proximal to the occluding embolus. Any fluids infused proximal to the

pulmonary artery occlusion will make only evanescent contact with the edge of the thrombus, and the fluid is washed into the nonoccluded ipsilateral and contralateral pulmonary arteries. Following embolus fragmentation, the infused fluid is carried completely into the formerly occluded artery. These flow studies possibly explain why thrombolytic agents administered via a catheter positioned adjacent to the embolus may have no more effect than systemically infused agents. The enhanced local effect, observed in other vascular territories, is precluded by the rapid washout into the nonoccluded pulmonary arteries followed by systemic dilution of the drug (Figure 56–21). These results support the practice of direct intrathrombotic injection of thrombolytic drugs or the local infusion following embolus fragmentation techniques, despite the lack of clinical evidence of superiority of one technique over the other. However, a greater number of such patients would possibly benefit from an algorithm that used spiral CT for diagnosis of PE, followed by IV thrombolytic therapy, leading to more rapid treatment in most hospitals, mainly in the ones where catheter-directed thrombolysis is not immediately available.

Catheter fragmentation followed by intrapulmonary thrombolytic infusion is an adequate and, in the author's opinion, underused technique to achieve rapid resolution of the thrombus, improving hemodynamic conditions in most patients. Simple fragmentation with an angiographic catheter may be highly beneficial. The use of larger angioplasty balloons for clot fragmentation is also a simple and immediately available technique to most budgets and angiographic laboratories (42). As discussed above, the association of fragmentation, mechanical thrombectomy, and thrombolytic therapy is desirable for potentially improving outcomes. In fact, it is likely that most of the devices will be more effective if thrombolytic therapy is used in association with the

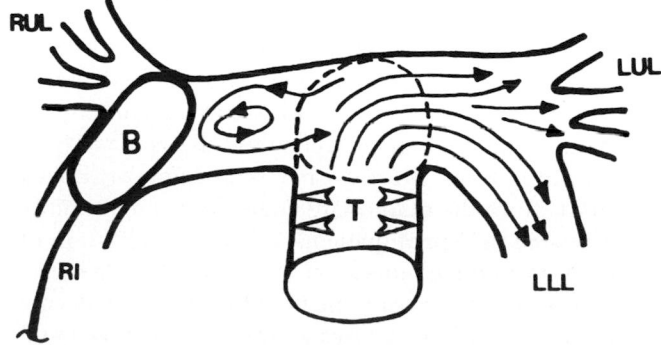

Figure 56–21 Schematic drawing of the flow model, showing vortex formation immediately proximal to the level of obstruction. Note that most of the fluid is washed into the nonoccluded left pulmonary artery and the vortex close to the occlusion, with only minimal flow of fluid making evanescent contact with an occluding embolus (B). RUL, right upper lobe; LUL, left upper lobe; LLL, left lower lobe; RI, right intermediate artery; T, pulmonary artery trunk; B, balloon. (Reproduced with permission from Schmitz-Rode T, Kilbinger M, Günther RW. Simulated flow pattern in massive pulmonary embolism: significance for selective intrapulmonary thrombolysis. Cardiosvasc Intervent Radiol 1998;21:199–204.)

thrombectomy device. There are, however, situations that make patients unsuitable for thrombolysis, either systemic or intrapulmonary.

For high-risk PE patients, unsuitable for pharmacological thrombolysis or open embolectomy, modern catheter thrombectomy technology may be employed. In acute massive PE, the main purpose of the treatment should be the rapid restoration of the pulmonary blood flow to increase pulmonary perfusion, improve oxygenation, and reduce pulmonary pressure and cardiac failure. When thrombolysis is contraindicated or inadvisable, mechanical intervention using some of the available devices should be considered (Table 56–2). The specific device and strategy that is selected to manage the patient with massive PE will depend on the expertise of the interventional radiologist and the availability of the equipment. Each procedure and technique may have particular advantages and disadvantages. At this time, it is difficult to point out the best catheter intervention alternative. Catheter intervention, however, should be considered when heparin alone is insufficient and when thrombolysis is not feasible, while systemic arterial pressure is preserved and before pressor dependence ensues (47).

It is common knowledge that the currently available thrombolytic therapy, mechanical thrombectomy, and fragmentation devices are more useful and successful when dealing with fresher thrombus. Three weeks is, in general, the age limit of thrombus when considering the option of a mechanical or rheolytic thrombectomy device. Based on the history, angiographic findings, outcomes, and follow-up of patients undergoing pulmonary thrombectomy with the ATD, three groups of patients have been identified (15). Type I patients, with fresh clots that have recently embolized, should respond well to mechanical thrombectomy with increased peripheral flow and oxygenation. Type II patients, with old, more organized clots that have recently embolized, respond less effectively to the thrombectomy, and although more residual clots are likely to remain, there is a good chance for improvement of pulmonary flow. Type III patients, with a history of old, organized chronic PE with recent worsening secondary to recurrent PE, do not respond well to the effects of mechanical thrombectomy. Devices that scrape the organized thrombus from the pulmonary artery walls are certainly more desired in Type III patients. Acute recanalization of the main pulmonary arteries can also be obtained with stent placement and improvement of blood flow, reducing pulmonary resistance in cases with more organized and treatment-resistant thrombi. As a general rule, smaller fragmented thrombi positioned inside the pulmonary artery, even when causing massive proximal occlusion, are more likely to be fresher clots, as demonstrated in Figures 56–2 and 56–17, while larger nonfragmented thrombi, occluding the main bifurcation of the pulmonary artery, are more likely to represent older, more organized thrombi, as demonstrated in Figures 56–6 and 56–18. However, older thrombi originated in smaller peripheral, tibial, and peroneal veins may appear angiographically as smaller fragments within the pulmonary artery.

The advent of more aggressive interventional treatments and techniques for the management of massive PE has a tremendous potential for saving lives. Nevertheless, the new technology that became available in the past few years requires the close participation of the skilled interventional radiologist as a member of the interdisciplinary team in charge of identification and treatment of those patients. The development and implementation of protocols for treatment of massive PE, tailored for each institution, is mandatory and may improve outcomes, saving patients' lives. However, no easy or final solution is currently available for the management of the difficult problems faced when treating patients with massive PE, and it is likely that the new devices and the available thrombolytic techniques will be used in association rather than individually.

REFERENCES

1. Dalen JE, Alper JS. Natural history of pulmonary embolism. Prog Cardiovasc Dis 1975;17:259–270.
2. Uflacker R. Interventional therapy for pulmonary embolism. J Vasc Interv Radiol 2001;12:147–164.
3. Olin JW. Pulmonary embolism. Rev Cardiovasc Med 2002;3: S68–S75.
4. Brotman DJ, Jaffer A. "Coach class thrombosis": Is the risk real? What do we tell our patients? Cleve Clin J Med 2002;69:832–837.
5. Lapostolle F, Surget V, Borron SW, et al. Severe pulmonary embolism associated with air travel. N Engl J Med 2001;345: 779–783.
6. Barritt DW, Jordan SE. Anticoagulant drugs in the treatment of pulmonary embolism: a controlled trial. Lancet 1960;1:1309–1312.
7. Elliot CG. Pulmonary physiology during pulmonary embolism. Chest 1992;101(suppl):163S–171S.
8. Lilienfeld DE, Chan E, Ehland J, et al. Mortality from pulmonary embolism. Prog Cardiovasc Dis 1975;17:259–270.
9. Kearon C. Diagnosis of pulmonary embolism. CMAJ 2003;168: 183–194.
10. Mastora I, Remy-Jardin M, Masson P, et al. Severity of acute pulmonary embolism: evaluation of a new spiral CT angiographic score in correlation with echocardiographic data. Eur Radiol 2003;13:29–35.
11. Haage P, Piroth W, Krombach G, et al. Pulmonary embolism: comparison of angiography with spiral CT, MRA and real-time MR imaging. Am J Respir Crit Care Med 2002;167:729-734.
12. Pruszczyk P, Bochowicz A, Torbicki A, et al. Cardiac troponin T monitoring identifies high-risk group of normotensive patients with acute pulmonary embolism. Chest 2003;123:1947–1952.
13. De Gregorio MA, Gimeno MJ, Mainar A, et al. Mechanical and enzymatic thrombolysis for massive pulmonary embolism. J Vasc Interv Radiol 2002;13:163–169.
14. Konstantinides S, Geibel A, Olschewski M, et al. Association between thrombolytic treatment and the prognosis of hemodynamically stable patients with major pulmonary embolism: results of a multicenter registry. Circulation 1997;96:882–888.
15. Uflacker R, Strange C, Vujic I. Massive pulmonary embolism. Preliminary results of treatment with the Amplatz thrombectomy device. J Vasc Interv Radiol 1996;7:519–528.
16. Moser KM. Pulmonary embolism. In: Braunwald E, Fauci A, Kasper D, et al., eds. Harrison's Principles of Internal Medicine. New York: McGraw-Hill, 2002:1214–1220.
17. Jones TK, Barnes RW, Greenfield LJ. Greenfield vena cava filter: rationale and current indications. Ann Thorac Surg 1986;42: S48–S55.
18. Carson JL, Kelley MA, Duff A, et al. The clinical course of pulmonary embolism. N Engl J Med 1993;326:1240–1245.

19. Hull RD, Raskob GE, Hirsh J, et al. Continuous intravenous heparin compared with intermittent subcutaneous heparin in the initial treatment of proximal-vein thrombosis. N Engl J Med 1986; 315.1109–1114.

20. Curry N, Bardana EJ, Pirofsky B. Enoxaparin: a low-molecular-weight heparin. Med Letter 1993;35:75–76.

21. Aguilar D, Goldhager SZ. Clinical uses of low-molecular-weight heparins. Chest 1999;115:1418–1423.

22. Quader MA, Stump LS, Sumpio BE. Low molecular weight heparins: current use and indications. J Am Coll Surg 1998;187: 641–658.

23. Howard PA. Dalteparin: a low-molecular-weight heparin. Ann Pharmacother 1997;31:192–203.

24. Samama MM, Cohen AT, Darmon J-Y, et al. A comparison of enoxaparin with placebo for the prevention of venous thromboembolism in acutely ill medical patients. N Engl J Med 1999;341:793–800.

25. Haas SK. Treatment of deep venous thrombosis and pulmonary embolism. Current recommendations. Med Clin North Am 1998;82:495–510.

26. Ranze O, Ranze P, Magnani HN, et al. Heparin-induced thrombocytopenia in paediatric patients—a review of the literature and a new case treated with danaparoid sodium. Eur J Pediatr 1999;158:S130–S133.

27. Mullen MP, Thomas KC, McGowan FX, et al. Heparin induced thrombocytopenia in pediatric patients undergoing cardiopulmonary bypass surgery. American Heart Association Abstract.

28. Almeida JI, Coats R, Liem TK, et al. Reduced morbidity and mortality rates of the heparin-induced thrombocytopenia syndrome. J Vasc Surg 1998;27:309–314.

29. Ridker PM, Goldhaber SZ, Danielson E, et al. Long-term, low-intensity warfarin therapy for the prevention of recurrent venous thromboembolism. N Engl J Med 2003;348:1425–1434.

30. Urokinase pulmonary embolism trial: Phase 1 results: a cooperative study. JAMA 1970;214:2163–2172.

31. Urokinase-streptokinase embolism trial. Phase 2 results: a cooperative study. JAMA 1974;229:1606–1613.

32. Schwarz F, Stehr H, Zimmerman R, et al. Sustained improvement of pulmonary hemodynamics in patients at rest and during exercise after thrombolytic therapy of massive pulmonary embolism. Circulation 1985;71:117–123.

33. Agnelli G, Becattini C, Kirschstein T. Thrombolysis vs heparin in the treatment of pulmonary embolism: a clinical outcome-based meta-analysis. Arch Intern Med 2002;162:2537–2541.

34. Konstantinides S, Geibel A, Heusel G, et al. Heparin plus alteplase compared with heparin alone in patients with submassive pulmonary embolism. N Engl J Med 2002;347:1143–1150.

35. Gunn NA, Tierney LM. Letter to the editor. N Engl J Med 2002; 348:357–358.

36. Goldhaber SZ. Thrombolytic therapy for pulmonary embolism. Semin Vasc Surg 1992;5:69–75.

37. Verstraete M, Miller GAH, Bounameaux H, et al. Intravenous and intrapulmonary recombinant tissue-type plasminogen activator in the treatment of acute massive pulmonary embolism. Circulation 1988;77:353–360.

38. Raschke RA, Reilly BM, Guidry JR, et al. The weight-based heparin dosing nomogram compared with a "standard of care" nomogram: a randomized controlled trial. Ann Intern Med 1993;119: 874–881.

39. Molina HE, Hunter DW, Yedlicka JW, et al. Thrombolytic therapy for postoperative pulmonary embolism. Am J Surg 1992;163: 375–381.

40. Gonzalez-Juanatey JR, Valdes L, Amaro A, et al. Treatment of massive pulmonary thromboembolism with low intrapulmonary dosages of urokinase. Short-term angiographic and hemodynamic evolution. Chest 1992;102:341–346.

41. Vujic I, Young JWR, Gobien RP, et al. Massive pulmonary embolism treatment with full heparinization and topical low-dose streptokinase. Radiology 1983;148:671–675.

42. Fava M, Loyola S, Flores P, et al. Mechanical fragmentation and pharmacologic thrombolysis in massive pulmonary embolism. J Vasc Interv Radiol 1997;8:261–266.

43. Goldhaber SZ, Markis JE, Meyrovitz MF, et al. Acute pulmonary embolism treated with tissue plasminogen activator. Lancet 1986;886–889.

44. Jamieson SW, Auger WR, Fedullo PF, et al. Experience and results of 150 pulmonary thromboendarterectomy operations over a 29-month period. J Thorac Cardiovasc Surg 1993;106:116–127.

45. Poletti GA, Actis Dato GM. Surgical treatment of massive pulmonary embolism. A case report. J Cardiovasc Surg 1999;40: 135–137.

46. Gulba DC, Schmid C, Borst HG, et al. Medical compared with surgical treatment for massive pulmonary embolism. Lancet 1994;343:576–577.

47. Goldhaber SZ. Integration of catheter thrombectomy into our armamentarium to treat acute pulmonary embolism. Chest 1998; 114:1237–1238.

48. Sharafuddin MJA, Hicks ME. Current status of percutaneous mechanical thrombectomy. Part I. General principles. J Vasc Interv Radiol 1997;8:911–921.

49. Sharafuddin MIA, Hicks ME. Current status of percutaneous mechanical thrombectomy. Part II. Devices and mechanisms of action. J Vasc Interv Radiol 1998;9:15–31.

50. Brady AJ, Crake T, Oakley CM. Percutaneous catheter fragmentation and distal dispersion of proximal pulmonary embolus. Lancet 1991;338:1186–1189.

51. Handa K, Sasaki Y, Kiyonaga A, et al. Acute pulmonary thromboembolism treated successfully by balloon angioplasty: a case report. Angiology 1988;8:775–778.

52. Girard P. Catheter fragmentation of pulmonary emboli. Chest 1999;115:1759.

53. Timsit JF, Reynaud P, Meyer G, et al. Pulmonary embolectomy by catheter device in massive pulmonary embolism. Chest 1991; 100:655–658.

54. Oakley CM. Conservative management of pulmonary embolism. Br J Surg 1968;55:801–805.

55. Greenfield LJ, Proctor MC, Williams DM, et al. Long-term experience with transvenous catheter pulmonary embolectomy. J Vasc Surg 1993;18:450–458.

56. Cela MC, Amplatz K. Nonsurgical pulmonary embolectomy. In: Cope C, ed. Current Techniques in Interventional Radiology. Philadelphia: Current Medicine, 1994.

57. Murphy JM, Mulvihill N, Mulcahy D, et al. Percutaneous catheter and guidewire fragmentation with local administration of recombinant tissue plasminogen activator as a treatment for massive pulmonary embolism. Eur Radiol 1999;9:959–964.

58. Stock KW, Jacob AL, Schnabel KJ, et al. Massive pulmonary embolism: treatment with thrombus fragmentation and local fibrinolysis with recombinant human-tissue plasminogen activator. Cardiovasc Intervent Radiol 1997;20:364–368.

59. Stein PD, Sabbah HN, Basha MA, et al. Mechanical disruption of pulmonary emboli in dogs with a flexible rotating-tip catheter (Kensey catheter). Chest 1990;98:994–998.

60. Reekers J, Kromhout J, van der Wall K. Catheter for percutaneous thrombectomy: first clinical experience. Radiology 1993;188: 871–874.

61. Michalis LK, Tsetis DK, Rees MR. Case report: percutaneous removal of pulmonary artery thrombus in a patient with massive pulmonary embolism using the Hydrolyser catheter: the first human experience. Clin Radiol 1997;52:158–161.

62. Koning R, Cribier A, Gerber L, et al. A new treatment for severe pulmonary embolism. Circulation 1997;96:2498–2500.

63. Voigtlander T, Rupprecht HJ, Nowak B, et al. Clinical application of a new rheolytic thrombectomy catheter system for massive pulmonary embolism. Catheter Cardiovasc Interv 1999;47:91–96.

64. Fontaine AB, Borsa JJ, Hoffer FK, et al. Type III heart block with peripheral use of the Angiojet thrombectomy system. J Vasc Interv Radiol 2001;12:1223–1225.

65. Schmitz-Rode T, Vorwerk D, Günther RW, et al. Percutaneous fragmentation of pulmonary emboli in dogs with the impeller basket catheter. Cardiovasc Intervent Radiol 1993;16:234–242.

66. Schmitz-Rode T, Günther RW. New device for percutaneous fragmentation of pulmonary emboli. Radiology 1991;180:135–137.

67. Schmitz-Rode T, Adam G, Kilbinger M, et al. Fragmentation of pulmonary emboli: in vivo experimental evaluation of two high-speed rotating catheters. Cardiovasc Intervent Radiol 1996;19:165–169.

68. Schmitz-Rode T, Günther RW, Pfeffer JG, et al. Acute massive pulmonary embolism: use of a rotatable pigtail catheter for diagnosis and fragmentation therapy. Radiology 1995;197:157–162.

69. Schmitz-Rode T, Janssens U, Schild HH, et al. Fragmentation of massive pulmonary embolism using a pigtail rotation catheter. Chest 1998;114:1427–1436.

70. Brown DB, Cardella JF, Wilson RP, et al. Evaluation of a modified Arrow-Trerotola percutaneous thrombolytic device for treatment of acute pulmonary embolus in a canine model. J Vasc Intervent Radiol 1999;10:733–740.

71. Rocek M, Peregrin J, Velimsky T. Mechanical thrombectomy of massive pulmonary embolism using an Arrow-Trerotola percutaneous thrombolytic device. Eur Radiol 1998;8:1683–1685.

72. Levison RM, Shure D, Moser KM. Reperfusion pulmonary edema after pulmonary artery thromboendarterectomy. Am Rev Respir Dis 1986;134:1241–1245.

73. Uflacker R, Rajagopalan PR, Vujic I, et al. Treatment of thrombosed dialysis grafts: randomized trial of surgical thrombectomy versus mechanical thrombectomy with the Amplatz device. J Vasc Interv Radiol 1996;7:185–192.

74. Houry D, Southall J, Manning M, et al. Use of the Amplatz thrombectomy device for severe deep venous thrombosis. South Med J 1999;92:915–917.

75. Uflacker R. Mechanical thrombectomy in acute and subacute thrombosis with use of the Amplatz device: arterial and venous applications. J Vasc Interv Radiol 1997;8:923–932.

76. Peuster M, Bertram H, Windhagen-Mahnert B, et al. Mechanical recanalization of venous thrombosis and pulmonary embolism with the Clotbuster thrombectomy system in a 12-year-old boy. Z Kardiol 1998;87:283–287.

77. Lang EV, Barnhart WH, Walton DL, et al. Percutaneous pulmonary thrombectomy. J Vasc Intervent Radiol 1997;8:427–432.

78. Schmitt H-E, Jäger KA, Jacob AL, et al. A new rotational thrombectomy catheter: system design and first clinical experiences. Cardiovasc Intervent Radiol 1999;22:504–509.

79. Haskal ZJ, Soulen MC, Huetti EA, et al. Life-threatening pulmonary emboli and cor pulmonale: treatment with percutaneous pulmonary artery stent placement. Radiology 1994;191:473–475.

80. Koizumi J, Kusano S, Akima T, et al. Emergent Z stent placement for treatment of cor pulmonale due to pulmonary emboli after failed lytic treatment: technical considerations. Cardiovasc Intervent Radiol 1998;21:254–255.

81. Schmitz-Rode T, Kilbinger M, Günther RW. Simulated flow pattern in massive pulmonary embolism: significance for selective intrapulmonary thrombolysis. Cardiosvasc Intervent Radiol 1998;21:199–204.

Interventional Radiology of Trauma

Arteriography and Transcatheter Treatment of Extremity Trauma

Michael D. Katz, Sue E. Hanks

Adverse consequences of arterial injury in extremity trauma include pseudoaneurysm, arteriovenous fistulae, ischemia, gangrene, limb loss, high-flow cardiac output, and differential limb growth in children. When traumatic injuries to vascular structures in the extremities are suspected, prompt and accurate diagnosis is essential to minimize these adverse sequelae. Limb salvage rates are routinely greater than 90% when rapid treatment is offered (1). Arteriography remains an important part of the management of patients with suspected vascular injury, both for diagnosis and for treatment.

HISTORY OF EXTREMITY TRAUMA MANAGEMENT

The principles of diagnosis and therapy for civilian trauma have evolved largely from military experience. During World War II, most extremity arterial injuries were treated by ligation. This treatment resulted in a high rate of limb amputation (2). During the Korean and Vietnam wars, primary vascular repair was performed for arterial injuries. This therapy markedly decreased the amputation rate, from 48–62% down to 7–13%, and a policy of mandatory surgical exploration was adopted (3,4).

This military experience with high-velocity extremity wounds was extrapolated to civilian trauma, leading to a large number of negative surgical explorations. Since the late 1970s, arteriography has replaced surgical exploration in most patients, reducing negative explorations from 84% to 3% (5). Accumulated experience has shown arteriography to be a safe and accurate means of diagnosing vascular injury (6–9). Concern now focuses on the resultant large number of negative arteriograms rather than on negative explorations. The precise indications for arteriography remain controversial.

PATIENT EVALUATION AND INDICATIONS FOR ARTERIOGRAPHY

The clinical situation, physical findings, and mechanism of injury play a large role in directing trauma management. In all forms of trauma—penetrating, iatrogenic, and blunt—physical examination is central to patient selection. Not all patients require arteriography for extremity trauma. For example, a patient with a through-and-through gunshot wound in the distal thigh, an expanding hematoma, and no distal pulses clearly has a superficial femoral artery injury, precisely localized by the wound. This injury requires prompt surgical repair rather than arteriography. Arteriography is indicated when an injury is suspected but not certain.

Significant clinical findings in extremity trauma that increase suspicion for arterial injury "hard signs" include pulse deficit, active bleeding, bruit, thrill, and an expanding hematoma. Pulse deficit, the most important finding, indicates arterial injury in 56–87% of cases (10–12). Although uncommon, the presence of a bruit or thrill, suggestive of an arteriovenous fistula (AVF), yields a positive arteriogram rate of nearly 100% (10,11). An expanding hematoma is associated with arterial injury in 38% of cases (11). Patients who present with these findings typically undergo immediate operative wound exploration and arterial repair. Emergency arteriography may be requested in these patients when a patient has multiple potential vascular injury sites, when the precise location of injury is not clear (for example, when it involves a long path through the limb), when surgical access is difficult (for example, at the thoracic outlet), when significant atherosclerosis limits the pulse exam, or when an injury might be amenable to transcatheter therapy (13).

"Soft signs" for extremity arterial trauma include injury to the anatomically related nerve, a small, stable hematoma, or a history of either hypotension or significant bleeding. A neurologic deficit has been found to be associated with a high percentage of vascular injuries in some studies, but this finding has not been confirmed by others (10,12,14,15). Other physical signs, such as long bone fracture or large areas of soft tissue injury, are of lesser yield (10,11). These patients may be observed for the interval development of hard signs, or urgent arteriography may be requested.

The greatest controversy exists as to the need for arteriography for wounds near major neurovascular bundles (15–26). A proximity wound is usually defined as being within 1 cm of the expected location of the vessels concerned. As many as 95% of arteriograms performed for proximity alone are negative (1). Efforts have been directed toward identifying subgroups of proximity wounds that are at higher risk for vascular injury. The Doppler-derived ankle-brachial index (ABI) or wrist-brachial index (WBI) has been adopted at several centers as an extension of the physical examination for this purpose (14,27,28). An ABI or WBI of less than 0.9 has been associated with a positive

arteriography rate of 30% (14). Such arteriograms need not be performed on an emergent basis but can be delayed as long as 24 hours unless surgical intervention is planned earlier for another indication (20). Doppler examinations miss lesions that do not decrease distal flow: branch arterial injuries, small AVFs, and nonobstructing arterial defects.

Other approaches have been reported for stable patients with suspicion of vascular injury. Alternate imaging modalities have been suggested to replace arteriography. Duplex ultrasound has been recommended as a screening tool to identify traumatic arterial injury. The sensitivity of ultrasound for detection of arterial injury has been reported from a poor 50% to an excellent 99% (29–33). Atherosclerotic disease, anatomic variants, and vasoconstriction resulting from hypotension may make interpretation difficult. The role of ultrasonography is somewhat limited for several additional reasons. It is an operator-dependent examination that is tedious when more than a single anatomic region needs evaluation. Open wounds and orthopedic hardware limit access for scanning.

A few authors have tried computerized tomographic (CT) angiography for the evaluation of extremity trauma because CT scanning is the cornerstone of trauma diagnosis elsewhere in the body (34–36). While CT scanning has been shown to be reliable for the diagnosis of injuries to large vessels, it is not useful for detection of injuries to small vessels of less than 2 mm in diameter. CT scanning is useful only for focal injuries because the contrast must be pretimed to the expected injury site.

Finally, limited arteriography performed in the emergency room has been recommended. A single, plain film is obtained following contrast injection, by hand, via a small needle (37). The advantage here is primarily the speed of diagnosis. Such an exam is limited to only one vascular territory, and injection timing errors could miss injuries.

The mechanism of injury is also an important factor in the decision to perform arteriography. All high-velocity wounds, such as those from assault weapons and rifles, should undergo exploration or arteriography because of the greater force and possibility of remote concussive damage. High-speed missiles are preceded by a shock wave and followed by an area of decreased pressure called the temporary cavity, which can produce extensive damage. Such high-velocity wounds have the highest incidence of arterial injury, followed in decreasing order by gunshot wounds and stab wounds, which must penetrate the vessel directly (19). Shotgun wounds have a high rate of arterial injury (46–62%) because of the multiplicity of projectiles and the larger area of trauma from pellet scatter (19). Recently, dog bites have been recognized as having a high rate of vascular injury. These wounds, a result of both blunt and penetrating trauma, are associated with a 24% rate of vascular injury (38).

Although in urban centers, most extremity arterial injuries are a result of penetrating trauma, blunt trauma can also cause significant vascular injuries, accounting for 17% of arterial injuries (39). Knee dislocations carry a 23–43% rate of popliteal artery injury (40–43). Dislocations produce stretch injuries, which may cause isolated intimal damage. As with other forms of trauma, it remains controversial whether arteriography is indicated in all patients with knee dislocation or only in those with physical or Doppler signs of injury (40–42). Open elbow dislocations and supracondylar humeral fractures also have a high incidence of vascular injury. Long bone fracture, however, is a poor indicator of arterial injury. Among patients with fractures requiring admission, the arterial injury rate is only 0.3% (39). Blunt injury to the distal extremities is more likely to produce significant arterial injury than more proximal injuries because of the smaller quantity of surrounding soft tissues. Complex fractures of the tibia and fibula are frequently associated with vascular injury. Blunt trauma may produce internal penetrating injury from fracture fragments. Identification of these injuries is important because isolated tibial arterial injuries, when associated with extensive soft tissue damage, should be repaired to avoid limb loss, nonunion of fractures, and poor wound healing (44).

Historically, all patients with abnormal arteriograms underwent surgical exploration without regard for the type of angiographic abnormality. Even small injuries were explored because of fear of subsequent thrombosis and possible distal embolization. Experience with angioplasty and anecdotal reports have brought into question such practices. Large and even multisegmental injuries heal after angioplasty, and small AVFs often close. Accordingly, doubt exists regarding the necessity to explore or treat small arterial injuries. Many of these asymptomatic injuries may not require surgical or radiologic intervention but rather can heal spontaneously (19,20,45,46). Minor arterial injuries are followed conservatively at many centers, and clinical deterioration has rarely occurred (45,47–49). The benign nature of these injuries remains unpredictable. Tufaro et al. have reported multiple significant delayed complications, which included major vessel thrombosis, following such observational management, and they advise caution (50).

When observation is the chosen management, clinical follow-up is essential because of the unpredictability of injury healing. Areas of segmental narrowing and small intimal flaps are best suited to such follow-up. Small pseudoaneurysms (<2–5 mm) and small AVFs can also be managed conservatively. Angiography is usually performed 1 to several weeks after the initial injury. Observation needs to be maintained until the injury completely heals or until definitive therapy is provided. Therefore, improving but incompletely healed or stable injuries require serial follow-up examinations (11,45,46). Platelet inhibitors may be used in these patients because of concern for thrombosis (46). An alternative method for follow-up in selected patients is color Doppler ultrasound (29,51). If an injury is to be treated expectantly and it can be well identified by ultrasound, this modality can be used to monitor wound healing.

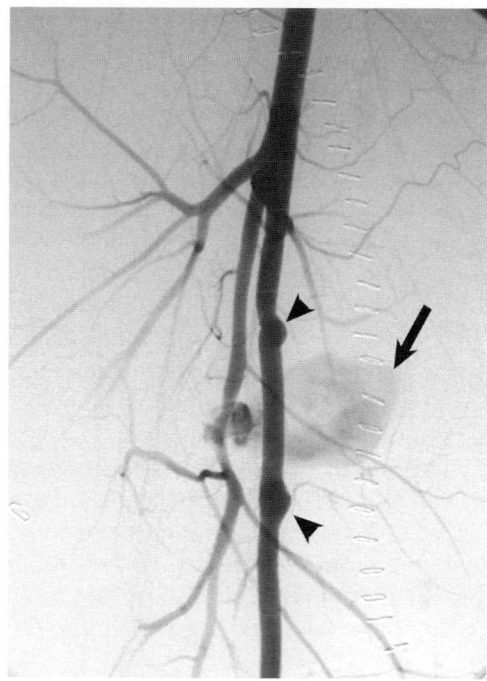

Figure 57–1   Patient following gunshot wound to thigh presents with a pulse deficit. Injury of the proximal superficial femoral artery was treated with surgical vein graft (*arrowheads*). A large pseudoaneurysm arising from the deep portion of the profunda femoris artery was missed (*arrow*). This injury was successfully treated by transcatheter embolization.

Alternatively, some trauma specialists believe that because major vascular injuries can result in limb loss and functional disability in characteristically young victims, diagnosis and repair of all injuries is critical. The cost and legal ramifications of a missed diagnosis motivate some surgeons to request arteriography on all penetrating trauma patients (17,52,53). Arteriography has been shown to be cost effective when the incidence of injury is greater than 1–2% (54).

Although arteriography is both sensitive (98%) and specific (98%), occult injuries do occur and may have a delayed presentation (6). Even surgical exploration does not identify all injuries (55,56) (Figure 57–1). Missed injuries requiring delayed intervention may not be as difficult to repair, nor complications as frequent, as previously thought (19,45). Although long-term delays in treatment may result in huge AVFs or large pseudoaneurysms, which would complicate treatment, most delays are of short duration, and definitive therapy is not usually more difficult (45,47).

TECHNIQUE OF ARTERIOGRAPHY

The site of arterial access depends on clinical evaluation of the patient. For isolated extremity trauma, the preferred access is femoral. With lower-extremity injuries, the contralateral common femoral artery is most often used to allow for possible transcatheter intervention. Occasionally, an axillary approach may be required. Digital subtraction arteriography is now a standard technique.

The arteriogram should include all potential sites of injury. Sequential images are essential, with early rapid images required to identify the site of a high-flow AVF, whereas delayed images are needed to identify sites of extravasation. Because each trauma site deserves attention in this manner, runoff-type filming should be avoided. At least two views, preferably orthogonal, should be obtained to exclude injury (Figure 57–2). When large foreign bodies are present, fluoroscopy and test injections can allow positioning of the vessel of interest away from obscuring metallic material. An area 10–15 cm proximal and distal to the potential injury site should be evaluated.

Careful positioning of the catheter is important so that all arteries in the potential injury path are evaluated. Knowledge of both the entrance and exit wounds, if present, is therefore required. The catheter should be positioned proximal enough to the injury site to allow for common anatomic variants (e.g., high takeoff of the radial artery).

Significant findings on extremity arteriography for trauma include arterial occlusion, extravasation, pseudoaneurysms, and AVFs. Occlusions may be caused by extrinsic vessel compression or by thrombosis associated with arterial laceration or intimal flap. Luminal narrowing may be secondary to arterial spasm, intramural hematoma, extrinsic compression, or atherosclerosis. Intraluminal filling defects indicate nonocclusive thrombi or intimal injuries. Intimal flaps appear as a thin strip or globule attached to the arterial wall in at least one view (57) (Figure 57–3). The vessel course may be altered because of hematoma or associated long bone fracture displacement. Slow flow is an important finding and may be the sole arteriographic indication of a compartment syndrome (57).

Of the many findings seen arteriographically, luminal narrowing is the most difficult to evaluate because vasospasm and intimal injury may be impossible to differentiate. Luminal narrowing may be a result of arterial spasm, which appears as a focal area of smooth concentric narrowing and is particularly prevalent in pediatric patients (58). Some authors recommend the use of vasodilators when such lesions are encountered to exclude more significant lesions.

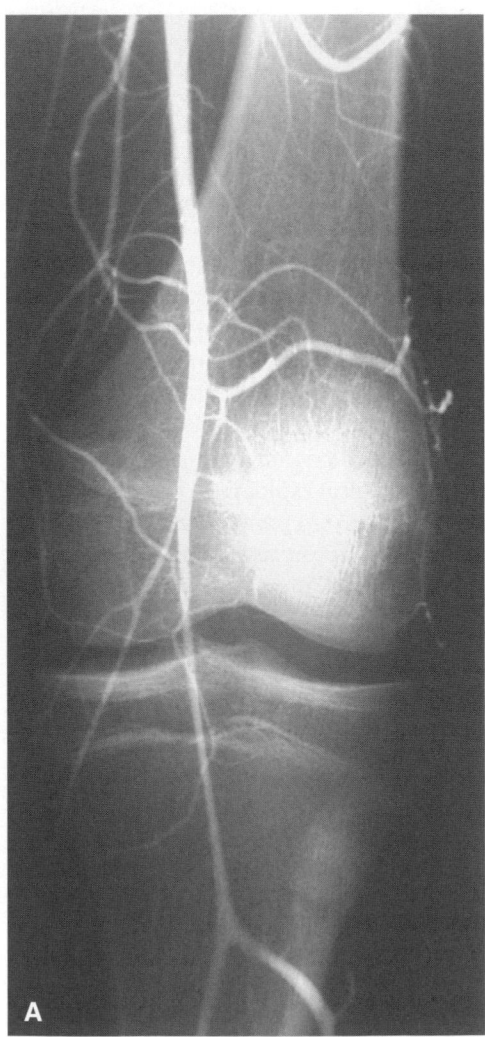
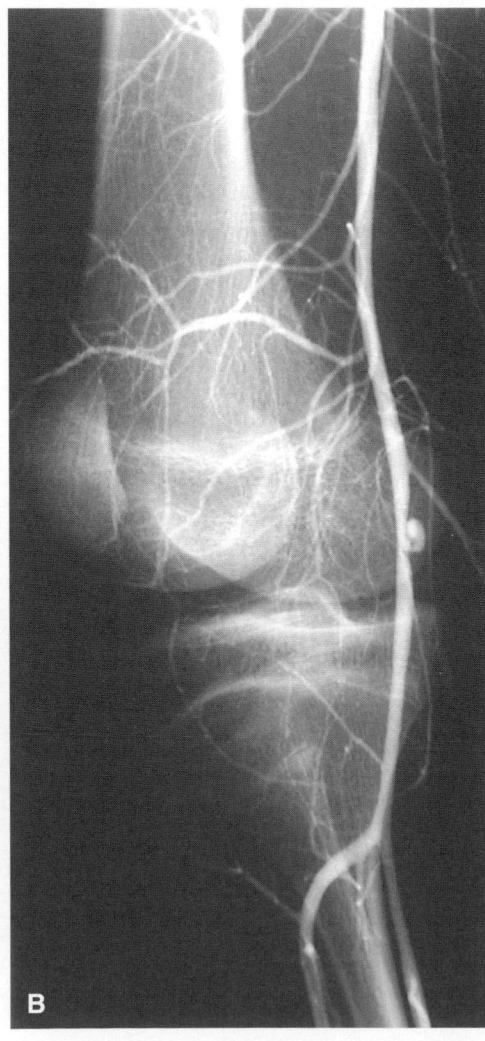

Figure 57–2 **A.** Frontal arteriogram after through-and-through gunshot wound to the knee reveals smooth tapering of the popliteal artery initially thought to be caused by spasm. **B.** The lateral view reveals a popliteal artery pseudoaneurysm and demonstrates the importance of orthogonal views.

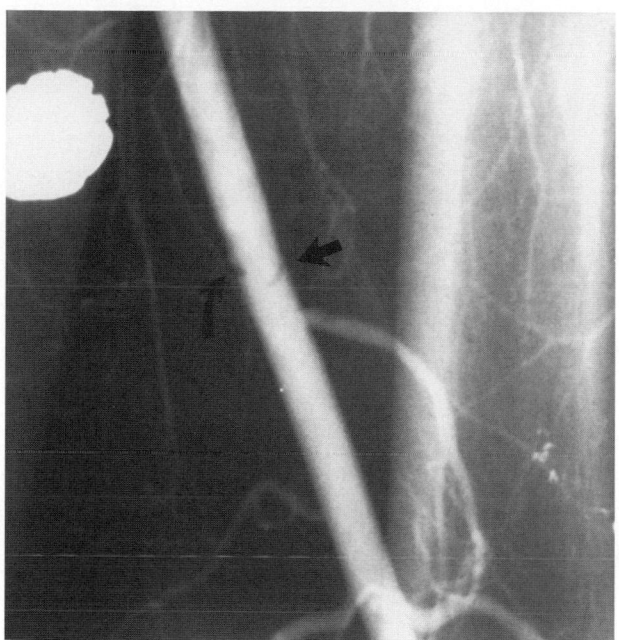

Figure 57–3 Two appearances of intimal flaps: a linear band (*arrow*) or a globule attached to the vessel wall (*curved arrow*). (Reprinted with permission from Hanks SE, Pentecost MJ. Angiography and transcatheter treatment of extremity trauma. Semin Intervent Radiol 1992;9: 20–25.)

Calcium channel blockers, nitroglycerin, as well as papaverine have been used as vasodilators, although their effectiveness is unreliable (46,58). Areas of narrowing that are not concentric should raise concern for intimal injury.

TRANSCATHETER MANAGEMENT OF ARTERIAL INJURIES: EMBOLOTHERAPY AND STENTS

Before undertaking transcatheter therapy for arterial lesions, it is important to understand the surgical alternatives for treatment and their risks and benefits. Arteries may be ligated, primarily repaired, patched by vein, bypassed by vein, or, rarely, bypassed by prosthetic graft. Percutaneous treatment includes embolization as well as transcatheter placement of bare or covered stents.

Until recently, radiologic management was primarily limited to embolotherapy, the intentional occlusion of a vessel. Vessels to be treated by this percutaneous means need to be expendable. These are vessels that are likely to be ligated surgically as an alternative treatment. Transcatheter embolization is usually used for nonaxial arteries (for example, profunda femoris artery, geniculate artery, etc.) or distal axial arteries that are multiple (for example, tibial arteries).

Each patient and each injury need to be considered individually with respect to treatment choice. Transcatheter embolization of significant injuries is preferable to surgical intervention in sites where surgical exposure and/or vascular control are difficult to acheive (for example, in distal profunda femoris arteries) (59). In such cases, surgical dissection may require division of important collateral vessels supplying the distal extremity. In older individuals, caution should be exercised to avoid obliterating such collaterals. It is fortunate that the majority of extremity trauma patients are young and without significant atherosclerosis.

The technique of embolization depends on the type and location of the vascular lesions. In general, the extremities have an extensive collateral network. It is important, therefore, to embolize both proximal and distal to the injury to prevent retrograde arterial filling or recruitment of collaterals (Figure 57–4). Occlusion of the proximal segment is satisfactory if the distal artery is thrombosed (Figure 57–5). For extremely peripheral branch arteries, embolization of the proximal portion of the injured artery may be sufficient (Figure 57–6).

A variety of materials is available for embolization. Choice of an agent is often based on personal preference and experience. In trauma, a temporary occluding agent such as gelatin sponge is theoretically advantageous because many of these lesions will heal. Alternatively, fibered coils, although permanent, offer the advantage of precise positioning. In the extremities, exact placement is usually of foremost concern, and, therefore, coils are favored. Standard coils are 0.038-inch or 0.035-inch steel or platinum wire segments, and microcoils are 0.018-inch or 0.010-inch platinum wire segments. These coils have polyester fibers attached to increase thrombogenicity and are available in multiple sizes and in straight, curved, and complex configurations. Detachable balloons and tissue adhesives, such as N-butyl cyanoacrylate, are possible alternatives but currently lack FDA approval for this indication. Regardless of the embolic agent chosen, the use of an arterial sheath is recommended to preserve arterial access in the event that embolic material lodges within the guiding catheter.

Embolization requires placement of a catheter at the injury site. After identification of an arterial injury suitable for transcatheter embolization, a diagnostic catheter must be manipulated to the target vessel. Achieving adequate catheter position can be the limiting factor for embolization success. Once the guiding catheter is in a good position for embolization, a soft guide wire should be passed to the catheter tip to check for stability. If the catheter is stable, coils of an appropriate size may be used.

It may be unsafe to embolize in too close proximity to essential arteries. If the target vessel is small or tortuous, or if the diagnostic catheter is unstable, a microcatheter can be placed coaxially. Microcatheters allow for rapid catheterization of branches that are unreachable by diagnostic catheters. They minimize vasospasm and the risk of nontarget embolization by providing added stability. Superselective coaxial systems maximize the amount of preserved blood supply (60–62).

Care should be taken in selecting the size of coils to match the target vessel. Too large a coil will not reform and

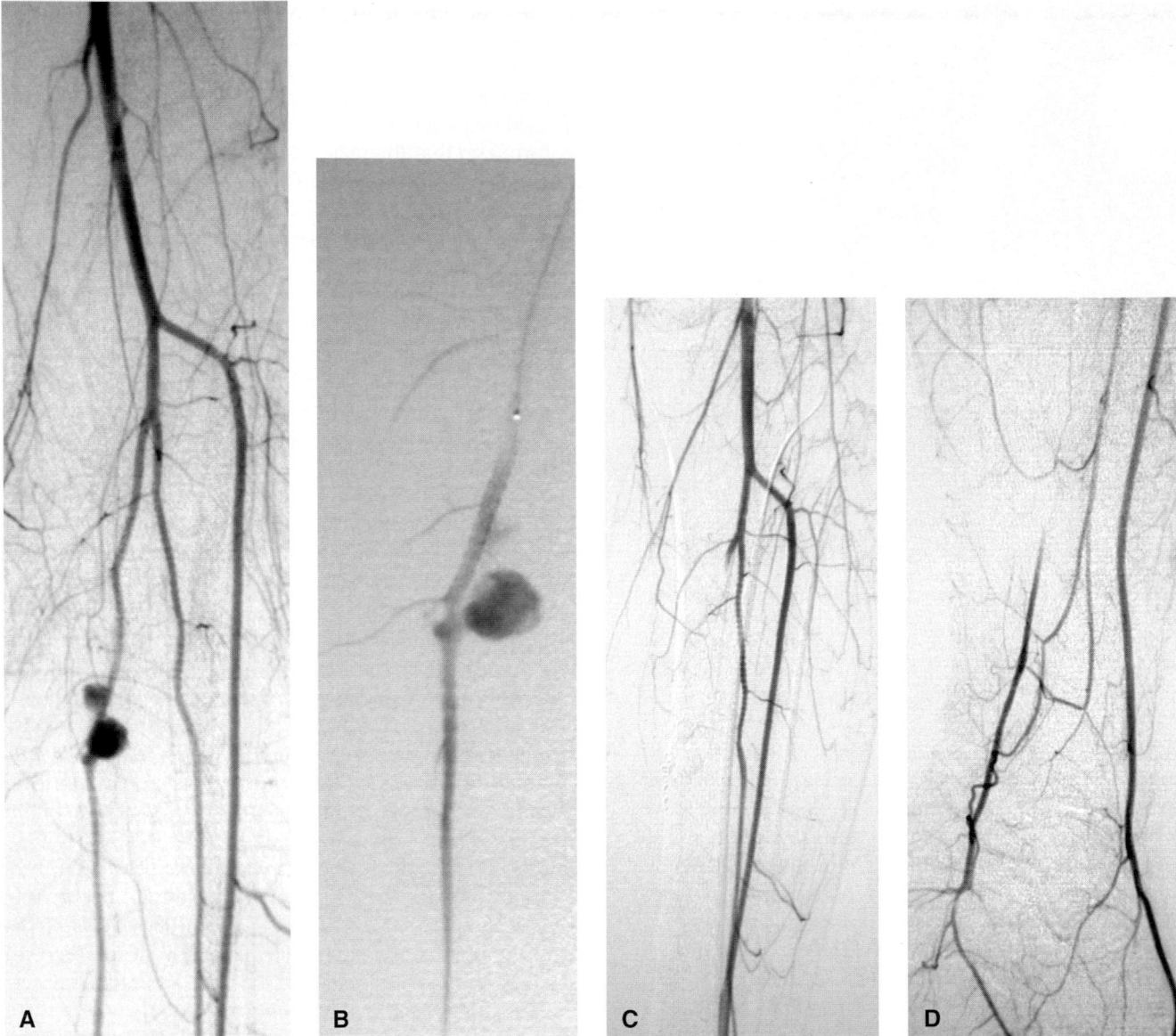

Figure 57–4   A. Leg arteriogram following stab wound reveals a pseudoaneurysm of the posterior tibial artery (PTA) with normal peroneal and anterior tibial arteries. **B.** Selective catheterization of the PTA with a microcatheter demonstrates that coils must be placed distal to the pseudoaneurysm to prevent retrograde filling of the pseudoaneurysm. **C.** Leg arteriogram after transcatheter embolization of the PTA with microcoils both proximally and distally to the injury site. The proximal PTA, including the pseudoaneurysm, no longer fills. **D.** Lateral foot arteriogram demonstrates that the distal portion of the PTA fills via the plantar arch.

will instead push the catheter out of the target vessel and risk embolization of a nontarget site. Too small a coil will pass too far distally, possibly compromising additional tissue or passing through an AVF, and will be ineffective at occluding the injured vessel at the appropriate site.

For AVFs or pseudoaneurysms, coils should be placed so that there are no arterial branches between the coils and the injury site. It is not necessary to occlude the pseudoaneurysm or AVF itself, but rather the artery proximal and distal to the injury (Figures 57–7 and 57–8). Coils may be placed directly

across the injury, beginning distally and progressing more proximally (Figure 57–9). Initial placement of a large coil can provide a network for retaining smaller coils (63). If the artery distal to the injury is patent and access to this distal segment cannot be achieved from the proximal vessel, alternative strategies should be employed to prevent distal retrograde filling. For pseudoaneurysms, small gelfoam pledgets can be used to occlude the distal arterial segment. For AVFs, a transvenous approach or direct percutaneous puncture of the distal artery can be performed (Figure 57–10).

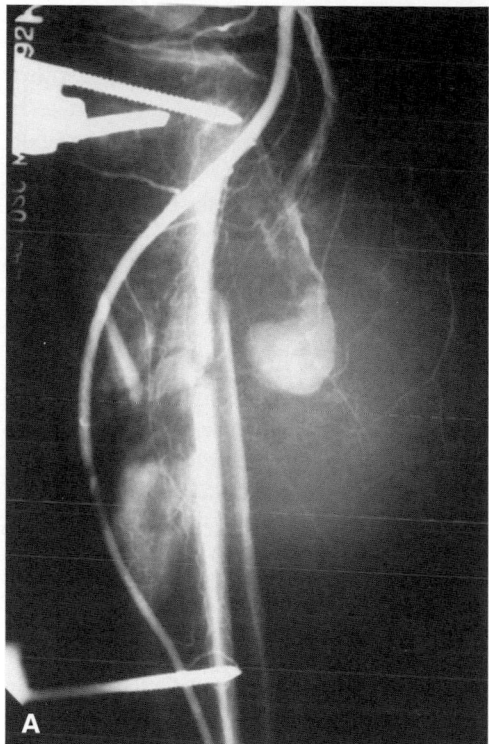
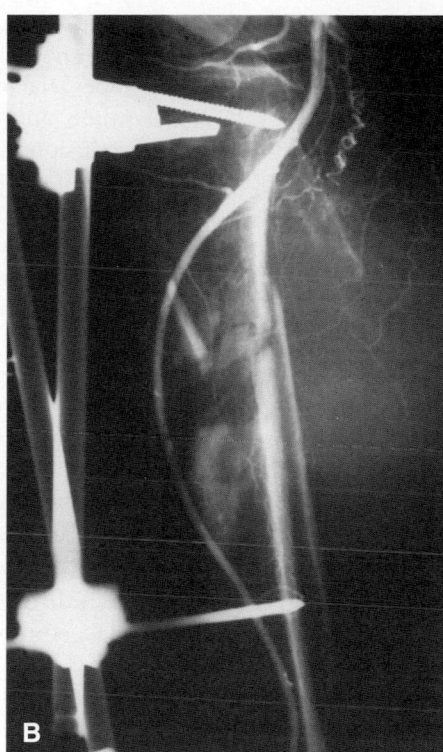

Figure 57–5 **A.** Lower-extremity arteriogram following gunshot injury demonstrates a large pseudoaneurysm of the tibioperoneal trunk with occlusion of the distal arterial segment. **B.** Successful embolization of the tibioperoneal trunk with steel coils only in the proximal arterial segment.

The success rate for transcatheter embolization has been reported to be between 85 and 100% (59,60,62,64,65). These high rates can safely be achieved with modern catheters and coaxial systems. Complications from transcatheter embolization are identical to those of diagnostic arteriography but also include nontarget embolization. With careful technique and, when necessary, the use of microcatheters and microcoils, nontarget embolization is infrequent (62,64). If coil maldeployment occurs, multiple retrieval devices have been developed to enable coil removal. Infection following embolization rarely occurs. Significant limb ischemia should not occur with appropriate lesion selection. Local infarction of tissue can be avoided by using gelatin sponge or coils rather than agents that permeate to the arteriolar or capillary level such as gelfoam powder or alcohol. Transcatheter embolization is

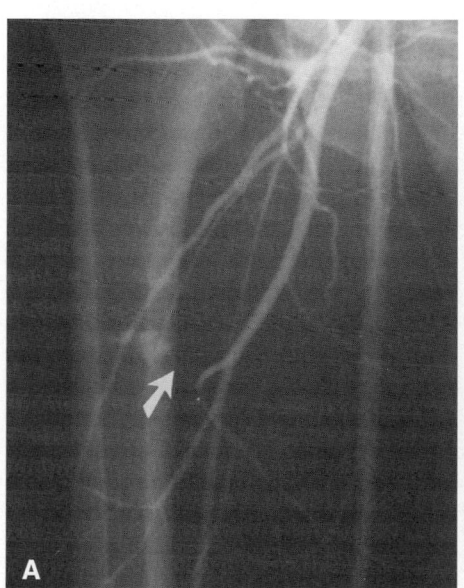
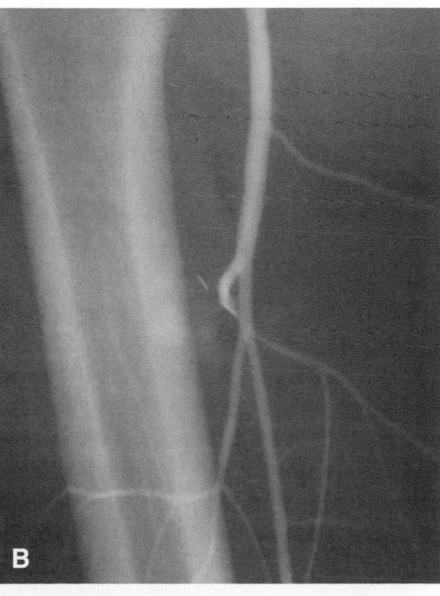

Figure 57–6 **A.** Lower-extremity arteriogram following thigh stab wound demonstrates extravasation from a distal branch of the profunda femoris artery (*arrow*). **B.** Successful superselective embolization of the bleeding muscular branch with two straight platinum microcoils.

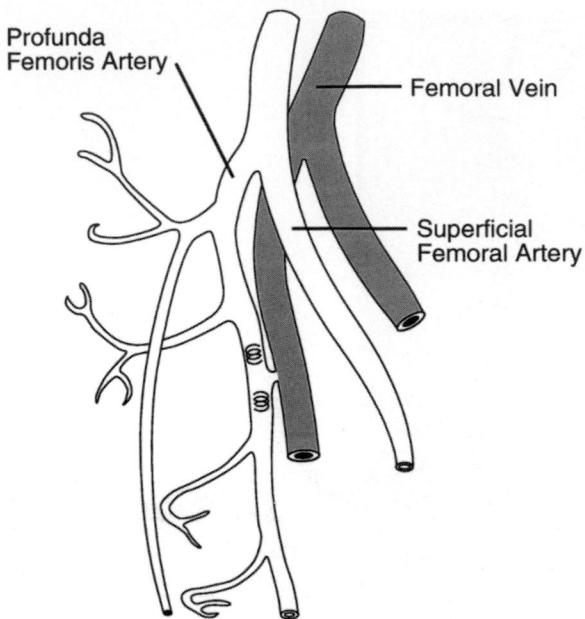

Figure 57–7   Diagrammatic representation of ideal coil placement for occlusion of an arteriovenous fistula. The coils are placed both distal and proximal to the AVF with no intervening arterial branches. (Reprinted with permission from Hanks SE, Pentecost MJ. Angiography and transcatheter treatment of extremity trauma. Semin Intervent Radiol 1992;9:20–25.)

effective and safe and can be definitive therapy for suitable arterial injuries.

For injuries to arteries that cannot be safely sacrificed by embolic occlusion, operative intervention remains the usual therapy. Occasionally, massive hemorrhage may be identified on an arteriogram from an essential artery (e.g., superficial femoral artery). If the clinical situation is appropriate, an occlusion balloon can be used for short-term occlusion to decrease blood loss during transit to the operating room (66).

Surgery can be avoided in some cases of injured axial vessels. The development of stents and covered stents has increased transcatheter therapy to include the management of arterial injuries in vessels that are essential conduits. These arteries may not be safely occluded. Recent case reports suggest that bare or, more frequently, covered stents can successfully treat injuries in axial vessels in which embolization would be inappropriate (67–75). Bare stents have been used to treat pseudoaneurysms and traumatic flow-limiting dissection. Metallic stents covered by polytetrafluoroethylene have been used to manage selected arterial injuries, including AVFs in the subclavian, axillary, brachial, iliac, common, and superficial femoral arteries (Figures 57–11 and 57–12).

Percutaneous treatment may be preferred in polytrauma patients because of associated major injuries or for patients in which vessels are difficult to access surgically, such as the subclavian arteries, which require thoracotomy. Treatment of these patients by placement of a bare or covered stent may be indicated. It remains early in the use of these devices for these applications, and long-term clinical outcomes have not yet been confirmed by prolonged follow-up.

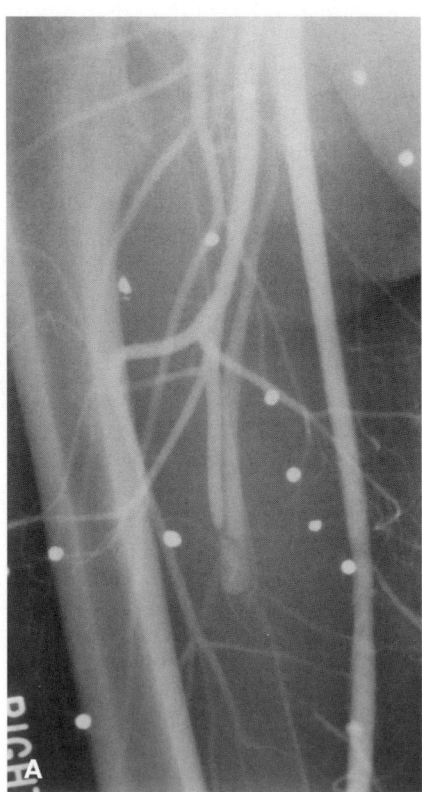

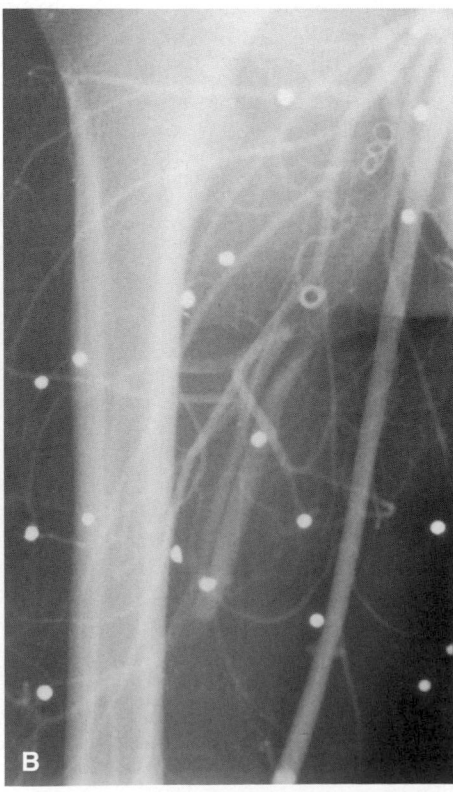

Figure 57–8   **A.** Lower-extremity arteriogram following shotgun injury demonstrates arteriovenous fistula from the distal profunda femoris artery. **B.** Arteriogram following poor placement of occlusion coils. Isolated proximal placement of the coils has allowed for distal reconstitution of the distal profunda femoris artery and persistence of the AVF. Distal occlusion could have been accomplished with a microcatheter. (Reprinted with permission from Hanks SE, Pentecost MJ. Angiography and transcatheter treatment of extremity trauma. Semin Intervent Radiol 1992;9:20–25.)

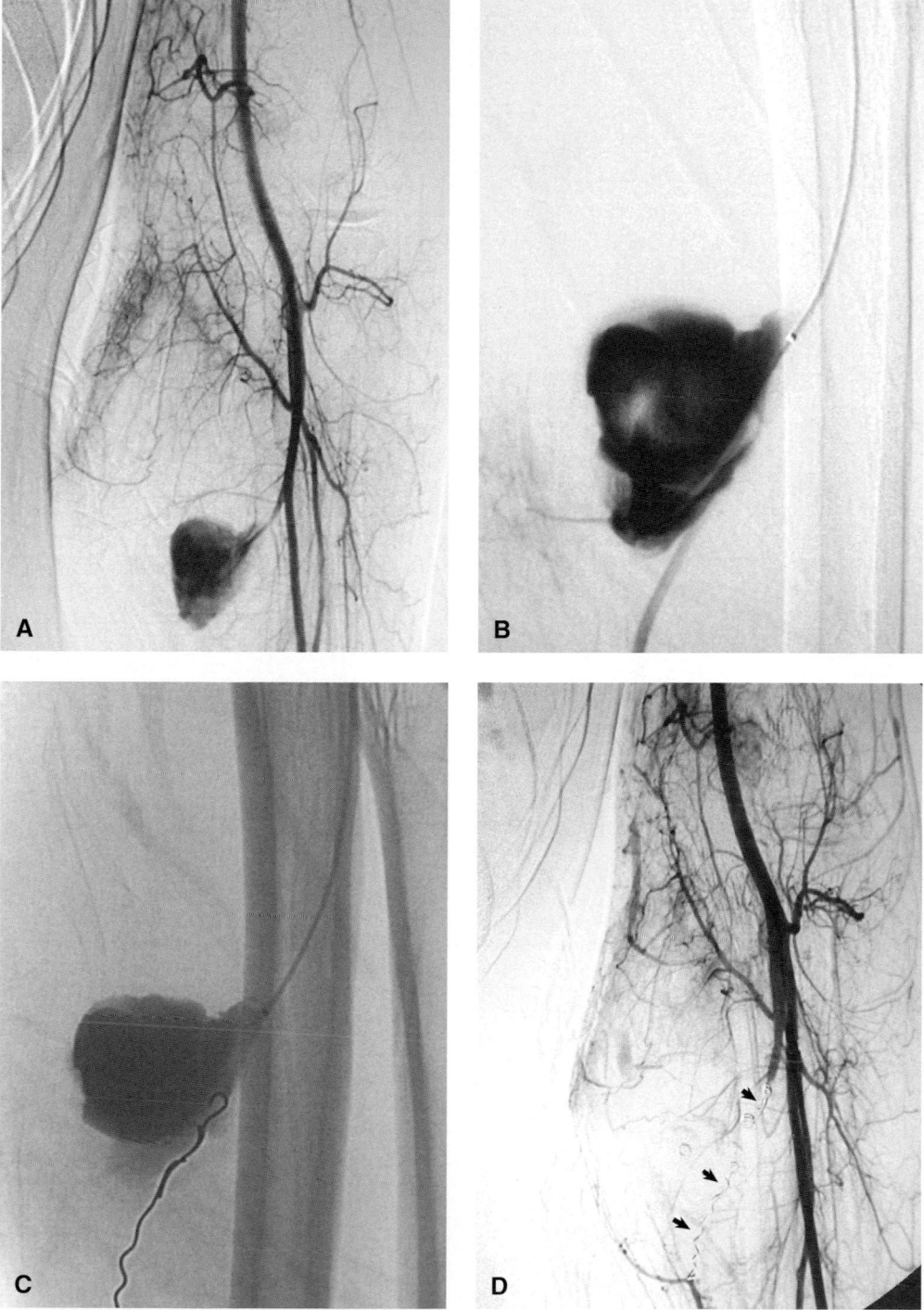

Figure 57–9   **A.** Patient with an enlarging forearm mass following gunshot wound. Upper-extremity arteriogram demonstrates a laceration of the radial artery with a large pseudoaneurysm (PA). The radial artery is not seen distal to the PA. **B.** Because surgical treatment would likely be radial artery ligation, transcatheter embolization of the radial artery was requested. Selective microcatheter placement at the site of injury reveals there is communication of the distal radial artery with the PA. The radial artery distal to the PA must be occluded to prevent retrograde filling. **C.** Occlusion of the distal segment has been achieved with the placement of platinum microcoils. **D.** Additional microcoils have been placed as the microcatheter was withdrawn across the injury (*arrows*). The proximal radial artery is now completely occluded. Flow to the hand is via the ulnar artery. There is no filling of the PA.

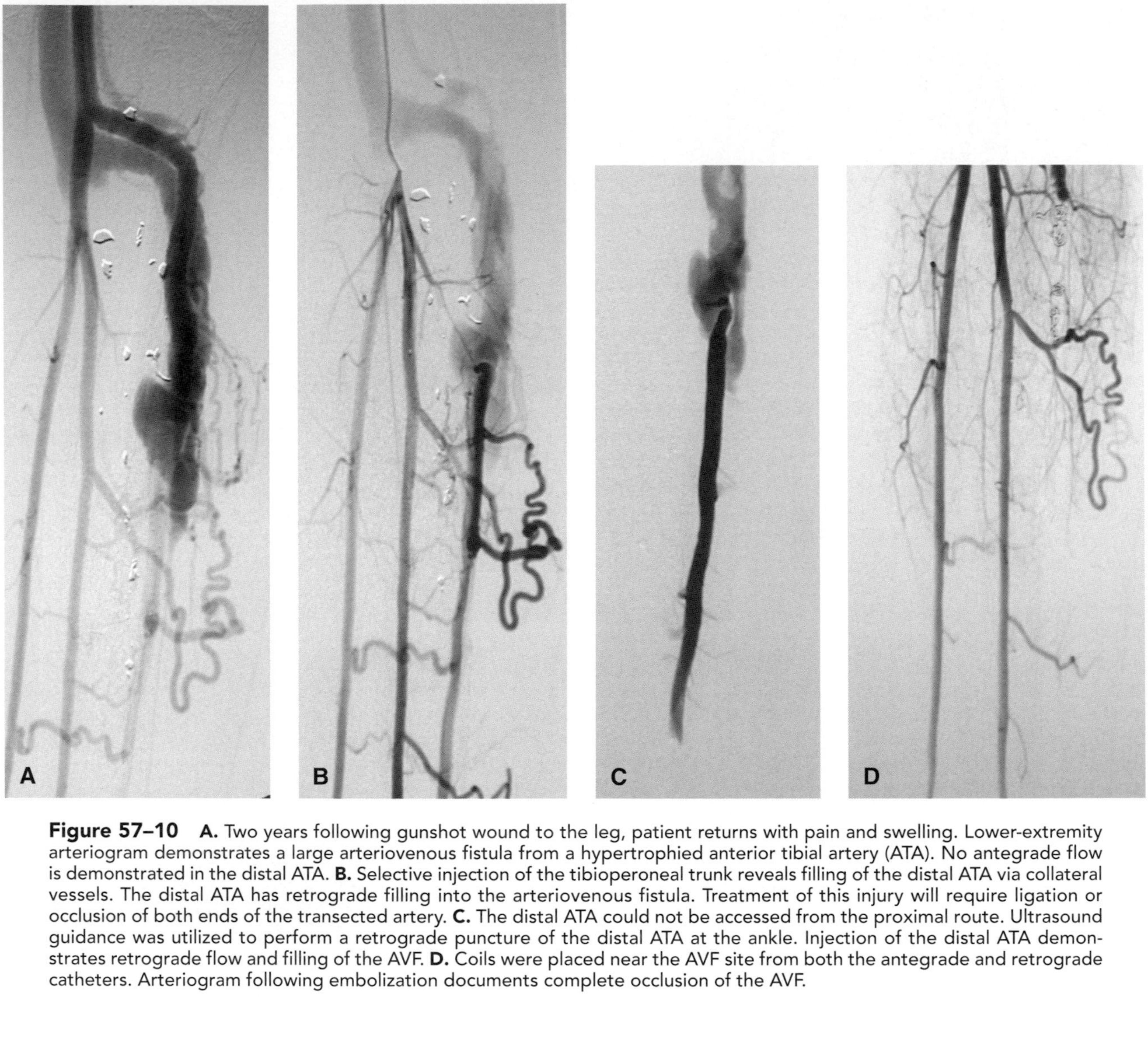

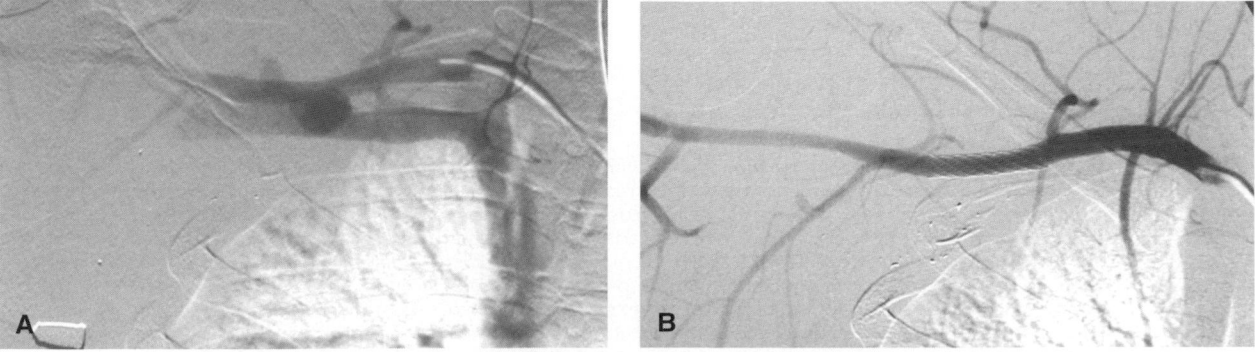

Figure 57–10 **A.** Two years following gunshot wound to the leg, patient returns with pain and swelling. Lower-extremity arteriogram demonstrates a large arteriovenous fistula from a hypertrophied anterior tibial artery (ATA). No antegrade flow is demonstrated in the distal ATA. **B.** Selective injection of the tibioperoneal trunk reveals filling of the distal ATA via collateral vessels. The distal ATA has retrograde filling into the arteriovenous fistula. Treatment of this injury will require ligation or occlusion of both ends of the transected artery. **C.** The distal ATA could not be accessed from the proximal route. Ultrasound guidance was utilized to perform a retrograde puncture of the distal ATA at the ankle. Injection of the distal ATA demonstrates retrograde flow and filling of the AVF. **D.** Coils were placed near the AVF site from both the antegrade and retrograde catheters. Arteriogram following embolization documents complete occlusion of the AVF.

Figure 57–11 **A.** Polytrauma patient with gunshots to the face, neck, chest, abdomen, and pelvis. Right subclavian arteriogram demonstrates a large arteriovenous fistula. It was advantageous to avoid thoracic surgery because this patient had already undergone multiple abdominal surgeries. **B.** Following placement of a covered stent from an axillary approach, arteriography confirms exclusion of the fistula from the circulation.

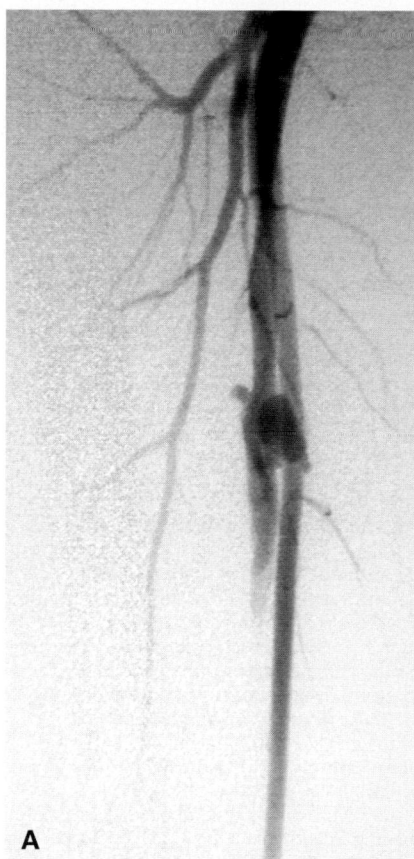

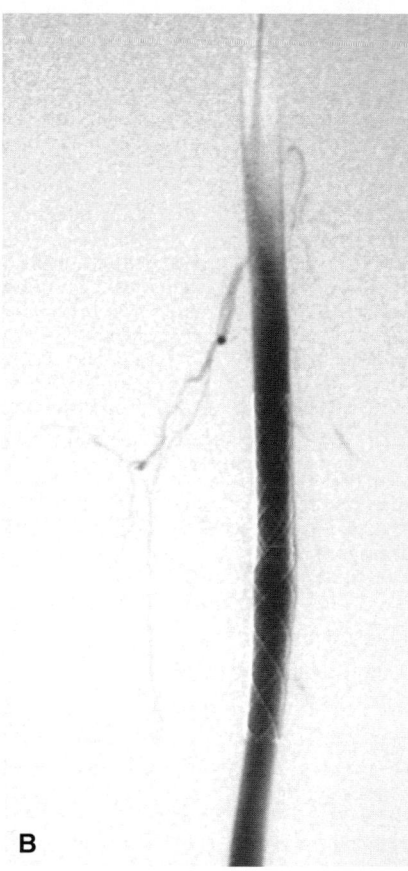

A   **B**

Figure 57–12 A. A midsuperficial femoral artery (SFA) pseudoaneurysm with associated AVF is present following gunshot to the thigh. **B.** A covered stent preserves SFA patency and prevents filling of the pseudoaneurysm and AVF.

SUMMARY

The management of extremity trauma continues to evolve as the natural history of nonsurgically explored arterial injuries is reported. Clinical findings form the basis for extremity trauma management. While arteriography is both sensitive and specific for the diagnosis of arterial injury, the indications for arteriography in extremity trauma remain controversial. Review of the recent literature indicates that, for most trauma specialists, proximity is no longer an indication for arteriography. Additionally, the increasing endorsement of expectant management of minor vascular injuries has caused surgeons and radiologists alike to question whether diagnosis of small injuries is necessary. By decreasing surgical and angiographic exploration, it is clear that additional arterial injuries will be missed regardless of the screening method. These injuries will be treated at the time of clinical manifestation. It remains unclear whether this triage is clinically sound, primarily because the natural history of such arterial lesions, particularly small injuries, is unknown. Resolution of this controversy depends on the difficult task of obtaining adequate follow-up in a largely noncompliant, unreliable patient population. The utility of arteriography, however, goes beyond diagnostic purposes. Arteriography can also be used therapeutically to guide transcatheter embolization or place a bare or covered stent. These interventions can be definitive therapy for suitable lesions.

REFERENCES

1. Frykberg ER. Advances in the diagnosis and treatment of extremity vascular trauma. Surg Clin North Am 1995;75:207–223.
2. DeBakey ME, Simeone FA. Battle injuries of the arteries in World War II: an analysis of 2,471 cases. Ann Surg 1946;123:534–579.
3. Inui FK, Shannon J, Howard JM. Arterial injuries in the Korean conflict: experiences with 111 consecutive injuries. Surgery 1955; 37:850–857.
4. Rich NM, Baugh JH, Hughes CW. Acute arterial injuries in Vietnam: 1,000 cases. J Trauma 1970;10:359–369.
5. Geuder JW, Hobson RW, Padberg FT, et al. The role of contrast arteriography in suspected arterial injuries of the extremities. Am Surg 1985;51:89–93.
6. Rose SC, Moore EE. Emergency trauma angiography: accuracy, safety, and pitfalls. AJR Am J Roentgenol 1987;148: 1243–1246.
7. Reid JDS, Redman HC, Weigelt JA, et al. Wounds of the extremities in proximity to major arteries: value of angiography in the detection of arterial injury. AJR Am J Roentgenol 1988;151: 1035–1039.
8. Snyder WH, Thal ER, Bridges RA, et al. The validity of normal arteriography in penetrating trauma. Arch Surg 1978;113:424–428.
9. Jebara VA, Haddad SN, Ghossain MA, et al. Emergency arteriography in the assessment of penetrating trauma to the lower limbs. Angiology 1991;42:527–532.
10. Weaver FA, Yellin AE, Bauer M, et al. Is arterial proximity a valid indication for arteriography in penetrating extremity trauma? A prospective analysis. Arch Surg 1990;125:1256–1260.
11. Trooskin SZ, Sclafani S, Winfield J, et al. The management of vascular injuries of the extremity associated with civilian firearms. Surg Gynecol Obstet 1993;176:350–354.
12. McCorkell SJ, Harley JD, Morishima MS, et al. Indications for angiography in extremity trauma. AJR Am J Roentgenol 1985; 145:1245–1247.

13. Lipchik EO, Kaebnick HW, Beres JJ, et al. The role of arteriography in acute penetrating trauma to the extremities. Cardiovasc Intervent Radiol 1987;10:202–204.
14. Schwartz MR, Weaver FA, Bauer M, et al. Refining the indications for arteriography in penetrating extremity trauma: a prospective analysis. J Vasc Surg 1993;17:116–124.
15. Henderson V, Nambisan R, Smith ME, et al. Angiographic yield in penetrating extremity trauma. West J Med 1991;155:253–255.
16. Kaufman JA, Parker JE, Gillespie DL, et al. Arteriography for proximity of injury in penetrating extremity trauma. J Vasc Intervent Radiol 1992;3:719–723.
17. King TA, Perse JA, Marmen C. Utility of arteriography in penetrating extremity injuries. Am J Surg 1991;162:163–165.
18. Anderson RJ, Hobson RW, Padberg FT, et al. Penetrating extremity trauma: identification of patients at high-risk requiring arteriography. J Vasc Surg 1990;11:544–548.
19. Dennis JW, Frykberg ER, Crump JM. New perspectives on the management of penetrating trauma in proximity to major limb arteries. J Vasc Surg 1990;11:84–93.
20. Frykberg ER, Crump JM, Vines FS, et al. A reassessment of the role of arteriography in penetrating proximity extremity trauma: a prospective study. J Trauma 1989;29:1041–1052.
21. Smyth SH, Pond GD, Johnson PL, et al. Proximity injuries: correlation with results of extremity arteriography. J Vasc Intervent Radiol 1991;2:451–456.
22. Modrall JG, Weaver FA, Yellin AE. Vascular considerations in extremity trauma. Orthop Clin North Am 1993;24:557–563.
23. Gonzalez RP, Falimirski ME. The utility of physical examination in proximity penetrating extremity trauma. Am Surg 1999;65:784–789.
24. Gahtan V, Bramson RT, Norman J. The role of emergent arteriography in penetrating limb trauma. Am Surg 1994;60:123–127.
25. Yilmaz AT, Arslan M, Demirkilic U, et al. Missed arterial injuries in military patients. Am J Surg 1997;173:110–114.
26. Reichard KW, Hall JR, Meller JL, et a1. Arteriography in the evaluation of penetrating pediatric extremity injuries. Pediatric Surg 1994;29:19–22.
27. Johansen K, Lynch K, Paun M, et al. Non-invasive vascular tests reliably exclude occult arterial trauma in injured extremities. J Trauma 1991;31:515–522.
28. Nassoura ZE, Ivatury RR, Simon RJ, et al. A reassessment of Doppler pressure indices in the detection of arterial lesions in proximity penetrating injuries of extremities: a prospective study. Am J Emerg Med 1996;14:151–156.
29. Schwartz M, Weaver F, Yellin A, et al. The utility of color flow Doppler examination in penetrating extremity arterial trauma. Am J Surg 1993;59:375–378.
30. Panetta TF, Hunt JP, Buechter KJ, et al. Duplex ultrasonography versus arteriography in the diagnosis of arterial injury: an experimental study. J Trauma 1992;33:627–636.
31. Bergstein JM, Blair JF, Edwards, et al. Pitfalls in the use of color-flow duplex ultrasound for screening of suspected arterial injuries in penetrated extremities. J Trauma 1992;33:395–402.
32. Kuzniec S, Kauffman P, Molnar LJ, et al. Diagnosis of limbs and neck arterial trauma using duplex ultrasonography. Cardiovascular Surg 1998;6:358–366.
33. Bynoe RP, Miles WS, Bell RM, et al. Noninvasive diagnosis of vascular trauma by duplex ultrasonography. J Vasc Surg 1991;14:346–352.
34. Busquets AR, Acosta JA, Colon E, et al. Helical computed tomographic angiography for the diagnosis of traumatic arterial injuries of the extremities. J Trauma 2004;56:625–628.
35. Soto JA, Munera F, Morales C, et al. Focal arterial injuries of the proximal extremities: helical CT arteriography as the initial method of diagnosis. Radiology 2001;218:188–194.
36. Soto JA, Munera F, Cardoso N, et al. Diagnostic performance of helical CT angiography in trauma to large arteries of the extremities. Comput Assist Tomogr 1999;23:188–196.
37. Itani KMF, Rotheberg SS, Brandt ML, et al. Emergency center arteriography in the evaluation of suspected peripheral vascular injuries in children. Pediatric Surg 1993;28:677–680.
38. Snyder KB, Pentecost MJ. Clinical and angiographic findings in extremity arterial injuries secondary to dog bites. Ann Emerg Med 1990;19:983–986.
39. Sturm JT, Bodily KC, Rothenberger DA, et al. Arterial injuries of the extremities following blunt trauma. J Trauma 1980;20:933–936.
40. Treiman GS, Yellin AE, Weaver FA, et al. Examination of the patient with a knee dislocation. Arch Surg 1992;127:1056–1063.
41. Kaufman SL, Martin LG. Arterial injuries associated with complete dislocation of the knee. Radiology 1992;184:153–155.
42. Applebaum R, Yellin AE, Weaver FA, et al. Role of routine arteriography in blunt lower-extremity trauma. Am J Surg 1990;160:221–225.
43. Bunt TJ, Malone JM, Moody M, et al. Frequency of vascular injury with blunt trauma-induced extremity injury. Am J Surg 1990;160:226–228.
44. Shah DM, Corson JD, Karmody AM, et al. Optimal management of tibial arterial trauma. J Trauma 1988;28:228–234.
45. Stain SC, Yellin AE, Weaver FA, et al. Selective management of nonocclusive arterial injuries. Arch Surg 1989;124:1136–1141.
46. Hoffer EK, Sclafani SJ, Herskowitz MM, et al. Natural history of arterial injuries diagnosed with arteriography. J Vasc Interv Radiol 1997;8:43–53.
47. Frykberg ER, Crump JM, Dennis JW, et al. Nonoperative observation of clinically occult arterial injuries: a prospective evaluation. Surgery 1991;109:85–96.
48. Frykberg ER, Vines FS, Alexander RH. The natural history of clinically occult arterial injuries: a prospective evaluation. J Trauma 1989;29:577–583.
49. Dennis JW, Frykberg ER, Veldenz HC, et al. Validation of nonoperative management of occult vascular injuries and accuracy of physical examination alone in penetrating extremity trauma: 5- to 10-year follow-up. J Trauma 1998;44:243–253.
50. Tufaro A, Arnaold T, Rummel M, et al. Adverse outcome of nonoperative management of intimal injuries caused by penetrating trauma. J Vasc Surg 1994;20:656–659.
51. Knudson MM, Lewis FR, Atkinson K, et al. The role of duplex ultrasound arterial imaging in patients with penetrating extremity trauma. Arch Surg 1993;128:1033–1038.
52. Cikrit DF, Dalsing MC, Bryant BJ, et al. An experience with upper-extremity vascular trauma. Am J Surg 1990;160:229–233.
53. Perry MO. Complications of missed arterial injuries. J Vasc Surg 1993;17:399–407.
54. Keen JD, Dunne PM, Keen RR, et al. Proximity arteriography: cost-effectiveness in asymptomatic penetrating extremity trauma. J Vasc Interv Radiol 2001;12:813–821.
55. Richardson JD, Vitale GC, Flint LM. Penetrating arterial trauma. Arch Surg 1987;122:678–683.
56. Feliciano DV, Cruse PA, Burch JM, et al. Delayed diagnosis of arterial injuries. Am J Surg 1987;154:579–584.
57. Rose SC, Moore EE. Angiography in patients with arterial trauma: correlation between angiographic abnormalities, operative findings, and clinical outcome. AJR Am J Roentgenol 1987;149:613–619.
58. Sclafani SJA, Cooper R, Shaftan GW, et al. Arterial trauma: diagnostic and therapeutic angiography. Radiology 1986;161:165–172.
59. Sclafani SJA, Shaftan GW. Transcatheter treatment of injuries to the profunda femoris artery. AJR Am J Roentgenol 1982;138:463–466.
60. Kaufman SL, Martin LG, Zuckerman AM. Peripheral transcatheter embolization with platinum microcoils. Radiology 1992;184:369–372.
61. Morse SS, Clark RA, Puffenbarger A. Platinum microcoils for therapeutic embolization: nonneuroradiologic applications. AJR Am J Roentgenol 1990;155:401–403.
62. Teitelbaum GP, Reed RA, Larsen D, et al. Microcatheter embolization of non-neurologic traumatic vascular lesions. J Vasc Interv Radiol 1993;4:149–154.
63. Butto F, Hunter DW, Castaneda-Zuniga W, et al. Coil-in-coil technique for vascular embolization. Radiology 1986;161:554–555.
64. Levey DS, Teitelbaum GP, Finck EJ, et al. Safety and efficacy of transcatheter embolization of axillary and shoulder arterial injuries. J Vasc Interv Radiol 1991;2:99–104.
65. Clark RA, Gallant TE, Alexander ES. Angiographic management of traumatic arteriovenous fistulas: clinical results. Radiology 1983;147:9–13.

66. Ben-Menachem Y. Embolotherapy in extremity trauma. In: Neal MP, Tisnado J, Cho SR, eds. Emergency Interventional Radiology, Boston: Little, Brown, 1989:79–90.

67. Marin ML, Veith FJ, Panetta TF, et al. Percutaneous transfemoral insertion of a stented graft to repair a traumatic femoral arteriovenous fistula. J Vasc Surg 1993;18:299–302.

68. Marin ML, Veith FJ, Cynamon J, et al. Transfemoral endoluminal repair of a penetrating vascular injury. J Vasc Interv Radiol 1994;5:592–594.

69. Marin ML, Veith FJ, Panetta TF, et al. Transluminally placed endovascular stented graft repair for arterial trauma. J Vasc Surg 1994;20:466–471.

70. Schmitter SP, Marx M, Bernstein R, et al. Angioplasty-induced subclavian artery dissection in a patient with internal mammary artery graft: treatment with endovascular stent and stent-graft. AJR Am J Roentgenol 1995;165:449–451.

71. Pfammatter T, Kunzli A, Hilfiker P, et al. Relief of subclavian venous and brachial plexus compression syndrome caused by traumatic subclavian artery aneurysm by means of transluminal stent-grafting. J Trauma 1998;45:972–974.

72. Althaus SJ, Keskey TS, Harker CP, et al. Percutaneous placement of self-expanding stent for acute traumatic arterial injury. J Trauma 1996;41:145–148.

73. Dinkel HP, Eckstein FS, Triller J, et al. Emergent axillary artery stent-graft placement for massive hemorrhage from an avulsed subscapular artery. J Endovasc Ther 2002;9:129–133.

74. Uflacker R, Elliott BM. Percutaneous endoluminal stent-graft repair of an old traumatic femoral arteriovenous fistula. Cardiovasc Intervent Radiol 1996;19:120–122.

75. Maynar M, Baro M, Qian Z, et al. Endovascular repair of brachial artery transection associated with trauma. J Trauma 2004;56:1336–1341.

Angiographic Management of Hemorrhage in Pelvic Fractures

58

John A. Kaufman, Arthur C. Waltman

Retroperitoneal arterial bleeding from pelvic trauma is ideally suited for management with angiographic embolization techniques. Uncontrolled pelvic hemorrhage is associated with a high mortality rate, despite aggressive transfusion (1,2). Open surgical procedures are extremely difficult because of the confined space of the pelvis and difficulty of localizing bleeding vessels in the presence of an extensive retroperitoneal hematoma (3–5). Proximal ligation of the hypogastric arteries is frequently unsuccessful because of the rich collateral arterial supply within the pelvis (1,6,7). Furthermore, incision of the retroperitoneum with evacuation of the hematoma can be counterproductive because release of the tamponading effect of the thrombus permits more bleeding and may predispose to infection (8).

Angiographic localization and embolization of pelvic arterial bleeding in blunt trauma were first described by Margolies et al. in 1972 (9). Angiography permits rapid, precise identification of arterial injury without disruption of the retroperitoneum. Transcatheter embolization effectively controls bleeding, with success rates that approach 90% (10–13). This technique is now generally accepted as the treatment of choice in patients with pelvic trauma and uncontrolled retroperitoneal bleeding (14–28).

HEMORRHAGE IN PELVIC FRACTURE

Exsanguination into the retroperitoneum has long been recognized as a major problem in patients with pelvic fractures (1,2). Historically, 60% of early deaths in patients with crush injuries of the pelvis were attributed to bleeding (2,19). Most patients with severe pelvic fractures can be managed successfully with pelvic fixation devices or binders, resulting in mortality rates that approach 10–20% (29–33). However, 5–15% of all patients with pelvic fractures continue to require angiographic intervention to control pelvic hemorrhage (14,15,34,35).

The etiology of retroperitoneal hemorrhage in patients with pelvic fracture is multifactorial. Bleeding may be from fractured cancellous bone, severed arterial and venous structures, or crushed soft tissues (14,36–38). Coagulopathic states induced by massive transfusion or iatrogenic lesions created during resuscitation of the patient can also contribute to bleeding (14,36–38).

Injury to arteries can occur from shearing against a fixed ligamentous structure, avulsion of a vessel attached to a displaced pelvic segment, or penetrating injury from a shard of bone (14). In a postmortem study of 27 individuals who had died from pelvic fractures, Huittinen et al. found retroperitoneal extravasation of contrast material from internal iliac artery injections in 23 cases (36). Leakage was unilateral in 6, bilateral in 17, and from multiple vessels in 14 (36). However, discrete sources of arterial extravasation could be identified at dissection in only 14 cases, and the remaining nine hematomas were attributed to bleeding from fractured cancellous bone (36).

Internal iliac artery ligation was suggested in the early 1960s in response to the dismal outcomes noted with supportive management of patients with obvious hemodynamic instability resulting from retroperitoneal hemorrhage (39). This technique was extrapolated from experience in elective pelvic surgery during which bilateral internal iliac artery ligation was performed with a low incidence of ischemic injury to the pelvic viscera or soft tissues (39–41). Successful outcomes were described in several small trauma series, but the technique did not achieve lasting popularity (15,39–41). Not only was the ligation difficult to perform in the setting of a massive retroperitoneal hematoma and active bleeding, but serious concerns were expressed regarding the utility of the technique and the morbidity of disturbing the retroperitoneal hematoma (4,42,43). In particular, critics of proximal ligation of both internal iliac arteries argued that it would not stop hemorrhage from vessels that had uninterrupted collateral supply from lumbar, femoral, and inferior mesenteric arteries, and that the risk of infection of the pelvic hematoma was increased (6).

The potential value of angiography in the evaluation and management of hemodynamically unstable patients with pelvic trauma was suggested in 1971 and described in a small series in 1972 (9,44). In the first reported case, autologous blood clot was used to embolize the right obturator artery after a pitressin infusion failed to control bleeding in an elderly patient (9). Although two of the three patients in this series died of multiorgan system failure, there was dramatic hemodynamic stabilization immediately after embolization (9). The clinical utility of the technique was confirmed in a larger series from the same institution, which showed that early embolization markedly reduced transfusion requirements in patients with pelvic fractures (22). Embolization was successfully applied by several other authors with similarly encouraging results (8,10,23–27). In some centers, angiographic evaluation assumed an early and primary role in the management of patients with pelvic fractures (20). However, it was recognized that angiographic techniques had limitations in that the bleeding sites could not be identified in as many as 29% of patients, and embolizations could not be performed in 10% of patients in whom bleeding was visualized because of technical difficulties (10,20).

Early stabilization of pelvic fractures to control pelvic bleeding and facilitate recuperation was proposed because of evidence suggesting that a large amount of the bleeding was a result of fractured cancellous bone (36). This technique has since become a basic component of the management of pelvic fractures. Initial studies employed the pneumatic antishock garment (the "MAST-suit" or "G-suit") (17). This apparatus was supplanted in the 1980s by externally or internally applied fixation devices (29–32). More recently, pelvic binders and C-clamps have been utilized to provide simple and rapid means for stabilization. Early stabilization is believed to reduce the bleeding associated with pelvic fractures by reapproximating bone fragments and reducing the volume of the bony pelvis (14,15). A 3-cm diastasis of the symphysis pubis is estimated to double the potential volume of the pelvis to 8 liters (14). In addition to reducing transfusion requirements, pelvic fixation has other benefits, such as early and simpler mobilization of the patient, which decreases overall morbidity (31,32). Rapid stabilization of the pelvis has dramatically improved the mortality and morbidity rates associated with pelvic fracture when compared with the conservative management techniques of the 1960s.

Despite the application of early pelvic stabilization, some patients continue to exsanguinate from their fractures. Between 5 and 20% of all patients with pelvic fractures will still have uncontrolled retroperitoneal bleeding after pelvic fixation (14,15,18,34,35). Several studies have suggested that the patients at risk for continued bleeding can be identified by the mechanism of pelvic fracture (15,34,35,45). Pelvic fractures are caused by (a) lateral compression, (b) anteroposterior compression, (c) vertical shear, and (d) combined mechanisms (15,35,44). In civilian trauma, the mechanism of injury in 65% of patients is lateral compression (14,44). Lateral compression fractures are graded on a scale of 1–3, with higher grades indicative of increased severity of injury (35). With the application of lateral force, the side of the pelvis folds inward, preserving the pelvic ligaments (44). In general, this is a stable injury with a *reduced* pelvic volume and intact ligaments that contain the retroperitoneal hematoma (34). Transfusion requirements are usually low, with angiographic intervention needed in only 1% of patients, most of whom have grade 2 or 3 fractures (35). An uncommon but severe form of lateral compression injury in which the contralateral side of the pelvis rotates externally, the so-called wind-swept pelvis, typically results in greater blood loss, with embolization necessary in 7% of instances (35).

Anteroposterior compression, vertical shear, and combined force injuries to the pelvis are less common than lateral compression fractures but typically result in more unstable injuries (15,34,35,44). Anteroposterior injuries may involve disruption of the sacrotuberous, sacrospinous, and sacroiliac ligaments in addition to widening of the symphysis pubis and/or pubic rami fractures (35). These are also graded on a scale of 1–3, with grade 2 and 3 injuries most likely to require transfusion (46,47). Vertical shear injuries involve symphysial diastasis or fracture of the pubic rami, rupture of the sacroiliac ligaments and/or a vertical fracture through the sacrum or ilium, and vertical displacement of the affected hemipelvis (44). Combined injuries involve multiple force vectors, but usually one predominates (35). Vertical shear and combined injuries require angiographic intervention more often than do lateral or anterior compression injuries (12,47).

Patients with these mechanisms of injury are more likely to be hemodynamically unstable than patients with lateral compression fractures (34). The potential volume of the pelvis is increased because of the disrupted ligaments, allowing unchecked retroperitoneal bleeding (14). As a group, these patients have a higher transfusion requirement than patients with lateral compression fractures (34). Percutaneous embolization is required in addition to early pelvic fixation in 18–28% of patients with anteroposterior compression, vertical shear, and combined force injuries (12,15,34,35).

The current management of hemodynamically unstable patients with pelvic fractures involves vigorous fluid resuscitation, rapid assessment to determine the sources of bleeding, and rapid intervention (4,14). Survival of patients with severe pelvic fractures can be predicted by transfusion requirements, with risk of death increasing 62% for each 1 U/hour increase in blood transfusion during the initial resuscitation (48). This process is complicated by the fact that patients with severe pelvic fractures are frequently multiply injured because of the high energy of the trauma (4,5,15,18,20,49). Because associated intra-abdominal injury is found in as many as 31% of these patients, peritoneal lavage, or more often abdominal computed tomography (CT) or ultrasound, is performed early in the evaluation of patients with pelvic fractures (1,50). Conventional contrast-enhanced CT has an 80% sensitivity and 98% specificity for identification of bleeding from pelvic fractures based on visualization of a large hematoma or extravasation of contrast (51). The sensitivity improves to 90% with single-channel helical CT and will likely improve further with multichannel scanners (52). If bleeding is suspected from a primarily intra-abdominal source such as a liver laceration, the patient proceeds to emergent laparotomy (4,10,14). Patients with massive pelvic bleeding should undergo angiographic evaluation and embolization prior to laparotomy because opening the abdomen results in decompression of the peritoneal cavity and increased retroperitoneal bleeding. Patients who are more stable undergo pelvic stabilization as soon as possible (31,32). If the patient has a persistent transfusion requirement that exceeds 4–6 units in 24 hours, angiography is performed emergently as both a diagnostic and therapeutic procedure (10,14,15,22). In all unstable patients, an important reason for early angiography is that the embolization can be performed before the patient develops a coagulopathic diathesis secondary to massive transfusion (15,22). When angiography is delayed, mortality can exceed 18% despite successful embolization.

ANGIOGRAPHY

Angiography in hemodynamically unstable patients with pelvic fractures has two goals: (a) rapid but thorough diagnostic evaluation of potential sources of arterial bleeding, and (b) expeditious embolization of bleeding vessels. Whenever possible, plain films and CT scans of the pelvis should be reviewed to identify the location of fractures and potential ligamentous injuries. The sites of arterial trauma may be suggested by the pattern of pelvic fracture and the location of hematomas (Figure 58–1) (18,34,35,53). Frank extravastion or a pseudoanuerysm may be seen on the CT scan (Figure 58–2). Abdominal and chest studies, if available, should also be reviewed to determine whether angiographic evaluation of the abdomen or thorax is also indicated (Figure 58–3). Angiography is indicated in the absence of a fracture in patients with blunt pelvic trauma if there is CT and/or clinical evidence of uncontrolled retroperitoneal bleeding. Arterial injury in the pelvis without bony injury has been reported (54–56).

The internal iliac branches that are most commonly injured are (in descending order of frequency) the superior gluteal; the internal pudendal; the obturator; the inferior gluteal; the lateral sacral; and the iliolumbar arteries (Figures 58–4 through 58–6) (15,20,22). Complete transection of the internal iliac artery trunk occurs less frequently than injury to a branch vessel (20). Less common bleeding sites include lumbar arteries (particularly in patients with vertical shear injuries); branches of the inferior epigastric artery such as accessory or replaced obturator and external pudendal arteries; and the iliac circumflex arteries (22). Spasm is commonly observed in the external iliac artery as a result of either vasoconstriction or trauma, but the predominant injury to this vessel is intimal tear rather than transection (20,57).

The full range of arterial injuries occurs in patients with pelvic trauma, including complete transection, partial transection, intimal disruption, intramural hematoma, acute arteriovenous communication, and spasm. These injuries manifest angiographically as free extravasation, contained extravasation or pseudoaneurysm, abrupt vessel occlusion, intimal flap, arteriovenous fistula, and focal arterial spasm (Figures 58–7 and 58–8).

Angiography should be performed from the femoral approach if possible (15–28). The short distance from the femoral access site to the internal iliac arteries facilitates selective catheterization. In some patients, a femoral pulse may not be palpable because of overlying soft tissue swelling, vasospasm, or hypotension. In these instances, ultrasonographically guided puncture is usually successful. If the femoral vein is inadvertently punctured, an angiographic guide wire should be inserted. This guide wire can then be used as an indirect guide to fluoroscopically localize the femoral artery for a more lateral puncture. The axillary approach may be necessary in patients

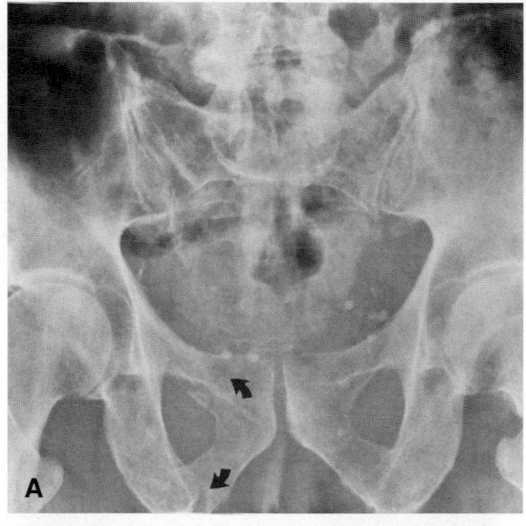

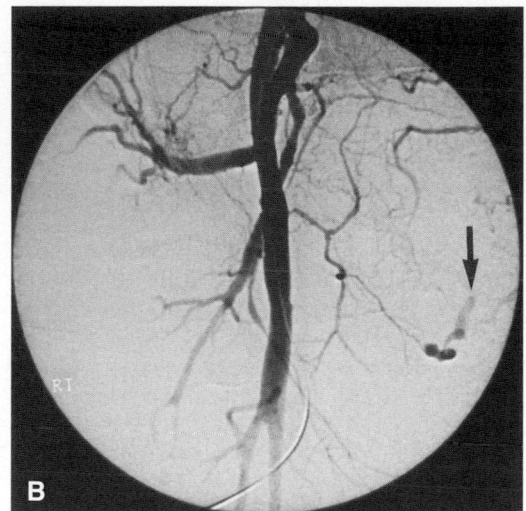

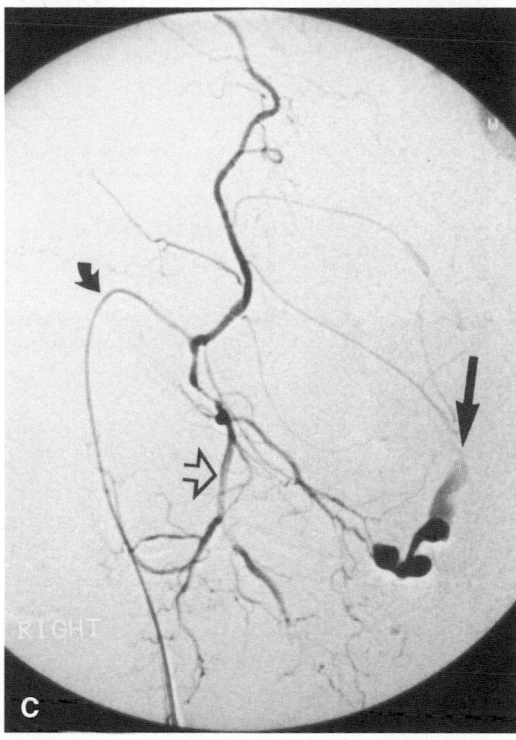

Figure 58–1 Examination of the plain films may predict the site of bleeding. Elderly man with a stable pelvic fracture but a massive pelvic hematoma. **A.** Plain film of the pelvis shows fractures of the right pubic rami (*arrows*). **B.** Digital subtraction angiogram of the right common iliac artery (left posterior oblique) shows extravasation in the region of the fractures (*arrow*). **C.** Selective right inferior epigastric artery injection shows extravasation from the external pudendal artery (*straight arrow*). In this patient, the obturator artery is replaced to the inferior epigastric artery (*open arrow*). The injection was performed through a 5 French Cobra-2 catheter from the ipsilateral approach (*curved arrow*).

with extensive soft tissue trauma to the groins (15,21,28). In this instance, the left axillary approach is preferred to minimize the risk to the great vessels and to provide the most direct access to the descending thoracic aorta. Regardless of the approach, insertion of an angiographic sheath is recommended early in the procedure to protect the arterial access during catheter exchanges and the embolization procedure (15).

Drainage of the bladder by a Foley catheter or a cystostomy tube is helpful to prevent a contrast-filled bladder from obscuring the pelvic vessels during the angiogram. However, this may not be feasible before angiography in hemodynamically unstable patients with suspected urethral

injury. The potentially lifesaving angiographic procedure should not be delayed in order to drain the patient's bladder (15,21,22).

An initial pelvic arteriogram should be performed with a 5 or 6 French pigtail catheter positioned above the aortic bifurcation to fill the lower lumbar and pelvic arteries. Contrast material should be injected at a rate of 8–12 mL per second for 3–4 seconds. The purpose of the pelvic arteriogram is to determine the arterial anatomy and to detect extravasation. Therefore, adequate volumes of contrast and extended filming are essential. Important arterial variants, such as obturator arteries replaced to the inferior epigastric artery and occlusive disease in older patients,

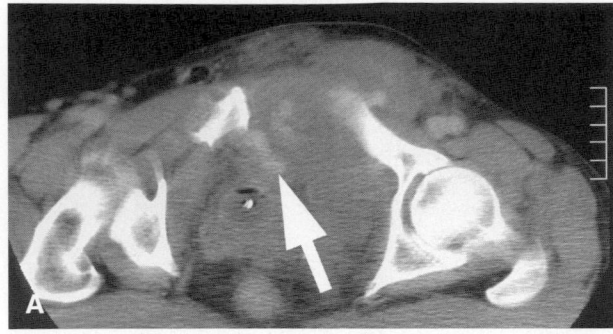

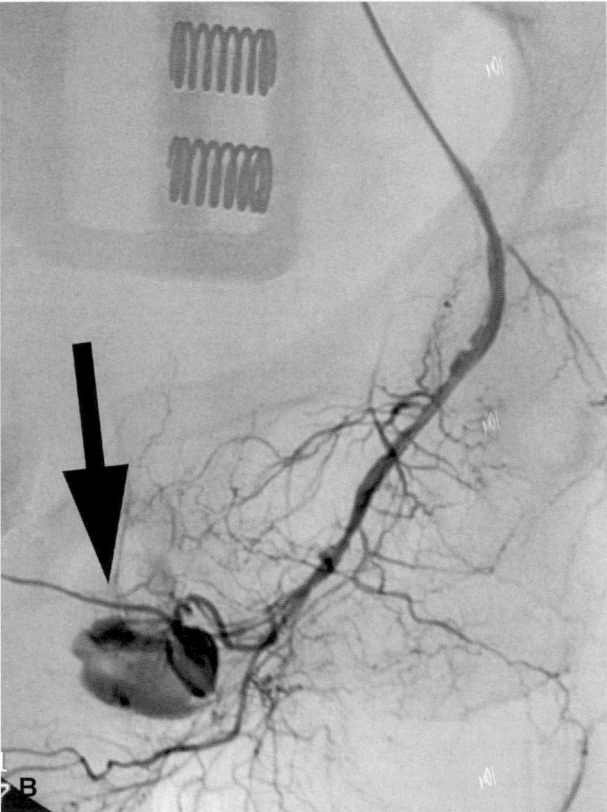

Figure 58–2 Patient with hypotension following motorcycle accident. **A.** Contrast enhanced CT image showing diastasis of the pubic symphysis and extravasation of contrast (*arrow*) in the pelvis. **B.** Selective left internal pudendal angiogram showing extravasation (*arrow*).

may be detected on the pelvic arteriogram. Brisk arterial bleeding from an internal iliac artery branch can frequently be visualized from injection in the distal aorta, but an absence of this finding on the pelvic angiogram does not exclude its presence.

Selective bilateral internal and external iliac artery angiograms should then be routinely performed in patients with pelvic trauma (15). A selective catheter should be positioned in the proximal internal iliac artery most closely associated with the fracture or hematoma. Angiograms in both the posterior and anterior oblique projections should be obtained, with injection of contrast material at a rate of 5–8 mL per second for 3 seconds. In some cases, selective

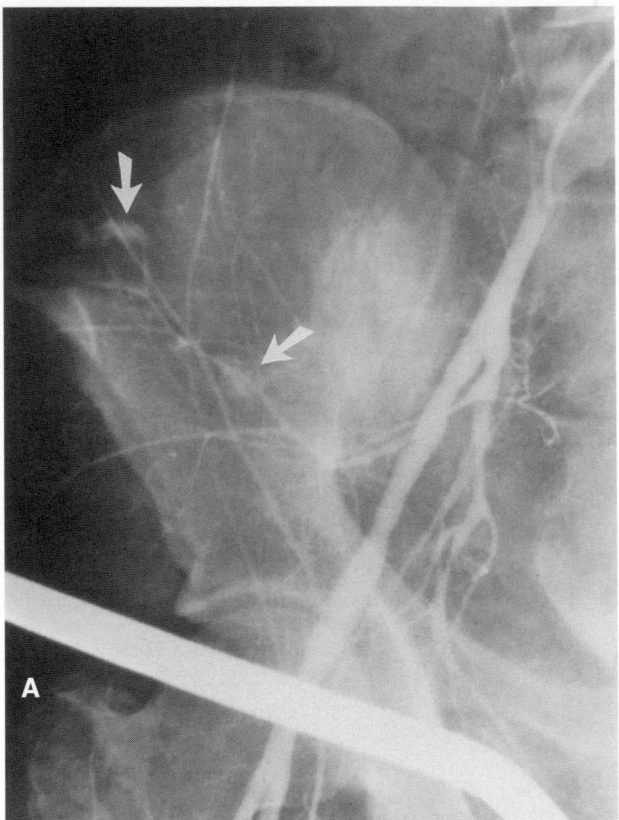

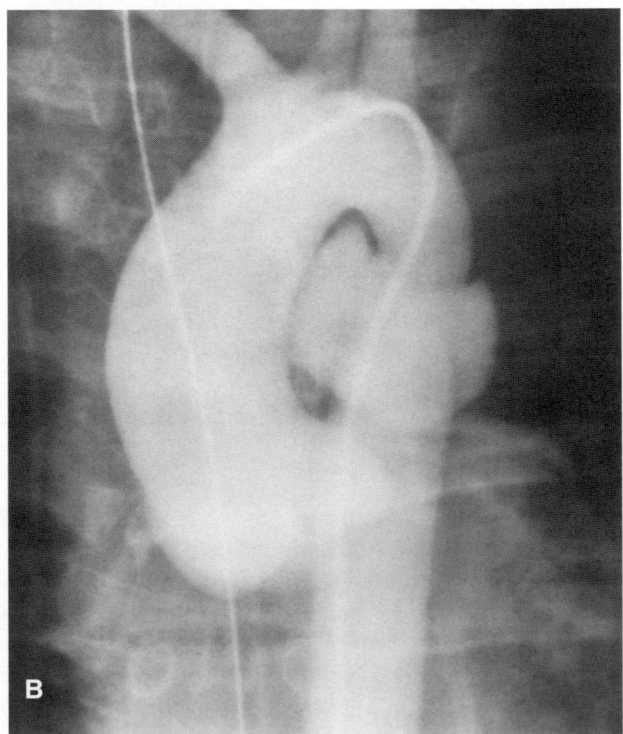

Figure 58–3 Patients with pelvic fractures frequently have multiple injuries. Young man involved in a high-speed motor vehicle accident with pelvic fractures and a widened mediastinum on chest radiograph. **A.** Right common iliac artery angiogram shows diffuse spasm and multiple sites of extravasation in the region of the right iliac fracture (*arrows*). These were successfully embolized with Gelfoam pledgets. **B.** Thoracic aortogram in the same patient performed after the embolization shows an aortic transection.

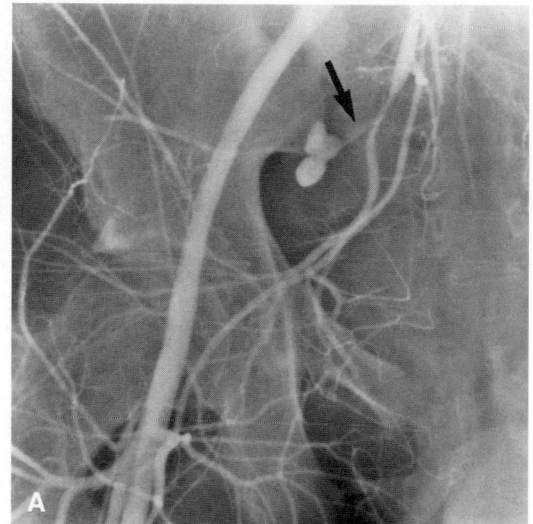

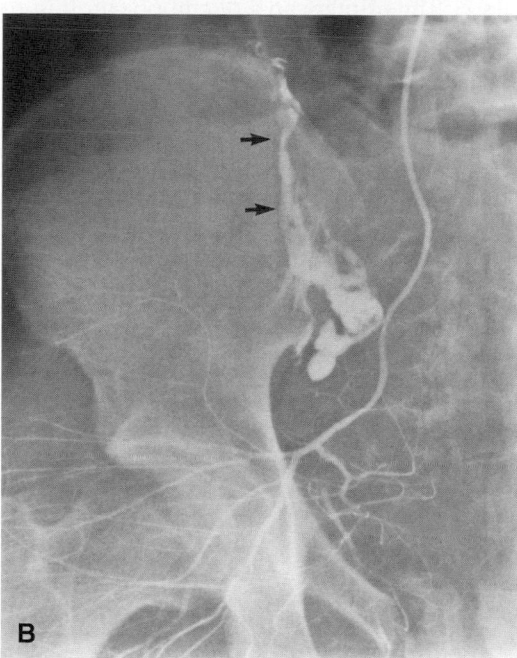

Figure 58–4 Patient with fractures of the right pubic rami and right ilium. **A.** Extravasation is present from a transected right superior gluteal artery (*arrow*). **B.** Selective injection of the gluteal arteries shows massive extravasation (*arrows*).

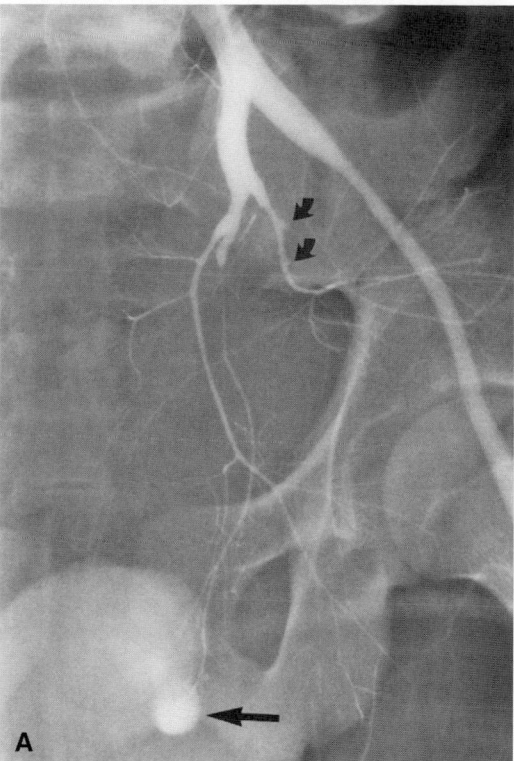

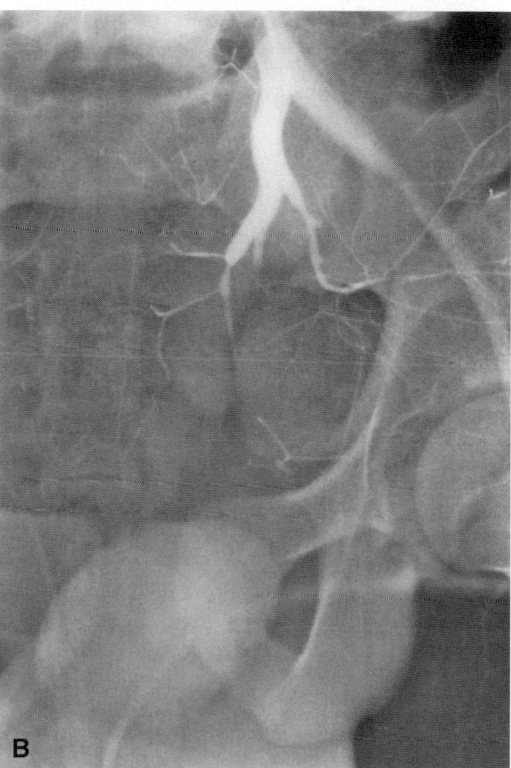

anterior and posterior division branch injections may be required to evaluate questionable areas of extravasation. Multiple views are commonly necessary to completely evaluate patients with metallic external pelvic fixation because of the bulky metal components of the device.

The importance of selective angiography in patients with pelvic trauma cannot be overstated. Selective arteriography is necessary before embolization when extravasation is present on the initial pelvic angiogram to precisely localize the bleeding. When extravasation is not demonstrated on the initial pelvic angiogram, selective arteriography is essential to conclusively exclude arterial injury (Figure 58–8).

Figure 58–5 Young man with pelvic injury including disruption of the symphysis pubis and left sacroiliac joint. **A.** Left common iliac angiogram shows generalized spasm of the hypogastric artery, occlusion of the branches of the superior gluteal artery (*curved arrows*), and extravasation from the inferior pudendal artery (*straight arrow*). The external iliac artery is narrowed because of spasm, extrinsic compression by hematoma, or both. **B.** After successful embolization with Gelfoam, both the internal pudendal and the inferior gluteal arteries are occluded.

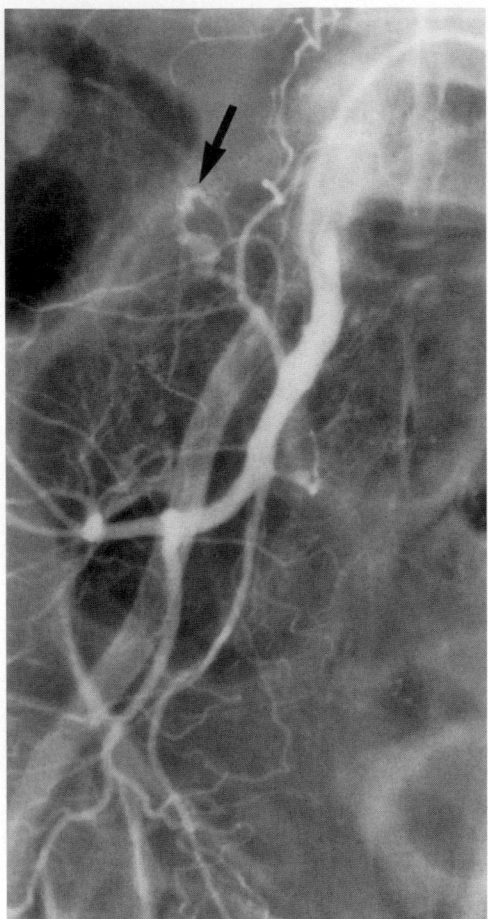

Figure 58–6   Extravasation from the right iliolumbar artery (*arrow*) in a patient with a pelvic fracture.

Finally, selective injections are required to evaluate extravasation that occurs in a site supplied by multiple vessels such as the sacrum and the iliac wing (Figure 58–9).

Several techniques can be used for performing selective internal iliac artery angiography (10,15,21,28). From the femoral approach, the authors favor a 5 French braided Cobra-2 catheter and an angled hydrophilic guide wire for both the ipsilateral and contralateral arteries (10). A loop is formed for catheterization of the ipsilateral iliac arteries. The precise torque control and cephalad angle of the tip of the looped catheter permit rapid selection of the internal iliac artery trunk and the branches of the anterior and posterior divisions. Alternatively, an angled or recurved selective catheter can be used to select the ipsilateral internal iliac artery directly. In elderly patients with a steep aortic bifurcation or tortuous iliac arteries, a long, curved sheath placed over the aortic bifurcation improves the stability and control of the selective catheter for the contralateral arteries. Bilateral femoral artery punctures with bilateral selection of the contralateral internal iliac artery may be required in patients with tortuous or diseased iliac arteries. The catheterization from the axillary approach requires a long, angled catheter such as a Headhunter 1 (28).

Extended filming may be necessary to visualize pelvic arterial extravasation (21,28) (Figure 58–10). Digital subtraction angiography (DSA) allows for rapid examination of hemodynamically unstable patients (18). An important pitfall of DSA is pseudoextravasation caused by misregistration artifacts from bowel gas, ureteral peristalsis, and patient movement. Careful selection of the mask, pixel shifting, or review of the unsubtracted digital angiogram may reveal the true nature of the suspected extravasation. Neither the normal uterine blush in menstruating women nor the stain at the base of the penis in males should be confused with extravasation (58).

Embolization

Once bleeding has been identified, a selective catheter should be securely positioned to allow embolization of the target vessel. The primary goal of embolization in patients with pelvic fractures is to expeditiously decrease or arrest the flow of arterial blood to the injured vessel to allow hemostasis to occur (15). Superselective catheterization should be used judiciously in patients who are unstable because the time spent manipulating a microcatheter into a small vessel may unnecessarily prolong the procedure and limit the operator to small embolic materials. Rapid embolization of the entire anterior or posterior division is preferable to an elegant but long superselective embolization. Complete occlusion of the internal iliac artery is an acceptable alternative to exsanguination.

The embolic material should be easy to use, widely available, and able to rapidly occlude medium-size arteries. Temporary occlusion on the order of several weeks is ideal because this allows recanalization of the vessel after healing of the injury (15). Materials that are difficult to use, such as tissue adhesives, are inappropriate because of the emergent nature of the procedure. Materials that embolize the terminal arterial branches, such as Gelfoam powder or other fine particles, should not be used because of the risk of ischemia to the pelvic viscera, soft tissues, and nerves (59,60). Absolute alcohol is contraindicated because of tissue necrosis and poor control of the liquid embolic agent within the richly anastomotic pelvic circulation. The original pelvic embolizations for trauma employed autologous blood clot formed in a sterile bowl during the procedure (9). Formation of clot can take a long time in coagulopathic patients, requiring the use of topical thrombin (25). This is no longer a firstline agent because it is difficult to control the size of the emboli and because recanalization can occur within days.

The agent of choice in pelvic trauma is Gelfoam cut into pieces to match the vessel to be embolized (10,15,20,21,28). Gelfoam is readily available, easy to use, quickly tailored to the individual patient, flow directed to the injured vessel when there is rapid extravasation, and a temporary agent that permits later recanalization. The dimensions of the pledget should be sized to the diameter of the vessel at the

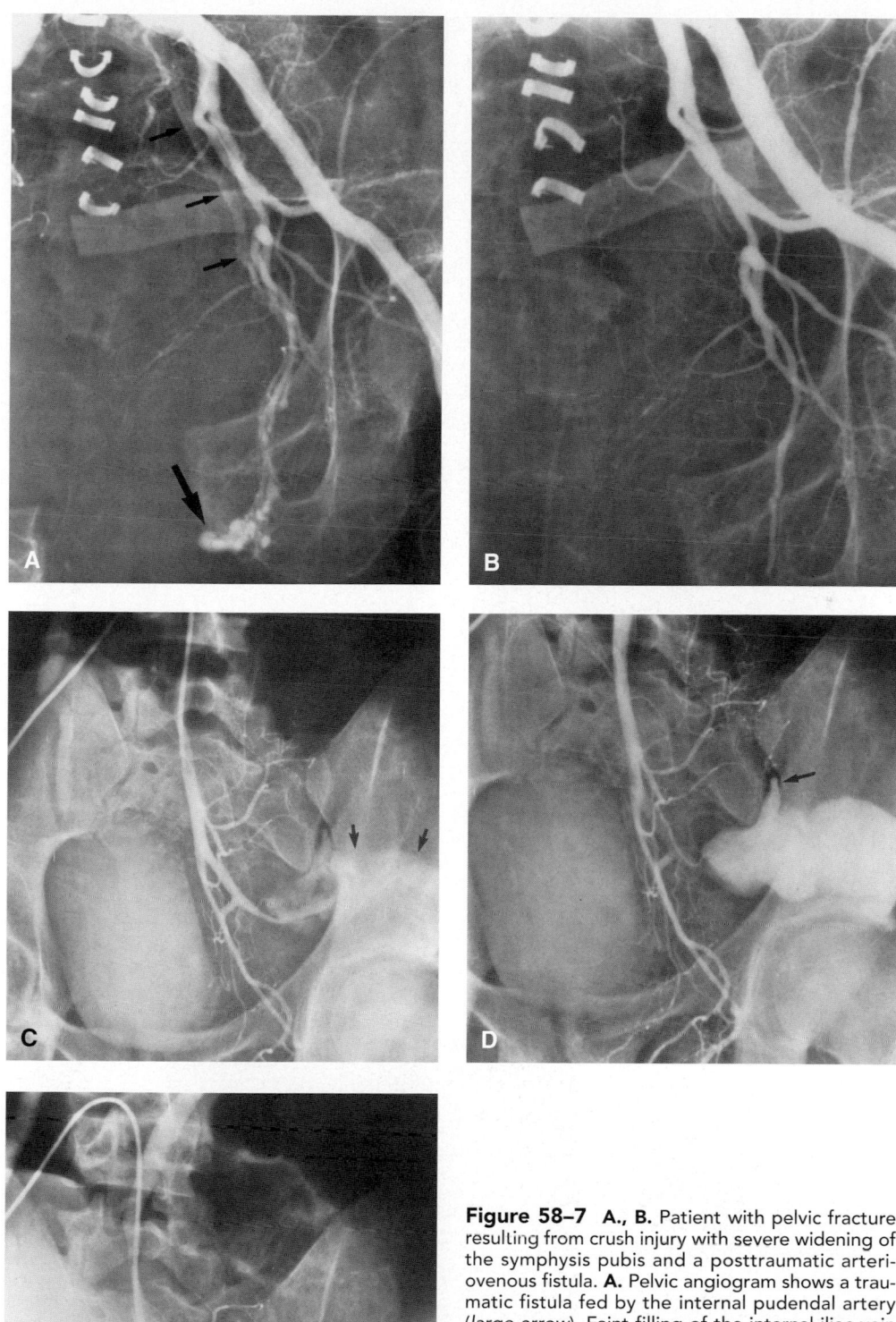

Figure 58–7 A., B. Patient with pelvic fracture resulting from crush injury with severe widening of the symphysis pubis and a posttraumatic arteriovenous fistula. **A.** Pelvic angiogram shows a traumatic fistula fed by the internal pudendal artery (*large arrow*). Faint filling of the internal iliac vein is present (*small arrows*). **B.** Postembolization angiogram shows occlusion of the fistula. **C., D., E.** Different patient with bilateral pelvic fractures and a large hematoma on the left. **C.** Left hypogastric artery angiogram shows filling of a large pseudoaneurysm (*arrows*) from the superior gluteal artery. Note the medial displacement of the hypogastric artery. **D.** Later image from the same injection shows extension of the pseudoaneurysm into the disrupted sacroiliac joint (*arrow*). **E.** Postembolization angiogram shows occlusion of the superior gluteal artery. The pseudoaneurysm does not opacify.

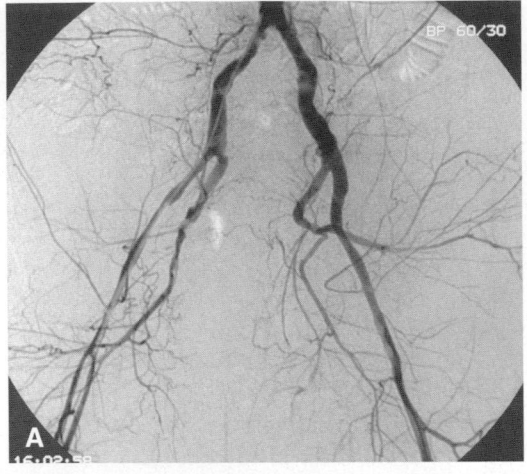
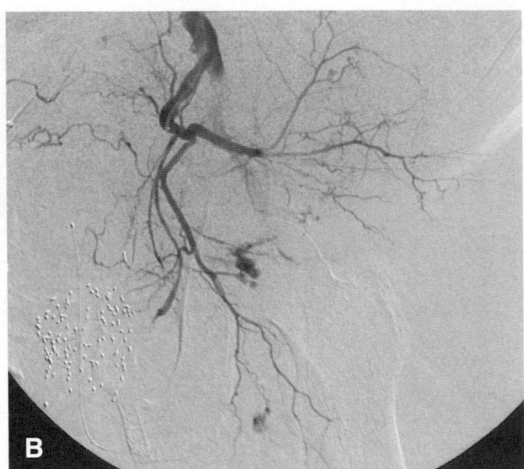
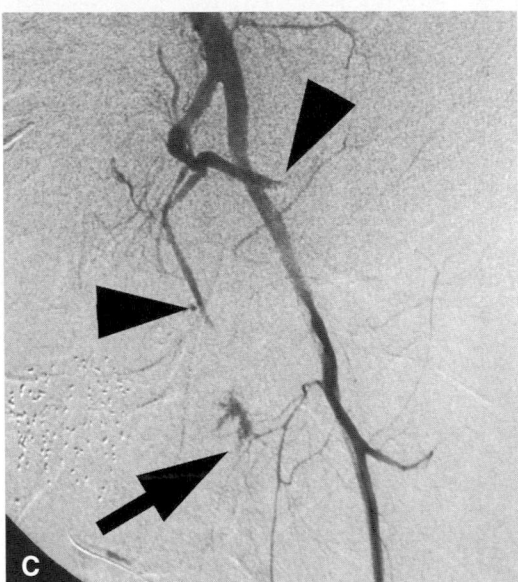

Figure 58–8 Selective internal iliac artery injections should be performed whenever possible when evaluating patients for posttraumatic pelvic bleeding. Patient with severe injury to the bony pelvis following a motor vehicle accident. **A.** Digital angiogram obtained while patient was hypotensive does not show extravasation. Patient was aggressively fluid resuscitated throughout the procedure. **B.** Selective left internal iliac artery injection shows extravasation from multiple arteries. **C.** Following embolization of the left internal iliac artery with Gelfoam, there is truncation of the branches (*arrowheads*). The patient's blood pressure improved dramatically. Extravasation (*arrow*) is now noted from an external pudendal branch from the external iliac artery.

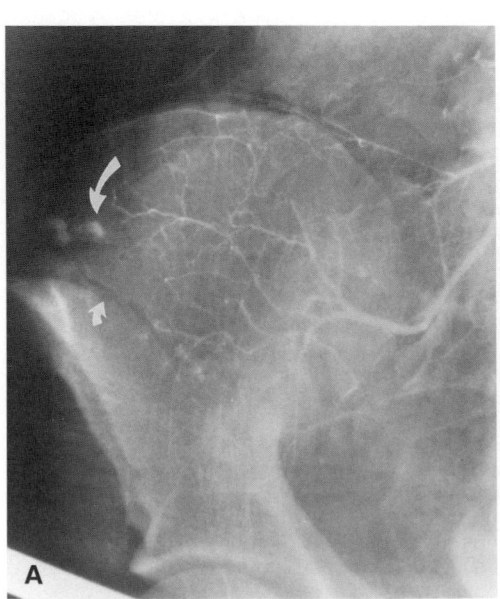
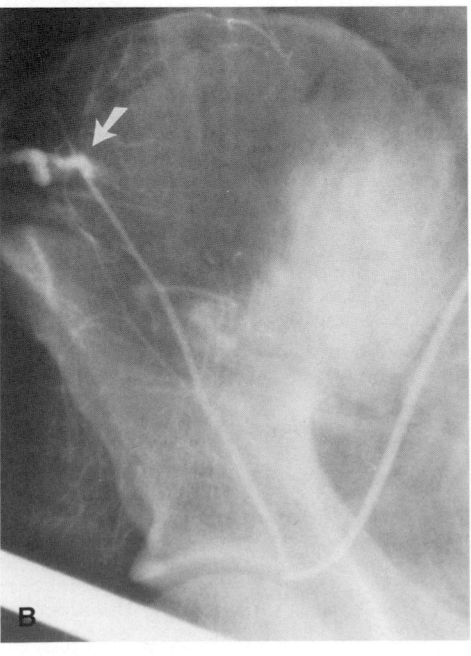

Figure 58–9 Selective injection of multiple vessels may be necessary to evaluate bleeding that occurs in territories with shared blood supply. Young man with right iliac wing pelvic fracture after a motor vehicle accident (same patient as in Figure 58–3). **A.** Selective injection of the iliolumbar artery shows extravasation of contrast (*long arrow*). The fracture of the iliac wing is also seen (*short arrow*). **B.** After embolization of the iliolumbar and superior gluteal arteries with Gelfoam pledgets, the patient had clinical evidence of continued bleeding. Injection of the right deep iliac circumflex artery showed extravasation in the same location as seen from the iliolumbar artery (*arrow*).

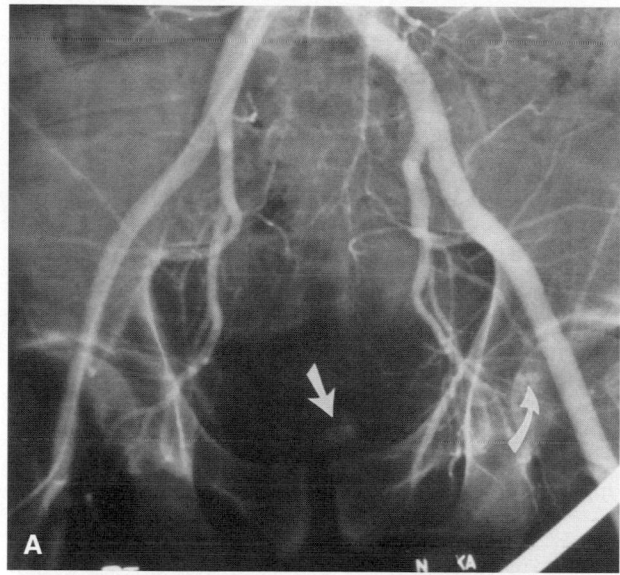

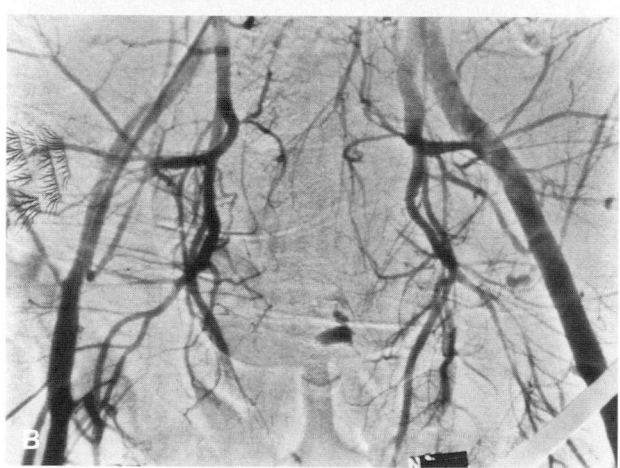

Figure 58–10 Subtraction techniques are useful in the evaluation of pelvic arterial trauma. Young man with a pelvic fracture after a motorcycle accident. **A.** Extravasation of contrast is seen faintly above the symphysis pubis (*straight arrow*) and over the femoral head (*curved arrow*) on the cut-film pelvic angiogram. **B.** The areas of extravasation are more obvious on the subtracted image. Digital subtraction angiography was not available at the time that this patient was studied but would have been similarly useful.

bleeding site. Proximal embolization of the vessel may allow continued bleeding via collateral supply. Typical pledget dimensions range from 1-mm cubes to 1 mm × 2 mm × 5 mm rectangles. Long Gelfoam strips up to 5 cm long may be necessary for large vessels (12). The Gelfoam pledget is first soaked in contrast and then loaded into a 1-mL Luer-Lok syringe. Embolization is accomplished by injection of the pledget through the selective catheter. Use of tuberculin syringes should be avoided because they lack Luer-Loks and dislodge from the catheter during injection of the embolus. Large strips of Gelfoam are injected using 5- to 10-mL Luer-Lok syringes and must be injected through 5 French or larger catheters (15). Multiple pledgets of varying sizes may be required, depending on the progress of the

embolization. Embolization continues until extravasation is no longer visualized.

When numerous bleeding sites are present or selection beyond the internal iliac trunk cannot be accomplished, the scatter technique described by Ben-Menachem et al. may be used (15) (Figure 58–8). Numerous 2-mm Gelfoam cubes suspended in contrast material are injected in a pulsatile fashion into the internal iliac artery, resulting in occlusion of multiple vessels (21). The low resistance within the bleeding vessels favors distribution of the Gelfoam emboli to these branches. Bilateral embolization is well tolerated and has been advocated as an empiric therapy in the absence of demonstrable extravasation for unstable patients with severe fractures (61).

Coils are useful adjuncts in pelvic embolization procedures. When large vessels are transected, the Gelfoam may be swept through the rent into the retroperitoneum. Coils can provide an intravascular substrate on which Gelfoam pledgets can be packed. In patients with pseudoaneurysms or arteriovenous fistulas, where a precise embolization may be desirable, coils are the embolic material of choice. In contrast to Gelfoam pledgets, which are injected in a relatively uncontrolled manner, coils can be pushed through the catheter with a floppy wire and deposited in a more deliberate fashion. In patients with pelvic hemorrhage, some authors have used proximal coil blockade to protect normal vessels during injection of small pieces of Gelfoam (10). This practice is suitable only in stable patients in whom the pace of the embolization can be slower, and is of unproven benefit. A variety of coil sizes and shapes are available for both standard selective and superselective microcatheters. In most cases, however, coils are not the primary embolization material in hemodynamically unstable patients because of the time needed for careful placement and occasional incomplete vascular occlusion (15).

Balloon occlusion catheters positioned in the internal iliac artery can temporarily control hemorrhage in exsanguinating patients (9,15,21,28,62). Embolization can then be performed through the lumen of the occlusion catheter using 3 French microcatheters. Balloon occlusion techniques may also be useful when hemorrhage is discovered from a vessel that cannot be safely embolized, such as the common or external iliac arteries. The balloon remains inflated while a stent graft is deployed or the patient is transferred to the operating room for open repair (63).

The role of embolization in the presence of traumatic occlusions of internal iliac artery branches is not well defined. These occlusions may represent thrombosed arterial transections or areas of spasm. Differentiation is impossible from the diagnostic angiograms because both lesions appear as abrupt arterial cutoffs. Probing of the occlusion with a guide wire is ill advised because of the risk of converting an intact but spastic artery into a perforated vessel.

Some authors recommend prophylactic embolization of the occluded vessels to prevent possible future hemorrhage, particularly in patients who are hemodynamically unstable (15,21). This may be technically difficult if only a short stump of the vessel remains patent. In this instance, placement of a coil is preferred to the less-controlled injection of Gelfoam pledgets. An alternative management strategy in hemodynamically stable patients is to follow transfusion requirements without embolization, with prompt return to the angiographic suite for evidence of resumed bleeding (transfusion of more than 4–6 units of packed red cells in fewer than 24 hours). Patients who are not embolized should be monitored carefully because the rate of clot lysis is unpredictable.

Successful embolization is frequently clinically evident with sudden improvement in the patient's hemodynamic status during the procedure. Angiographically, extravasation ceases, and vasospasm improves (Figure 58–11). Completion angiography is necessary to document cessation of bleeding and to screen for previously unsuspected sites of extravasation or collateral supply. A pelvic angiogram is mandatory. If extravasation was visualized with only selective injections, these should be repeated. Bilateral internal iliac angiograms should be performed if extravasation was from a midline vessel. When embolization in the pelvis is complete but the patient remains hemodynamically unstable, angiographic evaluation of the abdomen or thorax for another source of bleeding may be warranted (15).

The complications of percutaneous embolization of bleeding in pelvic trauma should be compared with the morbidity associated with attempted operative repair or conservative management with massive transfusion (27). Patients should never be considered "too unstable" to undergo this procedure if the suspected etiology of hemodynamic collapse is uncontrolled pelvic hemorrhage. Concerns regarding contrast material such as renal failure are legitimate but should never prevent the procedure. Patients who undergo angiography for diagnosis and treatment of pelvic bleeding are dying. Most complications are acceptable alternatives to exsanguinations.

Nontarget embolization is an important procedure-specific complication of pelvic embolization. Fortunately, the most common site of nontarget embolization is another branch of the internal iliac artery. This is usually of little clinical consequence because the bladder, rectum, and pelvic soft tissues have multiple sources of blood supply, including the opposite internal iliac artery and sources originating outside the anatomic boundaries of the pelvis. As long as the embolic material is of appropriate size and composition, ischemic complications are rare (59,60). Reflux of embolic material into the ipsilateral lower extremity can occur if the catheter is not well seated in the internal iliac artery or the pledget is injected with excessive force. Emboli that lodge in the profunda femoris artery or other muscular branches are usually clinically silent unless these are

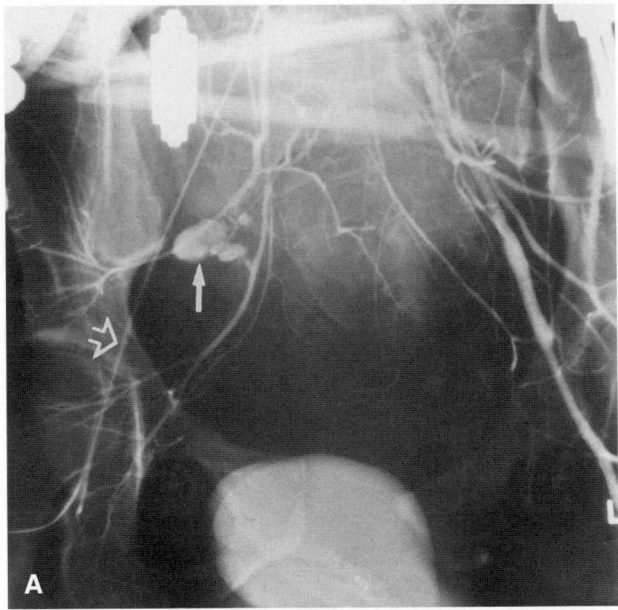

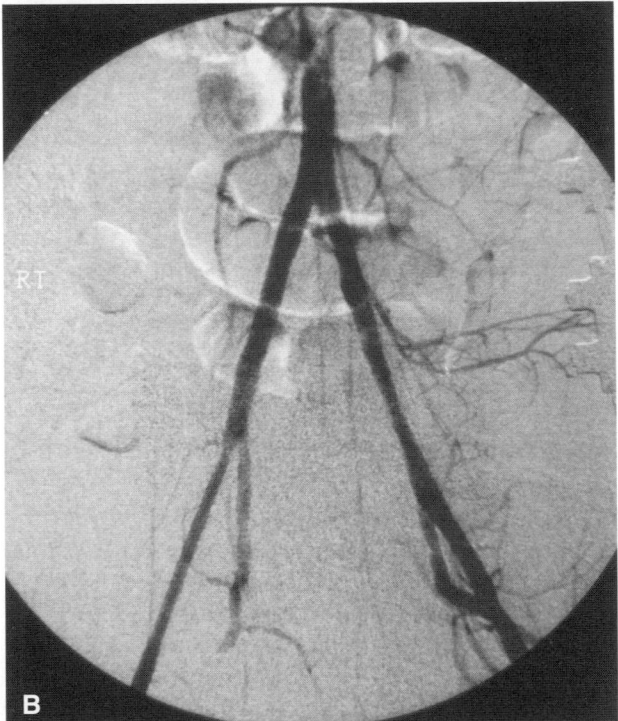

Figure 58–11   The hemodynamic status of the patient may improve dramatically after successful embolization. Young man with a pelvic fracture and persistent hemodynamic instability despite placement of an external fixation device. **A.** Cut-film angiogram of the pelvis shows massive extravasation from the right superior gluteal artery (*solid arrow*). There is severe spasm of the right external iliac artery (*open arrow*), which is virtually obturated by the 5 French catheter. **B.** Postembolization digital subtraction angiogram shows occlusion of most of the branches of the right hypogastric artery and marked improvement of the external iliac artery spasm. With embolization, the patient immediately became hemodynamically stable.

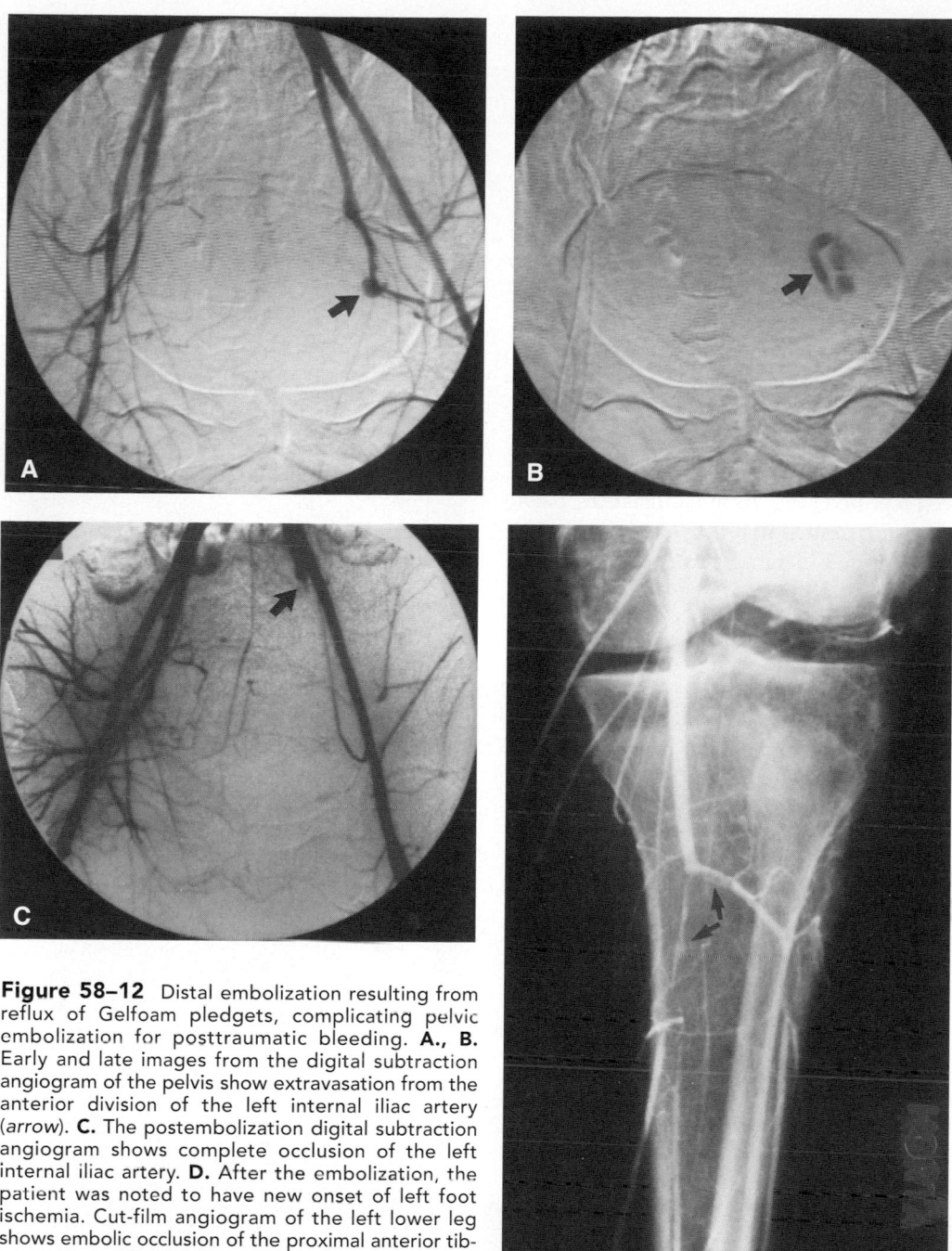

Figure 58–12 Distal embolization resulting from reflux of Gelfoam pledgets, complicating pelvic embolization for posttraumatic bleeding. **A., B.** Early and late images from the digital subtraction angiogram of the pelvis show extravasation from the anterior division of the left internal iliac artery (*arrow*). **C.** The postembolization digital subtraction angiogram shows complete occlusion of the left internal iliac artery. **D.** After the embolization, the patient was noted to have new onset of left foot ischemia. Cut-film angiogram of the left lower leg shows embolic occlusion of the proximal anterior tibial artery and the tibioperoneal trunk. Gelfoam strips and thrombus were recovered at surgery.

sources of collateral supply to the lower limb. Occlusion of a runoff vessel such as the superficial femoral or popliteal artery may result in a severely ischemic limb that requires urgent revascularization (Figure 58–12) (21). These complications can usually be quickly managed with suction embolectomy of Gelfoam or snare retrieval of coils.

Impotence in men and inability to achieve pregnancy in women may be perceived as potential complications of embolization by referring physicians. Before the widespread application of percutaneous embolization in pelvic trauma, impotence was closely linked to urethral injury, with an incidence of 30–50% (64,65). The etiologies of impotence following pelvic fracture are predominantly vascular and neurologic insults that occur at the time of the original trauma (66,67). In women, conception with successful pregnancies has been documented after surgical devascularization of the uterus and ovaries (68). The use of a temporary embolic agent such as Gelfoam may permit future recanalization of pudendal, uterine, and ovarian arteries (Figure 58–13). However, no studies prove that pelvic embolization in trauma does not cause impotence in men or infertility in women. These concerns should be weighed against the immediate needs of an exsanguinating patient.

OTHER APPLICATIONS

Retroperitoneal pelvic hemorrhage can occur after penetrating trauma, orthopedic surgery, obstetric procedures, and percutaneous interventions (7,21,28,69–71). The techniques and principles that apply to hemorrhage in pelvic fractures can be employed in these situations as well (Figure 58–14). Intraoperative embolization of the internal iliac artery to control bleeding from stab wounds and fractures has been reported (72). In most instances, pelvic embolization is best performed in a fully equipped angiographic suite with optimal imaging and the full range of angiographic materials.

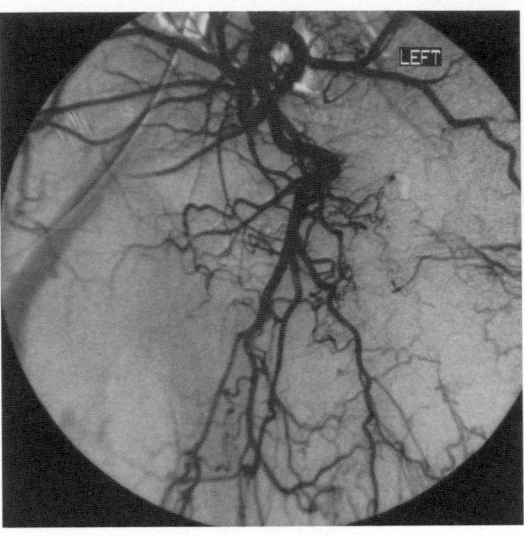

Figure 58–13   Recanalization of embolized vessels is common when temporary agents such as Gelfoam are used. Digital subtraction angiogram of the right hypogastric artery (right posterior oblique projection) of the same patient as in Figure 58–11 obtained 1 year later. The embolized vessel is now patent.

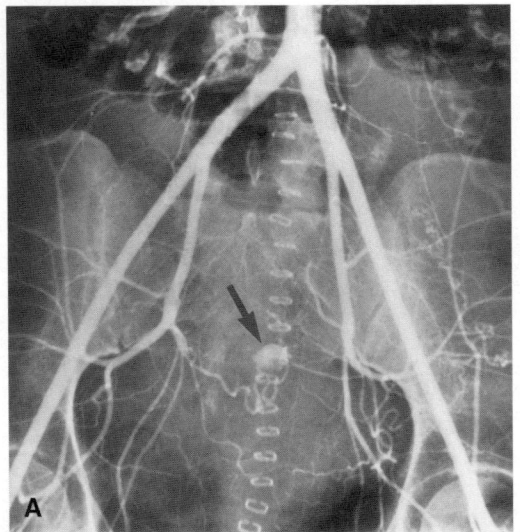

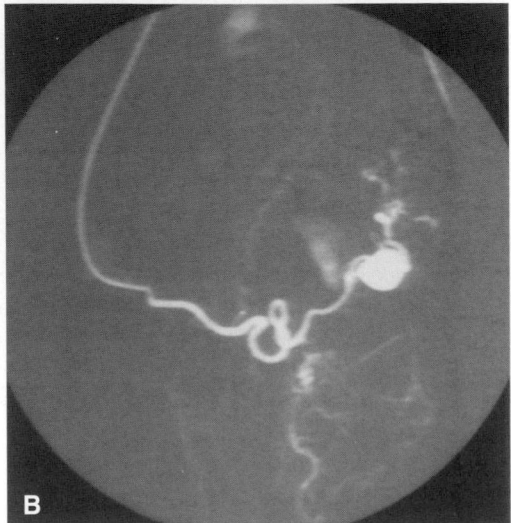

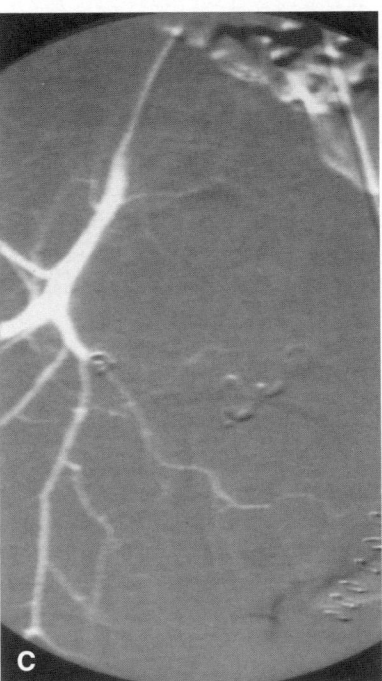

Figure 58–14   Embolization techniques used in pelvic fractures can be applied to hemorrhage from other types of pelvic trauma. Young woman with uterine bleeding after cesarean section. **A.** Cut-film angiogram of the pelvis shows extravasation of contrast centrally in the pelvis (*arrow*). **B.** Digital subtraction angiogram of the right uterine artery localizes the extravasation. **C.** Selective digital subtraction right internal iliac artery angiogram after embolization with Gelfoam pledgets and a single coil shows cessation of bleeding. (Courtesy of Edwin Kim, MD.)

SUMMARY

Percutaneous embolization of uncontrolled retroperitoneal pelvic hemorrhage is a lifesaving technique for which no adequate alternative procedure exists. Early intervention in hemodynamically unstable patients with pelvic fractures is essential to reduce the morbidity of the injury. Embolization can be quickly and safely performed using widely available embolic materials. Angiography is likely to continue to have an important role in the management of pelvic trauma.

REFERENCES

1. Patterson FP, Morton KS. The cause of death in fractures of the pelvis: with a note on treatment by ligation of the hypogastric (internal iliac) artery. J Trauma 1973;13:849–856.
2. Rothenberger DA, Fischer RP, Strate RG, et al. The mortality associated with pelvic fractures. Surgery 1978;84:356–361.
3. Ravitch MM. Hypogastric artery ligation in acute pelvic trauma. Surgery 1964;56:601–602.
4. Mucha P, Farnell MN. Analysis of pelvic fracture management. J Trauma 1984;24:379–386.
5. Reed RA, Teitelbaum GP, Katz MD, et al. Early management of the trauma patient with pelvic fracture: a medical perspective. Semin Intervent Radiol 1992;9:1–3.
6. Brotman S, Soderstrom CA, Oster-Granite M, et al. Management of severe bleeding in fractures of the pelvis. Surg Gynecol Obstet 1981;153:823–826.
7. Yellin AE, Lundell CJ, Finck EJ. Diagnosis and control of posttraumatic pelvic hemorrhage: transcatheter angiographic embolization techniques. Arch Surg 1983;118:1378–1383.
8. Ayella RJ, DuPriest RW Jr, Khaneja SC, et al. Transcatheter embolization of autologous clot in the management of bleeding associated with fractures of the pelvis. Surg Gynecol Obstet 1978;147:849–852.
9. Margolies MN, Ring EJ, Waltman AC, et al. Arteriography in the management of hemorrhage from pelvic fractures. N Engl J Med 1972;287:317–321.
10. Panetta T, Sclafani SJ, Goldstein AS, et al. Percutaneous transcatheter embolization for massive bleeding from pelvic fractures. J Trauma 1985;25:1021–1029.
11. Agolini S, Shah K, Jaffe J, et al. Arterial embolization is a rapid and effective technique for controlling pelvic fracture hemorrhage. J Trauma 1997;43:395–399.
12. Cook R, Keating J, Gillespie I. The role of angiography in the management of haemorrhage from major fractures of the pelvis. J Bone Joint Surg Br 2002;84:178–182.
13. Velmahos GC, Toutouzas KG, Vassiliu P, et al. A prospective study on the safety and efficacy of angiographic embolization for pelvic and visceral injuries. J Trauma 2002;53:303–308.
14. Agnew SG. Hemodynamically unstable pelvic fractures. Orthop Clin North Am 1994;25:715–721.
15. Ben-Menachem Y, Coldwell DM, Young JWR, et al. Hemorrhage associated with pelvic fractures: causes, diagnosis, and emergent management. AJR Am J Roentgenol 1991;157:1005–1014.
16. Brown JJ, Greene FL, McMillan RD. Vascular injuries associated with pelvic fractures. Am Surg 1984;50:150–154.
17. Evers BM, Cryer HM, Miller FB. Pelvic fracture hemorrhage: priorities in management. Arch Surg 1989;124:422–424.
18. Flint LW, Brown A, Richardson JD, et al. Definitive control of bleeding from severe pelvic fractures. Ann Surg 1979;189:709–714.
19. Gilliland MD, Ward RE, Barton RM, et al. Factors affecting mortality in pelvic fractures. J Trauma 1982;22:691–693.
20. Kam J, Jackson H, Ben-Menachem Y. Vascular injuries in blunt pelvic trauma. Radiol Clin North Am 1981;19:171–186.
21. Katz MD, Teitelbaum GP, Pentecost MJ. Diagnostic arteriography and therapeutic transcatheter embolization for post-traumatic pelvic hemorrhage. Semin Intervent Radiol 1992;9:4–12.
22. Matalon TS, Athanasoulis CA, Margolies MN, et al. Hemorrhage with pelvic fractures: efficacy of transcatheter embolization. AJR Am J Roentgenol 1979;133:859–864.
23. Maull KI, Sachatello CR. Current management of pelvic fractures: a combined surgical-angiographic approach to hemorrhage. South Med J 1976;69:1285–1289.
24. Poole GV, Ward EF, Muakkassa FF, et al. Pelvic fracture from major blunt trauma: outcome is determined by associated injuries. Ann Surg 1991;213:532–538.
25. Ring EJ, Athanasoulis CA, Waltman AC, et al. Arteriographic management of hemorrhage following pelvic fracture. Radiology 1973;109:65–70.
26. Ring EJ, Waltman AS, Athanasoulis CA, et al. Angiography in pelvic trauma. Surg Gynecol Obstet 1974;139:375–380.
27. Smith K, Ben-Menachem Y, Duke JH Jr, et al. The superior gluteal: an artery at risk in blunt pelvic trauma. J Trauma 1976;16:273–279.
28. Stock JR, Harris WH, Athanasoulis CA. The role of diagnostic and therapeutic angiography in trauma to the pelvis. Clin Orthop Relat Res 1980;151:31–40.
29. Davidson BS, Simmons GT, Williamson PR, et al. Pelvic fractures associated with open perineal wounds: a survivable injury. J Trauma 1993;35:36–39.
30. Riemer BL, Butterfield SL, Diamond DL, et al. Acute mortality associated with injuries to the pelvic ring: the role of early patient mobilization and external fixation. J Trauma 1993;35:671–677.
31. Latenser BA, Gentilello LM, Tarver AA, et al. Improved outcomes with early fixation of skeletally unstable pelvic fractures. J Trauma 1991;31:28–31.
32. Goldstein A, Phillips T, Sclafani SJ, et al. Early open reduction and internal fixation of the disrupted pelvic ring. J Trauma 1986;26:325–333.
33. Biffl WL, Smith WR, Morre EE, et al. Evolution of a multidisciplinary clinical pathway for the management of unstable patients with pelvic fractures. Ann Surg 2001;233:843–850.
34. Cryer HM, Miller FB, Evers BM, et al. Pelvic fracture classification: correlation with hemorrhage. J Trauma 1988;28:973–979.
35. Burgess AR, Eastridge BJ, Young JWR, et al. Pelvic ring disruptions: effective classification system and treatment protocols. J Trauma 1990;30:848–856.
36. Huittinen V-M, Slätis P. Postmortem angiography and dissection of the hypogastric artery in pelvic fractures. Surgery 1973;73:454–462.
37. Motsay GJ, Manlove C, Perry JF. Major venous injury with pelvic fracture. J Trauma 1969;9:343–346.
38. Ben-Menachem Y. Delayed, exsanguinating pelvic hemorrhage after blunt trauma without bony fracture: case report. J Trauma 1991;31:1018.
39. Seavers R, Lynch J, Ballard R, et al. Hypogastric artery ligation for uncontrollable hemorrhage in acute pelvic trauma. Surgery 1964;55:516–519.
40. Horton RE, Hamilton GI. Ligature of the internal iliac artery for massive haemorrhage complicating fracture of the pelvis. J Bone Joint Surg Br 1968;50:376–379.
41. Fleming WH, Bowen JC. Control of hemorrhage in pelvic crush injuries. J Trauma 1973;13:567–570.
42. Ger R, Condrea H, Steichen FM. Traumatic intrapelvic retroperitoneal hemorrhage: an experimental study. J Surg Res 1969;9:31–34.
43. Ravitch MM. Hypogastric artery ligation in acute pelvic trauma. Surgery 1964;56:601–602.
44. Athanasoulis CA, Duffield R, Shapiro JH. Angiography to assess pelvic vascular injury. N Engl J Med 1971;285:1539.
45. Young JW, Resnik CS. Fracture of the pelvis: current concepts and classification. AJR Am J Roentgenol 1990;155:1169–1175.
46. Eastridge B, Starr A, Minei JP, et al. The importance of fracture pattern in guiding therapeutic decision-making in patients with hemorrhagic shock and pelvic ring disruptions. J Trauma 2002;53:446–450.
47. Bassam D, Cephas GA, Ferguson KA, et al. A protocol for the initial management of unstable pelvic fractures. Am Surg 1998;64:862–867.
48. Wong YC, Wang LJ, Ng CJ, et al. Mortality after successful transcatheter arterial embolization in patients with unstable pelvic fractures: rate of blood transfusion as a predictive factor. J Trauma 2000;49:71–75.

49. Ochsner MG, Hoffman AP, DiPasquale D, et al. Associated aortic rupture-pelvic fracture: an alert for orthopedic and general surgeons. J Trauma 1992;33:429–434.

50. Demetriades D, Karaiskakis M, Toutouzas K, et al.Pelvic fractures: epidemiology and predictors of associated abdominal injuries and outcomes. J Am Coll Surg 2002;195:1–10.

51. Stephen DJ, Kreder HJ, Day AC, et al. Early detection of arterial bleeding in acute pelvic trauma. J Trauma 1999;47:638–642.

52. Pereira SJ, O'Brien DP, Luchette FA, et al. Dynamic helical computed tomography scan accurately detects hemorrhage in patients with pelvic fracture. Surgery 2000;128:678–685.

53. Blackmore CC, Jurkovich GJ, Linnau KF, et al. Assessment of volume of hemorrhage and outcome from pelvic fracture. Arch Surg 2003;138:504–508.

54. Brumback RJ. Traumatic rupture of the superior gluteal artery, without fracture of the pelvis, causing compartment syndrome of the buttock. A case report. J Bone Joint Surg 1990;72:134–137.

55. Baumgartner F, White GH, White RA, et al. Delayed, exsanguinating pelvic hemorrhage after blunt trauma without bony fracture: case report. J Trauma 1990;30:1603–1605.

56. Belley G, Gallix BP, Derossis AM, et al. Profound hypotension in blunt trauma associated with superior gluteal artery rupture without pelvic fracture. J Trauma 1997;43:703–705.

57. Birchard JD, Pichora DR, Brown PM. External iliac artery and lumbosacral plexus injury secondary to open book fracture of the pelvis: report of a case. J Trauma 1990;30:906–908.

58. Schrumpf JD, Sommer G, Jacobs RP. Bleeding simulated by the distal internal pudendal artery stain. AJR Am J Roentgenol 1978; 131:657–659.

59. Braf ZF, Koontz WW Jr. Gangrene of the bladder: complication of hypogastric artery embolization. Urology 1977;9:670–671.

60. Hare WS, Holland CJ. Paresis following internal iliac artery embolization. Radiology 1983;143:47–51.

61. Velmahos GC, Chahwan S, Hanks SE, et al. Angiographic embolization of bilateral internal iliac arteries to control life-threatening hemorrhage after blunt trauma to the pelvis. Am Surg 2000;66:858–862.

62. Paster SB, Van Houten FX, Adams DF. Percutaneous balloon catheterization: a technique for the control of arterial hemorrhage caused by pelvic trauma. JAMA 1974;230:573–575.

63. Balogh Z, Voros E, Suveges G, et al. Stent graft treatment of an external iliac artery injury associated with pelvic fracture. A case report. J Bone Joint Surg Am 2003;85:919–922.

64. Gibson GR. Impotence following fractured pelvis and ruptured urethra. Br J Urol 1970;42:86–88.

65. King J. Impotence following fractures of the pelvis. J Bone Joint Surg 1975;57:1107–1109.

66. Ellison M, Timberlake GA, Kerstein MD. Impotence following pelvic fracture. J Trauma 1988;28:695–696.

67. Sharlip ID. Penile arteriography in impotence after pelvic trauma. J Urol 1981;126:477–481.

68. Mengert WF, Burchell RC, Blumstein RW, et al. Pregnancy after bilateral ligation of the internal iliac and ovarian arteries. Obstet Gynecol 1969;34:664–666.

69. Mitty HA, Sterling KM, Alvarez M, et al. Obstetric hemorrhage: prophylactic and emergency arterial catheterization and embolotherapy. Radiology 1993;18:183–187.

70. Yamashita Y, Harada M, Yamamoto H, et al. Transcatheter arterial embolization of obstetric bleeding: efficacy and clinical outcome. Br J Radiol 1994;67:530–534.

71. Malden ES, Picus D. Hemorrhagic complication of transgluteal pelvic abscess drainage: successful percutaneous treatment. J Vasc Interv Radiol 1992;3:323–328.

72. Saueracker AJ, McCroskey BL, Moore EE, et al. Intraoperative hypogastric artery embolization for life-threatening pelvic hemorrhage: a preliminary report. J Trauma 1987;27:1127–1129.

Transcatheter Arterial Embolization in the Management of Splenic Trauma

59

Brian F. Stainken

The spleen, a small organ unaffected by most disease states, has been known for centuries to be uniquely vulnerable to blunt trauma. As with aortic rupture, injury to the spleen may also be clinically silent until the onset of massive hemorrhage. In both cases, waiting for the insult to manifest clinically may be waiting too long.

Splenectomy was first described as a solution for massive bleeding from splenic injury at the turn of the century (1). At the time, the procedure carried a 30% mortality rate, but it was far preferable to observation alone, which carried a threefold higher risk of death (2,3). Modern anesthesia techniques have reduced the risk of laparotomy and splenectomy dramatically, coincident with an increasing appreciation of the morbidity of large volume transfusion. The laparotomy became a diagnostic tool, and transfusion became something to be avoided. Aggressive efforts to identify the at-risk population through diagnostic peritoneal lavage and early splenectomy before the patient was exposed to potential transfusion complications became the standard. The spleen joined the gallbladder and appendix on the list of "unnecessary" organs to be removed whenever any doubt existed.

Greater understanding of the immunologic role of the spleen developed in parallel with physicians' skill with splenectomy. As early as 1919 (4), animal splenectomy models demonstrated the unique role the organ plays in clearing encapsulated (opsonized) bacteria from the bloodstream. While the overall risk of bacteremia from encapsulated organisms such as pneumococcus is relatively low (1–3%), the mortality rate of 50–80%, especially in the pediatric population is prohibitive and only partially protected by vaccination (5–7).

Increasing appreciation of the late risks associated with splenectomy has shifted surgical practice toward splenic preservation. Observation, surgical splenorrhaphy, and other approaches to salvage have grown in popularity. Largely, the focus has been on identifying a population that can be observed safely. A grading scale published in 1994 remains the standard by which injury is described and treatment approaches are defined (8) (Table 59–1).

In 1979, a technique for achieving splenic hemostasis through surgical ligation of the proximal splenic artery was described (9). The concept was translated into a percutaneous approach by Scalfani in 1981 (10). Today, proximal coil embolization of the splenic artery is a widely accepted lifesaving and laparotomy-saving solution.

TABLE 59-1

SPLENIC INJURY CLASSIFICATION

Splenic Hematoma Grade	Size	Capsule Intact	Active Bleeding	Expanding
I	Subcapsular <10% surface area	Y	N	N
II	Subcapcular 10–50% surface area; parenchymal <5 cm diameter	Y	N	N
III	Subcapsular >50% surface area or ruptured subcapsular;	Y/N	Y	Y
	parenchymal >5 cm diameter	Y	N	
IV	Parenchymal ruptured	N	Y	

Splenic Laceration Grade	Depth	Active Bleeding	Vessel Involved
I	<1 cm depth	N	N
II	1–3 cm depth (cannot involve a trabecular vessel)	Y	N
III	>3 cm depth or involving trabecular vessel	Y	Trabecular
IV	Major devascularization (>25% parenchyma)	Y	Segmental or Hilar
V	Shattered spleen Complete devascularization	Y	Hilar

Adapted with permission from the Organ Injury Scaling (OIS) Committee of the American Association for the Surgery of Trauma (AAST).
Moore EE, Cogbill TH, Jurkovich GJ, et al: Organ injury scaling: spleen and liver. J Trauma 1995;38:323.

THE SPLEEN

The spleen is a peritonealized sac of fluid suspended in the left upper quadrant by ligaments connected to the stomach, left kidney, colon, and diaphragm. Weighing 75–300 grams, it contains approximately 1 unit of blood and processes 200 cc per minute through a single end artery that courses through the gastrosplenic ligament along the superior and anterior aspect of the pancreatic body and tail.

The splenic artery divides before the hilum into a superior and inferior polar branch and subsequently divides into a series of horizontally oriented lobular parenchymal branches anastomosed across a sinusoidal space to a paired system of draining splenic portal vessels.

A rich network of collaterals may supply the spleen. The dorsal pancreatic artery (arising from any of the major mesenteric branches) may reconstitute the transverse pancreatic artery to the pancreatica magna that arises from the midsplenic artery. The pancreatica magna reconstitutes the caudal pancreatic artery that usually connects via the left gastroepiploic to the inferior polar branch of the distal splenic artery. In addition, the superior polar branch of the splenic artery contributes short gastric branches to the stomach funds that may collateralize to other celiac branches perfusing the region.

Ninety percent of the blood entering the splenic parenchyma perfuses the red pulp, an interstitial space communicating to the venous sinusoids through 0.5–2.5 μ pores. The relative stasis within the red pulp facilitates phagocytosis, immunoglobulin contact, and detection/ up-regulation of systemic immunoglobulin production. The red pulp is a unique low-flow environment that facilitates contact and clearance of opsinized (encapsulated) bacterial species. It accounts for 25% of the reticuloendothelial tissue in adults.

OPTIMIZING THERAPY

The decision-making process driving triage of patients for observation, embolization, or operation is not always clearcut. Clinical, laboratory, and radiographic criteria remain controversial and compromised by the lack of a predictive grading scheme that effectively integrates physiologic, imaging, and demographic criteria—not to mention institutional experience and resources. Some relative risk factors however are clear.

Age

The pediatric spleen, with a thicker capsule and greater elasticity than the adult spleen, is far more tolerant of blunt trauma and more amenable to conservative management in the setting of solitary organ injury regardless of the severity of the injury to the organ itself. Success rates for conservative therapy range from 87–98% (11–13). The adult spleen, however, though smaller, is progressively less elastic and more vulnerable to significant injury, especially after 50 years of age. In adults, reported success rates for patients who are managed conservatively vary widely (27–100%), depending on patient populations, selection criteria, and management approaches (14,16–19).

With increasing age, there is greater transfusion risk and compromised physiologic response to shock that compound the risk of splenic injury. The significance of age as a negative prognostic indicator for any form of trauma is reflected by its use as a final multiplier in the Trauma Injury and Severity Score (TRISS), a commonly used tool to assess survival probability. (15).

Injury Severity

It is reasonable to assume that one might be able to correlate a quantitative measure of parenchymal injury with outcomes, but an adequately predictive scoring system does not yet exist.

The most widely referenced standard was developed in 1987 by the Organ Injury Scaling (OIS) Committee of the American Association for the Surgery of Trauma (AAST) and last updated in 1994 (8) (Table 59–1). This system is useful as a common language to describe hematoma and laceration severity. The scale was developed to reflect surgical and autopsy data, and extrapolated to the computed tomography (CT) although the correlative accuracy of CT scoring is debated (20–23,27).

Further, a debate over the appropriate threshold values and predictive utility of this scale as a guide to triage remains active. In 1992 and 1996, Smith reported a splenic salvage rate of 58% with only 7% failing observation when surgery was reserved for injuries above grade 3 in patients under 55 years age (24,25). Failure rates for observant management described by others in the surgical literature range from 10–31% (14,26,28–29). Although it is generally accepted that there is an increasing probability of splenic hemorrhage associated with higher-grade injury, the scale alone is not sufficiently predictive of late splenic rupture to forego close in-hospital observation of all patients with diagnosed splenic injury.

Vascular Imaging

Given that the primary failure mode of observation is delayed rupture of the spleen, Scalfani et al. (30) theorized that direct visualization of an arterial injury as manifest by extracapsular or parenchymal contrast extravasation, vessel occlusion, arteriovenous fistula, or pseudoaneurysm might predict persistent pressurization of the splenic pulp and late rupture. Implicit affirmation of the concept rests in the dramatic decrease in late rupture seen in those patients treated with embolization.

Scalfani and colleagues suggested that, while CT was sensitive for detection of splenic injury, it was not sufficiently specific for splenic arterial injury. Arterial extravasation was rarely identified by single-slice CT. In the intervening 15 years, computed tomography-based vascular imaging tools have matured considerably, which begs a new question: Can data from multislice spiral CT with state-of-the art injectors be used alone to safely triage blunt splenic trauma? In 1998, Davis noted the appearance of splenic pseudoaneurysms on follow-up CT in 10% of his conservatively treated patients and determined that the finding predicted late rupture and reoperation in 67%

(31). Gavant et al. (32) similarly noted that contrast extravasation or vascular abnormality of the spleen was seen in 82% (9 of 11) of patients failing observation. Shanmuganathan et al. (33) compared findings of vascular injury on CT with angiography findings of vascular lesions in 16% of grade 1 and 2 injuries and 42% of grade 3–5 splenic injury. When compared to angiography, CT was 100% sensitive for contrast extravasation but was much less sensitive for pseudoaneurysm and arteriovenous (AV) fistula. Half of the CT findings were not identified by angiography. One patient with a negative angio and positive CT scan required late splenectomy, which suggests that the CT findings were more predictive of outcome. In two patients, angiography revealed findings of pseudoaneurysm and AV fistula that were believed to be truly discordant with CT. Importantly, both lesions were seen in grade 1 and 2 spleens (33).

It is not clear, however, that evidence for an arterial blush on CT should be an independent indicator for intervention. Omert et al. (34) reviewed 324 patients and found that the presence of a contrast blush that correlated with injury grade increased the likelihood of needed intervention ninefold, but it was not an independent predictor of outcome. Age, blood pressure, and splenic grade were more predictive (34). In his retrospective analysis of 133 pediatric splenic injuries, Lutz et al. (35) observed contrast extravasation in six, all with higher-grade (above 3) injury. Five were observed without incident. One child, with polytrauma, underwent laparotomy and splenectomy (35).

TECHNIQUE

The practical utility of splenic embolization in a single institution largely depends on the preparation of the intervention team. The greatest impact on care is realized when intervention is performed expeditiously in coordination with the trauma team's resuscitation efforts, thereby minimizing transfusion requirements.

Before the procedure, the CT should be reviewed closely. Discordant angiographic findings merit careful review and possible additional selective runs (33). The use of an oversized femoral sheath allows for arterial pressure monitoring through the side arm as well as additional large-bore access for resuscitation.

Celiac angiography should be performed using standard techniques, and the catheter should be advanced into the proximal splenic artery for anteroposterior (AP) and oblique views. Generally, a simple curved forward-seeking system is sufficient, with a hydrophilic guide wire/catheter or microcatheter reserved for difficult cases.

Proximal coil embolization (Figure 59–1) as a means of stabilizing splenic hemorrhage was described, refined, and popularized by Salvatore J. A. Scalfani during the early 1990s (30). The objective is to rapidly achieve a transient reduction in parenchymal perfusion to facilitate hemostasis. A high priority should be put on placing the coil embolus sufficiently proximal within the splenic artery to allow for collateral perfusion via the dorsal pancreatic-pancreatica magna arcade. Distal coil position in the region of the splenic hilum raises the risk of significant parenchymal infarction (36). Usually, the catheter will seat in a stable position 3–5 cm from the dorsal pancreatic origin.

To avoid coil reflux into the celiac trunk or distal embolization, one must choose the initial coils carefully. Generally, the first coil should be oversized, in the range of 8 mm, to allow for a stable embolus. Short coil lengths initially help position the embolus precisely and reduce the

risk of disengaging the delivery catheter. Smaller coils may be used subsequently to achieve a tight nest. On occasion, a single gelfoam pledget may be placed into the embolus to facilitate stasis. Dramatic improvement in hemodynamic parameters, commonly before the coil embolus is fully occlusive, is often the first indication of procedural success.

The completion angiogram is performed to demonstrate the collateral reconstitution of the distal splenic artery, and persisting evidence for parenchymal contrast blush is not unusual. It is unclear whether this predicts late failure (37).

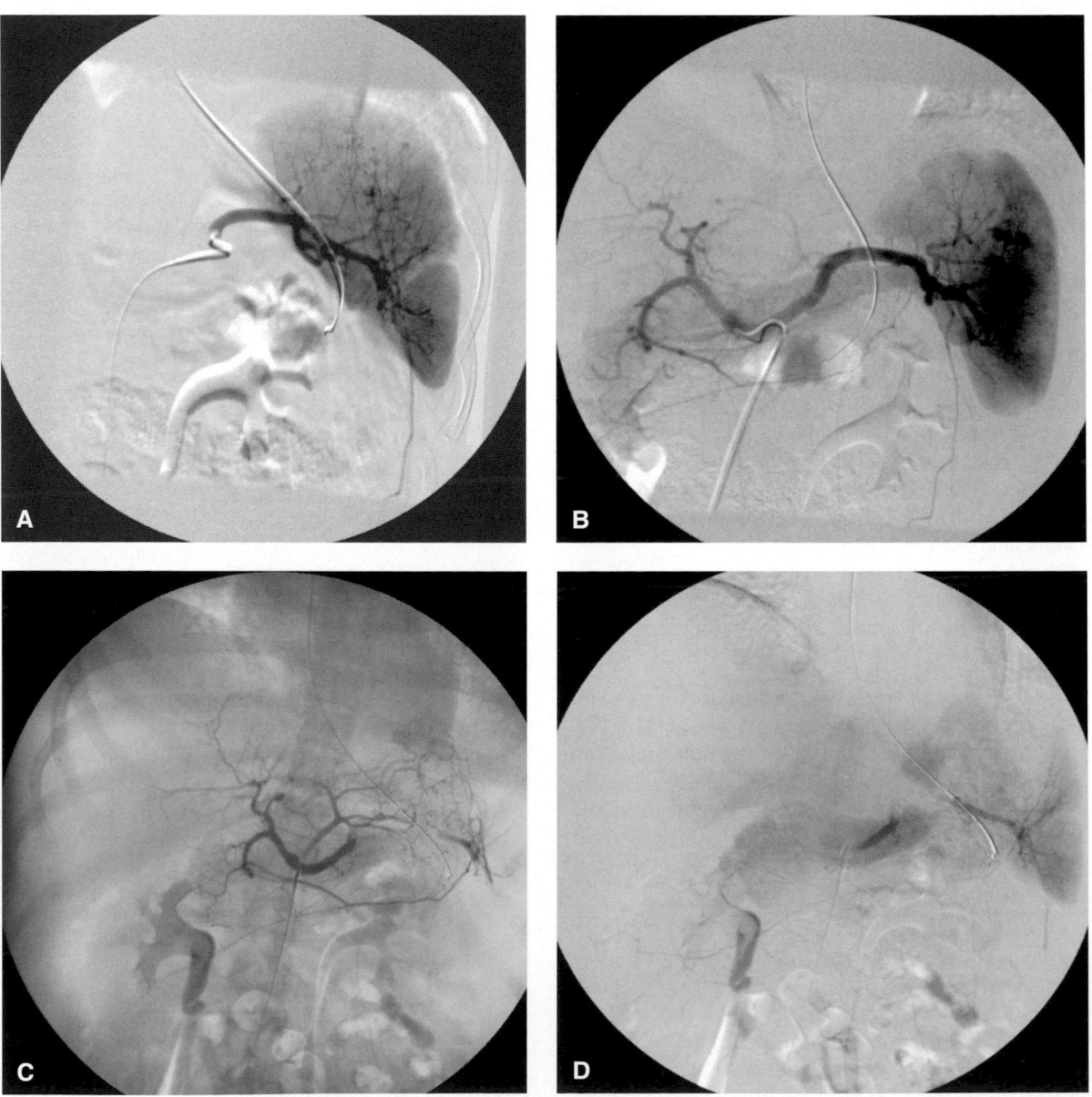

Figure 59–1   Proximal coil embolization. **A.** Arterial-phase splenic angiogram shows punctuate areas of extravascular contrast. **B.** Portal phase reveals persistent extravasation from the arterial injury. **C.** After embolization, left gastric and gastroepiploic collaterals reconstitute the splenic artery. **D.** Late arterial phase image shows preserved parenchymal flow without evidence for persistent arterial extravasation.

In most patients, proximal coil embolization is readily accomplished and dramatically effective. There are two situations in which a more selective approach, generally the use of a hydrophilic catheter or microcatheter, is warranted (Figure 59–2).

Massive extracapsular extravasation or extravasation from a major (interpolar) branch may present with dramatic bleeding. If the clinical infrastructure exists to resuscitate and rapidly access and monitor such a critically ill patient, superselective embolization may allow for even more rapid recovery.

AV fistula may only be detected at angiography. Careful inspection for paired opacified arterial and venous lumens and rapid-sequence imaging with sufficient contrast are necessary to demonstrate the lesion that should be addressed with superselective embolization to both sides of the fistulous communication.

While gelfoam scatter embolization is popular in pelvic trauma and has enjoyed transient use as a method of treatment for hypersplenism, the use of gelfoam slurry in the setting of blunt splenic trauma carries unnecessarily high risks of infection, infarction, and postoperative pain.

After embolization, patients will require intensive care unit monitoring. The sheath can be removed if coagulation parameters allow, although in many, the sheaths provide a useful tool for hemodynamic monitoring and elective removal, once the patient is warmed, and stabilized. Hemostatic devices may represent another useful option because many patients will transition from the angio suite to the OR for debridement, wound care, or orthopedic procedures.

All patients with blunt splenic trauma (Figure 59–3), regardless of intervention, require close observation for 5–7 days for evidence of late rupture. The use of CT scanning in the postoperative period may reveal findings such as enlarging hematoma or persistent arterial blush that may predict late failure and warrant a return to the angio suite to reassess the adequacy of embolization.

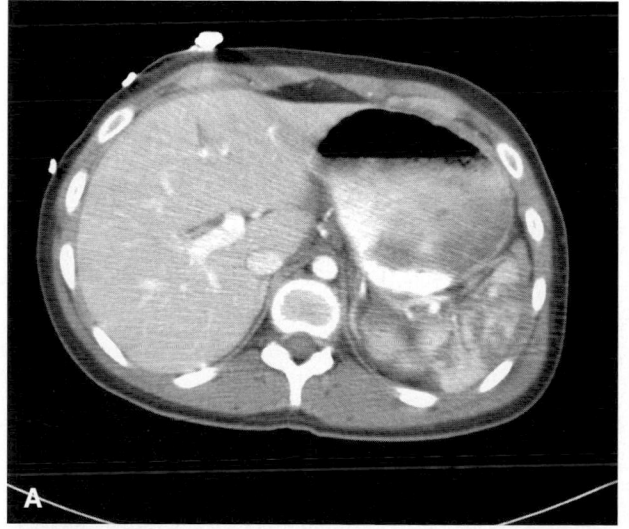

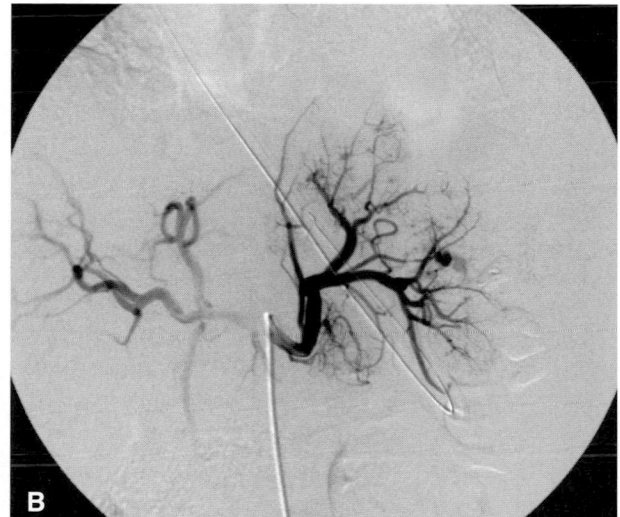

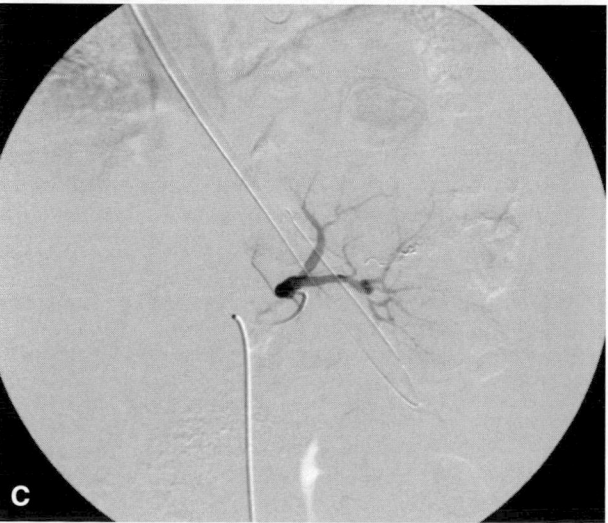

Figure 59–2 Selective splenic artery embolization. **A.** CT scan reveals grade 4/5 splenic injury with focal area of persistent contrast extravasation consistent with a pseudoaneurysm. **B.** Early image from selective splenic angiogram shows large pseudoaneurysm arising from lower pole interpolar artery. Note the superior polar artery arising from the proximal splenic artery (normal variant). **C.** Target branch occluded after selective embolization performed with a 4 French hydrophilic catheter and 3 mm fibered coils.

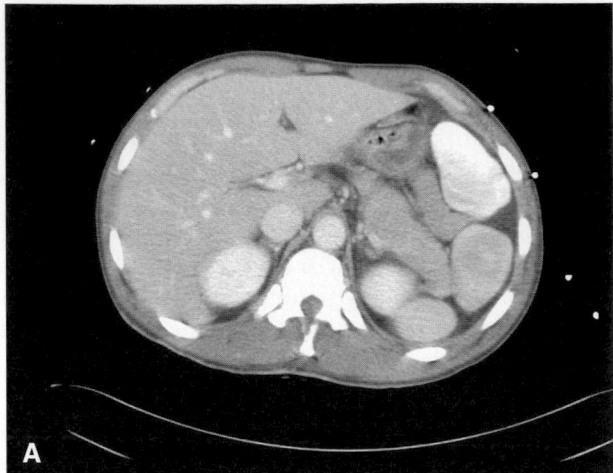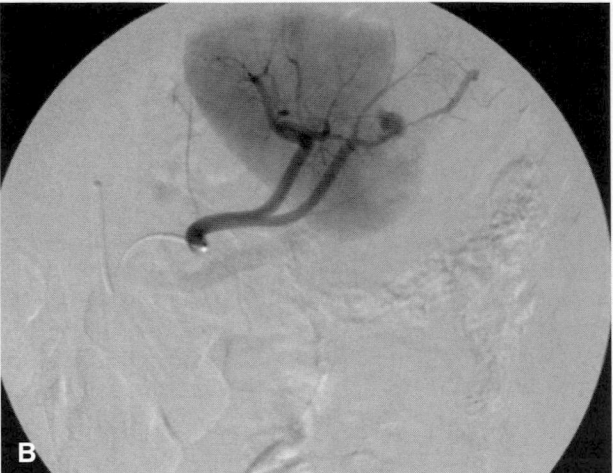

Figure 59–3 Splenic hematoma. **A.** CT image reveals low attenuation parenchymal hematoma with focal area of attenuation suggesting arterial extravasation. **B.** Angiogram shows proximal bifurcation of polar arteries with lower pole pseudoaneurysm.

RESULTS

The success of splenic arterial embolization is defined by the splenic salvage rate. Secondary endpoints might also include transfusion burden compared with an observed population. Ideally, the results of embolization should be sufficiently reliable to avoid a prolonged period of intensive observation for late rupture. The Society of Interventional Radiology quality improvement guidelines report a success rate between 87–100% (38). Cogbill et al. (39) described a 5% incidence of delayed hemorrhage 4 days after injury. Scalfani et al. (30) reported a splenic salvage rate of 97% in a group of 36 patients selected for observation or embolization based on angiography findings of arterial extravasation alone. Shanmuganathan et al. (33) increased his success rate from 93–97% when treatment was based on arterial extravasation seen either on CT screening or angiography.

Increasingly, splenic coil embolization is being used for higher-grade injuries in less stable patients at dedicated trauma centers. A recent large pooled series of 140 patients with splenic trauma reported an overall salvage rate of 87% with a surprisingly high 80% salvage rate in grade 4 and 5 spleens (40). A second prospective series of 15 patients, all of whom were hemodynamically unstable with a transient response to initial fluid resuscitation, produced a 100% salvage rate despite the fact that 13 of 15 had grade 4 or 5 injury (41).

SUMMARY

Proximal coil embolization of the splenic artery, described in the early 1990s, has become established as a mainstay in the modern management of blunt abdominal trauma. When combined with current CT technology in an integrated trauma care environment, it facilitates early stabilization, minimizes transfusion load, reduces the risk of observation, and maximizes splenic preservation.

REFERENCES

1. Reigner O. Ueber einen fall von exstirpation der traumatisach zerrissen milz. Berl Kiln Wochenschr 1893;30:177.
2. Foster JN, Prey D. Rupture of the spleen: an analysis of twenty cases. Am J Surg 1940;47:487.
3. Land-Sudden J. Observation on the surgery of the spleen. Br J Surg 1912;1:157.
4. Morris DH, Bullock FD. The importance of the spleen in resistance to infection. Ann Surg 1919;70:153.
5. Malangoni MA, Dillon LD, Klamer TW, et al. Factors influencing the risk of early and late serious infection in adults after splenectomy for trauma. Surgery 1984;96:775.
6. Green JB, Shackford SR, Sise MJ, et al. A prospective analysis of late septic complications in adult patients following splenectomy for trauma. J Trauma 1986;26:1999.
7. Gopal V, Bisno AL. Fulminant pneumococcal infections in "normal" asplenic hosts. Arch Intern Med 1977;137:1526.
8. Moore EE, Cogbill TH, Jurkovich GJ, et al: Organ injury scaling: spleen and liver. J Trauma 1995;38:323.
9. Keramidas DC. The ligation of the splenic artery in the treatment of traumatic rupture of the spleen. Surgery 1979;85:530–533.
10. Scalfani SJA. The role of angiographic hemostasis in salvage of the injured spleen. Radiology 1981;141:645.
11. Cogbill TH, Moore EE, Jurkovich GJ, et al: Nonoperative management of blunt splenic trauma: a multicenter experience. J Trauma 1989;29:1312.
12. Wesson DE, Filler RM, Ein SH, et al. Ruptured spleen—When to operate? J Pediatr Surg 1981;16:324.
13. Perl RH, Wesson De, Spence LJ, et al. Splenic injury: a five-year update with improved results and changing criteria for conservative management. J Pediatr Surg 1989;24:428.
14. Shackford SR, Molin M. Management of splenic injuries. Surg Clin North Am 1990;70:595.
15. Byd CR. Evaluating trauma care: the TRISS method. J Trauma 1989;29:623–629.
16. Elmore JR, Clark DE, Isler RJ, et al. Selective nonoperative management of blunt splenic trauma in adults. Arch Surg 1989;124:581–585.
17. Godley CD, Warren RL, Sheridan RL, et al. Nonoperative management of blunt splenic injury in adults: age over 55 years as a powerful indicator for failure. J Am Coll Surg 1996;183:133–139.

18. Smith JS Jr, Wengrovitz MA, DeLong BS. Prospective validation of criteria, including age, for safe, nonsurgical management of the ruptured spleen. J Trauma 1992;33:363–368.
19. Smith JS Jr, Cooney RN, Mucha P Jr. Nonoperative management of the ruptured spleen: a revalidation of criteria. Surgery 1996; 120:745–750;discussion 750–751.
20. Sutyak JP, Chiu WC, D'Amelio LF, et al. Computed tomography is inaccurate in estimating the severity of adult splenic injury. J Trauma 1995;39:514–518.
21. Mirvsi SE, Whitley NO, Gens D. Blunt splenic trauma in adults: CT-based injury classification and correlation with prognosis and treatment. Radiology 1989;171:27–32.
22. Malgione MA, Cue JI, Fallat ME, et al. Evaluation of splenic injury by computed tomography and its impact on treatment. Ann Surg 1990;211:592–599.
23. Resciniti A, Fink MP, Raptopoulos V, et al. Nonoperative treatment of adult splenic trauma: development of a computed tomographic scoring system that detects appropriate candidates for expectant management. J Trauma 1988;28:828–831.
24. Smith JS Jr, Wengrovitz MA, DeLong BS. Prospective validation of criteria, including age, for safe, nonsurgical management of the ruptured spleen. J Trauma 1992;33:363–368;discussion 368–369.
25. Smith JS Jr, Cooney RN, Mucha P Jr. Nonoperative management of the ruptured spleen: a revalidation of criteria. Surgery 1996; 120:745–750.
26. Myers JG, Dent DL, Stewart RM, et al. Blunt splenic injuries: dedicated trauma surgeons can achieve a high rate of nonoperative success in patients of all ages. J Trauma 2000;48:801–805.
27. Umlas SL, Cronan JJ. Splenic trauma: can CT grading systems enable prediction of successful nonsurgical treatment? Radiology 1991;178:481–487.
28. Molin MR, Shackford SR. The management of splenic trauma in a trauma system. Arch Surg 1990;125:840–843.
29. Feliciano PD, Mullins RJ, Trunkey DD, et al. A decision analysis of traumatic splenic injuries. J Trauma 1992;33:340–348.
30. Scalfani SJ, Weisberg A, Scalea TM, et al. Blunt splenic injuries: nonsurgical treatment with CT, arteriography, and transcatheter arterial embolization of the splenic artery. Radiology 1991;181: 189–196.
31. Davis KA, Fabian TC, Croce MA, et al. Improved success in nonoperative management of blunt splenic injuries: embolization of splenic artery pseudoaneurysms. J Trauma 1998;44:1008–1013.
32. Gavant ML, Schurr M, Flick P, et al. Predicting clinical outcome of nonsurgical management of blunt splenic injury: using CT to reveal abnormalities in the splenic vasculature. AJR Am J Roentgenol 1997;168:207–212.
33. Shanmuganathan K, Mirvis S, Boyd-Kranis R, et al. Nonsurgical management of blunt splenic injury: use of CT criteria to select patients for splenic arteriography and potential endovascular therapy. Radiology 2000;217:75–82.
34. Omert LA, Salyer D, Dunham CM, et al. Implications of the "contrast blush" finding on computed tomographic scan of the spleen in trauma. J Trauma 2001;51:272–277.
35. Lutz N, Mahboubi S, Nance ML, et al. The significance of contrast blush on computed tomography in children with splenic injuries. J Pediatr Surg 2004;39:491–494.
36. Killeen KL, Shanmuganathan K, Boyd-Kranis R, et al. CT findings after embolization for blunt splenic trauma. J Vasc Interv Radiol 2001;12:209–214.
37. Hagiwara A, Yukioka T, Ohta S, et al. Nonsurgical management of patients with blunt splenic injury: efficacy of transcatheter arterial embolization. AJR Am J Roentgenol 1996;167:159–166.
38. Drooz AT, Curtis AL, Allen TE, et al. Quality improvement guidelines for percutaneous transcatheter embolization. J Vasc Interv Radiol 2004;14:S237–S242.
39. Cogbill TH, Moore EE, Jurkovich GJ, et al. Nonoperative management of blunt splenic trauma: a multicenter experience. J Trauma 1989;29:1312–1317.
40. Haan JM, Biffl W, Knudson M. Splenic embolization revisited: a multicenter review. J Trauma 2004;56:542–547.
41. Hagiwara A, Fukushima H, Murata A, et al. Blunt splenic injury: usefulness of transcatheter arterial embolization in patients with a transient response to fluid resuscitation. Radiology 2005;235: 57–64.

Arteriography and Endovascular Management of Renal Trauma

60

Sue E. Hanks, Michael D. Katz

The radiological evaluation of patients with renal trauma is critical to their subsequent management. Computed tomography (CT) of the kidneys and adjacent structures is the cornerstone of the evaluation and provides essential anatomic and physiologic information needed to classify the severity of the injury according to the organ injury severity scales developed by the American Association for the Surgery of Trauma (AAST) (1). In addition, findings on the CT scan can determine those patients who may benefit from arteriography and therapeutic embolization of traumatic renal arterial injuries or other endovascular treatment methods (2). This chapter discusses the evaluation of renal trauma and the role of interventional radiology for both diagnosis and treatment.

ANATOMY

A thorough knowledge of renal and retroperitoneal anatomy is necessary to accurately stage renal injuries. The kidneys are retroperitoneal structures protected from injury by the lower ribs, Gerota fascia, and surrounding perirenal fat. At the level of the kidneys, the retroperitoneum may be divided into three compartments. The anterior pararenal space is bound anteriorly by parietal peritoneum and posteriorly by Gerota fascia. The perirenal space, surrounded by Gerota fascia, contains the kidney, adrenal gland, and perirenal fat. The posterior pararenal space is bound anteriorly by Gerota fascia and posteriorly by transversalis fascia (3,4).

CLASSIFICATION OF RENAL INJURIES

Renal injuries are classified according to the American Association for the Surgery of Trauma organ injury classification system (1). Class I injuries are minor in nature and include parenchymal contusions and nonexpanding subcapsular hematomas. Class II injuries are cortical lacerations <1.0 cm deep that do not extend into the collecting system. Class III injuries are cortical lacerations >1.0 cm deep without involvement of the collecting system. Class IV injuries are parenchymal lacerations involving the cortex, medulla, and, importantly, the collecting system. Class IV injuries also include vascular injuries to the main renal artery or vein that are contained, such as dissection flaps or small pseudoaneurysms. Class V injuries are completely shattered kidneys or avulsion of the renal hilum with devascularization (Figure 60–1).

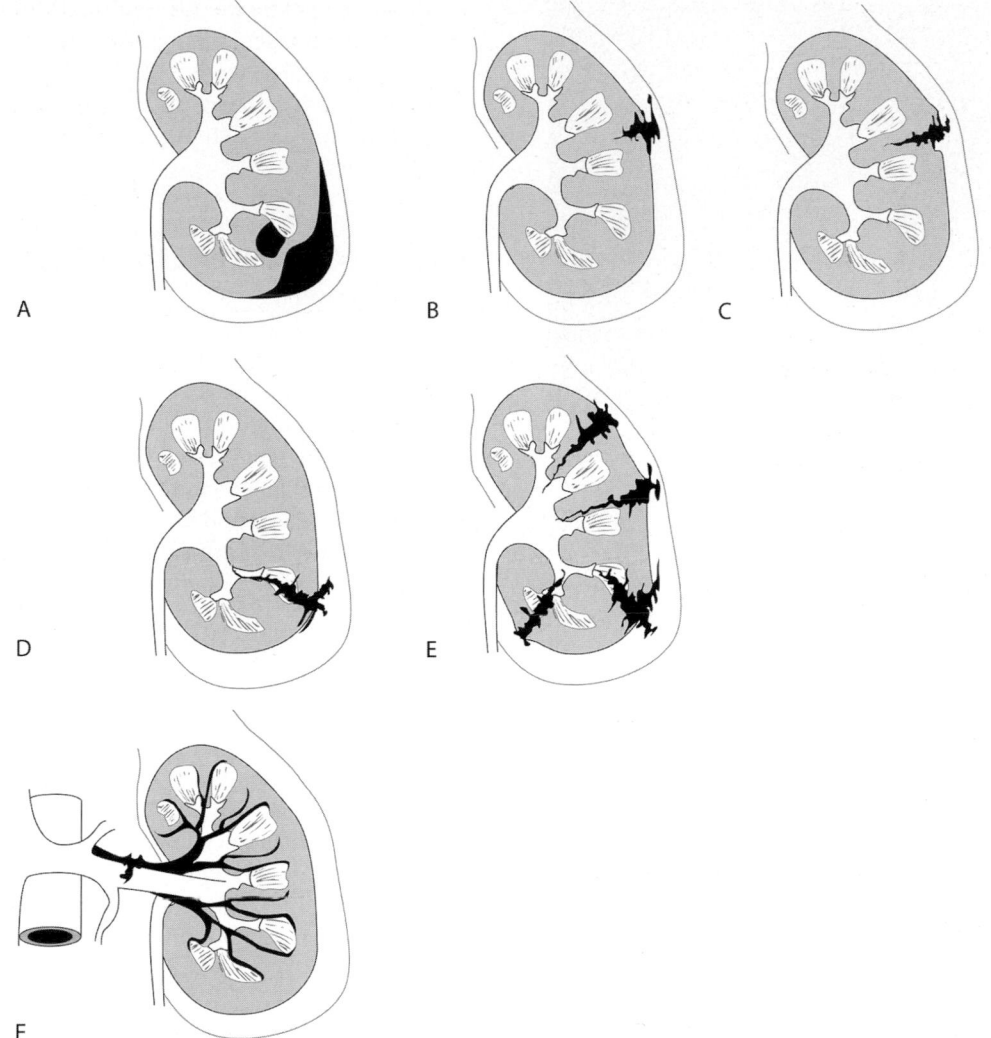

Figure 60–1   A. Class I renal injury. Subcapsular hematoma (*black*) with an underlying contusion (*dark gray*). **B.** Class II renal injury. Superficial cortical laceration less than 1 cm deep. **C.** Class III renal injury. Greater than 1 cm cortical laceration without involvement of the collecting system. **D.** Class IV renal injury. Cortical laceration with involvement of the collecting system **E., F.** Class V renal injury. Completely shattered kidney or vascular pedicle injury.

Renal trauma management is dictated by this classification system. Class I and II injuries are treated conservatively because almost all renal contusions and minor lacerations heal spontaneously. Many major injuries can be successfully managed expectantly as well. The trend is to be as conservative as possible and to closely monitor the patient for hypotension, dropping hematocrit, sepsis, or other signs that require intervention. Class V injuries require emergent surgical intervention. To successfully revascularize a renal pedicle injury, one should perform surgery within, at most, 12 hours (5). Even after successful surgical revascularization, the function of the repaired kidney is often quite poor, and it may not be to the patient's benefit to undergo a salvage operation with the attendant surgical and anesthetic risks (6).

MECHANISM OF RENAL INJURIES

Renal injuries must be categorized as blunt or penetrating in order to be properly evaluated and managed. Blunt renal trauma is much more common than penetrating trauma, except in a few urban trauma centers (7). Blunt injuries rarely require surgical exploration, with most series citing a less than 10% rate of surgical intervention. The mechanism of injury in blunt trauma may be a direct blow, laceration by adjacent ribs, or an acceleration–deceleration injury. Automobile accidents account for most blunt trauma. Because of the kidney's protected position, the force required to cause renal injury must be extreme; therefore, associated injuries are common and are found in approximately 20% of blunt trauma patients (8,9).

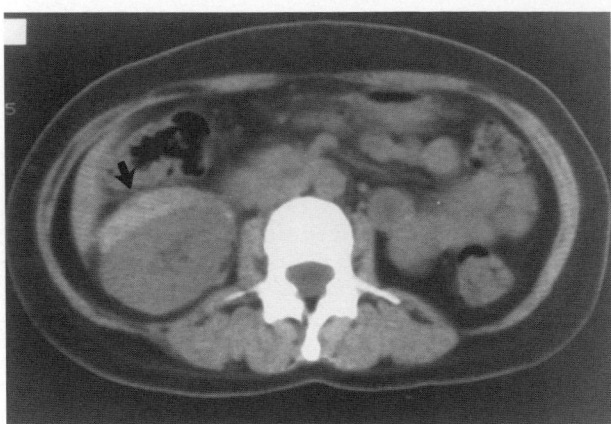

Figure 60–2   CT scan of high-density perirenal hematoma following a renal biopsy.

Penetrating injuries, such as gunshot and stab wounds, are much more likely to require intervention, with as many as 70% causing major injury. Penetrating injuries are frequently associated with injuries to adjacent organs. Some trauma surgeons still recommend surgical exploration for all patients with penetrating injuries, but others have found that a more conservative approach is also safe (8,10–12).

Iatrogenic trauma is a common cause of penetrating renal injury. Percutaneous renal biopsy causes some degree of hemorrhage in as many as 90% of cases (Figure 60–2) (13) and arteriovenous fistulas in as many as 15% of cases (14). The majority of these injuries can be managed conservatively. Serious vascular trauma occurs in 1–2% of percutaneous nephrostomy tube placements (15). Dilatation

of a tract for percutaneous nephrostolithotomy also may cause renal damage, ranging from arteriovenous fistulas to renal rupture (Figure 60–3) (16). The first report of transcatheter management of an arteriovenous fistula, by Bookstein and Goldstein, was in a patient following a renal biopsy (14).

RADIOLOGIC EVALUATION OF RENAL TRAUMA

The indications for radiologic workup in stable patients with blunt renal trauma has been controversial. In the past, all patients with hematuria underwent radiologic studies. Mee and McAninch reviewed this subject and compiled the results of several large series (17–19). Of 1,671 patients who had microhematuria and no history of shock, the researchers found only seven significant renal injuries. Five of these would have required radiologic studies for nonrenal injuries, and one minor laceration was managed conservatively. Thus, only one significant injury in 1,671 patients (0.05%) would have been missed. The authors advocate using either gross hematuria or microhematuria with a history of hypotension (systolic blood pressure <90 mm Hg) at any time after the injury as an indicator for radiologic studies.

The radiologic study of choice is contrast-enhanced CT for stable patients in need of imaging. Parenchymal disruption is better defined with this study compared with intravenous pyelography. The extent of a perirenal hematoma is also clearly demonstrated on CT, and small amounts of extravasation, either arterial or urinary, can be identified (20–22). In addition, the evaluation of the entire retroperitoneum and abdomen in those patients suspected of

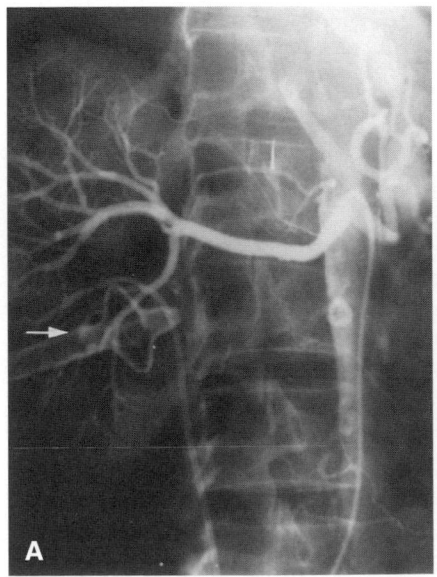
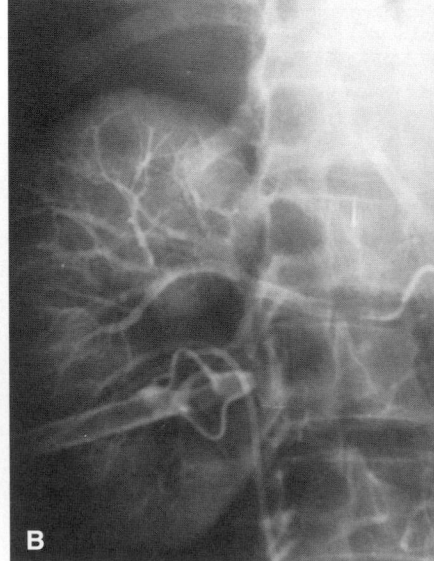
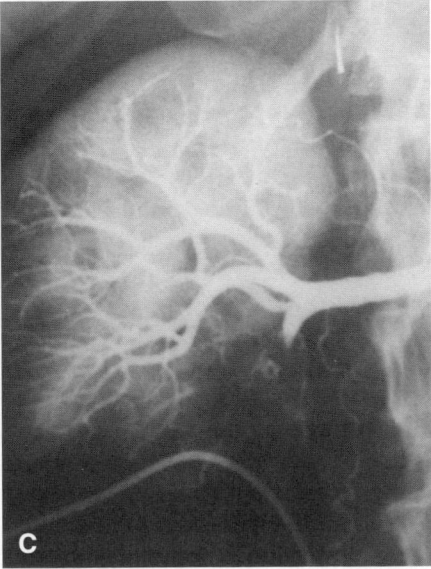

Figure 60–3   Early **A.** and late **B.** selective renal arteriograms demonstrate a pseudoaneurysm of a lower pole branch after placement of a 24 French Malecot catheter. **C.** Successful embolization of the injured lower pole branch with a single steel coil.

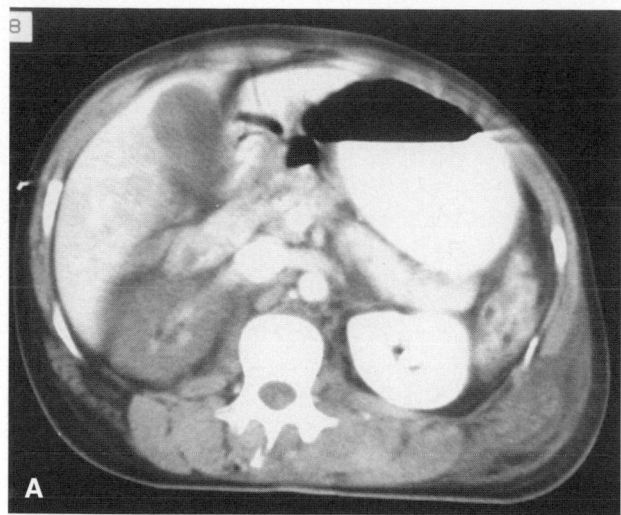 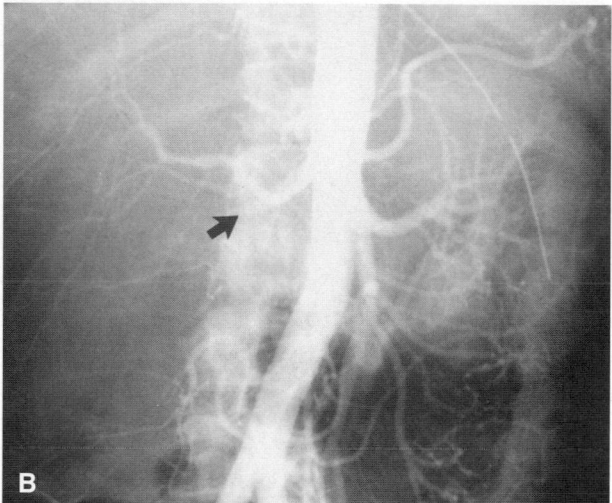

Figure 60–4 **A.** CT scan of a 25-year-old woman pedestrian who was struck by a train. The scan demonstrates nonfunction of the right kidney. **B.** Abdominal aortogram demonstrates occlusion of the main right renal artery (*arrow*).

having associated injuries can be invaluable (23). CT scanning can more accurately identify renal pedicle injuries by demonstrating nonvisualization of a kidney with or without a rim of enhancement from capsular collaterals (24) (Figure 60–4).

Additionally, CT scanning accurately delineates the nature of preexisting renal pathology (25). Preexisting conditions make a kidney more susceptible to blunt injury. Trivial trauma may cause hematuria out of proportion to the degree expected when an anomalous or abnormal kidney is present. Hydronephrosis, cysts, and tumors in normally positioned kidneys may become manifest after only minor trauma. Ectopic or horseshoe kidneys are less protected and, therefore, are more subject to lacerations (20,26). This is particularly true in pediatric patients, in whom as many as 20% with renal injuries have preexisting abnormalities (27,28).

Children are more susceptible to renal trauma, even without preexisting pathology. Almost 90% of renal pedicle injuries occur in children and young adults. In children, the kidney is one of the most frequently injured organs as a result of abdominal trauma (29). As in adults, conservative management is the preferred approach.

Penetrating trauma to the kidney differs considerably from blunt trauma. The number of associated injuries is much higher, especially after gunshot wounds. Surgical exploration is required in as many as 42% of stab wounds and 76% of gunshot wounds (8). If the wound is from the anterior abdomen, almost all patients require exploratory laparotomy to exclude bowel injuries. The trend is similar to blunt trauma in that a more conservative approach is considered appropriate and, when possible, surgical intervention is avoided, even in anterior wounds (10–12). Back and flank wounds do not always require urgent exploration, particularly if intraperitoneal injury has been excluded by peritoneal lavage and there are no peritoneal signs on physical

examination. CT should be used for evaluating stable patients because of the frequency of associated injuries.

In polytraumatized patients, from either blunt or penetrating trauma, emergent surgical exploration for abdominal injuries is often the required management. Radiological workup of renal trauma may then be limited to an abbreviated "one-shot" intravenous pyelogram (IVP) done in the operating room. The information gained from this procedure is enough to establish the position, perfusion, and functional status of the kidneys. The overriding concern for these patients is frequently the associated injuries, not the renal injury itself (30). Cass and Luxenberg correlated the severity of renal trauma with the number of associated injuries. They found that patients with more severe renal trauma often had more than two associated injuries, often requiring surgical interventions (31).

DIAGNOSTIC RENAL ARTERIOGRAPHY

The most frequent indications for renal arteriography are persistent or recurrent hematuria. Active extravasation identified on CT is an indication for emergent arteriography. A large retroperitoneal hematoma found during surgical exploration or seen on CT may also require arteriography. Occasionally, a preoperative arteriogram may be needed to define the arterial anatomy before a segmental renal resection. Evaluation of hypertension that has developed after renal trauma may include arteriography, although this is rare.

The initial arteriographic evaluation should begin with aortography for several reasons. Multiple renal arteries are common, occurring in approximately 30% of patients (32). Because associated injuries are also common, the additional information regarding adjacent structures may prove to be

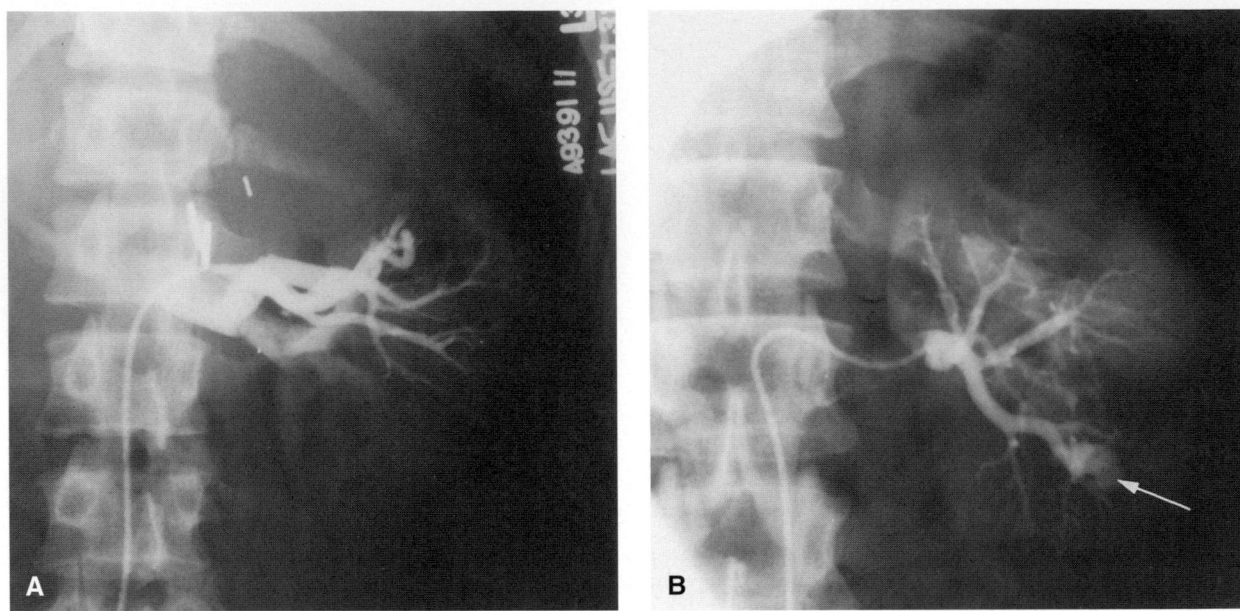

Figure 60–5   **A.** Arteriovenous fistula of an upper pole branch secondary to a stab wound in a patient with multiple renal arteries. **B.** Pseudoaneurysm of lower pole branch (*arrow*).

significant (33). For example, a retroperitoneal hematoma may be caused by a lumbar artery laceration. In addition, injury to the renal vascular pedicle can be identified on the aortogram, and selective catheterization of the injured vessel can then be avoided. Once the renal pedicle has been evaluated, variants in anatomy have been identified, and other major arterial injuries have been excluded, a selective renal arteriogram should be performed. An alternative approach is recommended by Sclafani and Stein, who advocate beginning the examination with a selective renal injection. Minimizing contrast in the collecting system helps one identify arteriocaliceal communication. With the advent of digital subtraction technology, beginning with a selective renal injection may not be as critical (34).

Selective renal arteriography is performed with a pre-shaped, curved catheter such as a Simmons I or Cobra catheter. Two or more projections are usually necessary to adequately evaluate the entire kidney. An ipsilateral anterior oblique projection shows the renal parenchyma to best advantage. Rapid filming sequences are necessary to identify arteriovenous fistulas or the vessel of origin of pseudoaneurysms, whereas delayed images are necessary to reveal subtle extravasation.

Findings that may be demonstrated on arteriography include intrarenal hematomas, which can be identified by displacement or splaying of vessels. Subcapsular hematomas may be demonstrated as concave or flattened areas of parenchyma best seen in the nephrogram phase. Perirenal hematomas may be large enough to cause significant displacement of the kidney. In blunt injury, in particular, there may be single- or multiple-branch artery occlusions. Follow-up

of these occlusions has shown them to be of little clinical consequence without development of complications such as hypertension (35).

Additional arteriographic findings include extravasation, arteriovenous fistulas, and pseudoaneurysms (Figure 60–5). Arterial extravasation may be difficult to distinguish from urinary extravasation, and careful examination of all phases of the arteriogram is necessary. Digital subtraction arteriography is helpful. Arteriovenous fistulas are identified by the presence of an early-draining vein. Pseudoaneurysms are demonstrated as focal areas of extravascular contrast that may show delayed washout. Identification of these renal injuries is particularly important because they may be appropriate for embolization. When the source of hemorrhage is a previously placed nephrostomy tube, it may require special maneuvers, such as repeat arteriography following removal of the catheter and exchange for a wire, to identify the injured branch (Figure 60–6).

TRANSCATHETER RENAL THERAPIES

Important factors to consider before embolizing any vessel include whether the vessel can be sacrificed and the alternative methods of treatment. The kidney is an end-artery organ with small collateral vessels from capsular branches. Occlusion of renal branch vessels will cause parenchymal infarction congruent to the size of the vessel. Accordingly, the embolization should be as selective as possible. Improvements in catheter technology and the availability of microcatheters now make it possible to cannulate 1- to 2-mm

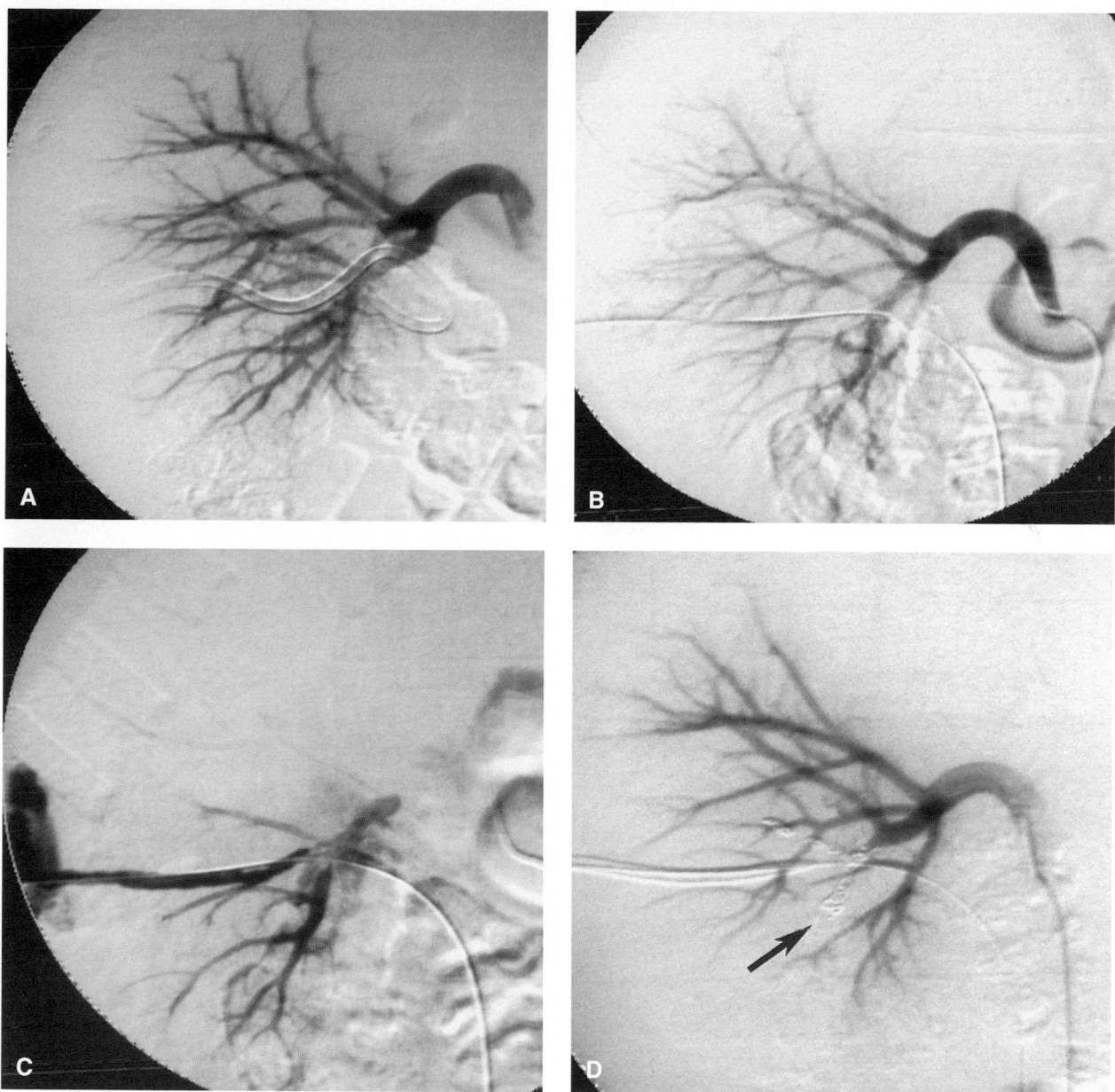

Figure 60–6 Forty-two-year-old man with persistent hematuria following nephrostomy tube placement for ureteral stones. **A.** Selective arteriography fails to identify the injured branch. **B.** Selective arteriography following removal of the nephrostomy tube, leaving only a 0.035-inch wire in place, again fails to identify the injury despite active bleeding from the tract. **C.** Injection of contrast directly into the skin tract fills several arterial branches. This image was compared with the selective arteriograms to identify the injured branch. This branch was then selectively catheterized transarterially with a microcatheter and embolized with microcoils. **D.** After successful coil embolization of the injured vessel. There is preservation of the majority of the parenchyma.

vessels. Although it may not be necessary in every case, the use of a coaxial microcatheter can facilitate cannulation of more distal or tortuous vessels, preserving the maximum amount of renal parenchyma (Figure 60–7). The alternative surgical treatment would result in at least equal and usually greater tissue loss (36,37). In addition, surgical treatment is much more invasive and has the associated

risks and morbidity of a major surgical procedure under general anesthesia.

Historically, many agents have been used to occlude abnormal vessels, including autologous clot (14), cotton pellets (33), detachable balloons (38), cyanoacrylate (39), and polyvinyl alcohol (40). Gelatin sponge (Gelfoam, Upjohn Co.) and coils are the most commonly used agents

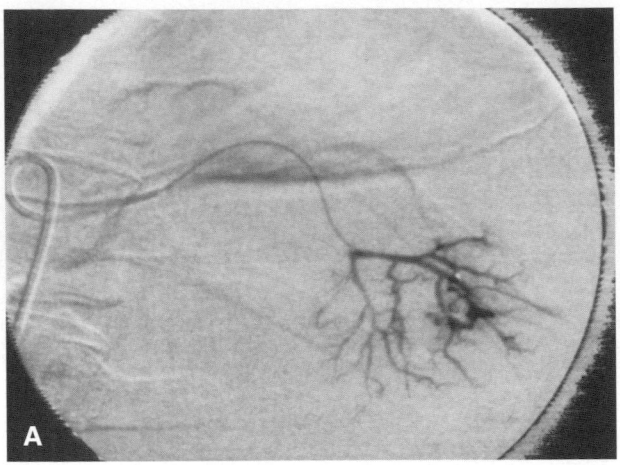 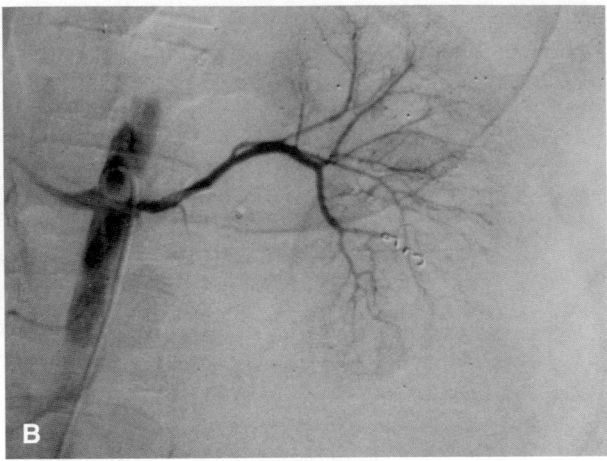

Figure 60–7   A. Digital arteriogram through a coaxial catheter demonstrates a pseudoaneurysm and extravasation from a distal renal artery branch following a biopsy. **B.** Postembolization arteriogram demonstrates occlusion of the injured branch by two microcoils placed distally.

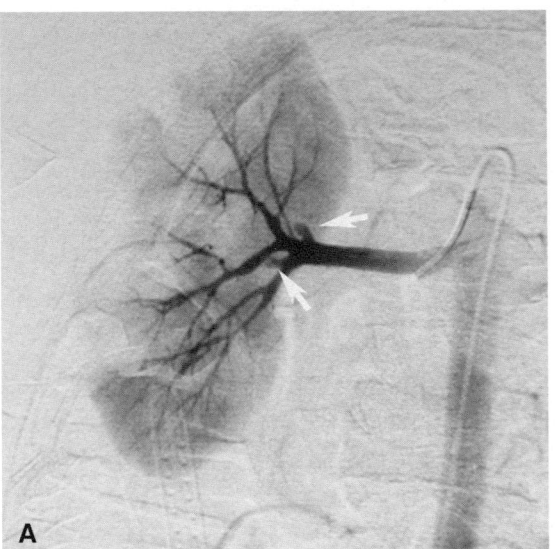 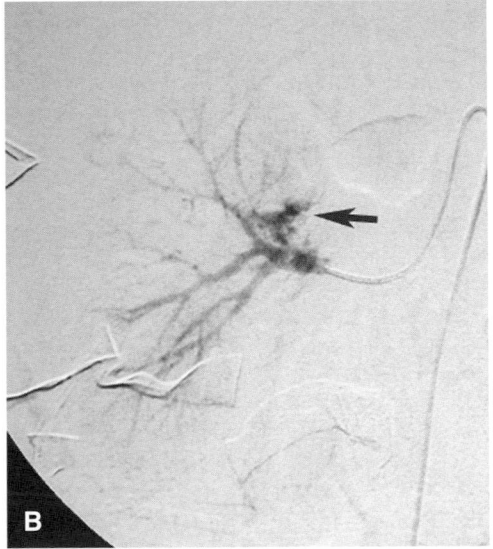

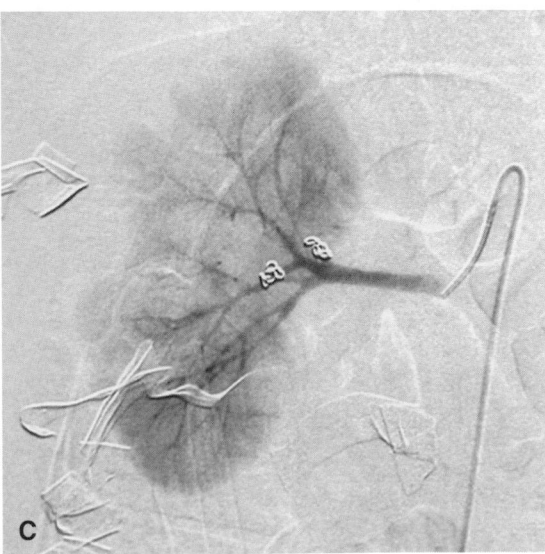

Figure 60–8   A. Sixteen-year-old boy after motor vehicle accident, with two proximal renal arterial branch occlusions (*arrows*). **B.** Selective arteriogram demonstrates active extravasation from one of the injured vessels. **C.** Successful occlusion of both injured branches with 0.035-inch coils.

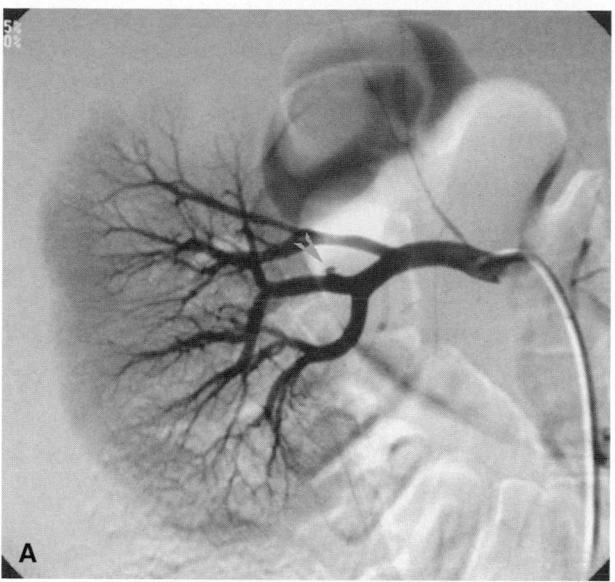 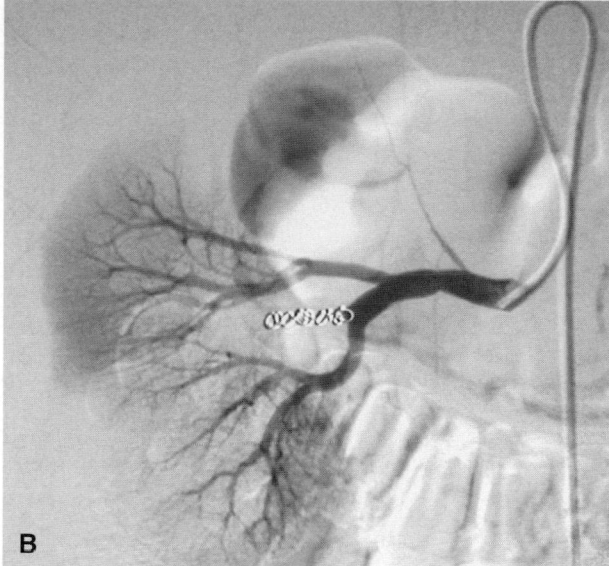

Figure 60–9   Twenty-year-old woman struck by a car. **A.** Selective renal arteriogram demonstrates a pseudoaneurysm of a renal artery branch (*arrow*). **B.** Successful embolization of this single injured branch artery.

(36,37,41–45). Gelfoam can be cut into pledgets that closely match the diameter of the vessel to be occluded and can be delivered through either diagnostic or coaxial catheter systems. Platinum microcoils may be used for distal small-vessel injuries; 0.035-inch coils deployed through diagnostic catheters work well in occluding more proximal arteriovenous fistulas and pseudoaneurysms (Figures 60–8 and 60–9). Particular care should be taken when choosing a coil to occlude an arteriovenous fistula. The coil size should match the vessel size as closely as possible or be slightly larger. If the coil chosen is too small, it could pass through the fistula and possibly embolize to the lungs. The position of the catheter should be as close to the injury as possible when deploying either coils or Gelfoam to minimize parenchymal infarction.

Transcatheter treatment of renal artery branch injuries has a high success rate. Studies report both radiologic and clinical success rates of 84–100% (36,41,42). The complication rate of transcatheter embolization is low. Nontarget embolization causes the greatest concern. The majority of studies report no incidents of coil misplacement (37,38, 41,45). There are few reports of nontarget embolization; however, there is one report of a case of embolization of the main renal artery that caused uncontrollable hypertension and that required nephrectomy (46). Should misplaced coils occur, they can be retrieved with snares designed for either microcoils or 0.035-inch coils (47,48). A complication unique to renal embolization is the rare occurrence of transient hypertension, which can be easily controlled with medication (35). Most studies do not report any cases of hypertension after embolization (35,36,38,45).

Approximately 10% of patients may develop postembolization syndrome, experiencing transient pain, leukocytosis, and low-grade fever. This condition is self-limited and resolves without treatment. Small infarcts are usually asymptomatic (49).

ADRENAL TRAUMA

The adrenal glands lie with the Gerota fascia adjacent to the kidneys. The adrenal glands are uncommonly injured, although the frequency increases with higher injury severity scores. Adrenal hematomas were identified in 1.9% of 2,692 patients who underwent a CT scan for trauma in one study. Patients with adrenal hematomas had a higher mortality rate than those in a control group without adrenal injuries (50–52). The literature contains little regarding the treatment of adrenal hemorrhage for trauma. Most reports involve anticoagulation and spontaneous hemorrhage. Traumatic adrenal hemorrhage can be diagnosed at the time of renal arteriography. Transcatheter embolization can be used as a treatment option for patients with active adrenal hemorrhage (Figure 60–10).

RENAL STENTS

As technology evolves, endovascular management of arterial trauma also includes use of vascular stents, covered and uncovered. Multiple case reports are available regarding the use of stents to repair traumatic dissections, arteriovenous

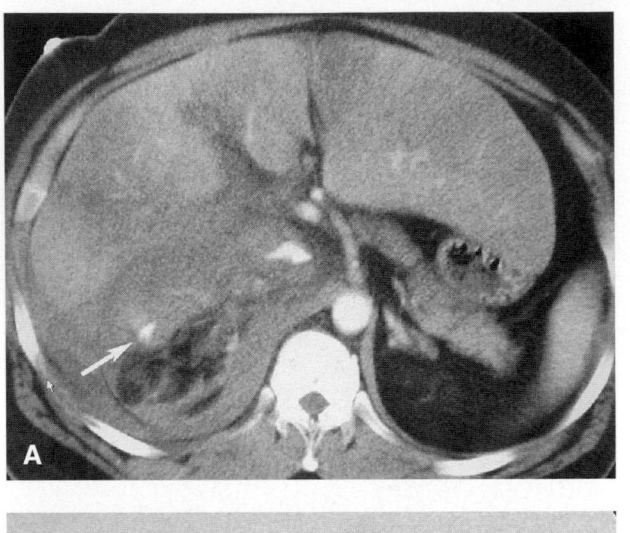

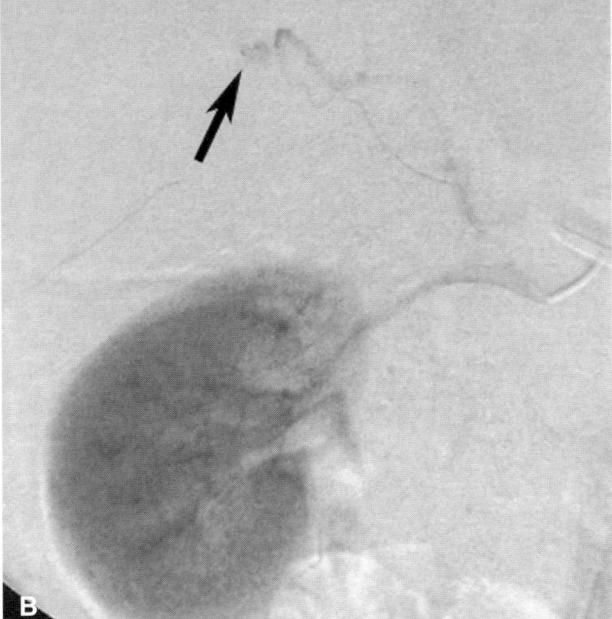

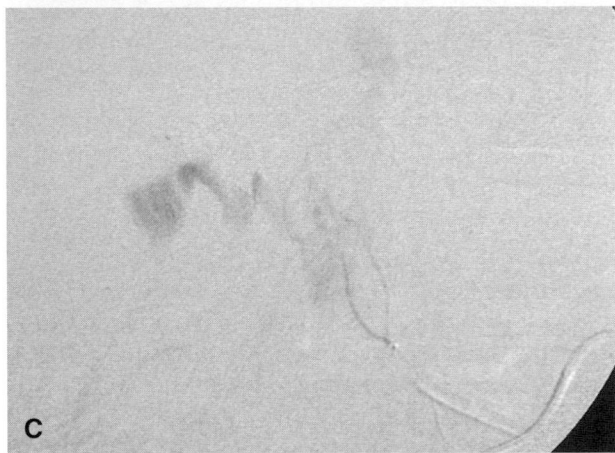

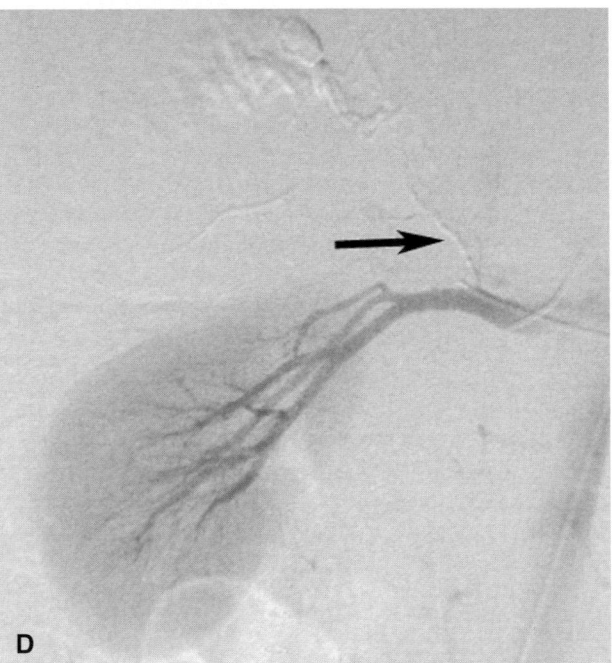

Figure 60–10   Thirty-one-year-old man following a two-story fall. **A.** CT scan demonstrates active extravasation of contrast into a large retroperitoneal hematoma (*arrow*). **B.** Selective right renal arteriogram demonstrates no renal injury but rather hemorrhage from the inferior adrenal artery (*arrow*). **C.** Selective microcatheter injection in the inferior adrenal artery demonstrates a brisk bleed. **D.** Selective renal arteriogram postembolization with N-butyl cyanoacrylate (glue). Subtraction artifact reveals a cast of glue within the inferior adrenal artery (*arrow*) and no further hemorrhage.

fistulae, and other injuries of the main renal artery (53–56). No systematic study of the use of stents in trauma has been published, but published case reports do indicate that endovascular techniques may offer an attractive alternative to surgical repair, particularly in polytraumatized patients. Vascular stents have been placed in patients as young as 15 years old with satisfactory initial results and short-term follow-up (57). The reports include use of both balloon-expandable and self-expanding stents (58–61). One should exercise caution

when crossing a complete occlusion because the precise nature of the underlying injury (dissection, transection, mural hematoma with thrombosis) is not known. The infrequency of these injuries will most likely never allow for a randomized study of the use of stents in trauma, but for select patients, the use of stents in main renal artery injuries should be weighed against the surgical treatment options. Stents may be the least invasive manner to treat a lesion that may otherwise result in complete loss of kidney function (Figure 60–11).

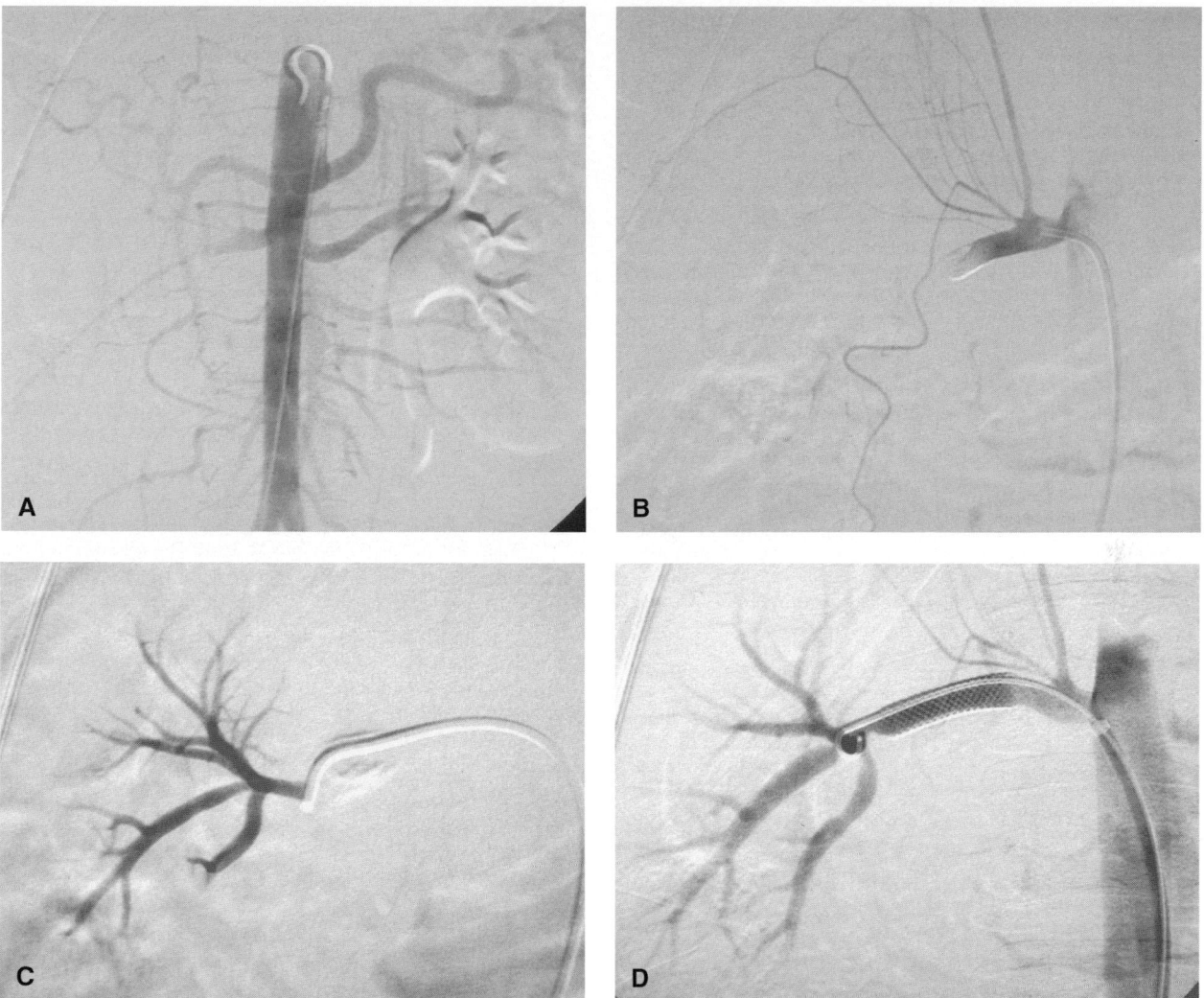

Figure 60–11   Thirty-two-year-old woman after motor vehicle accident. **A.** Abdominal aortagram demonstrates complete occlusion of the right renal artery. **B.** Selective right renal arteriogram demonstrates the stump of the right renal artery. **C.** Arteriogram of the distal right renal artery following manipulation across the complete occlusion. **D.** Injection of the vascular sheath demonstrates successful placement of a 7-mm × 4-cm Smart stent (Cordis Endovascular), recanalizing the occluded segment and restoring flow to peripheral branches. (Courtesy of Charles W. Nutting, MD.)

SUMMARY

Blunt, penetrating, or iatrogenic trauma may result in significant renal arterial injuries. The most conservative treatment possible is favored in managing an injured kidney. Arteriography is typically reserved for those patients who have failed conservative treatment and require intervention. This philosophy has resulted in an increased use of renal artery branch embolization to treat traumatic arterial injuries. Transcatheter embolization has a high success rate and a low complication rate and also minimizes parenchymal loss. The alternative surgical procedure frequently results in more parenchymal loss and is more invasive. Transcatheter embolization, therefore, is the preferred method of therapy in many patients with traumatic renal artery branch injuries. Further expansion of endovascular techniques in the treatment of renal trauma includes the use of vascular stents to repair main renal artery injuries. These techniques are highly complementary to the philosophy of conservative, nonoperative management of trauma patients that has been shown to be the preferred management strategy.

REFERENCES

1. Moore E, Cogbill TH, Malangoni MA, et al. Organ injury scaling. Surg Clin North Am 1995;75:293–303.
2. Nunez D Jr, Rivas L, McKenney K, et al. Helical CT of traumatic arterial injuries. AJR Am J Roentgenol 1998;170:1621–1626.
3. Love L, Meyers MA, Churchill RJ, et al. Computed tomography of extraperitoneal spaces. AJR Am J Roentgenol 1981;136:781–789.
4. Dodds WJ, Darweesh RM, Lawson TL, et al. The retroperitoneal spaces revisited. AJR Am J Roentgenol 1986;147:1155–1161.
5. Cass AS. Renovascular injuries from external trauma. Diagnosis, treatment, and outcome. Urol Clin North Am 1989;16:213–220.

6. Santucci RA, McAninch JW. Diagnosis and management of renal trauma: past, present, and future. J Am Coll Surg 2000;191: 443–451.
7. Peters PC, Sagalowsky AI. Genitourinary trauma. In: Walsh PC, Retik AB, Stamey TA, et al., eds. Campbell's Urology. 6th Ed. Philadelphia: WB Saunders, 1992:2571–2594.
8. McAninch JW, Carroll PR. Renal exploration after trauma. Indications and reconstructive techniques. Urol Clin North Am 1989;16:203–211.
9. Federle MP, Kaiser JA, McAninch JW, et al. The role of computed tomography in renal trauma. Radiology 1981;141:455–460.
10. Velmahos GC, Demetriades D, Cornwell EE 3rd, et al. Selective management of renal wounds. Br J Surg 1998;85:1121–1124.
11. Armenakas NA, Duckett CP, McAninch JW. Indications for non-operative management of renal stab wounds. J Urol 1999;161: 768–771.
12. Knudson MM, Maull KI. Nonoperative management of solid organ injuries. Past, present, and future. Surg Clin North Am 1999; 79:1357–1371.
13. Ralls PW, Barakos JA, Kaptein EM, et al. Renal biopsy-related hemorrhage: frequency and comparison of CT and sonography. J Comput Assist Tomogr 1987;11:1031–1034.
14. Bookstein JJ, Goldstein HM. Successful management of post-biopsy arteriovenous fistula with selective arterial embolization. Radiology 1973;109:535–536.
15. Cope C, Zeit RM. Pseudoaneurysms after nephrostomy. AJR Am J Roentgenol 1982;139:255–261.
16. Lang EK. Percutaneous nephrostolithotomy and lithotripsy: a multi-institutional survey of complications. Radiology 1987;162: 25–30.
17. Mee SL, McAninch JW. Indications for radiographic assessment in suspected renal trauma. Urol Clin North Am 1989;16: 187–192.
18. Cass AS, Luxenberg M, Gleich P, et al. Clinical indications for radiographic evaluation of blunt renal trauma. J Urol 1986;136: 370–371.
19. Hardeman SW, Husmann DA, Chinn HK, et al. Blunt urinary tract trauma: identifying those patients who require radiological diagnostic studies. J Urol 1987;138:99–101.
20. Harris AC, Zwirewich CV, Lyburn ID, et al. CT findings in blunt renal trauma. RadioGraphics 2001;21:S201–S214.
21. Sandler CM, Toombs BD. Computed tomographic evaluation of blunt renal injuries. Radiology 1981;141:461–466.
22. Pollack HM, Wein AJ. Imaging of renal trauma. Radiology 1989; 172:297–308.
23. Sclafani SJ, Becker JA, Shaftan GW, et al. Strategies for the radiologic management of genitourinary trauma. Urol Radiol 1985;7: 231–244.
24. Steinberg DL, Jeffrey RB, Federle MP, et al. The computerized tomography appearance of renal pedicle injury. J Urol 1984;132: 1163–1164.
25. Rhyner P, Federle MP, Jeffrey RB. CT of trauma to the abnormal kidney. AJR Am J Roentgenol 1984;142:747–750.
26. Brower P, Paul J, Brosman SA. Urinary tract abnormalities presenting as a result of blunt abdominal trauma. J Trauma 1978;18: 719–722.
27. Cass AS. Blunt renal trauma in children. J Trauma 1983;23: 123–127.
28. Mertz JH, Wishard WN Jr, Nourse MH, et al. Injury of the kidney in children. JAMA 1963;183:730–733.
29. Morse TS. Renal injuries. Pediatr Clin North Am 1975;22:379–391.
30. Morey AF, McAninch JW, Tiller BK, et al. Single shot intraoperative excretory urography for the immediate evaluation of renal trauma. J Urol 1999;161:1088–1092.
31. Cass AS, Luxenberg M. Conservative or immediate surgical management of blunt renal injuries. J Urol 1983;130:11–16.
32. Kadir S. Kidneys. In: Kadir S, ed. Atlas of Normal and Variant Angiographic Anatomy. Philadelphia: WB Saunders, 1991: 387–434.
33. Lang EK. Arteriography in the assessment of renal trauma: the impact of arteriographic diagnosis on preservation of renal function. J Trauma 1975;15:553–566.
34. Sclafani SJ, Stein K. Arteriographic management of traumatic arteriocalyceal fistula. Urol Radiol 1981;3:177–179.
35. Bertini JE Jr, Flechner SM, Miller P, et al. The natural history of traumatic branch renal artery injury. J Urol 1986;135:228–230.
36. Clark RA, Gallant TE, Alexander ES. Angiographic management of traumatic arteriovenous fistulas: clinical results. Radiology 1983;147:9–13.
37. Heyns CF, van Vollenhoven P. Increasing role of angiography and segmental artery embolization of renal stab wounds. J Urol 1992;147:1231–1234.
38. Kadir S, Marshall FF, White RI Jr, et al. Therapeutic embolization of the kidney with detachable silicone balloons. J Urol 1983; 129:11–13.
39. Kerber CW, Freeny PC, Cromwell L, et al. Cyanoacrylate occlusion of a renal arteriovenous fistula. AJR Am J Roentgenol 1977; 128:663–665.
40. Pilla TJ, Tantana S, Shields JB. Embolization of blunt trauma in the pediatric patient. Cardiovasc Intervent Radiol 1987;10: 153–156.
41. Uflacker R, Paolini RM, Lima S. Management of traumatic hematuria by selective renal artery embolization. J Urol 1984;132: 662–667.
42. Fisher RG, Ben-Menachem Y, Whigham C. Stab wounds of the renal artery branches: angiographic diagnosis and treatment by embolization. AJR Am J Roentgenol 1989;152:1231–1235.
43. Hagiwara A, Sakaki S, Goto H, et al. The role of interventional radiology in the management of blunt renal injury: a practical protocol. J Trauma 2001;51:526–531.
44. Richman SD, Green WM, Kroll R, et al. Superselective transcatheter embolization of traumatic renal hemorrhage. AJR Am J Roentgenol 1977;128:843–844.
45. Chuang VP, Reuter SR, Walter J, et al. Control of renal hemorrhage by selective arterial embolization. Am J Roentgenol Radium Ther Nucl Med 1975;125:300–306.
46. Eastham JA, Wilson TG, Larsen DW, et al. Angiographic embolization of renal stab wounds. J Urol 1992;148:266–270.
47. Cekirge S, Weiss JP, Foster RG, et al. Percutaneous retrieval of foreign bodies: experience with the nitinol Goose Neck snare. J Vasc Interv Radiol 1993;4:805–810.
48. Graves VB, Rappe AH, Smith TP, et al. An endovascular retrieving device for use in small vessels. AJNR Am J Neuroradiol 1993; 14: 804–808.
49. Kantor A, Sclafani SJ, Scalea T, et al. The role of interventional radiology in the management of genitourinary trauma. Urol Clin North Am 1989;16:255–265.
50. Rana AI, Kenney PJ, Lockhart ME, et al. Adrenal gland hematomas in trauma patients. Radiology 2004;230:669–675.
51. Wilms G, Marchal G, Baert A, et al. CT and ultrasound features of post-traumatic adrenal hemorrhage. J Comput Assist Tomogr 1987;11:112–115.
52. Murphy BJ, Casillas J, Yrizarry JM. Traumatic adrenal hemorrhage: radiologic findings. Radiology 1988; 169:701–703.
53. Bruce LM, Croce MA, Santaniello JM, et al. Blunt renal artery injury: incidence, diagnosis, and management. Am Surg 2001;67: discussion 555–556.
54. Lee JT, White RA. Endovascular management of blunt traumatice renal artery dissection. J Endovasc Ther 2002;9:354–358.
55. Sprouse LR 2nd, Hamilton IN Jr. The endovascular treatment of a renal arteriovenous fistula: placement of a covered stent. J Vasc Surg 2002;36:1066–1068.
56. Bates MC, Shamsham FM, Faulknier B, et al. Successful treatment of iatrogenic renal artery perforation with an autologous vein-covered stent. Catheter Cardiovasc Interv 2002;57:39–43.
57. Paul JL, Otal P, Perreault P, et al. Treament of posttraumatic dissection of the renal artery with endoprothesis in a 15-year-old girl. J Trauma 1999;47:169–172.
58. Whigham CJ, Bodenhamer JR, Miller JK. Use of the Palmaz stent in primary treatment of renal artery intimal injury secondary to blunt trauma. J Vasc Interv Radiol 1995;6:175–178.
59. Villas P, Cohen G, Putnam SG 3rd, et al. Wallstent placement in a renal artery after blunt abdominal trauma. J Trauma 1999;46: 1137–1139.
60. Inoue S, Koizumi J, Iino M, et al. Self-expanding metallic stent placement for renal artery dissection due to blunt trauma. J Urol 2004;171:347–348.
61. Bruce M, Kuan YM. Endoluminal stent-graft repair of a renal artery aneurysm. J Endovasc Ther 2002;9:359–362.

Embolotherapy of Hepatic Trauma

61

Michael D. Katz, Sue E. Hanks

The liver is the most commonly injured intra-abdominal organ. The mechanism of injury can be either blunt or penetrating trauma. The frequent use of diagnostic and therapeutic hepatic procedures also causes a number of iatrogenic hepatic injuries. Death from complex hepatic injury remains at least 10–15% and is typically caused by uncontrolled hemorrhage (1). The management of hepatic injuries has changed from one of routine surgical exploration to conservative observation of all hemodynamically stable patients. It is as an extension of such conservative management strategies that angiography and transcatheter therapies have their greatest utility.

CLASSIFICATION

Hepatic injuries are classified by the liver injury scale devised by the American Association for the Surgery of Trauma (AAST) (2) (Table 61-1). Grade I–II injuries are typically minor, although even these wounds can cause life-threatening hemorrhage. Grade III–VI injuries are considered major and/or complex.

TRIAGE

The triage of patients suffering abdominal trauma is based on both the mechanism of injury and the patient's hemodynamic status. Many penetrating trauma patients are surgically explored because of concern for bowel perforation. All unstable patients, regardless of mechanism, undergo emergency laparotomy. Massively traumatized patients may be treated by "damage-control" surgery solely for control of hemorrhage and enteric contamination (3).

Whereas unstable patients undergo emergency laparotomy, stable patients undergo radiologic evaluation. Computed tomography (CT) has the pivotal role in abdominal trauma triage and is the initial examination of choice for hemodynamically stable patients following blunt abdominal trauma. For patients who are hemodynamically stable or who can be stabilized with fluid resuscitation, contrast-enhanced CT is performed to assess for injuries. Other modalities, including ultrasound, scintigraphy, and arteriography, may be useful for select indications. Ultrasound may quickly demonstrate intraperitoneal blood (4). Scintigraphy is useful to evaluate for bile leaks. Abdominal arteriography is rarely used as the initial diagnostic modality but can be combined with emergency pelvic or thoracic arteriography in the polytrauma patient.

NONOPERATIVE MANAGEMENT

Operative management of complex hepatic injuries include hepatorrhapy, vessel ligation, omental packing, resectional debridement, perihepatic packing, and atriocaval shunts. Routine exploration of blunt hepatic injuries yields a nontherapeutic laparotomy rate as high as 50–70% (5). The majority of hepatic injuries stop bleeding by the time of laparotomy. Significant morbidity and mortality is associated with these negative operations. The goal of nonoperative management is to reduce nontherapeutic laparotomy. It consists of intensive care unit (ICU) observation with serial abdominal examinations and laboratory tests.

Both prospective and large retrospective series document the success of nonoperative management in blunt hepatic trauma to be 89–98%, with a complication rate less than 6% (6–9). Surprisingly, the grade of hepatic injury or degree of

TABLE 61-1

LIVER INJURY SCALE (1994 REVISION)

Grade[a]		Injury Description
I	Hematoma	Subcapsular, <10% surface area
	Laceration	Capsular tear, <1 cm parenchymal depth
II	Hematoma	Subcapsular, 10–50% surface area; intraparenchymal, <10 cm long
	Laceration	1–3 cm parenchymal depth, <10 cm long
III	Hematoma	Subcapsular, >50% surface area or expanding; ruptured subcapsular or parenchymal hematoma
		Intraparenchymal hematoma >10 cm or expanding
	Laceration	>3 cm parenchymal depth
IV	Laceration	Parenchymal disruption involving 25–75% of hepatic lobe or 1–3 Couinaud segments within a single lobe
V	Laceration	Parenchymal disruption involving >75% of hepatic lobe or >3 Couinaud segments within a single lobe
	Vascular	Juxtahepatic venous injuries, i.e., retrohepatic vena cava/central major hepatic veins
VI	Vascular	Hepatic avulsion

[a] Advance one grade for multiple injuries, up to grade III.
(Reprinted with permission from Table 2. Liver Injury Scale (1994 revision) in Organ injury scaling: spleen and liver. J of Trauma 1995;38:324.)

hemoperitoneum does not correlate with treatment success (10,11). Nonoperative management, originally utilized for only minor grade I–II injuries, has evolved to be applied to even grade III–V major and/or complex injuries (5). Arteriography and transcatheter embolization have increased the number of patients who can be managed without surgery by offering another method to control hepatic hemorrhage. Even patients whose hemodynamic status can be maintained only by continuous fluid or blood product replacement may be managed nonoperatively with transcatheter embolization (12). As many as 86% of patients with blunt hepatic trauma may be managed without open surgery (13).

Nonoperative management of blunt hepatic injuries is clearly the treatment of choice in all hemodynamically stable patients, irrespective of grade of injury or degree of hemoperitoneum. Patients treated without surgery have fewer septic complications, fewer transfusions, fewer ICU days, shorter hospitalizations, and lower mortality rates (1,13). Operative management is chosen, then, only when associated intra-abdominal injuries, such as bowel perforation, require operation or when there is persistent hemodynamic instability during resuscitation (13).

COMPLICATIONS OF HEPATIC INJURY

Morbidity related to hepatic injury remains high. Complications are common and, in fact, the norm, particularly with higher-grade injuries. These complications occur regardless of whether transcatheter embolization is performed (14). Persistent or recurrent hemorrhage occurs in

approximately 3% of patients and should be referred for arteriography and transcatheter embolization (15). Other complications include abscess, bile leak, and hepatic necrosis. The majority of these complications can be managed by percutaneous or endoscopic means (15). Posttraumatic or postoperative bilomas and/or abscesses can be successfully treated by percutaneous drainage in the majority. A potential late complication of hepatic injury is bile duct stricture, typically managed by stenting (Figure 61–1).

TREATMENT OF PENETRATING TRAUMA

Experience with management of blunt hepatic trauma has shown that even severe injuries can be managed conservatively in the hemodynamically stable patient. A limited number of carefully selected stab and gunshot injuries have been successfully managed with criteria similar to those for blunt trauma, including a mandatory lack of peritoneal signs, indicating possible perforation of a hollow viscus (16–19). As with blunt trauma, CT can be performed in stable victims of penetrating trauma. Angiography and embolization can be performed for identical indications with similar results (20,21) (Figure 61–2).

INDICATIONS FOR ARTERIOGRAPHY

Diagnostic hepatic arteriography is indicated when active hemorrhage is suspected. It is almost always performed with the intent to treat potential vascular injuries by therapeutic embolization. As with observational management, arteriography may be performed for all grades of hepatic injuries, in all patients who are hemodynamically stable or who can be stabilized with resuscitation (22–26). Hepatic arteriography may be performed based on CT evidence of hemorrhage or significant hepatic injury. It may be performed emergently, during or immediately following resuscitation, following a surgical procedure, or when delayed complications become apparent.

Advances in CT technology that allow for more rapid scanning (spiral and multidetector CT) have increased the frequency of identifying contrast extravasation within the liver and the peritoneal cavity (27). A characteristic focal high-density area, pooling of contrast material, reliably indicates active bleeding (28–30). These patients require additional intervention, either surgical or angiographic. Because active bleeding at CT can be identified before the development of hemodynamic instability, arteriographic intervention with transcatheter embolization can be attempted.

Fang et al. have described a classification system for extravasation on CT as intraparencyhmal, intraperitoneal, or combined, with the hope to differentiate patients who would be better served by immediate surgery rather than transcatheter embolization (31). No pattern of extravasation, however, has been confirmed to predict embolization failure (32).

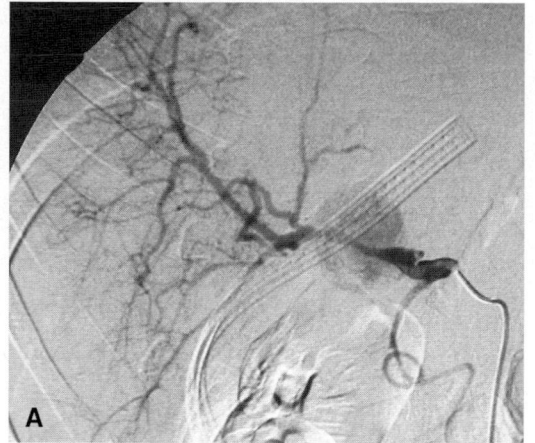
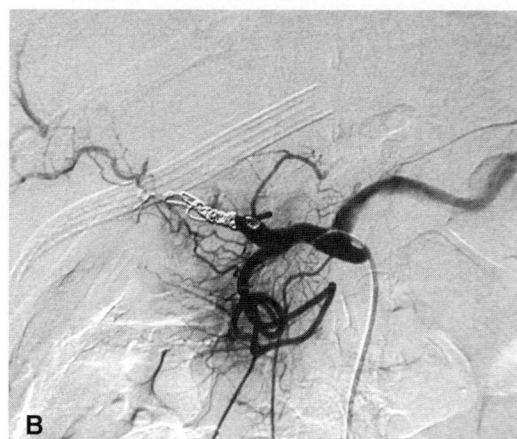
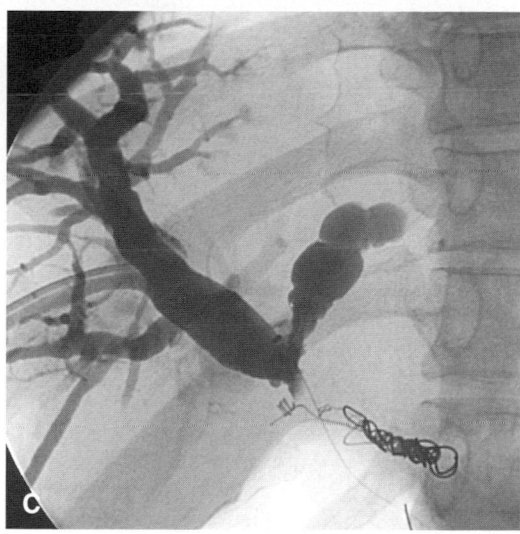

Figure 61–1 Hilar injury. **A.** Hepatic arteriogram following motor vehicle accident demonstrates a large pseudoaneurysm of the proper hepatic artery. **B.** Celiac arteriogram after coil embolization of the proper hepatic artery demonstrates successful occlusion of the proper hepatic artery with distal reconstitution via collaterals. The pseudoaneurysm no longer fills. **C.** Cholangiogram shows associated biliary injury with complete occlusion of the common hepatic duct.

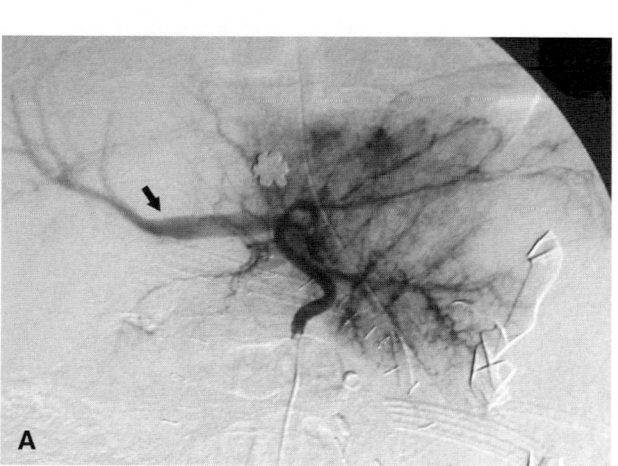
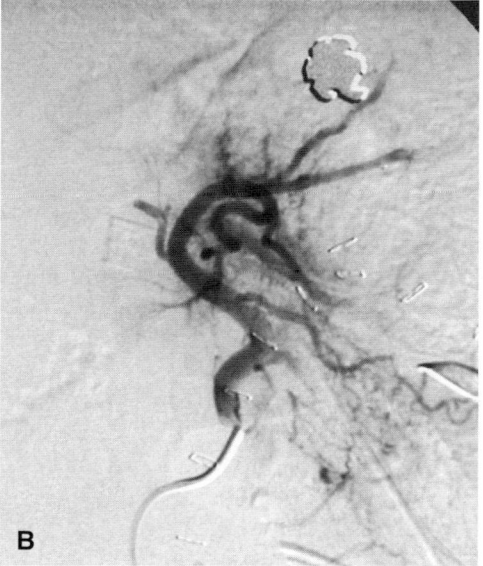

Figure 61–2 Arterioportal fistula. **A.** Emergency postoperative arteriogram for gunshot wound to the left lobe of the liver. The catheter is in the left hepatic artery. Abnormal prompt filling of the portal vein (*arrow*) is seen, indicating arterioportal fistula. **B.** Following Gelfoam slurry embolization there is pruning of the left hepatic arteries and no further filling of the arterioportal fistula.

When massive hemorrhage is found in the operative suite, the perihepatic space is packed at an abbreviated surgery (damage control). Damage-control surgery can be followed by damage-control arteriography. In those patients who continue to show signs of hemorrhage, an angiographic survey of all possible sites of injury should be performed (33). Immediate postoperative hepatic arteriography has been recommended in all patients with grade IV or V injuries (33). Arteriography and associated transcatheter embolization has emerged as the adjunctive therapeutic modality of choice.

Arteriography is also indicated for delayed complications of hepatic trauma. It is particularly good for bleeding from vessels deep within the hepatic parenchyma. It can obviate a return trip to the operating room in physiologically compromised patients. Hepatic arteriography and transcatheter embolization are standard treatment for iatrogenic injuries (34). Delayed hemorrhage may present as a falling hemoglobin, gastrointestinal bleeding from hemobilia, or fresh blood from an intra-abdominal drain.

ARTERIOGRAPHY TECHNIQUE

Arteriography to identify bleeding sites is undertaken as an exploration analogous to exploratory laparotomy. All potential sites of hemorrhage are examined. A global examination, abdominal aortography, is performed initially to rapidly identify massive bleeding and anatomic variants and to direct further therapy. Subsequently, more detailed selective arteriography is performed to better identify arterial injuries and for focused treatment, typically by embolization.

In the liver, arterial anatomic variations are common. Selective examination of the celiac and superior mesenteric arteries is often necessary. Common variants include the left hepatic artery arising from the left gastric artery and the right hepatic artery replaced to the superior mesenteric artery. It is important to scrutinize the arteriogram for defects in hepatic enhancement, which might alert one to the presence of anatomic variants or accessory vessels (Figure 61–3).

Typically, arteriography is performed using a preshaped 5 French selective catheter. Superselective catheterization may require use of 2–3 French microcatheters (35). Two or more projections should be obtained. Filming should be performed at 3–4 frames per second to identify arteriovenous fistulae and should be carried out to include the portal venous phase. Carbon dioxide may be a useful adjunct to conventional contrast if a discrepancy between CT findings and angiography exists (Figure 61–4). Arteriography should be performed quickly, thoroughly, and as early after trauma as possible because embolization still often requires an intact clotting cascade to achieve vessel occlusion.

It is clear that critical patients will be brought to the interventional radiology suite for angiography. Accordingly, aggressive resuscitative measures must continue in the interventional radiology area. The routine use of a patient

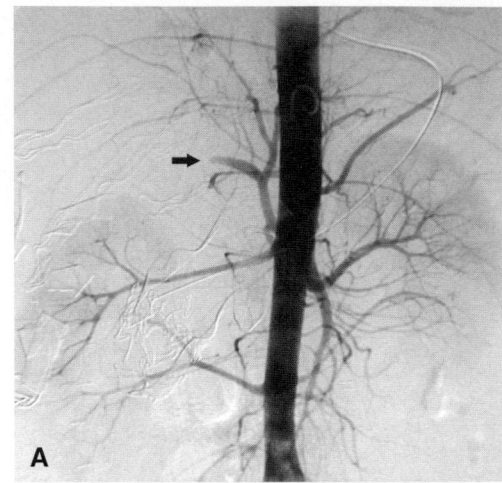

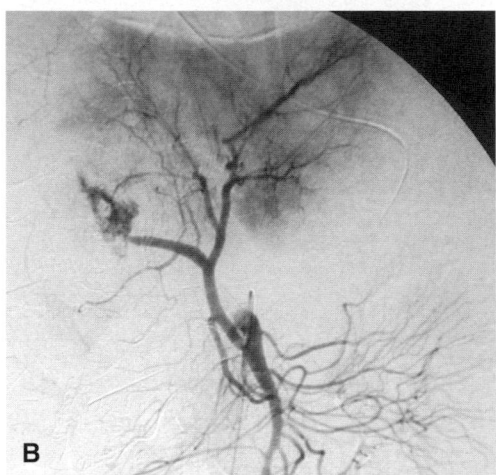

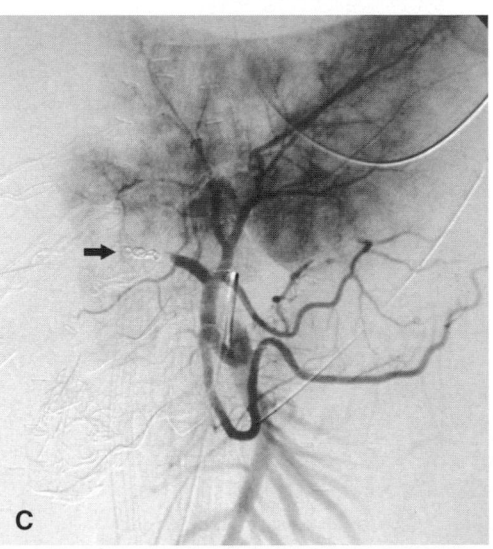

Figure 61–3   Variant hepatic anatomy. **A.** Postoperative abdominal aortogram following damage-control surgery for gunshot wound to the liver. Hemorrhage could not be controlled in the operating room. The right hepatic artery (*arrow*) appears to be occluded on this nonselective view. **B.** Selective superior mesenteric arteriogram (SMA) demonstrates variant anatomy with the common hepatic artery replaced to the SMA. The right hepatic artery is now actively bleeding, emphasizing the intermittent nature of arterial hemorrhage. **C.** Successful coil embolization of the right hepatic artery (*arrow*).

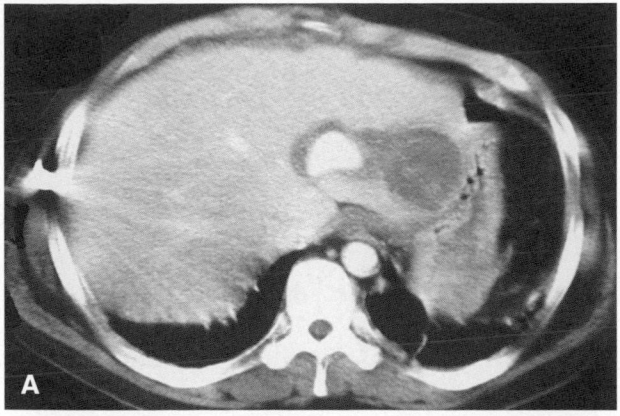

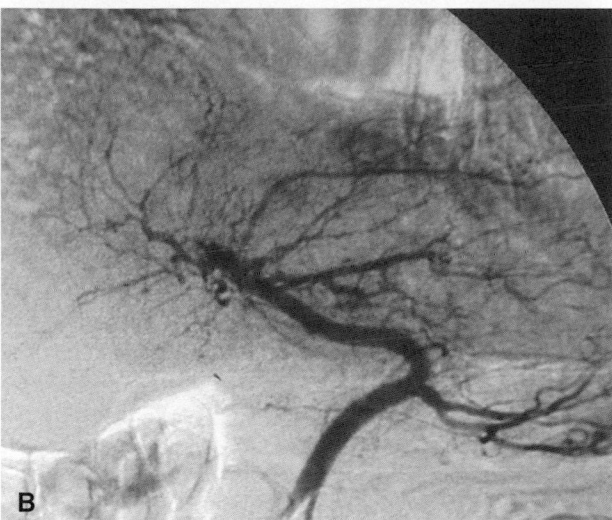

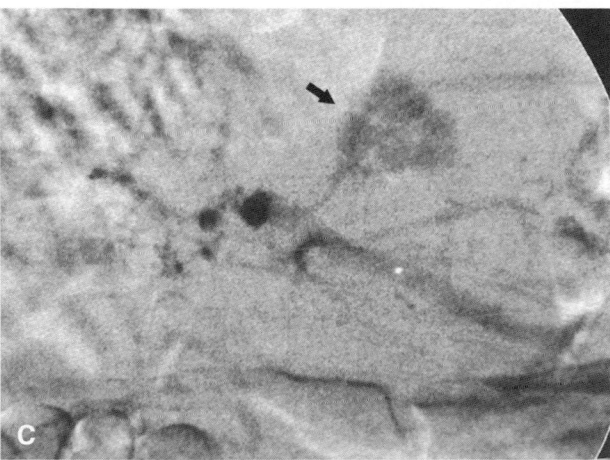

Figure 61–4 CO_2 angiography. **A.** CT scan for delayed complication (recurrent fever) following gunshot wound to the abdomen demonstrates a large pseudoaneurysm in the left lobe. **B.** The patient was referred for immediate hepatic arteriography. Conventional contrast left hepatic arteriogram fails to identify a lesion, despite multiple selective views. **C.** Superselective left hepatic arteriography utilizing CO_2 as the contrast agent demonstrates the pseudoaneurysm (*arrow*), localizing the injury not seen with conventional contrast material for transcatheter embolization.

warming unit (BairHugger, Arizant Heathcare) is advantageous. Collaboration with the ICU or surgical team can help manage fluid requirements, patient sedation, and patient rewarming (33).

EMBOLIZATION TECHNIQUE

Active extravasation, arteriovenous fistulae, pseudoaneurysms, and arteriobiliary fistulae are all amenable to treatment by embolization (36). The liver is well suited to transcatheter embolization because of its dual blood supply. Arterial embolization is unlikely to result in tissue infarction unless there is concomitant injury to the portal system. For focal injuries, it is preferable to place the embolic agent as close to the injury site as possible. Microcatheters may, therefore, speed treatment of selected injuries (35).

Once an arterial injury is identified, occlusion of the lesion with an embolic agent is performed. In trauma, the major considerations for selecting an embolic occluding agent are speed and reliability of delivery, duration of occlusive effect, location of the injury, and preservation of normal tissue. Two agents are frequently employed. Coils are ideal for single-vessel injuries, larger vessels, or instances in which the site of vessel occlusion must be precise. They provide controlled delivery with rapid occlusion and are available in a variety of sizes (Figure 61–5). Where injuries are multiple, or are distal in location or where numerous collateral pathways are present, the use of particulate agents is indicated. Gelfoam, because of its temporary occlusive effect, is the agent of choice. By using a temporary agent, vessel recanalization may occur later after wound healing. Gelfoam can be delivered as a slurry of small particles or as a larger single pledget (Figure 61–6). Additional embolic agents, which have occasionally been used, include microspheres, Ivalon, thrombin, and N-butyl cyanoacrylate (Figure 61–7). The final choice of embolic agent is dependent on the injury type and injury location, as well as individual anatomic considerations (Figure 61–8).

Transcatheter embolization is successful at stopping hemorrhage from hepatic arterial injuries in 83–88% of cases (32,37). Failures are most often related to inability to catheterize a bleeding artery. Recurrent bleeding does rarely occur and may be treated by repeat embolization. Reported complications of transcatheter embolization are few but include hepatic necrosis, abscess or biloma formation, nontarget embolization, and gallbladder infarction (14).

TREATMENT OF VENOUS INJURIES

Although most patients treated by percutaneous methods have arterial hemorrhage, occasionally venous hemorrhage can also be treated. Treatment of injuries to the perihepatic

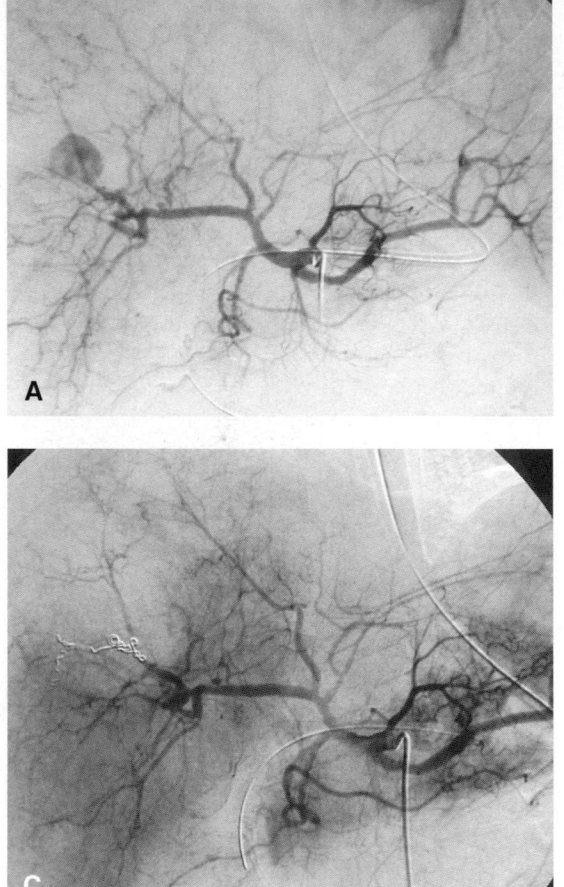

Figure 61–5   Coil embolization. **A.** Following a motor vehicle accident, selective celiac arteriogram demonstrates a large pseudoaneurysm within the right lobe. **B.** Superselective hepatic arteriogram shows that the pseudoaneurysm arises near the branch point of two arteries, requiring placement of coils into both vessels via a microcatheter. **C.** Postembolization celiac arteriogram demonstrates successful occlusion of the pseudoaneurysm, obviating the need for surgery in this patient.

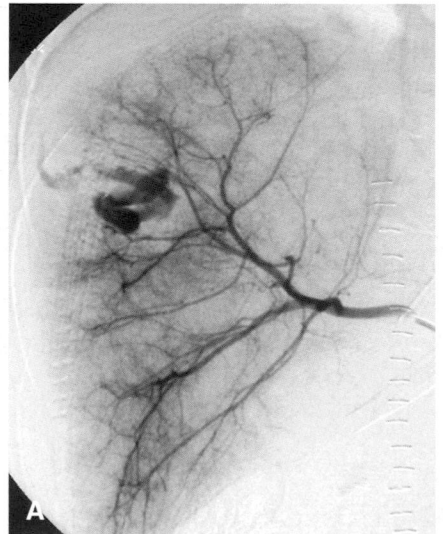
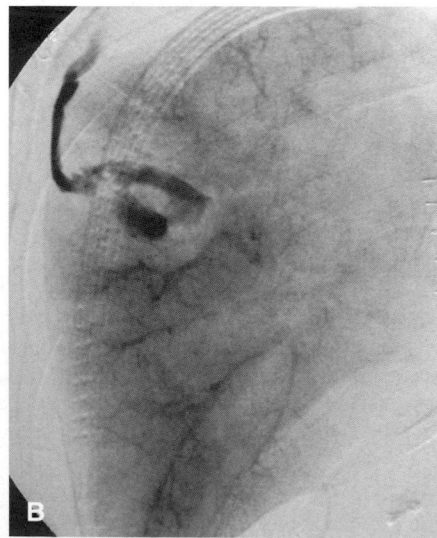
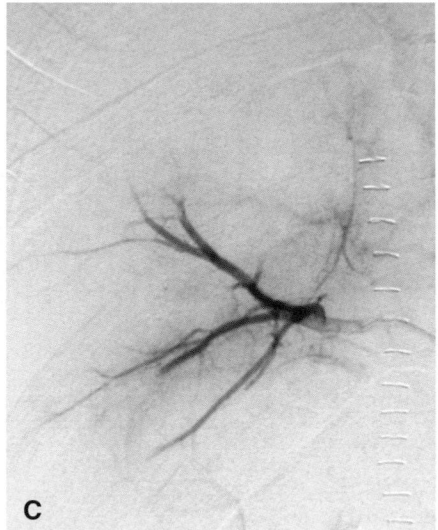

Figure 61–6   Gelfoam embolization. **A.** Following operative exploration for abdominal gunshot wound, arteriography was performed for decreasing hematocrit. Selective celiac arteriogram demonstrates brisk hemorrhage from the right lobe. **B.** Late arterial phase shows massive contrast extravasation into the perihepatic peritoneum. **C.** Gelfoam embolization of the right hepatic artery was quickly performed. Arteriography reveals occlusion of the branches of the right hepatic artery.

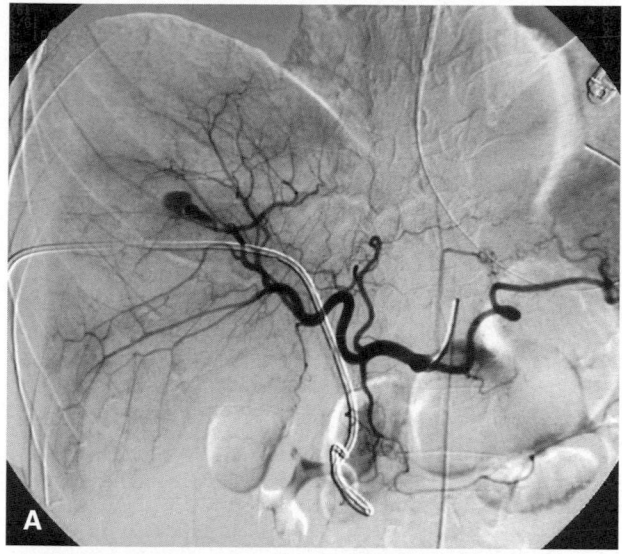

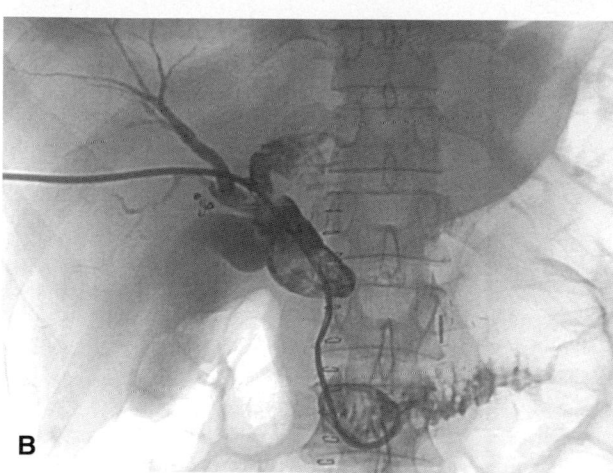

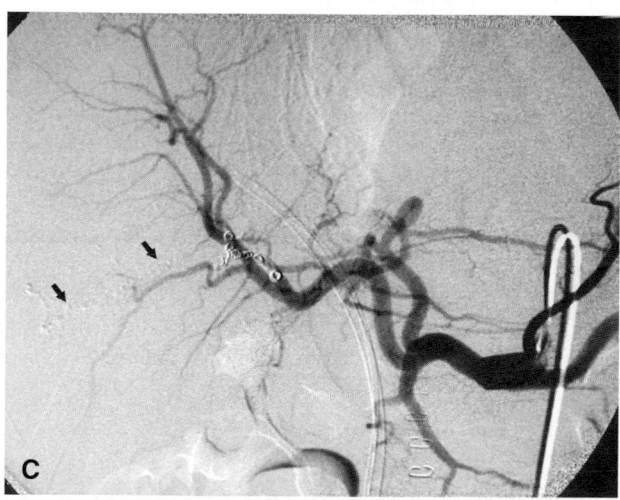

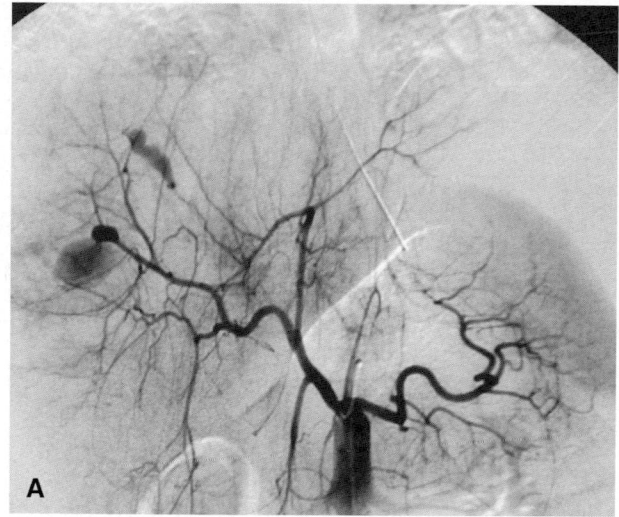

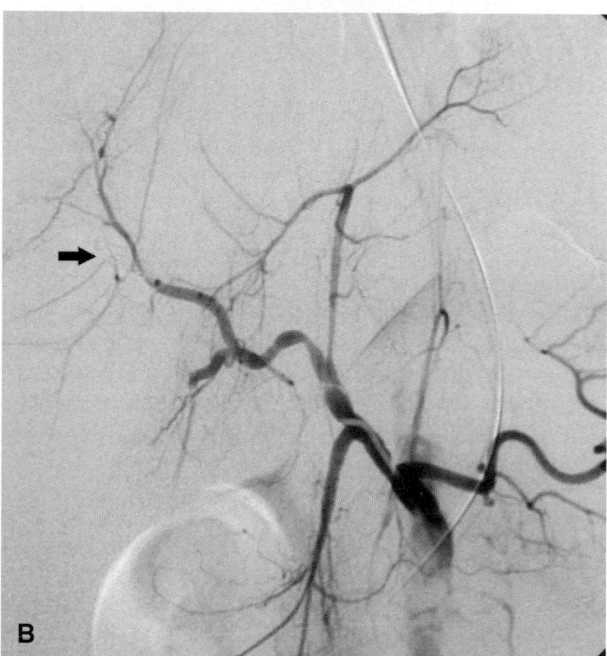

Figure 61-8 Multifocal hemorrhage. **A.** Celiac arteriogram following motor vehicle accident demonstrates active hemorrhage from at least two branches of the right hepatic artery. **B.** Gelfoam slurry followed by coils (*arrow*) was used to occlude the injured branches. Postembolization celiac arteriogram demonstrates successful embolization with a combination of agents.

Figure 61-7 Complex embolization for hemobilia. **A.** Celiac arteriogram for iatrogenic hemobilia following percutaneous biliary drain placement demonstrates extravasation from a right hepatic artery branch. **B.** Despite initially successful coil embolization, hemobilia recurred. Cholangiogram demonstrates recurrent clot in the common hepatic duct. **C.** The previously embolized artery had recanalized and was embolized again with Gelfoam, coils, and even thrombin injection into this right hepatic artery branch. Hemobilia returned yet again and was finally successfully treated by N-butyl cyanoacrylate embolization (*arrows*) of this branch.

vena cava or the hepatic veins is challenging, and these injuries are almost always lethal. Exsanguination can be rapid, and treatment is typically emergency surgical repair (38). Some investigators consider resuscitative fluid requirements in excess of 2 liters as suggestive of a venous injury (39). Arterial embolization, not surprisingly, does not work for hemorrhage from veins. Treatment of hepatic vein injury has been reported by transcatheter placement of bare or covered stents (40) (Figure 61-9). The role such treatments requires further investigation.

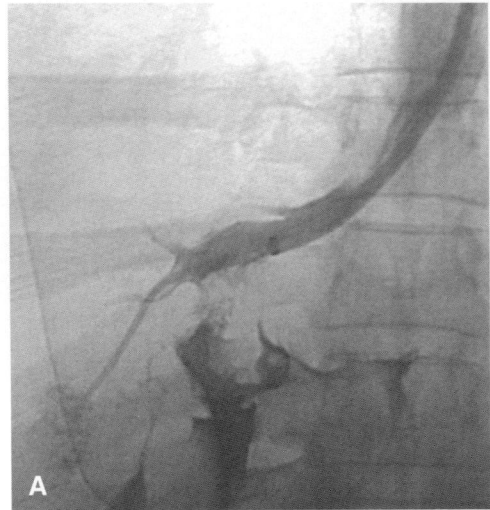 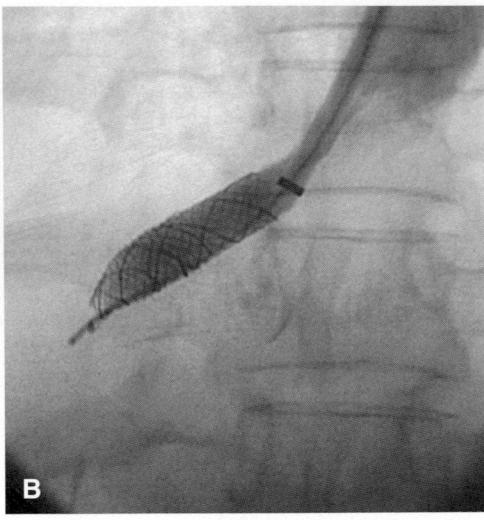

Figure 61–9 Hepatic vein injury. **A.** Hepatic venogram demonstrates a large laceration of the right hepatic vein with intraperitoneal extravasation in a cirrhotic patient undergoing a transjugular intrahepatic portosystemic shunt procedure. **B.** Following placement of two covered self-expanding stents in the right hepatic vein, no further extravasation of contrast is identified.

SUMMARY

Treatment of hemorrhage following trauma remains challenging and is crucial to optimizing patient outcomes. Both retrospective and prospective studies have confirmed that nonoperative management can be successful in a large number of cases of hepatic trauma. Transcatheter techniques are highly successful at stopping hepatic hemorrhage. Patients with ongoing hemorrhage, continued transfusion requirements, or CT-documented active bleeding can be treated by transcatheter embolization with likely success. The adjunctive use of transcatheter embolization increases the likelihood of overall nonoperative success. Such conservative management of organ injury decreases the mortality rate and morbidity associated with abdominal trauma.

REFERENCES

1. Cachecho R, Clas D, Gersin K, et al. Evolution in the management of the complex liver injury at a Level I trauma center. J Trauma 1998;45:79–82.
2. Moore EE, Cogbill TH, Jurkovich GJ, et al. Organ injury scaling: spleen and liver (1994 revision). J Trauma 1995;38:323–324.
3. Rotondo MF, Schwab CW, McGonigal MD, et al. `Damage control': an approach for improved survival in exsanguinating penetrating abdominal injury. J Trauma 1993;35:375–382.
4. McGahan JP, Wang L, Richards JR. From the RSNA refresher courses: focused abdominal US for trauma. Radiographics 2001; 21:S191–199.
5. Boone DC, Federle M, Billiar TR, et al. Evolution of management of major hepatic trauma: identification of patterns of injury. J Trauma 1995;39:344–350.
6. Pachter HL, Knudson MM, Esrig B, et al. Status of nonoperative management of blunt hepatic injuries in 1995: a multicenter experience with 404 patients. J Trauma 1996;40:31.
7. Pachter HL, Hofstetter SR. The current status of nonoperative management of adult blunt hepatic injuries. Am J Surg 1995;169: 442.
8. Croce MA, Fabian TC, Menke PG, et al: Nonoperative management of blunt hepatic trauma is the treatment of choice for hemodynamically stable patients. Results of a prospective trial. Ann Surg 1995;221:744.
9. Sherman HF, Savage BA, Jones LM, et al. Nonoperative management of blunt hepatic injuries: safe at any grade? J Trauma 1994; 37:616.
10. Datena SJ, Borzotta AP, Long WB, et al. Management of CT grade III, IV, V liver injury: early surgical intervention is rarely necessary. J Trauma 1999;46: 200.
11. Becker CD, Gal I, Baer HU, et al. Blunt hepatic trauma in adults: correlation of CT injury grading with outcome. Radiology 1996; 201:215–220.
12. Ciraulo DL, Luk S, Palter M, et al. Selective hepatic arterial embolization of grade IV and V blunt hepatic injuries: an extension of resuscitation in the nonoperative management of traumatic hepatic injuries. J Trauma 1998;45:353–359.
13. Brasel KJ, DeLisle CM, Olson CJ, et al. Trends in the management of hepatic injury. Am J Surg 1997;174:674–677.
14. Mohr AM, Lavery RF, Barone A, et al. Angiographic embolization for liver injuries: low mortality, high morbidity. J Trauma 2003;55: 1077–1082.
15. Carrillo EH, Spain DA, Wohltmann CD, et al. Interventional techniques are useful adjuncts in nonoperative management of hepatic injuries. J Trauma 1999;46:619–624.
16. Sclafani SJ, Shaftan GW, McAuley J, et al. Interventional radiology in the management of hepatic trauma. J Trauma 1984;24:256.
17. Renz BM, Feliciano DV. Gunshot wounds to the right thoracoabdomen: a prospective study of nonoperative management. J Trauma 1994;37:737.
18. Demetriades D, Rabinowitz B, Sofianos C. Nonoperative management of penetrative liver injuries: a prospective study. Br J Surg 1986;73:736.
19. Demetriades D, Charalambides D, Lakhoo M, et al. Gunshot wound of the abdomen: role of selective conservative management. Br J Surg 1991;78:220.
20. Velmahos GC, Demetriades D, Chahwan S, et al. Angiographic embolization for arrest of bleeding after penetrating trauma to the abdomen. Am J Surg 1999;367–373.
21. Munera F, Morales C, Soto JA, et al. Gunshot wounds of abdomen: evaluation of stable patients with triple-constrast helical CT. Radiology 2004;231:399–405.
22. Asensio JA, Demetriades D, Chahwan S, et al. Approach to the management of complex hepatic injuries. J Trauma 2000;48: 66–69.
23. Sriussadaporn S, Pak-art R, Tharavej C, et al. A multidisciplinary approach in the management of hepatic injuries. Injury 2002; 33:309–315.
24. Hagiwara A, Yukioka T, Ohta S, et al. Nonsurgical management of patients with blunt hepatic injury: efficacy of transcatheter arterial embolization. AJR Am J Roentgenol 1997;169:1151–1156.
25. Velmahos GC, Toutouzas KG, Vassiliu P, et al. A prospective study on the safety and efficacy of angiographic embolization for pelvic and visceral injuries. J Trauma 2002;52:303–308.

26. Hashimoto S, Hiramatsu K, Ido K, et al. Expanding role of emergency embolization in the management of severe blunt hepatic trauma. Cardiovasc Intervent Radiol 1990;13:193–199.

27. Yao DC, Jeffrey RB Jr, Mirvis SE, et al. Using contrast-enhanced helical CT to visualize arterial extravasation after blunt abdominal trauma: incidence and organ distribution. AJR Am J Roentgenol 2002;178:17–20.

28. Willmann JK, Roos JE, Platz A, et al. Multidetector CT: detection of active hemorrhage in patients with blunt abdominal trauma. AJR Am J Roentgenol 2002;179:437–444.

29. DiGiacomo JC, McGonigal MD, Haskal ZJ, et al. Arterial bleeding diagnosed by CT in hemodynamically stable victims of blunt trauma. J Trauma 1996;40:249.

30. Jeffrey RB, Cardoza JD, Olcott EW. Detection of active intraabdominal arterial hemorrhage: value of dynamic contrast-enhanced CT. AJR Am J Roentgenol 1991;156:725.

31. Fang JF, Chen RJ, Wong YC, et al. Classification and treatment of pooling of contrast material on computed tomographic scan of blunt hepatic trauma. J Trauma 2000;49:1083–1088.

32. Wahl WL, Ahrns KS, Brandt MM, et al. The need for early angiographic embolization in blunt liver injuries. J Trauma 2002;52:1097–1101.

33. Johnson JW, Gracias VH, Gupta R, et al. Hepatic angiography in patients undergoing damage control laparotomy. J Trauma 2002;52:1102–1106.

34. Savader SJ, Trerotola SO, Merine DS. Hemobilia after transhepatic biliary drainage: treatment with transcatheter embolotherapy. J Vasc Interv Radiol 1992;3:345–352.

35. Teitelbaum GP, Reed RA, Larsen D, et al. Microcatheter embolization of non-neurologic traumatic vascular lesions. J Vasc Interv Radiol 1993;4:149.

36. Forlee MV, Krige JEJ, Welman CJ, et al. Haemobilia after penetrating and blunt liver injury: treatment with selective hepatic artery embolisation. Injury 2004;35:23–28.

37. Schwartz RA, Teitelbaum GP, Katz MD, et al. Effectiveness of transcatheter embolization in the control of hepatic vascular injuries. J Vasc Interv Radiol 1993;4:359.

38. Chen RJ, Fang JF, Lin BC, et al. Surgical management of juxtahepatic venous injuries in blunt hepatic trauma. J Trauma 1995;38:886–890.

39. Hagiwara A, Murata A, Matsuda T, et al. The efficacy and limitations of transarterial embolization for severe hepatic injury. J Trauma 2002;52:1091–1096.

40. Denton JR, Moore EE, Coldwell DM. Multimodality treatment for grade V hepatic injuries: perihepatic packing, arterial embolization, and venous stenting. J Trauma 1997;42:964–968.

Pediatric Interventional Radiology

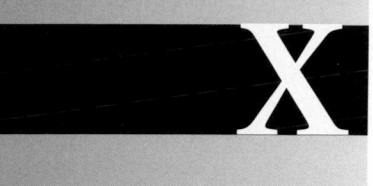

X

Pediatric Interventional Angiography

62

Josée Dubois, Laurent Garel, and J.A. Gordon Culham

Many of the newer vascular techniques are delayed in being applied to children because of the conservative nature of pediatric practitioners, the shortage of trained physicians, and the need for minification of equipment appropriate for pediatric use. In recent years, there has been tremendous growth in the field of pediatric vascular intervention, particularly in the treatment of vascular anomalies and in vascular access.

Interventional radiology in pediatrics differs from the practice in adult patients in several aspects. Interventional nonvascular, vascular, and cardiac procedures are usually confined to tertiary pediatric centers. In all pediatric patients, particularly neonates and infants, special consideration must be given to the choice of sedation or anesthesia, maintenance of temperature control, fluid balance, contrast dose, radiation safety, and equipment selection.

In pediatrics, patients range in weight from 500 grams to 60 kilograms, and the different pieces of equipment are not always suitable for all patients. Disease processes are also different in children; for example, atherosclerosis is, indeed, not a concern in this age group.

This review will cover the main indications of angiography and intervention in children, with the exclusion of neuroangiography and neurointervention.

THE IMPORTANCE OF A DEDICATED PEDIATRIC SUITE

A skilled and complementary team of personnel, including the pediatric radiology nurse, x-ray technologist, and hemodynamic technologist, is required to take care of the patient, prepare the room for the procedure, and assist the radiologist.

A high-resolution digital angiography system is necessary and helps in reducing the volume of contrast material and in speeding up the procedures. To reduce the radiation dose in children to a level below the usual radiation standards of angiography, fluoroscopy is performed at the lowest milliamp dose possible, pulsed at as low a rate as possible and performed without the scatter grid. In addition, rare earth filters should be installed in the x-ray tube to further reduce radiation. It is hoped that the recently developed flat-panel technology will contribute significantly to dose reduction.

CARE OF THE PEDIATRIC PATIENT

Consent

For all procedures, informed consent is obtained from the parent, guardian, or the patient if over 14 years of age. Care must be taken to provide an unbiased view of the procedure and to discuss alternative modalities of diagnosis or therapy. Serious complications must be mentioned, even if rare.

Laboratory Test

Routine bloodwork and coagulation studies are requested when a risk of bleeding is a concern clinically or from the procedure; a platelet count of less than 50,000/cu mm is associated with an increased risk of bleeding (1). Blood is matched only in case of possible significant blood loss.

Patient Preparation

Patients are kept NPO for an appropriate time as determined by age, alimentary requirements, type of sedation, and need for general anesthesia. Routine antibiotics are not prescribed except for splenic embolization and biliary intervention. Bacterial endocarditis prophylaxis is indicated for children with congenital heart defects who are undergoing percutaneous procedure (2). Anxious children may receive a preoperative sedative or anxiolytic agent.

Sedation is frequently used in pediatric radiology. The Committee on Drugs of the American Academy of Pediatrics (AAP) in 1992 issued guidelines for monitoring and management of pediatric patients during and after sedation for diagnostic and therapeutic procedures. The goals of sedation as stated are (a) to guard the patient's safety and welfare; (b) to minimize physical discomfort or pain; (c) to minimize psychologic responses to treatment by providing analgesia and to maximize the potential for amnesia; (d) to control behavior; and (e) to return the patient to a state in which safe discharge, as determined by recognized criteria, is possible (3). The close, continuous observation of the patient under sedation is crucial. Continuous pulse oximetry with an audible and visual signal is mandatory. Personnel and equipment for airway management and resuscitation with appropriate-size materials should be available within the angiography suite.

Sedative-Hypnotic Agents (2,4,5)

Chloral hydrate has no analgesic properties and has no use in the angiography suite. Similarly, pentobarbital (Nembutal, Abbott), methohexital, and thiopental are reserved for diagnostic procedures. Fentanyl (Sublimaze,

Janssen) is a short-acting opioid used for procedural analgesia. The disadvantage of fentanyl is the pruritis in the nasal area that may interfere with the procedure. Precautions are recommended for patients with impaired respiratory function or unstable or cyanotic cardiac disease. The effects of opioids can be reversed with the antagonist naloxone.

Ketamine induces a trancelike cataleptic condition characterized by intense somatic analgesia, amnesia, and immobility with minimal effects on ventilation or hemodynamics (2). The contraindications are uncontrolled hypertension, heart failure, increased intracranial and intraocular pressure, and the presence of psychiatric disorder.

Ketamine is more effective than most other drugs for performing painful procedures. Unpleasant hallucinations and bad dreams during the recovery period are known side effects of ketamine. Its use in association with midazolam prevents this "bad trip" phenomenon.

Midazolam hydrochloride (Versed, Hoffman-Laroche), a benzodiazepine, is the drug most commonly used in children for short procedures. Midazolam induces sedation, motion control, myorelaxation, and anxiolysis. It is reversible with flumazenil.

The Toronto mix is made of meperidine hydrochloride, promethazine hydrochloride, and chlorpromazine. This intramuscular cocktail (0.1 cc/kg, maximum dose 1.5 cc) was commonly used for long procedures but has been replaced by intravenous agents in most centers (Table 62–1).

General Anesthesia

Difficult interventions such as endovascular embolization, device implantation, or angioplasty are done under general anesthesia. Where resources are sufficient, there is a shift to more procedures being done under anesthesia. New, short-acting agents such as propofol can be useful for pediatric procedures. One drawback of these short-acting agents is the need to keep children still for several hours after an arterial procedure. Early postprocedure activity may lead to bleeding or hematoma at a groin puncture site. Often, these children are given longer-acting sedation after the short-acting anesthetic.

Patient Immobilization

Smaller children are immobilized on a restraining board. Older children have hand and leg restraints, but uncooperative or hyperactive patients are anesthetized.

Temperature/Fluid

Neonates and, in particular, premature babies are likely to become hypothermic if attention is not paid to maintaining a warm environment. The room temperature should be increased, Bair Hugger temperature management units must be installed on the table, and the head of the baby must be covered by a cap or a bag. Fluids, contrast material,

TABLE 62–1

THE MOST FREQUENTLY USED SEDATIVE-HYPNOTIC-ANTAGONIST AGENTS IN THE ANGIOGRAPHY SUITE

Drug	Dose	Time to Onset	Duration	Effects
Midazolam (IV) hydrochloride (Versed)	Age 0.5–5 yr: intially, 0.05–0.1 mg/kg adjusted to a max of 6 mg total Age 6–12 yr: 0.025–0.05 mg/kg adjusted to a max of 10 mg total	2–3 min	45–60 min	Sedation Motion control Anxiolysis No analgesia Reversible (Flumazenil)
Fentanyl (IV) (Citrate)	1.0 μg/kg/dose May be repeated Max dose 50 μg total	2–3 min	30–60 min	Analgesia–Sedative Reversible (Naloxone)
Ketamine (IV) (Ketalar)	1–1.5 mg/kg slowly over 1–2 min Half-dose may be repeated every 10 min as required	<1 min	15–60 min	Analgesia–Sedative Dissociation Amnesia Motion control Not reversible
Naloxone (IV) Hydrochloride (Narcan)	0.005 mg/kg Repeat 30 sec–1 min Max dose 0.02 mg/kg or 1 mg total (the smallest of the two)	1–2 min	20–40 min	Antagonist–Narcotic Opioids
Flumazenil (IV)	0.01 mg/kg Max dose 0.2 mg Repeat 45 sec–1 min Max dose 0.05 mg/kg or 1 mg total (the smallest of the two)	1–3 min	30–60 min	Antagonist–Benzodiazepine

and medications must be scaled to the patient size. The flush system must be included in the fluid count and the anesthetist informed of all injections.

Postprocedure Care

Monitoring should be continued until the patient is fully awake. Patients are often discharged the same day if the procedure went as planned, without residual pain. In case of long, difficult, painful, or complicated procedures, the patient will be discharged from the hospital once fully recovered, as evaluated by the physicians in charge.

Contrast Dose

The amount of contrast is a limiting factor in pediatrics. The dose of nonionic contrast should be limited to 5 cc/kg. The reported minor reactions rate is 0.9% for nonionic contrast media (6). Hydration should be maintained. The aspiration of the residual contrast in the catheter and connectors following the injection allows for a better control of the amount used.

Complications

Arterial spasm is frequent in this age group. A 4 or 5 French access sheath should be routine for all procedures. To prevent thrombosis, an initial bolus of heparin 100 units/kg is given, followed by subsequent injections in prolonged procedures (7). Ideally, activated clotting time (ACT) should be monitored during the procedure (8). Arterial spasm may be treated with direct intra-arterial injection of papaverine (1 mg/kg) or nitroglycerine (2–3 μg/kg, which may be repeated for three doses). Arterial thrombosis is treated first with an infusion of heparin and, if required, by an intravenous infusion of r-tPA. Such an infusion should be monitored in a critical care environment and supervised by staff knowledgeable in the use of r-tPA.

MAIN INDICATIONS FOR ANGIOGRAPHY IN CHILDREN

With the advancements in ultrasound and the development of computed tomographic (CT) angiography and magnetic resonance (MR) angiography, diagnostic angiography is rarely needed: gastrointestinal (GI) bleeding with a negative or inconclusive CT scan or MRI remains the main indication for diagnostic angiography. We will focus on the indications for endovascular interventions in children, discussing embolization and sclerotherapy, percutaneous transluminal angioplasty, vascular access, and foreign body retrieval.

Percutaneous transcatheter embolization is a common procedure in pediatric tertiary centers. It should be performed by specifically trained physicians experienced in the equipment and technical alternatives. Pediatric surgical backup is essential. Embolization competes with surgery for many clinical problems and provides a treatment alternative for patients for whom surgery has little to offer. Introducer sheaths should be used to preserve vascular access in the event that the delivery catheter has to be removed. They may also protect against thrombosis (9). Microcatheters allow access to small vessels and territories that were previously inaccessible. Coaxial systems with microcatheters are ideal for pediatric patients. Hydrophylic coated guide wires (Terumo) permit the catheterization of complex angles with less induced spasm than traditional guide wires. The embolic agents used in children are the same as in adults: Gelfoam, particles (polyvinyl alcohol), ethanol, sodium tetradecyl sulfate, cyanoacrylate, and coils. Angioplasty is performed with appropriate-size catheters and balloons. In the authors' judgment, stents should be used in small children only when there is no other therapeutic alternative.

EMBOLIZATION AND SCLEROTHERAPY

Vascular Anomalies

Terminology regarding the vascular anomalies remains confusing. Proper identification is essential to establish the correct diagnosis and define the appropriate treatment and follow-up. The authors follow the classification described initially by Mulliken and Glowacki (10) and accepted by the Workshop on Vascular Anomalies in Rome in June 1996. The vascular anomalies are divided into vascular tumors (hemangioma, hemangioendothelioma, and other vascular tumors) and vascular malformations. Hemangiomas are characterized by initial rapid growth of endothelial cells and subsequent slow involution. Vascular malformations consist of dysplastic vessels without cellular proliferation, and they never regress. These vascular malformations are subcategorized depending on flow (high- or low-flow malformations) and on predominant channel abnormality (arterial, venous, capillary, or lymphatic).

Hemangiomas

Hemangiomas appear on imaging as well-circumscribed masses, single or multiple, with intense, persistent tissue staining, organized in a lobular pattern, with enlarged branches of normal adjacent systemic arteries. In the majority of cases, no treatment is required because of the lesion's spontaneous resolution. Only 10–20% of hemangiomas need to be treated (11). Medical treatment is then the first choice, using steroids, interferon, or vincristin. Presenting symptoms include heart failure, uncontrollable bleeding, and functional impairment. Angiography with embolization is indicated only in cases of ineffective medical treatment. Embolization is mostly performed in cases of hepatic hemangioma with cardiac failure, uncontrolled proliferative hemangioma with functional disorder (e.g., tongue with feeding problem), and intramuscular hemangiomas (Figure 62–1).

The embolization provides control in the proliferative phase.

Kaposiform Hemangioendothelioma

Mueller (12) and Enjolras (13) reported that Kasabach-Merritt phenomenon (KMP) is caused by kaposiform hemangioendothelioma (KHE) or tufted angioma. The KMP consists of thrombocytopenia, microangiopathic hemolytic anemia, and localized consumption coagulopathy in association with rapid evolutive hemangioendothelioma. This syndrome requires aggressive treatment and carries a mortality rate of 20–30%.

Aspirine, dipyridamole antifibrinolytic agents, aminocaproic acid, corticosteroid, interferon, embolization, cyclophosphamide, pentoxifylline, radiotherapy, and antiplatelet aggregating agents have been tried with variable success (12–14). Mueller et al. (12) reported that heparin has been shown to boost the growth of KHE and worsen the clinical situation (15,16).

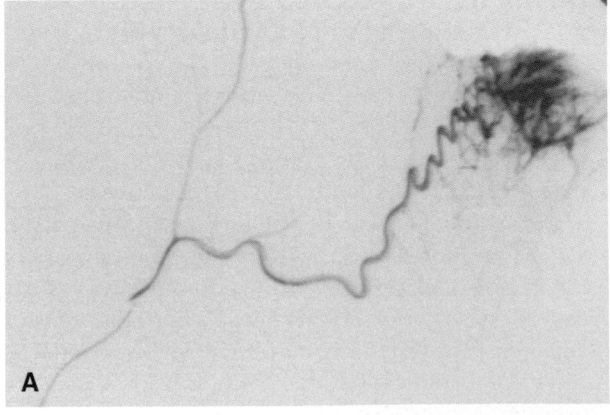
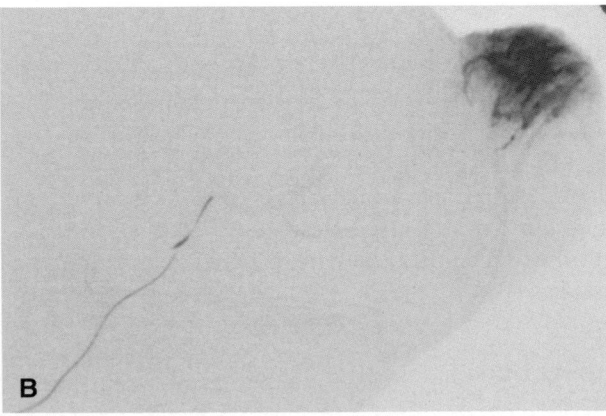

Figure 62–1   One-month-old infant with a hemangioma of the forehead. **A.** Selective catheterization of the superficial temporal artery shows a normal artery with a well-circumscribed lesion. **B.** Persistent tissue staining with a normal-draining vein is demonstrated on the late phase.

Embolization is performed to reduce the high flow. Embolization is performed by arterial approach using polyvinyl alcohol particles or alcohol.

Arteriovenous Malformations

Arteriovenous malformations (high-flow malformations) are abnormal communications between arteries and veins. Arteriovenous malformation (AVM) is the most difficult and dangerous type of vascular malformations to treat. If AVMs are quiescent, conservative management is suitable. In cases of bleeding, progression, or disfigurement, angiography is essential to provide the road map necessary for embolization. The angiographic characteristics of AVMs are dilatation and lengthening of afferent arteries, with early opacification

of enlarged efferent veins (17). To reach the nidus, a superselective catheterization with microcatheters is necessary combined with percutaneous puncture when feasible (18). The best agent to destroy the nidus and decrease the recurrence rate is dehydrated alcohol (Figure 62–2). In high-flow malformations, in which it is difficult to overcome the hemodynamic factors and flood the AVM nidus, ethanol is not diluted with contrast. Injection with a tuberculin syringe is sometimes necessary to overcome fast flow. The amount of ethanol and the pressure of injection are evaluated with contrast media test injections. The maximum dose is 1 mL/kg. Over this 1 mL/kg threshold, the elevated serum ethanol level puts the patient at risk of respiratory depression, cardiac arrhythmias, seizures, rhabdomyolysis, and hypoglycemia (19). The ethanol penetrates to the capillary

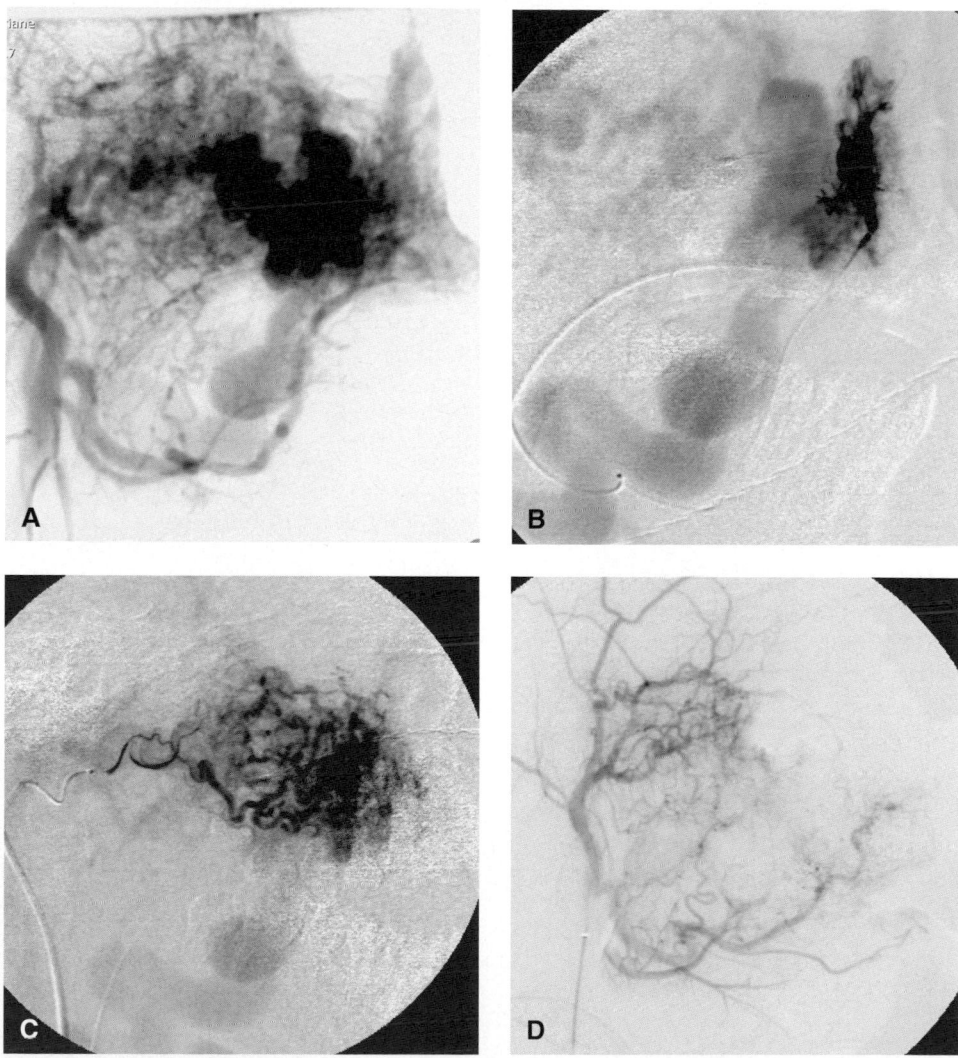

Figure 62–2 A 10-year-old girl with extensive arteriovenous malformation of the right hemiface presents with severe teeth bleeding. **A.** Arterial injection in the external carotid artery shows an important arteriovenous malformation with numerous arterial feeding branches, particularly from the facial artery and internal maxillary branches. **B.** Selective catheterization of the facial branch, and **C.** maxillary artery, was performed with a Tracker 18 in a coaxial system. Embolization was done with alcohol. Considering the numerous arterial feeders, embolization was completed with N-butyl cyanoacrylate, and percutaneous approach was also performed. **D.** External carotid control angiogram shows no residual fistula 1 month postembolization.

level and totally devitalizes normal tissues. If vascular occlusion is required to induce stasis, the authors use balloon occlusion, tourniquets, blood pressure cuffs inflated above systolic pressure, or a combination of these. Temporary compression of the venous drainage during the injection slows the blood flow and can prevent inadvertent washout into the distal venous outflow tract and pulmonary circulation. Dehydrated alcohol should be used with great precautions. Coagulation disturbances are reported in response to dehydrated alcohol that could increase the risk of bleeding, thrombosis, or hematoma. In these patients, in which the embolization is followed by surgery, the use of glue or coils as a substitute for dehydrated alcohol is recommended (20), but further studies are needed to evaluate the specific changes that occur with dehydrated alcohol. Occasionally, large arteriovenous connections are treated with N-butyl cyanoacrylate or coils.

Complications such as pulmonary embolus, cardiovascular collapse, neuropathy, skin blisters, radiculopathy, finger numbness, and focal skin necrosis have been reported (18,19). In cases of large AVM, arterial line monitoring and Swan-Ganz catheters are recommended (19). Occasionally,

large AV connections are treated with N-butyl cyanoacrylate or coils.

Liver Hemangiomas

Liver hemangiomas are the most common hepatic vascular tumors. The differential diagnosis includes hepatic angiosarcoma, hepatic epithelioid hemangioendothelioma, or metastatic disease such as neuroblastoma. Asymptomatic hepatic hemangiomas can be observed without treatment. The main indications for embolization are patients with congestive heart failure, patients who require mechanical ventilatory support, or patients who remain symptomatic after a reasonable trial of pharmacological therapy. Pre-embolization mapping is mandatory, assessing the possible involvement of intercostal or phrenic arteries in addition to the hepatic artery and the portal system (Figure 62–3) (21–23).

Five patterns of angiographic findings were described by Kassarjian et al. (24). The first type, the most classical appearance, is early filling of abnormal vascular channels, stagnation of contrast material, and no evidence of a direct shunting.

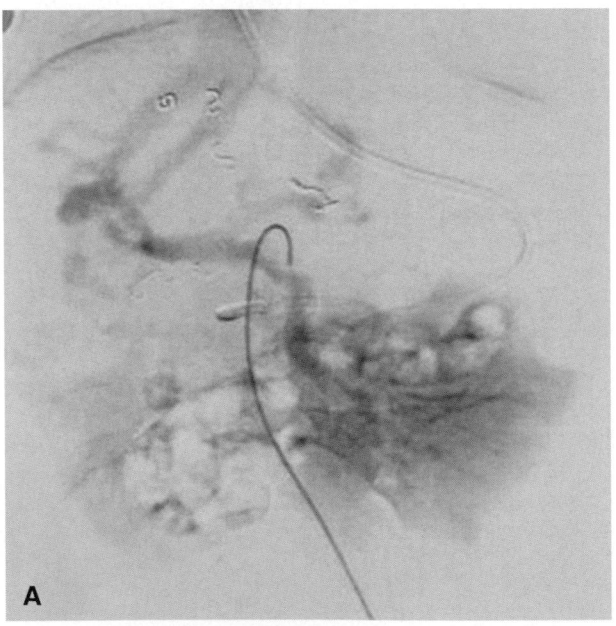

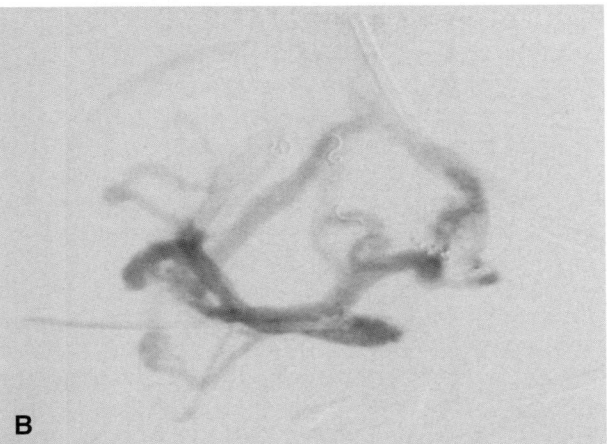

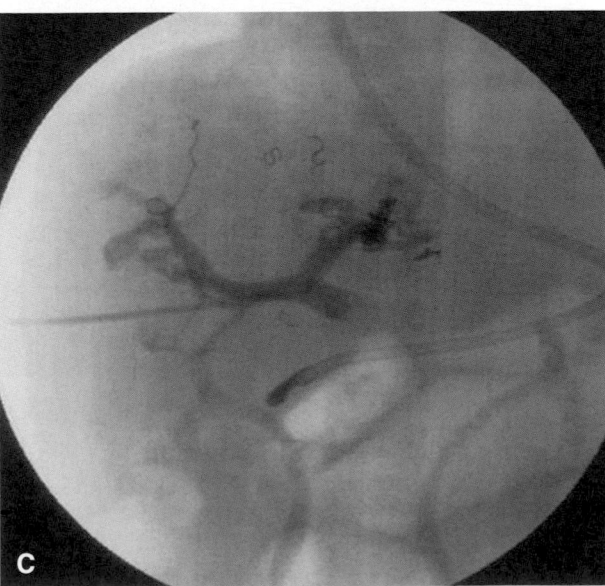

Figure 62–3 Newborn baby presenting with liver hemangioma and heart failure, resistant to medical treatment. Embolization with Gelfoam and coils was performed with persistent heart failure. **A.** Injection in the superior mesenteric artery shows portovenous shunts. **B.** Transhepatic portography displaying large direct shunts with the hepatic veins. **C.** The embolization was performed with coils. Control portography shows the occlusion of the shunts. Heart failure subsided.

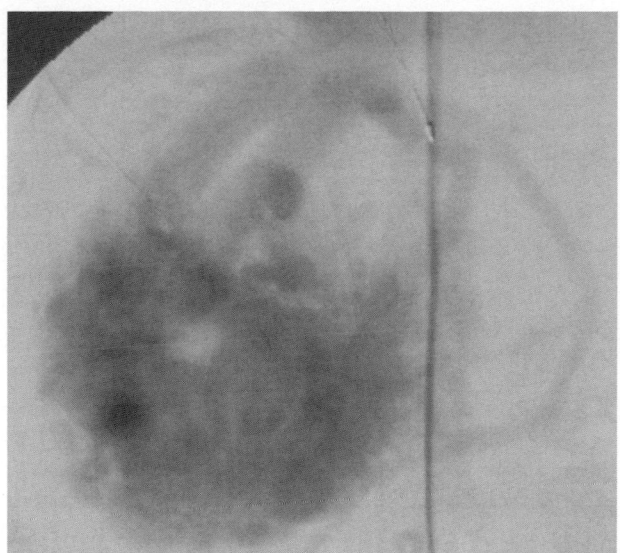

Figure 62–4 Newborn baby with liver hemangioma. Selective injection in the hepatic artery demonstrated an early filling of abnormal vascular channels with arteriovenous shunt (type 3).

Type 2 shows high-flow nodules without direct shunts. Type 3 is made of arteriovenous shunts (Figure 62–4), type 4 of portovenous shunt, and type 5 of the association of both arteriovenous and portovenous shunts.

The embolization is performed by the arterial approach for types 1, 2, 3, and 5 and by a transhepatic transvenous approach for portovenous shunt type 4.

The embolization material should be selected according to the vascular pattern of the shunts. Large particles can be used in types 1 and 2. Platinum fiber microcoils are generally safe in types 3, 4, and 5 and permit the occlusion of the shunt. Glue (N-butyl-2-cyanoacrylate) is the most effective device in patients with direct arteriovenous and arterioportal shunting arising from multiple sources (25). Medical antiangiogenesis drugs should be continued after embolization until nearly complete regression of the lesions is accomplished.

Vascular Malformations of the Liver

Arteriovenous malformation of the liver is rare. Embolization is recommended in case of congestive heart failure. Most AVMs are seen in hereditary hemorrhagic telangiectasia with hepatic ischemia, congestive heart failure, and portal hypertension. Embolization is not recommended in the diffuse lesions because of the risk of increasing the hepatic failure. Liver transplantation is the optimal treatment in such cases.

Arterioportal fistula can be treated by embolization in cases of hereditary hemorrhagic telangiectasia, Ehlers-Danlos syndrome, or patients with biliary artesia and cirrhosis.

Pure venous malformations are uncommon in children. Most of them are asymptomatic. These malformations are seen particularly in patients with blue rubber-bleb nevus syndrome, which is a familial condition with multiple venous malformations of the skin, musculoskeletal system, and viscera.

Venous Malformations

Venous malformations (VM), including capillary-venous malformations, are often misnamed as hemangioma, cavernoma, and phlebangioma. These malformations are characterized by a soft, compressible, nonpulsatile tissue mass. Doppler ultrasonography reveals low-flow lesions.

MRI is an excellent modality to define the extent of the lesions and their relationship to adjacent structures. Usually, VMs are hypointense or isointense on T_1-weighted sequences. In cases of hemorrhage or thrombosis, a heterogeneous signal can be observed on T_1 sequences. Abnormal veins can be observed in the area of the malformation. On T_2-weighted sequences, VMs display a bright signal. Areas of low signal can be observed related to thrombosis, septation within the malformation, or phleboliths. On T_2-weighted sequences, the extension of the malformation into adjacent structures is usually clearly delineated. T_1-weighted sequences after gadolinium infusion are useful to appreciate the circulating portion of the malformation (Figure 62–5) (26).

Arteriography is usually not required for the diagnosis of VMs. It can be normal or demonstrate dysmorphic veins on the late venous opacification phase. It can be useful in cases of complex malformations such as capillary-venous malformations or to demonstrate microfistulas. The physiopathology and clinical significance of these microfistulae are unclear. In most cases, peripheral limb phlebography is not helpful for the diagnosis of upper or lower limb VMs because most of them will not be opacified. In extensive lower limb malformations such as the Klippel-Trenaunay syndrome, the deep veins may be abnormal, and MR venography is needed prior to the treatment.

Direct percutaneous phlebography can be performed as a diagnostic procedure in cases of atypical VMs. It is frequently performed as the initial step during a sclerotherapy session. Direct puncture of the malformation is performed with a 25-gauge butterfly or 24-gauge sheath needle. Ultrasound can be useful for guiding the puncture, especially if the malformation is located deep in the soft-tissues. The needle is connected to a syringe through an extension tubing and is progressively withdrawn while applying slight aspiration. Once blood return is observed, a small amount of low osmolarity iodinated contrast is injected to display the lesion (27).

Three different phlebographic patterns can be observed during VM opacification: a cavitary pattern with late filling of venous drainage without evidence of abnormal veins (Figure 62–6), a spongy appearance with small honeycomb cavities and late venous drainage, or the rapid opacification of dysmorphic veins (Figure 62–7) (28).

No medical treatment is reported to be effective for VM. Prior to any intervention, the patient should be evaluated for low-grade disseminated intravascular coagulopathy. Enjolras et al. reported a high incidence of disseminated intravascular coagulation (DIC) in patients with VM (29). Conservative treatment with elastic stockings is helpful for comfort, protection of skin, and improvement of the coagulopathy. Treatment of VMs is indicated when they cause

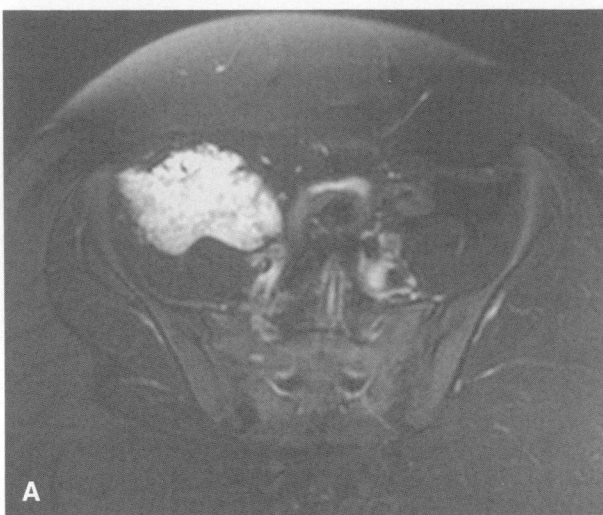
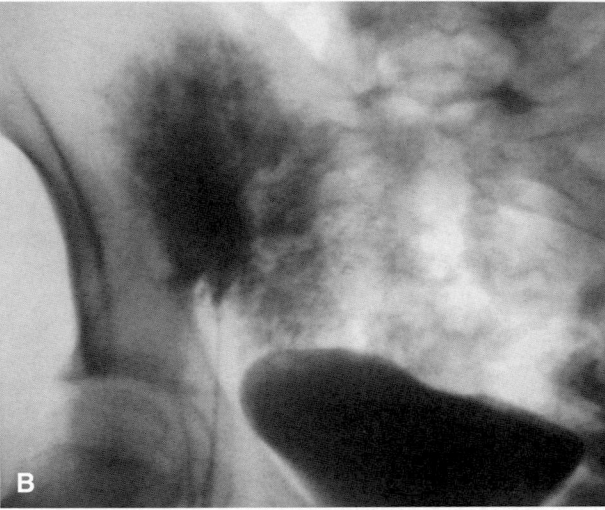

Figure 62–5   Venous malformation of the pelvis in a 15-year-old female. **A.** MR T$_2$-weighted image shows a hyperintense signal in the lesion and defines the extension. **B.** Phlebogram confirms the spongy appearance of the VM.

cosmetic problems, pain, or functional impairment. Absolute ethanol is the most commonly used agent (18,30,31). Ethibloc (Ethicon), a mixture of zein (a corn protein), alcohol, and contrast medium, is commonly used in Europe (32,33). The main drawback of this agent is its propensity to induce cutaneous fistulization with extrusion of the agent. In case of very superficial cutaneous or oromucosal lesions, sodium tetradecylsulfate is suitable to minimize the risk of superficial necrosis.

Sclerotherapy should be performed under fluoroscopic control by a skilled interventional radiologist. The amount of sclerosing agent required is evaluated by percutaneous phlebography. It is important to avoid the filling of draining veins with the sclerosing agent. Tourniquet or manual compression is useful to minimize

the passage of the sclerosing agent into the systemic circulation. A progressive decompression is then paramount to avoid pulmonary emboli. The authors tend to avoid tourniquet or manual compression. Sclerotherapy induces an inflammatory reaction, maximum during the week following the intervention. Analgesic and anti-inflammatory (NSAI or corticoids) medication must be given to alleviate the symptoms. A time span of 1–3 months should be recommended between subsequent sclerotherapy sessions.

Venous anomalies have a propensity for recanalization and recurrence. The authors have observed better results of sclerotherapy with cavitary lesions and dysmorphic veins. Spongy patterns, especially when intramuscular, are more difficult to treat.

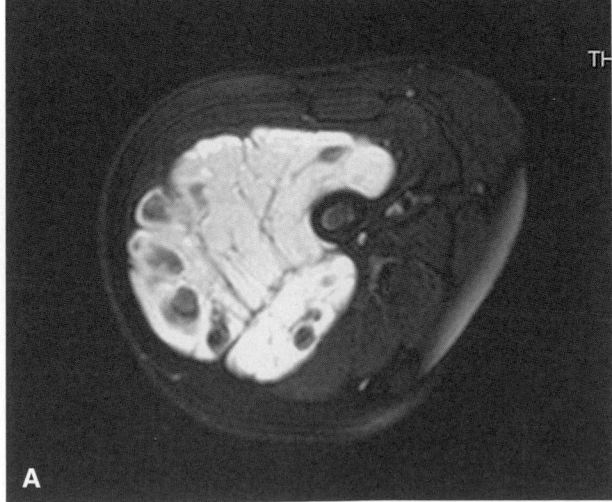
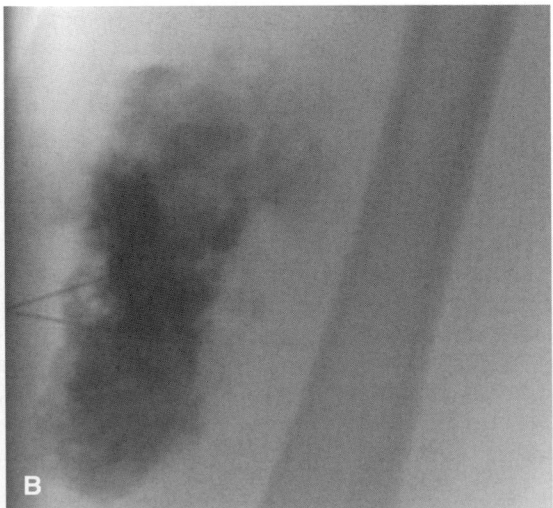

Figure 62–6   Venous malformation of the thigh in a 2-year-old boy. **A.** Spin-echo T$_2$-weighted image shows a hyperintense lesion within the muscle. **B.** Phlebogram displays the cavitary pattern with normal-draining vein.

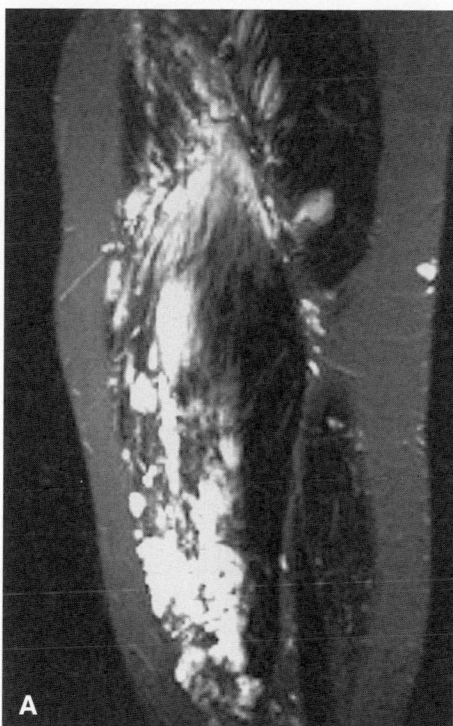
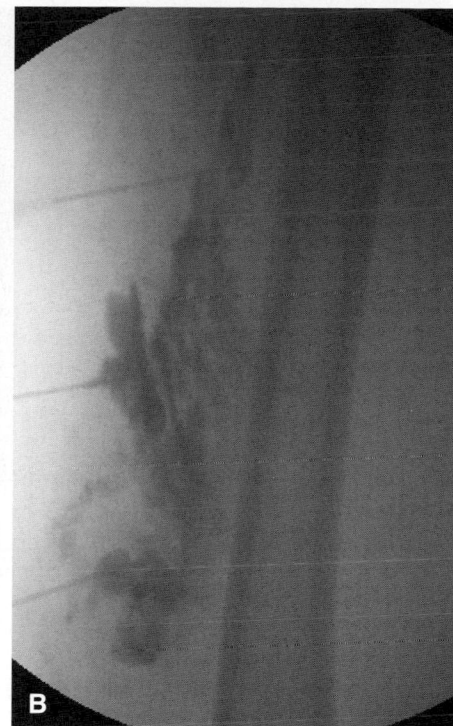

Figure 62–7 Venous malformation of the upper arm in a 16-year-old girl. **A.** Coronal T2-weighted MR image demonstrates dysmorphic veins. **B.** Phlebogram confirms the dysplasic veins.

The main complications of sclerotherapy are cutaneous necrosis and neural toxicity, especially when using alcohol. Systemic complications of alcohol are rare but severe, such as hemolysis with potential renal toxicity and cardiac arrest. The amount of absolute alcohol should be limited to 0.5–1.0 cc/kg.

Lymphatic Malformations

Lymphatic malformations are smooth, unilocular or multilocular soft-tissue masses. They are usually asymptomatic. Sudden enlargement occurs secondary to infection or bleeding. Lymphatic malformations can be subdivided in macrocystic, microcystic, and mixed types. Many authors still recommend a surgical excision, with a reported mortality rate of 2–6%, permanent nerve palsy in 12–13% of patients, and a recurrence rate between 11.8 and 52.9% (34). The authors favor a sclerosing percutaneous approach for the macrocystic and mixed types, with less recurrence and complications than surgery.

The technique is basically the same as for venous malformations. Under ultrasound guidance or palpation, direct puncture of the lesion is performed with a 22- or 24-gauge sheath needle. The opacification of the lesion is mandatory to determine its capacity (volume of contrast) and to verify the absence of draining veins. In most lymphangiomas, there are intercystic communications, and accordingly, a single puncture is all that is needed. Many sclerosing agents have been reported for the treatment of lymphangiomas (35): picibanil (OK-432), fibrin sealant, bleomycin, and tetracycline. The authors have elected to use Ethibloc because of its effectiveness and safety (Figure 62–8). From a practical standpoint, the amount of Ethibloc needed is 10% of the volume determined by the opacification with contrast. A recent report has described success with a combination of tetradecyl sodium, alcohol, and drainage (36).

Aneurysmal Bone Cysts

Aneurysmal bone cysts (ABC) are of unclear origin. Success of their treatment has improved. Treatment options include surgery, sclerotherapy, and arterial embolization. The main controversy regarding ABC is whether obtaining pathological proof is necessary. According to several authors and the authors' own experience and belief, pathological examination is not mandatory when the clinical presentation and radiological appearance are typical of ABC.

Surgery is the most definitive treatment of ABC, but the complications are numerous: growth plate injury, prolonged immobilization, hospitalization, and important bone loss. The recurrence rate is 18–59%.

Sclerotherapy is the primary treatment of ABC for several authors because it is safe, easy to perform, cost effective, and far less aggressive than surgery (Figure 62–9) (37,38). Complications include pulmonary emboli and osteomyelitis. Alcohol and alcoholic solution of zein (Ethnor Laboratories/Ethicon) are used. Steroids are not effective.

For ABCs close to the brain or spine, the authors prefer to use N-butyl cyanoacrylate (n-BCA) to avoid migration of the sclerosing agent into the surrounding veins with subsequent central nervous injury.

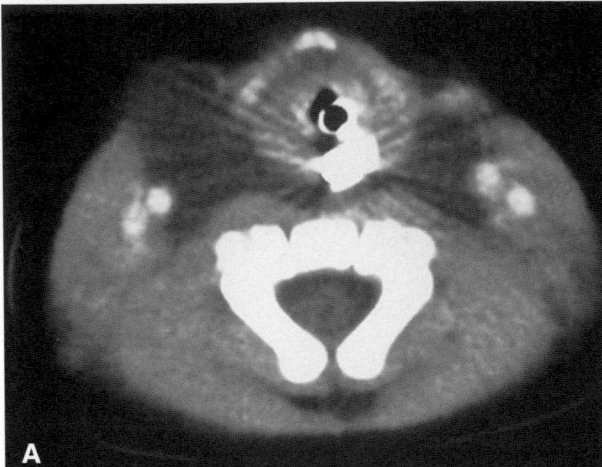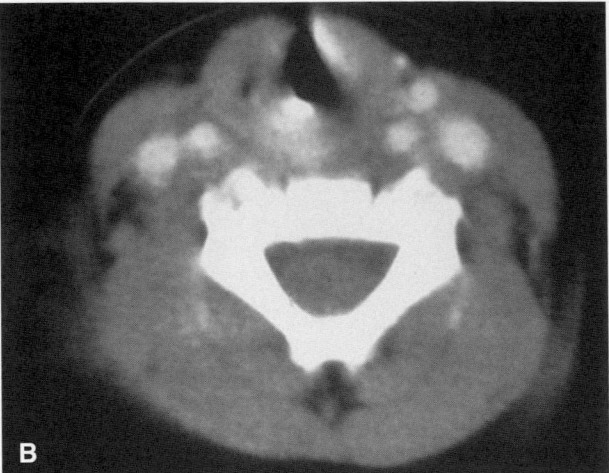

Figure 62–8 Newborn baby with an extensive lymphangioma of the neck extending behind the trachea. **A.** The initial CT scan displays a voluminous lymphangioma in both sides of the cervical region and behind the trachea. **B.** Six months after sclerosing treatment with Ethibloc, the control CT scan shows a complete regression of the lymphangioma.

In the authors' experience, 94% of cases show excellent regression following sclerotherapy without subsequent surgery, with only minor complications of local inflammation and leakage (39).The sclerosing treatment is particularly useful when surgery is technically impossible or not recommended in high-risk patients.

Epistaxis

The differential diagnosis of epistaxis in children includes trauma, foreign-body impaction, bleeding diathesis, vascular disorder, vascular anomalies (reported but rare in Sturge-Weber syndrome and nasal hemangioma), and neoplasms. The most common cause of epistaxis that needs an interventional approach is the nasopharyngeal angiofibroma.

Nasopharyngeal angiofibroma is a benign tumor most often encountered in the adolescent boy (age 10–17) who presents with recurrent epistaxis. Typically the mass originates from the sphenopalatine foramen and extends into the paranasal sinuses, the infratemporal fossa, the central and paracentral middle cranial fossa, intracranially, and into the orbit. The treatment of choice is preoperative embolization followed by radical surgical tumor removal (Figure 62–10). CT scan and MRI are essential for planning the angiographic workup and surgical approach.

Angiography shows that the arteries supplying the lesion arise from the external carotid artery (ECA) and internal carotid arteries (ICA) with minimal arterial dilatation. The tumor blush is intense and persistent. The draining veins appear during the late part of the venous phase. The contralateral ECA should be explored in all cases that reach the midline. The distal internal maxillary artery with its nasopharyngeal and nasal cavity branches is the first system investigated. Large tumors with an extension into the sphenoid sinus, infratemporal fossa, or parapharyngeal

space are supplied by the accessory meningeal, the ascending pharyngeal, and the ascending palatine arteries. It is important to perform a distal embolization because proximal occlusion results in revascularization of the tumor. For the intracranial extradural tumor extensions, the hemodynamics must be analyzed between the internal maxillary system and the internal carotid artery. Embolization is usually performed with particles or n-BCA. When the tumor has invaded the cavernous sinus, the pituitary fossa, or the suprasellar or intracranial intradural area, permanent preoperative balloon occlusion of the internal carotid artery should be considered (39,40).

Hemoptysis

Most patients referred for bronchial artery embolization are adolescents with cystic fibrosis and major hemoptysis. This procedure is usually performed under general anesthesia because of the need to control respiration to achieve ideal subtraction angiography. There have been concerns in the recent literature about the hazards of general anesthesia with positive pressure ventilation in such patients, with reports of fatal pulmonary hemorrhage during induction (41). The following technical features are widely recommended by all authors and are part of the authors' own protocol: femoral artery access, 5 French catheter, precise vascular mapping (descending thoracic aorta, looking for the bronchial arteries and any aberrant arteries, intercostal arteries, and subclavian arteries), coaxial technique with Tracker 18 catheters, secure catheter placement prior to performing embolization, and use of polyvinyl alcohol particles (size: 500–710 μ or 710–1,000 μ if microfistulas are observed) (Figure 62–11). Coils should be avoided because they hinder subsequent catheterization of the proximally

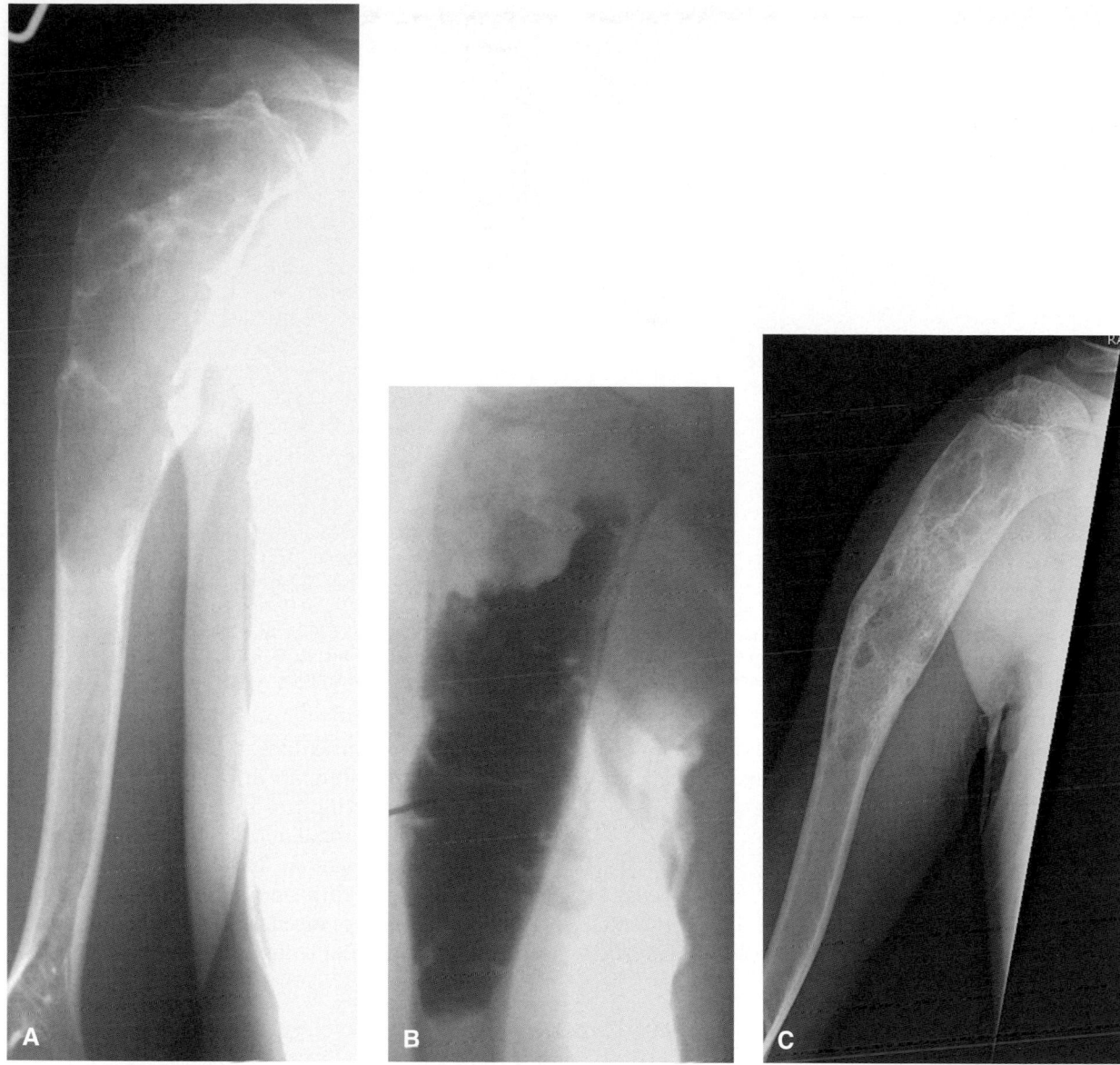

Figure 62–9 Aneurysmal bone cyst of the right humerus discovered in a 12-year-old boy presenting with a fracture. **A.** Plain radiograph shows an expansible lesion with septa involving the right humerus with a fracture. **B.** Percutaneous puncture was performed with a blood return from the lesion. Phlebogram shows the opacification of the cavities. Sclerosing treatment was done with Ethibloc. **C.** Eight months postsclerosing treatment. Plain radiograph shows reossification of the ABC.

occluded vessel. Surgical ligation of bronchial arteries is contraindicated for the same reason.

Careful attention should be paid to identifying spinal arteries arising from the bronchial arteries. In such cases, the operator faces two options: either to try to catheterize the bronchial artery distal to the take-off of the spinal branch or to use large enough particles for preventing any hazardous migration toward the spine. Another alternative when the operator does not know which vessel is bleeding is to avoid the vessel with spinal branches on the first procedure, treat the other bronchial arteries, and return if bleeding persists.

Bronchial artery embolization in cystic fibrosis patients is highly effective immediately. However, many patients (55% in a reported series) require repeated endovascular occlusion during the follow-up (42).

Performing emergency bronchoscopy during bleeding has been advocated to localize the site of hemorrhage and guide the embolization accordingly. In the authors' experience, endoscopy has not been useful.

Although severe complications of bronchial artery embolization have been reported (spinal infarction, myelitis, bronchial infarction, and bronchoesophageal fistula), the procedure has proved safe and effective if performed by

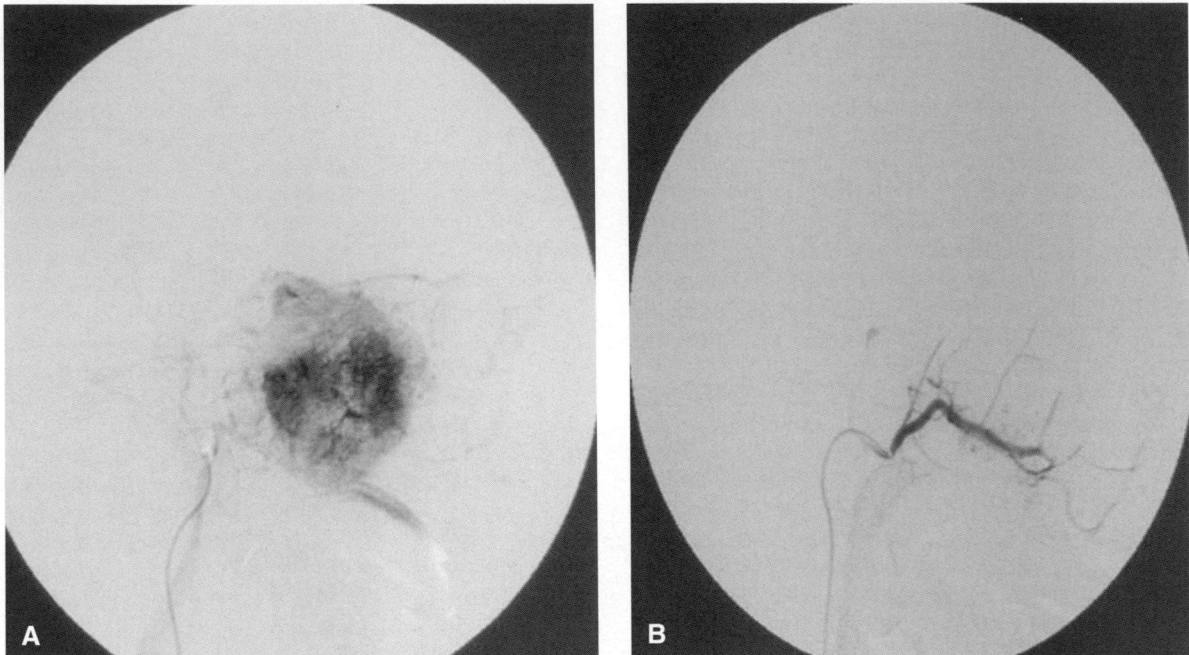

Figure 62–10 Juvenile nasopharyngeal angiofibroma in a 10-year-old boy. **A.** Preoperative embolization with particles of the arterial branches of the internal maxillary artery. **B.** Selective distal external carotid angiogram shows marked reduction in blood supply to this highly vascular tumor.

experienced angiographers. When obtaining consent for this procedure, the patient must know the rare but important risk of cord injury.

Gastrointestinal Bleeding

In children, localized gastrointestinal bleeding is usually secondary to duodenal ulcer and less frequently to gastric ulcer, Meckel's diverticulum, and vascular malformations. Diffuse bleeding can occur in vasculitis and coagulopathy.

Meckel's diverticulum is the most frequent congenital anomaly of the intestinal tract. It is related to the persistence of the omphalomesenteric duct, which is normally obliterated between the fifth and seventh weeks of gestation. Bleeding is a result of ulceration of ileal mucosa adjacent to ectopic gastric mucosa within the diverticulum.

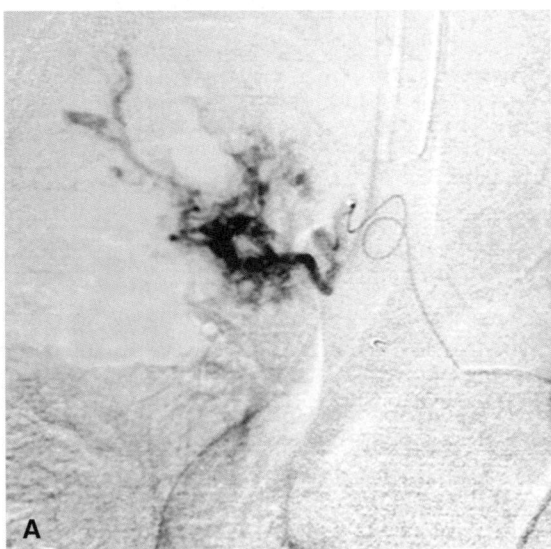
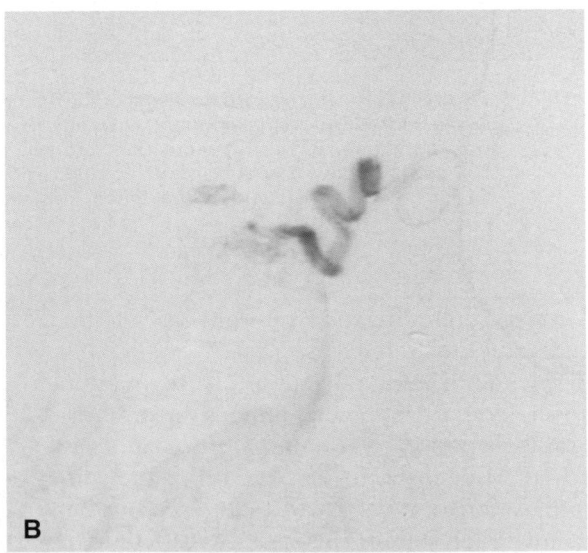

Figure 62–11 Hemoptysis in a 14-year-old child with cystic fibrosis. **A.** Selective catheterization shows the presence of a dilated and sinuous right intercostobronchial artery. **B.** Embolization with particles of 500–710 μ was performed. The angiographic control shows a complete occlusion. Hemoptysis was controlled.

On angiography, two small arteries arising from the antimesenteric side of the distal ileal artery can be seen surrounding the diverticulum (Figure 62–12). Mural enhancement of the diverticulum can be observed. No dilated vessels or arteriovenous fistulas are present.

Polyarteritis nodosa can involve mesenteric arteries. Small peripheral aneurysms are typically demonstrated. Stenosis or segmental thrombosis of small arterial branches are frequently encountered.

Gastrointestinal vascular anomalies (GIVA) are an uncommon cause of gastrointestinal bleeding. Confusing nomenclature has made objective comparisons of published cases difficult and has interfered with establishing a consensus regarding diagnosis and treatment. These benign vascular lesions are difficult to diagnose on barium studies and endoscopic examinations. A good knowledge of the different patterns encountered on CT, MR, and angiographic examinations is necessary to be able to diagnose and adequately classify GIVA (43). These anomalies are often associated with known syndromes such as Klippel-Trenaunay, Rendu-Osler-Weber disease, blue rubber-bleb nevus and Proteus syndrome. Therefore, the clinician must be aware of associated specific cutaneous or other systemic manifestations of these syndromes in order to make the correct diagnosis.

In our experience, venous malformations are the more common vascular anomaly encountered in cases of bleeding.

Angiography is the most useful examination to establish the nature and extent of vascular anomalies. Late opacification of dilated veins is characteristic of venous malformations (Figure 62–13). Preoperative angiography with superselective injection of methylene blue or indigo carmine is sometimes used to localize the bowel loop immediately prior to resection (44). Angiography of the specimen injected with diluted barium can be used to ensure that the venous malformation has been removed.

In children with gastrointestinal arteriovenous malformation, the angiographic examination confirms the diagnosis and the extent of the AVMs. Embolization is usually not recommended in small bowel and colonic lesions because of the risk of necrosis. Embolotherapy is sometimes considered preoperatively to lower the risk of operative bleeding.

Embolization/Sclerotherapy of Varicoceles

Varicoceles represent a frequent cause of male infertility. Already present in 15–20% of preadolescents and adolescents, variocele treatment in this age group remains controversial. Most authors, however, recommend the early treatment of grade 2 and grade 3 varicoceles, especially when coexisting with ipsilateral testicular growth arrest. Therapeutic alternatives can be subdivided into surgical or endoscopic techniques of cord vessels ligature, percutaneous radiological sclerotherapy or embolization of the internal spermatic vein, and mixed techniques (antegrade sclerotherapy via orchidotomy).

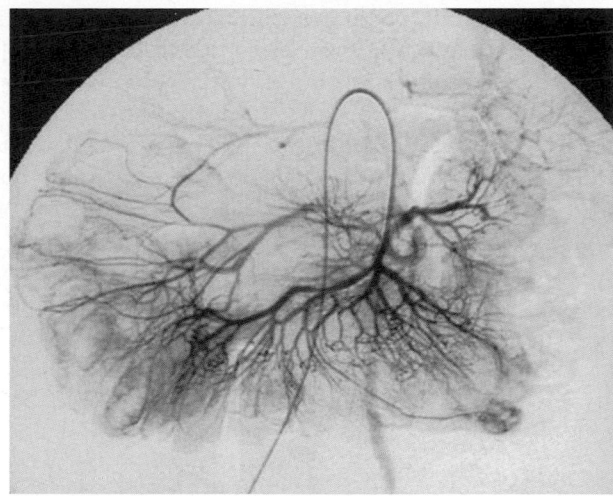

Figure 62–12   Five-year-old patient presenting with painless GI bleeding. Meckel's scan was negative. Selective superior mesenteric artery angiogram demonstrates the vitelline artery supplying a pediculated Meckel's diverticulum.

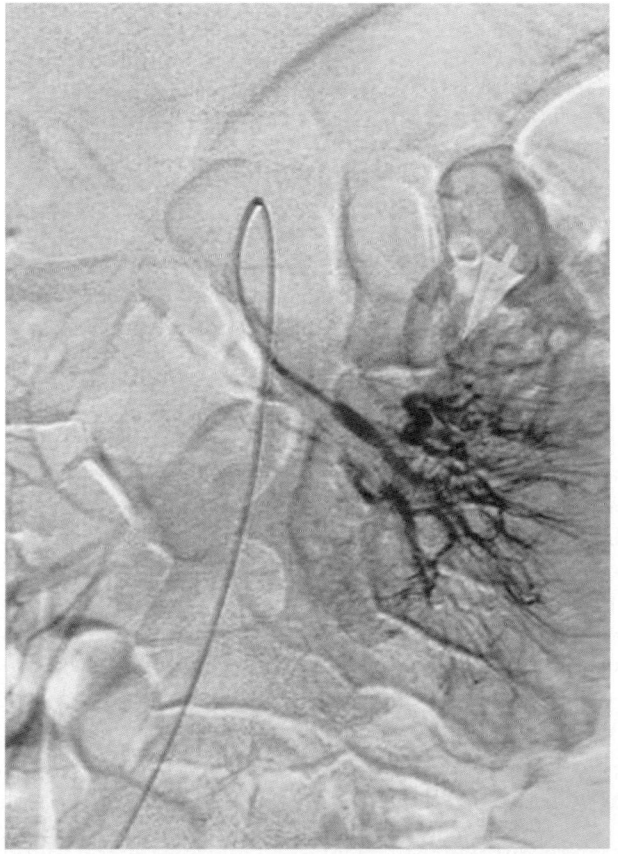

Figure 62–13   Sixteen-year-old boy with recurrent gastrointestinal bleeding. Superior mesenteric angiogram with selective catheterization of the second jejunal artery reveals dilated and tortuous draining veins. Methylene blue was injected just before the surgery for localizing the VM.

Most, if not all, paediatric varicoceles are left sided; the authors use the Bahren classification (45) of left varicocele anatomical variants: type I, single internal spermatique vein (ISV); type II, multiple ostia of ISV; type III, proximal branching of ISV; type IV, collaterals to ISV from segmental renal veins (IVa, incompetent ostial valve, IVb, competent ostial valve); and type V, double renal veins.

The authors' technical protocol for percutaneous endovascular occlusion of the ISV is as follows: IM or IV sedation by ketamine/midazolam, femoral vein approach, 7 French Cobra catheter with coaxial 3 French or Tracker 18 for distal sclerotherapy by sodium tetradecyl sulfate (STS) followed by more proximal coil occlusion, bed rest for 4 hours, and discharge 6 hours postprocedure. Follow-up consists of assessment of results by the referring surgeon 2 months later.

The authors' personal experience has shown a high incidence (44%) of anatomical variants in a pediatric population and specific technical difficulties of retrograde sclerotherapy in type IVb (12% of the authors' cases—failure rate, 50%) and in type V (14% of the authors' cases—failure rate, 33%). The authors' overall results (failure rate, 10%) are comparable with the recently reported pediatric series (46,47), either in the radiological or surgical literature. The debate about interventional radiology as the primary treatment is mostly correlated with the local availability of expertise and resources rather than with objective differences of results.

The surgical concern with retrograde sclerotherapy-related radiation has been addressed in the literature. An almost negligible gonad dose (0.01 m SV) is assured if the usual principles of radioprotection are observed.

Renal Artery Embolization and Trauma

Renal angiography is no longer needed for the diagnosis and grading of renal injuries, thanks to ultrasound, color Doppler ultrasound, and CT scan. Renal artery embolization can be indicated in two clinical situations: following blunt or penetrating trauma (including renal biopsy) or in relation to congenital vascular anomalies (AVM or aneurysm). In the authors' experience, most pediatric cases undergoing embolization are post-renal biopsy AV fistulas, either on native kidneys or on transplants. The authors favor a coaxial technique, allowing superselective catheterization and occlusion by microcoils, resulting in the sparing of all uninvolved renal branches (Figure 62–14).

Abdominal Trauma

A conservative management is the rule in pediatric abdominal trauma because most cases of splenic and hepatic vascular trauma resolve spontaneously. However, they require strict imaging follow-up until complete disappearance of these lesions.

Delayed or recurrent hemorrhage is the most common complication of trauma: 3–8% for hepatic injuries, 1.5% for liver–spleen, 6% for liver–spleen and pancreas, and 31% for pancreas (48). The bleeding is secondary to pseudoaneurysm with expanding hematoma and subsequent rupture.

This complication is suspected in a patient who needs transfusion, shows a drop in hemoglobin, or has persistent pain. If the patient is hemodynamically stable, a CT scan is indicated prior to angiography.

Ideally, embolization should be done as close as possible to the injury site to avoid functional parenchyma loss and to reduce the risk of secondary infection. The use of a coaxial microcatheter system (Tracker 18, Target Therapeutics) or 3 French focus microcatheter (Terumo) permits vessel occlusion close to the vascular lesion. A variety of embolic agents can be used: polyvinyl alcohol particles, isobutyl-2-cyanoacrylate, alcohol, and microcoils. The first choice for the occlusion of pseudoaneuryms is microcoil deposition on both sides of the pseudoaneurysm neck or particles (Figure 62–15) (48). Gelfoam is a temporary occluding agent and carries the risk of future recanalization. When the endoarterial route is difficult, a direct percutaneous approach under Doppler use is an option. The correct needle placement is confirmed by contrast injection. The most commonly used agent is thrombine (Thrombostat, Parke-Davis). The authors inject with a syringe of 1 cc containing 1,000 units. First, the authors inject 200 units under Doppler ultrasound, and if the flow is still present in the pseudoaneurysm, injection is repeated until reaching a maximum dose of 1,000 units. N-butyl cyanoacrylate, Gelfoam, or coils have also been injected percutaneously.

Splenic Embolization

In cases of hypersplenism, the hyperfunctioning spleen removes the red and white blood cells and the platelets from the circulation. The causes of hypersplenism are cirrhosis secondary to cystic fibrosis or biliary atresia, portal vein thrombosis, thalassemia, and idiopathic thrombocytopenic purpura. Hypersplenism is treated by surgical resection, which has an increased risk of infection in the pediatric age group. Partial splenic embolization is an alternative to splenectomy. Spigos developed a strict protocol for partial splenic embolization with a good response and few complications (49). The embolization is performed under general anesthesia in children with preprocedural and postprocedural antibiotic prophylaxis. A 5 French catheter is advanced through the femoral artery to the mid splenic artery. Subsequent catheterization into the intrasplenic arterial branches is performed either with the 5 French catheter or with a coaxial system with microcatheter if necessary. Embolization is carried out by injection of polyvinyl alcohol particles and antibiotic solution containing 0.2 mg of ampicillin. Splenic embolization is monitored angiographically during the procedure, and embolization is stopped after

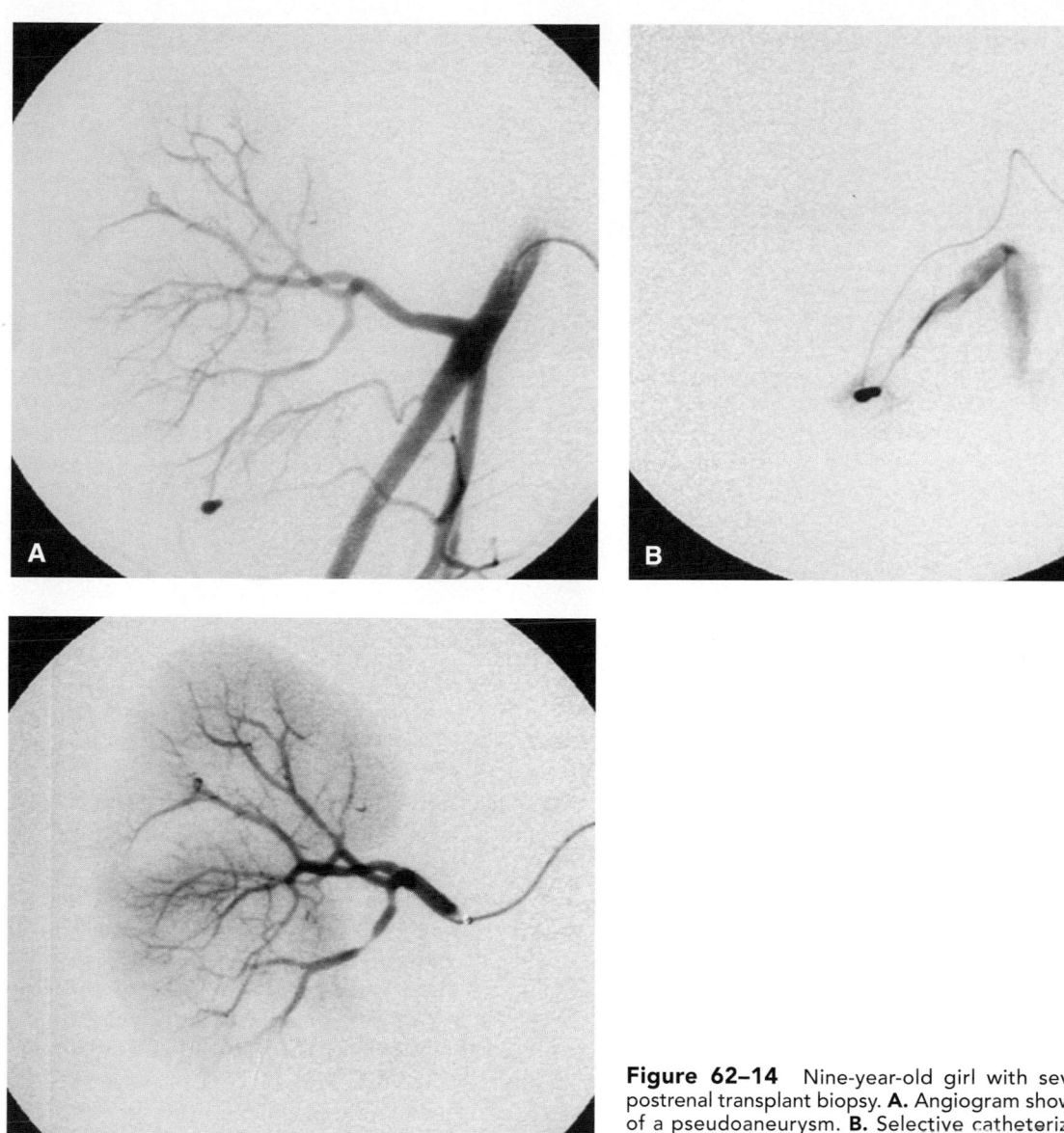

Figure 62–14 Nine-year-old girl with severe hematuria postrenal transplant biopsy. **A.** Angiogram shows the presence of a pseudoaneurysm. **B.** Selective catheterization was performed, and occlusion was done with a coil. **C.** Control angiogram shows complete exclusion of the pseudoaneurysm.

approximately 70% of the splenic parenchyma is devascularized. Aggressive pain control is needed for 7–10 days after the procedure. In children, Harned (50) demonstrated that 30–40% embolization of splenic blood flow is enough to improve the platelet count and white blood cells with a shorter hospitalization, faster recovery, and fewer complications. Fever, leucocytosis, pain, pleural effusion, splenic abscess, and peritonitis are known complications of splenic embolization. The long-term remission after partial splenic embolization has not been established. Kimura et al. (51) reported a 51% response to the initial embolization and the need for subsequent procedures in cases of chronic idiopathic thrombocytopenic purpura.

PERCUTANEOUS TRANSLUMINAL ANGIOPLASTY (PTA)

Renal Artery Stenosis

Renovascular disease (RVD) is the cause of hypertension in approximately 10% of children. RVD is associated with considerable morbidity and mortality.

Fibromuscular dysplasia is the most common cause of renal artery stenosis (RAS). In the pediatric age group, the investigations are crucial to define the precise underlying etiology and, accordingly, to provide the most adequate management.

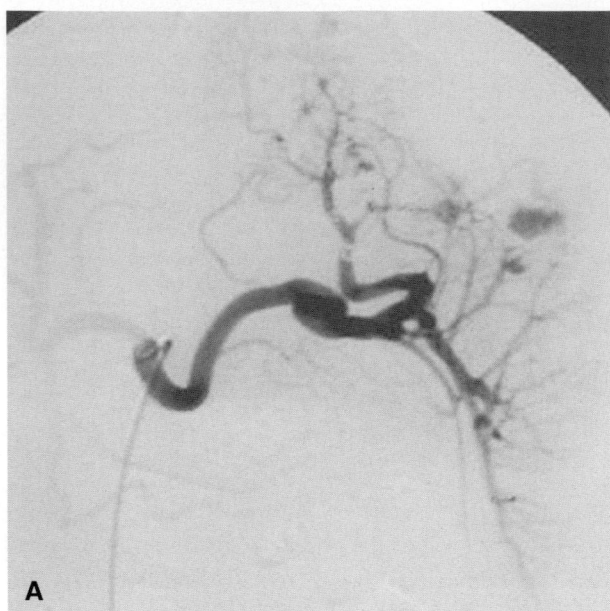
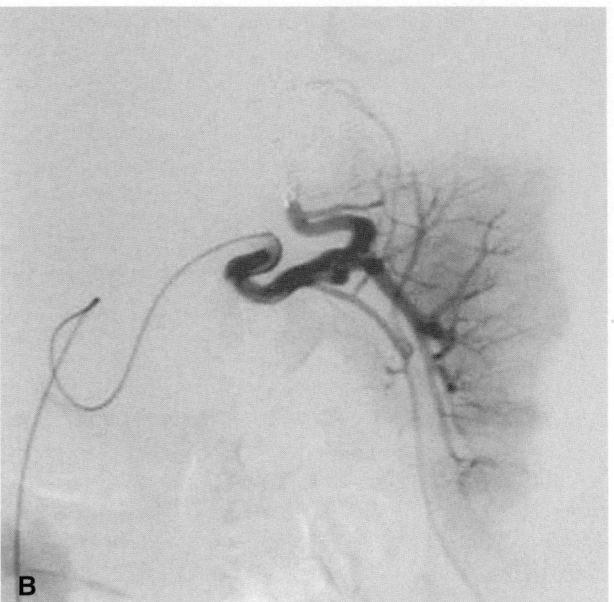

Figure 62–15   Splenic trauma in a 13-year-old boy. **A.** An angiogram demonstrates a laceration of the spleen with multiple pseudoaneurysms. **B.** Particles and coils were used to occlude the upper pole of the spleen.

Hypertension is defined as blood pressure above the ninety-fifth percentile for age, sex, and height (52). The recognition of RVD is theoretically based on the peripheral venous plasma renin activity (PRA). However, the PRA increase is seen in only 30–100% of cases, depending on series (53).

The accurate diagnosis of RVD in hypertensive children remains difficult. The initial imaging modality is always ultrasound, complemented by color Doppler. After having excluded diffuse parenchymal diseases (e.g., reflux nephropathy, glomerulopathies, hydronephrosis, etc.) and renal tumor or pheochromocytomas by ultrasound, the next investigation in pediatric hypertension is renal angiography and selective renin venous samplings. Contrast angiography is currently the only reliable way to diagnose renal artery stenosis. The correlation of vascular anatomy and renal venous assays is the rationale for offering endovascular, surgical, or medical treatment.

General anesthesia with control of respiration should be performed because it results in high-quality subtraction angiograms. An initial aortogram is performed, sometimes including oblique views. Selective renal artery injections are performed with AP and oblique views. It is important to verify by a careful analysis of the parenchymal phase that an accessory artery has not been overlooked.

Selective and superselective venous samplings are variably evaluated in the literature. In the authors' opinion, such samplings are highly useful in the pediatric age group. All drugs should be withheld prior to the procedure.

Venous samples are drawn at the same time as angiography. Samples are obtained from both kidneys as well as from the main renal vein and supra- and infrarenal inferior vena cava. Segmental samples are important for the assessment of segmental disease (54).

Fibromuscular dysplasia is the cause of renovascular hypertension in 40–70% of cases (55). The usual pattern is a weblike stenosis rather than the string of beads involving the main renal artery beyond its origin. Bilateral involvement is seen in 40% of cases. Small-vessel involvement occurs in 35% of fibromuscular dysplasia, and unilateral segmental involvement in 10%. Fifty percent of polar or intrarenal artery stenosis is found in children with fibromuscular dysplasia. Aneurysm can be associated with stenosis. The natural history is characterized by progression in 16–38% of patients within 10 years without resulting in complete occlusion (55). Exceptionally, disappearance of RAS with normalization of blood pressure has been reported.

Middle Aortoarteriopathy Syndrome (MAS)

This syndrome consists of severe stenosis of the descending thoracic and/or abdominal aorta, commonly including the ostia of the renal and visceral arteries, and it causes severe hypertension (Figure 62–16). The underlying etiologies are Takayasu arteritis, noninflammatory aortoarteriopathy, and, most commonly in North America, fibromuscular dysplasia and neurofibromatosis. This lesion is often referred to as abdominal coarctation. In MAS, percutaneous endoluminal angioplasty has been of limited success. Endovascular stenting has been used in the abdominal aorta.

The diagnosis of Takayasu arteritis theoretically relies on the association of multiple irregular and progressive

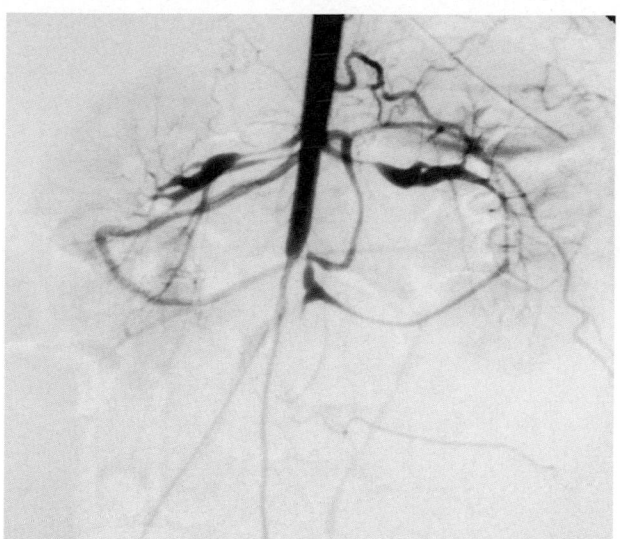

Figure 62–16 Middle aortic syndrome. Oblique abdominal aortography in an 18-month-old infant with middle aortic syndrome and Takayasu's arteritis. Multiple severe ostial stenoses are displayed along the renal arteries, coeliac trunk, and superior mesenteric artery.

stenotic abnormalities in the aorta and main branches, including renal arteries, and on inflammatory biological markers. The latter are rarely found when the arterial stenoses are displayed. McCulloch (56) reported a high incidence of fusiform and saccular aneurysms.

Neurofibromatosis type 1 is an autosomal dominant neurocutaneous syndrome with a developmental disorder of the neural crest. It is characterized by dysplastic and neoplastic lesions involving the neural and ectodermal tissues. The classic manifestations are café au-lait spots, cutaneous neurofibromas, axillary or inguinal freckling, sphenoid bone dysplasia, optic gliomas, iris hamartomas, and a dominant family history. One percent of patients with neurofibromatosis develop hypertension. McTaggart et al. (53) reported in their series of hypertensive Australian children that neurofibromatosis was the most common etiology (58% of patients) and that there were no cases of Takayasu arteritis. The radiological appearance of vascular neurofibromatosis was often identical to the appearance of either isolated fibromuscular dysplasia (FMD) or midaortic syndrome and was not helpful for the diagnostic recognition of neurofibromatosis (Figure 62–17).

Other pathology can cause renovascular hypertension in children. Williams syndrome is a congenital syndrome associated with a chromosomal deletion, characterized by mental retardation, ocular defect, hypercalcemia, and elfin facies. The cardiovascular anomalies consist of aortic supravalvular stenosis, abdominal aortic hypoplasia, and unilateral or bilateral renal artery stenosis. PTA is a failure in most (if not all) cases.

Pheochromocytomas are more often multiple in children than in adults. Renal artery stenosis associated with

pheochromocytoma is a result of direct arterial compression, fibrous bands that will need subsequent angioplasty, or catecholamine-induced vasospasm. Pheochromocytomas are diagnosed by laboratory workup, ultrasound, and CT.

Neuroblastoma and ganglioneuroblastoma can behave like pheochromocytoma and also be associated with coexisting RAS.

Periarteritis nodosa is another cause of RAS. The angiography pattern is characteristic with intrarenal microaneurysms of the small- and medium-size arteries. The presence of medium-size and large aneurysms is significantly associated with the presence of renal impairment and hypertension. Nonaneurysmal changes were detected more commonly on renal angiography than aneurysms in the PAN group reported by Brogan et al. (57). The most reliable nonaneurysmal signs were perfusion defects, the presence of collateral arteries, lack of crossing of peripheral renal arteries, and delayed emptying of small renal arteries. Aneurysms were also demonstrated on hepatic and mesenteric angiography. Renal artery stenosis has also been seen as a complication of Kawasaki disease.

Percutaneous transluminal angioplasty (PTA) or surgical revascularization is required for children with RAS to preserve renal function, prevent injury to other organs, and obviate or decrease the need for long-term antihypertensive medication.

In pediatric patients, percutaneous transluminal angioplasty (PTA) is feasible, with a low incidence of technical failure and a lower risk than surgery (Figure 62–18). According

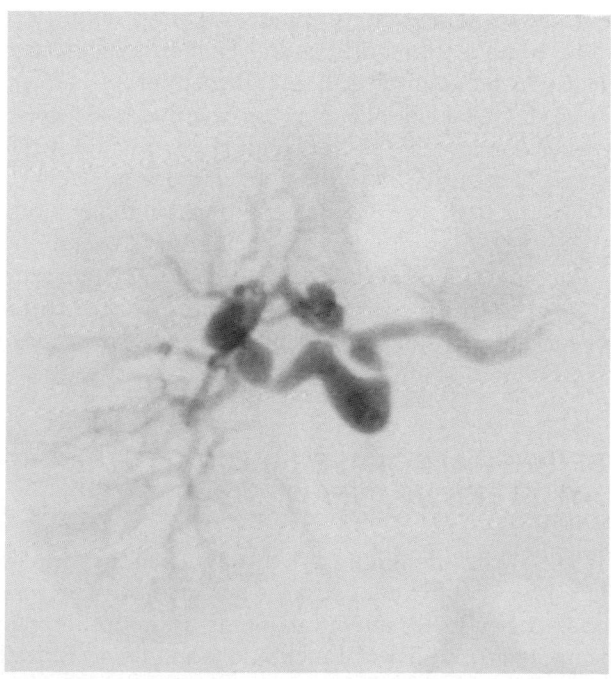

Figure 62–17 Neurofibromatosis. Selective right renal angiogram in a 14-year-old girl with neurofibromatosis. Multiple stenoses with poststenotic ectasias are displayed. Similar lesions were also demonstrated within the left kidney.

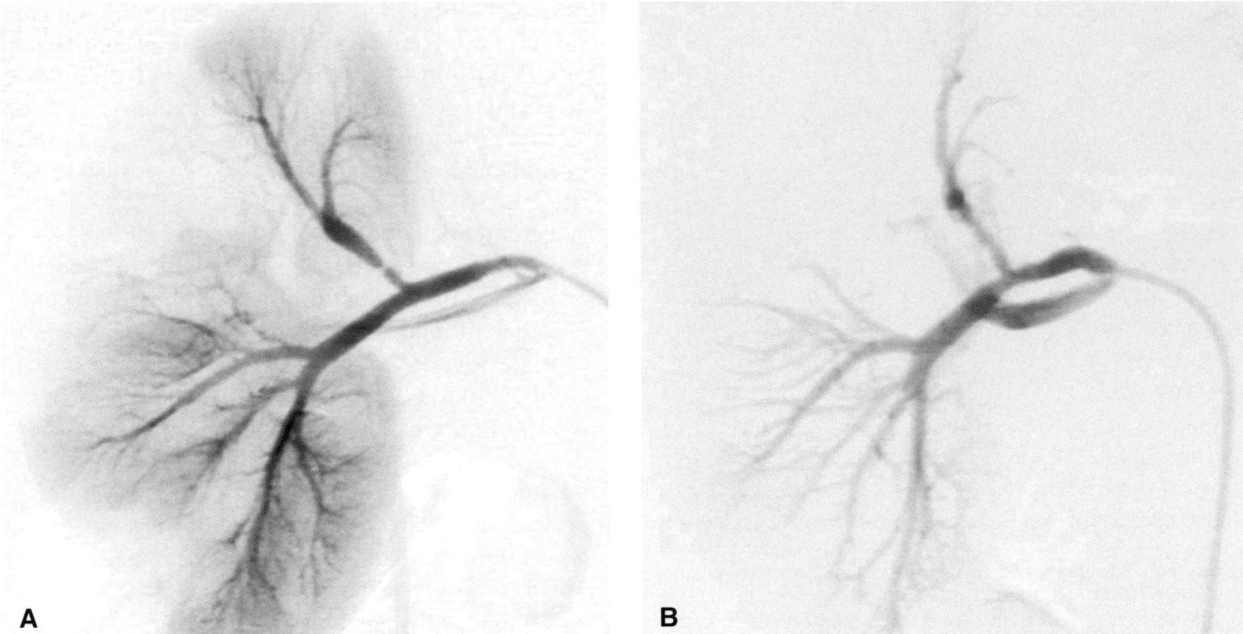

Figure 62–18   PTA. Four-year-old girl presenting with severe hypertension. **A.** Selective angiogram of the right renal artery: Evidence of fibromuscular dysplasia is seen within an intrarenal upper pole branch. **B.** Postangioplasty angiogram: No residual stenosis is shown. Blood pressure was normalized.

to the literature, PTA has a cure rate of 50% in FMD. Miranda et al. (58) reported a cure rate of 46 of 163, improvement in 45 of 163, and no change in 9. The authors' personal experience with PTA in FMD pediatric patients has been rewarding. The results are far better in cases of FMD compared with those in cases of neurofibromatosis (53) or vasculitis.

The complications of PTA are renal artery dissection, renal artery perforation, and local hematoma.

Selective renal embolization has been successful to treat hypertension in children but is not always totally effective because of the capacity of the kidney to develop collateral vessels. The best agent for selective renal embolization is alcohol. Intrarenal injection of alcohol can be complicated by death in relation either to the flow of alcohol in the adrenal artery, to cardiac toxicity, or to pulmonary hypertension.

Renal autotransplantation or bypass grafts are proposed mainly in MAS or after failure of PTA.

PERIPHERALLY INSERTED CENTRAL CATHETERS IN INFANTS

The use of peripherally inserted central venous catheters (PICC) for central venous access has markedly increased during the past decade. Outpatients on antibiotherapy, chemotherapy, or hyperalimentation, and the technically challenging inpatients needing a long or intermediate duration IV access account for such an increase in the insertion of PICC lines.

PICC lines are inserted by interventional radiologists, clinicians, residents, and nurse practitioners, depending on the institution. Many reports in the literature address the indications, the technique, and the complications. Most of the challenging PICC line insertions are related to low-birth-weight babies and infants with difficult vascular access. Described next is the authors' technique, which has proved useful in such cases.

Technique

No preprocedural routine laboratory tests or prophylactic antibiotics are needed. The authors recommend 3 hours NPO before the sedation.

PICC placement is performed in the angiography suite with a C-arm fluoroscopy under venographic guidance. Ultrasound guidance is difficult to use in infants because of the poor turgor and the mobility of the veins in this age group.

The patient's arms are prepared from the axilla to the hand using a Duraprep and draped in a standard sterile fashion. For the purpose of phlebography, the wrist veins are used most of the time, with a 27-gauge needle. Sometimes the authors puncture the finger veins. A sterile tourniquet is tightened below the shoulder.

Venous opacification is performed with nonionic contrast material, in a 3-cc syringe for small babies. Single- or double-wall venipuncture with a 24-gauge sheath needle is performed under fluoroscopy. When an intraluminal position is confirmed by return of blood, a 0.018-inch (0.46-mm) straight or angled guide wire is advanced to the superior vena cava (Glidewire, Terumo). The sheath is then withdrawn.

After local anesthesia (xylocaine 1% with bicarbonate), the puncture site is widened with a scalpel blade. The puncture site is dilated with a 4 French dilator over the guide wire. Occasionally, an intermediate dilatation with a 22-gauge sheath is useful.

The length of catheter is decided according to a local reference chart, depending on the entry vein and the side, or by draping the catheter externally along the patient.

The 18-gauge (3.5 F) polyurethane catheter is inserted over the guide wire (59). In babies weighing less than 1500 gm, the authors use a 20-gauge catheter with the same technique except for the use of a 0.014-inch guide wire.

The tip of the catheter is located at the junction of the superior vena cava and right atrium. T6 was reported to be the best landmark for an adequate location of the junction of superior vena cava and the right atrium in children (Figure 62–19) (60).

The catheter is flushed with heparin lock solution, and a short connector is attached to the hub of the PICC. Fixation is accomplished with skin-closure strips (Steri-Strip, 3M) covered by a moisture-responsive canula dressing (Opsite M3000, Smith and Nephew).

Technical Problems

In rare cases of failed access over the hand, a femoral vein approach can be used. When applying the tourniquet and performing the phlebogram in premature infants, the authors observe clinically numerous white spots over the skin and sometimes spots of contrast leaks resulting from the immaturity of the infant's vascular system. The authors have frequently noted these capillary leaks without sequelae.

Mechanical complications (dislodgment, cracks and fractures, lumen occlusion) occur in about 7% of all cases of PICC in children (61).

Pleural effusion related to vascular erosion by PICC line occurs through semicentral tip location (right and left brachiocephalic veins). Cardiac tamponade (including death) resulting from pericardial perforation is reported in the pediatric literature only in relation to blind bedside insertion (62). Paraplegia was also reported as a complication of inappropriate location of the catheter tip after blind bedside insertion through the great saphenous or femoral veins (63).

The authors favor the peripheral insertion over the central access to preserve central veins and to decrease the incidence of complications: mechanical complications, infection, and thrombosis. The overall frequency of central vein thrombosis after central access varies from 11–50%, and 30–86% of these are asymptomatic. PICC are associated with fewer complications (3.8%) than central lines or noncentrally placed catheters (28.8%) (64).

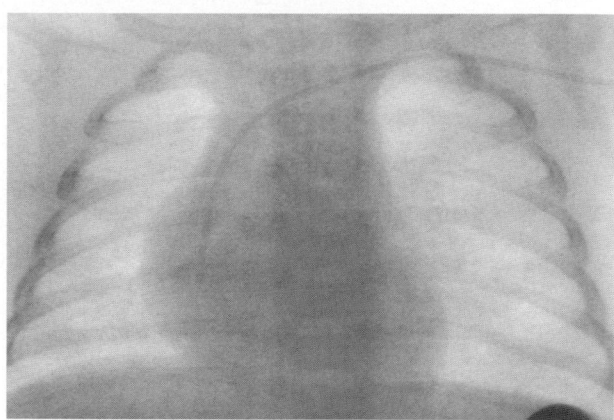

Figure 62–19 Chest radiograph after 18-gauge PICC placement in the left basilic vein of a 2.8-kg baby for hyperalimentation. The tip of the catheter projects at the T6 level, the landmark of SVC–RA junction.

MISCELLANEOUS VASCULAR PROCEDURES

Foreign Body Removal

Modern medicine, with its complex monitoring systems, indwelling catheters, and interventional radiology, is associated with an increase in intravascular foreign bodies. These vascular foreign bodies may be catheter fragments, pieces of guide wires, electrodes, or ventriculoatrial shunt tubing. Large intravascular fragments are believed to be a risk of thrombosis, hemorrhage, and arrhythmia. Snares, deflectable guide wires, wire baskets, and intravascular forceps may be used to retrieve these objects (65,66).

Transjugular Liver Biopsy

Transjugular liver biopsy is performed in children who are at risk for percutaneous biopsy resulting from coagulopathy. The technique is the same as in adults, and, unfortunately, current equipment sets preclude this procedure in extremely small children.

REFERENCES

1. MacPherson DS. Preoperative laboratory testing: should any tests be "routine" before surgery? Med Clin North Am 1993;77: 289–308.
2. Saker MC, Uejima T. Management of the pediatric patient for interventional radiologic procedures. Semin Intervent Radiol 2002;19:3–11.
3. American Academy of Pediatrics Committee on Drugs. Guidelines for monitoring and management of pediatric patients during and after sedation for diagnostic and therapeutic procedures. Pediatrics 1992;89:1110–1115.
4. Mason KP, Zurakowski D, Karian VE, et al. Sedatives used in pediatric imaging: comparison of IV pentobarbital with IV pentobarbital with midazolam added. AJR Am J Roentgenol 2001;177: 427–430.

5. Krauss B, Green SM. Sedation and analgesia for procedures in children. N Engl J Med 2000;342:938–945.
6. Committee on Drugs and Contrast Media of the American College of Radiology. Manual on contrast media. 4th Ed. Reston, VA: American College of Radiology, 1998.
7. Freed MD, Keane JF, Rosenthal A. The use of heparinization to prevent arterial thrombosis after percutaneous cardiac catheterization in children. Circulation 1974;50:565–569.
8. Andrew M. Anticoagulation and thrombolysis in children. Tex Heart Inst J 1992;19:168–177.
9. Burrows PE. Variations in the vascular supply to infantile hepatic hemangioendotheliomas. Radiology 1991;181:631–632.
10. Mulliken JB, Glowacki J. Hemangiomas and vascular malformations in infants and children: a classification based on endothelial characteristics. Plast Reconstr Surg 1982;69:412–422.
11. Enjolras O, Riche MC, Merland JJ, et al. Management of alarming hemangiomas in infancy: a review of 25 cases. Pediatrics 1990; 85:491–498.
12. Mueller BU, Mulliken JB. The infant with a vascular tumor. Semin Perinatol 1999;23:332–340.
13. Enjolras O, Wassef M, Mazoyer E, et al. Infants with Kasabach-Merritt syndrome do not have "true" hemangiomas. J Pediatr 1997;130:631–640.
14. Hu B, Lachman R, Phillips J, et al. Kasabach-Merritt syndrome-associated kaposiform hemangioendothelioma successfully treated with cyclophosphamide, vincristine, and actinomycin D. J Pediatr Hematol Oncol 1998;20:567–569.
15. Folkman J, Mulliken JB, Ezekowitz RAB. Antiangiogenic therapy of hemangiomas with interferon-alpha. In: Stuart-Harris R, Penny RD, eds. Clinical Applications of the Interferons. London: Chapman Hall–Medical, 1997:255–265.
16. Folkman J, Klagsbrun M, Sasse J, et al. A heparin-binding angiogenic protein—basic fibroblast growth factor—is stored within basement membrane. Am J Pathol 1988;130:393–400.
17. Burrows PE, Mulliken JB, Fellows KE, et al. Childhood hemangiomas and vascular malformations: angiographic differentiation. AJR Am J Roentgenol 1983;141:483–488.
18. Yakes WF, Luethke JM, Parker SH, et al. Ethanol embolization of vascular malformations. Radiographics 1990;10:787–796.
19. Mason KP, Michna E, Zurakowski D, et al. Serum ethanol levels in children and adults after ethanol embolization or sclerotherapy for vascular anomalies. Radiology 2000;217:127–132.
20. Mason KP, Neufeld EJ, Karian VE, et al. Coagulation abnormalities in pediatric and adult patients after sclerotherapy or embolization of vascular anomalies. AJR Am J Roentgenol 2001;177:1359–1363.
21. Burrows PE. Variations in the vascular supply to infantile hepatic hemangioendotheliomas. Radiology 1991;181:631–632.
22. McHugh K, Burrows PE. Infantile hepatic hemangioendotheliomas: significance of portal venous and systemic collateral arterial supply. J Vasc Interv Radiol 1992;3:337–344.
23. Fellows KE, Hoffer FA, Markowitz RI, et al. Multiple collaterals to hepatic infantile hemangioendotheliomas and arteriovenous malformations: effect on embolization. Radiology 1991; 181:813–818.
24. Kassarjian A, Dubois J, Burrows PE. Angiographic classification of hepatic hemangiomas in infants. Radiology 2002;222:693–698.
25. Burrows PE, Dubois J, Kassarjian A. Pediatric hepatic vascular anomalies. Pediatr Radiol 2001;31:533–545.
26. Dubois J, Garel L, Grignon A, et al. Imaging of hemangiomas and vascular malformations in children. Acad Radiol 1998;5: 390–400.
27. Dubois J, Soulez G, Oliva VL, et al. Soft-tissue venous malformations in adult patients: imaging and therapeutic issues. Radiographics 2001;21:1519–1531.
28. Claudon M, Upton J, Burrows PE. Diffuse venous malformations of the upper limb: morphologic characterization by MRI and venography. Pediatr Radiol 2001;31:507–514.
29. Enjolras O, Ciabrini D, Mazoyer E, et al. Extensive pure venous malformations in the upper or lower limbs: a review of 27 cases. J Am Acad Dermatol 1997;36:219–225.
30. Berenguer B, Burrows PE, Zurakowski D, et al. Sclerotherapy of craniofacial venous malformations: complications and results. Plast Reconstr Surg 1999;104:1–11.
31. Lee BB, Kim DI, Huh S. New experiences with absolute ethanol sclerotherapy in the management of a complex form of congenital venous malformation. J Vasc Surg 2001;33:764–772.
32. Riche MC, Hadjean E, Tran-Ba-Huy P, et al. The treatment of capillary-venous malformations using a new fibrosing agent. Plas Reconstr Surg 1983;71:607–614.
33. Dubois JM, Sebag GH, De Prost Y, et al. Soft-tissue venous malformations in children: percutaneous sclerotherapy with Ethibloc. Radiology 1991;180:195–198.
34. Hancock BJ, St-Vil D, Luks FI, et al. Complications of lymphangiomas in children. J Pediatr Surg 1992;27:220–224.
35. Dubois J, Garel L. Practical aspect of intervention in vascular anomalies in children. Semin Intervent Radiol 2002;19:73–87.
36. Shiels WE. Focused sclerotherapy of macrocystic lymphatic malformations. Presented at the annual meeting of the Society for Pediatric Radiology, San Francisco, 2003.
37. Guibaud L, Herbreteau D, Dubois J, et al. Aneurysmal bone cysts: percutaneous embolization with an alcoholic solution of zein—series of 18 cases. Radiology 1998;208:369–373.
38. Dubois J, Chigot V, Grimard G, et al. Sclerotherapy in aneurysmal bone cysts in children: a review of 17 cases. Pediatr Radiol 2003;33:365–372.
39. Lasjaunias P. Nasopharyngeal angiofibromas: hazards of embolization. Radiology 1980;136:119–123.
40. Valvanis A. Embolization of intracranial and skull base tumors, In: Valvanis A, ed. Interventional Neuroradiology. New York: Springer-Verlag 1993;77–83.
41. McDougall RJ, Sherrington CA. Fatal pulmonary haemorrhage during anaesthesia for bronchial artery embolization in cystic fibrosis. Paediatr Anaesth 1999;9:345–348.
42. Barben J, Robertson D, Olinsky A, et al. Bronchial artery embolization for hemoptysis in young patients with cystic fibrosis. Radiology 2002;224:124–130.
43. Fishman SJ, Burrows PE, Leichtner AM, et al. Gastrointestinal manifestations of vascular anomalies in childhood: varied etiologies require multiple therapeutic modalities. J Pediatr Surg 1998;33:1163–1167.
44. Frémond B, Yazbeck S, Dubois J, et al. Intestinal vascular anomalies in children. J Pediatr Surg 1997;32:873–877.
45. Bahren W, Lenz M, Porst H, et al. Side effects, complications and contraindications for percutaneous sclerotherapy of the internal spermatic vein in the treatment of idiopathic varicocele. Rofo 1983;128:172–179.
46. Lopez C, Serres-Cousine O, Averous M. Varicocele in adolescents. Treatment by sclerotherapy and percutaneous embolization: reflections on the method. Apropos of 23 cases. Prog Urol 1998;8:382–387.
47. Ficarra V, Porcaro AB, Righetti R, et al. Antegrade scrotal sclerotherapy in the treatment of varicocele: a prospective study. BJU Int 2002;89:264–268.
48. Goffette PP, Laterre PF. Traumatic injuries: imaging and intervention in post-traumatic complications (delayed intervention). Eur Radiol 2002;12:994–1021.
49. Spigos DG, Tan WS, Mozes MF, et al. Splenic embolization. Cardiovasc Intervent Radiol 1980;3:282–287.
50. Harned RK 2nd, Thompson HR, Kumpe DA, et al. Partial splenic embolization in five children with hypersplenism: effects of reduced-volume embolization on efficacy and morbidity.Radiology. 1998;209:803–806.
51. Kimura F, Itoh H, Ambiru S, et al. Long-term results of initial and repeated partial splenic embolization for the treatment of chronic idiopathic thrombocytopenic purpura. AJR Am J Roentgenol 2002;179:1323–1326.
52. Report of the second task force on blood pressure control in children—1987. Task force on blood pressure control in children. National Heart, Lung, and Blood Institute, Bethesda, Maryland.
53. McTaggart SJ, Gulati S, Walker RG, et al. Evaluation and long-term outcome of pediatric renovascular hypertension. Pediatr Nephrol 2000;14:1022–1029.
54. Garel L, Dubois J, Robitaille P, et al. Renovascular hypertension in children: curability predicted with negative intrarenal Doppler US results. Radiology 1995;195:401–405.

55. Youngberg SP, Sheps SG, Strong CG. Fibromuscular disease of the renal arteries. Med Clin North Am 1977;61:623–641.
56. McCulloch M, Andronikou S, Goddard E, et al. Angiographic features of 26 children with Takayasu's arteritis. Pediatr Radiol 2003;33:230–235.
57. Brogan PA, Davies R, Gordon I, et al. Renal angiography in children with polyarteritis nodosa. Pediatr Nephrol 2002;17:277–283.
58. Miranda F Jr, Perez M del C, Plavnik F, et al. Percutaneous transluminal angioplasty in the treatment of renovascular hypertension: sequential prospective study. Sao Paulo Med J 1998;116:1613–1617.
59. Dubois J, Garel L, Tapiero B, et al. Peripherally inserted central catheters in infants and children. Radiology 1997;204:622–626.
60. Connolly B, Mawson JB, McDonald CE, et al. Fluoroscopic landmark for SVC-RA junction for central venous catheter placement in children. Pediatr Radiol 2000;30:692–695.
61. Chait PG, Ingram J, Phillips-Gordon C, et al. Peripherally inserted central catheters in children. Radiology 1995;197:775–778.
62. Nadroo AM, Lin J, Green RS, et al. Death as a complication of peripherally inserted central catheters in neonates. J Pediatr 2001;138:599–601.
63. Chen CC, Tsao PN, Yau KI. Paraplegia: complication of percutaneous central venous line malposition. Pediatr Neurol 2001;24:65–68.
64. Racadio JM, Doellman DA, Johnson ND, et al. Pediatric peripherally inserted central catheters: complication rates related to catheter tip location. Pediatrics 2001;107:E28.
65. Selby JB, Tegtmeyer CJ, Bittner GM. Experience with new retrieval forceps for foreign body removal in the vascular, urinary, and biliary systems. Radiology 1990;176:535–538.
66. Yedlicka JW Jr, Carlson JE, Hunter DW, et al. Nitinol gooseneck snare for removal of foreign bodies: experimental study and clinical evaluation. Radiology 1991;178:691–693.

Abscess Drainage

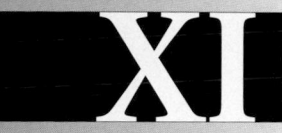

Percutaneous Treatment of Abdominal Abscesses

63

Debra A. Gervais, Steven L. Dawson

ETIOLOGY OF ABDOMINAL ABSCESSES

Abscess formation represents one of three possible outcomes in a patient with acute bacterial peritonitis (1). If the size of the bacterial innoculum is relatively small or the patient's host defense mechanisms are effective, then peritonitis may occur followed by complete resolution of the acute inflammatory process. If there is massive bacterial contamination or if the patient is immunocompromised, then fulminant peritonitis and death may occur. Abscess formation may be considered a "draw" between the host's defense mechanisms and the bacterial contaminants.

Abscess formation is the result of a specific set of events occurring within the abdomen. The physiologic flow of fluid spreads the contaminants throughout the abdomen and toward the diaphragm, allowing exposure to the greatest surface area of cell-mediated host defense mechanisms. As noted by Fry et al., the diaphragmatic fenestrations are the lymphatic channels by which macromolecules are resorbed from the peritoneum (1). If the volume of bacteria-laden fluid exceeds the body's capability for effective clearance, then the infected fluid gravitates toward well-defined regions within the abdomen, including the subphrenic, subhepatic, and pelvic spaces, thus explaining the most common locations for abdominal abscesses.

Approximately two thirds of abdominal abscesses occur after abdominal operations, and nearly one third are caused by a perforated viscus (2) (Figure 63–1).

THERAPY: SURGICAL AND MEDICAL

Traditionally, there have been two methods of therapy for intra-abdominal abscesses. Medical therapy based on antibiotic use alone is associated with a mortality rate above 50% (3). Although antibiotics play an important adjunctive role in the treatment of abdominal infection, they must not be the sole method of therapy and must not prevent primary surgical or radiologic drainage when signs of sepsis and clinical deterioration persist.

As noted by Gerzof et al. (4), "Percutaneous nonoperative catheter drainage is a significant departure from universally

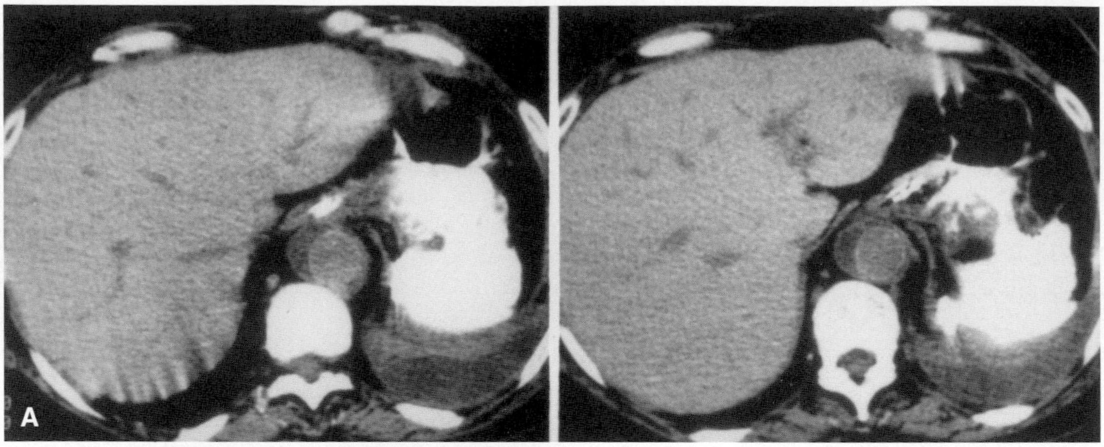

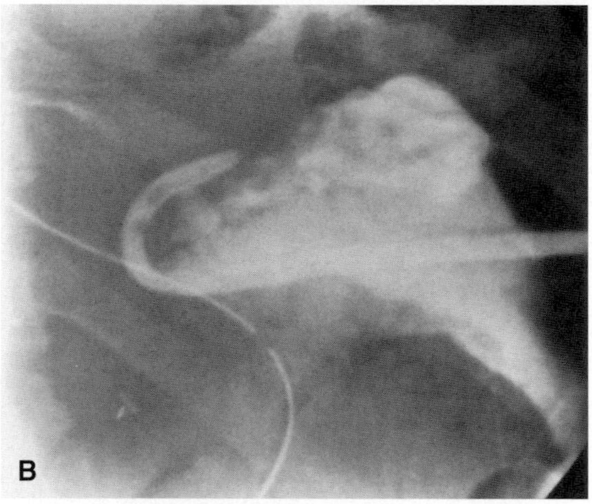

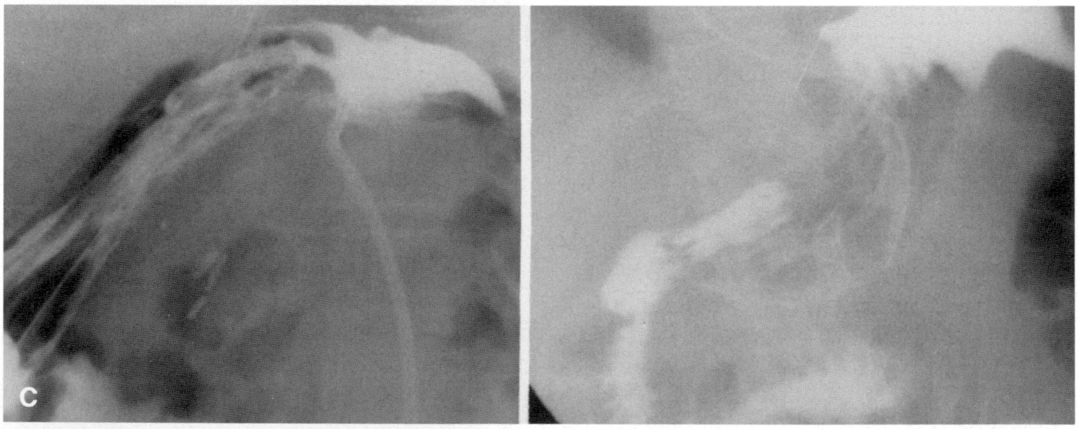

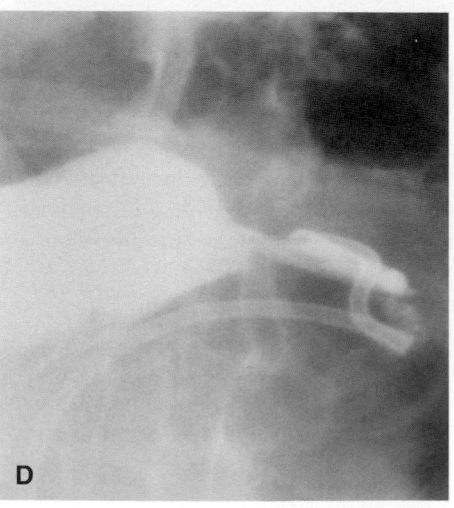

Figure 63–1 This 54-year-old woman developed a subphrenic abscess after repair of a thoracoabdominal aneurysm, with splenectomy. **A.** CT scans obtained 5 days after surgery. The left image shows contrast leaking from the gastric fundus into the subphrenic space. On the right, a widely patent gastric perforation is seen in the posterior fundal wall with accumulation of dense gastrograffin in the left subphrenic space. **B.** A 16 French catheter was placed into the collection, and contrast injection shows the left subphrenic space. **C.** Lateral (*left*) and anteroposterior (*right*) films after contrast injection show opacification of the stomach via the posterior fundal perforation, with the catheter in good position. The patient was maintained on bowel rest using hyperalimentation and nasogastric suction with subsequent gastrostomy tube placement. **D.** Right posterior oblique spot film, 3 months after the initial study, shows a smaller communication with the gastric fundus with no residual abscess collection in the subphrenic space. Drainage ceased, and the communication closed 10 days after this film. The catheter was removed.

accepted but heretofore unchallenged surgical methods of operative incision and drainage for therapy of abdominal abscess." The basic tenets of surgical abscess drainage were stated by Ochsner, DeBakey, and Murray in 1938—that drainage should be direct and simple, and it should avoid unnecessary contamination of uninvolved areas (5). Image-guided abscess drainage provides a rapid means of therapy (6), and percutaneous drainage routes usually closely parallel the specific operative approaches suggested for abscesses in similar locations.

Percutaneous catheter therapy and open surgical drainage should not be considered as two mutually exclusive therapies. Percutaneous drainage is the treatment of choice for abdominal abscesses, but when surgery will still be required, preoperative catheter drainage will allow improvements of the patient's condition to permit surgery in the most favorable physiologic condition.

PERCUTANEOUS THERAPY

Percutaneous therapy of abdominal abscesses begins with establishing the diagnosis of an abscess. Although this may seem obvious, it is not a simple matter, particularly in the postoperative patient, in whom signs and symptoms of infection from any of several anatomic sites are common and not specific. Computed tomography (CT) and ultrasound characteristics of abscesses are well known but not specific. In fact, the differential diagnosis may include other processes, such as hematoma, seroma, biloma, lymphocele, primary and secondary malignancies, pancreatic pseudocysts, and fluid-filled loops of bowel.

Fever and elevated white count are seen in postoperative infections in the immunocompetent patient. Physical examination may be localizing but can be limited because antibiotic therapy in the febrile patient with an elevated white count can mask findings of early infection, causing a delay in the clinical diagnosis (2).

Radiologic diagnosis of abdominal abscess has improved with the introduction of ultrasound, magnetic resonance imaging (MRI), and CT. However, conventional radiologic methods continue to be used in the patient with clinical suspicion of intra-abdominal infection. The plain abdominal film is of limited value but does provide important clinical information. One study has reported that more than 70% of upper abdominal abscesses in 82 patients were visible in retrospect on plain abdominal radiographs but were correctly diagnosed prospectively in only 51% (7). Upright views reveal the presence of intraperitoneal free air and may demonstrate extraluminal air-fluid levels. Additionally, abdominal films may demonstrate retroperitoneal air or an abdominal fluid collection with adjacent mass effect. Contrast examinations of the gastrointestinal tract are generally of limited usefulness.

The two most useful examinations to diagnose abdominal abscess are ultrasound and CT. Ultrasound has the advantages of being inexpensive, portable, quick, and free of ionizing radiation. Patients who are obese, who have an ileus, or who have extensive surgical wounds may be difficult to examine (2). Ultrasound is the screening modality of choice in thin patients and in children (8).

Sonographically, some abscesses appear anechoic with good posterior through transmission. However, bloody or cellular fluid can appear as mixed echogenicity, or the collection may actually appear highly echogenic (9).

Ultrasound is particularly useful in evaluating multiloculated collections. Real-time sonographic monitoring has been advocated to document complete or nearly complete evacuation of the abscess after initial drainage. In 33% of patients with complex or multiseptated abscesses, sonography revealed residual fluid that required an additional drainage catheter for complete evacuation (10).

Although ultrasound is particularly useful in selected cases, CT is the preferred method to diagnose abdominal abscesses. With complete bowel opacification, accurate diagnosis is possible in more than 95% of patients with abscesses (11). In addition, because CT allows for the guidance of percutaneous drainage, it is an important therapeutic tool.

The appearance of an abscess on CT depends to some extent on location. In the liver, for example, abscesses may be low attenuation with respect to either nonenhanced or enhanced liver parenchyma, with Hounsfield measurements ranging from 2 to 36, reflecting their varying contents (12). However, abscesses may appear of homogeneous soft tissue attenuation (13). In fact, the composition and maturity of any abdominal fluid collection are so variable that, unless an extraluminal air-fluid level is seen, there are no absolute indications that a collection is infected. Any extraluminal collection is potentially an abscess.

Imaging studies should be considered complementary to diagnostic needle aspiration. Needle aspiration can confirm the presence of a collection, determine whether that collection is infected, and determine whether the material present in the collection is amenable to catheter drainage (14).

As an example, consider the case of a large symptomatic hematoma (Figure 63–2). The ability to achieve successful catheter drainage depends on the fluidity of the blood, which may not be portrayed accurately by CT or ultrasound images. The decision to pursue catheter drainage must be based on the results of needle aspiration (14).

This chapter considers sites and etiologies of specific intra-abdominal abscesses and discusses interventional techniques specific to these conditions. Broadly applicable descriptions of the appropriate imaging guidance for abscess drainage, tools and techniques, catheter care, and management of fistulas can be found in Chapter 64, Percutaneous Drainage of Pelvic Abscesses and Fluid Collections.

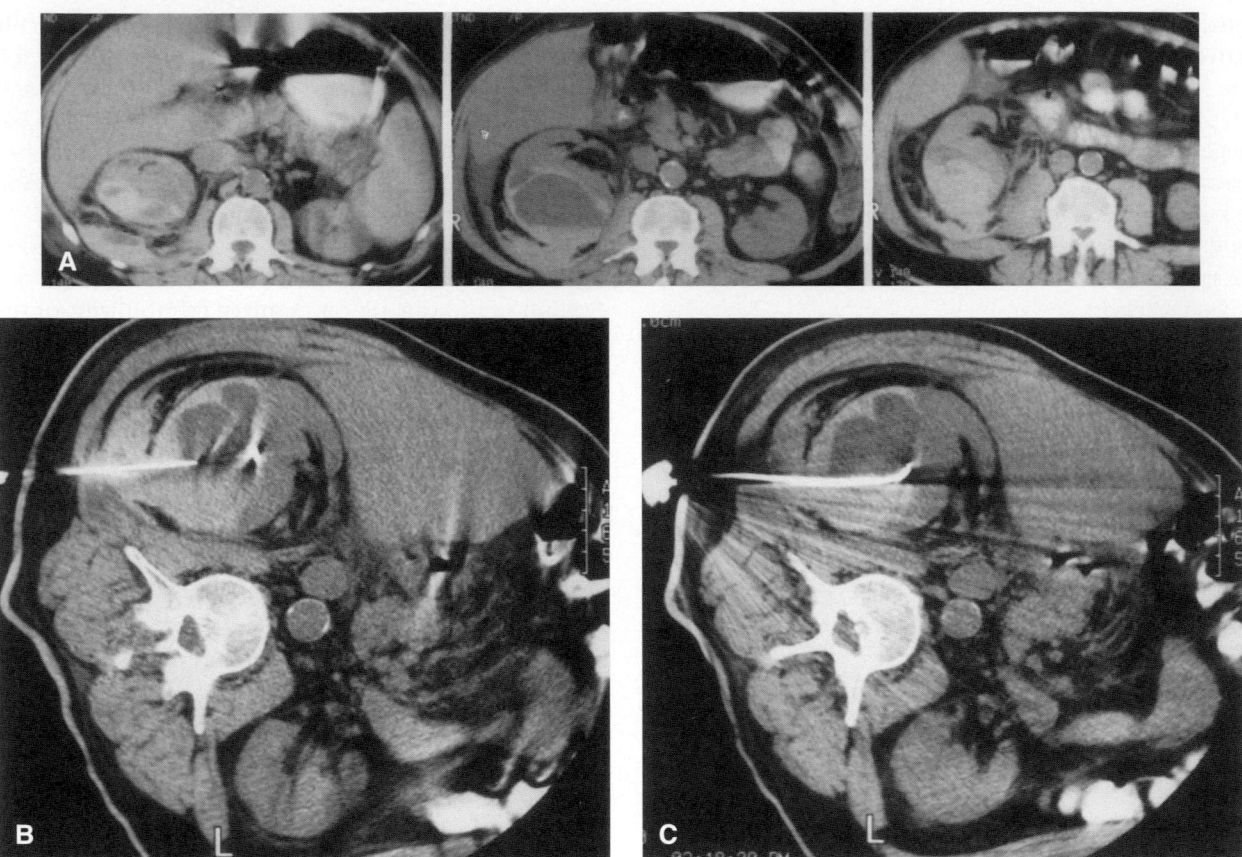

Figure 63-2 **A.** A 52-year-old patient on anticoagulants with complex right renal and posterior perirenal hematoma demonstrated on CT scan. The collection is loculated and consists of fluid and fresh blood components, with associated perirenal edema. Temperature and white count were elevated. **B.** With the patient in the left lateral decubitus position, the right renal cortical collection was aspirated using a 22-gauge needle, and frank pus was obtained. **C.** After diagnostic aspiration, a percutaneous drainage was performed via a posterolateral approach, with aspiration of bloody pus. Drainage continued for 8 days, after which the catheter was removed. (Courtesy of Michael J. Lee, MD.)

MORBIDITY AND MORTALITY: COMPARATIVE RESULTS

Despite the development and use of powerful antibiotics, intra-abdominal abscesses may still be associated with high morbidity and mortality. Delayed diagnosis and subsequent multisystem organ failure, inadequate localization of the abscess before drainage, and poor host defense mechanisms are cited as the etiologies for the failure of decline in morbidity and mortality (1). Clinical results of large published series indicate that percutaneous abscess drainage results in a better overall outcome with fewer complications, lower morbidity, and lower mortality compared with surgery. Johnson et al. evaluated 27 patients treated with percutaneous abscess drainage and 43 patients treated with surgical drainage and noted that the rate of complications (4% versus 16%), the rate of inadequate drainage (11% versus 21%), and the duration of drainage (17 versus 29 days) were lower in those patients treated percutaneously than in those treated surgically (15).

There are several reasons why percutaneous catheter drainage may be associated with a lower rate of complications and shorter postdrainage hospitalization than traditional open surgical drainage. As noted by Brolin et al. (3), patients treated with open surgical drainage had their abscesses diagnosed via imaging studies (CT or ultrasound) in only 51% of cases, as compared with 100% of those patients treated via percutaneous catheter drainage. In addition, open surgical drainage via midline incision has a greater potential for spreading contamination throughout the abdomen than does percutaneous drainage via the direct retroperitoneal approach suggested for treatment of subphrenic and other abdominal abscesses.

With percutaneous drainage, a shorter posthospitalization stay would also be anticipated. Patients are able to recuperate faster because they have not had general anesthesia and can be discharged from the hospital with small catheters in place, which can be cared for on an outpatient basis (3). Other contributing factors may include the more rapid institution of appropriate antibiotic regimens in those patients who have their abscesses diagnosed via percutaneous means (2,16).

LIVER ABSCESSES

In the 1938 review by Ochsner et al. (5), the most frequent cause of pyogenic hepatic abscess was pyelophlebitis secondary to acute appendicitis. Mortality was high because surgical drainage transgressed either the pleural or peritoneal space. Pyogenic liver abscess now more commonly results from prior abdominal surgery, trauma, neoplastic disease, biliary tract disease, or bacteremia in immunocompromised patients (17). Percutaneous therapy of pyogenic liver abscesses is considered the treatment of choice (15).

The ultrasound appearance of hepatic abscesses is variable, ranging from anechoic with marked posterior acoustic enhancement to echogenic with posterior shadowing. The walls may be well-defined or indistinct and may be irregular, thick, or imperceptible (18). Septations, fluid-fluid levels, and debris have all been noted.

The CT appearance is equally varied and may be nonspecific. Only when gas is detected within an intrahepatic fluid collection can a definitive imaging diagnosis of abscess be made, but this occurs in only approximately 19% of pyogenic liver abscesses (19,20). Pyogenic liver abscesses tend to be of lower attenuation than surrounding liver, but some peripheral enhancement may occur because of an inflammatory rind surrounding the abscess. The abscess may be detected more easily, and unsuspected additional abscesses may be discovered after contrast administration; however, according to Halvorsen et al. (19), no abscess was detected only on scans performed after contrast administration.

Immunosuppressed patients may have multifocal, tiny abscesses resulting from unusual organisms such as *Candida*. These collections generally are not amenable to percutaneous catheter drainage and typically are associated with a poor prognosis (21).

The differential diagnosis of hepatic abscess includes simple and complicated cysts, necrotic malignancies, echinococcal cysts, hematoma, and primary or metastatic cystadenocarcinoma (18).

Superficial abscesses in the left lobe and caudal aspect of the right lobe may be easily approached perpendicularly in the axial plane. Abscesses located high in the dome of the liver may require cephalocaudal angulation to avoid the pleura and may be approached with real-time ultrasound guidance or by CT using the triangulation approach (22). The entry site for aspiration and drainage is chosen according to the location of the abscess. Treatment begins with diagnostic needle aspiration using a 20- or 22-gauge needle. After the skin and subcutaneous tissue are infiltrated with 1% Xylocaine, the needle is inserted in a sterile fashion. A small amount of fluid is removed and sent for Gram stain, culture, and sensitivity. Gram stain should reveal both white blood cells and bacteria when an abscess is present. If

bowel has inadvertently been entered or if the patient is severely immunocompromised, bacteria without white blood cells will be seen on Gram stain. White cells without bacteria imply a "sterile abscess." These collections should be drained whenever they are symptomatic.

Once the presence of an abscess has been confirmed, catheter placement may be accomplished using either the modified Seldinger or trocar technique. If the Seldinger technique is chosen, a floppy-tipped guide wire is coiled within the cavity and the percutaneous tract is enlarged using fascial dilators. The trocar technique requires specifically designed catheters that include a sharp metal stiffener (Figure 63–3). Catheter insertion is monitored by CT, ultrasound, or fluoroscopy as the catheter is coiled within the abscess cavity in as dependent a position as possible (10).

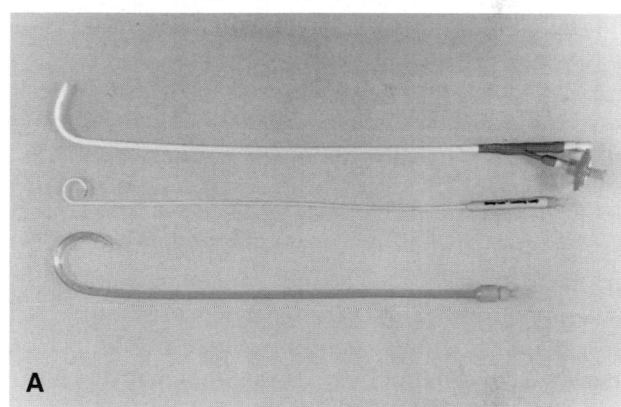

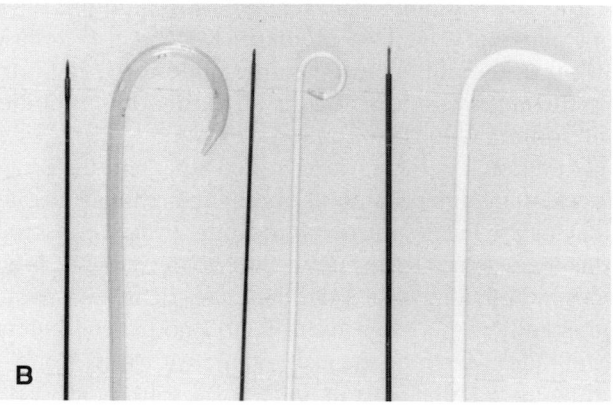

Figure 63–3 Representative catheters for percutaneous abscess drainage. **A.** (*top*) 14 French van Sonnenberg sump catheter (Medi-Tech). (*middle*) 8.5 French Dawson-Mueller drainage catheter (Cook, Inc.). (*bottom*) 16 French Dawson-Mueller drainage catheter (Cook, Inc.). **B.** Closeup of the catheter tips (*shown in* A) showing the design of the tip and the insertion stiffener and stylet used for trocar insertion. Each catheter is designed for primary trocar insertion but can be used in the Seldinger fashion in case of removal of the central needle. The van Sonnenberg catheter (*right*) is nonlocking, but it contains a sump lumen and is available in 12 French and 14 French sizes. The Dawson-Mueller catheter (*middle*) is a Cope loop self-retaining catheter and is currently available in 8.5–14 French sizes. The Dawson-Mueller catheter (*left*) is non–self-retaining and does not have a sump lumen. It is available in 8–16 French sizes.

To reduce inadvertent contamination of intervening spaces, all catheter side holes must be within the cavity. Pneumothorax and empyema may be avoided by locating the pleural reflection in its anterior and lateral margins (usually the eighth and tenth intercostal spaces, respectively) (17). Once the catheter is in satisfactory position, the cavity is lavaged gently with small aliquots of saline to remove residual debris. The catheter is then attached to gravity drainage.

An alternative form of therapy consisting of needle aspiration combined with systemic antibiotic treatment without the use of an indwelling drainage catheter was first described in 1953 and has more recently been proposed as an effective form of therapy for hepatic abscesses (23,24). In a series of 24 patients treated by this method, Baek et al. (23) reported that unilocular and mostly hypoechoic abscesses were more likely to heal completely (86% and 77%, respectively). Fifty-six percent of multiloculated abscesses were treated effectively in this way, although they required a slightly greater average number of aspirations than unilocular abscesses.

Although the duration of drainage is longer in hepatic abscesses that communicate with the biliary tree than in those without intrahepatic biliary communication, there is no significant difference in the cure rate between these groups of patients (25).

Numerous studies have demonstrated both the efficacy and safety of percutaneous catheter drainage for pyogenic hepatic abscess. Success rates range from 81% to 90% (26–28). Fifty percent of patients treated percutaneously have a shorter hospital stay than patients treated surgically (29). Many factors contribute to unsuccessful treatment, including the presence of large amounts of viscous material, attempted drainage of infected metastases (10), the presence of multiple intra-abdominal and intrahepatic abscesses, retained intrahepatic foreign bodies, and undrained loculated collections.

Numerous authors have noted that multiseptated abscesses are amenable to percutaneous drainage because many of the locules intercommunicate. In fact, true septations are believed to be rare in liver abscesses (27). In the series by Bernadino et al. (29), 83% of patients were treated successfully with a single catheter, and no patient required more than two simultaneously placed catheters. Mortality following percutaneous drainage of a solitary abscess is generally in the range of 3–4%. This figure compares favorably to that of surgery, which has an associated mortality of approximately 9% in the case of a solitary abscess and a 36% mortality rate for multiple abscesses (27).

ECHINOCOCCAL ABSCESSES

Echinococcus granulosus causes the most common form of hydatid disease in humans, resulting in benign cystic disease of the liver. Until recently, percutaneous treatment of echinococcal cysts was considered to be contraindicated because spillage or leakage of the cyst contents into the peritoneal cavity could result in anaphylactic shock or the dissemination of viable scolices throughout the peritoneum (13).

Because of the widespread occurrence of hydatid disease and the occasional absence of a pathognomonic imaging appearance (multiloculated cysts with daughter cysts and scolices), many inadvertent and intentional aspirations of hydatid cysts have occurred (30). Mueller et al. (31) first reported the successful drainage of a recurrent hepatic hydatid cyst.

Although aspiration and catheter drainage are not suggested as the primary means of diagnosis or treatment in hydatid disease, they may be indicated when there is suspicion of recurrent disease after surgery or in complex type IV lesions (30). Using ultrasound or CT for guidance, a transparenchymal approach should be used to minimize the chance of leakage of cyst contents. After microscopic demonstration of scolices, the cyst cavity may be gently aspirated and irrigated with a scolicidal agent such as hypertonic saline, 80% alcohol, or 0.5% silver nitrate (32). Formalin is not suggested as a sclerosant because of the risk of systemic toxicity and the risk of sclerosing cholangitis in the case of bile duct communication (30). Sclerotherapy has been performed successfully with 95% alcohol with no major complications and no cyst recurrence during a 12-month follow-up (33). Although hydatid cysts may be treated with needle aspiration and sclerosants, drainage catheters may be left in situ and removed when repeat cyst fluid analysis reveals no living parasites.

AMEBIC ABSCESSES

Amebic abscess, caused by the parasite Entamoeba, represents the most frequent nonenteric manifestation of amebiasis and is seen in up to 9% of patients with amebiasis (34), accounting for 42% of hospital admissions in this group. The diagnosis of amebiasis may be established with serologic studies in more than 90% of cases.

Medical therapy using metronidazole or chloroquine is effective therapy in most cases of hepatic amebic abscess (35). However, percutaneous drainage of amebic liver abscess may be done in the following situations: (a) to exclude pyogenic superinfection, (b) to treat pyogenic superinfection, (c) to treat a patient with a left lobe abscess where rupture into the pleura, bronchi, or pericardium may occur with a mortality rate of 30%, (d) to treat the 5–15% of patients refractory to medical therapy (36), or (e) to treat patients with persistent pain with imminent rupture (34). Many more than 90% of these patients may experience dramatic cure. An additional indication for percutaneous catheter therapy is in the patient with a perforated amebic abscess, which is associated with a mortality of 23–42% (37–39).

In pregnant patients, in whom antiamebic drugs are capable of crossing the placenta, the role of catheter drainage is uncertain because percutaneous drainage alone, without concurrent amebicidal therapy, has not been shown to be curative (35).

Fluid aspiration alone frequently is not diagnostic of amebic abscess. The classic anchovy paste-colored material is recovered in only 50% of patients, and purulent material is obtained in the remainder. Gram stain usually reveals abundant white cells without organisms, simulating a sterile pyogenic abscess. Biopsy of the wall may demonstrate active trophozoites in the capsule but not within the abscess cavity (34).

Amebicidal drugs are given to supplement catheter drainage. If the abscess is located cephalad within the right lobe, the most frequent site for a solitary amebic abscess, it may be safest to perform the drainage under CT guidance with the patient in the prone position using the triangulation technique to avoid transgressing the pleura (22).

SPLENIC ABSCESSES

Splenic abscess is a relatively uncommon clinical problem. Chun et al. (40) grouped the various etiologies into four categories: (1) pyogenic infections, most frequently related to endocarditis; (2) traumatic causes; (3) sickle cell disease; and (4) secondary to spread of inflammation from an adjacent focus. The clinical manifestations are nonspecific and include left upper quadrant pain and tenderness, splenomegaly, fever, and leukocytosis. Localizing signs may be present, but the classic triad of fever, splenic enlargement, and left upper quadrant pain is seen in less than 50% of cases. If the infectious process does not involve the capsule of the spleen, only vague symptoms may predominate.

The ultrasound and CT appearances of splenic abscesses are variable. On ultrasound, collections may be hypoechoic to hyperechoic (41). On CT, abscesses are usually low attenuation (42). Untreated splenic abscesses are associated with an 80–100% mortality rate (43,44). Surgical drainage or splenectomy is associated with a 14–30% mortality rate (42,45). Because of the concern about infection and subsequent sepsis in asplenic patients, percutaneous drainage is a desirable form of therapy because it preserves the spleen (46) (Figure 63–4).

Because of the vascularity of the spleen, clotting abnormalities should be corrected before interventional procedures are done (47). The access route must avoid transgressing surrounding structures such as colon, kidney, pleura, diaphragm, pancreas, and surrounding vascular structures. It is crucial to determine the position of the lung in full inspiration before drainage to avoid pleural

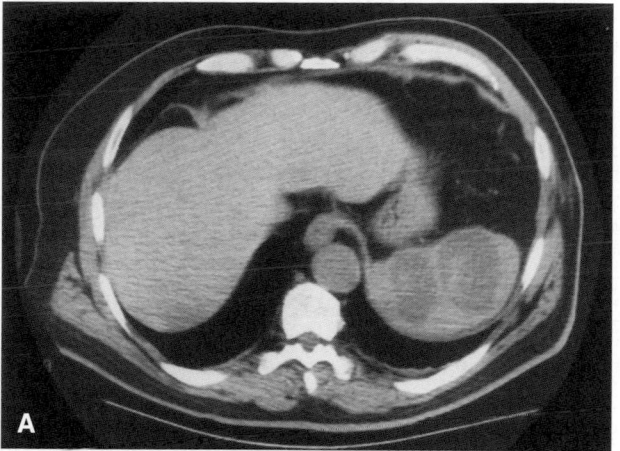

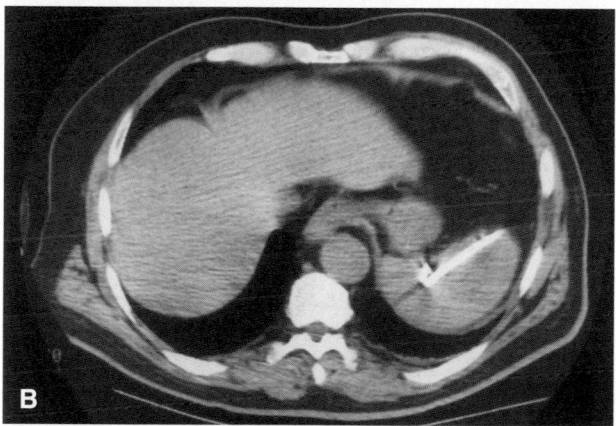

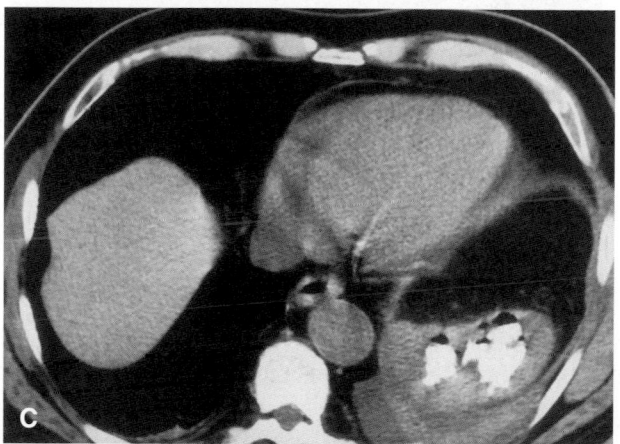

Figure 63–4 A 74-year-old man with severe bilateral carotid stenoses and three-vessel coronary disease. Fever to 106°F developed while he was awaiting carotid surgery. **A.** CT scan shows a bilobed central splenic collection. Diagnostic aspiration, without drainage, revealed Propionibacterium sp. The collection recurred within 4 days, and catheter drainage was performed using a transsplenic trocar technique. **B.** An 8.5 French self-retaining catheter was placed. **C.** CT image slightly cephalad to B obtained 5 days after drainage shows communication of the two locules. The patient did well, and the catheter was removed on the tenth postdrainage day. Carotid and coronary surgery was performed after the abscess resolved. The etiology of this unusual infection was hematogenous spread from psoriasis.

contamination or pneumothorax (41). In general, the route that is chosen should traverse the least amount of normal splenic tissue. However, if the collection is very peripheral, use of this approach may not provide secure catheter purchase; in such cases, aspiration using a small trocar catheter can still be performed.

After diagnostic aspiration, drainage may be accomplished with either the Seldinger or trocar technique. After a drainage catheter is placed, the abscess cavity may be manually decompressed and placed to gravity drainage. The catheter is removed when the drainage has decreased to 3–5 mL per day.

The rate of successful percutaneous drainage of the spleen is slightly lower than that reported for drainage in other organs (76% versus 80–90%). These lower rates may be related to multiloculation of the abscess and the associated phlegmon (47). Drainage of a unilocular hematogenous splenic abscess carries low morbidity. However, complex splenic abscesses more often require surgery for successful treatment (48). Microabscesses related to fungal disease in immunocompromised patients and tuberculosis are not amenable to percutaneous therapy, although diagnostic aspiration may be useful in identifying the underlying organism.

PANCREATIC DISEASE

One of the most serious complications of pancreatitis is sepsis resulting from infected parenchymal necrosis or secondary infection of a phlegmon, fluid collection, or pseudocyst (49). Mortality rates of 0% in patients treated surgically with less than 30% gland necrosis and up to 67% in patients with total or near total gland necrosis have been reported (50). The success of percutaneous drainage depends, to a large extent, on the form of complicated pancreatic disease present. There is little doubt that survival is unlikely in patients with extensive necrosis unless some form of operative intervention is undertaken (51), but patients with organized abscesses and pseudocysts are effectively treated with percutaneous drainage. However, in many cases, pancreatic abscess drainage improves the patient's status before subsequent surgery.

PSEUDOCYSTS

Percutaneous drainage of pseudocysts, which are reported to occur in 2–18% of cases of pancreatic inflammatory disease, remains controversial (52). Pseudocysts resolve spontaneously in up to 20% of cases, but the numbers decrease after the first 6 weeks after formation. Approximately 20% of patients may develop severe complications such as rupture, hemorrhage, infection, or obstruction. Infected pseudocysts are treated emergently and are considered abscesses associated with fistulas (53). Indications for draining noninfected pseudocysts are more complex but include persistent abdominal pain, biliary or intestinal obstruction, pseudocysts beyond 5 cm wide, and they increase in size or fail to decrease in size over a 2- to 6-week period of observation (52,54).

Imaging alone does not allow clear distinction between infected and uninfected collections. Infected pancreatic fluid collections and pseudocysts are well-marginated, homogeneous masses of low attenuation. Bubbles of gas may be seen in 50% of cases, but this does not necessarily signify infection because gas may arise from fistulization to the gastrointestinal tract (55). Whereas the thickness of the pseudocyst wall is of prognostic significance in surgical therapy, this is not true in percutaneous treatment, and a thin wall should not be considered a contraindication to percutaneous drainage.

Catheter insertion may be accomplished using either tandem needle trocar insertion or the Seldinger techniques. Broad-spectrum antibiotics are employed before or immediately after aspiration. Although most patients with pseudocysts can be treated effectively with a single catheter, the radiologist should not hesitate to place additional catheters when follow-up imaging studies reveal residual fluid collections (53) (Figure 63–5).

The choice of drainage route is controversial. The "conventional" route is a direct transperitoneal or retroperitoneal approach (56). However, pseudocysts are frequently surrounded by bowel, liver, spleen, kidney, and vascular structures that necessitate the use of other access routes. Numerous authors have demonstrated the safety and efficacy of the transgastric, transduodenal, transhepatic, and transsplenic routes for achieving prompt external decompression and drainage with equally successful drainage (53,57).

Various authors have performed "short-term drainage," defined as evacuation of pseudocyst contents without placement of an indwelling drainage catheter, in patients with both infected and noninfected pseudocysts. The recurrence rate of this technique ranges from 50–90%, and this is no longer advocated as a primary mode of therapy (52,58,59). In addition, simple aspiration may allow some pseudocyst fluid to leak from the puncture site, with resultant localized retroperitoneal, intraperitoneal, or pleural inflammatory reaction.

The success of long-term catheter drainage of pseudocysts varies from 67% to greater than 90% (52,53). Treatment failure may be attributed to undetected and undrained remote collections; subsequent development of new collections and unrecognized loculi (49); or an unrecognized pseudocyst-pancreatic duct fistula, resulting in recurrence after catheter removal. Freeny et al. (49) suggest that patients who are stable and being treated nonemergently should be evaluated with endoscopic retrograde cholangiopancreatography (ERCP) in an attempt to define the

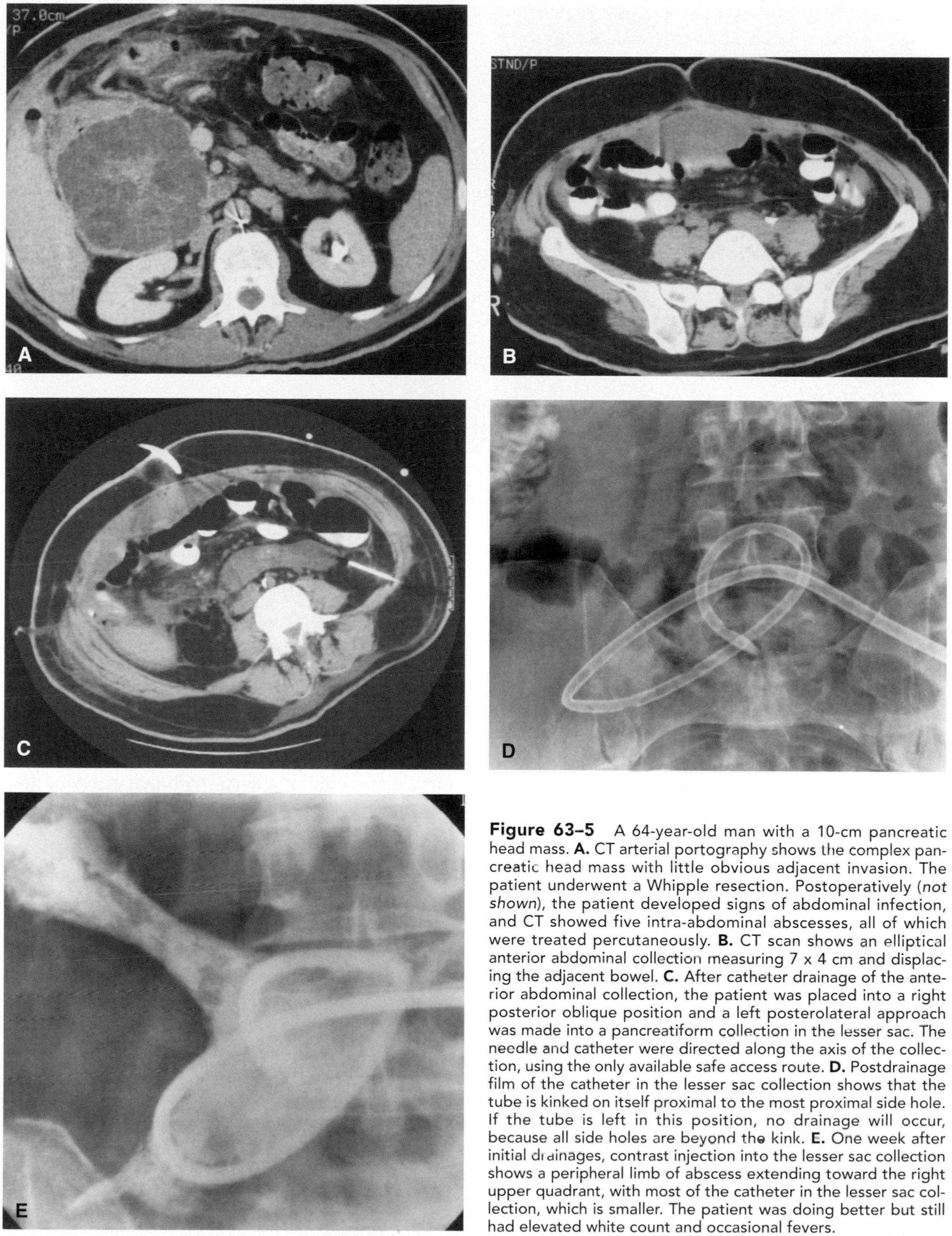

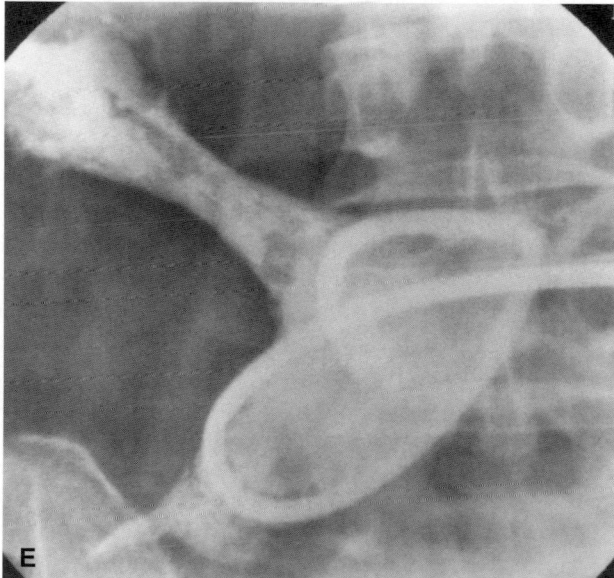

Figure 63–5 A 64-year-old man with a 10-cm pancreatic head mass. **A.** CT arterial portography shows the complex pancreatic head mass with little obvious adjacent invasion. The patient underwent a Whipple resection. Postoperatively (*not shown*), the patient developed signs of abdominal infection, and CT showed five intra-abdominal abscesses, all of which were treated percutaneously. **B.** CT scan shows an elliptical anterior abdominal collection measuring 7 x 4 cm and displacing the adjacent bowel. **C.** After catheter drainage of the anterior abdominal collection, the patient was placed into a right posterior oblique position and a left posterolateral approach was made into a pancreatiform collection in the lesser sac. The needle and catheter were directed along the axis of the collection, using the only available safe access route. **D.** Postdrainage film of the catheter in the lesser sac collection shows that the tube is kinked on itself proximal to the most proximal side hole. If the tube is left in this position, no drainage will occur, because all side holes are beyond the kink. **E.** One week after initial drainages, contrast injection into the lesser sac collection shows a peripheral limb of abscess extending toward the right upper quadrant, with most of the catheter in the lesser sac collection, which is smaller. The patient was doing better but still had elevated white count and occasional fevers.

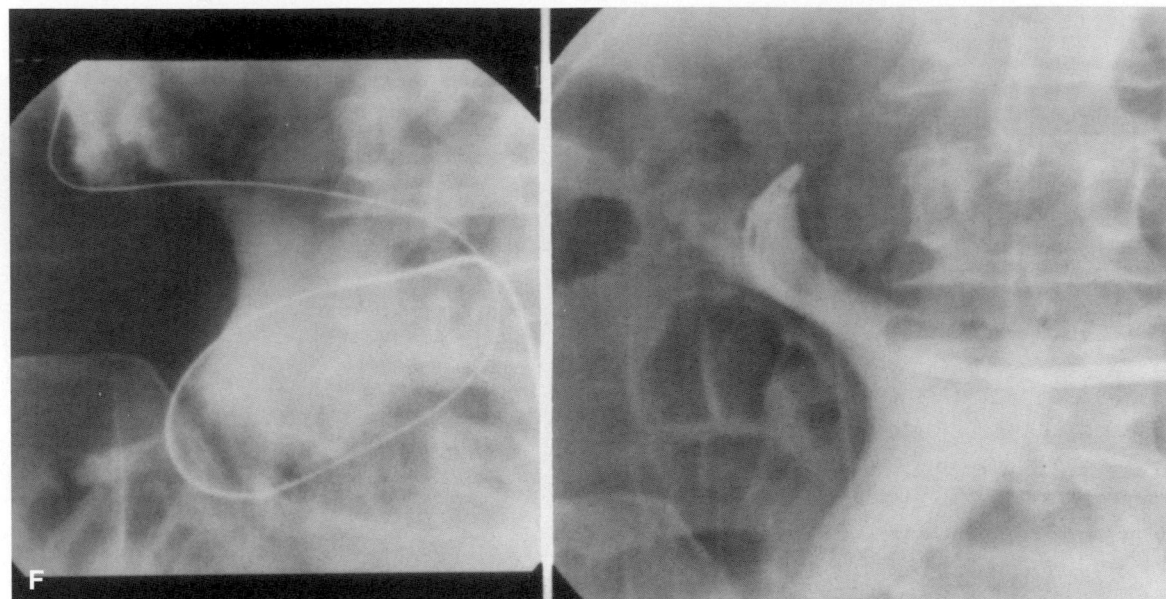

Figure 63–5 (*continued*)   **F.** Guide wire manipulation into the more superior portion of the lesser sac collection allows placement of the catheter into the most superior and dependent recess. The collection completely drained from this catheter position. This case demonstrates the value of aggressive management and close clinical follow-up by the interventional team to successfully treat a seriously ill patient who was deemed unfit for further surgical exploration after his original Whipple procedure and the development of multiple intra-abdominal abscesses.

relationship between the pancreatic duct and the fluid collection. Operative intervention is preferable when there is a high risk of pancreaticocutaneous fistula, such as when the fluid collection communicates with the pancreatic duct and the normal route of transpapillary drainage is compromised by stone or stricture.

Complications in pseudocyst drainage occur in approximately 13% of cases and consist of bacterial superinfection or colonization, minor bleeding, pleural effusion, empyema, and pneumothorax (49,52,53). These results compare favorably with those of surgery, which is associated with a mortality of 19–25% and a major complication rate of 46–75% in acutely ill patients treated with operative external drainage and a rate of 2–9% in those patients treated on an elective basis (54). The 10% rate of failed percutaneous catheter drainage compares favorably with the recurrence rate following surgery of 9–11% (53).

The timing of catheter removal depends on clinical as well as imaging criteria. If an uninfected pseudocyst does not communicate with the pancreatic duct and drainage is more than 10 mL per day, the tube is clamped for 2–3 days. If there is no reaccumulation, the catheter is removed (49,58).

PANCREATIC ABSCESSES

Pancreatic abscesses are the greatest challenge to successful percutaneous therapy. These collections are multiseptated and multilocular and are often associated with fistulas and

extensive necrotic debris (56). Some combination of percutaneous drainage and surgical debridement is usually necessary. The patient's overall clinical status may improve after drainage of infected fluid, allowing definitive surgery on an elective basis. Alternatively, surgery may be performed as the initial therapy with percutaneous drainage of residual or postoperative collections.

On CT, areas of decreased parenchymal enhancement following contrast administration correlate with surgically proven regions of necrotic pancreatic tissue (60). Needle aspiration of these areas is performed to evaluate for infection and to choose appropriate preoperative antibiotics. Patients with infected pancreatic necrosis should be treated surgically even in the presence of drainable fluid because the necrosis itself will not drain well through a catheter. In the subset of patients who are too ill for surgery, significant benefit may be derived from percutaneous catheter drainage (49).

The reported mortality rate from pancreatic abscess treated with extensive surgical debridement ranges from 0–67%, depending on the amount of necrotic pancreatic tissue present and the aggressiveness of surgical debridement (49,56,58). Postoperative recurrence approaches 19% (61). Factors such as acute respiratory distress syndrome (ARDS), pulmonary emboli, and pleural fluid collections contribute to the mortality associated with pancreatic abscess (62).

Numerous reasons exist for failure in percutaneous pancreatic abscess drainage. One of these is failure to differentiate between liquefied pancreatic abscess and more solid phlegmon. Percutaneous drainage should not be performed in the presence of phlegmon if a liquefied abscess is not present (63). Additional reasons for unsuccessful drainage include the use of an inadequate number of catheters to evacuate all of the loculated abscess compartments present. Lee et al. (64) noted that, in cases of complicated pancreatitis, patients required an average of 1.4 catheters during their course of treatment (a range of 1–10).

As noted by Steiner et al. (65), pancreatic abscesses may not only exist within the pancreatic bed itself but may extend into the lesser sac, peripancreatic, and pericolic areas. The rate of successful drainage depends on the location of the collection in relation to the pancreas. Primary percutaneous drainage in central areas such as the pancreas and lesser sac is associated with a success rate of 17%, compared to nearly 60% when the collection is in peripheral areas such as the pararenal space or paracolic gutter (64). The use of larger-bore catheters (24–28 French) is essential to allow adequate evacuation of the thick fluid, pus, and debris that may collect dependently in infected pancreatic collections (49). After surgical debridement, percutaneous drainage may be used in the event debridement is incomplete or whenever fluid reaccumulates.

Successful interventional treatment of infected pancreatic collections requires aggressive early therapy, diligence in follow-up care, and prompt evaluation of unfavorable clinical changes (64,65). Failure of percutaneous drainage of pancreatic abscesses results from inadequate drainage of all locules, incomplete liquefaction of the collection, or attempted drainage of the phlegmon that may not be associated with drainable fluid collection (63,64).

LESSER SAC ABSCESSES

Lesser sac abscesses can be therapeutically challenging because of the surrounding liver, stomach, spleen, and bowel (66). Because these structures surround a large potential space in which abscesses can sequester themselves, percutaneous drainage will usually require traversing one of these organs, preferably the liver (66).

Several principles guide transhepatic drainage of the lesser sac. The first is that the catheter should traverse the most peripheral portion of the liver, compatible with adequate drainage of fluid, preferably the left lobe. The second is that this access route should not be attempted in patients with obstructed bile ducts or in patients with large, dilated, tortuous vessels, as occur in portal hypertension. The third is that the cavity should be evacuated as completely as possible at the time of catheter placement, and the fourth is that care should be taken to ensure that all of the catheter's side holes are within the collection and none are within the hepatic parenchyma.

Adherence to these principles has allowed successful drainage of this anatomic space with no evidence of spread of infection to the liver parenchyma or of hematoma or biloma. It has also been used successfully in patients with lesser sac bowel and biliary fistulas.

PERIRENAL ABSCESSES

The perirenal space lies between the anterior and posterior portions of Gerota's fascia and contains the kidneys, adrenal glands, and associated connective tissues. Small perirenal abscesses may respond to antibiotic therapy alone, but large or persisting collections are best treated by percutaneous catheter drainage. In those few cases that do not respond completely to percutaneous management, surgery is often simplified by prior catheter placement (67).

Perirenal infection may arise from the kidney or from the spread of infection from adjacent structures (68). CT findings in perirenal infections include perirenal fluid and gas collections, distortion of the renal contour, and thickening of the Gerota fascia. Ultrasound may reveal a relatively sonolucent mass with low-level internal echoes and good through transmission. Occasionally, no through transmission is seen because of intra-abscess gas-fluid interfaces. Additionally, if a large number of small gas bubbles are present, the mass may be of increased echogenicity and appear solid (69). Ultrasound suffers from its inability to detect fascial thickening or subtle alteration in the perinephric fat (70).

Perirenal aspiration and drainage may be accomplished using fluoroscopy, ultrasound, CT, or a combination of these methods. A direct extraperitoneal approach will avoid contamination of the peritoneum (69). Lang et al. (67) noted that, in general, the size of the catheter required to adequately drain perirenal abscesses is larger than that required to treat intrarenal abscess because of the more viscous and debris-laden fluid present. However, the choice of catheter type and size is a matter of personal preference. One of the causes for failure in perirenal drainage is placement of an inadequate number of catheters in a septated abscess, but septation is no longer considered a contraindication to percutaneous treatment (68). Septa can be broken up with guide wires during initial catheter placement (71). Signs of complete drainage are resolution of fever and leukocytosis and reduction of output through a patent drainage catheter to less than 5–10 mL per day. In complicated collections, follow-up imaging should be performed before catheter removal.

PSOAS ABSCESSES

Psoas infections may present with nonlocalized abdominal pain, varied gastrointestinal complaints, and constitutional symptoms such as fever, chills, sweats, and malaise. Patients with psoas abscess may complain of pain referred to the hip, groin, or knee (72). Most commonly, patients complain of unilateral hip, back, or flank pain, which is exacerbated by extension of the ipsilateral leg because this causes stretching of the psoas muscle fibers. These vague signs combined with the relative rarity of psoas infection make the diagnosis of psoas abscess a difficult challenge to clinicians and radiologists (73).

The causes of psoas abscess are varied and may be related to direct extension from the kidneys, ureters, pancreas, and retroperitoneal portions of the bowel, or may be secondary to adjacent disk infections and spinal osteomyelitis (74). Diverticulitis and complicated appendicitis are reported as the most common etiologies of psoas abscess (74). Necrotic tumors may mimic true psoas abscesses (Figure 63–4).

Mueller et al. (75) noted that some pyogenic iliopsoas abscesses are related to suppuration of iliac lymph nodes that drain the peritoneum, buttocks, and pelvic areas. These nodes lie between the muscle bundles posteriorly and the peritoneum anteriorly within the iliac fossa.

CT is the best method to define psoas infection and to guide treatment. Asymmetrical muscular enlargement with a central low-attenuation collection is characteristic (75). In psoas hematomas, high-attenuation fresh blood may be seen. Drainage of fresh hematomas is usually not successful, but aspiration for culture and Gram stain can still be performed. If the collection is within the confines of the bony pelvis, aspiration and drainage are done from an anterior approach. The aspirating needle is directed over the anterior iliac spine and caudally and posteriorly into the psoas, taking care to avoid bowel. After the presence of pus is confirmed, a multi–side-hole, large-lumen catheter is inserted. If the collection is confined mostly to the lower lumbar regions as opposed to the pelvis, drainage may be performed using a posterior approach, which avoids transgressing the peritoneum (75). These collections tend to contain thick, viscous debris, necessitating the use of the largest drainage catheters available (75).

SUBPHRENIC ABSCESSES

Abscesses in the subphrenic spaces are unique in their proximity to the pleural space providing technical challenges especially when they track along a significant portion of the diaphragm (76). Right subphrenic collections are related most commonly to liver or gallbladder disease or surgery and may result from a bile leak. If a significant bile leak persists after percutaneous drainage, endoscopic sphincterotomy and stent placement have been advocated to promote antegrade flow of bile and closing of the leak (77). Left subphrenic collections are encountered after splenectomy or may be related to bowel perforation. Left subphrenic collections seen after surgery may be related to unsuspected pancreatitis or pancreatic duct leak, and demonstration of high amylase levels in the fluid will confirm this diagnosis.

Subphrenic abscesses that track along the diaphragm are drained from as caudal an approach as possible to minimize the chances of pleural transgression. Ultrasound guidance allows needle placement via a caudal approach. Subsequent use of Seldinger technique under fluoroscopic guidance allows manipulation of a wire and catheter so that the final catheter position rests along the long axis of the abscess thereby optimizing drainage. Drainage via a transpleural approach is associated with a higher risk of pleural complications but may be justified in some cases in which no other approach is feasible (78).

REFERENCES

1. Fry DE, Garrison RN, Heitsch RC, et al. Determinants of death in patients with intraabdominal abscess. Surgery 1980; 88:517–522.
2. Fry DE, Clevenger FW. Reoperation for intra-abdominal abscess. Surg Clin North Am 1991;71:159–173.
3. Brolin RE, Nosher JL, Leiman S, et al. Percutaneous catheter versus open surgical drainage in the treatment of abdominal abscesses. Am Surg 1984;50:102–108.
4. Gerzof SG, Robbins AH, Birkett DH, et al. Percutaneous catheter drainage of abdominal abscesses guided by ultrasound and computed tomography. AJR Am J Roentgenol 1979;133:1–8.
5. Ochsner A, DeBakey M, Murray S. Pyogenic abscess of the liver: II. An analysis of 47 cases with review of the literature. Am J Surg 1938;40:292–319.
6. Ferrucci JT. Percutaneous drainage of abdominal abscesses and fluid collections. M Sinai J Med 1984;51:547–551.
7. Connell TR, Stephens DH, Carlson HC, et al. Upper abdominal abscess: a continuing and deadly problem. AJR Am J Roentgenol 1980;134:759–765.
8. Nguyen KT, Sauerbrei EE, Nolan RL. The peritoneum and the diaphragm. In: Rumack CM, Wilson SR, Charboneau JW, eds. Diagnostic Ultrasound. St. Louis: Mosby-Year Book, 1991: 365–382.
9. Kressel HY, Filly RA. Ultrasonographic appearance of gas-containing abscesses in the abdomen. AJR Am J Roentgenol 1978; 130:71–73.
10. Jeffrey RB Jr, Wing VW, Laing FC. Real-time sonographic monitoring of percutaneous abscess drainage. AJR Am J Roentgenol 1985;144:469–470.
11. Knochel JQ, Koehler PR, Lee TG, et al. Diagnosis of abdominal abscesses with computed tomography, ultrasound, and ^{111}Indium leukocyte scans. Radiology 1980;137:425–432.
12. Baron RL, Freeny PC, Moss AA. The liver. In: Moss AA, Gamsu G, Genant HK, eds. Computed Tomography of the Body: With Magnetic Resonance Imaging. 2nd Ed. Philadelphia: W. B. Saunders, 1992:735–821.
13. Sones PJ. Percutaneous drainage of abdominal abscesses. AJR Am J Roentgenol 1984;142:35–39.
14. Mueller PR, van Sonnenberg E, Ferrucci JT Jr. Percutaneous drainage of 250 abdominal fluid collections. Part II. Current procedural concepts. Radiology 1984;151:343–347.
15. Johnson RD, Mueller PF, Ferrucci JT Jr, et al. Percutaneous drainage of pyogenic liver abscesses. AJR Am J Roentgenol 1985; 44:463–467.
16. Johnson WC, Gerzoff SG, Robbins AH. Treatment of abdominal abscesses: comparative evaluation of operative drainage versus percutaneous catheter drainage guided by computed tomography or ultrasound. Ann Surg 1981;194:510–519.
17. Silver S, Weinstein A, Cooperman A. Changes in the pathogenesis and detection of intrahepatic abscess. Am J Surg 1979;137: 608–610.
18. Kuligowska E, Connor SK, Shapiro JH. Liver abscess: sonography in diagnosis and treatment. AJR Am J Roentgenol 1982;138: 253–257.

19. Halvorsen RA, Korobkin M, Foster WL, et al. The variable CT appearance of hepatic abscesses. AJR Am J Roentgenol 1984;141: 941–946.
20. Robinson HA, Isikoff MB, Hill MC. Diagnostic imaging of hepatic abscesses: a retrospective analysis. AJR Am J Roentgenol 1980;135:735–740.
21. Bernadino ME. Space occupying lesions of the liver. In: Taveras J, Ferrucci JT Jr, eds. Radiology: Diagnosis, Imaging, Intervention. Philadelphia: Lippincott, 1992:1–13.
22. van Sonnenberg E, Wittenberg J, Ferrucci JT Jr, et al. Triangulation method for percutaneous needle guidance: the angled approach to upper abdominal masses. AJR Am J Roentgenol 1981;137: 757–761.
23. Baek SY, Lee MG, Cho KS, et al. Therapeutic percutaneous aspiration of hepatic abscesses: effectiveness in 25 patients. AJR Am J Roentgenol 1993;160:799–802.
24. McFadzean AJS, Chang KPS, Wong CC. Solitary pyogenic abscess treated by closed aspiration and antibiotics: fourteen consecutive cases with recovery. Br J Surg 1953;41:141–152.
25. Do H, Lambiase RE, Deyoe L, et al. Percutaneous drainage of hepatic abscesses: comparison of results in abscesses with and without intrahepatic biliary communication. AJR Am J Roentgenol 1991;157:1209–1212.
26. Bertel CK, van Heerden JA, Sheedy PF. Treatment of pyogenic hepatic abscesses: surgical versus percutaneous drainage. Arch Surg 1986;121:554–558.
27. Gerzof SG, Johnson WC, Robbins AH, et al. Intrahepatic pyogenic abscesses: treatment by percutaneous drainage. Am J Surg 1985;149:487–493.
28. Attar B, Levendoglu H, Causay NS. CT-guided percutaneous aspiration and catheter drainage of pyogenic liver abscesses. Am J Gastroenterol 1986;81:550–555.
29. Bernadino ME, Berkman WA, Plemmons M, et al. Percutaneous drainage of multiseptated hepatic abscess. J Comput Assist Tomogr 1984;8:38–41.
30. Bret PM, Fond A, Bretagnolle M, et al. Percutaneous aspiration and drainage of hydatid cysts in the liver. Radiology 1988;168: 617–620.
31. Mueller PR, Dawson SL, Ferrucci JT Jr, et al. Hepatic echinococcal cyst: successful percutaneous drainage. Radiology 1985;155: 627–628.
32. Acunas B, Rozanes I, Acunas G, et al. Hydatid cyst of the liver: identification of detached cyst lining on CT scans obtained after cyst puncture. AJR Am J Roentgenol 1991;156:751–752.
33. Simonetti G, Profili S, Sergiacomi GL, et al. Percutaneous treatment of hepatic cysts by aspiration and sclerotherapy. Cardiovasc Intervent Radiol 1993;16:81–84.
34. van Sonnenberg E, Mueller PR, Schiffman HR, et al. Intrahepatic amebic abscesses: indications for and results of percutaneous catheter drainage. Radiology 1985;156:631–635.
35. Ralls PW, Barnes PF, Johnson MB, et al. Medical treatment of hepatic amebic abscess: rare need for percutaneous drainage. Radiology 1987;165:805–807.
36. Thompson JE, Forlenza S, Verma R. Amebic liver abscess: a therapeutic approach. Rev Infect Dis 1985;7:171–179.
37. Eggleston FC, Handa AK, Verghese M. Amebic peritonitis secondary to amebic liver abscess. Surgery 1982;91:46–51.
38. Adams EB, MacLeod IN. Invasive amebiasis: amebic liver abscess and its complications. Medicine 1977;56:325–334.
39. Ken JG, van Sonnenberg E, Casola G, et al. Perforated amebic liver abscess: successful percutaneous treatment. Radiology 1989;170: 195–197.
40. Chun CH, Raff MJ, Conteras L, et al. Splenic abscess. Medicine 1980;59:50–65.
41. Chou YH, Hsu CC, Tiu CM, et al. Splenic abscess: sonographic and percutaneous drainage or aspiration. Gastrointest Radiol 1992;17:262–266.
42. van der Laan RT, Verbeeten B Jr, Smits NJ, et al. Computed tomography in the diagnosis and treatment of solitary splenic abscesses. J Comput Assist Tomogr 1989;13:71–74.
43. Lerner RM, Spataro RF. Splenic abscess: percutaneous drainage. Radiology 1984;153:643–645.
44. Karlson KB, Martin EC, Fankuchen EI, et al. Nonsurgical drainage of intraabdominal and mediastinal abscess: a report of 12 cases. Cardiovasc Intervent Radiol 1981;4:170–176.
45. Berkman WA, Harris SA, Bernadino ME. Nonsurgical drainage of splenic abscess. AJR Am J Roentgenol 1983;141:395–396.
46. Schwartz PE, Sterioff S, Mucha P, et al. Postsplenectomy sepsis and mortality in adults. JAMA 1982;248:2279–2283.
47. Quinn SF, van Sonnenberg E, Casola G, et al. Interventional radiology in the spleen. Radiology 1986;161:289–291.
48. Pruett TL, Simmons RL. Status of percutaneous catheter drainage of abscesses. Surg Clin North Am 1988;68:89–105.
49. Freeny PC, Lewis GP, Traverso LW, et al. Infected pancreatic fluid collections: percutaneous catheter drainage. Radiology 1988;167: 435–441.
50. Beger HG, Bittner R, Block S, et al. Bacterial contamination of pancreatic necrosis: a prospective study. Gastroenterology 1986; 91:433–438.
51. Bittner R, Block S, Buchler M, et al. Pancreatic abscess and infected pancreatic necrosis: different local septic complications in acute pancreatitis. In: Beger HG, Buchler M, eds. Acute Pancreatitis. Berlin: Springer-Verlag, 1987:216–223.
52. Torres WE, Evert MB, Baumgartner BR, et al. Percutaneous aspiration and drainage of pancreatic pseudocysts. AJR Am J Roentgenol 1986;147:1007–1009.
53. van Sonnenberg E, Wittich GR, Casola G, et al. Percutaneous drainage of infected and noninfected pancreatic pseudocysts: experience in 101 cases. Radiology 1989;170:757–761.
54. Matzinger FRK, Ho CS, Yee AC, et al. Pancreatic pseudocysts drained through a percutaneous transgastric approach: further experience. Radiology 1988;167:431–434.
55. Banks PA, Gerzof SG. Indications and results of fine needle aspiration of pancreatic exudate. In: Beger HG, Buchler M, eds. Acute Pancreatitis. Berlin: Springer-Verlag, 1987:171–174.
56. van Sonnenberg E, D'Agostino HB, Casola GC, et al. Percutaneous abscess drainage: current concepts. Radiology 1991;181:617–626.
57. Kuligowska E, Olsen WL. Pancreatic pseudocysts drained through a percutaneous transgastric approach. Radiology 1985;154:79–92.
58. van Sonnenberg E, Wittich GR, Casola G, et al. Complicated pancreatic inflammatory disease: diagnostic and therapeutic role of interventional radiology. Radiology 1985;155:335–340.
59. Grosso M, Gandini G, Cassinis MC, et al. Percutaneous treatment (including pseudocystogastrostomy) of 74 pancreatic pseudocysts. Radiology 1989;173:493–497.
60. Maier W. Early objective diagnosis and staging of acute pancreatitis by contrast-enhanced computed tomography. In: Beger HG, Buchler M, eds. Acute Pancreatitis. Berlin: Springer-Verlag, 1987: 132–140.
61. Altemeier WA, Alexander JW. Pancreatic abscess. Arch Surg 1963;87:80–89.
62. Bittner R, Block S, Buchler M, et al. Pancreatic abscess and infected pancreatic necrosis: difficult local septic complications in acute pancreatitis. Dig Dis Sci 1987;32:1082–1087.
63. Lang EK, Springer RM, Glorioso LW, et al. Abdominal abscess drainage under radiologic guidance: causes of failure. Radiology 1986;159:329–336.
64. Lee MJ, Rattner DW, Legemate DA, et al. Acute complicated pancreatitis: redefining the role of interventional radiology. Radiology 1992;183:171–174.
65. Steiner E, Mueller PR, Hahn PF, et al. Complicated pancreatic abscesses: problems in interventional management. Radiology 1988;167:443–446.
66. Mueller PR, Ferrucci JT Jr, Simeone JF, et al. Lesser sac abscesses and fluid collections: drainage by transhepatic approach. Radiology 1985;155:615–618.
67. Lang EK. Renal, perirenal, and pararenal abscesses: percutaneous drainage. Radiology 1990;174:109–113.
68. Sacks D, Banner MP, Meranze SG, et al. Renal and related retroperitoneal abscesses: percutaneous drainage. Radiology 1988;167:447–451.
69. Gerzof SG, Gale ME. Computed tomography and ultrasonography for diagnosis and treatment of renal and retroperitoneal abscesses. Urol Clin North Am 1982;9:185–193.
70. Hoddick W, Jeffrey RB, Goldberg HI, et al. CT and sonography of severe renal and perirenal infections. AJR Am J Roentgenol 1983; 140:517–520.
71. Lieberman RP, Hahn FJ, Imray, et al. Loculated abscesses: management by percutaneous fracture of septations. Radiology 1986;161:827–828.

72. Jeffrey RB, Callen PW, Federle MP. Computed tomography of psoas abscesses. J Comput Assist Tomogr 1980;4:639–641.

73. Ralls PW, Boswell W, Henderson R, et al. CT of inflammatory disease of the psoas muscle. AJR Am J Roentgenol 1980;134:767–770.

74. Mendez G Jr, Isikoff MB, Hill MC. Retroperitoneal processes involving the psoas demonstrated by computed tomography. J Comput Assist Tomogr 1980;4:78–82.

75. Mueller PR, Ferrucci JT Jr, Wittenberg J, et al. Iliopsoas abscess: treatment by CT-guided percutaneous catheter drainage. AJR Am J Roentgenol 1984;142:359–362.

76. Mueller PR, Simeone JF, Butch RJ, et al. Percutaneous drainage of subphrenic abscess: a review of 62 patients. AJR Am J Roentgenol 1986; 147:1237–1240.

77. Foutch PG, Harlan JR, Hoefer M. Endoscopic therapy for patients with a post-operative biliary leak. Gastrointest Endosc 1993;39:416–421.

78. McNicholas MM, Mueller PR, Lee MJ, et al. Percutaneous drainage of subphrenic fluid collections that occur after splenectomy: efficacy and safety of transpleural versus extrapleural approach. AJR Am J Roentgenol 1995;165:355–359.

Percutaneous Drainage of Pelvic Abscesses and Fluid Collections

64

Debra A. Gervais, Steven L. Dawson

Percutaneous drainage of pelvic abscesses was a late addition to the list of interventional procedures established in the 1980s. Before the revolutionary advances in cross-sectional imaging of the 1970s, the deep location and complicated anatomic relations of typical pelvic abscesses rendered them undiagnosable and undrainable except by laparotomy. Subsequently, they were able to be accurately characterized and localized, but safe access routes frequently were not recognized and the misconception persisted that abscesses complicated by fistulas were not suitable for percutaneous abscess drainage (PAD).

Only in the latter half of the 1980s were the indications for PAD widened to include "complicated" abscesses, and innovative access routes to deep pelvic abscesses were established. Percutaneous PAD in the pelvis is now accepted as a safe and effective therapy that may variously result in cure, delay of surgery in a seriously ill patient until the underlying medical condition has been stabilized, or "downstaging" of a subsequent surgical procedure. These benefits are achieved with lower morbidity and cost than traditional alternatives, success and complication rates that are at least similar, and greater patient acceptance.

COMMON SITES AND ETIOLOGIES

Pelvic fluid collections may be intraperitoneal or extraperitoneal. Knowledge of the anatomy of the pelvic peritoneum is necessary to understand the paths of dissemination of sepsis.

The pelvic peritoneal space extends from the pelvic brim, iliac vessels, and pelvic mesocolon superiorly to the peritoneal reflection from the anterior rectal wall inferiorly. The peritoneal reflection extends anteriorly to cover the seminal vesicles and bladder in men and the vagina, uterus, and bladder in women. In women, the reflection lies more caudally and is divided into the rectouterine and uterovesical fossae by the uterus, vagina, and broad ligament. Laterally, the peritoneum is reflected toward the pelvic wall and forms the shallow pararectal and paravesical fossae. There is free communication of the pelvic cavity with the abdominal peritoneum, including both its supracolic and infracolic portions. The most common site of pelvic abscess formation is the cul-de-sac, which is the most dependent portion of the abdominal cavity.

The pelvic extraperitoneal space and its compartments are more complex and are less well-known than their retroperitoneal counterparts (1). The anterior extraperitoneal fat is divided by the umbilicovesical fascia into the prevesical and perivesical spaces. The perivesical space contains the bladder, umbilical arteries, and urachus. The prevesical space, also known as the space of Retzius in its retropubic portion, is a large potential space extending superiorly to the umbilicus. Fluid in the prevesical space has a "molar-tooth" shape on axial scans, with the "roots" separating the bladder posteriorly from the cecum and sigmoid colon laterally (2). The "roots" are often asymmetric, resulting in displacement of the bladder from the midline. The prevesical space also communicates directly with the rectus sheath, femoral sheath, presacral space, and infrarenal peritoneal compartment, allowing for collections of fluid such as blood, urine, or pus from these sites of origin.

Common initiating causes of pelvic abscesses are surgery or trauma to the gastrointestinal tract. Appendicitis, diverticulitis, and Crohn disease are also frequent antecedents. Perianal abscesses may dissect into the retroperitoneum. These conditions share the common etiology of loss of integrity of the bowel wall as a barrier to the spread of infection. A different pathway exists in women, in whom tubo-ovarian abscesses may result from ascending sexually acquired infection of the genital tract.

Leakage of urine from surgery, trauma, or instrumentation of the lower urinary tract may result in very large collections that may become infected. Hematomas may result from trauma, surgery, anticoagulant medication, or angiography. Renal transplants may be complicated by various fluid collections, including urinoma, hematoma, lymphocele, abscess, or seroma. Pancreatic transplants may also be associated with pancreatitis or pseudocysts. Infected necrotic tumors are an uncommon but easily overlooked cause of pelvic abscess.

EFFICACY AND RATIONALE OF PELVIC PAD

Despite modern antibiotic therapy, undrained abdominal abscesses result in a distressingly high mortality rate of 50–80% (3).

The principles of therapy are as follows:

1. *Complete evacuation of pus.* Whether achieved surgically or radiologically, the major benefit of intervention occurs at the time of the procedure when the cavity contents are completely evacuated. This can result in the recovery of an unstable, critically ill patient in a matter of hours. Continued external drainage adds to the therapeutic effect, but the major benefit occurs immediately (4).
2. *Early diagnosis and intervention.* Early drainage forestalls the development of a multiorgan dysfunction syndrome, which is associated with a much worse prognosis.
3. *Accurate anatomic localization.* This allows a suitable access route to be chosen and defines loculations that will require a further drainage tube or more extensive surgery to prevent failure.
4. *Diagnosis of any underlying cause.* An underlying enteric connection must be identified and allowed to heal before the drainage tube can be successfully removed.
5. *Imaging follow-up to document resolution.* Minimal tube drainage alone does not necessarily equate with resolution because the tube may be blocked, malpositioned, or too small to drain the abscess contents.

Cross-sectional imaging techniques have revolutionized the treatment of abscesses by allowing assessment of these fundamentals. Success rates for PAD of selected unilocular uncomplicated abscesses range from 90–100%. Complicated abscesses in the pelvis result from factors such as recent surgery, urine leaks, or enteric communication. These abscesses have a lower cure rate than uncomplicated abscesses, in the range of 65–95%. Their management is more prolonged than for simple abscesses, often requiring CT at diagnosis and follow-up and multiple catheters for loculated abscesses. More than 90% of peridiverticular abscesses may be drained successfully percutaneously (5,6). Periappendiceal abscesses are drained successfully in approximately 90% of patients (7,8), and the success rate for PAD in Crohn disease is from 70–100% (9–11). Postoperative pelvic abscesses can be cured by PAD in 80–85% of cases (12).

Several studies have shown PAD to have a higher success rate with lower morbidity and mortality than surgical drainage (13,14). Johnson et al. (15), in a study comparing surgical and percutaneous drainage, found a mortality rate of 11% and a complication rate of 4% for percutaneous drainage, compared with 21% and 16%, respectively, for surgery. Other studies have shown no difference (16). Because a randomized prospective trial has never been performed, it is not valid to compare the success rates of PAD and surgical drainage. Such a trial would be unethical now that PAD has been so widely adopted as the initial therapy of choice.

Success rates for percutaneous drainage depend on the definition of cure. Cure is most completely defined as defervescence, disappearance of the abscess, avoidance of surgery, and lack of recurrence in the long term. However, even if all these objectives are not achieved, it does not mean the treatment has failed to be of benefit to the patient. Often the patient is gravely ill at the time of diagnosis for such reasons as advanced age, concurrent medical conditions, or recent surgery. Surgery in this setting may be life-threatening, particularly for complicated abscesses where the prognosis is dismal. PAD in this setting has a temporizing effect, delaying surgery until risks have been minimized.

PAD frequently reduces the extent of subsequent surgery. Once inflammation and mass effect have resolved, the task of the surgeon may be much easier than otherwise. More definitive surgery may be possible at the initial operation than would otherwise be contemplated. For example, in a patient with a pericolonic diverticular abscess, separate operations to drain the abscess and create a defunctioning colostomy, resect the diseased segment, and subsequently close the diversion may be unnecessary. Surgery may thus be "downstaged" from a two- or three-stage procedure to a one- or two-stage procedure. This is the major goal of PAD in enteric abscesses where subsequent surgery usually will be required (14).

To summarize, PAD is a nonoperative intervention performed under local anesthesia with success rates, morbidity, and mortality as good as or better than surgery, a major intervention that is accompanied by the risks of general anesthesia. PAD also encompasses the other major attributes of temporization and downstaging of subsequent surgery when this is required. Its role was summed up in an authoritative surgical review that referred to PAD as "clearly one of the great advances in abdominal surgery in the past few years" (15).

WHAT TO DRAIN AND WHAT NOT TO DRAIN

Management of abscesses will, in part, depend on the underlying disease.

Sigmoid Peridiverticular Abscesses

Sigmoid diverticulosis is a common entity in Western countries that may affect more than half of Americans over 60 years of age (16). Diverticulitis eventually develops in 15–30% of these cases, and in 1983 resulted in more than 200,000 hospitalizations and 50,000 surgical procedures in the United States (17,18).

Although uncomplicated acute diverticulitis will resolve with appropriate antibiotic therapy, surgery is indicated for bleeding, bowel obstruction, perforation with peritonitis, or abscess formation. The aims of pericolonic abscess surgery are to drain the abscess, resect the diseased segment, and restore colonic continuity (19–21). Depending on whether all these entities can be performed at the initial procedure, surgery may be performed as a one-stage procedure, two stages with delayed closure of the diverting colostomy, or three stages with delayed resection and delayed closure.

In a review of diverticular abscesses, Hinchey et al. (22) classified them according to size and containment. Type A abscesses are small and lie in the contiguous mesentery; type B abscesses result from a large perforation with a well-defined mesenteric or pelvic abscess; type C abscesses result from a free perforation into the adjacent mesentery or pelvis without fecal contamination; type D results from gross perforation with contamination of the peritoneum and pelvis from free fecal spillage. In type A abscesses, percutaneous drainage is unnecessary because the diseased segment can be removed en bloc in a single-stage procedure, whereas in type D percutaneous drainage is ineffective. PAD is best reserved for large localized abscesses in the mesentery or pelvis, without fecal contamination (types B and C).

The optimal timing of surgery after PAD is unclear. Frequently, the diseased segment is removed early—after the clinical signs have abated but with the catheter still in place. The patient may be sent home with the catheter still in place when early surgery is not contemplated. Surgery may not be necessary in all patients following successful PAD. Some elderly patients have not undergone subsequent resection and have remained well. Selection of suitable candidates for conservative follow-up may be possible with further experience (4).

Periappendiceal Abscesses

Periappendiceal abscesses may complicate acute appendicitis or appendectomy. Abscess formation complicates acute appendicitis in 2–3% of cases (21,22), resulting from a gangrenous or perforated appendix. Often, these patients present with a palpable "appendix mass," which may be the result of an abscess, a phlegmonous thickening of omentum and small bowel loops, or a combination of both. The differential diagnosis includes lymphadenitis, Meckel's diverticulitis, perforated cecum (including tumor, foreign body, and diverticulitis), Crohn disease, or ovarian pathology (8). Clinical diagnosis is imprecise, and 45% of a series of 42 patients undergoing surgical drainage for an appendix mass had phlegmons without significant abscess formation (23). There is also a high morbidity of 24–28% for attempted early appendectomy and drainage of periappendiceal abscesses, compared to only 5% when an unperforated appendix is removed intact (24,25). The more frequent complications include wound infection, abscess formation, fecal fistula, pylephlebitis, and intestinal obstruction (26,27).

CT with intravenous contrast can reliably stage complicated appendicitis and postappendectomy inflammation, allowing for rational selection of medical, surgical, or percutaneous therapy. A periappendiceal phlegmon is a mass of soft tissue density, 20 Hounsfield (HU) units or more, after contrast. A periappendiceal abscess is a well-defined fluid collection (<20 HU). The presence of a calcified appendicolith in the phlegmon or abscess is diagnostic of an inflammatory etiology and is detected much more frequently on CT than on plain radiographs (Figure 64–1).

Jeffrey et al. (28) reviewed 70 periappendiceal inflammatory masses in patients with clinically suspected appendiceal perforation. Patients with phlegmons or small abscesses less than 3 cm in diameter (category 1) responded rapidly to intravenous antibiotic therapy without surgical or percutaneous drainage. In these patients, CT-guided diagnostic aspiration may occasionally be useful for isolation of an organism for antibiotic sensitivity testing. Patients with larger well-defined abscesses (category 2) were treated with intravenous antibiotics in combination with percutaneous drainage. In both categories, the cure rate was approximately 90%. Fistulas to the tip of the appendix or cecum were demonstrated at routine sinography in 46% of category 2 patients. These required a longer period of catheter drainage, up to 3.5 weeks, but all fistulas closed. Patients were discharged from the hospital for outpatient follow-up and sinograms once their clinical signs had returned to normal.

Patients with extensive, poorly defined abscesses with pelvic, extraperitoneal, or interloop extension (category 3) were treated with early surgery in this study. Other causes of a periappendiceal inflammatory mass, such as perforated cecal lymphoma, diverticulitis, and ruptured ovarian cyst, were also present in this group, mimicking appendiceal abscess.

Patients with postappendectomy abscesses also respond favorably to PAD. Catheter drainage for several weeks is

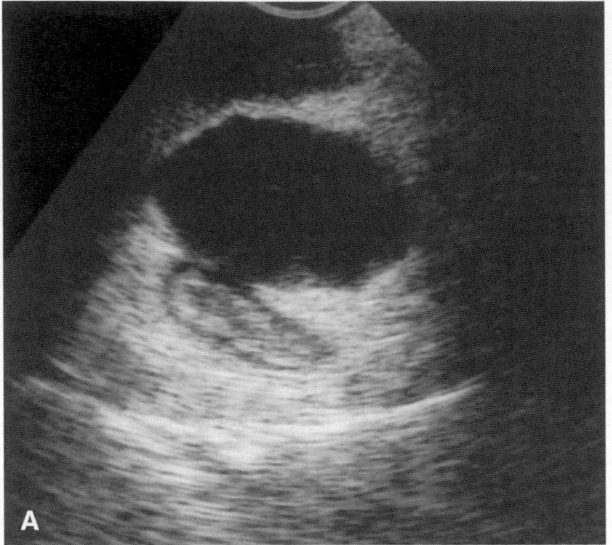

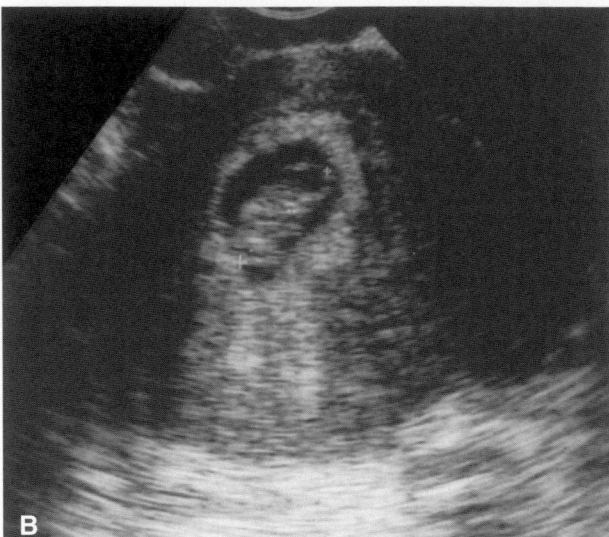

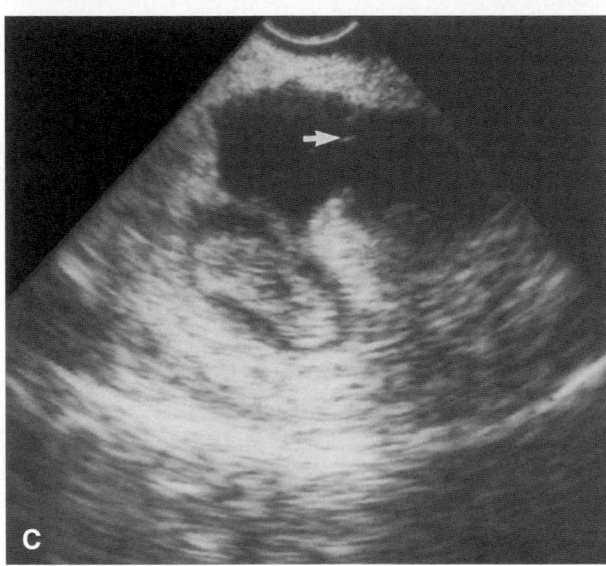

Figure 64–1   A 20-year-old pregnant woman with right lower quadrant pain, fever, and elevated white count. **A.** Transvaginal ultrasound shows a 5 x 3 cm collection between the vagina and a collapsed rectosigmoid. **B.** Transvaginal ultrasound of the uterus shows a single fetus of 9 weeks' gestational age. Fetal heart motion was seen. **C.** Transvaginal drainage of the cul-de-sac collection was performed using an 18-gauge needle inserted under direct ultrasound guidance through the vaginal vault into the collection (*arrow*). A guide wire and self-retaining catheter were placed into the collection and remained for 4 days, during which time the patient's clinical symptoms markedly improved, with no further collection identified on follow-up imaging. The pregnancy continued uneventfully, and the patient subsequently had interval appendectomy.

required in this group to allow the fistula that is usually present to heal (27).

Elective appendectomy may be unnecessary after PAD for a periappendiceal abscess (28). After surgical drainage of periappendiceal abscess without appendectomy, 80–95% of patients remain asymptomatic (29,30). If removed electively, the appendix frequently shows no sign of inflammation (31) or may be impossible to find, having been destroyed by inflammation at the time of the abscess (32,33). The 19% complication rate of interval appendectomy is also high in this situation (26).

The length of hospitalization for PAD for periappendiceal abscess averaged 8 days, comparing favorably with 6.5–17 days for operative therapy (8).

Crohn Disease

Crohn disease is complicated by abscess formation in 20–24% of patients, with approximately equal incidence

spontaneously and postoperatively (34,35). Mechanisms include direct extension from involved bowel, hematogenous seeding, and peritoneal contamination or anastomotic breakdown after surgery.

Diagnosis may be delayed because of masking or clinical signs by concurrent corticosteroid therapy, and CT is invaluable in making the diagnosis and differentiating abscess from phlegmon. Management by whatever means is fraught with difficulty, reflecting the transmural nature of the underlying disease. There is a high incidence of cutaneous fistula formation following surgical drainage, up to 85% (34). To avoid the considerable morbidity and mortality associated with bypass surgery in the presence of a coexisting abscess, a two-stage approach is advocated, consisting of abscess drainage and subsequent resection of the diseased segment and fistulectomy (when present) 6 weeks later.

The roles of PAD in Crohn disease are temporization and a decrease in the scope of subsequent surgery, with an increase in the proportion of patients undergoing a

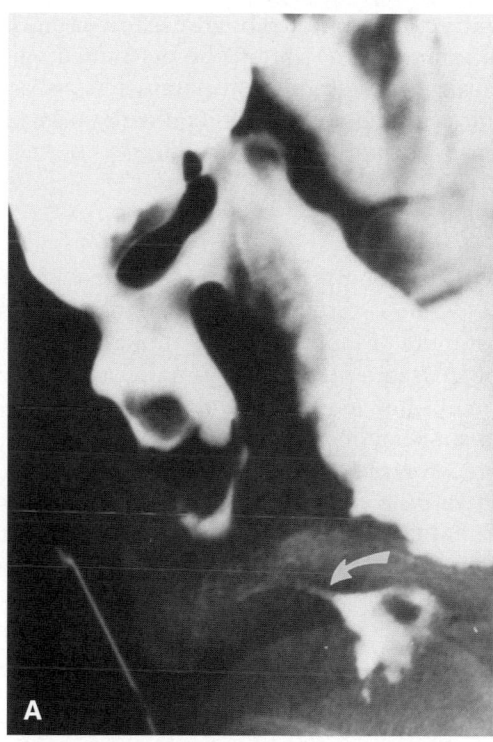

Figure 64–2 A 23-year-old woman with a 7-year history of Crohn disease. **A.** Spot film from a small bowel follow-through shows irregularity of the terminal ileum with narrowing of the cecum and a fistulous communication to a right lower quadrant collection (*curved arrow*). **B.** Three images from the CT examination show thickening of the cecum (*left image*), with air-fluid level and contrast opacifying the fistulous tract (*center image*). The collection tracks into the superficial right lower quadrant. Percutaneous drainage of Crohn abscesses and long-term management of fistulas is possible, but in this case the patient was managed surgically, and percutaneous drainage was not performed.

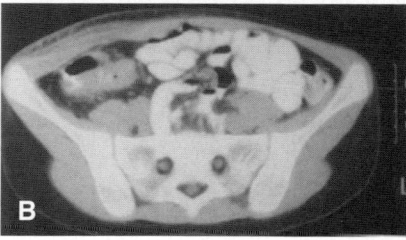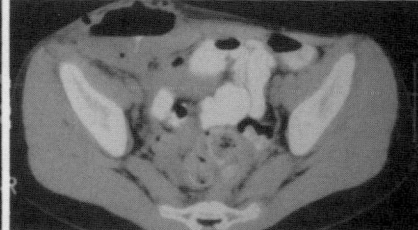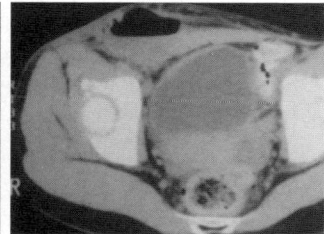

successful one-stage operation. Although both surgical and percutaneous drainages are well-tolerated, PAD is preferred as the less invasive technique (Figure 64–2).

In patients without enteric communication of the abscess, PAD has been shown to be an effective therapy (10). When communication is present, PAD is also effective in helping to resolve the abscess, although success rates are lower than when no communication exists, and a longer period is required for the fistula to close. Aggressive adjunctive medical therapy with intravenous antibiotics and total parenteral nutrition (TPN) is necessary and may allow resolution of the fistula. The fistula is likely to recur whenever the underlying bowel disease is severe and there are marked stenosis and strictures, and these patients benefit from elective resection. The recurrence rate is low in patients with mild underlying disease, and these patients may be observed. The extent of the underlying disease may be assessed with a barium study once resolution has occurred.

Postoperative abscesses in Crohn disease are because of an anastomotic leak and occur in 10–15% of patients. They respond well to PAD, in common with other postoperative abscesses with biliary or enteric communication, where there is an 80% cure rate (35–39).

Tubo-Ovarian Abscesses

Approximately 85,000 women develop tubo-ovarian abscesses (TOAs) each year in the United States (40). Management has traditionally been with intravenous antibiotics or surgery, which may range from colpotomy to total abdominal hysterectomy and bilateral salpingo-oophorectomy. Several series have documented success with PAD for TOAs, with cure rates of approximately 90% (41,42). Complications are few and minor. Some patients suffer recurrence some months after the initial abscess and require repeat PAD, but the long-term avoidance of surgery is more than 80%.

Although most TOAs are diagnosed with ultrasound, a diagnostic CT before drainage is useful to assess the entire extent of the abscess or abscesses and to exclude a diffuse peritoneal process that would be better suited for surgery. Organized abscesses, even when multiple, can be drained percutaneously. Access is obtained by the transabdominal, transgluteal, or transvaginal routes, depending on abscess location. CT is used for the transgluteal approach and often used for the transabdominal approach, but when the transvaginal route is selected, transvaginal ultrasound is used for guidance. A commercial or custom-made biopsy guide is used for needle insertion.

It has been suggested that abscesses larger than 7 cm may be best treated by a combination of antibiotics and PAD as initial therapy, but that smaller abscesses should be drained only in the event that medical treatment fails (41). Abscesses smaller than 3–4 cm in diameter can be aspirated but often cannot be catheterized, although needle aspiration alone can be therapeutic in this instance (42). The exact role and timing of aspiration, drainage, and surgery await further elucidation. PAD has the potential to reduce the early morbidity and mortality associated with major surgery, to reduce costs of hospital treatment, and to avoid surgical sterilization and premature menopause in young women.

Infected Tumors

Percutaneous drainage of infected tumors is an uncommon interventional procedure, constituting less than 1% of a series of more than 2,500 percutaneous abscess and fluid drainages (43). Central tumor necrosis occurs after a neoplasm outgrows its blood supply. Infection is more likely in debilitated patients (Figure 64–3).

Large catheters are effective in bringing about defervescence and clinical improvement in 75% of patients, but in most cases, the tumor persists with the relatively thick, nonpliable wall preventing collapse of the cavity. These patients require either surgery to resect the tumor or lifelong catheter drainage. Patients remained alive with catheter drainage for up to 1 year in the study (43). Catheter changes were usually performed every 2–3 months on an outpatient basis, affording significant palliation in patients who were unresectable.

Although the diagnosis of tumor usually has been established before the drainage procedure, infection may be the presenting manifestation of an underlying neoplasm. Clues that this is the case include nodularity of the wall, persistence of drainage, persistent hemorrhagic aspirate, failure of resolution, or recurrence following catheter withdrawal. Needle biopsy may be falsely negative for tumor, as has happened in all eight patients biopsied in the above series (43). However, cytology of aspirated fluid or image-guided biopsy of a mural nodule may be valuable in selected cases.

Fluid Collections

Patients who are febrile and have a new fluid collection or a collection of unknown duration require diagnostic aspiration with a small-bore needle. If the collection is determined to be infected by inspection or on Gram stain of the aspirate, PAD should be performed when a safe route exists and coagulation parameters are acceptable. Noninfected fluid collections require drainage only when they are believed to be symptomatic.

Lymphoceles

Lymphoceles complicate major abdominal vascular operations, up to 18% of renal transplantations (44), and 30% or more of radical pelvic lymphadenectomies (45). Although frequently asymptomatic and requiring no treatment, they may cause pain, tenesmus, urinary frequency, ureteral obstruction, compression of the vascular pedicle of renal transplants, bowel obstruction, leg edema, or deep venous thrombosis, or they may become infected (44,45). They result from leakage from lymphatics in the retroperitoneum or in the transplant, and typically do not manifest until 2–3 weeks after surgery. Heparin prophylaxis is an important promoter of lymphocele formation by preventing lymph coagulation. Corticosteroids, diuretics, extensive retroperitoneal dissection, and transplant rejection all increase lymph production and may also predispose to lymphocele formation, and immunosuppression significantly delays healing of transected lymphatics.

Surgery has been considered the therapy of choice in the past, with cure rates of more than 90% for peritoneal marsupialization. However, this is an extensive procedure with attendant risks, particularly in an immunosuppressed transplant recipient. Needle aspiration has a recurrence rate of 80–90% because of the persistence of leaking lymphatics. These require repeated aspirations, which are associated with an infection rate of 25–50% (46,47). Percutaneous catheter drainage alone has been shown to be successful, but drainage may be prolonged—more than 1 month in duration.

The duration of catheter drainage may be decreased and success rates increased to equal those of peritoneal marsupialization by the transcatheter installation of sclerosants, which inflame and seal the feeding lymphatics. These may be used whenever drainage persists after 1 week of catheter drainage alone (48). Agents used for sclerosis include povidone-iodine, ethanol, bleomycin, tetracycline, sodium salt solutions, bismuth, and talc. The lymphocele should not communicate with the peritoneal cavity when sclerosants are to be used. Multiple installation sessions are frequently required. Surgery should be reserved for patients in whom percutaneous therapy has failed repeatedly, because recurrences often respond to repeat drainage and sclerosis.

Renal biopsy should be performed when a lymphocele requires drainage in a renal transplant recipient because rejection frequently coexists, which when treated may facilitate resolution of the lymphocele (49,50,51). Cystic

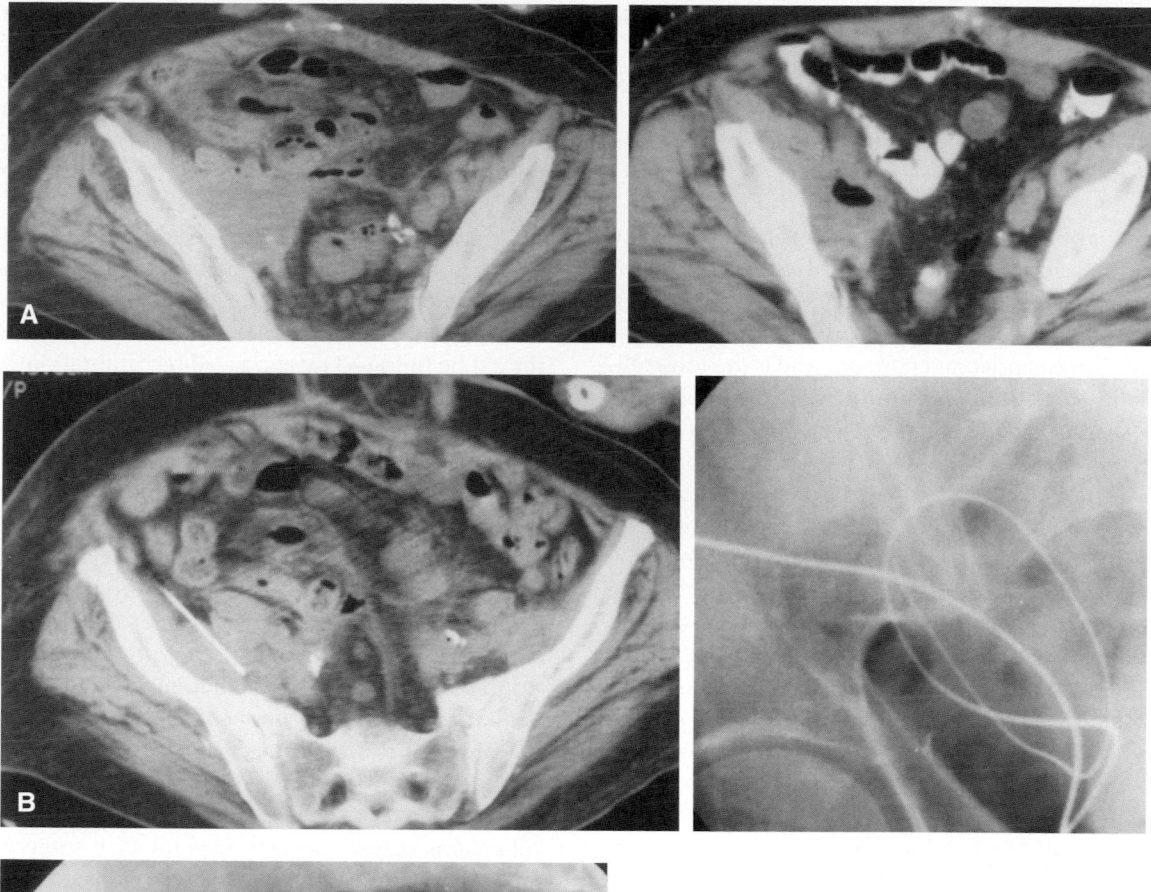

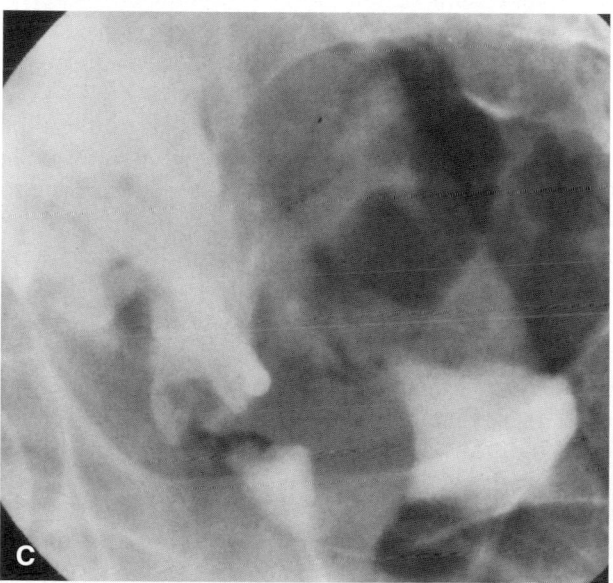

Figure 64–3 A 74-year-old man with a history of transitional cell carcinoma who presented to the emergency room with fever. **A.** CT scan shows a large air-containing fluid collection in the right iliacus muscle, with adjacent opacified and unopacified bowel. The preliminary diagnosis was diverticulitis with bowel communication and abscess. **B.** CT and fluoroscopic guidance were used to place a catheter into the iliacus muscle. The initial needle placement was performed under CT guidance, avoiding loops of bowel in the right lower quadrant. The patient was then transferred to fluoroscopy for further guide wire and catheter manipulations. **C.** After catheter placement, contrast injection shows a fistulous communication with a loop of bowel deep in the pelvis. Bacteriology showed mixed flora consistent with bowel communication. Cytology of the aspirated fluid showed transitional cell carcinoma metastatic to the iliacus. Because this collection represents necrotic metastasis with bowel communication, the catheter remained in place until the patient's death 5 months later.

ovarian neoplasms may be indistinguishable from lymphoceles on all imaging studies and on biochemical analysis of aspirate and may require a high index of suspicion for their recognition. For this reason, cytologic examination should be obtained on any aspirate from a pelvic cystic mass. Ovarian neoplasms are treated by resection and should not be aspirated because peritoneal dissemination may ensue.

Urinomas

Urinomas may occur in the setting of trauma, after surgery or renal transplantation, or because of obstruction, most commonly because of a ureteral calculus. Small urinomas resorb spontaneously once drainage of the urinary tract is established. Large urinomas or those causing obstruction or symptomatic compression require separate drainage as well. Resorption may be accompanied by elevation of the serum creatinine level.

CHOICE OF IMAGING METHOD FOR DIAGNOSIS AND DRAINAGE

Cross-sectional imaging has been responsible for the improved localization of abscesses and has been followed by an impressive reduction in their mortality (52,53). Ultrasound (US) is usually the most readily available modality, is relatively inexpensive and portable, and is the most reliable modality for the identification of fluid. For these reasons, it is particularly useful in intensive care or postoperative patients. However, an abscess may be obscured by overlying gas in the bowel or peritoneal cavity or sometimes within the abscess itself. Sinuses, stomas, wounds, or dressings may also impede US diagnosis. The examiner must be experienced and thorough, using a methodical technique such as that described by Baker et al. (52). An understanding of the anatomy of the peritoneal and extraperitoneal spaces will assist in the identification of abscesses remote from the site of original sepsis. A full bladder will be required if the pelvis is to be adequately examined transabdominally.

The classic US appearance of an abscess as an ovoid or round anechoic mass with posterior acoustic enhancement is only seen in half of all abdominal cases (53). Abscesses may contain internal echoes mimicking solid lesions or gas simulating a loop of bowel. The absence of typical features should not dissuade one from aspiration where it is otherwise indicated.

The advantages of US have led some to advocate its use as the initial diagnostic modality when an abdominal abscess is suspected (52). However, the superior sensitivity and specificity of CT have been documented in several studies (54) and approach 100%. Many also consider it to be the most cost-effective imaging investigation (3). It, too, has occasional pitfalls. Optimal opacification of the bowel with contrast material is necessary to distinguish between an unopacified loop and an abscess. Metallic hip prostheses and surgical clips may also hinder interpretation. The radiation dose burden is considerable and should be remembered in those requiring follow-up imaging. In practice, the choice between US and CT will depend on availability and the type of abscess suspected.

Radionuclide scanning is a sensitive method of detecting inflammation and abscesses, but it lacks the ability of CT and US to demonstrate exact anatomic relationships. Gallium 67 has been supplemented by the white blood cell-labeling agents [111]Indium and Tc-HMPAO. Gallium is inexpensive but requires 24–48 hours from administration for diagnostic imaging. Its interpretation may be difficult because of activity in the colon, liver, and spleen. Indium, unlike gallium, is not commonly taken up by tumors and, thus, is more specific for infective processes. Results are available in 3 hours. Tc-HMPAO is less well-established

than Indium as a white blood cell-scanning agent, and its interpretation is more difficult because of renal and biliary excretion. The labeling of white cells is time-consuming and requires skill, and false-negative results may occur when cells are damaged in labeling. False-positive uptake may occur in tumors, noninfected hematomas, and recent surgical wounds.

Isotope scanning is best reserved for the uncommon situation in which US and CT are negative but the clinical suspicion of an abscess remains high. In this instance, isotope scanning may reveal a focus of increased uptake, which should be followed by a targeted reexamination with US or CT under optimal conditions. An unsuspected focus remote from the pelvis may also be identified. However, "clinically useful serendipitous findings are rare" (55).

The choice of imaging modality for diagnosis also depends on the underlying pathologic condition. CT is indispensable in staging periappendiceal and peridiverticular abscesses and in determining the most appropriate therapy. US is frequently the preferred modality in the diagnosis of appendicitis and periappendiceal abscess in children, where it is desirable to avoid ionizing radiation. Similar considerations apply in assessing pelvic pathology in women of child-bearing age, where US is widely used in the diagnosis and follow-up of pelvic inflammatory disease (56). US is also widely used in the assessment of fluid collections complicating transplantation surgery. Without these specific indications, however, "CT is usually the only special radiologic test that should be performed to localize a suspected intra-abdominal abscess" (57).

MRI can detect abscesses, but, like other modalities, it is unable to differentiate between infected and noninfected fluid collections (58). Relatively long scan times, expense, inaccessibility of the patient inside the magnet, and metal-induced artifact from drainage needles have limited its use in PAD.

For guidance of PAD, US and especially CT allow a safe access route to be chosen. Deep abscesses may be obscured by overlying bowel gas on US, and collapsed loops of bowel may be difficult to recognize. US is most useful in guiding drainage of superficial abscesses or those that can be accessed by the transvaginal or transrectal routes, and at the bedside in intensive care or postoperative patients. The early approach to PAD as a two-step procedure with diagnosis at CT or US followed by fluoroscopically guided drainage has largely given way to one-step PAD, with the entire procedure performed expeditiously at CT or US. Postprocedure CT or US is performed immediately after evacuation of the cavity to confirm the adequacy of drainage or the need for catheter repositioning or additional catheters. The main role of fluoroscopy is to establish the presence of internal communication with bowel or other organs. This is best established at about 3 days after catheter insertion.

Barium studies may be required to exclude an underlying neoplasm in patients with a peridiverticular or periappendiceal abscess. These studies must be performed subsequent to CT and drainage; otherwise, valuable time may be lost waiting for barium to be cleared from the bowel before the diagnosis is made and drainage instituted. CT is the initial diagnostic imaging modality of choice in these adult patients.

TOOLS AND TECHNIQUES

The decision to proceed to PAD requires that a safe access route is available, that coagulation parameters are acceptable, and that appropriate parties give informed consent.

Consultation

Consultation with clinicians and surgeons involved in the care of the patient is important in making the decision to proceed to PAD. Ongoing communication is necessary for a satisfactory outcome, and the adjustment of catheter position, placement of additional catheters, or surgical intervention may need to be addressed.

Intravenous Drugs

Intravenous access should be established for the administration of antibiotics and analgesics. Broad-spectrum antibiotics covering multiple organisms, including anaerobes, can be administered during the procedure to combat bacteremia resulting from catheter manipulation and irrigation. They are continued until culture results permit selection of a more appropriate agent.

Adequate sedation is important for the safe and accurate placement of the drain and for patient comfort through the procedure. It is now possible to achieve IV sedation, which, in combination with the generous administration of local anesthetic, results in safe, reliable analgesia in virtually all patients, and amnesia for the procedure in most (59). This requires the presence of a specially trained and experienced nurse or doctor to administer frequent small intravenous doses of drugs such as midazolam and fentanyl in combination. The patient's vital signs, electrocardiogram (ECG), and blood oxygen saturation must be monitored continuously during the procedure and for a suitable period thereafter.

Diagnostic Aspiration

Diagnostic needle aspiration precedes catheter placement and achieves three purposes. It confirms the presence of a fluid collection, it determines whether the collection is infected, and it determines whether the viscosity of the contents is sufficiently low to allow successful drainage (4). Signs of an abscess such as the presence of gas or a hypervascular rim on contrast-enhanced CT are not frequently present, and drainable abscesses can appear "solid" on both CT and US, whereas lymphoma or fibrous scar can appear sonolucent.

The authors perform the initial aspiration with a 20- or 22-gauge needle because of its safety. If no fluid can be aspirated from the lesion, an 18-gauge needle is used. A Gram stain can be immediately performed if the fluid aspirated is not frankly purulent. If a layered collection is present, the dependent sediment should be sampled, because the supernatant fluid may yield false-negative results. Lack of free-flowing fluid aspirate through an 18-gauge needle indicates that a drainable collection is unlikely to be present. In this instance, biopsy for histologic examination may be performed when indicated.

Only 2–3 mL of fluid should be aspirated for Gram stain and culture. Withdrawal of larger volumes will result in partial collapse of the abscess, making insertion of a drainage catheter more difficult. Abscess fluid contains abundant leukocytes and bacteria on Gram stain. The presence of abundant leukocytes but no bacteria in a patient receiving prior antibiotic therapy indicates a sterile abscess, and drainage should proceed if the collection is causing symptoms. Abundant bacteria with scanty leukocytes indicate that bowel contents have been aspirated or that the patient has an abscess and is immunocompromised.

Choice of Access Route

Several routes have been described for pelvic abscess drainage.

Transabdominal

The advantages of transabdominal drainage are convenience for the operator, a comfortable position for the patient during the procedure, and easy and secure skin fixation (Figure 64–4). The disadvantages include the possibility of damage to the external iliac or inferior epigastric vessels because of the lateral approach required to avoid trangressing bowel, uterus, or bladder; the potential for contaminating the peritoneal cavity; and the length of the track. Despite CT guidance, this route is often not feasible in the pelvis.

Transgluteal

This route offers an alternative to surgery when a transabdominal approach is not possible. It requires precise catheter placement under CT guidance and a familiarity with the regional anatomy (Figure 64–5).

The greater sciatic foramen is crossed by the piriformis muscle, the sciatic nerve, the superior and inferior gluteal vessels, the superior gluteal nerve, the posterior cutaneous nerve of the thigh, the nerve to the obturator internis, and the internal pudendal vessels. The sciatic nerve is formed from the inferior continuation of the sacral plexus and exits the greater sciatic foramen in its anterior third, passing posterior to the sacrospinous ligament at its attachment to the ischial spine. The ideal trangluteal entry site to the pelvis is through the sacrospinous ligament medially, which avoids injury to the neurovascular structures of the greater sciatic foramen (Figure 64–6). The sacrospinous

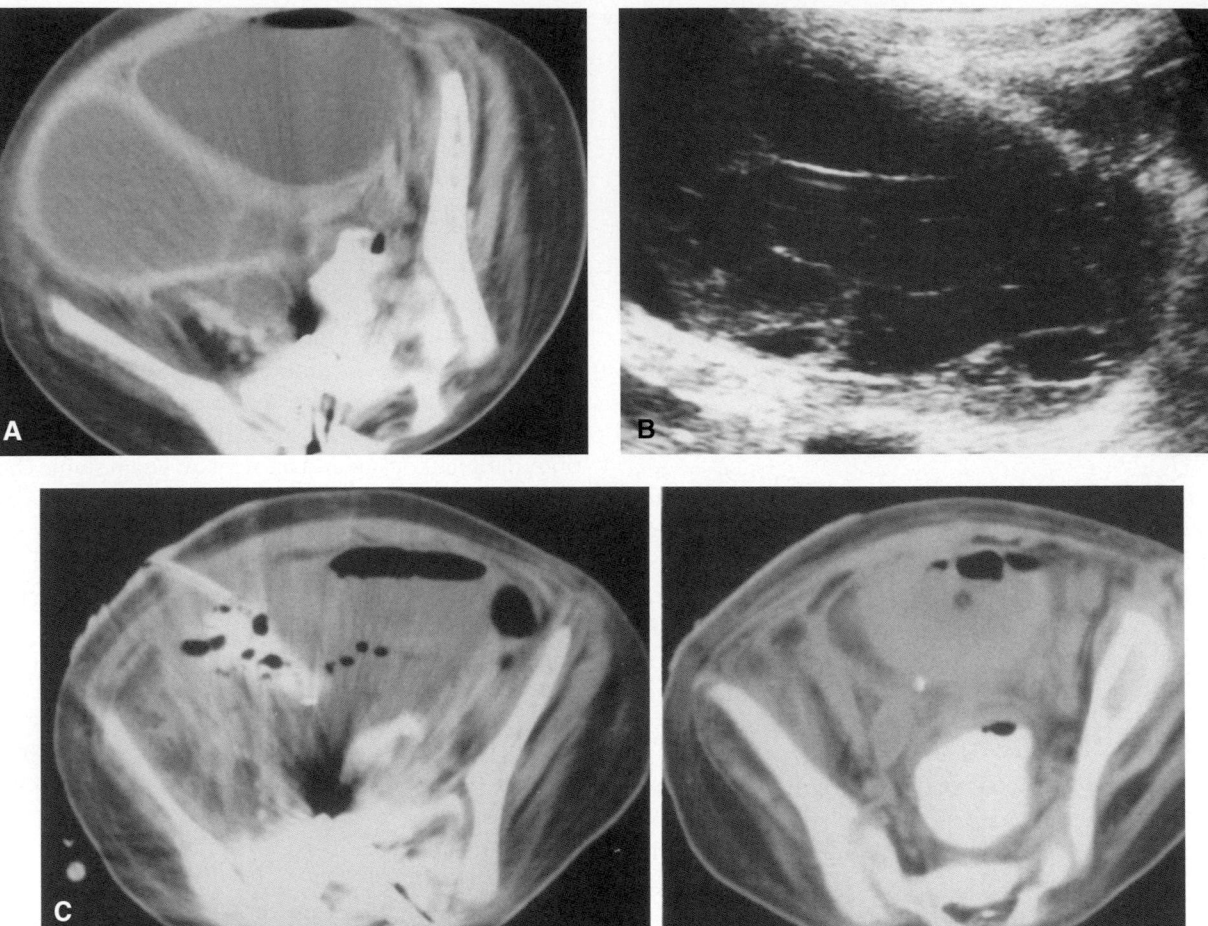

Figure 64–4 A 10-year-old child with cerebral palsy and spina bifida with an indwelling ventriculoperitoneal shunt. **A.** Pelvic CT scan shows an air-fluid level anteriorly within the bladder, with a right lower quadrant thick-walled, septated fluid density collection. **B.** Right lower quadrant ultrasound shows a large multiloculated superficial collection. No bowel is seen between the skin surface and the collection. Trocar catheter placement and drainage were performed. Laboratory studies revealed typical characteristics of a cerebral spinal fluid collection that had walled off at the tip of the ventriculoperitoneal shunt. **C.** Five days after catheter placement, no residual fluid collection is seen and the right lower quadrant is now filled with opacified bowel and minimal residual fatty inflammatory change. This case demonstrates the value of correlative imaging before abscess drainage. Although the CT scan appears to show a relatively simple collection, the multiple septa that were visible on the ultrasound could have deterred percutaneous treatment. However, all of the septa were broken easily with a guide wire during catheter placement, and the patient did well with percutaneous management and intravenous antibiotics. The shunt was subsequently replaced.

ligament is thin and is usually easily distinguished from the piriformis on CT. In a few patients, the location of the pelvic collection will necessitate puncture through the piriformis (60). The sacral plexus and sciatic nerve can still be avoided in these patients by entry as close to the sacrum as possible, although the gluteal vasculature may still be at risk. Major hemorrhage has been described in a patient undergoing transgluteal PAD through the greater sciatic foramen under guidance by fluoroscopy alone (61).

The most common complication of the transgluteal route is postprocedure pain, which may occur locally or deep in the pelvis or may radiate down the leg. It is associated with catheter placement through the piriformis and the sacral plexus, and in the authors' experience is most commonly mild and resolves within 24 hours. Soft catheters are better tolerated than those made from stiffer materials but are more difficult to insert through the large gluteal muscle bulk. Adequate dilation and dissection of the track help in this regard, as does the trocar technique, which increases stiffness of the catheter insertion system. Kinking of the catheter may occur in patients who lie supine or sit up.

Transvaginal

Surgical drainage of pelvic abscesses by the transvaginal route is well-established and of proven benefit (62), but it is limited in most instances to collections that displace the

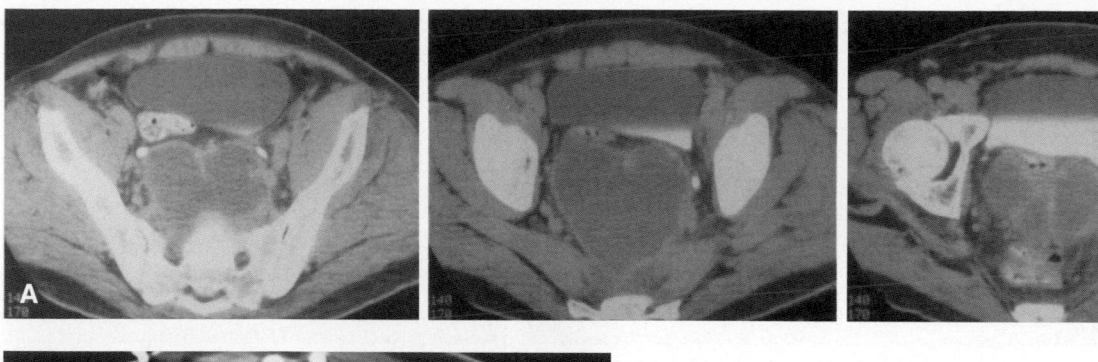

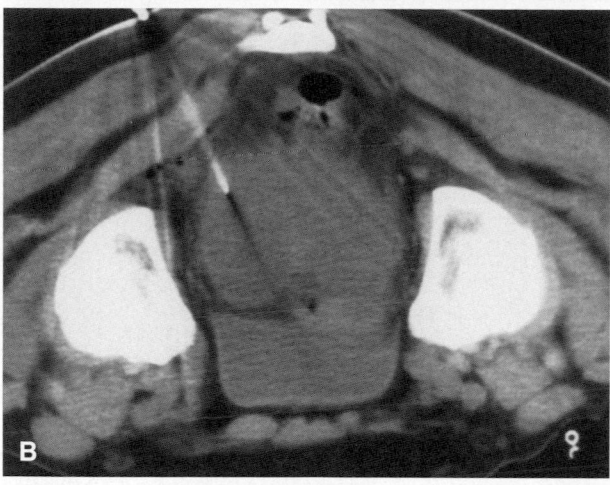

Figure 64–5 A 33-year-old HIV-positive man with a tender mass palpated on rectal examination. **A.** Three CT images through the pelvis following intravenous contrast and oral contrast administration show a septated thin-walled fluid collection in the pouch of Douglas. Anterior access routes are obscured by the iliac vasculature and the urinary bladder. **B.** The patient was placed prone, and a right transgluteal approach was made. Images of the initial needle can be seen in the pelvic musculature, but the tip of the needle used for drainage is seen within the cavity with the typical black artifact projecting from the tip. A relatively posterior approach is preferred for transgluteal drainage to avoid the sciatic nerve and neurovascular bundle, which are closely related to the ischial spine. **C.** Six days after percutaneous transgluteal drainage and after symptoms resolved, repeat scanning with the patient in a supine position shows no residual collection and normal position of the sigmoid and bladder.

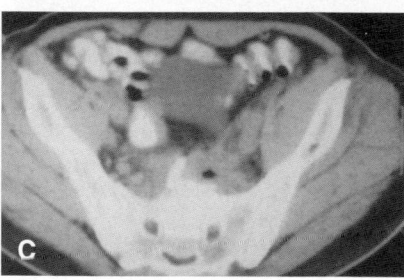 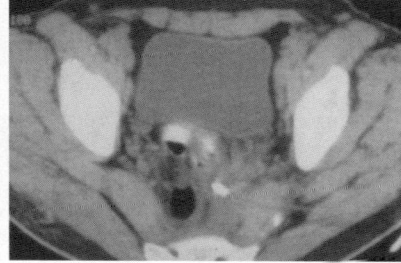 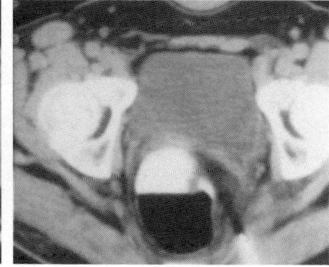

vaginal wall (63). Drainage may be readily performed under US guidance, which allows accurate needle or catheter placement within a collection that abuts but need not deform the vaginal vault.

Initial reports of transvaginal abscess drainage used transabdominal US for guidance (63–66). Transvaginal US, with its increased resolution, increases the sensitivity of diagnosis and allows for more precise catheter placement. It is not necessary to perform the procedure in the operating room, and the procedure may be combined with fluoroscopy to assist in catheter positioning if the Seldinger technique is used.

A vaginal speculum is unnecessary. The patient's bladder is emptied, she is placed in the lithotomy position, and the vagina is swabbed with a disinfectant solution, while the cervix is displaced and stabilized with a long clamp. Local anesthetic is administered directly through the long initial puncture needle. Intravenous sedation is also required. A biopsy guide is attached to the probe, although a plastic tube will suffice. A custom-made guide has been described.

If a drain has to be inserted, a small slit can made with a long scalpel in the vaginal vault, because penetrating the vaginal wall is sometimes difficult. Catheters with an inner metal stiffener are advantageous. A self-locking catheter eliminates the need for suturing to the vaginal wall or thigh for catheter retention.

In early studies and in the authors' own experience, transvaginal abscess drainage is safe and effective, with a success rate comparable to that of transabdominal drainage, if a little more difficult technically. It is relatively painless and well-tolerated. The place of needle aspiration alone in small nonviscous collections is yet to be determined (62–66).

Transrectal

Abscesses in contact with the rectum may be drained transrectally. Surgical drainage by the transrectal route is well-established but generally requires general anesthesia and an abscess that is palpable rectally. Image-guided drainage overcomes these problems and may be guided by a number

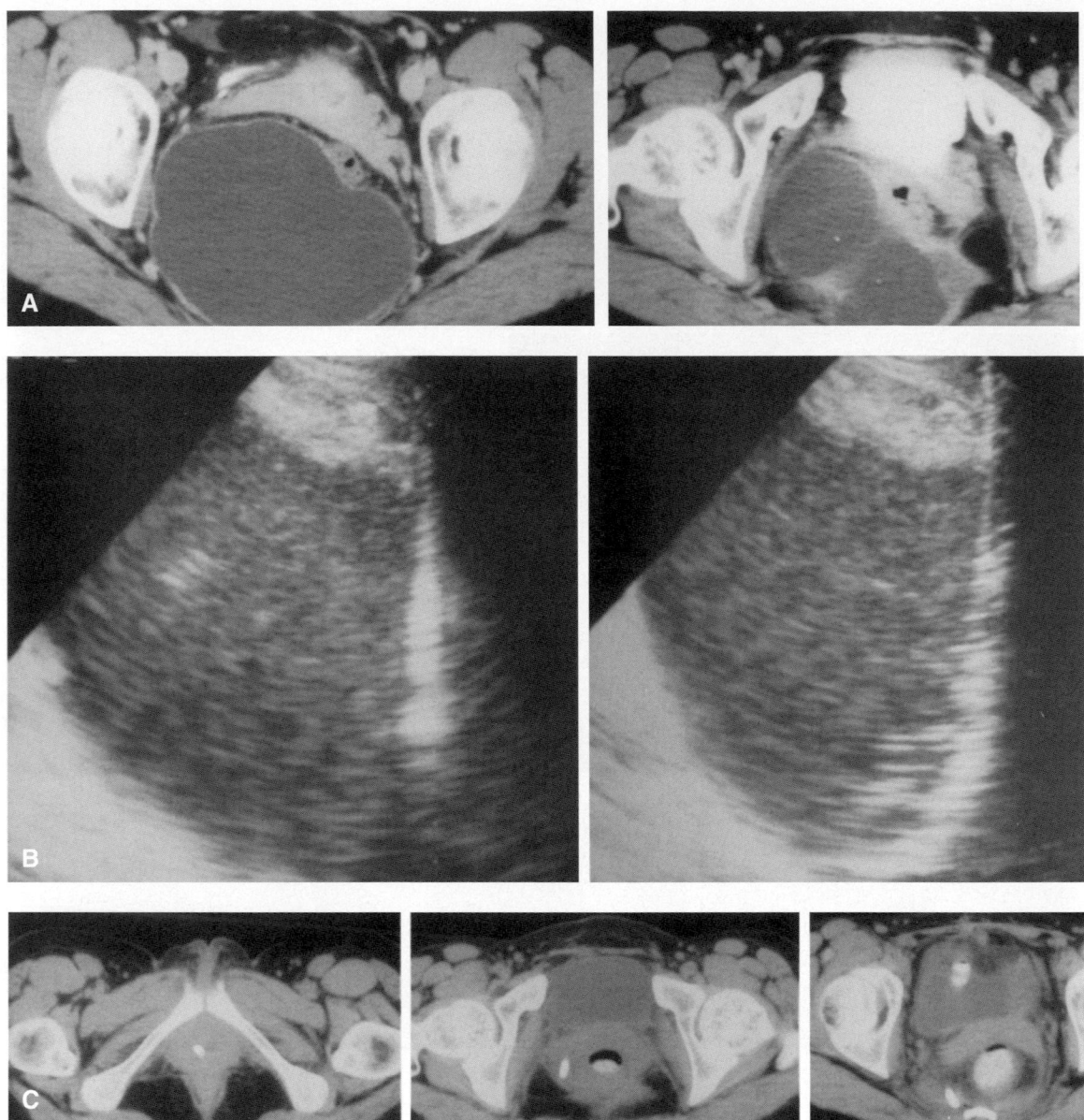

Figure 64–6 A 43-year-old woman with a 10-year history of benign presacral teratoma. Previous surgical resection attempts were unsuccessful and incurred large blood losses. Because of her religious beliefs, the patient refused further surgery, given the probable need for transfusion. **A.** CT scan shows a large loculated mass adherent to the sacrum, displacing the rectum and bladder anterolaterally. **B.** Transvaginal needle placement. The fluid shows uniform low-level echoes with bright linear echoes corresponding to the needle position. **C.** After complete aspiration of the collection and placement of a self-retaining 10 French catheter, follow-up CT shows no residual collection, with the catheter entering the presacral space via a right superior lateral transvaginal approach. Nine months later, the collection had recurred and was again treated with transvaginal drainage. The patient declined further surgery.

of modalities. Fluoroscopically guided drainage has been described with needle insertion through an anoscope (67) or a modified enema tip (68). CT guidance may also be used (69,70). Sonographic guidance was initially transabdominal (71), but more recently has been described transrectally and may be combined with fluoroscopy.

Abscesses anterior or posterior to the rectum may be drained transrectally. The abscess need not be palpable. The patient is placed in the left lateral decubitus position and the

needle, which is withdrawn a short distance into its sheath, is inserted into the rectum under imaging control. A gloved finger, plastic tube, or biopsy guide attached to a transrectal probe may be used to direct the needle, depending on the imaging method employed. The procedure is almost painless and is tolerated remarkably well. Local anesthesia and intravenous sedation are usually unnecessary. Skin fixation is unnecessary when locking catheters are used, but should be used whenever the patient is ambulatory.

A drawback of this technique is early expulsion of the catheter, which may occur during defecation. Reaccumulation of the abscess may result but usually is cured by repeat transrectal drainage. Lomas et al. (69) postulated that the use of large catheters will help maintain track patency in the event of catheter expulsion, but this is unproved. Overall success rates have been comparable with those of transabdominal drainage.

Catheter Selection

Large-bore catheters, such as the 12 French to 14 French van Sonnenberg sump (Medi-Tech) or the 16 French Mueller Drainage Catheter (Cook, Inc.) are used when the contents are viscous or the estimated volume exceeds 100 mL. The large lumen allows for drainage or aspiration of tenacious pus and particulate matter. The smaller lumen of sump catheters allows for circulation of room air to the collection through a filter, preventing adherence of the abscess wall to the side holes and allowing efficient introduction of irrigants. The efficiency of sump drainage is said to be 2–4 times that of closed drainage systems (72).

Medium-bore nonsump catheters include most standard biliary and nephrostomy catheters, such as the VTC Nephrostomy or Biliary Systems (Medi-Tech) or the Cope Biliary Loop (Cook, Inc.), and are suitable for drainage or nonviscous fluids. The smaller diameter of the lumen and side holes limits their effectiveness in patients with thick pus or necrotic material. Small-bore catheters (9 French and less), such as the Dawson-Mueller Ultrathane Drainage Catheter (Cook, Inc.) or the McGahan Multipurpose Catheter (Cook, Inc.) are effective for limited drainages of small nonviscous collections or as secondary catheters in tandem with double-lumen sumps for draining locules that are not decompressed by the main catheter.

Self-retaining catheters with locking loops or other devices to prevent dislodgment should be used where possible. They are particularly useful for transvaginal and transrectal drainages. Fixation of non–self-retaining catheters to the skin with sutures has given way to the use of various adhesive and locking devices that improve patient comfort and decrease the incidence of skin infection (73).

Catheter Insertion

The Seldinger technique may be used whenever the access route is difficult or the abscess is located immediately adjacent to a vital organ. It is particularly useful in drainages in which combined US-fluoroscopic guidance is used. Following diagnostic needle puncture, an 18-gauge sheathed needle is introduced into the abscess and a 0.038-inch wire is introduced through the outer sheath. A "single-stick" method using commercially available introducer systems, such as Accustik (Medi-Tech) or Neff (Cook), in which an 0.018-inch wire is initially passed through the diagnostic 22-gauge puncture needle may be used when additional safety is required.

When transabdominal or transgluteal catheter insertion is being performed via a safe percutaneous access path under CT guidance, many generally prefer the tandem trocar technique because of its speed and simplicity because the patient does not have to be moved to the fluoroscopy suite. The 22-gauge diagnostic needle is left in place to indicate the correct path, and the catheter with internal trocar and stiffener is placed alongside.

CATHETER MANAGEMENT

Catheter management optimizes the likelihood of successful drainage.

Cavity Lavage and Catheter Irrigation

Immediate cavity lavage is performed in the radiology department after aspiration of the drainable contents of the abscess. Multiple aliquots of normal saline are injected and aspirated until the irrigant is clear. The volume of fluid in each aliquot depends on the size of the collection that has been drained: 20- to 30-mL injections can be used in large cavities during the initial lavage, whereas 10-mL volumes are adequate in smaller cavities. A total volume of several hundred milliliters may be required.

Catheter irrigation is performed at the bedside. Initially, 10 mL of saline is injected every 8 hours by the patient's nurse and is tapered to once daily over a few days. Further irrigation is performed on interventional rounds if catheter blockage is suggested by persistent symptoms and unexpectedly low drainage.

Although low suction continues to be used in many institutions, continuous suction alone or through sump or double-catheter systems has not been convincingly shown to increase success rates over gravity drainage alone (74,75). Instillation of antibiotics has been unrewarding, and the proteolytic agent N-acetylcysteine lacks significant in vivo activity at the physiologic pH found within abscesses (76). However, intracavitary thrombolytics are of significant value in liquefying clot and increasing success rates in the drainage of infected hematomas that do not respond to catheter drainage alone. Thrombolytics also assist in breaking down fibrinous septations in other loculated collections resistant to drainage. For a large hematoma, abscess, or empyema, many use a schedule of 4–6 mg of tPA in 50 mL of normal saline, instilled every 12 hours for 3 days. The catheter is clamped, and the patient is placed in different positions for 30 minutes after instillation, following which drainage is resumed. Proportionately smaller volumes are used for smaller collections.

Catheter Withdrawal

Criteria for catheter withdrawal include the volume of daily drainage, the clinical status of the patient, the size of the abscess cavity, and the character of the drained fluid.

Satisfactory progress toward cure is indicated by a progressive decrease in the volume of drainage. Daily drainage should be less than 10 mL before the catheter is removed. Daily volumes that are not decreasing or that suddenly increase suggest the likelihood of internal fistulization. Similarly, the character of the drainage should progress from purulent to nonpurulent. A progressive change to resemble feces, urine, or lymph will be seen where a fistula exists and can be confirmed by chemical or microscopic examination of the fluid or definitively by abscessography.

Fever may continue for 4–5 days in certain patients, although defervesence typically occurs by 48 hours. Persistent sepsis at this time should prompt a search with CT for an undrained abscess or locule. If progress is satisfactory, follow-up imaging with abscessography or US can be performed to document resolution, but imaging is often not required in patients in whom the clinical response is appropriate and when the drained collection was simple. As experience is gained, less follow-up imaging is required, making PAD especially cost-effective. However, when in doubt, it is better to reimage than to prematurely remove a catheter and allow the patient to have a clinical recurrence. Although a small, infected collection may only require drainage for 3–4 days, a larger abscess may require 3–4 weeks. The drain should not be removed until drainage has effectively ceased and the patient's clinical condition has returned to normal.

Abscess-Fistula Association

Enteric abscesses occur in the setting of surgical enterotomy or anastomotic leakage or result from intestinal perforation in inflammatory disorders, particularly diverticulitis, appendicitis, and Crohn disease. Enteric communication, loosely termed *fistulization*, can be demonstrated in many of these patients. It is important to identify its presence because premature removal of the abscess drainage catheter will be followed by recurrence of the abscess unless the communication has been allowed to heal. Diagnosis of the communication is also important in determining the cause of the abscess, in providing correct catheter placement for healing of the communication, and in determining appropriate nutritional support. Enteric abscesses can be cured in 70–90% of cases with meticulous technique (73).

CT signs of enteric communication are the presence of gas, extraluminal oral or rectal contrast or a long gas-liquid level within the collection, proximity to bowel, and the presence of known gastrointestinal disease. Diagnosis is confirmed by abscessography at 3–5 days after catheter insertion, by which time the cavity can be distended with contrast without risk of bacteremia. Injection by appropriate positioning of the catheter and gentle probing of any areas of "beaking" of the cavity will often demonstrate a communication that would otherwise be overlooked (4). Occasionally, communications may not be apparent for up to 2 weeks.

Most enteric abscesses, including those resulting from postoperative bowel injury, anastomotic leaks, appendicitis,

and diverticulitis, are associated with a low-output "fistula" draining less than 100 mL per day. These abscesses respond well to PAD as long as the underlying bowel is healthy and capable of healing. The catheter should be placed with its side holes as close as possible to the opening of the communication, but the dependent portion of the abscess should also be drained. In most cases, this can be achieved with a single catheter, but sometimes two catheters will be necessary (37). Patients may be discharged once defervescence has occurred, and outpatient abscessograms may be obtained at 7- to 14-day intervals until the communication and abscess have healed. Patients should keep a record of catheter output while at home.

PAD of high-output "fistulas" requires a longer and more intensive period of therapy and is associated with a lower success rate. An underlying neoplastic cause must be ruled out, and distal bowel obstruction must be excluded with an appropriate luminal contrast study. Control of bowel secretions is obtained by gastrostomy or by nasogastric or nasojejunal intubation. Nutrition may be instituted enterally if the communication arises in the proximal small bowel and a jejunal feeding tube can be placed with its tip distal to the communication so that no reflux occurs into the fistula. Otherwise, total parenteral nutrition should be begun. Electrolyte balance and metabolic status must be closely monitored. PAD is achieved by placing a large-bore sump drain in a dependent portion of the cavity and another at the opening of the fistula, or preferably within it, occluding the tract. Subsequently, this catheter is replaced by smaller-bore catheters, which are slowly retracted to permit healing (75,76). A protracted period of catheter drainage will be required, with cure occurring as late as 12 weeks after drainage commenced. Patients with immunosuppression associated with solid organ transplantation can be successfully treated but usually require longer drainage times (77). In those patients in whom PAD is unsuccessful and surgery is required, worthwhile temporization and improvement of clinical status are still achieved.

Interventional Rounds

Catheter-related problems are common, occurring in 59% of inpatients in one study (78). Early identification of problems allows for their timely correction, maximizing the success rate of PAD and decreasing the length of hospital stay. The radiologist's familiarity with catheter problems, management, and imaging follow-up makes him or her the ideal person for the task.

The most common problem is that the catheter is not draining. This may be because of intrinsic obstruction, such as a blood clot, to extrinsic obstruction, such as kinking, or to inadequate drainage of the collection. Other problems are pericatheter leakage, improper catheter fixation, change in catheter position, local skin or wound complications, and distant complications such as peritonitis. Most of these problems can be managed successfully at the bedside. In the eyes of the referring physician, "increased participation in patient care elevates the status of the interventional radiologist from a technician to a valued consultant" (78).

Complications and Failures

Hemorrhage is usually minor and self-limiting but occasionally is major and life-threatening. Embolization of a perforated bleeding artery may rarely be necessary and has been described via the original needle track (61). Bacteremia with "shaking chills" is common, but septicemia with hypotension is rare. Both are minimized by using adequate cover with broad-spectrum antibiotics and by avoiding overdistention of the abscess with contrast or saline during irrigation, and both suggest an undrained locule or cavity when they persist.

Catheter insertion into or through the bowel should be avoided. Inadvertent diagnostic needle puncture of the bowel is usually innocuous, but a fistula has been described as a result of PAD of an interloop abscess. The fistula resolved with conservative management (79). Accidental catheter insertion into or through the bowel should be treated with the catheter left in situ for 1–2 weeks to allow the formation of a mature track, then slow withdrawal of it. In selected cases in which transgression of healthy bowel is recognized immediately, prompt removal of the catheter may be indicated with close observation.

Failure of PAD is avoidable in many cases. The principal cause of failure of both PAD and surgical drainage is incomplete recognition of the magnitude, extent, complexity, location, or response of the abscess. Meticulous preprocedural characterization of the abscess is necessary. Phlegmon and organized hematoma should be recognized as undrainable, whereas an underlying neoplasm can be treated by PAD if it is infected but cannot be cured. Undrained locules or abscesses and enteric communications should be pursued aggressively when the clinical course is indicative.

A common technical error is premature withdrawal of the catheter. Another is the improper selection of the route or entry site to the abscess, which results in the dependent portion remaining undrained. The catheter position should be corrected if it is unsatisfactory on follow-up imaging, as was the case in 26% of patients in one series (37). Additional catheters may be necessary, and multiple catheters were necessary in 31% of patients in that series.

While complications and failures are inevitable with PAD, guidelines are available for quality assurance purposes based on review of the literature. Overall success rates of PAD are reported to be approximately 85% (80). Complications, such as bacteremia or septic shock, may occur in 1–5% of cases (80). Hemorrhage, bowel transgression, and superinfection of sterile fluid are more rare, each with incidences of 1% or less (80). Pleural complications when working in the upper abdomen can run from 2–10% (80). Results will vary depending on the mix of underlying etiologies, comorbid conditions, and technical challenges encountered and quality assurance reviews can be triggered by thresholds set above these levels.

REFERENCES

1. Korobkin M, Silverman PM, Quint LE, et al. CT of the extraperitoneal space: normal anatomy and fluid collections. AJR Am J Roentgenol 1992;159:933–941.
2. Auh YH, Rubenstein WA, Schneider M, et al. Extraperitoneal paravesical spaces: CT delineation with US correlation. Radiology 1986;159:319–328.
3. Cook DE, Walsh JW. Computed tomography- and ultrasound-guided drainage of abscesses or other fluid collections. In: Pinson Neal M Jr, Tisnado J, Cho Shao-Lu, eds. Emergency Radiology. Boston: Little, Brown and Co., 1989:343–368.
4. Mueller PR, van Sonnenberg E, Ferrucci JT Jr. Percutaneous drainage of 250 abdominal abscesses and fluid collections: Part II. Current procedural concepts. Radiology 1984;151:343–347.
5. Neff CC, van Sonnenberg E, Casola G, et al. Diverticular abscesses: percutaneous drainage. Radiology 1987;163:15–18.
6. Mueller PR, Saini S, Wittenberg J, et al. Sigmoid diverticular abscesses: percutaneous drainage as an adjunct to surgical resection in 24 cases. Radiology 1987;164:321–325.
7. Jeffrey RB Jr, Tolentino CS, Federle MP, et al. Percutaneous drainage of periappendiceal abscesses: review of 20 patients. AJR Am J Roentgenol 1987;149:59–62.
8. van Sonnenberg E, Wittich G, Casola G, et al. Periappendiceal abscesses: percutaneous drainage. Radiology 1987;163:23–26.
9. Casola G, van Sonnenberg E, Neff CC, et al. Abscesses in Crohn disease: percutaneous drainage. Radiology 1987;163:19–22.
10. Safrit HD, Mauro MA, Jaques PF. Percutaneous abscess drainage in Crohn disease. AJR Am J Roentgenol 1987;148:859–862.
11. Saini S, Mueller PR, Wittenberg J, et al. Percutaneous drainage of diverticular abscess: an adjunct to surgical therapy. Arch Surg 1986;121:475–478.
12. Johnson CM. Drainage of retroperitoneal and pelvic abscesses and fluid collections. In: Kadir S, ed. Current Practice of Interventional Radiology. Philadelphia: Decker, 1991:727–734.
13. Glass CA, Cohn I Jr. Drainage of intra-abdominal abscesses: a comparison of surgical and computerized tomography-guided catheter drainage. Am J Surg 1984;147:315–317.
14. Aeder M, Jacqueline L, Wellman J, et al. Role of surgical and percutaneous drainage in the treatment of abdominal abscesses. Arch Surg 1983;118:273–280.
15. Johnson RD, Mueller PR, Ferrucci JT Jr, et al. Percutaneous drainage of pyogenic liver abscesses. AJR Am J Roentgenol 1985;144:463–467.
16. Olak J, Christou N, Stein LA, et al. Operative versus percutaneous drainage of intra-abdominal abscesses. Arch Surg 1986;121:141–146.
17. Welch CE, Malt RA. Abdominal surgery (three parts). N Engl J Med 1983;308.753–760.
18. Robbins SL. Robbins Pathologic Basis of Disease. Philadelphia: W.B. Saunders, 1989:884.
19. Williams I, Schnyder P. Diverticula. In: Margulis AR, Burhenne JH, eds. Alimentary Tract Radiology. 3rd Ed. St. Louis: Mosby, 1983:1090–1112.
20. Asch MJ, Markowitz AM. Diverticulitis coli: a surgical appraisal. Surgery 1967;62:239–247.
21. Jeffrey RB Jr. Enteric abscesses: imaging and intervention. Syllabus, Categorical Course in Interventional Radiology, 77th Scientific Assembly and Annual Meeting of the Radiological Society of North America, Chicago, 1991.
22. Hinchey EJ, Schaal PGH, Richards GK. Treatment of perforated diverticular disease of the colon. Adv Surg 1978;12:85–109.
23. Stafford ES, Sprong DH Jr. The mortality from acute appendicitis in the Johns Hopkins Hospital. JAMA 1940;115:1242–1245.
24. Cooperman M. Complications of appendectomy. Surg Clin North Am 1983;63:1233–1247.
25. Jordan JS, Kovalcic PJ, Schwab CW. Appendicitis with a palpable mass. Ann Surg 1981;193:227–229.
26. Bradley EL, Isaacs L. Appendiceal abscess revisited. Arch Surg 1978;113:130–132.
27. Paul DL, Bloom GP. Appendiceal abscess. Arch Surg 1982;117:1017–1019.
28. Jeffrey RB Jr, Federle M, Tolentino CS. Periappendiceal inflammatory masses: CT-directed management and clinical outcome in 70 patients. Radiology 1988;167:13–16.

29. Peer A, Strauss S. Percutaneous drainage of postappendectomy abscess complicated by enteric communication. Cardiovasc Intervent Radiol 1991;14:106–108.

30. Nunez D, Huber JS, Yrizarry JM, et al. Nonsurgical drainage of appendiceal abscesses. AJR Am J Roentgenol 1986;146:587–589.

31. Barnes BA, Behringer GE, Wheelock FC, et al. Treatment of appendicitis at the Massachusetts General Hospital, 1932–1959. JAMA 1962;180:122–126.

32. Mosegard A, Nielson OS. Interval appendectomy: a retrospective study. Acta Chir Scand 1979;145:109–111.

33. Homans J, Powers LH. Appendiceal abscess: treatment of the appendix. N Engl J Med 1928;199:319–321.

34. Greenstein AJ, Sacher DB, Greenstein RJ, et al. Intraabdominal abscess in Crohn's ileocolitis. Am J Surg 1982;143:727–730.

35. Keighley MRB, Eastwood D, Ambrose NS, et al. Incidence and microbiology of intraabdominal and pelvic abscess in Crohn's disease. Gastroenterology 1982;83:1271–1275.

36. Steinberg DM, Cooke WT, Alexander-Williams J. Abscess and fistulae in Crohn's disease. Gut 1973;14:865–869.

37. Papanicolaou N, Mueller P, Ferrucci JT, et al. Abscess-fistula association: radiologic recognition and percutaneous management. AJR Am J Roentgenol 1987;143:811–815.

38. Doemeny JM, Burke DR, Meranze SGO. Percutaneous drainage of abscesses in patients with Crohn's disease. Gastrointest Radiol 1988;13:237–241.

39. Millward SF, Ramswak W, Fitzsimons P, et al. Percutaneous abscess in Crohn's disease. Gastrointest Radiol 1986;11:289–290.

40. Ginsburg DS, Stern JL, Hamod KA, et al. Tubo-ovarian abscess: a retrospective review. Am J Obstet Gynecol 1980;138:1055–1058.

41. Tyrrel RT, Murphy FB, Bernadino ME. Tubo-ovarian abscesses: CT-guided percutaneous drainage. Radiology 1990;175:87–89.

42. Casola G, van Sonnenberg E, D'Agostino HB, et al. Percutaneous drainage of tubo-ovarian abscesses. Radiology 1992;182:399–402.

43. Mueller PR, White EM, Glass-Royal M, et al. Infected abdominal tumors: percutaneous catheter drainage. Radiology 1989;173:627–629.

44. Braun WE, Banowsky LH, Saffron RA, et al. Lymphoceles associated with renal transplantation: report of 15 cases and review of the literature. Am J Med 1974;57:714–729.

45. Ilacheran A, Monaghan JM. Pelvic lymphocyst—a 10-year experience. Gynecol Oncol 1988;29:333–336.

46. Gilliland JD, Spies JB, Brown SB, et al. Lymphoceles: percutaneous treatment with povidone-iodine sclerosis. Radiology 1989;171: 227–229.

47. Conte M, Panici PB, Guariglia L, et al. Pelvic lymphocele following radical para-aortic and pelvic lymphadenectomy for cervical carcinoma: incidence rate and percutaneous management. Obstet Gynecol 1990;76:268–271.

48. White M, Mueller PR, Ferrucci JT Jr, et al. Percutaneous drainage of postoperative abdominal and pelvic lymphoceles. AJR Am J Roentgenol 1985;145:1065–1069.

49. van Sonnenberg E, Wittich GR, Casola G, et al. Lymphoceles: imaging characteristics and percutaneous management. Radiology 1986;161:593–596.

50. van Sonnenberg E. Advances in percutaneous abscess drainage. Syllabus, Categorical Course in Interventional Radiology, 77th Scientific Assembly and Annual Meeting of the Radiological Society of North America, Chicago, 1991:56–72.

51. Cohan RH, Saeed M, Sussman SK, et al. Percutaneous drainage of pelvic lymphatic fluid collections in the renal transplant patient. Invest Radiol 1987;22:865–867.

52. Baker ME, Binder RA, Rice RP. Diagnostic imaging of abdominal fluid collections and abscesses. Crit Rev Diagn Imaging 1986; 25:233–278.

53. Saini S, Kellum JM, O'Leary MP, et al. Improved localization and survival in patients with intra-abdominal abscesses. Am J Surg 1983;145:136–142.

54. Schwerk WB, Durr HK. Ultrasound grayscale pattern and guided aspiration puncture of abdominal abscesses. J Clin Ultrasound 1981;9:389.

55. Dobrin PB, Gully PH, Greenlee HB, et al. Radiologic diagnosis of an intra-abdominal abscess: do multiple tests help? Arch Surg 1986;121:41–46.

56. Joseph AEA, Macvicar D. Ultrasound in the diagnosis of abdominal abscesses. Clin Radiol 1990;42:154–156.

57. Haaga JR. Imaging intra-abdominal abscesses and nonoperative drainage procedures. World J Surg 1990;14:204–209.

58. Brown JJ, van Sonnenberg E, Gerber KH, et al. Magnetic resonance relaxation times of percutaneously obtained normal and abnormal body fluids. Radiology 1985;154:727–731.

59. Lind LL, Mushlin PS. Sedation, analgesia and anesthesia for radiologic procedures. Cardiovasc Intervent Radiol 1987;10:247–253.

60. Butch RJ, Mueller PR, Ferrucci JT Jr, et al. Drainage of pelvic abscesses through the greater sciatic foramen. Radiology 1986; 158:487–491.

61. Malden ES, Picus D. Hemorrhagic complication of transgluteal pelvic abscess drainage: successful percutaneous treatment. J Vasc Intervent Radiol 1992;3:323–328.

62. Walker AP, Malangoni MA. Peritonitis and intra-abdominal abscesses. In: Schwartz SI, ed. Principles of Surgery. 5th Ed. New York: McGraw-Hill, 1989:1459–1489.

63. Nosher JL, Winchman HK, Needell GS. Transvaginal pelvic abscess drainage with US guidance. Radiology 1987;165:872–873.

64. Graham D, Sanders RC. Ultrasound-directed transvaginal aspiration biopsy of pelvic masses. J Ultrasound Med 1982;1:279–280.

65. VanDerKolk HL. Small deep pelvic abscesses: definition and drainage guided with an endovaginal probe. Radiology 1991; 181:283–284.

66. van Sonnenberg E, D'Agostino HB, Casola G, et al. US-guided transvaginal drainage of pelvic abscesses and fluid collections. Radiology 1991;181:53–56.

67. Mauro MA, Jaques PF, Mandell VS, et al. Pelvic abscess drainage by the transrectal catheter approach in men. AJR Am J Roentgenol 1985;144:477–479.

68. Bennett JD, Kozak RI, Taylor BM, et al. Deep pelvic abscesses: transrectal drainage with radiologic guidance. Radiology 1992; 185:825–828.

69. Lomas DJ, Dixon AK, Thomson HJ, et al. CT-guided drainage of pelvic abscesses: the perianal transrectal approach. Clin Radiol 1992;45:246–249.

70. Gazelle GS, Haaga JR, Stellato TA, et al. Pelvic abscesses: CT-guided transrectal drainage. Radiology 1991;181:49–51.

71. Nosher JL, Needell GS, Amorosa JK, et al. Transrectal pelvic abscess drainage with sonographic guidance. AJR Am J Roentgenol 1986; 146:1047–1048.

72. Casteñada-Zuniga WR, Tadavarthy SM, Letourneau JG, et al. Drainage of abdominal abscesses. In: Casteñada-Zuniga WR, Tadavarthy SM, eds. Interventional Radiology. 2nd Ed. Baltimore: Williams & Wilkins, 1992:1311–1356.

73. van Sonnenberg E, D'Agostino HB, Casola G, et al. Percutaneous abscess drainage: current concepts. Radiology 1991;181:617–626.

74. van Sonnenberg E, Schiffman HR, Casola G, et al. Simplified solvent infusion and drainage in closed systems: double-lumen single-catheter method. AJR Am J Roentgenol 1985;144:259–260.

75. Edwards KC, Katzen BT, Woods C. Continuous gentle suction apparatus for abscess drainage. Radiology 1982;145:537.

76. Dawson SD, Mueller PR, Ferrucci JT Jr. Mucomyst for abscesses: a clinical comment. Radiology 1984;151:342.

77. Schuster MR, Crummy AB, Wojtowycz MM, et al. Abdominal abscesses associated with enteric fistulas: percutaneous management. J Vasc Interv Radiol 1992;3:359–363.

78. Goldberg MA, Mueller PR, Saini S, et al. Importance of daily rounds by the radiologist after interventional procedures of the abdomen and chest. Radiology 1991;180:767–770.

79. Lambiase RE, Cronan JJ, Dorfman GS, et al. Postoperative abscesses with enteric communication: percutaneous treatment. Radiology 1989;171:497–500.

80. American College of Radiology. ACR Standards for specifications and performance of image-guided percutaneous drainage/aspiration of abscesses and fluid collections (PDAFC) in adults. In: ACR Standards 2001–2002. Reston: American College of Radiology, 2001:293–299.

Miscellaneous Applications of Interventional Radiology

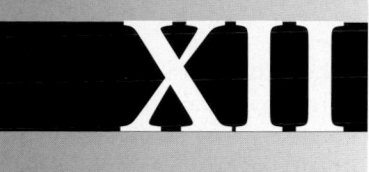

Interventional Radiology of Venous Insufficiency

65

Robert J. Min

Venous insufficiency is a widespread health problem affecting 25% of women and 15% of men in the United States (1). Incompetence of the superficial venous system is particularly common with risk factors such as female gender, pregnancy, hormones, aging, and prolonged standing or sitting (2,3). Although varicose veins can be visually unappealing, they are often associated with leg symptoms ranging from fatigue or heaviness to aching pain, night cramps and even restlessness (4–6). Without treatment, superficial venous insufficiency can lead to lower extremity swelling, eczema, pigmentation, hemorrhage, and ulceration (7). Despite the potentially disabling nature and the high socioeconomic cost of this prevalent condition, most patients suffering from venous insufficiency are poorly evaluated and often mismanaged. Fortunately, advancements in noninvasive testing, specifically duplex ultrasound, have improved the general understanding of venous insufficiency by allowing direct study of underlying pathways of reflux. Making a better diagnosis has led to better treatments. Compression sclerotherapy, widely practiced in Europe for decades, is finally gaining acceptance in the United States. Ambulatory phlebectomy, first practiced in the 1960s, is also experiencing an increase in popularity. The development of new minimally invasive techniques for ablation of incompetent veins, including radiofrequency and endovenous laser, now provide patients with excellent treatment options to surgery.

ANATOMY

The lower extremity venous system comprises deep and superficial veins that are interconnected by multiple perforating veins. The great saphenous vein (GSV) and the small saphenous vein (SSV) are the most important components of the superficial venous system. Driven by the calf muscle pump, one-way valves permit unidirectional flow of blood back to the heart against gravitational forces. Blood flow is directed from superficial to deep veins via valves at the saphenofemoral junction (SFJ), saphenopopliteal junction (SPJ), and within perforating veins.

Great Saphenous Vein

The GSV begins as the continuation of the dorsal venous arch in the foot, ascends medially in the leg, and ultimately drains into the deep system at the SFJ. It is characteristically found in the saphenous compartment, superficial to the muscular fascia and deep to the saphenous fascia. Two major tributaries feed into the GSV from below and above the knee. The GSV also receives blood from the superficial external pudendal, superficial inferior epigastric, and external circumflex iliac veins just before emptying into the femoral vein (Figure 65–1). An accessory saphenous vein can run parallel and anterior to the GSV acting as a duplicated GSV (8).

Small Saphenous Vein

The SSV is the other major superficial vein of the leg. Ascending behind the lateral malleolus and traveling up the dorsal aspect of the calf, the SSV has a singular junction with the popliteal vein just above the knee in two thirds of people. In the remaining population, the SSV has variant drainage into the deep system, most commonly into the posterior medial tributary of the GSV (as the vein of Giacomini), or into a deep vein in the thigh via a perforator (9), as illustrated in Figure 65–2. In many of these cases, a standard SPJ may also be present.

Deep Venous System

The deep veins are found below the muscular fascia and are familiar to most interventional radiologists in the context of deep venous obstruction. They include the plantar vein of the foot, three pairs of tibial veins in the calf, and the popliteal and femoral veins in the thigh. Numerous venous sinusoids, found within the muscles of the lower limb, are additional components of the deep venous system. Those in the calf are most important and include the soleal and gastrocnemial veins. These sinusoids drain into other deep veins via valved connecting veins. The deep veins are key elements of the pumping system, responsible for returning blood from muscles and blood collected from the superficial veins back to the heart.

Perforating Veins

Perforators course obliquely through the deep fascia connecting the superficial system with the sinusoidal, tibial,

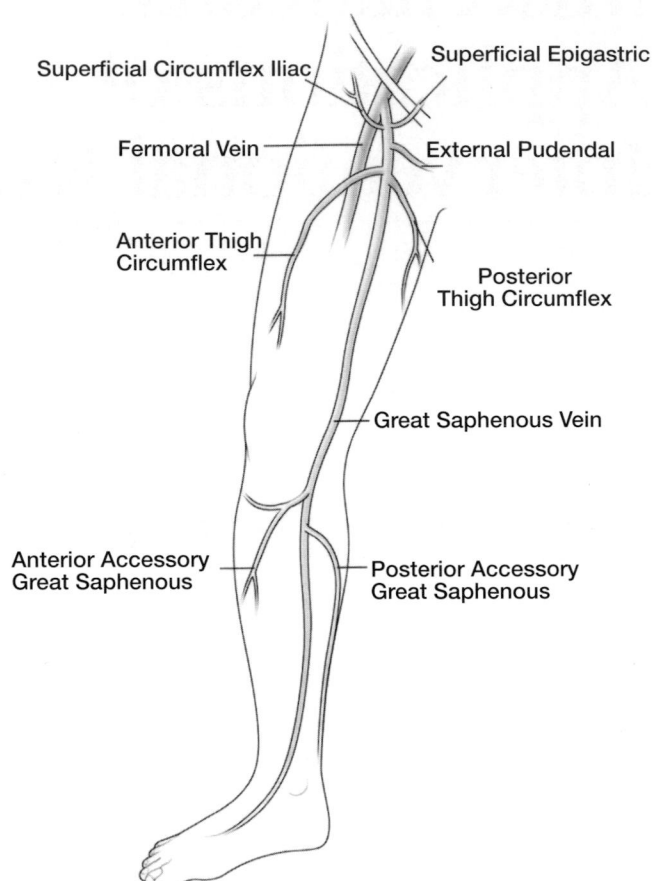

Figure 65–1   Anatomy of the great saphenous vein and its major tributaries.

popliteal, and femoral veins. Unidirectional valves within the perforating veins direct flow from the superficial to the deep veins. Clinically important, named perforating veins have been identified in typical locations as seen in Figure 65–3.

PATHOPHYSIOLOGY OF VENOUS INSUFFICIENCY

Incompetence of the Superficial Venous System

Several mechanisms have been postulated as the underlying cause of superficial venous reflux. Direct injury or superficial phlebitis may lead to valve failure. Congenital conditions may rarely be the etiology for weakened vein walls or abnormal valves. Hormonal influences, such as those in early pregnancy, may result in excessive distension of veins and valvular incompetence. No matter what the origin, superficial venous reflux is simply the inevitable result of the introduction of high pressures into superficial veins that are intended to function as a low-pressure system.

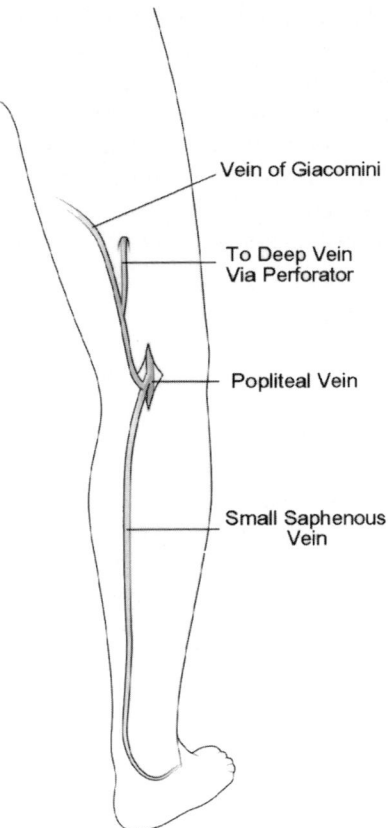

Figure 65–2 Anatomy of the small saphenous vein and its common variant terminations.

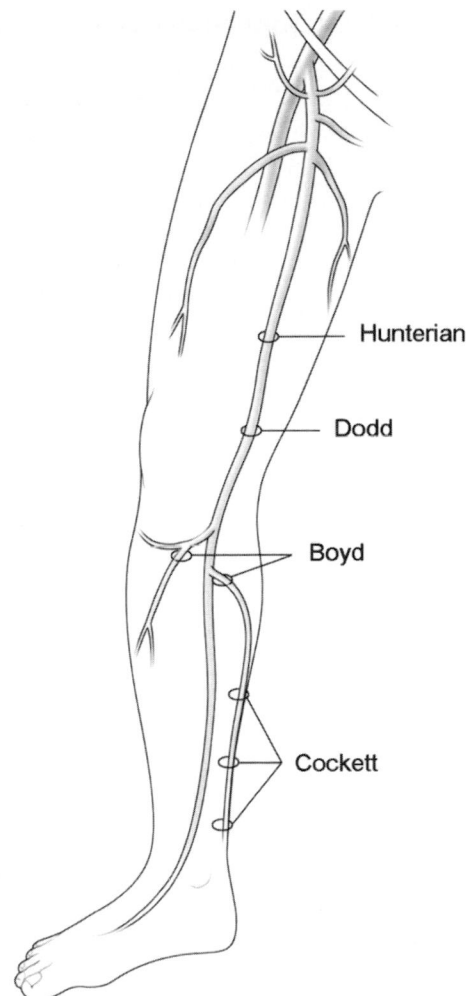

Figure 65–3 Approximate locations of named perforators along the great saphenous vein (above knee) and the posterior accessory GSV (below knee) where the superficial venous system connects with the deep venous system.

Incompetence of the venous valves occurs when the high pressures cause the normal superficial veins to dilate until the thin flaps of the valves no longer meet. Failure of valves at the saphenofemoral or saphenopopliteal junctions and within perforators represents the most significant routes for introduction of high pressures from the deep to superficial veins. Other characteristic patterns of venous disease can be the result of anterior thigh circumflex (ATC) or posterior thigh circumflex (PTC) reflux, with or without associated GSV insufficiency. Incompetent pudendal or gluteal varices, commonly seen in women during and after pregnancy, are also common causes of significant varicose veins.

CLINICAL EXAMINATION

Physicians who are unfamiliar with disorders of the superficial venous system often underestimate the complexity of the condition and the importance of a proper history and physical examination. Valuable information to be gathered includes the duration and evolution of the problem, presence and severity of symptoms, prior treatments, and the possibility of prior deep venous thrombosis (DVT). Physical examination is performed in the standing position, preferably on a platform. It consists of careful inspection,

palpation, and percussion. Examination should include not only the legs, but also the lower abdomen and pubic area. The purpose of clinical examination is to examine the main venous trunks to determine the location of primary or highest points of reflux. Additional diagnostic studies are then considered, and a treatment plan based upon the findings is devised.

DIAGNOSTIC EVALUATION: DUPLEX ULTRASOUND

Duplex ultrasound (DUS) examination of the superficial and deep venous systems has emerged as the most valuable tool in understanding the underlying sources of venous reflux. In the study of patients with venous insufficiency, the goal of DUS is to map out both the abnormal and normal venous pathways to identify the sources of incompetence and levels of obstruction when present (10).

Technique—Great Saphenous Vein

Unlike evaluation for DVT, DUS examination for superficial venous insufficiency is performed with the patient upright. The leg being studied is flexed and turned slightly outward. Evaluation is performed in a systematic manner, most commonly, beginning at the groin and proceeding peripherally. The entire length of the GSV is examined in axial projection with grayscale technique. Vein diameter is measured, and the major tributaries are followed and examined. Varicose tributaries are noted and followed for the purpose of determining their etiology.

The SFJ is assessed for the presence of reflux in longitudinal and short axis views. Color or power Doppler can rapidly facilitate the identification of reflux by movement of the probe along the vein during manual compression and release of peripheral venous segments. Reflux is most reliably identified, quantified, and documented with pulsed-wave Doppler (PWD) with similar techniques of distal compression and release.

Perforating Veins

Significant perforating veins associated with the GSV in the thigh and the posterior accessory GSV in the lower leg are sought and similarly examined. Transverse and oblique scanning planes are most helpful when evaluating perforators. Scanning with color Doppler or PWD following compression and release of the limb below the perforator tests valve competency.

Small Saphenous Vein

With the patient facing away, the knee is slightly flexed to prevent venous compression by the muscles or popliteal artery. The SSV is identified and examined in its entirety in the axial plane. Drainage of the SSV into the deep venous system is determined. The size, competency of the SSV and its junctions, and its relationship to posterior calf varicosities are assessed as was done with the GSV. Perforating veins connecting the SSV with the venous sinusoids are noted, including the level of inflow and competence of the gastrocnemial veins.

COMPRESSION SCLEROTHERAPY

Sclerosants

Only a few sclerosing agents are available today as appropriate choices for the safe treatment of varicose veins and telangiectasias. The most commonly used sclerosants are discussed below.

The Federal Drug Administration (FDA) has approved sodium morrhuate and ethanolamine oleate for sclerotherapy, but unacceptably high anaphylaxis risks make both poor choices for treatment of varicose veins and telangiectasias (11).

Hypertonic saline is not FDA-approved for sclerotherapy of leg veins, but it is often used for this purpose in the United States. Concentration varies from 11.7% or 23.4%, depending on vein size and responsiveness. It is widely available, inexpensive, and rarely allergenic; however, hypertonic saline causes burning pain; has a high risk of skin ulceration; and is quickly diluted, limiting the size of vein that can be treated.

Dextrose and hypertonic saline (25% dextrose, 10% sodium chloride) is produced in Canada under the trade name Sclerodex and is not FDA-approved in the United States. Its effects are similar to those of hypertonic saline, but given its lower saline concentration, Sclerodex is less painful and has lower risk of skin necrosis. It is used mainly for treatment of telangiectasias and reticular veins.

Polidocanol (hydroxypolyethoxydodecane) is not FDA-approved in the United States but is the most commonly used sclerosing agent in Europe. It is has an excellent safety profile with low risk of extravasation necrosis or allergic reaction and is painless upon injection. Polidocanol is used in concentrations of 0.25–4% to treat the whole range of veins from telangiectasias to incompetent saphenous veins.

Sodium tetradecyl sulfate (STS) is approved by the FDA and is the most widely used sclerosing agent in the United States to treat telangiectasias and varicose veins. It has a long history as a safe sclerosant and is effectively used to treat the whole spectrum of incompetent veins in concentrations of 0.1–3%.

General Principles

Although proper use of any of these sclerosants may yield the desired result, treatment efficacy will be maximized and complications minimized by following a few basic treatment principles. In general, the concentration of sclerosant depends on the type and diameter of vein to be treated (Table 65–1). It is best to start with the minimum sclerosant strength necessary to achieve effective sclerosis because collateral damage will occur when solutions too high in concentration are used. Injections usually proceed from central to peripheral and from larger to smaller veins. Although reflux can be present in a vein without an apparent underlying source, visible veins are often "fed" by other veins. Telangiectasias may be associated with refluxing reticular veins; incompetent saphenous veins, perforators, or truncal tributaries may be the cause of bulging varicose veins. These underlying sources will need to be addressed to achieve maximal treatment benefit.

Patient Selection

In addition to known allergy to the sclerosant, other relative contraindications to compression sclerotherapy include

TABLE 65-1

SCLEROSING AGENT VERSUS VEIN TYPE

Sclerosant	Telangiectasia	Reticular	Varicose	Saphenous
STS	0.1–0.3%	0.3–0.5%	0.5–2.0%	3.0%
Polidocanol	0.2–0.5%	0.5–1.0%	1.0–4.0%	4.0%
Hypertonic saline	11.7–23.4%	23.4%	N/A	N/A
Dextrose/HS	Full strength	Full strength	N/A	N/A

patients with known or suspected risk factors for DVT, such as a past history of DVT or pulmonary embolus; family history of hypercoagulability; air or other long-distance travel; prolonged bed rest; or inability to ambulate. Others who should not be treated with sclerotherapy are pregnant or nursing women; people with significant systemic illness, lymphedema, or nonpalpable pedal pulses; and those with unrealistic expectations. Although deep venous reflux is not necessarily a contraindication, sclerotherapy of superficial varicose veins should be avoided in patients with severe deep venous obstruction.

Sclerotherapy Technique

Injections are usually performed with the patient in the recumbent position. This allows injection of sclerosant into a relatively empty vein, minimizing mixing with blood while maximizing contact with the endothelium. Avoiding treatment in the upright position also lessens the incidence of vasovagal reactions. The overlying skin is wiped with isopropyl alcohol, and the vein is entered with either a 27-gauge or 30-gauge needle attached to a 3-mL syringe. Cannulation should be brisk, with the needle bevel facing up. When injecting telangiectasias, one can often feel entry into the vein and visualize the needle tip within the vein lumen. With gentle injection of a small amount of sclerosant, clearing of the telangiectasia will be noted as sclerosant displaces blood confirming intraluminal position. Injection should be immediately discontinued in the event that a bleb develops or the patient feels pain. Before injecting veins larger than telangiectasias, a small amount of blood should be aspirated into the needle hub to verify intravenous placement. As discussed previously, larger veins usually require higher concentrations and greater volumes for effective sclerosis. Telangiectasias require no more than a few drops of a mild sclerosant (0.2% STS, for example), reticular veins are injected with a few tenths of a milliliter of a slightly stronger solution (0.3–0.5% STS), and bulging varicose veins may be treated with 0.25–1 mL of a higher concentration sclerosant (0.5–1% STS). Injections are spaced at 3–5 mm intervals. In all cases, injections should be performed with minimal pressure and be painless when using polidocanol or STS.

Postsclerotherapy

Although it is generally agreed that some form of compression postsclerotherapy is beneficial, the exact amount is controversial. Following sclerotherapy treatment of telangiectasias and mild varicose veins, most physicians advocate wearing class I (20–30 mm Hg) graduated compression stockings for at least 5–7 days. In general, treatment of larger varicose veins requires tighter graduated compression (class II, for example) for longer periods of time postinjections. In theory, graduated compression improves treatment efficacy, minimizes adverse reactions such as "trapped blood" with resultant hyperpigmentation, and decreases the risk of DVT. Ambulation should be encouraged immediately following sclerotherapy to further minimize risks. Patients should avoid vigorous gym workouts, excessive sun or hot baths, and air travel for the first week following treatment.

Patients are seen 2–4 weeks after sclerotherapy for follow-up. Previously treated areas are examined, and areas of intravascular hematoma or "trapped blood" are expressed through an 18-gauge or 25-gauge needle puncture. Although eventually absorbed by the body over several months, removal of trapped blood in a timely fashion will minimize hyperpigmentation from hemosiderin staining of the overlying skin. Additionally, these areas of trapped blood are often tender and patients will experience immediate relief following removal. Additional sclerotherapy treatment can be performed at 4–6 week intervals, which allows adequate time for inflammation to subside and the benefits of the sclerosing process to be realized. Areas treated, amount injected, concentration used, and locations of trapped blood removed are recorded for each treatment session and adjustments are made at follow-up based on the clinical examination.

Ultrasound-Guided Sclerotherapy

Duplex ultrasound can be used to guide an injection of sclerosant into incompetent nonsurface veins, which are often the underlying cause for visible varicosities. Ultrasound-guided sclerotherapy (UGS) of the saphenous vein may be an alternative or complementary technique to surgery, endovenous laser, and radiofrequency ablation. It can also be used to treat an incompetent ATC, PTC, vein of Giacomini, neovascularization following surgery, or other significant nonsurface source of reflux in the superficial venous system. Injections can be done with sono-guided direct needle puncture or using transcatheter techniques (12).

Foam Sclerotherapy

Originally introduced decades ago, treatment of varicose veins with sclerosant foam has gained increased interest in recent years. Foam appears to increase the strength of a sclerosing agent by displacing blood and maximizing contact between sclerosant and endothelium. Increased efficacy in treating large incompetent veins with foam sclerotherapy compared to conventional liquid sclerotherapy has been suggested by a few nonrandomized studies (13–15). Unfortunately, displacing blood and remaining in the vein longer not only appears to increase sclerosant strength but also the incidence of adverse reactions, in particular DVT and visual disturbances. Various methods of producing and delivering foam with detergent sclerosants have been described in the literature (16–19). The long-term efficacy of foam sclerotherapy has yet to be determined.

Adverse Reactions and Complications

Hyperpigmentation following sclerotherapy is the most common side effect seen in 10–20% of patients following sclerotherapy. Hemosiderin deposition in the skin is believed to be the cause of the brownish discoloration along the course of a treated vein. In most cases, hyperpigmentation is temporary resolving in a matter of months but may occasionally persist for longer than a year (20). Although hyperpigmentation may result even with proper technique, too strong sclerosants and untreated underlying sources of reflux likely will increase the incidence of this aesthetically undesirable side effect. Removal of trapped blood following sclerotherapy should reduce the hemosiderin load and minimize skin discoloration. If hyperpigmentation does occur, management should include reassurance, protection from excessive sun, and time.

Telangiectatic matting or the appearance a fine network of tiny red blood vessels is another possible side effect of sclerotherapy. Matting is usually temporary, and in most cases, the treatment of choice is a tincture of time; however, if matting persists beyond a few months, a persistent underlying source of reflux should be searched for and treated. As with most unwanted side effects, the best treatment involves the use of meticulous technique to lessen the risk of developing matting. In particular, using the minimum effective sclerosant strength and injecting small volumes under low pressure are important preventive measures (21). Obesity and exogenous hormones seem to predispose patients to matting (22,23).

Ulceration of the skin is usually the result of extravasation of sclerosant or extraluminal injection. Any sclerosant can cause necrosis when it is too strong or improperly injected, but certain sclerosing agents (such as hypertonic saline) have higher risks of causing ulceration. Other factors that increase the incidence of this side effect are practitioners lacking adequate training or experience and certain anatomic injection danger zones, such as the ankle.

Although allergy to the most widely used sclerosing agents is uncommon, these reactions can occur and physicians performing sclerotherapy should be prepared to treat urticaria, rash, or anaphylaxis. Fortunately, intra-arterial injection is an extremely rare complication but has been reported. Extreme care must be exercised when performing sclerotherapy in the medial malleolar, saphenofemoral, and saphenopopliteal regions.

ENDOVENOUS LASER ABLATION

Great saphenous vein reflux is the most common underlying cause of significant varicose veins. Surgical ligation and stripping of the GSV has been the most commonly used and, until recently, the most durable treatment, but it is associated with significant morbidity. Initial attempts at less invasive treatment of incompetent GSVs resulted in limited success. Several practitioners have championed ultrasound-guided sclerotherapy with liquid or foam sclerosants, but studies have failed to demonstrate long-term recurrence rates equal to surgery (24–28). Early efforts of treatment by electrocoagulation involved creating thrombosis of the vein lumen, which ultimately resulted in recanalization (29–31). The first techniques using intraluminal radiofrequency (RF) energy to treat incompetent veins were associated with several complications, including skin burns, nerve injury, phlebitis, and infection (32).

More recently, a catheter-based bipolar RF device (VNUS Medical Technologies) has been used successfully to eliminate saphenous vein reflux. Preliminary results reported from a multicenter trial demonstrated an overall failure rate of 10% at a mean follow-up of 4.7 months (13% in patients treated with RF alone). Complications included skin paresthesias (thigh 9%, leg 51%), skin burns (3%), deep venous thromboses (3%) and one pulmonary embolus (33). Although liberal use of tumescent anesthesia has helped reduce the incidence of heat-related injury to adjacent nontarget tissues, there has been persistence of paresthesias (13–15%), clinical phlebitis (2–20%), thermal skin injury (4–7%), and rarely, DVT (1%) (34,35). Recent studies have demonstrated acceptable rates of continued closure of treated vein segments ranging from 73–90% at up to 24-month follow-up (34–37).

The latest minimally invasive technique to be developed to treat saphenous vein reflux is endovenous laser treatment (EVLT), which received FDA approval in January 2002. Endovenous laser involves delivery of laser energy directly into the blood vessel lumen (Figure 65–4) to produce endothelial and vein wall damage with subsequent fibrosis. Compared to other percutaneous techniques, such as UGS or RF, endovenous laser has the following potential advantages:

- Transmission of energy through a small diameter, flexible fiber permits a wider range of treatable veins with minimal access site size.
- Shallow depth of penetration of laser energy and faster withdrawal rates result in less thermal damage to surrounding nontarget perivenous tissue compared to RF.
- Patients with pacemakers are not excluded from endovenous laser.
- Eliminates risk of extravenous injection and lowers risk of anaphylaxis compared to UGS.

More reliable and thorough vein wall damage may lead to lower recanalization rates compared to UGS or RF

Patient Selection

Many of the contraindications described for sclerotherapy are also exclusion criteria for endovenous laser, including

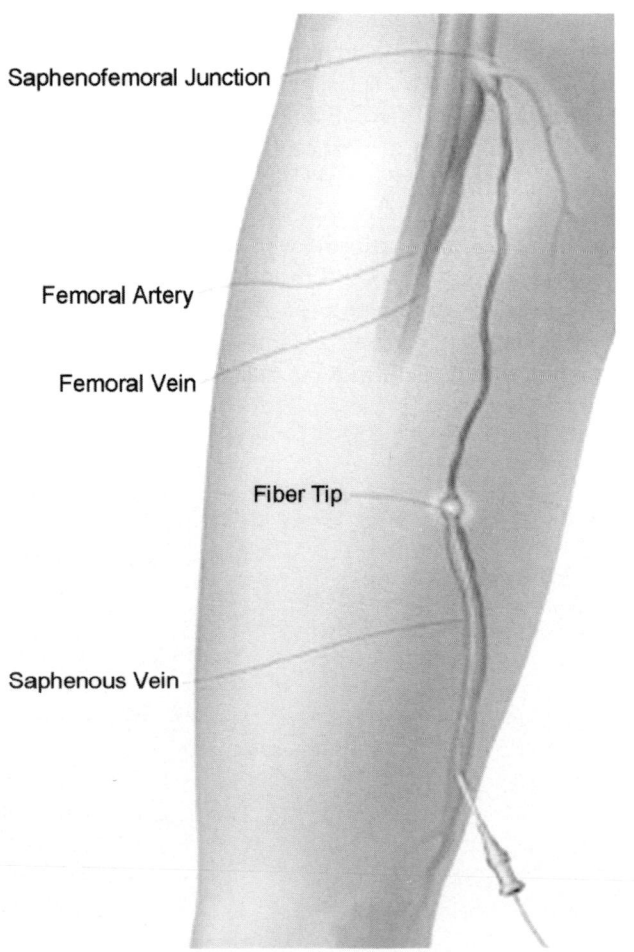

Figure 65–4 Illustration of endovenous laser ablation demonstrating delivery of intraluminal laser energy into the great saphenous vein as the laser fiber is withdrawn.

nonpalpable pedal pulses, inability to ambulate, DVT, general poor health, or women who are pregnant or nursing. An additional relative contraindication to all catheter-based endovenous ablation techniques is extremely tortuous target veins that would not allow passage of the laser fiber or RF catheter. Fortunately, this is an uncommon finding and should be recognized on pretreatment venous duplex ultrasound mapping.

Description of Technique

All incompetent venous pathways are mapped in the upright position with DUS. The course of the target vein is marked from the SFJ to the percutaneous entry point, which may be where reflux is no longer seen or where the GSV becomes too small to access (usually, just above or below knee level). Degree of tortuousity, areas of aneurysmal dilation, and significant perforator reflux are noted.

The GSV is punctured under ultrasound guidance and a 5 French introducer sheath is placed into the vein over a guide wire and advanced past the SFJ into the femoral vein. Intraluminal position within the GSV is verified by aspiration of nonpulsatile venous blood and visualization with ultrasound.

The sheath is flushed, and a 600-μ laser fiber (Diomed, Inc.) is inserted into the sheath and advanced up to the first site mark indicating that the distal tip of the laser fiber is at the end of the sheath. The distal 3 cm of the bare-tipped laser fiber is uncovered by withdrawal of the sheath to the second site mark. Both sheath and fiber are pulled back as a unit and positioned at the SFJ under ultrasound guidance as demonstrated in Figure 65–5A. Fiber tip location is confirmed by direct visualization of the red aiming beam of the laser fiber through the skin (Figure 65–5B).

Tumescent local anesthesia, consisting of 100–300 mL of 0.1% lidocaine neutralized with sodium bicarbonate, is administered along the perivenous space (distal to proximal) using ultrasound guidance. In addition to the anesthetic effects, this fluid, when properly delivered, serves two important functions: (1) It compresses and reduces the diameter of even the largest veins to maximize vein wall contact around the fiber tip with subsequent circumferential heating of the vein wall, and (2) it provides a "thermal heat sink" to minimize the possibility of heat-related damage to adjacent nontarget perivenous tissues (38). Figure 65–6 demonstrates the typical DUS cross-sectional appearance of the laser fiber located centrally within an enlarged GSV. Following delivery of adequate tumescent anesthesia, fluid should surround and compress the GSV against the laser fiber (as shown in Figure 65–6B). Trendelenburg positioning may also aid in reducing the vein diameter to further facilitate vein wall contact.

The tip of the laser fiber is repositioned within the GSV, 5–10 mm distal to the SFJ using ultrasound and verified with direct visualization of the red aiming beam through the skin. Laser energy—810 nm diode

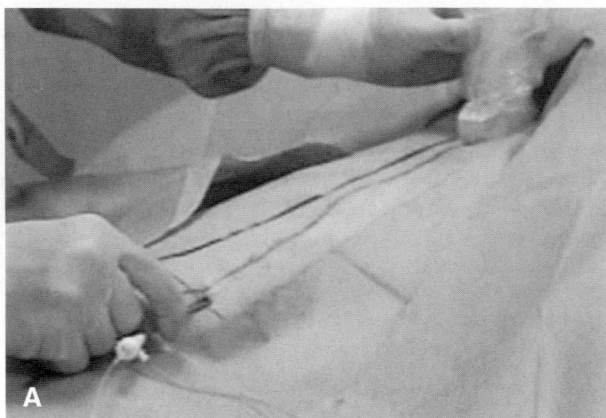
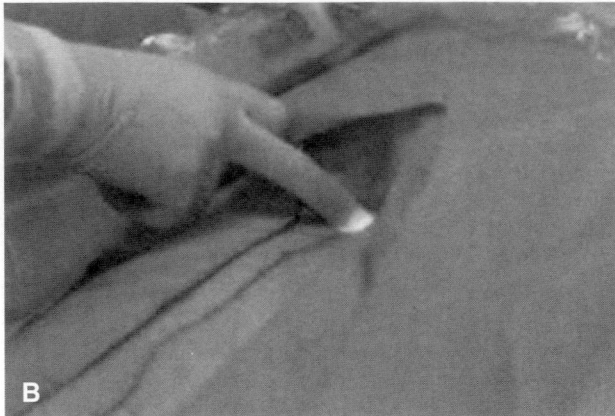

Figure 65–5 **A.** The laser fiber tip is positioned at the saphenofemoral junction using ultrasound guidance. **B.** With room lights turned down, fiber tip position is confirmed by direct visualization of the red aiming beam through the skin.

laser (Diomed, Inc.)—is delivered using 14 watts in continuous mode. The vein is treated from 5–10 mm below the SFJ to approximately 1 cm above the skin entry. The laser fiber is withdrawn at an average rate of 1–3 mm per second, slowest proximally and in larger vein segments.

A class II (30–40 mm Hg) full thigh graduated support stocking or panty hose is worn at all times (except to sleep or to take a shower) for at least 1 week following endovenous laser. Patients are encouraged to ambulate and to resume normal daily activities immediately. Clinical and DUS follow-up is obtained at 1 week, 1 month, 3 months, 6 months, 12 months, then yearly.

Varicose tributaries can be treated with concomitant ambulatory phlebectomy or compression sclerotherapy, starting 1 month following endovenous laser ablation of the GSV.

Duplex Ultrasound Imaging Findings

One to two weeks following successful endovenous laser, DUS should demonstrate a slightly smaller, noncompressible GSV with echogenic thickened vein walls and minimal to no flow seen within the occluded vein lumen. This appearance of postendovenous laser vein wall thickening (Figure 65–7A) should be differentiated from acute GSV thrombosis where the vein is also incompressible but the lumen is filled centrally with acute thrombus (Figure 65–7B). Several weeks after successful endovenous laser, resolution of acute inflammation in the vein wall will result in vein shrinkage, and after several months, most of the treated vein segments will fibrose and will be difficult to identify. Alternatively, superficial thrombophlebitis with GSV thrombus would result in recanalization of the vein.

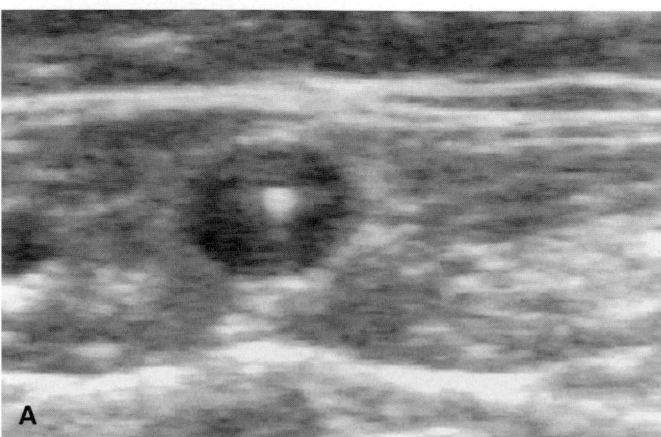
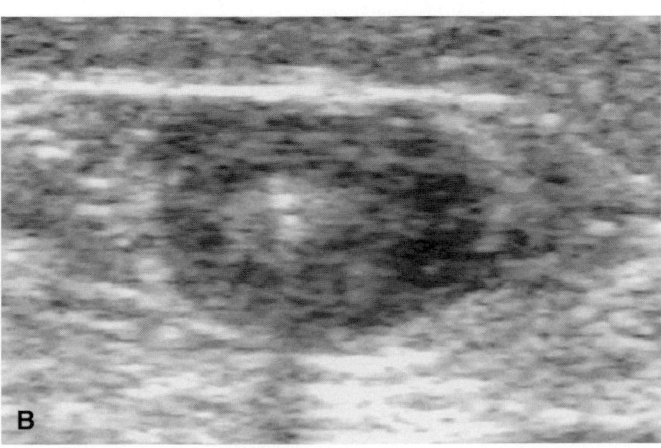

Figure 65–6 **A.** Echogenic laser fiber tip seen centrally within an enlarged GSV on axial DUS imaging. **B.** Following proper delivery of tumescent anesthesia, the previously enlarged GSV is now compressed around the laser fiber by surrounding fluid, ensuring maximal contact with the vein walls.

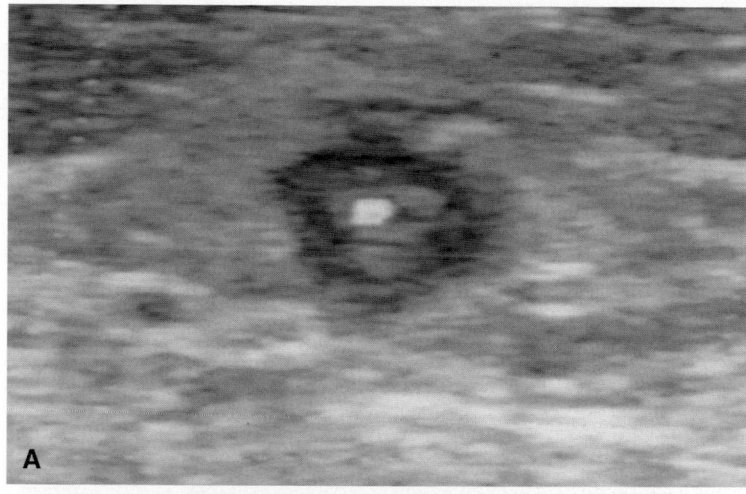

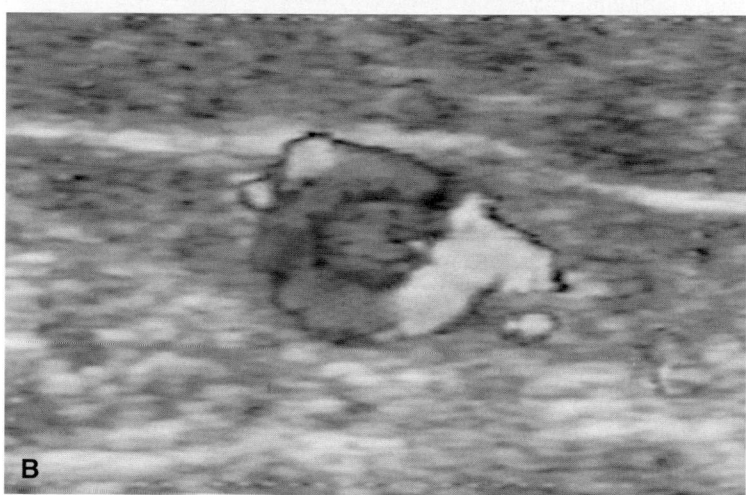

Figure 65–7 **A.** Color Doppler, 1 week after endovenous laser, demonstrating a slightly smaller, noncompressible GSV with echogenic thickened vein walls and minimal flow centrally within the vein lumen. **B.** Acute GSV thrombosis with central filling defect and flow within the periphery of the vein.

Results

Below are results on the first 701 limbs in 610 patients treated with endovenous laser (39). Most of the patients (85%) presented with aching leg pain as their primary complaint. Ninety-eight percent (686 of 701) of the veins treated with endovenous laser remained closed at 3–42-month follow-up (a mean of 20 months). Two hundred and twenty-three limbs have been followed for at least 2 years and remain closed. Success rates at various follow-up periods are illustrated in Table 65–2. Of note, most recanalizations have occurred early (prior to 9 months), which may indicate that these were not true recurrences but rather inadequate initial treatments. After 1 or 2 years, reopening of a successfully closed vein segment following endovenous laser is uncommon; however, patients may demonstrate progression of disease with reflux present within previously unrecognized and untreated accessory saphenous veins or truncal tributaries.

Clinical examination following successful endovenous laser should correlate to the DUS findings, and reduction in the size and number of visible branch varicosities should be noted. Remaining varicose veins can be removed with ambulatory phlebectomy or compression sclerotherapy. Most patients will note improvement in pretreatment leg symptoms following endovenous laser ablation even before the full restorative benefits of treatment are realized. Pretreatment and posttreatment photographs of a left lower extremity following endovenous laser and compression sclerotherapy are noted in Figure 65–8.

TABLE 65–2
ENDOVENOUS LASER ABLATION—RESULTS

Follow-Up	Closed/No. Treated	Continued Occlusion
<1 year	218/231	94%
1–2 years	245/247	99%
2–3 years	151/151	100%
>3 years	72/72	100%

701 total limbs followed 3–42 months (mean of 20 months)

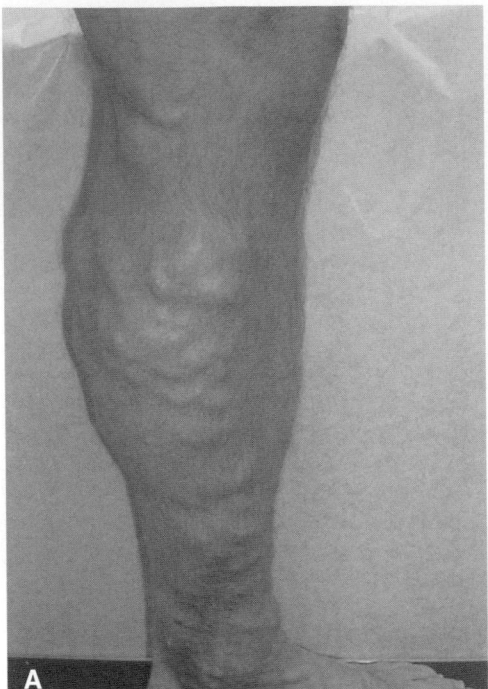
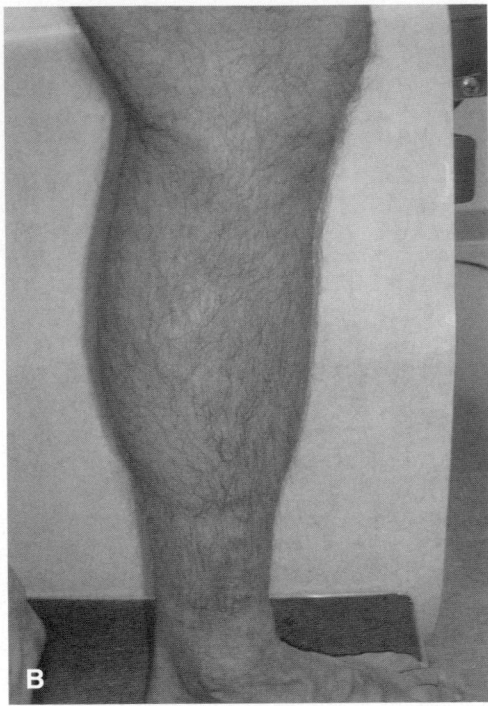

Figure 65–8   A. Left lower extremity with large varicose veins and venous stasis skin changes as a result of SFJ incompetence with GSV reflux. **B.** Marked improvement in appearance of the leg following endovenous laser ablation of the GSV and compression sclerotherapy of varicose tributaries.

Expected side effects following endovenous laser include bruising resulting from venopuncture during infiltration of tumescent anesthesia and delayed tightness peaking 4–7 days postlaser and lasting 3–10 days. This latter sensation is described as "pulling" along the course of the treated GSV and is likely the result of vein wall thickening and acute inflammation as seen on DUS imaging and histology. Infrequently, patients may develop superficial phlebitis of large varicose tributaries following endovenous laser occlusion of the GSV. Most cases require no treatment, although symptomatic patients can be treated with graduated compression stockings and over-the-counter anti-inflammatory medications. In more than 1,000 limbs treated with endovenous laser (810 nm) at our institution, there have been no skin burns, paresthesias, DVTs, or other heat-related complications.

SUMMARY

The understanding of venous disease has increased with tremendous speed over the past decade. Readily available DUS imaging now makes it possible for physicians to accurately diagnose abnormal venous pathways, identify all underlying points of incompetence, and preserve normal veins. New and improved minimally invasive techniques for treatment of incompetent veins provide patients with safe and effective options for managing the whole spectrum of superficial venous disease. Given these recent advances, many physicians—including interventional radiologists—will now be able to successfully diagnose and treat this extraordinarily common and often disabling medical condition.

REFERENCES

1. Callam MJ. Epidemiology of varicose veins. Br J Surg 1994;81: 167–173.
2. Rose SS. Anatomic observations on causes of varicose veins. In: Goldman MP, Weiss RA, Bergan JJ, eds. Varicose Veins and Telangiectasia: Diagnosis and Treatment. St. Louis: Quality Medical Publishing, 1999;12–17.
3. Goldman M. Pathophysiology of varicose veins. In: Goldman M, ed. Sclerotherapy: Treatment of Varicose and Telangiectatic Leg Veins. St. Louis: Mosby-Year Book, 1995;85–117.
4. Weiss R, Weiss M. Resolution of pain associated with varicose and telangiectatic leg veins after compression sclerotherapy. J Dermatol Surg Oncol 1990;16:333–336.
5. Wilder CS. Prevalence of selected chronic circulatory conditions. Vital Health Stat 1974;10:1–55.
6. Fegan WG, Lambe R, Henry M. Steroid hormones and varicose veins. Lancet 1967;2:1070–1071.
7. Widmer LK, Mall TH, Martin H. Epidemiology and social medical importance of diseases of the veins. MMW Munch Med Wochenschr 1974;116:1421–1426.
8. Ricci S, Caggiati A. Does a double long saphenous vein exist? Phlebology 1999;14:59–64.
9. Bergan JJ. Surgical management of primary and recurrent varicose veins. In: Gloviczki P, Yao JS, eds. Handbook of Venous Disorders: Guidelines of the American Venous Forum. 2nd Edition. London: Oxford University Press, 2001.
10. Min R, Khilnani N, Golia P. Duplex ultrasound evaluation of lower extremity venous insufficiency. J Vasc Interv Radiol 2003; 14:1233–1241.

11. Lewis KM. Anaphylaxis due to sodium morrhuate. JAMA 1936; 107:1298–1299.
12. Min RJ, Navarro L. Transcatheter duplex ultrasound-guided sclerotherapy for treatment of greater saphenous vein reflux: preliminary report. Dermatol Surg 2000;26:410–414.
13. Henriet JP. Expérience durant trois années de la mousse de polidocanol dans le traitement des varices réticulaires et des varicosités. Phlebologie 1999;52:277–282.
14. Cabrera J, Cabrera J Jr, Garcia-Olmedo MA. Treatment of varicose long saphenous veins with sclerosant in microfoam form: long-term outcomes. Phlebology 2000;15:19–23.
15. Frullini A, Cavezzi A. Sclerosing foam in the treatment of varicose veins and telangiectases: history and analysis of safety and complications. Dermatol Surg 2002;28:11–15.
16. Cabrera Garrido JR, Cabrera Garcia-Olmedo JR, Garcia-Olmedo Dominguez MA. Elargissement des limites de la schlérothérapie: noveaux produits sclérosants. Phlébologie 1997;50:181–188.
17. Monfreux A. Traitement sclerosant des troncs saphènies et leurs collatérales de gros calibre par le méthode mus. Phlébologie 1997;50:351–353.
18. Frullini A. New technique in producing sclerosing foam in a disposable syringe. Derm Surg 2000;26:705–706.
19. Tessari L, Cavezzi A, Frullini A. Preliminary experience with a new sclerosing foam in the treatment of varicose veins. Dermatol Surg 2001;27:58–60.
20. Georgiev M. Postsclerotherapy hyperpigmentation: a one-year follow-up. J Dermatol Surg Onc 1990;16:608–610.
21. Weiss RA, Feied CF, Weiss MA. Vein Diagnosis and Treatment. New York: McGraw-Hill, 2001.
22. Davis LT, Duffy DM. Determination of incidence and risk factors for postsclerotherapy telangiectatic matting of the lower extremity: a retrospective analysis. J Dermatol Surg Onc 1990;16:327–330.
23. Vin F, Allert FA, Levardon M. Influence of estrogens and progesterone on the venous system of the lower limbs in women. J Dermatol Surg Onc 1992;18:888–892.
24. Bishop CC, Fronek HS, Fronek A, et al. Real-time color duplex scanning after sclerotherapy of the greater saphenous vein. J Vasc Surg 1991;14:505–510.
25. Cornu-Thenard A, de Cottreau H, Weiss RA. Sclerotherapy: continuous-wave Doppler-guided injections. Dermatol Surg 1995; 21:867–870.
26. Kanter A. Clinical determinants of ultrasound-guided sclerotherapy outcome. Part I: The effects of age, gender, and vein size. Dermatol Surg 1998;24:131–135.
27. Kanter A. Clinical determinants of ultrasound-guided sclerotherapy outcome. Part II: The search for the ideal injectate volume. Dermatol Surg 1998;24:136–140.
28. Belcaro G, Nicolaides AN, Ricci A, et al. Endovascular sclerotherapy, surgery, and surgery plus sclerotherapy for superficial venous incompetence: a randomized 10-year follow-up trial—final results. Angiology 2000;51:529–534.
29. Politowski M, Szpak E, Marszalek Z. Varices of the lower extremities treated by electrocoagulation. Surgery 1964;56:355–360.
30. Watts GT. Endovenous diathermy destruction of internal saphenous. Br Med J 1972;4:53.
31. O'Reilly K. Endovenous diathermy sclerosis of varicose veins. Aust NZ J Surg 1977;47:393–395.
32. Politowski M, Zelazny, M. Complications and difficulties in electrocoagulation of varices of the lower extremities. Surgery 1966; 59:932–934.
33. Manfrini S, Gasbarro V, Danielsson G, et al. Endovenous management of saphenous vein reflux. J Vasc Surg 2000;32:330–342.
34. Merchant RF, DePalma RG, Kabnick LS. Endovascular obliteration of saphenous reflux: a multicenter study. J Vasc Surg 2002; 35:1190–1196.
35. Rautio T, Ohinmaa A, Perala, et al. Endovenous obliteration versus conventional stripping operation in the treatment of primary varicose veins: a randomized, controlled trial with comparison of the costs. J Vasc Surg 2002;35:959–965.
36. Rautio TT, Perala JM, Wiik HT, et al. Endovenous obliteration with radiofrequency-resistive heating for greater saphenous vein insufficiency: a feasibility study. J Vasc Interv Radiol 2002;13:569–575.
37. Weiss RA, Weiss MA. Controlled radiofrequency endovenous occlusion using a unique radiofrequency catheter under duplex guidance to eliminate saphenous varicose vein reflux: a 2-year follow-up. Dermatol Surg 2002;28:38–42.
38. Zimmet S, Min R. Endovenous laser treatment: assessing the risk for collateral damage. J Vasc Interv Radiol 2003;14:911–915.
39. Min R, Khilnani N, Zimmet. Endovenous laser treatment of saphenous vein reflux: long-term results. J Vasc Interv Radiol 2003;14:991–996.

Percutaneous Vertebroplasty

66

Mary E. Jensen, Avery J. Evans

Percutaneous vertebroplasty is an image-guided therapeutic procedure for the treatment of painful or unstable vertebral body compression fractures that are unresponsive to conservative medical therapy. The procedure involves the placement of a trocar into a fractured vertebral body followed by the application of an acrylic polymer to provide bone augmentation and prevent further collapse. The mechanism of pain relief is unclear, but it may be related to the "casting" of trabecular or endplate fractures, minimizing the movement of the fracture fragments. Although early reports focused mainly on the treatment of painful vertebral hemangiomas and bony metastases, most current literature has addressed osteoporotic crush fractures because these fractures respond particularly well to vertebroplasty. This chapter will focus primarily on the clinical and technical aspects of vertebroplasty in the osteoporotic patient.

HISTORY OF VERTEBROPLASTY IN OSTEOPOROTIC FRACTURES

In 1987, Galibert and Deramond (1) described the percutaneous application of acrylic polymer (polymethylmethacrylate, or PMMA) to vertebral body defects associated with painful hemangiomas, with resultant good control of pain. Other small series followed, with emphasis on the treatment of hemangiomas or metastases (2–4). In 1991, Debussche-Depriester (5) reported five patients suffering from painful osteoporotic vertebral compression fractures (VCF). All patients showed complete, immediate relief of pain after vertebroplasty with no or minimal residual discomfort. The first paper published in the North American literature described a small series from France (6) and included four patients with osteoporotic fractures, all of whom responded favorably.

Vertebroplasty was virtually unknown in North America until 1993 when a lecture on the topic was given at the annual meeting of the American Society of Neuroradiology. Dion and Jensen successfully treated the first patient in the United States at the University of Virginia later that year. The first paper focusing on the technical aspects of vertebroplasty was published in 1997 (7) and included 29 patients with 47 osteoporotic VCFs, showing acute pain relief in 90% as evidenced by patients' verbal expression of perceived pain and analgesic use. In 1998, Deramond and colleagues (8) reported the results of vertebroplasty on 80 patients with osteoporotic fractures, with rapid and complete relief of pain in more than 90% of cases. Follow-up of 1 month to 10 years showed prolonged analgesic effect and only a single complication was reported. Much of the ensuing literature consisted of case reports, small series, and in vitro biomechanical testing of various acrylic polymers used for bone augmentation. The first open prospective study was not published until 1999 (9); no control group was used, and the follow-up period ended at 6 months.

Vertebroplasty was enthusiastically accepted by interventional radiologists and embraced by older patients. Hands-on training courses were organized, and workshops and scientific sessions were included in national meetings as the technique expanded rapidly from the academic milieu to community practices. A competing technology, kyphoplasty (also known as "balloon-assisted vertebroplasty") rocketed to popularity primarily in the surgical community, primarily because of the positive outcomes seen with vertebroplasty. However, to date, no prospective, randomized controlled trial has been completed to show unequivocally that vertebroplasty is superior to medical therapy in the treatment of painful compression fractures.

VERTEBROPLASTY IN OSTEOPOROTIC VERTEBRAL BODY FRACTURES

In 1995, an estimated 700,000 vertebral fragility fractures occurred in older individuals (10). The lifetime risk of a clinically detected VCF is 15.6% for white women and 5% for white men (11). Estimates are that the incidence of hip fracture, and presumably other osteoporotic fractures, will increase fourfold worldwide by 2045 because of population increases and longevity gains (10). Clearly, osteoporosis of the spine and its clinical consequences are important health care issues that deserve attention.

Clinical Picture

Osteoporotic VCFs are most likely to occur in postmenopausal Caucasian and Asian women. Although most fractures result from age-related bone loss, certain conditions may be associated with the development of osteoporosis in 20% of women and 40% of men presenting with vertebral or hip fractures (12). Underlying factors that may contribute to osteoporosis include steroid therapy, early oophorectomy, hypogonadism in men, hyperthyroidism, chronic obstructive pulmonary disease, immobility, anticonvulsant use, smoking, and alcohol consumption. Low bone mass and a history of previous fracture independently predict the risk of subsequent fracture, with a sevenfold increased risk in women with low bone mass and a 25-fold risk in women with low bone mass and a single fracture (13).

A vertebral fracture may be defined as reduction in vertebral height by 15% or greater (34), or classified by degree and type of deformity, such as wedge, biconcavity, or compression (14). Compression fractures are most likely to occur at the T8, T12, L1 and L4 levels (15,16). The physiologic thoracic kyphosis places the greatest axial load at T8, and the thoracolumbar spinal junction is frequently affected because of the change in mobility between the relatively restricted thoracic spine and the more freely moving lumbar vertebrae (15).

Although many fractures are asymptomatic, clinically detected VCFs are associated with some degree of pain in 84% of patients (17). Most fractures occur spontaneously (59%) (15) or are associated with trivial strain or exertion (16). Pain is often described as intense and deep, localized to the level of the involved vertebra, and exacerbated by palpation over the affected site (16,17). Pain may be referred to adjacent levels, even as far away as four levels (16). It is often position-dependent with reduction or relief of pain when supine, while weight-bearing or bending causes the most discomfort. Pain may radiate to the flanks or anteriorly along the ribs, but frank radicular pain involving the legs is uncommon (16).

Pain associated with VCFs is usually self-limiting, lasting from 2 weeks to 3 months. For this reason, treatment of acute fractures has been largely conservative, with current therapy emphasizing pain control using narcotic medications, anti-inflammatories, and strict bed rest (18). Heating pads, ice packs, massage therapy, or trigger point injections may be useful. Other therapies, such as back bracing, physical therapy, and exercise, are introduced when the patient is capable of bearing weight. Preventive medical therapy (bisphosphonates, calcitonin, and, in some instances, hormonal replacement therapy—HRT) is encouraged to prevent new fractures. Surgery is rarely indicated, and internal fixation is reserved for the patient with gross deformity, instability, or neurologic deficits (19).

Quality of life and functional status are severely affected by vertebral osteoporosis. Older women with symptomatic fractures demonstrate significant performance impairments in physical, functional, and psychosocial testing when compared to a control group with no fractures (20). A late consequence of the disease is the development of progressive kyphosis, which may lead to chronic pain and disability, early satiety and weight loss, decreased exercise tolerance, fear of falling, and depression (17).

Consequences of Conservative Therapy

Before vertebroplasty, vertebral compression fractures were essentially the only fractures not treated orthopedically. Therapy was conservative, consisting of bed rest and analgesic administration, neither of which are benign or risk free (21,22). During bed rest, virtually every organ system is adversely affected, and these effects tend to be more pronounced in older patients who have less reserve than younger patients. In patients at bed rest, the incidence of deep vein thrombosis is 61% with proximal DVT occurring in 29%. Pulmonary embolism is seen in 2–12% of patients and is fatal in 0.5–10%. Muscle strength declines 1–3% per day or 10–15% per week. Bone density declines approximately 2% per week, a serious concern in patients already suffering from osteoporosis and unlikely ever to regain the lost bone mass. Gastrointestinal effects include reduced appetite, constipation, and fecal impaction, all exacerbated by the administration of narcotics. Cardiovascular effects include decreased stroke volume and cardiac output. Depending on the length of bed rest, it may take 20–72 days to restore pre-bedrest cardiac function. The lungs suffer from decreased ciliary clearance, less effective coughing, atelectasis, and a predilection for pneumonia. Patients are at increased risk of genitourinary calculus formation, incontinence, urinary tract infections, and urosepsis. Even the central nervous system is not immune; patients at bed rest exhibit higher levels of anxiety, depression, insomnia, and pain intolerance.

Patient Selection Criteria

The primary goal of vertebroplasty is to alleviate pain and improve mobility; vertebral body stabilization is a secondary goal. Treatment is directed toward affected patients who have failed a reasonable course of medical therapy but are still plagued by pain. The American College of Radiology (ACR) has published standards guidelines for the performance of percutaneous vertebroplasty, and selection criteria are outlined in detail. All practitioners should be familiar with the contents of this document (23). In short, appropriate candidates include: patients with painful VCF refractory to medical therapy, with failure defined as no or minimal pain relief following the administration of prescription analgesics for an unspecified time period; patients who are unable to ambulate because of the pain; painful VCF associated with osteonecrosis (Kümmell's disease) (24); and unstable VCF that demonstrates movement at the wedge deformity. Patients with multiple compression deformities who are at risk for pulmonary compromise, gastrointestinal dysfunction, or altered center of gravity (should further collapse occur) are also specified, although no data to support this position are available.

Absolute contraindications are few. Patients with asymptomatic stable fractures or who are clearly improving with conservative treatment are not candidates. No evidence exists to support prophylactic vertebroplasty in osteopenic patients with no acute fracture. Other contraindicated conditions include acute traumatic fractures in nonosteoporotic vertebrae, osteomyelitis of the targeted level, uncorrectable coagulopathies, and allergic sensitivity to any of the required components. Relative contraindications are not as well-defined and often operator-specific. Patients with significant spinal canal compromise from retropulsed fragments, vertebra plana, or chronic fractures may be candidates, but relief is variable. Radicular pain or radiculopathy involving the lower extremities is an infrequent finding with VCFs, and an appropriate search for other compressive pathology unrelated to the collapse should be performed before vertebroplasty.

Patient Screening and Evaluation

A clinical coordinator, such as a nurse or experienced assistant, is invaluable for the smooth operation of a busy vertebroplasty service. The coordinator can collect pertinent information such as a pain history, other relevant medical conditions or previous surgeries, current analgesic use, and radiologic studies, before scheduling an appointment. In many cases, noncandidates are discovered early on and can be redirected. Requiring a referral from an individual's primary care physician also helps to eliminate inappropriate patients who are self-referred.

Potential candidates for treatment should fulfill relevant clinical and radiologic criteria, and the information should be documented appropriately in the patient's chart.

History of Present Illness

A detailed history is obtained. It should concentrate on the patient's back pain, mobility, medication use (including analgesics, steroids, biphosphonates, calcitonin, and HRT), and general medical condition. Presenting symptoms, indications for the procedure, pertinent medical and surgical history, a list of current medications, history of allergies, and evidence of failed medical therapy are documented. Visual analog scales for determining pain level, dermatome drawings for pain localization, and questionnaires are useful for collecting data.

Patients with atypical back pain should be evaluated for a concomitant disease process. Any condition that results in bacteremia, such as urinary tract infection, may seed the spinal column resulting in diskitis or epidural abscess. Abdominal disease, such as posterior perforation of a gastric ulcer, also can cause unusual back pain. A high level of suspicion is required because older patients may not mount a vigorous immune response, resulting in an afebrile individual with nonspecific findings and a normal or mildly elevated white blood cell count and sedimentation rate (25).

Neurologic and Physical Examination

A focused physical and neurologic examination to identify painful vertebral levels and to evaluate for possible radicular symptoms or neurologic deficits is mandatory. Sites of point tenderness to percussion or palpation, and positional "trigger points" are identified, although a lack of preoperative spinous process tenderness does not preclude clinical success of vertebroplasty (26). Patients with diffuse or nonfocal pain, low back pain that radiates to the hip or iliac crest, or lumbar radiculopathy may have other pathology, such as facet or disk disease, that should first be excluded. Evaluation of the patient's ability to lie prone without pulmonary compromise is recommended. A detailed physical examination is indicated when significant concurrent illnesses are suspected.

Radiologic Evaluation

Osteoporotic postmenopausal women with a documented new or subacute fracture on a conventional radiograph and who meet the clinical criteria regarding pain pattern often proceed to vertebroplasty without undergoing other imaging. Adjunctive imaging is indicated in patients with single or multiple fractures of uncertain age (Figure 66–1), when serial conventional radiographs are unavailable, or when a marrow-replacement disease process is suspected. An example of this is multiple myeloma in an osteopenic male.

Bone scan imaging (Figure 66–1E and F) and MR imaging (Figure 66–1B, C, and D) are potentially useful in identifying active fractures (27) and predicting outcome (28). A limited MR study consisting of T1 and STIR (short-tau inversion recovery) sagittal images may be the only study needed to spot vertebral body edema. Although MR imaging is sensitive for the detection of acute compression fractures, the duration of vertebral body edema with respect to

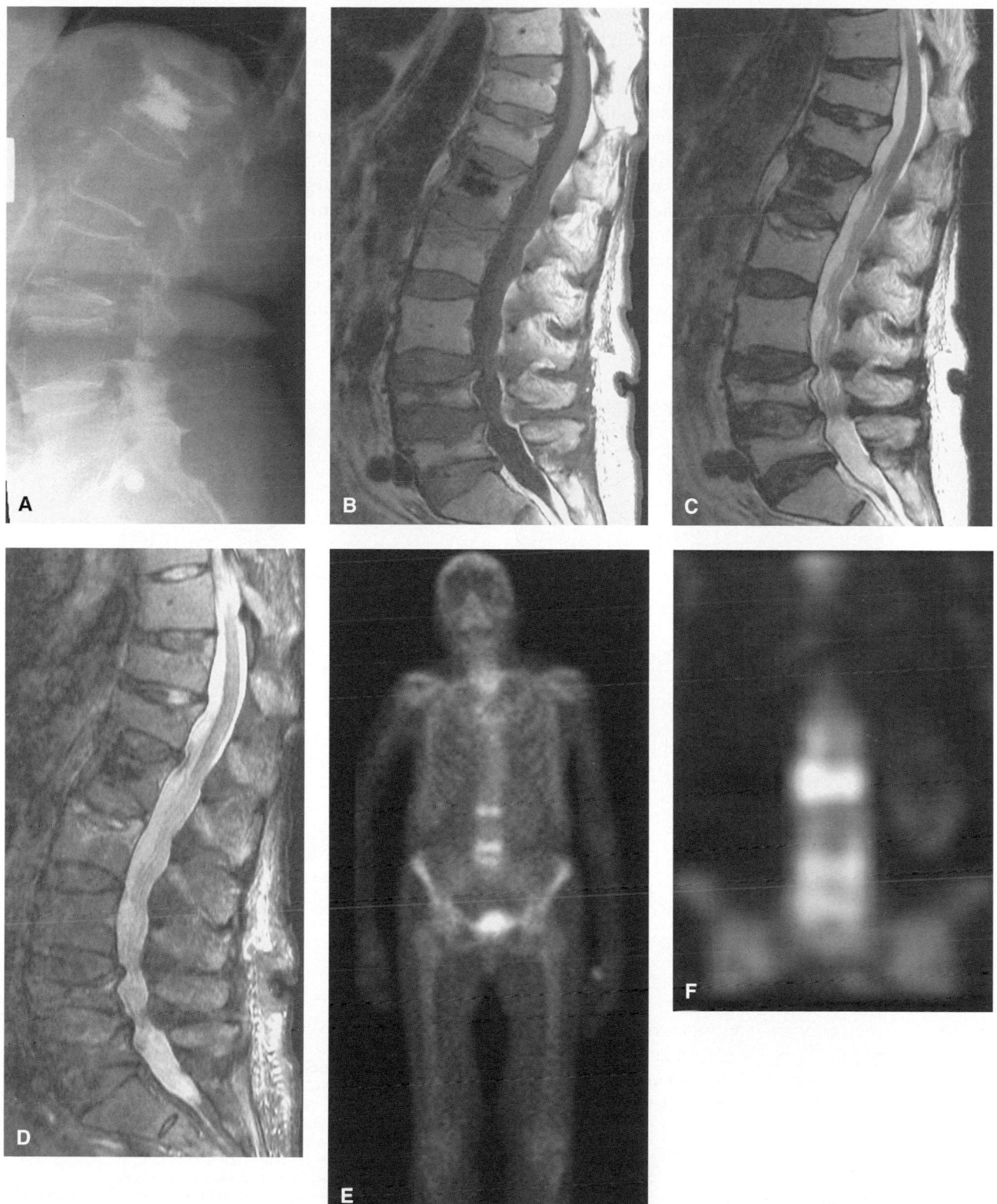

Figure 66–1   A. This 81-year-old female with osteoporosis underwent an L1 vertebroplasty for pain unresponsive to narcotics. She recovered well and was pain free for nearly 2 years when she developed new onset low back pain. **B.** T1- **C.** T2- and **D.** short-tau inversion recovery (STIR) MRI show multiple new lumbar compression fractures of L2, L4, and L5. Intraosseous edema is best seen on the STIR sequence, and the fluid-filled cavity located beneath the superior endplate of L2 is easily identified on both T2-weighted images and STIR. Note the hypointense appearance of the acrylic located within L1 on all sequences. The T11 and T12 compression fractures were known to be at least 6 months old by plain film. Bone scanning was performed to evaluate activity at all fracture levels. **E.** Wholebody bone scan and **F.** coronal SPECT studies show marked tracer activity in L2, L4, and L5. No uptake was noted in the thoracic vertebrae, which is consistent with healed fractures. The patient underwent a three-level vertebroplasty with resolution of pain.

the presence of pain is unknown. Subacute or chronic painful fractures may demonstrate normal (fatty) marrow signal intensity on T_1- and T_2-weighted images. In patients suspected of having active VCFs with no obvious acute fracture on MR, bone scintigraphy may be positive. In evaluating the use of scintigraphy in preprocedural evaluation of patients being considered for vertebroplasty, Maynard et al. (28) found that a high percentage of patients (94%) achieved nearly complete pain relief after treatment of those levels that showed increased uptake of tracer, even in patients with multiple fractures of uncertain age. However, one pitfall of bone scanning is that activity in chronic facet disease may be confused with activity in a partially collapsed

vertebral body on a routine scan. SPECT (single positron emission computed tomography) scanning can localize the tracer uptake within the vertebral body or the adjacent facet joints.

In patients with complex or severe fractures, CT before vertebroplasty may be used to evaluate the integrity of the posterior wall of the vertebral body, to locate fracture lines involving the vertebral body and pedicles, and to assess posterior displacement of fragments (Figure 66–2A, B, and C). Canal compromise from retropulsed bone is not considered an absolute contraindication, provided there is no cord or nerve root compression resulting in neurologic symptoms or dysfunction.

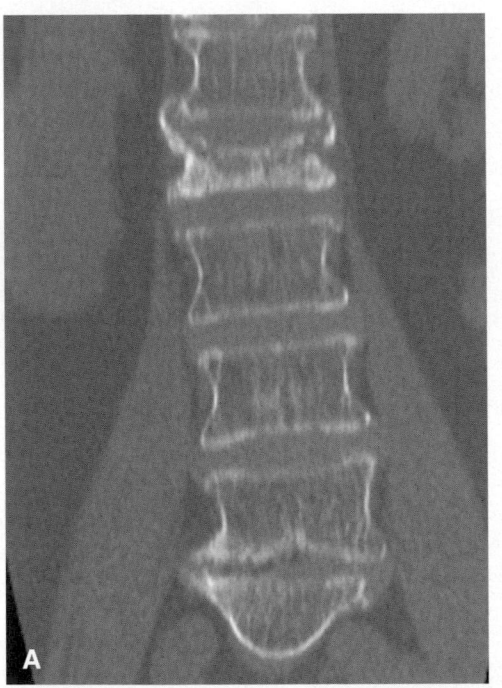
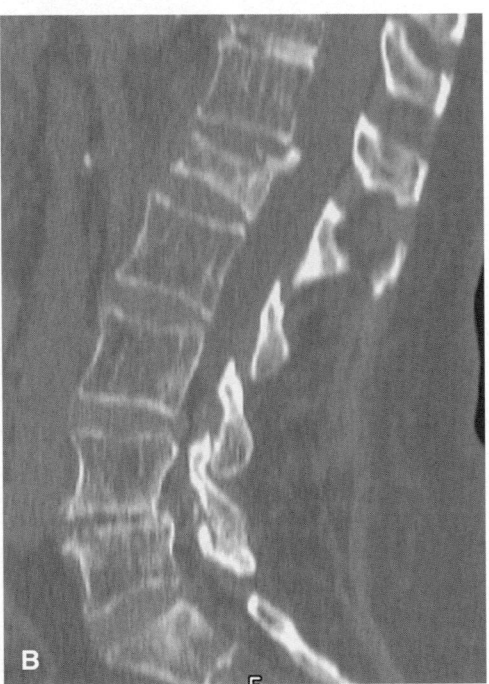
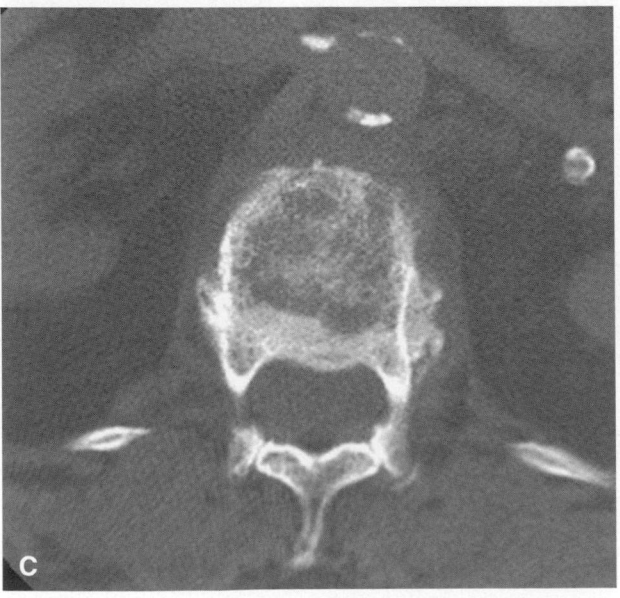

Figure 66–2   **A.** Coronal, **B.** sagittal, and **C.** axial images of a 70-year-old female with progressive compression of the L1 vertebral body. She had a pacemaker that precluded MRI. The fracture runs the length and breadth of the vertebral body inferior and parallel to the superior endplate and extends into the disc space at its posterior-most aspect. There is mild retropulsion of the superior posterior vertebral body corner that does not cause significant compromise of the canal or lateral recesses. The pedicles are not involved. She was found to be a suitable candidate for vertebroplasty and underwent an uneventful procedure.

In ambiguous cases, fluoroscopic examination of the painful sites may reveal an alternative explanation for back pain. Most common is the patient with low back pain radiating to the hip who demonstrates facet hypertrophy and point tenderness over the joint. Diagnostic facet injection can be performed first as part of the screening process.

Preprocedure Preparation and Counseling

Vertebroplasty is usually performed on an outpatient basis, so important preprocedure instructions should be given at the time of the evaluation. Patients are asked to remain NPO (nothing by mouth) after midnight and to avoid taking their morning analgesics. A responsible adult must be available to transport the patient home after a 2-hour observation period. Informed consent is obtained in all cases. Risks cited should include infection, bleeding, fracture, extravasation of acrylic into the surrounding epidural or paravertebral veins resulting in worsening pain or paralysis, pulmonary compromise, and death. The potential need for immediate surgical intervention should be discussed.

Older patients often have chronic conditions that require special consideration. When indicated, preprocedure laboratory testing is done, which may often include hemoglobin, hematocrit, electrolytes, and renal function tests, coagulation parameters, CBC (complete blood count) with differential, and sedimentation rate.

Individuals on Coumadin can be converted to enoxaparin (Lovenox), given subcutaneously once or twice a day, on an outpatient basis. Lovenox can be reversed with protamine sulfate at the time of the procedure and immediately reinstituted upon its completion, followed by resumption of Coumadin therapy. This process eliminates the need for a lengthy hospitalization but requires coordination with the patient's primary care physician.

Vertebroplasty should be avoided in patients with known infections, fevers, or elevated white blood count (unless the result of steroid use). Patients with chronic obstructive pulmonary disease (COPD) or asthma may have difficulty ventilating when lying prone, and anesthesia-managed conscious sedation may be required. General anesthesia is usually not indicated, except in the uncooperative patient or the patient in extreme pain.

Technical Aspects of Vertebroplasty

Different techniques have evolved based upon the predominant European (8,29,30) and North American (7,31–33) experiences. Descriptions of the procedure abound in the literature, but variations in technique are mostly minor and related to the availability of the products and equipment utilized and the operators' training and personal style. However, vertebroplasty is best learned in a hands-on training class, and interested operators are strongly encouraged to attend one of the many educational courses currently available.

Equipment Requirements and Operator Skills

Needle placement within the vertebral body has been described using standard fluoroscopy (7,8,29), CT-guidance (6,34), or CT fluoroscopy. Regardless of the modality used to position the needle, acrylic injection is a venous embolization and should always be performed under fluoroscopic observation. Operators should strive to use the highest quality fluoroscopy available, with multiple levels of magnification and small focal spot sizes. Use of a biplane digital angiography unit is ideal; biplane monitoring of fluoroscopic images decreases procedural time and enables orthogonal visualization of the acrylic injection. However, a high-quality single plane unit alone will suffice. Low-quality analog fluoroscopy portable units are to be avoided because the image quality is usually too poor for adequate visualization of bony landmarks and acrylic flow.

In addition to a high-quality imaging chain, the operator should possess appropriate cognitive and technical skills to ensure quality and safety of the study. These skills include but are not limited to knowledge of the radiographic anatomy of the spine and associated structures on both CT and fluoroscopy; formal training in radiation physics; use of equipment and techniques to minimize exposure to self and patient; performance of CT or fluoroscopic-guided biopsy procedures of the spine, such as radiographic triangulation; and experience with embolization techniques.

Patient Preparation and Monitoring

Vertebroplasty requires significant operator attention during the procedure; therefore, a dedicated nurse or other trained professional, should be the one whose primary responsibility is to establish and maintain venous access, administer conscious sedation, monitor the patient's physiologic status, and maintain the medical record. Of particular concern are those patients with decreased respiratory excursion when in the prone position, resulting in unsatisfactory oxygenation. Patients with respiratory compromise may require supplemental oxygen or anesthesia support during the procedure. Equipment and medications for emergency resuscitation should be immediately available.

Many patients are anxious about rolling into the prone position, and intravenous administration of 25–50 µg of fentanyl (Sublimaze, Abbott Labs), 5 minutes before positioning is useful. The patient is placed prone on the angiography table, and physiologic monitors such as EKG leads, pulse oximeter, and blood pressure cuff are attached, in addition to oxygen via nasal cannula. Additional conscious sedation may be given in the form of fentanyl and midazolam (Versed, Roche Pharma) in small increments.

To minimize infection risk, the procedure is performed under strict sterile conditions. All personnel wear surgical caps and masks, in addition to sterile gowns and gloves for the operators and personnel setting up the tray. The level to be treated is identified and marked under fluoroscopy, and the overlying skin surface is prepped and draped. The image intensifiers are also covered with sterile bags because they will be in close position to the operator and the vertebroplasty devices. Prophylactic antibiotic therapy, whether given intravenously or mixed with the acrylic polymer, has been advocated (7,8,31–33).

Pedicle Targeting

The pedicle to be punctured is isolated under AP (anteroposterior) fluoroscopy. In the simple "bulls-eye" approach to the pedicle, the fluoroscopic tube is either in a straight AP position or slightly obliqued. In this approach, the largest surface area of the pedicle is presented for targeting and its entire cortical circumference is easily seen. Advancement of the needle positions the tip in the midportion of the ipsilateral vertebral hemisphere (Figure 66–3A and B). If holovertebral filling is desired, a contralateral puncture will usually be necessary (Figure 66–4A, B, and C).

Puncture of the pedicle using the more oblique (20–30 degrees of ipsilateral angulation), "scotty-dog" view will result in a steeper lateral-to-medial needle track with the final needle position near the midline of the vertebral body (Figure 66–5). From this location, it is more likely that a single transpediculate injection will fill most of the vertebral body, minimizing the need for a contralateral puncture. This approach is more technically challenging because the pediculate cortex is not as clearly seen as it is in the bulls-eye view and the surface area is smaller, particularly in the thoracic spine. If the needle is positioned too

laterally, the transverse process may be fractured or the thoracic cavity may be entered. However, the unipediculate approach results in a shorter procedure time, diminished risk because only one pedicle is punctured, and better visualization as indwelling opacified acrylic is not present.

With either approach, the puncture site should avoid the medial and inferior borders of the pedicles. Tracks in these locations can result in a breach of the cortical wall and entry into the spinal canal or neural foramen.

Once the angle of approach is determined, the skin, subcutaneous soft tissues, and pediculate periosteum are anesthetized with 7–10 cc of 0.25% bupivacaine hydrochloride (Abbott Labs), using a 2-inch, 25-gauge spinal needle. Before removing this needle, AP and lateral fluoroscopy should show the tip of the needle approximating the same location on the pedicle in the superior-inferior plane (Figure 66–6A and B). If there is a discrepancy between the two and the patient is in the true lateral position, then the AP tube needs to be adjusted in either the cranial or caudal direction until the needle tip approximates the same location as on the lateral view. A small skin incision is made with a No. 11 scalpel blade to allow easy passage of the vertebroplasty needle.

Positioning of the Needle

A variety of disposable vertebroplasty needles, or trocars, are available for use, and no studies comparing performance among the different products exist to guide selection. These devices are generally listed as "bone biopsy" needles and range in size from 11–13 gauge; injection of acrylic is

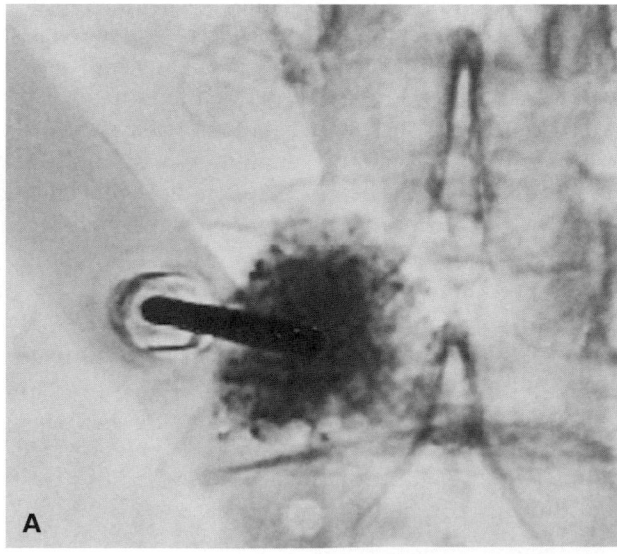
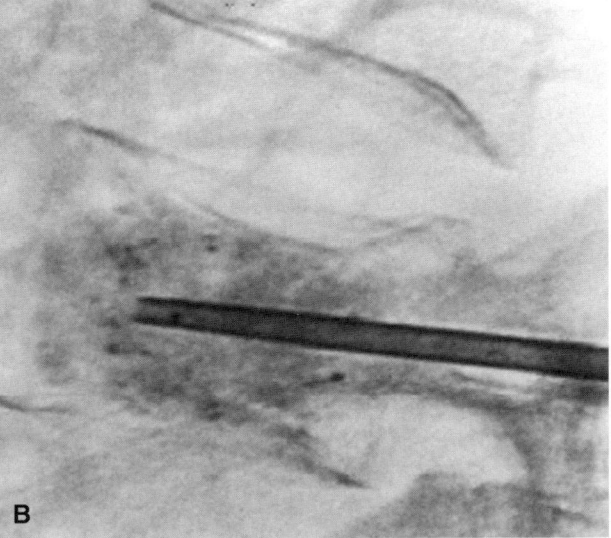

Figure 66–3 **A.** Anteroposterior (AP) and **B.** lateral views of a lumbar vertebroplasty using the "bulls-eye" approach. The needle approximates the midportion of the hemisphere on the AP view and is advanced to the anterior one third of the vertebral body on the lateral view. The vertebral hemisphere is well-filled from anterior to posterior but does not cross the midline. In the event that holovertebral filling is desired, the contralateral hemisphere will have to be punctured.

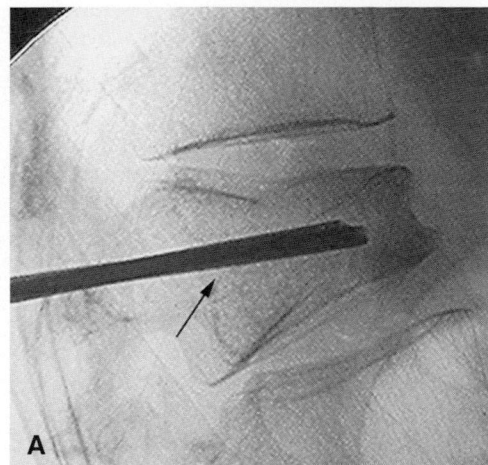
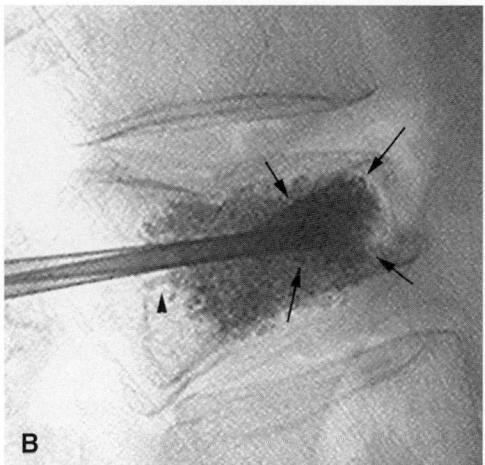

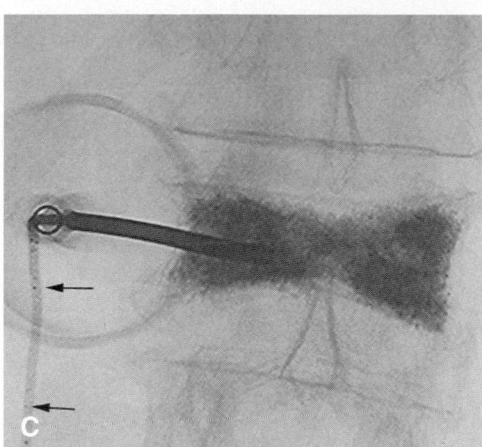

Figure 66–4   Lateral and AP views of a bipedic-ulate approach show placement of both needles before vertebroplasty. **A.** Note how the cannulas overlap and partially obscure the egress point of the basivertebral plexus (*arrow*). **B.** During injec-tion of the second hemivertebra, the overlapping acrylic boluses create a "double-density" effect (*arrows*), allowing the operator to monitor the injection in the lateral projection. Note the small amount of acrylic within the basivertebral plexus where it enters the spinal canal. **C.** On the AP view, holovertebral filling with containment of acrylic within the vertebral body is seen. The inho-mogeneous barium particles (*arrows*) within the PMMA (polymethylmethacrylate) allow easier visu-alization of acrylic flow. The use of injector tubing permits fluoroscopy in the AP view while keeping the operator's hands out of the field.

difficult through smaller gauge needles. Important features for consideration include the availability of different stylet tip shapes and cannula sizes and lengths, radiolucency of the handle, "locking" of the stylet within the cannula, and compatibility of the cannula Luer-lock hub with various injection devices and methacrylates. The reader should become familiar with the various products that are cur-rently available with these attributes in mind.

The needle is advanced until the stylet tip abuts the cor-tical surface in the superior to midpoint portion of the pedicle. Depending upon the shape of the pedicle, the nee-dle should enter at the widest point, away from the medial and inferior borders. The angle of approach on the lateral view is determined by the degree of endplate compression or anterior wedging (Figure 66–7A and B). Often, the course of the needle will parallel that of the superior end-plate; in which case, the stylet tip position will begin more superiorly on the pedicle. On the AP view, the needle should traverse the pedicle and vertebral body from lateral to medial (Figure 66–5C); otherwise, it may abut or exit the lateral wall of the vertebral body.

The stylet tip of the needle should be positioned pre-cisely before a cortical break is made. Positioning is best made with a diamond-point stylet, because beveled stylets have a tendency to slip off the pedicle. Once the track is started, repositioning becomes difficult because the stylet has a tendency to slide into the initial divot. A slight back-and-forth twisting motion is used to advance the tip through the cortex, with frequent fluoroscopic checks in both the AP and lateral planes as the needle traverses the pedicle. Alternatively, a small sterile orthopedic hammer can be used to tap gently on the needle handle, advancing the tip in small increments. Once within the trabecular bone, less pressure is required to advance the needle. Also, care must be taken not to pierce the endplates or vertebral wall. Use of the single-bevel stylet will allow deflection of the needle tip in the direction opposite to the bevel, allowing minor adjustments in either plane (Figure 66–8). The needle is advanced using continuous or intermittent lateral fluoroscopy until the stylet tip is placed in the ante-rior one third to one quarter of the vertebral body. The closer the tip is to the midline on the AP view, the fur-ther anterior it may be positioned on the lateral view (Figure 66–9). Because the stylet tip projects beyond the end of the cannula, the final cannula tip position will be slightly more posterior.

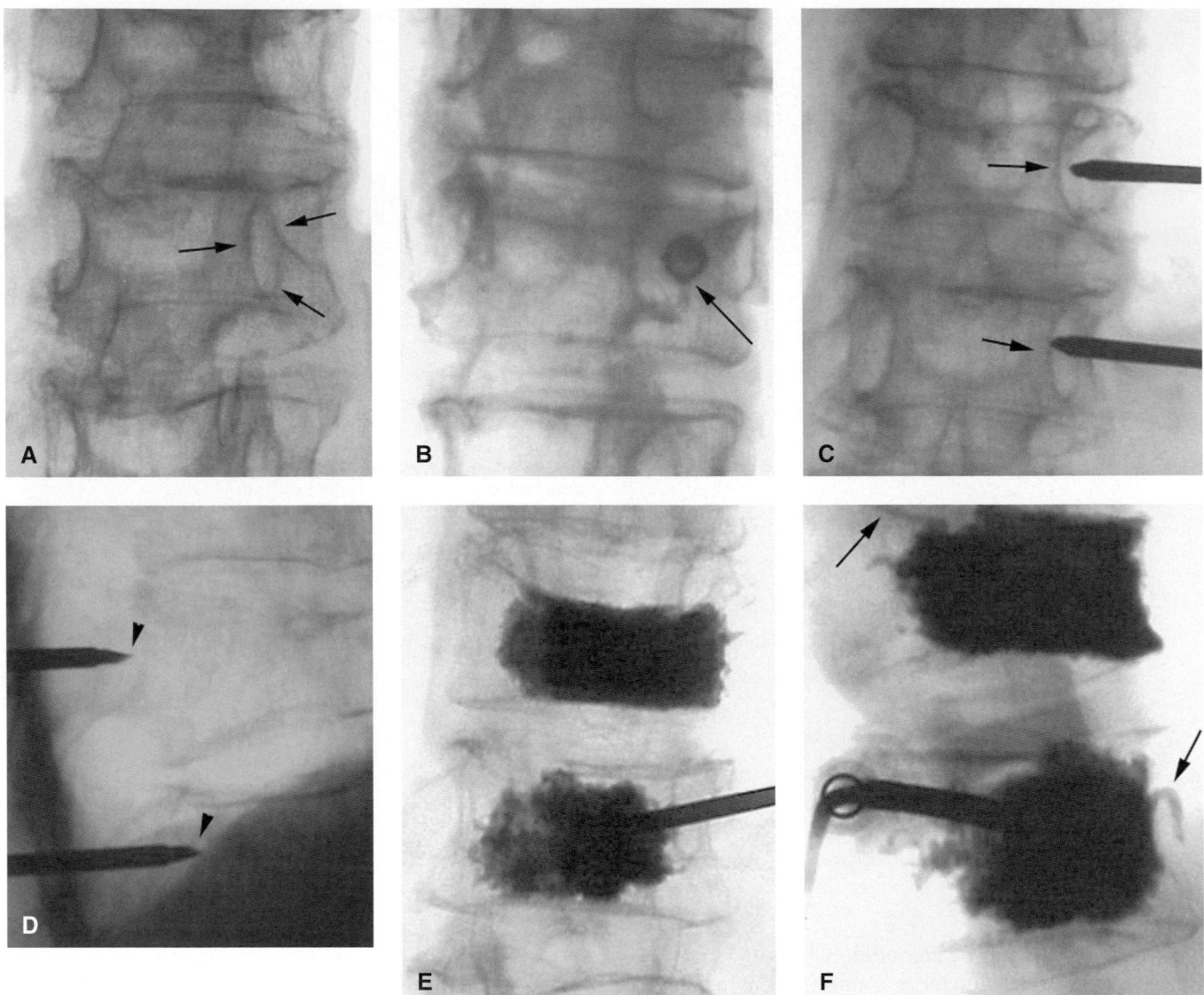

Figure 66–5   **A.** "Scotty-dog" oblique of the vertebral body shows the coronal diameter of the pedicle (*arrows*) to be smaller than on the corresponding AP view. **B.** The needle tip is positioned in the upper outer quadrant of the pedicle near its lateral border. **C.** As the needle is advanced, the tip travels from lateral to medial across the face of the pedicle in the AP view. **D.** When the stylet tip reaches the medial border of the pedicle, it should approximate the posterior border of the vertebral body on the lateral view (*arrowheads*). Otherwise, the needle may exit the pedicle and enter the spinal canal. **E.** Note the excellent vertebral filling from this single pedicle approach. **F.** Oblique view of the vertebral bodies during injection shows extravasation of acrylic into the paravertebral veins. Although this finding is usually of no clinical consequence, failure to recognize migration of acrylic into the paravertebral veins may lead to PMMA pulmonary embolism.

Placement of a Contralateral Needle

Many experienced practitioners position a single needle in the midportion of the vertebral body and perform only a single injection of acrylic, filling the midportion of the body (Figure 66–5). If the initial needle placement is within the lateral aspect of the hemivertebra, the acrylic will more than likely remain in the ipsilateral hemivertebra (Figure 66–3). Some operators prefer to fill the entire vertebra at a single sitting and will place a second needle when the initial fill

pattern is deemed unsatisfactory or incomplete. Whether this is necessary for a good clinical result is a matter of debate. An in vitro study by Tohmeh et al. (35) evaluating PMMA (polymethylmethacrylate) augmentation of osteoporotic vertebrae from a single or bipedicular approach showed no significant difference in height changes on compression testing between either augmented group; specifically, preferential deformation of the single-side augmented group was not noted. In a retrospective clinical study by Kim et al. (36), use of a unipediculate approach resulted in filling

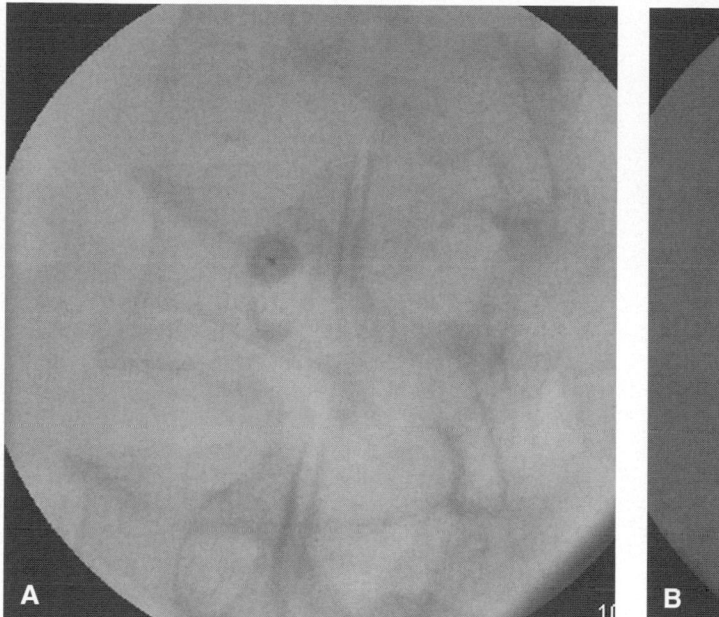
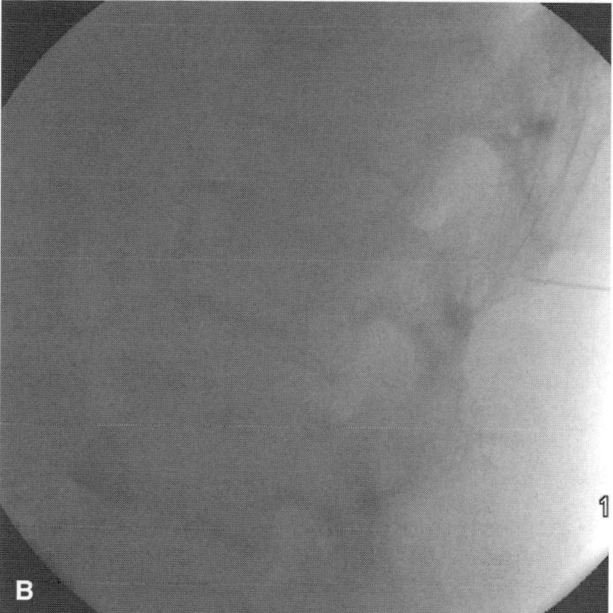

Figure 66–6   **A.** AP and **B.** lateral fluoroscopic images of the anesthetic needle shows its tip in the upper outer quadrant of the left pedicle on the AP view. This superior pediculate location corresponds to the needle tip location on the lateral view. Triangulation of the needle tip on the AP view may be difficult in patients with severe kyphosis or in vertebroplasty of the upper thoracic spine. In cases in which discrepancy appears between the two images, the AP tube should be angled in such a manner that the needle tip location corresponds to the lateral view.

of both vertebral halves from a single puncture site with no statistically significant difference in clinical outcome from that of bipediculate vertebroplasty.

When a bipediculate approach is used, the contralateral stylet is left in place during the initial ipsilateral acrylic injection; otherwise, the material will track through the trabecular

space and egress out the contralateral needle. The first needle may be removed before injection of the second hemivertebra. Another potential problem is the obscuration of the basivertebral plexus during injection by overlapping needles. One solution is to place the second needle after completion of the first injection. Visualization around the single

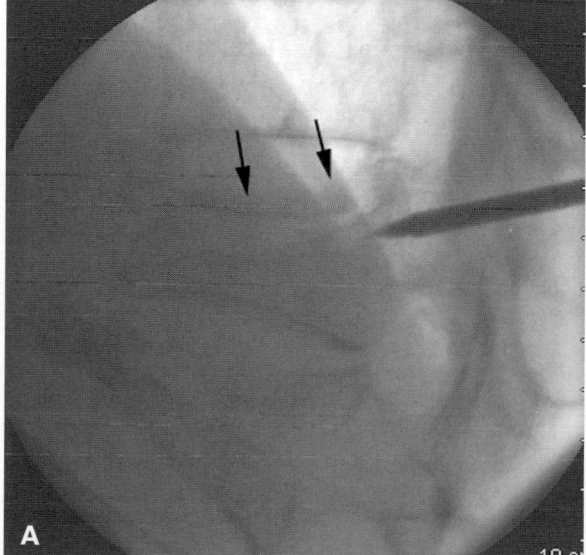
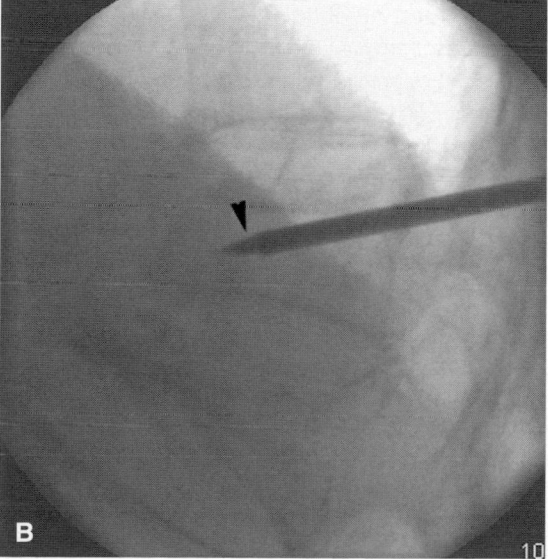

Figure 66–7   **A.** In this patient with a superior endplate fracture (*arrows*) and **B.** internal cavity (*arrowhead*), the needle is positioned higher on the pedicle so it will run parallel to the endplate rather than pierce it. The needle is also positioned so that the final cannula tip will be within the cavity rather than in the preserved trabecular space of the inferior vertebral body.

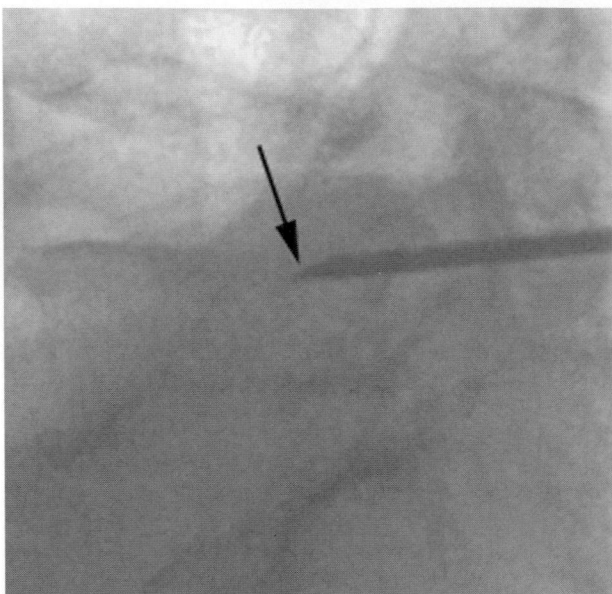

Figure 66–8   Deflection of the needle tip is accomplished with the use of the single-beveled stylet. With the beveled edge of the stylet pointing superiorly, the needle tip is deflected inferiorly to avoid piercing the superior endplate.

needle is easily done through a change of the lateral obliquity. Another technical difficulty is observing acrylic flow during contralateral injection because of the presence of PMMA in the ipsilateral hemisphere. Potential solutions include adding extra barium sulfate to the acrylic mixture used during the contralateral injection so it is seen through the ipsilateral acrylic cast (Figure 66–4); using final images of the ipsilateral injection as a guide by looking for acrylic extending outside the existing cast; or injecting under a combination of lateral and AP oblique views. Use of roadmapping technique is not advised because respiratory and bowel gas movement makes precise visualization impossible.

Vertebrography

The initial technical description of vertebroplasty (7) advocated the use of vertebrography before acrylic injection as a safety feature. Injection of small amounts of contrast into the vertebral body confirms the cannula location within the trabecular space; evaluates potential routes of acrylic extravasation; and clearly defines the location of the basivertebral plexus, which channels much of the vertebral venous outflow into the anterior internal epidural venous plexus (Figure 66–10). On the lateral view, the egress point of this plexus is seen as a bony depression located anterior to the posterior vertebral body margin between the pedicles, which may not be easily visualized in osteoporotic bone (Figure 66–4A). The location of this vascular junction is important information because extravasation of acrylic into the epidural veins is the major cause of neurologic complications in vertebroplasty.

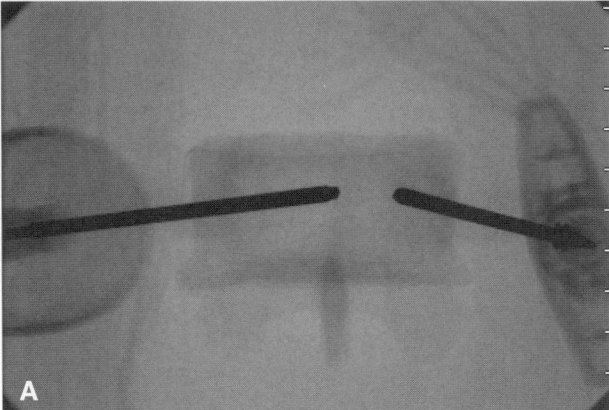

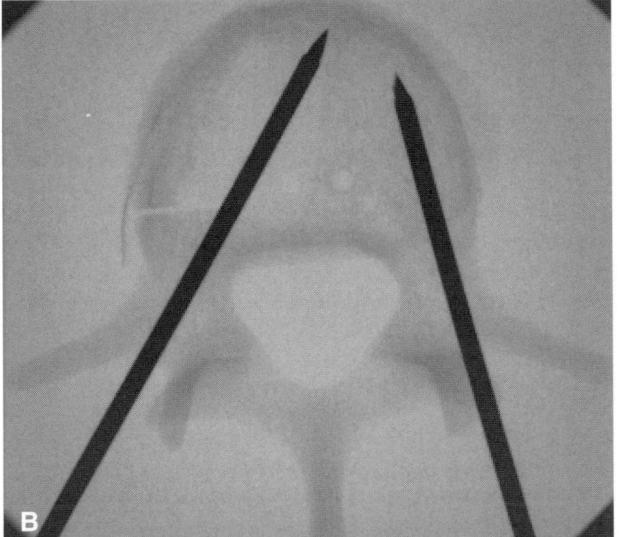

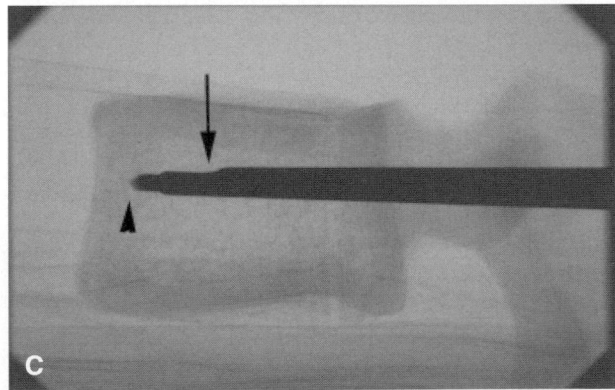

Figure 66–9   Styrofoam models in the **A.** AP, **B.** axial, and **C.** lateral views demonstrate the final location of the needle tips in the "scotty dog" oblique (*left side of image*) versus the straight AP approach. In the former approach, the needle tip reaches the midline and can be placed further anteriorly in the vertebral body without fear of transgressing the cortex. On the lateral view, the needle tip is almost to the inner cortex with the "scotty dog" approach (*arrowhead*), whereas the needle tip is closer to the junction of the anterior and mid–one third of the vertebral body with the straight AP approach (*arrow*).

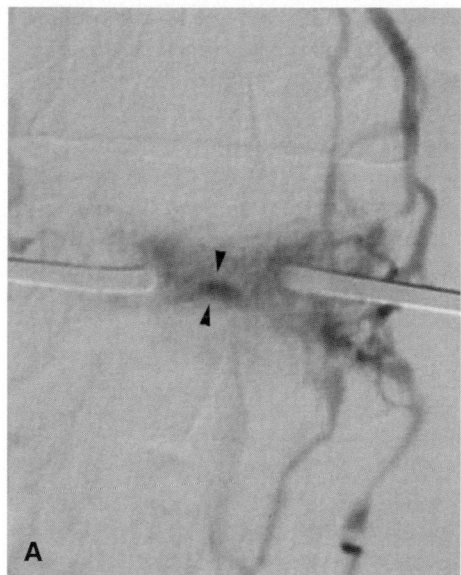
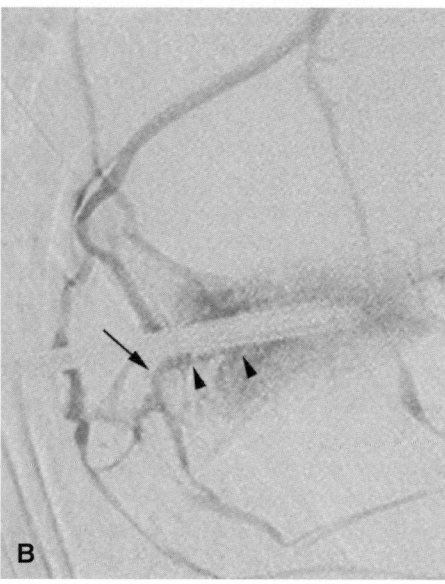

Figure 66–10 **A.** AP and **B.** lateral vertebrogram shows filling of the trabecular space with egress of contrast into the basivertebral plexus (*arrowheads*) and paravertebral veins that flow toward the azygous system. This vertebrogram precisely identified the entry point (*arrow*) of the plexus into the spinal canal and accurately predicted egress of acrylic into this structure (Figure 66–4B). Note that the needles parallel the basivertebral plexus, which may obscure visualization of this structure during acrylic injection.

Controversy exists over the need for vertebrography, particularly in the hands of experienced practitioners (37,38). Gaughen et al. (39) retrospectively evaluated the safety and efficacy of vertebroplasty performed in two patient populations; one in which venography was performed, and the other without venography. No significant differences between the two groups were found—either in frequency or amount of venous extravasation or in clinical outcome. However, this study was done at a major medical center by senior interventionalists with extensive experience, and its conclusions may not be valid for all practitioners.

In short, some operators may find the vertebrogram helpful because it easily identifies the exact point at which the basivertebral plexus exits the vertebral body, outlines the epidural and paraspinal venous system, and may predict PMMA flow characteristics and potential sites of egress (37). Detection of needle placement directly into a major venous structure allows the needle position to be readjusted, usually by advancement of the needle more anterior in the vertebral body before acrylic injection (7,32). Although no complications have been reported from vertebrography, contrast injected into a preexisting cavity or endplate fracture may be impossible to wash out, making it difficult to visualize the barium-opacified acrylic. Following vertebrography, residual contrast should be cleared from the needle with saline before acrylic injection.

Acrylic Preparation

Although a variety of bone filler substances have been used in the treatment of vertebral body disease, currently the only biomaterial approved for use in vertebroplasty in the United States is polymethylmethacrylate (PMMA). There are several commercially available PMMA products used for vertebroplasty, all with different handling characteristics. The injectable acrylic is created from two components: (1) a powdered polymer that may or may not contain an opacification agent and (2) a liquid monomer. When the two substances are combined, a slurry is formed and a chemical reaction begins that leads to progressive polymerization of the mixture to its solid state. Users should be familiar with PMMA before starting a vertebroplasty service. Bench testing is the recommended way to evaluate the material to ensure that the resultant mixture can be injected through a needle effectively and visualized fluoroscopically. This testing is best done at a formal course in which acrylic preparation and injection are performed on models or cadavers and a variety of materials and mixtures can be tried. Also, the literature on this substance is extensive, and the reader is encouraged to explore those biomaterials papers pertaining to its use in vertebroplasty. Of particular interest are reports concerning compressive strength of different PMMAs (40), the effects of the monomer-to-powder ratio on polymer strength (41), and in vitro temperature elevation from acrylic curing (42). Although the information is interesting, it has shown little clinical significance to date.

The major parameters of PMMA that have an impact on its use in vertebroplasty are polymerization time and opacification. The polymerization time, or curing rate, varies among the different products, and the slurry may be suitable for injection from as little as 5–20 minutes. The polymerization time of any PMMA can be prolonged by refrigeration of the powdered polymer pack and liquid monomer vial prior to their use or by placement of syringes filled with the prepared acrylic in an ice bath. For acrylics with longer curing times, the powdered polymer component needs to dissolve completely in the liquid monomer before injection. Otherwise, the powder may separate from the monomer in the needle during the injection, resulting in plugging of the cannula. The addition of a solvation time of approximately 1 minute after mixing and before injection is recommended by some manufacturers.

The second parameter of great significance is opacification. Because most clinically relevant complications are the result of PMMA migration into the extraosseous spaces, fluoroscopic visualization of the material during injection is of paramount importance. Visualization is influenced by the amount of barium sulfate within the product, the size of the patient, the location of the treated vertebral body, and the quality of the imaging chain. Therefore, all vertebroplasty practitioners must be familiar with the opacification characteristics of their chosen PMMA and should be prepared to supplement their mix with extra barium sulfate when necessary. Sterile barium sulfate for use in vertebroplasty is commercially available; any additional material should be thoroughly mixed with the powdered polymer before slurry preparation to guarantee homogenous opacification. Antibiotic powders for infection prophylaxis, such as tobramycin or vancomycin, also may be added to the powdered polymer. Any alteration of the manufacturers' product or mixing instructions through the addition of substances or a changing of the powder-to-liquid ratio may change the consistency and polymerization time of the material. Strictly speaking, altered material is no longer approved by the FDA.

Acrylic Injection

Injection of the acrylic slurry is performed using either 1-mL Luer-lock syringes or commercially available delivery systems. The 1-mL syringes are inexpensive, require minimal storage space, and allow exquisite tactile feedback during injection that improves acrylic flow control; however, their use places the operator's hands close to or within the radiation field. Commercially available injection devices are self-contained systems with a reservoir into which the PMMA is loaded, and a twist-type or trigger-activated plunger that advances the material. The system is attached to the cannula hub via high-pressure tubing. Each turn of the plunger or pull on the trigger delivers a consistent amount of acrylic into the cannula. Injection devices increase the distance between the operator and the x-ray tube, thus minimizing the dose to the hands especially in the AP plane (43). Only a single connection of the injector tubing to the cannula hub is necessary, resulting in less exposure of the acrylic to the atmosphere and of the hub's Luer-lock threads to the acrylic. Unfortunately, the tactile feedback is greatly diminished and the operator has to rely on visual cues, such as crowding of the barium particles in the cannula, to detect compromised acrylic flow. In addition, pressure buildup in the system, resulting in sudden expulsion of acrylic from the cannula tip, is more likely with injection devices than with 1-mL syringes. Regardless of the system used, operators should practice first on models or cadavers to become familiar with the tactile and visual cues used during acrylic injection.

The application of PMMA to the vertebral body is an embolization procedure, and all injections are visualized under fluoroscopic control. Lateral imaging is used primarily to ensure that epidural extravasation of cement does not occur; intermittent AP fluoroscopy monitors any lateral paravertebral extravasation. As the acrylic exits the cannula, it permeates the trabecular space, giving the appearance of a concentrically expanding cloud (Figure 66-11). Alternatively, it may seep along intraosseous cracks, leak through endplate fractures, or fill an internal cavity (Figure 66-12A, B, and C). In some instances, vertebral body expansion with reduction of kyphotic and wedge angulation will occur (Figure 66-13A, B, and C) (44-46). The cannula is withdrawn slightly whenever injection becomes difficult, creating a space for acrylic flow. When an injector is used, forward pressure is first alleviated to avoid sudden PMMA deposition into a new space. Typically, the injection is terminated when the acrylic reaches the posterior one quarter of the vertebral body to avoid embolization of the basivertebral plexus (Figure 66-11D). Good pain relief occurs with filling of two thirds of the vertebral body (36), and overzealous attempts at complete vertebral filling risks complication for little clinical gain.

Failure of the PMMA to egress from the cannula tip may be because of obstruction from bony trabeculae or from a blockage within the 1-mL syringe, injector tubing, or cannula. Acrylic compaction occurs when continued injection against a relative obstruction forces the liquid monomer out of the slurry. The resultant plug will obstruct the cannula lumen, necessitating its removal. Compaction is best identified by the lack of movement of PMMA into the vertebra, with crowding of the constrained barium particles within the cannula. If repositioning of the cannula tip slightly posteriorly does not result in acrylic flow, then the syringe or delivery system is disconnected and evaluated for plug formation. If no obstruction is present, the cannula is cleared with the stylet under fluoroscopic observation, and injection resumes.

Small acrylic leaks across endplate fractures are acceptable, but large amounts of PMMA within the disk space may act as a wedge, causing fracture of the adjacent vertebra (47). If the acrylic preferentially flows to a vein, the needle is repositioned more posteriorly and the material is allowed to thicken. Injection is terminated when continued venous filling occurs.

Before needle removal, a 360-degree twisting motion is performed to separate any stream of acrylic that may be attached to the material within the cannula dead space. Decompression of PMMA along the needle track has been seen with filling of large intraosseous cavities, and the needle should be removed cautiously. Any acrylic that remains in the subcutaneous soft tissues may become a source of pain or infection.

If inadequate filling of the vertebral body requires a contralateral puncture, then the procedure is repeated on the opposite side. Otherwise, the skin is cleaned and dressed with small adhesive bandages and the patient is transferred to the recovery room for further observation and care.

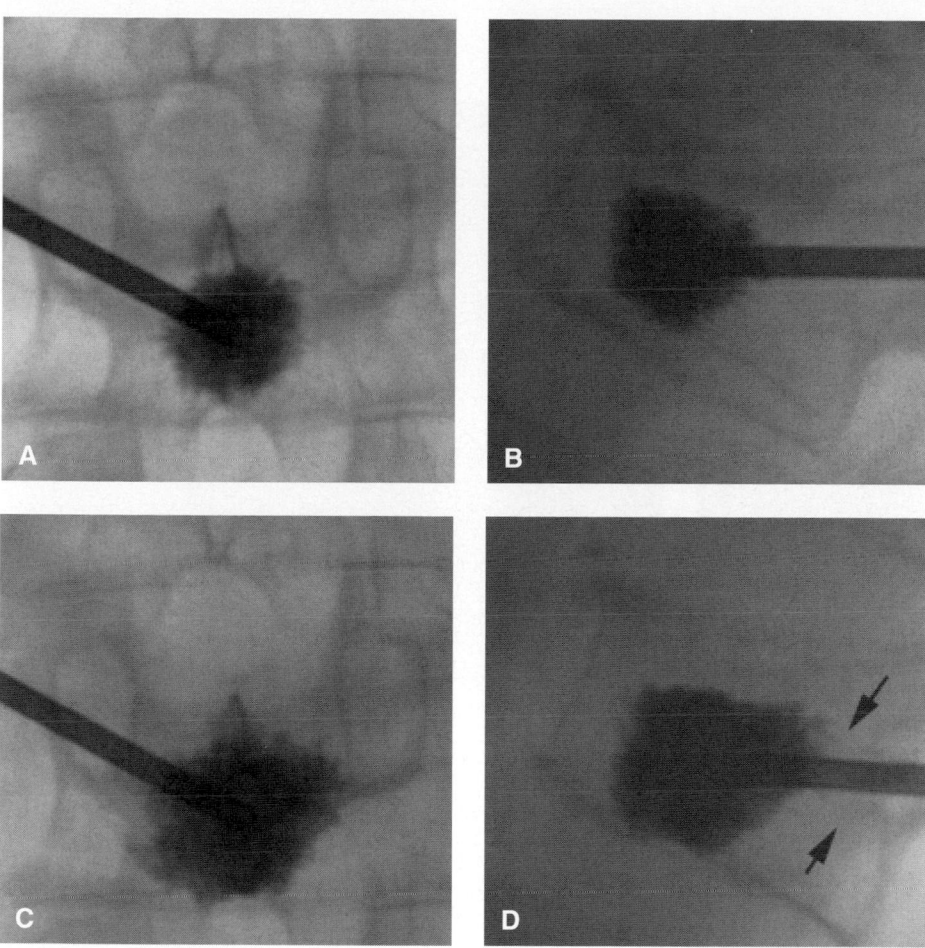

Figure 66–11 Selected images during an L3 vertebroplasty show the acrylic filling the **A.** trabecular space as a concentrically expanding "cloud." To better visualize the basivertebral plexus, **B.** the lateral tube is occasionally obliqued for the purpose of seeing around the cannula. **C.** The cannula remains in position during the injection and is withdrawn only when injecting the acrylic becomes difficult. **D.** When material is observed entering the posterior quarter of the vertebral body, the injection is terminated.

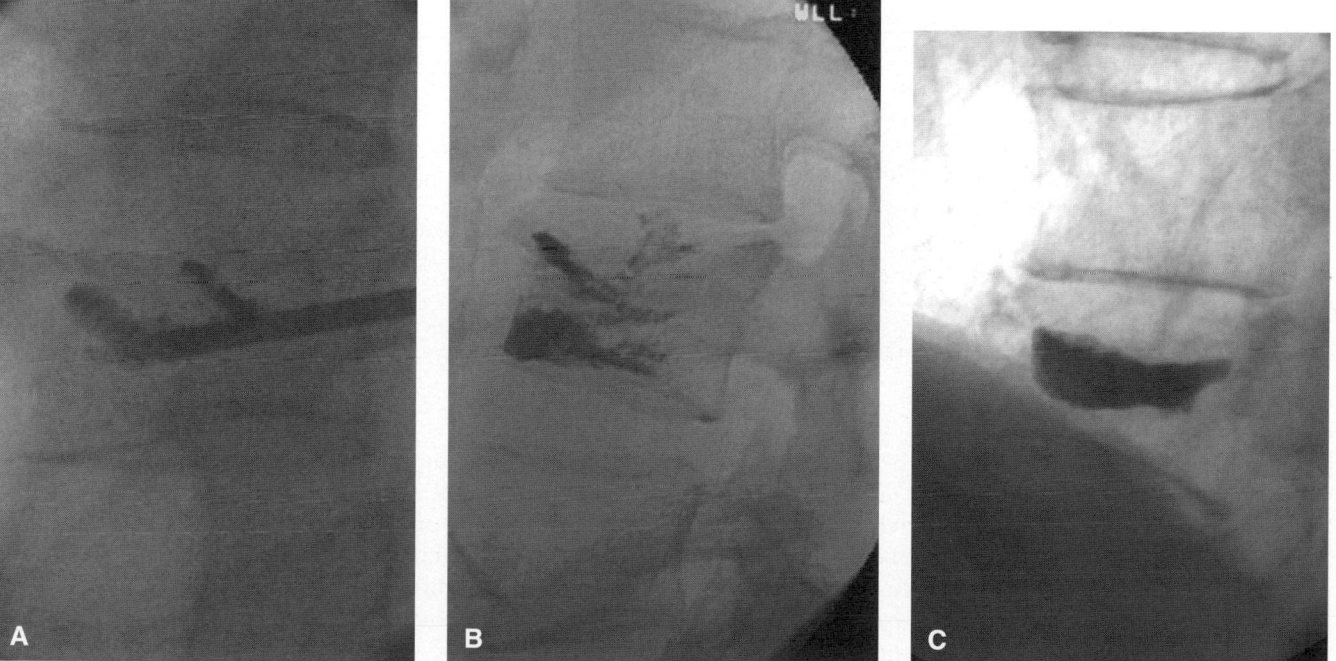

Figure 66–12 **A.** Vertebral body filling patterns are variable and include internal fractures that usually lead to the endplate, **B.** extravasation of acrylic into the disc space through an endplate rent, and **C.** contained cavities associated with osteonecrosis (Kümmell's disease).

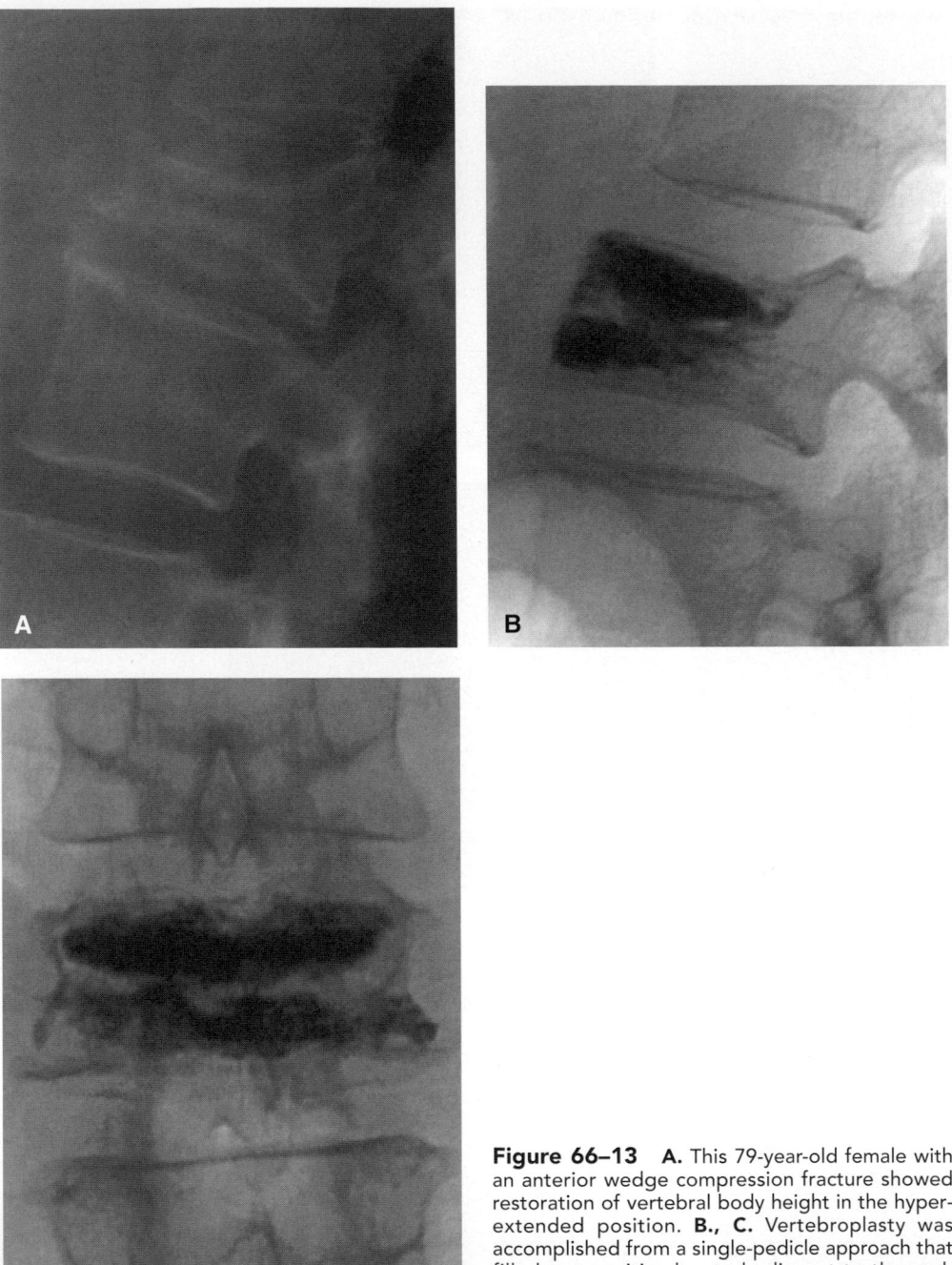

Figure 66–13 **A.** This 79-year-old female with an anterior wedge compression fracture showed restoration of vertebral body height in the hyperextended position. **B., C.** Vertebroplasty was accomplished from a single-pedicle approach that filled two cavities located adjacent to the endplates. Near complete height restoration is seen on the postvertebroplasty films.

Postprocedural Care

In the outpatient setting, most postvertebroplasty patients are observed for 2 hours before discharge. Individuals remain supine for 1 hour and are gradually allowed to sit up or stand over the next hour under direct nursing or physician supervision. Once recovered, ambulatory patients are discharged to the care of a responsible adult.

In many instances, patients experience some immediate pain relief, either from the residual effects of the local anesthetic or from the procedure or a combination of both. Patients are advised that focal pain at the puncture sites is common and may last up to 48 hours. Pain medication may be taken as needed; however, patients are encouraged to limit narcotic use so efficacy can be determined. Nonsteroidal, anti-inflammatory agents such as ibuprofen may be substituted.

Before discharge, patients are evaluated for chest or back pain, new neurologic dysfunction, dyspnea, or other potential complications of the procedure. Significant complications are the result of extraosseous acrylic deposition, and patients become symptomatic quickly. Early recognition is vital so that appropriate treatment can be instituted, and suspected complications should be treated as emergencies. For this reason, immediate access to CT scanning and surgical backup is an absolute requirement for any vertebroplasty service.

Small waterproof bandages placed over the puncture sites may be removed the next day, and skin incisions are kept clean and dry. Follow-up either by direct contact or telephone interview is done within 48 hours and at 7 days following the procedure. Patients are to notify the physician of redness or discharge at the operative site, recurrent or new back pain, chest pain or shortness of breath, or unexplained fever or neurologic symptoms. Any new symptom requires clinical evaluation and possible imaging. New back pain may indicate recurrent or new fracture, unrecognized facet pain, or epidural abscess. Chest pain may be the result of rib fractures or unsuspected pulmonary embolization of acrylic. All neurologic symptoms require immediate CT scanning to search for misplaced PMMA, and suspected osteomyelitis or abscess is best investigated with MRI.

For people who have been immobilized for a long period, a gradual increase of activity is recommended. Some individuals who feel better immediately try to return to full activity, only to fracture another vertebra, a hip, or a wrist. A short course of physical therapy with continued use of a brace may be helpful. Patients who are not receiving preventive medical therapy are referred to endocrinology or geriatrics for further evaluation and implementation of appropriate treatment.

COMPLICATIONS

Presently, a greater number of vertebroplasty procedures are being performed around the world, many by less experienced operators. As with any procedure, the complication rate will be highest during the operator's learning phase. Complications are best avoided through a thorough understanding of the factors that contribute to their occurrence. Often, it is the overzealous quest for complete vertebral body filling that results in complications, and practitioners new to the procedure must realize that "more" definitely is not "better" where vertebroplasty is concerned.

The primary cause of a symptomatic vertebroplasty complication is leakage of PMMA into adjacent structures—through fracture lines or cortical destruction, along the needle track, or into the epidural and paravertebral venous complexes (8,29,48–50). Acrylic material located within the epidural venous plexus or foraminal veins may cause spinal cord or nerve root compression, with resultant worsening pain or neurological dysfunction (Figure 66–14 and Figure 66–15A). Migration of small amounts of PMMA through the epidural or paravertebral venous system to the

pulmonary vasculature (Figure 66–15B) is usually without clinical significance, but symptomatic pulmonary embolus has been reported (51).

Perivertebral acrylic is usually asymptomatic, although dysphagia from esophageal compression after a cervical vertebroplasty has occurred (50). Acrylic within the disk space may decrease its cushioning ability, leading to focal fractures at adjacent endplates (47). Rarely, material within the disk space may cause disk extrusion resulting in acute myelopathy following vertebroplasty.

More often than not, PMMA leakage is asymptomatic, even in malignant lesions. Cotten et al. (49) demonstrated acrylic leaks by computed tomography, both venous and cortical, in 29 of 40 patients with osteolytic metastases or myeloma. Most of these leaks were asymptomatic, but two of eight foraminal leaks produced nerve root compression that required decompressive surgery. In a later series, Cotten et al. (29) reported 1 of 258 patients treated experienced spinal cord compression that required surgery. Of 13 patients with radicular pain, only three required surgical decompression, while 10 responded to local anesthetic infiltration or medical therapy. Deramond et al. (8) noted a single transient neurologic complication in 80 patients

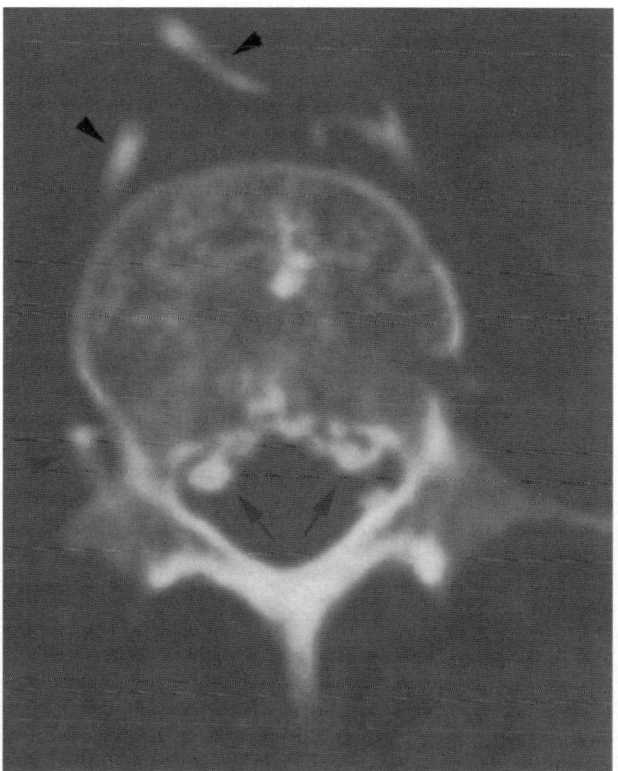

Figure 66–14 Selected CT axial image of an L3 vertebroplasty performed from the paravertebral approach. A cortical breach is seen along the left lateral wall of the vertebral body. Acrylic has decompressed into the epidural venous plexus (*arrows*) and migrated into the paravertebral veins (*arrowheads*) and the IVC. Acrylic was seen within the epidural venous plexus from L1–L4 and was noted to layer within the posterior aspect of the IVC (*not shown*).

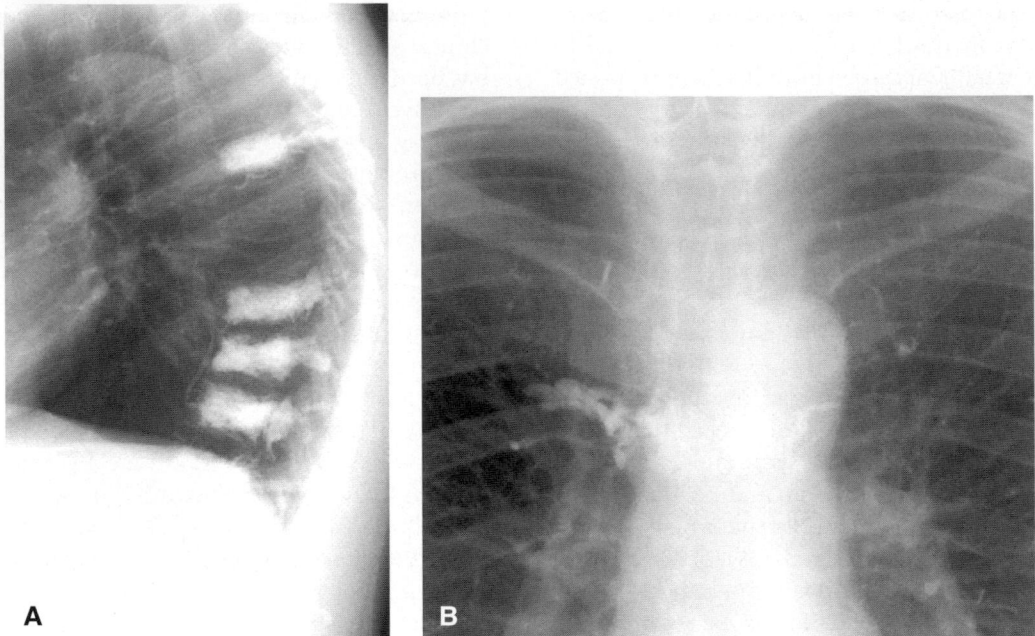

Figure 66–15 No clinical history was given on this chest radiograph that shows a multilevel vertebroplasty done outside the radiology department. **A.** Acrylic is seen within the spinal canal, paravertebral veins, and azygous system and **B.** the pulmonary vasculature. (Courtesy of Jonas Goldstein, MD.)

with osteoporotic fractures. Review of all major vertebroplasty series shows that the complication rate ranges from 1–10%; Murphy and Deramond (48) divide it further into 1.3% for osteoporosis, 2.5% for hemangiomas, and 10% for neoplastic disease. Fortunately, most patients with radicular symptoms respond to anti-inflammatory or narcotic analgesics or local anesthetic infiltration (Figure 66–16A and B), while surgical intervention is required only in a minority of cases. But, the small number of reported serious complications should not lull operators into a false sense of security. If significant neurologic compromise were to occur, surgical colleagues must be available for immediate consultation or intervention. Vertebroplasty should only be performed at sites where surgical backup is available.

Significant complications also may occur from inappropriate needle positioning. Improper placement of the cannula tip within or near the basivertebral plexus places the patient at risk for deposition of PMMA into the epidural venous plexus (Figure 66–17). Advancement of the needle through the anterior vertebral body wall could damage the aorta or inferior vena cava. Use of the paravertebral approach may injure the intercostal or lumbar artery. Transgression of the dura may lead to a symptomatic CSF leak or decompression of PMMA into the thecal sac after cannula removal (Figure 66–18A and B). Pneumothorax is a potential complication of thoracic vertebroplasty.

Other complications that have occurred include fracture of the transverse process or pedicle, paravertebral hematoma, epidural abscess (Figure 66–19), seizure or respiratory arrest from oversedation, and death. Severely osteoporotic patients

may sustain rib fractures from lying prone on the procedure table (7). Padding the table, performing the puncture with the patient in the decubitus position or advancing the needle through the bone with the use of a hammer may help to decrease the chance of a rib fracture.

Hemodynamic compromise has been associated with packing of the acetabulum with PMMA during hip replacement surgery. Transient systemic hypotension during acrylic injection in vertebroplasty has been reported (52), but a large retrospective study of the cardiovascular effects of PMMA in vertebroplasty found no generalized association between acrylic injection and systemic cardiovascular derangement (53).

One theoretical complication is thermal injury to adjacent neurologic structures during acrylic polymerization. There have been no clinical reports of this phenomenon, and its possibility appears unlikely based upon in vitro tests that showed no significant temperature rise in the spinal canal with vertebroplasty (42) and in vivo animal experiments that showed no spinal cord damage from PMMA located adjacent to the dural sac in dogs (54).

Injury to the medical staff from PMMA vapor exposure is an important concern. Occupational Safety and Health Administration (OSHA) limits for personnel are set at 100 ppm per 8-hour shift. Cloft et al. (55) showed exposure of less than 5 ppm to physicians performing vertebroplasty in a standard-ventilation angiography suite. Even though the exposure is negligible, some people may experience an idiosyncratic reaction or asthma exacerbation in response to the pungent smell of the material. The issue of increased risk

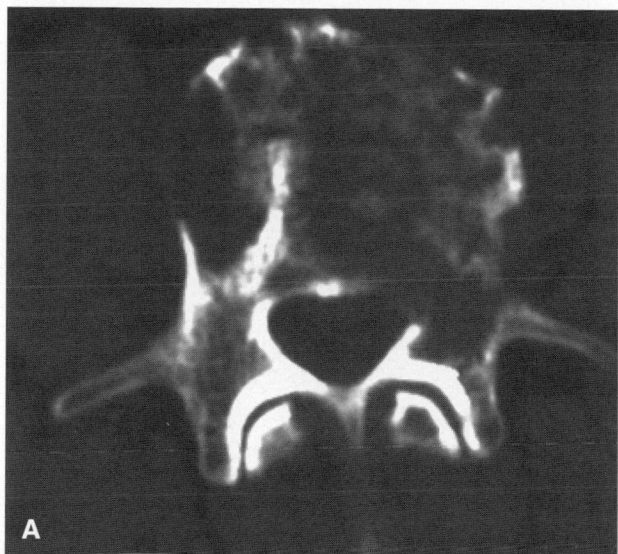

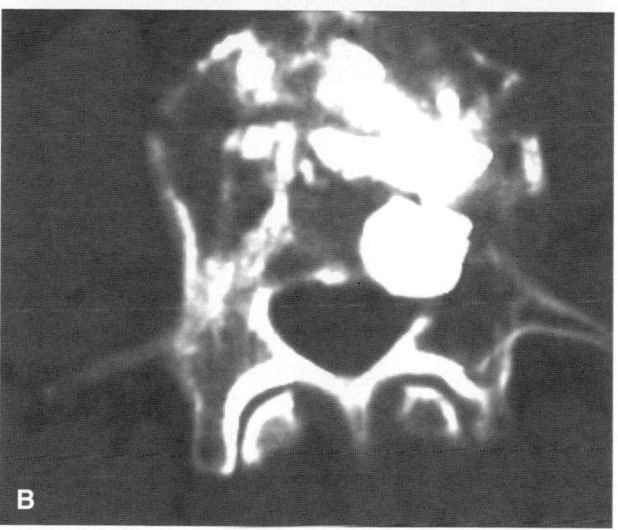

Figure 66–16 **A.** This 60-year-old male with renal cell metastasis to L4 was noted to have erosion of the posterior vertebral body wall along the left lateral recess, but no frank epidural tumor. **B.** Following vertebroplasty, the acrylic is filling the tumor in the left hemivertebral, including the portion impinging upon the spinal canal. The patient developed a transient left leg radiculopathy that resolved with a short course of steroids.

for fracture at an adjacent level has been raised in the literature. Grados and colleagues (56) found a slight but significantly increased risk of vertebral fracture in the vicinity of an augmented vertebra when compared to a vertebral fracture in the vicinity of an untreated fracture. Lin et al. (47) evaluated a small group of patients who developed adjacent endplate fractures following vertebroplasty and found a higher proportion than not had an acrylic leak into the adjacent disk space. These results must be considered with caution because association does not necessarily mean causation, and avoiding treatment of fractures that involve the endplate may change the clinical response (57). In addition, new fractures following vertebroplasty may actually represent

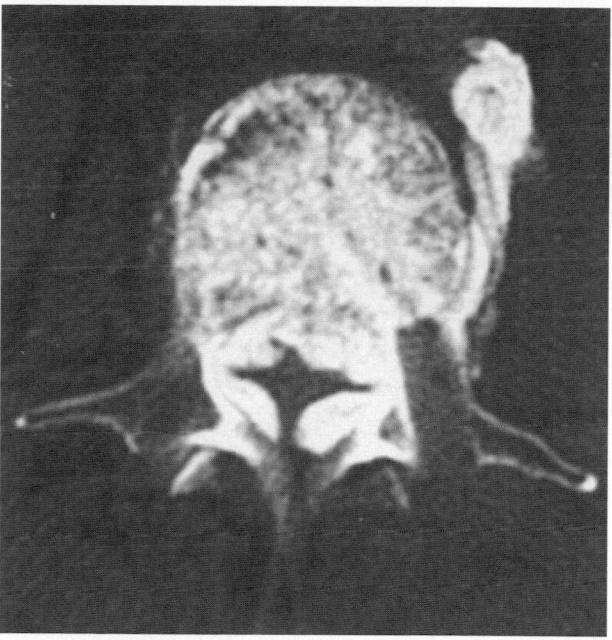

Figure 66–17 Placement of a large trocar in the posterior aspect of the vertebral body near the egress of the basivertebral plexus resulted in decompression of acrylic material into the epidural, intravertebral, and paravertebral veins with significant compression of the thecal sac. Leakage through a pediculate fracture into the spinal canal is another consideration as the defect left by the cannula approximates the diameter of the pedicle. (Courtesy of Rubin Sebben, MD.)

the natural history of osteoporosis rather than a complication of the procedure, and further study is necessary.

In summary, complications are most commonly associated with the following:

1. Poor visualization owing to inadequate fluoroscopic equipment, poor patient cooperation ("the moving target"), or unsatisfactory acrylic opacification
2. Operator error, such as inappropriate patient selection; lack of knowledge of the radiographic spinal anatomy, particularly bony and venous; poor fluoroscopic-triangulation skills; unfamiliarity with equipment, devices, and PMMA; and poor embolization technique
3. Lack of patient monitoring
4. Improper aseptic technique

By recognizing and avoiding these potential pitfalls and being thoroughly educated before performing vertebroplasty, operators will markedly decrease their chances of causing a significant complication.

CLINICAL OUTCOMES

More than 450 papers concerning vertebroplasty have been published in the last 20 years, with the bulk of these appearing in the 21st century. Among these papers, about 100 studies address the clinical outcomes of patients treated with percutaneous vertebroplasty. Without exception, these

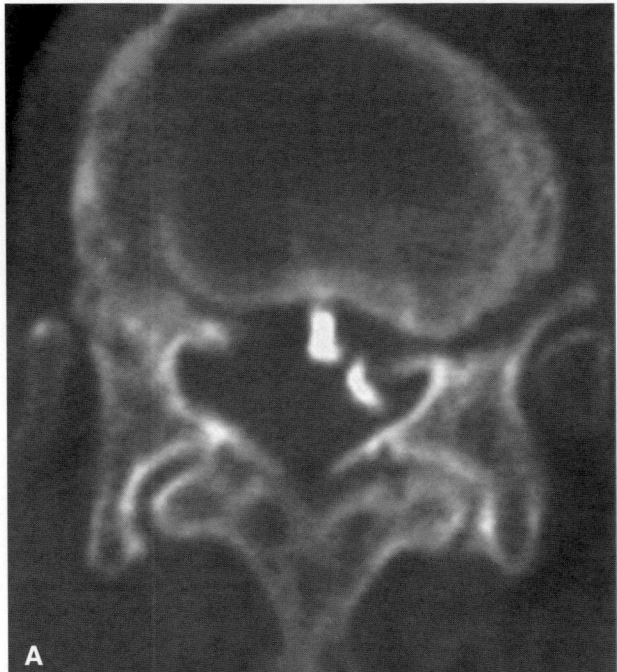

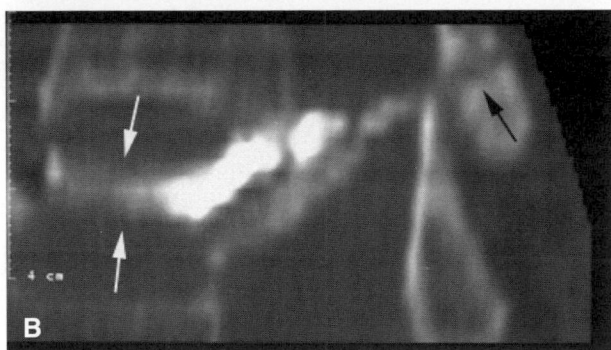

Figure 66-18 This 70-year-old lady presented with a new fracture following a vertebroplasty at an outside facility. She was noted to have bilateral hip flexor weakness on physical exam. **A.** Axial CT with sagittal reconstruction shows the needle's path through the spinal canal with decompression of acrylic along its course. **B.** The needle track is seen through the left lamina (*arrow*). In addition, the patient was an inappropriate candidate for vertebroplasty because the vertebral body was completely collapsed (*white arrows*).

reports describe vertebroplasty as a successful therapy for the relief of pain associated with vertebral compression fractures caused by either osteoporosis or tumor involvement. The earliest literature consisted of small, retrospective, uncontrolled case series introducing the technique and claiming excellent results for the patients involved (1–6). Since that time, larger case series have been published, but these too were retrospective and lacking controls (7,8,26,28,29,30,49,50,56, 58–60). Literature reviews on the efficacy of vertebroplasty have concluded that the procedure, when used in the setting of osteroporotic compression fractures, results in substantial and immediate pain relief, improved functional status, and minimal short-term complications (61–63). These reports also lack scientific

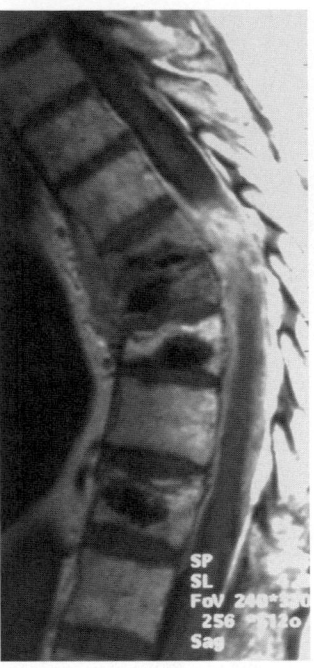

Figure 66-19 This 45-year-old male with a lung transplant developed multiple thoracic vertebral fractures because of chronic steroid use. A multilevel vertebroplasty was performed without difficulty. Tobramycin powder was mixed with the acrylic, but the patient did not receive intravenous antibiotics. Three weeks later, he complained of recurrent back pain. MRI shows a large epidural abscess adjacent to the most superior vertebroplasty level, which required surgical decompression.

merit. More encouraging are prospective reports that have now appeared (64–66); however, these too have lacked controls. Thus, despite the general endorsement in the literature of the procedure to date, published reports suffer from at least one of three primary methodologic limitations. These are (1) retrospective assessment of patient status (pain and functional ability); (2) assessment of patient status using either nonvalidated instruments, such as self-developed or validated instruments nonspecific to vertebral compression fractures; and (3) lack of control subjects. It is true that surgical therapies are rarely subjected to the same prospective randomized evaluation as medical therapies, but it must be noted that at this time, little actual scientific evidence exists to prove that vertebroplasty is an effective therapy. Two prospective, randomized trials—one sponsored by the NIH and one by industry—are currently underway that could answer this question.

KYPHOPLASTY

Recently, a new technique called *kyphoplasty*, or balloon-assisted vertebroplasty, has been described by investigators as being able to restore physiologic spinal column alignment and to provide pain relief. Kyphoplasty is a technique that, in principal, achieves similar results to vertebroplasty, an assertion supported by the literature (66,67). The vertebral body is accessed in a similar manner as vertebroplasty, but a balloon catheter is used to create a space within the hemivertebra before acrylic infusion. Theoretical advantages of kyphoplasty over vertebroplasty include the potential for vertebral body height restoration, reduction of kyphotic angulation of the spine, and lower rate of acrylic leakage into adjacent soft tissues. A few papers have been published on the clinical outcomes of patients treated with kyphoplasty (68–70), but they are hampered by the same methodologic flaws just described about the vertebroplasty literature. The positive clinical response rate is similar to vertebroplasty, but kyphoplasty proponents purport significant height restoration that theoretically benefits the patient, although data to support this belief are lacking. The vertebroplasty and kyphoplasty literature contain an approximately equal number of small case series that claim some degree of height restoration (44–46,67,69,70). Cadaveric studies support the assertion that vertebroplasty and kyphoplasty add structural integrity to a collapsed vertebral body; however, there is now evidence from biomechanical studies that vertebral bodies treated with kyphoplasty are more susceptible to further collapse than vertebral bodies treated with vertebroplasty (71).

Although the percentage of patients with cement leaks may be higher with vertebroplasty, the percentage of catastrophic complications is possibly higher with kyphoplasty (72). At this time, there is no compelling evidence that one technique is superior in clinical results or safer in the majority of patients. A multicenter prospective randomized trial is being organized that may shed light on this question.

SUMMARY

Percutaneous vertebroplasty has gone from an obscure technique reserved for a few special cases to a highly utilized procedure that consistently benefits a significant number of patients worldwide. The practice of vertebroplasty continues to grow in size and scope, fostering new developments, research, and products. Hopefully, conclusive data through randomized controlled trials will, in the near future, confirm what seems apparent—that vertebroplasty is safe and efficacious in the vast majority of treated individuals. It is vitally important to the growth of minimally invasive spine procedures that all interventional radiologists take an active interest in bringing this exciting technology to their patients and their practices.

REFERENCES

1. Galibert P, Deramond H, Rosat P, et al. [Preliminary note on the treatment of vertebral angioma by percutaneous acrylic vertebroplasty]. Neurochirurgie 1987;33:166–168.
2. Kaemmerlen P, Thiesse P, Bouvard H, et al. [Percutaneous vertebroplasty in the treatment of metastases. Technic and results]. J Radiol 1989;70:557–562.
3. Nguyen JP, Djindjian M, Pavlovitch JM, et al. [Vertebral hemangioma with neurologic signs. Therapeutic results. Survey of the French Society of Neurosurgery]. Neurochirurgie 1989;35:299–303, 305–308.
4. Dermond H, Darrason R, Gailibert P. Percutaneous vertebroplasty with acrylic cement in the treatment of aggressive spinal angiomas. Rachis 1989;1:143–153.
5. Debussche-Depriester C, Deramond H, Fardellone P, et al. Percutaneous vertebroplasty with acrylic cement in the treatment of osteoporotic vertebral crush fracture syndrome. Neuroradiology 1991;33(Suppl):149–152.
6. Gangi A, Kastler BA, Dietemann JL. Percutaneous vertebroplasty guided by a combination of CT and fluoroscopy. AJNR Am J Neuroradiol 1994;15:83–86.
7. Jensen ME, Evans AJ, Mathis JM, et al. Percutaneous polymethylmethacrylate vertebroplasty in the treatment of osteoporotic vertebral body compression fractures: technical aspects. AJNR Am J Neuroradiol 1997;18:1897–1904.
8. Deramond H, Depriester C, Galibert P, et al. Percutaneous vertebroplasty with polymethylmethacrylate. Technique, indications, and results. Radiol Clin North Am 1998;36:533–546.
9. Cortet B, Cotten A, Boutry N, et al. Percutaneous vertebroplasty in the treatment of osteoporotic vertebral compression fractures: an open prospective study. J Rheumatol 1999;26:2222–2228.
10. Riggs BL, Melton LJ. The worldwide problem of osteoporosis: insights afforded by epidemiology. Bone 1995;17(Suppl):505S–511S.
11. Melton LJ, Chrischilles EA, Cooper C, et al. Perspective. How many women have osteoporosis? J Bone Miner Res 1992;7:1005–1010.
12. Riggs BL, Melton LJ. Involutional osteoporosis. N Engl J Med 1986;314:1676–1686.
13. Ross PD, Davis SW, Epstein RS, et al. Preexisting fractures and bone mass predict vertebral fracture incidence in women. Ann Intern Med 1991;114:919–923.
14. Eastell R, Cedel SL, Wahner HW, et al. Classification of vertebral fractures. J Bone Miner Res 1991;6:207–215.
15. Cooper C, Atkinson EJ, O'Fallon WM, et al. Incidence of clinically diagnosed vertebral fractures: a population-based study in Rochester, Minnesota, 1985–1989. J Bone Miner Res;7:221–227.
16. Patel U, Skingle S, Campbell GA, et al. Clinical profile of acute vertebral compression fractures in osteoporosis. Br J Rheumatol 1991;30:418–421.
17. Silverman SL. The clinical consequences of vertebral compression fracture. Bone 1992;13:S27–S31.
18. Rapado A. General management of vertebral fractures. Bone 1996;18 (Suppl III):191S–196S.
19. Cohen LD. Fractures of the osteoporotic spine. Orthop Clin North Am 1990;21:143–150.
20. Lyles KW, Gold DT, Shipp KM, et al. Association of osteoporotic vertebral compression fractures with impaired functional status. Am J Med 1993;94:595–601.
21. Dittmer DK, Teasell R. Complications of immobilization and bed rest. Part 1: musculoskeletal and cardiovascular complications. Can Fam Physician 1993;39:1428–1432.
22. Teasell R, Dittmer DK: Complications of immobilization and bed rest. Part 2: other complications. Can Fam Physician 1993;39:1440–1442.
23. Barr JD, Mathis JM, Barr MS, et al. Standard for the performance of percutaneous vertebroplasty. In: American College of Radiology Standards 2000–2001. Reston, VA: American College of Radiology, 2000:441–448.
24. Do HM, Jensen ME, Marx WF, et al. Percutaneous vertebroplasty in vertebral osteonecrosis (Kümmell's spondylitis). Neurosurg Focus 1999;7:A1.
25. Stallmeyer MJ, Zoarski GH, Obuchoswski AM. Optimizing patient selection in percutaneous vertebroplasty. J Vasc Interv Radiol 2003;14:683–696.
26. Gaughen JR Jr, Jensen ME, Schweickert PA, et al. Lack of preoperative spinous process tenderness does not affect clinical success of percutaneous vertebroplasty. J Vasc Interv Radiol 2002;13:1135–1138.
27. Do HM. Magnetic resonance imaging in the evaluation of patients for percutaneous vertebroplasty. Top Magn Reson Imaging 2000;11:235–244.

28. Maynard AS, Jensen ME, Schweickert PA, et al. Value of bone scan imaging in predicting pain relief from percutaneous vertebroplasty in osteoporotic vertebral fractures. AJNR Am J Neuroradiol 2000;21:1807–1812.

29. Cotten A, Boutry N, Cortet B, et al. Percutaneous vertebroplasty: state of the art. Radiographics 1998;18:311–320.

30. Gangi A, Guth S, Imbert JP, et al. Percutaneous vertebroplasty: indications, technique, and results. Radiographics 2002;23:e10.

31. Mathis JM, Barr JD, Belkoff SM, et al. Percutaneous vertebroplasty: a developing standard of care for vertebral compression fractures. AJNR Am J Neuroradiol 2001;22:373–381. Review.

32. Jensen ME, Dion JE. Percutaneous vertebroplasty in osteoporotic compression fractures. Neuroimaging Clin N Am 2000; 10: 547–568. Review.

33. Kallmes DF, Jensen ME. Percutaneous vertebroplasty. Radiology 2003;229:27–36. Review.

34. Barr MS, Barr JD. Invited commentary. Radiographics 1998;18: 320–321.

35. Tohmeh AG, Mathis JM, Fenton DC, et al. Biomechanical efficacy of unipedicular versus bipedicular vertebroplasty for the management of osteoporotic compression fractures. Spine 1999;24:1772–1776.

36. Kim AK, Jensen ME, Dion JE, et al. Unilateral transpedicular percutaneous vertebroplasty: initial experience. Radiology 2002;222: 737–741.

37. McGraw JK, Heatwole EV, Strnad BT, et al. Predictive value of intraosseous venography before percutaneous vertebroplasty. J Vasc Interv Radiol 2002;13:149–153.

38. Vasconcelos C, Gailloud P, Beauchamp NJ, et al. Is percutaneous vertebroplasty without pretreatment venography safe? Evaluation of 205 consecutives procedures. AJNR Am J Neuroradiol 2002;23:913–917.

39. Gaughen JR Jr, Jensen ME, Schweickert PA, et al. Relevance of antecedent venography in percutaneous vertebroplasty for the treatment of osteoporotic compression fractures. AJNR Am J Neuroradiol 2002;23:594–600.

40. Belkoff SM, Maroney M, Fenton DC, et al. An in vitro biomechanical evaluation of bone cements used in percutaneous vertebroplasty. Bone 1999;25(Suppl II):23S–26S.

41. Jasper LE, Deramond H, Mathis JM, et al. The effect of monomer-to-powder ratio on the material properties of cranioplastic. Bone 1999;25(SupplII):27S–29S.

42. Deramond H, Wright NT, Belkoff SM. Temperature elevation caused by bone cement polymerization during vertebroplasty. Bone 1999;25(Suppl II):17S–21S.

43. Kallmes DF, O E, Roy SS, et al. Radiation dose to the operator during vertebroplasty: prospective comparison of the use of 1-cc syringes versus an injection device. AJNR Am J Neuroradiol 2003;24:1257–1260.

44. Teng MM, Wei CJ, Wei LC, et al. Kyphosis correction and height restoration effects of percutaneous vertebroplasty. AJNR Am J Neuroradiol 2003;24:1893–900.

45. Hiwatashi A, Moritani T, Numaguchi Y, et al. Increase in vertebral body height after vertebroplasty. AJNR Am J Neuroradiol 2003;24:185–189.

46. Dublin AB, Hartman J, Latchaw RE, et al. The vertebral body fracture in osteoporosis: restoration of height using percutaneous vertebroplasty. AJNR Am J Neuroradiol 2005;26:489–492.

47. Lin EP, Ekholm S, Hiwatashi A, et al. Vertebroplasty: cement leakage into the disc increases the risk of new fracture of adjacent vertebral body. AJNR Am J Neuroradiol 2004;25:175–180.

48. Murphy KJ, Deramond H. Percutaneous vertebroplasty in benign and malignant disease. Neuroimaging Clin N Am 2000;10: 535–545.

49. Cotten A, Dewatre F, Cortet B, et al. Percutaneous vertebroplasty for osteolytic metastases and myeloma: effects of the percentage of lesion filling and the leakage of methyl methacrylate at clinical follow-up. Radiology 1996;200:525–530.

50. Weill A, Chiras J, Simon J, et al. Spinal metastases: indications for and results of percutaneous injection of acrylic cement. Radiology 1996;199:241–247.

51. Padovani B, Kasriel O, Brunner P, et al. Pulmonary embolism caused by acrylic cement: a rare complication of percutaneous vertebroplasty. AJNR Am J Neuroradiol 1999;20:375–377.

52. Vasconcelos C, Gailloud P, Martin JB, et al. Transient arterial hypotension induced by polymethylmethacrylate injection during percutaneous vertebroplasty. J Vasc Interv Radiol 2001;12: 1001–1002.

53. Kaufmann TJ, Jensen ME, Ford G, et al. Cardiovascular effects of polymethylmethacrylate use in percutaneous vertebroplasty. AJNR Am J Neuroradiol 2002;23:601–604.

54. Wang GW, Wilson CS, Hubbard SL, et al. Safety of anterior cement fixation in the cervical spine: in vivo study of dog spine. South Med J 1984;77:178–179.

55. Cloft HJ, Easton DN, Jensen ME, et al. Exposure of medical personnel to methyl methacrylate vapor during percutaneous vertebroplasty. AJNR Am J Neuroradiol 1999;20:352–353.

56. Grados F, Depriester C, Cayrolle G, et al. Long-term observations of vertebral osteoporotic fractures treated by percutaneous vertebroplasty. Rheumatology (Oxford) 2000;39:1410–1414.

57. Jensen ME, Kallmes DF. Does filling the crack break more of the back? Am J Neuroradiol 2004;25:166–167.

58. Martin JB, Jean B, Sugiu K, et al. Vertebroplasty: clinical experience and follow-up results. Bone 1999;25(Suppl II):11S–15S.

59. Kaufmann TJ, Jensen ME, Schweickert PA, et al. Age of fracture and clinical outcomes of percutaneous vertebroplasty. AJNR Am J Neuroradiol 2001;22:1860–1863.

60. Evans AJ, Jensen ME, Kip KE, et al. Vertebral compression fractures: pain reduction and improvement in functional mobility after percutaneous polymethylmethacrylate vertebroplasty retrospective report of 245 cases. Radiology 2003;226:366–72.

61. Garfin SR, Yuan HA, Reiley MA. New technologies in spine: kyphoplasty and vertebroplasty for the treatment of painful osteoporotic compression fractures. Spine 2001;26: 1511–1515.

62. Levine SA, Perin LA, Hayes D, et al. An evidence-based evaluation of percutaneous vertebroplasty. Managed Care 2000;9:56–60, 63.

63. Watts NB, Harris ST, Genant HK. Treatment of painful osteoporotic vertebral fractures with percutaneous vertebroplasty or kyphoplasty. Osteoporos Int 2001;12:429–437.

64. Zoarski GH, Snow P, Olan WJ, et al. Percutaneous vertebroplasty for osteoporotic compression fractures: quantitative prospective evaluation of long-term outcomes. J Vasc Interv Radiol 2002;13: 139–148.

65. McGraw JK, Lippert JA, Minkus KD, et al. Prospective evaluation of pain relief in 100 patients undergoing percutaneous vertebroplasty: results and follow-up. J Vasc Interv Radiol 2002;13: 883–886.

66. Garfin SR, Reiley MA. Minimally invasive treatment of osteoporotic vertebral body compression fractures. Spine 2002; 2:76–80.

67. Lieberman IH, Dudeney S, Reinhardt MK, et al. Initial outcome and efficacy of "kyphoplasty" in the treatment of painful osteoporotic vertebral compression fractures. Spine 2001;26: 1631–1638.

68. Coumans JV, Reinhardt MK, Lieberman IH. Kyphoplasty for vertebral compression fractures: 1-year clinical outcomes from a prospective study. J Neurosurg 2003;Spine 99:44–50.

69. Phillips FM, Ho E, Campbell-Hupp M, et al. Early radiographic and clinical results of balloon kyphoplasty for the treatment of osteoporotic vertebral compression fractures. Spine 2003;28: 2260–2265.

70. Kasperk C, Hillmeier J, Noldge G, et al. Treatment of painful vertebral fractures by kyphoplasty in patients with primary osteoporosis: a prospective nonrandomized controlled study. J Bone Miner Res 2005;20:604–612.

71. Alamin T. Kyphoplasty versus vertebroplasty: behavior under repetitive loading conditions. [Abstract] Presented at the annual meeting of the North American Spine Society, Chicago, 2004.

72. Nussbaum DA, Gailloud P, Murphy K. A review of complications associated with vertebroplasty and kyphoplasty as reported to the Food and Drug Administration medical device related Web site. J Vasc Interv Radiol 2004;15:1185–1192.

Venous Thrombolysis and Stenting

67

Paul C. Lakin, Sean M. Carr

Obstruction of the superior vena cava (SVC) and inferior vena cava (IVC) and their major branches may be caused by a variety of benign and malignant pathologic conditions. Trauma, inflammatory lesions, and radiation may result in perivascular fibrosis. Neoplastic masses may either directly compress or invade major venous structures. In addition, indwelling catheters or local trauma may result in venous obstruction. Thrombosis may convert a partial obstruction into a venous occlusion. With the obstruction of major venous structures, various congestive syndromes may arise, depending upon the location of the obstruction, resulting in IVC or SVC syndrome or severe hepatic dysfunction.

Percutaneous interventional therapy is extremely useful in treating obstructions of large veins, and it frequently restores the patency of the vein while reversing the congestive symptoms. Because surgical repair or bypass of obstructed venous structures, particularly in malignant obstructions, is frequently difficult or impossible, interventional therapy is crucial in these patients and frequently provides effective long-term palliation in malignant obstructions. In benign obstructions in which conventional anticoagulation therapy is not effective, surgery may also be difficult, and percutaneous interventional therapy may provide long-term patency. Three interventional modalities can be used for the treatment of venous obstruction: local thrombolytic therapy, percutaneous transluminal angioplasty, and expandable stent placement. Although these modalities may be used alone, they are most often used in combination.

THROMBOLYSIS

In the 1970s, Charles Dotter was the first to describe a technique for regional infusion of fibrinolytic agents (1). Becker et al. (2) in 1983 described the use of local thrombolytic therapy for subclavian and axillary vein thrombosis. The perfusion of lytic agents directly into the thrombus using a catheter positioned in or near the offending clot resulted in excellent initial results, and in all cases, it demonstrated an underlying venous abnormality. Other reports followed with similar results (3,4).

Principles

When performing thrombolysis, there are essentially three agents from which to choose. Urokinase (Abbokinase, Abbott Laboratories) is a direct plasminogen activator with a plasma half-life of 15 minutes. The cost is approximately $380 for a 250,000 IU vial. Urokinase was removed from the market in 1999, and reintroduced in 2002, but production ceased in early 2005. The FDA currently approves it for the treatment of pulmonary embolism. Catheter-directed thrombolysis with urokinase is performed with an initial bolus of 250,000–500,000 units directly into the thrombus. Catheter infusion is then performed at a rate of 100,000 U/h. The infusion may be continued for 8–12 hours, at which point the progress should be reevaluated. Systemic heparinization is performed with an initial loading dose of 5,000 units. The patient is then kept on a dose sufficient to maintain the partial thromboplastin time (PTT) at approximately 1.5 times normal. The PTT is reevaluated 4 hours and 24 hours after the start of thrombolytic therapy.

Alteplase (Activase, Genentech) is a recombinant form of the naturally occurring tissue-type plasminogen activator enzyme. It has a plasma half-life of 4–6 minutes. The cost is approximately $1,100 per 50 mg vial. Alteplase (tPA) is currently FDA approved for acute myocardial infarction (MI), acute ischemic stroke, and acute massive pulmonary embolism. Alteplase is reconstituted with sterile water to a concentration of 1 mg/mL and should be used within 8 hours of preparation. Alteplase is typically further diluted to 0.2–0.5 mg/mL for infusion. Heparin should not be added directly to alteplase solution based on in vitro studies (5). Additionally, iodinated contrast agents may suppress the fibrinolytic activity of alteplase (6). An initial bolus dose of 5–10 mg tPA is administered with a multi–side-hole catheter. An infusion of tPA is administered at 0.5–1.0 mg/h. Repeat angiogram is performed at 4–8 hours to evaluate progression. All patients are treated systemically with heparin. After an initial loading dose of 5,000 units of heparin, the patient is placed on a dose sufficient to maintain the partial thromboplastin time (PTT) at approximately 1.5 times normal. The PTT is reevaluated 4 hours and 24 hours after the start of thrombolytic therapy (7).

Reteplase (Retavase, Centocor) is a genetically altered wild type r-tPA with a plasma half-life of 14–18 minutes. The cost is approximately $2,150 per 20 IU vial. Reteplase is currently FDA approved for acute MI. Reteplase is reconstituted with sterile water to a concentration of 1 U/mL. The drug can be further diluted with normal saline to concentrations no lower than 0.02 U/mL. Initial bolus is with 2–5 units followed with an infusion of 0.5–1.0 U/h. Heparinization is performed with an initial loading dose of 3,000 units of heparin, and the patient is then placed on an infusion of 500 U/h (7).

Criteria for choosing thrombolytic agents are not clear, and the decision generally depends on the operator. Comparison of urokinase to alteplase has been performed in several trials. The STILE (Surgery versus Thrombolysis for Ischemia of the Lower Extremity) trial in 1994 (8) showed no difference in the efficacy or safety of urokinase versus tPA in the thrombolytic arm of the trial. Sugimoto et al. (9), compared urokinase to tPA in 83 patients and found equal efficacy and safety of the two agents and concluded that tPA thrombolysis was faster and was less expensive overall than urokinase. In contrast, Ouriel et al. (10) compared the complication rates of urokinase to tPA and found a greater complication rate with the use of tPA. In the face of conflicting literature, the choice of thrombolytic becomes dependent upon the operator, availability, and familiarity.

As with arterial thrombolysis, venous thrombolysis is best performed via transcatheter regional infusion of thrombolytic agent directly into the area of involvement. This allows a higher concentration of the thrombolytic agent to reach the thrombus and thus results in more rapid lysis of the thrombus as well as reduced hemorrhagic complications when compared to systemic infusion. In patients with SVC, subclavian occlusions, or both, one or two catheters should be placed using the femoral, transjugular, or peripheral upper extremity approach.

After venography, a guide wire should be advanced through the thrombus with an appropriate multi–side-hole infusion catheter positioned with the side holes aligned within the thrombus.

Thrombolytic therapy is considered complete when: (1) at least 95% of the thrombus has been cleared, although complete clearing is optimal; (2) thrombolysis fails to progress at a high dosage level, or (3) a major bleeding complication occurs. At this point, it is necessary to make a decision regarding the treatment of the underlying lesion. Essentially all stenoses resulting from malignancies should be treated with stenting. In patients with an extrinsic constrictive process, such as fibrosing mediastinitis, retroperitoneal fibrosis, or fibrosis secondary to radiation therapy, percutaneous transluminal angioplasty (PTA) alone is frequently unsatisfactory, and stenting is required.

Complications

Hemorrhage is the major complication of thrombolysis. Ouriel et al. (10) evaluated 653 consecutive patients over a 9-year period for complications associated with the use of urokinase and tPA. Groin hematoma was the most common complication occurring in 169 patients, of which 32 patients required intervention, including surgery, compression, or thrombin injection. Fifteen percent (98 of 653) of patients required blood transfusion during the course of thrombolysis. The frequency of intracranial hemorrhage was 1.2% (8 of 653) and was fatal in 7 of 8 cases.

STENTING

There are many commercially available stents with most reported experience using three stents; the Gianturco Z stent (Cook Inc.), the Wallstent (Boston Scientific), and the Palmaz stent (Cordis).

The Gianturco Z stent is self-expanding and is the original stent used in venous stenting. It is constructed of stainless steel and possesses anchoring hooks that help prevent migration. It is available in diameters of 6–12 mm as a biliary stent or 15–30 mm as a tracheobronchial stent.

The Wallstent, which is also a self-expanding stent, has a low profile and probably now is the most commonly used stent for venous applications. A fine stainless-steel mesh construction allows greater flexibility and may deter tumor ingrowth. The Wallstent has FDA approval for venous stenting in hemodialysis grafts.

The Palmaz stent is the most commonly used balloon-expandable stent for venous applications. It is a rigid stent that, when the balloon expands, produces radial force against the vessel wall, a feature especially useful in stenosis caused by tumor and fibrosis. Balloon expansion allows greater accuracy in deployment, but it is also

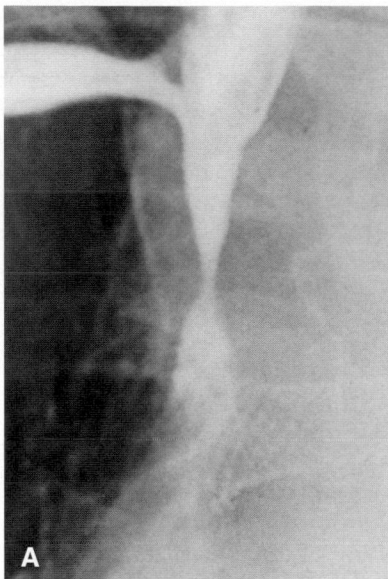 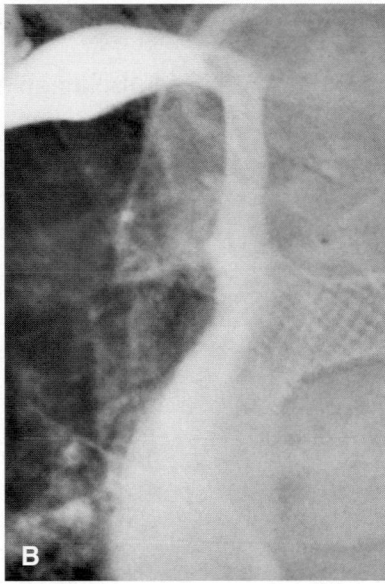 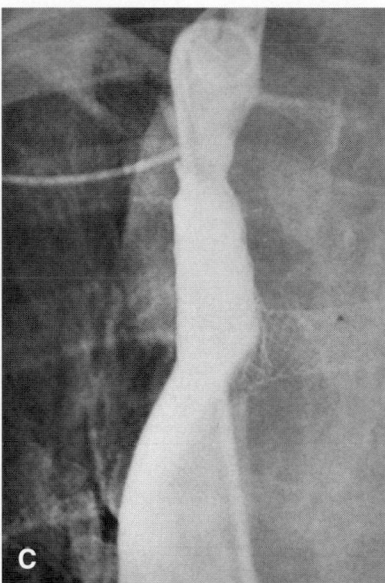

Figure 67–1   Right brachiocephalic vein stenosis related to a right percutaneous dialysis catheter. **A.** Right subclavian venogram in a 53-year-old woman with end-stage renal disease who had multiple previous percutaneously placed right subclavian and transjugular dialysis catheters. The venogram demonstrates a tight stenosis of the right brachiocephalic vein. Previously placed Wallstents, still patent, are identified in the left brachiocephalic vein. **B.** Angioplasty with a 12-mm balloon resulted in improvement. However, considerable recoil of the vein is evident, resulting in a lumen insufficient for the right arm dialysis fistula. **C.** A Palmaz stent was chosen to allow future access to the innominate vein from both the jugular and right subclavian approach and to provide minimal encroachment of the left brachiocephalic vein. After dilation of the stent to 12 mm, there is excellent flow through the right brachiocephalic vein. Washout by nonopacified blood from the left brachiocephalic vein is evident in the SVC.

less flexible (Figure 67–1). The Palmaz stent is FDA approved for use in the iliac and renal arteries and the biliary system.

Principles

Before a stent is placed, venography of the involved area is performed using either serial or digital radiography. Vessel diameter measurements of the involved area should be available. The stent should be of adequate length to cover the stenosis and, whenever the anatomy allows, to extend approximately 2 cm both proximal and distal to the stenosis. This is particularly true in malignant stenoses where overgrowth or extension of the neoplasm is anticipated. If thrombus is present, thrombolytic therapy is recommended, but is not absolutely necessary.

Complications

Complications that occur with venous stenting include stent fracture, migration, and infection. In a review of the literature, no large study could be found determining the exact complication rate with venous stenting.

Stent fracture may result from repetitive motion or extrinsic compression (Figure 67–2). Trerotola et al. (11)

reported stent migration and fracture when using self-expanding stents in the animal model. Meier et al. (12) reported subclavian stent breakage related to extrinsic bony compression. The use of self-expanding stents may reduce stent breakage in regions in which stent motion is anticipated.

Migration may occur immediately after stent placement because of undersizing of the stent or incomplete expansion. Stents may also be dislodged when they have not had adequate time to endothelialize and are subject to later manipulation. Migration of a venous stent can be treated by percutaneous snare removal when possible. Alternatively, a migrated stent can sometimes be redirected into an alternate vascular structure for safe reimplantation or surgical removal (13). Slonim et al. (14) reported a 96% success rate, following stent migration, with either percutaneous snare removal or intravascular repositioning in a small series of patients ($N = 27$) with a single major complication of tricuspid insufficiency.

Infection of an intravascular stent is very rare, although its exact frequency is unknown. Animal models have demonstrated stent infection following bacteremia (15). Once infected, an endovascular stent often requires surgical removal. However, one case of successful conservative

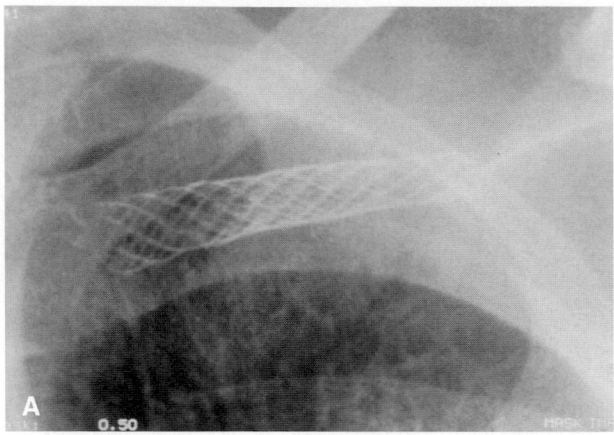

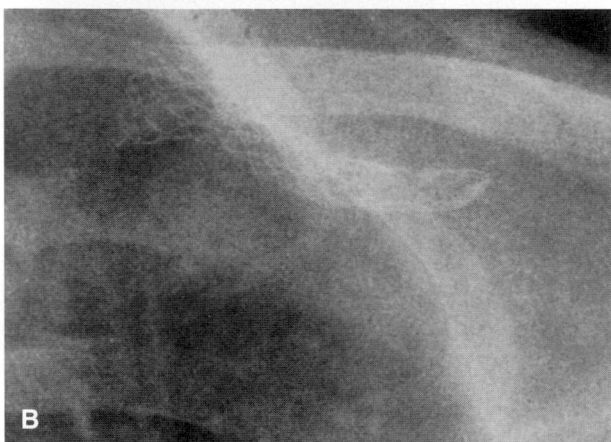

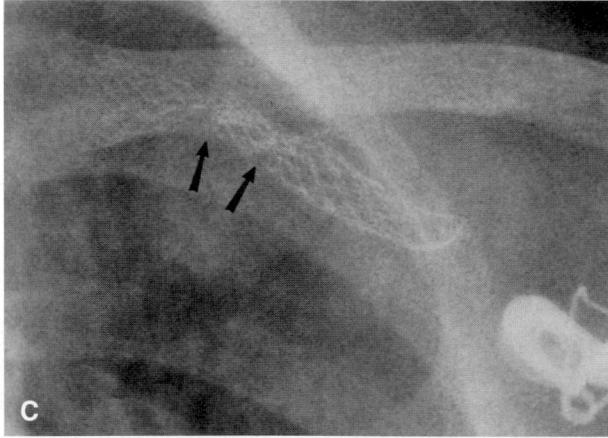

Figure 67–2   Compression of Palmaz stent. **A.** Two overlapping Palmaz stents were placed in this 32-year-old woman with hemodialysis fistula in the left upper extremity and an 85 % stenosis of the subclavian vein. **B.** A chest radiograph 2 weeks later demonstrates compression of the stents. The fistula in the left upper extremity was not functional. **C.** A chest radiograph 1 year later demonstrates further compression of the stents with fractures (*arrows*) of the stents. Complete disruption of the stent was confirmed fluoroscopically.

management with intravenous antibiotics has been reported (16). To avoid stent infection, rigorous sterile technique should be followed. The role of prophylactic antibiotics before stent placement is unclear (17).

CLINICAL APPLICATIONS

Subclavian Vein Stenosis

Occlusion of the subclavian and brachiocephalic veins may be the result of benign or malignant compression, inflammation, or trauma. The increased use of central venous catheters is held responsible for the increased prevalence of central venous occlusion (18). Upper extremity DVT is not as benign as once thought with pulmonary embolism from upper extremity DVT reaching as high as 7–20% in recent series (19). Thrombolysis and anticoagulation are the mainstays of treatment along with surgical correction of the underlying cause or condition.

Effort thrombosis, or Paget-Schroetter syndrome, is spontaneous thrombosis of the subclavian vein in young, active individuals following exercise. It is frequently associated with compression of the subclavian vein between the costocoracoid ligament and the subclavius muscle during downward and backward bracing of the shoulders (20). This syndrome most commonly occurs in young men, particularly bodybuilders, or after intense upper body exercise. Historically, therapy included operative thrombectomy followed by decompressive claviculectomy, scalenectomy, or first rib resection with continued oral anticoagulation (21). Adams et al. reported 23 patients with Paget-Schroetter syndrome who were treated conservatively. Ten percent of patients developed pulmonary embolism—one patient developed gangrene, and 70% had residual disability (22,23,24). With the advent of catheter-directed thrombolysis and angioplasty, there is an increasing role for endovascular treatment. Angioplasty alone to correct the underlying venous abnormality without surgical decompression is rarely successful (25,26), and surgical decompression is still indicated. The use of positional venography may aid in identifying patients in need of operative decompression (21). There appears to be a role for subclavian vein stenting in individuals who have undergone surgical decompression and have restenosis following angioplasty (27). Venous stenting without first rib resection has been reported, and increased incidence of stent fracture results (27).

There is also a role for subclavian vein stents in patients with malignant compression. However, patients with malignancy undergoing radiation or with indwelling central venous catheters may respond less favorably to stenting (25).

Hemodialysis Access

Treatment for a thrombosed dialysis arteriovenous (AV) graft can be performed with surgical thrombectomy or catheter-directed thrombolysis. Both surgical thrombectomy and catheter-directed thrombolysis produce an 85% immediate patency (28). The decision on which method to use is institutional-specific because they produce similar results. Regardless of the method employed, treatment of a thrombosed graft needs to be initiated promptly. Approximately 85–90% of AV access thromboses are associated with venous outflow stenosis. Thus, a postprocedural fistulagram should to be performed to reveal any underlying stenosis (28). Thrombosis of a native fistula is difficult to treat, and neither catheter-directed thrombolysis nor surgical thrombectomy provide good results.

Based on DOQI (Kidney Disease Outcomes Quality) 2000 guidelines (28), venous stenosis of an AV graft or fistula should be treated when the degree of stenosis exceeds 50% and clinical criteria are met. The choice between surgical revision and percutaneous angioplasty should be based on the expertise available at each institution. The long-term patency rate following PTA is well-established with published rates ranging from 40–50% at 6 months. The DOQI 2000 work group recommends that a venous stenosis that requires more then two PTAs in 3 months has failed therapy and should be corrected surgically. Stents are useful in select circumstances in which PTA fails because of elastic recoil and the lesions are surgically inaccessible. Studies have found that patency rates of stents are no better than PTA alone, excepting elastic stenosis (28).

SVC Obstruction

Superior vena cava (SVC) compression or occlusion affects approximately 15,000 people every year in the United States. Symptoms of arm or facial swelling, dyspnea, headache, and chest pain comprise the clinical entity of SVC syndrome. By far, the most common cause of SVC syndrome is malignancy, with lung cancer and lymphoma being the two most common causes; 80% and 10%, respectively (29). Radiation therapy and chemotherapy have been considered first line therapies in malignant SVC syndrome treatment. Approximately 70% of patients have symptomatic relief after 2 weeks of radiation treatment. However, there is a recurrence rate as high as 33% (29,30). Some cancers, especially small cell lung carcinoma, are exquisitely sensitive to chemotherapy, and responses as early as 7 days have been reported (30).

Rösch et al. (31) in 1992 reported a series of 22 patients who underwent stenting for SVC syndrome because of malignancy—all patients had symptomatic relief, with one patient developing stent thrombosis from tumor ingrowth. Since then, there have been hundreds of reports of SVC stenting. The Gianturco Z stent, the Wallstent, and the Palmaz stent are the most frequently used. High technical success rates have been reported for treatment of SVC obstruction with the Gianturco Z stent (81–100%) with similar results for the Wallstent (86–100%). Complete resolution of SVC syndrome occurs in 68–100% of patients following stenting, regardless of stent type (30). The long-term patency of SVC stents for both malignant and benign stenoses appears to be excellent. In patients with malignant disease, stents will likely remain patent for the patient's lifetime (Figure 67–3).

Benign causes of SVC occlusion include indwelling central venous catheters or pacemakers, inflammatory conditions such as mediastinitis, and benign tumors. A conservative approach to treating benign obstruction is to anticoagulate the patient and wait for venous collaterals to develop. With conservative therapy, 5–40% of patients will progress to develop symptoms of arm and face swelling. Surgical bypass has been performed successfully (30), although, many patients are not surgical candidates. The role of venous stents in benign SVC obstruction is debated, but it is usually considered after failed anticoagulation, thrombolysis, or angioplasty. However, the recurrence rate of stenosis following PTA alone is high in the SVC, and primary stenting provides an effective treatment (Figure 67–4). Qanadli et al. (32) reported successful stenting of 12 patients with benign SVC obstruction using primarily Wallstents for benign strictures related to indwelling catheters, postradiation fibrosis, pacemaker leads, and benign tumors. Rosenblum et al. (33) reported treating an additional six patients with Palmaz stents for strictures related to indwelling catheters. In both studies, there was a 100% technical success rate with complete resolution of symptoms. Stents remained patent in follow-up, which ranged from 1–36 months.

Catheter-directed thrombolysis is a useful adjunct in acute thrombosis of the SVC. Kee et al. (34) treated 27 patients with acute SVC syndrome using catheter-directed thrombolytic therapy. Five patients needed no further intervention, and 21 patients were subsequently treated with stenting with one patient failing thrombolytic therapy. Adjuvant thrombolysis is not without complication however, and several deaths have been reported (34,35).

IVC Obstruction

Stenosis of the inferior vena cava is symptomatic because of an elevated pressure gradient. It is unknown with certainty what reflects a significant caval gradient. Fletcher et al. (36) found that a caval-atrial gradient of 20 mm Hg was required to produce clinical symptoms. The placement of stents to treat caval stenosis provides effective symptomatic relief (Figure 67–5).

Occlusion of the inferior vena cava may be because of thrombus, extension of a tumor, extrinsic compression, or intrinsic caval disease (37). Caval obstruction may result in IVC syndrome; lower extremity pain and swelling, weakness, and venous ulceration. Liver and kidney function can decline as a result of infrahepatic caval or renal vein involvement (38). Acute thrombosis of the IVC has been successfully treated with transcatheter thrombolysis alone (39). Chronic occlusion of the IVC has been treated with a combination of mechanical recanulization, thrombolysis, and stent placement (38).

Anastomotic narrowing following liver transplantation in the inferior vena cava occurs in approximately 2% of the patients (40). Given the increased frequency of liver transplantation, one can assume the number of such

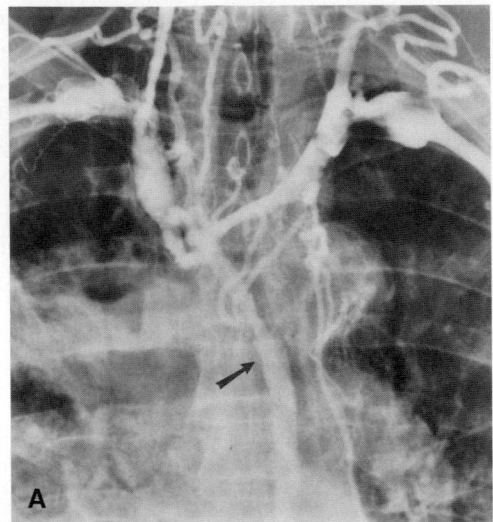

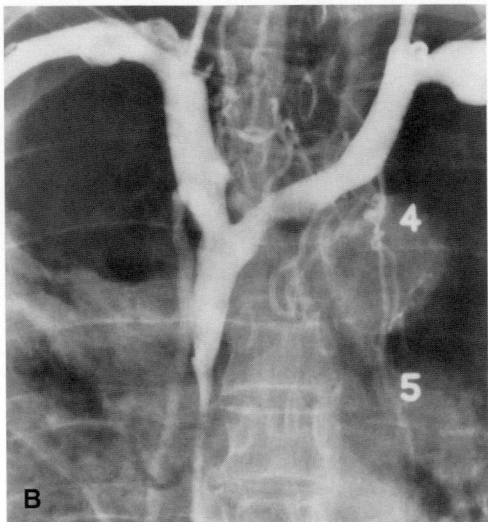

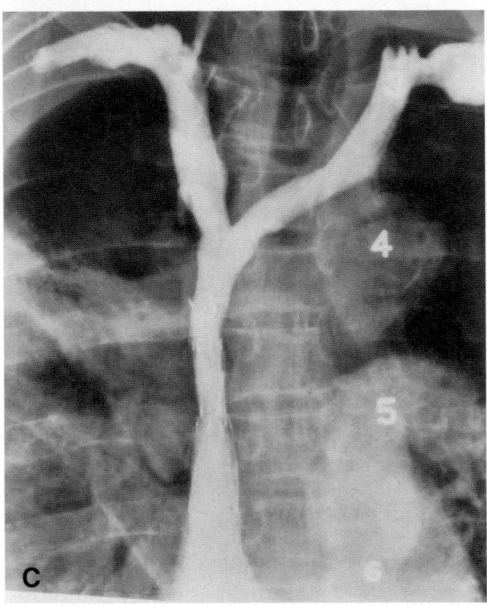

Figure 67–3 Thrombosed malignant SVC obstruction. **A.** The initial bilateral subclavian venogram in this 68-year-old man with pulmonary adenocarcinoma demonstrates complete obstruction of the SVC with collateral flow through the azygos vein (*arrow*). Extensive thrombus is present in both the brachiocephalic veins and the SVC. **B.** After thrombolytic therapy, there is complete thrombolysis of the brachiocephalic veins and SVC, with the underlying SVC stenosis revealed. **C.** The SVC has been stented with a triple-body GRZ stent, 18 mm in diameter and 6 cm in length. Note that the central body is centered on the stenosis (compare with Figure 67–4). The stent was fully expanded on a chest radiograph 2 weeks later.

abnormalities requiring treatment will increase. Weeks et al. (40) reported a series of patients (*n* = 9) who underwent Gianturco Z stent placement for hepatic transplant related anastomotic abnormalities. In all nine patients, placement of an IVC stent resulted in reduced caval pressure gradient, and eight of nine patients had improvement or resolution of symptoms.

Iliofemoral Stenosis (May-Thürner Syndrome)

In 1851, Virchow was the first to describe increased frequency of thrombosis within the left common iliac vein by an overlying right common iliac artery (41). One hundred years later, May and Thürner examined 430 cadavers and found 22% had obstructive "spurs" that histologically represent a chronic callus-type inflammatory response hypothesized to be from repetitive injury to the venous endothelium from iliac artery compression (42). Cockett

et al. (43) published the first clinical series of 57 patients with iliac vein thrombosis. Iliac compression syndrome (ICS) was used to describe patients with acute DVT, with sudden onset of leg pain and swelling usually following surgery, pregnancy, or bed rest. In the chronic phase, the patients presented with venous insufficiency, ulcers, varicose veins, or claudication (43). The recommended treatment of acute ICS was surgical thrombectomy, and the chronic phase was treated with venous bypass and concomitant mobilization of the right common iliac artery away from the vein.

Advances in endovascular technique and materials have made treatment with directed thrombolysis, PTA, and stenting viable alternatives (Figure 67–6). Patients presenting with acute ICS can be treated with direct thrombolysis, angioplasty, and placement of a Wallstent. O'Sullivan et al. (44) treated 19 patients with acute ICS using catheter-directed thrombolysis (120,000–180,000 IU UK/h) and

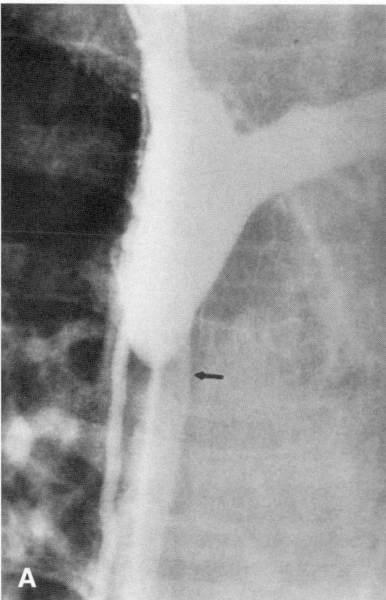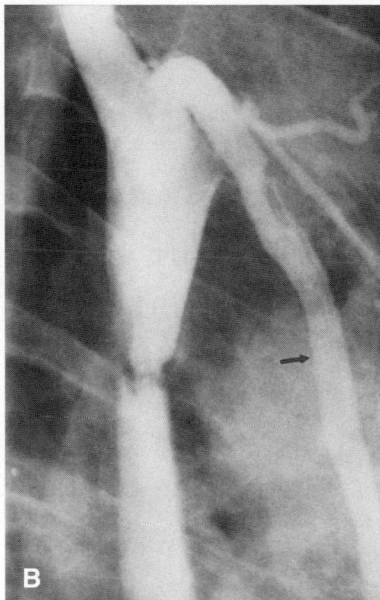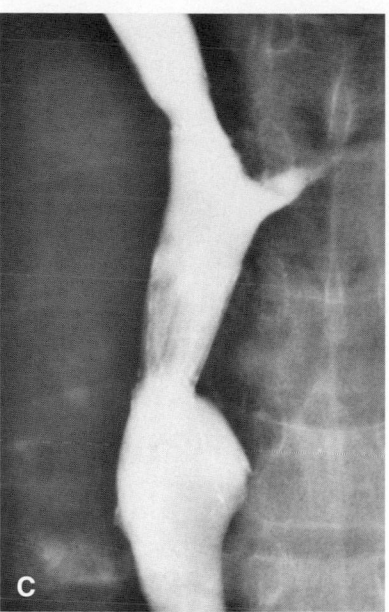

Figure 67–4 Benign idiopathic SVC stenosis in intravenous drug abuser. **A.** Transfemoral subclavian venogram in this 42-year-old man who presented with severe SVC syndrome demonstrates severe stenosis of the SVC. Opacification of the azygos vein (*arrow*) is evident. **B.** After percutaneous transluminal angioplasty (PTA) with a 12-mm balloon, there is improvement in the stenosis, although azygos collateral flow (*arrow*) remains. Symptoms recurred in 4 weeks and PTA was again performed, with similar results. **C.** Because of recurrence of symptoms, a double-body GRZ stent was placed, which completely resolved the symptoms. The patient remained asymptomatic until he was lost to follow-up.

angioplasty followed by stent (Palmaz or Wallstent) placement. The 1-day, 1-month, and 1-year patency rates were 100%, 93.1%, and 93.1% in the acute group. In 20 patients presenting with chronic ICS treatment, 12 underwent thrombolysis followed by PTA with stenting and eight had PTA with stenting (without thrombolysis). The 1-day, 1-month, and 1-year patency rates were 93.9%, 93.9%, and 93.9% in the chronic group. Patel et al. (45) reported treatment of 10 patients with acute ICS with catheter-directed thrombolysis (urokinase), PTA, and stenting (Wallstent). Initial technical success was 100% with complete resolution of symptoms. Ninety percent of patients remained asymptomatic with a mean follow-up of 14 months. Iliac vein stenoses secondary to extrinsic compression of other etiologies frequently respond well to stenting, particularly in patients with benign compression from retroperitoneal fibrosis or because of radiation therapy (Figure 67–7).

Budd-Chiari Syndrome

Budd-Chiari syndrome (BCS) is defined as abdominal pain, liver failure, and ascites that are the result of hepatic venous outflow obstruction. Obstruction may occur at the level of the hepatic veins or within the IVC between the liver and right atrium. Surgical therapies include decompressive shunts (46), thrombectomy, and orthotopic liver transplant (47). Medical therapy with diuretics and anticoagulants are also options (48). Warren et al. (49) in 1972 described the first successful use of systemic thrombolytics (streptokinase) in the treatment of acute BCS. Since then, there have been multiple attempts at treating BCS with a variety of percutaneous routes.

Many endovascular techniques have been used to treat Budd-Chiari syndrome. TIPS is a safe and effective treatment for BCS (50) and is often considered the first line endovascular therapy. Other endovascular therapies successfully described include the use of catheter-directed thrombolytics directly into the hepatic vein thrombus (51). Witte et al. (52) reported two cases with stents placed in the hepatic veins for treatment of BCS caused by hepatic venous outflow stenosis.

Portal Vein Obstruction

Portal vein obstruction accounts for 5–10% of all cases of portal hypertension (53). The complications of portal hypertension include variceal bleeding, ascites, and liver failure. Directed thrombolysis of the portal vein has been successfully performed (54,55). Access routes for thrombolysis include percutaneous-transhepatic, transjugular-intrahepatic, and superior mesenteric artery infusion. The long-term patency of the portal vein following thrombolysis is not clear.

Neoplasm accounts for 15–24% of extrahepatic portal vein occlusion (53). Portal venous stent placement for portal hypertension induced by malignant occlusion has been

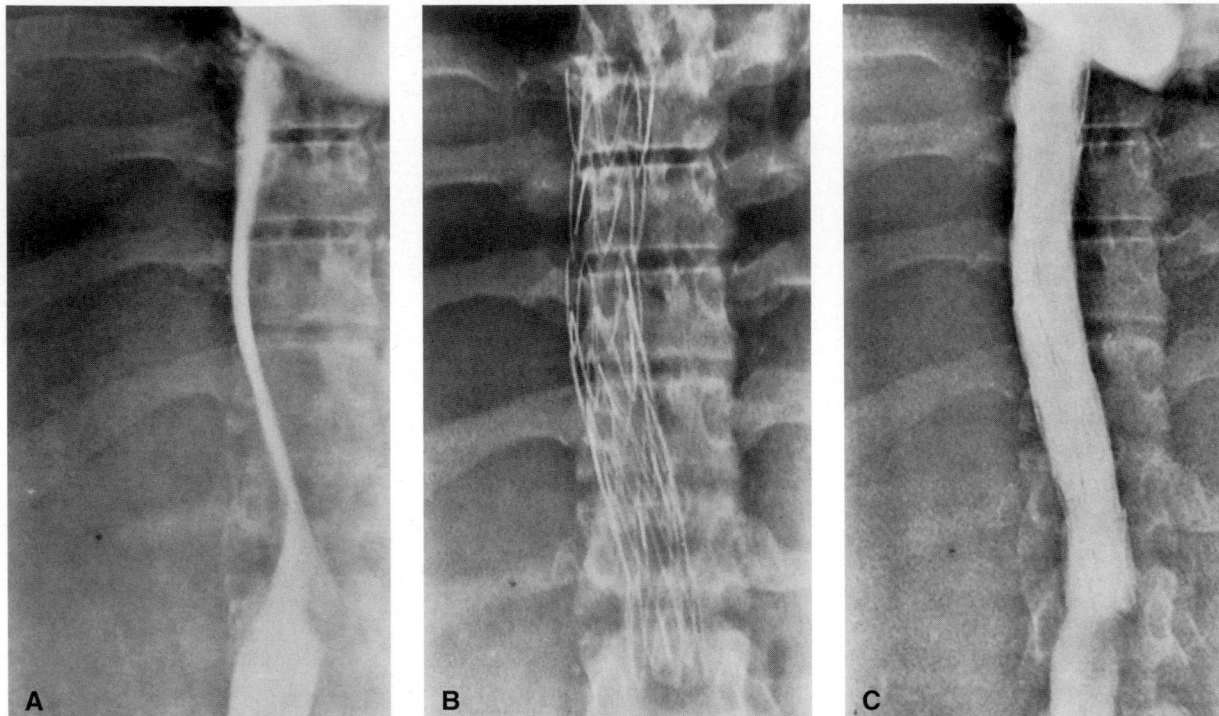

Figure 67–5   Intrahepatic IVC stenosis due to hepatic metastasis. **A.** The inferior vena cavogram in this 44-year-old woman with occular melanoma metastatic to the liver demonstrates severe stenosis of the intrahepatic portion of the IVC. The patient had recently developed severe peripheral edema and ascites. A 19-mm Hg gradient from the abdominal IVC to the right atrium was present. **B.** Because of the marked hepatomegaly and the extent of the stenosis, two overlapping multibody GRZ stents were placed. The initial central stent was a 20 mm x 10 cm multibody GRZ stent, and a 20 mm x 8 cm stent was then overlapped within the central stent to provide coverage of the lesion. **C.** Poststenting venogram demonstrates excellent flow through the IVC, and the gradient was reduced to 4 mm Hg. The patient had complete resolution of the leg edema at 7 days with marked improvement in her ascites. There was no recurrence of symptoms before her death 2 months after stent placement.

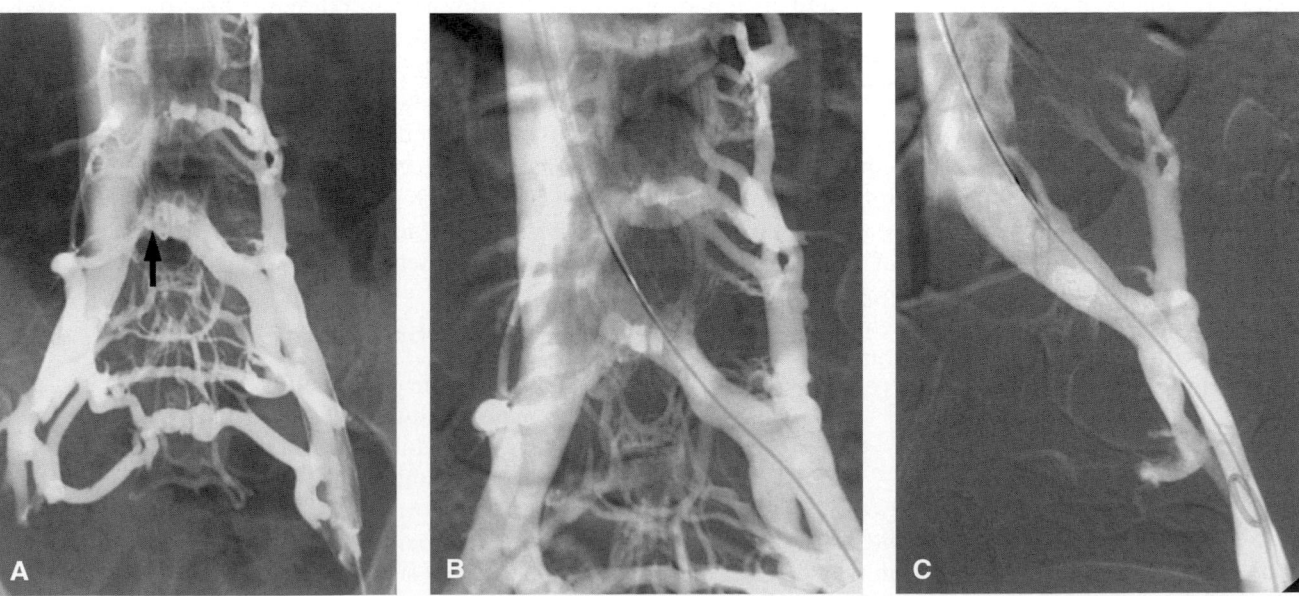

Figure 67–6   Iliofemoral stenosis (May-Thürner syndrome) in a 21-year-old female with longstanding swelling of the left leg. **A.** Left external iliac venogram demonstrates severe stenosis of the left common iliac vein (*arrow*) with extensive collaterals to the right iliac veins and through the ascending lumbar vein. **B.** Repeat left external iliac venogram with guide wire traversing the stenosis. **C.** Venogram following left common femoral vein angioplasty and placement of a 14-mm self-expanding stent demonstrates excellent flow in the left common iliac vein and essentially no filling of the collateral veins.

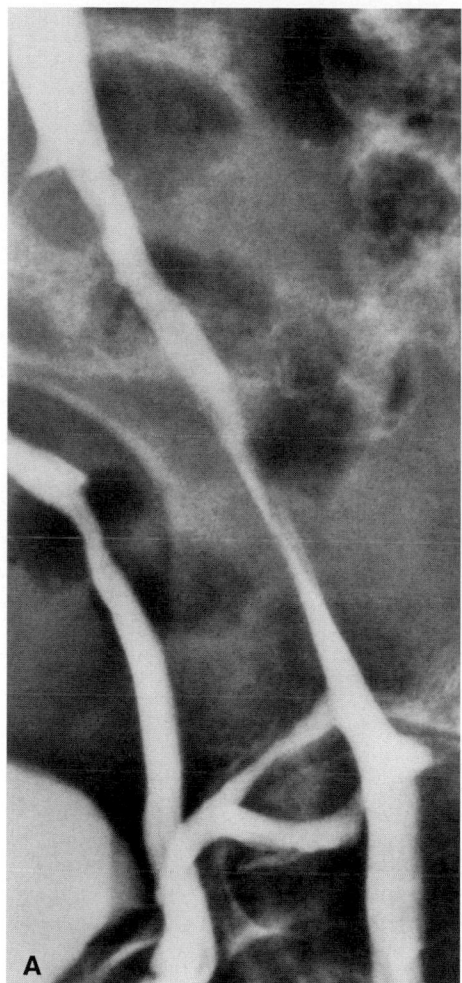
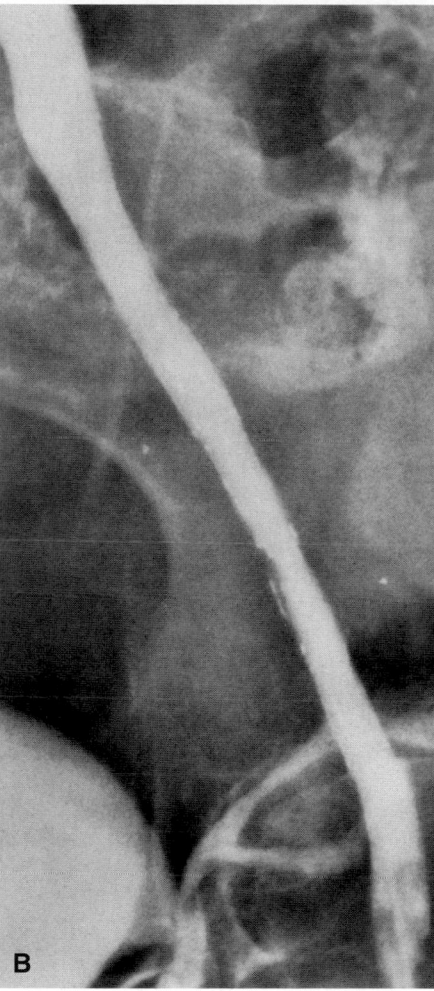

Figure 67–7 Iliac vein stenosis secondary to extrinsic compression. **A.** After radiation therapy of the abdomen and pelvis for lymphoma, this 66-year-old woman developed persistent left leg edema. The left iliac venogram demonstrates diffuse compression of the left iliac vein. **B.** After deployment of an 8 mm x 12 cm multibody GRZ stent, there is restoration of normal flow in the iliac vein. The patient became asymptomatic in 4 days and remained so.

found to be effective in reducing portal hypertension and resultant symptoms (56). Stent occlusion appears to be a major complication with a 40% occlusion rate, which occurred at a mean of 4 months. Splanchnic vein occlusion, severe hepatic dysfunction, and obstruction of the portal vein (such as from a bulky tumor mass) were factors affecting stent occlusion (53).

SUMMARY

The use of catheter-directed local fibrinolysis is an excellent treatment of venous thrombosis. PTA may be performed to treat the underlying lesion, although because of significant elastic recoil, this is frequently of limited benefit. Patients with malignant extrahepatic venous obstruction should be treated by local fibrinolytic therapy and primary stenting. Patients with malignant intrahepatic IVC obstruction have a short life expectancy even though a high patency rate can be expected.

In patients with subclavian stenosis associated with thoracic outlet obstruction, thrombolysis provides initial patency, but surgical intervention is frequently required.

Caval and iliac venous stenoses rarely respond to PTA alone, and stenting is frequently required. In patients with dialysis-associated stenoses or stenoses with significant elastic recoil following PTA, the stenoses should be stented but usually requires repeated interventions to maintain patency. Hemodialysis patients with nonelastic lesions may respond to PTA alone, but again, repeated interventions are usually required.

ACKNOWLEDGMENTS

I want to express my appreciation to Sheri Imai-Swiggart for her assistance with preparing the images for both this and the previous editions of this chapter.

REFERENCES

1. Dotter CT, Rosch J, Seaman AJ. Selective clot lysis with low-dose streptokinase. Radiology 1974;111(1):31–37.
2. Becker GJ, Holden RW, Rabe FE, et al. Local thrombolytic therapy for subclavian and axillary vein thrombosis: treatment of thoracic inlet syndrome. Radiology 1983;149:419–423.

3. Semba CP, Dake MD. Iliofemoral deep venous thrombosis: aggressive therapy with catheter directed thrombolysis. Radiology 1994;191(2): 487–494.

4. Chang R, Horne MK, Mayo DJ, et al. Pulse-spray treatment of subclavian and jugular venous thrombi with recombinant tissue plasminogen activator. J Vasc Interv Radiol 1996;7(6): 845–851.

5. Lam XM, Ward CA, DuMee CP. Stability and activity of altepase with injectable drugs commonly used in cardiac therapy. Am J Health Syst Pharm 1995;52:1904–1909.

6. Dehmer GJ, Gresalfi N, Daly D, et al. Impairment of fibrinolysis by streptokinase, urokinase, and recombinant tissue-type plasminogen activator in the presence of radiographic contrast agents. J Am Coll Cardiol 1995;25:1069–1075.

7. Valji K. Evolving strategies for thrombolytic therapy of peripheral vascular occlusion. J Vasc Interv Radiol 2000;11(4):411–420.

8. Results of a prospective randomized trial evaluating surgery versus thrombolysis for ischemia of the lower extremity. The STILE trial. Ann Surg 1994;220(3):251–266.

9. Sugimoto K, Hofmann LV, Razavi MK, et al. The safety, efficacy, and pharmacoeconomics of low-dose alteplase compared with urokinase for catheter-directed thrombolysis of arterial and venous occlusions. J Vasc Surg 2003;37(3):512–517.

10. Ouriel K, Gray B, Clair DG, et al. Complications associated with the use of urokinase and recombinant tissue plasminogen activator for catheter-directed peripheral arterial and venous thrombolysis. J Vasc Interv Radiol 2000;11(3):295–298.

11. Trerotola SO, Fair JH, Davidson D, et al. Comparison of Gianturco Z stents and Wallstents in a hemodialysis access graft animal model. J Vasc Interv Radiol 1995;6(3):387–396.

12. Meier GH, Pollak JS, Rosenblatt M, et al. Initial experience with venous stents in exertional axillary-subclavian vein thrombosis. J Vasc Interv Radiol 1996;24(6):974–983.

13. Gabelmann A, Kramer S, Gorich J. Percutaneous retrieval of lost or misplaced intravascular objects. AJR Am J Roentgenol 2001; 176(6):1509–1513.

14. Slonim SM, Dake MD, Razavi MK, et al. Management of misplaced or migrated endovascular stents. J Vasc Interv Radiol 1999;10(7): 851–859.

15. Thibodeaux LC, James KV, Lohr JM, et al. Infection of endovascular stents in a swine model. Am J Surg 1996;172(2):151–154.

16. Guest SS, Kirsch CM, Baxter R, et al. Infection of a subclavian venous stent in a hemodialysis patient. Am J Kidney Dis 1995; 26(2):377–380.

17. Dravid VS, Zegel HG, Morales AV, et al. Investigation of antibiotic prophylaxis usage for vascular and nonvascular interventional procedures. J Vasc Interv Radiol 1998;9(3):401–406.

18. Horrattas MC, Wright DJ, Fenton AH, et al. Changing concepts of deep venous thrombosis of the upper extremity-report of a series and review of the literature. Surgery 1988;104:561–567.

19. Sharafuddin MJ, Sun S, Hoballah JJ. Endovascular management of venous thrombotic disease of the upper torso and extremities. J Vasc Interv Radiol 2002;13(10):975–990.

20. Falconer MA, Weddell G. Costoclavicular compression of the subclavian artery and vein. Lancet 1943;2:539–544.

21. Azakie A, McElhinney DB, Thompson RW, et al. Surgical management of subclavian-vein effort thrombosis as a result of thoracic outlet compression. J Vasc Surg 1998;28(5):777–786.

22. Adams JT, DeWeese JA, Mahoney EB, et al. Intermittent subclavian vein obstruction without thrombosis. Surgery 1968;63:147–165.

23. Adams JT, DeWeese JA. "Effort" thrombosis of the axillary and subclavian veins. J Trauma 1971;11:923–930.

24. Adams JT, McEvoy RK, DeWeese JA. Primary deep venous thrombosis of upper extremity. Arch Surg 1965;91:29–42.

25. Beygui RE, Olcott C, Dlaman RJ. Subclavian vein thrombosis: outcome analysis based on etiology and modality of treatment. Ann Vasc Surg 1997;11:247–255.

26. Machleder HI. Evaluation of a new treatment strategy for Paget-Schroetter syndrome: Spontaneous thrombosis of the axillary-subclavian vein. J Vasc Surg 1993;17:305–317.

27. Meier GH, Pollak JS, Rosenblatt M, et al. Initial experience with venous stents in exertional axillary-subclavian vein thrombosis. J Vasc Surg 1996;24(6):974–983.

28. Section V. Management of Complications: Optimal Approaches for Treating Complications. Guidelines for Vascular Access, National Kidney Foundation Kidney Disease Outcome Quality Initiative (K/DOQI) Guidelines 2000. Available at http://www.kidney.org/professionals/kdoqi/guidelines_updates/doqi_uptoc.html#va. Accessed September 12, 2004.

29. Schindler N, Vogelzang RL. Superior vena cava syndrome. Endovasc Min Inv Vasc Surg 1999;79(3):683–694.

30. Yim DH, Sane SS, Bjarnason H. Superior vena cava stenting. Interv Chest Radiol 2000;38(2):409–424.

31. Rösch J, Uchida BT, Hall LD, et al. Gianturco-Rösch expandable Z-stents in the treatment of superior vena cava syndrome. Cardiovasc Intervent Radiol 1992;15(5):319–327.

32. Qanadli S, El HM, Mignon F, et al. Subacute and chronic benign superior vena cava obstruction: eEndovascular treatment with self-expanding metallic stents. AJR Am J Roentgenol 1999;172: 159–164.

33. Rosenblum J, Leef J, Messersmith R, et al. Intravascular stents in the management of acute superior vena cava obstruction of benign etiology. JPEN J Parenter Enteral Nutr 1994;18:362–366.

34. Kee S, Kinoshita L, Razavi M, et al. Superior vena cava syndrome: treatment with catheter-directed thrombolysis and endovascular stent placement. Radiology 1998;206:187–193.

35. Dyet J, Nicholson A, Cook A. The use of the Wallstent endovascular prosthesis in the treatment of malignant obstruction of the superior vena cava. Clin Radiol 1993;48:381–385.

36. Fletcher WS, Lakin PC, Pommier RF, et al. Results of treatment of inferior vena cava syndrome with expandable metallic stents. Arch Surg 1998;133(9):935–938.

37. Sonin AH, Mazer MJ, Powers TA. Obstruction of the inferior vena cava: a multiple-modality demonstration of causes, manifestations, and collateral pathways. Radiographics 1992;12(2): 309–322.

38. Razavi MK, Hansch EC, Kee ST, et al. Chronically occluded inferior vena cavae: endovascular treatment. Radiology 2000;214: 133–138.

39. Angle JF, Matsumoto AH, Shammari MA, et al. Transcatheter regional urokinase therapy in the management of inferior vena cava. J Vasc Interv Radiol 1998;9(6):917–925.

40. Weeks SM, Gerber DA, Jaques PF, et al. Primary Gianturco stent placement for inferior vena cava abnormalities following liver transplantation. J Vasc Inter Radiol 2000;11(2):177–187.

41. Virchow R. Uber die erweiterung kleiner gefasse. Arch Path Anat 1851;3:427.

42. May R, Thürner J. The cause of predominantly sinistral occurrence of thrombosis of the pelvic veins. Angiology 1957;8:419–427.

43. Cockett FB, Lea TM, Negus D. Iliac vein compression: its relation to iliofemoral thrombosis and the post-thrombotic syndrome. Br Med J 1967;2:14–19.

44. O'Sullivan GJ, Semba CP, Bittner CA, et al. Endovascular management of iliac vein compression (May-Thürner) syndrome. J Vasc Interv Radiol 2000;11(7):823–836.

45. Patel NH, Stookey KR, Ketcham DB, et al. Endovascular management of acute extensive iliofemoral deep venous thrombosis caused by May-Thürner syndrome. J Vasc Interv Radiol 2000; 11(10):1297–1302.

46. Henderson JM, Nagle A, Curtas S, et al. Surgical shunts and TIPS for variceal decompression in the 1990s. Surgery 2000;128(4): 540–547.

47. Ringe B, Lang H, Oldhafer KJ, et al. Which is best surgery for Budd-Chiari syndrome: venous decompression or liver transplantation? A single-center experience with 50 patients. Hepatology 1995;21(5):1337–1344.

48. Olzinski AT, Sanyal AJ. Treating Budd-Chiari syndrome: making rational choices from a myriad of options. J Clin Gastro 2000; 30(2):155–161.

49. Warren RL, Schlant RC, Wenger NK, et al. Treatment of Budd-Chiari syndrome with streptokinase. Gastroenterology 1972;62:200.

50. Blum U, Rossle M, Haag K, et al. Budd-Chiari syndrome: technical, hemodynamic, and clinical results of treatment with transjugular intrahepatic portosystemic shunt. Radiology 1995; 197(3):805–811.

51. Raju GS, Felver M, Olin JW, et al. Thrombolysis for acute Budd-Chiari syndrome: Case report and literature review. Am J Gastroenterol 1996;91(6):1262–1263.

52. Witte A, Kool L, Veenendal R, et al. Hepatic vein stenting for Budd-Chiari syndrome. Am J Gastroenterol 1997;92(3):498–501.
53. Yamakado K, Nakatsuka A, Tanaka N, et al. Malignant portal venous obstructions treated by stent placement: significant factors affecting patency. J Vasc Interv Radiol 2001;12(12):1407–1415.
54. Bilbao JI, Vivas I, Elduayen B, et al. Limitations of percutaneous techniques in the treatment of portal vein thrombosis. Cardiovasc Intervent Radiol 1999;22(5):417–422.
55. Lopera JE, Correa G, Brazzini A, et al. Percutaneous transhepatic treatment of symptomatic mesenteric venous thrombosis. J Vasc Surg 2002;36(5):1058–1062.
56. Yamakado K, Nakatsuka A, Tanaka N, et al. Portal venous stent placement in patients with pancreatic and biliary neoplasms invading portal veins and causing portal hypertension: initial experience. Radiology 2001;220(1):150–156.

Venous Access

68

Matthew A. Mauro, Susan M. Weeks

The indications for the placement of central venous catheters are continually expanding. The rapid growth of hemodialysis services, transplantation programs, and oncologic centers has contributed to the need for maintaining patients who require parenteral nutrition, hemodialysis, plasmapheresis, blood transfusions, blood sampling, and long-term chemotherapy for various neoplastic and infectious diseases. In addition, the desire for outpatient treatments has spurred the development of catheter materials that are compatible with long-term in-home use while being relatively free from infectious and thrombotic complications (1,2).

There are three basic categories of venous catheters: nontunneled catheters, tunneled catheters, and implantable subcutaneous ports. Nontunneled catheters are commonly placed via the central veins (subclavian and internal jugular) by blinded percutaneous techniques at the bedside. These catheters are sutured or taped into position and are primarily used for short-term access. Peripherally inserted central catheters (PICCs) are designed to be placed to the cavoatrial junction via an upper extremity vein—and may be placed at the bedside via a superficial vein—or may require imaging guidance for successful placement. PICCs and the nontunneled, nontapered, silicone centrally placed Hohn catheter (Bard Access Systems) are used for intermediate access (weeks to months).

Tunneled catheters are commonly constructed predominantly of either medical-grade silicone or polyurethane materials, with a Dacron cuff bonded to the catheter. This cuff is positioned in a subcutaneous tunnel for stabilization. These catheters are accessed externally and are designed for long-term home use. Tunneled and nontunneled catheters are available in single-, dual-, or triple-lumen varieties. Implantable subcutaneous ports use the same catheter materials as do tunneled catheters but are attached to a domed access reservoir (port) that is buried subcutaneously for stabilization. This type of device is accessed with a percutaneously placed noncoring needle and is intended for long-term use. Subcutaneous ports are available in single-port and dual-port configurations and may be placed either on the chest wall or the upper arm.

RADIOLOGIC PLACEMENT

Tunneled catheter and subcutaneous port placement have become one of the most commonly performed procedures in the interventional suite. Percutaneous radiologic placement of these long-term devices requires three basic procedural steps:

1. Establishment of central venous access and determination of appropriate intravascular catheter length
2. Formation of a subcutaneous tunnel or pocket
3. Placement of the catheter into the central venous system

Standard sites of venous access for central venous catheters include the internal jugular vein (IJV), the external jugular vein (EJV), subclavian vein (SCV), axillary vein, brachial vein, basilic vein, and common femoral vein (CFV). Unconventional access sites include the infrarenal inferior vena cava (IVC), the suprarenal IVC, hepatic veins (HV), and collateral veins. Long-term dialysis access via the renal vein has been reported (3). Additionally, recanalization of occluded veins may be required for successful catheter placement. The selection of venous access site depends not only on the catheter being placed but, more importantly, on the patency of venous pathways to the right heart.

VENOUS ACCESS TECHNIQUES

Some prefer sonographic guidance as a method for venous access when conventional and, when feasible, nonconventional sites are used. Ultrasound provides direct visualization of the target vessel to be accessed and the soft tissue pathway required to reach the target vessel. It also provides information concerning patency of the target vein; not just at the access site, but usually central to the access site. Visualization of neighboring arteries is possible, which almost completely ensures venous and not errant arterial access.

Internal Jugular Vein

Ultrasound Guidance

Ultrasound guidance is used routinely for IJV punctures. Using this system, successful entry is obtained on the first pass in most cases. A 7.5-MHz linear transducer is placed in transverse orientation just above the clavicle such that the IJV and the adjacent carotid artery are easily identified (4). The vein is easily differentiated from the artery by its compressibility and respiratory variation (Figure 68–1). Either an 18- or 21-gauge system is used. A 21-gauge system (Cope introducer kit or 4 French micropuncture set) is often preferred (Cook, Inc.). The skin and associated soft tissue pathway are infiltrated with 1% lidocaine with epinephrine, which can be performed under sonographic guidance. The 21-gauge needle is attached to short, flexible connector tubing and a 20 cc syringe. The tip of the needle is placed just superior to the midportion of the transducer directly over the vein. The side-to-side artery-vein orientation and the continuous visualization of the needle tip during advancement ensure that an inadvertent carotid puncture does not occur. The needle tip, IJV, and carotid artery are simultaneously imaged as the needle is advanced to indent the anterior wall of the vein. To enter the vein, a short, brisk thrust is made, with the needle tip clearly identified within the lumen of the vein. If the vein completely collapses during access, a through-and-through puncture may be made, requiring slow withdrawal of the needle back into the lumen, with simultaneous gentle aspiration applied to the attached syringe (4). Once free aspiration of venous blood is obtained, an 0.018-inch guide wire is advanced to the right heart under fluoroscopic guidance. Then, the needle is exchanged for a transitional dilator to secure venous access.

With respect to IJV access and the sternocleidomastoid muscle (SCM), either a low central approach between the two heads of the SCM or a posterior approach should be performed, depending upon the patients' anatomy. The low central approach will frequently allow for a gentler catheter course and should increase ease of future catheter manipulations. A posterior approach will require some angling of the transducer during puncture to ensure complete visualization of the needle tract through the soft tissues and to the venous access site. Puncture through the SCM muscle should be avoided whenever possible because this can cause discomfort to the patient and make future catheter manipulations difficult (5).

Standard Approach

Within the neck superiorly, the IJV is located medial to the SCM muscle; more inferiorly, the vein is found between the two heads of the SCM muscle. The classic anterior approach

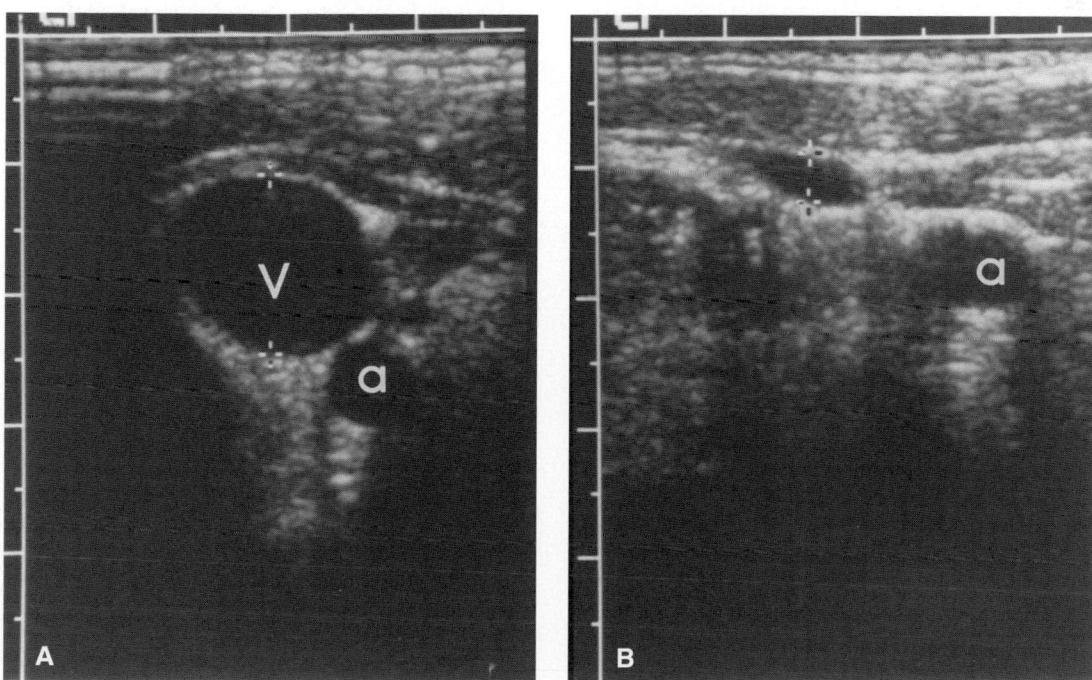

Figure 68–1   Internal jugular vein access. **A.** Transverse ultrasound image of internal jugular vein (V) without compression (carotid artery). **B.** Collapsed vein with mild compression (carotid artery). (Reprinted with permission from Mauro MA, Jaques PF. Radiologic placement of long-term central venous catheters: a review. J Vasc Interv Radiol 1993;4:127–137.)

is performed by identifying a site medial to the SCM muscle midway between the clavicle and the angle of the mandible. After appropriate administration of local anesthetic, the carotid pulse is localized, and the 21-gauge needle is inserted and directed inferolateral to the pulse, toward the ipsilateral nipple. After return of venous blood, guide wire insertion and venous catheterization proceed as usual.

Axillary and Subclavian Veins

In those patients who will require long-term venous access, maintaining central venous patency is a top priority. To that end, subclavian or axillary vein access should be avoided whenever possible with initial use of the IJV and EJV. In the dialysis population, SCV access should only be entertained when an upper extremity can no longer be used for long-term surgical dialysis access.

The axillary vein originates at the lateral border of the teres major muscle. It continues centrally to become the subclavian vein at the lateral margin of the first rib. The subclavian vein travels centrally between the first rib and clavicle, joining the IJV medial to the anterior scalene muscle to form the brachiocephalic vein. Peripherally, the paired subclavian and axillary arteries and veins lie in close proximity to one another, while centrally, the subclavian artery and vein are separated by the anterior scalene muscle. A peripheral venous entry minimizes the chance of a pneumothorax and ensures an intravenous catheter position peripheral to the space bordered by the clavicle and first rib, thereby avoiding potential catheter compression or fracture (6–8). Safe, peripheral entry requires a direct guidance technique. The needle, vein, and surrounding tissues are simultaneously imaged with ultrasound, and the needle can be seen directly entering the vein, thereby avoiding important surrounding structures.

Ultrasound Guidance

A 7.5-MHz linear transducer is most commonly used, but in larger patients, a 5-MHz probe may be needed for added penetration. The SCV is identified easily because of its easy compressibility and respiratory variation. The linear transducer can be used to image in either the transverse or longitudinal planes. When used in the transverse plane, the vein is centered within the visual field, the skin is infiltrated with 1% lidocaine, and a small dermatotomy is created. A 7-cm, 21-gauge needle is then advanced through the soft tissues toward the anterior wall of the vein. The needle path is imaged throughout its course via slow rocking of the transducer in the direction in which the needle is advanced. Once indentation of the anterior vein wall is evident, a short, sharp, thrusting motion ensures entrance into the vein.

Ultrasound-guided axillary vein access may also be performed in the longitudinal plane. Advantages of imaging in this plane include the ability to visualize the needle throughout its entire soft tissue course. However, in less experienced hands, following the needle may be more difficult because alignment may be slightly off center. Additionally, a longitudinal probe position requires a more lateral skin dermatotomy to allow safe venous access site peripheral to the clavicle. This may result in undesirable angulation of the resultant catheter course. When a longitudinal orientation is used, the probe is placed with its medial edge against the patient's clavicle. A skin dermatotomy is made at the lateral aspect of the linear transducer. A 7-cm, 21-gauge needle is inserted parallel to the transducer. The needle is advanced under real-time imaging, and when the needle indents the anterior wall of the vein, a short thrust is made for venous entry. Whenever a through-and-through puncture is performed, gentle aspiration is applied to the syringe while the needle is slowly withdrawn until free flow of venous blood occurs. Once venous access is documented, an 0.018-inch guide wire is inserted and guided into the right atrium. The needle is then exchanged for a transition-type catheter that is placed over the mandril guide wire and into the right atrium.

Standard Approach

The standard percutaneous access technique to the SCV uses an infraclavicular puncture approximately 2 cm inferior to the junction of the medial and middle thirds of the clavicle. The needle is advanced medially and cephalad to a point slightly behind a fingertip firmly placed in the suprasternal notch. The needle is advanced in a horizontal plane with respect to the table to minimize an inadvertent pleural puncture. A 7-cm, 21-gauge access needle (Cook, Inc.) is the choice for some, although 18-gauge needles are available in most commercial kits. The 21-gauge needle is attached to a 20-mL syringe with short flexible tubing. Intermittent gentle suction is applied during needle advancement. Once free blood is obtained, an 0.018-inch mandril guide wire is inserted and guided into the right atrium. After guide wire placement into the right atrium, the needle is removed and a transition dilator is placed.

Upper Extremity Veins

As mentioned previously, in the dialysis-dependent population, upper extremity venous access should be avoided whenever possible to maintain extremity veins and central venous patency for long-term surgical dialysis access.

Venous access devices inserted via the upper extremity use the basilic, cephalic, brachial, or axillary veins. Palpation may suffice whenever access to an antecubital median cephalic or basilic vein is desired. More commonly, access is preferred in the upper arm where simple palpation is not possible. In these cases, access can be guided by ultrasound or fluoroscopy with upper extremity contrast venography.

Ultrasound Guidance

Ultrasonography offers a safe and successful method for accessing the nonpalpable veins of the upper extremity. It is particularly useful in a swollen edematous arm where an initial venipuncture is impossible (4). Before prepping, a preliminary ultrasound of both extremities is performed to determine patency and size of veins. In those patients who have undergone multiple prior peripheral line placements, patency of the veins can be determined to the level of the axilla, minimizing unnecessary needle sticks. The basilic, cephalic, and brachial veins are interrogated, and the best site is determined. If needed, a tourniquet is applied to dilate the veins for more complete evaluation. Although it is usually easy to distinguish the veins from neighboring arteries, caution must be exercised to avoid inadvertent puncture of an aberrant radial artery originating from the axillary artery. After appropriate administration of local anesthetic and creation of a dermatotomy, a 21-gauge needle is advanced into the vein under ultrasound guidance until the tip of the needle is identified within the vein. An 0.018-inch guide wire is then advanced gently into the vein under fluoroscopic guidance. Alternatively, in those patients with excessive soft tissue, initial through-and-through access is often desirable; once the transducer is lifted from the patient's arm, there may be slight retraction of the needle out of the vein and into the soft tissues. A through-and-through access overcomes this. The needle is then slowly withdrawn under fluoroscopic guidance while gentle advancement of the mandril guide wire occurs. Once access is obtained, usual guide wire and catheter insertions are performed.

Venographic Guidance

For venographic guidance, a venipuncture is made within a superficial vein of the hand, forearm, or antecubital space. Contrast injection is then performed to identify an appropriate vein to access. Once the vein is fully opacified, a tourniquet can be placed to maximize venous opacification. The skin is anesthetized, and a 21-gauge needle is advanced into the vein under fluoroscopic guidance. Guide wire and catheter placement then is performed in the standard fashion. Whenever necessary, nitroglycerin in 100–200 mg aliquots may be given at the access site to avoid venospasm.

Femoral Venous Catheterization

Common femoral vein (CFV) catheterization can be performed with the use of either ultrasound guidance or standard techniques. Long-term catheter placement in the groin is not satisfactory, because it hinders free ambulation; promotes an increased likelihood of catheter trauma, kinking, or fracture; and is associated with an increased risk of catheter infection rates. However, CFV catheterization offers a safe, short-term alternative in those patients whose access sites are limited or in the patient who require quick venous access.

Ultrasound Guidance

Direct ultrasonographic visualization of the CFV during access is especially useful in those patients who have poorly palpable femoral arterial pulses or are coagulopathic. With the patient in the supine position, the common femoral artery (CFA) and vein are identified in the transverse projection overlying the femoral head. Local anesthetic is administered, and a small dermatotomy is created. The vein is accessed using either a 21- or 18-gauge needle with constant visualization of the needle tip as it is advanced through the soft tissues. As previously described, the needle will indent the anterior wall of the vein, after which a short thrusting motion is often required to access the vein. After venous blood is aspirated, usual guide wire and catheter placement follows.

Standard Technique

At the level of the femoral head, the CFA pulse is identified. The artery is protected with one hand, and an appropriate venous access site is determined over the femoral head—1 cm medial to the artery. The skin and subcutaneous tissues are infiltrated with 1% lidocaine, and an 18- or 21-gauge needle is then advanced toward the femoral head parallel with the course of the vein until venous return is evident. Alternatively, no blood flow may be visualized from the needle hub. In this case, the needle is advanced to the femoral head and slowly retracted while gentle suction is applied to aspirate venous blood. Usual guide wire and catheter placement then ensues.

Collateral Vein Catheterization

Today, placement of central venous catheters via collateral veins is commonly performed in the interventional suite (9–14). Suitable access sites include enlarged peripheral collateral veins, such as neck, chest wall, and thyrocervical, and intercostal veins.

Computed tomography venography (CTV) or magnetic resonance venography (MRV) can provide excellent preprocedural venous mapping in the more difficult access patient. In the event these techniques are not available, ultrasound-guided access of multiple peripheral sites with subsequent venography may be required to identify a suitable collateral vein for catheter placement. Once this vein is identified, standard catheter and guide wire techniques can be used to obtain central access with subsequent catheter placement (11). In these situations, once guide wire access into the right heart is achieved, it should obviously be maintained until catheter placement is successful. Successful catheter placement may require:

1. Back loading of the catheter over a guide wire
2. Placement of the catheter over the guide wire and through a peel away sheath
3. Placement of a long peel-away sheath to the target site, such as the right atrium, so that the catheter can be advanced safely through this sheath to the final resting place (15)

If these straightforward methods fail, venography can initially be performed from a peripheral site to identify a dominant collateral vein that communicates with the central circulation and is amenable to a percutaneous approach. Access into this vein may be accomplished in three ways. In all cases, use of a micropuncture system is recommended.

1. If the collateral vein is identified with ultrasound, direct guided puncture may be possible (12).
2. If ultrasonography of the target collateral access site is not feasible, the peripheral access can be advanced to the target collateral vein to be punctured, and the catheter may be exchanged for a goose neck snare (Microvena). The snare is then opened in the desired access vein and used as a target. Using fluoroscopy, a micropuncture needle is advanced into the target and through-and through-access is obtained (12–14).
3. Venography via the peripheral access can be performed to opacify the target collateral vessel, which is then directly punctured under fluoroscopic guidance (10).

Recanalization of Occluded Veins

Recanalization may be possible using either a straightforward antegrade approach or a combined antegrade and retrograde approach. Antegrade recanalization may include both access of an occluded vein, or crossing a more central occlusion in an effort to gain access to the right heart or azygous system. In the former case, complete interrogation of the vein using ultrasound should be performed to determine whether the vein is patent more peripherally. If a patent segment of vein can be identified peripherally, this segment should be accessed to allow a bit more working room while trying to cross the occlusion. An 0.018-inch system should initially be employed. If this proves inadequate, and if the vein is large enough at the chosen access site, an 18-gauge needle and 0.035-inch guide wire system may be used. It may then be possible to place a steerable catheter and a hydrophilic, torqueable guide wire (Terumo). Once the occlusion is successfully traversed, revascularization techniques including angioplasty and stenting may be required, and catheter placement can be completed. If antegrade guide wire traversal is possible, but complete revascularization cannot be performed solely from this initial access site, a second access (usually CFV) may be

necessary to introduce a snare used to grasp the wire and pull it inferiorly to maintain through-and-through access. Interventions including angioplasty and stenting can be performed from the groin, as can the gentle use of the snare to guide a catheter through the lesion to its desired final location (16,17).

In those patients in whom these straightforward recanalization methods are not successful, sharp recanalization may be necessary (18,19). This usually requires that both a CFV and the SVC can be catheterized successfully. Identification of an appropriate access site is determined using either multilocation venography or preprocedural CTV/MRV. Access into the vein is achieved, and venography is used to identify the proximal extent of the occlusion to be traversed. The CFV is then accessed, and catheterization of the right atrium is performed. Selective catheterization superiorly into the central vasculature as close to the site of obstruction as possible is completed, and venography is repeated from this access to identify the caudal aspect of the occlusion. The shorter and more inline the occlusion, the safer the recanalization. One access can then be exchanged for a small-bore needle system, such as a transjugular access kit (Angiodynamics), and the other access exchanged for a snare that is used as a target. Under fluoroscopic guidance, the needle is advanced carefully into the snare. If available, biplane fluoroscopy may be helpful to better localize the needle position in two planes as it is advanced toward the target. A guide wire is then advanced through the needle and snared; it is retracted inferiorly by the snare, and through-and-through access is secured. Catheter placement then follows.

Inferior Vena Cava

When central access via the SVC is no longer possible, catheter placement to the central venous system can still be accomplished via the IVC. Methods for accessing the IVC include a direct translumbar approach into the infrarenal IVC or a transhepatic approach into the suprarenal IVC (20–23). All conventional access routes should be reevaluated before an unconventional route is chosen because recanalization may occur quickly, particularly in children.

A translumbar IVC cannulation is somewhat analogous to translumbar aortography. A preprocedural CT scan is useful for determining patency of the cava—especially in patients with a long history of groin catheters—to detect any venous anomalies, to identify the location of the left renal vein, and to identify any structures (colon or ptotic kidney) that may be in the catheter path. The patient is placed in a prone or prone oblique position with the right side elevated 30–45 degrees. The L3 vertebral body on the right is the usual level of insertion. However, the CT scan may identify a more optimal site. A skin site is chosen to allow a 45-degree medial and slight cranial angulation of the needle. In average or thin patients, a 21-gauge diamond-tipped needle

(Cook, Inc.) is advanced until it hits the L3 vertebral body. The needle then is retracted and redirected anteriorly at increasing angles until a pass is made anterior to the vertebral body (20,22). At this time, the stylet is removed and the needle is withdrawn until blood is freely returned. Contrast injection can be used to confirm the needle's location, and this will be followed by an 0.018-inch mandril guide wire and transition catheter. In larger patients, a sturdier 18-gauge diamond-tipped or Turner needle may be used, which can be followed by a heavier-duty guide wire.

If the common femoral veins are patent, placing a guide wire via a transfemoral approach to serve as a fluoroscopic marker for the IVC is preferred. The patient is then placed prone, and the needle is inserted directly into the IVC using oblique fluoroscopic guidance (Figure 68–2). In very thin adults or children, the IVC is visualized easily with ultrasound using standard 3.0- or 3.5-MHz transducers. In these circumstances, an ultrasound biopsy guide can direct the entry. When necessary, computed tomography can also be used for initial caval access.

Suprarenal caval access can be performed when there is infrarenal IVC occlusion. A transhepatic approach is used by either a subcostal or intercostal approach. A subcostal approach using direct ultrasound guidance is a commonly preferred method for suprarenal caval access. In most patients, the liver and IVC can be imaged suitably with ultrasound and a subcostally positioned transducer. The initial ultrasound study is performed with an attached biopsy guide to determine the skin site that will allow a direct transhepatic approach to the IVC without traversal of major structures (24). Under direct real-time guidance, a 15-cm, 21-gauge, diamond-tipped needle can be advanced directly into the cava. The stylet is removed, and the needle is withdrawn until free flow of blood is returned. The mandril wire and transitional dilator are then placed. The subcostal approach avoids the pleura and rib space and is well-tolerated by patients. The intercostal approach is reserved for those patients with high-riding livers in whom safe access to the cava cannot be accomplished via a subcostal approach. In these cases, the needle is advanced via a right lateral approach under fluoroscopic control similar to that used for transhepatic cholangiography (21).

Hepatic Veins

An additional access pathway to the central venous system via the suprarenal IVC is by initial catheterization of a hepatic vein (25). In those patients with infrarenal caval occlusion, a transhepatic route may prove to be their final percutaneous access site (25,26). This approach has been used mostly in small children with short gut syndrome who require long-term venous access for nutrition. A hepatic vein entry maximizes the intravascular catheter length in these small children. With adequate nutrition, these children experience rapid growth, and catheters that are anchored externally may migrate out of the vascular system whenever a significant intravascular length is not placed.

For very young children, these procedures are performed under general anesthesia. Ultrasound is used for guidance, and with the patient in the supine position, an initial examination is performed to identify a suitable hepatic vein for entry. The middle hepatic vein is usually selected because of its relative anterior course within the main interlobar fissure of the liver. The right and left hepatic veins, however, may also be employed. A subcostal approach is again used to avoid the intercostal space, pleura, and lung. Using the biopsy guide, a 21-gauge diamond-tipped needle is inserted directly into the peripheral aspect of the hepatic vein. After successful aspiration of blood and contrast material documentation, a guide wire and transition catheter are placed in the standard fashion (25).

TUNNELING AND CATHETER PLACEMENT

Tunneled Catheters

Tunneled catheters are available in either an end-hole variety (Hickman-type catheters, Bard Access Systems) or a tip-occluded valved catheter (Groshong-type, Bard Access Systems). Both types are externally accessible catheters that require subcutaneous tunneling (27,28). Tunneling is performed as a second part of the procedure following venous access. Whenever the patient is to care for the catheter himself or herself, the skin exit site must be placed in an easily accessible position and must maximize patient comfort. Short, supraclavicular tunnels should be avoided, not only because of the risk of infection but because of discomfort from undergarments (25). For catheters placed via the IJV or EJV, an infraclavicular site on the upper chest wall is chosen. Those catheters accessing axillary or subclavian veins may exit at a parasternal site on the upper chest wall or an anterior chest wall site. For translumbar IVC catheters, the catheter exit site is usually placed on the lower anterior abdominal wall or the lower chest wall. If the tunnel is long, a two-step tunnel may be required. However, too long of a subcutaneous tunnel may make future catheter revisions difficult, requiring isolation of the catheter at the venous access site and creation of a new tunnel. For hepatic venous catheters, the exit site is usually formed superior and lateral to the venous entry site on the abdominal or chest wall. In those patients with a history of repeated accidental catheter removal, longer, more creative tunnels may be required to avoid inadvertent catheter removal.

The chosen skin exit site is infiltrated with local anesthesia, and a dermatotomy is made with a no. 11 blade scalpel. Hemostats are used to spread the skin and enter the subcutaneous space. The entire subcutaneous tunnel (skin exit site to venous access site) is then infiltrated

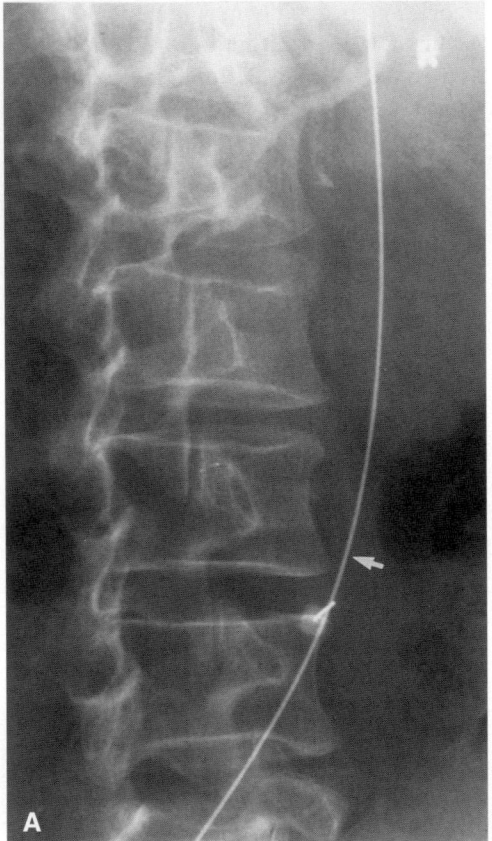

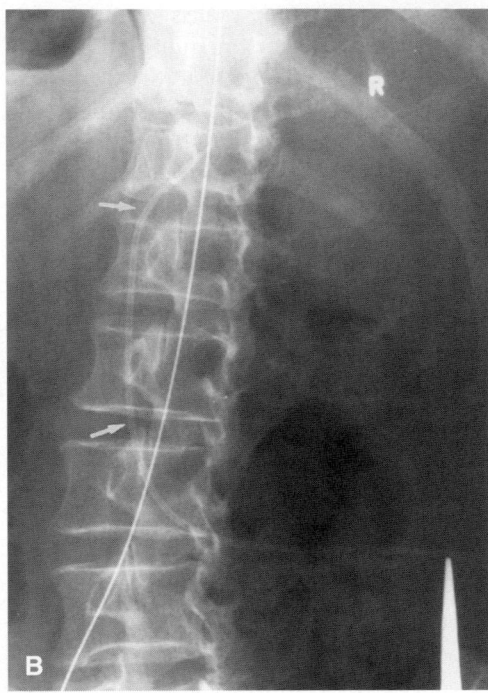

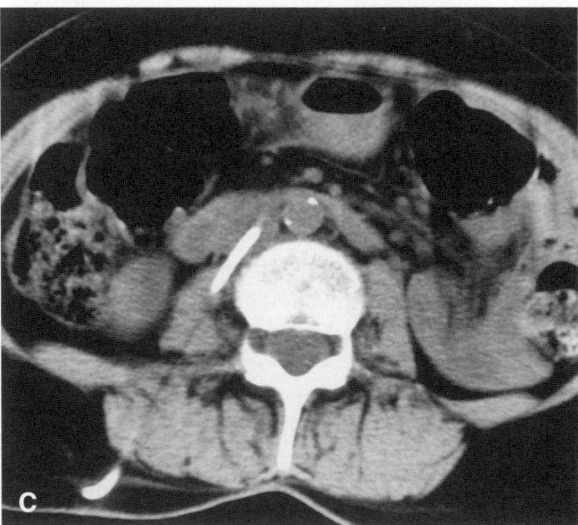

Figure 68–2 Translumbar IVC access. **A.** With a guide wire (*arrow*) inserted transfemorally into the IVC, a 21-gauge needle is inserted into the IVC with right posterior oblique fluoroscopy. **B.** Transition dilator (*arrows*) is inserted into the IVC with left posterior oblique fluoroscopy. Hemostat marks skin site. **C.** Postprocedural CT scan shows catheter entering the IVC. (Reprinted with permission from Mauro MA, Jaques PF. Radiologic placement of long-term central venous catheters: a review. J Vasc Interv Radiol 1993;4: 127–137.)

with local anesthesia using a 15-cm, 22-gauge Chiba-type needle. This needle must remain in the subcutaneous plane. For end-hole catheters, a tunneling tool (usually supplied in kit) is then inserted into the skin exit site and maneuvered through the subcutaneous tissues to the venous access site. With the Groshong-type catheter, the subcutaneous tunnel is formed in the reverse direction. The tunneling tool is inserted into the venous access site and is brought through to exit out of the skin exit site.

Both types of catheters have a Dacron cuff that should be positioned within the tunnel to allow stabilization once fibrosis occurs. This cuff can be positioned approximately 1–2 cm from the exit site to allow for easier subsequent catheter and cuff removal. Catheters are also available with a second cuff of silver-impregnated collagen (VitaCuff, Vitaphore), which serves as an antimicrobial barrier. When present, the VitaCuff is placed just within the skin exit site.

The correct intravascular catheter length (that length from the venous access site to its final tip position) is accurately determined by first inserting a guide wire through the indwelling venous catheter. The tip of the guide wire is placed at the cavoatrial junction or proximal right atrium, and the guide wire is kinked. Under fluoroscopic guidance, the guide wire is then withdrawn until its tip is at the venous access site, and a clamp is placed on the guide wire. The length between the kink and the clamp represents the required intravascular catheter length. Catheters placed more proximally into the brachiocephalic vein or proximal superior vena cava do not function as well, and they commonly cause venous stenoses. Distal placement deep into the right atrium may allow the catheter to contact the tricuspid valve and septum, which should be avoided.

With translumbar caval catheters, the tip ideally should be placed just inferior to the renal veins to help avoid renal vein thrombosis in the event that pericatheter thrombosis occurs. However, to ensure an adequate intravascular length of catheter, this is usually not possible. The catheter tip should then be placed at or just below the level of the hepatic veins. After measurement, the end-hole-type catheters are cut to the appropriate length. Groshong-type catheters should not be cut at their tips. The catheter length is adjusted after the catheter is placed into the venous system, and the catheter is trimmed from its proximal aspect.

After the tunnel is formed and hemostasis is achieved, a 0.038-inch guide wire is inserted through the transition catheter and functions as the final working wire. For axillary, subclavian, or jugular approaches, the guide wire should be placed well into the IVC when possible. Guide wire placement into the IVC adds stability to the system and eliminates the possibility of guide wire slippage into the right atrium during tract dilatation. The tract is dilated using a fascial dilator, and an appropriately sized peel-away sheath is then inserted (usually supplied in the kit). The dilator and guide wire are removed, followed immediately by insertion of the catheter into the venous system. The patient should carefully be instructed to suspend respirations during this step. For uncooperative patients, pinching the sheath between the fingertips between dilator removal and catheter insertion is necessary to avoid inadvertent air embolism. The final catheter placement is fluoroscopically checked, and, when satisfactory, the sheath is removed while a finger is placed on the catheter for stabilization. Minor adjustments to position can then be made. For the Groshong catheter, the proximal portion of the catheter is cut to length and an attachment is applied to assemble the hub (27) (Figure 68–3).

Following successful catheter placement, a skin suture is placed at the venous access site and the catheter exit site. The suture at the catheter exit site closes the skin but also is wrapped around the catheter for added initial stability. This suture should only gently dimple the catheter as it is being secured. The catheter is then heparinized, and an external dressing is applied.

Implantable Subcutaneous Ports

Implantable subcutaneous ports are available in the end-hole variety and are valved at the proximal catheter attachment

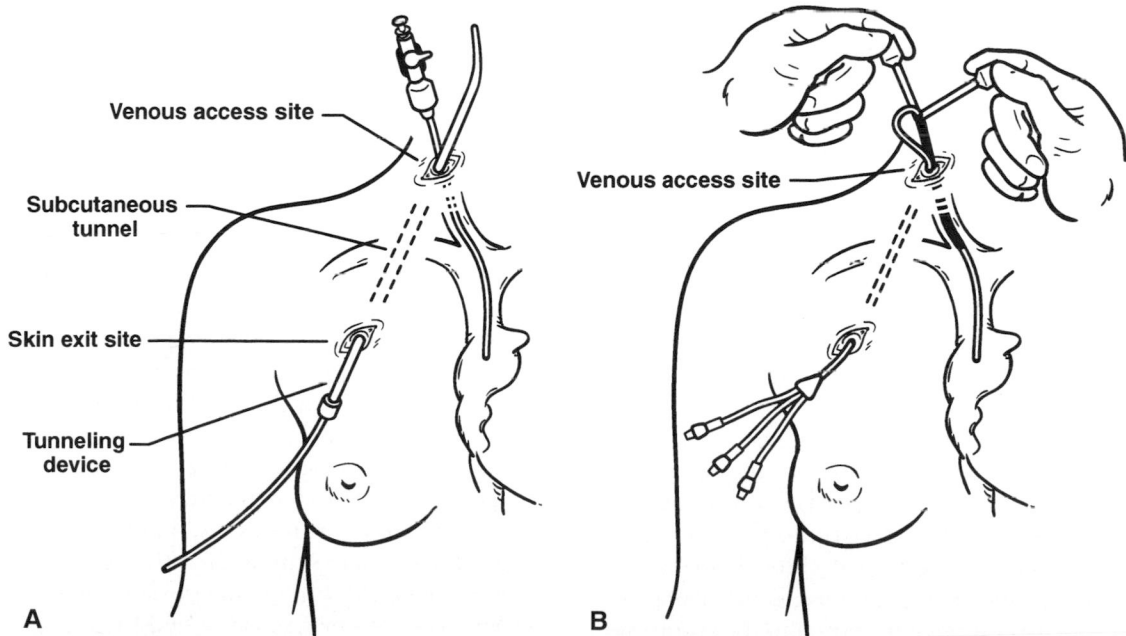

Figure 68–3 **A.** Schematic of tunneling tool for subcutaneous tunnel. **B.** Schematic of the Hickman catheter held in place while the sheath is split and peeled out. (Used with permission from Robertson LJ, Mauro MA, Jaques PF. Radiologic placement of Hickman catheters. Radiology 1989;170: 1007–1009.)

site or at the distal tip of the catheter. They may come pre-assembled, or they may require assembly at the time of the procedure. Following venous access, placement of implantable subcutaneous ports requires formation of a subcutaneous pocket (29). For chest wall ports, a site inferior and medial to the original venous access site is chosen where there is ample subcutaneous tissue to support the port. A cutdown tray contains all of the required surgical instruments. Lidocaine with epinephrine is used for local anesthesia. Depending upon the port size, an infraclavicular skin incision 2–4 cm long is made with a no. 15 blade scalpel and can be located inferior or superior to the subcutaneous pocket to be created. The incision is made through the dermis and into the subcutaneous space, which is easily identified by the presence of fatty tissue. The pocket is formed using blunt dissection. Fibrous bands within the subcutaneous space will need to be cut with small scissors. The subcutaneous pocket should be just large and deep enough to allow apposition of the skin margins at the incision adjacent to but not overriding the port. If the pocket is too large, port rotation is more likely to occur. In these cases, two or three absorbable sutures can be used to fixate the port to the deep fascia. When a snug fit is present, the stabilizing sutures may not be necessary. The pocket is visually inspected, and gauze pads are placed in the pocket to ensure that it is dry with no bleeding. A short, subcutaneous tunnel is then formed from the superior and lateral aspect of the subcutaneous pocket to the venous access site. The direction of tunneling will be determined by the type of catheter tip. After the catheter is brought through the tunnel, the port is situated into the pocket. At this time, the port can be accessed using the right-angled Huber needle (available in kit) attached via flexible tubing to a syringe with heparinized saline. Huber needle placement allows for stabilization of the port within the pocket during suturing and permits subsequent catheter flushing. The pocket is closed with interrupted absorbable subcutaneous sutures followed by interrupted skin sutures. The catheter is then cut to the appropriate length and inserted via a peel-away sheath into the appropriate final position as described earlier (24,29). Blood is withdrawn through the Huber needle and flushed. The venous access site can then be closed, and the port can be flushed with normal saline followed by heparin. When a Groshong catheter is chosen, the proximal end of the catheter is brought through the subcutaneous tunnel and the distal tip is positioned via the peel-away sheath into the venous system. The proximal end of the catheter is cut to length and secured to the port, which is placed into the pocket; the pocket is then closed. In patients with difficult access, port placement should similarly be performed, with initial placement of the catheter portion of the port into the venous system, through the peel-away sheath, with or without a guide wire. The tip of the catheter can be optimally placed using fluoroscopic guidance, and the external portion of the catheter cut to appropriate length and secured to the port.

For upper extremity ports, a small (2.5 cm) transverse incision is made at the site adjacent to the initial venous access that can accommodate the port. For upper arm placements, this incision often includes the initial skin nick. A small subcutaneous pocket is formed by blunt dissection. The catheter is then advanced to the cavoatrial junction via a peel-away sheath (contained in kit), cut to length, and attached to the port. If the subcutaneous pocket is placed away from the initial entry site, a short tunnel will be needed (24,30,31). Once the catheter is attached to the infusion port, the port is accessed, blood is aspirated, and the system is flushed. The port is then secured with a two-layered closure.

Dialysis Catheters

Dialysis catheters are dual-lumen catheters that are available in cuffed (tunneled) and noncuffed (nontunneled) varieties. They are therefore available in fixed lengths that are designed for access in the average adult or pediatric patient. As mentioned previously, in any patient in whom an upper extremity surgical dialysis access is a possibility, the subclavian veins are avoided at all cost and the catheter is placed preferably via the internal and external jugular routes. The subcutaneous tunnels ideally are formed down the neck and across the clavicle to exit on the upper chest wall. An appropriately sized catheter must be selected so that the tip can be placed in the appropriate location (for example, cavoatrial junction and proximal right atrium) and the cuff can be located in the tunnel, preferably near the catheter exit site, which allows easier removal.

A multitude of large-bore, dual-lumen, dialysis catheters are currently available. These catheters are predominantly comprised of either silicone or polyurethane, and they range in size from 13.5 French to 15.5 French. Catheters may have a staggered tip of various configurations (DuraFlow, Angiodynamics and Hickman, Bard), or may have a split tip (HemoSplit, Bard; Cannon Catheter, Arrow International; Split Cath, Split Stream, MedComp). Most catheters are preassembled as a single unit, but catheters are available that require assembly on the table (Tesio, Split Stream, Medcomp and Cannon Catheter, Arrow International). Advantages of the latter include: placement of the intravascular portion of the catheter often does not require a peel-away sheath; intravascular placement of the catheter as a first step allows precise tip placement; and tunnel length can be accurately determined before tunnel formation, so that the cuff will be placed 1–2 cm away from the catheter exit site. Additionally, back tunneling allows for a smaller skin incision (because the cuff does not need to be pulled through the incision), hopefully resulting in fewer catheters being inadvertently removed.

Although nontapered, many of these stiffer dialysis catheters may be placed without the use of a peel-away sheath, theoretically avoiding possible air embolism. When the tract is dilated with a dilator 1 French larger than the outer diameter of the catheter, the dialysis catheter can often be simply advanced over a stiff guide wire directly into the vein. Split-tip catheters are advanced over a single wire using the "guide wire weave insertion technique." When this is not possible, an appropriately sized peel-away sheath must be used in the standard fashion. All catheters should be heparinized according to manufacturers' recommendations because the amount of heparin varies with catheter length.

Nontunneled Catheters

Nontunneled catheters are available in tapered or nontapered varieties and can be placed via central or peripheral access. The standard tapered catheters placed via the central veins are for in-hospital use and are placed using standard needle and guide wire techniques.

Peripherally inserted central catheters (PICC) have working sizes of 3–5 French, available in end-hole, proximal valve (PASV valve, Boston Scientific) or Groshong-type tips. After venous access is achieved using techniques previously described, the length of catheter required is measured with an intravascular guide wire and the catheter is cut to an appropriate length (32). The catheter is then inserted via an appropriately sized peel-away sheath (included in the kit) and advanced to the cavoatrial junction. The catheter is then heparinized and secured to the skin.

CATHETER MANAGEMENT AND REMOVAL

A specialized nursing team that supervises routine catheter management has been shown to significantly reduce local and systemic infection and catheter thrombosis rates. Strict adherence to sterile techniques during catheter use, daily dressing changes, and proper heparinization are mandatory for successful long-term catheter survival and their importance cannot be overemphasized (33).

Catheter removal is the responsibility of the service that initially placed the catheter. For tunneled catheters, a local catheter prep is performed, and lidocaine is administered at the skin entry site and along the subcutaneous tunnel to the level of the cuff. Blunt dissection of the tissues surrounding the catheter and adherent to the cuff is completed, and in most cases, the catheter is then removed with gentle traction. Whenever the cuff remains within the soft tissues, complete removal will require a separate incision and local dissection at the level of the cuff. Both translumbar and transhepatic catheters can be removed in the same way because the catheters are accessing a low pressure venous system. However, if there is concern for bleeding from the transhepatic tract, catheter removal can be performed in the interventional suite following a full prep of the catheter and exit site. After lidocaine is administered, the cuff is dissected free, and a cutdown is performed

to localize the catheter at the venous access site. The extravascular portion of the catheter is removed, and the intravascular portion is exchanged over a guide wire for a similar-sized sheath. Pullback venography is completed to identify the hepatic venous exit site, and the parenchymal tract is then embolized using gelfoam torpedoes (Johnson and Johnson).

Removal of a subcutaneous port requires a more extensive dissection under a full sterile prep. For cosmetic purposes, the previous incision site is used. Long-term subcutaneous ports develop a white, tough fibrous capsule that must be incised for port removal. The subcutaneous pocket that is left behind must be closed with deep sutures to avoid the formation of a hematoma or seroma, which will increase the likelihood of a wound infection.

COMPLICATIONS

Procedural Complications

With the use of radiologic guidance, central venous catheters of all types can be successfully placed in more than 98% of cases (27,29,31). Blinded percutaneous placements have reported 5.0–8.9% access failures (6,34). A final catheter malposition complicates blinded insertion techniques in 1.2–2.5% of cases (6,34,35). During radiologic insertion, any malposition is immediately detected and corrected to ensure that virtually no patient leaves the suite with a malpositioned catheter.

The major procedural complications that may occur during radiologic catheter insertion include inadvertent arterial puncture and resultant hematoma, pneumothorax, air embolism, venous perforation, and early onset of infection. Hematomas may be the result of an inadvertent needle entry into the subclavian or axillary artery or bleeding within the subcutaneous tunnel or pocket in patients with bleeding disorders. The use of a 21-gauge needle and an ultrasonically directed peripheral puncture in a compressible region has virtually eliminated a clinically significant hematoma secondary to an arterial puncture (6,22,27,29). If there is any question as to whether an initial access is arterial, careful visualization of the guide wire course should allow one to determine whether the venous or arterial system has been entered. A venous puncture will direct the guide wire into the right atrium, whereas an inadvertent arterial puncture will have the guide wire proceed more centrally into the aorta. A simple injection of contrast can also be performed after needle entry to determine a proper puncture. Patients who are to receive tunneled catheters or implantable ports should have normal coagulation parameters, and, if abnormal, they should be corrected before catheter placement.

An ultrasound-guided peripheral puncture has lowered the pneumothorax rate to 2% or less (6,27,29). A pneumothorax may still occur with ultrasound guidance, particularly in cachectic patients, when visualization of the needle tip or target vein is lost and continued needle advancement occurs. Most pneumothoraces resulting from a 21-gauge needle are small, and they resolve spontaneously. When this does not occur, a small-bore tube can easily be placed in the apex under fluoroscopic guidance and connected to an underwater suction device.

Air embolism may occur in the event the patient takes a deep inspiration when the dilator of the peel-away sheath and guide wire are removed while the operator is preparing to pass the catheter into the venous system. This risk is minimized when the patient is instructed to stop breathing during this portion of the procedure and when the sheath is gently squeezed shut between removal of the dilator and insertion of the catheter (24). In the event an air embolism does occur, the air often will pass into the outflow tract of the right ventricle. The patient should be left in a supine position until the air is absorbed, which may take up to 20 minutes. Oxygen should be administered via face mask, and vital signs should be continuously monitored.

Venous perforation should not occur when line placement is performed with imaging guidance. This most commonly results when kinking of the guide wire occurs either during passage of a dilator or peel-away sheath. The kinked guide wire then acts like a trocar and pierces through the vein and into the surrounding tissues during advancement of the sheath. This can be avoided by advancing the dilator or peel-away sheath under fluoroscopic guidance and following the line of the wire. Alternatively, advancement of the sheath while applying gentle retraction on the guide wire should help avoid guide wire kinking. When it occurs, venous perforation is often asymptomatic. However, frequent vital signs and close procedural and postprocedural evaluation is strongly recommended.

Early infection is defined as a catheter-related infection occurring within 14 days of catheter placement and is believed to result from a breakdown in sterile technique during device placement. Infectious complications will be discussed fully in the next section.

Late Complications

Late complications following venous catheter placement include infection, catheter dysfunction, and venous stenosis and thrombosis. Delayed infectious complications are defined as occurring after 2 weeks following initial catheter placement. Anatomically, catheter-related infections include exit site infections, subcutaneous tunnel or pocket infections, and catheter-related bacteremias (27). Exit site infections are local infections manifested by local erythema, tenderness, induration or drainage confined to the catheter exit site. Induration, drainage, and tenderness extending into the subcutaneous tunnel or involving a pocket represent a tunnel or pocket infection, respectively. There should be no associated systemic symptoms in isolated exit site or tunnel infections. Patients with catheter-related

bacteremia may be asymptomatic or may present with fever or sepsis. Catheter-related bacteremias may result from primary infection of the catheter or secondary infection of the catheter from a peripheral site. This is suspected and assumed when persistent fevers exist without another source of infection, when there is resolution of fevers and leukocytosis after catheter removal, or when positive blood cultures are obtained for an organism not localized to another site. Quantitative cultures may lend weight to the diagnosis, when a 10-fold difference in bacterial growth is identified between a catheter-drawn specimen and a peripheral blood culture (36). It is definitively diagnosed when the same organism is isolated from both the catheter and peripheral blood (28, 37–39). External catheters, multilumen catheters, and increased duration of catheter placement increase the risk of catheter-related infections.

Treatment of catheter-related infections is multifactorial, but some general guidelines are applicable. In the patient with an intact immune system, every effort should be made to treat exit site and mild tunnel infections with local wound care and antibiotics in an attempt to avoid unnecessary catheter removal. When present, exudates should be cultured—with the knowledge that the culprit will likely be gram-positive skin flora. Commonly, in an effort to maintain an access site in the face of a simple tunnel infection, a cutdown can be performed at the venous access site, the tunnel excluded, and a temporary venous access device placed for 5–7 days. This device can then be exchanged for a new tunneled catheter placed through a newly fashioned subcutaneous tunnel, thereby salvaging the access site and allowing complete healing of the previously infected tunnel. For severe tunnel or pocket infections and those with accompanying bacteremia, incision and drainage of the tunnel or pocket will be required in addition to removal of the catheter.

Catheter-related bacteremias can be treated successfully in the immune-competent patient, often with intravenous antibiotics, salvaging the indwelling catheter. Bacteremias can be defined as complicated (associated with septic thrombophlebitis, endocarditis, or osteomyelitis) or uncomplicated (40). Complicated cases require prompt removal of the venous access device, and intravenous antibiotics for 4–8 weeks, depending on the site of infection (41–43). For uncomplicated bacteremias, 2 weeks of antibiotic coverage is recommended. If required, a single catheter exchange over a wire with sampling of the catheter tip is preferred. This will provide information about the infective nature of the catheter and can result in salvage of the access site. If bacteremia and leukocytosis persist despite appropriate antibiotic coverage and catheter exchange, then catheter removal is recommended.

Of note, catheter-related infection rates have been shown to be comparable and no higher for those procedures performed in a radiologic interventional suite than for those performed in the operating room (6,27–29,35,44–47). In addition to sterile insertion techniques, the quality of subsequent nursing care regarding wound and catheter management has been shown to be directly related to the rate of local and systemic infections (33).

Catheter dysfunction may be because of device migration, pericatheter fibrin sheath formation or intracatheter thrombus formation, catheter fracture, port rotation, or resultant venous stenosis and occlusion. Catheter malposition should not occur during initial device placement if imaging guidance is used. Delayed catheter migration may be because of normal head or arm motion or even coughing. In those cases in which the intravascular catheter length is appropriate and the catheter is simply malpositioned, appropriate repositioning may be performed via:

1. Forceful injection of saline via a small volume syringe
2. Repositioning via a second access site (usually the femoral vein) with the use of a snare
3. Repositioning of the catheter with a guide wire

If these techniques are unsuccessful, catheter exchange should be performed, maintaining the initial venous access site. In larger patients, especially those with significant chest wall soft tissues, marked catheter retraction may occur immediately following initial catheter placement when the patient assumes an upright position. If this occurs, the catheter will need to be exchanged for a longer one because repositioning via one of the three techniques mentioned earlier will not have a long-lasting effect. In this patient population, immediate catheter migration can be proactively avoided by using the IJ for access (rather than the SCV) and increasing the intravascular catheter length by 3–4 cm. Transhepatic catheters that become malpositioned because of respiratory motion are difficult to reposition and often require replacement.

Two basic types of catheter thrombosis occur: a circumferential fibrin-sleeve thrombosis that encircles the catheter and mural thrombosis that affects the catheter lumen and vein. Catheter thrombosis rates of radiologically inserted devices are similar to those inserted by surgeons (6,27–30, 44,45,48). The development of a circumferential fibrin sleeve occurs commonly on all catheter materials and may form as early as 24 hours after insertion (49–50). Catheter dysfunction resulting from fibrin sheath formation can occur in up to 57% of dialysis patients. Typically, blood cannot be aspirated through the catheter, but flushing is possible. The diagnosis is confirmed by catheter venography that usually is performed after the catheter has been withdrawn over a guide wire (Figure 68–4). Treatment of fibrin sheaths can be either pharmacologic or mechanical. Intracatheter thrombolytics, delivered by infusion or as a single administration, have been described (51,52). Mechanical means of disrupting fibrin sheaths include catheter exchange with disruption of the entire length of the fibrin sheath using an angioplasty balloon, and fibrin sheath stripping, most commonly via a femoral venous approach (53–55). Intracatheter thrombosis can be treated with endoluminal

brushing or instillation of a thrombolytic using either an infusion or dwell technique (56–58).

Catheters that lie outside the vein at the clavicle-first rib junction are subject to continuous trauma, which may result in compression, fracture, separation, and fragment embolization (8). This "pinch-off syndrome" can easily be avoided with a peripheral venous puncture to ensure an intravascular location at the clavicle-first rib junction. Patients experiencing pinch-off syndrome will present with catheter dysfunction, as the central portion of the catheter breaks free and migrates into the heart or pulmonary arterial tree. A second type of fragmentation that is not uncommonly seen is PICC line fracture following attempted

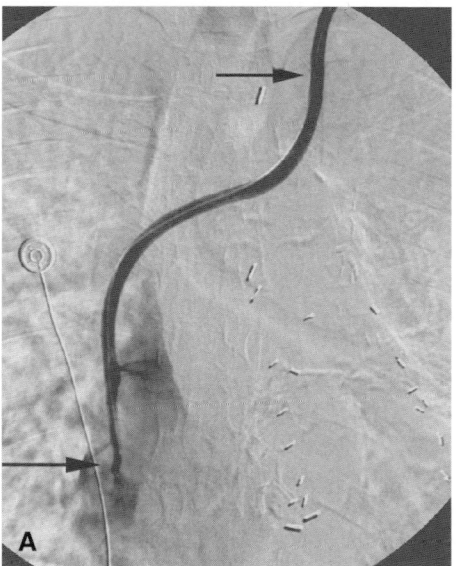

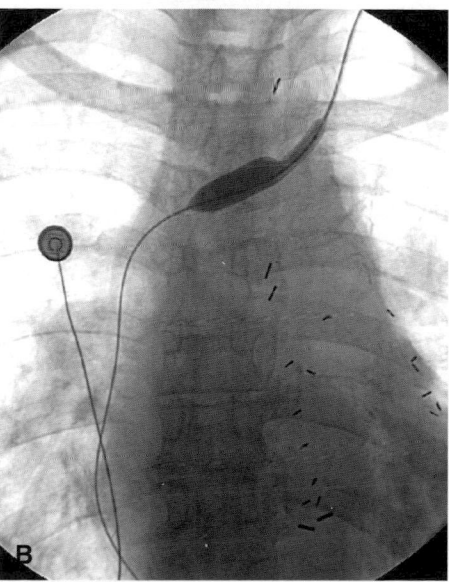

Figure 68–4   Fibrin sheath diagnosis and disruption. **A.** Initial venogram performed after withdrawal of a dialysis catheter to the level of the IJV demonstrates a long fibrin sheath extending from the IJV to the cavoatrial junction (*arrows*). **B.** Disruption of the entire fibrin sheath using a 10-mm angioplasty balloon.

removal. Venous spasm may occur in the access vein during attempted removal, and if not recognized, undue stretching of the catheter will result in shearing of the intravascular portion of the catheter. This can be avoided by initial recognition of the problem and subsequent application of heat to the access site for several minutes. If catheter removal is unsuccessful, nitrogycerin in 100 mg aliquots should relieve the spasm and allow for an uneventful catheter removal. Whatever the type of catheter involved, intravascular fragments should be removed using standard endovascular retrieval techniques.

Repeated clamp trauma at the hub of a catheter may eventually cause catheter fracture and leakage involving the external portion of the catheter. These fractures can often be repaired with commercially available kits. If this is unsuccessful, the catheter must be replaced.

Port rotation can be avoided by correct port pocket sizing and placement of bilateral stabilizing sutures around the port before pocket closure. A capacious pocket is more likely to result in port rotation than a smaller pocket in which the port snugly fits. If the port does indeed flip, rotating the port back to its normal position is often quite simple. Unfortunately, in the event rotation becomes a recurrent problem, the port should be exposed and stabilizing sutures applied.

The presence of a catheter within the venous system often leads to venous abnormalities including stenosis and thrombosis, which in turn results in catheter dysfunction. Venous stenosis may result from endothelial injury resulting from irritation by the catheter tip or other site at which the catheter touches the vessel wall or by irritation from an infusate (Figure 68–5). Venous thrombosis resulting from indwelling venous catheters is related to multiple interplaying factors including diameter of the catheter with respect to the vein, length of time the catheter is in place, composition of the catheter, position of the catheter tip, choice of access site, composition of the infusate, venous access history, and coagulation status (50,59,60). Although catheter-related central venous thrombosis is common, it frequently goes undiagnosed because of the development of a rich network of collaterals to compensate for the obstruction (Figure 68–6). Nonoccluding thrombus is generally asymptomatic, whereas an occlusive thrombus will be symptomatic in only approximately 30% of patients (27,61,62). The sudden onset of extremity, neck, or facial swelling should raise the possibility of acute venous thrombosis. Ultrasonography and possible venography can be performed for definitive diagnosis, and appropriate treatment can then be undertaken.

The treatment of catheter-related venous thrombosis heavily depends on the patient's presentation, need for access, access site, thrombus load, thrombus location, and availability of other sites. In the asymptomatic patient who no longer needs access, the catheter can be removed. Heparinization has been recommended to avoid possible

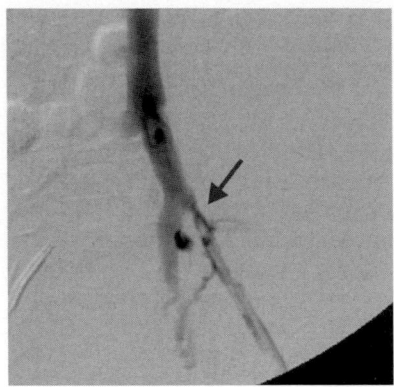

Figure 68–5   External iliac vein stenosis because of irritation of the vein by the indwelling catheter tip (*arrow*). Although the patient was asymptomatic, the catheter did not function appropriately. The patient has situs inversus.

pulmonary embolism (63); however, the location and thrombus load should be considered before initiating anticoagulation. In the asymptomatic patient who will require long-term venous catheterization, if the thrombosis is significant, thrombolytic therapy may be necessary to preserve future central access. In the symptomatic patient, if access is available elsewhere, the device can be removed, and the patient treated with anticoagulation or local thrombolytic therapy as the clinical course dictates. If access is limited, the initial access site can be maintained while local thrombolytic therapy is performed. A routine low-dose warfarin protocol may reduce the thrombotic complications associated with indwelling catheters (64).

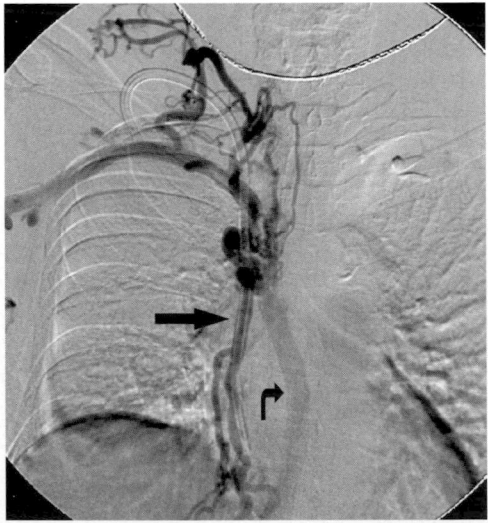

Figure 68–6   Asymptomatic central venous occlusion, with enlargement of the azygous vein (*curved arrow*). This is an indwelling right IJV dialysis catheter (*straight arrow*) with its tip in the right atrium via an occluded SVC.

SUMMARY

Traditionally, surgeons in operating rooms have performed the placement of long-term central venous catheters with acceptable procedural and late complication rates. However, surgical placement remains relatively expensive and often requires the services of both the operating surgeon and an anesthesiologist, in addition to costly operating room time. Moreover, operating room availability often limits prompt service. Procedural complication rates for radiologic placement are similar or lower when compared to surgical placement, and the use of imaging guidance in the interventional suite allows for exact catheter positioning. In most institutions, radiologic facilities can accommodate a request within 24 hours and do not carry the heavy overhead of the operating and recovery rooms or anesthesia facilities. Most cases can be completed within an hour, with minimal postoperative recovery period. These features result in a procedure that is significantly more cost-effective than standard surgical placement. However, catheter placement is only part of a radiologist's responsibility in patient care. The radiologist must become familiar with and involved in postprocedural catheter care, patient follow-up, and the management of complications.

REFERENCES

1. Hickman RO, Buckner CD, Clift RA, et al. A modified right atrial catheter for access to the venous system in marrow transplant recipients. Surg Gynecol Obstet 1979;148:871–875.
2. Broviac JW, Cole JJ, Scribner BS, Scribner BH. A silicone rubber atrial catheter for prolonged parenteral alimentation. Surg Gynecol Obstet 1973;136:602–606.
3. Murthy R, Arbabzadeh M, Lund G, et al. Percutaneous transrenal hemodialysis catheter insertion. J Vasc Interv Radiol 2002;13:1043–1045.
4. Jaques PF, Mauro MA, Keefe B. Ultrasonographic guidance for vascular access. J Vasc Interv Radiol 1992;3:427–430.
5. Sandhu J. Techniques for conventional access to central veins. J Vasc Interv Radiol 1998;1:125–132.
6. Laméris JS, Post PJM, Zonderland HM, et al. Percutaneous placement of Hickman catheters: comparison of sonographically guided and blind techniques. J Vasc Interv Radiol 1990;155:1097–1099.
7. Hinke DH, Zandt-Stastny DA, Goodman LR, et al. Pinch-off syndrome: a complication of implantable subclavian venous access devices. Radiology 1990;177:353–356.
8. Rubenstein RB, Alberty RE, Michels LG, et al. Hickman catheter separation. J Parent Ent Nutr 1985;9:754–757.
9. Meranze SG, McLean GK, Stein EJ, et al. Catheter placement in the azygos system: an unusual approach to venous access. AJR Am J Roentgenol 1985;144:1075–1076.
10. Solomon BA, Solomon J, Shlansky-Goldberg R. Percutaneous placement of an intercostal central venous catheter for chronic hyperalimentation guided by transhepatic venography. JPEN J Parenter Enteral Nutr 2001;25:42–44.
11. Kaufman JA, Crenshaw WB, Kuter I, et al. Percutaneous placement of a central venous access device via an intercostal vein. AJR Am J Roentgenol 1995;164:459–460.
12. Funaki B, Zaleski GX, Leef JA, et al. Radiologic placement of hemodialysis catheters in occluded neck, chest, or small thyrocervical collateral veins in central venous occlusion. Radiology 2001;218:471–476.
13. Hagen P, Yang JJ, Saibil EA. Use of an Amplatz Goose Neck Snare as a target for collateral neck vein dialysis catheter placement. J Vasc Interv Radiol 2001;12:493–495.
14. Ferral H, Bjarnason H, Wholey M, et al. Recanalization of occluded veins to provide access for central catheter placement. J Vasc Interv Radiol 1996;7:681–685.
15. Weeks S. Unconventional venous access. J Vasc Interv Radiol 2002;1:114–120.
16. Moriniere P, Rodary-Vautier R, Fillioux-Morfaux V, et al. Percutaneous recanalization of occlusion of central and proximal veins in chronic hemodialysis. Kidney Int 1997;52:1406–1411.
17. Nazarian GK, Myers TV, Bjarnason H, et al. Applications of the Amplatz Snare device during interventional radiologic procedures. AJR Am J Roentgenol 1995;165:673–678.
18. Farrell T, Lang EV, Barnhart W. Sharp recanalization of central venous occlusions. J Vasc Interv Radiol 1999;10:149–154.
19. Gupta H, Murphy TP, Soares GM. Use of a puncture needle for recanalization of an occluded right subclavian vein. Cardiovasc Intervent Radiol 1998;21:508–511.
20. Denny DF, Greenwood LH, Morse SS, et al. Inferior vena cava: translumbar catheterization for central venous access. Radiology 1989;170:1013–1014.
21. Kaufman JA, Greenfield AJ, Fitzpatrick GF. Transhepatic cannulation of the inferior vena cava. J Vasc Interv Radiol 1991;2:331–334.
22. Robertson LJ, Jaques PF, Mauro MA, et al. Percutaneous inferior vena cava placement of tunneled Silastic catheters for prolonged vascular access in infants. J Pediatr Surg 1990;25:596–598.
23. Lund GB, Lieberman RP, Haire WD, et al. Translumbar inferior vena cava catheters for long-term venous access. Radiology 1990;174:31–35.
24. Mauro MA, Jaques PF. Radiologic placement of long-term central venous catheters: a review. J Vasc Interv Radiol 1993;4:127–137.
25. Azizkhan RG, Taylor LA, Jaques PF, et al. Percutaneous translumbar and transhepatic inferior vena caval catheters for prolonged vascular access in children. J Pediatr Surg 1992;27:165–169.
26. Book WM, Raviele AA, Vincent RN. Transhepatic vascular access in pediatric cardiology patients with occlusion of traditional central venous sites. J Invasive Cardiol 1999;11:341–344.
27. Hull JE, Hunter CS, Luiken GA. The Groshong catheter: initial experience and early results of imaging-guided placement. Radiology 1992;185:803–807.
28. Robertson LJ, Mauro MA, Jaques PF. Radiologic placement of Hickman catheters. Radiology 1989;170:1007–1009.
29. Morris SL, Jaques PF, Mauro MA. Radiology-assisted placement of implantable subcutaneous infusion ports for long-term venous access. Radiology 1992;184:149–151.
30. Andrews JC, Walker-Andrews SC, William DE. Long-term central venous access with a peripherally placed subcutaneous infusion port: initial results. Radiology 1990;176:45–47.
31. Kahn ML, Barboza RB, Kling GA, et al. Initial experience with percutaneous placement of the PAS port implantable venous access device. J Vasc Interv Radiol 1992;3:459–461.
32. Andrews JC, Marx MV, Williams DM, et al. The upper arm approach for placement of peripherally inserted central catheters for protracted venous access. AJR Am J Roentgenol 1992;158:427–429.
33. Keohane PP, Jones BJ, Attrill H, et al. Effect of catheter tunnelling and a nutrition nurse on catheter sepsis during parenteral nutrition. A controlled trial. Lancet 1983;17:1388–1390.
34. Takasugi JK, O'Connell TX. Prevention of complications in permanent central venous catheters. Surg Gynecol Obstet 1988;167:6–11.
35. Delmore JE, Horbelt DV, Jack BL, et al. Experience with the Groshong long-term central venous catheter. Gynecol Oncol 1989;34:216–218.
36. Mauro M. Delayed complications of venous access. J Vasc Interv Radiol 1998;1:158–167.
37. Wechsler RJ, Spirn PW, Conant EF, et al. Thrombosis and infection caused by thoracic venous catheters: pathogenesis and imaging findings. AJR Am J Roentgenol 1993;160:467–471.
38. Corona ML, Peters SG, Narr BJ, et al. Subspecialty clinics: critical-care medicine (infections related to central venous catheters). Mayo Clin Proc 1990;65:979–986.

39. Norwood S, Ruby A, Civetta J, et al. Catheter-related infections and associated septicemia. Chest 1991;99:968–975.
40. Sitges-Serra A, Linares J, Garau J. Catheter sepsis: the clue is the hub. Surgery 1985;97:355–357.
41. Mermel LA, Farr BM, Sherertz RJ, et al. Guidelines for the management of intravascular catheter-related infections. Clin Infect Dis 2001;32:1249–1272.
42. Rupar DG, Herzog KD, Fisher MC, et al. Prolonged bacteremia with catheter-related central venous thrombosis. Am J Dis Child 1990;144:879–882.
43. Andes Dr, Urban AW, Acher CW et al. Septic thrombosis of the basilica, axillary, and subclavian veins caused by a peripherally inserted central venous catheter. Am J Med 1998;105:446–450.
44. Brothers TE, Von Moll LK, Niederhuber JE, et al. Experience with subcutaneous infusion ports in three hundred patients. Surg Gynecol Obstet 1988;166:295–301.
45. Harvey WH, Pick TE, Reed K, et al. A prospective evaluation of the Port-a-Cath implantable venous access system in chronically ill adults and children. Surg Gynecol Obstet 1989;169:495–500.
46. Guenier C, Ferreira J, Pector JC. Prolonged venous access in cancer patients. Eur J Surg Oncol 1989;15:553–555.
47. Greene FL, Moore W, Strickland G, et al. Comparison of a totally implantable access device for chemotherapy (Port-a-Cath) and long-term percutaneous catheterization (Broviac). South Med J 1988;81:580–583.
48. Ahmed N, Payne RF. Thrombosis after central venous cannulation. Med J Austr 1976;1:217–220.
49. Hoshal VL, Ause RG, Hoskins PA. Fibrin sleeve formation on indwelling subclavian central venous catheters. Arch Surg 1971;102:353–358.
50. Brismar B, Hardstedt C, Jacobson S. Diagnosis of thrombosis by catheter phlebography after prolonged central venous catheterization. Ann Surg 1981;194:779–783.
51. Savader SJ, Haikal LC, Ehrman KO, et al. Hemodialysis catheter associated fibrin sheaths: Treatment with a low-dose rt-PA infusion. J Vasc Interv Radiol 2000;11:1131–1136.
52. Haire WD, Atkinson JB, et al. Urokinase versus recombinant tissue plasminogen activator in thrombosed central venous catheters: a double-blinded, randomized trial. Thromb Haemost 1994;72:543–547.
53. Crain MR, Mewissen MW, Ostrowski GJ, et al. Fibrin sleeve stripping for salvage of failing hemodialysis catheters: technique and initial results. Radiology 1996;198:41–44.
54. Haskal ZJ, Leen VH, Thomas-Hawkins C, et al. Transvenous removal of fibrin sheaths from tunneled hemodialysis catheters. J Vasc Interv Radiol 1996;7:513–517.
55. Rockall AG, Harris A, Wetton CWN, et al. Stripping of failing hemodialysis catheters using the Amplatz gooseneck snare. Clin Radiol 1997;52:616–620.
56. Cox K, Vesely TM, Windus DW, et al. The utility of brushing dysfunctional hemodialysis catheters. J Vasc Interv Radiol 2000;11:979–983.
57. Bel'eed K, Kumar A, Asin M, et al. Endoluminal brushing of blocked indwelling haemodialysis catheters. Nephrol Dial Transplant 1999;14:241.
58. Farmer CK, Greenwood E, Goldsmith DJ, et al. Endoluminal brushing of blocked permanent indwelling haemodialysis catheters saves money. Nephrol Dial Transplant 1997;12:2040.
59. Namyslowski J. Management of catheter-induced venous thrombosis. J Vasc Interv Radiol 2002;5(2):85–88.
60. Jacobs MB, Yeager M. Thrombotic and infectious complications of Hickman-Broviac catheters. Arch Intern Med 1984;144:1597–1599.
61. Anderson AJ, Krasnow SH, Boyer MW, et al. Thrombosis: the major Hickman catheter complication in patients with solid tumor. Chest 1989;95:71–75.
62. Haire WD, Lieberman RP, Lund GB, et al. Thrombotic complications of silicone rubber catheters during autologous marrow and peripheral stem cell transplantation: prospective comparison of Hickman and Groshong catheters. Bone Marrow Transplant 1991;7:57–59.
63. Monreal M, Raventos A, Lerma R, et al. Pulmonary embolism in patients with upper extremity DVT associated to venous central lines: a prospective study. Thromb Haemost 1994;72:548–550.
64. Bern MM, Lokich JJ, Wallach SR, et al. Very low doses of warfarin can prevent thrombosis in central venous catheters. Ann Intern Med 1990;112:423–428.

Vena Cava Filters

69

Gregory M. Soares, Timothy P. Murphy

BACKGROUND AND EVOLUTION OF INFERIOR VENA CAVA FILTERS

The spectrum of disease that includes deep venous thrombosis and pulmonary embolism (PE) has been stated to be the third leading cause of death in the United States (1). Although detection and treatment of venous thromboembolic disease has improved, PE continues to be diagnosed in 355,000 patients yearly with a mortality rate of 120,000 –240,000 people per year in this country (2–4). Eighty-five to 95% of pulmonary emboli arise from the iliofemoral veins (5,6). Most of the remaining 10–15% arise from thrombi in the vena cava, ovarian veins, right atrium, or upper extremities (5,7,8). Untreated, proximal deep venous thrombosis or pulmonary embolism has a 30.5–50.0% chance of recurrent pulmonary embolism, with an 18–26% mortality rate (9–11). Anticoagulation is the initial treatment of pulmonary deep venous thromboembolic disease. Mechanical interruption of the pathway for thrombi traveling to the lungs is most often reserved for patients who cannot tolerate anticoagulation, who suffer pulmonary embolism during adequate anticoagulation, or who have extensive thrombosis above the inguinal ligament predisposing them to significant pulmonary embolism despite adequate anticoagulation (12,13).

Mechanical obstruction as a method to prevent lower extremity thrombi from traveling to the lungs was conceived only 8 years after Virchow's triad was postulated in 1860 (14–17). Homans recognized in 1944 that most symptomatic pulmonary emboli arise from the lower extremity and pelvic veins and that these proximal thrombi usually originate in the deep veins of the calf (5,18). Homans, DeBakey, and Ochsner advocated early femoral interruption in patients who had experienced pulmonary embolism (5,19). Vein ligations were often performed at the common femoral level, supplemented by suction thrombectomy of the iliac veins if thrombus was present in the common femoral vein on exploration (5).

After heparin became available for clinical use in 1935 (20) and warfarin became clinically available in 1948 (21,22), the use of anticoagulation paralleled vein interruption in the treatment of this disease process. In patients ineligible for or inadequtaely treated by anticoagulation, ligation of the inferior vena cava became popular as more peripheral ligations fell out of favor. Common femoral ligation was associated with an excessive incidence of lower extremity swelling, and superficial femoral vein ligation was inadequate for patients who had thrombus proximal to the junction of the superficial and deep femoral veins (5,23,24). By the early 1960s, evaluation of inferior vena cava ligation revealed a similar operative mortality rate to peripheral ligation and a significantly lower rate of recurrent pulmonary embolism (23,24). Most series reported mortality rates in the range of 12–15%, recurrent PE in 6%, and chronic venous stasis in 33% (25–29). Ligations were optimally performed directly below the renal veins to avoid venous stasis between the ligature and the renal veins, which could result in recurrent pulmonary embolism (24,26,30). Recurrent PE was also hypothesized to be a result of large collaterals that formed after ligation or embolism of clot from above the ligation (31). Severe leg swelling was also a debilitating sequela, occurring in 10–16% of patients (23,25).

In the late 1960s, the problems with inferior vena cava ligation were addressed with open surgical methods to preserve flow through the inferior vena cava while trapping or filtering out potentially harmful emboli. Stenosis, plication, or compartmentalization of the inferior vena cava lumen was performed with various sutures, staples, or clips (32–34) (Figures 69–1 and 69–2). Although partial interruption of the inferior vena cava demonstrated a significantly lower incidence of lower extremity morbidity than did complete caval interruption (46% versus 76%) (26), procedure-related mortality rates (12%) and recurrent pulmonary embolism rates (4%) remained similar to those resulting from caval interruption (35–37). Clips and suture

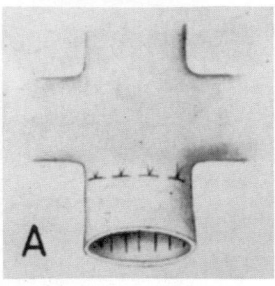

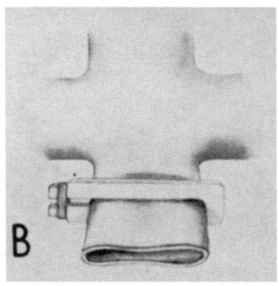

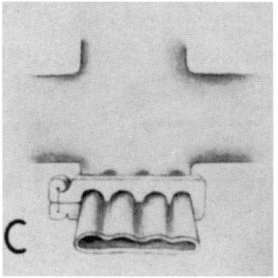

Figure 69–1 Drawing of early surgical approaches to partitioning of the vena cava. **A.** "Harp-string" grid method of surgical plication popularized by Spencer. **B.** Moretz clip. **C.** Miles clip. (Reprinted with permission from Adams JT, Feingold BE, DeWeese JA. Comparative evaluation of ligation and partial interruption of the inferior vena cava. Arch Surg 1971;103:272–276. Copyright 1971, American Medical Association.)

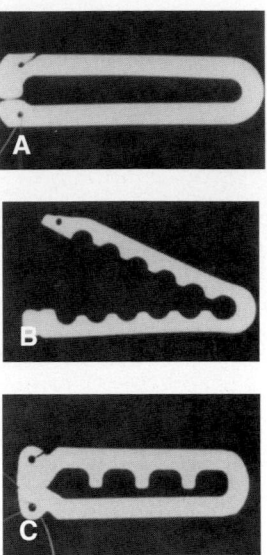

Figure 69–2 Photographs of the **A.** Moretz, **B.** Miles, and **C.** Adams-DeWeese vena cava clips. The Moretz clip narrows the lumen of the vena cava to 2.5 mm; the Miles and Adams-DeWeese clips compartmentalize the lumen of the vena cava into multiple channels between 3 and 4 mm in diameter. (Reprinted with permission from Eberlein TH, Carey LC. Comparison of surgical management for pulmonary emboli. Ann Surg 1974;179(6):836–841.)

plication of the vena cava were associated with a 30–40% incidence of inferior vena cava occlusion (17).

In 1967, the Mobin-Uddin umbrella (Edwards Laboratories) became the first endoluminal device for caval interruption (38). Because deployment utilized fluoroscopic guidance, procedures were usually performed in the angiography department. Using surgical exposure and right internal jugular venotomy, the device was delivered through a catheter-based carrier system with an inner diameter of 9 mm (27 French). The jugular approach was used to avoid potential iliocaval thrombus; a femoral carrier for the Mobin-Uddin umbrella did not exist.

The original version of this device, designed as an adjunct to anticoagulation in patients who experienced recurrent pulmonary embolism during adequate anticoagulation, was intended to result in occlusion of the inferior vena cava (38). This version consisted of six radiating spokes of stainless steel alloy connected by a fenestrated silicone membrane deployed with the apex of the umbrella directed

caudally. Cardiac output had been shown experimentally to decrease by 47% after inferior vena cava ligation (39). Fenestrations had been placed in the silicone membrane in an attempt to delay vena caval occlusion long enough for collaterals to develop and minimize these expected hemodynamic alterations (39). As experience with this device accumulated, it became evident that approximately one third of patients maintained patency of the vena cava after umbrella placement with no increase in the incidence of recurrent pulmonary embolism, which was reported as 3.6% in a review of 2,215 patients (40). The silicone membrane was subsequently heparin bonded in an attempt to improve caval patency rates (Figure 69–3).

Originally, the Mobin-Uddin umbrella had an expanded diameter of 23 mm. This was increased to 28 mm in the mid-1970s because of occasional reports of proximal migration of the 23-mm-diameter umbrella. The superiority of the transvenous method of inferior vena cava interruption as opposed to surgical methods was established by marked improvement in procedure-related mortality, which was negligible for transvenous placement (38,40–44), versus 8.0–14.2% for direct surgical methods of caval interruption (45,46). The Mobin-Uddin umbrella was removed from the market in 1986. The development of devices designed to maintain patency of the vena cava had been prompted by observations that patients with Mobin-Uddin umbrellas who maintained patency of the inferior vena cava had no increased incidence of recurrent pulmonary embolism (42,47) and a lower incidence of lower extremity sequelae

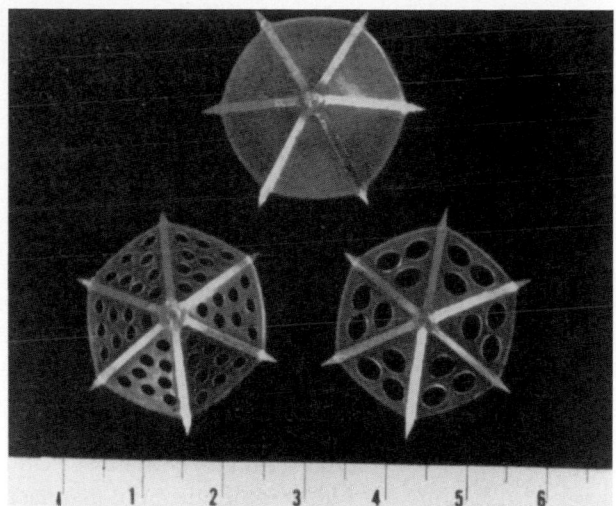

Figure 69–3 Axial view of three configurations of the Mobin-Uddin umbrella. The initial configuration consisted of six radial struts with a solid silicone membrane. The filter was later modified to contain fenestrations of 1.5 mm or 3.0 mm in the silicone membrane. (Reprinted with permission from Mobin-Uddin K, McLean R, Bolooki H, et al. Caval interruption for prevention of pulmonary embolism: long-term results of a new method. Arch Surg 1969;99:711–715. Copyright 1969, American Medical Association.)

(42,47). The first such device introduced was the Kimray-Greenfield filter, now known as the Greenfield filter.

The original Greenfield filter (Boston Scientific) was introduced in 1974. Though no longer commercially available and despite the proliferation of many low-profile filter systems, the original Greenfield filter remains the filter with which all others are compared. The original filter was placed by venotomy using a 29.5 French outer-diameter sheath. Percutaneous placement was first described by Tadavarthy in 1984 (48). The filter consisted of six radiating stainless steel struts crimped and angled so that the resulting filter was cone shaped. The cone apex was directed cephalad. Eighty percent of the cone's volume could be occupied by thrombus, with a corresponding reduction of cross-sectional area to 64% (17). This design demonstrated the ability to trap clinically significant emboli in vitro and in vivo (49,50). In clinical trials it demonstrated a rate of clinically evident recurrent pulmonary embolism of 4% while maintaining caval patency in 96%. These rates remain unchanged with more than 20 years clinical experience with the Greenfield filter and serve as the standard against which other devices are usually judged (51–53).

Percutaneous inferior vena cava filters have evolved since the early 1980s. Downsizing of introducer systems has been used to facilitate filter delivery and to reduce procedure time and patient blood loss. Initial reports of insertion-site thrombosis as high as 10–41% (54–57) also motivated development of lower-profile systems. Current insertion-site thrombosis rates are reported in the range of 2–14.3% for occlusive thrombosis (58–61). The effect that carrier systems as small as 6–9 French outer diameter have on access site thrombosis remains to be fully evaluated. Recent

developments in filter design and placement technique have included the introduction of temporary or retrievable devices and the use of alternative settings and imaging guidance for placement. Though endovascular filter placement has now existed for more than a quarter of a century, prospective direct comparisons of filter design and effectiveness are lacking. Because filters have been accepted as standard therapy for prevention of pulmonary embolism in the setting of anticoagulation contraindication or failure, prospective data may not be ethically attainable (62). Despite this, at least one prospective trial and several large retrospective studies have concluded that filters are effective in preventing life-threatening pulmonary embolism with acceptably low morbidity rates (63–65,52).

TECHNIQUE OF FILTER PLACEMENT

Percutaneous placement of vena cava filters is usually achieved after gaining access to a common femoral, internal jugular, or occasionally antecubital or brachial vein (66–68). A single-wall puncture is followed by tract dilatation with serial dilators exchanged over a guide wire. The final dilator is exchanged for a delivery sheath, which is left in the vena cava. The filter introducer system is passed through the sheath, and the filter is deployed. Balloon dilatation of the tract was shown to be less traumatic to the vein and to result in a lower incidence of insertion-site thrombosis than the serial dilatations required to create large-caliber tracts of the past (58,59,69,70). The smaller venotomies currently in use require far fewer, if any, serial dilators before sheath placement, and no similar studies have been performed. The safety of percutaneous access to the vein compared with surgical exposure of the vein has been demonstrated (71).

Imaging of the vena cava is routinely performed before filter placement to assess caval patency, anomalies, webs, or excessive narrowing of the intrahepatic portion (72). Location of renal veins must also be determined to ensure proper positioning of the filter. Finally, because approximately 3% of venae cavae are oversized (>28 mm in diameter) (73) and not suitable for many of the available filters, caval diameters are also routinely measured. The traditional and gold standard means of visualizing the vena cava is with iodinated contrast cavography performed in the angiography suite. Useful information is available in as many as 27% of cavograms performed before filter placement, and in 15% of cases this information significantly affects the performance of the procedure (72). Alternatives to iodinated contrast cavography have included carbon dioxide and gadolinium cavography. Both agents have been demonstrated to be safe alternatives for patients who are critically ill, have renal failure, or have had contrast reactions (74–77). CO_2 cavography may underestimate caval diameter, may be less sensitive for accessory renal veins, and has demontsrated interobserver interpretation variability (78,79,74). Imaging with intravascular ultrasound or duplex sonography has also been shown to be safe, accurate, and cost effective for intensive care unit populations who may be too ill for intrahospital transport (80–82).

Most percutaneous filter placements are done through the common femoral vein after the vena cava, iliac, and femoral veins are assessed. The majority of the remainder is placed by the jugular approach. Less frequently, antecubital access may be used. Complications of femoral access include site thrombosis and, rarely, pulmonary embolism resulting from inadvertent manipulation through iliac or caval thrombus. The jugular approach can cause pneumothorax and has resulted in death because of air embolization or trauma to the carotid or vertebral artery (70). Though increasing reliance on sonographic guidance for jugular access may decrease its risks, the femoral approach remains preferred when thrombus does not prohibit it. The left femoral approach was associated with a higher incidence of thrombosis of the insertion site than the right femoral approach when the large delivery system for the stainless steel Greenfield filter was used (83). This may have been a result of mechanical trauma caused by distortion of the more acutely angled left iliocaval junction during passage of the larger, stiffer delivery system. A higher incidence of thrombosis of the insertion site with placement by the left common femoral vein has not been confirmed with use of low-profile filter systems (84). Other access sites that have been used include the left internal jugular vein and the external jugular veins (85). Placement via antecubital vein access has been demonstrated to be safe and effective with the Simon nitinol and TrapEase filters (66–68). This approach also affords the option of inserting a peripherally inserted central catheter (PICC) via the same access.

Because most inferior vena cava filters are placed for lower extremity thrombus, infrarenal placement can usually be accomplished. When thrombus in the inferior vena cava or renal veins does not permit infrarenal placement, or, occasionally, in childbearing-age females with large ovarian veins or in pregnant females, suprarenal placement may be necessary. Though suprarenal inferior vena cava filter placement in the setting of advanced malignancy, preexisting renal vein thrombosis, and solitary kidney has been associated with fatal renal vein thrombosis (86), multiple larger retrospective evaluations have demonstrated the safety of suprarenal filters when required (65,87,88). These studies have revealed no significant incidence of permanent renal dysfunction, no significantly increased rate of recurrent pulmonary embolism, and no increase in rates of inferior vena caval occlusion. Use of upper extremity and jugular long-term central venous access has been accompanied by increasing recognition of upper extremity thromboembolic disease. In this setting, when anticoagulation has been ineffective or inappropriate, superior vena cava filter placement has been employed. Most reports describe use of Greenfield filters in the SVC, but multiple devices

have been placed in this location (89,90). Though small series of SVC filters suggest the safety and efficacy of this alternative, case reports of superior vena cava thrombosis exist (89–91) and should prompt caution.

INDICATIONS FOR FILTER PLACEMENT

Patients with absolute indications have thromboembolic disease. Thromboembolic disease and a contraindication to anticoagulation is the most frequent indication for vena cava filter placement, cited in 38–77% of patients (51,56,85,92–94). Absolute contraindications to anticoagulation include recent stroke or neurosurgical procedure (within 2 months), recent major surgery or trauma (within 2 weeks), active internal bleeding, intracranial neoplasm, recent ocular surgery, and heparin-induced thrombocytopenia (95–101). Coumadin is contraindicated in pregnancy because it crosses the placenta and can cause fetal anomalies (101). Relative contraindications include recent minor trauma (within 2 weeks), hematuria, occult blood in the stools, peptic ulcer disease, pericarditis, bacterial endocarditis, and unstable gait (95–101). Thromboembolic disease and complications of anticoagulation comprise the indication for filter placement in 6–17% of patients (51,85,93,94). Complications of anticoagulation occur in 5–60% of patients and include bleeding, heparin-induced thrombocytopenia, and warfarin-induced skin necrosis (95,99–107). Anticoagulation is associated with a 5–12% mortality rate (95,99–107). Recurrent or progressive thromboembolic disease while adequately anticoagulated is the indication for filter placement in 3–27% of patients (51,85,92–94). The risk of pulmonary embolism in patients with large, free-floating iliofemoral or caval thrombus is between 27% and 60% despite adequate anticoagulation (1,13). This situation also warrants placement of a vena cava filter, ideally as an adjunct to anticoagulation (85).

Patients with relative indications for filter placement may or may not have thromboembolic disease. The meaning of prophylactic filter placement has evolved since the advent of percutaneous filter placement (108). Though prophylaxis initially referred to filter placement in patients with deep venous thrombosis but without documented pulmonary embolism, prophylaxis now often means placement in patients without documented thromboembolic disease but at high risk for its development. Such clinical situations may include patients with poor pulmonary reserve with a cardiac index less than 1.5 liters per minute (11), patients undergoing pulmonary or lower extremity thrombolysis or thrombectomy (11,109), surgical and trauma patients (85,110–113), certain orthopedic patients, and patients with malignancy (114–119). In the setting of multitrauma, patients stratified at highest risk for thromboembolic disease have been further defined to include those with severe brain injury, spinal cord injury, particularly with para- or quadriplegia and long bone fracture, complex pelvic fracture, and multiple lower extremity long-bone fractures (120–126). Relative indications such as multitrauma and malignancy are not universal and need to be considered on an individual basis (127–129). Temporary or removable filters have now been applied in many of the above scenarios and will almost certainly modify and expand the indications for caval filtration in these and other clinical settings (130–133). Potential uses of nonpermanent filters include situations where pulmonary embolism risk is time limited. These patients may include multitrauma patients or others with temporary contraindications to anticoagulation, such as those proximal to major surgery, or other situations where indications for permanent filtration are relative. The Recovery filter (Bard) is currently the only device that is approved for "temporary" implantation or removal. The Günther Tulip filter (Cook) is designed to be removable but is FDA approved for permanent implantation, and retrieval is an "off-label" use.

EVALUATION AND COMPARISON OF VENA CAVA FILTERS

The majority of published filter data has relied on clinical follow-up (Table 69–1). Clinically significant adverse outcomes following filter placement, such as death, clinically apparent recurrent pulmonary embolism, and significant lower extremity swelling, are uncommon. Pulmonary embolism is often clinically silent with asymptomatic pulmonary emboli having been observed in 35–51% of patients with deep venous thrombosis (134,135). Thrombosis and occlusion of the inferior vena cava are also usually asymptomatic (5,23,24,40,136). Clinical follow-up, therefore, underestimates occurrence of both these events. Because patients with a history of lower extremity deep vein thrombosis are predisposed to postphlebitic syndrome, with as many as 79% developing lower extremity swelling resulting from damage to the valves in the deep veins of the legs, clinical evidence of inferior vena cava thrombosis is also dubious (137–140). Because instances of asymptomatic outcomes are more common than symptomatic ones, objective evaluation of such events with rigorous serial imaging might be more fruitful in pointing to real differences in filter performance. However, the magnitude and cost of such a study have prevented such an analysis of currently available filters (141). A recent meta-analysis of more than 6,500 filter insertions, though again suggesting the utility of filters in limiting clinically significant pulmonary emboli, failed to find evidence of superiority of any one device over the many others now available (142).

The self-limited risk of pulmonary embolism in most patients probably justifies the short duration follow-up data included in many early filter series. The acute period following filter placement is of most interest regarding recurrent pulmonary embolism, caval thrombosis (which probably always occurs because of trapped

TABLE 69–1

COMPARISON OF VENA CAVA FILTERS*

Filter	Recurrent Pulmonary Embolism	Inferior Vena Cava Patency	Insertion Site Thrombosis	Stability	Caval Penetration
Stainless steel Greenfield	4%	95%	0–41%	Excellent; occasional migrations to heart and pulmonary arteries reported	Rare, including penetration of adjacent organs
Bird's Nest	3%	97% clinical follow-up	Up to 33% (nonocclusive)	Case reports of migration to right atrium	Unknown
Titanium Greenfield	3%	100%	3.0–8.7%	11% >1 cm with new filter design	0.8% with new design
Simon nitinol	3%	79–86% imaging follow-up	10–11%	Rare; migration to heart and pulmonary arteries reported	25%, including aortic penetration in two patients
LGM (Vena Tech)	—	70–92% imaging follow-up	6–23%	14% migration >1cm; migration rarely significant	Not significant
Vena Tech LP	0%	100%	0%	0%	Unknown
TrapEase	0.5%	97.2%	0%	Case reports of migration to right atrium	Unknown
Günther Tulip	3.6%	93%	0%	Case reports of migration to right atrium	0%
Recovery	0% (53-day mean residence)	100% clinical follow-up	0%	Case report 4 cm cephalic migration	0%

*Summary of available data for the nine vena cava filters currently available. Comparison of published figures among filters in most cases is not reliable because of inconsistent methods of establishing outcomes. (See references 9, 10, 48, 49, 56–59, 85, 92, 94, 148, 160–163, 166–179, 182, 183, 187, and 193.)

emboli) (9,70,136), and insertion vein thrombosis. This is because thrombus is most likely to embolize in its acute form before it becomes adherent and incorporated into the vein wall, a process usually complete by 3–6 months (143). Because of the historical variations in filter outcomes evaluated, data collection, and reporting, documents have been created in attempts to standardize reporting and improve the quality of device use (144–146). Longer-term data and meta-analyses have continued to support earlier rates of recurrent pulmonary embolism, ranging from 2% to 5.6% (65,142,147–149). Caval thrombosis and insertion site thrombosis rates continue to range widely from 0% to 31% and from 2% to 35%, respectively. This is probably a result of the above-mentioned variation in data collected and reported. Most devices are associated with contemporary caval occlusion rates of less than 10% (142).

Currently, ten intracaval filter designs have been approved by the FDA in the United States. These include the stainless steel Greenfield filter (MediTech/Boston Scientific), which is no longer commercially available, the stainless steel over-the-wire Greenfield filter (MediTech), the titanium Greenfield filter (MediTech), the LGM Vena Tech filter (B. Braun), the Vena Tech LP filter (B. Braun), the Bird's Nest filter (Cook), the Simon nitinol filter (Bard), the TrapEase filter (Cordis), the Günther Tulip Vena Cava MREye filter (Cook), and the most recently approved Recovery vena cava nitinol filter (Bard). Filters differ in size, design, composition, and size of introducer. Criteria that are used to assess filters include rates of recurrent pulmonary embolism after filter placement, death rates resulting from pulmonary embolism after filter placement, occlusion of the filter and inferior vena cava, thrombosis of the insertion site, incidence significance of filter asymmetry, filter migration, potential sites of insertion, and ease of placement. An ideal vena cava filter should be biocompatible and nonthrombogenic, effectively filter all clinically significant emboli, result in minimal flow disturbance, be stable in the longitudinal and transverse planes within the vena cava, result in no injury to adjacent structures, be simply and safely placed, be affordable, and, if designed as such, be easily retrievable (150,151).

The ability of vena cava filters to trap experimental thrombi has been tested using in vitro and animal models of the human inferior vena cava (49,50,152–156). In Katsamouris's study, the Greenfield filter was relatively ineffective at trapping small emboli (<3 mm in diameter), particularly if tilted greater than 14 degrees off the caval long axis, whereas the Mobin-Uddin, Amplatz, Günther, Simon nitinol, and Bird's Nest filters were effective in filtering most of even the smallest emboli (2 mm in diameter) (49). Effectiveness in filtering emboli of all sizes was maintained with asymmetric postioning of the Amplatz, Günther, Simon nitinol, and Bird's Nest filters and with prolapse of the Bird's Nest filter's filaments (49). The Mobin-Uddin umbrella and the Kimray Greenfield filters were significantly less effective in filtering even large

thrombi (7 mm in diameter) when not oriented properly (49). However, another study using thrombi injected into the vena cava of sheep showed the Greenfield filter to remove 89% of emboli either 4 or 8 mm in diameter, with failures limited to emboli of the smaller sizes and no significant decrease in clot filtration with the filter tilted so that the apex was against the wall of the vena cava (50). Greenfield found that filtration by the Greenfield design was diminished as the downstream caval diameter increased and that asymmetry became important only in cavae with diameters greater than 22 mm (157). Others have debated the importance of filter tilt or asymmetry (158,159). Although trends suggesting increased risk of recurrent PE and IVC thrombosis with asymmetry have been shown, the use of clinical outcome parameters and insufficient follow-up data points have thwarted demonstration of statistical significance (158). The only consistent conclusion from these and other studies is that the Greenfield filter may be relatively less effective at filtering small emboli than other filter designs (49,50,152–154, 155,157,158). However, the importance of this conclusion is dubious because these small emboli may be clinically insignificant and the filter may have a higher patency rate because of fewer trapped emboli (153). Furthermore, none of these models duplicates the physiology of the inferior vena cava in humans.

Stainless Steel Greenfield Filter

The stainless steel Greenfield filter consists of six radiating struts projecting downward and outward from a central point, making the shape of a cone (Figure 69–4). The apex of the cone is directed cephalad in the vena cava. The filter is 4.4 cm in height. Each of the six legs of the filter is angled, taking a zigzag course from apex to base. At the base, each strut has a single barb or tine that anchors the filter within the vena cava. The filter is self-expanding and is deposited from the jugular or femoral vein usaually by percutaneous puncture. A hole in the apex of the filter permits placement over a guide wire. The filter is delivered through a 14.5 French delivery sheath.

The stainless steel Greenfield filter has been used since 1973 (56). In Greenfield and Michna's review of the first 12 years of experience with this device, they reported a 4% clinically suspected or confirmed rate of recurrent pulmonary embolism in 469 patients (51). A 20-year summary of experience with the design reported the same rate of recurrent pulmonary embolism and a caval patency rate of 96% (52). By comparison, the incidence of recurrent pulmonary embolism in patients not treated with anticoagulation is approximately 30% (9), and the mortality rate in patients with pulmonary embolism not treated with anticoagulation in 6 months is 25% (10), demonstrating the effectiveness of this device in preventing clinically significant pulmonary embolism. Separate reports by Greenfield and others have documented 95% caval patency rates using

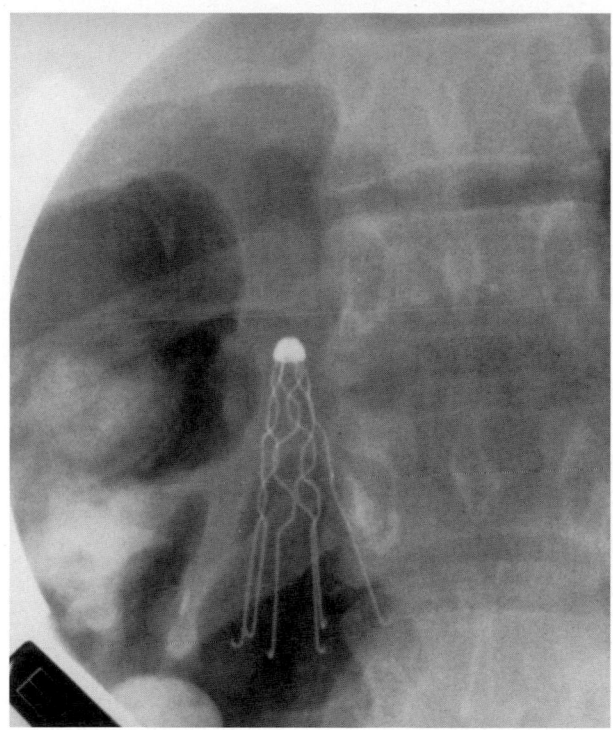

Figure 69–4   Radiograph of a suprarenal stainless steel Greenfield filter in a patient with thrombosis of the inferior vena cava extending to the renal veins.

contrast and radioisotope vena cavography (56,57,160). Periprocedural mortality is rare (51,52,56,57,160).

Percutaneous placement of the Greenfield filter was first reported in 1984 (48). It was achieved by puncture of either the jugular or femoral vein, placement of a guide wire in the vein through the needle, and subsequent dilatation of the tract using serial dilators, originally designed for urologic procedures. Tracts were dilated up to 24 French size, which was required to accommodate the delivery system (161). This approach obviated frustration inherent in coordinating vascular surgeons, operating instruments, and the radiologist with angiography equipment in the angiography suite necessary for earlier surgical methods of access (161). Hemostasis after removal of the delivery system was achieved by manual compression within 15–30 minutes (57,161). With the radiologist acting independently, it was found that placement of a vena cava filter lengthened the procedure time by only about 10 minutes after an inferior vena cavogram was performed (161). Tract dilatation using an angioplasty balloon saved time and trauma to the vein but has become largely historic with the advent of contemporary low-profile systems (58,59).

Bird's Nest Filter

The Bird's Nest filter (Cook) has been in use since 1982 (Figure 69–5) (92). This filter is unique in design. Filtration is achieved by a network of four 25-cm-long filaments 0.18 mm in diameter, which during deployment are wound

in such a way so that their relationship is fairly compact (92). These filaments are anchored to the vena cava by two sets of V-shaped struts, each composed of two legs connected to each other at one end with an acute angle at their junction. The legs have barbs and loops at their ends opposite their junction point to prevent movement within the vena cava and to limit penetration of the vena cava wall. One set of struts is deposited first, with the apex directed caudally. After these are anchored firmly within the vena cava, the filaments are deployed. The filaments are not visible fluoroscopically and only occasionally are seen with plain radiography. Manipulation of the introducer sheath, which is rotated 90 degrees four times during filament deployment, minimizes prolapse of the filaments beyond the anchoring struts (92). Finally, the second set of anchoring struts is deployed, with the apex or junction point of the legs directed cephalad, overlapping the first set of struts by at least 50%. The filter is placed through a 12 French sheath. Because the maximum expansion diameter between the free ends of the legs of the anchoring struts is 60 mm, this filter has been particularly useful in patients with venae cavae greater than 28 mm in diameter, which is the maximum acceptable diameter for placement of the Greenfield filter and several other currently available filters of similar design (162). This filter has been placed in venae cavae of as many as 42 mm in diameter and has demonstrated equal clot-trapping efficiency in an in vitro oversized vena cava model with less flow disturbance than with bilateral iliac placement of other filters (163).

Early results obtained with the Bird's Nest filter were reported in one of a larger series of filter patient studies published, 568 patients (92). Unfortunately, follow-up was almost exclusively clinical, with few imaging studies performed to document outcome (92). In addition, duration of follow-up was short, with a minimum required follow-up of 6 months and a maximum of 5 years (92). Twelve of 440 patients (2.7%) on whom 6-month follow-up information was available demonstrated clinically suspected recurrent pulmonary embolism, and 13 patients (2.9%) had clinical evidence of inferior vena cava thrombosis (92). Recurrent pulmonary embolism was confirmed in only two patients, and thrombosis of the inferior vena cava in seven patients. Of 27 follow-up vena cavograms performed, six demonstrated thrombosis; it is not stated in this report whether all these vena cavograms were obtained for symptoms. A 6-year, single-center review of the device in 267 patients found a 4.1% rate of recurrent pulmonary embolism (1.1% documented, 3.0% clinically suspected) and a 3% rate of access site thrombosis (164). A smaller, more recent 5-year series using clinical and imaging follow-up found rates of 1.3% for recurrent embolism and 4.7% for caval occlusion. The latter is interesting in that the rate of filament prolapse was reported to be 70% (165).

Because of migration of the filter in 5 of the first 422 patients with the original flexible 0.25-mm flexible struts, the struts were increased to 0.46 mm in diameter, and in

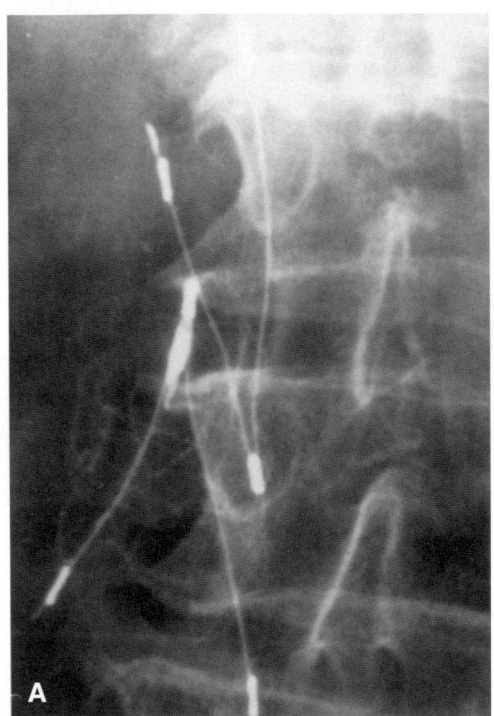

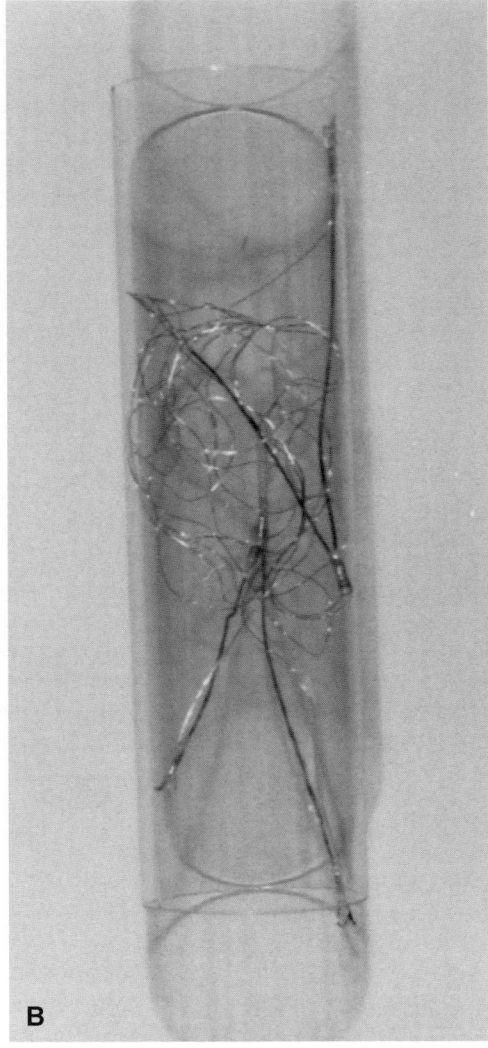

Figure 69–5 A. Radiograph of the Bird's Nest filter showing the stabilizing struts. The filaments that constitute the nest responsible for filtration are only faintly seen. **B.** Photograph of the filter in a model of the vena cava clearly shows the filaments.

the current model are rigid. This change required increasing the diameter of the insertion sheath from 8 French to 12 French. No migrations were reported in this series in the next 147 patients treated with the modified filter (92). A subsequent report described two patients treated with the modified filter who experienced cephalad migration of one set of anchoring struts, one to the intrahepatic inferior vena cava and the other to the right atrium (166). The Bird's Nest filter has been placed uneventfully in venae cavae with diameters of as much as 42 mm in one report of 18 patients with vena cava diameters greater than 28 mm (162). No filter migration was seen in the 10 patients who underwent plain radiographic follow-up in this group; the mean follow-up was 12 weeks (162).

Titanium Greenfield Filter

The titanium Greenfield filter is similar in design to the stainless steel Greenfield filter but is slightly longer at 4.7 cm and wider at the filter base at 38 mm (Figure 69–6)

(94,167). It is approximately half the weight of the stainless steel Greenfield filter and is placed using a 12 French carrier through a 14 French sheath (94,167). The filter is not placed over a guide wire. Titanium has demonstrated biocompatibility comparable with that of stainless steel (167).

The original version of the titanium Greenfield filter had hooks at the base of each filter strut, similar in design to those of the stainless steel Greenfield filter. However, this filter design was plagued by a high incidence of filter migration (27%) (94) as well as by unacceptably high rates of penetration of the cava or adjacent structures (13%) (94,167–169). Therefore, the filter hooks were modified by curving them to limit penetration and angling them 80 degrees to minimize migration (94). The modified design demonstrated improvement in the rates of migration 1 cm or greater and filter penetration of the cava to 11% and 0.8%, respectively (94).

Another concern with the titanium Greenfield design is the frequent crossing of one or more pairs of filter struts after deployment, reported in 7.4% of 181 cases in one

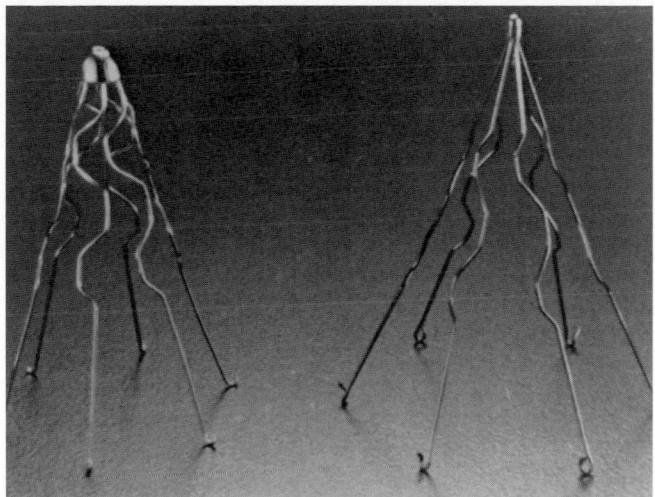

Figure 69–6 Photograph of the titanium Greenfield filter (*right*), with the stainless steel Greenfield filter (*left*) for comparison. (Reprinted with permission from Greenfield LJ, Cho KJ, Pais SO, et al. Preliminary clinical experience with the titanium Greenfield vena caval filter. Arch Surg 1989;124:657–659.)

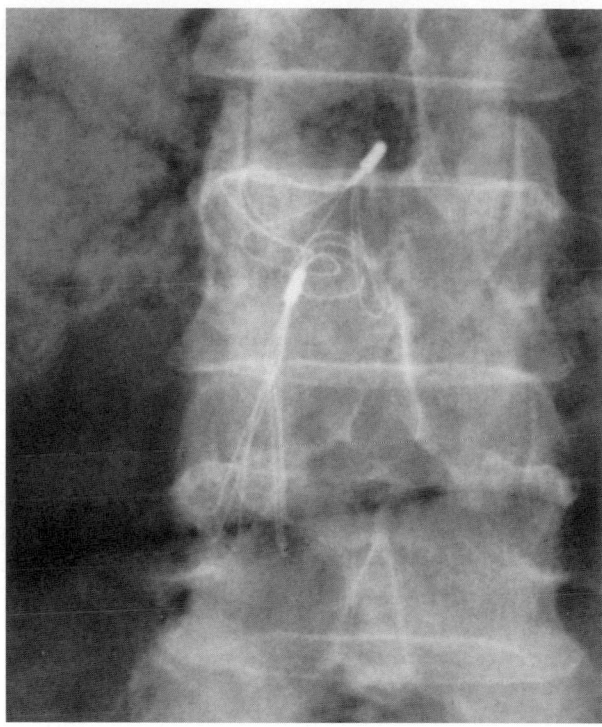

Figure 69–7 Radiograph of the Simon nitinol filter. The film demonstrates slight tilting of the filter petals compared with the longitudinal axis of the vena cava.

series (94). The crossing results in uneven segmentation of the vena cava and in some cases may be unsatisfactory, requiring placement of an additional filter. In the experience of one of the authors, crossing of the legs is less frequently seen with jugular placement, possibly because of the presentation of the filter struts on deployment, as opposed to the apical presentation with femoral placement.

In clinical trials, the titanium Greenfield filter has demonstrated similar clot-trapping effectiveness as the stainless steel Greenfield filter (94,167). Pulmonary embolism after filter placement was clinically suspected in 3% of 181 patients in one series (94). No patients were clinically suspected of having thrombosis of the inferior vena cava, although patients were followed for only 30 days in this study (94). Thrombosis of the insertion site has been reported in 3.0–8.7% of patients (94,167).

Simon Nitinol Filter

The Simon nitinol filter (Bard) is composed of a nickel–titanium alloy that has thermal memory (Figure 69–7). This filter is annealed in a predetermined shape at high temperature. When cooled, the filaments become pliable, and the filter can be straightened for introduction. Initially, the filter was cooled with iced saline as it was introduced. As it warmed on contact with blood, it assumed its molded configuration within seconds. Cooling with iced saline has since been found to be unnecessary, and the newer delivery system is simply flushed with room-temperature heparinized saline. The filter is 3.8 cm long, and the filter dome has a diameter of 28 mm (170). The filter is placed through a 9 French outer diameter introducer. It has six radiating legs projected from the center of the filter, each with a hook designed to minimize motion of the filter within the vena

cava. The filter has a second tier of struts located cranially to the anchoring struts consisting of seven wire loops arranged in the configuration of the petals of a flower for additional filtration.

In preliminary data from 103 patients with Simon nitinol filters placed at 17 centers, the recurrent pulmonary embolism rate was 3% (170). The same series reported occlusion of the inferior vena cava in 14% and insertion site thrombosis in 11%. Patient deaths resulting from pulmonary embolism or related to caval thrombosis with the use of the Simon nitinol filter have been described (106,171). Three cases of migration to the heart or pulmonary arteries have been published (172,173). Although tilting of the dome of the filter was observed in 55% of 44 patients, it has been stated that this does not affect filter effectiveness (170). In one of the largest series published to date, the number of patients undergoing objective testing for each of these outcomes is not specified.

Thrombosis of the vena cava after filter placement has been the major disadvantage of the Simon nitinol filter. Rates of caval occlusion as high as 21% of 24 patients were reported in one series (174). The possibility of more frequent occurrence of vena caval occlusion in patients with malignancies has been raised, although the number of patients on which this conclusion was based is small (174). Filter penetration has been documented by imaging studies in 5 of 20 patients (25%), including penetration of the aorta in two patients (172). Tilting of the cephalad cluster of loops in undersized venae cavae has been observed, and it has been postulated that this may impart excessive torque on the filter-anchoring struts, increasing the likelihood of penetration of the vena cava (172). This series confirmed the ability of this filter to prevent pulmonary embolism; no clinically suspected postfilter emboli were seen in 20 patients with mean follow-up of 14 months (172).

The relatively small delivery system and room-temperature flexibility of the Simon nitinol vena cava filter allows placement from virtually any access site, including the left jugular system and the antecubital veins The Simon nitinol filter is used at the authors' institution most frequently in patients who do not have traditional routes of venous access, in those in whom smaller access site diameters are preferred because of expected difficulty in obtaining hemostasis, or in those who require peripherally inserted central catheters for long-term venous access. In the final group, the delivery system, usually in the arm, is simply exchanged for the requested catheter at the end of the procedure.

LGM Vena Tech Filter

The LGM Vena Tech filter (B. Braun) is cone shaped and has six flat, radiating struts. It measures 38 mm high with a base width of 30 mm and is designed for cavae 28 mm or less in diameter (Figure 69–8). The filter is composed of an MRI-compatible stainless steel alloy called Elgiloy, which is stamped and point welded. Six longitudinal side rails are attached to the struts at the base of the filter parallel to the wall of the vena cava. They are designed to contact the wall

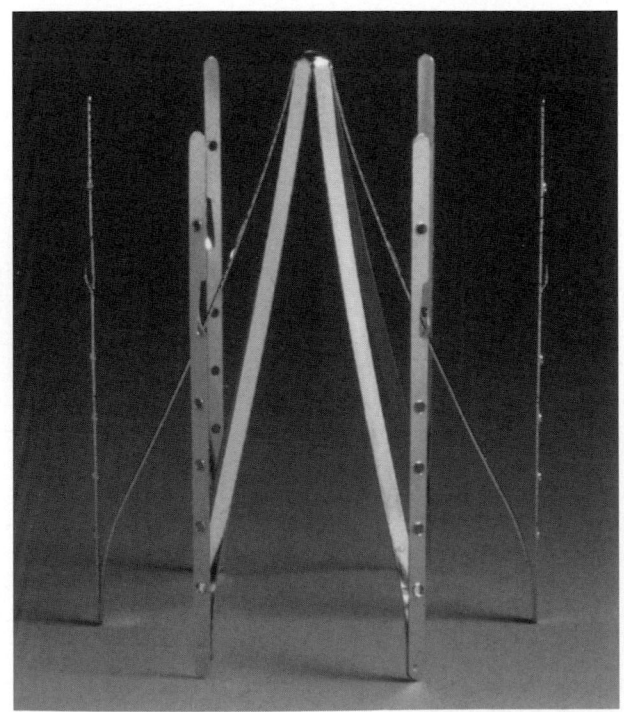

Figure 69–8   Lateral photograph of the LGM Vena Tech filter.

of the vena cava throughout their length, providing centering and transverse stability (85). The side rails were shorter than the diagonal struts in the original design. Hooks are punched from the metal at the cephalad ends of the side rails to provide longitudinal stability. The filter is inserted in the proper orientation (apex or base leading) into its delivery sheath with a syringe device, allowing flexibility of femoral or jugular use with one kit. The filter is deployed through a 14.6 French outer diameter sheath without a guide wire. This filter must be deployed rapidly from its constraining sheath because slow deployment may result in incomplete opening of the filter (85). After incomplete opening was reported in as many as 42% of filters placed by the jugular approach (175), the side rails were lengthened to nearly equal the height of the deployed filter. This was done to minimize crossing of the side rails with the diagonal struts during filter deployment, which could result in incomplete opening of the filter (85).

The LGM filter has been used in Europe since 1985 (176); use in the United States began in 1989 (85). This filter is one of the most thoroughly and objectively evaluated filters to date, with four large studies reporting mostly imaging-based follow-up (85,176–178). The filter is effective in preventing recurrent pulmonary embolism. In six large series involving a total of 704 patients, recurrent pulmonary embolism rates of 0–3.5% were reported (85,176–180).

Occlusion of the inferior vena cava (IVC) was studied in the first series by cavography in 90 patients 1 year after filter placement and was present in 7 (8%) (176). In the second series, 60 patients underwent routine imaging studies, and the probability of vena cava patency at 8 months was 92% (85). A higher rate of thrombotic occlusion of the vena cava was reported in the third series, seen by sonography or autopsy in 14 of 64 patients, for a rate of IVC occlusion of 22% (178). This result is considerably higher than that of other reports of short follow-up (85,176) and was not confirmed in other series, in which rates of IVC occlusion of 8% of 39 patients and 4.5% of 222 patients were reported (177,180). In a recently published series with 9-year follow-up, the patency of the inferior vena cava as documented by transabdominal duplex ultrasound or phlebocavography was 92% after 2 years but then continued to decrease by approximately 5% per year thereafter, to 66.8% at 9 years (179,181). Though these rates are lower than those reported for the stainless steel Greenfield filter, the difference may be attributable to closer scrutiny of the LGM filter with imaging studies, which were not used to document long-term stainless steel Greenfield patency. Because the filter material is biologically stable and the normal vena cava is a high-flow structure, spontaneous thrombosis is unlikely without constriction of the vein lumen (172). Narrowing of the filter base was highly correlated with thrombosis of the vena cava in these series (179,181). Although in previous experience this was felt to be a result of retraction of thrombus, it is possible that the filter side rails incite a hyperplastic or fibrotic response in the vein wall that results in narrowing and occlusion (179). Whether this feature is unique to the LGM filter awaits further study.

Thrombosis of the insertion site following placement of the LGM Vena Tech filter has been reported in 6% and 23% of patients in two series in which this was evaluated (85,178). Significant filter migration has been reported to occur at rates between 3.6% and 14% (85,176,177,180). One centimeter is assumed to be the minimum for significant migration when assessing filter stability because shorter migration cannot be reliably distinguished from perceived change resulting from parallax.

In combined data from several series, only 0.4–4.5% of patients demonstrated filter angulation greater than 15 degrees (85,177,178,180), which is the minimum angulation required to reduce filtration ability (49). This is attributed to the longitudinal side rails on the LGM Vena Tech filter, which provide transverse stability. One filter was noted to have spontaneously fractured on follow-up (177,182). Caval penetration of 2 and 5 mm was reported in one series, documented by computed tomography and ultrasound (178).

Vena Tech Low-Profile Filter

The Vena Tech Low-Profile (LP) filter is the second generation of the side-rail support system introduced by the Vena Tech LGM filter. Instead of six flat struts and side rails, the filter cone is fashioned from an Elgiloy wire, bent in a zigzag to create essentially eight cone struts with eight side-rail wires. Cephalad and caudally directed fixation hooks and an apical sleeve are then welded onto the device (Figure 69–9). As with the LGM Vena Tech device, Elgiloy is an MRI-compatible alloy. The filter is 43 mm high with a 40 mm base, meaning that although it is currently recommended for use in 28-mm cavae, it could potentially become

approved for vessels with a slightly larger diameter (34–35 mm). Its construction from thin, flexible wire allows insertion into a 9 French outer-diameter delivery sheath using a syringe-type plunger and passage from right or left sides. This makes a single kit applicable for femoral or jugular access. The brachial/subclavian system is pending FDA review. Limited published reports on the device are available.

TrapEase Filter

The TrapEase Filter (Cordis) is a symmetric, double-cone design fabricated from a nitinol alloy tube that is laser cut. It consists of opposing baskets, each formed by six diamond-shaped wire polygons joined at one end to form the cephalic and caudal apices and linked to the opposing basket by side rails at the other end (Figure 69–10). The filter length is dependent on the filter's expanded diameter and ranges between 50 and 60 mm, making it one of the longer devices. It is recommended for use in cavae 30 mm or less in diameter and can be delivered from either jugular, femoral, or antecubital access through its 8 French outer-diameter sheath. The device was approved for use by the FDA in 2000. Small series have demonstrated recurrent pulmonary embolism rates of 0–0.5% (183,184). Follow-up is limited, and outcome data have not been rigorously based on imaging criteria. In vitro evaluations have shown that the bilevel filtration provided by this design may be more effective at trapping small emboli (185). Case reports have raised concerns about inferior vena cava thrombosis rates, migration, and increased propensities for J-tipped guide wire entrapment (183,186,187). The device has fixation hooks on its connecting struts and is a permanent filter.

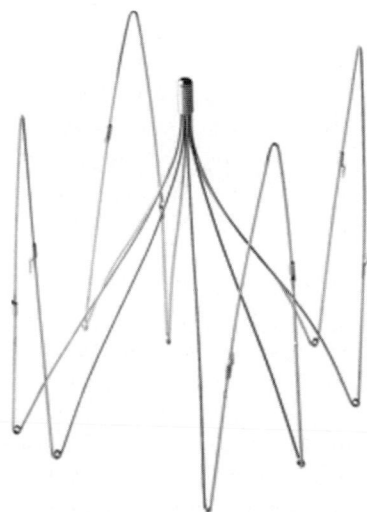

Figure 69–9 Lateral photograph of Vena Tech Low-Profile filter. (Reprinted with permission. © B. Braun Medical Inc.)

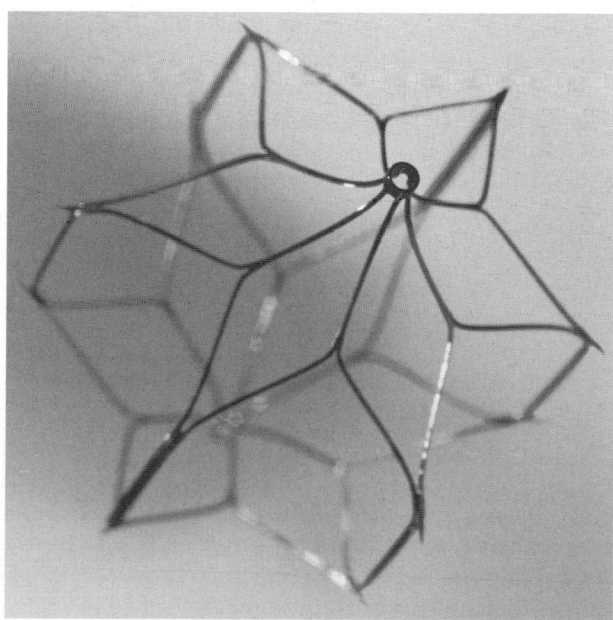

Figure 69–10 Photograph of the TrapEase filter, which utilizes cephalad and caudal baskets to provide dual-level filtration. (Reprinted with permission. © Cordis Corporation 2003.)

Günther Tulip Vena Cava MREye Filter

The Günther Tulip Vena Cava MREye filter (Cook) is cone shaped with four radiating struts projecting outward and downward from its apex to form an "x" when viewed on end. Each 0.45-mm strut has a wire loop wrapped around it several millimeters from its distal hooked end with the loop ends fixed to the cone apex. There is a cephalad-directed hook at the Elgiloy filter's apex. The design resembles an inverted tulip when postioned in the inferior vena cava. The filter is 45 mm high with a 30-mm base and is approved by the FDA for permanent placement in cavae of 28 mm or less diameter. The 8.5 French outer-diameter delivery sheath is 45 or 80 cm long for jugular or femoral access, respectively. Though used in the United States only since 2001, the device has been used in Europe since the early 1990s. In one multicenter study, the reported rate of recurrent pulmonary embolism with this device is similar to others, at 3.6%, as is the reported 9.6% rate of caval thrombosis (188).

The system is used as a permanent or retrievable filter in Europe and Canada (189,190) and is being evaluated for FDA approval for retrieval in the United States (190). Retrievability may be desirable in the patient with a transient contraindication to anticoagulation, such as recent trauma or recent or impending surgery. It is also a feature with intuitive appeal because deep venous and pulmonary thromboembolic disease is usually time limited and because of concerns about long-term durability and safety of permanent devices. Multiple reports describe successful Günther Tulip retrieval, which is performed using a goose-neck wire loop snare and 11 French sheath to remove the device via the right or left jugular vein (Figure 69–11). The manufacturer recommends removal within 10 days because endothelialization occurs between 12 and 14 days (191). Millward et al. reported 98% successful retrieval between 2 and 25 days after implantation (190), and Tay described repeated Günther Tulip repositioning within the inferior vena cava to allow extension of its implanation time to 19 days prior to closure of a patent foramen ovale (192). Like many contemporary filter designs, conclusions about the Tulip must be tempered by short-term follow-up and limited numbers reported.

Recovery Vena Cava Nitinol Filter

The Recovery vena cava nitinol filter (RNF) (Bard) is the most recently FDA approved device. It was approved for permanent placement in 2002 and in 2003 became the first design to be approved as a removable filter in the United States. The RNF is composed of twelve 0.13-inch nitinol wires that are joined at the apex of a two-tiered cone by a nitinol sleeve. The upper tier comprises six arms without fixation hooks. The lower tier is formed by six legs, each with a curved fixation hook at the end. The device is intended to function as a dual-level filter, similar to the Simon nitinol filter. Its base is 32 mm in diameter, its

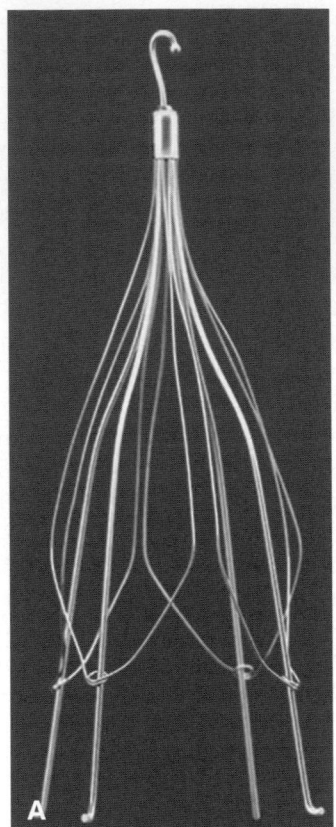

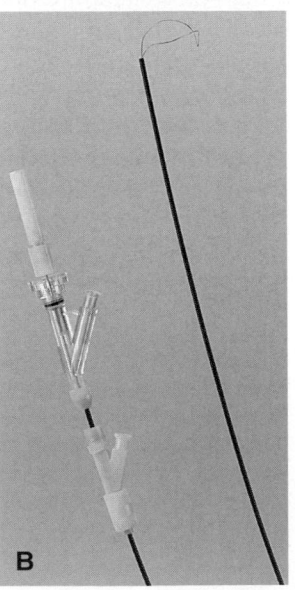

Figure 69–11   Though currently approved for permanent use in the United States, the Günther Tulip Vena Cava MREye is designed to be removable using its **A.** cephalic hook and **B.** a sheath-snare combination (Reprinted with permission. © Cook Inc. 2003.)

height is 40 mm, and it is recommended for placement in cavae of 28 mm or less in diameter. It is delivered through a 7 French delivery system and, like other contemporary designs fashioned from thermal-memory alloys, it requires flush only with standard, room-temperature heparinized

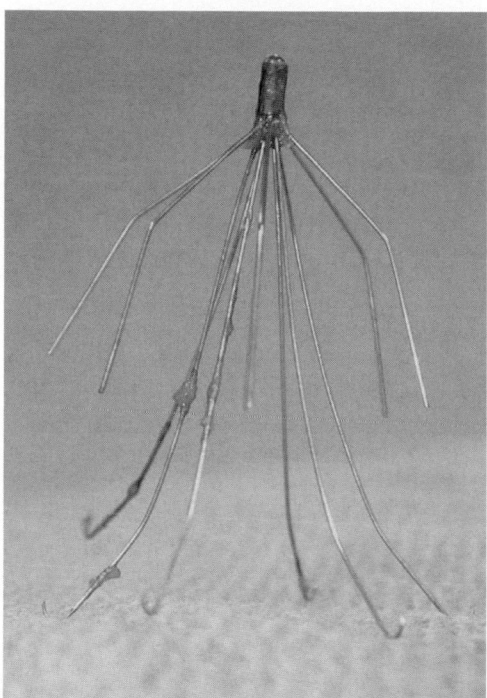

Figure 69–12 The Recovery filter is approved for permanent and temporary use. It has no recommended maximum implantation time. The above device was removed without complication at 134 days. (Reprinted with permission. © C.R. Bard Inc. 2003.)

saline. The device is removed via a 10 French jugular sheath using a retrieval cone consisting of nine metal claws with a urethane cover. A single published report described 0% documented recurrent pulmonary embolism, 0% documented vena caval thrombosis, 0% site thrombosis, and 100% successful retrieval after an average implantation time of 53 days (Figure 69–12). Though the study suggests the possibility of much longer temporary implantation, it was very small, comprising 32 patients in whom 24 filters were retrieved. Similar to most filter studies, it relied on clinical follow-up rather than serial imaging. The report did describe a 4 cm cephalad migration of one filter, which was found to have a large burden of trapped clot requiring removal through a 20 French sheath (193).

SUMMARY

Because of the high mortality rate for untreated thromboembolic disease, mechanical interruption of the inferior vena cava is necessary in patients with this condition who cannot be treated medically with anticoagulation, or in those who suffer pulmonary embolism or proximal propagation of thrombus while adequately anticoagulated. High-risk situations exist, such as large, free-floating iliac or vena cava thrombus or deep venous thromboembolism and poor cardiopulmonary reserve, that warrant caval interruption in addition to anticoagulation. Prophylactic indications may include patients who are without documented

thromboembolic disease but are at extremely high risk for its development and not good candidates for anticoagulation. Partial interruption of the vena cava by percutaneous placement of a vena cava filter is the method of choice for achieving this objective and is optimally performed with image guidance following imaging of the vena cava.

Nine vena cava filters are available in the United States: the stainless steel over-the-wire Greenfield filter, the titanium Greenfield filter, the Bird's Nest filter, the Simon nitinol filter, the LGM Vena Tech filter, the Vena Tech Low-Profile filter, the TrapEase filter, the Günther Tulip Vena Cava MREye filter, and the Recovery filter. Of these, the Greenfield filter design may be slightly less effective in removing small emboli from the bloodstream than the Bird's Nest, Simon nitinol, or TrapEase filters. However, it is equally effective in preventing clinically significant pulmonary embolism and may have a better rate of patency of the vena cava after placement, and it is the most extensively proven design clinically. The Bird's Nest and dual-level filters may be more efficient at trapping small emboli and therefore may be useful in patients unable to tolerate small pulmonary emboli, such as those with cor pulmonale or chronic lung disease. The Bird's Nest filter is ideal in patients with mega vena cava (>28 mm in diameter). The newer low-profile or flexible systems, including the Simon nitinol and TrapEase filters, may be more useful in patients without traditional routes of access for filter placement. Removable designs such as the Recovery and potentially Günther Tulip filters may expand and modify the indications for filter use and allow tailored implantation based on the temporally limited nature of thromboembolic risk in some patients. Because superiority of one filter design over the others has not been proved with significant differences in clinical outcome, it is likely that the actual differences are minor and that no filter is perfect for all patients. If and when a randomized clinical trial clearly elucidates the relative benefits of each of these devices, then the ideal filter for all scenarios may become evident. Until then, the choice of which filter to use remains best made on an individual basis.

REFERENCES

1. Evans AJ, Sostman HD, Knelson MH, et al. Detection of deep venous thrombosis: prospective comparison of MR imaging with contrast venography. AJR Am J Roentgenol 1993;161:131–139.
2. Ferris EJ. Deep venous thrombosis and pulmonary embolism: correlative evaluation and therapeutic implications. AJR Am J Roentgenol 1992;159:1149–1155.
3. Harmon B. Deep vein thrombosis: a perspective on anatomy and venographic analysis. J Thorac Imaging 1989;4:15–19.
4. Bick RL. Hereditary and acquired thrombophilia: preface. Semin Thromb Hemost 1999;25:251–253.
5. Homans J. Deep quiet venous thrombosis in the lower limb: preferred levels for interruption of veins; iliac sector or location. Surg Gynecol Obstet 1994;79:70–82.
6. Moser KM. Pulmnary embolism. Am Rev Respir Dis 1977;115:829–852.
7. Horattas MC, Wright DJ, Fenton AH, et al. Changing concepts of deep venous thrombosis of the upper extremity: report of a series and review of the literature. Surgery 1988;104:561–567.

8. Monreal M, Lafoz E, Ruiz J, et al. Upper-extremity deep venous thrombosis and pulmonary embolism: a prospective study. Chest 1991;99:280–283.

9. Barker NW, Nygaard KK, Walters W, et al. Statistical study of post-operative venous thrombosis and pulmonary embolism: time of occurrence during post-operative period. Proc Staff Meet Mayo Clin 1941;16:17–23.

10. Barritt DW, Jordan SC. Anticoagulant drugs in the treatment of pulmonary embolism: a controlled trial. Lancet 1960;1:1309–1312.

11. Rohrer MJ, Scheidler MG, Wheeler HB, et al. Extended indications for placement of an inferior vena cava filter. J Vasc Surg 1989;10:44–50.

12. Norris CS, Greenfield LJ, Herrmann JB. Free-floating iliofemoral thrombus: a risk of pulmonary embolism. Arch Surg 1985;120:806–808.

13. Radomski JS, Jarrell BE, Carabasi RA, et al. Risk of pulmonary embolus with inferior vena cava thrombosis. Am Surg 1987;53:97–101.

14. Virchow R, Chance F, trans. Cellular Pathology. New York: Dewitt, 1860.

15. Hoagland PM. Massive pulmonary embolus. In: Goldhaber SZ, ed. Pulmonary embolism and deep venous thrombosis. Philadelphia: Saunders, 1985:179.

16. Hunter J. Observation on inflammation of internal coat of veins. Trans Soc Improvement Med Chir Knowledge (London) 1793;1:18.

17. Greenfield LJ, DeLucia A. Endovascular therapy of venous thromboembolic disease. Surg Clin North Am 1992;72:969–989.

18. Bauer G. Venous thrombosis: early diagnosis with the aid of phlebography and abortive treatment with heparin. Arch Surg 1941;43:462.

19. DeBakey ME, Schroeder FG, Ochsner A. Significance of phlebography in phlebothrombosis. JAMA 1943;123:738–744.

20. Jaques LB. Addendum: the discovery of heparin. Semin Thromb Hemostas 1978;4:350–353.

21. Allen EV, Barker NW, Waugh JM. A preparation from spoiled sweet clover. JAMA 1942;120:1009–1015.

22. Seidman M, Robertson DN, Link KP. Studies on 4-hydroxy-coumarins: X. acyclation of 3-(alpha-phenyl-beta-acetylethyl)-4-hydrocycoumarin. J Am Chem Soc 1950;72:5193–5195.

23. Crane C. Femoral vs. caval interruption for venous thromboembolism. N Engl J Med 1964;270:819–821.

24. Mozes M, Adar R, Bogokowsky H, Agmon M. Vein ligation in the treatment of pulmonary embolism. Surgery 1964;55:621–629.

25. Nasbeth DC, Moran JM. Reassessment of the role of inferior vena cava ligation in venous thromboembolism. N Engl J Med 1965;273:1250–1253.

26. Adams JT, Feingold BE, DeWeese JA. Comparative evaluation of ligation and partial interruption of the inferior vena cava. Arch Surg 1971;103:272–276.

27. Amador E, Kai T, Crane C. Ligation of inferior vena cava for thromboembolism: clinical and autopsy correlations in 119 cases. JAMA 1968;206:1758–1760.

28. Garner AMN. Inferior vena caval interruption in prevention of fatal pulmonary embolism. Am Heart J 1972;84:537.

29. Piccone VA, Vidal E, Yarnoz M, et al. The late results of caval ligation. Surgery 1970;68:980–998.

30. Ferris EJ, Vittimberga FJ, Byrene JJ, et al. The inferior vena cava after ligation and plication. Radiology 1967;89:1–10.

31. Gurewich V, Thomas DP, Rabinov K. Pulmonary embolism after ligation of the inferior vena cava. New Engl J Med 1966;274:1350–1354.

32. Spencer FC, Quattlebaum JK, Sharp EH, et al. Plication of the IVC for pulmonary embolism: a report of 20 cases. Ann Surg 1962;155:827.

33. Miles RM, Elsea PW. Clinical evaluation of the serrate vena caval clip. Surg Gynecol Obstet 1971;132:581–587.

34. Eberlein TJ, Carey LC. Comparison of surgical management for pulmonary embolus. Ann Surg 1974;179:836–841.

35. Miles RM. Prevention of pulmonary embolism by the use of a plastic vena caval clip. Ann Surg 1966;163:192–198.

36. Moretz W, Rhode C, Shepard M. Prevention of pulmonary emboli by partial occlusion of the inferior vena cava. Ann Surg 1959;25:617.

37. Adams JT, DeWeese JA. Experimental and clinical evaluation of partial vein interruption in prevention of pulmonary embolism. Surgery 1965;57:82–102.

38. Mobin-Uddin K, McLean R, Bolooki H, Jude JR. Caval interruption for prevention of pulmonary embolism. Arch Surg 1969;99:711–715.

39. Maraan BM, Taber RE. The effects of inferior vena caval ligation on cardiac output: an experimental study. Surgery 1968;63:966–969.

40. Mobin-Uddin K, Utley JR, Bryant LR. The inferior vena cava umbrella filter. Prog Cardiovasc Dis 1975;17:391–399.

41. McIntyre AB, McCready RA, Hyde GL, et al. A ten-year follow-up study of the Mobin-Uddin filter for vena cava interruption. Surg Gynecol Obstet 1984;513–516.

42. Wingerd M, Bernhard VM, Maddison F, et al. Comparison of caval filters in the management of venous thromboembolism. Arch Surg 1978;113:1264–1271.

43. Gomez GA, Cutler BS, Wheeler HB. Transvenous interruption of the inferior vena cava. Surgery 1983;93:612–619.

44. Menzoian JO, LoGerfo FW, Weitzman AF, et al. Clinical experience with the Mobin-Uddin vena cava umbrella filter. Arch Surg 1980;115:1179–1181.

45. McConnel D, Mulder D, Buckberg G. The placement of vena cava umbrella filters: the value of phlebography. Arch Surg 1974;108:789–791.

46. Bernstein E. The place of venous interruption in the treatment of pulmonary thromboembolism. In: Moser K, Stein M, eds. Pulmonary thromboembolism. Chicago: Year Book, 1973:312–323.

47. Cimochowski GE, Evans RH, Zarins CK, et al. Greenfield filter versus Mobin-Uddin umbrella. J Thorac Cardiovasc Surg 1980;79:358–365.

48. Tadavarthy SM, Castaneda-Zuniga W, Salomonowitz E, et al. Kimray-Greenfield vena cava filter: percutaneous introduction. Radiology 1984;151:525–526.

49. Katsamouris AA, Waltman AC, Delichatsios MA, et al. Inferior vena cava filters: in vitro comparison of clot trapping and flow dynamics. Radiology 1988;166:361–366.

50. Thompson BH, Cragg AH, Smith TP, et al. Thrombus-trapping efficiency of the Greenfield filter in vivo. Radiology 1989;172:979–981.

51. Greenfield LJ, Michna BA. Twelve-year clinical experience with the Greenfield vena caval filter. Surgery 1988;104:706–712.

52. Greenfield LJ, Proctor MC. Twenty-year clinical experience with the Greenfield filter. Cardiovasc Surg 1995;3:199–205.

53. Greenfield LJ, Proctor MC, Cho KJ, et al. Extended evaluation of the titanium Greenfield vena caval filter. J Vasc Surg 1994;20:458–464.

54. Pais SO, Tobin KD. Percutaneous insertion of the Greenfield filter. AJR Am J Roentgenol 1989;152:933–938.

55. Kantor A, Glanz S, Gordon DH, et al. Percutaneous insertion of the Kimray-Greenfield filter: incidence of femoral vein thrombosis. AJR Am J Roentgenol 1987;149:1065–1066.

56. Pais SO, Tobin KD, Austin CB, et al. Percutaneous insertion of the Greenfield inferior vena cava filter: experience with ninety-six patients. J Vasc Surg 1988;8:460–464.

57. Rose BS, Simon DC, Hess ML, et al. Percutaneous transfemoral placement of the Kimray-Greenfield vena cava filter. Radiology 1987;165:373–376.

58. Shetty PC, Bok LR, Sharma RP. Balloon dilation of the femoral vein expediting percutaneous Greenfield vena caval filter placement. Radiology 1986;161:275.

59. Dorfman GS, Cronan JJ, Paolella LP, et al. Iatrogenic changes at the venotomy site after percutaneous placement of the Greenfield filter. Radiology 1989;173:159–162.

60. Ammann ME, Eibenberger K, Winkelbauer F, et al. Rate of thrombosis after cava filter implantation. Longterm results. (German) Ultraschall Med 1994;15:95–98.

61. Hicks ME, Middleton WD, Picus D, et al. Prevalence of local venous thrombosis after transfemoral placement of a Bird's Nest vena caval filter. J Vasc Interv Radiol 1990;1:63–68.

62. Becker DM, Philbrick JT, Selby JB. Inferior vena cava filters: indications, safety, effectiveness. Arch Intern Med 1992;152:1985–1994.

63. Decousus H, Leizorovicz A, Parent F, et al. A clinical trial of vena caval filters in the prevention of pulmonary embolism in patients with proximal deep-vein thrombosis. N Engl J Med 1998; 338:409–415.

64. Kazmers A, Jacobs LA, Perkins AJ. Pulmonary embolism in veterans affairs medical centers: is vena cava interruption underutilized? Am Surg 1999;65:1171–1175.

65. Athanasoulis CA, Kaufman JA, Halpern EF, et al. Inferior vena caval filters: review of a 26-year single-center clinical experience. Radiology 2000;216:54–66.

66. Engmann E, Asch MR. Clinical experience with the antecubital Simon nitinol IVC filter. J Vasc Interv Radiol 1998;9:774–778.

67. Stavropoulos SW, Clark T, Jacobs D, et al. Placement of a vena cava filter with an antecubital approach. Acad Radiol 2002;9:478–481.

68. Davison BD, Grassi CJ. TrapEase inferior vena caval filter placed via the basilic arm vein: a new antecubital access. J Vasc Interv Radiol 2002;13:107–109.

69. Dorfman GS, Esparza AR, Cronan JJ. Percutaneous large bore venotomy and tract creation: comparison of sequential dilator and angioplasty balloon methods in a porcine model, preliminary report. Invest Radiol 1988;23:441–446.

70. Pais SO, Mirvis SE, De Orchis DF. Percutaneous insertion of the Kimray-Greenfield filter: technical considerations and problems. Radiology 1987;165:377–381.

71. Roberts AC, Geller SC, Waltman AC, et al. Kimray-Greenfield inferior vena cava filter: safety of percutaneous insertion via the femoral vein. Radiology 1987;165(P):204.

72. Martin KD, Kempczinski RF, Fowl RJ. Are routine inferior vena cavograms necessary before Greenfield filter placement? Surgery 1989;106:647–651.

73. Prince MR, Novelline RA, Athanasoulis CA, et al. The diameter of the IVC and its implication for the use of vena cava filters. Radiology 1983;149:687–689.

74. Brown DB, Pappas JA, Vedantham S, et al. Gadolinium, carbon dioxide, and iodinated contrast material for planning inferior vena cava filter placement: a prospective trial. J Vasc Interv Radiol 2003;14:1017–1022.

75. Kaufman JA, Geller SC, Bazari H, Waltman AC. Gadolinium-based contrast agents as an alternative at vena cavography in patients with renal insufficiency—early experience. Radiology 1999;212:280–284.

76. Holtzman RB, Lottenberg L, Bass T, et al. Comparison of carbon dioxide and iodinated contrast for cavography prior to inferior vena cava filter placement. Am J Surg 2003;185:364–368.

77. Sing RF, Stackhouse DJ, Jacobs DG, et al. Safety and accuracy of bedside carbon dioxide cavography for insertion of inferior vena cava filters in the intensive care unit. J Am Coll Surg 2001;192:168–171.

78. Boyd-Kranis R, Sullivan KL, Eschelman DJ, et al. Accuracy and safety of carbon dioxide inferior vena cavography. J Vasc Interv Radiol 1999;10:1183–1189.

79. Dewald CL, Jensen CC, Park YH, et al. Vena cavography with CO(2) versus with iodinated contrast material for inferior vena cava filter placement: a prospective evaluation. Radiology 2000; 216:752–757.

80. Gamblin TC, Ashley DW, Burch S, et al. A prospective evaluation of a bedside technique for placement of inferior vena cava filters: accuracy and limitations of intravascular ultrasound. Am Surg 2003;69:382–386.

81. Ebaugh JL, Chiou AC, Morasch MD, et al. Bedside vena cava filter placement guided with intravascular ultrasound. J Vasc Surg 2001;34:21–26.

82. Conners MS 3rd, Becker S, Guzman RJ, et al. Duplex scan-directed placement of inferior vena cava filters: a five-year institutional experience. J Vasc Surg 2002;35:286–291.

83. Mewissen MW, Erickson SJ, Foley WD, et al. Thrombosis at venous insertion sites after inferior vena caval filter placement. Radiology 1989;173:155–157.

84. Molgaard CP, Yucel EK, Geller SC, et al. Access-site thrombosis after placement of inferior vena cava filters with 12–14F delivery sheaths. Radiology 1992;185:257–261.

85. Murphy TP, Dorfman GS, Yedlicka JW, et al. LGM vena cava filter: objective evaluation of early results. J Vasc Interv Radiol 1991;2:107–115.

86. Marcy PY, Magne N, Frenay M, et al. Renal failure secondary to thrombotic complications of suprarenal inferior venacava filter in cancer patients. Cardiovasc Intervent Radiol 2001; 24:257–259.

87. Greenfield LJ, Proctor MC. Suprarenal filter placement. J Vasc Surg 1998;28:432–438.

88. Matchett WJ, Jones MP, McFarland DR, et al. Suprarenal vena caval filter placement: follow-up of four filter types in 22 patients. J Vasc Interv Radiol 1998;9:588–593.

89. Ascher E, Hingorani A, Tsemekhin B, et al. Lessons learned from a 6-year clinical experience with superior vena cava Greenfield filters. J Vasc Surg 2000;32:881–887.

90. Spence LD, Gironta MG, Malde HM, et al. Acute upper extremity deep venous thrombosis: safety and effectiveness of superior vena caval filters. Radiology 1999;210:53–58.

91. Lidagoster MI, Widman WE, Chevinski AH. Superior vena caval occlusion after filter insertion. J Vasc Surg 1994;20:158–159.

92. Roehm JOF, Johnsrude IS, Barth MH, et al. The bird's nest inferior vena cava filter: progress report. Radiology 1988;168:745–749.

93. Epstein DH, Darcy MD, Hunter DW, et al. Experience with the Amplatz retrievable vena cava filter. Radiology 1989;172:105–110.

94. Greenfield LJ, Cho KJ, Proctor M, et al. Results of a multicenter study of the modified hook-titanium Greenfield filter. J Vasc Surg 1991;14:253–257.

95. Tobin KD, Pais SO, Austin CB. Reevaluation of indications for percutaneous placement of the Greenfield filter. Invest Radiol 1989;24:115–118.

96. Hirsh J. Treatment of pulmonary embolism. Annu Rev Med 1987;38:91–105.

97. Hayes SP, Bone RC. Pulmonary emboli with respiratory failure. Med Clin North Am 1983;67:1179–1191.

98. Mansour M, Chang AE, Sindelar WF. Interruption of the inferior vena cava for the prevention of recurrent pulmonary embolism. Am Surg 1985;51:375–380.

99. Carter BL, Jones ME, Waickman LA. Pathophysiology and treatment of deep-vein thrombosis and pulmonary embolism. Clin Pharmacol 1985;4:279–296.

100. Petitti DB, Strom BL, Melmon KL. Duration of warfarin anticoagulant therapy and the probabilities of recurrent thrombolism. Am J Med 1986;81:255–259.

101. Wessler S, Gitel SN. Warfarin from bedside to bench. N Engl J Med 1984;311:645–652.

102. Moore FD, Osteen RT, Karp DD, et al. Anticoagulants, venous thromboembolism, and the cancer patient. Arch Surg 1981;161:405–407.

103. Landfeld CS, Cook EF, Flatley M, et al. Identification and preliminary validation of predictors of major bleeding in hospitalized patients starting anticoagulant therapy. Am J Med 1987;82:703–713.

104. Mant MJ, O'Brien BD, Thong KL, et al. Haemorrhagic complications of heparin therapy. Lancet 1977;1:1133–1135.

105. Belt RJ, Leite C, Haas CD, et al. Incidence of hemorrhagic complication in patients with cancer. JAMA 1978;239:2571–2574.

106. Doyle DJ, Turpie AGG, Hirsh J, et al. Adjusted subcutaneous heparin or continuous intravenous heparin in patients with acute deep vein thrombosis. Ann Intern Med 1987;107:441–445.

107. King DJ, Kelton JG. Heparin-associated thrombocytopenia. Ann Intern Med 1984;100:535–540.

108. Proctor MC. Indications for filter placement. Semin Vasc Surg 2000;13:194–198.

109. Thery C, Asserman P, Amrouni N, et al. Use of a new removable vena cava filter in order to prevent pulmonary embolism in patients submitted to thrombolysis. Eur Heart J 1990;11:334–341.

110. Sevitt S, Gallagher N. Venous thrombosis and pulmonary embolism: a clinico-pathological study in injured and burned patients. Br J Surg 1961;48:475–489.

111. Kakkar VV, Howe CT, Flanc C, et al. Natural history of postoperative deep-vein thrombosis. Lancet 1969;2:230–233.

112. Jarrell BE, Posuniak E, Roberts J, et al. A new method of management using the Kimray-Greenfield filter for deep venous thrombosis and pulmonary embolism in spinal cord injury. Surg Gynecol Obstet 1983;157:316–320.

113. Lambie JM, Mahaffy RG, Barber DC, et al. Diagnostic accuracy in venous thrombosis. Br Med J 1970;2:142–143.

114. Cronan JJ, Froehlich JA, Dorfman GS. Image-directed Doppler ultrasound: a screening technique for patients at high risk to develop deep vein thrombosis. J Clin Ultrasound 1991;19:133–138.

115. Woolson ST, McCrory DW, Walter JF, et al. B-mode ultrasound scanning in the detection of proximal venous thrombosis after total hip replacement. J Bone Joint Surg 1990;72:983–987.

116. Leyvraz PF, Richard J, Bachmann F, et al. Adjusted versus fixed-dose subcutaneous heparin in the prevention of deep-vein thrombosis after total hip replacement. N Engl J Med 1983;309:954–958.

117. Marcy PY, Magne N, Gallard JC, et al. Cost-benefit assessment of inferior vena cava filter placement in advanced cancer patients. Support Care Cancer 2002;10:76–80.

118. Schwarz RE, Marrero AM, Conlon KC, et al. Inferior vena cava filters in cancer patients: indications and outcome. J Clin Oncol 1996;14:652–657.

119. Lossef SV, Barth KH. Outcome of patients with advanced neoplastic disease receiving vena caval filters. J Vasc Interv Radiol 1995;6:273–277.

120. Shackford SR, Davis JW, Hollingsworth-Fridlung P, et al. Venous thromboembolism in patients with major trauma. Am J Surg 1990;159:365–369.

121. Khansarinia S, Dennis JW, Veldenz HC, et al. Prophylactic Greenfield filter placement in selected high-risk trauma patients. J Vasc Surg 1995;22:231–236.

122. Rogers FB, Strindberg G, Shackford SR, et al. Five-year follow-up of prophylactic vena cava filters in high-risk trauma patients. Arch Surg 1998;133:406–412.

123. Duperier T, Mosenthal A, Swan KG, et al. Acute complications associated with Greenfield filter insertion in high-risk trauma patients. J Trauma 2003;54:545–549.

124. Rogers FB, Cipolle MD, Velmahos G, et al. Practice management guidelines for the prevention of venous thromboembolism in trauma patients: the EAST practice management guidelines work group. J Trauma 2002;53:142–164.

125. Maxwell RA, Chavarria-Aguilar M, Cockerham WT, et al. Routine prophylactic vena cava filtration is not indicated after acute spinal cord injury. J Trauma 2002;52:902–906.

126. Langan EM 3rd, Miller RS, Casey WJ 3rd, et al. Prophylactic inferior vena cava filters in trauma patients at high risk: follow-up examination and risk/benefit assessment. J Vasc Surg 1999;30:484–488.

127. Jarrett BP, Dougherty MJ, Calligaro KD. Inferior vena cava filters in malignant disease. J Vasc Surg 2002;36:704–707.

128. Ihnat DM, Mills JL, Hughes JD, et al. Treatment of patients with venous thromboembolism and malignant disease: should vena cava filter placement be routine? J Vasc Surg 1998;28:800–807.

129. Rosen MP, Porter DH, Kim D. Reassessment of vena cava filter use in patients with cancer. J Vasc Interv Radiol 1994;5:501–506.

130. Offner PJ, Hawkes A, Madayag R, et al. The role of temporary inferior vena cava filters in critically ill surgical patients. Arch Surg 2003;138:591–594.

131. Watanabe SI, Shimokawa S, Moriyama Y, et al. Clinical experience with temporary vena cava filters. Vasc Surg 2001;35:285–290.

132. Millward SF, Bhargava A, Aquino J Jr, et al. Günther Tulip filter: preliminary clinical experience with retrieval. J Vasc Interv Radiol 2000;11:75–82.

133. Linsenmaier U, Rieger J, Schenk F, et al. Indications, management, and complications of temporary inferior vena cava filters. Cardiovasc Intervent Radiol 1998;21:64–69.

134. Dorfman GS, Cronan JJ, Tupper TB, et al. Occult pulmonary embolism: a common occurrence in deep venous thrombosis. AJR Am J Roentgenol 1987;148:263–266.

135. Huisman MV, Buller HR, ten Cate JW, et al. Unexpected high prevalence of silent pulmonary embolism in patients with deep venous thrombosis. Chest 1989;95:498–502.

136. Moran JM, Kahn PC, Callow AD. Partial versus complete caval interruption for venous thromboembolism. Am J Surg 1969;117:471–479.

137. Strandness DE, Langlois Y, Cramer M, et al. Long-term sequelae of acute venous thrombosis. JAMA 1983;250:1289–1292.

138. Lindner DJ, Edwards JM, Phinney ES, et al. Long-term hemodynamic and clinical sequelae of lower extremity deep vein thrombosis. J Vasc Surg 1986;4:436–442.

139. Browse NL, Clemenson G, Thomas ML. Is the postphlebitic leg always postphlebitic? Relation between phlebographic appearances of deep-vein thrombosis and late sequelae. Br Med J 1980;281:1167–1170.

140. Mudge M, Hughes LE. The long term sequelae of deep vein thrombosis. Br J Surg 1978;65:692–694.

141. Athanasoulis CA. Complications of vena cava filters. Radiology 1993;188:614–615.

142. Streiff MB. Vena caval filters: a comprehensive review. Blood 2000;95:3669–3677.

143. Murphy TP, Cronan JJ. Evolution of deep venous thrombosis: a prospective evaluation with US. Radiology 1990;177:543–548.

144. Grassi CJ, Swan TL, Cardella JF, et al. Quality improvement guidelines for percutaneous permanent inferior vena cava filter placement for the prevention of pulmonary embolism. J Vasc Interv Radiol 2001;12:137–141.

145. Greenfield LJ, Rutherford RB. Recommended reporting standards for vena caval filter placement and patient follow-up. J Vasc Surg 1999;30:573–579.

146. Levy JM, Duszak RL Jr, Akins EW, et al. Inferior vena cava filter placement. American College of Radiology. ACR appropriateness criteria. Radiology 2000;215:981–997.

147. Grassi CJ. Inferior vena caval filters: analysis of five currently available devices. AJR Am J Roentgenol 1991;156:813–821.

148. Rousseau H, Perreault P, Otal P, et al. The 6-F nitinol TrapEase inferior vena cava filter: results of a prospective multicenter trial. J Vasc Interv Radiol 2001;12:299–304.

149. Greenfield LJ, Proctor MC. The percutaneous Greenfield filter: outcomes and practice patterns. J Vasc Surg 2000;32:888–893.

150. Yune HY. Inferior vena cava filter: search for an ideal device. Radiology 1989;172:15–16.

151. Grassi CJ. Inferior vena caval filters: analysis of five currently available devices. AJR Am J Roentgenol 1991;156:813–821.

152. Palestrant AM, Prince M, Simon M. Comparative in vitro evaluation of the nitinol inferior vena cava filter. Radiology 1982;145:351–355.

153. Millward SF, Marsh JI, Pon C, et al. Thrombus-trapping efficiency of the LGM (Vena Tech) and titanium Greenfield filters in vivo. J Vasc Interv Radiol 1992;3:103–106.

154. Xian ZY, Roy S, Hosaka J, et al. Multiple embolic and filter function: an in vitro comparison of three vena cava filters. J Vasc Interv Radiol 1995;6:887–893.

155. Qian Z, Yasui K, Nazarian GK, et al. In vitro and in vivo experimental evaluation of a new vena caval filter. J Vasc Interv Radiol 1994;5:513–518.

156. Simon M, Rabkin DJ, Kleshinski S, et al. Comparative evaluation of clinically available inferior vena cava filters with an in vitro physiologic simulation of the vena cava. Radiology 1993;189:769–774.

157. Greenfield LJ, Proctor MC. Experimental embolic capture by asymmetric Greenfield filters. J Vasc Surg 1992;16:436–444.

158. Greenfield LJ, Proctor MC, Cho KJ, et al. Limb asymmetry in titanium Greenfield filters: clinically significant? J Vasc Surg 1997;26:770–775.

159. Kinney TB, Rose SC, Weingarten KW, et al. IVC filter tilt and asymmetry: comparison of the over-the-wire stainless-steel and titanium Greenfield IVC filters. J Vasc Interv Radiol 1997;8:1080–1082.

160. Greenfield LJ, Peyton R, Crute S, et al. Greenfield vena caval filter experience: late results in 156 patients. Arch Surg 1981;116:1451–1456.

161. Denny DF, Cronan JJ, Dorfman GS, et al. Percutaneous Kimray-Greenfield filter placement by femoral vein puncture. AJR Am J Roentgenol 1985;145:827–829.

162. Reed RA, Teitelbaum GP, Taylor FC, et al. Use of the bird's nest filter in oversized inferior venae cavae. J Vasc Interv Radiol 1991;2:447–450.

163. Korbin CD, Reed RA, Taylor FC, et al. Comparison of filters in an oversized vena caval phantom: intracaval placement of a bird's nest filter versus biliac placement of Greenfield, Vena Tech-LGM, and Simon nitinol filters. J Vasc Interv Radiol 1992;3:559–564.

164. Wojtowycz MM, Stoehr T, Crummy AB, et al. The Bird's Nest inferior vena caval filter: review of a single-center experience. J Vasc Interv Radiol 1997;8:171–179.

165. Nicholson AA, Ettles DF, Paddon AJ, et al. Long-term follow-up of the Bird's Nest IVC Filter. Clin Radiol 1999;54:759–764.

166. Rogoff PA, Hilgenberg AD, Miller SL, et al. Cephalic migration of the bird's nest inferior vena caval filter: report of two cases. Radiology 1992;184:819–822.

167. Greenfield LJ, Cho KJ, Pais SO, et al. Preliminary clinical experience with the titanium Greenfield vena caval filter. Arch Surg 1989;124:657–659.

168. Teitelbaum GP, Jones DL, van Breda A, et al. Vena caval filter splaying: potential complication of use of the titanium Greenfield filter. Radiology 1989;173:809–814.

169. Ramchandani P, Koolpe HA, Zeit RM. Splaying of titanium Greenfield inferior vena caval filter. AJR Am J Roentgenol 1990; 155:1103–1104.

170. Simon M, Athanasoulis CA, Kim D, et al. Simon nitinol inferior vena cava filter: initial clinical experience. Radiology 1989;172: 99–103.

171. Dorfman GS. Percutaneous inferior vena caval filters. Radiology 1990;174:987–992.

172. McCowan TC, Ferris EJ, Carver DK, et al. Complications of the nitinol vena caval filter. J Vasc Interv Radiol 1992;3:401–408.

173. LaPlante JS, Contractor FM, Kiproff PM, et al. Migration of the Simon nitinol vena cava filter to the chest. AJR Am J Roentgenol 1993;160:385–386.

174. Grassi CJ, Matsumoto AH, Teitelbaum GP. Vena caval occlusion after Simon nitinol filter placement: identification with MR imaging in patients with malignancy. J Vasc Interv Radiol 1992; 3:535–539.

175. Reed RA, Teitelbaum GP, Taylor FC, et al. Incomplete opening of LGM (Vena Tech) filters inserted via the transjugular approach. J Vasc Interv Radiol 1991;2:441–445.

176. Ricco JB, Crochet D, Sebilotte P, et al. Percutaneous transvenous caval interruption with the "LGM" filter: early results of a multi-center trial. Ann Vasc Surg 1988;2:242–247.

177. Taylor FC, Awh MH, Kahn CE, et al. Vena Tech vena cava filter: experience and early follow-up. J Vasc Interv Radiol 1991;2: 435–440.

178. Millward SF, Marsh JI, Peterson RA, et al. LGM (Vena Tech) vena cava filter: clinical experience in 64 patients. J Vasc Interv Radiol 1991;2:429–433.

179. Crochet DP, Stora O, Ferry D, et al. Vena Tech-LGM filter: long-term results of a prospective study. Radiology 1993;188:857–860.

180. Ricco JB, Dubreuil F, Reynaud P, et al. The LGM Vena-Tech caval filter: results of a multicenter study. Ann Vasc Surg 1995;9(Suppl): S89–S100.

181. Crochet DP, Brunel P, Trogrlic S, et al. Long-term follow-up of Vena Tech-LGM filter: predictors and frequency of caval occlusion. J Vasc Interv Radiol 1999;10:137–142.

182. Awh MH, Taylor FC, Lu C. Spontaneous fracture of a Vena Tech inferior vena caval filter. AJR Am J Roentgenol 1991;157: 177–178.

183. Schutzer R, Ascher E, Hingorani A, et al. Preliminary results of the new 6F TrapEase inferior vena cava filter. Ann Vasc Surg 2003;17:103–106.

184. Rousseau H, Perreault P, Otal P, et al. The 6-F nitinol TrapEase inferior vena cava filter: results of a prospective multicenter trial. J Vasc Interv Radiol 2001;12:299–304.

185. Lorch H, Dallmann A, Zwaan M, et al. Efficacy of permanent and retrievable vena cava filters: experimental studies and evaluation of a new device. Cardiovasc Intervent Radiol 2002; 25:193–199.

186. Stavropoulos SW, Itkin M, Trerotola SO. In vitro study of guide wire entrapment in currently available inferior vena cava filters. J Vasc Interv Radiol 2003;14:905–910.

187. Porcellini M, Stassano P, Musumeci A, et al. Intracardiac migration of nitinol TrapEase vena cava filter and paradoxical embolism. Eur J Cardiothorac Surg 2002;22:460–461.

188. Neuerburg JM, Günther RW, Vorwerk D, et al. Results of a multi-center study of the retrievable Tulip vena cava filter: early clinical experience. Cardiovasc Intervent Radiol 1997;20:10–16.

189. Millward SF. Günther Tulip retrievable filter: why, when and how? Can Assoc Radiol J 2001;52:188–192.

190. Millward SF, Oliva VL, Bell SD, et al. Günther tulip retrievable vena cava filter: results from the registry of the Canadian inter-national radiology association. J Vasc Interv Radiol 2001;12: 1053–1058.

191. Burbridge BE, Walker DR, Millward SF. Incorporation of the Günther temporary inferior vena cava filter into the caval wall. J Vasc Interv Radiol 1996;198:765–767.

192. Tay KH, Martin ML, Fry PD, et al. Repeated Günther Tulip infe-rior vena cava filter repositioning to prolong implantation time. J Vasc Interv Radiol 2002;13:509–512.

193. Asch MR. Initial experience in humans with a new retrievable inferior vena cava filter. Radiology 2002;225:835–844.

Percutaneous Vascular and Nonvascular Foreign Body Retrieval

70

Christoph A. Binkert, Frederick S. Keller, Josef Rösch

The first percutaneous foreign body removal was described in 1964 by Thomas et al. (1). A broken segment of a steel spring guide was removed from the right atrium and inferior vena cava using a bronchoscopic forceps that was inserted through a saphenous vein cutdown. In 1968, Henley and Ballard removed a foreign body from the heart percutaneously (2). Three years later, Dotter published the first series of 29 transvascular foreign-body retrievals, six of which were done percutaneously (3). In 1978, 180 cases of nonsurgical retrieval of intracardiac foreign bodies were reported in an international survey (4). Eighty percent of foreign bodies were central venous catheters cut by a needle. To this day, dislodged central venous catheters remain the majority of retrieved objects (Figure 70–1). With the introduction of many new devices, successful interventional retrieval of misplaced or subsequently displaced devices has become more frequent. Several reports of successfully retrieved vascular stents and coils have been published (5–10).

GENERAL CONSIDERATIONS

There are certain prerequisites to attempting percutaneous foreign body retrieval. First, the object should be visible. Because most retrievals are performed under fluoroscopic guidance, the object should be radiopaque. In certain instances, a nonradiopaque object can be visualized as a filling defect; for example, in the biliary tree or in the collecting system of the kidney. In the vascular territory, indirect filling requires a significant amount of contrast and is therefore less suitable. Alternatively, a different guidance modality such as ultrasound or magnetic resonance imaging could be considered. Second, the object size can limit percutaneous retrieval. Most lost foreign bodies, including wires and catheters, are introduced percutaneously through small holes and, therefore, have a small diameter. Other objects, such as vena cava filters, have the ability to collapse and can be used for successful percutaneous retrieval. In addition to the size, the object should not have sharp edges that could damage the vessel during the retrieval process. Third, the foreign body has to be in a location accessible by the percutaneous route. This requires that at least a portion of the foreign body be within the blood vessel, the collecting system of the kidney, or the biliary tree. Foreign bodies generally travel to a location where they become wedged. In the arterial system, typical locations are bifurcations or large branch vessels (Figure 70–2). In the venous system, the cut end of a catheter fragment is most commonly located either in front of the right ventricle—superior vena cava or right atrium (Figure 70–1)—or has traveled through the right ventricle to the pulmonary artery (4). Fourth, the object should not be incorporated in the vessel wall. Chronically retained foreign bodies could adhere to the vessel wall and, therefore, may not be amenable for retrieval. A catheter

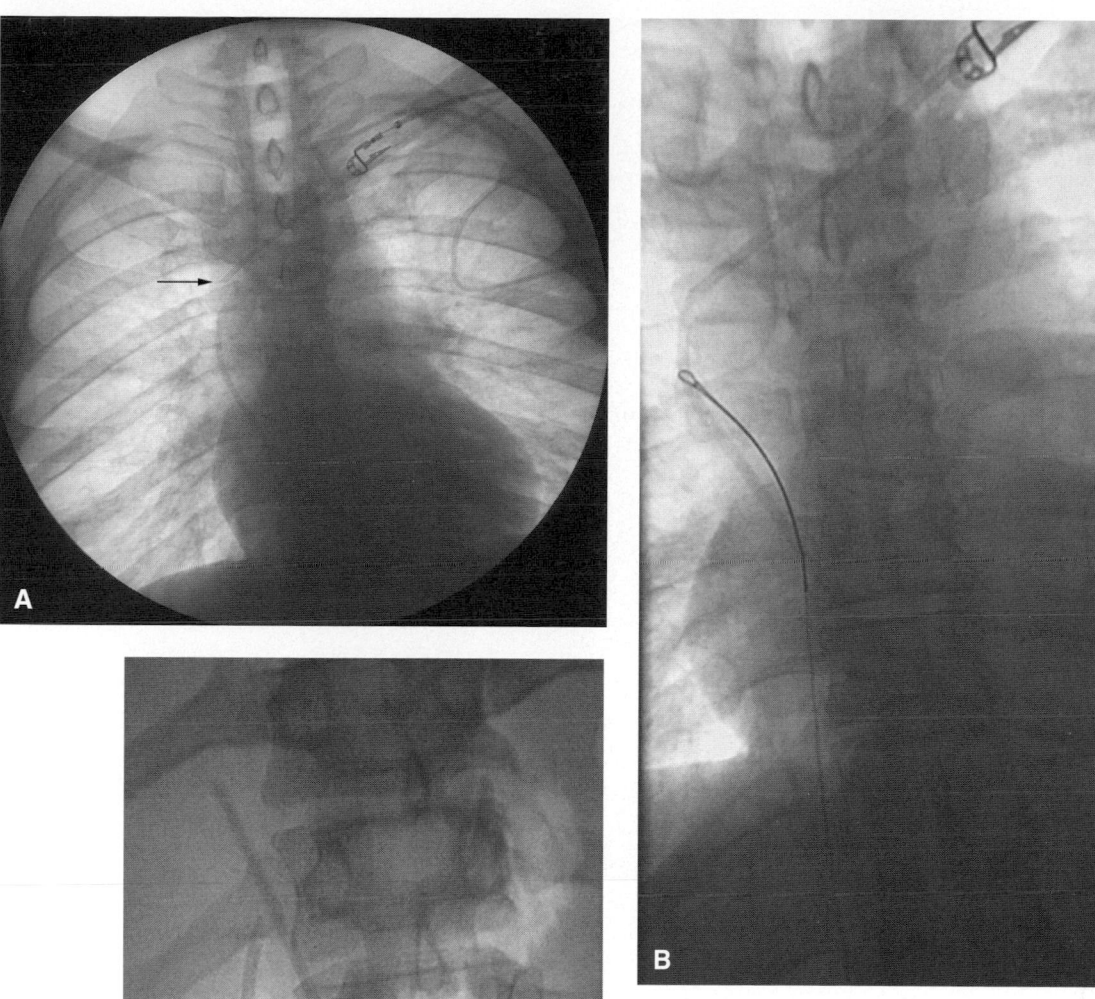

Figure 70–1 A. Broken central venous catheter (*arrow*) with central part of the catheter dislodged into the superior vena cava. **B.** Successful snaring of the broken catheter and pulling of the catheter segment into the **C.** inferior vena cava and into the 10 French sheath.

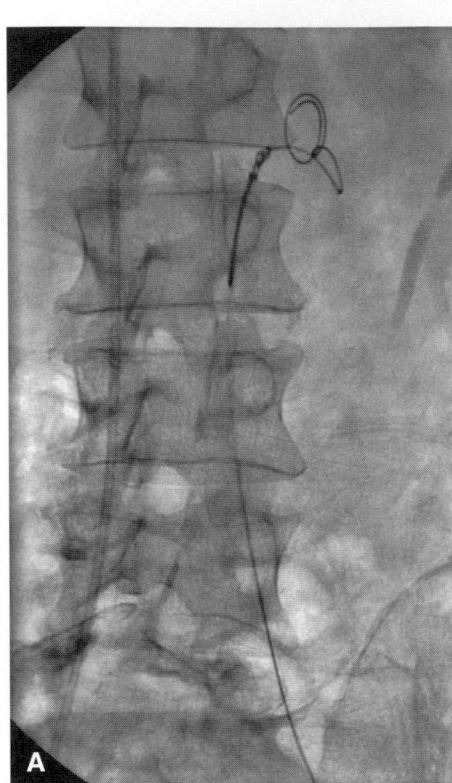

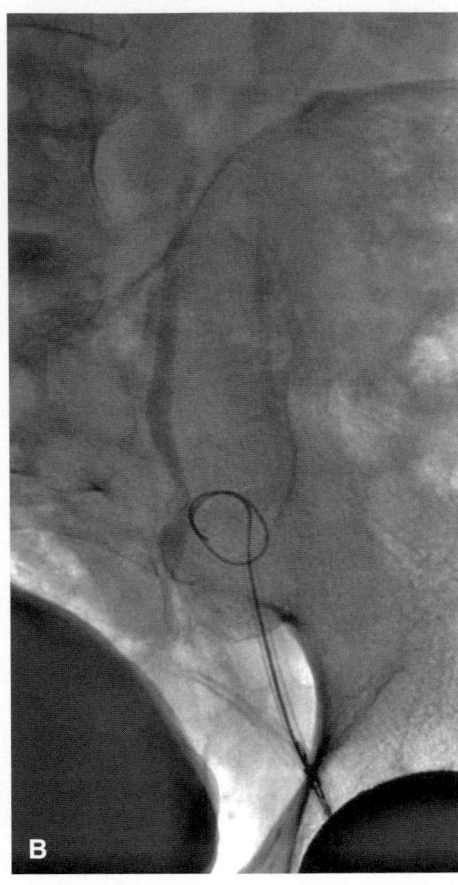

Figure 70–2 Lost coil during embolization of a large pulmonary arteriovenous malformation. The coil stopped at the left renal artery. **A.** Successful snaring and retrieval through a 6 French sheath in the **B.** left common femoral artery.

fragment indwelling for 6 years was found partially incorporated into the vessel wall (11). Recently, however, Savage et al. (12) reported a 100% success rate for retrieval of six chronically retained foreign bodies (5–90 days). One case report described a successful retrieval of a catheter fragment that had been lost for 11 years (13). Therefore, percutaneous foreign body removal can be attempted even for objects that are known to have been inside the patient for a long time. Lack of flotation under fluoroscopy can be an indirect sign that the foreign body is adherent to the vessel, but the reliability of this scenario is not proven.

TECHNIQUES AND TOOLS

The techniques and tools for any retrieval procedure must be chosen according to the individual circumstances. Certain principles however apply to every retrieval procedure. At the beginning of any retrieval procedure, an appropriate access site and sheath size must be selected. For foreign bodies in the arterial system, the common femoral artery is usually approached in either retrograde or antegrade fashion depending on the location of the foreign body. For retrievals in the venous system or the pulmonary

circulation, either the internal jugular vein or the common femoral vein can be used. Concerning the size of the access sheath, there is a simple rule: the bigger the better, especially for venous access. A 10 French sheath should be the minimal size for venous access. Upsizing of access during the procedure can be cumbersome, and there exists the potential drawback of losing a foreign body that already had been captured. After achieving access, the appropriate retrieval device must be navigated to the foreign body using standard angiographic technique.

From a technical point of view, there are two main situations regarding how a foreign body can present. Either one end of the foreign body is free or both ends are abutted against the wall. The use of a loop snare is the preferred technique of most interventionalists to grab the free end. The most commonly used snare is the nitinol "gooseneck" snare (Microvena). This snare has a 90-degree loop in different sizes ranging from 2–35 mm. For best performance, it is important to match the snare size to the vessel diameter. Within limits, if one loop could do it, more loops can do it sooner, especially when poor visibility impedes precise 3D control of the snaring maneuver. Following this rationale, the EN-Snare (Medical Device Technology) was designed with three nitinol loops (Figure 70–3). The EN-Snare loop ranges in size from 2–45 mm.

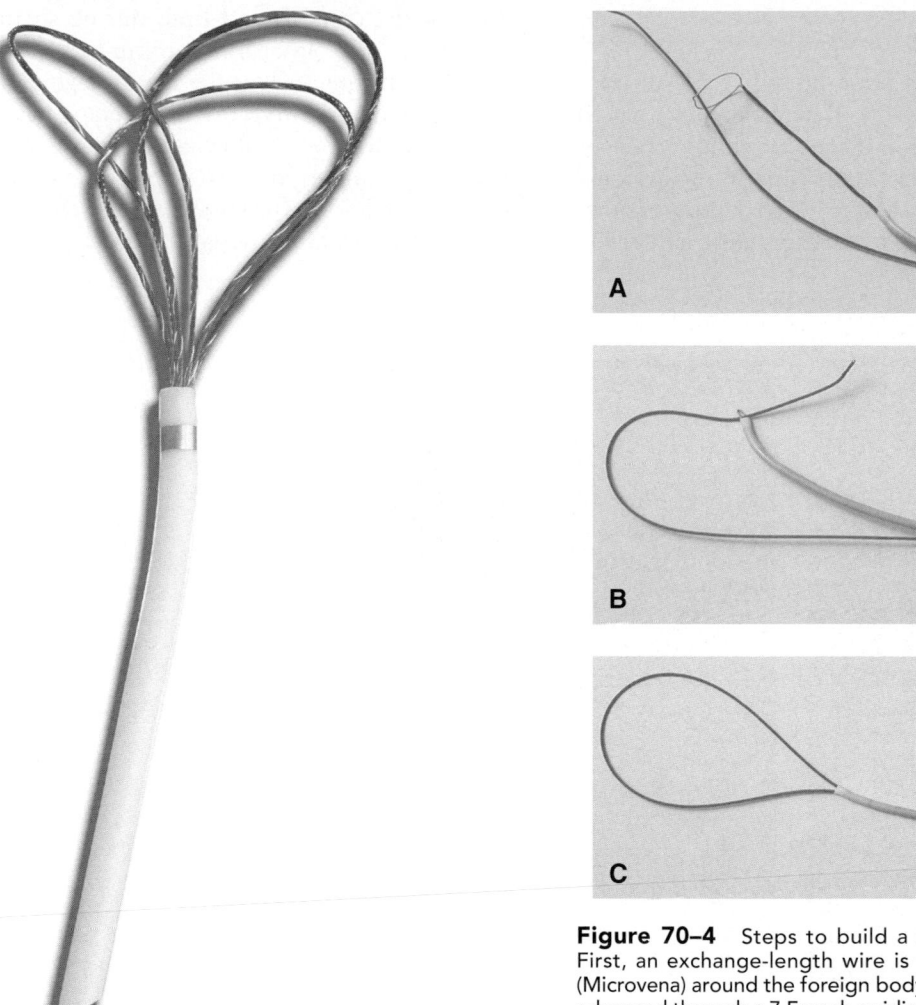

Figure 70–3   Three-dimensional loop snare consisting of three nitinol loops for easy grasping of foreign bodies (Medical Device Technology).

Figure 70–4   Steps to build a snare around a foreign body: First, an exchange-length wire is snared by a gooseneck snare (Microvena) around the foreign body. **A., B.** The gooseneck snare is advanced through a 7 French guiding catheter which itself is placed alongside the guide wire through a 10 French sheath. **C.** Then, the snared end of the guide wire is pulled out through the sheath, and the guiding catheter is readvanced over both wire ends creating a loop around the foreign body.

These closed-loop snares are unlikely to be effective when there is no free end to snare. In that situation, when no free end is available, there are two possible approaches. Either an attempt is made to free one end of the foreign, then it is snared as described earlier, or the object is grabbed directly. Different tools are available to free one end: hook-tip guide wires, pigtail catheters (preferably in 6 French or 7 French in size for better stability), or deflecting wires. These tools may be used alone or in combination. A suitable combination is a pigtail catheter and a deflecting wire: the pigtail can be spun around the object, while the deflecting wire adds the necessary strength to pull on the object. Alternatively, the object may be grabbed directly using a basket retriever system or forceps (3).

An elegant way to overcome the lack of a free end is to build a snare around the object (Figure 70–4). Because this approach is somewhat cumbersome, freeing one end to allow easy snaring should be attempted first.

In certain circumstances, special techniques may be required. Seong et al. (14) described a coaxial snare technique to retrieve tubular foreign bodies. This technique uses a monorail approach of a snare over a guide wire and is, therefore, especially useful when a guide wire is already through the lost object.

Sometimes, the foreign body cannot be removed percutaneously. However, a percutaneous approach can help move an object to a more favorable location. El Feghaly et al. (7) reported a successful dislodgment of a migrated stent from the right ventricle into the iliac vein using an angioplasty balloon allowing easy surgical removal. Whenever removal is not possible, a lost object may be moved to a safe location and placed there permanently. Such an approach is described by Meisel et al. (15) who have successfully moved dislodged stents from the coronary artery into the iliac artery. The stents were deployed in the iliac artery and secured by another peripheral stent.

DISCUSSION

The number of foreign body retrievals is likely to increase because of the increased number of percutaneously placed devices and the increased use of central venous catheters. While classic foreign body retrieval is performed for any lost object, snaring techniques have been adapted for other applications. Examples include snaring of the guide wire through the contralateral limb during aortic stent-graft placement or to establish continuity of an interrupted tubular structure, such as the ureter (Figure 70–5). Newer developments in interventional therapy have introduced techniques to remove intravascular devices intentionally. The best examples are retrievable filters that are placed with the intention to be removed when clinically no longer needed. Different filter designs allow either removal with a

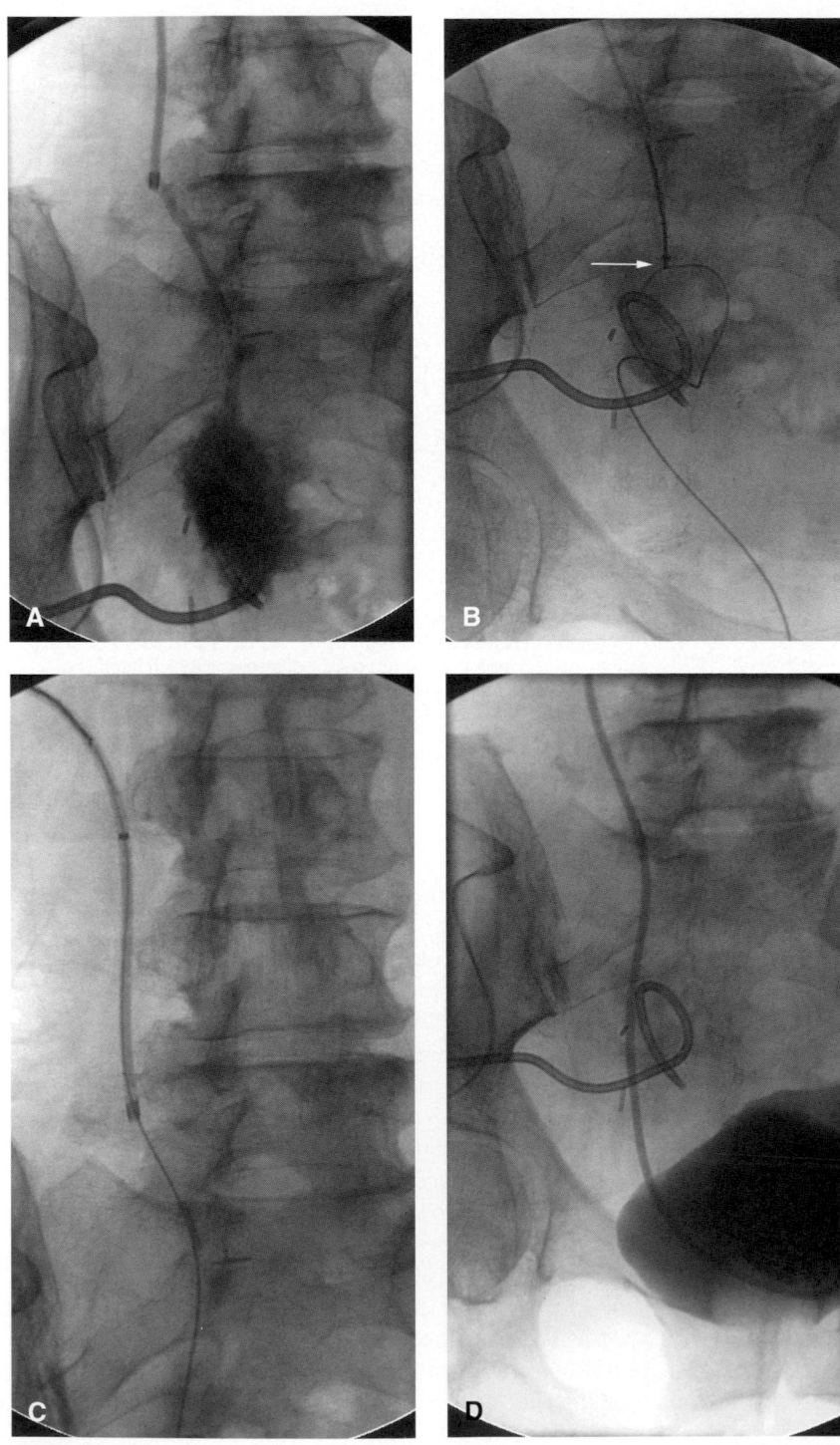

Figure 70–5   A. Postsurgical interruption of right ureter with contrast extravasation and transabdominal pigtail catheter placed for drainage. Recanalization of the ureter either from above or from below was not possible. **B.** Using a combined approach, a guide wire inserted via the distal ureter was snared from above (*arrow*). **C.** After pulling the guide wire through the nephrostomy, **D.** a ureteral stent was successfully placed.

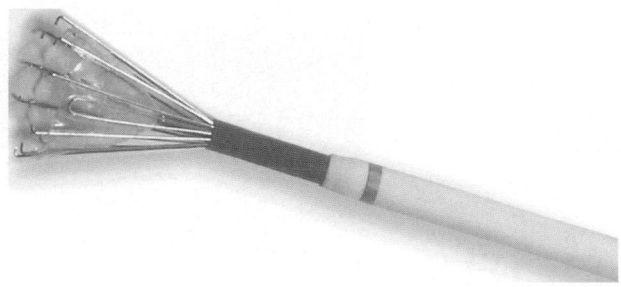

Figure 70–6 Recovery cone (peripheral vascular, BARD) specifically designed to retrieve BARD recovery filter.

standard loop snare, including the Tulip (Cook, Inc.) (16) and Optease (Cordis), or require a special retrieval cone, such as the Recovery filter (Bard peripheral) (Figure 70–6) (17). These temporary devices will also increase the number of retrieval procedures over the next few years.

Foreign body retrieval procedures, especially the classic retrieval of an accidentally lost foreign body, are different from other interventions in the sense that the procedure differs from case to case depending on the location and size of the foreign body. There is no standard or uniformly accepted retrieval procedure. Individual planning of every case is necessary. Basic strategies for a successful retrieval are described in the section about tools and techniques.

A high success rate, between 89.5% (6) and 97% (8), has been reported for percutaneous foreign body retrieval. With the development of dedicated retrieval devices such as the EN-Snare (Figure 70–3) or the Recovery cone (Figure 70–6), the rate of successful retrieval is likely to even climb. The complication rate for retrieval procedures is minimal. The biggest risk of foreign body retrieval is failure to remove it. Minor complications, such as transient arrhythmias while pulling an object from the pulmonary artery through the right ventricle, can occur. One case of mild, self-limiting hemoptysis has also been reported (12). Based on the high success rate and low morbidity, the percutaneous approach should be the treatment of choice for objects lost in the human body. Surgery is much more invasive and should, therefore, be reserved for cases in which the percutaneous approach is not feasible or has failed.

In summary, understanding foreign body retrieval is certainly important, but it should be remembered that preventing loss of objects in the human body by proper handling of intravascular devices and catheters is better.

REFERENCES

1. Thomas J, Sinclair-Smith B, Bloomfield D, et al. Non-surgical retrieval of a broken segment of steel spring guide from the right atrium and inferior vena cava. Circulation 1964;30:106–108.
2. Henley FT, Ballard JW. Percutaneous removal of flexible foreign body from the heart. Radiology 1969;92:176.
3. Dotter CT, Rösch J, Bilbao, MK. Transluminal extraction of catheter and guide fragments from the heart and great vessels: 29 collected cases. Am J Roentgenol Radium Ther Nucl Med 1971; 111:467–472.
4. Bloomfield DA. The nonsurgical retrieval of intracardiac foreign bodies—an international survey. Cathet Cardiovasc Diagn 1978;4:1–14.
5. Slonim SM, Dake MD, Razavi MK, et al. Management of misplaced or migrated endovascular stents. J Vasc Interv Radiol 1999;10:851 859.
6. Gabelmann A, Kramer S, Gorich J. Percutaneous retrieval of lost or misplaced intravascular objects. AJR Am J Roentgenol 2001; 176:1509–1513.
7. El Feghaly M, Soula P, Rousseau H, et al. Endovascular retrieval of two migrated venous stents by means of balloon catheters. J Vasc Surg 1998;28:541–546.
8. Egglin TK, Dickey KW, Rosenblatt M, et al. Retrieval of intravascular foreign bodies: experience in 32 cases. AJR Am J Roentgenol 1995;164:1259–1264.
9. Ashar RM, Huettl EA, Halligan R. Percutaneous retrieval of a Wallstent from the pulmonary artery following stent migration from the iliac vein. J Interv Cardiol 2002;15:101–106.
10. Davies RP, Voyvodic F. Percutaneous retrieval of a partially expanded iliac artery stent: case report. Cardiovasc Intervent Radiol 1992;15:120–122.
11. Reynen K. 14-year follow-up of central embolization by a guide wire. N Engl J Med 1993;329:970–971.
12. Savage C, Ozkan OS, Walser EM, et al. Percutaneous retrieval of chronic intravascular foreign bodies. Cardiovasc Intervent Radiol 2003;28:28.
13. Thanigaraj S, Panneerselvam A, Yanos J. Retrieval of an IV catheter fragment from the pulmonary artery 11 years after embolization. Chest 2000; 117:1209–1211.
14. Seong CK, Kim YJ, Chung JW, et al. Tubular foreign body or stent: safe retrieval or repositioning using the coaxial snare technique. Korean J Radiol 2002;3:30–37.
15. Meisel SR, DiLeo J, Rajakaruna M, et al. A technique to retrieve stents dislodged in the coronary artery followed by fixation in the iliac artery by means of balloon angioplasty and peripheral stent deployment. Catheter Cardiovasc Interv 2000;49:77–81.
16. Neuerburg JM, Gunther RW, Vorwerk D, et al. Results of a multicenter study of the retrievable Tulip Vena Cava Filter: early clinical experience. Cardiovasc Intervent Radiol 1997;20:10–16.
17. Asch MR. Initial experience in humans with a new retrievable inferior vena cava filter. Radiology 2002;225:835–844.

Hemangiomas and Vascular Malformations

71

Robert J. Rosen, Francine Blei

Vascular malformations have been described since antiquity but remain one of the most commonly misdiagnosed and mismanaged conditions in clinical medicine. Part of the difficulty lies in the relative rarity of these lesions, so few clinicians have gained adequate expertise in their diagnosis and management. Even clinicians with significant experience have discovered that these malformations are often difficult and frustrating disorders to manage. This is one area where the caveat "do no harm" is particularly applicable.

The first step, and possibly the most important, is correctly classifying a lesion encountered clinically. This is not merely an academic exercise; these lesions can resemble one another clinically but fall into several distinct categories, each of which has its own prognostic and therapeutic implications. Some can be predicted to involute spontaneously and require little or no intervention, while others progress relentlessly and may result in life-threatening complications. A review of the literature compounds the problem because various terms have been applied to these lesions over the years, resulting in confusion when attempting to interpret the results of various therapies (1). Many systems of classification have been described. For practical purposes, it is helpful to divide the lesions into five major categories: hemangioma (and other nonmalignant proliferative vascular lesions), arteriovenous fistula, arteriovenous malformation, venous malformation, and lymphatic malformation. Although this categorization is not exhaustive or based on pathogenesis, it is most helpful in prognostic and therapeutic terms. Each of these lesions is distinctive enough to be discussed separately.

HEMANGIOMA

The general consensus among experts in the field of vascular malformations is that the term *hemangioma* be applied to only a specific lesion. This lesion is the benign vascular neoplasm of endothelial cells generally encountered in infancy, characteristically progressing to a proliferative phase followed by spontaneous involution in most cases. The natural history and pathology of this lesion are therefore clearly different from true vascular malformations. The distinguishing features of the true hemangioma have been emphasized by Mulliken and Glowacki and are presented in Table 71–1 (2).

Hemangiomas are relatively common in infancy, occurring in approximately 10% of children in the first year of life (3). Hemangiomas may be present at birth or become manifest shortly thereafter and may be multiple in 20% of cases (4). Beginning as a small area of reddish discoloration, hemangiomas typically enter a proliferative phase in which growth can be dramatic. Pathologically, endothelial cell proliferation accounts for the rapid growth; this pattern of actual neoplastic cellular growth is not seen in true vascular malformations. Another distinguishing feature is the marked female to male predominance (3:1) as opposed to the equal distribution seen in vascular malformations.

The clinical course of the lesion during the proliferative phase depends largely on the location of the lesion. Superficial lesions may be quite disfiguring and may also show ulceration, bleeding, or infection (Figure 71–1). Lesions involving respiratory, visual, or digestive structures can present serious management problems. Very large lesions, particularly in the liver, can be associated with

TABLE 71–1

DISTINGUISHING FEATURES OF HEMANGIOMAS AND ARTERIOVENOUS MALFORMATIONS

Hemangioma	Arteriovenous Malformations
Neoplasm	Congenital anomaly
30% present at birth; remainder present in first 3 months	90% present at birth, although many not manifest
Proliferative phase: first year	Female:male is 1:1
Female:male is 5:1	No cellular proliferation
Endothelial proliferation	No growth in tissue culture
Growth in tissue culture	No mast cells
Cellular Stroma	No spontaneous involution— growth with individual
Increased mast cells	May or may not require treatment
Spontaneous involution in 95% by age 7	
No treatment required in vast majority	

Data from Mulliken JB, Glowacki J. Hemangiomas and vascular malformations in infants and children: a classification based on endothelial characteristics. Plast Reconstr Surg 1982;69:412.

high-output congestive heart failure (5). Many physicians are not aware that early referral to subspecialists can decrease morbidity and improve outcome for infants with proliferative hemangiomas. Unfortunately, it is still common to see deprivational amblyopia secondary to ptosis, unnecessary tracheotomies, and other unnecessary interventions resulting from inadequate information (6–8).

The most interesting (and fortunate) aspect of the natural history of the hemangioma is its tendency toward spontaneous regression. Fully 70% of these lesions will show substantial involution by the age of 7 years without treatment. The remainder of children show continued resolution until the age of 12 (9). It is apparent that many treatments described in the past owed their success to this tendency toward spontaneous involution. Involution may be complete, or there may be complete residual discoloration or redundant skin, in some cases requiring plastic surgical intervention.

Hemangioma Research

The unique nature of hemangiomas has made them an area of intense interest in the fields of angiogenesis, molecular biology, and genetics. Using DNA microarrays, Ritter and colleagues identified insulinlike growth factor 2 (IGF2) as a potentially important regulator of hemangioma growth (10,11). IGF2 was highly expressed during the proliferative phase and decreased during involution. This finding was confirmed at the messenger RNA level and at the protein level. Additionally, several angiogenesis-related factors (e.g., integrins $\alpha(v)\beta3$ and $\alpha5\beta1$) were

identified in proliferating hemangiomas, and an increase in several interferon-induced genes was observed in the involuting phase. These studies identify potential regulators of hemangioma growth and involution and provide a foundation on which to build further mechanistic investigations into angiogenesis. Other recent studies have identified endothelial precursor cells within hemangioma tissue as well as in the circulation of patients with hemangiomas. Ideally, studies of this nature could be designed to provide the molecular signature of those hemangiomas that warrant aggressive medical therapy.

The vast majority of hemangiomas appear to be sporadic, with a 3:1 predilection for females, more frequently involving the craniofacial regions, and seen commonly in premature infants. Complex hemangiomas are even more frequently seen in females, far above the expected 3:1 female to male ratio (12–14).

Sasaki et al. reported increased levels of circulating estradiol in patients with hemangiomas (15), and increased estrogen receptor expression was detected in hemangioma tissue. Lui et al. detected estrogen, progesterone, and androgen receptors in hemangioma tissues (16); however, recent findings are contradictory (17). The significance of these observations remains unclear but raises the question of the relationship between hormones and/or genetic factors in the pathophysiology of these lesions.

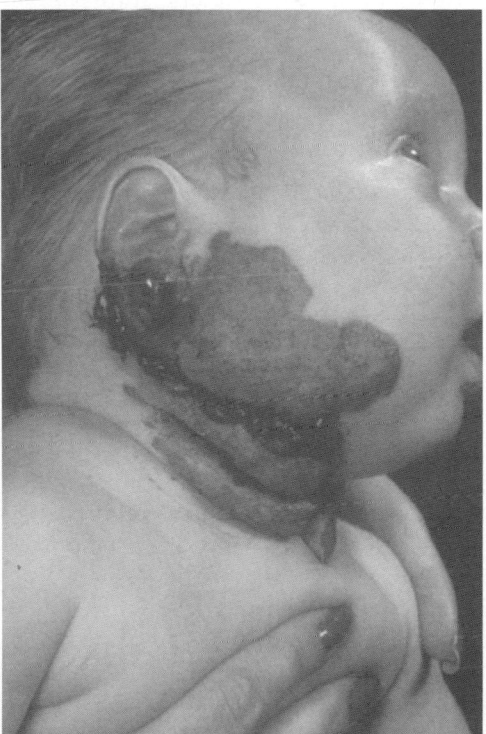

Figure 71–1 Extensive hemangioma in 6-month-old female during proliferative phase. Lesion is complicated by superficial ulceration and bleeding.

Loss of heterozygosity has been demonstrated in hemangioma tissues, suggesting clonality of sporadic hemangiomas (18,19). Furthermore, Walter et al. recently identified two unique somatic mutations in hemangioma specimens—in the vascular endothelial growth factor receptor (VEGFR) genes VEGFR2 (FLK-1/KDR) and VEGFR3 (FLT-4) (20).

Genetic mutations and inheritance patterns have been clearly identified in several hereditary vascular syndromes (21). Hereditary hemorrhagic telangiectasia (HHT) is associated with mutations of endoglin, or ALK-1, the activin receptor kinase gene, members of the TGF-receptor family (22).

Patients with the endoglin mutation appear predisposed to pulmonary arteriovenous malformations. At least three different loci for genetic mutations have been associated with familial cerebral cavernous malformations (CCM) (23,24,25).

One of the CCM genes (CCM1) maps to chromosome 7q and has been identified as KRIT1, a gene involved in G-protein signal transduction (25–29).

Glomus tumors may be of the paraganglionoma or glomangioma type. Although most cases occur sporadically, rare familial glomangiomas have been reported for both types. Paraganglionomas originate from the APUD cell system, and the underlying genetic defect has been mapped to chromosome 11q23 (30).

Glomangiomas are benign uni- or multifocal cutaneous vascular tumors involved in temperature regulation and are linked to chromosome 1p21-p22 in familial cases (31,32). The gene for hereditary lymphedema has been linked to distal chromosome 5q, an area to which vascular endothelial growth factor C receptor (FLT4) has been mapped (33,34). Additionally, the FLT4 gene has been identified as a marker for lymphatic endothelium during development, and VEGF-CR has been detected in lymphatic vasculature (35,36).

A mutation causing an activating mutation in the kinase domain of tie-2 was reported in two families with multiple members having mucosal venous vascular malformations (37).

Not only does this genetic information provide us with etiologic clues for vascular anomalies, but it also demonstrates which genes are important in normal vascular development. However, many questions remain—why are patients with Turner syndrome prone to lymphedema, why are hemangiomas more common in females, and why are hemangiomas so rare in the Black population?

Although most hemangiomas are sporadic, there are published reports of rare kindreds with "familial hemangiomas." A primary genetic alteration may lead to hemangioma development. Six families were recently reported with multiple generations affected by hemangiomas or vascular malformations. In contrast to the generally accepted gender ratio of 3–4:1 female to male seen in sporadic hemangiomas, the "hemangioma families" demonstrated a 2:1 ratio. Additionally, vascular malformations and hemangiomas were present in different members of the same family. The vascular lesions appeared to be transmitted in an autosomal dominant fashion with moderate to high penetrance. Genetic linkage analysis within hemangioma kindreds suggests a germline mutation with autosomal dominant segregation and linkage to chromosome 5q31–33 in some of these kindreds (38,39).

Important exceptions to the typical hemangioma growth/regression pattern are two recently recognized entities: rapidly involuting congenital hemangiomas (RICH), which are generally present in full form at birth (or even detected prenatally) and undergo rapid regression (40–43), and noninvoluting congenital hemangiomas (NICH), which are histologically and immunophenotypically different from typical hemangiomas of infancy (44).

Diagnosis

Most hemangiomas can be diagnosed on physical examination, particularly when the lesion is followed over a period of time (Figure 71–2). Superficial lesions, sometimes referred to as "strawberry birthmarks," are bright red, while deeper lesions may show only a bluish discoloration or simply a soft tissue mass that may require a biopsy for diagnosis (Figure 71–3A). On palpation, these lesions are firm and spongy, reflecting the dense cellular stroma that is found pathologically. As stated, these lesions are usually single but can be multiple, particularly in children

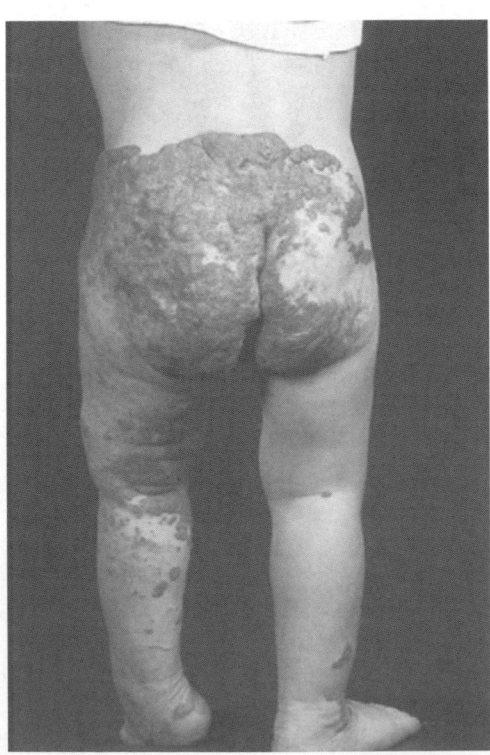

Figure 71–2 Extensive hemangioma starting to involute. Lesions initially become lighter centrally; after involution is complete, skin may be pale and atrophic.

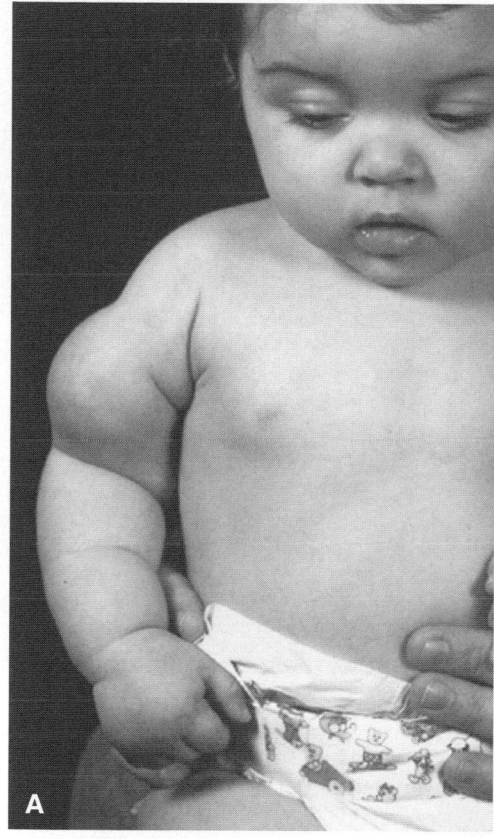

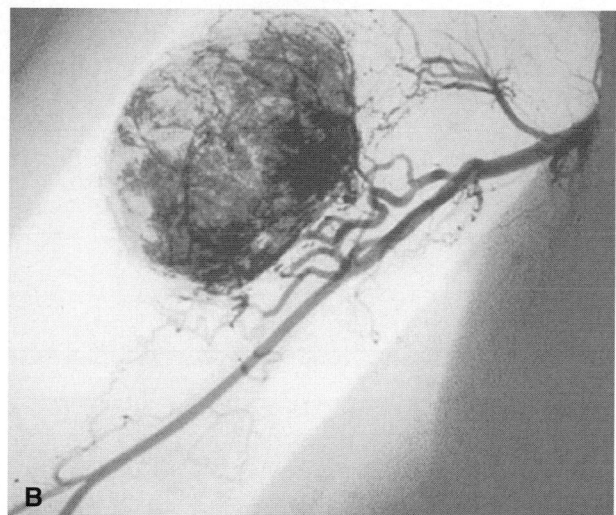

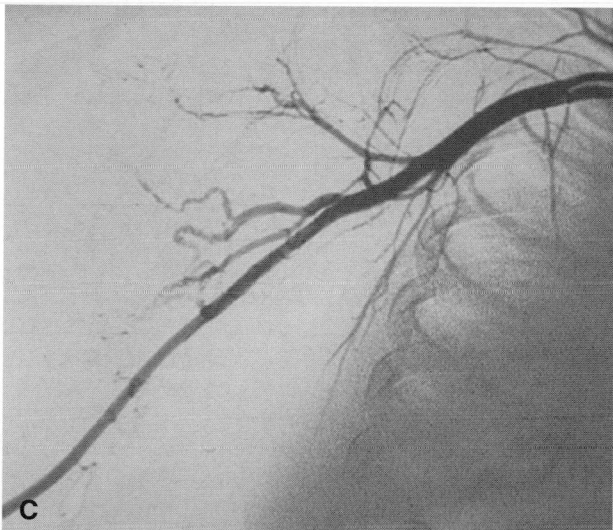

Figure 71–3 A. Hemangiomas located more deeply may present as a nonspecific soft tissue mass. Angiography is not normally necessary because cross-sectional imaging is usually sufficient for diagnosis. **B.** Nonspecific findings in this case led to angiogram, which demonstrates uniform intense vascularity of well-defined mass. **C.** Embolization was performed prior to biopsy; embolization is rarely necessary for simple hemangiomas, but it does appear to accelerate involution.

with hemangiomatosis of the liver. These latter children will also demonstrate hepatomegaly, bruits over the liver, and in some cases, evidence of high-output congestive heart failure (45). Some lesions cannot be differentiated clinically from true vascular malformations at the time of presentation, but the characteristic progression of the lesion over time will generally clarify the diagnosis (46). When the process of involution begins (toward the second half of the first year), the color of the lesion becomes duller, the lesion becomes softer, and it starts to show shrinkage generally beginning at the center and progressing toward the periphery. Ultimately, the skin over the lesion may be lighter in color than the surrounding normal skin.

Radiologic studies are generally not required for superficially located lesions but may be helpful in evaluating deep visceral lesions. Angiography demonstrates a diffusely hypervascular mass with enlarged feeding arteries, and a lobular pattern is often present (Figure 71–3B). CT and MR scanning will show a well-defined mass that shows dense enhancement after contrast is administered (Figure 71–4A) (47).

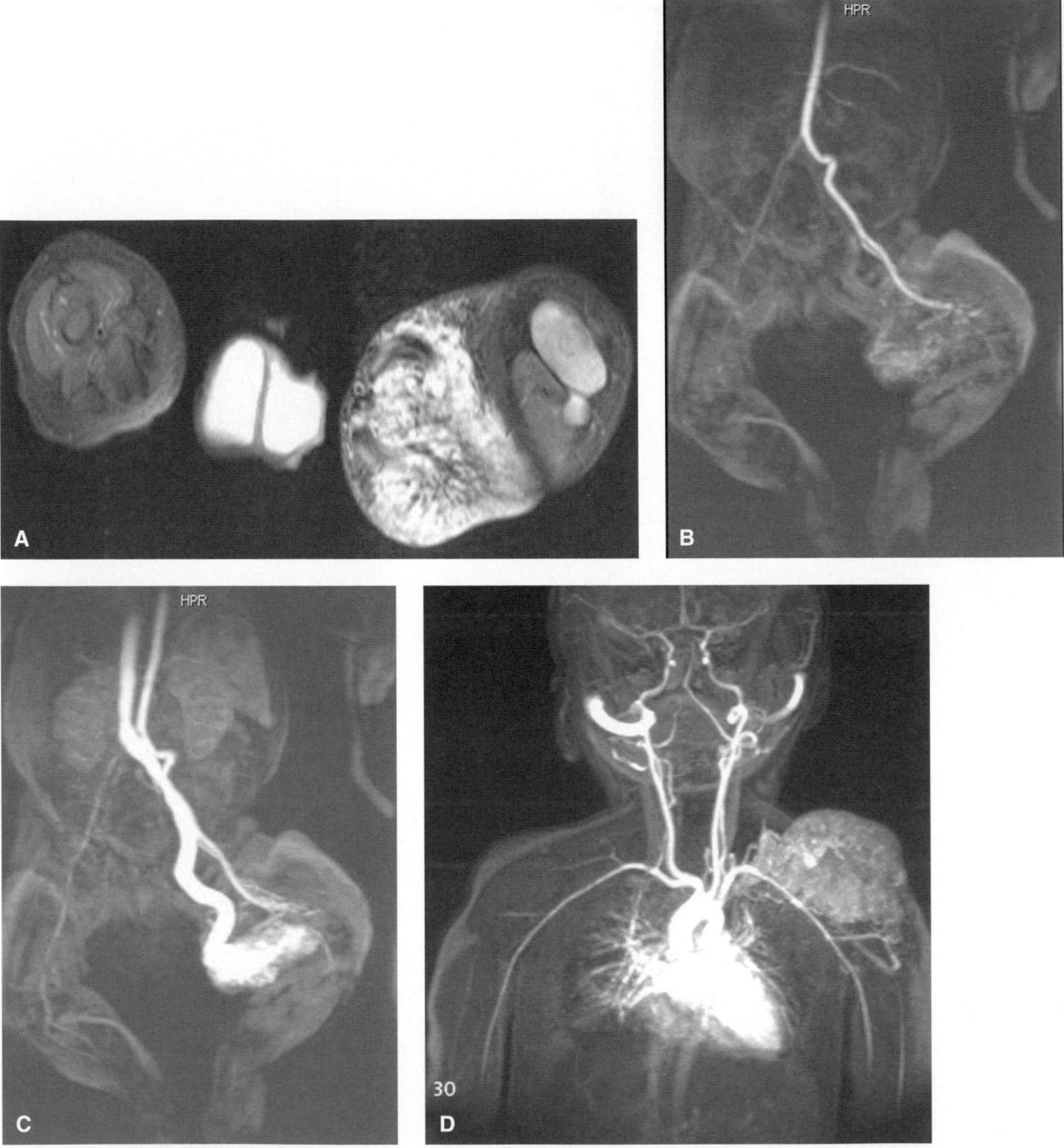

Figure 71–4   A. Cross-sectional MRI study of infant with extensive left thigh hemangioma demonstrating typical findings of densely hypervascular mass. **B., C.** MR angiogram of same infant shows vascular mass with enlarged feeding artery and shunting into dilated vein. **D.** Another infant with a large left-shoulder hemangioma showing similar findings.

Treatment

Because these lesions characteristically involute spontaneously, conservative management should be the rule in most cases. Parents may find this difficult to accept during the proliferative phase, but they should be reassured as to the natural history of the condition.

In a few situations, treatment must be attempted because of bleeding, high-output failure, or interference with respiratory or visual structures (Figure 71–5) Treatment is difficult at best; the primary methods described are pharmacologic therapy, surgery, and embolization.

The mainstay of pharmacologic therapy is corticosteroids, which can produce marked shrinkage of the lesion.

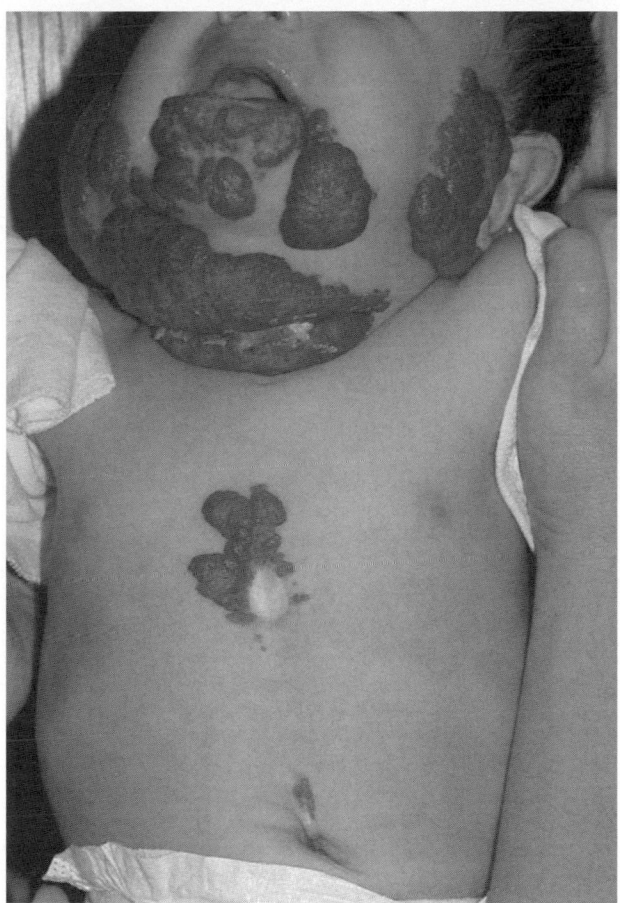

Figure 71–5 Infant with PHACES syndrome. Hemangioma involves midline structures including neck, where airway management may present a clinical problem.

Generally a 2- to 3-month course of oral prednisone is given during the proliferative phase (48). Steroids used during infancy can cause significant problems, including irritability, gastric upset, delayed linear growth, and hirsuitism, all of which remit after therapy is disconintued (49,50).

Decreased resistance to infection may also present a problem in some patients. This therapy has therefore generally been reserved for complicated lesions or those involving critical anatomic structures and/or documented or protential morbidity. The use of chemotherapeutic agents has also been reported in occasional cases of life-threatening hemangiomas (51).

Like most rapidly proliferating tissues, hemangiomas are quite sensitive to radiation, which has been used in their treatment. However, as a result of concerns over long-term carcinogenesis, particularly in the head and neck region, this modality is rarely employed (52). Surgical resection of hemangiomas is technically difficult and, until recently, was rarely performed except in lesions interfering with breathing, feeding, or sensory development (53). A growing opinion in the plastic surgery community is that some disfiguring lesions should be addressed surgically in early childhood rather than waiting

it out, because of the severe impact these lesions may have on the child's psychosocial development (54).

Embolization therapy has been used in certain cases where specific treatment of the lesion is required. Preoperative embolization may facilitate surgical resection by significantly reducing blood loss (55). Selective hepatic embolization has also been used in infants with high-output congestive heart failure resulting from extensive hepatic hemangiomatosis (6,56). This is a devastating clinical problem, carrying a mortality rate of up to 80% resulting from the intractable congestive failure. These infants characteristically present with multiple cutaneous hemangiomas, hepatomegaly associated with a bruit, and severe congestive heart failure. In the absence of cutaneous lesions, the problem may be initially misdiagnosed as a congenital heart defect. Note that, like the cutaneous lesions, hepatic hemangiomas will show eventual spontaneous involution if congestive heart failure can be controlled during the proliferative phase.

Surgical ligation of the hepatic artery was employed in the past to reduce the degree of shunting, but this should rarely be necessary with the availability of embolization. Good results have been reported with gelfoam pledgets, PVA particles, and acrylic adhesives; proximal hepatic artery embolization using coils has also been reported to be effective (5). Gelfoam powder and absolute ethanol should not be used because of the risk of hepatic necrosis.

Kaposiform Hemangioendothelioma (KHE)

Trapping of platelets and other blood elements (Kasabach-Merritt phenomenon—KMP) has been known to occur in association with some vascular anomalies since it was first described in 1940 (Figure 71–6) (57). Perhaps one of the most surprising observations in the past decade has been that KMP is not associated with common hemangiomas of infancy but with kaposiform hemangioendotheliomas (KHE) (58,59).

The diagnostic features of KHE on biopsy are spindled endothelial cells resembling Kaposi sarcoma but not associated with HIV infection. On examination, the lesion is often edematous, smooth, and ecchymotic (Figure 71–7). Anatomic predilection is for the chest wall and shoulder, groin extending down the leg, retroperitoneum, or face. The gender distribution tends to be equal, in contrast to hemangiomas, which have a predilection for females. There may be residual KHE tumor after resolution of hematologic abnormalities.

Kaposiform hemangioendothelioma can be a medical emergency. Unfortunately, the medical literature contains only scattered case reports, and management is often by trial and error. There may be a role for stratification of these lesions by age at presentation and histologic, hematologic, and other criteria, to better tailor treatment protocols. Current therapies include corticosteroids, vincristine and cyclophsophamide, interferon, epsilon aminocaproic acid (Amicar), compression therapy, and, occasionally, embolization (Figure 71–8).

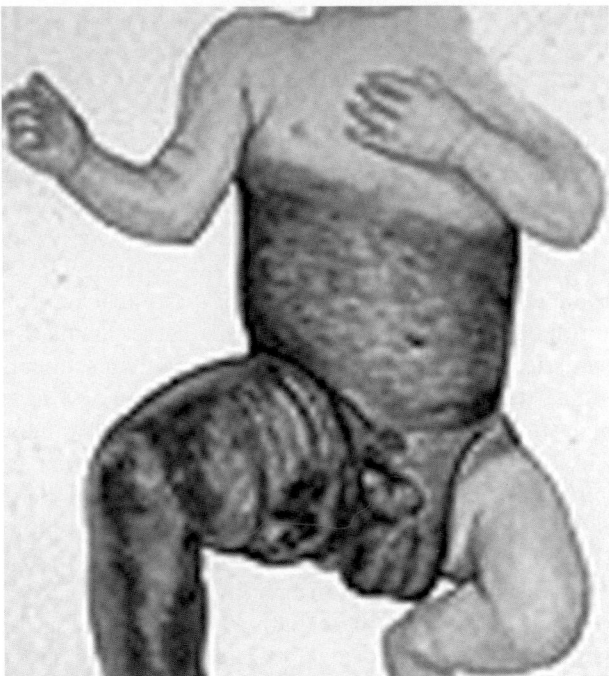

Figure 71–6 Original illustration from paper by Kasabach and Merritt describing coagulopathy secondary to platelet trapping in "hemangioma." It now appears that this phenomenon is associated specifically with Kaposiform hemangioendothelioma (KHE), a distinct pathologic entity.

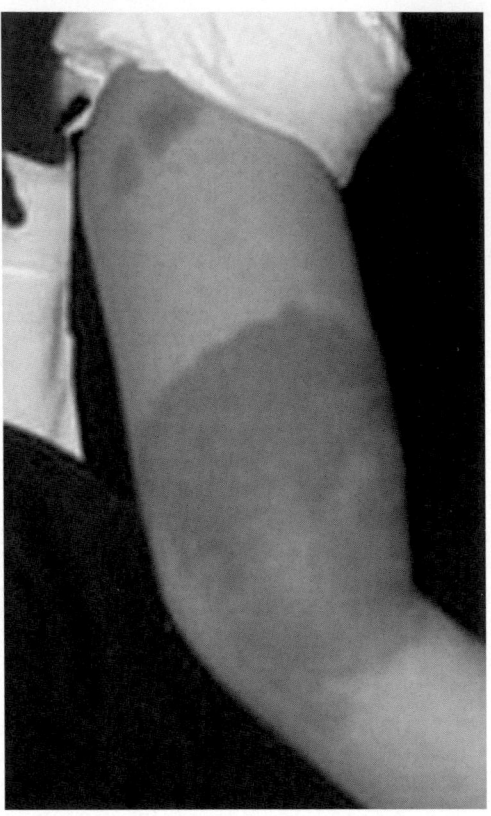

Figure 71–7 Clinical case of KHE involving broad area of thigh with thickened erythematous skin. This type of lesion may progress rapidly and present life-threatening complications; aggressive treatment is often necessary.

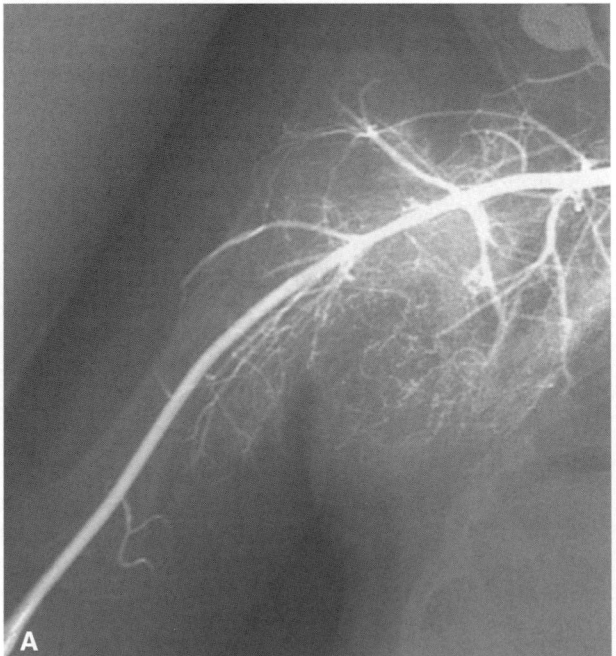

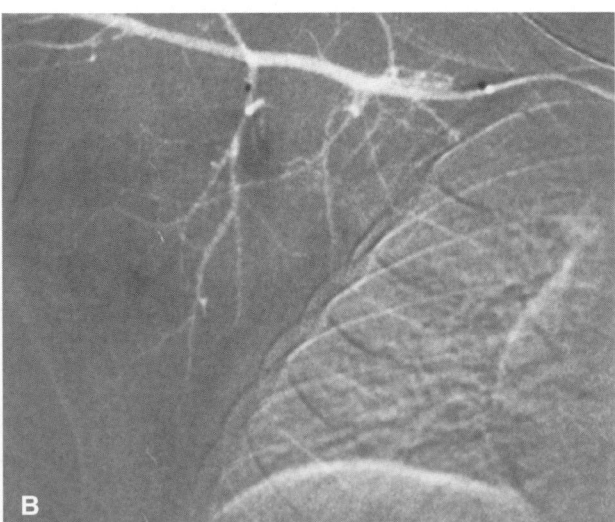

Figure 71–8 **A.** Axillary angiogram of infant with KHE of shoulder with rapid progression and coagulopathy. **B.** Selective embolization was performed, which along with aggressive medical treatment and compression therapy accelerated the process of involution.

ARTERIOVENOUS FISTULAS

An arteriovenous (AV) fistula is, by definition, a direct connection between an artery and a vein. The vast majority of these lesions are acquired, usually the result of trauma. Other causes include surgery or other invasive procedures, infection, tumor erosion, and rupture of an artery into an adjacent venous structure (e.g., carotid-cavernous fistula).

The first descriptions of arteriovenous fistulas were recorded more than 200 years ago, related to penetrating injuries or following bloodletting procedures (60). Attempts to repair these lesions constituted the earliest efforts in vascular surgery, and the results of these efforts were decidedly mixed. Initially, treatment consisted of ligation of the feeding artery, which nearly always resulted in either recurrence of the fistula or gangrene of the extremity (61,62). Subsequently, the procedure was extended to include "quadruple ligation and excision," referring to the afferent and efferent arteries and veins (63). While this procedure was effective for chronic fistulas with well-developed collaterals, ischemic complications developed in most acute lesions. For this reason, it became accepted practice to allow fistulas to mature for a period of months prior to excision (64).

Following Carrel's description of vascular anastomosis in 1902, reconstruction of the vessels with restoration of the normal circulation became the goal, although this often proved impossible in practice, even through World War II. Using modern reconstructive techniques, this goal can be achieved in most cases. Unfortunately, cases are still encountered on a regular basis in which the same mistakes made 200 years ago still occur, with the same poor clinical result.

An understanding of the architecture and physiology of the arteriovenous fistula is essential to planning proper treatment, whether by surgery or interventional radiologic technique. The most complete description of the pathophysiology of arteriovenous connections was provided by Emile Holman, beginning in the 1920s (65,66). Holman described the local, distal, and systemic effects of acute and chronic fistulas. Once these effects are appreciated, the difficulties in treating these lesions are much more easily understood, and certain common mistakes can be avoided. Diagramatically, the physiology of an AV fistula is shown in Figure 71–9. The basic phenomenon is the creation of a low-pressure sump; various authors have made analogies to plumbing systems or electrical circuits to explain subsequent events (67,68). Briefly, flow through the fistula will depend on the size and length of the AV connection, with the highest flow encountered in direct side-to-side fistulas. The connection tends to enlarge over time, although small traumatic fistulas occasionally close spontaneously, such as those seen after renal biopsy. As flow in the feeding artery increases, the feeding vessel tends to dilate and elongate. If the resistance across the fistula is lower than in the artery distal to it, a steal will develop, with eventual ischemic changes in the distal tissues. This is particularly pronounced in extremity lesions, where claudication, skin and muscle

atrophy, and frank gangrene may ultimately develop. (Figure 71–10) If the pressure gradient across the fistula is low enough, reversal of flow in the artery beyond the fistula will occur, further worsening the ischemia.

It is well established that an arteriovenous fistula is the most powerful stimulus known for the development of collateral arteries and veins, much more so than an atherosclerotic occlusion (69). These collaterals can, in some cases, compensate for the steal through the fistula, although they may also show eventual reversal of flow. These extensive collaterals explain the predictability of recurrence of the fistula if only proximal ligation of the feeding artery is performed. Indeed, these recurrences can show such complex patterns of circulation that the original underlying fistula cannot be identified, the angiographic appearance becoming indistinguishable from a complex congenital vascular malformation (Figure 71–11). It can readily be appreciated what a disservice this type of proximal ligation represents, whether performed surgically or by an embolization coil. Subsequent treatment often becomes impossible by any modality.

Other pathologic changes occur on the venous side of the fistula, including venous hypertension and enlargement of draining veins with eventual valvular incompetence and reversal of venous flow. The elevated venous pressures result in distal changes that resemble chronic venous insufficiency, with extensive varicosities, edema, thickening of tissues, and venous ulcerations. In many cases, these secondary venous abnormalities are the presenting findings. Extensive venous varicosities confined to one extremity should at least raise the question of an underlying arteriovenous fistula or malformation.

Finally, there are the systemic effects of the fistula. A detailed description of this physiology is beyond the scope of this chapter, but briefly, the changes consist of the cardiovascular effects of a left-to-right shunt. These effects include a decrease in peripheral vascular resistance with a secondary increase in cardiac output through an increased heart rate and stroke volume. This phenomenon can be demonstrated on physical examination by eliciting the so-called Branham-Nicoladoni sign, which consists of slowing of the heart rate when the fistula is occluded by manual compression, a reflex that is probably vagally mediated (70,71). Blood volume is also increased in the presence of a significant fistula.

Over time, the increased circulatory work caused by the shunt leads to secondary cardiac changes, including hypertrophy and eventual dilatation. Ultimately, high-output congestive failure may develop in the presence of a large fistula. It is interesting and important to note that while these generalized cardiovascular effects are commonly associated with large arteriovenous fistulas, they are rarely seen in connection with congenital vascular malformations, even large ones. The reason for this difference is not entirely understood but appears to be related to the preservation of peripheral vascular resistance by the complex connections

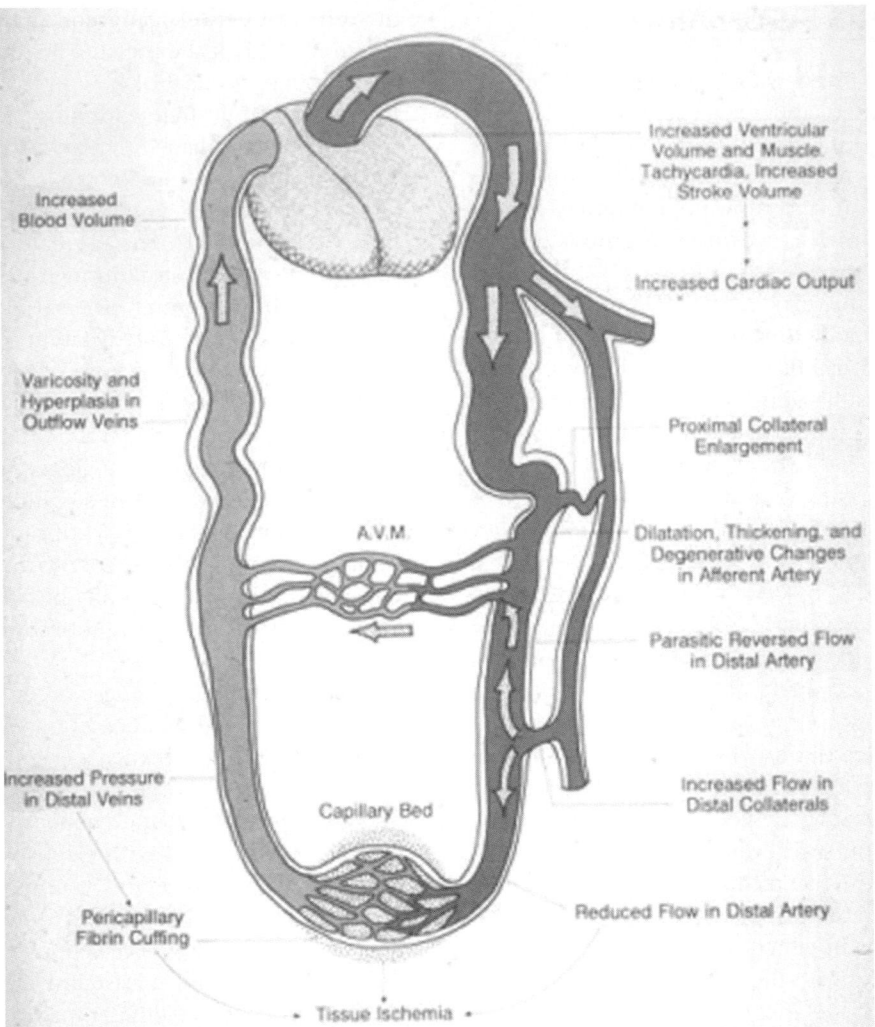

Increased
Blood Volume

Increased Ventricular
Volume and Muscle.
Tachycardia. Increased
Stroke Volume

Increased Cardiac Output

Varicosity and
Hyperplasia in
Outflow Veins

Proximal Collateral
Enlargement

Dilatation, Thickening, and
Degenerative Changes
in Afferent Artery

A.V.M.

Parasitic Reversed Flow
in Distal Artery

Increased Pressure
in Distal Veins

Capillary Bed

Increased Flow in
Distal Collaterals

Pericapillary
Fibrin Cuffing

Reduced Flow in Distal Artery

Tissue Ischemia

Figure 71–9   (after Holman) Diagram of pathophysiology of a fistulous arteriovenous communication. Most of these phenomena are also seen to a lesser degree in high-flow congenital vascular malformations.

of the malformation as opposed to the low resistance presented by the arteriovenous fistula (72). This difference provides a strong justification for early intervention in fistulas and reason for conservatism in treating malformations.

From the preceding discussion, it is apparent that the treatment of arteriovenous fistulas must be directed at obliteration of the fistula itself, with preservation of distal flow whenever possible. In certain situations, particularly in extremity trauma, early surgical intervention will provide the best result. This is because of the fact that these fistulas are usually side to side or quite short, and in a large percentage of cases are associated with traumatic pseudoaneurysms. The introduction of endovascular grafting now allows a significant number of these lesions to be treated nonsurgically, occluding the fistula while preserving distal flow (73) (Figure 71–12). In young patients, the long-term durability of these devices must be considered when deciding on the best approach. In other types of lesions, embolization has clearly become the initial treatment of choice, such as in

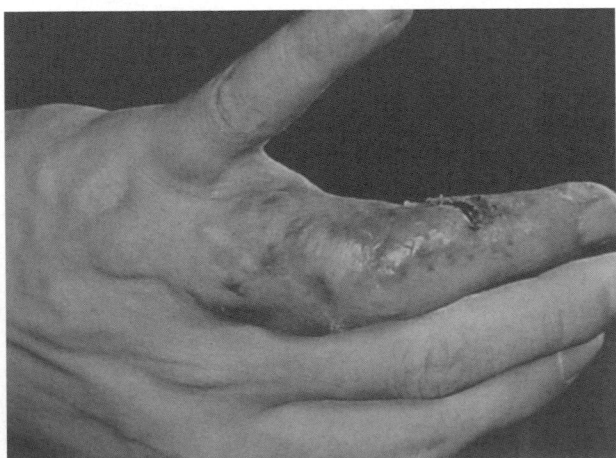

Figure 71–10   Arteriovenous fistulas often cause clinical manifestations distal to the actual vascular lesion. In this 35-year-old male, the fistula is in the metacarpal region, but venous hypertension and the steal phenomenon results in pain, swelling, distal atrophy, and ulceration of the finger.

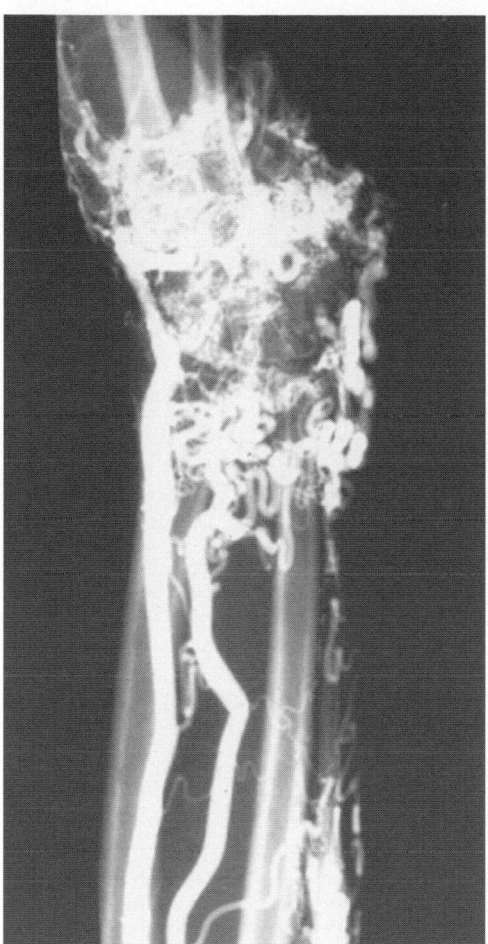

Figure 71–11 Arteriogram of forearm of 52-year-old patient who originally had a traumatic arteriovenous fistula in the palm of the hand from a penetrating injury. Several proximal surgical ligations resulted in resupply of the lesion by collaterals and ischemia, requiring amputation of a portion of the hand. At this time, the lesion is nearly indistinguishable from a complex congenital lesion and almost impossible to treat.

carotid-cavernous fistulas and some visceral lesions. The embolization procedure can be directed at occluding the fistula itself (the ideal) or at isolating the segment of artery from which the fistula originates.(Figure 71–13). The choice of embolic device or material will be determined by the anatomic situation, but generally, macroscopic occluding devices such as coils or detachable balloons are effective, balloons having the advantage of being flow directed and the ability to be repositioned for optimal placement (74). The use of Gelfoam or other reabsorbable materials is inadvisable, and particulate materials will obviously be shunted through the arteriovenous connection. In some cases, acrylic adhesive has been used to seal a small fistulous tract with preservation of the parent artery and vein.

After an arteriovenous fistula has been occluded, a cure can generally be anticipated, and recurrences are rare. This is unlike vascular malformations, where the patterns of supply are much more complex and recurrences common. As previously noted, however, an improperly treated fistula can become as difficult to manage as a complex congenital lesion.

ARTERIOVENOUS MALFORMATIONS

Arteriovenous malformations (AVMs) are congenital anomalies that represent a focal failure of vascular differentiation in utero, generally between the fourth and tenth week of development. They are nearly always isolated lesions in otherwise healthy individuals and are not genetically transmitted in most cases. An exception is the Rendu-Osler-Weber syndrome, in which the lesions are multiple and there tends to be a strong family history.

Because these are developmental anomalies and not neoplasms, they tend to grow at the same rate as the individual, unlike the pattern of rapid growth and involution seen in hemangiomas. Depending on the size and location, AVMs can remain asymptomatic and undetected throughout life or represent a severe clinical problem. In the past and, unfortunately, the present as well, these lesions have often been misdiagnosed and mistreated, sometimes with disastrous results (Figure 71–14). Because these tend to be stable, slow-growing lesions, conservative management is advisable in many cases, with treatment reserved for lesions causing significant signs and symptoms.

Clinical Features

AVMs can occur anywhere in the body, although certain anatomic sites seem more commonly affected, including the central nervous system, the pelvis, and the lower extremities. If the malformation is in a location accessible to physical examination, it generally presents as a pulsatile, nontender mass. Often the arterial pulses in the region will be bounding, and bruits or a continuous flow murmur may be audible on auscultation. Draining veins may be prominent and may also be pulsatile. In the extremities, there is often evidence of long-standing venous hypertension, including thickening of the skin, edema, hyperpigmentation, and, in some cases, venous ulceration. Depending on the degree of steal, there may be distal ischemic changes such as atrophy or even ischemic ulceration. It is important to note that the major clinical manifestations of these lesions are often located downstream rather than over the lesion itself. When extremity lesions present in childhood, limb length may be affected, usually by overgrowth, but occasionally by shortening. Focal gigantism of digits or hands and feet may also occur (Figure 71–15). Some of these abnormalities are undoubtedly a result of regional mesodermal developmental problems associated with, but not necessarily caused by, the vascular malformation itself.

Deep lesions of the trunk may be clinically silent, in which case they may be detected as a pulsatile mass on routine examination or as a vascular mass found incidentally on radiologic examination. If symptoms are present,

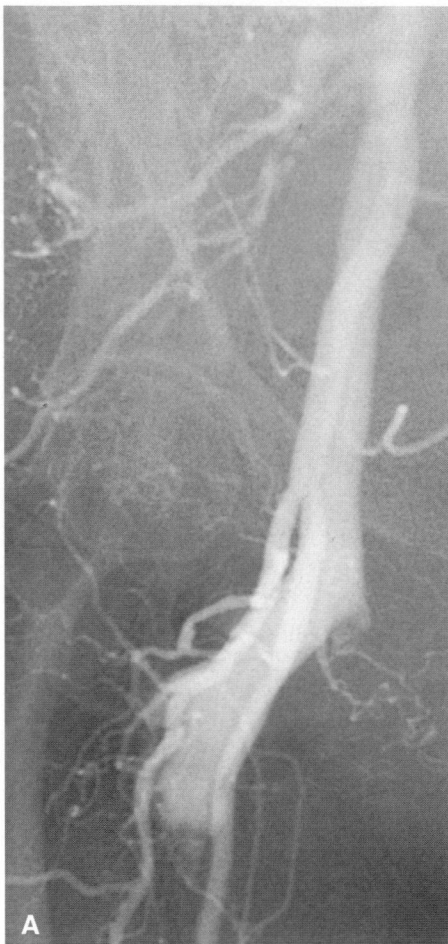

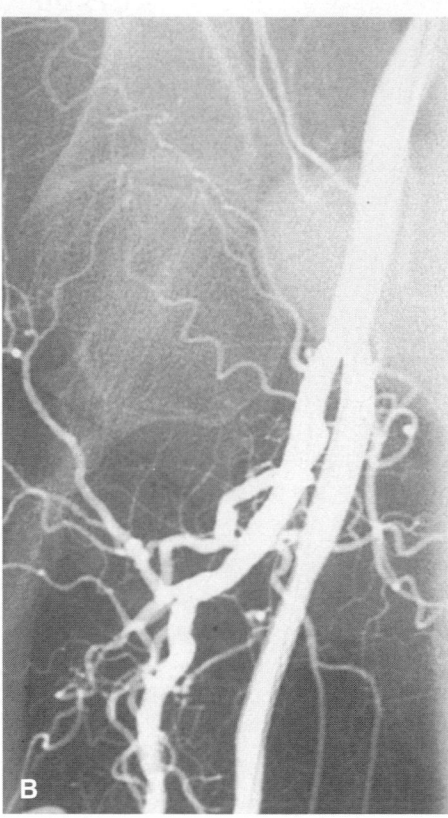

Figure 71–12 A. Direct femoral arteriovenous fistula several months following cardiac catheterization. **B.** These side-to-side fistulas may now be treated using covered stents.

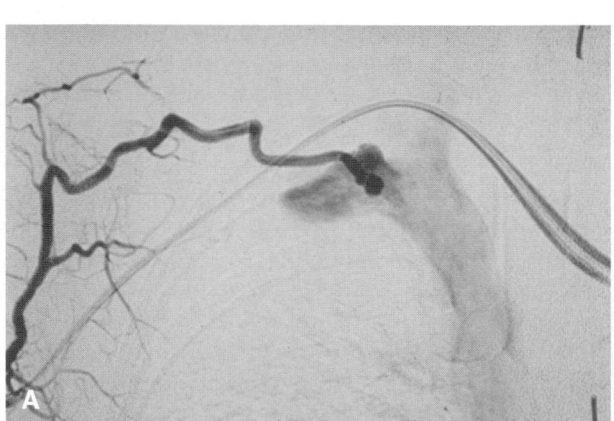

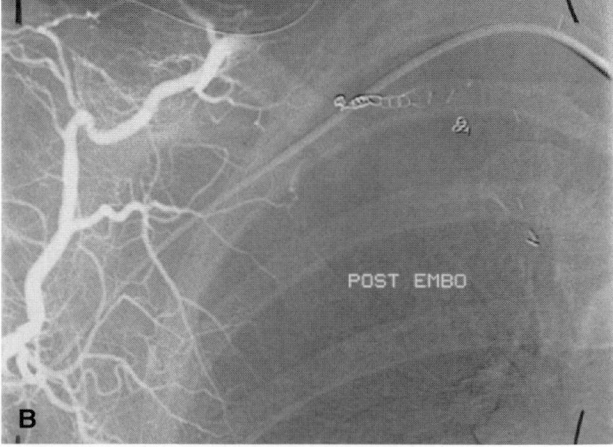

Figure 71–13 A. Arteriovenous fistula between axillary artery branch and right subclavian vein following central line placement. **B.** A permanent cure can be expected following embolization (in this case, using microcoils), but it is imperative to occlude the actual site of the fistula, or proximal branches will resupply the lesion.

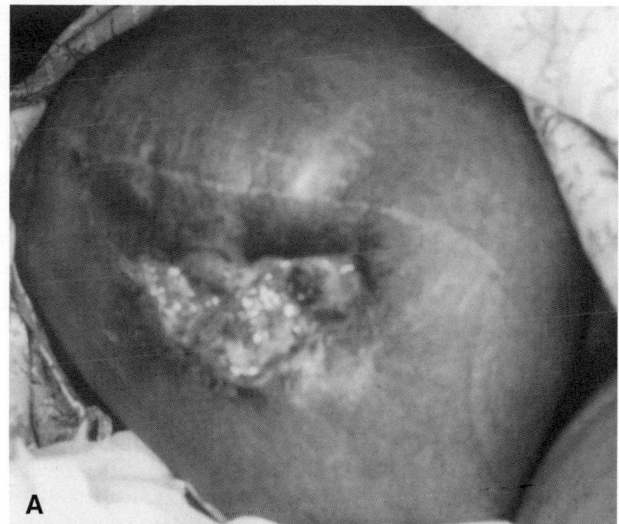

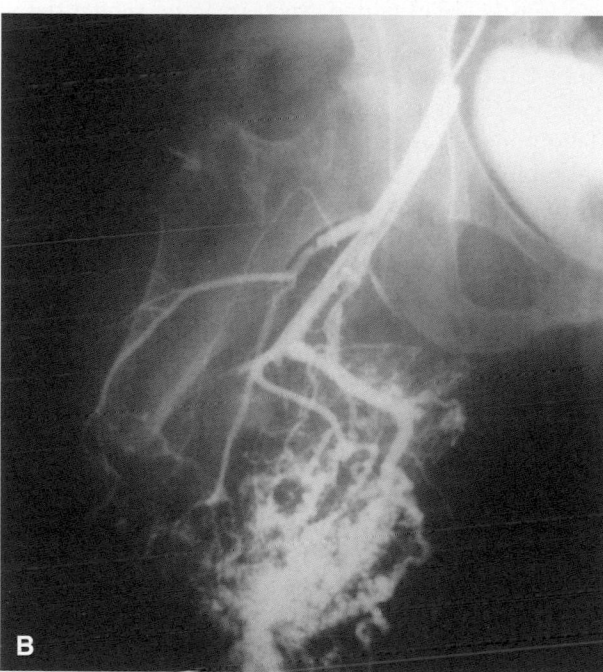

Figure 71–14 A. This 20-year-old woman, otherwise healthy, underwent a series of surgical ligations and amputations for what began as a localized AVM of the right foot starting at age 12. At this time, she shows breakdown of her high thigh amputation stump. **B.** Arteriogram demonstrates significant residual AVM. Such catastrophic results are not uncommon after misguided attempts at treatment of high-flow vascular malformations.

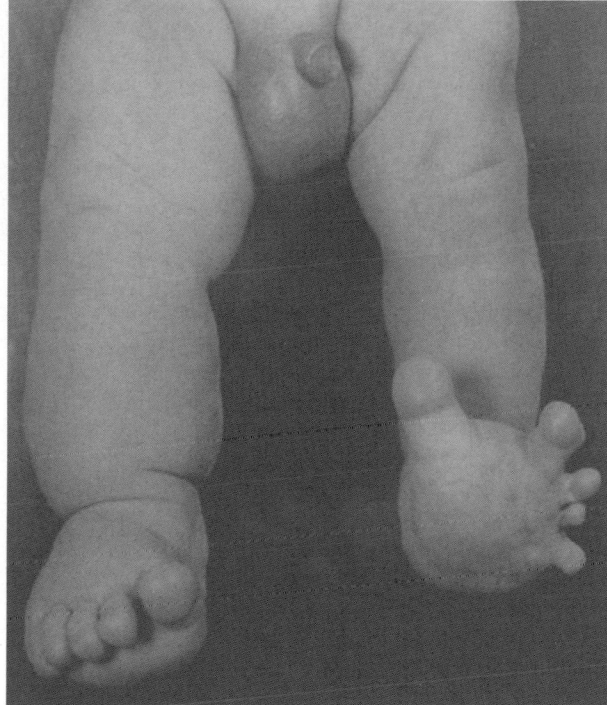

Figure 71–15 Overgrowth, undergrowth, and focal gigantism may be associated with extremity vascular malformations. Some of these abnormalities are a result of altered blood flow, and others appear to be associated mesodermal defects associated with, but not caused by, the vascular anomaly.

enlargement. The two primary settings in which this occurs are (a) in response to a change in the hormonal environment and (b) following unsuccessful attempts at surgical or interventional treatment. In female patients, there is an unpredictable but definite association between menarche, pregnancy, and the clinical course of a previously stable AVM (75,76). Young patients who have significant vascular malformations should be advised that pregnancy may be associated with progression of the lesion, sometimes to a marked degree. The progression does not involve any cellular proliferation but represents enlargement of existing channels and recruitment of new collaterals. In the second setting, after attempted treatment, it appears that mechanically disturbing a stable lesion can result in significant worsening, again most likely resulting from the development of new collaterals. This is more likely to occur following ligation or proximal embolization of feeding arteries or incomplete excision. It is for this reason that all treatment should be undertaken with extreme caution.

Diagnostic Studies

Lesions accessible to physical examination have characteristic findings that should permit the diagnosis to be made on clinical grounds, although the authors see at least two or three patients per year who have undergone biopsies or

they can cover an almost unlimited spectrum, depending on the size and location of the lesion. As stated previously, generalized cardiovascular effects from an AVM are distinctly uncommon. In the authors' own series of more than 700 cases, only two patients with extensive pelvic vascular malformations and two patients with congenital intrarenal lesions demonstrated high-output states (Figure 71–16).

While these lesions tend to grow slowly, in proportion to the individual, some lesions do exhibit periods of rapid

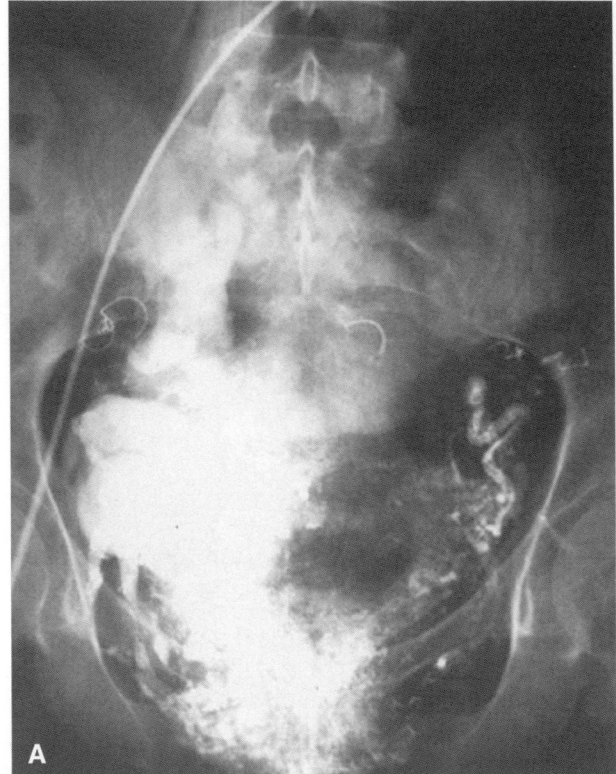

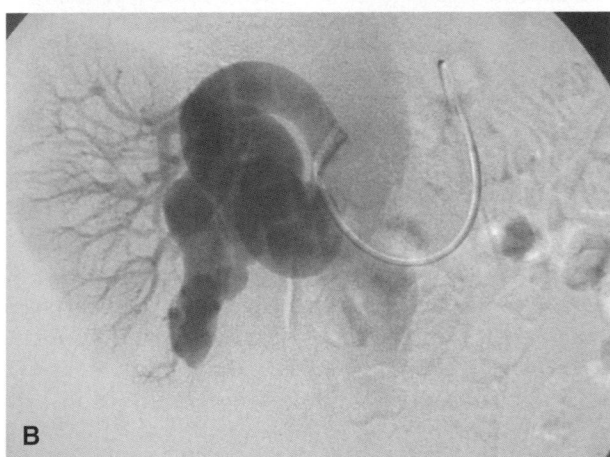

Figure 71–16 High-output cardiac states are actually quite uncommon in adult patients with vascular malformations despite this being a major concern of referring clinicians. This complication is most often associated with either **A.** high-flow pelvic lesions or **B.** congenital fistula-like lesions in the kidney. The former lesions are extremely difficult to treat, whereas the latter can usually be cured with embolization.

attempted excisions of misdiagnosed vascular malformations. Noninvasive studies (ultrasound, color-flow Doppler) will clearly demonstrate a high-flow lesion with enlarged feeding and draining vessels (77,78). Isotope studies using particles to demonstrate arteriovenous shunting have been described but are not widely used (79). Plain radiographs are generally uninformative, although venous lesions may show phleboliths and high-flow lesions will occasionally

show bone erosion, demineralization, or, rarely, a permeative pattern that can resemble tumor involvement. Disturbances in bone growth or development may also be noted in some cases.

Computed tomography and particularly MRI are extremely valuable modalities in evaluating vascular malformations (80,81) (Figure 71–17). They demonstrate the true extent of the lesion, which is often much larger than can be appreciated on physical examination or even angiography. MRI and MRA studies provide excellent anatomic detail as well as characterizing flow within the lesion. High-flow lesions will show flow voids on T_2 sequences and enlarged feeding arteries and draining veins on MR angiograms performed with gadolinium. These techniques also clearly show the relationship of the lesion to surrounding structures; commonly, a lesion that was felt to be localized and resectable on clinical examination is clearly not when these studies are obtained. Such imaging modalities are also quite valuable as an objective baseline that can be repeated at intervals or after intervention. Because even noninvasive imaging studies (MRI, CT) require the use of sedation or anesthesia in infants and young children, the authors obtain these studies only when the clinical diagnosis is in doubt or when treatment is required.

Angiography provides the most detailed depiction of vascular anatomy, although these findings can also be misleading without the additional information provided by cross-sectional studies. Nonselective studies are of limited value beyond confirming the diagnosis and giving an overview of the vascular supply. Detailed selective studies are not necessary until intervention is planned. The angiographic findings include enlargement and tortuosity of

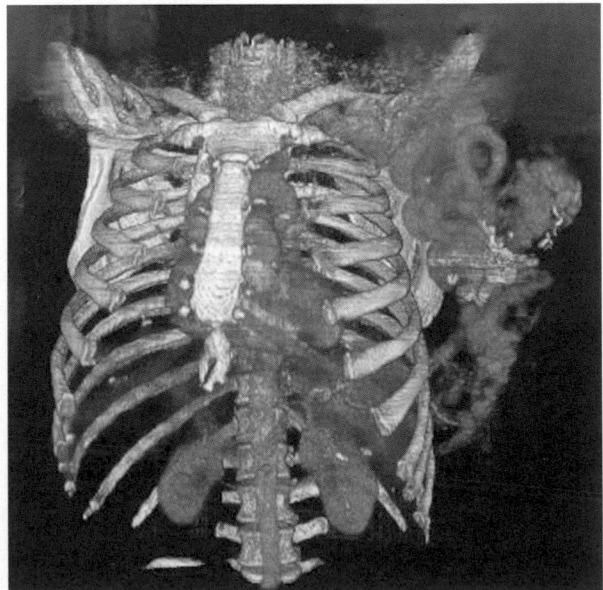

Figure 71–17 Spiral CT scan with 3D reconstruction of 47-year-old male with large high-flow AVM in left axillary region. CT and MR studies are now the mainstay of initial diagnosis and follow-up studies in patients with vascular malformations.

feeding arteries, a dense nidus of malformation that can range from innumerable small vessels to a few large ones, and early opacification of draining veins that may show marked dilatation. Most malformations demonstrate a primary feeding artery and multiple smaller secondary feeders. If the primary feeding artery is occluded, the secondary vessels will resupply the nidus of the lesion almost immediately.

Treatment

Unlike hemangiomas, which involute spontaneously, and fistulas, which can usually be permanently cured, true vascular malformations are notoriously difficult to treat. Surgeons long ago discovered that complete resection of the lesion is rarely possible and is often associated with blood loss that can be uncontrollable. A minority of AVMs can be completely resected, but when this can be accomplished, it probably represents the best chance of a complete cure. The apparently more conservative approach of ligating feeding vessels ("skeletonization") virtually always results in recurrence, sometimes within months (Figure 71–18). These recurrences may be more symptomatic than the original lesion and are invariably more complex anatomically, with numerous feeding vessels. This is not to imply that surgery has no role in the management of these lesions, only that such surgery must be carefully planned with realistic goals in mind. Planning includes careful radiologic study, consisting of both cross-sectional and angiographic examinations. It must also include provision for tourniquet control and large-volume blood replacement, such as cell-saver devices. In some cases, preoperative embolization can convert a lesion from unresectable to resectable with an acceptable blood loss.

Transcatheter embolization has now assumed a primary role in the management of congenital vascular malformations. An endovascular approach to this type of lesion makes a great deal of sense, but the apparent ease of catheterizing a feeding artery and depositing embolic materials must not tempt the interventionalist into making the same surgical mistakes that were made in the past. Specifically, proximal occlusion of feeding vessels, whether performed by surgical ligation or an endovascular device, will produce the same poor clinical result with virtually guaranteed recurrence. Because these are benign lesions in relatively young patients, a long-term view of results is always necessary. A large number of these patients require only a correct diagnosis and reassurance, and the temptation to intervene must be tempered with a realistic assessment of the long-term prospects of treatment. Although complete cures can be accomplished in only a minority of cases, control of clinical symptoms can often be achieved with minimal morbidity. Both the physician and the patient should be prepared for the likelihood of repeated future procedures.

There are few conditions in which a team approach to treatment is more important than in vascular malformations.

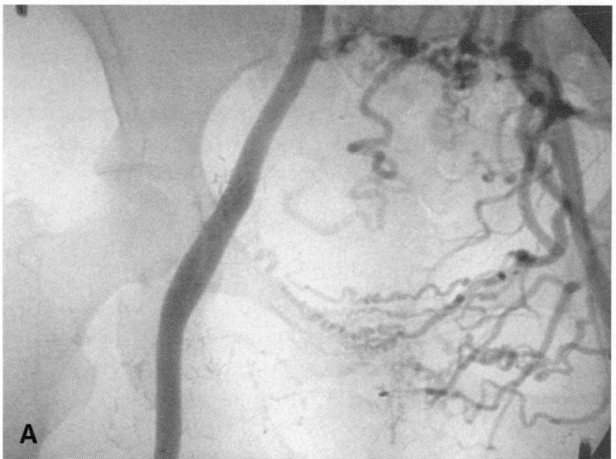

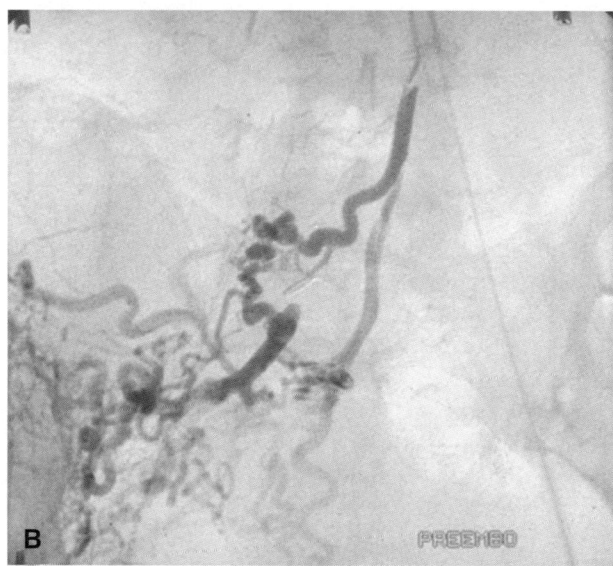

Figure 71–18 Surgical ligation or proximal coil embolization of feeding arteries rarely produces a satisfactory long-term result in patients with vascular malformations because of rapid collateral recruitment. **A.** This 30-year-old female with a pelvic AVM underwent a 14-hour surgical "skeletonization" procedure with ligation of every branch of the iliac and femoral arteries. She returned with recurrent symptoms of pelvic pain 4 months later. **B.** A selective study of the middle sacral artery demonstrates extensive collateral resupply of the original lesion, making subsequent treatment even more difficult.

Members of the team should include internists, pediatricians, plastic surgeons, interventional radiologists, vascular surgeons, dermatologists, orthopedists, and psychiatrists and/or social workers. A multidisciplinary conference at which cases are presented on a regular basis can facilitate managment and decision making as well as maximizing the experience of the group in dealing with these relatively unusual conditions.

The authors perform virtually all embolization procedures under general anesthesia. They feel that the increased risk, time, and expense are justified by the length of these procedures and the discomfort involved in numerous superselective studies, particularly in the extremities.

A variety of embolization techniques and materials have been described over the past 30 years. Dramatic advances have also occurred in vascular imaging and catheterization. Among the most significant in the realm of treating AVMs has been the introduction and rapid refinement of digital angiography and road mapping. The development of coaxial microcatheters and steerable guide wires has made possible superselective catheterization of vessels that would have been difficult to image a few years ago. There is no question that the availability of better embolic materials has lagged considerably behind our ability to reach even the smallest vascular bed. There is still no embolic agent that is ideal for treating vascular malformations, meaning one that has proven long-term safety, ease of handling and delivery, permanence, and the ability to reach and occlude the nidus of the malformation. Each of the devices or agents that is currently in use will be briefly discussed individually.

Gelfoam

Gelfoam is an absorbable gelatin sponge and is available in several forms. The most commonly used in embolization are the pledget and powdered forms. Gelfoam pledgets are generally cut into small strips or cubes and suspended in contrast for injection. While this material is quite useful in treating acute hemorrhage and in preoperative embolization, its large size and reabsorption over a period of days or weeks makes it unsuitable for treating most AVMs. This agent is sometimes useful for protecting normal vessels from distal embolization by occluding them proximally when other agents are used.

Gelfoam powder consists of particles as small as 40 μ in size, permitting this material to reach capillary level and presenting a definite risk of tissue ischemia. Except when tissue infarction is intended, as in treating neoplasms, this material should generally be avoided.

Coils

Stainless steel coils were among the first devices designed specifically for transcatheter vascular occlusion. They cause thrombosis by creating a mechanical blockade of the vessel, with thrombosis promoted by the incorporation of Dacron fibers. Coils have the advantages of being an approved device and are easy to use; they come in a wide variety of shapes and sizes and can be passed through standard selective angiographic catheters. More recently, miniaturized platinum coils (microcoils) have become available. They can be introduced through 2 and 3 French microcatheters into extremely small arteries. Microcoils are available in unfibered and fibered types, the latter being much more effective occluding devices. Detachable coils, using either mechanical or electrothermal means, may be useful in some high-flow situations in which the ability to reposition the device is desirable.

Despite their advantages, coils are unsuitable for treating most vascular malformations because of their size. An exception would be certain AVMs with a simple fistula-like architecture (pulmonary AVM, some high-flow renal lesions). The proximal occlusion caused by these devices is equivalent to surgical ligation, a technique that is known to be ineffective. As with Gelfoam, coils may be of use as proximal protective devices or to redistribute flow during embolization with other more penetrating agents.

Detachable Balloons

Detachable balloons are useful in situations in which flow guidance, reversible occlusion, and repositioning are required. Examples include high-flow lesions (such as carotid-cavernous fistulas) and pulmonary AVMs. In these situations, they provide unique advantages that may justify their complexity and cost. Their use is not justified as simple proximal occluding devices and would offer little advantage over coils in nonfistulous vascular malformations.

Particles and Microspheres

Ivalon, or polyvinyl alcohol (PVA) sponge, was first introduced as an embolic material in 1975 (82). It is generally used in particulate form, with particle sizes ranging from 150 μ to 1,000 μ. Newer preparations of PVA in the form of uniform microspheres are now available; they are easier to use and have theoretical advantages over the irregular particles. This agent is usually injected as a suspension through standard-size catheters or microcatheter systems. The particles will follow the flow of blood until they lodge in a vessel too small to allow further passage. Thus, different particle sizes can be selected based on the size of the vascular matrix to be occluded.

Because PVA is considered a permanent (nonreabsorbable) material and can be deposited deeply into vascular beds, it was hoped that this would be a suitable agent for treating AVMs. Indeed, PVA embolization can produce an impressive immediate angiographic result, with a gradual pruning of vessels and slowing of flow until stasis is reached. Unfortunately, these initial results are often followed by recurrence of the lesion, often within a period of months. Further investigation has demonstrated that this is primarily a result of recanalization around the irregular particles (83); it is possible that the newer microspheres will have less tendency to permit recanalization. In any case, PVA may be effective as a preoperative embolic agent and may also be useful as a trial agent to determine the effect of embolization on a lesion clinically; if there is significant benefit, proximal access to feeding vessels will not have been sacrificed, and more permanent agents can then be used in the event of recurrence.

Absolute Ethanol

Absolute (95%) ethanol is a highly potent embolic agent that causes vascular occlusion by a combination of direct toxic effect on the vessel wall and clumping of damaged erythrocytes and denatured proteins. It was initially used as an embolic agent in the treatment of renal tumors, where its marked tissue toxicity was desirable. This agent also has the advantages of being readily available, inexpensive, and easy to deliver through virtually any catheter system. Its use in treating AVMs was first described by Sasaki in 1984 (84) and popularized by Yakes (85,86). While some series have reported excellent results, absolute ethanol must be used with a great deal of caution because of its toxicity. It is capable of causing considerable damage to normal tissues, particularly when used in vessels supplying mucosal surfaces, skin surfaces, and neural structures (Figure 71–19). One must therefore be certain of all structures supplied by a feeding vessel in addition to considering how distribution of the agent may change abruptly as occlusion occurs. The difficulty in making this agent radiopaque without losing its effectiveness as a sclerosing agent adds to the risk.

The authors have found alcohol and other sclerosants to be more applicable in the treatment of venous malformations by direct injection, where the risk of tissue damage is much lower. This technique is discussed in detail in the section on venous malformations.

Acrylic Adhesives

Cyanoacrylates, a group of rapidly polymerizing adhesives, have been used for a variety of clinical applications over the past 40 years and specifically for intravascular occlusion for nearly 30 years (87). Its use has been controversial over the years in that a wide variety of tissue reactions have been described, causing concern over long-term toxicity or even carcinogenicity. In an exhaustive review of the histotoxicity of cyanoacrylates, Vinters in 1985 concluded that there was no evidence of carcinogenicity but that more work was neeed in evaluating tissue reactions to these agents (88). In most series where pathologic studies have been carried out, a chronic inflammatory reaction with foreign body giant cells, mural inflammation, and eventual fibrosis are demonstrated. A gradual reduction in the amount of acrylic adhesive within an embolized lesion has also been documented and correlates with radiographic observations of shrinkage or disappearance of the opaque material over time (89). Whether this is a result of phagocytosis or another mechanism is not entirely clear, but this phenomenon can be associated with recurrence of AVMs following embolization with acrylic adhesives.

Despite these problems, the authors have seen better long-term results using acrylic adhesives in AVMs than with any of the alternative agents. This embolic material rapidly polymerizes on contact with any ionic medium, including the mildly basic bloodstream. The material is generally combined with oily contrast (Pantopaque or ethiodol), which adds radiopacity and slows the polymerization time to allow more controllability (90). Powdered tantalum metal may also be added to further increase radiopacity. This mixture is then delivered as close as possible to the nidus of the malformation, generally through a coaxial microcatheter. Extremely small depositions are used, generally ranging from 0.2 to 0.6 cc, delivered as a continuous injection or with a "push" of nonionic D5W (Figure 71–20). These small depositions polymerize rapidly, incorporating blood elements to produce a significantly larger cast than the volume of the agent itself. The

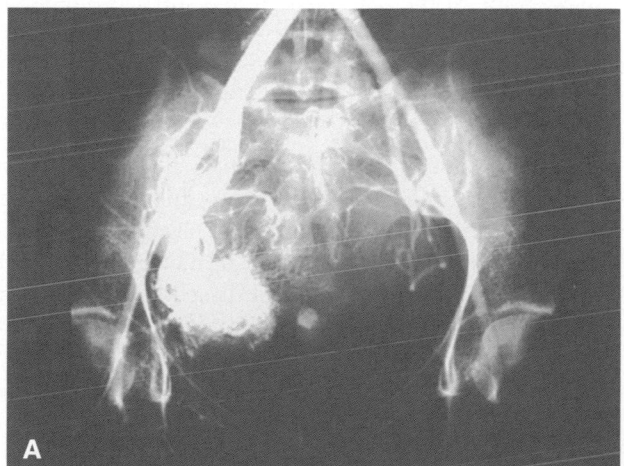
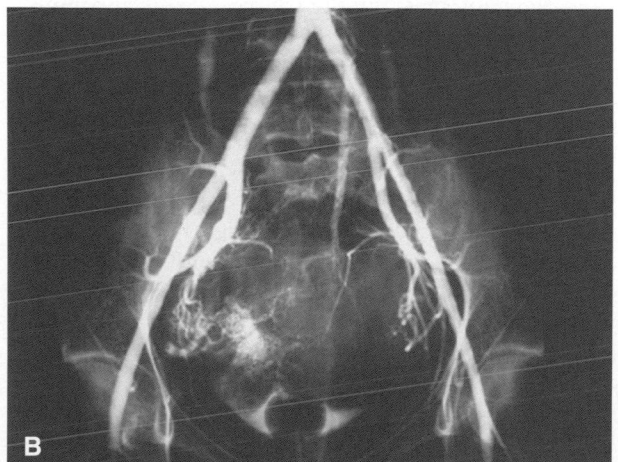

Figure 71–19 Pelvic angiogram of 28-year-old female with pelvic pain resulting from high-flow right pelvic AVM. **A.** Selective embolization of multiple feeders, including the IMA and hypogastric branches, was performed using absolute ethanol. **B.** Postembolization study shows marked reduction in flow through lesion, but complications included perineal skin sloughing, colon perforation, leg neuropathy, and neurogenic bladder. Ethanol is an effective but highly tissue-toxic agent that carries significant risk when used intra-arterially.

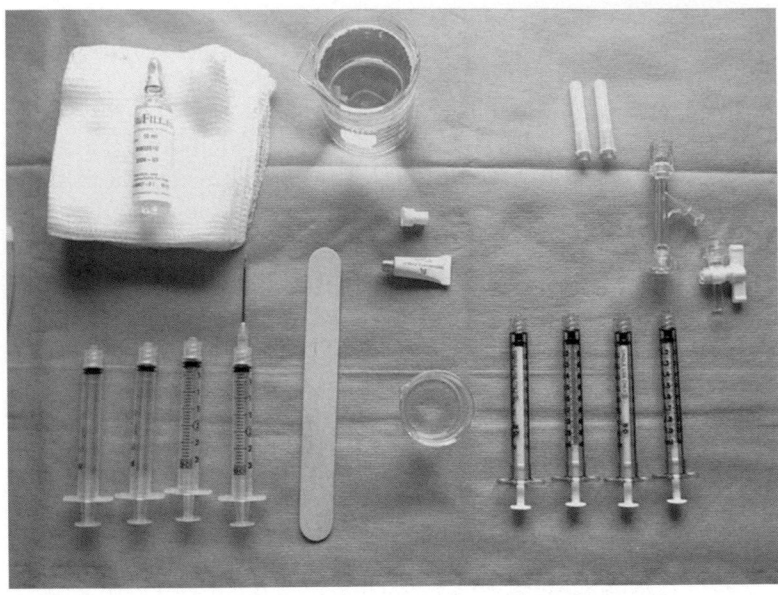

Figure 71–20 Typical arrangement of "glue table" for NBCA adhesive. A strict nonionic environment must be maintained when preparing the glue, with D5W used as a flush solution. The glue is mixed with ethiodol, an oily contrast agent, which adds radiopacity and slows polymerization to make the embolization more controllable.

goal, which cannot always be acheived, is to create a "cast" of the nidus of the lesion (Figure 71–21). This should theoretically obliterate the low-pressure sump that is the stimulus for the development of new collaterals and recurrences. Clinically observed tissue toxicity has been minimal in the authors' experience, with no evidence of mucosal damage, tissue necrosis, or nerve damage.

Specific Clinical Lesions

Pulmonary AVMs

Pulmonary AVMs constitute a distinct category of vascular malformation because of the presence of right-to-left shunting, which is generally the source of clinical complications. This entity is discussed in detail elsewhere in this volume (Chapter 53).

Renal AVMs

Vascular malformations in the kidney are generally of the high-flow type, ranging from small angiomatous lesions causing hematuria to fistula-like lesions with massive arteriovenous shunting. Treatment of the small-vessel type is relatively straightforward, as the renal circulation consists of end arteries, and recruitment of collaterals is unusual (91). Particles, microspheres, or adhesive agents are all suitable embolic agents in this situation (Figure 71–22). A so-called postembolization syndrome is to be expected, consisting of flank pain, fever, and other abdominal symptoms because of the infarction of a variable amount of normal renal parenchyma, which is usually unavoidable.

The fistulous type of renal AVM is an entirely different lesion, consisting of a direct connection between a proximal renal arterial branch and the corresponding vein, which dilates massively because of the arterialized flow

(Figure 71–23) These patients may be intially misdiagnosed as having giant intrarenal aneurysms. This is one of the few lesions that cause a generalized high-output state in the adult patient. Manifestations can include an abdominal bruit, cardiomegaly, marked dilatation of the suprarenal inferior vena cava, and in extreme cases, high-output failure. The authors have treated 11 patients with remarkably similar lesions and clinical presentations, all but one in the right kidney. Treatment can be challenging because of the size and torrential flow through the fistula; losing embolic materials or devices into the pulmonary circulation is a distinct possibility, even with the largest coils. The authors have had satisfactory results in their series using a combination of large coils, detachable balloons, and acrylic adhesives. None of the patients required surgical intervention, and all were cured completely with embolization (92).

Pelvic AVMs

The pelvis is one of the more common locations for AVMs to occur. The complex blood supply to this region, as well as the numerous organs that may be involved, combine to produce an extremely difficult clinical management problem.

The anatomic distribution of these lesions is quite variable, ranging from focal lesions confined to the broad ligament of the uterus to extensive lesions involving the bladder, bowel, uterus, ovaries, muscle, nerves, and even bone. The blood supply may be equally complex, the most common feeding vessels consisting of the hypogastric, middle sacral, lumbar, inferior mesenteric, and common femoral artery branches.

These lesions are most often encountered in young female patients. Presenting features may include local or referred pain, leg edema, abnormal menstrual bleeding or hematuria, and, rarely, high-output congestive failure. In males, the anatomic distribution tends to be simpler, often

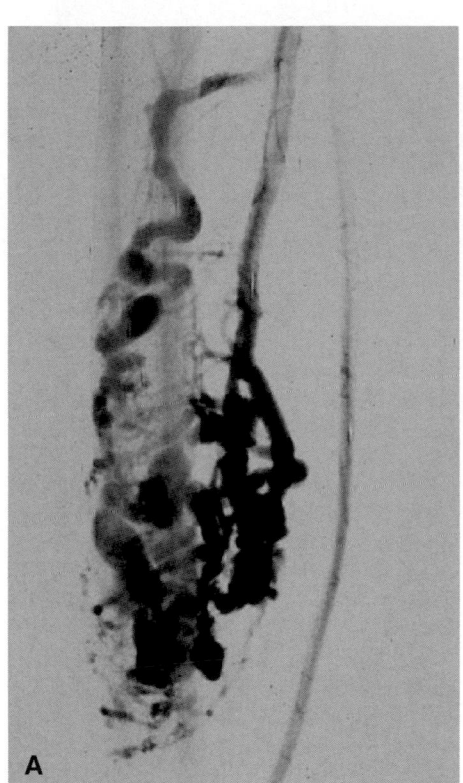

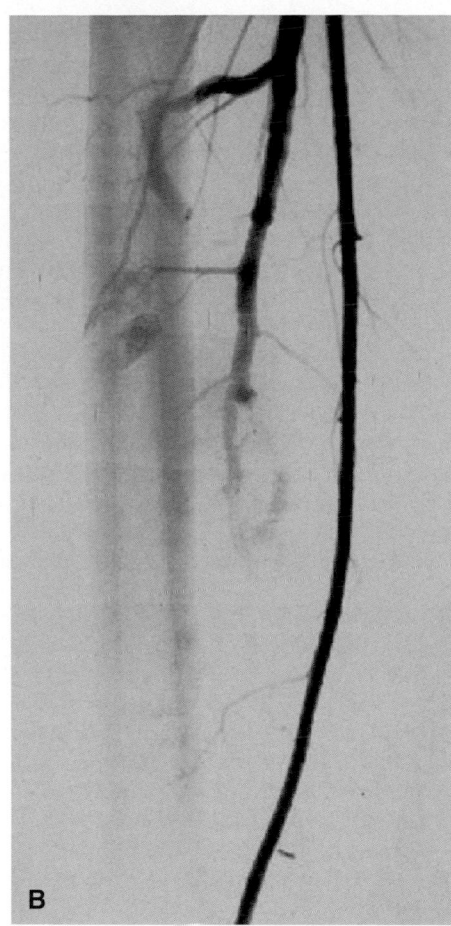

Figure 71–21 The goal of any AVM embolization is occlusion of the nidus of the lesion. High-flow malformation in thigh supplied by profunda **A**. before and **B**. after selective embolization using NBCA tissue adhesive.

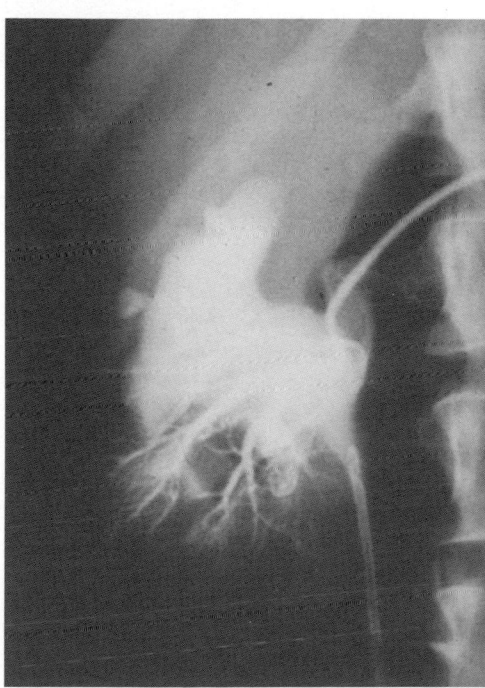

Figure 71–22 Angiogram of lower pole renal vessels in 36-year-old woman with intermittent gross hematuria shows small vessel malformation. Because the renal circulation is end-vessel, this type of lesion is generally curable using a variety of agents. In this case, PVA particles were used.

with a single hypogastric artery feeder and drainage through hugely dilated veins, which are primarily responsible for the symptoms of pain, disturbed bowel and or bladder function, and occasional bleeding (75) (Figure 71–24). In both male and female patients, these lesions may be asymptomatic and discovered incidentally on physical or radiologic examination.

Treatment of pelvic AVMs, particularly in females, is extremely difficult. Complete cures are the exception, and recurrences are common. Thus, the decision to initiate treatment must be tempered by a realistic assessment of the goals and risks involved. Surgical resection may be quite successful for lesions confined to the broad ligament; this is one of the few situations where radiologic studies may actually overestimate the difficulty of surgical treatment. Although the lesion may draw feeders from multiple sources, the nidus itself is localized and can often be completely removed. Other lesions may be confined to the uterus, curable by hysterectomy. The authors have embolized 14 patients who presented with severe menorrhagia resulting from a uterine AVM (93) (Figure 71–25). Hysterectomy was avoided in all cases, and three patients subsequently carried full-term pregnancies uneventfully.

Unfortunately, most pelvic lesions are not so localized, and surgical resection is not feasible with an acceptable degree of morbidity. Palliation of symptoms, and in some

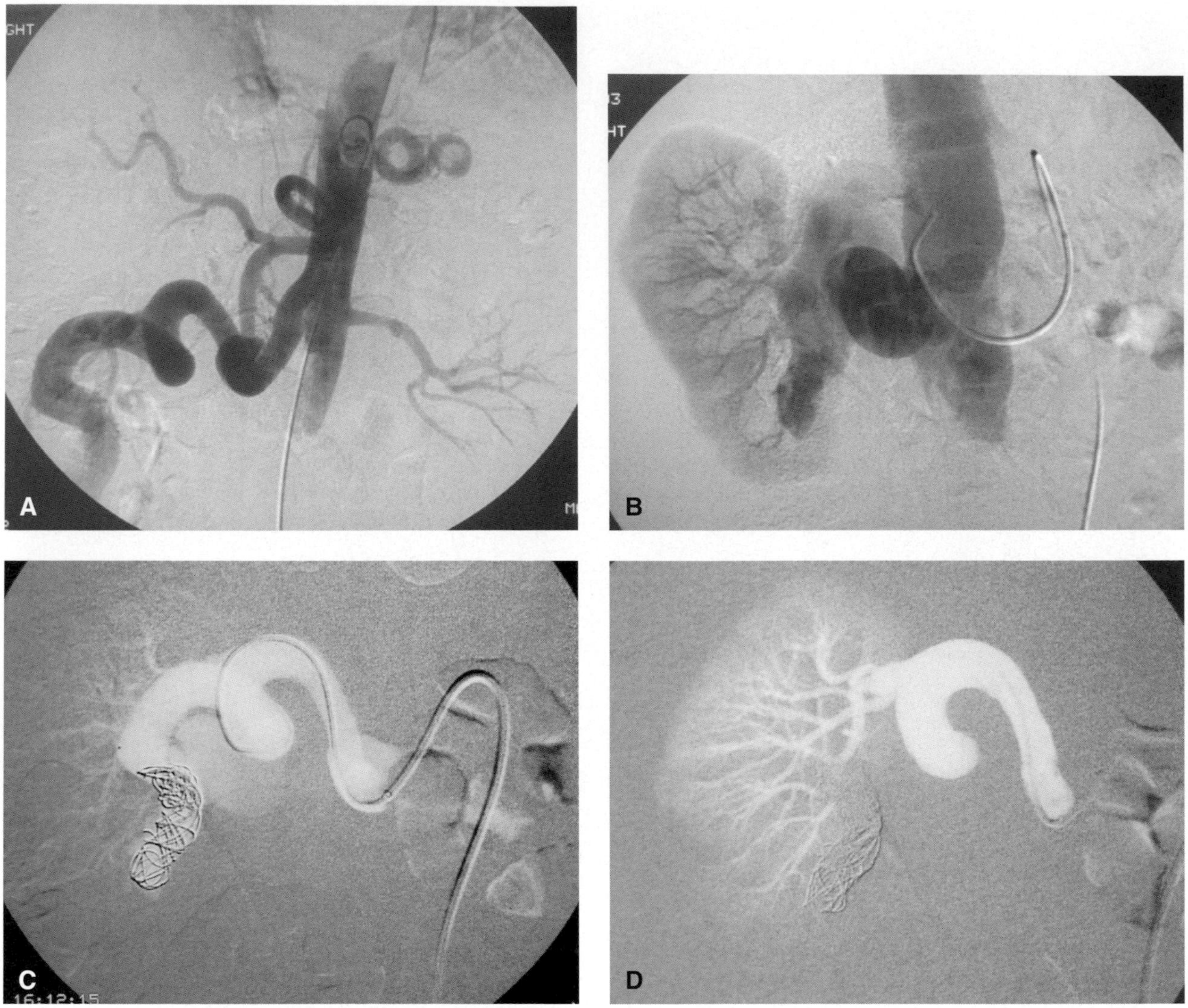

Figure 71–23   Extremely high-flow fistula-like lesions are also encountered in the kidney. **A.** Note the marked dilatation and tortuosity of the feeding artery as well as **B.** dilatation of the inferior vena cava above the renal vein inflow. Some of these lesions are discovered incidentally while others present with hypertension, hematuria, and high-output cardiac states. **C., D.** These lesions are generally curable by embolization, in this case using large coils but extreme care must be used to avoid loss of embolic materials into the pulmonary circulation.

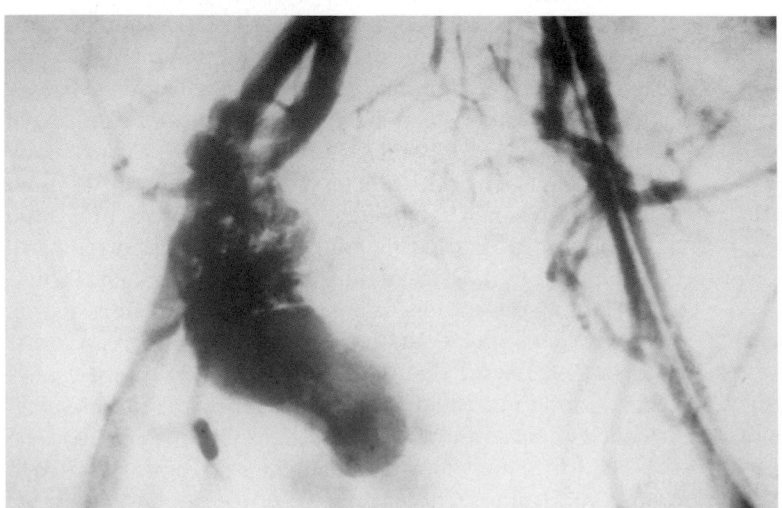

Figure 71–24   A 22-year-old man with complaints of pelvic pain and urinary retention. Rectal examination revealed a pulsatile mass. Pelvic arteriogram demonstrates a "male" pattern AVM, with a single hypogastric artery supply wrapped around a massively dilated draining vein, which is responsible for the symptoms.

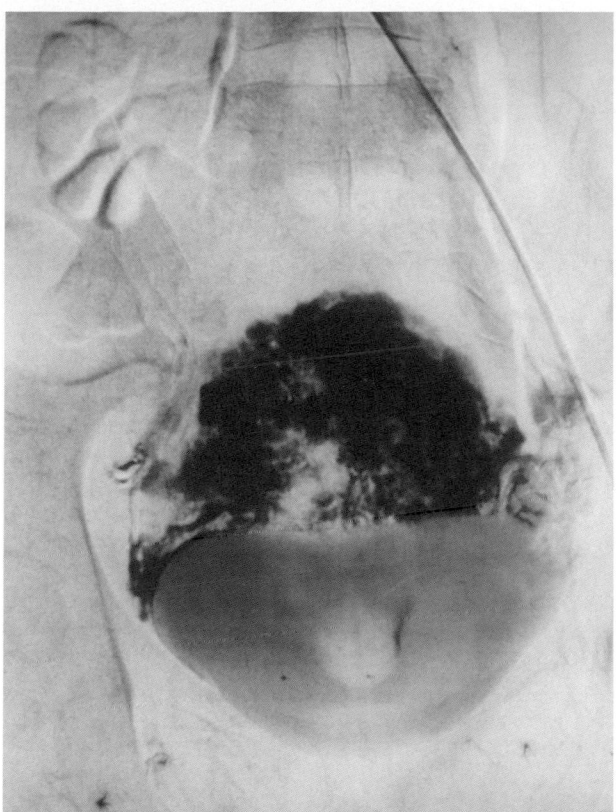

Figure 71–25 A 27-year-old woman with severe menorrhagia found to have a vascular malformation confined to the uterus. This was successfully managed with embolization.

cases cure, can be achieved by embolization in these patients. As always, the goal should be obliteration of the nidus of the lesion rather than occluding feeders. Most of these cases will require multiple staged procedures because of the complexity of the blood supply. Branches of the hypogastric arteries are usually the primary feeding vessels, but all the regional arteries should be studied to evaluate other sources of supply or likely routes of recurrence. Ischemic complications have been extremely rare, even when embolizing branches of the inferior mesenteric artery (Figure 71–26). Extreme caution must be used when employing tissue-toxic agents such as absolute alcohol, which may cause tissue necrosis, mucosal injury, or permanent nerve damage.

The simpler blood supply of most male pelvic AVMs renders them much more treatable. If the nidus supplied by a single hypogastric artery can be occluded, the large draining veins will collapse or thrombose, and excellent long-term results have been encountered (Figure 71–27).

Extremity Lesions

Extremity lesions are among the most difficult malformations to treat. They more often interfere with function than truncal or visceral lesions because of edema, muscle and nerve involvement, and distal ischemia. These lesions are also more subject to trauma during normal activity. From the standpoint of surgery or embolization, it may be difficult to determine which vessels can be sacrificed without compromising perfusion of normal tissues.

As with other vascular malformations, proximal ligation is worse than useless, resulting in recurrence with a more complex pattern of supply. Newer microsurgical techniques,

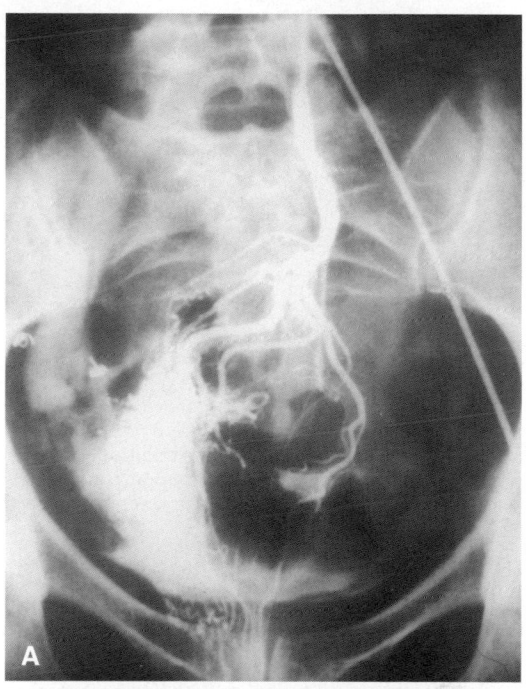

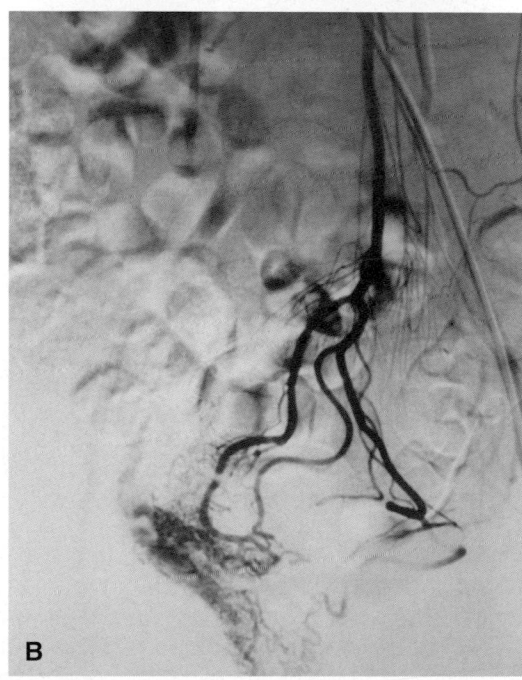

Figure 71–26 Examples of women with pelvic AVMs partially supplied by branches of the inferior mesenteric artery. This type of involvement is occasionally associated with rectal pain or bleeding. Superselective embolization of the involved branches has been performed without ischemic complications.

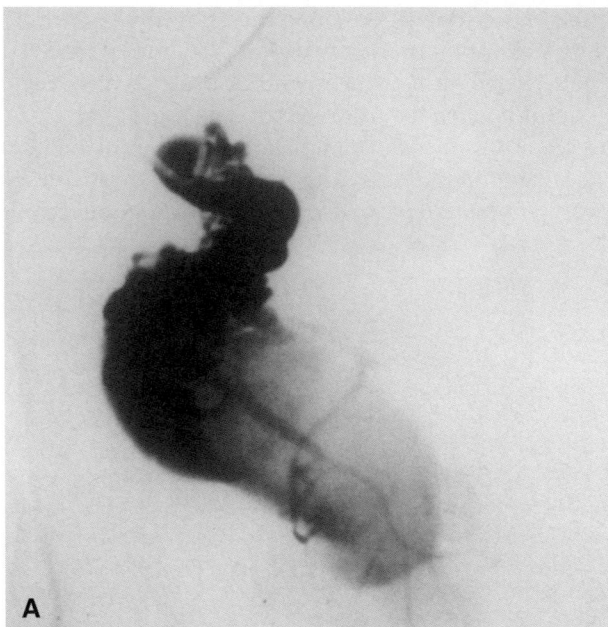
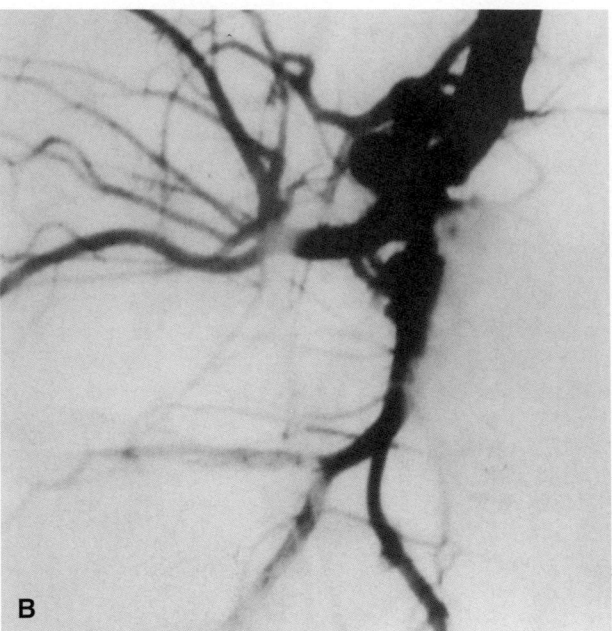

Figure 71–27 **A.** Pelvic arteriogram demonstrates a "male" pattern AVM, with a single hypogastric artery supply wrapped around a massively dilated draining vein, which is responsible for the symptoms. **B.** After embolization with acrylic adhesive, the lesion has been occluded with preservation of the normal hypogastric branches. This patient remained asymptomatic and without radiologic evidence of recurrence 8 years after embolization.

with or without preoperative embolization, have been successfully used in some of the more localized lesions. The availability of microcatheter systems and digital imaging has permitted superselective embolization of many lesions that would have been untreatable in the past (Figure 71–28). Especially after previous ligations or embolizations, transvascular access to the lesion may be impossible or present an unacceptable risk of occluding normal vessels. Direct puncture techniques, using either adhesives or alcohol, may be

technically easier and safer (Figure 71–29). The risks of intra-arterial alcohol have been discussed but are particularly significant in the extremities, where the compartments containing the malformation also contain nerves and muscles that can be damaged by this agent.

Ischemic pain, atrophy, or even tissue loss is commonly encountered with extremity AVMs. Even when the lesion cannot be eradicated completely, reducing the shunt by embolization will improve distal perfusion and can often

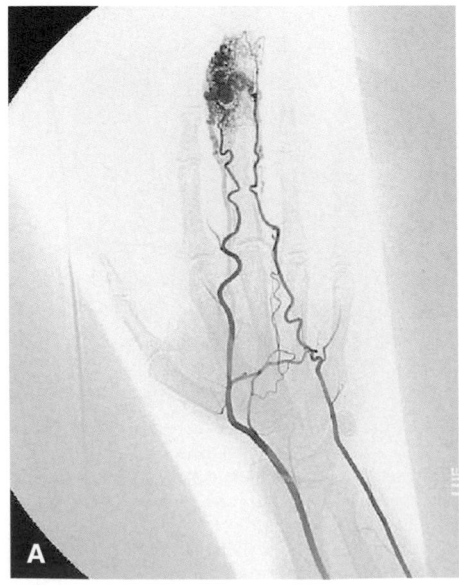
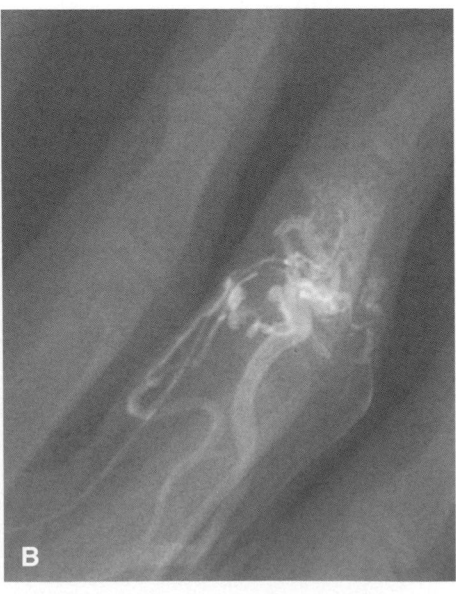

Figure 71–28 Although digital roadmapping and microcatheter technology now permit extremely distal catheterization, distal extremity AVMs are difficult to treat because of the size of the vessels and the difficulty in determining which branches can be sacrificed without impairing viability.

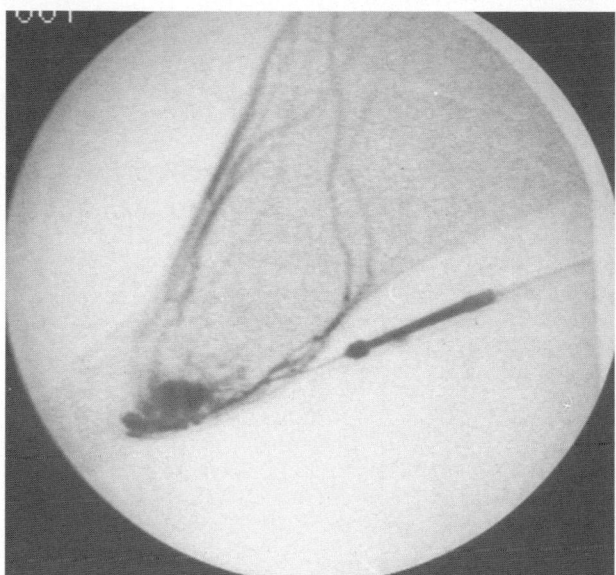

Figure 71–29 Some distal lesions are best approached by direct puncture, as in this 19-year-old female with a high-flow lesion on the plantar aspect of the foot. Direct puncture provides direct access to the nidus without endangering normal regional vessels and may be the only access possible when there have been previous ligations or embolizations.

be quite effective in relieving the most distressing clinical symptoms (Figure 71–30). Treatment should generally be undertaken in stages, with assessment of the clinical result at least 3 months following each procedure before continuing. The patient should also be aware that the lesion is unlikely to be completely eradicated and that repeated procedures may be required. Judgments as to the necessity and timing of treatment are particularly difficult in the pediatric population. Except in life- or limb-threatening situations, the authors try to avoid performing procedures on children under 5 years of age. At this point, the natural history of the lesion can be observed, and there is less risk to normal vessels in older children.

VENOUS MALFORMATIONS

Venous (low-flow) malformations are much more common than arteriovenous (high-flow) malformations and range from anomalies of venous anatomy to focal cavernous lesions. There is also a category of "mixed" lesions, which are primarily composed of venous elements but demonstrate an arterial component when studied angiographically. As with other vascular malformations, these are not neoplastic lesions and generally show growth commensurate with growth of the individual.

Cavernous Venous Malformations

This is the prototypical venous lesion, in the past referred to as cavernous hemangioma. These lesions may occur

anywhere in the body and are composed of irregular venous spaces with slow flow under low pressure. When they are located close to the skin surface, they have a characteristic bluish appearance and a soft nonpulsatile compressible consistency (Figure 71–31). They can be actively emptied by manual compression or passively by elevation of the affected part. Conversely, they can become tense and painful when engorgement occurs after activity, in the dependent position in extremity lesions, and during increased intrathoracic or intra-abdominal pressure in truncal lesions. (e.g., Valsalva maneuver, crying in children). Venous lesions that infiltrate skeletal muscle can cause disabling pain after activity but often show virtually no physical findings and are often misdiagnosed for years until an MR study is performed and the characteristic findings are seen (94). These lesions are usually nontender unless there is superimposed acute thrombosis. Very superficial lesions may show marked thinning of the overlying skin, which may even show breakdown with spontaneous bleeding.

Plain radiographs may be normal or may demonstrate phleboliths, pathognomonic for a venous lesion. Ultrasound studies show irregular, fluid-filled spaces with slow flow. MRI is the single most valuable study in confirming the diagnosis and delineating the true extent of the lesion, which may involve a much larger territory than is evident clinically (80,81). On a T2 fat saturation or inversion recovery sequence, the lesion will show a striking, bright signal, representing slow flow (Figure 71–32). This examination should be obtained prior to any surgical or interventional treatment.

Arteriography is typically unimpressive, demonstrating normal-caliber regional arteries that may show late venous staining on delayed films after high-volume contrast injections (Figure 71–33). Occasionally, a lesion that appears purely venous clinically will turn out to have an arterial component, which may alter treatment significantly (Figure 71–34).

Standard venography often fails to show any filling of the lesion from normal venous structures, although associated venous anomalies may be present. Direct puncture or "closed-space" venography is a much more effective technique for outlining these lesions; the abnormal venous structure is entered directly with a sheathed needle and then filled with contrast under fluoroscopic control (95) (Figure 71–35). The lesion may be composed of a single irregular chamber or demonstrate multiple noncommunicating compartments. Intramuscular venous malformations show a typical striated appearance on direct puncture studies (Figure 71–36). When the capacity of the lesion is reached, opacification of small draining veins is typically observed, with eventual drainage into the normal venous system. This direct puncture technique has been extended into a therapeutic modality, as described below.

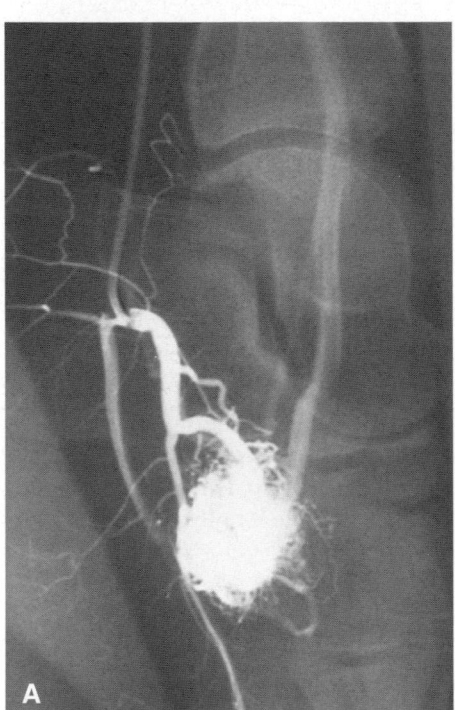

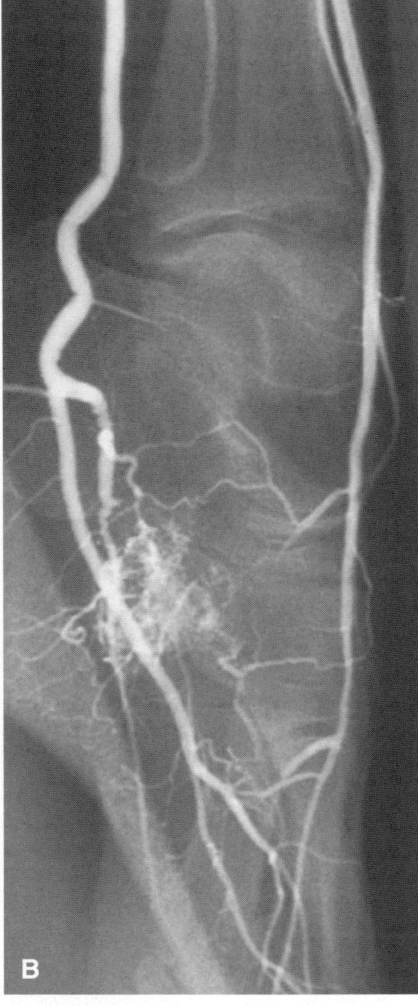

Figure 71–30 Presenting signs and symptoms in extremity AVMs are often distal to the lesion itself, related to distal ischemia from the proximal "steal" or chronic skin changes related to venous hypertension. **A.** This 35-year-old male presented with ischemic ulceration at the base of the toes distal to this high-flow malformation deep in the posterior plantar aspect of the foot. **B.** Postembolization angiogram shows minimal residual AVM, and the patient healed chronic ulcers within 4 weeks. Even if the nidus cannot be completely obliterated, a reduction in flow will often resolve the presenting complaint.

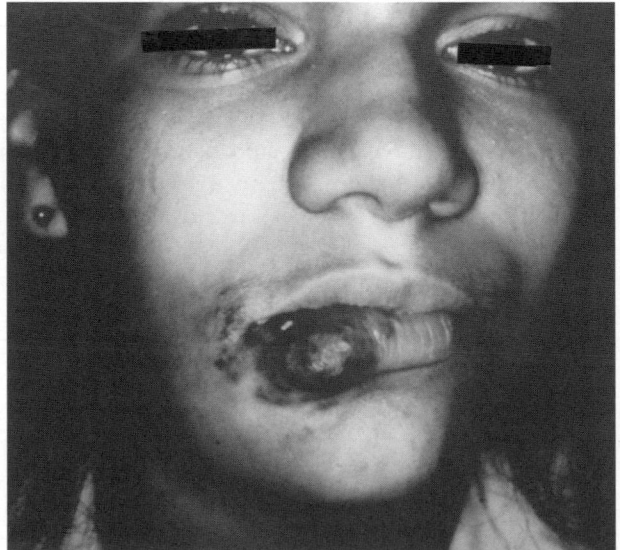

Figure 71–31 Typical cavernous venous malformation. When close to a skin surface, these lesions are soft, nonpulsatile, and compressible with a bluish discoloration. The overlying skin may be thinned to the point of spontaneous breakdown with bleeding.

Treatment

As with any vascular malformation, venous lesions require treatment only if they are significantly symptomatic or disfiguring. Once the diagnosis is clear, patients can be reassured that these lesions generally change little over time and rarely bleed spontaneously. A more common problem is local pain resulting from distention of the lesion or superimposed thrombosis. The pain of distention can often be reduced by positioning or compression (e.g., support stockings or elastic bandages). Local thrombosis is managed in the same way as any superficial phlebitis, with elevation, anti-inflammatory agents, and warm soaks. Anticoagulation is rarely indicated in this setting. On occasion, cavernous lesions may show the same type of progression at menarche and during pregnancy as is seen with other vascular malformations.

Complete surgical resection may be possible for localized lesions, but their true extent should first be carefully evaluated by imaging studies and direct puncture venography, as the visible component of the lesion may be only the tip of the iceberg. Partial resections are generally associated with significant blood loss and a high likelihood of recurrence.

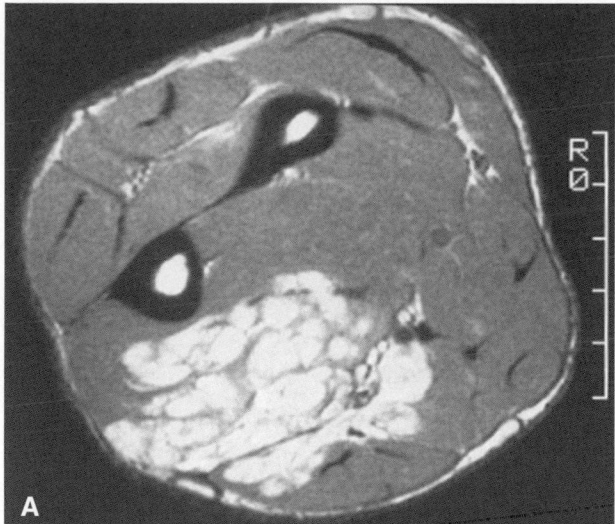

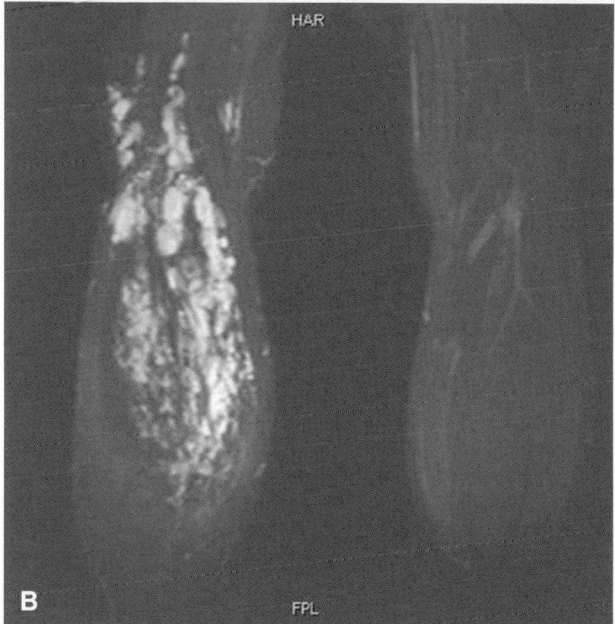

Figure 71–32 Two MRI studies (*sequence x*) of intramuscular venous malformations, one in the forearm (**A**. *axial view*) and one in the calf (**B**. *sagittal view*). MR studies will often clearly demonstrate a deep venous lesion that is inapparent by any other imaging modality. These lesions are often misdiagnosed for prolonged periods of time because of the lack of physical findings and the relatively nonspecific symptoms, which typically include muscle pain on activity or a "heavy" sensation in the involved limb.

Embolization of regional arterial branches in an effort to decompress these lesions was attempted in the past with little success. Lesions that appear venous on physical examination and have ultrasound and MR findings consistent with a low-flow malformation do not routinely require arteriography prior to treatment, although arteriograms will occasionally be performed if there is any question of an arterial component. This type of mixed lesion is uncommon but may benefit from combined arterial and venous embolization. Direct puncture embolization or sclerotherapy

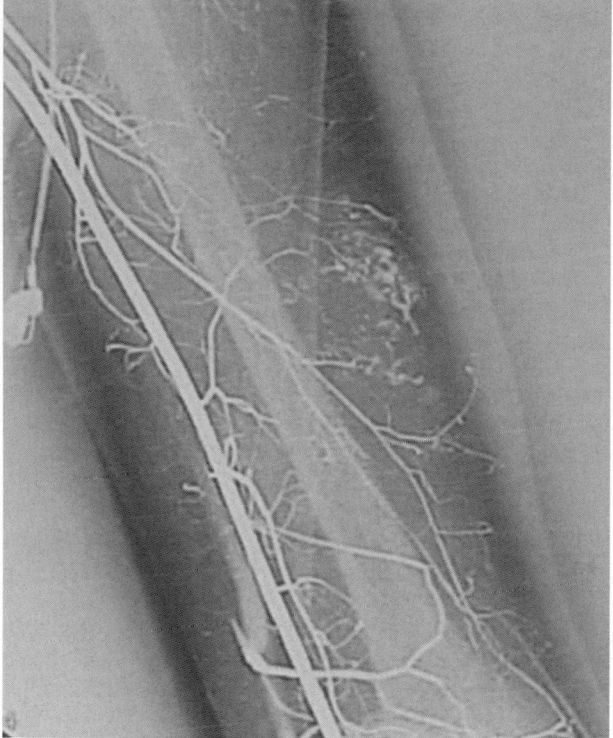

Figure 71–33 Typical unimpressive angiographic findings in venous malformations include normal arterial branches and faint late-phase blush of venous "staining."

is a fairly simple technique that has proved effective in treating cavernous venous lesions. This is an extension of the closed space venography technique, involving direct puncture of the lesion using a sheathed needle inserted through the adjacent normal skin, usually under anesthesia (Figure 71–37). The lesion can be localized by palpation, ultrasound, prior opacification by venography, CT, or MRI (Figure 71–38). MRI guidance is somewhat cumbersome but useful because of the clear visualization of venous malformations that may not be well seen by any other modality; deep lesions may be especially suited to this technique, which requires the use of MR-compatible titanium needles. After venous blood return is observed, contrast (iodinated or gadolinium in the case of MR guidance) is slowly hand injected until the capacity of the lesion is reached; this can be judged by observing small draining veins begin to fill from the periphery of the lesion toward normal regional veins. The lesion is then allowed to empty passively (active compression will often dislodge the catheter), after which the lesion is refilled with a smaller volume of 95% ethanol. Various techniques have been described for keeping the sclerosant solution confined to the malformation, including tourniquet control and direct compression of draining veins. A variation of this technique has recently been described (double-needle sclerotherapy) that may be effective in prolonging endothelial surface contact of the agent while reducing the likelihood of extravasation and toxicity

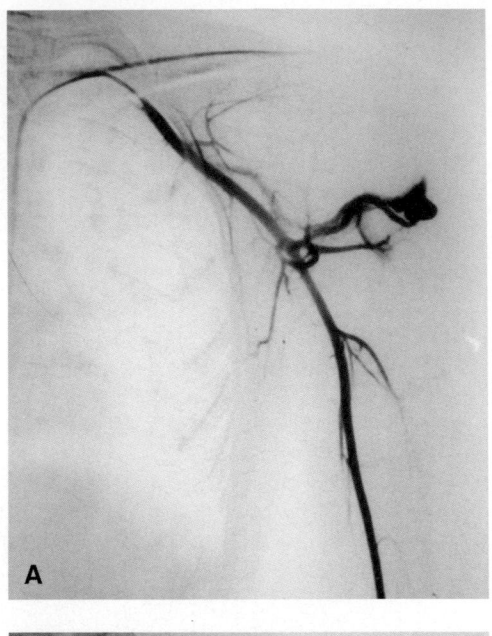

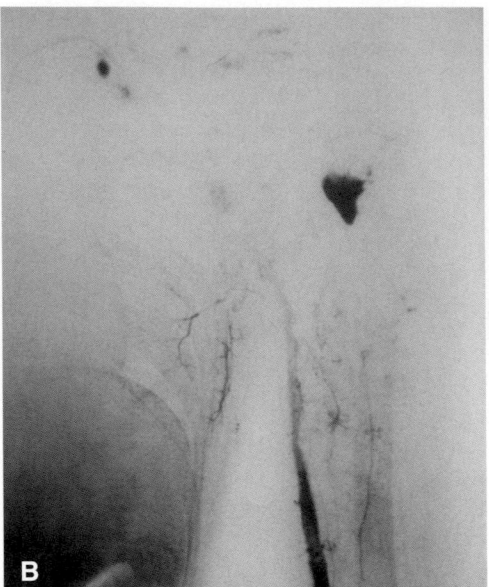

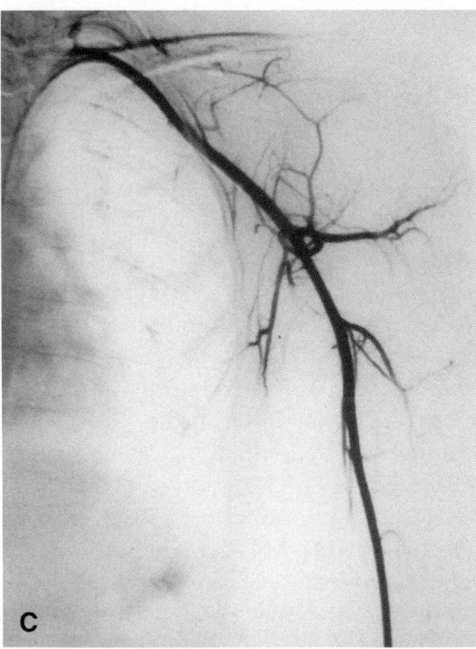

Figure 71–34 An 8-year-old girl with what appeared clinically to be a purely venous malformation involving the shoulder and upper arm. **A.** Left subclavian arteriogram demonstrates an unexpected fistula from the axillary artery branch. **B.** Later-phase film demonstrates filling of cavernous venous spaces. This lesion is typical of Parkes Weber syndrome. **C.** Embolization of the arterial component produced dramatic decompression and shrinkage of the lesion.

(96). Other sclerosing agents such as sodium tetradecyl sulfate (Sotradecol) have also been used with good results and what appears to be less risk of nerve injury and ulceration. This agent is available in 1% and 3% solutions and can be injected alone or mixed with a small amount of contrast to enable fluoroscopic visualization. This agent can also be prepared as a foam, which will fill a larger volume and has a more potent sclerosing effect (97). Lesions with multiple noncommunicating compartments will require multiple sites of injection. The alcohol or other sclerosant is left in place, causing clotting of the blood and damage to the vascular endothelium lining the venous spaces. As thrombosis develops, the lesion will become enlarged and firm. A small amount (approximately 1 cc) of a collagen suspension is injected along the tract as the catheter is withdrawn to prevent bleeding and tracking of the agent to the skin surface, where it may cause ulceration.

Signs of thrombosis (inflammation, pain, swelling) will persist for 2–3 weeks, and it will often require 6–8 weeks to observe shrinkage of the lesion. Depending on the size of the lesion, multiple treatments over time may be necessary.

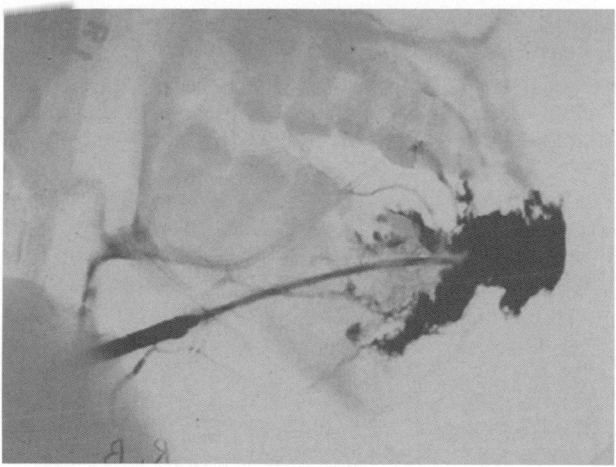

Figure 71–35 Direct puncture study of cavernous venous malformation involving lower lip demonstrates irregular venous space much more extensive than the clinicially visible lesion. Note filling of small veins around the periphery of the lesion that drain into normal regional veins. (Image coutesy of Alex Berenstein, MD.)

Klippel-Trénaunay Syndrome

Klippel-Trénaunay (K-T) syndrome is probably the most frequent major venous malformation encountered clinically. Although the lesion is congenital, there is usually no associated family history. The major components of the syndrome, first described in 1900, consist of (a) extensive venous varicosities usually involving a single limb, (b) hypertrophy of the entire limb, including bones and soft tissues, and (c) a large irregular birthmark (actually a superficial capillary or venular malformation) over the affected

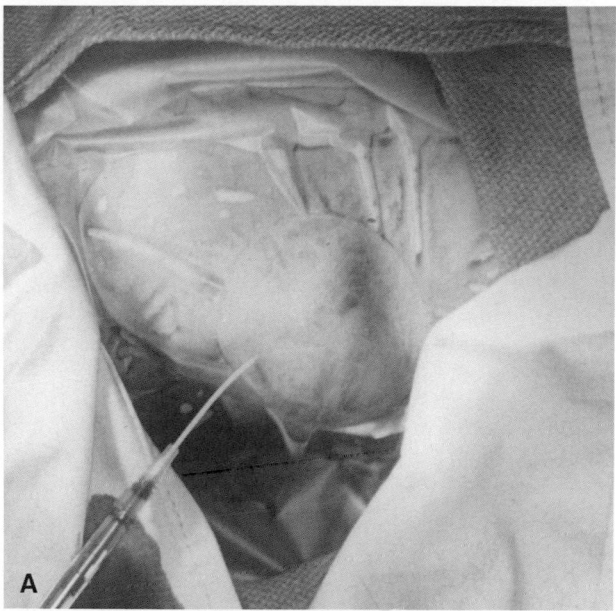

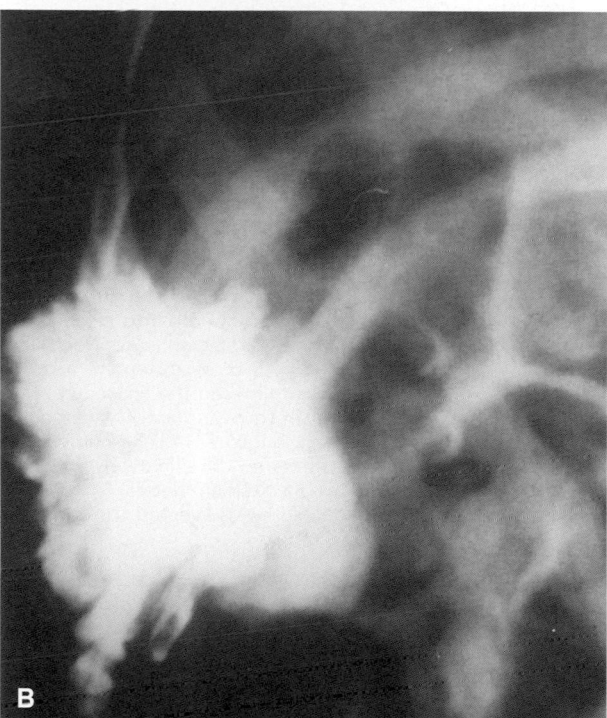

Figure 71–37 Direct puncture embolization of cavernous venous malformation is a fairly simple technique. **A.** Under anesthesia, the lesion is entered through the adjacent normal skin using a sheathed needle. **B.** After blood return is obtained, the lesion is filled with contrast to determine its capacity. The contrast is then permitted to drain passively, and the lesion is refilled with a smaller volume of opacified absolute ethanol under fluoroscopic control. The alcohol is left in place, and the tract is occluded with collagen suspension as the sheath is withdrawn to prevent bleeding and tracking of alcohol to the skin surface.

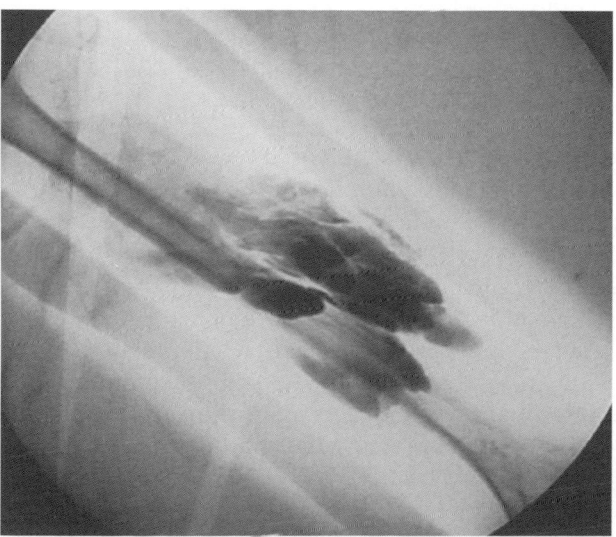

Figure 71–36 Direct puncture study of extensive intramuscular venous malformation of upper arm. Distension of these spaces after activity results in diffuse pain that may last for hours.

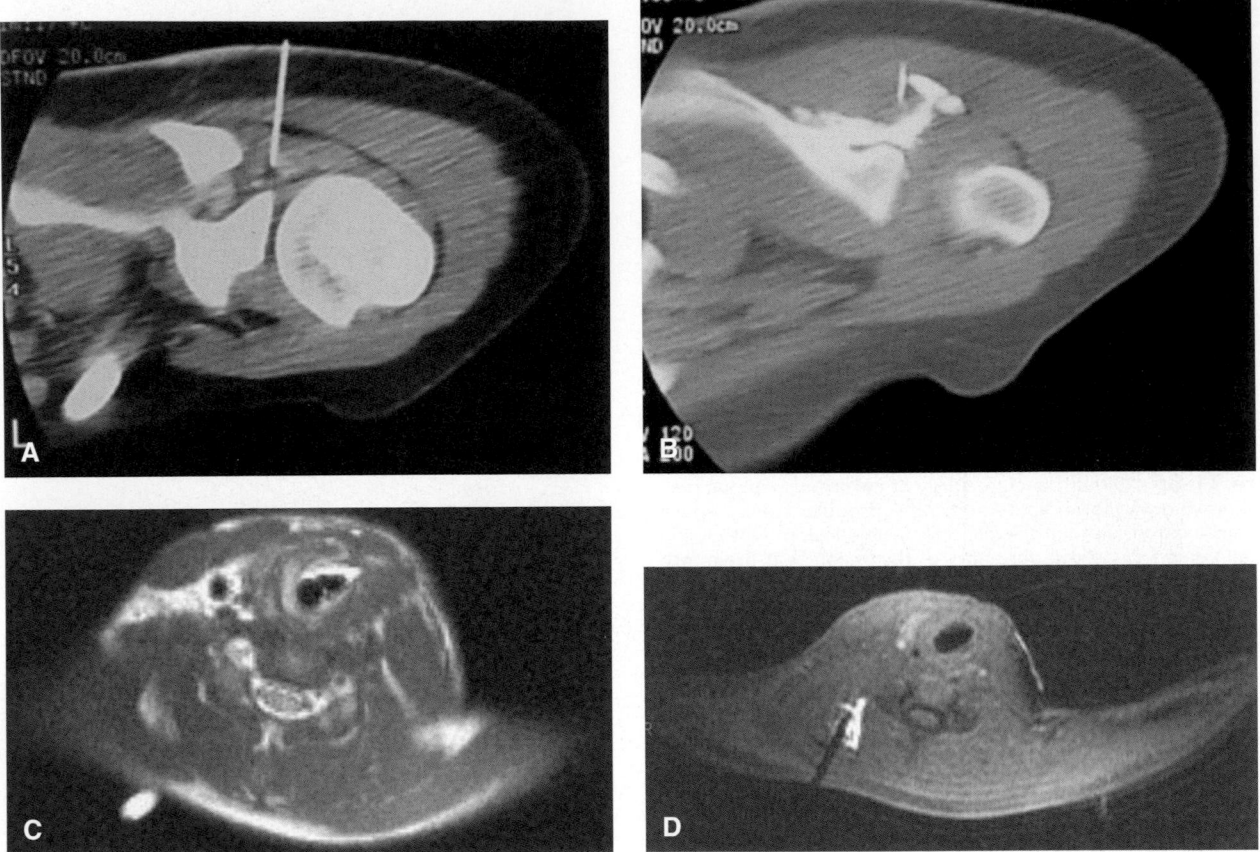

Figure 71–38 Some venous malformations are relatively difficult to access and may require cross-sectional imaging by CT or MRI for direct puncture embolization. **A.** Demonstrates CT-guided placement of 22-gauge needle into small painful venous lesion posterior to the glenoid. **B.** A small amount of dilute radiographic contrast is injected to confirm distribution throughout the lesion This was followed by 5 cc of absolute ethanol, which resulted in complete resolution of the symptoms several weeks following the procedure. **C.** Another patient, a 17-year-old male athlete with severe right neck pain following activity, demonstrates small intramuscular venous malformation deep in the right neck on axial HASTE MRI image following intravenous gadolinium injection. (A vitamin E capsule is affixed to the skin overlying the painful atrea.) **D.** Following puncture of the lesion with an MR-compatible titanium needle (*dark linear artifact*), a small amount of sotradecol opacified with dilute gadolinium was injected. The patient's symptoms resolved completely within days.

extremity (98). The vast majority of these cases involve the lower limb and are unilateral, a finding which suggests this diagnosis rather than simple varicose veins (Figure 71–39). The varicosities are typically extensive and associated with changes of long-standing venous hypertension, including edema, skin thickening, hyperpigmentation, ulceration, and often areas of superficial phlebitis. In young patients, limb length discrepancies and difficulty in fitting shoes may present significant problems. Some patients will present with recurrent hemarthrosis when the malformation involves the joint space, particularly the knee; the resulting degenerative changes may resemble the joint pathology seen in hemophilia (Figure 71–40).

A significant number of these patients will demonstrate an anomalous deep venous system on venography, sometimes showing hypoplastic deep veins with marked hypertrophy of the varicose superficial veins (including a

characteristic "lateral embryonic vein"), which may carry the bulk of venous return from the leg (Figure 71–41). It is essential to be aware of the status of the deep venous system prior to performing any interventional or surgical procedures on the varicosities or other associated venous malformations. Most cases are confined to a single extremity, but there are severe cases that extend into the pelvis and abdomen, sometimes associated with hematuria or gastrointestinal bleeding (99). Plain films may show phleboliths scattered over a wide anatomic region in these patients (Figure 71–42).

Most patients with K-T syndrome are best managed conservatively, using support stockings, leg elevation at night, and symptomatic treatment for episodes of superficial phlebitis (100–102). Although there have been reported series of successful surgical treatment (103–105), patients may actually become worse after these procedures. If there

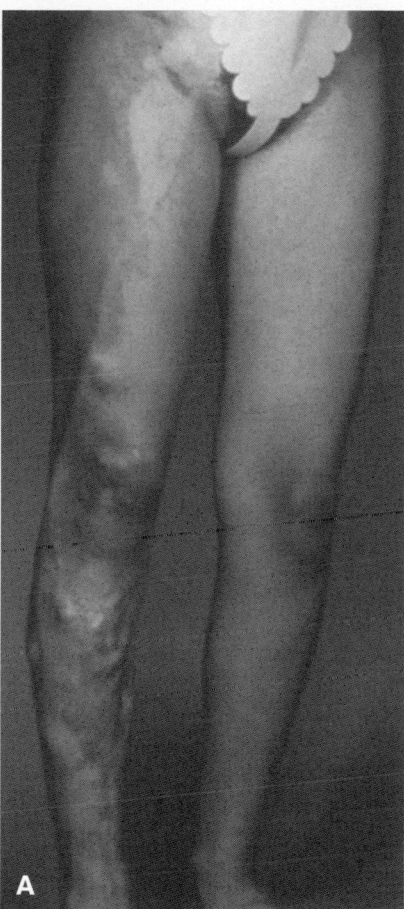

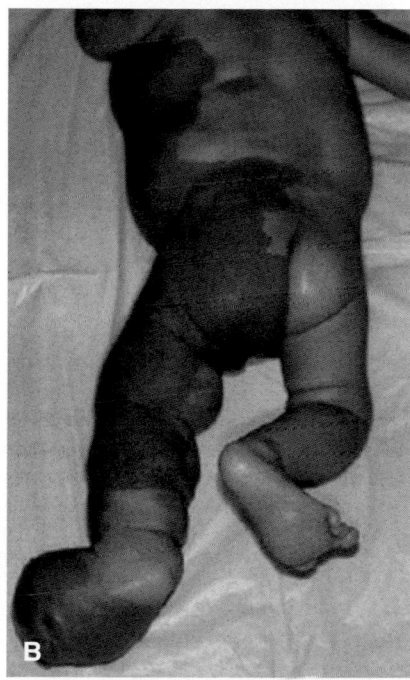

Figure 71–39 Young adult female patient with Klippel-Trénaunay syndrome. **A.** Demonstrates typical findings of severe unilateral varicose veins, overlying pigmented skin lesion (capillary venous malformation), and leg length discrepancy. **B.** Severe forms, such as in this infant, are much less common and represent difficult management problems.

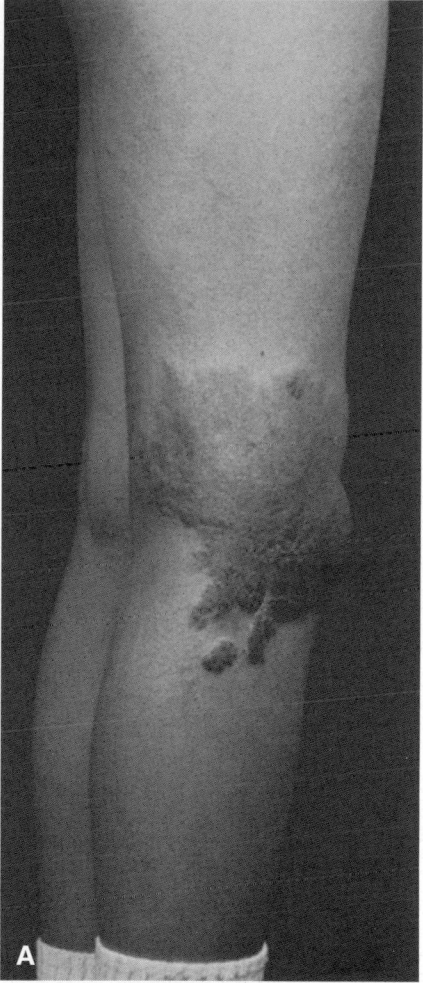

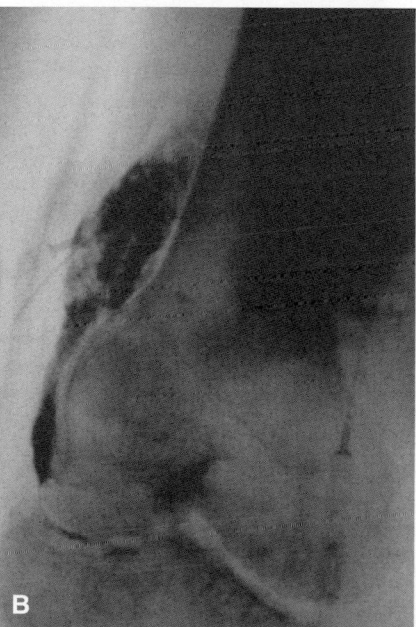

Figure 71–40 A. This 12-year-old girl has Klippel-Trénaunay syndrome involving the right knee, demonstrating overlying cutaneous venous lesion. **B.** Recurrent bleeding from the deep venous malformation into the knee joint results in degenerative arthritis similar to that seen in hemophilia.

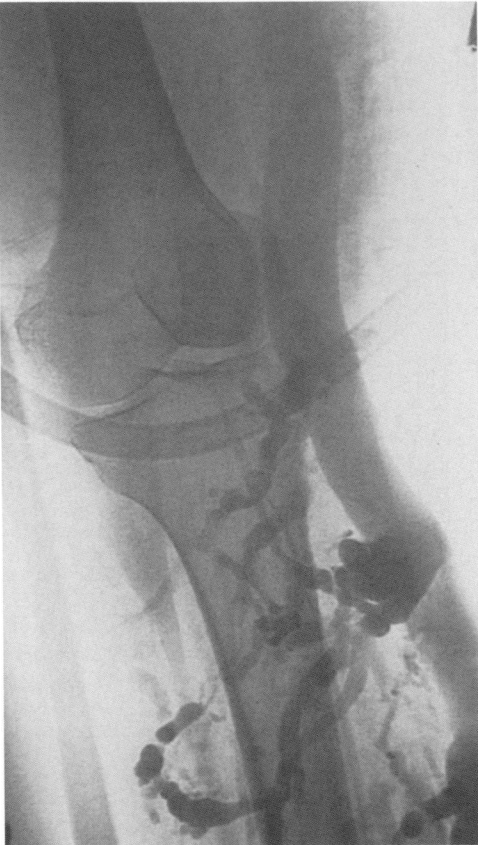

Figure 71–41 Venographic findings in Klippel-Trénaunay syndrome are highly variable, commonly showing a large anomalous superficial vein (lateral embryonic vein) with or without aplasia or hypoplasia of the normal deep venous system. The status of the deep veins should always be determined prior to any intervention in these patients.

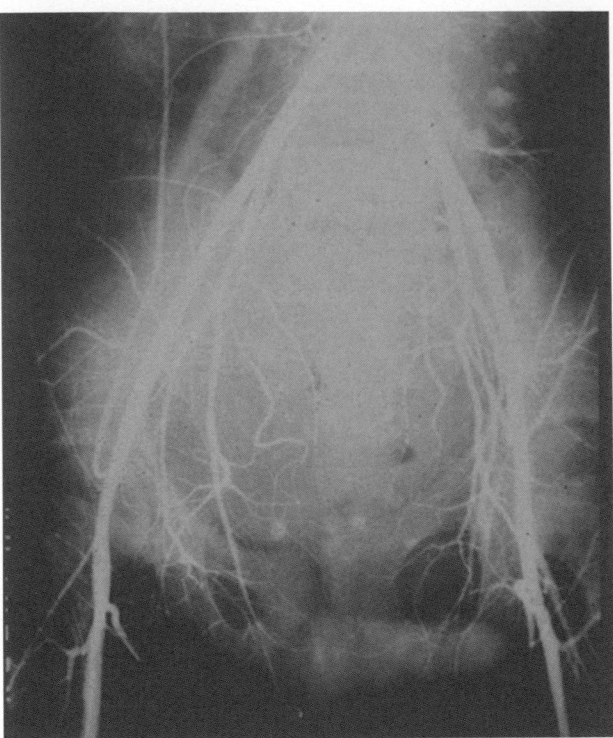

Figure 71–42 Rarely, Klippel-Trénaunay syndrome can involve the trunk as well as an extremity, in some cases causing GI bleeding and hematuria. Note the scattered phleboliths and splaying of the iliac vessels in this 10-year-old boy with extensive venous malformation throughout the retroperitoneum.

is hypoplasia of the deep venous system, removal of superficial veins may result in acute venous insufficiency with intractable leg swelling. Careful venographic evaluation should therefore be performed prior to any invasive treatment, and only localized symptomatic veins should be stripped. Some of the newer endovenous techniques (laser and radiofrequency ablation) may have a role to play in treating these patients. Some of these patients will also demonstrate associated cavernous venous lesions that may be amenable to direct embolization. In some patients, the superficial venous components causing cosmetic problems may be amenable to laser treatment (106).

A variant of Klippel-Trénaunay syndrome is Parkes Weber syndrome, which is clinically almost identical but on angiography demonstrates arteriovenous fistulas (107). Some of these patients will show significant improvement with embolization of these fistulous connections, often with dramatic decompression of the venous structures (Figure 71–43).

LYMPHATIC MALFORMATIONS

Some of the most frustrating cases are those of lymphatic malformations. Abnormal growth of lymphatic circulation encompasses overdevelopment (in lymphangiodysplasias, lymphangiomas, and lymphangiomatosis) and/or underdevelopment of lymphatic vasculature. Disorders of the lymphatic circulation are common, diverse, and often devastating in their functional consequences. Clinical issues common to lymphatic anomalies reflect the tendency of these malformations to develop: (a) local (and systemic) infections/cellulitis (infectious and aseptic); (b) leakage (e.g., superficial blebs, chylous ascites, chylothorax, peritonitis, and pleural effusions) (Figure 71–44); (c) malabsorptive syndromes with significant metabolic consequences; (d) craniofacial distortion interfering with swallowing and sensory organs or significant visceral dysfunction; (e) recurrences or complications after surgery; and/or (f) swelling of the affected limb or body part, with extremely limited lifestyles. At present, lymphatic diseases lack highly efficacious therapies. Therapy is generally limited to sclerotherapy when possible, complete decompressive massage, compression, and pneumatic therapy (108–121).

64. Shumacker HB Jr. The problem of maintaining the continuity of the artery in the surgery of aneurysms and arteriovenous fistulae: notes on the development and clinical application of methods of arterial suture. Ann Surg 1948;127:207.

65. Holman E. Arteriovenous aneurysm: clinical evidence correlating size of fistula with changes in the heart and proximal vessels. Ann Surg 1924;80:801.

66. Holman E. Arteriovenous Aneurysm: Abnormal Communications Between the Arterial and Venous Circulations. New York: Macmillan, 1937.

67. Holman E. The anatomic and physiologic effects of an arteriovenous fistula. Surgery 1940;8:362.

68. Sumner DS. Hemodynamics and pathophysiology of arteriovenous fistulas. In: Rutherford R, ed. Vascular Surgery. Philadelphia: Saunders, 1989:1007,1015.

69. John HT, Warren R. The stimulus to collateral circulation. Surgery 1961;49:14.

70. Nicoladoni C. Phlebarteriectasie der rechten oberen Extremitat. Arch Klin Chir 1875;18:252.

71. Branham HH. Aneurismal varix of the femoral artery and vein following a gunshot wound. Int J Surg 1890;3:250.

72. Szilagyi DE, Elliot JP, DeRusso FJ, et al. Peripheral congenital arteriovenous fistulas. Surgery 1965;57:61.

73. Criado E, Marston WA, Ligush J, Mauro MA, Keagy BA. Endovascular repair of peripheral aneurysms, pseudoaneurysms and arteriovenous fistulas. Ann Vasc Surg 1997;11:256–263.

74. Berenstein A, Kricheff I. Catheter and material selection for transarterial embolization: II. Materials. Radiology 1979;132:631.

75. Natali J, Jue-Denis P, Kieffer E, et al. Arteriovenous fistulae of the internal iliac vessels. J Cardiovasc Surg 1984;25:165.

76. Rosen RJ, Riles TS. Arteriovenous malformations. In: Strandness D, van Breda A, eds. Vascular Diseases: Surgical and Interventional Therapy. New York: Churchill-Livingstone, 1994:1126.

77. Rutherford RB. Congenital vascular malformations: diagnostic evaluation. Semin Vasc Surg. 1993 Dec;6(4):225–232.

78. Paltiel HJ, Burrows PE, Kozakewich HP, Zurakowski D, Mulliken JB: Soft-tissue vascular anomales: utility of US for diagnosis. Radiology 2000;214:747–754.

79. Rutherford RB. Noninvasive testing in the diagnosis and assessment of arteriovenous fistula. In: Berenstein EF, ed. Noninvasive Diagnostic Techniques in Vascular Disease. St. Louis:Mosby, 1982:430–442.

80. Rinker B, Karp NS, Margiotta M, et al. The role of magnetic resonance imaging in the management of vascular malformations of the trunk and extremities. Plast Reconstr Surg 2003;112:504–510.

81. Herborn CU, Goyen M, Lauenstein TC, et al. Comprehensive time-resolved MRI of peripheral vascular malformations. AJR Am J Roentgenol 2003;181:729–735.

82. Tadavarthy SM, Moller JH, Amplatz K. Polyvinyl alcohol (Ivalon): a new embolic material. AJR Am J Roentgenol 1975:125:609–616.

83. Lasjaunias P, Berenstein A. Technical aspects of surgical neuroangiography. In: Surgical Neuroangiography, vol 2. Berlin: Springer-Verlag, 1987.

84. Sasaki M, Tadokeoro S, Kimura S, et al. Two cases of renal arteriovenous fistula treated by transcatheter embolization with absolute ethanol. Hinyokika Kiyo 1984;30:295–298.

85. Yakes WF, Haas DK, Parker SH, et al. Symptomatic vascular malformations: ethanol embolotherapy. Radiology 1989;170:1059–1066.

86. Yakes WF, Rossi P, Odink H. How I do it. Arteriovenous malformation management. Cardiovasc Intervent Radiol. 1996;19:65–71.

87. Kerber C. Intracranial cyoanacrylate: a new catheter therapy for arteriovenous malformation. Invest Radiol 1975;10:536–538.

88. Vinters HV, Galil KA, Lundie MJ, et al. The histotoxicity of cyanoacrylates. A selective review. Neuroradiology 1985;27:279–291.

89. Rao VR, Mandalam KR, Gupta AK, et al. Dissolution of isobutyl 2-cyanoacrylate on long-term follow-up. AJNR Am J Neuroradiol 1989;10:135–141.

90. Sadato A, Wakhloo AK, Hopkins LN. Effects of a mixture of a low concentration of n-butylcyanoacrylate and ethiodol on tissue reactions and the permanence of arterial occlusion after embolization. Neurosurgery 2000;47:1197–1203;discussion.

91. Takebayashi S, Hosaka M, Kubota Y, et al. Transarterial embolization and ablation of renal arteriovenous malformations; efficacy and damages in 30 patients with long-term followup. J Urol 1998;159:696–701.

92. Steckman DA, Chaft JE, Blei F, et al. Diagnosis and management of giant congenital intrarenal arteriovenous fistulas. J Urol in press, 2003.

93. Markoff G, Quagliarello J, Rosen RJ, et al. Uterine arteriovenous malformation successfully embolized with a liquid polymer, isobutyl 2-cyanoacrylate. Am J Obstet Gynecol 1986;55:659–660.

94. Hein KD, Mulliken JB, Kozakewich HP, et al. Venous malformations of skeletal muscle. Plast Reconstr Surg 2002;110:1625–1635.

95. Boxt LM, Levin DC, Fellows KE. Direct puncture angiography in congenital venous malformations. AJR Am J Roentgenol 1983;140:135.

96. Puig S, Aref H, Brunelle F. Double-needle sclerotherapy of lymphangiomas and venous angiomas in children: a simple technique to prevent complications. AJR Am J Roentgenol 2003;180:1399–1401.

97. Hsu TS, Weiss RA. Foam sclerotherapy: a new era. Arch Dermatol. 2003;139:1494–1496.

98. Klippel M, Trenaunay P. Du naevus variqueux osterhypertrophique. Arch Gen Med (Paris) 1900;3:611.

99. Servelle M, Bastin R, Lougue J, et al. Hematuria and rectal bleeding in the child with Klippel Trenaunay syndrome. Ann Surg 1976;183:418.

100. Jacob AG, Driscoll DJ, Shaughnessy WJ, et al. Klippel-Trenaunay syndrome: spectrum and management. Mayo Clin Proc 1998;73:28–36.

101. Al-Salman MM. Klippel-Trenaunay syndrome: clinical features, complications, and management. Surg Today 1997;27:735–740.

102. Baskerville PA, Ackroyd JS, Lea Thomas M, et al. The Klippel-Trenaunay syndrome: clinical, radiological and haemodynamic features and management. Br J Surg 1985;72:232–236.

103. Servelle M. Klippel and Trenaunay's syndrome: 768 operated cases. Ann Surg 1985;201:365.

104. Noel AA, Gloviczki P, Cherry KJ, et al. Surgical treatment of venous malformations in Klippel-Trenaunay syndrome. J Vasc Surg 2000;32:840–847.

105. McCarthy R, Lytle J, Van Devanter S. The use of total circulatory arrest in the surgery of giant hemangioma and Klippel-Trenaunay syndrome in neonates. Clin Orthop Relat Res 1993;289:237–242.

106. Waner M. Recent developments in lasers and the treatment of birthmarks. Arch Dis Child 2003;88:372–374.

107. Parkes Weber F. Haemangiectatic hypertrophy of the limbs: congenital phlebarterietasis and so-called congenital varicose veins. Br J Child Dis 1918;15:13.

108. Lakshman R, Finn A. Lymphopenia in lymphatic malformations. Arch Dis Child 2000;83:276.

109. Witte MH, Way DL, Witte CL, et al. Lymphangiogenesis: mechanisms, significance and clinical implications. Exs 1997;79:65–112.

110. Foldi E, Sauerwald A, Hennig B. Effect of complex decongestive physiotherapy on gene expression for the inflammatory response in peripheral lymphedema. Lymphology 2000;33:19–23.

111. Witte CL, Witte MH. Diagnostic and interventional imaging of lymphatic disorders. Int Angiol 1999;18:25–30.

112. Witte CL, Witte MH. An imaging evaluation of angiodysplasia syndromes. Lymphology 2000;33:158–166.

113. Child AH, Beninson J, Sarfarazi M. Cause of primary congenital lymphedema. Angiology 1999;50:325–326.

114. Foldi M. Lymphology in the second millennium. Lymphology 2001;34:12–21.

115. Foldi E. Treatment of lymphedema and patient rehabilitation. Anticancer Res 1998;18:2211–2212.

116. DeLuca L, Guyuron B, Najem RW. Management of an extensive cervicofacial lymphovenous malformation of the maxillofacial region. Ann Plast Surg 1996;36:644–648.

117. Fishman SJ, Burrows PE, Upton J, et al. Life-threatening anomalies of the thoracic duct: anatomic delineation dictates management. J Pediatr Surg 2001;36:1269–1272.

118. Fliegelman LJ, Friedland D, Brandwein M, et al. Lymphatic malformation: predictive factors for recurrence. Otolaryngol Head Neck Surg 120;123:706–710.

119. Pandit SK, Rattan KN, Budhiraja S, et al. Cystic lymphangioma with special reference to rare sites. Indian J Pediatr 2000;67: 339–341.

120. Yavuzer R, Latifoglu O, Ataoglu O, et al. Lymphatic malformation or lymphovenous malformation. Plast Reconstr Surg 1999;104:1579–1580.
121. Greinwald JH Jr, Burke DK, Sato Y, et al. Treatment of lymphangiomas in children: an update of Picibanil (OK-432) sclerotherapy. Otolaryngol Head Neck Surg 1999;121:381–387.
122. Witte MH, Way DL, Witte CL, et al. Lymphangiogenesis: mechanisms, significance and clinical implications. Exs 1997;79:65–112.
123. Szuba A, Skobe M, Karkkainen MJ, et al. Therapeutic lymphangiogenesis with human recombinant VEGF-C. Faseb J 2002;16:1985–1987.

124. Saaristo A, Karkkainen MJ, Alitalo K. Insights into the molecular pathogenesis and targeted treatment of lymphedema. Ann N Y Acad Sci 2002;979:94–110.
125. Alitalo K, Carmeliet P. Molecular mechanisms of lymphangiogenesis in health and disease. Cancer Cell 2002;1:219–227.
126. Baldwin ME, Stacker SA, Achen MG. Molecular control of lymphangiogenesis. Bioessays 2002;24:1030–1040.
127. Rockson SG. Preclinical models of lymphatic disease: the potential for growth factor and gene therapy. Ann N Y Acad Sci 2002;979:64–75.

Recanalization of Dialysis Fistulas

72

Anne Roberts

The maintenance of hemodialysis access is an important, but sometimes frustrating, challenge. Large numbers of patients depend on hemodialysis; approximately 300,000 individuals in the United States are receiving hemodialysis for end-stage renal disease (ESRD) (1). The survival rate of patients with ESRD has been steadily increasing. There has been a trend toward treating older patients, and there are increasing numbers of patients with diabetes (1). As a result, the prevalence of treated ESRD is growing at approximately 5% per year. The number of older patients treated with hemodialysis has also increased dramatically. Since 1992, the overall incidence rate for ESRD has doubled in patients over the age of 65 (1). Those age 75 and older now make up more than a quarter of the ESRD population, up from only 8% in 1980 (1).

Because older patients are less likely to be candidates for renal transplantation, the number of patients on hemodialysis will increase even more dramatically as the population continues to age. In some centers, as few as 10% of the patients on dialysis are transplant candidates (2). Even those patients who are transplant candidates may need dialysis access for a considerable period of time because of the limited availability of donor organs. The percentage of patients transplanted within 3 years is 19%; however, in patients over 60, the percentage is only 6.0%. The number of patients awaiting transplantation has continued to increase steadily. In 2002, almost 50,000 patients were awaiting transplantation, double the number awaiting transplants in 1995 (1). Thus, for patients with ESRD who are either awaiting transplants or are not transplant candidates, their hemodialysis access is their "lifeline."

The frustrations with access maintenance result from the many problems associated with hemodialysis fistulas and grafts. The most common problem for fistulas is the failure of the fistula to mature; with grafts it is the development of stenoses and eventual thrombosis. Vascular access placement and the complications associated with vascular access still account for a significant number of admissions and hospitalization days for hemodialysis patients. Despite this, the rate of hospitalization for grafts, fistulas, and catheters has diminished markedly over the last 10 years as more of the procedures are being performed as outpatients (1).

The placement of a hemodialysis access is the first challenge. An endogenous arteriovenous (AV) fistula is the preferred access because it provides the greatest chance for long-term function. The National Kidney Foundation—Dialysis Outcomes Quality Initiative (DOQI) guidelines set a goal that 50% of all new patients requiring hemodialysis receive an AV fistula, so that ultimately at least 40% of hemodialysis patients will have a native AV fistula (3). The Brescia-Cimino fistula is constructed with a side-to-side anastomosis of the cephalic vein and radial artery at the wrist. Such fistulas should be placed 3–4 months before being used for dialysis so there is time for wound healing, resolution of edema, dilation of the vein, and hypertrophy of the vein wall. Other fistulas include a brachiocephalic fistula (between the brachial artery and the cephalic vein), the brachiobasilic fistula (between the brachial artery and basilic vein), and a fistula between the femoral artery and saphenous vein (4). Creation of an autologous fistula may be difficult or impossible in a substantial number of patients. However, progress has been made in increasing the number of patients with AV fistulas. Failures continue to be particularly common in elderly and diabetic patients. As the number of these patients in the dialysis population has increased, an increased percentage of patients with obstacles to the creation of an AV fistula has occurred. Consequently, less than 30% of the dialysis population nationwide currently has a native AV fistula (1).

Patients who are not candidates for an endogenous AV fistula have fistulas created from polytetrafluoroethylene (PTFE) graft material. The PTFE grafts mature in only 2 weeks, which allows for earlier dialysis than with endogenous fistulas. However, these grafts are plagued by relatively frequent failures, with primary patency rates at 1 year of approximately 40% (5). The most common reason for failure is the development of a stenosis in the outflow veins and subsequent thrombosis of the graft.

Vascular access patency and adequate flow for dialysis depend on fistula blood flow, which may reach as high as 850 mL per minute in normal grafts, at least 300 mL per minute is essential for successful long-term dialysis (6). Insufficient graft flow increases the risk of thrombosis and decreases dialysis efficacy by limiting extracorporeal blood flow. As neointimal hyperplasia and subsequent stenoses begin to develop, the graft flow decreases and the risk of thrombosis increases.

SURVEILLANCE OF GRAFTS AND FISTULAS

Dialysis grafts and, to a lesser degree, fistulas are at continuous risk for malfunction. Thrombosis is the most common cause of vascular access loss and is almost always associated with stenoses, usually in the venous outflow tract. The veins (which are subject to the turbulence, high flows, and pressures caused by the arteriovenous fistula) develop neointimal hyperplasia, which leads to stenoses. Occasionally, venous stenoses develop rapidly within the first month (7), but usually thrombosis occurring in the first weeks to a month after placement of the access is because of a technical error in the creation of the fistula/graft. Thrombosis developing later than 1 month is most commonly due to stenosis in the venous outflow. Less frequently, arterial inflow stenoses are responsible for thrombosis, but in one series, this occurred in less than 2% of thrombosed grafts (8). Rarely, no underlying anatomic lesion can be identified; these patients may have had excessive post-dialysis compression, hypotension, hypovolemia, compression of the graft because of sleeping position, or a hypercoagulable state, any of which may lead to thrombosis (9).

Neointimal hyperplasia occurring in the venous outflow leads to the development of venous stenoses. The phenomenon of neointimal hyperplasia is complex and not well understood. The hyperplasia and resulting stenoses develop near the venous anastomosis most likely as a response to turbulent blood flow and vibration resulting from placement of the fistula (10,11). Other mechanical factors, such as compliance mismatch between graft materials and the vein (12); wall shear rates (13); or angulation and stretching of the vein may be important (14). When treated with either angioplasty or surgical revision, stenoses inevitably recur, because the conditions that caused the original stenoses are unchanged (15,16). These lesions are the most common cause for thrombosis of the dialysis grafts, and the long-term durability of any procedure to improve the venous outflow is constrained by the development of such stenoses.

The DOQI guidelines are an attempt to improve monitoring of the grafts and fistulas to identify those at risk for thrombosis. An organized monitoring approach is recommended with regular assessment of clinical parameters of the AV access and dialysis adequacy (3). Asymptomatic but hemodynamically significant stenoses can usually be detected through several surveillance techniques (17). The methods preferred for monitoring include evaluating sequential intra-access flow (3,18,19) or static venous dialysis pressures (3,20). Other methods that can be used are dynamic venous pressures (20–22), measurement of recirculation (23), unexplained decreases in the measured amount of hemodialysis delivered (3), and duplex ultrasound with color flow technique (3).

Physical examination of the graft/fistula is also useful. Persistent swelling of the arm, prolonged bleeding after needle withdrawal, difficulty with needle placement, or changes in the characteristics of the thrill within the graft are all findings that may herald graft failure (2,3,24,25). Auscultation of the graft, particularly at the region of the venous anastomosis, can be very informative. When a stenosis is present, there is often a high-pitched, harsh, or discontinuous bruit at the site of the stenosis. Palpation of a discontinuous or water-hammer pulse within the graft usually indicates an outflow stenosis. If an abnormality is found on physical examination, approximately 90% of patients will be found to have an angiographically significant abnormality (26).

Fistula surveillance uses many of the same methods as grafts. Physical examination is very helpful and may be even more informative than with grafts. Ultrasound evaluation is helpful in evaluating fistula maturation (27). The other measures of access function also are important in fistulas, but the thresholds for abnormality are not as well delineated as they are for grafts (3). This is because the stenoses tend to occur more centrally, in the outflow tract at areas of vein bifurcation, pressure points, and venous valves (3). As a result, collateral veins draining the fistula develop, preventing a marked increase in pressure (28). Thus, indirect measures of flow are less predictive of thrombosis and access failure, although measurement of recirculation may be more helpful in the evaluation of fistulas (3).

When surveillance indicates developing problems in the graft/fistula, then venography should be performed to evaluate the graft and correct the underlying lesion. Correction of the lesion improves patency and decreases the incidence of thrombosis (3,19,29,30).

TREATMENT OF GRAFT/FISTULA DYSFUNCTION

Because access sites for dialysis access are limited, it is important to extend the life of each access as long as possible. Therapeutic interventions for hemodynamically significant stenoses reduce the rate of thrombosis and graft loss and prolong the life of the access (29,30). Patency will appear to be improved when stenoses are treated before thrombus formation rather than when treatment of the patient occurs after occlusion of the access (3). The DOQI guidelines suggest that each center should determine whether angioplasty or surgical revision is best for the patient based on the expertise at that center (3). The guidelines do indicate that surgical revision should be held to a higher standard than angioplasty because surgical revision usually extends the access farther up the extremity by the use of a jump graft. Thus, more vein is used in surgical revisions than in angioplasty (3). A primary patency rate of 50% at 1 year following surgical revision should be expected (3).

Angioplasty for venous stenosis is widely performed. There are only a few studies comparing the treatment of venous stenoses by angioplasty versus surgical revision, and the results have been contradictory (3,31–33). The patency rates for angioplasty of venous stenosis are 40–50% at 6 months (15,16). Angioplasty preserves the vein, leaving it available for subsequent revision when angioplasty is no longer feasible. The graft is also immediately available for dialysis, avoiding the need for temporary dialysis catheters. Although the stenoses will recur following balloon angioplasty, patients are much more willing to accept repeated angioplasty rather than repeated surgery. Grafts referred to angiography because of potential stenoses that are treated with angioplasty have an excellent technical success rate, in one study reported as 98% (26). The primary patency at 1 year was 23%, but repeated angioplasty significantly improved the patency rates with a primary assisted patency rate of 68% at 1 year and 51% at 2 years. A combination of thrombolysis and repeated angioplasty further improved patency, with secondary patency rates at 1 year of 82% and at 2 years of 65% (26). Aggressive therapy for failing dialysis grafts appears useful, and periodic redilations allow continued graft use for months or years (2). Gaining these months of patency can be extremely valuable to dialysis patients

Treatment of a dysfunctional AV fistula is different than with a graft. In AV fistulas, failure of maturation is a more common problem. The fistula may not have developed a major venous outflow. Instead, multiple outflow veins are present, none of which is large enough to support dialysis. In some cases, this is because of a stenosis in the major outflow vein that causes the collaterals to form. Treatment of the stenosis will allow the flow to proceed in the major outflow, decreasing the collaterals and allowing development of a major outflow (34). Alternatively, the fistula may

have developed but has decreased flow with a flat appearance of the major outflow vein. This indicates an arterial anastomotic inflow problem. If the major outflow vein is dilated but then becomes flat farther up the arm, there is likely to be an outflow stenosis. The presence of multiple stenoses in a fistula is not uncommon. Ultrasound may be helpful in evaluating the fistula and identifying the problem area (34).

When evaluating either a graft or fistula for possible intervention, the entire venous outflow to the superior vena cava and the inflow artery should be studied. The possibility of measuring flow during percutaneous procedures may help to identify both inflow and outflow lesions (35,36). Use of this type of device allows for quantitative measurements that can guide therapy and determine whether adequate angioplasty has been performed, or it may suggest the existence of other lesions. This is particularly useful in AV fistulas. There are specific high-risk areas that should be studied carefully during any evaluation of a graft or fistula:

Venous Anastomotic Stenoses

Significant narrowing in the venous outflow is present in 75–90% of failed grafts, either alone or in combination with other sources for thrombosis (8,37–39). Because these types of stenoses are so common, it is important to carefully evaluate the venous anastomotic site. In the case of multiple outflow channels, the offending stenosis may not be visualized easily and a number of different angiographic projections may be required for visualization. The presence of multiple collaterals is a clue to the presence of a significant venous outflow obstruction. Venous stenoses respond relatively well to balloon dilatation, at least in the short term (Figure 72–1). Selection of the proper balloon size is based on the diameter of the PTFE graft and the size of the draining vein. In most cases, a 6-mm balloon is appropriate, but sizes from 5–8 mm are not uncommon. The high-pressure balloon (15–30 mm Hg) is centered across the stenosis and inflated. An inflation device is helpful to maintain the high-pressure inflation. Prolonged inflations for 2–5 minutes may be useful for resistant lesions. Multiple inflations may be required to completely expand the balloon at the site of stenosis. In some cases in which a very resistant lesion is present, a cutting balloon may be helpful (40–44). The cutting balloon has small blades embedded in the balloon; when the balloon is inflated across the stenosis, these blades make microincisions in the wall. A smaller cutting balloon (4–5 mm) may be used, followed by reinsertion of the larger high-pressure balloon to complete the dilation (41,43).

In other cases, the balloon will inflate completely but a stenosis remains after the inflation. This type of stenosis is referred to as elastic. However, it may represent under treatment from using a balloon that was too small. If the patient

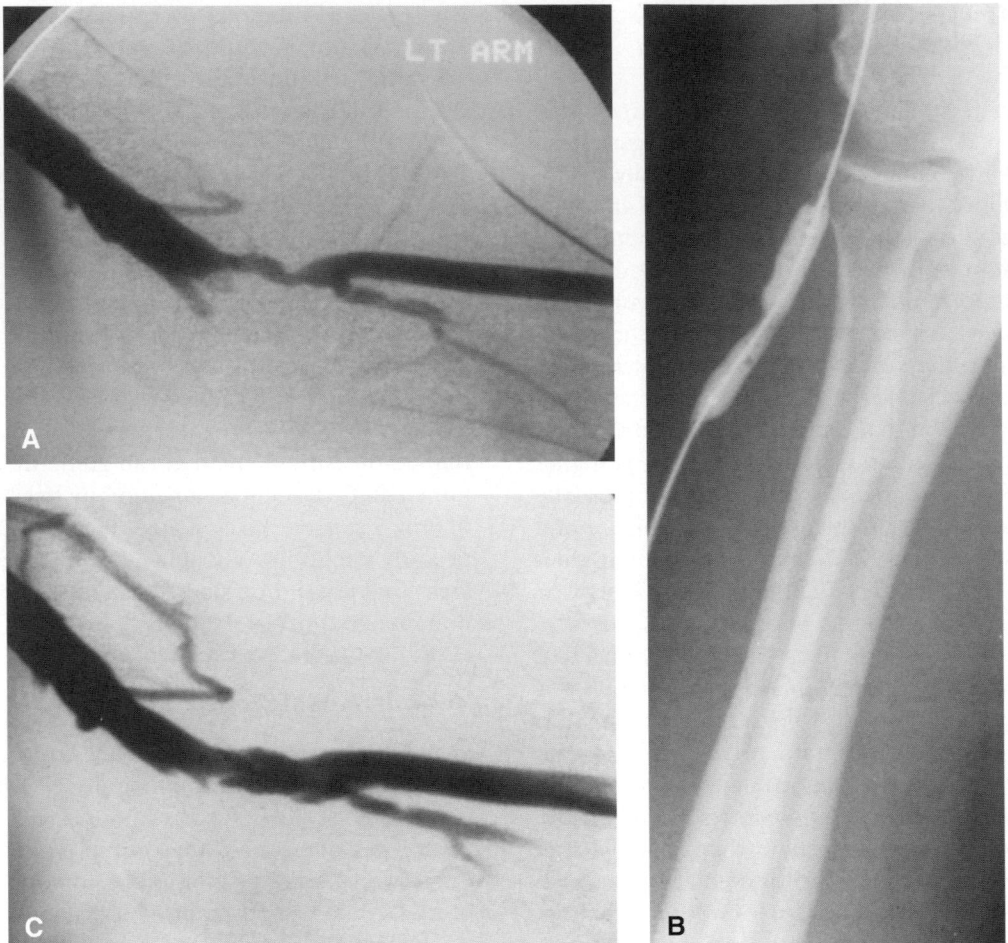

Figure 72–1   A. Tight stenosis of outflow vein, just at the venous anastomosis. **B.** Balloon inflation. Balloons should be fully inflated for 2 minutes. Inflation usually is repeated at least once. **C.** After dilatation. Although the appearance is slightly irregular, the vein remained patent for approximately 15 months.

has had minimal or no pain with the angioplasty, then a larger balloon should be tried to achieve a better result.

The use of stents in dialysis venous stenoses should be extremely selective. Appropriate indications for stents are vein rupture and, in some cases, elastic recoil or restenosis. The initial results from stent placement may appear satisfying, but restenosis is almost inevitable. The restenosis following stent placement commonly is much more extensive than the initial problem, with intimal hyperplasia occurring within the stent and at both ends of the stent. This requires further angioplasty, occasionally with additional stenting. Placement of stents should take into consideration whether the placement would jeopardize surgical revision of the graft. One of the advantages of percutaneous transluminal angioplasty is that it does not preclude surgery at a later date. Areas of bending, such as at the elbow joint, are usually not stented because of the potential strain on the stent. An important complication reported related to the migration of two stents to the pulmonary artery after placement of a

central line into the stented subclavian vein (45). The DOQI guidelines state that stents should generally be reserved for surgically inaccessible stenoses that fail angioplasty because the unassisted patency of the stents in hemodialysis access is no better than that of angioplasty, with the exception of truly elastic lesions (3,46). Vein rupture is probably the best indication for stent placement because the stent can salvage this complication (47). With the advent of covered stents, there are case reports of small series of patients being treated with covered stents (34,48–50). The usual indication is rupture of the vein following angioplasty (34,49) but covered stents have also been used to treat patients with degenerating grafts and pseudoaneurysms (50–52). These covered stents are approved by the FDA for tracheal/bronchial applications and are used off-label in the vascular system.

The evaluation of a malfunctioning fistula requires a different approach than one would use for a graft, particularly if the problem is poor maturation of the fistula. The entire fistula needs to be evaluated, preferably without puncturing the fistula because spasm can result that makes evaluation difficult (34). To study a forearm fistula, the brachial artery can be punctured at the elbow with a 22-gauge sheathed needle (34), or a micropuncture needle and the small inner dilator of the micropuncture set (Cook, Inc.) is used to access the artery. Angiography is then performed, which allows evaluation of the palmar arch and evaluation of antegrade or retrograde filling of the distal artery feeding the fistula (34). Once the diagnostic study has been performed, the fistula can be accessed appropriately, usually from a retrograde approach. Venous stenoses should be dilated, attempting to achieve at least a 5 mm lumen. In a poorly developed fistula with a very small draining vein, it may be wise to start with small balloons (3–4 mm) and perform serial dilatations using progressively larger balloons. This may avoid potential rupture of a small, undilated vein.

Arterial Inflow Stenoses

Significant stenoses in the feeding artery requiring treatment are found in less than 15% of treated grafts (8,16,53). However, these lesions often result in inadequate flow for dialysis or in early rethrombosis. To visualize the arterial anastomosis, the catheter directed toward the arterial anastomosis is advanced until it is positioned just at the anastomosis, and an injection of contrast is made at that position. If good flow has been reestablished, visualization of the proximal artery may be difficult. Visualization can be improved by briefly compressing the graft or by inflating a blood pressure cuff above the shunt to occlude outflow. Because of the geometry of the anastomosis, multiple views may be necessary to adequately assess the anastomosis and the arterial inflow. If a significant stenosis is identified, balloon angioplasty may be an effective alternative to surgical revision. It is often possible to pass a wire through the anastomosis from the graft and to perform an angioplasty in the same session as the thrombolysis. If angioplasty cannot be done from the venous side of the graft because of an unfavorable angle at the anastomosis, direct puncture of the supplying artery can be performed.

If an inflow lesion is suspected that is not visualized by refluxing into the artery from the graft, an angiographic evaluation of the entire length of the feeding artery should be performed. This should visualize the artery from its origin to the artery-graft anastomosis. Many of the dialysis patients are elderly, diabetic, or both and are prone to the development of atherosclerosis anywhere along the course of the supplying artery. If such a lesion is identified, it can usually be successfully treated with angioplasty.

Intragraft Stenoses

Significant intragraft stenoses are uncommon. The cause of these stenoses is not clear. They may represent hypertrophy of the neointima that lines the luminal surface of

PTFE grafts (54) or may represent organized mural thrombus lining the graft, particularly in the area of multiple previous punctures. Such stenoses often can be treated with balloon angioplasty. Usually, the balloon should be the same diameter or, at the most, 1 mm larger than the graft diameter.

Central Venous Stenoses

The venous outflow should be examined to the level of the superior vena cava because stenoses may develop anywhere along the venous outflow. The most common site of stenoses is the venous anastomosis site, but stenoses may develop in the axillary region and as far proximal as the subclavian and brachiocephalic veins. Subclavian stenoses are most often the result of venous injury from previous dialysis access catheters (3,55–57) (Figure 72–2). Although a subclavian stenosis or occlusion may negatively impact the efficiency of dialysis, such a stenosis is not commonly the cause of dialysis access thrombosis. When a graft thromboses, a careful search should be made for an anastomotic stenosis that is much more likely to be the cause of the thrombosis. Subclavian stenoses can be treated with balloon angioplasty if they are causing graft dysfunction (39,58). The use of stents should be reserved for treatment of central venous occlusions or elastic central vein stenoses or whenever a stenosis recurs in a 3-month period (3,39,59,60–62). If stents are placed in the central veins, stents should not bridge the internal jugular vein or contralateral brachiocephalic vein that may be needed for dialysis catheters (63).

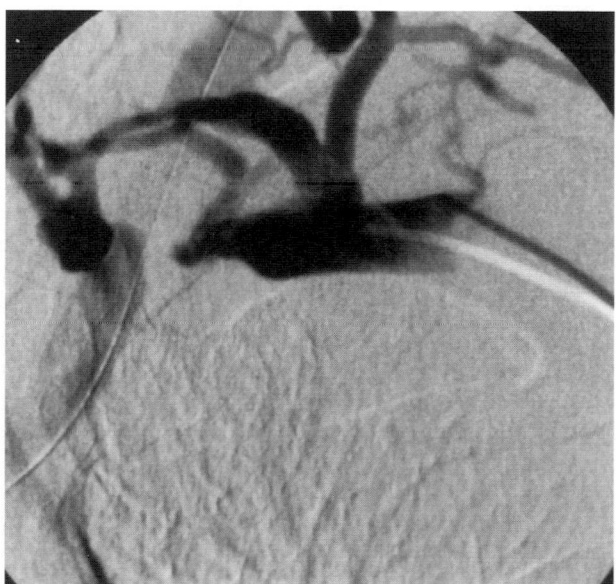

Figure 72–2 Occlusion of left subclavian vein after subclavian catheter placement for hemodialysis. The patient had developed massive arm swelling after placement of an upper arm graft.

TREATMENT OF GRAFT/FISTULA THROMBOSIS

The surgical therapy for thrombosis has been thrombectomy with graft revision as necessary. Thrombectomy alone is generally not curative because the thrombosis is usually a consequence of a stenosis, most frequently at the venous end of the graft. Therefore, if a surgical approach is used to treat thrombosed grafts, a patch angioplasty or interposition graft must be performed to ensure prolonged patency. When the graft is treated operatively, an intraoperative angiogram or blind exploration is essential after thrombectomy to identify the cause of thrombosis. Graft longevity after operative repair is significantly reduced; the 1-year primary patency for revised PTFE grafts is 17–50% (32,64). The DOQI guidelines set a goal of a 50% unassisted patency at 6 months and a 40% unassisted patency at 1 year for surgical therapy (3). Revision of the outflow is limited by anatomic considerations because there is limited vein available for sequential revisions. If grafts are replaced rather than revised, the possible vascular access sites will be rapidly exhausted.

Because of the significant drawbacks to the surgical management of dialysis grafts, percutaneous treatment has become an important therapeutic option. Thrombosed dialysis grafts are uniquely suited to percutaneous therapy. The grafts are readily accessible and are easily punctured directly. The clot within the graft is fresh because patients are usually no longer than 2–3 days from their last dialysis session. This fresh clot is well-treated with pharmacologic or mechanical thrombolytic therapy. The closed system of the graft, with only a single inflow and outflow, means that the thrombolytic agent administered into the clot will be less likely to diffuse into the systemic circulation until lysis has been achieved.

There has been an interest in performing thrombolysis of occluded dialysis shunts and grafts for more than 30 years (65–67). The equipment, techniques, and approaches to malfunctioning grafts and fistulas have continued to improve. Refinements of techniques for treating thrombosed grafts/fistulas include the development of the crossed two-catheter technique, which allows for deposition of thrombolytic agent throughout the graft (68); clot maceration, which increases the surface area available to the thrombolytic agent; and early angioplasty of the usual venous stenosis, which improves the speed of lysis and prevents rethrombosis (68). Other techniques include pulse-spray catheters, which permitted more homogeneous intrathrombic infusion, increasing the area of interface between clot and fibrinolytic agent (69). Higher concentrations of thrombolytics more rapidly administered directly into the graft increases the speed of lysis.

Methods of thrombolysis have evolved from prolonged infusions to pulse-spray thrombolysis using a crossed-catheter technique to "lysis and wait" and "lysis and go," and includes mechanical thrombectomy devices.

The pulse-spray technique is characterized by the high-pressure delivery of small aliquots of highly concentrated thrombolytic agents via a multi–side-hole catheter. This allows for the homogeneous and simultaneous distribution of concentrated thrombolytic agent throughout the entire length of the occlusion. It enhances the diffusion of activator into the clot, and the mechanical disruption of the clot matrix increases the surface area exposed to the thrombolytic agent. Because almost all the fibrinolytic agent is incorporated into the clot and not freely circulating, the risk of bleeding complications is decreased. The technique results in the rapid restoration of graft patency with a minimal dose of thrombolytic agent.

The "lysis and wait" and "lysis and go" techniques are very similar. The "lysis and wait" technique was described by Cynamon (70,71) as an injection of thrombolytics through a standard intravenous catheter inserted within the venous limb of the graft. The graft is manually compressed at the arterial and venous anastomoses while the thrombolytic mixture is infused over 1 minute into the graft. This portion of the procedure can be performed in a holding area outside the interventional radiology suite. After at least 30 minutes, the patient is transferred to the interventional radiology suite, and the declotting procedure is continued with angioplasty of the venous stenosis and mobilization of the arterial plug. Introducing the thrombolytic mixture into the graft before bringing the patient into the interventional radiology suite results in the declotting portion of the procedure requiring little or no room time and avoiding the expense of an infusion catheter. The "lysis and go" technique is very similar, but the thrombolytic is injected when the patient is in the angiographic room. The patient is then prepped and draped and the procedure started without any waiting period.

PATIENT SELECTION

Thrombosed PTFE grafts are the most common type of vascular access treated with the percutaneous approach, but thrombosed endogenous AV fistulas can also be treated with this technique. AV fistulas more commonly present with dialysis difficulties, such as problems with punctures or increased venous pressure, and are less likely to present with thrombosis. Thrombosis of a recently constructed graft (<1 month) is usually because of a technical problem. Although thrombolysis can be performed to establish the nature of the problem, a surgical revision of the graft usually will be required.

The criteria for excluding a patient from pharmacologic thrombolysis are the same as those for any pharmacologic thrombolytic procedure. Absolute contraindications to thrombolytic therapy are recent neurologic processes, including intracranial bleeding, stroke, or neurologic surgery, and the presence of active gastrointestinal bleeding. Relative contraindications include recent major surgery, severe hypertension, and pregnancy. Mechanical thrombolysis does not have such constraints. However, a contraindication that is more unique to thrombosed dialysis access and also a contraindication to mechanical thrombolysis is the presence of a graft infection. This requires primary surgical therapy. Infected clot is relatively resistant to thrombolysis. More importantly, lysis of infected thrombus is potentially life threatening because it may precipitate bacteremia and lethal sepsis (68).

Determining infection in a graft may be difficult. The classic signs of infection or inflammation include redness, tenderness, warmth, and fluctuance around the graft. These signs may be blunted in uremic patients. A fever or the presence of leukocytosis may be of diagnostic help, but some patients may not manifest such a response. Purulent discharge or skin breakdown around the graft is a clear sign of an infectious process but is rarely present. Gram stain and culture from a needle aspirate of graft clot or perigraft fluid collections found on ultrasound evaluation may be helpful in diagnosing graft infections (72). Any patient with signs of infection must be treated with antibiotics and referred for surgical removal of the graft.

TECHNIQUE OF THROMBOLYSIS

Access

A cross-catheter technique can be used in patients undergoing thrombolysis of dialysis grafts (37,53). Although this is now considered an older technique and perhaps not as fashionable, it provides the basis for other techniques and, for the beginning practitioner, has a very short learning curve because it uses standard angiographic techniques and fluoroscopic guidance. This approach can serve as a backup when there are problems with other techniques.

The cross-catheter technique allows for simultaneous access to both the arterial and venous ends of the graft. The graft is first punctured with a one-wall needle or micropuncture needle (Cook, Inc.) at the arterial end of the graft directed toward the venous end of the graft (Figure 72–3A). The graft is grasped between the thumb and index finger and held as the needle punctures the graft. When the graft has been punctured, there is usually a popping sensation as the needle traverses the PTFE material. Successful entry into the graft is indicated by easy passage of a guide wire through the graft or sometimes by the return of a small amount of dark blood. The guide wire should go through the graft quite easily despite the presence of clot. Injection of contrast material to determine whether the graft has been entered should be avoided. If the needle is not in the graft, the contrast agent is injected into the soft tissues, often with a misleading appearance. Early in the injection, it may appear as if the graft has been entered, but with continued injection, it will become evident that the contrast material is in the tissues and not within the graft.

Unfortunately, by this point, the graft is often obscured and remains obscured for the remainder of the procedure.

After the guide wire has been placed into the graft, a 5 French dilator or catheter is passed over the guide wire. The guide wire is then used to traverse the venous anastomosis (Figure 72–3B). The venous anastomosis is occasionally difficult to cross because of the presence of a venous stenosis. In such cases, an angled Glidewire (Terumo, Inc.) can be very useful. It is important to confirm the passage of a wire into the venous outflow before proceeding with further punctures or thrombolysis. If the venous outflow cannot be cannulated, thrombolysis is not performed. Thrombolysis without venous outflow results in reestablished blood flow with no outlet for the blood except through puncture sites. This leads to bleeding from previous puncture sites and possibly the development of hematomas. Patients in whom the venous anastomosis cannot be crossed are referred for surgical thrombectomy and revision of the anastomosis.

The dilator or a catheter is placed over the wire into the outflow tract. While small amounts of contrast material are injected, the catheter is withdrawn until the venous extent of the thrombosis is identified. The length of the thrombosed segment can be estimated. The length of the occlusion determines the length of the subsequent pulse-spray catheter side-hole segment. A second puncture is then made in the venous end of the graft, and the guide wire is directed toward the arterial end (Figure 72–3C). The length of this occluded segment is determined and a catheter is placed with the length of the side-hole segment corresponding to the length of the occlusion. The end-hole of the catheter is again placed just beyond the clot. The crisscross nature of the catheterization allows the entire clot to be treated simultaneously and permits access to both sides of the graft for possible angioplasty or other transcatheter therapy (Figure 72–3D). It is important that catheter or wire manipulations are done gently at the arterial end of the graft because vigorous movement of the wire or forceful contrast injections can cause the embolization of clot from the arterial anastomosis into the artery.

This procedure is identical for both straight and loop grafts. In the loop graft (Figure 72–4), there will be more overlap of the catheters, and the catheters may need to be repositioned during the pulse-spray procedure so that the entire graft receives the thrombolytic agent.

The technique of "lyse and wait" also begins with the puncture of the graft as close as possible to the arterial end with the angiocatheter directed toward the venous end. The puncture is performed directly into the graft, and it is important to get at least a small amount of blood back into the angiocatheter to verify that the angiocatheter is within the graft. If the catheter is not in the graft, then injection of the thrombolytic will result in the thrombolytic being instilled into the soft tissues, which can result in a hematoma and, obviously, no thrombolysis of the graft. The arterial and venous anastomosis should be compressed

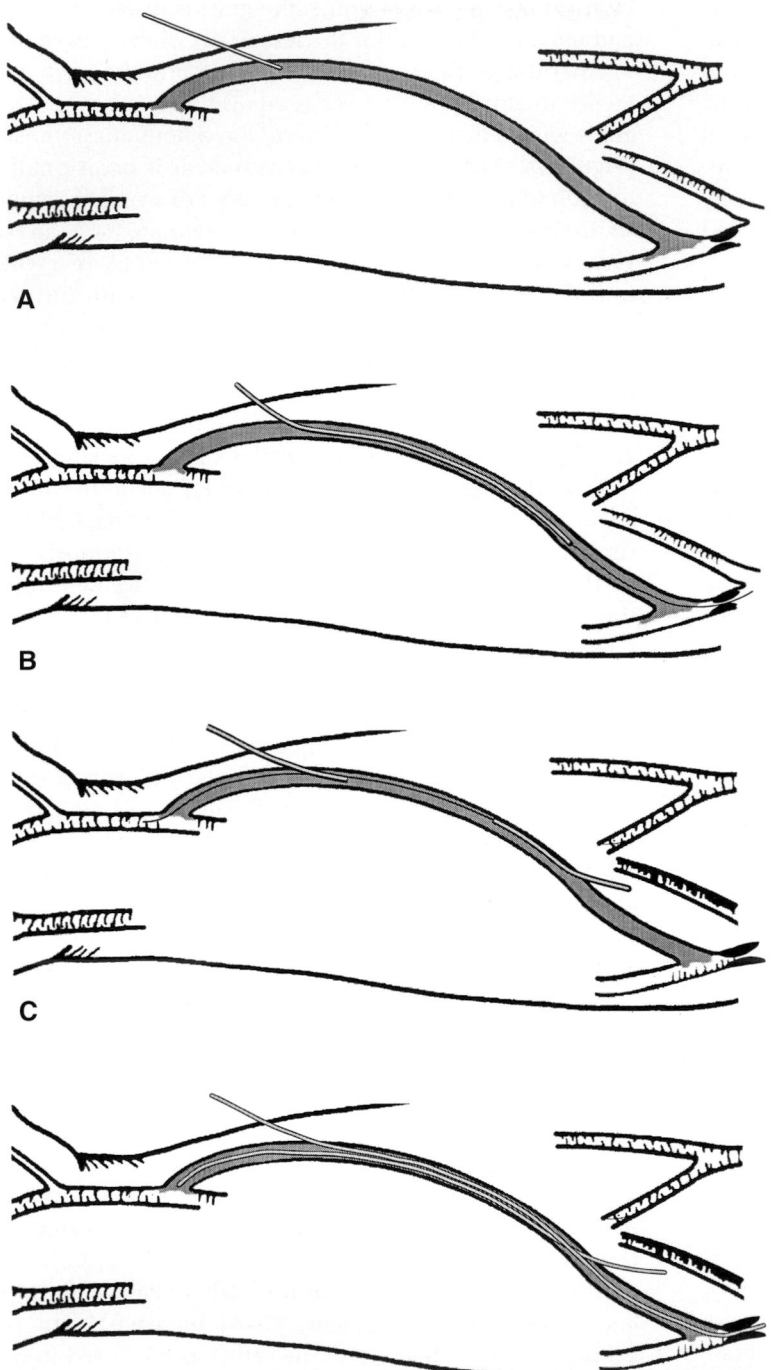

Figure 72–3 **A.** The graft is punctured with a one-wall needle at the junction of the proximal and middle thirds of the graft (the arterial end of the graft) and directed toward the venous end of the graft. **B.** The guide wire is placed through the needle, and the needle is exchanged for a 5 French dilator or catheter. The guide wire is then used to traverse the venous anastomosis. **C.** A second puncture is then made at the junction of the middle third and the distal third of the graft (the venous end of the graft), and the guide wire is directed toward the arterial end. **D.** Crisscross catheters allow the entire clot to be treated simultaneously and permit access to both sides of the graft for possible angioplasty or other transcatheter therapy.

while the thrombolytic agent is being slowly injected. This traps the thrombolytic agent in the graft but also helps to avoid displacement of thrombus out of the graft (particularly important on the arterial end). The procedure then begins with the angiocatheter being exchanged over a guide wire for a sheath or catheter to allow intervention at the venous outflow. One downside of this method is there is no initial evaluation of whether a wire can traverse the venous

outflow. This means, potentially, the thrombus could be lysed without the venous outflow being able to be opened, leading to failure of the procedure and increased potential for bleeding complications. After the venous outflow is addressed, the graft is punctured with a needle in the venous portion of the graft directed towards the arterial end, and there is placement of a sheath or catheter for treatment of the arterial anastomosis.

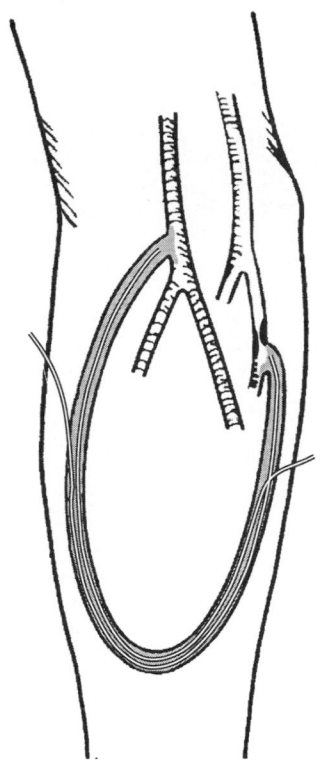

Figure 72–4 Loop grafts are accessed in a similar manner. Because of the length of the graft, there is more overlap of the catheters.

Equipment

Several different commercial pulse-spray catheter systems suitable for use in clotted dialysis grafts are available. The catheters used most often are the multi–side-hole infusion catheter (Cook, Inc.) and the side-slit catheter (Angiodynamics, Inc.). These catheters have multiple, tiny side holes or slits over a length of 4–30 cm. A wire with a bead is used to occlude the end-hole of the catheter. These systems come prepackaged with a hemostatic Y adapter to allow injections around the wire.

A suitable delivery system can also be fashioned from standard angiographic materials. Multiple side holes are created in a 5 French polyethylene catheter by puncturing the catheter every 5 mm with the tip of a 27- or 30-gauge needle. The side holes are placed in a spiral pattern around the catheter, and the length of the segment with side holes varies with the length of the occlusion. With this type of catheter, the length of the side-hole segment should probably not exceed 15 cm. The catheter end-hole is occluded by a wire and a hemostatic Touhy-Borst or Y adapter is placed over the wire and attached to the catheter. The gasket of the adapter is tightened down over the end of the wire, and a three-way stopcock is placed on the side arm of the adapter.

Thrombolytic Agents

Urokinase had been the most commonly used thrombolytic agent until its production was halted by the FDA in 1999. It returned to the market, but the manufacturer is planning to withdraw it. For readers who still have access to urokinase, the contents of a 250,000-unit vial of urokinase (Abbokinase, Abbott Laboratories) is dissolved in 9 mL of saline with 1 mL of heparin (in a dilution of 5,000 units/mL). This yields a concentration of 25,000 units of urokinase and 500 units of heparin per milliliter of solution. For the "lyse and wait" technique a 250,000 unit vial of urokinase is diluted in 5 mL of saline with 1 mL of heparin (5,000 units/mL) (71).

Tissue plasminogen activator (tPA) (alteplase, Genentech) is now the most commonly used thrombolytic (73–75). For pulse-spray application, 2 mg of tPA is dissolved in 5–10 mL of saline. The manufacturer of tPA states that there is a concern for possible precipitation if heparin is combined with tPA. However, the benefit of intrathrombic heparin may outweigh the theoretical concern for precipitation, and 3,000–5,000 units of heparin may be combined with tPA (73,76). Reteplase (RPA) has also been used in dialysis grafts in a dosage of 1–3 units/10 mL (77,78). For the "lyse and wait" technique 2 mg of tPA is diluted in 4 mL of saline with 5,000 units of heparin (5,000 units/mL) (73) or 2–5 mg of tPA is diluted with 5 mL of saline, with 5,000 units of heparin being given systemically (71).

For all thrombolytic procedures anticoagulation and antiplatelet agents are important. A 2,000- to 3,000-unit bolus of heparin is usually given intravenously when the thrombolytic procedure begins. If the procedure extends for longer than an hour, heparin is administered at a rate of 1,000 units per hour. If the patient has no contraindications to aspirin therapy, a soluble aspirin tablet (325 mg) is administered orally before the procedure is begun.

Thrombolytic Procedure

After the pulse-spray catheters have been positioned and their end-holes securely occluded, the hemostatic valves are tightened around the wires. The thrombolytic solution is divided equally into two syringes. One syringe is attached to a port on the one-way valve system attached to the Y adapter on each pulse-spray catheter. A 1 mL syringe is connected to the other port and is used to inject the thrombolytic solution, in 0.2-mL increments, as forcefully as possible through the catheter. This forceful injection is designed to maximize the penetration of thrombolytic into the clot. Injections are repeated every 10–15 seconds (Figure 72–5A). When the active catheter length is shorter than the length of clot to be treated, the catheter is advanced or withdrawn as needed to expose the entire clot to the pulse spray (Figure 72–5B). After the thrombolytic agent has been injected into the graft, contrast material is used to

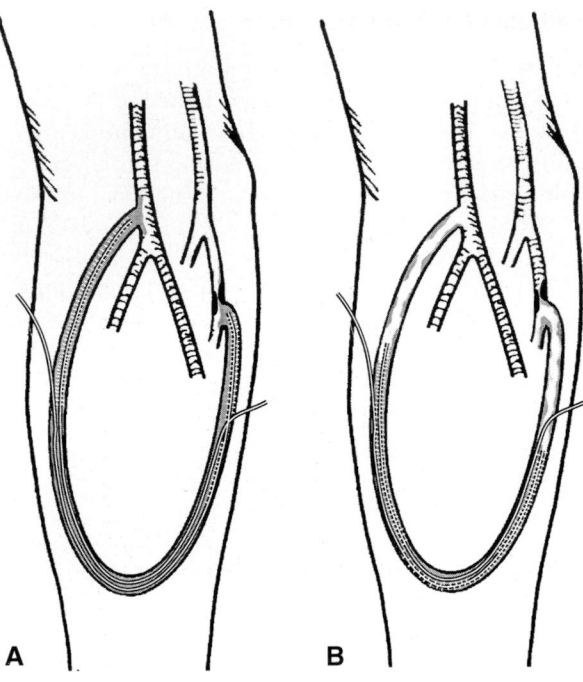

Figure 72–5 **A.** After the catheters are positioned, pulse-spray thrombolysis is begun with a tuberculin syringe to make forceful injections through the catheters. **B.** When the active catheter length is shorter than the length of clot to be treated, the catheter is withdrawn as needed to expose the entire clot to urokinase.

assess clot dissolution. Contrast agent is injected through the catheter directed toward the arterial anastomosis. The contrast injection evaluates the graft for residual clot and usually demonstrates an anatomic abnormality, most commonly a venous stenosis, which is responsible for the thrombosis.

In most cases, clot lysis is almost complete after the thrombolytic has been delivered. However, graft flow may be slow and the graft pulse may be faint. Several possibilities should be considered in this situation. If a critical venous anastomotic stenosis preventing outflow is present, balloon angioplasty will be required before clot lysis is completed. Other causes for poor flow include resistant thrombus at the arterial anastomosis, incomplete delivery of thrombolytic to the entire thrombus, inadequate heparin administration, or infected thrombus that is resistant to lysis.

Once the thrombolytic has been placed into the clot, either with pulse-spray technique or with the "lyse and wait" technique, relatively aggressive methods can be used to reestablish flow. Attention should first be directed to the venous outflow. A venous anastomotic stenosis is often found. If a stenosis is present, the first intervention should be dilatation with an angioplasty balloon (Figure 72–6). Relatively small amounts of residual clot in the graft can then be compressed and broken up with the same angioplasty balloon catheter (Figure 72–7). If a large clot burden remains, further therapy with thrombolytic will be required. Early venous angioplasty is also necessary if bleeding develops around the catheters or through recent dialysis puncture sites. The reestablishment of inflow in the setting of a tight venous outflow stenosis invariably leads to bleeding from puncture sites in the graft. This is usually handled by dilatation of the venous stenosis and gentle compression of the bleeding sites.

After lysis, with either the pulse-spray or "lyse and wait" technique, a residual plug of lysis-resistant clot may remain at the arterial anastomosis (Figure 72–8A and Figure 72–9A). In one series, these plugs were present in almost 60% of patients treated with PMPST (53), and they have also been noted by surgeons performing graft embolectomy (79). These plugs

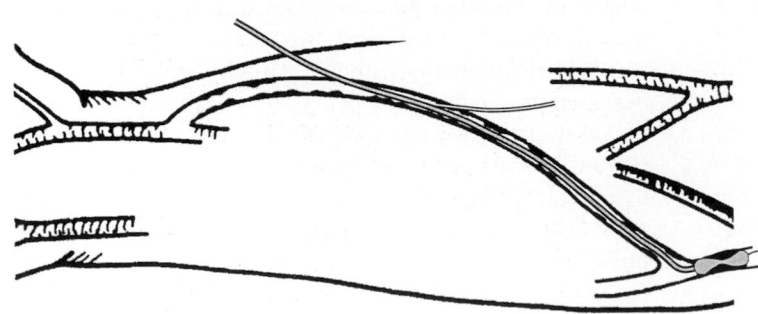

Figure 72–6 After initial pulse-spray thrombolysis, contrast is injected and the graft is evaluated. A venous anastomotic stenosis is usually present, and the first intervention should be dilatation with an angioplasty balloon.

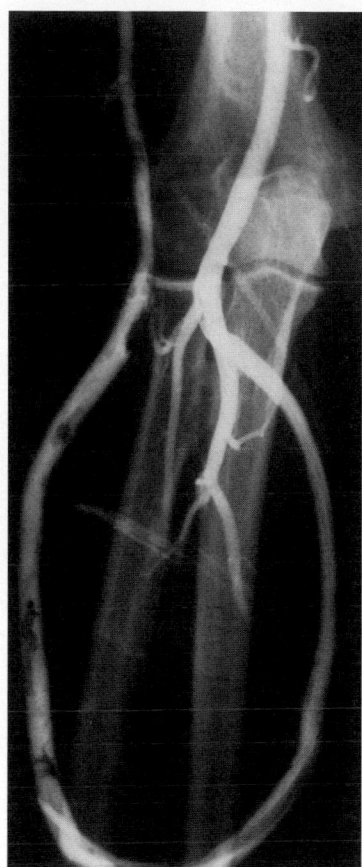

Figure 72–7 Relatively small amounts of residual clot in the graft can then be compressed and broken up with the same angioplasty balloon catheter.

have a consistency different from that of clot removed from the remainder of the graft. They are believed to represent platelet-rich "white clots" formed because of persistent exposure of the leading edge of clot to arterial blood flow and tend to be relatively resistant to thrombolysis (80). These plugs may be partially treated by the thrombolytic agent and appear to be stenoses. They should not be treated, at least initially, as stenoses with balloon dilatation, because this may cause the clot to be displaced into the artery. Because this material tends to be more resistant to thrombolysis, a potentially more hazardous embolization may occur. Instead, a thrombectomy type procedure should be performed. Following the thrombectomy, the stenotic appearance usually resolves.

The plugs can usually be removed with an 8.5-mm occlusion balloon catheter (Boston Scientific Inc.). The thrombolysis catheter, which is directed toward the arterial anastomosis, is exchanged for an occlusion balloon catheter (Figure 72–8B). The catheter is positioned with the balloon beyond the clot in the distal artery. Using dilute contrast material, the balloon is inflated and the catheter is pulled back, dragging the clot into the graft. It is important not to overinflate the balloon while it is in the native artery. As the balloon is pulled up against the clot, the balloon is more firmly inflated to dislodge the clot. If the clot is not dislodged on the initial pass (Figure 72–9B), repeated passes can be performed as needed (Figure 72–9C). If the displaced clot becomes trapped in the graft (Figure 72–9D), it can be crushed with an angioplasty balloon.

Angiographic evaluation is then performed to assess the arterial inflow, the body of the graft, and the venous outflow to the level of the superior vena cava. After the treatment of

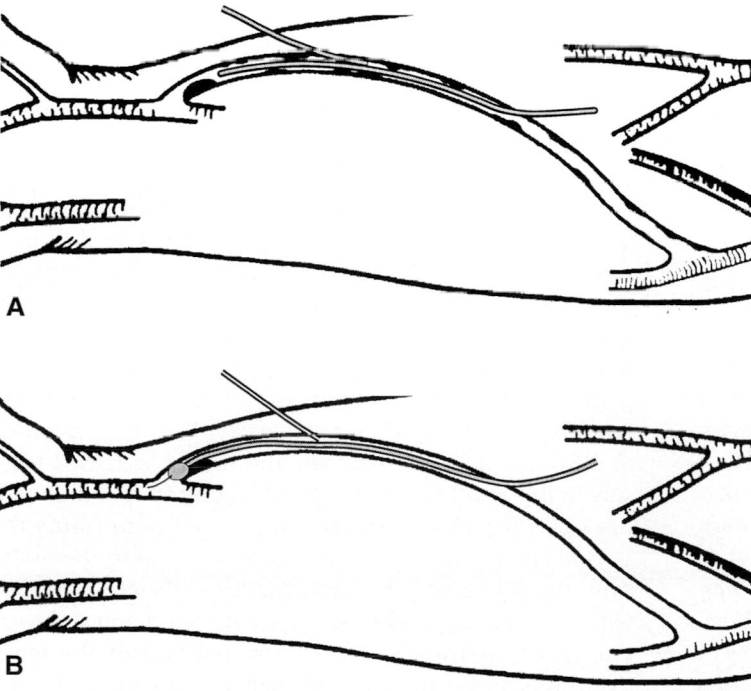

A

B

Figure 72–8 A. After lysis, a residual plug of lysis-resistant clot may remain at the arterial anastomosis. **B.** The thrombolysis catheter is exchanged for an occlusion balloon catheter. The catheter is positioned with the balloon beyond the clot in the distal artery. Using dilute contrast material, the balloon is inflated and the catheter is pulled back, dragging the clot into the graft.

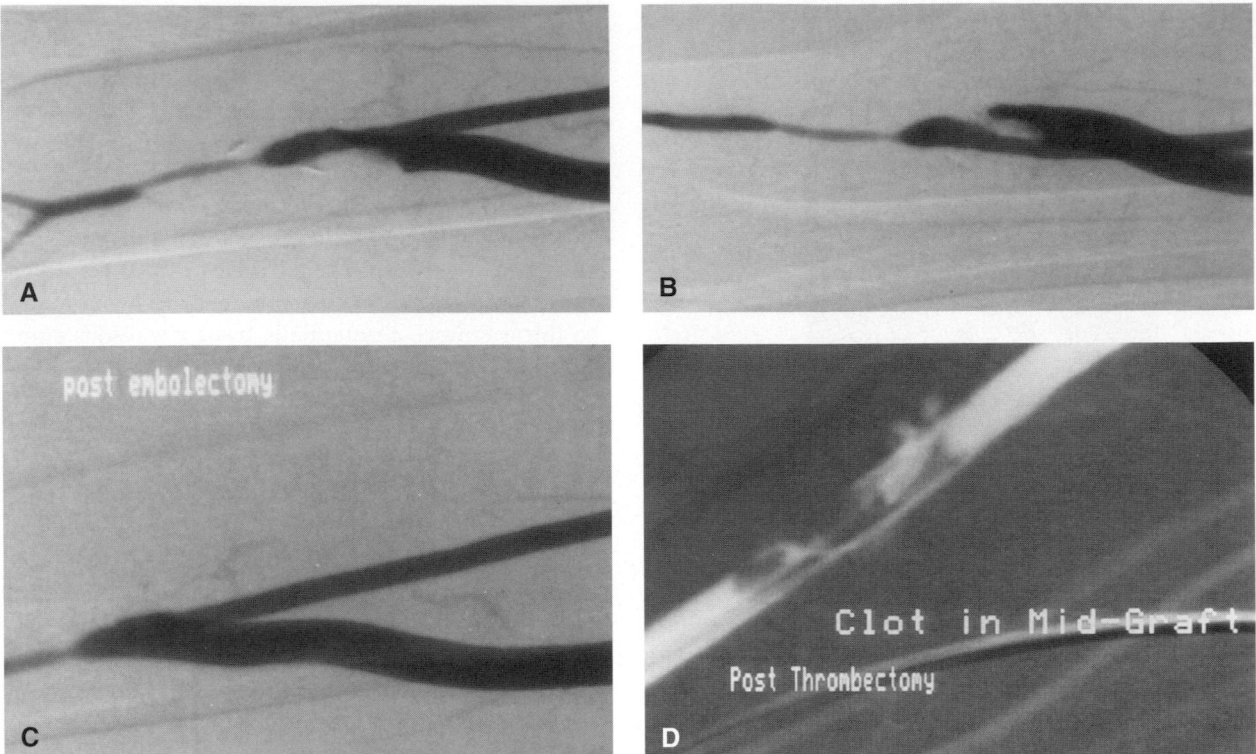

Figure 72–9 **A.** Residual clot at the arterial anastomosis. **B.** After the first pass with the occlusion balloon, there is an improved appearance, but residual thrombus remains. **C.** Second pass with occlusion balloon and clearing of plug. **D.** The clot is now caught in the midgraft and treated with an angioplasty balloon.

any underlying abnormalities, a final angiogram is obtained to document graft patency and flow. To assess the anticoagulation status, an activated clotting time (ACT) may be obtained before the catheters are removed. When the catheters are removed, gentle digital compression is applied to the puncture sites until hemostasis is obtained. Upon completion of the procedure, the patients are sent to the dialysis unit or are discharged home. Patients are continued on daily aspirin (325 mg) if they have no contraindications to such therapy.

MECHANICAL THROMBECTOMY

The other approach to removing thrombus from a dialysis graft is a mechanical thrombectomy. Several different thrombectomy devices are available for treating dialysis grafts. These include the Amplatz thrombectomy device (ATD), also known as the Helix Clot Buster, (Microvena); the AngioJet (Possis Medical); the Arrow-Trerotola percutaneous thrombectomy device (PTD) (Arrow International); the Cragg and Castaneda thrombolytic brushes (Microtherapeutics); the Oasis catheter (Boston Scientific); the X-Sizer (EV3); the Hydrolyser (Cordis); and others. These thrombectomy devices have different mechanisms of action. Some cause clot fragmentation by the creation of a

vortex by the rotation at high speed of an impeller or basket. Others work by a Venturi effect, which draws thrombus into an opening of the device where it is macerated and removed through an exhaust lumen (81). All of these devices are capable of removing clot, and the experience of the operator is the most important determinant of success. Whichever device is chosen, it is important that the operator becomes familiar with the device and understands its capabilities, characteristics, and the problems that may occur with the individual device.

The approach to using these devices is similar to the pulse-spray thrombolytic approach. An initial needle puncture is made into the arterial end of the graft directed toward the venous portion. A wire followed by an angiographic catheter is advanced through the venous anastomosis. A diagnostic venogram is performed to evaluate the graft and the venous outflow, including the central veins. Some operators will then angioplasty the venous stenosis to allow outflow and decrease the risk of increased pressure in the graft leading to arterial emboli (82). Others will not open the venous stenosis until after performing the thrombectomy to avoid embolization of clot to the lungs. After the venogram, the angiographic catheter is replaced with a sheath to provide access for the mechanical device. The device is then used as indicated within the graft. Contrast can be injected through the sheath while the thrombectomy is performed to visualize the clot and assess the progress of the procedure. After the clot is removed, the venous stenosis is dilated if that has not been previously performed. After the venous angioplasty, the venous end of the graft is punctured with the needle directed toward the arterial end. The thrombectomy device is then advanced to clear the clot at the arterial end. An occlusion balloon is then placed to dislodge the arterial plug. Following this maneuver, the graft is assessed with contrast to determine whether the procedure is complete or whether there are other areas that require therapy. Some operators will pull the arterial plug back into the graft early in the procedure, before treating the venous stenosis, so the plug can be fragmented by the mechanical device (82). An alternative method for accessing a loop graft is to perform a single access approach using the apex of a loop graft as the access. From that single access point, all of the catheters, thrombectomy devices, and balloons are directed toward whichever part of the graft requires treatment.

When using mechanical devices, it is important not to forget anticoagulation and antiplatelet agents. Heparin and aspirin are important adjuncts to the use of these devices. Heparin (2,000–5,000 units) is commonly infused through the sheath before placement of the thrombectomy device (82). If heparin is not given through the access sheath, it should be given intravenously. Aspirin is important because the use of devices in the clot, as well as the lysis of clot, will lead to platelet aggregation and new clot formation.

COMPLICATIONS

Complications of the thrombolytic procedures, whether pharmacologic or mechanical, are uncommon. Most of the complications involve bleeding from the puncture sites or from previous needle punctures. Usually, these hematomas require no further therapy. Arterial embolization can occur in up to 10% of procedures (83). Other complications are embolic or associated with angioplasty, such as venous rupture.

Arterial embolization is caused by the dislodgement of the arterial plug into the feeding artery. It seems to be somewhat more common with the forearm loop grafts, perhaps because of the size of the brachial artery and the geometry of the anastomosis. Prevention is the ideal, and careful technique with gentle manipulation of guide wires and catheters at the arterial anastomosis is important. Angioplasty of clot directly at the arterial anastomosis should be avoided. Thrombolysis is not usually effective, because the clot tends to be lysis resistant. Placement of an occlusion balloon past the clot and gentle displacement of the clot back into the graft is a possible approach. This embolectomy technique is similar to a surgical embolectomy. Performing this maneuver in the angiographic suite has the advantage of fluoroscopic guidance, an embolectomy catheter that is placed over a wire, and immediate

angiographic evaluation, which is preferable to a blind operative procedure. If the graft is patent, the "backbleeding" technique can be tried (84). A balloon catheter is placed into the arterial inflow, just above the anastomosis, on the upstream side. The balloon is inflated, and the patient exercises his or her hand for about 1 minute. The balloon is deflated, and an arteriogram is performed to evaluate the results. A successful procedure will dislodge the embolus from its position in the artery below the anastomosis and move it into the graft (85).

Small pulmonary emboli are produced with all percutaneous declotting techniques (86–91). This raises some concern regarding mechanical devices that allow the clot to fragment and pass through the graft to the lungs. Patients with cardiopulmonary compromise are a group that may be at particular risk from even small emboli (86). It is unclear whether a repeated declotting procedure could cause respiratory difficulties. It is possible that the use of thrombolytics diminishes the risk of emboli (91). Although symptomatic pulmonary embolism is rare, there have been fatal pulmonary emboli reported after mechanical thrombectomy (using an occlusion balloon to pull the clot through the graft) where the entire clot burden of a graft was delivered to the lungs (86,92).

RESULTS

Thrombolysis, either pharmacologic or mechanical, in conjunction with balloon angioplasty allows for rapid, consistent, and safe restoration of graft patency. Almost all grafts can be effectively treated when the anastomoses can be traversed with a wire so that angioplasty can be performed. With improved techniques, such as rapid administration of thrombolytics, early angioplasty of the venous anastomosis and prompt displacement of the arterial plug with procedure times can be decreased usually in <2 hours (73,75,93). Mechanical thrombectomy devices are relatively comparable in terms of time, between types of devices (94), and in comparison to the thrombolytic approach (74,95). Technically successful lysis can be achieved in almost all cases (pharmacologic or mechanical), with a clinical success rate (defined as the ability to dialyze) of >90% (74,95–97). The time required for a procedure and the success of the procedure are highly correlated to operator experience (73).

The patency of clotted dialysis grafts treated with percutaneous therapy seems to be similar between pharmacologic thrombolysis and mechanical thrombolysis when evaluated at 1 month, 3 months, and 6 months (74,95–98). The long-term patency rate of thrombosed dialysis grafts is relatively poor no matter how the grafts are treated. Studies comparing thrombolysis to surgical thrombectomy demonstrate similar long-term patency rates (79,99–101). Primary patency rates of thrombosed grafts at 1 year are 11–26% (100,102,103), with secondary patency rates of 57–69% (83). Patency rates of thrombosed grafts are decreased when compared to grafts that have not thrombosed but have been treated with balloon angioplasty. Thrombosed grafts have a 6-month primary patency of 18–39% while nonthrombosed grafts have a 6-month primary patency rate of 38–63% (83). At 12 months, the secondary patency rate for thrombosed grafts is 57–69% compared with a rate of 81–82% for nonthrombosed grafts (83). These findings suggest that the method for opening the graft is less important than the underlying cause of the thrombosis. The poor long-term patency rates indicate that recurrent therapeutic procedures will be required. The need for repeated treatments does not indicate failure of the technique, but rather, it represents the chronic physiologic abnormality that produces restenosis. Although the patency rates may not be as good with thrombosed grafts, it is reasonable to keep treating them because the reocclusion rates are similar following multiple declotting procedures, and this allows the graft function to be preserved as long as possible (104). Even when the grafts have early rethrombosis (within 1 month), aggressive retreatment, commonly with larger angioplasty balloons or occasionally stent placement, will allow salvage of the grafts without significantly decreased patency rates (105).

AV FISTULA THROMBOLYSIS

The approach to a thrombosed AV fistula is much more challenging than to a thrombosed dialysis graft. It was a commonly held belief that AV fistulas, when thrombosed, could not be salvaged percutaneously. This perception was in part because of the relative infrequency of AV fistula thrombosis, but probably was also the lack of experience in treating these thromboses. As the number of AV fistulas has increased, experience with thrombosed fistulas has also increased (and there has been a change in attitude). Although the fistula anatomy tends to make thrombolysis somewhat more complicated, fistulas can be successfully treated and percutaneous attempts should be made to restore flow (106,107).

In some cases, something that appears to be a thrombosis actually is a stenosis that is causing poor flow and flattening of the outflow vein of the fistula. If there is a thrombosis, then pharmacologic thrombolysis may have less risk of damaging the venous endothelium than would a mechanical device (108). Obtaining access to the fistula may be aided by placing a tourniquet or using ultrasound guidance (34,109). Multiple thrombolytic techniques have been used in fistulas including pulse-spray, "lyse and wait" (107), and thrombectomy devices (110–112). Direct thromboaspiration of the fistula has also been successful (34,111,113). This technique uses a 7 French or 8 French thin-walled catheter and a 20-mL syringe to provide the aspiration suction (81,107).

The technical success rates for treating AV fistulas are lower than for grafts, ranging from 75–100%. The primary patency rates are probably better, with rates of 36–70% at

3 months and 18–60% at 6 months (107). The assisted primary patency rates at 6 months are 60–80% (107). These rates indicate that when one can restore flow, the fistula has a good chance of remaining patent as long as careful surveillance is performed.

SUMMARY

The repeated failure of dialysis access remains a frustrating problem. However, there have been enormous advances in our understanding and approach to grafts and fistulas. The emphasis on surveillance of dialysis access is of critical importance. This identifies at-risk grafts, which then allows scheduled evaluation and therapy for the inevitable venous stenosis. This is faster and more convenient for the patient, the interventional radiologist, and the dialysis center. The adequacy of angioplasty of lesions in grafts and fistulas can be evaluated more quantitatively with the use of catheters that measure flow. Lysis of thrombosed grafts is faster and more economical than it was previously, and operators today have the ability to achieve excellent technical success. The lysis of thrombosed fistulas is also now widely accepted. However, long-term success continues to be elusive, and there is a need to continue to refine approaches to dialysis access. Ultimately, the ability to achieve long-term success with dialysis access depends upon advances in mechanisms to prevent neointimal hyperplasia and subsequent restenosis. Once that process can be controlled, many of the present frustrations will merely become of historical interest.

REFERENCES

1. USRDS 2004 annual data report. Am J Kidney Dis 2005;45:8–280.
2. Ziegler TW, Safa A, Amarillis K, et al. Prolonging the life of difficult hemodialysis access using thrombolysis, angiography and angioplasty. Adv Ren Replace Ther 1995;2:52–59.
3. III. NKF-K/DOQI Clinical Practice Guidelines for Vascular Access: update 2000. Am J Kidney Dis 2001;37:S137–181.
4. Chin AI, Chang W, Fitzgerald JT, et al. Intra-access blood flow in patients with newly created upper-arm arteriovenous native fistulae for hemodialysis access. Am J Kidney Dis 2004;44:850–858.
5. Huber TS, Buhler AG, Seeger JM. Evidence-based data for the hemodialysis access surgeon. Semin Dial 2004;17:217–223.
6. Beathard GA. Physical examination of AV grafts. Semin Dial 1992;5:74.
7. Zeit RM. The problems and management of hemodialysis accesses. In: Castañeda-Zuniga W, Tadavarthy S, eds. Interventional Radiology: Williams & Wilkins, 1992;422–437.
8. Roberts AC, Valji K, Bookstein JJ, et al. Pulse-spray pharmacomechanical thrombolysis for treatment of thrombosed dialysis access grafts. Am J Surg 1993;166:221–225; discussion 225–226.
9. Fan PY, Schwab SJ. Vascular access: concepts for the 1990s. J Am Soc Nephrol 1992;3:1–11.
10. Fillinger M, Reinitz E, Schwartz R, et al. Graft geometry and venous intimal-medial hyperplasia in arteriovenous loop grafts. J Vasc Surg 1990;11:556–566.
11. Liu SQ. Focal expression of angiotensin II type 1 receptor and smooth muscle cell proliferation in the neointima of experimental vein grafts: relation to eddy blood flow. Arterioscler Thromb Vasc Biol 1999;19:2630–2639.

12. Windus DW. Permanent vascular access: a nephrologist's view. Am J Kidney Dis 1993;21:457–471.

13. Keynton RS, Evancho MM, Sims RL, et al. The effect of graft caliber upon wall shear within *in vivo* distal vascular anastomoses. J Biomech Eng 1999;121:79–88.

14. Malchesky P, Koshino I, Pennza P, et al. Analysis of the segmental venous stenosis in blood access. Trans Am Soc Artif Intern Organs 1975;21:310–319.

15. Turmel-Rodrigues L, Pengloan J, Blanchier D, et al. Insufficient dialysis shunts: improved long-term patency rates with close hemodynamic monitoring, repeated percutaneous balloon angioplasty, and stent placement. Radiology 1993;187:273–278.

16. Kanterman RY, Vesely TM, Pilgram TK, et al. Dialysis access grafts: anatomic location of venous stenosis and results of angioplasty. Radiology 1995;195:135–139.

17. D'Cunha PT, Besarab A. Vascular access for hemodialysis: 2004 and beyond. Curr Opin Nephrol Hypertens 2004;13:623–629.

18. Lopot F, Nejedly B, Sulkova S, et al. Comparison of different techniques of hemodialysis vascular access flow evaluation. Int J Artif Organs 2003;26:1056–1063.

19. Schwarz C, Mitterbauer C, Boczula M, et al. Flow monitoring: performance characteristics of ultrasound dilution versus color Doppler ultrasound compared with fistulography. Am J Kidney Dis 2003;42:539–545.

20. Besarab A. Advances in end-stage renal diseases 2000. Access monitoring methods. Blood Purif 2000;18:255–259.

21. Besarab A, Lubkowski T, Frinak S, et al. Detection of access strictures and outlet stenoses in vascular accesses. Which test is best? ASAIO J 1997;43:543–547.

22. Besarab A, Lubkowski T, Frinak S, et al. Detecting vascular access dysfunction. ASAIO J 1997;43:M539–543.

23. Basile C, Ruggieri G, Vernaglione L, et al. A comparison of methods for the measurement of hemodialysis access recirculation. J Nephrol 2003;16:908–913.

24. Beathard GA. Physical examination of AV grafts. Semin Dial 1996;5:74–76.

25. Trerotola SO, Scheel PJ, Jr., Powe NR, et al. Screening for dialysis access graft malfunction: comparison of physical examination with US. J Vasc Interv Radiol 1996;7:15–20.

26. Safa AA, Valji K, Roberts AC, et al. Detection and treatment of dysfunctional hemodialysis access grafts: effect of a surveillance program on graft patency and the incidence of thrombosis. Radiology 1996;199:653–657.

27. Robbin ML, Chamberlain NE, Lockhart ME, et al. Hemodialysis arteriovenous fistula maturity: US evaluation. Radiology 2002;225:59–64.

28. Polkinghorne KR, Kerr PG. Predicting vascular access failure: a collective review. Nephrology (Carlton) 2002;7:170–176.

29. Cayco AV, Abu-Alfa AK, Mahnensmith RL, et al. Reduction in arteriovenous graft impairment: results of a vascular access surveillance protocol. Am J Kidney Dis 1998;32:302–308.

30. McCarley P, Wingard RL, Shyr Y, et al. Vascular access blood flow monitoring reduces access morbidity and costs. Kidney Int 2001;60:1164–1172.

31. Marston WA, Criado E, Jaques PF, et al. Prospective randomized comparison of surgical versus endovascular management of thrombosed dialysis access grafts. J Vasc Surg 1997;26:373–380; discussion 380–371.

32. Bitar G, Yang S, Badosa F. Balloon versus patch angioplasty as an adjuvant treatment to surgical thrombectomy of hemodialysis grafts. Am J Surg 1997;174:140–142.

33. Dougherty MJ, Calligaro KD, Schindler N, et al. Endovascular versus surgical treatment for thrombosed hemodialysis grafts: a prospective, randomized study. J Vasc Surg 1999;30:1016–1023.

34. Turmel-Rodrigues L, Mouton A, Birmele B, et al. Salvage of immature forearm fistulas for haemodialysis by interventional radiology. Nephrol Dial Transplant 2001;16:2365–2371.

35. Khan FA, Vesely TM. Arterial problems associated with dysfunctional hemodialysis grafts: evaluation of patients at high risk for arterial disease. J Vasc Interv Radiol 2002;13:1109–1114.

36. Vesely TM, Gherardini D, Gleed RD, et al. Use of a catheter-based system to measure blood flow in hemodialysis grafts during angioplasty procedures. J Vasc Interv Radiol 2002;13:371–378.

37. Valji K, Bookstein JJ, Roberts AC, et al. Pulse-spray pharmaco-mechanical thrombolysis of thrombosed hemodialysis access grafts: long-term experience and comparison of original and current techniques. AJR Am J Roentgenol 1995;164:1495–1500; discussion 1501–1493.

38. Trerotola SO, Lund GB, Scheel PJ, et al. Thrombosed dialysis access grafts: percutaneous mechanical declotting without urokinase. Radiology 1994;191:721–726.

39. Beathard GA. Thrombolysis versus surgery for the treatment of thrombosed dialysis access grafts. J Am Soc Nephrol 1995;6:1619–1624.

40. Vorwerk D, Adam G, Muller-Leisse C, et al. Hemodialysis fistulas and grafts: use of cutting balloons to dilate venous stenoses. Radiology 1996;201:864–867.

41. Bittl JA, Feldman RL. Cutting balloon angioplasty for undilatable venous stenoses causing dialysis graft failure. Catheter Cardiovasc Interv 2003;58:524–526.

42. Song HH, Kim KT, Chung SK, et al. Cutting balloon angioplasty for resistant venous stenoses of Brescia-Cimino fistulas. J Vasc Interv Radiol 2004;15:1463–1467.

43. Sreenarasimhaiah VP, Margassery SK, Martin KJ, et al. Cutting balloon angioplasty for resistant venous anastomotic stenoses. Semin Dial 2004;17:523–527.

44. Singer-Jordan J, Papura S. Cutting balloon angioplasty for primary treatment of hemodialysis fistula venous stenoses: preliminary results. J Vasc Interv Radiol 2005;16:25–29.

45. Gray RJ, Horton KM, Dolmatch BL, et al. Use of Wallstents for hemodialysis access-related venous stenoses and occlusions untreatable with balloon angioplasty. Radiology 1995;195:479–484.

46. Beathard GA. Gianturco self-expanding stent in the treatment of stenosis in dialysis access grafts. Kidney Int 1993;43:872–877.

47. Funaki B, Szymski GX, Leef JA, et al. Wallstent deployment to salvage dialysis graft thrombolysis complicated by venous rupture: early and intermediate results. AJR Am J Roentgenol 1997;169:1435–1437.

48. Lin PH, Johnson CK, Pullium JK, et al. Transluminal stent graft repair with Wallgraft endoprosthesis in a porcine arteriovenous graft pseudoaneurysm model. J Vasc Surg 2003;37:175–181.

49. Quinn SF, Kim J, Sheley RC. Transluminally placed endovascular grafts for venous lesions in patients on hemodialysis. Cardiovasc Intervent Radiol 2003;26:365–369.

50. Silas AM, Bettmann MA. Utility of covered stents for revision of aging failing synthetic hemodialysis grafts: a report of three cases. Cardiovasc Intervent Radiol 2003;26:550–553.

51. Najibi S, Bush RL, Terramani TT, et al. Covered stent exclusion of dialysis access pseudoaneurysms. J Surg Res 2002;106:15–19.

52. Ryan JM, Dumbleton SA, Doherty J, et al. Technical innovation. Using a covered stent (wallgraft) to treat pseudoaneurysms of dialysis grafts and fistulas. AJR Am J Roentgenol 2003;180:1067–1071.

53. Valji K. Transcatheter treatment of thrombosed hemodialysis access grafts. AJR 1995;164:823–829.

54. Puckett J, Lindsay S. Midgraft curettage as a routine adjunct to savage operations for thrombosed polytetrafluoroethylene hemodialysis access grafts. Am J Surg 1988;156:139.

55. Davis D, Peterson J, Feldman R, et al. Subclavian vein stenosis: a complication of subclavian dialysis. JAMA 1984;252:3404.

56. Schwab SJ, Quarles LD, Middleton JP, et al. Hemodialysis-associated subclavian vein stenosis. Kidney Int 1988;33:1156–1159.

57. Schwab SJ, Beathard G. The hemodialysis catheter conundrum: hate living with them, but can't live without them. Kidney Int 1999;56:1–17.

58. Schwab SJ, Raymond JR, Saeed M, et al. Prevention of hemodialysis fistula thrombosis. Early detection of venous stenoses. Kidney Int 1989;36:707–711.

59. Quinn SF, Schuman ES, Hall L, et al. Venous stenoses in patients who undergo hemodialysis: treatment with self-expandable endovascular stents. Radiology 1992;183:499–504.

60. Vogel PM, Parise C. SMART stent for salvage of hemodialysis access grafts. J Vasc Interv Radiol 2004;15:1051–1060.

61. Gunther RW, Vorwerk D, Bohndorf K, et al. Venous stenoses in dialysis shunts: treatment with self-expanding metallic stents. Radiology 1989;170:401–405.

62. Haage P, Vorwerk D, Piroth W, et al. Treatment of hemodialysis-related central venous stenosis or occlusion: results of primary Wallstent placement and follow-up in 50 patients. Radiology 1999;212:175–180.

63. Turmel-Rodrigues L, Bourquelot P, Raynaud A, et al. Primary stent placement in hemodialysis-related central venous stenoses: the dangers of a potential "radiologic dictatorship." Radiology 2000;217:600–602.

64. Marston WA, Beathard GAS. Surgical management of thrombosed dialysis access grafts. Am J Kidney Dis 1998;32:168–171.

65. Hartley LC, Ellis FG, Rendall M, et al. The use of urokinase in Scribner shunts. Br J Urol 1972;42:246–249.

66. Hargrove WI, CF B, HD B, et al. Treatment of acute peripheral arterial and graft thromboses with low-dose streptokinase. Surgery 1982;92:981–993.

67. Zeit R. Clearing of clotted dialysis shunts by streptokinase injection at multiple sites. AJR 1983;141:1053–1054.

68. Davis GB, Dowd CF, Bookstein JJ, et al. Thrombosed dialysis grafts: efficacy of intrathrombic deposition of concentrated urokinase, clot maceration, and angioplasty. AJR Am J Roentgenol 1987;149:177–181.

69. Bookstein J, Fellmeth B, Roberts A, et al. Pulsed-spray pharmacomechanical thrombolysis: preliminary clinical results. AJR Am J Roentgenol 1989;152:1097–1100.

70. Cynamon J, Lakritz PS, Wahl SI, et al. Hemodialysis graft declotting: description of the "lyse and wait" technique. J Vasc Interv Radiol 1997;8:825–829.

71. Cynamon J, Pierpont CE. Thrombolysis for the treatment of thrombosed hemodialysis access grafts. Rev Cardiovasc Med 2002;3:S84–S91.

72. Valji K, Roberts A, Bookstein J. Thrombosed hemodialysis access grafts: management with pulse-spray thrombolysis and balloon angioplasty. In: Strandness D, Van Breda A, eds. Vascular Diseases: Surgical and Interventional Therapy. New York: Churchill Livingstone, 1994;1087–1095.

73. Falk A, Guller J, Nowakowski FS, et al. Reteplase in the treatment of thrombosed hemodialysis grafts. J Vasc Interv Radiol 2001;12:1257–1262.

74. Vogel PM, Bansal V, Marshall MW. Thrombosed hemodialysis grafts: lyse and wait with tissue plasminogen activator or urokinase compared to mechanical thrombolysis with the Arrow-Trerotola percutaneous thrombolytic device. J Vasc Interv Radiol 2001;12:1157–1165.

75. Sofocleous CT, Hinrichs CR, Weiss SH, et al. Alteplase for hemodialysis access graft thrombolysis. J Vasc Interv Radiol 2002;13:775–784.

76. Semba CP, Murphy TP, Bakal CW, et al. Thrombolytic therapy with use of alteplase (rt-PA) in peripheral arterial occlusive disease: review of the clinical literature. The Advisory Panel. J Vasc Interv Radiol 2000;11:149–161.

77. Benenati J, Shlansky-Goldberg R, Meglin A, et al. Thrombolytic and antiplatelet therapy in peripheral vascular disease with use of reteplase and/or abciximab. The SCVIR Consultants' Conference; May 22, 2000; Orlando, FL. Society for Cardiovascular and Interventional Radiology. J Vasc Interv Radiol 2001;12:795–805.

78. Semba CP, Sugimoto K, Razavi MK. Alteplase and tenecteplase: applications in the peripheral circulation. Tech Vasc Interv Radiol 2001;4:99–106.

79. Etheredge E, Haid S, Maeser M, et al. Salvage operations for malfunctioning polytetrafluroethylene hemodialysis access grafts. Surgery 1983;94:464–470.

80. Winkler TA, Trerotola SO, Davidson DD, et al. Study of thrombus from thrombosed hemodialysis access grafts. Radiology 1995;197:461–465.

81. Morgan R, Belli AM. Percutaneous thrombectomy: a review. Eur Radiol 2002;12:205–217.

82. Vesely TM. Techniques for using mechanical thrombectomy devices to treat thrombosed hemodialysis grafts. Tech Vasc Interv Radiol 1999;2:208–216.

83. Aruny JE, Lewis CA, Cardella JF, et al. Quality improvement guidelines for percutaneous management of the thrombosed or dysfunctional dialysis access. J Vasc Interv Radiol 2003;14:S247–253.

84. Tretotola S, M.D. J, Shah H, Namyslowski J. Backbleeding technique for treatment of arterial emboli resulting from dialysis graft thrombolysis. J Vasc Interv Radiol 1998;9:141–143.

85. Beathard GA. Management of complications of endovascular dialysis access procedures. Semin Dial 2003;16:309–313.

86. Swan TL, Smyth SH, Ruffenach SJ, et al. Pulmonary embolism following hemodialysis access thrombolysis/thrombectomy. J Vasc Interv Radiol 1995;6:683–686.

87. Beathard GA, Welch BR, Maidment HJ. Mechanical thrombolysis for the treatment of thrombosed hemodialysis access grafts. Radiology 1996;200:711–716.

88. Trerotola SO, Johnson MS, Schauwecker DS, et al. Pulmonary emboli from pulse-spray and mechanical thrombolysis: evaluation with an animal dialysis-graft model. Radiology 1996;200:169–176.

89. Smits HF, Van Rijk PP, Van Isselt JW, et al. Pulmonary embolism after thrombolysis of hemodialysis grafts. J Am Soc Nephrol 1997;8:1458–1461.

90. Petronis JD, Regan F, Briefel G, et al. Ventilation-perfusion scintigraphic evaluation of pulmonary clot burden after percutaneous thrombolysis of clotted hemodialysis access grafts. Am J Kidney Dis 1999;34:207–211.

91. Kinney TB, Valji K, Rose SC, et al. Pulmonary embolism from pulse-spray pharmacomechanical thrombolysis of clotted hemodialysis grafts: urokinase versus heparinized saline. J Vasc Interv Radiol 2000;11:1143–1152.

92. Soulen MC, Zaetta JM, Amygdalos MA, et al. Mechanical declotting of thrombosed dialysis grafts: experience in 86 cases. J Vasc Interv Radiol 1997;8:563–567.

93. Falk A, Mitty H, Guller J, et al. Thrombolysis of clotted hemodialysis grafts with tissue-type plasminogen activator. J Vasc Interv Radiol 2001;12:305–311.

94. Smits HF, Smits JH, Wust AF, et al. Percutaneous thrombolysis of thrombosed haemodialysis access grafts: comparison of three mechanical devices. Nephrol Dial Transplant 2002;17:467–473.

95. Barth KH, Gosnell MR, Palestrant AM, et al. Hydrodynamic thrombectomy system versus pulse-spray thrombolysis for thrombosed hemodialysis grafts: a multicenter prospective randomized comparison. Radiology 2000;217:678–684.

96. Trerotola SO, Vesely TM, Lund GB, et al. Treatment of thrombosed hemodialysis access grafts: Arrow-Trerotola percutaneous thrombolytic device versus pulse-spray thrombolysis. Arrow-Trerotola Percutaneous Thrombolytic Device Clinical Trial. Radiology 1998;206:403–414.

97. Sofocleous CT, Cooper SG, Schur I, et al. Retrospective comparison of the Amplatz thrombectomy device with modified pulse-spray pharmacomechanical thrombolysis in the treatment of thrombosed hemodialysis access grafts. Radiology 1999;213:561–567.

98. Gibbens DT, Triolo J, Yu T, et al. Contemporary treatment of thrombosed hemodialysis grafts. Tech Vasc Interv Radiol 2001;4:122–126.

99. Summers S, Drazan K, Gomes A, et al. Urokinase therapy for thrombosed hemodialysis access grafts. Surg Gynecol Obstet 1993;176:534–538.

100. Sands JJ, Patel S, Plaviak DJ, et al. Pharmacomechanical thrombolysis with urokinase for treatment of thrombosed hemodialysis access grafts. A comparison with surgical thrombectomy. ASAIO J 1994;40:M886–888.

101. Schuman E, Quinn S, Standage B, et al. Thrombolysis versus thrombectomy for occluded hemodyalisis grafts. Am J Surg 1994;167:473–476.

102. Valji K, Bookstein JJ, Roberts AC, et al. Pharmacomechanical thrombolysis and angioplasty in the management of clotted hemodialysis grafts: early and late clinical results. Radiology 1991;178:243–247.

103. Cohen MA, Kumpe DA, Durham JD, et al. Improved treatment of thrombosed hemodialysis access sites with thrombolysis and angioplasty. Kidney Int 1994;46:1375–1380.

104. Mansilla AV, Toombs BD, Vaughn WK, et al. Patency and lifespans of failing hemodialysis grafts in patients undergoing repeated percutaneous declotting. Tex Heart Inst J 2001;28:249–253.

105. Murray SP, Kinney TB, Valji K, et al. Early rethrombosis of clotted hemodialysis grafts: graft salvage achieved with an aggressive approach. AJR Am J Roentgenol 2000;175:529–532.

106. Zaleski GX, Funaki B, Kenney S, et al. Angioplasty and bolus urokinase infusion for the restoration of function in thrombosed Brescia-Cimino dialysis fistulas. J Vasc Interv Radiol 1999;10:129–136.

107. Rajan DK, Clark TW, Simons ME, et al. Procedural success and patency after percutaneous treatment of thrombosed autogenous arteriovenous dialysis fistulas. J Vasc Interv Radiol 2002;13: 1211–1218.

108. Cooper SG, Gaetz H, Sofocleous CT, et al. Hemodialysis graft mechanical thrombolysis with use of the Amplatz Thrombectomy Device: histopathologic evaluation of extracted myointimal tissue. J Vasc Interv Radiol 1999;10:285–288.

109. Turmel-Rodrigues L, Raynaud A, Louail B, et al. Manual catheter-directed aspiration and other thrombectomy techniques for declotting native fistulas for hemodialysis. J Vasc Interv Radiol 2001;12:1365–1371.

110. Pattynama PM, van Baalen J, Verburgh CA, et al. Revascularization of occluded haemodialysis fistulae with the Hydrolyser thrombectomy catheter: description of the technique and report of six cases. Nephrol Dial Transplant 1995;10:1224–1227.

111. Overbosch EH, Pattynama PM, Aarts HJ, et al. Occluded hemodialysis shunts: Dutch multicenter experience with the hydrolyser catheter. Radiology 1996;201:485–488.

112. Rocek M, Peregrin JH, Lasovickova J, et al. Mechanical thrombolysis of thrombosed hemodialysis native fistulas with use of the Arrow-Trerotola percutaneous thrombolytic device: our preliminary experience. J Vasc Interv Radiol 2000;11: 1153–1158.

113. Turmel-Rodrigues L, Sapoval M, Pengloan J, et al. Manual thromboaspiration and dilation of thrombosed dialysis access: mid-term results of a simple concept. J Vasc Interv Radiol 1997; 8:813–824.

Index

Adenomyositis, imaging of, 803, 804
Adenosine, 14
Adenosine diphosphate receptor agonists, 336
Adenosine-induced transient cardiac asystole, 419
Adjuvant medications, for cancer pain, 33–34
ADMIRAL (Abciximab before Direct Angioplasty and Stenting in Myocardial Infarction Regarding Acute and Long-term Follow-up) trial, 336
Admission privileges, 3
Adolescents. See Pediatric patients
Adrenal glands
    biopsy of, 274–275
    metastasis, 275
    nonfunctioning, 275
    opacification, 492
    pregnancy-related hemorrhage, 827
    traumatic injury to, 1033
Adrenocarcinomas, 274
Adson forceps, 140
Advanced cardiovascular life support (ACLS), 8, 19, 23
Aethoxysclerol (hydroxypolyaethoxydode-canol), 791
Agatston score equivalents (ASEs), 89
Age/aging. See also Elderly patients; Infants; Pediatric patients
    atherosclerotic disease and, 282
    Crohn disease and, 547
    dialysis fistulas and, 1213
    splenic anatomy and, 1020–1021
Aggrastat (tirofiban), 230, 286, 336, 475
Agratoban, 229
Ahlberg NE, 832
Ahmad T, 643
Ahmadi R, 342
AIDS-related cholangiopathy, 550
Air emboli, 270, 678, 1151
Airway obstruction, 20
Airway stenosis, 957, 959
Airway supplies, 21
Ajani JA, 529
Akinesia, 845
Al-Shahi R, 862
Alavi A, 493
Albala DM, 705
Albiero R, 215
Albuterol, 15
Alcohol. See Ethanol
Alcohol consumption, 1111
Alcohol-induced gastritis, 500
Aldosterone, 363
Alexander MJ, 881
Alginate hydrogels, 173
Aliasing (wraparound artifacts), 130
ALK-1 gene, 1182
Allergic reactions. See also Anaphylactoid reactions
    to contrast agents, 1159
    data collection and, 8
    to local anesthetics, 11
    management of, 14–15
    preparation, 6

prevention of, 19
    prophylactic antibiotics, 7
    to sclerotic agents, 1104
    signs of, 20
Alpha$_2$-antiplasmin, 225
Alpha$_2$-macroglobulin, 225
5-alpha-reductase inhibitors, 736
Alric P, 857
Alteplase (Activase, r-tPA), 224, 1131
    dosage, 968, 969
    heparin with, 968
    for peripheral fibrinolysis, 297
    in pulmonary embolization, 250
Alvarado R, 544
Alves A, 538
AMATC (Amplatz maceration aspiration thrombectomy catheter), 985–986
Amebiasis, 1074
Amebic abscesses, 1074–1075
Amenorrhea, 815
American Academy of Pediatrics, 1048
American Association for the Surgery of Trauma (AAST), 1021, 1026, 1037, 1038
American College of Cardiology, 472
American College of Radiology (ACR), 676
American College of Rheumatology (ACR), 1112
American Heart Association
    estimate of PTCA procedures, 471
    guidelines
        ACLS, 23
        angioplasty, 330, 332
        antibiotic, 680
        for aortoiliac disease, 306
        for carotid endarterectomy, 850
        CPR, 21–22
        elective coronary angioplasty, 472
American Pain Society, 33
American Society for Reproductive Medicine (ASRM), 796
American Society of Anesthesiologists, 8
American Urological Association (AUA), 698, 705, 720, 735, 796
AMI (acute mesenteric ischemia), 398, 401–402
Aminocaproic acid (Amicar), 497, 1050, 1185
Aminophylline, 15
Amiodarone, 23
Ampicillin, 7, 1060
Amplatz coronary angiographic curves, 473
Amplatz injectors, 165
Amplatz KA, 165
Amplatz maceration aspiration thrombec-tomy catheter (AMATC), 985–986
Amplatz needles, 725, 728
Amplatz thrombectomy devices (ATDs), 299, 982–984, 1224
Amplatzer ASD occlusion device, 184
Amplatzer PDA occlusion device, 183
Amplatzer PFO occlusion device, 184
Amplatzer vascular plugs, 183, 184
Amytal Sodium (sodium amobarbital), 866
Analgesia, 9, 33–34. See also Specific drugs
Anaphylactoid reactions, 14–15. See also Allergic reactions

Anaphylaxis. See Anaphylactoid reactions
Anastomoses
    aortic, 423
    bile duct
        choledochojejunostomy, 550, 561–562
        leaks, 566
        in liver transplantation, 561–562
        obstruction, 567
    Billroth II, 506
    choledochojejunostomy, 550, 561–562
    continent urinary diversions, 760
    femoropopliteal grafts, 353
    hepatic arteries, 561
    inferior vena cava suprahepatic, 560–561
    infrahepatic inferior vena cava, 561
    liver transplantation, 1135
    lung transplantation, 957
    portal veins, 562–563
    pulmonary, 911
    renal allograft artery, 388
    Roux stricture, 573
    ulcers, 503–504, 506
    ureteroenteral, 762
    ureteroilial, 758, 759
    venous stenoses, 1215–1217
Anatomy exclusion artifacts, 128–129
Anatomy for interventional radiologists, 142–146
Androgen receptors, 1182
Anesthesia. See also Specific agents; Specific procedures
    complications, 717
    epidural, 147
    general, 147
    inhaled, 147
    local, 11–12, 147
    nerve blocks, 147
    overview, 147
    in pediatric patients, 1048
    of the pharynx, 628
    regional, 147
    spinal, 147
Aneurx endografts, 86
Aneurysmal bone cysts (ABCs), 1055–1056, 1057
Aneurysms. See also Endovascular aneurysm repair; Thoracic aortic aneurysms
    after coarctation repair, 415
    Aneurx endograft repair, 86
    aortic, 92, 93 (See also Abdominal aortic aneurysms)
    atherosclerotic disease and, 421
    basilar tip, 102
    cavernous segment, 897
    cerebral, 876
    classification of, 421
    endoleaks, 461–466
    follow-up, 461
    formation of, 322
    fusiform, 420, 421, 879–881
    graft rejection and, 133
    infrarenal, 98, 100
    intracranial, 876–882
        balloon angioplasty, 878–879
        balloon-assisted technology, 878–879
        endovascular embolization therapy, 877–878